ALSO BY FRANCESCO CORDASCO

A JUNIUS BIBLIOGRAPHY.
With a Preliminary Essay on the Political Background, Text, and Identity.
A Contribution to 18th Century Constitutional and Social History
(1949; rev. ed., 1974)

A REGISTER OF 18TH CENTURY BIBLIOGRAPHIES (1950)

AN INTRODUCTION TO 18TH CENTURY MEDICAL BIBLIOGRAPHY (1950)

THE BOHN LIBRARIES:
A History and A Checklist (1951)

DANIEL COIT GILMAN AND THE PROTEAN Ph.D.:
The Shaping of American Graduate Education (1959; rev. ed., 1972)

A BIBLIOGRAPHY OF ROBERT WATT, M.D.,
Author of the Bibliotheca Britannica (1968)

ITALIANS IN THE CITY:
Health and Related Needs (1975)

USEFUL SPANISH FOR MEDICAL AND HOSPITAL PERSONNEL:
With a Bibliography on Hispanic Peoples in the United States (1977)

TOBIAS GEORGE SMOLLETT, M.D.:
A Bibliographical Guide (1978)

MEDICAL EDUCATION IN THE UNITED STATES (1980)

AMERICAN MEDICAL IMPRINTS, 1820-1910

AMERICAN MEDICAL IMPRINTS, 1820-1910

ALSO BY FRANCESCO CORDASCO

A JUNIUS BIBLIOGRAPHY.
With a Preliminary Essay on the Political Background, Text, and Identity.
A Contribution to 18th Century Constitutional and Social History
(1949; rev. ed., 1974)

A REGISTER OF 18TH CENTURY BIBLIOGRAPHIES (1950)

AN INTRODUCTION TO 18TH CENTURY MEDICAL BIBLIOGRAPHY (1950)

THE BOHN LIBRARIES:
A History and A Checklist (1951)

DANIEL COIT GILMAN AND THE PROTEAN Ph.D.:
The Shaping of American Graduate Education (1959; rev. ed., 1972)

A BIBLIOGRAPHY OF ROBERT WATT, M.D.,
Author of the Bibliotheca Britannica (1968)

ITALIANS IN THE CITY:
Health and Related Needs (1975)

USEFUL SPANISH FOR MEDICAL AND HOSPITAL PERSONNEL:
With a Bibliography on Hispanic Peoples in the United States (1977)

TOBIAS GEORGE SMOLLETT, M.D.:
A Bibliographical Guide (1978)

MEDICAL EDUCATION IN THE UNITED STATES (1980)

FRANCESCO CORDASCO

AMERICAN MEDICAL IMPRINTS, 1820-1910

A CHECKLIST OF PUBLICATIONS ILLUSTRATING THE HISTORY AND PROGRESS OF MEDICAL SCIENCE, MEDICAL EDUCATION, AND THE HEALING ARTS IN THE UNITED STATES

A PRELIMINARY CONTRIBUTION

Foreword
by
James Tait Goodrich, M.D., Ph.D.

Volume I

1985

ROWMAN & LITTLEFIELD, PUBLISHERS
TOTOWA, NEW JERSEY

JUNIUS-VAUGHN PRESS, INC.
FAIRVIEW, N.J. & LONDON

Library of Congress Cataloging in Publication Data

Cordasco, Francesco, 1920-
American medical imprints, 1820-1910.

Bibliography: p.
Includes index.
1. Medicine—United States—Bibliography. 2. Medicine—Bibliography. 3. Medicine—United States—History—19th century—Sources—Bibliography. 4. United States—Imprints. I. Title. [DNLM: 1. Bibliography of Medicine—United States. ZWB 100 C794a 1820-1910]
Z6661.U5C67 1984 [R152] 016.61'0973 84-11829
ISBN 0-8476-7338-3 Set
ISBN 0-8476-7422-3 Vol. I
ISBN 0-8476-7423-1 Vol. II

First published in the United States 1985 by:

Rowman & Littlefield, Publishers
81 Adams Drive
Totowa, New Jersey 07512 USA
****
[Junius Vaughn Press, Inc.]
PO Box 85, Fairview, New Jersey 07022 USA
St. John's Road, London SW11 U.K.

Printed & bound in the United States of America

FOR MY WIFE
EDNA MAE VAUGHN CORDASCO
AND
IN MEMORY OF MY MOTHER
CARMELA MADORMA CORDASCO (1883–1962)

The theme which I have selected for my discourse is, "The Progress of American Medical Literature during the last Century;" a theme which, while it may, I think, incite your ambition, will afford us an opportunity of discharging a debt of gratitude to our predecessors and contemporaries; men who have advanced the interests of the profession and surrounded it with a halo of glory. I have undertaken this task, difficult as it is, the more willingly because my entrance into the profession fifty years ago was coeval with the birth of our medical literature. . . . We have medical literature, based upon a broad and solid foundation; a literature full of vigor and inspiration, honorable alike to the profession and to the nation. I have portrayed to you, perhaps too feebly, one of the noble legacies bequeathed to us by our forefathers. Let us, their heirs, cherish their memories, and strive to render ourselves worthy of our inheritance.

Samuel D. Gross,
History of American Medical Literature
(1876)

FOREWORD

BY JAMES TAIT GOODRICH, M.D., Ph.D.

I

Bibliography is a noble and ancient art and only with its evolution has come systematic access to the literature: with its development the interested writer is able now to trace a theme, subject, or author. Anyone who has ever attempted even so simple a task as a bibliography for publication will appreciate the work, endurance and scholarship that go into a study such as this. Many a student, bibliophile, antiquarian, and librarian will thank Dr. Francesco Cordasco for providing this bibliography of American medical imprints. "Learning, as with water, is never more fair, pure and simple than at its source." (Naude)

Bibliography has an ancestral and honorable design. The subject of bibliography dates at least to the great library of Alexandria when listings were provided with references to authors and subjects. The great Pergamite, Galen (130-200 A.D.) compiled two classified bibliographies of his own writings, this in the 2nd century A.D. (*De libris propriis and De oridine librorum suorum ad Eugenianum*). In these works, Galen classified his writings into seventeen various categories. Fulton called this the "... first attempt at classified bibliography by a medical writer."[1] In recent history, the first systematization of the literature of medicine and science was the *Bibliotheca universalis* ... (1545) by Conrad Gesner (1516-1565).[2] Gesner, while only in his twenties, compiled a "universal dictionary" which listed the writings of all authors, famous, obscure, ancient, and modern, each entry with a brief resume and all this done in three languages, Latin, Greek, and Hebrew. This work laid the foundation of modern medical bibliography and was listed as the first work of medical bibliography in Garrison-Morton.[3] The irony was that while twenty-one books were to be published, in actual

[1] Fulton, J. F. *The Great Medical Bibliographers*. Philadelphia: The University of Pennsylvania Press, 1951, p. 1.

[2] Gesner, Conrad. *Bibliotheca universalis ... in tribus linguis. Tiguri*, apud C. Froschouerum, 1545-1555.

[3] Morton, T. *A Medical Bibliography* (Garrison-Morton) ... Edinburgh: Deutsch 1970. See G. M. citation 6743.

fact only twenty were. The twenty-first book on medicine was never completed. This left the first systematic medical bibliography to Pascal Lecoq[4] (1567-1632) who published his *Bibliotheca medica . . .* in 1590, a listing of 1224 authors. Further significant works in medical bibliography were issued by Linden[5] (1609-1664) *De Scriptus medicis . . .* (1637) and by Lipen[6] (1630-1692) *Bibliotheca realis medica . . .* (1679). This last work contained an elaborate subject analysis, numerous cross references, author and subject indices. With the 18th century came the great father of medical bibliography, Albrecht von Haller (1708-1777), an extraordinary man, physician, scientist and man of letters who continued Gesner's great effort. Haller's intellectual powers and feats of memory are legend. Fulton[7] notes that at the age of four, Haller could repeat the Scriptures at great length to the family servants. At age eight, he succeeded in writing two thousand brief biographies of great historical figures. At age ten, he completed a Greek lexicon with supplements in Hebrew and Chaldee—certainly an awesome mind by any standard. Haller went on to complete four great bibliographies on botany, anatomy, surgery, and medicine. With a classified analysis of over 52,000 publications of all countries, this compendium formed the most complete reference work of its time. The bibliographies are still in use today.

The practice of medical bibliography continued, even though it could be "... dry, dusty, tedious, accursed, hateful"[8] as described by James Atkinson (1759-1839). Works by James Douglas (1675-1742), *Bibliographiae anatomicae . . .* (Londini: G. Sayes, 1715); Herman Boerhaave (1668-1738) *Methodus discendi medicinam* (London, 1726); J. F. Blumenbach (1752-1840) *Medicinische Bibliothek* (Göttingen, J. C. Dieterich, 1783-1788) were with others to round out the 18th century. The 19th century was to see a virtual explosion of works in medical bibliography by Hain, Choulant, Forbes, The Royal Society of London, Gross, and finally the spectacular work of Billings.

John Shaw Billings (1839-1913) provided a work unique in the history of medical bibliography, a work that William Henry Welch (1850-1934) proclaimed one of the four greatest contributions that the United States has made to medicine. The *Index-Catalogue,*[9] for the first time in a medical bibliography, provided author and subject indices in one alphabet. Titles of books and periodicals were included. William Osler (1849-1919) commented

---

[4] Lecoq, Pascal. *Bibliotheca medica. Sive catalogus illorum, qui ex professo artem medicam in hunc usque annum scriptis illustrarunt.* Basileae: C. Waldkirch, 1590.

[5] Linden, J. A. *De scriptis medicis, libri duo.* Amstelredami: J. Blaeu, 1637.

[6] Lipen, M. *Bibliotheca realis medica, omnium materiarum, rerum, et titulorum, in universa medicina occurrentium.* Francofurti ad Moenum, J. Friderici, 1679.

[7] Fulton, J. F. *The Great Medical Bibliographers.* Philadelphia: The University of Pennsylvania Press, 1951. p. 39.

[8] *Ibid.*, p. 52.

[9] Billings, J. S. *Index-Catalogue of the Library of the Surgeon-General's Office.* Washington: GPO, 1880-1961.

on this work: "No undertaking in bibliography of the same magnitude dealing with a special subject had ever been issued, and its extraordinary value was at once appreciated all over the world."[10] While this work was intended as a catalogue of the Surgeon-General's Library (SGL) holdings, in actual fact, because of Billings determined efforts to compile a "complete" medical library, it became a comprehensive index to the world literature as it existed then. The first series of sixteen volumes was completed in 1895. By the time of completion of the fourth series, some three million books, journal articles, and pamphlets had been catalogued.

Billings built this collection and bibliography from almost nothing. In 1860 the Surgeon-General's Library, the precursor to the present National Library of Medicine, had a total of 304 volumes in its collection. When Billings took charge in 1865, the collection had expanded to a grand sum of 2,253 books, journals, and pamphlets.[11] Billings determined that this country needed a medical library, central in location, to house the medical works of the world. We had no Bibliothèque Nationale, British Museum, or the like to turn to for medical information. In 1872 Billings issued a short-title catalogue of the holdings and, by this point, the SGL collection had grown to 13,300 volumes; by 1878 the card catalogue held over 400,000 subject cards. Billings, long a historian, realized the value of bibliography and approached Congress on the funding of a catalogue listing of the SGL collection. He was successful in obtaining support; and in 1880 the first volume of the *Index-Catalogue of the Library of the Surgeon-General* was published with over 50,000 volumes and 60,000 pamphlets listed. To put the size of the SGL collection in perspective, consider that the oldest library in the country, Pennsylvania Hospital, listed 1200 volumes in 1876.[12] The College of Physicians of Philadelphia listed 19,000 volumes; Harvard University had 7000 volumes. The Manchester Medical Library in England listed 130,000 volumes. Personal collections of physicians in the United States had varying numbers, *e.g.,* Samuel D. Gross (1805-1884)–4500; Robley Dunglison (1799-1869)–5000; David Hosack (1769-1835)–2500; Samuel Smith Purple (1822-1900)–6000. The enormity and rapidity at which the SGL collection evolved was such that by 1895, when Billings retired from the SGL, sixteen volumes of his first series of the *Index-Catalogue* had been published. The SGL collection now totaled some 116,847 books and 191,598 pamphlets. Today, the National Library of Medicine stands as the largest repository of biomedical literature in the world, attesting to this man's genius and foresight for gathering together these written dictates of medicine, both old and new. William Henry Welch

[10] Fulton, J. F. *The Great Medical Bibliographers.* Philadelphia: The University of Pennsylvania Press, 1951, p. 74.

[11] National Library of Medicine. *John Shaw Billings Centennial.* 1965. See page 2.

[12] Gross, S. D. *History of American Medical Literature, from 1776 to the Present Time.* Philadelphia: Collins, 1876. See p. 74.

considered the *Index-Catalogue* to be the "most important American contribution to medical science in the 19th century."[13]

II

A review of Professor Cordasco's bibliography shows that mediocrity was not necessarily a result of 19th century medical education. Imperfect as the system may have been, physicians of distinction were produced, eminent in the art of practicing medicine. Personalities are, by and large, self-made; the ability to persevere is a major key to success. It is a person's intrinsic drive and intellectual delights that subserve genius. An education, no matter what the design, cannot create talent nor compel taste: "You may, indeed, give it opportunity, but you cannot force it."[14]

A look at the early American medical literature, as cited in Guerra[15] and Austin[16] shows the earliest literature dealt with the local medical experience of our founders and contained mostly medical observations. Medicine, as practiced in this early period, was mostly an ancillary preoccupation, usually involving the clergy. Clergy received some medical education as part of their training; hence, it was they who provided the earliest medical writings. An example of a clergy-physician was Thomas Thacher (1620-1678) who provided the first known medical publication in a broadside: *A Brief Rule to Guide the Common People of New England on How to Order Themselves and Theirs in the Small-pox and Measles* (Boston: J. Foster, 1678).

With the rise of the first two medical schools in Philadelphia and New York City in the late 18th century, the rate at which medical literature appeared accelerated. Two influential papers by Samuel Bard[17] (1742-1821) and John Morgan[18] (1735-1789) signify the early influence American medicine was to have. Both the high standard of conduct, as outlined by Bard, and the course of education with topics in anatomy, materia medica, chemistry, and botany, as outlined by Morgan were discussed in these germinal works.

In the post-Revolutionary War era, a new development took place: the introduction of the American medical journal, long a familiar item in England and the Continent, but conspicuously lacking here. With this new medium the practitioner could now publish his observations for wide public distribution. Prior to this period the medical writer could only disseminate

[13] *John Shaw Billings Centennial*, p. v.
[14] Bigelow, H. J. *Medical Education in American* ... Cambridge: Welch, Bigelow, and Company, 1871. p. 14.
[15] Guerra, F. *American Medical Bibliography 1639-1783*. New York: Lathrop and Harper, 1962.
[16] Austin, R. *Early American Medical Imprints 1668-1820*. Washington: GPO, 1961.
[17] Bard, S. *A Discourse upon the Duties of a Physician*. New York: A. and J. Robertson, 1769.
[18] Morgan, J. *A Discourse upon the Institution of Medical Schools in America* ... Philadelphia: William Bradford, 1765.

his works by bearing the expense of publishing his own pamphlet or broadside. It is interesting to note that before 1800, only one journal was in print, but by 1850 there were over 117 journals. This number does not even begin to account for those that opened and failed.[19]

In discussing 19th century American medicine, many authors have shown this era as being essentially devoid of extensive research efforts, either applied or pure. This comparison is inevitable when one looks at the work of the British and the Continentals. While this may be true in pure numbers of original efforts, one only has to consult Professor Cordasco on American papers and realize that in actual fact there was a tremendous effort being undertaken, albeit by a few. While American physicians were "practical" in their outlook, this by the very design of the land and their pioneering heritage, they produced several significant and important original contributions, *e.g.,* works by Oliver Wendell Holmes (1809-1894) on puerperal fever,[20] Austin Flint (1812-1886) on cardiac disease,[21] William Beaumont (1785-1853) on physiology of digestion,[22], S. Weir Mitchell (1829-1914) on diseases of the nervous system, Samuel D. Gross (1805-1884) on surgery,[23] and John Shaw Billings in bibliography. Examination of Cordasco entries reflects a developmental theme: American physicians were making their major contributions in the field of differential diagnosis and clinical observation. Without the extensive didactic education of the Europeans, the Americans made their studies by doing what they could do best—observation of the patient. Journals of this era are replete with reports of diseases presented in the descriptive sense. From this, one sees that the American physician reflected upon his profession as an "art" versus a "science." This development was all a result of the style of education the American physician was exposed to here versus his European counterpart.

What was this "style" of education for the 19th century physician? Prior to 1800 American physicians were heavily dependent on European and English authors for their texts. After 1800 this was to change with the dominance of the early New York and Philadelphia schools. It was these sources along with a growing number of medical periodicals that were to influence 19th century American medical men. In the first half of the 19th century, Americans were under the influence of the French, German, and English schools. German medical sciences emerged from an *a priori* 18th century speculative science to 19th century Baconian reasoning. The Germans substituted rigorous deduction from ascertained

[19] Shaftel, N. "The Evolution of American Medical Literature." In *History of American Medicine. A Symposium*. Edited by Felix Marti-Ibanez. New York: MD Publication, 1959, pp. 95-118. See p. 103.

[20] Holmes, O. W. "The Contagiousness of Puerperal Fever." *New England Quarterly Journal of Medical Surgery,* 1842-43. 1:503-30.

[21] Flint, A. "On Cardiac Murmurs." *American Journal of Medical Science,* 1862, n.s. 44:29-54.

[22] Beaumont, W. *Experiments and Observations on the Gastric Juice, and the Physiology of Digestion*. Plattsburgh: F. P. Allen, 1833.

[23] Gross, S. D. *A System of Surgery*. Philadelphia: Blanchard & Lea, 1859.

facts for vain discussion and ignored in turn the earlier flatulent pedantry enunciated from the magisterial chairs.[24] With exact observation the German schools laid a foundation for a new style of science. Their neighbors, the French were, at the same time, providing the most prominent educational schools of the period for Americans. With personalities like Laennec (1781-1826), Magendie (1783-1855), Bouillard (1796-1881), Corvisart (1755-1821) and others, the physical diagnostic art was introduced on a firm ground. Across the channel in England great strides were being made by the works and investigations of Bright (1789-1858), Addison (1793-1860), Hodgkin (1798-1866), Watson (1792-1882) and others. Americans, at this time, were more involved with internal and external strife and with shifting transportation routes. As a result of this American medical schools developed along their separate themes.

How evident these various themes were can be seen by reviewing Professor Cordasco's bibliography: homeopathy, eclectic, Thomasonian, botanic, allopathic. In discussing the state of American medicine in the early 19th century, the president of the New York State Medical Society commented in 1818: "With a few, honorable exceptions . . . the practitioners were ignorant, degraded and contemptible."[25] Medical licensure at this time was in a ludicrous state. While there were medical societies in nearly all the states by 1830, few were compelled to give rigorous exams. Just the opposite was occurring in Europe and Great Britain where medical boards were being set up to establish and enforce uniform standards of medical practice.[26] In this American era there was a plethora of new and dubious schools opening (1810-1840, twenty-six new schools; 1840-1875, forty-seven new schools). These schools were mostly proprietary in style with loosely defined requirements where professors were supported by students' fees, hardly a pedantic playground. These schools for profit followed many a philosophy depending upon the mountebank character leading the forum. An enterprising student could study homeopathy, eclectic, botanic, Thomasonian, to name but a few; and, of course, these competed with the "regular" or allopathic schools of medicine.

By 1900 the ratio of doctors to patients in America had exceeded England by about two to one: In the United Kingdom the ratio was 1:1100 and in the United States it was 1:600.[27] Shryock did an analysis on the education of "practitioners" in eastern Tennessee in 1850 and found that there were 201 "physicians" serving a population of 164,000. In analyzing their educational achievements, it was noted, of these 35 (17%) were graduates of some sort of regular school; 42 (20%) said they had "taken

---

[24] Anderson, W. *British Journal of Medicine*. 2:351, 1895.

[25] Shryock, R. H. *Medical Licensing in America, 1650-1965*. Baltimore: Johns Hopkins Press, 1967. p. 4.

[26] *Ibid*., p. 27.

[27] *Ibid*., p. 30. See footnote #44.

one course of lectures," but had not graduated; and 27 (13%) were "botanic and steamers." The rest (some 50%) had received no other education other than some reading, most likely as apprentices.[28] To appreciate what some people thought of an average medical student, consider the following quote which appeared in an editorial in *The New York Sun* in 1861; when describing a Southern medical student one editor observed ". . . a long haired, lantern-jawed verdant youth afflicted with chronic salivation and inveterate profanity . . . deriving his ideas of morals, grammar, and behavior from his negro nurse . . . he becomes in New York a puzzle to professors, a terror to landladies, and a munificient patron of grog shops"[29] – not exactly flowery praise. But then one must also appreciate this was a Northerner writing about a Southerner in 1861. Nevertheless, this was probably not too far from an accurate description of medical students at some of the schools of this era.

William Henry Welch, educator, pathologist, and a founder of Johns Hopkins could only describe native medical education in the United States in 1878 as "simply horrible."[30] This unflattering view does unfortunately detract from the many good students and physicians in practice at this time. A study of Professor Cordasco's bibliography graphically illustrates the logarithmic increases in American medical literature as the 19th century progressed. A good deal of this came from physicians traveling abroad and returning with new information, which was then published locally (Shryock reports that some 15,000 American physicians traveled abroad between 1875 and 1914).[31] In the latter half of the 19th century, American physicians began to introduce their own "systems" of medicine, detailed in example by Pepper[32] and Osler.[33] In this period the American Medical Association and its president, Nathan S. Davis (1817-1904) were demanding educational reform with pre-clinical education requirements, minimum medical school and hospital clinical experience. Improved licensing examinations by state boards and improved medical schools were advocated.[34]

Out of this came the great Hopkins experiment and a paradigm for future medical education. Founded by a philanthropist, patterned after the German medical institutions, and led by the medical greats of this era, a revolution in medical education occurred with the Hopkins experience.

[28] Shryock, R. H. *Medical Licensing in America, 1650-1965*. Baltimore: Johns Hopkins Press, 1967. p. 4.

[29] *Ibid.*, p. 36.

[30] *Ibid.*, p. 43.

[31] *Ibid.*, p. 4.

[32] Pepper, W. *A System of Practical Medicine by American Authors*. Philadelphia: Lea Brothers, 1885-1886. 5 vols.

[33] Osler, W. and T. McCrae. *Modern Medicine, Its Theory and Practice. In Original Contributions by American and Foreign Authors*. Philadelphia and New York: Lea Brothers, 1907-1910. 7 vols.

[34] Shryock, R. H. *Medical Licensing in America, 1650-1965*. Baltimore: Johns Hopkins Press, 1967. p. 47.

For the first time there were strict pre-medical requirements; a four-year graded course, full-time pre-clinical professors, and emphasis on both teaching and research. In 1900 the United States Office of Education reported 151 active medical schools in the United States of which eight were eclectic and physiomedical and twenty-two homeopathic. In 1910 Flexner issued *Bulletin #4*, a now well-known and heavily cited work which devastated the medical profession at this time. The "Flexner Report"[35] was undertaken by Abraham Flexner on behalf of the Carnegie Foundation. In 1908 Henry Pritchett had read *The American College*, a criticism of the elective and lecture system.[36] Pritchett discussed with Flexner a study which would analyze American medical education from the perspective of educational theory and practice: the rest is history. After Flexner's work, many of the worst medical schools closed. By the end of the Great War the epoch of European research had slowed, and the Americans headed to the forefront.

From this brief foreword, it can be seen how appropriate it was for Dr. Cordasco to select a bibliographic period crucial to American medicine—a period embryonic for American physicians. No medical man can practice in a chronological vacuum for our methods today were developed yesterday. In this wonderful work of Professor Cordasco, we see a compendium of our past. The lapse of centuries has removed the amulet from the physician's sanctum, the bleeding lancets from our bags, and added anesthesia and antiseptics to our surgical techniques. Professor Cordasco has outlined it all here, a crucial period in our development of medical knowledge. Professor Cordasco's work will rank with the great studies of Billings, Evans, Sabin, Austin, and Guerra. Happy the student, be he physician, historian, librarian, or antiquarian dealer, who pulls this work from the shelf for he will now be able to locate, with ease and leisure, the works of this most important era in American medicine. This bibliographic repository will stand as an enduring tribute to Dr. Francesco Cordasco for his experience, erudition, and multitudinous talents. By returning to the original descriptions of diseases, clinical pictures are etched more deeply in the mind of the student, practitioner, and the researcher. Here, uninterrupted over a period of 90 years, lies our medical heritage. *Pigmei gigantum humeris imposit plusauam ipsi gigantes vident.*[37]

Acknowledgment: The author would like to express his sincere thanks to Karen Hall, Historical Librarian, Columbia University Health Science Library for her assistance and guidance.

---

[35] Flexner, A. *Medical Education in the United States and Canada. Bulletin Number Four*. The Carnegie Foundation for the Advancement of Learning, 1910.

[36] Kaufman, M. *American Medical Education. The Formative Years 1765-1910*. Westport: Greenwood Press, 1976. p. 167.

[37] "A Dwarfe standing on the shoulders of a giant may see farther than a giant himselfe." From: Burton, R. *The Anatomy of Melancholy* . . . Oxford: John Lichfield and James Short for Henry Cripps A°Dom, 1624. p. 7.

PREFACE

The genesis of this work lies in those expectant and exciting years in the 1930's when I was an undergraduate student in New York City's Columbia College, a formidable citadel of learning, and of social privilege in an America, at that time, wrenched by economic privation. For the most part excluded (by the lack of money, and by blatantly undisguised discrimination) from the round of social activities found in any collegial environment (and at the Columbia of my time predicated on the money and social privilege of its national and international student constituency), I turned to the wondrous resources of the city: to its libraries and museums, to the exploration of its ethnic communities, and the contemplation of its historic monuments; and, out of these contemplative wanderings, with a kind of fated inevitability, I discovered, fortuitously, a fabled antiquarian book market which extended from the John Wanamaker emporium off Astor Place north along Fourth Avenue to 14th Street and Union Square. Although, it is long since gone, part of a vanished era, it remains, for me, as real as yesterday.

The Fourth Avenue book bazaar (truly, a *bazaar* in seemingly inexhaustible stocks spilling out of its shops onto outside tables and shelving, disordered and overseen by idiosyncratic, impecunious entrepreneurs whose penury was exceeded only by their amiable arrogance) for me, was a vertiginous source of continuing excitement; it was here that I spent all of my free time; reading, browsing, talking to shopkeepers, and in day-dreaming reveries which magically provided me with all the money needed to buy any (and all) of the wares which had captured my fancy.

I did acquire a multitude of volumes (*belles-lettres*, history, social sciences) for nickels and dimes (and an occasional dollar), and as token payment for a wide range of chores for shopkeepers: and from the earliest sojourns my attention was drawn to the ubiquitously scattered 19th century medical textbooks, with few exceptions, disdained by both the shopkeepers and buyers. My preoccupation with the medical texts (more often than not enormously thick non-descripto, teutonic shape, tub-model tomes) was not altogether fortuitous: at Columbia, I was a pre-medical student, and a mentor at the University (whose influence I can only inadequately acknowledge) was the medical sociologist, Bernhard J. Stern, whose *Society and Medical Progress* (1941) and *American Medical Practice* (1945) have become prophetically classic statements.

Professor Stern was a tragic figure, denied promotion at a WASPish Columbia because he was a Jew and a reputed Marxist (it would appear); to me, Professor Stern was a source of sustained inspiration and encouragement who marvelled over the medical texts I brought him from Fourth Avenue for examination; it was Professor Stern who first explained to me the 19th century social contexts out of which Austin Flint, Sr., Samuel D. Gross, Charles D. Meigs, and J. Marion Sims (with a multitude of others) emerged, and *pari passu*, related them to the evolving history of American medicine and its social relationships.

The nucleus of the medical titles described in *American Medical Imprints, 1820-1910* is my collection of some 2500 19th century medical textbooks, some 1500 of which derive from my excursions to the Fourth Avenue enchanted book "bazaar" of the 1930's, and assembled with Professor Stern's encouragement. In a sense, then, *American Medical Imprints, 1820-1910* has been in progress for over forty years.

In the last ten years, I have worked steadily toward the work's completion. Using my collection as a core-base, I articulated a practicable framework, defined bibliographical descriptive canons, and established criteria for entry inclusion. It has been a one-man task, and however formidable, it has not been objectionable or onerous: painful, at times, to be sure, yet a continuing source of delight and wonder as it evolved, with little attention to mounting costs and little expectation of even modest remuneration. I am reminded of Samuel D. Gross's plaintive lamentation on the meagre financial gains from his monumental *System of Surgery* (1859; 6th ed., 1882): "What compensation does the reader think I obtained for this hard work, this excessive toil of my brain, including original composition, the correction and improvement of new editions, and the proof-reading, in itself a horrible task, death to brain and eyes, extending over a period certainly not less than fifteen years? Eighty-five cents a copy, all told, and no extra dividends! Two dollars and a half ought to have been the price, or, what would have been more equitable, an equal distribution of the profits from the sale of the work. No wonder authors are poor and publishers are rich!" (*Autobiography*, I, 141)

American Medical Imprints, 1820-1910 includes over 36,000 entries. Its subtitle calls it "a preliminary contribution," and, hopefully, critics will remain mindful of this caveat. I am not unaware of the carping criticisms which have purused Francisco Guerra's *American Medical Bibliography, 1639-1783* (1962) and Robert B. Austin's *Early American Medical Imprints . . . , 1668-1820* (1961), and I am resigned to the inevitable critical prattle which will greet *American Medical Imprints, 1820-1910* and dog its heels. Of the work's value, I have no doubt; and, given the bibliographical canons and inclusion-criteria, the work is honest to its task. Completeness is not proposed, and any such pretension would be palpably both presumptuous and ludicrous: anyone familiar with the byzantine bibliographical history of 19th century America (and for that matter, of the entire history of American book publishing) recognizes the virtue of modest affirmations.*

I welcome constructive criticism, and look forward to receiving notices of corrections, additions, and ancillary emendations. I have a special fondness for *American Medical Imprints, 1820-1910*: not only because, of its long gestation, or because, like a petulant offspring, it has made such heavy demands on my time: its titles gather together a multiplicity of themes which I have explored in other books, themes not incongruent with an expanding America and its evolving social institutions. It is only with reluctance (but with unconcealed glee) that an author recalls Samuel Johnson's caustic commentary on launching his *Dictionary*: "I have protracted my work till most of those whom I wished to please, have sunk into the grave, and success and miscarriage are empty sounds: I therefore dismiss it with frigid tranquillity, having little to fear or hope from censure or from praise." G. Thomas Tanselle, with a touching magnanimity, is closer to the mark in his *Guide to the Study of United State Imprints* (1971) with this plaintive observation: "Bibliographers traditionally end their introductory remarks with a reference to the inevitable omissions which will be discovered in their work, and sometimes their tone suggests a grudging acceptance of an unfortunate fact. They should rather feel pleased that their work is being used and that it is serving to stimulate the recording of additional relevant material. Margaret B. Stillwell, recalling the time when she took her 'first plunge into the study of Americana,' says in her preface to *Incunabula and Americana,* 'I felt often haunted by a questioning fear. Had I not overlooked the obvious?' If a checklist is to allay such fears on the part of its users, it must be constructed through a collaborative effort in which additional information can be gathered in a meaningful way; it provides a framework into which the community of workers in a field can place further references in an organized fashion. Not until the additions and corrections to this book begin to flow in, therefore, can it be thought of as fulfilling its true function." (I, iii)

There is, of course, a serious concern to be addressed. Of what value is retrospective bibliography? *American Medical Imprints, 1820-1910* is a retrospective bibliography consciously predicated on retrieval systems imbedded in and dependent on traditional deposit libraries with vast and continuously expanding holdings. In a new printing of her seminal *The*

*John Tebbel, in contemplating the fortunes of his *A History of Book Publishing in the United States* (1972-1981, 4v.) spoke to this issue: "Whatever their considerable virtues, none of these volumes offers a detailed view of publishing in America that even approaches the comprehensive. While I agree with Professor [G. Thomas] Tanselle that individual scholars will still confront the necessity of doing a host of small-scale studies before the pieces can be put together in a general publishing history of the kind he envisions, I disagree with him that what has been done to date is adequate as even a first step in synthesis and generalization. I intend the volumes on which I have embarked to be that first step, and make no more claims for them than that. (I, xv)

Development of Medical Bibliography (1954; rep. 1982), Estelle Brodman presciently observes that "The growth of automation from the first fumbling attempts to use punched cards and sorting and printing machines to the present on-line systems of bibliographical control has been a revolution all of whose effects have still not been understood." Of this there is no doubt; and it may well be that the traditional library, as we have known it, will be ineluctably changed with the continuing advance of a technology whose advocates predict the replacement of paper and print by electronic recording: all remains uncertain.

The new technology (with promise of protean videotext capabilities), and its multitudinous applications, has proven to be both blessing and bane. Medical bibliography presents special problems, and, in the main, the caution expressed by Scott Adams is judicious: "In the last analysis, there is only one thing which can be said with any degree of certainty about the future forms and content of biomedical bibliography; they will continue to be responsive to the socio-political-technological changes in the society they serve. Since such changes interact with each other, it would take a brave person to predict the results of three forces whose directions are only partially understood." (*Medical Bibliography In An Age of Discontinuity*, [1981], 186). And these sentiments are echoed in Frank B. Roger's prognostications in a centennial tribute to the *Index Medicus*, the companion to the *Index-Catalogue of the Library of the Surgeon-General's Office*: "I do not foresee the demise of a printed version of the *Index Medicus* store; I do, however, believe that inevitably we must see radical changes in the periodicity of publication, and at the same time marked changes in the shape and configuration and relationships of the *Index Medicus* family membership—the *Index Medicus* siblings and all the *Index Medicus* children, and the cousins, too. It is bound to happen that some of them are going to have their lease on printed life rescinded, and will remain only as ghosts within the machine." (*Centenary of Index Medicus 1879-1979* [1980], 59)

I remain confident that *American Medical Imprints, 1820-1910* will, for a long time, meet the needs I had in mind when I compiled it. Above all else, it adds to the corpus of systematic and enumerative bibliography which evolves into a national form: and this is adequate reason, alone, for its compilation.* It affords, also, easy access to a multifarious literature

*The *doyen* of bibliographers, Theodore Besterman (1904-1976), saw no need to justify *American Medical Imprints, 1820-1910* as anything more than systematic and enumerative bibliography, a part of an evolving national bibliographical register. In long discursive bibliothecal discussions with Dr. Besterman while preparing the publication of the *Supplement* (1977, 2v.) to his *World Bibliography of Bibliographies* (4th ed., 1965-1966, 5v.), Dr. Besterman applauded the design of the *American Medical Imprints, 1820-1910*, and encouraged its completion. He scoffed at the electronic threat to libraries, and predicted that the libraries would shape and adapt the new technology to *their* needs, not the other way around. Dr. Besterman's prediction is congruent with the historical patterns of societal and institutional change: libraries are not immune to axiomatic phenomenon.

integrally coincident with the age out of which it emerges and of which it is a dimensional representation. It incorporates the archives out of which the sociologist and cultural historian recreate a vanished era which explain both the genesis and transformation of contemporary reality; and for the medical historian and investigator, *American Medical Imprints, 1820-1910* affords limitless opportunities to explore, in its thousands of entries, the evolution and formation of the profession. The history of medicine and its archives, of course, go far beyond antiquarian pursuits and systematic bibliography. Owsei Temkin's *obiter dicta* are not inappropriate. "Indeed, why turn to new fields to study the moral nature of man? We can behold truth only in the form of samples, and if the historiography of medicine is to comprise 'all that is historical in medicine, as well as all that is medical in history,' it constitutes a sample of considerable size. It is also a good sample, I believe. Hippocrates, Galen, Avicenna, Averröes, Maimonides, Paracelsus, Rabelais, Haller, Virchow, Claude Bernard, and Freud were among the intellectual leaders of mankind. Physicians have been both praised and ridiculed in novels and on the stage. Health and disease have been subjects of religious and philosophical meditation, and as metaphors they are to be found in politics, science, and literature. The human body in the glory of health and in the wretchedness of sickness has been depicted in art. Man has speculated over the meaning of his disease for himself and for his community. Medicine is not only a science and an art; it is also a mode of looking at man with compassionate objectivity. Why turn elsewhere to contemplate man's moral nature?" (*The Double Face of Janus* [1977], 37)

In a centennial review of the state of American medical publishing, John S. Billings (1838-1913), the creator of the Surgeon General's library and architect of its *Index Catalogue*, proudly observed: "In the retrospective reviews, historical sketches, and centennial addresses which have, during the past year, been devoted to American medicine, our most important contributions to the healing art have been duly pointed out and, for the most part, sufficiently eulogized. That the United States has a medical literature, has been cumulatively demonstrated, even to the extent of raising a suspicion of the existence of a doubt upon this point; and that this literature contains many valuable original contributions to the art, if not to the science, of medicine may be considered and unanimously affirmed and admitted." (*A Century of American Medicine, 1776-1876* [1876], 291-292). *American Medical Imprints 1820-1910* documents Billings's proud affirmations.

FRANCESCO CORDASCO
West New York, New Jersey
December, 1983

ACKNOWLEDGMENTS

Over the years, I have incurred many obligations while preparing *American Medical Imprints, 1820-1910*. Many of these obligations cannot be acknowledged, lost as they are in the hundreds of fortuitous encounters in libraries and institutions where my questions were answered, and resources placed at my disposal by countless but nameless individuals always courteous and helpful. However anonomously, they figure in the history of this work. I salute and applaud this library phalanx and the institutions they serve: The Yale University School of Medicine; Library of Congress; National Library of Medicine; John Crerar Library; Health Sciences Library, University of Louisville; Rudolph Matas Medical Library, Tulane University; Boston Public Library; The Francis A. Countway Library of Medicine; William H. Welch Medical Library, Johns Hopkins University; New York Public Library; Health Sciences Library, Columbia University; New York Academy of Medicine; Lloyd Library and Museum; Cleveland Health Sciences Library, Case Western Reserve University; College of Physicians of Philadelphia; Hahnemann University of the Health Sciences; Scott Memorial Library, Jefferson Medical College; Library of the School of Medicine, University of Pennsylvania; Richmond Academy of Medicine.

I owe a special debt to Dr. James Tait Goodrich of the College of Physicians and Surgeons, Columbia University, who graciously prepared a foreword to the work; and to R. Kenneth Bussy, executive editor at Lea & Febiger of Philadelphia, who made available to me the rich resources of the 19th century premier medical publisher, now on the threshold of its third century. Special thanks are due: Stanly B. Burns, M.D.; Heidi E. Duda, Francis A. Countway Library of Medicine; Ellen G. Gartrell, College of Physicians of Philadelphia; John B. Griggs and Rebecca A. Perry, Lloyd Library and Museum; Miriam Mandelbaum and Anne M. Pascarelli, New York Academy of Medicine; Alice Kennedy, Library of the School of Medicine, University of Pennsylvania; Caroline Morris, Pennsylvania Hospital Medical Library; and Barbara Williams, Hahnemann University of the Health Sciences.

American Medical Imprints, 1820-1910 could not have been done without Mrs. Chalmers Morehead who brought to the task those bountiful skills which disciplined a project always on the verge of tumbling out of control; Mary Faith Daly attended to a constellation of needs which brought the work to completion and for these services, I am grateful; and special thanks are due Edna Cordasco, Carmela Cordasco, Michael Cordasco and Gaetana Cordasco for a multitude of tasks cheerfully performed. My bibliographical assistant, John M. Macagne, made his way back and forth through the formidable "Mansell" in his continuing pursuit of evasive and perplexing entries, and his tireless efforts contributed to the completion of this work.

TABLE OF CONTENTS

INTRODUCTION

American Medical Imprints, 1820-1910 is intended as a checklist of publications illustrating the history and progress of medical science, medical education, and the healing arts in the United States. It continues the work of Robert B. Austin, *Early American Medical Imprints, 1668-1820* (1961), and not unlike Austin's work, *American Medical Imprints, 1820-1910* is a *genre* checklist, to use the felicitous classification described by G. Thomas Tanselle: "A second basic category of imprint lists consists of those checklists which attempt to record all the items of a particular type printed within a specified area and period." (Guide to the *Study of United States Imprints* [1971], I, xx).

TERMINI A QUO ET AD QUEM

The opening date, 1820, needs no justification; concluding the work with 1910, might be justified by reference to the publication that year of Abraham Flexner's *Medical Education in the United States and Canada* (1910), but the date would be somewhat arbitrarily chosen. There is little question of the importance of Flexner's *Medical Education*, but Flexner's report may well have been the attestation of change in American medicine rather than its cause. Paul Starr's judicious assessment in his *The Social Transformation of American Medicine* (1982) epitomizes the dramatic changes in American medicine by 1910: "Well before Flexner's report was published in 1910, the number of medical schools had begun to decline, dropping from a high point of 162 in 1906 to 131 four years later, a loss of almost one fifth. The turnabout came as the steadily rising requirements set by state licensing boards and other authorities gradually altered the economics of medical education for students and schools alike. The new requirements extending the length of medical training imposed increasingly large opportunity costs on prospective physicians. The academic year, time almost wholly lost for earnings, went from four to eight or nine months, and the total period of training from two years, possibly without high school, to four, then five, and eventually more than eight years beyond high school. Under the emerging system, young doctors could scarcely hope to make a living on their own before age thirty. Higher tuition fees added to the change. The combined rise in indirect and direct costs produced a long-term decline in the number of medical students. This was especially evident among many schools of the second and third rank that later became extinct. They could ill afford losses of enrollment. Medical schools were then facing greatly increased expenses under the new requirements for modern laboratories, libraries, and clinical facilities. No institution could defray all these costs out of their tuition charges, and since the commercial schools had no other source of income, they went under. These changing economic realities, rather than the Flexner report, were what killed so many medical schools in the years after 1906." (118)

Why, then, conclude *American Medical Imprints, 1820-1910* at 1910? Lester S. King has argued, convincingly, that "If we had to find a single date to distinguish the old medicine from the new, the year 1886 would serve quite well. Of the innumerable events that occurred in that year, I would regard two as especially symbolic: the death of Austin Flint, Sr. (1812-1886) and the founding of the American Association of Physicians." (JAMA 249, 1983: 1897) King cogently frames a context, with 1886 as a base-line, in which one could look back across the medical advances of the 19th century, and look forward fifty years into the future: and he uses as one of his sources Austin Flint's *Medicine of the Future* (1886), read posthumously before the British Medical Association by Flint's son, Austin Flint, Jr. (1836-1915), the distinguished physiologist. But a case can be made for the end-date, 1910, with reference to interrelated complex factors in the larger society.

By 1910, a world on the threshold of war, was entering the last phase that tied it inextricably to the 19th century which had given it definition and form: in a few years this world was to vanish. In the first decade of the 20th century, American medicine achieved a maturity singularly its own: the German influence was in decline (a decline accelerated during the years of the 1914-1918 war), and if American medicine was still largely pragmatic, it had developed theoretic and research orientations which heralded the new maturity.

In their bicentennial history, *Two Centuries of American Medicine, 1776-1976* (1976), James Bordley and A. McGehee Harvey succintly note: "Great reforms in medicine coincided with the great sociopolitical reforms of the early twentieth century. The connection between the two movements is not easy to discern; either might have occurred without the other. Nevertheless, both were impelled by similar forces: (1) a more broadly educated citizenry; (2) extraordinary advances in science and technology; (3) a pent-up need to break away from entrenched and long-outmoded traditions; and (4) enlightened, bold leadership." (110)

In the annals of American publishing, the early 20th century marked the achievement of both maturity and stability. In 1900, the trade organ, *Publishers Weekly*, commenting on the end of the 19th century, boastfully observed: "One hundred years ago the total number of books in circulation in this country amounted to less than fourteen hundred separate works, mostly of foreign origin, published by less than fifty booksellers or printers. In the year just closed, upwards of seven thousand separate works, chiefly by American writers, have been published by nearly six hundred publishers. In the year 1813, Mathew Carey, then president of the Philadelphia Company of Booksellers, issued a circular in which he warned the trade against the folly of printing so large an edition as 4,000 copies of any book. During the last year of the century, more than one of the six best-selling books has required an edition fifty times greater than an edition considered extravagantly large a century ago. . . ." (December 29, 1900, p. 1819)

Medical publishing (with Philadelphia as its center) had, by the advent of the 20th century, grown to enormous size. The field, by 1910, was dominated by a handful of firms. Lea & Febiger (1907) has evolved out of the multiplicity of Lea imprints which had originated in the firm founded by Mathew Carey in 1785. (See, *infra*, "19th Century American Medical Literature: A Gallery of Lea Titles") With Lea & Febiger in Philadelphia were P. Blakiston's Son & Company whose origins went back to 1825; J. B. Lippincott Company whose antecedents went back to 1792; F. A. Davis Company which had entered medical publishing in 1879; and W. B. Saunders Company whose medical publications began in 1888 with Hobart Amory Hare's *Essentials of Physiology*, the first of twenty-four question-and-answer compendia whose sales were to exceed a quarter million. In New York, William Wood & Company (founded by Samuel Wood in 1804) had, by the 19th century's end, become a major medical publisher. In 1874, William Wood & Company undertook the publication in translation of H. W. von Ziemssen's *Cyclopedia of the Practice of Medicine* (22 vs.) which was sold on a subscription basis; and Wood's *Library of Standard Medical Authors* began publication in January, 1879, publishing a volume each month: the issuance of the series continued for eight years with an enormous sale. (For a checklist of titles, see Appendix, *infra*) D. Appleton & Company of New York (presently Appleton-Century-Crofts) had entered medical publishing in 1852 with J. A. Swett's *Treatise on the Diseases of the Chest*, and although never exclusively a medical publisher, D. Appleton & Company maintained a distinguished medical list which included Sir William Osler's *Principles and Practice of Medicine* (1892).

In 1881, *Publishers Weekly* began a yearly report of book production. Although the figures are not accurate (and it is impossible to measure the margin of error), the production lists furnish a valuable profile of the growth of medical publishing. The medical book figures for 1880-1910 are subjoined:

Year	*Medical Titles*	*Year*	*Medical Titles*
1880	114	1883	211
1881	190	1884	209
1882	188	1885	188

Year	*Medical Titles*	*Year*	*Medical Titles*
1886	177	1899	120
1887	171	1900	146
1888	151	1901	186
1889	157	1902	207
1890	117	1903	257
1891	108	1904	186
1892	128	1905	349
1893	129	1906	294
1894	118	1907	309
1895	141	1908	266
1896	119	1909	613
1897	129	1910	369
1898	143		

It is an impressive record, unmatched anywhere in the world at the time.*

DESIGN OF THE WORK

American Medical Imprints, 1820-1910 is a systematic and enumerative bibliography (*i.e.*, a checklist) arranged in nine *alpha* modalities (each comprehending a decade): each *alpha* modality is an entity in itself, independent of the others, but an integral part of the chronological continuum which the nine *alpha* components, together, constitute. Such an arrangement made practicable the management of over 36,000 bibliographical entries, with the added advantage of easy decennial review.

A two digit identification of the decade, followed by four or five digits for entry numbering provide the framework and basic design of the checklist:

Years	*Entry Numbers*
1820-1829	20-0001-20-0645
1830-1839	30-0001-30-0976
1840-1849	40-0001-40-1406
1850-1859	50-0001-50-2042
1860-1869	60-0001-60-2061
1870-1879	70-0001-70-4148
1880-1889	80-0001-80-7070
1890-1899	90-0001-90-10378
1900-1910	00-0001-00-7886

Total Number of Entries: 36,612

*The data are conveniently gathered in John Tebbel, *A History of Book Publishing in the United States* (1975), II, 675-701.

I have, also, provided "A Handlist of Selected Bibliographies, Catalogues and Related Reference Materials" which constitutes those works (most, not all) which were consulted during the compilation of *American Medical Imprints, 1820-1910*; and I have included "19th Century American Medical Literature: A Gallery of Lea Titles," originally written for the bicentennial of the Philadelphia publishers, in which I was able to sketch (using the Lea imprint as a point of continuing reference) the evolution of an indigenous American medical literature. For quick reference, I have appended "Wood's Library of Standard Medical Authors: A Checklist" in which the individual volumes in the series are arranged in the order in which they were published, with originally assigned volume numbers.

The *Index of Names* is keyed to entry numbers; beyond authors, editors, compilers, it includes all substantival references within the titles and annotations. However useful (and with considerable effort, practicable) a *Subject Index* presented difficulties I chose not to confront.

ENTRY DESIGN

As far as possible, the bibliographical design of the entry includes what appears on the title page of the work described, with a minimal modification. With few exceptions, only major pagination is recorded. Each entry incorporates from one to four locations for the item described. The location symbols are the conventional symbols found in *The National Union Catalog, Pre-1956 Imprints* and other catalogues, but these have been modified where necessary to meet more delimited needs. (See "Key to Locations," *infra*) Annotations have been provided where they are appropriate.

A few sample entries are subjoined:

ROSA, Storm (1794?-1864)
History of medical science. An introductory lecture delivered before the class of the Cincinnati Eclectic Institute, 1850. Cincinnati, O.: J. D. Thorpe, 1850. 20p. DNLM; PPHa
50-1595

LUDLOW, John Livingston (1819-1888)
A manual of examinations upon anatomy, physiology, surgery, practice of medicine, chemistry, obstetrics, materia medica, pharmacy, and therapeutics. Especially designed for students of medicine. To which is added a medical formulary. A new ed. Philadelphia: Henry C. Lea, 1865. 816p. DNLM; MBM; NNNAM; PPC
60-1137

AMERICAN ACADEMY OF DENTAL SCIENCE, BOSTON
A history of dental and oral science in America. Prepared under direction of the American Academy of Dental Science. Philadelphia: S. S. White, 1876. 271p. DLC; DNLM; PPC
[Edited by James E. Dexter]
70-0046

AMERICAN ECLECTIC MEDICAL COLLEGE OF OHIO, AT CINCINNATI
Private circular to the graduates [soliciting their cooperation in securing a large class for the next session, offering ten dollars cash for every student they may induce to attend the lectures in this college. Signed W. Nicely, M.D.] Cincinnati, 1879. 1 sheet. DNLM
70-0048

ADDRESSES at the inauguration of William Pepper as provost of the University of Pennsylvania, Feb. 22, 1881. Philadelphia: Collins, 1881. 62p. DNLM; PPC; PHi; PU
80-0027

GEAR, Frank J., Company (Boston)
Illustrated catalogue of invalid and sick room supplies, also surgical and electric apparatus and physicians' supplies. Boston, [*c.* 1890]. 44p. MBM
90-2690

These entries are illustrative of governing captions which include authors, institutions, firms, associations, societies, academies, etc. For uncaptioned entries, the first word (or substantive) of the title is in capital letters. Birth and death dates of authors (or birth or death date, alone) have been provided when available.*

CRITERIA FOR INCLUSION

I have chosen to define the coverage of *American Medical Imprints, 1820-1910* very broadly. Within the comprehensively framed sub-title (*A Checklist of Publications Illustrating the History and Progress of Medical Science, Medical Education, and the Healing Arts in the United States*), I have acted very freely to include any item which could legitimately be related to the medical arts and their progress in the United States.

As in Austin's *Early American Medical Imprints, 1668-1820*, I have interpreted medicine "in its wider sense to include nursing, pharmacy, dentistry, child care, hygiene, first aid, education and psychology." A few titles on veterinary medicine have been included, but this *genre* deserves a separate bibliography. Only a very selective range of works in botany and chemistry have been included beyond those botanical works specifically related to the materia medica, or those works in chemistry intended for the medical student or physician. Annual reports (with very few exceptions) have been excluded. Periodicals, and periodical literature, have not been included. It is important to note that I have recorded a particular work and its subsequent *different* editions, but I have excluded separate notices of reprintings (without change) of any of the editions.

Within the broad patterns of inclusion, one criterion has been inflexibly applied: to be included a printed item must have had an independent,

*An invaluable biographical resource for medical biography is Lisabeth M. Holloway, Medical Obituaries: *American Physicians' Biographical Notices in Selected Medical Journals Before 1907* (New York: Garland Publishing, 1981) which includes 17,355 entries. In a review, Edward C. Atwater defines the scope of the work: "Who will be found in the book and who will not? What is the scope and bias of the sample? The United States federal census provides an enumeration of physicians starting in 1850. The Massachusetts census offers death rate data by age cohort, although the sexes are combined. From these sources, one may calculate as an estimate that about 55,000 American physicians died between 1850 and 1907. Extrapolating the curve backward to 1800 would add perhaps another 12,000, giving a total of 67,000 physician deaths between 1800-1907. Since the census included a broad spectrum of healers under the appellation "physician," this figure is probably a generous one. The national medical directories published by R. H. Polk and Company in 1886 and in 1896 give figures for the physician population that are 7 to 14 percent lower than those of the census. Of the 67,000 figure, the present book offers a 25 percent sample. A somewhat lower percentage was derived by an alternate computation. Eighty-seven (or 21 percent) of 409 American physicians who are known to have died in 1858 are listed. So, the whole sample is on the order of 20 to 25 percent." (*Bulletin of the History of Medicine* 56, 1982: 281)

separate pagination.* This criterion has allowed the inclusion of the vast *off-print* literature which is an important and integral part of 19th century medical publishing; technically, an *off-print* is a separate printing of the work (article) out of the periodical in which is appeared, with title page, usually in small print-runs for the author's personal distribution. Unlike the *extract* out of the periodical literature, the *off-print* is almost invariably independently paginated, and, thus, a bibliographical entity in its own right.

Off-print literature is, by its very nature, ephemeral, and cataloguing and storing have always been troublesome. For many years, libraries (*e.g.*, the New York Academy of Medicine; the Surgeon-General's Library, *i.e.*, the National Library of Medicine) frequently bound groups of pamphlets and assigned the volumes chronological numbers for easy retrieval. For example, a study of the subjoined entry (Index Catalogue of the Library of the Surgeon-General's Office, Series I, 4: 650) indicates that one copy was catalogued as a separate item and one additional copy was bound in Vol. 751 of the pamphlet collection:

> **Ferguson, (Edward J.)** Observations on the nervous system and the neuroses; being the subject of a course of lectures. 16pp. 8°. [Buffalo], C.F.S. Thomas, [1843].
> [*Also*, in P., v. 751.]

Unfortunately, this reprint-ephemera, in their slip-cases or pamphlet-collection volumes, present difficulties: many individual pieces disappear from slip-cases, or are misplaced, and their arrangement has always posed problems to librarians.

BIBLIOGRAPHICAL SOURCES

Vast resources exist for the study of American imprints. For the period 1820-1910, the coverage is unusually good, with the exception of the period 1835 through 1875. A number of works attempt to record all imprints during a given period. These include: Sabin, *Bibliotheca Americana* (1868-1936) for the period through 1850 [. . . 1876]; Evans, *American Bibliography* (1903-1934, 1955) for the period through 1800; Shaw and Shoemaker, *American Bibliography* (1958-1966) for 1801-1819; Shoemaker, *Checklist of American Imprints* (1964-) for 1820-1875 (at present completed through

*Theodore Besterman addressed this issue in the introduction to his *World Bibliography of Bibliographies* (4th ed., 1965-1966): "My bibliography is limited to separately published bibliographies, as are in effect the three we have considered. This rule I have not only established, but, unlike my predecessors, I have adhered to it rather strictly. Let me make quite clear what I mean by a separately published work. For our present purpose I define such a work as one having separate pagination. Exception has been made for a few bibliographies not separately paginated, where there is definite evidence that they were published in that form, as for instance, in the case of separate works which also form part of series. From this definition it is clear that no bibliography in a book is included unless it forms the bulk, or at least the principal purpose, of that book." (I, 23-25)

1834); Roorbach, *Bibliotheca Americana* (1852-1861) for 1820-1861; Kelly, *American Catalogue* (1866-1871) for 1861-1871; *The American Catalogue* (1876-1910) for 1876-1910; and these can be supplemented by reference to *Publishers Weekly* (1872-); *Publisher's Trade List Annual* (1874-); U.S. Copyright Office, *Copyright Entries* (1891-); *The United States Catalogue* (1899-1928), and the *Cumulative Book Index* (1899-).

Roorbach's *Bibliotheca Americana* and Kelly's *American Catalogue* are too incomplete to serve as useful guides, but this deficiency will be corrected with the completion of the ongoing *Checklist of American Imprints*. The timeframe of *American Medical Imprints, 1820-1910*, and its bibliographical sources are outlined in the following schematic overview of United States national bibliography:

NATIONAL BIBLIOGRAPHY: UNITED STATES
A GRAPHIC OVERVIEW

Reference Work	*Time Period Covered*
Sabin,	← 1639——1840 . . . 1876
Evans,	1639—1800
Shaw and Shoemaker,	1801–1819
Roorbach,	1820—1860
Shoemaker,	1820–[1875]
Kelly,	1861–71
Publishers' Weekly,	1872 ——→
Publishers' Trade List Annual,	1874 ——→
The American Catalogue of Books,	1876—1910
U.S. Copyright Office, *Copyright Entries*,	1891 ——→
United States Catalogue,	1899—1928
Cumulative Book Index,	1899 ——→

All of these have, in differing degrees, been used in compiling *American Medical Imprints, 1820-1910*, and they have been supplemented by reference to library catalogues, both general and specialized.

The most important of the specialized library catalogues is the *Index-Catalogue of the Library of the Surgeon-General's Office, United States Army*, Series 1-5 (61 v.), 1880-1961, which is an index of the collection of what is now the National Library of Medicine and which is the major guide to medical publication from the beginning of printing to 1950. It was issued in four alphabetical series with a supplementary fifth series: Series 1, v. 1-16, 1880-1895; Series 2, v. 1-21, 1896-1916; Series 3, v. 1-10, 1918-1932; Series 4, v. 1-11, 1936-1955; Series 5, v. 1-3, 1959-1961.

Periodical articles, in addition to books, are listed in Series 1-4, but only under subjects, whereas books, theses and pamphlets, are listed under authors, editors and translators, as well as subjects. Each volume, with some exceptions, covers the publications in its part of the alphabet which had been catalogued by the National Library of Medicine (formerly called the Library of the Surgeon-General's Office, the Army Medical Library and the Armed Forces Medical Library) since the similar volume in the preceding series. Series 4 ceased with v. 2 "Mh-mn," 1955, because the backlog of unpublished references was growing at an uncontrollable rate. The supplementary fifth Series contains the remaining entries for only books, theses and project reports through 1950. Series 5, v. 1, 1959, completes the author listing of books; v. 2 and 3, 1961, complete their subject listing.

I have used Series 1 and Series 2 of the *Index Catalogue*, and have incorporated into *American Medical Imprints, 1820-1910* from Series 1 and Series 2 all *Index Catalogue* items which meet my inclusion criteria.

Other specialized library catalogues consulted include those of the Francis A. Countway Library of Medicine, Boston; and the New York Academy of Medicine. (See *A Handlist of Selected Bibliographies . . . . infra.*)

The completion of the *National Union Catalog, Pre-1956 Imprints* (London: Mansell, 1968-1981, 754 vs.) made possible the use of an invaluable bibliographical resource. The *NUC, Pre-1956*, probably the last mammoth-scale, non-automated bibliographic project that will be undertaken, includes over 11 million author entries. William J. Welsh, Deputy Librarian of Congress, has, quite correctly, attested to the significance of the completion of the monumental *NUC, Pre-1956*: "The uses of the pre-1956 catalog are many and are still being discovered. For that matter, we know that its very existence is still being discovered. There is an educational task ahead. Like the 'post-1956' portion of the *NUC*, the earlier portion greatly assists librarians in acquisitions, cataloging, bibliography, interlibrary loan, reference, and research. But its uses, present and potential, go far beyond the walls of any single institution, whether it be library, university, bookstore, or think-tank. As Gordon Williams commented in 1968 when the first volumes appeared, the publication of the retrospective volumes of the national union catalog vastly increases the historical and scholarly resources available for research in this country and around the world. Its publication enables 'every library, wherever it is, to locate promptly and to provide its patrons with access to the millions of volumes it could never afford to acquire and house in its own collection.' " (*American Libraries*, 1981, 468)

As far as proved practicable, I have examined each of the items listed in *American Medical Imprints, 1820-1910*; only one item has eluded me, whose existence I do not doubt: the 5th edition (1875?) of William Alexander Hammond's *Treatise on Diseases of the Nervous System* (Entry 70-1492). There is no entry in *NUC, Pre-1956* for the Hammond title, and no copy has been found in the major medical libraries: it may be that the 5th edition was wholly or partly destroyed (fire?), and the 6th edition (1876) was quickly prepared to meet the continuing demand for Hammond's popular treatise.

For the most part, I have encountered few difficulties in compiling *American Medical Imprints, 1820-1910*. The Hammond case was an exception. Most questions were, with some diligent effort, resolved: for example, it would appear that the Lea announcements (beginning in the mid-1880s and continuing into the early 1890s) of the forthcoming publication of Virgil Pendleton Gibney's *Orthopedic Surgery: For the Use of Practitioners and Students* were never implemented. For whatever reasons, the work was never published.

Even the seemingly endless pirating of English medical works by American publishers remained traceable, although the furtive activities of Blakiston of Philadelphia invited special scrutiny. (Blakiston issued English medical works, numbering editions as it saw fit, and very often simply tipped in its own title-page, leaving the work in all other respects unchanged, and its origins unacknowledged.) Other publishers were guilty of the same practices, but not on the scale of Blakiston: whatever the ethics of those American publishers who imaginatively (and profitably) raided English publishers' lists, the chief beneficiaries were American physicians and the profession. These problems largely disappeared with the advent of international copyright in the early 1890s.

A final word. *American Medical Imprints, 1820-1910* is intended as a functional checklist whose first concern is with the use and availability of the materials it describes. It is not intended as an antiquarian depository. The first concern must be the *availability* of primary source materials. Edwin Clarke and B. I. Williams have eloquently addressed this issue: "The prime requisite for any historian is ready access to the primary sources which constitute the essential raw materials of his subject. Their provision is clearly his central problem, for like the chemist he must be able to analyze before he can synthesise. This is especially true in the history of medicine where many kinds of people write on its various aspects. One of the commonest failings of many of them is a tacit willingness to accept another author's citation from primary material or his interpretation of it, without having seen the original. A great deal of the so-called historical writing in medicine is, in fact, based upon secondary, tertiary or even more remote sources. There is today in some countries a conception of the historian of medicine as a multilingual expert on rare books, working exclusively in an antiquarian library and thus entirely divorced from modern medicine. There are probably several reasons for this apart from the natural need that the medical historian has for early works. The most important is the influence of such men as Osler and his disciples, who encouraged all those around them to think of the history of medicine as mainly an antiquarian, library-based study. This possibly accounts for the more frequent occurrence of this interpretation in Britain and in the United States of America, whereas in Germany, for example, where the Oslerian tradition is much less, it is rare." (*Modern Methods in the History of Medicine* [1971], 306-307) Over a decade later, the cogency of their observations remains unquestioned.

19TH CENTURY AMERICAN MEDICAL LITERATURE: A GALLERY OF LEA TITLES

I

When Austin Flint (1812-1886), Professor of Medicine, Bellevue Hospital Medical College, completed the 5th edition of his *Treatise on the Principles and Practice of Medicine* (Henry C. Lea's Son & Co., 1884), he wrote in its Preface: "The author . . . tenders his thanks to the present publishers for a continuance of the courtesy and kindness which rendered most agreeable his relations, for a quarter of a century, with their predecessors, Blanchard & Lea, and Henry C. Lea."

The sentiments were reaffirmed in the Preface to the 6th edition (Lea Brothers & Co., 1886) of the *Principles and Practice* by Austin Flint, *fils* (1836-1915), himself a distinguished clinician, and the sentiments were expanded: "In the Preface to the fifth edition the author 'tenders his thanks to the present publishers for a continuance of the courtesy and kindness which rendered most agreeable his relations, for a quarter of a century, with their predecessors, Blanchard & Lea and Henry C. Lea.' Judging by the popular criterion of commercial success, the publishers can certainly testify to the appreciation, on the part of the profession, of the completeness with which each one of the preceding five editions has been made to represent the actual condition of medical knowledge at the time of its publication; and it may be safely asserted that during the last twenty years no systematic work on the Principles and Practice of Medicine, printed in the English language, has been more extensively circulated and read, and has had a greater influence on the practice of English-speaking physicians, than has the present treatise."

The long life of the *Principles and Practice*, whose first edition had appeared in 1866 (Lea & Blanchard), ended with its 7th edition in 1894 (Lea Brothers & Co.); its seven editions chronicled the evolution of modern clinical medicine over the course of the later part of the 19th century: Austin Flint, *fils*, noted that his father's text derived from "an unbroken series of records of cases in private practice and in hospitals, begun in 1833 and continued for more than half a century, covering sixteen thousand nine hundred and twenty-two folio pages of manuscript, written with the author's own hand. These records embrace carefully-written histories of cases in all departments of practical medicine, observed under varied conditions of life, climate, and general surroundings. Soldiers in camp and barracks; the rich and the poor; those affected with diseases incident to lives of ease and luxury and paupers in hospitals; the pioneers of Western New York and the inhabitants of the metropolis; patients in the wards of the almshouse and hospitals of Buffalo, of the Marine Hospital in Louisville, Kentucky, the great Charity Hospital in New Orleans, Louisiana, the Bellevue Hospital, the Charity Hospital, the dispensaries, and similar institutions in the city of New York; cases observed in the experience of a quarter of a century as a general practitioner, and of more than another quarter of a century as a consulting physician, including the epidemics which have occurred in this country within the last fifty years, the experience derived from these various sources of observation, carefully recorded, studied, and analyzed, was finally used in the composition of this treatise, the first edition of which appeared in 1866." An extraordinary history, indeed.

In another frame of reference, Austin Flint's *Principles and Practice* epitomized the history and development of an indigenous American medical literature; and in this history, as it evolved in 19th century America, the descendants of Mathew Carey played an important part.* The eminent 19th century surgeon, Samuel D. Gross (1805-1884), was keenly aware of the importance of Mathew Carey and his descendants. In an introductory address (1875) to the Fifty-First Course of Lectures in the Jefferson Medical College, Gross had sketched (with the impending centennial of the nation at hand) *The History of American Medical Literature from 1776 to the Present Time* (Henry C. Lea, 1876): in this overview of an indigenous medical literature, Professor Gross opined: "The great publishing house, however, of the country was that originally of the Careys, descendants of Mathew Carey, an Irish gentleman of great intelligence and enterprise, who was himself engaged in the book business from 1783 till 1822. He then formed a partnership with his sons, which expired in 1825, when Carey, Lea & Carey came upon the stage, then Carey & Lea; Carey, Lea & Blanchard; Lea & Blanchard; and Blanchard & Lea, who, after a reign of fourteen years, were succeeded by Mr. Henry C. Lea, the eminent medical book publisher, who has ever since been his own master. From these respective firms a large majority of our native and reprinted medical works have emanated, and it affords me pleasure to add that they all have been fully rewarded for their labor and the investment of their capital." (p. 72)

*The reader may find a Lea & Febiger chronology-schema useful:

Mathew, Carey, 1785-1817
M. Carey & Son, 1817-1821
M. Carey & Sons, 1821
H. C. Carey & I. Lea, 1822-1827
Carey, Lea & Carey, 1827-1829
Carey & Lea, 1829-1832
Carey, Lea & Blanchard, 1833-1838
Lea & Blanchard, 1838-1851
Blanchard & Lea, 1851-1865
Lea & Blanchard, 1865
Henry C. Lea, 1865-1880
Henry C. Lea's Son & Co., 1880-1885
Lea & Brothers & Co., 1885-1907
Lea & Febiger, 1907 to date

Henry C. Lea, who published Gross's long essay for distribution among his [Gross's] "professional brethren," was clearly unashamed of the essay's historical judgments. And Gross's judgment was reaffirmed a near-century later by the historian of American book publishing who (in a notice of Henry C. Lea) stated flatly: "By 1875, Lea had made his firm the largest publisher of medical, surgical and scientific books in the world, and in addition published four important medical periodicals." (John Tebbel, *A History of Book Publishing in the United States*. New York: R. R. Bowker, 1972-81, 4 vols. I, 372)

Writing in *A Century of American Medicine, 1776-1876* (Henry C. Lea, 1876),* John S. Billings (1838-1913), the creator of the Surgeon General's Library and the architect of its *Index Catalogue*, surveyed the state of American medical publishing. Billings made use of "statistics obtained from a nearly complete list of the medical books published in this country from 1776 to the present," and from which "it may be considered certain that no important work has been omitted." The books which he counted were classified as follows: I. Systematic treatises and monographs by physicians residing in this country, including reports of hospitals, corporations, and government department; II. Reprints and translations of foreign medical books; III. Medical journals; IV. Transactions of medical societies. The first, third, and fourth classes include what Billings regarded as American medical literature. And he illustrated his findings with an invaluable schematic graph:

Table showing number of Medical Books printed in the United States from January 1, 1776, *to January* 1, 1876.

		1775 to 1799	1800 to 1809	1810 to 1819	1820 to 1829	1830 to 1839	1840 to 1849	1850 to 1859	1860 to 1869	1870 to 1875	Total
	CLASS I.										
American	No. 1st edition	39	24	51	48	83	96	101	157	130	729
Medical	No. later editions	9	4	14	17	34	49	80	85	44	336
Books	No. Vols. Total	51	31	77	86	136	162	197	256	180	1176
	CLASS II.										
Reprints	No. 1st edition	28	39	64	72	145	135	99	104	81	767
and	No. later editions	11	23	28	33	36	67	76	64	50	388
Trans.	No. Vols. Total	49	76	111	135	192	214	184	160	137	1274
	CLASS III.										
Medical	No. Journs. com'ced	1	5	6	17	18	26	52	38	32	195
Journals	" " discont'd	...	3	5	10	18	14	31	36	20	137

*This collection of papers appeared originally in the *American Journal of the Medical Sciences* (itself a Lea publication whose origins go back to Mathew Carey's founding of the *Philadelphia Journal of the Medical and Physical Sciences* in 1820) and includes Edward H. Clarke, "Practical Medicine"; Henry J. Bigelow, "A History of the Discovery of Modern Anaesthesia"; Samuel D. Gross, "Surgery"; T. Gaillard Thomas, "Obstetrics and Gynaecology"; and John S. Billings, "Literature and Institutions."

Table showing number of Medical Books printed in the United States from January 1, 1776, *to January* 1, 1876. (continued)

	1775 to 1799	1800 to 1809	1810 to 1819	1820 to 1829	1830 to 1839	1840 to 1849	1850 to 1859	1860 to 1869	1870 to 1875	Total
"A."										
Original: No. Vols. com'nced	2	21	27	85	104	173	376	292	296	1376
Original: No. Vols. compl'ted	2	20	27	79	98	166	366	271	283	1312
"B."										
Reprints: No. Journals	...	...	1	4	...	5	1	3	3	17
Reprints: No. Volumes	...	...	9	20	20	46	71	51	32	258
CLASS IV.										
Transactions Med. Societies: No. Volumes	7	3	2	5	17	27	76	88	111	336

Billings subjected his statistics to careful analyses, primarily seeking answers to two questions: Where had the works been published? By whom had they been published? His findings were not unanticipated. Philadelphia was the acknowledged center of medical publishing; and the Lea imprint was the dominating presence. "Of Class one (I) we find that three hundred and seventy-three (373) first editions were published in Philadelphia, one hundred and seventy-three (173) in New York, eighty-one (81) in Boston, twenty-four (24) in Cincinnati, sixteen (16) in New Orleans, and fifteen (15) in Baltimore, leaving ninety-six (96) published elsewhere. If each edition be reckoned as a separate work, we find that six hundred and thirteen (613) have appeared in Philadelphia, two hundred and twenty-six (226) in New York, ninety-six (96) in Boston, and eighteen (18) in Baltimore. Of the reprints and translations, six hundred and eighteen (618) books, or seven hundred and fifty-three (753) editions have been issued from Philadelphia, one hundred and seventy-seven (177) books, or two hundred and nineteen (219) editions from New York, eighty (80) from Boston, and ninety-four (94) from elsewhere. It appears then that more than one-half of our medical books have been published in Philadelphia, and about one-fifth in New York. The firm of Carey, Lea & Carey, now H. C. Lea, has published nearly six hundred editions of medical works; and those of Lindsay and Blakiston, and Lippincott, each between one and two hundred. In New York, the principal publishing house is that of S. S. & W. Wood, now Wm. Wood & Co., which has issued about one hundred and fifty (150) editions." (*A Century of American Medicine*, 327-328) Six hundred titles! The ubiquity of the Lea imprint helps explain the observation of Professor Gross noted earlier, and its reaffirmation by John Tebbel a century later. The Carey descendants had, indeed, become "the largest publisher of medical, surgical and scientific books in the world."

A selection of titles out of this overwhelming Lea presence is a difficult task: it is made somewhat easier if the criteria of selection use as a guide works of the stature of Austin Flint's *Principles and Practice of Medicine* whose importance was attested by revision, reissue, and the acclaim of continuing use. But even with this delimitation (however arbitrary), only a handful of works will be noted in a few broadly representative fields, *e.g.*, surgery; the practice of medicine; and obstetrics and gynaecology.

II

Surgery

In the annals of surgical literature, the historical importance of Samuel D. Gross's *System of Surgery* (Blanchard & Lea, 1859, 2 vols.) is unchallenged. Garrison called it the most important surgical treatise of its time. (Garrison-Morton, No. 5607)* For a quarter-century it stayed in print, its last (6th edition) appearing in 1882 (Henry C. Lea's Son & Co., 2 vols.); and in his *Autobiography* (1887; posthumously edited by his sons), Gross recaptured its genesis and initial appearance:

> I had commenced the composition of my Surgery several years before I left Kentucky, and I now set vigorously to work to complete it. I had sketched the plan and adopted a title, both of which met with the approval of Messrs. Blanchard & Lea, who had agreed to publish it. . . . I generally spent from five to eight hours a day upon my manuscript, subject of course to frequent and sometimes annoying interruptions by patients. In the winter I commonly sat up till eleven and half past eleven o'clock at night. I then closed my study, and almost invariably took a walk down Chestnut Street as far as the State House, in order to obtain a little fresh air and to shake off my mind the subject upon which I had been so assiduously engaged. By this means I generally succeeded in obtaining a good night's rest with sound and refreshing sleep. Unless I was greatly interrupted, I seldom wrote less than from ten to fifteen pages of foolscap in the twenty-four hours, and I rarely retired until they were carefully corrected. It was not often I rewrote anything, although I not unfrequently interlined. In the winter, during the continuance of the lectures, my pen was less active than in the recess, but I nevertheless seldom failed to do a good day's work. I jogged along in this manner until early in the spring of 1859, when, the manuscript being ready, the printers commenced their task, and I the hard one of proof-reading. The preface was dated July 8th, 1859. Soon after, the work was issued in two portly octavo volumes, numbering, in the aggregate, two thousand three hundred and sixty pages, and profusely illustrated by engravings on wood. The mechanical execution was highly creditable to the publishers, printers, and artists. The edition comprised two thousand copies, and cost a large sum of money, enough, as Blanchard & Lea assured me, to have enabled them to open a respectable mercantile house on Market Street. (I, 138-139)

**A Medical Bibliography: An Annotated Check-List of Texts Illustrating the History of Medicine* (Philadelphia: J. B. Lippincott Co., 1970).

Samuel D. Gross published considerably more under the Lea imprints. His *Elements of Pathological Anatomy* (1836) appeared in a 3rd revised edition in 1857 (Blanchard & Lea). The *Elements* was "the first exhaustive study in English of the subject." (Garrison-Morton, No. 2292) His *Practical Treatise on the Diseases, Injuries and Malformations of the Urinary Bladder, the Prostate Gland, and the Urethra* was published in 1851 (Blanchard & Lea; 2nd ed., 1855; 3rd ed., Henry C. Lea, 1876); and his *Practical Treatise on Foreign Bodies in the Air Passages* appeared in 1854 (Blanchard & Lea), "the first systematic study of the subject." (Garrison-Morton, No. 3264) The elder Gross was joined by his son, Samuel Weissel Gross (1837-1889) as a Lea author. Gross, *fils*, published *A Practical Treatise on Impotence, Sterility and Allied Disorders of the Male Sexual Organs* (Henry C. Lea's Son & Co., 1881) which went through four editions, the last appearing in 1890. (Lea Brothers & Co.) S. W. Gross also assisted his father in the later editions of the great *System of Surgery*.

A vast number of works in surgical literature appeared under the Lea imprints of the 19th century, ranging from the works of English surgeons published in the early century, to the great multi-volumed systems published toward the century's close. The *Principles of Surgery* (Lea & Blanchard, 1845) and the *Practice of Surgery* (Lea and Blanchard, 1846) of James Miller (1812-1864), are representative of the early English works; and these are joined by the still earlier *Institutes and Practice of Surgery* (Carey, Lea & Carey, 1827) of William Gibson (1788-1868), and the *Principles and Practice of Surgery* (H. C. Carey & I. Lea, 1825) of Sir Astley Paston Cooper (1768-1841).

The early English authors are the precursors of a continuing appearance under the Lea imprints of English and Scots physicians. Even with the emergence of a strong indigenous American medical literature by mid-century, the English connection is not abandoned. And, joining S. D. Gross's *System of Surgery* (1859) in the mid-century are the Scots surgeon, William Pirrie (1807-1882), *Principles and Practice of Surgery* (Blanchard & Lea, 1852); and the London surgeons, Robert Druitt (1814-1883), *Principles and Practice of Modern Surgery* (Blanchard & Lea, 1852); Frederick Carpenter Skey (1798-1872), *Operative Surgery* (Blanchard & Lea, 1851); and John Eric Erichsen (1818-1896), *The Science and Art of Surgery* (Blanchard & Lea, 1854), "the most popular text-book on the subject for many years." (Garrison-Morton, No. 5602) Erichsen was Holme Professor of Clinical Surgery at University College Hospital, London, where Lister served as his house surgeon.

In a class by itself is the work of the London anatomist, Joseph Maclise, whose *Surgical Anatomy*, in "large imperial quarto, with 68 large and splendid plates," Lea and Blanchard published in 1859. The Maclise volume represents a supreme artistic achievement in anatomical illustration, and it anticipates the work of the Johns Hopkins medical illustrator, Max Brödel (1870-1941).

Beyond S. D. Gross, the major American surgeons in the Lea canons include John Ashhurst (1839-1900), whose *Principles and Practice of Surgery* (Henry C. Lea, 1871) went through six editions, the last published in 1893 (Lea Brothers & Co.); Stephen Smith (1823-1922), *Principles and Practice of Operative Surgery* (Lea Brothers & Co., 1887); and Lewis A. Stimson (1844-1917), *A Manual of Operative Surgery* (Henry C. Lea, 1878), whose 4th edition appeared in 1900 (Lea Brothers & Co.). In the related surgical specialties, the *Practical Treatise on Fractures and Dislocations* (Blanchard & Lea, 1860; 8th ed., Lea Brothers & Co., 1891) of Frank Hastings Hamilton (1813-1886) remained a leading text, asserting Hamilton's preeminence as a surgeon. (Garrison-Morton, 1742, 4420, 5747) Frederic S. Dennis (1850-1934), Professor of Surgery, Bellevue Hospital Medical School, served as general editor of the mammoth *System of Surgery* whose four volumes appeared between 1895 and 1896 (Lea Brothers & Co.). Tucked away in its 1st volume (pp. 17-144) is an invaluable "History and Literature of Surgery," prepared by John S. Billings. A companion work was *A Treatise on Surgery by American Authors* (Lea Brothers & Co., 1896, 2 vols.; condensed edition with revisions, 1899) edited by Roswell Park (1852-1914), longtime Professor of Surgery at the University of Buffalo. A synthesis of American surgical technique, as it evolved across the 19th century, is available in John Bingham Roberts (1852-1924), *A Manual of Modern Surgery*, a compact volume of 800 pages (Lea Brothers & Co., 1890; 2nd ed., 1899); and in the still more concise *Surgery* (Lea Brothers & Co., 1893) of Bern Budd Gallaudet (1860-1934).

The adaptation of English works to the needs of American practitioners was skillfully pursued, and an excellent example was the publication of the giant *System of Surgery, Theoretical and Practical* (Henry C. Lea's Son & Co., 1881-1882, 3 vols.) edited by Timothy Holmes (1825-1907), Hunterian Professor of Surgery at the Royal College of Surgeons. This work was "thoroughly revised and much enlarged" by John H. Packard (1832-1907), an eminent surgeon and member of the College of Physicians of Philadelphia.

One of the most prolific surgical authors of the late 19th century was the Englishman, Sir Frederick Treves (1853-1923) of "elephant-man" fame. He was an important author in the Lea lists, and among his works were *Surgical Applied Anatomy* (Henry C. Lea's Son & Co., 1883; 2nd ed., 1883; 3rd ed., Lea Brothers & Co., 1888); *Manual of Operative Surgery* (Lea Brothers & Co., 1892, 2 vols.); and his *Students' Handbook of Surgical Operations* (Lea Brothers & Co., 1892). Treves acquired world fame by his operation on King Edward VII for appendicitis in 1902. Lea was the American publisher of his celebrated Jacksonian Prize Essay on *Intestinal Obstruction* (Henry C. Lea's Son & Co., 1884). (Garrison-Morton, No. 3482)

The Practice of Medicine

Mention has been made of Austin Flint's *Principles and Practice of Medicine*. In a very real sense, Professor Flint was the quintessential Lea author, producing a score of works for the Lea presses. The supreme diagnostician (Samuel D. Gross: "I know of no one who is so well entitled as Austin Flint to be regarded as the American Laennec."), Flint first described the murmur (the "Austin Flint murmur") present at the apex beat in aortic regurgitation (Garrison-Morton, No. 2764); and his *Treatise on the Diagnosis, Pathology, and Treatment of Diseases of the Heart* (Blanchard & Lea, 1859; 2nd ed., Henry C. Lea, 1870) has an important place in the annals of American cardiology. The range of Austin Flint's works (beyond those already noted) in American medical practice is best suggested by the short-title subjoined list:

Physical Exploration and Diagnosis of Diseases Affecting the Respiratory Organs (Blanchard & Lea, 1856; 2nd ed., Henry C. Lea, 1866)
Phthisis: Its Morbid Anatomy, Aetiology . . . Treatment and Physical Diagnosis (Henry C. Lea, 1875)
A Manual of Percussion and Auscultation . . . (Henry C. Lea, 1876; 5th ed., Lea Brothers & Co., 1890)
Clinical Medicine . . . (Henry C. Lea, 1879)

The long and excellent relationship of Austin Flint and his publisher is attested by Henry C. Lea's publication of his *Essays on Conservative Medicine and Kindred Topics* (1874), an eloquent plea for rational therapeutics, and a classic in the history of American medical practice.

Representative of the early practices of medicine is *General Therapeutics; or Principles of Medical Practice* (Carey, Lea & Blanchard, 1836; 6th edition, Blanchard & Lea, 1857) of the Englishman Robley Dunglison (1798-1869) whom Thomas Jefferson had summoned to the University of Virginia. Dunglison, who was to spend most of his professional career at Jefferson Medical College in Philadelphia, was a Lea stalwart, producing a variety of influential and long-lived texts. His *Human Physiology* (Carey & Lea, 1832; 8th ed., Blanchard & Lea, 1856), in Samuel D. Gross's words "accomplished for [physiology] in America in the nineteenth century what Albert von Haller's great work accomplished for physiology in Europe in the eighteenth." (*Autobiography* II, 330) Dunglison's *Medical Lexicon: A New Dictionary of Medical Science* appeared under the Lea imprint in 1839 (Lea & Blanchard) and its 23rd edition, edited by his son, Richard J. Dunglison (1834-1901) appeared in 1893 (Lea Brothers & Co.). Robley Dunglison's *Practice of Medicine; or a Treatise on Special Pathology and Therapeutics* (Lea & Blanchard, 1842; 3rd ed., Lea & Blanchard, 1848) which anticipates "Huntington's Chorea" in its description of chronic hereditary chorea in adults (Garrison-Morton, No. 4691), is the *facile princeps* of the plethora of 19th century American practices, affording both model and substantive form. It clearly influenced Samuel H. Dickson's *Elements of Medicine; A Compendious View of Pathology and Therapeutics* (Blanchard & Lea, 1855; 2nd ed., Blanchard & Lea, 1859). Dickson (1798-1872) was a colleague of Robley Dunglison at Jefferson Medical College.

Amid a multitude of duties, Dunglison found time to edit and revise *The Cyclopaedia of Practical Medicine* . . . (Lea & Blanchard, 1845, 4 vols.) jointly edited by John Forbes (1787-1861) and Alexander Tweedie (1794-1884), redoubtable Scotsmen, whose *Cyclopaedia* had appeared between 1832-1835. The posthumous publication of Robley Dunglison's *Autobiographical Ana* (American Philosophical Society, 1963) reveals the mutual trust and respect which characterized the relationship between Dunglison and his publishers. It is best illustrated in Dunglison's account (in the *Autobiographical Ana*) of some of the fortunes of his phenomenal *Medical Lexicon*:

> In the year 1851, it became necessary to prepare an eighth edition of the *Dictionary*, and propositions were made to me by my publishers to have it stereotyped. To this I objected for some time, but ultimately consented, provided that I should have the privilege of having the plates destroyed after a short period, so that the work should not suffer materially by its recomposition being delayed a little longer than had, thus far, been the case. The following arrangement was therefore entered into.
>
> Philadelphia April 12th, 1851
>
> Professor Dunglison
>
> Dear Sir,
>
> It is understood, that we are to stereotype your revised copy of the *Medical Dictionary* and that you are not to require us to destroy or modify the plates, nor are we to require you to revise the work for a new edition, for a period of five years from the publication of the first fifteen hundred copies, (unless the said steel plates are accidentally injured or destroyed). Should we not have printed and sold *ten thousand copies* from the plates, at the expiration of the said five years, then, the understanding exists until the quantity of *ten thousand copies* are sold. The existing contract for this work, of accounting for each fifteen hundred copies, and other matters, are not affected by stereotyping it.
> Yours very truly,
>
> Blanchard and Lea
>
> P.S. It is understood, that our selling price of the edition is not to be increased.
>
> * * * * *
>
> The following is an account of the number of copies and of the copy money paid to me for the *Dictionary* up to this date (June 1852):

Edition	Number of Copies	Copy Money
1833 First-	1000	$ 1250
1839 Second-	1500	$ 600
1842 Third-	1500	$ 900
1844 Fourth-	1500	$ 900
1845 Fifth-	1500	$ 900
1846 Sixth-	3750	$ 2250
1848 Seventh-	5000	$ 3000
1851 Eighth-	1500	$ 900
	17250	$10700

(*Ana*, p. 47)

Note should also be made of Dunglison's *Elements of Hygiene* (Carey, Lea & Blanchard, 1835; 2nd ed., Lea & Blanchard, 1844); and his *New Remedies: The Method of Preparing and Administering Them* (Lea & Blanchard, 1839; 7th ed., Blanchard & Lea, 1856), both influential works; and attention called to his *The Medical Student or Aids to the Study of Medicine* (Carey, Lea & Blanchard, 1837; 2nd ed., Lea & Blanchard, 1844), an early example in a *genre* of medical literature which has continued to the present.

Two English titles adapted to American practice proved to be very popular. Sir Thomas Watson (1792-1882), Professor at King's College, London, published his lectures in 1843; Lea & Blanchard reprinted these the next year (*Lectures on the Principles and Practice of Physic*, 1844; 5th ed., Henry C. Lea, 1872): the 2nd, 3rd and 4th editions of the Lea Watson were revised and enlarged by the American pediatrician, D. Francis Condie (1796-1875); and the 5th edition updated by the Philadelphia physician-scientist Henry Hartshorne (1823-1897). Watson's *Lectures* "formed the most important treatise of medicine for a quarter-century." (Garrison-Morton, No. 2219) Charles J. B. Williams (1805-1889), first president of the [London] Pathological Society, was the author of *Principles of Medicine* (1843) which Lea & Blanchard issued "with additions and notes by Meredith Clymer" in 1844 (5th ed., Blanchard & Lea, 1864). Appearing somewhat later, and as popular as the American editions of Watson and Williams, was the *Treatise on the Theory and Practice of Medicine* (1876) by John Syer Bristowe (1827-1895), a president of the Medical Society of London. Henry C. Lea published the *Treatise* "with notes and additions" by James Howell Hutchinson (1834-1889), sometime editor of the "Philadelphia Medical Times," in 1877, and a 7th edition appeared in 1890 (Lea Brothers & Co.).

The American counterpart to the adapted English works was represented by the work of Henry Hartshorne (1823-1897) who had updated Watson's *Lectures*. Hartshorne's *Essentials of the Principles and Practice of Medicine* (Henry C. Lea, 1867) went through five editions, the last appearing in 1881 (Henry C. Lea's Son & Co.); and it was Hartshorne whom Henry C. Lea invited to superintend the American editions of J[ohn] Russell Reynolds' elaborate *System of Medicine* (Henry C. Lea, 1880, 3 vols.). Reynolds (1828-1896), Professor of Medicine at University College, London, planned and edited one of the first systems of medicine in English; under the Lea imprint in America it proved immensely popular. The very popularity of Reynolds' *System* led to *A System of Practical Medicine by American Authors* (Lea Brothers & Co., 1885-1886, 5 vols.), a mammoth work under the general editorship of William Pepper (1843-1898), Provost of the University of Pennsylvania and pioneer investigator of pernicious anaemia. (Garrison-Morton, No. 3125) Pepper was assisted by Louis Starr (1849-1925), Clinical Professor of the Diseases of Children at the University of Pennsylvania. The publisher's prospectus proudly announced: "In this great work American medicine is for the first time reflected by its worthiest teachers, and presented in the full development of the practical utility which is its preeminent characteristic. The most able men—from the East and the West, from the North and the South, from all the prominent centres of education, and from all the hospitals which afford special opportunities for study and practice—have united in generous rivalry to bring together this vast aggregate of specialized experience."

A successor to the Pepper work was *A System of Practical Medicine by American Authors* (Lea Brothers & Co., 1897-1898, 4 vols.) edited by Alfred L[ebbens] Loomis (1831-1895), Professor of Medicine at New York University, and an associate of Edward L. Trudeau (1848-1915) in the battle against tuberculosis; Loomis was assisted in editing the *System* by William Gilman Thompson (1856-1927). The supreme achievement in the massive multi-volumed *System genre* remains *Modern Medicine, Its Theory and Practice, in Original Contributions by American and Foreign Authors* (Lea Brothers & Co. [& Lea & Febiger], 1907-1910, 7 vols.), edited by Sir William Osler (1849-1919), assisted by Thomas McCrae (1870-1935).

Obstetrics and Gynaecology

In the Preface to his *On the Nature, Signs, and Treatment of Childbed Fevers* (Blanchard & Lea, 1854), Charles D. Meigs (1792-1869), long-time Professor of Obstetrics at Jefferson Medical College, observed: "I believe that the only American work on the subject of Obstetrics that was in existence, when I began to study Medicine, was the small duodecimo *Compendium of Midwifery* by the venerable Dr. Samuel Bard, of New York. We had, at that day, reprints of Denman's *Mifwifery* and the two volumes of Burns, edited by Dr. James, the London Practice, pirated from Dr. Clark, and a very much razed copy of Baudelocque's two fine volumes. I apprehend that, at that period, few of our American practitioners possessed more obstetric works than those I have above named, and not many, all, even of these. Since that time, we have had the benefit of Dr. Dewees's contributions, and some few others of less note than his, among them my own. There is a ground, then, in this little progress, to hope that we shall gradually obtain an American medical literature on this branch, as well as in other branches of our science."

Historically, the early development of an American literature on midwifery and obstetrics (and in a related frame of reference on paediatrics) can be traced in the work of Charles D. Meigs and William Potts Dewees (1768-1841). Dewees, whose *Treatise on the Physical and Medical Treatment of Children* (H. C. Carey & I. Lea, 1825; 11th ed., Blanchard & Lea, 1858) was the "first American text-book on paediatrics" (Garrison-Morton, No. 6331), more than any other shaped the character of early American obstetric practice. His *Compendious System of Midwifery* (Carey & Lea, 1824, 12th ed., Blanchard & Lea, 1852) was preceded by the tentative enquiries in

Essays on Various Subjects Connected with Midwifery (H. C. Carey and I. Lea, 1823); and dimensionally expanded by his *Treatise on the Diseases of Females* (H. C. Carey & I. Lea, 1826; 11th ed., Blanchard & Lea, 1860). Of Dewees, Samuel D. Gross wrote: "As an obstetric practitioner Dewees was one of the most popular men of his day. No woman of any social position in Philadelphia considered herself safe if she could not have Dewees in her confinement." (*Autobiography*, II, 248)

Charles D. Meigs, who "drew attention to embolism as a cause of sudden death in childbed" (Garrison-Morton, No. 6177), continued the Dewees tradition. His *Females and Their Diseases* (Lea & Blanchard, 1848; 4th ed., Blanchard & Lea, 1859) was followed by his *Obstetrics: The Science and the Art* (Lea & Blanchard, 1849; 3rd ed., Blanchard & Lea, 1856), and *A Treatise on Acute and Chronic Diseases of the Neck of the Uterus* (Blanchard & Lea, 1854), distinguished by a set of 22 finely embellished plates. Despite his vast obstetric experience, Meigs rejected the contagion doctrine in puerperal fever. Samuel D. Gross, who knew Meigs well as a colleague at Jefferson reminisced: "Meigs was all his life a non-believer in the infectious nature of puerperal fever, notwithstanding that for a time numerous facts demonstrative of the incorrectness of his belief almost daily stared him in the face. One Philadelphia obstetric practitioner alone had during one season in rapid succession nearly thirty cases of this disease, traceable from one house to another, the result beyond question of direct inoculation. Although Meigs saw some of these cases in consultation, he could not perceive the relation of cause and effect between this sequence and infectious communication; but the attending physician did, and he was obliged to leave the city in search of another field. Professor Oliver Wendell Holmes's admirable monograph on this disease failed to convince him, and he finally died a non-contagionist." (*Autobiography*, II, 341-42)

The English tradition in obstetrics and gynaecology continued in America across the 19th century, and this despite the continuing development of an American practice: the reasons are complex, and are not unrelated to the ease of availability of proven English works. Samuel Ashwell (1798-1857), the London obstetrician, is represented by his *Practical Treatise on the Diseases Peculiar to Women* (Lea & Blanchard, 1845; 3rd ed., Blanchard & Lea, 1855); and Edward Rigby (1804-1860) with his *System of Midwifery* (Lea & Blanchard, 1841; 2nd ed., Lea & Blanchard, 1851) exerted a wide influence. But the commanding English presence at mid-century was Fleetwood Churchill (1808-1878), an expatriate Englishman (and staunch supporter of the Episcopal Church in Ireland)in practice in Dublin where he was a Fellow of the College of Physicians. Churchill was the author of *On the Theory and Practice of Midwifery* (Lea & Blanchard, 1843; 4th ed., Blanchard & Lea, 1860) which the "Charleston Medical Journal" called "the most popular work on midwifery ever issued from the American press"; and this work was paired with *Diseases of Females* (Lea & Blanchard, 1843; 5th ed., Blanchard & Lea, 1857). Churchill's work was comprehensively augmented by his *Diseases of Infants and Children* (Lea & Blanchard, 1850; 2nd ed., Blanchard & Lea, 1856) and his *Essays on Puerperal Fever* (Lea & Blanchard, 1850). The popular *Theory and Practice of Midwifery* was "edited, with notes and additions" by D. Francis Condie (1796-1875), the Philadelphia pediatrician, whose *Practical Treatise on the Diseases of Children* (Lea & Blanchard, 1844, 6th ed., Henry C. Lea, 1868) was the accepted authority until superseded by the work of Meigs.

Two other English authors at mid-century deserve notice. Charles West (1816-1898) whose *Lectures on the Diseases of Infancy and Childhood* (Lea & Blanchard, 1850; 5th ed., Henry C. Lea, 1874) was "in its day . . . the best English work on the subject" (Garrison-Morton, No. 6334) was also author of *Lectures on the Diseases of Women* (Blanchard & Lea, 1857-58; 3rd ed., Henry C. Lea, 1867), and delivered the prestigious Croonian lectures for 1854, *An Inquiry into the Pathological Importance of Ulceration of the Os Uteri* (Blanchard & Lea, 1854). Francis H. Ramsbotham (1801-1868), obstetric physician to the London Hospital, produced *The Principles and Practice of Obstetric Medicine and Surgery* (Lea & Blanchard, 1842; 6th ed., Blanchard & Lea, 1855), an imperial octavo volume, opulently illustrated with figures and lithographic plates.

There are other English authors who continue the influence on American practice to the end of the 19th century and beyond. The more important include William Leishman (1834-1894), *A System of Midwifery* (Henry C. Lea, 1873; 4th ed., Lea Brothers & Co., 1888); William S. Playfair (1836-1903), *The Science and Practice of Midwifery* (Henry C. Lea, 1876; 7th ed., Lea Brothers & Co., 1898); Arthur W. Edis (1840-1893), *Diseases of Women* (Henry C. Lea's Son & Co., 1882); and Robert Barnes (1817-1907), *A System of Obstetric Medicine and Surgery* (Lea Brothers & Co., 1885).

The continuing assertion of the American practice is seen in a number of indigenous authors. Hugh Lenox Hodge (1796-1873), who "invented the Hodge pessary" (Garrison-Morton, No. 6185) wrote the *Principles and Practice of Obstetrics* (Blanchard & Lea, 1864) and an earlier *Diseases Peculiar to Women* (Blanchard & Lea, 1860; 2nd ed., Henry C. Lea, 1868). Thomas Addis Emmet (1828-1919), an ardent advocate of Irish home rule and an associate of J. Marion Sims (1813-1883) at the Women's Hospital in New York City, published *Principles and Practice of Gynaecology* (Henry C. Lea, 1879; 3rd ed., Henry C. Lea's Son & Co., 1884). T[heodore] Gaillard Thomas (1831-1903), who described the first vaginal ovariotomy (Garrison-Morton, No. 6061), and whose *Practical Treatise on Diseases of Women* (Henry C. Lea, 1868, 6th ed., Lea Brothers & Co., 1891) "was the outstanding work on the subject" (Garrison-Morton, No. 6060) was a major figure. Thomas wrote the bicentennial review of American obstetrics and gynaecology in *A Century of American Medicine, 1776-1876* (Henry C. Lea, 1876). Theophilus Parvin (1829-1899) and Albert F. A. King (1841-1914) deserve notice. Parvin's *The Science and Art of Obstetrics* (Lea Brothers & Co., 1886, 4th ed., 1895) proved a popular textbook; and King's

A Manual of Obstetrics (Henry C. Lea's Son & Co., 1882; 11th ed., Lea & Febiger, 1910) served as a worthy competitor.

But the crowning achievements of the 19th century were *The American Systems of Gynaecology and Obstetrics*. The *System of Gynaecology by American Authors* (Lea Brothers & Co., 1887-1888, 2 vols.) was edited by Matthew D[arbyshire] Mann (1845-1921); and the *System of Obstetrics by American Authors* (Lea Brothers & Co. 1888-1889, 2 vols.) was edited by Barton Cooke Hirst (1861-1925). The four large octavo volumes comprised 3612 pages, with 1092 engravings and colored plates, and represented a synthesis of the medical science of the time.

III

Our self-imposed limitation to the areas of surgery, practice, and obstetrics/gynaecology, invites brief notice of titles in other fields. The Lea imprints covered all medical fields, and Lea catalogues (very often in a 32-page signature-form appended to 19th century texts) included listings in all medical areas; the Lea Brothers & Co.'s "Classified Catalogue of Medical and Surgical Publications for 1885" adopted the following reading captions: Periodicals; Manuals; Dictionaries; Anatomy; Physics; Physiology; Chemistry; Pharmacy; Materia Medica; Therapeutics; Pathology; Histology; Practice of Medicine; Clinical Medicine; Hygiene; Electrical Practice; Throat, Heart, Lungs; Nervous and Mental Diseases; Surgery, Ophthalmology; Otology; Dentistry; Urinary and Renal Diseases; Venereal Diseases; Diseases of the Skin; Diseases of Women; Midwifery; Diseases of Children; Medical Jurisprudence; Miscellaneous. This is an extraordinary coverage, itself congruent with 19th century optimism and encyclopedism, but still instructive to the present age. A few titles, of particular significance, will be noted.

Henry Gray (1827-1861) and his *Anatomy Descriptive and Surgical* (Blanchard & Lea, 1859; 29th ed., Lea & Febiger, 1973) must be accorded a centerpiece position in 19th century medicine. It was originally published in London in 1858 by J. W. Parker & Son (Garrison-Morton, No. 418: "Gray's text-book of anatomy remains today a standard work on the subject in the English-speaking world."); and soon thereafter Blanchard & Lea made arrangements with Parker for its publication in the United States. It has remained a Lea publication since. Charles Mayo Goss (editor of the 25-27th American editions of the *Anatomy*), in a centennial notice of the text's publication in America, observed: "We take the book for granted now, but having thrice edited it I can vouch for the enormous amount of drudgery that must have gone into the preparation of the text and the dissections which necessarily accompanied its writing. The plan of the book could not have been conceived without a phenomenal grasp of the entire subject."*

*Charles Mayo Goss, *A Brief Account of Henry Gray, F.R.S., and His Anatomy, Descriptive and Surgical During A Century of Its Publication in America* (Lea & Febiger, 1959), p. 21.

The first Lea editor of the *Anatomy* was Richard J. Dunglison (1834-1901) who had served as editor of the later editions of his father's *Medical Lexicon*, whose 23 editions occupied an illustrious place in the Lea canons. Dunglison, *fils*, edited the first five editions of the *Anatomy* (1859, 1862, 1870, 1878, 1883); he was succeeded by the Jefferson Medical College anatomist, William W. Keen (1837-1932) who edited the 6th edition (1887); it was Keen who attended President James A. Garfield in 1881 when he was shot by a disappointed office seeker; Bern Budd Gallaudet (1860-1934) of Columbia University who edited the 7th and 8th editions (1893, 1896); and J. Chalmers Da Costa (1863-1933) of Jefferson Medical College whose 9th edition (1901) carried the *Anatomy* into the 20th century.

There were many other Lea anatomy titles. Two were of extraordinary merit (beyond a general didactic use). Harrison Allen (1841-1897), Professor of Physiology at the University of Pennsylvania (and who had performed the autopsy on the celebrated Siamese twins, Chang and Eng Bunker in 1875) prepared *A System of Human Anatomy, Including Its Medical and Surgical Relations* (Henry C. Lea's Son & Co., 1884; in six sections in portfolio) which included "about 825 double-columned quarto pages, with 380 illustrations on 109 full page lithographic plates, many of which are in colors, and 241 engravings in the text." Its sumptuousness was matched by the work of John C. Dalton (1825-1889) on *The Topographical Anatomy of the Brain* (Lea Brothers & Co., 1885, 3 vols.) in three imperial quarto volumes "comprising about 200 pages of descriptive text . . . illustrated with forty-eight life-size photographic plates of brain sections, with a like number of outline explanatory plates, as well as many carefully-executed woodcuts through the text." Dalton, who was Professor of Physiology at Columbia University's College of Physicians and Surgeons, "was the first American to devote his time exclusively to that subject." (Garrison-Morton, Nos. 1401, 1571-72)

In all of the medical disciplines, there were outstanding achievements. In materia medica there was the *National Dispensatory* (Henry C. Lea, 1879; 5th ed., Lea Brothers & Co., 1894, 1896) of Alfred Stillé (1813-1900) and John M. Maisch (1831-1893), and its continuation, *The National Standard Dispensatory* (Lea Brothers & Co., 1905), edited by Hobart Amory Hare (1862-1931) whose *Text-Book of Practical Therapeutics* (Lea Brothers & Co., 1890; 13th ed., Lea & Febiger, 1903) was the leading text of his time.

In pathology, there is an unbroken continuity extending from the *Physiological and Pathological Anatomy* (H. C. Carey & I. Lea, 1824) of John Davidson Godman (1794-1830) to the *Practical Pathology* (Henry C. Lea's Son & Co., 1884) of G[erman] Sims Woodhead (1855-1921); a singular event in mid-century had been the publication of the *Atlas of Pathological Histology* (Blanchard & Lea, 1853) of Gottlieb Glüge (1812-1898), translated from the German by Joseph Leidy (1823-1891), anatomist at the University of Pennsylvania, and first engaged in the experimental transplantation of malignant tumors. (Garrison-Morton, No. 2614) The

Glüge *Atlas* was a very large imperial quarto, with 320 copper-plate figures, plain and colored, with descriptive letter-press.

Representative of dermatology texts was that of J[ames] Nevins Hyde (1840-1910), responsible for the naming of "prurigo nodularis" and the eponym "Hyde's disease" (Garrison-Morton, No. 4076), of the Rush Medical College of Chicago, whose *Practical Treatise on Diseases of the Skin* (Henry C. Lea's Son & Co., 1883; 6th ed., Lea Brothers & Co., 1901) was joined by English works of which the *Skin Diseases* (Henry C. Lea, 1880) of Malcolm Morris (1849-1924) is typical. Central to clinical description and enquiry was the great *Atlas of Venereal Diseases* (Henry C. Lea, 1868) of Auguste Cullerier (1805-1874) which was translated with additions by Freeman J. Bumstead (1826-1879) whose *Pathology and Treatment of Venereal Diseases* (Blanchard & Lea, 1861; 5th ed., Henry C. Lea's Son & Co., 1883) continued as the standard text in the field.

In pediatrics, the development of the specialty, traditionally linked to midwifery, can be traced in the early work of D[avid] Francis Condie (1796-1875), *A Practical Treatise on the Diseases of Children* (Lea & Blanchard, 1844; 6th ed., Henry C. Lea, 1868), through the continuing labors of J[ob] Lewis Smith (1827-1897) whose *Treatise on the Diseases of Infancy and Childhood* (Henry C. Lea, 1869; 8th ed., Lea Brothers & Co., 1896) was the leading text for a quarter-century. And John M[arie] Keating (1852-1893), a young and energetic 19th century Dr. Benjamin Spock, prepared *The Mother's Guide in the Management and Feeding of Infants* (Henry C. Lea's Son & Co., 1881) which went through countless printings, and of which the "New York Medical Journal and Obstetrical Review" (February, 1882) remarked: "A book small in size, written in pleasant style, in language which can be readily understood by any mother, and eminently practical and safe; in fact, a book for which we have been waiting a long time, and which we can most heartily recommend to mothers as *the* book on this subject."

Two authors, both of Philadelphia, have been left for final attention. Very much different, they exercise a continuing fascination. The aristocratic, reclusive René La Roche (1795-1872) is the very antithesis of the genial and amiable novelist-physician S[ilas] Weir Mitchell (1829-1914). Both were Lea authors, and in their very idiosyncratic differences and interests illustrate the scope and range of the Lea influence.

René La Roche, the son of a French physician, was born in Philadelphia, took his M.D. at the University of Pennsylvania (1820), and spent his entire professional life in the city. A founder of the Monday Evening Club (said to be the first medical club in the United States), and a member of the Philadelphia College of Physicians, he was an accomplished musician and an aesthete, and one of the most erudite physicians of his time. Samuel D. Gross, who knew La Roche for many years, speaks of him affectionately: "Dr. La Roche had an expressive and intellectual countenance, a handsome eye, and a good forehead, although his head was not very large. His highly-organized and well-balanced brain enabled him to perform a vast amount of labor. In his habits he was retiring; and he never seemed so happy as when he was in his library up to his elbow in his manuscripts. He was fond of his friends, and his friends were fond of him; and they can never forget his pleasant social visits, enlivened as they were by agreeable conversation and the recital of pertinent anecdotes, of which he had a supply of rare value. He was a charming conversationalist, always instructive, and free from affectation and pedantry. He was a great reader of light literature, was well informed respecting passing events, and could talk well upon almost any subject." (*Autobiography*, II, 375-376)

Like most Philadelphians, La Roche was both terrified and obsessed by the "malarial fevers" out of which the dreaded yellow fever seemed to derive, and to these morbid agencies he directed most of his researches. Out of his investigations came two works: *Pneumonia: Its Supposed Connection . . . with Autumnal Fevers, Including An Inquiry into the Existence and Morbid Agency of Malaria* (Blanchard & Lea, 1854) and his *magnum opus*, the 1500 page *Yellow Fever, Considered in its Historical, Pathological, Etiological, and Therapeutical Relations, Including a Sketch of the Disease as It Has Occurred in Philadelphia from 1699 to 1854* (Blanchard & Lea, 1855, 2 vols.). More than a medical treatise, this is a kaleidoscopic social history, in which La Roche placed "before the reader an exposé of the whole subject; in a word, a comprehensive treatise on the yellow fever, in which every point of interest is fully examined." Gross has testified to the work's importance: "As a work of profound erudition, at once complete and exhaustive, written in a scholarly style, and evincing the most patient and extraordinary research, the monograph on Yellow Fever, by Dr. La Roche, is without a rival in any language. The author was at great pains and expense in obtaining everything that had been written upon the subject, and, as he himself expresses it, neglected no opportunity of rendering himself practically familiar with the disease of which he thus became the distinguished historian. The facts borrowed from the numerous writers consulted by him seem to have been verified in every instance by personal reference to their works, a task in itself of immense labor—enough, indeed, to cause the eye and brain to ache and the hand to tremble. This, assuredly, is high praise, but it is deserved. His library on yellow fever embraced the literature of all countries—the United States, Cuba, Mexico, South America, Spain, the East and West Indies, France, Germany, Italy, and Great Britain." (*Autobiography*, II, 376) It is a curious irony that it remained for the descendants of Mathew Carey (who had himself written a book on the yellow fever scourge in Philadelphia) to publish the monumental *Yellow Fever* of René La Roche.

S. Weir Mitchell was a long-time friend and associate of Henry C. Lea (1825-1909); for a time he served as Lea's personal physician. The son of a noted physician (John Kearsley Mitchell, 1793-1858), Mitchell took his M.D. at Jefferson Medical College (1850), and devoted most of his attention to clinical neurology. His manner of writing is engaging and easy, personal but not idiosyncratic, and unpretentious, the very opposite of René La Roche, whose scholarship is, at times, overwhelming. These very qualities of Mitchell may explain his success not only as a therapeutist, but as a novelist-storyteller. Mitchell inspires confidence, and the ameliorative effects of his "rest-treatment" may have well been due as much to his manner as to his prescriptive tonic remedies. His importance as a neurologist is attested by a wide range of citations in Garrison-Morton (Nos. 1367, 1404, 2167, 2706, 4544-4545, 4551-4555). For over forty years, Mitchell was physician to the Philadelphia Orthopaedic Hospital which under his influence became a center for the treatment of nervous disorders.

In the Lea canons, Mitchell is represented by *Lectures on Diseases of the Nervous System, Especially in Women* (Henry C. Lea's Son & Co., 1881; 2nd ed., Lea Brothers & Co., 1885), and *Clinical Lessons on Nervous Diseases* (Lea Brothers & Co., 1897); and by dozens of reprints extracted out of the Lea medical journals (and individually paginated) of which "Physiologic Studies of the Knee-Jerk, and of Reactions of Muscles under Mechanical and Other Excitants" (Lea Brothers & Co., 1886) is an example.

The *Lectures on Diseases of the Nervous System* proved more successful than most other works published under the Lea imprint in the same field*; and this may have been due more to Mitchell's unpretentious and confidence-inspiring manner in a field which invited general skepticism. An excerpt from the *Lectures* illustrates Mitchell's easy manner, so compelling in its sincerity:

> What it is convenient to call the nervous temperament, or that state which may be acquired, and which I like to describe as general nervousness, is a fertile field for simulated maladies, because in it, as in hysteria, the qualities which we all possess are apt to take on a morbid development, and to get out out of the limits of rational control.
>
> Of the individual share taken by each of these causes I shall by and by speak. Before, however, I pass on to lesser premises, I would like to digress in order to say a few words in explanation of what I mean by general nervousness. You will find this term used over and over in these lectures, and also in the annual statement of diseases treated at the Infirmary for diseases of the nervous system. I used to try to classify these cases under other heads, but came at last to see that there is a state which is best labelled thus, and that after eliminating all the cases which can be otherwise classed, a small residuum is left to which no other name applies. Some of them are more or less neurasthenic people, easily tired in brain or body; but others without this, or with this peculiarity but slightly developed, are merely tremulous nervous folks, easily agitated, over-sensitive, emotional, and timid. This state falls on man or woman or child, and

*Other Lea texts include: G[eorge] Fielding Blanford (1829-1911), *Insanity and Its Treatment* (Henry C. Lea, 1871); Thomas Smith Clouston (1840-1915), *Clinical Lectures on Mental Diseases* (Henry C. Lea's Son & Co., 1884); Allan McLane Hamilton (1848-1919), *Nervous Diseases: Their Description and Treatment* (Henry C. Lea, 1878; 2nd ed., Henry C. Lea's Son & Co., 1881); James Ross (1837-1892), *Handbook of Diseases of the Nervous System* (Lea Brothers & Co., 1885); and George H. Savage, *Insanity and Allied Neuroses* (Henry C. Lea's Son & Co., 1884).

> is not hysteria. It is with some people a morbid birth-gift, with some an inheritance, and in its worst shapes it is made or acquired by misuse of alcohol or tobacco, or tea or coffee. Naturally you may think that such a state must be slowly created, and usually it is; but also it is true that a very permanent state of general nervousness may be evolved by the accident of a moment, when precedent conditions favor it. In a lecture on general nervousness in the male, I mentioned examples of this kind, and last week we saw at my clinic a case in which a moment of intense terror, owing to the fall of a house wall, caused in a healthy girl a state of general nervousness, alike serious and lasting. However acquired, the condition I have outlined highly favors the mimicry of disease. (51-53)

Yet, the empiric soundness of Mitchell's methods is attested by modern clinicians: "Most of his [Mitchell's] ideas arose from his clinical experience. He was one of the first American examples of the class of investigators who have the ability to weld together their laboratory observations and their clinical experience in such a way as to benefit their patients while they are advancing science."* This is high praise, indeed.

---

*James Bordley and A. McGehee Harvey, *Two Centuries of American Medicine*. (Philadelphia: W. B. Saunders Co., 1976), p. 709.

A HANDLIST OF SELECTED BIBLIOGRAPHIES, CATALOGUES AND RELATED REFERENCE MATERIALS

Abbott, L. T. "Medical and Dental Diploma Mills in Vermont in the 1880's and 1890's." Vermont History 37 (Summer (1960): 194-206.

Abrahams, H. J. The Extinct Medical Schools of Baltimore, Maryland. Baltimore: Maryland Historical Society, 1969.

__________ . Extinct Medical Schools of Nineteenth Century Philadelphia. Philadelphia: University of Pennsylvania Press, 1966.

__________ . "Extinct Medical Schools of Nineteenth Century Philadelphia. VI. The Eclectic Medical College of Philadelphia and Philadelphia University of Medicine and Surgery. VII. Last Days of the Bogus Schools. VIII. Summary and Conclusions." Transactions of the College of Physicians of Philadelphia 31 (1964): 231-74, 307-43; 32 (1964): 41-48.

Adams, George W. Doctors in Blue: The Medical History of the Union Army in the Civil War. New York: Abelard-Schuman, 1952. Rep. New York: Collier Books, 1966.

Initially a doctoral dissertation at Harvard University, the author deals with "the medical sciences of that period, . . . [and] continuing problems of military medicine."

Adams, J. H. History of the Life of D. Hayes Agnew. Philadelphia: Davis, 1892.

Adams, Scott. Medical Bibliography in an Age of Discontinuity. Chicago: Medical Library Association, 1981.

Examines development of medical bibliography in relation to the political, social, scientific and technological changes in the United States, focusing on the information requirements of biomedical research.

Adams, S. S. "The Evolution of Pediatric Literature in the United States. Washington, D.C., 1897." Transactions of the American Pediatrics Society 9 (1897): 5-31; Archives of Pediatrics 14 (1897): 401-29.

Albert, Daniel M., and Harold G. Scheie. A History of Ophthalmology at the University of Pennsylvania. Springfield, IL: Charles C. Thomas, 1965.

Allen, J. G. "Daniel Drake and His Friends on Medical Education." Archives of Surgery (Chicago) 92 (1960): 428-44.

American Book Publishing Record Cumulative, 1876-1949. New York: R. R. Bowker, 1980. 15v.

The American Book Publishing Record: Author/Title/Subject Indexes on Microfiche, 1876-1981. New York: R. R. Bowker, 1982.

Multiple access index to some 1.7 million titles, from the inception of LC cataloging to the present. 750 fiche, 42x.

The American Catalogue of Books. Or English Guide to American Literature, Giving the Full Title of Original Works Published in the United States Since the Year 1800. . . . London: S. Low, Son & Co., 1856.

American College of Surgeons. A Catalogue of the H. Winnett Orr Collection and Other Rare Books in the Library. Chicago: 1960.

Contains 2,289 items in classified arrangement, with index of names and selected titles. Incudes early imprints and classics (468 items), important nineteenth- and twentieth-century medical works, especially in surgery, orthopedics, and military medicine; and medical history and biography.

American Journal of the Medical Sciences (1820-1969). Philadelphia: Lea & Febiger, 1820-1969. Quarterly, 1820-87; monthly, 1887-1969.

Originally founded by Mathew Carey as the Philadelphia Journal of the Medical and Physical Sciences in 1820. An invaluable repository of medical history and the biomedical sciences. See Robert E. Turner, "Lea & Febiger," Spectrum 11 (September-October 1963): 64-66.

American Medical Association. Digest of Official Actions, 1846-1958. Compiled by Susan Crawford. Chicago: 1959. Supplement (1959-63), 1966.

Arranged alphabetically by broad subjects with actions in chronological order, and with reference to documents or publications. Subject index.

American Otological Society. History of the American Otological Society, Inc., 1868-1968, Five Score Years of Progress. New York: 1968.

"Anatomical Illustrations from the Fothergill Collection at the Pennsylvania Hospital, with a Foreword by Florence M. Greim." What's New, April 1952, pp. 10-16.

Annan, Gertrude L. "The Academy of Medicine of New York, 1825-1830, and Its Contemporary, the New York Medical Academy." Bulletin of the Medical Library Association 36 (1948): 117-23.

__________ . "Medical Libraries and Medical History." Bulletin of the New York Academy of Medicine 21 (1945): 163-67.

__________ . "The Medical Library Association in Retrospect, 1937-1967." Bulletin of the Medical Library Association 55 (October 1967): 379-89.

__________ . "Outstanding Acquisitions of Rare Books in Medical Libraries of the United States in the Last Decade." Bulletin of the Medical Library Association 45 (1957): 291-300.

__________ . "The Rare Book and History of Medicine Department in the New York Academy of Medicine." Bulletin of the Medical Library Association 39 (1951): 6-8.

__________ . "Recent Trends in Medical Historical Libraries of the United States." LIBRI 3 (1954): 67-74.

Anson, Barry J. "The History of Anatomy in Medical Education." Quarterly Bulletin of the Northwestern University Medical School 30 (1956): 80-94.

Appleton's Cyclopaedia of American Biography. Ed. by J. G. Wilson and John Fiske. New York: Appleton, 1894-1900. 7v. Rep. Detroit, Gale, 1968.

Arrington, George E. A History of Ophthalmology. New York: M. D. Publications, 1959.

Ash, Lee, comp. Serial Publications Containing Medical Classics: An Index to Citations in Garrison-Morton. New Haven, CT: Antiquarium, 1961.
See also his "Corrections to Ash's 'Serial Publications Containing Medical Classics,' " Journal of the History of Medicine 21 (April 1966): 185-87.

Ashhurst, Astley P. C. "The Centenary of Lister (1827-1927): A Tale of Sepsis and Antisepsis." Annals of Medical History 9 (1927): 205-11.

Ashhurst, John, ed. Transactions of the International Medical Congress of Philadelphia, 1876. Philadelphia: Centennial Medical Commission, 1877.
Samuel D. Gross was the president of the Centennial Medical Commission which convened this historic congress. Speakers included Lord Lister, Austin Flint, Henry I. Bowditch, J. M. Toner, N. S. Davis, Lewis Sayre, Washington L. Atlee, Isaac Ray, and others of note. Eleven opening addresses (pp. 1-304) are historical; other sections are devoted to medicine, biology, surgery, dermatology, obstetrics, ophthalmology, otology, sanitary sciences, and mental diseases.

Astbury, Effie C. Casey A. Wood (1856-1942): Ophthalmologist, Bookman, Ornithologist. A Bibliography. Montreal: McGill University Graduate School of Library Sciences, 1981.

Atkinson, William B. The Physicians and Surgeons of the United States. Philadelphia: Robson, 1878.
Includes less well-known men and is especially valuable for the nineteenth century. Many portraits. Arrangement is haphazard; the work is well indexed by name, locality, and subject. A second edition, entitled A Biographical Dictionary of Contemporary American Physicians and Surgeons (Philadelphia: Brinton, 1880), has some new biographies and revisions of others.

Austin, Robert B. "Plans for a Check-List of Medical Americana." Bulletin of the Medical Library Association 40 (1952): 144-46.

___________ . Early American Medical Imprints: A Guide to Works Printed in the United States 1668-1820. Washington, DC: U.S. Department of Health, Education and Welfare, 1961. Rep. Arlington, MA: Printer's Devil, 1977.
Includes 2,105 items alphabetically by author with notices of locations. Titles listed include books, pamphlets, theses, and broadsides.

Ayer, Hugh M. "Nineteenth Century Medicine." Indiana Magazine of History 48 (1952): 233-54.

Baird, Nancy D. David Wendel Yandell: Physician of Old Louisville. Lexington: University of Kentucky Press, 1978.

Ballard, James F. "Boston Medical Library. Oliver Wendell Holmes Exhibit." Bulletin of the Medical Library Association 32 (1944): 240-42.

Ballard, James F. "Historical Source Materials in the Boston Medical Library." Bulletin of the Medical Library Association 39 (1951): 13-15.

Bartholow, Roberts. Medical Education and the Jefferson Medical College of Philadelphia. Philadelphia: W. F. Fell, 1886.

Bauer, Edward L. Doctors Made in America. Philadelphia: J. B. Lippincott, 1963.

Bauer, Louis H., ed. Seventy-Five Years of Medical Progress, 1878-1953. Philadelphia: Lea & Febiger, 1954.

Beecher, Henry K., and Mark D. Altschule. Medicine at Harvard: The First Three Hundred Years. Hanover, NH: University Press of New England, 1977.

Bell, Whitfield J., Jr. "An American Medical Plutarch (James Thacher)." Journal of the American Medical Association 204 (1 April 1968): 11-14.

__________ . "Lives in Medicine: The Biographical Dictionaries of Thacher, Williams, and Gross." Bulletin of the History of Medicine 42 (March-April 1968): 101-20.

Besterman, Thomas. Medicine: A Bibliography of Bibliographies. Totowa, NJ: Rowman and Littlefield, 1971.

Extracted from the author's A World Bibliography of Bibliographies (4th ed., 1965-66).

Bick, Edgar M. "French Influences on Early American Medicine and Surgery." Journal of the Mount Sinai Hospital 24 (1957): 499-509.

Bierring, Walter L. "References of Early American Medicine Available in the Iowa State Medical Library." Journal of Iowa State Medical Society 30 (1940): 40-41.

Billingham, R. E., and H. Koprowski. "The Wistar Institute of Anatomy and Biology, Philadelphia." Nature 184 (1959): 6-10.

Billings, John S. "The Medical Journals of the United States." Boston Medical and Surgical Journal 100 (1879): 1-14.

__________ . "The History and Literature of Surgery." In System of Surgery, edited by Frederic S. Dennis, vol. 1, pp. 17-144. Philadelphia: Lea, 1895.

Blake, John Ballard and Charles Roos. Medical Reference Works, 1679-1966: A Selected Bibliography. Chicago: Medical Library Association, 1967.

Supersedes the bibliographies published as part of the Medical Library Association's Handbook of Medical Library Practice (1956). Lists more than 2,700 titles in classed arrangement with three main sections: medicine, general; history of medicine; and special subjects.

__________ . Supplement 1. Compiled by Mary Virginia Clark. Chicago: Medical Library Association, 1970.

Follows the pattern of the main work, but excludes references on the history of medicine. Includes some three hundred entries.

__________ . Supplement 2, 1969-72. Chicago: Medical Library Association, 1973.

The second Supplement is computer-produced from the National Library of Medicine Current Catalog data base and includes about five hundred citations arranged by author and by subject.

Blake, John Ballard and Charles Roos. Supplement 3. Compiled by Joy S. Richmond. Chicago: Medical Library Association, 1975.

The third Supplement is computer-produced from the National Library of Medicine Current Catalog and includes 244 annotated citations.

Blake, John Ballard, ed. Centenary of Index Medicus, 1879-1979. Bethesda, MD: National Library of Medicine, 1980.

Blanton, Wyndham B. Medicine in Virginia . . . 17th-19th Centuries. Richmond, VA: Garrett & Massie, 1931-33. 3v.

An exhaustive history with a wealth of information, bibliographic references, and lists of Virginia surgeons in the Revolutionary and Civil Wars, medical fees, and acts of the assembly concerning medicine.

Bloomfield, Arthur L. A Bibliography of Internal Medicine; Communicable Diseases. Chicago: University of Chicago Press, 1958.

__________ . A Bibliography of Internal Medicine; Selected Diseases. Chicago: University of Chicago Press, 1960.

Bond, Earl D. Dr. Thomas Story Kirkbride and His Mental Hospital. Philadelphia: J. B. Lippincott, 1947.

Bonner, Thomas N. "Dr. Nathan Smith Davis and the Growth of Chicago Medicine, 1850-1900." Bulletin of the History of Medicine 26 (July-August 1952): 360-74.

__________ . American Doctors and German Universities: A Chapter in International Intellectual Relations, 1870-1914. Lincoln: University of Nebraska Press, 1963.

Deals with the "influences which German study and travel exerted on several generations of American physicians."

__________ . The Kansas Doctor: A Century of Pioneering. Lawrence: University of Kansas Press, 1959.

__________ . Medicine in Chicago, 1850-1950: A Chapter in the Social and Scientific Development of a City. Madison, WI: American History Research Center, 1957.

Bordley, James and Harvey A. McGehee. Two Centuries of American Medicine, 1776-1976. Philadelphia: W. B. Saunders Co., 1976.

A sumptuous bicentennial history intended as "an account of the extraordinary advances in medical education and in the prevention and treatment of disease that have taken place during the two centuries of this nation's political independence."

Bowditch, Henry I. Public Hygiene in America. Boston: Little, Brown, 1877. Rep. New York: Arno Press, 1972.

Bowker's Medical Books in Print. Subject Index, Author Index, Title Index. New York: R. R. Bowker, 1972-. Annual.

Some 25,000 titles currently available in the United States. Classified by subject with author and title indexes. Over 5,000 subject categories in medicine, dentistry, nursing, and veterinary medicine.

Bracken, M. C. "An Analysis of the Evolution of the National Library of Medicine: Implications for the Development of Scientific and Technical Information Networks." Ph.D. dissertation, American University, 1971.

Bradford, Thomas L. Homeopathic Bibliography of the United States, From the Year 1825 to the Year 1891, Inclusive. Philadelphia: Boericke & Tafel, 1892.

Lists books and pamphlets (including many reprints), journals, directories, institutions: a classified compilation, alphabetically by author, with occasional annotations.

__________. The Pioneers of Homeopathy. Philadelphia: Boericke & Tafel, 1897.

Biographical sketches of some five hundred homeopathic physicians of all countries who were practitioners prior to 1835.

Bradley, Edward Sculley. Henry Charles Lea, A Biography. Philadelphia: University of Pennsylvania Press, 1931.

Brieger, Gert H., ed. Medical America in the Nineteenth Century: Readings from the Literature. Baltimore: Johns Hopkins Press, 1972.

A collection of original materials drawn from the nineteenth century on medical education, medical literature, medical practice, surgery, psychiatry, hospitals, and hygiene.

Brodman, Estelle. The Development of Medical Bibliography. Baltimore: Medical Library Association, 1954. Rep. 1982.

An historical study which includes a list of 255 medical bibliographies published since 1500.

Bullough, Vern, and Bonnie Bullough. The Care of the Sick: The Emergence of Modern Nursing. New York: Science History Publications, 1978.

A history of the development of nursing, with historical and contemporary data.

Burke, Margaret N. "The Miller Collection in the Library of the Richmond Academy of Medicine." Bulletin of the History of Medicine 19 (1946): 200-225, 319-44.

Burns, Stanley B. Early Medical Photography in America (1839-1883), Part I, History of Photographic Processes. New York State Journal of Medicine, 79, No. 5 (April 1979): 788-795.

__________. Early Medical Photography in America (1839-1883), Part II, Physicians and Early Photography. New York State Journal of Medicine, 79, No. 6 (May 1979): 943-947.

__________. Early Medical Photography in America (1839-1883), Part III, The Daguerrean Era. New York State Journal of Medicine, 79, No. 8 (July 1979): 1256-1268.

__________. Early Medical Photography in America (1839-1883), Part IV, Early Wet-Plate Era, New York State Journal of Medicine, 79, No. 12 (November 1979): 1931-1938.

__________. Early Medical Photography in America (1839-1883), Part V, Beginnings of Psychiatric Photography. New York State Journal of Medicine, 80, No. 2 (February 1980): 270-282.

__________. Early Medical Photography in America (1839-1883), Part VI, Civil War Medical Photography. New York State Journal of Medicine, 80, No. 9 (August 1980): 1444-1469.

__________. Early Medical Photography in America (1839-1883), Part VII, American Medical Publications with Photographs. New York State Journal of Medicine, 81, No. 8 (July 1981): 1226-1264.

Caldwell, C., M.D., Autobiography. Preface, notes, and appendix by H. W. Warner. Philadelphia: Lippincott, Grambo & Co., 1855.

Calhoun, Daniel H. Professional Lives in America: Structure and Aspiration 1750-1850. Cambridge, MA: Harvard University Press, 1965.

Camac, Charles N. B., ed. Epoch-Making Contributions to Medicine, Surgery, and the Allied Sciences: Being Reprints of Those Communications Which First Conveyed Epoch-Making Observations to the Scientific World, Together with Biographical Sketches of the Observers. Philadelphia: W. B. Saunders, 1909. Rep. New York: Dover, 1959.

Contains texts in English of Twelve papers, by Lister, Harvey, Auenbrugger, Laennec, Jenner, Morton, Warren Simpson, and Holmes.

Carmichael, Emmett B. "J. Marion Sims: Inventor, Physician, Surgeon." Journal of the International College of Surgeons 33 (1960): 756-62.

Cary, John. Joseph Warren: Physician, Politician, Patriot. Urbana: University of Illinois Press, 1961.

A Catalogue of Books Represented by Library of Congress Printed Cards. Ann Arbor, MI: Edwards Brothers, 1942-1946. 167v. Also: Supplement, Ann Arbor, MI: J. W. Edwards, 1948. 42v.; Library of Congress Author Catalog, 1948-1952. Ann Arbor, MI: J. W. Edwards, 1953. 24v.; and the National Union Catalog, A Cumulative Author List, 1953-1957. Ann Arbor, MI: J. W. Edwards, 1958. 28v.

Cathell, D. W. The Physician Himself and What He Should Add to His Scientific Requirements. 2d. ed. Baltimore: Cushings & Bailey, 1882. Rep. with an introduction by Charles E. Rosenberg. New York: Arno Press/New York Times, 1972.

The first edition appeared in 1881, and the last revision in 1922. Intended as a manual for the medical practitioner, and an accurate "index to the problems and aspirations of American medical men for several decades."

Cavanagh, G. S., ed. Early American Medical Imprints in the Library of Duke University Medical Center. Durham, NC: Duke University Medical Center, 1966.

A Century of Service: Boericke & Tafel, 1835-1935. Philadelphia: Boericke & Tafel, 1935.

Chaff, Sandra L., *et al.* Women in Medicine: A Bibliography of the Literature on Women Physicians. Metuchen, NJ: Scarecrow Press, 1977.

Comprehensive coverage of the literature about women physicians in all parts of the world, with some 4,000 largely annotated entries. Most of the material cited is in the Florence A. Moore Library of Medicine at the Medical College of Pennsylvania. Formerly the Female Medical College of Pennsylvania (1850-66) and the Women's Medical College of Pennsylvania (1867-1969), this institution has been a leader in the medical education of women.

Chapman, C. B. "The Flexner Report by Abraham Flexner." Daedalus 103 (Winter 1974): 105-17.

Chen, K. K., ed. The American Society for Pharmacology and Experimental Therapeutics, Incorporated; The First Sixty Years 1908-1969. Washington, DC: Judd & Detwiler, 1969.

Chicago Medical Society. History of Medicine and Surgery and Physicians and Surgeons of Chicago. Chicago: Biographical Publishing Corp., 1922.
Includes biographies of 172 physicians (1803-1922), with historical accounts of medical colleges, hospitals, medical societies, and the health department.

Churchill, Edward D. "The Harvard Medical School, 1906-1956." New England Journal of Medicine 255 (1956): 1035-41.

Cincinnati University. Medical College Library. David A. Tucker, Jr. Library of the History of Medicine: A Bibliography. Cincinnati: 1959.

Clark, J. Henry. The Medical Men of New Jersey in Essex District From 1666 to 1866. Newark, NJ: Evening Courier, 1867.

Clarke, E. H., ed. A Century of American Medicine. 1776-1876. Philadelphia: Lea, 1876. Rep. New York: Burt Franklin, 1973.
Contains chapters by E. H. Clarke, "Practical Medicine"; H. J. Bigelow, "Discovery of Modern Anesthesia"; S. D. Gross, "Surgery"; T. G. Thomas, Obstetrics and Gynaecology"; and J. S. Billings, "Literature and Institutions." No index. First published in the American Journal of the Medical Sciences, 1876.

Cleave, Egbert. Biographical Cyclopaedia of Homeopathic Physicians and Surgeons. Philadelphia: Galaxy Publishing Co., 1873.

College of Physicians of Philadelphia. Transactions of the College of Physicians of Philadelphia, Centennial Volume. Philadelphia: 1887.

Cooper, Gayle. A Checklist of American Imprints for [date]. Metuchen, NJ: 1972-.
Continues Richard H. Shoemaker's A Checklist of American Imprints for the Year 1830 and After. Arrangement and entries follow the practice of Shoemaker.

Cordasco, Francesco, ed. Italians in the City: Health and Related Needs. New York: Arno Press/New York Times, 1975.
On Italian immigrant health problems and needs, 1903-34.

Cordasco, Francesco and David N. Alloway. Medical Education in the United States: A Guide to Information Sources. Detroit: Gale Research Co., 1980.

Cordell, Eugene F. The Medical Annals of Maryland. 1799-1899. Baltimore: Medical and Chirurgical Faculty, 1903.
Prepared for the centennial of the Medical and Chirurgical Faculty. Includes history, chronology (1608-1902), and some 2,400 biographical sketches.

Corner, G. W. Two Centuries of Medicine: A History of the School of Medicine, University of Pennsylvania. Philadelphia: J. B. Lippincott, 1965.

Coulter, Harris L. "Political and Social Aspects of Nineteenth-Century Medicine in the United States: The Formation of the American Medical Association and Its Struggle with Homeopathic and Eclectic Physicians." Ph.D. disseration, Columbia University, 1969.

Crowley, C. George. Dental Bibliography: A Standard List of Books on Dentistry Published throughout the World from 1536 to 1885. Arranged Chronologically, and Supplemented with a Complete Cross-Reference to Authors. Philadelphia: The S. S. White Dental Mfg. Co., 1885.

The Cumulative Book Index: A World List of Books in the English Language. New York: H. W. Wilson Co., 1898-. Title and Frequency have varied;

published monthly (except August), with tri-monthly and annual cumulations. From 1928 to 1968 appeared also in 2-, 4-, and 5-yr cumulations.

Annual volumes provide a single-alphabet author-title-subject list which attempts to include all books written in English and published anywhere in the world, excepting only limited editions, local publications, government documents, pamphlets, reprints. Main entries are under author's name and include full name (pseudonyms are identified), complete title, series, edition, number of pages, imprint, ISBN code, LC card number, and price. Provides a directory of publishers.

Cushing, Harvey. The Life of Sir William Osler. New York: Oxford University Press, 1940. (orig., 2v., 1925).

Da Costa, Jacob M. Biographical Sketch of Professor Samuel D. Gross. Philadelphia: Times Printing House, 1884.

Dana, C. L. "The Seguins of New York: Their Careers and Contributions to Science and Education." Annals of Medical History 6 (1924): 475-79.

Darling, Louise, ed. Handbook of Medical Library Practice. 4th ed. Chicago: Medical Library Association, 1982-1983. 3v.

Davis, Loyal. Fellowship of Surgeons: A History of the American College of Surgeons. Springfield, IL: Charles C. Thomas, 1960.

Davis, Nathan Smith. History of Medical Education and Institutions in the United States. Chicago: S. C. Griggs and Co., 1851.

____________ . History of the American Medical Association from Its Organization up to January, 1855. Philadelphia: Lippincott, Grambo, and Co., 1855.

Denny-Brown, D., *et al.* Centennial Anniversary Volume of the American Neurological Association, 1875-1975. New York: Springer, 1975.

[Dental History.] A Catalogue of the Rare Book Collection in the Northwestern University Dental School Library. Chicago: Dental School Library, Northwestern University, 1976.

Dictionary of American Biography. Ed. Allen Johnson and Dumas Malone. 20 vols. plus Index. New York and London: Scribner's 1928-37. Supplement One (to Dec. 31, 1935), 1944. Rptd. in 22 vols. with corrigenda in vol. 1, 1946. Supplement Two (to Dec. 31, 1940), 1958. Supplement Three (to Dec. 31, 1945), 1973; Supplement Four (to Dec. 31, 1950) 1974.

A collection of biographies of deceased Americans who lived from colonial times to the present. The 23 volumes published so far contain 14,443 biographical articles. Articles are relatively long and can include all the kinds of information found in full-length biographies. Bibliographies of sources used in preparing the biography are provided at the end of each article. Arrangement is alphabetical by name of biographee. The Index for the original 20 vols. consists of 6 separate lists: (1) biographees, alphabetically by name, (2) contributors, alphabetically by name, (3) biographees, by state (or country) and city of birth, (4) biographees, by schools and colleges attended, (5) biographees, by occupation or activity (*e.g.*, abolitionist, writer), and (6) topics and subjects, including titles of literary works. The Concise Dictionary of American Biography (2nd. ed. 1977), is an epitome of the DAB and its supplements; it provides some 16,000 biographical articles averaging about 1/14 the length of the originals.

Dictionary of National Biography. Ed. Leslie Stephen and Sidney Lee. 63 vols. London: Smith, Elder 1885-1900. Supplement 3, vols., 1901. Errata, 1904. The original 63 vols. plus the 3 vol. supplement rptd. in 22 vols., London, 1921. 'Compact Edition' (with reading glass), 2 vols., 1975. Decennial supplements cover the period 1901-1960.

Biographies of deceased residents of Great Britain and the colonies from the beginning of history to the present. Arranged alphabetically by biographees' names. Entries are relatively full (some extend to more than 100 pages) and can include all the kinds of information found in full-length biographies. Bibliographies of sources used in preparing the biography are provided at the end of each article. Indexing varies. The original 66 vols. are not indexed. The first 21 vols. of the 1921 reprint each contain an index that supplies references to vol. 22 which is a reprint of the original 3 vol. supplement of 1901. The supplementary vols. covering the period 1901-1960 have cumulating indexes; the supplement (for the years 1951-60) includes an index to all the supplements for 1901-1960. The Concise Dictionary of National Biography, 2 vols. 1903, (1961) is an epitome of the DNB and its supplements, in which entries are reduced to about 1/14 of the original.

Drake, Daniel. A Systematic Treatise, Historical, Etiological, and Practical, on the Principal Diseases of the Interior Valley of North America, As They Appear in the Caucasian, African, Indian and Esquimaux Varieties of Its Population. Cincinnati: W. B. Smith & Co., 1850. Rep. New York: Plenum, 1969.

Duffy, John. The Rudolph Matas History of Medicine in Louisiana. Baton Rouge: Louisiana State University Press, 1958-62. 2v.

__________ . "The Changing Image of the American Physician." Journal of the American Medical Association 200 (3 April 1967): 30-34.

__________ . A History of Public Health in New York City, 1625-1866. New York: Russell Sage Foundation, 1968.

__________ . "Medical Practice in the Ante-Bellum South." Journal of Southern History 25 (1959): 53-72.

__________ . "A Note on Ante-Bellum Southern Nationalism and Medical Practice." Journal of Southern History 34 (May 1968): 266-76.

__________ . "Slavery and Slave Health in Louisiana, 1766-1825." Bulletin of the Tulane Medical Faculty 26 (1967); 1-6.

Dunglison, Richard J. The Public Medical Libraries of Philadelphia. Philadelphia: J. B. Lippincott, 1871.

Dunglison, Robley. A Dictionary of Medical Science. 23 eds. Philadelphia: Lea, 1833-1903.

Includes biographies, and bibliographies for some name and subject entries. Some patent medicines listed under proprietors' names. First edition has title A New Dictionary of Medical Science and Literature; 1839-66 editions have title Medical Lexicon; 1874-1900 editions revised by Richard J. Dunglison; 1903 edition revised by Thomas L. Stedman.

Durbin, Paul T., ed. A Guide to the Culture of Science, Technology, and Medicine. New York: Free Press, 1980.

Earle, A. Scott, ed. Surgery in America: Selected Writings. Philadelphia: W. B. Saunders, 1965.

Includes source materials from the colonial era to the twentieth century.

Ebaugh, Franklin G. "The History of Psychiatric Education in the United States from 1844 to 1944." American Journal of Psychiatry 100 (1944): 151-60.

Ebert, Myrl. "The Rise and Development of the American Medical Periodical, 1797-1850." Bulletin of the Medical Library Association 40 (July 1952): 243-76.

Eckenhoff, J. E. Anesthesia from Colonial Times: A History of Anesthesia at the University of Pennsylvania. Montreal: Lippincott, 1966.

The Evan Bedford Library of Cardiology: Catalogue of Books, Pamphlets and Journals. London. Royal College of Physicians, 1977.

Evans, A. S. "Austin Flint and His Contributions to Medicine." Bulletin of the History of Medicine 32 (1958): 224-41.

Fay, M. S. "Ann Preston: Dean of the Women's Medical College of Philadelphia, 1866-1872." Transactions of the College of Physicians of Philadelphia 33 (1965): 43-48.

Fellman, Anita C. and Michael Fellman. Making Sense of Self: Medical Advice Literature in Late Nineteenth-Century America. Philadelphia: University of Pennsylvania Press, 1981.

Fishbein, Morris. "Centennial of the American Medical Association." British Medical Journal 1 (1947): 795-98.

__________ . "Centennial of the American Medical Association and Its Fundamental Motivations." Hygeia 25 (1947): 423-25.

__________ . "History of the American Medical Association." Journal of the American Medical Association 132 (1946): 636-38, passim; 133 (1947): 23-26, passim.

__________ . A History of the American Medical Association, 1847 to 1947; With Biographies of the Presidents . . . By Walter Bierring; and With the Histories of the Publications, Councils, Bureaus and Other Official Bodies [by Various Authors]. Philadelphia: W. B. Saunders, 1947.

Fleming, Donald. William H. Welch and the Rise of Modern Medicine. Boston: Little, Brown, 1954.

Flexner, Abraham. "Medical Education, 1909-1924." Journal of the American Medical Association 82 (15 March 1924): 833-38.

__________ . Medical Education in the United States and Canada. 1910. Rep. New York: Carnegie Foundation, 1960.

Commissioned by the Carnegie Foundation for the Advancement of Teaching, the Flexner Report generated massive reforms in medical education. As a result of the agitation for reform set in motion by the report, seventy-six medical schools went out of existence between 1910 and 1920 either by ceasing to function or by merging with stronger institutions. The Flexner Report is in two parts. Part 1 gives a history of medical education in the United States, describes its status, and makes recommendations for its improvement. Part 2 presents, state by state, a description of each medical school; included are data on 155 medical schools, 7 of which were in Canada. Of the 148 in the United States, 116 were of the regular type, 15 were homeopathic, 8 were osteopathic, and 1 was physiomedical.

Flexner, Abraham. I Remember. New York: Simon and Schuster, 1940. Rev. ed., 1960.

Flexner, James T. Doctors on Horseback: Pioneers of American Medicine. New York: Viking, 1937. Rep. New York: Macmillan, 1962.

Biographies of John Morgan, Benjamin Rush, Ephraim McDowell, Daniel Drake, William Beaumont, and a sketch of the discovery of ether anesthesia.

Flexner, Simon. A Half Century of American Medicine. Founders' Day Address. University of Louisville, 3 April 1937. Louisville, KY: University of Louisville, 1937.

Flexner, Simon, and James Thomas. William Henry Welch and the Heroic Age of American Medicine. New York: Viking, 1941.

"The Francis A. Countway Library of Medicine." Harvard Library Bulletin 14 (1960): 307-8.

Francis. A. Countway Library of Medicine, Boston. Author-Title Catalog of the Francis A. Countway Library of Medicine for Imprints through 1959. Boston: G. K. Hall, 1973. 10v.

The Francis A. Countway Library of Medicine was established in 1965 and houses the merged collections of the Boston Medical Library and the Harvard Medical Library. This catalog lists imprints from before 1960, and is basically an historical collection.

Francis, Samuel W. Biographical Sketches of Distinguished Living New York Surgeons. New York: John Bradburn, 1866.

Fulton, John F. The Great Medical Bibliographers: A Study in Humanism. Philadelphia: University of Pennsylvania Press, 1951.

Garrison, Fielding H. "Available Sources and Future Prospects of Medical Biography." Bulletin of the New York Academy of Medicine 4 (1928): 586-607.

Lists works which include biographic material, arranged by countries; also general medical biographic collections, biographies of individual men, and dictionaries of anonymous and pseudonymous works. Reprinted in his Contributions to the History of Medicine . . . 1925-1935 (New York: Hafner, 1966), pp. 698-718.

__________ . "Revised Students' Check-List of Texts Illustrating the History of Medicine, with References for Collateral Reading." Bulletin of the History of Medicine 1 (1933): 333-434.

__________ . An Introduction to the History of Medicine, With Medical Chronology, Suggestions for Study and Bibliographic Data. 4th. ed. Philadelphia: W. B. Saunders, 1960.

The standard English-language reference history. Classified bibliography (pp. 884-922) with references throughout. The first edition appeared in 1914.

__________ . A Medical Bibliography [Garrison and Morton]: An Annotated Check-List of Texts Illustrating the History of Medicine. 3d ed. Compiled by Leslie T. Morton. Philadelphia: J. B. Lippincott; [London]: Andre Deutsch, [1970].

Includes 7,534 largely annotated entries, arranged by subject. "Under each subject the important works showing the development of that subject are arranged in chronological order." Includes index of personal names and an index of subjects.

Gayley, James F. History of the Jefferson Medical College of Philadelphia. Philadelphia: Joseph M. Wilson, 1858.

Gemmill, C. L. "Robley Dunglison's Dictionary of Medical Science, 1833." Bulletin of the New York Academy of Medicine 48 (June 1972): 791-98.

Gibbon, J. H. "Samuel D. Gross." Annals of Medical History 8 (1926): 136-40.

__________ . "Thomas Dent Mütter, Professor of Surgery, Jefferson Medical School, 1841-1856." Annals of Medical History 7 (1925): 237-41.

Gibney, R. Gibney of the Ruptured and Crippled. Edited by A. R. Shands, New York: Appleton-Century-Crofts, 1969.

Gilbert, Judson, B. A Bibliography of Articles on the History of American Medicine Compiled from "Writings on American History," 1902-1937. New York: New York Academy of Medicine, 1951.

Some 650 references, mainly on the United States. Valuable for indexing of local history and other nonmedical journals.

Gillespie, Charles C., ed. Dictionary of Scientific Biography. New York: Scribner's 1970-1980. 16v.

A vast biographical compendium of scientists of all regions and periods which includes biographies of many American physicians and medical scientists.

Goodwin, E. Medical Education in Brooklyn 1860-1960: The First Hundred Years. New York: State University of New York, 1973.

Goss, C. M. A Brief Account of Henry Gray, F.R.S. and His "Anatomy, Descriptive and Surgical," During a Century of Its Publication in America. Philadelphia: Lea & Febiger, 1959.

A centenary notice of the American edition of the celebrated Anatomy by Henry Gray (1827-61). The first American edition was published in Philadelphia by Blanchard and Lea in 1859.

Gould, G. M. Jefferson Medical College of Philadelphia, 1826-1904. Chicago: Lewis Publishing Co., 1904. 2v.

Green, Samuel A. History of Medicine in Massachusetts. Boston: Williams, 1881.

__________ . "Notes on the Earliest Teaching of Medicine in Massachusetts." Proceedings of the Massachusetts Historical Society, 2d ser., (1884-85): entire issue.

Greenwood, R. D. "Nathan Smith Davis: Medical Educator." Journal of the Kansas Medical Society 79 (January 1975): 13-16.

Grob, Gerald N. Edward Jarvis and the Medical World of Nineteenth-Century America. Knoxville: University of Tennessee Press, 1978.

Edward Jarvis (1803-94), a physician alienist, and statistician, was a major figure in nineteenth-century medicine, notable for his reform of procedures in the United States census.

Gross, Samuel D. History of American Medical Literature from 1776 to the Present Time. Philadelphia: Collins, 1875. Rep. New York: Burt Franklin, 1972.

A bibliographical survey dealing with textbooks, translations, reprints, periodicals, and book publishers. Presented as a series of lectures at Jefferson Medical College in 1875.

Gross, Samuel D. Autobiography of Samuel D. Gross. Philadelphia: George Barrie, 1887. 2v. Rep. New York: Arno Press, 1972.

Samuel David Gross (1805-84), professor of surgery in the Jefferson Medical College of Philadelphia, was one of the most famous medical teachers of the nineteenth century. His System of Surgery (Philadelphia: Lea, 1859, 2 vols.) went into six editions. His Autobiography, edited and published posthumously by his sons, is an invaluable repository of information on nineteenth-century medical practice and teaching.

__________ . A Discourse on the Life, Character, and Services of Daniel Drake. Louisville, KY: Louisville Journal, 1853.

__________ . Memoir of Robley Dunglison. Philadelphia: Collins, 1869.

__________ . Memoir of Valentine Mott, M.D. New York: D. Appleton, 1868.

__________ . Memorial Oration in Honor of Ephraim McDowell, Louisville: Kentucky State Medical Society, 1879.

__________ , ed. Lives of Eminent American Physicians and Surgeons of the Nineteenth Century. Philadelphia: Lindsay & Blakiston, 1861.

Guerra, Francisco. American Medical Bibliography 1639-1783; A Chronological and Critical and Bibliographical Study of Books, Pamphlets, Broadsides, and Articles in Periodical Publications Relating to the Medical Sciences: Medicine, Surgery, Pharmacy, Dentistry, and Veterinary Medicine; Printed in the Present Territory of the United States of America During the British Dominion and the Revolutionary War. New York: L. C. Harper, 1962.

Lists and describes books, pamphlets, broadsides, almanacs, magazines and newspapers.

Hall, Courtney R. "The Rise of Professional Surgery in the United States, 1800-1865." Bulletin of the History of Medicine 26 (1952): 231-62.

Haller, John S. American Medicine in Transition, 1840-1910. Urbana: University of Illinois Press, 1981.

Hamlin, P. G. "Aesculapius in Charlottesville: Robley Dunglison, M.D." Virginia Cavalcade 22 (1972): 14-21.

Hanaway, J. "William Osler: The Man and the Influence of the History of Medicine on His Career." Virginia Medical Monthly 97 (May 1970): 282-93.

Harrington, T. F. The Harvard Medical School: A History, Narrative and Documentary. New York: Lewis, 1905. 3v.

Hartshorne, H. "Memoir of George B. Wood. Read before the American Philosophical Society. October 11, 1880." Proceedings of the American Philosophical Society 19 (1880): 118-52.

Harvard Medical School Faculty. The Harvard Medical School, 1782-1906. Boston: Harvard Medical School Faculty, 1906.

Harvey, A. McGehee, and Victor A. McKiesick, eds. Osler's Textbook Revisited. New York: Appleton-Century-Crofts, 1967.

Selections, with commentaries, from Sir William Osler's Principles and Practice of Medicine (1892), the sixteenth edition of which appeared in 1947. Selections are from the seventh edition (1909), the last edition which Osler did unaided.

Haymaker, W. E., and F. Schiller, eds. The Founders of Neurology: One Hundred and Forty-Six Biographical Sketches by Eighty-Eight Authors. 2d ed. Springfield, IL: Charles C. Thomas, 1970.

Health Science Books, 1876-1982. New York: R. R. Bowker, 1982. 4v.

Lists some 100,000 health science books published in the United States since the inception of Library of Congress cataloging.

Heirs of Hippocrates: The Development of Medicine in a Catalogue of Historic Books in the Health Sciences Library, University of Iowa. Iowa City: Friends of the University of Iowa Libraries, 1980.

Descriptions of 1196 books in the John Martin Rare Book Room in Health Sciences Library, University of Iowa.

Henkel, Herman H., ed. Catalog of the Clifford G. Grulle Collection on Pediatrics. Chicago: John Crerar Library, 1959.

__________ . "The Physician as Book Collector. Notes on Famous Libraries." Journal of the International College of Surgeons 34 (1960): 107-17.

Henry, Frederick P., ed. Standard History of the Medical Profession of Philadelphia. Chicago: Goodspeed, 1897.

Includes biographical sketches, data on institutions and literature, accounts of works of important authors, and an annotated chronology of forty-five journals.

Hirsch, Rudolph, ed. A Catalogue of the Manuscripts and Archives in the Francis Clark Wood Institute of the College of Physicians of Philadelphia. Philadelphia: University of Pennsylvania Press, 1981.

Hollenbeck, Z. J., and J. I. Hollenbeck. Profiles in Surgery, Gynecology, and Obstetrics: Bibliographical Sketches of Famous Personalities. New York: Medical Examination Publishing Co., 1973.

Holloway, Lisabeth, ed. Medical Obituaries: American Physicians' Biographical Notices in Selected Medical Journals Before 1907. New York and London: Garland Publishing, 1981.

Holmes, Oliver Wendell. The Medical Profession in Massachusetts. Boston: John Wilson and Son, 1869.

Honan, James H. Honan's Handbook to Medical Europe. Philadelphia: P. Blakiston's Son, 1912.

Hooker, Worthington. Physician and Patient: Or a Practical View of the Mutual Duties, Relations and Interests of the Medical Profession and the Community. New York: Baker and Scribner, 1849. Rep. New York: Arno Press, 1972.

Howard, J. W. "Nineteenth Century Medicine." Delaware Medical Journal 48 (October 1976): 581-82.

Hubbell, Alvin A. The Development of Ophthalmology in America, 1800-1870. A Contribution to Ophthalmologic History and Biography. Chicago: American Medical Association, 1908.

Hun, Henry. A Guide for American Medical Students in Europe. New York: William Wood & Co., 1883.

Index Medicus: A Monthly Classified Record of the Current Medical Literature of the World. Compiled under supervision of John S. Billings and

Robert Fletcher. Washington, DC: Carnegie Institution of Washington, 1879-99. 21v.

A second series (81 volumes), edited by Fletcher and F. H. Garrison, appeared from 1903 to 1920; a third series (6 volumes), edited by Garrison, from 1921 to 1927. In 1927 the Quarterly Cumulative Index to Current Medical Literature (12 vols., 1916-26) was amalgamated with the Index Medicus to form Quarterly Cumulative Index Medicus (1927-56) which, with number 21, was superseded in 1960 by a new monthly Index Medicus with an annual Cumulated Index Medicus. The gap 1900-1902 was filled by Bibliographia Medica (3 vols.), edited by C. Potain and C. Richet.

Ivy, R. H. "Personal Recollections of Holders of the John Rhea Barton Professorship of Surgery at the University of Pennsylvania School of Medicine." Transactions and Studies of the College of Physicians of Philadelphia 42 (January 1975): 239-62.

Jacobi, Abraham. "The New York Medical College, 1882-1906." Annals of Medical History 1 (December 1917): 368-73.

Johns Hopkins University. The Johns Hopkins University School of Medicine 1893-1943. Baltimore: Johns Hopkins University Press, 1943.

Juettner, Otto. Daniel Drake and His Followers. Cincinnati: Harvey Publishing Company, 1909.

Kampmeier, Otto F. "Nathan Smith Davis, 1817-1904." Journal of Medical Education 34 (May 1959): 496-508.

Katz, A. L. "Samuel D. Gross, M.D." The Pennsylvania German Society Proceedings and Addresses 39 (12 October 1928): 1-20.

Kauffman, James L. Dr. George McClellan (1796-1847) and His Jefferson Medical College and Medical Center. New York: Newcomer Society in North America, 1950.

Kaufman, Martin. American Medical Education: The Formative Years, 1765-1910. Westport, CT: Greenwood Press, 1976.

An examination of the "major trends and developments" in medical education, and its relationship "to the social and cultural milieu, to scientific developments, and to problems within the medical profession itself."

Keen, William W. Samuel David Gross: The Lesson of His Life and Labors. Philadelphia: Jefferson Medical College, 1910.

Kelly, Howard A., and Walter L. Burrage. Dictionary of American Medical Biography. New York: Appleton, 1928. Rep. Boston: Milford House, 1971.

Published in 1912 as Cyclopedia of American Medical Biography (Philadelphia: W. B. Saunders, 2 vols.) and in 1920 as American Medical Biographies (Baltimore: Norman, Remington Co., 1,320 p.). Comprehensive biographies, with bibliographies, of 2,049 deceased American physicians and surgeons from Colonial days to 1927. Although each edition includes new biographical sketches, some material is dropped from each, and the earlier editions continue to be useful.

Kelly, James. The American Catalogue of Books (Original and Reprints) Published in the United States . . . with Date of Publication, Size, Price, and Publisher's Name. 2 vols. New York: J. Wiley & Sons, 1866-71. Rptd., New York: Peter Smith, 1938; rptd. in 1 vol., Metuchen, NJ: Scarecrow Press, 1967.

A continuation of Roorbach's Bibliotheca Americana for the period Jan., 1861 to Jan., 1871. Arranged as a single-alphabet author-title list, entries provide information on date, format, price, and publisher. The first volume supplies items omitted by Roorbach.

Kett, Joseph F. The Formation of the American Medical Profession: The Role of Institutions, 1780-1860. New Haven, CT: Yale University Press, 1968.

A chronological study of aspects "connected with the formation of the profession." Kett has sought " to go beyond an institutional approach; my method has been to use social and intellectual currents as manifested in sectarianism to evaluate the role of institutions."

Kilgour, Frederick G. The Library of the Medical Institution of Yale College and Its Catalogue of 1865. New Haven, CT: Yale University Press, 1960.

King, Lester S. The Growth of Medical Thought. Chicago: University of Chicago Press, 1974.

Chapters on successive periods, with emphasis on selected individuals representing trends in medical science and theories of disease. First issued in 1963.

King, William H., ed. History of Homeopathy and Its Institutions in America. New York: Lewis, 1905. 4v.

Largely a compilation, with notices of state histories, biographies, and accounts of medical colleges, hospitals, societies, and periodicals.

Krumbhaar, E. B. "Days at the Pennsylvania Hospital During Its First Century." American Journal of Medicine 11 (1951): 540-45.

__________ . "The Pennsylvania Hospital." Annals of Internal Medicine 34 (1951): 1280-83.

__________ . "The Pennsylvania Hospital." Transactions of the American Philosophical Society 43 (1953): 237-46.

Lamb, Albert R. The Presbyterian Hospital and the Columbia-Presbyterian Medical Center, 1868-1943: A History of a Great Medical Adventure. New York: Columbia University Press, 1956.

Landis, H. R. M. The History of the Development of Medical Science in America. Philadelphia: Lea Brothers, 1901.

[Lea & Febiger.] One Hundred and Fifty Years of Publishing, 1785-1935. Philadelphia: 1935.

A brief history of the medical publishing house founded by Mathew Carey (1759-1939) whose pioneering efforts established medical publishing in America on a sound basis. The firm published the first American edition of Gray's Anatomy (1859) and all subsequent editions of the text (29th American ed., 1978), and many other famous works by Samuel D. Gross, Austin Flint, Robley Dunglison, William Pepper, and other distinguished medical figures.

Henry Charles Lea, 1825-1909. (Philadelphia: Privately Printed, 1910.)

Lebenson, J. E., ed. An Anthology of Ophthalmic Classics. Baltimore: Williams & Wilkins, 1969.

Levinson, Abraham. Pioneers of Pediatrics. 2d ed. New York: Froben Press, 1943.

[Leypoldt, F(rederick), L(ynds) E. Jones, *et al.*] The American Catalogue of Books in Print and For Sale . . . 1876-1910. New York: Publishers'

Weekly Office, 1880-1911. 21v. in 15. Rep. New York: Peter Smith, 1941. 9v. in 15. Also: Annual American Catalogue, 1886-1910. New York: Publishers' Weekly Office, 1887-1911. 25v.

Litoff, Judy B. American Midwives, 1860 to the Present. Westport, CT: Greenwood Press, 1978.

A general overview of the history of American midwifery in the context of the development of obstetrics and American medical education and care.

Lloyd, J. U., *et al.* Catalogue of the Pharmacopoeias, Dispensatories, Formularies and Allied Publications (1943-1957) in Lloyd Library. Cincinnati: Lloyd Library and Museum, 1957.

Ludmerer, Kenneth M. "Reform at Harvard Medical School, 1869-1909." Bulletin, History of Medicine, 1981, 55: 343-370.

Lyons, Albert S., and R. Joseph Petrucelli. Medicine: An Illustrated History. New York: Harry N. Abrams, 1978.

A sumptuous large history which includes over 1,000 illustrations, 250 in full color. Includes a bibliography and is fully indexed.

MacCallum, W. G. William Stewart Halsted—Surgeon. Baltimore: Johns Hopkins University Press, 1930.

MacFarlane, Catharine. "The Woman's Medical College of Pennsylvania: The First Hundred Years." Journal of the American Medical Women's Association 5 (1950): 194-95.

McDaniel, W. B. II. "Expanding the Use of the Library's Historical Collections." Transactions and Studies of the College of Physicians of Philadelphia 23 (1956): 135-40.

__________ . "Historical Source Material of All Classes in All Types of Medical Libraries." Bulletin of the Medical Library Association 39 (1951): 9-11.

__________ . Index to the William G. Leaman, Jr., Collection of Lantern Slides in the Library of the College of Physicians of Philadelphia on Medical History. Philadelphia: College of Physicians of Philadelphia, 1955.

McGovern, J. P., and G. C. Roland, eds. William Osler: The Continuing Education. Springfield, IL: Charles C. Thomas, 1969.

Consists of essays by Osler with commentaries by W. G. Anlyan, W. B. Bean, W. K. Beatty, M. M. Cummings, G. T. Harrell, H. E. MacDermot, W. Penfield, R. D. Pruitt, H. G. Taylor, W. L. Wells, W. C. Wescoe, and S. G. Wolf.

Major, Ralph H. A History of Medicine. Springfield, IL: Charles C. Thomas, 1954. 2v.

Marion, John F. Philadelphia Medica: Being a Guide to the City's Historical Places of Health Interest. Philadelphia: Smith-Kline Corp., 1975.

Marks, G., and W. K. Beatty. The Story of Medicine in America. New York: Charles Scribner's Sons, 1973.

Marshall, Clara. Woman's Medical College of Pennsylvania. An Historical Outline. Philadelphia: Blakiston, 1897.

Massie, F. M., and M. D. Eiseman. "History of the Transylvania Medical School: The Heritage of Medical Education in Lexington, Kentucky." American Surgeon 31 (1965): 298-306.

Matas, Rudolph. "Biographic Annotations Appended to the Pictorial Gallery of the Editors and Builders of the New Orleans Medical and Surgical Journal Since Its Birth in May, 1844, to the Close of the First Century of Its Service to the Medical Profession, under the Auspices and Ownership of the Louisiana State Medical Society on May 4, 1944." New Orleans Medical and Surgical Journal 96 (1944): 519-22.

__________ . "The New Orleans Medical and Surgical Journal, One Hundred Years of Medical Journalism in Louisiana May, 1844-May, 1944, A Message from Dr. Matas." New Orleans Medical and Surgical Journal 96 (1944): 489-96.

Mathews, Joseph M. How to Succeed in the Practice of Medicine. Philadelphia: W. B. Saunders, 1905. Rep. New York: Arno Press, 1972.

Mears, J. Ewing. Sketch of the Life of Professor Samuel D. Gross. Philadelphia: William J. Dornan, 1885.

"Medical Biography: Recently Published Sources and Guides." Annals of Internal Medicine 76 (March 1972): 517-21.

Meier, Richard Y. The Joseph H. Kiefer Catalog of History of Urology and Medicine. Chicago: Library of Health Sciences, University of Illinois at the Medical Center, 1982. (Over 1800 items from 1496.)

Meigs, J. F. A History of the First Quarter of the Second Century of the Pennsylvania Hospital. Philadelphia: Collins, 1877.

Mettler, Cecilia C. History of Medicine, A Correlative Text, Arranged According to Subjects. Edited by Fred A. Mettler. Philadelphia: Blakiston, 1947.

Arranged by broad subject sections, with excerpts from original writings. Extensive bibliographical materials are included.

Miles, Wyndham D. A History of the National Library of Medicine. Washington: Government Printing Office, 1982.

Miller, Genevieve, ed. Bibliography of the History of Medicine of the United States and Canada, 1939-1960. Baltimore: Johns Hopkins Press, 1964.

A consolidation of the annual bibliographies reprinted from the Bulletin of the History of Medicine, covering the years 1939 through 1960.

Minot, George R. "James Jackson as a Professor of Medicine." New England Journal of Medicine 208 (2 February 1933): 254-58.

Monk, George H. "Selections from the Medical Writings and Sayings of Dr. Oliver Wendell Holmes." Boston Medical and Surgical Journal 197 (26 January 1928): 1385-94.

Morton, T. G., and F. Woodbury. The History of Pennsylvania Hospital, 1751-1895. Philadelphia: Times Printing House, 1895.

Myers, G. W. History of the Massachusetts General Hospital—June, 1872 to December, 1900. Boston: Griffith-Stilling Press, 1929.

Nation, Earl F., *et al.* An Annotated Checklist of Osleriana. Kent, OH: Kent State University Press, 1977.

National Union Catalog; Pre-1956 Imprints. A Cumulative Author List Representing Library of Congress Printed Cards for Books, Pamphlets,

Maps, Atlases, Music, and Periodicals, and Titles Reported by Other North American Libraries. [London]: Mansell, 1968-1981. 754v.

The National Cyclopaedia of American Biography. New York: White, 1892-. Index. New York, 1971.

Published in two series whose total volumes now include over 55,000 entries. The "Permanent" series vols. are numbered; these provide biographies of deceased Americans from colonial times to the present. Entries are arranged in chronological order, and each vol. includes an alphabetical index of biographee's names. The "Current" series vols. are lettered and provide biographies of living Americans. The Index (1971) is a comprehensive name and subject index to vols. 1-52 of the "Permanent" series and vols. A-K of the "Current" series.

Nelson, Bonnie R. A Guide to Published Library Catalogs. Metuchen, N.J. & London: The Scarecrow Press, 1982.

New York Academy of Medicine. Library. Author Catalog. Boston G.K. Hall, 1969. 43v., Suppl., 4v (1974).

__________ . Catalog of Biographies. Boston: G. K. Hall, 1960.

A photographic reproduction of the library's shelflist, containing "single biographies of physicians and scientists, with a few autobiographies, family histories and occasional biographies written by physicians."

__________ . Illustration Catalog. 2d ed., enl. Boston: G. K. Hall, 1965.

Photographic reproduction of an Index to illustrative material in medical works. Arranged by subject. A total of 21,625 illustrations are cataloged.

__________ . Portrait Catalog. Boston, G. K. Hall, 1960. 5v.

Reproduction of the catalog cards listing the 10,784 separate portraits (paintings, woodcuts, engravings, photographs) in the academy and 151,792 entries of portraits appearing in books and journals.

__________ . Portrait Catalog: First Supplement, 1959-1965. Boston: G. K. Hall, 1965.

"Contains 1,073 separate portraits (paintings, woodcuts, engravings, photographs in the Academy, and also 35,976 portraits) appearing in books and journals . . . in addition to those listed in the original five-volume catalog published in 1960."

__________ . Portrait Catalog: Second Supplement, 1965-1971. Boston: G. K. Hall, 1971.

__________ . Subject Catalog. Boston: G. K. Hall, 1969. 34v., Suppl., 4v. (1974).

New York Hospital. Society of the New York Hospital Commemorative Exercises. 150th Anniversary. New York: New York Hospital, 1921.

Norwood, William F. "American Medical Education from the Revolutionary War to the Civil War." Journal of Medical Education 32 (June 1957): 433-48.

__________ . "Critical Incidents in the Shaping of Medical Education in the U.S." Journal of the American Medical Association 194 (1965): 715-18.

__________ . "Early Medical Education in the United States. Excerpts from 'A History of Medical Education in the United States Before the Civil War.' " Journal of the American Medical Association 118 (1942): 759.

Norwood, William F. "A History of Medical Education in the United States Before the Civil War." Harveian Review, August 1941, p. 27.

__________ . "The Mainstream of American Medical Education, 1765-1965." Annals of the New York Academy of Sciences 128 (27 September 1965): 463-72.

__________ . Medical Education in the United States Before the Civil War. Philadelphia: University of Pennsylvania Press, 1944. Rep. New York: Arno Press, 1971.

Novotny, Ann and Carter Smith, eds. Images of Healing: A Portfolio of American Medical and Pharmaceutical Practice in the 18th, 19th, and Early 20th Centuries. New York: Macmillan, 1980.

Numbers, Ronald L. "The Making of an Eclectic Physician: Joseph M. McElhinney and the Eclectic Medical Institute of Cincinnati." Bulletin of the History of Medicine 47 (March-April 1973): 155-66.

__________ , ed. The Education of American Physicians: Historical Essays. Berkeley: University of California, 1980.

Olcott, C. T. "Pathology at the New York Hospital, 1810-1932." Bulletin of the History of Medicine 34 (1960): 137-47.

O'Malley, C. D., ed. The History of Medical Education. Los Angeles: University of California Press, 1970.

The published proceedings of an international symposium on the history of medical education held at Bio-Medical Library, 5-9 February 1968. See, particularly, chapters by William F. Norwood, "Medical Education in the U.S. Before 1900" (pp. 463-500), and John Field, "Medical Education in the U.S.: Late 19th and 20th Centuries" (pp. 501-30).

One Hundred Years. Philadelphia: The Blakiston Co., 1943.

One Hundred Years of Medical Progress: A History of the New York Medical College, Flower and Fifth Avenue Hospitals. Springfield, IL: Charles C. Thomas, 1967.

One Hundred Years of Publishing, 1804-1904. A Brief Historical Account of the House of William Wood & Company. New York: William Wood & Co., 1904.

The Osler Library. Montreal: Osler Library, McGill University, 1979.

Osler, Sir William. Bibliotheca Osleriana: A Catalogue of Books Illustrating the History of Medicine and Science. Collected, arranged, and annotated by Sir William Osler, and bequeathed to McGill University. Oxford: Clarendon Press, 1929.

Includes 7,965 items, with extensive annotations. Arranged in groups as bibliotheca prima; bibliotheca secunda; bibliothecae litteraria, historica, biographica, and bibliographica; incunabula and manuscripts; and Oriental books. Author, subject, and selective title index.

Overton, Grant Martin. Portrait of a Publisher, and the First Hundred Years of the House of Appleton, 1825-1925. New York: Appleton & Co., 1925.

Packard, Francis R. History of Medicine in the United States. 2d ed. New York: Hoeber, 1931. 2v. New York: Hafner Press, 1963, 1973.

The first edition appeared in 1901. Francis R. Packard (1870-1950) also served as editor of Annals of Medical History (25 vols., 1917-42). The Hafner reprint includes a valuable introduction by John B. Blake, and a bibliography (II, 1243-66). See memoir of Packard by W. B. McDaniel II, in Bulletin of the History of Medicine 25 (1951): 66-85.

———— . Some Account of the Pennsylvania Hospital, From Its First Rise to the Beginning of the Year 1938. With a Continuation of the Account to the Year 1956 by F. M. Greim. Philadelphia: Pennsylvania Hospital, 1957.

Payne, L. M. "Materials for Medical Biography." In Proceedings of the Third International Congress of Medical Librarianship, Amsterdam, 5-9 May, 1969, edited by Davis K. Ellison and W. D. Sweeney, pp. 251-57. Amsterdam: Excerpta Medica, 1970.

Pearson, William A. "The Hahnemann Medical College of Philadelphia, 1898-1948." Hahnemannian Monthly 82 (1947): 412-14.

Pepper, William. Higher Medical Education, the True Interest of the Public and the Profession. An Address Introductory to the 112th Course of Lectures of the Medical Department of the University of Pennsylvania. Philadelphia: Collins, 1877.

Postell, William D. Applied Medical Bibliography for Students. Springfield, IL: Charles C. Thomas, 1955.

An introductory handbook in three sections: historical bibliography; modern bibliography, including the organization of the medical library and recommendations for a basic reference collection; and methods of bibliography, including an introduction to the principles of scientific investigation and procedures to be followed for writing papers.

———— . The Development of Medical Literature. New Orleans: Louisiana State University, 1942.

———— . "The History of Medicine Collection in the Louisiana State University School of Medicine Library." New Orleans Medical and Surgical Journal 103 (1951): 533-36.

———— , "Rudolph Matas Medical Library. An Opportunity for Service." Bulletin of the Tulane Medical Faculty 19 (1960): 99-105.

Publishers' Trade List Annual. 1- (1874-).

An annual collection of current publishers' catalogues bound together. There are usually several volumes for each year. Arrangement is alphabetical by publisher's name; an alphabetical list of publishers' names is usually given at the beginning of the first volume. Presently includes about 2500 publishers' catalogues.

Publishers' Weekly. 1- (1872-).

A weekly journal of the American book trade, including lists of newly published books and announcements of forthcoming publications. Lists are usually arranged alphabetically by author. The weekly lists are now cumulated in American Book Publishing Record, 1- (1960-), in lists arranged by Dewey Decimal classes with an author-title index. The lists of forthcoming books are supplemented by Forthcoming Books, 1- (1966-) which is an author-title index and Subject Guide to Forthcoming Books, 1- (1967-) which provides a subject index; both are bi-monthly publications.

Quinan, John R. Medical Annals of Baltimore From 1608 to 1880, Including Events, Men and Literature. Baltimore: Friedenwald, 1884.

Includes a chronology, 1608 to 1880; a record of public services of Baltimore physicians, 1730 to 1880; and a bio-bibliography of Baltimore physicians, 1730 to 1880, with a subject index.

Radbill, Samuel X. The Autobiographical Ana of Robley Dunglison. Philadelphia: American Philosophical Society, 1963.

__________. "David Hayes Agnew, M.D. (1818-1892)." Transactions of the College of Physicians of Philadelphia 33 (1966): 252-60.

__________. "John Eberle: A Pennsylvania Dutch Pioneer in American Medical Education." Bulletin of the Institute of the History of Medicine 4 (February 1936): 121-36.

__________. "The College of Physicians of Philadelphia." Transactions and Studies of the College of Physicians of Philadelphia 32 (1965): 116-21.

Rauch, John H. Medical Education, Medical Colleges, and the Regulation of the Practice of the Medicine in the United States and Canada, 1765-1891. Illinois State Board of Health. Springfield, IL: H. W. Rokker, 1891.

Ravitch, Mark M., ed. A Century of Surgery, 1880-1980. Philadelphia: J. B. Lippincott, 1981. 2 vols.

Selected papers, with commentary, from the "Transactions" of the American Surgical Association.

Redenbaugh, Mary Y. The Biography of Ephraim McDowell. New York: Charles L. Webster, 1890.

Rees, Alan M. and Susan Crawford, eds. Directory of Health Sciences Libraries in the United States, 1979. Cleveland: The Cleveland Health Sciences Library, Case Western Reserve University, 1980.

Ricci, James V. One Hundred Years of Gynaecology, 1800-1900. Philadelphia: Blakiston, 1945.

Robinson, Victor. "The Life of A. Jacobi." Medical Life 35 (1928): 213-58, 262-306.

__________. "The Myth of Benjamin Rush." Medical Life 36 (September 1929): 445-48.

Rogers, Fred B. "Nicholas Romayne, 1756-1817: Stormy Petrel of American Medical Education." Journal of Medical Education 35 (March 1960): 258-63.

__________. Selected Papers of John Shaw Billings. Compiled with "Life of Billings." Chicago: Medical Library Association, 1965. 300 p.

__________. "William Osler: Teacher." Transactions and Studies of the College of Physicians of Philadelphia 42 (July 1974): 94-97.

__________. "William Pepper, 1843-1898." Journal of Medical Education 34 (September 1959): 885-89.

Rohrer, C. W. G. "Professor Samuel D. Gross: America's Foremost Surgeon." Bulletin of the Johns Hopkins Hospital 23 (1912): 83-94.

Roland, G. C. *et al.* "William Osler, 1849-1919—Commemorative Issue." Journal of the American Medical Association 210 (1969): 2213-71.

Romaine, Lawrence B. A Guide to American Trade Catalogs—1744-1900. New York: R. R. Bowker, 1960.

Classified lists include medical and surgical instruments, dental supplies, and pharmaceuticals; important collections are located; annotated.

Roorbach, Orville Augustus. Bibliotheca Americana: Catalogue of American Publications, Including Reprints and Original Works, from 1820 to 1852, Inclusive, Together with a List of Periodicals Published in the United States. New York: Roorbach, 1952. Supplements, 1852-60, 3 vols., 1855-61. Rptd. in 2 vols., New York: Peter Smith, 1939; and Metuchen, NJ: Scarecrow Press, 1967.

A list of books published in the United States 1820-1860. Each volume is a single-alphabet author-title list; entries give publisher, format, price and (sometimes) date.

Roper, Fred W., and Jo Anne Boorkmàn. Introduction to Reference Sources in the Health Sciences. Chicago: Medical Library Association, 1980.

Rosenberg, Charles E. "Social Class and Medical Care in Nineteenth-Century America: The Rise and Fall of the Dispensary." Journal of the History of Medicine and Allied Science 29 (January 1974): 32-54.

__________, ed. The Cholera Bulletin. New York: Arno Press, 1972.

Reprints numbers 1-24 (1832) of the Cholera Bulletin, a triweekly newspaper published in New York by a group of physicians during the outbreak of the cholera epidemic.

__________. The Cholera Years: The United States in 1832, 1849, and 1866. Chicago: University of Chicago Press, 1962.

__________. Medicine and Society in America. 47 vols. New York: Arno Press, 1972.

Intended as a source collection of basic materials illustrating the rise of the medical profession and its responses to American societal needs. Reprints works by William A. Alcott, George M. Beard, Catharine E. Beecher, Elizabeth Blackwell, Wyndham B. Blanton, Henry Bowditch, A. A. Brill, D. W. Cathell, Edward H. Clarke, William Currie, Charles B. Davenport, Michael M. Davis, Pliny Earle, I. S. Falk, Bernard C. Faust, Abraham Flexner, Samuel D. Gross, Worthington Hooker, S. G. Howe, James Jackson, Samuel K. Jennings, Joseph McD. Mathews, Benjamin W. McCready, S. Weir Mitchell, T. L. Nichols, Sir William Osler, George Rosen, Samuel Royce, Benjamin Rush, Lemuel Shattuck, Stephen Smith, Andrew T. Still, Horatio R. Storer, Edgar Sydenstricker, Samuel Thomson, Caleb Ticknor, and William A. White.

__________. Origins of Public Health in America: Selected Essays, 1820-1855. 4 vols. in 1. New York: Arno Press, 1972.

Includes reprints of the following reports: Henry G. Clark, An Address Delivered Before the Suffolk District Medical Society (1852); Bennet Dowler, Researches Upon the Necropolis of New Orleans (1850); John H. Griscom, Anniversary Discourse Before the New York Academy of Medicine (1854); and David Hosack, Observations on Febrile Contagion and on the Means of Improving the Medical Police of the City of New York (1820).

__________. The Physician and Child Bearing. Two Guides: 1809-1894. 2 vols. in 1. New York: Arno Press, 1972. 66 p.

A reprint of William Buchan, Advice to Mothers (1809); and L. Emmett Holt, The Care and Feeding of Children (1894).

Rosner, David. A Once Charitable Enterprise: Hospitals and Health Care in Brooklyn and New York, 1885-1915. New York: Cambridge University Press, 1982.

Rothstein, William G. American Physicians in the 19th Century. Baltimore: Johns Hopkins University Press, 1972.

An historical and sociological examination of the development of the medical profession in the nineteenth century.

Ruschenberger, W. S. W. An Account of the Institution and Progress of the College of Physicians of Philadelphia, During a Hundred Years, From January, 1787. Philadelphia: W. J. Dornan, 1887.

Sabin, Joseph, Wilberforce Eames and R. W. G. Vail. A Dictionary of Books Relating to America, From Its Discovery to the Present Time. Half-Title: Bibliotheca Americana. 29 vols. New York: Sabin, 1868-92; Bibliographical Society of America, 1928-1936. Rptd., Amsterdam, N. Israel, 1961-62.

A single-alphabet author list (anonymous works by title and, sometimes, under "the most obvious subject.") Attempts to include all books which had been written in the Western Hemisphere or written about it. The scope and *terminus ad quem* were changed in the course of publication: see vol. 29, pp. x-xi for details. The 106,413 entries give title, imprint, format, and number of pages. Some entries also include notes on content and other matters such as editions, review citations, and location of copies. Author-title index to Sabin, comp. J. E. Molnar, Metuchen, NJ: Scarecrow Press, 1975.

Saffron, Morris H. Collection of Books on Historical Medicine: A Short Title Catalogue. Newark: George F. Smith Library of the Health Sciences. College of Medicine and Dentistry of New Jersey, 1980.

Sanborn, F. B., ed. Memoirs of Pliny Earle, M.D. With Extracts From His Diary and His Letters (1830-1892) and Selections From His Professional Writings. Boston: Damrell & Upham, 1898. Rep. New York: Arno Press, 1973.

Schachner, August. Ephraim McDowell, "Father of Ovariotomy" and Founder of Abdominal Surgery. Philadelphia: J. B. Lippincott, 1921.

Scull, Andrew, ed. Madhouses, Mad-Doctors, and Madmen: The Social History of Pyschiatry in the Victorian Era. Philadelphia: University of Pennsylvania Press, 1981.

Senn, Nicholas. Four Months Among the Surgeons of Europe. Chicago: American Medical Association, 1887.

Shafer, Henry B. The American Medical Profession, 1783 to 1850. New York: Columbia University Press, 1936.

Examines medical practices in America during the years 1783 through 1850, and traces the history of the American medical profession. "As such, it is concerned with the regular, or allopathic physician; other practitioners are discussed only incidentally as they impinge upon the development of the regular profession."

Shaftel, Norman. "The Evolution of American Medical Literature." International Record of Medicine 171 (1958): 431-54.

__________ . "Austin Flint, Sr. (1812-1886): Educator of Physicians." Journal of Medical Education 35 (1960): 1122-35.

Sharpe, W. D. "The Confederate States Medical and Surgical Journal: 1864-1865." Bulletin of the New York Academy of Medicine 52 (March-April 1976-): 373-418.

Shastid, Thomas H. Ophthalmology, History of. In Casey A. Wood, ed., The American Encyclopedia and Dictionary of Ophthalmology (Chicago: Cleveland Press, 1913-21), vol. 11 (1917), pp. 8524-8904.

Shoemaker, Richard H. A Checklist of American Imprints for [date]. Metuchen, NJ: Scarecrow Press, 1967-1971. 10v.

Lists of American publications for the years 1820-1829; each vol. covers a single year. Arrangement is alphabetical by author, with anonymous works by title. More complete than Roorbach for the years covered. There are two separately published indexes compiled by M. Frances Cooper, A Checklist of American Imprints 1820-1829: Title Index, Metuchen, NJ: Scarecrow Press, 1972, and A Checklist of American Imprints 1820-1829: Author Index, Corrections and Sources, Metuchen, NJ: Scarecrow Press, 1973.

Shrady, John, ed. The College of Physicians and Surgeons, New York: New York: Lewis Publishing Co., 1903.

Shryock, Richard H. "The American Physician in 1846 and in 1946. A Study in Professional Contrasts." Journal of the American Medical Association 134 (1947): 417-24.

__________ . "Changing Outlooks in American Medicine Over Three Centuries." Sudhoffs Archiv Für Geschichte Der Medizin Und Der Naturwissenschaften 37 (1953): 377-88.

__________ . Medical Licensing in America, 1650-1965. Baltimore: Johns Hopkins Press, 1967.

__________ . "The Medical Profession and the Public, 1840-1940." J. A. M. Students 4 (1940): 139-42, 158-59.

__________ . Medicine and Society in America, 1660-1860. New York: New York University Press, 1960.

Traces rise of medical profession, and changes in medical thought, practice, and public health.

__________ . "Medicine and Society in the Nineteenth Century." Journal of World History 5 (1959): 1.

__________ . Medicine in America: Historical Essays. Baltimore: Johns Hopkins Press, 1966.

A brief general survey, followed by special studies reprinted from various journals (1930-62).

__________ . "Relations between Medicine and Society in the Nineteenth Century." Cahiers D'Histoire Mondiale 5 (1959): 116-46.

__________ . "The Academic Profession in the United States," American Association of University Professors." Bulletin 38 (1952): 32-70.

__________ . "American Indifference to Basic Science during the Nineteenth Century." Archives Internationales d'Histoire des Sciences 28 (1948): 50-65.

__________ . American Medical Research Past and Present. New York: Commonwealth Fund, 1947.

Shryock, Richard H. "Before and After: A Medical Drama of 1849 and 1949." Bulletin of the History of Medicine 23 (1949): 554-76.

__________ . The Development of Modern Medicine. New York: Alfred A. Knopf, 1947.

__________ . "Eighteenth Century Medicine in America." Proceedings of the American Antiquarian Society 59 (1949): 275-92.

__________ . "Factors Affecting Medical Research in the United States, 1800-1900." Bulletin of the Society of Medical History of Chicago 5 (1943): 1-18.

__________ . The History of Nursing: An Interpretation of the Social and Medical Factors Involved. Philadelphia: W. B. Saunders, 1959.

__________ . "Medical Progress during the Past Century." Virginia Medical Monthly 74 (1947): 543-46.

__________ . "The Significance of Medicine in American History." American Historical Review 62 (1957): 81-91.

__________ . The Unique Influence of The Johns Hopkins University on American Medicine. Copenhagen: Munksgaard, 1953.

Sims, J. Marion. The Story of My Life. New York: D. Appleton & Co., 1884. Rep. New York: Da Capo Press, 1968.

Autobiography of James Marion Sims (1813-83), a major gynecologist whose Clinical Notes on Uterine Surgery (1866) was a significant factor in formation of the nascent specialty of gynecology.

Smit, Pieter. History of the Life Sciences: An Introductory Guide to the Literature of the History of Biology and Medicine. New York: Hafner Press, 1974.

Smith, Emily A. The Life and Letters of Nathan Smith. New Haven, CT: Yale University Press, 1914.

Smith, Stephen. Doctor in Medicine: And Other Papers on Professional Subjects. New York: William Wood, 1872. New York: Arno Press, 1972.

__________ . "The Evolution of American Surgery." In American Practice of Surgery, vol. 1, pp. 3-67. New York: Wood, 1906-11.

Snyder, Charles. "The Lucien Howe Library of Ophthalmology." Harvard Library Bulletin 9 (1955): 128-31.

Sonnedecker, Glenn. Kremers & Urdang's History of Pharmacy. 4th ed. Philadelphia: J. B. Lippincott, 1976.

Steiner, P. E. Medical-Military Portraits of Union and Confederate Generals. Philadelphia: Witmore, 1968.

__________ . Physician-Generals in the Civil War: A Study in Nineteenth Century American Medicine. Springfield, IL: Charles C. Thomas, 1966.

Still, Andrew T. Autobiography of Andrew T. Still. Kirksville, MO: 1897. Rep. New York: Arno Press, 1972.

Stone, Richard F., ed. Biography of Eminent American Physicians and Surgeons. Indianapolis: Carlon & Hollenbeck, 1894.

Striker, Cecil, ed. Medical Portraits. Cincinnati: Academy of Medicine of Cincinnati, 1963.

Biographical sketches of seventy-nine Ohio physicians.

Szymanski, F. J. Centennial History of the American Dermatological Association, 1876-1976. Chicago: American Dermatological Association, 1976.

Tanselle, G. Thomas. Guide to the Study of United States Imprints. Cambridge, MA: Harvard University Press, 1971. 2v.

A bibliographic guide to American publishing. Arranged as a classified bibliography with categories covering (1) basic imprint lists (regional, genre, and author), (2) related lists for copyright records, catalogues, and book trade directories, (3) lists of supplementary studies of individual printers etc. Author-title-subject index.

Taylor, F. L. Crawford W. Long, and the Discovery of Ether Anaesthesia. New York: Hoeber, 1928.

Tebbel, John. A History of Book Publishing in the United States. New York: R. R. Bowker, 1972-1981. 4v. (V.I: The Creation of an Industry, 1630-1865; V.II: The Expansion of an Industry, 1865-1919; V.III: The Golden Age Between the Two Wars, 1920-1940; V.IV: The Great Change, 1940-1980.)

Thacher, James. American Medical Biography. New introduction and bibliography by Whitfield J. Bell, Jr. New York: Da Capo, 1967. 2v.

Thacher's work appeared originally in 1828 (Boston: Richardson, 2 vols.), and he was the first American medical historian.

Thompson, Lawrence S. The New Sabin: Books Described by Joseph Sabin and His Successors, Now Described Again on the Basis of Examination of Originals, and Fully Indexed by Title, Subject, Joint Authors, and Institutions and Agencies. Vol. 1- . Troy, NY: White, 1974- .

Not a revision of Sabin's Bibliotheca Americana but an entirely new work. Individual vols. are each arranged as a separate A-Z author list with accompanying separately published index. For an analysis of the weaknesses of this work, see the review in Choice, 11 (October, 1974), 1114.

Thomson, Samuel. A Narrative of the Life and Medical Discoveries of Samuel Thomson Containing an Account of His System of Practice and the Manner of Curing Disease with Vegetable Medicine. Boston: E. G. House, 1822. Rep. New York: Arno Press, 1972.

Thornton, John L. A Select Bibliography of Medical Biography: With an Introductory Essay on Medical Biography. 2d ed. London: Library Association, 1970.

__________ . Medical Books, Libraries and Collectors; A Study of Bibliography and the Book Trade in Relation to the Medical Sciences. 2d ed. Introduction by Sir Geofrey Keynes. London: Deutsch, 1966. Rep. Boulder, CO: Westview Press, 1977.

Narrative chronological bibliography of important contributions to medical knowledge, with chapters on medical societies, periodicals, bibliographies, and libraries.

Traub, E. F. "New York Dermatological Society 1869 to 1969. The Fountainhead of Dermatology in the Americas." Archives of Dermatology (Chicago) 99 (May 1969): 513-20.

Truax, R. The Doctors Warren of Boston: First Family of Surgery. Boston: Houghton Mifflin, 1968.

Tucker, D. A., Jr. "Daniel Drake and the Origin of Medicine in the Ohio Valley." Ohio Archives of History 44 (1935): 451-68.

Uhlenhuth, Eduard. "The Collection of Classics of Anatomical Literature in the Library of the Department of Anatomy." Bulletin of the School of Medicine, University of Maryland 41 (1956): 1-11.

United States Catalog. 1st. ed. 1900; 2nd ed. 1903; 3rd ed. 1912; 4th ed. 1928.

Lists of books in print. The first ed. cited books in print for 1899 and was arranged in two lists: (1) author-title and (2) subjects. The 4th ed. is arranged as a single-alphabet author-title-subject list. Entries give publisher and price information. Continued by the Cumulative Book Index.

U.S. Copyright Office. Catalog of Copyright Entries. New Series, 1891-1946. Series 3, 1947- . Washington, DC: 1891- .

Records of books deposited for copyright with the United States Copyright Office. The Copyright Office publishes lists of all materials copyrighted, with separate lists for books, pamphlets, periodicals, works of art, music, etc. For discussion of U.S. Copyright records, see G. Thomas Tanselle's "Copyright Records and the Bibliographer," Studies in Bibliography, 22 (1969), 77-124.

U.S. War Department. Surgeon General's Office. Index-Catalogue of the Library of the Surgeon-General's Office. 61 vols. 1st. ser., 16 vols.; 2d ser., 21 vols.; 3d ser., 10 vols.; 4th ser., 11 vols.; (A-Mn). 5th ser., 3 vols. Washington, DC: Government Printing Office, 1880-1961.

Series 1 through 4 index about three million books, journal articles, and pamphlets. In series 5 only monographs and theses are included. The name of the library was changed to Armed Forces Medical Library in 1952; it became the National Library of Medicine in 1956.

Van Ingen. Philip. The New York Academy of Medicine: Its First Hundred Years. New York: Columbia University Press, 1949.

Chronological account with brief biographies of the presidents.

Viets, Henry R. "The Bibliography of Medicine." Bulletin of the Medical Library Association 27 (1938): 105-17.

Descriptive accounts of medical bibliographies from the fifteenth century to the Index Catalogue.

__________ . "Cushing's Library." New England Journal of Medicine 230 (1944): 440.

__________ . Museum in a Medical Library. Read at the Dedication of the Howard Dittrick Museum of Historical Medicine, Cleveland Medical Library Association, October 6, 1945. Boston: Privately printed, 1945.

__________ . "A Passing Era in Medical History (Book Collecting–Osler, Welch, Harvey Cushing, Klebs, Casey Wood, Streeter)." New England Journal of Medicine 237 (1947): 106-7.

Vogel, Morris J. and Charles E. Rosenberg, eds. The Therapeutic Revolution: Essays in the Social History of American Medicine. Philadelphia: University of Pennsylvania Press, 1979.

Vogel, Morris J. The Invention of the Modern Hospital. Boston, 1870-1930. Chicago: University of Chicago Press, 1980.

Waite, Frederick C. The Story of a Country Medical College. A History of the Clinical School of Medicine and the Vermont Medical College, Woodstock, Vermont, 1827-1856. Montpelier: Vermont Historical Society, 1945.

Waite, Frederick C. Western Reserve University Centennial History of the School of Medicine, Cleveland, Ohio. Cleveland: Western Reserve University Press, 1946.

__________ . "The Beginning of Institutional Medical Education in Cleveland." Bulletin of the Academy of Medicine of Cleveland 31 (July 1946): 9-11, 16.

__________ . "Changes in the Medical Education Program in Ohio from 1890 to 1910." Ohio State Medical Journal 45 (1949): 1083-88.

__________ . "The First Medical College in Northern Ohio: The Medical Department of Willoughby University of Lake Erie." Bulletin of the Academy of Medicine of Cleveland 28 (August 1943): 9-10, 19.

__________ . "The First Medical College in Vermont." Bulletin of the History of Medicine 21 (1947): 788-94.

__________ . History of the New England Female Medical College: 1848-1874. Boston: Boston University School of Medicine, 1950.

__________ . "Medical Education in Ohio." Ohio State Medical Journal 49 (1953): 623-26.

Walsh, James J. History of Medicine in New York: Three Centuries of Medical Progress. New York: National Americana Society, 1919. 5v. Contains extensive data, incomplete in some areas, and very little documentation. Volume 1 is a general survey, with accounts of specialties; volume 2 is mainly on medical schools; volume 3, on societies and hospitals; and volumes 4 and 5 include biographies (with lists of publications).

Waring, Edward John. Bibliotheca Therapeutica, or Bibliography of Therapeutics: London: New Sydenham Society, 1878-1879. 2v.

Warner, Harriot W., ed. Autobiography of Charles Caldwell. Philadelphia: Lippincott, Grambo and Co., 1855.

Warren, Edward. The Life of John Collins Warren. Boston: Ticknor and Fields, 1860. 2v.

Watson, Irving A., ed. Physicians and Surgeons of America . . . A Collection of Biographical Sketches of the Regular Medical Profession. Concord, NH: Republican Press Association, 1896.

Weiskotten, Herman G. "Nicholas Romayne: Pioneer in Medical Education in the United States." New York State Journal of Medicine 66 (15 August 1966): 2158-77.

Whorton, James C. Crusaders for Freedom: The History of American Health Reformers. Princeton: Princeton University Press, 1982.

Williams, Stephen W. American Medical Biography: Or, Memoirs of Eminent Physicians, Embracing Principally Those Who Have Died Since the Publication of Dr. Thacher's Work. Greenfield, MA: Merriam, 1845.

Wolfe, Gerald. The House of Appleton: The History of a Publishing House and Its Relationship to the Cultural, Social, and Political Events that Helped Shape the Destiny of New York City. Metuchen, NJ and London: The Scarecrow Press, 1981.

Women in Medicine Collection. Florence A. Moore Library of Medicine. Medical College of Pennsylvania, Philadelphia.

Comprehensive repository of published and unpublished material about women physicians (ca. 1850-). Includes the Kate Hurd Mead and American Medical Women's Association Collections, also 300 monographs, 3,500 photographs, and papers of several medical women's associations. Numerous personal collections of women physicians, including Martha Tracy (1876-1942), Ellen Culver Potter (1871-1958), Emiline Horton Cleveland (1829-78), and Catharine Macfarlane (1877-1969) are found here, as well as nineteenth-century M.D. theses, and the archives of the college (formerly Woman's Medical College of Pennsylvania).

Woollcott, J. Classics in Medical Literature from the University of Pennsylvania, 1765-1965. Philadelphia: University of Pennsylvania Press, 1965.

Yale University. Yale Medical Library Historical Library. The Harvey Cushing Collection of Books and Manuscripts. New York: Henry Schuman, 1943.

Short-title author catalog of 7,959 manuscripts. Orientalia, incunabula, general works, and Cushing memorabilia in Yale Medical Library.

KEY TO LOCATION SYMBOLS

AU . . . . University of Alabama. University, Alabama

CLM . . . . Los Angeles County Medical Association. Los Angeles, California

CSmH . . . . Henry E. Huntington Library. San Marino, California

CU-M . . . . University of California Medical Center. San Francisco, California

CtHi . . . . Connecticut Historical Society. Hartford, Connecticut

CtY-M . . . . . . Yale University School of Medicine. New Haven, Connecticut

DLC . . . . Library of Congress. Washington, D.C.

DNLM . . . . . . National Library of Medicine. Bethesda, Maryland

GU . . . . Medical College of Georgia. Augusta, Georgia

ICJ . . . . John Crerar Library. Chicago, Illinois

ICRM . . . . Rush Medical College. Chicago, Illinois

ICU . . . . Joseph Regenstein Library. University of Chicago. Chicago, Illinois

IEN-M . . . . . . Northwestern University. Medical Library. Chicago, Illinois

IU-M . . . . University of Illinois at the Medical Center. Library of the Health Sciences. Chicago, Illinois

InHi . . . . Indiana Historical Society. Indianapolis, Indiana

KU . . . . Science Library. University of Kansas. Lawrence, Kansas

KyLoJM . . . . . Health Sciences Library. University of Louisville. Louisville, Kentucky

LNT-M . . . . . . Tulane University. Rudolph Matas Medical Library. New Orleans, Louisiana

MA . . . . Amherst College. Amherst, Massachusetts

MB . . . . Boston Public Library. Boston, Massachusetts

MBAt . . . . Boston Athenaeum. Boston, Massachusetts

MBM .... The Boston Medical Library. The Francis A. Countway Library of Medicine. Boston, Massachusetts

MdBM ...... Medical and Chirurgical Faculty of Maryland. Baltimore, Maryland

MH .... Widener Library. Harvard University. Cambridge, Massachusetts

MH-M .... Harvard Medical Library. The Francis A. Countway Library of Medicine. Boston, Massachusetts

MHi .... Massachusetts Historical Society. Boston, Massachusetts

MSaE .... Essex Institute. Salem, Massachusetts

MWA .... American Antiquarian Society. Worcester, Massachusetts

MWiW .... Williams College. Williamstown, Massachusetts

MdHi .... Maryland Historical Society. Baltimore, Maryland

MdBJ-W ..... William H. Welch Medical Library. Johns Hopkins University. Baltimore, Maryland

MdU-D ...... University of Maryland. Health Sciences Library. Baltimore, Maryland

N .... New York State Library. Albany, New York

NBM .... Library. State University of New York. Downstate Medical Center. Brooklyn, New York

NHi .... New York Historical Society. New York City, New York

NIC .... Cornell University. Ithaca, New York

NN .... New York Public Library. New York City, New York

NNC .... Health Sciences Library. Columbia University. New York City, New York

NNNAM ..... New York Academy of Medicine. Library. New York City, New York

NNS .... New York Society Library. New York City, New York

NNU-M ...... Frederick L. Ehrman Medical Library. New York University Medical Center. New York City, New York

NcD .... School of Medicine. Library. Duke University. Durham, North Carolina

NcU .... Health Sciences Library. University of North Carolina. Chapel Hill, North Carolina

Nh .... New Hampshire State Library. Concord, New Hampshire

NjR . . . . University of Medicine and Dentistry of New Jersey. Smith Library. Newark, New Jersey; and Rutgers University Library of Science and Medicine. Piscataway, New Jersey

OC . . . . Medical Center Libraries. University of Cincinnati. Cincinnati, Ohio

OCHP . . . . Historical and Philosophical Society of Ohio. Cincinnati, Ohio

OCLloyd . . . . Lloyd Library and Museum. Cincinnati, Ohio

OCIM . . . . Cleveland Health Sciences Library. Case Western Reserve University. Cleveland, Ohio

OCIWHi . . . . . Western Reserve Historical Society. Cleveland, Ohio

PHi . . . . Historical Society of Pennsylvania. Philadelphia, Pennsylvania

PLF . . . . Franklin and Marshall College. Library. Lancaster, Pennsylvania

PMA . . . . Allegheny College. Meadville, Pennsylvania

PP . . . . Free Library of Philadelphia. Philadelphia, Pennsylvania

PPAmP . . . . . . American Philosophical Society. Philadelphia, Pennsylvania

PPC . . . . College of Physicians of Philadelphia. Philadelphia, Pennsylvania

PPF . . . . Franklin Institute. Philadelphia, Pennsylvania

PPG . . . . German Society of Pennsylvania. Philadelphia, Pennsylvania

PPHa . . . . Hahnemann University of the Health Sciences. Philadelphia, Pennsylvania

PPJ . . . . Scott Memorial Library. Thomas Jefferson University. Jefferson Medical College. Philadelphia, Pennsylvania

PPPH . . . . Pennsylvania Hospital. Medical Library. Philadelphia, Pennsylvania

PPL . . . . Library Company of Philadelphia. Philadelphia, Pennsylvania

PPPrHi . . . . . . Presbyterian Historical Society. Philadelphia, Pennsylvania

PU . . . . The Library of the School of Medicine. University of Pennsylvania. Philadelphia, Pennsylvania

RHi . . . . Rhode Island Historical Society. Providence, Rhode Island

RPB . . . . Brown University. Providence, Rhode Island

RPJCB . . . . . . John Carter Brown Library. Providence, Rhode Island

RPM . . . . Rhode Island Medical Society. Providence, Rhode Island

ScC . . . . Charleston Library Society. Charleston, South Carolina

ScCM .... Library. Medical University of the State of South Carolina. Charleston, South Carolina

ScMS .... Medical Society of the State of South Carolina. Charleston, South Carolina

ScU .... University of South Carolina. Columbia, South Carolina

ViRA .... Richmond Academy of Medicine. Richmond, Virginia

VtHi .... Vermont Historical Society. Montpelier, Vermont

I. AMERICAN MEDICAL IMPRINTS, 1820-1829

The objects of this work are, 1st, to teach those who have the charge of children, either as parent or guardian, the most approved methods of securing and improving their physical powers. This is attempted by pointing out the duties which the parent or the guardian owes for this purpose, to this interesting but helpless class of beings, and the manner by which their duties shall be fulfilled. And 2d, to render available a long experience to these objects of our affection when they become diseased. In attempting this, the author has avoided as much as possible, "technicality"; and has given, if he does not flatter himself too much, to each disease of which he treats, its appropriate and designating characters, with a fidelity that will prevent any two being confounded together, with the best mode of treating them, that either his own experience or that of others has suggested.

William Potts Dewees,
The Physical and Medical Treatment of Children
(1825)

ABERNETHY, John (1764-1831)
The surgical and physiological works of John Abernethy.... From the 6th London ed. London: Pr. by Longman, Hurst, Rees, Orme & Brown; Hartford: Rep. by O. D. Cooke & Co., 1825. 2v. CU-M; MB; OC **20-0001**

ABERNETHY, John (1764-1831)
Lectures on anatomy, surgery, and pathology; including observations on the nature and treatment of local diseases.... Boston: B. Perkins & Co., 1828-29. 2v. DLC; DNLM; MB; PPC **20-0002**

ACCUM, Friedrich Christian (1769-1838)
A treatise on adulterations of food, and culinary poisons. Exhibiting the fraudulent sophistications of bread, beer, wine, spiritous liquors, tea, coffee, cream, confectionery, vinegar, mustard, pepper, cheese, olive oil, pickles, and other articles employed in domestic economy. And method of detecting them.... Philadelphia: Ab'm Small, 1820. 269p. CtY-M; DLC; DNLM; ICJ **20-0003**

ADVICE to the young mother in the management of herself and infant. By a member of the Royal College of Surgeons. Philadelphia: H. C. Carey & I. Lea, 1822. 96p. PPL **20-0004**

AKERLY, Samuel (1785-1845)
Deafness, and other diseases of the organ of hearing, attended to by Dr. Samuel Akerly, Physician to the New York Institution for the Instruction of the Deaf and Dumb. New York: E. Conrad, 1820. 4 p. NNNAM **20-0005**

AKERLY, Samuel (1785-1845)
Elementary exercises for the deaf and dumb. New York: Pr. by E. Conrad, 1821. 374p. DLC; NN; DNLM; GU **20-0006**

AKERLY, Samuel (1785-1845)
Observations and correspondence on the nature and cure of deafness, and other diseases of the ears. New York, 1821. 20p. MH-M **20-0007**

AKERLY, Samuel (1785-1845)
Observations and correspondence on the nature and cure of deafness, and other diseases of the ears. [Philadelphia]: Pr. by E. Conrad, 1824. 20p. DNLM; MWA; PPC **20-0008**

ALDEN, Ebenezer (1788-1881)
An address, delivered in Hanover, N.H., before the Dartmouth Medical Society, on their first anniversary, Dec. 28th, 1819.... Boston: James Loring, 1820. 16p. DLC; DNLM; IEN-M; MBM **20-0009**

ALLEN, Jonathan Adams (1787-1848)
A synopsis of pharmacology.... Middlebury [Vt.]: Pr. by J. W. Copeland, 1823. 66p. DLC; DNLM; IEW-M; NNNAM **20-0010**

ALLEN, Jonathan Adams (1787-1848)
A system of pharmacology; designed for a practical compendium of materia medica and pharmacy and as a text book for students attending medical lectures. Middlebury: Ovid Miner, 1828. 56p. NNNAM **20-0011**

ALLEN, Stephen (1767-1852)
Letter of the Hon. Stephen Allen, Mayor of the City of New York, to Joseph Bayley.... in relation to the cases of yellow fever, at the quarantine ground in 1821, and Dr. Bayley's report thereon. Published by order of the Board of Health. [New York]: Van Pelt & Spear, 1822. 37p. DLC; MB; MBM; NN **20-0012**

ALLEN, William (1784-1868)
An address occasioned by the death of Nathan Smith, M.D., first lecturer in the Medical School of Maine at Bowdoin College, delivered by appointment of the faculty of Medicine, March 26, 1829. Brunswick: G. Griffin, pr., 1829. 31p. DLC; DNLM; MWA; OC **20-0013**

[ANATOMY]
Address to the community on the necessity of legalizing the study of anatomy. By order of the Massachusetts Medical Society. Boston: Perkins & Marvin, 1829. 27p. MB; MBM; MH; MH-M **20-0014**

[ANATOMY-DISSECTION]
On the importance of the study of anatomy. From the Westminster Review, with some additional remarks. Boston: Wells & Lilly, 1825. 12p. MB; MBM **20-0015**

ANDERSON, William
System of surgical anatomy. Part first. On the structure of the groin, pelvis, and perineum, as connected with inguinal and femoral hernia; tying the iliac arteries; and the operation of lithotomy. Illustrated by nine copper-plate engravings. New York: J. V. Seaman, 1822. 199p. DLC; DNLM; GU; IU-M **20-0016**

ARISTOTLE [pseud.]
Aristotle's complete masterpiece, in two parts: displaying the secrets of nature in the generation of man.... To which is added, A treasure of health; or The family physician; being choice and approved remedies for all the several distempers incident to the human body. New England: Printed for the publishers, and sold by the principal booksellers in the United States, 1820. 71p. DNLM; MWA **20-0017**

ARMSTRONG, John (1784-1829)
The art of preserving health. Philadelphia: R. Wright, 1821. 72p. DLC; PPC; PPF; PPHa **20-0018**

ARMSTRONG, John (1784-1829)
Practical illustrations of typhus fever, of the common continued fever, and of inflammatory diseases, &c, &c. 1st American from 3rd English ed. Philadelphia: J. Webster, 1821. 468p. DLC; DNLM; ICJ; PPAmP **20-0019**

ARMSTRONG, John (1784-1829)
Practical illustrations of typhus fever, of the common continued fever, and of inflammatory diseases, etc. etc. With Notes critical and explanatory by Nathaniel Potter. 2nd American from the 3rd English ed. Philadelphia: J. Webster, 1822. 434p. PHi; PP; PPC; PPHa **20-0020**

ARMSTRONG, John (1784-1829)
Facts, observations and practical illustrations, relative to puerperal fever, scarlet fever, pulmonary consumption, and measles. A general view of the pathology and treatment of chronic diseases: with illustrations of the utility of sulpherous waters, and observations on the efficacy of the balsam of copaiva in inflammation of the mucous membranes. 1st American from the 2nd London ed. Hartford: O. D. Cooke & Sons, 1823. 120p; 216p; 11p; 80p. DLC; DNLM; ICJ; MdBM **20-0021**

ARMSTRONG, John (1784-1829)
Practical illustrations of typhus fever, of the common continued fever, and of inflammatory diseases, etc. From the last London ed. New York: Pub. by Everet Duyckinck, George Long, Collins and Co., and Collins and Hannay. W. E. Dean, pr., 1824. 432p. DNLM; IEN-M; MB; PPC
20-0022

ARMSTRONG, John (1784-1829)
Facts, observations and practical illustrations relative to puerperal fever, scarlet fever, pulmonary consumption, and measles. 2nd American from the 2nd London ed. Philadelphia: J. Grigg, H. C. Carey & I. Lea, Towar & Hogan, T. Desilver, E. Parker, U. Hunt, Marot & Walter, R. Desilver, J. G. Auner, B. & T. Kite, and J. J. Woodward: And E. Duyckinck, Collins & Hannay, Collins & Co., and H. Stevenson, New York, 1826. [Philadelphia, Pr. by Samuel Parker] 120, 216, 80p. CU-M; ICJ; PP; PPC **20-0023**

ARMSTRONG, John (1784-1829)
A treatise on sulphureous waters. . . . Staunton, Va.: Printed at the Spectator office, 1826. 24p. DLC; DNLM; ScU; ScMS
20-0024

ARMSTRONG, John (1784-1829)
Facts, observations and practical illustrations relative to puerperal fever, scarlet fever, pulmonary consumption, and measles. . . . 1st American, from the 2nd London ed. Hartford: O. D. Cooke, 1826. 120, 216, 80p. MB; MBM; MH
20-0025

ARMSTRONG, John (1784-1829)
Practical illustrations of typhus and other fevers: of pulmonary consumption, measles, &c, &c. From the last London editions, with notes, by P. Washington Leland. Boston: T. Bedlington, 1829. 559p. IEN-M; NIC; NN; PPC **20-0026**

ARNOTT, Neil (1788-1874)
Elements of physics; or, natural philosophy, general and medical explained independently of technical mathematics, and containing new disquisitions and practical suggestions. . . . 1st American from the 3rd London ed., with additions by Isaac Hays. . . . Philadelphia: Carey, Lea & Carey, 1829. 552 p. GU; ICJ; MB; NNNAM **20-0027**

AVERILL, Charles
A short treatise on operative surgery, describing the principal operations as they are practiced in England and France, designed for the use of students in operating on the dead body. . . . 1st American ed., with additions by John Bell. Philadelphia: H. C. Carey and I. Lea; Boston: Wells and Lilly, 1823. 230p. DLC; DNLM; PPC; PU **20-0028**

AYRE, Joseph (1781-1860)
Practical observations on the nature and treatment of marasmus. And of those disorders allied to it, which may be strictly denominated bilious. Northampton, Mass.: Pub. by Simeon Butler. J. Metcalf, Printer, 1822. 219p. MB; PPL
20-0029

BACON, John
Directions for using the medicines, &c contained in the family medicine chest. Boston, 1820. 32p. MWA **20-0030**

BAILEY, Rufus William (1798-1863)
An address, delivered at the annual commencement of the Berkshire Medical Institution. Pittsfield, December 23, 1824. . . . Pittsfield [Mass.]: Printed by P. Allen, 1825. MH-M; MHi
20-0031

BAILLIE, Matthew (1761-1823)
The morbid anatomy of some of the most important parts of the human body. . . . 3rd American from the 5th London ed. Philadelphia: Hickman and Hazzard, 1820. 288p. CtY-M; DNLM; ICJ; IEN-M **20-0032**

BALFOUR, William
Illustrations of the power of emetic tartar, in the cure of fever, inflammation, and asthma; and in preventing consumption and apoplexy. From the 2nd Edinburgh ed., Lexington, Ky.: James W. Palmer, 1823. 84p. DNLM; PPC **20-0033**

[BALTIMORE]
A series of letters and other documents relating to the late epidemic or yellow fever; comprising: the correspondence of the mayor of the city, the board of health, the executive of the State of Maryland, and the reports of the faculty and District Medical Society of Baltimore. Also, essays of the physicians, in answer to the mayor's circular requesting information for the use of the city council in relation to the causes which gave origin to this disease—To which is added, the late ordinance reorganizing the board of health, &c, &c. Published by authority of the mayor with the consent of the authors for the benefit of the Baltimore Second Dispensary. . . . Baltimore: William Warner, 1820. 212p. CtY-M; DLC; DNLM; IEN-M
20-0034

[BALTIMORE]
Report of the Health committee and accompanying documents of the board of physicians appointed to direct the vaccination of the city. Laid before the city council of Baltimore, January session, 1822. Baltimore: Pr. by J. Murphy, 1822. 15p. MdBJ-W; MdU-D **20-0035**

BANCROFT, Edward Nathaniel (1772-1842)
An essay on the disease called yellow fever; with observations concerning febrile contagion typhus fever, dysentery, and the plague, partly delivered as the Gulstonian Lectures, before the College of Physicians, in the years 1806 and 1807. Baltimore: Pr. by J. Robinson, for Cushing & Jewett, 1821. 526p. DLC; DNLM; IEN-M; NNNAM **20-0036**

BARBER, William
The improved system of botanic medical practice. . . . New York: Pr. at no. 2 Frankfort Street, November, 1829. 108p. ICJ; NNNAM **20-0037**

BARNES, John
Jefferson Medical College: a representation of the conduct of the Trustees and members of the faculty, and circumstances connected therewith, in relation to John Barnes, M.D. Philadelphia, 1828. 38p. PPJ **20-0038**

BARTLETT, Benjamin D.
An address delivered at Brunswick, before the Medical Society of Maine, at their annual meeting, Sept. 4, 1827. Bath: Joseph G. Torrey, 1827. 17p. PU **20-0039**

BARTLETT, John Stephen
Physician's pocket synopsis: affording a concise view of the symptoms and treatment of the medical and surgical diseases incident to the human frame. . . . Boston: Munroe and Francis, 1822. 396p. MB; MBM; OC; RPB **20-0040**

BARTON, John Rhea (1794-1871)
On the treatment of anchylosis, by the formation of artificial joints. Philadelphia: J. Harding, pr., 1827. 17p. DNLM; NNNAM; OC PPL **20-0041**

BARTON, William Paul Crillon (1786-1856)
Memorial from the professor of botany in the University of Pennsylvania, to the Trustees of that institution; praying for the removal of the professorship from the faculty of natural science, into the medical faculty; and to render it a requisite branch for the attainment of a medical degree. Philadelphia: Robert P. M'Culloh, 1820. 26p. DNLM; MBM; PHi; PPAmP
20-0042

BARTON, William Paul Crillon (1787-1856)
Outlines of lectures on materia medica and botany, delivered in Jefferson Medical College, Philadelphia.... Philadelphia: J. G. Auner, 1827. 2 v. DLC; DNLM; ICJ; KU
20-0043

BARTON, William Paul Crillon (1787-1856)
Outlines of lectures on materia medica and botany, delivered in Jefferson Medical College, Philadelphia. Philadelphia: Pub. by Jos. G. Auner, T. Town, pr., 1828. 246p. MB; ScCM
20-0044

BATCHELDER, John Putnam (1784-1868)
Memoir of the fracture of the lower extremity of the radius. Pittsfield: Argus office, 1827. 4p. DNLM; NNNAM
20-0045

BATCHELDER, John Putnam (1784-1868)
Case of tumor at the angle of the jaw. [New York, 1829] 8p. DNLM **20-0046**

BATCHELDER, John Putnam (1784-1868)
2nd Edition of "An Advertisement" by C. B. Coventry, M.D., with "A Candid Exposition of Facts." Utica, N.Y.: Dauby and Maynard, 1829. 16p. NHi; NN **20-0047**

A **BRIEF** memoir of the late Thomas Batemen, M.D., physician to the public dispensary, Carey Street; and to the Fever Institution ... who died 9th April, 1821. 1st American from the 5th London ed. New York: Mahlon Day, 1822. 34p. PHi; PPL
20-0048

BATEMAN, Thomas (1778-1821)
A practical synopsis of cutaneous diseases, according to the arrangement of Dr. Willan, exhibiting a concise view of the diagnostic symptoms and the method of treatment.... Philadelphia: James Crissy, 1824. 320p. DNLM; IEN-M; PPC
20-0049

BATES, Joshua (1776-1854)
Address, delivered in Castleton, December 2, 1823, at the commencement of the Vermont Academy of Medicine. [Poultney] Pr. by Smith and Shute 1824. DNLM; MB; NNNAM; PU **20-0050**

BAUDELOCQUE, Jean Louis (1745-1810)
An abridgement of Mr. Heath's translation of Baudelocque's midwifery. With notes by William P. Dewees.... Philadelphia: Published by Thomas Desilver; Clark & Raser, printers, 1823. GU; ICJ; PU; RPB **20-0051**

BAYLE, Antoine Laurent Jessé (1799-1858)
A manual of general anatomy, containing a concise description of the elementary tissues of the human body. From the French of A. L. J. Bayle and H. Hollard. By S. D. Gross. Philadelphia: J. Grigg, 1828. x, 272p. DLC; DNLM; ICJ; OC
20-0052

BEATTIE, Francis Smith (1794-1841)
Statement of proceedings on the part of the members of the faculty and the trustees of the Jefferson Medical College against Francis S. Beattie.... Philadelphia, 1826. 39p. DLC; DNLM; PHi; PU **20-0053**

BECK, John Brodhead (1794-1851)
An introductory lecture, delivered at the College of Physicians and Surgeons of the City of New York, November 6, 1829. New York: Charles S. Francis [Sleight & Robinson, prs.] 1829. 30p. DLC; MH; MdBM; NNC **20-0054**

BECK, Paul (1760?-1844)
A proposal for altering the eastern front of the city of Philadelphia, with a view to prevent the recurrence of malignant disorders, on a plan conformable to the original design of William Penn. By a citizen of Philadelphia. Philadelphia: William Fry, 1820. 11p. DLC; DNLM; PHi; PPAmP
20-0055

BECK, Theodoric Romeyn (1791-1855)
Elements of medical jurisprudence. Albany: Websters and Skinners, 1823. 2 v. CU-M; DLC: DNLM; PPL
20-0056

BECK, Theodoric Romeyn (1791-1855)
On the utility of country medical institutions; an introductory lecture, delivered at the College of Physicians and Surgeons of the Western District of the State of New York, Dec. 13, 1824. ... Albany: Websters and Skinners, 1825. 20p. DLC; NN; OC
20-0057

BECK, Theodoric Romeyn (1791-1855)
Annual address delivered before the Medical Society of the State of New York. Februay 6, 1828. Albany: Pr. by Websters and Skinners, 1828. 23p. DLC; MB; MWA; N
20-0058

BECK, Theodoric Romeyn (1791-1855)
Statistical notices of some of the lunatic asylums of the United States. New York [1829] 25p. NN; NNNAM
20-0059

BECK, Theodoric Romeyn (1791-1855)
Annual address delivered before the Medical Society of the State of New York, February 4, 1829. Albany: Pr. by Websters and Skinners, 1829. 20p. DNLM; MB; NNNAM
20-0060

BECLARD, Pierre Auguste (1785-1825)
Additions to the general anatomy of Xavier Richart. Transl. from the French, by George Hayward.... Boston: Published by Richardson and Lord; J. H. A. Frost, printer, 1823. 328p. DLC; ICJ; PPHa; PU **20-0061**

BEDINGFIELD, James
A compendium of medical practice ... with notes by Stephen W. Williams. 1st American from the last London ed. Greenfield, Mass.: Phelps, 1823. 192p. MB; MBM; MH-M; MWA
20-0062

BEGIN, Louis Jacques (1793-1859)
The French practice of medicine; being a translation of L. J. Bégin's treatise on therapeutics, with occasional notes and observations illustrative of the treatment of diseases in the climate of North America.... 1st ed. New York: E. Bliss, 1829. 2 v. in 1. CU-M; DNLM; ICJ; PPC **20-0063**

BELL, Charles (1774-1842)
An exposition of the natural system of the nerves of the human body. . . . Philadelphia: H. C. Carey & I. Lea, 1825. 165p. DNLM; ICJ; IEN-M **20-0064**

BELL, John (1763-1820)
The anatomy and physiology of the human body. . . . 4th American from the 4th English ed. . . . New York: Collins & Co., 1822. 3 v. IEN-M; MdBM; PPC **20-0065**

BELL, John (1763-1820)
The anatomy and physiology of the human body. By John and Charles Bell. The whole more perfectly systematized and corrected by Charles Bell. . . . The 5th American ed. (repr. from the 6th London ed. of 1826). The text revised . . . by John D. Goodman. . . . New York: Collins & Co., 1827. 2 v. DLC; DNLM; MB; NNC **20-0066**

BELL, John (1796-1872)
On the influence of medicine. An oration delivered before the Philadelphia Medical Society, pursuant to appointment. . . . February 9, 1828. Pub. by the Society. Philadelphia: Mifflin and Parry, prs., 1828. 36p. DNLM; MB; MWA; NNNAM **20-0067**

BELL, John (1796-1872)
An address introductory to a course of lectures of the institutes of medicine and medical jurisprudence. Philadelphia: Pr. by James Kay, Jr. & Co., prs. to the Philadelphia Medical Society, 1829. 24p. DNLM; NNNAM; PHi **20-0068**

[BENEZET, Anthony A.]
The family physician; comprising rules for the prevention and cure of diseases; calculated particularly for the inhabitants of the western country, and for those who navigate its waters. With a dispensatory and appendix. . . . By a graduate of the Pennsylvania University, and honorary member of the Medical Society of Philadelphia. Cincinnati: Pr. and pub. by W. Hill Woodward [1826]. 562p. NN; OC; OCHP; OCLloyd **20-0069**

BICHAT, Xavier (1771-1802)
General anatomy, applied to the physiology and medicine. . . . Transl. from the French. By George Hayward. . . . Boston: Richardson and Lord, 1822. 3 v. DLC; DNLM; OC; ScCM **20-0070**

BICHAT, Xavier (1771-1802)
Pathological anatomy. The last course of Xavier Bichat, from an autographic manuscript of P. A. Beclard; with an account of the life and labours of Bichat, by F. G. Boisseau. . . . Transl. from the French by Joseph Togno. . . . Philadelphia: J. Grigg, 1827. 234p. DLC; MBM; NcU; PU **20-0071**

BICHAT, Xavier (1771-1802)
Physiological researches on life and death; transl. from the French by F. Gold . . . with notes by F. Magendie. . . . The notes transl. by George Hayward, M.D. Boston: Richardson and Lord, 1827. 334p. DLC; GU; ICJ; PU **20-0072**

BIGELOW, Jacob (1787-1879)
American medical botany, being a collection of the native medicinal plants of the United States, containing their botanical history and chemical analysis, and properties and uses in medicine, diet and the arts, with coloured engravings. . . . Boston: Published by Cummings and Hilliard; [Cambridge] University Press, Hilliard and Metcalf, 1817-20 [i.e., 1817-21]. 3 v. 60 col. plates. Issued in 6 parts. CU-M; CtY-M; DLC; DNLM **20-0073**

BIGELOW, Jacob (1787-1879)
A treatise on the materia medica, intended as a sequel to the Pharmacopoeia of the United States. . . . Boston: C. Ewer, 1822. 424p. CU-M; ICJ; PPC **20-0074**

BIGELOW, Jacob (1787-1879)
Florula Bostoniensis. A collection of plants of Boston and its vicinity, with their generic and specific characters, principal synonyms, descriptions, places of growth, and time of flowering, and occasional remarks. 2nd ed., greatly enlarged. . . . Boston: Cummings, Hilliard, 1824. 422p. MBM; MH; OCLloyd; PHi **20-0075**

BLACKALL, John (1771-1860)
Observations on the nature and cure of dropsies, and particularly on the presence of the coagulable part of the blood in dropsical urine; to which is added, an appendix, containing several cases of angina pectoris, with dissections, &c. . . . 1st American, from the 3rd London ed. Philadelphia: James Webster, 1820. 274p. CLM; CU-M; CtY-M; DLC **20-0076**

BLACKALL, John (1771-1860)
Observations on the nature and cure of dropsies. . . . 2nd American from 4th London ed., with an additional appendix. Philadelphia: J. Webster, 1825. 319p. DNLM; MB **20-0077**

BLANE, Gilbert (1749-1834)
Elements of medical logic, illustrated by practical proofs and examples. . . . 1st American from 2nd London ed. Hartford: Huntington and Hopkins, 1822. 319p. ICJ; MB; MBM; PPC **20-0078**

BOND, Henry (1790-1859)
Practical and surgical anatomy. Philadelphia, Nov. 1, 1822. 1p. [Prospectus of Dr. Bond's Anatomical Rooms.] PHi **20-0079**

[BOSTON]
An interesting account of the plague, yellow fever, &c as they have prevailed in different countries. Printed at the request of the Boston Board of Health. Boston: James Loring, 1820. [An address made to the legislature of Louisiana and communicated to the Boston Board of Health, which authorized its printing.] 24p. DNLM; MBM; MWA **20-0080**

BOWDOIN COLLEGE, Brunswick, Maine
Catalogue of the library of the Medical School of Maine, at Bowdoin College, February, 1823. Brunswick: Joseph Griffin, printer, 1823. 24p. MH; MWA; PPAmP **20-0081**

BOWDOIN COLLEGE, Brunswick, Maine
Appendix to the catalogue of the medical library of Bowdoin College. The books and plates, mentioned in this appendix, have been added to the medical library since the publication of the catalogue in February, 1823. December, 1823. Brunswick: Joseph Griffin, printer, 1823. 16p. DLC; CtY-M; MBM **20-0082**

BOWDOIN COLLEGE, Brunswick, Maine
Catalogue of the library of the Medical School of Maine, at Bowdoin College. February, 1825. Brunswick: J. Griffin, pr., 1825. 62p. MH **20-0083**

BRODIE, Benjamin Collins (1783-1862)
Pathological and surgical observations on diseases of the joints. Philadelphia: Pr. by Frankish, for Benjamin Warner, 1821. 329p. ICJ; IEN-M; MBM; MdBM **20-0084**

BROOKS, John
An address, delivered before the Second Medical Society of the State of Vermont, at their annual meeting in Dummerston, January 12, 1820. Brattleboro: Printed by John Holbrook [1820]. 15p. DLC; MBM **20-0085**

BROUSSAIS, François Joseph Victor (1772-1838)
A treatise on physiology applied to pathology. Transl. from the French, by John Bell, . . . and R. LaRoche. Philadelphia: Carey & Lea, Mifflin & Parry, prs., 1826. 599p. CU-M; KU; MB; PPC **20-0086**

BROUSSAIS, François Joseph Victor (1772-1838)
A treatise on physiology applied to pathology. . . . Transl. from the French by John Bell and R. LaRoche. 2nd American ed. Philadelphia: Carey, Lea & Carey, publishers, Skerrett, pr., 1828. 600p. IEN-M; MdBM; PPC; PU **20-0087**

BROWN, Stephen
A dissertation on smallpox, varioloid, and vaccination. . . . New Brunswick [N.J.]. December 5, 1828. 99p. [Medical Prize Essay] NjR; NNNAM **20-0088**

BROWN, Stephen
Syllabus of a course of lectures on materia medica and pharmacy. . . . New York College of Pharmacy. New York: Vanderpool & Cole, prs., 1829. 13p. NNNAM **20-0089**

BROWN, Thomas
The ethereal physician, or The medical powers of electricity demonstrated . . . in the prevention and cure of a great variety of diseases. . . . Albany: Printed for the authors, by E. and E. Hosford, 1823. 152p. NNNAM; PPC **20-0090**

BUCHAN, William (1729-1805)
Domestic medicine. . . . Boston: Phelps and Farnham, 1825. 652p. DNLM [*Vel subseq.*] **20-0091**

BUCHAN, William (1729-1805)
Domestic medicine, or A treatise on the prevention and cure of diseases. . . . From the 22nd English ed., with considerable additions, and notes. Exeter: J. & B. Williams, 1828. 495p. DLC; MA; NcU **20-0092**

BUCHAN, William (1729-1805)
The domestic medicine . . . with advice to mothers in promoting the health of their offspring. To which is annexed, the family receipt book. . . . New York: T. Kinnersley, [1829]. 224p. NNAM **20-0093**

BUCKELEW, Frederick
A treatise on fever. New York: Pr. by Charles N. Baldwin, 1821. 40p. DLC **20-0094**

BURLINGAME, Josiah
The poor man's physician, the sick man's friend; or, Nature's botanic garden exibited to view. . . . Norwich, N.Y.: Pr. by Wm. G. Hyer, for the author, 1826. 293p. CSmH **20-0095**

BURNS, Allan (1781-1813)
Observations on the surgical anatomy of the head and neck, illustrated by cases and engravings. . . . 1st American ed. With a life of the author; and additional cases and observations. By Granville Sharpe Pattison. . . . Baltimore: F. Lucas, Jr., E. J. Coale, and Cushing & Jewett; Philadelphia: H. Carey & I. Lea, 1823. 512p; CtY-M; ICU; PU **20-0096**

BURNS, John (1774-1850)
The principles of midwifery; including the diseases of women and children. . . . The 5th American, from the 3rd London ed., greatly enl. With improvements and notes, by Thomas C. James. . . . Philadelphia: Published by Benjamin & Thomas Kite [etc.] J. R. A. Skerrett, printer, 1820-21. 2 v. CtY-M; NdBM; MBM; NNNAM **20-0097**

BURNS, John (1774-1850)
The principles of midwifery; including the diseases of women and children. 4th American from 3rd London ed., greatly enl. With imp. and notes, by Thomas C. James. Philadelphia: Benjamin Warner, Edward Parker, Mathew Carey & Son, Benjamin & Thomas Kite, Solomon W. Conrad and Anthony Finley, 1821. 406p. PPC; PPHa **20-0098**

BURNS, John (1774-1850)
The principles of midwifery; including the diseases of women and children. . . . From the 5th London ed., enlarged, with improvements and notes by T. C. James. . . . Philadelphia: Published by Edward Parker, J. H. Cunningham, printer, 1823. 2 v. IEN-M; MdBM; NNNAM; OC **20-0099**

CABANIS, Pierre Jean Georges (1757-1808)
An essay of the certainty of medicine. . . . Philadelphia: Robert Desilver, 1823. 119, 108p. DNLM; ICJ; NN; PPHa **20-0100**

CALDWELL, Charles (1772-1853)
An address to the committees on education of both houses of the legislature of Kentucky, on the state of the school of medicine of Transylvania University. . . . Published by order of the committees. Lexington, Ky.: T. Smith, 1820. 23p. DNLM **20-0101**

CALDWELL, Charles (1772-1853)
Outlines of a course of lectures on the institutes of medicine. Lexington, Ky.: Pr. by William Tanner, 1823. 188p. DLC; ICU; MH; NcD **20-0102**

CALDWELL, Charles (1772-1853)
Elements of phrenology. . . . Lexington, Ky.: Printed for the author by T. T. Skillman, 1824. 100p. DLC; DNLM; OCIM **20-0103**

CALDWELL, Charles (1772-1853)
Analysis of fever. An analysis of fever. . . . Lexington, Ky.: Printed for the author by T. T. Skillman, 1825. 97p. DLC; DNLM **20-0104**

CALDWELL, Charles (1772-1853)
Correspondence between Dr. Charles Caldwell of the medical school of Transylvania University, and Dr. James Fishback, pastor of the first Baptist Church of Lexington. Lexington, Ky.: Pr. by Thomas T. Skillman, 1825. 40p. ICU; KU; OC **20-0105**

CALDWELL, Charles (1772-1853)
Medical and physical memoirs. . . . Lexington: Pr. at the office of the Kentucky Whig, 1826. 224p. DLC; MHi; NN; OC
20-0106

CALDWELL, Charles (1772-1853)
Medical and physical memoirs. . . . Lexington, Ky.: Pr. by A. G. Meriwether, 1827. 85p. ICU; MB **20-0107**

CALDWELL, Charles (1772-1853)
Elements of phrenology. (2nd ed., greatly enl.) With a preliminary discourse in vindication of the science against an attack on it by Francis Jeffrey, Esq.; and a concluding essay in proof of its usefulness as the true philosophy of the human intellect, and applicable to the most important purposes of life. . . . Lexington, Ky.: Printed by A. G. Meriwether, 1827. 279p. DLC; NcD; OC **20-0108**

CAPEN, Nahum, ed. (1804-1886)
The friend to health, being a selection of valuable truths relating to the preservation of health, from the works of Thatcher, Franklin, Thompson, Salzmann, etc. Boston: Marsh and Capen, 1826. 107p. CtY-M; MB; NN **20-0109**

CARMICHAEL, Richard (1779-1849)
An essay on venereal diseases, and the uses and abuses of mercury in their treatment. . . . Philadelphia: J. Dobson (agent), and A. Sherman, J. Harding, pr., 1825. 360p. CtY-M; MB; PPL **20-0110**

CARPENTER, George Washington (1802-1860)
Observations and experiments in the pharmaceutical preparations and constituent principles of opium. . . . Philadelphia, 1827. 16p. DLC; PLF; PP; PPC **20-0111**

CAZENAVE, Pierre Louis Alphée (1795-1877)
A practical synopsis of cutaneous diseases, from the most celebrated authors, and particularly from documents afforded by the clinical lectures of Dr. Biett. By A. Cazenave and H. E. Schedel. Transl. from the French, with notes. Philadelphia: Carey, Lea & Carey [Skerrett, pr.] 1829. 400p. DLC; IU-M; PPJ **20-0112**

[CHANNING, Walter] (1786-1876)
Remarks on the employment of females as practitioners in midwifery. By a physician. Boston: Cummings and Hilliard, 1820. 22p. DLC; DNLM; MBM; MH-M **20-0113**

CHAPMAN, Nathaniel (1780-1853)
Correspondence between Mr. Granville Sharpe Pattison and Dr. N. Chapman. [Philadelphia? 1820]. 16p. DLC; DNLM; NNNAM; NNU-M **20-0114**

CHAPMAN, Nathaniel (1780-1853)
Correspondence between Mr. Granville Sharpe Pattison and Dr. N. Chapman. 2nd ed. with explanatory remarks. [Philadelphia, 1821]. 44p. DLC; MB; MH; RPB **20-0115**

CHAPMAN, Nathaniel (1780-1853)
Correspondence between Mr. Granville Sharpe Pattison and Dr. N. Chapman. 2nd ed. [Philadelphia, 1821]. 35p. PPL [variant ed.] **20-0116**

CHAPMAN, Nathaniel (1780-1853)
Elements of therapeutics and materia medica. . . . 2nd ed., enl. and revised. Philadelphia: M. Carey & Sons, 1821-22. 2 v. MB; MH-N; NNNAM; ScCM **20-0117**

CHAPMAN, Nathaniel (1780-1853)
Elements of therapeutics and materia medica. . . . 3rd ed., enlarged and revised. Philadelphia: H. C. Carey & I. Lea, 1823-24. 2v. ICJ; MdBM; PPHa **20-0118**

CHAPMAN, Nathaniel (1780-1853)
Elements of therapeutics and materia medica. To which are prefixed two discourses on the history and improvement of the materia medica, originally delivered as introductory lectures. . . . 4th ed., enl. and revised. Philadelphia: H. C. Carey and I. Lea, 1825. 2 v. NjR; PPC; PPJ **20-0119**

CHAPMAN, Nathaniel (1780-1853)
Elements of therapeutics and materia medica. To which are prefixed two discourses on the history and improvement of the materia medica, originally delivered as introductory lectures. . . . 5th ed., enl. and revised. Philadelphia: Carey, Lea, and Carey, 1827. 2 v. DLC; DNLM; PPC; PU
20-0120

CHAPMAN, William
Impediments of speech. Mr. & Mrs. Chaptman's institution for the cure of impediments of speech. No. 187 Pine Street, Philadelphia, continues open for the reception of those ladies and gentlemen, who are oppressed with any kind of hesitancy, stuttering or stammering. . . . [Philadelphia, 1825]. 1p. DLC
20-0121

CHARLESTON, S.C., Medical College of the State of South Carolina
Medical college of South Carolina. Charleston, S.C.: Wm. Riley, 1825. 8p. DLC **20-0122**

CLARKE, Charles Mansfield (1782-1857)
Observations on those diseases of females which are attended by discharges. . . . Philadelphia: H. C. Carey and I. Lea, 1824. 222p. IEN-M; MB; NNNAM; PPC **20-0123**

CLARKE, Charles Mansfield (1782-1857)
Observations on those diseases of females which are attended by discharges. 2nd American ed. Boston: Wells & Lilly; Philadelphia: H. C. Carey and I. Lea, 1826. 306p. CU-M; MdBM; OCIM; PU **20-0124**

COFFIN, John Gorham
A discourse on medical education and on the medical profession. Boston: J. W. Ingraham, 1822. 46p. MBM; MN; MWA
20-0125

COFFIN, John Gorham
Domestic medicine; or, A Treatise on the prevention and cure of diseases by regimen and simple medicines. Boston: Pub. by Phelps and Farnham, 1825. 652p. IEN-M; MB; MWA; NNNAM
20-0126

COFFIN, John Gorham
Discourses on cold and warm bathing; with remarks on the effects of drinking cold water in warm weather. . . . 2nd ed. Boston: Cummings, Hilliard, and Co. [Cambridge, from the University Press, by Hilliard & Metcalf], 1826. 70p. DLC; MB; MWA; NjR **20-0127**

COLLEGE OF PHYSICIANS, Philadelphia
Address to the citizens of the city and county of Philadelphia. . . . Pub. by Board of Trustees. [Philadelphia, 1826]. 7p. MWA
20-0128

COLLES, Abraham (1773-1843)
A treatise on surgical anatomy. Part the first. . . . Philadelphia: J. Maxwell, 1820. 179p. CU-M; CtY-M; DNLM; MBM. [No more published.] **20-0129**

COLLIN, Victor
Manual for the use of the stethoscope. A short treatise on the different methods of investigating the diseases of the chest. Transl. from the French . . . by W. N. Ryland. From the 3rd London ed. Boston: Benjamin Perkins & Co. [Pr. by Peirce & Williams] 1829, xv[1], 133p. DLC; DNLM; PPC **20-0130**

COMBE, George (1788-1858)
Essays on phrenology, or An inquiry into the principles and utility of the system of Drs. Gall and Spurzheim, and into the objections made against it. . . . With notes and additions, comprehending memoirs on the anatomy of the brain, and on insanity. Philadelphia: H. C. Carey and I. Lea, 1822. 463p. DLC; MB; MBM; ScC **20-0131**

COMBE, George (1788-1858)
Elements of phrenology. . . . 1st America ed., with notes from the second Edinburgh, imp. and enl. Philadelphia: E. Littell, Clark & Raser, prs., 1826. 221p. CSmH; GU; MdBM; PPC **20-0132**

COMSTOCK, John Lee (1789-1858)
An examination of essays on fevers, and other medical subjects, by Thomas Miner and William Tully, with some observations on their doctrines and practice. Hartford: Huntington & Hopkins, P. Canfield, pr., 1824. 64p. MBM **20-0133**

CONDIE, David Francis (1796-1875)
A course of examinations on anatomy and physiology, surgery, chemistry, materia medica, midwifery, and the practice of medicine. 2nd ed. with additions and improvements. Philadelphia: J. Webster [etc. etc.], 1824. 205p. DNLM; MdBM; NNNAM; OC **20-0134**

CONNECTICUT MEDICAL SOCIETY
Proceedings of the president and fellows . . . at their annual convention in May, 1828. . . . Weathersfield: A. Francis, pr., 1828. 14p. CtHi **20-0135**

COOKE, Charles Turner
Observations on the efficacy of white mustard seed in affections of the liver, internal organs and nervous system. . . . 1st American from the 4th English ed. New York: G. & C. Carvill [etc.] [Sleight & George, prs., Jamaica, L.I.], 1827. 116p. DLC; DNLM; ICJ; MB **20-0136**

COOKE, Charles Turner
Observations on the efficacy of white mustard seed, in affections of the liver, internal organs, and nervous system. . . . 2nd American from 4th English ed. New York: G. & C. Carvill, W. E. Dean, pr., 1828. 116p. DLC; MBM; NNNAM **20-0137**

COOKE, John
A treatise on nervous diseases. Boston: Wells and Lilly; and H. C. Carey and I. Lea, Philadelphia, 1824. 432p. DLC; DNLM; PPC **20-0138**

COOKE, John Esten (1783-1853)
A treatise of pathology and therapeutics. In three volumes. Lexington, Ky. [S. H. Davis, pr., Winchester, Va.], 1828. 2 v. [v. 3 not pub.] DLC; DNLM; ICJ; NNNAM **20-0139**

COOKE, John Esten (1783-1853)
Essays on the autumnal and winter epidemics. [Lexington, Ky.]: Transylvania Press. Pr. by J. G. Norwood, pr. to the university, 1829. 188p. DLC; DNLM; MB; NN **20-0140**

COOPER, Astley Paston (1768-1841)
Surgical essays. Parts 1 and 2. 1st American from 3rd London ed. Philadelphia: Pr. by J. Robinson for David Hanna, 1821. 409p. ICJ; IEN-M; OC **20-0141**

COOPER, Astley Paston (1768-1841)
Surgical essays. Parts 1 and 2. 1st American from 3rd London ed. Philadelphia: Pr. by J. Robinson, for James Webster, 1821. 409p. MBM; MH-M; NBM; PPC **20-0142**

COOPER, Astley Paston (1768-1841)
A treatise on dislocations and on fractions of the joints. . . . Philadelphia: H. C. Carey & I. Lea, 1824. 425p. PPHa **20-0143**

COOPER, Astley Paston (1768-1841)
The lectures of Sir Astley Cooper . . . on the principles and practice of surgery. . . . 1st American from the 3rd London ed. Philadelphia: H. C. Carey & I. Lea, 1825. 425, [46]p., xxi pl. OCIM; PPC **20-0144**

COOPER, Astley Paston (1768-1841)
A treatise on dislocations and on fractions of the joints. 1st American, from the 3rd London ed. Boston: Wells & Lilly, 1825. vii, 425p. CU-M; MB; NNNAM **20-0145**

COOPER, Astley Paston (1768-1841)
The lectures of Sir Astley Cooper . . . on the principles and practice of surgery. . . . Boston: Wells & Lilly, 1825-28. 3 v. CtY-M; MB; OC; RPM **20-0146**

COOPER, Astley Paston (1768-1841)
The lectures of Sir Astley Cooper . . . on the principles and practice of surgery, with additional notes and cases. By Frederick Tyrrell. . . . Philadelphia: A. Sherman, 1826. 3 v. CU-M; IU-M; NjR; PPC **20-0147**

COOPER, Samuel (1780-1848)
The first lines of the practice of surgery, designed as an introduction for students, and a concise book of reference for practitioners. . . . From the 4th London ed. Corr. and enl. New York: James V. Seaman, James and John Harper, printers, 1822. 2 v. CU-M; MBM; NNNAM; OC **20-0148**

COOPER, Samuel (1780-1848)
A dictionary of practical surgery. . . . With notes and an appendix, by William Anderson. . . . From the 4th London ed. New York: Pub. by Collins and Hannay, J. & J. Harper, printers, 1822. 2 v. CU-M; MB; MdBM; PPC **20-0149**

COOPER, Samuel (1780-1848)
A dictionary of practical surgery. . . . With notes and an appendix, by William Anderson. . . . From the 4th London ed. New York: Pub. by Collins & Hannay, J. & J. Harper, prs., 1823. 2 v. MdBM; NNNAM; PPL **20-0150**

COOPER, Samuel (1780-1848)
First lines of practice of surgery. 3rd American ed. from the 3rd London ed., rev. & cor. with practical notes and observations. Boston: T. Bedlington, 1828. 447p. GU; ICJ; NNNAM **20-0151**

COOPER, Samuel (1780-1848)
First lines of practice of surgery. 3rd American ed. from the 5th London ed., rev. & cor. with practical notes and observations. With notes by Alexander H. Stevens. . . . Philadelphia: T. Desilver & H. Cowperthwait, J. R. Bailey, pr., 1828. 2 v. MdBM; NNNAM; PPC **20-0152**

COOPER, Thomas (1759-1839)
An address delivered before the Medical Board of S. Carolina, at Columbia, December, 1821. Columbia: Pr. at the Gazette office, 1821. 16p. ScC; ScCM **20-0153**

COOPER, Thomas (1759-1839)
A treatise of domestic medicine, intended for families, in which the treatment of common disorders is alphabetically enumerated. To which is added, a practical system of domestic cookery. . . . Also, the art of preserving all kinds of animal and vegetable substances for many years, by M. Appert. Reading: C. Getz, 1824. 128p. CSmH; DLC; ScU **20-0154**

COOPER, Thomas (1759-1839)
A view of the metaphysical and physiological arguments in favour of materialism. By a physician. . . . Philadelphia, 1824. 67p. MB; PPL **20-0155**

CORNARO, Luigi (1467-1566)
An abridgement of the writings of Lewis Cornaro, a nobleman of Venice, on health and long life. By Herman Daggett. . . . Andover: Pub. by Mark Newman [Pr.: Flagg and Gould] 1824. [7], 68p. MBM; RPB; RPM **20-0156**

COSTER, Jacques (1795-1868)
Manual of surgical operations; containing the new methods of operating, devised by Lisfranc. Philadelphia: H. C. Carey & I. Lea, 1825. 265p. IEN-M; MdBM; OC; PPHa **20-0157**

COXE, John Redman (1773-1864)
The American dispensatory . . . together with the operations of pharmacy: illustrated and explained, according to the principles of modern chemistry . . . 5th ed. Philadelphia: H. C. Carey and I. Lea. Wm. Fry, printer, 1822. 816p. DLC; MB; MdBM; PPC **20-0158**

COXE, John Redman (1773-1864)
The American dispensatory . . . 4th ed. . . . Philadelphia: Pub. by Thomas Dobson and Son, William Fry, printer, 1823. 735p. NNNAM; OCLloyd **20-0159**

COXE, John Redman (1773-1864)
The American dispensatory . . . illustrated and explained . . . the arrangement simplified . . . 6th ed. Philadelphia: [H. C. Carey & I. Lea; J. R. A. Skerrett, pr.], 1825. 766p. CtY-M; MdBM; PPC **20-0160**

COXE, John Redman (1773-1864)
The American dispensatory . . . 7th ed. Philadelphia: H. C. Carey & I. Lea, 1827. iv, 780p. ICJ; ICRM; PPC; ScCM **20-0161**

CULLEN, William (1710-1790)
First lines of the practice of physic . . . 2nd ed., rev. and enl. Philadelphia: E. Parker, 1822. 2 v. DLC; DNLM; IEN-M; NBM **20-0162**

CULPEPER, Nicholas (1616-1654)
The English physician enl., containing three hundred and sixty-nine receipts for medicines made from herbs. Taunton: Pr. by Samuel W. Mortimer, 1826. 259p. DLC; NN; PPC **20-0163**

DANIELL, William C.
Observations upon the autumnal fevers of Savannah. Savannah: W. T. Williams; New York: Collins & Hannay, 1828. 152p. MB; NN; PPAmP **20-0164**

DAVIDGE, John Beale
Physical sketches, or Outlines of correctives, applied to certain modern errours in physick. . . . Baltimore: Pr. by J. Robinson, 1823. 2 v. DLC; MdHi **20-0165**

De La MOTTA, Jacob
An oration, on the causes of mortality among strangers, during the late summer and fall. Pronounced before the Georgia Medical Society, and citizens of Savannah, on January 1st, 1820. Being the anniversary of the Society. . . . Savannah: Kappel & Bartlett [1820]. 16p. DNLM; MBM; NHi; NNNAM **20-0166**

DENMAN, Thomas (1733-1815)
An introduction to the practice of midwifery. . . . From the last London ed., rev. by the author. With notes and emendations by J. W. Francis. New York: E. Bliss & E. White, 1821. 683p. DNLM; ICJ; MBM; PMA **20-0167**

DENMAN, Thomas (1733-1815)
Aphorisms on the application and use of the forceps and vectis; on preternatural labours; on labours attended with hemorrhage, and with convulsions. From the 7th London ed. Boston: Wells & Lilly, 1822. 95p. DNLM; MB; MdBM **20-0168**

DENMAN, Thomas (1733-1815)
An introduction to the practice of midwifery. From the last London ed. With notes and emendations, by John W. Francis, M.D. New York: Pub. by E. Bliss and E. White. Sleight & Tucker, prs., Jamaica, 1825. 684p. 16 pls. MA; MB; PPC **20-0169**

DENMAN, Thomas (1733-1815)
An introduction to the practice of midwifery. From the 6th London ed., with a biographical sketch of the author. 3rd American ed. . . . New York: G. & C. & H. Carvill [J. Seymour, pr.], 1829. 776p. DLC; DNLM; ICJ; MdBM **20-0170**

DEWEES, William Potts (1768-1841)
Essays on various subjects connected with midwifery. Philadelphia: H. C. Carey & I. Lea, 1823. 479p. IEN-M; MB; PPAmP; PPC **20-0171**

DEWEES, William Potts (1768-1841)
A compendious system of midwifery, chiefly designed to facilitate the inquiries of those who may be pursuing this branch of study. . . . Philadelphia: Carey & Lea, 1824. 602p. DLC; DNLM; ICJ; MdBM **20-0172**

DEWEES, William Potts (1768-1841)
A treatise on the physical and medical treatment of children. Philadelphia: H. C. Carey & I. Lea, 1825. 496p. DNLM; ICJ; MB; NNNAM **20-0173**

DEWEES, William Potts (1768-1841)
A compendious system of midwifery.... 2nd ed., with additions, etc. Philadelphia: H. C. Carey & I. Lea, 1826. 612p. DLC; ICJ, IU-M; PPHa **20-0174**

DEWEES, William Potts (1768-1841)
A treatise on the physical and medical treatment of children. ... 2nd ed., with corrections, &c. Philadelphia: H. C. Carey & I. Lea, 1826. 508p. PPL **20-0175**

DEWEES, William Potts (1768-1841)
A treatise on the diseases of females. Philadelphia: H. C. Carey & I. Lea, L. R. Bailey, pr., 1826. 557p. DNLM; MB; MH; OCIM **20-0176**

DEWEES, William Potts (1768-1841)
A treatise on diseases of females. 2nd ed. Philadelphia: Carey, Lea and Carey, 1827. 538p. PPHa **20-0177**

DEWEES, William Potts (1768-1841)
A treatise on the diseases of females. 2nd ed. rev. and corr. Philadelphia: Carey, Lea and Carey [I. Ashmead & Co., prs.], 1828. 542p. DNLM; MdBM; RPM **20-0178**

DEWEES, William Potts (1768-1841)
A compendious system of midwifery, chiefly designed to facilitate the inquiries of those who may be pursuing this branch of study. . . . 3rd ed. with additions. Philadelphia: Carey, Lea & Carey, 1828. Skerrett, Philadelphia, pr. 644p. CU-M; RPM; ScCm **20-0179**

DEWEES, William Potts (1768-1841)
A treatise on the physical and medical treatment of children. 3rd ed., with corr. Philadelphia: Carey, Lea & Carey, Skerrett, pr., 1829. xiv, [2] [9]-528p. DNLM; ICJ; PPC; RPM **20-0180**

DICKINSON, J.
A syndesmological chart, or, A table of the ligaments of the human skeleton. 1st American from the 1st London edition of 1821. Philadelphia, Baltimore: J. Webster [1822]. NNNAM **20-0181**

DICKSON, Samuel Henry (1798-1872)
Introductory lecture, delivered at the commencement of the second session of the Medical College of South Carolina, November, 1825. Charleston: W. Riley, 1826. 31p. DLC; MH **20-0182**

DICKSON, Samuel Henry (1798-1872)
Introductory lecture delivered at the commencement of the fourth session of the Medical College of South Carolina, November, 1827. Charleston: Pr. by W. Riley, 1828. 24p. NBM; ScMS; ScU **20-0183**

DISPENSATORIES, eclectic and general, comprehending a system of pharmacy, materia medica, etc. By an American physician. Philadelphia: Towar & Hogan, 1827, 627p. MdBJ-W **20-0184**

THE DOMESTIC physician, travellers' medical companion. Compiled from the practice of the most eminent physicians and surgeons, viz.: Sir Astley Cooper, Sir Henry Halford, Drs. Baillie, Latham, Heberden, Saunders, Babington, Birckbeck, &c. &c. &c. . . . By a physician. 1st American from 2nd London ed.... New York: Elam Bliss, 1827. 316p. OCLloyd **20-1085**

DONALDSON, Peter
A review of the present systems of medicine and chirurgery of Europe and America . . . viewed in connexion with the most refined principles and demonstrations of anatomy, physiology, pathology, nosology, pharmacy, chemistry, materia medica, medical jurisprudence and philosophy. . . . New York: The author, 1821. 440p. DLC; MBM; MH-M **20-0186**

DONALDSON, Peter
A dissertation on the history and curation of the obstruction of the intestines in all their modifications and combinations . . . together with some cases of these diseases, subjoined in confirmation of the success of the method proposed for the general benefit of man. New York: N. B. Holmes, 1821. 43p. CtY-M; DLC; NNNAM **20-0187**

DONALDSON, Peter
Medical advice to European emigrants, residing in the Continent of America. New York: The author, 1822. 12p. NN **20-0188**

DONALDSON, Peter
The natural history of the rise, progress and termination of the epidemic inflammation, commonly called yellow malignant fever, which prevailed in the city of New York, during the autumn of 1822. . . . New York: The author. 1822. 36p. CtY-M; DLC; NNNAM; NNU-M **20-0189**

DORSEY, John Syng (1783-1818)
Elements of surgery: for the use of students . . . with notes by J. Randolph. . . . 3rd ed. Philadelphia: Pub. by Edward Parker, William Brown, pr., 1823. 2 v. DNLM; ICJ; IEN-M; PMA **20-0190**

DOUCET, Francis O.
Lecture on the medical systems . . . before the City and County Medical Society of New York. New York: Pr. by J. Seymour, 1829. 26p. NNNAM **20-0191**

DRAKE, Daniel (1785-1852)
An inaugural discourse on medical education; delivered at the opening of the Medical College of Ohio, in Cincinnati, November 11th, 1820. . . . Cincinnati, Ohio: Looker, Palmer and Reynolds, 1820. 31p. CtY-M; DNLM; LNT-M; MWA **20-0192**

DRAKE, Daniel (1785-1852)
A narrative of the rise and fall of the Medical College of Ohio. Cincinnati, Ohio: Looker & Reynolds, printers, 1822. 42p. DLC; DNLM; MH; NNNAM **20-0193**

DRAKE, Daniel (1785-1852)
Introductory lecture on the necessity and value of professional industry; delivered in the chapel of Transylvania University, November 7, 1823. Lexington, Ky.: William Tanner, 1823. 31p. RPJCB; OCIWHi; KU; KyLoJM **20-0194**

[DRAKE, Daniel] (1785-1852)
The people's doctors; a review, by 'The People's Friend.' Cincinnati, Ohio: Pr. and pub. for the use of the people, 1829. 60p. CSmH; DLC; MB; PPL **20-0195**

DUCACHET, Henry William (1796-1865)
A biographical memoir of Samuel Bard, M.D., LL.D., late president of the College of Physicians and Surgoens of the University of the State of New York, &c. Philadelphia, 1821. 27p. DLC; MB; NNC; NNNAM **20-1096**

DUCAMP, Theodore Joseph (1792?-1823?)
A treatise on the retention of urine, caused by strictures in the urethra; and of the means by which obstructions of this canal may be effectually removed. . . . New York: S. Wood & Sons, 1827. 219p. v pl. CU-M; DLC; ICJ; NN **20-0197**

DUNBAR, John Richard Woodcock (1805-1871)
An essay on the structure, functions, and diseases of the nervous system. . . . Philadelphia: J. Dobson, 1828. 80p. MB; NNNAM; PHi **20-0198**

DUNGLISON, Robley (1798-1869)
Syllabus of the lecture on the medical jurisprudence and on the treatment of poisoning & suspended animation. Delivered in the University of Virginia. . . . Pr. for the use of the students. University of Virginia: Pr. by Clement P. M'Kennie, 1827. 142p. DLC; MdBM; PPC **20-0199**

EBERLE, John (1787-1838)
A treatise of the materia medica and therapeutics. . . . Philadelphia: J. Webster, 1822-23. 2 v. IEN-M; NBM; PPC; PPHa **20-0200**

EBERLE, John (1787-1838)
A treatise on the materia medica and therapeutics. . . . 2nd ed., with corrections. Baltimore: S. & W. Meeteer; Philadelphia: J. Webster, 1825. 2 v. MdHi; MdBJ-W; MdU-D; NcD **20-0201**

EBERLE, John (1787-1838)
A reply to certain calumnious statements uttered and published by Francis S. Beattie, M.D. Philadelphia: R. Wright, 1826. 8p. DNLM **20-0202**

EBERLE, John (1787-1838)
Notes of lectures on the theory and practice of medicine delivered in the Jefferson Medical College at Philadelphia. Philadelphia: Pub. by J. G. Auner, Lydia R. Bailey, pr., 1827. 252p. MdBM; PPC; PPHa **20-0203**

THE ECLECTIC and general dispensatory: comprehending a system of pharmacy, materia medica, the formulae of the London, Edinburgh, and Dublin pharmacopoeias, prescriptions of many eminent physicians, and receipts for the most common empirical medicines: collated from the best authorities, by an American physician. Philadelphia: Towar & Hogan, Mifflin & Parry, prs., 1827. 627p. DNLM; ICJ; IEN-M; OC **20-0204**

EDWARDS, Henry Milne (1800-1885)
A manual of surgical anatomy. . . . Transl., with notes, by Wm. Coulson. . . . 1st American from the 1st London ed. rev. and cor. with additional notes, by James Webster. . . . Philadelphia: T. Desilver, Pr. by L. R. Bailey, 1828. 382p. NNAM; PPC; ScCM **20-0205**

EDWARDS, Henry Milne (1800-1885)
A manual of materia medica and pharmacy, comprising a concise description of the articles used in medicine. . . . Transl. from the French, with numerous additions and corrections, and adapted to the practice of medicine and the art of pharmacy in the United States by Joseph Togno . . . and E. Durand. . . . Philadelphia: Carey, Lea & Carey [Skerrett, pr.] 1829. 523, [1]p. NNAM; NjR; PPC **20-0206**

ELIOT, Ephraim
Medicine boxes, for any voyages, with directions suitable to their contents, are prepared by Ephraim Eliot. . . . [Boston, ca. 1820]. 6p. MBM **20-0207**

ELLIOTT, Stephen (1771-1830)
An address delivered at the opening of the Medical College, in Charleston, S.C. on Monday, the 13th of November, 1826. Pub. by the Hon. City Council of Charleston. Charleston: A. E. Miller, 1826. 23p. DLC; DNLM; NcU; ScC **20-0208**

ELLIS, Benjamin (1798-1831)
The medical formulary; being a collection of prescriptions, derived from the writings and practice of many of the most eminent physicians in America and Europe. . . . Philadelphia: H. C. Carey & I. Lea, 1826. Skerrett, pr. 148p. ICJ; KyLoJM; MdBM; PPC **20-0209**

ELLIS, Benjamin (1798-1831)
The medical formulary: being a collection of prescriptions, derived from the writings and practice of many of the most eminent physicians in America and Europe. To which is added, an appendix, containing the usual dietetic preparations and antidotes for poisons. The whole accompanied with a few brief pharmaceutic and medical observations. . . . 2nd ed., with additions. Philadelphia: Carey, Lea & Carey, 1829. 214p. ICJ; MB; OCLloyd; PPC **20-0210**

EVERETT, Jesse
A synopsis of rules and directions for exciting electricity . . . as a remedy for diseases. . . . New York: Pr. by P. and H. Van Pelt, June, 1825. 54p. NNNAM **20-0211**

EWELL, James (1773-1832)
The medical companion, or Family physician treating of the diseases of the United States. . . . 6th ed. rev. and enl. Baltimore: Pr. for the Proprietors, by B. Edes, 1822. 792p. MdBJ-W; MdU-D **20-0212**

[EWELL, James] (1773-1832)
The medical companion, or family physician: treating of the diseases of the United States, with their symptoms, causes, cure, and means of prevention. . . . [7th ed. Philadelphia, 1827] 852p. DLC; DNLM; PU **20-0213**

[EWELL, James] (1773-1832)
The medical companion, or family physician: treating of the diseases of the United States, with their symptoms, causes, cure, and means of prevention . . . 7th ed., rev., enl. and very considerably improved. Washington: Pr. for the proprietors, 1827. 862p. OCLloyd; PPC **20-0214**

EWELL, Thomas (1785-1826)
American family physician. . . . With an appendix, containing hints respecting the treatment of domestic animals. . . . Georgetown, D.C.: J. Thomas, 1824. 480p. MdHi; MdBJ-W; MdU-D **20-0215**

EWELL, Thomas (1785-1826)
American family physician. . . . Georgetown, D.C. Pub. by James Thomas, 1826. 503p. MA **20-0216**

FAITHORN, John
Facts and observations on liver complaints, and bilious disorders in general; and on those derangements of that important organ, and of its immediate or intimate connections, which most sensibly influence the biliary secretion . . . connected by an appropriate and successful mode of treatment. . . . First American edition. Philadelphia: Hickman & Hazzard [etc., etc.] 1820. 158p. CtY-M; DNLM; ICJ; MBM **20-0217**

FARRAR, John (1779-1853)
An experimental treatise on optics, comprehending the leading principles of the science. . . . Cambridge, N.E.: Pr. by Hilliard & Metcalf, 1826. 350p. ICJ; IU-M; NNC; PPL
20-0218

FARRAR, John (1779-1853)
Elements of electricity, magnetism and electro-magnetism. . . . Cambridge, N.E.: Pr. by Hilliard & Metcalf, 1826. 395p. MB; MH; PPF; PU **20-0219**

FAUST, Edwin D.
A sketch of medical chemistry. . . . Columbia: Pr. by D. and J. M. Faust, 1828. 337p. NNNAM; PPF **20-0220**

FERNALD, Joseph
Medical deception and imposition upon the public. Discovered, detected and exposed. Portland, Me.: A. Shirley, pr., 1824. 16p. MB; MWA **20-0221**

FISHER, John Dix (1797-1850)
Description of the distinct, confluent and inoculated smallpox, varioloid disease, cow pox and chicken pox. Boston: Wells and Lilly, publisher; Dutton & Wentworth, prs., 1829. 73p. MB; NNNAM; OCIM; PPC **20-0222**

FITCH, Samuel Sheldon
Remarks on the importance of the teeth, on their diseases and modes of cure; with directions for forming regular and beautiful sets of teeth, and for the preservation of their health and beauty. Philadelphia: Jesper Harding, pr. 1828. 27p. NjR; PPL
20-0223

FITCH, Samuel Sheldon
A system of dental surgery: in three parts. New York: G. & C. & H. Carvill [R. & C. S. Wood, prs.] 1829. 568p. CU-M; MdBM; NBM; RPB **20-0224**

FLAGG, Josiah Foster (1789-1853)
The family dentist; containing a brief description of the structure, formation, diseases, and treatment of the human teeth. . . . Boston: J. W. Ingraham, 1822. 82p. CU-M; MB; MBM; OC **20-0225**

FLINT, Joseph Henshaw (1786?-1846)
A dissertation, on the prophylactic management of infancy and early childhood. Read before The Massachusetts Medical Society, at their annual meeting June 7, 1826. Northampton: Pr. by T. Watson Shepard, 1826. 20p. DLC; MWA
20-0226

FORDYCE, George (1736-1802)
Five dissertations on fever. . . . 2nd American ed., from the latest English edition of each respective dissertation. Boston: Pub. by T. Bedlington and C. Ewer, 1823. Goodale, Glazier & Co., prs., Hallowell. 442p. CU-M; DNLM; MB; PU
20-0227

FRICK, George (1793-1870)
A treatise on the disease of the eye; including the doctrines and practice of the most eminent modern surgeons. . . . Baltimore: F. Lucas, jun., 1823. 320p. IEN-M; MB; MBM; OC
20-0228

GALL, Franz Joseph (1758-1828)
Outlines of phrenology, or The philosophy of man, founded by Drs. Gall and Spurzheim. Designed to accompany the bust. From the Edinburgh edition, with alterations. Philadelphia: J. Harding, pr., 1824. 32p. DLC **20-0229**

GALLUP, Joseph Adams (1769-1849)
Pathological reflections on the supertonic state of disease. Read before the Vermont Medical Society, convened at Montpelier, October 10, 1822. Montpelier: Pr. by E. P. Walton, 1822. 26p. MBM; NNNAM; OC **20-0230**

GIBSON, William (1788-1868)
Strictures on "Mr. Pattison's reply to certain oral and written criticisms." . . . Philadelphia: James Maxwell, 1820. 56p. DNLM; MdBJ-W; NHi; NNNAM **20-0231**

GIBSON, William (1788-1868)
Strictures on "Mr. Pattison's reply to certain oral and written criticisms." . . . 2nd ed. Philadelphia: James Maxwell, 1820. 48p. DLC; DNLM; NNNAM; PHi **20-0232**

GIBSON, William (1788-1868)
The institutes and practice of surgery: being the outlines of a course of lectures. . . . Philadelphia: Pub. by Edward Parker, Clark & Raser, prs., 1824-25. 2 v. MB; NNNAM; PPC; PPHa
20-0233

GIBSON, William (1788-1868)
The institutes and practice of surgery: being the outlines of a course of lectures. . . . 2nd ed., with additions. . . . Philadelphia: Carey, Lea & Carey, 1827. 2 v. DLC; PPC; PPJ; PU
20-0234

GIDNEY, Eleazer
A treatise on the structure, diseases, and management of the human teeth. 1st ed. Utica: Pr. for the author by Augustine G. Dauby, 1824. 144p. MWA; NN; NNNAM
20-0235

GIRAUD, John James (1759-1839)
Memoir on the discovery of a specific medicine, for the cure and prevention of the yellow fever, plague, malignant and pestilential fevers, with documents. . . . Baltimore: Pr. by Wm. Wooddy, 1825. 23p. MWA; OC; PPAmP
20-0236

GODMAN, John Davidson (1794-1830)
Analytic anatomy. A lecture introductory to a course delivered in the Philadelphia anatomical rooms, session of 1823-4. Philadelphia: W. Brown, pr., 1824. 23p. MdBM; NNNAM; PHi
20-0237

GODMAN, John Davidson (1794-1830)
Anatomical investigations, comprising descriptions of various fasciae of the human body. . . . To which is added an account of some irregularities of structure and morbid anatomy. . . . Philadelphia: H. C. Carey & I. Lea, 1824. 134p. PPC; PPL; PU; PPHa **20-0238**

GODMAN, John Davidson (1794-1830)
Contributions to physiological and pathological anatomy; containing the observations made at the Philadelphia anatomical rooms during the session of 1824-5. Philadelphia: H. C. Carey & I. Lea, Wm. Fry, pr., 1825. 86p. IEN-M; PHi; PPC; PU **20-0239**

GODMAN, John Davidson (1794-1830)
Monitions to the students of medicine. A lecture introductory to the course delivered in the Philadelphia anatomical rooms, session of 1824-5. Philadelphia: Pr. by J. R. A. Skerrett, 1825. 20p. MB; PHi; PC **20-0240**

GODMAN, John Davidson (1794-1830)
Anatomy taught by analysis. A lecture introductory to the course delivered in the Philadelphia anatomical rooms, 5th session, 1825-6. Philadelphia: Pr. by Wm. Fry, 1826. 23p. MB; MdBM; OC; PPHa **20-0241**

GODMAN, John Davidson (1794-1830)
Professional reputation. An oration delivered before the Philadelphia Medical Society. Pursuant to appointment, Feb. 8, 1826. Pub. by order of the Society. Philadelphia: Benj. & Thomas Kite, J. R. A. Skerrett, pr., 1826. 24p. ICJ; NNNAM; PU **20-0242**

GODMAN, John Davidson (1794-1830)
Introductory lecture to a course of anatomy and physiology in Rutgers Medical College, New York, delivered Nov. 11, 1826. New York: Pub. for the students of Rutgers College by H. Stevenson, J. Seymour, pr., 1826. 44p. MB; NNNAM; NjR **20-0243**

GODMAN, John Davidson (1794-1830)
Introductory lecture to the course of anatomy and physiology. Rutgers Medical College, New York, delivered, Nov. 11, 1826. 2nd ed. New York: Pub. by H. Stevenson [J. Seymour, pr.] 1827. 44p. NNNAM **20-0244**

GODMAN, John Davidson (1794-1830)
American natural history. . . . Part 1.—Mastology. Philadelphia: H. C. Carey & I. Lea, 1826-28. 3 v. CSmH; KU; PHi; PPAmP **20-0245**

GODMAN, John Davidson (1794-1830)
Lecture introductory to the course of anatomy and physiology in Rutgers Medical College, delivered on Friday, Nov. 2, 1827. Published by the class. New York: W. A. Mercein, 1827, 24p. MH; NNNAM; NjR; PHi **20-0246**

GOOD, John Mason (1764-1827)
A physiological system of nosology; with a corrected and simplified nomenclature. Boston: Wells and Lilly, 1823. 443p. CU-M; ICJ; MB; PU **20-0247**

GOOD, John Mason (1764-1827)
The study of medicine. Boston: Wells & Lilly, 1823. 4 v. IU-M; MH; PU; RPM **20-0248**

GOOD, John Mason (1764-1827)
The study of medicine with a physiological system of nosology. . . . 2nd American ed. Philadelphia: Bennett & Walton [etc., etc.] 1824. 5 v. MdBM; PPC; PPHa; PU **20-0249**

GOOD, John Mason (1764-1827)
The study of medicine, with a physiological system of nosology. 4th American ed. Philadelphia: H. C. Carey & I. Lea, E. Parker, Marot & Walter, and T. Desilver; and Collins & Hannay, New York [Pr. by Wm. Brown] 1825. 5 v. IU-M; NNNAM; PPC **20-0250**

GOOD, John Mason (1764-1827)
The study of medicine. . . . 4th American ed. Repr. from the last London ed., greatly imp. & enl. Boston: Wells and Lilly, 1826. 5 v. ICU; KyLoJM; PP; PPC **20-0251**

GOOD, John Mason (1764-1827)
The study of medicine. 5th American ed., repr. from the last London ed., greatly imp. and enl. New York: Collins and Hannay, J. & J. Harper, pr., 1827. 5 v. ICJ; PPC **20-0252**

GOOD, John Mason (1764-1827)
The study of medicine. . . . Containing all the author's final corrections and improvements. From the last London ed., with much additional modern information on physiology, practice, pathology, and the nature of diseases in general. By Samuel Cooper. . . . Boston: Pub. by Wells and Lilly and J. & J. Harper, New York, 1829. 5 v. CU-M; ICJ; PPC; PPL **20-0253**

GRAHAM, Thomas John (1795?-1876)
Sure methods of improving health, and prolonging life; or, A treatise on the art of living long and comfortably, by regulating the diet and regimen. . . . By a physician. 1st American ed., with additions. Philadelphia: Carey, Lea & Carey; New York: G. & C. Carvill [etc., etc.] 1828. 248p. DLC; PPC; PPJ; PU **20-0254**

GREGG AND HOLLIS, Firm, Druggists, Boston
Medicine chests carefully prepared for all climates, with directions for using the medicines, and treatment of diseases incident to seaman. Boston: Pr. by Moore & Prowse, 1826. 17, [3] p. MB **20-0255**

GREGORY, George (1790-1853)
Treatise on the theory and practice of physic. With notes and additions, adapted to the practice of the United States, by Nathaniel Potter. . . . and S. Calhoun. . . . Philadelphia: Towar & Hogan, Pr. by J. H. Cunningham, 1826. 2 v. ICJ; MB; PPHa **20-0256**

GREGORY, George (1790-1853)
Elements of the theory and practice of physic. . . . With notes and additions, adapted to the practice of the United States by Nathaniel Potter . . . and S. Colhoun. . . . 2nd American from the 3rd London ed., with numerous additions and amendments. Philadelphia: Towar & Hogan, 1829. 2 v. IEN-M; NBM; NNNAM **20-0257**

GREGORY, Olinthus Gilbert (1774-1841)
Memoirs of the life, writings, and character, literary, professional, and religious of the late John Mason Good, M.D. . . . With the sermon occasioned by his death, by Charles Jerram, M.A. Boston: Crocker & Brewster; New York: J. Leavitt, 1829. 344p. MWA; PPC **20-0258**

HALE, Enoch (1790-1848)
Boylston medical prize dissertations for the years 1819 and 1821. Experiments and observations on the communication between the stomach and the urinary organs, and on the propriety of administering medicine by injection into the veins. Boston: O. Everett & J. W. Ingraham, 1821. 135p. DLC; IEN-M; MA; MHM **20-0259**

HALL, Marshall (1790-1857)
A descriptive, diagnostic and practical essay on disorders of the digestive organs and general health . . . and a second edition of the essay On the mimoses, with additions. Keene, N.H.: J. Prentiss, 1823. 192p. DLC; IEN-M; MB **20-0260**

HAMERSLEY, Andrew
An essay on the remote and proximate causes of phthisis pulmonalis, being the essay to which the prize was adjudged for the year 1825 by the New York State Medical Society. . . . Philadelphia: Webster, 1825. 54p. DNLM; MB; MH; NNNAM **20-0261**

HAMERSLEY, Andrew
A dissertation on the remote and proximate causes of phthisis pulmonalis; to which the prize was adjudged for the year 1825, by the New York State Medical Society. 2nd ed., rev. and corr. New York: E. Bliss & E. White, 1827. 99p. DNLM; ICJ; MB; MdBM **20-0262**

HAMILTON, James, Jr.
Observations on the use and abuse of mercurial medicines in various diseases. New York: E. Bliss & E. White, 1821. 216p. DLC; IEN-M; PPC **20-0263**

HAMILTON, James (1749-1835)
Observations on the utility and administration of purgative medicines in several diseases. . . . 2nd American ed. Philadelphia: James Webster, publisher. Wm. Brown, pr. 1823. 122, 168p. MdBM; NNNAM; PPC **20-0264**

HAMILTON, James (1749-1835)
Observations on the utility and administration of purgative medicines in several diseases. From the 5th Edinburgh ed. Philadelphia: Thos. Kite, 1829. 126, 138p. MdBM; PPC; PPHa **20-0265**

HAND, William M.
The house surgeon and physician; designed to assist heads of families, travellers, and sea-faring people, in discerning, distinguishing, and curing diseases; with concise directions for the preparation and use of a numerous collection of the best American remedies; together with many of the most approved, from the shop of the apothecary. All in plain English. . . . 2nd ed., rev. and enl. New Haven: Printed by S. Converse, for Silas Andrus, Hartford, 1820. 288p. CtY-M; DLC; MBM **20-0266**

HARDIE, James (1750?-1826?)
An account of the yellow fever, which occurred in the city of New York, in the year 1822. . . . New York: Pr. by Samuel Marks, 1822. 120p. DLC; ICJ; MB; PPC **20-0267**

HARE, Robert (1781-1858)
Minutes of the course of chemical instruction in the medical department of the University of Pennsylvania. . . . Philadelphia: William Brown, printer, 1822-3. 3 pts. in 1. DNLM; PPAmP; PPC; PU **20-0268**

HARE, Robert (1781-1858)
Minutes of the course of chemical instruction in the medical department of the University of Pennsylvania, or the use of his pupils; reprinted, with corrections and additions. Philadelphia: Clark & Raser, pr., 1824-25. 3 v. in 1. DLC; DNLM; NcU; PU **20-0269**

HARE, Robert (1781-1858)
Minutes of the course of chemical instruction in the medical department of the University of Pennsylvania. For the use of his pupils. Repr. with corr. and additions. Philadelphia: Clark & Raser, 1825. 96, 69, 56, [12]p. ICU. OCLloyd; PP; PU **20-0270**

HARE, Robert (1781-1858)
A compendium of the course of chemical instruction in the medical department of the University of Pennsylvania. . . . Philadelphia: J. G. Auner, Carey, Lea & Carey. Clark & Raser, prs., 1827. 310, 46p. DNLM; PPL **20-0271**

HARE, Robert (1781-1858)
A compendium of the course of chemical instruction in the medical department of the University of Pennsylvania. . . . For the use of his pupils. Philadelphia: J. G. Auner [etc.] 1828. xiv, 2, 310, 46p. DNLM; IEN-M; KU; OCLloyd **20-0272**

[HARLAN, Richard] (1796-1843)
An inquiry into the functions of the brain in man and in the lower order of animals. Delivered as a lecture before the Academy of Natural Sciences of Philadelphia, by a physician. . . . Philadelphia, 1824. 24p. DLC; MWA; PHi **20-0273**

HARLAN, Richard (1796-1843)
Documents relating to the late election of the professor of surgery in the University of Maryland. . . . [Philadelphia, 1827]. [8]p. NHi; NNC **20-0274**

HARRISON, John P[ollard] (1796-1849)
Remarks on the influence of the mind upon the body. . . . Louisville, Ky.: Pr. by W. W. Worsley, 1827. 16p. OC **20-0275**

HARVARD UNIVERSITY. Boylston Medical Society
Catalogue of the members of the Boylston Medical Society of Harvard University, Oct. 1825. Boston: True & Greene, 1825. 8p. MHi **20-0276**

HARVARD UNIVERSITY. Medical School
Some account of the medical school in Boston, and of the Massachusetts General Hospital. Boston: Pr. by Phelps and Farnham, 1824. 16p. DLC; DNLM; IEN-M; MB **20-0277**

HASTINGS, Charles (1794-1866)
An experimental inquiry of the general nature of inflammation. 1st American from the 1st London ed. Philadelphia: J. Webster, 1821. 68p. DLC; DNLM; MB; PPC **20-0278**

HATIN, Jules (ca. 1800-1839)
A manual of practical obstetrics: arranged so as to afford a concise and accurate description of the management of preternatural labours; preceded by an account of the mechanism of natural labour. . . . With an appendix, containing a physiological memoir upon the brain. From the French of M. Magendie, by Joseph Gardner, M.D. Philadelphia: J. Grigg, 1828. 198p. DLC; DNLM; NNNAM; OCIM **20-0279**

HATIN, Jules (ca. 1800-1839)
Compendium of operative midwifery. . . . New York: Charles S. Francis; Munroe and Francis, Boston, [George H. Evans, pr.] 1828. 171p. DLC; DNLM; PPC **20-0280**

HENCHMAN, Daniel
Medicine chests of all kinds, with directions suitable to their contents, are carefully put up. . . . Boston: Bellamy, 1825. 16p. MBM; MWA **20-0281**

HENDERSON, Thomas (1789-1854)
A Lecture Delivered at the Opening of the Medical Department of the Columbia College, Introductory to a Course on the Theory and Practice of Medicine. Washington, D.C.: Gales and Seaton, 1825. 23p. DLC; DNLM **20-0282**

HENDERSON, Thomas (1789-1854)
A lecture delivered at the opening of the medical department of the Columbian College. [Philadelphia, 1826?] 8p. DLC; MHi; PPL **20-0283**

HENDERSON, Thomas (1789-1854)
An epitome of the physiology, general anatomy, and pathology of Bichat. Philadelphia: Carey, Lea & Carey, 1829. 326p. DLC; ICJ; OCIM; PPC **20-0284**

HENRY, William (1774-1836)
The elements of experimental chemistry. . . . 2nd American from the 8th London ed., with an account of Dr. Wollaston's scale of chemical equivalents. . . . Also, a substitute for Woulfe's or North's apparatus, and a theory of Galvanism by Robert Hare. Philadelphia: R. Desilver, 1822. 2 v. 16 Plates. DNLM; NNNAM; ICU; KU **20-0285**

HEUSTIS, Jabez Wiggins (1784-1841)
Medical facts and inquiries, respecting the causes, nature, prevention and cure of fever. . . . Cahawba: Pr. by Wm. B. Allen, 1825. 434p. DLC; DNLM; OCIM **20-0286**

HILDENBRAND, Johann Valentin von (1763-1818)
A treatise on the nature, cause, and treatment of contagious typhus. From the German of J. Val de Hildenbrand. . . . By S. D. Gross, M.D. New York: Elam Bliss [Pr. by Gray & Bunce], 1829. 175p. IU-M; MdBM; PPC **20-0287**

HOGAN, Robert
Strictures on the present state of the medical profession among the foreign practitioners in Havana. New York: Pr. by J. Seymour, 1824. 37p. DLC; NNNAM **20-0288**

HOHMAN, Johann Georg
Der lange verborgene Freund: oder: Getreuer und christlicher Unterricht für jedermann, enthaltend: wunderbare und probmässige Mittel und Künste, sowohl für die Menschen als das Vieh. . . . Reading: Gedruckt für den Verfasser, 1820. 100p. PPL **20-0289**

HOHMAN, Johann Georg
Der lange verborgene Freund, oder: Getreuer und christlicher Unterricht für jedermann, enthaltend: wunderbare und probmässige Mittel und Künste, sowohl für die Menschen als das Vieh. . . . 2. und verbesserte Aufl. [Reading? ca. 1820]. 87p. DLC **20-0290**

HOOPER, Robert (1773-1835)
Lexicon-medicum; or, Medical dictionary, containing an explanation of the terms in anatomy, physiology, etc. . . . From the 4th London ed. New York: Pub. by E. Bliss and E. White, J. and J. Harper, printers, 1822. viii, 953p. DLC; PPC **20-0291**

HOOPER, Robert (1773-1835)
Lexicon-medicum; or, Medical dictionary, containing an explanation of the terms in anatomy, physiology, etc. . . . From the 4th London ed. New York: Pub. by E. Duyckinck, Collins & Co., Collins & Hannay, and Samuel Wood & Sons, J. & J. Harper, printers, 1822. 953p. IU-M **20-0292**

HOOPER, Robert (1773-1835)
Lexicon-medicum; Medical dictionary; containing an explanation of the terms in anatomy, physiology. . . . 2nd American from the 4th London ed. New York: Pub. by E. Duyckinck, E. Bliss & E. White, Collins & Hannay, Collins & Co. and James V. Seaman, J. & J. Harper, prs., 1824. 952p. MB; PPC; PU **20-0293**

HOOPER, Robert (1773-1835)
Lexicon-medicum; or, Medical dictionary. . . . The 4th American ed., from the 5th London, very considerably enl. New York: Pr. by J. & J. Harper, 1826. 1026p. ICJ; MB; PPC **20-0294**

HOOPER, Robert (1773-1835)
Lexicon medicum; or, Medical dictionary. . . . 4th American, from the last London ed., with additions from American authors . . . by Samuel Akerly. . . . New York: Pr. by J. and J. Harper, 1829. 2 v. DLC; DNLM; OCIM; PPC **20-0295**

HOOPER, Robert (1773-1835)
Examinations in anatomy, physiology, practice of physic, surgery, chemistry, materia medica, and pharmacy. . . . New York: Collins & Co., publisher [W. E. Dean, pr.] 1829. 182p. DNLM; NNNAM **20-0296**

HOPPIN, George W.
Medicine chest and instructive advice, with directions for ships and family use. . . . Providence, R.I.: John Miller, pr. 1823. 21p. RHi **20-0297**

HORNER, William Edmonds (1793-1853)
Lessons in practical anatomy, for the use of dissectors. Philadelphia: Pub. by Edward Parker, William Brown, pr., 1823. 505p. DLC; PPAmP; PPC **20-0298**

HORNER, William Edmonds (1793-1853)
Report on the state of the Anatomical museum of the University of Pennsylvania, 30th June, 1824 by W. E. Horner. . . . Philadelphia: R. Wright, pr., 1824. 36p. PHi; PPL **20-0299**

HORNER, William Edmonds (1793-1853)
Description of a small muscle at the internal commissure of the eyelids. Philadelphia: Pr. by Wm. Fry, 1824. 14p. MWA; NNNAM **20-0300**

HORNER, William Edmonds (1793-1853)
A treatise on special and general anatomy. Philadelphia: H. C. Carey & I. Lea. Wm. Brown, pr., 1826. 2 v. DNLM; NjR; PPC; PU **20-0301**

HORNER, William Edmonds (1793-1853)
Lessons in practical anatomy, for the use of dissectors, 2nd ed. Philadelphia: H. C. Carey & I. Lea, 1827. 500p. IEN-M; PPC **20-0302**

HORNER, William Edmonds (1793-1853)
An inquiry into the anatomical characters of infantile follicular inflammation of the gastro-intestinal mucous membrane. Philadelphia: Pr. by Joseph R. A. Skerrett, 1829. 15p. NNNAM **20-0303**

HORNER, William Edmonds (1793-1853)
A treatise on pathological anatomy. Philadelphia: Carey, Lea and Carey [Griggs & Dickinson, prs.] 1829. 460p. DNLM; MB; PPL **20-0304**

HOSACK, David (1769-1835)
A biographical memoir of Hugh Williamson, M.D., LL.D. . . . Delivered on the first of November, 1819, at the request of the New York Historical Society. . . . New York: C. S. Van Winkle, 1820. 91p. DNLM; ICJ; IEN-M; MBM
20-0305

HOSACK, David (1769-1835)
Course of studies designed for the private medical school established in New York by David Hosack. . . . New York: C. S. Van Winkle, 1820. 7p. MBM; NHi; NNNAM
20-0306

HOSACK, David (1769-1835)
Observations on febrile contagion, and on the means of improving the medical police of the Çity of New York. Delivered as an introductory discourse, in the hall of the College of Physicians and Surgeons, on the sixth of November, 1820. New York: Published by Elam Bliss, J. Seymour, printer, 1820. 79p. CtY-M; DNLM; MBM; NWA
20-0307

HOSACK, David (1769-1835)
A biographical memoir of Hugh Williamson, M.D., LL.D. delivered on the first of November, 1819, at the request of the New York Historical Society. New York: Pr. by J. Seymour, for E. Bliss and E. White, 1821. 78p. DLC; NN; NNC; PPAmP
20-0308

HOSACK, David (1769-1835)
A system of practical nosology. . . . 2nd ed., cor. and enl. New York: Pr. by C. S. Van Winkle, 1821. 386p. MBM; NjR; PMA; PPC **20-0309**

HOSACK, David (1769-1835)
Observations on cruritis, or phlegmasia dolens. . . . New York: Pr. by C. S. Van Winkle, printer to the University. 1822. 7p. DNLM; NNNAM; NNU-M **20-0310**

HOSACK, David (1769-1835)
Observations on ergot; communicated in a letter to James Hamilton, M.D., F.R.S.E. New York: Pr. by C. S. Van Winkle, 1822. 7p. DNLM; MH-M; NNNAM; NBM
20-0311

HOSACK, David (1769-1835)
Observations on the use of emetics in constipation of the bowels. Communicated in a letter to John B. Beck. New York: C. S. Van Winkle, 1822. 8p. DLC; MH-M; NNNAM; NNU-M
20-0312

HOSACK, David (1769-1835)
Essays on various subjects of medical science. New York: Pr. by J. Seymour, 1824. 3 v. DLC; MB; PPC; PPL
20-0313

HOSACK, David (1769-1835)
An inaugural address delivered before the Medical Society of the County of New York, on the 12th day of July, 1824. New York: J. Seymour, 1824. 24p. NNNAM; PPL
20-0314

HOSACK, David (1769-1835)
An introductory lecture, delivered in the College of Physicians and Surgeons, at the opening of the winter session, on the 7th of November, 1825. . . . New York: Pr. by J. Seymour, 1825. 61, [27] p. DLC; DNLM; NNNAM; OC
20-0315

HOSACK, David (1769-1835)
Observations on the medical character, addressed to the graduates of the College of Physicians & Surgeons of New York at the commencement April 4, 1826. New York: J. Seymour, pr., 1826. 38p. DLC; DNLM; MB; MdBM
20-0316

HOSACK, David (1769-1835)
An inaugural discourse, delivered at the opening of Rutgers Medical College, in the city of New York, on Monday, the 6th day of November, 1826. New York: Pr. by J. Seymour, 1826. 176p. DLC; DNLM; IEN-M; MB
20-0317

HOWSHIP, John
Practical observations on the symptoms, discrimination, and treatment, of some of the most important diseases of the lower intestines and anus. . . . 1st American from the 2nd London ed. Philadelphia: Pr. by Frankish for Benjamin Warner, and sold also at his stores in Richmond, Va. and Louisville, Ky., and by W. P. Bason, Charleston, S.C., 1821. 240p. DLC; DNLM **20-0318**

HUFELAND, Christoph Wilhelm (1762-1836)
A treatise on the Schrofulous disease. . . . Transl. from the French of M. Bonsquet by Charles D. Meigs. . . . Philadelphia: Pr. by Charles D. Meigs. . . . Philadelphia: Pr. by James Kay, Jr. & Co. for Carey, Lea & Carey, John Grigg, Towar & Hogan, Uriah Hunt, J. G. Auner, H. Cowperthwait. New York: Elam Bliss, Collins & Co., C. S. Francis, Collins & Hannay, White, Gallaher & White, E. Duyckinck, O. H. Roorbach. Boston. Richardson & Lord, 1829. 215p. DLC; DNLM; MB
20-0319

HULL, Amos Gerald (1810-1859)
Esplicacion practica de la naturaleza de la hernia. . . . Escrito en ingles por su inventor Dr. Amos G. Hull . . . con privilegio esclusivo. New York: Impreso pro Henrique Spear, 1824. 27p. DLC; NNNAM **20-0320**

HULL, Amos Gerald (1810-1859)
Practical elucidation of the nature of hernia, together with some remarks on the unfit instruments hitherto used for its confinement. . . . New York: Pr. by Henry Spear, 1824. 28p. DLC; NNNAM **20-0321**

HULL, Amos Gerald (1810-1859)
Practical elucidation of the nature of hernia, together with some remarks on the unfit instruments hitherto used for its confinement. . . . With an explanation of the experienced utility and effectual cures of the instrument now recommended. . . . New York: Pr. by H. Spear, 1824. 24p. CtY-M; DNLM; NNNAM **20-0322**

HUNTER, John (1728-1793)
A treatise on the blood, inflammation, and gunshot wounds. 2nd American ed. Philadelphia: Pub. by James Webster, William Brown, pr. 1823. 480p. CU-M; DLC; ICJ; PPC
20-0323

HUTIN, Philippe
Manual of the physiology of man; or A concise description of the phenomena of his organization. Transl. from the French, with notes, by Joseph Togno. . . . Philadelphia: Carey, Lea & Carey, 1828. 309p. DNLM; ICJ; NBM; ScCM
20-0324

AN ILLUSTRATION of the present pernicious mode of fashionable practice of medicine. With plates. Accompanied with A dialogue, between an apothecary and a physician, on the subject of the statute regulating the practice of physic and surgery. After which is added a few brief anecdotes. Albany, 1828. 36p. DNLM **20-0325**

ILLUSTRATIONS of the principal regions of the human body, in relation to surgical anatomy: Twelve plates, accompanied by letter press explanations. New York: Charles S. Francis; Munroe & Francis, Boston, 1829. [2]p, 12 pls. DNLM; NNNAM **20-0326**

IRELAND, William Matthews
Advice to mothers, on the management of infants, and young children, with directions how to distinguish and prevent their complaints. New York: B. Young, 1820. 39p. NNNAM **20-0327**

IRVINE, Matthew (ca. 1755-1827?)
Irvine's Treatise on the yellow fever. [Charleston, S.C., 1820]. 57p. DLC; DNLM; NHi; NNNAM **20-0328**

JACKSON, James (1777-1868)
Textbook of a course of lectures on the theory and practice of physic. Boston: Wells & Lilly, 1825. 2 v. DNLM; PPC; RPM **20-0329**

JACKSON, James (1777-1868)
An address delivered at the funeral of John Gorham, M.D. on the 31st day of March, 1829, by the appointment of the Boston Medical Association, and published at their request. Boston: Press of the Boston Daily Advertiser, W. L. Lewis, pr., 1829. 16p. DLC; MB; MH **20-0330**

JACKSON, Samuel (1787-1872)
An oration, delivered before the Philadelphia Medical Society, on the 22nd of February, 1820. . . . Published at the request of the Society. Philadelphia: M. Carey and Son, 1820. 38p. DNLM; MBM; MWA; NNNAM **20-0331**

JACKSON, Samuel (1787-1872)
An introductory lecture to the institutes of medicine. . . . Published by request of the medical class. Philadelphia: Carey, Lea & Carey, Mifflin & Parry, prs., 1827. 41p. CSmH; DLC; MWA **20-0332**

JAMESON, Horatio Gates (1778-1855)
An introductory lecture . . . at the opening of Washington Medical College of Baltimore, 1827. Baltimore: R. J. Matchett, 1828. 18p. DLC **20-0333**

JEFFERSON MEDICAL COLLEGE. Philadelphia
The memorial of the medical faculty of Jefferson College, in reply to the memorial of the trustees of the University of Pennsylvania. Philadelphia: R. Wright, pr., 1826. 7p. PPJ **20-0334**

JEFFERSON MEDICAL COLLEGE. Philadelphia
Jefferson Medical College: a representation of the conduct of the trustees and members of the faculty, and circumstances connected therewith, in relation to John Barnes, M.D. . . . Philadelphia, 1828. 38p. DLC; DNLM; PHi; PPC **20-0335**

JEWELL, William
An inaugural dissertation, on the medical topography of Shepherdsville, and its vicinity. . . . Danville: James Armstrong, 1820. 47p. KU; KyLoJM **20-0336**

JOHNSON, James (1777-1845)
The influence of civic life, sedentary habits, and intellectual refinement, on human health, and human happiness; including an estimate of the balance of enjoyment and suffering in the different gradations of society. . . . 1st American from the London copy. Philadelphia: Printed for Thomas Hope, Published by Mathew Carey and Son [etc.], T. Town, printer, 1820. 110p. DLC; DNLM; MBM; NNNAM **20-0337**

JOHNSON, James (1777-1845)
The influence of civic life, sedentary habits, and intellectual refinement, on human health, and human happiness; including an estimate of the balance of enjoyment and suffering in the different gradations of society. . . . 2nd American ed., from the London copy. Philadelphia: Printed for Thomas Hope, Published by Mathew Carey and Son [etc.], T. Town, Printer, 1820. 110p. CU-M; DLC; DNLM; MBM **20-0338**

JOHNSON, James (1777-1845)
Practical researches on the nature, cure and prevention of gout. . . . Philadelphia: T. Dobson, 1821. 2 v. DNLM **20-0339**

JOHNSON, James (1777-1845)
The influence of tropical climates on European constitutions. From the latest London edition, greatly improved. Philadelphia: Pr. by J. Harding, for Thomas Dobson & Son, 1821. 2 v. DNLM; MBM; OC; PPC **20-0340**

JOHNSON, James (1777-1845)
A treatise on derangements of the liver, internal organs, and nervous system; pathological and therapeutical. . . . 1st American from the 3rd London ed. Philadelphia: H. C. Carey & I. Lea, 1825. 223p. MdBM; NNNAM; OC **20-0341**

JOHNSON, James (1777-1845)
A treatise on derangements of the liver, internal organs, and nervous system; pathological and therapeutical. . . . 2nd American, from 3rd London ed., rev. and imp. Philadelphia: H. C. Carey & I. Lea, 1826. 223p. DLC; DNLM; ICJ; IEN-M **20-0342**

JOHNSON, James (1777-1845)
A treatise on derangements of the liver, internal organs, and nervous system; pathological and therapeutical. . . . 2nd American from the 3rd London ed., rev. & imp. Philadelphia: L. B. Clark, 1826. 223p. NNNAM; PPC; PU **20-0343**

JOHNSON, James (1777-1845)
The influence of tropical climates on European constitutions: being a treatise on the principal diseases incidental to Europeans in the East and West Indies, Mediterranean, and coast of Africa. From the 3rd London ed., greatly enl. New York: E. Duyckink, G. Long [etc., etc.] W. E. Dean, pr., 1826. 416p. DLC; ICJ; ICU; MWA **20-0344**

JOHNSON, James (1777-1845)
An essay on morbid sensibility of the stomach and bowels, as the proximate cause, or characteristic condition of indigestion. . . . Philadelphia: B. & T. Kite, 1827. 154p. DLC: DNLM; OC; PPC **20-0345**

JOHNSON, James (1777-1845)
An essay on morbid sensibility of the stomach and bowels. . . . Philadelphia: Pub. by Thos. Kite, 1828. 155p. DNLM; RPM; ScCM **20-0346**

JOHNSON, Joseph (1776-1862)
Letters addressed to the Agricultural Society of South Carolina, on the means of improving the health of the lower country. With corr. and additions. Charleston: Pr. and for sale by A. E. Miller, 1827. 12p. CSmH
20-0347

JONES, Alexander
An oration, delivered before the Central Medical Society of Georgia, at its annual meeting in Milledgeville, on 2nd Dec., 1828. Augusta: Pr. at Lawson's Job Office, 1829. 22p. NcD
20-0348

JONES, Alexander
An essay on the non-existence of malaria read before the Central Medical Society of Georgia Dec. 3, 1828. Augusta, 1829. 35p. CtY-M; DLC **20-0349**

JONES, Charles Williams
A series of lectures, on the most approved principles and practice of modern surgery. . . . 1st American ed., from the 2nd London ed. Boston: C. Ewer, 1823. 456p. DLC; DNLM; MB; PPC **20-0350**

JOURDAN, Antoine Jacques Louis (1788-1848)
Historical and critical observations on syphilis. . . . Transl. from the French by R. La Roche. Philadelphia: R. Desilver, 1823. 108p. MH; NNNAM; PPC; PPL
20-0351

KITCHINER, William (1775?-1827)
The art of invigorating and prolonging life . . . and peptic precepts. . . . From the 3rd London ed. Philadelphia: H. C. Carey & I. Lea, 1823. 281p. DLC; MB; OC; ScC
20-0352

[KITCHINER, William] (1775?-1827)
The art of invigorating and prolonging life . . . and peptic precepts. . . . From the 3rd London ed. Lexington, Ky.: Pr. by W. W. Worsley, 1823. 117p. DLC; DNLM; MB; PPL
20-0353

KITTREDGE, Jacob
A report on the medical virtues of Secale cornutum, ergot, or spurred rye, in parturition. Read before the Strafford District of the N.H. Medical Society, Feb. 14, 1821. Portsmouth: Pr. by S. Whidden [1821] 12p. CSmH; DNLM; Nh
20-0354

KNAPP, Moses L. (1799-1879)
An inaugural dissertation on the properties of the apocynum cannabinum (Indian hemp) submitted to the faculty of Jefferson Medical College. Philadelphia: Wright, 1826. 24p. DNLM; NNNAM; PPJ; PU **20-0355**

KNIGHT, Jonathan (1789-1864)
An eulogium on Nathan Smith, M.D., late professor of the theory and practice of physic and surgery, in the medical institution of Yale College; pronounced at his funeral. . . . New Haven: Pr. by H. Howe, 1829. 28p. DLC; MB; MH; NNNAM **20-0356**

KOECKER, Leonard (1785-1850)
On the treatment of denuded nerves of the teeth. [Philadelphia, 1821] 12p. DLC; DNLM; MB; MBM
20-0357

KOECKER, Leonard (1785-1850)
An essay on the devastation of the gums and the alveolar processes. [Philadelphia: H. C. Carey & I. Lea, Chesnut Street, William Fry, printer, 1822] 15p. MB; MBM; NNNAM
20-0358

KOECKER, Leonard (1785-1850)
An essay on the diseases of the jaws, and their treatment; with observations on the amputation of a part or the whole of the inferior maxilla; tending to prove that such operation is seldom, if ever, necessary. . . . Philadelphia: H. C. Carey & I. Lea, 1828. 95p. DLC; PPC; PPJ; ScCM
20-0359

LAENNEC, René Théophile Hyacinthe (1781-1826)
A treatise of the diseases of the chest. . . . 1st American ed. Philadelphia: J. Webster, William Brown, pr., 1823. 319p. [8 plates]. CU-M; DLC; ICJ; MB
20-0360

La ROCHE, René (1795-1872)
An oration delivered before the Philadelphia Medical Society, pursuant to appointment. . . . February 3, 1827. Published by the society. Philadelphia: Mifflin and Parry, printers, 1827. 31p. DLC; PPC **20-0361**

LARREY, Dominique Jean (1766-1842)
Surgical essays. . . . Baltimore: N. G. Maxwell, 1823. 335p. MB; MdBM; PPC; PU **20-0362**

LAWRENCE, William (1783-1867)
Lectures on physiology, zoology, and the natural history of man, delivered at the Royal College of Surgeons. . . . Salem: Pr. and pub. by Foote & Brown, 1828. 495p. CSmH; NcD; PPL **20-0363**

LIEUTAUD, Joseph (1703-1780)
Synopsis of the universal practice of medicine. Exhibiting a concise view of all diseases, both internal and external: illustrated with complete commentaries. Transl. from the Latin, by Edwin A. Atlee, M.D. Philadelphia: Edward and Richard Parker, 1820. 641p. NNNAM **20-0364**

LOBSTEIN, Johann Friedrich Daniel (1777-1835)
Researches and observations on the use of phosphorus, in the treatment of various diseases. Philadelphia: The Author; R. Wright, pr., 1825. 114p. DLC; DNLM; ICJ; OCLloyd
20-0365

LOBSTEIN, Johann Friedrich Daniel (1777-1835)
Dr. L. has the honour to inform the physicians and literati of the U.S. that he is writing a new work, entitled, Treatise on the semeiology of the eye. [New York? 1829] 8p. DLC
20-0366

LOGAN, George (1778-1861)
A biographical sketch of Tucker Harris, M.D. delivered on the first of September, 1821, at the request of the Medical Society of Charleston, South Carolina. Charleston: Pr. by William Cox Young, 1821. 15p. DLC; MWA; ScC
20-0367

LOGAN, George (1778-1861)
Practical observations on diseases of children, comprehending a description of complaints & disorders, incident to the early states of life, and method of treatment. Charleston: Pr. by A. E. Miller, 1825. 218p. DLC; DNLM; ICJ; PPC
20-0368

The LONDON practice of midwifery; to which are added, instructions for the treatment of lying-in women, and the principal diseases of children, chiefly designed for students and early practitioners. 1st American, from the 4th London, edition corrected and improved. New York: Published by James V. Seaman, J. & J. Harper, printers, 1820. 303p. DNLM; OCIM **20-0369**

The LONDON practice of midwifery; to which are added, instructions for the treatment of lying-in women, and the principal diseases of children, chiefly designed for students and early practitioners. 1st American, from the 4th London, edition corrected and improved. New York: Published by Samuel Wood & Sons, and Samuel S. Wood & Co.; Baltimore: J. & J. Harper, printers, 1820. 303p. DNLM; OCIM **20-0370**

The LONDON practice of midwifery; to which are added, instructions for the treatment of lying-in women, and the principal diseases of children, chiefly designed for students and early practitioners. 1st American, from the 4th London, edition corrected and improved. New York: Published by James V. Seaman, Samuel Wood & Sons, and Samuel S. Wood & Co.; Baltimore: J. & J. Harper, printers, 1820. 303p. CtY-M; DLC; DNLM; IEN-M **20-0371**

The LONDON practice of midwifery; including the treatment during the puerperal state, and the infantile diseases. To which is added notes, plates and Denman's Aphorisms. By an American practitioner. 6th ed., much enl. and improved. Concord, N.H.: Pr. by I. Hill, 1826. 335p. DLC; DNLM; PPC; RPM **20-0372**

LOWELL, Charles (1793-1858)
An authentic report of a trial before the Supreme Judicial Court of Maine, for the County of Washington, June term, 1824. Charles Lowell vs. John Faxon and Micajah Hawks, surgeons and physicians, in an action of trespass on the case, for ignorance and negligence in their professional treatment of the plff's dislocated hip. . . . Portland: Pr. for the author, 1825. 29p. DLC; MB **20-0373**

LOWELL, Charles (1793-1858)
Report of the trial of an action Charles Lowell against John Faxon and Micajah Hawks, doctors of medicine, defendants, for malpractice in the capacity of physicians and surgeons, at the Supreme Judicial Court of Maine holden at Machias for the County of Washington — June term, 1824. Before the Hon. Nathan Weston, Jun. justice of the court. Portland: Pr. for James Adams, Jr. by David and Seth Paine, 1825. 124p. DLC; IEN-M; MB **20-0374**

LYNCH, David
A candid and unvarnished view of a small part of Dr. Lynch's practice in cancer complaints, and in the art of healing generally. . . . [New York, Totten, 1829] 24p. DNLM **20-0375**

LYON, Isaac
A short statement of the excellency of Doctor Horwitz's antibilious pills. 2nd ed., enl. Frederick-Town, Md.: Ritchie and Magill, 1823. 15p. NN **20-0376**

MACAULAY, Patrick
An anniversary discourse delivered before the medical and chirurgical faculty of Maryland, Tuesday, Juen 3, 1823, on medical improvement. Baltimore: F. Lucas, Jr., and E. J. Coale, 1824. 38p. MdHi; MdU-D **20-0377**

MacCULLOCH, John (1773-1835)
Malaria; an essay on the production and propagation of this poison, and on the nature and localities of the places by which it is produced. . . . Philadelphia: Pr. and pub. by Thos. Kite, 1829. 219p. CSmH; ICJ; MdBM; PU **20-0378**

MACKENTOSH, John
Receipts for the cure of most diseases incident to the human family. By the celebrated Indian doctor John Mackentosh, of the Cherokee Nation; none of which have ever before been communicated to the world. New York: Pr. for the pub. [i.e., Seth Holderwell] 1827. 12p. MWA; NN; NNNAM; PPL **20-0379**

MACLEAN, Charles
Evils of quarantine laws, and non-existence of pestilential contagion. Deduced from the phenomena of the plague of Levant, the yellow fever in Spain, and the cholera morbus of Asia. Philadelphia: Carey & Lea [etc., etc.] 1824. 444p. DLC; PPPH; ScC **20-0380**

MACNEVEN, William James (1763-1841)
. . . Outline of the lecture and demonstrations of William James Macneven, M.D., as professor of chemistry and materia medica. New York: George Long, 1820. 7p. DNLM **20-0381**

MAGENDIE, François (1783-1855)
Physiological and chemical researches on the use of the prussic or hydrocyanic acid in the treatment of diseases of the breast, and particularly in phthisis pulmonialis. . . . Transl. from the French, with notes, &c. by James G. Percival. New Haven: Howe & Spalding [etc.] 1820. 86p. CtY-M; DLC; ICJ; MBM **20-0382**

MAGENDIE, François (1783-1855)
A summary of physiology. Transl. from the French by John Revere. . . . Baltimore: E. J. Coale & Co., 1822. John D. Toy, printer. 430p. DLC; ICJ; MB; NcU **20-0383**

MAGENDIE, François (1783-1855)
An elementary compendium of physiology; for the use of students. Philadelphia: Pub. by James Webster, 1824. 496p. DLC; ICJ; PPC; PU **20-0384**

MAGENDIE, François (1783-1855)
Formulary for the preparation and mode of employing several new remedies. . . . Revised and corr. by a physician of Philadelphia. With an appendix. Philadelphia: J. Webster, 1824. 286p. DLC; ICJ; MB **20-0385**

MAGENDIE, François (1783-1855)
A summary of physiology. . . . Transl. from the French by John Revere. . . . 2nd ed. Baltimore: E. J. Coale, 1824. 444p. ICJ; MB; PU; ViRA **20-0386**

MAGENDIE, François (1783-1855)
Formulary for the preparation and employment of many new medicines. . . . Transl. from the 5th ed., rev., and additions. New York: G. H. Evans and Co., 1827. xii, 138, [2]p. MB; NNNAM **20-0387**

MAGENDIE, François (1783-1855)
Formulary for the preparation and employment of many new medicines . . . by F. Magendie. . . . Transl. from the 5th ed., rev. and augm., by John Baxter. . . . With notes and additions. 2nd ed. New York: G. H. Evans, 1828. x, 138, [2]p. MB; OCIM; PPC **20-0388**

MAGENDIE, François (1783-1855)
A physiological memoir upon the brain, read in a public sitting of the Royal Academy of Sciences, on the 16th of June, 1828. From the French, by Joseph Gardner [Philadelphia, 1828]. 198p. MdBM; RPM **20-0389**

MAGENDIE, François (1783-1855)
Formulary for the preparation and employment of several new remedies. . . . Transl. from the 6th ed. of the Formulaire of M. Magendie, pub. in Paris, Oct. 1827. London: T. and G. Underwood; New York: Repr. by J. & J. Harper, for F. and N. G. Carnes, 1829. 145, 18p. DLC; ICJ; NNNAM; PPL **20-0390**

MAGILL, Alfred Thruston (1804-1837)
An essay on the history, causes, and treatment of typhus fever: to which the annual prize for the year 1828 was awarded by the Medical Society of the State of New York. New York: C. S. Francis, 1829. 69p. DLC; NNNAM **20-0391**

MANLEY, James Robert (1781-1851)
An inaugural address delivered before the Medical Society of the State of New York . . . on the 8th day of February, 1826. New York: J. Seymour, 1826. 28p. DLC; DNLM; NNC; NNNAM **20-0392**

MARRYAT, Thomas (1730-1792)
Dr. Marryat's therapeutics, or The art of healing. . . . 21st English, and 1st American ed.; carefully rev., corr., and considerably enl. by the proprietor. To which are added, a glossary, explaining all the difficult words; with recipes for several popular medicines now in use. New York: Pub. by Hugh Evans, surgeon; and may be purchased at the principal book stores in New York, Albany, & Utica, 1828. 240 [i.e., 224] p. ScMS **20-0393**

MARTINET, Louis (1795-1875)
Manual of pathology containing the symptoms, diagnosis and morbid characteristics of diseases. . . . Transl. with notes and additions, by Jones Quain. Philadelphia: Carey, Lea & Carey, 1827. 310p. MB; PMA; PPC **20-0394**

MASSACHUSETTS CHARITABLE EYE AND EAR INFIRMARY, Boston
Statement of a committee of the Eye and Ear Infirmary, Boston. Boston: T. R. Marvin, pr., 1828. 8p. DLC; DNLM; MB **20-0395**

MASSACHUSETTS MEDICAL SOCIETY
A catalogue of books, belonging to the Massachusetts Medical Society, 17th June, 1822. 12p. [Boston, 1822]. MB; MH-M; MHi; NNNAM **20-0396**

MASSACHUSETTS MEDICAL SOCIETY
Medical dissertations delivered at the annual meeting of the Massachusetts Medical Society. Pub. by the Society. 3rd vol. Boston: Pr. by Joseph W. Ingraham, 1822. 469p. DLC; IU-M; MBM; MH-M **20-0397**

MASSACHUSETTS MEDICAL SOCIETY
Address to the community, on the necessity of legalizing the study of anatomy. By Order of the Massachusetts Medical Society. Boston: Perkins & Marvin, 1829. 27p. MBM; MHi; MWA **20-0398**

MASSACHUSETTS MEDICAL SOCIETY
Memoir of Edward A. Holyoke, M.D., LL.D. Prepared in compliance with a vote of the Essex South District Medical Society, and published at their request. Boston: Pub. by Perkins & Marvin, 1829. 80p. DLC; ICJ; MB; MH **20-0399**

McMURTRIE, Henry (1793-1865)
The gentleman's medical vademecum and travelling companion. . . . Philadelphia: Pub. by A. R. Poole, 1824. 239p. NNNAM; PPL **20-0400**

McVICKAR, John (1787-1868)
A domestic narrative of the life of Samuel Bard, M.D., LL.D., late president of the College of Physicians and Surgeons of the University of the State of New York. . . . New York: The literary rooms [Columbia College], A. Paul, printer, 1822. 244p. DLC; DNLM; ICJ; PU **20-0401**

MEAD, Elijah
An experimental inquiry into the botanical history, chemical properties and medicinal virtues of the Spirea tomentosa of Linneus. New York: Pr. by William A. Mercein, 1821. 26p. DNLM; MH; NNC; PHi **20-0402**

The MEDICAL practitioner's pocket companion; or, A key to the knowledge of diseases, and of the appearances that denote recovery or danger. . . . Philadelphia: Pub. by James Webster; Wm. Brown, printer, 1822. 64, [4] p. DLC; DNLM **20-0403**

MEDICAL SOCIETY OF THE COUNTY OF NEW YORK
Report of the committee of the Medical Society of the City and County of New York, explanatory of the causes and character of the epidemic fever, which prevailed in Bancker Street and its vicinity, in the summer and autumn of 1820. Published by order of the Society. New York: James V. Seaman, 1820. 38p. DNLM; MBM; MdBJ-W; NHi **20-0404**

MEDICAL SOCIETY OF THE COUNTY OF NEW YORK
Reports of the Medical Society of the City of New York, on nostrums, or secret medicines. Part I. Published by order of the Society, under the direction of the Committee on Quack remedies. New York: Pr. by E. Conrad, 1827. 52p. DLC; DNLM; MH **20-0405**

MEDICAL SOCIETY OF ORANGE COUNTY [NEW YORK]
Report of the committee appointed by the Orange County Medical Society, to analyze the waters of Chechunk Spring, in the town of Goshen. Goshen: T. B. Crowell, 1820. 24p. MBM; MWA; NHi; NNNAM **20-0406**

MEDICAL SOCIETY OF SOUTH CAROLINA
To the inhabitants of South Carolina. Charleston: Pr. by A. E. Miller, 1821. 12p. NNNAM **20-0407**

MEIGS, Charles Delucena (1792-1869)
The Philadelphia practice of midwifery. Philadelphia: James Kay, Jun. & brother; Pittsburg: John I. Kay & Co., 1828. 370p. KyLoJM **20-0408**

MEIGS, Charles Delucena (1792-1869)
An oration delivered before the Philadelphia Medical Society, February 18, 1829. . . . Philadelphia: Pr. by James Kay, Jun. & Co., prs. to the Philadelphia Medical Soceity, 1829. 28p. DLC; DNLM; NN; NNNAM **20-0409**

MEMORIA medica, a common place book, with an alphabetical index of the most common terms occurring in practice, carefully selected and arranged by a fellow of the Massachusetts Medical Society. Boston: Carter & Hendee, 1829. 20p. NBM **20-0410**

MILES, Charles
A new and improved system of medical botanical practice. Also, a concise view of anatomy and surgery. . . . Cleveland: Pr. for the author, 1829. 228p. NNNAM; PMA **20-0411**

MILLER, Henry (1800-1874)
An inaugural thesis on the relation between the sanguiferous and nervous systems, submitted to the examination of the Rev. Horace Holley, A.M.; A.A.S. President, the trustees and medical professors of Transylvania University, on the 12th day of March, 1822. For the degree of Doctor of Medicine. Lexington, Ky.: Pr. by William Gibbes Hunt, 1822. 46p. CSmH; DLC; DNLM; NNNAM **20-0412**

MILLER, Nathaniel (1784?-1863)
A dissertation, read before the Massachusetts Medical Society, on the importance and manner of detecting deep seated matter. . . . Boston: Pr. by John G. Scobie, 1827. 16p. NNNAM; RPB **20-0413**

MILNER, Thomas (1777-1841)
Essay on fevers and other medical subjects. Middletown, Conn.: E. & H. Clark, 1823. 484p. CU-M; CtHi; PPC; PU **20-0414**

MILNER, Thomas (1777-1841)
An examination of the strictures in the New England Journal for October for 1823, and in the North American Review for October, 1823, on essays on fevers, &c. By Thomas Milner and William Tully. Middletown, Conn.: Pr. by E. & H. Clark, 1823. 32p. CtHi; DLC; MH; RPM **20-0415**

MILNER, Thomas (1777-1841)
Typhus syncopalis, sinking typhus, or the spotted fever of New England, as it appeared in the epidemic of 1823, in Middletown, Conn. Middletown: Pr. for the author, 1825. 48p. DLC; MB; MdBM; NNNAM **20-0416**

MITCHELL, John Kearsley (1798-1858)
An oration delivered before the Philadelphia Medical Society, pursuant to appointment. . . . Philadelphia: Pr. by I. Ashmead & Co., 1825. 28p. MH; PHi; PPL **20-0417**

MITCHILL, Samuel Latham (1764-1831)
Address to the officers composing the medical staff, by Samuel L. Mitchill. . . . Surgeon General of the Militia, in the State of New York. New York: E. Conrad, 1820. 8p. DNLM; MBM; NHi; NNC **20-0418**

MITCHILL, Samuel Latham (1764-1831)
A discourse on the life and character of Samuel Bard, M.D. & LL.D., late president of the New York College of Physicians and Surgeons. . . . New York: Pr. by D. Fanshaw, 1821. 40p. DLC; ICJ; MB; MWA **20-0419**

MITCHILL, Samuel Latham (1764-1831)
A discourse on the life and character of Thomas Addis Emmet. . . . New York: Printed by E. Conrad, 1828. 26p. NHi; NN; NNU-M **20-0420**

MOBILE, ALABAMA
Committee on Causes and Extent of the Late Extraordinary Sickness and Mortality in the Town. Report of the committee appointed to investigate the causes and extent of the late extraordinary sickness and mortality in the town of Mobile. Philadelphia: S. Potter and Co., 1820. 12p. DLC; DNLM **20-0421**

MONROE, John
The American botanist, and family physician: In which the medical virtues of the mineral, animal and vegetable productions of North America are exhibited; . . . Compiled by Silas Gaskill. Wheelock, Vt.: Jonathan Morrison, 1824. 203p. CSmH; ICJ; MB **20-0422**

MORAND, J.
Memoir on acupuncturation, embracing a series of cases, drawn up under the inspection of M. Julius Cloquet; by M. Morand. . . . Paris, 1825. Transl. from the French, by Franklin Bache. . . . Philadelphia: R. Desilver, Clark & Raser, prs., 1825. [5], 87p. DLC; PPC; PPL; PU **20-0423**

MORGAGNI, Giovanni Battista (1682-1771)
The seats and causes of diseases, investigated by anatomy; containing a great variety of dissections, and accompanied with remarks. Abridged, and elucidated with copious notes, by Wm. Cooke. . . . Boston: Wells and Lilly; Philadelphia: H. C. Carey & I. Lea, 1824. 2 v. GU; MB; NNNAM **20-0424**

MOTT, Valentine (1785-1865)
Successful ligature of the common iliac artery. [Philadelphia, 1827] 8p. NNNAM **20-0425**

MOTT, Valentine (1785-1865)
A biographical memoir of Wright Post, M.D., late professor of anatomy and physiology, and president of the College of Physicians and Surgeons in the City of New York. Delivered as an introductory lecture, on the 4th of November, 1828. . . . New York: Printed by E. Conrad, 1829. 32p. DLC, NNNAM **20-0426**

MOULTRIE, James (1793-1869)
An eulogium on Dr. Samuel Wilson read before the Medical Society of South Carolina, and published at their request. . . . Charleston: A. E. Miller, 1827. 14p. DLC **20-0427**

MURRAY, John (*d.* 1820)
A system of materia medica and pharmacy . . . from the 4th and last Edinburgh ed. With notes . . . by John B. Beck, M.D. New York: Pub. by Evert Duyckinck, Geo. Long, Collins & Co., and Collins & Hannay. W. E. Dean, pr., 1824. 560p. NNNAM; NcU; PPC; PU **20-0428**

MURRAY, John (*d.* 1820)
A system of materia medica and pharmacy including translations of the Edinburgh, London, and Dublin pharmacopoeias by John Murray, M.D. from 4th and last Edinburgh editions with notes and additions by John Beck, M.D. New York: Pub. by Evert Duyckinck and others, W. E. Dean, pr., 1828. 2 v. in 1 v. CU-M; ICJ; NIC; ScCM **20-0429**

MUSSEY, Reuben Dimond (1780-1866)
An address on ardent spirit, [sic] read before the New Hampshire Medical Scoeity at their annual meeting, June 5, 1827. . . . Boston: Perkins & Marvin, 1829. 16p. MB; MH; NNNAM **20-0430**

NEWELL, Daniel
The guide to health. Designed to promote the health, happiness, and longevity of students and all others in sedentary life, especially invalids. Boston: S. T. Farren, 1825. 84p. DLC; MH
20-0431

NEW ORLEANS. PHYSICO-MEDICAL SOCIETY
Report of the committee of the Physico-Medical Society of New Orleans, on the epidemic of 1820. New Orleans: Pr. by C. W. Duhy, 1821. 16p. LNT-M; NNNAM
20-0432

[NEW YORK CITY]
A statement of facts relative to the late fever which appeared in Bancker Street and its vicinity. New York: E. Bliss, 1821. 28, 16p. DLC; MB; MH-M; NNNAM
20-0433

[NEW YORK CITY]
Address of the Board of Health of the city of New York, to their fellow citizens. P. & H. Van Pelt, prs. [New York, 1826] 16p. KU; NNNAM **20-0434**

NEW YORK CITY TEMPERANCE SOCIETY
An address to physicians, by the executive committee of the board of managers of the New York City Temperance Society. New York: Pr. by J. & J. Harper, 1829. 22p. DNLM; MB; NNNAM; PPC **20-0435**

NEW YORK. COLLEGE OF PHYSICIANS AND SURGEONS
Catalogue of the anatomical museum, in the College of Physicians and Surgeons, New York, By F. G. King. New York: J. W. Palmer & Co., prs., 1825. 43p. DLC; NNNAM
20-0436

NEW YORK. COLLEGE OF PHYSICIANS AND SURGEONS
Outlines of the lectures on chemistry, delivered in the College of Physicians and Surgeons of the University of the State of New York. Pr. by A. Ming, [New York?] 1828. 12p. DNLM; NNC; NNNAM **20-0437**

NEW YORK HOSPITAL
Address by the governors of the New York Hospital, to the public, relative to the asylum for the insane at Bloomingdale. New York: Pr. by Mahlon Day, May 10, 1821. 8p. DLC; DNLM; NNNAM **20-0438**

NEW YORK HOSPITAL
An account of the New York Hospital. New York: Mahlon Day, 1820. 62p. DLC; DNLM; MWA; NNNAM
20-0439

NEW YORK INSTITUTION FOR THE INSTRUCTION OF THE DEAF AND DUMB
Address of the directors of the New York Institution for the Instruction of the Deaf and Dumb, to their fellow citizens. New York: Pr. by E. Conrad, 1821. 8p. DLC; NNNAM; NNU-M **20-0440**

NEW YORK STATE. COLLEGE OF PHYSICIANS AND SURGEONS
Outlines of the lectures of chemistry, delivered in the College of Physicians and Surgeons of the University of the State of New York. 2nd ed. New York: J. Post, 1829. 114p. NNNAM; PPF **20-0441**

NEW YORK STATE. MEDICAL SOCIETY
Transactions of the Medical Society of the State of New York . . . with the annual address, by T. Romeyn Beck, M.D. . . . Albany: Pr. by Websters and Skinners, 1828. 64p. NjR; NN; NNNAM **20-0442**

NILES, Nathaniel (1791-1869)
Medical statistics; or A comparative view of the mortality in New York, Philadelphia, Baltimore, and Boston, for a series of years, including comparisons of the mortality of whites and blacks in the two former cities; and of whites, free blacks, and slaves, in Baltimore. New York: Pub. by Elam Elias, J. Seymour, pr., 1827. 10p. DLC; NNNAM; PHi; PPL; PU
20-0443

NOUVELLE ORLÉANS. SOCIÉTÉ MEDICALE
Rapport publié an nom de la Société medicale de la Nouvelle-Orleans sur la fièvre jaune, qui y a régné épidémiquement, durant l'été et l'automne de 1819. Lu et approuvé dans sa séance du 21 mai 1820, en présence de Mr. Roufignac, maire. Nouvelle-Orléans: James M'Karaher [1820]. 60p. DNLM; LNT-M; MBM; NNNAM **20-0444**

O'FLAHERTY, Thomas J.
A medical essay on drinking. Hartford: W. Hudson and L. Skinner, pr., 1828. 46p. MWA; OC; NjR
20-0445

OLIVER, Samuel Clark
An essay on the causes which prevent the progress and usefulness of medical science in the United States. Philadelphia: M'Carty & Davis, 1820. 16p. DLC; PPAmP
20-0446

ONDERDONK, John
An inaugural address delivered before the Medical Society of the County of New York, on the 8th day of August, 1825. New York: Pr. by J. Seymour, 1825. 23p. DLC; MH; MWA; NNNAM **20-0447**

ORFILA, Matthieu Joseph Bonaventure (1787-1853)
A practical treatise on poisons and asphyxies adapted to general use. Followed by directions for the treatment of burns, and for the distinction of real from apparent death. . . . Transl. from the French, with notes and additions, by J. G. Stevenson, M.D. with an appendix. . . . Boston: Hilliard Gray, Little and Wilkins, 1826. xii, 240p. DLC; ICJ; MB; NcD
20-0448

OSGOOD, Daniel (1776-1852)
A letter on the yellow fever of the West Indies. . . . New York: Published by Elam Bliss; J. Seymour, printer, 1820. 72p. CtY-M; DLC; DNLM; MBM **20-0449**

PARIS, John Ayrton (1785-1856)
Pharmacologia; or, The history of medicinal substances. . . . From the last London ed., with a general English index. New York: F. & R. Lockwood, 1822. 426p. ICJ; MB; MBM; PPC
20-0450

PARIS, John Ayrton (1785-1856)
Pharmacologia; comprehending the art of prescribing upon fixed and scientific principles. . . . New York: F. & R. Lockwood; J. & J. Harper, pr., 1823-24. 2 v. DLC; ICJ; PPC
20-0451

PARIS, John Ayrton (1785-1856)
Pharmacologia . . . the art of prescribing . . . with the history of medicinal substances. 2nd American from the 5th London ed. With additions . . . by Ansel W. Ives, M.D. New York: F. & R. Lockwood, J. & J. Harper, prs., 1824. 2 v. NIC; NNNAM; PPC **20-0452**

PARIS, John Ayrton (1785-1856)
The elements of medical chemistry. . . . New York: Collins & Hannay, 1825. 471p. ICJ; NNC; NNNAM; RPM **20-0453**

PARIS, John Ayrton (1785-1856)
Pharmacologia: corrected and extended, in accordance with the London pharmacopoeia of 1824, and with the generally advanced state of chemical science. 3rd American, from the 6th London ed. Embracing a history of the most important medicinal substances of the United States, by Ansel W. Ives. . . . New York: S. Wood & Sons [etc.]; Baltimore; S. S. Wood & Co., 1825. 2 v. MB; PPC **20-0454**

PARIS, John Ayrton (1785-1856)
Pharmacologia. 3rd American, from the 6th London ed. Corrected and extended, in accordance with the London pharmacopoeia of 1824, and with the generally advanced state of chemical science. New York: E. Duyckinck [etc.], 1825. 552p. CU-M; DLC; PPC **20-0455**

PARIS, John Ayrton (1785-1856)
A treatise on diet: with a view to establish on practical grounds, a system of rules for the prevention and cure of the diseases incident to a disordered state of the digestive functions. Philadelphia: Robert H. Small, 1826. 210p. GU; ICJ; PPAmP; PPC **20-0456**

PARIS, John Ayrton (1785-1856)
Pharmacologia. 3rd American from the 6th London ed., corr. and extended, in accordance with the London pharmacologia of 1824, and with the generally advanced state of chemical science. . . . New York: E. Duyckinck, Collins & Co. [etc.] [W. C. Dean, pr.] 1828. 544p. MB; NNNAM; PPC; PPF **20-0457**

PARIS, John Ayrton (1785-1856)
A treatise on diet: with a view to establish, on practical grounds, a system of rules for the prevention and cure of the diseases incident to a disordered state of the digestive functions. New York: E. Duyckinck, Collins & Co., Collins & Hannay, and O. A. Roorbach, 1828. [W. E. Dean, pr.] 210p. ICJ; MA; OC **20-0458**

PARMLY, Eleazar (1797?-1874)
An essay on the disorders and treatment of the teeth. 3rd ed. Pr. for the author; and published by Henry Durell and Co., New York and T. and G. Underwood, Medical Booksellers, Fleet St., London, 1822. 88p. IEN-M; MBM; NNC; PPL **20-0459**

PARMLY, Levi Spear (1790-1859)
Lectures on the natural history and management of the teeth; the cause of their decay; the art of preventing its accession; and various operations, never hitherto suggested, for the preservation of such teeth as it is too frequently considered necessary to extract. . . . New York: Published for the author by Kirk and Mercein, Broderick & Ritter, printers, 1820. 99p. DNLM; IU-M; LNT-M; MBM **20-0460**

PARMLY, Levi Spear (1790-1859)
Lectures on the natural history and management of the teeth. 2nd ed. New York: E. B. Clayton for the author, 1821. 101p. ICJ; IEN-M; MBM; NNNAM **20-0461**

PARR, Bartholomew (1750-1810)
The London medical directory. . . . Philadelphia: Published by Gilbert Marshall; William Brown, printer, 1820. 2 v. DLC; NNNAM **20-0462**

PARSONS, Usher (1788-1868)
Sailor's physician, exhibiting the symptoms, causes and treatment of diseases incident to seamen and passengers in merchant vessels, with directions for preserving their health in sickly climates: intended to afford medical advice to such persons while at sea, where a physician cannot be consulted. Cambridge [Mass.]: Hilliard and Metcalf, 1820. 204p. IEN-M; MBM; MH-M; MWA **20-0463**

PARSONS, Usher (1788-1868)
Sailor's physician, containing medical advice for seamen and other persons at sea on the treatment of diseases and on the preservation of health in sickly climates. 2nd ed. Providence: Barnum Field and Co., prs., 1824. 203p. NNC; PPC; PPL; RPB **20-0464**

PARSONS, Usher (1788-1868)
The importance of the sciences of anatomy and physiology as a branch of general education; being an introduction to a course of lectures to the upper classes in Brown University. . . . Cambridge: Pr. by Hilliard & Metcalf, 1826. 31p. MH; NNNAM; RHi **20-0465**

PATTISON, Granville Sharp (1791-1851)
A reply to certain oral and written criticisms, delivered against an essay on lithotomy, published in the January number of the American medical recorder. . . . Inserted in the American medical recorder for July, 1820. Philadelphia: James Webster, 1820. 23p. DNLM; PPL; PU **20-0466**

PATTISON, Granville Sharp (1791-1851)
A refutation of certain calumnies published in a pamphlet, entitled, "Correspondence between Mr. Granville Sharpe Pattison and Dr. Nathaniel Chapman" . . . Baltimore: J. Robinson, 1820. 64p. DNLM; MBM; MH-M; MWA **20-0467**

PATTISON, Granville Sharp (1791-1851)
An answer to a pamphlet entitled "Strictures on Mr. Pattison's reply to certain oral and written criticisms, by W. Gibson" . . . Baltimore: Printed by Richard J. Matchett, 1820. 52p. DNLM; MdBJ-W; NNNAM; NNU-M **20-0468**

PATTISON, Granville Sharp (1791-1851)
An answer to a pamphlet entitled "Strictures on Mr. Pattison's reply to certain oral and written criticisms, by W. Gibson" . . . 2nd ed. Baltimore: Richard J. Matchett, 1820. 32p. CtY-M; DNLM; MBM; MH-M **20-0469**

PATTISON, Granville Sharp (1791-1851)
Experimental observations on the operation of lithotomy; with the description of a fascia of the prostate gland, which appears to explain anatomically the cause of urinal infiltrations, and consequent death. . . . [Philadelphia: James Webster, 1820]. 24p. DNLM **20-0470**

PEABODY, Nathaniel
The art of preserving teeth. Salem, [Mass.]: Pr. by Joshua and John D. Cushing, 1824. 31p. MH-M; MSaE
20-0471

PEABODY, Nathaniel
The art of preserving teeth. 2nd ed. Salem: Pr. by W. and S. B. Ives, 1828. 28p. MSaE **20-0472**

PEIRSON, Abel Lawrence (1794-1853)
Medical dissertation on the diagnosis and treatment of pertussis or chin-cough, which obtained the Boylston Premium for 1822. Pub. by Whipple & Lawrence. Salem, W. & S. B. Ives, prs., 1824. 51p. NNNAM; NjR; PPL; OC [See **20-0496**]
20-0473

PENNELL, Richard [1799?-1861)
An inaugural essay on the bilious typhus which prevailed in Bancker Street and its vicinity, in the city of New York, in the summer and autumn of 1820. New York: E. Bliss and E. White, 1821. 72p. MB; MBM; NNNAM; PHi
20-0474

PENNOCK, Caspar Wister (1799-1867)
Observations and experiments on the efficacy and modus operandi of cupping-glasses, in preventing and arresting the effects of poisoned wounds. Philadelphia: Pr. by J. R. A. Skerrett, 1828. 20p. PPL **20-0475**

PERCIVAL, Anthony
Extracts from the Medical ethics of Dr. Percival. Philadelphia: [T. Town, pr.] 1829. 24p. PHi **20-0476**

PERCIVAL, Thomas (1740-1804)
Extracts from the medical ethics, or a code of institutes and precepts, adapted to the professional conduct of physicians & surgeons. . . . Lexington: Pr. by T. Smith, at the Reporter Office, 1821. 15p. KU; KyLoJM **20-0477**

PERCY, Pierre François (1754-1825)
Report made to the Institute of France on the 22nd of March, 1824, by Baron Percy and Chev. Chaurrier, on a memoir presented by M. Chiviale, M.D. of the faculty of Paux: entitled A new method of destroying the stone in the bladder, without the operation of lithotomy. Philadelphia: Pr. by J. Harding, 1824. 38p. DLC; NNNAM; PU **20-0478**

The **PHARMACOPOEIA** of the United States of America. 1820. By the authority of the medical societies and colleges. Boston: Printed by Wells and Lilly for Charles Ewer, 1820. 272p. CU-M; DLC; DNLM; IEN-M **20-0479**

The **PHARMACOPOEIA** of the United States of America. By the authority of the medical societies and colleges. 2nd ed. Boston: C. Ewer, 1828. 272p. NNNAM; PU; RPB
20-0480

PHILADELPHIA. ALMSHOUSE
A catalogue of the medical library belonging to the Philadelphia Almshouse, prepared agreeably to a resolution of the Board of Managers. . . . Philadelphia: Pr. for the Almshouse, 1824. 52p. PPF **20-0481**

PHILADELPHIA. COLLEGE OF PHARMACY
The druggists manual, being a price current of drugs, medicines, paints, dyestuffs, glass, patent medicines, etc., compiled by direction of the Philadelphia College of Pharmacy. Philadelphia: Pr. for the College by Solomon W. Conrad, 1826. 119p. ICJ; OCLloyd; PPL **20-0482**

PHILADELPHIA. FRIENDS' ASYLUM FOR THE INSANE
An account of the asylum for the insane. [Philadelphia, 1825] 34p. MdBM **20-0483**

PHILADELPHIA MEDICAL SOCIETY
First report of the Committee of the Philadelphia Medical Society on quack medicines. Read on the 15th December, 1827, and ordered to be published by the Society. Philadelphia: Judah Dobson, Agent, 1826. 37p. DLC; MHi; PP; ScC
20-0484

PHILADELPHIA. PENNSYLVANIA HOSPITAL
Catalogue of the medical library of the Pennsylvania Hospital. Philadelphia: T. A. Conrad, printer, 1825. 426p. PPPH
20-0485

PHILADELPHIA. PENNSYLVANIA HOSPITAL
Some account of the origin, objects, and present state of the Pennsylvania Hospital. Philadelphia: Pr. by Thos. Kite, 1828. 24p. IEN-M; MB; PHi; PU **20-0486**

PHILADELPHIA. PENNSYLVANIA HOSPITAL.
Catalogue of the medical library of the Pennsylvania Hospital. Philadelphia: T. A. Conrad, printer, 1829. 322p. DLC; PPPH; PU **20-0487**

PHILADELPHIA. PENNSYLVANIA INFIRMARY FOR DISEASES OF THE EYE AND EAR
The Pennsylvania Infirmay for Diseases of the Eye and Ear established at Philadelphia. Philadelphia: Pr. by order of the Society, William Fry, printer, 1822. 6p. PHi, PPAmP; PPC
20-0488

PHILADELPHIA. UNIVERSITY OF PENNSYLVANIA MEDICAL SCHOOL
Department of medicine. [Catalog of the anatomical museum and a report to the committee on Wistar Institute by W. E. Horner, Philadelphia, 1824] 36p. MdBM
20-0489

PHILIP. Alexander Philip Wilson (1770-1851)
A treatise on indigestion and its consequences, called nervous and bilious complaints. . . . Philadelphia: H. C. Carey & I. Lea; Harrisburg: Pr. by Wm. Greer, 1822. 205p. IU-M; MB; MBM; PPC **20-0490**

PHILIP, Alexander Philip Wilson (1770-1851)
A treatise on indigestion and its consequences, called nervous and bilious complaints. . . . Philadelphia: Benjamin & Thomas Kite, 1822. 205p. PPC; PPJ; PU; ScCM
20-0491

PHILIP, Alexander Philip Wilson (1770-1851)
A treatise on indigestion and its consequences, called nervous and bilious complaints; with observations on the organic diseases, in which they sometimes terminate. 3rd ed., with some additional observations. Philadelphia: H. C. Carey and I. Lea, J. Crissy & G. Goodman, prs., 1823. 195p. ICJ; MdBM; PPAmP **20-0492**

PHILIP, Alexander Philip Wilson (1770-1851)
A treatise on indigestion and its consequences, called nervous and bilious complaints . . . 4th ed. with some additional observations. Philadelphia: James Crissy; J. Crissy & G. Goodman, prs., 1824. 195p. ICJ; NNNAM **20-0493**

PHILIP, Alexander Philip Wilson (1770-1851)
A treatise on indigestion and its consequences, called nervous and bilious complaints . . . 4th ed. with some additional observations. New York: Pub. by Evert Duyckinck and Geo. Long, W. E. Dean, pr., 1824. 192p. MB; MdBM; PPC
20-0494

PHILIP, Alexander Philip Wilson (1770-1851)
Treatise on indigestion & its consequences called nervous & bilious complaints. . . . 5th ed. Philadelphia: James Crissy, 1825. 195p. MB; NNNAM; PPC **20-0495**

PIERSON, A. L. (1794-1853)
Medical dissertation on the diagnosis and treatment of pertussis or chin-cough, which obtained the Boylston Premium for 1822. Salem: Whipple & Lawrence, 1824. 51p. MSaE; MWA
20-0496

PLANTOU, Anthony
Observations on the yellow fever, with an account of a new mode of treatment & cure for putrid & malignant diseases in general. . . . Philadelphia, 1822. 58p. NNNAM; PPAmP; PU
20-0497

PLANTOU, Anthony
Observations on the yellow fever, with an account of a new mode of treatment and cure for the same, as well as for putrid and malignant diseases in general. . . . 2nd ed. Philadelphia, 1822. 58p. DLC; PPC; ScCM **20-0498**

POPULAR directions for the prevention and cure of headaches, colds, and indigestion. . . . Philadelphia: James E. Moore, J. Harding, pr., 1823. 135p. DLC; MdBM **20-0499**

POTTER, W. W.
First letter of W. W. Potter, to the committee of the Philadelphia Medical Society, on quack medicines. Read on the 12th February, 1828. Philadelphia, 1828. 7p. NIC
20-0500

PROUT, William (1785-1850)
An inquiry into the nature and treatment of diabetes, calculus. . . . From the 2nd London ed., with notes and additions by S. Colhoun, M.D. . . . Philadelphia: Pub. by Towar & Hogan, W. Brown, pr., 1826. 308p. ICJ; PPC; PPL
20-0501

PROUT, William (1785-1850)
An inquiry into the nature and treatment of diabetes, calculus, and other affections of the urinary organs: with remarks on the importance of attending to the state of the urine in organic diseases of the kidney and bladder. . . . From the 2nd London ed., rev. and much enlarged: With notes and additions by S. Calhoun. Philadelphia: Pub. by Towar & Hogan, W. Brown, pr., 1828. 308p. ViRA **20-0502**

RAFINESQUE, Constantine Samuel (1783-1840)
Medical flora: or, Manual of the medical botany of the United States of North America . . . Philadelphia: Pr. & pub. by Atkinson & Alexander, 1828-30. 2 v. DLC; PPAmP; PPC; PU
20-0503

RAFINESQUE, Constantine Samuel (1783-1840)
. . . The pulmist; or, Introduction to the art of curing and preventing the consumption or chronic phthisis; a medical essay, including a new and better distinction of its causes, kinds, remedies, diets, and other peculiarities. Philadelphia: Pr. for the author by C. Alexander, 1829. 72p. KU; MH; NNNAM; PPC **20-0504**

RAMSBOTHAM, John
Practical observations on midwifery. . . . With notes by William P. Dewees. Philadelphia: H. C. Carey and I. Lea, 1822. 379p. ICJ; MBM; NNNAM; OC **20-0505**

RAMSBOTHAM, John
Practical observations in midwifery. . . . With notes by William P. Dewees. Philadelphia: Pub. by H. C. Carey and I. Lea, 1826. 379p. DLC; DNLM **20-0506**

REESE, David Meredith (1800-1861)
Strictures on health; or, An investigation into the physical effects of intemperance upon the public health. . . . New York: N. Bangs and J. Emory, Azor Hoyt, pr., 1828. 160p. OC
20-0507

RHEES, B. Rush
An address delivered March 8, 1825, in the Hall of the Medical Faculty of Jefferson College, located in Philadelphia. Philadelphia: Stavely and Bringhurst, 1825. 30p. PPC; PPJ; PU
20-0508

RHODE ISLAND. MEDICAL SOCIETY
Stat Nominis Umbra [pseud.]
A discourse on the object and utility of the Rhode Island Medical Society. . . . Providence, 1823. 15p. DLC; RPM
20-0509

RICHARDSON, Josiah
The New England farrier and family physician. . . . Exeter: Josiah Richardson, 1828. 444, 24p. CSmH; DNLM; MWA
20-0510

RICHERAND, Anthelme Balthaser (1779-1840)
Elements of physiology; from the 5th London edition, rev. and corr. and enl. Transl. from the French by G. J. M. de Lys . . . with notes by Nathaniel Chapman. . . . Philadelphia: Pr. by Jespar Harding, 1821. 554p. MB; MBM; MdBM; PMA
20-0511

RICHERAND, Anthelme Balthasar (1779-1840)
Elements of physiology. . . . From the 5th London ed., rev., corr. and enl. Transl. from the French, by G. J. M. Delys, M.D. Philadelphia: Pub. by James E. Moore, J. Harding, pr., 1823. 621p. DLC; MdBM; PPC; PU **20-0512**

RICHERAND, Anthelme Balthasar (1779-1840)
Elements of physiology. Transl. from the French by G. J. M. de Lys . . . From the last London ed., with annotations by N. Chapman . . . copious notes and an appendix, by James Copland . . . and additional notes, by John D. Godman. . . . 5th American from the last London ed. Philadelphia: H. C. Carey & I. Lea, 1825. 448, 111p. NNNAM; PPC; PU
20-0513

RICHERAND, Anthelme Balthasar (1779-1840)
Elements of physiology. Transl. from the French by G. J. M. de Lys. . . . From the last London ed. with notes and a copious appendix, by James Copland. . . . New York: Pr. by W. E. Dean, 1825. 407, 94p. ICJ; NcU; PPC
20-0514

RICHERAND, Anthelme Balthasar (1779-1840)
Elements of therapeutics and materia medica. . . . 4th ed., enl. and rev. Philadelphia: H. C. Carey and I. Lea, 1825. 2 v. PPC; PPHa; PPJ **20-0515**

RICKMAN, William
Explanations of an engraved plan for an establishment for the reception of individuals in a state of mental derangement. . . . Drawn in outline. Washington City: Pr. by Duff Green, 1829. 12p. PPL **20-0516**

RISHEL, Jonas
The Indian physician, containing a new system of practice, founded on medical plants. . . . Together with a description of their properties, localities and method of using, and preparing them. . . . New Berlin, Penn.: Pr. for the author and proprietor, by Jos. Miller, 1828. 132p. ICJ; IEN-M **20-0517**

ROBERTSON, Archibald
Conversations on anatomy, physiology, and surgery. Philadelphia: Towar & Hogan, publishers, 1828. 2 v. NNNAM; OC; PPC **20-0518**

ROBINSON, Samuel
A course of fifteen lectures on medical botany, denominated Thomson's new theory of medical practice; in which the various theories that have preceded it, are reviewed and compared; delivered in Cincinnati, Ohio. . . . Columbus: H. Howard, 1829. 199p. DLC; DNLM; OCHP; OCIM **20-0519**

RODGERS, John Kearney (1793-1851)
Report of surgeons of New York Eye Infirmary [from . . . 1820-1821.] [New York, 1821] 8p. DNLM **20-0520**

ROGERS, David
The American physician: being a new system of practice founded on botany. Rochester, N.Y.: Pr. for the author by H. Leavenworth, 1824. 130p. NNNAM **20-0521**

ROGERS, J. Smyth
Syllabus of a course on medical examinations. . . . New York: Pr. by T. and J. Swords, 1823. 7p. NNC; NNNAM **20-0522**

RUSH, Benjamin (1746-1813)
An inquiry into the effects of ardent spirits upon the human body and mind: with an account of the means of preventing, and of the remedies for curing them. 8th ed., with additions. Boston: Pub. by James Loring, 1823. Pr. by Manning & Loring. 36p. DLC; NN; PHi; PPL **20-0523**

RUSH, Benjamin (1746-1813)
Extracts from Dr. Benjamin Rush's inquiry into the effects of ardent spirits upon the human body and mind. Philadelphia: To be had of Benjamin & Thomas Kite, and for sale by Solomon W. Conrad, Kimber & Sharpless, 1823. 16p. PP; PPAmP; PPC; PPHa **20-0524**

RUSH, Benjamin (1745-1813)
Extracts from Dr. Benjamin Rush's inquiry into the effects of ardent spirits upon the human body and mind. Philadelphia: To be had of Benjamin & Thomas Kite, 1827. 16p. PPC; PPHa **20-0525**

RUSH, Benjamin (1745-1813)
Medical inquiries and observations, upon the diseases of the mind. 3rd ed. Philadelphia: J. Grigg, 1827. 365p. DNLM; OC; PPC; PPL **20-0526**

RUSSELL, Henry P., comp.
An official register of the deaths which occurred among the white population in the city of Savannah, during the extraordinary season of sickness and mortality which prevailed in the summer and fall months of the year 1820. To which is annexed a list of the persons (so far as they could be ascertained) who died out of the city, after retreating from it. Also, the aggregate amount of deaths among the people of color. Savannah: Henry P. Russell, 1820. 24p. DNLM; MWA; NNNAM; PHi **20-0527**

SAISSY, Jean Antoine (1756-1822)
An essay on diseases of the internal ear. . . . Transl. from the French by Nathan R. Smith . . . with a supplement on diseases of the external ear, by the translator. Baltimore: Hatch & Dunning, 1829. 228p. DLC; DNLM; NjR; PP **20-0528**

SANBORN, P. E.
The Sick Man's Friend, being a plain practical medical work; designed for the use of families and individuals on vegetable or botanical principles. Taunton, Mass., 1825. 252p. MBM; MH-M; MWA **20-0529**

SAUNDERS, John Cunningham (1773-1810)
The anatomy of the human ear, illustrated by a series of engravings of the natural size; with a treatise on the diseases of that organ, the causes of deafness, and their proper treatment. 1st American from the 2nd London ed. With notes and additions by Wm. Price. . . . Philadelphia: B. Warner, 1821. 128p. DNLM; KyLoJM; MdBM; RPM **20-0530**

SAUNDERS, John Cunningham (1773-1810)
A treatise on some practical points relating to the diseases of the eye. . . . A new ed. with additions. Philadelphia: Pub. by Benjamin Warner, and sold also at his stores in Richmond, Va. and Louisville, Ken. and by W. P. Bason, Charleston, S.C., 1821. 232p. DNLM; ICJ; MBM; OC **20-0531**

SEDGWICK, Elijah
The plain physician, giving directions for the preservation of health, and the cure of disease. Rochester: Pr. by E. F. Marshall, 1827. 48p. DLC; NNNAM **20-0532**

SEWALL, Thomas (1786-1845)
A lecture delivered at the opening of the medical department of the Columbian College. . . . Washington City: Pr. at the Columbian office, 1825. 80p. DLC; MB; MH; PHi **20-0533**

SEWALL, Thomas (1786-1845)
A lecture, delivered at the opening of the medical department of the Columbian College, in the District of Columbia. . . . Washington City: Pr. at the Columbian office, 1826. 44p. DLC; DNLM; NjR; OC **20-0534**

SEWALL, Thomas (1786-1845)
A charge delivered to the graduating class of the Columbian College, D.C., at the medical commencement, March 22, 1827. . . . Washington: Pr. by D. Green, 1828. 12p. DLC; DNLM; IEN-M; MH **20-0535**

SHAW, Charles
An inaugural dissertation on the non-specific nature, and non-mercurial treatment of venereal affections. . . . Lexington, Ky.: Pr. at the Transylvania Press, by J. G. Norwood, 1829. 16p. NN; OC **20-0536**

SHERRILL, Hunting (1783-1866)
A review of the diseases of Dutchess County, from 1809 to 1825; being the subject of two addresses read before the Medical Society at their annual meetings in 1819 and 1825. Published by S. C. Schenk, New York. Pr. by J. Seymour, 1826. 134p. MB; MH; NBM; PPHa **20-0537**

SIMONS, Thomas Young (1798-1857)
Observations on mental alienation and the application of its phenomena to the illustration of subjects connected with medical jurisprudence. Charleston [S.C.]: A. F. Cunningham, 1828. 50p. CSmH; DLC; NN; ScCM **20-0538**

SIMONS, Thomas Young (1798-1857)
An address to the graduates of the Medical College of South Carolina; delivered on March 23rd, 1829, after conferring the degree of doctor of medicine. Charleston: Pr. by A. E. Miller, 1829. 20p. ScCM; ScMS **20-0539**

SLACK, Elijah
A key to the technical language, and a few other difficulties of chemistry, or chemical nomenclature. Together with a concise view of the doctrine of definite proportions and chemical equivalents. For the use of students in the Medical College of Ohio. Cincinnati: Pr. by G. T. Williamson, 1828. 25p. OCHP **20-0540**

SMITH, Elias (1769-1846)
The medical pocket-book, family physician, and sick man's guide to health; containing a short description of vegetable medicines. . . . Boston: Bowen, 1822. 168p. MB; MH-M; PPC **20-0541**

SMITH, Elias (1769-1846)
The American physician, and family assistant, in four parts. . . . Boston: E. Bellamy, pr., 1826. 216p. DLC; DNLM; MBM **20-0542**

SMITH, James (1771-1841)
The National Vaccine Institution. To the citizens of the United States. . . . Baltimore, 1822. [2] p. DNLM **20-0543**

SMITH, John Rubens
A compendium of picturesque anatomy, adapted to the arts of designing, painting, sculpture and engraving, on four folio lithographic plates. . . . Boston: Pub. by the author, 1827. 8p., 4 pl. ICJ **20-0544**

SMITH, Joseph Mather (1789-1866)
Elements of the etiology and philosophy of epidemics. New York: Pr. by and for J. & J. Harper, 1824. 223p. MdBM; NNC; PPC **20-0545**

SMITH, Nathan (1762-1829)
A practical essay on typhus fever. New York: Pub. by E. Bliss & E. White, Gray & Bunce, prs. 1824. 88p. CU-M; PPC; RPM **20-0546**

SMITH, Nathan Ryno (1797-1877)
A physiological essay on digestion. . . . New York: Pub. by E. Bliss, and E. White [Dodd and Manter, prs.] 1825. 93p. DLC; NNNAM; PU **20-0547**

SMITH, Nathan Ryno (1797-1877)
An address pronounced before the medical graduates of the University of Maryland, April 7, 1828. Baltimore: Benjamin Edes, 1828. 21p. MdHi; MdBJ-W; MdU-D **20-0548**

SMITH, Nathan Ryno (1797-1877)
An address pronounced before the medical graduates of the University of Maryland, April 6th, 1829. Baltimore: Hatch & Dunning [Lucas & Deaver, prs.] 1829. 23p. MdHi; NNNAM **20-0549**

SMITH, W.
A physician at hand, or A collection of receipts and cures, to heal diseases and wounds of various kinds. Published by Dr. W. Smith, 1829. J. Barr, pr., Wooster. 7p. DLC; MWiW; MSaE **20-0550**

STEARNS, John (1770-1848)
An address delivered before the Medical Society of the State of New York, and the members of the legislature, at the capitol in the city of Albany, the 2nd of February, 1820, on the influence of the mind upon the body in the production and cure of diseases. . . . Albany: E. and E. Hosford, 1820. 19p. DNLM; MWA; NNNAM; NNS **20-0551**

STEARNS, John (1770-1848)
Observations on the secale cornutum, or ergot. . . . 1822. 8p. NNNAM **20-0552**

STEEL, John Honeywood (1780-1838)
An analysis of the mineral waters of Saratoga and Ballston, with practical remarks on their use in various diseases containing observations on the geology and mineralogy of the surrounding country with a geological map. 2nd ed., imp. Saratoga Springs, 1828. 118p. MWA; RPM **20-0553**

STEWARD, William
The first edition of Steward's Healing art, corrected and improved by the original hand. To which he has added, all his late improvements and new discoveries, both in physick and surgery, from the year 1812, to the year 1826, including his whole system upon physick and surgery. To which he has added a concise herbal, containing a full description of herbs, roots. Saco, Maine: Pr. by Putnam & Blake, 1827. 126, 40, 22p. CSmH; PPHa **20-0554**

STRANG, John
A short account of the smallpox which prevailed at Bridgeport . . . with remarks on vaccination. Bridgeport, 1826. PPPH **20-0555**

STAUGHTON, James M[artin] (1800-1833)
Charge addressed to the graduates at the medical commencement of the Columbia College, D.C. Mar. 11, 1829. Washington City: Pr. by Stephen C. Ustick, 1829. 11p. OC; PPPrHi **20-0556**

STROBEL, B. B.
An experimental enquiry into the medical properties of the Aralie spinosa, or, prickly ash. Charleston: Gray and Ellis, 1826. 45p. DNLM; NNNAM; ScC **20-0557**

SUCKLEY, John L.
Secretion; the source of pleasurable sensations. A thesis. . . . New York: J. & J. Harper, prs., 1823. 49p. NN; NNC; NNNAM **20-0558**

SUMNER, George (1793-1855)
A compendium of physiological and systematic botany. . . . Hartford: Oliver D. Cooke, 1820. 300p. MWA; MWiW; PPC; OCLloyd **20-0559**

[SWAIM, William]
A treatise on Swaim's panacea; being a recent discovery for the cure of scrofula, or king's evil, mercurial diseases, deep-seated syphilis. Philadelphia: Clark & Raser, 1822. 138p. IEN-M; PPL
20-0560

[SWAIM, William]
A treatise on Swaim's panacea; being a recent discovery for the cure of scrofula, or king's evil, mercurial disease, deep-seated syphilis. Philadelphia: Clark & Raser, printers, 1822. 84p. NNNAM; PPL **20-0561**

SWAIM, William
A treatise on Swaim's panacea, being a recent discovery for the cure of scrofula or king's evil, mercurial disease, deep-seated syphilis, rheumatism, and all disorders arising from a contaminated or impure state of the blood. Philadelphia: Clark and Raser, prs., 1824. 159p. NNNAM; PHi; PMA **20-0562**

[SWAIM, William]
The case of Nancy Linton, illustrative of the efficacy of Swaim's panacea. Philadelphia: Pr. by Clark & Raser, 1827. 12p. PPL **20-0563**

[SWAIM, William]
Cases of cures performed by the use of Swaim's panacea. Philadelphia, 1827. 84p. PPL **20-0564**

[SWAIM, William]
Some remarks upon a publication by the Philadelphia Medical Society concerning Swaim's panacea. . . . Philadelphia, 1828. 52p. DLC; MB; NNNAM; PHi **20-0565**

SWAIM, William
Cases of cures performed by the use of Swaim's panacea. Philadelphia, 1829. 98p. PPL **20-0566**

SWEET, Waterman
An essay on the sciences of bone setting. . . . Providence: Marshall & Hammond, 1829. 16p. RPB **20-0567**

SWEETSER, William (1797-1875)
Dissertations on cynanche trachealis or croup; and on the functions of the extreme capillary vessels in health and diseases . . . Boston: Cummings, Hilliard & Co., 1823. 123p. DLC; MB; NNNAM; PPC **20-0568**

TALBOTT, John
A collection of theoretical and practical observations on medicine. Portsmouth, O.: Pr. at the office of the Western Times, 1826. 10p. DLC **20-0569**

TAVERNIER, Alphonse
Elements of operative surgery. Transl. from the French of A. Tavernier. Ed. by S. D. Gross. . . . Philadelphia: J. Grigg, [etc.]; New York: Collins & Hannay [etc.] 1829. xxx, 448p. DLC; IEN-M; PU **20-0570**

THACHER, James (1754-1844)
The American new dispensatory. . . . 4th ed. Boston: Pub. by Thomas B. Wait, Joseph W. Ingraham, printer, 1821. 736p. IEN-M; NNNAM; PPC; PPJ **20-0571**

THACHER, James (1754-1844)
American modern practice; or A simple method of prevention and cure of diseases, according to the latest improvements and discoveries. . . . Boston: Pub. by Cotton & Barnard. John Cotton, pr., 1826. viii, 796p. DLC; GU; ICJ; RPM
20-0572

THACHER, James (1754-1844)
American medical biography; or, Memoirs of eminent physicians who have flourished in America. Boston: Richardson & Lord, [etc.] 1828. 2 v. in 1. CSmH; DNLM; ICU; MB
20-0573

THOMAS, Robert (1753-1835)
The modern practice of physic, exhibiting the characters, causes, symptoms, prognostics, morbid appearances, and improved method of treating the diseases of all climates. . . . The 5th American, from the 6th London ed., rev. and considerably enl. by the addition of much important matter, as well as by an English translation of the formulae or prescriptions. . . . With an Appendix, by David Hosack. . . . New York: Published by Collins and Co., J. & J. Harper, printers, 1820. 1016p. DNLM; MBM; NNNAM; OCIM **20-0574**

THOMAS, Robert (1753-1835)
A treatise on domestic medicine. . . . 1st American ed. rev. by David Hosack. New York: Collins & Co., A Paul, printer, 1822. 500p. ICJ; IEN-M; OCLloyd; PPC **20-0575**

THOMAS, Robert (1753-1835)
The modern practice of physic. . . . 6th American from the 7th London ed. New York: Collins & Co., J. & J. Harper, printers, 1822. 1050p. DLC; ICJ; IEN-M; PPC **20-0576**

THOMAS, Robert (1753-1835)
The modern practice of physic, 7th American from the last London ed., rev. and considerably enl. With an appendix by David Hosack. New York: S. B. Collins & Collins & Co., 1824. 1058p. CU-M; MB; NNNAM; PPC **20-0577**

THOMAS, Robert (1753-1835)
The modern practice of physic. . . . 8th American, from the last London ed. With an appendix by David Hosack. New York: S. B. Collins, and Collins & Co., 1825. 1072p. MB; NNNAM **20-0578**

THOMAS, Robert (1753-1835)
Modern domestic medicine: being a treatise divested of professional terms on the nature, causes, symptoms, and treatment of the diseases of men, women, and children. . . . New York: Collins & Co., W. E. Dean, pr., 1829. 499p. NNNAM; OCIM
20-0579

THOMSON, Anthony Todd (1778-1849)
A conspectus of the pharmacopoeias of the London, Edinburgh and Dublin college of physicians; being a practical compendium of materia medica and pharmacy. 1st American from the 5th London ed.; improved by the additions of the United States Pharmacopoeia, Magendie's Formulary, and other new pharmaceutical preparations. New York: E. Bliss & E. White, 1825. 220p. DLC; PPC **20-0580**

THOMSON, John (1765-1846)
An account of the varioloid epidemic which has lately prevailed in Edinburgh and other parts of Scotland; with observations on the identity of chicken-pox, in a letter to Sir James McGrigor. Philadelphia: Carey & Lea, 1824. 418p. ICJ; MH; MdBM; PU
20-0581

THOMSON, John
A vindication of the Thomsonian system of the practice of medicine on botanical principles. . . . Albany: Pr. by Webster & Wood, 1825. 76p. MB; NNNAM; OCLloyd
20-0582

THOMSON, Samuel (1769-1843)
A brief sketch of the causes and treatment of disease; addressed to the people of the United States. . . . Boston: Pr. for the author, by E. G. House, 1821. 36p. MBM; MH; MH-M
20-0583

THOMSON, Samuel (1769-1843)
New guide to health; or, Botanic family physician. Containing a complete system of practice, upon a plan entirely new; . . . Boston: Pr. for the author, by E. G. House, 1822. 300p. MB; MBM; MH; OCLloyd **20-0584**

THOMSON, Samuel (1769-1843)
A narrative of the life and medical discoveries of Samuel Thomson. . . . Boston: Pr. for the author, by E. G. House, 1822. 204p. ICJ; OCIWHi; PPL **20-0585**

THOMSON, Samuel (1769-1843)
An earnest appeal to the public, showing the misery caused by the fashionable mode of practice of the doctors at the present day. . . . Boston: Pr. for the author by E. G. House, 1824. 36p. NjR; OCIWHi **20-0586**

THOMSON, Samuel (1769-1843)
Address to the public on the causes and treatment of disease; showing the bad consequences of administering poison as medicine, and the advantages of following the course pointed out by nature, using vegetable substances only. Boston: E. G. House, 1825. 48p. MB **20-0587**

THOMSON, Samuel (1769-1843)
A narrative of the life and medical discoveries of Samuel Thomson. . . . Boston: Pr. for the author by E. G. House, 1825. 224p. DLC; MB: OCIM; OCLloyd **20-0588**

THOMSON, Samuel (1769-1843)
New guide to health; or, Botanic family physician . . . to which is prefixed a narrative of the life and medical discoveries of the author. 2nd ed. Boston: E. H. House, 1825. 192, 132p. MH; MdBM; NNNAM; OCIM **20-0589**

THOMSON, Samuel (1769-1843)
New guide to health; or Botanic family physician. . . . 3rd ed. Columbus: Horton Howard, 1827. 115p. IU-M
20-0590

THOMSON, Samuel (1769-1843)
A narrative of the life and medical discoveries of Samuel Thomson; . . . to which is added an introduction to his new guide to health, or botanic family physician; . . . Horton Howard, 1827. 188p. OCLloyd; PHi **20-0591**

THOMSON, Samuel (1769-1843)
Eine beschreibung von dem leben und medicinischen erfindungen von Samuel Thomson, enthaltend eine erklarüng seines systems in seinem praxis, oder gewohneit, und die art und weise um krankheiten zu kuriren mit gekräuter-medicinen, auf einen ganz neuen plan. . . . 1. deutsche, von der 4. englischen ausg. Geschrieben von ihm selbst. Lancaster, O.: Gedruckt für H. Howard, bey J. Herman, 1828. 228p. DLC; DNLM **20-0592**

THOMSON, Samuel (1769-1843)
Neue anweisung zur Gesundheit; oder, botanischer familien arzt, ethaltend ein vellständiges system von practistren, auf einen ganz neuen plan. . . . Erste Deutsche, von der vierten Englischen ausgabe. Lancaster, O.: Gedruckt für Horton Howard, bey Johann Herman, 1828. 144p. PPL
20-0593

THOMSON, Samuel (1769-1843)
A narrative of the life and medical discoveries of Samuel Thomson; containing an account of his system of practice, and the manner of curing disease with vegetable medicine. . . . 5th ed. St. Clairsville, [O].: Horton Howard. Howard & Little, prs., 1829. 188p. CSmH; OCIWHi; PPC **20-0594**

THOMSON, Samuel (1769-1843)
New guide to health; or, Botanic family physician. Containing a complete system of practice, upon a plan entirely new: with a description of the vegetables made use of, and directions for preparing and administrating them to cure disease. . . . 5th ed. St. Clairsville: Pub. by Horton Howard. Howard & Little, prs., 1829. 115p. DNLM; OCIWHi; PPL **20-0595**

The **THOMSONIAN** practice revealed: in which the secret medicine and nostrums of the most ignorant and bare-faced set of quacks that ever have infested the world are fully developed. New York, 1829. 8p. NN; NHi **20-0596**

TOGNO, Joseph
Experiments to establish a peculiar physico-organic action inherent in the animal tissues, called endosmose and exosmose. Philadelphia: Pr. by J. R. A. Skerrett, 1829. 23p. DLC
20-0597

TOOLEY, Henry (1773-1848)
History of the yellow fever, as it appeared in the city of Natchez, in the months of August, September and October, 1823. Natchez: Pr. by F. Baker, 1823. 29p. DLC; DNLM; NHi **20-0598**

TOOLEY, Henry (1773-1848)
History of the yellow fever, as it appeared in the city of Natchez, in the months of August, September, and October, 1823. 2nd ed. Washington, Miss.: A. Marschalk, 1823. 23p. DNLM; DLC **20-0599**

TOWER, David
Four lectures on the Thomsonian practice of medicine. . . . Canandaigua: Pr. by Bemis, Morse and Ward (for the author) 1828. 72p. DLC **20-0600**

[TOWNSEND, Peter Solomon] (1796?-1849)
Remarks on the Report of the committee of the Medical Society of this city, on the "Epidemic fever of Bancker Street and its vicinity, in the summer and autumn of 1820." [New York, 1820] 16p. DNLM; NHi; NNNAM
20-0601

TOWNSEND, Peter Solomon (1796?-1849)
An account of the yellow fever, as it prevailed in the city of New York, in the summer and autumn of 1822. New York: O. Halsted, 1823. 383p. ICJ; MH; MdBM; PPC
20-0602

TOWNSEND, Peter Solomon (1796?-1849)
Case of three remarkable tumors extirpated from the nose. New York: Pr. by J. Seymour, 1825. 8p. MB; NNNAM; OC
20-0603

TOWNSEND, Peter Solomon (1796?-1849)
Memoir on the topography, weather, and diseases of the Bahama Islands. . . . New York: J. Seymour, pr., 1826. 80p. NNNAM; PPAmP; PPC; PPL **20-0604**

TRANSYLVANIA UNIVERSITY
Report on the Transylvania University and Lunatic Asylum. [Lexington, ky.? 1824?] 50, 2p. KU **20-0605**

TRAVERS, Benjamin (1783-1858)
A synopsis of the diseases of the eye, and their treatment. . . . New York: E. Bliss & E. White, 1825. 474p. MdBM; NNNAM; RPB **20-0606**

TRAVERS, Benjamin (1783-1858)
An inquiry concerning that disturbed state of the vital functions usually denominated constitutional irritation. New York: Pub. for the author, by H. Stevenson, J. Seymour, pr., 1826. 374p. ICRM; IU-M; PPC; RPM **20-0607**

A TREATISE on the diseases most prevalent in the United States with directions for medicine chests. . . . Philadelphia: J. R. A. Skerrett, 1821. 24p. PHi; RPB **20-0608**

A TREATISE on the diseases most prevalent in the United States, with directions for medicine chests. . . . Philadelphia: Pr. by J. R. A. Skerrett, 1825. 36p. NNNAM **20-0609**

A TREATISE on the diseases most prevalent in the United States, with directions for medicine chests, designed for the use of families. . . . Philadelphia: Pr. by J. R. A. Skerrett, 1827. 36p. NNNAM **20-0610**

TRENOR, John
A physiological inquiry into the structure, organization, and nourishment to the human teeth. . . . J. Seymour, pr., New York, 1828. 25p. NNNAM **20-0611**

TYTLER, James (1747?-1805)
An interesting account of the dreadful effects of the plague and yellow fever, at London, in 1665, at Athens in the time of the Peloponesian war, at Constantinople in the time of Justinian, and at Marseilles, in 1720, &c., 1st American from the 21st London ed. Boston: Rutter, 1824. 568p. ICJ; MB; OC **20-0612**

VACHÉ, Alexander F. (1800-1857)
On surgical anatomy of the groin, as connected with hernia of the abdomen. . . . New York: Pr. by William Grattan, 1825. 52p. NNNAM **20-0613**

VETHAKE, John W.
A discourse on the western autumnal disease, read before the Tenth District Medical Society of Ohio; at Chillicothe, May 30th, 1826. Chillicothe: Pr. by John Bailhache & Co., 1826. 39p. DLC; DNLM; OCHP; PHi **20-0614**

VOUGHT, John G.
A treatise on bowel complaints: intended for the use of physicians, families, parents, masters of vessels, &c. in the United States. Rochester, N.Y.: Pr. for the author, by E. Peck & Co., 1823. 216p. DLC **20-0615**

[VOUGHT, John G.]
Medical notice. To parents, masters of ships, and such physicians as do not prepare and compound their own prescriptions. The New York Infirmary for Diseases of the Bowels, is removed to Masonic Hall, no. 316 Broadway, opposite the New York Hospital. [New York, 1829] 8p. NN **20-0616**

WARE, John (1795-1864)
Medical dissertations on hemoptysis or the spitting of blood, and on suppuration, which obtained the Boylston premiums for the years 1818 & 1820. . . . Boston: Cummings and Hilliard, 1820. 95p. DLC; RPB; RPJCB **20-0617**

WARREN, John Collins (1778-1856)
Description of an Egyptian mummy, presented to the Massachusetts General Hospital. . . . [Boston, 1821] 34p. NN **20-0618**

WARREN, John Collins (1778-1856)
A comparative view of the sensorial and nervous systems in men and animals. Boston: J. W. Ingraham, 1822. 159p. CU-M; DLC; IU-M; ScCM **20-0619**

WARREN, John Collins (1778-1856)
A letter to the Hon. Isaac Parker, Chief Justice of the Supreme Court of the State of Massachusetts, containing remarks on the dislocation of the hip joint, occasioned by the publication of a trial which took place at Machias, in the State of Maine, June, 1824. Cambridge: Pr. by Hilliard & Metcalf, 1826. viii, 142p. DLC; ICU; IEN-M; RPM **20-0620**

WASHINGTON: PHRENOLOGICAL SOCIETY
A report submitted to the Phrenological Society of the City of Washington on the 14th of March, 1828 and printed by order. Washington: E. DeKrafft, pr. [1828] 8p. DLC **20-0621**

WATERHOUSE, Benjamin (1754-1846)
Cautions to young persons concerning health in a public lecture delivered at the close of the medical course in the chapel at Cambridge, Nov. 20, 1804; containing the general doctrine of chronic diseases; showing the evil tendency of the use of tobacco upon young persons; more especially the pernicious effects of smoking cigars; with observations on the use of ardent and vinous spirits in general. 5th ed. With additional notes. Cambridge: University Press, 1822. 40p. IEN-M; MdBM; N; NNNAM **20-0622**

WATERHOUSE, Benjamin (1754-1846)
An essay concerning tussis convulsiva, or, whooping-cough, with observations on the diseases of children. Boston: Munroe and Francis, 1822. 152p. ICJ; MB; MBM; PPC **20-0623**

WEBB, Jonathan (1795-1832)
Medicine chests, with particular directions, prepared by Jonathan Webb, apothecary, Salem. [Salem]: W. Palfray, Jr. 1820. 8p. MWA **20-0624**

WEBSTER, James (1803-1854)
An essay on medical jurisprudence. Philadelphia: Wm. Brown, 1824. 52p. PHi; PPAmP; PPC; PU **20-0625**

WEBSTER. James (1803-1854)
A card, During the last winter. Dr. John Eberle published a certain pamphlet. . . . [Philadelphia, 1827] 8p. MB; PPL **20-0626**

WETHERILL, Samuel P. & Co.
A treatise on the diseases of seamen. Medicine chests carefully put up by Samuel P. Wetherill & Co. chemists and druggists. No. 65 North Front Street, Philadelphia. Philadelphia: Mifflin and Parry, prs., 1828. 24p. PHi **20-0627**

WHILLDIN, John Galloway
An essay on the nature and treatment of that state of disorder generally called dropsy. . . . Philadelphia: Printed for the author by William Fry, 1820. 35p. DNLM; MBM; PPAmP; PPC **20-0628**

WHITLAW, Charles
Reply of Dr. Hosack's inaugural address delivered before the Medical Society of the County of New York, on the 12th day of July, 1824. Philadelphia, 1825. 48p. DLC; MB: PHi; ScC
20-0629

WHITRIDGE, J. B.
Remarks on fractures, embracing a description of an improved apparatus for their treatment. . . . Boston: Wells & Lilly, 1827. 21p. NNNAM **20-0630**

WILLIAMS COLLEGE. BERKSHIRE MEDICAL INSTITUTION
[Course of study] Pittsfield: Pr. by Phinehas Allen [1823] 12p. DLC **20-0631**

WILLIAMS, John
Dr. John Williams' last legacy; or, The useful family herbal. Pr. for the vendor. Little Falls, N.Y.: Griffing's Press, 1829. 22p. NHi; PPC **20-0632**

WILLIAMS, Stephen West (1790-1855)
A biographical memoir of Josiah Goodhue, M.D., late president of the Berkshire Medical Institution, delivered at the close of an introductory lecture, on the 20 of November, 1829. Pittsfield: Pr. by Phinehas Allen & Son [1829?] 20p. MWA
20-0633

WILLISON, John
The afflicted man's companion, or A directory for persons and families afflicted with sickness or any other distress. New York: American Tract Society, 1827. 343p. NN; NHi
20-0634

WILSON, John T. J.
An address to the KA Society of Hippocrates; delivered January 6th, 1823. Lexington, Ky.: Pr. by Thomas T. Skillman, 1823. 11p. KU; KyLoJM **20-0635**

WISTAR, Caspar (1761-1818)
A system of anatomy for the use of students of medicine. . . . 3rd ed. With notes and additions by William E. Horner . . . pub. by Moore; Philadelphia: Pr. by J. Harding, 1823. 2 v. ICJ; PPC; PU **20-0636**

WISTAR, Caspar (1761-1818)
A system of anatomy for the use of students of medicine. 3rd ed. Philadelphia: Pub. by H. C. Carey & I. Lea, 1825. 2 v. MA; MB; MdBM; PPC **20-0637**

WISTAR, Caspar (1761-1818)
A system of anatomy for the use of students of medicine. . . . 4th ed. Philadelphia: Carey, Lea & Carey, 1827. 2 v. ICJ; NNNAM; PPC **20-0638**

WOOD, George B[acon] (1797-1879)
A oration delivered before the Philadelphia Medical Society. . . . Feb. 14, 1824. Philadelphia: Pub. by order of the Society, Jesper Harding, pr. 1824. 32p. IEN-M; N; NNNAM; PHi
20-0639

YOUNG, David
The New York medical almanac, and repository of useful science and amusement for 1825. New York: John C. Totten [1824] 18p. MWA **20-0640**

YOUNG, David
The New York medical almanac, and repository of useful science and amusement for 1826. New York: Samuel Marks [1825] 18p. MWA **20-0641**

YOUNG, David
The New York medical almanac, and repository of useful science and amusement for 1827. New York: Samuel Marks [1826] 18p. MWA; NjR **20-0642**

YOUNG, David
The Pennsylvania medical almanac and repository of useful science for 1827. Philadelphia: Pr. for the proprietor [1826] 18p. MWA **20-0643**

ZOLLICKOFFER, William (1793-1853)
A treatise on the use of Prussiate of iron, (or, Prussian blue) in intermitting and remitting fevers. Frederick, Md.: Pr. by Samuel Barnes, 1822. 32p. MdBM; N; PPAmP
20-0644

ZOLLICKOFFER, William (1793-1853)
A materia medica, of the United States, systematically arranged. . . . 2nd ed., with emendations, &c. Baltimore: J. Lovegrove, 1827. Wm. Wooddy, pr. 245p. MdBM; PPC; PU
20-0645

II. AMERICAN MEDICAL IMPRINTS, 1830-1839

The present undertaking was suggested by the frequent complaints, made by the author's pupils, that they were unable to meet with information on numerous topics of professional inquiry, —especially of recent introduction, —in the medical dictionaries accessible to them.

It may, indeed, be correctly affirmed, that we have no dictionary of medical subjects and terms which can be looked upon as adapted to the state of the science. In proof of this the author need but to remark, that he has found occasion to add several thousand medical terms, which are not to be met with in the only medical lexicon at this time in circulation in the country.

Robley Dunglison,
*Dictionary of Medical
Science and Literature*
(1833)

ABERCROMBIE, John (1780-1844)
Pathological and practical researches on diseases of the stomach, the intestinal canal, the liver, and other viscera of the abdomen. Philadelphia: Carey & Lea; E. & G. Merriam, printer, 1830. 416p. CU-M; DNLM; ICJ; MB
30-0001

ABERCROMBIE, John (1780-1844)
Pathological and practical researches on diseases of the brain and the spinal cord. . . . 1st American from the 2nd Edinburgh ed., enl. Philadelphia: Carey & Lea, 1831. 464p. DLC; ICJ; MH
30-0002

ABERCROMBIE, John (1780-1844)
Pathological and practical researches on the diseases of the stomach, the intestinal canal, the liver, and other viscera of the abdomen. 3rd American from the 2nd London ed., enl. Philadelphia: Carey, Lea and Blanchard, 1838. 320p. DLC; GU; PPC; NIC **30-0003**

ABERNETHY, John (1764-1831)
Lectures on the theory and practice of surgery. New York: C. S. Francis. . . . Munroe & Francis; Boston [Clayton & Van Norden, printer] 1830. 191p. PU **30-0004**

ABERNETHY, John (1764-1831)
Surgical observations on the constitutional origin and treatment of local diseases and on aneurisms. Boston: Stimpson & Clapp, 1832. 140p. MBM **30-0005**

ACADEMIE DE MEDECINE, PARIS
Report of the Royal Academy of Medicine, to the Minister of the Interior, upon the cholera-morbus. Pub. by order of the French Government. Transl. from the French by John W. Sterling. . . . New York: Samuel Wood and Sons, 1832. 234p. DLC; MBM; NNNAM **30-0006**

ACKERLY, George
On the management of children in sickness and in health. 2nd ed., enl. New York: Published for the author by Bancroft & Holley, 1836. 78p. DNLM; NN; NNU-M
30-0007

ACKERLY, George
On the management of children in sickness and in health. 3rd ed. New York: Published for the author by Bancroft & Holley, 1836. 78p. DLC; NN; NNU-M; OCHP
30-0008

AFFECTING scenes; being passages from the diary of a physician. New York: J. and J. Harper, 1833. 2 v. MH; MWA; NN
30-0009

ALCOTT, William Andrus (1798-1859)
The young mother, or Management of children in regard to health. . . . 2nd ed. Boston: Light & Stearns, 1836. 322p. DLC; KU; MBM; PPC **30-0010**

ALCOTT, William Andrus (1798-1859)
An address delivered before the American Physiological Society, March 7, 1837. Boston: Light & Stearns, 1837. 36p. MBM; MH-M; MWA **30-0011**

ALCOTT, William Andrus (1798-1859)
Vegetable diet: as sanctioned by medical men, and by experience in all ages. . . . Boston: Marsh, Capen & Lyon, 1838. 276p. CU-M; MBM; MH-M; PPC **30-0012**

ALCOTT, William Andrus (1798-1859)
Dosing and drugging; or destroying by inches. Boston: New York: G. W. Light, 1839. 52p. DLC; NN; NNNAM; PU
30-0013

ALCOTT, William Andrus (1798-1859)
Breathing bad air. . . . Boston: G. W. Light, 1839. 56p. DNLM
30-0014

The AMERICAN gentleman's medical pocket-book and health adviser . . . by the author of The lady's medical pocket-book. Philadelphia: J. Kay, Jr. and Brother; Pittsburgh: J. I. Kay and Co., 1833. 254p. CSmH; NNC **30-0015**

The AMERICAN lady's medical pocket-book, and nursery-adviser: containing rules for preserving the health of unmarried females; directions to pregnant and lying-in-women; and an account of their diseases; together with instructions for the rearing of children from the hour of their birth; and an account of the diseases of infancy. By the author of The gentleman's medical pocket-book. Philadelphia: J. Kay, Jr. and Brother; Pittsburgh: J. I. Kay and Co., [c1833]. 296p. DLC; IEN-M; MBM
30-0016

AMUSSAT, Jean Zuléma (1796-1856)
Amussat's lessons on retention of urine, caused by strictures of the urethra, and on the diseases of the prostate. Ed. by A. Petit. . . . Transl. from the French, by James P. Jervey, M.D. With notes. Charleston, S.C.: D. J. Dowling, printer, 1836. 246p. DLC; ScC; ScM **30-0017**

[ANATOMY]
The pocket anatomist: being a summary description of the muscles; with a tabular view of the arteries and nerves. Concordant with "The Dublin Dissector" and "Harrison on the Arteries." Philadelphia: J. Kay, Jr. & Bro., 1836. 63p. DNLM; PPHa; PPJ **30-0018**

ANDERSON, Thomas A.
The practical monitor, for the preservations of health, and the prevention of diseases. 1st ed. Pub. and sold by Z. Jayne, of Philadelphia, Monroe County, Tennessee. Knoxville, T[enn.]: F. S. Heiskell, 1831. 253p. CtY-M; DLC; DNLM
30-0019

ANDERSON, Thomas A.
The female's practical monitor, or Guide to health. . . . 1st ed. Pub. and sold by Z. Jayne, of Philadelphia, Monroe County, T. Nelson & Harding, prs. Knoxville, T., 1832. 118p. LNT-M; KU; KyLoJM; MBM **30-0020**

ANDERSON, Thomas A.
An outline of the various means and methods heretofore used for the radical cure of hernia: with an account of a new operation and plan of cure, illustrated with cases. Madisonville: Johnston & Edwards, 1835. 31p. DNLM; OClWHi
30-0021

ANDRAL, Gabriel (1797-1876)
A treatise on pathological anatomy. . . . Transl. from the French by Richard Townsend . . . and William West. . . . New York: S. Wood & Sons, 1832. 2 v. DLC; MH; Nh; PP
30-0022

ANDRAL, Gabriel (1797-1876)
The medical clinic. . . . Condensed and translated by D. Spillan; containing diseases of the encephalon, with extracts from Ollivier's work on diseases of the spinal chord and its membranes. [Dunglison's American Medical Library] Philadelphia: Barrington & Haswell, 1838. 299p. DNLM
30-0023

ANNAN, Samuel (1797-1868)
An address delivered to the graduates of Washington Medical College, Baltimore, at the annual commencement, March 17, 1834. Baltimore: J. D. Toy, 1834. 14p. DNLM
30-0024

ARMSTRONG, John (1784-1829)
Lectures on the morbid anatomy, nature, and treatment, of acute and chronic diseases; . . . Edited by Joseph Rix. . . . 1st American ed.: with an account of the life and writings of Dr. Armstrong, by John Bell. . . . Philadelphia: Desilver, Thomas & Co., 1837. 2 v. DLC; DNLM; MBM; PPC
30-0025

ARMSTRONG, John (1784-1829)
Lectures on the morbid anatomy, nature, and treatment of acute and chronic diseases. . . . Edited by Joseph Rix. . . . Philadelphia: Haswell & Barrington, 1837. 687p. DNLM
30-0026

ARNOTT, Neil (1788-1874)
Elements of physics or natural philosophy, general and medical. . . . 1st American from the 3rd London ed., with additions by Isaac Hays. Illustrated. Philadelphia: Carey & Lea, 1831. 2 v. DNLM; PPC; PPJ; ScC **30-0027**

ARNOTT, Neil (1788-1874)
Elements of physics or natural philosophy, general and medical. . . . 3rd American from the last London ed. Philadelphia: Lea and Blanchard, 1838. 2 v. DNLM; PPC; PPJ; ScC
30-0028

ATKINS, Dudley (1798-1845)
Reports of hospital physicians, and other documents in relation to the epidemic cholera of 1832. . . . New York: G. & C. & H. Carvill, 1832. 200p. CtY-M; DLC; MBM
30-0029

ATKINS, Dudley (1798-1845)
Medical and surgical cases and observations. . . . New York: P. Hill, 1834. 127p. DLC; NN; NNNAM
30-0030

ATKINSON, James (1759-1839)
Medical bibliography. New York: Gazette office. Bellerby, 1833. 379p. DLC; NN **30-0031**

AVERY, S. W.
The dyspeptic's monitor; or The nature, causes , and cure of the diseases called dyspepsia, indigestion, liver complaint . . . etc. New York: E. Bliss, 1830. 152p. GU; MWA; PPC
30-0032

AVERY, S. W.
The dyspeptic's monitor; or the nature, causes and cure of the diseases called dyspepsia, indigestion, liver complaint . . . etc. 2nd ed. New York: E. Bliss, 1830. 164p. MA
30-0033

AYDELOTT, B[enjamin] P[arham]
The medical student's danger and means of safety; A discourse preached in Christ Church, Cincinnati, January 9, 1831. . . . Cincinnati: Pr. by J. Whetstone, Jr., 1831. 12p. NNNAM; ScCM **30-0034**

BAKER, Joseph
The natural physician's book of remedies, containing a patent right for doctoring. 2nd ed. Chillicothe, O.: 1832. 172, 16p. N; OCLloyd; OCIWHi **30-0035**

BAKER, Samuel George (1814-1841)
. . . An introductory lecture, delivered before the medical class of the University [Maryland], November, 1837. Baltimore: J. D. Toy, 1837. 32p. DNLM **30-0036**

BAKER, William N. (1811-1841)
A lecture introductory to a course on anatomy, physiology, . . . delivered November 21, 1834. Baltimore: Carey, Hart & Co., 1834. 22p. DNLM; MdU-D; PPL
30-0037

BALDWIN, Loammi
Report on the subject of introducing pure water into the city of Boston. Boston: J. H. Eastburn, 1834. 78p. DNLM; MWA
30-0038

BARBER, Jonathan (1784-1864)
An address delivered before the Boston Phrenological Society, on the evening of its organization. . . . Boston: Marsh, Capen & Lyon, 1833. 44p. DLC; MBAt; MWA
30-0039

[BARTLETT, Elisha] (1804-1855)
Sketches of the character and writings of eminent living surgeons and physicians of Paris. Translated from the French of J[ean] L[ouis] H[ippolyte] P[eisse]. Boston, 1831. 131p. CtY-M; MB; MBM; PPC **30-0040**

BARTLETT, Elisha (1804-1855)
The "laws of sobriety," and "the temperance reform": an address delivered before the Young men's temperance society in Lowell, March 8, 1835. . . . Published by the Society. Lowell: Printed by Dearborn & Bellows [1835]. 23p. DLC; MA; MB; MWA **30-0041**

BARTLETT, Elisha (1804-1855)
Obedience to the laws of health, a moral duty. A lecture, delivered before the American Physiological Society, January 30, 1838. . . . Boston: J. A. Noble [1838]. 24p. DLC; MB; MBM; MH **30-0042**

BARTLETT, Elisha (1804-1855)
An address delivered at the anniversary celebration of the birth of Spurzheim, and the organization of the Boston Phrenological Society, January 1, 1838. . . . Boston: Marsh, Capen and Lyon, 1838. 28p. DLC; MB; MBM; MH
30-0043

BARTLETT, John Stephen
The Physician's pocket synopsis: conveying an accurate and concise view of the history, character, symptoms, and treatment of the various medical and surgical diseases incident to the human frame. . . . 2nd ed., revised, and brought down to the present time by Henry Coley. New York: G. & C. & H. Carvill, 1833. 709p. DNLM; MB **30-0044**

BARTLETT, John Stephen
A letter to the president, counsellors, and fellows of the Massachusetts Medical Society on their anniversary, May 31, 1837. Boston, 1834. 12p. DNLM **30-0045**

BARTLEY, Horatio
Illustrations of cholera, asphyxia in its different stages. Selected from cases treated at the cholera hospital, Rivington Street. New York: S. H. Jackson, 1832. 11p. DNLM; NN **30-0046**

BARTON, Edward H[all] (*d.* 1859)
Account of the epidemic yellow fever which prevailed in New Orleans during the autumn of 1833. Philadelphia: J. R. A. Skerrett, 1834. 52p., 13 tab. DNLM; LNT-M; PPC; PU **30-0047**

BARTON, Edward H[all] (*d.* 1859)
Introductory lecture on acclimation, delivered at the opening of the third session of the Medical College of Louisiana. Published at the request of the class. New Orleans: Com. Bulletin Print., 1837. 17p. DNLM; LNT-M **30-0048**

BARTON, J. Rhea (1794-1871)
New treatment for certain cases of anchylosis. Philadelphia: E. G. Dorsey, 1838. 8p. DNLM **30-0049**

BARTON, William P. C. (1787-1856)
Prodrome of a work to aid teaching of the vegetable materia medica, by the natural families of plants, in the Therapeutic Institute of Philadelphia. 1833. 104p. DNLM **30-0050**

BAUDELOCQUE, Auguste César (1795-1851)
Treatise on puerperal peritonitis, . . . to which was awarded the prize by the Royal Society of Medicine of Bordeaux. Translated from the French by G. S. Bedford. . . . New York: Pr. by Elliott & Palmer for Collins and Hannay [etc.] 1831. 480p. DLC; MA; RPM **30-0051**

BAYLE, Antoine Laurent Jeané (1799-1858)
An elementary treatise on anatomy. Transl. from the 4th ed of the French. By A. Sidney Doane. . . . New York: Harper & Brothers, 1837. 470p. MWA; PPL; N; ViRA **30-0052**

BEACH, Wooster (1794-1868)
The American Practice of Medicine; being a treatise on character, causes, symptoms, morbid appearances and treatment of disease, on vegetable and botanic principles. . . . New York: Betts and Anstice, 1832. 3 v. PPHa **30-0053**

BEACH, Wooster (1794-1868)
The American Practice of Medicine; being a treatise on the character, causes, symptoms, morbid appearances and treatment of the diseases of men, women and children . . . the vegetable or botanical principles. . . . New York: Betts and Anstice, 1833. 3 v. DNLM; PPHa; PPL **30-0054**

BEAUMONT, William (1785-1853)
The physiology of digestion with experiments on the gastric juice. . . . Plattsburgh, N.Y.: Chauncey Goodrich, 1833? 280p. MWA; N; NN **30-0055**

BEAUMONT, William (1785-1853)
Experiments and observations on the gastric juice and the physiology of digestion. Plattsburgh, N.Y.: F. P. Allen, 1833. 280p. CU-M; ICJ; KyLoJM **30-0056**

BEAUMONT, William (1785-1853)
Experiments and observations on the gastric juice, and the physiology of digestion. . . . Boston: Lilly, Wait, and Company, 1834. 280p. DLC; MBM; MH; MWA **30-0057**

BECK, John Brodhead (1794-1851)
An introductory lecture, delivered at the College of Physicians and Surgeons of the City of New York, Nov. 5, 1830. New York: G. & C. & H. Carvill, 1830. 30p. DLC; DNLM; MdBM; NNNAM **30-0058**

BECK, John Brodhead (1794-1851)
A letter on the establishment of a new medical school in connection with Columbia College. . . . New York: Pr. by G. P. Scott & Co., successors to J. Seymour, 1832. 8p. MB; NNN **30-0059**

BECK, John Brodhead (1794-1851)
Researches in medicine and medical jurisprudence. . . . 2nd ed. New York: E. Bliss, 1835. 258p. DLC; DNLM; ICJ; PPC **30-0060**

BECK, John Brodhead (1794-1851)
Valedictory address to the students in medicine of the College of Physicians and Surgeons of the University of the State of New York. New York: W. E. Dean, 1839. 24p. DNLM; NNNAM **30-0061**

BECK, Lewis C. (1798-1853)
A manual of chemistry . . . intended as a text book for medical schools. 3rd ed. New York: W. E. Dean, 1838. 482p. DNLM; NNNAM **30-0062**

BECK, Theodoric Romeyn (1791-1855)
Elements of medical jurisprudence. By Theodoric Romeyn Beck . . . and John B. Beck. . . . 5th ed. . . . Pub. by O. Steele [etc.] Albany; R. and G. S. Wood [etc.] New York; Desilver and Thomas, Philadelphia. Albany: Printed by Packard and Van Benthuysen, 1835. 2 v. DLC; N; NN **30-0063**

BECK, Theodoric Romeyn (1791-1855)
Statistics of the medical colleges of the United States. Albany: J. Munsell, 1839. 64p. N; NN; NNNAM **30-0064**

BÈCLARD, Pierre Auguste (1785-1825)
Elements of general anatomy; or, A description of every kind of organ composing the human body. . . . Preceded by a critical biographical memoir of the life and writings of the author, by Oliver, M.D. Transl. from the French, with notes by Joseph Togno. Philadelphia: Carey & Lea, 1830. 541p. ICJ; KU; PPC **30-0065**

BEDFORD, Gunning S. (1806-1870)
Eulogy on the late James M. Pendleton, M.D. Delivered by appointment of the New York City and County Medical Society, in the hall of Columbia College, February 9th, 1832. . . . New York: Pr. by J. Watt, 1832. 16p. DLC; NN; OCHP **30-0066**

BEDFORD, Gunning S. (1806-1870)
An address introductory to a course of lectures delivered in the hall of the Medical College of South Carolina, before the trustees and faculty, the students of medicine, and the public generally, at the opening of the session of 1833-4. Charleston: J. S. Burges, 1833. DLC; MH-M; PU; ScC
30-0067

BEDFORD, Gunning S. (1806-1870)
An address, introductory to a course of lectures delivered in Clinton Hall, New York, November 8, 1834. New York: J. M. Elliott, 1834. 29p. DLC; NN; NNNAM
30-0068

BEDFORD, Gunning S. (1806-1870)
An address, introductory to a course of lectures. . . . 2nd ed. New York: J. M. Elliott, 1835. 29p. DNLM; NNNAM
30-0069

BEDFORD, Gunning S. (1806-1870)
An address, introductory to a course of lectures November 15, 1835. New York: J. M. Elliott, 1836. 32p. DNLM; NNNAM
30-0070

BEDFORD, Gunning S. (1806-1870)
Introductory lecture before the Albany Medical College, delivered October 1, 1839. Albany: J. Munsell, 1839. 23p. N; NN; NNU-M; PPAmP **30-0071**

BÉGIN, Louis Jacques (1793-1859)
Application of the physiological doctrine to surgery: . . . Transl. from the French by Wm. Sims Reynolds. Charleston: Printed by E. J. Van Brunt, 1835. 227p. CU-M; DLC; PPHa; ScCM **30-0072**

BELINAYE, Henry George
Sources of health & disease in communities; or, Elementary views of hygiene, illustrating its importance to legislators, heads of families, etc. Boston: Allen & Ticknor, 1833. 160p. CtY-M; DLC; PPJ **30-0073**

BELL, Charles (1774-1842)
Engravings of the arteries, illustrating the second volume of the anatomy of the human body, and serving as an introduction to the surgery of the arteries. Third American ed., corrected. Philadelphia: A. Finley, 1833. 64p. CU-M; MH; RPM
30-0074

BELL, Charles (1774-1842)
The nervous system of the human body; embracing the papers delivered to the Royal Society on the subject of the nerves. . . . Washington: Stereotyped by D. Green, for the Register and Library of medical and chirurgical science, 1833. 230p. DLC; NN; PPC **30-0075**

BELL, Charles (1774-1842)
The hand, its mechanism and vital endowments as evincing design. . . . Philadelphia: Carey, Lea & Blanchard, 1833. 213p. (Half-title: The Bridgewater treatise on the power, wisdom, and goodness of God as manifested in the creation. Treatise IV). DLC; PP; PPC **30-0076**

BELL, Charles (1774-1842)
A series of engravings explaining the course of the nerves. . . . With an address to young physicians on the study of the nerves. 2nd American ed. Philadelphia: A Finley, 1834. 47p. DNLM **30-0077**

BELL, Charles (1774-1842)
The hand, it mechanism and vital endowments, as evincing design. . . . New ed. Philadelphia: Carey, Lea & Blanchard, 1836. 147p. (Half-title: The Bridgewater treatise on the power, wisdom and goodness of God, as manifested in the creation. Treatise IV). DLC; MH; NNC; NcD **30-0078**

BELL, John (1796-1872)
An address delivered at Nashville, T., October 5, 1830, being the first anniversary of the Alumni Society of the University of Nashville. Nashville: Hunt, Tardiff & Co., 1830. 37p. DNLM **30-0079**

BELL, John (1796-1872)
On baths and mineral waters. . . . Philadelphia: H. H. Porter, 1831. 582p. DLC; ICRM; PPC; PU
30-0080

BELL, John (1796-1872)
All the material facts in the history of epidemic cholera: being a report of the College of Physicians of Philadelphia, to the Board of Health; and a full account of the causes, post mortem appearances, and treatment of the disease. By John Bell . . . and by D. Francis Condie. . . . Philadelphia: T. Desilver, Jr., 1832. 127p. PU; RPM **30-0081**

BELL, John (1796-1872)
All the material facts in the history of epidemic cholera: being a report of the College of Physicians of Philadelphia, to the Board of Health: and a full account of the causes, post mortem appearances, and treatment of the disease. By John Bell . . . and by D. Francis Condie. . . . 2nd ed. Philadelphia: Thomas Desilver, Jr., 1832. DLC; KU; NcD; PP
30-0082

BELL, John (1796-1872)
An address to the Medical students' temperance society, of the University of Pennsylvania, . . . [Philadelphia, 1833?] 10p. NN; PPPrHi; PHi **30-0083**

BELL, John (1796-1872)
Health and beauty. An explanation of the laws of growth and exercise; through which a pleasing contour, symmetry of form, and graceful carriage of the body are acquired. . . . Philadelphia: E. L. Carey & A. Hart, 1838. 253p. DLC; PPC; PPHa; PPPH **30-0084**

BELL, John (1763-1820) and Charles BELL (1774-1842)
The anatomy and physiology of the human body, containing the anatomy of the bones, muscles, and joints, and the heart and arteries, by John Bell; and the anatomy and physiology of the brain and nerves, the organs of the senses, and the viscera, by Charles Bell. The 6th American from the last London ed. . . . Ed. by John D. Godman. New York: Collins & Co., 1834. 2 v. DNLM; NNNAM **30-0085**

BELL, Luther Vose (1806-1862)
A dissertation on the Boylston prize question for 1835: "What diet can be selected which will ensure the greatest probable health and strength to the laborer in the climate of New England? Quantity and quality, and the time and manner of taking it, to be considered." . . . Boston: D. Clapp, Jr., 1836. 46p. DLC; MA; MB; MBM **30-0086**

BELL, Luther Vose (1806-1862)
An attempt to investigate some obscure and undecided doctrines in relation to small-pox, varioloid and vaccination. . . . Boston: Marsh, Capen and Lyon, 1836. 72p. DLC; MB; MBM; MWA **30-0087**

BELL, Thomas (1792-1880)
The anatomy, physiology and diseases of the teeth. Philadelphia: Carey and Lea [William Sharpless, pr.] 1830. 352p. CU-M; MdBJ-W; NNNAM **30-0088**

BELL, Thomas (1792-1880)
The anatomy, physiology and diseases of the teeth. 2nd ed. . . . Philadelphia: Carey & Lea, 1831. 351p. MB; MH **30-0089**

BELL, Thomas (1792-1880)
The anatomy, physiology and diseases of the teeth. 3rd American ed., with numerous plates. Philadelphia: Carey, Lea & Blanchard, 1837. 351p. DNLM; NNNAM; MdBJ-W **30-0090**

BERTIN, René Joseph Hyacinthe (1757-1828)
Treatise on the diseases of the heart and great vessels. . . . Ed. by Jean Bouillaud. . . . Transl. from the French by C. W. Chauncy. Philadelphia: Carey, Lea & Blanchard, 1833. 449p. DLC; NcD **30-0091**

BIGELOW, Jacob (1787-1879)
A discourse on self-limited diseases. Delivered before the Massachusetts Medical Society, at their annual meeting, May 27, 1835. . . . Boston: N. Hale, 1835. 48p. DLC; MB; MBM; MH **30-0092**

BILLARD, Charles Michel (1800-1832)
A treatise on the diseases of infants, founded on recent clinical observtions and investigations in pathological anatomy, made at the Hospice des enfans-trouvés: with a dissertation on the viability of the child. . . . With notes, by Dr. Ollivier. . . . Transl. from the 3rd French ed., with an appendix, by James Stewart, M.D. New York: G. Adlard; [etc., etc.] 1839. 620p. DLC; MBAt; PPPrHi; ScU **30-0093**

BILLING, Archibald (1791-1881)
First principles of medicine. Philadelphia: Pr. by O. S. Cooke & Co., 1831. 246p. DNLM; PU; ScC **30-0094**

BINAGHI, O. A.
Opinion upon the epidemic choleramorbus observed at Warsaw. Transl. from the Italian by Wm. Sampson, New York: P. Hill, 1832. 27p. DLC; NN; RPM; ScU **30-0095**

BIRD, F. William (1809-1894)
Physiological reform. An address. . . . Boston: Marsh, Capen & Lyon, 1837. 48p. DNLM; MBM **30-0096**

BLAKE, Andrew
A practical essay on the disease generally known under the denomination of delirium tremens. . . . Washington: D. Green, 1834. 24p. DNLM **30-0097**

BLANE, Gilbert (1749-1834)
Elements of medical logick. . . . Hartford: Huntington & Hopkins, 1832. 319p. DLC; MH-M; MdU-D **30-0098**

BLOEDE, Karl August
Dr. F. J. Gall's system of the function of the brain. New York: 1830. 92p. NNC; NNNAM; PHi **30-0099**

BLUNDELL, James (1790-1878)
The principles and practice of obstetricy, as at present taught. . . . To which are added, notes and illustrations. By Thomas Castle. . . . Washington, D. Green, 1834. 520p. DLC; MdBJ-W; NNNAM **30-0100**

BOISSEAU, François Gabriel (1791-1836)
A treatise on cholera morbus; or, Researches on the symptoms, nature, and treatment of the disease; and on the different means of avoiding it. . . . Transl. from the French, by G. S. Bedford. . . . New York: Collins & Co., 1832. 148p. IEN-M; IU-M; LNT-M; MBM **30-0101**

BOISSEAU, François Gabriel (1791-1836)
Physiological pyretology; or, A treatise on fevers: according to the principles of the new medical doctrine. [1st American from the 4th French ed. Transl. by J. R. Knox.] . . . Philadelphia: Carey & Lea, 1832. 504p. CU-M; GU; NjR; PPC **30-0102**

The BOOK of health; a compendium of domestic medicine, deduced from the experience of the most eminent modern practitioners. . . . 1st American from the second London ed. Boston: Richardson, Lord & Holbrook, 1830. 9, 179p. ICJ; MB; MWA; NNNAM **30-0103**

BOUILLAUD, Jean Baptiste (1796-1881)
New researches on acute articular rheumatism in general; and especially on the law of coincidence of pericarditis and endocarditis with this disease, as well as on the efficacy of the method of treating it by repeated bloodlettings at short intervals. . . . Transl. by James Kitchen, M.D. Philadelphia: Haswell, Barrington, and Haswell, 1837. 64p. DLC; PPC; PU **30-0104**

BOURGERY, Jean Marc (1797-1849)
A treatise on lesser surgery, or, the minor surgical operations. Transl. from the French with notes and appendix by William C. Roberts and James B. Kissam. New York: C. S. Francis, 1834. 367p. MBM; PPHa; ScC **30-0105**

BOWEN, Isaac
A dissertation read before the Medical Society of Augusta, Georgia. On the mechanism and practicability of a new surgical bed-stead. Together with the report of a select committee on the subject. [Augusta, 1833]. 4p. GU; MH-M **30-0106**

BRICHETEAU, Isidore (1789-1862)
Medical clinics of the Hospital Necker, on researches and observations on the nature, treatment, and physical causes of disease. Transl. for the American Medical Library. Philadelphia: A. Waldie, 1837. 141p. DNLM; PPC; PU **30-0107**

BRIGHAM, Amariah (1798-1849)
A treatise on the epidemic cholera; including an historical account of its origin and progress, to the present period. Comp. from the most authentic sources. . . . Hartford: H. and F. J. Huntington, 1832. 368p. CtY-M; DLC; ViRa **30-0108**

BRIGHAM, Amariah (1798-1849)
Remarks on the influence of mental cultivation and mental excitement upon health. Hartford: F. J. Huntington, 1832. 116p. MB; PPC; RPJCB **30-0109**

BRIGHAM, Amariah (1798-1849)
Remarks on the influence of mental cultivation and mental excitement upon health. 2nd ed. Boston: Marsh, Capen & Lyon, 1833. 130p. MB; MBM; PPC; RPJCB **30-0110**

BRIGHAM, Amariah (1798-1849)
Observations on the influence of religion upon the health and physical welfare of mankind. Boston: Marsh, Capen & Lyon, 1835, 331p. MBM; MH; MWA; NN **30-0111**

BRODIE, Benjamin Collins (1783-1862)
Pathological and surgical observations on the diseases of the joints. . . . 3rd ed., with alterations and additions. Washington: D. Green, 1834. 131p. DLC; MdBJ-W; PPC; PU
30-0112

BROUSSAIS, François Joseph Victor (1772-1838)
On irritation and insanity; a work, wherein the relations of the physical with the moral conditions of man, are established on the basis of physiological medicine. . . . transl. by Thomas Cooper . . . to which are added two tracts on materialism, and an outline of the association of ideas. By Thomas Cooper. . . . Columbia, S.C.: Pr. by S. J. M'Morris, 1831. 408p. MBM; PU; ScU **30-0113**

BROUSSAIS, François Joseph Victor (1772-1838)
History of Chronic phlegmasiae or inflammations founded on clinical experience and pathological anatomy . . . transl. from the French of the 4th ed. by Isaac Hays . . . and R. Eglesfeld Griffith. Philadelphia: Carey & Lea, 1831. 2 v. PU; ScC
30-0114

BROUSSAIS, François Joseph Victor (1772-1838)
A treatise on physiology applied to pathology. . . . Transl. from the French, by John Bell, M.D. . . . and R. LaRoche, M.D. 3rd American ed. Philadelphia: Carey & Lea, 1832. DLC; MBM; OCHP; ViRA **30-0115**

BROUSSAIS, François Joseph Victor (1772-1838)
Principles of physiological medicine, in the form of propositions; embracing physiology, pathology, and therapeutics, with commentaries on those relating to pathology. . . . Transl. from the French by Isaac Hays, M.D., and R. Eglesfeld Griffith. . . . Philadelphia: Carey & Lea, 1832. 594p. ICJ; PPC
30-0116

BROUSSAIS, François Joseph Victor (1772-1838)
Cholera. Two clinical lectures upon the nature, treatment and symptoms, of spasmodic cholera. . . . Delivered during the prevalence of the disease in Paris. [Transl. by John S. Bartlett] New York: W. Stodart, 1832. 28p. IEN-M; MB; NNN
30-0117

BROWN, Benjamin Boyer
Notes on various subjects connected with medicine. . . . Philadelphia, 1830. [Philadelphia] 1832. 185 [29]p. DLC; PU; PPF **30-0118**

BROWN, John A.
Quackery Exposed!!! or a few Remarks on the Thomsonian System of Medicine; consisting of Testimonies and Extracts from various writers. With Introductory Remarks. . . . Boston, 1833. 22p. DLC; ICJ; MWA; OCHP **30-0119**

BROWN, John A.
The family guide to health, containing a description of the botanic Thomsonian system of medicine. With a biographical sketch of the author. . . . Providence: B. T. Albro, printer, 1837. 234p. DLC; RHi; RPB; RPM **30-0120**

BROWN, John A.
Supplement to the Family guide to health: containing directions for compounding botanic medicines. Also some remarks on the subject of midwifery. . . . Providence: B. T. Albro, printer, 1837. 32p. DLC; DNLM; PPHa; ScC
30-0121

BROWN, John Ball (1784-1862)
Two letters on curvature of the spine. Boston: D. Clapp, Jr., 1838. 12p. DNLM; MBM **30-0122**

BROWN, John Ball (1784-1862)
Remarks on the operation for the cure of club-feet, with cases. Also, letters to John C. Warren on curvature of the spine. Boston: D. Clapp, Jr., 1839. 27p. DNLM; MBM; MH-M
30-0123

BROWN, Matthew (1776-1853)
Address to the graduates of Jefferson College, delivered on the day of commencement, September 27, 1838. . . . Washington: Printed by U. W. Wise, 1839. 10p. DLC; PPJ
30-0124

BROWN, Solyman (1790-1876)
Dentologia, a poem on the diseases of the teeth, and their proper remedies. With notes, practical, historical, illustrative, and explanatory, by Eleazer Parmly. New York: Peabody & Co., 1833. 176p. CSmH; RPB **30-0125**

BRUNNOW, Ernest Georg
A concise view of the principles of homeopathia, with introductory remarks in presenting this exposition, in English, to the New York Homoeopathic Society, by John L. Sullivan. New York: H. Ludwig. 1835. 34pp. DLC; PPHa [See **30-0861**]
30-0126

BRYANT, Thomas Sydenham
Examinations in anatomy and physiology; being a complete series of quotations and answers . . . to which are annexed, tables of the bones, muscles, and arteries. . . . Philadelphia: Printed for the author, 1835. 404p. DLC; PPC; PU
30-0127

BUCHAN, William (1729-1805)
Domestic Medicine, or A treatise on the prevention and cure of diseases, by regimen and simple medicines: . . . Exeter: J. & B. Williams, 1832. 495p. NN; Nh **30-0128**

BUCHAN, William (1729-1805)
Domestic medicine, or A treatise on the prevention and cure of diseases, by regimen and simple medicines: with observations on sea-bathing, and the use of the mineral waters. To which is annexed, a dispensatory for the use of private practitioners. From the 22nd English ed., with considerable additions, and notes. Exeter [N.H.]: J. & B. Williams, 1834. 495p. DLC; MH; MSaE; MWA **30-0129**

BURDEKIN, Richard
An historical account of the plague and other pestilential distempers, which have appeared in Europe, more especially England, from the earliest period. . . . New York [1832] 78p. MBM **30-0130**

BURNS, John (1774-1850)
The principles of midwifery: including the diseases of women and children. . . . From the 7th London ed., rev. and enl., with additions. . . . New York: C. S. Francis; Boston: Munroe & Francis, 1831. 754p. DLC; NNNAM; PPC
30-0131

BURNS, John (1774-1850)
The principles of midwifery: including the diseases of women and children. . . . From the 7th London edition, revised and enlarged with improvements and notes by T. C. James. New York: C. S. Francis, 1831. 798p. GU; NNNAM; NNU-M
30-0132

BURNS, John (1774-1850)
Principles of midwifery; including the diseases of women and children. With improvements and notes by T. C. James. From 5th London ed. Philadelphia: Parker, 1832. 592p. PPC
30-0133

BURROUGH, M.
[On spasmodic cholera, in two letters]; 1. Letter addressed to David Hosack, M.D.; 2. Letter addressed to the Board of Health of Philadelphia. [Philadelphia, 1831] 8p. DNLM; MWA **30-0134**

BUSHE, George Macartney (1797?-1836)
An essay on the operation for cleft palate. New York: W. Jackson, 1835. 18p., 2 plates. DNLM NNNAM
30-0135

BUSHE, George Macartney (1797?-1836)
A treatise on the malformations, injuries, and diseases of the rectum and anus. . . . New York: French & Adlard, 1837. 209p. DLC: MBM; NN; NNNAM **30-0136**

BUSHE, George Macartney (1797?-1836)
Plates illustrating a treatise on the malformations, injuries, and diseases of the rectum and anus. . . . New York: French & Adlard, 1837. 10p., 9 plates. DLC; NN; NNNAM; NNU-M
30-0137

BUSHE, George Macartney (1797?-1836)
A catalogue of the valuable library of the late Dr. Geo. M. Bushe, comprising a selection of the best works on anatomy, surgery, and medicine, published in England, France, and the United States . . . which will be sold by auction, by Cooley & Bangs . . . July 13, 1837, and following evening. . . . [New York: W. Osborn, printer, 1837] 23p. DLC; NN
30-0138

BUTLER, Samuel Worcester (1823-1874)
A biographical sketch of the late Nathaniel Chapman, M.D., Reprinted from the New Jersey Medical Reporter. Philadelphia: Joseph M. Wilson, [T. K. and P. G. Collins, prs., 183-?] NNNAM **30-0139**

BYRNE, Barnard Myles (1807-1860)
An essay to prove the contagious character of malignant cholera; with brief instructions for its prevention and cure. . . . Baltimore: Carey, Hart & Co.; Philadelphia: E. L. Carey & A. Hart, 1833. 156p. DLC; MB; OCHP
30-0140

CALDWELL, Charles (1772-1853)
Thoughts on the original unity of the human race. New York: E. Bliss, 1830. DNLM **30-0141**

CALDWELL, Charles (1772-1853)
Thoughts on febrile miasms, intended as an answer to the Boylston medical prize question, for the year 1830, "whether fever is produced by the decomposition of animal or vegetable substances, and if by both, their comparative influence?" [n.p., 1830] 63p. DNLM **30-0142**

CALDWELL, Charles (1772-1853)
A valedictory address on some of the duties and qualifications of a physician, delivered to the graduates of the medical department of Transylvania University, on the 17th day of March, 1830. [Lexington: The University, 1830] 22p. DLC; KyLoJM **30-0143**

CALDWELL, Charles (1772-1853)
Essays on Malaria and Temperament. . . . Lexington, Ky.: Pr. by N. L. Finnell & J. F. Herndon, 1831. 300p. OC; PU
30-0144

CALDWELL, Charles (1772-1853)
. . . An essay upon the nature and sources of the malaria or noxious miasma, from which originate the family of diseases usually known by the denomination of bilious diseases; together with the best means of preventing the formation of malaria. . . . Offered as a "prize essay," according to the conditions prescribed by "The Medical and surgical faculty of Maryland, at their annual convention held in the city of Baltimore, on the 7th and 8th of June, 1830." . . . Philadelphia: Carey & Lea, 1831. 80p. DLC; PPC; PPJ; PU
30-0145

CALDWELL, Charles (1772-1853)
Thoughts on the means of preserving health in hot climates; being an introductory lecture, delivered on the 6th day of November, 1832. MdBJ-W; NN; PU **30-0146**

CALDWELL, Charles (1772-1853)
Thoughts on the true mode of improving the condition of man. Read to the Lexington Medical Society, and printed at its request. Lexington, Ky.: H. Savary & Co., 1833. 44p. DNLM; IU; PPL **30-0147**

CALDWELL, Charles (1772-1853)
An address on the vice of gambling; delivered to the medical pupils of Transylvania University, November 4, 1834. Lexington, Ky.: J. Clarke & Co., 1834. 37p. DNLM; KyLoJM
30-0148

CALDWELL, Charles (1772-1853)
Thoughts on the impolicy of multiplying schools of medicine. Lexington, Ky.: J. Clarke & Co., 1834. 35p. KU; KyLoJM; PU
30-0149

CALDWELL, Charles (1772-1853)
Thoughts on physical education: being a discourse delivered to a convention of teachers in Lexington, Ky., on the 6th & 7th of Nov., 1833. . . . Boston: Marsh, Capen & Lyon, 1834. 133p. DLC; MBM; MH **30-0150**

CALDWELL, Charles (1772-1853)
Thoughts on quarantine and other sanitary systems, being an essay which received the prize of the Boylston medical committee, of Harvard University in August, 1834. . . . Boston: Marsh, Capen & Lyon, 1834. 72p. DLC; MBM; MH; MWA
30-0151

CALDWELL, Charles (1772-1853)
Phrenology vindicated, in a series of remarks, physiological, moral and critical, on article VII, of the November number, 1834, of the "Christian Examiner," headed "Pretensions of Phrenology Examined." . . . Lexington, Ky.: J. Clarke & Co., printers, 1835. 93p. DLC; MH; OCHP
30-0152

CALDWELL, Charles (1772-1853)
A report made to the Legislature of Kentucky, on the Medical Department of Transylvania University, February 15th, 1836. Lexington, Ky.: J. Clarke & Co., 1836. 34p. KU; KyLoJM; ScMS **30-0153**

CALDWELL, Charles (1772-1853)
An inaugural address to the College of Physicians and Surgeons of the city of Lexington and the County of Fayette. Lexington, Ky.: J. Clarke & Co., 1836. 38p. DNLM; KyLoJM
30-0154

CALDWELL, Charles (1772-1853)
Thoughts on schools of medicine, their means of instruction, and modes of administration, with references to the schools of Louisville and Lexington. . . . Louisville [Ky.]: Prentice and Weissinger, 1837. 31p. DLC; GU; KU; KyLoJM
30-0155

CALDWELL, Charles (1772-1853)
A succinct view of the influence of mental cultivation of the destinies of Louisville. An introductory lecture, delivered at the opening of the Louisville Medical Institute, October 31, 1837. Louisville, Ky.: Prentice & Weissinger, 1838. 34p. DNLM; KyLoJM **30-0156**

CALDWELL, Charles (1772-1853)
A discourse commemorative of Philip Syng Physick, M.D., prepared by appointment of the faculty and class of the Louisville Medical Institute, and delivered January 12th, 1838. . . . Published by request. Louisville, Ky.: Prentice & Weissinger, 1838. 41p. DLC; DNLM; KU; KyLoJM
30-0157

CALDWELL, Charles (1772-1853)
Phrenology vindicated, and anti-phrenology unmasked. . . . New York: S. Colman, 1838. 156p. DLC: NN; NNNAM
30-0158

CALVERT, George Henry, ed. (1803-1889)
Illustrations of phrenology; being a selection of articles from the Edinburgh phrenological journal, and the Transactions of the Edinburgh phrenological society. With twenty-six wood cuts. . . . With an introduction by the editor. Baltimore: W. & J. Neal, 1832. 192p. CSmH; GU; IEN-M; PP
30-0159

[CALVERT, George Henry] (1803-1889)
A summary of phrenology, to accompany the bust approved by Dr. Spurzheim. Cambridge [Mass.] Printed by Charles Folsom, 1833. 11p. DLC; DNLM; MB; MH
30-0160

CAREY, Mathew (1760-1839)
A brief account of the malignant fever which prevailed in Philadelphia, in the year 1793. . . . 5th ed., improved. Philadelphia: Clark & Raser, prs., 1830. [13]-97p. CU-M; PHi; PPL; PU **30-0161**

CARPENTER, George W. (1802-1860)
Essays on some of the most important articles of the materia medica . . . to which is added a catalogue of medicines, surgical instruments. . . . Philadelphia: G. W. Carpenter, 1831. 226p. DLC; PU; RPM **30-0162**

CARPENTER, George Washington (1802-1860)
Essays on some of the most important articles of the materia medica, comprising a full account of all the new proximate principles . . . with remarks on the most eligible form of their exhibition; to which is added, a Catalogue of medicines, surgical instruments, &c. &c., adapted for a physician at the outset of his practice, with the doses and effects attached to each medicine, &c. &c. . . . 2nd ed. rev. and enl. Philadelphia: G. W. Carpenter, 1834. 320p. DLC; NIC; OC; PPPH
30-0163

CARPENTER, George Washington (1802-1860)
Carpenter's family medicine chest dispensatory, containing a select catalogue of drugs, chemicals, and family medicines, with the properties and doses of each article most approved of in domestic medicine. To which is appended, a concise description of diseases, with directions for the treatment of such as are unattended with serious consequences. . . . Philadelphia: G. W. Carpenter's Chemical Warehouse, 1835. 327p. DLC; PPC; PP; PPHa **30-0164**

CARSON, Joseph (1808-1876)
Address delivered to the graduates of the Philadelphia College of Pharmacy. Philadelphia: Merrihew & Thompson, 1839. 16p. DNLM **30-0165**

CARTER, Jesse
Observations on mania a potu . . . Extracted from the American Journal of the Medical Sciences, for August, 1830. Philadelphia: Pr. by Joseph R. A. Skerrett, 1830. 18p. PHi
30-0166

CARTER, Richard
Valuable vegetable medical prescriptions, for the cure of all nervous and putrid disorders. Cincinnati: Pub. by Nathaniel Lewis. Lodge, L'Hommedieu & Hammond, prs., 1830. 178p. DNLM; OCLloyd **30-0167**

CARTWRIGHT, Samuel Adolphus (1793-1863)
Some account of the Asiatic cholera, cholera asphyxia or pulseless plague; with a sketch of its pathology and treatment from the best authors, and some original remarks; also, advice, relative to its prevention on plantations, and its mitigation, premonitory symptoms and treatment should it occur. . . . Natchez, Miss.: Printed at "The Natchez" office, 1832. 34p. DLC; MB; MBM; NNNAM **30-0168**

CARTWRIGHT, Samuel Adolphus (1793-1863)
Some additional observations relative to the cholera, and a prescription for the treatment of that disease in all its stages; . . . Printed at the Natchez courier office, 1833. 8p. DLC; MB; MBM; MH-M **30-0169**

CASTLE, Thomas, ed. (1804?-1870?)
A Manual of Surgery, founded upon the principles and practice lately taught by Sir Astley Cooper, Bart. F.R.S and Joseph Henry Green, Esq. F.R.S. 4th ed., considerably enlarged, containing many additional notes from the writings of other distinguished surgeons. . . . Boston: Republished by Munroe & Francis, and Joseph H. Francis; New York: Charles S. Francis, 1831. 467p. DLC; DNLM; ScC; ViRA
30-0170

CASTLE, Thomas, ed. (1804?-1870?)
A manual of surgery, founded upon the principles and practice lately taught by Sir Astley Cooper. 3rd ed. . . . Boston: Repub. by Munroe and Francis and Charles S. Francis, 1832. 463p. GU; MBM; MH-M; NNNAM
30-0171

CAZENAVE, Pierre Louis Alphée (1795-1877)
A practical synopsis of cutaneous diseases, from the most celebrated authors, and particularly from documents afforded by the clinical lectures of Dr. Biett. . . . By A. Cazenave . . . & H. E. Schedel. . . . Transl. from the French, with notes, 2nd American ed. Philadelphia: Carey & Lea, 1832. 400p. CtY-M; NcD; PPC **30-0172**

CHANNING, William
The reformation of medical science, demanded by inductive philosophy: a discourse delivered before the "New York physicians' society," on their anniversary, November 21, 1838. . . . New York: Wiley & Putnam, 1839. 58p. DLC; MBM; NN
30-0173

CHANNING, William
The reformation of medical science demanded by inductive philosophy. . . . 2nd ed. New York: Wiley & Putnam, 1839. 58p. DNLM; NN **30-0174**

CHAPMAN, Nathaniel (1780-1853)
Elements of therapeutics and materia medica; to which are prefixed two discourses on the history and improvement of the materia medica. . . . 6th ed., enl. and rev. Philadelphia: Carey & Lea, 1831. 2 v. ICJ; MBM; PPC **30-0175**

CHAPMAN, Nathaniel (1780-1853)
Observations on a letter from Dr. N. Chapman, of Philadelphia, to Dr. W. B. Tyler, of Frederick, Md., on the subject of cholera, as appearing in Philadelphia, August, 1832. Repr. fr. Frederick Herald, 1833. 48p. MB; MBM; PHi **30-0176**

CHAPMAN, Nathaniel (1780-1853)
An introductory lecture to a course of lectures on the theory and practice of medicine, in the University of Pennsylvania: delivered at the opening of the session of 1838-39. Philadelphia: J. G. Auner, 1838. 19p. DNLM; PHi; PPL
30-0177

CHASE, Heber
Treatise on the radical cure of hernia by instruments. . . . Philadelphia: J. G. Auner, 1836. 195p. DNLM; PPC; PU
30-0178

CHASE, Heber
The final report of the committee on the Philadelphia Medical Society, on the construction of instruments and their mode of action in the radical cure of hernia. . . . Philadelphia: J. G. Auner, 1837. 243p. DNLM; NNNAM; PPC; ViRA
30-0179

CHASE, Heber
Improved surgeon's trusses, for the radical cure of hernia, or rupture. Philadelphia, 1838. 47p. DNLM; PPJ
30-0180

CHEWNING, Francis B.
Remarks on the importance of the teeth; on the diseases of the teeth and gums; and on diseases produced by diseased teeth; with their modes of cure; . . . Richmond: Printed at the Office of the Religious Herald, 1833. 12p. CSmH
30-0181

CHILDS, Henry Halsey (1783-1868)
Eulogy on the death of John Doane Wells, M.D., late professor in the Berkshire Medical Institution, delivered before the faculty and medical class, September, 1830. Pittsfield: Phinehas Allen & Son [1830] 14p. MH; NBM **30-0182**

CHITTY, Joseph (1776-1841)
A practical treatise on medical jurisprudence, with so much of anatomy, physiology, pathology, and the practice of medicine and surgery, as are essential. . . . 1st American ed., with notes and additions adapted to American works and judicial decisions. Part I. Philadelphia: Carey, Lea & Blanchard, 1835. 509p. DLC; PPC; PPJ; PU [No more published]
30-0183

[CHOLERA]
Report of deaths of cholera, that have occurred in Cincinnati, from the 24th of September, to the 14th of November. Alphabetically arranged by an attentive observer. Cincinnati: Pr. by Wood & Stratton, 1832. 18p. OCHP
30-0184

[CHOLERA]
An account of the rise and progress of the Indian or spasmodic cholera. With a particular description of the symptoms attending the disease. Illustrated by a map, showing the route and progress of the disease from Jessore near the Ganges, in 1817, to Great Britain in 1831. New Haven: L. H. Young, 1832. 48p. DLC; DNLM; MB; MWA **30-0185**

[CHOLERA]
A full account of the operation of injecting the veins with aqueous and saline liquids, for the cure of malignant cholera, in the most hopeless cases. . . . New York: Peter Hill, 1832. 13(1)p. MB; MH; NN; NNNAM **30-0186**

[CHOLERA]
Sanitary precepts, in relation to epidemic cholera morbus, published by the Hamburg Council of Health. Transl. and repub. with an appendix. By John G. Kettner. Philadelphia, 1832. 9p. PPHa **30-0187**

[CHOLERA]
Remarks on the cholera, embracing facts and observations collected at New York. . . . 2nd ed. Providence: W. Marshall & Co., 1832. 34p. MWA **30-0188**

[CHOLERA]
Remarks on the cholera, embracing facts, and observations collected at New York. . . . 3rd ed. Providence: Pr. by W. Marshall & Co., 1832. 34p. MWA **30-0189**

CHRISTISON, Robert (1797-1882)
Manual of practical toxicology: condensed from Dr. Christison's Treatise on poisons. With notes and additions by J. T. Ducatel. . . . Baltimore: W. & J. Neal, 1833. 341p. DLC; MB; PPAmP **30-0190**

CHRISTISON, Robert (1797-1882)
. . . On granular degeneration of the kidneys, and its connection with dropsy, inflammations, and other diseases. . . . [Dunglison's American Medical Library]. Philadelphia: A. Waldie, 1839. 146p. DLC; DNLM; PPC; PPL
30-0191

CHURCHILL, Fleetwood (1808-1878)
. . . Outlines of the principal diseases of females. Chiefly for the use of students. . . . [Dunglison's American Medical Library] Philadelphia: A. Waldie, 1839. 302p. DLC; PPC; PPJ; PU **30-0192**

CLARK, James (1788-1870)
A treatise on pulmonary consumption; comprehending an inquiry into the causes, nature, prevention, and treatment of tuberculosis and scrofulous diseases in general. Philadelphia: Carey, Lea & Blanchard, 1835. 296p. DNLM; PPC; PU
30-0193

CLOQUET, Hippolyte (1787-1840)
A system of human anatomy, transl. from the fourth edition of the French of H. Cloquet. . . . With notes and a corrected nomenclature, by Robert Knox. . . . Boston: Wells & Lilly, [etc.] 1830. 836p. MB; NNNAM; NjR; PPC
30-0194

CLUTTERBUCK, Henry (1767-1856)
Lectures on bloodletting. . . . [Dunglison's American Medical Library] Philadelphia: Haswell, Barrington, & Haswell, 1839. 120p. DNLM; MBM; PPC **30-0195**

COATES, Benjamin Hornor (1797-1881)
An oration on certainty in medicine. Delivered before the Philadelphia Medical Society, February 10, 1830. Philadelphia: Pr. by James Kay, Jr. & Co., 1830. 29p. DLC; DNLM; MWA; PHi **30-0196**

COATES, Benjamin Hornor (1797-1881)
A biographical sketch of the late Thomas Say. Read before the Academy of Natural Sciences of Philadelphia. Philadelphia: W. P. Gibbons, 1835. 31p. DNLM; PPC; PU **30-0197**

COATES, Reynell (1802-1886)
Oration on the defects in the present system of medical instruction in the United States. Read before the Philadelphia Medical Society, November 21, 1835. . . . Philadelphia: J. Kay, Jr. and Brother [1835]. 32p. DLC; PPC; PPJ; PU **30-0198**

COATES, Reynell (1802-1886)
Popular medicine; or, Family adviser. . . . Philadelphia: Carey, Lea & Blanchard, 1838. 614p. DLC; PPC; PU **30-0199**

COLEY, Henry
A treatise on medical jurisprudence. Part I. Comprising the consideration of poisons and asphyxia. . . . New York: W. Stodart, 1832. 72p. MBM; PPC **30-0200**

COLLINS, Robert (1801-1868)
A practical treatise on midwifery, containing the result of sixteen thousand six hundred and fifty-four births, occurring in the Dublin Lying-in-Hospital, during a period of seven years, commencing November, 1826. Philadelphia: Haswell, Barrington & Haswell, 1838. 264p. DNLM; PPC **30-0201**

COMBE, Andrew (1797-1847)
Observations on mental derangement: being an application of the principles of phrenology to the elucidation of the causes, symptoms, nature, and treatment of insanity. . . . 1st American ed., with notes and bibliography, by an American physician. Boston: Marsh, Capen & Lyon, 1834. 336p. CtY-M; DLC; MBM; MH-M **30-0202**

COMBE, Andrew (1797-1847)
The principles of physiology applied to the preservation of health, and to the improvement of physical and mental education. . . . New York: Harper & Brothers, 1834. 291p. DLC; MdBJ-W; NcD; PU **30-0203**

COMBE, Andrew (1797-1847)
The physiology of digestion, considered with relation to the principles of dietetics. . . . 1st American ed. Boston: Marsh, Capen & Lyon, 1836. 328p. DLC; MBM; PPC; PPHa **30-0204**

COMBE, George (1788-1858)
Constitution of man considered in relation to external objects. 2nd American ed. Boston: Allen, 1833. 313p. MB; ScU **30-0205**

COMBE, George (1788-1858)
Elements of phrenology. . . . 2nd American ed., improved and enl., from the 3rd Edinburgh, by the author. . . . Boston: Marsh, Capen & Lyon, 1834. 204p. DLC; DNLM; NIC; PPC **30-0206**

COMBE, George (1788-1858)
The constitution of man considered in relation to external objects. With an additional chapter on the harmony between phrenology and revelation by Joseph A. Warne. 9th American ed. Boston: W. D. Ticknor, 1839. 412p. DNLM; MH; MWA **30-0207**

COMSTOCK, John Lee (1789-1858)
Outlines of physiology, both comparative and human; . . . Second edition. New York: Robinson, Pratt, 1837. 310p. DLC; PP; ScMS; NBM **30-0208**

COOKE, John Esten (1783-1853)
Remarks on some of the diseases incident to a state of pregnancy. Read before the Lexington Medical Society, and published by their request. Lexington, Ky.: J. Clarke, 1833. DLC; MBM; NN **30-0209**

COOKE, John Esten (1783-1853)
An introductory lecture, delivered to the medical class of Transylvania University in 1835. [Lexington, Ky., 1835] 12p. DNLM; KyLoJM **30-0210**

COOPER, Astley Paston (1768-1841)
The lectures of Sir Astley Cooper, Bart., F.R.S. Surgeon to the King, &c., on the principles and practice of surgery. With additional notes and cases by Frederick Tyrrell, Esq. 3rd American from the last London ed. Boston: Lilly & Wait, 1831. 3 v. ICJ; NNNAM **30-0211**

COOPER, Astley Paston (1768-1841)
Treatise on dislocations on fractures of the joints. . . . 2nd American from 6th London ed., rev. and greatly improved. . . . Boston: Lilly & Wait and Carter & Hendee [etc. etc.] 1832. 516p. DLC; KU; MBM **30-0212**

COOPER, Astley Paston (1768-1841)
The lectures of Sir Astley Cooper . . . on the principles and practice of surgery with additional notes and cases by Frederick Tyrrell. . . . 5th American from the last London ed. Philadelphia: Haswell, 1839. 580p. DLC; DNLM; NNNAM **30-0213**

COOPER, Samuel (1780-1848)
The first lines of the practice of surgery designed as an introduction for students and a concise book of reference for practitioners, . . . With notes by Alexander H. Stevens, and additional notes by Samuel McClellan. 3rd American from the 5th London ed. Philadelphia: Pub. by John Grigg; L. H. Bailey, pr., 1830. 2 v. CtY-M; ICJ; PPC **30-0214**

COOPER, Samuel (1780-1848)
. . . A dictionary of practical surgery; comprehending all the most interesting improvements from the earliest times down to the present period. . . . From the 6th London ed., rev., corr. & enl. with numerous notes . . . embracing improvements . . . by American surgeons . . . by David Meredith Reese. New York: J. & J. Harper, 1830. 2 v. DLC; ICJ; OCIM; PPC **30-0215**

COOPER, Samuel (1780-1848)
A dictionary of practical surgery, comprehending all the most interesting improvements, from the earliest times down to the present period. . . . With numerous notes and additions, by David Meredith Reese, M.D. From the 6th London ed., rev., cor. and enl. New York: J. & J. Harper, 1832. 2 v. in 1. KU; NcD; ScCM **30-0216**

CORBYN, Frederick
A treatise on the epidemic Cholera, as it has prevailed in India, together with the reports of the medical officers, made to the medical boards of the presidencies of Bengal, Madras, and Bombay. . . . Calcutta: Pr. at the Baptist mission press; Philadelphia: Carey, Lea & Carey, 1832. 389p. DLC; ICJ; MB; OCIM **30-0217**

CORNARDO, Luigi (1467-1566)
Discourses on a sober and temperate life, wherein is demonstrated by his own example, the method of preserving health to extreme old age. New ed. With introd. and notes, by Sylvester Graham [New York: Day, 1832]. vi, 90p. MB; RPB **30-0218**

CORNARDO, Luigi (1467-1566)
Discourses on a sober and temperate life, wherein is demonstrated, by his own example, the method of preserving health to extreme old age. . . . Transl. from the Italian original. A new ed., corr. Middletown, N.J.: G. H. Evans, 1836, vi. 90p. DNLM; NjR **30-0219**

COSTER, Jacques (1795-1868)
The practice of medicine, according to the principles of the physiological doctrine. . . . Transl. from the French. Philadelphia: Carey & Lea, 1831. 319p. ICJ; RPM **30-0220**

COXE, John Redman (1773-1864)
The American dispensatory containing the natural, chemical, pharmaceutical, and medical history of the different substances employed in medicine; together with the operations of pharmacy; . . . 8th ed. imp. and greatly enl. Philadelphia: Carey & Lea [Skerrett] 1830. 808p. IEN-M; MdBJ-W; PPC **30-0221**

COXE, John Redman (1773-1864)
The American dispensatory, containing the natural, chemical, pharmaceutical and medical history of the different substances employed in medicine; together with the operations of pharmacy; illustrated and explained, according to the principles of modern chemistry. . . . 9th ed. By John Redman Coxe. . . . Philadelphia: H. C. Carey & I. Lea, 1831. 832p. CSmH; MH; NN; PP **30-0222**

COXE, John Redman (1773-1864)
An inquiry into the claims of Doctor William Harvey to the discovery of circulation of the blood; with a more equitable retrospect of that event. To which is added, an introductory lecture, delivered on the third of November, 1829, in vindication of Hippocrates from sundry charges of ignorance preferred aginst him by the late Professor Rush. . . . Philadelphia: C. Sherman & Co., 1834. 258p. DLC; PPC; PU **30-0223**

COXE, John Redman (1773-1864)
An inquiry into the claims of Doctor William Harvey to the discovery of the circulation of the blood; with a more equitable retrospect of that event. To which is added, an introductory lecture, delivered on the third of November, 1829, in vindication of Hippocrates from sundry charges of ignorance preferred against him by the late Professor Rush. . . . Philadelphia: E. L. Carey & A. Hart [etc.] 1834. 258p. DLC; MBM; PPC; PPJ **30-0224**

COXE, John Redman (1773-1864)
An appeal to the public, and especially to the medical public, from the proceedings of the trustees of the University of Pennsylvania, vacating the chair of materia medica and pharmacy. . . . Philadelphia: The author [G. Sherman & Co., printers] 1835. 68p. DLC; PU **30-0225**

COXE, John Redman, ed. (1773-1864)
A short account of the occurrences which led to the removal of Dr. John Redman Coxe from the chair of materia medica & pharmacy, in the University of Pennsylvania. Presented with Dr. Coxe's respects. [Philadelphia, 1835] 12p. DLC; PU **30-0226**

CRABB, George (1778-1851)
A family encyclopaedia; or, an explanation of words and things connected with all the arts and sciences. . . . Enlarged and improved. . . . New York: C. S. Dunning, 1831. 412p. DLC; MH; NN; PP **30-0227**

CROSERIO, Camille (1786-1855)
On homoeopathic medicine, illustrating its superiority over the other medical doctrines, with an account of the regimen to be followed during the treatment of diseases. . . . Transl. from the French, with notes, containing the opinions of Brera, Broussais, &c., on homoeopathia. By C. Neidhard, M.D. Philadelphia: Kiderlen & Stollmeyer, 1837. 89p. DLC; PPHa **30-0228**

CROSS, James Conquest
Thoughts on the policy of establishing a school of medicine in Louisville, together with a sketch of the present condition and future prospects of the Medical Department of Transylvania University. Lexington, Ky.: N. L. Finnell, 1834. 113p. DLC; KU; KyLoJM; OCIWHi **30-0229**

CROSS, James Conquest
An inaugural discourse on medical eclectism. . . . Cincinnati: Printed by Kendall and Henry, 1835. 20p. DLC; OCHP; OCIWHi **30-0230**

CROSS, James Conquest
An inaugural discourse on the value of time, and the importance of study to the physician. . . . Lexington, Ky.: Finnell & Zimmerman, printers, 1837. 34p. DLC; KU; KyLoJM; OCHP **30-0231**

CURIE, Paul F.
Domestic homoeopathy. . . . With additions and improvements by Gideon Humphrey, M.D. Philadelphia: Printed by Jasper Harding, 1839. 250p. DLC; PPHa **30-0232**

CURLING, Thomas Blizard
A treatise on tetanus [Jacksonian Prize Essay for 1834] . . . . Philadelphia: Haswell, Barrington & Haswell, 1837. 126p. DNLM; PPC; PPJ; PU **30-0233**

CURTIS, Alva (1797-1881)
Discussions between several members of the regular medical faculty and the Thomsonian botanic physicians, on the comparative merits of their respective systems. Columbus: J. Phillips, 1836. 400p. DNLM; KU; ICU
30-0234

CURTIS, Alva (1797-1881)
Lectures on midwifery and the forms of disease peculiar to women and children, delivered to the members of the Botanico-Medical School, at Columbus, Ohio. Columbus: J. Phillips, 1837. 398p., 1 pl. DNLM; OC
30-0235

CUTBUSH, Edward (1772-1843)
A discourse delivered at the opening of the Medical Institution of Geneva College, State of New York, February 10, 1835. Geneva: John Greves and Co., 1835. 24p. DLC; N; NHi; NNC
30-0236

CUTLER, Thomas
The surgeon's practical guide in the dressing, and in the methodic application of bandages. Philadelphia: Haswell & Co., 1838. 92p. DNLM; NNNAM; PPC; PU
30-0237

DARRACH, William (1796-1865)
Drawings of the anatomy of the groin, with anatomical remarks. Philadelphia: Littell; James Kay, Jr. & Co., prs., 1830. 28p. MdBM; OCIM; PPC; PU **30-0238**

DAVIES, John (1796-1872)
. . . Selections in pathology and surgery; or, An exposition of the nature and treatment of local disease; exhibiting new pathological views, and pointing out an important practical improvement. Illustrated by cases. . . . [Dunglison's American Medical Library] Philadelphia: A. Waldie, 1839. 119p. DLC; DNLM; PPF; PPHa **30-0239**

DAVIS, Samuel W.
A refutation of sundry unfounded accusations, contained in letters and communications from Dr. Daniel Drake, to a committee of the third district medical society. [Cincinnati, 1833?] 8p. IEN-M; OC; OCIWHi **30-0240**

DAY, L. Meeker
The botanic family physician; or, The secret of curing all diseases on improved hygeian principles. . . . New York, 1833. 24p. DLC; OCLloyd **30-0241**

DAY, L. Meeker
The improved American family physician; or, Sick man's guide to health: containing a complete theory of the botanic practice of medicine, on the Thomsonian and hygeian system, with alterations and improvements. To which is appended a concise formula for compounding medicines. . . . Also, a complete digest on midwifery. . . . New York, 1833. 120p. CtY-M; DLC
30-0242

DELAFIELD, Edward (1794-1875)
Introductory address to the students in medicine of the College of Physicians and Surgeons of the University of the State of New York. Delivered Nov. 7, 1837. . . . New York: Scatcherd & Adams, 1837. 44p. DLC; NN; NNC; NNNAM
30-0243

DE LANCEY, William Heathcote (1797-1865)
A Charge addressed to the graduates in medicine of the University of Pennsylvania at the public commencement held in the College Hall, on Thursday, March 24th, 1831. . . . Pub. at the request of the graduates. Philadelphia: Pr. by Joseph R. A. Skerrett, 1831. 16p. CSmH; MWA; PPPrHi; PU
30-0244

DENDY, Walter Cooper (1794-1871)
The book of the nursery: precepts for the management of infants, and for the prevention and domestic treatment of the diseases incidental to childhood. New York: Jackson, 1833. 148p. MB; MBM; PPC **30-0245**

DESRUELLES, Henri Marie Joseph (1791-1858)
Memoir on the treatment of venereal diseases without mercury, employed at the military hospital of the Val-de-Grace. Transl. from the French. . . . To which is added, Observations on the treatment of the venereal disease without mercury. By G. J. Guthrie. . . . Philadelphia: Carey & Lea, 1830. 217p. IEN-M; NNNAM; NjR; PPC **30-0246**

DEWEES, William Potts (1768-1841)
A compendious system of midwifery. Chiefly designed to facilitate the inquiries of those who may be pursuing this branch of study. Illustrated by occasional cases. With many engravings. 4th ed., with additions, and improvements. Philadelphia: Carey & Lea, 1830. 640p. KU; NNNAM; RPM
30-0247

DEWEES, William Potts (1768-1841)
A practice of physic, comprising most of the diseases not treated of in "Diseases of females," and "Diseases of children." . . . Philadelphia: Carey & Lea [Skerrett, pr.] 1830. 2 v. DNLM; NNNAM; PPC; RPM **30-0248**

DEWEES, William Potts (1768-1841)
A treatise on the physical and medical treatment of children. . . . 4th ed., with cor. Philadelphia: Blanchard & Lea, 1832. 560p. ICJ; NcD; PU **30-0249**

DEWEES, William Potts (1768-1841)
A compendious system of midwifery chiefly designed to facilitate the inquiries of those who may be pursuing this branch of study. Illustrated by occasional cases. With many engravings. 5th ed., with additions and improvements. . . . Philadelphia: Lea & Carey, 1832. 2 v. DLC; PPC
30-0250

DEWEES, William Potts (1768-1841)
A treatise on the physical and medical treatment of children. . . . Philadelphia: Carey, Lea and Blanchard, 1833. 560p; MBM; PPC; PU **30-0251**

DEWEES, William Potts (1768-1841)
A practice of physic, comprising most of the diseases not treated in "Diseases of females," and "Diseases of children." . . . 2nd ed., with additions and improvements. Philadelphia: Carey, Lea & Blanchard, 1833. 819p. GU; MB; PU
30-0252

DEWEES, William Potts (1768-1841)
A treatise on the diseases of females. 4th ed., rev. and cor. Philadelphia: Carey, Lea & Blanchard, 1833. 563p. CtY-M; CU-M; PPC **30-0253**

DEWEES, William Potts (1768-1841)
A compendious system of midwifery, chiefly designed to facilitate the inquiries of those who may be pursuing this branch of study. Illustrated by occasional cases. 6th ed., with additions and improvements. Philadelphia: Carey, Lea & Blanchard, 1833. 650p. DLC; PU; RPM
30-0254

DEWEES, William Potts (1768-1841)
A treatise on the physical and medical treatment of children. . . . 6th ed., with corrections. Philadelphia: Carey, Lea & Blanchard, 1836. 548p. DNLM; PPC; PPJ
30-0255

DEWEES, William Potts (1768-1841)
A compendious system of midwifery, chiefly designed to facilitate the inquiries of those who may be pursuing this branch of study. Illustrated by occasional cases, and with many engravings. 8th ed., with additions and improvements. . . . Philadelphia: Carey, Lea & Blanchard, 1837. 600p. DLC; PPC; PPHa; PU **30-0256**

DEWEES, William Potts (1768-1841)
A treatise on the physical and medical treatment of children. . . . 7th ed., with corrections. Philadelphia: Carey, Lea & Blanchard, 1838. 548p. DLC; PPC; PPJ; PU
30-0257

DICKSON, Samuel Henry (1798-1872)
Syllabus of part of the course of lectures of S. Henry Dickson, M.D., Professor of the Institutes and Practice of Medicine. In the Medical College of South Carolina. Charleston: Pr. by James S. Burges, 1830. 106p. ScCM **30-0258**

DICKSON, Samuel Henry (1798-1872)
Address before the South Carolina society for the promotion of temperance, April 6th, 1830. . . . To which is annexed the constitution of the South Carolina temperance society, and the report of the Columbia temperance society. Charleston [S.C.]: Observer Office Press [1830]. 72p. DLC; ScC; ScCM; ScU
30-0259

DICKSON, Samuel Henry (1798-1872)
Introductory lecture, delivered on the eleventh of November, 1833. . . . Charleston, S.C.: Published by the students, 1833. 30p. DLC; NNNAM; NcD; ScC **30-0260**

DICKSON, Samuel Henry (1798-1872)
Introductory lecture delivered at the opening of the Medical College of the State of South Carolina, November 12, 1838. Charleston: A. E. Miller, 1838. 26p. DNLM; ScCM
30-0261

DICKSON, Samuel Henry (1798-1872)
On dengue: its history, pathology, and treatment. Philadelphia: Haswell, Barrington, and Haswell, 1839. 347p. DLC; DNLM; PPJ; ScMS **30-0262**

DICKSON, Samuel Henry (1798-1872)
Manual of pathology and practice, being the outline of the course of lectures delivered . . . in the Medical College of the State of South Carolina. Charleston [S.C.]: Observer Office Press, 1839. 204p. DLC; PPC; ScC; ScCM
30-0263

DICTIONARY of chemistry. . . . Transl. from "Le dictionnaire de chemie, approuvé par Vauquelin." With additions and notes by Mrs. Almira H. Lincoln. New York: G. & C. & H. Carvill, 1830. 531p. DNLM; MH; NN; NNNAM **30-0264**

DIXON, Edward H. (1808-1880)
An eulogy on the life and character of the late Abel J. Starr. New York, 1836. 16p. DNLM; NN; NNC
30-0265

DIXON, Edward H. (1808-1880)
. . . To Valentine Mott, M.D. . . . this case of osteo-sarcoma is presented by his obliged pupil. New York: G. A. C. Van Buren, 1838. 8p. DNLM; NNNAM **30-0266**

DORSEY, John Syng (1783-1818)
Elements of Surgery: for the use of students; with plates. . . . Philadelphia: Edward Parker, Kimber & Conrad, 1831. 2 v. DLC; PPC; PPHa **30-0267**

DRAKE, Daniel (1785-1852)
An oration on the causes, evils, and preventives of intemperance. Columbus: Olmsted & Bailhache, 1831. 21p. DNLM
30-0268

DRAKE, Daniel (1785-1852)
Practical essays on medical education, and the medical profession in the United States. . . . Cincinnati, O.: Roff & Young, 1832. 104p. KyLoJM; OCIWHi; PPL; ScU
30-0269

DRAKE, Daniel (1785-1852)
A practical treatise on the history, prevention, and treatment of epidemic cholera, designed both for the profession and the people. . . . Cincinnati: Corey & Fairbank, 1832. 180p. DLC; MH; OCHP **30-0270**

DRAKE, Daniel (1785-1852)
An account of the epidemic of cholera, as it appeared in Cincinnati. . . . Cincinnati, Ohio: Pr. at the Chronicle office, E. Deming, 1832. 46p. ICJ; MH; NNNAM; ScU
30-0271

DRAKE, Daniel (1785-1852)
A practical treatise on the history, prevention, and treatment of epidemic cholera, designed both for the profession and the people. . . . Cincinnati: Corey and Fairbank, 1832. 180p. DLC; NcD; OCHP **30-0272**

DRAKE, Daniel (1785-1852)
The "war of extermination." [Cincinnati? 1839.] 15p. [Contains correspondence relating to controversy between the Medical College of Ohio and the Cincinnati College concerning admission of the students and professors of the latter institution to the Commercial Hospital and Lunatic Asylum, Cincinnati.] DLC **30-0273**

DRAPER, Alexander C.
Observations on abortion, with an account of the means, both medicinal and mechanical, employed to produce that effect, together with advice to females. Philadelphia, 1839. 44p. DNLM **30-0274**

DRAPER, John William (1811-1882)
Some experimental researches to determine the nature of capillary attraction. . . . Philadelphia: J. Harding, 1834. 21p. PP; PPC **30-0274A**

DUCATEL, Julius Timoleon (1796-1849)
Introductory lecture delivered 31 Oct., 1832, in the Chemical Hall of the University of Maryland. Baltimore, 1833. 31p. CtY-M; DNLM; MdBM **30-0275**

DUDLEY, Benjamin W. (1785-1870)
Observations on the nature and treatment of calculous diseases. Lexington, Ky.: J. Clarke & Co., 1836. 40p. DNLM; KyLoJM
30-0276

DUFFIN, Edward Wilson (1800-1874)
The influence of modern physical education of females; in producing and confirming deformity of the spine. New York: Chas. S. Francis; Boston: Clayton & Van Norden, prs., 1830. 140p. MWA; NNNAM; PPC **30-0277**

DUNGLISON, Robley (1798-1869)
Human physiology. . . . Philadelphia: Carey & Lea, 1832. DLC; GU; NN; PP **30-0278**

DUNGLISON, Robley (1798-1869)
A lecture, delivered to the medical class of the University of Virginia, at the conclusion of the course, and on the occasion of his leaving the institution; . . . July 9th, 1833. Published by the class. Charlottesville: Printed by Watson & Tompkins, 1833. 18p. MdBM; PPPAmP **30-0279**

DUNGLISON, Robley (1798-1869)
An introductory lecture, delivered to the medical class of the University of Maryland, on Friday, October 31st, 1833. . . . Baltimore: J. D. Toy, printer, 1833. 23p. DLC; NNNAM; PPC; PPL **30-0280**

DUNGLISON, Robley (1798-1869)
A new dictionary of medical science and literature, containing a concise account of the various subjects and terms; with the synonyms in different languages; and formulae for various officinal and empirical preparations, &c. &c. . . . Boston: C. Bowen, 1833. 2 v. CtYM; DLC; MBM; PU
30-0281

DUNGLISON, Robley (1798-1869)
An address, delivered to the graduates in medicine, at the annual commencement of the University of Maryland, on Wednesday, March 19th, 1834. . . . Baltimore: W. Wooddy, printer, 1834. 23p. DLC; MdU-D; PPJ **30-0282**

DUNGLISON, Robley (1798-1869)
On the influence of atmosphere and locality; change of air and climate; seasons; food; clothing; bathing; exercise; sleep; corporeal and intellectual pursuits, &c. &c. on human health; constituting elements of hygiene. . . . Philadelphia: Carey, Lea & Blanchard, 1835, 514p. DLC; PPC; PPJ; PU
30-0283

DUNGLISON, Robley (1798-1869)
Human physiology. . . . 2nd ed. Philadelphia: Carey, Lea & Blanchard, 1836. 2 v. DNLM; NN; PPC; PP
30-0284

DUNGLISON, Robley (1798-1869)
General therapeutics; or, Principles of medical practice; with tables of the chief remedial agents, and their preparations; and of the different poisons and their antidotes. . . . Philadelphia: Carey, Lea & Blanchard, 1836. 580p. CU-M; DLC; PPJ; PU
30-0285

DUNGLISON, Robley (1798-1869)
Address to the medical graduates of the Jefferson Medical College. Delivered March 11, 1837. . . . Philadelphia: Printed by A. Waldie, 1837. 20p. DLC; PPJ
30-0286

DUNGLISON, Robley (1798-1869)
The medical student; or, Aids to the study of medicine, including a glossary of the terms of the science, and of the mode of prescribing,—bibliographical notices of medical works; the regulations of different medical colleges of the Union, &c. &c. . . . Philadelphia: Carey, Lea & Blanchard, 1837. 323p. DLC; PPC; PPJ; PU **30-0287**

DUNGLISON, Robley (1798-1869)
Human physiology. . . . 3rd ed., with numerous additions and modifications. . . . Philadelphia: Carey, Lea & Blanchard, 1838. 2 v. DLC; PPC; PPJ; PU **30-0288**

DUNGLISON, Robley (1798-1869)
Medical lexicon. A new dictionary of medical science, containing a concise account of the various subjects and terms; with a vocabulary or synonyms in different languages, and formulae for various officinal and empirical preparations, &c. 2nd ed., with numerous modifications and additions. . . . Philadelphia: Lea & Blanchard, 1839. 821p. DLC; PPC; PPJ; PU
30-0289

DUNGLISON, Robley (1798-1869)
Introductory lecture to the course of institutes of medicine, and materia medica, in Jefferson Medical College, of Philadelphia. For the session of 1839-40. . . . Philadelphia: W. F. Geddes, 1839. 20p. DLC; PPJ **30-0290**

DUNGLISON, Robley (1798-1869)
. . . New remedies: the method of preparing and administering them; their effects on the healthy and diseased economy, &c. . . . [Dunglison's American Medical Library] . . . Philadelphia: A. Waldie, 1839. 429p. DLC; PPC; PPJ; PU
30-0291

DUPUYTREN, Guillaume (1778-1835)
Clinical lectures on surgery, delivered at Hotel Dieu, in 1832. . . . Published by an association of physicians. Transl. from the French, by A. Sidney Doane, . . . New York: Collins & Hannay, 1833. 312p. CtY-M; PPC; MH
30-0292

DUPUYTREN, Guillaume (1778-1835)
Clinical lectures on surgery, delivered at the Hotel Dieu in 1832. . . . Boston: Carter, Hendee, & Co., 1833. 312p. DNLM; MH; PPC **30-0293**

EARLE, Pliny (1809-1892)
A visit to thirteen asylums for the insane in Europe, with statistics. Philadelphia: T. K. & P. G. Collins, 1839. 38p. DNLM; PPL; MWA; MBAt **30-0294**

EBERLE, John (1787-1838)
A treatise of the materia medica and therapeutics. . . . 3rd ed., enl. and corr. Philadelphia: John Grigg; William Brown, pr., 1830. 2 v. DLC; NNNAM; OCHP; PPC
30-0295

EBERLE, John (1787-1838)
A treatise on the practice of medicine. Philadelphia: John Grigg, William Brown, pr., 1830. 2 v. DNLM; GU; LNT-M; PPC **30-0296**

EBERLE, John (1787-1838)
A treatise on the practice of medicine. . . . 2nd ed., rev. and enl. Philadelphia: John Grigg, 1831. 2 v. CU-M; ICJ; RPM
30-0297

EBERLE, John (1787-1838)
A treatise on the diseases and physical education of children, . . . Cincinnati: Corey & Fairbank, 1833. 559p. OCHP; PP; PPHa **30-0298**

EBERLE, John (1787-1838)
A treatise of the materia medica and therapeutics. . . . 4th ed. Philadelphia: Grigg & Elliot, 1834. 2 v. DNLM; OCHP; OCLloyd **30-0299**

EBERLE, John (1787-1838)
Notes of lectures on the theory and practice of medicine, delivered in the Jefferson Medical College, at Philadelphia. 2nd ed., cor. . . . Cincinnati: Corey & Fairbank, 1834. 218p. DLC; OCHP; PPC; PU **30-0300**

EBERLE, John (1787-1838)
A treatise on the diseases and physical education of children. . . . 2nd ed. Cincinnati: Corey & Fairbank, 1834. 558p. OC; MdBM; NjR **30-0301**

EBERLE, John (1787-1838)
A treatise on the practice of medicine. . . . 3rd ed. Philadelphia: Grigg & Elliot, 1835. 2 v. DNLM; PPC; PPJ **30-0302**

EBERLE, John (1787-1838)
A treatise on the diseases and physical education of children. . . . 3rd ed. Philadelphia: Grigg & Elliott, 1837. 555p. DLC; DNLM; PPC; PU **30-0303**

EBERLE, John (1787-1838)
A treatise on the practice of medicine. . . . 4th ed., rev. and enl. Philadelphia: Grigg & Elliot, 1838. 2 v. DLC; KyLoJM; PPAmP; ViRA **30-0304**

ELKINTON, John A[braham] (1801-1853)
Notes on the practice pursued with cholera patients at the hospitals in New York; Facts and observations of a practical nature. . . . Read before the Sanitary Committee of the Northern Liberties, August 2nd, 1832, by John A. Elkinton, M.D., who visited New York, during the prevalence of epidemic cholera, and spent one week among the hospitals while the disease was at its height. [Philadelphia, 1831] 12p. DLC; DNLM; NNNAM **30-0305**

ELLIS, Benjamin (1798-1831)
The medical formulary; being a collection of prescriptions. . . . 3rd ed. Philadelphia: Carey & Lea, 1831. 231p. CtY-M; DLC; ICJ; ScMS **30-0306**

ELLIS, Benjamin (1798-1831)
The medical formulary; being a collection of prescriptions. . . . 4th ed. Philadelphia: Carey, Lea & Blanchard, 1834. 231p. DNLM; OCLloyd **30-0307**

ELLIS, Benjamin (1798-1831)
The medical formulary; being a collection of prescriptions. . . . 5th ed. Philadelphia: Carey, Lea & Blanchard, 1838. 231p. CtY-M; PPC; PPHa; PPL **30-0308**

EMERSON, Gouverneur (1796-1874)
Medical statistics; consisting of estimates relating to the population of Philadelphia, with its changes as influenced by the deaths and births, during ten years, viz., from 1821 to 1830, inclusive. . . . Philadelphia: Printed by J. R. A. Skerrett, 1831. 32p. DLC; ICJ; LNT-M **30-0309**

EUSTAPHIEVE, Alexander
Homoeopathia revealed. A brief exposition of the whole system, adapted to general comprehension, with a notice of psora and Dr. Duringe's objections. New York: G. & C. Carvill & Co., 1837. 77p. DLC; MB; MH-M; PPHa **30-0310**

EVANS, Thomas
Condensed view of the cholera in Europe, with its introduction in America; to which is added forty-seven days' experience in a cholera hospital. With a list of names of those who were admitted and who died. By Thomas Evans and James C. Kent. New York, the Authors, 1832. 21p. DLC; MH-M; NN **30-0311**

EVANSON, Richard T.
A practical treatise on the management and diseases of children. By Richard T. Evanson . . . and Henry Maunsell. . . . Philadelphia: Haswell, Harrington, and Haswell, 1838. 300p. CU-M; DLC; PPC; PU **30-0312**

EVE, Joseph A. (1805-1886)
Introductory address, delivered at the opening of the session of the Medical College of Georgia. Augusta: W. T. Thompson, 1838. 24p. DNLM; GU **30-0313**

EVE, PAUL Fitzsimmons (1806-1877)
An address delivered at the Medical College of Georgia. Augusta, Ga.: Guion & Thompson, 1838. 14p. DNLM; GU **30-0314**

EVEREST, Thomas Roupell
A popular view of homoeopathy. . . . Allentown, Pa.: Academical Book Store; Philadelphia [etc.]: J. G. Wessellhoeft, 1835. 75p. DLC; DNLM; PPHa **30-0315**

EVERS, P.
The student's compendium of comparative anatomy. [Dunglison's American Medical Library] Philadelphia: A. Waldie, 1839. 112p. DNLM; PPC **30-0316**

FERGUS, John Freeland (1810-1838)
History and treatment of the malignant cholera, as it prevailed at Vienna. . . . From the London Lancet of June, 1832. . . . New York: Charles S. Francis, 1832. 23p. MH; NN; PU **30-0317**

FERRIS, Floyd T.
A treatise on epidemic cholera, as observed in the Duane Street Cholera Hospital, New York, during its prevalence there in 1834. . . . New York: Harper & Brothers, 1835. 70p. 4 col. plates. DLC; NNNAM; NNU-M; PP **30-0318**

FISHER, John D. (1797-1850)
Description of the distinct, confluent, and inoculated small pox, varioloid disease, cow pox, and chicken pox. . . . 2nd ed. Boston: Lilly, Wait & Co., 1834. 73p. 13 col. plates. DLC; MBM; MH; MH-M **30-0319**

FISHER, William R.
Introductory lecture, delivered in the chemical hall of the University of Maryland. Philadelphia: Merrihew & Gunn, 1837. 24p. DNLM; MdU-D **30-0320**

FITCH, Samuel Sheldon
Remarks on the importance of the teeth. On their diseases and modes of cure; with direction for forming regular and beautiful sets of teeth, and for the preservation of their health and beauty. . . . 3rd ed. Philadelphia: Carey & Lea, 1830. 24p. DLC; PPC; PPL; PHi **30-0321**

FITCH, Samuel Sheldon
A system of dental surgery. . . . 2nd ed., rev., cor., and imp., with new plates. . . . Philadelphia: Carey, Lea & Blanchard, 1835. 528p. DLC; OClWHi; PPC **30-0322**

FITCH, Samuel Sheldon
The influence of intellectual cultivation. . . . A lecture introductory to a course of lectures on anatomy and physiology. . . . Philadelphia: T. K. & P. G. Collins, 1838. 24p. PHi; PPC **30-0323**

FITZ-GIBBON, Maurice
An experimental and analytical essay on the powers by which the blood is circulated in the veins. Philadelphia: J. R. A. Skerrett, 1833. 21p. DNLM **30-0324**

FLINT, Joshua B. (1801-1864)
Address delivered to the students of the Louisville Medical Institute. Louisville, Ky.: Prentice & Weissenger, 1838. 31p. DNLM; ICJ; KyLoJM **30-0325**

FONERDEN, William Henry
The institutes of Thomsonism. . . . Philadelphia: Printed at the office of the Botanic Sentinel, 1837. 123p. DLC; OCHP; OCLloyd; PPHa **30-0326**

FOSTER, Theodore
Practical phrenology simplified. . . . Philadelphia: O. Rogers, 1838. 106p. DLC; PHi; PP; PPAmP **30-0327**

FOWLER, Orin (1791-1852)
A disquistion on the evils of using tobacco, and the necessity of immediate and entire reformation. 2nd ed. Boston: W. Pierce, 1835. 24p. DNLM; MWA **30-0328**

FOWLER, Orson Squire (1809-1887)
Phrenological chart; presenting a synopsis of the science of phrenology. . . . Baltimore: J. W. Woods, printer, 1836. 16p. DLC; MdBJ-W; MdU-D **30-0329**

FOWLER, Orson Squire (1809-1887)
Phrenology proved, illustrated, and applied, accompanied by a chart . . . together with a view of the moral and theological bearing of the science. By O. S. & L. N. Fowler . . . assisted by Samuel Kirkham. . . . New York: Printed for the authors, by W. H. Colyer, 1837. 323p. DLC; NN; NNNAM; NNU-M **30-0330**

FRANCIS, John Wakefield (1789-1861)
An address delivered on the anniversary of the Philolexian Society of Columbia College, May 15, 1831. New York: G. & C. & H. Carvill, 1831. 43p. DNLM; NN; NNC **30-0331**

FRANCIS, John Wakefield (1789-1861)
Letter on the cholera asphyxia, now prevailing in the city of New York: addressed to James Bond Read. . . . New York: Printed by G. P. Scott & Co., 1832. 35p. DLC; IEN-M; MB; MHi **30-0332**

FRANCIS, John Wakefield (1789-1861)
Observations on the mineral waters of Avon, Livingston County, New York. . . . New York: Printed by G. P. Scott & Co., 1834. 16p. DLC; N; NHi; NNC **30-0333**

FRECKLETON, George
Outlines of general pathology. . . . Philadelphia: Haswell, Barrington, & Haswell, 1839. 151p. DLC; PPC; PPPH; PU **30-0334**

FROST, Henry Rutledge (1790-1866)
Syllabus of a course of lectures on the materia medica. . . . Charleston: Pr. by A. E. Miller, 1830. 64p. NNNAM; ScCM **30-0335**

FROTHINGHAM, N. L.
A sermon preached to the First Church, after the death of J. G. Stevenson, M.D. Boston: I. R. Butts, 1835. 15p. DNLM; MWA; MBAt **30-0336**

FULLER, Jacob (*d.* 1839)
Delirium tremens, its causes and treatment. Fiske Fund prize dissertation of the Rhode Island Medical Society. No. IV, June, 1837. Boston: D. Clapp, 1837. 16p. DLC; DNLM; MH; RPJCB **30-0337**

GALL, Franz Joseph (1758-1828)
Manual of phrenology: being an analytical summary of the system of Dr. Gall, on the faculties of man and the functions of the brain. Transl. from the 4th French ed. Philadelphia: Carey, Lea & Blanchard, 1835. 257p. 5 plates. DLC; GU; MB; PU **30-0338**

GALL, Franz Joseph (1758-1828)
Works of. . . . Transl. from the French by Winslow Lewis. [The Phrenological Library] Boston: Marsh, Capen & Lyon, 1835. 6 v. DNLC; MB; MBM; MWA [Each volume has special title page] **30-0339**

GALLUP, Joseph Adams (1769-1849)
Outlines of an arrangement of medical nosology; founded on the physiology of the diseased system. Woodstock: Pr. by David Watson, 1831. 87p. MBM; MH **30-0340**

GALLUP, Joseph Adams (1769-1849)
Outlines of the institutes of medicine; founded on the philosophy of the human economy, in health, and in disease. Boston: Otis, Broaders & Co., 1839. 2 v. DNLM; MBM; MH **30-0341**

GEDDINGS, Eli (1799-1878)
Introductory lecture, delivered on the fifteenth of November, 1830. . . . Charleston: J. S. Burges, 1830. 22p. NNNAM **30-0342**

GEDDINGS, Eli (1799-1878)
Valedictory address to the graduates of the University of Maryland. Delivered at the commencement held on the 21st of March, 1833, by E. Geddings. Baltimore: Lucas & Deaver, 1833. 20p. NcD **30-0343**

GEDDINGS, Eli (1799-1878)
Introductory lecture, delivered at the opening of the session of the Medical College of the State of S. Carolina, on the second Monday of November, 1837. Charleston [S.C.]: Published by the class, 1838. 38p. NcD **30-0344**

The GENTLEMAN's medical pocket-book and health-adviser; containing a concise statement of the modes of curing every disease to which he is liable, with direction for his conduct in case of accidents on the road or at sea. By a medical practitioner. Philadelphia: J. Kay, Jr. & Co.; Pittsburgh: J. I. Kay & Co. [1832]. 160p. DLC; PHi; PP; PPAmP **30-0345**

GERHARD, William Wood (1809-1872)
Observations on the endermic application of medicines. . . . Philadelphia: Pr. by James Kay, Jr. & Co., 1830. 27p. NNNAM; PHi; PPL **30-0346**

GERHARD, William Wood (1809-1872)
On the diagnosis of diseases of the chest; based upon the comparison of their physical and general signs. . . . Philadelphia: Key & Biddle, 1836. 183p. CtY-M; DLC; MH-M; PU
30-0347

GERHARD, William Wood (1809-1872)
Clinical guide, and syllabus of a course of lectures, on clinical medicine and pathology. . . . Philadelphia: J. G. Auner, 1837. 37p. CU-M; DLC; MBM; PU 30-0348

GIBSON, John Mason
A condensation of matter upon the anatomy, surgical operations and treatment of diseases of the eye. . . . Baltimore: W. R. Lucas, 1832. 204p. ICJ; NNNAM; PU
30-0349

GIBSON, William (1788-1868)
The institutes and practice of surgery: being the outlines of a course of lectures. . . . 3rd ed., with additions. Philadelphia: Carey & Lea, 1832. 2 v. CtY-M; GU; MBM; ScC
30-0350

GIBSON, William (1788-1868)
The institutes and practice of surgery: being the outlines of a course of lectures. . . . 4th ed., greatly enl. . . . Philadelphia: Carey, Lea & Blanchard, 1835. 2 v. CtY-M; DLC; IU-M; PPC
30-0351

GIBSON, William (1788-1868)
A sketch of lithotripsy, with cases. [Philadelphia, 1836] 30p. DNLM 30-0352

GIBSON, William (1788-1868)
The institutes and practice of surgery: being the outline of a course of lectures. . . . 5th ed., greatly enl. . . . Philadelphia: Carey, Lea & Blanchard, 1838. 2 v. DNLM; PPC; PPHa; PU
30-0353

GIBSON, William (1788-1868)
Sketches of prominent surgeons of London and Paris, introductory to a course of surgical lectures. Philadelphia: Office of the Medical Examiner, 1839. 17p. DNLM; NNNAM; PPC; PU 30-0354

GILMAN, Charles R.
Hints to the people on the prevention and early treatment of spasmodic cholera. . . . New York: Charles S. Francis, 1832. 15p. NjR; NNNAM 30-0355

GILMAN, J.
A treatise on epidemic cholera, including an historical account of its origin and progress up to the present time; . . . Hartford: H. & F. J. Huntington, 1833. 368p. MBM; MH-M; MWA
30-0356

GODDARD, Paul B[eck] (1811-1866)
Plates of the cerebro-spinal nerves, with references; for the use of medical students. Philadelphia: J. G. Auner, 1837. 60p. 12 plates. DNLM; MBM; NNNAM; PPC
30-0357

GODMAN, John D. (1794-1830)
American natural history. . . . 2nd ed. Philadelphia: Key & Mielke, 1831. 3 v. DNLM; MB; MH; NN
30-0358

GOOCH, Robert (1784-1830)
An account of some of the most important diseases peculiar to women. . . . From the 2nd London ed. Philadelphia: E. L. Carey & A. Hart, 1832. 326p. ICJ; KyLoJM; NcD
30-0359

GOOCH, Robert (1784-1830)
A practical compendium of midwifery; being the course of lectures on midwifery, and on the diseases of women and infants, delivered at St. Bartholomew's Hospital, . . . Prepared for publication by George Skinner. . . . Philadelphia: E. L. Carey & A. Hart, 1832. 319p. DLC, ICJ; ViRA
30-0360

GOOCH, Robert (1784-1830)
An account of some of the most important diseases peculiar to women. . . . From the 2nd London ed. Philadelphia: E. Barrington & G. D. Haswell, 1836. 326p. DLC; PPC; PPU
30-0361

GOOD, John Mason (1764-1827)
The book of nature. . . . From the last London ed. To which is now prefixed, a sketch of the author's life. New York: J. & J. Harper, 1831. 467p. DNLM; NN; NNNAM
30-0362

GOOD, John Mason (1764-1827)
The study of medicine. . . . improved from the author's manuscripts, and by reference to the latest advances in physiology, pathology, and practice. By Samuel Cooper. . . . 6th American, from the last English ed. With notes, by A. Sidney Doane . . . to which is prefixed, A sketch of the history of medicine, from its origin to the commencement of the nineteenth century. By J. Bostock. . . . New York: Harper & Brothers, 1836. 2 v. DLC; NjR; OC; PPPrHi 30-0363

GOODE, Thomas
The invalid's guide to the Virginia hot springs. Richmond: P. D. Bernard, 1839. 44p. DNLM; ViRA 30-0364

GOODLETT, A. G.
The family physician, or every man's companion, being a compilation from the most approved medical authors, adapted to the Southern and Western climates. . . . Nashville, Tenn.: Smith & Nesbit, 1838. 792p. DNLM; KyLoJM; OC
30-0365

GOUPIL, Jean Martin Auguste (1800-1837)
An exposition of the principles of the new medical doctrine, with an analysis of the theses sustained on its different parts. Transl. from the French of J. M. A. Goupil . . . by Josiah C. Nott, M.D. To which is appended a short essay on leeches, by the translator. Columbia [S.C.]: Printed at the Times and Gazette Office, 1831. 371p. DLC; GU; KyLoJM; LNT-M
30-0366

GRAHAM, Sylvester (1794-1851)
A lecture on epidemic diseases generally and particularly the spasmodic cholera. . . . With an appendix, containing several testimonials, —rules of the Graham boarding house, &c. . . . New York: Mahlon Day, 1833. CSmH; DLC; MH-M; MdBJ-W
30-0367

GRAHAM, Sylvester (1794-1851)
The Aesculapian tablets of the nineteenth century. . . . Providence: Printed by Weeden and Corey, 1834. 95p. DLC; RHi
30-0368

GRAHAM, Sylvester (1794-1851)
A lecture on epidemic diseases generally, and particularly the spasmodic cholera, delivered in the city of New York, March, 1832, and repeated June, 1832, and in Albany, July 4, 1832, and in New York, June, 1833. With an appendix, containing several testimonials, and a review of Beaumont's experiments on the gastric juice. New ed., rev. and enl. . . . Boston: D. Cambell, 1838. 125p. DLC; MBM; MH-M; MWA
30-0369

GRAHAM, Sylvester (1794-1851)
Lectures on the science of human life. . . . Boston: Marsh, Capen, Lyon & Webb, 1839. 2 v. DNLM; MBM; MH
30-0370

[GRAHAM, Thomas John] (1795?-1876)
The manual for invalids. By a physician. Boston: Wells and Lilly, 1830. 232p. DLC; DNLM; ICJ
30-0371

GRAHAM, Thomas John (1795?-1876)
A treatise on indigestion. With observations on some painful complaints originating in indigestion, as tic douloureux, nervous disorder, &c. . . . 1st American, from the last London ed. rev. and enl. with notes; and an appendix . . . by an American physician. Philadelphia: Key and Mielke, 1831. 206p. DLC; PPC; MB **30-0372**

GRANGER, J. L.
Homoeopathic treatment for chronic and acute diseases. New York: Bradbury, Printer, 1837. 16p. DLC; MBM; PPHa
30-0373

GRANGER, Ralph
Introductory lecture delivered at the Willoughby Medical College of the Willoughby University of Lake Erie, 1837-1838. Painesville: Howe & Jaques, 1837. 16p. DNLM; OCIM; OCIWHi
30-0374

GRANVILLE, Augustus Bozzi (1783-1871)
Counter-irritation, its principles and practice; illustrated by one hundred cases of the most painful and important diseases effectually cured by external applications. [Dunglison's American Medical Library] Philadelphia: A. Waldie, 1838. 172p. DNLM; PPC; PPJ; PU **30-0375**

GRAVES, Robert James (1796-1853)
. . . Clinical lectures delivered during the sessions of 1834-5 and 1836-7. . . . [Dunglison's American Medical Library] Philadelphia: A. Waldie, 1838. 405p. CtY-M; DLC; PPC; PPJ
30-0376

GRAY, John F[ranklin] (1804-1882)
The policy of chartering colleges of medicine; being an introductory lecture to a course of the theory and practice of physic, delivered Monday, November 5, 1832. . . . New York: Henry Ludwig, 1832. 31p. CU-M; NN; NNNAM; NNU-M
30-0377

GREEN, Jacob (1790-1841)
Advantages of chemistry; an introductory address. Philadelphia: W. Brown, 1834. 30p. DNLM **30-0378**

GREEN, James D.
An address delivered at the anniversary celebration of the birth of Spurzheim, and the organization of the Boston Phrenological Society, December 30, 1836. Boston: Marsh, Capen & Lyon, 1837. 27p. DNLM; MH; MBAt; MWA
30-0379

GREEN, Jonas (1798?-1868)
A familiar exposition of homoeopathia; or, the new mode of curing diseases; illustrating its superiority over the prevalent system of medicine. "Magna est veritas, praevalabit." Printed and sold by J. G. Wesselhoeft, Philadelphia, 9 Broad Street, near Arch. New York: Pearl near Chatham Street; Baltimore: 29 Point Market, 1836. 24p. DLC; PPHa
30-0380

GREEN, Jonathan (1788?-1864)
. . . A practical compendium of the diseases of the skin, including a particular consideration of the more frequent and intractable forms of these affections; with cases. . . . [Dunglison's American Medical Library] From the 2nd London ed. Philadelphia: A. Waldie, 1838. 252p. DLC; PPC; PPHa; ScU **30-0381**

GREEN, Jonathan (1788?-1864)
A practical compendium of the diseases of the skin, including a particular consideration of the more frequent and intractable forms of these affections; with cases. . . . From the 2nd London ed. Philadelphia: Thomas, Cowperthwait & Co., 1839. 252p. DLC; GU; LNT-M; PU **30-0382**

GREEN, Jonathan (1788?-1864)
A practical compendium of the diseases of the skin, including a particular consideration of the more frequent and intractable forms of these affections; with cases. . . . Boston: Stimpson & Clapp, 1839. 252p. DLC; MBM; MH; MH-M
30-0383

GREENHOW, Thomas Michael (1791-1881)
Cholera, as it recently appeared in the towns of Newcastle and Gateshead; including cases illustrative of its physiology and pathology, with a view to the establishment of sound principles of practice. . . . Philadelphia: Carey & Lea, 1832. 168p. MB; PPC **30-0384**

GREGORY, George (1790-1853)
Elements of the theory and practice of physic, designed for the use of students. 1st New York from 3rd London ed. New York: M. Sherman, 1830. 738p. ICJ; KyLoJM; PPC; RPM
30-0385

GREGORY, George (1790-1853)
Elements of the theory and practice of physic; . . . with notes and additions adapted to the practice of the United States, by Nathaniel Potter, M.D., professor of the practice of physic in the University of Maryland, and S. Colhoun, M.D. . . . Philadelphia: Towar, J. & D. M. Hogan; Pittsburgh: Hogan & Co., 1831. 2 v. MBM; PMA **30-0386**

GREGORY, George (1790-1853)
Gregory on vaccination, republished with notes, by J. M. Cosgrave. . . . Philadelphia: Printed by W. F. Geddes, 1835. 28p. DLC; PU **30-0387**

GRIFFITH, Robert Eglesfeld (1798-1850)
Lecture introductory to the course on pathology and practice of medicine, in the University of Virginia, for the session of 1837-1838. Published by the members of the class. Charlottesville: J. Alexander, 1837. 16p. DNLM; ViRA
30-0388

GRISCOM, John Hoskins (1809-1874)
Observations on the Apocynum cannabinum. Philadelphia: J. R. A. Skerrett, 1833. 19p. DNLM; PPC
30-0389

GROSS, Samuel David (1805-1884)
The anatomy, physiology, and diseases of the bones and joints. Philadelphia: John Grigg, 1830. 389p. NNNAM; PU **30-0390**

GROSS, Samuel D[avid] (1805-1884)
Elements of pathological anatomy. Boston: Marsh, 1839. 2 v. DLC; PPJ; PU; ScCM **30-0391**

GUNN, John C. (1800-1863)
Gunn's domestic medicine, or Poor man's friend. In the hours of affliction, pain and sickness, this book points out, in plain language, free from Doctor's terms the diseases of men, women and children, and the latest and most approved means used in their cure, and is expressly written for the benefit of families in the western and southern states. Knoxville: Pr. under the immediate superintendence of the Author, a physician of Knoxville, 1830. 440p. MBM; KyLoJM; ScC **30-0392**

GUNN, [John C.] (1800-1863)
Gunn's Domestic Medicine or Poor Man's Friend. Showing the diseases of men, women and children, and expressly intended for the benefit of families. Containing a description of the medicinal roots, and herbs and how they are to be used in the cure of disease. Arranged of a new and simple plan. 2nd ed. Knoxville: F. S. Heiskell, 1831. 500p. DLC; KU; MBM **30-0393**

GUNN, [John C.] (1800-1863)
Gunn's domestic medicine, or poor man's friend. Showing the diseases of men, women and children, and expressly intended for the benefit of families. Containing a description of the medicine roots and herbs, and how they are to be used in the cure of diseases. Arranged on a new and simple plan. . . . 2nd edition, Knoxville, Tenn.: Printed by F. S. Heiskell, 1833. 552p. CSmH; ICJ; MWA **30-0394**

GUNN, [John C.] (1800-1863)
Gunn's domestic medicine, or poor man's friend, in the hours of affliction, pain, and sickness. . . . 12th ed. Louisville [Ky.]: C. Pool, 1838. 768p. DLC; KU; KyLoJM **30-0395**

GUTHRIE, George James (1785-1856)
Clinical lectures on compound fractures of the extremities, on excision of the head of the thigh-bone, the arm-bone and the elbow-joint. On the diseases of the Peninsula, and on several miscellaneous subjects. Delivered at the Westminster Hospital. . . . Philadelphia: A. Waldie, 1839. 90p. DLC; PPC; PPHa; PU **30-0396**

HAHNEMANN, Samuel Christian F. (1755-1843)
Organon of homoeopathic medicine. . . . 1st American from the British transl. of the 4th German ed., with improvements and additions from the 5th, by the North American Academy of the Homoeopathic Healing Art, Allentown, Pa. Published at the Academical Bookstore, 1836. 212p. DLC; PPHa **30-0397**

HALL, Marshall (1790-1857)
Researches principally relative to the morbid and curative effects of loss of blood. . . . Philadelphia: E. L. Carey and A. Hart; Thomas Kite, pr., 1830. 173p., fold. tab. IU-M; MdBM; PP **30-0398**

HALL, Marshall (1790-1857)
Researches, principally relative to the morbid and curative effects of loss of blood. 2nd American ed. Philadelphia: E. L. Carey & A. Hart, 1835. 254p. DNLM; PPC; PU **30-0399**

HALL, Marshall (1790-1857)
The principles of diagnosis. . . . 2nd ed., entirely re-written. New York: D. Appleton & Co., 1835. 463p. DLC; NNNAM; NNU-M **30-0400**

HALL, Marshall (1790-1857)
Principles of the theory and practice of medicine. . . . 1st American ed. Rev. and much enl., by Jacob Bigelow . . . and Oliver Wendell Holmes. . . . Boston: C. C. Little and J. Brown, 1839. DLC; MBM; MH; MH-M **30-0401**

HALL, Marshall (1790-1857)
The principles of diagnosis. . . . 2nd American ed., with notes by John A. Swett. New York: D. Appleton & Co., 1839. 458p. DLC; NN; NNNAM **30-0402**

HALSTED, Oliver
A full and accurate account of the new method of curing dyspepsia, discovered and practiced by O. Halsted. With some observation on diseases of the digestive organs. New York: O. Halsted [Browns, prs.] 1830. 155p. DLC; IU-M; PPC **30-0403**

HALSTED, Oliver
A full and accurate account of the new method of curing dyspepsia, discovered and practiced by O. Halsted. With some observations on diseases of the digestive organs. 2nd ed., with plates and explanatory notes. New York: O. Halsted, 1831. 155p. GU; NjR **30-0404**

HALSTED, Oliver
A full and accurate account of the new method of curing dyspepsia discovered and practiced by O. Halsted with some observations on diseases of the digestive organs. 2nd ed., with plates and explanatory notes. New York: O. Halsted, 1832. 155p. MWA; NN; NNNAM **30-0405**

HAMILTON, Frank Hastings (1813-1886)
Introductory address and catalogue of students attending the annual course of lectures on anatomy and surgery. Auburn: Oliphant & Skinner, 1837. 16p. DNLM; NHi **30-0406**

HAMILTON, Frank Hastings (1813-1886)
Discourse on the importance of a general diffusion of a knowledge of anatomy, physiology, and hygiene. Auburn: Oliphant & Skinner, 1838. 20p. DNLM **30-0407**

HAMILTON, Frank Hastings (1813-1886)
Introductory lecture before the surgical class of the College of Physicians and Surgeons, Fairfield, New York, delivered December 3, 1839. Albany: Hoffman, White, and Company, 1839. 22p. DLC; NN; NNNAM **30-0408**

HAMILTON, James, Jr.
Practical observations on various subjects relating to midwifery. [Dunglison's American Medical Library] Philadelphia: A. Waldie, 1837. 102p. DNLM; PPC; NNNAM **30-0409**

HANCE, William
An address and lectures, delivered before the Botanic Society in Columbus, Ohio. 2nd ed. Columbus, Ohio: Horton Howard, pr. by Charles Scott, 1830. 42p. DLC; OC; OClWHi; PPC **30-0410**

HANCE, William
An appeal to the citizens of Ohio; showing the unconstitutionality, injustice, and impolicy of the medical law. Columbus: Pr. by Charles Scott, 1830. 20p. DNLM **30-0411**

HARE, Robert (1781-1858)
Essays on electricity. Being a portion of his compendium of the course of chemical instruction in the medical department of the University of Pennsylvania. Published in advance for the use of students. Philadelphia, 1830. 23p. PPC
30-0412

HARLAN, Richard (1796-1843)
Medical and physical researches; or, Original memoirs in medicine, surgery, physiology, geology, zoology, and comparative anatomy. . . . Philadelphia: Printed by Lydia R. Bailey, 1835. 653p. 39 plates. DLC; PPC; PPJ; PU
30-0413

HARLOW, Samuel
The botanist & physician; containing a description of the principal active medicinal plants found in the middle and northern states of America. . . . Kingston, N.Y.: Pr. by Wm. Culley, 1831. 151p. CSmH; DLC; NNNAM
30-0414

HARRIS, Chapin Aaron (1806-1860)
The dental art, a practical treatise on dental surgery. . . . Baltimore: Armstrong & Berry, 1839. 384p. 3 plates. DLC; MdHi; MdU-D **30-0415**

HARRIS, Thomas (1784-1861)
An oration delivered before the Philadelphia Medical Society. Philadelphia: J. Kay, Jr., & Co., 1831. 28p. DNLM
30-0416

HARRIS, Thomas (1784-1861)
An oration delivered before the Philadelphia Medical Society, February 19, 1831. . . . Philadelphia: Pr. by J. Kay, Jr. & Co., for the Society, 1831. 28p. MH-M; PU
30-0417

HARRISON, John Pollard (1796-1849)
Lectures on the responsibilities of the medical profession. . . . Louisville, Ky.: Pr. by W. W. Worsley, 1831. 11p. CSmH; DNLM **30-0418**

HARRISON, John Pollard (1796-1849)
Address delivered before the Louisville Medical Society, at their annual meeting, January 1, 1833. . . . Louisville: Printed at the Herald office, 1833. 12p. DLC; KU; KyLoJM; NN
30-0419

HARRISON, John Pollard (1796-1849)
Essays and lectures on medical subjects. . . . Philadelphia: J. Crissy, 1835. 192p. DLC; DNLM; PPC; PU
30-0420

HARRISON, Robert (1796-1858)
The Dublin dissector, or Manual of anatomy: comprising a concise description of the bones, muscles, vessels, nerves and viscera, also the relative anatomy of the different regions of the human body; for the use of students in the dissecting room. By a member of the Royal College of Surgeons in Ireland. 1st American from the 2nd Dublin ed. Washington [D.C.]: D. Green, 1835. DLC; MdBJ-W; MdU-D
30-0421

[HARTFORD, Connecticut]
Society for the Relief of the Insane. The Institute located at Hartford, in Connecticut. Annual Meeting at Hartford, 2nd Wednesday of May. Hartford: Hudson & Skinner, 1832. 35p. CtHi; CtY-M; MBM **30-0422**

HASKELL, Benjamin
A lecture, introductory to the first course of lectures on popular physiology, instituted by the American Physiological Society, October 10, 1837. . . . Published by request. Boston: Office of the Graham Journal, 1838. 24p. DLC
30-0423

HAXALL, Robert William (1802-1872)
Prize essay on fistula lachrymalis. Richmond: J. H. Nash, 1832. 41p. DNLM; ViRA **30-0424**

HAXALL, Robert William (1802-1872)
A dissertation on the importance of physical signs in the various diseases of the abdomen and thorax. . . . Boston: Printed by Perkins & Marvin, 1836. 106p. [Harvard University. Boylston Medical Society Prize Dissertations] DLC; MBM; MH; MWA **30-0425**

HAYS, Isaac, ed. (1796-1879)
Select medico-chirurgical transactions; a collection of the most valuable memoirs read to the medico-chirurgical societies of London and Edinburgh. . . . Philadelphia: E. L. Carey and A. Hart, 1831. 420p. CtY-M; MdBM **30-0426**

HAYS, Isaac, ed. (1796-1879)
The American Cyclopaedia of Practical Medicine and Surgery, a digest of medical literature. . . . Philadephia: Carey, Lea & Blanchard, 1833-1834. Parts I-III. DNL; PPC: PPJ; PPHa
30-0427

HAYWARD, George (1791-1863)
A lecture on some of the diseases of a literary life, delivered before the American Institute August 23, 1832; . . . Boston: Carter, Hendee & Co., 1833. 20p. DLC; MB: MHi
30-0428

HAYWARD, George (1791-1863)
Outlines of human physiology; designed for the use of higher classes in common schools. Boston: Marsh, Capen & Lyon, 1834. 217p. DNLM; MWA; MBAt
30-0429

HAYWARD, George (1791-1863)
A discourse on some of the diseases of the knee-joint. Boston: Whipple & Damrell, 1837. 28p. DNLM; MBM
30-0430

HAYWARD, George (1791-1863)
Report of the surgical cases and operations that occurred in the Massachusetts General Hospital, from May 12, 1837 to May 12, 1838. Boston: D. Clapp, Jr., 1838. 32p. DNLM; MBM **30-0431**

HAYWARD. George (1791-1863)
Remarks on some of the medicinal springs of Virginia. Boston: D. Clapp, Jr., 1839. 11p. DNLM; MWA; MBAt
30-0432

HECKER, Justus Friedrich Karl (1795-1850)
The epidemics of the middle ages. [No. 2]. The dancing mania. Transl. by B. G. Babington. Philadelphia: Haswell, Barrington & Haswell, 1837. 84p. DNLM; PU
30-0433

HECKER, Justus Friedrich Karl (1795-1850)
The epidemics of the middle ages. [No. 2] The black death in the fourteenth century. Transl. by B. G. Babington. Philadelphia: Haswell, Barrington & Haswell, 1837. 74p. DNLM; PU
30-0434

HECKER, Justus Friedrich Karl (1795-1850)
The epidemics of the middle ages: from the German of J. F. K. Hecker. . . . Transl. by B. G. Babington. . . . Philadelphia: Haswell, Barrington, & Haswell, 1837. 2 v. in 1. DLC: PPC; PU **30-0435**

HENDERSON, Thomas (1789-1854)
The physician's first steps in professional life: an address delivered at the medical commencement in Washington, March 7, 1832. . . . Washington, 1832. 16p. DNLM **30-0436**

HENNEN, John (1779-1828)
Principles of military surgery; comprising observations on the arrangement, police and practice of hospitals, and on the history, treatment and anomalies of variola and syphilis. . . . 1st American from the 3rd London ed. With life of the author, by his son, Dr. John Hennen. Philadelphia: Carey & Lea [Griggs & Dickinson, prs.], 1830. 452p. DLC; NN; OC **30-0437**

HENRY, John Flourney (1793-1873)
A letter on the cholera as it occurred in Cincinnati, Ohio, in October, 1832, addressed to Dr. Short of Lexington, Ky. [Lexington, Ky., 1832] 29p. DNLM; OC **30-0438**

HENRY, John Flourney (1793-1873)
An exposure of the conduct, of the trustees and professors of the Medical College of Ohio. . . . Cincinnati: Wood & Stratton, Printers, 1833. 20p. CSmH; DLC; IEN-M **30-0439**

HERING, Constantine (1800-1880)
Kurze Uebersicht der homoeopathischen Heilkunst, ihrer allmalingen Enstehung und jezigen Ausbildung, von Dr. Constantin Hering, praktischen Arzte in Philadelphia. Vorgetragen in der Hahnemannischen Gesellschaft zu Philadelphia den 18 April, 1833. Philadelphia: J. G. Wesselhoeft, 1833. 30p. DLC; PPHa **30-0440**

HERING, Constantine (1800-1880)
A concise view of the rise and progress of homoeopathic medicine. Transl. from the German by Charles F. Matlack, M.D. Delivered before the Hahnemannian Society in Philadelphia the 18th day of April, 1833. No. 1. Printed for the Hahnemannian Society in Philadelphia. 1833. Young, printer, Black Horse Alley. 29p. DLC; PPHa **30-0441**

HERING, Constantine (1800-1880)
Proposals for publishing by subscription "The Library of Homoeopathia." A circular. By Drs. Hering and J. G. Wesselhoeft. Philadelphia, 1833. 8p. DLC; PPHa **30-0442**

HERING, Constantine (1800-1880)
The Homoeopathist or Domestic Physician. By C. Hering, M.D., Professor in the College of Homoeopathic Medicine at Allentown, Pa. First Part. Sold by J. G. Wesselhoeft, Philadelphia, No. 9 Broad Street, near Arch. Allentown, Pa., at the Academical Bookstore, 1835-1838. 2 v. DLC; PPHa **30-0443**

HERING, Constantine (1800-1880)
Homöopathischer hausarzt. Für die deutschen burger der Vereinigten Staaten nach den besten vaterländischen werken und eignen erfabrungen bearb. von C. Hering. . . . Allentaun an der Lecha, J. Behlert. Philadelphia: Gedruckt bei J. G. Wesselhoeft, 1837. 352p. DLC; PPHa **30-0444**

HERING, Constantine (1800-1880)
Wirkungen des Schlangengiftes, zum ärztlichen Gebrauche vergleichend zusammengestellt. Mit einer Einleitung über das Studium der homöopathischen Arzneimittellehre. Allentown, Pa.: A. & W. Blumer, 1837. 116p. DNLM; PPHa **30-0445**

HERRICK, N. N.
The cheap physician, and guide to health. . . . Penn Yan [N.Y.]: Printed by Bennett, 1838. 28p. DLC; N; NN **30-0446**

HERSEY, Thomas
The midwife's practical directory; or the woman's confidential friend . . . with an appendix. The whole designed by the special use of the botanic friends in the United States. 2nd ed. Baltimore: Sands & Neilson, 1836. 336p. 11 plates. DNLM; MdU-D **30-0447**

HIBBARD, David R.
A treatise on cow-pox. In which the existence of small-pox, or varioloid in any form, subsequent to vaccination, is shown to arise from some imperfection in its performance, and not the result of inefficacy on the part of the vaccina to shield the system entirely from these diseases. . . . New York: Printed by Harper & Brothers, 1835. 69p. DLC; NN; NNNAM **30-0448**

HILDRETH, Charles T.
Case of notencephale. Boston, 1834. 16p. 2 plates. DNLM **30-0449**

HILDRETH, Samuel Prescott (1783-1863)
Address of . . . president of the third medical convention of Ohio, delivered at Cleveland, May 14th, 1839. Cleveland: Penniman & Bemis, 1839. 33p. DNLM; OCIM; OCIWHi **30-0450**

HITCHCOCK, Edward (1793-1864)
An essay on alcoholic and narcotic substances, as articles of common use; addressed particularly to students. Amherst: J. S. & C. Adams & Co., 1830. 48p. DNLM; MA **30-0451**

HITCHCOCK, Edward (1793-1864)
Dyspepsy forestalled & resisted: or, Lectures on diet, regimen, & employment; delivered to the students of Amherst College; spring term, 1830. Amherst: J. S. & C. Adams and Co.; New York: J. Leavitt; [etc., etc.] 1830. 360p. DLC; MB; MH; PPC **30-0452**

HITCHCOCK, Edward (1793-1864)
Dyspepsy forestalled and resisted; or, Lectures on diet, regimen, and employment; delivered to the students of Amherst College, Spring term, 1830. . . . 2nd ed. corr. and enl. by the addition of an address delivered before the Mechanical Association in Andover Theological Institution, Sept. 21, 1830, and an appendix of notes. Amherst: J. S. & C. Adams; New York: J. Leavitt; [etc., etc.] 1831. 452p. DLC; MB; PPC **30-0453**

HOBSON, Samuel J.
An essay on the history, preparation & therapeutic uses of iodine. Philadelphia, 1830. 60p. DLC; MWA; NNNAM; PPC **30-0454**

HODGE, Hugh Lenox (1796-1873)
Essay on the pathology and therapeutics of cholera maligna. American Journal of the Medical Society, Aug. 1833. Philadelphia: Skerrett, Pr., 1833. 48p. CtY-M; DLC; DNLM
30-0455

HODGE, Hugh Lenox (1796-1873)
A lecture introductory to the course on obstetrics, and diseases of women and children, in the University of Pennsylvania. Philadelphia: J. G. Auner, 1835. 19p. DNLM; PU
30-0456

HODGE, Hugh Lenox (1796-1873)
An introductory lecture to the course on obstetrics, and diseases of women and children, in the University of Pennsylvania, for the session of 1836-1837. Philadelphia: T. B. Town, 1836. 20p. DNLM; PU **30-0457**

HODGE, Hugh Lenox (1796-1873)
An introductory lecture to the course on obstetrics, and diseases of women and children, delivered in the University of Pennsylvania, November 7, 1838. Philadelphia: J. G. Auner, 1838. 23p. DNLM; PU **30-0458**

HODGE, Hugh Lenox (1796-1873)
Foeticide, or criminal abortion: a lecture. Philadelphia: Lindsay & Blakiston, 1839. 44p. DNLM; PPHa; PU
30-0459

HODGE, Hugh Lenox (1796-1873)
An introductory lecture to the course of obstetrics, and diseases of women and children, delivered in the University of Pennsylvania November 6, 1839. Philadelphia: Lydia R. Bailey, 1839. 20p. DNLM; PU **30-0460**

HOLLAND, Henry (1788-1873)
Medical notes and reflections. Philadelphia: Haswell, Barrington & Haswell, 1839. 383p. DNLM; NjR; PPC; PU
30-0461

HOLMES, Oliver Wendell (1809-1894)
Dissertations on the question How far are the external means of exploring the condition of the internal organs to be considered useful and important in medical practice: For which premiums were adjudged by the Boylston Medical Committee of Harvard University, 1836. By Oliver W. Holmes; Robert W. Haxall, and Luther V. Bell, M.D. Boston: Printed by Perkins & Marvin, 1836. 288p. DLC; MH; MBM; MH-M
30-0462

HOLMES, Oliver Wendell (1809-1894)
Boylston prize dissertations for the years 1836 and 1837. . . . Boston, C. C. Little and J. Brown, 1838. 371p. DLC; MH; MH-M; MHi **30-0463**

HOOKER, Charles (1799-1863)
An essay on the relation between the respiratory and circulating functions. Boston: D. Clapp, Jr., 1838. 47p. DNLM; MBM **30-0464**

HOOPER, Robert (1773-1835)
Examinations in anatomy, physiology, practice of physic, surgery, chemistry, obstetrics, materia medica, and pharmacy; For the use of students. New York: Pub. by Collins and Co. [W. E. Dean, pr.] 1830. 182p. CtY-M; DLC; PPL
30-0465

HOOPER, Robert (1773-1835)
Examinations in anatomy, physiology, practice of physic, surgery, chemistry. obstetrics, materia medica, pharmacy and poisons . . . from last London ed. New York City: Collins and Co., 1832. 190p. MdBM; Nh; PU; RPB
30-0466

HOOPER, Robert (1773-1835)
. . . Lexicon medicum; or medical dictionary. . . . The 4th American, from the last London ed., with additions from American authors . . . by Samuel Akerly. . . . New York: Printed by J. and J. Harper, 1833. 2 v. in 1. OCIM
30-0467

HOPKINSON, John P.
Remarks on the pathology and treatment of the disease termed malignant cholera. . . . Philadelphia: Pr. by Jos. R. A. Skerrett, 1832. 16p. NNNAM; PPL; ScU **30-0468**

HOPKINSON, John P.
Engravings of the arteries. Philadelphia: Gibbons, 1832. 15p. Plates. DLC; MH-M; PPC **30-0469**

HORNER, Gustavus R. B. (1804-1892)
Medical and topographical observations upon the Mediterranean; and upon Portugal, Spain, and other countries. . . . Philadelphia: Haswell, Barrington, & Haswell, 1839. 212p. DLC; PPC; PP; PU **30-0470**

HORNER, William Edmonds (1793-1853)
A treatise on special and general anatomy. . . . 2nd ed., rev. and corr. Philadelphia: Carey and Lea [Griggs & Dickinson, pr.] 1830. 2 v. DNLM; GU; PPC; RPM **30-0471**

HORNER, William Edmonds (1793-1853)
Introductory to a course of anatomy in the University of Pennsylvania, delivered November 7th, 1831. . . . Philadelphia: J. G. Auner, 1831. 28p. DLC; OCIWHi; PHi
30-0472

HORNER, William Edmonds (1793-1853)
Catalogue of the anatomical museum of the University of Pennsylvania, with a report to the museum committee of the trustees Nov. 1832. 2nd ed. Philadelphia: Bailey, 1832. 51p. DLC; NNNAM; IEN-M; PHi **30-0473**

HORNER, William Edmonds (1793-1853)
A treatise on special and general anatomy . . . 3rd ed., rev. and corr. Philadelphia: Carey, Lea & Blanchard, 1834. 2 v. DNLM; PPC; PU **30-0474**

HORNER, William Edmonds (1793-1853)
On the anatomical characters of Asiatic cholera, with remarks on the structure of the mucous coat of the alimentary canal. Philadelphia: J. R. A. Skerrett, 1835. 45p. 2 plates. DNLM; DLC; PPC **30-0475**

HORNER, William Edmonds (1793-1853)
A treatise on special and general anatomy. . . . 4th ed., rev. and improved. Philadelphia: Carey, Lea & Blanchard, 1836. 2 v. DLC; PPC; PPJ; PU **30-0476**

HORNER, William Edmonds (1793-1853)
Lessons in practical anatomy for the use of dissectors. 3rd ed. Philadelphia: J. G. Auner, 1836. 503p. DNLM; PPC; PU
30-0477

HORNER, William Edmonds (1793-1853)
Necrological notice of Dr. Philip Syng Physick. Philadelphia: Haswell, Barrington & Haswell, 1838. 32p. DNLM; PPC; PPJ
30-0478

HOSACK, Alexander E[ddy] (1805-1871)
A memoir upon staphyloraphy; with cases and a description of the instruments requisite for the operation. New York: J. & J. Harper, 1833. 20p. 1 plate. DNLM; NNNAM
30-0479

HOSACK, David (1769-1835)
Lectures on the theory and practice of physic, delivered in the College of Physicians and Surgeons of the University of the State of New York. . . . With an introductory letter, by Nathaniel Chapman. . . . Ed. by his friend and former pupil, Henry W. Ducachet. . . . Philadelphia: H. Hooker, 1838. 699p. DLC; PPC; PPJ; PU **30-0480**

HOWARD, Horton
A treatise on the complaints peculiar to females: embracing a system of midwifery; the whole in conformity with the improved system of botanic medicine. . . . Columbus: Pr. by Chas. Scott, for the author, 1832. 172p. IEN-M; OCHP; PU
30-0481

HOWARD, Horton
An improved system of botanic medicine. founded upon correct physiological principles, embracing a concise view of anatomy and physiology; together with an illustration of the new theory of medicine. . . . Columbus: The Author, 1832. 2 v. DLC; KyLoJM; RPM **30-0482**

HOWARD, Horton
An improved system of botanic medicine, founded upon correct physiological principles; together with an illustration of the new theory of medicine. . . . In three volumes. 2nd edition; revised and corrected. Columbus, Ohio: Published by the author, 1833. 3 v. CtY-M; KU; MBM
30-0483

HOWARD, Horton
An improved system of botanic medicine; founded upon correct physiological principles; embracing a concise view of anatomy and physiology; together with an illustration of the new theory of medicine. To which is added, a treatise on female complaints, midwifery, and the diseases of children. . . . 3rd ed. rev. and cor. Columbus, O.: Published by the proprietors, 1836. 3 v. in 2. Plates. DLC: OCLloyd; NjR; OCIWHi
30-0484

HOWE, Samuel Gridley (1801-1870)
An address delivered at the anniversary celebration of the Boston Phrenological Society, December 28, 1835. Boston: Marsh, Capen & Lyon, 1836. 27p. DNLM; MBM; MWA
30-0485

HOWE, Samuel Gridley (1801-1870)
A discourse on the social relations of man, delivered before the Boston Phrenological Society. Boston: Marsh, Capen & Lyon, 1837. 40p. DNLM; MBM; MWA
30-0486

HULL, Amos Gerald (1810-1859)
Dr. Hull's patent truss. Extracts from the opinions of distinguished surgeons, and late medical authors . . . of Dr. Hull's newly invented instrument for . . . disease of hernia, or rupture. [New York: Philip French, 1832] 8p. NNNAM
30-0487

HULL, Amos Gerald (1810-1859)
A brief account of the application and uses of the utero-abdominal supporter, a new instrument for the relief and cure of procidentia and prolapsus uteri invented by the late A. G. Hull, M.D. of New York. New York: D. Murphy, 1836. 11p. NNNAM **30-0488**

HULL, Amos Gerald (1810-1859)
. . . A plain account of the application and uses of A. G. Hull's utero-abdominal supporter. New York: W. Plows, 1839. 16p. DNLM; NNNAM **30-0489**

HULL, Laurens (1779-1865)
Annual address delivered before the Medical Society of the State of New York: Albany: J. Munsell, 1839. 14p. DNLM; N; NHi **30-0490**

HUN, Thomas (1808-1896)
Introductory lecture before the Albany Medical College. Delivered Nov. 12, 1839. . . . Albany: Printed by H. D. Stone and Co., 1839. 30p. DLC; N; NHi; NN
30-0491

HUNTER, John (1728-1793)
A treatise on the venereal disease. . . . With notes by George G. Babington. . . . [American Medical Library] Philadelphia: Haswell, Barrington, and Haswell, 1839. 347p. 6 plates. DLC; PPC; PU **30-0492**

HUNTER, John (1728-1793)
Lectures on the principles of surgery. . . . With notes by James F. Palmer. . . . Philadelphia: Haswell, Barrington, and Haswell, 1839. 400p. 3 plates. DLC; PPC; PPJ; PU
30-0493

HUNTER, John (1728-1793)
The natural history of the human teeth. Explaining their structure, use, formation, growth, and diseases. . . . With notes, by Eleazar Parmly. New York: 1839. 2 v. in 1. Plates. DLC; NN; NNNAM **30-0494**

HUNTER, John (1728-1793)
Treatise on the natural history and diseases of the human teeth: explaining their structure, use, formation, growth, and diseases. . . . With notes by Thomas Bell. . . . Philadelphia: Haswell, Barrington, and Haswell, 1839. 127p. 5 plates. DLC; MBM; PPC; PU **30-0495**

HUNTT, Henry (1792-1838)
Observations on a change of climate in pulmonary consumption. Read before the Columbian Institute in 1826, and published in the Medical and Surgical Journal. With additional remarks on the Red Sulphur Springs of Virginia. . . . Washington, D.C.: Printed by J. Gideon, Jr., 1834. 22p. DLC; MdU-D
30-0496

HUNTT, Henry (1792-1838)
A visit to the Red Sulphur Spring of Virginia, during the summer of 1837: with observations on the waters. . . . Washington City: J. Gideon, 1838. 27p. DLC; PPC; NNNAM
30-0497

HUNTT, Henry (1792-1838)
A visit to the Red Sulphur Spring of Virginia, during the summer of 1837: with observations on the waters. . . . With an introduction, containing notices of routes, &c., by an annual visitor. Boston: Dutton and Wentworth, printers, 1839. 40p. DLC; MB; MBM; MWA **30-0498**

IMPROVED American family physician, or sick man's guide to health, containing a complete theory of the botanic practice of medicine on the Thomsonian and hygeian system . . . also a complete digest of midwifery. New York, 1833. 120, 24p. DLC; NN; NNNAM; NjR **30-0499**

[INFLUENZA]
An account of the origin, symptoms, and cure of the influenza or epidemic catarrh; with some hints respecting common colds and incipient pulmonary consumption. Philadelphia: H. H. Porter, 1832. 80p. DLC; PHi; PP **30-0500**

INGALLS, William (1769-1851)
An essay on the ganglionary system of nerves in the cavity of the cranium, and its use. Boston: Marsh, Capen & Lyon, 1832. 15p. DLC; MB; MH-M; DNLM **30-0501**

INGALLS, William (1769-1851)
On scarlatina, in a letter addressed to his son. . . . Also, observations on the various therapeutic agents that have been employed in the treatment of scarlatina. Boston: Otis, Broaders & Co., 1837. 39p. MB; MBM; MH **30-0502**

INGALLS, William (1769-1851)
On scarlatina, in a letter addressed to his son. . . . Also, observations on the various therapeutic agents that have been employed in the treatment of scarlatina. 2nd ed. With an appendix. Boston: B. H. Greene, 1839. 40p. MB; MBM; MH **30-0503**

INGALLS, William (1769-1851)
A lecture on the subject of: phrenology not opposed to the principles of religion, nor the precepts of Christianity. Boston: Dutton & Wentworth, 1839. 50p. MB; MBM; MH; MWA **30-0504**

IRVING, C.
A catechism of practical chemistry; being a familiar introduction . . . 5th American ed., rev. and corrected by John Griscom. New York: Collins, Keese & Co., 1837. 81p. 1 plate. DNLM **30-0505**

JACKSON, James (1777-1867)
A memoir of James Jackson, Jr., M.D., with extracts from his letters to his father; and medical cases, collected by him. . . . Boston: Printed by I. R. Butts, 1835. 444p. DLC; MA; MH-M; NN **30-0506**

[JACKSON, James] (1777-1867)
Memoir of James Jackson, Jr., M.D., written by his father, with extracts from his letters, and reminiscences of him, by a fellow student. For the Warren Street Chapel. . . . Boston: Hilliard, Gray & Co., 1836. 228p. DLC; MB; MBM; MWA **30-0507**

JACKSON, James (1777-1867)
A report founded on the cases of typhoid fever, or the common continued fever of New England, which occurred in the Massachusetts General Hospital from 1821-1835. . . . Boston: Whipple and Damrell, 1838. 95p. ICJ; MBM; MHi; MH-M **30-0508**

JACKSON, James. Jr. (1810-1834)
Cases of cholera collected at Paris, in the month of April, 1832, in the wards of MM. Andral and Louis, at the hospital, La Pitié. . . . Boston: Carter, Hendee & Co., 1832. 212p. DLC; MB; PPAmP **30-0509**

JACKSON, Samuel (1787-1872)
Introductory lecture to the institutes of medicine. Philadelphia: W. Sharpless, 1830. 35p. DLC; NBM; PHi **30-0510**

JACKSON, Samuel (1787-1872)
Observations on delirium tremens. Philadelphia: J. R. A. Skerrett, 1831. 24p. DNLM; PU **30-0511**

JACKSON, Samuel (1787-1872)
The Principles of Medicine, founded on the structure and functions of animal organism. . . . Philadelphia: Carey & Lea, 1832. 630 [28] p. DLC; PU; ViRA **30-0512**

JACKSON, Samuel (1787-1872)
Lecture on medical education, introductory to the course of the institutes of medicine in the University of Pennsylvania for the session, 1833-1834. Published by request of the class. Philadelphia, 1833. 32p. DLC; IEN-M; NjR; PHi **30-0513**

JACKSON, Samuel (1787-1872)
A lecture introductory to the course of institutes of medicine, in the University of Pennsylvania, for the session of 1835-6. . . . Published by members of the class. Philadelphia: Printed by T. B. Town, 1835. 23p. DLC; DNLM; PPC; PU **30-0514**

JACKSON, Samuel (1787-1872)
Introductory lectures to the course of the institutes of medicine, in the University of Pennsylvania, November 6, 1837. Philadelphia: J. G. Auner, 1837. 30p. DNLM; PU **30-0515**

JACKSON, Samuel (1787-1872)
On the methods of acquiring knowledge. An introductory lecture to the course of institutes of medicine for the session 1838-1839. Philadelphia: J. G. Auner, 1838. 32p. DNLM; PPC; PU **30-0516**

JAHR, Gottlieb Heinrich Georg (1800-1875)
G. H. G. Jahr's Manual of Homoeopathic Medicine. Translated from the German by authority of the North American Academy of the Homoeopathic Healing Art, with an introduction and some additions by C. Hering. Allentown, Pa., at the Academical Book Store. In commission by J. G. Wesselhoeft. Philadelphia, 9 Broad St., 1836-1838. 2 parts [I, 419p. II, 180p]. DLC; PPHa **30-0517**

JAMESON, Horatio Gates (1778-1855)
An epitome of the epidemic cholera; in which is exhibited an inquiry into the character, nature and prevention of the disease, its treatment. . . . Baltimore: Pr. by W. Wooddy, 1832. 78p. MdBJ-W; MdU-D **30-0518**

JEANES, Jacob (1800-1877)
Homoeopathic practice of medicine. . . . Philadelphia: A. Waldie, 1838. 391p. DNLM; DLC; MBM; PPHa **30-0519**

JOHNSON, James (1777-1845)
Change of air, or The philosophy of travelling, being autumnal excursions through France, Switzerland, Italy, Germany, and Belgium; with observations and reflections on the moral, physical, and medicinal infuence of travelling-exercise, change of scene, foreign skies, and voluntary expatriation. To which is prefixed, Wear and tear of modern Babylon. . . . New York; S. Wood and Sons, 1831. 326p. DLC; DNLM; PPPH **30-0520**

JOHNSON, James (1777-1845)
An essay on indigestion; or morbid sensibility of the stomach and bowels, as the proximate cause or characteristic condition of dyspepsy, nervous irritability, mental despondency, hypochondriasis. . . . To which are added, observations on the diseases & regimen of invalids on their return from hot and unhealthy climates. . . . 3rd Philadelphia, from the 6th London ed., much enl. Philadelphia: Nathan Kite, 1831. 194p. GU; IE-M; PPC **30-0521**

JOHNSON, James (1777-1845)
A treatise on derangements of the liver, internal organs, and nervous system, pathological and therapeutical. Concord: H. Hill & Co., 1832. 234p. DNLM; MBM; MH-M **30-0522**

JOHNSON, James (1777-1845)
The economy of life; or the stream of human life from the cradle to the grave. . . . New York: Harper & Bros., 1837. 283p. DNLM; MBM; NN; NNNAM **30-0523**

JOHNSTONE, James
A therapeutic arrangement and syllabus of materia medica. Philadelphia: Haswell, Barrington & Haswell, 1837. 71p. DNLM; PPC; PPJ; PU **30-0524**

JONES, Thomas P.
Charge addressed to the graduates in medicine, at the commencement of the Medical Department of the Columbian College, D.C. March 10, 1830. Washington: Gales & Seaton, 1830. 12p. DNLM; PPL **30-0525**

JOSLIN, Benjamin Franklin (1796-1861)
Observations on vision. Philadelphia: J. R. A. Skerrett, 1831. 8p. DNLM; PPC **30-0526**

JOSLIN, Benjamin Franklin (1796-1861)
The physiology of respiration and chemistry of the blood, applied to epidemic cholera. [1835] 32p. DNLM; PPC **30-0527**

JOSLIN, Benjamin Franklin (1796-1861)
Physiological explanation of the beauty of form. Albany: E. W. & C. Skinner, 1837. 29p. DNLM; N; NHi **30-0528**

JUDSON, H. T.
Alphabet of phrenology. A short sketch of that science, for the use of beginners. . . . New York: C. S. Francis; Boston: Munroe & Francis, 1833. 47p. DLC; PU **30-0529**

KAIN, John H.
An oration, pronounced before the Medical Society of the State of Tennessee, May 3rd, 1831. On medical emulation. . . . Nashville: Pub. by the Society, 1831. 13-29p. CtY-M; MHi **30-0530**

KIDD, John (1775-1851)
On the adaptation of external nature to the physical condition of man, principally with reference to his supply of wants, and the exercise of his intellectual faculties. Philadelphia: Carey, Lea & Blanchard, 1833. 280p. DNLM; PPC; PU **30-0531**

KING, David (1812-1882)
Purpura haemorrhagica, its causes and treatment. (Fiske Fund Prize Dissertation, No. 2, June, 1836.) Boston: D. Clapp, 1837. 38p. DNLM; MBM; MH **30-0532**

KING, David (1812-1882)
Cholera infantum, its causes and treatment. (Fiske Fund Prize Dissertation, No. 3, June, 1837.) Boston: D. Clapp, 1837. 22p. DNLM; MBM; MH **30-0533**

KINMONT, Alexander
Twelve lectures on the natural history of man. . . . With a biographical sketch of the author. Cincinnati: U. P. James, 1839. 355p. DNLM; OC **30-0534**

KIRK, James Bladerstone
Practical observations on cholera asphyxia. Communicated in a report to the Greenock Board of Health, as the result of a mission to the infected districts. New York: P. Hill, 1832. 72p. DNLM; NNNAM **30-0535**

KISSAM, Richard S. (1808-1861)
A dissertation on iritis. Submitted to the public examination of the trustees and professors of the College of Physicians and Surgeons in the University of the State of New York. For the degree of Doctor of Medicine, April 6th, 1830. New York: J. & J. Harper, 1830. 27p. CSmH; NNNAM **30-0536**

KITCHINER, William (1775?-1827)
Directions for invigorating and prolonging life; or, The invalid's oracle. Containing peptic precepts, pointing out agreeable and effectual methods to prevent and relieve indigestion, and to regulate and strengthen the action of the stomach and bowels. . . . From the 6th London ed.; rev. and improved, by T. S. Barrett. . . . New York: J. & J. Harper, 1833. 256p. DLC; LNT-M; MdHi; PMA **30-0537**

KNIGHT, Jonathan (1789-1864)
A lecture, introductory to the course of instruction in the medical institution of Yale College, delivered Nov. 2, 1838. . . . New Haven: Printed by B. L. Hamlen, 1838. 27p. CtY-M; DLC; MH; MBM **30-0538**

KRAMER, Wilhelm (1801-1876)
. . . Nature and treatment of diseases of the ear. . . . 2nd ed. of the author's treatise on chronic deafness, much improved and enlarged. Transl. from the German, with the latest improvements of the author since the last London ed., by James Risdon Bennett. . . . Philadelphia: A. Waldie, 1838. 204p. DLC; PPC; PPHa; PPJ **30-0539**

KRAMER, Wilhelm (1801-1876)
Nature and treatment of diseases of the ear. . . . 2nd ed. of the author's treatise on chronic deafness, much improved and enlarged. Transl. from the German, with the latest improvements of the author since the last London ed., by James Risdon Bennett. . . . Philadelphia: Thomas, Cowperthwait & Co., 1838. 250p. DLC; PPC; PU **30-0540**

LABARRAQUE, Antoine Germain (1777-1850)
Method of using the chlorides of soda, either for dressing ill-conditioned sores, or as a means of purifying unhealthy places, and of disinfecting animal substances. Transl. by Jacob Porter. New Haven: H. Howe, 1830. 7p. CtY-M; DNLM **30-0541**

LABARRAQUE, Antoine Germain (1777-1850)
Method of using the chloride of soda, either for dressing ill-conditioned sores, or as a means of purifying unhealthy places, and of disinfecting animal substances. . . . Transl. by Jacob Porter, 2nd ed. Northampton: Printed by J. Metcalf, 1833. 7p. DLC; DNLM; MWA; ScU **30-0542**

LACOMBE, Dr.
Homoeopathia explained; being an exposition of the doctrine of Hahnemann according to the opinions published by the principal physicians of the Faculty of Paris. New York: James E. Betts, 1835. 24p. DLC; PPHa **30-0543**

LAËNNEC, Mériadec
A manual of percussion and auscultation. Composed from the French. . . . By James Birch Sharpe. . . . New York: S. Wood & Sons, 1832. 120p. DNLM; MA; PPC; RPM **30-0544**

LAENNEC, René Théophile Hyacinthe (1781-1826)
A treatise on the diseases of the chest and on mediate auscultation. Transl. from the latest French ed., with notes and a sketch of the author's life, by John Forbes. . . . From the 3rd rev. London ed., with additional notes. New York: S. Wood & Sons [etc.] [R. & G. S. Wood, pr.]; Philadelphia: J. Grigg [etc.] 1830. 736p. DNLM; MdBM; NNNAM; PU **30-0545**

LAENNEC, René Théophile Hyacinthe (1781-1826)
A treatise on the diseases of the chest, and on mediate auscultation. Transl. from the 3rd French ed. by John Forbes. To which are added the notes of Professor Andral contained in the 4th and latest French ed., transl. and accompanied with observations on cerebral auscultation by John Fisher. New York: S. Wood & Sons, 1838. 784p. DLC; NNNAM; PPC; ScC **30-0546**

LA ROCHE, René (1795-1872)
Medical education and institutions. An account of the origin, progress, and present state of the Medical School of Paris. Parts I-III. [16, 18, 72p] Philadelphia, 1831-1832. DNLM; PPC; PPJ; PU **30-0547**

LARREY, Dominique Jean (1766-1842)
Observations on wounds, and their complications by erysipelas, gangrene and tetanus. . . . Transl. by E. F. Rivinus, M.D. Philadelphia: Key, Mielke & Biddle, 1832. 332p. CtY-M; KyLoJM; PU **30-0548**

LARREY, Dominique Jean (1776-1842)
Surgical memoirs of the campaigns of Russia, Germany and France. . . . Transl. from the French by John C. Mercer. . . . Philadelphia: Carey & Lea, 1832. 293p. CtY-M; DNLM; KyLoJM; PU **30-0549**

LATHAM, Peter Mere (1789-1875)
Lectures on subjects connected with clinical medicine: comprising diseases of the heart. Philadelphia: Barrington & Haswell, 1837. 154p. DLC; MBM; PPC; PU **30-0550**

LAVATER, Johann Casper (1741-1801)
The pocket Lavater; or, The science of physiognomy to which is added an inquiry into the analogy existing between brute and human physiognomy, from the Italian of Porta. Hartford: Andrus & Judd, [1832]. 116p. DLC; DNLM; PPC **30-0551**

LAWRENCE, William (1783-1867)
Treatise on the diseases of the eye. Washington [D.C.]: D. Green, 1835. 582p. DLC; DNLM; OCIM; PPC **30-0552**

LEE, Edwin
Observations on the principal medical institutions and practice of France, Italy and Germany; with notices of the universities and cases from hospital practice. To which is added an appendix on animal magnetism and homoeopathy. Philadelphia: Haswell, Barrington & Haswell, 1837. 102p. DLC; PPHa **30-0553**

LEO-WOLF, Joseph
Observations on the prevention and cure of hydrophobia. According to the latest and popular publications in Germany. Read before the New York Medical and Philosophical Society. New York: Carvill, 1831. 31p. MH-M; PPL **30-0554**

LEO-WOLF, William
Remarks on the abracadabra of the nineteenth century; or on Dr. Samuel Hahnemann's homoeopathic theory of medicine, with particular reference to Dr. Constantine Hering's Concise View of the Rise and Progress of Homoeopathic Medicine (1833). Philadelphia: Carey, Lea & Blanchard, 1835. 272p. MBM; DLC; PPHa **30-0555**

LEROY, Louis
Curative medicine, or purgation, directed against the cause of diseases, discovered by Doctor Leroy, of Paris. Transl. from the 12th ed. by Gabriel Paul of St. Louis. . . . St. Louis: Pub. by G. Paul from the Republican Press, 1830. 169p. DNLM; DLC; NN **30-0556**

LINCOLN, Benjamin (1802-1835)
Hints on the present state of Medical education and the influence of medical schools in New England. . . . Burlington [Vt.]: Printed for the author, 1833. 76p. IEN-M; MB; PPC **30-0557**

LINCOLN, Benjamin (1802-1835)
An exposition of certain abuses, practiced by some of the medical schools in New England, and particularly of the agent sending system, as practiced by Theodore Woodward, M.D. Burlington: Printed for the author, 1833. 76p. IEN-M; MH **30-0558**

LINDSLY, Harvey (1804-1889)
An essay on the origin and introduction into medical practice . . . of ardent spirits. Washington: D. Green, 1835. 130p. DNLM **30-0559**

LISFRANC, Jacques (1790-1847)
Diseases of the uterus; a series of clinical lectures delivered at the Hospital La Pitié. Ed. by H. Pauly, M.D. Transl. from the French by G. Henry Lodge, M.D. Boston: W. D. Ticknor, 1839. 401p. DNLM; MB: MBM; MH **30-0560**

LISTON, Robert (1794-1847)
Elements of surgery. . . . Philadelphia: Haswell, Barrington & Haswell, 1837. 540p. DNLM; PPC; PPJ; PPHa **30-0561**

LISTON, Robert (1794-1847)
Practical Surgery with notes and additional illustrations by G. W. Norris. Philadelphia: Adam Waldie, 1838. 374p. GU; PPC; PPJ; PU **30-0562**

LISTON, Robert (1794-1847)
Practical Surgery. With notes and additional illustrations by George W. Norris. Philadelphia: Crissy, 1838. 374p. CSmH; DLC; IU-M; PPC **30-0563**

LITTELL, Squire (1803-1866)
A Manual of the Diseases of the Eye. . . . Philadelphia: Published by John S. Littell, 1837. 255p. DLC; PPC; PPJ; PU
30-0564

LOBSTEIN, Johann Georg (1777-1840)
A treatise upon the semeiology of the eye, for the use of physicians; and the countenance, for criminal jurisprudence. . . . New York: C. S. Francis; Philadelphia: Towar & Hogan, [etc., etc.] J. Seymour, pr., 1830. 175p. DNLM; ICJ; PU
30-0565

LOBSTEIN, Johann Georg (1777-1840)
A treatise on the structure, functions and diseases of the human sympathetic nerve. . . . Transl. from the Latin with notes, by Joseph Pancoast, M.D. Philadelphia: J. C. Auner, 1831. 157p. ICJ; NjR **30-0566**

LOBSTEIN, Johann Georg (1777-1840)
Remarks on the pernicious effects and fatal consequences of blood-letting. New York: W. Mitchell, 1832. 16p. DNLM; NNNAM **30-0567**

LOBSTEIN, Johann Georg (1777-1840)
Dialogues between patients and the physician on the several principal diseases in this country. . . . New York: the Author, 1839. 143p. DNLM; NNNAM **30-0568**

LOUIS, Pierre Charles Alexandre (1787-1872)
Anatomical, pathological and therapeutic researches upon the disease known under the name of gastro-enterite, putrid, adynamic, ataxic, or typhoid fever, etc., compared with the most common acute diseases. . . . Transl. from the original French, by Henry I. Bowditch. . . . Boston: I. R. Butts, 1836. 2 v. DLC; MB; MB: MH-M **30-0569**

LOUIS, Pierre Charles Alexandre (1787-1872)
Researches on the effects of bloodletting in some inflammatory diseases, and on the influence of tartarized antimony and vesication in pneumonitis. . . . Transl. by C. G. Putnam, M.D. With preface and appendix by James Jackson. . . . Boston: Hilliard, Gray & Company, 1836. 171p. DLC; MBM; MH-M; NcD **30-0570**

LOUIS, Pierre Charles Alexandre (1787-1872)
Pathological researches on phthisis. . . . Transl. from the French, with introduction and notes, and an essay on treatment; rev. and altered by Henry I. Bowditch. Boston: Hilliard, Gray & Co., 1836. 550p. DNLM; MBM; NN; PPC
30-0571

LOUIS, Pierre Charles Alexandre (1787-1872)
Pathological researches on phthisis. . . . Transl. from the French, with introduction, notes, additions, and an essay on treatment. By Charles Cowan. . . . Washington [D.C.]: D. Green, 1836. 293p. DLC; MdBJ-W; MdU-D; PPC
30-0572

LOUIS, Pierre Charles Alexandre (1787-1872)
An essay on clinical instruction; memoir on the proper method of examining a patient, and of arriving at facts of a general nature. Transl. from the French by H. I. Bowditch. [Dunglison's American Medical Library] Philadelphia: A. Waldie, 1838. [149]-187p. DNLM; PPC; PPJ; PU
30-0573

LOUIS, Pierre Charles Alexandre (1787-1872)
Anatomical, pathological and therapeutic researches on the yellow fever of Gibraltar of 1828; . . . From observations taken by himself and M. Trousseau, as members of the French commission at Gibraltar. Transl. from the manuscript by G. C. Shattuck, Jr. . . . Boston: C. C. Little and J. Brown, 1839. 374p. DLC; MBM; MH; NNNAM **30-0574**

MACKENZIE, William (1791-1868)
A practical treatise on diseases of the eye. . . . From the last London ed. Boston: Carter, Hendee & Co., 1833. 719p. ICJ; MWA; PPC; RPM **30-0575**

MACKINTOSH, John
Principles of pathology and practice of physic. . . . 1st American from the 3rd London ed. Washington [D.C.]: Stereotyped by D. Green, for the Register and library of medical and chirurgical science, 1834. 744p. DLC; DNLM; MA; MBM **30-0576**

MACKINTOSH, John
Principles of pathology, and practice of physic. . . . From the last London ed., with notes and additions, by Samuel George Morton. . . . Philadelphia: Key & Biddle, 1836. 2 v. CSmH; DLC; KU; PPC **30-0577**

MACKINTOSH, John
Principles of pathology, and practice of physic. . . . 2nd American from the 4th London ed., with notes and additions by Samuel George Morton. . . . Philadelphia: E. C. Biddle, 1837. 2 v. DNLM; DLC; PPC; PU
30-0578

MACNISH, Robert (1802-1834)
The philosophy of sleep. New York: D. Appleton & Co., 1834. 296p. NN; NNC; NNNAM; PP **30-0579**

MACNISH, Robert (1802-1834)
The philosophy of sleep. [Also:] The anatomy of drunkenness. New York: W. Pearson & Co., 1835. 96p. DNLM; NN
30-0580

MAGENDIE, François (1783-1855)
Formulary for the preparation and employment of several new remedies. . . . Transl. from the 6th ed. of the Formulaire of Mr. Magendie. . . . New York: Repr. by J. J. Harper for F. & N. G. Carnes, 1830. 145, 18p. ViRA
30-0581

MAGENDIE, François (1783-1855)
Formulary for the preparation and employment of several new remedies. . . . Transl. from the 6th ed., with an appendix, containing the experience of British practitioners, with many of the new remedies, by J. Houlton. Philadelphia: E. L. Carey & A. Hart, 1834. 164p. DNLM; PPC **30-0582**

MAGENDIE, François (1783-1855)
Lectures on the blood, and on the changes which it undergoes during disease. Delivered at the College of France in 1837-1838. Philadelphia: Haswell, Barrington & Haswell, 1839. 276p. DNLM; PPHa. [Also, in: Dunglison's American Medical Library] **30-0583**

MAGILL, Alfred T[hruston] (1804-1837)
An introductory lecture, on physiology, delivered to the medical class of the University of Virginia; . . . October 19th, 1833. Published by the medical class. Charlottesville: Printed by Watson & Tompkins, 1833. 15p. DLC; DNLM
30-0584

MAGILL, Alfred T[hruston] (1804-1837)
An essay on the history, causes, and treatment of typhus fever. . . . Charlottesville: Moseley & Tompkins, 1834. 64p. DNLM; GU; ViRA **30-0585**

MAGILL, Alfred T[hruston] (1804-1837)
Three lectures on the origin and properties of malaria or marsh miasma. . . . Charlottesville: Watson & Tompkins, 1834. 70p. DNLM; ViRA **30-0586**

MALIN, William Gunn
Some account of the Pennsylvania Hospital, its origin, objects and present state. . . . Philadelphia: Pr. by Thomas Kite, 1831. 46p. DLC; MH; PHi; PU **30-0587**

MANEC, Pierre-Joseph
The cerebro-spinal axis of man. With the origin and first division of its nerves. From the French of M. Manec. . . . Transl. and rev. by J. Pancoast, M.D. Philadelphia: Pub. by Towar and Hogan, Adam Waldie, pr. [1830]. Wall map, fol. DNLM; PPL **30-0588**

MANEC, Pierre-Joseph
Great sympathetic nerve. Transl. and corrected by J. Pancoast. Philadelphia: A. Waldie [1838?] Wall map, fol. DNLM **30-0589**

MANESCA, John (1774-1837?)
Strictures on phrenological doctrines upon the human intellect, in a letter address to Dr. Spurzheim. . . . New York: Butts & Anstice, 1832. 28p. DNLM; MB; NN; PPAmP **30-0590**

MANLEY, Joseph R. (1781-1851)
Letters addressed to the Board of Health, and to Richard Riker, Recorder of the City of New York, on the subject of his agency in constituting a special medical council. New York: P. Van Pelt, 1832. 27p. DNLM; NNNAM **30-0591**

MANLEY, Joseph R. (1781-1851)
An address delivered before the Medical Society of the County of New York, July 25, 1836. New York, 1836. 24p. DNLM; NNNAM **30-0592**

MANN, Edwin John
The Deaf and Dumb; Or, a collection of articles relating to the condition of deaf mutes; their education, and the principal asylums devoted to their instruction. Boston: Hitchcock, 1836. 312pp. MA; MBM; MHi; MWA **30-0593**

MARCH, Alden (1795-1830)
A lecture on the expediencey of establishing a medical college and hospital in the city of Albany. Delivered January 11, 1830; introductory to a course on anatomy and operative surgery. Albany: L. G. Hoffman, 1830. 20p. DNLM; N; NN; NNNAM **30-0594**

MARTINET, Louis (1795-1875)
Manual of pathology; containing the symptoms, diagnosis, and morbid characters of diseases. . . . Transl. with notes and additions, by Jones Quain. . . . 2nd American ed. Philadelphia: Carey and Lea; [Brookfield, Mass.: E. & G. Merriam, prs.] 1830. 275p. MdBM; PPC; PPF **30-0595**

MARTINET, Louis (1795-1875)
Manual of therapeutics. . . . Transl. with alterations and additions, by Robert Norton, M.D. . . . New York: C. S. Francis [Clayton & Van Norden, prs.] 1830. 278p. DLC; DNLM; MWA; RPM **30-0596**

[MARYLAND. UNIVERSITY OF MARYLAND, School of Medicine, Baltimore]
Address of the trustees of the University of Maryland, concerning the Medical Department of the institution. . . . Baltimore: John D. Troy, 1836. 15p. DNLM; MdBJ-W; MdU-D **30-0597**

MASSACHUSETTS GENERAL HOSPITAL
Report of surgical cases and operations that occurred in the . . . from May 12, 1837 to May 12, 1838. By George Hayward. Boston: D. Clapp, Jr., 1838. 32p. DNLM; MBM; MHi **30-0598**

MASSACHUSETTS MEDICAL SOCIETY
Library of practical medicine; published by order of the. . . . Boston, Cambridge, New York, Philadelphia, 1831-1838. vs. 1-14; 17-19; 21-25. 22 v. [See Index-Catalogue, Library of Surgeon-General's Office, 1st Series, VIII (1887), 663] **30-0599**

MASSACHUSETTS MEDICAL SOCIETY
A report on spasmodic cholera; prepared by a committee under the direction of the counsellors of the. . . . Boston: Carter & Hendee, 1832. 190p. DNLM; MBM; MH-M; MHi **30-0600**

MAURAN, Joseph (1796-1873)
Remarks on the Cholera, embracing facts and observations collected at New York, during a visit to the city expressly for that purpose. Providence: Pr. by W. Marshall & Co., 1832. 34p. DLC; MB; MH; NNNAM **30-0601**

MAURAN, Joseph (1796-1873)
Remarks on the Cholera, embracing facts and observations collected at New York, during a visit to the city expressly for that purpose. Pr. by W. Marshall & Co., 1832. 32p. NNU-M; RPB **30-0602**

MAYGRIER, Jacques Pierre (1771-1835)
The anatomists' manual; or, A treatise on the manner of preparing all the parts of anatomy, followed by a complete description of these parts. . . . Transl. from the 4th French ed. by Gunning S. Bedford. . . . New York: Collins & Co., 1832. 2 v. in 1. PU; OCIM; RPM **30-0603**

MAYGRIER, Jacques Pierre (1771-1835)
Midwifery illustrated. Transl. from the French, with notes by A. Sidney Doane. New York: J. K. Moore, 1833. 186p. 80 plates. DNLM; NNNAM; NNU-M **30-0604**

MAYGRIER, Jacques Pierre (1771-1835)
Midwifery illustrated. Transl. from the French, with notes by A. Sidney Doane. 3rd ed. New York: Harper & Bros., 1834. 179p. 81 plates. DNLM; NNNAM; NNU-M **30-0605**

MAYHEW, Horace (1816-1872)
The Toothache imagined, by Horace Mayhew. Boston: Bradford [1831]. 3p. MBM **30-0606**

MAYO, Herbert (1796-1852)
Observations on injuries and diseases of the rectum. . . . Washington: D. Green, 1834. 61p. DLC; DNLM; MBM; MdBJ-W **30-0607**

MAYO, Herbert (1796-1852)
Outlines of human pathology. . . . Philadelphia: Printed by Adam Waldie, 1839. 364p. NjR; PPC; PU **30-0608**

MAYO, Thomas (1790-1871)
Elements of pathology of the human mind. [Dunglison's American Medical Library] Philadelphia: A. Waldie, 1839. 73p. DNLM; PPC; PPJ **30-0609**

McALLISTER, A.
A dissertation on the medical properties and injurious effects of the habitual use of tobacco. . . . Utica: Press of W. Williams, 1830. 24p. DLC; NN; NNNAM **30-0610**

McALLISTER, A.
A dissertation on the medical properties and injurious effects of the habitual use of tobacco: read, according to appointment, before the Medical Society of the County of Oneida, at their semi-annual meeting, January 5, 1830. . . . 2nd ed., imp. and enl., with an introductory preface, by Moses Stuart. Boston: Peirce & Parker; New York: H. C. Sleight, 1832. 36p. IEN-M; MH; PPPrHi **30-0611**

McCLELLAN, George (1796-1847)
Valedictory address delivered to the graduates of the Jefferson Medical College. . . . March, 1836. Philadelphia: Printed by W. S. Martien, 1836. 16p. DLC; PPJ **30-0612**

MacCULLOCH, John (1773-1835)
An essay on the remittent and intermittent diseases, including, generically, marsh fever and neuralgia. . . . Philadelphia: Carey & Lea, 1830. 474p. GU; PPC; PPPH; PPPrHi **30-0613**

McDOWELL, Joseph Nash (1803-1868)
A valedictory address, delivered by appointment, before the Medical and Philosophical Society of Ohio, at the close of its winter session, February 27, 1830. Cincinnati: March, 1830. 16p. OCHP **30-0614**

McDOWELL, Joseph Nash (1803-1868)
An introductory lecture, on the causes obstructing the progress of medical science. . . . Published at the request of his class. Cincinnati: Williamson & Wood, prs., 1830. 19p. CSmH; OCHP **30-0615**

McDOWELL, Joseph Nash (1803-1868)
An introductory lecture . . . on anatomy and surgery. Pub. by his class. Cincinnati: Pr. at the office of the Cincinnati Chronicle, 1832. 16p. CSmH; MH-M **30-0616**

McNAUGHTON, James (1796-1874)
An enquiry into the present system of medical education, in the state of New York. . . . By an observer. Albany: Pr. by Websters and Skinners, 1830. 16p. MH; N; NN; NNNAM **30-0617**

McNAUGHTON, James (1796-1874)
A discourse delivered at the anniversary meeting of the Kappa Alpha Phi Society of the College of Physicians and Surgeons of the Western District. Albany: Pr. by Websters and Skinners, 1830. 23p. DLC; MB; N **30-0618**

McNAUGHTON, James (1796-1874)
Address delivered before the Medical Society of the State of New York, February 8, 1837. Albany: E. W. & C. Skinner, 1837. 40p. DNLM; N; NHi **30-0619**

MEASE, James (1771-1846)
On the causes, cure and means of preventing the sick headache. 3rd ed. Philadelphia: H. H. Porter, 1831. 52p. DNLM; PPAmP; PPL; PU **30-0620**

MEASE, James (1771-1846)
On the causes, cure and means of preventing the sick headache. 4th ed. Philadelphia: H. H. Porter, 1832. 52p. DNLM; PPAmP **30-0621**

MEASE, James (1771-1846)
On the causes, cure and means of preventing the sick headache. 5th ed. Philadelphia: H. H. Porter, 1832. 80p. DNLM; PPAmP; PPL; PU **30-0622**

MEIGS, Charles Delucena (1792-1869)
The Philadelphia practice of midwifery. . . . Philadelphia: J. Kay, Jr. & Brother; Pittsburgh: J. I. Kay & Co., 1838. 370p. Plates. DLC; IU-M; PPC; PU **30-0623**

MEREDITH, W.
A comprehensive minute commemorative of Philip Syng Physick. Philadelphia, 1838. 14p. DNLM **30-0624**

MICKEL, Johann Friedrich (1781-1833)
Manual of general, descriptive, and pathological anatomy. . . . Transl. from German into French, with additions and notes, by A. J. L. Jeurdan . . . and G. Breschet. Transl. from the French with notes by A. Sidney Doane. . . . New York: H. C. Sleight [etc.] 1831-2. 3 v. NjR **30-0625**

MIGUET, E.
Chemical and medical researches on kreosote, its preparation, properties and use. . . . Transl. from the French, by William Wetherill. . . . Philadelphia: J. Dobson, 1835. 49p. DLC; PPC; PPHa; PU **30-0626**

MILLER, Henry (1800-1874)
On the true value of experience in medicine; an introductory lecture. Louisville, Ky.: Prentice & Weissinger, 1838. 21p. DNLM; KyLoJM **30-0627**

MILLER, James H[enry] (1788-1853)
"Thomsonalgia." Report to the trustees of the Baltimore County Alms House. . . . [Baltimore, 1836], 19p. DNLM **30-0628**

MILLINGEN, John Gideon (1782-1862)
Curiosities of medical experience. . . . Philadelphia: Haswell, Barrington, & Haswell, 1838. 372p. DLC; PPC; PPF; PPJ **30-0629**

MITCHELL, C. L[eeds] (1813-1888)
A synoptical table of thoracic percussion and auscultation. Arranged from the works of Laennec, Hope, Louis, Piorry, Williams and others. . . . New York. 1839. 1 sheet. Folio. DNLM **30-0630**

MITCHELL, John Kearsley (1798-1858)
On the penetrativeness of fluids. . . . Philadelphia: Pr. by Joseph R. A. Skerrett, 1830. 34p. DNLM; PHi; PPL **30-0631**

MITCHELL, John Kearsley (1798-1858)
On a new practice in acute and chronic rheumatism. Philadelphia: J. R. A. Skerrett, 1831. 12p. DNLM; PPC **30-0632**

MITCHELL, John Kearsley (1798-1858)
Further cases and observations relative to rheumatism. Philadelphia: J. R. A. Skerrett, 1833. 15p. DNLM; PU **30-0633**

MITCHELL, John Kearsley (1798-1858)
The value of a great medical reputation, with suggestions for its attainment: a lecture, introductory to the summer course of the Medical Institute. . . . Philadelphia: Printed by J. R. A. Skerrett, 1834. 20p. DLC; PPC; PPHa; PU
30-0634

MITCHELL, John Kearsley (1798-1858)
A lecture on some of the means of elevating the character of the working classes. Philadelphia: J. Harding, 1834. 17p. DNLM **30-0635**

MITCHELL, John Kearsley (1798-1858)
The value of the practical interrogation of nature: a lecture. Philadelphia: J. R. A. Skerrett, 1834. 22p. DNLM
30-0636

MITCHELL, John Kearsley (1798-1858)
On the liquefaction and solidification of carbonic acid. [Philadelphia, 1838], 8p. 1 plate. DNLM
30-0637

MITCHELL, Thomas Duché (1791-1865)
Elements of chemical philosophy on the basis of Reid, comprising the rudiments of that science. . . . Cincinnati: Corey & Fairbank, 1832. 553p. 2 plates. DNLM; OCIM; OCIHWi
30-0638

MITCHELL, Thomas Duché (1791-1865)
Hints on the connexion of labor with study, as a preventive of diseases peculiar to students. . . . Cincinnati: Corey, Fairbank & Co., 1832. 85p. DNLM; OCIM **30-0639**

MITCHELL, Thomas Duché (1791-1865)
The annual oration of the Ohio Medical Lyceum: delivered in the Medical College of Ohio, January 1, 1834. . . . Cincinnati: Published by order of the Lyceum, by Truman, Smith, & Co., 1834. 32p. DLC; OCIM; OCIWHi **30-0640**

MITCHELL, Thomas Duché (1791-1865)
A cursory view of the history of chemical science, and some of its more important uses to the physician . . . being an introductory to the course of lectures for the session 1837-1838. Lexington: Finnell & Zimmermann, 1837. 22p. DNLM
30-0641

MITCHELL, Thomas Duché (1791-1865)
Annual address to the College of Physicians and Surgeons of Lexington. . . . Lexington: Noble & Dunlop, 1839. 32p. DNLM
30-0642

MITCHELL, Thomas Duché (1791-1865)
The pains and pleasures of a medical life, being an introductory to a course of lectures on materia medica and therapeutics. Lexington, Ky.: J. Virden, 1839. 23p. DNLM; OCLloyd
30-0643

MITCHELL, Thomas Duché (1791-1865)
Annual address to the College of Physicians and Surgeons of Lexington; in which the principles and practice of medical ethics are illustrated. . . . Lexington: Noble & Dunlop, 1839. 32p. DNLM **30-0644**

MOFFAT, William B.
The medical manual; containing accurate information concerning the most prevalent diseases and the most approved remedies. . . . New York: The author, 1839. 64p. DLC; NN; NNNAM; NNU-M **30-0645**

MONTGOMERY, William Fetherston (1797-1859)
An exposition of the signs and symptoms of pregnancy, the period of human gestation, and the signs of delivery. . . . Philadelphia: A. Waldie, 1839. 220p. DNLM; PPC; PPJ; PU
30-0646

MOORE, Samuel W. (1786-1854)
A memoir of the life and character of John Watts, M.D., late president of the College of Physicians and Surgeons. With an address to the gentlemen who were graduated doctors of medicine at the annual commencement of the College of Physicians and Surgeons, held April 5th, 1831. New York: G. & C. & H. Carvill, 1831. 28p. DNLM; MBAt; ICU; ScC
30-0647

MORGAN, George T.
An outline of inflammation and its effects; being the first principles of surgery. [Dunglison's American Medical Library] Philadelphia: A. Waldie, 1838. 134p. DNLM; PPC: ViRA
30-0648

MORGAN, James (1770-1840)
An essay, or tract, on the vitality of the warm blood and air. . . . Ed. and republished by Elisha North. . . . New York: Printed for the author, 1835. 29p. DLC; NN; NNNAM; NNU-M **30-0649**

MORTON, Samuel George (1799-1851)
Introductory lecture to a course of demonstrative anatomy; delivered December 11th, 1830. . . . Philadelphia: Pr. by Mifflin & Parry, 1831. 16p. DNLM; PHi; PU
30-0650

MORTON, Samuel George (1799-1851)
Illustrations of pulmonary consumption, its anatomical characters, causes, symptoms and treatment. With twelve plates, drawn and coloured from nature. . . . Philadelphia: Key & Biddle, 1834. 183p. DLC; PPC; PPHa; PU
30-0651

MORTON, Samuel George (1799-1851)
Illustrations of pulmonary consumption, its anatomical characters, causes, symptoms and treatment. To which are added, some remarks on the climate of the United States, the West Indies, . . . 2nd ed. Philadelphia: E. C. Biddle, 1837. 349p. 13 plates. DNLM; PPC; PU **30-0652**

MORTON, Samuel George (1799-1851)
Crania Americana; or a comparative view of the skulls of various aboriginal nations of North and South America. . . . Philadelphia: J. Dobson, 1839. 296p. 78 plates. 1 map. DNLM; LNT-M; MBM; NN **30-0653**

MOTT, Valentine (1785-1865)
Case of aneurism of the right subclavian artery, in which that vessel was tied within the scaleni muscles. . . . Philadelphia: Printed by J. R. A. Skerrett, 1833. 8p. NNNAM
30-0654

MOULTRIE, James (1793-1869)
An eulogium on Stephen Elliott, M.D., professor of natural history, and botany in the Medical College of S.C. Delivered by appointment of the faculty, and the philosophical society, at the opening of the college on 8th November,1830. Charleston: Pr. by A. E. Miller, 1830. 46p. MB; MH; PPAmP; RPB **30-0655**

MURRAY, John (*d.* 1820)
A system of materia medica and pharmacy, including translations of the Edinburgh, London, and Dublin pharmacopoeias. . . . 6th ed. Adapted to the present state of chemical and medical science. . . . With notes and additions by John B. Beck. . . . New York: Collins and Hannay, and J. B. Collins, 1834. 584p. DLC; NNNAM; OCLloyd **30-0656**

MUSSEY, Reuben Dimond (1780-1866)
Essay on ardent spirits and its substitutes as a means of invigorating health. Washington: D. Green, 1835. 65p. DNLM **30-0657**

MUSSEY, Reuben Dimond (1780-1866)
An essay on the influence of tobacco upon life and health. 48p. Boston: Perkins & Marvin, 1836. DNLM; MBM **30-0658**

MUSSEY, Reuben Dimond (1780-1866)
An essay on the influence of tobacco upon life and health. A new ed., enlarged by the author. New York: American Tract Society, [1836]. 64p. DNLM; NNNAM **30-0659**

MUSSEY, Reuben Dimond (1780-1866)
An essay on the influence of tobacco upon life and health. 3rd ed. Cincinnati: G. L. Weed, 1839. 48p. DNLM **30-0660**

MÜTTER, Thomas Dent (1811-1859)
A lecture on loxarthrus or club-foot. Philadelphia: Hooker & Claxton, 1839. 104p. DNLM; NjR **30-0661**

NUTTALL, Thomas (1786-1859)
An introduction to systematic and physiological botany. . . . 2nd ed. Cambridge: Pub. by Hilliard & Brown [E. W. Metcalf & Co., prs.] 1830. 362p. DLC; MH; PP; ScC **30-0662**

O'BEIRNE, James (1786-1862)
New views on the process of defecation, and their application to the pathology and treatment of diseases of the stomach, bowels, and other organs, together with an analytical correction of Sir Charles Bell's views respecting the nerves of the face. Washington: D. Green, 1834. 142p. DNLM; IU-M; LNT-M; PPC **30-0663**

OBSERVATIONS on the mineral waters in the southwestern part of Virginia. In a series of letters. By a physician of Philadelphia. Philadelphia: J. Thompson, 1834. 30p. DNLM; ViRA **30-0664**

OHIO. MEDICAL COLLEGE
An inquiry into the causes which have retarded the prosperity of the Medical College of Ohio. [Cincinnati, 1835?] 42p. DNLM **30-0665**

OLIVER, Daniel (1787-1842)
An address delivered before the Temperance Society of the medical class in Dartmouth College, October 31, 1832. Windsor: Chronicle Press [1832] 16p. MB; MH; ScMS **30-0666**

OLIVER, Daniel (1787-1842)
An address delivered before the New Hampshire Medical Society at Concord June 4, 1833. . . . Concord: Marsh, Capen & Lyon, 1833. 23p. DNLM; MB; MWA; NNNAM **30-0667**

OLIVER, Daniel (1787-1842)
First lines of physiology; designed for the use of students of medicine. Boston: Marsh, Capen & Lyon, 1835. 520p. DNLM; MBM **30-0668**

OTTLEY, Drewry
The life of John Hunter. [Dunglison's American Medical Library] Philadelphia: Haswell & Co., 1839. 139p. DNLM; PPC; PU **30-0669**

PAINE, Martyn (1794-1877)
Letters on the cholera asphyxia, as it has appeared in the city of New York; addressed to John C. Warren, M.D. of Boston, and originally published in that city, together with other letters, not before published. . . . New York: Collins & Hannay, 1832. 160p. DNLM; LNT-M; PU; RPM **30-0670**

PAINE, Martyn (1794-1877)
Lecture on the improvement of medical education in the United States; introductory to a course of lectures in the University of New York. . . . [New York, 1832] 16p. DLC; DNLM; MB **30-0671**

PALMER, David (1790-1873)
Anniversary address to the class of graduates of the Vermont Medical College, in Woodstock. Woodstock, 1839. 12p. DNLM; VtHi **30-0672** •

PANCOAST, Joseph (1805-1882)
An introductory lecture delivered at the commencement of the winter course of anatomy for 1834-1835. Philadelphia: W. B. Gibbons, 1835. 18p. DNLM; PPJ **30-0673**

PANCOAST, Joseph (1805-1882)
A lecture introductory to the course of surgery in the Jefferson Medical College. Philadelphia: W. F. Geddes, 1839. 16p. DNLM; PPJ **30-0674**

PANCOAST, Joseph (1805-1882)
The art of prolonging life briefly considered. A lecture delivered before the Athenian Institute. Philadelphia: A. Waldie, 1839. 40p. DNLM **30-0675**

PARIS, John Ayrton (1785-1856)
Pharmacologia. . . . 4th American from 7th London ed. . . . With notes and add. by John B. Beck, M.D. . . . New York: Pr. by W. E. Dean, for Collins & Hannay and White, Gallaher & White, 1831. 550p. DLC; PPC **30-0676**

PARKER, Langston (1805?-1871)
. . . The stomach in its morbid states; being a practical enquiry into the nature and treatment of diseases of that organ; and into the influence they exercise upon the origin, progress, and termination of diseases of the liver, heart, lungs, and brain. . . . [Dunglison's American Medical Library] Philadelphia: A. Waldie, 1839. 194p. CtY-M; DLC; NN; NNNAM **30-0677**

PARRISH, Isaac (1811-1852)
Remarks on spinal irritation as connected with nervous diseases, with cases. . . . Philadelphia: J. R. A. Skerrett, 1832. 24p. MBM; NNNAM; PHi **30-0678**

PARRISH, Joseph (1779-1840)
Practical observations on strangulated hernia, and some of the diseases of the urinary organs. . . . Philadelphia: Key & Biddle, 1836. 330p. 4 plates. CtY-M; DLC; NIC; PPHa
30-0679

PARSONS, Usher (1788-1868)
On the comparative influence of vegetable and animal decomposition as a cause of fever. . . . Philadelphia: Pr. by Joseph R. A. Skerrett, 1830. 36p. DLC; MB; NNNAM; PPPrHi
30-0680

PARSONS, Usher (1788-1868)
Directions for making anatomical preparations formed on the basis of Pole, Marjolin and Breschet. . . . 1st ed. Philadelphia: Carey & Lea, 1831. 316p. 4 plates. CU-M; MB; PU
30-0681

PARSONS, Usher (1788-1868)
Boylston prize dissertations on: (1) Inflammation of the periosteum; (2) Eneuresis irritata; (3) Cutaneous diseases; (4) Cancer of the breast; Also remarks on malaria. Boston: Little & J. Brown, 1839. 248p. DNLM; MBM 30-0682

PASCALIS OUVIERE, Felix
Eulogy on the life and character of the Hon. Samuel Latham Mitchell, M.D. Delivered at the request of the New York City and County Medical Society. . . . New York: From the American Argus Press, 1831. 25p. MB; MH; NjR; PMA
30-0683

PATTISON, Granville Sharp (1791-1851)
A discourse delivered on commencing the lectures in Jefferson Medical College, session of 1832-1833. . . . Philadelphia: French & Perkins, 1832. 39p. DLC: MB; NNNAM; PPC 30-0684

PATTISON, Granville Sharp (1791-1851)
Letter on cholera, from Professor Pattison, to Dr. Carmichael, of Virginia. Originally published in the Washington Telegraph. Philadelphia: Wm. F. Geddes, 1832. 16p. DNLM; NNNAM
30-0685

PATTISON, Granville Sharp (1791-1851)
A lecture delivered in Jefferson Medical College, Philadelphia . . . on the question "Has the parotid gland ever been extirpated?" Philadelphia: Published by the students of Jefferson Medical College, 1833. 16p. DNLM; PPJ; PU; ScU
30-0686

PATTISON, Granville Sharp (1791-1851)
The introductory lectures of Profs. Pattison & Revere, delivered in Jefferson Medical College, Philadelphia, on commencing the lectures for the session, 1832-1833. Philadelphia: W. F. Geddes, 1833. 20, 4p. DNLM; MH-M; NNNAM; OC 30-0687

PATTISON, Granville Sharp (1791-1851)
Jefferson Medical College. Professor Pattison's introductory lecture. Session 1838-9. Philadelphia: Pub. by order of the Committee, A. Waldie, 1838. 19p. DLC; DNLM; PPJ
30-0688

PAXTON, James (1786-1860)
An introduction to the study of human anatomy. . . . 1st American ed., with additions, by Winslow Lewis, Jr. . . . Boston: Carter & Hendee, 1832-1834. 2 v. DLC; DNLM; MBM
30-0689

PAXTON, James (1786-1860)
An introduction to the study of human anatomy. . . . 2nd American ed., with additions by Winslow Lewis, Jr. . . . Boston: W. D. Ticknor, 1835. 2 v. DLC; MBM; MH-M; PU
30-0690

PAXTON, James (1786-1860)
An introduction to the study of human anatomy. . . . 3rd American ed., with additions by Winslow Lewis, Jr. Boston: W. D. Ticknor, 1837-1840. 2 v. DNLM; MBM
30-0691

PEARSON, John (1758-1826)
Principles of surgery. . . . Boston: Stimpson & Clap, 1832. 263p. DLC; DNLM; ICJ; MWA 30-0692

PEERS, Benjamin O.
Inaugural address delivered at the opening of Morrison College, Lexington, Kentucky, November 4, 1833. Lexington: J. Clarke & Co., 1833. 30p. DNLM 30-0693

PEIRSON, Abel Lawrence (1794-1853)
Remarks on puerperal fever. . . . [Salem, 1831] 30p. DNLM; MSaE 30-0694

PEIRSON, Abel Lawrence (1794-1853)
Remarks on puerperal fever. . . . Boston: Pr. by W. L. Lewis, from N. Hale's steampower press, 1831. 30p. NjR
30-0695

PEISSE, Jean-Louis Hippolyte (1803-1880)
Sketches of the character and writing of eminent living surgeons & physicians of Paris, transl. from the French of J. L. H. Peisse by Elisha Bartlett. . . . Boston: Carter, Hendee & Babcock, 1831. 131p. CU-M; ICJ; MB; NcD
30-0696

PEIXOTTO, Daniel L. M.
Address delivered before the Medical Society . . . city and county of New York on the 25th day of July, 1831. . . . New York: Pr. by J. Seymour, 1831. 30p. PU
30-0697

PEIXOTTO, Daniel L. M.
Introductory lecture delivered at the Willoughby Medical College of the Willoughby University of Lake Erie, 1836-1837. Cleveland: Canfield and Spencer, 1837. 31p. DLC; DNLM; OCIM; OCIWHi 30-0698

PEMBERTON, Christopher Robert (1765-1822)
A practical treatise on various diseases of the abdominal viscera. With notes by John Hayes, M.D. . . . Richmond: Pr. by Peter Cottom, and for sale at his book store, 1830. 196p. DNLM; MB; NNNAM 30-0699

PENNOCK, Caspar Wistar (1799-1867) and W. W. GERHARD
Observations on the cholera of Paris. Philadelphia: J. R. A. Skerrett, 1832. 76p. DNLM; PPC 30-0700

PERRY, John
The household physician: or, An easy and natural method of curing most diseases. Compiled from the Rev. John Wesley's Primitive physic; Nicholas Culpepper's English physician enlarged; and the Goodrich encyclopedia. . . . Providence: B. T. Albro, printer, 1838. 125p. CU-M; DLC; RPB; RPJCB
30-0701

PETER, Robert (1805-1894)
. . . On the mode of collecting and preserving objects of natural history, with a view to the formation of a cabinet, or to their transportation. Read before the Medical Society of Lexington, and pub. at its request. [n.p., 1833?] [133]-149p. CtY-M; KyLoJM 30-0702

PETER, Robert (1805-1894)
Thoughts on some of the applications of chemistry to medicine. Read before the [Lexington Medical] Society, November 14, 1834. [Lexington, 1836] 24p. DNLM
30-0703

PETER, Robert (1805-1894)
On the application of galvanic electricity to medicine. Read before the [Lexington Medical] Society, December 2, 1836. [Lexington, 1836] 19p. DNLM **30-0704**

PETER, Robert (1805-1894)
On the influence of caloric on the living animal body. [Lexington, 1838] 22p. DNLM **30-0705**

PETER, Robert (1805-1894)
Thoughts on medical education in America. An introductory lecture, delivered in the chapel of Morrison College to the medical students of Transylvania University on the 11th November, 1838. . . . Lexington, Ky.: Printed at the observer & reporter office, 1838. 22p. DLC; DNLM; KyLoJM; OCHP
30-0706

The **PHARMACOPOEIA** of the United States of America, by the authority of "The General convention for the formation of the American pharmacopoeia," held in 1830. 2nd ed., from the 1st ed., pub. in 1820, with additions and corrections. New York: S. Converse [D. Fanshaw, pr.] 1830. 176p. CU-M; DLC; ICJ; NcD **30-0707**

The **PHARMACOPOEIA** of the United States of America. By authority of the National Medical Convention held at Washington, A.D. 1830. 1st ed. rev. Philadelphia: John Grigg, 1831. 268p. MHi; OCLloyd; PU
30-0708

PHILADELPHIA. COLLEGE OF PHYSICIANS
Report of the College of Physicians of Philadelphia, to the Board of Health, on epidemic cholera. Philadelphia: T. Desilver, Jr., 1832. 36p. DLC; PPC; PU
30-0709

PHILADELPHIA. PENNSYLVANIA HOSPITAL
Supplement to the catalogue of the medical library of the Pennsylvania Hospital published in 1829. Philadelphia: J. and W. Kite, printers, 1837. [323-426p]. DLC; PU
30-0710

PHILADELPHIA. PHILADELPHIA HOSPITAL (Blockley Almshouse)
A catalogue of the medical library of the Philadelphia Almshouse. Prepared agreeably to a resolution of the board of managers. By E. F. Rivinus. [Philadelphia, 1831] vii, 174p. DNLM; PPPH; PU **30-0711**

PHILADELPHIA. UNIVERSITY OF PENNSYLVANIA
Examination of certain charges preferred against the medical class of the University of Pennsylvania, during the session of 1834-1835. [Philadelphia, 1835] 24p. PPJ; PU
30-0712

PHILIP, Alexander Philip Wilson (1770-1851?)
A treatise on the nature and cure of those diseases, either acute or chronic, which precede change of structure; with a view to the preservation of health, and, particularly, the prevention of organic diseases. . . . With notes and appendices, by J. H. Miller. . . . Baltimore: E. J. Coale; Washington City: Cole & Co., 1831. 328p. DLC; DNLM; ICJ; PU
30-0713

PHILIP, Alexander Philip Wilson (1770-1851?)
Observations on the nature of malignant cholera, with a view to establish correct principles of its prevention and treatment. . . . Washington: D. Green, 1834. 60p. DNLM
30-0714

PHILIP, Alexander Philip Wilson (1770-1851?)
On the influence of minute doses of mercury, combined with the appropriate treatment of various diseases. . . . Washington, D. Green, 1834. 60p. DNLM **30-0715**

[PHYSICK, Philip Syng (1768-1837)]
Examination of a pamphlet, entitled A brief review of Dr. Horner's Necrological notice of Philip Syng Physick, M.D. Philadelphia [1838?] 11p. DLC; PPC
30-0716

PINKNEY, Ninian (1811-1877)
The nervous system of the human body; embracing a dissertation delivered to the medical profession of Philadelphia, and students of the two universities, on the subject of the nerves, brain, and organs of sense. . . . Philadelphia: Printed by W. F. Geddes, 1839. 32p. DLC; DNLM; PPC; PP
30-0717

PLEASANTS, James A.
Treatise on the functions, disorders and treatment of the teeth, designed for the use of individuals and private families. New York: Elliott, 1832, 48p. DLC; PU
30-0718

PLUMBE, Samuel
A practical treatise on the diseases of the skin, arranged with a view to their constitutional causes and local characters: including the substance of the essay to which the Royal College of Surgeons awarded the Jacksonian prize, and all such valuable facts as have been recorded by continental authors on these subjects to the present time. . . . From the last London ed., rev., cor., considerably enl., and with additional engravings. Philadelphia: Haswell, Barrington, & Haswell, 1837. 396p. 4 plates. DLC; PPC; PPPH; PU **30-0719**

[PORTER, Henry H.]
The catechism of health; or, Plain and simple rules for the preservation of the health and vigour of the constitution from infancy to old age. Ladies ed. Philadelphia: Journal of Health and Journal of Law, 1831. 195p. DNLM; MWA; OC; RPM
30-0720

[PORTER, Henry H.]
An account of the origin, symptoms, and cure of influenza or epidemic catarrh; with some hints respecting common colds and incipient pulmonary consumption. Philadelphia: H. H. Porter, 1832. 80p. DNLM **30-0721**

PORTER's health almanac for 1832; calculated generally for all parts of the U.S. . . . the calculations by Wm. Collom. Philadelphia: Henry H. Porter, 1832. 80p. MWA; PHi; PP
30-0722

POTTER, Nathaniel (1770-1843)
Notes on the Locusta septentrionalis americanae decem septima. 27p. Baltimore: J. Robinson, 1839. DNLM
30-0723

PRACTICAL proofs of the soundness of the Hygeian System of Physiology. 3rd ed. [New York, 1832] 202p. MBM; MWA
30-0724

PRICHARD, James Cowles (1786-1848)
A treatise on insanity and other disorders affecting the mind. . . . Philadelphia: Haswell, Barrington, & Haswell, 1837. 337p. DLC; DNLM; ICU; PPC **30-0725**

PRICHARD, James Cowles (1786-1848)
A treatise on insanity and other disorders affecting the mind. . . . Philadelphia: E. L. Carey & A. Hart, 1837. 339p. DLC; MH-M; PU; ViRA **30-0726**

PROUT, William (1785-1850)
Chemistry, meterology, and the function of digestion. . . . New ed. Philadelphia: Carey, Lea & Blanchard, 1836. 276p. [Bridgewater Treatises, No. 5] DLC; MB; NN; NNC **30-0727**

RACIBORSKI, Adam (1809-1871)
An elementary treatise on auscultation and percussion, or the application of acoustics to the diagnosis of diseases, with a synoptical table. . . . Tranls. with notes. &c., by Minturn Post, M.D. New York: Collins, Keese & Co., 1839. 261p. 1 plate. CU-M; DLC; DNLM; NNNAM **30-0728**

RALPH, Joseph
A domestic guide to medicine, by which individuals, both male and female, are enabled to treat their own complaints with perfect safety. . . . [New York, 1834] 116p. DNLM; NNNAM **30-0729**

RALPH, Joseph
A plain treatise on cholera: (being a chapter extracted from Dr. Ralph's guide to domestic medicine). Intended for the use of private individuals; showing its nature, cause and symptoms, with directions for its treatment, &c. . . . To this is added—a list of articles to be kept in readiness by every family, and by every person going on a journey. Also—directions for avoiding an attack of cholera. . . . New York: Sold by J. Leavitt [etc.] 1834. 16p. DLC; NN; NNNAM **30-0730**

RALPH, Joseph
A domestic medical treatise on the nature, causes, and cure of dyspepsia and liver disease. Intended for the perusal and guide of every dyspeptic individual. . . . New York: Sold at the general office of the Domestic medicine. . . , 1835. 40p. DLC; NN; NNC; NNNAM **30-0731**

[RALPH, Joseph]
A domestic guide to medicine, by which individuals both male and female, are enabled to treat their own complaints. . . . New York: Sold by the author, 1835. 210p. DLC; NN; NNC; NNU-M **30-0732**

RALPH, Joseph
A private treatise on veneral disease, gonorrhea. . . . [New York: J. & W. Sandford, printers, 1836] 100p. CU-M; DLC; NNNAM; NNU-M **30-0733**

RAMADGE, Francis Hopkins (1793?-1867)
Consumption curable. The manner in which nature and remedial art operate in effecting a healing process in cases of consumption. . . . From the 3rd London ed. New York: J. M. Howe [1839]. 48p. DNLM; NNNAM **30-0734**

RAMADGE, Francis Hopkins (1793?-1867)
Consumption curable, and the manner in which nature as well as remedial art operates in effecting a healing process in cases of consumption. . . . With an introduction by the publisher. 1st American from the 3rd London ed. New York: J. M. Howe, 1839. 160p. CSmH; DNLM; NcD; NNNAM **30-0735**

RANDOLPH, Jacob (1796-1848)
Some remarks on morbus coxarius, with an account of P. S. Physick's method of treating this disease. Philadelphia: J. R. A. Skerrett, 1831. 12p. 1 plate. DNLM **30-0736**

RANDOLPH, Jacob (1796-1848)
Account of six cases of stone in the bladder, in which the operation of lithotripsy was successfully performed. [Philadelphia, 1834] 19p. DNLM **30-0737**

RANDOLPH, Jacob (1796-1848)
An account of seven additional cases of stone in the bladder, in which the operation of lithotripsy was successfully performed. [Philadelphia, 1836] 13p. DNLM **30-0738**

RANDOLPH, Jacob (1796-1848)
A memoir of the life and character of Philip Syng Physick, M.D. Philadelphia: T. K. and P. G. Collins, 1839. 114p. DLC; PPC; PU; RPJCB **30-0739**

RATIER, Felix Severin (1797-1866)
A practical formulary of the Parisian hospitals; exhibiting the prescriptions employed by the physicians and surgeons of those establishments. . . . Transl. from the 3rd ed. of the French . . . by R. D. McLellan. . . . New York: C. S. Francis; Boston: Munroe & Francis [Clayton & Van Norden, pr.] 1830. 262p. PPL; PU **30-0740**

RATIER, Felix Severin (1797-1866)
A practical formulary of the Parisian hospitals; exhibiting the prescriptions employed by the physicians and surgeons of those establishments. With remarks illustrative of their doses, mode of administration, and appropriate application. . . . Transl. from the 3rd ed. of the French, with notes and illustrations, by R. D. McLellan. New York: Pr. by Clayton & Van Norden, for F. & N. G. Carnes, 1831. 262p. MB **30-0741**

RAY, Isaac (1807-1881)
A treatise on the medical jurisprudence of insanity. . . . Boston: C. C. Little and J. Brown, 1838. . . . 480p. DLC; MBM; MH; NNNAM **30-0742**

RAY, Joseph
Inaugural dissertation on some of the abuses of blood letting. . . . Cincinnati, 1831. 33p. OC **30-0743**

REECE, Richard (1775-1831)
Lady's medical guide; being a popular treatise on the causes, prevention & mode of treatment of the diseases to which females are particularly subject. Philadelphia: Carey, Lea & Blanchard, 1833. 144p. DLC; DNLM; MBM; OCIM **30-0744**

REED, Sampson
Observations on the growth of the mind; with remarks on some other subjects. Boston: O. Clapp, 1838. 192p. DNLM; MBAt; MWA **30-0745**

REED, Thomas C.
A discourse on the character of the late Chester Averill. 70p. Schenectady: S. S. Riggs, 1837. DNLM **30-0746**

REESE, David Meredith (1800-1861)
A plain and practical treatise on the epidemic cholera, as it prevailed in the city of New York, in the summer of 1832. . . . To which is added by way of appendix, a brief essay on the medical use of ardent spirits. New York: Conner & Cooke, 1832. 110p. NN; NNU-M; OCHP **30-0747**

REESE, David Meredith (1800-1861)
A plain and practical treatise on the epidemic cholera, as it prevailed in the city of New York, in the summer of 1832; including its nature, causes, treatment and prevention. . . . New York: Conner & Cooke; Boston: Lilly, Wait, & Co., 1833. 110p. DNLM; ICJ; ScU **30-0748**

REESE, David Meredith (1800-1861)
Phrenology, known by its fruits, being a brief review of Doctor Brigham's late work, entitled "Observations on the influence of religion upon the health and physical welfare of mankind." New York: Howe & Bates, 1836. 195p. DNLM; N; NN; NNNAM **30-0749**

REESE, David Meredith (1800-1861)
Humbugs of New York, being a remonstrance against popular delusion, whether in science, philosophy, or religion. . . . New York: J. S. Taylor; Boston: Weeks, Jordan & Co., 1838. 22p. NNNAM, NjR; MBM **30-0750**

REESE, David Meredith (1800-1861)
Introductory lecture delivered at the opening of the Albany Medical College, in the anatomical theatre, January 2, 1839. . . . Albany: Printed by Hoffman & White, 1839. 44p. DLC; N; NN; NNNAM **30-0751**

REESE, David Meredith (1800-1861)
Introductory lecture before the Albany Medical College, delivered October 1, 1839. . . . Albany: Printed by J. Munsell, 1839. 22p. DLC; N; NHi; PPL **30-0752**

The **REFORMED** practice of medicine as taught at the reformed medical colleges in the city of New York, at Worthington, Ohio, and all the reformed schools in the United States. Containing all the practice of Dr. Beach of New York, of the celebrated Dr. Bone of New Jersey, and other celebrated botanic practitioners. Boston, 1831. 2 v. in 1. DNLM; MBM **30-0753**

REMARKS relative to the pay of the medical staff of the Army of the United States. [Washington, 1834] 7p. DNLM **30-0754**

RENWICK, James (1790-1863)
Syllabus of lectures on chemistry . . . in Columbia College. New York: G. F. Hopkins & Son, 1831. 55p. DLC; NNC **30-0755**

REVERE, John (1787-1847)
A discourse introductory to the course of lectures on the theory and practice of physic in Jefferson Medical College, session 1832-1833. Philadelphia, 1832. 24p. DNLM; PPJ **30-0756**

REVERE, John (1787-1847)
A lecture delivered at Jefferson Medical College, Philadelphia, January 8, 1834. Philadelphia: T. K. Collins & Co., 1834. 16p. DNLM; PPJ **30-0757**

REYNOLDS, Edward (1793-1881)
On the importance of a knowledge of the principles of physiology to parents and teachers. Boston: I. R. Butts, 1833. 31p. DNLM; MH; MWA **30-0758**

[RHINELANDER, John R.]
Catalogue of anatomical preparations in the museum of John R. Rhinelander, M.D. (Founded by Professor Bailley of Columbia College and enlarged by Dr. Post.) New York, 1833. 28p. MH; NNNAM **30-0759**

RICHERAND, Anthelme Balthasar (1779-1840)
Elements of physiology, by A. Richerand. . . . Transl. from the French by G. J. M. De Lys, M.D. 5th ed. Carefully rev. after the 9th and latest French ed., and supplied with notes and a copious appendix by James Copland. . . . 2nd ed. New York: W. E. Dean . . . , 1833. 386p. MB; NBM; PPC **30-0760**

RILLIET, Frédéric (1814-1861) and E. BARTHEZ
A treatise on the pneumonia of children. Transl. from the French by S. Parkman. Philadelphia: A. Waldie, 1839. 100p. DNLM; NjR **30-0761**

RIVINUS, Edward Florens (1802-1873)
On the operation of physical causes upon the constitution, the health, and diseases of man. Philadelphia: J. R. A. Skerrett, 1831. 26p. DNLM; DLC; PHi; ScC **30-0762**

RIVINUS, Edward Florens (1802-1873)
A catalogue of the medical library of the Philadelphia Almshouse, prepared agreeably to a resolution of the Board of Managers. . . . [Philadelphia, 1831] 174p. DNLM; PPL **30-0763**

ROBINSON, Samuel
A course of fifteen lectures on medical botany, denominated Thomson's new theory of medical practice; in which the various theories that have preceded it are reviewed and compared. Delivered in Cincinnati, Ohio. . . . With introductory remarks by the proprietor. Boston: Pr. by Jonathan Howe, 1830. 192p. DLC; DNLM; PPC; PPL **30-0764**

ROBINSON, Samuel
A course of fifteen lectures on medical botany, denominated Thomson's new theory of medical practice; in which the various theories that have preceded it are reviewed and compared. Delivered in Cincinnati, Ohio. . . . With introductory remarks by the proprietor. 2nd ed. Columbus: Pub. by Horton Howard. Charles Scott, pr., 1830. 162p. DLC; DNLM; NNNAM **30-0765**

ROBINSON, Samuel
A course of fifteen lectures, on medical botany, denominated Thomson's new theory of medical practice; in which the various theories that have preceded it are reviewed and compared. Delivered in Cincinnati, Ohio. . . . With introductory remarks by the proprietor. Columbus: Pub. by Pike, Platt and Co., 1832. 206p. DNLM; GU; RPM **30-0766**

ROBINSON, Samuel
A lecture, introductory a course, on the science of life, organization. . . . [Columbus, 1832] 13p. DNLM; RPM **30-0767**

ROBINSON, Samuel
A course of fifteen lectures, on medical botany, denominated Thomson's new theory of medical practice; in which the various theories that have preceded it are reviewed and compared. Delivered in Cincinnati, Ohio. . . . Boston: J. Howe, printer, 1834. DLC; OCHP; OCLloyd; PU **30-0768**

ROBINSON, Samuel
A course of fifteen lectures, on medical botany, denominated Thomson's new theory of medical practice; in which the various theories that have preceded it are reviewed and compared. Delivered in Cincinnati, Ohio. . . . Boston: J. Q. Adams, printer, office of the Investigator, 1835. DLC; DNLM; GU; NBM **30-0769**

ROGERS, David L. (1799-1877)
Description of a new instrument for excising enlarged tonsils. [New York]: Clayton & Van Norden [1831] 3p. 1 plate. DNLM **30-0770**

ROGERS, Henry
Directions for a family medicine chest, put up and sold by Henry Rogers, chemist and druggist, Charleston, Kanawha County, Virginia. [Laidly & Co., prs., 1830?] 9p. DNLM; MWA; ViRA **30-0771**

ROGET, Peter Mark (1779-1869)
Animal and vegetable physiology considered with reference to natural theology. Philadelphia: Carey, Lea & Blanchard, 1836. 2 v. [Bridgewater Treatises, No. 7] DLC; MB; NN; NNNAM **30-0772**

ROGET, Peter Mark (1779-1869)
Outlines of physiology: with an appendix on phrenology. . . . 1st American ed., rev., with numerous notes. Philadelphia: Lea & Blanchard, 1839. 516p. CtY-M; DLC; DNLM; PPC **30-0773**

ROSENSTEIN, J. G.
Treatise upon a new manner of medical practice, called homoeopathic, elucidated by comparing the high station of homoeopathic with the usual mode of practice called allopathic. Albany: Lackard & Van Benthuysen, 1836. 16p. DNLM; NNNAM **30-0774**

RUSH, Benjamin (1745-1813)
The effects of ardent spirits upon the human body and mind. New York: Pub. by the American Tract Society [1830?] 8p. NNNAM **30-0775**

RUSH, Benjamin (1745-1813)
Medical inquiries and observations upon the diseases of the mind. 4th ed. Philadelphia: John Grigg, 1830. 365p. GU; KU; PPC **30-0776**

[RUSH, Benjamin, 1745-1813]
Extracts from Dr. Benjamin Rush's inquiry into the effects of ardent spirits upon the human body and mind. Philadelphia: Tract Association of Friends, 1833. 16p. OClWHi **30-0777**

RUSH, James (1786-1869)
The philosophy of the human voice: embracing its physiological history. . . . 2nd ed., enl. Philadelphia: Grigg & Eliott, 1833. 432p. DLC; DNLM; PU **30-0778**

RUSH, William
Introductory lecture delivered before the class of the Philadelphia School of Medicine. Philadelphia: W. Stavely, 1833. 12p. DNLM; PPC **30-0779**

RYAN, Michael (1800-1841)
A manual of medical jurisprudence, compiled from the best medical and legal works: being an analysis of a course of lectures on forensic medicine, annually delivered in London. . . . 1st American ed., with notes and additions, by R. Eglesfeld Griffith. . . . Philadelphia: Carey & Lea, 1832. 327p. CSmH; DLC; ICJ; MB **30-0780**

RYAN, Michael (1800-1841)
A manual of midwifery, or Compendium of gynecology and paidonosology; comprising a new nomenclature of obstetric medicine, with a concise account of the symptoms and treatment of the most important diseases of women and children, and the management of the various forms of parturition. . . . 1st American from the 3rd London ed. Burlington [Vt.]: Smith & Harrington, 1835. 520p. DNLM; IU-M; PPC; VtHi **30-0781**

RYAN, Michael (1800-1841)
Lectures on population, marriage and divorce; comprising an account of the causes and treatment of impotence and sterility, of the morbid and curative effects of marriage, and on the diseases produced by onanism. . . . 1st American from the last London ed., Baltimore: W. R. Lucas & R. N. Wright, 1835. 95p. CU-M; DLC:KU; KyLoJM **30-0782**

SARLANDIÈRE, Jean-Baptiste (1787-1838)
Systematized anatomy, or human organography, in synoptical tables, with numerous plates. . . . Transl. from the French by W. C. Roberts. New York: J. & E. Bisbee, 1835. 19 l. 16 plates. DNLM **30-0783**

SARLANDIÈRE, Jean-Baptiste (1787-1838)
Systematized anatomy, or human organography, in synoptical tables, with numerous plates. . . . Transl. from the French by W. C. Roberts. New York: J. S. Rohrer & G. Hills, 1837. 17 l. 15 plates. DNLM **30-0784**

SAWYER, Matthias Enoch
A treatise on primitive or secondary disguised or misplaced fever, as a single disease; with the varieties, cause, and treatment, as it appears in most of the particular forms of fever recognized by nosologists. . . . New York: Peabody & Co., 1831. 307p. DLC; MH; MWA **30-0785**

SCOTT, John Witherspoon (1800-1892)
The Cholera, God's Scourge for the chastisement of the nations: A discourse delivered on the occasion of a fast observed in reference to the approach of the epidemic, Oxford, Ohio, August 16th, 1833. . . . Oxford, Ohio: W. W. Bishop, 1833. 15p. CSmH; DNLM; OCHP; PPPrHi **30-0786**

SCOUTETTEN, Raoul Henri Joseph (1799-1871)
A medical and topographical history of the cholera morbus, including the mode of prevention and treatment. . . . With a report read at the Royal Academy of Medicine, at Paris, September 17, 1831. Transl. from the French by A. Sidney Doane. Boston: Carter & Hendee, 1832. 100p. 1 map. DLC; DNLM; GU; PPAmP **30-0787**

SEARS, William
A treatise on the physiology and pathology of the digestive organs, with introductory remarks. . . . New York: I. W. Bell, 1834. 35p. DNLM; NNNAM **30-0788**

SEE, John
Family medicine. . . . New York: Printed for the Author, 1833. 51p. DLC; NNN **30-0789**

SEEGER, Charles L. (1763-1848)
A lecture on the epidemic cholera, delivered in Springfield on the 2nd of August, and in Northampton on the 9th of August, and published at the request of a number of inhabitants of both places. Boston: Carter & Hendee, 1832. 26p. MB; MBM; NNNAM **30-0790**

SEWALL, Thomas (1786-1845)
An address delivered before the Washington City Temperance Society, November 15, 1830. Washington, W. Greer, 1830. 24p. DNLM; NN; PPL **30-0791**

SEWALL, Thomas (1786-1845)
An eulogy on Dr. Godman, being an introductory lecture, delivered November 1, 1830. Washington: W. Greer, 1830. 24p. DNLM; PPL **30-0792**

SEWALL, Thomas (1786-1845)
An eulogy on Dr. Godman, being an introductory lecture, delivered November 1, 1830. Printed at Washington; reprinted at Manchester: Harrison & Crossfield, 1832. 24p. DNLM; PPL **30-0793**

SEWALL, Thomas (1786-1845)
An euology on Dr. Godman, being an intorductory lecture, delivered November 1, 1830. New York: B. Waugh & T. Mason, 1832. 24p. DNLM; PPC; PPL **30-0794**

SEWALL, Thomas (1786-1845)
Memoir of Dr. John D. Godman, professor of anatomy, author of "Anatomical Illustrations," who died at Philadelphia, April 17, 1830. From an introductory lecture. . . . New York: American Tract Society [1834?]. 2, 20, 3-[4]p. DNLM; NHi; NN; NNC **30-0795**

SEWALL, Thomas (1786-1845)
An examination of phrenology; in two lectures, delivered to the students of the Columbian College, District of Columbia, February, 1837. Washington City: B. Homans, 1837. 70p. DNLM; InHi; NN **30-0796**

SEWALL, Thomas (1786-1845)
An examination of phrenology; in two lectures, delivered to the students of the Columbian College, District of Columbia, February, 1837. 2nd ed. Boston: D. S. King, 1839. 110p. DNLM; MWA **30-0797**

SHELTON's American medicine; or, improvement in uniting his new steam system and the old practice of medicine, in which doctors' terms are explained and the complaints of men, women, and children are treated of. . . . The valuable practice and preparations of Dr. Isaac Wright, of Tennessee, are fully developed in this work. Madisonville, Tenn.: W. Harvey, 1834. 400p. DNLM **30-0798**

SHERRILL, Hunting (1783-1866)
An essay on epidemics, as they appeared in Dutchess County, from 1809 to 1825; also a paper on diseases of the jaw-bones: with an appendix, containing an account of the epidemic cholera, as it appeared in Poughkeepsie in 1832. . . . New York: Pr. by Booth & Smith, 1832. 184p. DNLM; MH; RPM **30-0799**

SHERRILL, Hunting (1783-1866)
On the pathology of epidemic cholera, with some preliminary observations in the history of the disease and the general cause and nature of epidemics; containing an approved plan of treatment, the means of prevention and rules for corporations and individuals to pursue. New York: Sam'l Wood & Sons, 1835. 198p. DLC; LNT-M; NN; NNNAM **30-0800**

SHERWOOD, Henry Hall
New or electric symptoms of chronic diseases, or Chronic tubercula of the organs and limbs . . . and their natural or electric remedies . . . Including all the forms of scrofula. . . . Cincinnati: James & Gazlay, printers, 1836. 58p. DLC; DNLM; OCHP; OClWHi **30-0801**

SHERWOOD, Henry Hall
New or electric symptoms of chronic diseases, or chronic tubercula of the organs and limbs . . . and their natural or electric remedies. . . . Including all the forms of scrofula. . . . 2nd ed. Cincinnati: F. Surguy, 1837. 70p; DNLM; OClWHi **30-0802**

SHERWOOD, Henry Hall
Electro-galvanic symptoms and electro-magnetic remedies, in chronic diseases of the class hypertrophy, or chronic enlargements of the organs and limbs, including all forms of scrofula, with illustrative diagrams and cases. New York: J.-W. Bell, 1837. 88p. DNLM; NNNAM; NNU-M **30-0803**

SHORT, Charles Wilkins (1794-1863)
A biographical memoir of H. Hulbert Eaton . . . (delivered Nov. 10th, as an introductory address to the medical class, at the opening of the session of 1832-3). [Lexington? Ky., 1832-3] 15p. NN; NNC **30-0804**

SHORT, Charles Wilkins (1794-1863)
Instructions for the gathering and preservation of plants for herbaria; in a letter to a young botanist. Lexington: J. Clarke, 1833. 16p. DNLM; OCLloyd **30-0805**

[SHURTLEFF, Nathaniel Bradstreet] (1810-1874)
An epitome of phrenology; being an outline of the science as taught by Gall, Spurzheim and Combs; to accompany a chart delineated according to this system, or the marked bust approved by Dr. Spurzheim. . . . Boston: Marsh, Capen & Lyon, 1835. 128p. DLC; MBM; MH; MWA **30-0806**

SIMONS, Thomas Young (1798-1857)
The annual address to the graduates of the Medical College of South Carolina, delivered March 23, 1830, after conferring the degree of Doctor of Medicine. Charleston: A. F. Cunningham, 1830, 13p. DLC; MB; NcD **30-0807**

SIMONS, Thomas Young (1798-1857)
An introductory letter delivered in the Medical College of South Carolina. Charleston: T. A. Hayden, 1835. 16p. DNLM; ScCM **30-0808**

SIMONS, Thomas Young (1798-1857)
Introductory lecture delivered at the opening of the session of the Medical College of South Carolina. Charleston: E. C. Councell, 1838. 25p. 1 plate. DNLM; ScCM **30-0809**

SIMONS, Thomas Young (1798-1857)
A report on the history and causes of the strangers' or yellow fever of Charleston. Charleston: W. Riley, 1839. 23p. DNLM; ScCM; ScMS **30-0810**

SINCLAIR, Elijah
Address to the graduates of the Medical College of Georgia. Augusta: W. T. Thompson & Co., 1838. 11p. DNLM; GU **30-0811**

SMITH, Ashbel (1805-1886)
The cholera spasmodica, as observed in Paris in 1832: comprising its symptoms, pathology, and treatment. Illustrated by cases. . . . New York: P. Hill, 1832. 80p. DLC; OCHP; PPAmP **30-0812**

SMITH, Ashbel (1805-1886)
An account of the yellow fever which appeared in the city of Galveston, republic of Texas, in the autumn of 1839, with cases and dissections. . . . Galveston: H. Stuart; Houston: Cruger & Moore . . . . , 1839. 78p. DLC; LNT-M; NcD; PPHA **30-0813**

SMITH, A. F.
The Indian doctor's dispensatory; or, every man his own physician, by A. F. Smith & J. Merwin. Hamilton, N.Y.: Printed at the Wesleyan Office, J. Hogan, Printer, 1833. 181p. OCLloyd **30-0814**

SMITH, David S. C. H. (1796-1859)
Suggestions with regard to the general treatment of fractures, with the description and mode of application of a new kind of splinting composed of felt. Boston: Carter, Hendee & Babcock, 1831. 11p. 3 plates. DNLM; MBM **30-0815**

SMITH, Elias (1769-1846)
The American physician, and family assistant: in four parts. . . . 3rd ed. Boston: H. Bowen's Print, 1832. 198p. DNLM; MB; MBM **30-0816**

SMITH, Elias (1769-1846)
An address to the citizens of Boston, and the people of the United States, on poison, health, disease, vegetable medicine, and manner of curing the sick. Boston: B. True, 1836. 72p. DNLM; MBM; MH-M **30-0817**

SMITH, Elias (1769-1846)
The American physician, and family assistant: in five parts. . . . 4th ed. Boston: B. True, 1837. 306p. DLNM; MBM; MH-M **30-0818**

SMITH, Elisha
The botanic physician: being a compendium of the practice of physic, upon botanical principles. . . . New York: Murphy & Bingham, prs., 1830. 624p. DLC; ICJ; IEN-M; NNNAM **30-0819**

SMITH, Jerome Van Crowinshield (1800-1879)
The class-book of anatomy, designed for schools, explanatory of the first principles of human mechanism, as the basis of physical education. Boston: Allen & Ticknor, 1834. 280p. DNLM; MH; MWA **30-0820**

SMITH, Jerome Van Crowinshield (1800-1879)
The class-book of anatomy, designed for schools, explanatory of the first principles of human mechanism, as the basis of physical education. 2nd ed. Boston: R. S. Davis, 1836. 286p. DNLM; ICU; MH; NN **30-0821**

SMITH, John
The curiosities of common water; on the advantage thereof in curing cholera, intemperance, and other maladies. . . . 5th ed. Salem: Whipple & Lawrence, 1832. 54p. DNLM; MB; NNNAM; MWA **30-0822**

SMITH, Joseph Mather (1789-1866)
A discourse on the epidemic of cholera morbus of Europe and Asia; delivered as an introductory lecture, at the College of Physicians and Surgeons in the city of New York, November 9, 1831. . . . New York: Pr. by J. Seymour, 1831. 36p. DNLM; MB; MBM; MH-M **30-0823**

SMITH, Nathan (1762-1829)
Medical and surgical memoirs. . . . Edited with addenda, by Nathan R. Smith, M.D. . . . Baltimore: Pr. by Wm. A. Francis, 1831. 374p. DNLM; DLC; ICJ; PU **30-0824**

SMITH, Nathan Ryno (1797-1877)
Surgical anatomy of the arteries, with plates and illustrations. . . . Baltimore: J. D. Toy & W. R. Lucas [J. D. Toy, pr.] 1830. 104p. DNLM; MdHi; PPC **30-0825**

SMITH, Nathan Ryno (1797-1877)
Surgical anatomy of the arteries, with plates and illustrations. . . . 2nd ed. Baltimore: W. R. Lucas & R. N. Wright, 1835. 133p. DNLM; MdHi **30-0826**

SMITH, Nathan Ryno (1797-1877)
An address, introductory to a course of lectures on the theory and practice of medicine. Lexington, Ky.: Observor & Reporter Office, 1838. 24p. DNLM; KyLoJM **30-0827**

SMITH, [Thomas] Southwood (1788-1861)
A treatise on fever. Philadelphia: Carey & Lea, publishers, I. Ashmead & Co., prs., 1830. 448p. DNLM; NjR; OC; PPC **30-0828**

SMITH, [Thomas] Southwood (1788-1861)
A treatise on fever. . . . Boston: Stimpson and Clapp, 1831. 412p. DLC; MBM; PPC; PU **30-0829**

SMITH, [Thomas] Southwood (1788-1861)
A treatise on fevers. 3rd American ed. Philadelphia: Carey, Lea & Blanchard, 1835. 326p. DNLM; PPC; PPJ; PU **30-0830**

SMITH, William G.
An inaugural dissertation on opium. . . . [New York] 1832. 23p. DNLM; NNC; NNNAM **30-0831**

SNELL, James
A practical guide to operations on the teeth. To which is prefixed a historical sketch of the rise and progress of dental surgery. . . . Philadelphia: Carey & Lea, 1832. 207p. CU-M; DNLM; ICJ; PPHa **30-0832**

SOUTH CAROLINA. MEDICAL SOCIETY
Exposition of the affairs of the Medical Society of South Carolina, so far as they appertain to the establishment of the Medical College in Charleston, and the subsequent division of the latter into two schools of medicine. Charleston: E. J. Van Brunt, 1833. 40p. DNLM; ScC; ScCM; ScMS **30-0833**

SPENCER, Thomas (1793-1857)
. . . Practical observations on epidemic diarrhoea, known as the epidemic cholera, spasmodic cholera, . . . with a brief outline of its treatment, founded on the pathology of the disease. . . . Utica: Pr. by E. A. Maynard, 1832. 7p. DNLM; CSmH; MB; NNNAM **30-0834**

SPENCER, Thomas (1793-1857)
An essay on the nature of the epidemic usually called Asiastic cholera . . . and an attempt to found the treatment upon the pathology of the disease. Being the annual communication to the Medical Society of the State of New York, February 5th, 1833. . . . Albany: Printed by Webster and Skinners, 1833. 131p. DNLM; ICJ; MB; NNNAM **30-0835**

SPOONER, Shearjashub (1809-1859)
An inaugural dissertation on the physiology and diseases. Of the teeth. . . . New York: J. & W. Sandford, printers, 1835. 32p. DLC; DNLM; NN; NNNAM **30-0836**

SPOONER, Shearjashub (1809-1859)
Guide to sound teeth, or A popular treatise on the teeth illustrating the whole judicious management of these organs from infancy to old age. . . . New York: Wiley & Long, 1836. 207p. DLC; DNLM; NNNAM; NNU-M **30-0837**

SPOONER, Shearjashub (1809-1859)
Guide to sound teeth, or A popular treatise on the teeth, illustrating the whole judicious management of these organs from infancy to old age. . . . 2nd ed. New York: Collins, Keese & Co., 1838. 207p. DLC; NNNAM; NjR; OC **30-0838**

SPURZHEIM, Johann Gaspar (1776-1832)
Outlines of phrenology; being also a manual of reference for the marked bust. Boston: Marsh, Capen and Lyon, 1832. 96p. DLC; DNLM; RPB; ScC **30-0839**

SPURZHEIM, Johann Gaspar (1776-1832)
Phrenology; or, The doctrine of the mental phenomena; 1st American ed., greatly imp. by the author, from 3rd London ed. Boston: Marsh, 1832. 2 v. MBM; PPC **30-0840**

SPURZHEIM, Johann Gaspar (1776-1832)
Sixty phrenological specimens, described by Dr. Spurzheim. Boston: Marsh, Capen & Lyon, 1832. 16p. DLC; MH; MHi **30-0841**

SPURZHEIM, Johann Gaspar (1776-1832)
Examination of the objections made in Britain against the doctrines of Gall and Spurzheim. . . . With notes by J. G. Spurzheim. . . . 1st American ed., with improvements by Dr. Spurzheim. Boston: Marsh, Capen & Lyon, 1833. 99, 4, 112p. DNLM; PPPH; RPB **30-0842**

SPURZHEIM, Johann Gaspar (1776-1832)
Observations on the deranged manifestations of the mind, or Insanity. . . . 1st American ed., with notes, improvements, and plates. With an appendix by A. Brigham. . . . Boston: Marsh, Capen & Lyon, 1833. 260p. DLC; DNLM; IU-M; ScCM **30-0843**

SPURZHEIM, Johann Gaspar (1776-1832)
Outlines of phrenology; being also a manual of reference for the marked bust. 2nd ed. Boston: Marsh, Capen & Lyon, 1833. 96, ivp. MH; OC; RPB **30-0844**

SPURZHEIM, Johann Gaspar (1776-1832)
Phrenology, or The doctrine of the mental phenomena. . . . 2nd American ed., greatly improved by the author, from the 3rd London ed. Boston: Marsh, Capen & Lyon, 1833. 2 v. DLC; MBM; MWA; NBM **30-0845**

SPURZHEIM, Johann Gaspar (1776-1832)
Phrenology, in connexion with the study of physiognomy. 1st American ed. improved. To which is prefixed a biography of the author, by Nahum Capen. Boston: Marsh, Capen & Lyon, 1833. 191p. DLC; DNLM; MH; MdBJ-W **30-0846**

SPURZHEIM, Johann Gaspar (1776-1832)
The anatomy of the brain, with a general view of the nervous system. . . . Transl. from the unpublished French ms. by R. Willis. . . . With an appendix, and eighteen plates. 1st American ed., rev. by Charles H. Stedman. . . . Boston: Marsh, Capen & Lyon, 1834. 244p. DLC; MBM; MH; MWA **30-0847**

SPURZHEIM, Johann Gaspar (1776-1832)
Phrenology; or, The doctrine of the mental phenomena. . . . 3rd American ed. greatly improved by the author, from the 3rd London ed. Boston: Marsh, Capen & Lyon, 1834. 2 v. DLC; MBM; MH; MWA **30-0848**

SPURZHEIM, Johann Gaspar (1776-1832)
Observations on the deranged manifestations of the mind, or Insanity. . . . 2nd American ed., with notes, improvements, and plates. With an appendix, by A. Brigham. . . . Boston: Marsh, Capen & Lyon, 1835. 272p. CSmH; DLC; MBM; MBAt **30-0849**

SPURZHEIM, Johann Gaspar (1776-1832)
Observations on the deranged manifestations of the mind, or Insanity. . . . 3rd American ed., with notes, improvements and plates. With an appendix, by A. Brigham. . . . Boston: Marsh, Capen & Lyon, 1836. 272p. DLC; MBM; MWA **30-0850**

SPURZHEIM, Johann Gaspar (1776-1832)
The anatomy of the brain, with a general view of the nervous system. Transl. from the unpublished French Ms. by R. Willis. . . . With an appendix and eighteen plates. 2nd American ed., rev. by Charles H. Stedman. Boston: Marsh, Capen & Lyon, 1836. 244p. DNLM; MBM; MWA **30-0851**

STEEL, John H[oneywood] (1780-1838)
An analysis of the mineral waters of Saratoga and Ballston, containing some general remarks on their use in various diseases. Together with observations on the geology and mineralogy of the surrounding country. . . . An entire new work. Saratoga Springs: G. M. Dawson, 1831. 203p. DNLM **30-0852**

STEELE, Oliver (1800-1861)
A catalogue of theological, medical, classical, miscellaneous and school books for sale by Oliver Steele, Nos. 433 & 437 South Market Street, [Albany]: G. J. Loomis, 1830. 85p. CSmH; N **30-0853**

STEVENS, Alexander Hodgdon (1789-1869)
Familiar instructions for the prevention of cholera, prepared for a family about leaving the city, New York, 5th July, 1832. New York: W. A. Mercein, 1832. 8p. DNLM; NNNAM **30-0854**

STEVENS, Alexander Hodgdon (1789-1869)
A clinical lecture on the primary treatment of injuries, delivered at the New York Hospital, November 22nd, 1837. . . . New York: Adlard & Saunders, 1837. 34p. DLC; NNNAM **30-0855**

STEVENS, Alexander Hodgdon (1789-1869)
Lectures on lithotomy, delivered at the New York Hospital, December, 1837. . . . New York: Adlard & Saunders, 1838. 93p. DLC; NNNAM **30-0856**

STEVENS, William (1786-1868)
[Dr. Stevens's] treatise on the cholera, extracted from his work entitled "Observations on the healthy and diseased properties of the blood." New York: G. & C. & H. Carvill, 1832. 63p. MB; ScU **30-0857**

STILLÉ, Alfred (1813-1900)
An examination of certain charges preferred against the medical class of the University of Pennsylvania during the session of 1834-1835. [Philadelphia, 1835] 24p. DLC; PU **30-0858**

STOKES, William (1804-1878)
Lectures on the theory and practice of physic. 1st American ed. Philadelphia: A. Waldie, 1837. 407p. DNLM; PPC; ViRA **30-0859**

STOKES, William (1804-1878)
. . . A treatise on the diagnosis and treatment of diseases of the chest. Part 1. Diseases of the lung and windpipe. . . . [Dunglison's American Medical Library] Philadelphia: A. Waldie, 1837. 300p. CtY-M; DLC; MBM; PU **30-0860**

SULLIVAN, John L.
A concise view of the principles of homoeopathia. By the Baron de Brunnow, of Dresden; with introductory remarks in presenting this exposition in English to the New York Homoeopathic Society. Published by the Society. New York: Henry Ludwig, 1835. 34p. DLC; NN; PPHa **30-0861**

SULLIVAN, John L.
Homoeopathia, the science of specific remedies; showing the consistency of the homoeopathic treatment of consumption, with that of Dr. Ramage, of the London Lung Hospital; and that, combined, they constitute a complete system of remedial means for its cure. The substance of a dissertation read October 2, 1839, before the New Haven County Medical Society. Published in reference to a passage in Dr. Miner's printed address to the medical class, February 26, 1839. New Haven: Babcock & Galpin, 1839. 60p. DLC; MBM; MH-M; PPHa **30-0862**

SWAIM, William
A collection of cases, illustrating the restorative and sanative properties of Swaim's panacea, in variety of diseases. . . . Philadelphia, 1831. 120p. DLC; DNLM; PPC; PU **30-0863**

SWAIM, William
A collection of cases illustrating the restorative and sanative properties of Swaim's panacea, in a variety of diseases. . . . Philadelphia, 1832. 132p. DLC; DNLM; MH; MdBJ-W **30-0864**

SWAIM, William
A treatise on the alternative and curative virtues of Swaim's panacea, and its application to the different diseases of the human system. Philadelphia: J. Bioren, 1833. 161p. DLC; DNLM; PPL **30-0865**

SWAIM, William
Plain and practical observations upon diseases resulting from worms; with remarks upon the utility of Swaim's vermifuge in cholera morbus and many other diseases originating in debility of the digestive organs. Philadelphia: H. Dickinson, 1833. 12p. DNLM; PPHa **30-0866**

SWAIM, William
Coleccion de casos, en ilustracion de las propiendades restauratives y sanativas de la panacea de Swaim, en varias enfermedades. Filadelfia, 1837. 124p. DNLM; PPC; PPHa **30-0867**

SWEET, Waterman
An essay on the science of bone-setting. Schenectady: Reprinted for the author by S. S. Riggs, 1833. 75p. RHi **30-0868**

SWEETSER, William (1797-1875)
A treatise on consumption; embracing an inquiry into the influence exerted upon it by journeys, voyages and change of climate. With directions for the consumptive visiting the south of Europe, and remarks upon its climate. Adapted for general readers. . . . Boston: T. H. Carter, 1836. 254p. DLC; DNLM; ICRM; VtHi **30-0869**

SWEETSER, William (1797-1875)
A treatise on digestion, and the disorders incident to it, which are comprehended under the term dyspepsia. Adapted for general readers. . . . Boston: T. H. Carter, 1837. 359p. DLC; MA; MBM; MWA **30-0870**

SYME, James (1799-1870)
The principles of surgery. . . . Philadelphia: Carey & Lea, 1832. [29], 375p. GU; MBM; MH; Nh **30-0871**

SYME, James (1799-1870)
On diseases of the rectum. . . . [Philadelphia, 1839?] 42p. DNLM **30-0872**

TANNER, Henry S. (1786-1858)
A geographical and statistical account of the epidemic cholera, from its commencement in India to its entrance into the United States. . . . Philadelphia: the Author, 1832. 35p. DNLM; PPL; PU; ScC **30-0873**

TANNER, John
The homoeopathist's pocket reference. Transl. from the German. Compiled and arranged, with considerable additions and improvements. Philadelphia: Published by the Author, 104 Chestnut St., 1838. 158p. DLC; MBM; PPHa; PU **30-0874**

TATE, George
A treatise on hysteria. . . . Philadelphia: E. L. Carey & A. Hart, 1831. 134p. OCIM; RPM **30-0875**

TEALE, Thomas Pridgin (1801?-1868)
A treatise on neuralgic diseases, dependent upon irritation of the spinal marrow and ganglia of the sympathetic nerve. . . . Concord: Pub. by Horatio Hill & Co. [1830?] 120p. DLC; DNLM; PPPrHi; MBAt **30-0876**

TEALE, Thomas Pridgin (1801?-1868)
A treatise on neuralgic diseases, dependent upon irritation of the spinal marrow and ganglia of the sympathetic nerve. . . . Philadelphia: E. L. Carey & A. Hart, 1830. 120p. DNLM; PPC; PU **30-0877**

TEALE, Thomas Pridgin (1801?-1868)
A treatise on neuralgic diseases, dependent upon irritation of the spinal marrow and ganglia of the sympathetic nerve. Concord: H. Hill & Co., [1832?]. 120p. DNLM
30-0878

TEALE, Thomas Pridgin (1801?-1868)
A treatise on neuralgic diseases, dependent upon irritation of the spinal marrow and ganglia of the sympathetic nerve. . . . Woodstock, Vt.: N. Haskell, 1834. 120p. DNLM; VtHi
30-0879

THERAPEUTIC INSTITUTE OF PHILADELPHIA
Program . . . of instruction by William Barton. Philadelphia, 1832. 10p. MH 30-0880

THOMSON, John
A historical sketch of the Thomsonian system of the practice of medicine on botanical principles, as originated by Samuel Thomson, and continued by his coadjutors. Albany: B. N. Packard & Co., 1830. 59p. DNLM; N; NHi; NN
30-0881

THOMSON, John
A view of science and quackery. . . . Albany, N.Y.: Pr. by S. Southwick, 1831. 48p. N; NHi; NN; NcD
30-0882

THOMSON, John
A philosophical theory of an "empiric," proved practically, compared with doubtful science and known quackery, as practiced by the regular physicians during the prevalence of the cholera in this city. . . . Albany: [the Author], 1833. 59p. DNLM; N; NHi; NN 30-0883

THOMSON, John (1765-1846)
Lectures on inflammation, exhibiting a view of the general doctrines, pathological and practical, of medical surgery. . . . 2nd American from the last London ed. Philadelphia: Pr. by C. Sherman & Co., for Carey & Lea, 1831. 526p. PP; PU
30-0884

THOMSON, Samuel (1769-1843)
New guide to health, or, Botanic family physician. Containing a complete system of practice on a plan entirely new. 3rd ed. Boston: J. Howe, 1831. 156p. PPL; PHi 30-0885

THOMSON, Samuel (1769-1843)
New guide to health; or Botanic family physician. Containing a complete system of practice on a plan entirely new: with a description of the vegetables made use of, and directions for preparing and administering them, to cure disease. . . . 3rd ed. Boston: Pr. by J. Howe, for the author, 1832. 2 v. in 1. MB; OC 30-0886

THOMSON, Samuel (1769-1843)
New guide to health; or Botanic family physician. Containing a complete system of practice on a plan entirely new: with a description of the vegetables made use of, and directions for preparing and administering them to cure disease. . . . 8th ed. by Samuel Thomson: Columbus, O.: Pike Platt & Co., 1832. 208p. OCHP; OCLloyd 30-0887

THOMSON, Samuel (1769-1843)
A narrative of the life and medical discoveries of Samuel Thomson: containing an account of his system of practice, and the manner of curing disease with vegetable medicine upon a plan entirely new. . . . Columbus, O.: Pike, Platt & Co., 1832. 290p. MH; OCIWHi 30-0888

THOMSON, Samuel (1769-1843)
A narrative of the life, and medical discoveries of Samuel Thomson; containing an account of his system of practice, and the manner of curing disease with vegetable medicine: upon a plan entirely new. Written by himself. 9th ed. Columbus, O.: Pike & Co., 1833. 256p. CSmH; MH
30-0889

THOMSON, Samuel (1769-1843)
New guide to health; or, Botanic family physician, containing a complete system of practice upon a plan entirely new. With a description of the vegetables made use of, and directions for preparing and administering them to cure disease. 10th ed. Columbus, [Ohio]: Jarvis Pike & Co., 1833. 219p. CSmH; DLC 30-0890

THOMSON, Samuel (1769-1843)
New guide to health; or, Botanic family physician, containing a complete system of practice upon a plan entirely new. With a description of the vegetables made use of, and directions for preparing and administering them to cure disease. 9th ed. Columbus, O.: Jarvis & Co., 1833. 229p. DLC; MH; PU
30-0891

THOMSON, Samuel (1769-1843)
A narrative of the life, and medical discoveries of Samuel Thomson; containing an account of his system of practice, and the manner of curing disease with vegetable medicine: upon a plan entirely new. 10th ed. Columbus, O.: Jarvis Pike & Co., 1833. 256p. DLC; OCIWHi 30-0892

THOMSON, Samuel (1769-1843)
Learned quackery exposed; or, Theory according to art; as exemplified in the practice of the fashionable doctors of the present day. . . . 36p. [n.p., 1834?]. DLC
30-0893

THOMSON, Samuel (1769-1843)
New guide to health; or Botanic family physician. Containing a complete system of practice on a plan entirely new: with a description of the vegetables made use of, and directions for preparing and administering them, to cure disease. To which is prefixed, a narrative of the life and medical discoveries of the author. . . . Boston: Printed for the author, J. Q. Adams, printer, 1835. 2 v. in 1. DLC; MBM; MH; OCLloyd
30-0894

THOMSONIAN BOTANICAL CONVENTION OF THE UNITED STATES [1832]
Proceedings of the United States Thomsonian Convention; . . . Troy [O.]: E. P. G. Sutherland, Printer, 1833. 50p. CSmH; NN 30-0895

The THOMSONIAN's manual and vade mecum; being a synopsis of the theory and principles on which is based the botanic practice of medicine, as promulgated to the world by Doctor Samuel Thomson. . . . Philadelphia: J. Kay, Jr., & Brother, 1835. 64, 2p. DNLM; OCLloyd 30-0896

TICKNOR, Caleb Bingham (1804-1840)
A popular treatise on medical philosophy; or, An exposition of quackery and imposture in medicine. (Read before the Phi Beta Kappa Society of Union College, at its anniversary meeting, and, in conformity with a resolution, pub. as a part of its Transactions.) . . . New York: Gould & Newman, 1838. 273p. DLC; NHi; NN; NNNAM 30-0897

TICKNOR, Caleb Bingham (1804-1840)
A guide for mothers and nurses in the management of young children; with reference to hereditary, or family disease; and advice to the pregnant, and lying-in female. Compiled, in part, from the best English and American writers. . . . New York: Taylor & Dodd, 1839. 244p. CSmH; DLC; NNC; PP
30-0898

TISSOT, Samuel Auguste Andre David (1728-1797)
A treatise on the diseases produced by onanism. Transl. from a new ed. of the French, with notes and an appendix. New York: Collins & Hannay, 1832. 132p. ICJ; NNN; RPM; ScCM
30-0899

TORREY, Jesse (1787-1834)
A dissertation on the causes, preventatives and remedies of plague, yellow fever, cholera, dysentery, and other pestilential, epidemic, or contagious diseases. . . . Philadelphia: J. Grigg, 1832. 80p. KyLoJM; MBM; PHi **30-0900**

TOWER, David
Four lectures on the Thomsonian practice of medicine. . . . Canandaigua [N.Y.]: Pr. by Bemis, Morse & Ward (for the author) 1828; Poughkeepsie [N.Y.]: Repr. by Thos. S. Ranney, by a resolution of the Dutchess Botanic Medical Society, 1832. 71p. CSmH **30-0901**

TOWNSEND, P[eter] S[olomon] (1796?-1849)
Result of observations made upon the black vomit, or yellow fever, at Havana and New York . . . read to the Board of Health, New York, and pub. in the New York Medical Journal . . . 1831. New York: Clayton, 1831. 65p. NjR; PPC
30-0902

A TREATISE on the diseases most prevalent in the United States, with directions for medicine chests, designed for the use of families. Compiled from the most approved medical writers. Philadelphia: Printed by J. R. A. Skerrett, 1833. 36p. ICJ
30-0903

TREATMENT of the premonitory symptoms of the cholera, by a citizen of New York. New York: Morgan & Burger, 1832. 20p. MB; NNNAM **30-0904**

TROUSSEAU, Armand (1801-1867)
. . . A practical treatise on laryngeal phthisis, chronic laryngitis, and diseases of the voice by A. Trousseau and H. Belloc. . . . Transl. by J. A. Warder. [Dunglison's American Medical Library] Philadelphia: A. Waldie, 1839. 186p. DLC; PPHa; PPC; PU **30-0905**

TURNBULL, Alexander
An investigation into the remarkable medicinal effects resulting from the external application of veratria. Washington: D. Green, 1834. 46p. DNLM; OCLloyd **30-0906**

TURNBULL, Alexander
On the medicinal properties of the natural order Ranunculaceae, and more particularly on the uses of sabadilla seeds. . . . Philadelphia: Haswell, Barrington & Haswell, 1838. 72p. DNLM; OCLloyd **30-0907**

TURNBULL, William (1729?-1796)
A popular treatise on health. . . . From the last London ed. . . . New York: J. K. Porter, 1831. 92p. MB; OCLloyd
30-0908

TWEEDIE, Alexander (1794-1884)
Clinical illustrations of fever comprising a report of the cases treated at the London fever hospital, 1828-1829. . . . Philadelphia: Carey & Lea, 1831. 152p. DNLM; PP; PPC; ViRA
30-0909

VANHOOK, C.
The sick man's companion, or, The preserver of health, treating diseases common to this country, according to the most successful practice. To which is added a short and comprehensive description of the medicines used in the practice, and their doses. . . . Vincennes, Ind.: Pr. by E. Stout, at the office of the "Western Sun," 1832. 76p. GU; InHi; MBM
30-0910

VELPEAU, Alfred Armand Louis Marie (1795-1867)
A treatise on surgical anatomy; or, The anatomy of regions, considered in its relations with surgery. . . . Transl. from the French, with additional notes, by John W. Sterling. . . . New York: S. Wood & Sons, 1830. 2 v. 14 fold. plates. DLC; PPC; PU **30-0911**

VELPEAU, Alfred Armand Louis Marie (1795-1867)
An elementary treatise on midwifery: or Principles of tokology and embryology. . . . Transl. from the French by Ch. D. Meigs. . . . Philadelphia: J. Grigg, 1831. 584p. DLC; ICJ; PU; RPM
30-0912

VELPEAU, Alfred Armand Louis Marie (1795-1867)
An elementary treatise on midwifery. . . . Philadelphia: Pr. by James Kay, Jr., & Co., 1831. 585p. IU-M; PPC; PU; ScC
30-0913

VELPEAU, Alfred Armand Louis Marie (1795-1867)
New elements of operative surgery; with an atlas of nearly three hundred engravings, representing the principal operative processes, and a great number of surgical instruments. . . . With an appendix of notes, by Granville Sharp Pattison. . . . Washington: D. Green, 1835. 912p. CU-M; DLC; GU; MBM
30-0914

VELPEAU, Alfred Armand Louis Marie (1795-1867)
An elementary treatise on midwifery: or Principles of tokology and embryology. . . . Transl. from the French by Ch. D. Meigs. . . . 2nd American ed. Philadelphia: Grigg & Elliot, 1838. 592p. DNLM; PPC; PPJ; PU **30-0915**

WAITE, George
The surgeon-dentist's anatomical and physiological manual. . . . Philadelphia: E. L. Carey and A. Hart [Thomas Kite, pr.] 1830. 210p. DNLM; CSmH **30-0916**

WAITE, George
The gums, with late discoveries on their structure, growth, connections, diseases, and sympathies. Philadelphia: Barrington & Haswell, 1838. 80p. DNLM; MdU-D
30-0917

WALKER, Alexander
Intermarriage, or the mode in which, and the causes why, beauty, health, and intellect result frm certain unions, and deformity, disease, and insanity from others. New York: J. & H. G. Langley, 1839. 384p. 8 plates. DNLM; NNNAM
30-0918

WALLACE, William Clay
The structure of the eye with reference to natural theology. New York: Wiley & Long, 1836. 52p. DNLM; NNNAM
30-0919

WALLACE, William Clay
A treatise on the eye. Containing discoveries of the causes of near and far sightedness, and of the affections of the retina, with remarks on the use of medicines as substitutes for spectacles. . . . 2nd ed. New York: S. Colman, 1839. 88p. DLC; DNLM; NN; PPHa **30-0920**

WARE, John (1795-1864)
Remarks on the history and treatment of delirium tremens. . . . Boston: Pr. by W. L. Lewis on N. Hale's Stream Power Press, 1831. 61p. DNLM; ICJ; MH-M **30-0921**

WARE, John (1795-1864)
An introductory lecture delivered before the medical class in Harvard University, on the 16th day of October, 1833. Boston: Hilliard, Gray & Co., 1833. 40p. DNLM; MH **30-0922**

WARNER, Augustus L[ockman] (*d.* 1847)
An introductory lecture, delivered to the medical class of the University of Virginia, at the commencement of the course on anatomy, physiology, and surgery. Charlottesville: Moseley & Tompkins, 1834. 16p. DNLM; ViRA **30-0923**

WARREN, Edward (1804-1878)
Sketch of the progress of the malignant or epidemic cholera, from its arrival in America. With tables illustrative of its progress in the principal cities it has visited. . . . Boston: Carter, Hendee & Co., 1832. 40p. DLC; DNLM; MHi; MWA **30-0924**

WARREN, John Collins (1778-1856)
Surgical observations on tumours, with cases and operations. . . . Boston: Crocker & Brewster, 1837. 607p. 16 plates. DLC; DNLM; MH-M; MWA **30-0925**

[WARREN, Samuel], 1807-1877
. . . Affecting scenes; being passages from the diary of a physician. . . . New York: J. & J. Harper, 1831. 2 v. MB **30-0926**

[WARREN, Samuel], 1807-1877
The diary of a late physician. . . . New York, 1832. 2 v. MWA **30-0927**

WARREN, Samuel (1807-1877)
Passages from the diary of a late physician. From the 5th London ed. New York: J. & J. Harper [1837]. 3 v. DLC; NN; PPAmP **30-0928**

WARRINGTON, Joseph (1805?-1888)
An oration on the improvements in medicine, delivered before the Philadelphia Medical Society, 1837. Philadelphia: J. & W. Kite, 1837. 28p. DNLM; PPC **30-0929**

WARRINGTON, Joseph (1805?-1888)
The nurse's guide. Containing a series of instructions to females who wish to engage in the important business of nursing mother and child in the lying-in chamber. Philadelphia: T. Cowperthwait & Co., 1839. 131p. DNLM; PPC; PPJ; ViRA **30-0930**

WATERVLIET, N.Y. UNITED SOCIETY
Catalogue of medicinal plants and vegetable medicines, prepared in the United Society. Watervliet, N.Y. . . . Orders to be directed to Watervliet, N.Y. Albany: Pr. by Packard & Van Benthuysen, 1830. 8p. OClWHi **30-0931**

WEATHERFORD, Hardin M.
A treatise on cholera, with the causes, symptoms, mode of prevention and cure, on a new and successful plan. . . . Louisville, Ky.: Printed by C. Settle, Book & Job Printer, 1833. 48p. OC **30-0932**

WEATHERHEAD, George Hume (1790-1853)
A practical treatise on the principal diseases of the lungs, considered especially in relation to particular tissues affected. Illustrating the different kinds of cough. Philadelphia: Haswell, Barrington & Haswell, 1837. 89p. DNLM; PPC; PPJ; PU **30-0933**

WEBB, Ezekiel
The philosophy of medicine, deduced from a series of self-evident propositions, developing self-evident principles for illustrating the medical sciences to intuitive demonstration. . . . Philadelphia: Carey, Lea & Blanchard, 1833. 232p. DNLM; IEN-M; MB; NcU **30-0934**

WEBB, Ezekiel
The philosophy of medicine, deduced from a series of self-evident propositions, developing self-evident principles for illustrating the medical sciences to intuitive demonstration. . . . With the addition of preliminary observations. . . . 2nd ed. New York: the Author, 1834. xxix, 232, xvp. DNLM; MBM; NNNAM **30-0935**

WELLS, Horace (1815-1848)
An essay on teeth, comprising a brief description of their formation, diseases, and proper treatment. . . . Hartford: Printed for the author, 1838. 70p. DLC; DNLM; MBM; MH **30-0936**

WELLS, William Charles (1754-1817)
An essay on dew and several appearances connected with it. Philadelphia: Haswell, Barrington & Haswell, 1838. 71p. DNLM **30-0937**

WEYER, A.
The family physician, or Poor man's friend, and married lady's companion: containing a great variety of valuable medical recipes, designed to assist heads of families, travellers, and seafaring people in curing diseases. . . . St. Clairsville, O.: Pr. by H. J. Howard, for the author, 1831. 216p. DLC; IEN-M **30-0938**

WHITE, Thomas
Treatise on the diseases of the teeth, and the cause of those diseases, with directions for preventing their occurrence. Lexington, Ky.: Savary & Co., 1832. 23p. DLC; KU; KyLoJM **30-0939**

WHITELAW's patent medicated vapor baths. New York: H. R. Piercy, 1834. 8p. DNLM **30-0940**

WHITING, Henry (1788-1851)
An address to the public, on the importance of restoring health to the sick. . . . New York: D. Murphy, 1831. 14p. NN; NNNAM **30-0941**

WHITNEY, Daniel H.
The family physician, and guide to health, in three parts: Part I. Contains the theory and practice of physic. Part II. Diseases of women and children, and the botanic practice. Part III. Dispensatory, anatomy, and the practice of surgery; together with the history, causes, symptoms and treatment of the Asiatic cholera: a glossary explaining the most difficult words that occur in medical science, and a copious index; to which is added an appendix. . . . Penn Yan, [N.Y.]: Printed by H. Gilbert, 1833. 509p. DLC; NBM; NNNAM; PMA
30-0942

WICKHAM, William John (1798-1864)
Practical treatise on diseases of the joints. Winchester: Jacob & Johnson, 1833. 178p. DLC; DNLM; PPC
30-0943

WIGHT, Danforth Phipps
Seaman's medical guide . . . with advice on the preservation of health in hot climates. . . . Boston: Russell, Odiorne and Metcalf, 1834. 172p. DLC; DNLM; MBM; MH-M
30-0944

WILLIAMS, Charles James Blasius (1805-1889)
A rational exposition on the physical signs of the diseases of the lungs and pleura; illustrating their pathology, and facilitating their diagnosis. Philadelphia: Carey & Lea, 1830. 203p. DLC; ICJ; IU-M; PPC **30-0945**

WILLIAMS, Charles James Blasius (1805-1889)
A rational exposition of the physical signs of the diseases of the lungs and pleura; illustrating their pathology, and facilitating their diagnosis. 2nd American ed. Philadelphia: Carey, Lea & Blanchard, 1834. 203p. 2 plates. DNLM; PPC; PU
30-0946

WILLIAMS, Charles James Blasius (1805-1889)
Lectures on the physiology and diseases of the chest, including the principles of physical and general diagnosis. Delivered during the Spring Sessions of 1836 and 1837 at the Anatomical School. Philadelphia: Haswell, Barrington & Haswell, 1839. 347p. [Dunglison's American Medical Library] DLC; DNLM; MH; PPC **30-0947**

WILLIAMS, Stephen West (1790-1855)
A catechism of medical jurisprudence; being principally a compendium of the opinions of the best writers upon the subject. With a preliminary discourse upon the importance of the study of forensic medicine. Designed for physicians, attorneys, coroners and jurymen. . . . Northampton: J. H. Butler; Boston: Hilliard, Gray & Co., 1835. 205p. DLC; DNLM; MB; MBM **30-0948**

WILLIS, Robert (1798-1878)
Urinary diseases, and their treatment. [Dunglison's American Medical Library] Philadelphia: Haswell, Barrington & Haswell, 1839. 232p. DLC; DNLM; PPJ; PPHa
30-0949

WINSLOW, George Erving
Essay on the nature, symptoms, and treatment of Asiatic cholera. New York: Sleight & Robinson, 1832. 70p. DNLM; OCHP; ScC **30-0950**

WISTAR, Caspar (1761-1818)
A system of anatomy for the use of students of medicine. . . . 5th ed. With notes and additions by William Edmonds Horner. . . . Philadelphia: Carey & Lea, 1830. 2 v. NNNAM; PPC; PU; RPM **30-0951**

WISTAR, Caspar (1761-1818)
A system of anatomy for the use of students of medicine. . . . 6th ed. With notes and additions. . . . Philadelphia: Carey, Lea & Blanchard, 1835. 2 v. NjR; PPC; PU
30-0952

WISTAR INSTITUTE OF ANATOMY AND BIOLOGY. PHILADELPHIA
Catalogue of the Anatomical Museum of the University of Pennsylvania, with a report to the Museum committee of the trustees. November, 1832. By W. E. Horner. . . . 2nd ed. Philadelphia: Printed by L. R. Bailey, 1832. 51p. DLC; PU
30-0953

WOOD, George Bacon (1797-1879)
The dispensatory of the United States of America. By George B. Wood . . . and Franklin Bache. Philadelphia: Grigg & Elliot, 1833. 1073p. DNLM; OCLloyd; PPC; PU
30-0954

WOOD, George Bacon (1797-1879)
The dispensatory of the United States of America. By George B. Wood . . . and Franklin Bache. . . . 2nd ed., enl. and carefully rev. Philadelphia: Grigg & Elliot, 1834. 1162p. DLC; OCLloyd; PU **30-0955**

WOOD, George Bacon (1797-1879)
The history of the University of Pennsylvania from its origin to the year 1827. Philadelphia: McCarty & Davis, 1834. 112p. DNLM; PU **30-0956**

WOOD, George Bacon (1797-1879)
Lecture introductory to the course of materia medica and pharmacy in the University of Pennsylvania. Philadelphia: T. B. Town, 1835. 20p. DNLM; PU
30-0957

WOOD, George Bacon (1797-1879)
The dispensatory of the United States of America. By George B. Wood . . . and Franklin Bache. . . . 3rd ed., enl. and carefully rev. Philadelphia: Grigg & Elliot, 1836. 1171p. DLC; OCLloyd; PU **30-0958**

WOOD, George Bacon (1797-1879)
Lecture introductory to the course of materia medica and pharmacy in the University of Pennsylvania. Philadelphia: T. B. Town, 1836. 20p. DNLM; PU **30-0959**

WOOD, George Bacon (1797-1879)
Address to the medical graduates of the University of Pennsylvania, delivered March 26, 1836. . . . Philadelphia: Printed by L. R. Bailey, 1836. 36p. DLC; PPC; PU **30-0960**

WOOD, George Bacon (1797-1879)
Introductory lecture to the course of materia medica, delivered in the University of Pennsylvania. Philadelphia: J. G. Auner, 1837. 24p. DNLM; PU **30-0961**

WOOD, George Bacon (1797-1879)
Syllabus of the course of lectures on materia medica and pharmacy, delivered in the University of Pennsylvania. Philadelphia: L. R. Bailey, 1838. 69p. DNLM; PU
30-0962

WOOD, George Bacon (1797-1879)
The dispensatory of the United States of America. By George B. Wood . . . and Franklin Bache. . . . 4th ed., enl. and carefully rev. Philadelphia: Grigg & Elliot, 1839. 1249p. DLC; OCLloyd; PU **30-0963**

WOODWARD, Samuel B. (1787-1850)
Essays on asylums for inebriates. [Worcester, Mass., 1838] 38p. DNLM; MBM; MH-M; MWA **30-0964**

[WORCESTER LUNATIC HOSPITAL]
Reports and other documents relating to the State Lunatic Hospital at Worcester, Mass. Printed by the Order of the Senate. Boston: Dutton & Wentworth, 1837. 200p. MBM; MHi; MWA **30-0965**

WORTHINGTON, OHIO. REFORMED MEDICAL COLLEGE
The reformed practice of medicine as taught at the reformed medical colleges. . . . By professors and members of the reformed medical colleges in New York and Worthington, Ohio. Boston, 1831. 2 v. in 1. MH; NBM; RPM; PPPH **30-0966**

WRIGHT, Isaac
Wright's family medicine, or system of domestic practice. Containing the improvements suggested by an experience of forty years. Madisonville, Tenn.: J. F. Grant, Printer, 1833. 276p. DLC; NcD **30-0967**

WRIGHT, Marmaduke Burr (1803-1879)
A lecture on the physiological and therapeutical uses of water, delivered to the students of the Ohio Medical College, at the opening of the session of 1839-1840. [1839] 23p. DNLM **30-0968**

YANDELL, Lunsford Pitts (1805-1878)
An introductory lecture on the advantages and pleasures of the study of chemistry. Lexington: N. L. Finnell & J. F. Herndon, 1831. 26p. DNLM; ICRM; IEN-M **30-0969**

YANDELL, Lunsford Pitts (1805-1878)
An account of spasmodic cholera, as it appeared in the City of Lexington in June, 1833. [Lexington, 1833] 32p. DNLM **30-0970**

YANDELL, Lunsford Pitts (1805-1878)
Remarks on dyspepsia. Read to the Lexington Medical Society, December 12, 1834. [Lexington, 1834] 64p. DNLM **30-0971**

YANDELL, Lunsford Pitts (1805-1878)
Chemistry as affording evidence of the wisdom of God. An introductory lecture. Lexington: J. Clarke & Co., 1835. 27p. DNLM **30-0972**

YANDELL, Lunsford Pitts (1805-1878)
A narrative of the dissolution of the medical faculty of Transylvania University. . . . Nashville: W. H. Hunt, printer, 1837. 31, 10p. DLC; DNLM; KU; KyLoJM **30-0973**

YANDELL, Lunsford Pitts (1805-1878)
An address delivered before the Medical Society of Tennessee, at its eighth annual meeting. Louisville: Prentice & Weissinger, 1838. 23p. DNLM; KyLoJM **30-0974**

YATES, Christopher C. (*d.* 1848)
Observations on the epidemic now prevailing in the city of New York, called Asiatic or spasmodic cholera; with advice to the planters of the South, for the medical treatment of their slaves. . . . New York: G. P. Scott & Co., 1832. 43p. DNLM; NN; NNNAM **30-0975**

YATES, Christopher C. (*d.* 1848)
Observations of the epidemic now prevailing in the city of New York, called the Asiatic or spasmodic cholera; with advice to the planters of the South, for the medical treatment of their slaves, 2nd ed. . . . New York: Collins & Hannay, 1832. 57p. DNLM; MWA; NjR; PU **30-0976**

III. AMERICAN MEDICAL IMPRINTS, 1840-1849

Many medical men, and along with them a major part of the unthinking, unreasoning public, looking in vain for rationales of the cause of childbed fever, endeavor to satisfy their hankering after knowledge on that point, by adopting the notion that the cause of *epidemic* childbed fever is a contagion.

The Student will naturally be desirous to learn, if childbed fever be really a contagious disease, what the principle of that contagion is; and I apprehend that here, as in the instance of the epidemic malady, he shall have to rest content with the *sound* of the word contagion, a word which, being interpreted, means communicable from person to person, or by individual to individual. This is the whole meaning of the word; for, as to how, and the what, no man hath yet obtained the least definite notion, since no man hath known or can know what a miasm or a contagion is. Miasm and contagion are words, nothing more, they represent no precise material idea of the mind.

Charles D. Meigs,
Obstetrics: The Science and the Art
(1849)

ABERNETHY, John (1764-1831)
Abernethy's family physician; or ready prescriber in cases of illness and accident. . . . 2nd American from the 30th London ed. rev. and enl. by H. Bostwick. New York: Stringer & Townsend, 1849. 132p. DNLM; NNNAM
40-0001

ACTON, William (1813-1875)
A complete treatise on venereal diseases, and their immediate and remote consequences. . . . 2nd American ed., with additional illustrations and colored plates. New York: J. S. Redfield, 1848. 334p. CSmH; DNLM; NNNAM
40-0002

ALCOTT, William Andrus (1798-1859)
Health in common schools. Boston: G. W. Light, 1840. 31p. MB; NN **40-0003**

ALCOTT, William Andrus (1798-1859)
The mother's medical guide in children's diseases. . . . Boston: T. H. Marvin, 1842. 314p. DLC; MBA; PPC; PU
40-0004

ALCOTT, William Andrus (1798-1859)
The teacher of health, and the laws of the human constitution. Boston: King, 1843. 384p. MB; NN **40-0005**

ALCOTT, William Andrus (1798-1859)
Vegetable diet: as sanctioned by medical men, and by experience in all ages. Including a system of vegetable cookery. 2nd ed. New York: Fowler & Wells, 1849. 312p. DNLM; NNNAM
40-0006

ALLEN, Isaac J.
Address introductory to the lectures on medical jurisprudence, before the medical class of the Willoughby University, January, 1846. Willoughby, Ohio, 1846. 23p. DNLM; IEN-M; IU-M
40-0007

ALLEN, J.
Refutation and vindication of the charges alleged against him before the American Society of Dental Surgeons. . . . Cincinnati: M. Bemiss, 1847. 8p. DNLM; OC
40-0008

ALLEN, Nathan (1813-1889)
An essay on the connection of mental philosophy with medicine. Philadelphia: A. Waldie, 1841. 32p. DNLM; PPC; PPHa
40-0009

ALLEN, Richard I. (1808-1873)
A historical, chemical and therapeutical analysis of the principal mineral fountains at Saratoga Springs; together with general directions for their use. . . . Saratoga Springs: B. Huling; New York: W. H. Graham, 1844. 71p. DLC; DNLM; N; NHi **40-0010**

AMERICAN MEDICAL ALMANAC FOR 1848. Philadelphia: Lindsay and Blakiston, 1847. 224p. DLC; PPC
40-0011

[AMERICAN MEDICAL ASSOCIATION]
A defense of the "six months lecture term." Report of a special committee of the American Medical Association. . . . Philadelphia: T. K. & P. G. Collins, 1849. 14p. DLC; PPC; PU
40-0012

AMES, S.
Some account of an epidemic cerebrospinal meningitis, which prevailed in Montgomery, Ala., in the winter and spring of 1848. Montgomery, Ala. [1848?] 58p. DNLM
40-0013

AMUSSAT, Jean Zuléma (1796-1856)
Amussat's lessons on retention of urine, caused by strictures of the urethra, and on diseases of the prostate. Ed. by A. Petit. . . . Transl. from the French by James P. Jervey, M.D. with notes. Philadelphia: Haswell, Barrington & Haswell, 1840. 103p. DNLM; PPC; PU **40-0014**

[ANATOMY]
The anatomical remembrancer; or Complete pocket anatomist. . . . From the 2nd London ed., rev. New York: S. S. & W. Wood, 1845. 245p. DLC; MBM; NNNAM
40-0015

[ANATOMY]
The pocket anatomist: being a summary description of the muscles; with a tabular view of the arteries and nerves. Concordant with "The Dublin Dissector," and "Harrison on the Arteries." 4th ed. Philadelphia: J. Kay, Jr. & Bro., 1844. 63p. DNLM **40-0016**

ANDERSON, Robert M.
The student's review, or examinations on therapeutics, materia medica, and pharmacy. Adapted especially to the course of lectures delivered in the University of Pennsylvania. Richmond: H. K. Ellyson, 1845. 296p. DNLM; PU; PPJ; ViRA
40-0017

ANDRAL, Gabriel (1797-1876)
Medical clinic: diseases of the abdomen. . . . Condensed and translated, with observations, by D. Spillan. . . . Philadelphia: E. Barrington & G. D. Haswell; New York: J. & H. G. Langley, 1843. 420p. DNLM; NNNAM; ViRA **40-0018**

ANDRAL, Gabriel (1797-1876)
Medical clinic: diseases of the chest. . . . Condensed and transl. with observations, by D. Spillan. . . . Philadelphia: E. Barrington & G. D. Haswell; New York: J. & H. G. Langley, 1843. 406p. DNLM; NNNAM; PPC; PPJ
40-0019

ANDRAL, Gabriel (1797-1876)
Pathological hematology. An essay on the blood in disease. . . . Transl. from the French by J. F. Meigs, M.D., and Alfred Stillé M.D. . . . Philadelphia: Lee & Blanchard, 1844. 129p. DNLM; PPC; PU **40-0020**

ANDRAL, Gabriel (1797-1876)
Lectures on the grippe, or epidemic influenza. Transl. from the French by Thos. F. Betton. [Philadelphia, 1844?] 3 l. DNLM; PPC **40-0021**

ANDRY, Felix
A manual of diagnosis of the diseases of the heart; preceded by clinical researches for the study of these afflictions. Transl. by S. Kneeland, Jr. Boston: Wm. D. Ticknor & Co., 1846. 168p. DNLM; MH-M; MdBJ-W **40-0022**

ANDRY, Felix
A manual of diagnosis of the diseases of the heart: preceded by clinical researches, calculated to facilitate the study of these afflictions. Transl. by W. S. Chipley and R. P. Hunt. Cincinnati: Robinson & Jones, 1847. 144p. DNLM; OC; OCIM; ViRA
40-0023

ARNOTT, Neil (1788-1874)
Elements of physics, or natural philosophy, general and medical. . . . A new edition, revised and corrected from the last English edition. With additions, by Isaac Hays. Philadelphia: Lea & Blanchard, 1848. 486p. DNLM; PPC; PU
40-0024

ARTHUR, Robert (1819-1880)
A popular treatise on the teeth: embracing a description of their structure, the disease to which they are subject, and their treatment, both for the prevention and cure of those diseases; together with an account of the usual methods of inserting artificial teeth. . . . New York, Philadelphia: E. Ferrett & Co., 1845. 187p. CtY-M; DLC; NNNAM; PPC
40-0025

ASHWELL, Samuel (1798-1857)
On incision in cases of occlusion, and rigidity of the uterus. [Dunglison's American Medical Library] Philadelphia: A. Waldie, 1840. 90-104p. DNLM; PPC; PPHa; PU
40-0026

ASHWELL, Samuel (1798-1857)
On incision in cases of occlusion and rigidity of the uterus. Philadelphia: Carey & Hart, 1841. 15p. DNLM; PPJ; PPL
40-0027

ASHWELL, Samuel (1798-1857)
A practical treatise on the diseases peculiar to women, illustrated by cases, derived from hospital and private practice. . . . Boston: Press of T. B. Marvin, 1843. 312p. DLC; MBM; NNNAM **40-0028**

ASHWELL, Samuel (1798-1857)
A practical treatise on the diseases peculiar to women, illustrated by cases, derived from hospital and private practice. . . . 1st complete American from the last London ed. With notes, by Paul B. Goddard. . . . Philadelphia: Lea & Blanchard, 1845. 520p. DLC; NNNAM; PPC; PU [2nd ed., Lea & Blanchard, 1845. 520p.] **40-0029**

ATLEE, Washington Lemuel (1808-1878)
Lecture introductory to the course of medical chemistry, Pennsylvania College, for the session, 1844-1845. Philadelphia: William I. Young, 1844. 16p. DNLM; PU **40-0030**

ATLEE, Washington Lemuel (1808-1878)
Tabular view and analysis (of 240 cases of ovariotomy). [1844?] 4 sheets, broadside fol. DNLM; PPC
40-0031

ATLEE, Washington, Lemuel (1808-1878)
Case of extirpation of a bilocular ovarian cyst by the large peritoneal section. Read before "The Lancaster City and County Medical Society," April 17th, 1844. Philadelphia: T. K. & P. G. Collins, 1844. 29p. DNLM; PPC
40-0032

ATLEE, Washington Lemuel (1808-1878)
The chemical relations of the human body with surrounding agents. A lecture introductory to a course on medical chemistry, in the medical department of Pennsylvania College, for the session of 1845-1846. Philadelphia: Barrett & Jones, 1845. 16p. DNLM; PU **40-0033**

ATLEE, Washington Lemuel (1808-1878)
Valedictory address to the graduates of the medical department of Pennsylvania College, session of 1846-1847. Philadelphia, 1847. 19p. DNLM; PU **40-0034**

BACHE, Franklin (1792-1864)
Introductory lecture to the course of chemistry delivered in Jefferson Medical College, November 3, 1841. Philadelphia: Merrihew & Thompson, 1841. 16p. DNLM; PPJ
40-0035

BACHE, Franklin (1792-1864)
Introductory lecture to the course of chemistry in Jefferson Medical College, November 6, 1843. Philadelphia: Merrihew & Thompson, 1843. 25p. DNLM; PPJ
40-0036

BACHE, Franklin (1792-1864)
Introductory lecture to the course of chemistry. Philadelphia: B. E. Smith, 1844. 24p. DNLM; PPJ
40-0037

BACHE, Franklin (1792-1864)
Introductory lecture to the course of chemistry, delivered in Jefferson Medical College, October 18th, 1848. . . . Published by the class. Philadelphia: C. Sherman, printer, 1848. 20p; DLC; DNLM; PPJ **40-0038**

BACHE, Franklin (1792-1864)
Introductory lecture to the course of chemistry, delivered in Jefferson Medical College, October 16, 1849. Philadelphia: C. Sherman, 1849. 20p. DNLM; PPJ **40-0039**

BAGLEY, George K.
The family instructor, or Guide to health; containing the names and description of the most useful herbs and plants that are now in use, with their medicinal qualities annexed. . . . [Montpelier, Vt.]: Published for the author, 1848. 72p. DLC; VtHi **40-0040**

BAILEY, M. J.
Report of the practical operation of the law relating to the importation of adulterated and spurious drugs, medicines. . . . New York: D. Fanshaw, 1849. 20p. DNLM; NNNAM
40-0041

BAKER, Elisha
Essays on ulceration of the fangs of the teeth and the best method of cure. New York: American Society of Dental Surgeons, 1841. 11p. DNLM; NNNAM
40-0042

BALLARD, Edward, and Alfred B. GARROD
Elements of materia medica and therapeutics with additions and alterations by R. Eglesfeld Griffith. Philadelphia: Hogan & Thompson, 1846. 516p. DNLM; OCLloyd; PPC; PPJ
40-0043

BANNING, Edmund Prior
Popular lectures on the mechanical nature and physical cure of chronic diseases of the human trunk. . . . New Haven: Patten & Co., printers, 1843. 59p. DLC; MBM; MH-M
40-0044

BANNING, Edmund Prior
Popular lectures on the mechanical nature and physical cure of chronic diseases of the human trunk. . . . Boston: Printed by S. N. Dickinson, 1844. 58p. DNLM; MBM
40-0045

BANNING, Edmund Prior
Common sense on chronic diseases; or, A rational treatise on the mechanical cause and cure of most chronic affections of the truncal organs of both male and female systems. Embracing the author's views on physical education, and the present popular system of artificial life. . . . 6th ed. New York: Paine & Burgess, 1846. 199p. 10 plates. DLC; MBA; NNNAM
40-0046

BANNING, Edmund Prior
Dr. Banning's patent lace, or body brace, for the relief of vocal, pulmonary, nervous and spinal, digestive, female and locomotive debility. . . . Cincinnati: Printed by E. Shepard [1849]. 32p. DLC; OC; KyLoJM **40-0047**

BARRETT, Moses (1816-1873)
Address delivered before the Genesee County Medical Society, at its annual meeting, held at Batavia, January 12, 1847. LeRoy, N.Y.: C. B. Thomson, 1847. 16p. N; NHi; NN
40-0048

BARTH, Jean Baptiste Philippe (1806-1877)
A manual of auscultation and percussion. By M. Barth . . . and M. Henry Roger. . . . Transl. with additions, by Francis G. Smith. . . . Philadelphia: Lindsay & Blakiston, 1845. 160p. DLC; PPC; PPHa **40-0049**

BARTH, Jean Baptiste Philippe (1806-1877)
A practical treatise on auscultation. Transl. with notes by Patrick Newbigging. With an appendix by L. M. Lawson. Lexington, Ky.: Scugham & Dunlop, 1847. 312p. DNLM; KyLoJM **40-0050**

BARTH, Jean Baptiste Philippe (1806-1877)
A manual of auscultation and percussion by M. Barth . . . and M. Henry Roger. Transl. with additions by Francis G. Smith. . . . 2nd ed. Philadelphia: Lindsay & Blakiston, 1849. 167p. DNLM; PPC; PPJ **40-0051**

BARTLETT, Elisha (1804-1855)
An introductory lecture on the objects and nature of medical science. [Medical Dept. of Transylvania University] Lexington, Ky.: N. L. & J. W. Finnell, 1841. 18p. DNLM; KyLoJM
40-0052

BARTLETT, Elisha (1804-1855)
The history, diagnosis, and treatment of typhoid and of typhus fever; with an essay on the diagnosis of bilious remittant and of yellow fever. . . . Philadelphia: Lea & Blanchard, 1842. 393p. DLC; PPC; MBM; ViRA **40-0053**

BARTLETT, Elisha (1804-1855)
An essay on the philosophy of medical science. . . . Philadelphia: Lea & Blanchard, 1844. 312p. DLC; DNLM; PPC
40-0054

BARTLETT, Elisha (1804-1855)
The history, diagnosis, and treatment of the fevers of the United States. . . . [2nd ed.] Philadelphia: Lea & Blanchard, 1847. 547p. DLC; DNLM; PPC **40-0055**

BARTLETT, Elisha (1804-1855)
An inquiry into the degree of certainty in medicine; and into the nature and extent of its power over disease. . . . Philadelphia: Lea & Blanchard, 1848. 84p. DLC; DNLM; NNNAM
40-0056

BARTLETT, Elisha (1804-1855)
A brief sketch of the life, character, and writing of William Charles Wells, M.D., F.R.S. An address delivered before the Louisville Medical Society, December 7th, 1849. . . . Louisville, Ky.: Prentice & Weissinger, 1849. 32p. DLC; DNLM; OCIM
40-0057

BARTON, William P. C. (1787?-1855)
Report. [To the Secretary of the Navy, on the condition of the Medical Department of the Navy.] Navy Department [n.p.], 1842. 9p. DNLM **40-0058**

BARWELL, Louisa Mary (Bacon) (1800-1885)
Infant treatment: with directions to mothers for self-management before, during, and after pregnancy. Addressed to mothers and nurses. . . . 1st American ed. Rev., enl., and adapted to habits and climate in the United States, by a physician of New York. . . . New York: J. Mowatt & Co., 1844. 148p. DLC; NNNAM **40-0059**

BATCHELDER, John Putnam (1784-1868)
Inflammation: its symptoms, causes, and treatment philosophically considered. New York: H. G. Langley, 1848. 66p. DNLM; NNNAM **40-0060**

BATCHELDER, John Putnam (1784-1868)
Cholera: its causes, symptoms, and treatment, considered and explained. New York: Dewitt & Davenport, 1849. 45p. DNLM; NNNAM **40-0061**

BAUMES, Jean Baptiste Timothée
A treatise on first dentition and the frequently serious disorders which depend upon it. Transl. by Thomas E. Bond, Jr. New York: Fraetas & Kelly, 1841. 159. DNLM; NNNAM; OCIM **40-0062**

BEACH, Wooster (1794-1868)
A treatise on pulmonary consumption (phthisis pulmonalis) with remarks on bronchitis. [New York?]: J. B. Allee, 1840. 24p. DNLM; NNNAM **40-0063**

BEACH, Wooster (1794-1868)
A treatise on anatomy, physiology, and health, designed for students, schools, and popular use. Illustrated with numerous plates. . . . New York: The author, 1847. 220p. DLC; NNNAM
40-0064

BEACH, Wooster (1794-1868)
Medical and botanical dictionary, giving a definition of the terms used in the various branches of medical science. . . . New York: Baker & Scribner, 1848. 258p. DLC; NN; NNNAM
40-0065

BEACH, Wooster (1794-1868)
The American practice condensed, or the family physician; being the scientific system of medicine, on vegetable principles, designed for all classes. 14th ed. New York: J. McAlister, 1848. 800p. 21 plates. DNLM; NNNAM **40-0066**

BEAUMONT, William (1785-1853)
The physiology of digestion, with experiments on the gastric juice. . . . 2nd ed.: cor. by Samuel Beaumont, M.D. Burlington [Vt.]: C. Goodrich, 1847. 303p. DLC; DNLM; NNNAM; PPC
40-0067

BECK, John Brodhead (1794-1851)
Observations on ergot, read before the Medical Society of the State of New York. Albany: J. Munsell, 1841. 16p. DNLM; N; NNNAM **40-0068**

BECK, John Brodhead (1794-1851)
Observations on ergot, read before the Medical Society of the State of New York. New York: W. E. Dean, 1841. 16p. DNLM
40-0069

BECK, John Brodhead (1794-1851)
An historical sketch of the state of American medicine before the revolution; being the annual address delivered before the Medical Society of the State of New York, February 1st, 1842. . . . Albany: Printed by J. Munsell, 1842. 35p. DLC; DNLM; N; NNNAM **40-0070**

BECK, John Brodhead (1794-1851)
The effects of blisters on the young subject. New York: J. & H. G. Langley, 1847. 10p. DNLM; NNNAM
40-0071

BECK, John Brodhead (1794-1851)
Essays on infant therapeutics: to which are added observations on ergot, an account of the origin of the use of mercury in inflammatory complaints. New York: W. E. Dean, 1849. 117p. DNLM; NNNAM; NNU-M **40-0072**

BECK. Lewis C. (1798-1853)
Adulterations of various substances used in medicine and the arts, with means of detecting them. New York: S. S. & W. Wood, 1846. 333p. DNLM; NNNAM; OCLloyd
40-0073

BECKER, Alexander C. (1815-1849)
Diseases of the eye, treated homoeopathically. From the German. New York: William Radde, 1847. 77p. DNLM; PPHa
40-0074

BECKER, Alexander C. (1815-1849)
Consumption treated homoeopathically. From the German. New York: William Radde, 1847. 86p. DNLM; PPHa
40-0075

BECKER, Alexander C. (1815-1849)
Dentition according to some of the best and latest German authorities; intended for domestic use. New York: William Radde, 1848. 82p. DNLM **40-0076**

BECKER, Alexander C. (1815-1849)
Constipation. New York: William Radde, 1848. 128p. PPHa
40-0077

BECKER, Alexander C. (1815-1849)
Allopathy, Hahnemannism and rational homoeopathy. Compiled from the German of Dr. Griesselich. . . . New York: William Radde, 1848. 24p. DNLM; PPHa
40-0078

BECKLARD, Eugène
Physiological mysteries and revelations in love, courtship and marriage. . . . Transl. from the 3rd Paris ed. by Philip M. Howard. New York, 1842. 192p. MB; ICU; NN; KU
40-0079

BECKLARD, Eugène
The physiologist: an infallible guide to health and happiness, for both sexes. . . . Being physiological information concerning love, courtship, marriage, and many other things, which were treated of by the famous philosopher Aristotle. . . . Transl. from the 4th Paris ed., with corrections and additions, by M. Sherman Wharton, M.D. 2nd ed. Boston, 1844. 108p. DLC; NN; OCIM **40-0080**

BEDFORD, Gunning S. (1806-1870)
A valedictory address. (New York University, Medical Department.) New York: J. H. Jennings, 1845. 20p. DNLM; NNU-M
40-0081

BEDFORD, Gunning S. (1806-1870)
An introductory lecture. Session 1845-1846, New York University, Department of Medicine. New York: Herald Job Office, 1845-1846. 18p. DNLM; NNU-M
40-0082

BEDFORD, Gunning S. (1806-1870)
Lecture introductory to a course on obstetrics and the diseases of women and children. New York: Press of the New York University, 1846. 26p. DNLM; NNU-M **40-0083**

BEDFORD, Gunning S. (1806-1870)
A lecture introductory to a course on obstetrics and the diseases of women and children, in the University of New York, session 1847-1848. New York: J. H. Jennings, 1847. 27p. 2 plates. DNLM; NNU-M **40-0084**

BEDFORD, Gunning S. (1806-1870)
A lecture introductory to a course on obstetrics and the disease of women and children, delivered November 5, 1848. New York: J. H. Jennings, 1848. 25p. DNLM; NNU-M
40-0085

BELL, Charles (1774-1842)
The hand, its mechanism and vital endowments, as evincing design. New York: Harper & Brothers, 1840. 313p. DNLM; MBM; NNNAM; PPC **40-0086**

BELL, Charles (1774-1842)
Institutes of surgery: arranged in the order of the lectures delivered in the University of Edinburgh. [Dunglison's American Medical Library] Philadelphia: Adam Waldie, 1840. 446p. DNLM; MBM; PPC; ViRA **40-0087**

BELL, Charles (1774-1842)
Institutes of surgery: arranged in the order of the lectures delivered in the University of Edinburgh. Philadelphia: Barrington & Haswell, 1843. 448p. CSmH; DNLM; MBM; NNNAM **40-0088**

BELL, John (1796-1872)
. . . A practical dictionary of materia medica: including the composition, preparation, and uses of medicines. . . . On the basis of Brande's Dictionary of materia medica and practical pharmacy. . . . Philadelphia: Haswell, Barrington & Haswell; New York: J. & H. Langley, 1841. 479p. DLC; NNNAM; PPC; PPL **40-0089**

BELL, John (1796-1872)
On regimen and longevity: comprising materia alimentaria, national dietetic usages, and the influence of civilization on health and the duration of life. . . . Philadelphia: Haswell & Johnson, 1842. 420p. DLC; PPC; PU; ViRA
40-0090

BELL, John (1796-1872) and William STOKES
Lectures on the theory and practice of physic. 3rd ed. Philadelphia: E. Barrington & G. D. Haswell, 1845. 2 v. DNLM; PPC; PPJ; PU **40-0091**

BELL, John (1796-1872) and William STOKES
Lectures on the theory and practice of physic. 4th ed., rev. and enl. Philadelphia: Barrington & Haswell, 1848. 2 v. DNLM; PPC; PU; ScC **40-0092**

BELL, Luther Vose (1806-1862)
The practical methods of ventilating buildings, being the annual address before the Massachusetts Medical Society, May 31, 1848. With appendix on heating by steam and hot water. . . . Boston: Damrell & Moore, 1848. 131p. DLC; MBM; MH; MHi **40-0093**

BENNET, James Henry (1816-1891)
A practical treatise on inflammation, ulceration, and induration of the neck of the uterus: with remarks on the value of leucorrhoea and prolapsus uteri as symptoms of uterine disease. Philadelphia: Lea & Blanchard, 1847. 146p. CtY-M; DNLM; PPC; ViRA **40-0094**

BERDMORE, Thomas
A treatise on the disorders and deformities of the teeth and gums, explaining the most rational methods of treating their diseases. Baltimore: American Society of Dental Surgeons, 1844. 87p. DNLM; MdU-D; NNU-M; NcD **40-0095**

BIEGLER, Augustus P.
Anatomy and physiology of the brain and nervous system, an essay read to the Albany Phrenological Society, April 3, 1840. . . . Albany: Printed by C. Van Benthuysen, 1840. 22p. DLC; DNLM; NNNAM **40-0096**

BIGELOW, Henry Jacob (1818-1890)
Manual of orthopedic surgery, being a dissertation which obtained the Boylston prize for 1844, on the following question: "In what cases, and to what extent is the division of muscles, tendons, or other parts proper for the relief of deformity or lameness?" . . . Boston: W. D. Ticknor & Co., 1845. 211p. DNLM; MBM; PPC; PU **40-0097**

BIGELOW, Henry Jacob (1818-1890)
Fragments of medical science and art. An address delivered before the Boylston Medical Society of Harvard University. Boston: W. D. Ticknor & Co., 1846. 54p. DNLM; MBM; NNNAM; PPC **40-0098**

BIGELOW, Henry Jacob (1818-1890)
Ether and chloroform: a compendium of their history and discovery. Boston: D. Clapp, 1848. 27p. DNLM; MH; MBM; PPC **40-0099**

BIGELOW, Henry Jacob (1818-1890)
Ether and chloroform: their discovery and physiological effects. Boston: D. Clapp. 1848. 27p. DNLM; MH; MBM; NNNAM **40-0100**

BIGELOW, Henry Jacob (1818-1890)
On the employment of a new agent in the treatment of strictures of the urethra. Boston: D. Clapp. 1849. 8p. DNLM; MH; MBM; ViRA **40-0101**

BIGELOW, John Milton (1804-1878)
A list of the medicinal plants of Ohio (not embraced in Wood & Bache's U.S. dispensatory), containing, as far as known, a brief account of their properties. . . . Columbus: J. H. Riley & Co., 1849. 47p. DLC; DNLM; OCIM; OCLloyd **40-0102**

BIGGS, A.
The botanico-medical reference book, comprising the fundamental principles of life, the true theory of fever and inflammation. . . . Also the theory and practice of medicine, upon botanico-medical principles, a materia medica, containing a description of the various articles used. Pharmacy—teaching the mode of preparing, compounding, and preserving medicines, with a number of recipes. . . . Memphis: Wells & Carr, print., 1847. 603p. DLC; LNT-M; OCLloyd; PPC **40-0103**

BILLARD, Charles Michel (1800-1832)
A treatise on the diseases of infants, founded on recent clinical observations and investigations in pathological anatomy, made at the Hospice des enfans-trouvés: with a dissertation on the viability of the child. . . . With notes by Dr. Ollivier. . . . 2nd American, transl. from the 3rd French ed., with an appendix, by James Stewart. . . . New York: J. & H. G. Langley, 1840. 620p. CtY-M; CU-M; DLC; MBM **40-0104**

BIRD, Golding (1814-1854)
Urinary deposits: their diagnosis, pathology, and therapeutical indications. Philadelphia: Lea & Blanchard, 1845. 227p. DNLM; PPC; PPJ; PPHa **40-0105**

BIRD, Robert M[ontgomery] (1803-1854)
The difficulties of medical science. An inaugural lecture. Philadelphia, 1841. 24p. DNLM; PPC **40-0106**

BIRD, Robert M[ontgomery] (1803-1854)
Valedictory address delivered before the graduates of Pennsylvania Medical College, session of 1842-1843. Philadelphia: Merrihew & Thompson, 1843. 11p. DNLM; PPC; PU **40-0107**

BLAKE, Robert
An essay on the structure and formation of the teeth in man and various animals, being principally a translation of his inaugural dissertation. Rev. and corrected with notes by C. O. Cone. Baltimore: American Society of Dental Surgeons, 1848. 128p. DNLM; MdU-D; PU **40-0108**

BLAKISTON, Peyton (1801-1878)
Practical observations on certain diseases of the chest and on the principles of auscultation. Philadelphia: Lea & Blanchard, 1848. 384p. DNLM; PPC; PU; ScMS **40-0109**

BLANDIN, Philippe-Frederic (1798-1849)
Anatomy of the dental system, human and comparative. Transl. from the French by Robert Arthur. Baltimore: American Society of Dental Surgeons, 1845. 140p. DNLM; MdU-D; PU **40-0110**

BLATCHFORD, Thomas Windeatt (1794-1866)
Homoeopathy; an address delivered before the Rensselaer County Medical Society at the annual meeting June 14, 1842. Published by the Society, 1842. 16p. N; NHi; PPHa **40-0111**

BLATCHFORD, Thomas Windeatt (1794-1866)
Homoeopathy illustrated. 2nd ed. rev. and enl. Albany: J. Munsell, 1843. 81p. DNLM; PPHa **40-0112**

BLATCHFORD, Thomas Windeatt (1794-1866)
Two addresses before the Medical Society of the State of New York. In session at Albany, February 1 & 2, 1848. . . . Published by order of the Society. Albany: Printed by J. Munsell, 1848. 28p. DNLM; DLC; N; NHi **40-0113**

BLUNDELL, James (1790-1878)
Observations on some of the more important diseases of women. Edited by Thomas Castle. Philadelphia: A. Waldie, 1840. 215p. DNLM; PPC; ScCM; ViRA **40-0114**

BLUNDELL, James (1790-1878)
Lectures on the principles and practice of midwifery. Edited by Charles Severn. Philadelphia: E. Barrington & G. D. Haswell, 1842. 442p. DLC; DNLM; PPC; PU **40-0115**

BOARDMAN, Andrew
An essay on the means of improving medical education and elevating medical character. (Presented to the faculty of Geneva Medical College, January 1840.) Philadelphia: Haswell, Barrington & Haswell, 1840. 23p. DNLM; PPC **40-0116**

BOARDMAN, G. S.
An address delivered in Waterville before the Oneida County Temperance Society. Rome, N.Y.: H. N. Bill, 1844. 18p. DNLM; N; NN **40-0117**

BOARDMAN, H. A.
The claims of religion upon medical men. Philadelphia, 1844. 24p. DNLM **40-0118**

BOENNINGHAUSEN, C. von (1785-1864)
Boenninghausen's essay on the homoeopathic treatment of intermittent fevers. Transl. and edited by Charles Julius Hempel, M.D. New York: William Radde, 1845. 56p. DNLM; PPHa **40-0119**

BOENNINGHAUSEN, C. von (1785-1864)
Boenninghausen's therapeutic pocketbook for homoeopathists; to be used at the bedside of the patient, and in the study of the materia medica. Edited by A. Howard Okie, M.D. Boston: Otis Clapp, 1847. 483p. PPHa; OCLloyd **40-0120**

BOENNINGHAUSEN, C. von (1785-1864)
Therapeutic pocket-book for homoeopathic physicians; to be used at the bedside of the patient, and in studying the materia medica pura. . . . Edited by Charles J. Hempel, M.D. New York: William Radde, 1847. 504p. PPHa; OCLloyd **40-0121**

BOND, Henry (1790-1859)
Biographical notice of the late John Ruan, M.D.; read (by appointment) before the College of Physicians of Philadelphia, September 2, 1845. Philadelphia: W. F. Geddes, 1845. 8p. DNLM; PPC **40-0122**

BOND, Joseph B.
The master-mariner's guide in the management of his ship's company, with respect to their health; being designed to accompany a ship's medicine chest. Boston: W. Crosby & H. P. Nichols, 1847. 71p. DNLM; MBM; MWA **40-0123**

BOND, Thomas Emerson (1813-1872)
A dissertation on the varieties of mankind; being an address read before the Cuvierian and Physiological Societies of Wesleyan University, August 2, 1843. . . . Middletown, Conn.: The Societies, 1843. 40p. CtY-M; DLC; NN **40-0124**

BOND, Thomas Emerson (1813-1872)
An introductory lecture, delivered before the class of the Medical Department of the Washington Unversity, November 11th, 1848. . . . Baltimore: J. W. Woods, printer, 1849. 23p. DLC; MdU-D; NNNAM **40-0125**

BOSTWICK, Homer
Medical quackery: its origin, cause and cure; with hints to young physicians, in relation to the important subject of consultation. . . . New York: T. Smith, 1847. 12p. DLC; NNNAM **40-0126**

BOSTWICK, Homer
A complete practical work on the nature and treatment of venereal diseases, and other affections of the genito-urinary organs of the male and female. . . . New York: Burgess, Stringer & Co., 1848. 348p. 35 plates. DLC; DNLM; NNNAM **40-0127**

BOSTWICK, Homer
A treatise on the nature and treatment of seminal diseases, impotency, and other kindred affections. 2nd ed. New York: Burgess, Stringer & Co., 1848. 251p. 13 plates. DNLM; MBM; NNNAM **40-0128**

BOWDITCH, Henry Ingersoll (1808-1892)
Remarks relative to Dr. Paine's commentaries upon the writings of M. Louis. Boston: D. Clapp, Jr., 1840. 32p. DNLM; MBM; MH **40-0129**

BOWDITCH, Henry Ingersoll (1808-1892)
The ether controversy. Vindication of the hospital report of 1848. Boston: J. Wilson, 1848. 32p. DNLM; MBAt; MWA **40-0130**

BOWDITCH, Henry Ingersoll (1808-1892)
The young stethoscopist; or, The student's aid to auscultation. . . . 2nd ed. New York: S. S. & W. Wood, 1848. 306p. 42 plates. DLC; DNLM; NNNAM; PPC **40-0131**

BOWEN, William
Address delivered before the Stark County Medical Society, May 2, 1843. . . . Massillon, O.: John P. Worstell, 1843. 16p. DNLM **40-0132**

BOWER, Mark Noble
Memoranda on anatomy, surgery, and physiology. . . . Cor. and enl. by an American physician. New York: S. S. & W. Wood, 1848. 328p. DLC; NNNAM **40-0133**

BOWERS, Benjamin Franklin (1796-1875)
Reasons why homoeopathy should receive an impartial investigation from the medical profession and the public. New York: William Radde, 1846. 24p. PPHa **40-0134**

BRAINARD, Daniel (1812-1866)
A lecture introductory to the course of anatomy and surgery, delivered at the opening of the Rush Medical College, December 4, 1843. Chicago: Ellis & Fergus, 1843. 17p. DNLM; ICRM **40-0135**

BRAINARD, Daniel (1812-1866)
Address to the graduating class of Rush Medical College: Chicago: Duzan, Davisson & Co., 1849. 15p. DNLM; ICRM **40-0136**

BRAINARD, Dyar Throop (1790-1863)
The annual address to the candidates for degrees and licenses, in the medical institution of Yale College, January 21, 1840. . . . Published at the request of the class. New Haven: Printed by B. L. Hamlen, 1840. 16p. CtY-M; DLC; DNLM
40-0137

BRANDRETH, Benjamin
Purgation: or, The Brandrethian method of treating diseases and curing them with one and the same universal medicine, the efficacy of which has been fully tested, beyond the power of malice or misrepresentation to dispute, with an attempt to explain the cause and origin of all diseases. . . . New York: Pub. by the author, 1840. 39p. DLC; DNLM; NNNAM
40-0138

BRIGHAM, Amariah (1798-1849)
An inquiry concerning the diseases and fucntions of the brain, the spinal cord, and the nerves. . . . New York: G. Adlard, 1840. 327p. DLC; NNNAM **40-0139**

BRIGHAM, Amariah (1798-1849)
Remarks on the influence of mental cultivation and mental excitement upon health. 3rd ed. Philadelphia: Lea & Blanchard, 1845. 204p. DNLM; PPC; PPJ; PU
40-0140

BRIGHAM, Amariah (1798-1849)
The Asylum souvenir. Utica, N.Y., 1849. 64p. DNLM; MWA
40-0141

BROACKES, William
Diseases of the alimentary canal, and constipation, treated homoeopathically. . . . With preface and notes by Gideon Humprehy, M.D. Also an essay on homoeopathic diet [by P. Curie] Philadelphia: J. Dobson, 1841. 134p. DLC; PPHa
40-0142

BROACKES, William
Diseases of the digestive organs, and constipation, treated homoeopathically. . . . 2nd American, from the 3rd London ed. With preface and additions, by A. C. Becker, M.D. New York: W. Radde, 1848. 128p. DLC; DNLM; MBM; NNNAM
40-0143

BRODIE, Benjamin Collins (1783-1862)
Pathological and surgical observations on the diseases of the joints. . . . With alterations and additions. From the 4th London ed. Boston: Press of T. R. Marvin, 1842. 343p. DLC; MBM; NNNAM; ViRA **40-0144**

BRODIE, Benjamin Collins (1783-1862)
Lectures on the diseases of the urinary organs. From the 3rd London ed., with alterations and additions. Philadelphia: Lea & Blanchard, 1843. 214p. DNLM; PPC; PU; ViRA
40-0145

BRODIE, Benjamin Collins (1783-1862)
Pathological and surgical observations on diseases of the joints. From the 4th London ed., with the author's alterations and additions. Philadelphia: Lea & Blanchard, 1843. 216p. DNLM; PPC; PPJ; PU **40-0146**

BRODIE, Benjamin Collins (1783-1862)
Clinical lectures on surgery, delivered at St. George's Hospital. . . . Philadelphia: Lea & Blanchard, 1846. 352p. CtY-M; DLC; GU; ICJ **40-0147**

BRODIE, Benjamin Collins (1783-1862)
Lectures on the diseases of the urinary organs. . . . 2nd American, from the last London ed. With the alterations and additions of the author. Philadelphia: Lea & Blanchard, 1847. DLC; PPC; NNNAM; ViRA **40-0148**

BRODIE, Benjamin Collins (1783-1862)
Select surgical works of Sir Benjamin Brodie containing clinical lectures on surgery, surgical observations on the diseases of the joints and the diseases of the urinary organs [in one volume]. Philadelphia: Lea & Blanchard, 1847. 352, 172, 194p. DLC; PPC; PU **40-0149**

BROWN, Abner H.
An address delivered before the Rush Medical Society, connected with the Willoughby Medical College, December 17, 1845. [n.p.], 1846. 24p. DNLM; ICRM; ICU
40-0150

BROWN, Buckminster (1819-1891)
On the pathological and physiological effects of etherial inhalation, with an appendix containing an additional case and experiments. Boston: D. Clapp, 1847. 170. DNLM; MWA
40-0151

BROWN, Buckminster (1819-1891)
The treatment and cure of cretins and idiots; with an account of a visit to the institution on the Abendberg. Boston: W. D. Ticknor & Co., 1847. 19p. DNLM; MWA
40-0152

BROWN, John Ball (1784-1862)
Reports of cases in the Boston Orthopedic Institution. Boston: D. Clapp, Jr., 1844. 39p. DNLM; MBM; MH-M
40-0153

BROWN, John Ball (1784-1862)
Reports of cases in the Boston Orthopedic Institution. With some preliminary observations on spinal curvature, distortions of the chest, and spinal irritation. Boston: D. Clapp, Jr., 1845. 35p. DNLM; MBM; MH-M **40-0154**

BROWN, Joseph
Introductory lecture on chemistry, delivered to the class in the Botanico-Medical College. [n.p.], 1845. 11p. DNLM
40-0155

BROWN, Solyman (1790-1876)
Essay on the most direct methods by which a dental practitioner may succeed. . . . New York: J. W. Oliver, 1842. 8p. DNLM; NNNAM **40-0156**

BRUCKHAUSEN, Caspar (1806?-1891)
Allopathia and homoeopathia. A popular essay, briefly illustrating the prevailing medical doctrines and especially the medical system of Samuel Hahnemann. New York: W. E. Dean, 1841. 18p. DNLM; PPHa **40-0157**

BRYAN, James (1810-1881)
An introductory lecture. To a course on the principles and practice of surgery. Delivered in the Vermont Academy of Medicine: March 12th, 1840. . . . [Rutland: H. T. White & Co., printers] 1840. 12p. DLC; DNLM; VtHi
40-0158

BRYAN, James (1810-1881)
Report on the state of the lying-in-hospitals in Europe. . . . Philadelphia: King & Baird, 1845. 23p. DNLM; PPC; PU
40-0159

BRYAN, James (1810-1881)
An essay on strictures of the urethra, with an account of the mode of curing stricture by cutting. . . . Philadelphia: J. G. Auner; New York: Burgess, Stringer & Co., 1847. 21p. DLC; NNNAM; NNU-M; NcD **40-0160**

BRYAN, James (1810-1881)
Introductory lecture to a course on surgery to the medical class of Geneva College, on the life and character of Baron Larrey. Geneva, N.Y.: I. & S. H. Parker, 1848. 20p. DLC; DNLM; N; NHi **40-0161**

BUCHAN, William (1729-1805)
Buchan's Domestic medicine: or the family physician. . . . Hartford: S. W. Slater, 1840. 442p. CtY-M [Also: Boston: Otis, 1846. 495p.] **40-0161A**

BUCHAN, William (1729-1805)
A treatise on the prevention and cure of diseases, by regimen and simple medicines. . . . Cincinnati: J. A. James, 1841. 863p. ICJ; NcD **40-0161B**

BUCHANAN, Joseph Rodes (1814-1899)
Sketches of Buchanan's discoveries in neurology. Louisville: Eliot, 1842. 120p. KyLoJM; OCIM **40-0162**

BUCHANAN, Joseph Rodes (1814-1899)
Report of three lectures in defense of neurology, against charges recently adduced by Rev. N. L. Rice, D.D. . . . Cincinnati: Herald of Truth print, 1848. 48p. DLC; DNLM; OC; KyLoJM **40-0163**

BUCHANAN, Joseph Rodes (1814-1899)
The "vanguard of the army." An introductory lecture, delivered at the Eclectic Medical Institute, November 7, 1849. Cincinnati: J. W. Thorpe, 1849. 24p. DNLM; KyLoJM; OC **40-0164**

BUCKINGHAM, Charles E. (1821-1877)
Circumstances affecting individual and public health. Boston: W. Chadwick, 1848. 31p. DNLM; MBM; MWA **40-0165**

BUELL, P. L.
A guide to phrenology . . . together with the adaptation of each of the organs and a phrenological chart, in seven degrees of development with numerous combinations. . . . By P. L. Buell & N. Sizer, phrenologists. 1st ed. Woodstock, Vt.: Printed by Haskell & Palmer, 1842. 184p. DCL; VtHi **40-0166**

BUELL, P. L.
A phrenological chart, giving a description of the phenomena of the human mind, as manifested through the brain by its various organs, in seven degrees of development; also, the character produced by the combination of the faculties. . . . By P. L. Buell & N. Sizer. . . . 1st ed. Woodstock, Vt.: Printed by Haskell & Palmer, 1842. 84p. DLC; VtHi **40-0167**

BULL, Thomas
The maternal management of children, in health and disease; . . . From the 3rd London ed. Philadelphia: Lindsay & Blakiston, 1849. 406p. DLC; PPC; PPF; ScCM **40-0168**

BULLITT, Henry M[assie] (*d.* 1880)
Introductory lecture delivered before the class of the medical department of the Saint Louis University, session of 1846-1847. Saint Louis: Chambers & Knapp, 1846. 19p. DNLM **40-0169**

BULLITT, Henry M[assie] (*d.* 1880)
Introductory lecture, addressed to the medical class of Transylvania University, session of 1849-1850. Lexington, Ky.: Kentucky Statesman Office, 1849. 23p. DNLM; KyLoJM **40-0170**

BURDELL, John
Teeth, their structure, disease and treatment, with numerous illustrative engravings. New York: Fowlers & Wells, 1848. 72p. DNLM; NNNAM **40-0171**

BURDEN, Jesse R.
Introductory lecture delivered at the winter session of the Philadelphia College of Medicine, November 1847. Philadelphia: John H. Gihon, 1847. 9p. DNLM; PPJ; PU **40-0172**

BUSH, James M[iles] (1808-1875)
An introductory lecture, to the dissecting class of Transylvania University, Lexington, Nov. 9, 1840. Lexington, Ky.: N. L. & W. Finnell, 1840. 12p. DNLM **40-0173**

BUSH, James M[iles] (1808-1875)
Observations on the operations of lithotomy; illustrated by cases from the practice of Professor B. W. Dudley. [1842?] 21p. DNLM **40-0174**

BYRNE, D. P.
An exposition, of the medical treatment, of S. M. Watson. [Boston, May, 1841]. 36p. MBM; MH; MWA; MWiW **40-0175**

CALDWELL, Charles (1772-1853)
Facts in mesmerism, and thoughts on its causes and uses. Louisville, Ky.: Prentice & Weissinger, 1842. 132p. DNLM; KyLoJM **40-0176**

CALDWELL, Charles (1772-1853)
Physiology vindicated, in a critique on Liebig's animal chemistry. Jeffersonville, Ind.: A. S. Tilden, 1843. 95p. DNLM **40-0177**

CALDWELL, Charles (1772-1853)
A lecture introductory to a course of lectures by the faculty of medicine of the medical department of the University of Louisville. Louisville: Prentice & Weissinger, 1846. 34p. DNLM; KyLoJM **40-0178**

CALDWELL, Charles (1772-1853)
Thoughts on the effects of age on the human constitution. A special introductory. Louisville: J. C. Noble, 1846. 27p. DNLM; KyLoJM **40-0179**

CALDWELL, Charles (1772-1853)
Thoughts on the impolicy and injustice of capital punishment; on the rationale or philosophy crime; and on the best system of penitentiary discipline and moral reform. An address. Louisville, Ky.: G. H. Monsarrat & Co., 1848. 64p. DNLM; KyLoJM **40-0180**

CALDWELL, Charles (1772-1853)
Thoughts on the education, qualifications, and duties of the physicians of the United Stats. A valedictory address. Louisville, Ky.: Courier Office, 1849. 39p. DNLM; KyLoJM
40-0181

CARNOCHAN, John Murray (1817-1887)
On the pathology of congenital dislocation of the head of the femur upon the dorsum of the ilium. New York: H. G. Langley, 1848. 14p. DNLM; NNNAM **40-0182**

CARPENTER, William Benjamin (1813-1885)
Inaugural dissertation on the physiological inferences to be deducted from the structure of the nervous system in the invertebrated classes of animals. Prize thesis. [Dunglison's American Medical Library] Philadelphia: A. Waldie, 1840. 137-188p. DNLM; PPC; PPJ **40-0183**

CARPENTER, William Benjamin (1813-1885)
Inaugural dissertation on the physiological inferences to be deducted from the structure of the nervous system in the invertebrated classes of animals. Prize thesis. Philadelphia: Carey & Hart, 1841. 52p. DNLM; NNNAM; ViRA
40-0184

CARPENTER, William Benjamin (1813-1885)
Principles of human physiology, with their chief applications to pathology, hygiene, and forensic medicine. Especially designed for the use of students. . . . 1st American ed., with additions by the author, and notes and additions by Meredith Clymer. . . . Philadelphia: Lea & Blanchard, 1843. 618p. DLC; PPC; PPJ; RPM **40-0185**

CARPENTER, William Benjamin (1813-1885)
Principles of human physiology, with their chief applications to pathology, hygiene, and forensic medicine. Especially designed for the use of students. . . . 2nd American, from the last London ed. With notes and additions, by Meredith Clymer. . . . Philadelphia: Lea & Blanchard, 1845. DLC; PPC; PU; ScCM **40-0186**

CARPENTER, William Benjamin (1813-1885)
Elements of physiology, including physiological anatomy. Philadelphia: Lea & Blanchard, 1846. 566p. 2 plates. DNLM; PPC; PU **40-0187**

CARPENTER, William Benjamin (1813-1885)
Principles of human physiology, with their chief applications to pathology, hygiene, and forensic medicine. Especially designed for the use of students. . . . 3rd American from the last London ed., with notes and additions by Meredith Clymer. Philadelphia: Lea & Blanchard, 1847. 752p. DNLM; GU; ICJ; ICRM **40-0188**

CARR, Ezra S[locum] (1819-1894)
An introductory lecture delivered in the Castleton Medical College at the opening of the fall session, 1843. Albany: Van Benthuysen & Co., 1843. 20p. DNLM
40-0189

CARSON, Joseph (1808-1876)
Address to the graduates of the Philadelphia College of Pharmacy delivered April 15, 1846. . . . Published by request of the Board of Trustees. Philadelphia: Merrihew & Thompson, printers, 1846. 14p. DLC; DNLM; PPC
40-0190

CARSON, Joseph (1808-1876)
Illustrations of medical botany: consisting of coloured figures of the plants affording the important articles of the materia medica. And descriptive letterpress. . . . The drawings on stone by J. H. Colen. Philadelphia: R. P. Smith, 1847. 2 v. DLC; DNLM; PU **40-0191**

CARSON, Joseph (1808-1876)
An essay on scammony, with an examination into the qualities of the drug found in the market. [1848?] 15p. DNLM; PPC
40-0192

CARTWRIGHT, Samuel Adolphus (1793-1863)
Statistical medicine: or, Numerical analysis applied to the investigation of morbid actions; a lecture, delivered to the medical class of the University of Louisville, and furnished for publication at their request. . . . Louisville: Prentice & Weissinger, 1848. 24p. DLC; DNLM; KyLoJM
40-0193

CARTWRIGHT, Samuel Adolphus (1793-1863)
The pathology and treatment of cholera: with an appendix containing his latest instructions to planters and heads of families . . . in regard to its prevention and cure. . . . New Orleans: Printed at Spencer & Middleton's "Magic press" office, 1849. 40p. DLC; DNLM; LNT-M
40-0194

CASSELS, J. Lang (1808-1879)
An introductory lecture delivered before the medical department of the Western Reserve College, in Cleveland. Cleveland: Younglove, 1846. 16p. OCIM **40-0195**

CATOR, Harvey Hull (1815-1882)
An address delivered before the Homoeopathic Medical Society of Western New York, at Waterloo, October 2nd, 1845. [Waterloo, N.Y., 1846], 9p. PPHa **40-0196**

CAZENAVE, P.-L.-Alphée (1795-1877)
Manual of diseases of the skin. Transl. from the French, with notes and additions by Thomas H. Burgess. Rev. and corrected, with additional notes by H. D. Bulkley. New York: J. & H. G. Langley, 1846. 341p. DNLM; NNNAM; NNU-M
40-0197

CHAILLY-HONORÉ, Nicolas Charles (1805-1866)
A practical treatise on midwifery. . . . A work adopted by the Royal Council of Public Instructions. Transl. from the French and ed. by Gunning S. Bedford. . . . New York: Harper & Brothers, 1844. 530p. 1 plate. DLC; DNLM; NNNAM
40-0198

CHAILLY-HONORÉ, Nicolas Charles (1805-1866)
A practical treatise on midwifery. . . . A work adopted by the Royal Council of Public Instruction. Transl. from the French and ed. by Gunning S. Bedford. . . . 3rd ed. New York: Harper & Brothers, 1846. 530p. 1 plate. DNLM; NNNAM
40-0199

CHAMBERS, Reuben
The Thomsonian practice of medicine; containing the names, and a description of the virtues and uses of the medicines belonging to this system of practice; also, directions for giving the proper quantity of each article for a dose: together with the names and symptoms of the different forms of disease. . . . Berthania, Pa., 1842. 449p. DLC **40-0200**

CHAMBERS, Reuben
The Thomsonian practice of medicine; containing the names, and a description of the virtues and uses of the medicines belonging to this system of practice. . . . Bethania, Pa., 1843. 449p. DLC **40-0201**

CHANNING, Walter (1786-1876)
A plea for pure water: being a letter to Henry Williams, Esq., with an address to the citizens of Boston, by Mr. H. Williams. [Boston: S. N. Dickinson, 1844] 39p. DNLM; MWA **40-0202**

CHANNING, Walter (1786-1876)
Of the medical profession, and of its preparation. An introductory lecture, read before the medical class of Harvard University, November 5, 1845. . . . Boston: D. Clapp, Jr., 1845. 32p. DLC; MBM; MH-M **40-0203**

CHANNING, Walter (1786-1876)
Six cases of inhalation of ether in labor. . . . Boston: White & Potter, 1847. 33p. DLC; MBM; MWA **40-0204**

CHANNING, Walter (1786-1876)
Cases of inhalation of ether in labor. 2nd ed. Boston: White & Potter, 1847. 44p. DNLM; MBM; MWA **40-0205**

CHANNING, Walter (1786-1876)
The late John Revere, M.D. [Boston, 1847]. 5p. DNLM; MBAt **40-0206**

CHANNING, Walter (1786-1876)
Memoir of the late Enoch Hale, M.D. . . . Boston: D. Clapp, printer, 1848. 12p. DLC; MBAt **40-0207**

CHANNING, Walter (1786-1876)
A treatise on etherization in childbirth. Illustrated by five hundred and eighty-one cases. . . . Boston: W. D. Ticknor and Company, 1848. 400p. DLC; MBM; MBAt **40-0208**

CHANNING, Walter (1786-1876)
On etherization in childbirth. Read to the Boston Society for Medical Improvement. [1849?] 8p. DNLM; MBM **40-0209**

[CHAPIN, John R.]
Description of Dr. Chapin's instrument for the treatment of prolapsus uteri, by external support. New York, 1840. 6p. DNLM; NNNAM **40-0210**

CHAPIN, Joshua Bicknell (1814-1881)
Asthma; its causes and treatment. Boston: T. H. Webb & Co., 1843. 19p. [Fiske Fund Prize Dissertation] DNLM; MWA **40-0211**

CHAPIN, William
Report on the benevolent institutions of Great Britain and Paris, including the schools and asylums for the blind, deaf and dumb, and the insane. . . . Columbus: C. Scott & Co., 1846. 61p. DNLM; OC **40-0212**

CHAPMAN, Nathaniel (1780-1853)
Essays on practical medicine and surgery. . . . Philadelphia: Lea & Blanchard, 1841. 2 v. DLC; DNLM; PHi; PU **40-0213**

CHAPMAN, Nathaniel (1780-1853)
Lectures on the more important eruptive fevers, hemorrhages and dropsies, and on gout and rheumatism. Delivered in the University of Pennsylvania. . . . Philadelphia: Lea & Blanchard, 1844. 448p. DLC; DNLM; PPC; PU **40-0214**

CHAPMAN, Nathaniel (1780-1853)
Lectures on the more important diseases of the thoracic and abdominal viscera. Delivered in the University of Pennsylvania. . . . Philadelphia: Lea & Blanchard, 1844. 383p. CU-M; DLC; DNLM; GU **40-0215**

CHAPMAN, Nathaniel (1780-1853)
Notes on Dr. Chapman's lectures, in the University of Pennsylvania, with an appendix, containing a few remarks on Asiatic cholera and yellow fever, by a physician. Philadelphia: W. S. Young, printer, 1845. 131p. DLC; DNLM; PPL **40-0216**

CHAPMAN, Nathaniel (1780-1853)
A compendium of lectures on the theory and practice of medicine, delivered by Professor Chapman. . . . Prepared . . . from Dr. Chapman's manuscripts. . . . By N. D. Benedict. . . . Philadelphia: Lea & Blanchard, 1846. 258p. DLC; DNLM; MBM; PPC **40-0217**

CHASE, Heber
Cases of club foot, treated by mechanical means alone. Philadelphia: Lea & Blanchard, 1841. 14p. DNLM; PPC; PU **40-0218**

CHASE, Heber
Cases of incomplete anchylosis of the knee joint, treated by mechanical means without the aid of tenotomy. Philadelphia: Lea & Blanchard, 1842. 18p. DNLM; PPC; PU **40-0219**

CHASE, Heber
The medical student's guide; being a compendious view of the collegiate and clinical and medical schools, the courses of private lectures, the hospitals, and almshouses and others. . . . Philadelphia: J. G. Auner, 1842. 106p. ICJ; ICRM; MBM; PPC **40-0220**

CHASE, Heber
Announcement of the private lectures of . . . with a catalogue of the classes, from their commencement in 1838. For the session of 1843-1844. Philadelphia: G. G. Dorsey, 1843. 11p. DNLM; PPC; PPJ **40-0221**

CHAVASSE, Pye Henry (1810-1879)
Advice to mothers on the management of their offspring. During the periods of infancy, childhood, and youth. . . . From the 3rd English ed. New York: D. Appleton & Co.; Philadelphia: G. S. Appleton, 1844. 153p. DLC; NNNAM; NNU-M **40-0222**

CHELIUS, Maximillian Joseph von (1794-1876)
A system of surgery. . . . Transl. from the German, and accompanied with additional notes and observations by John F. South. . . . Philadelphia: Lea & Blanchard, 1847. 3 v. DLC; DNLM; PPC; ViRA **40-0223**

CHEPMELL, Edward C.
A domestic homoeopathy, restricted to its legitimate sphere of practice, together with rules for diet and regimen. 1st American ed., with additions and improvements by Samuel B. Barlow, M.D. New York: William Radde, 1849. 224p. NNNAM; PPHa **40-0224**

CHILDS, Henry Halsey (1783-1868)
Philosophy of general principles: an introductory lecture delivered before the medical class of the Berkshire Medical Institution. Pittsfield, Mass.: C. Montague, 1844. 32p. DNLM
40-0225

CHRISTIE, A. H.
The wonders of galvanism and its application as a remedial agent. New York: D. C. Morehead, 1848. 8p. DNLM; NNNAM
40-0226

CHRISTISON, Robert (1797-1882)
A treatise on poisons in relation to medical jurisprudence, physiology, and the practice of physic. . . . 1st American, from the 4th Edinburgh ed. Philadelphia: E. Harrington & G. D. Haswell, 1845. 2 v. DNLM; DLC; MBM; MdBM
40-0227

CHRISTISON, Robert (1797-1882)
A dispensatory; or Commentary on the pharmacopoeias of Great Britain (and the United States). . . . 2nd ed. rev. and improved, with a supplement, containing the most important new remedies. With copious additions . . . by R. Eglesfeld Griffith. . . . Philadelphia: Lea & Blanchard, 1848. 1008p. DLC; DNLM; ICJ; ICU **40-0228**

CHURCHILL, Fleetwood (1808-1878)
Observations on the diseases incident to pregnancy and childbed. [Dunglison's American Medical Library] Philadelphia: A. Waldie, 1840. 290p. DNLM; PPC; PU
40-0229

CHURCHILL, Fleetwood (1808-1878)
On the theory and practice of midwifery. . . . With notes and additions, by Robert M. Huston. . . . Philadelphia: Lea & Blanchard, 1843. 519p. DLC; PPC; PPJ
40-0230

CHURCHILL, Fleetwood (1808-1878)
The diseases of females: including those of pregnancy and childbed. . . . 2nd American ed. With notes by Robert M. Huston. . . . Philadelphia: Lea & Blanchard, 1843. 575p. DLC; MBM; MH-M; PPC **40-0231**

CHURCHILL, Fleetwood (1808-1878)
The diseases of females: including those of pregnancy and childbed. . . . 3rd American ed. . . . With notes by Robert M. Huston. . . . Philadelphia: Lea & Blanchard, 1844. 571p. DLC; ICJ; IU-M; ViRA **40-0232**

CHURCHILL, Fleetwood (1808-1878)
On the theory and practice of midwifery. . . . With notes and additions, by Robert M. Huston. . . . 2nd American ed. . . . Philadelphia: Lea & Blanchard, 1846. 525p. DLC; PPC; PU
40-0233

CHURCHILL, Fleetwood (1808-1878)
The diseases of females: including those of pregnancy and childbed. 4th American ed. With illustrations. With notes by R. M. Huston. . . . Philadelphia: Lea & Blanchard, 1847. 601p. DNLM; NNNAM; PPC; ScMS **40-0234**

CHURCHILL, Fleetwood (1808-1878)
On the theory and practice of midwifery. . . . With notes and additions, by Robert M. Huston. . . . 3rd American ed. Rev. and improved by the author. . . . Philadelphia: Lea & Blanchard, 1848. 525p. DLC; PPC; PPJ; PU
40-0235

CLARIDGE, R. T.
Hydropathy; or, The cold water cure, as practiced by Vincent Priessnitz, at Graefenberg, Silesia, Austria. . . . 1st American, from the 3rd London ed. With notes by Dr. P. Lapham. New York: Pub. by the proprietor, 1843. 285p. DLC; NNNAM
40-0236

CLARIDGE, R. T.
Every man his own doctor. The cold water, tepid water, and friction cure, as applicable to every disease to which the human frame is subject. And also the cure of disease in horses and cattle. . . . New York: J. Wiley, 1849. 212p. DLC; NNNAM
40-0237

CLARK, James (1788-1870)
. . . The sanative influence of climate: with an account of the best places of resort for invalids in England, the south of Europe, &c. . . . From the 3rd London ed. [Dunglison's American Medical Library] Philadelphia: A. Waldie, 1841. 196p. DLC; DNLM; PPC; PU **40-0238**

CLYMER, Meredith, ed. (1817-1902)
Fevers: their diagnosis, pathology, and treatment. Prepared and ed., with large additions, from the essays on fever in Tweedie's library of practical medicine. . . . Philadelphia: Lea & Blanchard, 1846. 604p. DLC; PPC; PU **40-0239**

COATES, Reynell (1802-1886)
Syllabus of a course of popular lectures on physiology, with an outline of the principles which govern the gradual development of the faculties of mind and body. . . . Philadelphia: C. Sherman & Co., printers, 1840. 23p. DLC; MBM; PPC; PU
40-0240

COATES, Reynell (1802-1886)
Syllabus of a course of popular lectures on physiology. . . . Philadelphia: T. K. & P. G. Collins, 1840. 270. DNLM; PPC
40-0241

COGSWELL, William H.
The annual address to the candidates for degrees and licenses, in the medical institution of Yale College, January 21, 1846. . . . New Haven: Printed by W. H. Stanley, 1846. 15p. CtY-M; MWA **40-0242**

COLBY, Benjamin
A guide to health, being an exposition of the principles of the Thomsonian system of practice, and their mode of application in the cure of every form of disease; embracing a concise view of the various theories of ancient and modern practice. . . . 3rd ed., enl. and rev. . . . Milford, N.H.: J. Burns, 1846. 181p. DLC; DNLM **40-0243**

COLEY, James Millman
A practical treatise on the diseases of children. . . . Philadelphia: E. Barrington & G. D. Haswell, 1846. 414p. DLC; PPC; PPJ **40-0244**

COLLES, Abraham (1773-1843)
Lectures on the theory and practice of surgery. Edited by Simon McCoy. . . . Philadelphia: E. Barrington & G. D. Haswell, 1845. 420p. DNLM; NNNAM; PPC; PU **40-0245**

COLLINS, Robert (1801-1868)
A practical treatise on midwifery, containing the result of sixteen thousand, six hundred and fifty-four births, occurring in the Dublin lying-in hospital, during a period of seven years, commencing November, 1826. . . . Boston: W. D. Ticknor, 1841. 320p. DLC; MBM; MH-M **40-0246**

COLOMBAT, Marc (1797-1851)
A treatise upon diseases and hygiene of the organs of the voice. Transl. by J. F. W. Lane, M.D. Boston: Otis, Broaders & Co., 1845. 220p. 1 plate. DNLM; MBM **40-0247**

COLOMBAT, Marc (1797-1851)
A treatise on the diseases and special hygiene of females. . . . Transl. from the French, with additions. By Charles D. Meigs. . . . Philadelphia: Lea & Blanchard, 1845. 703p. DLC; NDLM; PPJ; PU **40-0248**

COMBE, Andrew (1797-1847)
A treatise on the physiological and moral management of infancy. For the use of parents. . . . With notes by John Bell. . . . Philadelphia: Carey & Hart, 1840. 307p. PPC; PU **40-0249**

COMBE, Andrew (1797-1847)
The principles of physiology, applied to the preservation of health and to the improvement of physical and mental education. New York: Harper & Brothers, 1843. 396p. DNLM; NNNAM; PPC **40-0250**

COMBE, Andrew (1797-1847)
The physiology of digestion, considered with relation to the principles of dietetics. From the 3rd Edinburgh ed. New York: Wm. H. Colyer, 1845. 287p. DNLM; NNNAM **40-0251**

COMBE, Andrew (1797-1847)
A treatise on the physiological and moral management of infancy. For the use of parents. . . . From the 4th Edinburgh ed. New York: W. H. Colyer; Boston: Phillips & Sampson, 1846. 296p. CtY-M; DLC; MBM **40-0252**

COMBE, Andrew (1797-1847)
The principles of physiology applied to the preservation of health, and to the improvement of physical and mental education. . . . With five wood-cuts. To which is added, notes and observations, by O. S. Fowler. . . . From the 7th Edinburgh ed. Enl. and improved. New York: Fowler & Wells, 1846. 320p. CU-M; DLC; IU-M; MBM **40-0253**

COMBE, George (1788-1858)
Lectures on phrenology . . . including its application to the present and prospective condition of the United States. With notes, an introductory essay, and an historical sketch by Andrew Boardman, M.D. 3rd ed., with corrections and additions. . . . New York: J. P. Giffing, 1841. 391p. DLC; NNNAM **40-0254**

COMBE, George (1788-1858)
Notes on the United States of North America during a phrenological visit in 1838, 1839, 1840. Philadelphia: Carey & Hart, 1841. 2 v. MBM; MBAt; MWA **40-0255**

COMBE, George (1788-1858)
Elements of phrenology. From the 5th Edinburgh ed. New York: Wm. H. Colyer, 1845. 256p. 6 plates. DNLM; NNNAM; MBM; PPC **40-0256**

COMBE, George (1788-1858)
A system of phrenology. . . . New York: Harper & Bros., 1849. 516p. ICU; MBM; NN; NNC **40-0257**

COMBE, George (1788-1858)
The constitution of man considered in relation to external objects. With an additional chapter on the harmony between phrenology and revelation, by Joseph A. Warne. Hartford: S. Andrus & Son, 1849. 60p. DNLM; MBM; MWA **40-0258**

COMFORT, John W.
Practice of medicine on Thomsonian principles. . . . And a materia medica adapted to the work. Philadelphia: A. Comfort, 1843. 514p. DLC; DNLM; PPC **40-0259**

COMFORT, John W.
Thomsonian practice of midwifery, and treatment of complaints peculiar to women and children. . . . Philadelphia: A. Comfort, 1845. 215p. DLC; PPC; PU **40-0260**

CONDIE, David Francis (1796-1875)
A practical treatise on the diseases of children. . . . Philadelphia: Lea & Blanchard, 1844. 651p. DLC; PPC; PPJ; PU **40-0261**

CONDIE, David Francis (1796-1875)
Annual oration delivered before the Philadelphia Medical Society, by appointment, at the opening of its session of 1844-1845. . . . Published by order of the Society. Philadelphia: King & Baird, printers, 1845. 24p. DLC; PPC **40-0262**

COOK, George W. (1806-1849)
The mariner's physician and surgeon; or, a guide to the homoeopathic tratment of those diseases to which seamen are liable, comprising the treatment of syphilitic diseases. . . . New York: J. T. S. Smith. 1848. 105p. NNNAM; PPHa **40-0263**

COOK, Simeon A. (1803-1873)
Address delivered before the Medical Society of the County of Rensselaer, New York. Troy, N.Y.: Printed at the Budget Office [1844]. 31p. DNLM **40-0264**

COOMBE, Frederick
Coombe's popular phrenology; exhibiting the exact phrenological admeasurements of above fifty distinguished and extraordinary personages, of both sexes, with skulls of the various nations of the world. . . . Boston: Printed for the author, 1841. 130p., plates. DLC; MWA; MBAt **40-0265**

COOPER, Astley Paston (1768-1841)
A treatise on dislocations and fractures of the joints. . . . A new ed., much enl. Ed. by Bransby B. Cooper. . . . With additional observations, and a memoir of the author. Philadelphia: Lea & Blanchard, 1844. 490p. DLC; PPC; PPJ; PU **40-0266**

COOPER, Astley Paston (1768-1841)
The anatomy and surgical treatment of abdominal hernia. . . . From the 2nd London ed. By C. Aston Key. . . . Philadelphia: Lea & Blanchard, 1844. 427p. DLC; MBM; MH-M; PPC **40-0267**

COOPER, Astley Paston (1768-1841)
The anatomy and diseases of the breast. . . . To which are added, his various surgical papers, now first published in a collected form. Philadelphia: Lea & Blanchard, 1845. 130, 63, 188p. 36 plates. CtY-M; DLC; PPC; PU **40-0268**

COOPER, Astley Paston (1768-1841)
Observations on the structure and diseases of the testis. . . . From the 2nd London ed. Edited by Bransby B. Cooper. . . . Philadelphia: Lea & Blanchard, 1845. 247p. 24 plates. CtY-M; DLC; PPJ; PU **40-0269**

COOPER, Astley Paston (1768-1841)
The anatomy of the thymus gland. . . . From the last London ed. Philadelphia: Lea & Blanchard, 1845. 37p. 5 plates. DLC; DNLM; GU; PPC **40-0270**

COOPER, J. W.
The experienced botanist, or Indian physician; being a new system of practice founded on botany. . . . Lancaster: The author, 1840. 303p. DNLM; OCLloyd **40-0271**

COOPER, Samuel (1780-1848)
A dictionary of practical surgery. . . . from the 7th London ed., rev., cor., and enl. With numerous notes and additions, embracing all the principal improvements and greater operations introduced and performed by American surgeons, together with a Supplementary index, in which the science of surgery is brought down to the present period, including all the recent improvements in Europe and America. . . . By David Meredith Reese. . . . New York: Harper & Brothers, 1842. 506, 170p. DLC; NNNAM; PPC; PU **40-0272**

COOPER, Samuel (1780-1848)
The first lines of the theory and practice of surgery; including the principal operations. . . . With notes and additions, by Willard Parker. . . . 4th American, from the 7th London ed. New York: S. S. and W. Wood, 1844. 2 v. DLC; DNLM; NNNAM; PPC **40-0273**

CORNARO, Luigi (1467-1566)
The discourses and letters of Louis Cornaro on a sober and temperate life; with a biography of the author, by Piero Moroncelli, and notes and an appendix by John Burdell. New York: Fowlers & Wells [1842]. 228p. DNLM; NN; NNC; ICU **40-0274**

CORNELL, William M[ason] (1802-1895)
Consumption forestalled and prevented. Boston: J. French, 1846. 120p. DNLM; MBM; MH-M **40-0275**

COVENTRY, Charles B. (1801-1875)
Address to the graduates of the medical institution of Geneva College. Utica: Democrat Office, 1842. 16p. DNLM **40-0276**

COVENTRY, Charles B. (1801-1875)
A lecture introductory to the course of obstetrics in Geneva Medical College: Geneva: Merrell, 1843. 22p. DNLM **40-0277**

COVENTRY, Charles B. (1801-1875)
Report on epidemic cholera. [Utica, N.Y., 1848] 13p. DNLM **40-0278**

COVENTRY, Charles B. (1801-1875)
Epidemic cholera: its history, cause, pathology, and treatment. Buffalo: G. H. Derby & Co., 1849. 119p. DNLM; NNNAM **40-0279**

COX, Abraham L[idden] (1800-1864)
The rejected article, in reply to Dr. S. P. White's "Case of tumor of the shoulder," in the May number of the "New York Journal of Medicine and the Collateral Sciences." With introductory remarks containing a true statement of the facts in relation to that case. . . . New York: Printed for the author, 1845. 35p. DLC; DNLM; NNNAM **40-0280**

COX, Abraham L[idden] (1800-1864)
The patnology and treatment of Asiatic cholera, so called. . . . 2nd ed. New York: J. Wiley, 1849. 77p. DLC; DNLM; NNNAM **40-0281**

COXE, Edward Jenner (1801-1862)
A practical treatise on medical inhalation: with numerous cases. . . . Philadelphia: J. Dobson, 1841. 108p. DNLM; PPL; PU; ScC **40-0282**

COXE, John Redman (1773-1864)
The writings of Hippocrates and Galen, epitomized from the Latin original translations. . . . Philadelphia: Lindsay & Blakiston, 1846. 681p. DNLM; ICU; MB; NN **40-0283**

CRAIN, E.
Remarks on disease of the spine, with directions for applying [his] spino-abdominal supporter. [Springfield, Vt., 1844] 8p. DNLM; VtHi **40-0284**

CROSS, James Conquest
An appeal to the medical profession of the United States: together with an analysis and refutation of the "statements of facts in relation to the expulsion of James C. Cross from Transylvania University." 2nd ed. Louisville: Prentice & Weissinger, 1846. 39p. DNLM; KyLoJM **40-0285**

CROSS, James Conquest
An analysis and refutation of the "statements of facts in relation to expulsion of James C. Cross from Transylvania University," recently published by Dudley, Mitchell, and Peter. Louisville: Prentice & Weissinger, 1846. 39p. DNLM; KyLoJM **40-0286**

CROSS, James Conquest
An appeal to the medical profession of the United States. Cincinnati: Daily Atlas, 1846. 63p. DNLM; KyLoJM **40-0287**

CROSS, James Conquest
An inaugural discourse on the policy of establishing a school of medicine in the city of Memphis, Tennessee. Memphis, 1847. 47p. DNLM **40-0288**

CROSS, James Conquest
An essay on scarlatina. . . . [Memphis, 1847?] 48p. DNLM **40-0289**

CROSSMAN, T. J.
A catalogue of the names of upwards of nine hundred persons operated on for the cure of strabismus, or squinting. Cincinnati: Shepard & Co., 1843. 31p. DNLM; OCIM **40-0290**

CRUVEILHIER, Jean (1791-1874)
The anatomy of the human body. . . . The 1st American, from the last Paris ed. Ed. by Granville Sharp Pattison. . . . New York: Harper & Brothers, 1844. 907p. DLC; NNNAM; ViRA **40-0291**

CULVERWELL, Robert James (1802-1852)
Guide to health and long life: or, What to eat, drink, and avoid; what exercise to take, how to control and regulate the passions and appetites. . . . To which is added, a popular exposition of Liebig's theory of life, health, and disease. . . . New York: J. S. Redfield, 1848. 71p. DLC; DNLM; NNNAM
40-0292

CULVERWELL, Robert James (1802-1852)
Guide to health and long life: or What to eat, drink, and avoid; what exercise to take, how to control and regulate the passions and appetites; and on the general conduct of life, whereby health may be secured, and a happy and comfortable old age attained. . . . To which is added, a popular exposition of Liebig's theory of life, health, and disease. . . . New York: J. S. Redfield, 1849. 71p. DLC **40-0293**

CULVERWELL, Robert James (1802-1852)
Guide to health and long life . . . to which is added, a popular exposition of Liebig's theory of life, health, and disease. Cincinnati: U. P. James [1849?] 71p. DNLM; OC
40-0294

CULVERWELL, Robert James (1802-1852)
Porneio-pathology. A popular treatise on venereal and other diseases of the male and female genital system. New York: J. S. Redfield, 1849. 215p. DNLM; NNNAM **40-0295**

CULVERWELL, Robert James (1802-1852)
Diseases of winter. On consumption, coughs, . . . New York: J. S. Redfield, 1849. 91p. DNLM; NNNAM
40-0296

[CUNNINGHAM, A. C.]
The mystery of diseases revealed; or guide to the inexperienced. New York: the Author, 1845. 101p. DNLM; NNNAM
40-0297

CURLING, Thomas Blizard
A practical treatise on the diseases of the testis, and of the spermatic cord and scrotum. Ed. by P. B. Goddard. Philadelphia: Carey & Hart, 1843. 568p. DNLM; PPC; PPJ; PU
40-0298

CURTIS, Alva (1797-1881)
A synopsis of lectures on medical science; embracing the principles of medicine, or physiology, pathology, and therapeutics, as discovered in nature; and the practice according to those principles as applied by art. . . . 5th ed. Carefully rev., and much enl. New York: A. J. Graham, [1846]. 428p. DLC; DNLM; OCIM **40-0299**

CURTIS, Alva (1797-1881)
Lectures on midwifery and the forms of disease peculiar to women and children, delivered to the members of the Botanico-Medical School, at Columbus, Ohio. 3rd ed. Cincinnati: C. Nagle, 1846. 446p. DNLM; OCIM
40-0300

CURTIS, Alva (1797-1881)
A synopsis of a course of lectures on medical science, delivered to the students of the Botanico-Medical College of Ohio. Cincinnati: Edwin Shepard, 1846. 464p. DLC; OCIM
40-0300A

CURTIS, Alva (1797-1881)
Introductory lecture, delivered to the students of the Botanico-Medical College of Ohio, November 3, 1945. [Columbus, 1846?] 5p. DNLM; OCIM **40-0301**

CURTIS, Alva (1797-1881)
Lectures on medical science. Delivered to the students of the Botanico-Medical College of Ohio. [Columbus, 1846?] 48p. DNLM; OCIM **40-0302**

CURTIS, Alva (1797-1881)
A synopsis of lectures on medical science, embracing the principles of medicine. . . . 5th ed. New York: A. J. Graham, [1848?]. 428p. DNLM; NNNAM **40-0303**

CURTIS, John Harrison
Curtis on the preservation of sight, the diseases of the eye, and the use, abuse, and choice of spectacles, reading-glasses, &c.; being practical observations for popular use. . . . 1st American, from the 2nd London ed. New York: Burgess & Stringer, 1844. 48p. DLC; NNNAM **40-0304**

CURTIS, Joseph T. and J. LILLIE
An epitome of homoeopathic practice. Compiled chiefly from Jahr, Rueckert, Beauvais, Boenninghausen. . . . New York: William Radde, 1843. 153p. PPHa **40-0305**

CURTIS, Josiah (1816-1883)
Brief remarks on hygiene of Massachusetts, but more particularly of the cities of Boston and Lowell: being a report to the American Medical Association: submitted, as member for Massachusetts of the Committee on Public Hygiene, at their annual meeting in Boston, May 1849. . . . Philadelphia: T. K. and P. G. Collins, printers, 1849. 70p. DLC; PPC; PU
40-0306

CUTTER, Calvin (1807-1872)
Practical remarks upon the treatment and cure of burns, scalds, sprains, ruptures or hernia, diarrhoea, dysentery, colic, cholera morbus, costiveness, piles, indigestion, coughs, colds, recovery of drowned persons, stoppage of blood, fresh cuts and wounds, fainting, injuries of the head, management of sick rooms, &c. . . . Springfield [Mass.]: Printed by Wood & Rupp, 1844. 48p. DLC; MBAt; MBM; MWA **40-0307**

CUTTER, Calvin (1807-1872)
Anatomy and physiology. . . . With one hundred and fifty engravings. Boston: S. N. Dickinson & Co., 1845. 262p. DLC; MB; MBM **40-0308**

CUTTER, Calvin (1807-1872)
Common school physiology. . . . 1st stereotype ed., with over one hundred engravings. Boston: B. B. Mussey; New York: S. S. and W. Wood, 1846. 226p. DLC; NN; NNNAM
40-0309

CUTTER, Calvin (1807-1872)
Anatomy and physiology. . . . 2nd ed., with two hundred engravings. Boston: B. B. Mussey; Springfield. G. and C. Merriam, 1846. 322p. DLC; ICU; MB; MBM
40-0310

CUTTER, Calvin (1807-1872)
First book on anatomy and physiology. . . . with eighty-four engravings. Stereotype ed. New York: Clark & Austin; Boston: B. B. Mussey & Co. [etc., etc.] 1847. 144p. DLC; DNLM
40-0311

CUTTER, Calvin (1807-1872)
First book on anatomy and physiology. . . . with eighty engravings. Boston: B. B. Mussey & Co.; New York: Clark & Austin, 1847. 139p. DLC; NN; NNNAM **40-0312**

CUTTER, Calvin (1807-1872)
First book of anatomy and physiology, for grammar schools. . . . With eighty-four engravings. Stereotype ed. Boston: B. B. Mussey & Co.; New York: Clark & Austin, 1848. 144p. DLC; ICU; NIC; NN **40-0313**

CUTTER, Calvin (1807-1872)
A treatise on anatomy, physiology, and hygiene. . . . With one hundred and fifty engravings. Stereotype ed. Boston: B. B. Mussey & Co.; New York: Clark, Austin, & Co., 1849. 458p. DLC; MB; NN; NNC **40-0314**

DAILY, William
The Indian doctor's practice of medicine . . . giving the symptoms of diseases and a vegetable treatment of the diseases of men, women, and children. Louisville: N. H. White, 1848. 224p. DNLM; KyLoJM **40-0315**

DARRACH, William (1796-1865)
Drawings of the anatomy of the groin; with anatomical remarks. . . . Philadelphia: Lindsay & Blakiston, 1844. 127p. DLC; DNLM; PPC; PU **40-0316**

DARRACH, William (1796-1865)
Lecture introductory to the course of theory and practice of medicine in the medical department of Pennsylvania College, Philadelphia. Philadelphia: W. S. Young, 1844. 16p. DNLM; PPC; PU **40-0317**

DARRACH, William (1796-1865)
Lecture on medical obedience. . . . Philadelphia: Barrett & Jones, 1845. 15p. DNLM; PPC; PU
40-0318

DARRACH, William (1796-1865)
Lecture, introductory to the course of the theory and practice of medicine, in the Medical Department of Pennsylvania College, Session of 1846-1847. . . . Philadelphia: King & Baird, printers, 1846. 24p. DLC; DNLM; PPC; PPJ
40-0319

DARRACH, William (1796-1865)
Memoir of George McClellan. A lecture. Philadelphia: King & Baird, 1847. 40p. DNLM; PPC; PPJ
40-0320

DAVIDSON, William
. . . Essays on the sources and mode of action of fever. By . . . and Alfred Hudson. . . . [Dunglison's American Medical Library] Philadelphia: A. Waldie, 1841. 178p. CtY-M; DLC; DNLM; PPC **40-0321**

DAVIDSON, William
. . . Essays on the sources and mode of action of fever. By . . . and Alfred Hudson. . . . Philadelphia: E. Barrington & G. Haswell, 1843. 178p. DNLM; PPC; PPJ; PU
40-0322

DAVIES, John (1796-1872)
Selections in pathology and surgery. . . . Philadelphia: Carey & Hart, 1841. 119p. DNLM; NNNAM; PPC; ViRA
40-0323

DAVIES, William
Good advice, or The family companion: containing an account of the beneficial nature of mustard seed, in the prevention and cure of disease; together with many valuable recipies. . . . Philadelphia: Printed for the author, 1842. 96p. DLC; PPC **40-0324**

DAVIS, Daniel
The medical application of electricity. Boston: D. Davis, Jr., 1846. 24p. DNLM; MBM; MWA **40-0325**

DAVIS, David Daniel (1777-1841)
. . . Acute hydrocephalus, or water in the head, an inflammatory disease, and curable equally by the same means with other diseases of inflammation. . . . [Dunglison's American Medical Library] Philadelphia: Printed by A. Waldie, 1840. 126p. DLC; DNLM; NNNAM; PPC **40-0326**

DAVIS, Nathan Smith (1817-1904)
Address on free medical schools, introductory to the session of 1849-1850 in Rush Medical College: Chicago: Printed for the class, 1849. 16p. DNLM; ICRM; IU-M
40-0327

DAWSON, John (1810-1866)
An account of epidemic erysipelas as it prevailed in some parts of Ohio. [1845]. 62p. DNLM **40-0328**

DAY, George Edward (1815-1872)
A practical treatise on the domestic management and most important diseases of advanced life. With an appendix, containing a series of cases illustrative of a new and successful mode of treating lumbago and other forms of chronic rheumatism, sciatica and other neuralgic affections, and certain forms of paralysis. . . . Philadelphia: Lea & Blanchard, 1849. 226p. DLC; DNLM; PPC **40-0329**

DELABARRE, Christophe-François (1787-1862)
A treatise on second dentition and the natural method of directing it; followed by a summary of stomatic semeology. . . . Baltimore: Published by the American Society of Dental Surgeons, 1845. 171p. DNLM; MdU-D; PU
40-0330

DEMING, Elizur H. (1797-1855)
An address at the opening of the session of 1847-1848 of the Indiana Medical College. La Porte, Indiana: W. & J. Millikan, 1848. 15p. DNLM **40-0331**

DENDY, Walter Cooper (1794-1871)
. . . Practical remarks on the diseases of the skin, on the external signs of disorder, and on the constitutional peculiarities during infancy and childhood. . . . [Dunglison's American Medical Library] Philadelphia: A. Waldie, 1841. 88p. DLC; DNLM; PPC; PU **40-0332**

[DESIRABODE et ses fils]
The science and art of dentistry; with an historical and chronological notice of works on the art of dentistry from Hippocrates to our time. 2nd ed. Transl. for the American Library of Dental Science. . . . Baltimore: American Society of Dental Surgeons, 1847. 552p. DNLM; MdU-D; PU
40-0333

DESLANDES, Léopold
A treatise on the diseases produced by onanism, masturbation, self-pollution, and other excesses. . . . Transl. from the French, with many additions. 3rd ed. Boston: Otis, Broaders & Company, 1841. 252p. DNLM; MBM; MH-M; NNNAM
40-0334

DESLANDES, Léopold
Manhood; the causes of its premature decline. . . . Boston: Otis, Broaders & Co., 1842. 252p. DNLM; MBM; MH; MH-M **40-0335**

DETMOLD, William Ludwig (1808-1894)
An essay on club foot, and some analogous diseases. New York: G. Adlard, 1840. 64p. 4 plates. DNLM; NNNAM
40-0336

DEWEES, William Potts (1768-1841)
A compendious system of midwifery. . . . 7th ed. Philadelphia: Lea & Blanchard, 1840. 591p. DNLM; PPC; PPJ; PU
40-0337

DEWEES, William Potts (1768-1841)
A treatise on the physical and medical treatment of children. . . . 8th ed. with the author's last improvements and corrections. Philadelphia: Lea & Blanchard, 1842. 548p. DLC; PPC; PPHa; PU **40-0338**

DEWEES, William Potts (1768-1841)
A compendious system of midwifery. . . . 8th ed. Philadelphia: Lea & Blanchard, 1847. 562p. PPC; PPJ; PU
40-0339

DEWEES, William Potts (1768-1841)
A treatise on the physical and medical treatment of children. 9th ed. with the author's last improvements and corrections. Philadelphia: Lea & Blanchard, 1847. 501p. DLC; PPC; PPL; PU **40-0340**

DEWEES, William Potts (1768-1841)
A treatise on the diseases of females. . . . 9th ed. Philadelphia: Lea & Blanchard, 1847. 532p. DNLM; PPC; PPJ; PU
40-0341

DICKSON, Samuel (1802-1869)
The principles of the chrono-thermal system of medicine, with the fallacies of the faculty, in a series of lectures; containing also an introduction by William Turner. 2nd American from the 5th London ed. New York: H. Long & Bro., 1848. 224p. DNLM; NNNAM **40-0342**

DICKSON, Samuel (1802-1869)
Revelations on cholera; or its causes and cure. Ed. by Wm. T. Turner. New York: H. Long & Bro., 1849. 72p. DNLM; NNNAM **40-0343**

DICKSON, Samuel Henry (1798-1872)
Annual report to the President and Board of Trustees of the Medical College of the State of South Carolina. With the valedictory address to the class. Charleston: Burges & James, 1841. 12p. PPC; ScC; ScCM; ScU **40-0344**

DICKSON, Samuel Henry (1798-1872)
Address delivered at the opening of the new edifice of the Charleston apprentices' library society on the evening of the 13th January, 1841. . . . Charleston: W. Riley, printer, 1841. 37p. DLC; ScC; ScU **40-0345**

DICKSON, Samuel Henry (1798-1872)
Manual of pathology and practice, being the outline of the course of lectures. Charleston, 1842. 240p. DNLM; ScCM; ScMS **40-0346**

DICKSON, Samuel Henry (1798-1872)
A few remarks on "the principle of life." . . . Printed at the request of an association of gentlemen, before whom they were read. Charleston: Observer office press, 1843. 21p. DLC; ScU
40-0347

DICKSON, Samuel Henry (1798-1872)
Essays on pathology and therapeutics, being the substance of the course of lectures delivered by. . . . Charleston: McCarter & Allen, 1845. 2 v. DLC; ScCM; ScMS
40-0348

DICKSON, Samuel Henry (1798-1872)
Essays on pathology and therapeutics, being the substance of the course of lectures delivered by. . . . New York: S. S. & W. Wood, 1845. 2 v. DNLM; NNNAM; PPC; ScCM
40-0349

DICKSON, Samuel Henry (1798-1872)
A lecture introductory to the course on the theory and practice of medicine, in the University of New York: New York: J. H. Jennings, 1847. 19p. DNLM; NNNAM; NNU-M
40-0350

DICKSON, Samuel Henry (1798-1872)
Hygiene; an introductory lecture, delivered at the New York University medical department. New York: J. H. Jennings, 1848. 24p. DNLM; NNNAM; MBM **40-0351**

DIX, Dorothea Lynde (1802-1887)
Memorial soliciting a State hospital for the insane, submitted to the legislature of Pennsylvania, February 3, 1845. Harrisburg: J. M. G. Lescure, 1845. 59p. DNLM; PPC; PU
40-0352

DIX, Dorothea Lynde (1802-1887)
Memorial soliciting a State hospital for the insane submitted to the legislature of Pennsylvania. . . . With the act to establish an asylum for the insane poor. Philadelphia: J. Ashmead, 1845. 52p. DNLM; PU **40-0353**

DIX, Dorothea Lynde (1802-1887)
Memorial soliciting an appropriation for the State hospital for the insane, at Lexington; and also urging the necessity for establishing a new hospital in the Green River country. Frankfurt: A. G. Hodges, 1846. 14p. DNLM
40-0354

DIX, Dorothea Lynde (1802-1887)
Memorial of D. L. Dix, praying a grant of land for the relief and support of the indigent curable and incurable insane in the United States 30th Cong., 1st sess., June 27, 1848. [Washington: Tippin & Streeper, 1848] 32p. DNLM
40-0355

DIX, John Homer (1813?-1884)
Treatise on strabismus, or squinting and the new mode of treatment. Boston: D. Clapp, Jr., 1841. 105p. DNLM; MBM; MH-M **40-0356**

DIX, John Homer (1813?-1884)
Treatise upon the nature and treatment of morbid sensibility of the retina, or weakness of sight. Being the dissertation to which the Boylston medical prize for 1848 was awarded upon the following question: "What is the nature and best mode of treatment of that affection of the eyes, commonly called morbid sensibilty of the retina?" . . . Boston: W. D. Ticknor & Company, 1849. 146p. DLC; DNLM; MBM; MH-M
40-0357

DIXON, Edward H. (1808-1880)
A treatise on diseases on the sexual organs; adapted to popular and professional reading, and the exposition of quackery, professional and otherwise. New York: W. Taylor, 1845. 260p. 4 plates. DNLM; NNNAM **40-0358**

DIXON, Edward H. (1808-1880)
A treatise on diseases of the sexual organs; adapted to popular and professional reading, and the exposition of quackery, professional and otherwise. xii, 260p. 2 plates. New York: C. H. Ring. 1847. DNLM; NNNAM **40-0359**

DIXON, Edward H. (1808-1880)
Women, and their diseases, from the cradle to the grave. New York: For the author, 1847. 309p. DNLM; NNNAM **40-0360**

DIXON, Edward H. (1808-1880)
A treatise on diseases of the sexual organs; adapted to popular and professional reading, and the exposition of quackery, professional and otherwise. 6th ed. New York: C. H. Ring, 1847. 260p. 2 plates. DNLM; NNNAM **40-0361**

DIXON, Edward H. (1808-1880)
A treatise on diseases of the sexual system; adapted to popular and professional reading, and the exposition of quackery. . . . 8th ed. New York: Dewitt & Davenport, 1849. 260p. 4 plates. DNLM; NNNAM **40-0362**

DOANE, George Bartlett (1793-1842)
[List of works of the library of the late Dr. . . . presented to the Boston Society for Medical Improvement.] [Boston, 1843] 4p. DNLM; MBM **40-0363**

DOUGLAS, James S. (1801-1878)
Homoeopathy. A lecture before the Hygeian Society of the Hamilton Literary and Theological Institution, delivered in the Chapel of the Institution, April, 1845. Published by request. Hamilton, N.Y.: Waldron & Baker [1845]. 29p. NNNAM; PPHa **40-0364**

DOUGLAS, Robert (1820-1844)
Adventures of a medical student. . . . With a memoir of the life of the author. . . . New York: Burgess, Stringer & Co., 1848. 2 v. in 1. DLC; MH; NN; NNC **40-0365**

DOWLER, Bennet (1797-1879)
Experimental researches on the post-mortem contractility of the muscles, with observations on the reflex theory. . . . New York: R. Craighead, printer, 1846. 39p. DLC; DNLM; NNNAM **40-0366**

DOWLER, Bennet (1797-1879)
Criticisms and controversies relating to the nervous and muscular systems. . . . New Orleans: J. Cohn, printer, 1847. 69p. DLC; LNT-M **40-0367**

DOWLER, Bennet (1797-1879)
Contributions to physiology. New Orleans, 1849. 25p. DNLM; LNT-M **40-0368**

DOWLER, Bennet (1797-1879)
Researches, critical and experimental, on the capillary circulation. New Orleans: J. Cohn, 1849. 25p. DNLM; LNT-M **40-0369**

DRAKE, Daniel (1785-1852)
An introductory discourse to a course of lectures on clinical medicine and pathological anatomy. Louisville, Ky.: Prentice & Weissinger, 1840. 16p. DNLM; OCHP **40-0370**

DRAKE, Daniel (1785-1852)
A memoir on the disease called by the people the trembles, and the sick stomach or milk-sickness, as they appear in the Virginia military district in the state of Ohio. Louisville, Ky.: J. Maxwell, Jr., 1841. 57p. DNLM; OCIM **40-0371**

DRAKE, Daniel (1785-1852)
The northern lakes, a summer residence for invalids of the South. Louisville, Ky.: J. Maxwell, Jr., 1842. 29p. DNLM; KyLoJM **40-0372**

DRAKE, Daniel (1785-1852)
. . . An introductory lecture, on the means of promoting the intellectual improvement of the students and physicians, of the valley of the Mississippi. Delivered in the Medical Institute of Louisville, November 4th, 1844. . . . Published by the class. Louisville, Ky.: Printice & Weissinger, 1844. 24p. DLC; OCIM; OCWHi **40-0373**

DRAKE, Daniel (1785-1852)
Strictures on some of the defects and infirmities of intellectual and moral character, in students of medicine: an introductory lecture, delivered in the University of Louisville, November 1st, 1847. . . . Published by the class. Louisville, Ky.: Prentice & Weissinger, 1847. 16p. DLC; KyLoJM; OCIM; OCWHi **40-0374**

DRAKE, Daniel (1785-1852)
An introductory lecture at the opening of the thirtieth session of the Medical College of Ohio, delivered at the request of the faculty, November 5, 1849. . . . Published by the class. Cincinnati: Morgan & Overend, printers, 1849. 16p. DLC; OCHP; OCIM **40-0375**

DRAPER, John William (1811-1882)
Introductory lecture to the course of chemistry, University of New York, medical department. New York: Hopkins & Jennings, 1841. 15p. DNLM; NNNAM **40-0376**

DRAPER, John William (1811-1882)
Introductory lecture to the course of chemistry, University of New York, medical department. 2nd ed. New York: Hopkins & Jennings, 1841. 15p. DNLM; NNNAM **40-0377**

DRAPER, John William (1811-1882)
University of New York. Medical department. A valedictory lecture, delivered by Professor Draper. Session 1841-1842. New York: Hopkins & Jennings, printers, 1842. 14p. DLC; DNLM; NNNAM **40-0378**

DRAPER, John William (1811-1882)
. . . Introductory lecture, to the course of chemistry: delivered by Professor Draper, on the relations of atmospheric air to animals and plants. Session. 1844-1845. New York: Printed for the medical class of the University, by J. H. Jennings, 1844-1845. 16p. DLC; DNLM; NNC; NNNAM **40-0379**

DRAPER, John William (1811-1882)
. . . Introductory lecture, to the course of chemistry: delivered by Professor Draper, on the relations and nature of water. Session 1845-1846. New York: Printed for the medical class of the University, at the Herald job office, 1845-1846. 15p. DLC; DNLM; NNNAM **40-0380**

DRAPER, John William (1811-1882)
An introductory lecture on the history of chemistry. New York, 1846. 15p. DNLM; NN; NNC **40-0381**

DRAPER, John William (1811-1882)
An introductory lecture on phosphorus. New York: J. H. Jennings, 1847. 14p. DNLM; NN; NNC **40-0382**

DRAPER, John William (1811-1882)
An introductory lecture on oxygen gas. New York: J. H. Jennings, 1848. 15p. DNLM; NN; NNC **40-0383**

DRUITT, Robert (1814-1883)
The principles and practice of modern surgery. . . . From the 2nd London ed. . . . With notes and comments, by Joshua B. Flint. . . . Philadelphia: Lea & Blanchard, 1842. 534p. DLC; PPC; PU **40-0384**

DRUITT, Robert (1814-1883)
The principles and practice of modern surgery. . . . 3rd American from the last London ed. . . . Philadelphia: Lea & Blanchard, 1847. 540p. DNLM; PPC; PPJ; PU **40-0385**

DRUITT, Robert (1814-1833)
The principles and practice of modern surgery. . . . A new American from the last and improved London ed. Ed. by F. W. Sargent. . . . Philadelphia: Lea & Blanchard, 1848. 576p. DLC; PPJ; PU **40-0386**

DUDLEY, Benjamin W. (1785-1870)
Statements of facts in relation to the expulsion of James C. Cross from the Transylvania University, Ky. Lexington, Ky.: Scrugham & Dunlop, 1846. 19p. DNLM; KyLoJM **40-0387**

DUDLEY, Ethelbert L.
Valedictory address to the medical class of Transylvania University. Lexington, Ky.: Observor and Reporter Print., 1849. 15p. DNLM; KyLoJM **40-0388**

DUFTON, William
The nature and treatment of deafness and diseases of the ear, and the treatment of the deaf and dumb. Philadelphia: Lea & Blanchard, 1848. 120p. DNLM; PPC; PU **40-0389**

DUGAS, Louis Alexander (1806-1884)
An address to the class of the Medical College of Georgia . . . containing a sketch of the improvements in medicine during the present century. Augusta: J. McCafferty, 1846. 16p. DNLM; GU; MdBM **40-0390**

DUGAS, Louis Alexander (1806-1884)
Malformation of the genito-urinary apparatus. [Augusta, 1849] 8p. DNLM **40-0391**

DUNGLISON, Robley (1798-1869)
Human physiology. . . . 4th ed. Philadelphia: Lea & Blanchard, 1841. 2 v. CtY-M; NNNAM; PPC; ViRA **40-0392**

DUNGLISON, Robley (1798-1869)
New remedies: the method of preparing and administering them; their effects on the healthy and diseased economy, . . . 3rd ed., with numerous modifications and additions. . . . Philadelphia: Lea & Blanchard, 1841. 541p. DLC; DNLM; PPC; PU **40-0393**

DUNGLISON, Robley (1798-1869)
An introductory lecture to the course of institutes of medicine, delivered in Jefferson Medical College, November 1, 1841. . . . Published by the class. Philadelphia: Merrihew & Thompson, printers, 1841. 24p. CtY-M; DLC; PPC; PPJ **40-0394**

DUNGLISON, Robley (1798-1869)
Medical lexicon; a new dictionary of medical science. . . . 3rd ed. Philadelphia: Lea & Blanchard, 1842. 749p. DNLM; MBM; NNNAM; PPC **40-0395**

DUNGLISON, Robley (1798-1869)
On certain medical delusions, an introductory lecture to the course of institutes of medicine in Jefferson Medical College of Philadelphia. Delivered November 4, 1842. . . . Philadelphia: Merrihew & Thompson, printers, 1842. 34p. DLC; PPJ; PU **40-0396**

DUNGLISON, Robley (1798-1869)
The practice of medicine; or, A treatise on special pathology and therapeutics. . . . Philadelphia: Lea & Blanchard, 1842. 2 v. DLC; PPC; PPJ; PU **40-0397**

DUNGLISON, Robley (1798-1869)
New remedies: pharmaceutically and therapeutically considered. 4th ed. with extensive modifications and additions. . . . Philadelphia: Lea & Blanchard, 1843. 625p. DLC; MBM; PPC; ViRA **40-0398**

DUNGLISON, Robley (1798-1869)
An introductory lecture to the course of institutes of medicine . . . in the Jefferson Medical College. Philadelphia: Merrihew & Thompson, 1843. 28p. DNLM; PPC; PPJ **40-0399**

DUNGLISON, Robley (1798-1869)
General therapeutics and materia medica, adapted for a medical text book. . . . Philadelphia: Lea & Blanchard, 1843. 2 v. DLC; PPC; PPJ **40-0400**

DUNGLISON, Robley (1798-1869)
Human physiology. . . . 5th ed. Philadelphia: Lea & Blanchard, 1844. 2 v. DNLM; NNNAM; PPC; ViRA **40-0401**

DUNGLISON, Robley (1798-1869)
Medical lexicon; a new dictionary of medical science. . . . 4th ed. Philadelphia: Lea & Blanchard, 1844. 771p. DNLM; PPC; PPJ; PPHa **40-0402**

DUNGLISON, Robley (1798-1869)
The medical student; or, aids to the study of medicine. A revised and modified edition. Philadelphia: Lea & Blanchard, 1844. 311p. DNLM; PPC; PPL; PU **40-0403**

DUNGLISON, Robley (1798-1869)
The practice of medicine: a treatise on special pathology and therapeutics. . . . 2nd ed. . . . Philadelphia: Lea & Blanchard, 1844. 2 v. DLC; NNNAM; PPC; PPJ **40-0404**

DUNGLISON, Robley (1798-1869)
An introductory lecture to the course of institutes of medicine, in Jefferson Medical College, delivered Nov. 4, 1844. . . . Published by the class. Philadelphia: B. E. Smith, pr., 1844. 31p. DLC; PPC; PPJ **40-0405**

DUNGLISON, Robley (1798-1869)
Human health; or The influence of atmosphere and locality; change of air and climate seasons; food; clothing; bathing and mineral springs; exercise; sleep; corporeal and intellectual pursuits, &c. &c. on healthy man; constituting elements of hygiene. . . . A new ed. with many modifications and additions. Philadelphia: Lea & Blanchard, 1844. 464p. DLC; PPC; PPJ; ViRA **40-0406**

DUNGLISON, Robley, ed. (1798-1869)
The cyclopaedia of practical medicine; comprising treatises on the nature and treatment of diseases, materia medica and therapeutics, medical jurisprudence, . . . edited by John Forbes . . . Alexander Tweedie . . . John Conolly . . . thoroughly revised with numerous additions. . . . Philadelphia: Lea and Blanchard, 1845. 4 v. DLC; DNLM; NNNAM; PPC **40-0407**

DUNGLISON, Robley (1798-1869)
Medical lexicon; a new dictionary of medical science. . . . 5th ed. Philadelphia: Lea & Blanchard, 1845. 771p. CU-M; PPC; ViRA **40-0408**

DUNGLISON, Robley (1798-1869)
An introductory lecture, delivered before the class of institutes of medicine, in Jefferson Medical College, November 3, 1845. . . . Philadelphia: The class, 1845. 24p. DLC; PPC; PPJ **40-0409**

DUNGLISON, Robley (1798-1869)
Medical lexicon; a new dictionary of medical science. . . . 6th ed. Philadelphia: Lea & Blanchard, 1846. 808p. CtY-M; MBM; PPC; PPJ **40-0410**

DUNGLISON, Robley (1798-1869)
New remedies; the methods of preparing and administering them, their effects on the healthy and diseased economy. . . . 5th ed. Philadelphia: Lea & Blanchard, 1846. 639p. DNLM; MBM; NNNAM; PPC **40-0411**

DUNGLISON, Robley (1798-1869)
General therapeutics and materia medica, adapted for a medical text book. . . . 3rd ed., rev. and imp. Philadelphia: Lea & Blanchard, 1846. 2 v. DNLM; MBM; NNNAM; PPC **40-0412**

DUNGLISON, Robley (1798-1869)
An introductory lecture . . . in Jefferson Medical College. Philadelphia: Merrihew & Thompson, 1847. 24p. DNLM; PPC; PPJ **40-0413**

DUNGLISON, Robley (1798-1869)
Charge to the graduates of Jefferson Medical College of Philadelphia; delivered March 25, 1847. With a list of the graduates. Philadelphia: J. C. Clark, 1847. 20p. DNLM; PPC; PPJ **40-0414**

DUNGLISON, Robley (1798-1869)
Medical lexicon; a new dictionary of medical science. . . . 7th ed. Philadelphia: Lea & Blanchard, 1848. 912p. DNLM; PPC; NNNAM; ViRA **40-0415**

DUNGLISON, Robley (1798-1869)
The practice of medicine, or a treatise on special pathology and therapeutics. 3rd ed. Philadelphia: Lea & Blanchard, 1848. 2 v. DNLM; PPC; PPJ; PU **40-0416**

DUNGLISON, Robley (1798-1869)
An introductory lecture delivered to the class of institutes of medicine, in Jefferson Medical College, October 19th, 1848. . . . Published by the class. Philadelphia: C. Sherman, printer, 1848. 20p. DLC; PPC; PPJ **40-0417**

DUNSFORD, Harris F. (1808-1847)
The practical advantages of homoeopathy, illustrated by numerous cases. Dedicated by permission to Her Majesty Queen Adelaide. . . . Philadelphia: J. Pennington, 1842. 201p. DLC; PPC; PPHa **40-0418**

DURLACHER, Lewis
A treatise on corns, bunions, the diseases of nails, and the general management of the feet. . . . Philadelphia: Lea & Blanchard, 1845. 134p. DLC; PPC; PU **40-0419**

DURLACHER, Lewis
A treatise on corns, bunions, the diseases of the nails, and the general management of the feet. . . . Philadelphia: Lea & Blanchard, 1845. 134p. DLC; PPC; PU [Designated as 2nd ed.] **40-0420**

DUVAL, Jacques Réné (1758-1854)
. . . The youth's dentist; or, The way to have sound and beautiful teeth. Designed for the more intelligent orders of parents and guardians and containing some useful hints to the faculty. . . . Transl. and supplied with notes by J. Atkinson. . . . Baltimore: The American Society of Dental Surgeons, 1848. 102p. DLC; MdU-M; MBM **40-0421**

DWINELLE, William H.
The casket and the ribbon, or the honors of ether. Baltimore: J. W. Woods, 1849. 26p. DNLM; MdU-D **40-0422**

EARLE, Pliny (1809-1892)
A visit in thirteen asylums for the insane in Europe; to which are added a brief notice of similar institutions in transatlantic countries and in the United States, and an essay on the causes, duration, termination and moral treatment of insanity. With copious statistics. . . . Philadelphia: J. Dobson, 1841. 144p. DLC; DNLM; PPC; PU **40-0423**

EARLE, Pliny (1809-1892)
A visit to thirteen asylums for the insane in Europe; to which are added a brief notice of similar institutions in transatlantic countries and in the United States, and an essay on the causes, duration, termination, and moral treatment of insanity with copious statistics. New York: Egbert, Hovey & King, 1845. 82p. DNLM; MBM; NNNAM **40-0424**

EARLE, Pliny (1809-1892)
History, description and statistics of the Bloomingdale asylum for the insane. . . . New York: Egbert, Hovey & King, printers, 1848. 136p. DLC; DNLM; NNNAM **40-0425**

EASTMAN, Buell
A practical treatise on diseases peculiar to women and girls: to which is added an eclectic system of midwifery. Also the treatment of diseases of children, and the remedies used in the cure of diseases; particularly adapted to the use of heads of families and midwives. . . . Connersville, 1845. 182p. DLC **40-0426**

EATON, Horace (1810-1883)
The field and the work of the medical profession. An address delivered before the Associated Alumni of Castleton Medical College, at their annual meeting, June 18, 1845. . . . Albany: Printed by C. Van Benthuysen & Co., 1845. 31p. DLC; DNLM; N **40-0427**

EBERLE, John (1787-1838)
Notes of lectures on the theory and practice of medicine, delivered in the Jefferson Medical College, at Philadelphia. 3rd ed. Philadelphia: Grigg & Elliot, 1840. 248p. DNLM; PPJ; PU; ViRA **40-0428**

EBERLE, John (1787-1838)
A treatise on the materia medica and therapeutics. 5th ed. Philadelphia: Grigg & Elliot, 1841. 2 v. DNLM; PPC; PU **40-0429**

EBERLE, John (1787-1838)
Notes of lectures on the theory and practice of medicine, delivered in the Jefferson Medical College, at Philadelphia. . . . 4th ed. Philadelphia: Grigg & Elliot, 1844. 248p. DLC; PPJ; PU **40-0430**

EBERLE, John (1787-1838)
A treatise on the diseases and physical education of children. 3rd ed. Philadelphia: Grigg & Elliot, 1845. 548p. DNLM; PPC; ViRA **40-0431**

EDWARDS, F. O.
Report of the Secretary of the Treasury, with the report of Dr. Edwards, on the practical operation of the law for the prevention of the importation of spurious and adulterated drugs and medicines. 30th Cong. 2nd sess. Senate Exec. Doc. No. 16. Jan. 23, 1849. 11p. [Washington, 1849]. DNLM **40-0432**

EDWARDS, H. Milne (1800-1885)
Outlines of anatomy and physiology, transl. from the French by J. F. W. Lane. Boston: Charles C. Little & James Brown, 1841. 312p. MBM; MH-M **40-0433**

ELLIOT, William
On scientific medicine, and its relations to, and claims upon society at large; an address. With an appendix. Carlisle: S. Jefferson, 1840. 44p. DNLM **40-0434**

ELLIOTSON, John (1791-1868)
Numerous cases of surgical operations without pain in the mesmeric state; with remarks upon the opposition of many members of the Royal Medical and Chirurgical Society and others to the reception of the inestimable blessings of mesmerism. . . . Philadelphia: Lea & Blanchard, 1843. 56p. DLC; DNLM; PPC; PU **40-0435**

ELLIOTSON, John (1791-1868)
The principles and practice of medicine. . . . Ed. by Nathaniel Rogers . . . and Alexander Cooper Lee. 1st American from the 2nd London ed., greatly enlarged and improved. With notes and additions by Thomas Stewardson. . . . Philadelphia: Carey & Hart, 1844. 1046p. DLC; PPC; ViRA **40-0436**

ELLIS, Benjamin (1798-1831)
The medical formulary: being a collection of prescriptions, derived from the writings and practice of many of the most eminent physicians in America and Europe. To which is added an appendix, containing the usual dietetic preparations and antidotes for poisons. The whole accompanied with a brief pharmaceutic and medical observations. . . . 6th ed., rev. and extended. By Samuel George Morton, M.D. Philadelphia: Lea & Blanchard, 1842. 262p. DLC; PPHa; PPJ **40-0437**

ELLIS, Benjamin (1798-1831)
The medical formulary: being a collection of prescriptions, derived from the writings and practice of many of the most eminent physicians in America and Europe. To which is added an appendix, containing the usual dietetic preparations and antidotes for poisons. The whole accompanied with a brief pharmaceutic and medical observations. . . . 7th ed., revised and extended by Samuel George Morton. Philadelphia: Lea & Blanchard, 1843. 263p. DNLM; PPC; PU **40-0438**

ELLIS, Benjamin (1798-1831)
The medical formulary: being a collection of prescriptions, derived from the writings and practice of many of the most eminent physicians in America and Europe. To which is added an appendix, containing the usual dietetic preparations and antidotes for poisons. The whole accompanied with a few brief pharmaceutic and medical observations. . . . 8th ed. [much improved and extended] with numerous additions. By Samuel George Morton, M.D. Philadelphia: Lea & Blanchard, 1846. 272p. DLC; OCLloyd; PPC **40-0439**

ELLIS, Benjamin (1798-1831)
The medical formulary: being a collection of prescriptions, derived from the writings and practice of many of the most eminent physicians in America and Europe. To which is added an appendix, containing the usual dietetic preparations and antidotes for poisons. The whole accompanied with a few brief pharmaceutic and medical observations. . . . 9th ed., corrected and extended by Samuel George Morton. Philadelphia: Lea & Blanchard, 1849. 267p. DNLM; GU; PPC; PPHa **40-0440**

ELLIS, George W.
Synopsis of phrenology: presenting general principles of the science, a description of the mental organs, and their location; also a combination, showing the manner in which they assist or counteract each other. . . . 4th ed., rev. Boston: Printed by A. J. Wright, 1844. 48p. DLC; MWA; MBAt **40-0441**

EMMONS, E[benezer] (1799-1863)
Introductory address, delivered before the class of the Albany Medical College. Albany: Carroll & Cook, 1845. 24p. DNLM **40-0442**

EPPS, John (1805-1869)
Domestic homoeopathy; or, Rules for the domestic treatment of the maladies of infants, children, and adults, and for the conduct and the treatment during pregnancy, confinement, and suckling. . . . 1st American ed. Boston: Otis Clapp, 1843. 200p. PPHa; PPPH **40-0443**

EPPS, John (1805-1869)
Domestic homoeopathy; or, Rules for the domestic treatment of the maladies of infants, children, and adults, and for the conduct and the treatment during pregnancy, confinement, and suckling. . . . 2nd American, from 4th London ed. Boston: Otis Clapp, 1845. 239p. PPHa **40-0444**

EPPS, John (1805-1869)
An answer to the question: "What is homoeopathy?" . . . Republished by E. H. Clapp, M.D. Columbus, O.: Hazewell & Co., 1846. 16p. PPHa; PPH **40-0445**

EPPS, John (1805-1869)
Domestic homoeopathy; or, Rules for the domestic treatment of the maladies of infants, children, and adults, and for the conduct and the treatment during pregnancy, confinement, and suckling. . . . 3rd American, from 4th London ed. Edited and enlarged by George W. Cook, M.D. Boston: Otis Clapp, 1848. 287p. PPHa; PPH **40-0446**

EPPS, John (1805-1869)
What is homoeopathy? From the 3rd London ed. New York: J. T. S. Smith [1848?] 16p. DNLM; PPHa **40-0447**

ESQUIROL, Jean Etienne Dominique (1772-1840)
On mental diseases. . . . Philadelphia, 1840. 30p. DNLM **40-0448**

ESQUIROL, Jean Etienne Dominique (1772-1840)
Mental maladies. A treatise on insanity. . . . Transl. from the French, with additions, by E. K. Hunt, M.D. Philadelphia: Lea & Blanchard, 1845. 496p. DLC; DNLM; PPC **40-0449**

EUSTAPHIEVE, Alexis
Homoeopathia revealed. A brief exposition of the whole system adapted to general comprehension. 2nd ed. with a sketch of isopathia. Inscribed to John Forbes, M.D. New York: D. Fanshaw, 1846. 91p. DNLM; PPHa **40-0450**

EVANS, Charles (1802-1879)
Account of the Asylum for the relief of persons deprived of the use of their reason, near Frankford, Pennsylvania; with the statistics of the institution from its foundation to the 31st 12th month, 1838. Philadelphia: J. Rakestraw, 1846. 14p. DNLM; PPC **40-0451**

EVANS, J. P.
Popular address, delivered before the Medical Society of East Tennessee. Together with rules of medical etiquet [sic] . . . . Knoxville, Tenn.: H. & I. E. Barry, 1847. 14p. DNLM **40-0452**

EVANS, John (1824-1897)
Observations on the spread of Asiatic cholera, and its communicable nature. [Chicago, 1849] 43p. DNLM **40-0453**

EVANSON, Richard T.
A practical treatise on the management and diseases of children. By Richard T. Evanson . . . and Henry Maunsell. . . . 2nd American, from the 4th Dublin ed., with notes, by D. Francis Condie. . . . Philadelphia: E. Barrington & G. D. Haswell, 1843. 372p. DLC; DNLM; PPC; ViRA **40-0454**

EVANSON, Richard T.
A practical treatise on the management and diseases of children. By R. T. Evanson, M.D., and H. Maunsell, M.D. . . . From the 5th Dublin ed. Boston: Press of T. R. Marvin, 1848. 430p. DLC; DNLM; MBM; NNNAM **40-0455**

EVE, Joseph Adams (1805-1886)
Introductory lecture, delivered in the Medical College of Georgia, at the opening of the annual session, November 6th, 1848. . . . [Published by the class] Augusta, Ga.: Printed by J. McCafferty, 1848. 23p. DLC; DNLM; GU **40-0456**

EVE, Paul Fitzsimmons (1806-1877)
The present position of the medical profession in society. An introductory lecture. Augusta: J. M. McCafferty, 1849. 24p. DNLM; GU **40-0457**

EVEREST, Thomas Roupell
A popular view of homoeopathia. From the 2nd ed. With annotations and a brief survey of the progress and present state of homoeopathia in Europe. By A. Gerald Hull. New York: W. Raddle, 1842. 243p. DNLM; PPHa **40-0458**

EVERETT, Edward (1795-1865)
Address delivered at the opening of the new Medical College in North Grove Street, Boston, November 6, 1846. And the introductory lecture by George Hayward. Boston: William D. Ticknor & Co., 1846. 36p. DNLM; MBM; MHi **40-0459**

EVERY man's doctor: containing a condensed description of the various causes and symptoms of diseases; with an appendix, showing the medical properties of the most valuable roots and herbs. . . . New York: J. K. Wellman, 1844. 72p. DLC; NNNAM **40-0460**

EWELL, James (1773-1832)
The medical companion, or Family physician: treating of the diseases of the United States, with their symptoms, causes, cure, and means of prevention. . . . 10th ed., rev., enl., and very considerably improved. . . . Philadelphia: Thomas, Cowperthwait & Co., 1847. 692p. DLC; PPC; PPJ; PPL **40-0461**

EWELL, James (1773-1832)
The medical companion, or family physician: treating of the diseases of the United States, with their symptoms, causes, cure, and means of prevention. . . . 10th ed., rev., enl., and very considerably improved. . . . Philadelphia: Pub. by Crissy & Markley, for J. A. Geer, 1848. 692p. DLC; PPC; PPJ; PU **40-0462**

FERGUSON, Edward J.
Observations on the nervous system, and the neuroses; being the subject of a course of lectues. [Buffalo] : C. F. S. Thomas [1843], 16p. DNLM **40-0463**

FERGUSSON, William (1808-1877)
A system of practical surgery. . . . With two hundred and forty-six illustrations, from drawings by Bagg. . . . With notes and additional illustrations, by George W. Norris. . . . Philadelphia: Lea & Blanchard, 1843. 629p. DLC; PPC; NNNAM; ViRA **40-0464**

FERGUSSON, William (1808-1877)
A system of practical surgery. . . . With two hundred and fifty-two illustrations, from drawings by Bagg, engraved by Gilbert. 2nd American ed. With notes and additional illustrations, by George W. Norris. . . . Philadelphia: Lea & Blanchard, 1845. 639p. DLC; DNLM; ICU; PPPH **40-0465**

FERGUSSON, William (1808-1877)
A system of practical surgery. . . . 3rd American from the last English ed. With two hundred and seventy-four illustrations by Bagg, engraved by Gilbert. Philadelphia: Lea & Blanchard, 1848. 630p. DLC; NBM; PPC; PPJ **40-0466**

FEUCHTWANGER, Lewis
The mad dog: or Hydrophobia, with all its various symptoms, causes, and remedies, minutely described. . . . New York: W. Applegate, 1840. 16p. 1 plate. DLC; DNLM; NNNAM **40-0467**

FISHER, William R.
Introductory lecture delivered at the Philadelphia College of Pharmacy. Philadelphia: Merrihew & Thompson, 1842. 21p. DNLM; PPC; PPHa **40-0468**

FITCH, G. N.
Valedictory to the graduates of Rush Medical College, Chicago. Chicago: W. Ellis, 1847. 22p. DNLM; ICRM; ICU **40-0469**

FITCH, Samuel Sheldon
Diseases of the chest. A treatise on the uses of the lungs and on the cause and cure of pulmonary consumption. . . . Philadelphia: Hooker & Agnew, 1841. 175p. DNLM; NcD; PPC; PU **40-0470**

FITCH, Samuel Sheldon
Six lectures on the uses of the lungs: and cure of pulmonary consumption, asthma, and diseases of the heart: on the laws of longevity. . . . New York: H. Carlisle, 1847. 324p. DLC; DNLM; NNNAM **40-0471**

FITCH, Samuel Sheldon
Manual for persons using the remedies of S. S. Fitch. New York: C. M. Fitch [1848]. 74p. CtY-M; DLC; DNLM; MBM **40-0472**

FITCH, Samuel Sheldon
Guide to invalids; for persons using the remedies of Samuel Sheldon Fitch. With remarks on the cure of consumption. . . . New York: Fitch [1849]. 48p. DNLM; MB: NNNAM **40-0473**

FLEMING, L. D.
Self-pollution the cause of youthful decay; showing the dangers and remedy of venereal exercise. New York: J. K. Wellman, 1846. 70p. DNLM; PPC **40-0474**

FLEMING, L. D.
A popular lecture on the philosophy and claims of homoeopathy. Boston: O. Clapp, 1848. 11p. DNLM; PPHa **40-0475**

FLINT, Austin (1812-1886)
The reciprocal duties and obligations of the medical profession and the public: a public introductory lecture delivered at the Rush Medical College, commencement 1844-1845. Chicago: Z. Eastman, 1844. 24p. DNLM; ICRM; NNNAM **40-0476**

FOLTZ, Jonathan Messersmith (1810-1877)
The endemic influence of evil government, illustrated in a view of the climate, topography, and diseases, of the Island of Minorca, with medical statistics of a voyage of circumnavigation of the globe, and an account of other service, both ashore and afloat. . . . New York: J. & H. G. Langley, 1843. 65p. DNLM; NNNAM; PPL **40-0477**

FOLTZ, Jonathan Messersmith (1810-1877)
Report on the scorbutus as it appeared on board the United States squadron, blockading the ports in the Gulf of Mexico, in the summer of 1846. Philadelphia: T. K. & P. G. Collins, 1848. 23p. DNLM; PPF; PPL **40-0478**

FOOTE, John
Ophthalmic memoranda respecting those diseases of the eye which are more frequently met within practice. New York: S. S. & W. Wood, 1848. 135p. DNLM; NNNAM; MBM; PPC **40-0479**

FORBES, John (1787-1861)
Homoeopathy, allopathy, and young physic. Philadelphia: Lindsay & Blakiston, 1846. 121p. DLC; DNLM; PPHa **40-0480**

FORBES, John (1787-1861)
Homoeopathy, allopathy, and young physic. New York: William Radde, 1846. 58p. DNLM; PPHa **40-0481**

FORBES, John (1787-1861)
Review of hydropathy, or the water-cure. Also the opinions of Magendie, Bichat, Forbes, and others. [Troy, N.Y.]: W. A. Hamilton, 1848. 24p. DNLM **40-0482**

FORBES, John, Alex. Tweedie, John Conolly, eds.
The cyclopedia of practical medicine, comprising treatises on the nature and treatment of diseases, materia medica and therapeutics, medical jurisprudence . . . thoroughly revised with numerous additions by Robley Dunglison. Philadelphia: Blanchard & Lea, 1845. 4 v. CtY-M; DLC; DNLM; PPC **40-0483**

FORD, Lewis D. (1801-1883)
An introductory lecture delivered in the Medical College of Georgia, at the opening of the session of 1842-1843. Augusta. James McCafferty, 1843. 23p. GU **40-0484**

FORDYCE, George (1736-1802)
Five dissertations on fever. . . . 2nd American ed., with an introduction. Philadelphia: E. Barrington & G. D. Haswell, 1846. 403p. DLC; DNLM; PPC; PU **40-0485**

FORMAN, Jacob Gilbert
Elements of phrenology applied to the human character. . . . Cincinnati: Printed by W. L. Mendenhall, 1844. 50p. DLC; MH; MBAt **40-0486**

FORRY, Samuel (1811-1844)
The climate of the United States and its endemic influences. Based chiefly on the records of the Medical Department and Adjutant General's Office, United States Army. 2nd ed. New York: J. & H. G. Langley, 1842. 378p. 2 plates. DNLM; MBM; NNNAM **40-0487**

FORT, Tomlinson (1787-1859)
A dissertation on the practice of medicine. Containing an account of the causes, symptoms and treatment of diseases: and adapted to the use of physicians and families. . . . Milledgeville, Ga.: Printed at the Federal Union Office, 1849. 740p. DNLM; GU; MBM; NNNAM **40-0488**

FOWLER, Lorenzo Niles
Marriage: its history and ceremonies; with a phrenological and physiological exposition of the functions and qualifications for happy marriages. New York: Fowler & Wells, 1848. 216p. DNLM; NNNAM **40-0489**

FOWLER, Orson Squire (1809-1887)
A lecture on temperance considered physiologically and phrenologically . . . ; or the laws of life. . . . 2nd ed. Philadelphia, 1841. 32p. DNLM; PPC **40-0490**

FOWLER, Orson Squire (1809-1887)
Tight lacing, or the evils of compressing the organs of animal life. New York: O. S. & L. N. Fowler [1844?] 16p. DNLM **40-0491**

FOWLER, Orson Squire (1809-1887)
Education and self-improvement, founded on physiology and phrenology: or, What constitutes good heads and bodies, and how to make them good, by enlarging deficiencies and diminishing excesses. . . . New York: O. S. & L. N. Fowler; Boston: Saxton & Peirce, 1844-1846. 3 v. in 2. DLC; MBM; NNNAM **40-0492**

FOWLER, Orson Squire (1809-1887)
Fowler's practical phrenology: giving a concise elementary view of phrenology. . . . With references to . . . pages of "Phrenology proved, illustrated, and applied." . . . 22nd ed., enl. and improved. New York: O. S. & L. N. Fowler; Boston: Saxton & Peirce's phrenological depot, 1845. 71p. DLC; MBM; NNNAM **40-0493**

FOWLER, Orson Squire (1809-1887)
Tight lacing, or the evils of compressing the organs of animal life. New York: Fowler & Wells, 1846. 16p. DNLM; NNNAM **40-0494**

FOWLER, Orson Squire (1809-1887)
Temperance, founded on phrenology and physiology: or, The laws of life, and the principles of the human consitution, as developed by the sciences of phrenology and physiology, applied to total abstinence from all alcoholic and intoxicating drinks. . . . 24th ed., enl. and improved. . . . New York: Fowler's & Wells' phrenological cabinet; Boston: Saxton & Kelt, 1846. 32p. DLC; MBM; NNNAM **40-0495**

FOWLER, Orson Squire (1809-1887)
Physiology, animal and mental: applied to the preservation and restoration of health of body, and power of mind. . . . New York: Fowler & Wells, 1847. 312p. DLC; NNNAM **40-0496**

FOWLER, Orson Squire (1809-1887)
Maternity: or the bearing and nursing of children. Including female education and beauty. New York: Fowler & Wells, 1848. 221p. NN; NNNAM **40-0497**

FOWNES, George (1815-1849)
Chemistry, as exemplifying the wisdom and beneficence of God. (Actonian prize essay.) New York & Philadelphia: Wiley & Putnam, & J. W. Moore, 1844. 158p. DNLM; OCIM; PPC; ViRA **40-0498**

FOWNES, George (1815-1849)
Elementary chemistry, theoretical and practical. Ed. with additions by Robert Bridges. A new ed. Philadelphia: Lea & Blanchard, 1847. 460p. DNLM; PPC; PPJ; PU **40-0499**

FOX, Joseph
The natural history and diseases of the human teeth. . . . 1st American from the 3rd London ed. Edited by Chapin A. Harris. Philadelphia: E. Barrington, 1846. 440p. MBM; NNNAM; PU; ViRA **40-0500**

FRANCIS, John Wakefield (1789-1861)
A discourse; delivered upon the opening of the new hall of the New York Lyceum of Natural History. New York: H. Ludwig, 1841. 93p. DNLM; NN; NNNAM **40-0501**

FRANCIS, John Wakefield (1789-1861)
Anniversary discourse before the New York Academy of Medicine. Delivered in the Broadway Tabernacle, November 10th, 1847. . . . New York: Printed by H. Ludwig, 1847. 112p. DLC; DNLM; NNNAM **40-0502**

FRANCIS, John Wakefield (1789-1861)
An inaugural address, delivered before the New York Academy of Medicine, Feb. 2nd, 1848. . . . New York: H. Ludwig & Co., 1848. 23p. DLC; DNLM; NNNAM **40-0503**

FRANCIS, John Wakefield (1789-1861)
Address of . . . , late president of the New York Academy of Medicine, on the 7th of February, 1849. To the president-elect, Valentine Mott, M.D. New York: Printed by H. Ludwig & Co., 1849. 8p. DLC; NNNAM **40-0504**

FRAZEE, L. J[acob] (1819-1905)
The medical student in Europe. Maysville, Ky.: R. H. Collins, 1849. 297p. 1 plate. DNLM; KyLoJM **40-0505**

GALT, John Minson (1819-1862)
Practical medicine; illustrated by cases of the most important diseases. Philadelphia: Barrington & Haswell, 1843. 328p. DNLM; PPC; PPJ; PU **40-0506**

GANNAL, Jean Nicolas (1791-1852)
History of embalming, and of preparations in anatomy, pathology, and natural history; including an account of a new process for embalming. . . . Transl. from the French, with notes and additions. By R. Harlan, M.D. Philadelphia: J. Dobson, 1840. 264p. DLC; DNLM; PPC; PU **40-0507**

GARDETTE, Emile B[laise] (1803-1887)
Biographical notice of [the late] James Gardette, dentist, of Philadelphia. Philadelphia, 1847. 22p. DNLM; PU **40-0508**

GARDETTE, Emile B[laise] (1803-1887)
Valedictory address to the graduating class of the Baltimore College of Dental Surgery. Baltimore: J. W. Woods, 1849. 24p. DNLM; MdBM; MdU-D **40-0509**

GARDNER, D. P.
An introductory lecture on the relations of chemistry to the vital force. Philadelphia: J. H. Gihon, 1847. 11p. DNLM; PPC; PPL **40-0510**

GARDNER, D. P.
An introductory lecture on the chemical relations of plants to animals. Philadelphia: J. H. Gihon, 1848. 18p. DNLM; PPF; PPL **40-0511**

GARDNER, D. P.
Medical chemistry for the use of students and the profession. Philadelphia: Lea & Blanchard, 1848. 396p. DNLM; PPC; PPJ; PU **40-0512**

GARIOT, J. B.
. . . Treatise on diseases of the mouth. . . . Transl. by J. B. Savier. Baltimore: American Society of Dental Surgeons, 1843. 162p. DNLM; MdU-D; PU **40-0513**

GAY, Martin (1804?-1850)
A statement of the claims of Charles T. Jackson, M.D., to the discovery of the applicability of sulphuric ether to the prevention of pain in surgical operations. Boston: D. Clapp, 1847. 29p. DNLM; MBM; NcD; NNNAM **40-0514**

GEIB, W.
An essay on homoeopathy. A synopsis of the history and principles of the science, with the author's opinion of palliative remedies. Designed principally for lay readers. Philadelphia: J. Dobson, 1842. 24p. PPHa **40-0515**

GERHARD, William Wood (1809-1872)
Lectures on the diagnosis, pathology, and treatment of the diseases of the chest. . . . Philadelphia: Haswell & Barrington, 1842. 157p. 1 plate. DLC; DNLM; PCC; PU **40-0516**

GERHARD, William Wood (1809-1872)
Lectures on the diagnosis, pathology, and treatment of the diseases of the chest. . . . 2nd ed. Philadelphia: Barrington & Haswell, 1846. 288p. DNLM; PPC; PPJ; PU **40-0517**

GERRISH, Andrew
A synopsis on the prevention and cure of disease. Boston: Saxton & Peirce, 1841. 208p. DNLM; MBM; MH-M; MWA **40-0518**

GIBBES, Robert Wilson (1809-1866)
A lecture on the magnetism of the human body. Columbia, S.C. Dubose & Johnston, 1843. 37p. DNLM; ScCM; ScMS **40-0519**

GIBBONS, Henry, Sr. (1808-1884)
Valedictory address to the graduating class of the Philadelphia College of Medicine. Philadelphia: J. H. Gihon, 1848. 16p. DNLM; PU **40-0520**

GIBBONS, Henry, Sr. (1808-1884)
Introductory lecture to the summer course of 1849 in the Philadelphia College of Medicine. Philadelphia: Merrihew & Thompson, 1849. 24p. DNLM; PU **40-0521**

GIBERT, Camille-Melchior
Changes of the blood in disease. Transl. from the French by John H. Dix. [Dunglison's American Medical Library] Philadelphia: Barrington & Haswell, 1843. 59p. DNLM; PPC; PU **40-0522**

GIBSON, William (1788-1868)
Institutes and practice of surgery: being outlines of a course of lectures. . . . 6th ed., much enl. and improved. . . . Philadelphia: J. Kay, Jr. & Brother; Pittsburgh: C. H. Kay & Co., 1841. 2 v. 34 plates. DLC; DNLM; PPC; PU **40-0523**

GIBSON, William (1788-1868)
Lecture introductory to a course on the principles and practice of surgery in the University of Pennsylvania. Philadelphia: N. B. Manning, 1841. 34p. DNLM; PPC; PU **40-0524**

GIBSON, William (1788-1868)
Rambles in Europe, in 1839. With sketches of prominent surgeons, physicians, medical schools, hospitals, literary personages, scenery. . . . Philadelphia: Lea & Blanchard, 1841. 309p. DLC; DNLM; PPC; ViRA **40-0525**

GIBSON, William (1788-1868)
Lecture, introductory to a course on the principles and practice of surgery, in the University of Pennsylvania, delivered November 6, 1843. . . . Philadelphia: King & Baird, printers, 1843. 24p. DLC; DNLM; PPC; ScCM **40-0526**

GIBSON, William (1788-1868)
Introductory lecture before the medical class of the University of Pennsylvania, delivered Nov. 4, 1844. . . . Philadelphia: I. Ashmead, printer, 1844. 25p. DLC; DNLM; PU; ScMS **40-0527**

GIBSON, William (1788-1868)
Institutes and practice of surgery: being outlines of a course of lectures. . . . 7th ed., improved and altered. . . . Philadelphia: J. Kay, Jr. and Brother; Pittsburgh: C. H. Kay, 1845. 2 v. DLC; DNLM; NNNAM; PPC **40-0528**

GIBSON, William (1788-1868)
Valedictory address, to the class of medical graduates of the University of Pennsylvania, on the third of April, 1846. . . . Published by request of the class. Philadelphia: L. R. Bailey, printer, 1846. 16p. DLC; DNLM; PPC; PU **40-0529**

GIBSON, William (1788-1868)
Lecture, introductory to a course, on surgery, in the University of Pennsylvania, containing a short account of eminent British surgeons, physicians, scientific and literary men; delivered October 22, 1847. . . . Philadelphia: J. G. Auner, 1847. 32p. DLC; PPC; ScCM; ViRA **40-0530**

GIBSON, William (1788-1868)
Lecture, correlative to a course, on surgery, in the University of Pennsylvania, embracing a short account of eminent Belgian surgeons, physicians, . . . Philadelphia: J. G. Auner, 1848. 32p. DNLM; PPC; PU **40-0531**

GILBERT, David (1803-1868)
Lecture introductory to the course of principles and practice of surgery in the medical department of Pennsylvania College, Philadelphia. Philadelphia: W. S. Young, 1844. 12p. DNLM; PPC; PU **40-0532**

GILBERT, David (1803-1868)
Valedictory address to the graduating class of the medical department of Pennsylvania College. Philadelphia: King & Baird, 1846. 14p. DNLM; PU **40-0533**

GILBERT, David (1803-1868)
Introductory lecture to the course on the principles and practice of surgery, in the medical department of Pennsylvania College. Philadelphia: King & Baird, 1846. 18p. DNLM; PU **40-0534**

GILBERT, David (1803-1868)
An introductory lecture to the course of the principles and practice of surgery in the medical department of Pennsylvania College. Philadelphia, [1849]. 16p. DNLM; PU **40-0535**

GOLDSMITH, Alban (*b.* 1788)
Lithotripsy; or, The breaking of stone in the bladder. . . . New York: Printed by J. F. Birch, 1843. 24p. DLC: DNLM; NNNAM **40-0536**

GOLDSMITH, Middleton (1818-1887)
An introductory lecture delivered in the Castleton Medical College at the opening of the fall session, 1846. Whitehall, N.Y.: Democrat Print., 1846. 15p. DNLM; MBM; NNC
40-0537

GOOCH, Robert (1784-1830)
An account of some of the most important diseases peculiar to women. . . . 2nd ed. Philadelphia: E. Barrington & G. D. Haswell, 1848. 322p. PPJ; PTC; PU; ViRA
40-0538

GOOD, Peter P.
The family flora and materia medica botanica, containing the botanical analysis, natural history, and chemical and medical properties of plants. Illustrated by colored engravings of original drawings, copied from nature. Elizabethtown, N.J., 1847. 2 v. 52 plates. DNLM; NjR; OCLloyd
40-0539

GORMAN, John B.
Philosophy of animated existence; or, sketches of living physics, with discussions of physiology philosophical. To which is added a brief medical account of the middle regions of Georgia. Philadelphia: Sorin & Ball, 1845. 570p. DNLM; GU; PPC **40-0540**

GOVE, Mary S.
Lectures to ladies on anatomy and physiology. Boston: Saxton & Peirce, 1842. 300p. DNLM; MB; MBM; MH
40-0541

GRAETER, Francis
Hydriatics; or, a manual of the water cure. . . . 3rd ed. New York: W. Radde, 1843. 198p. 1 plate. DNLM; NNNAM
40-0542

GRAETER, Francis
Hydriatics; Or, a manual of the water cure. . . . 4th ed. New York: W. Radde, 1844. 198p. 1 plate. DNLM; NNNAM
40-0543

GRANT, Geo. R.
An introductory address, delivered at the opening of the session of 1847-1848, to the students of the Memphis Medical College, November 1, 1847. Memphis, 1847. 18p. DNLM; KyLoJM **40-0544**

GRANT, William R. (1811-1853)
An introductory lecture to the course of anatomy and physiology in the medical department of Pennsylvania College, Philadelphia: Barrett & Jones,1845. 15p. DLC; DNLM; PU
40-0545

GRANT, William R. (1811-1853)
Valedictory address to the graduating class of the medical department of Pennsylvania College. Philadelphia, 1848. 14p. DNLM; PU **40-0546**

GRAVES, Robert James (1796-1853)
Sketch of the origin and progress of Asiatic cholera. Philadelphia: Carey & Hart, 1841. 55p. DNLM; PPC: PPJ; PU
40-0547

GRAVES, Robert James (1796-1853)
Clinical lectures. . . . 2nd American ed., with notes and a series of lectures, by W. W. Gerhard. . . . Philadelphia: E. Barrington & G. D. Haswell; New York: J. & H. G. Langley [etc., etc.] 1842. 560p. DLC; IEN-M; MBM; PPC **40-0548**

GRAVES, Robert James (1796-1853)
A system of clinical medicine. . . . With notes and a series of lectures, by W. W. Gerhard. 3rd American ed. Philadelphia: E. Barrington & G. D. Haswell, 1848. 751p. CtY-M; DLC; DNLM; PPC **40-0549**

GRAVIORA, Manent (pseud.)
Letters on the College of Physicians and Sugeons. New York: A. S. Gould, 1841. 16p. DNLM; NN; NNC; NNNAM
40-0550

GRAY, S. C.
The human teeth, their development, importance to health, and means of preservation. Cincinnati: Dumas & Lawyer [1849?]. 12p. DNLM; OC **40-0551**

GREEN, Horace (1802-1866)
A treatise on diseases of the air passages: comprising an inquiry into the history, pathology, causes, and treatment of those affections of the throat called bronchitis, chronic laryngitis, clergyman's sore throat. . . . New York & London: Wiley & Putnam, 1846. 276p. DNLM; MBM; NNNAM; ViRA
40-0552

GREEN, Horace (1802-1866)
A treatise on diseases of the air passages: comprising an inquiry into the history, pathology, causes, and treatment, of those affections of the throat called bronchitis, chronic laryngitis, clergyman's sore throat. . . . 2nd ed., rev. and enl. New York: G. P. Putnam; London: Putnam's American Agency, 1849. 306p. DLC; MBM; NNNAM; PPC **40-0553**

GREEN, Horace (1802-1866)
Observations on the pathology of croup: with remarks on its treatment by topical medications. . . . New York: J. Wiley, 1849. 115p. DLC; DNLM; NNNAM
40-0554

GREEN, James Mercer
A case of carotid aneurism, and some remarks on the diagnosis of that disease; with Dr. Paul F. Eve's comments thereon, and a reply. Macon: B. F. Griffin, 1848. 56p. DNLM; GU
40-0555

GREEN, John Orne (1799-1885)
The factory system in its hygienic relations. An address. Boston: W. S. Damrell, 1846. 34p. DNLM; MH
40-0556

GREEN, Jonas (1798?-1868)
A familiar exposition of homoeopathy, or the new system of curing diseases. Illustrating its superiority over the prevalent system of medicine. . . . Washington: J. & G. S. Gideon, printers, 1845. 12p. DLC; DNLM; PPHa
40-0557

GREGORY, Holly
The Rubicon; or unfortunates' friend and pocket medical companion; detailing the origin, progress and circumstances of venereal disease, with instructions for its treatment. New York, 1840. 59p. DNLM; NNNAM
40-0558

GREGORY, Samuel (1813-1872)
Man-midwifery exposed and corrected; or, The employment of men to attend women in childbirth, and in other delicate circumstances, shown to be a modern innovation, unnecessary, unnatural, and injurious to the physical welfare of the community, and pernicious in its influence on professional and public morality; and the whole proved by numerous facts, and the testimony of the most eminent physicians, in Boston, New York, and other places; and the education and employment of midwives recommended: together with remarks on the use and abuse of ether, and Dr. Channing's "Cases of inhalation of ether in labor." . . . Boston: G. Gregory; New York: Fowlers and Wells, 1848. 50p. DLC; DNLM; MBM; NNNAM
40-0559

GRIFFITH, John William
A practical manual, containing a description of the general chemical and microscopical characters of the blood, and secretions of the human body. . . . Philadelphia: Lea & Blanchard, 1848. 182p. 4 plates. DNLM; PPC; PU
40-0560

GRIFFITH, Robert Eglesfeld (1798-1850)
Medical botany; or, Descriptions of the more important plants used in medicine, with their history, properties, and mode of administration. . . . With upwards of three hundred illustrations. Philadelphia: Lea & Blanchard, 1847. 704p. DLC; DNLM; OCLloyd; PPC **40-0561**

GRISCOM, John Hoskins (1809-1874)
Spinal irritation; its history, diagnosis, pathology, and treatment, illustrated by cases. An essay read before the New York Medical and Surgical Society, November, 1839. . . . New York: Printed by Hopkins & Jennings, 1840. 52p. DLC; DNLM; NNNAM **40-0562**

GRISCOM, John Hoskins (1809-1874)
The sanitary condition of the laboring population of New York. With suggestions for its improvement. New York: Harper & Bros., 1845. 58p. DNLM; NNC; NN; NNNAM
40-0563

GROSS, Samuel D[avid] (1805-1884)
Experimental and critical inquiry into the nature and treatment of wounds of the intestines. Louisville: Prentice & Weissinger, 1843. 219p. 1 plate. DNLM; MBM; PPC; PPJ
40-0564

GROSS, Samuel David (1805-1884)
Elements of pathological anatomy. . . . 2nd ed., thoroughly rev. and greatly enl. Philadelphia: E. Barrington & G. D. Haswell, 1845. 822p. 6 plates. DLC; DNLM; MBM; PPJ
40-0565

GUNN, John C. (1800-1863)
Domestic medicine; or, poor man's friend in the hours of affliction, pain, and sickness. . . . It also contains descriptions of the medicinal roots and herbs of the United States, and how they are to be used in the cure of diseases. The last revised ed. Louisville: A. Mygatt, 1840. 893p. 10 plates. DNLM; OCIM **40-0566**

GUNN, John C. (1800-1863)
Domestic medicine. . . . Arranged on a new and sure plan, by which the practice of medicine is reduced to principles of common sense. First revised ed., enlarged in 1840. Philadelphia: B. J. Webb & Bro., 1844. 893p. 3 plates. DNLM; PPC; PU **40-0567**

GUTHRIE, George James (1785-1856)
On the anatomy and diseases of the urinary and sexual organs. Containing the anatomy of the bladder and of the urethra, and the treatment of the obstructions to which these passages are liable. . . . From the 3rd London ed. Philadelphia: Lea & Blanchard, 1845. 150p. DLC; DNLM; MBM; PPC
40-0568

GUY, William Augustus (1810-1885)
Principles of forensic medicine. . . . 1st American ed. With notes and additions, by Charles A. Lee. . . . New York: Harper & Brothers, 1845. 711p. DLC; DNLM; ICRM; IEN-M
40-0569

GUY, William Augustus (1810-1885)
. . . Principles of medical jurisprudence, with so much of anatomy, physiology, pathology, and the practice of medicine and surgery as are essential to be known by lawyers, coroners, magistrates, officers of the army and navy. . . . 1st American ed. Edited by C. A. Lee, M.D., who has added 200 pages of original matter, adapting the work to the wants of the medical and legal professions in the United States. . . . New York: Harper & Brothers, 1845. 711p. DLC; MBM; PU
40-0570

HAHNEMANN, Samuel (1755-1843)
Organon of homoeopathic medicine. . . . 2nd American ed. New York: William Radde, 1843. 212p. NNNAM; PPHa
40-0571

HAHNEMANN, Samuel (1755-1843)
The chronic diseases; their specific nature and homoeopathic treatment. Transl. and ed. by Charles J. Hempel, with a preface by Constantine Hering. New York: William Radde, 1845-1846. 5 v. DNLM; PPHa **40-0572**

HAHNEMANN, Samuel (1755-1843)
Materia medica pura. . . . Transl. and ed. by C. J. Hempel. New York: W. Radde, 1846. 4 v. in 1. DNLM; PPHa
40-0573

HAHNEMANN, Samuel (1755-1843)
Samuel Hahnemann's organon of homoeopathic medicine. . . . 3rd American ed., with improvements and additions from the last German ed., and Dr. C. Hering's introductory remarks. . . . New York: W. Radde, 1849. 230p. DLC; DNLM; PPHa
40-0574

HALL, Charles Radclyffe
Mesmerism; its rise, progress, and mysteries in all ages and countries, being a critical inquiry into its assumed merits and history of its mock marvels, hallucinations, and frauds. 1st American ed. New York: Burgess, Stringer & Co., 1845. 166p. DNLM; MB; MH; NN **40-0575**

HALL, William W. (1810-1876)
Consumption a curable disease, illustrated in the treatment of one hundred and fifty cases. Pittsburgh, 1845. 100p. DNLM
40-0576

HALL, William W. (1810-1876)
Observations on the curability of consumption; by a new, safe and painless mode of treatment; illustrated in selections from three hundred and ten late cases. 5th ed. [n.p.], 1847. 184p. DNLM **40-0577**

HAMILTON, Frank Hastings (1813-1886)
Introductory lecture before the surgical class of Geneva Medical College. Delivered December 1, 1840. . . . Geneva, N.Y.: Printed by I. Merrell, 1840. 20p. DLC; DNLM
40-0578

HAMILTON, Frank Hastings (1813-1886)
Introductory address, delivered in the theatre of Geneva Medical College. Geneva, N.Y.: I. Merrell, 1841. 18p. DNLM
40-0579

HAMILTON, Frank Hastings (1813-1886)
Lecture on phrenology. Rochester: Shepard & Strong, 1841. 32p. DNLM **40-0580**

HAMILTON, Frank Hastings (1813-1886)
Valedictory to the graduates of Geneva Medical College, delivered January 22, 1843. Rochester: E. Shepard, 1843. 25p. DNLM **40-0581**

HAMILTON, Frank Hastings (1813-1886)
Monograph on strabismus, with cases. Buffalo: Thomas & Co., 1845. 69p. DNLM **40-0582**

HAMILTON, Frank Hastings (1813-1886)
Fracture tables. Showing the results of treatment in one hundred and thirty-six cases. Buffalo: Jewett, Thomas & Co., 1849. 8p. DNLM **40-0583**

HANCORN, James Richard (1808-1861)
Medical guide for mothers, in pregnancy, accouchement, suckling, weaning, . . . and in most of the important diseases of children. . . . From the 2nd London ed. New York: Saxton & Miles; Philadelphia: G. B. Zeiber & Co., 1844. 117p. DLC; NNNAM **40-0584**

HAND, William M.
The house surgeon and physician: designed to assist heads of families, travellers, and sea-faring people, in discerning, distinguishing, and curing disease; with concise directions for the preparation and use of a numerous collection of the best American remedies. . . . With an introduction, by J. L. Comstock, M.D. 3rd ed., rev. and improved. Hartford: S. Andrus & Son, 1847. 256p. CtY-M; DLC; MBM
40-0585

HANDY, Washington R. (1811-1857)
Valedictory address delivered before the Baltimore College of Dental Surgery. Baltimore: Woods & Crane, 1842. 16p. DNLM; MdU-D; MdBJ-W **40-0586**

HARBERT, Samuel C.
A practical treatise on the operations of surgical and mechanical dentistry. Philadelphia: Barrett & Jones, 1847. 206p. 4 plates. DNLM; MdU-D; PPC; PU **40-0587**

HARD, Nicholas (1818-1851)
A lecture on atresia vaginae. La Port: W. & J. Millikan, 1848. 14p. DNLM **40-0588**

HARE, Robert (1781-1858)
A compendium of the course of chemical instruction in the medical department of the University of Pennsylvania. For the use of his pupils. In 2 pts. 4th ed. with amendments and additions. Philadelphia: J. G. Auner, 1840-1843. 605p. 20 plates. DNLM; MB; MH; PU **40-0589**

HARE, Robert (1781-1858)
Lecture, introductory to a course on chemistry, in the University of Pennsylvania. Philadelphia: Barrett & Jones, 1843. 21p. DNLM; PU **40-0590**

HARRIS, Chapin Aaron (1806-1860)
A physiological and pathological inquiry concerning the physical characteristics of the human teeth and gums. . . . Baltimore: Armstrong & Berry, 1841. 119p. DNLM; MdU-D
40-0591

HARRIS, Chapin Aaron (1806-1860)
Dissertation on the diseases of the maxillary sinus. Philadelphia: Lea & Blanchard, 1843. 165p. DNLM; MdU-D; PU
40-0592

HARRIS, Chapin Aaron (1806-1860)
Address delivered before the American Society of Dental Surgeons, at the opening of its fourth annual meeting; Baltimore, July 18th, 1843. . . . Published by order of the society. Baltimore: Woods & Crane, printers, 1843. 22p. DLC; MdU-D; PPC **40-0593**

HARRIS, Chapin Aaron (1806-1860)
The principles and practice of dental surgery. . . . 2nd ed., rev., modified, and greatly enlarged. . . . Philadelphia: Lindsay & Blakiston, 1845. 600p. DLC; MdU-D; PU
40-0594

HARRIS, Chapin Aaron (1806-1860)
Valedictory address, delivered before the Baltimore College of Dental Surgery . . . February 17, 1846. . . . Baltimore: J. W. Woods, printer, 1846. 22p. DLC; MdU-D
40-0595

HARRIS, Chapin Aaron (1806-1860)
The principles and practice of dental surgery. . . . 3rd ed., rev., modified, and greatly enlarged. . . . Philadelphia: Lindsay & Blakiston, 1848. 752p. DLC; MdU-D; PU
40-0596

HARRIS, Chapin Aaron (1806-1860)
A dictionary of dental science, biography, bibliography and medical terminology. . . . Philadelphia: Lindsay & Blakiston, 1849. 780p. DLC; MBM; PPC; PU **40-0597**

HARRIS, William (1792-1861)
Lectures on puerperal fevers. . . . Philadelphia: T. & G. Town, 1845. 50p. DLC; DNLM; NNNAM; PPC
40-0598

HARRIS, William (1792-1861)
Lecture introductory to a course, on obstetrics and the diseases of women and children, delivered April 10, 1848. Philadelphia: T. K. & P. G. Collins, 1848. 24p. DNLM; PPC; PU
40-0599

HARRISON, John Hoffman (1808-1849)
Essay towards a correct theory of the nervous system. Philadelphia: Lea & Blanchard, 1844. 292p. DNLM; PPC; PPJ; ViRA **40-0600**

HARRISON, John Pollard (1796-1849)
An introductory lecture before the students of the Medical College of Ohio. Cincinnati: J. & C. H. Brough, 1841. 11p. DNLM; OC **40-0601**

HARRISON, John Pollard (1796-1849)
Moral exposures of the medical profession: an introductory lecture, delivered in the Medical College of Ohio; November 10th, 1842. . . . Cincinnati: Printed by R. P. Donough, 1842. 15p. DLC; DNLM; OCIM **40-0602**

HARRISON, John Pollard (1796-1849)
The sources, evils, and correctives of pride of intellect; an address. Cincinnati: J. B. & R. P. Donough, 1842. 22p. DNLM; OC **40-0603**

HARRISON, John Pollard (1796-1849)
A lecture, on the best mode of discouraging empiricism; delivered before the Ohio Medical Lyceum, January, 1843, by . . . . Cincinnati: Printed by R. P. Donough, 1843. 12p. DLC; DNLM; OCIM **40-0604**

HARRISON, John Pollard (1796-1849)
The benefits accruing to society from the medical profession. An introductory lecture. Cincinnati: R. P. Donough, 1843. 16p. DNLM **40-0605**

HARRISON, John Pollard (1796-1849)
On the formation of professional character. An introductory lecture. Cincinnati: R. P. Donough, 1844. 15p. DNLM; OC **40-0606**

HARRISON, John Pollard (1796-1849)
Medical ethics. A lecture. Cincinnati: Enquirer & Message Print, 1844. 20p. DNLM **40-0607**

HARRISON, John Pollard (1796-1849)
Elements of materia medica and therapeutics. Cincinnati: Desilver & Burr; Philadelphia: Thomas Cowperthwait & Co., 1845. 2 v. DNLM; OC; OCHP; OCLloyd **40-0608**

HARRISON, John Pollard (1796-1849)
Sources, evils, and correctives of professional discontent. An introductory lecture. Cincinnati: Ben Franklin Print. Off., 1845. 16p. DNLM; OCIM **40-0609**

HARRISON, John Pollard (1796-1849)
An introductory lecture on the reciprocal obligations of the medical profession and society. . . . Professor of materia medica in the Medical College of Ohio. Delivered November 2, 1846. Cincinnati: Printed by Looker & Co., 1846. 28p. DLC; DNLM; OCIM **40-0610**

HARRISON, John Pollard (1796-1849)
An address on the bonds of professional union, delivered before the medical association of Adams, Brown, and Clermont Counties, Ohio, at Batavia, October 30, 1847. . . . Cincinnati: Atlas Job Room Print, 1847. 27p. DLC; DNLM; OCIM **40-0611**

HARRISON, John Pollard (1796-1849)
An introductory lecture, delivered to the students of the Medical College of Ohio. Cincinnati: Collins & Van Wagner, 1847. 16p. DNLM; OCIM **40-0612**

HARRISON, John Pollard (1796-1849)
Valedictory address on the sources and benefits of professional earnestness. Delivered March 3, 1849, to the graduates of the Medical College of Ohio. . . . Cincinnati: Printed at the office of the "Western Lancet," 1849. 15p. DLC; DNLM; OCIM **40-0613**

HARRISON, Robert (1796-1858)
The Dublin dissector, or manual of anatomy; comprising a description of the bones, muscles, vessels, nerves, and viscera; also the relative anatomy of the different regions of the human body, together with the elements of pathology. . . . 1st American, from the 5th enl. Dublin ed. With additions by Robert Watts, Jr. . . . New York: J. & H. G. Langley; Philadelphia: Haswell, Barrington & Haswell, 1840. 541p. DLC; DNLM; MBM; ViRA **40-0614**

HARRISON, Robert (1796-1858)
The Dublin dissector, or manual of anatomy; comprising a description of the bones, muscles, vessels, nerves, and viscera; also the relative anatomy of the different regions of the human body, together with the elements of pathology. . . . 2nd American, from the 5th enl. Dublin ed. With additions by Robert Watts, Jr. . . . New York: J. & H. G. Langley; Philadelphia: Haswell, Barrington & Haswell [etc., etc.], 1843. 541p. DLC; DNLM; NNNAM; PPC **40-0615**

HARRISON, Robert (1796-1858)
The Dublin dissector, or manual of anatomy; comprising a description of the bones, muscles, vessels, nerves, and viscera; also the relative anatomy of the different regions of the human body, together with the elements of pathology. . . . 2nd American, from the 5th enl. Dublin ed., with additions by Robert Watts, Jr. . . . New York: J. & H. G. Langley, 1845. 541p. DLC; PPC; ScCM; ViRA **40-0616**

HARRISON, Robert (1796-1858)
A text-book of practical anatomy. . . . With additions, by an American physician. New York: S. S. & W. Wood, 1848. 720p. CU-M; DLC; DNLM; NNNAM **40-0617**

HARTMANN, Franz (1796-1853)
Practical observations on some of the chief homoeopathic remedies. Transl. from the German, with notes by A. Howard Okie, M.D., of Philadelphia. First series: aconite, bryonia, mercurius sol. Hahn., merc. subl., corr., merc. praec. ruber., merc. dulcis and chamomilla. Philadelphia: J. Dobson, 1841. 171p. DNLM; PPHa **40-0618**

HARTMANN, Franz (1796-1853)
Practical observations on some of the chief homoeopathic remedies. Transl. from the German, with notes by A. Howard Okie, M.D., Translator of Hartmann's Remedies, Part 1. Ruoff's Repertory, etc. 2nd and last series, containing: Belladonna, Nux vomica, etc. New York: William Radde, 1846. 192p. DNLM; PPHa **40-0619**

HARTMANN, Franz (1796-1853)
Hartmann's theory of acute diseases, and their homoeopathic treatment. 3rd German ed., revised and considerably enlarged by the author. Transl. with additions, and adapted to the use of the American profession, by Charles J. Hempel, M.D. New York: William Radde, 1847-1848. 2 v. DNLM; PPHa **40-0620**

HARTMANN, Franz (1796-1853)
Hartmann's theory of chronic diseases and their homoeopathic treatment. 3rd German ed., revised and considerably enlarged by the author. Transl. with additions and adapted to the American profession, by Charles J. Hempel, M.D. New York: William Radde, 1849. 2 v. DNLM; PPHa **40-0621**

HARTSHORNE, Henry (1823-1897)
Water versus hydropathy; or, An essay on water, and its true relations to medicine. . . . Philadelphia: L. P. Smith, 1847. 131p. DLC; DNLM; PPC; PU **40-0622**

HARVARD UNIVERSITY. MEDICAL SCHOOL
Annual circular of the Massachusetts Medical College, with a history of the medical department of Harvard University, a catalogue of graduates, &c. Boston: Printed by D. Clapp, 1846. 32p. MH; MH-M **40-0623**

HARVARD UNIVERSITY. MEDICAL SCHOOL
A list of books belonging to the library of the Massachusetts Medical College. Boston: D. Clapp, 1847. 23p. DNLM; MH; MH-M; MBAt **40-0624**

HASSE, Charles Ewald
An anatomical description of the diseases of the organs of circulation and respiration. Transl. and ed. by W. E. Swaine. Philadelphia: Lea & Blanchard, 1846. 377p. MBM; NNNAM; PPC; PU **40-0625**

HASTINGS, John
Lectures on yellow fever, its causes, pathology & treatment, by. . . . Philadelphia: Lindsay & Blakiston, 1848. 69p. DLC; DNLM; PPC; PPJ **40-0626**

HAWTHORNE, George Stuart
Cholera, its cure and prevention. The true pathological nature of cholera. . . . With introductory remarks by D. C. Morehead. From the 2nd London ed. New York: W. H. Graham, 1849. 48p. DNLM; NNNAM **40-0627**

HAWTHORNE, George Stuart
The prevention and treatment of epidemic cholera, and its true pathological nature, in a series of letters. Cleveland: M. C. Younglove & Co., 1849. 47p. DNLM; OCIM; OCIWHi **40-0628**

HAYWARD, George (1791-1863)
Some account of the first use of sulphuric ether by inhalation in surgical practice. [Boston, 1847] 8p. DNLM; MBM **40-0629**

HEBERDEN, William (1710-1801)
Commentaries on the history and cure of diseases. From the last London ed. Philadelphia: E. Barrington & G. D. Haswell, 1845. [Dunglison's American Medical Library] 214p. DNLM; PPC; PU; ViRA **40-0630**

HEMPEL, Charles Julius (1811-1879)
On eclecticism in medicine; or, a critical review of the leading medical doctrines: an inaugural thesis presented at the New York University on the first of March, 1845. New York: William Radde, 1845. 45p. DLC; PPHa **40-0631**

HEMPEL, Charles Julius (1811-1879)
A treatise on the use of arnica in cases of contusions, wounds, strains, sprains, lacerations of the solids, concussions, paralysis, rheumatism, soreness of the nipples, etc. With a number of cases illustrative of the use of that drug. New York: William Radde, 1845. 16p. DNLM; PPHa **40-0632**

HEMPEL, Charles Julius (1811-1879)
The homoeopathic domestic physician. New York: William Radde, 1846. 184p. PPHa **40-0633**

HENDERSON, Thomas (1789-1854)
Hints on the medical examination of recruits for the army; and on the discharge of soldiers from the service on surgeon's certificate. Adapted to the service of the United States. . . . Philadelphia: Haswell, Barrington, & Haswell, New Orleans: J. J. Haswell & Co., 1840. 82p. DLC; DNLM; LNT-M; PPC **40-0634**

HENDERSON, William (1810-1872)
Letter to John Forbes, M.D., F.R.S., editor of the "British & Foreign Medical Review," on his article entitled "Homoeopathy, Allopathy, and Young Physic," contained in the number of the Review for January, 1846. . . . New York: W. Radde; Boston: O. Clapp, 1846. 66p. DLC; DNLM; NNNAM; PPHa **40-0635**

HENDERSON, William (1810-1872)
An inquiry into the homoeopathic practice of medicine. . . . New York: W. Radde; Boston: O. Clapp, 1846. 154p. DLC; NNNAM; PPHa **40-0636**

HERING, Constantine (1800-1880)
The homoeopathist; or, domestic physician. 2nd American with additions from the 4th German ed. Philadelphia, 1844. Sold by Jacob Behlert and J. N. Bauersachs, No. 260 Market Street. 217p. PPHa **40-0637**

HERING, Constantine (1800-1880)
C. Hering's domestic physician. 3rd American ed., comprising the former editions of The homoeopathist, or domestic physician, rev., with additions from the author's manuscript of the 5th German ed., together with the additions of Drs. Goullon, Gross & Stapf, to which is added a chapter on the diseases of women. Philadelphia: C. L. Rademacher's Homoeopathic Book & Medicine Store; New York: W. Radde, 1845. 412p. DLC; PPHa **40-0638**

HERING, Constantine (1800-1880)
C. Hering's domestic physician. 4th American ed., revised, with additions, from the author's manuscript of the 6th German ed. The part relating to the diseases of females and children, by Walter Williamson, M.D. Philadelphia: C. L. Rademacher, 1848. 415p. PPHa **40-0639**

HILL, H. W.
Introductory lectures delivered to the students of the Botanico-Medical College of Ohio, on the circulation of the blood, and the unphilosophical practice of blood-letting for the cure of disease. [n.p.], 1845. 16p. DNLM **40-0640**

The HISTORY, pathology, and treatment of puerperal fever and crural phlebitis: I. A treatise on the epidemic puerperal fever of Aberdeen, by Alex. Gordon. II. A treatise on the puerperal fever; illustrated by cases which occurred in Leeds and its vicinity in the years 1809-1812, by Wm. Hey. III. Facts and observations relative to the fever commonly called puerperal, by John Armstrong. IV. On puerperal fever and crural phlebitis, by Robt. Lee. With an introductory essay by Charles D. Meigs. Philadelphia: E. Barrington & G. D. Haswell, 1842. 338p. DNLM; PPC; PU; ViRA **40-0641**

HITCHCOCK, David K.
Preservation of the teeth; a family guide. Boston: Ives & Dennet; New York: Gould, Newman & Saxton, 1840. 96p. DNLM; MBM; NNNAM **40-0642**

HITT, J. D.
Hitt's electro-dynamics, or electricity the universal cause of motion in matter; illustrative of the diagnosis and treatment of all diseases, the motion of the planetary system, the laws of gravity, polarization of the needle, climate, and physiology. Philadelphia: J. H. Jones, 1848. 142p. 2 plates. DNLM; PPC; PU **40-0643**

HOCKEN, Edward Octavius
A treatise on amaurosis and amaurotic affections. Philadelphia: Haswell & Johnson, 1842. 201p. DNLM; PPC; PU **40-0644**

HODGE, Hugh Lenox (1796-1873)
An introductory lecture to the course of obstetrics, the diseases of women and children, delivered at the University of Pennsylvania, November 2, 1840. Philadelphia: T. K. & P. G. Collins, 1840. 16p. DNLM; PPC; PU **40-0645**

HODGE, Hugh Lenox (1796-1873)
An eulogium on William P. Dewees. Philadelphia: Merrihew & Thompson, 1842. 58p. DNLM; PPC; PPJ; PU **40-0646**

HODGE, Hugh Lenox (1796-1873)
A memoir of Thomas C. James, M.D. Read before the College of Physicians of Philadelphia. . . . Philadelphia: T. K. & P. G. Collins, printers, 1843. 25p. DLC; PPC **40-0647**

HODGE, Hugh Lenox (1796-1873)
An introductory lecture to the course on obstetrics, and diseases of women and children, delivered in the University of Pennsylvania. Philadelphia: W. S. Young, 1846. 15p. DNLM; PPC; PU **40-0648**

HOFFENDAHL, C[arl] F[riedrich]
On the homoeopathic treatment of cholera. . . . Boston: D. Clapp, 1849. 20p. DLC; DNLM; PPHa **40-0649**

HOLLICK, Frederick (*b.* 1818)
Neuropathy; or, The true principles of the art of healing the sick. Being an explanation of the action of galvanism. electricity, and magnetism, in the cure of disease. . . . [6th ed.] Philadelphia: National Publishing Company, 1847. 193p. DLC; DNLM; PPC **40-0650**

HOLLICK, Frederick (*b.* 1818)
The diseases of woman, their causes and cure familiarly explained; with practical hints for their prevention, and for the preservation of female health. . . . New York: Burgess, Stringer & Co., 1847. 294p. DLC; NNNAM **40-0651**

HOLLICK, Frederick (*b.* 1818)
Practical facts in the medical application of galvanism and electromagnetism; showing the results of their application, and explaining the most efficient manner for their successful use in the cure of disease, with descriptions of the various instruments employed, and the mode of using them. . . . New York: Burgess, Stringer & Co., 1848. 143p. DLC; NNNAM **40-0652**

HOLLICK, Frederick (*b.* 1818)
The matron's manual of midwifery, and the diseases of women during pregnancy and in child bed. New York: American News Co., 1848. 450p. NNNAM **40-0653**

HOLMES, Oliver Wendell (1809-1894)
Homoeopathy, and its kindred delusions; two lectures delivered before the Boston Society for the Diffusion of Useful Knowledge. Boston: W. D. Ticknor, 1842. 72p. DNLM; MBM; PPHa **40-0654**

HOLMES, Oliver Wendell (1809-1894)
The contagiousness of puerperal fever. . . . [Read before the Boston Society for Medical Improvement, and published at the request of the Society.] Boston, 1843. 28p. DNLM; MBM; MH; MH-M [See No. 50-0899] **40-0655**

HOLMES, Oliver Wendell (1809-1894)
The position and prospects of the medical student. An address delivered before the Boylston Medical Society of Harvard University, January 12, 1844. Boston: John Putnam, 1844. 28p. DNLM; MH; MBM; MBAt **40-0656**

HOLMES, Oliver Wendell (1809-1894)
An introductory lecture delivered at the Massachusetts Medical College. Boston: W. D. Ticknor & Co., 1847. 38p. DNLM; MBM; MH; MWA **40-0657**

HOLT, Daniel (1810-1883)
Views of homoeopathy; with reasons for examining and admitting it as a principle in medical science. . . . New Haven: J. H. Benham, 1845. 48p. DNLM; PPHa **40-0658**

HOLT, Daniel (1810-1883)
Cholera and its homoeopathic treatment, with an account of its success in Europe and America, and remarks upon its symptoms, preventive means, early management. . . . Published by request. Lowell: B. H. Penhallow, 1849. 12p. PPHa **40-0659**

HOMOEOPATHIC ASSOCIATION OF CINCINNATI
A report read before the Homoeopathic Association of Cincinnati, October 2, 1849. Cincinnati: Bradley & Anthony, 1849. 48p. DLC; OCHP; PPHa [Report of a Committee to inquire into complaints against the report of the practice of certain homoeopathic doctors in the cholera epidemic of 1849. The "Addenda" (pp. [29]-48) include reports from several homoeopathic physicians of Cincinnati, Rev. Mr. Barrett's letter to Dr. Hering, from the Philadelphia Evening Bulletin, and Dr. Hahnemann's letter to Hufeland, translated by Geddes M. Scott, on the necessity of a reform in medical practice.] **40-0660**

[HOMOEOPATHY]
The family guide to the administration of homoeopathic remedies. New York: William Radde, 1843. 44p. NNNAM; PPHa **40-0661**

[HOMOEOPATHY]
A manual of homoeopathic cookery. Designed chiefly for the use of such persons as are under homoeopathic tratment. By the wife of a homoeopathic physician; with additions by the wife of an American homoeopathic physician. New York: William Radde, 1846. 176p. NNNAM; PPHa **40-0662**

HOOKER, Charles (1799-1863)
An essay on intestinal auscultation. Boston: D. Clapp, 1849. 14p. DNLM; MBM **40-0663**

HOOKER, Worthington (1805-1867)
Dissertation on the respect due to the medical profession, and the reasons why it is not awarded by the community. Norwich: J. G. Cooley, 1844. 28p. DNLM **40-0664**

HOOKER, Worthington (1805-1867)
Physician and patient; or, A practical view of the mutual duties, relations and interests of the medical profession and the community. . . . New York: Baker & Scribner, 1849. 453p. DLC; MBM; NNNAM; ViRA **40-0665**

HOOPER, Robert (1773-1835)
Examinations in anatomy, physiology, practice of physic, surgery, chemistry, materia medica, and pharmacy; for the use of students. New York: J. & H. G. Langley, 1846. 252p. MBM; NNNAM; PPC **40-0666**

HOOPER, Robert (1773-1835)
Dr. Hooper's physician's vade-mecum: or, A manual of the principles and practice of physic. Considerably enlarged and improved, with an outline of general pathology and therapeutics, by Wm. Augustus Guy. . . . With additions, by James Stewart. . . . New York: Harper & Brothers, 1846. 541p. DLC; NNNAM; PU; ViRA **40-0667**

HOPE, James (1801-1841)
A treatise on the diseases of the heart and great vessels, and on the affections which may be mistaken for them. . . . First American from the third London ed. With notes and a detail of recent experiments, by C. W. Pennock. Philadelphia: Lea & Blanchard, 1842. 572p. 9 plates. DNLM; PPPH; ViRA **40-0668**

HOPE, James (1801-1841)
Principles and illustrations of morbid anatomy; adapted to the elements of Andral, and to the Cyclopaedia of Practical Medicine. . . . 1st American ed., edited by L. M. Lawson. Philadelphia: Lindsay & Blakiston, 1845. 359p. 260 plates. DNLM; MBM; PPC; PU **40-0669**

HOPE, James (1801-1841)
A treatise on diseases of the heart, and great vessels, and on the affections which may be mistaken for them. . . . 2nd American from the 3rd London ed. With notes and a detail of recent experiments by C. W. Pennock. Philadelphia: Lea & Blanchard, 1846. 572p. 6 plates. DNLM; PPC; PPJ; PU **40-0670**

HORNER, Gustavus R. B. (1804-1892)
Medical topography of Brazil and Uruguay. . . . Philadelphia: Lindsay & Blakiston, 1845. 296p. DLC; DNLM; PPC **40-0671**

HORNER, William Edmonds (1793-1853)
A treatise on special and general anatomy. 5th ed. Philadelphia: Lea & Blanchard, 1840. 2 v. DNLM; NNNAM; PPC; ViRA **40-0672**

HORNER, William Edmonds (1793-1853)
Introductory lecture . . . , University of Pennsylvania. Philadelphia: Merrihew & Thompson, 1841. 20p. DNLM; PU **40-0673**

HORNER, William Edmonds (1793-1853)
Introductory lecture before the medical class of the University of Pennsylvania, delivered November 19, 1843. Philadelphia: Merrihew & Thompson, 1843. 26p. DNLM; PU **40-0674**

HORNER, William Edmonds (1793-1853)
Special anatomy and histology. 6th ed. Philadelphia: Lea & Blanchard, 1843. 2 v. DNLM; PPC; PU **40-0675**

HORNER, William Edmonds (1793-1853)
Special anatomy and histology. . . . 7th ed. . . . Philadelphia: Lea & Blanchard, 1846. 2 v. DLC; DNLM [First edition, 1826; first five editions issued under title: A treatise on special and general anatomy.] **40-0676**

HORNER, William Edmonds (1793-1853)
The United States dissector, or, Lessons in practical anatomy. . . . 4th ed. . . . Edited by Henry H. Smith. . . . Philadelphia: Lea & Blanchard, 1846. 444p. DLC; DNLM; PPC; PU **40-0677**

HORNER, William Edmonds (1793-1853)
Introductory lecture before the anatomical class of the University of Pennsylvania. Philadelphia: T. K. & P. G. Collins, 1848. 32p. DNLM; PU **40-0678**

HOSACK, Alexander Eddy (1805-1871)
Extirpation of a tumor of the parotid; with observations upon the pathology of that gland. [New York, 1844.] 6p. 1 plate. DNLM; NNNAM **40-0679**

HOSACK, Alexander Eddy (1805-1871)
Cases illustrative of the beneficial effects of ether. New York: G. F. Nesbitt, 1847. 8p. DNLM; NNNAM **40-0680**

HOSACK, Alexander Eddy (1805-1871)
Case of popliteal aneurism cured by compression with a new instrument. [New York, 1848.] 4p. 1 plate. DNLM; NNNAM **40-0681**

HOUGH, Lewis Sylvester (1819-1903)
The science of man, applied to epidemics: their cause, cure, and prevention. . . . Boston: B. Marsh, 1849. 290p. DLC; DNLM; MBM **40-0682**

HOWARD, Henry (1792-1874)
A synopsis of medical jurisprudence, from the latest and best authorities, forming the basis of lectures on the science. . . . 4th ed. Charlottesville, [Va.]: Printed by O. S. Allen & Co., 1849. 157p. DLC; ViRA **40-0683**

HOWARD, Richard L. (1809-1854)
Introductory to the course in the Starling Medical College of Columbus. Columbus: Scott & Bascom, 1849. 25p. DNLM **40-0684**

HOWE, J. M[offatt] (1806-1885)
To consumptives. Information respecting the practice of F. H. Ramadge, containing an account of several cases in relation to this practice. . . . New York: Published by the author, 1846. 72p. DNLM; NNNAM **40-0685**

HOWE, Samuel Gridley (1801-1870)
Insanity in Massachusetts. Boston: J. H. Eastburn, 1843. 20p. DNLM; MBM **40-0686**

HOWE, Samuel Gridley (1801-1870)
An essay on separate and congregate systems of prison discipline; being a report made to the Boston Prison Discipline Society. Boston: W. D. Ticknor, 1846. 90p. DNLM; MB; MH; MWA **40-0687**

HOWE, Samuel Gridley (1801-1870)
Idiots. Report in part, to which is appended a letter on the school for idiots in Paris, by George Sumner. [House Doc. 152]. Boston, 1847. 17p. DNLM; MWA; MBAt
40-0688

HOWE, Samuel Gridley (1801-1870)
Report made to the legislature of Massachusetts on idiocy. Boston: Coolidge & Wiley, 1848. 100, 46p. DNLM; MBM; MWA **40-0689**

HUGHES, Henry Marshall (1805-1858)
A clinical introduction to the practice of auscultation and other modes of physical diagnosis: intended to simplify the study of the diseases of the lungs and heart. . . . Philadelphia: Lea & Blanchard, 1846. 270p. DLC; PPC; PU
40-0690

HUMPHREY, Gideon (1776-1872)
An address to the public on the subject of the regular practice of medicine. Burlington: E. Morris, 1848. 15p. DNLM; PPHa
40-0691

HUMPHREYS, Frederick (1816-1900)
The cholera and its homoeopathic treatment. New York: William Radde, 1849. 72p. DNLM; PPHa
40-0692

HUN, Thomas (1808-1896)
Medical systems, medical science, and empiricism; an introductory lecture. Albany: J. Munsell, 1849. 46p. DNLM
40-0693

HUNTER, John (1728-1793)
A treatise on venereal disease. With notes by James F. Palmer. [Dunglison's American Medical Library] Philadelphia: Haswell, Barrington & Haswell, 1840. 611p. DNLM; PPC; PPJ; PU
40-0694

HUNTER, John (1728-1793)
Observations on certain parts of the animal oeconomy. . . . [Dunglison's American Medical Library] Philadelphia: Haswell, Barrington & Haswell, 1840. 479p. DNLM; MBM; PPC
40-0695

HUNTER, John (1728-1793)
A treatise on the blood, inflammation, and gunshot wounds. . . . With notes by James F. Palmer. . . . Philadelphia: Haswell, Barrington & Haswell; New Orleans: J. J.Haswell & Co., 1840. 611p. DLC; MBM; PPC; ViRA **40-0696**

HUSSEY, Zimri
A comprehensive and practical treatise on the prevention and cure of epidemic cholera. Cincinnati: Wright, Fisher & Co., 1849. 11p. DNLM; OCIM **40-0697**

HUSTON, Robert Mendenhall (1795-1864)
Introductory lecture to the course of obstetrics and diseases of women and children, in the Jefferson Medical College of Philadelphia. Philadelphia: W. F. Geddes, 1840. 22p. DNLM; PPJ **40-0698**

HUSTON, Robert Mendenall (1795-1864)
An introductory lecture delivered before the class of Jefferson Medical College. Philadelphia: Merrihew & Thompson, 1846. 24p. DNLM; PPJ **40-0699**

HUSTON, Robert Mendenhall (1795-1864)
Charge to the graduates of Jefferson Medical College of Philadelphia . . . with a list of the graduates. Philadelphia: Merrihew & Thompson, 1849. 15, 4p. DNLM; PPJ **40-0700**

INGALLS, William (1769-1851)
A treatise on malignant fever and vomito priesto. . . . Boston: W. D. Ticknor & Co., 1847. 108p. DLC; DNLM; MBM
40-0701

INGALLS, William (1769-1851)
A case of typhus or ship fever, with remarks. . . . Boston: D. Clapp, printer, 1848. 28p. DLC; DNLM; MBM
40-0702

JACKSON, John Barnard Swett (1806-1878)
A descriptive catalogue of the monstrosities in the cabinet of the Boston Society for Medical Improvement. Boston: Freeman & Bolles, 1847. 88p. 10 plates. DNLM; MBM; MH-M
40-0703

JACKSON, John Barnard Swett (1806-1878)
A descriptive catalogue of the anatomical museum of the Boston Society for Medical Improvement. Boston: Ticknor, 1847. 352p. 10 plates. DNLM; MBM; MH-M
40-0704

JACKSON, John Barnard Swett (1806-1878)
Review of Dr. M. Gay's statement of Dr. Charles T. Jackson's claims to the discovery of the inhalation of sulphuric ether, as a preventive of pain. [Boston, 1847.] 8p. DNLM; MBM
40-0705

JACKSON, John Barnard Swett (1806-1878)
An introductory lecture, delivered at the Massachusetts Medical College. Boston: W. D. Ticknor & Co., 1848. 30p. DNLM; MBM; MH-M **40-0706**

JACKSON, Samuel (1787-1872)
Address to the medical graduates of the University of Pennsylvania. Philadelphia: T. K. & P. G. Collins, 1840. 21p. DNLM; PU **40-0707**

JACKSON, Samuel (1787-1872)
The introductory lecture to the course of the institutes of medicine, in the University of Pennsylvania, for 1841-1842. . . . Published by the class. Philadelphia: Merrihew & Thompson, printers, 1841. 24p. DLC; DNLM; PU
40-0708

JACKSON, Samuel (1787-1872)
Introductory lecture to the course of medical institutes in the University of Pennsylvania. Philadelphia: Merrihew & Thompson, 1842. 26p. DNLM; PU **40-0709**

JACKSON, Samuel (1787-1872)
Lecture introductory to a course on the institutes of medicine in the University of Pennsylvania. Philadelphia: King & Baird, 1844. 28p. DNLM; PU **40-0710**

JACKSON, Samuel (1787-1872)
Lecture introductory to a course on the institutes of medicine in the University of Pennsylvania. Philadelphia: J. Young, 1845. 32p. DNLM; PU **40-0711**

JACKSON, Samuel (1787-1872)
An introductory address delivered before the medical class of the University of Pennsylvania. Philadelphia: W. S. Young, 1846. 15p. DNLM; PU **40-0712**

JACKSON, Samuel (1787-1872)
Lecture introductory to a course on the institutes of medicine in the University of Pennsylvania. Philadelphia: J. Young, 1847. 23p. DNLM; PU **40-0713**

JACKSON, Samuel (1787-1872), et al.
A defense of the "six months lecture term," report of a special committee of the American Medical Association. Philadelphia: T. K. & P. G. Collins, 1849. 14p. PPC; PU **40-0714**

JAHR, Gottlieb Heinrich Georg (1800-1875)
Jahr's new manual of homoeopathic practice. Edited with annotations by A. Gerald Hull, M.D. 2nd American from the 3rd, or Paris edition. New York: William Radde, 1841-1842. 2 v. DNLM; PPHa **40-0715**

JAHR, Gottlieb Heinrich Georg (1800-1875)
New homoeopathic pharmacopoeia and posology, or The preparation of homoeopathic medicines and the administration of doses. . . . Transl. with additions, by James Kitchen, M.D. Philadelphia: J. Dobson; New York: W. Radde, 1842. 306p. DLC; DNLM; PPHa **40-0716**

JAHR, Gottlieb Heinrich Georg (1800-1875)
Short elementary treatise upon homoeopathia, and the manner of its practice, with some of the most important effects of ten of the principal homoeopathic remedies; for the use of all honest men who desire to convince themselves by experiment of the truth of the doctrine. 2nd French ed., corrected and enlarged. Transl. by Edward Bayard, M.D. New York: William Radde, 1845. 90p. PPHa **40-0717**

JAHR, Gottlieb Heinrich Georg (1800-1875)
Jahr's new manual (or Symptomen-codex). Transl. with extensive additions from various sources, by Charles Julius Hempel, M.D., aided by James M. Quin, M.D. With a preface by Dr. C. Hering, revisions and clinical notes by Dr. J. F. Gray, contributions from Drs. A. Gerald Hull, G. W. Cook . . . [and others]. New York: W. Radde; Boston: O. Clapp, 1848-1853. 3 v. DLC; PPHa **40-0718**

JARVIS, Edward (1803-1884)
Insanity and insane asylums. Louisville, Ky.: Prentice & Weissinger, 1841. 40p. DNLM; KyLoJM **40-0719**

JARVIS, Edward (1803-1884)
What shall we do with the insane of the Western country? [Louisville, 1842] 45p. DNLM **40-0720**

JARVIS, Edward (1803-1884)
Insanity among the coloured population of the free states. . . . Philadelphia: T. K. & P. G. Collins, printers, 1844. 15p. DLC; MBM; PPC; ViRA **40-0721**

JARVIS, Edward (1803-1884)
Practical physiology for the use of schools and families. Philadelphia: Thomas Cowperthwait & Co., 1848. 396p. DNLM; ICJ; MB; PPC **40-0722**

JARVIS, Edward (1803-1884)
Production of vital force. A discourse delivered before the Massachusetts Medical Society, at their annual meeting, May 30, 1849. . . . Boston: Printed by D. Clapp, 1849. 77p. DLC; MBM; MH-M; MWA **40-0723**

JARVIS, George Ogelvie (1795-1875)
To the medical profession. Remarks on the advantages of Dr. Jarvis's surgical adjuster, in the treatment of fractures and dislocations. New York: J. Meakim, agent, 1844. 12p. DLC; DNLM; NNNAM **40-0724**

JARVIS, George Ogelvie (1795-1875)
The surgical adjuster, for reducing dislocations, adjusting fractures, and maintaining coaptation. [Middletown, Conn.: C. H. Pelton], 1846. 80p. DNLM **40-0725**

JARVIS, George Ogelvie (1795-1875)
Lectures on fractures and dislocations, together with concise instructions in the use of the "surgical adjuster." Derby, Conn.: H. & G. Kellogg, 1846. 80p. 12 plates. DNLM **40-0726**

JARVIS, George Ogelvie (1795-1875)
Lectures on fractures and dislocations, together with concise instructions in the use of the "surgical adjuster." 3rd ed. Boston: D. Clapp, 1847. 93p. 12 plates. DNLM; MBM **40-0727**

JARVIS, George Ogelvie (1795-1875)
Lectures on fractures and dislocations, together with concise instructions in the use of the "surgical adjuster." 4th ed. Boston: D. Clapp, 1847. 93p. DNLM; MBM **40-0728**

JARVIS, George Ogelvie (1795-1875)
Lectures on fractures and dislocations, together with concise instructions in the use of the "surgical adjuster." 5th ed. Birmingham: T. M. Newson, 1848. 92p. 12 plates. DNLM **40-0729**

JARVIS, George Ogelvie (1795-1875)
Treatise on dislocations of the shoulder. Together with important cases illustrating the benefits of the adjuster. Compiled by George Kellogg. Birmingham, Conn.: T. M. Newson, 1848. 32p. 3 plates [Folio] DNLM **40-0730**

JEANES, Jacob (1800-1877)
Address delivered before the American Institute of Homoeopathy at its fifth anniversary meeting, held at New York, June 14, 1848. Philadelphia: North American Print., 1848. 20p. PPHa **40-0731**

JENNINGS, Isaac
Medical reform. A treatise on man's physical being and disorders; embracing an outline of a theory of human life, and a theory of disease, its nature, cause and remedy. Oberlin, O.: Fitch & Jennings, 1847. 375p. DNLM; PPHa **40-0732**

JENNINGS, Samuel Kennedy (1771-1854)
A compendium of medical science, or fifty years' experience in the art of healing. . . . Tuskaloosa, Ala.: M. J. Slade, printer, 1847. 592p. DLC; AU **40-0733**

JEWELL, Wilson (1800-1867)
Statistics on cholera; with the sanitary measures adopted by the board of health prior to, and during the prevalence of, the epidemic in Philadelphia, in the summer of 1849, chronologically arranged. Philadelphia: The Sanitary Committee, 1849. 62p. DNLM; PPC; PU **40-0734**

JOBSON, David Wemyss
A treatise on the anatomy and physiology of the teeth, . . . their diseases and treatment with practical observations on artificial teeth, and rules for their construction. Baltimore: American Society of Dental Surgeons, 1844. 133p. DNLM; MdU-D **40-0735**

JOHNSON, Charles P.
A treatise on animal magnetism. New York: Burgess & Stringer, 1844. 96p. DNLM; MB; MH; NNC **40-0736**

JOHNSON, Edward
Results of hydropathy, or constipation not a disease of the bowels; indigestion not a disease of the stomach. . . . New York: J. Wiley, 1849. 181p. DNLM; NNNAM **40-0737**

JOHNSON, Edward
The domestic practice of hydropathy. New York: J. Wiley, 1849. 467p. DNLM; NNNAM **40-0738**

JOHNSON, James (1777-1845)
A treatise on derangements of the liver, internal organs, and nervous system, pathological and therapeutical. From the 3rd London ed. Concord: J. F. Brown, 1847. 234p. DNLM; MBM; NNNAM **40-0739**

JOHNSTON, William Edwin (1822-1886)
An inaugural dissertation on spermatorrhoea, pathologically and therapeutically considered. New York: G. F. Nesbitt, 1847. 42p. DNLM; NNNAM **40-0740**

JONES, Henry
Mesmerism examined and repudiated, as "the sin of witchcraft," etc.; especially in its mysteries of clairvoyance; with an appendix of mesmeric phenomena witnessed by William H. Beecher. 2nd ed. New York: J. S. Redfield, 1846. 24p. DNLM; MB; MH; NN **40-0741**

JONES, Thomas Wharton (1808-1891)
The principles and practice of ophthalmic medicine and surgery. . . . Ed. by Isaac Hays. . . . Philadelphia: Lea & Blanchard, 1847. 509p. DLC; DNLM; PPC; NNNAM **40-0742**

JOSLIN, Benjamin Franklin (1796-1861)
Address before the New York Homoeopathic Physicians' Society, December 3, 1845. [New York, 1846] 4p. DNLM; PPHa **40-0743**

JOSLIN, Benjamin Franklin (1796-1861)
On the limit of subdivision by trituration and solution, and the principles on which the limit may be indefinitely extended. [New Haven, 1847] 8p. DNLM; PPHa **40-0744**

JOSLIN, Benjamin Franklin (1796-1861)
Discourse on the evidence of the power of small doses and attenuated medicines, including a theory of potentization. Read before the New York Homoeopathic Physicians' Society, March 9, 1847. New York: C. G. Dean, 1847. 18p. DLC; PPHa **40-0745**

JOSLIN, Benjamin Franklin (1796-1861)
On the use of chemical and mechanical means, and large doses in connection with homoeopathic practice. A report to the American Institute of Homoeopathy at its fifth annual session, June, 1848. New York: C. G. Dean, 1848. 8p. PPHa **40-0746**

JOSLIN, Benjamin Franklin (1796-1861)
On the limit of subdivision by trituration. . . . Evidences of the power of small doses. Nashua, N.H.: Murray & Kimball, 1848. 32p. DNLM; PPHa **40-0747**

JOSLIN, Benjamin Franklin (1796-1861)
Causes and homoeopathic treatment of the cholera, including repertories for this disease, and for vomiting, diarrhoea, cholera infantum and dysentery. New York: William Radde, 1849. 144p. DLC; DNLM; PPHa **40-0748**

JOSLIN, Benjamin Franklin (1796-1861)
Homoeopathic treatment of diarrhoea, cholera morbus and the cholera, with repertories for these diseases. 2nd ed. New York: William Radde, 1849. 144p. DLC; DNLM; PPHa **40-0749**

JOURDAIN-BERCHILLET, Anselme-Louis Bernard (1734-1816)
A treatise on the diseases and surgical operations of the mouth, and parts adjacent. . . . Transl. from the French. Baltimore: Published by the American Society of Dental Surgeons, 1849. 410p. DNLM; MdU-D; PU **40-0750**

JUDKINS, Jesse P. (1815-1867)
Introductory lecture to a course on descriptive and surgical anatomy. Cincinnati: H. C. & J. B. McGrew, 1845. 12p. DLC; DNLM; OCHP **40-0751**

JUDKINS, Jesse P. (1815-1867)
Introductory lecture to a course on anatomy. Cincinnati: H. C. McGrew, 1846. 15p. DNLM; OCHP **40-0752**

KANE, Elisha Kent (1820-1857)
Experiments on kiesteine; with remarks on its application to the diagnosis of pregnancy. Philadelphia, 1842. 26p. DNLM; PPC **40-0753**

KANE, Robert John (1810-1878)
Elements of chemistry, including the most recent discoveries and applications of the science to medicine and pharmacy, and to the arts. Am. ed. by John Wm. Draper. New York: Harper & Bros., 1848. 704p. DNLM; NNNAM; OCIM; PPC **40-0754**

KELLEY, E. G. (1813?-1881)
A popular treatise on the human teeth and dental surgery, [etc.]. Boston: J. Munroe & Co., 1843. 196p. DNLM; MBM **40-0755**

KELLEY, J. Clawson (1793?-1863)
Key to medical science. New York: J. A. Fraetas & J. W. Kelley, 1842. 239p. DNLM; NNNAM [Cover marked "Second uniform edition, New York, J. W. Kelley, 1844."] **40-0756**

KELLEY, J. Clawson (1793?-1863)
A new philosophy of medical science, based upon analytical principles; the cause, symptoms, and treatment of the most prevalent diseases, to which are appended tests of their curability. New York: J. A. Fraetas & Co., 1847. 48p. DNLM; NNNAM **40-0757**

KENNEDY, Evory
Observations on obstetric auscultation, with an analysis of the evidences of pregnancy, and an inquiry into the proofs of the life and death of the foetus in utero. With an appendix containing legal notes by John Smith. With notes and additional illustrations, by Isaac E. Taylor. New York: J. & H. G. Langley, 1843. 311p. DNLM; MBM; NNNAM; ViRA **40-0758**

KENWORTHY, Charles James
Lecture introductory to the annual course of lectures, in the Medical College of Petersburg, Virginia, session 1848-1849. Petersburg: Republican Office, 1849. 13p. DNLM; ViRA
40-0759

A KEY to the science of electrical biology. All its secrets explained, with full and comprehensive instructions in the mode of operation and its application to disease. . . . By a professor of the science. Cleveland: Smead & Cowles, 1849. 15p. DNLM; OCIM **40-0760**

KING, Edward
Cholera, a scourge to the negligent. Ten propositions . . . comprising the means for prevention and cure, forming the substance of a lecture. . . . [Philadelphia, 1849?] 18p. DNLM
40-0761

KIRKBRIDE, Thomas Story (1809-1883)
Remarks on the construction and arrangements of hospitals for the insane. . . . Philadelphia: Printed by T. K. and P. G. Collins, 1847. 19p. 2 plates. DLC; DNLM; PPJ; PPHa
40-0762

KIRKES, William Senhouse (1823-1864)
Manual of physiology. . . . Assisted by James Paget. . . . With one hundred and eighteen illustrations on wood. Philadelphia: Lea & Blanchard, 1849. 552p. DLC; DNLM; PPC; PU
40-0763

KNAPP, Moses L. (1799-1879)
Address delivered to the graduating class of the Indiana Medical College, at the public commencement, February 18, 1847. Chicago, 1847. 23p. DNLM
40-0764

KNAPP, Moses L. (1799-1879)
An address delivered at the opening of the Rock Island Medical School. Chicago: Campbell & Fuller, 1849. 20p. DNLM; ICRM **40-0765**

KNEELAND, Samuel (1821-1888)
On the contagiousness of puerperal fever and its connection with epidemic erysipelas. Philadelphia: Lea & Blanchard, 1846. 42p. DNLM; PPC; PPJ; PU **40-0766**

KNIGHT, Jonathan (1789-1864)
On the propagation of communicable diseases. An introductory lecture to the course of 1849-1850, in the medical institution of Yale College. New Haven: B. L. Hamlen, 1849. 20p. CyT-M; DNLM **40-0767**

KNOX, Franklin
A vindication of character, and an examination of the accusations contained in Dr. I. Reyburn's supplement to the "St. Louis Medical and Surgical Journal," Sept. 18, 1846. St. Louis: Office of the St. Louis "Union," 1846. 21p. DNLM
40-0768

KREBS, John M.
The reciprocal relations of physicians and clergymen. New York: H. Ludwig, 1847. 10p. DNLM
40-0769

LALLEMAND, Claude François (1790-1854)
A practical treatise on the causes, symptoms, and treatment of spermatorrhea. Transl. and edited by Henry J. McDougall. . . . Philadelphia: Lea & Blanchard, 1848. 320p. DNLM; MBM; PPC; PU **40-0770**

LATHAM, Peter Mere (1789-1875)
Lectures on subjects connected with clinical medicine: comprising diseases of the heart. . . . Philadelphia: E. Barrington & G. D. Haswell, 1847. 365p. DLC; DNLM; PPC
40-0771

LATHAM, Peter Mere (1789-1875)
Lectures on subjects connected with clinical medicine. . . . 2nd ed. Philadelphia: Barrington & Haswell, 1847. 158p. DLC; DNLM; PPC; PPJ **40-0772**

LATTA, Samuel Arminius (1804-1852)
Homoeopathy vs. The Expositor. [1849]. 40p. DNLM
40-0773

LAURIE, Joseph (*d.* 1865)
Homoeopathic domestic medicine. Edited, with additions, by A. Gerald Hull, M.D. New York: William Radde, 1843. 230p. PPHa **40-0774**

LAURIE, Joseph (*d.* 1865)
Homoeopathic domestic medicine. . . . 2nd American ed. Enlarged and improved. New York: William Radde, 1844. 244p. PPHa **40-0775**

LAURIE, Joseph (*d.* 1865)
Homoeopathic domestic medicine. Arranged as a practical work for students. Containing a glossary of medical terms. 3rd American ed., enlarged and improved by A. Gerald Hull, M.D. New York: William Radde, 1846. 438p. DLC; PPHa
40-0776

LAURIE, Joseph (*d.* 1865)
Homoeopathic domestic medicine. Latest American ed., enlarged and improved by A. Gerald Hull, M.D. New York: William Radde, 1849. 264p. PPHa
40-0777

LAWRENCE, William (1783-1867)
A treatise on ruptures, containing an anatomical description of each species; with an account of its symptoms, progress and treatment. From the 5th London ed. Philadelphia: Lea & Blanchard, 1843. 480p. DNLM; PPC; PU
40-0778

LAWRENCE, William (1783-1867)
A treatise on the diseases of the eye. . . . From the last London ed., with numerous additions, and sixty-seven illustrations, by Isaac Hays. . . . Philadelphia: Lea & Blanchard, 1843. 778p. DLC; DNLM; NNNAM; PPC **40-0779**

LAWRENCE, William (1783-1867)
A treatise on the diseases of the eye. . . . A new ed. Edited, with numerous additions and one hundred and seventy-six illustrations, by Isaac Hays. . . . Philadelphia: Lea & Blanchard, 1847. 858p. 1 plate. DLC; MBM; NNNAM; ViRA
40-0780

LAWSON, Leonidas Merion (1812-1864)
A review of homoeopathy, allopathy, and young physic. Lexington, Ky.: Scruyham & Dunlop, 1846. DNLM; KyLoJM; PPHa **40-0781**

LAWSON, Leonidas Merion (1812-1864)
An introductory address delivered in the Medical College of Ohio. Cincinnati: J. A. Robinson & Co., 1847. 22p. DNLM; OCIM **40-0782**

LAWSON, Leonidas Merion (1812-1864)
The nature and treatment of cholera, including a historical sketch of the disease, the causes which produce it, mode of propagation, pathology. . . . Cincinnati: Robinson & Jones, 1848. 58p. DNLM; OCIM **40-0783**

LAWSON, Leonidas Merion (1812-1864)
Cholera, its nature and treatment. Cincinnati: Robinson & Jones, 1848. 58p. DNLM; OCIM **40-0784**

LAYCOCK, Thomas (1812-1876)
An essay on hysteria: Being an analysis of its irregular and aggravated forms; including hysterical hemorrhage, and hysterical ischuria. With numerous illustrative cases. . . . Philadelphia: Haswell, Barrington, & Haswell; New Orleans: J. J. Haswell & Co., 1840. 192, 30p. DLC; DNLM; LNT-M; PPC **40-0785**

Le CONTE, John (1818-1891)
The philosophy of medicine. An address delivered before the graduates of the Medical College of Georgia. Augusta, 1849. 21p. DNLM; GU **40-0786**

LECTURES on diseases of the uterus, by Waller, Lisfranc and Ingleby, and aphorisms on insanity, by J. G. Millingen, M.D. Philadelphia: E. Barrington & G. D. Haswell, 1841. 2 v. in 1. DLC; IEN-M; NNNAM; PPC **40-0787**

LEE, Charles Alfred (1801-1872)
An introductory discourse on medical education, delivered to the students of Geneva Medical College, October 1, 1844. . . . Geneva, N.Y.: Merrell, 1844. 40p. DLC; DNLM **40-0788**

LEE, Charles Alfred (1801-1872)
Remarks on the character and writings of Hahnemann. New York: J. & H. G Langley, 1847. 14p. DNLM; NNNAM **40-0789**

LEE, Charles Alfred (1801-1872)
Address to the graduates of Geneva Medical College, delivered in the Presbyterian Church, Geneva, January 26, 1847. . . . Published by request of the graduates. New York: S. W. Benedict, 1847. 23p. DLC; DNLM; NNNAM **40-0790**

LEE, Charles Alfred (1801-1872)
A catalogue of the medical plants, indigenous and exotic, growing in the state of New York. With a brief account of their composition and medical properties. . . . New York: J. & H. G. Langley, 1848. 64p. DLC; DNLM; OCLloyd **40-0791**

LEE, Charles Alfred (1801-1872)
Valedictory address to the medical class of the Medical School of Maine, delivered at Brunswick, March 21st, 1849. . . . Published by request of the class. Buffalo: Steam Press of Jewett, Thomas & Co., 1849. 30p. DLC; DNLM **40-0792**

LEE, Charles Alfred (1801-1872)
Valedictory address, to the medical class of Geneva Medical College, delivered at Geneva, June 9th, 1849. . . . Geneva, N.Y.: Hollett & Van Volkenburgh, printers, 1849. 20p. DLC; DNLM **40-0793**

LEE, Charles Alfred (1801-1872)
Valedictory address to the graduating class of Geneva Medical College at the commencement. Buffalo, Jewett, Thomas & Co., 1849. 32p. DNLM **40-0794**

LEE, Edwin
Hydropathy and homoeopathy impartially appreciated. With an appendix of notes illustrative of the influence of the mind over the body. New York: H. Long & Bro., 1848. 94p. DNLM; PPHa **40-0795**

LEE, Henry
Reflections on the principles and practice of homoeopathy. New Haven, Conn.: W. Storer, Printer, 1845. 12p. PPHa **40-0796**

LEE, Robert (1793-1877)
On puerperal fever and crural phlebitis. With an introductory essay by Charles D. Meigs. Philadelphia: E. Barrington & G. D. Haswell, 1842. 118p. DNLM; MBM; NNNAM; PPC **40-0797**

LEE, Robert (1793-1877)
Lectures on the theory and practice of midwifery. Delivered in the theatre of St. George's Hospital. . . . Philadelphia: E. Barrington & G. D. Haswell, 1844. 540p. CU-M; DLC; DNLM; PPC **40-0798**

LEE, Robert (1793-1877)
Clinical midwifery. Comprising the histories of five hundred and forty-five cases of difficult, preternatural, and complicated labour. With commentaries. . . . 1st American from the 2nd London ed. Philadelphia: Lea & Blanchard, 1849. 238p. DLC; DNLM; ICRM; PPC **40-0799**

LEE, Samuel H. P.
Remarks on the stone and gravel in the kidneys and bladder, with an account of the discovery of a solvent remedy, now used with universal success, and commonly known as Dr. Lee's gravel specific. New York: F. Hart, 1846. 35p. DNLM; NNNAM **40-0800**

LEE, William (1778-1863)
. . . The excellent properties of brandy and salt, as an efficacious medicine, in several dangerous diseases incident to mankind. Published by William Lee, Esq., of Leeds, for the benefit of the community. With a preface by a clergyman of the Church of England. Philadelphia: Reprinted from the English edition, by C. A. Elliott, 1840. 8p. DLC; DNLM; PPC; PU **40-0801**

LEFOULON, J.
A new treatise on the theory and practice of dental surgery. Transl. from the French for the American Library of Dental Science, by Thomas E. Bond. Baltimore: Published by the American Society of Dental Surgeons, 1844. 295p. DNLM; MdU-D; NNNAM; PPC **40-0802**

LEIDY, Joseph (1823-1891)
Researches into the comparative structure of the liver. Philadelphia, 1848. 18p. 3 plates. DNLM; PPC **40-0803**

LEIDY, Joseph (1823-1891)
On the intimate structure and history of the articular cartilages. . . . [Philadelphia, 1849]. 18p. DLC; DNLM; PPC **40-0804**

LEVER, John Charles Weaver (1811-1858)
A practical treatise on organic diseases of the uterus: being the prize essay to which the Medical Society of London awarded the Fothergillian Gold Medal for 1843. . . . 2nd thousand. Newburgh, N.Y.: D. L. Proudfit; New York: C. S. Francis & Co., 1846. 240p. DLC; DNLM; MBM; NNNAM **40-0805**

LEVER, John Charles Weaver (1811-1858)
A practical treatise on organic diseases of the uterus: being the prize essay to which the Medical Society of London awarded the Fothergillian Gold Medal for 1843. . . . New York: Wiley & Putnam, 1846. 240p. DNLM; NNNAM **40-0806**

LIEBIG, Justus von (1803-1873)
Organic chemistry in its applications to agriculture and physiology. Edited from the manuscript of the author by Lyon Playfair. 2nd American ed., with an introduction, notes, and appendix by John W. Webster. Cambridge: J. Owen, 1841. 424p. DNLM; ICU; MH; NNC **40-0807**

LIEBIG, Justus von (1803-1873)
Organic chemistry in its applications to agriculture and physiology. Edited from the manuscript of the author by Lyon Playfair. 3rd American from 2nd English ed., with notes and appendix, by John W. Webster. Cambridge: J. Owen, 1842. 430p. AU; DNLM; CLM; MH **40-0808**

LIEBIG, Justus von (1803-1873)
Animal chemistry; or, Organic chemistry in its application to physiology and pathology. . . . Ed. from the author's manuscript, by William Gregory. . . . With additions, notes, and corrections, by Dr. Gregory, and others by John W. Webster. Cambridge [Mass.]: J. Owen; New York: D. Appleton & Company, 1842. 347p. DLC; DNLM; GU; NN **40-0809**

LIEBIG, Justus von (1803-1873)
Animal chemistry, or Organic chemistry in its application to physiology and pathology. . . . Ed. from the author's manuscript, by William Gregory. . . . New York: J. Winchester [1842]. 48p. DLC; DNLM; ICU; NN **40-0810**

LIEBIG, Justus von (1803-1873)
Organic chemistry in its applications to agriculture and physiology. Edited from the manuscript of the author by Lyon Playfair. From the London ed. Philadelphia: J. M. Campbell & Co., 1843. 135p. DNLM; MB; MH-M; PPC **40-0811**

LIEBIG, Justus von (1803-1873)
Familiar letters on chemistry, and its relation to commerce, physiology, and agriculture. Edited by John Gardner. New York: J. Winchester, 1843. 53p. AU; DNLM; GU; NN **40-0812**

LIEBIG, Justus von (1803-1873)
Familiar letters on chemistry, and its relation to commerce, physiology, and agriculture. Edited by John Gardner. Philadelphia: J. M. Campbell & Co., 1843. 55p. DNLM; LNT-M; MB; NN **40-0813**

LIEBIG, Justus von (1803-1873)
Animal chemistry, or Organic chemistry in its application to physiology and pathology. . . . Ed. from the author's manuscript, by William Gregory. . . . With additions, notes, and corrections, by Dr. Gregory, and others by John W. Webster. . . . 2nd ed. Cambridge [Mass.]: J. Owen; New York: D. Appleton & Company, 1843. 347p. DLC; DNLM; MH; NN **40-0814**

LIEBIG, Justus von (1803-1873)
Animal chemistry, or Organic chemistry in its applications to physiology and pathology. . . . Ed. from the author's manuscript, by William Gregory. . . . Philadelphia: J. M. Campbell, New York: Saxton & Miles, 1843. 111p. DLC; DNLM; ICJ; NN **40-0815**

LIEBIG, Justus von (1803-1873)
Animal chemistry, or Organic chemistry in its application to physiology and pathology. . . . Ed. from the author's manuscript, by William Gregory. . . . Philadelphia: J. M. Campbell, 1845. 111p. DLC; DNLM; NN; PU **40-0816**

LIEBIG, Justus von (1803-1873)
Organic chemistry in its applications to agriculture and physiology. Edited from the manuscript of the author by Lyon Playfair. [From the last London ed.] Philadelphia: T. B. Peterson, 1847. 135p. DNLM; GU; MA; NNNAM **40-0817**

LIEBIG, Justus von (1803-1873)
Animal chemistry, or Organic chemistry in its applications to physiology and pathology. . . . Edited from the author's manuscript, by William Gregory. . . . Philadelphia: T. B. Peterson, 1847. 111p. DLC; DNLM; MB; NN **40-0818**

LIEBIG, Justus von (1803-1873)
Animal chemistry, or Organic chemistry in its application to physiology and pathology. . . . Ed. from the author's manuscript, by William Gregory. . . . With additions, notes, and corrections, by Dr. Gregory, and others by John W. Webster. . . . From the 3rd London ed. New York: J. Wiley, 1848. 173p. DNLM; KU; MB; NN **40-0819**

LILLIE, James
. . . Homoeopathy vindicated. In a letter to J. V. C. Smith, M.D., editor of the Boston Medical and Surgical Journal, containing a reply to his views of Drs. C. and L.'s "Epitome of homoeopathic practice," with the acceptance of Dr. J. V. C. Smith's and Dr. C. A. Lee's challenges, and the consequences. . . . New York: W. G. Boggs, printer [1843]. 8p. DLC; NNNAM; PPHa **40-0820**

LINDSLY, Harvey (1804-1889)
Medical science and the medical profession in Europe and the United States. An introductory lecture. . . . November, 1840. Washington: P. Force, 1840. 35p. DLC; DNLM **40-0821**

LINTON, Moses L. (1808-1872)
An introductory lecture delivered in the hall of the medical department of St. Louis University, November 4, 1845. St. Louis, 1845. 20p. DNLM; OCIM **40-0822**

LINTON, Moses L. (1808-1872)
Introductory address delivered before the class of the medical department of the St. Louis University. St. Louis: Casamayon & Hill, 1849. 16p. DNLM **40-0823**

LISFRANC, Jacques (1790-1847)
Lectures on diseases of the uterus and its appendages. Philadelphia: E. Barrington & G. D. Haswell, 1841. 56p. DNLM; GU; ICRM; PPC **40-0824**

LISFRANC, Jacques (1790-1847)
Diseases of the uterus, a series of clinical lectures, delivered at the hospital La Pitié, by M. Lisfranc, and edited by H. Pauly, M.D. Transl. from the French by G. Henry Lodge. . . . Boston: W. D. Ticknor & Company, 1846. 401p. DLC; DNLM; MBM; MH-M **40-0825**

LISTON, Robert (1794-1847)
Elements of surgery. . . . From the 2nd London ed. with copious notes and additions, by Samuel D. Gross. . . . Philadelphia: E. Barrington & G. D. Haswell; New York: J. & H. G. Langley [etc., etc.], 1842. 640p. DLC; DNLM; PPC; PU **40-0826**

LISTON, Robert (1794-1847)
Practical surgery. With additional notes and illustrations by George W. Norris. 2nd American from the 3rd London ed. Philadelphia: Thomas, Cowperthwait & Co., 1842. 588p. DNLM; PPC; PPJ; ViRA **40-0827**

LISTON, Robert (1794-1847)
Lectures on the operations of surgery, and on diseases and accidents requiring operations. With numerous additions by Thomas D. Mütter. Philadelphia: Lea & Blanchard, 1846. 565p. DLC; DNLM; IEN-M; PPC **40-0828**

LISTON, Robert (1794-1847)
Elements of surgery. 4th American from the last London ed., with copious notes and additions, by Samuel D. Gross. Philadelphia: Ed. Barrington & Geo. D. Haswell; Louisville, Ky.: James Maxwell, Jr., 1846. 664p. CU-M; PPC: PPJ; PU **40-0829**

LITTELL, Squire (1803-1866)
A manual of diseases of the eye. . . . 2nd ed., revised and enlarged. Philadelphia: Hogan & Thompson, 1846. [25], 372p. DNLM; PPC; PU **40-0830**

LITTON, Abram (1814-1901)
An introductory lecture, to the course of chemistry and pharmacy, in the medical department of the St. Louis University. . . . St. Louis: Printed by Chambers & Knapp, 1844. 32p. DLC; OCIM **40-0831**

LOCKE, John (1792-1856)
A lecture on toxicology; delivered before the class of the Medical College of Ohio. 3rd ed. Cincinnati: J. A. Robinson & Co., 1848. 14p. DNLM; OCIM **40-0832**

LONGSHORE, Joseph Skelton (1809-1879)
The principles and practice of nursing, or a guide to the inexperienced. . . . Philadelphia: Printed by Merrihew & Thompson, 1842. 238p. DLC; DNLM; PPC **40-0833**

LORD, John
Important discovery! Cure for cancers, scrofula and tumors, abscesses, felons, boils, corn . . . , with a plaster, healing-salves, and internal medicines. Portland: W. Nichols & Co., 1849. 41p. DNLM **40-0834**

LORD, Joseph L., and Henry C. LORD
A defense of Dr. Charles T. Jackson's claims to the discovery of etherization. Containing testimony disproving the claims set up in favor of Mr. W. T. G. Morton, in the report of the trustees of the Massachusetts General Hospital, and in no. 201 of Littell's Living Age. . . . Boston: Office of Littell's Living Age, 1848. 37p. DLC; DNLM; MWA **40-0835**

LORD, Joseph L.
Memorial addressed to the trustees of the Massachusetts General Hospital, in behalf of Charles T. Jackson, in relation to the discovery of etherization. By his attorneys. Boston: Thurston, Torry & Co., 1849. 27p. DLC; DNLM; MWA **40-0836**

LOUISVILLE, KENTUCKY. MEDICAL INSTITUTE
Introductory lecture, on the means of promoting the intellectual improvement of the students and physicians, of the valley of Mississippi. (Delivered in the Medical Institute of Louisville, November 4, 1844.) Louisville: Prentice & Weissinger, 1844. 24p. DNLM; KyLoJM **40-0837**

LUDLOW, John Livingston (1819-1888)
A manual of examinations upon anatomy and physiology, surgery, practice of medicine, chemistry, materia medica, obstetrics, etc. Designed for the use of students of medicine throughout the United States. . . . Philadelphia: E. Barrington & G. D. Haswell, 1844. 615p. DLC; PPC; PPJ; PU **40-0838**

LUDLOW, John Livingston (1819-1888)
A manual of examinations upon anatomy and physiology, surgery, practice of medicine, chemistry, obstetrics, materia medica, pharmacy, and therapeutics; to which is added, a medical formulary. . . . 2nd ed., rev. and enl. Philadelphia: E. Barrington & G. D. Haswell, 1846. 689p. DLC; MBM; NNNAM; PPC **40-0839**

McALISTER, James
Enchiridion medicum, in syphiliticum. A treatise setting forth the signs, symptoms and treatment of syphilis, in all its forms and stages. . . . With full directions how to use the only infallible remedy known or discovered for the cure of syphilis. . . . The accompanying medicine sold only. . . . New York, 1847. 36p. DLC; NNNAM **40-0840**

MACARTNEY, James
A treatise on inflammation. . . . Philadelphia: Haswell, Barrington & Haswell, 1840. 117p. DNLM; PPC; PU; ViRA **40-0841**

McCLELLAN, George (1796-1847)
Principles and practice of surgery. . . . Ed. by his son, John H. B. McClellan, M.D. Philadelphia: Grigg, Elliot & Co., 1848. 432p. DLC; DNLM; PPJ; PU **40-0842**

McCLINTOCK, James (1809-1881)
Introductory lecture to the winter course of anatomy in the Philadelphia School of Anatomy. Philadelphia: C. A. Elliott, 1840. 16p. DNLM; PPC: PPJ; PU **40-0843**

McCLINTOCK, James (1809-1881)
Annual lecture. Introductory lecture to the course on anatomy and physiology, in the Vermont Academy of Medicine. Delivered April 7, 1841. . . . Castleton [Vt.]: Printed by L. R. H. Robinson, 1841. 12p. DLC; DNLM; VtHi **40-0844**

McCLINTOCK, James (1809-1881)
Annual lecture. Introductory lecture delivered in the Castleton Medical College, March 8, 1842. . . . Castleton, Vt.: Robinson & Southmayd, printers, 1842. 14p. DLC; DNLM; VtHi **40-0845**

McCLINTOCK, James (1809-1881)
An introductory lecture, delivered in the Castleton Medical College on the 10th April, 1843. . . . Albany: Printed by C. Van Benthuysen & Co., 1843. 28p. DLC; DNLM; VtHi **40-0846**

McCLINTOCK, James (1809-1881)
Introductory lecture, delivered in the Philadelphia College of Medicine. Session of 1847-1848. . . . Published by the class. Philadelphia: J. H. Gihon, printer, 1847. 9p. DLC; PPC; PU **40-0847**

McDOWELL, Joseph Nash (1803-1868)
An address delivered on laying the cornerstone of the medical department of Kemper College, St. Louis, June 11, 1840. St. Louis: Churchill & Harris, 1840. 16p. DNLM **40-0848**

McDOWELL, Joseph Nash (1803-1868)
. . . An address to the graduates at the commencement of the college, March, 1841. St. Louis: Chambers & Knapp, 1841. 32p. DNLM **40-0849**

McDOWELL, William Adair (1795-1853)
A demonstration of the curability of pulmonary consumption, in all its stages. Comprising an inquiry into the nature, causes, symptoms, treatment and prevention of tuberculous diseases in general. . . . Louisville, Ky.: Prentice & Weissinger, 1843. 269p. DLC; DNLM **40-0850**

McDOWELL, William Adair (1795-1853)
Reply of William A. McDowell to Dr. Yandell's rejoinder, in a controversy relative to cure of consumption. Louisville, Ky.: Prentice & Weissinger, 1844. 30p. DLC; DNLM **40-0851**

McDOWELL, William Adair (1795-1853)
Answer to a review of his treatise on consumption, by Dr. Y[andell]. [Louisville, 1844] 3p. DNLM **40-0852**

MACGOWAN, Daniel J.
Claims of the missionary enterprise on the medical profession; an address. New York: W. Osborn, 1842. 24p. DNLM **40-0853**

McGOWN, Thompson
A practical treatise on the most common diseases of the South: exhibiting their peculiar nature, and the corresponding adaptation of treatment. To which is added an appendix, containing some miscellaneous matter. Also a glossary, explaining the meaning of the technicalities, or medical phrases, used in this work. . . . Philadelphia: Grigg, Elliot & Co., 1849. 441p. DLC; DNLM; PPC; ViRA **40-0854**

McILHENNY, J. J.
A treatise on the disease called the milksickness, or trembles. . . . Springfield, [O.]: Gallagher & Halsey, printers, 1843. 22p. DLC; DNLM **40-0855**

MACKALL, Louis (1802-1876)
Outlines of a new system of physiology: Washington: T. Barnard, 1848. 15, 3p. DNLM **40-0856**

MACKINTOSH, John
Principles of pathology and practice of medicine. . . . 4th American, from the last London ed. With notes and additions, by Samuel George Morton. . . . Philadelphia: Lindsay & Blakiston, 1844. 892p. DLC; DNLM; PPC; PU **40-0857**

McLEAN, John
Valedictory lecture delivered before the class of Rush Medical College on January 2, 1847. Chicago: R. Fergus, 1847. 12p. DNLM; ICU **40-0858**

McNAIR, Alexander H.
Suggestions to parents and others on the physical and medical treatment of children, also diseases of females, together with a practical account of all the diseases to which the human body is liable, and more particularly of diseases of the spine, consumption of the lungs, dyspepsy, and nervous affections. Philadelphia: The author, 1841. 496p. DNLM; PPC; PU **40-0859**

MACNISH, Robert (1802-1834)
The philosophy of sleep. [Also:] The anatomy of drunkenness. Hartford: S. Andrus & Son, 1849. 96p. DNLM **40-0860**

MACROBIN, John (1804-1879)
An introduction to the study of practical medicine; being an outline of the leading facts and principles of the science, as taught in a course of lectures, delivered in the Marischal College of Aberdeen. . . . 1st American ed. . . . [Dunglison's American Medical Library] Philadelphia: A. Waldie, 1841. 127p. DLC; DNLM; PPC **40-0861**

MACROBIN, John (1804-1879)
An introduction to the study of practical medicine; being an outline of the leading facts and principles of the science, as taught in a course of lectures, delivered in the Marischal college of Aberdeen. . . . Philadelphia: Haswell & Johnson, 1842. 127p. DNLM; PPC; PPJ; PU **40-0862**

MACROBIN, John (1804-1879)
An introduction to the study of practical medicine; being an outline of the leading facts and principles of the science, as taught in a course of lectures delivered in the Marischal College of Aberdeen. . . . Philadelphia: E. Barrington & G. D. Haswell, 1843. 127p. DLC; PPC **40-0863**

McVICKAR, John Augustus (1812-1892)
Homoeopathia; a principle in medicine and not an exclusive system, in a letter to Alban Goldsmith, M.D. New York: J. S. Taylor & Co., 1841. 45p. DNLM; PPHa **40-0864**

MAGENDIE, François (1783-1855)
An elementary treatise on human physiology, on the basis of the Précis élémentaire de physiologie. Transl., enlarged, and illustrated . . . by John Revere. New York: Harper & Bro., 1844. 539p. 1 plate. DNLM; MdBM; NNNAM **40-0865**

MANLEY, James R. (1781-1851)
Letters on the College of Physicians and Surgeons, by Graviora manent [pseud.]. New York: Printed by A. S. Gould, 1841. 16p. DLC; NNNAM **40-0866**

MANLEY, James R. (1781-1851)
Exposition on the conduct and character of Dr. John Augustus Smith, president of the College of Physicians and Surgeons in the city of New York; as exhibited in the session of 1839-1840. New York, 1841. 48p. DNLM; NNNAM **40-0867**

MANLEY, James R. (1781-1851)
Anniversary discourse before the New York Academy of Medicine. Delivered November 8, 1848. New York: H. Ludwig & Co., 1849. 36p. DNLM; NNNAM **40-0868**

A MANUAL on beauty and health; containing useful remarks on the proper treatment of the human system. . . . To which is added: Dr. Gregory's legacy to his daughters. . . . Providence: B. T. Albro, 1848. 96p. DNLM **40-0869**

MARCH, Alden (1795-1869)
Account of an operation for the removal of an ovarian tumor. [1849] 8p. DNLM **40-0870**

MARKOE, Thomas Masters (1819-1901)
An introductory lecture delivered in the Castleton Medical College. Troy, N.Y.: J. C. Kneeland & Co., 1847. 19p. DNLM
40-0871

MARWICK, Alfred
A guide to the examination of the urine in health and disease, for the students. . . . Philadelphia: Lea & Blanchard, 1848. 113p. DNLM; PPC; PPJ; PU **40-0872**

MARSHALL, Warren W.
Views of the origin, nature, symptoms and progress of cancer, fistula, etc., derived from practical knowledge, together with certificates of some of the cures perfected. Richmond: I. Lyon, 1842. 24p. DNLM; ViRA **40-0873**

MARTINEAU, Harriet (1802-1876)
Life in the sick room. Essays by an invalid. With an introduction to the American ed. by Eliza L. Follen. 2nd American ed. Boston: W. Crosby, 1845. 196p. DNLM; AU; MA; NN
40-0874

MARTINEAU, Harriet (1802-1876)
Letters on mesmerism. New York: Harper & Brothers, 1845. 27p. DNLM; GU; ICU; NNC **40-0875**

MASON, Augustus (1822-1882)
The quackery of the age: a satire on the times. Boston: White, Lewis & Potter, 1845. 44p. DNLM; MB; MWA; MBAt
40-0876

MASON, Augustus (1822-1882)
The cholera. Brief hints for the prevention of cholera, with a plain account of the symptoms, the proper preventive measures, and the management of its early stages. Sanctioned by the Medical Faculty of Lowell. Lowell: B. H. Penhallow, 1849. 8p. DNLM; MBM **40-0877**

MASON, Augustus (1822-1882)
Social ethics as connected with the business of the physician. The mutual duties of physicians and society; being the annual address delivered before the Middlesex District Medical Society. Lowell: J. Atkinson, 1849. 27p. DNLM; MBAt; MBM; MWA **40-0878**

MASSE, Joseph Nicholas
A pocket atlas of the descriptive anatomy of the human body. Transl. from the last Paris ed. and edited by G. Sharp Pattison. New York: Harper & Bros., 1845. 56 l. 112 plates. DNLM; MBM; NNNAM; PPC **40-0879**

MATTHEWS, William
A treatise on domestic medicine and kindred subjects, embracing anatomical and physiological sketches of the human body. Indianapolis: J. D. Defrees, 1848. 196p. DNLM
40-0880

MATTSON, Morris
The American vegetable practice, or a new and improved guide to health, designed for the use of families. In 6 pts. Boston: D. L. Hale, 1841. 2 v. in 1. DNLM; MBM
40-0881

MAUNSELL, Henry (1806-1879)
The Dublin practice of midwifery. With notes and additions by Chandler R. Gilman. New York: LeBlanc, 1842. 292p. NNNAM **40-0882**

MAURICEAU, A.M.
The married woman's private medical companion, embracing the treatment of menstruation, or monthly turns, during their stoppage, irregularity, or entire suppression. Pregnancy, and how it may be determined; with the treatment of its various diseases. Discovery to prevent pregnancy; its great and important necessity where malformation or inability exists to give birth. To prevent miscarriage or abortion. When proper and necessary to effect miscarriage, when attended with entire safety. Causes and mode of cure of barrenness, or sterility. New York, 1847. 238p. DNLM; NNNAM
40-0883

MAURY, [J. C.] F. [M.]
Treatise on the dental art, founded on actual experience. Transl. from the French, with notes and additions, by J. B. Savier. Philadelphia: Lea & Blanchard, 1843. 324p. 20 plates. DNLM; MdU-D; PPC; PU **40-0884**

MAYNARD, J. P[arker] (1817?-1898)
History of the discovery and mode of application of the liquid adhesive plaster or ethereal solution of prepared cotton. Boston: Maynard & Noyes, 1848. 19p. DNLM; MBM
40-0885

MAYNE, John
A dispensatory and theapeutical remembrancer with a full and distinct version of every practical formula, as authorized by the London, Edinburgh and Dublin Royal College of Physicians, in the latest editions of their several pharmacopoeias. . . . Rev. with the addition of the formulae of the United States pharmacopoeia, etc. By R. Eglesfeld Griffith. . . . Philadelphia: Lea & Blanchard, 1848. 329p. DLC; DNLM; OCLloyd; PPC
40-0886

MAYO, Herbert (1796-1852)
Outlines of human pathology. . . . From the last London ed. Philadelphia: Carey & Hart, 1841. 436p. DLC; DNLM; PPC; PU **40-0887**

MAYO, Thomas (1790-1871)
Elements of the pathology of the human mind. Philadelphia: Carey & Hart, 1841. 73p. DNLM; MBM; PPC; ViRA
40-0888

MEANS, A.
An address delivered before the Medical College of Georgia at the opening of its annual session. Augusta: J. M. McCafferty, 1847. 31p. DNLM; GU **40-0889**

MEDICAL application of electricity, with descriptions of apparatus and institutions for its use. [By Daniel Davis, Jr.] Boston: D. Davis, Jr., 1846. 24p. DNLM [3rd ed., 1848; no change]
40-0890

MEDICAL INSTITUTE OF PHILADELPHIA
An account of the . . . with a list of pupils for 1844 [and a table of the classes from 1819 to 1843]. Philadelphia: J. C. Clark, 1845. 15p. DNLM; PPC **40-0891**

MEDICAL INSTITUTE OF PHILADELPHIA
Announcement for the year 1847. Philadelphia: United States Printing Office, 1847. 18p. [List of students from 1819 to 1845, in: Announcement for 1847. Founded as a summer school in 1817. Conferred no degrees, being intended only to afford continuous instruction to those who remained in the city after the winter sessions.] DNLM; PPC
40-0892

MEIGS, Charles Delucena (1792-1869)
Introductory lecture to a course on obstetrics, delivered in Jefferson Medical College, November 4, 1841. . . . Published by the class. Philadelphia: Merrihew & Thompson, printers, 1841. 18p. DLC; DNLM; PPJ **40-0893**

MEIGS, Charles Delucena (1792-1869)
The Philadelphia practice of midwifery. . . . 2nd ed., improved and enl. Philadelphia: J. Kay, Jr. & Brother; Pittsburgh: C. H. Kay & Co., 1842. 408p. 53 plates. DLC; DNLM; PPJ **40-0894**

MEIGS, Charles Delucena (1792-1869)
A lecture introductory to the course of obstetrics in Jefferson Medical College. Philadelphia: Merrihew & Thompson, 1842. 31p. DNLM; PPC; PPJ; ViRA **40-0895**

MEIGS, Charles Delucena (1792-1869)
Lecture introductory to his course of lectures for 1843-1844. Philadelphia: Merrihew & Thompson, 1843. 31p. DNLM; PPC; PPJ; PPL **40-0896**

MEIGS, Charles Delucena (1792-1869)
Introductory lecture [Jefferson Medical College]. Philadelphia: Merrihew & Thompson, 1846. 24p. DNLM; PPJ **40-0897**

MEIGS, Charles Delucena (1792-1869)
Lecture on some of the distinctive characteristics of the female. Philadelphia: Collins, 1847. 20p. DNLM; PPC; PPJ; ScCM **40-0898**

MEIGS, Charles Delucena (1792-1869)
An introductory lecture [Jefferson Medical College]. Philadelphia: C. Sherman, 1848. 20p. DNLM; PPJ **40-0899**

MEIGS, Charles Delucena (1792-1869)
Females and their diseases; a series of letters to his class. . . . Philadelphia: Lea & Blanchard, 1848. 670p. DLC: DNLM; PPJ; ViRA **40-0900**

MEIGS, Charles Delucena (1792-1869)
Obstetrics: the science and the art. . . . Philadelphia: Lea & Blanchard, 1849. 685p. DLC; DNLM; PPJ; ScCM **40-0901**

MEIGS, Charles Delucena (1792-1869)
Remarks on spasmodic cholera. . . . Philadelphia, 1849. 68p. DLC; DNLM; PPC; PPJ **40-0902**

MEIGS, John Forsyth (1818-1882)
A practical treatise on the diseases of children. . . . Philadelphia: Lindsay & Blakiston, 1848. 575p. DLC; DNLM; NcD; PPC **40-0903**

MENDENHALL, George (1814-1874)
The medical student's vade mecum, or manual of examinations upon anatomy, physiology. . . . 2nd edition, revised and greatly enlarged. Philadelphia: Lindsay & Blakiston, 1847. 574p. CtY-M; DNLM; PPC; PU **40-0904**

MERRICK, Frederick
Introductory lecture delivered to the class of the Starling Medical College. Columbus: Legg & Murray, 1848. 16p. DNLM; OCIM; OCIWHi **40-0905**

METCALF, John George (1801-1892)
The physiology of the skin. A lecture. Boston: Marsh, Capen & Co., 1840. 23p. DNLM; MBM **40-0906**

MICHEL, Middleton (1822-1894)
On organogeny. Charleston: Burges & James, 1846. 21p. DNLM; ScCM **40-0907**

MILLER, Henry (1800-1874)
An examination of the claims of homoeopathy, as a system of medical doctrine and practice: being a lecture delivered before the Medical Society of Louisville on the 14th December, 1847. . . . Published by the Society. Louisville, Ky.: Printed by G. H. Monsarrat & Co. [1847]. 24p. DLC; DNLM; PPHa **40-0908**

MILLER, Henry (1800-1874)
A theoretical and practical treatise on human parturition. . . . Louisville: J. V. Cowling & G. C. Davies; New York: A. A. Barnes & Co., 1849. 463p. DLC; NNNAM **40-0909**

MILLER, James (1812-1864)
The principles of surgery. . . . Philadelphia: Lea & Blanchard, 1845. 525p. DLC; DNLM; PPC; PPJ **40-0910**

MILLER, James (1812-1864)
The practice of surgery. Philadelphia: Lea & Blanchard, 1846. 496p. DNLM; PPC; PPJ; PU **40-0911**

MILLER, Thomas (1806-1873)
Introductory lecture on anatomy. . . . professor of anatomy and physiology. Columbian College, D.C. Delivered on Thursday, the 5th of November, 1840. Washington: Printed by J. Gideon, Jr., 1840. 20p. DLC; DNLM **40-0912**

MILLER, Thomas (1806-1873)
An address to the graduates of the medical department of Columbian College. . . . Delivered March 2, 1842. Washington: Blair & Rives, printers, 1842. 31p. DLC; DNLM **40-0913**

MILLINGEN, J. G.
Aphorisms on the treatment and management of the insane; with considerations on public and private lunatic asylums, pointing out the errors in the present system. Philadelphia: Barrington & Haswell, 1842. 91p. DNLM; MBM; NNNAM; PPC **40-0914**

MITCHELL, C. L[eeds] (1813-1888)
Introductory lecture to the fall session of lectures in the Castleton Medical College. Albany: C. Van Benthuysen & Co., 1844. 16p. DNLM **40-0915**

MITCHELL, John Kearsley (1798-1858)
On the usefulness of the medical profession, beyond the limits of the profession. A lecture, introductory to the course of the practice of medicine in Jefferson Medical College. Philadelphia: Merrihew & Thompson, 1842. 30p. DNLM; PPJ **40-0916**

MITCHELL, John Kearsley (1798-1858)
Lecture introductory to the course of the practice of medicine in the Jefferson Medical College, delivered November 2, 1847. Philadelphia: Merrihew & Thompson, 1847. 24p. DNLM; PPJ **40-0917**

MITCHELL, John Kearsley (1798-1858)
Introductory lecture to the course of the practice of medicine, delivered in Jefferson Medical College, October 16th, 1849. . . . Published by the class. Philadelphia: C. Sherman, printer, 1849. 24p. DLC: DNLM; PPJ **40-0918**

MITCHELL, John Kearsley (1798-1858)
On the cryptogamous origin of malarious and epidemic fevers. . . . Philadelphia: Lea & Blanchard, 1849. 137p. DLC; DNLM; PPJ **40-0919**

MITCHELL, Thomas Duché (1791-1865)
The good physician; being an introduction to the course of lectures on materia medica and therapeutics in the medical department of Transylvania University. Lexington, Ky., 1842. 18p. DNLM **40-0920**

MITCHELL, Thomas Duché (1791-1865)
The reciprocal obligations of professors and pupils; an introductory lecture. Lexington: N. L. Finnell, 1845. 16p. DNLM **40-0921**

MITCHELL, Thomas Duché (1791-1865)
The character of Rush, an introductory to the course on the theory and practice of medicine, in the Philadelphia College of Medicine. . . . Philadelphia: J. H. Gihon, printer, 1848. 23p. DLC; DNLM **40-0922**

MITCHELL, Thomas Duché (1791-1865)
Lecture on epidemic cholera, delivered in the hall of the Philadelphia College of Medicine, in May, 1849, at the request of the medical class. . . . Philadelphia: Craig & Young, printers, 1849. 22p. DLC; DNLM **40-0923**

MITCHELL, Thomas Duché (1791-1865)
The study of medicine: an introductory lecture, delivered in the hall of the Philadelphia College of Medicine, October 15th, 1849. . . . Philadelphia: Craig & Young, printers, 1849. 24p. DLC; DNLM; PPC; PU **40-0924**

MOHR, Francis, and Theophilus REDWOOD
Practical pharmacy; the arrangements, apparatus, and manipulations of the pharmaceutical shop and laboratory. Edited, with extensive additions, by William Procter, Jr. Philadelphia: Lea & Blanchard, 1849. 576p. DNLM; OCIM; OCLloyd; PPC **40-0925**

MONDAT, Vincent Marie
On sterility in the male and female, its causes and treatment. . . . Transl. from the 5th French ed. . . . New York: J. S. Redfield; Boston: Saxton, Peirce & Co., 1844. 248p. DLC; DNLM; NNNAM **40-0926**

MONELL, Gilbert Chichester (1816-1881)
Rheumatism, acute and chronic. A prize essay. . . . (Published by order of the Orange County Medical Society.) New York: H. G. Langley, 1845. 144p. DLC; DNLM; NNNAM **40-0927**

MONROE COUNTY MEDICAL SOCIETY
Report of a committee on the subject of medical legislation to the Monroe County Medical Society, Rochester, Nov. 9, 1842. [Rochester, 1842.] 15p. DNLM **40-0928**

MONTGOMERY, William Fetherston (1797-1859)
An exposition of the signs and symptoms of pregnancy, the period of human gestation, and the signs of delivery. . . . Philadelphia: Carey & Hart, 1841. 220p. DNLM; MdBM; MBM; PPC **40-0929**

MOORE, George (1803-1880)
The use of the body in relation to the mind. New York: Harper & Bros., 1847. 356p. DNLM; NNNAM **40-0930**

MOORMAN, John J. (*d.* 1885)
Water from the White Sulphur Springs, Greenbrier County, Va. With practical remarks on its medical properties, and applicability to particular diseases. [1840]. DNLM **40-0931**

MOORMAN, John J. (*d.* 1885)
A brief notice of a portion of a work by Wm. Burke, entitled, "The Mineral Spings of Western Virginia." . . . Philadelphia: Merrihew & Thompson, 1843. 52p. DNLM; PPL **40-0932**

MOORMAN, John J. (*d.* 1885)
The Virginia springs with their analysis . . . and an account of the different routes to the springs. Philadelphia: Lindsay & Blakiston, 1847. 219p. map. DNLM; PP; PPL **40-0933**

MOREAU, François-Joseph (1789-1862)
A practical treatise on midwifery; exhibiting the present advanced state of the science. Transl. from the French by Thos. Forrest Betton, and edited by Paul B. Goddard. Philadelphia: Carey & Hart, 1844. 235p. 80 plates. DNLM; PPC; PU; ViRA **40-0934**

MORFIT, Campbell (1820-1897)
Chemical and pharmaceutic manipulations: a manual of the mechanical and chemico-mechanical operations of the laboratory. . . . For the use of chemists, druggists, teachers, and students. . . . Assisted by Alexander Mucklé. . . . With four hundred and twenty-three illustrations. Philadelphia: Lindsay & Blakiston, 1849. 452p. plates. DLC; OCLloyd **40-0935**

MORGAN, George T.
An outline of inflammation and its effects; being the first principles of surgery. Philadelphia: Carey & Hart, 1841. 134p. DNLM; NNNAM; PPC; ViRA **40-0936**

MORISON, Benjamin
The treatment, cure and prevention of hemorrhoids or piles, upon scientific principles. . . . Philadelphia, 1842. 16p. DLC; PPC **40-0937**

MORISON, Benjamin
Dr. Morison's remedy for diarrhea, cholera, and all affections of the bowels attended with inordinate discharges, especially those of hot and bilious climates . . . with a description of the nature and comon causes of the diseases. . . . Philadelphia, 1842. 7p. DLC; PPJ; PU **40-0938**

MORLEY, Charles
Elements of animal magnetism; or process and application for relieving human suffering. New York: Fowler & Wells, 1847. 27p. DNLM; NNNAM **40-0939**

MORROW, T. V.
A few thoughts on the necessity of medical reformation, in a lecture delivered before the class of the Reformed Medical School of Cincinnati, Ohio, November 6, 1843. Cincinnati: A. Derrough, 1844. 16p. DNLM; OCIM **40-0940**

MORROW, T. V.
Introductory address, delivered before the class of the Eclectic Medical Institute, Cincinnati, Ohio, at the commencement of the session, November, 1847. Cincinnati, 1847. 20p. DNLM; OCIM **40-0941**

MORTON, Samuel George (1799-1851)
Catalogue of skulls of man, and the inferior animals, in the collection of. . . . Philadelphia: Turner & Fisher, 1840. 48p. DNLM; MWA; NIC **40-0942**

MORTON, Samuel George (1799-1851)
A memoir of William Maclure, Esq., late president of the Academy of Natural Sciences of Philadelphia. Philadelphia: T. K. & P. G. Collins, 1841. 37p. 1 plate. DNLM; PPL **40-0943**

MORTON, Samuel George (1799-1851)
Brief remarks on the diversities of the human species, and on some kindred subjects; being an introductory lecture delivered before the class of Pennsylvania Medical College. Philadelphia: Merrihew & Thompson, 1842. 24p. DNLM; PPF **40-0944**

MORTON, Samuel George (1799-1851)
A memoir of William Maclure, Esq., late president of the Academy of Natural Sciences of Philadelphia. 2nd ed. [Philadelphia, 1844] 33p. DNLM; PPL **40-0945**

MORTON, Samuel George (1799-1851)
An inquiry into the distinctive characteristics of the aboriginal race of America. 2nd ed. Philadelphia: J. Penington, 1844. 48p. DNLM; PPL; MWA **40-0946**

MORTON, Samuel George (1799-1851)
Biographical notice of the late George McClellan, M.D. [Philadelphia, 1849] 10p. DNLM; PPJ **40-0947**

MORTON, Samuel George (1799-1851)
Catalogue of skulls of man, and the inferior animals, in the collection. . . . 3rd ed. Philadelphia: Merrihew & Thompson, 1849. 37p. DNLM; NN; ViRA **40-0948**

MORTON, Samuel George (1799-1851)
An illustrated system of human anatomy, special, general, and microscopic. Philadelphia: Grigg, Elliot & Co., 1849. 642p. DNLM; MBM; PPC; PPH **40-0949**

[MORTON, William T. G.] (1819-1868)
Circular. Morton's letheon. [Cautioning those who attempt to infringe upon his legal rights.] Boston: Dutton & Wentworth [1846]. 14p. DNLM; MB; MWA **40-0950**

MORTON, William T. G. (1819-1868)
Remarks on the proper mode of administering sulphuric ether by inhalation. Boston: Dutton & Wentworth, 1847. 44p. DNLM; MH; MHi; MWA **40-0951**

MORTON, William T. G. (1819-1868) and Francis WHITMAN
On the loss of the teeth and the modern way of restoring them, as practiced by. . . . Boston: Damrell & Moore, 1847. 23p. 1 plate. DNLM; MBM; MH; MWA **40-0952**

MORTON, William T. G. (1819-1868)
On the loss of the teeth, and the modern way of restoring them, as practiced by. . . . 2nd ed. Boston: W. A. Hall, 1848. 32p. DNLM; MH; MBM; MWA **40-0953**

MOSHER, Alanson
Learned quackery exposed, or the difference shown between poisons and medicines. Schoharie: Gallup & Lawyer, 1846. 37p. DNLM **40-0954**

MOTT, Lucretia (1793-1880)
A sermon to the medical students, delivered by . . . , at Cherry Street Meeting House, Philadelphia, on first-day evening, second month 11th, 1849. Rev. phonographic report. Philadelphia: W. B. Zeiber [etc.], 1849. 21p. DLC; DNLM; PPC **40-0955**

MOTT, Valentine (1785-1865)
Travels in Europe and the East. . . . In the years 1834, '35, '36, '37, '38, '39, '40, and '41. . . . New York: Harper & Brothers, 1842. 452p. DLC; DNLM; ICU; NN **40-0956**

MOTT, Valentine (1785-1865)
A biographical memoir on the late John Revere, M.D., professor of the theory and practice of medicine in the University of New York. . . . Delivered at the request of the medical faculty of the University. New York: J. H. Jennings, printer, 1847. 40p. DLC; DNLM; NNNAM **40-0957**

MOTT, Valentine (1785-1865)
An inaugural address, delivered before the New York Academy of Medicine, February 7, 1849. . . . to which is prefixed, an address by Dr. J. W. Francis, to the president elect. Published by order of the Academy. New York: Printed by H. Ludwig & Co., 1849. 24p. DLC; DNLM; NNNAM **40-0958**

MOULTRIE, James (1793-1869)
On the organic function of animals. Charleston: Burges & James, 1844. 20p. DNLM; ScCM **40-0959**

MÜLLER, Johannes (1801-1858)
Elements of physiology. . . . Transl. from the German, by Wm. Baly. . . . Arranged from the 2nd London ed., by John Bell. . . . Philadelphia: Lea & Blanchard, 1843. 886p. DNLM; MBM; PPC; PU **40-0960**

MUNSELL, Henry
The Dublin practice of midwifery. With notes and additions by Chandler R. Gilman. New York: W. E. Dean, 1845. 292p. DNLM; MH-M; NNNAM; PPC **40-0961**

MUSSEY, Reuben Dimond (1780-1866)
Animalcula in the atmosphere of cholera patients. [Cincinnati], 1849. 4p. DNLM **40-0962**

MÜTTER, Thomas Dent (1811-1859)
The salt sulphur springs, Monroe County, Va. Philadelphia: T. K. & P. G. Collins, 1840. 32p. DNLM; ViRA **40-0963**

MÜTTER, Thomas Dent (1811-1859)
On recent improvements in surgery. An introductory lecture to the course on the principles and practice of surgery in Jefferson Medical College. Philadelphia: Merrihew & Thompson, 1842. 52p. DNLM; PPC; PPJ **40-0964**

MÜTTER, Thomas Dent (1811-1859)
Cases of deformity from burns, successfully treated by plastic operations. Philadelphia: Merrihew & Thompson, printers, 1843. 23p. DNLM; PPC; PPJ **40-0965**

MÜTTER, Thomas Dent (1811-1859)
A report on the operations for fissures of the palatine vault. Philadelphia: Merrihew & Thompson, 1843. 28p. DNLM; PPC; PPJ **40-0966**

MÜTTER, Thomas Dent (1811-1859)
Syllabus of the course of lectures on the principles and practice of surgery, delivered in the Jefferson Medical College, Philadelphia. Pts. 1-3. Philadelphia: Merrihew & Thompson, 1843. 206p. DNLM; PPC; PPJ **40-0967**

MÜTTER, Thomas Dent (1811-1859)
Cases of deformity of various kinds successfully treated by plastic operations. Philadelphia: Merrihew & Thompson, 1844. 38p. 2 plates. DNLM; PPC; PPJ; PU **40-0968**

MÜTTER, Thomas Dent (1811-1859)
Introductoy for 1844-1845, on the present position of some of the most important of the modern operations of surgery. Philadelphia: Merrihew & Thompson, 1844. 34p. DNLM; PPC; PPJ; PU **40-0969**

MÜTTER, Thomas Dent (1811-1859)
Syllabus of the course of lectures on the principles and practice of surgery, delivered in the Jefferson Medical College, Philadelphia. Pts. 1-3. Philadelphia: Barrett & Jones, 1846. 206p. DNLM; PPJ **40-0970**

MÜTTER, Thomas Dent (1811-1859)
Lecture introductory to a course on the principles and practice of surgery in the Jefferson Medical College. Philadelphia: Merrihew & Thompson, 1847. 26p. DNLM; PPC; PPJ **40-0971**

MÜTTER, Thomas Dent (1811-1859)
Syllabus of the course of lectures on the principles and practice of surgery, delivered in the Jefferson Medical College, Philadelphia. . . . Philadelphia: J. H. Jones, printer, 1848. 212p. DLC; DNLM; PPJ **40-0972**

NASMYTH, Alexander
Researches on the development, structure, and diseases of the teeth. Baltimore: Published by the American Society of Dental Surgeons, 1842. 116p. DNLM; MdU-D; PPC; PU **40-0973**

NEIDHARD, Charles (1809-1895)
An answer to the homoeopathic delusions of Dr. Oliver Wendell Holmes. Philadelphia: J. Dobson, 1842. 36p. DNLM; PPHa **40-0974**

NEILL, John (1819-1880)
Outlines of the nerves, with short descriptions. Philadelphia: E. Barrington & G. D. Haswell, 1845. 30p. 9 plates. DNLM; PPC **40-0975**

NEILL, John (1819-1880)
Outlines of the arteries; with short descriptions. Philadelphia: E. Barrington & G. D. Haswell, 1845. 30p. 6 plates. DNLM; PPC; PPJ; PU **40-0976**

NEILL, John (1819-1880)
Outlines of the veins and lymphatics; with short descriptions. Designed for the use of medical students. Philadelphia: E. Barrington & G. D. Haswell, 1847. 29p. 8 plates. DNLM; PPC **40-0977**

NEILL, John (1819-1880) and Francis Gurney SMITH
A handbook of surgery; being a portion of an analytical compend of the various branches of medicine. Philadelphia: Lea & Blanchard, 1848. 122p. DNLM; MBM; PPC; ViRA **40-0978**

NEILL, John (1819-1880) and Francis Gurney SMITH
A handbook of anatomy. . . . Being a portion of an analytical compend of the various branches of medicine. Philadelphia: Lea & Blanchard, 1848. 180p. DNLM; PPC; PU **40-0979**

NEILL, John (1819-1880) and Francis Gurney SMITH
A handbook of chemistry. . . . Being a portion of an analytical compend of the various branches of medicine. Philadelphia: Lea & Blanchard, 1848. 115p. DNLM; PPC; ViRA **40-0980**

NEILL, John (1819-1880) and Francis Gurney SMITH
An analytical compendium of the various branches of medical science, for the use and examination of students. . . . Philadelphia: Lea & Blanchard, 1848. 7 v. in 1. PPC; PPJ; PU **40-0981**

NELIGAN, John Moore (1815-1863)
Medicines. Their uses and mode of administration; including a complete conspectus of the three British pharmacopoeias, an account of all the new remedies, and an appendix of formulae. . . . With notes and additions, conforming it to the pharmacopoeia of the United States. . . by David Meredith Reese. . . . New York: Harper & Brothers, 1844. 453p. DNLM; NNNAM; PPC; ViRA **40-0982**

NEWMAN, John B.
The home doctor: or, Family manual, giving the causes, symptoms, and treatment of diseases. . . . New York: J. S. Husted & Co., 1847. 98p. DLC; NNNAM **40-0983**

NICHOLS, Mary S. Gove
Experience in water-cure. A familiar exposition of the principles and results of water treatment in the cure of acute and chronic diseases, illustrated by numerous cases . . . , with an explanation of water-cure processes, advice on diet and regimen, and particular directions to women in the treatment of female diseases, water treatment in childbirth, and the diseases of infancy. New York: Fowler & Wells, [1849]. 108p. DNLM; NNNAM **40-0984**

NORRIS, George W. (1808-1872)
Biographical memoir of Jacob Randolph, M.D. Philadelphia: W. F. Giddes, 1848. 12p. DNLM; PPC **40-0985**

NORRIS, George W. (1808-1872)
Introductory lecture to the course of clinical instruction in surgery, at the Pennsylvania Hospital; delivered Nov. 1st, 1848. Philadelphia: King & Baird, 1848. 15p. DNLM; PU **40-0986**

NORTH, M. L[inus] (1790-1856)
Analysis of Saratoga waters; also of Sharon, Avon, Virginia, and other mineral waters of the United States. With directions for invalids. New York: Saxton & Miles, 1846. 72p. DNLM; NN; NNNAM **40-0987**

NOTES on Dr. Chapman's lectures, in the University of Pennsylvania, with an appendix, containing a few remarks on Asiatic cholera and yellow fever, by a physician. Philadelphia: W. S. Young, 1845. 131p. DNLM; PPC; PU **40-0988**

NUNNELEY, Thomas (1809-1870)
A treatise on the nature, causes, and treatment of erysipelas. 1st American ed. Philadelphia: Barrington & Haswell, 1844. 235p. DNLM; PPC; PPJ; ViRA **40-0989**

OBSTINATE, inveterate, and habitual constipation (costiveness) . . . totally overcome . . . by a natural, simple, agreeable, and infallible means recently discovered in France. [Warton's ervalenta.] 5th English ed. from the 22nd French ed. New York: J. Smith, 1844. 129p. DNLM; NNNAM **40-0990**

OKIE, Abraham Howard (*d.* 1882)
Homoeopathy explained and objections answered. . . . Philadelphia: J. Dobson, 1841. 24p. PPHa **40-0991**

OKIE, Abraham Howard (*d.* 1882)
Homoeopathy, with particular reference to a lecture by O. W. Holmes, M.D. Boston, Mass.: Otis Clapp, 1842. 48p. DNLM; PPHa **40-0992**

OLCOTT, Thomas W.
Address delivered before the Albany Phrenological Society at its meeting, April 2, 1840. Albany: J. Munsell, 1840. 10p. DNLM **40-0993**

OLIVER, Daniel (1787-1842)
First lines of physiology; designed for the use of students of medicine. Philadelphia: H. Hooker, 1840. 514p. DNLM; PPC; ViRA **40-0994**

OLIVER, Daniel (1787-1842)
First lines of physiology; designed for the use of students of medicine. 2nd ed. Philadelphia: Hooker & Agnew, 1841. 514p. DNLM; PPJ; PU **40-0995**

OLIVER, Daniel (1787-1842)
First lines of physiology; designed for students of medicine. 3rd ed. Boston: W. D. Ticknor & Co., 1844. 517p. DNLM; MBM; MH-M **40-0996**

OSGOOD, Charles (1808-1881)
The causes, treatment and cure of fever and ague, and other diseases of bilious climates. 11th ed. New York, 1847. 14p. DNLM; NNNAM **40-0997**

PACKARD, Frederick A.
Memorandum of a late visit to some of the principal hospitals, prisons, etc., in France, Scotland, and England. Embraced in a letter to the acting committee of the Philadelphia Society for Alleviating the Miseries of Public Prisons. Philadelphia: E. G. Dorsey, 1840. 33p. DNLM; PU **40-0998**

PAIGE, A.
The electropathic guide: devoted to electricity and its medical applications. Boston, 1849. 129p. DNLM; MBM **40-0999**

PAINE, Martyn (1794-1877)
A reply to an attack by Henry I. Bowditch, M.D., upon the essay On the principal writings of P. Ch. A. Louis, M.D., as contained in the medical and physiological commentaries, by the author. . . . Boston: Republished from the Medical and Surgical Journal, 1840. 56p. DLC; DNLM; MBM **40-1000**

PAINE, Martyn (1794-1877)
Medical and physiological commentaries. . . . New York: Collins, Keese & Co., 1840-1844. 3 v. DLC: DNLM; NNNAM; PPC **40-1001**

PAINE, Martyn (1794-1877)
Notice of reviews by the British and Foreign Medical Review and the Medico-Chirurgical Review (April, 1841) of the Medical and Physiological Commentaries, as contained in the Boston Medical and Surgical Journal of September, 1841. Boston: D. Clapp, Jr., 1841. 8p. DNLM; MBM **40-1002**

PAINE, Martyn (1794-1877)
Supplement second to the "Humoral Pathology." New York, 1841. 5p. DNLM **40-1003**

PAINE, Martyn (1794-1877)
An examination of a review, contained in the British and Foreign Medical Review, of the medical and physiol. commentaries, by the author. . . . New York: Hopkins & Jennings, printers, 1841. 96p. DLC; NNNAM **40-1004**

PAINE, Martyn (1794-1877)
Answer to circular letters by Drs. Carpenter and Forbes. Boston: D. Clapp, Jr., 1842. 8p. DNLM; MBM **40-1005**

PAINE, Martyn (1794-1877)
A therapeutical arrangement of the materia medica, or, The materia medica arranged upon physiological principles . . . New York: J. & H. G. Langley, 1842. 271p. DLC; DNLM; OCLloyd **40-1006**

PAINE, Martyn (1794-1877)
Essays on the philosophy of vitality as contradistinguished from chemical and mechanical philosophy, and on the modus operandi of remedial agents. . . . New York: Printed for the author by Hopkins & Jennings, 1842. 70p. DLC; DNLM; NNNAM **40-1007**

PAINE, Martyn (1794-1877)
A discourse introductory to a course of lectures on the institutes of medicine and materia medica, delivered before the medical class of the University of New York, at the session of 1841-1842. . . . Boston: D. Clapp, Jr., printer, 1842. 33p. DLC; DNLM; MBM **40-1008**

PAINE, Martyn (1794-1877)
A lecture on the improvement of medical education in the United States, introductory to a course of lectures in the University of New York. New York: A. Craighead, 1843. 16p. DNLM; NNNAM **40-1009**

PAINE, Martyn (1794-1877)
A defense of an introductory lecture on the "improvement of medical education in the United States," against an attack by the Medico-Chirurgical Review. Boston: D. Clapp, Jr., 1844. 4p. MBM; NNNAM **40-1010**

PAINE, Martyn (1794-1877)
A lecture on the physiology of digestion, introductory to a course of lectures on the institutes of medicine and materia medica. Delivered before the medical class of the University of the City of New York, at the session of 1844-1845. . . . New York: Printed for the medical class of the University, by J. H. Jennings, 1844-1845. 24p. DLC; DNLM; NNNAM **40-1011**

PAINE, Martyn (1794-1877)
A lecture on the physiology of digestion, introductory to a course of lectures on the institutes of medicine and materia medica. Delivered before the medical class of the University of the City of New York, at the session of 1844-1845. . . . 2nd ed. New York: Printed for the medical class of the University, by J. H. Jennings, 1844-1845. 24p. DLC; DNLM; NNNAM
40-1012

PAINE, Martyn (1794-1877)
A lecture on the physiology of digestion, introductory to a course of lectures on the institutes of medicine and materia medica. Delivered before the medical class of the University of the City of New York, at the session of 1844-45. 3rd ed. New York: Printed for the medical class of the University, by J. H. Jennings, 1844-1845. 24p. NNNAM
40-1013

PAINE, Martyn (1794-1877)
A lecture on the physiology of digestion, introductory to a course of lectures on the institutes of medicine and materia medica. Delivered before the medical class of the University of the City of New York, at the session of 1844-45. 4th ed. New York: Printed for the medical class of the University, by J. H. Jennings, 1844-1845. 24p. DNLM; NNNAM
40-1014

PAINE, Martyn (1794-1877)
A lecture on the philosophy of medicine, introductory to a course of lectures on the institutes of medicine and materia medica. New York, 1844-1846. 19p. DNLM; NNNAM
40-1015

PAINE, Martyn (1794-1877)
A defense of the medical profession of the United States; being a valedictory address to the graduating class at the medical commencement of the University of New York, delivered March 11, 1846. . . . New York: Burgess, Stringer & Co., 1846. 24p. DLC; DNLM; NNNAM **40-1016**

PAINE, Martyn (1794-1877)
A defense of the medical profession of the United States; being a valedictory address to the graduating class at the medical commencement of the University of New York, delivered March 11, 1846. . . . 2nd ed. New York: Burgess, Stringer & Co., 1846. 24p. DNLM; NNNAM **40-1017**

PAINE, Martyn (1794-1877)
A defense of the medical profession of the United States; being a valedictory address to the graduating class at the medical commencement of the University of New York, delivered March 11, 1846. . . . 3rd ed. New York: Burgess, Stringer & Co., 1846. 24p. NNNAM **40-1018**

PAINE, Martyn (1794-1877)
A defense of the medical profession of the United States; being a valedictory address to the graduatng class at the medical commencement of the University of New York, delivered March 11, 1846. . . . 4th ed. New York: Burgess, Stringer & Co., 1846. 24p. NNNAM **40-1019**

PAINE, Martyn (1794-1877)
A defense of the medical profession of the United States; being a valedictory address to the graduating class at the medical commencement of the University of New York, delivered March 11, 1846. . . . 5th ed. New York: Burgess, Stringer & Co., 1846. 24p. DNLM; NNNAM **40-1020**

PAINE, Martyn (1794-1877)
A defense of the medical profession of the United States; being a valedictory address to the graduating class at the medical commencement of the University of New York, delivered March 11, 1846. . . . 6th ed. New York: Published for the author, by S. S. & W. Wood, 1846. 24p. DLC; DNLM; NNNAM
40-1021

PAINE, Martyn (1794-1877)
A defense of the medical profession of the United States; being a valedictory address to the graduating class at the medical commencement of the University of New York, delivered March 11, 1846. . . . 7th ed. New York: Published for the author, by S. S. & W. Wood, 1846. 24p. DNLM; NNNAM
40-1022

PAINE, Martyn (1794-1877)
A defense of the medical profession of the United States; being a valedictory address to the graduating class at the medical commencement of the University of New York, delivered March 11, 1846. . . . 8th ed. New York: Published for the author, by S. S. & W. Wood, 1846. 24p. NNNAM
40-1023

PAINE, Martyn (1794-1877)
A defense of the medical profession of the United States; being a valedictory address to the graduating class at the medical commencement of the University of New York, delivered March 11, 1846. . . . 9th ed. New York: Published for the author, by S. S. & W. Wood, 1846. 24p. DNLM; NNNAM
40-1024

PAINE, Martyn (1794-1877)
A defense of the medical profession of the United States; being a valedictory address to the graduating class at the medical commencement of the University of New York, delivered March 11, 1846. . . . 10th ed. New York: Published for the author, by S. S. & W. Wood, 1846. 24p. DNLM; NNNAM
40-1025

PAINE, Martyn (1794-1877)
The institutes of medicine. . . . New York: Harper & Brothers, 1847. 826p. DLC; DNLM; NNNAM **40-1026**

PAINE, Martyn (1794-1877)
. . . A lecture, introductory to a course on the institutes of medicine and materia medica, for the session of 1847-1848. . . . New York: J. H. Jennings, printer, 1847. 20p. DLC; DNLM; NNNAM **40-1027**

PAINE, Martyn (1794-1877)
Contributions in physiology; the circulation. New York, 1848. 8p. DNLM **40-1028**

PAINE, Martyn (1794-1877)
Materia medica and therapeutics. . . . New York: S. S. & W. Wood, 1848. 411p. DLC. DNLM; NNNAM; PPC
40-1029

PAINE, Martyn (1794-1877)
A discourse on the soul and the principle of instinct, as physiologically distinguished from materialism. New York: J. H. Jennings, 1848. 40p. DNLM; NN; NNNAM
40-1030

PAINE, Martyn (1794-1877)
A discourse on the soul and instinct, physiologically distinguished from materialism, introductory to the course of lectures on the institutes of medicine and materia medica, in the University of the City of New York. Delivered . . . Nov. 2, 1848. . . . [Published originally by the medical class.] Enl. ed. New York: E. H. Fletcher, 1849. 230p. DLC; NNNAM
40-1031

PANCOAST, Joseph (1805-1882)
Introductory lecture to the course of general, descriptive, and surgical anatomy, in Jefferson Medical College, delivered Nov. 8, 1843. . . . Published by the class. Philadelphia: Merrihew & Thompson, printers, 1843. 21p. DLC; DNLM
40-1032

PANCOAST, Joseph (1805-1882)
A treatise on operative surgery: comprising a description of the various processes of the art, including all new operations. . . . Philadelphia: Carey & Hart, 1844. 380p. CU-M; DNLM; PPC; ViRA **40-1033**

PANCOAST, Joseph (1805-1882)
Introductory lecture to the course of general, descriptive, and surgical anatomy, in Jefferson Medical College. Philadelphia: Merrihew & Thompson, 1845. 23p. DNLM; PPJ
40-1034

PANCOAST, Joseph (1805-1882)
A treatise on operative surgery; comprising a description of the various processes of the art, including all the new operations; exhibiting the state of surgical science in its present advanced condition; with eighty plates, containing four hundred and eighty-six separate illustrations. 2nd ed., rev. and enl. . . . Philadelphia: Carey & Hart for G. N. Loomis, 1846. 389p. 80 plates. CtY-M; DLC; DNLM; PPC **40-1035**

PANCOAST, Joseph (1805-1882)
Charge to the graduates of Jefferson Medical College of Philadelphia, delivered March 29, 1848. With a list of the graduates. Philadelphia: Frick, Kelly & Co., 1848. 20p. DNLM; PPJ
40-1036

PANCOAST, Joseph (1805-1882)
Introductory lecture to the course of anatomy, delivered in Jefferson Medical College. Philadelphia: C. Sherman, 1849. 20p. DNLM; PPJ **40-1037**

PARIS, John Ayrton (1785-1856)
. . . A treatise on diet: with a view to establish, on practical grounds, a system of rules for the prevention and cure of the diseases incident to a disordered state of the digestive functions. . . . [Dunglison's American Medical Library] Philadelphia: A. Waldie, 1841. 220p. DLC; DNLM; MBM; PPC
40-1038

PARIS, John Ayrton (1785-1856)
Pharmacologia, being an extended inquiry into the operations of medicinal bodies, upon which are founded the theory and art of prescribing. . . . From the 9th London ed. Rewritten in order to incorporate the latest discoveries in physiology, chemistry, and materia medica. With notes by Charles A. Lee. . . . New York: Harper & Brothers, 1844. 353p. DLC; DNLM; OCLloyd **40-1039**

PARISH, Charles W. (1793-1856)
Address, delivered at the annual meeting of the Chester County Medical Society, May 1st, 1849. West Chester, Pa., 1849. 18p. DNLM **40-1040**

PARKER, Langston (1805?-1871)
. . . The modern treatment of syphilitic diseases, both primary and secondary: comprising an account of the new remedies, with numerous formulae for their preparation, and mode of administration. . . . [Dunglison's American Medical Library] Philadelphia: Printed by A. Waldie, 1840. 94p. DLC; DNLM; PPC; PU **40-1041**

PARKER, Langston (1805?-1871)
. . . The stomach in its morbid states, and the modern treatment of syphilitic diseases. Philadelphia: Carey & Hart, 1841. 194, 94p. DNLM; PPC; PPJ; ViRA **40-1042**

PARKMAN, Samuel (1816-1854)
Introductory lecture to the spring session of lectures in Castleton Medical College. Whitehall, N.Y.: Southmayd and Watkins, 1845. 15p. DNLM **40-1043**

PARMLY, Eleazar (1797?-1874)
Address to the graduating class of the Baltimore College of Dental Surgery. Baltimore: J. W. Woods, 1847. 30p. DNLM; MdU-D **40-1044**

PARMLY, Eleazar (1797?-1874)
Properties and effects of amalgam examined. In a letter to Charles A. Lee, M.D., and published by him in the New York Journal of Medicine and the Collateral Sciences. New York: H. Ludwig, 1847. 26p. DNLM; NNNAM
40-1045

PARMLY, Eleazar (1797?-1874)
Address delivered at the eighth annual commencement of the Baltimore College of Dental Surgery. Baltimore: J. W. Woods, 1848. 21p. DNLM; MdU-D **40-1046**

PARRISH, Isaac (1811-1852)
Biographical memoir of John C. Otto, M.D., late vice president of the College of Physicians; read before the college by appointment, March 4th, 1845. . . . Printed by order of the college. Philadelphia: W. F. Geddes, printer, 1845. 20p. DLC; DNLM; PPC **40-1047**

PARRISH, Isaac (1811-1852)
The sanitary condition of Philadelphia, from the report of the committee on public hygiene of the American Medical Association, read at the annual meeting in Boston, May 5, 1849. Philadelphia: T. K. & P. G. Collins, 1849. 32p. DNLM; MBM
40-1048

PARSONS, Charles William (1823-1893)
. . . An essay on the question, vis medicatrix naturae, how far is it to be relied on in the treatment of diseases? . . . [Fiske Fund Prize Dissertation of the Rhode Island Medical Society, No. 11, 1848] Boston: The Society, 1849. 18p. DLC; DNLM; RHi **40-1049**

PARSONS, Usher (1788-1868)
A lecture on the connexion and reciprocal influence, between the brain and stomach; delivered before the American Institute of Instruction at Providence, 1840. . . . Providence: B. Cranston & Co., 1841. 16p. DLC; DNLM
40-1050

PARSONS, Usher (1788-1868)
Physician for ships; containing medical advice for seamen and other persons at sea, on the treatment of diseases, and on the preservation of health in sickly climates. . . . 3rd ed. Boston: C. C. Little and J. Brown, 1842. 216p. DLC; DNLM; MBM
40-1051

PARSONS, Usher (1788-1868)
. . . Spinal diseases, both structural and functional, their causes and treatment. . . . Boston: T. H. Webb & Co., 1843. 56p. DLC; DNLM; MBM **40-1052**

PARSONS, Usher (1788-1868)
Prize dissertations on 1. Inflammation of the periosteum. 2. Eneuresis irritata. 3. Cutaneous diseases. 4. Cancer of the breast. 5. Malaria. 6. Spinal diseases. . . . 2nd ed. Providence: Printed by B. T. Albro, 1849. 248, 56p. DLC; MBM; MH-M **40-1053**

PATTERSON, A. W.
The radical cure of hernia. Cincinnati: E. Shepard, 1849. 22p. DNLM **40-1054**

PATTERSON, Henry S. (1815-1854)
Valedictory address, delivered before the graduates of the medical department of Pennsylvania College, session 1843-1844. Philadelphia: Barrett & Jones, 1844. 14p. DNLM; PPC **40-1055**

PATTERSON, Henry S. (1815-1854)
Lecture introductory to the course of materia medica and pharmacy in the medical department of Pennsylvania College, Philadelphia, for the session 1844-1845. Philadelphia: W. S. Young, 1844. 16p. DNLM; PU **40-1056**

PATTERSON, Henry S. (1815-1854)
Lecture introductory to the course of materia medica and pharmacy in the medical department of Pennsylvania College, session of 1846-1847. Philadelphia: King & Baird, 1846. 20p. DNLM; PPC **40-1057**

PATTERSON, Henry S. (1815-1854)
Introductory lecture to the course of materia medica and therapeutics in the medical department of Pennsylvania College, for the session of 1848-1849. Philadelphia: King & Baird, 1848. 16p. DNLM; PPC; PU **40-1058**

PATTERSON, Henry S. (1815-1854)
Valedictory address to the graduating class of the medical department of Pennsylvania College at the annual commencement, March 7, 1849. Philadelphia: King & Baird, 1849. 24p. DNLM; PPC; PU **40-1059**

PAYNE, William E[lisha] (1815-1877)
Report of a committee appointed by the American Institute of Homoeopathy, in 1848, to report on the employment of emetics and cathartics by homoeopathic physicians. June, 1848. 10p. PPHa **40-1060**

PEASLEE, Edmund Randolph (1814-1878)
A synopsis of lectures on general and human physiology in the New Hampshire Medical Institution (Dartmouth College). Pt. 1. Hanover, 1848. 54p. DNLM **40-1061**

PEASLEE, Edmund Randolph (1814-1878)
The elements of medical eminence. An introductory address, delivered before the medical class of the Medical School of Maine, March 13, 1848. Brunswick, Me.: J. Griggin, 1848. 24p. DNLM **40-1062**

PEET, Harvey Prindle (1794-1873)
Address delivered at the New York Institution for the Instruction of the Deaf and Dumb, December 2, 1846. With an appendix containing the proceedings at the dedication of the chapel. New York: Egbert, Hovey & King, 1847. 40p. DNLM; NNNAM **40-1063**

PEIRCE, E. D.
Five lectures upon the cause, prevention, and cure of disease; the mysteries and fallacies of the faculty; and upon the origin, design, benefit, and phenomena of animal magnetism, with an appendix, containing many interesting facts on magnetism or mesmerism, and clairvoyance . . . recipes for making their appropriate medicines, [etc.]. 1st ed. Rochster, N.Y., 1847. 103p. DNLM **40-1064**

PEIRSON, Abel L. (1794-1853)
On physical education. A lecture delivered before the American Institute of Instruction. Boston: Marsh, Capen, 1840. 26p. DNLM; MH; MWA **40-1065**

PENDLETON, Hester
The parents' guide for the transmission of desired qualities to offspring, and childbirth made easy. New York: Fowlers & Wells, 1848. 212p. DNLM; NNNAM **40-1066**

PEREIRA, Jonathan (1804-1853)
A treatise on food and diet; with observations on the dietetical regimen suited for disordered states of the digestive organs; and an account of the dietaries of some of the principal metropolitan and other establishments for paupers, lunatics, criminals, children, the sick, &c. . . . Ed. by Charles A. Lee, M.D. New York: J. & H. G. Langley, 1843. 325p. DLC; DNLM; PPC; PU **40-1067**

PEREIRA, Jonathan (1804-1853)
A treatise on food and diet: with observations on dietetical regimen suited for disordered states of the digestive organs; and an account of the dietaries of some of the principal metropolitan and other establishments for paupers, lunatics, criminals, children, the sick. . . . Ed. by Charles A. Lee, M.D. New York and Boston: Fowlers & Wells, 1843. 320p. DLC; MBM; NNNAM; PPC **40-1068**

PEREIRA, Jonathan (1804-1853)
The elements of materia medica; comprehending the natural history, preparation, properties, composition, effects, and uses of medicines. From the 2nd London ed. . . . with notes and additions by Joseph Carson. Philadelphia: Lea & Blanchard, 1843. 2 v. DNLM; OCLloyd; PPC; PPJ

40-1069

PEREIRA, Jonathan (1804-1853)
The physiology of health: being a view of some of the more important functions of the human body; with practical observations on their management. To which is added, a dietical regimen for dyspeptics. . . . New York: Wilson & Company, 1844. 64p. DLC; MBM; NNNAM; PPC **40-1070**

PEREIRA, Jonathan (1804-1853)
A treatise on food and diet, with observations on the dietetical regimen suited for disordered states of the digestive organs; and an account of the dietaries of some of the principal metropolitan and other establishments for paupers, lunatics, criminals, children, the sick, etc. New York: Wilson & Co., 1847. 318p. DNLM; NNNAM **40-1071**

PERKINS, Joseph (1798-1872)
Introductory lecture to the spring session of lectures in Castleton Medical College. Albany: C. Van Benthuysen & Company, 1844. 16p. DNLM **40-1072**

PERKINS, Joseph (1798-1872)
An address, delivered at the Castleton Medical College, introductory to the spring session of 1848. Troy, N.Y. J. C. Kneeland & Co., 1848. 16p. DNLM **40-1073**

PETER, Robert (1805-1894)
Review of Dr. Caldwell's pamphlet, entitled: Physiology vindicated, in a critique on Liebig's Animal Chemistry. Cincinnati: R. P. Donough, 1843. 45p. DNLM; OCIM
40-1074

PETER, Robert (1805-1894)
Chemical examination of the urinary calculi, in the museum of the medical department of Transylvania University. Lexington: Scurgham & Dunlop, 1846. 37p. DLC; DNLM
40-1075

PETTIGREW, Thomas Joseph (1791-1865)
On superstitions connected with the history and practice of medicine and surgery. . . . Philadelphia: E. Barrington & G. D. Haswell, 1844. 213p. DLC; DNLM; ICU; NNC
40-1076

The PHARMACOPOEIA of the United States of America. By authority of the National Medical Convention, held at Washington, A.D. 1840. Philadelphia: Grigg & Elliot, 1842. 279p. DLC; DNLM; OCLloyd **40-1077**

PHILADELPHIA. UNIVERSITY OF PENNSYLVANIA/ JEFFERSON MEDICAL COLLEGE
Portraits of the professors in the medical department of the University of Pennsylvania and in the Jefferson Medical College. Philadelphia: V. F. Harrison, 1846. 2 v. 14 plates. DNLM; PPJ; PU **40-1078**

PHILIP, Alexander Philip Wilson (1770?-1851?)
A treatise on protracted indigestion and its consequences; being the application to the practical department of medicine of the results of an inquiry into the laws of the vital functions: addressed by the author on his retirement from the medical profession, both to the members of that profession, and to the well-educated public, particularly parents. . . . Philadelphia: Lea & Blanchard, 1843. 156p. DLC; DNLM; PPC
40-1079

PHILLIPS, Benjamin (1805-1861)
Scrofula; its nature, its causes, it prevalence, and the principles of treatment. Philadelphia: Lea & Blanchard, 1846. 350p. 1 plate. DNLM; NNNAM; PPC **40-1080**

[A PHYSICIAN]
A temperance method of treating epidemic cholera. New York, 1849. 20p. DNLM **40-1081**

PIERCE, George E.
An address to the graduating class of the Medical College of Georgia. Augusta, Ga., 1844. 11p. DNLM; GU
40-1082

PIERCE, George E.
A plea for stability and permanence in institutions of learning; delivered before the trustees, officers, and students of the Cleveland Medical College, February 26, 1845. Cleveland: Younglove, 1845. 16p. DNLM; OCIM
40-1083

The POCKET anatomist: being a summary description of the muscles; with a tabular view of the arteries and nerves. Concordant with "The Dublin Dissector," and "Harrison on the Arteries." 4th ed. Philadelphia: J. Kay, Jr., & Bro., 1844. 63p. DNLM; PPC **40-1084**

POPE, Charles A. (1818-1870)
Introductory lecture delivered before the class of the medical department of the St. Louis University. St. Louis: Chambers & Knapp, 1847. 22p. DNLM **40-1085**

POPE, Charles A. (1818-1870)
Congenital inversion of the bladder. St. Louis, 1848. 1 plate with description. DNLM **40-1086**

PORCHER, Francis Peyre (1825-1895)
A medico-botanical catalogue of the plants and ferns of St. John's, Berkly, South Carolina. . . . Charleston [S.C.]: Printed by Burges & James, 1847. 55p. DLC; OCLloyd; ScMS; ScU
40-1087

PORCHER, Francis Peyre (1825-1895)
A sketch of the medical botany of South Carolina; being a report made to the American Medical Association, at its sessions held in Baltimore and Boston. . . . Philadelphia: T. K. & P. G. Collins, printers, 1849. 677p. DLC; OCLloyd; ScMS; ScU **40-1088**

POST, Alfred Charles (1806-1886)
Observations on the cure of strabismus. . . . With an appendix on the new operation for the cure of stammering. New York: C. S. Francis, 1841. 67p. DLC; DNLM; NNNAM
40-1089

POST, Alfred Charles (1806-1886)
An introductory address to the students of Castleton Medical College, at the commencement of a course of lectures on ophthalmic anatomy and surgery, for 1843. . . . Published by the class. Rutland [Vt.]: Printed by H. T. White, 1843. 13p. DLC; DNLM; VtHi **40-1090**

POST, Alfred Charles (1806-1886)
Anniversary oration, before the New York Academy of Medicine, delivered in the chapel of the University of the City of New York, November 14th, 1849. . . . New York: Printed for the Academy by H. Ludwig & Co., 1849. 70p. DLC; DNLM; NNNAM **40-1091**

POWELL, James William
The eye: its imperfections and their prevention; comprising a familiar description of the anatomy and physiology, of the organ of vision: rules for the preservation, improvement, and restoration of sight, with remarks on near sight and aged sight; on optics, and the use and abuse of spectacles, with directions for their selection. . . . New York: The author, 1847. 139p. 1 plate. DLC; DNLM; NNNAM; PPC
40-1092

POWELL, James William
The eye: its diseases and cure; comprising a familiar description of the anatomy and physiology, of the organ of vision: rules for the preservation, improvement, and restoration of sight, with remarks on optics, on near sight and aged sight; and the use and abuse of spectacles, with directions for their selection. . . . 3rd ed. New York: The author, 1849. 156p. DLC; DNLM; NNNAM; PPC **40-1093**

POWELL, William (1813-1852)
Lecture, introductory to a course on the theory and practice of medicine, delivered in the University of Maryland. [Baltimore]: J. Robinson, 1846. 23p. DNLM; MdU-D
40-1094

The PRESCRIBER's pharmacopoeia, containing all the medicines in the British Pharmacopoeia arranged in classes according to their action, with their composition and doses. Revised and edited. . . . By a practicing physician. Altered to correspond with the United States Dispensatory. Revised and improved by an American physician. 2nd American from the 3rd London ed. New York: S. S. & W. Wood, 1846. 144p. DNLM; OCLloyd; NNNAM **40-1095**

PROUT, William (1785-1850)
On the nature and treatment of stomach and urinary diseases; being an inquiry into the connexion of diabetes, calculus, and other affections of the kidney and bladder, with indigestion. From the 4th rev. London ed. Philadelphia: Lea & Blanchard, 1843. 465p. 6 plates. DNLM; PPC: PPJ; PU **40-1096**

[PUNCH]
The physiology of the London medical student and curiosities of medical experience. Philadelphia: Carey & Hart, 1844. 96, 94, 72, 62p. 14 plates; [1 col. fold-out plate]. CtY-M; DNLM; PPC; PU **40-1097**

PURPLE, Samuel Smith (1822-1900)
Corpus luteum: its value as evidence of conception, and its relation to legal medicine; with the characteristics of the true and false. Being an attempt to reconcile the conflicting opinion of writers by the recent discoveries in the physiology of the ovaries. New York: J. & H. G. Langley, 1846. 13p. DNLM; NNNAM **40-1098**

PURPLE, William D. (1802-1886)
The influence of dress in the production of disease in females. Read before the Chenango County Medical Society, June 10th, 1847. Albany: J. Munsell, 1848. 11p. DNLM **40-1099**

QUAIN, Jones (1796-1865)
A series of anatomical plates; with references and physiological comments. . . . and W. J. E. Wilson. American ed. rev., with additional notes, by Joseph Pancoast. . . . Philadelphia: G. N. Loomis, 1842. 445p. 200 plates. DLC; DNLM; MBM; PPC **40-1100**

QUAIN, Jones (1796-1865)
Human anatomy. . . . Ed. by Richard Quain, and William Sharpey. . . . 1st American, from the 5th London ed., ed by Joseph Leidy. . . . With over five hundred illustrations. . . . Philadelphia: Lea & Blanchard, 1849. 2 v. DLC; DNLM; MBM; NNNAM **40-1101**

RALPH, Joseph
A private treatise on venereal disease. In two parts. The first on gonorrhea, vulgarly called clap. The second on venereal, properly so called. Adapted to the use of every one, but more especially designed for those who are delicately circumstanced and require a private as well as a speedy cure. 2nd ed. New York, [1840]. 259p. DNLM; NNNAM **40-1102**

RALPH, Joseph
. . . A practical private treatise on the diseases of the genital organs. 6th ed. New York: Stearns & Co., 1848. 342p. DNLM; NNNAM **40-1103**

RALPH, Joseph
. . . A plain treatise on cholera, intended for the use of private individuals. . . . To which is added Rules for the preservation of health in the four seasons. . . . New York: H. Long & Bro., 1848. 16p. DLC; DNLM; NNNAM **40-1104**

RAMSBOTHAM, Francis H. (1801-1868)
The principles and practice of obstetric medicine and surgery, in reference to the process of parturition. 1st American ed., revised. Philadelphia: Lea & Blanchard, 1842. 458p. 52 plates. CtY-M; DNLM; PPC; ViRA **40-1105**

RAMSBOTHAM, Francis H. (1801-1868)
The principles and practice of obstetric medicine and surgery, in reference to the practice of parturition. . . . A new ed., from the enlarged and rev. London ed. . . . Philadelphia: Lea & Blanchard, 1845. 519p. 55 plates. CU-M; DLC; PPC; ScCM **40-1106**

RAMSEY, Frank A.
. . . Cholera; a series of letters communicated to "The Standard and Reformer." Knoxville, Tenn.: J. E. & W. T. Helms, 1849. 30p. DNLM **40-1107**

RASPAIL, François Vincent (1794-1878)
Annual diary of health, or family physician and druggist; containing the necessary theoretical and practical manner of preparing medicines and preserving or curing yourself of disease, at small cost and with promptitude, of all curable evils, and of giving relief to those who labor under chronic or incurable diseases. Transl. from the Paris ed. of 1846 by A. Fortier. New Orleans, 1846. 106p. DNLM; LNT-M **40-1108**

RAU, Gottlieb Martin W. L. (1779-1840)
Organon of the specific healing art. Transl. from the German, with an essay on the present internal condition of the Homoeopathic School, by Charles Julius Hempel. New York: William Radde, 1847. 200p. DNLM; PPHa **40-1109**

RAY, Isaac (1807-1881)
A treatise on the medical jurisprudence of insanity. . . . 2nd ed. With additions. Boston: W. D. Ticknor & Co., 1844. 490p. DLC; MBM; PPC **40-1110**

RAYNER, John
Cod-liver oil: its uses, mode of administration, etc. Compiled from the best and latest authorities, British and foreign. 2nd American ed. New York: Rushton, Clark & Co., 1849. 16p. DNLM; NNNAM [Preface says "3rd ed."] **40-1111**

REDFIELD, J. W.
Outlines of a new system of physiognomy. Illustrated by numerous engravings, indicating the location of the signs of the different mental faculties. New York: J. S. Redfield, 1849. 96p. DNLM; NNNAM **40-1112**

REES, George Owen (1813-1889)
On the analysis of the blood and urine, in health and disease; and on the treatment of urinary diseases. From the 2nd London ed. Philadelphia: Lea & Blanchard, 1848. 165p. 1 plate. DNLM; PPC; PU **40-1113**

REESE, David Meredith (1800-1861)
A plea for the intemperate. New York: J. S. Taylor & Co., 1841. 86p. DNLM; NNNAM **40-1114**

REESE, David Meredith (1800-1861)
Introductory lecture delivered before the medical class in Castleton Medical College, at the opening of the fall session: 1842. . . . Castleton, Vt.: Robinson & Southmayd, printers, 1842. 14p. DLC; DNLM; VtHi **40-1115**

REESE, David Meredith (1800-1861)
Rudiments of vegetable physiology. For use in schools and in private instruction. Revised and improved. (No. 3, Dr. Reese's improved edition of Chamber's Educational Course.) Philadelphia: Sorin & Ball, [1846]. 162p. DNLM; PP; PPG; PPL **40-1116**

REESE, David Meredith (1800-1861)
Ship fever at the Bellevue Hospital. New York: J. & H. G. Langley, 1847. 8p. DNLM; NNNAM **40-1117**

REESE, John James (1818-1892)
An analysis of physiology: being a condensed view of most important facts and doctrines. Designed especially for the use of students. . . . Philadelphia: J. Auner, 1847. 314p. DLC; DNLM; PPC; PU **40-1118**

REMARKS on the use of alcohol for the preparation of medicines. Boston: J. Wilson, 1849. 8p. DNLM **40-1119**

REVERE, John (1787-1847)
An introductory lecture on the comparative state of the profession of medicine, and of medical education, in the United States and Europe, session 1846-1847. (University of the City of New York.) New York: Herald Job Office, 1846-1847. 18p. NNNAM **40-1120**

REYBURN, Thomas (1819-1857)
A supplement to the July number of the St. Louis Medical and Surgical Journal (containing an examination of the testimony appended to the "Remarks of Dr. Thos. J. White," published in said number of that journal). [St. Louis: Keemle & Field, 1846.] 32p. DNLM **40-1121**

REYNOLDS, Edward (1793-1881)
An address on the present condition, prospects and duties of the medical profession, delivered before the members of the Massachusetts Medical Society, at the annual meeting, May 26, 1841. . . . Boston: Whipple & Damrell,1841. 50p. DLC; DNLM; MBM **40-1122**

RICHARDSON, Charles
The cholera: its cause, prevention, and cure. By. . . . New York: D. Appleton & Company; Philadelphia: G. S. Appleton, 1849. 32p. DLC; DNLM; PPC **40-1123**

RICHARDSON, Samuel B.
Observations on tenotomy or section of the tendons, as a remedy for club-foot and other deformities. . . . Louisville, Ky.: Prentice & Weissinger, 1840. 41p. 1 plate. DLC **40-1124**

RICORD, Philippe (1799-1889)
A practical treatise on venereal diseases . . . with a therapeutical summary and special formulary. Transl. from the French by Henry Pilkington Drummond. Philadelphia: Lea & Blanchard, 1843. 256p. DNLM; PPC; PPJ; ViRA **40-1125**

RICORD, Philippe (1799-1889)
A practical treatise on venereal diseases . . . with a therapeutical summary and special formulary. Transl. from the French by A. Sidney Doane. 2nd ed. New York: J. S. Redfield, 1844. 339p. DNLM; NNNAM **40-1126**

RICORD, Philippe (1799-1889)
A practical treatise on venereal diseases . . . with a therapeutical summary and special formulary, 4th ed. New York: J. S. Redfield, 1849. 339p. DNLM; NNNAM **40-1127**

RIGBY, Edward (1804-1860)
A system of midwifery. . . . With notes and additional illustrations. Philadelphia: Lea & Blanchard, 1841. 491p. DLC; DNLM; PPC; NNNAM **40-1128**

RIGBY, Edward (1804-1860)
Memoranda for young practitioners in midwifery. . . . 2nd American ed., enl. and improved. Boston: W. D. Ticknor & Co., 1847. 62p. DLC; MBM; NNNAM **40-1129**

RILLIET, Frédéric (1814-1861) and E. BARTHEZ
A treatise on the penumonia of children. Transl. from the French by S. Parkman. [Dunglison's American Medical Library] Philadelphia: Carey & Hart, 1841. 100p. DNLM; PPC; PU **40-1130**

RITTER, Thomas
A medical manual and medicine chest companion, for popular use in families and on ship board, for the treatment of the ordinary diseases of the human system. . . . 4th ed., rev. and enl. New York: S. W. Benedict, 1849. 384p. DLC; NNNAM **40-1131**

RIVERS, Henry Wheaton (1814-1868)
Accidents: popular directions for their immediate treatment; with observations on poisons and their antidotes. Boston: Webb, 1845. 108p. MBM **40-1132**

ROBERTSON, F. K.
The book of health, or Thomsonian theory and practice of medicine, including the latest views of physiology, pathology, and therapeutics. . . . Bennington, Vt.: J. I. C. & A. S. C. Cook, 1843. 304p. DNLM; VtHi **40-1133**

ROBERTSON, William
A practical treatise on the human teeth: showing the causes of their destruction, and the means of their preservation. Philadelphia: Lea & Blanchard, 1841. 229p. 6 plates. DNLM; PPC; PU **40-1134**

RODGERS, John Kearny (1793-1851)
Ligature of the left subclavian artery within the scalenus muscle for aneurism. [New York, 1846] 8p. DNLM **40-1135**

RODGERS, M. M.
Physical education and medical management of children, for the use of families and teachers. New York: E. Darrow, 1848. 144p. DNLM **40-1136**

ROGERS, David L. (1799-1877)
Surgical essays and cases in surgery. . . . Newark, N.J.: Printed at the Daily Advertiser Office, 1849. 151p. DLC; DNLM; NjR **40-1137**

ROKITANSKY, Carl von (1804-1878)
A treatise on pathological anatomy. Pt. 1. Containing the abnormal conditions of the organs of respiration. Transl. from the German, with additions on diagnosis from Schoenlein, Skoda, and others. By John C. Peters. New York: W. Radde, 1845. 164p. DNLM; NNNAM [A translation of pp. 1-152 of v. 3 of his Handbook, 1842.] **40-1138**

ROSA, Storm (1794?-1864)
Homoeopathy and allopathy compared, together with some of the reasons for adopting the former. With an appendix. Painesville, O.: Telegraph Press, 1846. 32p. PPHa **40-1139**

ROSE, Jacob Servoss
Consumption curable, a practical treatise to prove consumption a manageable disease; with cases successfully treated, under a new mode in this country. Philadelphia: Crolius & Gladding, and J. G. Auner, 1841. 170p. DNLM; PPC; PU
40-1140

ROSE, Jacob Servoss
The reformed practice of medicine, based upon the principles of the chrono-thermal system practiced by the celebrated Dr. Dickson, of London. Philadelphia & New York: J. Pennington, 1845. 268p. 4 plates. DNLM; NNNAM; PPC
40-1141

ROSENSTEIN, J. G.
Theory and practice of homoeopathy. First Part. Containing a theory of homoeopathy, with dietetic rules. . . . Louisville, Ky.: Henkle & Logan, 1840. 288p. DNLM; OCIM; PPHa
40-1142

ROSS, Joel H.
Remarks on hot air and vapour bathing, shampooing, etc. [New York, 1845.] 8p. DNLM; NNNAM
40-1143

ROSS, Joel H.
Golden rules of health and hints to dyspeptics, with special reference to diet, exercise, air, temperature, ventilation, hygrometry, influence of domestic habits, together with remarks on allopathy, hydropathy, aeropathy, thermopathy, psychropathy, homoeopathy, thumpingpathy, healingpathy, killingpathy, [etc.]. New York: The author, 1849. 165p. DNLM; NNNAM **40-1144**

ROYLE, John Forbes (1799?-1858)
Materia medica and therapeutics. . . . Ed. by Joseph Carson. . . . Philadelphia: Lea & Blanchard, 1847. 689p. DLC; DNLM; OCLloyd; PPC **40-1145**

RUECKERT, Ernst Ferdinand
Homoeopathic therapeutics; or, Outlines of successful homoeopathic cures, collected from the best homoeopathic periodicals. Transl. and edited by C. J. Hempel, M.D. New York: William Radde, 1846. 496p. DNLM; PPHa
40-1146

RUECKERT, Ernst Ferdinand
Consumption treated homoeopathically. From the German, by A. C. Becker. New York: W. Radde, 1847. 86p. DNLM; PPHa **40-1147**

RUOFF, A. Jos. Fredericus
Ruoff's repertory of homoeopathic medicine, nosologically arranged. Transl. from the German by A. H. Okie . . . with additions and improvements by Gideon Humphrey, M.D. Philadelphia: J. Dobson, Kay & Bros. & H. Hooker, 1840. 254p. DNLM; PPHa **40-1148**

RUOFF, A. Jos. Fredericus
Ruoff's repertory of homoeopathic medicine, nosologically arranged. . . . 2nd American edition, carefully amended and revised, with additions. New York: William Radde, 1845. 251p. DNLM; NNNAM; PPHa **40-1149**

RUSH, George
Mesmer and Swedenborg; or the relation of the developments of mesmerism to the doctrines and discloures of Swedenborg. New York: J. Allen, 1847. 288p. DNLM; MA; MH; NN
40-1150

RUSH, William
Valedictory address to the graduates of the medical department of Pennsylvania College. Philadelphia: F. F. Grund, 1840. 16p. DNLM; PPC **40-1151**

RUSSELL, David
The invalid's friend, being a plain, practical work designed for the use of familes and individuals, on vegetable and botanical principles. In four parts. [Andover, Mass.], 1843. 208p. DNLM; MBM **40-1152**

ST. JOHN, Samuel (1813-1876)
An introductory lecture delivered before the medical department of the Western Reserve College. Cleveland: Younglove, 1846. 16p. DNLM; OCIM **40-1153**

SAPPINGTON, John (1776-1856)
The theory and treatment of fevers. . . . Revised and corrected by Ferdinando Stith. . . . Arrow Rock [Missouri]: Published by the author, 1844. 216p. CtY-M; DNLM; NNNAM; PPC
40-1154

SARGENT, F. W. (1820-1889)
On bandaging and other operations of minor surgery. Philadelphia: Lea & Blanchard, 1848. 379p. CtY-M; DNLM; PPC; ViRA **40-1155**

SAYRE, Lewis Albert (1820-1900)
Extracts from my note-book. New York: D. Fanshaw, 1849. 11p. DNLM; NNNAM **40-1156**

SCHIEFERDECKER, Christian Charles
Vincenz Priessnitz; or the wonderful power of water in healing the diseases of the human body. After Rause. Philadelphia: Burgess & Zieber, 1843. 140p. DNLM; PPC; PPHa
40-1157

SCHIEFERDECKER, Christian Charles
Vincenz Priessnitz; or, the wonderful power of water in healing the diseases of the human body. . . . 2nd ed. Philadelphia: Printed for the author, 1844. 140p. DLC; DNLM; PPC
40-1158

SCHIEFERDECKER, Christian Charles
Short essay on the invariably successful treatment of cholera with water. Philadelphia: J. W. Moore, 1849. 32p. DNLM; PPC **40-1159**

SCOUTETTEN, Henri (1799-1871)
Memoir on the radical cure of club-foot. . . . With six plates. Transl. from the French. By F. Campbell Stewart. . . . [Dunglison's American Medical Library] Philadelphia: Printed by A. Waldie, 1840. 54p. DLC; DNLM; PPC
40-1160

SEATON, John Simpson
A treatise on the cause of the disease called by the people the milk-sickness; as it occurs in the western and southern states. . . . Louisville, Ky.: Prentice & Weissinger, 1841. 49p. DLC; DNLM; OCIM **40-1161**

SEMPLE, Matthew
Introductory lecture in the Homoeopathic Medical College of Pennsylvania, November 25, 1849. Philadelphia: Merrihew & Thompson, 1849. 14p. PPHa **40-1162**

SENTER, Issac (1753?-1799)
The journal of Isaac Senter, physician and surgeon to the troops detached from the American army encamped at Cambridge, Mass., on a secret expedition against Quebec, under the command of Col. Benedict Arnold, in September, 1775. Philadelphia: Historical Society of Pennsylvania, 1846. 40p. DLC; PP. PPAmP; PU **40-1163**

SHATTUCK, Lemuel (1793-1859)
The vital statistics of Boston; containing an abstract of the bills of mortality for the last twenty-nine years, and a general view of the population and health of the city at other periods of its history. Philadelphia: Lea & Blanchard, 1841. 35p. DNLM; MH; MBM; MWA **40-1164**

SHAW, Edward B. L.
The medical remembrancer, or book of emergencies; in which are concisely pointed out the immediate remedies to be adopted in the first moments of danger from poisoning, drowning, apoplexy, burns, and other accidents; with the tests for the principal poisons, and other useful information. Revised and improved by an American physician. New York: S. S. & W. Wood, 1845. 112p. DNLM; NNNAM; MBM; PPC **40-1165**

SHERRILL, Hunting (1783-1866)
A manual of homoeopathic prescriptions, with a full and improved repertory, in which diseases are alphabetically arranged, with the remedy for them connected. An introduction, in which the doctrine and nature of the homoeopathic system is explained. Also a complete catalogue of poisons, with the most certain antidotes and remedies for them. With directions for diet and regimen during the use of homoeopathic treatment. New York: William Radde, 1845. 181p. DLC; DNLM; PPHa; PPC **40-1166**

SHERRILL, Hunting (1783-1866)
An essay on the temperance method of treating epidemic cholera. 2nd ed. New York, 1849. 30p. DNLM; PPHa **40-1167**

SHERWOOD, Henry Hall
The motive power of the human system, with the symptoms and treatment of chronic diseases. . . . New York: Printed by J. W. Bell, 1840. 120p. DLC; NNNAM **40-1168**

SHERWOOD, Henry Hall
The motive power of organic life, and magnetic phenomena of terrestrial and planetary motions, with the application of the ever-active and all-pervading agency of magnetism, to the nature, symptoms, and treatment of chronic diseases. . . . New York: H. A. Chapin & Co., 1841. 196p. plates. DLC; NNNAM **40-1169**

SHERWOOD, Henry Hall
Motive power of organic life, and the symptoms and treatment of chronic diseases. 2nd ed.-enl. . . . New York: Wiley & Putnam, 1844. 268p. plates. DLC; DNLM; NNNAM **40-1170**

SHERWOOD, Henry Hall
Manual for magnetizing, with the rotary and vibrating magnetic machine, in the duo-dynamic treatment of diseases. New York: Wiley & Putnam, 1847. 388p. DNLM; NNNAM **40-1171**

SHERWOOD, Henry Hall
The motive power of the human system, with the symptoms and treatment of chronic diseases. New York: Wiley & Putnam, 1847. 216p. DNLM; NNNAM **40-1172**

SHERWOOD, Henry Hall
The magnetic organization of the human system, and its application to the cure of chronic diseases. . . . Abridged from his larger works by H. H. Sherwood's successors. . . . New York: Tribune Steam Printing Office, 1849. 16p. DLC; NNNAM **40-1173**

SHEW, Joel (1816-1855)
Hydropathy; or, The water-cure: its principles, modes of treatment, &c. . . . New York: Wiley & Putnam, 1844. 304p. DLC; DNLM; NNNAM; PPC **40-1174**

SHEW, Joel (1816-1855)
Hand-book of hydropathy, or, a popular account of the treatment and prevention of diseases by means of water. New York: Wiley & Putnam, 1844. 144p. DNLM; NNNAM **40-1175**

SHEW, Joel (1816-1855)
Facts in hydropathy, or water-cure; a collection of cases, with details of treatment, showing the safest and most effectual known means to be used in gout, rheumatism, indigestion, hypochondriasis, fevers, consumption, etc., from various authorities. New York: Burgess, Stringer & Co., 1844. 108p. DNLM; NNNAM **40-1176**

SHEW, Joel (1816-1855)
Facts in hydropathy, or water-cure; a collection of cases, with details of treatment, showing the safest and most effectual known means to be used in gout, rheumatism . . . &c. &c., from Sir Charles Scudmore, Drs. Wilson, Gully . . . and others. To which is prefixed Bulwer's celebrated letter. . . . Cooperstown, N.Y.: H. & E. Phinney, 1847. 93p. DLC; DNLM; NNNAM **40-1177**

SHEW, Joel (1816-1855)
The cholera, its causes, prevention, and cure: showing the inefficacy of drug-treatment, and the superiority of the water-cure, in this disease. . . . New York: Fowlers & Wells, 1849. 98p. DLC; DNLM; NNNAM **40-1178**

SHEW, Joel (1816-1855)
Tobacco: its history, nature, and effects on the body and mind. New York: Fowlers & Wells, 1849. 116p. DNLM; NN; NNC; NNNAM **40-1179**

SHIPMAN, A. B. (1803-1868)
An introductory lecture to a course on surgery in the Indiana Medical College, session 1847-1848. La Porte, Ind.: W. & J. Millikan, 1848. 24p. DNLM **40-1180**

SHIPMAN, A. B. (1803-1868)
Valedictory address to the medical class and graduates of the Indiana Medical College (La Porte University). Syracuse: Barns, Smith & Cooper, 1848. 26p. DNLM **40-1181**

SHIPMAN, George Elias (1820-1893)
Homoeopathia worthy of examination. Addressed to the graduating class of Rush Medical College, February 17, 1848. Together with evidences of the power of small doses and attenuated medicines, including a theory of potentization by J. F. Joslin. Chicago: B. H. Bartlett, 1848. 48p. DNLM; PPHa **40-1182**

SHIPMAN, George Elias (1820-1893)
Cholera. An extra of the Northwestern Journal of Homoeopathia. Chicago: Davis & Haddock, 1849. 28p. PPHa
40-1183

SHORT, Charles Wilkins (1794-1863)
Duties of medical students during attendance on lectures. An introductory address, delivered at the opening of the sesssion 1845-1846, in the Medical Institute of Louisville, Nov. 3rd, 1845. Louisville, Ky.: Morton & Griswold, 1845. 24p. DNLM; OCIM **40-1184**

SIMON, I. Franz
Animal chemistry, with reference to the physiology and pathology of man. . . . Transl. and edited by George E. Day. . . . Part I. Philadelphia: Lea & Blanchard, 1845. 292p. ICU; PPC; PU; ScCM **40-1185**

SIMONS, J. Hume
The planters' guide, and family book of medicine, for the instruction and use of planters, families, country people, and all others who may be out of the reach of physicians or unable to employ them. With particular directions respecting Asiatic cholera, by a Charleston physician. Charleston, S.C.: McCarter & Allen, [1848]. 210p. 2 plates. DNLM; ScC; ScCM
40-1186

SIMPSON, James Young (1811-1870)
Remarks on the superinduction of anaesthesia in natural and morbid parturition: with cases illustrative of the use and effects of chloroform in obstetric practice. . . . With an appendix. Boston: W. B. Little & Co., 1848. 48p. DLC; DNLM; MBM; NNNAM **40-1187**

SIMPSON, James Young (1811-1870)
Anaesthesia, or the employment of chloroform and ether in surgery, midwifery, etc. . . . Philadelphia: Lindsay & Blakiston, 1849. 248p. DLC; DNLM; PPC; ViRA **40-1188**

SIMS, James Marion (1813-1883)
An essay on the pathology and treatment of trismus nascentium or lock-jaw of infants. Philadelphia: Lea & Blanchard, 1846. 21p. DNLM; NNNAM; PPC; PPJ
40-1189

SMALL, Alvan Edmond (1811-1886)
Remarks upon the utility of specific remedies; addressed to the candid and reflecting. Philadelphia: Barrett & Jones, 1846. 20p. PPHa **40-1190**

SMALL, Alvan Edmond (1811-1886)
An address delivered to the Homoeopathic Medical College of Pennsylvania, as a preliminary to the course of 1849-1850. Boston: Otis Clapp, 1849. 19p. DNLM; PPHa
40-1191

SMALL books on great subjects. No. 2. On the connection between physiology and intellectural science. (From the 2nd London ed.) Philadelphia: Lea & Blanchard, 1846. 85p. DNLM; PPC; PU **40-1192**

SMILEY, Thomas T[ucker] (1795-1879)
The physician's pocket dose-book, and student's manual: comprising all the important articles of the materia medica, with their appropriate doses. . . . Philadelphia: Printed by L. R. Bailey, 1843. 54p. DLC; PPU; PU **40-1193**

SMITH, Elisha
The botanic physician: being a compendium of the practice of physic upon botanical principles; containing all the principal branches necessary to the study of medicine, as anatomy, physiology, surgery, causes, symptoms, and cure of diseases, midwifery, materia medica, pharmacy, botany, etc.; together with a great variety of useful recipes. Revised, corrected, and improved by Isaac S. Smith. New York: D. Adee, 1844. 508p. DNLM; OCIM; NNNAM **40-1194**

SMITH, Gibson
Lectures on clairmativeness, or human magnetism. With an appendix. New York: Searing & Prall, 1845. 40p. DNLM; NN; NNNAM **40-1195**

SMITH, Henry Foster
An essay on human magnetism, or the infant magnetism enrobed in its true panoply. 2nd ed. Philadelphia: W. S. Young, 1844. 96p. DNLM; PPC; PU **40-1196**

SMITH, Henry Hollingsworth (1815-1890)
Minor surgery; or, Hints on the every-day duties of the surgeon. . . . Philadelphia: E. Barrington & G. D. Haswell, 1843. 303p. DLC; DNLM; PPC **40-1197**

SMITH, Henry Hollingsworth (1815-1890)
Anatomical atlas, illustrative of the structure of the human body. . . . Under the supervision of William E. Horner. . . . Philadelphia: Lea & Blanchard, 1844. 14p. 634 fig. on 183 leaves. DLC; DNLM; PPC; ViRA **40-1198**

SMITH, Henry Hollingsworth (1815-1890)
Minor surgery, or hints on the every-day duties of the surgeon. . . . 2nd ed., with numerous additions. Philadelphia: E. Barrington & G. D. Haswell, 1846. 384p. DNLM; PPC; PU
40-1199

SMITH, Henry Hollingsworth (1815-1890)
Minor surgery; or, Hints on the every-day duties of the surgeon. . . . 3rd ed., with numerous additions. Illustrated by 247 engravings. Philadelphia: E. Barrington & G. D. Haswell, 1846. 456p. DLC; DNLM; PPC; PU **40-1200**

SMITH, Jerome Van Crowinshield (1800-1879)
The class book of anatomy, designed for schools, explanatory of the first principles of human mechanism, as the basis of physical education. 4th ed. Boston: R. S. Davis, 1840. 286p. DNLM; MH; NN; RPJCB **40-1201**

SMITH, John Augustine (1782-1865)
Select discourses on the functions of the nervous system in opposition to phrenology, materialism, and atheism. To which is prefixed a lecture on the diversities of the human character arising from physiological peculiarities. New York: D. Appleton & Co., 1840. 210p. DNLM; NNNAM
40-1202

SMITH, Joseph Mather (1789-1866)
A discourse on the public duties of medical men, delivered as an introductory lecture at the College of Physicians and Surgeons in the City of New York. New York: D. Adee, 1846. 30p. DNLM; NNNAM **40-1203**

SMITH, Joseph Mather (1789-1866)
A discourse on the influence of diseases on the intellectual and moral powers, delivered as an introductory lecture at the College of Physicians and Surgeons, in the city of New York, October 30th, 1848. . . . New York: D. Adee, printer, 1848. 35p. DLC; DNLM; NNNAM **40-1204**

SMITH, Mayo G.
A popular treatise on the teeth: containing a history of the dental art, with anatomical descriptions of the mouth and its appendages, and accounts of chemical and physiological experiments on the teeth; also a full and accurate account of the history of ether or letheon, for the prevention of pain, with directions for use. Designed for the use of families, and as a manual for the student and the practical dentist. Boston: J. P. Jewett & Co., 1848. 316p. 1 plate. DNLM; MBM
40-1205

SMITH, Mayo G.
A treatise on the inhalation of ether for the prevention of pain. Boston: J. P. Jewett & Co., 1848. 107p. DNLM; MBM; MWA
40-1206

SMITH, Samuel Hanbury (1810-1894)
An introductory address delivered in the Cincinnati Medical Institute, April 3, 1848. Cincinnati: Robinson & Jones, 1848. 22p. DNLM; OCIM **40-1207**

SMITH, William Tyler (1815-1873)
Parturition, and the principles and practice of obstetrics. Philadelphia: Lea & Blanchard, 1849. 395p. ICRM; DNLM; PPC; PU **40-1208**

SOLLY, Samuel (1805-1871)
The human brain: its structure, physiology and diseases. With a description of the typical forms of brain in the animal kingdom. From the 2nd London ed. Philadelphia: Lea & Blanchard, 1848. 496p. CtY-M; PPC; PU; ViRA
40-1209

SOME account of the origin and present condition of the Medical Institute of Louisville, with remarks on a late rejected report. Louisville: Prentice & Weissinger, 1842. 30p. DNLM; OCIM
40-1210

SPENCER, Thomas (1793-1857)
Address to the graduates of the medical institution of Geneva College, delivered Jan. 21, 1840. Geneva (N.Y.): Stow & Frazee, 1840. 20p. DNLM **40-1211**

SPENCER, Thomas (1793-1857)
Introductory lecture to the course of instruction in the medical institution of Geneva College, Geneva, N.Y.: Merrell, 1842. 19p. DNLM **40-1212**

SPENCER, Thomas (1793-1857)
Vital chemistry. Lectures on animal heat. Geneva, N.Y.: I. & S. H. Parker, 1845. 114p. DNLM **40-1213**

STANLEY, Edward (1791-1862)
A treatise on diseases of the bones. Philadelphia: Lea & Blanchard, 1849. 286p. DNLM; MBM; NNNAM; PPC
40-1214

STAPF, Joannes Ernest
Additions to the materia medica pura. Translated by C. J. Hempel. New York: William Radde, 1846. 292p. DNLM; PPHa
40-1215

STEARNS, John (1770-1848)
An address, delivered on the occasion of assuming the chair as president, at the first regular meeting of the New York Academy of Medicine, February 3rd, 1847. New York: H. Ludwig, 1847. 13p. DNLM; NNNAM
40-1216

STEVENS, Alexander Hodgdon (1789-1869)
An address to the class of graduates of the College of Physicians and Surgeons of the University of the State of New York. New York: H. Ludwig, 1847. 16p. DNLM; NNNAM
40-1217

STEVENS, Alexander Hodgdon (1789-1869)
Address, delivered before the state Agricultural Society, members of the Legislature, and of the Medical Society of the State of New York, on the food of plants. Albany: C. Van Benthuysen, 1848. 22p. DNLM; N **40-1218**

STEVENS, Alexander Hodgdon (1789-1869)
A plea of humanity in behalf of medical education; the annual address delivered before the New York State Medical Society. Albany: J. Munsell, 1849. 20p. DNLM **40-1219**

STEVENS, Alexander Hodgdon (1789-1869)
A plea of humanity in behalf of medical education: the annual address delivered before the New York State Medical Society, and members of the Legislature, at the Capitol, February 6, 1849. . . . Printed by order of the Assembly. Albany: Weed, Parsons & Co., public printers, 1849. 28p. DLC; NNNAM
40-1220

STEVENS, Alexander Hodgdon (1789-1869)
A plea of humanity in behalf of medical education: the annual address delivered before the New York State Medical Society, and members of the Legislature, at the capitol, February 6, 1849. . . . 4th ed. New York: H. Ludwig & Co., printers, 1849. 44p. DLC; DNLM; NNNAM **40-1221**

STEWART, Ferdinand Campbell (1815-1899)
The hospitals and surgeons of Paris. An historical and statistical account of the civil hospitals of Paris; with miscellaneous information, and biographical notices of some of the most eminent of the living Parisian surgeons. . . . New York: J. & H. G. Langley; Philadelphia: Carey & Hart, 1843. 432p. DLC; DNLM; MBM; PPC **40-1222**

STEWART, Ferdinand Campbell (1815-1899)
Eminent French surgeons, with a historical and statistical account of the hospitals of Paris; together with miscellaneous information and biographical notices of the most eminent of the living Parisian surgeons. Buffalo: A. Burke, [1845?] 432p. DNLM; NNNAM **40-1223**

STEWART, Ferdinand Campbell (1815-1899)
Anniversary address to the New York Medical and Surgical Society. New York, 1846. 31p. DNLM; NNNAM
40-1224

STEWART, James (1799-1864)
A practical treatise on the diseases of children. . . . New York: Wiley & Putnam, 1841. 547p. DLC; DNLM; NNNAM; PPC
40-1225

STEWART, James (1799-1864)
The lungs: their uses and the prevention of their diseases; with practical remarks on the use of remedies by inhalation. New York: W. H. Graham, 1848. 139p. DNLM; NNNAM
40-1226

STILLÉ, Alfred (1813-1900)
An address delivered before the class of the Philadelphia Medical Association at the close of the session of 1845. (Published by the class.) Philadelphia: J. C. Clark, 1845. 16p. DNLM; PPC; PU **40-1227**

STILLÉ, Alfred (1813-1900)
Medical education in the United States: An address, delivered to the students of the Philadelphia Association for Medical Instruction, at the close of the session, 1846. Philadelphia: Isaac Ashmead, 1846. 39p. DNLM; PPC; PPF; PPL
40-1228

STILLÉ, Alfred (1813-1900)
Elements of general pathology. . . . Philadelphia: Lindsay & Blakiston, 1848. 483p. DLC; DNLM; PPC; ViRA
40-1229

STOKES, William (1804-1878)
Lectures on the theory and practice of physic. . . . 2nd American ed. With numerous notes, and twelve additional lectures, by John Bell. . . . Philadelphia: Haswell, Barrington, & Haswell; New York: J. & H. G. Langley; [etc., etc.], 1840. 672p. DLC; DNLM; NNNAM; PPC
40-1230

STOKES, William (1804-1878)
Lectures on the theory and practice of physic. By William Stokes . . . and by John Bell. . . . 2nd ed. . . . Philadelphia: E. Barrington & G. D. Haswell; New York: J. & H. G. Langley [etc., etc.], 1842. 2 v. DLC; NNNAM; PPC
40-1231

STOKES, William (1804-1878)
A treatise on the diagnosis and treatment of diseases of the chest. Diseases of the lung and windpipe. . . . 2nd ed., with an introduction and numerous notes, by the American editor. Philadelphia: E. Barrington & G. D. Haswell, 1844. 528p. DLC; DNLM; PPC **40-1232**

STOKES, William (1804-1878)
Lectures on the theory and practice of physic. By John Bell . . . and by William Stokes. . . . 4th ed., rev. and enl. . . . Philadelphia: E. Barrington & G. D. Haswell, 1848. 2 v. DLC; PPC; PU; ViRA **40-1233**

STONE, C. H.
The history of the mild yellow fever which prevailed in the city of Natchez in 1848, with observations respecting its character and natural mode of cure; to which is appended from various authors descriptions and notices of that disease, of dengue and of inflammation of the stomach and bowels. Vidalia, La.: Concordia Intell. Off., 1849. 6, 549-593, 18p. DNLM; LNT-M
40-1234

STUART, J. P.
Essays on neurology; or an account of the new discoveries in phrenology, and animal magnetism. New York: E. C. Church, 1843. 36p. DNLM; NNNAM **40-1235**

SUNDERLAND, La Roy (1802-1885)
Confessions of a magnetiser exposed! Exhibiting the folly and falsehood of a recent pamphlet with the above title, with remarks, showing the falsity of the notions hitherto prevalent in regard to what has been denominated "mesmerism," and giving the outlines of the author's new theory of mind. Boston: Redding & Comp., 1845. 47p. DNLM; MBM
40-1236

SUNDERLAND, La Roy (1802-1885)
Book of health for the million, with practical remarks on bathing, diet, exercise, disease, and the water cure. Boston: White & Potter, 1847. 108p. MBM
40-1237

SUTTON, W. L.
Prize essay on scrofula: submitted to the Medical Society of Tennessee, May 1846. . . . Louisville: Prentice & Weissinger, 1846. 63p. DLC; DNLM **40-1238**

SWEET, Waterman
Views of anatomy and practice of natural bone-setting; by a mechanical process, different from all book knowledge. Schenectady: I. Riggs, 1844. 124p. DNLM
40-1239

SWEETSER, William (1797-1875)
Mental hygiene, or an examination of the intellect and passions, designed to illustrate their influence on health and duration of life. New York: J. & H. G. Langley, 1843. 270p. DLC; DNLM; NNNAM **40-1240**

SWEETSER, William (1797-1875)
An address delivered at the Castleton Medical College, introductory to the autumnal session of 1847. Troy, N.Y.: J. C. Kneeland & Co., 1847. 15p. DNLM **40-1241**

SWEET, John Appleton (1808-1854)
Eulogy on James Macdonald, delivered before the New York Medical and Surgical Society. New York: D. Fanshaw, 1849. 7p. DNLM; NNNAM **40-1242**

TABB, John Prosser
Statistics of the causes of death in the Philadelphia Hospital, Blockley, during a period of twelve years. [Philadelphia, 1844.] 12p. DNLM; PPC; PU **40-1243**

TAFT, Alphonso
A report read before the Homoeopathic Association of Cincinnati, 1849. Cincinnati: Bradley & Anthony, 1849. 48p. PPHa **40-1244**

TAMPLIN, Richard William (1814-1875)
Lectures on the nature and treatment of deformities delivered at the Royal Orthopaedic Hospital, Bloomsbury Square. . . . Philadelphia: Ed. Barrington & Geo. D. Haswell, 1846. 311p. DNLM; PPC; PPJ **40-1245**

TANNER, John
Circular prospectus addressed to the homoeopathic physicians and the friends of homoeopathy throughout the United States, Canada, etc. . . . Philadelphia: Printed by T. B. Town, 1843. 16p. PPHa; PPC **40-1246**

TANQUEREL DES PLANCHES, L. (1809-1862)
Lead diseases. A treatise from the French; with notes and additions on the use of lead pipe and its substitutes, by Samuel L. Dana. Lowell: Bixby & Co., 1848. 441p. DNLM; MB; MBM
40-1247

TARBELL, John A[dams] (1810-1864)
The pocket homoeopathist and family guide. Boston: Otis Clapp, 1849. 67p. MBM; PPHa **40-1248**

TAYLOR, Alfred Swaine (1806-1880)
Medical jurisprudence. . . . Ed. with notes and additions by R. Eglesfeld Griffith. . . . Philadelphia: Lea & Blanchard, 1845. 539p. DLC; DNLM; PPC; ViRA **40-1249**

TAYLOR, Alfred Swaine (1806-1880)
On poisons, in relation to medical jurisprudence and medicine. . . . Ed., with notes and additions, by R. Eglesfeld Griffith. . . . Philadelphia: Lea & Blanchard, 1848. 687p. DLC; DNLM; PPC; PPJ **40-1250**

TAYLOR, Jane
Physiology for children. Revised and corrected. New York: G. F. Cooledge & Bro., 1847. 91p. DNLM; MH; NN; NNC
40-1251

TESTE, Alphonse (*b.* 1814)
A practical manual of animal magnetism: containing an exposition of the methods employed in producing the magnetic phenomena; with its application to the treatment and cure of diseases. Transl. from the 2nd ed. by Dr. Spillan. 1st American ed. Philadelphia: Brown, Bicking & Gilbert, 1844. 321p. PPHa
40-1252

THOMSON, Anthony Todd (1778-1849)
The domestic management of the sickroom, necessary, in aid of medical treatment, for the cure of diseases. 1st American from the 2nd London ed. Revised, with additions, by R. E. Griffith. Philadelphia: Lea & Blanchard, 1845. 353p. DNLM; PPC; PPJ; PU **40-1253**

THOMSON, Anthony Todd (1778-1849)
A conspectus of the pharmacopoeias of the London, Edinburgh, and Dublin colleges of physicians, and of the United States Pharmacopoeia; being a practical compendium of materia medica and pharmacy. 3rd American ed. Edited by Charles A. Lee (from the 13th English ed.) New York: H. C. Langley, 1845. 313p. 1 tab. DNLM; OCLloyd; NNNAM; PPC
40-1254

THOMSON, Robert Dundas (1811-1864)
Experimental researches on the food of animals, and the fattening of cattle; with remarks on the food of man; based upon experiments undertaken by order of the British Government. From the last London ed. New York: Appleton & Co., 1846. 172p. 1 diag. DNLM; NN; NNC; PU
40-1255

THOMSON, Samuel (1769-1843)
The Thomsonian materia medica; or, Botanic family physician: comprising a philosophical theory, the natural organization and assumed principles of animal and vegetable life: to which are added the description of plants and their various compounds. . . . 12th ed., enl., cor., rev. and improved. Albany: Printed by J. Munsell, 1841. 834p. DLC; DNLM; OCLloyd; PPC
40-1256

THOMSON, William (1802-1852)
Historical notices on the occurrence of inflammatory affections of the internal organs after external injuries and surgical operations. . . . Philadelphia: Haswell, Barrington, & Haswell; New Orleans: J. J. Haswell & Co., 1840. 31p. DLC; DNLM; LNT-M; PPC **40-1257**

THOMSON, William (1802-1852)
A practical treatise on the diseases of the liver and biliary passages. . . . Also, clinical illustrations of diseases of the liver and spleen. By William Twining. . . . Philadelphia: E. Barrington & G. D. Haswell; New York: J. & H. G. Langley [etc., etc.], 1842. 339p. DLC; DNLM; NNNAM; PPC
40-1258

TICKNOR, Caleb Bingham (1804-1840)
Letter to the Hon.— —, with reasons for examining and believing the fundamental principles of homoeopathy. New York: H. Ludwig, 1840. 31p. DNLM; NNNAM
40-1259

[TICKNOR, Caleb Bingham] (1804-1840)
Quacks and quackery; or, A popular treatise on medical philosophy and imposture in medicine. By a physician of New York. New York: M. H. Newman, 1844. 278p. DLC; NNNAM
40-1260

TICKNOR, Luther (1790-1846)
The annual address to the candidates for degrees and licenses in the medical institution of Yale College, January 20, 1841. New Haven: B. L. Hamlen, 1841. 16p. CtY-M; DNLM; MBM
40-1261

TICKNOR, [William D.] & Co.
Catalogue of medical books, comprising all the late publications. . . . Boston, 1844-1845. 35, 12p. DNLM; MWA
40-1262

TICKNOR, [William D.] & Co.
Catalogue of medical books. Boston, 1847. 64p. DNLM; MH; MWA **40-1263**

[TILLET, Auguste]
Treatise on the dental art, founded on actual experience. Illustrated by two hundred and forty-one figures in lithography, and fifty-four wood cuts. By F. Maury [pseud.] . . . Transl. from the French, with notes and additions, by J. B. Savier. . . . Philadelphia: Lea & Blanchard, 1848. 324p. 20 plates. DLC; PPC; PPJ; PU **40-1264**

TOWNSHEND, Chauncy Hare (1800-1868)
Facts in mesmerism, or animal magnetism, [etc.]. 1st American ed., with an appendix, by Robert H. Collyer. Boston: C. C. Little & J. Brown, 1841. 539p. DNLM; MH; MHi; MSaE
40-1265

TOWNSHEND, Chauncy Hare (1800-1868)
Animal magnetism, or mesmerism; its history, phenomena, and present condition; containing practical instructions and the latest discoveries in the science. Principally derived from a recent work by William Lang. With a supplement, containing new and important facts never before published in the United States. New York: J. Mowatt & Co., 1844. 144p. DNLM; NN; NNNC; NNNAM **40-1266**

TRAILL, Thomas Stewart (1781-1862)
Outlines of a course of lectures on medical jurisprudence. . . . 1st American, from the 2nd Edinburgh, ed. Revised with numerous notes. Philadelphia: Lea & Blanchard, 1841. 234p. DLC; DNLM; NNNAM; PPC **40-1267**

TROUSSEAU, Armand (1801-1867)
. . . A practical treatise on laryngeal phthisis, chronic laryngitis, and diseases of the voice. By A. Trousseau and H. Belloc. Pathology and surgery; or, An exposition of the nature and treatment of local disease. By John Davies. . . . Philadelphia: Carey & Hart, 1841. 186p. DLC; DNLM; PPC; PU **40-1268**

TUCKER, David H[unter] (1815-1871)
Elements of the principles and practice of midwifery. Philadelphia: Lindsay & Blakiston, 1848. 405p. DNLM; PPC; PPJ; PU
40-1269

TUCKER, George (1775-1861)
Memoir of the life and character of John P. Emmet, M.D., professor of chemistry and materia medica in the University of Virginia. Delivered before the visitors, faculty, and alumni of the University, on the fourth of July, 1845. . . . Published by order of the faculty. Philadelphia: C. Sherman, printer, 1845. 31p. DLC; PPC; PU; ViRA **40-1270**

TURNER, Edward (1796-1837)
Elements of chemistry, including the actual state and prevalent doctrines of the science. Including history of the imponderables and the inorganic chemistry of the late. . . . 7th ed., and the outlines of organic chemistry by William Gregory, with notes and additions, by James B. Rogers and Robert E. Rogers. Philadelphia: Thomas Cowperthwait & Co., 1846. 848p. DNLM; PPC; PPJ; PU **40-1271**

TURNER, William
Triumphs of "Young Physic": or, chrono-thermal facts. New York: Burgess, Stringer & Co., 1847. 31p. DNLM; NNNAM **40-1272**

TURNER, William
A letter on cholera; its causes and cure. Addressed to the editors of the New York Sun. [New York, 1849.] 4p. DNLM; NNNAM **40-1273**

TWEEDIE, Alexander (1794-1884), ed.
A system of practical medicine comprised in a series of original dissertations. Arranged and ed. by Alexander Tweedie. . . . Philadelphia: Lea & Blanchard, 1840-1841. 5 v. CtY-M; DLC; PPC; PU **40-1274**

TWEEDIE, Alexander (1794-1884), ed.
A system of practical medicine comprised in a series of original dissertations. Arranged and ed. by Alexander Tweedie. . . . With notes and additions by W. W. Gerhard. . . . The 2nd American ed. . . . Philadelphia: Lea & Blanchard, 1842. 3 v. DLC; ICRM; PPC; ViRA **40-1275**

UNDERWOOD, Michael (1737-1820)
A treatise on the diseases of children, with general directions for the management of infants from the birth. From the 9th English ed., with notes, by S. Merriman and Marshall Hall. With notes, by John Bell. Philadelphia: E. Barrington & G. D. Haswell, 1841. 368p. DNLM; MBM; PPC; PU **40-1276**

UPHAM, Thomas C.
Outlines of imperfect and disordered mental action. New York: Harper Bros., 1840. 399p. DNLM; NN; NNC; NNNAM **40-1277**

VAIDEN, Thomas J.
The commencement of a practical system of medicine, to meet the premonitions of disease, and to secure on rational principles more uniform popular benefit, on the immediate and absolute requirements of nature, through her earliest cooperation, with permanent and satisfactory pledges, as to the medicine used in all the departments of fevers of general character. Mobile: Off. Daily Advertiser, 1845. 33p. DNLM **40-1278**

VAN AMRINGE, William Frederick
An investigation of the theories of the natural history of man, by Lawrence, Prichard, and others, founded upon animal analogies and an outline of a new natural history of man, founded upon history, anatomy, physiology and human analogies. New York: Baker & Scribner, 1848. 739p. DNLM; MH; NN; NNC **40-1279**

VANDERBURGH, F[ederal] (1788-1868)
An appeal for homoeopathy; or, remarks on the decision of the late Judge Cowen, relative to the legal rights of homoeopathic physicians. New York: W. Radde, 1844. 29p. DNLM ; NNNAM; PPHa **40-1280**

VAN DYKE, Rush (1813-1882)
Introductory lecture delivered in the Philadelphia College of Medicine. Philadelphia: J. H. Gilhon, 1848. 15p. DNLM; PPC; PU **40-1281**

VAN DYKE, Rush (1813-1882)
Valedictory address to the graduates of the Philadelphia College of Medicine. Philadelphia: J. H. Jones, 1849. 15p. DNLM; PPC; PU **40-1282**

VELPEAU, Alfred Armand Louis Marie (1795-1867)
A treatise on diseases of the breast. Transl. from the French by S. Parkman. Philadelphia: A. Waldie, 1840. 83p. DNLM; PPC; PPJ; PU **40-1283**

VELPEAU, Alfred Armand Louis Marie (1795-1867)
An elementary treatise on midwifery; or, principles of tokology and embryology. . . . Transl. from the French, by Charles D. Meigs. . . . 3rd American ed., with notes and additions, by William Harris. . . . Philadelphia: Lindsay & Blakiston, 1845. 600p. CtY-M; DLC; NNNAM; PPC **40-1284**

VELPEAU, Alfred Armand Louis Marie (1795-1867)
New elements of operative surgery . . . carefully rev., entirely remodelled, and augm. with a treatise on minor surgery. Illustrated by over 200 engravings, incorporated with the text: accompanied with an atlas in quarto of twenty-two plates, representing the principal operative processes, surgical instruments, &c. 1st American from the last Paris ed. Transl. by P. S. Townsend. . . . Augm. by the addition of several hundred pages of entirely new matter, comprising all the latest improvements and discoveries in surgery, in America and Europe, up to the present time. Under the supervision of, and with notes and observations by Valentine Mott. . . . New York: S. S. & W. Wood, 1847. 3 v., atlas. 23 plates. CtY-M; DLC; DNLM; PPC **40-1285**

VOGEL, Julius (1814-1880)
The pathological anatomy of the human body. . . . Transl. from the German with additions, by George E. Day. . . . Illustrated by upwards of one hundred plain and coloured engravings. Philadelphia: Lea & Blanchard, 1847. 534p. 10 plates. DLC; DNLM; PPC; PPJ **40-1286**

WAITE, G.
A critical inquiry into a few facts connected with the teeth. Baltimore: J. W. Woods, 1846. 23p. DNLM; MdU-D **40-1287**

WAKLEY, Thomas (1795-1862)
The mother's medical adviser, on the diseases and management of children. With recipes. From 10th London ed. New York: Wilson & Co., 1844. 64p. DNLM; NNNAM **40-1288**

WALKER, Alexander
Woman physiologically considered, as to mind, morals, marriage, matrimonial slavery, infidelity and divorce. With an appendix containing notes and additions; edited by an American physician. New York: J. & H. G. Langley, 1840. 432p. DNLM; NNNAM **40-1289**

WALKER, Alexander
Pathology, founded on the natural system of anatomy and physiology; a philosophical sketch, in which the natural classification of diseases and the distinction between morbid and curative symptoms, afforded by pain or its absence, are pointed out, as well as the errors of homoeopathy and other hypotheses. New York: J. & H. G. Langley, 1842. 186p. DNLM; PPHa **40-1290**

WALKER, Benjamin B.
The Indian practice of medicine . . . on the nature, causes, symptoms, and treatment of diseases of men, women and children; with appropriate prescriptions in English. Louisville: J. C. Noble, 1847. 120p. DNLM; OCIM
40-1291

WALKER, William Johnson (1789-1865)
An essay on the treatment of compound and complicated fractures, being the annual address before the Massachusetts Medical Society, May 28, 1845. Boston: Crocker & Brewster, 1845. 46p. DNLM; MBM **40-1292**

WALLACE, William Clay
Accommodation of the eye to distances. [Boston, 1844.] 10p. DNLM; MH-M **40-1293**

WALLER, Charles (1802-1862)
Diseases of the uterus. . . . Philadelphia: E. Barrington & G. Haswell, 1842. 92p. DNLM; PPC; PU
40-1294

WALSHE, Walter Hayle (1812-1892)
The physical diagnosis of diseases of the lungs. Philadelphia: Lea & Blanchard, 1843. 306p. DNLM; NNNAM; PPC; PPJ
40-1295

WALSHE, Walter Hayle (1812-1892)
The anatomy, physiology, pathology, and treatment of cancer. . . . With additions by J. Mason Warren. . . . Boston: W. D. Ticknor & Company, 1844. 351p. DLC; DNLM; MBM
40-1296

WARDLAW, Ralph (1779-1853)
Lectures on magdalenism: its nature, extent, effects, guilt, causes, and remedy. New York: J. S. Redfield, 1843. 172p. DNLM; MH; NN; NNC **40-1297**

WARE, John (1795-1864)
Contributions to the history and diagnosis of croup. [Boston, D. Clapp, 1842.] 18p. DNLM; MBM
40-1298

WARE, John (1795-1864)
Discourses on medical education, and on the medical profession. . . . Boston: J. Munroe & Company, 1847. 113p. DLC; DNLM; MBM **40-1299**

WARNER, Augustus L[ockman] (*d.* 1847)
An introductory lecture delivered before the medical class of Hampden-Sidney College, November 4, 1842. Richmond: P. D. Bernard, 1842. 20p. DNLM; ViRA
40-1300

WARREN, Edward (1804-1878)
Boyleston prize dissertations for the years 1838 and 1839 on scrofula, rheumatism, and erysipelatous inflammation. Philadelphia: A. Waldie, 1840. 122p. DNLM; PPC; PPJ; PU
40-1301

WARREN, Edward (1804-1878)
Some account of the letheon; or, who was the discoverer? 2nd ed. Boston: Dutton & Wentworth, 1847. 79p. DNLM; MBM; MWA **40-1302**

WARREN, Edward (1804-1878)
Some account of the letheon; or who was the discoverer? 3rd ed. Boston: Dutton & Wentworth, 1847. 88p. DNLM
40-1303

WARREN, John Collins (1778-1856)
Inhalation of ethereal vapor for the prevention of pain in surgical operations. [Boston, 1846.] 4p. DNLM; MBM; MWA
40-1304

WARREN, John Collins (1778-1856)
Physical education and the preservation of health. . . . Boston: W. D. Ticknor & Company, 1846. 90p. DLC; DNLM; MBM
40-1305

WARREN, John Collins (1778-1856)
Etherization with surgical remarks. . . . Boston: W. D. Ticknor & Company, 1848. 100p. DLC; DNLM; MBM
40-1306

WARREN, John Collins (1778-1856)
Effects of chloroform and of strong choloric ether, as narcotic agents. Boston: William B. Ticknor, 1849. 66p. DNLM; MBM
40-1307

WARREN, Jonathan Mason (1811-1867)
Rhinoplastic operations, with some remarks on the autoplastic methods usually adopted for the restoration of parts lost by accident or disease. Boston: D. Clapp, 1840. 28p. DNLM; MBM **40-1308**

WARREN, Jonathan Mason (1811-1867)
Ligature of both carotid arteries for a remarkable erectile tumor of the mouth, face and neck. Boston, 1846. 11p. 2 col. plates. DNLM; MBM **40-1309**

WARREN, Jonathan Mason (1811-1867)
Foreign bodies in the air passages. [Boston, 1847.] 8p. DNLM; MBM **40-1310**

WARREN, Jonathan Mason (1811-1867)
Inhalation of ether. [Boston, 1847.] 18p. DNLM; MBM; MWA **40-1311**

WARREN, Jonathan Mason (1811-1867)
Operation for fissure of the soft and hard palate, with the result of twenty-four cases. Boston: D. Clapp, 1848. 12p. DNLM; MBM **40-1312**

WARREN, Jonathan Mason (1811-1867)
Operation for artificial anus. Boston: D. Clapp, 1849. 7p. DNLM; MH-M **40-1313**

WARREN, Jonathan Mason (1811-1867)
Ligature of the left subclavian artery for subclavian aneurism; with a remarkable deviation of the vessel and consequent change of its relations. [Philadelphia, 1849.] 7p. DNLM; PPC
40-1314

WARREN, Jonathan Mason (1811-1867)
Lithotrity and lithotomy, with the use of ether in those operations. Boston: D. Clapp, 1849. 15p. DNLM; MBM
40-1315

WARRINGTON, Joseph (1805?-1888)
The obstetric catechism. . . . Philadelphia: J. G. Auner, 1842. 350p. DLC; DNLM; PPC; PPJ **40-1316**

WATERSTON, Robert Classie
The condition of the insane in Massachusetts. Boston: J. Munroe & Co., 1843. 23p. DNLM; MA; MB; MBM
40-1317

WATSON, John (1807-1863)
A lecture on practical education in medicine, and on the courses of instruction at the New York Hospital. New York: J. & H. G. Langley, 1846. 19p. DNLM; NNNAM
40-1318

WATSON, Thomas (1792-1882)
Lectures on the principles and practice of physic; delivered at King's College, London. Philadelphia: Lea & Blanchard, 1844. 920p. DNLM; MBM; PPC; ViRA **40-1319**

WATSON, Thomas (1792-1882)
Lectures on the principles and practice of physic; delivered at King's College, London. . . . 2nd American, from the 2nd London ed. Rev. with additions, by D. Francis Condie. . . . Philadelphia: Lea & Blanchard, 1845. 1000p. CtY-M; DLC; LNT-M; PPC **40-1320**

WATSON, Thomas (1792-1882)
Lectures on the principles and practice of physic; delivered at King's College, London. . . . 3rd American from the last London ed. Rev., with additions, by D. Francis Condie. . . . Philadelphia: Lea & Blanchard, 1847. 1040p. DLC; DNLM; IEN-M; IU-M **40-1321**

WEBER, Moritz Ignaz (1795-1875)
Explanation of the anatomical atlas of the human body in natural size. New York: G. Endicott, 1844. 54p. DNLM; MBM; NNNAM **40-1322**

WEBSTER, James (1803-1854)
Lecture introductory to the course on anatomy and physiology in Geneva Medical College, Oct., 1840. Geneva, N.Y.: Stow & Frazee, 1840. 21p. DNLM **40-1323**

WEBSTER, James (1803-1854)
Address to the graduates of Geneva Medical College. Rochester: Shepard & Strong, 1841. 16p. DNLM **40-1324**

WEBSTER, James (1803-1854)
Introductory to the course on anatomy in Geneva Medical College, session 1842-1843. Geneva, N.Y.: Scrotten Merrell & Stow, 1842. 20p. DNLM **40-1325**

WEBSTER, James (1803-1854)
Address to the graduates of Geneva Medical College. Geneva, N.Y.: Scotten & Van Brunt, 1844. 18p. DNLM
40-1326

WEBSTER, James (1803-1854)
To the medical profession to the city of New York. [Difficulties between Geneva Medical College and the medical department of the University of the City of New York, in reference to a paragraph contained in the annual circular for 1846, of the latter, on the subject of practical anatomy. Nov. 14, 1846.] [New York, 1846.] 4p. DNLM; NNNAM
40-1327

WELCH, Archibald (1794-1865)
The annual address to the candidates for degrees and licenses, in the medical institution of Yale College, January 17, 1844. New Haven: B. L. Hamlen, 1844. 22p. CtY-M; DNLM
40-1328

WELLS, Horace (1815-1848)
A history of the discovery of the application of nitrous oxide gas, ether, and other vapors, to surgical operations. Hartford: J. G. Wells, 1847. 25p. DNLM; MB; MBAt; MBM
40-1329

WESSELHOEFT, Robert
Some remarks on Dr. O. W. Holmes's lectures on homoeopathy and its kindred delusions. Boston: O. Clapp, 1842. 59p. DNLM; MBM; MH **40-1330**

WESTCOTT, A[mos] (1815-1873)
An introductory lecture, delivered before the class of the Baltimore College of Dental Surgery, at the session of 1846-1847. . . . Baltimore: J. W. Woods, printer, 1846. 32p. DLC; DNLM; MdU-D **40-1331**

WHEELER, John
A treatise on Asiatic cholera. New York: [G. Mitchell], 1849. 71p. DNLM; NNNAM **40-1332**

WHITE, James Platt (1811-1881)
Remarks on the construction of obstetrical forceps, with a description of an instrument. [Buffalo: Jewett, Thomas & Co., 1849.] 7p. 1 plate. DNLM **40-1333**

WHITE, Samuel (1777-1845)
Address on insanity, delivered before the New York State Medical Society. Albany: J. Munsell, 1844. 20p. DNLM
40-1334

WHITEHEAD, James (1812-1885)
On the causes and treatment of abortion and sterility: being the result of an extended practical inquiry into the physiological and morbid conditions of the uterus, with reference especially to leucorrhoeal affections and the diseases of menstruation. . . . Philadelphia: Lea & Blanchard, 1842. 368p. DLC; DNLM; PPC; PPJ **40-1335**

WIGAND, Henry
Croup and its specific remedy. Boston: O. Clapp, 1846. 24p. DNLM; MH-M **40-1336**

WIGAND, Henry
Homoeopathy explained and objections answered, with additional articles, viz.: (1) The effects of mercury. (2) Physics and purging. (3) Laudanum and paregoric. (4) Coffee, tea, liquors, and tobacco. Sandusky City, 1847. 14p. DNLM
40-1337

WIGAND, Henry
A letter to the allopathic doctors of Dayton. Dayton: Wilson & Decker, 1849. 12p. DNLM **40-1338**

WILLARD, Emma (1787-1870)
A treatise on the motive powers which produce the circulation of the blood. New York & London: Wiley & Putnam, 1846. 170p. CtY-M; DNLM; MBM; NNNAM **40-1339**

WILLARD, Emma (1787-1870)
Respiration and its effects; more especially in relation to Asiatic cholera, and other sinking diseases. New York: Huntington & Savage, 1849. 64p. DNLM; MBM; NNNAM
40-1340

WILLIAMS, B. B[rown] (1815?-1894)
A treatise upon the electrical philosophy and cure of cholera. Richmond: Christian Advocate Office, 1849. 44p. DNLM; ViRA **40-1341**

WILLIAMS, C[harles] D[raper]
A review of Prof. C. B. Coventry's introductory lecture delivered before the class of medical students of Geneva College. Geneva: I. Merrell, 1844. 24p. DNLM; PPHa
40-1342

WILLIAMS, Charles James Blasius (1805-1889)
Principles of medicine: comprising general pathology and therapeutics, and a brief general view of etiology, nosology, semeiology, diagnosis, and prognosis. . . . With numerous additional notes, explanatory and critical, by the editor of the Science medical library and Bulletin of medical science [John Bell]. Philadelphia: E. Barrington & G. D. Haswell, 1844. 395p. DNLM; DNLM; PPC; PPJ **40-1343**

WILLIAMS, Charles J[ames] B[lasius] (1805-1889)
Principles of medicine: comprising general pathology and therapeutics. . . . With additions and notes by Meredith Clymer. . . . Philadelphia: Lea & Blanchard, 1844. 383p. DLC; DNLM; PPC; ViRA **40-1344**

WILLIAMS, Charles James Blasius (1805-1889)
A practical treatise on the diseases of the respiratory organs: including diseases of the larynx, trachea, lungs and pleura. . . . With numerous additions and notes, by Meredith Clymer. . . . Philadelphia: Lea & Blanchard, 1845. 508p. DLC; DNLM; NcD; PPC **40-1345**

WILLIAMS, Charles James Blasius (1805-1889)
Principles of medicine: comprising general pathology and therapeutics. . . . Ed., with additions, by Meredith Clymer. . . . 3rd American from the 2nd and enl. London ed. Philadelphia: Lea & Blanchard, 1848. 440p. CtY-M; DLC; OCIM; PPC **40-1346**

WILLIAMS, Stephen West (1790-1855)
American medical biography: or, Memoirs of eminent physicians, embracing principally those who have died since the publication of Dr. Thacher's work on the same subject. . . . Greenfield, Mass.: L. Merriam & Co., 1845. 664p. DLC; DNLM; ICRM; PPC **40-1347**

WILLIAMSON, Walter (1811-1870)
A short domestic treatise on the homoeopathic treatment of the diseases of females and children, originally published as Chapters 11 and 12 of the American ed. of Dr. Hering's domestic medicine. Philadelphia: C. L. Rademacher, 1848. 80p. DNLM; PPHa **40-1348**

WILLOUGHBY UNIVERSITY. MEDICAL DEPARTMENT
Catalogue of the officers, alumni, and students of the Willoughby Medical College [from 1835 to 1846]. Painesville, 1847. 16p. DNLM; OCIM [Chartered in 1834-1835. Ceased to exist Jan. 29, 1848 by the voluntary transfer of the medical faculty of the University to the Starling Medical College.] **40-1349**

WILSON, Erasmus (1809-1884)
A system of human anatomy, general and special. . . . American ed., edited by Paul B. Goddard. . . . With one hundred and seventy illustrations by Gilbert, from the 2nd London ed. Philadelphia: Lea & Blanchard, 1843. 576p. DLC; DNLM; PPC; PU **40-1350**

WILSON, Erasmus (1809-1884)
A practical and theoretical treatise on the diagnosis, pathology, and treatment of diseases of the skin, arranged according to a natural system of classification, and preceded by an outline of the antomy and physiology of the skin. . . . Philadelphia: Lea & Blanchard, 1843. 370p. DLC; DNLM; NNNAM; PPC **40-1351**

WISLON, Erasmus (1809-1884)
A system of human anatomy, general and special. . . . 2nd American ed., edited by Paul B. Goddard from the 2nd London ed. Philadelphia: Lea & Blanchard, 1844. 607p. DNLM; PPC; PPJ; PU **40-1352**

WILSON, Erasmus (1809-1884)
The dissector, or, Practical and surgical anatomy. . . . With one hundred and six illustrations. Modified and re-arranged by Paul B. Goddard. . . . Philadelphia: Lea & Blanchard, 1844. 444p. CU-M; DLC; DNLM; PPC **40-1353**

WILSON, Erasmus (1809-1884)
A practical treatise on healthy skin; with rules for the medical and domestic treatment of cutaneous diseases. New York: D. Appleton & Co., 1846. 263p. 6 plates. DNLM; NNNAM; OCIM; PPC **40-1354**

WILSON, Erasmus (1809-1884)
A practical treatise on healthy skin; with rules for the medical and domestic treatment of cutaneous diseases. With notes by S. F. Lambert. New York: Leavitt, Trow & Co., 1847. 100p. DNLM; NNNAM **40-1355**

WILSON, Erasmus (1809-1884)
On diseases of the skin. 2nd American, from the 2nd London ed. Philadelphia: Lea & Blanchard, 1847. 439p. DNLM; PPC; PPJ; PU **40-1356**

WILSON, Erasmus (1809-1884)
A system of human anatomy, general and special. . . . 3rd American ed. from the 3rd London ed. Edited by Paul B. Goddard. Philadelphia: Lea & Blanchard, 1847. 610p. 1 plate. DNLM; NNNAM; MBM; PPC **40-1357**

WILSON, Erasmus (1809-1884)
A system of human anatomy, general and special. . . . 4th American from the last London ed. Ed. by Paul B. Goddard. . . . With two hundred and fifty-one illustrations by Gilbert. Philadelphia: Lea & Blanchard, 1848. 576p. CtY-M; ICRM; MdBM; PPPH **40-1358**

WILTBANK, John (1806-1860)
The peculiarities of the female. A lecture introductory to the course on obstetrics in the medical department of Pennsylvania College. Philadelphia: Barrett & Jones, 1845. 16p. DNLM; PPC **40-1359**

WILTBANK, John (1806-1860)
Valedictory address to the graduating class of the medical department of Pennsylvania College for the session of 1844-1845. Philadelphia: Getz & Smith, 1845. 15p. DNLM; PU **40-1360**

WILTBANK, John (1806-1860)
An introductory lecture to the course of midwifery, and the diseases of women and children, in the medical department of Pennsylvania College. Philadelphia: King & Baird, 1848. 16p. DNLM; PU **40-1361**

WILTBANK, John (1806-1860)
A plea for obstetrics. Introductory lecture to the course of midwifery, in the medical department of Pennsylvania College. Philadelphia: King & Baird, 1848. 16p. DNLM; PPC; PU **40-1362**

WING, Joel A. (1788-1852)
An address delivered before the Medical Society of the State of New York, February 3, 1845. Albany: Munsell & Tanner, 1845. 42p. DNLM **40-1363**

WINSLOW, Forbes Benignus (1810-1874)
The plea of insanity in criminal cases. . . . Boston: C. C. Little & J. Brown, 1843. 111p. DNLM; MBM **40-1364**

WINSLOW, Forbes Benignus (1810-1874)
The plea of insanity, in criminal cases. . . . Philadelphia: J. S. Litttell, 1843. 42p. DLC; PPC; PPJ; PU **40-1365**

WINSLOW, Forbes Benignus (1810-1874)
Physic and physicians: a medical sketch book, exhibiting the public and private life of the most celebrated medical men of former days; with memoirs of eminent living London physicians and surgeons. In two parts. . . . Philadelphia: G. B. Zieber & Co., 1845. 2 v. in 1. DLC; DNLM; PPC; PU **40-1366**

WISHART, J[ohn] (1781-1864)
An inquiry into the origin of epidemics, and a physical and chemical analysis of their specific cause, on a new theory of matter and form. [St. Louis, 1848.] 16p. DNLM; OCIM **40-1367**

WISTAR, Caspar (1761-1818)
A system of anatomy for the use of students of medicine. . . . With notes and additions by William E. Horner. . . . 9th ed. Entirely remodeled, and illustrated by more than two hundred engravings. By J. Pancoast. . . . Philadelphia: Thomas Cowperthwait & Co., 1846. 2 v. CtY-M; DLC; MBM; PPC **40-1368**

WOOD, George Bacon (1797-1879)
Introductory lecture to the course of materia medica in the University of Pennsylvania. Philadelphia: Haswell, Barrington & Haswell, 1840. 30p. DNLM; PPC; PU **40-1369**

WOOD, George Bacon (1797-1879)
A memoir of the life and character of the late Joseph Parrish, M.D., read before the Medical Society of Philadelphia, October 23rd, 1840. . . . Philadelphia: L. R. Bailey, printer, 1840. 72p. DLC; DNLM; PPC; PU **40-1370**

WOOD, George Bacon (1797-1879)
Syllabus of the course of lectures on materia medica and pharmacy, delivered in the University of Pennsylvania. Philadelphia: L. R. Bailey, 1840. 69p. DNLM; PPC; PU **40-1371**

WOOD, George Bacon (1797-1879)
An address to the class of medical graduates of the University of Pennsylvania. Philadelphia: L. R. Bailey, 1841. 21p. DNLM; PPC; PU **40-1372**

WOOD, George Bacon (1797-1879)
Introductory lecture to the course of materia medica in the University of Pennsylvania. Philadelphia: Merrihew & Thompson, 1842. 27p. DNLM; PPC; PU **40-1373**

WOOD, George Bacon (1797-1879)
Syllabus of the course of lectures on materia medica and pharmacy, delivered in the University of Pennsylvania. Philadelphia: L. R. Bailey, 1842. 70p. DNLM; PU **40-1374**

WOOD, George Bacon (1797-1879)
The dispensatory of the United States of America. By George B. Wood . . . and Franklin Bache. . . . 5th ed., enl. and carefully rev. Philadelphia: Grigg & Elliot, 1843. 1368p. DLC; DNLM; OCLloyd, PPHa **40-1375**

WOOD, George Bacon (1797-1879)
Syllabus of the course of lectures on materia medica and pharmacy, delivered in the University of Pennsylvania. Philadelphia: L. R. Bailey, 1844. 70p. DNLM; PPC; PU **40-1376**

WOOD, George Bacon (1797-1879)
Introductory lecture to the course of materia medica in the University of Pennsylvania. Philadelphia: J. Young, 1845. 21p. DNLM; PPC; PU **40-1377**

WOOD, George Bacon (1797-1879)
The dispensatory of the United States of America. By George B. Wood . . . and Franklin Bache. . . . 6th ed., carefully rev. Philadelphia: Grigg & Elliot, 1845. 1368p. DLC; DNLM; OCLloyd; PPC **40-1378**

WOOD, George Bacon (1797-1879)
The dispensatory of the United States of America. By George B. Wood . . . and Franklin Bache. 7th ed., rev. Philadelphia: Grigg, Elliot, & Co., 1847. 1368p. DLC; DNLM; OCLloyd; PPJ **40-1379**

WOOD, George Bacon (1797-1879)
Introductory lecture to the course of materia medica in the University of Pennsylvania. Philadelphia: J. Young, 1847. 24p. DNLM; PPC; PU **40-1380**

WOOD, George Bacon (1797-1879)
A treatise on the practice of medicine. . . . Philadelphia: Grigg, Elliot & Co., 1847. 2 v. DLC; DNLM; PPC; PU **40-1381**

WOOD, George Bacon (1797-1879)
Introductory lecture to the course of materia medica and pharmacy in the University of Pennsylvania. Philadelphia: T. K. & P. G. Collins, 1848. 23p. DNLM; PU **40-1382**

WOOD, George Bacon (1797-1879)
Syllabus of the course of lectures on materia medica and pharmacy, delivered in the University of Pennsylvania. Philadelphia: L. R. Bailey, 1848. 70p. DNLM; PU **40-1383**

WOOD, George Bacon (1797-1879)
The dispensatory of the United States of America. By George B. Wood . . . and Franklin Bache. . . . 8th ed., carefully rev. Philadelphia: Grigg, Elliot & Co., 1849. 1380p. DLC; DNLM; OCLloyd; ViRA **40-1384**

WOOD, George Bacon (1797-1879)
A treatise on the practice of medicine. . . . 2nd ed. . . . Philadelphia: Grigg, Elliot & Co., 1849. 2 v. DLC; DNLM; PPC; PPJ **40-1385**

WORCESTER, Noah (1812-1847)
A synopsis of the symptoms, diagnosis, and treatment of the more common and important diseases of the skin. Philadelphia: T. Cowperthwait & Co., 1845. 292p. 7 plates. DNLM; PPC; PPJ; PU **40-1386**

WORTHINGTON, Wilmer (1804-1873)
Annual address to the Chester County Medical Society. West Chester, 1848. 35p. DNLM **40-1387**

WORTHY, A. N.
A treatise on the botanic theory and practice of medicine, compiled from various sources, with revision and additions. Forsyth, Ga.: C. R. Hanleiter, 1842. 631p. DNLM; GU; PPC; ViRA **40-1388**

WRIGHT, Marmaduke Burr (1803-1879)
A lecture delivered to the students of the Medical College of Ohio at the opening of the session, 1841-1842. Cincinnati: J. & C. H. Brough, 1841. 14p. DNLM; OCHP; OCIM **40-1389**

WRIGHT, Marmaduke Burr (1803-1879)
A lecture on drunkenness and insanity. Cincinnati, O., 1845. 20p. DNLM; OCIM **40-1390**

WRIGHT, Marmaduke Burr (1803-1879)
A lecture delivered to the students of the Medical College of Ohio, at the opening of the session, 1843-1844. Cincinnati: R. P. Donogh, 1844. 16p. DNLM; OCIM **40-1391**

WRIGHT, Marmaduke Burr (1803-1879)
A lecture on the exhumation and dissection of human bodies. Cincinnati: Printed by J. A. Robinson & Co., 1846. 19p. DNLM; OCIM **40-1392**

WRIGHT, Marmaduke Burr (1803-1879)
An introductory address, delivered to the students of the Medical College of Ohio, November, 1847. Cincinnati: Clark & Collins, 1847. 16p. OC; OCHP; OCIM **40-1393**

WRIGHT, Thomas Lee (1825-1893)
Notes on the theory of human existence. Comprising remarks on vitality, the mind, and, incidentally, the soul. The whole being an exposition of the nature, powers, and destiny of man. Cincinnati: Collins & Van Wagner, 1848. 37p. DNLM; OCHP; OCIM **40-1394**

WYMAN, Jeffries (1814-1874)
Twelve lectures on comparative physiology, delivered before the Lowell Institute, in Boston, January and February, 1849. Phonographic report by James W. Stone. (Originally reported and published in the Boston Daily Evening Traveller.) Boston: H. Flanders & Co., 1849. 72p. DNLM; MBM; MH **40-1395**

WYMAN, Jeffries (1814-1874)
Twelve lectures on comparative physiology, delivered before the Lowell Institute, in Boston, January and February, 1849. Phonographic report by James W. Stone. (Originally reported and published in the Boston Daily Evening Traveller.) New York: Dewitt & Davenport, 1849. 72p. DNLM; NNNAM **40-1396**

YANDELL, David W[endell] (1826-1898)
Notes on medical matters and medical men in London and Paris. Louisville, Ky.: Prentice & Weissinger, 1848. 309p. DNLM; OCIM **40-1397**

YANDELL, Lunsford Pitts (1805-1878)
A prize essay on bilious fever. Louisville: Prentice & Weissinger, 1841. 46p. DNLM; OCIM **40-1398**

YANDELL, Lunsford Pitts (1805-1878)
An address on the improvement of the medical profession; delivered before the Medical Society of Tennessee. Louisville: Prentice & Weissinger, 1841. 18p. DNLM; OCIM **40-1399**

YANDELL, Lunsford Pitts (1805-1878)
A reply to a critique on Liebig's animal chemistry. Louisville: Prentice & Weissinger, 1843. 34p. DNLM; OCIM **40-1400**

YANDELL, Lunsford Pitts (1805-1878)
A review of Harrison's materia medica. [1845]. 14p. DNLM **40-1401**

YANDELL, Lunsford Pitts (1805-1878)
On etherization. Louisville: Prentice & Weissinger, 1848. 36p. DNLM; OCIM **40-1402**

YANDELL, Lunsford Pitts (1805-1878)
An introductory lecture to the medical class of the University of Louisville. . . . Louisville, October 16, 1848. Louisville, Ky.: Prentice & Weissinger, 1848. 28p. DLC; DNLM; KyLoJM; OCIM **40-1403**

YANDELL, Lunsford Pitts (1805-1878)
On the progress of etherization. [Louisville, 1849.] 36p. DNLM; OCIM **40-1404**

YELLOTT, George
The Thompsonian quack, or The miraculous cure and marvellous metamorphosis: a satire on somebody, by Nathan Nobody [pseud.]; with a critique by Billy Booby [pseud.]. . . . Baltimore: W. Taylor, publisher for the author, 1848. 70p. DLC **40-1405**

YOUNG, William
Marriage. Pocket Aesculapius, or every one his own physician: being observations on marriage, medically and philosophically considered, as manhood's early decline, with directions for its perfect cure, [etc.]. Philadelphia, 1848. 184p. 2 plates. DNLM; PPC; PU **40-1406**

IV. AMERICAN MEDICAL IMPRINTS, 1850-1859

But the work, though treating more especially of the yellow fever of Philadelphia, aims at something of a more enlarged and important character. By means of a constant comparison of facts observed here with those noticed elsewhere, on every point connected with the disease, the author has been enabled to lay before the reader an *exposé* of the whole subject; in a word, a comprehensive treatise on the yellow fever, in which every point of interest is fully examined. The fever of Philadelphia is used, in what follows, as a kind of foundation to a full consideration of the disease, as observed in different places, at home and abroad, where it has occurred—as a central point, towards which facts connected with the fever, as manifested elsewhere, converge, in other words, to use a homely expression, as a hook upon which to hang a dissertation on yellow fever generally—its symptomatology, its anatomical characters, its pathology, its treatment, its etiology, and the laws by which it is governed.

René La Roche, *Yellow Fever, Historical, Pathological, Etiological, and Therapeutical Relations* (1855)

ADAMS, Horatio (1801-1861)
On the action of water on lead pipes, and the diseases proceeding from it. Philadelphia: T. K. & P. G. Collins, 1852. 76p. DNLM; PPC; PU **50-0001**

ADAMS, R. E. W.
A lecture introductory to the first session of the Homoeopathic College of Missouri, delivered at the College Hall, November 2, 1859. St. Louis: Strong & Co., 1859. 23p. DNLM; PPHa **50-0002**

An **ADDRESS** to the friends of homoeopathy in New York, from the trustees of the New York Homoeopathic Dispensary Association. New York: W. C. Bryant & Co., 1852. 17p. DNLM; NNNAM **50-0003**

AGNEW, D[avid] Hayes (1818-1892)
Practical anatomy; a new arrangement of the London dissector, with numerous modifications and additions, containing a concise description of the muscles, blood vessels, nerves, viscera, and ligaments of the human body as they appear on dissection. Philadelphia: J. B. Lippincott & Co., 1856. 310p. DNLM; PPC; ViRA **50-0004**

AGNEW, David Hayes (1818-1892)
Valedictory address to the anatomical class of Philadelphia School of Anatomy, on Tuesday evening, February 19th, 1856. Published by the class. Philadelphia: J. B. Chandler, Printer, 1856. 16p. DNLM; PU **50-0005**

AGNEW, D[avid] Hayes (1818-1892)
Valedictory address to the anatomical class of the Philadelphia School of Anatomy, delivered Thursday evening, February 19th, 1857. Philadelphia: T. K. & P. G. Collins, 1857. 20p. DNLM; PPC; PU **50-0006**

AGNEW, D[avid] Hayes (1818-1892)
Valedictory address to the anatomical class of the Philadelphia School of Anatomy, delivered on Tuesday evening, February 16, 1858. Published by the class. Philadelphia: T. K. & P. G. Collins, 1858. 20p. DNLM; PPC; PU **50-0007**

AGNEW, David Hayes (1818-1892)
Valedictory address to the anatomical class of the Philadelphia School of Anatomy, delivered on Friday evening, February 18, 1859. . . . Published by the class. Philadelphia: W. S. Young, Printer, 1859. 24p. DNLM; PPC; PU **50-0008**

AGNEW, David Hayes (1818-1892)
An introductory lecture delivered in the Philadelphia School of Anatomy, October 17th, 1859. Philadelphia: J. M. Wilson, 1859. 16p. DNLM; PPC; PU **50-0009**

ALCOTT, William Andrus (1798-1859)
Vegetable diet: as sanctioned by medical men, and by experience in all ages. Including a system of vegetable cookery. . . . 2nd ed., rev. and enl. New York: Fowlers & Wells, 1851. 312p. DLC; NNNAM; ViRA **50-0010**

[ALCOTT, William Andrus] (1798-1859)
The physiology of marriage. By an old physician. Boston: J. P. Jewett & Co.; New York: Shelden, Lamport & Blakeman; [etc., etc.], 1856. 259p. DLC; MBM; NNNAM **50-0011**

ALCOTT, William Andrus (1798-1859)
Forty years in the wilderness of pills and powders; or the cogitations and confessions of an aged physician. Boston: J. P. Jewett & Co.; New York: C. M. Saxton & Co. . . . , 1859. 384p. CtY-M; MBM; MH; NN **50-0012**

ALCOTT, William Andrus (1798-1859)
The young woman's book of health. . . . New York: C. M. Saxton, 1859. 311p. DLC; NNNAM **50-0013**

ALDEN, Ebenezer (1788-1881)
The early history of the medical profession in the county of Norfolk, Mass.: an address delivered before the Norfolk District Medical Society, at its annual meeting, May 10, 1823. Boston: S. K. Whipple & Co., 1853. 48p. DNLM; MBAt **50-0014**

ALLEN, J[ohn]
A new method of constructing artificial dentures, combining cleanliness, strength, natural expression, and restoration of the form of the face. New York: Holman, Gray & Co., 1854. 12p. DNLM; NNNAM **50-0015**

ALLEN, John R.
Introductory address delivered to the medical class of Transylvania University, March 17, 1851. Lexington, Ky., 1851. 15p. DNLM **50-0016**

ALLEN, John R.
Introductory address, delivered to the class in the medical department of Iowa State University [etc.], 1855-1856. Keokuk, 1855. 15p. DNLM **50-0017**

ALLEN, Jonathan Adams (1825-1890)
Introductory address to the third session of the College of Medicine and Surgery, of the University of Michigan, October, 1852. 2nd ed. Detroit: G. E. Pomeroy & Co., 1852. 25p. DNLM **50-0018**

ALLEN, Jonathan Adams (1825-1890)
Observations on the medical platform. An introductory lecture. Session of 1853-1854. Detroit, 1853. 29p. DNLM **50-0019**

ALLEN, Jonathan Adams (1825-1890)
Steps to the medical platform. An address. Ann Arbor: Cole & Gardiner, 1854. 32p. DNLM **50-0020**

ALLEN, Jonathan Moses (1815-1867)
Lecture introductory to the course on anatomy, in the medical department of Pennsylvania College, for 1852-1853. Philadelphia: J. Richards, 1852. 24p. DNLM; PU **50-0021**

ALLEN, Jonathan Moses (1815-1867)
Address to the graduates of the medical department of Pennsylvania College. (With a list of the graduates.) Philadelphia: King & Baird, 1855. 18p. DNLM; PU **50-0022**

ALLEN, Jonathan Moses (1815-1867)
The practical anatomist; or, The student's guide in the dissecting-room. . . . With two hundred and sixty-six illustrations. Philadelphia: Blanchard & Lea, 1856. 631p. DLC; DNLM; PPC; PU **50-0023**

ALLEN, Nathan (1813-1889)
An essay on the opium trade, including a sketch of its history, extent, effects, etc., as carried on in India and China. Boston: John P. Jewett & Co., 1850. 68p. DNLM; MBM; MH; MWA
50-0024

ALLEN, Nathan (1813-1889)
An essay on the opium trade, including a sketch of its history, extent, effects, etc., as carried on in India and China. 2nd ed. Boston: J. B. Jewett & Co., 1850; Lowell: James P. Walker, 1853. 80p. DNLM; MBAt; MWA **50-0025**

ALLEN, R. A.
The diagnosis and treatment of venereal diseases; New York: H. Bailliere, 1855. 84p. DNLM; NNNAM **50-0026**

ALLEN, Richard I. (1808-1873)
A historical, chemical and therapeutical analysis of the principal mineral fountains at Saratoga Springs, together with general directions for their use. . . . 3rd ed., rev. . . . Saratoga Springs: B. Huling, 1853. 72p. DLC; DNLM **50-0027**

ALLEN, Richard I. (1808-1873)
An analysis of the principal mineral fountains at Saratoga Springs, embracing an account of their history; their chemical and curative properties; together with general directions for their use; also, some remarks upon the natural history, and objects of general interest in the county of Saratoga. . . . New York: Ross & Tousey, 1858. 113p. plates. DLC; DNLM; NNNAM **50-0028**

ALLPORT, W. W[ebb] (1824-1893)
Diseases of the teeth; a paper read before the Cook Co. Medical Society at Chicago. Chicago: Barnet & Clarke, 1853. 19p. DNLM **50-0029**

ALLPORT, W. W[ebb] (1824-1893)
An address to the graduates of the Ohio College of Dental Surgery, session of 1858-1859. [1858.] 16p. DNLM
50-0030

AMERICAN and European druggists' directory, 1858-1859. New York: Michels & Elder, [1858]. 2 vs. in 1 v. (358, 70p.) NN; NNNAM; OCIM; OCLloyd [Names and places of business of the wholesale and retail druggists in the U.S. and Territories, Canada, New Brunswick, Nova Scotia . . . Mexico, Central America, West Indies, South America, Europe, Russia, etc.]
50-0030A

AMERICAN INSTITUTE OF HOMOEOPATHY
Materia medica of American provings. By C. Hering, M.D., J. Jeanes, M.D., C. B. Matthews, M.D., W. Williamson, M.D., C. Neidhard, M.D., S. Dubs, M.D. [and] C. Bute, M.D. . . . Collected and arranged by the American Institute of Homoeopathy. With a repertory, by W. B. Earey, M.D. . . . Philadelphia: Rademacher & Sheek, 1853. 299p. DLC; DNLM; PPHa
50-0031

AMERICAN MEDICAL ASSOCIATION
Report on the epidemics of Ohio, Indiana, and Michigan, for the years 1852 and 1853. [By. Geo. Mendenhall, chairman of the committee.] [1854] 132p., 1 map, 3 diag. DNLM; PU
50-0032

AMERICAN MEDICAL ASSOCIATION
Memorial of the . . . by the chairman of the committee to investigate the etiology and pathology of epidemic cholera. 34 Cong., 1st session. Mis. Doc. 142. Aug. 5, 1856. [Washington, D.C., 1856.] 9p. DNLM; PPC; PU **50-0033**

AMERICAN MEDICAL ASSOCIATION
Report on a uniform plan for registration reports of births, marriages, and deaths. Philadelphia, 1859. 50p. DNLM; PU
50-0034

AMERICAN PHARMACEUTICAL ASSOCIATION
Report on weights and measures, read before the Pharmaceutical Association at their eighth annual session, held in Boston, Sept. 15, 1859. By Alfred B. Taylor, chairman. Boston: G. C. Rand & Avery, 1859. 104p. DNLM; MBM; NNNAM
50-0035

AMES, S.
On the treatment of pneumonia. Montgomery, Ala. [1855?] 25p. 1 tab. DNLM **50-0036**

AMUSSAT, Alphonse-Auguste (1821-1878)
On the employment of water in surgery. . . . Transl. from the French by Frank H. Hamilton. . . . Buffalo: Steam Press of Jewett, Thomas & Co., 1851. 62p. DLC; DNLM; PPC
50-0037

[ANATOMY]
The pocket anatomist: being a summary description of the muscles; with a tabular view of the arteries and nerves. Concordant with "The Dublin Dissector," and "Harrison on the Arteries." Buffalo: G. H. Derby & Co., 1850. 61p. DNLM
50-0038

[ANATOMY]
The anatomical remembrancer, or, Compete pocket anatomist: containing a concise description of the structure of the human body. 2nd American, from the 4th London ed. With corrections and additions by C. E. Isaacs. New York: S. S. & W. Wood, 1855. 265p. DLC; DNLM; NNNAM; PPC
50-0039

ANDREWS, C. N.
Divinity, law, and medicine. Anniversary address of the Illinois State Medical Society. Delivered before the Society, and citizens of Jacksonville, June 3, 1852. Peoria: B. Foster, 1852. 24p. DNLM **50-0040**

ANDREWS, Edmund (1824-1904)
Report on the functions of the cerebellum. Philadelphia: T. K. & P. G. Collins, 1858. 19p. DNLM; PPC
50-0041

ANNAN, Samuel (1797-1868)
An introductory lecture delivered at the opening of the Kentucky School of Medicine. Louisville: W. N. Haldeman, 1850. 15p. DNLM; KyLoJM **50-0042**

An **APPEAL** in behalf of the medical education of women. New York, 1856. 16p. DLC; DNLM **50-0043**

An **APPEAL** to the public, by members of the medical profession, in New York. [In behalf of Dr. Morton.] New York: G. F. Nesbitt & Co., 1858. 20p. DNLM; NNNAM
50-0044

An **APPEAL** to the public, by members of the medical profession, in New York. [In behalf of Dr. Morton.] New York: W. C. Bryant & Co., 1859. 44p. DNLM; NNNAM
50-0045

ARMOR, Samuel Glasgow (1819-1885)
Prize essay, on the zymotic theory of essential fevers and other disordered conditions of the blood; together with an appendix on medical theories and vital statistics. Read before the Ohio State Medical Society. Dayton: B. P. Dubois & Co., 1853. 26p. DNLM; OCIM **50-0046**

ARMOR, Samuel Glasgow (1819-1885)
Valedictory lecture delivered to the students of the Medical College of Ohio, Feb. 17, 1857. Cincinnati: Moore, Wilstach, Keys & Co., 1857. 18p. DNLM; OCIM **50-0047**

ARMSBY, James H. (1810-1875)
Hospitals, their rise and progress; an address delivered before the Albany County Medical society . . . at its semi-annual session, November, 1851. Albany: C. van Benthuysen, printer, 1852. 21p. DLC; NNNAM **50-0048**

ARMSBY, James H. (1810-1875)
Hospitals. Annual address delivered before the Albany County Medical Society, November, 1852. . . . Communicated by the Society. Albany [N.Y.]: C. van Benthuysen, printer, 1853. 23p. DLC; DNLM **50-0049**

ARMSTRONG, George Dodd (1813-1890)
The summer of the pestilence. A history of the ravages of the yellow fever in Norfolk, Virginia, A.D. 1855. . . . Philadelphia: J. B. Lippincott & Co., 1856. 192p. DLC; PPC **50-0050**

ARMSTRONG, George Dodd (1813-1890)
The summer of the pestilence. A history of the ravages of the yellow fever in Norfolk, Virginia, A.D. 1855. . . . 2nd ed. Philadelphia: J. B. Lippincott & Co., 1856. 192p. DLC; DNLM; PPC **50-0051**

ARNOLD, J[ohn] L.
Arnold's lectures on anatomy, physiology and hygiene; and disease, its cause, prevention, and cure. . . . Cincinnati: H. M. Rulison; Philadelphia: D. Rulison, 1856. 2pts. in 1 v. DLC; PPC **50-0052**

ARNOLD, J[ohn] L.
Arnold's lectures on the structure and laws of the human body; adapted to the capacity of youth. . . . Cincinnati: H. M. Rulison; Philadelphia: D. Rulison, 1856. 165p. DLC; PPJ; PU **50-0053**

ARNOLD, John L.
Arnold's medical companion for young men; containing the laws of physiology and health, and a history of every disease; its cause, prevention, and cure. Also, a special lecture on organic generation; its philosophy, singularities, and derangements; containing many strange and useful facts on the subject of procreation. . . . Cincinnati: M. H. Rulison; Philadelphia: D. Rulison, 1856. 187p. DLC; PPC **50-0054**

ARNOLD, Richard D. (1808-1876)
The reciprocal duty of physicians and of the public towards each other. An address, delivered before the Medical Society of the State of Georgia at its second annual meeting, held at Atlanta on the 9th of April, 1851. Published by order of the society. Savannah: J. B. Cubbedge, printer, 1851. 30p. DNLM; GU **50-0055**

ARNOLD, Richard D. (1808-1876)
An essay upon the relation of bilious and yellow fever, prepared at the request of, and read before, the Medical Society of the State of Georgia. With addendum. Augusta, Ga., 1856. 24p. 3 col. plates. DNLM; GU **50-0056**

ARNOLD, Richard D. (1808-1876)
Dengue, or break-bone fever, as it appeared in Savannah in the summer and fall of 1850. Savannah, Ga.: N. Nichols, 1858. 16p. DNLM; GU **50-0057**

ARNOLD, Richard D. (1808-1876)
The identity of dengue, or break-bone fever, and yellow fever. Savannah, 1858-1859. 19p. DNLM; GU **50-0058**

ARTHUR, Robert (1818-1880)
Treatment of dental caries complicated with disorders of the pulp. . . . Philadelphia, New York [etc.]: Jones, White & McCurdy, 1853. 121p. DLC; NNNAM; PPC **50-0059**

ARTHUR, Robert (1819-1880)
An argument against professional patents. Baltimore: J. W. Woods, 1853. 23p. DNLM; MdU-D **50-0060**

ARTHUR, Robert (1819-1880)
Valedictory address delivered before the graduating class of the Philadelphia College of Dental Surgery, session 1854-1855. Philadelphia: J. H. Jones & Co., 1855. 40p. DNLM; PPC; PU **50-0061**

ARTHUR, Robert (1819-1880)
A treatise on the use of adhesive gold foil. . . . Philadelphia: Jones, White & McCurdy, 1857. 86p. DLC; MdU-D; PPC **50-0062**

ASHWELL, Samuel (1798-1857)
A practical treatise on the diseases peculiar to women. Illustrated by cases derived from hospital and private practice. . . . 3rd American from the 3rd and rev. London ed. Philadelphia: Blanchard & Lea, 1855. 528p. CtY-M; DLC; ICRM; PPC **50-0063**

ASKEW, Henry F[ord] (1805-1876)
An address delivered before the Medical Society at Dover, June 8, 1852. Wilmington, Del.: H. Eckel & Co., printers, 1852. 24p. DNLM **50-0064**

ATLEE, Walter Franklin (1828-1910)
Notes on M. Bernard's lectures on the blood; with an appendix. Philadelphia: Lippincott, Grambo & Co., 1854. 224p. DNLM; PPC **50-0065**

ATLEE, Washington Lemuel (1808-1878)
An introductory address to the class of the Medical Department of Pennsylvania College. Philadelphia: B. Mifflin, 1850. 16p. PPC; PU **50-0066**

ATLEE, Washington Lemuel (1808-1878)
Physical education, the only solid foundation of moral and intellectual culture and development: an address delivered before the Linnaean Association of Pennsylvania College, Gettysburg, Pa., at the annual commencement, Sept. 19th, 1851. Gettysburg: H. C. Heinstedt, 1851. 18p. DNLM **50-0067**

ATLEE, Washington Lemuel (1808-1878)
A table of all the known operations of ovariotomy. From 1701 to 1851. Comprising two hundred and twenty-two cases: including their synoptical history and analysis. Philadelphia: T. K. & P. G. Collins, 1851. 37p. DNLM; PPC
50-0068

ATLEE, Washington Lemuel (1808-1878)
Memoir of William R. Grant, with a notice of his theory of the foetal circulation, read to the College of Physicians of Philadelphia, March 2, 1853. Written and printed by order of the College. Philadelphia: Lippincott, Grambo & Co., 1853. 22p. DNLM; PPC; PU **50-0069**

ATLEE, Washington Lemuel (1808-1878)
Prize essay. The surgical treatment of certain fibrous tumours of the uterus, heretofore considered beyond the resources of art. Philadelphia: T. K. & P. G. Collins, 1853. 99p. DNLM; PPC **50-0070**

ATLEE, Washington Lemuel (1808-1878)
Correction of the erroneous statements of Henry H. Smith, published in the Medical Examiner, January, 1855, in relation to a case of gastrotomy, which occurred in the practice of. . . . Philadelphia: James H. Bryson, 1855. 32p. DNLM; PPC
50-0071

ATLEE, Washington Lemuel (1808-1878)
Report of a case of hydrophobia, extracted from the report of T. W. Blatchford, M.D., in transactions of the American Medical Association, for the year 1856. With an appendix, containing the report of a committee of citizens of Lancaster, Pa., on the efficacy of Stoy's cure for hydrophobia. Philadelphia: T. K. & P. G. Collins, 1856. 38p. DNLM; PPC
50-0072

AUSTEN, Philip H. (1822-1878)
Valedictory delivered before the graduating class of the Baltimore College of Dental Surgery, Marcy 25, 1853. Baltimore: J. W. Woods, 1853. 24p. DNLM; MdU-D
50-0073

AYRES, Daniel (1822-1892)
Contributions to practical surgery. New York: Miller & Holman, 1857. 29p. 2 fig. DNLM; NNNAM
50-0074

AYRES, Daniel (1822-1892)
Congenital exstrophy of the urinary bladder, and its complications, successfully treated by a new plastic operation. New York: Hall, Clayton & Co., 1859. 14p. 4 fig. DNLM; NNNAM
50-0075

BACHE, Franklin (1792-1864)
An obituary notice of Thomas T. Hewson, M.D., late president of the Philadelphia College of Physicians. . . . Read before the College, November 6, 1849, and pub. by its direction. Philadelphia: Printed by W. F. Geddes, 1850. 15p. DLC; DNLM; PPC **50-0076**

BACHE, Franklin (1792-1864)
Introductory lecture to the course of chemistry, delivered in Jefferson Medical College, October 13th, 1852. Philadelphia: T. K. & P. G. Collins, 1852. 16p. DNLM; PPJ
50-0077

BACHE, Franklin (1792-1864)
Valedictory address to the graduates of Jefferson Medical College of Philadelphia, delivered at the public commencement, held March 9, 1853. . . . Published by the graduating class. Philadelphia: T. K. & P. G. Collins, printers, 1853. 20p. DLC; PPJ **50-0078**

BACHE, Franklin (1792-1864)
Valedictory address to the graduates of Jefferson Medical College of Philadelphia, delivered at the public commencement, held March 15, 1859. Philadelphia: J. M. Wilson, 1859. 16p. DNLM; PPJ **50-0079**

BACKUS, Henry
Essay on "unity of disease." Selma, Ala., 1853. 46p. AU; DNLM **50-0080**

BACKUS, Henry
Medicine a science, or disease a unit. Selma, Ala.: J. Hardy, 1855. 46p. DNLM **50-0081**

BACKUS, Henry
Disease a unit; or, Medicine a science. Selma, Ala.: Printed at the Selma Reporter Job Printing Office, 1857. 66p. AU; DLC; DNLM **50-0082**

BACON, John
Introductory address delivered to the medical class of Harvard University, November 3, 1858. Boston: D. Clapp, 1858. 19p. DNLM; MH-M **50-0083**

BALCH, Henry W.
The seamen's medical guide: a treatise on various diseases, with directions for treatment. . . . Boston: Sargent & Brown, 1851. 95p. DNLM; MH-M **50-0084**

BALDWIN, William Owen (1818-1886)
Physic and physicians. The annual address delivered before the Alabama State Medical Association. Montgomery: Job Office of Alabama Journal, 1850. 43p. AU; DNLM **50-0085**

BALL, Alonzo S[pafford] (1800-1893)
The present position of the two schools of medicine. An address delivered in the Assembly Chamber, Albany, before the Homoeopathic Medical Society of the State of New York, at its annual meeting, February 14, 1851. Albany, N.Y.: Munsell, 1854. 25p. PPHa **50-0086**

BANNING, Edmund Prior
An essay on the prevention and cure of vocal, pulmonary, dyspeptic, nervous, spinal, female, uterine, and child-bed weaknesses, and also of hernia, piles, and prolapsus-ani, etc., by mechanical supports. New York, 1850. 32p. DNLM; NNNAM **50-0087**

BANNING, Edmund Prior
Explanation of the principles and action of Dr. Banning's braces, spinal supporters, [etc.]. New York: Bauer & Palmer, 1850, 32p. DNLM; NNNAM **50-0088**

BANNING, Edmund Prior
Common sense on the mechanical pathology and treatment of chronic diseases of the male and female systems. . . . 14th ed. rev. enl. . . . Together with two lectures by the author: I.—His lecture on the philosophy of the human voice, containing important hints to public speakers and singers. II.—His lecture on dress, laying down the rules for the regulation of male and female attire. . . . New York: Wilson & Co. [1852]. 333p. DLC; DNLM; NNNAM **50-0089**

BARCLAY, Andrew Whyte (1817-1884)
A manual of medical diagnosis: being an analysis of the signs and symptoms of disease. . . . Philadelphia: Blanchard & Lea, 1858. 423p. DLC; PPC; PU; ViRA **50-0090**

BARKER, Fordyce (1818-1891)
Remarks on puerperal fever before the New York Academy of Medicine, October 7, 1857. . . . (Phonographically reported by Dr. Geo. F. Shrady. . . .). . . . New York: E. P. Allen, 1857. 23p. DLC; DNLM; NNNAM **50-0091**

BARKER, Fordyce (1818-1891)
A case of fibrous tumor of the uterus, accompanied with excessive hemorrhage, successfully treated by excision. . . . [New York, 1857]. 8p. DLC; DNLM; NNNAM **50-0092**

BARKER, Fordyce (1818-1891)
On the comparative use of the ergot and the forceps, in labor. Read by appointment before the Medical Society of the State of New York. . . . New York: H. B. Price, 1858. 16p. DLC; DNLM; NNNAM **50-0093**

BARKER, Fordyce (1818-1891)
Remarks on puerperal fever before the New York Academy of Medicine, Oct. 6, 1858. New York: Printed for the publishers, 1858. 16p. DNLM; NNNAM **50-0094**

BARNES, George William (1825-1890)
Homoeopathy and allopathy. A contrast. Cincinnati: B. Chapman, 1859. 48p. DNLM; PPHa **50-0095**

BARNES, John
Valedictory address to the class of graduates of the Missouri Medical College, at the annual commencement of the session of 1857-1858. St. Louis, Mo.: Printed by "Missouri Democrat," 1858. 17p. DNLM **50-0096**

BARTLETT, Elisha (1804-1855)
The history, diagnosis, and treatment of edematous laryngitis. Louisville: Prentice & Weissinger, 1850. 34p. DNLM; KyLoJM **50-0097**

BARTLETT, Elisha (1804-1855)
A discourse on the times, character and writings of Hippocrates. Read before the trustees, faculty and medical class of the College of Physicians and Surgeons, at the opening of the term of 1852-1853. . . . Published by the class. New York, London: H. Bailliere, 1852. 72p. DLC; DNLM; MH-M; NNNAM **50-0098**

BARTLETT, Elisha (1804-1855)
The history, diagnosis, and treatment of the fevers of the United States. . . . 3rd ed., rev. Philadelphia: Blanchard & Lea, 1852. 595p. DLC; DNLM; MH-M; NNNAM **50-0099**

BARTLETT, Elisha (1804-1855)
The history, diagnosis, and treatment of the fevers of the United States. 4th ed., revised by A. Clark. Philadelphia: Blanchard & Lea, 1856. 610p. DNLM; PPC; PPJ; PU **50-0100**

BARTON, Edward H[all] (*d.* 1859)
Report to the Louisiana State Medical Society, on the meteorology, vital statistics, and hygiene of the State of Louisiana. . . . To which is added an appendix, showing the experience of life insurance companies in Louisiana, with tables of mortality for the use of such companies, and the laws of probability of life (English calculation); also, the experience of the London life insurance offices, etc., by H. G. Heartt. . . . New Orleans: Davies, Son & Co., 1851. 69p. 3 folding charts. DLC; LNT-M **50-0101**

BARTON, Edward H[all] (*d.* 1859)
An address before the Louisiana State Medical Society. . . . late president of the society. . . . (on retiring from the chair). Pub. by the Society. New Orleans: Printed at H. Spencer's [1852?] 16p. DLC; LNT-M **50-0102**

BARTON, Edward H[all] (*d.* 1859)
The cause and prevention of yellow fever, contained in the report of the sanitary commission of New Orleans. Philadelphia: Lindsay & Blakiston, 1855. 282p. 7 tables, 1 map. DNLM; LNT-M; PPC; PU **50-0103**

BARTON, Edward H[all] (*d.* 1859)
The cause and prevention of yellow fever at New Orleans and other cities in America; and notices of the report of the sanitary commission, dated New Orleans, December 12, 1854. 3rd ed. New York: H. Bailliere, 1857. 282p. 6 maps. DNLM; NNNAM; LNT-M **50-0104**

BARWELL, Louisa Mary (Bacon) (1800-1885)
Advice to mothers on the treatment of infants: with directions for self-management before, during, and after pregnancy. Addressed to mothers and nurses. . . . Rev., enl., and adapted to habits and climate in the United States, by a physician of New York, under the approval and recommendation of Valentine Mott, M.D. Philadelphia: J. & J. L. Gihon, 1850. 148p. DLC; NNNAM; PPC **50-0105**

BATCHELDER, John Putnam (1784-1868)
An inaugural address delivered before the New York Academy of Medicine February 3rd, 1858. New York, 1858. 18p. DNLM; NNNAM **50-0106**

BAUER, Louis (1814-1898)
Some observations on hip-joint disease and its rational treatment. [1853.] 23p. DNLM **50-0107**

BAUER, Louis (1814-1898)
Outlines of the principles and practice adopted in the Orthopaedic Institution of Brooklyn; by Louis Bauer . . . and Richard Barthelmess. . . . New York: L. W. Schmidt, 1854. 39p. DLC; DNLM; NNNAM **50-0108**

BAUER, Louis (1814-1898)
A critical examination of a pathological specimen of softening of the intervertebral fibro-cartilages. New York: Holman, Gray & Co., 1854. 7p. DNLM; NNNAM **50-0109**

BAUER, Louis (1814-1898)
Hip disease: a lecture delivered at the Long Island Hospital of Brooklyn. . . . New York: W. H. Tinson, printer and stereotyper, 1859. 42p. DLC; DNLM; NNNAM **50-0110**

BAYARD, Edward (1806-1889)
Obligation of the world to homoeopathia; an address delivered before the American Institute of Homoeopathy at its annual session at Cleveland Ohio, June 9, 1853. Philadelphia: H. Duffield, 1853. 24p. DNLM; OCIM **50-0111**

BAYARD, Edward (1806-1889)
Homoeopathia and nature against allopathia and art. The annual address delivered by the President, before the New York County Homoeopathic Medical Society, on the anniversary of Hahnemann's birthday, April 10, 1858. New York: H. Ludwig, 1858. 17p. DNLM; OCIM
50-0112

BAYLESS, George Wood (1816-1873)
Some of the rewards of medicine. An introductory address delivered in the Kentucky School of Medicine, October 30, 1858. Louisville, Ky.: Morton & Griswold, 1858. 24p. DNLM; KyLoJM **50-0113**

BEACH, Wooster (1794-1868)
An improved system of midwifery, adapted to the reformed practice of medicine: illustrated by numerous plates. To which is annexed, a compendium of the treatment of female and infantile diseases, with remarks on physiological and moral elevation. . . . New York: C. Scribner, 1851. 272p. DLC; DNLM; NNNAM; PPC **50-0114**

BEACH, Wooster (1794-1868)
Beach's family physician and home guide for the treatment of the diseases of men, women and children, on reform principles. . . . Illustrated with nearly two hundred engravings. Forty-fifth thousand, rev. and enlarged, with an appendix, from eminent writers, giving the laws of health. . . . Cincinnati: Moore, Wilstach, Keys & Co., 1859. 992p. DLC; NNNAM; OCIM **50-0115**

BEAKLEY, Jacob (1812?-1872)
Valedictory address, delivered at the sixth annual commencement of the Homoeopathic Medical College of Pennsylvania, March 1, 1854. Philadelphia: C. Sherman, 1854. 16p. DNLM; PPHa **50-0116**

BEAKLEY, Jacob (1812?-1872)
Introductory lecture to the class of the Homoeopathic Medical College of Pennsylvania, October 14, 1859. Philadelphia: J. E. Potter, 1859. 23p. DNLM; NNNAM
50-0117

BECK, John Brodhead (1794-1851)
An historical sketch of the state of medicine in the American colonies, from their first settlement to the period of the revolution. . . . 2nd ed. Albany: C. Van Benthuysen, printer, 1850. 63p. DLC; DNLM **50-0118**

BECK, John Brodhead (1794-1851)
Lectures on materia medica and therapeutics, delivered in the College of Physicians and Surgeons of the University of the State of New York. . . . Prepared for the press, by his friend, C. R. Gilman. . . . New York: S. S. & W. Wood, 1851. 581p. DLC; DNLM; NNNAM; PPC **50-0119**

BECK, John Brodhead (1794-1851)
Essays on infant therapeutics. To which are added, observations on ergot; history of the origin of the use of mercury in inflammatory complaints; together with the statistics of the deaths from poisoning in New York in the years 1841-1842-1843. . . . 2nd ed., enl. and rev. New York: W. E. Dean, 1852. 168p. CtY-M; DLC; NNNAM; PPC **50-0120**

BECK, Theodoric Romeyn (1791-1855)
Elements of medical jurisprudence. By Theodoric Romeyn Beck . . . and John B. Beck. . . . 10th ed. . . . Albany: Little & Company, 1850-1851. 2 v. CtY-M; DLC; NNNAM; PPC
50-0121

BEDFORD, Gunning S. (1806-1870)
Clinical lectures on the diseases of women and children. 4th ed. New York: Sam'l. S. and Wm. Wood, 1856. 602p. DNLM; NNNAM; NNU-M **50-0122**

BEECH, John Henry (1819-1878)
Report on the topography and epidemic diseases of Michigan. Philadelphia: T. K. & P. G. Collins, 1859. 27p. DNLM; PPC
50-0123

BEECHER, Catharine E[sther] (1800-1878)
Letters to the people on health and happiness. New York: Harper & Bros., 1855. 192, 29p. DNLM; ICU; MH; NN
50-0124

BEECHER, Catharine E[sther] (1800-1878)
Physiology and calisthenics for schools and families. New York: Harper & Bros., 1856. 58p. DNLM; MH; NN; NNC
50-0125

BELCHER, George E[lisha] (1818-1890)
Inaugural address before the Hahnemann Academy of Medicine, January 7, 1857. New York: H. Ludwig, 1857. 21p. DNLM; NNNAM **50-0126**

BELL, Agrippa Nelson (1820-1911)
Quarantine. New York: G. W. Wood, 1856. 14p. DNLM; NNNAM **50-0127**

BELL, John (1796-1872)
Dietetical and medical hydrology. A treatise on baths; including cold, sea, warm, hot, vapour, gas, and mud baths; also, on the water regimen, hydropathy, and pulmonary inhalation; with a description of bathing in ancient and modern times. . . . Philadelphia: Barrington & Haswell, 1850. 658p. CtY-M; DLC; DNLM; PPC **50-0128**

BELL, John (1796-1872)
An introductory lecture, delivered at the opening of the thirty-first session, of the Medical College of Ohio, November 4th, 1850. . . . Cincinnati: Printed at The Daily Commercial Office, 1850. 28p. DLC; DNLM **50-0129**

BELL, John (1796-1872)
Memorial to the trustees of the medical department of the University of Pennsylvania [on the necessity of an increase in the number of branches to be taught, and an extension of the lecture term. Aug. 10, 1850.] Philadelphia: E. Barrington & G. D. Haswell, 1850. 16p. DNLM; PPC; PU
50-0130

BELL, John (1796-1872)
The mineral and thermal springs of the United States and Canada. . . . Philadelphia: Parry & McMillan, 1855. 394p. DLC; NNC; PU **50-0131**

BELL, John (1796-1872)
Report on the importance and economy of sanitary measures to cities. New York: E. Jones & Co., 1859. 243p. DNLM; ICU; NNNAM **50-0132**

BELL, John (1796-1872)
Medical heroism. Address before the Philadelphia County Medical Society, delivered February 24, 1859. Philadelphia: T. K. & P. G. Collins, 1859. 38p. DNLM; PPC; PU
50-0133

BELL, John (1796-1872)
Water, as a perservative of health, and a remedy in disease. A treatise on baths . . . also on hydropathy and pulmonary inhalation. . . . 2nd ed. Philadelphia: Lindsay & Blakiston, 1859. 658p. CtY-M; DLC; PPC; PU
50-0134

BELL, Theodore S[tout] (1807-1884)
Introductory lecture in the medical department of the University of Louisville, session, 1859-1860. Louisville, Ky.: L. A. Civill, 1859. 30p. DNLM; KyLoJM
50-0135

BEMAN, Henry D.
An address delivered at the laying of the corner stone of the Atlanta Medical College, July 21, 1855. Atlanta, Ga., 1855. 22p. DNLM; GU **50-0136**

BEMISS, S. M. (1821-1884)
Report on influence of marriages of consanguinity upon offspring. Philadelphia: T. K. & P. G. Collins, 1858. 109p. DNLM; PPC **50-0137**

BENNET, James Henry (1816-1891)
A practical treatise on inflammation, ulceration, and induration of the neck of the uterus: with remarks on the value of leucorrhoea and prolapsus uteri as symptoms of uterine disease. 2nd American, from 2nd London ed. Philadelphia: Lea & Blanchard, 1850. 355p. DNLM; PPC; PU; ViRA
50-0138

BENNET, James Henry (1816-1891)
A practical treatise on inflammation of the uterus and its appendages and on ulceration and induration of the neck of the uterus. 3rd American from the 2nd London ed. Philadelphia: Blanchard & Lea, 1852. 373p. CtY-M; PPC; PU; ViRA
50-0139

BENNET, James Henry (1816-1891)
Practical treatise on inflammation of the uterus, its cervix and appendages, and on its connection with uterine disease. . . . 4th American from the 3rd and revised London ed. To which is added a review of the present state of uterine pathology. Philadelphia: Blanchard & Lea, 1856. 430p. CU-M; OCIM; PPC; PU **50-0140**

BENNET, James Henry (1816-1891)
A review of the present state of uterine pathology. Philadelphia: Blanchard & Lea, 1856. 75p. DNLM; PPC; PPJ; PU
50-0141

BENNETT, John Hughes (1812-1875)
The pathology and treatment of pulmonary tuberculosis; and on the local medication of pharyngeal and laryngeal diseases frequently mistaken for, or associated with, phthisis. . . . Philadelphia: Blanchard & Lea, 1854. 130p. DLC; DNLM; PPC; PU **50-0142**

BENNETT, John Hughes (1812-1875)
Clinical lectures on the principles and practice of medicine. . . . 2nd ed., with four hundred and sixty-eight illustrations on wood. New York: S. S. & W. Wood, 1858. 951p. CtY-M; DLC; NNNAM; ViRA **50-0143**

BENSON, J. W.
Introductory address in the medical department of the University of Louisville, session, 1858-1859. Louisville, Ky.: Hanna & Co., 1858. 27p. DNLM; KyLoJM
50-0144

BENTLEY, Joseph
Health made easy for the people; or, physical training, to make their lives, in this world, long and happy. 1st American ed. Philadelphia: J. L. Gihon, 1854. 171p. DNLM; PPC; PU
50-0145

BERKLEY, Helen
Sketch of Hahnemann and his wife; together with a homoeopathic dietary and a list of popular works on the principles and practice of homoeopathy. New York: W. Radde, 1850. 34p. DNLM; NNNAM **50-0146**

BERNARD, Claude (1813-1878)
Illustrated manual of operative surgery and surgical anatomy, by MM. Cl. Bernard . . . and Ch. Huette, ed. with notes and additions, and adapted to the use of the American medical student, by W. H. Van Buren . . . and C. E. Isaacs. . . . Illustrated with steel engravings, from drawings after nature, by M. J. Léveillé, designed to serve as a companion to the ordinary text books of surgery. New York and London: H. Bailliere; [etc., etc.] 1852. 513p. 107 col. plates. CtY-M; DLC; OCIM; NNNAM **50-0147**

BERNARD, Claude (1813-1878)
On the alteration of the taste in paralysis of the facial nerve. . . . [Richmond, Va.: G. A. Otis, Jr., 1853]. 10p. DLC; DNLM; ViRA **50-0148**

BERNARD, [Claude] (1813-1878)
Notes of M. Bernard's lectures on the blood; with an appendix. By Walter F. Atlee, M.D. Philadelphia: Lippincott, Grambo & Co., 1854. 224p. DLC; DNLM; PPC; PU
50-0149

BICKLEY, George W. L.
Introductory address. Eclectic Medical Institute, November 10, 1853. [1853?] 12p. DNLM **50-0150**

BICKLEY, George W. L.
Review of the pretended "Report of Eclectic Physicians." Cincinnati: Abbott & Bentley, 1853. 16p. DNLM
50-0151

BIDDLE, John Barclay (1815-1879)
Review of materia medica, for the use of students. . . . Philadelphia: Lindsay & Blakiston, 1852. 322p. DLC; DNLM; OCLloyd; PPC **50-0152**

BIDDLE, John Barclay (1815-1879)
Valedictory address to the graduates of the medical department of Pennsylvania College, March 5, 1856. Philadelphia: Brown, 1856. 18p. DNLM; PPC; PU
50-0153

BIDDLE, John Barclay (1815-1879)
An address delivered before the Linnaean Association of Pennsylvania College, September 16, 1857. . . . Gettysburg: Printed by H. C. Neinstedt, 1857. 16p. DLC; DNLM; PU
50-0154

BIGELOW, Henry Jacob (1818-1890)
Dr. Harlow's case of recovery from the passage of an iron bar through the head. Philadelphia: T. K. & P. G. Collins, 1850. 12p. DNLM; MH-M **50-0155**

BIGELOW, Henry Jacob (1818-1890)
An introductory lecture delivered at the Massachusetts Medical College, November 6th, 1849. . . . Boston: D. Clapp, printer, 1850. 24p. DLC; DNLM; MH; MH-M **50-0156**

BIGELOW, Henry Jacob (1818-1890)
Notes from clinical lectures on surgery. Boston: D. Clapp, 1851. 34p. DNLM; MBM **50-0157**

BIGELOW, Henry Jacob (1818-1890)
Science and success. A valedictory address delivered to the medical graduates of Harvard University, at the annual commencement, Wednesday, March 9, 1859. . . . Boston: D. Clapp, 1859. 24p. DLC; DNLM; MH **50-0158**

BIGELOW, Jacob (1787-1879)
An introductory lecture on the treatment of disease, delivered before the medical class at the Massachusetts Medical College, November 3, 1852. Boston: Ticknor, Reed & Fields, 1853. 28p. DNLM; MH-M **50-0159**

BIGELOW, Jacob (1787-1879)
Nature in disease, illustrated in various discourses and essays. To which are added miscellaneous writings, chiefly on medical subjects. . . . Boston: Ticknor & Fields, 1854. 391p. DLC; MH; MH-M; NNNAM **50-0160**

BIGELOW, Jacob (1787-1879)
Brief expositions of rational medicine: to which is prefixed The paradise of doctors, a fable. . . . Boston: Phillips, Sampson & Company, 1858. 69p. CtY-M; DLC; MH-M; NNNAM **50-0161**

BIGELOW, Jacob (1787-1879)
Nature in disease; illustrated in various discourses and essays. To which are added miscellaneous writings, chiefly on medical subjects. . . . 2nd ed., enlarged. Boston: Phillips, Sampson & Company, 1859. 410p. CtY-M; DLC; DNLM; MH-M **50-0162**

BILLING, Archibald (1791-1881)
First principles of medicine. . . . 2nd American, from the rev. and improved 5th London ed. Philadelphia: Lea & Blanchard, 1851. 246p. DLC; DNLM; NNNAM; PPC **50-0163**

BILLINGS, John T.
Rheumatism, gout, neuralgia, and their cure. Lowell: S. N. Merrill, 1859. 12p. DNLM **50-0164**

BIRD, Golding (1814-1854)
Urinary deposits; their diagnosis, pathology, and therapeutical indications. A new American ed. from the 4th revised and enlarged London ed. Philadelphia: Blanchard & Lea, 1854. 371p. DNLM; PPC; PU; ViRA **50-0165**

BLACKMAN, George C. (1819-1871)
Reduction of strangulated hernia in mass. New York: J. F. Trow, 1851. 62p. DNLM; NNNAM **50-0166**

BLACKMAN, George C. (1818-1871)
On the claims of priority in exsection and disarticulation of the lower jaw; with an appendix containing the report of several operations. New York: Van Norden & Ackerman, 1852. 18p. DNLM; NNNAM **50-0167**

BLACKMAN, George C. (1818-1871)
An account of chronic hydrocephalus and of a case in which paracentesis was performed, and on the statistics of this operation. New York: Holman, Gray & Co., 1854. 31p. DNLM; NNNAM **50-0168**

BLACKWELL, Elizabeth (1821-1910)
The laws of life with special reference to the physical education of girls. . . . New York: G. P. Putnam, 1852. 180p. DLC; DNLM; MH; NN **50-0169**

BLAIR, George H.
A popular treatise concerning homoeopathy; to which is prefixed a brief glance at the fallacies of the old school of medicine. Columbus: Osgood & Pierce, 1857. 37p. OCIM; PPHa **50-0170**

BLANCHARD & LEA. PHILADELPHIA
Illustrated catalogue of medical, surgical and scientific publications. Philadelphia: Blanchard & Lea, 1854. 64p. DNLM; PPC **50-0171**

BLANDY, Alfred A.
Cheoplastic process, an improvement in mechanical dentistry. Baltimore: Woods, [1857]. 25p. DNLM; MdU-D **50-0172**

BLATCHFORD, Thomas Windeatt (1794-1866)
Homoeopathy illustrated: an address first delivered before the Rensselaer County Medical Society, at the annual meeting in the city of Troy, June 14th, and by request repeated before a popular audience, June 18, 1842. . . . [2nd ed.] Albany: C. Van Benthuysen, printer, 1851. 76p. DNLM **50-0173**

BLATCHFORD, Thomas Windeatt (1794-1866)
Cases of hydrophobia. . . . [Boston, 1854]. 8p. DLC; DNLM; MH-M **50-0174**

BLATCHFORD, Thomas Windeatt (1794-1866)
Report on rest and the abolition of pain in the treatment of disease, prepared by appointment of the New York State Medical Society . . . and read at the annual meeting, February, 1856. Albany: C. Van Benthuysen, printer, 1856. 20p. DLC; DNLM **50-0175**

BLATCHFORD, Thomas Windeatt (1794-1866)
Hydrophobia: its origin and development, as influenced by climate, season, and other circumstances. Being the report of the special committee appointed by the American Medical Association, and read at the meeting in Detroit, Michigan, May, 1856. . . . Philadelphia: T. K. & P. G. Collins, printers, 1856. 104p. DLC; DNLM; PPC **50-0176**

BLATCHFORD, Thomas Windeatt (1794-1866)
Eulogy on Samuel McClellan, M.D., prepared by order of the Medical Society of the State of New York, and read at the annual meeting in Albany, February 3, 1857. . . . Albany: C. Van Benthuysen, printer, 1857. 23p. DLC; DNLM **50-0177**

BLYTHE, James E.
Address to the graduates of the Medical College of Evansville. Evansville: A. H. Sanders, 1850. 32p. DNLM; ICRM; IEN-M **50-0178**

BODENHAMER, William (1808-1905)
A few brief and desultory remarks on anal fistula: being a defense of the author against the slanders and the misrepresentations of Drs. B. L. Hill, Wooster Beach, and others, relative to the treatment of this disease. . . . Louisville: Prentice & Weissinger, 1850. 44p. DLC; DNLM **50-0179**

BODENHAMER, William (1808-1905)
Practical observations on some of the diseases of the rectum, anus, and contiguous textures; giving their nature, seat, causes, symptoms, consequences, and prevention; especially addressed to the non-medical reader. . . . 2nd ed. New York: Published for the author, by J. S. Redfield, 1855. 257p. DLC; DNLM; NNNAM **50-0180**

BOECKER, Friedrich Wilhelm
Medical chemistry, for physicians and students of medicine, or practical instructions. . . . Transl. and arranged by A. Zumbrock. Philadelphia: Boericke & Tafel, 1855. 58p. PPC; PPHa; PU **50-0181**

BOENNINGHAUSEN, C. Von (1785-1864)
The sides of the body and drug affinities. Homoeopathic exercises. Edited by Charles J. Hempel, M.D. . . . Philadelphia: Rademacher & Sheek, 1854. 28p. CtY-M; PPC; PPHa; ViRA **50-0182**

BOLING, William M. (1811-1859)
Valedictory address to the graduating class of the medical department of Transylvania University at the annual commencement, March 1, 1850. Lexington, Ky.: N. L. Finnell, 1850. 20p. DNLM **50-0183**

BOLING, William M. (1811-1859)
Valedictory address to the graduating class of the medical department of the Pennsylvania University. 1850. 26p. DNLM; PU **50-0184**

BOLING, William M. (1811-1859)
Essay on the mechanism and management of parturition, in the shoulder presentation. Charleston: Walker & James, 1854. 91p. DNLM; ScCM **50-0185**

BOND, Thomas Emerson (1813-1872)
Address before the graduates of Washington University of Baltimore. Baltimore: Sherwood & Co., 1851. 19p. DNLM; MdU-D **50-0186**

BOND, Thomas Emerson (1813-1872)
A practical treatise on dental medicine, being a compendium of medical science, as connected with the study of dental surgery. . . . Philadelphia: Lindsay & Blakiston, 1851. 307p. DLC; DNLM; PPC; PU **50-0187**

BOND, Thomas Emerson (1813-1872)
A practical treatise on dental medicine, being a compendium of medical science as connected with the study of dental surgery. . . . Philadelphia: Lindsay & Blakiston, 1851. 324p. DLC; MdU-D; PPC **50-0188**

BOND, Thomas Emerson (1813-1872)
A practical treatise on dental medicine, being a compendium of medical science as connected with the study of dental surgery: to which is appended an inquiry into the use of chloroform, and other anesthetic agents. 2nd ed., rev., cor., and enl. . . . Philadelphia: Lindsay & Blakiston, 1852. 366p. DLC; DNLM; MdU-D; PPC **50-0189**

[BOSTON DISPENSARY]
A history of the Boston Dispensary. Compiled by one of the Board of Managers [William R. Lawrence]. Boston: J. Wilson & Son, 1859. 244p. DNLM; MBM **50-0190**

BOSTWICK, Homer
An inquiry into the cause of natural death, or death from old age. . . . New York: Stringer & Townsend, 1851. 152p. DNLM; NNNAM **50-0191**

BOWDITCH, Henry Ingersoll (1808-1892)
Memoir of Amos Twitchell, M.D., with an appendix, containing his addresses. . . . Boston: Printed by J. Wilson & Son, 1851. 212p. DLC; MH-M **50-0192**

BOWDITCH, Henry Ingersoll (1808-1892)
On paracentesis thoracis, with an analysis of cases. . . . Philadelphia: T. K. & P. G. Collins, printers, 1852. 35p. DLC; DNLM; MH-M; PPC **50-0193**

BOWDITCH, Henry Ingersoll (1808-1892)
A treatise on diaphragmatic hernia; being an account of a case observed at the Massachusetts General Hospital; followed by a numerical analysis of all the cases of this affection, found recorded in the writings of medical authors, between the years 1610 and 1846. . . . Buffalo: Printed by Jewett, Thomas & Co., 1853. 77p. DLC; DNLM; MH-M; NNNAM **50-0194**

BOWDITCH, Henry Ingersoll (1808-1892)
Cases of anomalous development of tubercles, commencing at the base of the lung and gradually extending upward; with the physical signs of pneumonia. Analysis of the cases: diagnosis, prognosis, pathology; read before the Boston Society for Medical Observation, February 20, 1855. New York: E. P. Allen, 1855. 32p. DNLM; MH-M **50-0195**

BOWDITCH, Henry Ingersoll (1808-1892)
Paracentesis thoracis. An analysis of twenty-five cases of pleuritic effusions in which this operation was performed. New York: Baker, Godwin & Co., 1855. 14p. DNLM; NNNAM **50-0196**

BOWDITCH, Henry Ingersoll (1808-1892)
On paracentesis thoracis. Boston, 1857. 8p. DNLM **50-0197**

BOWDITCH, Henry Ingersoll (1808-1892)
An address on the life and character of James Deane, M.D. Greenfield: H. D. Minick & Co., 1858. 45p. DNLM **50-0198**

BOWDITCH, Nathaniel Ingersoll (1805-1861)
A history of the Massachusetts General Hospital. Boston: J. Wilson & Son, 1851. 442p. 1 plate. DNLM; MB; MBM; MH **50-0199**

BOWLING, William K. (1808-1885)
Lecture introductory to the second course in the medical department of the University of Nashville. Nashville, Tenn.: J. T. S. Fall, 1852. 23p. DNLM **50-0200**

BOWLING, William K. (1808-1885)
Character and writings of Sydenham. An introductory lecture. Nashville: Cameron & Fall, 1854. 18p. DNLM **50-0201**

BOWLING, William K. (1808-1885)
"Catchings" for "Catchings," to show what is caught; being a special undertaking in the way of "Catchings," according to a proposition in the Nashville Medical Journal for May, 1855. Nashville, 1855. 24p. DNLM **50-0202**

BOWLING, William K. (1808-1885)
A reply to the St. Louis Medical and Surgical Journal by the editor of the Nashville Journal of Medicine and Surgery. [On an editorial in the former headed "Nashville vs. Philadelphia and the rest of creation."] Nashville: Cameron & Fall, 1855. 20p. DNLM **50-0203**

BOWLING, William K. (1808-1885)
Nashville Journal of Medicine and Surgery, extra [from the August No. for 1858]. American Medical Association and North American Medical Review. [On Dr. S. D. Gross's review of Dr. P. F. Eve's address before the American Med. Assoc., at Washington.] [Nashville, 1858.] 15p. DNLM
50-0204

BOWMAN, John E. (1819-1854)
A practical handbook of medical chemistry. 2nd American from the 3rd and revised London ed. Philadelphia: Blanchard & Lea, 1855. 287p. CtY-M; DNLM; NNNAM; PPC
50-0205

BOWRON, John S.
Observations on planetary and celestial influences in the production of epidemics, and on the nature and treatment of diseases. New York: J. S. Taylor, 1850. 72p. DNLM; ICU; MB; NNNAM **50-0206**

BOZEMAN, Nathan (1825-1905)
Remarks on vesico-vaginal fistule, with an account of a new mode of suture and seven successful operations. Louisville, 1856. 26p. DNLM **50-0207**

BOZEMAN, Nathan (1825-1905)
Remarks on vesico-vaginal fistule, with an account of a new mode of suture, and seven successful operations. . . . Montgomery [Ala.]: Barrett & Wimbish, book and job printers, 1856. 29p. DLC; DNLM **50-0208**

BOZEMAN, Nathan (1825-1905)
Urethro-vaginal and vesico-vaginal fistules: remarks upon their peculiarities, and complications: their classification and treatment: modifications of the button suture: report of cases successfully treated. . . . Montgomery [Ala.]: Barrett & Wimbish, book and job printers, 1857. 59p. DLC; DNLM
50-0209

BRADFORD, George W. (1796-1883)
Historical and biographical address, delivered before the Cortland County Medical Society, at the fiftieth anniversary meeting, August 10, 1858. . . . Published at the request of the Society. Homer [N.Y.]: J. R. Dixon, printer, 1858. 27p. DLC; DNLM **50-0210**

BRADFORD, J. Taylor (1818-1871)
Selections from a report on ovariotomy, read before the Kentucky State Medical Society, at its annual meeting at Louisville, April, 1857. [1857.] 56p. DNLM
50-0211

BRAINARD, Daniel (1812-1866)
Essay on a new method of treating serpent bite and other poisoned wounds, being the annual address delivered before the Illinois State Medical Society. Chicago: J. F. Ballantyne, 1854. 26p. 2 plates. DNLM; ICRM; IU-M **50-0212**

BRAINARD, Jehu (1807-1878)
Valedictory address. Delivered at the close of the third annual session of the Western College of Homoeopathic Medicine, at Cleveland, Ohio, February 28, 1853. Cleveland: Harris & Fairbanks, 1853. 24p. DNLM **50-0213**

BRAINARD, Jehu (1807-1878)
A lecture upon narcotic stimulants delivered to the students of the Western Homoeopathic College, December 14, 1858. Cleveland: Steam Press of Fairbanks, Benedict & Co., 1858. 18p. DNLM **50-0214**

BRAUN, Carl R. (1822-1891)
The uraemic convulsions of pregnancy, parturition, and childbed. Transl. from the German, with notes by J. Matthews Duncan. New York: S. S. & W. Wood, 1858. 182p. DNLM; NNNAM; NNU-M **50-0215**

BRECK, Samuel
A short biography of Robert M. Patterson, M.D. Philadelphia: J. C. Clark & Son, 1854. 16p. DNLM; PPC; PU
50-0216

BRECKINRIDGE, Robert J. (1828-1867)
Address to the graduates of the Kentucky School of Medicine, session 1853-1854. Louisville: Courier job rooms, 1854. 16p. DNLM; KyLoJM **50-0217**

BRIERRE-de-BOISMONT, Alexandre, J. F.
Hallucinations; or, the rational history of apparitions. . . . 1st American from the 2nd Paris ed. Philadelphia: Lindsay & Blakiston, 1853. 553p. DNLM; NNC; PPC; PU
50-0218

BRIERRE-de-BOISMONT, Alexandre J. F.
A history of dreams, visions, apparitions, ecstasy, magnetism, and somnambulism. 1st American from the 2nd enlarged and improved Paris ed. Philadelphia: Lindsay & Blakiston, 1855. 553p. DNLM; MH; NN; PPC **50-0219**

[BRIGHAM, Amariah] (1798-1849)
Biographical sketch of Amariah Brigham, late superintendent of the New York Asylum, Utica, N.Y. Utica: W. O. McClure, 1858. 84p. DNLM **50-0220**

BRILLAT-SAVARIN, Anthelme (1755-1826)
The physiology of taste; or transcendental gastronomy. . . . Transl. from the last Paris ed. by Fayette Robinson. Philadelphia: Lindsay & Blakiston, 1854. 347p. DNLM; MH; NN; NNC
50-0221

BRINSMADE, Thomas C. (1802-1868)
Annual address delivered before the Rensselaer County Medical Society. Albany: C. Van Benthuysen, 1851. 31p. DNLM
50-0222

BRINSMADE, Thomas C. (1802-1868)
Annual address delivered before the Medical Society of the State of New York. Albany: C. Van Benthuysen, 1859. 28p. DNLM **50-0223**

BRINSMADE, Thomas C. (1802-1868)
Inaugural address at the convening of the Medical Society of the State of New York, February 1, 1859. Albany: C. Van Benthuysen, 1859. 9p. DNLM **50-0224**

BRINTON, John Hill (1832-1915)
On a new method of preserving anatomical and pathological specimens. [1854?] 4p. DNLM **50-0225**

BRINTON, John Hill (1832-1915)
Description of a valve at the termination of the right spermatic vein in the vena cava, with remarks on its relations to varicocele. Philadelphia, 1856. 8p. 1 plate. DNLM; PPC
50-0226

BROCA, Pierre-Paul (1824-1880)
A classification of tumours confounded under the name of cancer. [Transl. from Monit. d. hop., Par., 1854.] [Richmond, 1855.] 11p. 1 plate **50-0227**

BRODIE, Benjamin Collins (1783-1862)
Mind and matter: or physiological inquiries. In a series of essays, intended to illustrate the mutual relations of the physical organization and the mental faculties. . . . With additional notes by an American editor. New York: G. P. Putnam & Co., 1857. 279p. DLC; MH-M; NNNAM; PPC
50-0228

BRODIE, Benjamin Collins (1783-1862)
Mind and matter: or physiological inquiries. In a series of essays, intended to illustrate the mutual relations of the physical organization and the mental faculties. . . . With additional notes by an American editor. New York: S. S. & W. Wood, 1858. 279p. DNLM; NNNAM; PPC; PU
50-0229

BROWN, Buckminster (1819-1891)
A case of extensive disease of the cervical vertebrae, with clinical observations on this and some other forms of caries of the spine. Also, a report of an operation for neuralgia. Boston: J. Wilson & Son, 1853. 20p. DNLM; MBM
50-0230

BROWN, Buckminster (1819-1891)
Ectopia cordis: cardiac displacement. Boston: D. Clapp, 1855. 8p. DNLM **50-0231**

BROWN, Buckminster (1819-1891)
Talipes varus. [Bostin, 1858.] 3p. DNLM
50-0232

BROWN, Buckminster (1819-1891)
Spinal caries, or angular curvature. [1858.] 8p. DNLM
50-0233

BROWN, Buckminster (1819-1891)
Cases of talipes, or club-foot. Boston: D. Clapp, 1858. 8p. DNLM **50-0234**

BROWN, Henry James
A voice from the pious dead of the medical profession; or, Memoirs of eminent physicians who have fallen asleep in Jesus; with a preliminary dissertation on the cross, as the key to all knowledge. . . . Philadelphia: Higgins & Perkinpine, 1855. 320p. DLC; DNLM; PU **50-0235**

BROWN, Isaac Baker (1812-1873)
On some diseases of women admitting of surgical treatment. . . . Illustrated by twenty-four wood engravings. Philadelphia: Blanchard & Lea, 1856. 276p. DLC; DNLM; PPC; PU
50-0236

BROWN, Moses
Consumption, and its spontaneous cure. Newburyport: Herald Job Press, 1859. 36p. DNLM **50-0237**

BROWN, William Symington
The capability of women to practice the healing art. A lecture delivered before the Ladies' Medical Academy, Nov. 9, 1859. Boston: Ripley & Co., 1859. 15p. DNLM; MBM
50-0238

BROWN-SÉQUARD, Charles-Edouard (1817-1894)
Experimental and clinical researches on the physiology and pathology of the spinal cord and some other parts of the nervous centres. Richmond: Colin & Nowlan, 1855. 66p. DNLM; ViRA **50-0239**

BROWN-SÉQUARD, Charles-Edouard (1817-1894)
Researches on epilepsy; its artificial production in animals, and its etiology, nature and treatment in man. First part of a new series of experimental and clinical researches applied to physiology and pathology. Boston: D. Clapp, 1857. 82p. DNLM; MBM; MH-M **50-0240**

BRYAN, James (1810-1881)
A short history of medicine, from the earliest periods, up to the revival of literature; an introductory lecture, delivered March 28th, 1850, in the Philadelphia College of Medicine. . . . Published by the class. Philadelphia: A. Scott, printer, 1850. 29p. DLC; DNLM; PPC; PU **50-0241**

BRYAN, James (1810-1881)
Progress of medicine during the first half of the nineteenth century. Being an introductory lecture to the spring session in the Philadelphia College of Medicine. Delivered March 17, 1851. . . . Published by the class. Philadelphia: Grattan & McLean, 1851. 28p. DLC; DNLM; PPC; PU
50-0242

BRYAN, James (1810-1881)
A treatise on the anatomy, physiology and disease of the human ear. . . . Philadelphia: Published by the author, 1851. 124p. DLC; DNLM; PPC; PU **50-0243**

BRYAN, James (1810-1881)
A historical sketch of surgery, from the revival of literature, to the end of the seventeenth century, being an introductory lecture to a course on surgery, in Geneva Medical College, N.Y. . . . Geneva: Cleveland and Look, printers, 1851. 26p. DLC; DNLM **50-0244**

BRYAN, James (1810-1881)
Certainty in medicine, being an introductory lecture delivered before the Philadelphia Medical College, session of 1852-1853. . . . Philadelphia: Brown's Steam Power Book and Job Printing Office, 1852. 23p. DLC; DNLM; PPC: PU
50-0245

BRYAN, James (1810-1881)
Introductory lecture before the class of the Philadelphia College of Medicine, October 8, 1855. . . . Philadelphia: The class, 1855. 16p. DLC; DNLM; PPC: PU
50-0246

BRYAN, James (1810-1881)
The medical profession and its claims. . . . Being an introductory lecture to the winter session of the New York Medical College of 1859-1860. . . . Delivered October 18th, 1859. New York: Published by the class, 1859. 25p. DLC; DNLM; NNNAM **50-0247**

BRYANT, Henry (1820-1867)
The radical cure of inguinal hernia; being a dissertation which obtained the Boylston prize for 1847, on the following questinn: "Is there any certain and safe manner of accomplishing the cure of common inguinal hernia?" . . . Boston: Printed by W. Chadwick, 1851. 70p. DLC; DNLM; MH-M
50-0248

BRYANT, Joel (1813-1868)
The pocket manual, or repertory of homoeopathic medicine, alphabetically and nosologically arranged; which may be used as the physicians' vade-mecum, the traveller's medical companion, or the family physician; containing the principal remedies for the most important diseases, symptoms, sensations, characteristics of diseases, with the principal pathogenetic effects of the medicines on the most important organs and functions of the body; together with diagnosis, explanation of technical terms, directions for the selection and exhibition of the remedies, rules of diet, . . . Compiled from the best authorities. New York: William Radde, 1851. 352p. NNNAM; OCIM; PPHa; PU **50-0249**

BRYANT, John Delavan (1811-1877)
The epidemic of yellow fever in Norfolk and Portsmouth, Virginia, during the summer and fall of 1855. . . . Philadelphia: T. K. & P. G. Collins, printers 1856. 39p. DLC; DNLM; PPC; ViRA **50-0250**

BUCHAN, William (1729-1805)
New and enlarged edition of Dr. Buchan's Domestic medicine. . . . 29th American from the last London ed. . . . Philadelphia: W. A. Leary & Co., 1852. 495p. ICJ; PPHa; PPC [Also: Philadelphia: Leary & Getz, 1854. 495p.; New York: Derby, 1857. 442p.] **50-0250A**

BUCHANAN, A. H. (1808-1863)
An address on scientific and practical medicine. Nashville: Cameron & Fall, 1857. 29p. DNLM; KyLoJM **50-0251**

BUCHANAN, A. H. (1808-1863)
Amputation at the hip-joint. Nashville: J. T. S. Fall, 1859. 8p. 1 plate. DNLM **50-0252**

BUCHANAN, Joseph Rodes (1814-1899)
American eclecticism; an introductory lecture. [1850.] 15p. DNLM **50-0253**

BUCHANAN, Joseph Rodes (1814-1899)
Eclecticism and exclusivism. Introductory lecture. Cincinnati: W. M. Naudain, 1851. 32p. DNLM; OCIM **50-0254**

BUCHANAN, Joseph Rodes (1814-1899)
Free collegiate education. A public lecture . . . together with a statement of the measures adopted by the trustees and faculty of the E. M. Institute for the establishment of a free medical college, [etc.]. Cincinnati: W. M. Naudain, 1852. 16p. DNLM; OCIM **50-0255**

BUCHANAN, Joseph Rodes (1814-1899)
Second era of medical reform. An introductory lecture. Cincinnati: Eclectic Med. Publishing Office, 1852. 13p. DNLM; OCIM **50-0256**

BUCHANAN, Joseph Rodes (1814-1899)
Introductory lecture on the subject of elevating the medical profession; delivered November 15, 1853, at the Eclectic Medical Institute. [1854?] 12p. DNLM **50-0257**

BUCHANAN, Joseph Rodes (1814-1899)
Medical sectarianism. An introductory lecture . . . before the eclectic medical class, in Greenwood Hall, November 6, 1854. Cincinnati: Printed by G. H. Lawyer, 1854. 16p. DLC; DNLM; OCIM **50-0258**

BUCHANAN, Joseph Rodes (1814-1899)
Outlines of lectures on the neurological system of anthropology, as discovered, demonstrated and taught in 1841 and 1842. . . . Cincinnati: Printed at the office of Buchanan's Journal of Man, 1854. 384p. DLC; DNLM; OCIM **50-0259**

BUCKLER, Thomas Hepburn (1812-1901)
A history of epidemic cholera, as it appeared at the Baltimore city and county alms-house, in the summer of 1849, with some remarks on the medical topography and diseases of this region. . . . Baltimore: Printed by J. Lucas, 1851. 45p. 2 tables. DLC; DNLM; MdU-D **50-0260**

BUCKLER, Thomas Hepburn (1812-1901)
On the etiology, pathology, and treatment of fibro-bronchitis and rheumatic pneumonia. . . . Philadelphia: Blanchard & Lea, 1853. 150p. DLC; DNLM; PPC; PU **50-0261**

BUCKLY, J. Gillis
An epitome of phrenology and temperamental physiology. . . . Cincinnati: Printed for the author, and for sale by Longley Brothers, 1857. 144p. DLC; OCIM **50-0262**

BUDD, George (1808-1882)
On the organic diseases and functional disorders of the stomach. . . . Philadelphia: Blanchard & Lea, 1856. 252p. DLC; DNLM; PPC; PU **50-0263**

BULL, Thomas
Hints to mothers, for the management of health during the period of pregnancy, and in the lying-in room; with an exposure of popular errors in connexion with those subjects. . . . From the 3rd London ed., with additions by an American physician; to which is added, the ladies' perpetual calendar. New York: J. Wiley, 1852. 242p. DLC; DNLM; NNNAM; PPC **50-0264**

BULL, Thomas
The maternal management of children, in health and disease. . . . 2nd ed. Philadelphia: Lindsay & Blakiston, 1853. 424p. DLC; DNLM; NNNAM; PPC **50-0265**

BULLITT, Henry M[assie] (*d.* 1880)
Introductory lecture addressed to the class of the Kentucky School of Medicine, session 1853-1854. Louisville: Courier Print, 1853. 19p. DNLM; KyLoJM **50-0266**

BULLITT, Henry M[assie] (*d.* 1880)
An address on the life and character of the late Coleman Rogers, M.D. Louisville: Hull & Bros., 1855. 36p. DNLM; KyLoJM **50-0267**

BULWER-LYTTON, Edward (1803-1873) and John FORBES
On the water treatment; a compilation of papers on the subject of hygiene and rational hydropathy. Edited with additional matter by R. S. Houghton. New York: Fowler & Wells, 1851. 258p. DNLM; NNNAM **50-0268**

BULWER-LYTTON, Edward (1803-1873), John FORBES, and Roland S. HOUGHTON
On the water treatment: a compilation of papers on the subject of hygiene and national hydropathy; edited with additional matter by Roland S. Houghton. New and revised ed., with additions and improvements. New York: Fowler & Wells, 1855. 258p. DNLM; NNNAM **50-0269**

BURDEN, Jesse R.
Valedictory address to the graduates of the spring session, 1850 [Philadelphia College of Medicine]. Philadelphia, 1850. 20p. DNLM; PU **50-0270**

BURGE, J. H. Hobart (1823-1901)
Remarks on extension and counter-extension, in the treatment of fractured thigh; with description and illustrations of a new apparatus, and report of cases. New York: W. R. Plunkett, 1857. 8p. 2 fig. DNLM; NNNAM **50-0271**

BURGE, J. H. Hobart and William J. BURGE
Observations on the treatment of fractures on the femur with a new apparatus, and report of seventeen cases. Brooklyn: W. Wilton, 1859. 45p. DNLM; NBM; NNNAM **50-0272**

BURKE, William
The mineral springs of Virginia. . . . A new work. Richmond: Morris & Brother, 1851. 348p. DNLM; ViRA **50-0273**

BURKE, William
The Virginia mineral springs. 2nd ed., improved and enlarged. Richmond, Va.: Ritchies & Dunnavant, 1853. 376p. DNLM; ViRA **50-0274**

BUSH, Lewis Potter (1812-1892)
Address before the Medical Society of Delaware, delivered at its annual meeting, held at Dover, June, 1855. Wilmington, Del.: H. Eckell & Co., 1856. 20p. DNLM **50-0275**

BUTLER, David P.
The phrenological delineator. A compendium of phrenology; including recent discoveries in relation to the brain, temperaments, and other conditions of body which affect mentality. Together with a chart of the phrenological developments. . . . Boston: Fowler, Wells & Co., 1856. 32p. plates. DLC; NN; MB **50-0276**

BUTLER, David P.
The phrenological delineator. A compendium of phrenology; including recent discoveries in relation to the brain, temperaments, and other conditions of body which affect mentality. Together with a chart of the phrenological developments. . . . 5th ed., rev. Boston: D. P. Butler, 1859. 32p. plates. DLC; NN; MB; MWA **50-0277**

BUTLER, Robert O.
Report of cases in the surgical practice of the Brooklyn City Hospital. Joseph C. Hutchison, attending surgeon. New York: Holman, 1857. 7p. DNLM; NNNAM **50-0278**

BUTLER, Samuel Worcester (1823-1874)
Doctors' commons. An ethic address, delivered before the District Medical Society, for the county of Burlington, January 10, 1854. . . . Published by order of the society. Burlington [N.J.]: Printed by J. Rodgers, 1854. 12p. DLC; DNLM; NjR **50-0279**

BUTLER, Samuel Worcester (1823-1874)
A biographical sketch of the late Nathaniel Chapman, M.D. Philadelphia: J. M. Wilson, [1855]. 11p. DNLM; PPC: PPJ; PU **50-0280**

BYFORD, William Heath (1817-1890)
Physiology, pathology, and therapeutics of muscular exercise; a paper read before the Cook County Medical Society, and published at their request. . . . Chicago: J. Barnet, book, job and card printer, 1858. 26p. DLC; DNLM; ICRM **50-0281**

BYRN, Marcus Lafayette
The anatomy, physiology, and diseases of the hair, with directions for their treatment and cure. . . . New York: M. L. Byrn, 1857. 99p. DLC; NNNAM **50-0282**

BYRNE, Barnard M. (1807-1860)
An essay to prove the contagious character of malignant cholera; with brief instructions for its prevention and cure. . . . 2nd ed., with additional notes by the author. . . . Philadelphia: Childs & Peterson, 1855. 160p. DLC; DNLM; PPC **50-0283**

BYRNE, Barnard M. (1807-1860)
Proceedings of a court martial for the trial of Surgeon B. M. Byrne, held at Fort Moultrie, S.C., on March 24th, 1859. Charleston: Walker, Evans & Co., 1859. 130p. DLC; DNLM; ScCM **50-0284**

CABELL, James L[awrence] (1813-1889)
Syllabus of the lectures on physiology and histology, including the outlines of comparative anatomy, delivered at the University of Virginia. University of Virginia: McKennie & Son, 1853. 114p. DNLM; ViRA **50-0285**

CADWELL, Frederick A.
Treatise on the eye and ear: rules for the preservation and restoration of sight; deafness, its causes and progress explained; new discoveries in treatment. . . . 5th ed. Chicago: S. P. Rounds' book and job printing house, 1859. 279p. DLC; DNLM; ICRM **50-0286**

CALDWELL, Charles (1772-1853)
Autobiography of Charles Caldwell, M.D., with a preface, notes, and appendix, by Harriot W. Warner. Philadelphia: Lippincott, Grambo & Co., 1855. 454p. DLC; DNLM; ICU; MH **50-0287**

CALHOUN, George R.
Report of the consulting surgeon on spermatorrhoea. Philadelphia: Printed for the Howard Association, 1858. 23p. DNLM; PPC **50-0288**

CALKINS, Marshall (1828-1922)
A valedictory lecture, delivered before the students in the Eclectic Medical College of Pennsylvania. Worcester: C. Hamilton, 1856. 25p. DNLM; PPC **50-0289**

CALKINS, Marshall (1828-1922)
An introductory address delivered in the Eclectic Medical College of Pennsylvania. Philadelphia: Bryson, 1857. 12p. DNLM; PPC **50-0290**

CALKINS, Marshall (1828-1922)
Thoracic diseases: their pathology, diagnosis and treatment. In 4 pts. With the posthumous writings of Calvin Newton, A.M., M.D., and a biographical sketch of the life and character of Professor Calvin Newton. 2nd ed., revised. Philadelphia: H. Cowperthwait & Co., 1858. 545p. DNLM; NNNAM; PPC; PPJ **50-0291**

CAMPBELL, Henry Fraser (1824-1891)
The difficulties and the privileges of the medical profession. An address delivered before the Medical Society of the State of Georgia. Augusta: J. McCafferty, 1852. 19p. DNLM; GU
50-0292

CAMPBELL, Henry Fraser (1824-1891)
An inquiry into the nature of typhoidal fevers. Based upon a consideration of their history and pathology. Presented to the American Medical Association, at its session of May, 1853. Philadelphia: T. K. & P. G. Collins, 1853. 60p. DNLM; PPC
50-0293

CAMPBELL, Henry Fraser (1824-1891)
Croup and its treatment with anti-periodic doses of quinine. [1853?] 4p. DNLM **50-0294**

CAMPBELL, Henry Fraser (1824-1891)
A claim of priority in the discovery and naming of the excito-secretory system of nerves. . . . Augusta, Ga.: McCafferty's Office—J. Morris, printer, 1857. 18p. DLC; DNLM; GU
50-0295

CAMPBELL, Henry Fraser (1824-1891)
. . . Essays on the secretory and the excito-secretory system of nerves in their relations to physiology and pathology. Comprising I. A new classification of febrile diseases. II. An exposition of the "ganglionic pathology" of all continued fevers, as illustrated in typhus and typhoid fever. III. The prize essay on the excito-secretory system of nerves in its relation to physiology and pathology. IV. A letter to Dr. Marshall Hall, of London, claiming priority in the discovery and naming of the excito-secretory system of nerves. . . . Philadelphia: J. B. Lippincott & Co., 1857. 135p. DLC; DNLM; PPC; PU
50-0296

CAMPBELL, Robert
An essay on empirical remedies, read before the Medical Society of the State of Georgia, April, 1852. Augusta, Ga.: J. McCafferty, 1852. 17p. DNLM; GU
50-0297

CAMPBELL, Robert
Dysentery: its pathology and treatment. Clinical lectures. Augusta, Ga.: J. Morris, 1858. 65p. DNLM; GU
50-0298

CAMPBELL, Robert
Letter on the treatment of typhoid fever. In answer to inquiries. Augusta, Ga.: J. Morris, 1858. 9p. DNLM; GU
50-0299

CARNOCHAN, John Murray (1817-1887)
A treatise on the etiology, pathology and treatment of congenital dislocations of the head of the femur. New York: S. S. & W. Wood, 1850. 235p. DNLM; NNNAM; PPC
50-0300

CARNOCHAN, John Murray (1817-1887)
Elephantiasis Arabum of the right inferior extremity; successfully treated by ligature of the femoral artery. New York: J. F. Trow, 1852. 13p. 1 plate. DNLM; NNNAM
50-0301

CARNOCHAN, John Murray (1817-1887)
Remarks on amputation of the lower jaw. [New York, 1852.] 3p. DNLM; NNNAM **50-0302**

CARNOCHAN, John Murray (1817-1887)
Amputation of the entire lower jaw; with disarticulation of both condyles. New York: Van Norden & Ammerman, 1852. 11p. 2 plates. DNLM; NNNAM **50-0303**

CARNOCHAN, John Murray (1817-1887)
Remarks on double capital amputations; with two cases and plates. 1853. 7p. DNLM; NNNAM **50-0304**

CARNOCHAN, John Murray (1817-1887)
Remarks on osteo-aneurism; with a case involving the condyles of the left femur. New York: D. Fanshaw, 1853. 15p. 1 plate. DNLM; NNNAM **50-0305**

CARNOCHAN, John Murray (1817-1887)
Exsection of the entire ulna. New York: Baker, Godwin & Co., 1854. 11p. 1 plate. DNLM; NNNAM
50-0306

CARNOCHAN, John Murray (1817-1887)
Case of penetrating gun-shot wound of the heart; life protracted for eleven days; bullet found embedded and encysted in the substance of the heart. New York: E. P. Allen, 1855. 6p. 1 plate. DNLM; NNNAM **50-0307**

CARNOCHAN, John Murray (1817-1887)
A case of encysted sanguineous tumor of the neck, successfully removed. [New York, 1856.] 6p. DNLM; NNNAM
50-0308

CARNOCHAN, John Murray (1817-1887)
A case of exsection of the entire os calcis. New York: Baker & Godwin, 1857. 8p. 2 col. plates. DNLM; NNNAM
50-0309

CARNOCHAN, John Murray (1817-1887)
Address on the study of science, delivered in the New York Medical College. New York: Wynkoop, Hallenbeck & Thomas, 1857. 43p. DNLM; NNNAM **50-0310**

CARNOCHAN, John Murray (1817-1887)
Contributions to operative surgery, and surgical pathology. Philadelphia: Lindsay & Blakiston, 1857. 77p. 4 plates. DNLM; NNNAM; PPC; PU **50-0311**

CARPENTER, William Benjamin (1813-1885)
On the use and abuse of alcoholic liquors, in health and disease. Prize essay. Philadelphia: Lea & Blanchard, 1850. 204p. DNLM; PPC; PU **50-0312**

CARPENTER, William Benjamin (1813-1885)
On the use and abuse of alcoholic liquors, in health and disease. Prize essay. Boston, Mass.: Temperance Society, 1851. 264p. MH-M; MWA; PPL **50-0313**

CARPENTER, William Benjamin (1813-1885)
. . . On the use and abuse of alcoholic liquors, in health and disease. . . . With a preface, by D. F. Condie. . . . Philadelphia: Blanchard & Lea,1853. 178p. DLC; DNLM; PPC; PU
50-0314

CARPENTER, William Benjamin (1813-1885)
Principles of human physiology, with their chief applications in psychology, pathology, therapeutics, hygiene, and forensic medicine. . . . 5th American from the 4th and enl. London ed. . . . Ed., with additions by Francis Gurney Smith. . . . Philadelphia: Blanchard & Lea, 1853. 1091p. 2 plates. DLC; NNNAM; PPC; ViRA **50-0315**

CARPENTER, William Benjamin (1813-1885)
Principles of comparative physiology. . . . A new American from the 4th and rev. London ed. Philadelphia: Blanchard & Lea, 1854. 752p. DLC; DNLM; MH-M; PPC
50-0316

CARPENTER, William Benjamin (1813-1885)
Principles of human physiology, with their chief applications to psychology, pathology, therapeutics, hygiene, and forensic medicine. . . . A new American from the last London ed. . . . Edited, with additions, by Francis Gurney Smith. . . . Philadelphia: Blanchard & Lea, 1855. 902p. 2 plates. DLC; DNLM; PPC; PU **50-0317**

CARPENTER, William Benjamin (1813-1885)
The microscope: and its revelations. . . . With an appendix containing the applications of the microscope to clinical medicine, etc. By Francis Gurney Smith. . . . Philadelphia: Blanchard & Lea, 1856. 724p. DLC; DNLM; PPC; PU
50-0318

CARROLL, Thomas (1795-1871)
Observations on the Asiatic cholera, as it appeared in Cincinnati in 1849-1850. . . . [Cincinnati? 1854?] 75p. DLC; DNLM; OCIM **50-0319**

CARSON, Joseph (1808-1876)
Lecture introductory to the course on materia medica and pharmacy, in the University of Pennsylvania. . . . Delivered October 10, 1950. Published by the class. Philadelphia: Merrihew & Thompson, printers, 1850. 18p. DLC; DNLM; PU **50-0320**

CARSON, Joseph (1808-1876)
Synopsis of the course of lectures on materia medica and pharmacy, delivered in the University of Pennsylvania. . . . Philadelphia: Blanchard & Lea, 1851. 204p. DLC; DNLM; OCLloyd; PPC **50-0321**

CARSON, Joseph (1808-1876)
A memoir of the life and character of James B. Rogers, M.D., professor of chemistry in the University of Pennsylvania. . . . Delivered by request of the faculty, October 11, 1852, and published by the class. Philadelphia: T. K. & P. G. Collins, printers, 1852. 23p. DLC; DNLM; PPC; PU
50-0322

CARSON, Joseph (1808-1876)
Synopsis of the course of lectures on materia medica and pharmacy, delivered in the University of Pennsylvania. 2nd ed. Philadelphia: Blanchard & Lea, 1855. 196p. DNLM; NNNAM; PPC; PU **50-0323**

CARSON, Joseph (1808-1876)
Introductory lecture on the claims of the materia medica, delivered in the University of Pennsylvania, October 10th, 1859. . . . Published by the class. Philadelphia: Collins, printer, 1859. 23p. DLC; DNLM; PPC; PU **50-0324**

CARTER, Francis (1814-1881)
Introductory lecture to the class of Starling Medical College, at the opening of the session of 1851-1852. Columbus: S. Medary, 1851. 30p. DNLM; OCIM **50-0325**

CARTWRIGHT, Samuel Adolphus (1793-1863)
A few remarks on haematokinety. [New Orleans, 1853.] 3p. DNLM **50-0326**

CARTWRIGHT, Samuel Adolphus (1793-1863)
Ethnology of the Negro or prognathous race. [1857.] 15p. DNLM **50-0327**

CARTWRIGHT, Samuel Adolphus (1793-1863)
Malum Egyptiacum, cold plague, diphtheria, or black tongue. New Orleans: Bulletin Office, 1859. 11p. DNLM; LNT-M **50-0328**

CASPARI, Carl (1798-1828)
Dr. Caspari's homoeopathic domestic physician. Edited by F. Hartmann, M.D. . . . Transl. from the 8th German edition, and enriched by a treatise on anatomy and physiology, by W. P. Esrey, M.D. with additions and a preface by C. Hering, M.D. Containing also a chapter on mesmerism and magnetism; directions to enable patients living at a distance from a homoeopathic physician, to describe their symptoms; a tabular index of the medicines, and the diseases in which they are used; and a sketch of the biography of Samuel Hahnemann. . . . Philadelphia: Rademacher & Sheek, 1852. 475p. DNLM; PPHa **50-0329**

CASSELBERRY, Isaac (1821-1873)
The use of water in the treatment of fever. Philadelphia: T. K. & P. G. Collins, 1857. 21p. DNLM; NNNAM; PPC; PU
50-0330

CASSELBERRY, Isaac (1821-1873)
Quinine in fever. [1857?]. 13p. DNLM
50-0331

CASSELS, J. Lang (1808-1879)
Address introductory to the opening of the session of Cleveland Medical College. Cleveland: Plain Dealer Book and Job Printing House, 1851. 19p. OCIM
50-0332

CATHERS, John
A positive cure for cancer, without the use of caustic or the knife. . . . Baltimore, [1856]. 32p. DNLM
50-0333

CATLIN, Benjamin Hopkins (1801-1880)
The annual address delivered before the Connecticut Medical Society. Hartford: Case, Lockwood & Co., 1858. 29p. CtY-M; DNLM **50-0334**

CAZEAUX, Pierre (1808-1862)
A theoretical and practical treatise on midwifery, including the diseases of pregnancy and parturition. . . . Transl. from the 2nd French ed., with occasional notes and a copious index, by Robert P. Thomas. Philadelphia: Lindsay & Blakiston, 1850. 765p. 11 plates. DLC; OCIM; PPC; PU **50-0335**

CAZEAUX, Pierre (1808-1862)
A theoretical and practical treatise on midwifery, including the diseases of pregnancy and parturition, and the attentions required by the child from birth to the period of weaning. . . . 2nd American, transl. from the 5th French ed., by Wm. R. Bullock. . . . Philadelphia: Lindsay & Blakiston, 1857. 962p. 4 plates. DLC; PPC; PU; ViRA **50-0336**

CAZENAVE, Pierre Louis Alphée (1802?-1877)
Manual of diseases of the skin, from the French of MM. Cazenave and Schedel, with notes and additions by Thomas H. Burgess. . . . 2nd American ed., enl. and cor. from the last French ed., with additional notes by H. D. Bulkley. . . . New York: S. S. & W. Wood, 1852. 348p. DLC; NNNAM; PPC; ViRA **50-0337**

CHABERT, J. Xavier
Observations on the origin, treatment, and cure of Asiatic cholera and cholera morbus; and the result of an experience of forty-five years during a residence in Asia, Europe, and America. New York: W. Marks, 1852. 24p. DNLM; NNNAM
50-0338

CHAILLÉ, Stanford E[merson] (1830-1911)
Anniversary oration of the Physico-Medical Society. Delivered Dec. 1, 1855. [New Orleans, 1856.] 16p. DNLM; LNT-M
50-0339

CHAMBERS, Thomas King (1818-1889)
Digestion and its derangements. New York: S. S. & W. Wood, 1856. 441p. DNLM; NNNAM **50-0340**

CHANDLER, Charles F[rederick] (1836-1925)
Miscellaneous chemical researches. [Göttingen.] Albany: C. Van Benthuysen, 1857. 52p. DNLM
50-0341

CHANNING, Walter (1786-1876)
Sketch of the life and character of John D. Fisher, M.D. [Boston, 1850]. 7p. DNLM; MBM **50-0342**

CHANNING, Walter (1786-1876)
Professional reminiscences of foreign travel. Boston, 1852. 32p. DNLM; ICU; MH; NNC **50-0343**

CHANNING, Walter (1786-1876)
Cases of polypus of the womb, with remarks. Boston: D. Clapp, 1855. 21p. DNLM; MBM **50-0344**

CHANNING, Walter (1786-1876)
On some of the diseases of the female urethra. . . . [Boston, 1856]. 12p. DLC; MH-M **50-0345**

CHANNING, Walter (1786-1876)
A physician's vacation; or, a summer in Europe. Boston: Ticknor & Fields, 1856. 564p. MH; NN; ICU; NNNAM
50-0346

CHANNING, William
The reformation of medical science demanded by inductive philosophy. 2nd ed. New York: Angell, Engel & Hewitt, 1851. 71p. DNLM; NNNAM **50-0347**

CHAPMAN, Chandler Burnell (1815-1877)
An introductory lecture to the class of the Ohio College of Dental Surgery; session of 1856-1857. . . . Cincinnati: Wrightson & Co., printers, 1856. 16p. DLC; DNLM
50-0348

CHAPMAN, Nathaniel (1780-1853)
. . . Catalogue of the medical library of Dr. N. Chapman, dec'd., late professor in the University of Pennsylvania, embracing rare and valuable authors, in the various departments of medical science, the whole to be sold on Friday and Saturday evenings, January 27th & 28th, 1854. . . . M. Thomas & Sons, auct'rs. . . . Philadelphia: Printed by Wm. Y. Owen, 1854. 19p. PHi; PPC **50-0349**

[CHEEVER, Charles] (1793-1852)
Extracts from the writings of . . . with a memoir by A. P. Peabody. Printed for private circulation. Boston: Wilson, 1854. 309p. MB; MH **50-0350**

CHEW, Samuel (1806-1863)
Oration delivered before the Medical and Chirurgical Faculty of Maryland, at their annual meeting in Baltimore, June 3, 1858. Baltimore: Hedian & Piet, 1858. 21p. DNLM; MdBM
50-0351

CHILDS, Timothy (1748-1821)
Rational medicine: its past and present; its true relations to specialists, to the partisans of exclusive systems, and to empirics. Boston: D. Clapp, 1859. 29p. DNLM; MBM
50-0352

CHURCHILL, Fleetwood (1808-1878)
The diseases of females; including those of pregnancy and childbed. . . . A new American ed., rev. by the author. With notes of Robert M. Huston. Philadelphia: Lea & Blanchard, 1850. 632p. DLC; OCIM; PPC; PU **50-0353**

CHURCHILL, Fleetwood (1808-1878)
On the diseases of infants and children. . . . Philadelphia: Lea & Blanchard, 1850. 636p. CU-M; DLC; ICRM; PPC
50-0354

CHURCHILL, Fleetwood, ed. (1808-1878)
. . . Essays on the puerperal fever and other diseases peculiar to women. Selected from the writings of British authors previous to the close of the eighteenth century. . . . Philadelphia: Lea & Blanchard, 1850. 444p. DLC; PPC; PPJ; PU
50-0355

CHURCHILL, Fleetwood (1808-1878)
On the theory and practice of midwifery. . . . With notes and additions, by D. Francis Condie. . . . New American from the last improved Dublin ed. Philadelphia: Blanchard & Lea, 1851. 510p. DLC; PPC; PU; ViRA **50-0356**

CHURCHILL, Fleetwood (1808-1878)
On the diseases of women, including diseases of pregnancy and childbed. . . . A new American ed., rev. by the author. With notes and additions by D. Francis Condie. . . . Philadelphia: Blanchard & Lea, 1852. 683p. DLC; MH-M; NNNAM; PPC
50-0357

CHURCHILL, Fleetwood (1808-1878)
On the diseases of infants and children. . . . 2nd American ed., enl. and rev. by the author. Ed. with additions, by William V. Keating. . . . Philadelphia: Blanchard & Lea, 1856. 735p. DLC; DNLM; PPC; PU **50-0358**

CHURCHILL, Fleetwood (1808-1878)
On the diseases of women; including those of pregnancy and childbed. . . . A new American ed., rev. by the author. With notes and additions by D. Francis Condie. Philadelphia: Blanchard & Lea, 1857. 768p. DLC; DNLM; PPC; ScCM
50-0359

CHURCHILL, John Francis
Treatise on the immediate cause, and the specific treatment of pulmonary phthisis, and tubercular diseases. . . . Transl. from the French by a physician. New York: J. Winchester [1859]. 111p. DLC; DNLM; NNNAM; PPC
50-0360

CLAPP, Asahel (1792-1863)
A synopsis, or, systematic catalogue of the medical plants of the United States. . . . Philadelphia: T. K. & P. G. Collins, printers, 1852. 222p. DLC; DNLM; OCLloyd; PPC
50-0361

CLAPP, Sylvanus (1815-1879)
Diabetes mellitus. An address read before the Rhode Island Medical Society, at their annual meeting, Providence, R.I., June 7, 1854. . . . R. Sherman, printer, 1854. 38p. DLC
50-0362

CLARK, Alonzo (1807-1887)
The claims of the medical profession. The annual address delivered before the New York State Medical Society, 1853. . . . Albany: C. Van Benthuysen, 1853. 29p. DNLM; N; NNNAM **50-0363**

CLARK, Alonzo (1807-1887)
The claims of the medical profession. The annual address delivered before the New York State Medical Society, 1853. 2nd ed. . . . Albany: C. Van Benthuysen, 1853. 24p. DNLM; NNNAM **50-0364**

CLARK, Henry Grafton (1804-1892)
Ship fever, so called; its history, nature, and best treatment. The Fiske Fund Prize Dissertation for 1849. Printed by order of the Rhode Island Medical Society. Boston: Ticknor, Reed & Fields, 1850. 48p. DNLM; MH-M; MWA
50-0365

CLARK, Henry Grafton (1804-1892)
Superiority of sanitary measures over quarantines. An address delivered before the Suffolk District Medical Society, April 24, 1852. Printed by request of the society. Boston: Thurston, Torry & Emerson, 1852. 40p. DNLM; MH-M
50-0366

CLARK, Henry Grafton (1804-1892)
Draft of a metropolitan sanitary code. (Reported to the committee on internal hygiene.) [Boston: G. C. Rand & Avery, 1859.] 23p. DNLM; MH-M **50-0367**

CLARK, James Henry (1814-1869)
. . . Sight and hearing, how preserved, and how lost. . . . New York: C. Scribner, 1856. 351p. DLC; DNLM; NNNAM
50-0368

CLARK, Rufus Wheelwright (1813-1886)
A discourse delivered before the Boston Society for the Prevention of Pauperism, on its nineteenth anniversary, Jan. 8, 1854. Boston: J. Wilson & Son, 1854. 23p. DNLM; MB: MH; MWA **50-0369**

CLARKE, Edward Hammond (1820-1877)
The relation of drugs to treatment. An introductory lecture before the medical class of 1856-1857 of Harvard University. Boston: D. Clapp, 1856. 28p. DNLM; MH-M
50-0370

CLEAVELAND, Charles Harley (1820-1863)
Galvanism; its application as a remedial agent. New York: S. W. Benedict, 1853. 96p. DNLM; NNNAM
50-0371

CLEAVELAND, Charles Harley (1820-1863)
Are the mercurials anti-syphilitics? Cincinnati, 1857. 30p. DNLM **50-0372**

CLEAVELAND, Charles Harley (1820-1863)
Imponderables. A lecture to the students of the Eclectic College of Medicine. Cincinnati, 1857. 8p. DNLM
50-0373

CLEVELAND, Emeline H. (1829-1878)
Introductory lecture to the class of the Female Medical College of Pennsylvania for the session of 1858-1859. Philadelphia: Merrihew & Thompson, 1858. 16p. DNLM; PPC
50-0374

CLIFTON SPRINGS water-cure. Report of the addresses and sermon at the dedication, July 25, 1856. Geneva & Canadaigua: National New York Press, 1857. 16p. DNLM
50-0375

COALE, William Edward (1816-1865)
A treatise on the causes, constitutional effects and treatment of uterine displacements. Boston: D. Clapp, 1852. 52p. DNLM; MH-M **50-0376**

COALE, William Edward (1816-1865)
Hints on health, with familiar instructions for the treatment and preservation of the skin, hair, teeth, eyes. . . . Boston: Phillips, Sampson, 1852. 207p. MB; MH-M
50-0377

COATES, Benjamin Hornor (1797-1881)
Biographical notice of Charles Caldwell. Read before the American Philosophical Society. Philadelphia: T. K. & P. G. Collins, 1855. 31p. DNLM; PPAmP; PPL; PPC
50-0378

COCK, Thomas (1782-1869)
Inaugural address, delivered before the New York Academy of Medicine, April 7th, 1852. . . . To which is added the annual report of 1851, for the recording secretary, John G. Adams. . . . New York: Printed for the Academy by R. Craighead, 1852. 30p. DLC; DNLM; NNNAM **50-0379**

COCK, Thomas Ferris (1819-1896)
A manual of obstetrics. . . . New York: S. S. & W. Wood, 1853. 250p. DLC; DNLM; NNC; NNNAM **50-0380**

COCK, Thomas Ferris (1819-1896)
Cases in midwifery, with remarks. . . . New York: S. S. & W. Wood, 1855. 40p. DLC; NNNAM; PPC; PU
50-0381

COCKBURN, Samuel
Medical reform: being an examination into the nature of the prevailing system of medicine; and an exposition of some of its chief evils, with allopathic revelations. A remedy for the evil. 1st American edition. Philadelphia: Rademacher & Sheek, 1857. 180p. DNLM; PPHa **50-0382**

COCKE, William I.
The theory and practice of medicine. New York: Holman, Gray & Co., 1853. 366p. DNLM; NNNAM; OCIM
50-0383

COE, Grover (1825-1860)
Concentrated organic medicines: being a practical exposition of the therapeutic properties and clinical employment of the combined proximate medicinal constituents of indigenous and foreign plants. . . . New York: B. Keith & Co., 1858. 432p. DLC; MBM; MWA; NNNAM **50-0384**

COFFIN, Amory
Anniversary oration delivered before the South Carolina Medical Association at the annual meeting in Charleston, held on 31st January, 1853. Charleston, S.C.: Walker & James, 1853. 15p. DNLM; ScMS **50-0385**

COLES, L. B.
Philosophy of health. . . . Revised and enlarged. Boston: Brown, Taggard & Chase, 1857. 312p. MH-M
50-0386

COLES, L. B.
The beauties and deformities of tobacco using or its ludicrous and its solemn realities. Boston: Brown, Taggard & Chase, 1857. 312p. MH-M **50-0387**

COLGAN, Joseph P.
Diseases of the ear. An essay on the present state of aural medicine and surgery. Read before the Medico-Chirurgical Society, August 24, 1857. Brooklyn, W. H. Hogan, 1858. 49p. DNLM; NNU-M **50-0388**

COLLINS, John D.
Valedictory address to the graduating class of the Eclectic Medical Institute, May 19, 1855. Cincinnati: Ben Franklin Steam Printing House, 1855. 16p. DNLM
50-0389

COLOMBAT, Marc (1797-1851)
A treatise on the diseases and special hygiene of females. . . . Transl. from the French, with additions, by Charles D. Meigs. . . . A new ed., rev. Philadelphia: Lea & Blanchard, 1850. 720p. DLC; PPC; PPJ; PU **50-0390**

COLOMBAT, Marc (1797-1851)
A treatise upon diseases and hygiene of the organs of the voice. Transl. by J. F. W. Lane, M.D. 2nd ed. Boston: Redding & Co., 1857. 220p. 1 plate. DLC; MBM; NNNAM; PPC
50-0391

COMBE, Andrew (1797-1847)
A treatise on the physiological and moral management of infancy. For the use of parents. With notes and a supplementary chapter by John Bell. 6th ed. New York: Fowlers & Wells, 1853. 307p. DNLM; NNNAM
50-0392

COMBE, George (1788-1858)
Essay on the constitution of man, and its relations to external objects. With an additional chapter on the harmony between phrenology and revelation by Joseph A. Warne. 20th ed. New York: Fowlers & Wells, 1852. 436p. DNLM; NNNAM
50-0393

COMBE, George (1788-1858)
The constitution of man considered in relation to external objects. Philadelphia: Leary & Getz, 1854. 371p. PPL; PU
50-0394

COMFORT, John W.
Practice of medicine on Thomsonian principles . . . and a materia medica adapted to the work. Philadelphia: A. Comfort, 1850. 578p. NNNAM; MH-M; OCIM **50-0395**

CONDIE, David Francis (1796-1875)
A practical treatise on the diseases of children. . . . 4th ed., rev. and augm. Philadelphia: Blanchard & Lea, 1853. 732p. DLC; PPC; PU; ViRA **50-0396**

CONDIE, David Francis (1796-1875)
Address delivered before the Philadelphia County Medical Society. Philadelphia: T. K. & P. G. Collins, 1856. 20p. DNLM; PPC; PU **50-0397**

CONDIE, David Francis (1796-1875)
A practical treatise on the diseases of children. 5th ed., rev. and enlarged. Philadelphia: Blanchard & Lea, 1858. 762p. DNLM; PPC; PU; ViRA **50-0398**

CONE, Edmund
A synopsis of the treatment of fever and febrile diseases, indigestion, neuralgia and tubercular diseases: with remarks on the effects of blood-letting, emetics, purgatives, mercury, diet, etc. in diseases. . . . Columbus: Printed by Follett, Foster & Company, 1858. 71p. DLC; OCIM **50-0399**

CONKLING, Frederick Augustus (1816-1891)
Remarks on the bill for the promotion of medical science. Albany. Weed Parsons & Company, 1854. 13p. DNLM
50-0400

COOK, William H[enry] (1832-1899)
The questions of life and death; a review of allopathy and defense of physico-medicalism. Cincinnati: Cook & Gallinger, [1857?]. 28p. DNLM **50-0401**

COOK, William H[enry] (1832-1899)
A treatise on the principles and practice of physio-medical surgery. Cincinnati: Moore, Wilstach, Keys & Co., 1858. 714p. 133 figs. DNLM; OCIM **50-0402**

COOKE, George
Professional experience in various climates: a complete practical treatise on genital maladies; with pathological observations on the philosophy of reproduction . . . together with the more successful management of diseases of women and children, as adopted at the present day. 2nd ed. . . . Albany, N.Y.: The author, 1852. 312p. DLC; MBM; NNNAM
50-0403

COOPER, Bransby Blake (1792-1853)
Lectures on the principles and practice of surgery. . . . Philadelphia: Blanchard & Lea, 1852. 771p. DLC: DNLM; NNNAM; PPC **50-0404**

COOPER, Elisha Samuel (1822-1862)
Report of an operation for removing a foreign body from beneath the heart. Published by the San Francisco County Medico-Chirurgical Association as an additional paper to its transactions for the year 1857. San Francisco: Whilton, Towne & Co., 1857. 8p. DNLM **50-0405**

CORNELL, William Mason (1802-1895)
Consumption curable, and its treatment. Boston: W. Crosby & H. P. Nichols, 1850. 101p. DNLM; MBM; NNNAM
50-0406

CORNELL, William Mason (1802-1895)
Practical observations on the inhalation of various vapors and powders in diseases of the air tubes and lungs. Boston: D. Clapp, 1850. 22p. DNLM; MH-M **50-0407**

CORNELL, William Mason (1802-1895)
An introductory lecture delivered to the class of the Female Medical College. Philadelphia: G. S. Harris, 1852. 16p. DNLM; PPC; PU **50-0408**

CORNELL, William Mason (1802-1895)
Observations on epilepsy, its pathology and treatment. Boston: Fetridge & Co., 1854. 44p. DNLM; MH-M
50-0409

CORNELL, William Mason (1802-1895)
The ship and shore physician and surgeon. Boston: C. Stone, 1858. 88p. DNLM; MH-M **50-0410**

CORSON, John W. (1816-1882)
Functional and sympathetic affections of the heart: a paper read before the Society of Statistical Medicine.... New York: Holman, Gray & Co., 1854. 31p. DLC; DNLM; NNNAM **50-0411**

CORSON, John W. (1816-1882)
A paper on protracted valvular disease of the heart. New York: Holman & Gray, 1855. 29p. DNLM; NNNAM **50-0412**

CORSON, John W. (1816-1882)
A paper on the effects of lead on the heart. [New York]: Miller & Holman, 1856. 24p. DNLM; NNNAM **50-0413**

CORSON, John W. (1816-1882)
A paper on the management of the shoulders in examinations of the chest, including a new physical sign. New York: H. Bailliere, 1859. 32p. DNLM; NNNAM **50-0414**

COTTING, Benjamin Eddy (1812-1897)
Nature in disease. An address. Boston: D. Clapp, 1852. 12p. DNLM; MH-M **50-0415**

COTTING, Benjamin Eddy (1812-1897)
An obituary notice of the late Timothy Wellington, of West Cambridge. Boston: J. Wilson & Son, 1853. 6p. DNLM; MH-M **50-0416**

COTTING, Benjamin Eddy (1812-1897)
Statistics of consumption in Roxbury . . . with an appendix. Boston: D. Clapp, 1854. 24p. DNLM; MH-M **50-0417**

COTTING, Benjamin Eddy (1812-1897)
Diphtheritis or the membranous disease, commonly called membranous croup as it appears in Roxbury and the vicinity of Boston. . . . Boston: D. Clapp, 1859. 19p. DLC; DNLM; MH-M **50-0418**

COVENTRY, Charles B. (1801-1875)
Medicine a science and an art. A lecture introductory to the course in the medical institution of Geneva College. Geneva: I. & S. H. Parker, 1850. 24p. DNLM **50-0419**

COVENTRY, Charles B. (1801-1875)
Report on the medical jurisprudence of insanity. Philadelphia: Collins, 1858. 56p. DNLM; PPC; PU **50-0420**

COVENTRY, Charles B. (1801-1875)
Nature and art in the cure of disease. Utica: Roberts, 1859. 22p. DNLM; NNNAM **50-0421**

COX, Abraham L[idden] (1800-1864)
An address, delivered on the first public exhibition of the edifice of the New York Medical College, and the inauguration of its faculty, October 16, 1850. . . . New York: J. F. Trow, printer, 1850. 28p. DLC; DNLM; NNNAM **50-0422**

COX, Abraham L[idden] (1800-1864)
Practical remarks on enlarged tonsils, with a new apparatus for their removal. [New York, 1853?] 8p. DNLM **50-0423**

COX, Henry G[eorge] (1818-1866)
Placenta praevia. . . . New York: Baker, Godwin & Co., 1854. 13p. DLC; NNNAM **50-0424**

COXE, Edward Jenner (1801-1862)
Remarks on cholera, more especially in reference to the treatment proper for its different stages. [New Orleans, 1850.] 16p. DNLM; LNT-M **50-0425**

COXE, Edward Jenner (1801-1862)
A practical treatise on medical inhalation; or, the direct and local application of remedies to the air passages. With cases. . . . 3rd ed. Philadelphia: G. T. Stockdale, 1854. 115p. DNLM; PPC; PU **50-0426**

COXE, Edward Jenner (1801-1862)
Practical remarks on yellow fever, having special reference to the treatment. New Orleans: J. C. Morgan, 1859. 108p. DNLM; LNT-M **50-0427**

COXE, John Redman, Jr. (1799-1863)
Introductory lecture to the class of the Homoeopathic Medical College of Pennsylvania. Delivered October 14, 1858. Published by the class. Philadelphia: J. E. Potter, 1858. 19p. DNLM; PPHa **50-0428**

COXE, John Redman, Jr. (1799-1863)
Valedictory address delivered at the eleventh annual commencement of the Homoeopathic Medical College of Pennsylvania, March 3, 1859. Philadelphia: King & Baird, 1859. 18p. DNLM; PPHa **50-0429**

CRAGIN, John (1812-1877)
Homoeopathy explained; or, the old and new systems of medicine compared. Mobile, Ala.: Forsyth & Harris, 1855. 28p. PPHa **50-0430**

CRAIGIE, David (1793-1866)
Elements of general and pathological anatomy, presenting a view of the present state of knowledge in these branches of science. . . . 2nd ed., enl., rev., and improved. Philadelphia: Lindsay & Blakiston, 1851. 1072p. DLC; DNLM; PPC; PU **50-0431**

CRAWFORD, S. P.
The physician and his profession. An address to the graduating class of the medical department of the University of Nashville. Nashville: Cameron & Fall, 1858. 18p. DNLM **50-0432**

CRENSHAW, E. A.
An essay on animal magnetism, or mesmerism. Yorkville, S.C.: Chronicle Office, 1857. 15p. DNLM; ScMS **50-0433**

CRENSHAW, E. A.
A short account of the motive-power of man together with the symptoms and treatment of disease. Yorkville, S.C.: Chronicle Office, 1857. 8p. DNLM; ScMS **50-0434**

CROPPER, Charles
Cholera and its homoeopathic treatment. Cincinnati, O., 1856. 16p. OCIM; PPHa **50-0435**

CROSERIO, Camille (1786-1855)
Homoeopathic manual of obstetrics: or, A treatise on the aid of the art of midwifery may derive from homoeopathy. . . . From the French, by M. Coté. Cincinnati: Moore, Anderson, Wilstach & Keys, 1853. 153p. DLC; DNLM; OCIM; PU
50-0436

CULVER, C[harles] P[ost]
A guide to mothers and nurses in directing first & second dentition, with hints to the adult for the preservation of their teeth. . . . Louisville: Hull & Brother, printers, 1855. 62p. DLC; OCIM **50-0437**

CULVERWELL, Robert James (1802-1852)
Guide to health and long life; or What to eat, drink, and avoid; what exercise to take, how to control and regulate the passions and appetites; and on the general conduct of life, whereby health may be secured, and a happy and comfortable old age attained. . . . To which is added, a popular exposition of Liebig's theory of life, health, and disease. . . . New York: J. S. Redfield, 1850. 71p. DLC; DNLM; NNNAM
50-0438

CURRY, James H[art] (1827?-1900)
A valedictory address delivered to the graduating class of the medical institution of Yale College. Boton: D. Clapp, 1852. 12p. CtY-M; DNLM; MBM **50-0439**

CURTIS, Alva (1797-1881)
A fair exposition of allopathy; or the pathological system of medicine, with its kindred systems and branches. Cincinnati: Campbell & Miller, 1850. 48p. DNLM; OCIM **50-0440**

CURTIS, Alva (1797-1881)
A fair examination and criticism of all the medical systems in vogue; . . . Cincinnati: Printed for the proprietor, 1855. 208p. DLC; DNLM; OCIM **50-0441**

CURTIS, Joseph Thomas
The relations of homoeopathy to chemistry; an inaugural address, delivered before the Hahnemann Academy of Medicine, January 14, 1852. Published by order of the Academy. New York: Angell, Engel & Hewitt, 1852. 20p. DNLM; PPHa **50-0442**

CUTTER, Calvin (1807-1872)
A treatise on anatomy, physiology, and hygiene. . . . With one hundred and fifty engravings. Stereotype ed. Boston: B. B. Mussey & Co.; New York: Clark, Austin & Co.; [etc., etc.], 1850. 458p. DLC; DNLM; NN **50-0443**

CUTTER, Calvin (1807-1872)
First book on anatomy, physiology, and hygiene . . . with eighty-three engravings. . . . Stereotype ed. Boston: B. B. Mussey & Co.; New York: Clark & Austin [etc., etc.], 1850. 180p. DLC; ICU; NN; OC **50-0444**

CUTTER, Calvin (1807-1872)
First book on anatomy, physiology, and hygiene, for grammar schools and families. With eighty-three engravings. . . . Rev. stereotype ed. Boston: B. B. Mussey & Co.; New York: Clark & Austin [etc., etc.], 1852. 191p. AU; DLC; MA; MB
50-0445

CUTTER, Calvin (1807-1872)
A treatise on anatomy, physiology, and hygiene. . . . With one hundred and fifty engravings. Rev. stereotype ed. Boston: B. B. Mussey & Co.; New York: Clark, Austin, & Co. [etc., etc.], 1854. 466p. DLC; MH; NN; PU **50-0446**

CUTTER, Calvin (1807-1872)
First book on anatomy, physiology, and hygiene. For grammar schools and families. With eighty-three engravings. . . . Rev. stereotype ed. Philadelphia: J. B. Lippincott & Co. [1854]. 191p. DLC; GU; MB; NN **50-0447**

DA COSTA, Jacob Mendez (1833-1900)
An inquiry into the pathological anatomy of acute pneumonia. Philadelphia: T. K. & P. G. Collins, 1855. 19p. 1 plate. DNLM; PPC; PU **50-0448**

DA COSTA, Jacob Mendez (1833-1900)
The physicians of the last century. A lecture introductory to the course at the Philadelphia Association for Medical Instruction. Philadelphia: H. D. Ashmead, 1857. 32p. DNLM; PPC; PU **50-0449**

DA COSTA, Jacob Mendez (1833-1900)
Cancer of the pancreas. [Philadelphia, 1858.] 27p. DNLM; PPC **50-0450**

DA COSTA, Jacob Mendez (1833-1900)
On the morbid anatomy and symptoms of cancer of the pancreas. Philadelphia: J. B. Lippincott & Co., 1858. 29p. DNLM; PPC; PU **50-0451**

DAKE, C. M. (1816-1872)
Popular exposé and defense of medicine. An address, at the first session of the Livingston County Homoeopathic Med. Society. [Geneseo, N.Y., 1857.] 12p. DNLM
50-0452

DAKE, Jabez Philander (1827-1894)
The sources of the materia medica. An introductory lecture to the class of the Homoeopathic Medical College of Pennsylvania, delivered October 10, 1855. Philadelphia: O. P. Glessner, 1855. 18p. DNLM; PPHa **50-0453**

DAKE, Jabez Philander (1827-1894)
Valedictory address delivered at the ninth annual commencement of the Homoeopathic Medical College of Pennsylvania, February 27, 1857. Philadelphia: King & Baird, 1857. 16p. DNLM; PPHa **50-0454**

DAKE, Jabez Philander (1827-1894)
Acute diseases, and their homoeopathic treatment. Also, directions for the treatment of injuries received by accidents and from poisons. . . . Pittsburgh: J. G. Backofen & Son [1859]. 77p. DLC; DNLM; PPHa **50-0455**

DALTON, John Call (1825-1889)
. . . On the corpus luteum of menstruation and pregnancy. . . . Philadelphia: T. K. & P. G. Collins, printers, 1851. 100p. DLC; DNLM; PPC; PU **50-0456**

DALTON, John Call (1825-1889)
Introductory address, delivered at the College of Physicians and Surgeons, New York, October 16, 1855. . . . New York: J. J. Schroeder, 1855. 29p. DLC; DNLM; NNC; NNNAM
50-0457

DALTON, John Call (1825-1889)
On the constitution and physiology of the bile. [Philadelphia, 1857.] 20p. DNLM; NNNAM **50-0458**

DALTON, John Call (1825-1889)
Anatomy of the placenta. [New York, 1858.] 14p. DNLM; NNNAM **50-0459**

DALTON, John Call (1825-1889)
A treatise on human physiology. . . . Philadelphia: Blanchard & Lea, 1859. 608p. DLC; DNLM; NNNAM; PPC
50-0460

DALTON, S. W.
Letters of Cenci, written four years ago, on the sanitary reforms needed in New Orleans, and republished by order of the city council. New Orleans: I. T. Hinton, 1853. 27p. DNLM; LNT-M **50-0461**

DANIELS, E.
A synoptical view of the mechanical relations of muscles of the lower limbs, with an application of the mechanical principles deducible therefrom to the treatment of fractures of those bones; and an account of a new apparatus. Binghamton: Republican Office, 1856. 20p. 1 plate. DNLM
50-0462

DARBY, John Thompson (1836-1879)
Anatomy, physiology, and pathology of the supra-renal capsules. Presented as a thesis for graduation at the University of Pennsylvania. Charleston, S.C.: James & Williams, 1859. 18p. DNLM; PU **50-0463**

DARLINGTON, William (1782-1863)
Address to the Chester County Medical Society. Westchester, Pa.: Reg. & Exam. Office, 1852. 9p. DNLM **50-0464**

DARRACH, William (1796-1865)
Charge to the graduates of the Medical Department of Pennsylvania College, at the public commencement, March 6th, 1851. . . . Published by order of the faculty. Philadelphia: Printed by King & Baird [1851]. 20p. DLC; DNLM; PPC; PU
50-0465

DARRACH, William (1796-1865) and John WILTBANK
Reply to a pamphlet entitled "A statement of the facts connected with the late re-organization of the faculty of the medical department of Pennsylvania College, together with a documentary history of said department, from its origin to the present time." Philadelphia: King & Baird, 1855. 68p. DNLM; PPC; PU **50-0466**

DAVIS, Daniel
A manual of magnetism, including galvanism, magnetism, electro-magnetism, magneto-electricity, electro-dynamics, and thermo-electricity. 4th ed. Boston: D. Davis, Jr., 1852. 322p. DNLM; MB; MH **50-0467**

DAVIS, Henry Gassett (1807-1896)
Special exercises in the treatment of diseases of the lungs. New York: Hall, Clayton & Co., 1858. 12p. DNLM; NNNAM
50-0468

DAVIS, Henry Gassett (1807-1896)
On the effect of pressure upon ulcerated vertebrae, and in morbus coxarius, and the relief afford by mechanical remedies, with cases. . . . New York: T. Holman, printer, 1859. 8p. DLC; DNLM; NNNAM **50-0469**

DAVIS, Nathan Smith (1817-1904)
History of medical education and institutions in the United States, from the first settlement of the British colonies to the year 1850; with a chapter on the present condition and wants of the profession, and the means necessary for supplying those wants, and elevating the character and extending the usefulness of the whole profession. . . . Chicago: S. C. Griggs & Co., 1851. 228p. DLC; DNLM; ICRM; PPC **50-0470**

DAVIS, N[athan] S[mith] (1817-1904)
Address to the Mechanics' Institute, at the close of the fourth annual fair, October 13, 1851. . . . With the reports of the committees of examination, and the awards by the Board of Directors. Chicago: Whitmarsh & Fulton, printers, 1851. 20p. DLC; ICRM; IUM **50-0471**

DAVIS, Nathan Smith (1817-1904)
A lecture on the effects of alcoholic drinks on the human system, and the duties of medical men in relation thereto. Delivered in the lecture room of Rush Medical College, on Christmas day, 1854, in compliance with the request of the class attending the college. . . . Chicago: J. F. Ballantyne, book and job printer [1855]. 31p. DLC; ICRM
50-0472

DAVIS, Nathan Smith (1817-1904)
History of the American Medical Association from its organization up to January, 1855 . . . to which is appended biographical notices. . . . Ed. by S. W. Butler, M.D. Philadelphia: Lippincott, Grambo & Co., 1855. 191p. DLC; DNLM; NNNAM; PPC
50-0473

DAVIS, Nathan Smith (1817-1904)
Report on the changes in the composition and properties of the milk of the human female, produced by menstruation and pregnancy. Philadelphia: T. K. & P. G. Collins, 1856. 13p. DNLM; PPC **50-0474**

DAVIS, Nathan Smith (1817-1904)
Inaugural address delivered at the opening of the medical department of Lind University. Chicago: W. Cravens & Co., 1859. 26p. DNLM; IU-M **50-0475**

DAVIS, Phebe B.
Two years and three months in the New York Lunatic Asylum at Utica; together with the outlines of twenty years' peregrinations in Syracuse. Syracuse: The author, 1855. 87p. DNLM; NN; NNC **50-0476**

DAVIS, R.
Cox's companion to the sea medicine chest, and compendium of domestic medicine. . . . 1st American from the 33rd London ed. New York: S. S. & Wm. Wood, 1851. 216p. DNLM; NNNAM **50-0477**

DAYTON, A. B[ailey] (1812-1870)
A brief history of the past and present relations of the Medical Society of New Jersey to the State; more especially as regards legislative enactments. Burlington, 1855. 17p. DNLM; NjR
50-0478

DEAN, Amos (1803-1868)
Principles of medical jurisprudence: designed for the professions of law and medicine. . . . Albany: Gould, Banks & Gould; New York: Banks, Gould & Co., 1850. 664p. DLC; NN; NNC; NNNAM **50-0479**

DEANE, James (1801-1858)
On the hygienic condition of the survivors of ovariotomy. Boston: J. Wilson & Son, 1855. 11p. DNLM; MH-M
50-0480

[DEE, Dr.]
The family medical scrap book. Dayton, O.: Ellis, Marguis, 1855. 160p. OCIM **50-0481**

DELAFIELD, Edward (1794-1875)
Biographical sketch of J. Kearny Rodgers. . . . Read before the New York Academy of Medicine on Wednesday, October 6th, 1852, and published under its authority. New York: G. A. C. Van Beuren, printer, 1852. 28p. DLC; DNLM; NNNAM
50-0482

DELAFIELD, Edward (1794-1875)
An address at the dedication of the new building of the New York Eye Infirmary, April 25, 1856. New York: G. A. C. Van Beuren, 1856. 47p. DNLM; NNNAM
50-0483

DELAMATER, Jacob J.
Introductory address delivered at the opening of the session of the Cleveland Medical College. Cleveland: Harris, Fairbanks & Co., 1850. 32p. DNLM; OCIM **50-0484**

DEVOTION, John L.
Observations on bilious diseases, comp. from the works of the ablest members of the medical profession, with remarks on the extraordinary virtues of Devotion's lexipyreta, in the treatment and cure of fever and ague. . . . New York, 1852. 16p. DLC; NNNAM **50-0485**

DEWEES, H. P[hillips] (1810-1879)
Rheumatism of the epithelial and non-epithelial fibrous tissues; its sequence to scarlatina and other exanthemata. On rheumatic gout, chorea. . . . New York: E. P. Allen, 1857. 32p. DNLM; NNNAM **50-0486**

DEWEES, William Potts (1768-1841)
A compendious system of midwifery, chiefly designed to facilitate the inquiries of those who may be pursuing this branch of study. . . . Philadelphia [1852]. 562p. DLC; NNNAM; PPC; ViRA **50-0487**

DEWEES, William Potts (1768-1841)
A treatise on the physical and medical treatment of children. . . . 10th ed., with the author's last improvements and corrections. Philadelphia: Blanchard & Lea, 1853. 481p. DLC; PPC; PPJ; PU **50-0488**

DEWEES, William Potts (1768-1841)
A treatise on the physical and medical treatment of children. . . . 11th ed., with the author's last improvements and corrections. Philadelphia: Blanchard & Lea, 1858. 281p. CU-M; DLC; ICRM; PPC **50-0489**

DICKSON, Samuel (1802-1869)
The principles of the chronothermal system of medicine . . . , containing also an introduction and notes by William Turner. 14th ed. New York: Long & Bros., 1850. 224p. DNLM; NNNAM **50-0490**

DICKSON, Samuel (1802-1869)
The principles of the chronothermal system of medicine . . . , containing also an introduction and notes by William Turner. 15th ed. New York: J. S. Redfield, 1852. 224p. DNLM; NNNAM **50-0491**

DICKSON, Samuel (1802-1869)
The "destructive art of healing"; or facts for families. . . . To which is added a word to women by Lydia Jane Pierson. 1st American from the 2nd London ed. New York: S. French [1853]. 72p. DNLM; NNNAM **50-0492**

DICKSON, Samuel Henry (1798-1872)
Lecture introductory to the course on the institutes and practice of medicine in the Medical College of the State of South Carolina. Charleston, S.C.: J. Russell, 1850. 24p. DNLM; ScCM **50-0493**

DICKSON, Samuel Henry (1798-1872)
Manual of pathology and practice of medicine. . . . New York: Jennings & Harrison, printers, 1850. 251p. DLC; MBM; NNNAM; PPC **50-0494**

DICKSON, Samuel Henry (1798-1872)
Essays on life, sleep, pain. . . . Philadelphia: Blanchard & Lea, 1852. 301p. DLC; PPJ; PPC; PU **50-0495**

DICKSON, Samuel Henry (1798-1872)
Medical progress: a lecture introductory to the course on the institutes and practice of medicine. Charleston: Walker & James, 1854. 23p. DNLM; ScCM **50-0496**

DICKSON, Samuel Henry (1798-1872)
Elements of medicine; a compendious view of pathology and therapeutics; or, The history and treatment of diseases. . . . Philadelphia: Blanchard & Lea, 1855. 752p. CtY-M; DLC; NNNAM; PPC **50-0497**

DICKSON, Samuel Henry (1798-1872)
Lecture introductory to the course of institutes and practice of medicine in the Medical College of the State of South Carolina. Charleston: Walker, Evans & Co., 1856. 19p. DNLM; ScCM **50-0498**

DICKSON, Samuel Henry (1798-1872)
Address of Dr. S. H. Dickson, delivered at the inauguration of the public school, fourth of July, 1856. . . . Charleston, S.C.: Walker, Evans & Co., stationers and printers, 1856. 24p. DLC; ScC; ScCM **50-0499**

DICKSON, Samuel Henry (1798-1872)
The late Prof. J. K. Mitchell, M.D. Inaugural lecture to the course on the practice of medicine in the Jefferson Medical College of Philadelphia, delivered October 12, 1858 . . . preceded by preliminary remarks to an introductory lecture to the course on the institutes of medicine, delivered October 11, 1858, by Prof. Robley Dunglison. . . . Published by the class. Philadelphia: J. M. Wilson, 1858. 40p. DLC; PPJ; PPC; PU
50-0500

DICKSON, Samuel Henry (1798-1872)
Elements of medicine: a compendious view of pathology and therapeutics; or the history and treatment of diseases. 2nd ed. Philadelphia: Blanchard & Lea, 1859. 768p. DNLM; MH-M; NNNAM; PPC **50-0501**

DIX, Dorothea Lynde (1802-1887)
Memorial to the honorable the general assembly in behalf of the insane of Maryland [Feb. 25, 1852]. [Annapolis, 1852.] 20p. DNLM **50-0502**

DIXON, Edward H. (1808-1880)
Scenes in the practice of a New York surgeon. . . . With eight illustrations by Darley. . . . New York: DeWitt & Davenport, [1855]. 407p. plates. DLC; NNNAM **50-0503**

DIXON, Edward H. (1808-1880)
A treatise on diseases of the sexual system adapted to popular instruction. . . . 9th ed., with an appendix. New York: O. A. Roorback, Jr., 1855. 285p. DLC; NNNAM
50-0504

DODS, John Bovee (1795-1872)
The philosophy of electrical psychology. In a course of nine lectures. Stereotype ed. New York: Fowlers & Wells, 1850. 168p. NNNAM **50-0505**

DODS, John Bovee (1795-1872)
Spirit manifestations examined and explained. Judge Edmonds refuted: Or, an exposition of the involuntary powers and instincts of the human mind. New York: DeWitt & Davenport, [1854]. 252p. NNNAM **50-0506**

DONNÉ, Alfred (1801-1878)
Mothers and infants, nurses and nursing. Transl. from the French of a treatise on nursing, weaning, and the general treatment of young children. . . . Boston: Phillips, Sampson & Company, 1859. 303p. DLC; MH-M; NNNAM **50-0507**

DOUGHERTY, Alexander N. (1822-1883)
Surgical notes. Newark, N.J.: S. C. Atkinson, 1859. 8p. DNLM; NjR **50-0508**

DOUGLAS, James S. (1801-1878)
Homoeopathic treatment of intermittent fevers. New York: William Radde, 1853. 108p. DNLM; PPHa **50-0509**

DOUGLAS, James S. (1801-1878)
Homoeopathy. A lecture before the faculty and students of Madison University, New York, April, 1845. Published by request. 2nd ed. Milwaukee: Starr's Printers, 1854. 40p. DNLM; PPHa **50-0510**

DOUGLAS, James S. (1801-1878)
Practical homoeopathy for the people; adapted to the comprehension of the non-professional and for reference by the young practitioner, including a number of the most valuable new remedies. 10th ed. Milwaukee: Douglas & Perrine, [1858?]. 132p. DNLM **50-0511**

DOWLER, Bennet (1797-1879)
Researches upon the necropolis of New Orleans, with brief allusions to its vital arithmetic. . . . New Orleans: Printed by Bills & Clark, 1850. 30p. DLC; LNT-M **50-0512**

DOWLER, Bennet (1797-1879)
Researches on the natural history of a death. New Orleans, 1850. 22p. DNLM; LNT-M **50-0513**

DOWLER, Bennet (1797-1879)
Review of Dr. Drake's work on the principal diseases of the interior valley of North America. New Orleans: W. A. Bills, 1850. 16p. DNLM; LNT-M **50-0514**

DOWLER, Bennet (1797-1879)
Experimental researches, illustrative of the functional oneness, unity, and diffusion, of nervous action; in opposition to the anatomical assumption, of four sets of nerves, and a fourfold set of functions, and transmitted impressions; with a brief exposition of the philosophy of vivisection, and of sensation. . . . New Orleans: Printed by J. Cohn [1851]. 34p. DLC; LNT-M **50-0515**

DOWLER, Bennet (1797-1879)
Contributions to experimental physiology, showing that the ligation of the trachea, the divisions of the spinal cord in the cervical and dorsal regions . . . do not prevent intelligence, sensation, and motions which are accurate in design, perfect in execution, being simultaneous and altogether, voluntary in all parts of the body, even though connected only by the muscles; also experiments on the roots of the spinal cord. . . . New Orleans: Printed by J. Cohn, 1852. 19p. DLC; LNT-M **50-0516**

DOWLER, Bennet (1797-1879)
Tableau of the yellow fever of 1853, with topographical, chronological, and historical sketches of the epidemics of New Orleans since their origin in 1796, illustrative of the quarantine question. . . . New Orleans: Printed at the office of the Picayune, 1854. 65p. DLC; LNT-M **50-0517**

DOWLER, Bennet (1797-1879)
Progress of discovery in the nervous system and in medical ethics. (From the New Orleans Medical and Surgical Journal, March, 1856.) [New Orleans, 1856]. 4p. DLC; LNT-M **50-0518**

DOWLER, Bennet (1797-1879)
Contributions to the pathological anatomy of the large intestine, including pathological remarks, followed by a translation from the French, on the faecal retention. . . . [New Orleans, 1858?] 43-60p. DLC; LNT-M **50-0519**

DRAKE, Daniel (1785-1852)
A systematic treatise, historical, etiological and practical, on the principal diseases of the interior valley of North America, as they appear in the Caucasian, African, Indian, and Esquimaux varieties of its population. . . . Cincinnati: W. B. Smith & Co.; New York: Mason & Law, 1850. 878p. tables, maps. DLC; MH-M; NNNAM; PPC **50-0520**

DRAKE, Daniel (1785-1852)
Discourses delivered by appointment, before the Cincinnati Medical Library Association, January 9th and 10th, 1852. . . . Cincinnati: Pub. for the Association, by Moore & Anderson, 1852. 93p. DLC; NNNAM; OCIM; PPC **50-0521**

DRAKE, Daniel (1785-1852)
A systematic treatise, historical, etiological, and practical, on the principal diseases of the interior valley of North America, as they appear in the Caucasian, African, Indian, and Esquimaux varieties of its population. . . . Ed. by S. Hansbury Smith . . . and Francis G. Smith. . . . 2nd ser. Philadelphia: Lippincott, Grambo & Co., 1854. 985p. tables. DLC; OCIM; NNNAM; PPC **50-0522**

DRAKE'S patent artificial legs, hands, arms. . . . Boston [1859]. 48p. DNLM **50-0523**

DRAPER, John William (1811-1882)
The influence of physical agents on life: being an introductory lecture. New York: J. A. Gray, 1850. 14p. DNLM; NNNAM **50-0524**

[DRAPER, John William] (1811-1882)
Petition of the medical faculty of the University of the City of New York, to . . . the Senate and Assembly of New York, for the legalization of anatomy. Also, an introductory lecture, delivered at the opening of the medical department of the University, for session 1853-1854, entitled An appeal to the people of the state, to legalize the dissection of the dead. . . . New York: The Faculty, 1853. 12p. NN; NNNAM
50-0524A

DRAPER, John William (1811-1882)
Human physiology, statistical and dynamical; or, the conditions and course of the life of man. New York: Harper & Brothers, 1856. 649p. DNLM; MBM; NNNAM; PPC
50-0525

DRUITT, Robert (1814-1883)
The principles and practice of modern surgery. New American from the last and improved London ed., edited by F. W. Sargent. Philadelphia: Blanchard & Lea, 1852. 576p. DNLM; PPJ; PPC; PU **50-0526**

DU BOUCHET, Charles A.
The family dentist; including the surgical, medical, and mechanical treatment of the teeth.... Philadelphia: Lippincott, Grambo & Co., 1850. 167p. DLC; MdU-D; PPC; PU **50-0527**

DUGAS, Louis Alexander (1806-1884)
A case of urinary calculus, attended with peculiar circumstances, and treated by lithotrity. [Augusta, 1851.] 8p. DNLM; GU **50-0528**

DUGAS, Louis Alexander (1806-1884)
Report on a new principle of diagnosis in dislocations of the shoulder-joint. Philadelphia: T. K. & P. G. Collins, 1857. 7p. DNLM; PPC **50-0529**

DUGAS, Louis Alexander (1806-1884)
Remarks upon fractures of the scapula, with cases presenting striking peculiarities; read before the Medical Society of the State of Georgia, at their annual meeting in Augusta, April 8, 1857. Augusta, Ga.: J. Morris, 1857. 22p. DNLM; GU
50-0530

DUNGLISON, Richard J[ames] (1834-1901)
Observations on the deaf and dumb. Philadelphia: J. B. Lippincott & Co., 1858. 31p. DNLM; PPC; PPF; PPL
50-0531

DUNGLISON, Robley (1798-1869)
New remedies: with formulae for their administration.... 6th ed., with extensive additions. . . . Philadelphia: Blanchard & Lea, 1851. 755p. DLC; DNLM; OCIM; PPC **50-0532**

DUNGLISON, Robley (1798-1869)
Medical lexicon. A dictionary of medical science. . . . 8th ed., rev. and greatly enl. Philadelphia: Blanchard & Lea, 1851. 927p. DLC; NNNAM; OCIM; PPC **50-0533**

DUNGLISON, Robley (1798-1869)
Medical lexicon. A dictionary of medical science. . . . 9th ed., rev. and greatly enlarged. Philadelphia: Blanchard & Lea, 1852. 927p. MBM; NNNAM; PPC; ViRA **50-0534**

DUNGLISON, Robley (1798-1869)
Medical lexicon. A dictionary of medical science. . . . 10th ed., rev. and greatly enlarged. Philadelphia: Blanchard & Lea, 1853. 927p. LNT-M; NNNAM; OCIM; PPC **50-0535**

DUNGLISON, Robley (1798-1869)
Medical lexicon. A dictionary of medical science. . . . 11th ed., rev. Philadelphia: Blanchard & Lea, 1854. 927p. DLC; DNLM; PPJ; PPC **50-0536**

DUNGLISON, Robley (1798-1869)
Medical lexicon. A dictionary of medical science. . . . [12th ed.] Philadelphia: Blanchard & Lea, 1854. 927p. DNLM; NNNAM; OCIM; PPC **50-0537**

DUNGLISON, Robley (1798-1869)
Clinical report on Robert Bates's cure for stammering. (Reported by J. Aitken Meigs.) [With report of the committee on science and the arts of the Franklin Institute of the State of Pennsylvania on Robert Bates's instruments for the cure of stammering.] [Philadelphia, 1854.] 8p. DNLM; PPC
50-0538

DUNGLISON, Robley (1798-1869)
On the blind, and institutions for the blind, in Europe. A letter to the president of the board of managers of the Pennsylvania Institution for the Instruction of the Blind. . . . Printed by order of the board of managers. Philadelphia: J. C. Clark & Son, printers, 1854. 24p. DLC; PP; PPC; PPL
50-0539

DUNGLISON, Robley (1798-1869)
Charge to the graduates of Jefferson Medical College of Philadelphia, delivered March 11, 1854. Philadelphia: T. K. & P. G. Collins, 1854. 20p. DNLM; PPC; PPJ
50-0540

DUNGLISON, Robley (1798-1869)
Recollections of Europe in 1854. An introductory lecture. . . . Jefferson Medical College. Philadelphia: T. K. & P. G. Collins, 1854. 28p. DNLM; PPC; PPJ; PU **50-0541**

DUNGLISON, Robley (1798-1869)
Medical lexicon. A dictionary of medical science. . . . [13th ed.] Philadelphia: Blanchard & Lea, 1855. 927p. NNNAM; MBM; OCIM; PPC **50-0542**

DUNGLISON, Robley (1798-1869)
Medical lexicon. A dictionary of medical science. . . . [14th ed.] Rev. and very greatly enlarged. Philadelphia: Blanchard & Lea, 1856. 927p. CU-M; IEN-M; IU-M; PPC
50-0543

DUNGLISON, Robley (1798-1869)
New remedies; the method of preparing and administering them, their effects on the healthy and diseased economy. . . . 7th ed. Philadelphia: Blanchard & Lea, 1856. 769p. DNLM; OCIM; PPJ; PU **50-0544**

DUNGLISON, Robley (1798-1869)
Medical lexicon. A dictionary of medical science. . . . [15th ed.] Rev. and very greatly enl. Philadelphia: Blanchard & Lea, 1857. 992p. DLC; NNNAM; OCIM; PPC
50-0545

DUNGLISON, Robley (1798-1869)
General therapeutics and materia medica. 6th ed. rev. and improved. . . . Adapted for a medical text-book. . . . Philadelphia: Blanchard & Lea, 1857. 2 v. CU-M; DLC; OCIM; PPC
50-0546

DUNGLISON, Robley (1798-1869)
A brief memorial of the late Judge John K. Kane, senior vice-president of the Pennsylvania Institution for the Instruction of the Blind. [Philadelphia, 1858.] 4p. DNLM; PPC
50-0547

DURKEE, Silas
A treatise on gonorrhoea and syphilis. Boston: J. P. Jewett & Co., 1859. 442p. 8 col. plates. DNLM; MH-M
50-0548

DWINELLE, William H.
A treatise on the use of A. J. Watt's crystal gold. Utica: Roberts, 1855. 32p. 1 plate. DNLM **50-0549**

EARL, William
The illustrated silent friend; being a complete guide to health, marriage, and happiness, [etc.]. New York, 1858. 304p. 1 plate **50-0550**

EARLE, Pliny (1809-1892)
European institutions for idiots. [Utica, N.Y.: W. Saunderson, printer, 1852]. 22p. DLC; NNNAM **50-0551**

EARLE, Pliny (1809-1892)
Institutions for the insane, in Prussia, Austria and Germany. . . . Utica: Printed at the New York State Lunatic Asylum, 1853. 29p. DLC; DNLM; NNNAM **50-0552**

EARLE, Pliny (1809-1892)
Institutions for the insane in Prussia, Austria, and Germany. New York: S. S. & W. Wood, 1854. 229, 16p. DNLM; OCIM; NNNAM; PPC **50-0553**

EARLE, Pliny (1809-1892)
An examination of the practice of blood-letting in mental disorders. New York: S. S. & W. Wood, 1854. 126p. DNLM; MBM; NNNAM; PU **50-0554**

EARLE, Pliny (1809-1892)
Medical opinion in the Parish will case. New York: J. F. Trow, 1857. 50p. DNLM; NNNAM **50-0555**

EBERLE, John (1787-1838)
A treatise on the diseases and physical education of children. 4th ed., with notes and large additions by Thomas D. Mitchell. Philadelphia: Lippincott, Grambo & Co., 1850. 768p. DNLM; MBM; NNNAM; PPC **50-0556**

ELDRIDGE, Joseph
A discourse delivered in Norfolk, Conn., at the funeral of Benjamin Welch, M.D. New York: E. O. Jenkins, 1850. 16p. DNLM; NNNAM **50-0557**

ELIOT, Johnson (1815-1883)
A valedictory to the graduating class of the medical department of Georgetown College. Washington: H. Polkinhorn, 1856. 14p. DNLM **50-0558**

ELLIOTT, Ezekiel Brown (1823-1888)
Deductions from Prussian vital statistics. [1856?] 4p. DNLM
50-0559

ELLIOTT, Stephen (1771-1830)
An address, delivered at the opening of the first session of the Savannah Medical College. Savannah: G. N. Nichols, 1853. 16p. DNLM; GU **50-0560**

ELLIS, Benjamin (1798-1831)
. . . The medical formulary: being a collection of prescriptions, derived from the writings and practice of many of the most eminent physicians in America and Europe. Together with the usual dietetic preparations and antidotes for poisons. To which is added an appendix, on the endermic use of medicines, and on the use of ether and chloroform. The whole accompanied with a few brief pharmaceutical and medical observations. . . . 10th ed. rev. [to 1854] and much extended. By Robert P. Thomas. . . . Philadelphia: Blanchard & Lea, 1854. 296p. DLC; DNLM; MBM; PPC **50-0561**

ELY, J. W. C[oleman] (1820-1906)
On fatty degeneration. Annual discourse before Rhode Island Medical Society, 1853. Philadelphia: T. K. & P. G. Collins, 1854. 28p. DNLM; PPC; PU **50-0562**

EMMET, Thomas Addis (1828-1919)
On oedema glottidis resulting from typhus fever. Philadelphia: T. K. & P. G. Collins, 1856. 20p. DNLM; NNNAM; PPC; PPJ
50-0563

EPPS, John (1805-1869)
Domestic homoeopathy; or rules for the domestic treatment of maladies of infants, children, and adults, and for the conduct and the treatment during pregnancy, confinement, and suckling. 5th American, from the 4th London edition. Edited and enlarged by John A. Tarbell, M.D. Boston: D. Clapp, 1853. 382p. MBM; PPHa **50-0564**

ERICHSEN, John Eric (1818-1896)
The science and art of surgery. . . . Ed. by John H. Brinton. . . . Philadelphia: Blanchard & Lea, 1854. 908p. DLC; DNLM; MBM; PPC **50-0565**

ERICHSEN, John Eric (1818-1896)
The science and art of surgery. Being a treatise on surgical injuries, diseases, and operations. . . . An improved American ed. from the 2nd enl. and carefully rev. London ed. Illustrated by four hundred and seventeen engravings on wood. Philadelphia: Blanchard & Lea, 1859. 996p. DLC; DNLM; OCIM; PPC
50-0566

ERNI, Henri
On food, or upon what does man live? Knoxville, Tenn.: Kinsloe & Rice, 1857. 15p. DNLM **50-0567**

ERNI, Henri
Introductory lecture, delivered before the medical class of the University of Vermont, May 12, 1857. Burlington: D. A. Danforth, 1857. 16p. DNLM **50-0568**

ESREY, William P. (1818-1854)
A treatise on anatomy and physiology, with 30 illustrations. Philadelphia: Rademacher & Sheek, 1851. 195p. DNLM; PPHa
50-0569

AN ESSAY on the summer and autumnal fevers of south Alabama, as they appear in Sumter County; to which is appended some remarks on the diagnosis and treatment of typhoid fever. By a member of the Sumter County Medical Society. Mobile: Dade, Thompson & Co., 1853. 60p. DNLM
50-0570

EVANS, John (1824-1897)
The obstetrical extractor. Chicago, 1850. 51p. DNLM; ICRM; IEN-M **50-0571**

EVANS, John (1824-1897)
Address to the graduating class of Rush Medical College, on the nature, utility, and obligations of the medical profession. Chicago: C. A. Swan, 1850. 16p. DNLM; ICRM
50-0572

EVE, Joseph Adams (1805-1886)
A report on diseases of the cervix uteri; read before the Medical Society of the State of Georgia, at the annual meeting in Augusta, April, 1857. . . . Augusta, Ga.: McCafferty's Office —J. Morris, printer, 1857. 42p. DLC; DNLM; GU
50-0573

EVE, Paul Fitzsimmons (1806-1877)
The claims of medicine to be regarded a science. An introductory lecture delivered at the opening of the third session in the Medical Department of the University of Nashville (31st October, 1853). . . . Published by the class. Nashville, Tenn.: Printed at the office of the Nashville Med. Journal, 1853. 32p. DLC; DNLM **50-0574**

EVE, Paul Fitzsimmons (1806-1877)
Treatment of structure of the urethra by rapid and free dilatation. Illustrated with cases. Nashville, Tenn.: J. T. S. Fall, 1853. 15p. DNLM **50-0575**

EVE, Paul Fitzsimmons (1806-1877)
Removal of a nail from the lungs by tracheotomy. Nashville, Tenn.: J. T. S. Fall, 1853. 16p. DNLM
50-0576

EVE, Paul Fitzsimmons (1806-1877)
Professional letters from Europe, written during the summer of 1852. Nashville: J. T. S. Fall, 1854. 45p. DNLM; OCIM
50-0577

EVE, Paul Fitzsimmons (1806-1877)
An address to the graduating class of the medical department of the University of Nashville. Nashville: Cameron & Fall, 1855. 22p. DNLM **50-0578**

EVE, Paul Fitzsimmons (1806-1877)
History of the ligature applied to the brachio-cephalic artery; with statistics of the operation. (Paper read before the Tennessee State Medical Society, May, 1856.). . . . Nashville: Cameron & Fall, book and job printers, 1856. 24p. DLC; DNLM **50-0579**

EVE, Paul Fitzsimmons (1806-1877)
A collection of remarkable cases of surgery. . . . Philadelphia: J. B. Lippincott & Co., 1857. 858p. DLC; NNNAM; PPC; PU
50-0580

EWELL, James (1773-1832)
The medical companion, or family physician, treating of the diseases of the United States, with their symptoms, cause, cure, and means of prevention. . . . 11th ed., greatly enl. and improved . . . with new treatises upon neuralgia, fevers, female complaints, and other diseases common in the United States, to all which is added, with numerous illustrations, a complete American materia medica, and also an account of homoeopathic, hydropathic, and chronothermal treatment. Philadelphia: C. Desilver; Chicago: Keen & Lee, 1856. 720p. col. plates. DLC; DNLM; OCIM; PPC **50-0581**

FAGET, Jean-Charles (1818-1884)
Etudes sur les bases de la science médicale et exposition sommaire de la doctrine traditionnelle. . . . Nouvelle-Orléans: H. Méridier, 1855. 444p. DNLM; LNT-M **50-0582**

FAGET, Jean-Charles (1818-1884)
Etude médicale de quelques questions importantes pour la Louisiane, et exposé succinct d'une endemie paludéenne de forme catarrhale, qui a sévi a la Nouvelle-Orleans, particulièrement sur les enfants, pendant l'épidémie de fièvre jaune de 1858. Nouvelle-Orleans: Imp. Franco-Américaine, 1859. 112p. DNLM; LNT-M **50-0583**

FAGET, Jean-Charles (1818-1884)
Extraits de quelques-unes des lettres sur la fièvre jaune. Nouvelle-Orleans, [1859-1861]. 14, 20, 18, 20, 9p. DNLM; LNT-M **50-0584**

The **FAMILY** and ship medicine chest companion: being a compendium of domestic medicine, surgery, and materia medica. . . . By a practicing physician. Philadelphia: Lindsay & Blakiston, 1851. 416p. DLC; PPC; PU
50-0585

The **FAMILY** guardian. Containing a brief treatise on some of the principal diseases of North America, and suggestions for their treatment and cure. With a biographical sketch of James McClintock, A.M., M.D. New York: Cushman Co., [1855]. 91p. DNLM; NNNAM **50-0586**

The **FAMILY** doctor: a counsellor in sickness, pain and distress, for childhood, manhood and old age. . . . Philadelphia: J. E. Potter, 1857. 308p. DLC; PPC; PU **50-0587**

The **FAMILY** doctor, or, The home book of health and medicine. A popular treatise on the means of avoiding and curing diseases, and of preserving the health and vigor of the body to the latest period. . . . By a physician of Philadelphia: New York: C. M. Saxton, Barker & Co., 1859. 630p. DLC; NNNAM
50-0588

FARRAR, S. C.
Remarks on the medicinal properties of Bailey's Spring, Lauderdale County, Ala., and Cooper's Well, Hinds County, Miss. Jackson: F. C. Jones, 1854. 24p. DNLM
50-0589

FEMALE MEDICAL EDUCATION SOCIETY
Report of the Female Medical Education Society, from November, 1848, to December, 1850; containing the charter, constitution, by-laws, names of officers and members, together with information respecting the Boston Female Medical School and the proposed clinical hospital which is to form a part of the institution, etc. Boston, 1851. 16p. DNLM; MBM
50-0590

FEMALE physicians. [Boston, 1856.] 8p. DNLM; MBM
50-0591

FENNER, Erasmus Darwin (1807-1866)
Southern medical reports; consisting of general and special reports on the medical topography, meterology, and prevalent diseases in the following States: Louisiana, Alabama, Mississippi, North Carolina, South Carolina, Georgia, Florida, Arkansas, Tennessee, Texas, California. 1849-1850. New Orleans: B. M. Norman, D. Davies & Son, 1850-1851. 2 v. DNLM; LNT-M; NcD; NcU **50-0592**

FENNER, Erasmus Darwin (1807-1866)
History of the epidemic yellow fever at New Orleans, La., in 1853. New York: Hall, Clayton & Co., 1854. 84p. DNLM; LNT-M; NNNAM; PU **50-0593**

FENNER, Erasmus Darwin (1807-1866)
On yellow fever of Norfolk and Portsmouth, Va., 1855. New Orleans: Daily Delta Print, 1855. 8p. DNLM; LNT-M
50-0594

FENNER, Erasmus Darwin (1807-1866)
Report on the epidemics of Louisiana, Mississippi, Arkansas, and Texas, for the years 1854-1855, to the American Medical Association. Philadelphia, 1856. 104p. DNLM; PPC; PU
50-0595

FERGUSSON, William (1808-1877)
A system of practical surgery. 4th American edition from the 3rd and enlarged London edition. Philadelphia: Blanchard & Lea, 1853. 621p. DNLM; PPC; PPJ; PU
50-0596

FISHER, J. W.
Memoir of A. Clarkson Smith, M.D. Columbus, Pa.: S. Greene, ptr., 1855. 16p. DNLM **50-0597**

FISKE FUND PRIZE ESSAYS
The effects of climate on tuberculous disease. By Edwin Lee. (Being the dissertation to which the Fiske Fund Prize was awarded June 6, 1855); *Bound with*: The influence of pregnancy on the development of the tubercles. By Edward Warren (Being the dissertation to which the Fiske Fund Prize was awarded June 4, 1856). Philadelphia: Blanchard & Lea, 1857. 73p., 42p. DNLM; PPC; PU **50-0598**

FITCH, James C[lark] (1792-1884)
Case of fracture of the skull, with loss of a portion of the substance of the brain; recovery. [With remarks by S. W. Butler.] [Burlington, 1852?] 7p. DNLM
50-0599

FITCH, Samuel Sheldon
Six lectures on the uses of the lungs; and causes, prevention and cure of pulmonary consumption, asthma, and diseases of the heart. New York: Carlisle, 1850. 324p. DNLM; NNNAM; PPC **50-0600**

FITCH, Samuel Sheldon
Health almanac. . . . [New York? 1852]. 60p. MHi; NNNAM; PPL **50-0601**

FITCH, Samuel Sheldon
Six lectures on the uses of the lungs: and causes, prevention, and cure of pulmonary consumption, asthma, and diseases of the heart. . . . New edition. . . . New York: S. S. Fitch, 1852. 368p. NNNAM; PPC; PU **50-0602**

FITCH, Samuel Sheldon
Health almanac for 1853, and guide to invalids; or, Directions for the treatment of consumption, asthma, heart diseases, bronchitis, dyspepsia, custiveness, diarrhoea, dysentery, falling of the bowels, piles, salt rheum, and scrofula, female diseases, &c. &c. . . . New York: S. S. Fitch & Co., [1853?] 48p. NNC; NNNAM **50-0603**

FITCH, Samuel Sheldon
Six discourses on the functions of the lungs; and causes, prevention, and cure of pulmonary consumption, asthma, and diseases of the heart; on the laws of life; and on the mode of preserving male and female health to an hundred years. New York: S. S. Fitch, 1853. 368p. CtY-M; DNLM; NNNAM
50-0604

FITCH, Samuel Sheldon
Six discourses on the functions of the lungs; and causes, prevention, and cure of pulmonary consumption, asthma, and diseases of the heart: on the laws of life and on the mode of preserving male and female health to an hundred years. New York, 1855. 324p. NNNAM; OCIM; PPC
50-0605

FITCH, Samuel Sheldon
Six lectures on the functions of the lungs, and causes, prevention, and cure of pulmonary consumption, asthma, and diseases of the heart; on the laws of life; and on the mode of preserving male and female health to an hundred years. Also a treatise on medicated inhalation. With 30 illustrations. . . . Twenty-fourth edition. . . . New York: S. S. Fitch & Co.; [etc., etc.], 1856. 384p. DNLM; ICJ; PPL; MWA
50-0606

FITCH, Samuel Sheldon
A friendly letter of counsel and advice to consumptives and other invalids. Also, prescriptions with special directions for the cure of chills and fever. [New York, 1857] 50p. DNLM; NNNAM **50-0607**

FITCH, Samuel Sheldon
A treatise on health, its aids and hindrances; containing an exposition of the causes and cure of diseases, and the laws of life. . . . New York: Pudney & Russell, 1857. 522p. DLC; DNLM; NNNAM **50-0608**

FITCH, Samuel Sheldon
A popular treatise upon diseases of the heart, dyspepsia, and other chronic diseases, with proofs of their curability. Also, rules for preventing disease, and preserving health (especially after forty) to one hundred years. . . . New York, 1859. 112p. CtY-M; DNLM; NNNAM; PPC **50-0609**

FITCH, Samuel Sheldon
Six lectures on the functions of the lungs, and causes, prevention, and cure of pulmonary consumption, asthma, and diseases of the heart; on the laws of life; and on the mode of preserving male and female health to an hundred years. Also a treatise on medical inhalation. 24th ed. New York: S. S. Fitch, 1859. 384p. MBM; NNNAM; OCIM; PPC
50-0610

FLAGG, J. F. B.
Ether and chloroform; their employment in surgery, dentistry, midwifery, therapeutics. . . . Philadelphia: Lindsay & Blakiston, 1851. 189p. DNLM; PPC: PPJ; PU
50-0611

FLINT, Austin (1812-1886)
Prize essay. On variations of pitch in percussion and respiratory sounds, and their application to physical diagnosis. Buffalo: Jewett, Thomas & Co., 1852. 47p. DNLM
50-0612

FLINT, Austin (1812-1886)
Clinical reports on continued fever, based on analyses of one hundred and sixty-four cases; with remarks on the management of continued fever, the identity of typhus and typhoid fever, relapsing fever, diagnosis, etc.; to which is added a memoir on the transportation and diffusion by contagion of typhoid fever, as exemplified in the occurrence of the diseases at North Boston, Erie County, N.Y. Buffalo: G. H. Derby & Co., 1852. 390p. DNLM **50-0613**

FLINT, Austin (1812-1886)
Clinical report on chronic pleurisy, based on an analysis of forty-seven cases. . . . Buffalo: Printed by Jewett, Thomas & Co., 1853. 58p. DLC; DNLM **50-0614**

FLINT, Austin (1812-1886)
Clinical report on dysentery, based on an analysis of forty-nine cases, with remarks on the causation, pathology, and management of the disease. Buffalo: Jewett, Thomas & Co., 1853. 90p. DNLM **50-0615**

FLINT, Austin (1812-1886)
Address at the opening of the session for 1854-1855 in the medical department of the University of Louisville. Louisville: Ky.: J. F. Brennan, 1854. 15p. DNLM **50-0616**

FLINT, Austin (1812-1886)
Clinical reports on continued fever, based on analyses of one hundred and sixty-four cases; with remarks on the management of continued fever, the identity of typhus and typhoid fever, relapsing fever, diagnosis, etc.; to which is added a memoir on the transportation and diffusion by contagion of typhoid fever, as exemplified in the occurrence of the disease at North Boston, Erie County, N.Y. Philadelphia: Lindsay & Blakiston, 1855. 390p. DNLM; MBM; PPC; PU **50-0617**

FLINT, Austin (1812-1886)
Physical exploration and diagnosis of diseases affecting the respiratory organs. . . . Philadelphia: Blanchard & Lea, 1856. 636p. DLC; DNLM; PPC; PU **50-0618**

FLINT, Austin (1812-1886)
A practical treatise on the diagnosis, pathology, and treatment of diseases of the heart. . . . Philadelphia: Blanchard & Lea, 1859. 473p. DLC; DNLM; PPC; PU **50-0619**

FLINT, Joshua B. (1801-1864)
A discourse delivered to the class of the Kentucky School of Medicine, introductory to a course on surgery. Louisville: Haldeman & Co., 1852. 36p. DNLM **50-0620**

FLINT, Joshua B. (1801-1864)
Sketches of military surgery. An introductory discourse delivered to the Kentucky School of Medicine. Louisville: Haldeman & Co., 1852. 36p. DNLM **50-0621**

FLINT, Joshua B. (1801-1864)
Report of the standing committee on surgery, read before the Kentucky State Medical Society. Louisville: Morton & Griswold, 1853. 51p. DNLM **50-0622**

FLINT, Joshua B. (1801-1864)
A lecture, introductory to the course of surgical instruction in the Kentucky School of Medicine. Louisville: Morton & Griswold, 1854. 31p. DNLM **50-0623**

FLINT, Joshua B. (1801-1864)
A discourse introductory to a course of clinical surgery. Louisville: Morton & Griswold, 1856. 46p. DNLM **50-0624**

FLINT, Joshua B. (1801-1864)
A discourse addressed to the Kentucky State Medical Society. Louisville, Ky.: Hanna & Co., 1859. 23p. DNLM **50-0625**

FLINT, William
An address delivered before the Erie County Medical Society, January 7, 1851. . . . Erie, Penn.: Printed at the office of the Chronicle, 1851. 33p. DLC; DNLM **50-0626**

FONDEY, John
A brief and intelligible view of the nature, origin, and cure of tubercular or scrofulous disease. . . . Including, also, a manual for the application of electro-magnetism in this disorder. . . . Philadelphia: W. C. & J. Neff, 1855. 209p. DLC; DNLM; PPC; PU **50-0627**

FOOTE, George F[ranklin] (1817-1889)
An address upon the subject of life insurance. New York: N. York Life Insurance Co., [1858]. 23p. DNLM **50-0628**

FOOTE, Henry E. (1825-1871)
Introductory address; delivered to the students of the Medical College of Ohio. Cincinnati: Wrightson & Co., 1858. 24p. DNLM; OCIM **50-0629**

FOOTE, John
The practitioner's pharmacopoeia and universal formulary; containing 2,000 classified prescriptions, [etc.]. With corrections and additions by an American physician. New York: S. S. & W. Wood, 1855. 390p. DNLM; MBM; NNNAM; PPC **50-0630**

FORBES, John (1787-1861)
Nature and art in the cure of disease. From the 2nd London edition. New York: S. S. & W. Wood, 1858. 261p. DNLM; PPHa **50-0631**

FORD, Henry A. (1820?-1858)
Observations on the fevers of the west coast of Africa. New York: E. O. Jenkins, 1856. 48p. DNLM; NNNAM **50-0632**

FORD, John P[ryor] (1810-1865)
The difficulties, duties, and rewards of the physician. An address to the graduating class . . . of the University of Nashville. Nashville: Cameron & Fall, 1856. 16p. DNLM **50-0633**

FOREMAN, Richard
The Cherokee physician; or, Indian guide to health, as given by . . . comprising a brief view of anatomy, with general rules for preserving health without the use of medicines. . . . To which is added a short dispensatory, by Jas. W. Mahoney, 3rd ed. New York: J. M. Edney, 1857. 304p. DLC; DNLM; NNNAM **50-0634**

FORREST, William S.
The great pestilence in Virginia; being an historical account of the origin, general character, and ravages of the yellow fever in Norfolk and Portsmouth in 1855; together with sketches of some of the victims. . . . New York: Derby & Jackson; Philadelphia: J. B. Lippincott & Co. [etc., etc.], 1856. 326p. DLC; DNLM; NNNAM; PPC **50-0635**

FORSTER, J. J.
Consumption and scrofula; some important discoveries relative to their cause, nature and cure. New York: R. C. Valentine, 1856. 58p. DNLM; NNNAM **50-0636**

FOULKE, William Parker
Discourse in commemoration of the founding of the Academy of Natural Sciences of Philadelphia. Philadelphia: Printed for the Academy, 1854. 58p. DNLM; PP; PPL
50-0637

FOWLER, Orson Squire (1809-1887)
Maternity; or the bearing and nursing of children. Including female education and beauty. New York: Fowlers & Wells, 1856. 221p. DNLM; NNNAM **50-0638**

FOWNES, George (1815-1849)
Elementary chemistry. . . . Edited by R. Bridges. Philadelphia: Blanchard & Lea, 1855. 555p. DNLM; OCIM; PPC; PU
50-0639

FRANCIS, John Wakefield (1789-1861)
New York during the last half century. A discourse in commemoration of the fifty-third anniversary of the New York Historical Society, and of the dedication of their new edifice. New York: J. F. Trow, 1857. 232p. DNLM; NNNAM
50-0640

FRANCIS, John W[akefield] (1789-1861)
. . . Address on the commencement of the winter course on clinical instruction at Bellevue Hospital, October 19th, 1857. . . . [New York; 1857]. 16p. DLC; NNNAM
50-0641

FRANCIS, John Wakefield (1789-1861)
Introductory discourse to the several courses of clinical instruction at Bellevue Hospital, New York. New York: J. F. Trow, 1858. 55p. DNLM; NNNAM **50-0642**

FRANCIS, John Wakefield (1789-1861)
Remarks introductory to the course of lectures delivered on behalf of the Kane monument in New York. New York: J. F. Trow, 1859. 8p. DNLM; NNNAM **50-0643**

FRANCIS, John Wakefield (1789-1861)
Reminiscences of Samuel Lathan Mitchell, M.D., LL.D. . . . Enlarged from Valentine's City manual. New York: J. F. Trow, printer, 1859. 31p. DLC; NNNAM **50-0644**

FRANCIS, Valentine Mott
A thesis on hospital hygiene, for the degree of doctor of medicine in the University of New York. New York: J. F. Trow, 1859. 217p. 3 plates. DNLM; NNNAM; NNU-M
50-0645

FRAZER, E. S.
Valedictory address to the class of graduates of the Missouri Medical College. St. Louis, Mo., 1857. 21p. DNLM
50-0646

FRELIGH, Martin (1813-1889)
A brief treatise on the pathology and cure of consumption. New York: Harrison, 1851. 12p. NNNAM; PPHa
50-0647

FRELIGH, Martin (1813-1889)
Homoeopathic practice of medicine: embracing the history, diagnosis and treatment of disease in general, including those peculiar to females; and the management of children. Designed as a text-book for the student, as a concise book of reference for the profession, and simplified and arranged for domestic use. . . . New York: Lamport, Blakeman & Law, 1853. 576p. DLC; NNNAM **50-0648**

FRELIGH, Martin (1813-1889)
Homoeopathic practice of medicine: embracing the history, diagnosis and treatment of disease in general, including those peculiar to females; and the management of children. Designed as a text-book for the student, as a concise book of reference for the profession, and simplified and arranged for domestic use. . . . New ed., revised and enlarged. New York: Sheldon, Lamport & Blakeman, 1855. 593p. DNLM; NNNAM
50-0649

FRELIGH, Martin (1813-1889)
Homoeopathic practice of medicine. . . . 6th ed. New York: H. W. Law, 1856. 602p. DNLM; NNNAM; PPHa
50-0650

FRELIGH, Martin (1813-1889)
The homoeopathic pocket companion, or a simplified abridgement of the Homoeopathic Practice of Medicine, designed expressly for the use of families and travellers. New York: H. W. Law, 1856. 291p. NNNAM; PPHa
50-0651

FRELIGH, Martin (1813-1889)
Homoeopathic practice of medicine: embracing the history, diagnosis and treatment of diseases in general, including those peculiar to females: and the management of children. 8th ed., rev. and enl. . . . New York: T. Hurlburt; Boston: O. Clapp [etc., etc.], 1859. 620p. DLC; MBM; NNNAM; PPHa
50-0652

FRELIGH, Martin (1813-1889)
Homoeopathic materia medica: being a summary of the curative action of the principal remedial agents employed in the homoeopathic practice. Comp. from Hahnemann, Jahr . . . and other distinguished members of the profession, together with additions, references, and notes. . . . New York: C. T. Hurlburt; Boston: O. Clapp [etc., etc.], 1859. 201p. DLC; OCLloyd; MBM; NNNAM **50-0653**

FRICK, Charles (1823-1860)
Renal affections; their diagnosis and pathology. Philadelphia: Lea & Blanchard, 1850. 189p. DNLM; OCIM; PPC; PU
50-0654

FRICK, Charles (1823-1860)
Valedictory address to the graduates of the Maryland College of Pharmacy, delivered March 6, 1857. With a list of the graduates. Baltimore: J. W. Woods, 1857. 25p. DNLM; MdU-D
50-0655

FROST, Henry Rutledge (1790-1866)
Outlines of a course of lectures on the materia medica. . . . 4th ed. Charleston, S.C.: Walker & James, 1851. 384p. DNLM; OCLloyd, ScCM **50-0656**

FROST, Henry Rutledge (1790-1866)
Outlines of a course of lectures on the materia medica. . . . 5th ed. Charleston, S.C.: James & Williams, 1858. 318p. DNLM; ScCM **50-0657**

FULLER, Henry William (1820-1873)
On rheumatism, rheumatic gout, and sciatica, their pathology, symptoms, and treatment. . . . New York: S. S. & W. Wood, 1854. 322p. DLC; OCIM; NNNAM; PPC
50-0658

FUSSELL, Edwin (1813-1882)
Valedictory address to the graduating class of the Female Medical College of Pennsylvania, for the session 1856-1857. . . . Published by the class. Philadelphia: A. Ketterlinus, printer, 1867. 15p. DLC; PPC **50-0659**

GAILLARD, Edwin Samuel (1827-1885)
An essay on intermittent and bilious remittent fevers: with their pathological relation to ozone. . . . Charleston [S.C.]: Walker & Evans, Stationers and Printers, 1856. 59p. DNLM; ScCM **50-0660**

GALT, John Minson (1819-1862)
Essay on asylums for persons of unsound mind. Richmond: H. K. Ellyson, 1850. 22p. DNLM; ViRA **50-0661**

GALT, John Minson (1819-1862)
Essays on asylums for persons of unsound mind. Richmond, Va.: Ritichies & Dunnavant, 1853. 44p. DNLM; ViRA **50-0662**

GALT, John Minson (1819-1862)
A lecture on idiocy. Richmond, Va., 1859. 37p. DNLM; ViRA **50-0663**

GANNETT, Ezra S.
The physician; a sermon delivered after the death of Marshall Sears Perry. Boston: Crosby, Nichols & Co., 1859. 20p. DNLM; MBM **50-0664**

GARDETTE, Emile B[laise] (1803-1887)
The professional education of dentists. [Philadelphia, 1852.] 12p. DNLM; PPC **50-0665**

GARDINER, William A.
Introductory lecture to the class of the Homoeopathic Medical College of Pennsylvania, delivered October 16, 1851. Published by the Class. Philadelphia: King & Baird, 1851. 15p. DNLM; PPHa **50-0666**

GARDINER, William A.
Introductory lecture to the class of the Homoeopathic Medical College of Philadelphia. Philadelphia, 1853. 16p. DNLM; PPHa **50-0667**

GARDINER, William A.
Valedictory address delivered at the commencement of the Homoeopathic Medical College of Philadelphia. Philadelphia: King & Baird, 1855. 16p. DNLM; PPHa **50-0668**

GARDNER, Augustus Kinsley (1821-1876)
Report of a committee appointed by the Academy of Medicine, upon the comparative value of milk, formed from the slop of distilleries and other food, with chemical and microscopical analyses. . . . Read March 1, 1848. . . . New York: R. Craighead, Printer, 1851. 19p. DLC; NNNAM **50-0669**

GARDNER, Augustus Kinsley (1821-1876)
A history of the art of midwifery: a lecture delivered at the College of Physicians and Surgeons, November 11th, 1851, introductory to a course of private instruction on operative midwifery; showing the past inefficacy and present natural incapacity of females in the practice of obstetrics. . . . New York: Stringer & Townsend, 1852. 32p. DLC; NNNAM; PU **50-0670**

GARDNER, Augustus Kinsley (1821-1876)
The causes and curative treatment of sterility, with a preliminary statement of the physiology of generation. . . . New York: De Witt & Davenport, [1856]. 170p. 5 col. plates. DLC; NNNAM; PU **50-0671**

GASKELL, John
Sense and sound, as they reciprocally form any sign of mind. Philadelphia: T. K. Collins, Jr., 1854. 32p. DNLM; PPL **50-0672**

GASSETT, Helen M.
Categorical account of the Female Medical College, to the people of New England States. Boston, 1855. 139p. DNLM; MH-M; MWA **50-0673**

GAY, George H[enry] (1823?-1878)
Surgical cases, communicated to the Boston Society for Medical Improvement. Boston: D. Clapp, 1856. 24p. 3 plates. DNLM; MBM **50-0674**

GAY, George H[enry] (1823?-1878)
Membranous croup. [Boston, 1859]. 10p. DNLM; MBM **50-0675**

GAYLEY, James Fyfe (1818-1894)
A history of the Jefferson Medical College of Philadelphia . . . with biographical sketches of the early professors. . . . Philadelphia. J. M. Wilson, 1858. 59p. DNLM; PPC; PPJ; PU **50-0676**

GEDDINGS, Eli (1799-1878)
Valedictory address to the graduating class of the Medical College of the State of South Carolina, delivered . . . on the 12th of March, 1852. Charleston, S.C.: Steam Power Press of Walker & James, 1852. 27p. CtY-M; DLC: DNLM; ScCM **50-0677**

GEDDINGS, Eli (1799-1878)
Report of the committee of the South Carolina Medical Association of the medical topography of the State of South Carolina. Charleston: Walker, Richards & Co., 1852. 23p. DLC; DNLM; ScCM **50-0678**

GEDDINGS, Eli (1799-1878)
Outlines of a course of lectures on the principles and practice of surgery, delivered. . . . Prepared by Thos. S. Waring . . . and Samuel Logan . . . from notes taken during the course. Published with the consent of, and revised by Professor Geddings. Charleston [S.C.]: S. G. Courtenay & Co. 1858. 560p. CtY-M; DNLM; PU; ScCM **50-0679**

GEORGETOWN UNIVERSITY. WASHINGTON, D.C. GEORGETOWN UNIVERSITY SCHOOL OF MEDICINE
Annual announcements for the sessions of 1851-2 (2.); 1854-5 (5.); 1861-2 (12.); 1863-4 to 1866-7 (14.-17.); 1869-70 (21.); 1871-2 to 1900-1901 (23.-52.) Washington, 1851-1900. DNLM. [Organized in 1850. First session commenced in May, 1850. List of alumni from 1852 to 1884, in announcement for 1884-5. Held two sessions in 1851, and two commencements in 1865.] **50-0680**

GERHARD, William Wood (1809-1872)
The diagnosis, pathology, and treatment, of the diseases of the chest. . . . 3rd ed., rev. and enl. Philadelphia: E. Barrington and G. D. Haswell, 1850. 351p. DLC; MBM; PPC; PU **50-0681**

GERONDALO, R.
Homoeopathy; its early history, character and tendency. Wilkesbarre: Times Office, 1854. 18p. PPHa
50-0682

GIBBONS, Henry, Sr. (1808-1884)
Annual address before the San Francisco County Medical Society. San Francisco: Whitton, Towne & Co., 1857. 16p. DNLM **50-0683**

GIBSON, Chas. Bell (1815-1865)
Statement of facts in a case of dislocation of the femur into the foramen ovale, probably complicated with fracture of the acetabulum, and presenting unusual difficulties in diagnosis. Richmond: Colin & Nowlan, 1855. 7p. DNLM; ViRA
50-0684

GIBSON, William (1788-1868)
Institutes and practice of surgery: being outlines of a course of lectures. . . . 8th ed. improved and altered. . . . Philadelphia: J. Kay, Jr. & Brother; Pittsburgh: Kay & Co., 1850. 2 v. 34 plates. DNLM; OCIM; PPC; PU **50-0685**

GIBSON, William (1788-1868)
Three lectures, preliminary to a course on the principles and practice of surgery, delivered on the 4th, 8th, and 9th of October, 1849. Before the medical class of the University of Pennsylvania. . . . Published by the class. Philadelphia: Grattan & McLean, 1850. 57p. DLC; DNLM; PPC; PU
50-0686

GILBERT, David (1803-1868)
Valedictory address to the graduates of the medical department of Pennsylvania College. Philadelphia: King & Baird, 1852. 19p. DNLM; PPC; PU **50-0687**

GILBERT, David (1803-1868), et al.
A refutation of the misstatements contained in a pamphlet recently issued by W. Darrach, M.D., and J. Wiltbank, M.D., in reference to the medical department of Pennsylvania College. Philadelphia: Merrihew & Thompson, 1855. 64p. DNLM; PPC; PU **50-0688**

GILBERT, David (1803-1868)
Adhesive plaster the best counter-extending means in fractures of the thigh. [Philadelphia, 1858.] 5p. DNLM
50-0689

GILBERT, David (1803-1868)
Valedictory address to the graduates of the medical department of Pennsylvania College. Philadelphia: Merrihew & Thompson, 1859. 15p. DNLM; PPC; PU
50-0690

GILBERT, John P.
A treatise on deafness and diseases of the eye and ear, with remarks on their nature and cure; illustrated with cases. Albany: Munsell & Rowland, 1858. 16p. DNLM
50-0691

GLEIWITZ, George
Homoeopathy; its nature and principles. Bridgeport, Conn.: Pomeroy & Morse, 1857. 48p. PPHa
50-0692

GLEIWITZ, George
The realities of homoeopathy. Boston: A. H. Copeland, 1859. 52p. PPHa **50-0693**

GLENN, James
The venereal disease, its primary cause explained; and the possibility of its being fully prevented, described. To which is added a few remarks on the laws regarding seduction, adultery, and prostitution. [New York, 1857.] 12p. DNLM; NNNAM
50-0694

GLUCK, Isidor
Amaurosis. Clinical lectures on some of the principal diseases of the eye. New York: E. P. Allen, 1855. 16p. DNLM; NNNAM **50-0695**

GLUGE, Gottlieb (1812-1898)
Atlas of pathological histology. Transl. from the German by Joseph Leidy. Philadelphia: Blanchard & Lea, 1853. 100p. 12 plates. DLC; DNLM; PPC; PU **50-0696**

GOBRECHT, William H. (1828-1901)
An inaugural address introductory to the course on anatomy delivered in the medical department of Pennsylvania College. Philadelphia: Collins, 1859. 23p. DNLM; NNNAM; PPC; PU
50-0697

GOLDSMITH, Alban (1788?-186?)
Diseases of the genito-urinary organs. . . . New York: Wiley & Halsted, 1857. 96p. 5 plates. DNLM; NNNAM
50-0698

GOLLMAN, William
The homoeopathic guide in all diseases of the urinary and sexual organs, including the derangements caused by onanism and sexual excesses; with a strict regard to the present demands of medical science, and accompanied by an appendix on the use of electro-magnetism in the treatment of these diseases. . . . Transl., with additions, by Charles J. Hempel, M.D. Philadelphia: Rademacher & Sheek, 1855. 309p. MBM; NNNAM; PPC; PPHa **50-0699**

GOOD, Peter P. (1789?-1875)
A materia medica animalia, containing the scientific analysis, natural history, and chemical and medical properties and uses of the substances that are the products of beasts, birds, fishes, or insects. Cambridge, Mass.: Metcalf & Co., [1853]. 55p. 25 col. plates. DNLM; MBM; NNNAM; OCLloyd
50-0700

GOODE, S.
Some account of the medicinal properties of the Hot Springs, Virginia; also an analysis of the water. . . . Richmond: C. Wynne, 1857. 48p. DNLM; ViRA **50-0701**

GOODRICH, Jesse W. (1803-1857)
The phrenological organs; the phrenological character: (as marked, and given by Prof. O. S. Fowler) together with the Maelstroom Wreck: the Pyramids: the Battle of Bunker Hill; a Colloquy in the Clouds; the Bridal Flounces; and some other occasional poems, and prose writings. Worcester, 1855. 50p. ICU; MH; NN; NNC **50-0702**

GOULD, Augustus Addison (1805-1863)
Search out the secrets of nature. The annual discourse before the Massachusetts Medical Society at Springfield, June 27, 1855. Boston: J. Wilson & Son, 1855. 56p. DNLM; MH-M
50-0703

GOULD, John Stanton (1810-1874)
A report on food and diet, with observations on the dietetical regimen suitable for almshouses, prisons, and hospitals; also on heating, ventilation, etc., with practical recommendations, prepared at the request of the board of commissioners of emigration, and the board of governors of the New York Almshouse Department. New York: W. C. Bryant & Co., 1852. 90p. DNLM; NN; NNNAM **50-0704**

GRAHAM, Sylvester (1794-1851)
Chastity, in a course of lectures to young men; intended also for the serious consideration of parents and guardians. With an appendix by R. T. Trall. New York: Fowler & Wells, 1857. 76p. DNLM; NNNAM **50-0705**

GRANT, C.
The fallacy of a supposed vis medicatrix naturae, being an inquiry into the true nature of disease. Cincinnati: Wright, Ferris & Co., 1850. 11p. DNLM; OC; OCIM **50-0706**

GRANT, G.
A case of necrosis, occurring during intermittent fever, and operation. . . . Newark, N.J.: P. C. Atkinson, 1859. 6p. DNLM; NjR **50-0707**

GRANT, George R.
The vital statistics and sanitary condition of Memphis, Tenn.; an anniversary address. New Orleans: J. Cohn, 1852. 19p. DNLM; LNT-M **50-0708**

GRANT, Henry Allen (1813-1884)
The annual address to the candidates for the degree of doctor of medicine in the medical institution of Yale College. New Haven: W. H. Stanley, 1850. 18p. CtY-M; DNLM **50-0709**

GRANT, William Robertson (1811-1852)
Lecture introductory to a course on anatomy and physiology in the medical department of Pennsylvania College, delivered October 13, 1851. Philadelphia: J. Royer, 1852. 12p. DNLM; PPC **50-0710**

GRAY, Henry (1827-1861)
Anatomy, descriptive and surgical . . . The drawings by H. V. Carter . . . The dissections jointly by the author and Dr. Carter. . . . Philadelphia: Blanchard & Lea, 1859. 754p. [First American edition] DLC; DNLM; NNNAM; PPC **50-0711**

GRAY, John Franklin (1804-1882)
The duty of the state in relation to homoeopathy. An inaugural address delivered before the Hahnemann Academy of Medicine, New York, January 9, 1850. Published by order of the Academy. New York: Angell, Engel & Hewitt, 1850. 28p. NNNAM; PPHa **50-0712**

GREELEY, S. S. N.
The aims, duties, responsibilities and elements of success in medical practice. An address delivered at the 34th commencement of the Berkshire Medical College, Pittsfield, Mass. . . . Pittsfield: Chickering & Davis, 1856. 21p. DNLM **50-0713**

GREEN, Horace (1802-1866)
An introductory address delivered before the students and trustees of the New York Medical College. New York: Baker, Godwin & Co., 1850. 24p. DNLM; NNNAM **50-0714**

GREEN, Horace (1802-1866)
The prospective progress of medicine in America: a valedictory address, delivered before the graduating class at the first annual commencement of the New York Medical College. . . . New York: Baker, Godwin & Co., printers, 1851. 23p. DLC; NNNAM **50-0715**

GREEN, Horace (1802-1866)
A treatise on diseases of the air passages: comprising an inquiry into the history, pathology, causes, and treatment, of those affections of the throat, called bronchitis, chronic laryngitis, . . . 3rd ed., revised and enlarged. New York: G. P. Putnam, 1852. 314p. DLC; MBM; NNNAM; PPC **50-0716**

GREEN, Horace (1802-1866)
On the surgical treatment of polypi of the larynx, and oedema of the glottis. . . . New York: G. P. Putnam, 1852. 124p. 4 plates. DLC; NNNAM; PPC; PU **50-0717**

GREEN, Horace (1802-1866)
On the subject of priority in the medication of the larynx and trachea. New York: Baker, Godwin & Co., 1854. 17p. DNLM; NNNAM **50-0718**

GREEN, Horace (1802-1866)
Remarks on croup and its treatment. New York: Baker, Godwin & Co., 1854. 21p. DNLM; NNNAM **50-0719**

GREEN, Horace (1802-1866)
Epidemics and quarantine: a lecture, introductory to the winter course, at the New York Medical College, for the session of 1855-1856. . . . (Published by request of the class.) New York: E. P. Allen, 1855. 22p. DLC; NNNAM **50-0720**

GREEN, Horace (1802-1866)
On injection of the bronchial tubes, and tubercular cavities of the lungs. New York: E. P. Allen, 1855. 20p. DLC; DNLM; NNNAM **50-0721**

GREEN, Horace (1802-1866)
Report on the use and effect of applications of nitrate of silver to the throat, either in local or general disease. New York: E. P. Allen, 1856. 42p. DLC; DNLM; NNNAM **50-0722**

GREEN, Horace (1802-1866)
Bronchial injections: a report, with a statistical table, of one hundred and six cases of pulmonary diseases treated by bronchial injections. . . . New York: E. P. Allen, 1856. 40p. DLC; NNNAM; PU **50-0723**

GREEN, Horace (1802-1866)
On the difficulties and advantages of catheterism of the air-passages in diseases of the chest. [1857?] 24p. DNLM; NNNAM **50-0724**

GREEN, Horace (1802-1866)
On the introduction of the sponge-armed probang into the larynx and trachea. [New York, 1857.] 14p. DNLM; NNNAM **50-0725**

GREEN, Horace (1802-1866)
Lesions of the epiglotic [sic] cartilage. . . . New York: E. P. Allen, 1857. 28p. DLC; NNNAM **50-0726**

GREEN, Horace (1802-1866)
Selections from favorite prescriptions of living American practitioners. New York: Wiley & Halsted, 1858. 206p. DNLM; MBM; NNNAM; PPC **50-0727**

GREEN, Horace (1802-1866)
Observations on the pathology of croup: with remarks on its treatment by topical medications. . . . [2nd ed.] New York: J. Wiley, 1859. 198p. DLC; MBM; NNNAM; PPC **50-0728**

GREEN, James Mercer
Cases of inflammation and ulceration of the cervix uteri. Charleston: Walker & James, 1853. 58p. DNLM; ScCM **50-0729**

GREEN, James Mercer
Case of acute ovarian abscess, supervening upon chronic disease of the ovarium, in which the tumor, after pointing in the left iliac region, moved completely over to the right. [1854?] 6p. DNLM **50-0730**

GREENE, Reuben (*b.* 1817)
Indianopathy. Or science of Indian medicine . . . whereby he is enabled to successfully treat cancers, tumors, scrofula, ulcers, and all chronic diseases. 14th ed. Boston, 1858. 80p. DNLM; MBM **50-0731**

GREGG, Rollin Robinson (1828-1886)
Phthisis pulmonalis; or, consumption shown to be the result of a perverted secretion of the mucous membranes; and its cure established by homoeopathic remedies under the law, similia similibus curantur. Canandaigua, N.Y.: N. J. Milliken, Printer, 1859. 56p. PPHa **50-0732**

GREGORY, George (1790-1853)
Lectures on the eruptive fevers; as now in the course of delivery at St. Thomas's Hospital, in London. . . . 1st American ed. With numerous additions and amendments by the author, comprising his latest views. With notes and an appendix. . . . By H. D. Bulkley. . . . New York: S. S. & W. Wood, 1851. 379p. 4 col. plates. DLC; MBM; NNNAM; PPC **50-0733**

GREGORY, George
Medical morals, illustrated with plates and extracts from medical works; designed to show the pernicious social and moral influence of the present system of medical practice, and the importance of establishing female medical colleges, and the educating and employing female physicians for their own sex. New York: Published by the Author, 1853. 48p. DNLM; MBM; NNNAM; PPC **50-0734**

GREGORY, Samuel (1813-1872)
Letter to ladies, in favor of female physicians. . . . Boston: The Society, 1850. [American Medical Education Society] 48p. DLC; DNLM; MBM **50-0735**

GREGORY, Samuel (1813-1872)
Letter to ladies in favor of female physicians for their own sex. . . . 2nd ed. Boston: [Female Medical Education] Society, 1854. 48p. DLC; DNLM; MBM **50-0736**

GREGORY, Samuel (1813-1872)
Facts and important information for young women, on the self-indulgence of the sexual appetite, its destructive effects on health, exciting causes, prevention, and cure. Boston: G. Gregory, 1857. 66p. DNLM; MBM **50-0737**

GRIFFITH, Robert Eglesfeld (1798-1850)
A universal formulary: containing the methods of preparing and administering officinal and other medicines. The whole adapted to physicians and pharmaceutists. . . . Philadelphia: Lea & Blanchard, 1850. 567p. DLC; MBM; OCLloyd; PPC **50-0738**

GRIFFITH, Robert Eglesfeld (1798-1850)
A universal formulary: containing the methods of preparing and administering officinal and other medicines. The whole adapted to physicians and pharmaceutists. . . . A new ed. carefully rev. and much extended by Robert P. Thomas. . . . Philadelphia: Blanchard & Lea, 1859. 651p. DLC; MBM; OCLloyd; PPC **50-0739**

GRIFFITHS, Thomas J.
Thoughts on homoeopathy; or, facts for the people. Louisville, Ky.: Printed for the Author, 1852. 11p. PPHa; OCIM **50-0740**

GRIMES, J. Stanley (1807-1903)
Etherology; or the philosophy of mesmerism and phrenology . . . with a review of the pretensions of neurology and phreno-magnetism. Revised and edited by W. G. LeDuc. Boston: J. Munroe & Co., 1850. 251, 121p. DNLM; MBM; MWA **50-0741**

GRIMES, J. Stanley (1807-1903)
Compend of the phreno-philosophy of human nature. Boston & Cambridge: J. Munroe & Co., 1850. 121p. DNLM; MB **50-0742**

GRIMES, J. Stanley (1807-1903)
Phreno-geology; the progressive creation of man. . . . Boston & Cambridge: J. Munroe & Co., 1851. 216p. DNLM; MB **50-0743**

GRIMES, J. Stanley (1807-1903)
The mysteries of human nature explained by a new system of nervous physiology. . . . Buffalo: R. M. Wanzer, 1857. 432p. DNLM **50-0744**

GRINDLE, Wesley
A late important discovery in medicine. Consumption positively cured. . . . New York, 1855. 12p. DLC; NNNAM **50-0745**

GRINDLE, Wesley
A practical treatise on the pathology and treatment of pulmonary consumption. . . . New York, 1858. 24p. DLC; NNNAM **50-0746**

GRINDLE, Wesley
A practical treatise on the pathology and treatment of pulmonary consumption. . . . New York, 1859. 32p. DLC; NNNAM **50-0747**

GRINDLE, Wesley
A practical treatise on the pathology and treatment of pulmonary consumption; also, remarks upon the most effectual treatment of all scrofulous diseases, catarrhal affections, [etc.]. New York: Rennie, Shea & Lindsay, 1859. 32p. DNLM; NNNAM **50-0748**

GRISCOM, John Hoskins (1809-1874)
The uses and abuses of air: showing its influence in sustaining life, and producing disease; with remarks on the ventilation of houses, and the best methods of securing a pure and wholesome atmosphere inside of dwellings, churches, courtrooms, workshops, and buildings of all kinds. . . . 2nd ed. New York: J. S. Redfield, 1850. 252p. plates. DLC; NNNAM
50-0749

GRISCOM, John Hoskins (1809-1874)
Hospital hygiene illustrated. New York, 1853. 12p. DNLM; NNNAM **50-0750**

GRISCOM, John Hoskins (1809-1874)
The uses and abuses of air; showing its influence in sustaining life and producing disease, with remarks on the ventilation of houses, etc. 3rd ed. New York: Redfield, 1854. 249p. DNLM; NNNAM **50-0751**

GRISCOM, John Hoskins (1809-1874)
Animal mechanism and physiology; being a plain and familiar exposition of the structure and functions of the human system. . . . New York: Harper & Bros., 1855. 357p. DNLM; MB; MH; MBM **50-0752**

GRISCOM, John Hoskins (1809-1874)
Anniversary discourse before the New York Academy of Medicine. New York: R. Craighead, 1855. 58p. DNLM; NNNAM **50-0753**

GRISCOM, John Hoskins (1809-1874)
A history, chronological and circumstantial, of the visitations of yellow fever at New York. New York, 1858. 36p. DNLM; NNNAM **50-0754**

GROSS, Samuel David (1805-1884)
A practical treatise on the diseases and injuries of the urinary bladder, the prostate gland, and the urethra. . . . Philadelphia: Blanchard & Lea, 1851. 726p. DLC; DNLM; MBM; PPC
50-0755

GROSS, S[amuel] D[avid] (1805-1884)
Report on Kentucky surgery; read before the Kentucky State Medical Society at its annual meeting at Louisville, Oct. 20, 1852. Louisville: Webb, 1853. 194p. PPJ **50-0756**

GROSS, S[amuel] D[avid] (1805-1884)
On the results of surgical operations in malignant diseases. Philadelphia: T. K. & P. G. Collins, 1853. 161p. PPJ
50-0757

GROSS, Samuel David (1805-1884)
A discourse on the life, character, and services of Daniel Drake, M.D. Delivered, by request, before the faculty and medical students of the University of Louisville, January 27, 1853. . . . Louisville: Printed at the office of the Louisville Journal, 1853. 92p. DLC; DNLM; PPJ; PPC
50-0758

GROSS, S[amuel] D[avid] (1805-1884)
A practical treatise on foreign bodies in the air-passages. . . . Philadelphia: Blanchard & Lea, 1854. 468p. DLC; PPC; PPJ; PU **50-0759**

GROSS, Samuel David (1805-1884)
A practical treatise on the diseases, injuries, and malformations of the urinary bladder, the prostate gland, and the urethra. . . . 2nd ed., rev. and much enl. . . . Philadelphia: Blanchard & Lea, 1855. 925p. DLC; DNLM; PPJ; PPC **50-0760**

GROSS, Samuel D[avid] (1805-1884)
Inaugural address introductory to the course on surgery in the Jefferson Medical College of Philadelphia, delivered October 17, 1856. Philadelphia: J. M. Wilson, 1856. 36p. PPJ
50-0761

GROSS, Samuel D[avid] (1805-1884)
Report on the causes which impede the progress of American medical literature. . . . Philadelphia: T. K. & P. G. Collins, printers, 1856. . . . 24p. DLC; DNLM; PPJ; PU
50-0762

GROSS, Samuel David (1805-1884)
Elements of pathological anatomy. . . . 3rd ed., modified and thoroughly rev. . . . Philadelphia: Blanchard & Lea, 1857. 771p. DLC; PPC; PPJ; PU **50-0763**

GROSS, Samuel David (1805-1884)
Practical observations on the nature and treatment of tuberculosis of the hip-joint. Philadelphia: J. B. Lippincott & Co., 1858. 43p. DNLM; PPJ **50-0764**

GROSS, Samuel David (1805-1884)
A system of surgery; pathological diagnostic, therapeutic, and operative. Philadelphia: Blanchard & Lea, 1859. 2 v. DNLM; PPC; PPJ; PU **50-0765**

GROSS, Samuel Weissell (1837-1889)
A case of aneurism of the right femoral artery, cured by digital compression, with remarks and a statistical report of twenty-two other cases treated by this method. Philadelphia: J. B. Lippincott & Co., 1859. 15p. DNLM; PPC; PPJ
50-0766

GUERNSEY, Egbert (1823-1903)
Homoeopathic domestic practice; containing also chapters on anatomy, physiology, hygiene and an abridged materia medica. New York: William Radde, 1853. 581p. PPHa
50-0767

GUERNSEY, Egbert (1823-1903)
Homoeopathic domestic practice; containing also chapters on anatomy, physiology, hygiene and an abridged materia medica. 2nd enlarged, revised and improved edition. New York: William Radde, [1854?] PPHa **50-0768**

GUERNSEY, Egbert (1823-1903)
The gentleman's hand book of homoeopathy; especially for travellers and for domestic practice. Boston: O. Clapp, 1855. 255p. PPHa **50-0769**

GUERNSEY, Egbert (1823-1903)
The gentleman's hand book of homoeopathy; especially for travellers and for domestic practice. 2nd ed. New York: William Radde, 1857. 255p. PPHa **50-0770**

GUILBERT, Edward Augustus (1826-1900)
Valedictory address to the graduating class of the Western Homoeopathic College, Cleveland, Ohio. Delivered at the annual commencement, February 27, 1856. Dubuque, Ia.: Daily Northwest Printers, 1858. 19p. PPHa
50-0771

GUNN, John C. (1800-1863)
Gunn's domestic medicine, or Poor man's friend, in the hours of affliction, pain, and sickness. . . . New rev. ed.—improved and enl. New York: C. M. Saxton; Philadelphia: T. Cowperthwait & Co.; [etc., etc.], 1853. 896p. DLC; NNNAM; PPC **50-0772**

GUNN, John C. (1800-1863)
Gunn's new domestic physician: or, Home book of health. . . . Cincinnati: Moore, Wilstach, Keys & Co., 1857. 791p. DLC; OCIM **50-0773**

GUNN, John C. (1800-1863)
Gunn's new domestic physician: or, Home book of health. . . . With an appendix on anatomy, physiology, etc., etc. [by J. H. Jordan]. Cincinnati: Moore, Wilstach, Keys & Co., 1859. 1046p. DLC; OCIM **50-0774**

GUNN, Moses (1822-1887)
Luxations of hip and shoulder. Ann Arbor: E. B. Pond, 1855. 11p. DNLM **50-0775**

GUNN, Moses (1822-1887)
Luxations of the hip and shoulder joints, and the agents which oppose their reduction. Detroit: Barns, French & Way, 1859. 16p. DNLM **50-0776**

HABERSHON, Samuel Osborne (1825-1889)
Pathological and practical observations on diseases of the alimentary canal, oesophagus, stomach, caecum and intestines. . . . Philadelphia: Blanchard & Lea, 1859. 312p. DNLM; PPC; PPJ; PU **50-0777**

HAHNEMANN ACADEMY OF MEDICINE
Schedule of prices for medical services adopted by the members. January 1, 1855. [New York, 1855]. 2p. DNLM **50-0778**

HAHNEMANN, Samuel (1755-1843)
The lesser writings of Samuel Hahnemann. Collected by R. E. Dudgeon. With a preface and notes by E. E. Marcy. . . . New York: William Radde, 1852. 784p. PPC; PPHa; NNNAM **50-0779**

[HAHNEMANN, Samuel, 1755-1843]
Address and poem delivered before the Massachusetts Homoeopathic Medical Society, in the Tremont Temple, Boston, on the occasion of the centennial birthday of Doctor Samuel Hahnemann, April 10, 1855. Address by W. E. Payne. Poem by Henry C. Preston. Boston: O. Clapp, 1855. 52p. MBM; MWA **50-0780**

HALE, Edwin M[oses] (1829-1899)
Homoeopathy and its principles, explained and defended. . . . Published by the Author, 1858. 8p. PPHa **50-0781**

HALL, Alfred G.
Views of the new theory of disease and of treatment and cure, based upon the nutritive principle; illustrative of the science of fluid physiology and the chemical properties of the blood. For the people. 4 pts. in 1 v. Washington, D.C.: The author, 1852. 135p. DNLM **50-0782**

HALL, William Whitty (1810-1876)
The nature, causes, symptoms, and cure of diseases of the throat and lungs. Cincinnati: J. D. Thorpe, 1850. 40p. DNLM **50-0783**

HALL, William Whitty (1810-1876)
Throat-ail, bronchitis, consumption; their causes, symptoms, and cure, in language adapted to common readers. 6th ed. New York: J. S. Redfield, 1851. 40p. DNLM; NNNAM **50-0784**

HALL, William Whitty (1810-1876)
Bronchitis and kindred diseases, in language adapted to common readers. . . . 7th ed. New York: J. S. Redfield, 1852. 350p. DLC; OCIM; NNNAM; PPC **50-0785**

HALSEY, William S.
A valedictory address delivered to the graduating class of the Philadelphia College of Medicine, at the semi-annual commencement, July 1, 1857. . . . Philadelphia: T. K. & P. G. Collins, printers, 1857. 14p. DLC; DNLM; PPC; PU **50-0786**

HALSTED, H.
Exposition of motorpathy; a new system of curing diseases, by statuminating, vitalizing motion. Rochester, N.Y.: Curtis & Butts, 1853. 171p. DNLM **50-0787**

HALSTED, H.
Motion-life; or the demon of the age and means of its exorcism. North Hampton, Mass.: Hopkins, Bridgman & Co., 1856. 69p. DNLM **50-0788**

HALSTED, O.
Method of curing dyspepsia, biliousness, etc. Cincinnati: J. Hart, 1852. 15p. DNLM; OCIM **50-0789**

HAMILTON, Frank Hastings (1813-1886)
Life of Nathaniel T. Otis, Jr., being part of an introductory lecture, delivered before the medical class of the University of Buffalo. Buffalo: G. Reese & Co., 1850. 14p. DNLM **50-0790**

HAMILTON, Frank Hastings (1813-1886)
Vegetable malaria one of the exciting causes of Asiatic cholera: being a report on the immediate . . . cause of the Asiatic cholera, which appeared in . . . Buffalo, July 26, 27, and 28, 1852. Read before the "Buffalo Medical Association," August 2, 1852. . . . Also the report of a committee appointed . . . "to investigate the relation of upturning of the soil to the causation of the cholera." Read Sept. 8, 1852. . . . Buffalo: Press of Jewett, Thomas & Co., 1852. 36p. map. DLC **50-0791**

HAMILTON, Frank Hastings (1813-1886)
New views on provisional callus. Bufflao: Jewett, Thomas & Co., 1853. 15p. DNLM **50-0792**

HAMILTON, Frank Hastings (1813-1886)
Fracture tables. Showing the results of treatment in one hundred and thirty-six cases. With a supplement compiled from Dr. Hamilton's notes, by John Boardman, comprising in all an analysis of 461 cases of fractures. Buffalo: Jewett, Thomas & Co., 1853. 36p. DNLM **50-0793**

HAMILTON, Frank Hastings (1813-1886)
Address to the graduates in medicine at the University of Buffalo, April 27, 1853. . . . Buffalo: Printed by Jewett, Thomas & Co., 1853. 15p. DLC **50-0794**

HAMILTON, Frank Hastings (1813-1886)
Elkoplasty, or anaplasty applied to the treatment of old ulcers. Also, a new mode of treatment for delayed or non-union of a fractured humerus. New York: Holman, Gray & Co., 1854. 19p. DNLM; NNNAM **50-0795**

HAMILTON, Frank Hastings (1813-1886)
New mode of treatment for delayed or non-union of a fractured humerus, read before the Medical Society of the County of Erie, June, 1854. [1854.] 6p. DNLM **50-0796**

HAMILTON, Frank Hastings (1813-1886)
Elkoplasty, or anaplasty applied to the treatment of old ulcers. (A reply to Dr. Watson's reclamation.) New York: Holman & Co., 1855. 14p. DNLM; NNNAM **50-0797**

HAMILTON, Frank Hastings (1813-1886)
Deformities after fractures. Philadelphia: T. K. & P. G. Collins, 1855. 99p. DNLM; PPC; PU **50-0798**

HAMILTON, Frank Hastings (1813-1886)
Eulogy on the life and character of Theodric Romeyn Beck, M.D., LL.D. delivered before the Medical Society of the State of New York. . . . Pub. by order of the Senate. Albany: Printed by C. Van Benthuysen, 1856. 96p. DLC **50-0799**

HAMILTON, Frank Hastings (1813-1886)
Compound dislocation of the long bones: considered with especial reference to the value of resection. Philadelphia: T. K. & P. G. Collins, 1857. 16p. DNLM; PPC; PU **50-0800**

HAMILTON, Frank Hastings (1813-1886)
Hygiene. Being the substance of a "charge" given February, 1859, to the graduating class in the medical department of the University of Buffalo. [1859.] 15p. DNLM **50-0801**

HAMMOND, N. J.
Address delivered at a supper given by the faculty to the students of the Atlanta Medical College, Aug. 13, 1855. Atlanta, Ga.: C. R. Hauleiter & Co., [1855]. 18p. DNLM **50-0802**

HAMMOND, William Alexander (1828-1900)
The relations existing between urea and uric acid. [Philadelphia, 1855.] 5p. DNLM **50-0803**

HAMMOND, William Alexander (1828-1900)
The physiological effects of alcohol and tobacco upon the human system. [Philadelphia, 1856.] 16p. DNLM; PPC **50-0804**

HAMMOND, William Alexander (1828-1900)
Experimental researches relative to the nutritive value and physiological effects of albumen, starch, and gum, when singly and exclusively used as food. Being the prize essay of the American Medical Association for 1857. . . . Philadelphia: T. K. & P. G. Collins, printers, 1857. 79p. DLC; PPC **50-0805**

HAMMOND, William Alexander (1828-1900)
On the action of certain vegetable diuretics. [Philadelphia, 1858.] 4p. DNLM **50-0806**

HAMMOND, William Alexander (1828-1900)
On the alterations induced by intermittent fever in the physical and chemical qualities of the urine, and on the action of the disulphate of quinine. [Philadelphia, 1858.] 5p. DNLM **50-0807**

HAMMOND, William Alexander (1828-1900)
On the injection of urea and other substances into the blood. [Philadelphia, 1858.] 7p. DNLM **50-0808**

HAMMOND, William Alexander (1828-1900) and S. Weir MITCHELL
Experimental researches relative to corroval and vao, two new varieties of woorara, the South American arrow poison. [Philadelphia, 1859.] 48p. DNLM **50-0809**

HAMPDEN-SIDNEY COLLEGE. RICHMOND, VIRGINIA
Address to the public in regard to the affairs of the Medical Department of Hampden-Sidney College. By several physicians of the City of Richmond. Richmond: Ritchies & Dunnavant, 1853. 59p. DNLM; ViRA **50-0810**

HANDY, Washington R. (1811-1857)
A text-book of anatomy and guide in dissections, for the use of students of medicine and dental surgery. Philadelphia: Lindsay & Blakiston, 1854. 810p. DNLM; OCIM; PPC; ViRA **50-0811**

HARLAN, Caleb
Lecture on allopathy and homoeopathy. Philadelphia: King & Baird, 1855. 13p. DNLM; PPHa **50-0812**

HARRIS, Chapin Aaron (1806-1860)
The principles and practice of dental surgery. . . . 4th ed.: rev., modified and greatly enlarged. . . . Philadelphia: Lindsay & Blakiston, 1850. 803p. DLC; OCIM; NNNAM; PPC **50-0813**

HARRIS, Chapin Aaron (1806-1860)
The principles and practice of dental surgery. . . . 5th ed.: rev., modified and greatly improved. . . . Philadelphia: Lindsay & Blakiston, 1853. 811p. DLC; MdU-D; PPC **50-0814**

HARRIS, Chapin Aaron (1806-1860)
The principles and practice of dental surgery. . . . 6th ed.: enl. and improved. With two hundred and fifty-seven illustrations. Philadelphia: Lindsay & Blakiston, 1855. 828p. DLC; MdU-D; OCIM; PPC **50-0815**

HARRIS, Chapin Aaron (1806-1860)
Dictionary of medical terminology, dental surgery, and the collateral sciences. . . . 2nd ed. Carefully rev. and enl. Philadelphia: Lindsay & Blakiston, 1855. 800p. DLC; MBM; NNNAM; PPC **50-0816**

HARRIS, Chapin Aaron (1806-1860)
The principles and practice of dental surgery. . . . 7th ed.: enl. and improved. With two hundred and seventy illustrations. Philadelphia: Lindsay & Blakiston, 1858. 802p. DLC; MdU-D; PPC; PU **50-0817**

HARRIS, Chapin Aaron (1806-1860)
Syllabus of the course of lectures delivered in the Baltimore College of Dental Surgery. Baltimore: Cushings & Bailey, 1859. 172p. DNLM; MdU-D **50-0818**

HARRIS, Elisha (1824-1884)
The annual report of the physician-in-chief of the marine hospital at quarantine. Albany, N.Y., 1857. 63p. 1 map. DNLM **50-0819**

HARRIS, Elisha (1824-1884)
Pestilential diseases, and the laws which govern their propagation. A letter from Elisha Harris . . . in reply to inquiries addressed by the quarantine commissioners. Transmitted to the Legislature by the governor, March 10, 1858. Albany: C. Van Benthuysen, printer, 1858. 23p. DLC **50-0820**

HARRIS, James C.
An essay on the climate and fevers of the Southwestern, Southern Atlantic, and Gulf States. New Orleans: The Bulletin Book Office, 1858. 32p. DNLM; LNT-M **50-0821**

HARRISON, James S.
Valedictory address to the graduating class of the Indiana Central Medical College. Indianapolis: J. D. Defrees, 1850. 15p. DNLM **50-0822**

HARRY, Samuel H.
Address delivered before the "Chester County Medical Society." West Chester: J. Hodgson, 1851. 8p. DNLM **50-0823**

HARSHA, David A.
The principles of hydropathy, or the invalid's guide to health and happiness; being a plain familiar exposition of the principles of the water-cure system. Albany: E. H. Pease & Co., 1852. 52p. DNLM; N; NHi **50-0824**

HARTMANN, Franz (1796-1853)
Dr. Franz Hartmann's diseases of children and their homoeopathic treatment. Transl. with notes, and prepared for the use of the American and English profession, by Charles J. Hempel, M.D. New York: William Radde, 1853. 516p. DNLM; PPHa **50-0825**

HARTSHORNE, Henry (1823-1897)
On animal decomposition as the chief promotive cause of cholera. Philadelphia: Lindsay & Blakiston, 1855. 12p. DNLM; PPC **50-0826**

HARTSHORNE, Henry (1823-1897)
Valedictory to the graduating class of the Philadelphia College of Medicine. Philadelphia: Inquirer Printing Office, 1856. 21p. DNLM; PPC **50-0827**

HARTSHORNE, Henry (1823-1897)
On the arterial circulation; its physiology and chief pathological relations. Philadelphia: T. K. & P. G. Collins, 1856. 61p. DNLM; PPC; PU **50-0828**

HARTSHORNE, Henry (1823-1897)
An introductory lecture on medical education. Delivered at the Philadelphia College of Medicine. Philadelphia: T. K. & P. G. Collins, 1857. 14p. DNLM; PPC; PU **50-0829**

HARTSHORNE, Henry (1823-1897)
Medical record for private medical statistics. Prepared under the sanction of the Medical Society of the State of Pennsylvania, and of the biological department of the Philadelphia Academy of Natural Sciences. Philadelphia: C. J. Price & Co., 1859. 30 l. DNLM; PPC **50-0830**

HARVARD UNIVERSITY. MEDICAL SCHOOL
An introductory lecture delivered at the Massachusetts Medical College, Nov. 6, 1849. Boston: D. Clapp, 1850. 24p. MBM **50-0831**

HARVARD UNIVERSITY. MEDICAL SCHOOL
Practical views on medical education, submitted to the members of the American Medical Association, by the medical faculty of Harvard University. Boston: D. Clapp, 1850. 7p. DNLM; MH-M **50-0832**

HASKELL, Benjamin
Essays on the physiology of the nervous system, with an appendix on hydrophobia. . . . Gloucester: J. S. E. Rogers, 1856. 87p. DLC **50-0833**

HASKINS, E. B.
On the chemical analysis of the Tennessee collection of urinary calculi. Clarksville: C. O. Faxon, 1855. 24p. 2 plates. DNLM **50-0834**

HASKINS, E. B.
Therapeutic cultivation; its errors and its reformation; an address delivered to the Tennessee Medical Society. Nashville: Cameron & Fall, 1857. 28p. DNLM **50-0835**

HASKINS, E. B.
The subjective and the objective influences of medicine. An address. Nashville, Tenn., 1859. 23p. DNLM **50-0836**

HASSALL, Arthur Hill (1817-1894)
The microscopic anatomy of the human body, in health and disease. . . . With additions to the text and plates, and an introduction, containing instructions in microscopic manipulation, by Henry Van Arsdale. . . . New York: Pratt, Woodford & Co.; [etc., etc.] 1851. 2 v. DLC; MBM; NNNAM; PPC **50-0837**

HASSALL, Arthur Hill (1817-1894)
The microscopic anatomy of the human body, in health and disease. With additions to the text and plates, and an introduction, containing instructions in microscopic manipulation, by Henry Van Arsdale. New York: S. S. & W. Wood, 1855. 2 v. DNLM; NNNAM; PU **50-0838**

HASTINGS, John (1805-1874)
The practice of surgery: embracing minor surgery and the application of dressings, etc. . . . Philadelphia: Lindsay & Blakiston, 1850. 479p. 1 plate. DLC; MBM; PPC; PU **50-0839**

HAYES, Isaac I. (1832-1881)
Observations upon the relations existing between food and the capabilities of men to resist low temperatures. Philadelphia, 1859. 5p. DNLM **50-0840**

HAYES, J. J.
Yellow fever; its prevention and cure. The fever as an epidemic checked in a day or two; as a disease, cured in an hour or two. New Orleans, 1858. 43p. DNLM; LNT-M **50-0841**

HAYES, J. J.
Yellow fever; its prevention and cure. The fever as an epidemic checked in a day or two; as a disease, cured in a hour or two. New Orleans: Rea's Rotary Press, 1858. 17p. DNLM; LNT-M **50-0842**

HAYWARD, George (1791-1863)
Statistics of the amputation of large limbs that have been performed at the Massachusetts General Hospital, from its establishment, to Jan. 1, 1850. . . . Boston: D. Clapp, printer, 1850. 16p. DLC; DNLM; MH-M **50-0843**

HAYWARD, George (1791-1863)
Remarks on the comparative value of the different anaesthetic agents. Boston: D. Clapp, 1850. 11p. DNLM; MH-M **50-0844**

HAYWARD, George (1791-1863)
Cases of vesico-vaginal fistula, treated by operation. Boston: D. Clapp, 1851. 21p. DNLM; MH-M **50-0845**

HAYWARD, George (1791-1863)
Permanent cure of reducible hernia. Philadelphia: T. K. & P. G. Collins, 1852. 25p. DNLM; PPC **50-0846**

HAYWARD, George (1791-1863)
Case of hydrophobia. . . . Boston: Printed by D. Clapp. 1854. 11p. DLC; DNLM; MH-M **50-0847**

HAYWARD, George (1791-1863)
Surgical reports, and miscellaneous papers on medical subjects. . . . Boston: Phillips, Sampson & Co. [etc., etc.], 1855. 452p. DLC; DNLM; MH-M; PU **50-0848**

HEADLAND, Frederick William (1830-1875)
The action of medicines in the system; or, "on the mode in which therapeutic agents introduced into the stomach produce their peculiar effects on the animal economy." Philadelphia: Lindsay & Blakiston, 1853. 560p. DNLM; OCIM; MBM; PPC **50-0849**

HEADLAND, Frederick William (1830-1875)
The action of medicines in the system; or, "on the mode in which therapeutic agents introduced into the stomach produce their peculiar effects on the animal economy." 2nd ed. Philadelphia: Lindsay & Blakiston, 1856. 540p. DLC; MBM; NNNAM; PU **50-0850**

HEADLAND, Frederick William (1830-1875)
The action of medicines in the system; or, "on the mode in which therapeutic agents introduced into the stomach produce their peculiar effects on the animal economy." 3rd ed., revised and enlarged. Philadelphia: Lindsay & Blakiston,1859. 463p. NNNAM; PPC; PU **50-0851**

HEATON, George (1808-1879)
A review of a report of a committee of the American Medical Association on the permanent cure of reducible hernia or rupture. Boston: W. Chadwick, 1853. 31p. DNLM; MBM **50-0852**

HELMUTH, William Sheaff (1801-1880)
Valedictory address delivered at the second annual commencement of the Homoeopathic Medical College of Pennsylvania, March 2, 1850. Philadelphia: Merrihew & Thompson, 1850. 16p. DNLM; PPHa **50-0853**

HELMUTH, William Sheaff (1801-1880)
Introductory lecture to the class of the Homoeopathic Medical College of Pennsylvania. Philadelphia, 1852. 19p. DNLM; PPHa **50-0854**

HELMUTH, William Tod (1833-1902)
Surgery and its adaptation into homoeopathic practice. . . . Illustrated with numerous engravings on wood. Philadelphia: Moss & Brother, 1855. 651p. DLC; DNLM; PPHa; PU **50-0855**

HEMPEL, Charles Julius (1811-1879)
New homoeopathic pharmacopoeia and posology, or the mode of preparing homoeopathic medicines, and the administration of doses. Compiled and translated from the German works of Buchner and Gruner, and the French work of Jahr. With original contributions by . . . New York: William Radde, 1850. 359p. DNLM; NNNAM; PPHa **50-0856**

HEMPEL, Charles Julius (1811-1879)
The homoeopathic domestic physician. 2nd ed. Revised and considerably enlarged by the author. New York: William Radde, 1850. 216p. NNNAM; PPHa **50-0857**

HEMPEL, Charles Julius (1811-1879)
The homoeopathic domestic physician. German ed. New York: William Radde, 1853. 133p. PPHa **50-0858**

HEMPEL, Charles Julius (1811-1879)
Compete repertory of the homoeopathic materia medica. New York: William Radde, 1853. 1224p. NNNAM **50-0859**

HEMPEL, Charles Julius (1811-1879)
Nouvelle Homoeopathie Domestique, avec une Explication Introductoire du principe Homoeopathique, et une Description Detaillée des Remedes, dont on a besoin dans toutes les maladies ordinaires des Hommes, Femmes et Infants, et une indication particuliere des Doses requises dans chaque cas de Maladie. New York: William Radde, 1854. 151p. NNNAM **50-0860**

HEMPEL, Charles Julius (1811-1879)
Organon of specific homoeopathy; or, an inductive exposition of the principles of the homoeopathic healing art; addressed to physicians and intelligent laymen. Philadelphia: Rademacher & Sheek, 1854. 216p. DLC; PPC **50-0861**

HEMPEL, Charles Julius (1811-1879)
An introductory address delivered in the Homoeopathic Medical College of Pennsylvania, October 20, 1857. Philadelphia: King & Baird, 1857. 32p. DNLM; PPHa **50-0862**

HEMPEL, Charles Julius (1811-1879) and Jacob BEAKLEY
Manual of homoeopathic theory and practice; with an elementary treatise on the homoeopathic treatment of surgical diseases. Designed for students and practitioners of medicine, and as a guide for families and an intelligent public generally. New York: William Radde, 1858. 1088p. NNNAM; PPHa **50-0863**

HEMPEL, Charles Julius (1811-1879)
A new and comprehensive system of materia medica and therapeutics; arranged upon a physiologico-pathological basis, for the use of practitioners and students of medicine. New York: William Radde, Jr., 1859. 1202p. NNNAM **50-0864**

HENDERSON, Thomas (1789-1854)
Hints on the medical examination of recruits for the Army, and on the discharge of soldiers from the service on surgeon's certificate. Adapted to the service of the United States. A new ed., revised by Richard H. Coolidge. Philadelphia: J. B. Lippincott & Co., 1856. 211p. DNLM; NNNAM; PPC; PU **50-0865**

HENDERSON, William (1810-1872)
Homoeopathy fairly represented. A reply to Professor Simpson's "Homoeopathy" misrepresented. 1st American from the last Edinburgh ed. Philadelphia: Lindsay & Blakiston. 1854. 302p. DNLM; PPC; PPHa **50-0866**

HENLE, Jakob (1809-1885)
A treatise on general pathology. . . . Transl. from the German, by Henry C. Preston. . . . Philadelphia: Lindsay & Blakiston, 1853. 391p. DLC; OCIM; MBM; PPC **50-0867**

HERING, Constantine (1800-1880)
C. Hering's domestic physician, revised, with additions, from the author's manuscript of the 7th German edition. Containing also a tabular index of the medicines and the diseases in which they are used. 5th American ed. Philadelphia: Rademacher & Sheek, 1851. 515p. DNLM; PPHa **50-0868**

HERING, Constantine (1800-1880)
C. Hering's domestic physician, revised, with additions, from the author's manuscript of the 7th German edition. Containing also a tabular index of the medicines and the diseases in which they are used. 5th American edition. Philadelphia: Rademacher & Sheek, 1851. 515p. DNLM; PPHa **50-0869**

HERING, Constantine (1800-1880)
The voluntary system of medical education. Instituted by the Independent Medical School of Pennsylvania, chartered May 8, 1854. Philadelphia: King & Baird, 1854. 20p. PPHa **50-0870**

HERING, Constantine (1800-1880)
The homoeopathic domestic physician. 6th American edition by the author himself thoroughly revised and reformed from the original, and augmented by numerous additions from the forthcoming 11th German edition. Philadelphia: Ig. Kohler, 1858. 393p. DNLM; PPHa **50-0871**

HERING, Constantine (1800-1880)
The homoeopathic domestic physician. 7th American edition. By the author himself thoroughly revised and reformed from the original, and augmented by numerous additions from the forthcoming 11th German edition. Philadelphia: Ig. Kohler, 1859. 393p. PPHa **50-0872**

HEWSON, Addinell (1828-1889)
On the prominence of the eye-ball, with sinking of the caruncle and semilunar fold following the ordinary operation for strabismus. With an account of a pair of scissors for performing the sub-conjunctival operation. Philadelphia: J. B. Lippincott & Co., 1858. 23p. DNLM; PPC; PU **50-0873**

HILGARD, T. C[harles] (1828-1875)
Contributions to the physiology of sight. Cambridge. Metcalf & Co., 1856. 23p. DNLM; MBM **50-0874**

HILL, Benjamin L[ord] (1813-1871)
Lectures on the American eclectic system of surgery. . . . Cincinnati: W. Phillips & Company, 1850. 671p. DLC; OCIM **50-0875**

HILL, Benjamin L[ord] (1813-1871)
The homoeopathic practice of surgery, together with operative surgery, illustrated by two hundred and forty engravings. By B. L. Hill . . . and Jas. G. Hunt. . . . Cleveland: O. J. B. Cobb & Company, 1855. 431p. DLC; OCIM **50-0876**

HILL, Benjamin L[ord] (1813-1871)
An epitome of the homoeopathic healing art, containing the new discoveries and improvements to the present time; designed for the use of families, for travelers on their journey, and as a pocket companion for the physician. . . . Cleveland, O.: J. Hall; Chicago, Ill.: Halsey & King [1859]. 160p. DLC; OCIM **50-0877**

HISTORY of the yellow fever in New Orleans, during the summer of 1853. A complete and authentic record of that fatal epidemic. By a physician of New Orleans. Philadelphia & St. Louis: C. W. Kenworthy, 1854. 104p. DNLM; LNT-M; PPC **50-0878**

HITCHCOCK, Alfred (1813-1874)
Unwritten studies and duties of the physician. Anniversary address before the Worcester North District Medical Society. Fitchburg: E. & J. F. D. Garfield, 1859. 24p. DNLM **50-0879**

HITCHINGS, D.
Elements of human nature. Utica, N.Y.: De W. C. Grove, printer, 1856. 25p. DNLM **50-0880**

HITCHMAN, William
Consumption; its nature, prevention, and homoeopathic treatment (with illustrations of homoeopathic practice). Philadelphia: W. Radde, 1859. 184p. DNLM; PPHa; PPC **50-0881**

HOBLYN, Richard Dennis (1803-1886)
A dictionary of scientific terms. . . . New York: D. Appleton & Co.; Philadelphia: G. S. Appleton, 1850. 386p. DLC; NNNAM; PPC **50-0882**

HOBLYN, Richard Dennis (1803-1886)
A dictionary of terms used in medicine and the collateral sciences. . . . A new American from the last London ed. Revised, with numerous additions, by Isaac Hays. . . . Philadelphia: Blanchard & Lea, 1855. 522p. DLC; IU-M; MBM; PPC **50-0883**

HODGE, Hugh Lenox (1796-1873)
A valedictory address to the graduates of the University of Pennsylvania, delivered April 6, 1850. . . . Philadelphia: L. R. Bailey, printer, 1850. 24p. DLC; DNLM; PU **50-0884**

HODGE, Hugh Lenox (1796-1873)
On the non-contagious character of puerperal fever; an introductory lecture. Philadelphia: T. K. & P. G. Collins, 1852. 32p. DNLM; PPC **50-0885**

HODGE, Hugh Lenox (1796-1873)
On criminal abortion. A lecture. Philadelphia: T. K. & P. G. Collins, 1854. 20p. DNLM; PPC **50-0886**

HODGEN, John Thompson (1826-1882)
The influence of surroundings; an address delivered at the beginning of the course of lectures in Missouri Medical College. St. Louis: G. Knapp & Co., 1859. 20p. DNLM **50-0887**

HODGES, Richard Manning (1827-1896)
Practical dissections. Cambridge: J. Bartlett, 1858. 254p. MBM **50-0888**

HOLCOMBE, William Henry (1825-1893)
The scientific basis of homoeopathy. . . . Cincinnati: H. W. Derby & Co., 1852. 304p. DNLM; OCIM **50-0889**

HOLCOMBE, William Henry (1825-1893)
Yellow fever and its homoeopathic treatment. . . . New York: W. Radde; Philadelphia: Rademacher & Sheek [etc., etc.], 1856. 71p. DLC; DNLM; NNNAM; PPHa **50-0890**

HOLCOMBE, William Henry (1825-1893)
Nature and limitations of the homoeopathic law. New York: Ludwig, Printer, 1858. 16p. DNLM; NNNAM; PPHa **50-0891**

HOLLAND, Henry (1788-1873)
Medical notes and reflections. From the 3rd London edition. Philadelphia: Blanchard & Lea, 1857. 493p. DNLM; PPC; PU **50-0892**

HOLLICK, Frederick (*b.* 1818)
The marriage guide, or natural history of generation. . . . New York: T. W. Strong, [1850]. 428p. NNNAM
50-0893

HOLLICK, Frederick (*b.* 1818)
A popular treatise on venereal diseases, in all their forms, embracing their history and probable origin; their consequences, both to individuals and to society and the best modes of treating them. Adapted for general use. . . . New York: T. W. Strong [1852]. 413p. DLC; NNNAM
50-0894

HOLLICK, Frederick (*b.* 1818)
The diseases of woman, their causes and cure familiarly explained. . . . 53rd[?] ed., much enl. and improved. New York: T. W. Strong, [1855?]. 466p. 2 col. plates. DLC; NNNAM
50-0895

HOLLICK, Frederick (*b.* 1818)
The male generative organs, in health and disease, from infancy to old age. . . . 120th ed., much enl. and improved. New York: T. W. Strong, [1855]. 467p. 2 col. plates. DLC; NNNAM
50-0896

HOLLINGSWORTH, Samuel L[overing] (1816-1872)
Memoir of Moreton Stillé, M.D., read before the College of Physicians of Philadelphia. Philadelphia: T. K. & P. G. Collins, 1856. 35p. 1 plate. DNLM; PPC **50-0897**

HOLMES, Oliver Wendell (1809-1894)
The benefactors of the Medical School of Harvard University; with a biographical sketch of the late Dr. George Peckman. An introductory lecture delivered at the Massachusetts Medical College, November 7, 1850. . . . Boston: Ticknor, Reed & Fields, 1850. 37p. DLC; MH; MH-M **50-0898**

HOLMES, Oliver Wendell (1809-1894)
Puerperal fever, as a private pestilence. . . . Boston: Ticknor & Fields, 1855. 60p. MB; MBM; MH; MWA [An enlargement of his "The contagiousness of puerperal fever," *New Engl. Quart. J. Med. & Surgery*, I (1842-1843):503-30; probably the rarest of all 19th century medical classics.] **50-0899**

HOLMES, Oliver Wendell (1809-1894)
Valedictory address, delivered to the medical graduates of Harvard University, at the annual commencement, Wednesday, March 10, 1858. . . . Boston: D. Clapp, 1858. 15p. DLC; MH; MH-M **50-0900**

HOLSTON, John G. F. (1809-1874)
Address before the National Medical College on the opening of that institution. Washington: H. Polkinhorn, 1858. 16p. DNLM
50-0901

HOMANS, Charles D[udley] (1826-1886)
A case of hydrophobia. Read before the Boston Society for Medical Observation, March 6, 1854. [Boston, 1854]. 7p. DLC; DNLM; MBM **50-0902**

HOMOEOPATHY exposed, being a review of Dr. Henderson's defense of Hahnemann. . . . [Charleston, S.C., 1855]. 26p. DLC **50-0903**

HOMOEOPATHY; its testimony against itself. Boston: D. Clapp, 1857. 28p. DNLM; MBM **50-0904**

HOOKER, Charles (1799-1863)
Report on the diet of the sick; submitted to the American Medical Association, May, 1855. Philadelphia: T. K. & P. G. Collins, 1855. 48p. DNLM; PPC; PU **50-0905**

HOOKER, Worthington (1806-1867)
. . . Lessons from the history of medical delusions. . . . [Rhode Island Medical Society. Fiske Fund]. New York: Baker & Scribner, 1850. 105p. DNLM; DLC; NNNAM
50-0906

HOOKER, Worthington (1806-1867)
Report of the committee on medical education. Philadelphia: T. K. & P. G. Collins, 1851. 42p. DNLM; PPC
50-0907

HOOKER, Worthington (1806-1867)
Report of the committee on medical education in relation to "demonstrative midwifery." Philadelphia: T. K. & P. G. Collins, 1851. 8p. DNLM; PPC **50-0908**

HOOKER, Worthington (1806-1867)
. . . Homoeopathy: an examination of its doctrines and evidences. . . . [Rhode Island Medical Society. Fiske Fund. Prize dissertation[s] No. XIII. 1851]. New York: C. Scribner, 1851. 146p. DLC; DNLM; NNNAM **50-0909**

HOOKER, Worthington (1806-1867)
. . . Homoeopathy: an examination of its doctrines and evidences. . . . [Rhode Island Medical Society. Fiske Fund. Prize dissertation[s] no. XIV. 1851]. 2nd ed. New York: C. Scribner, 1852. 162p. DLC; NNNAM **50-0910**

HOOKER, Worthington (1806-1867)
The present mental attitude and tendencies of the medical profession. Inaugural address of Worthington Hooker, M.D., a professor of the theory and practice of medicine, in Yale College, delivered in the college chapel, October 2, 1852. New Haven: T. J. Stafford, printer, 1852. 28p. CtY-M; DLC; DNLM; MH-M **50-0911**

HOOKER, Worthington (1806-1867)
The treatment due from the medical profession, to physicians who become homoeopathic practitioners. Norwich, Conn.: J. G. Cooley, 1852. 11p. DNLM **50-0912**

HOOKER, Worthington (1806-1867)
. . . Rational therapeutics; or, The comparative value of different curative means, and the principles of their application. . . . Boston: Printed by J. Wilson & Son, 1857. 70p. DLC; MBM
50-0913

HOOPER, Robert (1773-1835)
A new medical dictionary . . . with the formulas of the principal pharmacopoeias, and valuable practical articles on the treatment of disease. On the basis of Hooper and Grant. . . . By D. Pereira Gardner. . . . New York: Harper & Brothers, 1851. 686p. CtY-M; DLC; NNNAM; PPC
50-0914

HOOPER, Robert (1773-1835)
Hooper's physician vade-mecum; or a manual of the principles and practice of physic. . . . With additions by James Stewart. Philadelphia: E. Barrington & G. D. Haswell, 1853. 533p. DNLM; PPC; PPHa; PPJ **50-0915**

HOOPER, Robert (1773-1835)
Lexicon medicum; or, Medical dictionary. . . . 16th American, from the last London ed., with additions from American authors . . . by Samuel Akerly. . . . New York: Harper & Brothers, 1858. 2 v. in 1. DLC; MBM; NNNAM; PPC
50-0916

HORNER, Gustavus R. B. (1804-1892)
Diseases and injuries of seamen: with remarks on their enlistment, naval hygiene, and the duties of medical officers. . . . Philadelphia: Lippincott, Grambo & Co., 1854. 252p. 4 plates. DLC; PPC; PU **50-0917**

HORNER, William Edmonds (1793-1853)
Medical commencement of the University of Pennsylvania, held on Saturday, April 5, 1851; with a valedictory. 2nd ed. Philadelphia: L. R. Bailey, 1851. 31p. DNLM; PU
50-0918

HORNER, William Edmonds (1793-1853)
Special anatomy and histology. . . . 8th ed. Philadelphia: Blanchard & Lea, 1851. 2 v. CtY-M; DLC; PPC; PU
50-0919

HORNER, William Edmonds (1793-1853)
Introductory lecture. Philadelphia: T. K. & P. G. Collins, 1852. 23p. DNLM; PPC **50-0920**

HORNER, William Edmonds (1793-1853)
The United States dissector: or, Lessons in practical anatomy . . . 5th ed., carefully rev. and entirely remodelled by Henry H. Smith . . . with one hundred and seventy-seven new illustrations. Philadelphia: Lippincott, Grambo & Co.. 1854. 519p. DLC; DNLM; PPC; PU **50-0921**

HORNOR, S. Stockton
The medical student's guide in extracting teeth. With numerous cases in the surgical branch of dentistry. With illustrations. . . . Philadelphia: Lindsay & Blakiston, 1857. 76p. DLC; DNLM; MdU-D; PPC **50-0922**

HORSELL, William
Hydropathy for the people: with plain observations on drugs, diet, water, air, and exercise. With notes and observations, by R. T. Trall, M.D. New York: Fowlers & Wells, 1850. 250p. [Water Cure Library, v. 3] NNNAM; OCIM; OCLloyd; PPC
50-0923

HOSACK, Alexander Eddy (1805-1871)
History of the case of the late John Kearny Rodgers, M.D., addressed to the profession. New York: S. W. Benedict, 1851. 47p. DNLM; NNNAM **50-0924**

HOSMER, William
Appeal to husbands and wives in favor of female physicians. New York: G. Gregory, 1853. 24p. DNLM; NNNAM
50-0925

HOUGH, Lewis Sylvester (1819-1903)
The cholera, physiologically explained; showing its nature, cause, cure and prevention. . . . Philadelphia: Printed at Frankford Herald Office, 1854. 16p. DLC; PPC; PU
50-0926

HOWARD ASSOCIATION OF NEW ORLEANS
Report, with addenda. Epidemic of 1853. New Orleans: Sherman & Wharton, 1853. 28, 36p. DNLM; LNT-M
50-0927

HOWARD ASSOCIATION OF NORFOLK, VIRGINIA
Report to all contributors who gave valuable aid in behalf of the sufferers from epidemic yellow fever during the summer of 1855. Philadelphia: Inquirer Printing Office, 1857. 108p. DNLM; PPC **50-0928**

HOWARD, Henry (1792-1874)
A synopsis of medical jurisprudence, from the latest and best authorities, forming the basis of lectures on the science. 5th ed. Charlottesville: J. Alexander, 1851. 182p. DNLM; ViRA
50-0929

HOWARD, Horton
An improved system of botanic medicine; founded upon correct physiological principles . . . to which is added a treatise on female complaints, midwifery, and the diseases of children. Cincinnati: J. Kost, 1852. 542p. DNLM; MBM; OCIM; OCLloyd **50-0930**

HOWARD, Horton
A treatise on midwifery and the diseases of women and children; adapted to the use of heads of families, and females particularly. . . . To which is added, a brief collection of medical plants, illustrated with plates, describing such remedies as are recommended in the work. Cincinnati: Kost, Bigger & Hart, 1853. 223p. DLC; IEN-M; OCIM; PPC **50-0931**

HOWARD, Horton
Howard's domestic medicine: being a revised edition of Horton Howard's anatomy and physiology, and midwifery, diseases of women and children. Practice of medicine and materia medica. . . . New enl. ed. . . . Three volumes in one. Cincinnati: H. M. Rulison; Philadelphia: D. Rulison, 1859. 989p. plates. DLC; OCIM; PPC; PU **50-0932**

HOWARD, Horton
Dr. Howard's private medical companion, and complete midwife's guide. . . . Cincinnati: H. M. Rulison [1859]. 15, 17p. DLC; OCIM **50-0933**

HOWE, Samuel Gridley (1801-1870)
Dr. Howe's report on idiocy, 1850. Massachusetts, Senate, No. 38. [Boston, 1850]. 72p. DNLM; MBM
50-0934

HOWE, Samuel Gridley (1801-1870)
A letter to the governor of Massachusetts upon his veto of a bill providing for an increase of State beneficiaries at the School for Idiotic Children. Boston: Ticknor & Fields, 1857. 24p. DNLM; MBM; MWA **50-0935**

HUBBARD, George H[arris] (1823-1876)
An address delivered before the graduating class at the Dartmouth Medical College. Manchester, N.H.: Fisk & Gage, 1857. 14p. DNLM; Nh **50-0936**

HUBBARD, George H[arris] (1823-1876)
Report of the committee on surgery [to New Hampshire Medical Society, 1857]. [1858.] 15p. DNLM; Nh
50-0937

HUBBARD, Silas
Chart of phrenology, and the phrenological developments of ——— as given by ———. [Form.] Buffalo: G. Reese & Co., 1852. 15p. DNLM **50-0938**

HUBBARD, Silas
Theories of the production of males and females. [Buffalo, 1854?] 7p. DNLM **50-0939**

HUDSON, A. S.
Lecture introductory to the course on materia medica and therapeutics in the medical department of the Iowa State University. Keokuk, 1851. 11p. DNLM
50-0940

HUDSON, William N.
An anti-calomel lecture; being the substance of an address, written by appointment of the Medical Association of Meigs County, Ohio. . . . Pomeroy, O., 1854. 14p. DNLM; OCIM
50-0941

HUFF, Gershom
Electro-physiology: a scientific, popular, and practical treatise on the prevention, causes, and cure of disease; or, Electricity as a curative agent, supported by theory and fact. . . . 2nd ed. . . . New York: D. Appleton & Company [etc.], 1853. 385p. DLC; NNNAM **50-0942**

HUGHES, J. C[lokey] (1821-1881)
Introductory address at the opening of the session of 1852-1853, of the College of Physicians and Surgeons of the Iowa University. Keokuk, 1852. 13p. DNLM **50-0943**

HUGHES, J. C[lokey] (1821-1881)
Reply to a certain document published by John F. Sanford, exposing his base falsehoods and dark designs against the medical department of Iowa State University. [1855?] 24p. DNLM **50-0944**

HUMPHREYS, Frederick (1816-1900)
Homoeopathic treatment of diseases of the sexual system, being a complete repertory of all the symptoms occurring in the sexual system of the male and female; adapted to the use of physicians and laymen; translated, arranged and edited, with additions and improvements, by F. Humphreys, M.D. New York: William Radde, 1850. 144p. PPHa; NNNAM
50-0945

HUMPHREYS, Frederick (1816-1900)
The materia medica. An address delivered before the Central New York Homoeopathic Society, at Syracuse, at its second semi-annual meeting, June 3, 1851. Published by vote of the Society. Utica, N.Y.: H. H. Curtis, printer, 1851. 19p. PPHa; NNNAM **50-0946**

HUMPHREYS, Frederick (1816-1900)
Introductory lecture to the class of the Homoeopathic Medical College of Pennsylvania, delivered October 12, 1853. Published by the class. Philadelphia, 1853. 16p. PPHa
50-0947

HUMPHREYS, Frederick (1816-1900)
Dysentery and its homoeopathic treatment. Containing also a repertory and numerous cases. New York: William Radde, 1853. 87p. DNLM; PPHa; NNNAM **50-0948**

HUMPHREYS, Frederick (1816-1900)
Humphreys' manual of specific homoeopathy for the administration of medicine and cure of disease. Auburn, N.Y. 1856. 148p. PPHa **50-0949**

HUMPHREYS, Frederick (1816-1900)
Humphreys' manual of specific homoeopathy for the administration of medicine and cure of disease. New York: Humphreys Specific Homoeopathic Medicine Co., 1858. 148p. PPHa [There have been ten revised editions. The first editions were from 10,000 to 20,000 annually. For ten years the issue has been from 500,000 to 2,500,000 annually. The present rate of issue is 3,000,000 per annum; of this book 15,000,000 copies have been distributed in the English, German, French, Spanish, and Portuguese languages, of which about 12,000,000 have been distributed in the United States. Bradford, p. 167, *Homoeopathic Bibliography* (1892).] **50-0950**

HUMPHREYS, Frederick (1816-1900)
Manual of specific homoeopathy, for the administration of medicine and cure of disease. . . . New York: J. A. Gray, printer, 1859. 106p. DLC; NNNAM **50-0951**

HUNT, Ezra Mundy (1830-1894)
A physician's counsels to his professional brethren. By a practicing physician. Philadelphia: Presbyterian Board of Publication [1859]. 103p. DLC; PPrHi; PPC
50-0952

HUNT, Sanford B. (1825-1884)
Report of the committee on the hygrometrical state of the atmosphere in various localities, and its influence on health. Philadelphia: T. K. & P. G. Collins, 1855. 22p. DNLM; PPC
50-0953

HUNT, Sanford B. (1825-1884)
Medical policy. Valedictory charge to the graduates in medicine of the University of Buffalo. Buffalo: Thomas & Lathrops, 1855. 15p. DNLM **50-0954**

HUNTER, John (1728-1793)
A treatise on the venereal disease. . . . With copious additions, by Dr. Philip Ricord. . . . Ed., with notes, by Freeman J. Bumstead. . . . Philadelphia: Blanchard & Lea, 1853. 520p. 8 plates. DLC; DNLM; PPC; PU **50-0955**

HUNTER, John (1728-1793)
A treatise on the venereal disease. . . . With copious additions, by Dr. Philip Ricord. . . . Transl. and ed., with notes, by Freeman J. Bumstead. . . . 2nd ed., rev., containing a résumé of Ricord's recent lectures on chancre. Philadelphia: Blanchard & Lea, 1859. 552p. 8 plates. DLC; MBM; PPC; PU
50-0956

HUNTT, Henry (1792-1838)
A visit to the Red Sulphur Springs of Virginia, during the summer of 1837; with observations on the waters. Philadelphia: W. S. Young, 1853. 16p. DNLM; PPC
50-0957

HUSSEY, Zimri
Brief instructions in the use of the perfect adjuster. Cincinnati: Marshall & Langtry, 1854. 20p. DNLM; OCIM
50-0958

HUSTON, Robert Mendenhall (1795-1864)
Introductory lecture delivered in Jefferson Medical College of Philadelphia. Philadelphia: T. K. & P. G. Collins, 1850. 16p. DNLM; PPJ **50-0959**

HUSTON, Robert Mendenhall (1795-1864)
Lecture introductory to the course of materia medica and general therapeutics, in the Jefferson Medical College of Philadelphia. Philadelphia: T. K. & P. G. Collins, 1852. 20p. DNLM; PPJ **50-0960**

HUSTON, Robert Mendenhall (1795-1864)
Reminiscences of Great Britain in the summer of 1855. A lecture introductory to the course of materia medica and general therapeutics, in the Jefferson Medical College of Philadelphia. Philadelphia: J. M. Wilson, 1855, 16p. DNLM; PPJ **50-0961**

HUSTON, Robert Mendenhall (1795-1864)
Charge to the graduates of Jefferson Medical College of Philadelphia, delivered at the public commencement, March 8, 1856. With a list of the graduates. Published by the graduating class. Philadelphia: J. M. Wilson, 1856. 16p. PPJ **50-0962**

HUTCHINSON, David
What are the causes of that disease, incident to pregnancy and lactation, characterized by inflammation and ulceration of the mouth and fauces, usually accompanied by anorexia, emaciation, and diarrhoea; and what is the best mode of treatment. Fiske Fund Prize Essay. Philadelphia, 1857. 18p. DNLM; PPC; PU **50-0963**

HUTCHISON, Joseph Chrisman (1827-1887)
Vaccination and the causes of prevalence of small-pox, in New York in 1853-1854. New York: Holman, Gray & Co., 1854. 18p. DNLM; NNNAM **50-0964**

HUTCHISON, Joseph Chrisman (1827-1887)
History and observations on Asiatic cholera in Brooklyn, N.Y., in 1854. . . . New York: Holman, Gray & Co., printers, 1855. 24p. DLC; NNNAM **50-0965**

HUTCHISON, Joseph Chrisman (1827-1887)
Brooklyn City Hospital. [Cases]. Reported by Robert O. Butler. [Brooklyn, 1857.] 7p. DNLM; NBM **50-0966**

HUTCHISON, Joseph Chrisman (1827-1887)
The Brooklyn City Hospital in 1858, and the address by . . . , one of the attending surgeons. Delivered at the inauguration of the Pathological Hall, on the 25th of November, 1858. Brooklyn: J. Van Anden, 1859. 38p. 1 plate. DNLM; NBM **50-0967**

HYDE, Frederick (1807-1887)
Address to the graduates of Geneva Medical College. New York: E. F. Gould, 1856. 15p. DNLM; NNNAM **50-0968**

THE INVALID's own book; a collection of recipes from various books and various countries by the Honourable Lady [Mary Anne] Cust. New York: D. Appleton & Co., 1853. 144p. DNLM; NNNAM **50-0969**

ISAACS, Charles Edward (1811-1860)
On the extent of the pleura above the clavicle. [New York?, 1857.] 19p. DNLM; NNNAM **50-0970**

IVES, Charles L. (1831-1879)
A sketch of human embryology. New Haven, 1858. 14p. CtY-M; DNLM **50-0971**

JACKSON, James, Sr. (1777-1867)
Letters to a young physician just entering upon practice. . . . Boston: Phillips, Sampson & Company; New York: J. C. Derby, 1855. 344p. DLC; NNNAM; PPC; PU **50-0972**

JACKSON, James C[aleb] (1811?-1895)
Hints on the reproductive organs; their diseases, causes, and cure on hydropathic principles. New York: Fowlers & Wells, 1853. 48p. DNLM; NNNAM **50-0973**

JACKSON, John Barnard Swett (1806-1878)
Address on morbid anatomy, delivered before the Massachusetts Medical Society. Boston: J. Wilson & Son, 1853. 32p. DNLM; MBM **50-0974**

JACKSON, Samuel (1787-1872)
An introductory lecture preliminary to a course on the institutes of medicine. Philadelphia, 1850. 20p. DNLM; PPC; PU **50-0975**

JACKSON, Samuel (1787-1872)
A review of the memorial of Dr. John Bell, to the trustees of the University of Pennsylvania. Philadelphia: S. Mifflin, 1850. 24p. DNLM; PPC; PU **50-0976**

JACKSON, Samuel (1787-1872)
Lecture introductory to the course on the institutes of medicine in the University of Pennsylvania. . . . Published by the class. Philadelphia: Merrihew & Thompson, printers, 1851. 32p. DLC; DNLM; PPC; PU **50-0977**

JACKSON, Samuel (1787-1872)
The organizing of the American Medical Association. Read before the Philadelphia County Medical Society, Feb., 1852, by the president, Samuel Jackson. . . . Philadelphia: The Society, 1852. 11p. DLC; DNLM; PPC **50-0978**

JACKSON, Samuel (1787-1872)
The annual discourse before the Philadelphia County Medical Society. Philadelphia: Published by the Society, 1852. 23p. DNLM; PPC **50-0979**

JACKSON, Samuel (1787-1872)
Medical commencement of the University of Pennsylvania . . . with a valedictory. Philadelphia: L. R. Bailey, 1852. 31p. DNLM; PPC; PU **50-0980**

JACKSON, Samuel (1787-1872)
Memoir of Isaac Parrish, M.D., read to the College of Physicians of Philadelphia. February 2, 1853. . . . Written and printed by order of the College. Philadelphia: T. K. & P. G. Collins, printers, 1853. 27p. DLC; DNLM; PPC **50-0981**

JACKSON, Samuel (1787-1872)
Medical education: The annual discourse before the Philadelphia County Medical Society. Delivered December 29, 1852. Philadelphia: T. K. & P. G. Collins, 1853. 32p. DNLM; PPC; PU **50-0982**

JACKSON, Samuel (1787-1872)
A discourse commemorative of the late William E. Horner, M.D., professor of anatomy. Delivered before the faculty and students of the University of Pennsylvania, October 10, 1853. . . . Published by the class. Philadelphia: T. K. & P. G. Collins, printers, 1853. 46p. DLC; DNLM; PPC **50-0983**

JACKSON, Samuel (1787-1872)
A discourse commemorative of Nathaniel Chapman, M.D., late professor of the theory and practice of medicine and of clinical medicine. Delivered before the trustees, the medical faculty, and students of the University of Pennsylvania. . . . October 13, 1854. Philadelphia: T. K. & P. G. Collins, printers, 1854. 28p. DLC; DNLM; PPC; PU **50-0984**

JACKSON, Samuel (1787-1872)
Introductory lecture to the course of the institutes of medicine in the University of Pennsylvania. Philadelphia: Published by the Class, 1855. 25p. DNLM; PPC; PU **50-0985**

JACKSON, Samuel (1787-1872)
On the fundamental laws of the organic molecular action of the animal organism, identical with those of rational mechanics. An introductory lecture. Philadelphia: T. K. & P. G. Collins, 1856. 20p. DNLM; PU **50-0986**

JACKSON, Samuel (1787-1872)
Introductory lecture to the course on the institutes of medicine. Philadelphia: Published by the Class, 1859. 29p. DNLM; PU **50-0987**

JAHR, Gottlieb Heinrich Georg (1800-1875)
New homoeopathic pharmacopoeia and posology, or the mode of preparing homoeopathic medicines, and the administration of doses. Compiled and transl. from the German works of Buchner, Gruner, and the French work of Jahr, by Charles J. Hempel, M.D., with original contributions. New York: William Radde, 1850. 359p. NNNAM; PPHa **50-0988**

JAHR, Gottlieb Heinrich Georg (1800-1875)
Alphabetical repertory of the skin symptoms and external alterations of substance, together with the morbid phenomena observed in the glandular, osseous, mucous and circulatory systems, arranged with pathological remarks on the diseases of the skin. Edited by C. J. Hempel, M.D. New York: William Radde, 1850. 515p. DNLM; NNNAM; PPHa **50-0989**

JAHR, Gottlieb Heinrich Georg (1800-1875)
Jahr's clinical guide or pocket repertory. For the treatment of acute and chronic diseases. Transl. and edited, with annotations, by Charles J. Hempel, M.D. New York: William Radde, 1850. 409p. DNLM; NNNAM; PPHa **50-0990**

JAHR, Gottlieb Heinrich Georg (1800-1875)
Jahr's new manual of homoeopathic medicine. Edited, with annotations, by A. Gerald Hull. Repertory. 3rd American, from the 4th, or Paris edition. New York: William Radde, 1850. 837p. PPHa **50-0991**

JAHR, Gottlieb Heinrich Georg (1800-1875)
Jahr's new manual of homoeopathic medicine. Symptomatology. 3rd American edition. New York: William Radde, 1851. 1025p. NNNAM; PPHa **50-0992**

JAHR, Gottlieb Heinrich Georg (1800-1875)
Jahr's and Possart's new manual of the homoeopathic materia medica, with Possart's additions, arranged with reference to well authenticated observations at the sick-bed; and accompanied by an alphabetical repertory, to facilitate and secure the selection of a suitable remedy in any given case. 4th edition, revised and enlarged by the author. Transl. and edited by Chas. J. Hempel, M.D. New York: William Radde, 1853. 923p. NNNAM; PPHa **50-0993**

JAHR, Gottlieb Heinrich Georg (1800-1875)
Nervous derangements and mental diseases; being the fifth volume of Hartmann's Therapie. Transl. by Charles J. Hempel, M.D. New York: William Radde, 1856. 400p. DNLM; NNNAM **50-0994**

JAHR, Gottlieb Heinrich Georg (1800-1875)
The homoeopathic treatment of diseases of females, and infants at the breast. Transl. from the French, by Charles J. Hempel, M.D. Philadelphia: Rademacher & Sheek, 1856. 422p. DNLM; NNNAM; PPHa **50-0995**

JAHR, Gottlieb Heinrich Georg (1800-1875)
Jahr's new manual of the homoeopathic materia medica, with Possart's additions; arranged with reference to well authenticated observations at the sick-bed, and accompanied by an alphabetical repertory, to facilitate and secure the selection of a suitable remedy in any given case. 5th ed., revised and enlarged by the author. Transl. and edited by Chas. J. Hempel, M.D. Symptomatology and repertory. New York: William Radde, 1859. 923p. NNNAM; PPHa **50-0996**

JAMESON, Horatio Gates (1778-1855)
A treatise on epidemic cholera. Philadelphia: Lindsay & Blakiston, 1855. 286p. CU-M; DNLM; NNNAM; PPC **50-0997**

JARVIS, Edward (1803-1884)
On the comparative liability of males and females to insanity, and their comparative curability and mortality when insane. . . . Utica, N.Y.: State Lunatic Asylum, 1850. 22p. DLC; MBM; NNNAM **50-0998**

JARVIS, Edward (1803-1884)
Primary physiology, for schools. Philadelphia: Thomas Cowperthwait & Co., 1850. 168p. CtY-M; DNLM; PPC: PU **50-0999**

JARVIS, Edward (1803-1884)
On the causes of insanity. . . . [1851.] 17p. DLC **50-1000**

JARVIS, Edward (1803-1884)
On the supposed increase of insanity. . . . [Utica: W. Saunderson, printer, 1852]. 36p. DLC **50-1001**

JARVIS, Edward (1803-1884)
Practical physiology; or, Anatomy and physiology applied to health. . . . Rev. ed. . . . Philadelphia: Thomas Cowperthwait & Co.; New York: G. F. Cooledge & Bro.; [etc., etc.], 1852. 427p. DLC; MBM; NNNAM; PPC **50-1002**

JARVIS, Edward (1803-1884)
Memoir of the life and character of George Cheyne Shattuck. Read before the American Statistical Association, April 12, 1854. [1854.] 7p. DNLM **50-1003**

JARVIS, Edward (1803-1884)
Insanity and idiocy in Massachusetts. . . . Report of the Commission on Lunacy. . . . Boston: Wright & Potter, printers, 1855. 313p. DLC; DNLM; MBM; OCHP **50-1004**

JARVIS, Edward (1803-1884)
Address delivered at the laying of the corner stone of the insane hospital at Northampton, Massachusetts. . . . Northampton, [Mass.]: Printed by J. & L. Metcalf, 1856. 39p. DLC **50-1005**

JARVIS, Edward (1803-1884)
Criminal insane; insane transgressors and insane convicts. Utica: S. H. Sankey, 1857. 39p. DLC
50-1006

JARVIS, Edward (1803-1884)
Tendency of misdirected education and the unbalanced mind to produce insanity. [1858.] 11 l. DLC; DNLM
50-1007

JARVIS, Edward (1803-1884)
The law of insanity, and hospitals for the insane in Massachusetts. Boston: G. C. Rand & Avery, 1859. 24p. DNLM; MH-M
50-1008

JARVIS, George Ogelvie (1795-1875)
Lectures on fractures and dislocations. Explaining new modes of treatment, founded on anatomy, physiology, and the laws of mechanics; together with concise instructions in the use of the adjuster. . . . 9th ed. New Haven: Printed by J. H. Benham, 1852. 67p. CtY-M; DLC; MBM **50-1009**

JEFFERSON MEDICAL COLLEGE. PHILADELPHIA
A catalogue of all the graduates from 1826 to 1856. With announcement for 1856-1857. Philadelphia: T. K. & P. G. Collins, 1856. 32p. DNLM; PPJ **50-1010**

JENKINS, J. Foster (1826-1882)
Puerperal mania, has it connection with toxaemia? Yonkers, N.Y., 1857. 7p. DNLM **50-1011**

JENKINS, J. Foster (1826-1882)
Report on spontaneous umbilical hemorrhage of the newly-born. Philadelphia: T. K. & P. G. Collins, 1858. 58p. DNLM; PPC **50-1012**

JENNINGS, Isaac
The philosophy of human life; with especial design to develop the true idea of disease. . . . Cleveland, O.: Jewett, Proctor & Worthington; Boston: J. P. Jewett & Company, 1852. 276p. DLC; MBM; OCIM; PU **50-1013**

JENNINGS, Thomas Reed (1805-1874)
An introductory lecture, delivered before the class of the medical department of the University of Nashville, October 30, 1854. . . . Nashville: Cameron & Fall, book and job printers, 1854. 39p. DLC; OCIM **50-1014**

JENNINGS, Thomas Reed (1805-1874)
Valedictory address to the graduates of the medical department of the University of Nashville, delivered February 28, 1857. . . . Published by request of the faculty and the class. Nashville, Tenn., 1857. 43p. DLC; OCIM
50-1015

JEWELL, Wilson (1800-1867)
Report of the committee of the Northern Medical Association of Philadelphia on public hygiene. Philadelphia, [1851]. 18p. DNLM; PPC **50-1016**

JEWELL, Wilson (1800-1867)
Yellow or malignant bilious fever in the vicinity of South Street wharf, Philadelphia, 1853. With an appendix. Philadelphia: T. K. & P. G. Collins, 1853. 40p. 1 map. DNLM; PPC; PU **50-1017**

JEWELL, Wilson (1800-1867)
Historical sketches of quarantine. Address delivered before the Philadelphia County Medical Society. Philadelphia: T. K. & P. G. Collins, 1857. 32p. DNLM; PPC; PU
50-1018

JOHNS, Montgomery (1830?-1871)
A clinical phrase book; in English and German, containing the usual questions & answers employed in examining and prescribing for patients . . . with an English-German and German-English pronouncing lexicon . . . grammatical appendix, table of idioms, &c. . . . Philadelphia: Lindsay & Blakiston, 1853. 308p. DLC; NNNAM; PPC; PU **50-1019**

JOHNSON, Alexander Bryan (1786-1867)
The physiology of the senses; or, how and what we see, hear, taste, feel, and smell. New York: Derby & Jackson, 1856. 214p. DNLM; MH; NN; NNC **50-1020**

JOHNSON, Charles Earl (1812-1876)
An address before the Medical Society of North Carolina at its second annual meeting. Raleigh, N.C.: S. Gales, 1851. 32p. DNLM; NcD **50-1021**

JOHNSON, Charles Earl (1812-1876)
An address before the Medical Society of North Carolina. . . . Raleigh: Southern Weekly Post, 1854. 70p. DNLM; NcU
50-1022

JOHNSON, Edward (1785-1862)
Life, health, and disease. New York: J. Wiley, 1850. 172p. DNLM; NNNAM **50-1023**

JOHNSON, Edward (1785-1862)
The theory and principles of hydropathy shown to be in strict accordance with the most recent discoveries of science. . . . New York: Fowler & Wells, 1854. 181p. DNLM; NNNAM
50-1024

JOHNSON, Edward (1785-1862)
The domestic practice of hydropathy. . . . With a form of a report for the assistance of patients in consulting their physician by correspondence. New York: Fowler & Wells, 1854. 467p. DNLM; NNNAM **50-1025**

JOHNSON, Isaac D. (1827-1911)
A lecture on homoeopathy. New London, Pa.: Crushfield, Printer, 1856. 15p. PPHa; PU **50-1026**

JOHNSON, James (1777-1845)
The economy of health; or, the stream of human life, from the cradle to the grave. . . . New York: Harper & Bros., 1858. 283p. DNLM; NN; NNC; NNNAM **50-1027**

JOHNSON, John George
On intra-capsular fractures of the cervix femoris. College of Physicians and Surgeons, University of the State of New York. New York: Miller & Holman, 1857. 32p. DNLM; NNNAM
50-1028

JOHNSTON, Christopher (1822-1891)
Oration before the Medical and Surgical Society of Baltimore, at their third anniversary, January 18, 1858. Baltimore: D. Toy, 1858. 19p. DNLM; MdU-D; MdBJ-W
50-1029

JOHNSTON, William Patrick (1811-1876)
Valedictory address to the graduating class of the National Medical College. Washington: Gideon & Co., 1850. 16p. DNLM **50-1030**

JONES, Charles Handfield (1819-1890)
A manual of pathological anatomy. By C. Handfield Jones . . . and Edward H. Sieveking. . . . 1st American ed., rev. Philadelphia: Blanchard & Lea, 1854. 733p. DLC; PPC; PPJ; PU **50-1031**

JONES, Elijah U[tley] (1826-1893)
Dry cough; or, tussis sicca. Philadelphia: Rademacher & Sheek. New York; William Radde, 1854. 16p. NNNAM; PPHa **50-1032**

JONES, H[enry] J.
The chrono-thermal manual; containing a list of the doses of the principal medicines both mineral and vegetable; and most of the latest pharmaceutical preparations; also, the Latin, French, German and English nomenclature. . . . Louisville, Ky.: Printed at the "Varieties" office, 1851. 19p. DLC; OCIM **50-1033**

JONES, Ichabod Gibson (1807-1857)
The American eclectic practice of medicine. To which are appended the posthumous writings of T. V. Morrow. Cincinnati: Moore, Anderson & Co., 1853-4. 2 v. DNLM; OCIM **50-1034**

JONES, Ichabod Gibson (1807-1857)
The American eclectic practice of medicine. Revised by William Sherwood. Cincinnati: Moore, Wilstach, Keys & Co., 1857-8. 2 v. DNLM; OCIM **50-1035**

JONES, John W.
An address delivered at the opening exercises of the Atlanta Medical College on the 7th of May, 1855. Atlanta, Ga.: C. R. Hanleiter & Co., 1855. 15p. DNLM; GU **50-1036**

JONES, Joseph (1833-1896)
Abstract of experiments upon the physical influences exerted by living, organic and inorganic membranes upon chemical substances, passing through them by endosmose. Philadelphia: Merrihew & Thompson, 1855. 8p. 1 plate. DNLM; PPC **50-1037**

JONES, Joseph (1833-1896)
Investigations, chemical and physiological, relative to certain American vertebrata. Washington: Smithsonian Institution, 1856. 137p. DNLM; PU **50-1038**

JONES, Joseph (1833-1896)
. . . Case of diabetes mellitus. Treated by Joseph Jones . . . [Augusta, Ga., 1858]. 25p. DLC; GU **50-1039**

JONES, Joseph (1833-1896)
Observations on some of the physical, chemical, physiological and pathological phenomena of malarial fever. . . . Philadelphia: T. K. & P. G. Collins, Printer, 1859. 419p. DLC; PPC; PU **50-1040**

JONES, Lorenzo E.
Introductory lecture, delivered in the hall of the Eclectic Medical Institute. Cincinnati: J. A. & U. P. James. 1850. 16p. DNLM; OCIM **50-1041**

JONES, Lorenzo E., and A. H. BALDRIDGE
An exposition of the character of Prof. J. R. Buchanan, in reply to his defamatory attack upon L. E. Jones. [1853.] 24p. DNLM; OCIM **50-1042**

JONES, Lorenzo E.
The American eclectic materia medica and therapeutics. By L. E. Jones . . . and John M. Scudder. . . . Cincinnati: Moore, Wilstach, Keys & Co., printers, 1858. 311p. DLC; OCLloyd; OCIM **50-1043**

JONES, Thomas Wharton (1808-1891)
The principles and practice of ophthalmic medicine and surgery. . . . With one hundred and ten illustrations. 2nd American ed., with additions, from the 2nd and rev. London ed. Philadelphia: Blanchard & Lea, 1856. 500p. 4 plates. DLC; DNLM; PPC; PU **50-1044**

JONES, Thomas Wharton (1808-1891)
Defects of sight and hearing; their nature, causes, prevention, and general management. Edited, with additions, by Laurence Turnbull. Philadelphia: C. J. Price & Co., 1859. 247p. DNLM; PPC; PPJ; PU **50-1045**

JORDAN, J[ohnson] H.
Anatomy, physiology, and the laws of health. . . . Cincinnati: Moore, Wilstach, Keys & Co.; St. Louis and Chicago: J. H. Jordan & Co., 1857. 88p. DLC; ICRM; OCIM **50-1046**

JOSLIN, Benjamin Franklin (1796-1861)
Principles of homoeopathy. In a series of five lectures. New York: William Radde, 1850. 185p. NNNAM; PPHa **50-1047**

JOSLIN, Benjamin Franklin (1796-1861)
Discovery of curatives by observation. An address delivered in the Assembly Chamber, Albany, before the Homoeopathic Medical Society of the State of New York, at its annual meeting, February 8, 1853. Albany: J. Munsell, 1853. 24p. PPHa **50-1048**

JOSLIN, Benjamin Franklin (1796-1861)
Homoeopathic treatment of epidemic cholera. 3rd edition, with additions. New York: William Radde, 1854. 252p. NNNAM; PPHa **50-1049**

JOSLIN, Benjamin Franklin (1796-1861)
The character of Hahnemann. An address. Philadelphia: King & Baird, 1855. 8p. PPHa; PPC **50-1050**

JOSLIN, Benjamin Franklin (1796-1861)
Letter to the homoeopathic physicians of the United States. [New York, 1855.] 7p. DNLM; PPHa **50-1051**

KANE, John K. (1795-1858)
An obituary notice of the late Robert Maskell Patterson. [Philadelphia, 1855.] 12p. DNLM **50-1052**

KELLEY, J. Clawson (1793?-1863)
The analytical system of medicine, or the treatment of disease according to the principles and requirements of nature. New York: J. P. Prall, 1854. 120p. DNLM; NNNAM **50-1053**

KELLEY, J. Clawson (1793?-1863)
History and practical illustrations of the foundation and progress of the analytical system of medicine, embracing a memoir of the author. New York, 1858. 66p. DNLM; NNNAM
50-1054

KELLOGG A. O[tis] (1818-1888)
The physical tendencies of medical science. [1858.] 12p. DNLM **50-1055**

KEMP, William Miller (1814-1886)
Obstetrical notes, based on 1,000 cases of delivery. Read at the annual session of "The medical and chirurgical faculty of Maryland," in June, 1859, as the report of the Committee on obstetrics. . . . [New York, 1859.] 51p. DLC; DNLM; MdBM; NNNAM **50-1056**

KENDALL, George W.
"American dental patents." A vindication of the truth of certain articles in the American Journal of Dental Science, entitled a "Sketch of American dental patents," and a refutation of the charges made against them, by the "Dental Register." Cincinnati, 1854. 26p. DNLM **50-1057**

KENNEDY, Alfred L. (1818-1896)
Practical chemistry, a branch of medical education; considered in a brief letter to his class. Philadelphia: B. Mifflin, 1852. 11p. DNLM; PPC; PPL; PU **50-1058**

KENNEDY, Duncan (1809-1887)
A clergyman's idea of a model physician. An address delivered at the commencement of the Albany Medical College. Albany: Munsell & Rowland, 1858. 24p. DNLM
50-1059

KING, Daniel (1791-1864)
Quackery unmasked; or, a consideration of the most prominent empirical schemes of the present time, with an enumeration of some of the causes which contribute to their support. Boston: D. Clapp, 1858. 334p. DNLM; MBM
50-1060

KING, Edward
Glimpses of an improved medical philosophy. Philadelphia: J. Harding, 1850. 32p. DNLM; PPC **50-1061**

KING, John (1813-1893)
An introductory lecture, delivered before the eclectic medical class, Nov. 10, 1852. Cincinnati: Eclectic Med. Publ. Office, 1852. 15p. DNLM; OCIM **50-1062**

KING, John (1813-1893)
The American eclectic dispensatory. . . . Cincinnati: Moore, Wilstach & Keys, 1852. 708p. OCIM; OCLloyd; NNNAM; PU
50-1063

KING, John (1813-1893)
The American eclectic dispensatory. . . . Cincinnati: Moore, Wilstach & Keys, 1854. 1391p. DLC; OCLloyd
50-1064

KING, John (1813-1893)
Introductory lecture. [Cincinnati, 1854?] 15p. DNLM
50-1065

KING, John (1813-1893)
American eclectic obstetrics. . . . Cincinnati: Moore, Wilstach, Keys & Co., 1855. 741p. DLC; IU-M; OCIM; PPC
50-1066

KING, John (1813-1893)
Table of urinary deposits, with their microscopical and medical tests, for clinical examinations. Cincinnati: C. F. O'Driscoll, [1855]. 1 sheet. DNLM **50-1067**

KING, John (1813-1893)
The American eclectic dispensatory. 3rd ed. Cincinnati: Moore, Wilstach, Keys & Co., 1856. 1391p. DNLM; OCLloyd; PU
50-1068

KING, John (1813-1893)
The American eclectic dispensatory. . . . 4th ed. Cincinnati: Moore, Wilstach, Keys & Co., 1857. 1391p. DNLM; OCLloyd; PPC **50-1069**

KING, John (1813-1893)
The American family physician; or, Domestic guide to health. For the use of physicians, families, plantations, ships, travelers, etc. . . . Cincinnati: Longely Brothers, 1857. 798p. DLC; NNNAM; OCIM; PPC **50-1070**

KING, John (1813-1893)
Women: their diseases and their treatment. . . . Cincinnati: Longley Brothers, 1858. 366p. DLC; ICRM; IEN-M; OCIM
50-1071

KING, John (1813-1893)
The American dispensatory. . . . 5th ed., rev. and enl. from "The American eclectic dispensatory." Cincinnati: Moore, Wilstach, Keys & Co., 1859. 1475p. DLC; OCLloyd; PU
50-1072

KING, John (1813-1893)
The microscopist's companion; a popular manual of practical microscopy. . . . To which is added a glossary of the principal terms used in microscopic science. . . . Cincinnati: Rickey, Mallory & Co., 1859. 308p. DLC; DNLM; OCIM; PPC
50-1073

KINLOCH, R[obert] A[lexander] (1826-1891)
A brief description of the yellow fever, as it prevailed at Mt. Pleasant and in Charleston harbor during the summer of 1857. Charleston: Walker, Evans & Co., 1858. 34p. DNLM; ScCM
50-1074

KINNE, William W.
Magneto-electricity, or electro-magnetism, medically applied for the cure of disease. Designed to accompany Kinne's magneto-electric and electro-magnetic machine. . . . New York: Printed by B. R. Barlow, 1852. 112p. DLC; DNLM; NNNAM **50-1075**

KIRBY, Stephen R[eynolds] (1801-1876)
Inaugural address delivered before the Hahnemann Academy of Medicine, January 8, 1851. New York, 1851. 9p. DNLM; NNNAM **50-1076**

KIRBY, Stephen R[eynolds] (1801-1876)
An address on homoeopathia, delivered in the Assembly Room, Baltimore, Md., on Wednesday evening, May 19, 1852. Published by order of the American Institute of Homoeopathy. New York: Angell, Engel & Hewitt, 1852. 16p. DNLM; NNNAM; PPHa **50-1077**

[KIRKBRIDE, Thomas Story] (1809-1883)
Letter to the regents of the South Carolina Hospital for the insane. Philadelphia: T. K. & P. G. Collins, printers, 1854. 8p. DLC; PPC **50-1078**

KIRKBRIDE, Thomas Story (1809-1883)
On the construction, organization, and general arrangements of hospitals for the insane. . . . Philadelphia: Lindsay & Blakiston, 1854. 80p. DLC; PPC; PU; ViRA
50-1079

KIRKES, William Senhouse (1823-1864)
Manual of physiology. By William Senhouse Kirkes . . . assisted by James Paget. . . . 2nd American, from the 2nd London ed. With one hundred and sixty-five illustrations. Philadelphia: Blanchard & Lea, 1853. 568p. DLC; MBM; NNNAM; PPC
50-1080

KIRKES, William Senhouse (1823-1864)
Manual of physiology. . . . A new and rev. American, from the last London ed. With two hundred illustrations. Philadelphia: Blanchard & Lea, 1857. 584p. DLC; MdBJ-W; NNNAM; PPC
50-1081

KNAPP, C. S.
A short essay on the teeth; showing the value and importance of these organs, and their effects upon the constitution, when diseased; with directions for their proper management, in order to secure sound and healthy teeth, or restore them to health and usefulness when decayed. Jackson, Miss.: Dobson & Dickey, 1851. 32p. DNLM **50-1082**

KNAPP, Moses L. (1799-1879)
Discovery of the cause, nature, cure and prevention of epidemic cholera. . . . Cincinnati: H. W. Derby, 1855. 48p. DLC; OCIM **50-1083**

KNAPP, Moses L. (1799-1879)
Essay on cholera infantum. . . . Cincinnati: H. W. Derby, 1855. 96p. DLC; OCIM **50-1084**

KNAPP, Moses L. (1799-1879)
Inquiry into the cause and nature of nursing sore mouth. Philadelphia: Robb, Pile & McElroy, 1856. 312p. DNLM; PPC; PU **50-1085**

KNAPP, Moses L. (1799-1879)
Researches on primary pathology and the origin and laws of epidemics, deducing from the phenomena observed . . . the inane cause, scorbutic nature, and essential unity of disease. Philadelphia, 1857-1858. 2 v. DNLM; PPC; PU
50-1086

KNIGHT, Jonathan (1789-1864)
A lecture, introductory to the course of lectures in the medical institution of Yale College. New Haven: W. H. Stanley, 1853. 19p. CtY-M; DNLM **50-1087**

KNOWLES, F.
The duties of the medical student. Introductory address, on the commencement of the session of the medical department of the Iowa State University, for the year 1854-1855. Keokuk: Daily Whig, 1854. 20p. DNLM **50-1088**

KNOX, Robert (1791-1862)
The races of men; a fragment. Philadelphia: Lea & Blanchard, 1850. 323p. DNLM; ICU; MH; NN **50-1089**

KOST, J[ohn] (1819-1904)
The elements of materia medica and therapeutics, adapted to the American reformed and eclectic practice. . . . New ed. rev. and enl. Cincinnati: Moore, Wilstach, Keys & Co., 1858. 829p. DLC; IU-M; OCIM; OCLloyd **50-1090**

KOST, John (1819-1904)
Domestic medicine. A treatise on the practice of medicine, adapted to the reformed system, comprising a materia medica, with numerous illustrations. Cincinnati: J. W. Sewell, 1859. 624p. DNLM; IEN-M; OCIM; PPC **50-1091**

KREUSSLER, Emilius
The homoeopathic treatment of acute and chronic diseases. Transl. from the German, with important additions and revisions. Philadelphia: Rademacher & Sheek, 1854. 190p. PPHa **50-1092**

LAFON, Thomas (1802-1876)
Review of the homoeopathic controversy. Delivered before the Homoeopathic Medical Society of the State of New Jersey, March 4, 1856. Newark, N.J.: A. S. Holbrook, 1856. 24p. PPHa **50-1093**

LALLEMAND, Claude François (1790-1854)
A practical treatise on the causes, symptoms, and treatment of spermatorrhoea, Transl. and edited by Henry J. McDougall. 2nd American ed. Philadelphia: Blanchard & Lea, 1853. 328p. DNLM; MBM; NNNAM; PPC **50-1094**

LAMB, John Ferguson (1791-1869)
The annual address before the Philadelphia County Medical Society. Philadelphia: T. K. & P. G. Collins, 1854. 16p. DNLM; PPC **50-1095**

LAMBE, William (1765-1847)
Water and vegetable diet in consumption, scrofula, cancer, asthma, and other chronic diseases. . . . With notes and additions by John Shew. Fowler & Wells, 1850. 258p. DNLM; NNNAM **50-1096**

LAMBERT, Thomas Scott (1819-1897)
Popular anatomy and physiology, adapted to the use of students and general readers. New York: Leavitt & Co., 1850. 408p. 5 col. plates. DNLM; NNNAM **50-1097**

LAMBERT, Thomas Scott (1819-1897)
Practical anatomy, physiology, and pathology: hygiene and therapeutics. . . . Portland: Sanborn & Carter; New York: Leavitt & Co., 1851. 257p. 5 col. plates. DLC; MBM; NNNAM
50-1098

LAMBERT, Thomas Scott (1819-1897)
Human anatomy, physiology and hygiene. . . . Hartford: Brockett, Hutchinson & Co.; New York: Ivison & Phinney; [etc., etc.], 1854. 456p. 8 plates. CtY-M; DLC; NNNAM
50-1099

LA ROCHE, René (1795-1872)
Pneumonia: its supposed connection, pathological and etiological, with autumnal fevers; including an inquiry into the existence and morbid agency of malaria. . . . Philadelphia: Blanchard & Lea, 1854. 502p. DLC; DNLM; PPC; PU **50-1100**

LA ROCHE, René (1795-1872)
Yellow fever, considered in its historical, pathological, etiological and therapeutical relations. Including a sketch of the disease as it has occurred in Philadelphia from 1699 to 1854. . . . Philadelphia: Blanchard & Lea, 1855. 2 v. CtY-M; DLC; DNLM; PPC **50-1101**

LA ROCHE, René (1795-1872)
An address delivered before the Medical Society of the State of Pennsylvania. Philadelphia: T. K. & P. G. Collins, 1857. 51p. DNLM; PPC **50-1102**

LATTA, Samuel Arminius (1804-1852)
The cholera in Cincinnati: or a connected view of the controversy between the homoeopathists and the Methodist expositor. Also, a review of the report read before the Homoeopathic Association. Cincinnati: Morgan & Overend, printers, 1850. 40p. DLC; OCIM **50-1103**

LAURIE, Joseph (*d.* 1865)
Homoeopathic domestic medicine. . . . Arranged as a practical work for students. Containing a glossary of medical terms. 6th American ed., enl. and improved. By A. Gerald Hull, M.D. New York: W. Radde; Philadelphia: Rademacher & Sheek; [etc., etc.], 1850. 568p. DLC; NNNAM; PPHa **50-1104**

LAURIE, Joseph (*d.* 1865)
Elements of homoeopathic practice of physic. An appendix to Dr. A. G. Hull's Laurie's homoeopathic domestic medicine, arranged as a practical work for students. Containing also the diseases of the urinary and genital organs. New York: William Radde, 1850. 372p. NNNAM; PPHa **50-1105**

LAURIE, Joseph (*d.* 1865)
Elements of homoeopathic practice of physic, by Dr. J. Laurie, with additions by A. G. Hull, M.D., and an appendix on intermittent fever, by Dr. Douglas, of Milwaukee. New York: William Radde, 1852. 939p. PPHa **50-1106**

LAURIE, Joseph (*d.* 1865)
Elements of homoeopathic practice of physic. 1st American from the 2nd London edition. Philadelphia: Matthew & Houard, 1852. 642p. PPC; PPHa **50-1107**

LAURIE, Joseph (*d.* 1865)
Elements of homoeopathic practice of physic. 2nd American edition, enlarged and improved, by A. Gerald Hull, M.D., and an appendix on intermittent fever, by J. S. Douglas, A.M., M.D. New York: William Radde, 1853. 939p. PPC; PPHa **50-1108**

LAURIE, Joseph (*d.* 1865)
The parent's guide; containing the diseases of infancy and childhood and their homoeopathic treatment, to which is added a treatise on the method of rearing children from their earliest infancy; comprising the essential branches of moral and physical education. Edited, with additions, by W. Williamson, M.D. Philadelphia: Rademacher & Sheek, 1854. 458p. DLC; PPC; PPHa **50-1109**

LAWRENCE WATER-CURE, Brattleboro, Vt.
Prospectus of the opening of the Lawrence water-cure, May 15, 1853; containing a few remarks on the general effects of the water treatment on healthy and disordered bodies; also, a description of the establishment, with its rules and regulations. New York: Curran, Dinsmore & Co., 1853. 20p. DNLM; NNNAM **50-1110**

LAWRENCE, William (1783-1867)
A treatise on the diseases of the eye. . . . A new ed. Edited, with numerous additions, and two hundred and forty-three illustrations, by Isaac Hays. . . . Philadelphia: Blanchard & Lea, 1854. 948p. DLC; PPC; PPJ; PU **50-1111**

[LAWRENCE, William Richards]
A history of the Boston Dispensary. Boston: J. Wilson & Sons, 1859. 244p. DNLM; MBM **50-1112**

LAWSON, Leonidas Merion (1812-1864)
The incentives, means, and rewards of study; an introductory address delivered at the opening of the thirty-third annual course of lectures in the Medical College of Ohio, Nov. 1, 1852. Cincinnati: Published by the Class, 1852. 31p. DLC; DNLM; OCIM **50-1113**

LAWSON, Leonidas Merion (1812-1864)
An introductory lecture delivered at the opening of the thirty-eighth course of lectures in the Medical College of Ohio. Cincinnati: Wrightson & Co., 1857. 22p. DNLM; OCIM **50-1114**

LAWTON, A. G.
The science of medicine and the science of life and theory of disease, comprising a condensed view of the theory of disease and the application of remedies and medical hygiene. La Salle, Ill.: Kirkpatrick & Bowen, 1857. 64p. DNLM **50-1115**

LAYCOCK, Thomas (1812-1876)
Lectures on the principles and methods of medical observation and research, for the use of advanced students and junior practitioners. . . . Philadelphia: Blanchard & Lea, 1857. 200p. DLC; DNLM; PPC; PU **50-1116**

LAZARUS, M. Edgeworth
The human trinity; or three aspects of life: the passional, the intellectual, the practical sphere. New York: Fowler & Wells, 1851. 141p. DNLM; NN; NNC **50-1117**

LAZARUS, M. Edgeworth
Homoeopathy; a theoretic demonstration, with social applications. New York: William Radde, 1851. 69p. DNLM; NNNAM; PPHa **50-1118**

LAZARUS, M. Edgeworth
Passional hygiene and natural medicine; embracing the harmonies of man with his planet. New York: Fowler & Wells, 1852. 436p. DNLM; NNNAM **50-1119**

LAZARUS, M. Edgeworth
Involuntary seminal losses; their causes, effects, and cure. New York: Fowler & Wells, 1852. 96p. DNLM; NNNAM **50-1120**

LEA, John
Cholera, with reference to the geological theory: a proximate cause, a law by which it is governed, a prophylactic. Cincinnati: Wright, Ferris & Co., 1850. 25p. DNLM; OCIM **50-1121**

LEA, John
Cholera: the geological theory. Cincinnati, 1851. 7p. DNLM; OCIM **50-1122**

LEE, Charles Alfred (1801-1872)
Address to the graduating class of Geneva Medical College. Geneva: S. H. Parker, 1852. 24p. DNLM **50-1123**

LEE, Charles Alfred (1801-1872)
Homoeopathy; an introductory address to the students of Starling Medical College. Columbus, Ohio, 1853. 40p. OCIM PPHa **50-1124**

LEE, Edwin (*d.* 1870)
Hydropathy and homoeopathy impartially appreciated. With an appendix of notes illustrative of the influence of the mind over the body. 2nd ed. from the 3rd London ed. Cincinnati: W. Phillips & Co., 1851. 46p. DNLM; PPHa
50-1125

LEE, Edwin (*d.* 1870)
Homoeopathy impartially appreciated, with an appendix of notes illustrative of the influence of the mind on the body. . . . 2nd American, from the 3rd London ed. Cincinnati: W. Phillips & Co., 1851. 40p. DLC; OCIM **50-1126**

LEE, Edwin
The effects of climate on tuberculous disease. [Fiske Fund Prize Essay.] Philadelphia: Blanchard & Lea, 1857. 73p. CtY-M; DNLM; PPC; PU **50-1127**

LEE, James
Diseases of Saratoga County. Albany: C. Van Benthuysen, 1859. 27p. DNLM **50-1128**

LEE, Samuel H. P.
Remaks on the stone and gravel in the kidneys and bladder, with the account of the discovery of a solvent remedy, now used with universal success, and commonly known as Dr. Lee's gravel specific. 7th ed. New York, 1852. 48p. DNLM
50-1129

LEE, William (1778-1863)
The use of brandy and salt, as a remedy for inflammation, illustrated and explained by the discoverer. Boston: C. C. P. Moody, 1851. 35p. DNLM; MBM; MWA
50-1130

LEEDS, G. F.
A new and important discovery. The quinine substitute, or nerve tonic, a certain remedy for fever and ague, etc., and preventive of bilious, Chagres, Panama, and yellow fevers. New York: G. F. Nesbitt & Co., 1858. 15p. DNLM; NNNAM
50-1131

LEHMANN, Carolus Gotthelf (1812-1863)
Physiological chemistry. Transl. from the 2nd ed. by George E. Day. Edited by R. E. Rodgers. Philadelphia: Blanchard & Lea, 1856. 2 v. CtY-M; DNLM; IEN-M; PPC
50-1132

LEHMANN, Carolus Gotthelf (1812-1863)
Manual of chemical physiology. . . . Trans. with notes and additions by J. Cheston Morris, with an introductory essay on vital force by Samuel Jackson. Philadelphia: Blanchard & Lea, 1856. 331p. DNLM; PPC; PU; ViRA
50-1133

LEIDY, Joseph (1823-1891)
Lecture introductory to the course of anatomy in the University of Pennsylvania. Philadelphia: T. K. & P. G. Collins, 1853. 22p. DNLM; PU **50-1134**

LEIDY, Joseph (1823-1891)
Valedictory address to the class of medical graduates of the University of Pennsylvania, delivered at the public commencement, March 27th, 1858. . . . Philadelphia: T. K. & P. G. Collins, 1858. 32p. DLC; PU **50-1135**

LEIDY, Joseph (1823-1891)
Introductory lecture to the course on anatomy. Philadelphia, 1859. 23p. DNLM; PU **50-1136**

LEIDY, Joseph (1823-1891)
Lecture introductory to the course of anatomy in the University of Pennsylvania. Philadelphia: T. K. & P. G. Collins, 1859. 20p. DNLM; PU **50-1137**

LEIGH, E[dwin] (1815-1890)
Respiration subservient to nutrition. [Harvard.] Boston: Ticknor, Reed & Fields, 1853. 20p. DNLM; MH-M
50-1138

LEIGH, E[dwin] (1815-1890)
The philosophy of medical science, considered with special reference to Dr. Elisha Bartlett's "Essay on the philosophy of medical science." (Boylston Prize Essay, 1849.) Boston: Ticknor, Reed & Fields, 1853. 23p. DNLM; MBM
50-1139

LENTE, Frederick Divoux (1823-1883)
A statistical account of the fractures of the skull, occurring in the New York Hospital, during the twelve years elapsing between the first of January, 1839, and the first of April, 1851. New York: Van Norden & Amerman, 1852. 38p. DNLM; NNNAM **50-1140**

A LETTER to clergymen on the perservation of health and the use of Peruvian syrup, or protected solution of protoxide of iron combined as a medicinal agent. Boston: N. L. Clark & Co., [1859]. 48p. DNLM; MBM **50-1141**

LIEBIG, Justus von (1803-1873)
Familiar letters on chemistry, and its relations to commerce, physiology, and agriculture. Edited by John Gardner. New York: Fowler & Wells, 1850. 54p. DNLM; NNNAM; ViRA
50-1142

LIEBIG, Justus von (1803-1873)
Researches on the motion of the juices in the animal body; and the effect of evaporation in plants. Together with an account of the origin of the potato-disease; with full and ingenious directions for the protection and entire prevention of the potato-plant against all diseases. Edited from the manuscript of the author, by William Gregory. Philadelphia: T. B. Peterson, [1850]. 47p. DNLM; PPC; PU
50-1143

LINDSLEY, John Berrien (1822-1897)
An address on the life and character of Robert M. Porter, M.D., late professor of anatomy in the University of Nashville. . . . Delivered at Nashville, Nov. 8, 1856. Pub. by the class. Nashville, Tenn.: Printed by E. Vallette, 1856. 47p. DLC; OCIM **50-1144**

LINDSLEY, John Berrien (1822-1897)
An address on the lfe and character of Robert M. Porter, M.D., late professor of anatomy in the University of Nashville. . . . Delivered at Nashville, Nov. 8, 1856. Pub. by the class. Nashville, Tenn.: E. Vallette, 1857. 52p. DNLM; OCIM
50-1145

LINDSLEY, John Berrien (1822-1897)
On medical colleges. An introductory lecture, to the course of 1858-59, in the medical department of the University of Nashville. . . . Pub. by the class. Nashville: Printed by J. T. Bell & Co., 1858. 32p. DLC; OCIM **50-1146**

LINDSLY, Harvey (1804-1889)
Address. From the minutes of the twelfth annual meeting of the American Medical Association. Philadelphia: Collins, 1859. 12p. DNLM; PPC; PU **50-1147**

LINTON, Moses L. (1808-1872)
The outlines of general pathology. St. Louis: Republican Office, 1851. 205p. DNLM **50-1148**

LINTON, Moses L. (1808-1872)
The unity of mankind. An introductory lecture delivered before the class of the medical department of the St. Louis University. St. Louis: Missouri Democrat Office, [1855]. 26p. DNLM **50-1149**

LINTON, Moses L. (1808-1872)
Medical science and common sense. A lecture introductory to the session 1858-1859 of the St. Louis Medical College. St. Louis: G. Knapp & Co., 1858. 29p. DNLM **50-1150**

LINTON, Moses L. (1808-1872)
Medical science and common sense. A lecture introductory to the session 1858-1859 of the St. Louis Medical College. 2nd ed., revised. St. Louis: Knapp & Co., 1859. 28p. DNLM **50-1151**

LIPPE, Adolph (1812-1888)
Key to the materia medica; or, Comparative pharmacodynamic. . . . Philadelphia: H. Duffield; New York: J. T. S. Smith; [etc., etc.], 1854. 144p. DLC; NNNAM; PPC **50-1152**

LITTELL, Squire, Jr. (1803-1886)
On the influence of electrical fluctuations as a cause of disease. [1857?] 27p. DNLM **50-1153**

LITTON, Abram (1814-1901)
An address to the graduates of the medical department of the St. Louis University. St. Louis: Missouri Republican, 1851. 18p. DNLM **50-1154**

LIVEZEY, Abraham (1821-1896) and J. Emerson KENT
A new compendium of the principles and practice of medicine. New York: J. S. Redfield, 1853. 239p. DNLM; MBM; NNNAM; PU **50-1155**

LIVINGSTON, C. E.
A treatise on displacement of the womb, with suggestions for treatment. Toledo, O.: The B. F. Wade Co. [1852?] 20p. DNLM **50-1156**

LIZARS, John (1878?-1860)
Anatomy of the brain, from the celebrated dissections of John Lizars . . . comprising fifteen engravings (colored after nature) with accompanying explanations. Ed. by Landon Rives. Cincinnati: H. W. Derby, 1854. 2 p. 15 col. plates. DLC; OCIM; NNNAM; PPC **50-1157**

LIZARS, John (1787?-1860)
The use and abuse of tobacco. From the 8th Edinburgh ed. Philadelphia: Lindsay & Blakiston, 1859. 138p. DNLM; PPC; PU **50-1158**

LOCHRANE, O. A.
An address delivered before the Southern Reform Medical Association at their annual meeting in Macon, March 2, 1858. Macon, Ga.: Telegraph Press, 1858. 16p. DNLM; GU **50-1159**

LOGAN, Joseph P[ayne] (1820-1891)
Address introductory to the fifth course of lectures in Atlanta Medical College. Atlanta: J. L. Miller & Co., 1859. 30p. DNLM; GU **50-1160**

LONGSHORE, Joseph Skelton (1809-1879)
An introductory lecture delivered before the class, at the opening of the Female Medical College of Pennsylvania, Oct. 12, 1850. Philadelphia: J. Young, 1850. 28p. DNLM; PPC; PU **50-1161**

LONGSHORE, Joseph Skelton (1809-1879)
A valedictory address . . . at the first annual commencement of the Female Medical College of Pennsylvania, Dec. 30, 1851. Philadelphia, 1852. 14p. DNLM; PPC **50-1162**

LONGSHORE, Joseph Skelton (1809-1879)
The practical importance of female medical education; an introductory lecture. Philadelphia, 1853. 15p. DNLM; PPC; PU **50-1163**

LONGSHORE, Joseph Skelton (1809-1879)
Medical institution for women. A letter to the ladies of the United States, on the medical education of women. Broadside. [Philadelphia, 1854] DNLM **50-1164**

LONGSHORE, Joseph Skelton (1809-1879)
Valedictory address to the graduating classes of Penn Medical University of Philadelphia, delivered May 30, 1857, with announcement and catalogue for 1857-1858. Philadelphia: M. P. Williams & Co., 1857. 32p. DNLM; PPC; PU **50-1165**

LOOMIS, I. M.
Lobelia; being a refutation of the many falsehoods uttered and published respecting the poisonous and deleterious properties of that valuable plant. Macon: B. F. Griffin, [1855]. 3p. DNLM; GU **50-1166**

LORD, John Chase (1805-1877)
Medical science and materialism. A discourse delivered before the faculty and students of the Buffalo Medical College on Sabbath, the 12th February, 1854. . . . Published by request. Buffalo: Jewett, Thomas & Co., printers, 1854. 29p. DLC; DNLM **50-1167**

LOVET, H. T.
Treatise on the human hair; with particular reference to greyness and baldness, giving the origin of, and remedies for, these common complaints, with special directions for the preservation of the color, health, and beauty of the hair to old age. New York, 1851. 23p. DNLM; NNNAM **50-1168**

LUDLAM, Reuben (1831-1899)
On the relations of general pathology to homoeopathic therapeutics. Read before the Chicago Homoeopathic Medical Society. New York: H. Ludwig, 1858. 17p. NNNAM; PPHa **50-1169**

LUDLAM, Reuben (1831-1899)
On the sources and benefits of professional earnestness; being an address delivered in Jacksonville, November 2, 1859, before the Illinois Homoeopathic Medical Association. Chicago: Halsey & King, 1859. 15p. PPHa **50-1170**

LUDLOW, John Livingston (1819-1888)
Reply to a pamphlet entitled "Correction of the erroneous statements of Henry H. Smith, M.D., published in the Medical Examiner, January, 1855, in relation to a case of gastrotomy which occurred in the practice of Washington L. Atlee." Philadelphia: T. K. & P. G. Collins, 1855. 22p. DNLM; PPC **50-1171**

LUDLOW, John Livingston (1819-1888)
A manual of examinations upon anatomy, physiology, surgery, practice of medicine, chemistry, obstetrics, materia medica, pharmacy, and therapeutics. . . . To which is added, a medical formulary. . . . A new ed., thoroughly rev. and much enl. With three hundred and seventy illustrations. Philadelphia: Blanchard & Lea, 1857. 816p. DLC; PPF; PPC; PU
50-1172

LYMAN, George
A discourse commemorative of the life and religious experience of the late David S. C. H. Smith, M.D., of Providence, R.I. Worcester: E. R. Fiske, 1859. 23p. DNLM; MB; MH
50-1173

LYMAN, George H[inckley] (1819-1891)
Non-malignant diseases of the uterus. An essay which obtained the Boylston prize for 1854. Boston: Ticknor & Fields, 1854. 76p. DNLM; MBM **50-1174**

LYMAN, George H[inckley] (1819-1891)
The history and statistics of ovariotomy, and the circumstances under which the operation may be regarded as safe and expedient. Boston: J. Wilson & Son, 1856. 146p. DNLM; MBM **50-1175**

MABEY, Jerome A.
What is homoeopathy? Its position defined and contrasted with allopathy. A lecture. Albany, N.Y.: Munsell & Rowland, 1858. 31p. PPHa **50-1176**

McCALL, John (1787-1867)
[Progress in medicine.] Communications presented by . . . at the annual meeting of the society, held in February, 1853. [Albany, 1853.] 11p. DNLM **50-1177**

McCALL, John (1787-1867)
Needs, duties, and privileges of the medical profession. [Albany, 1855.] 12p. DNLM **50-1178**

McCLINTOCK, James (1809-1881)
Introductory lecture to the winter course of instruction in the Philadelphia College of Medicine, delivered on Monday at 5 o'clock p.m., October 14, 1850. . . . Published by the class. Philadelphia: Hughes & Gaskill, printers, 1850. 15p. DLC; DNLM; PPC; PU **50-1179**

McCOY, E. Halley
Inhalation a valuable remedy for pulmonary diseases, including laryngitis, or clergyman's sore throat, bronchitis, asthma, pulmonary irritation, and incipient consumption. New Philadelphia, O.: Tuscarawas Advocate Office, 1854. 32p. DNLM
50-1180

McCREADY, Benjamin William (1813-1892)
A lecture introductory to the course on materia medica and pharmacy; for the term of 1850-51. [College of Pharmacy of the City of New York] . . . . Published by the College. New York: B. R. Barlow, printer, 1850. 16p. DLC; NNNAM
50-1181

McCREADY, Benjamin William (1813-1892)
Memoir of John A. Swett, M.D. . . . Read before the New York Medical and Surgical Society, and published by its order. New York: D. Appleton & Company, 1855. 36p. DLC; DNLM; NNNAM **50-1182**

McDOWELL, Joseph Nash (1803-1868)
An address delivered on laying the corner stone of the medical department of Kemper College, St. Louis . . . and the valedictory charge to the class of graduates in 1854, by John Barnes. St. Louis, 1854. 30p. DNLM **50-1183**

McDOWELL, Joseph Nash (1803-1868)
[Valedictory address, before the graduating class of the medical department of the University of the State of Missouri, of the session of 1855-1856.] [St. Louis, 1856.] 15p. DNLM
50-1184

[MACKALL, Louis] (1802-1876)
Oak Hill Cemetery, or, A treatise on the fatal effects resulting from the location of cemeteries in the immediate vicinity of towns. By a physician. Washington: Printed by H. Polkinhorn, 1850. 24p. DLC **50-1185**

MACKALL, Louis (1802-1876)
Notes on Carpenter's human physiology, containing some original views of the economy of nature. Washington: Gideon & Co., 1852. 127p. DNLM; MBM; OCIM; PPC
50-1186

MACKALL, Louis (1802-1876)
An essay on the life in nature. Washington: H. Polkinhorn, 1855. 12p. DNLM **50-1187**

MACKALL, Louis (1802-1876)
An essay on the law of muscular action. Washington, D.C.: H. Polkinhorn, 1859. 23p. 2 plates. DNLM
50-1188

MACKENZIE, William (1791-1868)
A practical treatise on the diseases of the eye. . . . To which is prefixed, an anatomical introduction explanatory of a horizontal section of the human eyeball. By Thomas Wharton Jones. . . . From the 4th rev. and enl. London ed. With notes and additions, by Addinell Hewson. Philadelphia: Blanchard & Lea, 1855. 1027p. 2 plates. DLC; DNLM; NNNAM; PPC
50-1189

MACKIE, Andrew (1794-1871)
Medical education. Address read at annual meeting of the Massachusetts Medical Society, May 20, 1850. [1850?] 36p. MBM **50-1190**

MACLEAN, George Macintosh
Elements of somatology; a treatise on the general properties of matter. New York: J. Wiley, 1859. 124p. DNLM; ICU; MH; NN **50-1191**

MACLISE, Joseph
Surgical anatomy. Philadelphia: Lea & Blanchard, 1859. 156p. 68 plates. DNLM; ICRM; PPC; NNNAM
50-1192

McNEIL, A.
Treatise on the cure of consumption at the North. New York: J. Egbert, 1859. 14p. DNLM; NNNAM
50-1193

McPHEETERS, William M[arcellus] (1815-1905)
The legitimate goal of professional ambition. An address. St. Louis: M. Niedner, 1853. 16p. DNLM
50-1194

McQUILLEN, John Hugh (1826-1879)
Valedictory address delivered before the graduating class of the Pennsylvania College of Dental Surgery. Philadelphia: J. H. Jones & Co., 1859. 12p. DNLM; PPC; PU
50-1195

McSHERRY, Richard (1817-1885)
A lecture on gunshot wounds; prepared to be read before Prof. Dunbar's private class. Baltimore: J. Murphy & Co., 1852. 28p. DNLM; MdU-D **50-1196**

McVICKAR, John Augustus (1812-1892)
The social position of medicine. An inaugural address, delivered before the "Hahnemann Academy of Medicine," January 20, 1853. New York: Angell, Engel & Hewitt, 1853. 18p. DNLM; NNNAM; PPHa **50-1197**

McWHINNIE, Andrew Melville (1808-1866)
Malformation of the bladder. Account of the history and dissection of a case of malformation of the urinary bladder. [With an additional case of congenital inversion of the bladder, reported by Dr. Chas. A. Pope.] [Boston, 1854.] 12p. DNLM; MBM **50-1198**

MADDEN, Henry Ridewood
Uterine diseases, with an appendix, containing an abstract of 180 cases of uterine diseases and their treatment, together with analytical tables of results, ages, symptoms, etc., to which is added a clinical record of interesting cases, treated in the Manchester Homoeopathic Hospital. . . . New York: W. Radde; Philadelphia: Rademacher & Sheek; [etc., etc., 1852]. 111p. DLC; NNNAM; PPHa; PPC **50-1199**

MADDOCK, Alfred Beaumont
Pulmonary consumption, bronchitis, asthma, chronic cough, and various diseases of the lungs, air-passages, throat, and larynx, successfully treated by medicated inhalations. Illustrated with cases. With notes and additions by Charles Greene. Philadelphia: C. W. Vanhorn & Co., 1855. 146p. DNLM; PPC; PPJ; PU **50-1200**

MALAN, H. V. (1817-1879)
The family guide to the administration of homoeopathic remedies. New York: William Radde, 1852. 112p. NNNAM; PPHa **50-1201**

MALAN, H. V. (1817-1879)
Family guide to the administration of homoeopathic remedies. Philadelphia: Boericke & Tafel, 1852. 112p. PPC; PPHa
50-1202

MALGAIGNE, Joseph François (1806-1865)
Operative surgery, based on normal and pathological anatomy. . . . Transl. from the French, by Frederick Brittan. Philadelphia: Blanchard & Lea, 1851. 565p. DLC; DNLM; MBM; PPC
50-1203

MALGAIGNE, J[oseph] F[rançois] (1806-1865)
A treatise on fractures. . . . Transl. from the French, with notes and additions, by John H. Packard. Philadelphia: J. B. Lippincott & Co., 1859. 683p. 16 plates. DLC; DNLM; NNNAM; PPC **50-1204**

MANSFIELD, Edward D[eering] (1801-1880)
Memoirs of the life and services of Daniel Drake, M.D., physician, professor, and author; with notices of the early settlement of Cincinnati, and some of its pioneer citizens. Cincinnati: Applegate & Co., 1855. 408p. DNLM; OCHP; OCIM; PP
50-1205

MANSON, Otis Frederick (1822-1888)
Pneumonia cut short. [Richmond, 1859.] 7p. DNLM; ViRA
50-1206

MARCH, Alden (1795-1869)
On coxalgia, or hip disease. Philadelphia: T. K. & P. G. Collins, 1853. 31p. DNLM; PPC **50-1207**

MARCH, Alden (1795-1869)
Paper read before the Medical Society of the State of New York, on, first, penetrating wounds of the abdomen, with punctured wound of the intestines; and, second, penetrating wounds of the larynx, and their treatment, with cases for illustration. Albany: C. Van Benthuysen, 1854. 15p. DNLM
50-1208

MARCH, Alden (1795-1869)
Improved forceps for hare-lip operation, and fatal result of an operation for the removal of a tumor from the neck. 1855. 19p. DNLM **50-1209**

MARCH, Alden (1795-1869)
Encysted osseous tumors, or a thin secreting membranous cyst, developed on cancellous structure of bone and surrounded by a thin bony wall. Albany: Van Benthuysen, 1856. 18p. 1 plate. DNLM **50-1210**

MARCH, Alden (1795-1869)
Semi-centennial address delivered before the Medical Society of the State of New York. Albany: C. Van Benthuysen, 1857. 20p. DNLM **50-1211**

MARCH, Alden (1795-1869)
On intra-capsular fracture of cervix femoris with bony union; and an interesting case of urinary calculi. . . . Albany: Van Benthuysen, printer, 1858. 26p. DLC
50-1212

MARCY, Erastus Edgerton (1815-1900)
The homoeopathic theory and practice of medicine. "Similia Similibus Curantur." New York: William Radde, 1850. 631p. NNNAM; PPHa **50-1213**

MARCY, Erastus Edgerton (1815-1900)
Homoeopathy and allopathy. Reply to "An Examination of the Doctrines and Evidences of Homoepathy, by Worthington Hooker, M.D." New York: William Radde, 1852. 144p. MBM; PPHa **50-1214**

MARSH, Seymour N.
Rupture and its radical cure; with a full description of the parts involved. Also, of falling of the womb, varicocele, enlarged veins of the legs, piles, curved spine, spermatorrhea or nocturnal emissions from self-abuse, and its cure by pressure. New York: Marsh & Co., 1853. 63p. DNLM; NNNAM
50-1215

MARSH, Seymour N.
. . . Rupture and its radical cure: with a full description of the parts involved, also, of falling of the womb, varicocele, enlarged veins of the legs, piles, curved spine, bow-legs, club-feet, and other deformities. . . . New York and Cincinnati, O.: Marsh and Company, 1855. 72p. plates. DLC; OCIM; NNNAM
50-1216

MARSH, W. R.
Medical department of the Iowa State University. Introductory address. Keokuk, Iowa: Daily Post, 1856. 19p. DNLM
50-1217

MARTIN, Henry Austin (1824-1884)
Bretonneau and Husband's method of preserving and using fluid vaccine lymph. Roxbury, 1859. 4p. DNLM
50-1218

MARYLAND. MEDICAL AND CHIRURGICAL FACULTY
Catalogue of books belonging to the library of the medical and chirurgical faculty, of Maryland. Baltimore: J. W. Woods, 1852. 66p. DLC; MdBM **50-1219**

MARYLAND. MEDICAL AND CHIRURGICAL FACULTY
Report of the committee [W. Chew Van Bibber, Chas. O'Donovan, and G. Morgan] upon obstetrics, June, 1855. Baltimore: J. Lucas & Sons, 1855. 33p. DNLM; MdBM
50-1220

MARYLAND. MEDICAL AND CHIRURGICAL FACULTY
Report on the progress of medical chemistry. Read June 8, 1855, by Lewis H. Steiner, chariman of committee on chemistry. Baltimore: J. Lucas & Son, 1855. 27p. DNLM; MdBM
50-1221

[MASSACHUSETTS]
Report on insanity and idiocy in Massachusetts by the Commission on Lunacy under resolve of the legislature of 1854. Boston: Wm. White, 1855. 215p. MBM; MH; MWA
50-1222

MASSACHUSETTS MEDICAL SOCIETY
Fellows of the Massachusetts Medical Society, 1787-1854. Alphabetically arranged. Boston: Printed by J. Wilson & Son, 1855. 50p. DLC; MBM; MH; MWA **50-1223**

MASSIE, J. Cam
A treatise on the eclectic southern practice of medicine. . . . Philadelphia: Thomas Cowperthwait & Co.; St. Louis: A. H. Shultz & Co.; [etc., etc.], 1854. 720p. DNLM; PPC; PU; ViRA **50-1224**

MATHEWS, J. M.
An address before the Association of the Alumni of the University of the City of New York. New York: D. Fanshaw, 1856. 26p. DNLM; NN; NNS; NNU-M **50-1225**

MATTHES, F.
Letter to Worthington Hooker, of Norwich, in relation to so much of his book, entitled, "Physician and Patient," as has reference to homoeopathy. Boston: O. Clapp, 1850. 16p. DNLM; MBM; MH **50-1226**

MATTHEWS, C. Bentley (1801?-1851)
Introductory lecture, in the Homoeopathic College of Pennsylvania. Philadelphia: Barnard & Co., 1850. 30p. DNLM; PPHa
50-1227

MATTSON, Morris
Manual of directions for the employment of injections in various diseases, with remarks upon the nature and treatment of habitual constipation; preceded by a treatise on the intestinal canal, its structure, functions, etc. . . . Boston: Printed for the author, 1852. 164p. plates. DLC; MBM; NNNAM
50-1228

MAUPIN, S(ocrates) (1808-1871)
Address to the graduates of the Medical Department of the Hampden-Sidney College at the commencement, March 14, 1853. Richmond: Collin & Nowlan, 1853. 16p. DNLM; ViRA
50-1229

MAURICEAU, A. M.
The married woman's private medical companion. . . . [New York, 1854]. 228p. NNNAM **50-1230**

MEADS, Orlando
An address to the class of graduates of the Albany Medical College, delivered December 26, 1854. Albany: J. Munsell, 1855. 19p. DNLM; N **50-1231**

MEIGS, Charles Delucena (1792-1869)
Introductory lecture. . . . Published by the class. Philadelphia: T. K. & P. G. Collins, printers, 1850. 20p. DLC; DNLM; PPC; PPJ **50-1232**

MEIGS, Charles Delucena (1792-1869)
Observations on certain of the diseases of young children. . . . Philadelphia: Lea & Blanchard, 1850. 215p. DLC; DNLM; PPC; PU **50-1233**

MEIGS, Charles Delucena (1792-1869)
A memoir of Samuel George Morton, M.D., late president of the Academy of Natural Sciences of Philadelphia. . . . Read November 6, 1851, and published by direction of the Academy. Philadelphia: T. K. & P. G. Collins, printers, 1851. 48p. DLC; DNLM; PPC; PU **50-1234**

MEIGS, Charles Delucena (1792-1869)
Woman; her diseases and remedies. A series of letters to his class. . . . 2nd ed. rev. and enl. Philadelphia: Lea & Blanchard, 1851. 690p. DLC; PPC; PPJ; PU **50-1235**

MEIGS, Charles Delucena (1792-1869)
Obstetrics: the science and art. 2nd ed. Philadelphia: Blanchard & Lea, 1852. 752p. OCIM; PPC; PPJ **50-1236**

MEIGS, Charles Delucena (1792-1869)
Charge to the graduates of Jefferson Medical College, delivered March 6, 1852. Philadelphia: T. K. & P. G. Collins, 1852. 15p. DNLM; PPJ **50-1237**

MEIGS, Charles Delucena (1792-1869)
A biographical notice of Daniel Drake, M.D., of Cincinnati. Prepared by appointment of the College of Physicians of Philadelphia. . . . Read at the meeting, July, 1853. Philadelphia: Lippincott, Grambo & Co., 1853. 38p. DLC; DNLM; PPC; PU **50-1238**

MEIGS, Charles Delucena (1792-1869)
Introductory lecture to the class of midwifery. Philadelphia: T. K. & P. G. Collins, 1854. 24p. DNLM; PPJ
50-1239

MEIGS, Charles Delucena (1792-1869)
On the nature, signs, and treatment of childbed fevers; in a series of letters addressed to the students of his class. . . . Philadelphia: Blanchard & Lea, 1854. 362p. DLC; DNLM; NNNAM; PPC **50-1240**

MEIGS, Charles Delucena (1792-1869)
Woman: her diseases and remedies. A series of letters to his class. 3rd ed. Philadelphia: Blanchard & Lea, 1854. 672p. DNLM; MBM; OCIM; PPC **50-1241**

MEIGS, Charles Delucena (1792-1869)
A treatise on acute and chronic diseases of the neck of the uterus. . . . Philadelphia: Blanchard & Lea, 1854. 116p. 22 plates. DLC; DNLM; NNNAM; PPC
50-1242

MEIGS, Charles Delucena (1792-1869)
Obstetrics: the science and the art. 3rd ed., rev. Philadelphia: Blanchard & Lea, 1856. 751p. DNLM; OCIM; NNNAM; PPC
50-1243

MEIGS, Charles Delucena (1792-1869)
Charge to the graduating class of Jefferson Medical College. (With a list of the graduates.) Philadelphia: T. K. & P. G. Collins, 1858. 16p. DNLM; PPJ **50-1244**

MEIGS, Charles Delucena (1792-1869)
Woman; her diseases and remedies. A series of letters to his class. 4th ed. Philadelphia: Blanchard & Lea, 1859. 706p. DNLM; PPC; PPJ; PU **50-1245**

MEIGS, Charles Delucena (1792-1869)
Introductory lecture to the course on midwifery, and diseases of women and children, in Jefferson Medical College, delivered October 12, 1859. . . . Published by the class. Philadelphia: J. M. Wilson, 1859. 21p. DLC; DNLM; PPJ
50-1246

MEIGS, James Aitken (1829-1879)
A brief notice of Dr. Martyn Paine's work on the "Institutes of medicine"; with some remarks on the theory of the correlation of the physical and vital forces. [Philadelphia, 1853.] 19p. DNLM; PPC; PU **50-1247**

MEIGS, James Aitken (1829-1879)
Essay on the relation of atomic heat to crystalline form. Philadelphia: Merrihew & Thompson, 1855. 32p. DNLM; PPC
50-1248

MEIGS, James Aitken (1829-1879)
Catalogue of human crania, in the collection of the Academy of Natural Science of Philadelphia: based upon the third edition of Dr. Morton's "Catalogue of Skulls," etc. Philadelphia: J. B. Lippincott & Co., 1857. 112p. DNLM; PPC; PPF; PU **50-1249**

MEIGS, James Aitken (1829-1879)
Hints to craniographers, upon the importance and feasibility of establishing some uniform system by which the collection and promulgation of craniological statistics and the exchange of duplicate crania may be promoted. . . . Philadelphia: Merrihew & Thompson, printers, 1858. 6p. DLC; DNLM; PPC; PPL **50-1250**

MEIGS, James Aitken (1829-1879)
Valedictory address to the graduating class of the Philadelphia College of Medicine, at the annual commencement, March 2nd, 1859. . . . Philadelphia: Bryson's Printing Rooms, 1859. 16p. DLC; PPC; PU **50-1251**

MEIGS, James Aitken (1829-1879)
Some remarks on the methods of studying and teaching physiology. Philadelphia: J. B. Lippincott & Co., 1859. 36p. DNLM; PPC **50-1252**

MEIGS, John Forsyth (1818-1882)
A practical treatise on the diseases of children. . . . 2nd ed., rev. and enl. Philadelphia: Lindsay & Blakiston, 1858. 711p. DLC; DNLM; PPC; PU **50-1253**

MEIGS, John Forsyth (1818-1882)
A practical treatise on the diseases of children. . . . 3rd ed., carefully rev. Philadelphia: Lindsay & Blakiston, 1858. 724p. DLC; DNLM; OCIM; PPC **50-1254**

MELVILLE, Henry
The modern treatment of pulmonary consumption and other diseases of the respiratory organs, being suggestions to invalids on the most rational method of cure. New York, 1859. 76p. DNLM; NNNAM **50-1255**

MEMOIR of John W. Francis, Jr. [New York, 1855.] 3p. DNLM; NNC; NNNAM **50-1256**

MENDENHALL, George (1814-1874)
Report of the committee on the epidemics of Ohio. Philadelphia: T. K. & P. G. Collins, 1858. 6p. DNLM; PPC
50-1257

MENDENHALL, George (1814-1874)
Report on the epidemics of Ohio, Indiana, and Michigan, for the years 1852 and 1853. [Philadelphia, 1858.] 132p. 1 map, 3 diag. DNLM; OCIM; PPC; PU **50-1258**

MERCIER, J.-J.-C.-Alfred
Oration delivered before the Physico-Medical Society of New Orleans, at their University meeting, held December, 1854. New Orleans, 1854. 22p. DNLM; LNT-M
50-1259

MERRILL, A. P[hillips] (1793-1873)
Medical essays. New Orleans: J. Cohn, 1851. 24p. DNLM; LNT-M **50-1260**

MERRILL, A. P[hillips] (1793-1873)
A public lecture on medical ethics, and the mutual relations of patients and physician. Memphis, 1857. 18p. DNLM
50-1261

MERRITT, A. T. B., *et al.*
An address to the public of the Medical Department of Hampden-Sidney College. Richmond: Ritchies & Dunnavant, 1853. 59p. ViRA **50-1262**

METCALF, James W.
Homoeopathy and its requirements of the physician; an address delivered before the Homoeopathic Medical Society of the State of New York: New York: Angell, Engel & Hewitt, 1852. 24p. DNLM; NNNAM; PPHa **50-1263**

METCALF, James W.
Homoeopathic provings. Containing the Vienna provings of colocynth and thuja occidentalis, and the symptoms of aethusa cynapium, alcohol sulphuris, amphisbaena vermicularis, anagallis arvensis, apis mellifica, aristolochia milhomens, arsenicum metallicum, artemisia vulgaris, asterias rubens, cinnabaris, turpethum, coccus cacti. . . . New York: William Radde, 1853. 417p. NNNAM; PPHa **50-1264**

METCALF, John George (1801-1892)
The study and practice of midwifery; a discourse read before the Massachusetts Medical Society. Boston: J. Wilson & Son, 1856. 123p. DNLM; MBM **50-1265**

MICHEL, Middleton (1822-1894)
Poisoning by ergot in attempting criminal abortion; with reflections upon some of the causes of sudden death. Charleston: C. Canning, 1850, 30p. DNLM; ScCM
50-1266

MICHEL, Middleton (1822-1894)
Introductory address, delivered before the class of the Medical College of South Carolina, Nov. 1, 1851. Charleston: J. B. Nixon, [1851]. 31p. DNLM; ScCM; ScMS **50-1267**

MICHEL, Middleton (1822-1894)
Microscopic researches on the black vomit of yellow fever. Charleston: Walker & James, 1853. 26p. 1 plate. DNLM; ScCM **50-1268**

MILES, Mason M., and David S. FOGG
Boston Vapor Bathing Institution, conducted by. . . . Boston: W. D. Ticknor & Co., 1850. 24p. DNLM; MH-M **50-1269**

MILLER, Adam (1810-1901)
Review of Dr. S. A. Latta's pamphlet, entitled "The cholera in Cincinnati, or a connected view of the controversy between the homoeopathists and the Methodist Expositor; also, a review of the report read before the Homoeopathic Association." Cincinnati, 1850. 16p. DNLM; OCIM **50-1270**

MILLER, Henry (1800-1874)
Report of the obstetric committee on anaesthesia in midwifery, and the speculum uteri. Louisville: Webb & Levering, 1853. 29p. DNLM **50-1271**

MILLER, Henry (1800-1874)
Lectures in reply to the Croonian lectures for 1854, of Charles West, of London, on the pathological importance of ulceration of the os uteri. Louisville, Ky.: I. F. Brennan, 1855. 71p. DNLM; OCIM **50-1272**

MILLER, Henry (1800-1874)
Lectures on inflammation and ulceration of the cervix uteri. [Louisville? 1855.] 71p. DNLM **50-1273**

MILLER, Henry (1800-1874)
The principles and practice of obstetrics, including the treatment of chronic inflammation of the uterus, considered as a frequent cause of abortion. . . . Philadelphia: Blanchard & Lea, 1858. 624p. DLC; MBM; OCIM; PPC **50-1274**

MILLER, Henry (1800-1874)
Two cases of encysted tumor of the ovary successfully treated by excision; and an attempt to justify the opertion of ovariotomy under certain circumstances. Philadelphia, 1859. DNLM; PPC **50-1275**

MILLER, James (1812-1864)
The principles of surgery. . . . 3rd American from the 2nd and enl. Edinburgh ed.. . . Rev., with additions, by F. W. Sargent. . . . Philadelphia: Blanchard & Lea, 1852. 751p. DLC; PPC; PU; ViRA **50-1276**

MILLER, James (1812-1864)
The practice of surgery. . . . 3rd American, from the 2nd Edinburgh ed. Ed., with additions, by F. W. Sargent. . . . Illustrated by three hundred and nineteen engravings on wood. Philadelphia: Blanchard & Lea, 1853. 720p. CtY-M; DLC; OCIM; PPC **50-1277**

MILLER, James (1812-1864)
The principles of surgery. 4th American from the 3rd and revised English ed. Philadelphia: Blanchard & Lea, 1856. 696p. DNLM; PPC; PPJ; PU **50-1278**

MILLER, James (1812-1864)
The practice of surgery. . . . Rev. by the American editor. 4th American, from the last Edinburgh ed. Illustrated by three hundred and sixty-four engravings on wood. Philadelphia: Blanchard & Lea, 1857. 682p. DLC; MBM; PPC; PU **50-1279**

MILLER, James (1812-1864)
Alcohol; its place and power. (From the 19th Glasgow ed.) Philadelphia: Lindsay & Blakiston, 1859. 179p. DNLM; MBM; NNNAM; PPC **50-1280**

"MILO" [pseudon.]
Error of position; being a discussion of the ultra medical policy of the American Medical Association, as advocated by medical professors, Medicus and others; showing the policy to be adverse to the great interests and institutions of society, and the peace and prosperity of the nation. [In 4 numbers, No. 1.] Nashville: W. F. Bang & Co., 1854. 46p. DNLM **50-1281**

"MILO" [pseudon.]
"Catchings" for "catchings" to show what is caught; being a special undertaking in the way of "catchings," according to a proposition in the Nashville Medical Journal for May, 1855. Nashville, 1855. 24p. DNLM **50-1282**

MILTENBERGER, George W[arner] (1819-1905)
Oration before the Medical and Surgical Society of Baltimore, at their anniversary meeting, January 21, 1856. Baltimore: J. W. Woods, 1856. 17p. DNLM; MdU-D **50-1283**

MITCHELL, John Kearsley (1798-1858)
Charge to the graduates of Jefferson Medical College, of Philadelphia, delivered at public commencement, held March 9, 1850. Philadelphia: C. Sherman, 1850. 24p. DNLM; PPJ **50-1284**

MITCHELL, John Kearsley (1798-1858)
Impediments to the study of medicine; a lecture, introductory to the course of practice of medicine. . . . Delivered on the 18th of November, 1850. Philadelphia: T. K. & P. G. Collins, printers, 1850. 28p. DLC; DNLM; PPJ **50-1285**

MITCHELL, J[ohn] K[earsley] (1798-1858)
On the progress of recent science, a lecture, introductory to the course of practice of medicine. . . . Delivered November 13, 1851. Philadelphia: T. K. & P. G. Collins, printers, 1851. 23p. DLC; DNLM; PPJ **50-1286**

MITCHELL, John Kearsley (1798-1858)
Charge to the graduates of Jefferson Medical College. . . . With a list of the graduates. Philadelphia: T. K. & P. G. Collins, 1857. 16p. DNLM; PPJ **50-1287**

MITCHELL, John Kearsley (1798-1858)
Five essays: [1. On the cryptogamous origin of malarious and epidemic fevers; 2. On animal magnetism; 3. On the penetrativeness of fluids; 4. On the penetration of gases; 5. On a new practice in acute and chronic rheumatism.] Edited by S. Weir Mitchell. Philadelphia: J. B. Lippincott & Co., 1859. 371p. DLC; DNLM; PPC; PU **50-1288**

MITCHELL, Thomas Duché (1791-1865)
Valedictory to the graduating class of the Philadelphia College of Medicine. Philadelphia: T. K. & P. G. Collins, 1852. 16p. DNLM; PPC; PU **50-1289**

MITCHELL, Thomas Duché (1791-1865)
The past, the present, and the future of the medical profession in the United States of America; being a general introductory to the course of lectures in the third session of the Kentucky School of Medicine. Louisville: Haldeman & Co., 1852. 23p. DNLM; KyLoJM; OCIM **50-1290**

MITCHELL, Thomas Duché (1791-1865)
Materia medica and therapeutics; with ample illustrations of practice in all the departments of medical science, and very copious notes of toxicology, suited to the wants of medical students, practitioners, and teachers. Philadelphia: J. B. Lippincott & Co., 1857. 820p. CtY-M; DNLM; NNNAM; PPC **50-1291**

MITCHELL, Thomas Duché (1791-1865)
A lecture introductory to the course on materia medica and therapeutics in the Jefferson Medical College of Philadelphia: Philadelphia: J. M. Wilson, 1857. 31p. DNLM; PPJ **50-1292**

MONROE COUNTY MEDICAL SOCIETY
Report of a committee on Dr. Lovejoy's alleged new remedies. Rochester: A. Strong & Co., 1858. 15p. DNLM **50-1293**

MONTGOMERY, William Fetherston (1797-1859)
An exposition of the signs and symptoms of pregnancy, the period of human gestation, and the signs of delivery. From the 2nd London ed. Philadelphia: Blanchard & Lea, 1857. 568p. 2 col. plates. DNLM; NNNAM; PPC; ViRA **50-1294**

MONUMENT to Jenner. Considerations and suggestions in its favor. [With the report of committee, appointed by the Suffolk District Medical Society, to receive subscriptions. Boston, Sept. 1, 1851.] [Boston, 1851.] 3p. DNLM; MWA **50-1295**

MOORE, George (1803-1880)
Health, disease, and remedy familiarly and practically considered in a few of their relations to the blood. New York: Harper & Bros., 1850. 320p. DNLM; NNNAM **50-1296**

MOORE, George (1803-1880)
The power of the soul over the body, considered in relation to health and morals. New York: Harper & Bros., 1859. 270p. DNLM; NNNAM **50-1297**

MOORMAN, John J. (*d.* 1885)
The Viriginia springs . . . with remarks on the nature and medical applicability of each. 2nd ed. . . . Richmond: J. W. Randolph, 1857. 204p. 2 maps. 6 plates. DNLM **50-1298**

MOORMAN, John J. (*d.* 1885)
The Virginia springs, and springs of the South and West. Philadelphia: J. B. Lippincott & Co., 1859. 403p. 5 plates. DNLM; PU **50-1299**

MOORMAN, John J. (*d.* 1885)
The Ohio White Sulphur Springs, with observations at the Ohio White Sulphur, in 1858, by W. W. Dawson. Cincinnati: Moore, Wilstach, Keys & Co., 1859. 72p. 1 plate, 1 map. DNLM **50-1300**

MORFIT, Campbell (1820-1897)
Chemical and pharmaceutical manipulations: a manual of the mechanical chemico-mechanical operations of the laboratory. For the use of chemists, druggists, manufacturers, teachers, and students. 2nd and enl. ed. By Campbell Morfit . . . and Clarence Morfit. . . . Philadelphia: Lindsay & Blakiston, 1857. 626p. DLC; PPC; PU **50-1301**

MORGAN, James Ethelbert (1822-1889)
Introductory to the course of medical lectures, delivered in the medical department of Georgetown College, session, 1856-57. Washington. T. McGill, 1857. 14p. DNLM **50-1302**

MORGAN, John
A warning against quackery, with a brief narrative of the sufferings of the author. Boston: G. B. Rand, 1851. 32p. DNLM; MB; MWA **50-1303**

MORGAN, William
The homoeopathic treatment of indigestion, constipation and haemorrhoids. Edited, with notes and annotations, by A. E. Small, M.D. Philadelphia: Rademacher & Sheek, 1854. 166p. PPC; PPHa; PU **50-1304**

MORLAND, William Wallace (1818-1876)
Diseases of the urinary organs. A compendium of their diagnosis, pathology, and treatment. Philadelphia: Blanchard & Lea, 1858. 579p. DNLM; MBM; NNNAM; PPC **50-1305**

MORRIS, Caspar (1806-1884)
Appeal on behalf of the sick. Philadelphia: Lindsay & Blakiston, 1851. 48p. DNLM; PPC **50-1306**

MORRIS, Caspar (1806-1884)
Lectures on scarlet fever. Philadelphia: Lindsay & Blakiston, 1851. 104p. DNLM; PPC **50-1307**

MORRIS, Caspar (1806-1884)
An essay on the pathology and therapeutics of scarlet fever. Philadelphia: Lindsay & Blakiston, 1858. 192p. CtY-M; PPC; PU; ViRA **50-1308**

MORRIS, Richard L[ewis] (1805-1880)
Memoir of the late Francis U. Johnston, read . . . before the New York Academy of Medicine. . . . New York, 1858. 20p. DNLM; NNNAM **50-1309**

MORTON, Samuel George (1799-1851)
Additional observations on hybridity in animals and on some collateral subjects; being a reply to the objections of the Rev. John Bachman, D.D. Charleston: Walker & James, 1850. 53p. DNLM; ScCM **50-1310**

MORTON, Samuel George (1799-1851)
Letter to the Rev. John Bachman, D.D., on the question of hybridity in animals, considered in reference to the unity of the human species. Charleston, 1850. 18p. DNLM; ScMS; ScU **50-1311**

MORTON, Samuel George (1799-1851)
Notes on hybridity, designed as a further supplement to a memoir on that subject in a former number of this journal. Being a second letter to the editors of the Charleston Medical Journal and Review. Charleston, 1851. 8p. DNLM; ScU **50-1312**

MORTON, William T. G. (1819-1868)
On the physiologicl effects of sulphuric ether, and its superiority to chloroform. Boston: D. Clapp, 1850. 24p. DNLM; MBM; MWA **50-1313**

[MORTON, William T. G.] (1819-1868)
(Report of) the select committee to whom was referred the memorial of Dr. William T. G. Morton, asking remuneration from Congress for the discovery of the anaesthetic or pain-subduing properties of sulphuric ether. . . . Thirty-second Congress, First Session, House of Representatives, 1852. 128p. 2 plates. DLC; DNLM; MBM; MWA
50-1314

MOTT, Alexander Brown (1826-1889)
Surgical operations. Series No. 1. [New York], 1856-1857. 26p. 3 plates. DNLM; NNNAM **50-1315**

MOTT, Valentine (1785-1865)
An introductory discourse, delivered in the University of New York, session 1849-1850. New York: Jennings & Harrison, 1850. 32p. DNLM; NNNAM
50-1316

MOTT, Valentine (1785-1865)
Reminiscences of medical teaching and teachers in New York. An address introductory to a course of lectures, at the College of Physicians and Surgeons, New York Session, 1850-1851. New York: Joseph H. Jennings, 1850. 32p. DNLM; NNNAM
50-1317

[MOTT, Valentine] (1785-1865)
Catalogue of the surgical and pathological museum of Valentine Mott, and of his son, Alexander B. Mott. New York: W. M. Taylor, 1858. 78p. DNLM; NN; NNNAM
50-1318

MOULTRIE, James (1793-1869)
Introductory lecture to the course of physiology in the Medical College of the State of South Carolina. Charleston: Walker, Evans & Co., 1856. 15p. ScCM **50-1319**

MÜLLER, Johannes (1801-1858)
Elements of human physiology . . . (unabridged ed.), chiefly from Baly's English translation; . . . Edited by T. S. Lambert. Portland [Me.]: Sanborn & Carter; New York: Leavitt & Company, 1852. 142p. DNLM; MBM; NNNAM [no more published] **50-1320**

MUNDE, Carl
Hydriatic treatment of scarlet fever in its different forms. . . . New York: W. Radde, 1857. 92p. DNLM; NNNAM
50-1321

MURE, B[enoit] Jules (1809-1858)
Dr. B. Mure's materia medica; or, provings of the principal animal and vegetable poisons of the Brazilian Empire, and their application in the treatment of diseases. Transl. from the French and arranged according to Hahnemann's method, by C. J. Hempel, M.D. New York: William Radde, 1854. 220p. NNNAM; PPHa **50-1322**

MURPHY, John A[lexander] (1824-1900)
An introductory address, delivered to the students of the Miami Medical College, of Cincinnati, Oct. 30, 1854. Cincinnati: T. Wrightson & Co., 1855. 24p. DNLM; OCIM
50-1323

MUSSEY, Reuben Dimond (1780-1866)
An introductory lecture delivered at the opening of the thirty-second session of the Medical College of Ohio, October 15, 1851. Cincinnati: Marshall & Langtry, 1852. 23p. DNLM; OCIM **50-1324**

MUSSEY, Reuben Dimond (1780-1866)
The trials and rewards of the medical profession; an introductory lecture delivered at the opening of the first session of the Miami Medical College, at Cincinnati, October 3, 1852. Cincinnati: T. Wrightson, 1853. 24p. DNLM; OCIM
50-1325

MUSSEY, Reuben Dimond (1780-1866)
Surgical cases. Aneurismal tumors upon the ear, successfully treated by the ligation of both carotids. Recto-vaginal fistula cured by operation. [1853.] 6p. DNLM
50-1326

MUSSEY, Reuben Dimond (1780-1866)
Alcohol in health and disease. A lecture introductory to the fourth annual course of the Miami Medical College, at Cincinnati, October 15, 1855. Cincinnati: T. Wrightson & Co., 1856. 19p. DNLM; OCIM **50-1327**

MUSSEY, Reuben Dimond (1780-1866)
Fracture of the neck of the thigh bone. [1857.] 19p. DNLM
50-1328

MUSSEY, William Heberden (1818-1882)
Anaesthesia. Non-fatal accidents from anaesthetic agents, with observations. Cincinnati, 1853. 8p. DNLM; OCIM
50-1329

MUSSEY, William Heberden (1818-1882)
Vesico-vaginal fistula complicated with vesical calculus, cured by operation. Cincinnati, 1854. 3p. DNLM; OCIM
50-1330

MUSSEY, William Heberden (1818-1882)
Surgical cases. Cases of polypi of the larynx cured by operation. [Cincinnati, 1856.] 4p. DNLM; OCIM
50-1331

MÜTTER, Thomas Dent (1811-1859)
Charge to the graduates of Jefferson Medical College of Philadelphia. Delivered March 8, 1851. With a list of the graduates. Philadelphia: T. K. & P. G. Collins, 1851. 28p. DNLM; PPJ
50-1332

MÜTTER, Thomas Dent (1811-1859)
Syllabus of the course of lectures on the principles and practice of surgery, delivered in the Jefferson Medical College, Philadelphia, Pts. 1-3. Philadelphia: J. H. Jones & Co., 1855. 212p. DNLM; PPJ **50-1333**

[MÜTTER, Thomas Dent] (1811-1859)
Catalogue of the pathological museum of Prof. T. D. Mütter. Philadelphia, 1856. 60p. DNLM; PPJ
50-1334

NEIDHARD, Charles (1809-1895)
Homoeopathy in Germany and England in 1849, with a glance at alloeopathic men and things. Being two preliminary discourses, delivered in the Homoeopathic Medical College of Pennsylvania. Boston: O. Clapp, 1850. 45p. DNLM; MBM; PPHa **50-1335**

NEIDHARD, Charles (1809-1895)
An address delivered before the Rhode Island Homoeopathic Society, at its annual meeting, May 7, 1851. Providence: Sayles & Miller, [1851]. 28p. DNLM
50-1336

NEIDHARD, Charles (1809-1895)
On homoeopathic medical education and the present state of homoeopathy. An introductory lecture to a course on clinical medicine delivered to the students of the Homoeopathic Medical College of Pennsylvania. Philadelphia, 1852. 18p. PPHa **50-1337**

NEILL, John (1819-1880)
Observations on the occipital and superior maxillary bones of the African cranium. [Philadelphia, 1850.] 5p. DNLM; PPC **50-1338**

NEILL, John (1819-1880)
Outlines of the arteries; with short descriptions. 2nd ed. Philadelphia: E. Barrington & G. D. Haswell, 1852. 28p. 7 plates. DNLM; PPC **50-1339**

NEILL, John (1819-1880) and Francis Gurney SMITH
An analytical compendium of the various branches of medical science, for the use and examination of students. 2nd ed., revised and improved. Philadelphia: Blanchard & Lea, 1852. 7 pts. in 1 v. DNLM; MBM; PPC; PU **50-1340**

NEILL, John (1819-1880)
A hand-book of anatomy: with one hundred and fifty-nine illustrations. Being a portion of an analytical compendium of the various branches of medicine. By John Neill . . . and Francis Gurney Smith. . . . 2nd ed., rev. and improved. Philadelphia: Blanchard & Lea, 1852. 192p. DLC; OCIM; PPC; PU **50-1341**

NEILL, John (1819-1880)
A hand-book of chemistry: with nineteen illustrations. Being a portion of an analytical compendium of the various branches of medicine. By John Neill . . . and Francis Gurney Smith. . . . 2nd ed., rev. and improved. Philadelphia: Blanchard & Lea, 1852. 106p. DLC; NNNAM; PPC; PU **50-1342**

NEILL, John (1819-1880)
A hand-book of materia medica and therapeutics: with twenty-nine illustrations. Being a portion of an analytical compendium of the various branches of medicine. By John Neill . . . and Francis Gurney Smith. . . . 2nd ed., rev. and improved. Philadelphia: Blanchard & Lea, 1852. 130p. CtY-M; DLC; PPC; PPHa **50-1343**

NEILL, John (1819-1880)
New means for making extension and counter-extension in fractures of the leg and thigh. Philadelphia: Merrihew & Thompson, 1855. 7p. DNLM; PPC **50-1344**

NEILL, John (1819-1880) and Francis Gurney SMITH
An analytical compendium of the various branches of medical science, for the use and examination of students. . . . A new edition, revised and improved. With three hundred and seventy-four illustrations. Philadelphia: Blanchard & Lea, 1856. 974p. DLC; OCIM; NNNAM; PPC **50-1345**

NEILL, John (1819-1880)
On the structure of the mucous membrane of the human stomach. [Philadelphia, 1857.] 16p. 1 plate. DNLM; PPC **50-1346**

NEILL, John (1819-1880)
Valedictory address before the medical department of Pennsylvania College, March 6, 1858. (With a list of graduates.) Philadelphia: Sherman & Son, 1858. 19p. DNLM; PPC; PU **50-1347**

NÉLATON, [Auguste] (1807-1873)
Clinical lectures on surgery. . . . From notes taken by Walter F. Atlee. . . . Philadelphia: J. B. Lippincott & Co., 1855. 755p. DLC; DNLM; PPC; PU **50-1348**

NELIGAN, John Moore (1815-1863)
Medicines; their uses and modes of administration, including a complete conspectus of the three British pharmacopoeias, an account of all the new remedies, and an appendix of formulae. With notes and additions conforming it to the Pharmacopoeia of the United States, by D. M. Reese. New York: Harper & Brothers, 1851. 453p. DNLM; OCLloyd; PPC; PU **50-1349**

NELIGAN, John Moore (1815-1863)
A practical treatise on diseases of the skin. . . . Philadelphia: Blanchard & Lea, 1852. 333p. DLC; MBM; OCIM; PPC **50-1350**

NELIGAN, John Moore (1815-1863)
A practical treatise on diseases of the skin. 2nd American ed. Philadelphia: Blanchard & Lea, 1857. 333p. DNLM; MBM; NNNAM; PPC **50-1351**

NELIGAN, John Moore (1815-1863)
A practical treatise on diseases of the skin. 3rd American ed. Philadelphia: Blanchard & Lea, 1859-1860. 333p. atlas; 16 plates. DNLM; MBM; NNNAM; PPC **50-1352**

NELKEN, Michel (1811-1861)
Sea-sickness; its cause, nature, symptoms, and treatment, derived from experience and strict observation. New York: Stringer & Townsend, 1856. 32p. DNLM; NNNAM **50-1353**

NEW, C. B.
Cholera. Observations on the management of cholera on plantations, and method of treating the disease, as practiced by. . . . Rodney, Miss.: R. N. Fetherston'h & Co., [1850]. 8p. DNLM **50-1354**

NEWARK MEDICAL ASSOCIATION
Statement in reference to a diploma granted by the New York Medical College. Presented to the American Medical Association,. May 4, 1858. Newark, N.J.: Newark Mercury Office, 1858. 13p. DNLM **50-1355**

NEWMAN, Albert
Croup: its history, nature, and treatment. Fiske fund prize dissertation of the Rhode Island Medical Society. Philadelphia: T. K. & P. G. Collins, 1855. 28p. DNLM; RHi **50-1356**

NEWMAN, James M.
Congestion of the brain in cholera; its etiology, diagnosis, and treatment. A paper read before the Buffalo Medical Association, October 3, 1854. Buffalo: Thomas & Lathrops, 1854. 25p. DNLM **50-1357**

NEWMAN, James M.
Report on the sanitary policy of cities. Presented to the American Medical Association, May, 1856. Philadelphia: T. K. & P. G. Collins, 1856. 53p. DNLM; PPC **50-1358**

NEW ORLEANS
The epidemic summer. List of interments in all the cemeteries of New Orleans, from the first of May to the first of November, 1853, together with names and ages of deceased, places of nativity, causes of deaths, date of interment and name of cemetery in which interred. . . . New Orleans: Pub. by the Proprietor of the True Delta, 1853. 67p. DLC; LNT-M
50-1359

NEW ORLEANS [YELLOW FEVER]
History of the yellow fever in New Orleans, during the summer of 1853. A complete and authentic record of the fatal epidemic. By a physician of New Orleans. Philadelphia & St. Louis: C. W. Kenworthy, 1854. 104p. DNLM; LNT-M
50-1360

NEWTON, Calvin (1800-1853)
Thoracic diseases: their pathology, diagnosis and treatment. By Calvin Newton . . . and by Marshall Calkins. . . . With a biographical sketch of the life and character of Professor Calvin Newton. Worcester: D. and M. Calkins, 1854. 439p. DLC; MBM; NNNAM; PU **50-1361**

NEWTON, Calvin (1800-1853)
Thoracic diseases: their pathology, diagnosis and treatment. . . . By Marshall Calkins. . . . With the posthumous writings of Calvin Newton. . . . And a biographical sketch of the life and character of Professor Calvin Newton. 2nd ed., rev. and greatly enl. Philadelphia: H. Cowperthwait & Co., 1858. 546p. DLC; MBM; PPC; PU **50-1362**

NEW YORK CITY. EASTERN DISPENSARY
Vaccine. Information upon the subject of the prevention of small-pox, by vaccination, etc. New York: J. Egbert, 1859. 8p. DNLM; NNNAM **50-1363**

NICHOLS, Thomas L[ow] (1815-1901)
The curse removed. A statement of facts respecting the efficacy of water-cure in the treatment of uterine diseases, and the removal of the pains and perils of pregnancy and childbirth. New York: Office of the Water-Cure Journal, 1850. 20p. DNLM; NNNAM **50-1364**

NICHOLS, Thomas L[ow] (1815-1901)
An introduction to the water-cure. A concise exposition of the human constitution, the conditions of health, etc. Founded in nature and adapted to the wants of man. New York: Fowler & Wells, 1850. 40p. DNLM; NNNAM **50-1365**

NICHOLS, Thomas L[ow] (1815-1901)
Esoteric anthropology. Port Chester, New York, 1853. 482p. DNLM **50-1366**

NIESZ, John
The family guide to health and husbandry, containing essays on homoeopathic and other medical preparations, for the cure of diseases of men, horses, cattle and sheep, and imparting useful information to the dairyman and woolgrower. Canton, O.: David Schell, M.D., Publisher, 1851. 376p. NNNAM; PPHa
50-1367

NIESZ, John
A short treatise on the use of arnica, and a few other useful homoeopathic preparations to heal contusions, wounds, strains, sprains, lacerations, concussions, paralysis, rhematism, pains, soreness of the nipples, and to give ease before, in, and after parturition, etc.: with a number of cases illustrating the use of several drugs. Compiled from the best authors. Canton, O.: D. Schell, 1851. 376p. OCIM; PPHa **50-1368**

NOEGGERATH, Emil Jacob (1827-1895)
Remarks on the employment of pessaries; with the description of a new instrument. New York: G. Tiemann & Co., 1858. 20p. DNLM; NNNAM **50-1369**

NOEGGERATH, Emil Jacob (1827-1895) and Abraham JACOBI
Contributions to midwifery, and diseases of women and children; with a report on the progress of obstetrics, and uterine and infantile pathology in 1858. New York: Bailliere Brothers, 1859. 475p. DNLM; MBM; NNNAM; PPC
50-1370

NORTH, M. L[inus] (1790?-1856)
Analysis of Saratoga waters; also of Sharon, Avon, Virginia, and other mineral waters of the United States. With directions for invalids. 7th ed. with an appendix. Saratoga Springs: B. Huling, 1858. 72p. DNLM **50-1371**

NORWOOD, Wesley C.
The therapeutical powers and properties of *Veratrum viride*. . . . New York: Kneeland, Printer, 1854. 40p. DLC; NNNAM
50-1372

NORWOOD, Wesley C.
The therapeutical powers and properties of *Veratrum viride*. . . . 2nd ed. New York: D. Bedford & Co., Printers, 1856. 24p. DLC; NNNAM **50-1373**

NORWOOD, Wesley C.
The therapeutical powers and properties of *Veratrum viride*. 3rd ed. New York: J. D. Bedford & Co., [1857]. 22p. DNLM; NNNAM **50-1374**

NORWOOD, Wesley C.
The therapeutical powers and properties of *Veratrum viride*. 4th ed. Albany: Van Benthuysen, 1858. 24p. DNLM
50-1375

NOTTINGHAM, Curtis B[ell] (1818-1876)
The annual address delivered to the graduates of the Atlanta Medical College at the commencement, Sept. 2, 1858. Atlanta: G. P. Eddy & Co., 1858. 16p. DNLM; GU
50-1376

NUTTING, J. H.
An essay on some of the principles of medical delusion. Boston: D. Clapp, 1853. 36p. MBM; PPHa
50-1377

OBSTETRIC INSTITUTE OF PHILADELPHIA
[Under the charge of Joseph Warrington] Announcement and catalogue for 1851. Philadelphia: H. Evans, 1851. 13p. [Established 1837.] DNLM; PPC; PU [Contains list of students from September term, 1837, to May 1851]
50-1378

OEHME, Ferdinand Gustave (*b.* 1826)
The homoeopathic domestic physician and traveller's medical companion. Concord, N.H.: E. C. Eastman, 1859. 124p. PPHa
50-1379

OKIE, Abraham Howard (*d.* 1882)
An address delivered before the Rhode Island Homoeopathic Society. Providence: G. H. Whitney, 1850. 28p. DNLM; RHi; RPB **50-1380**

OLIVER, W. G.
Electrical anesthesia, comprising a brief history of its discovery, a synopsis of experiments, also full directions for its application in surgical and dental operations. Buffalo: Murray, Rockwell & Co., 1858. 25p. DNLM
50-1381

OLMSTEAD, Adolphus
Elements of electropathy, with rules and directions for the application of Olmstead's improved voltaic arrangement, patented 17th April, A.D. 1849, for medical, chemical, and philosophical purposes. New York, 1850. 40p. DNLM; NNNAM **50-1382**

O'REILLY, John (1813-1868)
The connection of the nervous centres of animal and organic life. [New York, 1859.] 10p. DNLM; NNNAM
50-1383

OWEN, Richard (1804-1892)
The principal forms of the skeleton and of the teeth. Philadelphia: Blanchard & Lea, 1854. 329p. CtY-M; DNLM; PPC; PU
50-1384

PACKARD, John H[ooker] (1832-1907)
The present state of microscopical science medically considered. Philadelphia: J. B. Lippincott & Co., 1859. 43p. DNLM; PPC; PU **50-1385**

PAGET, James (1814-1899)
Lectures on surgical pathology. . . . Hypertrophy, atrophy, repair, inflammation, mortification, specific disease, and tumors. Philadelphia: Lindsay & Blakiston, 1854. 699p. DNLM; MBM; OCIM; PPC **50-1386**

PAIGE, A.
Mental and physical electropathy, or electricity; its physiological relations and medical applications. Philadelphia: Brown, 1852. 32p. DNLM; PPC **50-1387**

PAIGE, A.
The medical advantages of Dr. Paige's perpetual electrometers and galvanic supporters; with directions for their use. Boston, 1852. 16p. DNLM; MBM **50-1388**

PAIGE, A.
The electropathic guide; devoted to electricity and its medical applications. New York: Chatterton & Bros., 1854. 129p. DNLM; NNNAM **50-1389**

PAINE, Martyn (1794-1877)
The institutes of medicine. . . . New York: Harper & Brothers, 1858. 1095p. DLC; DNLM; NNNAM; PPC
50-1390

PAINE, Martyn (1794-1877)
The institutes of medicine. . . . 5th ed. New York: Harper & Brothers; [etc., etc.], 1859. 1109p. DLC; ICRM; MBM; PPC
50-1391

PAINE, William (*b.* 1821)
Introductory lecture delivered in the hall of the Eclectic Medical College, October 14, 1856. Philadelphia: J. Richards, 1856. 11p. DNLM; PPC **50-1392**

PAINE, William (*b.* 1821)
An epitome of the American eclectic practice of medicine, surgery, obstetrics, diseases of women and children, materia medica, and pharmacy; with glossary, designed for physicians, the student of medicine, and as a domestic practice for families. Philadelphia: J. Gladding, 1859. 716p. 2 plates. DNLM; PPC; ViRA **50-1393**

PAJOT, Charles (1816-1896)
Obstetric tables. Transl. from the French, and arranged by O. A. Crenshaw and J. B. McCaw. With three additional tables on the mechanism of natural, unnatural, and complex labor, by N. P. Rice. Richmond: J. W. Randolph, 1856. 1p. 8 tables. DNLM; PPC; ViRA **50-1394**

PALLEN, [Montrose] A[nderson] (1836-1892)
Vision, and some of its anomalies, as revealed by the ophthalmoscope. Prize essay. Philadelphia: T. K. & P. G. Collins, 1858. 78p. 4 plates. DNLM; PPC
50-1395

PALLEN, Moses Montrose (1810-1876)
Introductory address delivered before the class of the Medical Department of the Saint Louis University, session of 1850-1851. . . . Published by request of the class. Saint Louis: Printed by W. B. Foster, 1850. 21p. DLC
50-1396

PALLEN, Moses Montrose (1810-1876)
An address to the graduates of the Medical Department of the St. Louis University. Delivered March 1, 1853. . . . St. Louis: Printed by Charles & Hammond, 1853. 19p. DLC
50-1397

PALLEN, Moses Montrose (1810-1876)
Introductory address delivered before the St. Louis Medical College, November 1, 1856. St. Louis, Mo., 1856. 20p. DNLM
50-1398

PALMER, Alonzo Benjamin (1815-1887)
Observations on the cause, nature, and treatment of epidemic cholera. . . . Detroit: Printed by G. E. Pomeroy & Co., 1854. 37p. DLC; DNLM **50-1399**

PALMER, Alonzo Benjamin (1815-1887)
Lectures on sulphate of quinia; delivered in the regular course of the medical department of the University of Michigan. [Four lectures.] Detroit, Mich.: Fleming & Davis, 1858. 59p. DNLM **50-1400**

PALMER, Alonzo Benjamin (1815-1887)
Report of the committee on medical literature. Philadelphia: T. K. & P. G. Collins, 1858. 62p. DNLM **50-1401**

PALMER, B. Frank (*fl.* 1845-1870)
Glances at operative surgery and subsidiary science. [Testimonials.] [1855.] 32p. DNLM **50-1402**

PALMER, Benjamin Rush (1813-1866)
An introductory address, delivered before the faculty and students of the Medical Department of the University of Louisville, at the opening of the session of 1853-1854. . . . Louisville: W. Tanner, 1853. 23p. DLC; DNLM
50-1403

PANCOAST, Joseph (1805-1882)
A treatise on operative surgery . . . exhibiting the state of surgical science in its present advanced condition. . . . 3rd ed., rev. and enl. . . . Philadelphia: A. Hart, late Carey & Hart, 1852. 389p. 80 col. plates. DLC; OCIM; NNNAM; PPC
50-1404

PANCOAST, Joseph (1805-1882)
Charge to the graduates of Jefferson Medical College of Philadelphia, delivered March 10, 1855. With a list of the graduates. Philadelphia: T. K. & P. G. Collins, 1855. 15, 4p. DNLM; PPJ **50-1405**

PANCOAST, Joseph (1805-1882)
Professional glimpses abroad. A lecture, introductory to the course on anatomy, in the Jefferson Medical College of Philadelphia, delivered October 17, 1856. . . . Published by the class. Philadelphia: J. M. Wilson, 1856. 31p. DLC; DNLM; PPJ
50-1406

PANCOAST, Joseph (1805-1882)
A discourse commemorative of the late Professor T. D. Mütter . . . being the introductory lecture to the course of anatomy in the Jefferson Medical College of Philadelphia, delivered October 14, 1859. . . . Philadelphia: J. M. Wilson, 1859. 28p. DLC; DNLM; PPJ **50-1407**

PANCOAST, Seth (1823-1889)
An original treatise on the curability of consumption by medical inhalation and adjunct remedies, agreeably to the new pathological doctrines and curative treatment, as founded and solely employed by. . . . Philadelphia, 1855. 196p. DNLM; PPC
50-1408

PANCOAST, Seth (1823-1889)
Onanism, spermatorrhoea. Porneio-kalogynomia, pathology. Boyhood's perils and manhood's curse. An earnest appeal to the young of America. Philadelphia, 1858. 225p. 9 plates. DLC; DNLM; PPC **50-1409**

PANCOAST, Seth (1823-1889)
. . . The ladies' medical guide and marriage friend. . . . Philadelphia: The author [1859]. 584p. plates. DLC; PPC; PU
50-1410

PARKER, Amasa J[unius] (1807-1890)
An address delivered before the graduating class of the Albany Medical College, January 21, 1851. . . . Albany: E. H. Pease & Co., 1851. 32p. DLC; DNLM **50-1411**

PARKER, Edward Hazen (1823-1896)
Is the practice of medicine based on science? A lecture, introductory to the session of the New York Medical College for the winter of 1854-1855. New York: Baker, Godwin & Co., 1854. 12p. DNLM; NNNAM **50-1412**

PARKER, Edward Hazen (1823-1896)
Results of the quantitative and qualitative analysis of homoeopathic medical preparations. [1856.] 8p. DNLM; PPHa
50-1413

PARKER, Edward Hazen (1823-1896)
Cholera, infantum, diarrhoea, and enterocolitis; their relations to each other, their pathology, and their treatment. New York: E. P. Allen, 1857. 16p. DNLM; NNNAM
50-1414

PARKER, Edward Hazen (1823-1896)
The mother's handbook: A guide in the care of young children. New York: E. P. Allen, 1857. 250p. NNNAM
50-1415

PARKER, Edward Hazen (1823-1896)
A monograph on scarlet fever. New York: Hall, Clayton & Co., 1859. 32p. DNLM; NNNAM **50-1416**

PARKER, Joel (1799-1873)
The beloved physician: a tribute to the memory of James C. Bliss, M.D. A discourse on the combined influence of the gospel and the medical profession in forming the character. . . . Published by the Kappa Lambda Society. New York: S. S. & W. Wood, 1856. 29p. DLC; DNLM; NNNAM
50-1417

PARKER, Langston (1805?-1871)
The modern treatment of syphilitic diseases, both primary and secondary; comprising the treatment of constitutional and confirmed syphilis by a safe and successful method; with numerous cases, formulae, and clinical observations. . . . From the 3rd, and entirely re-written London ed. Philadelphia: Blanchard & Lea, 1854. 316p. DLC; DNLM; PPC; ScCM
50-1418

PARKMAN, Samuel (1816-1854)
The present tendency of investigation in medicine. An address delivered before the Suffolk District Medical Society. Boston: D. Clapp, 1851. 40p. DNLM; MBM **50-1419**

PARKMAN, Samuel (1816-1854)
The relations of the medical witness with the law and the lawyer. Philadelphia: T. K. & P. G. Collins, 1852. 11p. DNLM; PPC **50-1420**

PARRISH, Edward (1822-1872)
An introduction to practical pharmacy: designed as a textbook for the student, and as a guide to the physician and pharmaceutist. With many formulas and prescriptions. . . . Philadelphia: Blanchard & Lea, 1856. 544p. DLC; DNLM; PPC; PU **50-1421**

PARRISH, Edward (1822-1872)
An introduction to practical pharmacy: designed as a textbook for the student, and as a guide to the physician and pharmaceutist. With many formulas and prescriptions. . . . 2nd ed. Philadelphia: Blanchard & Lea, 1859. 720p. DNLM; PPC; PJ; PU **50-1422**

PARRISH, Joseph (1818-1891)
The influence of the uterus on the female constitution. An address delivered before the Burlington County Medical Society. Burlington, S.C.: Atkinson, 1850. 15p. DNLM; ScCM
50-1423

PARSONS, Charles William (1823-1893)
Neuralgia, its history, nature, and treatment. . . . The dissertation to which the Fisk fund prize was awarded. Published by request of the Rhode Island Medical Society. Philadelphia: T. K. & P. G. Collins, printers, 1854. 35p. DLC; PPC; RPM
50-1424

PARSONS, John A.
A lecture on the human body. . . . New York: C. Shepard & Company, 1854. 51p. DLC; NNNAM
50-1425

PARSONS, Usher (1788-1868)
Report of the committee on medical sciences, presented at the third annual meeting of the American Medical Association, Cincinnati, May, 1850. Philadelphia: T. K. & P. G. Collins, 1850. 53p. DLNM; PPC **50-1426**

PARSONS, Usher (1788-1868)
Sketches of Rhode Island physicians, deceased prior to 1850: ...for the Rhode Island Medical Society. Providence: Knowles, Anthony & Co., printers, 1859. 64p. DLC; DNLM; RHi; RPM **50-1427**

PATERSON, T. V.
Medical schools, medical educations, and medical teachers, exemplified in the past and present career of that mutual admiration society, yclept the New York Medical College. [Prospectus]. New York: Literary Bureau and Agency, 185-? 4p. DLC; DNLM **50-1428**

PATON, George
On the perceptive power of the spinal cord, as manifested by experiments on cold-blooded animals. [Philadelphia, 1858.] 16p. DNLM **50-1429**

PATTERSON, Henry S. (1815-1854)
Lecture introductory to the course of materia medica and therapeutics in the medical department of Pennsylvania College, session 1850-1851. Philadelphia: B. Mifflin, 1850. 16p. DNLM; PPC; PU **50-1430**

PATTERSON, Henry S. (1815-1854)
Lecture introductory to the course of materia medica and therapeutics in the medical department of Pennsylvania College, for the session of 1851-1852. Philadelphia: J. Royer, 1851. 16p. DNLM; PU **50-1431**

PATTERSON, Henry S. (1815-1854)
Notice of the life and professional services of William R. Grant, M.D. A discourse at the opening of the lectures in the medical department of Pennsylvania College, for the session of 1852-1853. Philadelphia: King & Baird, 1852. 16p. DNLM; PPC **50-1432**

PATTISON, Granville Sharp (1792-1851)
Letter on cholera, to Dr. Carmichael, of Virginia. Philadelphia: W. F. Geddes, 1852. 16p. DNLM; PPC; PU **50-1433**

PATTON, William N.
A notice of the healing springs in Bath County, Virginia: Lewesburg: Mauzy & Gilmer, 1853. 21p. DNLM **50-1434**

PAUL, James (1798-1852)
The food and the teeth; observations on the inorganic constituents of the food of children, as connected with the decay of the teeth, and the physical constitution of woman in America. Particularly addressed to parents. Philadelphia: Grattan & McLean, 1850. 21p. DNLM; MdU-D; PPC **50-1435**

PAYNE, F. R[ice] (1821-1873)
Public address on the intellectual, moral, and physical training necessary to constitute the true physician, delivered before the Aesculapian Medical Society, at its semi-annual session held in Marshall, Ill., May 31, 1854. Marshall: E. Callahan & Co., 1854. 14p. DNLM **50-1436**

PAYNE, William E[lisha] (1815-1877)
An address delivered at the 11th session of the American Institute of Homoeopathy, held in Albany, N.Y., June 7, 1854. New York: Samuel T. Callahan, 1854. 25p. NNNAM; PPHa **50-1437**

PAYNE, William E[lisha] (1815-1877) and Henry C. PRESTON
Address and poem delivered before the Massachusetts Homoeopathic Medical Society, on the occasion of the centennial birthday of Doctor Samuel Hahnemann, April 10, 1855. Boston: O. Clapp, 1855. 52p. DNLM; MBM **50-1438**

PEABODY, Elizabeth Palmer (1804-1894)
Memorial of Dr. William Wesselhöft. To which is added his last address to the Homoeopathic Association. Boston: N. C. Peabody, 1859. 54p. DNLM; MBM; MH; MWA **50-1439**

PEARSON, Clement (1819-1886)
Is there a system of medicine? A lecture delivered in reply to the proceedings of the Iowa State Medical Society, June 17th, 1858. Mount Pleasant: H. L. Robinson, 1858. 23p. DNLM **50-1440**

PEASE, Calvin
Address delivered before the graduating class in the medical department of the University of Vermont, June 4, 1856. [Burlington, 1856] 35p. DNLM; VtHi **50-1441**

PEASLEE, Edmund Randolph (1814-1878)
Comparative intellectual standing of the medical profession. An introductory address to the class in the Medical School of Maine, Brunswick, March, 1851. Concord, N.H.: McFarland & Jenks, 1851. 29p. DNLM **50-1442**

PEASLEE, Edmund Randolph (1814-1878)
The moral character of the medical profession. An address introductory to the course of public lectures in the New York Medical College, session of 1852-1853. Published by the class. New York: Baker, Godwin & Co., 1852. 24p. DNLM; NNNAM **50-1443**

PEASLEE, Edmund Randolph (1814-1878)
A case of amputation at the shoulder-joint. New York: J. F. Trow, 1853. 14p. 1 plate. DNLM; NNNAM **50-1444**

PEASLEE, Edmund Randolph (1814-1878)
A monograph on the foetal circulation. New York: Baker, Godwin & Co., 1854. 26p. DNLM; NNNAM **50-1445**

PEASLEE, Edmund Randolph (1814-1878)
A monograph on the pathology and the rational treatment of infantile laryngo-tracheitis or croup. New York: Baker, Godwin & Co., 1854. 31p. DNLM; NNNAM **50-1446**

PEASLEE, Edmund Randolph (1814-1878)
Human histology in its relations to descriptive anatomy, physiology, and pathology. Philadelphia: Blanchard & Lea, 1857. 616p. DNLM; OCIM; MBM; PPC **50-1447**

PEASLEE, Edmund Randolph (1814-1878)
The progress and the spirit of medical science. An anniversary discourse delivered before the New York Academy of Medicine, November 15, 1858. New York, 1859. 104p. DNLM; NNNAM **50-1448**

PEEBLES, J. F. (*d.* 1853)
On displacements of the non-gravid uterus; their local and constitutional effects. (Fiske fund prize essay, 1852.) Philadelphia: T. K. & P. G. Collins, 1853. 47p. DNLM; PPC; PU **50-1449**

PEET, Harvey Prindle (1794-1873)
Statistics of the deaf and dumb. A paper read before the Medical Society of the State of New York, June 25, 1852. [Published by order of the Society.] New York: J. Egbert, 1852. 44p. DNLM; NNNAM **50-1450**

PEIRCE, C[harles] H[enry] (1814-1855)
Examinations of drugs, medicines, chemicals, etc., as to their purity and adulterations. Cambridge: J. Bartlett, 1852. 264p. DNLM; MH; MBM **50-1451**

PENNSYLVANIA COLLEGE, GETTYSBURG. MEDICAL DEPARTMENT, PHILADELPHIA
Annual announcement for the session of 1852-1853. (14.). Philadelphia: D. Mifflin, 1852. 15p. DNLM **50-1452**

PENNSYLVANIA HOSPITAL. PHILADELPHIA
An address on the occasion of the centennial celebration of the founding of the . . . delivered June 10, 1851, by George B. Wood, M.D. [With appendices, containing: I. Charter. II. Abstract of the rules now in force. III. Managers and treasurers from the commencement to the present time. IV. Physicians and surgeons who have served in the institution. V. Stewards and matrons. VI. Contributors. VII. Legacies. VIII. Donations. IX. Deposits. X. Total number of patients admitted from its foundation to fourth month, April 26, 1851.] Published by order of the board of managers. Philadelphia: T. K. & P. G. Collins, 1851. 141p. 2 plates. DNLM; PPPH; PU **50-1453**

PENROSE, R[ichard] A[lexander] F. (1827-1908)
Introductory lecture to a course of obstetrics. Philadelphia: T. K. & P. G. Collins, 1859. 21p. DNLM; PPC **50-1454**

PEPPER, William (1810-1864)
On the use of bebeerine and cinchonia in the treatment of intermittent fever. . . . Philadelphia: T. K. & P. G. Collins, printers, 1853. 14p. DLC; PPC **50-1455**

PEREIRA, Jonathan (1804-1853)
A treatise on food and diet, with observations on the dietetical regimen suited for disordered states of the digestive organs; and an account of the dietaries of some of the principal metropolitan and other establishments for paupers, lunatics, criminals, children, the sick. . . . New York: Fowlers & Wells, 1850. 318p. DNLM; MBM; NNNAM; PPC **50-1456**

PEREIRA, Jonathan (1804-1853)
The elements of materia medica and therapeutics. . . . 3rd American ed., enl. and improved by the author. Including notices of most of the medicinal substances in use in the civilized world, and forming an encyclopaedia of materia medica. Edited by Joseph Carson. . . . Philadelphia: Blanchard & Lea, 1852-1854. 2 v. 2 plates. DLC; DNLM; OCLloyd; PPC **50-1457**

PEREIRA, Jonathan (1804-1853)
The physician's prescription book; containing list of terms, phrases, contractions, and abbreviations used in prescriptions, with explanatory notes; also, the grammatical construction of prescriptions, etc. To which is added a key, containing the prescriptions in an unabbreviated form, with a literal translation, intended for the use of medical and pharmaceutical students. 2nd American from the 12th London ed. Philadelphia: Lindsay & Blakiston, 1857. 282p. DNLM; MBM; OCLloyd; PPC **50-1458**

PERKINS, Joseph (1798-1872)
Valedictory address, delivered to the graduating class at the fiftieth commencement of Castleton Medical College. Rutland: G. A. Tuttle & Co., 1854. 14p. DNLM; VtHi **50-1459**

PERKINS, Joseph (1798-1872)
An address delivered before the Medical Society of the State of Vermont, October 22, 1856. Rutland: G. A. Tuttle & Co., 1857. 14p. DNLM; VtHi **50-1460**

PERKINS, Roger G.
Insanity in its legal relations. New York: H. Ludwig, 1858. 24p. DNLM; NNNAM **50-1461**

PERKINS, S. G[ridley] (1826-1862)
Valedictory address to the graduating class, at the fifty-second commencement of the Castleton Medical College, Rutland: G. A. Tuttle & Co., 1855. 18p. DNLM; VtHi **50-1462**

PERRINE, George W. (1816-1872)
Address delivered before the New York State Homoeopathic Society. New York: H. Ludwig, 1855. 30p. NNNAM; PPHa **50-1463**

PERRY, Bela C.
A treatise on the human hair, and its diseases. . . . New Bedford, Mass.: C. Taber & Co., 1859. 192p. DLC; DNLM; MBM; NNNAM **50-1464**

PERRY, Marshall Sears (1805?-1859)
Case of Hon. Charles Sumner. Communicated to the Boston Society for Medical Improvement, Dec. 8, 1856. [Boston, 1856.] 7p. DNLM; MBM; MH **50-1465**

PERRY, Marshall Sears (1805?-1859)
The principles and objects of the Massachusetts Medical Society, delivered at their annual meeting, June 3, 1857. Boston: J. Wilson & Son, 1857. 28p. DNLM; MBM **50-1466**

PETER, Robert (1805-1894)
A brief sketch of the history of Lexington, Kentucky, and of Transylvania University, delivered as an introductory lecture to the winter course in the medical department of Transylvania University, Nov. 6th, 1854. Lexington, Ky.: D. C. Wickliffe, 1854. 23p. DNLM; OCIM **50-1467**

PETERS, John Charles (1819-1893)
A treatise on headaches: including acute, chronic, nervous, gastric, dyspeptic, or sick headaches; also, congestive, rheumatic, and periodical headaches, based on Th. J. Rueckert's "Clinical Experience in Homoeopathy," with introduction, appendix, synopsis, notes, directions for doses and fifty additional cases. New York: William Radde, 1853. 135p. NNNAM; PPHa **50-1468**

PETERS, John Charles (1819-1893)
A treatise on apoplexy. With an appendix on softening of the brain and paralysis. Based on Th. J. Rueckert's "Clinical Experience in Homoeopathy." New York: William Radde, 1853. 164p. DNLM; PPHa **50-1469**

PETERS, John Charles (1819-1893)
A treatise on the diseases of females. Disorders of menstruation. New York: William Radde, 1854. 165p. DLC; DNLM; NNNAM **50-1470**

PETERS, John Charles (1819-1893)
A treatise on the diseases of married females, including the disorders of pregnancy, parturition and lactation. New York: Philadelphia and London: William Radde, 1854. 192p. NNNAM; PPHa **50-1471**

PETERS, John Charles (1819-1893)
The diseases of females and married females. 2nd edition. Two parts in 1 v. New York: William Radde, 1854. 356p. NNNAM; PPHa **50-1472**

PETERS, John Charles (1819-1893)
A treatise on diseases of the eyes; including diseases of the eyelids, inflammation of the conjunctiva, sclerotica and cornea; also catarrhal, rheumatic, scrofulous and purulent ophthalmia. Based on Theodore J. Rueckert's "Clinical Experience in Homoeopathy." New York: William Radde, 1854. 172p. NNNAM; PPHa **50-1473**

PETERS, John Charles (1819-1893)
A treatise on the inflammatory and organic diseases of the brain. Including irritation, congestion, inflammation of the brain and its membranes, tuberculous meningitis, hydrocephaloid disease, hydrocephalus, atrophy and hypertrophy, and cancer of the brain. Based upon Th. J. Rueckert's "Clinical Experience in Homoeopathy." New York: William Radde, 1855. 156p. NNNAM; PPHa **50-1474**

PETERS, John Charles (1819-1893)
A treatise on internal diseases of the eyes, including diseases of the iris, crystalline lens, choroid, retina and optic nerve. Based on Th. J. Rueckert's "Clinical Experience in Homoeopathy." New York: William Radde, 1856. 128p. NNNAM; PPHa **50-1475**

PETERS, John Charles (1819-1893)
A treatise on the principal diseases of the eyes, including diseases of the eyelids, conjunctiva, cornea, sclerotica, crystalline lens, choroid, retina, and optic nerve. Based on Th. J. Rueckert's "Clinical Experience in Homoeopathy." New York: William Radde, 1856. 291p. NNNAM; PPHa **50-1476**

PETERS, John Charles (1819-1893)
A complete treatise on headaches and diseases of the head. 1. The nature and treatment of headaches; 2. the nature and treatment of apoplexy; 3. the nature and treatment of mental derangement; 4. the nature and treatment of irritation, congestion and inflammation of the brain and its membranes. Based on Th. J. Rueckert's "Clinical Experience in Homoeopathy." New York: William Radde, 1856. [Parts separately paged.] DNLM; NNNAM; PPHa **50-1477**

PETERS, John Charles (1819-1893)
The science and art or the principles and practice, of medicine. Vol. 1, No. 1. New York: William Radde, 1859. 96p. DNLM; NNNAM; PPHa **50-1478**

THE PHARMACOPOEIA OF THE UNITED STATES OF AMERICA
By authority of the National Medical Convention, held at Washington, A.D. 1850. Philadelphia: Lippincott, Grambo & Co., 1851. 317p. DLC; DNLM; OCLloyd **50-1479**

THE PHARMACOPOEIA OF THE UNITED STATES OF AMERICA
By authority of the National Medical Convention. . . . 2nd ed. Philadelphia: Lippincott, Grambo & Co., 1855. 317p. DNLM; OCIM; OCLloyd; PPC **50-1480**

PHILADELPHIA COUNTY MEDICAL SOCIETY
Sanitary, meteorological and mortuary report of the Philadelphia County Medical Society, for 1855. By Wilson Jewett. With an account of the prevalent diseases in the consolidated city during the year; . . . presented to the State Society at its annual session, held in Philadelphia, May, 1856. Philadelphia: T. K. & P. G. Collins, 1856. 64p. DNLM; PPC; PU **50-1481**

PHILADELPHIA. PENNSYLVANIA HOSPITAL FOR INSANE
Reports of the Pennsylvania Hospital for the Insane, with a sketch of its history, buildings, and organization. By Thomas S. Kirkbride, physician to the institution. Published by order of the Board of Managers. Philadelphia, 1851. [Report of first to tenth reports, 1841-1850. Each report paged separately, with special half-title.] 437p. 2 plates. 3 plans. DNLM; PPC; PU **50-1482**

PHILADELPHIA. PENNSYLVANIA HOSPITAL FOR THE INSANE
Proceedings on the occasion of laying the corner stone of the new Pennsylvania Hospital for the Insane, at Philadelphia. Including the address by George B. Wood. . . . Published by request of the Board of Managers. Philadelphia: T. K. & P. G. Collins, 1856. 30p. DLC; DNLM; PU **50-1483**

PHILADELPHIA. PENNSYLVANIA HOSPITAL. LIBRARY
Catalogue raisonné of the medical library of the Pennsylvania Hospital. By Emil Fischer. . . . Philadelphia: Printed by T. K. & P. G. Collins, 1857. 750p. DLC; DNLM; PU **50-1484**

THE PHYSICIAN'S prescription book; containing list of terms, phrases, contractions, and abbreviations used in prescriptions, with explanatory notes, also the grammatical construction of prescriptions, etc. To which is added a key containing the prescriptions in an unabbreviated form, with a literal translation, intended for the use of medical and pharmaceutical students. -1st American from the 10th London ed. Philadelphia: Lindsay & Blakiston, 1852. 288p. DNLM; MBM; NNNAM; PPC **50-1485**

PIERCE, C. H.
Examination of drugs, medicines, chemicals, etc., as to their purity and adulterations. Philadelphia: Bairds, 1853. 264p. DNLM; OCLloyd; PPC **50-1486**

PIPER, R. U[ston] (1816-1897)
Operative surgery illustrated: containing more than nineteen hundred engravings; including two hundred original and fifty colored drawings, with explanatory text. . . . Also, a chapter upon the use of ether in surgery, from the transactions of the American Medical Association, written at the request of a surgical committee of that body, by Henry J. Bigelow. . . . Boston: Ticknor, Reed & Fields, 1852. 384p. DNLM; MBM; NNNAM; PPC **50-1487**

PIRRIE, William (1807-1882)
The principles and practice of surgery. . . . Ed., with additions, by John Neill. . . . Philadelphia: Blanchard & Lea, 1852. 784p. DLC; DNLM; PPC; PU **50-1488**

THE POCKET anatomist: being a summary description of the muscles; with a tabular view of the arteries and nerves; Concordant with "The Dublin Dissector" and "Harrison on the Arteries." Bufflao: G. H. Derby & Co., 1850. 61p. DNLM; MBM; NNNAM **50-1489**

A POCKET MANUAL, or repertory of homoeopathic medicine, alphabetically and nosologically arranged. . . . 3rd ed. . . . New York: Boericke & Tafel, [1851]. 352p. DNLM; NNNAM; PPC; PU **50-1490**

POMEROY & CO.
Catalogue of the grand anatomical museum or national academy of natural, anatomical, and pathological science, No. 300 Broadway. New York: S. J. Reed, 1852. 94p. DNLM; NNNAM **50-1491**

POMEROY, T.
Female complaints: a brief examination of the pathology of uterine diseases, together with an exposition of the principle and method of their treatment. Utica: H. H. Curtiss, 1851. 8p. DNLM **50-1492**

POMEROY, T.
Female complaints: a brief examination of the pathology of uterine diseases with an exposition of the principle and method of their treatment. 2nd ed., enl. Utica: Curtiss & White, 1854. 12p. DNLM **50-1493**

POPE, Charles (1818-1870)
An address to the graduates of the medical department of the St. Louis University. St. Louis, 1852. 27p. DNLM **50-1494**

POPE, Charles (1818-1870)
The topical uses of water in surgery. Philadelphia: T. K. & P. G. Collins, 1852. 24p. DNLM; PPC **50-1495**

POPE, Charles (1818-1870)
An address introductory to the course of lectures in the St. Louis Medical College. St. Louis, Mo., 1855. 22p. DNLM; OCIM **50-1496**

PORCHER, Francis Peyre (1825-1895)
The medicinal, poisonous, and dietetic properties, of the cryptogamic plants of the United States. Being a report made to the American Medical Association, at its sessions held in Richmond, Va., and St. Louis, Mo. . . . New York: Baker, Godwin & Co., printers, 1854. 126p. DLC; DNLM; NNNAM; PPC **50-1497**

POTTER, J. F[itch] (1808-1868)
Letter to Prof. R. D. Mussey [Refutation of charges.] Cincinnati: J. A. & U. P. James, 1850. 14p. DNLM; OCIM **50-1498**

POTTER, J. Hamilton
The consumptive's guide to health; or, the invalid's five questions, and the doctor's five answers. A comprehensive practical treatise on pulmonary consumption, its preventive and curative treatment, etc., addressed in popular language to non-medical readers, and incidentally to physicians and students. 2nd ed. New York: J. S. Redfield, 1852. 176p. DNLM; MBM; NNNAM; PPC **50-1499**

POTTER, S. Hollister
Notes of lectures on the American practice of medicine, delivered in the American Medical College, at Cincinnati, Ohio. Syracuse, N.Y.: Potter & Voak, 1855. 311p. DNLM; MBM; OCIM; PPC **50-1500**

POWELL, Llewellyn
An address to the medical class of the Kentucky School of Medicine, delivered at the opening of its second session, Nov. 4, 1851. Published by request of the class. Louisville: Harney & Hughes, 1851. 16p. DNLM; OCIM **50-1501**

POWELL, Thomas Spencer (1826-1895)
A pocket formulary and physician's manual, embracing the art of combining and prescribing medicines to the best advantage; with many valuable recipes, tables, etc. adapted to the profession throughout the United States. . . . Savannah: W. T. Williams, 1855. 181p. DLC; DNLM; GU **50-1502**

POWELL, William Byrd (1799-1866) and Robert S. NEWTON
The eclectic practice of medicine. Cincinnati: H. W. Derby, 1854. 1084p. DNLM; OCIM **50-1503**

POWELL, William Byrd (1799-1866) and Robert S. NEWTON
The eclectic practice of medicine. (Diseases of children.) Cincinnati: Rickey, Mallory & Co., 1858. 610p. DNLM; OCIM **50-1504**

THE PRESCRIBER's pharmacopoeia. Containing all the medicines in the London Pharmacopoeia. . . . Altered to correspond with the U.S. Dispensatory. Revised, with additions. 3rd American from the 4th London ed., by Thomas F. Cock. New York: S. S. & W. Wood, 1853. 178p. DNLM; NNNAM; OCLloyd; PPC **50-1505**

PRESTON, Ann (1813-1872)
Introductory lecture, to the course of instruction in the Female Medical College of Pennsylvania, for the session 1855-1856. . . . Philadelphia: Printed by A. E. McDowell, 1855. 14p. DLC; PPC; PU **50-1506**

PRESTON, Ann (1813-1872)
Valedictory address to the graduating class of the Female Medical College of Pennsylvania, for the session of 1857-1858. Philadelphia: A. Ketterlinus, 1858. 16p. DNLM; PPC **50-1507**

PRESTON, Ann (1813-1872)
Introductory lecture to the class of the Female Medical College of Pennsylvania. Philadelphia: A. Ketterlinus, 1859. 14p. DNLM; PPC; PU **50-1508**

PRESTON, Henry Canfield
Inaugural address delivered before the Rhode Island Homoeopathic Medical Society, November 3, 1852. Published by the Society. Providence, R.I.: Sayles & Miller, 1852. 44p. PPHa; RPM **50-1509**

PRICE, James W.
An essay upon the practice of medicine. New York: W. L. S. Harrison, 1858. 14p. DNLM; NNNAM **50-1510**

PRICE, James W.
Reply to Dr. Coe's essay on the modus operandi of calomel. Atlanta, Ga.: Miller & Co., 1859. 15p. PPHa; GU **50-1511**

PROCTER, William, Jr. (1817-1874)
Valedictory address to the graduates of the Philadelphia College of Pharmacy. With a list of the graduates. Philadelphia: Merrihew & Thompson, 1852. 31p. DNLM; PPC; PU
50-1512

PROCTER, William, Jr. (1817-1874)
Valedictory charge to the graduates of the Philadelphia College of Pharmacy. With a list of the graduates. Philadelphia: Kite & Watton, 1855. 18p. DNLM; PPC; PU **50-1513**

PROCTER, William, Jr. (1817-1874)
Valedictory charge to the graduates of the Philadelphia College of Pharmacy. With a list of the graduates. Philadelphia, 1858. 16p. DNLM; PPC **50-1514**

PROCTER, William, Jr. (1817-1874)
Syllabus of a course of study, intended as an aid to students of pharmacy who cannot avail themselves of regular instruction, being a report made to the American Pharmaceutical Association. Philadelphia: Merrihew & Thompson, 1858. 66p. DNLM; PPC; PPJ; PU **50-1515**

PULTE, Joseph Hippolyte (1811-1884)
Homoeopathic domestic physician; containing the treatment of diseases; with popular explanations on anatomy, physiology, hygiene, and hydropathy; also, an abridged materia medica. . . . Cincinnati: H. W. Derby & Co. [etc.]; New York: A. S. Barnes & Co., 1850. 556p. DLC; OCIM; NNNAM; PPC
50-1516

PULTE, Joseph Hippolyte (1811-1884)
Homoeopathic domestic physician; containing the treatment of diseases; with popular explanations on anatomy, physiology, hygiene, and hydropathy; also, an abridged materia medica. . . . 2nd ed., rev. and enl. Cincinnati: H. W. Derby & Co.; New York: G. P. Putnam [etc.], 1851. 540p. DLC; OCIM; NNNAM; PPC **50-1517**

PULTE, J[oseph] H[ippolyte] (1811-1884)
Reply to the article of Dr. J. W. Metcalf, contained in the North American Journal of Homoeopathy, No. II, purporting to be a criticism of my "Domestic physician." Cincinnati: H. W. Derby & Co., 1851. 23p. DNLM; OCIM
50-1518

PULTE, Joseph Hippolyte (1811-1884)
. . . Homoeopathic domestic physician; containing the treatment of diseases; with popular explanations of anatomy, physiology, hygiene, and hydropathy: also an abridged materia medica. . . . Enl. with special hydropathic directions, and illustrated with anatomical plates. [3rd ed.] Eighth thousand. Cincinnati: Moore & Anderson; New York: Newman & Ivison [etc., etc.], 1852. 576p. DLC; OCIM; NNNAM; PPC
50-1519

PULTE, J[oseph] H[ippolyte] (1811-1884)
The science of medicine. An introductory lecture delivered before the Western College of Homoeopathic Medicine. Cleveland: Harris, Fairbanks & Co., 1852. 23p. DNLM; OCIM
50-1520

PULTE, Joseph Hippolyte (1811-1884)
Woman's medical guide; containing essays on the physical, moral, and educational development of females, and the homoeopathic treatment of their diseases. . . . Cincinnati: Moore, Anderson, Wilstach & Keys; New York: Newman & Ivison; [etc., etc.], 1853. 336p. DLC; DNLM; OCIM; NNNAM
50-1521

PULTE, Joseph Hippolyte (1811-1884)
Homoeopathic domestic physician. Containing the treatment of diseases with popular explanations on anatomy, physiology; hygiene and hydropathy; also an abridged materia medica. 4th edition. Enlarged, with special hydropathic directions and illustrated with anatomical plates. 12th thousand. Cincinnati: Moore, Anderson & Co., 1853. 576p. DNLM; OCIM
50-1522

PULTE, Joseph Hippolyte (1811-1884)
Homoeopathic domestic physician. Containing the treatment of diseases with popular explanations on anatomy, physiology, hygiene and hydropathy; also an abridged materia medica. 5th ed. . . . Cincinnati: Moore, Anderson & Co., 1854. 576p. DNLM; OCIM **50-1523**

PULTE, Joseph Hippolyte (1811-1884)
Homoeopathic domestic physician. Containing the treatment of diseases with popular explanations on anatomy, physiology, hygiene and hydropathy; also an abridged materia medica. 6th ed. . . . Cincinnati: Moore, Anderson & Co., 1854. 576p. DNLM; OCIM **50-1524**

PULTE, Joseph Hippolyte (1811-1884)
Woman's medical guide; containing essays on the physical, moral and educational development of females, and the homoeopathic treatment of their diseases in all periods of life, together with directions for the remedial use of water and gymnastics. . . . 2nd ed., rev. Cincinnati: Moore, Wilstach, Keys & Co., 1859. 336p. DLC; MBM; OCIM; PPC
50-1525

PURPLE, Samuel Smith (1822-1900)
A literary and practical sketch of acrania, brainless, or pseudo-encephalous monsters. New York: S. S. & W. Wood, 1850. 32p. DNLM; NNNAM **50-1526**

PURPLE, Samuel Smith (1822-1900)
Observations on some of the remedial properties of Simaba cedron, and on its employment in intermittent fever. New York: S. S. & W. Wood, 1854. 16p. DNLM; NNNAM
50-1527

PURPLE, Samuel Smith (1822-1900)
Statistics of injuries of the heart: observations on wounds of the heart, and their relations to forensic medicine, with a table of forty-two recorded cases. New York: S. S. & W. Wood, 1855. 32p. DNLM; NNNAM **50-1528**

QUACKENBUSH, John Van Pelt (1819-1876)
An address delivered before the students of the Albany Medical College, introductory to the course on obstetrics. Albany: B. Taylor, 1855. 21p. DNLM **50-1529**

QUACKENBUSH, John Van Pelt (1819-1876)
Inversion of the uterus. A report submitted to the N. Y. State Medical Society. Albany: C. Van Benthuysen, 1859. 10p. DNLM **50-1530**

QUINTARD, Charles Todd
An address delivered before the graduating class of the Medical College of Georgia, March, 1851. Augusta: J. McCafferty, 1851. 20p. DNLM; GU **50-1531**

QUINTARD, Charles Todd
The true physician. An address to the graduating class of the Memphis Medical College, session 1851-1852. Memphis, 1852. 15p. DNLM **50-1532**

QUINTARD, Charles Todd
A report on the health and mortality of the city of Memphis, Tenn., for the year 1852. Memphis: Moseley, Finnie & Pryor, 1853. 30p. DNLM **50-1533**

RALPH, Joseph
. . . A practical private treatise on the diseases of the genital organs. 14th ed., rev. and corr. New York: H. Long & Brother, 1852. 342p. 8 plates. DNLM; NNNAM **50-1534**

RALPH, Joseph
A practical treatise on the diseases and abuses of the sexual system. . . . 18th ed., rev. and cor. New York: E. D. Long, 1857. 255p. DLC [1st ed. published 1836 under title: A private treatise on venereal disease, gonorrhea, &c.] **50-1535**

RAMSAY, H. A.
Contributions to obstetrics, with tabular views and miscellaneous practical observations. Philadelphia: W. S. Young, 1851. 16p. DNLM; PPC; PU **50-1536**

RAMSAY, H. A.
To the medical profession. (A statement with regard to a controversy with Dr. F. M. Robertson.) Raysville, Ga., 1851. 24p. DNLM **50-1537**

RAMSAY, H. A.
The necrological appearances of Southern typhoid fever in the Negro, with hints upon its prophylaxis and therapeutic management; together with observations upon the mental and physical peculiarities of the Ethiopian, [etc.]. Columbia County, Ga., 1852. 23p. DNLM **50-1538**

RAMSAY, H. A.
To the members of the Georgia State Medical Society. [Answer to a charge of violation of "code of ethics."] Thompson, Ga., 1853. 1 l. DNLM **50-1539**

RAMSAY, H. A.
Letter to Dr. James Bryan, on the Southern Negro, etc. Philadelphia: A. Hughes & Co., 1853. 8p. DNLM **50-1540**

RAMSAY, H. A.
An essay on Southern typhoid fever. Plattsburgh, N.Y., 1853. 32p. DNLM **50-1541**

RAMSBOTHAM, Francis Henry (1801-1868)
The principles and practice of obstetric medicine and surgery, in reference to the process of parturition. . . . A new American ed., rev. by the author, with notes and additions, by William V. Keating. . . . Philadelphia: Blanchard & Lea, 1855. 648p. 64 plates. CtY-M; DLC; OCIM; PPC **50-1542**

RAMSEY, Frank A.
Report of a case read before the Medical Society of East Tennessee . . . in which the diagnosis was disease of the kidney. Knoxville, Tenn.: H. Barry, 1850. 36p. DNLM **50-1543**

RAMSEY, Frank A.
Letter addressed to the mayor and aldermen of the city of Knoxville [on cholera]. Knoxville: Kinsloe & Bros., 1854. 87p. DNLM **50-1544**

RAND, Benjamin Howard (1827-1883)
Charge to the graduating class of the Philadelphia College of Medicine. Philadelphia, 1857. 12p. DNLM; PU **50-1545**

RAPOU, Augustus
A treatise on typhoid fever and its homoeopathic treatment. Transl. from the French by Arthur Alleyn Granville. New York: William Radde, 1853. 96p. NNNAM; PPHa **50-1546**

RAPOU, Augustus
Typhoid fever and its homoeopathic treatment. Transl. by M. Coté, M.D. Cincinnati: Moore, Anderson & Co., 1853. 114p. NNNAM; PPHa **50-1547**

RAY, Isaac (1807-1881)
Education in its relation to the physical health of the brain. A lecture delivered before the Rhode Island Institute of Instruction, October 18, 1850. Boston: Ticknor, Reed & Fields, 1851. 52p. DLC; DNLM; RPM **50-1548**

RAY, Isaac (1807-1881)
Hints to the medical witness in questions of insanity. Utica: New York State Lunatic Asylum, [1851]. 15p. DNLM **50-1549**

RAY, Isaac (1807-1881)
The popular feeling towards hospitals for the insane. [n.p.], W. Saunderson, [1852]. 30p. DNLM **50-1550**

RAY, Isaac (1807-1881)
Insanity of King George III. Utica, 1855. 31p. DNLM **50-1551**

RAYNER, John
Cod-liver oil; its uses, mode of administation, etc. Compiled from the best and latest authorities, British and foreign. 4th American ed. New York: Ruston, Clark & Co., 1850. 16p. DNLM; MBM; NNNAM; PPC **50-1552**

READ, E.
An address read before the Esculapian Society of the Wabash Valley, held at Paris, Illinois, on the 29th of October, 1857. Chicago: Barnet & Clark, 1858. 24p. DNLM; ICRM; IEN-M; IU-M **50-1553**

REDFIELD, J. W.
The twelve qualities of mind; or, outlines of a new system of physiognomy. No. 2. New York: J. S. Redfield, 1850. 96p. DNLM; NNNAM **50-1554**

REED, William A[shton] (1827-1895)
Valedictory address delivered at the tenth annual commencement of the Homoeopathic Medical College of Pennsylvania. Philadelphia: King & Baird, 1858. 15p. DNLM; PPHa; PPC **50-1555**

REED, William B[radford] (1806-1876)
Address before the alumni of the University of Pennsylvania, Nov. 13, 1849. Philadelphia: H. Longstreth, 1850. 40p. DNLM; PPC **50-1556**

REESE, David Meredith (1800-1861)
Medical lexicon of modern terminology; being a complete vocabulary of definitions, including all the technical terms employed by writers and teachers of medical science at the present day, and comprising several hundreds of words not found in any other dictionary. Designed for the use of students and practitioners. 3rd ed. New York: S. S. & W. Wood, 1855. 233p. DNLM; ICRM; MBM; PPC **50-1557**

REESE, David Meredith (1800-1861)
Report on infant mortality in large cities, the source of its increase, and means for its diminution. Philadelphia: T. K. & P. G. Collins, 1857. 19p. DLC; DNLM; PPC
50-1558

REESE, David Meredith (1800-1861)
Report on moral insanity in its relations to medical jurisprudence. Philadelphia: T. K. & P. G. Collins, 1858. 26p. DNLM; PPC **50-1559**

REESE, John James (1818-1892)
The American medical formulary; based upon the United States and British pharmacopoeias; including also numerous standard formulae, derived from American and European authorities. Together with the medical properties and uses of medicines; poisons, their antidotes, tests, etc. Philadelphia: Lindsay & Blakiston, 1850. 357p. DLC; DNLM; OCLloyd; PPC **50-1560**

REESE, John James (1818-1892)
An analysis of physiology: being a condensed view of its most important facts and doctrines. Designed especially for the use of students. 2nd ed. Philadelphia: Lindsay & Blakiston, 1852. 368p. DNLM; NNNAM; PPC; PU **50-1561**

REESE, John James (1818-1892)
Chemistry: its importance to the physician. An introductory to the course of lectures on medical chemistry and pharmacy in the medical department of Pennsylvania College. Philadelphia: J. Richards, 1852. 27p. DNLM; PPC; PU
50-1562

REESE, John James (1818-1892)
Valedictory address to the graduates of the medical department of Pennsylvania College. Philadelphia: Brown's Steam Press, 1854. 24p. DNLM; PU **50-1563**

REESE, John James (1818-1892)
Syllabus of the course of lectures on medical chemistry, delivered in the medical department of Pennsylvania College. . . . Philadelphia: Lindsay & Blakiston, 1857. 198p. DLC; PPC; PU **50-1564**

REEVES, James Edmund (1829-1896)
A practical treatise on enteric fever; its diagnosis and treatment; being an analysis of 130 consecutive cases, derived from private practice, and embracing a partial history of the disease in Virginia. Philadelphia: J. B. Lippincott & Co., 1859. 199p. DLC; DNLM; PPC; PU **50-1565**

REFORM MEDICAL COLLEGE OF GEORGIA
The reform medical practice, with a history of medicine, from the earliest period to the present time, and a synopsis of principles on which the new practice is founded. By the faculty of the. . . . 1st ed. Macon, Ga.: M. S. Thompson, 1857. 1120p. DNLM; GU **50-1566**

REFUTATION of the misstatements contained in a pamphlet recently issued by W. Darrach, M.D., and John Wiltbank, M.D. in reference to the Medical Department of Pennsylvania College. Philadelphia: Merrihew & Thompson, 1855. 64p. DNLM; PU **50-1567**

RENOUARD, Pierre Victor (*b.* 1798)
History of medicine, from its origin to the nineteenth century, with an appendix, containing a philosophical and historical review of medicine to the present time. . . . Transl. from the French by Cornelius G. Comegys. . . . Cincinnati: Moore, Wilstach, Keys & Co.; New York: Miller, Orton & Mulligan; [etc., etc.], 1856. 719p. DLC; MH; OCIM; NNNAM
50-1568

REPLY to a pamphlet entitled "A Statement of the Facts Connected with the Late Re-organization of the Faculty of the Medical Department of Pennsylvania College, together with a Documentary of Said Department, from its Origin to the Present Time." Philadelphia: King & Baird, 1855. 68p. DNLM; PU **50-1569**

REPORT of the origin of the yellow fever in Norfolk during the summer of 1855. Made to city councils by a committee of physicians. Richmond, Va.: Ritchie & Dunnavant, 1857. 44p. DNLM; ViRA **50-1570**

REVIEW of the memorial of Doctor John Bell, to the Trustees of the University of Pennsylvania. Philadelphia: B. Mifflin, 1850. 24p. DNLM; PU **50-1571**

REYBURN, Thomas (1819-1857)
Report on the diseases of Missouri and Iowa. Philadelphia: T. K. & P. G. Collins, 1855. 243p. 3 diagrams. DNLM; MBM; OCIM; PPC **50-1572**

REYNOLDS, Edward (1793-1881)
Address at the dedication of the new building of the Massachusetts Eye and Ear Infirmary, July 3, 1850. Boston: C. C. P. Moody, 1850. 40p. 1 plate. DLC; DNLM; MBM
50-1573

RICE, C. D[arwin] (1810-1853)
Illustrations of physiology. Boston: O. Clapp, 1851. 212p. DNLM; MH **50-1574**

RICE, Nathan P.
Trials of a public benefactor, as illustrated in the discovery of etherization. [With inscription written by Dr. Bigelow for the Norton monument.] New York: Pudney & Russell, 1859. 460p. 3 plates. DNLM; MBM; MH; MWA
50-1575

RICHARDSON, Charles
An essay on cholera infantum; with some few observations on inflammation, local blood-letting, and the action of epispastics. . . . Baltimore: Taylor & Co., 1851. 40p. DLC; MdU-D; PPC
50-1576

RICHARDSON, John W. (1809-1872)
An address upon the difficulties and responsibilities of the physician. Delivered to the graduates in the medical department of the University of Nashville, Feb. 24, 1853. Nashville, Tenn.: J. T. S. Fall, 1853. 18p. DNLM; KyLoJM
50-1577

RICHARDSON, Tobias Gibson (1827-1892)
Elements of human anatomy: general, descriptive, and practical. . . . Philadelphia: Lippincott, Grambo & Co., 1854. 734p. DLC; DNLM; PPC; PPJ **50-1578**

RICORD, Philippe (1799-1889)
A practical treatise on venereal diseases . . . with a therapeutical summary and special formulary. Transl. from the French by Henry Pilkington Drummond. 7th ed. New York: Redfield, 1853. 339p. DNLM; MBM; NNNAM; PPC
50-1579

RIDDLE, S.
Every man his own physician, or The best mode of preserving health and curing disease. Also a number of the most valuable recipes. . . . Ashland, O.: L. J. Sprengle & Co., printers, 1857. 15p. DLC; OCIM **50-1580**

RIGBY, Edward (1804-1860)
A system of midwifery. . . . With notes and additional illustrations. 2nd American ed. Philadelphia: Lea & Blanchard, 1851. 422p. DLC; DNLM; PPC; PU **50-1581**

RIGBY, Edward (1804-1860)
On the constitutional treatment of female diseases. . . . Philadelphia: Blanchard & Lea, 1857. 256p. DLC; DNLM; NNNAM; PPC **50-1582**

ROBERTSON, F. M[arion] (1806-1872)
To the members of the American Medical Association. (Correspondence of Dr. H. A. Ramsay.) [n.p., 1851.] 12p. DNLM
50-1583

ROCHESTER. NEW YORK
Report of the board of health on cholera, as it appeared in Rochester, New York, in 1852. Rochester: Curtis, Falls & Co., 1852. 61p. DNLM **50-1584**

RODGERS, M. M.
Causes of contagious and epidemic diseases, with hints for their prevention and reform in medical police. Rochester: Darrow & Bro., 1851. 31p. DNLM **50-1585**

RODMAN, William W[oodbridge] (1817-1900)
Letter to the members of the Connecticut Medical Society. Waterbury, Conn.: American Office Print, 1851. 8p. DNLM; PPHa **50-1586**

RODMAN, William W[oodbridge] (1817-1900)
An examination of the evidence in regard to infinitesimal doses. Waterbury, Conn.: Wm. Patton, 1851. 99p. DNLM; PPHa **50-1587**

RODMAN, William W[oodbridge] (1817-1900)
Letter to a member of the Connecticut Medical Society. Waterbury, Conn.: E. B. Cook & Co., 1856. 28p. PPHa
50-1588

ROGERS, David L. (1799-1877)
Surgical essays and cases in surgery. . . . New York: J. Westall, printer, 1850. 160p. DLC; DNLM; NNNAM
50-1589

ROGERS, Lewis (1812-1875)
Introductory lecture before the medical class of the University of Louisville, delivered Nov. 4, 1850. Louisville: Morton & Griswold, 1850. 24p. DNLM; OCIM **50-1590**

ROGERS, Lewis (1812-1875)
A lecture on sanitary reform. Louisville, Ky., 1851. 42p. DNLM; OCIM **50-1591**

ROGERS, William C.
An address on the registration of diseases, reprinted, with additions, from the Transactions of the N.Y. State Medical Society, for the year 1859. . . . Troy, N.Y.: D. H. Jones, printer, 1859. 23p. DLC; DNLM; NNNAM
50-1592

ROKITANSKY, C. von (1804-1878)
A manual of pathological anatomy. . . . Transl. by W. E. Swaine, Edward Sieveking, C. H. Moore, and G. E. Day. Philadelphia: Blanchard & Lea, 1855. 4 v. in 2 v. CtY-M; DNLM; MH; PPC **50-1592A**

ROOT, Harmon Knox
The people's medical lighthouse; a series of popular and scientific essays on the nature, uses, and diseases of the lungs, heart, liver, stomach, kidneys, womb and blood. . . . . New York: Pub. by the proprietor, 1852. 470p. DLC; DNLM; NNNAM **50-1593**

ROOT, Harmon Knox
The lover's marriage lighthouse; a series of sensible and scientific essays on the subjects of marriage and free divorce, and on the uses, wants, and supplies of the spiritual, intellectual, affectional, and sexual natures of man and woman; being a key to the causes, prevention, remedies, and cure of mental and physical uncongenialities. . . . New York, 1858. 511p. DNLM; NNNAM **50-1594**

ROSA, Storm (1794?-1864)
History of medical science. An introductory lecture delivered before the class of the Cincinnati Eclectic Institute, 1850. Cincinnati, O.: J. D. Thorpe, 1850. 20p. DNLM; PPHa
50-1595

ROSCH, D.
Chronic diseases; especially the nervous diseases of women. Transl. from the German by Charles Dummig. New York: Fowler & Wells, 1850. 61p. DNLM; NNNAM
50-1596

ROSS, Joel H.
Remarks on hot air and vapour bathing. . . . Hints and helps to health and happiness, or long life and little physic. 2nd ed. Auburn, N.Y.: Derby & Miller, 1851. 303p. DNLM; NNNAM
50-1597

ROWELL, Charles S.
A manual of dental economy; or practical instruction on the physiology and treatment of teeth, in order to check their diseases, repair their injuries, and insure their preservation. New York: C. Scribner, 1855. 158p. DNLM; NNNAM
50-1598

ROWLAND, James S.
Principles and progress of homoeopathy. Hopkinsville, Ky.: McCarroll, Printer, 1853. 40p. PPHa **50-1599**

RUSHTON, Frederick V.
Rushton's treatise on cod-liver oil, giving its curative properties and uses in various diseases. New York: F. V. Rushton, 1855. 60p. DNLM; NNNAM **50-1600**

ST. JOHN, Samuel (1813-1876)
An introductory address delivered at the opening of the annual course of lectures of the College of Physicians and Surgeons, in the city of New York, October 19th, 1857. New York: Wynkoop, Hallenbeck & Thomas, 1858. 24p. DNLM; NNNAM
50-1601

SANBORN, E[ben] K. (1827-1862)
Successful treatment of a case of ligamentous union of fractured radius and ulna by drilling and wiring after failure by other means. [Rutland, Vt., 1859.] 6p. DNLM
50-1602

SANBORN, Guilford D.
On the inhalation of cold medicated vapors in phthisis pulmonalis, and the use of showering syringes in laryngeal and catarrhal diseases. New York: Baker, Godwin & Co., 1855. 16p. DNLM; NNNAM **50-1603**

SANBORN, Guilford D.
The nature, causes, and symptoms of diseases of the lungs and throat; with their treatment by the use of cold medicated inhalation. New York: the author, 1856. 120p. DNLM; NNNAM **50-1604**

SANBORN, Guilford D.
Letters upon the effects of alcohol as a preventive to tubercular formations and deposits. Rochester: Curtis & Butts, 1856. 18p. DNLM **50-1605**

SANDERSON, J. M.
A letter on the treatment of hernia. New York: Hood Truss Office, 1852. 12p. DNLM; NNNAM **50-1606**

SANFORD, E.
Homoeopathy and homoeopathic practitioners in Europe. Boston: O. Clapp, 1857. 28p. DNLM; MBM
50-1607

SANGER, William W[allace] (1819-1872)
The history of prostitution; its extent, causes, and effects throughout the world. [Being an official report to the board of alms-house governors of the city of New York.] New York: Harper & Bros., 1858. 685p. DNLM; MB; MH; NN
50-1608

SARGENT, F[itzwilliam] W. (1820-1889)
On bandaging, and other operations on minor surgery. New edition, revised and enlarged, with one hundred and eighty-one illustrations. Philadelphia: Blanchard & Lea, 1856. 359p. CtY-M; DNLM; MBM; PPC **50-1609**

SAUNDERS, D. L.
Woman's own book; or, a plain and familiar treatise on all complaints and diseases peculiar to females. Also a full system of midwifery, well adapted to the use of common readers. For the ladies themselves. Little Rock: J. D. Butler, 1858. 133p. 1 plate. DNLM **50-1610**

SAYRE, Lewis Albert (1820-1900)
Case of the perforation of the rectum and extensive faecal abscess. . . . New York: Holman, Gray & Co., printers, 1854. 14p. DLC; DNLM; NNNAM **50-1611**

SAYRE, Lewis Albert (1820-1900)
Exsection of the head of the femur, and removal of the upper rim of the acetabulum, for morbus coxarius. New York: Holman, Gray & Co., 1854. 15p. DNLM; NNNAM
50-1612

SCHAEFFER, George C[hristian] (1815-1893)
Introductory address to the students of the medical department of Georgetown College. . . . Washington, H. Polkinhorn, printer, 1856. 22p. DLC; DNLM
50-1613

SCHAEFFER, George C[hristian] (1815-1893)
Valedictory address to the graduating class of the medical department of Georgetown College, delivered March 18, 1858. Washington: T. McGill, 1858. 15p. DNLM
50-1614

SCHIEFERDECKER, Christian Charles
A short guide for the rational treatment of children, in health and disease, by water. . . . Philadelphia: J. W. Moore, 1852. 299p. DLC; PPC; PU **50-1615**

SCHIEFERDECKER, Christian Charles
Dr. C. G. G. Nittinger's evils of vaccination. Philadelphia, 1856. 88p. DNLM; PPC; PU **50-1616**

SCHIEFERDECKER, Christian Charles
The scientific foundation of water-cure. Pamphlet 1. Baltimore: J. Robinson, 1859. 32p. DNLM
50-1617

SCHMIDT, Jacob (1813-1880)
A letter to Thos. E. Bond, A.M., M.D., on homoeopathy. Occasioned by the publication of his address to the graduates at Washington University on March 3, 1851. Baltimore: Sands & Mills, 1851. 21p. DNLM; PPHa **50-1618**

SCUDDER, John Milton (1829-1894)
A practical treatise on the diseases of women. Illustrated by colored plates and numerous wood engravings. . . . With an introduction by Geo. W. L. Bickley. . . . And a paper on the diseases of the breasts, by Robert S. Newton. . . . Cincinnati: Moore, Wilstach, Keys & Co., printers, 1857. 525p. DLC; OCIM; NNNAM; PPC **50-1619**

SEMPLE, Matthew
Valedictory address delivered at the fifth annual commencement of the Homoeopathic Medical College of Pennsylvania, March 1, 1853. Philadelphia: C. Sherman, 1853. 20p. DNLM; PPHa **50-1620**

SEYMOUR, David L. (1803-1867)
Address, delivered before the friends and patrons of the Troy Hospital, February 12, 1850. Also, the remarks of Maj. Gen. Wool, and Rev. Peter Havermans, on the occasion of the laying of the corner stone of the above institution. Troy, N.Y.: Johnson & Davis, 1851. 32p. DNLM **50-1621**

SEYMOUR, William P[ierce] (1825-1893)
The two ways: an address to the graduating class of Castleton Medical College, delivered November 24, 1858. Rutland: G. A. Tuttle & Co., 1858. 32p. DNLM; VtHi
50-1622

SHANKS, L[ewis] (1801-1861)
A brief history of the commencement and progress of the yellow fever in Memphis, Tenn., in 1855, with some account of its symptoms, treatment, and fatality. Memphis, 1856. 41p. DNLM **50-1623**

SHARP, William (1805-1896)
Tracts on homoeopathy. No. 4. The small dose of homoeopathy. New York: W. Radde, 1855. 23p. DNLM; NNNAM
50-1624

SHARP, William (1805-1896)
Tracts on homoeopathy. No. 6. The advantages of homoeopathy. New York: W. Radde, 1856. 19p. DNLM; NNNAM
50-1625

SHARP, William (1805-1896)
Tracts on homoeopathy. No. 7. The principles of homoeopathy. New York: W. Radde, 1856. 19p. DNLM; NNNAM
50-1626

SHATTUCK, George Cheyne, Jr. (1813-1893)
An introductory lecture before the medical class of 1857-1858 of Harvard University. Boston: D. Clapp, 1857. 29p. DNLM; MH-M **50-1627**

SHATTUCK, Lemuel (1793-1859)
Contributions to the vital statistics of the State of New York. [Communicated to T. Romeyn Beck, M.D.] [Boston, 1850.] 28p. DNLM; MBM; NNNAM **50-1628**

SHATTUCK, Lemuel (1793-1859)
Memorial in relation to the small-pox. City doc. No. 30. March 13, 1856. [Boston, 1856.] 13p. DNLM; MBM
50-1629

SHAW, Benjamin S[hurtleff] (1827-1893)
Colored prismatic crystals in blood-globules. [Analysis of blood; a new method of separating the blood-globules from the coagulum.] Philadelphia, 1853. 3p. DNLM **50-1630**

SHERRILL, Hunting (1773-1866)
Suggestions on an improved mode of prevention and cure of small-pox and varioloid; delivered before the Hahnemann Academy of Medicine. New York: E. Varey, 1852. 12p. NNNAM; PPHa **50-1631**

SHERRILL, Hunting (1773-1866)
A treatise on homoeopathic practice of medicine: complete in a repertory for prescribing, adapted to domestic or professional use. 3rd ed., improved and enl.... New York: W. Radde, 1854. 428p. DLC; NNNAM; PPHa **50-1632**

SHERRILL, Hunting (1773-1866)
A temperance medical lecture on the injurious and dangerous effects of stimulants and alcohol in many states of disease. New York, 1859. 48p. DNLM; NNNAM; PPHa
50-1633

SHERWOOD, Henry Hall
Manual for magnetizing, with the vibrating magnetic machine, and for the magnetic or duodynamic treatment of diseases. . . . 14th ed. Rev. by H. H. Sherwood's successors. . . . New York: Fowlers & Wells, 1850. 375p. DLC; NNNAM
50-1634

SHERWOOD, Henry Hall
The motive power of the human system with the duodynamic symptoms and treatment of chronic diseases. . . . Rev. by H. H. Sherwood's successor, William Larned. . . . 16th ed., enl. New York: Pub. by the proprietor, 1850. 206p. 16 plates. DNLM; NNNAM **50-1635**

SHERWOOD, Henry Hall
The magnetic organization of the human system, and its application to the cure of chronic diseases. Abridged from the works of the late Henry Hall Sherwood, by William Larned. New York: Tribune Steam Printing Office, 1850. 16p. DNLM; NNNAM **50-1636**

SHERWOOD, William
Medical education for the people and the profession. An introductory lecture delivered before the eclectic medical class, Nov. 10, 1852. Cincinnati, 1852. 15p. DNLM; OCIM
50-1637

SHERWOOD, William
The only true and accurate announcement, by themselves, of the character and ability of the spurious faculty, who now pretend to represent the Eclectic Medical Institute. Compiled from the manuscripts and publications of said faculty, with a running commentary. [Cincinnati, 1856?] 14p. DNLM; OCIM
50-1638

SHERWOOD, William
History of the expulsion of Drs. R. S. Newton and Z. Freeman from the Eclectic Medical Institute, with the causes which rendered it necessary, and an exposition of the slanderous and factious course which has been pursued by the off-casts from the institute. [Oct. 11, 1856.] [Cincinnati, 1856?] 18p. DNLM; OCIM **50-1639**

SHEW, Joel (1816-1855)
Hydropathy, or the water-cure: its principles, processes, and modes of treatment. . . . 4th ed. New York, 1850. 360p. DNLM; NNNAM **50-1640**

SHEW, Joel (1816-1855)
The water-cure manual: a popular work, embracing descriptions of the various modes of bathing, the hygienic and curative effects of air, exercises, clothing. . . . Illustrated with cases of treatment and cure, containing also a fine engraving of Priessnitz. Tenth thousand, improved. New York: Fowlers & Wells, 1850. 282p. DNLM; NNNAM **50-1641**

SHEW, Joel (1816-1855)
Hydropathy, or The water-cure: its principles, processes, and modes of treatment. Compiled in part from the most eminent authors, ancient and modern, on the subject: together with an account of the latest methods adopted by Priessnitz. Illustrated with numerous cases of cure. . . . 4th ed., improved and enl. New York: Fowlers & Wells, 1851. 360p. DLC; NNNAM
50-1642

SHEW, Joel (1816-1855)
Consumption; its prevention and cure by the water treatment; with advice concerning hemorrhage from the lungs, coughs, colds, asthma, bronchitis, and sore throat. New York: Fowlers & Wells, 1851. 288p. DNLM; NNNAM
50-1643

SHEW, Joel (1816-1855)
Children, their hydropathic management in health and disease; a descriptive and practical work, designed as a guide for families and physicians. Illustrated with numerous cases. . . . New York [etc.]: Fowlers & Wells, 1852. 432p. DLC; DNLM; NNNAM **50-1644**

SHEW, Joel (1816-1855)
Midwifery and the diseases of women, a description and practical work showing the superiority of water-treatment in menstruation and its disorders, chlorosis, leucorrhea, fluor albus, prolapsus uteri, hysteria, spinal diseases, [etc.]. New York: Fowlers & Wells, [1852]. 432p. DNLM; NNNAM
50-1645

SHEW, Joel (1816-1855)
The hydropathic family physician; a ready prescriber and hygienic adviser with reference to the nature, causes, prevention, and treatment of diseases, accidents, and casualties of every kind. . . . Illustrated with nearly three hundred engravings. New York, London [etc.]: Fowlers & Wells, 1854. 816p. DLC; DNLM; NNNAM **50-1646**

SHEW, Joel (1816-1855)
The water-cure in pregnancy and childbirth. Illustrated with cases showing the remarkable effects of water in mitigating the pains and perils of the parturient state. New York, 1855. 122p. DNLM; NNNAM **50-1647**

SHIPMAN, A. B. (1803-1868)
An introductory lecture to the students in the Indiana Medical College, session 1849-1850. Laporte: W. & J. Millikan, 1850. 13p. DNLM **50-1648**

SHIPMAN, George Elias (1820?-1893)
Homoeopathy, allopathy and the City Hospital; a legend of the nineteenth century. Addressed in form of a letter to N. S. Davis, M.D. Published by the Chicago Homoeopathic Medical Society, 1857. 28p. ICJ; ICRM; IU-M; PPHa **50-1649**

SICHEL, Jules (1802-1868)
Spectacles: their uses and abuses in long and short sightedness, and the pathological conditions resulting from their irrational employment. Transl. from the French by H. W. Williams. Boston: Phillips, Sampson & Co., 1850. 202p. DNLM; MBM; NNNAM; PPC **50-1650**

SIMON, John (1816-1904)
General pathology, as conducive to the establishment of rational principles for the diagnosis and treatment of disease. A course of lectures delivered at St. Thomas's Hospital during the summer session of 1850. Philadelphia: Blanchard & Lea, 1852. 211p. CU-M; DNLM; OCIM; PPC **50-1651**

SIMONDS, J. C.
An address on the sanitary condition of New Orleans, as illustrated by its mortuary statistics. New Orleans: D. Davies, Son & Co., 1851. 56p. DNLM; LNT-M **50-1652**

SIMONDS, J. C.
An address on the sanitary condition of New Orleans, as illustrated by its mortuary statistics. Revised for the Charleston Medical Journal and Review. Charleston, S.C.: Walker & James, 1851. 71p. DNLM; ScCM; ScMS **50-1653**

SIMONS, Thomas Young (1798-1857)
An essay on the yellow fever, as it has occurred in Charleston, including its origin and progress up to the present time. Charleston, S.C.: Walker & James, 1851. 30p. DNLM; ScCM **50-1654**

SIMPSON, James Young (1811-1870)
Homoeopathy, its tenets and tendencies, theoretical, theological, and therapeutical. . . . 1st American from the 3rd Edinburgh ed. Philadelphia: Lindsay & Blakiston, 1854. 304p. DLC; PPC; PPJ; PU **50-1655**

SIMPSON, James Young (1811-1870)
The obstetric memoirs and contributions of James Y. Simpson . . . Edited by W. O. Priestley . . . and Horatio R. Storer. . . . Philadelphia: J. B. Lippincott & Co., 1855-1856. 2 v. DLC; DNLM; PPC; PU **50-1656**

SIMS, James Marion (1813-1883)
On the treatment of vesico-vaginal fistula. Philadelphia: Blanchard & Lea, 1853. 28p. DNLM; PPC; PPJ; PU **50-1657**

SIMS, James Marion (1813-1883)
Silver sutures in surgery. . . . New York: S. S. & W. Wood, 1858. 79p. DLC; DNLM; NNNAM; PPC **50-1658**

SINGLETON, James William (1829-1881)
An address delivered before the eighth graduating class of the medical department of the University of Nashville. Nashville: J. T. S. Fall, 1859. 28p. DNLM; OCIM **50-1659**

SKETCH of the proceedings of the Medical and Chirurgical Faculty of Maryland, at the annual session in June and special session in July, 1853. Baltimore: J. W. Woods, 1853. 14p. DNLM; MdBM **50-1660**

SKEY, Frederic Carpenter (1798-1872)
Operative surgery. Philadelphia: Blanchard & Lea, 1851. 661p. DNLM; MBM; NNNAM; PPC **50-1661**

SLADE, Daniel Denison (1823-1896)
Some observations on the treatment of narrow and irritable structure of the urethra. Boston: D. Clapp, 1858. 8p. DNLM; MBM **50-1662**

SLADE, Daniel Denison (1823-1896)
To what affections of the lungs does bronchitis give origin? Prize essay. [Boston, 1859.] 75p. DNLM; MBM **50-1663**

SMALL, Alvan Edmond (1811-1886)
Address delivered before the American Institute of Homoeopathy at its annual meeting in Albany in 1850. Boston: Otis Clapp, 1850. 42p. MBM **50-1664**

SMALL, Alvan Edmond (1811-1886)
Valedictory address delivered at the 4th annual commencement of the Homoeopathic Medical College of Pennsylvania, March 1, 1852. Philadelphia: C. Sherman, 1852. 20p. DNLM; PPHa **50-1665**

SMALL, Alvan Edmond (1811-1886)
Eulogium on the life and character of Joseph G. Loomis, M.D. Delivered in the Homoeopathic Medical College of Pennsylvania, January 12, 1854. By the faculty. 1854. 16p. PPHa; PPC **50-1666**

SMALL, Alvan Edmond (1811-1886)
Manual of homoeopathic practice, for the use of families and private individuals. Philadelphia: Rademacher & Sheek, 1854. 815p. DNLM; PPHa; PPC **50-1667**

SMALL, Alvan Edmond (1811-1886)
The pocket manual of homoeopathic practice, abridged from the manual of homoeopathic practice by Jacob F. Sheek. Philadelphia: Rademacher & Sheek, 1855. 126p. DNLM; PPHa; PPC **50-1668**

SMALL, Alvan Edmond (1811-1886)
Manual of homoeopathic practice for the use of families and private individuals. 3rd enlarged ed. Philadelphia: Rademacher & Sheek, 1855. 831p. DNLM; PPC; PPHa; PU **50-1669**

SMALL, Alvan Edmond (1811-1886)
Diseases of the nervous system, to which is added a treatise on the diseases of the skin, by Dr. C. E. Toothaker. Philadelphia: Rademacher & Sheek, 1856. 208p. DNLM; PPHa **50-1670**

SMALL, Alvan Edmond (1811-1886)
Manual of homoeopathy practice for the use of families and private individuals. 4th enlarged ed. Philadelphia: Rademacher & Sheek, 1856, 831p. DNLM; NNNAM; PPHa
50-1671

SMALL, Alvan Edmond (1811-1886)
Handbuch der homöopathie für familien und das publikum im allgemeinen. . . . 4. verm. ausg. in's deutsche ubersetzt von doctor Karl Julius Hempel. . . . Philadelphia: Rademacher und Sheek; New York: W. Radde, 1856. 572p. DLC; NNNAM; PPG; PPHa **50-1672**

SMALL, Alvan Edmond (1811-1886)
Manual of homoeopathic practice, for the use of families and private individuals. 6th ed. Philadelphia: Rademacher & Sheek, 1857. 831p. DNLM; PPHa **50-1673**

SMALL, Alvan Edmond (1811-1886)
Manual of homoeopathic practice for the use of families and private individuals. 7th enlarged ed. Philadelphia: Rademacher & Sheek, 1857. 831p. DNLM; PPC: PPHa **50-1674**

SMALL, E.
A treatise on inflammatory disease of the uterus and its appendages, and on ulceration and enlargement of the neck of the uterus, in which the morbid uterine manifestations and functional derangements are explained and illustrated. 2nd ed. Boston: Sanborn, Carter & Bazin, 1856. 263p. DNLM; MBM
50-1675

SMEE, Alfred (1818-1877)
Accidents and emergencies: a guide containing directions for treatment in bleeding, cuts, stabs, bruises, sprains, ruptures, [etc.]. With alterations, corrections, and appendix, by Dr. R. T. Trall. New York: Fowler & Wells, [1850]. 43p. DNLM; NNNAM **50-1676**

SMEE, Alfred (1818-1877)
Principles of the human mind, deduced from physical laws; together with a lecture on electro-biology, or the voltaic mechanism of man. New York: Fowler & Wells, 1852. 64p. DNLM; NNNAM **50-1677**

SMITH, Francis Gurney (1818-1878)
A hand-book of obstetrics. . . . Being a portion of an analytical compendium of the various branches of medicine. By Francis Gurney Smith . . . and John Neill. . . . 2nd ed., rev. and impr. Philadelphia: Blanchard & Lea, 1852. 123p. DLC; DNLM; PPC; PU **50-1678**

SMITH, Francis Gurney (1818-1878)
A hand-book of physiology: with forty-three illustrations. Being a portion of an analytical compendium of the various branches of medicine. By Francis Gurney Smith . . . and John Neill. . . . 2nd ed., rev. and improved. Philadelphia: Blanchard & Lea, 1852. 143p. DLC; NNNAM; PPC; PU
50-1679

SMITH, Francis Gurney (1818-1878)
Valedictory address to the graduates of the Medical Department of Pennsylvania College. Delivered at the public commencement, March 5, 1853. Philadelphia: C. Sherman, 1853. 24p. DNLM; PPC; PU **50-1680**

SMITH, Francis Gurney (1818-1878)
Experiments upon digestion. . . . Philadelphia: Merrihew & Thompson, printers, 1856. 18p. DLC; DNLM; PPC; PU
50-1681

SMITH, Hamilton L[anphere] (1819-1903)
The scientific relations of homoeopathy. An introductory lecture delivered before the Western College of Homoeopathic Medicine. Cleveland: Harris, Fairbanks & Co., 1851. 30p. DNLM; OCIM **50-1682**

SMITH, Henry Hollingsworth (1815-1890)
Minor surgery; or, Hints on the every-day duties of the surgeon. . . . 2nd ed., with numerous additions. Illustrated by 227 engravings. Philadelphia: E. Barrington & G. D. Haswell, 1850. 384p. DLC; DNLM; NNNAM; PPC **50-1683**

SMITH, Henry Hollingsworth (1815-1890)
A system of operative surgery: based upon the practice of surgeons in the United States: and comprising a bibliographical index and historical record of many of their operations, during a period of two hundred years. . . . Philadelphia: Lippincott, Grambo & Co., 1852. 698p. 80 plates. DLC; DNLM; PPC; PU
50-1684

SMITH, Henry Hollingsworth (1815-1890)
Anatomical atlas, illustrative of the structure of the human body. . . . Under the supervision of William E. Horner. . . . Philadelphia: Blanchard & Lea, 1854. 200p. DLC; MBM; NNNAM; PPC **50-1685**

SMITH, Henry Hollingsworth (1815-1890)
On the treatment of ununited fracture by means of artificial limbs, which combine the principle of pressure and motion at the seat of fracture, and lead to the formation of an ensheathing callus; illustrated by the history of four cases of false joint in the femur, eight in the leg, and two in the humerus. Philadelphia: T. K. & P. G. Collins, 1855. 20p. DLNM; PPC
50-1686

SMITH, Henry Hollingsworth (1815-1890)
Syllabus of the lectures on the principles and practice of surgery, delivered in the University of Pennsylvania. . . . Printed for the use of the class. Philadelphia: T. K. & P. G. Collins, printers, 1855. 115p. DLC; DNLM; PPC; PU
50-1687

SMITH, Henry Hollingsworth (1815-1890)
A system of operative surgery: based upon the practice of surgeons in the United States: with a bibliographical index and historical record of many of their operations, during a period of two hundred and thirty-four years. . . . 2nd ed., with numerous additions in both the text and illustrations. . . . Philadelphia: Lippincott, Grambo & Co., 1855. 2 v. 80 plates. DLC; DNLM; PPC; PU **50-1688**

SMITH, Henry Hollingsworth (1815-1890)
A professional visit to London and Paris. Introductory lecture to the course on the principles and practice of surgery. Delivered in the University of Pennsylvania, October 9, 1855. Philadelphia: T. K. & P. G. Collins, 1855. 24p. DNLM; PPC; PU **50-1689**

SMITH, Henry Hollingsworth (1815-1890)
The medical, literary, and social influence of the alumni of the medical department of the University. An introductory lecture. Philadelphia: C. Sherman & Son, 1856. 32p. DNLM; PPC; PU **50-1690**

SMITH, Henry Hollingsworth (1815-1890)
The medical, literary, and social influence of the alumni of the medical department of the University. An introductory lecture. Philadelphia: J. M. Wilson, 1856. 32p. DNLM; PU
50-1691

SMITH, Henry Hollingsworth (1815-1890)
A treatise on the practice of surgery. . . . Philadelphia: B. Lippincott & Co., 1856. 828p. DLC; DNLM; PPC; PU **50-1692**

SMITH, Henry Hollingsworth (1815-1890)
Address delivered at the University of Pennsylvania, before the Society of the Alumni, on the occasion of their 100th annual celebration, November 30th, 1858. Philadelphia: King & Baird, 1859. 32p. DNLM; PPC; PU **50-1693**

SMITH, Henry Hollingsworth (1815-1890)
The moral and legal responsibilities of a surgeon. Introductory lecture to the course on the principles and practice of surgery, delivered in the University of Pennsylvania, October 10, 1859. Philadelphia, 1859. 29p. DNLM; PPC; PU **50-1694**

SMITH, Henry Hollingsworth (1815-1890)
Minor surgery; or, hints on the everyday duties of the surgeon. Reprinted from the 3rd ed. Philadelphia: Blanchard & Lea, 1859. 456p. DNLM; OCIM; PPC; PU **50-1695**

SMITH, Henry Hollingsworth (1815-1890)
Valedictory address in the class of medical graduates of the University of Pennsylvania. Philadelphia: T. K. & P. G. Collins, 1859. 28, 4p. DNLM; PPC; PU **50-1696**

SMITH, Henry M[itchell] (*d.* 1901)
Smith's homoeopathic directory of the United States. New York: Smith's Homoeopathic Pharmacy [J. T. S. Smith], 1856. 28p. NNNAM; PPHa **50-1697**

SMITH, Henry M[itchell] (*d.* 1901)
Smith's homoeopathic directory of the United States. . . . New York: J. T. S. Smith, 1857. 95p. DLC; NNNAM; PPHa **50-1698**

SMITH, J[ames] Dickson
A few facts in relation to the lobelia and pepper practice: its prospects and policy; as challenged by "Professor" M. S. Thomson, in his recent pamphlet. [Macon, Georgia]: Telegraph Steam Print. House, 1859. 16p. DNLM; GU **50-1699**

SMITH, J[ames] Dickson
Rational medicine and Thomsonianism. An essay on rational vs. routine and book practice of medicine, reviewed by Dr. M. S. Thomson and vindicated by . . . of Macon, Ga. [Macon, Ga.]: Telegraph Steam Print. House, 1859. 56p. DNLM; GU **50-1700**

SMITH, John
The curiosities of common water, or the advantages thereof in preventing and curing many distempers. Gather'd from the writings of several eminent physicians, and also from more than forty years experience. To which are added some rules for preserving health by diet. From the 5th London ed., . . . With additions by Joel Shew. New York: Fowler & Wells, 1851. 92p. DNLM; NNNAM **50-1701**

SMITH, John
Fruits and farinacea the proper food of man; being an attempt to prove from history, anatomy, physiology and chemistry, that the original, natural and best diet of man is derived from the vegetable kingdom. With notes and illustrations, by R. T. Trall. From the 2nd London ed. New York, Boston & Philadelphia: Fowlers & Wells, 1854. 314p. DNLM; NNNAM; PPC **50-1702**

SMITH, J[ohn] Lawrence (1818-1883)
On some of the thermal waters of Asia Minor. [New Haven, 1851.] 20p. CtY-M; DNLM; MB **50-1703**

SMITH, John Lawrence (1818-1883)
Analysis of Jackson County Springs, at Lynchburg, Miss. New Orleans: Magic Press Office, 1852. 10p. DNLM **50-1704**

SMITH, John Lawrence (1818-1883)
The inverted microscope (a new form of microscope). With the description of a new eye-piece micrometer, and a new form of goniometer for measuring the angles of cyrstals under the microscope. [New Haven, 1852.] 9p. CtY-M; DNLM; MB; MBM **50-1705**

SMITH, John Lawrence (1818-1883)
Du Pont's artesian well, Louisville, Kentucky. Report, analysis, and medical properties of its water. With remarks upon the nature of artesian wells. Louisville, 1859. 23p. 1 plate. DNLM **50-1706**

SMITH, J[onathan] D.S. (*b.* 1830)
Medical electricity. New York: Couch & Johnston, [1859?] 16p. port. DNLM **50-1707**

SMITH, Joseph M[ather] (1789-1866)
Anniversary discourse, before the New York Academy of Medicine . . . November 13th, 1850. . . . New York: The Academy, 1851. 56p. DNLM; NNNAM **50-1708**

SMITH, Joseph Mather (1789-1866)
An address delivered on the occasion of the inauguration of the new south building of the New York Hospital, on the 18th of April, 1855. New York: T. Callahan & Co., 1855. 42p. 8 plates. DNLM; NNNAM **50-1709**

SMITH, Joseph Mather (1789-1866)
Puerperal fever; its causes and modes of propagation. New York: T. Holman, 1857. 29p. DNLM; NNNAM **50-1710**

SMITH, Lyndon Arnold (1795-1856)
Report on the topography and epidemic diseases of New Jersey, and the treatment thereof. Philadelphia: T. K. & P. G. Collins, 1858. 14p. DNLM; NjR; PPC **50-1711**

SMITH, Robert K.
Introductory lecture to the clinical course of the Philadelphia Hospital. Philadelphia: King & Baird, 1855. 15p. DNLM; PPC **50-1712**

SMITH, Robert K.
Introductory lecture to the clinical course at the Philadelphia Hospital, 1858-1859. Philadelphia: Published by the Board, 1858. 20p. DNLM; PPC **50-1713**

SMITH, Robert William (1807-1873)
A treatise on fractures in the vicinity of joints, and on certain forms of accidental and congenital dislocations. Philadelphia: Lea & Blanchard, 1850. 314p. DNLM; NNNAM; PPC; PU **50-1714**

SMITH, Robert William (1807-1873)
A treatise on fractures in the vicinity of joints, and on certain forms of accidental and congenital dislocations. Dublin: Hodges & Smith; New York: S. S. & W. Wood, 1854. 312p. DNLM; MBM; NNNAM; PPC **50-1715**

SMITH, Samuel B.
The medical application of electro-magnetism. 2nd ed. New York, 1852. 80p. DNLM; NNNAM **50-1716**

SMITH, Samuel B.
The medical application of electro-magnetism. 4th ed. New York, 1853. 92p. DNLM; NNNAM **50-1717**

SMITH, Samuel Hanbury (1810-1894)
A discourse pronounced before the class of Starling Medical College at the opening of the winter session of 1850-1851. Columbus: S. Medary, 1850. 32p. DNLM; OCIM **50-1718**

SMITH, Samuel Hanbury (1810-1894)
Some remarks on medicinal mineral waters, natural and artificial; their efficacy in the treatment of chronic diseases, and rules for their employment; especially those of Carlsbad, Ems, Kissingen, Marienbad, Pyrmont, Pullna, Seidschutz, and Heilbrunn. Hamilton, O.: D. W. Halsey, 1855. 40p. DNLM; OCHP **50-1719**

SMITH, Samuel Hanbury (1810-1894)
Medicinal mineral waters, natural and artificial; their efficacy in the treatment of chronic diseases; and rules for their employment, especially those of Carlsbad, Ems, Vichy, Kissingen, Marienbad, Pyrmont, Egra, Pullna, Seidschutz, and Heilbrunn. Hamilton, O.: D. W. Halsey, 1856. 70p. DNLM; OCHP **50-1720**

SMITH, Stephen (1823-1922)
A contribution to the statistics of rupture of the urinary bladder; with a table of seventy-eight cases. New York: J. F. Trow, 1851. 43p. DNLM; NNNAM **50-1721**

SMITH, Truman (1791-1884)
Anaesthesia! The greatest discovery of the age! Who is entitled to the credit of it? [New York, 1858.] 16p. DNLM; NNNAM **50-1722**

SMITH, Truman (1791-1884)
An examination of the question of anaesthesia, arising on the memorial of Charles Thomas Wells, presented to the United States Senate, second session, 32nd Congress, [etc.]. New York: J. A. Gray, 1858. 135p. DLC; DNLM; NNNAM **50-1723**

SMITH, Truman (1791-1884)
An examination of the question of anaesthesia, arising on the memorial of Charles Thomas Wells, presented to the United States Senate, second session, 32nd Congress, [etc.]. New York: J. A. Gray, 1859. 154p. DLC; DNLM; NNNAM **50-1724**

SMITH, William F.
Valedictory to the graduating class attending the course of lectures at the Reformed Medical Institute, February 29th, 1852. Philadelphia: Fairbanks & Glessner, 1852. 16p. DNLM; PPC **50-1725**

SMITH, William Tyler (1815-1873)
The modern practice of midwifery. A course of lectures on obstetrics: delivered at St. Mary's Hospital, London. With an introductory lecture on the history of the art of midwifery, and copious practical annotations by Augustus K. Gardner. 2nd ed. New York: R. M. DeWitt, [1858]. 760p. DNLM; NNNAM; PPC **50-1726**

SMITH, William Tyler (1815-1873)
The modern practice of midwifery. A course of lectures on obstetrics: delivered at St. Mary's Hospital, London. With an introductory lecture on the history of the art of midwifery, and copious practical annotations by Augustus K. Gardner. 3rd American ed. Philadelphia: P. Blakiston, Son & Co., [1859?]. 760p. DNLM; NNNAM; PPC; PU **50-1727**

SNOW, Edwin Miller (1820-1888)
Statistics and causes of Asiatic cholera, as it prevailed in Providence, in the summer of 1854. Being a letter addressed to the mayor of Providence. City doc. no. 5. Providence: Knowles, Anthony & Co., 1855. 20p. DNLM; RPJCB; RPM **50-1728**

SNOW, Edwin Miller (1820-1888)
History of the Asiatic cholera in Providence. [Providence, 1858.] 8p. DNLM **50-1729**

SNOW, Edwin Miller (1820-1888)
Report on the small-pox in the city of Providence from January to June, 1859. Providence: Knowles, Anthony & Co., 1859. 22p. DNLM; RPM; RPJCB **50-1730**

SPENCER, C. L.
A lecture on the philosophy and claims of homoeopathy, delivered at Nantucket, Mass., June 30, 1856. New York: H. Ludwig [For the Author], 1857. 24p. NNNAM; PPHa **50-1731**

SPRATT, George
Obstetric tables: comprising graphic illustrations. 1st American from the 4th and greatly improved London ed., carefully revised, and with additional notes and plates. Philadelphia: J. A. Bill, 1850. 13p. 15 plates. DNLM; PPC; PU **50-1732**

STATEMENT of the facts connected with the late re-organization of the faculty of the Medical Department of the Pennsylvania College, together with a documentary history of said department from its origin to the present time. Philadelphia: Brown's Steam Power Books and Job Printing Office, 1855. 64p. DLC; PPC; PU **50-1733**

STEARNS, Frederick
Upon improvements in rendering medicinal preparations pleasing to the eye and taste, and agreeable to use. Detroit, 1857. 12p. DNLM **50-1734**

STEEL, John H[oneywood] (1780-1838)
Analysis of the Congress Spring, with practical remarks on its medical properties. Revised and corrected by John L. Perry. New York: W. Rose, 1856. 35p. 1 plate. DNLM; NNNAM **50-1735**

STEINER, Lewis Henry (1827-1892)
Lecture, introductory to the course on chemistry and pharmacy, in the National Medical College, Washington, D.C. . . . Delivered October 31st, 1853. Chambersburg, Pa.: Printed by M. Kieffer & Co., 1853. 21p. DLC; DNLM; PPC; PPHa **50-1736**

STEINER, Lewis Henry (1827-1892)
Paracelsus and his influence on chemistry and medicine. Chambersburg, Pa.: M. Kieffer & Co., 1853. 18p. DNLM; PPHa; PPC **50-1737**

STEINER, Lewis Henry (1827-1892)
Henry Cavendish and the discovery of the chemical constitution of water. A lecture. New York: E. P. Allen, 1855. 24p. DNLM; PPHa; PPC **50-1738**

STEINER, Lewis H[enry] (1827-1892)
Report on the progress of medical chemistry. Read before the Medical & Chirurgical Faculty of Maryland, June 8, 1855. . . . Baltimore: Printed by J. Lucas & Son, 1855. 27p. DLC; DNLM; MdBM; PPHa **50-1739**

STEINER, Lewis H[enry] (1827-1892)
The medical profession and modern chemistry. An oration delivered before the Medical and Chirurgical Faculty of Maryland, at its annual convention, June 4, 1856. . . . Baltimore: Printed by J. Lucas & Son, 1856. 26p. DLC; DNLM; MdBM; PPHa **50-1740**

STEINER, Lewis Henry (1827-1892)
The utility of colleges of pharmacy. An address . . . before the Maryland College of Pharmacy, November 3, 1856. [Baltimore: Printed by F. A. Hanzsche, 1856?] 23p. DLC; DNLM; MdU-D; PPHa **50-1741**

STEINER, Lewis Henry (1827-1892)
Report on strychnia: its physiological properties, and chemical detection. . . . Philadelphia: T. K. & P. G. Collins, printers, 1856. 19p. DLC; DNLM; PPHa; PPC **50-1742**

STEINER, Lewis Henry (1827-1892)
Report on the recent contributions of chemistry to the medical profession. Richmond, Va.: Ritchie & Dunnavant, 1857. 44p. DNLM; ViRA **50-1743**

STEINER, Lewis Henry (1827-1892)
The human body and disease, considered from the Christian standpoint. . . . Chambersburg, Pa.: Printed by M. Kieffer & Co., 1858. 32p. DLC; DNLM; PPHa; PPC **50-1744**

STEINER, Lewis Henry (1827-1892)
Oration before the Medical and Surgical Society of Baltimore, at its fourth anniversary meeting, January 17, 1859. . . . Baltimore: Printed by J. D. Toy, 1859. 22p. DLC; DNLM; MdU-D; PPHa **50-1745**

STEINER, Lewis H[enry] (1827-1892)
Valedictory address delivered at the third annual commencement of the Maryland College of Pharmacy March 15, 1859. . . . Baltimore: Printed by F. A. Hanzsche, 1859. 21p. DNLM; MdU-D; PPC **50-1746**

STEPHENSON, Mark (1803?-1865)
Syllabus of a course of lectures on ophthalmic medicine and surgery. 2nd ed. New York: D. Fanshaw, 1855. 22p. DNLM; NNNAM **50-1747**

STEPHENSON, Mark (1803?-1865)
An essay on the treatment of cataract. . . . Read before the American Medical Association, at the city of Washington, May 6, 1858. Philadelphia: T. K. & P. G. Collins, Printer, 1858. 26p. 2 col. plates. DLC; DNLM; PPC **50-1748**

STEVENS, Alexander Hodgdon (1789-1869)
Annual address delivered before the New York State Medical Society. Albany: C. Van Benthuysen, 1850. 31p. DNLM **50-1749**

STEVENS, William Bacon (1815-1887)
A sermon preached before the students of the several medical colleges of the city of Philadelphia, on Sunday evening, December 5, 1852, in St. Andrew's Church. Philadelphia: King & Baird, 1852. 34p. DNLM; PPC **50-1750**

STEVENS, William Bacon (1815-1887)
The religious teachings of medical science. A sermon delivered before the medical students of the several colleges of Philadelphia, in St. Andrew's Church, November 7th, 1856, and repeated, by request, in the same place, December 6th, 1857. Philadelphia: C. Sherman & Son, 1858. 40p. DNLM; PPC **50-1751**

STEWART, Ferdinand Campbell (1815-1899)
Anniversary discourse, before the New York Academy of Medicine. New York, 1853. 48p. DNLM; NNNAM **50-1752**

STEWART, James (1799-1864)
A practical treatise on the diseases of children. Including an introductory chapter, in the management of infants in health. 4th ed. New York: Harper & Bro., 1854. 555p. DNLM; MBM; NNNAM; PPC **50-1753**

STEWART, James (1799-1864)
Essay on cholera infantum, for which the prize of the New York Academy of Medicine was awarded, March 5th, 1856. . . . New York: Baker & Godwin, book and job printers, 1856. 66p. DLC; NNAM **50-1754**

STILES, R. Cresson (1830-1873)
An introductory lecture to the course of instruction in the medical department of the University of Vermont. Burlington: Free Press Print., 1858. 22p. DNLM; VtHi **50-1755**

STILLÉ, Alfred (1813-1900)
An introductory lecture delivered at the Pennsylvania College, medical department. Philadelphia: King & Baird, 1854. 16p. DNLM; PPC; PU **50-1756**

STILLÉ, Alfred (1813-1900)
The unity of medicine. An introductory lecture to the course of theory and practice of medicine, in the Medical Department of Pennsylvania College. Delivered Oct. 14, 1856. . . . Published by the class. Philadelphia: T. K. & P. G. Collins, printers, 1856. 39p. DLC; DNLM; PPC; PU **50-1757**

STILLÉ, Alfred (1813-1900)
Valedictory address to the graduates of the Medical Department of Pennsylvania College. Philadelphia: T. K. & P. G. Collins, 1857. 22p. DNLM; PPC; PU **50-1758**

STILLÉ, Alfred (1813-1900)
Humboldt's life and character. An address before the Linnaean Association of Pennsylvania College. Philadelphia: T. K. & P. G. Collins, printers, 1859. 38p. DNLM; PPC; PU **50-1759**

STILLÉ, Alfred (1813-1900), Samuel JACKSON and John BELL
Circular addressed to the Medical Colleges of the United States, by a committee of the American Medical Association. . . . Philadelphia: T. K. & P. G. Collins, 1856. 12p. PPC; PU **50-1760**

STOKES, William (1804-1878)
The diseases of the heart and the aorta. Philadelphia: Lindsay & Blakiston, 1854. 689p. DNLM; IEN-M; IU-M; PPC
50-1761

STOKES, William (1804-1878)
The diseases of the heart and the aorta. Philadelphia: Lindsay & Blakiston, 1855. 710p. DNLM; MdBM; NNNAM; PPC
50-1762

STORER, David Humphreys (1804-1891)
Statistics of the Boston Lying-in Hospital. Philadelphia: T. K. & P. G. Collins, 1850. 24p. DNLM; MBM; PPC; PPJ
50-1763

STORER, David Humphreys (1804-1891)
Report of the committee on obstetrics of the American Medical Association. Philadelphia: T. K. & P. G. Collins, 1851. 63p. DNLM; PPC **50-1764**

STORER, David Humphreys (1804-1891)
An address on medical jurisprudence: its claims to greater regard from the student and the physician: delivered before the fellows of the Massachusetts Medical Society, at the annual meeting, May 28, 1851. . . . Boston: Printed by J. Wilson & Son, 1851. 48p. DLC; DNLM; MBM; NNNAM
50-1765

STORER, David Humphreys (1804-1891)
An address delivered at the first medical commencement of the Massachusetts Medical College, March 7, 1855. Boston: J. Wilson & Son, 1855. 15p. DNLM; MH-M
50-1766

STORER, David Humphreys (1804-1891)
An introductory lecture before the medical class of 1855-1856 of Harvard University. Boston: D. Clapp, 1855. 32p. DNLM; MBM; MH-M **50-1767**

STRINGFELLOW, T[hornton]
Two letters on cases of cure at Fauquier White Sulphur Springs; embracing, also, mineral waters in general. Washington: Union Office, 1851. 16p. DNLM **50-1768**

SUNDERLAND, La Roy (1802-1885)
Theory of nutrition. The treatment of disease, and philosophy of healing, without medicine. . . . Boston: B. Marsh; New York: Stearns & Co. [etc.], 1855. 216p. DLC; DNLM; MBM; NNNAM **50-1769**

THE SURGICAL adjuvant and reporter of artificial limbs. Published by Palmer & Co., July 1859. No. ix. New York & Boston, 1859. 48p. DNLM **50-1770**

SUTTON, George (1812-1886)
A report to the Indiana State Medical Society on Asiatic cholera as it prevailed within the State of Indiana during the years 1849, 1850, 1851, and 1852. With observations on the laws which govern its progress. Indianapolis: Elder & Harkness, 1854. 69p. DNLM **50-1771**

SUTTON, W. Loftus (1797-1862)
A history of the disease usually called typhoid fever, as it has appeared in Georgetown and its vicinity, with some reflections as to its causes and nature. . . . Louisville: Maxwell & Co., 1850. 127p. DLC; DNLM; OCIM **50-1772**

SUTTON, W. Loftus (1797-1862)
Report on the epidemics of Tennessee and Kentucky. Philadelphia: T. K. & P. G. Collins, 1852. 42p. DNLM; PPC
50-1773

SUTTON, W. Loftus (1797-1862)
Report on a uniform plan for registration reports of births, marriages, and deaths. Philadelphia: T. K. & P. G. Collins, 1859. 50p. DNLM; PPC **50-1774**

SWAZEY, George W.
Life, disease, and the law of cure. An address delivered June 11, 1851, before the American Institute of Homoeopathy, at New Haven, Conn., with a list of members. Published by request. Springfield, 1852. 48p. DNLM; PPHa
50-1775

SWEETSER, William (1797-1875)
Mental hygiene; or, An examination of the intellect and passions. Designed to show how they affect and are affected by the bodily functions, and their influence on health and longevity. . . . 2nd ed., re-written and enl. New York: G. P. Putnam, 1850. 390p. DLC; NNNAM **50-1776**

SWEETSER, William (1797-1875)
Valedictory address, delivered to the graduating class, at the Castleton Medical College. Castleton, 1853. 20p. DNLM
50-1777

SWETT, John Appleton (1808-1854)
A treatise on the diseases of the chest: being a course of lectures delivered at the New York Hospital. New York: D. Appleton & Co., 1852. 585p. 2 plates. DNLM; MBM; NNNAM; PPC **50-1778**

SWETT, John Appleton (1808-1854)
A treatise on diseases of the chest: being a course of lectures delivered at the New York Hospital 3rd ed. New York: D. Appleton & Co., 1856. 585p. 2 plates. DNLM; NNNAM
50-1779

SWIFT, H. S.
Observations on exhaustion from the effects of heat (coup de soleil). New York: Holman, Gray & Co., 1854. 15p. DNLM; NNNAM **50-1780**

SWINBURNE, John (1820-1889)
Treatment of fractures of the femur by simple extension. Albany: C. Van Benthuysen, 1859. 9p. DNLM
50-1781

TAFT, Alphonse
Address delivered on the occasion of the opening of the Cincinnati House of Refuge, Oct. 7, 1850. Cincinnati: Wright, Ferris & Co., 1850. 26p. DNLM; OCIM **50-1782**

TAFT, J[onathan] (1820-1903)
Crystal gold for filling teeth. [Cincinnati, 1854.] 8p. DNLM
50-1783

TAFT, Jonathan (1820-1903)
A practical treatise on operative dentistry. . . . With eighty illustrations. Philadelphia: Lindsay & Blakiston, 1859. 383p. DLC; MdU-D; PPC; PU **50-1784**

TALCOTT, Alvan (1804-1891)
The annual address to the graduating class in the medical institution of Yale College, January 15, 1852. New Haven: W. H. Stanley, 1852. 18p. CtY-M; DNLM **50-1785**

TANNER, Thomas Hawkes (1824-1871)
A manual of clinical medicine and physical diagnosis. To which is added the code of ethics of the American Medical Association. Philadelphia: Blanchard & Lea, 1855. 252p. DNLM; PPC; PPJ; PU **50-1786**

TANNER, Thomas Hawkes (1824-1871)
A manual of clinical medicine and physical diagnosis. 2nd American ed. Philadelphia: Blanchard & Lea, 1856. 252p. DNLM; MBM; NNNAM; PPC **50-1787**

TANNER, Thomas Hawkes (1824-1871)
The practice of medicine. . . . 1st American from the 3rd revised and improved London ed. Philadelphia: Lindsay & Blakiston, 1858. 398p. DNLM; OCIM; PPC; PU **50-1788**

TANQUEREL DES PLANCHES, L. (1809-1862)
Lead diseases. A treatise from the French; with notes and additions . . . by Samuel L. Dana. Boston: Tappan, Whittemore & Mason, 1850. 441p. DNLM; MBM **50-1789**

TAPPAN, Henry P[hilip] (1805-1881)
The mutual responsibilities of physicians and the community, being an address to the graduating class of the medical college of the University of Michigan. Detroit, Mic.: Free Press Print, 1856, 25p. DNLM **50-1790**

TARBELL, John Adams (1810-1864)
Sources of health and the prevention or mental and physical hygiene. Boston: Otis Clapp, 1850. 170p. PPHa **50-1791**

TARBELL, John Adams (1810-1864)
Homoeopathy simplified, or domestic practice made easy; containing explicit directions for the treatment of disease, the management of accidents and the preservation of health. Boston: Otis Clapp, 1856. 360p. DNLM; PPHa **50-1792**

TARBELL, John Adams (1810-1864)
Homoeopathy simplified, or domestic practice made easy; containing explicit directions for the treatment of disease, the management of accidents and the preservation of health. 4th ed. Boston: Otis Clapp, 1859. 360p. DNLM; MBM **50-1793**

TAYLOR, Alfred B[ower] (1824-1898)
Report on weights and measures, read before the Pharmaceutical Association. Boston: G. C. Rand & Avery, 1859. 104p. DNLM; MBM; OCLloyd **50-1794**

TAYLOR, Alfred Swaine (1806-1880)
Medical jurisprudence. . . . 2nd American, from the 3rd London ed. With notes and additions by R. Eglesfeld Griffith. . . . Philadelphia: Lea & Blanchard, 1850. 670p. DLC: OCIM; NNNAM; PPC **50-1795**

TAYLOR, Alfred Swaine (1806-1880)
Medical jurisprudence. . . . 3rd American, from the 4th London ed. Ed., with additions, by Edward Hartshorne. . . . Philadelphia: Blanchard & Lea, 1853. 621p. DLC: ICRM; NNNAM; PPC **50-1796**

TAYLOR, Alfred Swaine (1806-1880)
Medical jurisprudence. . . . 4th American from the fifth and improved London ed. Ed. with additions. By Edward Hartshorne. . . . Philadelphia: Blanchard & Lea, 1856. 697p. DLC; MBM; NNNAM; PPC **50-1797**

TAYLOR, Alfred Swaine (1806-1880)
On poisons in relation to medical jurisprudence and medicine. . . . 2nd American from the 2nd and rev. London ed. Philadelphia: Blanchard & Lea, 1859. 755p. DLC; OCIM; NNNAM; PPC **50-1798**

TAYLOR, Charles Fayette (1827-1899)
The movement cure. [New York, 1857.] 16p. DNLM; NNNAM **50-1799**

TAYLOR, Charles Fayette (1827-1899)
The treatment of paralysis of motion. [New York, 1858.] 15p. DNLM **50-1800**

TAYLOR, Charles Fayette (1827-1899)
The movement cure; with cases. New York: J. A. Gray, 1858. 16p. DNLM; NNNAM **50-1801**

TAYLOR, Charles Fayette (1827-1899)
The pathology and treatment of some of the diseases incident to women. New York, 1859. 16p. DNLM; NNNAM **50-1802**

TAYLOR, Charles Fayette (1827-1899)
The treatment of lateral curvature of the spine by special exercises. New York: H. Ludwig, 1859. 16p. DNLM; NNNAM **50-1803**

TAYLOR, George H. (1821-1896) and Charles Fayette TAYLOR
Principles and practice of hygeio-medical science. New York, 1857. 16p. DNLM **50-1804**

TAYLOR, George H. (1821-1896)
The treatment of consumption by the compressed air-bath; embracing a sketch of the causes and pathology of pulmonary affections, and the proper hygiene to be observed for their cure. New York: J. A. Gray, 1858. 16p. DNLM; NNNAM **50-1805**

TAYLOR, Isaac E[benezer] (1812-1889)
Case of obstinate regurgitation of the contents of the stomach, treated by the inhalation of chloroform, with remarks on regurgitation. New York: Miller & Holman, 1856. 15p. DNLM; NNNAM **50-1806**

TAYLOR, Isaac Ebenezer (1812-1889)
The sunburnt appearance of the skin as an early diagnostic symptom of supra-renal capsule disease. New York: Miller & Holman, 1856. 21p. 3 plates. DNLM; NNNAM **50-1807**

TAYLOR, Jane
Wouldst know thyself! or the outlines of human physiology. New York: G. F. Cooledge, [1858]. 64p. DNLM; NN; NNC **50-1808**

TAYLOR, Jeremiah
The medical profession; its positions and claims. . . . Middletown, Conn.: C. H. Pelton, 1857. 22p. DNLM **50-1809**

TAYLOR, Othniel Hart (1803-1869)
Medical reform and the present system of medical instruction. An address. Camden, N.J.: Gray & Elliott, 1850. 20p. DNLM; PPC **50-1810**

TAYLOR, Othniel Hart (1803-1869)
Relations of popular education with the progress of empiricism. Annual address. Burlington: Gazette Office, 1853. 23p. DNLM **50-1811**

TAYLOR, T. K.
The medical pocket companion, or domestic adviser; designed for both married and single; containing a brief description of the causes, symptoms, and treatment of the most common and obstinate diseases which affect humanity; together with many valuable hints upon the preservation of health and the proper management of infancy and childhood. New stereotype ed. Boston: The Author, 1858. 222p. DNLM; MBM; NNNAM
50-1812

TEMPLE, John Taylor (1803-1877)
Dr. J. T. Temple's reply to Prof. Pallen's attack on homoeopathy, in his valedictory before the St. Louis University. Published by particular request. St. Louis, Mo.: T. W. Ustick, 1853. 16p. DNLM; PPHa **50-1813**

TEMPLE, John Taylor (1803-1877)
Anniversary address before the Illinois State Homoeopathic Medical Association, Chicago, December 1, 1858. St. Louis, Mo.: T. W. Ustick, 1859. 16p. DNLM; PPHa
50-1814

TESSIER, Jean-Paul (1811-1862)
Clinical remarks concerning the homoeopathic treatment of pneumonia: preceded by a retrospective view of the allopathic materia medica, and an explanation of the homoeopathic law of cure. . . . Transl. by Charles J. Hempel, M.D. New York: William Radde, 1855. 131p. PPHa **50-1815**

TESSIER, Jean-Paul (1811-1862)
Clinical researches concerning the homoeopathic treatment of Asiatic cholera. Preceded by a review on the abuse of the numerical method in medicine. Transl. by Charles J. Hempel, M.D. New York: William Radde, 1855. 109p. DNLM; NNNAM
50-1816

TESTE, Alphonse (*b.* 1814)
The homoeopathic materia medica, arranged systematically and practically by A. Teste. Transl. from the French, and edited by Charles J. Hempel, M.D. Philadelphia: Rademacher & Sheek, 1854. 634p. DLC; DNLM **50-1817**

TESTE, Alphonse (*b.* 1814)
A homoeopathic treatise on the diseases of children. Transl. from the French by Emma H. Coté. Cincinnati: Moore, Wilstach, Keys & Co., 1854. 342p. DLC
50-1818

TESTE, Alphonse (*b.* 1814)
A homoeopathic treatise on the diseases of children. . . . Transl. from the French, by Emma H. Coté. 2nd ed. Rev. by J. H. Pulte. . . . Cincinnati: Moore, Wilstach, Keys & Co., 1857. 342p. DLC; DNLM; OCIM **50-1819**

TEWKSBURY, Samuel Henry (1819-1880)
Remarks on the bill for the promotion of medical science; also, an appeal to the members of the legislature in behalf of the Maine Medical Association, in the senate chamber, Feb. 27, 1855. Portland, Maine: Peck & Ayer, 1855. 25p. DNLM
50-1820

THAYER, Henry
Trial for malpractice. Boston, 1856. 17p. DNLM
50-1821

THAYER, William Henry (1822-1897)
An address before the Vermont Medical College, introductory to the lectures of 1855. Woodstock, Vt.: Haskell & Palmer, 1855. 17p. DNLM **50-1822**

THAYER, William Henry (1822-1897)
Address to the graduates of the Vermont Medical College of the class of 1856. Keene, N.H., 1856. 16p. DNLM
50-1823

THE THIRD anniversary oration for the New York Academy of Medicine, which was not delivered before that remarkable body, but ought to have been, at their annual meeting, held in the chapel of the university, November 14th, 1849, by the physician who was not elected for that occasion. [Published without the knowledge or consent of the Academy.] New York, 1850. 28p. DNLM; NNNAM **50-1824**

THOMAS, Daniel Golden (1806-1880)
Address, delivered at the semi-centennial celebration of the Oneida County Medical Society, held at Utica, Tuesday, July 8, 1856. Utica: N. D. Jewell, 1856. 23p. DNLM
50-1825

THOMAS, John H.
An address on success in the medical profession, delivered before the class in the Eclectic Medical College of Pennsylvania, October 20th, 1859. Philadelphia: W. S. Young, 1859. 16p. DNLM; PPC; PU **50-1826**

THOMAS, Robert Pennell (1821-1864)
Valedictory address to the graduates of the Philadelphia College of Pharmacy . . . with a list of the graduates. Philadelphia: Stavely & McCalla, 1851. 19p. DNLM; PPC
50-1827

THOMAS, Robert Pennell (1821-1864)
Valedictory charge to the graduates of the Philadelphia College of Pharmacy. With a list of the graduates. Philadelphia: T. K. & P. G. Collins, 1857. 19p. DNLM; PPC
50-1828

THOMAS, T[heodore] Gaillard (1832-1903)
The hymen. An essay. [New York, 1859.] 21p. DNLM; NNNAM **50-1829**

THOMAS, Theodore Gaillard (1832-1903)
A lecture on the prevention of post-partum haemorrhage. Charleston, S.C.: James & Williams, 1859. 16p. DNLM; ScCM
50-1830

THOMPSON, Caroline M.
Petition of . . . to the legislature of New York in aid of the Woman's Hospital. Albany: Weed, Parsons & Co., 1857. 8p. DNLM **50-1831**

THOMPSON, M. La Rue P.
A sermon preached by request before the medical class of the university in the city of Buffalo, December 28, 1851. Buffalo: E. A. Maynard, 1852. 28p. DNLM **50-1832**

THOMPSON, Theophilus (1808-1860)
Clinical lectures on pulmonary consumption. Philadelphia: Lindsay & Blakiston, 1854. 259p. 2 plates. CtY-M; DNLM; MBM; PPC **50-1833**

THOMPSON, T. D.
Facts for the people relating to the teeth; showing their influence upon the health, speech, and looks; with directions for their care and preservation. Boston: B. B. Mussey & Co., 1854. 251p. DNLM; MBM **50-1834**

THOMSON, Anthony Todd (1778-1849)
A conspectus of the Pharmacopoeias of the London, Edinburgh, and Dublin Colleges of Physicians, and of the United States Pharmacopoeia; being a practical compendium of the materia medica and pharmacy. 6th American ed., much enlarged and improved. Edited by Charles A. Lee. New York: S. S. & W. Wood, 1852. 322p. DNLM; OCLloyd; PPC; PU
50-1835

THOMSON, M. S.
A lecture, being one of a course on materia medica, delivered before the students of the Reform Medical College of Georgia. Macon: Telegraph Steam Press, 1857. 15p. DNLM; GU
50-1836

THOMSON, M.S.
Medical reform and allopathy; being a vindication of the doctrines, principles, and practices of the former from an attack made upon them by the latter in a recent pamphlet by J. Dickson Smith, of Macon, Ga. Together with a review of two essays on medical abuses from the same author. Macon: Telegraph Printing House, 1859. 80p. DNLM; GU
50-1837

THOMSON, Spencer (1808-1883)
A dictionary of domestic medicine and household surgery.... 1st American from the last London ed. Rev., with additions, by Henry H. Smith. . . . Philadelphia: Lippincott, Grambo & Co., 1853. 582p. DLC; DNLM; PPC; PU
50-1838

TIEDEMANN, Henry
On dysentery and its treatment. . . . Philadelphia: R. Stein, printer, 1857. 29p. DLC; PPHa; PPC
50-1839

TILDEN & COMPANY. NEW YORK
A catalogue of pure medicinal extracts prepared in vacuo. New York: Tilden & Co., 1854. 32p. DNLM; NNNAM
50-1840

TILDEN & COMPANY. NEW YORK
Formulae for making tinctures, infusions, syrups, wines, mixtures, pills, etc., simple and compound, from the fluid and solid extracts, prepared at the laboratory of Tilden & Company. [New York, 1858.] 162, 32p. DNLM; NNNAM
50-1841

TILT, Edward John (1815-1893)
On diseases of menstruation and ovarian inflammation, in connexion with sterility, pelvic tumours, and affections of the womb. . . . New York: S. S. & W. Wood, 1851. 286p. DLC; DNLM; NNNAM; PPC **50-1842**

TILT, Edward John (1815-1893)
Elements of health, and principles of female hygiene. . . . Philadelphia: Lindsay & Blakiston, 1853. 436p. DLC; DNLM; MBM; PPC **50-1843**

TIMBERLAKE, J.
Dr. C. J. B. Williams and others, on the principles of the water cure; with comments and explanatory remarks. Designed chiefly to point out or delineate the safest, the most efficient, and the most beneficial modes of bathing as to all, but more especially for invalids, or the delicate and the weak. Richmond, Va.: J. W. Randolph, 1853. 129p. DNLM; ViRA
50-1844

TODD, Robert Bentley (1809-1860)
Clinical lectures on certain diseases of the urinary organs and on dropsies. Philadelphia: Blanchard & Lea, 1857. 283p. DNLM; NNNAM; OCIM; PPC **50-1845**

TODD, Robert Bentley (1809-1860)
The physiological anatomy and physiology of man by Robert Bentley Todd . . . and William Bowman. . . . With two hundred and ninety-eight illustrations. Philadelphia: Blanchard & Lea, 1857. 926p. DLC; OCIM; PPC; PU **50-1846**

TOOTHAKER, Charles Everett (1805-1890)
A treatise on diseases of the skin. Philadelphia: Rademacher & Sheek, 1856. 64p. DNLM; PPHa **50-1847**

TOWNSEND, C.
Improved phreno-chart; containing a survey of the constitution, and an estimate of the various powers of mind, and traits of the character, of *Lydia I. King*, as given *Feb. 2nd, 1854*, by *Charles Frentz*, examiner. Arranged according to Grimes's New System of Phrenology. Boston: White & Potter, 1853. 76p. DNLM **50-1848**

TOWNSEND, Elisha (*d.* 1858)
Address delivered before the graduating class of the Baltimore College of Dental Surgery. Baltimore: J. D. Toy, 1850. 11p. DNLM; MdU-D **50-1849**

TOWNSEND, Elisha (*d.* 1858)
Opening address delivered before the Society of the Alumni of the Baltimore College of Dental Surgery. Baltimore: J. D. Toy, 1850. 23p. DNLM; MdU-D **50-1850**

TOWNSEND, Elisha (*d.* 1858)
Valedictory to the graduating class of the Philadelphia College of Dental Surgery. Philadelphia: J. H. Jones, 1854. 11p. DNLM; PPC; PU **50-1851**

TOWNSEND, Howard (1823-1867)
An introductory lecture delivered before the students of the Albany Medical College. Albany: J. Munsell, 1853. 18p. DNLM
50-1852

TOWNSEND, John F[ondey] (1810?-1874)
Relations between the professions of law and medicine. Albany: J. Munsell, 1854. 20p. DNLM **50-1853**

TRALL, Russell Thacher (1812-1877)
The hydropathic encyclopedia; a system of hydropathy and hygiene in eight parts. Designed as a guide to families and students, and a textbook for physicians. [v. 1] New York: Fowler & Wells, [1851]. 504p. 5 plates. DNLM; NNNAM
50-1854

TRALL, Russell Thacher (1812-1877)
The new hydropathic cook-book; with recipes for cooking on hygienic principles, [etc.]. New York: Fowlers & Wells, [1853]. 226p. DLC; NNNAM **50-1855**

TRALL, Russell Thacher (1812-1877)
Home-treatment for sexual abuses. . . . New York: Fowler & Wells, 1853. 118p. DLC: DNLM; NNNAM
50-1856

TRALL, Russell Thacher (1812-1877)
The hydropathic encyclopedia: a system of hydropathy and hygiene. . . . New York: Fowlers & Wells, 1853. 2 v. DLC; NNNAM **50-1857**

TRALL, Russell Thacher (1812-1877)
The illustrated family gymnasium; containing the most improved methods of applying . . . exercises to the development of bodily organs. . . . New York: Fowler & Wells, [1857]. 215p. 6 plates. DNLM; NNNAM **50-1858**

TRIPLER, Charles Stuart (1806-1866)
Delirium tremens: its nature and treatment. [Cincinnati, 1857.] 29p. DNLM **50-1859**

TRIPLER, Charles Stuart (1806-1866)
Manual of the medical officer of the Army of the United States. Part 1. Recruiting and the inspection of recruits. Cincinnati: Wrightson & Co., 1858. 117p. DNLM; OCIM **50-1860**

TRIPLER, Charles Stuart (1806-1866)
The duties of physicians in relation to medical delusions. An address. Covington, Ky.: S. G. Cobb, 1859. 32p. DNLM **50-1861**

TURNBULL, Laurence (1821-1900)
Hooping cough: its history, nature, and successful treatment. Philadelphia: Lindsay & Blakiston, 1855. 18p. DNLM; PPC **50-1862**

TURNBULL, Laurence (1821-1900)
Biographical sketch of the late John K. Mitchell. Philadelphia, 1858. 5p. DNLM; PPC: PPJ **50-1863**

TURNER, William
Petition against blood-letting. To the legislature of the State of New York, March 17, 1851. [New York, 1851.] 8 l. DNLM **50-1864**

TYLER, Grafton (1811-1884)
Medicine as a science and an art; its philosophy, influences, purposes and results, its past and present condition and future prospects. Being an address before the Medical Society of the District of Columbia, delivered by appointment, at the hall of the Smithsonian Institution, January, 1852. . . . Washington: R. A. Waters, 1852. 35p. DLC; DNLM; ViRA **50-1865**

TYLER, Grafton (1811-1884)
Valedictory address, delivered at the commencement of the National Medical College, Washington, D.C. in the hall of the Smithsonian Institution, March 5th, 1853. . . . Washington: R. A. Waters, printer, 1853. 23p. DLC; DNLM; ViRA **50-1866**

TYLER, John Eugene (1819-1878)
An address to the graduates of the New Hampshire Medical Institution, at the medical commencement, November, 1853. [Concord, 1853] 19p. DNLM **50-1867**

TYSON, James Lawrence (1813-1898)
Diary of a physician in California; being the results of actual experience, including notes of the journey by land and water, and observations on the climate, soil, resources of the country, etc. . . . New York: D. Appleton & Company; Philadelphia: G. S. Appleton, 1850. 92p. DLC; DNLM; NNNAM **50-1868**

UPDEGRAFF, J. T. (*d.* 1882)
An essay on the mutual claims of the public and the medical profession on each other. Bridgeport, O.: J. G. Affleck, 1855. 15p. DNLM **50-1869**

UPHAM, J. Baxter (1820?-1902)
Records of maculated typhus, or ship fever, with suggestions of treatment. Being the result of a series of observations made during the prevalence of this disease at South Boston and Deer Island Hospitals in 1847-1848. New York: J. F. Trow, 1852. 60p. 2 plates. DNLM; NNNAM **50-1870**

UPHAM, J. Baxter (1820?-1902)
Illustrations of typhus fever in Great Britain, the result of personal observations made in the summer of 1853, with some remarks as to its origin, habits, symptoms, and pathology; to which is appended a brief account of the re-appearance of typhus in Boston in the winter of 1857-1858. Boston: D. Clapp, 1858. 46p. DNLM; MBM **50-1871**

VACHÉ, Alexander F. (1800-1857)
Letters on yellow fever, the cholera, and quarantine, addressed to the legislature of the State of New York; with an appendix, containing correlative correspondence, and an act of the legislature of the state, relative to the public health, with suggested amendments. 2nd ed. New York: J. W. Bell & Son, 1854. 106p. DNLM; NNNAM **50-1872**

VANDERBURGH, Federal (1788-1868)
Letter to Valentine Mott, in reply to his valedictory address to the members of the New York Academy of Medicine, New York, June 3rd, 1850. New York: Angell & Engel, 1850. 8p. DNLM; NNNAM **50-1873**

VANDERBURGH, Federal (1788-1868)
Annual address delivered in Albany before the Academy of Medicine of the State of New York, February 19, 1851. Published by order of the Society. New York: Angell, Engel & Hewitt, 1851. 29p. DNLM; NNNAM; PPHa **50-1874**

VAN DEUSEN, E. H. (1829-1909)
A biographical sketch of T. Romeyn Beck. New York: Holman & Gray, 1856. 23p. 1 plate. DNLM; NNNAM **50-1875**

VAN DYKE, Rush (1813-1882)
Lecture introductory to the course of the 11th session of the Philadelphia College of Medicine. Philadelphia: Jared Craig, 1852. 40p. DNLM; PPC; PU **50-1876**

VATTIER, John Loring (1808-1881)
To the physicians of the state of Ohio. [Reply to a letter of Dr. Marmaduke B. Wright.] . . . . [Cincinnati, 1850.] 8p. DNLM **50-1877**

VATTIER, John Loring (1808-1881)
Memoir of John T. Shotwell, late professor of anatomy in the Medical College of Ohio. An address. Cincinnati: J. Ernst, 1851. 16p. DNLM **50-1878**

VELPEAU, Alfred Armand Louis Marie (1795-1867)
A complete treatise on midwifery: or, The theory and practice of tokology: including the diseases of pregnancy, labor, and the puerperal state. . . . Transl. from the French, by Charles D. Meigs. . . . 4th American, with the additions from the last French ed., by Wm. Byrd Page. . . . Philadelphia: Lindsay & Blakiston, 1852. 652p. 12 plates. DLC; DNLM; PPC; PU **50-1879**

VELPEAU, Alfred Armand Louis Marie (1795-1867)
New elements of operative surgery. . . . With an appendix of notes by Granville Sharp Pattison. Transl. by P. S. Townsend . . . with notes and observations by Valentine Mott. 4th ed., with additions by G. C. Blackman. New York: S. S. & W. Wood, 1856. 3 v. atlas, 23 plates. DNLM; NNNAM; PPC; PU **50-1880**

WAINWRIGHT, Daniel Wadsworth (*d.* 1863)
Pustule maligne. New York: Billin & Bro., 1855. 32p. DNLM; NNNAM **50-1881**

WALKER, Alexander
Woman physiologically considered, as to mind, morals, marriage, matrimonial slavery, infidelity and divorce. With an appendix containing notes and additions; edited by an American physician. New ed. Hartford: S. Andrus & Son, 1851. 432p. CtY-M; DNLM; MBM **50-1882**

WALLACE, William Clay
Accommodation of the eye to distances. New York: J. Wiley, 1850. 36p. DNLM; NNNAM **50-1883**

WALLACE, William Clay
An attempt to show that light, heat, electricity, and magnetism are effects of the law of gravitation. New York: D. Fanshaw, 1854. 15, 2p. DNLM; NNNAM **50-1884**

WALSH, Joseph (1806-1879)
Address delivered before the regular meeting of the Pharmaceutical Association, D.C., on the first July, 1857. Washington: H. Polkinhorn, 1858. 13p. DNLM **50-1885**

WALSHE, Walter Hayle (1812-1892)
A practical treatise on the diseases of the lungs and heart, including the principles of physical diagnosis. Philadelphia: Blanchard & Lea, 1851. 512p. CtY-M; DNLM; PPC; PU **50-1886**

WALTON, Henry Haynes (1816-1889)
A treatise on operative ophthalmic surgery. 1st American ed. from the 1st London ed. Edited by S. Littell. Philadelphia: Lindsay & Blakiston, [1853]. 599p. DNLM; OCIM; NNNAM; PPC **50-1887**

WARD, Isaac Moreau (1806-1895)
Introductory lecture to the class of the Homoeopathic Medical College of Pennsylvania, delivered October 11, 1854. Philadelphia: Rademacher & Sheek, 1854. 16p. DNLM; PPHa **50-1888**

WARD, Isaac Moreau (1806-1895)
Valedictory address delivered at the 8th annual commencement of the Homoeopathic Medical College of Pennsylvania, March 1, 1856, and, also, the 9th annual announcement for the session of 1856-1857. Philadelphia: King & Baird, 1856. 16p. DNLM; PPHa **50-1889**

WARE, John (1795-1864)
Hints to young men on the true relation of the sexes. Boston: Tappan, Whittemore & Mason, 1850. 64p. DNLM; MH; NN; NNC **50-1890**

WARE, John (1795-1864)
Contributions to the history, diagnosis, and treatment of croup. Boston: D. Clapp, 1850. 29p. DNLM; MBM **50-1891**

WARE, John (1795-1864)
Success in the medical profession. An introductory lecture delivered at the Massachusetts Medical College, November 6, 1850. Boston: D. Clapp, 1851. 28p. DLC; DNLM; MH-M **50-1892**

WARE, John (1795-1864)
Farewell address delivered to the medical graduates of Harvard University, at the annual commencement, Wednesday, March 12, 1856. Boston: D. Clapp, 1856. 18p. DLC; DNLM; MH **50-1893**

WARNER, Harriot W., ed.
Autobiography of Charles Caldwell. Philadelphia: Lippincott, Grambo, & Company, 1855. 454p. OCIM; MH; NN; NNC **50-1894**

WARREN, Edward (1828-1893)
The influence of pregnancy on the development of tubercles. Being the dissertation to which the Fisk fund prize was awarded, June 4, 1856. Philadelphia: Blanchard & Lea, 1857. 42p. DNLM; PPC; PU **50-1895**

WARREN, Ira (1806-1864)
The household physician; for the use of families, planters, seamen, and travellers. . . . Boston: Higgins, Bradley, & Dayton, 1859. 728p. col. plates. DLC; DNLM; MBM; PU **50-1896**

WARREN, John Collins (1778-1856)
Address before the American Medical Association, at the anniversary meeting in Cincinnati, May 8, 1850. . . . Boston: Printed by J. Wilson, 1850. 65p. DLC; DNLM; MH-M **50-1897**

WARREN, John Collins (1778-1856)
On the prevention of constipation. [Philadelphia, 1850.] 8p. DNLM; PPC **50-1898**

WARREN, John Collins (1778-1856)
Address to the Boston Society of Natural History. Boston: J. Wilson & Son, 1853. 48p. DNLM; MB; MBAt **50-1899**

WARREN, John Collins (1778-1856)
The preservation of health. With remarks on constipation, old age, use of alcohol in the preparation of medicines. . . . Boston: Ticknor, Reed & Fields, 1854. 140p. DLC; MB; MBM **50-1900**

WARREN, Jonathan Mason (1811-1867)
Cases of occlusion of the vagina, with retention of the catamenia, relieved by an operation. Boston: J. Wilson & Son, 1853. 28p. DNLM; MH-M **50-1901**

WARREN, Jonathan Mason (1811-1867)
Supposed encephaloid testicle. hermaphrodism. [Philadelphia, 1859.] 6p. 1 plate. DNLM; PPC **50-1902**

WARREN, Jonathan Mason (1811-1867)
Amputation at the hip-joint for a large osteo-sarcomatous tumor of the femur. [Boston, 1859.] 7p. 1 plate. DNLM; MBM **50-1903**

WARRINGTON, Joseph (1805?-1888)
The obstetric catechism; containing two thousand three hundred and forty-seven questions and answers on obstetrics proper. . . . Philadelphia: E. Barrington & G. D. Haswell, 1853. 445p. DLC; PPC; PPJ; PU **50-1904**

WATSON, John (1807-1863)
Thermal ventilation and other sanitary improvements, applicable to public buildings, and recently adopted at the New York Hospital. New York: W. W. Rose, 1851. 41p. DNLM; NNNAM **50-1905**

WATSON, John (1807-1863)
The medical profession in ancient times. An anniversary discourse delivered before the New York Academy of Medicine. New York, 1856. 222p. DNLM; NNNAM **50-1906**

WATSON, John M[cClaran] (1796-1866)
A treatise on the history, etiology, and prophylaxis of trismus nascentium. 2nd ed. Nashville: J. T. S. Fall, 1851. 30p. DNLM; OCIM **50-1907**

WATSON, John McClaran (1796-1866)
An address read before the Tennessee Medical Society, at its twenty-third session. Nashville: J. T. S. Fall, 1852. 14p. DNLM; OCIM **50-1908**

WATSON, John McClaran (1796-1866)
An introductory lecture on the subject of early marriage, etc., October 31, 1854. Nashville: W. F. Bang & Co., 1854. 16p. DNLM; OCIM **50-1909**

WATSON, John McClaran (1796-1866)
An introductory address, delivered before the class of the medical department of the University of Nashville, Oct. 30th, 1855. Nashville: Cameron & Fall, 1855. 29p. DNLM; OCIM **50-1910**

WATSON, Thomas (1792-1882)
Lectures on the principles and practice of physic; delivered at King's College, London. . . . A new American, from the last rev. and enl. English ed. With additions by D. Francis Condie. . . . Philadelphia: Blanchard & Lea, 1853. 1224p. DLC; DNLM; PPC; PU **50-1911**

WATT, George (1820-1893)
An essay on dental surgery, for popular reading. Prize essay of the Mississippi Valley Association of Dental Surgeons. Cincinnati: T. Wrightson & Co., 1855. 56p. DNLM; OCHP **50-1912**

WATT, George (1820-1893)
An essay on dental surgery, for popular reading. Prize essay of the Mississippi Valley Association of Dental Surgeons. Cincinnati: Miss. Valley Ass. Dent. Surg., 1856. 72p. DNLM **50-1913**

WATT, George (1820-1893)
An essay on dental surgery, for popular reading. Prize essay of the Mississippi Valley Association of Dental Surgeons. [2nd ed.] Cincinnati: Miss. Valley Ass. Dent. Surg., 1858. 72p. DNLM **50-1914**

WATTERS, J. H.
An essay on organic or life force. Philadelphia: Lippincott, Grambo & Co., 1851. 36p. DNLM; PPC; PU **50-1915**

WATTERS, J. H.
Knowledge the only guide to action. An address to the graduates of the St. Louis College, delivered Feb. 28, 1857. [St. Louis], 1857. 16p. DNLM **50-1916**

WATTERS, J. H.
An essay on inflammation. [St. Louis, 1858.] 32p. DNLM **50-1917**

WATTERS, J. H.
Method of education. An address introductory to the session 1859-1860 of the St. Louis Medical College. St. Louis: G. Knapp & Co., 1859. 20p. DNLM **50-1918**

WEAVER, G[eorge] S[umner] (1818-1908)
Lectures on mental science, according to the philosophy of phrenology. Delivered before the Anthropological Society of the Western Liberal Institute of Marietta, Ohio, in the autumn of 1851. New York: Fowler & Wells, 1854. 245p. DNLM; NNNAM **50-1919**

WEIR, Robert Fulton (1838-1927)
Hernia cerebri. First prize essay of the College of Physicians and Surgeons, March 10, 1859. New York: T. Holman, 1859. 19p. 1 tab. DNLM; NNNAM **50-1920**

WELCH, Benjamin (1798-1873)
Surgeons' splints and improved apparatus for fractures. New York: E. O. Jenkins, 1852. 23p. 2 plates. DNLM; NNNAM **50-1921**

WELFORD, Beverley Randolph (1797-1870)
An address delivered before the Medical Society of Virginia. Richmond: Ritchies & Dunnavant, 1852. 38p. DNLM; ViRA **50-1922**

WELFORD, Beverley Randolph (1797-1870)
An address delivered before the Medical Society of Virginia. Richmond: Ritchies & Dunnavant, 1852. 62p. DNLM; ViRA. [Pages 39-62 contain: Proceedings of the Medical Society of Virginia at its 29th annual meeting.] **50-1923**

WELLING, D. S.
Information for the people; or the asylums of Ohio. With miscellaneous observations on health, diet, and morals, and the causes, symptoms, and proper treatment of nervous diseases and insanity. Pittsburgh: G. Parkin & Co., 1851. 376p. DNLM **50-1924**

[WELLS, Horace] (1815-1848)
Discovery by the late Dr. Horace Wells of the applicability of nitrous oxyd gas, sulphuric ether and other vapors in surgical operations nearly two years before the patented discovery of Drs. Charles T. Jackson and W. T. G. Morton. Hartford: Case, Tiffany & Co., 1850. 39p. DNLM; MBM; MWA **50-1925**

[WELLS, Horace] (1815-1848)
Discovery by the late Dr. Horace Wells of the applicability of nitrous oxyd gas, sulphuric ether and other vapors in surgical operations nearly two years before the patented discovery of Drs. Charles T. Jackson and W. T. G. Morton. Hartford: E. Geer, 1852. 40p. DNLM; MBM; MWA **50-1926**

[WELLS, Horace] (1815-1848)
An examination of the question of anesthesia, arising on the memorial of Charles Thomas Wells, presented to the U.S. Senate, 2nd Session, 32nd Congress, and referred to a select committee, of which the Hon. Isaac P. Walker is Chairman. Prepared for the information of said committee by the Hon. Truman Smith. New York: Gray, 1858. 135p. NNNAM **50-1927**

WEST, Charles (1816-1898)
Lectures on the diseases of infancy and childhood. Philadelphia: Lea & Blanchard, 1850. 451p. DNLM; PPC: PPJ; PU
50-1928

WEST, Charles (1816-1898)
Lectures on the diseases of infancy and childhood. . . . 2nd American from the 2nd and enl. London ed. Philadelphia: Blanchard & Lea, 1854. 486p. DLC; MBM; NNNAM; PPC
50-1929

WEST, Charles (1816-1898)
An inquiry into the pathological importance of ulceration of the os uteri. Being the Croonian lectures for the year 1854. . . . Philadelphia: Blanchard & Lea, 1854. 88p. DLC; DNLM; PPC; PU **50-1930**

WEST, Charles (1816-1898)
How to nurse sick children: intended especially as a help to the nurses at the hospital for sick children; but containing directions which may be found of service to all who have the charge of the young. New York: S. S. & W. Wood, 1855. 69p. DLC; DNLM; MBM; NNNAM **50-1931**

WEST, Charles (1816-1898)
Lectures on the diseases of women. Part I: Diseases of the uterus. Philadelphia: Blanchard & Lea, 1857. 316p. DNLM; NNNAM; PPC; PU **50-1932**

WEST, Charles (1816-1898)
Lectures on the diseases of women. . . . Philadelphia: Blanchard & Lea, 1858. 500p. DLC; OCIM; NNNAM; PPC
50-1933

WESTMORELAND, John G. (1816-1887)
A syllabus of lectures on materia medica and therapeutics, delivered in the Atlanta Medical College. Atlanta, Ga.: G. P. Eddy & Co., printers, 1857. 100p. DNLM; GU
50-1934

WESTMORELAND, Willis Foreman (1828-1890)
Address introductory to the fourth course of lectures in the Atlanta Medical College. Atlanta, Ga.: G. P. Eddy & Co., printers, 1858. 15p. DNLM; GU **50-1935**

WHARTON, Francis (1820-1889)
A monograph on mental unsoundness. Philadelphia: Kay & Bro., 1855. 228p. DNLM; PPC; PU **50-1936**

WHARTON, Francis (1820-1889) and Moreton STILLÉ
A treatise on medical jurisprudence. Philadelphia: Kay & Bro., 1855. 815p. CtY-M; DNLM; PPC; PPJ **50-1937**

WHAT to observe at the bed-side and after death in medical cases. Published under the authority of the London Medical Society of Observation. 2nd American, from the 2nd and enl. London ed. Philadelphia: Blanchard & Lea, 1859. 228p. DNLM; NNNAM; PPC; PU **50-1938**

WHITE, Anthony (1782-1849)
An inquiry into the proximate cause of gout, and its rational treatment. 1st American from 2nd London ed. New York: Nesbitt & Co., 1852. 24p. DNLM; NNNAM
50-1939

WHITE, Anthony (1782-1849)
An inquiry into the proximate cause of gout, and its rational treatment. 2nd American from 2nd London ed. Boston: J. Burnett, 1854. 24p. DNLM; MBM **50-1940**

WHITE, Daniel
A new and accurate method of diagnosing pulmonary consumption: being a treatise on the faucal symptoms, discovered and arranged. Springfield: Bailbache & Baker, 1858. 8p. DNLM
50-1941

WHITE, J. D.
On the treatment of exposed dental pulp, preparatory to the operation of filling. Philadelphia: J. H. Jones, 1853. 22p. DNLM; PPC **50-1942**

WHITE, James Platt (1811-1881)
Remarks at the annual meeting of the Erie County Medical Society, in relation to the formation of a society for the relief of widows and orphans of medical men. Buffalo: Thomas & Lathrops, 1856. 7p. DNLM **50-1943**

WHITE, Octavius Augustus (1826-1903) and William Hudson FORD
Bradycrote treatment of yellow fever, by veratrum viride and gelseminum sempervirens. [Charleston, 1858.] 7p. DNLM; ScMS **50-1944**

WHITE, Octavius A[ugustus] (1826-1903)
Description of a new hysterotome for the cure of dysmenorrhoea. Charleston, S.C.: James & Williams, 1859. 7p. DNLM; ScMS **50-1945**

WHITE, Thomas
The true cause of the cholera explained, with appropriate directions relative to diet, treatment, and disinfectants; also, the cause of the potato-rot explained, with directions how to prevent it. Cincinnati: J. A. & U. P. James, 1850. 48p. DNLM; OCIM **50-1946**

WHITHEAD, James (1812-1885)
On the causes and treatment of abortion and sterility: being the result of an extended practical inquiry into the physiological and morbid conditions of the uterus, with reference specially to leucorrhoeal affections, and the diseases of menstruation. . . . 2nd American ed. Philadelphia: Blanchard & Lea, 1854. 320p. DLC; NNNAM; PPC; PU
50-1947

WHITRIDGE, Joshua Barker (1789-1865)
An address to the candidates for the degree of doctor of medicine, delivered at the annual commencement of the Medical College of South Carolina, March 15, 1837. 3rd ed. Boston: White & Potter, 1850, 23p. DNLM; MBM; ScMS
50-1948

WICKES, Stephen (1813-1889)
Medical topography of Orange, N. Jersey. Newark, N.J.: S. C. Atkinson, 1859. 8p. 1 map. DNLM; NjR
50-1949

WIGAND, Henry
The complete physician, surgeon, and accoucheur; containing the symptoms, causes, and the allopathic, homoeopathic, hydropathic, and eclectic treatments of all known diseases of the human body; poisons and their antidotes; accidents and their treatment. Cincinnati: J. M. Parks, 1856. 731p. DNLM; OCIM **50-1950**

WILDE, William Robert Wills (1815-1876)
Practical observations on aural surgery, and the nature and treatment of diseases of the ear. Philadelphia: Blanchard & Lea, 1853. 475p. DNLM; MBM; NNNAM; PPC
50-1951

WILKINSON, James John Garth (1812-1899)
The human body and its connection with man. Illustrated by the principal organs. Philadelphia: Lippincott, Grambo & Co., 1851. 411p. DNLM; PPHa; PU **50-1952**

WILKINSON, James John Garth (1812-1899)
War, cholera and the ministry of health. An appeal to Sir Benjamin Hall and the British people. "Pro Civibus Servandis." From the London ed. Boston: Otis Clapp and Crosby, Nichols & Co., 1855. 80p. DNLM; MBM **50-1953**

WILKINSON, James John Garth (1812-1899)
The homoeopathic principles applied to insanity. A proposal to treat lunacy by spiritualism. Reprinted from the London ed. Boston: O. Clapp, 1857. 18p. DNLM; MBM **50-1954**

WILLARD, Sylvester D[avid] (1825-1865)
Biographical memoirs of physicians of Albany County. An address. Albany, N.Y.: J. Munsell, 1857. 22p. DNLM; N **50-1955**

WILLARD, S[ylvester] D[avid] (1825-1865)
Eulogy upon the life and character of Hiram Augustus Edmonds. Albany, N.Y.: J. Munsell, 1857. 20p. DNLM; N **50-1956**

WILLARD, S[ylvester] D[avid] (1825-1865)
Historical address. Delivered before the Medical Society of the County of Albany, November 11, 1856. Albany: C. Van Benthuysen, 1857. 28p. DNLM; N **50-1957**

WILLARD, S[ylvester] D[avid] (1825-1865)
Biographical memoir of Thomas Spencer. Albany: C. Van Benthuysen, 1858. 14p. DNLM; N **50-1958**

WILLARD, S[ylvester] D[avid] (1825-1865)
Diphtherite: its prevalence in Albany. Albany: C. Van Benthuysen, 1859. 6p. DNLM; N **50-1959**

WILLARD, S[ylvester] D[avid] (1825-1865)
Annual address before the Medical Society of the County of Albany. Albany: Munsell & Rowland, 1859. 18p. DNLM **50-1960**

WILLARD, S[ylvester] D[avid] (1825-1865)
Gun shot wound within the cavity of the thorax. Albany: C. Van Benthuysen, 1859. 6p. DNLM; N **50-1961**

WILLIAMS, B. Brown (1815?-1894)
A treatise on mental alchemy, electro-psychology, biology, magnetism, and mesmerism, with the cards of classes, editorials, etc. (making known their importance and remedial tendencies). Brooklyn, N.Y.: Shannon & Co., 1852. 91p. DNLM; NNNAM **50-1962**

WILLIAMS, B. Brown (1815?-1894)
A treatise on the mind, nervous system, psychology, magnetism, mesmerism, and diseases. New York: Fowlers & Wells, 1853. 180p. DNLM; NNNAM **50-1963**

WILLIAMS, Charles Draper
General introductory address before the class of the Western College of Homoeopathic Medicine. Cleveland, O.: Smead & Cowles, 1850. 16p. DNLM; PPHa **50-1964**

WILLIAMS, Charles Draper
The reviewer reviewed. An address delivered before the class of the Western College of Homoeopathic Medicine. Cleveland, O.: Gray & Wood, 1852. 28p. OCIM **50-1965**

WILLIAMS, Charles James Blasius (1805-1889)
The pathology and diagnosis of diseases of the chest; illustrated especially by a rational exposition of their physical signs; with new researches on the sounds of the heart. . . . Edited, with additions, by Meredith Clymer. 4th American ed., revised. Philadelphia: Blanchard & Lea, 1853. 476p. DNLM; OCIM; PPC; PU **50-1966**

WILLIAMS, Charles James Blasius (1805-1889)
Principles of medicine: comprising general pathology and therapeutics, and a brief general view of etiology, nosology, semeiology, diagnosis, prognosis, and hygienics. . . . Ed., with additions, by Meredith Clymer. . . . 4th American ed., rev. Philadelphia: Blanchard & Lea, 1853. 476p. DLC; MBM; PPC; PU **50-1967**

WILLIAMS, Charles James Blasius (1805-1889)
Principles of medicine. An elementary view of the causes, nature, treatment, diagnosis and prognosis of disease. New American from the 3rd and revised London ed. Philadelphia: Blanchard & Lea, 1857. 486p. NNNAM; PPC; PPJ; PU **50-1968**

WILLIAMS, Henry W[illard] (1821-1895)
An address delivered before the Suffolk District Medical Society, Boston, April 30, 1853. Boston: D. Clapp, 1853. 32p. DNLM; MBM **50-1969**

WILLIAMS, Henry Willard (1821-1895)
On the treatment of iritis without mercury. Boston: D. Clapp, 1856. 24p. DNLM; MBM **50-1970**

WILLIAMS, Stephen West (1790-1855)
Notice of some of the medical improvements and discoveries of the last half century, and more particularly in the United States of America. New York: Van Norden & Amerman, 1852. 36p. DNLM; NNNAM **50-1971**

WILLIAMSON, Walter (1811-1870)
Valedictory address delivered at the third annual commencement of the Homoeopathic Medical College of Pennsylvania. Philadelphia, 1851. 20p. DNLM; PPHa **50-1972**

WILLIAMSON, Walter (1811-1870)
Diseases of females and children, and their homoeopathic treatment; containing also a full description of the dose of each medicine. Philadelphia: Rademacher & Sheek, 1854. 256p. DNLM; PPHa; PPC; PU **50-1973**

WILSON, B. O. and G. C. WILSON
Botanic materia medica, or the physician's guide to the remedies of the botanic kingdom. Embracing the principal articles in use, with a brief account of their medicinal properties. Boston: J. Putnam, 1850. 80p. DNLM; MBM; OCLloyd **50-1974**

WILSON, Erasmus (1809-1884)
A system of human anatomy, general and special. 4th American from last London ed. Edited by Paul B. Goddard. Philadelphia: Lea & Blanchard, 1850. 576p. DNLM; MBM; NNNAM; PPC **50-1975**

WILSON, Erasmus (1809-1884)
The dissector; or, practical and surgical anatomy. Edited by Paul B. Goddard. 2nd ed. Philadelphia: Blanchard & Lea, 1851. 458p. DNLM; MBM; OCIM; PPC **50-1976**

WILSON, Erasmus (1809-1884)
On diseases of the skin. 3rd American from the 3rd London ed. Philadelphia: Blanchard & Lea, 1852. 483p. CU-M; DNLM; OCIWHi; PPC **50-1977**

WILSON, Erasmus (1809-1884)
On syphilis, constitutional and hereditary, and on syphilitic eruptions. Philadelphia: Lea & Blanchard, 1852. 284p. 4 col. plates. CU-M; DNLM; PPC; ViRA **50-1978**

WILSON, Erasmus (1809-1884)
Healthy skin: a popular treatise on the skin and hair, their preservation and management. 2nd American from 4th and revised London ed. Philadelphia: Blanchard & Lea, 1854. 291p. DNLM; OCIM; MBM; PPC **50-1979**

WILSON, Erasmus (1809-1884)
Hufeland's art of prolonging life. . . . Boston: Ticknor, Reed & Fields, 1854. 328p. MB; MBAt **50-1980**

WILSON, Erasmus (1809-1884)
The dissector's manual of practical and surgical anatomy. . . . The 3rd American from the last rev. London ed. Illustrated with one hundred and fifty-four wood engravings. Edited by William Hunt. . . . Philadelphia: Blanchard & Lea, 1856. 583p. DLC; DNLM; PPC; PU **50-1981**

WILSON, Erasmus (1809-1884)
A system of human anatomy, general and special. . . . 4th American, from the last London ed. Edited by Paul B. Goddard. . . . With two hundred and fifty-one illustrations by Gilbert. Philadelphia: Blanchard & Lea, 1856. 576p. DLC; DNLM; NNNAM; PPC **50-1982**

WILSON, Erasmus (1809-1884)
On diseases of the skin. . . . 4th American, from the 4th and enl. London ed. Philadelphia: Blanchard & Lea, 1857. 649p. atlas. DLC; DNLM; PPC; PU **50-1983**

WILSON, Erasmus (1809-1884)
Plates illustrative of Wilson on diseases of the skin. 4th ed. Philadelphia: Blanchard & Lea, 1857. 20p. 19 plates. CtY-M; DNLM; PPC; ViRA **50-1984**

WILSON, Erasmus (1809-1884)
A system of human anatomy, general and special. . . . A new and improved American, from an enl. London ed. Ed. by William H. Gobrecht. . . . With three hundred and ninety-seven illustrations on wood. Philadelphia: Blanchard & Lea, 1858. 616p. DLC; DNLM; OCIM; PPC **50-1985**

WILSON, J. A[rthur] (1795-1882)
An essay on follicular diseases of the throat and air passages. Memphis: Moseley & Finnie, 1853. 11p. DNLM **50-1986**

WILSON, William
The practice of medicine on Thomsonian principles; containing a treatise on animal life, cause and effect, with the names given to diseases and symptoms described, including prescriptions for practice, selected from different authors, [etc.]. Memphis: Eagle & Enquirer Press, 1855. 510p. DNLM; OCLloyd **50-1987**

WILTBANK, John (1806-1860)
Address to the graduates of the medical department of Pennsylvania College. Philadelphia: King & Baird, 1850. 14p. DNLM; PPC **50-1988**

WILTBANK, John (1806-1860)
The introductory lecture to the course of midwifery, in the medical department of Pennsylvania College, for the session of 1853-1854. Philadelphia: E. Grattan, 1854. 17p. DNLM; PPC **50-1989**

WINSTON, Charles K. (1811-1882) and Paul F. EVE
Addresses delivered by Professors Winston and Eve at the opening of the Medical Department of the University of Nashville, on the third day of November, 1851. Nashville: Eastman, Boyers & Co., 1851. 34p. DNLM; OCIM **50-1990**

WINSTON, Charles K. (1811-1882)
Ninth annual introductory address delivered before the class of the Medical Department of the University of Nashville, November 7, 1859. Nashville: J. T. S. Fall, 1859. 22p. DNLM **50-1991**

WISTAR ANATOMICAL MUSEUM OF THE UNIVERSITY OF PENNSYLVANIA
Catalogue of the Wistar Anatomical Museum of the University of Pennsylvania, by W. E. Horner. 3rd ed. Philadelphia: L. R. Bailey, 1850. 82p. DNLM; PPC; PU **50-1992**

WOLF, C. W.
Apis mellifica; or, the poison of the honey-bee, considered as a therapeutic agent. Philadelphia: W. Radde, 1858. 80p. DNLM; PPC **50-1993**

WOMEN'S MEDICAL COLLEGE OF PENNSYLVANIA. PHILADELPHIA
Annual announcements for the sessions of 1850-1851 to 1857-1858 (1.-8.); 1859-1860 (10.); 1862-1863 (13.); 1865-1866 to 1890-1891 (16.-41.). Philadelphia, 1850-1890. DNLM [Chartered March 11, 1850. List of students and graduates for the years 1850-1851 to 1855-6, 1858-9, 1864-5 to 1889-90, in announcements for subsequent year. List of alumnae from 1852 to 1890 in announcement for 1890-91. Chartered March 11, 1850, as the "Female Medical College of Pennsylvania."] **50-1994**

WOOD, George Bacon (1797-1879)
Introductory to the course of lectures on the theory and practice of medicine in the University of Pennsylvania. Philadelphia: Merrihew & Thompson, 1850. 23p. DNLM; PPC; PU **50-1995**

WOOD, George Bacon (1797-1879)
An address on the occasion of the centennial celebration of the founding of the Pennsylvania Hospital. Philadelphia: T. K. & P. G. Collins, 1851. 60p. DNLM; PPPH **50-1996**

WOOD, George Bacon (1797-1879)
The dispensatory of the United States of America. By George B. Wood . . . and Franklin Bache. . . . 9th ed., carefully rev. Philadelphia: Lippincott, Grambo & Co., successors to Grigg, Elliot & Co., 1851. 1456p. DLC; DNLM; OCLloyd; PPC **50-1997**

WOOD, George Bacon (1797-1879)
A treatise on the practice of medicine. 3rd ed. Philadelphia: Lippincott, Grambo & Co., 1852. 2 v. in 4. CtY-M; DNLM; MBM; PPC **50-1998**

WOOD, George Bacon (1797-1879)
Introductory lecture to the course on the theory and practice of medicine in the University of Pennsylvania. Philadelphia: T. K. & P. G. Collins, 1853. 26p. DNLM; PPC; PU **50-1999**

WOOD, George Bacon (1797-1879)
A biographical memoir of Samuel George Morton. Philadelphia: T. K. & P. G. Collins, 1853. 19p. DNLM; PPC **50-2000**

WOOD, George Bacon (1797-1879)
The dispensatory of the United States of America. By George B. Wood . . . and Franklin Bache. 10th ed., carefully rev. Philadelphia: Lippincott, Grambo & Co., 1854. 1480p. DLC; DNLM; OCLloyd; PPC **50-2001**

WOOD, George Bacon (1797-1879)
A treatise on the practice of medicine. . . . 4th ed. . . . Philadelphia: Lippincott, Grambo & Co., 1855. 2. v. DLC; DNLM; NNNAM; PPC **50-2002**

WOOD, George Bacon (1797-1879)
A treatise on therapeutics, and pharmacology, or materia medica. . . . Philadelphia: J. B. Lippincott & Co.; [etc., etc.], 1856. 2 v. DLC; MBM; NNNAM; PPC **50-2003**

WOOD, George Bacon (1797-1879)
An address to the class of medical graduates of the University of Pennsylvania. Philadelphia: T. K. & P. G. Collins, 1856. 16p. 1 plate. DNLM; PPC; PU **50-2004**

WOOD, George Bacon (1797-1879)
Address delivered at the late meeting of the American Medical Association, in Detroit, May 6, 1856. Philadelphia: T. K. & P. G. Collins, 1856. 14p. DNLM; PPC **50-2005**

WOOD, George B[acon] (1797-1879)
A treatise on the practice of medicine. . . . 5th ed. . . . Philadelphia: J. B. Lippincott & Co., 1858. 2 v. DLC; DNLM; MBM; PPC **50-2006**

WOOD, George Bacon (1797-1879)
Introductory to the course of lectures on the theory and practice of medicine, in the University of Pennsylvania. Philadelphia: T. K. & P. G. Collins, 1858. 22p. DNLM; PPC; PU **50-2007**

WOOD, George Bacon (1797-1879)
The dispensatory of the United States of America. By George B. Wood . . . and Franklin Bache. 11th ed., carefully rev. Philadelphia: J. B. Lippincott & Co., 1858. 1588p. DLC; DNLM; OCLloyd; PPC **50-2008**

WOOD, George Bacon (1797-1879)
Introductory lectures and addresses, on medical subjects, delivered chiefly before the medical classes of the University of Pennsylvania. . . . Philadelphia: J. B. Lippincott & Co., 1859. 460p. DLC; NNNAM; PPC; PU **50-2009**

WOOD, Isaac (1793-1868)
An inaugural address, delivered before the New York Academy of Medicine, February 6th, 1850. [To which is prefixed a valedictory address by Valentine Mott.] New York: H. Ludwig & Co., 1850. 26p. DNLM; NNNAM **50-2010**

WOOD, Jacob A. (1810-1879)
Pott's disease; or angular curvature of the spine. Cases successfully treated. New York: Holman, 1857. 7p. DNLM; NNNAM **50-2011**

WOOD, James Rushmore (1816-1883)
Spontaneous dislocation of the head of the femur into the ischiatic notch, occurring in morbus coxarius. [New York, 1854.] 4p. DNLM; NNNAM **50-2012**

WOOD, James Rushmore (1816-1883)
Removal of the entire lower jaw for necrosis caused by phosphoric acid gas. New York: Miller & Holman, 1856. 21p. 2 plates. DNLM; NNNAM **50-2013**

WOOD, James Rushmore (1816-1883)
Early history of the operation of ligature of the primitive carotid artery, with a report of forty-eight unpublished cases, and a summary of forty-four cases, with remarks by Valentine Mott. New York: H. Bailliere, 1857. 59p. DNLM; NNNAM **50-2014**

WOOD, T[homas] (1813-1880)
A compendium of anatomy, designed to accompany the anatomical chart. Cincinnati: F. Bly, [1857?]. 24p. DNLM; OCIM **50-2015**

WOOD, William B.
A report of the yellow fever at Centreville, in the year 1855; with some remarks on the disease, as it appeared in the parish of St. Mary, in 1853, 1854, and 1855. [New Orleans, 1856.] 12p. DNLM; LNT-M **50-2016**

WOOD, William Maxwell (1809-1880)
Hints to the people upon the profession of medicine. . . . Buffalo: G. H. Derby, 1852. 67p. DNLM **50-2017**

WOOD, William Maxwell (1809-1880)
A shoulder to the wheel of progress; being essays, lectures, and miscellanies upon themes of the day. [With hints to the people upon the profession of medicine.] Buffalo: Derby [and others], 1853. 291p. DNLM **50-2018**

WOODWARD, Samuel B[ayard] (1787-1850)
Hints for the young in relation to the health of body and mind. Boston: G. W. Light; Cleveland, O.: Jewett, Proctor & Worthington, 1856. 65p. DNLM; OCIM **50-2019**

WOOSTER, David (*b.* 1827)
An essay on diphtheria, with cases. San Francisco, 1859. 32p. DNLM **50-2020**

WOOTEN, H. V.
Character. A valedictory address to the graduating class of the Memphis Medical College. Memphis, 1853. 24p. DNLM **50-2021**

WRAGG, William T.
Remarks on the efficiency of quarantine as a means of prevention to the spread of epidemic diseases in cities and other populous communities; being the anniversary oration before the South Carolina Medical Association for 1854. Charleston, 1854. 20p. DNLM; ScCM **50-2022**

WRAGG, William T.
Physician's report on closing the Roper Hospital after the yellow fever epidemic of 1854, made to the trustees of the institution. Charleston: James, Williams & Gitsinger, 1855. 21p. DNLM; ScCM **50-2023**

WRIGHT, Charles W.
The means by which the eye adapts itself to distinct vision, at different distances. Louisville, Ky.: I. T. Cavins & Co., 1859. 14p. DNLM **50-2024**

WRIGHT, Marmaduke Burr (1803-1879)
Late controversy in relation to the Medical College of Ohio. Cincinnati, 1850. 4p. DNLM; OCHP **50-2025**

WRIGHT, Marmaduke Burr (1803-1879)
The memorial in relation to the Medical College of Ohio. The official misconduct of its trustees; the maladministration of its affairs, and the dangerous position of the Commercial Hospital. Made to the forty-ninth general assembly. Columbus: S. Medary, 1851. 29p. DNLM **50-2026**

WRIGHT, Marmaduke Burr (1803-1879)
Difficult labors and their treatment. (Prize essay, Ohio State Medical Society.) Cincinnati: Jackson, White & Co., 1854. 32p. DNLM; OCIM **50-2027**

WRIGHT, Marmaduke Burr (1803-1879)
An address on the life and character of the late Professor John Locke, delivered at the request of the Cincinnati Medical Society. Cincinnati: Moore, Wilstach, Keys & Co., 1857. 72p. DNLM; OCHP **50-2028**

WRIGHT, Marmaduke Burr (1803-1879)
Drunkenness, its nature and cure; or asylums for inebriates. An address delivered before the Ohio State Medical Society. Columbus: Follet, Foster & Co., 1859. 22p. DNLM; OCHP **50-2029**

WRIGHT, Thomas Lee (1825-1893)
A disquisition on the ancient history of medicine; comprising critical notices of the origin of medical science, its vicissitudes in the remotest times, and of its reconstruction and final establishment by the Greeks. . . . Cincinnati: Power Press of C. F. Bradley & Co., 1855. 84p. CtY-M; DLC; DNLM; OCIM **50-2030**

WYNNE, James (1814-1871)
Importance of the study of legal medicine: a lecture introductory to the course on medical jurisprudence at the New York Medical College. New York: H. Bailliere, 1859. 16p. DNLM; NNNAM **50-2031**

WYOMING WATER-CURE INSTITUTE
A report of the Wyoming Water-Cure Institute, including cases treated at Greenwood Springs Water-Cure, comprising a synoptical view of 377 cases. Buffalo: Jewett, Thomas & Co., 1853. 48p. DNLM **50-2032**

WYTHE, Joseph Henry (1822-1901)
The microscopist; or, A complete manual on the use of the microscope. . . . Philadelphia: Lindsay & Blakiston, 1851. 191p. DLC; DNLM; PPC; PU **50-2033**

WYTHE, Joseph H[enry] (1822-1901)
The microscopist; or, A complete manual on the use of the microscope. . . . 2nd ed., impr. and enl. . . . Philadelphia: Lindsay & Blakiston; London: Trubner & Co., 1853. 212p. DLC; DNLM; PPC; ViRA **50-2034**

YANDELL, Lunsford Pitts (1805-1878)
A reply to the attacks of Dr. Charles Caldwell. Louisville: Prentice & Weissinger, 1850. 9p. DNLM **50-2035**

YANDELL, Lunsford Pitts (1805-1878)
History of the Medical Department of the University of Louisville; an introductory lecture. Louisville, 1852. 38p. DNLM; KyLoJM **50-2036**

YANDELL, Lunsford Pitts (1805-1878)
History of the Medical Department of the University of Louisville: an introductory lecture, delivered November 1st 1852. . . . Louisville: Printed at the Office of the Journal, 1852. 38p. DLC; OCIM **50-2037**

YEOMAN, Thomas Harrison
Consumption of the lungs, or decline; the causes, symptoms, and rational treatment. With the means of prevention. Revised by a Boston physician. Boston: J. Monroe & Co., 1850. 107p. DNLM; MBM **50-2038**

YOUMANS, Edward L[ivingston] (1821-1887)
Alcohol and the constitution of man; being a popular scientific account of the chemical history and properties of alcohol, and its leading effects upon the healthy human constitution. New York: Fowlers & Wells, 1853. 127p. DNLM; NNNAM **50-2039**

YOUNG, Noble (1808-1883)
Valedictory address to the graduating class of the medical department of Georgetown College. Washington: T. McGill, 1857. 14p. DNLM **50-2040**

DR. YOUNG'S practice in the cure of chronic and other diseases, containing three hundred practical receipts, examined and approved by eminent American professors of medicine. 2nd ed. Cincinnati: E. Shepard, 1852. 120p. DNLM; OCIM **50-2041**

ZENDER, J[oachim] D. L.
Andronomy, or magneto-physiogonomico-craniology. . . . Improved from the systems of Messmer, Puysegur, Gall, Lavater, Spurzheim, etc. . . . New York, 1859. 108p. DNLM; NNNAM; PU **50-2042**

V. AMERICAN MEDICAL IMPRINTS, 1860-1869

Cholera infantum, or, as it is sometimes called, choleriform diarrhoea, is a disease of the summer months; and, with exceptional cases, of the cities. It receives the name, which designates it, from the violence of its symptoms, which closely resemble those in Asiatic cholera. It is, however, quite distinct in its nature, occurring independently of the epidemics of that disease. Post-mortem examinations establish the fact that it is a non-inflammatory diarrhoea, but on account of the violence and striking character of its symptoms, and its great mortality, it is proper to describe it as a distinct disease.

I have elsewhere stated that as regards at least this city, the term cholera infantum has been so extended as to embrace a large part of the diarrhoeal maladies affecting infants in the summer months. Some physicians apply it even to mild but protracted cases of ordinary non-inflammatory or inflammatory diarrhoea occurring in the season mentioned. I employ it, and it should, in my opinion, only be employed to designate that form of infantile diarrhoea in which there are frequent watery, perhaps serous stools, accompanied by vomiting and rapid and great emaciation. Moreover, when the disease ceases to be of this character, the term cholera infantum should no longer be applied to it, but it should receive another name indicative of the pathological state which has supervened. Intestinal inflammation frequently succeeds cholera infantum, and some writers describe it as a state of that disease. Properly, the inflammation should be regarded as a distinct affection, just as the enteritis, which sometimes results from cholera morbus, is not considered as a state of that disease, but as a disease itself.

J. Lewis Smith, *A Treatise on the Diseases of Infancy and Childhood*
(1869)

AN ACCOUNT of the medicinal properties of the Healing Springs, Bath Co., Va. . . . Richmond: Printed by J. D. Hammersley, 1868. 28p. DNLM; ViRA **60-0001**

ADAMS, John G[lover] (1807-1884)
Memoir of Jacob Harsen, M.D., read before the New York Academy of Medicine, June 1, 1864. With testimonials. [1864?] 34p. DNLM; NNNAM **60-0002**

ADDRESS of the pharmaceutists to the people of Philadelphia. 1 broadside. Philadelphia, 1860. DNLM **60-0003**

AGNEW, Cornelius R. (1830-1888)
. . . Preliminary report of the operations of the Commission during the present campaign in northern Virginia. [New York, 1864.] 12p. United States Sanitary Commission. [No. 76] DNLM; NNNAM **60-0004**

AGNEW, Cornelius Rea (1830-1888)
A method of operating for divergent squint. [New York, 1866.] 4p. DNLM; NNNAM **60-0005**

AGNEW, D[avid] Hayes (1818-1892)
Classification of the animal kingdom. A lecture introductory to the course of anatomy, in the Philadelphia School of Anatomy . . . on October 10, 1860. Philadelphia: J. M. Wilson, 1860. 16p. DNLM; PPC; PU **60-0006**

AGNEW, D[avid] Hayes (1818-1892)
Valedictory address to the anatomical class of the Philadelphia School of Anatomy, delivered on Friday evening, February 17, 1860. [Philadelphia, 1860.] 20p. DNLM; PPC; PU **60-0007**

AGNEW, D[avid] Hayes (1818-1892)
Baron Larrey: A lecture. Published for the class [at the Philadelphia School of Anatomy]. Philadelphia: Lindsay & Blakiston, 1861. 59p. PPC **60-0008**

AGNEW, D[avid] Hayes (1818-1892)
Valedictory lecture delivered to the anatomical class of the Philadelphia School of Anatomy, February 28, 1861. [Philadelphia, 1861.] 14p. PPC **60-0009**

AGNEW, D[avid] Hayes (1818-1892)
Lecture on the medical history of the Philadelphia Alms House. Delivered at the opening of the clinical lectures, October 15, 1862. Published by the request of the Board of Guardians. Philadelphia: Holland & Edgar, 1862. 52p. DNLM; PPC **60-0010**

AGNEW, D[avid] Hayes (1818-1892)
Vesico-vaginal fistula: its history and treatment. Philadelphia: Office of the Medical and Surgical Reporter, 1867. 42p. DNLM; PPC; PU **60-0011**

AGNEW, D[avid] Hayes (1818-1892)
Laceration of the female perineum; its history and treatment. [Philadelphia, 1868.] 45p. PPC **60-0012**

AGNEW, D[avid] Hayes (1818-1892)
Practical anatomy: a new arrangement of the London dissector; with numerous modifications and additions, containing a concise description of the muscles, blood vessels, nerves, viscera, and ligaments of the human body as they appear on dissection. 2nd ed. Philadelphia: J. B. Lippincott & Co., 1868. 307p. DNLM; PPC; PU **60-0013**

AITKEN, William (1825-1892)
The science and practice of medicine. From the 4th London ed., with additions by Meredith Clymer. Philadelphia: Lindsay & Blakiston, 1866. 2 v. DNLM; PPC; PU **60-0014**

AITKEN, William (1825-1892)
The science and practice of medicine. 2nd American from the 5th, enl. and carefully rev., London ed., adopting the new nomenclature of the Royal College of Physicians of London. With large additions by Meredith Clymer. Philadelphia: Lindsay & Blakiston, 1868. 2 v. PPC; PPJ; PU; ViRA **60-0015**

AITKIN, William E. A.
Valedictory address to the graduates of the University of Maryland. Baltimore: W. M. Innes, 1864. 20p. DNLM; MdU-D **60-0016**

ALBANY MEDICAL COLLEGE
Historical sketches of the medical college, the law school, and the Dudley Observatory of the University of Albany. Also, a sketch of the Albany Hospital. Albany: J. Munsell, 1867. 31p. DNLM; NNNAM **60-0017**

ALBANY MEDICAL SOCIETY
Annals of the Medical Society of the County of Albany, 1806-1851. With biographical sketches of deceased members. By Sylvester D. Willard. Albany: J. Munsell, 1864. 368p. DNLM; NNNAM **60-0018**

ALCOTT, Louisa May (1832-1888)
Hospital sketches. Boston: J. Redpath, 1863. 102p. ICU; N; NN; NNC **60-0019**

[ALCOTT, William Andrus] (1798-1859)
The physiology of marriage. . . . By a physician of many years' experience. Boston: W. H. Piper & Co.; New York: O. S. Felt, 1868. 259, 308p. DLC; MBM; NNNAM; PPC **60-0020**

ALDEN, Ebenezer (1788-1881)
Medical uses of alcohol. [Boston, 1869?] 16p. DNLM; MBM **60-0021**

ALLEN, Harrison (1841-1897)
Modern methods of investigation. [Cincinnati, 1869.] 8p. DNLM **60-0022**

ALLEN, Harrison (1841-1897)
Outlines of comparative anatomy and medical zoology. . . . Philadelphia: J. B. Lippincott & Co., 1869. 190p. DLC; DNLM; PPC; PU **60-0023**

ALLEN, J[ohn]
Teeth. An improved method of constructing artificial dentures. Combining five important points not heretofore attained. . . . New York: B. Urner, printer, 1860. 38p. 2 plates. DLC; DNLM; NNNAM **60-0024**

ALLEN, Jonathan Adams (1825-1890)
Professional success. Valedictory to the graduates of Rush Medical College, February 27th, 1861. [1861?] 20p. DNLM; ICRM **60-0025**

ALLEN, Jonathan Adams (1825-1890)
Medical examinations for life insurance. . . . Chicago: Horton & Leonard, printers, 1867. 143p. DLC; DNLM; ICRM **60-0026**

ALLEN, Jonathan Adams (1825-1890)
Medical examination for life insurance. 2nd ed. Chicago: Horton & Leonard, 1867. 143p. DNLM; ICRM; IEN-M
60-0027

ALLEN, Jonathan Adams (1825-1890)
Medical examinations for life insurance. 3rd ed. Chicago: Clarke & Co., [1867]. 143p. DNLM; ICRM **60-0028**

ALLEN, Jonathan Adams (1825-1890)
Medical examinations for life insurance. Revised and enlarged ed., with new introductory chapter and an extensive appendix. Chicago: J. H. & C. M. Goodsell, 1869. 181p. DNLM; IU-M; NNNAM; PU **60-0029**

ALLEN, Jonathan Adams (1825-1890)
Valedictory address to the graduates of the Medical Department of Pennsylvania College. Delivered at the public commencement. . . . Published by the class. Philadelphia: King & Baird, printers, 1865. 18p. DLC; PPC; PU
60-0030

ALLEN, Paul W.
Eclectic medicine; the lessons of its past and the duties of its future. Annual address, before the Eclectic Medical Society of the State of New York. Albany: C. Van Benthuysen & Sons, 1868. 24p. DNLM; N **60-0031**

ALLEY, James T. (1831?-1878)
The small doses of homoeopathy, confirmed by the teachings of physiology and pathology. New York: John T. S. Smith & Sons, 1860. 20p. DNLM; NNNAM **60-0032**

AMERICAN MEDICAL ASSOCIATION
Protection from small-pox by means of vaccination and revaccination. [Resolutions adopted by the . . . and report of the central committee appointed June, 1864, to carry them out.] [Philadelphia, 1864.] 10p. DNLM; OCIM; PPC
60-0033

AMERICAN MEDICAL ASSOCIATION
Report of the committee of medical ethics on specialties. By Worthington Hooker. Also, minority report, by Henry I. Bowditch. Philadelphia: Collins, 1866, 16p. DNLM; PPC; PU
60-0034

AMERICAN MEDICAL ASSOCIATION
Report of the committee on medical education. Philadelphia: Collins, 1869. 30p. DNLM; PPC; PU **60-0035**

AMERICAN POPULAR LIFE INSURANCE COMPANY. NEW YORK CITY
Sources of longevity, and its indications. New York: William Wood & Co., 1869. 112, 25, 9, 58, 16p. DNLM; NNNAM
60-0036

AMERICAN POPULAR LIFE INSURANCE COMPANY. NEW YORK CITY
Sources of longevity, its indications and practical applications. Pts. I & II. 2nd ed. New York: William Wood & Co., 1869. 42, 25, 9, 22p; 82, 64, 14, 4, 15p. DNLM; NNNAM
60-0037

AMORY, Robert (1842-1910)
Experiments upon the physiological action of bromide of potassium and ammonium (as determined on man and the lower animals); selected paper read before the Massachusetts Medical Society, June 1, 1869. Boston: D. Clapp & Son, 1869. 49p. DNLM; MBM **60-0038**

AMORY, Robert (1842-1910)
Atropine. Its physiological action and its use in tetanus, with experiments. Boston: D. Clapp & Son, 1869. 24p. DNLM; MBM **60-0039**

AMORY, Robert (1842-1910)
A contribution to the physiological study of veratrum viride and veratria (with experiments on lower animals, made at La Grange St. Laboratory, 1869) by Robert Amory [and] S. G. Webber. . . . Boston: Printed by D. Clapp & Son, 1869. 66p. DLC; DNLM; MBM **60-0040**

AMORY, Thomas C., Jr.
An address delivered at the dedication of the City Hospital May 24, 1864. Boston: J. E. Farwell and Co., 1864. 45p. DNLM; MBM **60-0041**

AMSBY, James H. (1810-1875)
History of the Albany City Hospital and extracts from addresses delivered in its behalf, in 1851-1852. Albany: J. Munsell, 1868. 47p. DNLM **60-0042**

ANDERSON, James (1798-1886)
An inaugural address, delivered before the New York Academy of Medicine, January 16, 1861. . . . Published by order of the Academy. New York: W. A. Wheeler, stationer and printer, 1861. 11p. DLC; DNLM; NNNAM **60-0043**

ANDERSON, James (1798-1886)
Address on retiring from the presidential chair of the New York Academy of Medicine. Delivered January 16, 1867. New York, 1869. 34p. DNLM; NNNAM
60-0044

ANDREW, John Albion (1818-1867)
An address to the graduating class of the Medical School in the University of Cambridge, on Wednesday, March 9, 1864. . . . Boston: Ticknor & Fields, 1864. 28p. DLC; DNLM; MH-M
60-0045

ANDREWS, Edmund (1824-1904)
Complete record of the surgery of the battles fought near Vicksburg, December 27, 28, 29, & 30, 1862. . . . Chicago: G. H. Fergus, book and job printer, 1863. 48p. DLC; DNLM
60-0046

ANDREWS, Edmund (1824-1904)
Report of the Committee on Military Hygiene. Philadelphia: Collins, 1864. 15p. DNLM; PPC **60-0047**

ANDREWS, E[dmund] (1824-1904)
The primary surgery of Gen. Sherman's campaigns. By E. Andrews . . . and J. M. Woodworth. . . . Chicago: G. H. Fergus, printer, 1866. 20p. DLC; OCIM; NNNAM
60-0048

ANDREWS, Judson B. (1834-1894)
The physiological action and therapeutic uses of the "acidum phosphoricum dilutum." [Utica, N.Y., 1869.] 17p. DNLM
60-0049

ANNANDALE, Thomas (1838-1907)
The malformations, diseases, and injuries of the fingers and toes, and their surgical treatment. [The Jackson prize essay for the year 1864.] Philadelphia: J. B. Lippincott & Co., 1866. 292p. 12 plates. DNLM; PPC; PU **60-0050**

ANSTIE, Francis Edmund (1833-1874)
Stimulants and narcotics, their mutual relations: with special researches on the action of alcohol, ether and chloroform on the vital organism. . . . Philadelphia: Lindsay & Blakiston, 1865. 414p. DLC; DNLM; PPC; PU **60-0051**

ANSTIE, Francis Edmund (1833-1874)
Notes on epidemics. For the use of the public. . . . 1st American ed. Philadelphia: J. B. Lippincott & Co., 1866. 95p. DLC; DNLM; PPC; PU **60-0052**

ARLT, Carol. Ferdinand, von (1812-1887)
Retinitis myctalopica. From "Der Bericht über die Augenklinik." Transl. by J. F. Weightman. Philadelphia: Lindsay & Blakiston, 1868. 23p. DNLM; PPC; PU **60-0053**

ARLT, Carol. Ferdinand, von (1812-1887)
Treatment of lachrymal affections. Transl. by J. F. Weightman. Philadelphia: Lindsay & Blakiston, 1869. 30p. 1 plate. DNLM; PPC; PU **60-0054**

ARMOR, Samuel Glasgow (1819-1885)
Medical logic: an introductory lecture to the medical department of the University of Michigan, session of 1863-1864. Detroit: Free Press, 1863. 21p. DNLM **60-0055**

ARNOLD, Edmund Samuel Foster (1820-1907)
On medical provision for railroad accidents, in a letter to the American Medical Times, with a postscript, by a country surgeon. Yonkers: Examiner Print, 1861. 12p. DLC; DNLM **60-0056**

ARNOLD, Edmund Samuel Foster (1820-1907)
On medical provision for railroads as a humanitarian measure, as well as a source of economy, to the companies. Read before the State Medical Society. . . . Printed by permission. Albany: N.Y.: Weed, Parsons & Company, printers, 1862. 20p. DLC **60-0057**

ARNOLD, Edmund Samuel Foster (1820-1907)
On medical provision for railroads as a humanitarian measure as well as a source of economy to the companies. In two papers. Read, respectively, before the New York State Medical Society, Feb. 5, 1862, and the surgical section of the New York Academy of Medicine, Oct. 28, 1862. New York: Bailliere Brothers, 1862. 47p. DLC; DNLM; NNNAM **60-0058**

ARNOLD, Edmund Samuel Foster (1820-1907)
On the uses of opium in managing the shock and reaction of severe surgical injuries. . . . New York: M. B. Brown & Co., 1863. 30p. DLC; DNLM **60-0059**

ARNOLD, Richard D. (1808-1876)
An address before the Georgia Medical Society, on its sixty-fourth anniversary, January 8, 1868. Savannah, Ga.: Purse, 1868. 16p. DNLM; GU **60-0060**

ARROWSMITH, Wm. L.
Introductory address to the 20th Annual Session of the Homoeopathic Medical College of Pennsylvania. Philadelphia: King & Baird, 1867. 26p. PPHa; PPC **60-0061**

ARTHUR, Robert (1819-1880)
Some suggestions concerning the nature and treatment of decay of the teeth. . . . Baltimore: J. Murphy & Co., 1867. 70p. DLC; DNLM; MdU-D **60-0062**

ASHHURST, John (1839-1900)
Injuries of the spine. With an analysis of nearly four hundred cases. . . . Philadelphia: J. B. Lippincott & Co.; [etc., etc.], 1867. 127p. DLC; DNLM; PPC; PU **60-0063**

AVERY, Henry N[ewell] (1838-1898)
Hand-book for consumptives. A practical guide for the invalid and student, embracing all the recent discoveries applicable to the consumptive in climate, hygiene, food and treatment. New York: S. P. Hermance & Son, 1869. 34p. PPHa; NNNAM **60-0064**

BACHE, Franklin (1792-1864)
General introductory to the course of instruction in Jefferson Medical College of Philadelphia, for the session of 1861-1862. Delivered Oct. 14th, 1861. Philadelphia: Collins, 1861. 20p. DNLM; PPJ **60-0065**

[BACHE, Thomas Hewson]
Some practical observations on yellow fever, published for the use of surgeons of the volunteer forces in the Department of the Gulf. New Orleans, 1862. 20p. DNLM; LNT-M **60-0066**

BACKUS, Henry
Pathological phenomena generalized. Selma, Ala.: Shelley & Williams, 1860. 42p. AU; DNLM **60-0067**

BACKUS, Henry
Pathological phenomena generalized. Montevallo, Ala., 1867. 59p. AU; DNLM **60-0068**

BACON, Leonard (1802-1881)
The beloved physician. A discourse delivered in First Church in New Haven, at the interment of Jonathan Knight, M.D. New Haven: T. I. Stafford, 1864. 28p. CtY-M; DNLM **60-0069**

BAEHR, Bernhard
The science of therapeutics according to the principles of homoeopathy. Transl. and enriched with numerous additions from Kafka and other sources. By Charles J. Hempel, M.D. New York: Boericke & Tafel, 1869. 2 v. NNNAM; PPHa **60-0070**

BALDWIN, David A.
The family pocket homoeopathist, a concise manual of homoeopathic practice, for families and travelers. . . . Rochester, N.Y.: E. Darrow & Brother, 1864. 142p. DLC **60-0071**

BALDWIN, William Owen (1818-1886)
Physic and physician. The annual address delivered before the Alabama State Medical Association, at the Capitol. . . . Printed by order of the Association. Cambridge [Mass.]: Printed at Riveside Press, 1866. 88p. DLC; MBM **60-0072**

BALDWIN, W[illiam] O[wen] (1818-1886)
Annual address . . . before the American Medical Association, at New Orleans, La., May 4, 1868. Louisville, Ky.: Bell & Co., 1869. 29p. DNLM; OCIM **60-0073**

BALDWIN, William Owen (1818-1886)
An address delivered before the American Medical Association. Philadelphia: Collins, 1869. 28p. DNLM; PPC **60-0074**

BANNING, E[dmund] P[rior] (*b.* 1810)
Uterine displacements. Philadelphia, 1867. 7p. DNLM
60-0075

BANNING, E[dmund] P[rior] (*b.* 1810)
A rational treatise on the trunkal muscles, elucidating the mechanical cause of chronic spinal, pelvic, abdominal, and thoracic affections ... with the rationale of their cure by mechanical support. . . . New York: W. A. Townsend & Adams, 1868. 352p. DLC; NNNAM **60-0076**

BANNING, E[dmund] P[rior] (*b.* 1810)
Spinal symmetry and deformity. [New York, 1868.] 44p. DNLM **60-0077**

BANTING, William (1797-1878)
Letter on corpulence, addressed to the public. 3rd ed., with addenda, and remarks by Mr. Harvey. New York: Mohun, Ebbs & Hough, 1864. 36p. DNLM; NNNAM
60-0078

BANTING, William (1797-1878)
Letter on corpulence, addressed to the public. 3rd ed., with addenda. New York: Mohun, Ebbs & Hough, 1864. 22p. DNLM; NNNAM **60-0079**

BANTING, William (1797-1878)
Letter on corpulence, addressed to the public. . . . 4th ed., with addenda. New York: Mohun, Ebbs & Hough, Booksellers & Importers, 1864. 36p. DLC; NNNAM
60-0080

BANTING, William (1797-1878)
Letter on corpulence; addressed to the public. 5th ed., with addendas and remarks by Mr. Harvey. New York: Mohun & Ebbs, 1865. 31p. DNLM; NNNAM **60-0081**

BANTING, William (1797-1878)
Letter on corpulence; advice to the public. 6th ed. Philadelphia: J. B. Lippincott & Co., 1868. 51p. DNLM; PPC
60-0082

BARCLAY, Andrew Whyte (1817-1884)
A manual of medical diagnosis being an analysis of the signs and symptoms of disease. Philadelphia: Blanchard & Lea, 1864. 451p. CtY-M; DNLM; MBM; NNNAM
60-0083

BARKER, [Benjamin] Fordyce (1818-1891)
On the comparative use of ergot and the forceps in labor. [1860?] 16p. DNLM **60-0084**

BARKER, George T. (1836-1878)
Instructions in the preparation, administration, and properties of nitrous oxide, protoxide of nitrogen, or laughing gas. Philadelphia: Rubencame & Stockton, 1866. 61p. DNLM; PPC; PU **60-0085**

BARLOW, Samuel Bancroft (1798-1876)
Valedictory address delivered at the sixth annual commencement of the Homoeopathic Medical College of New York, February 24, 1866. New York: Gray & Green, 1866. 22p. DNLM; NNNAM **60-0086**

BARLOW, Samuel Bancroft (1798-1876)
A brief history of the materia medica. Boston: A. Mudge & Son, 1869. 15p. DNLM; MBM **60-0087**

BARTH, Jean Baptiste Philippe (1806-1877)
A manual of auscultation and percussion, as applied to the diagnosis of diseases of the heart and lung, and to pregnancy; transl. from the French of MM. Barth and Roger, by J. H. Pottenger. . . . St. Louis: R. P. Studley & Co., printers, 1860. 161p. DLC; OCIM; NNNAM **60-0088**

BARTH, Jean Baptiste Philippe (1806-1877)
A manual of auscultation and percussion. By M. Barth, and M. Henri Roger. . . . Transl. from the 6th French ed. Philadelphia: Lindsay & Blakiston, 1866. 161p. DLC; NNNAM; PPC
60-0089

BARTHOLOW, Roberts (1831-1904)
A manual of instruction for enlisting and discharging soldiers. With special reference to the medical examination of recruits, and the detection of the disqualifying and feigned diseases. Philadelphia: J. B. Lippincott & Co., 1863. 276p. CtY-M; DNLM; MH-M; PPC **60-0090**

BARTHOLOW, Roberts (1831-1904)
Experimental investigations into the action and uses of the bromide of potassium. . . . Cincinnati: A. Moore, printer, 1865. 16p. DLC; DNLM; OCIM **60-0091**

BARTHOLOW, Roberts (1831-1904)
Observations, pathological and experimental, on cholera; being a report to the board of health [Cincinnati], with an addendum. Cincinnati: A. Moore, 1866. 14p. DNLM; OCIM
60-0092

BARTHOLOW, Roberts (1831-1904)
On spermatorrhoea. New York: William Wood & Co., 1866. 112p. CU-M; DNLM; NNNAM; PPC **60-0093**

BARTHOLOW, Roberts (1831-1904)
On the progressive locomotor ataxia. Cincinnati: R. Clarke & Co., 1866. 27p. DNLM; OCIM **60-0094**

BARTHOLOW, Roberts (1831-1904)
The principles and practice of disinfection. Cincinnati: R. W. Carroll & Co., 1867. 111p. DLC; DNLM; OCIM; PPC
60-0095

BARTHOLOW, Roberts (1831-1904)
On spermatorrhoea. 2nd ed. New York: William Wood & Co., 1868. 112p. DNLM; ICRM; NNNAM; PU
60-0096

BARTHOLOW, Roberts (1831-1904)
Case of Davis B. Lawler. Amnesia of written language, etc. . . . [Cincinnati: R. Clarke & Co., 1869] 8p. DLC
60-0097

BARTHOLOW, Roberts (1831-1904)
The physiological effects and therapeutical uses of atropia and its salts. Prize essay. Philadelphia: Collins, 1869. 48p. DNLM; PPC; PU **60-0098**

BARTHOLOW, Roberts (1831-1904)
Manual of hypodermic medication. . . . Philadelphia: J. B. Lippincott & Co., 1869. 150p. 3 fold. diagr. DLC; DNLM; NNNAM; PPC **60-0099**

BARWELL, Richard (1827-1916)
A treatise on diseases of the joints. Philadelphia: Blanchard & Lea, 1861. 463p. CtY-M; MBM; NNNAM; PPC
60-0100

BAUDENS, J. B. Lucien (1804-1857)
On military and camp hospitals, and the health of troops in the field. Transl. by Franklin B. Hough. New York: Bailliere Brothers, 1862. 260p. NNNAM; OCIM; PU
60-0101

BAUER, Louis (1814-1898)
Lectures on orthopedic surgery. Delivered at the Brooklyn Medical and Surgical Institute. . . . Philadelphia: Lindsay & Blakiston, 1864. 108p. DLC; DNLM; NNNAM; PPC
60-0102

BAUER, Louis (1814-1898)
Lectures on causes, pathology, and treatment of joint diseases. New York: William Wood & Co., 1868. 96p. DNLM; MBM; NNNAM; PC **60-0103**

BAUER, Louis (1814-1898)
Remarks on Dr. Sayre's paper entitled: "A new operation for artificial hip-joint in bony anchylosis." New York: D. Appleton & Co., 1869. 15p. DNLM; NNNAM
60-0104

BAYES, William
Plain directions for the treatment of cholera and epidemic diarrhoea, and for their prevention. Enlarged and improved edition. New York: William Radde, 1866. 8p. DNLM; PPHa
60-0105

BAYLESS, George Wood (1816-1873)
Reminiscences of the medical college: being an introductory lecture delivered before the medical department of the University of Louisville. Louisville: Courier Printing Establishment, 1866. 50p. DNLM; KyLoJM **60-0106**

BEACH, Wooster (1794-1868)
The American practice condensed. Or, The family physician: being the scientific system of medicine: on vegetable principles, designed for all classes. . . . This work embraces the character, causes, symptoms, and treatment of the diseases of men, women, and children of all climates. . . . Illustrated with nearly two hundred engravings. 56th ed., rev., with the latest improvements. Cincinnati: Moore, Wilstach & Moore, 1869. 873p. 4 col. plates. DLC; OCIM **60-0107**

BEAKLEY, Jacob (1812?-1872)
Valedictory address. Delivered at the first annual commencement of the Homoeopathic College of New York. New York: Francis Hart & Co., 1861. 32p. DNLM; NNNAM
60-0108

BEARD, George Miller (1839-1883)
The medical use of electricity. . . . By George M. Beard and A. D. Rockwell. New York: William Wood & Co., 1867. 65p. DLC; NNNAM **60-0109**

BEARD, George Miller (1839-1883)
The medical use of electricity, in the form of general electrization. New York: N.Y. Print. Co., 1868. 16p. DNLM; NNNAM
60-0110

BEARD, George M[iller] (1839-1883)
Our home physician: a new and popular guide to the art of preserving health and treating disease; with plain advice for all the medical and surgical emergencies of the family. . . . New York: E. B. Treat & Co.; Chicago, Ill.: C. W. Lilley; [etc., etc.], 1869. 1066p. DLC; IEN-M; IU-M; NNNAM
60-0111

BECK, John Brodhead (1794-1851)
Lectures on materia medica and therapeutics. Prepared for the press by C. R. Gilman. 3rd ed. New York: S. S. & W. Wood, 1861. 563p. DNLM; NNNAM; PU
60-0112

BECK, Theodoric Romeyn (1791-1855) and John B. BECK
Elements of medical jurisprudence. 11th ed. With notes by an association of the friends of Drs. Beck. The whole revised by C. R. Gilman. Philadelphia: J. B. Lippincott & Co., 1860. 2 v. DNLM; NNNAM; PPC; PU **60-0113**

BECK, Theodoric Romeyn (1791-1855) and John B. BECK
Elements of medical jurisprudence. 12th ed. . . . Philadelphia: J. B. Lippincott & Co., 1863. 2 v. CtY-M; DNLM; PPC; PU
60-0114

BECKER, Alexander R.
Gunshot wounds, particularly those caused by newly-invented missiles. [Fiske Fund Prize Essay for 1864]. 1865. 33p. DNLM; MH-M **60-0115**

BECKER, P. J.
Ten lectures, on medical electricity. Embracing the system of electropathic treatment, as taught by Dr. Paige, of Boston, together with extracts from various works, giving the view of Dr. Golding Bird, of London, Dr. Channing, of Boston, and others. . . . Auburn, [N.Y.]: 1862. 48p. DLC
60-0116

BECKWITH, Simeon W.
Electrical treatment of diseases. [1864?] 15p. DNLM
60-0117

BECKWITH, Simeon W.
Electricity, in its various modifications for the treatment of chronic diseases. Philadelphia: H. A. Ashmead, 1866. 15p. DLC; DNLM; PPC **60-0118**

BEDFORD, Gunning S. (1806-1870)
The principles and practice of obstetrics. New York: S. S. & W. Wood, 1861. 731p. 4 plates. DNLM; NNNAM; PPC; PU
60-0119

BEDFORD, Gunning S. (1806-1870)
The principles and practice of obstetrics. 2nd ed. New York: William Wood & Co., 1862. 731p. 4 plates. DNLM; NNNAM; NNU-M; PPC **60-0120**

BEDFORD, Gunning S. (1806-1870)
The principles and practice of obstetrics. 3rd ed. New York: William Wood & Co., 1863. 743p. 4 plates. DNLM; NNNAM; NNU-M; PU **60-0121**

BEDFORD, Gunning S. (1806-1870)
Clinical lectures on the diseases of women and children. 8th ed., revised and enlarged. New York: William Wood & Co., 1866. 667p. CtY-M; DNLM; NNNAM; NNU-M
60-0122

BEDFORD, Gunning S. (1806-1870)
The principles and practice of obstetrics. 4th ed. New York: William Wood & Co., 1868. 763p. DNLM; NNNAM; NNU-M; PU **60-0123**

BEDORTHA, N.
Practical medication, or The invalid's guide; with directions for the treatment of disease. . . . Albany, N.Y.: Munsell & Rowland, 1860. 281p. DLC **60-0124**

BEEBE, Gaylord D. (1835-1877)
Introductory address, delivered in the Hahnemann Medical College of Chicago, October 10, 1864. Chicago: Calhoun, 1864. 16p. IEN-M; PPHa **60-0125**

BEEBE, Gaylord D. (1835-1877)
Valedictory address to the graduating class of Hahnemann Medical College of Chicago, February 27, 1867. Chicago: Beach & Barnard, 1867. 14p. IEN-M; PPHa **60-0126**

BEECHER, Catharine Esther (1800-1878)
The American woman's home: or, principles of domestic science . . . by Catharine E. Beecher and Harriet Beecher Stowe. New York: J. B. Ford & Co., 1869. 500p. NN **60-0127**

BELL, Agrippa Nelson (1820-1911)
Malignant pustule in the United States. Albany: C. Van Benthuysen, 1862. 25p. DNLM **60-0128**

BELL, Agrippa Nelson (1820-1911)
Disinfection of vessels. New York: G. W. Wood, 1863. 12p. DNLM; NNNAM **60-0129**

BELL, Agrippa Nelson (1820-1911)
[Merritt H. Cash Prize Essay]. How complete is the protection of vaccination, and what are the dangers of communicating other diseases with the vaccinia? Albany, 1864. 27p. DNLM **60-0130**

BELL, James Bachelder (1838-1914)
The homoeopathic therapeutics of diarrhoea, dysentery, cholera, cholera morbus, cholera infantum and all other loose evacuations of the bowels. Philadelphia: A. J. Tafel, 1869. 168p. PPHa; PPC **60-0131**

BELL, John (1796-1872)
Report on the importance and economy of sanitary measures to cities. . . . Board of Councilmen, November 28, 1859. Document no. 20. New York: E. Jones & Co., Printers, 1860. 243p. DLC; NNNAM **60-0132**

BELL, John (1796-1872)
Report of the committee on the relations of alcohol to medicine. Philadelphia: Collins, 1869. 120p. DNLM; PPC **60-0133**

BELL, Theodore Stout (1807-1884)
[On] E. S. Gaillard, M.D., editor of the Richmond and Louisville Medical Journal. . . . Nashville, Tenn.: W. H. F. Ligon, 1869. 21p. DNLM **60-0134**

BELL, Theodore Stout (1807-1884)
Medical and surgical science, as expounded by E. S. Gaillard. [Louisville, 1869.] 36 [38], 27, 4p. DNLM **60-0135**

BELL, Theodore Stout (1807-1884)
A pseudo-critic unmasked, in a review of the writings of E. S. Gaillard, M. D., ex-professor of three medical schools. 2nd ed. Louisville, Ky.: Bradley & Gilbert, 1869. 36 [38], 27, 4p. DNLM **60-0136**

BELLEVUE HOSPITAL MEDICAL COLLEGE. NEW YORK CITY
Inauguration of the . . . at the first annual session, Oct., 1861. New York: Baker & Godwin, 1862. 15p. DNLM; NNNAM; NNU-M **60-0137**

BELLOWS, Albert J[ones] (1804-1869)
"Currents and counter-currents in medical science." Oliver Wendell Holmes, M.D., reviewed in an address delivered before the Boston Academy of Homoeopathic Medicine. 2nd ed. Boston: J. M. Hewes, 1860. 27p. DNLM; MH-M **60-0138**

BELLOWS, Albert J[ones] (1804-1869)
A memorial to the trustees of the Free City Hospital, with statistics and facts showing the comparative merits of homoeopathy and allopathy, as shown by treatment in European hospitals. Boston: O. Clapp, 1863. 26p. DNLM; MBM **60-0139**

BELLOWS, Henry W[hitney] (1814-1882)
Address before the "College of Physicians and Surgeons" at their annual commencement, March 14, 1867. New York: J. F. Trow & Co., 1867. 12p. DNLM; NNNAM **60-0140**

BEMISS, S. M. (1821-1884), C. L. BICKHAM, and B. A. POPE
Memoranda of cases treated before the medical class in the session of 1866-1867. New Orleans: L. Graham, 1867. 51p. DNLM; LNT-M **60-0141**

BENNETT, John Hughes (1812-1875)
Clinical lectures on the principles and practice of medicine. From the last Edinburgh ed. New York: S. S. & Wm. Wood, 1860. 952p. DNLM; NNNAM; PPC; PU **60-0142**

BENNETT, John Hughes (1812-1875)
Clinical lectures on the principles and practice of medicine. 2nd American from the last Edinburgh ed. New York: William Wood & Co., 1863. 952p. DNLM; MdBM; MH-M; NNNAM **60-0143**

BERJEAU, Jean P[hilibert] (1809-1891)
The homoeopathic treatment of syphilis, gonorrhoea, spermatorrhoea and urinary diseases. . . . Revised, with numerous additions, by J. H. P. Frost, M.D., late professor of physiology and pathology in the Homoeopathic Medical College of Pennsylvania. Philadelphia: A. J. Tafel, 1869. 256p. PPC; PPHa; PU **60-0144**

BERNARD, Claude (1813-1878)
Lecture on the physiology of the heart, and its connections with the brain, delivered at a meeting at the Sorbonne, the 27th March, 1865. . . . Transl. by J. S. Morel. . . . Savannah: Purse & Son, 1867. 47p. DLC; GU; LNT-M; PPC **60-0145**

BERRIDGE, Edward W.
A repertory to the materia medica. . . . Philadelphia: De Armond & Goodrich, 1869. 220p. PPHa; OCLloyd **60-0146**

BIDDLE, John Barclay (1815-1879)
Introductory lecture delivered before the class of Jefferson Medical College . . . October 9, 1865. Philadelphia: H. B. Ashmead, 1865. 19p. DNLM; PPJ **60-0147**

BIDDLE, John Barclay (1815-1879)
Materia medica, for the use of students. . . . [2nd ed.] Philadelphia: Lindsay & Blakiston, 1865. 359p. DLC; PPC; PU **60-0148**

BIDDLE, John Barclay (1815-1879)
Materia medica, for the use of students. . . . 3rd ed. enl. . . . Philadelphia: Lindsay & Blakiston, 1868. 384p. DLC; OCLloyd; PPC; PU **60-0149**

BIGELOW, Henry Jacob (1818-1890)
Ununited fracture successfully treated, with remarks on the operation. . . . With abstracts from Dr. Bigelow's clinical lectures on the subject, and cases. (Reported by Richard H. Derby.) Boston: D. Clapp & Son, 1867. 25p. DLC; MBM
60-0150

BIGELOW, Henry Jacob (1818-1890)
Practical views of the treatment of fractures and dislocations of the elbow-joint, and on the general impropriety of passive motion. An abstract of remarks made at a clinical lecture delivered at the Massachusetts Medical College, March 2, 1868. Reported by Henry H. A. Beach. [Boston, 1868.] 3p. DNLM; MBM **60-0151**

BIGELOW, Henry Jacob (1818-1890)
The mechanism of dislocation and fracture of the hip, with the reduction of the flexion method. Philadelphia: H. C. Lea, 1869. 150p. DNLM; NNNAM; PPC; PU
60-0152

BIGELOW, Jacob (1787-1879)
Modern inquiries: classical, professional, and miscellaneous. Boston: Little, Brown & Co., 1867. 379p. DNLM; MB; MBM; NN **60-0153**

BIRD, Golding (1814-1854)
Urinary deposits; their diagnosis, pathology, and therapeutical indications. Edited by Edmund Lloyd Birkett. A new American from the last London ed. Philadelphia: Blanchard & Lea, 1863. 382p. DNLM; NNNAM; PPC; PU
60-0154

BLACKMAN, George Curtis (1819-1871)
A case of removal of the lower jaw, for osteo-sarcoma of immense size. [1860] 8p. DNLM **60-0155**

BLACKMAN, George C[urtis] (1819-1871)
Physiological effects produced upon the brain by the ligature of both primitive carotid arteries, with the statistics of this operation. Cincinnati: S. G. Cobb, 1863. 12p. DNLM
60-0156

BLACKMAN, George Curtis (1819-1871)
A few thoughts on strangulated hernia. Illustrated. Cincinnati: S. G. Cobb, 1863. 10p. DNLM **60-0157**

[BLACKWELL, Elizabeth] (1821-1910)
Medicine as a profession for women. New York: Trustees of the New York Infirmary for Women, 1860. 24p. DLC; NNNAM **60-0158**

BLACKWELL, Elizabeth (1821-1910) and Emily BLACKWELL
Address on the medical education of women. Read before a meeting held at the New York Infirmary, December 19, 1863. New York: Baptist and Taylor, 1864. 16p. DLC; DNLM; NNNAM **60-0159**

BLAKE, John B.
A biographical sketch of the late Dr. William Jones. Washington, D.C.: McGill & Witherow, 1867. 16p. DNLM
60-0160

BLANEY, James Van Zandt (1820-1874)
Opening lecture at the twenty-third annual course of lectures of Rush Medical College. Chicago: J. W. Bailey, 1865. 11p. DNLM; ICRM **60-0161**

BLATCHFORD, Thomas Windeatt (1794-1866)
Our alma mater fifty years ago. An oration delivered before the Alumni Association of the College of Physicians and Surgeons, Medical Department of Columba College, New York, at the spring commencement, March 14, 1861. . . . Troy, N.Y.: Printed by A. W. Scribner & Co., 1861. 44p. DLC; DNLM; NNC **60-0162**

BLOOR, Alfred J[anson] (1828-1917)
Letters from the Army of the Potomac, written during the month of May, 1864, to several of the supply correspondents of the U.S. Sanitary Commission. Washington: McGill & Witherow, 1864. 67p. [No. 80. U.S. San. Com. Documents, 1861-1865] DNLM **60-0163**

BODENHAMER, William (1808-1905)
A practical treatise on the etiology, pathology, and treatment of the congenital malformation of the rectum and anus. . . . New York: S. & W. Wood, 1860. 368p. 16 plates. DLC; NNNAM **60-0164**

BODENHAMER, William (1808-1905)
Practical observations on the etiology, pathology, diagnosis, and treatment of anal fissure. . . . New York: William Wood & Co., 1868. 199p. DLC; NNNAM **60-0165**

BODLEY, Rachel L. (1831-1888)
Introductory lecture to the class of the Woman's Medical College of Pennsylvania. . . . Delivered at the opening of the nineteenth annual session, Oct. 15, 1868. . . . Philadelphia: Merrihew & Son, printers, 1868. 20p. DLC; PPC
60-0166

BOND, Thomas Emerson (1813-1872)
A practical treatise on dental medicine, being a compendium of medical science, as connected with the study of dental surgery. . . . 3rd ed., rev., cor. and enl. Philadelphia: Lindsay & Blakiston, 1863. 411p. DLC; DNLM; NNNAM; PPC
60-0167

BOSSANGE, FIRM, BOOKSELLERS, PARIS.
HECTOR BOSSANGE ET FILS (1860)
Catalogue of anatomy, comprising 1. Museum of pathological and normal anatomy of docteur Thibert, continued by docteur Léger. 2500 pieces modelled in relief and painted from nature. 2. Preparations of clastic anatomy of docteur Auzoux. 3. Models of anatomy in wax. 4. Human osteology. 5. Pieces of anatomy mounted upon natural bones. 6. Artificial human eyes, movable, in enamel. 7. Comparative anatomy. 8. Bibliography. Paris: H. Bossange & Son; New York: P. Bossange, 1860. 1495-1589p. DLC; NN; NNNAM
60-0168

BOTH, Carl
A sketch of the theory and cure of phthisis (tuberculous consumption). Boston: A. Williams & Co., 1864. 32p. DNLM
60-0169

BOTH, Carl
Questions asked in "The Boston Medical and Surgical Journal," under the heading, "Irregular and quackish advertisements," answered. Boston, 1864. 12p. DNLM **60-0170**

BOTH, Carl
A new and effective method of treating consumption (phthisis pulmonalis) through artificial calcification, with explanatory cases and drawings. Boston: E. P. Dutton & Co., 1868. 46p. 2 plates. DNLM; MBM **60-0171**

BOUCHARD, Charles J[acques] (1837-1915)
Secondary degenerations of the spinal cord. . . . Transl. from the French by Edward R. Hun. Utica, N.Y.: Roberts, Book and Job Printer, 1869. 104p. plate, fold. tab. DLC: DNLM; NN; PPC **60-0171A**

BOUCHARDAT, Apollinaire (1806-1886)
Annual abstract of therapeutics, materia medica, pharmacy and toxicology, for 1867; followed by an original memoir on gout, gravel, and urinary calculi. . . . Transl. and ed. by M. J. De Rosset. . . . Philadelphia: Lindsay & Blakiston, 1868. 314p. DLC; PPC; PU **60-0172**

BOWDITCH, Henry Ingersoll (1808-1892)
Consumption in New England: or, Locality one of its chief causes. An address delivered before the Massachusetts Medical Society. . . . Boston: Ticknor & Fields, 1862. 104p. maps. DLC; MBM **60-0173**

BOWDITCH, Henry Ingersoll (1808-1892)
An apology for the medical profession, as a means of developing the whole nature of man. A valedictory address . . . Harvard University, March 11, 1863. With additional remarks on a topic of importance at the present hour. Boston: Ticknor & Fields, 1863. 52p. DNLM; MBM **60-0174**

BOWDITCH, Henry Ingersoll (1808-1892)
A brief plea for an ambulance system for the army of the United States, as drawn from the extra sufferings of the late Lieut. Bowditch and a wounded comrade. . . . Boston: Ticknor & Fields, 1863. 28p. DLC; MBM **60-0175**

BOWDITCH, Henry Ingersoll (1808-1892)
Paracentesis thoracis: a résumé of twelve years' experience. [1863.] 5p. DNLM; MBM **60-0176**

BOWDITCH, Henry Ingersoll (1808-1892)
Sketch of the life and character of Nathaniel Bowditch. Boston: J. E. Farwell & Co., 1863. 17p. DNLM; MBM **60-0177**

BOWDITCH, Henry Ingersoll (1808-1892)
Is consumption ever contagious, or communicated by one person to another in any manner? A paper prepared for the Boston Society for Medical Observation. . . . Boston: Printed by D. Clapp, 1864. 14p. DLC; DNLM; MBM **60-0178**

BOWDITCH, Henry Ingersoll (1808-1892)
Case of thoracic aneurism; autopsy. Remarks on the treatment of internal aneurism. Boston, 1866. 12p. DNLM; MBM **60-0179**

BOWDITCH, Henry Ingersoll (1808-1892)
Hippophagy. New York: D. Appleton & Co., [1868]. 29p. DNLM; NNNAM **60-0180**

BOWDITCH, Henry Ingersoll (1808-1892)
Consumption in New England and elsewhere; or soil-moisture one of its chief causes. Boston: David Clapp & Sons, 1868. 17p. DNLM; MBM **60-0181**

BOWDITCH, Henry Ingersoll (1808-1892)
Report of the committee on climatology and epidemics in Massachusetts, 1868-1869. Philadelphia: Collins, 1869. 14p. DNLM; MBM; PPC **60-0182**

BOWKER, H. L.
Dyphtheria, its cause and cure. Boston: J. J. Dyer & Co., 1864. 24p. DNLM; MBM **60-0183**

BOWLING, William K. (1808-1885)
Eulogy on the life and character of the late John M. Watson, in an introductory lecture. Nashville: W. H. F. Ligon, 1866. 19p. DNLM **60-0184**

BOWLING, William K. (1808-1885)
Cholera, as it appeared in Nashville in 1849, 1850, 1854, and 1866. Nashville, Tenn.: W. H. F. Ligon, 1866. 27p. DNLM **60-0185**

BOWLING, William K. (1808-1885)
Historical address to the graduating class of 1868, in the medical department of the University of Nashville. 2nd ed. Nashville: W. H. F. Ligon, 1868. 31p. DNLM **60-0186**

BOWLING, William K. (1808-1885)
Mercury and cinchona shown to be therapeutically allied. Nashville: W. H. F. Ligon, 1868. 23p. DNLM **60-0187**

BOWLING, William K. (1808-1885)
Lying facts; or a revelation of a new use for the organs of locomotion. Nashville: W. H. F. Ligon, 1868. 15p. DNLM **60-0188**

BOWLING, William K. (1808-1885)
Incidents of travel to the American Medical Association, at New Orleans, May, 1869. Nashville: W. H. F. Ligon, 1869. 20p. DNLM **60-0189**

BOWMAN, John E[ddowes] (1819-1854)
A practical handbook of medical chemistry. Edited by Charles L. Bloxam. 4th American from the 4th and revised London ed. Philadelphia: Henry C. Lea, 1866. 351p. DNLM; NNNAM; PPC; PU **60-0190**

BOZEMAN, Nathan (1825-1905)
Urethro-vaginal, vesico-vaginal, and recto-vaginal fistules: general remarks; report of cases treated with the button suture in this country, and in London, Edinburgh, Glasgow, and Parisian hospitals. New Orleans, 1860. 56p. DNLM; LNT-M **60-0191**

BOZEMAN, Nathan (1825-1905)
Application of the button suture to the treatment of varicose dilation of veins. New Orleans: Bulletin Office, 1860. 8p. DNLM; LNT-M **60-0192**

BOZEMAN, Nathan (1825-1905)
Operation of vesico-vaginal fistule without the aid of assistants; with a view of the relativve merits of the clamp, interrupted silver, and button sutures. . . . New York: D. Appleton & Company, 1869. 26p. DLC; NNNAM **60-0193**

BRADFORD, George W. (1796-1883)
Memoir of Hon. John Miller, M.D., late of Truxton, Cortland County, N.Y. . . . Albany: Steam Press of C. Van Benthuysen, 1862. 14p. DLC **60-0194**

BRADFORD, J. Taylor (1818-1871)
Complete rupture of the perineum, of ten years' standing, successfully operated on. Cincinnati: A. Abraham, 1869. 8p. DNLM **60-0195**

BRADLEY, W. Lockwood (1837-1903)
Alcohol as a dressing for wounds. New Haven: Tuttle & Co., 1866. 7p. CtY-M; DNLM **60-0196**

BRAINARD, Daniel (1812-1866)
Address on "Dental specialties," before the American Dental Association, Chicago, July 27, 1865. [1865] 14p. DNLM
60-0197

BRANDE, William Thomas (1788-1866) and Alfred Swaine TAYLOR
Chemistry. Philadelphia: Blanchard & Lea, 1863. 696p. DNLM; PPC; PPJ; PU **60-0198**

BRANDE, William Thomas (1788-1866) and Alfred Swaine TAYLOR
Chemistry. 2nd American ed. Philadelphia: Henry C. Lea, 1867. 764p. DNLM; NN; PPC; PU **60-0199**

BRANDRETH, Benjamin (1807-1880)
The guide to prevent premature death. . . . Bleeding always improper! . . . Part I. . . . New York: Excelsior Medical College [1861]. 12p. DLC; NNNAM **60-0200**

BRANDRETH, Benjamin (1807-1880)
The doctrine of purgation. Curiosities from ancient and modern literature. A collection of quotations on the use of purgatives, from Hippocrates, and other medical writers . . . proving purgation is the corner-stone of all curatives. . . . New York: Baker & Godwin, printers, 1867. 224p. DLC; NNNAM
60-0201

BRANSTON, Thomas F.
The pharmaceutist's and druggist's practical receipt book, with a glossary of medical terms. Philadelphia: Lindsay & Blakiston, 1865. 307p. DNLM; MBM; NNNAM; PPC
60-0202

BREYFOGLE, William L. (*b.* 1845)
Epitome of homoeopathic medicines. Philadelphia: F. E. Boericke, 1869. 383p. PPHa **60-0203**

BRICKELL, Daniel Warren (1824-1881)
Biographical sketch of Erasmus D. Fenner, M.D. New Orleans: Bouvain & Lewis, 1866. 23p. DNLM **60-0204**

A BRIEF description of James A. Foster's patent union artificial limbs. Philadelphia, Cincinnati, Detroit & Rochester, [1864]. 42p. DNLM **60-0205**

BRIGHAM, Charles B[rooks] (1845-1903)
Diabetes mellitus. [Boylston prize essay for 1868.] Boston: A. A. Kingman, 1868. 55p. DNLM; MBM **60-0206**

BRIGHAM HALL. CANANDAIGUA, N.Y.
Announcement of Brigham Hall, a hospital for the insane, Canandaigua, N.Y., Jan., 1860. [Being a history and description of the institution.] Canandaigua: N. J. Milliken, 1860. 16p. DNLM [Commenced in 1855, for the purpose of establishing a hospital of the independent class for the insane of both sexes. Opened Oct. 3, 1855, and named "Brigham Hall," in honor of Dr. Amariah Brigham. Incorporated April 10, 1859.] **60-0207**

BRIGHAM HALL. CANANDAIGUA, N.Y.
[Circular of the managers to the public stating the necessity and merits of the institution, Oct., 1860.] Canandaigua, 1860. 8p. DNLM **60-0208**

BRIGHT, W. C.
Valedictory address to the graduating class of 1868, in the medical department of the University of Nashville. Nashville: W. H. F. Ligon, 1868. 11p. DNLM **60-0209**

BRINSMADE, Thomas C. (1802-1868)
Record of private practice for the year 1858-1859, and mortuary record of the city of Troy (N.Y.) for the years 1858 and 1859. Albany: C. Van Benthuysen, 1860. 43p. DNLM
60-0210

BRINTON, John Hill (1832-1907)
Consolidated statement of gun-shot wounds. [Washington, 1863.] 11p. DNLM **60-0211**

BRINTON, William (1823-1867)
Lectures on the diseases of the stomach, with an introduction on its anatomy and physiology. From the 2nd English ed. Philadelphia: Lea & Blanchard, 1865. 302p. DNLM; MBM; NNNAM; PPC **60-0212**

BRITTAN, S. B.
Man and his relations: illustrating the influence of the mind on the body; the relations of the faculties to the organs, and to the elements, objects, and phenomena of the external world. New York: C. W. Bean, 1865. 578p. DNLM; NNNAM
60-0213

BROADBENT, Charles R.
A medical treatise on the causes and curability of consumption, laryngeal chronic catarrh, and diseases of the air-passages. . . . Boston: Damrell & Welch, 1862. 227p. DNLM; MBM
60-0214

BROCKWAY, J.
An introductory lecture delivered before the Third District Dental Association of the State of New York, Jan. 12, 1869. [Synopsis of dentistry as it was, as it is, and as it ought to be.] Albany, N.Y.: J. Munsell, 1869. 23p. DNLM
60-0215

BRONSON, Henry (1804-1893)
The annual address to the candidates for the degree in medicine, in the Medical Institution of Yale College, Jan. 15, 1863. New Haven: W. H. Stanley, 1863. 19p. CtY-M; DNLM
60-0216

BRONSON, Henry (1804-1893)
Biographical notice of Prof. Eli Ives, M.D. New Haven: Tuttle, Morehouse & Taylor, 1867. 12p. CtY-M; DNLM
60-0217

BROOKS. Silas Swift (1817-1871)
Valedictory address delivered to the graduating class of the Homoeopathic Medical College of Pennsylvania, at the fifteenth annual commencement, March 3, 1863. Philadelphia: Bryson, 1863. 20p. PPHa **60-0218**

BROWN, Buckminster (1819-1891)
Femoral aneurism treated by immediate compression. [1866.] 4p. DNLM; MBM **60-0219**

BROWN, Buckminster (1819-1891)
Cases of orthopedic surgery. Boston: D. Clapp & Son, 1868. 23p. 8 plates. DNLM; MBM **60-0220**

BROWN, D. Tilden (1822-1889)
An address delivered before the Alumni Association of the College of Physicians and Surgeons, medical department of Columbia College, New York, at the spring commencement. New York: J. A. Gray, 1862. 43p. DNLM; NNNAM
60-0221

BROWN, Francis H. (1835-1917)
Hospital construction. Boston: D. Clapp, 1861. 13p. DNLM; MBM **60-0222**

BROWN, Francis H. (1835-1917)
The medical register for the cities of Boston, Cambridge, Charlestown, and Chelsea. For the years 1866, 1873, 1875. Boston, 1866-75. 3 v. DNLM; MBM; MH; MWA **60-0223**

BROWN, John
Health: Five lay sermons to working people. New York: R. Carter & Bros., 1862. 90p. DNLM; NNNAM **60-0224**

BROWN, O. Phelps
The complete herbalist, or the people their own physicians by the use of nature's remedies; showing the great curative properties of all herbs, gums, balsams, barks, flowers, and roots; how they should be prepared; when and under what influences selected; at what times gathered, and for what diseases administered, [etc.]. Jersey City, 1867. 407p. 12 plates. DNLM; NjR **60-0225**

BROWNE, Gardner S[hepard] (1810-1879)
Annual inaugural address delivered at the semi-annual meeting of the Connecticut Homoeopathic Medical Society, at Bridgeport, November 28, 1865. Hartford: Coburn & Clark, 1865. 42p. PPHa **60-0226**

BROWN-SEQUARD, Charles Edouard (1817-1894)
Course of lectures on the physiology and pathology of the central nervous system. Delivered at the Royal College of Surgeons of England, in May, 1858. Philadelphia: Collins, 1860. 276p. DLC; DNLM; PPC; PU **60-0227**

BROWN-SEQUARD, Charles Edouard (1817-1894)
Lectures on the diagnosis and treatment of the principal forms of paralysis of the lower extremities. . . . Philadelphia: J. B. Lippincott & Co., 1861. 118p. DLC; PPC; PU **60-0228**

BROWN-SEQUARD, Charles Edouard (1817-1894)
Advice to students: an address delivered at the opening of the medical lectures of Harvard University, Nov. 7, 1866. Cambridge: J. Wilson & Son, 1867. 33p. DLC; DNLM; MBM; MH **60-0229**

BROWN-SEQUARD, Charles Edouard (1817-1894)
Lectures on the diagnosis and treatment of functional nervous affections. Philadelphia: J. B. Lippincott & Co., 1868. 89p. DLC; DNLM; NNNAM; PPC **60-0230**

BUCHANAN, John
The treatment of the venereal disease. Philadelphia: W. B. Selheimer, 1865. 139p. DNLM; PPC; PPJ; PU **60-0231**

BUCHANAN, John
A practical treatise on the diseases of children, adapted to the use of families and physicians. Philadelphia:J. Buchanan, 1866. 104p. DNLM; PPC; PU **60-0232**

BUCHANAN, John
The eclectic practice of medicine and surgery. Designed as a text-book for the student, and as a guide for the physician and surgeon; containing the latest improvements in medicine and surgery. 3rd ed. Philadelphia: J. Buchanan, 1867. 860p. DNLM; NNNAM; PPC; PU **60-0233**

BUCHANAN, John
The American practice of medicine. Philadelphia: J. Buchanan, 1868. 400p. DNLM; PPC; PU **60-0234**

BUCK, Gurdon (1807-1877)
History of a case of partial reconstruction of the face. Albany: Van Benthuysen, 1864. 16p. 7 plates. DNLM **60-0235**

BUCK, Gurdon (1807-1877)
Case of destruction of the body of the lower jaw, and extensive disfiguration of the face from a shell wound. Reparative autoplastic operation. Albany: Van Benthuysen, 1866. 5p. DNLM **60-0236**

BUCK, Gurdon (1807-1877)
Description of an improved extension apparatus for the treatment of fracture of the thigh, in use in the New York Hospital for the past six years, and in the United States Army general hospitals during the civil war. New York: William Wood & Co., 1867. 10p. 2 plates. DNLM; NNNAM **60-0237**

BUCK, Gurdon (1807-1877)
A new method of reconstructing the lower lip after its removal for disease; illustrated by two cases of epithelioma. Philadelphia: Collins, 1868. 10p. 6 plates. DNLM; PPC **60-0238**

BUCKINGHAM, Charles E. (1821-1877)
Introductory lecture to the students of the medical school of Harvard University. Nov. 4th, 1868. Boston: A. A. Kingman, 1868. 24p. DNLM; MBM; MH **60-0239**

BULKLEY, Henry D. (1804-1872)
Address delivered before the New York County Medical Society, January 29, 1861. New York: H. S. Taylor, 1861. 15p. DNLM; NNNAM **60-0240**

BULL, Thomas
Hints to mothers, for the management of health during the period of pregnancy, and in the lying-in room; with an exposure of popular errors in connexion with those subjects. From the 3rd London ed., with additions by an American physician. To which is added the ladies' perpetual calendar. New York: J. Wiley & Son, 1868. 268p. DNLM; MBM; NNNAM; PPC **60-0241**

BULLARD, Ebenezer Waters (1809-1896)
The good physician. A sermon preached in Royalston, Mass., at the funeral of Isaac P. Willis, M.D., June 30th, 1863. . . . Winchendon [Mass.]: F. W. Ward, printer, 1863. 10p. DLC **60-0242**

BULLITT, Henry M[assie] (*d.* 1880)
Lecture introductory to the course of the Kentucky School of Medicine, delivered October 3, 1865. Louisville: Bradley & Gilbert, 1865. 20p. DNLM; KyLoJM **60-0243**

BULLITT, Henry M[assie] (*d.* 1880)
Introductory lecture delivered at the opening of the session of the medical department of the University of Louisville, October 14, 1867. Louisville, Ky.: C. Y. Duncan, 1867. 31p. DNLM; KyLoJM **60-0244**

BULLOCK & CRENSHAW. PHILADELPHIA
Catalogue of drugs, pharmaceutical preparations, utensils, apparatus, surgical instruments, anatomical preparations, etc. Philadelphia, 1860. 111p. DNLM; PPC; PU **60-0245**

BUMSTEAD, Freeman Josiah (1826-1879)
The pathology and treatment of venereal diseases: including the results of recent investigations upon the subject.... Philadelphia: Blanchard & Lea, 1861. 686p. DLC; DNLM; PPC; PU **60-0246**

[BUMSTEAD, Freeman Josiah] (1826-1879)
... Report of a committee of the associate medical members of the Sanitary Commission on the subject of venereal diseases, with special reference to practice in the army and navy. New York: J. F. Trow, printer, 1862. 17p. [U.S. Sanitary Commission, Medical and Surgical Monographs, H]. DLC; NNNAM **60-0247**

[BUMSTEAD, Freeman Josiah] (1826-1879)
... Report of a committee of the associate medical members of the Sanitary Commission, on the subject of venereal diseases, with special reference to practice in the army and navy. Washington: McGill, Witherow & Co., printers, 1862. 19p. [U.S. Sanitary Commission, Medical and Surgical Monographs, H]. DLC; DNLM **60-0248**

BUMSTEAD, Freeman Josiah (1826-1879)
The pathology and treatment of the venereal diseases. A new and revised ed. Philadelphia: Blanchard & Lea, 1864. 640p. CU-M; DNLM; IU-M; PPC **60-0249**

BURKE, William
Red Sulphur Springs, Monroe County, Virginia. Wytheville: D. A. St. Clair, 1860. 24p. DNLM **60-0250**

BURRALL, Frederick Augustus
Asiatic cholera. . . . New York: William Wood & Co., 1866. 155p. NNNAM **60-0251**

BURROWES, George (1811-1894)
A discourse delivered at the funeral of James Couper, M.D., at New Castle, Del. Philadelphia: Collins, 1865. 20p. DNLM; PPC **60-0252**

BURT, William H. (1836-1897)
Monograph upon polyporus officinalis and polyporus pinicola, their physiologico-pathological effects, together with their uses in diseases. Detroit: Lodge's Homoeopathic Pharmacy, 1867. 55p. DNLM; PPHa **60-0253**

BURT, William H. (1836-1897)
Monograph on ustilago maidis, its physiologico-pathological effects, together with its uses in disease. Detroit: Lodge's Homoeopathic Pharmacy, 1868. 35p. DNLM; PPHa **60-0254**

BURT, William H. (1836-1897)
Characteristic materia medica. . . . Philadelphia: A. J. Tafel, 1869. 460p. DLC; OCLloyd; PPC; PPHa **60-0255**

BUTLER, David P.
Butler's system of improved gymnastics. Strength and health culture for men, women, and children, as taught and applied by D. P. Butler. . . . Boston: Wright & Potter, 1865. 15p. DLC **60-0256**

BUTLER, David P.
Butler's system of health-exercise. The lifting cure: a scientific application of the laws of motion or mechanical action to physical culture and the cure of disease. . . . Boston: D. P. Butler; New York: J. W. Leavitt [etc.], 1868. 23p. DLC; DNLM **60-0257**

[BUTLER, David P.]
Butler's system of physical training. The lifting cure: an original, scientific application of the laws of motion or mechanical action to physical culture and the cure of disease. With a discussion of true and false methods of physical training. . . . Boston: D. P. Butler, 1868. 104p. DLC; DNLM **60-0258**

BYFORD, William Heath (1817-1890)
A treatise on the chronic inflammation and displacements of the unimpregnated uterus. . . . Philadelphia: Lindsay & Blakiston, 1864. 215p. DLC; DNLM; PPC; PU **60-0259**

BYFORD, William Heath (1817-1890)
The practice of medicine and surgery applied to the diseases and accidents incident to women. . . . Philadelphia: Lindsay & Blakiston, 1865. 566p. DLC; DNLM; PPC; PU **60-0260**

BYFORD, William Health (1817-1890)
The practice of medicine and surgery applied to diseases and accidents incident to women. . . . 2nd ed., enl. Philadelphia: Lindsay & Blakiston, 1867. 616p. DLC; NNNAM; PPC; PU **60-0261**

BYFORD, William H[eath] (1817-1890)
An intra-mural fibrous tumor removed from the anterior wall of the uterus. [Chicago, 1869.] 8p. DNLM **60-0262**

BYRN, Marcus Lafayette
The physiology of marriage and philosophy of generation, being a confidential and reliable friend for medical and scientific consultation, on subjects of vital importance. . . . New York: M. L. Byrn, 1863. 144p. DLC; NNNAM **60-0263**

BYRN, Marcus Lafayette
The art of beautifying the hair, with rules for promoting its growth . . . and preservation. . . . New York: M. L. Byrn, 1866. 97p. DLC; NNNAM **60-0264**

BYRN, M[arcus] Lafayette
The family physician, and household companion; being a treatise, in plain language, on the art of preserving health and prolonging life. . . . New York: M. L. Byrn, 1867. 377p. DLC; NNNAM **60-0265**

BYRN, Marcus Lafayette
The guide to health; or How to live a hundred years. . . . New York: M. L. Byrn, 1867. 41p. DLC; NNNAM **60-0266**

BYRN, Marcus Lafayette
The mystery of medicine explained; a family physician and household companion; prepared for the use of families, plantations, ships, travelers, etc. New York: M. L. Byrn, 1869. 12p. DNLM; NNNAM **60-0267**

BYRNE, John (1825-1902)
Researches and observations on pelvic haematocele. New York: William Wood & Co., 1862. 44p. DNLM; NNNAM **60-0268**

BYRNE, John (1825-1902)
Contributions to gynaecology. No. 3. A case of retroversion of the uterus, of eighteen years' standing, successfully treated by elytrorrhaphia. With clinical remarks. To which is added a supplemental history of the same case. New York: W. A. Townsend & Adams, 1869. 22p. DNLM; NNNAM
60-0269

CADWELL, Frederick A.
Treatise on the eye and ear: rules for the preservation and restoration of sight. 6th ed. Chicago, 1861. 279p. 1 plate. DNLM; ICRM; IU-M; NNNAM **60-0270**

CADWELL, Frederick A.
Treatise on the eye and ear; rules for the preservation and restoration of sight; deafness, its causes and progress explained; new discoveries in treatment, illustrated with numerous cases and engravings. 7th ed. New York: [Holt Bros.], 1869. 276p. DNLM; ICRM; NNNAM **60-0271**

CALKINS, Marshall (1828-1922)
Diseases of the lungs, heart and blood, scrofula, consumption, bronchitis; their causes, prevention, and cure, with the posthumous writings of Calvin Newton. Philadelphia: H. Cowperthwait & Co., 1860. 546p. DNLM; PPC; PC
60-0272

CALKINS, Marshall (1828-1922)
Essays on the preventable diseases of summer and autumn. No. 1. Epidemic cholera. Its causes, phenomena, and mode of propagation; together with the means of prevention and proper treatment. . . . Springfield, Mass.: Bickford & Bullock, 1866. 30p. DLC; DNLM **60-0273**

CAMPBELL, Henry Fraser (1824-1891)
Caffeine as an antidote in the poisonous narcotism of opium. Augusta, Ga.: Chronicle & Sentinel, 1860. 12p. DNLM; GU
60-0274

CAMPBELL, J. B.
The electro-hydric practice, combining all the virtues of electricity and water, electric herbs, and magnetic remedies. . . . Cincinnati, O.: Printed at the Central Printing Office, 1861. 240p. DLC; OCIM **60-0275**

CAMPLIN, John M[ussendine]
On diabetes and its successful treatment. From the 2nd London ed. New York: S. S. & W. Wood, 1861. 87p. DNLM; NNNAM **60-0276**

CANNIFF, William (1830-1910)
A manual of the principles of surgery, based on pathology. . . . Philadelphia: Lindsay & Blakiston, 1866. 402p. CU-M; DLC; DNLM; IEN-M **60-0277**

CARLETON, Charles M. (1836-1886)
The use and abuse of spectacles. New Haven: Tuttle, Morehouse & Taylor, 1869. 29p. CtY-M; DNLM; MBM
60-0278

CARPENTER, William Benjamin (1813-1885)
. . . On the use and abuse of alcoholic liquors, in health and disease. . . . With a preface by D. F. Condie. . . . Philadelphia: Blanchard & Lea, 1860. 178p. DLC; PPC; PU
60-0279

CARROLL, Alfred Ludlow (1833-1893)
Hygiene, in its relations to therapeusis. A paper read before the N.Y. Medical Journal Association, June 25th, 1869. . . . New York: Turner & Mignard, 1869. 37p. DLC; DNLM; NNNAM
60-0280

CARSON, Joseph (1808-1876)
Medical commencement of the University of Pennsylvania . . . valedictory address. Philadelphia: Collins, 1860. 28p. DNLM; PPC; PU **60-0281**

CARSON, Joseph (1808-1876)
Introductory lecture on the opening of the session of 1860-1861 in the Medical Department of the University of Pennsylvania, delivered October 8, 1860. . . . Published by the class. Philadelphia: Wallace, Printer, 1860. 28p. DLC; PPC; PU
60-0282

CARSON, Joseph (1808-1876)
Address before the Philadelphia County Medical Society. Delivered January 30, 1862 . . . at the close of his official term as president. . . . Philadelphia: Collins, Printer, 1862. 15p. DLC; DNLM; PPC; PU **60-0283**

CARSON, Joseph (1808-1876)
Synopsis of the course of lectures on materia medica and pharmacy, delivered in the University of Pennsylvania: with three lectures on the modus operandi of medicines. . . . 3rd ed., rev. Philadelphia: Blanchard & Lea, 1863. 244p. DLC; PPC; PU
60-0284

CARSON, Joseph (1808-1876)
A history of the Medical Department of the University of Pennsylvania, from its foundation in 1765. With sketches of the lives of deceased professors. . . . Philadelphia: Lindsay & Blakiston, 1869. 227p. DLC; DNLM; PPC; PU
60-0285

CARTER, Charles L.
A treatise on general pathology and its relation to practical medicine. . . . St. Louis: G. Knapp & Co., 1867. 149p. DLC; OCIM; PPC **60-0286**

CATE, Shadrach M.
Correct observation in medicine. An address delivered before the Massachusetts Homoeopathic Medical Society, at the annual meeting in Boston, April, 1864. . . . Boston: J. Wilson & Son, 1866. 26p. DNLM; PPHa; MBM
60-0287

CATE, Shadrach M.
Some suggestions on hydro-thorax. A report to the American Institute of Homoeopathy. Boston: A. Mudge & Son, 1869. 32p. PPHa; MMB **60-0288**

CATLIN, George (1796-1872)
The breath of life; or mal-respiration, and its effects upon the enjoyments and life of man. New York: J. Wiley, 1861. 76p. DNLM; NNNAM **60-0289**

CAZEAUX, Pierre (1808-1862)
A theoretical and practical treatise on midwifery, including the diseases of pregnancy and parturition, and the attentions required by the child from birth to the period of weaning. 2nd American, transl. from the 5th French ed. by William R. Bullock. Philadelphia: Lindsay & Blakiston, 1863. 992p. 4 plates. DNLM; NNNAM; PPC; PU **60-0290**

CAZEAUX, Pierre (1808-1862)
A theoretical and practical treatise on midwifery, including the diseases of pregnancy and parturition, and the attentions required by the child from birth to the period of weaning. . . . 3rd American, transl. from the 6th French ed. by Wm. R. Bullock, M.D. with one hundred and forty illustrations. Philadelphia: Lindsay & Blakiston, 1864. 971p. 4 plates. DLC; NNNAM; PPC; PU **60-0291**

CAZEAUX, Pierre (1808-1862)
A theoretical and practical treatise on midwifery. . . . 4th American from the 6th French ed. by Wm. R. Bullock. Philadelphia: Lindsay & Blakiston, 1866. 987p. 4 plates. DNLM; PPC; PU **60-0292**

CAZEAUX, Pierre (1808-1862)
A theoretical and practical treatise on midwifery, including the diseases of pregnancy and parturition. . . . Rev. and annotated by S. Tarnier. . . . 5th American from the 7th French ed. By Wm. R. Bullock. . . . Philadelphia: Lindsay & Blakiston, 1868. 1124p. 5 plates. DLC; NNNAM; PPC **60-0293**

CHAILLÉ, Stanford Emerson (1830-1911)
Life and death in New Orleans from 1787 to 1869, and more especially during the five years 1856 to 1860. New Orleans, 1869. 66p. DNLM; LNT-M **60-0294**

CHAMBERLAIN, William Baker (1827-1889)
The origin of homoeopathy and reasons for preferring it to the common system of medical treatment; with the by-laws of the Worcester County Homoeopathic Medical Society. Worcester, Mass.: Worcester Homoeopathic Pharmacy, 1868. 12p. PPHa **60-0295**

CHAMBERS, Thomas King (1818-1889)
The renewal of life. Lectures: chiefly clinical. . . . From the 3rd London ed. Philadelphia: Lindsay & Blakiston, 1865. 638p. DLC; NNNAM; PPC **60-0296**

CHAMBERS, Thomas King (1818-1889)
The renewal of life: clinical lectures illustrative of the restorative system of medicine given at Saint Mary's Hospital. 2nd American from the 4th London ed. Philadelphia: Lindsay & Blakiston, 1866. 646p. DNLM; PPC; PU **60-0297**

CHAMBERS, Thomas King (1818-1889)
The indigestions; or, diseases of the digestive organs functionally treated. 2nd ed., from the 2nd and revised London ed. Philadelphia: Henry C. Lea, 1868. 319p. DNLM; NNNAM; PPC; PU **60-0298**

CHANDLER, Thomas Henderson (*d.* 1895)
Address before the Massachusetts Dental Society, at its fourth annual meeting, May 21, 1868. . . . Boston: W. H. Chandler, printer, 1868. 16p. DLC; MBM **60-0299**

CHANNING, Walter (1786-1876)
Review of Elwell's medico-legal treatise on malpractice and medical evidence. [1860?]. 26p. DNLM; MBM **60-0300**

CHANNING, Walter (1786-1876)
Bed case: its history and treatment. Boston: Ticknor & Fields, 1860. 52p. DNLM; MBM **60-0301**

CHAPIN, John Bassett (1829-1918)
Tubercle of the brain. Utica, N.Y., 1862. 13p. DNLM **60-0302**

CHAPIN, John Bassett (1829-1918)
Report on provision for the chronic insane. . . . Canandaigua [N.Y.]: Printed at the Times Office, 1868. 17p. DLC **60-0303**

CHAPMAN, Edwin Nesbit (1819-1888)
A selection of remarkable cases occurring in a practice of eighteen years. Philadelphia: King & Baird, 1863. 17p. DNLM; PPC **60-0304**

CHAPMAN, Edwin Nesbit (1819-1888)
Essay on the pyrophosphate of iron, with notices of its combinations and forms of preparations, etc., by Caswell, Mack & Co. New York: J. A. Gray & Green, 1865. 12p. DNLM; NNNAM **60-0305**

CHAPMAN, Edwin Nesbit (1819-1888)
Essay on the pyrophosphate of iron, with notices of its combinations, and forms of preparations, &c., &c. By Caswell, Mack & Co., family and dispensing chemists. New York: Gray & Green, 1866. 12p. DNLM; NNNAM **60-0306**

CHAPMAN, John (1822-1894)
Diarrhoea and cholera: their origin, proximate cause, and cure, through the agency of the nervous system, by means of ice. Philadelphia: J. B. Lippincott & Co., 1866. 57p. DLC; DNLM; PPC **60-0307**

CHASE, Alvin Wood (1817-1885)
Dr. Chase's recipes: or, Information for every body; an invaluable collection of about six hundred practical recipes. . . . 8th ed., rev., illustraated and enl. . . . Ann Arbor, Mich.: The author, 1860. 224p. DLC; OCIM **60-0308**

CHASE, Alvin Wood (1817-1885)
Dr. Chase's recipes; or, Information for every body; an invaluable collection of about eight hundred practical recipes. . . . 10th (stereotype) ed., carefully rev., illustrated and much enl., with remarks and full explanations. Ann Arbor, Mich.: Chase & Stelle, 1863. 384p. DNLM **60-0309**

CHAVASSE, Pye Henry (1810-1879)
Advice to a mother on the management of her offspring. . . . Reprinted from the 6th London ed. New York: Bailliere Brothers, 1862. [With this are bound The young mother, or Management of children in regard to health. By W. A. Alcott. 2nd ed. Boston, 1836; and Medical guide for mothers, in pregnancy, accouchement, suckling, weaning, etc. and in most of the important diseases of children. By J. R. Hancorn. From the 2nd London ed. New York, 1844.] 172p. DLC; NNNAM **60-0310**

CHAVASSE, Pye Henry (1810-1879)
Advice to a mother on the management of her children, and on the treatment on the moment of some of their more pressing illnesses and accidents. . . . 9th ed. Philadelphia: J. B. Lippincott & Co.; [etc., etc.], 1869. 408p. DLC; DNLM; PPC; PU **60-0311**

CHEEVER, David Williams (1831-1915)
The value and the fallacy of statistics in the observation of disease. Boston: D. Clapp, 1861. 36p. DNLM; MBM **60-0312**

CHEEVER, David Williams (1831-1915)
Lectures on hernia. [1866.] 27p. DNLM; MBM **60-0313**

CHEEVER, David Williams (1831-1915)
Two cases of oesophagotomy for the removal of foreign bodies; with a history of the operation. Boston: D. Clapp & Son, 1867. 42p. DNLM; MH-M **60-0314**

CHEEVER, David Williams (1831-1915)
Surgical cases in 1867. . . . [Boston? 1867?] 37p. DLC; MH-M **60-0315**

CHEEVER, David W[illiams] (1831-1915)
Surgical cases. . . . Boston: Printed for the author, D. Clapp & Son, 1869. 33p. DLC; MH-M **60-0316**

CHEW, Samuel (1806-1863)
Valedictory discourse, delivered at the annual commencement of the school of medicine, in the University of Maryland, March 1, 1862. Baltimore: Published by the class, 1862. 22p. DNLM; MdU-D **60-0317**

CHEW, Samuel (1806-1863)
Lectures on medical education, or on the proper method of studying medicine. Philadelphia: Lindsay & Blakiston, 1864. 152p. DNLM; PPC **60-0318**

CHEW, Samuel Claggett (1837-1915)
Valedictory address to the graduates of the University of Maryland, school of medicine. Baltimore: Kelly & Piel, 1866. 15p. DNLM; MdU-D **60-0319**

CHILD, Linus
Synopsis of facts and argument, presented to the joint standing committee on education, in behalf of the remonstrants against the petition of I. J. Wetherbee and others, for an act to incorporate "The Boston Dental College," May 5, 1868. Boston: Wright & Potter, 1868. 16p. DNLM; MBM **60-0320**

CHILDS, Timothy (1748-1821)
Rational medicine: its past and present. . . . New York: Baker & Godwin, 1863. 31p. DNLM; NNNAM **60-0321**

CHISOLM, Julian John (1830-1903)
A manual of military surgery, for the use of surgeons in the Confederate army, with an appendix of the rules and regulations of the medical department of the Confederate army. . . . Richmond, Va.: West & Johnston, 1861. 447p. forms. DLC; DNLM; PPC; ViRA **60-0322**

CHISOLM, Julian John (1830-1903)
A manual of military surgery, for the use of surgeons in the Confederate States army; with an appendix of the rules and regulations of the medical department of the Confederate States army. . . . 2nd ed.—rev. and improved. Richmond, Va.: West & Johnson, 1862. 514p. forms. DLC; DNLM; PPC; ViRA **60-0323**

CHISOLM, Julian John (1830-1903)
A manual of military surgery, for the use of surgeons in the Confederate State army; with explanatory plates of all useful operations. . . . 3rd ed.—carefully rev. and improved. Columbia: Evans & Cogswell, 1864. 592p. 26 plates. DLC; NNNAM; ViRA **60-0324**

CHISOLM, Julian John (1830-1903)
Introductory lecture to the course of military surgery delivered in the University of Maryland, October 20, 1868. Baltimore: Published by the class, 1868. 16p. DNLM; MdU-D **60-0325**

[CHOLERA]
The origin, history, cause, prevention, and cure of cholera, with an account of its progress and ravages through the world, and the latest and most successful treatment, endorsed and approved by the medical faculty. By a New York physician. New York: G. Munro & Co., [1865]. 86p. DNLM; NNNAM **60-0326**

CHOPPIN, Samuel Paul (1828-1880)
Removal of the uterus and its appendages in a case of procidentia uteri, by means of the ecraseur. . . . New Orleans: Bouvain & Lewis, book and job printers, 1867. 4p. DLC; LNT-M **60-0327**

CHURCH, William Henry (1826-1866)
Resection at the hip-joint for morbus coxarius. Enchondroma, or cartilaginous tumors. New York: Hilton, Gallaher & Co., 1860. 38p. DNLM; NNNAM **60-0328**

CHURCHILL, Fleetwood (1808-1878)
On the theory and practice of midwifery. . . . With additions by D. Francis Condie. . . . A new American from the 4th cor. and enl. English ed. Philadelphia: Blanchard & Lea, 1860. 655p. DLC; MBM; NNNAM; PPC **60-0329**

CHURCHILL, John Francis
Treatise on the immediate cause, and the specific treatment of pulmonary phthisis, and tubercular diseases. . . . Transl. from the French by a physician. 2nd ed., with appendix. New York: J. Winchester, 1860. 144p. DLC; DNLM; NNNAM; PPC **60-0330**

CHURCHILL, John Francis
Treatise on the immediate cause, and the specific treatment of pulmonary phthisis, and tubercular diseases. . . . Transl. from the French by a physician. 3rd American ed., with appendix. New York: J. Winchester, 1861. 147p. DLC; NNNAM **60-0331**

CHURCHILL, John Francis
Treatise on the immediate cause, and the specific treatment of pulmonary phthisis, and tubercular diseases. . . . Transl. from the French by a physician. 4th American ed. With an Appendix. New York: J. Winchester, 1861. 150p. DNLM; NNNAM **60-0332**

CLARK, Daniel (1835-1912)
Practical principles of medical electricity, with an appendix, exemplifying the principles by particular instructions for the treatment of sundry diseases. . . . Joliet, Ill.: C. F. Gritzner, 1866. 71p. DLC; OCIM **60-0333**

CLARK, Daniel (1835-1912)
A newly discovered system of electrical medication. . . . Chicago: Rounds & James, book and job printers, 1869. 141p. DLC; DNLM **60-0334**

CLARK, E. A. (1836?-1871)
Interdental splint for treating fractures of the inferior maxilla. St. Louis: Levison & Blythe, [1869]. 7p. 1 figure. DNLM **60-0335**

CLARK, Henry Grafton (1804?-1892)
Outlines of a plan for a free city hospital. Boston: G. C. Rand, 1860. 18p. 2 plates. DNLM; MBM **60-0336**

CLARK, Henry Grafton (1804?-1892)
Department of special inspection of the general hospitals of the army. First report to the commission by . . . inspector in chief, Nov. 18, 1862. New York: W. C. Bryant & Co., 1862. 15p. DNLM; NNNAM; [No. 56, U.S. San. Com. documents, 1861-1865.] **60-0337**

CLARK, Henry Grafton (1804?-1892)
Department of special inspection of the general hospitals of the army. Second report to the committee, Jan. 21, 1863. Washington: McGill & Witherow, 1863. 10p. DNLM [No. 65, U.S. San. Com. documents, 1861-1865.] **60-0338**

CLARK, Henry Grafton (1804?-1892)
Department of the special inspection of the general hospitals, U.S.A. Third (preliminary) report to the committee, May, 1863. New York: W. C. Bryant & Co., 1864. 41p. DNLM [No. 79, U.S. San Com. documents, 1861-1865.] **60-0339**

CLARK, Henry Grafton (1804?-1892)
Sanitary code for cities. Revised and adopted by the National Quarantine and Sanitary Convention. Boston: G. C. Rand & Avery, [1865]. 48p. DNLM; MBM **60-0340**

CLARK, Henry Grafton (1804?-1892)
Boards of health. Boston: G. C. Rand & Avery, 1866. 13p. DNLM; MBM **60-0341**

CLARK, Henry Grafton (1804?-1892)
Inspection of the slaughter-houses of Brighton, April 30, 1866. Boston: J. E. Farwell & Co., 1866. 12p. 1 map. DNLM; MBM **60-0342**

CLARK, Henry Grafton (1804?-1892)
Medical jurisprudence. Boston: D. Clapp & Sons, 1868. 27p. DNLM; MH-M **60-0343**

CLARK, James Henry (1814-1869)
The medical topography of Newark, N.J. New York: J. A. Gray, printer, 1861. 25p. DLC; DNLM; NjR; NNNAM **60-0344**

CLARK, James Henry (1814-1869)
The medical men of New Jersey, in Essex district, from 1666 to 1866. . . . Newark, N.J.: Pub. for the author, printed at the Evening Courier Office, 1867. 104p. DLC; NjR; NNNAM **60-0345**

CLARK, Rufus Wheelwright (1813-1886)
The sources of a physician's power. An address delivered at the commencement of the Albany Medical College, May 28, 1863. Albany: C. Van Benthuysen, 1863. 30p. DNLM **60-0346**

CLARK, Rufus Wheelwright (1813-1886)
A discourse on the life and character of Howard Townsend, M.D. Albany: S. R. Gray, 1867. 18p. DNLM **60-0347**

CLARKE, Edward Hammond (1820-1877)
The value of a diploma. A valedictory address delivered before the medical graduates of Harvard University, at the Massachusetts Medical College in Boston, Wednesday, March 7, 1860. Boston: David Clapp, 1860. 20p. DNLM; MH-M **60-0348**

CLARKE, E[dward] H[ammond] (1820-1877)
Recent progress in materia medica. Boston: D. Clapp & Son, 1864. 19p. DNLM; MBM **60-0349**

CLARKE, Edward Hammond (1820-1877)
Observations on the nature and treatment of polypus of the ear. Boston: Ticknor & Fields, 1867. 71p. DNLM; MBM **60-0350**

CLARKE, Henry Bradford (1827-1888)
Clinical homoeopathy. The annual address delivered before the Massachusetts Homoeopathic Medical Society, April 12, 1865. Cambridge: J. Wilson & Son, 1867. 14p. MBM; PPHa **60-0351**

CLARKE, Henry Bradford (1827-1888)
The homoeopathic idea in therapeutics. Annual address delivered before the American Institute of Homoeopathy, at its twenty-first session, St. Louis, June 3, 1868. Boston: Mudge & Son, 1869. 20p. MBM; PPHa **60-0352**

CLEAVELAND, Charles Harley (1820-1863)
Causes and cure of diseases of the feet, with practical suggestions as to their clothing. Cincinnati: Bradley & Webb, 1862. 111p. DNLM; OCIM **60-0353**

CLEAVELAND, Charles Harley (1820-1863)
Pronouncing medical lexicon, containing the correct pronunciation and definition of most of the terms used by speakers and writers on medicine and the collateral sciences. With addenda. Philadelphia: Lindsay & Blakiston, 1865. 302p. DNLM; NNNAM; PPC; PU **60-0354**

CLEVELAND, Emeline H. (1829-1878)
Valedictory address to the graduating class of the Female Medical College of Pennsylvania. Philadelphia: Crissy & Markley, 1863. 15p. DNLM; PPC **60-0355**

CLEVELAND, Emeline H. (1829-1878)
Valedictory address to the graduating class of the Woman's Medical College of Pennsylvania. Philadelphia: J. B. Rodgers, 1868. 12p. DNLM; PPC **60-0356**

CLOUD, J. A[lbert] (1841-1900)
Homoeopathy: Its difficulties and some of the principal errors against it, with hints on dietetics, viewed in relation to the laws of digestion. Also, the practice of homoeopathic medicine simplified for the use of families; and a history of the Cincinnati Homoeopathic Medical Dispensary. Cincinnati: V. C. Tidball, 1869. 82p. OCIM; PPHa **60-0357**

CLYMER, Meredith (1817-1902)
Review of Circular No. 6. Surgeon-General's Office, Nov. 1, 1865. [1866.] 33p. DNLM **60-0358**

COATES, Benjamin Horner (1797-1881)
Annual address [to] the Philadelphia County Medical Society. Philadelphia: Collins, 1860. 28p. DNLM; PPC; PU **60-0359**

COATES, Reynell (1802-1886)
Introductory lecture to the class of the Female College of Pennsylvania. Philadelphia: Merrihew & Thompson, 1861. 16p. DNLM; PPC **60-0360**

COCHRAN, James
Manual of anatomy. A new and revised ed. Philadelphia: J. Buchanan, 1868. 203p. DNLM; PPC; PU **60-0361**

COCHRAN, Jerome (1831-1896)
Administration of chloroform by deglutition. Nashville: W. H. F. Ligon, 1867. 26p. DNLM; OCIM **60-0362**

CODMAN, Benjamin S. (1816?-1894) and Ashahel M. SHURTLEFF
Illustrated catalogue of surgical instruments. . . . Boston: Ripley & Co., [1860?]. 32p. DNLM; MBM **60-0363**

COHEN, Jacob [da Silva] Solis (1838-1927)
Inhalation: its therapeutics and practice. A treatise on the inhalation of gases, vapors, nebulized fluids, and powders, including a description of the apparatus employed. . . . Philadelphia: Lindsay & Blakiston, 1867. 305p. DLC; DNLM; PPC; PU **60-0364**

COLBURN, George F. J.
Popular dentistry. Practical knowledge of the teeth, that should be possessed by every one. In order to preserve these organs from infancy to old age. . . . [Newark, N.J.], 1861. 15p. DLC; NNNAM **60-0365**

COLES, Walter (1839-1892)
Progressive locomotor ataxia. Being extracts from two papers on "Progressive locomotor ataxia, with special reference to its differential diagnosis," read before the Wood County Medical Association, Parkersburg, W. Va., in May and June, 1867. [Louisville, 1868.] 48p. DNLM **60-0366**

COLLEGE OF PHARMACY OF THE CITY OF NEW YORK
Annual prospectuses for the session of 1868-1869 to 1879-1880 (39.-50.); 1881-1882 to 1897-1898 (52.-68.). New York, 1868-1897. DNLM. [List of students and graduates for 1867-1868 to 1879-1879; 1880-1881 to 1896-1897, in prospectuses for subsequent years. Graduates' roll from 1831 to 1894, in prospectus for 1849-1895.] **60-0367**

COLLINS, G. T.
The cholera: a familiar treatise on its history. . . . [New York & Cincinnati, 1866]. 162p. DNLM; NNNAM; OCIM **60-0368**

COLTON, D. Alphonso (1821?-1891)
Valedictory address to the graduating class of Hahnemann Medical College, February 25, 1864. Chicago: Beach & Bernard, 1864. 12p. ICRM; PPHa **60-0369**

COLUMBIA COLLEGE. NEW YORK CITY
Catalogue embracing the names of its trustees, officers, and graduates. . . . From 1754 to 1867 [including graduates in medicine from 1769 to 1810; 1860 to 1867]. New York: D. Van Nostrand, 1868. 143p. DNLM; NN; NNC **60-0370**

COMEGYS, Cornelius George (1816-1896)
Introductory address. Session of 1866-1867. Medical College of Ohio. Cincinnati, 1866. 21p. DNLM; OCIM **60-0371**

COMFORT, J. W.
The practice of medicine on Thomsonian principles, adapted as well to the use of families as to that of the practitioner, containing a biographical sketch of Dr. Thomson, propositions illustrative of the philosophy of Thomsonianism; a brief history of the symptoms, peculiarities, and general course of disease in its different forms and varieties; with practical directions for administering the Thomsonian medicines, including the various methods of administering vapour baths, emetics, etc., and a materia medica, adapted to the work. 6th ed. Philadelphia: Lindsay & Blakiston, 1863. 588p. DNLM; NNNAM; PPC; PU **60-0372**

COMINGS, B. N[ewton] (1816-1899)
Class-book of physiology; for the use of schools and families. Comprising the structure and functions of the organs of man, illustrated by comparative reference to those of inferior animals. 2nd ed., with an appendix. Memphis: Cleaves & Vaden, 1860. 324p. DNLM **60-0373**

CONANT, David Sloan (1825-1865)
The science, causes, and anatomical peculiarities of human monstrosities. Read before the New York Academy of Medicine, Jan. 15, 1862. New York: William Wood & Co., 1862. 29p. NNNAM **60-0374**

CONDIE, David Francis (1796-1875)
Biographical notice of Henry Bond, M.D. Philadelphia: Collins, 1860. 22p. DNLM; PPC; PU **60-0375**

CONDIE, David Francis (1796-1875)
A practical treatise on the diseases of children. . . . 6th ed., rev. and enl. Philadelphia: Henry C. Lea, 1868. 783p. DLC; NNNAM; PPC; PU **60-0376**

CONDIE, David Francis (1796-1875)
Report on the diseases of Pennsylvania. Philadelphia: Collins, 1868. 13p. DNLM; PPC; PU **60-0377**

CONNECTICUT STATE DENTAL ASSOCIATION
Transactions, 1864-1865. Hartford: Wiley, Waterman & Eaton, 1866. [All published.] 102p. DNLM **60-0378**

CONQUEST, John Tricker (1789-1866)
What is homoeopathy? And is there any, and what amount of truth in it? 2nd American ed. Philadelphia: W. Radde, Jr., 1861. 18p. DNLM; PPHa **60-0379**

COOK, A. A.
An address before the Massachusetts Dental Society. Boston: The Society, 1869. 20p. DNLM; MBM **60-0380**

COOK, A. B[rown] (1828-1895)
Joined twins; the obstetrical and surgical management. Louisville: Bell & Co., 1869. 26p. 1 plate. DNLM **60-0381**

COOK, E. G[eorge] (1817-1893)
The cause of tuberculosis; a review of Dr. Rollin R. Gregg's hypothesis. Read before the Erie County Homoeopathic Medical Society. [Buffalo, N.Y., 1869.] 16p. DNLM **60-0382**

COOK, George
Remarks on the care and treatment of the chronic insane poor. Canandaigua: N. J. Milliken, 1867. 6p. DNLM **60-0383**

COOKE, Nicholas Francis (1829-1885)
Valedictory address to the graduating class of Hahnemann Medical College, delivered February 15th, 1865. . . . Chicago: Printed by Beach & Barnard, 1865. 16p. DLC; PPHa **60-0384**

COOKE, Nicholas Francis (1829-1885)
Extract from an address delivered before Hahnemann Medical College, and homoeopathy and allopathy statistically compared. Published by order of the Homoeopathic Medical Society of Chester, Delaware, and Lancaster Counties. West Chester Republican and Democrat Office, Pa., 1866. 15p. PPHa **60-0385**

COOKE, Nicholas Francis (1829-1885)
Annual address before the American Institute of Homoeopathy at its 20th session held in New York, June 4th, 5th, 6th, 7th, 1867. [1868.] 14p. NNNAM **60-0386**

COOKE, Nicholas Francis (1829-1885)
Valedictory address to the graduating class of Hahnemann Medical College, February 25, 1869. Chicago: Beach & Barnard, 1869. 18p. PPHa **60-0387**

COOLEY, Arnold James
The toilet and cosmetic arts in ancient and modern times . . . including instructions and cautions respecting the selection and use of perfumes, cosmetics, and other toilet articles, and a comprehensive collection of formulae and directions for their preparation. Philadelphia: Lindsay & Blakiston, 1866. 804p. DNLM; PU **60-0388**

COOMBS, Frederick
Coombs' popular phrenology: exhibiting the phrenological admeasurements of above fifty distinguished and extraordinary personages, of both sexes. With skulls of the various nations of the world. Embellished with above fifty engravings. . . . New York, Boston [etc.]: Fowler & Wells, 1865. 106p. DLC; NNNAM **60-0389**

COTTING, Benjamin Eddy (1812-1897)
Vesico-vaginal fistula—spontaneous relief. "The American operation." Boston: D. Clapp, 1861. 7p. DNLM; MBM **60-0390**

COTTING, Benjamin Eddy (1812-1897)
Cholera—its management and medical treatment. [Boston, 1866.] 7p. DNLM; MBM **60-0391**

COTTING, Benjamin Eddy (1812-1897)
Disease, a part of the plan of creation. The annual discourse before the Massachusetts Medical Society, May 31, 1865. . . . Boston: D. Clapp & Son, 1866. 45p. DLC; DNLM; MBM **60-0392**

COTTING, B[enjamin] E[ddy] (1812-1897)
Dr. Sayre's cases of artificial hip-joint. Boston, 1869. 2 l. DNLM **60-0393**

COVENTRY, Charles B. (1801-1875)
Annual address before the Medical Society of the County of Oneida. Utica, N.Y.: Roberts, 1865. 18p. DNLM **60-0394**

COVENTRY, Charles B. (1801-1875)
Spotted or congestive fever. Albany: Van Benthuysen & Sons, 1867. 18p. DNLM **60-0395**

[COXE, John Redman] (1773-1863)
Catalogue of the extensive and valuable medical, theological and miscellaneous library of the late. . . . Philadelphia: W. B. Selheimer, 1864. 153p. DNLM **60-0396**

CRICCA, Anacleto
Cholera in the Orient and its successful treatment and prophylaxis, in the epidemic of 1865. . . . New edition, revised and corrected. Transl. by John Davies. Chicago: C. S. Halsey, 1868. 35p. PPHa **60-0397**

CROSBY, Alpheus Benning (1832-1877)
Memorial address. Prof. David S. Conant, M.D. . . . With remarks and resolutions from other sources. Burlington: Times Book and Job Office, 1866. 30p. DNLM **60-0398**

CROSBY, Alpheus Benning (1832-1877)
An address commemorative of Reuben Dimond Mussey, M.D., LL.D. Manchester: J. B. Clarke, 1869. 23p. DNLM **60-0399**

CROSERIO, Camille (1786-1855)
Homoeopathic manual of obstetrics. From the French, by M. Côté. Cincinnati: Moore, Wilstach & Baldwin, 1866. 153p. DNLM; OCIM **60-0400**

CROWELL, James M. (*b.* 1827)
In memoriam. A discourse at the funeral of William Harris, M.D., delivered in the Seventh Presbyterian Church, Philadelphia, March 6, 1861. Philadelphia: W. S. & A. Martien, [1861.]. 16p. DNLM; PPC **60-0401**

CULBERTSON, Howard (1828-1890)
A prosecution for infanticide; with remarks. [Cincinnati, 1862.] 23p. DNLM **60-0402**

CULBERTSON, Howard (1828-1890)
Prize essay on the use of anaesthetics in obstetrics. Cincinnati: S. G. Cobb, 1862. 55p. DNLM **60-0403**

CULLERIER, August, i.e., Adrien Fidèle Auguste (1805-1874)
Atlas of venereal diseases. . . . Transl. from the French, with notes and additions, by Freeman J. Bumstead. . . . Philadelphia: Henry C. Lea, 1868. 328p. 26 col. plates. DLC; NNNAM; PPC; PU [French original published in 1861-66 under title: Précis iconographique des maladies vénériennes.] **60-0404**

CURTIS, Alva (1797-1881)
Synopsis of lectures on obstetrics and the forms of disease peculiar to women and children, delivered to the students of the Physio-Medical College of Ohio. Cincinnati: The author, 1862. 447p. DNLM; OCIM **60-0405**

CURTIS, Alva (1797-1881)
Lectures on midwifery and the diseases peculiar to women and children, delivered to the members of the Botanico-Medical School, at Columbus, Ohio. [Columbus, O., 1864?] 398p. DNLM; OCIM **60-0406**

CURTIS, Alva (1797-1881)
A fair examination and criticism of all the medical systems in vogue; . . . 3rd ed. Cincinnati: Printed for the proprietor, 1866. 208p. DLC; OCIM **60-0407**

CURTIS, Alva (1797-1881)
Allopathy and physio-medication contrasted. Cincinnati, 1867. 7p. DNLM **60-0408**

CURTIS, Charles R. S.
The nature and treatment of diphtheria; with a report of three cases of tracheotomy. . . . Keokuk, Ia.: Rees' Book Printing Office, 1866. 42p. DLC **60-0409**

CURTIS, Edward (1838-1912)
Catalogue of the microscopical section of the United States Army Medical Museum. Prepared under the direction of the Surgeon-General, U.S. Army. Washington: Govt. Print. Office, 1867. 160p. 1 plate. DNLM [Bound with: Catalogue of the medical section, Washington, 1867.] **60-0410**

CURTIS, George Ticknor (1812-1894) and S. D. LAW
Argument of . . . in the United States Circuit Court for the southern district of New York, before Justice Nelson, on behalf of the dentists as to their right to use hard rubber vulcanite in the manufacture of bases for artificial teeth, in the suits of H. B. Goodyear *et al. vs.* Thomas G. Wait, brought for an alleged infringement of the Goodyear patents, and to restrain the use of hard rubber for such purpose. New York, 1867. 157p. DNLM; NNNAM **60-0411**

CURWEN, John (1821-1901)
Address delivered before the Medical Society of the State of Pennsylvania, at its annual session, June, 1869. . . . Extracted from the Transactions of the Medical Society of the State of Pennsylvania. Philadelphia: Collins, Printer, 1869. 20p. DLC; PPC **60-0412**

CURWEN, John (1821-1901)
Address [on insanity] delivered before the Medical Society of the State of Pennsylvania. Philadelphia: Collins, Printer, 1869. 20p. DNLM; PPC **60-0413**

CUSHING, A[lvin] M[atthew] (*b.* 1829)
Monograph on Dioscorea villosa and dioscorein; their physiological effects, together with their use in disease. Detroit, Mich.: Published at Lodge's Homoeopathic Pharmacy, [1869]. 52p. DNLM; PPHa **60-0414**

CUTTER, Ephraim (1832-1917)
Veratrum viride as a therapeutical agent. Cambridge, Mass.: Riverside Press, 1862. 31p. DNLM; MBM **60-0415**

CUTTER, Ephraim (1832-1917)
Report of the zymoses of 1857, as they occurred in the Middlesex East District Medical Society. [1864.] 10p. 1 tab. DNLM; MH-M **60-0416**

CUTTER, Ephraim (1832-1917)
The anterior splint of Dr. Nathan R. Smith, of Baltimore, Md. [1869.] 6p. DNLM **60-0417**

DA COSTA, Jacob Mendes (1833-1900)
Medical diagnosis, with special reference to practical medicine. A guide to the knowledge and discrimination of diseases. . . . Philadelphia: J. B. Lippincott & Co., 1864. 690p. DLC; DNLM; PPC; PU **60-0418**

DA COSTA, Jacob Mendes (1833-1900)
On inhalations in the treatment of diseases of the respiratory passages, particularly as affected by the use of atomized fluids. New York: J. Medole, 1866. 41p. DNLM; NNNAM **60-0419**

DA COSTA, Jacob Mendes (1833-1900)
Medical diagnosis, with special reference to practical medicine. A guide to the knowledge and discrimination of diseases. . . . 2nd ed., rev. Philadelphia: J. B. Lippincott & Co., 1866. 784p. DLC; DNLM; NNNAM; PPC **60-0420**

DA COSTA, Jacob Mendes (1833-1900)
Inhalations in the treatment of diseases of the respiratory passages, particularly as affected by the use of atomized fluids. . . . Philadelphia: J. B. Lippincott & Co., 1867. 86p. DLC; DNLM; PPC; PU **60-0421**

DALTON, Edward Barry (1834-1872)
Report [as sanitary superintendent of the Metropolitan Board of Health, New York City]. Albany: Van Benthuysen & Sons, 1867. 36p. DNLM **60-0422**

DALTON, John C[all] (1825-1889)
An introductory address to the medical class of 1860-1861 of the College of Physicians and Surgeons. New York: Baker & Godwin, 1860. 24p. DNLM; NNNAM **60-0423**

DALTON, John C[all] (1825-1889)
A treatise on human physiology. . . . 2nd ed. Philadelphia: Blanchard & Lea, 1861. 700p. MBM; NNNAM; OCIM; PPC **60-0424**

DALTON, John C[all] (1825-1889)
Observations on trichina spiralis. New York: Bailliere Brothers, 1864. 18p. DNLM; NNNAM **60-0425**

DALTON, John Call (1825-1889)
A treatise on human physiology. . . . 3rd ed., rev. and enl. . . . Philadelphia: Blanchard & Lea, 1864. 706p. DLC; NNNAM; PPC; PU **60-0426**

DALTON, John Call (1825-1889)
A treatise on physiology and hygiene. New York: Harper Brothers, 1866. 424p. MBM; NNNAM; PPC; PU **60-0427**

DALTON, John Call (1825-1889)
A treatise on human physiology. . . . 4th ed., rev. and enl. Philadelphia: Henry C. Lea, 1867. 695p. MBM; NNNAM; OCIM; PPC **60-0428**

DALTON, John Call (1825-1889)
. . . Vivisection; what it is, and what it has accomplished. . . . New York: Bailliere Brothers; [etc., etc.], 1867. 40p. DLC; NNNAM **60-0429**

DALTON, John Call (1825-1889)
A treatise on physiology and hygiene. . . . With illustrations. New York: Harper & Brothers; London: S. Low, Son, & Marston, 1868. 399p. CtY-M; DLC; MBM; NNNAM **60-0430**

DAMON, Howard F. (1833-1884)
Leucocythemia. Boston: De Vries, Ibarra & Co., 1864. 93p. 3 phot. DNLM; MH-M **60-0431**

DAMON, Howard F. (1833-1884)
The neuroses of the skin; their pathology and treatment. Philadelphia: J. B. Lippincott & Co., 1868. 114p. DNLM; PPC; PPJ; PU **60-0432**

DAMON, Howard F. (1833-1884)
The structural lesions of the skin; their pathology and treatment. Philadelphia: J. B. Lippincott & Co., 1869. 255p. 5 plates. DNLM; MBM; NNNAM; PPC **60-0433**

D'AVIGNON, F. J.
Annual address delivered before the Medical Society of Clinton County. Plattsburgh: J. W. Tuttle, 1860. 18p. DNLM **60-0434**

DAVIS, Henry Gassett (1807-1896)
Medical testimony in regard to the proper mechanical treatment of joint disease. New York: Hall, Clayton & Medole, [1862]. 12p. DNLM **60-0435**

DAVIS, Henry Gassett (1807-1896)
On the pathological basis of the treatment of joint diseases. New York: Hall, Clayton & Medole, [1862]. 16p. DNLM **60-0436**

DAVIS, Henry Gassett (1807-1896)
The American method of treating joint diseases and deformities. . . . Philadelphia: Collins, Printer, 1863. 32p. DLC; PPC
60-0437

DAVIS, Henry Gassett (1807-1896)
. . . Medical testimony in regard to Dr. Davis's new mode of treating joint diseases. New York: Hall, Clayton & Medole, [1863]. 19p. DNLM; NNNAM **60-0438**

DAVIS, Henry Gassett (1807-1896)
Curability of pulmonary consumption. New York: C. A. Alvord, 1866. 24p. DNLM; NNNAM **60-0439**

DAVIS, Henry Gassett (1807-1896)
Conservative surgery, as exhibited in remedying some of the mechanical causes that operate injuriously both in health and disease. With illustrations. . . . New York: D. Appleton & Company, 1867. 314p. DLC; MBM; NNNAM; PPC
60-0440

DAVIS, James J. (*d.* 1876)
A guide to health designed for families and others. Containing a short and concise mode of treatment for most forms of disease to which man is liable, with sanative agents. . . . New York: Oakley & Mason, 1868. 190p. DLC; NNNAM
60-0441

DAVIS, Nathan Smith (1817-1904)
How far do the facts accompanying the prevalence of epidemic cholera in Chicago, during the summer and autumn of 1866, throw light on the etiology of that disease? Presented to the Section on meteorology, medical topography, and epidemic diseases of the American Medical Association, May, 1867. . . . [Chicago, 1867]. 19p. fold; map. DLC; ICRM; IEN-M
60-0442

DAVIS, T. J[efferson]
A treatise on the artificial human eyes, made from a new material, on an improved principle. New York, 1863. 34p. DLC; NNNAM **60-0443**

DAVIS, William B[ramwell] (1832-1893)
Carbolic acid, its surgical and therapeutical uses. Cincinnati: A. Abraham, 1869. 13p. DNLM **60-0444**

DAWES, Ebenezer (1825-1892)
A sermon preached . . . at the funeral of Joseph Emmons Briggs, M.D., May 12, 1867. Cambridge: Welch, Bigelow & Co., 1867. 34p. DNLM; MH **60-0445**

DAWSON, Charles Carroll (*b.* 1833)
Saratoga: its mineral waters, and their use in preventing and eradicating disease, and as a refreshing beverage. . . . New York: [Russell Bros.], 1868. 64p. DLC; NNNAM
60-0446

DAWSON, W. W[irt] (1828-1893)
Fibro-cystic tumor attached to the fundus of the uterus, seventeen other tumors in the cavity of the abdomen, with some account of abdominal section for the relief of such and similar cases. Cincinnati: A. Abraham, 1869. 15p. DNLM
60-0447

DAY, Albert (*d.* 1894)
Methomania: a treatise on alcoholic poisoning. With an appendix by Horatio R. Storer. Boston: James Campbell, 1867. 70p. DNLM; MH-M **60-0448**

[DAY, Horace, ed.]
The opium habit, with suggestions as to the remedy. New York: Harper & Brothers, 1868. 342p. NN; NNNAM
60-0449

DAYFOOT, Herbert M. (1846-1894)
Homoeopathy for the people. Mount Morris, New York, 1868. 16p. DNLM **60-0450**

DEAN, John (1831-1888)
Microscopic anatomy of the lumbar enlargement of the spinal cord. Cambridge: Welch, Bigelow, 1861. 21p. 4 plates. MBM
60-0451

DEAN, John (1831-1888)
The gray substance of the medulla oblongata and trapezium. Washington: Smithson. Inst., 1864. 75p. 14 plates. DNLM [*also*: 75p. 16 plates] **60-0452**

DE GERSDORFF, Ernest Bruno (1820-1893)
Conservatism in its relation to homoeopathy. Annual address delivered before the Massachusetts Homoeopathic Medical Society, April 10, 1867. Cambridge: John Wilson & Son, 1868. 24p. MH-M; PPHa **60-0453**

DERBY, George (1819-1874)
Geographical distribution of consumption in Massachusetts. Boston, 1867. 17p. DNLM; MBM **60-0454**

DERBY, George (1819-1874)
An inquiry into the influence of anthracite fires upon health; with remarks upon artificial moisture, and the best modes of warming houses. 2nd ed., enlarged. Boston: A. Williams & Co., 1868. 76p. DNLM; MH-M **60-0455**

DERBY, George (1819-1874)
An inquiry into the influence, upon health, of anthracite coal, when used as fuel for warming dwelling-houses; with some remarks upon special evaporating apparatus. Boston: A. Williams & Co., 1868. 46p. DNLM; MBM
60-0456

A DESCRIPTION of the newly invented elastic tourniquet, for the use of armies and employment in civil life. New York: G. T. Nesbitt & Co., 1862. 31p. DNLM; NNNAM
60-0457

DESORMEAUX, Antonin Jean (*d.* 1894)
The endoscope, and its application to the diagnosis and treatment of affections of the genito-urinary passages. Lessons given at Necker Hospital. . . . Transl. by R. P. Hunt. . . . Chicago: R. Fergus' Sons, printers, 1867. 108p. DLC; ICRM; OCIM **60-0458**

DEWEES, William Potts (1768-1841)
A treatise on the diseases of females. . . . 11th ed., with the author's last improvements and corrections. Philadelphia: Blanchard & Lea, 1860. 536p. 12 plates. DLC; PPC; PPJ; PU
60-0459

DICKSON, Samuel Henry (1798-1872)
Valedictory address delivered before the graduating class of Jefferson Medical College of Philadelphia. Philadelphia: Collins, 1862. 23p. DNLM; PPJ **60-0460**

DICKSON, Samuel Henry (1798-1872)
Introductory address delivered before the students of Jefferson Medical College, Philadelphia. Philadelphia: H. B. Ashmead, 1863. 31p. DNLM; PPJ **60-0461**

DICKSON, Samuel Henry (1798-1872)
On certain morbid conditions of the sensorial system. [Richmond, 1867]. 44p. DNLM **60-0462**

DICKSON, Samuel Henry (1798-1872)
Studies in pathology and therapeutics. . . . New York: William Wood & Co., 1867. 201p. DLC; NNNAM; PPC; PU **60-0463**

DICKSON, Samuel Henry (1798-1872)
On the causation of diseases. [Richmond, 1867.] 30p. DNLM **60-0464**

DICKSON, Samuel Henry (1798-1872)
Therapeutics. [Richmond, 1867.] 30p. DNLM **60-0465**

DICKSON, Samuel Henry (1798-1872)
Valedictory address to the graduates at the forty-fourth annual commencement of the Jefferson Medical College of Philadelphia. Philadelphia, 1869. 22p. DNLM; PPJ **60-0466**

DICKSON, Samuel Henry (1798-1872)
Necrology. (Obituary of Dr. Robley Dunglison.) [Philadelphia, 1869.] 3p. DNLM; PPJ **60-0467**

DILLENBACK, H. P.
Consumption, bronchitis, asthma, catarrh and clergyman's sore throat successfully treated by medical inhalations comprising all the recent improvements in this mode of practice with the remedies used. Boston: Published by the author, 1866. 336p. MBM **60-0468**

DIRIX, M.E.
Woman's complete guide to health. New York: W. A. Townsend & Adams, 1869. 342p. DNLM; NNNAM **60-0469**

DIXON, Edward H. (1808-1880)
Woman and her diseases, from the cradle to the grave; adapted exclusively to her education in the physiology of her system, and all the diseases of her critical periods. 10th ed. Philadelphia: J. W. Bradley, 1860. 318p. DNLM; PPC; PU **60-0470**

DIXON, Edward H. (1808-1880)
The organic law of the sexes. Positive and negative electricity, and the abnormal conditions that impair virility. . . . New York: J. S. Redfield, [1861]. 36p. DLC; DNLM; NNNAM **60-0471**

DIXON, Edward H. (1808-1880)
Some abnormal conditions of the sexual and pelvic organs, which impair virility. New York: A. Brentano, [1861]. 40p. DNLM; NNNAM **60-0472**

DIXON, Edward H. (1808-1880)
Back-bone; photographed from "The Scalpel." New York: R. M. De Witt, [1866]. 396p. DNLM; NNNAM **60-0473**

DIXON, Edward H. (1808-1880)
A treatise on diseases of the sexual system, adapted to popular instruction. . . . 10th ed., with an appendix. New York: R. M. De Witt, [1867]. 312p. DLC; MBM; NNNAM; PPC **60-0474**

DIXON, James (1813-1896)
A guide to the practical study of diseases of the eye; with an outline of their medical and operative treatment. From the 2nd London ed. Philadelphia. Lindsay & Blakiston, 1860. 435p. DNLM; NNNAM; PPC; PU **60-0475**

DOBELL, Horace (1828-1917)
Report on "pancreatic emulsion of fat." Greenpoint, N.Y.: C. Etheridge, [1867]. 4 l. DNLM **60-0476**

DONALDSON, Francis (1823-1891)
Physiology the true basis of rational medicine. An introductory lecture. Baltimore: Kelly & Piet, 1866. 19p. DNLM; MdU-D **60-0477**

DONALDSON, Francis (1823-1891)
Medicine an aggregate of progressive sciences. Valedictory address at the commencement of the University of Maryland. Baltimore: Kelly & Piet, 1867. 28p. DNLM; MdU-D **60-0478**

DOUGLAS, James S. (1801-1878)
Practical homoeopathy, for the people, adapted to the comprehension of the non-professional, and for reference by the young practitioner, including a number of most valuable new remedies and improvements in the treatment of numerous diseases not in general use. . . . Milwaukee: Daily Wisconsin Printing House, 1860. 84p. DLC **60-0479**

DRAPER, John Christopher (1835-1885)
A text-book on anatomy, physiology, and hygiene. . . . New York: Harper & Brothers, 1866. 300p. DLC; NN; NNC; NNNAM **60-0480**

DRAPER, John William (1811-1882)
The historical influence of the medical profession. An anniversary discourse delivered before the New York Academy of Medicine, December 10, 1863. . . . Pub. by order of the Academy. New York: Bailliere Brothers; [etc., etc.], 1863. 32p. DLC; NNNAM **60-0481**

DRAPER, John William (1811-1882)
A text-book on physiology. . . . Being an abridgement of the author's larger work on human physiology. . . . Illustrated with nearly 150 wood engravings. New York: Harper & Brothers, 1866. 376p. DLC; NN; NNC; NNNAM **60-0482**

DRAPER, John William (1811-1882)
Lecture, introductory to the course of 1869-1870, in the medical department of the University of New York. New York: J. Sarell, [1869]. 16p. DNLM; NNNAM **60-0483**

DRUITT, Robert (1814-1883)
The principles and practice of modern surgery. . . . A new and rev. American from the 8th enl. and improved London ed. With four hundred and thirty-two illustrations. Philadelphia: Blanchard & Lea, 1860. 695p. DLC; DNLM; PPC; PU **60-0484**

DUCHENNE, Guillaume Benjamin (1806-1875)
The nature, causes and treatment of nervous deafness, translated from the French of "Duchenne," with additions, by Laurence Turnbull. . . . Philadelphia: Lindsay & Blakiston, 1863. 119p. DLC; NNNAM; PPC; PU **60-0485**

DUFFIELD, Samuel P[earce]
A new process for the manufacture of the medicinal extracts. Detroit: W. Graham, [1866]. 10p. DNLM
60-0486

DUNCAN, James Matthews (1826-1890)
Researches in obstetrics. New York: William Wood & Co., 1868. 467p. DNLM; NNNAM; OCIM; PPC
60-0487

DUNCAN, James Matthews (1826-1890)
A practical treatise on perimetritis and parametritis. New York: William Wood & Co., 1869. 249p. DLC; MBM; NNNAM; PPC **60-0488**

DUNGLISON, Richard James (1834-1901)
Statistics of insanity in the United States. Philadelphia: J. B. Lippincott & Co., 1860. 40p. DNLM; PPC; PPJ; PU
60-0489

DUNGLISON, Robley (1798-1869)
Introductory lecture. . . . Jefferson Medical College. Philadelphia: J. M. Wilson, 1860. 30p. DNLM; PPJ
60-0490

DUNGLISON, Robley (1798-1869)
Medical lexicon. A dictionary of medical science; containing a concise explanation of the various subjects and terms of anatomy, physiology, pathology, hygiene, therapeutics, pharmacology, pharmacy, surgery, obstetrics, medical jurisprudence, and dentistry; notices of climate, and of mineral waters; formulae for officinal, empirical, and dietetic preparations; with the accentuation and etymology of the terms. And the French and other synonyms; so as to constitute a French as well as English medical lexicon. . . . Thoroughly rev. and very greatly modified and augm. Philadelphia: Blanchard & Lea, 1860. 992p. DNLM; MBM; NNNAM; PPC
60-0491

DUNGLISON, Robley (1798-1869)
An obituary notice of George W. Bethune. Read before the American Philosophical Society. Philadelphia: C. Sherman & Son, 1862. 20p. DNLM; PPJ **60-0492**

DUNGLISON, Robley (1798-1869)
An obituary notice of George Tucker, read before the American Philosophical Society. [Philadelphia, 1862.] 7p. DNLM **60-0493**

DUNGLISON, Robley (1798-1869)
An exhortation to the graduates of the Jefferson Medical College of Philadelphia. Philadelphia: Collins, 1864. 20p. DNLM; PPJ **60-0494**

DUNGLISON, Robley (1798-1869)
Medical lexicon. A dictionary of medical science; containing a concise explanation of the various subjects and terms of anatomy, physiology, pathology, hygiene, therapeutics, pharmacology, pharmacy, surgery, obstetrics, medical jurisprudence, and dentistry; notices of climate, and of mineral waters; formulae for officinal, empirical, and dietetic preparations; with the accentuation and etymology of the terms. And the French and other synonyms; so as to constitute a French as well as English medical lexicon. . . . Thoroughly rev. and very greatly modified and agum. Philadelphia: Henry C. Lea, 1866. 1047p. DLC; DNLM; PPC; PU
60-0495

DUNHAM, Carroll (1828-1877)
Address delivered at the semi-annual meeting of the Homoeopathic Medical Society of the State of New York. Albany: February 10, 1863. Albany: C. Van Benthuysen, 1863. 26p. PPHa **60-0496**

DUNHAM, Carroll (1828-1877)
Homoeopathy the science of therapeutics. New York: J. T. S. Smith & Sons, 1863. 68p. NNNAM; PPHa
60-0497

DUNHAM, Carroll (1828-1877)
Cholera. . . . New York: J. T. S. Smith & Sons, 1866. 24p. DLC; DNLM; NNNAM **60-0498**

DUNLAP, Alexander (1815-1894)
Ovariotomy; a paper read before the Ohio State Medical Society. Cincinnati: A. Abraham, pr., 1868. 22p. DNLM
60-0499

DUNLAP, Alexander (1815-1894)
Address delivered at the twenty-fourth annual meeting of the Ohio State Medical Society. Columbus: Nevins & Myers, 1869. 13p. DNLM **60-0500**

DURKEE, Silas
A treatise on gonorrhoea and syphilis. 2nd ed., revised and enlarged. Philadelphia: Lindsay & Blakiston, 1864. 446p. 8 plates. DNLM; MBM; NNNAM; PPC
60-0501

DUTTON, George (*b.* 1830)
Life and health, or how to restore health and prolong life on rational principles. Rutland: Warner & McLean, 1864. 28p. DNLM **60-0502**

DUTTON, George (*b.* 1830)
Hygienic manual, or how to restore health and secure longevity on rational principles. Rutland: McLean & Robbins, 1867. 84p. DNLM **60-0503**

DWIGHT, Thomas, Jr. (1843-1911)
The intracranial circulation. Cambridge: University Press, 1867. 28p. 1 plate. DNLM; MH-M **60-0504**

DWINELLE, Justin
Domestic practice of medicine; an entirely new and original work, containing a minute and faithful description of the causes, symptoms, and treatment of diseases and designed for the especial use of heads of families, planters, emigrants, sailors, and all others who are deprived of the immediate services of a physician. Syracuse, N.Y., 1861. 372p. DNLM
60-0505

EARLE, Pliny (1809-1892)
The psychopathic hospital of the future: an address delivered at the laying of the corner stone of the general hospital for the insane of the state of Connecticut, June 20, 1867. . . . Utica, N.Y.: Roberts, Printer, 1867. 15p. DLC; DNLM
60-0506

EARLE, Pliny (1809-1892)
An address delivered before the Berkshire Medical Institute, November 24, 1863. . . . Utica, N.Y.: Roberts, Book and Job Printer, 1867. 25p. DLC; DNLM **60-0507**

EARLE, Pliny (1809-1892)
Prospective provision for the insane. . . . Utica, N.Y.: Roberts, Printer, 1868. 17p. DLC; DNLM **60-0508**

EASTMAN, Sandford (1821-1874)
Introductory lecture to the students of the medical department of the University of Buffalo. Buffalo: Jos. Warren & Co., 1868. 14p. DNLM **60-0509**

EATON, Horace (1810-1883)
The great physician: a sermon on occasion of the death of Alexander McIntyre, M.D., delivered in the Presbyterian Church, Palmyra, N.Y., July 24, 1859. . . . New York: Printed by J. F. Trow, 1860. 20p. DLC; NNNAM **60-0510**

EDES, Robert T. (1838-1923)
The part taken by nature and time in the cure of diseases. [Prize diss.] Boston: D. Clapp & Sons, 1868. 44p. DNLM; MBM **60-0511**

EDES, Robert T. (1838-1923), J. F. HIBBERD, and J. SPARE
Dissertations on the part performed by nature and time in the cure of diseases; for which prizes were awarded by the Massachusetts Medical Society. Boston: D. Clapp & Son, 1868. 155p. DNLM; MBM; NNNAM **60-0512**

EDES, Robert T. (1838-1923)
The physiology and pathology of the sympathetic or ganglionic nervous system. [O'Reilly prize essay.] New York: William Wood & Co., 1869. 152p. 1 plate. DNLM; NNNAM **60-0513**

EDWARDS, Arthur Mead
Note on a point in the habits of diatomaceae and desmidiaceae. [Boston, 1868.] 2 l. DNLM **60-0514**

ELDRIDGE, C. S.
Self enervation; its consequences and treatment. With an introduction by Joseph Hooper. Chicago: C. S. Halsey, 1869. 64p. DNLM **60-0515**

ELIOT, Charles W. (1834-1926) and Frank H. STORER
A manual of inorganic chemistry, arranged to facilitate the experimental demonstration of the facts and principles of the science. 2nd ed., revised. New York: Ivison, 1868. 605p. DNLM; MH; NN; NNC **60-0516**

ELIOT, Johnson (1815-1883) and William C. TILDEN
Addresses delivered at the eighteenth commencement of the medical department of Georgetown College. Washington: W. H. Moore, 1867. 12p. DNLM **60-0517**

ELIOT, Samuel (1821-1898)
Address before the American Social Science Association. To which are added lists of papers, members, etc. Boston: Wright & Potter, 1867. 14p. DNLM; MH; MWA **60-0518**

ELIOT, Samuel (1821-1898)
Address at the commencement of the medical school of Harvard University, March 11, 1868. Boston: D. Clapp & Son, 1868. 21p. DNLM; MH-M **60-0519**

ELLIOTT, Ezekiel Brown (1823-1888)
Preliminary report on the mortality and sickness of the volunteer forces of the United States Government during the present war. New York: W. C. Bryant & Co., 1862. 28p. 9 diag. DNLM; NNNAM **60-0520**

ELLIOTT, George Thomson, Jr. (1827-1871)
Address delivered before the alumni of the medical department of the University of the City of New York. New York: Trow & Smith Co., 1868. 19p. DNLM; NNNAM **60-0521**

ELLIOTT, George Thomson, Jr. (1827-1871)
Obstetric clinic: a practical contribution to the study of obstetrics and the diseases of women and children. New York: D. Appleton & Co., 1868. 458p. CtY-M; DLC; MBM; NNNAM **60-0522**

ELLIOTT, George Thomson, Jr. (1827-1871)
Description of a new midwifery forceps, having a sliding pivot to prevent compression of the foetal head. [With cases.] [1869?] 24p. DNLM **60-0523**

ELLIS, Benjamin (1798-1831)
. . . The medical formulary: being a collection of prescriptions, derived from the writings and practice of many of the most eminent physicians in America and Europe. Together with the usual dietetic preparations and antidotes for poisons. To which is added an appendix, on the endermic use of medicines, and on the use of ether and chloroform. . . . 11th ed., carefully rev. [to 1864] and much extended, by Robert P. Thomas. . . . Philadelphia: Blanchard & Lea, 1864. 341p. DLC; MBM; NNNAM; PPC **60-0524**

ELLIS, Benjamin (1798-1831)
The medical formulary: being a collection of prescriptions derived from the writings and practice of many of the most eminent physicians in America and Europe, together with the usual dietetic preparations and antidotes for poisons. To which is added an appendix, on the endermic use of medicines, and on the use of ether and chloroform. The whole accompanied with a few brief pharmaceutical and medical observations. . . . 12th ed. carefully rev. and much improved by Albert H. Smith. . . . Philadelphia: Henry C. Lea, 1868. 374p. CtY-M; DLC; NNNAM; PPC **60-0525**

ELLIS, Calvin (1826-1883)
Tubercle; its pathology, and especially in relation to inflammation. Boylston prize essay. [Boston, 1860.] 20p. DNLM; MBM **60-0526**

ELLIS, Erastus R[anney] (1832-1914)
Homoeopathic family guide, and information for the people. . . . [Detroit: O. S. Gulley, book and job printer, 1868]. 144p. DLC; OCIM; PPHa **60-0527**

ELLIS, John (1815-1896)
The avoidable causes of disease, insanity and deformity. . . . A book for the people as well as for the profession. . . . New York: The author, 1860. 348p. DLC; DNLM; NNNAM **60-0528**

ELLIS, John (1815-1896)
The avoidable causes of disease, insanity, and deformity. . . . A book for the people as well as the profession. . . . New York: Mason Brothers, 1860. 348p. DLC; NNNAM **60-0529**

ELLIS, John (1815-1896)
Family homoeopathy. . . . 6th ed. New York: C. T. Hulburt; Boston: O. Clapp; [etc., etc.], 1867. 404p. DLC; MBM; NNNAM **60-0530**

ELLIS, John (1815-1896)
The avoidable causes of disease, insanity and deformity. By . . . A book for the people as well as for the profession. . . . 5th ed. New York: S. R. Wells, 1868. 348p. DLC; NNNAM **60-0531**

ELLIS, Thomas T.
Leaves from the diary of an army surgeon; or, Incidents of field, camp, and hospital life. . . . New York: J. Bradburn, 1863. 312p. DLC; DNLM; NNNAM **60-0532**

ELSBERG, Louis (1836-1885)
The domain of medical police. [New York], 1862. 16p. DNLM; NNNAM **60-0533**

ELSBERG, Louis (1836-1885)
Laryngoscopal medication; or, the local treatment of the diseases of the throat, larynx, and neighboring organs, under sight. New York: William Wood & Co., 1864. 38p. DNLM; OCIM; NNNAM **60-0534**

ELSBERG, Louis (1836-1885)
Laryngoscopal surgery illustrated in the treatment of morbid growths within the larynx. Being the prize essay to which the American Medical Association awarded the gold medal for 1865. Philadelphia: Collins, 1866. 56p. 4 plates. DNLM; PPC; PU **60-0535**

EMERSON, George Barrell (1797-1881)
Letter to Samuel C. Cobb, relative to a site for a new lunatic hospital. City doc. No. 113. Dec. 9, 1869. [Boston, 1869.] 5p. DNLM; MBM; MWA **60-0536**

EMMET, Thomas Addis (1828-1919)
A radical operation for procidentia. New York: J. M. Bradstreet & Son, 1865. 17p. 2 plates. DNLM; NNNAM **60-0537**

EMMET, Thomas Addis (1828-1919)
Treatment of dysmenorrhoea and sterility resulting from anteflexion of the uterus. . . . Rev., with additions. New York: Press of J. M. Bradstreet & Son, 1865. 23p. DLC; DNLM; NNNAM **60-0538**

EMMET, Thomas Addis (1828-1919)
Reduction of inverted uteri by a new method. New York: Bradstreet Press, 1866. 15p. DNLM; NNNAM **60-0539**

EMMET, Thomas Addis (1828-1919)
Accidental and congenital atresia of the vagina, with a mode of operating for successfully establishing the canal. . . . New York: Bradstreet Press, 1866. 17p. DLC; DNLM; NNNAM **60-0540**

[EMMET, Thomas Addis] (1828-1919)
Catalogue of the library belonging to Thomas Addis Emmet, M.D. New York: Bradstreet Press, 1868. 371p. DLC; DNLM; NNNAM **60-0541**

EMMET, Thomas Addis (1828-1919)
Vesico-vaginal fistula from parturition and other causes; with cases of recto-vaginal fistula. . . . New York: William Wood & Co., 1868. 250p. DLC; DNLM; MBM; NNNAM **60-0542**

EMMET, Thomas Addis (1828-1919)
Surgery of the cervix in connection with the treatment of certain uterine diseases. New York: J. M. Bradstreet & Son, 1869. 23p. DNLM; NNNAM **60-0543**

. . . EPIDEMIC cholera: its mission and mystery, haunts and havocs, pathology and treatment. With remarks on the question of contagion, the influence of fear, and hurried and delayed interments. By a former surgeon in the service of the Honorable East India Company. New York: Carleton, 1866. 120p. DLC; NNNAM **60-0544**

ERICHSEN, John Eric (1818-1896)
The science and art of surgery. Being a treatise on surgical injuries, diseases, and operations. Improved American from 2nd London ed. Philadelphia: Blanchard & Lea, 1860. 996p. DNLM; MBM; NNNAM; PPC **60-0545**

ERICHSEN, John Eric (1818-1896)
On railway and other injuries of the nervous system. . . . Philadelphia: Henry C. Lea, 1867. 103p. CtY-M; DLC; DNLM; PPC **60-0546**

ERICHSEN, John Eric (1818-1896)
The science and art of surgery. Being a treatise on surgical injuries, diseases, and operations. . . . From the 5th enl. and carefully rev. London ed. Illustrated with six hundred and thirty engravings on wood. With additions, by John Ashhurst. . . . Philadelphia: Henry C. Lea, 1869. 1228p. CtY-M; DLC; MH-M; PPC **60-0547**

ERNI, Henri
A systematic outline for the qualitative analysis of urine, with illustrative lithographic plates. Nashville, Tenn.: A. A. Stitt, 1860. 31p. DNLM **60-0548**

ERNI, Henri
Quantitative analysis of urine. Nashville: A. A. Stitt, 1860. 35p. DNLM **60-0549**

[EVANS, John]
Memorial of Dr. John Evans, praying the establishment of a system of quarantine regulations for the prevention of the spread of cholera. 39th Congress, 1st sess., Senate Mis. Doc. No. 66, Feb., 1866. Washington: Government Printing Office, 1866. 14p. DNLM **60-0550**

EVANS, Warren Felt (1817-1889)
The mental-cure, illustrating the influence of the mind on the body, both in health and disease, and the psychological method of treatment, by . . . 9th ed. Boston: Banner of Light Publishing Co. [1869]. 364p. DLC; MB; MH; NN **60-0551**

EVANS, Warren Felt (1817-1889)
The mental-cure, illustrating the influence of the mind on the body, both in health and disease, and the psychological method of treatment. . . . Boston: H. H. & T. W. Carter, 1869. 364p. DLC; MB; MBM; NN **60-0552**

EVE, Paul Fitzsimmons (1806-1877)
Fractures of the patella, treated by a ring; with cases. Nashville, Tenn.: W. H. F. Ligon, 1867. 7p. DNLM **60-0553**

EVE, Paul Fitzsimmons (1806-1877)
Report of seven operations for stone in thirty-three days. Nashville, Tenn.: W. H. F. Ligon, 1867. 13p. DNLM **60-0554**

EVE, Paul Fitzsimmons (1806-1877)
A contribution to the history of the hip-joint operations performed during the late civil war; being the statistics of twenty cases of amputations and thirteen of resections at this articulation, in the Southern service. Philadelphia: Collins, Printer, 1867. 17p. DNLM; PPC; PU **60-0555**

EVE, Paul Fitzsimmons (1806-1877)
The proper definition of the word cure, as applied to medicine. Nashville, [1868?] 4p. DNLM **60-0556**

EVE, Paul Fitzsimmons (1806-1877)
A consideration of some of the many popular errors in regard to medicine and medical practitioners. An introductory to the course of lectures in the Missouri Medical College, delivered in the hall of the Polytechnic Institute, Oct. 11, 1869. [St. Louis] : Levison & Blythe, 1869. 22p. DNLM **60-0557**

EVE, Paul Fitzsimmons (1806-1877)
Successful application of the trephine over the right lateral sinus of the brain. Nashville, [1869?] 4p. DNLM **60-0558**

EWER, F. C[artwright] (1826-1883)
Public health of the city of New York: Remarks before the Sanitary Association. With appendix. New York: E. Jones & Co., 1861. 33p. DNLM; NNNAM **60-0559**

FAGET, J[ean] C[harles] (1818-1884)
Considérations générales sur les mesures à prendre pour mettre la Nouvelle-Orléans à l'abri de la fièvre jaune. Nouvelle-Orléans, [1864]. 23p. DNLM; LNT-M **60-0560**

FAGET, J[ean] C[harles] (1818-1884)
Parallèle des deux fièvres étudiées dans ce travail. [Nouvelle-Orléans, 1864]. 13p. DNLM **60-0561**

FAGET, J[ean] C[harles] (1818-1884)
Mémoires et lettres sur la fièvre jaune et la fièvre paludéenne. Nouvelle-Orléans: Imp. du Propagateur Catholique, 1864. 40p. DNLM; LNT-M **60-0562**

FAGET, J[ean] C[harles] (1818-1884)
Fièvre paludéenne hémorrhagique. Premier mémoire de la fièvre paludéenne hemorrhagique, observée à la Nouvelle-Orléans. Second mémoire. Monographie sur une des variétés (la variété hématémesique) de la fièvre muqueuse grave de certains pays chauds, marécageux et humides. [Nouvelle-Orléans, 1864.] 72p. DNLM; LNT-M **60-0563**

FAHNESTOCK, William Baker
Artificial somnambulism, hitherto called mesmerism; or, animal magnetism. Containing a brief historical survey of Mesmer's operations, and the examination of the same by the French commissioners. Phreno-somnambulism; or, the exposition of phreno-magnetism and neurology, a new view and division of the phrenological organs into functions, with descriptions of their nature and qualities. . . . Together with an account of several obstetrical cases delivered while in this state; the proper method of preparing subjects for surgical operations; their management during and after the same, and the latest and best method of curing diseases, etc., in those persons who are in that condition. Philadelphia: Barclay & Co., [1869]. 328p. DNLM; PPC; PC **60-0564**

THE FAMILY adviser and guide to the medicine chest. A concise hand-book of domestic medicine. By a physician. Philadelphia: J. Wyeth and Brother, 1868. 104p. DLC; PPC **60-0565**

FARNSWORTH, Theodore H.
A treatise on venereal diseases, including syphilis, gonorrhea, stricture, gleet, and spermatorrhea; together with a number of female diseases. . . . Indianapolis, Ind.: [Ben Franklin Print], 1866. 34p. DLC **60-0566**

FARNSWORTH, Theodore H.
A treatise on spermatorrhea, its causes and effects. . . . [Indianapolis, Ind.]: Ben Franklin Print, 1867. 14p. DLC **60-0567**

FARNSWORTH, Theodore H.
A plain and familiar treatise on female complaints, and diseases peculiar to both married and single, old or young. . . . Indianapolis, Ind., 1869. 60p. DLC **60-0568**

FINCKE, A.
Homoeopathics. What it is and the logic of it. Philadelphia: A. J. Tafel, 1865. 15p. PPHa **60-0569**

FINCKE, Bernhard
On high potencies and homoeopathics. Clinical cases and observations. . . . With an appendix containing Hahnemann's original views and rules on the homoeopathic dose, chronologically arranged. . . . Philadelphia: A. J. Tafel, 1865. 131p. DLC; PPHa **60-0570**

FISHER, Alexander (1804-1882)
Report on the use of the sulphites of lime and soda in the treatment of hospital gangrene, phlebitis, erysipelas, and other zymotic diseases. Philadelphia: Collins, 1865. 28p. DNLM; PPC **60-0571**

FISHER, George J[ackson] (1825-1893)
Biographical sketches of the deceased physicians of Westchester County, N.Y. Being the annual address before the Westchester County Medical Society, at its session held in White Plains, June 1, 1858. . . . Pub. by order of the Society. New York: Hall, Clayton & Co., Printers, 1861. 52p. DLC; NNNAM **60-0572**

FISHER, George Jackson (1825-1893)
On the animal substances employed as medicines by the ancients. . . . New York: Hall, Clayton & Medole, printers [1862]. 16p. DLC; NNNAM **60-0573**

FISHER, George Jackson (1825-1893)
Diploteratology. An essay on compound human monsters, comprising the history, literature, classification, description and embryology of double and triple formation; including parasitic monsters, foetus in foetu, and supernumerary development. . . . Albany: Van Benthuysen's Steam Printing House, 1865[-68]. 39, 92, 131-165p. 33 plates. DLC; DNLM **60-0574**

FITCH, Samuel Sheldon
A popular treatise on the diseases of the heart, palsy, rheumatism, dyspepsia, dysentery, dysentery of children, cholera infantum, cholera and cholera morbus, bilious cholic, costiveness, yellow fever, diphtheria, putrid sore throat, with proofs of their curability; and how to treat the diseases of the elderly and old people; with medical prescriptions for nine of the complaints; also rules for preventing sickness and preserving health to one hundred years. New York: B. S. Fitch & Co., 1860. 168p. NNNAM **60-0575**

FITCH, Samuel Sheldon
Popular treatise on diseases of the heart, palsy, rheumatism, dyspepsia, etc. New York, 1862. 168p. MWA; NNNAM
60-0576

FITCH, Samuel Sheldon
Guide to the healthy in preserving their health, and to the sick in recovering it. New York, 1864. 50p. DNLM; MB
60-0577

FITCH, Samuel Sheldon
Family physician. . . . Boston: S. S. Fitch, 1866. 76p. DLC; DNLM; MBM **60-0578**

FITCH, Samuel Sheldon
Family physician. New York, 1868. 89p. DNLM; NNNAM
60-0579

FLEMING, Andrew
Blood stains in criminal trials. Pittsburgh: W. S. Haven, 1861. 69p. DNLM **60-0580**

FLEMING, L. D.
The air cure; or, atmospheric therapeutics, its philosophy, pathology and results, being a new discovery in medical science. Rochester, New York: W. S. Falls, 1867. 39p. PPHa
60-0581

FLINT, Austin (1812-1886)
Conservative medicine. New York, 1862. 24p. DNLM; NNNAM; PPC; PU **60-0582**

[FLINT, Austin] (1812-1886)
. . . Report of a committee of the associate medical members of the Sanitary Commission on the subject of pneumonia. Washington: McGill, Witherow & Co., Printers, 1862. 24p. DLC; DNLM; NNNAM; PPC [United States Sanitary Commission. (Medical and surgical monographs.)] **60-0583**

FLINT, Austin (1812-1886)
Compendium of percussion and auscultation, and of the physical diagnosis of diseases affecting the lungs and heart. 2nd ed. New York: William Wood & Co., 1865. 12p. DNLM; NNNAM **60-0584**

FLINT, Austin (1812-1886)
A treatise on the principles and practice of medicine; designed for the use of practitioners and students of medicine. . . . Philadelphia: Henry C. Lea, 1866. 867p. DLC; MBM; NNNAM; PPC **60-0585**

FLINT, Austin (1812-1886)
A practical treatise on the physical exploration of the chest, and the diagnosis of diseases affecting the respiratory organs. 2nd ed. Philadelphia: Henry C. Lea, 1866. 595p. DLC; DNLM; NNNAM; PPC **60-0586**

FLINT, Austin (1812-1886)
A treatise on the principles and practice of medicine. Designed for the use of practitioners and students of medicine. 2nd ed., revised and enlarged. Philadelphia: Henry C. Lea, 1867. 967p. CtY-M; NNNAM; OCIM; PPC **60-0587**

FLINT, Austin, ed. (1812-1886)
Contributions relating to the causation and prevention of disease, and to camp diseases; together with a report of the diseases, etc., among the prisoners at Andersonville, Ga. . . . New York: Published for the U.S. Sanitary Commission, by Hurd & Houghton, 1867. 667p. DNLM **60-0588**

FLINT, Austin (1812-1886)
A treatise on the principles and practice of medicine; designed for the use of practitioners and students of medicine. . . . 3rd ed., thoroughly rev. Philadelphia: Henry C. Lea, 1868. 1002p. DLC; NNNAM; PPC; PU **60-0589**

FLINT, Austin (1812-1886)
Compendium of percussion and auscultation, and of the physical diagnosis of diseases affecting the lungs and heart. . . . 4th ed. New York: William Wood & Company, 1869. 36p. DLC; NNNAM; OCIM; PU **60-0590**

FLINT, Austin, Jr. (1836-1915)
Experimental researches into a new excretory function of the liver; consisting in the removal of cholesterine from the blood, and its discharge from the body in the form of stercorine (the seroline of Boudet). [New York, 1862?] 61p. 3 plates. DNLM; NNNAM **60-0591**

FLINT, Austin, Jr. (1836-1915)
The physiology of man; designed to represent the existing state of physiological science, as applied to the functions of the human body. Introduction; the blood; circulation; respiration. New York: D. Appleton & Co., 1866. 502p. DNLM; MBM; NNNAM; PU **60-0592**

FLINT, Austin, Jr. (1836-1915)
The physiology of man; designed to represent the existing state of physiological science as applied to the functions of the human body. . . . New York: D. Appleton & Company, 1866-75. 5 v. CtY-M; DLC; NNNAM; OCIM **60-0593**

FLINT, Austin, Jr. (1836-1915)
The physiology of man. . . . Alimentation; digestion; absorption; lymph and chyle. New York: D. Appleton & Co., 1867. 556p. DNLM; NNNAM; PPC; PU **60-0594**

FLINT, Austin, Jr. (1836-1915)
Experiments undertaken for the prupose of reconciling some of the discordant observations upon the glycogenic function of the liver. [New York, 1869.] 11p. DNLM; NNNAM
60-0595

FOLSOM, James
The mariner's medical guide; designed for the use of ships, families, and plantations; containing the symptoms and treatment of diseases; also a list of medicines, their uses, and the mode of administering, when a physician cannot be procured. Selected from standard works. 3rd ed. Boston: J. Folsom, 1864. 189p. 1 plate. DNLM; MBM; MWA
60-0596

FOLSOM, Norton (1842-1903)
An essay on the senses of smell and taste; to which was awarded the prize of the Boylston Medical Society in 1863. Boston: D. Clapp, 1863. 8p. DNLM; MBM
60-0597

FONDA, Sebastian F.
Analysis of Sharon waters, Schoharie County; also of Avon, Richfield, and Bedford mineral waters. With directions for invalids. New York: Craighead, 1860. 96p. DNLM
60-0598

FOOTE, Edward Bliss (1829-1906)
Medical common sense; applied to the causes, prevention and cure of chronic diseases and unhappiness in marriage. . . . Rev. and enl. ed. New York: Pub. by the author, 1863. 390p. DLC; NNNAM **60-0599**

FOOTE, Edward Bliss (1829-1906)
. . . Comfort and cure for the ruptured. . . . New York: E. B. Foote, 1865. 24p. DLC; DNLM; NNNAM **60-0600**

FOOTE, Edward Bliss (1829-1906)
. . . Cold feet: the cause, prevention, and cure, together with other valuable advice. . . . New York, 1867. 6p. DLC; NNNAM **60-0601**

FOOTE, Elial T[odd] (1796-1877)
Inaugural address and transactions of the Connecticut Homoeopathic Medical Society, 1864-1865. New Haven: J. T. Stafford, 1866. 32p. CtY-M; PPHa **60-0602**

FOOTE, George F[ranklin] (1817-1889)
Homoeopathic insane asylum [argument in favor of]. [New York, 1869?] 7p. DNLM **60-0603**

FORBES, W. S[mith] (1831-1905)
History of the anatomy act of Pennsylvania. Philadelphia, 1867. 23p. DNLM; PPC **60-0604**

FORD, Corydon L. (1813-1894)
Questions in osteology. Ann Arbor, Mich., 1861. 16p. DNLM **60-0605**

FORD, Corydon L. (1813-1894)
Questions on anatomy, for the use of students. Ann Arbor: A. W. Chase, 1865. 64p. DNLM **60-0606**

FORD, Corydon L. (1813-1894)
Questions on histology and physiology, on the plan on "Questions on anatomy." Ann Arbor, Mich., 1869. 64p. DNLM **60-0607**

[FORMAN, Jacob Gilbert]
The Western Sanitary Commission; a sketch of its origin, history, labors for the sick and wounded of the western armies, and aid given to freedmen and Union refugees, with incidents of hospital life. St. Louis: Pub. for the Mississippi Valley Sanitary Fair, R. P. Studley & Co., 1864. 144p. DLC; DNLM **60-0608**

FOSTER, Samuel Conant (1816-1878)
The physician's knowledge. An oration delivered before the New York Academy of Medicine, at its fifteenth anniversary, November 11, 1862. . . . Published by order of the Academy. New York, 1863. 29p. DLC; DNLM; NNNAM **60-0609**

FOUNTAIN, Ezra James (1828-1861)
An essay on the treatment of phthisis by the chlorate of potash; with observations on oxygen as a therapeutic agent, and the exposition of a new theory of the formation of ozone. Read before the American Medical Association at its thirteenth annual session, held at New Haven, June, 1860. . . . New York: Hall, Clayton & Co., printers, 1860. 23p. DLC; NNNAM **60-0610**

FOWLER, Edward Payson (1833-1914)
Prevention and treatment of Asiatic cholera. New York: Smith & Sons, 1866. 8p. NNNAM; PPHa **60-0611**

FOWLER, Orson Squire (1809-1887)
. . . Offspring, and their hereditary endowment: or, Paternity, maternity, and infancy; including sexuality; its laws, facts, impairment, restoration, and perfection, as taught by phrenology and physiology, together with warning and advice to youth. . . . Boston: O. S. Fowler, [1869]. 278p. DLC; MBM **60-0612**

FOWNES, George (1815-1849)
Elementary chemistry. . . . From the 7th revised and corrected London ed. Edited by R. Bridges. Philadelphia: Blanchard & Lea, 1862. 600p. DNLM; MH; NN; PU **60-0613**

[FRANCIS, John Wakefield] (1789-1861)
. . . Catalogue of the . . . library, both medical and miscellaneous, of the late Dr. John W. Francis, LL.D. The . . . books . . . will be sold at auction . . . by Bangs, Merwin & Co. . . . N.Y. . . . N[ew] Y[ork]: C. Shelley, Printer, 1862. 126p. DLC; NNNAM [3159 entries] **60-0614**

FRANCIS, Samuel Ward (1835-1886)
Report of Professor Valentine Mott's surgical cliniques in the University of New York, session 1859-1860. . . . New York: S. S. & W. Wood, 1860. 209p. 2 plates. DLC; NNNAM; NNU-M **60-0615**

FRANCIS, Samuel Ward (1835-1886)
Water: its history, characteristics, hygienic and therapeutic uses. . . . New York: S. S. & W. Wood, 1861. 47p. DLC; NNNAM **60-0616**

FRANCIS, Samuel Ward (1835-1886)
Memoir of the life and character of Prof. Valentine Mott, facile princeps. . . . New York: W. J. Widdleton, 1865. 32p. DLC; NNNAM; NNU-M **60-0617**

FRANCIS, Samuel Ward (1835-1886)
Memoir of the life and character of Prof. Valentine Mott, facile princeps. . . . 2nd ed. New York: W. J. Widdleton, 1865. 32p. DLC; NNNAM; NNU-M **60-0618**

FRANCIS, Samuel Ward (1835-1886)
Biographical sketches of distinguished living New York surgeons. . . . New York: J. Bradburn, 1866. 220p. DLC; NN; NNNAM; NNC **60-0619**

FRANCIS, Samuel Ward (1835-1886)
Biographical sketches of distinguished living New York physicians. . . . New York: G. P. Putnam & Son, 1867. 228p. DLC; NN; NNC; NNNAM **60-0620**

FRANKLIN, Edward C. (1822-1885)
Statistics of homoeopathic and allopathic hospitals. St. Louis: H. C. G. Luyties, Homoeopathic Pharmacy, 1864. 8p. DNLM; PPHa **60-0621**

FRANKLIN, Edward C. (1822-1885)
Statistics of homoeopathic and allopathic hospitals. St. Louis Homoeopathic Pharmacy, T. W. Ustick, 1864. 8p. PPHa **60-0622**

FRANKLIN, Edward C. (1822-1885)
Valedictory address to the graduating class of the Homoeopathic Medical College of Missouri. Detroit: Lodge's Homoeopathic Pharmacy, 1866. 14p. DNLM **60-0623**

FRANKLIN, Edward C. (1822-1885)
The science and art of surgery, embracing minor and operative surgery; compiled from standard allopathic authorities, and adapted to homoeopathic therapeutics, with a general history of surgery from the earliest periods to the present time, for the use of practitioners and students of the homoeopathic practice of medicine. . . . Illustrated by new and copious engravings, and many original cuts from the author's private museum. St. Louis: Missouri Democrat Book and Job Print, 1867-1873. 2 v. DNLM **60-0624**

FRANKLIN, Edward C. (1822-1885)
Osteo-sarcoma of the inferior maxillary. Operation for its removal. Albany: Van Benthuysen & Sons, 1868. 6p. 2 plates. PPHa **60-0625**

FRANKLIN, Edward C. (1822-1885)
Hypertrophy of the tarso-phalangeal portion of the foot. Operation for its removal. Albany: Van Benthuysen & Sons, 1868. 5p. PPHa **60-0626**

FRASER, Edwin J.
Medical electricity; a treatise on the nature of vital electricity in health and disease, with plain instructions in the uses of artificial electricity as a curative agent. Chicago, Ill.: C. S. Halsey, 1863. 56p. OCIM; PPHa **60-0627**

FRAZEE, L. J[acob] (1819-1905)
Valedictory address to the graduating class of the medical department, University of Louisville. Louisville, Ky.: J. F. Morton & Co., 1867. 30p. DNLM; OCIM **60-0628**

FRELIGH, Martin (1813-1889)
The homoeopathic pocket companion; or, A simplified abridgement of the "Homoeopathic practice of medicine." Designed expressly for the use of families and travellers. . . . 7th ed. New York: C. T. Hurlburt, 1867. 291p. DLC; NNNAM; PPHa **60-0629**

FRELIGH, Martin (1813-1889)
Homeopatia familiar. Compendio simplificado de la "Práctica homeopática de la medicina." Adaptado al uso de familias y viajeros. . . . New York: C. T. Hurlburt, 1869. 319p. DLC; NNNAM **60-0630**

FRICK, Charles (1823-1860)
General remarks on diuretic remedies. Baltimore: J. W. Wood, [1860]. 26p. DNLM; MdU-D **60-0631**

FROST, James H. P. (1825-1875)
Introductory address delivered at the opening of the eighteenth annual session of the Homoeopathic Medical College of Pennsylvania, October 10, 1865. Philadelphia: King & Baird, 1865. 24p. DNLM; PPHa **60-0632**

FULLER, Henry William (1820-1873)
On diseases of the lungs and air-passages: their pathology, physical diagnosis, symptoms, and treatment. . . . From the 2nd and rev. London ed. Philadelphia: Henry C. Lea, 1867. 479p. DLC; OCIM; PPC; PU **60-0633**

FUSSELL, Edwin (1813-1882)
Valedictory address to the graduating class of the Female Medical College of Pennsylvania, at the tenth annual commencement, March 13th, 1861. . . . Published by the class. Philadelphia: J. B. Chandler, printer, 1861. 16p. DLC; PPC; PU **60-0634**

GAGE, Thomas H[ovey] (1826-1909)
A case of hydrophobia: with remarks. (Paper read before the Medical Society meeting, January, 1865). Worcester, Mass.: Worcester District Medical Society. 26p. MBM **60-0635**

GAILLARD, Edwin Samuel (1827-1885)
Ozone: its relations to health and disease. An essay which received the Fiske fund premium of the Rhode Island Medical Society, June, 1861. . . . [Boston, 1864.] 53p. DLC; DNLM; MBM **60-0636**

GAILLARD, Edwin Samuel (1827-1885)
Diphtheria: a prize essay. Richmond, Va.: Richmond Medical Journal Office, 1867. 114p. DNLM **60-0637**

GAILLARD, Edwin Samuel (1827-1885)
The medical and surgical lessons of the late war. The introductory address delivered before the medical class of the Kentucky School of Medicine, Louisville, Ky., Oct. 5, 1868. . . . Louisville, Ky.: Louisville Journal Job Print, 1868. 16p. DLC; DNLM; OCIM **60-0638**

GANOT, A[dolphe] (1804-1887)
Elementary treatise on physics, experimental and applied. Transl. and edited by E. Atkinson. 3rd ed. New York: William Wood & Co., 1868. 861p. DNLM; NNNAM **60-0639**

GARDETTE, Emile B[laise] (1803-1887)
Biographical memoir of William Draper Brinkli, M.D. Philadelphia: C. Sherman, Son & Co., 1863. 54p. DNLM; PPC **60-0640**

GARDINER, D. Pereira
A new medical dictionary. . . . On the basis of Hooper and Grant. New York: Harper & Brothers, 1864. 686p. DNLM; MBM; NNNAM; PPC **60-0641**

GARDNER, Augustus Kinsley (1821-1876)
Eulogy on John W. Francis, M.D., LL.D., delivered before the New York Medico-Chirurgical College, March 7, 1861. . . . New York: Hall, Clayton & Co., printers, 1861. 24p. DLC; DNLM; NNNAM **60-0642**

GARDNER, Augustus Kinsley (1821-1876)
Eulogy on Richard Sharp Kissam, A.M., M.D., read before the New York Academy of Medicine, December 3rd, 1862. . . . New York: C. A. Alvord, printer, 1863. 28p. DLC; NNNAM **60-0643**

GARDNER, Augustus Kinsley (1821-1876)
Gonorrhoea; a non-specific disease. New York, 1864. 11p. DNLM; NNNAM **60-0644**

GARRATT, Alfred Charles (1813?-1891)
Electro-physiology and electro-therapeutics; showing the best methods for the medical uses of electricity. . . . Boston: Ticknor & Fields, 1860. 708p. DLC; DNLM; MH-M; NNNAM **60-0645**

GARRATT, Alfred Charles (1813?-1891)
Electro-physiology and electro-therapeutics; showing the best methods for the medical uses of electricity. . . . 2nd ed., with additions. Boston: Ticknor & Fields, 1861. 716p. DLC; MBM; NNNAM; PPC **60-0646**

GARRATT, Alfred Charles (1813?-1891)
Medical electricity: embracing electro-physiology and electricity; as a therapeutic, with special reference to practical medicine: showing the most approved apparatus, methods and rules, for the medical uses of electricity in the treatment of nervous diseases. . . . 3rd ed., rev. and illustrated. 1108p., fold. diagr. DLC; MBM; OCIM; PPC **60-0647**

GARRATT, Alfred Charles (1813?-1891)
Guide for using medical batteries: (being a compendium from his larger work on medical electricity and nervous diseases), showing the most approved apparatus, methods and rules, for the medical employment of electricity in the treatment of nervous diseases. . . . Philadelphia: Lindsay & Blakiston, 1867. 180p. DLC; DNLM; PPC; PU **60-0648**

GARRETSON, James E[dmund] (1828-1895)
A treatise on the diseases and surgery of the mouth, jaws, and associate parts. Philadelpia: J. B. Lippincott & Co., 1869. 700p. DNLM; PPC; PPJ; PU **60-0649**

GARROD, Alfred B[aring] (1819-1907)
On gout and rheumatism, their differential diagnosis, and the nature of so-called rheumatic gout. New York: William Wood & Co., 1865. 439p. DNLM; OCIM; NNNAM; PPC **60-0650**

GAUSE, Owen B[everly] (1825-1895)
Valedictory address delivered at the annual commencement of the Hahnemann Medical College of Philadelphia, March 4, 1868. Philadelphia: King & Baird, 1868. 16p. PPHa; PPC **60-0651**

GAY, Charles Curtis Fenn (1821-1886)
Puerperal eclampsia. [Buffalo, 1869.] 11p. DNLM **60-0652**

GAY, Charles Curtis Fenn (1821-1886)
Venesection as one of the means for the arrest of unavoidable hemorrhage. [Philadelphia, 1869.] 8p. DNLM; PPC **60-0653**

GAY, George H[enry] (1823?-1878)
A few remarks on the primary treatment of wounds received in battle; a report to the Surgeon-General of Massachusetts. Boston: D. Clapp, 1862. 8p. DNLM; MH-M **60-0654**

GEARY, John Fitzgibbon (1814-1883)
Epidemic cholera; its modes of treatment, their respective results, with directions for prevention and what to do in cases of sudden emergency. San Francisco: H. H. Bancroft & Co., 1866. 54p. OCIM; PPHa **60-0655**

GEBHARD, Lewis P. (1791-1873)
Address before the Philadelphia County Medical Society. Delivered February 8, 1865 . . . at the close of his official term as president. Philadelphia: Collins, Printer, 1865. 53p. DLC; PPC; PU **60-0656**

GEORGIA MEDICAL SOCIETY. SAVANNAH
Report of the committee of the Georgia Medical Society, on the hygienic condition of the city of Savannah, and surrounding country, made to the Society, and adopted May 16, 1866. Savannah, Ga.: C. E. O'Sullivan, printer, 1866. 12p. DLC; DNLM **60-0657**

GERHARD, William W. (1809-1872)
Lectures on the diagnosis, pathology, and treatment of the diseases of the chest. 4th ed. Philadelphia: J. B. Lippincott & Co., 1860. 448p. 1 plate. DNLM; NNNAM; PPC; PU **60-0658**

GETCHELL, F. H[orace] (1836-1907)
The material management of infancy. For the use of parents. Philadelphia: J. B. Lippincott & Co., 1868. 67p. DNLM; OCIM; NNNAM; PPC **60-0659**

THE GETTYSBURG Spring, its remarkable history, embracing statements of physicians and the people, of its wonderful cures. New York: J. K. Van Slyke & Co., 1868. 23p. DNLM; NNNAM **60-0660**

GIBBONS, Henry, Sr. (1808-1884)
University of the Pacific. Fifth annual announcement of the medical department, session of 1862-1863; also valedictory address. San Francisco: Towne & Bacon, 1862. 29p. DNLM **60-0661**

GIBBONS, Henry. Sr. (1808-1884)
Tobacco and its effects. A prize essay, showing that the use of tobacco is a physical, mental, moral, and social evil. New York: Carlton & Lanahan, 1868. 48p. DNLM; NNNAM **60-0662**

GIBBONS, Henry, Sr. (1808-1884)
Annual address before the San Francisco Medical Society, delivered pursuant to appointment, November 9, 1869. . . . San Francisco: Clarke, Book and Job Printer, 1869. 22p. DLC **60-0663**

GIBBS, O. C. (1824?-1871)
A report on epidemics and endemics. Read before the Medical Society of Southwestern New York. Philadelphia: J. B. Lippincott & Co., 1861. 44p. DNLM; PPC **60-0664**

GIFFORD, J. B.
Manual of specific homoeopathy: being a treatise on the common diseases of life. . . . Also directions for treatment with Gifford's homoeopathic remedies. . . . New York: P. Lee, [1861]. 88p. DLC; NNNAM; PPHa **60-0665**

GILCHRIST, J. Grant (1842-1906)
Rules for the finding and tying of the principal arteries. Chicago: C. S. Halsey, 1867. 16p. OCIM; PPHa **60-0666**

GLONINGER, D. S[tanley] (1827-1889)
The medical examiner's manual. . . . Philadelphia: Claxton, Remsen, and Haffelfinger, 1869. 52p. DLC; PPC; PU **60-0667**

GOBRECHT, William H. (1828-1901)
Valedictory address to the graduates of the medical department of Pennsylvania College. Philadelphia: Collins, 1860. 16p. DNLM; PPC **60-0668**

GOBRECHT, William H. (1828-1901)
Salutatory to the class of the Medical College of Ohio. Cincinnati: R. W. Carroll & Co., 1867. 20p. DNLM; OCIM **60-0669**

GOLDSMITH, Middleton (1818-1887)
The compound solution of bromine. Formula and direction for use. Louisville, 1863. 1 sheet. fol. DNLM **60-0670**

GOLDSMITH, Middleton (1818-1887)
A report on hospital gangrene, erysipelas and pyaemia, as observed in the departments of the Ohio and the Cumberland. Louisville: Bradley & Gilbert, 1863. 95p. 1 table. DNLM **60-0671**

GOODMAN, J[ohn] (1837-1912)
A new method of conducting the after-treatment in the operation for vesico-vaginal fistula. Louisville: Bell & Co., 1869. 8p. DNLM **60-0672**

GOODWIN, E. J.
The special treatment of syphilis, chronic rheumatism, and scrofula. Richmond: Gary & Clemmitt, 1866. 28p. DNLM **60-0673**

GOSSE, Philip H.
Evenings at the microscope; or, researches among the minuter organs and forms of animal life. . . . New York: D. Appleton & Co., 1860. 480p. NN; NNC; NNU-M
60-0674

GOULD, Benjamin Apthorp (1824-1896)
Investigations in the military and anthropological statistics of American soldiers. New York: United States Sanitary Commission, 1869. 655p. 7 tables. DNLM; MH; NN; NNNAM
60-0675

GOULEY, John W. S. (1832-1920)
On external perineal urethrotomy, or an improved method of external division of the urethra in perinaeo, for the relief of obstinate stricture. With remarks on the preparatory- and after-treatment. New York: D. Appleton & Co., 1869. 32p. 1 fig. DNLM; NNNAM; PPC; PU **60-0676**

GRACE, William
The army surgeon's manual, for the use of medical officers, cadets, chaplains, and hospital stewards, containing the regulations of the Medical Department, all general orders from the War Department, and circulars from the Surgeon-General's Office . . . 1861, to . . . 1864. . . . New York: Bailliere Brothers, 1864. 200p. DLC; MBM; NNNAM; PPC
60-0677

GRACE, William
The army surgeon's manual, for the use of medical officers, cadets, chaplains, and hospital stewards, containing the regulations of the Medical Department, all general orders from the War Department, and circular from the Surgeon-General's office . . . to . . . 1865. . . . 2nd ed. . . . New York: Bailliere Brothers, 1865. 225p. DLC; NNNAM; OCIM; PPC
60-0678

GRAY, Henry (1827-1861)
Anatomy, descriptive and surgical. The drawings by H. V. Carter. The dissections jointly by the author and Dr. Carter. 2nd American from the revised and enlarged London ed. Philadelphia: Blanchard & Lea, 1862. 816p. DNLM; MH-M; NNNAM; PPC **60-0679**

GRAY, John Franklin (1804-1882)
The early annals of homoeopathy in New York. A discourse before the Homoeopathic Societies of New York and Brooklyn, on the 10th of April, 1863, the anniversary of the birthday of Hahnemann. New York: Published by the Homoeopathic Medical Society of the County of New York, 1863. 30p. NNNAM; PPHa **60-0680**

GRAY, John Franklin (1804-1882)
Homoeopathy in New York, and the late Abraham D. Wilson, A.M., M.D. By his early friend, John F. Gray. New York: Published by request of the Homoeopathic Medical Societies of the County and State of New York. William S. Dorr, Printer, 1865. 39p. DNLM **60-0681**

GRAY, John P[erdue] (1825-1886)
General paresis, or incomplete progressive paralysis. Albany: C. Van Benthuysen, 1866. 33p. DNLM
60-0682

GRAY, John P[erdue] (1825-1886)
Inaugural address before the Medical Society of the State of New York, February 4, 1868. Albany: C. Van Benthuysen & Sons, 1868. 12p. DNLM **60-0683**

GRAY, John P[erdue] (1825-1886)
Annual address before the Medical Society of the State of New York. Utica, N.Y.: Roberts, 1868. 30p. DNLM
60-0684

GREEN, Horace (1802-1866)
On the difficulties and advantags of catheterism of the air-passages in diseases of the chest. [New York, 1860.] 24p. DNLM; NNNAM **60-0685**

GREEN, Horace (1802-1866)
Selections from favorite prescriptions of living American practitioners. New York: J. Wiley, 1860. 214p. DNLM; NNNAM; OCIM; PPC **60-0686**

GREEN, Horace (1802-1866)
A practical treatise on pulmonary tuberculosis. Embracing its history, pathology, and treatment. . . . New York: J. Wiley, 1864. 355p. col. plates. DLC; DNLM; MH-M; NNNAM
60-0687

[GREEN, Horace] (1802-1866)
Death of Dr. Horace Green [1802-1866]. [New York, 1867.] 3p. DNLM; NNNAM **60-0688**

GREEN, John (1835-1913)
City hospitals. . . . Boston: Little, Brown, & Company, 1861. 66p. DLC; DNLM; MBM **60-0689**

GREEN, John (1835-1913)
Case of fracture of the thigh treated by immovable apparatus of gypsum. Boston, 1863. 3p. DNLM; MBM
60-0690

GREEN, John (1835-1913)
On amputation of the thigh. [Boston, 1863.] 34p. DNLM; MBM **60-0691**

GREEN, John (1835-1913)
Mechanical ulcer of stump. Boston, 1863. 3p. DNLM; MBM
60-0692

GREEN, John
On the detection and measurement of astigmatism. [Philadelphia, 1867.] 11p. DNLM; PU **60-0693**

GREEN, John Orne (1799-1885)
A memorial of John C. Dalton, M.D. (Delivered before the Middlesex North District Medical Society, April 27, 1864.) Cambridge: University Press, 1864. 35p. MBM; NNNAM
60-0694

GREEN, Traill (1813-1897)
The true physician a student of nature, and medical science in harmony with divine law. An address. Philadelphia: Collins, 1868. 23p. DNLM; PPC **60-0695**

GREENE, William Warren (1831-1881)
Significance of a diploma; a valedictory address. Berkshire Medical College. Pittsfield, Mass.: H. Chickering, 1862. 8p. DNLM **60-0696**

GREENE, William Warren (1831-1881)
Cases of ovariotomy, with some remarks upon the operation. [Boston, 1868.] 8p. DNLM; MBM **60-0697**

GREENHOW, E. Headlam (1814-1888)
On diphtheria. New York: Bailliere Brothers, 1861. 160p. DNLM; NNNAM **60-0698**

GREENLEAF, Charles R[avenscroft] (1838-1911)
A manual for the medical officers of the United States Army. Philadelphia: J. B. Lippincott & Co., 1864. 199p. DNLM; NNNAM **60-0699**

GREGG, Rollin R[obinson] (1828-1886)
Synopsis of a forthcoming work upon consumption and its numerous kindred maladies; with tracings of their causes, and of their cures under homoeopathic treatment. . . . Buffalo: Printing House of Matthews & Warren, 1865. 33p. DLC; DNLM **60-0700**

GREGG, Rollin R[obinson] (1828-1886)
The physical evils of alcohol. [Buffalo, 1869.] 24p. DNLM **60-0701**

[GREGORY, Samuel] (1813-1872)
Female physicians. [Boston: N. E. Female Medical College, 1864.] 8p. DLC; MBM **60-0702**

GREGORY, Samuel (1813-1872)
The war against the New England Female Medical College. Circular to members of the Massachusetts legislature. Boston: A. Mudge & Son, 1866. 27p. DNLM; MBM **60-0703**

GREGORY, Samuel (1813-1872)
Doctor or doctress? Boston, 1868. 8p. DNLM; MBM **60-0704**

GRINDLE, Wesley
The sexual system, and medical companion. . . . Philadelphia: [Printed by Smith & Peters], 1864. 377p. DLC; NNNAM; PPC **60-0705**

GRISCOM, John Hoskins (1809-1874)
Sanitary legislation, past and future; the value of sanitary reform, and the true principles for its attainment. New York: E. Jones & Co., 1861. 37p. DNLM; NNNAM **60-0706**

GRISCOM, John Hoskins (1809-1874)
An improved method of house ventilation. With evidences of its efficacy and general applicability. New York: G. F. Nesbitt & Co., 1862. 12p. DNLM; NNNAM **60-0707**

GRISCOM, John Hoskins (1809-1874)
Case of diarrhoea adiposa. Philadelpha: Collins, 1863. 12p. DNLM **60-0708**

GRISCOM, John Hoskins (1809-1874)
A history, chronological and circumstantial, of the visitations of yellow fever at New York. [New York, 1864?] 36p. DNLM **60-0709**

GRISCOM, John Hoskins (1809-1874)
The physiological and dietetic relations of phosphorus. Philadelphia: Collins, 1864. 20p. DNLM **60-0710**

GRISCOM, John Hoskins (1809-1874)
The where, the when, the why, and the how of the first appearance and greatest prevalence of cholera in cities. . . . [New York, 1866.] 21p. DLC; NNNAM **60-0711**

GRISCOM, John Hoskins (1809-1874)
Report of sub-committee of the New York Academy of Medicine on ventilation. June 6, 1866. New York: New York Printing Co., 1866. 10p. DNLM; NNNAM **60-0712**

GRISCOM, John Hoskins (1809-1874)
Essay on the therapeutic value of certain articles of the materia medica of recent introduction. Albany: C. Van Benthuysen & Son, 1868. 19p. DNLM **60-0713**

GRISCOM, John Hoskins (1809-1874)
Prison hygiene; an essay prepared at the request of the Prison Association of New York for insertion in their twenty-third annual report, and reprinted by their order. Albany: C. Van Benthuysen & Sons, 1868. 23p. DNLM **60-0714**

GROSS, Reuben Herman
Doctor R. H. Gross' comparative materia medica. Edited by Constantine Hering. Philadelphia: F. E. Boericke, 1867. 520p. DLC; PPC; PPHa; PU **60-0715**

GROSS, Samuel D[avid] (1805-1884)
Valedictory address to the graduates of the Jefferson Medical College of Philadelphia. Delivered at the public commencement, held March 12, 1860. Published by the graduating class. Philadelphia: J. M. Wilson, 1860. 16, 4p. PPJ **60-0716**

GROSS, Samuel D[avid] (1805-1884)
Practical observations upon the nature and treatment of prostatorrhoea. Philadelphia: J. B. Lippincott & Co., 1860. 9p. DNLM; PPJ **60-0717**

GROSS, S[amuel] D[avid] (1805-1884)
Remarkable case of melanosis or black cancer. Philadelphia: J. B. Lippincott & Co., 1860. 7p. PPJ **60-0718**

GROSS, Samuel D[avid] (1805-1884)
A sketch of the life, character, and services of Ambrose Paré. . . . Philadelphia: J. B. Lippincott & Co., 1861. 27p. DLC; PPC; PPJ; PU **60-0719**

GROSS, Samuel D[avid] (1805-1884)
Necrological notice of Jedediah Cobb. Philadelphia, 1861. 8p. PPJ **60-0720**

GROSS, Samuel D[avid], ed. (1805-1884)
Lives of eminent American physicians and surgeons of the nineteenth century. . . . Philadelphia: Lindsay & Blakiston, 1861. 836p. DLC; NNNAM; OCIM; PPC **60-0721**

GROSS, Samuel D[avid] (1805-1884)
A manual of military surgery; or, Hints on the emergencies of field, camp and hospital practice. Illustrated with wood-cuts. . . . Philadelphia: J. B. Lippincott & Co., 1861. 186p. DLC; MBM; NNNAM; PPJ **60-0722**

GROSS, Samuel D[avid] (1805-1884)
A manual of military surgery; or, Hints on the emergencies of field, camp and hospital practice. Illustrated with wood-cuts. . . . [2nd ed.] . . . Philadelphia: J. B. Lippincott & Co., 1862. 186p. DLC; NNNAM; PPC; PPJ **60-0723**

GROSS, Samuel D[avid] (1805-1884)
A manual of military surgery; or, Hints on the emergencies of field, camp and hospital practice. . . . Richmond, Va.: J. W. Randolph, 1862. 96p. DLC; PPC; PU; ViRA **.60-0724**

GROSS, Samuel D[avid] (1805-1884)
A system of surgery; pathological, diagnostic, therapeutic and operative. . . . Illustrated by twelve hundred and twenty-seven engravings. 2nd ed., much enl. and carefully rev. . . . Philadelphia: Blanchard & Lea, 1862. 2 v. DLC; NNNAM; PPC; PPJ **60-0725**

GROSS, Samuel D[avid] (1805-1884)
System of surgery; pathological, diagnostic, therapeutic and operative. . . . 3rd ed. Philadelphia: Blanchard & Lea, 1864. 2 v. MBM; NNNAM; PPC; PPJ **60-0726**

GROSS, Samuel D[avid] (1805-1884)
Biographical sketch of Charles Wilkins Short. [Philadelphia, 1865.] 31p. DNLM **60-0727**

GROSS, Samuel D[avid] (1805-1884)
A system of surgery; pathological, diagnostic, therapeutic, and operative. . . . 4th ed. Philadelphia: Henry C. Lea, 1866. 2 v. DNLM; NNNAM; PPC; PPJ **60-0728**

GROSS, S[amuel] D[avid] (1805-1884)
Then and now: a discourse introductory to the forty-third course of lectures in the Jefferson Medical College of Philadelphia. . . . Philadelphia: Collins, Printer, 1867. 44p. DLC; PPJ **60-0729**

GROSS, Samuel D[avid] (1805-1884)
The live physician. Charge to the graduates at the forty-third annual commencement of the Jefferson Medical College of Philadelphia. Philadelphia: Collins, 1868. 24p. DNLM; PPJ **60-0730**

GROSS, Samuel D[avid] (1805-1884)
Memoir of Valentine Mott, M.D., LL.D., professor of surgery in the University of the City of New York; member of the Institute of France. . . . New York: D. Appleton & Co.; Philadelphia: Lindsay & Blakiston, 1868. 96p. front. (port.). DLC; NNNAM; PPC; PPJ **60-0731**

GROSS, Samuel D[avid] (1805-1884)
Address; [before the American Medical Association]. Philadelphia: Collins, 1868. 20p. PPJ **60-0732**

GROSS, Samuel D[avid] (1805-1884)
Remarks on the training of nurses. Read originally as a report before the American Medical Association at its meeting at New Orleans, May, 1869, and referred by it to the several state medical societies. Philadelphia, 1869. 15p. DNLM; PPJ; PPC; PU **60-0733**

GROSS, S[amuel] D[avid] (1805-1884)
Memoir of Robley Dunglison, M.D., LL.D. Read before the College of Physicians at a special meeting held October 20th, 1869. Philadelphia: Collins, 1869. 22p. DNLM; PPC; PPJ; PU **60-0734**

GROSS, Samuel W[eissell] (1837-1889)
Case of poisoning by three grains of atropia. Philadelphia: Collins, 1869. 10p. DNLM; PPJ **60-0735**

GUERNSEY, Egbert (1823-1903)
Homoeopathic domestic practice, containing also chapters on physiology, anatomy, and an abridged materia medica. 5th ed. New York: W. Radde, 1862. 653p. 5 plates. DNLM; OCIM; NNNAM; PPC **60-0736**

GUERNSEY, Egbert (1823-1903)
Valedictory address at the fourth annual commencement of the New York Homoeopathic Medical College. New York: Harper & Brothers, 1864. 16p. DNLM; NNNAM **60-0737**

GUERNSEY, Egbert (1823-1903)
Address before the Ulster County Homoeopathic Medical Society. New York: J. A. Gray & Green, 1867. 16p. DNLM; NNNAM **60-0738**

GUERNSEY, Henry Newell (1817-1885)
Valedictory address delivered to the graduating class of the Homoeopathic Medical College of Pennsylvania, at the sixteenth annual commencement, March 2, 1864. Philadelphia: C. Sherman, Son & Co., 1864. 29p. DLC; PPHa **60-0739**

GUERNSEY, Henry Newell (1817-1885)
An introductory lecture comprising the principles of obstetrics and the diseases of women and children, as taught in the Homoeopathic Medical College of Pennsylvania. . . . Philadelphia: King & Baird, 1865. 14p. PPHa **60-0740**

GUERNSEY, Henry Newell (1817-1885)
Report on obstetrics to the American Institute of Homoeopathy. Philadelphia: King & Baird, 1867. 8p. PPHa **60-0741**

GUERNSEY, Henry Newell (1817-1885)
The application of the principles and practice of homoeopathy to obstetrics and the disorders peculiar to women and young children. . . . With nearly one hundred illustrations. Philadelphia: F. E. Boericke, 1867. 752p. DLC; PPHa **60-0742**

GUERNSEY, Henry Newell (1817-1885)
The bandage after parturition. Philadelphia: Sherman & Co., 1868. 20p. PPHa **60-0743**

GUERNSEY, Henry Newell (1817-1885)
Reproduction, physically, physiologically, and spiritually considered. Read before the Philadelphia Homoeopathic Medical Society, November 12, 1868. Philadelphia: Sherman & Co., 1868. 15p. PPHa **60-0744**

GUILD, J. H.
A practical treatise on spasmodic asthma, its causes, symptoms, and the various methods of its treatment; together with a full description of the only rational mode of cure, fully attested and approved after a most thorough trial in over 10,000 cases. Rutland: Tuttle & Co., 1869. 23p. DNLM **60-0745**

GUNN, John C. (1800-1863)
Gunn's new domestic physician: or, Home book of health. . . . With supplementary treatises on anatomy, physiology, and hygiene, and on nursing the sick, and the management of the sick room. . . . Cincinnati: Moore, Wilstach, Keys & Co., 1863. 1129p. plates. DLC; OCIM **60-0746**

GUNN, John C. (1800-1863)
. . . Gunn's new family physician: or, Home book of health; forming a complete household guide. . . . With supplementary treatises on anatomy, physiology, and hygiene, on domestic and sanitary economy, and on physical culture and development. Newly illustrated, and re-stereotyped. Cincinnati: Moore, Wilstach & Baldwin, 1864. 1213p. DLC; OCIM **60-0747**

GUNN, John C. (1800-1863)
Gunn's neuer hausarzt, oder Handbuch der gesundheit. Ein vollständiger leitfaden für familien. . . . Nach der 17. stereotyp. aufl. des englischen originals für das deutsche publikum bearb. von dr. C. A. Rodin, unter mitwirkung von Johann Eggers. . . . Cincinnati: Moore, Wilstach & Baldwin, 1864. 1088p. plates. DLC; NNNAM; OCIM **60-0748**

GUNN, Moses (1822-1887)
Luxations of the hip and shoulder joints, and the agents which oppose their reductions. 2nd ed. Chicago: R. Fergus' Sons, 1869. 20p. DNLM **60-0749**

GUNNING, Thomas Brian
Treatment of fracture of the lower jaw by interdental splints. New York: J. Medole, 1866. 36, 3p. DNLM; NNNAM **60-0750**

GUNNING, Thomas Brian
On the physiological action of the muscles concerned in the movements of the lower jaw. New York: H. Ludwig, 1868. 21p. 1 plate. DNLM; NNNAM **60-0751**

GUTHRIE, George James (1785-1856)
. . . Directions to army surgeons on the field of battle. By G. J. Guthrie, surgeon general to the British forces during the Crimean War. Adopted by the Commission and printed for the use of U.S.A. surgeons. By order: Fred. Law Olmsted, secretary. (2nd ed.). [Washington, 1861]. 9p. DLC [U.S. Sanitary Commission, Documents, No. 14]. **60-0752**

GUTHRIE, George James (1785-1856)
. . . Directions to army surgeons on the field of battle. By G. J. Guthrie, surgeon general to the British forces during the Crimean War. Adopted by the Commission and printed for the use of U.S.A. surgeons. By order: Fred. Law Olmsted, secretary. (3rd ed.). [New York, 1861]. 8p. DLC [U.S. Sanitary Commission, Medical and Surgical Monographs, B] **60-0753**

GUTHRIE, George James (1785-1856)
Commentaries on surgery of the war in Portugal, Spain, France, and the Netherlands, from the battle of Rolica, in 1808, to that of Waterloo in 1815, with additions relating to those in Crimea in 1854-1855. 6th ed. Philadelphia: J. B. Lippincott & Co., 1862. 614p. DNLM; NNNAM; PPC; PU **60-0754**

GUTMANN, Edward
A treatise on baths and vapor baths. [Transl. from the German.] New York: Koppel Bros., [1863]. 32p. 1 plate. DNLM; NNNAM **60-0755**

HAGNER, Daniel R[andall] (1830-1893)
. . . Essay on vaccination and revaccination. . . . Washington, D.C.: Gibson Brothers, Printers, 1864. 16p. DLC **60-0756**

HAHNEMANN MEDICAL COLLEGE AND HOSPITAL OF CHICAGO
Annual announcements for the sessions of 1863-1864 (4.); 1866-1867 (7.); 1868-1869 (9.); 1881-1882 to 1900-1901 (22.-41.). Chicago, 1863-1900. DNLM [The words "and Hospital" added to the title in 1873. List of students and graduates for 1862-1863; 1865-1866; 1867-1868; 1868-1869; 1880-1881 to 1899-1900, in announcements for subsequent years. List of alumni from 1861 to 1888, in announcement for 1888-1889.] **60-0757**

HAHNEMANN MEDICAL COLLEGE AND HOSPITAL. PHILADELPHIA
Catalogue of the museum and library of the Hahnemann Medical College of Philadelphia, no. 1105 Filbert Street. C. M. Thomas . . . curator of museum and librarian. Philadelphia: W. P. Kildare, Printer, 1869. 45p. DLC; DNLM; PPHa **60-0758**

HAHNEMANN, Samuel Christian Friedrich (1755-1843)
Organon of homoeopathic medicine. . . . 4th American edition. New York: William Radde 1860. 229p. DNLM; NNNAM; PPHa **60-0759**

HALE, Edwin Moses (1829-1899)
On the homoeopathic treatment of abortion, its causes and consequences; with some suggestions and indications for the use of the new remedies, with a prefatory letter by R. Ludlam. Chicago: Halsey & King, 1860. 22p. PPHa **60-0760**

HALE, Edwin Moses (1829-1899)
The soldiers' and travellers' manual: a guide for the administration of homoeopathic medicine. . . . Detroit, Mich.: E. A. Lodge; New York: C. T. Hurlburt; [etc., etc.], 1862. 31p. DLC; OCIM **60-0761**

HALE, Edwin Moses (1829-1899)
A monograph upon gelseminum: its therapeutic and physiological effects together with its uses in disease. . . . With an introductory letter by J. S. Douglas. . . . Detroit: Dr. Lodge; New York: W. Radde; [etc., etc.], 1862. 55p. DLC; DNLM **60-0762**

HALE, Edwin Moses (1829-1899)
The therapeutics of retroflexion and retroversion of the uterus. With plates. Chicago: C. S. Halsey, 1864. 22p. PPHa **60-0763**

HALE, Edwin Moses (1829-1899)
Valedictory addresses to the graduating class of Hahnemann Medical College, February 25, 1864. By E. M. Hale and D. A. Colton. Chicago: Beach & Barnard, 1864. 8p. PPHa **60-0764**

HALE, Edwin Moses (1829-1899)
The law of dose; based on the primary and secondary action of drugs. Chicago, 1864. 16p. PPHa **60-0765**

HALE, Edwin Moses (1829-1899)
New remedies. Their pathogenetic effects and therapeutcial application in homoeopathic practice. Detroit, Mich.: E. A. Lodge, Homoeopathic Pharmacy, 1864. 448p. PPHa **60-0766**

HALE, Edwin Moses (1829-1899)
A systematic treatise on abortion. . . . Chicago: C. S. Halsey, 1866. 347p. 2 col. plates. DLC; OCIM **60-0767**

HALE, Edwin Moses (1829-1899)
The great crime of the nineteenth century. [Criminal abortion.] Chicago: C. S. Halsey, 1867. 40p. DNLM **60-0768**

HALE, Edwin Moses (1829-1899)
Pathogenesis of kali bromatum (bromide of potassium). Detroit: Published at Lodge's Pharmacy, [1867?]. 36p. DNLM **60-0769**

HALE, Edwin Moses (1829-1899)
Homoeopathic materia medica of the new remedies; their botanical description, medical history, pathogenetic effects and therapeutical application in homoeopathic practice. . . . 2nd ed., rev. and enl. Detroit, Mich.: E. A. Lodge; New York: W. Radde [etc., etc.], 1867. 1142p. 4 col. plates. DLC; OCLloyd **60-0770**

HALE, Edwin Moses (1829-1899)
A systematic treatise on abortion and sterility. 2nd ed. Revised. Chicago: C. S. Halsey, 1868. 361p. PPHa **60-0771**

HALE, Edwin Moses (1829-1899)
Pathogenesis of Myrica cerifera. Detroit: E. A. Lodge, 1868. 14p. DNLM **60-0772**

HALL, A. D.
On extraction of soft cataract by suction. [Philadelphia?]: Oakwood Press, 1867. 8p. DNLM **60-0773**

HALL, Alfred G.
Institutes of medical jurisprudence. An exposition of the new theory of medical science on the nutritive principle. Boston: J. B. Chisholm, 1860. 576p. DNLM; MBM **60-0774**

HALL, John B.
American directory of homoeopathic physicians. [Proof copy.] John B. Hall, publisher, St. Paul, Minn. Cleveland: Nevins Print, 1867. 103p. OCIM; PPHa **60-0775**

HALL, R. P., & Co.
A treatise on the hair. Nashua, N.H.: R. P. Hall & Co., 1866. 24p. DNLM **60-0776**

HALL, William Whitty (1810-1876)
Soldier-health. . . . New York: H. B. Price, 1861. 127p. DLC; NNNAM **60-0777**

HALL, William Whitty (1810-1876)
Soldier-health. 3rd ed. . . . [New York: The author], 1862. 31p. DLC; NNNAM **60-0778**

HALL, William Whitty (1810-1876)
Soldier-health. 5th ed. . . . [New York: The author], 1863. 160p. DLC; NNNAM **60-0779**

HALL, William Whitty (1810-1876)
Sleep. . . . 4th ed., rev., with additions. New York: W. J. Widdleton, 1864. 349p. DLC; NNNAM **60-0780**

HALL, William Whitty (1810-1876)
Bronchitis, and kindred diseases. 10th edition. New York: W. J. Widdleton, 1865. 397p. NNNAM **60-0781**

HALSEY & KING. CHICAGO
The homoeopathic family guide, for the use of twenty-five principal remedies in the treatment of the more simple forms of disease. Comp. from the best authorities, for Halsey & King. Chicago, Ill.: Dunlop, Sewell & Spalding, printers, 1861. 156p. DLC; OCIM **60-0782**

HALTON, Richard J.
Large abdominal-uterine tumor, extirpated by John O'Reilly. Reported by Richard J. Halton. New York: R. Craighead, 1863. 8p. DNLM; NNNAM **60-0783**

HAMILTON, Frank Hastings (1813-1886)
A practical treatise on fractures and dislocations. . . . Philadelphia: Blanchard & Lea, 1860. 757p. DLC; NNNAM; PPC; PU **60-0784**

HAMILTON, Frank Hastings (1813-1886)
A practical treatise on military surgery. . . . New York: Bailliere Brothers, [etc., etc.], 1861. 234p. DLC; MBM; NNNAM; PPC **60-0785**

HAMILTON, Frank Hastings (1813-1886)
A practical treatise on fractures and dislocations. . . . 2nd ed., rev. and improved. . . . Philadelphia: Blanchard & Lea, 1863. 751p. CtY-M; NNNAM; PPC; PU **60-0786**

HAMILTON, Frank Hastings (1813-1886)
A treatise on military surgery and hygiene. . . . Illustrated with 127 engravings. New York: Bailliere Brothers; London: H. Bailliere; [etc., etc.], 1865. 648p. DLC; DNLM; NNNAM; PU **60-0787**

HAMILTON, Frank Hastings (1813-1886)
A practical treatise on fractures and dislocations. . . . 3rd ed., rev. and improved. Illustrated with two hundred and ninety-four wood-cuts. Philadelphia: Henry C. Lea, 1866. 777p. DLC; MBM; NNNAM; OCIM **60-0788**

HAMILTON, George (1808-1885)
Address before the Philadelphia County Medical Society. Philadelphia, 1869. 24p. DNLM **60-0789**

HAMILTON, Robert
Dr. Hamilton's medical and surgical institute for the treatment and entertainment of ladies and gentlemen, and the cure of female lung and chronic diseases, Saratoga Springs, N.Y. Boston: J. M. Usher, 1866. 44p. DNLM; MBM **60-0790**

HAMLIN, Cyrus (1811-1900)
Cholera and its treatment. Boston: H. Hoyt, [1866]. 15p. DNLM; MH-M **60-0791**

HAMLIN, Cyrus (1811-1900)
Treatment and cure of cholera. Washington: Intelligencer Printing Office, 1866. 12p. DNLM **60-0792**

HAMLIN, Cyrus (1811-1900)
Dr. Hamlin's essay on the cholera: preparation for its prevention and cure. . . . and other eminent men, who treated the cholera with unparalleled success in Europe and America, in 1848, 1855, and 1865. . . . New York: American News Company, 1866. 24p. DLC; NNNAM **60-0793**

HAMMACK, E[lijah] B.
The family physician and guide to health. . . . Including a treatise on midwifery and the diseases peculair to women. . . . St. Louis: Southwestern Book and Publishing Co., 1869. 648p. DLC; OCIM **60-0794**

HAMMOND, William Alexander (1828-1900)
On uraemic intoxication. Philadelphia: Collins, 1861. 31p. DNLM; PPC **60-0795**

[HAMMOND, William Alexander] (1828-1900)
. . . Two reports on the condition of military hospitals at Grafton, Va., and Cumberland, Md. . . . New York: W. C. Bryant & Co., Printers, 1862. 40p. DLC; NNNAM [U.S. Sanitary Commission Documents, No. 41] **60-0796**

HAMMOND, William Alexander (1828-1900)
Physiological memoirs. . . . Philadelphia: J. B. Lippincott & Co., 1863. 348p. DLC; MBM; OCIM; PPC
60-0797

HAMMOND, William Alexander (1828-1900)
A treatise on hygiene, with special reference to the military service. . . . Philadelphia: J. B. Lippincott & Co., 1863. 604p. double plate. DLC; NNNAM; PPC; PU **60-0798**

HAMMOND, William Alexander, ed. (1828-1900)
Military medical and surgical essays, prepared for the United States Sanitary Commission. . . . Philadelphia: J. B. Lippincott & Co., 1864. 552p. DLC; NNNAM; PPC; PU
60-0799

HAMMOND, William Alexander (1828-1900)
Lectures on venereal disease. . . . Philadelphia: J. B. Lippincott & Co., 1864. 287p. DLC; OCIM; PPC; PU
60-0800

[HAMMOND, William Alexander] (1828-1900)
Reply of the Judge Advocate to the defense of the accused before a general court-martial for the trial of Brig. Gen. William A. Hammond, Surgeon-General, U.S.A. Washington: Government Printing Office, 1864. 64p. DNLM
60-0801

[HAMMOND, William Alexander] (1828-1900)
A statement of the causes which led to the dismissal of Surgeon-General William A. Hammond from the army; with a review of the evidence adduced before the court. [New York, 1864]. 73p. DLC: DNLM; NNNAM **60-0802**

HAMMOND, William Alexander (1828-1900)
On sleep and insomnia. . . . [New York, 1865]. 36p. DLC; NNNAM **60-0803**

HAMMOND, William Alexander (1828-1900)
Insanity in its medico-legal relation. Opinion relative to the testamentary capacity of the late James C. Johnston. New York: Baker, Voorhis & Co., 1866. 72p. DNLM
60-0804

HAMMOND, William Alexander (1828-1900)
On wakefulness. With an introductory chapter on the physiology of sleep. . . . Philadelphia: J. B. Lippincott & Co., 1866. 93p. DLC; NNNAM; PPC **60-0805**

HAMMOND, William Alexander (1828-1900)
Sleep and its derangements. . . . Philadelphia: J. B. Lippincott & Co., 1869. 318p. DLC; MBM; OCIM; PPC
60-0806

HAMMOND, William Alexander (1828-1900)
The physiology and pathology of the cerebellum. New York: D. Appleton & Co., 1869. 38p. DNLM; NNNAM
60-0807

HARLOW, John M.
Recovery from the passage of an iron bar through the head. Boston: D. Clapp & Son, 1869. 20p. 1 plate. DNLM; MBM
60-0808

HARRIS, Chapin Aaron (1806-1860)
The principles and practice of dental surgery. . . . 8th ed.: enl. and rev., with three hundred and twenty illustrations. Philadelphia: Lindsay & Blakiston, 1863. 869p. DLC; MBM; NNNAM; PPC **60-0809**

HARRIS, Chapin Aaron (1806-1860)
The principles and practice of dental surgery. 9th ed. Philadelphia: Lindsay & Blakiston, 1866. 869p. DNLM; MdU-D; NNNAM; PPC **60-0810**

HARRIS, Chapin Aaron (1806-1860)
A dictionary of medical terminology, dental surgery, and the collateral sciences. . . . 3rd ed., carefully rev., and enl., by F. J. S. Gorgas. . . . Philadelphia: Lindsay & Blakiston, 1867. 743p. DLC; NNNAM; PPC; PU **60-0811**

HARRIS, Charles T[aylor] (1818-1890)
A review of four lectures on homoeopathy, delivered in Ann Arbor, Michigan, on the 28th to the 31st of December, 1868, by A. B. Palmer. . . . Detroit: William Graham's Steam Presses, 1869. 16p. OCIM; PPHa **60-0812**

HARRIS, Elisha (1824-1884)
The utility and application of heat as a disinfectant. Boston: G. C. Rand & Avery, 1860. 22p. DNLM; MBM
60-0813

[HARRIS, Elisha] (1824-1884)
. . . Hints for the control and prevention of infectious diseases in camps, transports, and hospitals. New York: W. C. Bryant & Co., printers, 1863. 36p. DLC; NNNAM [U.S. Sanitary Commission. Medical and Surgical Monographs, S]
60-0814

HARRIS, Elisha (1824-1884)
Cholera prevention: examples and practice: and a note on the present aspects of the epidemic. (Communicated to the Metropolitan Board of Health, August 8, 1867.). . . . New York: D. Appleton & Company, 1867. 50p. DLC; DNLM; NNNAM
60-0815

HARRIS, Elisha (1824-1884)
The vital statistics and sanitary condition of the hospitals and other institutions in which medical care is systematically provided, in the metropolitan sanitary district. New York: C. S. Westcott & Co., 1868. 16p. DNLM; NNNAM
60-0816

HARRIS, Elisha (1824-1884)
Sanitary qualities of the water supply of New York and Brooklyn, with chemical analyses, by C. F. Chandler. New York: C. S. Westcott & Co., 1868. 16p. DNLM; NNNAM
60-0817

HARRIS, Robert (1796-1858)
A text-book of practical anatomy, with additions by an American physician. New York: S. S. & W. Wood, 1860. 720p. DNLM; MBM; NNNAM; PPC **60-0818**

HART, John (1824?-1873)
The hydroconion and its success in the treatment of diseases of the respiratory organs. Catarrh, inflammations and ulcers of the throat, loss of the voice, hoarseness, [etc.]. Boston: H. Vossnack, 1865. 18p. DNLM; MBM
60-0819

HARTSHORNE, Edward (1818-1885)
Remarks on the treatment of oblique fracture of the clavicle, and especially on the application (with support of the adjoining limb) of pressure to the lower angle and blade of the scapula, as the ruling indication. Also the suggestion of new forms of apparatus for this purpose. Philadelphia: Sherman & Co., 1869. 35p. DNLM; PPC; PU **60-0820**

HARTSHORNE, Henry (1823-1897)
A discourse on speculative and inductive medicine, being the introductory lecture delivered in the medical department of Pennsylvania College. Philadelphia: Collins, 1860. 19p. DNLM; PPC **60-0821**

HARTSHORNE, Henry (1823-1897)
Memoranda medica; or, Note-book of medical principles. . . . Philadelphia: J. B. Lippincott & Co., 1860. 190p. DLC; NNNAM; PPC; PU **60-0822**

HARTSHORNE, Henry (1823-1897)
A monograph on glycerin and its uses. Philadelphia: J. B. Lippincott & Co., 1865. 68p. DNLM; PPC; PU **60-0823**

HARTSHORNE, Henry (1823-1897)
Cholera: facts and conclusions as to its nature, prevention, and treatment. . . . Philadelphia: J. B. Lippincott & Co., 1866. 79p. DLC; PPC; PU **60-0824**

HARTSHORNE, Henry (1823-1897)
Essentials of the principles and practice of medicine. A handy-book for students and practitioners. . . . Philadelphia: Henry C. Lea, 1867. 417p. DLC; NNNAM; PPC; PU **60-0825**

HARTSHORNE, Henry (1823-1897)
A hand-book of human anatomy and physiology. For the use of students. . . . Philadelphia: Henry C. Lea, 1869. 312p. DLC; DNLM; PPC; PU **60-0826**

HARTSHORNE, Henry (1823-1897)
A conspectus of the medical sciences; comprising manuals of anatomy, physiology, chemistry, materia medica, practice of medicine, surgery, and obstetrics. For the use of students. . . . With three hundred and ten illustrations. Philadelphia: Henry C. Lea, 1869. 1002p. DLC; NNNAM; OCIM; PPC **60-0827**

HARTSHORNE, Henry (1823-1897)
Essentials of the principles and practice of medicine. 2nd ed. Philadelphia: Henry C. Lea, 1869. 452p. MBM; NNNAM; PPC; PU **60-0828**

HARVARD UNIVERSITY. DENTAL SCHOOL (BOSTON)
Annual announcements for the sessions of 1868-1869 to 1876-1877 (1.-9.); 1880-1881 to 1883-1884 (13.-16.). Boston & Cambridge, 1868-1883. DNLM; MH **60-0829**

HAWLEY, J. S.
The use of pepsine in the diarrhoea of infants. Greenpoint, Long Island, [1869]. 12p. DNLM **60-0830**

HAWLEY, J. S.
The use of pepsine in the diarrhoea of infants. Brooklyn, N.Y., [1869]. 16p. DNLM **60-0831**

HAYS, Issac (1796-1879)
[Cataract.] [Philadelphia, 1863.] 5p. DNLM **60-0832**

HAYWARD, John W[arren] (1841-1905)
Taking cold the cause of half our diseases; its nature, causes, prevention and cure; its frequency as a cause of other diseases, and the diseases of which it is a cause. . . . New York: William Radde, 1866. 20p. DNLM **60-0833**

HAYWOOD, E[dmund] Burke (1825-1894)
Valedictory address, delivered before the Medical Society of the State of North Carolina at its sixteenth annual meeting, held at Salisbury, N.C., May 12, 1869. Raleigh, 1869. 20p. DNLM **60-0834**

HEADLAND, Frederick William (1830-1875)
The action of medicines in the system. . . . 4th American ed. . . . Philadelphia: Lindsay & Blakiston, 1863. 448p. PPC; PU **60-0835**

HEADLAND, Frederick William (1830-1875)
On the action of medicines in the system. . . . 5th American ed. . . . Philadelphia: Lindsay & Blakiston, 1867. 431p. NNNAM; OCIM; PPC; PU **60-0836**

HEADLAND, Frederick William (1830-1875)
On the action of medicines in the system. . . . 6th American from the 4th London ed. Philadelphia: Lindsay & Blakiston, 1867. 431p. DNLM; NNNAM; PPC; PU **60-0837**

HEARD, T. J[efferson] (1814-1899)
Report on medical topography, meteorology, and epidemic diseases of Texas. Philadelphia: Collins, 1868. 39p. DNLM **60-0838**

HELMUTH, William Tod (1833-1902)
Valedictory address to the graduating class of the Homoeopathic Medical College of Missouri, St. Louis, Mo.: R. P. Studley & Co., 1861. 18p. PPHa **60-0839**

HELMUTH, William Tod (1833-1902)
A treatise on diphtheria; its nature, pathology and homoeopathic treatment. St. Louis: Luyties & Co., 1862. 125p. DLC **60-0840**

HELMUTH, William Tod (1833-1902)
A treatise on diphtheria; its nature, pathology and homoeopathic treatment. 2nd ed., revised and corrected. St. Louis Homoeopathic Pharmacy: H. C. C. Luyties, 1864. 136p. PPHa **60-0841**

HELMUTH, William Tod (1833-1902)
Medical pomposity; or, the doctor's dream. A satire. Detroit, Mich.: E. A. Lodge, 1866. 15p. DLC **60-0842**

HELMUTH, William Tod (1833-1902)
The annual address before the American Institute of Homoeopathy for the session of 1866, held at Pittsburgh, Pa. To which is added a report of the Bureau on Surgery for that year. Boston: Rand & Avery, 1867. 40p. MBM **60-0843**

HELMUTH, William Tod (1833-1902)
An essay on cleft palate. Illustrated with nine colored lithographic plates. St. Louis, Mo.: Van Benthuysen & Son, 1867. 29p. PPHa **60-0844**

HELMUTH, William Tod (1833-1902)
Valedictory address to the class of the Homoeopathic Medical College of Missouri. Delivered March 3rd, 1868. [1868.] 14p. PPHa **60-0845**

HEMPEL, Charles Julius (1811-1879)
Homoeopathy, a principle in nature. Its scientific universality unfolded; its development and philosophy explained; and its applicability to the treatment of diseases shown. . . . Philadelphia: King & Baird, Printers, 1860. 248p. DNLM **60-0846**

HEMPEL, Charles Julius (1811-1879)
A new and comprehensive system of materia medica and therapeutics; arranged upon a physiologico-pathological basis, for the use of practitioners and students of medicine. 2nd ed. Revised and considerably enlarged. New York: William Radde, Jr., 1865. 2 v. DNLM **60-0847**

HEMPEL, Charles Julius (1811-1879)
A lecture on homoeopathy, delivered before the legislature of Michigan. Detroit, 1867. 40p. DNLM **60-0848**

HEMPEL, Charles Julius (1811-1879)
The new remedies; their description, pathogenetic effects, and their therapeutical application in homoeopathic practice. New York: William Radde, 1868. 72p. DNLM **60-0849**

HENDERSON, E. C.
Guide, for acute diseases, to the use of forty leading homoeopathic remedies, designed for the use of families.... Rochester, N.Y.: Benton & Andrews, printers, 1868. 19, 6, 4p. DLC **60-0850**

HERING, Constantin (1800-1880)
Cistus canadensis; its pathogenesis. Philadelphia: A. J. Tafel, 1866. 16p. DNLM **60-0851**

HERING, Constantin (1800-1880)
Introductory lecture to the course at Hahnemann Medical College, Philadelphia, 1867-1868. Detroit: Lodge, 1868. 13p. DNLM **60-0852**

HERING, Constantin (1800-1880)
The last events of 1867. The tele-microscope of Gottlieb Juntz, and the oranopathy of Wm. Sharp, M.D., F.R.S. Philadelphia: F. E. Boericke, 1868. 22p. DNLM; PPC **60-0853**

HERING, Constantin (1800-1880)
Heaven for homoeopathy; an historical document. Philadelphia, 1869. 5p. DNLM **60-0854**

HERSEY, Thomas
The midwife's practical directory; or woman's confidential friend. . . . Philadelphia: Stone, 1861. 336p. DNLM; PPC; PU **60-0855**

HEWITT, Henry S[tuart] (1825-1873)
The relations and reciprocal obligations between the medical professor and the educated and cultivated classes. An oration delivered before the Alumni Association of the medical department of the University of the City of New York. New York, 1869. 16p. DNLM; NNNAM **60-0856**

HEWITT, [William Morse] Graily (1828-1893)
The diagnosis, pathology and treatment of diseases of women, including the diagnosis of pregnancy. First American from the 2nd London ed., rev. and enlarged. Philadelphia: Lindsay & Blakiston, 1868. 707p. DNLM; NNNAM; PPC; PU **60-0857**

HEWSON, Addinell (1828-1889)
On localized galvanism as a remedy for the photophobia of strumous ophthalmia. [Philadelphia, 1860.] 5p. DNLM **60-0858**

HEWSON, Addinell (1828-1889)
On the influence of the weather over the results of surgical operations, and on the value of the barometer as a guide in the choice of the time for and the prognosis in such operations, as shown by the results of "immediate amputations" during a period of thirty years in the Pennsylvania Hospital. Philadelphia: Sherman & Co., 1868. 19p. DNLM; PPC **60-0859**

HIBBARD, John B.
American practical physician. . . . A condensed treatment with new principles for acute, chronic, and surgical diseases, by clinical experience of more than twenty-five years, without poisons. . . . New York: Printed by P. G. Bergen & Tripp, 1860. 204p. DLC; NNNAM **60-0860**

HILDRETH, E. A[ugustus] (1821-1885)
Report on topography, climatology, and epidemic diseases of West Virginia. Philadelphia: Collins, 1868. 36p. 2 tables. DNLM **60-0861**

HILDRETH, Joseph S. (*d.* 1870)
Report on the use of pressure in the treatment of gonorrhoeal and purulent ophthalmia. New York: J. Medole, 1865. 15p. DNLM; NNNAM **60-0862**

HILDRETH, Joseph S. (*d.* 1870)
Entropion and trichiasis of the upper lid; their radical treatment, by an operation, without division of the skin. Chicago: G. H. Fergus, 1866. 6p. DNLM **60-0863**

HILDRETH, Joseph S. (*d.* 1870)
Report of the committee on ophthalmology of the American Medical Association at Washington, D.C., session of 1868. Chicago: Church, Goodman & Donnelly, 1869. 8p. DNLM **60-0864**

HILL, Benjamin L. (1813-1871)
Illustrated midwifery; or Lectures on obstetrics, and the diseases of women and children. . . . Rev. by S. S. Oslin. . . . Cincinnati: J. W. Sewell & Co., 1860. 300p. 43 plates. DLC; OCIM **60-0865**

HILL, Benjamin L. (1813-1871)
An epitome of the homoeopathic healing art, containing the new discoveries and improvements to the present time; designed for the use of families, for travelers on their journey, and as a pocket companion for the physician. Cleveland: Hall, 1860. 160p. OCIM **60-0866**

HILL, [Matthew] Berkeley (1834-1892)
Syphilis and local contagious disorders. Philadelphia: Henry C. Lea, 1869. 467p. DNLM; MBM; NNNAM; PPC **60-0867**

HILL, Thomas (1818-1891)
An address delivered to the graduating class at the Massachusetts Medical College. Boston: D. Clapp & Son, 1865. 14p. DNLM; MH **60-0868**

HILLER, Frederick (*b.* 1820)
Common sense vs. allopathic humbuggery; or, chloroform and apoplexy duly considered in connections with certain allopathic luminaries. Virginia City, Nev.: Enterprise Printing Office, 1868. 15p. DNLM **60-0869**

HILLER, Frederick (*b.* 1820)
Medical truths and light for the million, or Homoeopathy vs. allopathy. Virginia City, Nev.: Enterprise Printing Office, 1869. 16p. PPHa **60-0870**

HILLIER, Thomas (1831-1868)
Hand-book of skin diseases for students and practitioners. . . . Philadelphia: Blanchard & Lea, 1865. 353p. DLC; NNNAM; PPC; PU [2nd ed. Philadelphia: H. C. Lea, 1870. 353p.]
60-0871

HINTON, James (1822-1866)
Dr. Watters' doctrines of life. Letter from . . . 3 l. St. Louis, [1868]. DNLM **60-0872**

HISTORY and medical description of the two-headed girl. Told in "her own peculiar way," by "one of them." Buffalo, N.Y.: Warren, Johnson & Co., 1869. 32p. DNLM
60-0873

HITCHENS, Peter S.
An introductory to the sixteenth annual course of lectures in the Homoeopathic Medical College of Pennsylvania; delivered October 12, 1863. Published by the class. Philadelphia: J. A. Wagenseller, 1863. 16p. PPHa
60-0874

HOBLYN, Richard Dennis (1803-1886)
A dictionary of terms used in medicine and the collateral sciences. A new American from the last London ed. Revised, with numerous additions, by Isaac Hays. Philadelphia: Henry C. Lea, 1865. 522p. DNLM; MBM; NNNAM; PPC
60-0875

HODGE, Hugh Lenox (1796-1873)
On diseases peculiar to women, including displacements of the uterus. . . . Philadelphia: Blanchard & Lea, 1860. 469p. DLC; DNLM; NNNAM; PPC [2nd rev. ed. Philadelphia: H. C. Lea, 1868. 531p.] **60-0876**

HODGE, Hugh Lenox (1796-1873)
The principles and practices of obstetrics. . . . Philadelphia: Blanchard & Lea, 1864. 550p. 32 plates. DLC; DNLM; MBM; PPC **60-0877**

HODGEN, John Thompson (1826-1882)
The treatment of stumps with retracted flaps and protruded bones. [St. Louis, 1864.] 4p. DNLM
60-0878

HODGEN, John Thompson (1826-1882)
Man's relations to the physical universe. An address. St. Louis: G. Knapp & Co., 1865. 19p. DNLM **60-0879**

HODGEN, John Thompson (1826-1882)
Treatment of cholera by atropine and saline solutions. [St. Louis, 1866.] 5p. DNLM **60-0880**

HODGEN, John T[hompson] (1826-1882)
An apparatus for suspending the superior extremities in case of extensive injuries about the wrist, fore-arm, and elbow. [Leavenworth, 1868.] 1 l. DNLM **60-0881**

HODGES, Richard Manning (1827-1896)
The excision of joints. . . . Boston, Mass., 1861. 204p. DLC; DNLM; MBM **60-0882**

[HODGES, Richard Manning] (1827-1896)
. . . Report of a committee of the associate medical members of the Sanitary Commission on the subject of excision of joints for traumatic cause. Cambridge: Welch, Bigelow, & Company, 1862. 23p. DLC; DNLM; MBM; [U.S. Sanitary Commission. Medical and Surgical Monographs, L]
60-0883

HODGES, Richard Manning (1827-1896)
Excision of joints for traumatic cause. Cambridge: Welch, Bigelow & Co., 1862. 23p. DNLM; MBM
60-0884

HODGES, Richard Manning (1827-1896)
Practical dissections. . . . Philadelphia: Henry C. Lea, 1867. 286p. DNLM; MBM; NNNAM; PPC
60-0885

HODGES, Richard Manning (1827-1896)
An introductory lecture delivered before the medical and dental schools of Harvard University. Boston: D. Clapp & Son, 1869. 32p. DNLM; MH **60-0886**

HOFFMANN, Frederick (1832-1904)
Annual report on the progress of pharmacy. Philadelphia: Merrihew & Son, 1869. 163p. DNLM; PPC; PPJ; PU
60-0887

HOLCOMBE, William Henry (1825-1893)
What is homoeopathy? A new exposition of a great truth. New Orleans, 1864. 32p. DNLM **60-0888**

HOLCOMBE, William Henry (1825-1893)
What is homoeopathy? A new exposition of a great truth. . . . Chicago: C. S. Halsey, 1865. 24p. DLC
60-0889

HOLCOMBE, William Henry (1825-1893)
How I become a homoeopath. . . . Chicago: C. S. Halsey, 1866. 30p. DLC; DNLM **60-0890**

HOLCOMBE, William Henry (1825-1893)
The philosophy of homoeopathy. [1868?] 20p. DNLM
60-0891

HOLCOMBE, William Henry (1825-1893)
What is homoeopathy? A new exposition of a great truth. . . . 6th ed. Chicago, Buffalo: C. S. Halsey, 1869. 24p. DLC
60-0892

HOLCOMBE, William Henry (1825-1893)
Report on the yellow fever of 1867; made by request, to the American Institute of Homoeopathy. New Orleans: A. Eyrich, 1869. 22p. DNLM **60-0893**

HOLDEN, Luther (1815-1905)
A manual of the dissection of the human body. . . . With notes and additions by Erskine Mason. . . . New York: R. M. De Witt, [1868]. 588p. DLC; NNNAM; PPC; PU
60-0894

HOLLICK, Frederick (*b.* 1818)
The marriage guide, or natural history of generation; a private instructor for married persons and those about to marry, both male and female, in everything concerning the physiology and relations of the sexual system and the production or prevention of offspring; including all new discoveries, never before given in the English language. 200th ed. New York: T. W. Strong, [1860]. 483p. 4 plates. DNLM; NNNAM
60-0895

HOLLICK, Frederick (*b.* 1818)
Los organos generativos masculinos; en estado de salud y en el de enfermedad; desde la ynfancia á la vejez. . . . Trad. de D. E. de Tabares. Nueva York: T. W. Strong, [1863]. 428p. 9 plates. DNLM; NNNAM **60-0896**

HOLLICK, Frederick (*b.* **1818)**
Datos para los debilitados, ó Apuntes y notas facultativas, sacadas de las consultas mas estrañas, sobre las peculiaridades, impotencia y distintas formas de descaecimiento del sistema secsual. . . . [New York, 1863]. 119p. DLC; NNNAM
60-0897

HOLMES, H. J.
Remarks on diseases of the womb. Atlanta, 1869. 24p. DNLM; GU **60-0898**

HOLMES, Oliver Wendell (1809-1894)
Currents and counter-currents in medical science. An address delivered before the Massachusetts Medical Society. Boston: Ticknor & Fields, 1860. 48p. DNLM; MBM; MH
60-0899

HOLMES, Oliver Wendell (1809-1894)
Currents and counter-currents in medical science. With other addresses and essays. . . . Boston: Ticknor & Fields, 1861. 406p. DLC; DNLM; MBM; MH **60-0900**

HOLMES, Oliver Wendell (1809-1894)
Border lines of knowledge in some provinces of medical science. An introductory lecture, delivered before the medical class of Harvard University, Nov. 6, 1861. . . . Boston: Ticknor & Fields, 1862. 80p. DLC; DNLM; MBM; MH
60-0901

HOLMES, Oliver Wendell (1809-1894)
Teaching from the chair and at the bedside. An introductory lecture delivered before the medical class of Harvard University. Boston: D. Clapp & Son, 1867. 45p. DNLM; MH-M
60-0902

HOLMES, Oliver Wendell (1809-1894)
The medical profession in Massachusetts. A lecture of a course by members of the Massachusetts Historical Society, delivered before the Lowell Institute, Jan. 29, 1869. . . . Boston: Press of J. Wilson & Son, 1869. 45p. DLC; DNLM; MBM; MH
60-0903

HOLMES, T[imothy] (1825-1907)
The surgical treatment of the diseases of infancy and childhood. 2nd ed. Philadelphia: Lindsay & Blakiston, 1869. 687p. 9 plates. DNLM; NNNAM; PPC; PU **60-0904**

H[OLSTEIN], [Anna M.]
Three years in field hospitals of the Army of the Potomac. Philadelphia: J. B. Lippincott & Co., 1867. 131p. DNLM; PPC; PU **60-0905**

HOMBERGER, Julius
Batpaxomyomaxia: a fight on "ethics." New Orleans, 1869. 20p. DNLM **60-0906**

THE HOMOEOPATHIC family guide, for the use of twenty-five principal remedies in the treatment of the more simple forms of disease; compiled from the best authorities. Chicago: Halsey & King, 1861. 156p. DNLM; IEN-M; OCIM
60-0907

HOMOEOPATHIC MEDICAL COLLEGE OF MISSOURI FOR MEN AND WOMEN. ST. LOUIS
Annual announcements for the sessions of 1868-1869 (7.); 1875-1876 (17.); 1876-1877 (18.); 1881-1882 (23.); 1882-1883 (24.); 1884-1885 (26.); 1889-1890 (31.); 1891-1892 (33.); 1892-1893 (34.); 1894-1895 (36.); 1895-1896 (38.); 1898-1899 (41.). St. Louis, 1868-1898. DNLM [List of students and graduates for 1866-1867; 1867-1868; 1870-1871; 1871-1875; 1875-1876; 1880-1881; 1881-1882; 1883-1884; 1888-1889; 1890-1891; 1891-1892; 1893-1894; 1894-1895; 1897-1898 in announcements for subsequent years. In 1880 a portion of the faculty seceded and re-established the St. Louis College of Physicians and Surgeons, but after the second session (1881-1882) it and the Hering Medical College were consolidated with this school.] **60-0908**

HOMOEOPATHIC MEDICAL COLLEGE. PHILADELPHIA
[Circular letter of the president to homoeopathic physicians, requesting their advice and assistance in the foundation and endowment of a hospital for the treatment and cure of the sick poor on the homoeopathic principle.] Aug. 30, 1868. [Philadelphia, 1868.] 1 l. DNLM; PPHa **60-0909**

HOOKER, Worthington (1805-1867)
Human physiology: designed for colleges and the higher classes in schools, and for general reading. New York: Sheldon & Co., 1862. 454p. DNLM; NN; NNC; NNNAM **60-0910**

HOOKER, Worthington (1805-1867)
First book in physiology. For the use of schools and families. . . . New York: Sheldon & Co., 1863. 191p. NN; NNC; NNNAM **60-0911**

HOOKER, Worthington (1805-1867) and Henry L. BOWDITCH
Report of the committee of medical ethics on specialties. Philadelphia: Collins, 1866. 12p. DNLM; PPC
60-0912

HOOPER, Joseph
Homoeopathy; what are its claims on public confidence? A popular tractate. Detroit, Mich.: E. A. Lodge, 1866. 8p. PPHa
60-0913

HOOPER, Joseph
Popular fallacies concerning homoeopathy refuted. . . . Detroit, Mich.: E. A. Lodge, 1866. 8p. DNLM **60-0914**

HOOPER, Joseph
Sketch of the life of Hahnemann. Detroit, Mich.: E. A. Lodge, 1866. 16p. PPHa **60-0915**

HOPKIN'S chalybeate water, its chemical constituents and curative and healing properties; with a brief notice of the sanitary effects derived from the use of chalybeates. Baltimore: J. F. Wiley, 1860. 15p. DNLM **60-0916**

[HOSACK, David] (1769-1835)
. . . Catalogue of the entire medical library of the late Dr. David Hosack. . . . To be sold at auction on . . . March 4th, 5th and 6th, 1867, by Bangs, Merwin & Co. . . . New York. . . . New York: C. C. Shelley, printer, 1867. 39p. DLC; DNLM; NNNAM **60-0917**

HOSKINS, Thomas H.
What we eat; an account of the most common adulterations of food and drink, with simple tests by which many of them may be detected. Boston: T. O. H. P. Burnham, 1861. 218p. DNLM; MB **60-0918**

HOSMER, George W[ashington] (1804-1881)
Report of delegates from the General Aid Society for the Army, at Buffalo (N.Y.), to visit the government hospitals and the agencies of the United States Sanitary Commission. Buffalo, 1862. 16p. DNLM **60-0919**

HOSPITAL transports. . . . . A memoir of the embarkation of the sick and wounded from the Peninsula of Virginia in the summer of 1862. Compiled and published at the request of the Sanitary Commission. Boston: Ticknor & Fields, 1863. 167p. DNLM; MBM; NNNAM **60-0920**

HOT SPRINGS, Bath County, Virginia; with some account of their medicinal properties and an analysis of the waters, with cases of cure of gout, rheumatism, diseases of the liver, paralysis, neuralgia, chronic diarrhoea, enlarged glands, old injuries, deafness, etc. S. C. Tardy & Co., proprietors. Richmond: Gary, Clemmitt & Jones, 1869. 92p. 1 map. DNLM **60-0921**

HOUGH, Franklin Benjamin (1822-1885)
Prize essay on medical and vital statistics. Albany: C. Van Benthuysen & Sons, 1867. 37p. 1 plate. DNLM **60-0922**

HOUGH, Franklin Benjamin (1822-1885)
Clinical charts. [Albany, N.Y.: J. Munsell, 1867.] 1 l. DNLM **60-0923**

HOUGH, Franklin Benjamin (1822-1885)
Biographical notice of Dr. Charles Milford Crandall. Albany: C. Van Benthuysen's Sons, 1868. 6p. DNLM **60-0924**

HOUGH, Lewis Sylvester (1819-1903)
Insurance against cholera. . . . Philadelphia: Ringwalt & Brown, printers, 1867. 32p. DLC; DNLM; PPC **60-0925**

HOWARD, Benjamin (*d.* **1900)**
Plain rules for the restoration of persons apparently dead from drowning. New York: E. B. Treat & Co., 1869. 3 l. DNLM; NNNAM **60-0926**

HOWARD UNIVERSITY, WASHINGTON. MEDICAL DEPARTMENT
Annual announcements for the sessions of 1868-1869 to 1873-1874 (1.-6.); 1875-1876 to 1882-1883 (8.-15.). Washington, 1868-1882. DNLM [List of students for the sessions 1868-1869 to 1872-1873; 1880-1881: 1881-1882, in announcements for subsequent years.] **60-0927**

HOWARD, W. J.
The valedictory address, delivered . . . at the annual commencement of the School of Medicine, in the University of Maryland. Baltimore: Kelly & Piet, 1868. 17p. DNLM **60-0928**

HOWE, J. M[offatt] (1806-1885)
Consumption curable. Information respecting the practice of F. H. Ramadge . . . ; containing an account of several cases in relation to this practice in which it has been beneficial in this country, with other corroborative testimony. New York, 1867. 96p. DNLM; NNNAM **60-0929**

HOWE, Samuel Gridley (1801-1870)
A letter on the sanitary condition of the troops in the neighborhood of Boston, addressed to his excellency the governor of Massachusetts. Washington: Government Printing Office, 1861. 16p. DNLM **60-0930**

HOWE, Samuel G[ridley] (1801-1870)
Address delivered at the ceremony of laying the corner-stone of the New York State Institution for the Blind, at Batavia, September 6, 1866. Boston: Walker, Fuller & Co., 1866. 51p. DNLM **60-0931**

HOWE, Samuel Gridley (1801-1870)
Remarks upon the education of deaf mutes; in defense of the doctrines of the second annual report of the Massachusetts Board of State Charities, and in reply to the charges of the Rev. Collins Stone, principal of the American Asylum at Hartford. Boston: Walker, Fuller & Co., 1866. 58p. DNLM; MBM **60-0932**

HOWE, Samuel Gridley (1801-1870)
Perkins Institution and Massachusetts Asylum for the Blind. [Special report to the trustees, recommending changes and improvements in the premises. Also, in favor of the family system in preference to the congregate. April 12, 1868.] [Boston, 1868.] 23p. DNLM; MBM **60-0933**

HOYNE, Temple S[toughton] (1841-1899)
Classification of a few of the "New remedies," according to the parts of the body acted upon, after the plan of Bonninghausen. . . . St. Louis, Mo.: H. C. G. Luyties, 1868. 70p. DLC; DNLM **60-0934**

HOYNE, Temple S[toughton] (1841-1899)
Monograph on fevers. Detroit: E. Lodge, 1868. 16p. DNLM **60-0935**

HUDSON, Alfred (1808-1880)
Lectures on the study of fever. Philadelphia: Henry C. Lea, 1869. 316p. DNLM; NNNAM; PPC; PU **60-0936**

HUDSON, E[rasmus] D[arwin] (1805-1880)
The surgical adjuvant, and reporter of surgical apparatus, artificial limbs, etc. . . . New York, [1862?] 20p. DLC; NNNAM **60-0937**

HUDSON, Erasmus Darwin (1805-1880)
Save the arm. Remarks on exsections. New York, 1864. 16p. DNLM **60-0938**

HUDSON, Erasmus Darwin (1805-1880)
Artificial limbs for the United States Army and Navy. [New York, 1865.] 32p. DNLM **60-0939**

HUDSON, Erasmus Darwin (1805-1880)
Mechanical surgery. Artificial limbs, apparatus for resections. . . . New York: Baker & Godwin, printers, [1867?] 43p. DLC; NNNAM **60-0940**

HUGHES, Richard
A manual of pharmacodynamics. . . . 2nd ed. Mostly rewritten. New York: William Radde, 1868. 590p. DNLM **60-0941**

HUGHES, Richard
A manual of therapeutics. New York: William Radde, 1869. 540p. NNNAM **60-0942**

HUMPHREYS, Frederick (1816-1900)
Humphreys' manual. Specific homoeopathy for the administration of medicine and cure of disease. . . . New York: Humphreys' Specific Homoeopathic Medicine Co., [1869]. 144p. DLC; NNNAM **60-0943**

HUNT, E[zra] M[undy] (1830-1894)
The patients' and physicians' aid; or, how to preserve health; what to do in sudden attacks, or until the doctor comes; and how best to profit by his directions when given. New York: C. M. Saxton, Barker & Co., 1860. 365p. DNLM; NNNAM **60-0944**

HUNT, Ezra Mundy (1830-1894)
The mind and nervous system in their relation to disease. New York: J. A. Gray, 1861. 18p. DNLM; NNNAM **60-0945**

HUNT, Ezra Mundy (1830-1894)
The medical profession, its position and its claims as a science, a business and an art. An address . . . at the ninety-ninth annual meeting, held at Burlington, January 24th, 1865. New York: F. Somers, printer, [1865]. 34p. DLC; DNLM; NNNAM **60-0946**

HUTCHINSON, James H[owell] (1834-1889)
Hypodermic injection of sulphate of morphia in the treatment of sunstroke; with a table containing a list of the cases treated at the [Pennsylvania] Hospital during June and July, 1867. [1867.] 7p. DNLM **60-0947**

HUTCHISON, Joseph Chrisman (1827-1887)
An address on the life and character of the late Charles Edward Isaacs, M.D., delivered to the graduates of Long Island College Hospital, Brooklyn, N.Y. New York: Hall, Clayton & Medole, 1862. 16p. DNLM; NNNAM **60-0948**

HUTCHISON, Joseph Chrisman (1827-1887)
Annual address before the Medical Society of the State of New York. Albany: C. Van Benthuysen & Sons, [1867]. 20p. DNLM **60-0949**

HUTCHISON, Joseph Chrisman (1827-1887)
Acupressure. An essay to which was awarded the Merrit H. Cash prize, by the Medical Society of the State of New York, February, 1869. Albany: Weed, Parsons & Co., 1869. 22p. 15 plates. DNLM **60-0950**

IVES, Charles L. (1831-1879)
The prophylaxis of phthisis pulmonalis. The annual dissertation read before the convention of the Conn. Medical Society, May 24, 1866. New Haven: Tuttle, Morehouse & Taylor, 1866. 21p. CtY-M; DNLM **60-0951**

IVES, Charles L. (1831-1879)
An inquiry into the therapeutic value of mercury and its preparations. A prize essay. New Haven: Tuttle, Morehouse & Taylor, 1866. 22p. CtY-M; DNLM **60-0952**

JACKSON, Charles Thomas (1805-1880)
A manual of etherization: containing directions for the employment of ether, chloroform, and other anaesthetic agents, by inhalation, in surgical operations, intended for military and naval surgeons . . . also a brief history of the discovery of anaesthesia. . . . Boston: Published for the Author, by J. B. Mansfield, 1861. 134p. DNLM; MBM; MWA; PU **60-0953**

JACKSON, James, Sr. (1777-1867)
Memoir on the last sickness of General Washington and its treatment by the attendant physicians. . . . Boston: Priv. print., 1860. 31p. DLC; DNLM; MH; MBM **60-0954**

JACKSON, James, Sr. (1777-1867)
Another letter to a young physician: to which are appended some other medical papers. . . . Boston: Ticknor & Fields, 1861. 179p. DLC: DNLM; MBM **60-0955**

JACKSON, James Caleb (1811-1895)
The sexual organism, and its healthful management. Boston: B. L. Emerson, 1862. 279p. MBM; MH **60-0956**

JACKSON, James Caleb (1811-1895)
Consumption: how to prevent it, and how to cure it. Boston: B. L. Emerson (1862). 400p. DNLM; MBM; NNNAM **60-0957**

JACKSON, James Caleb (1811-1895)
How to get well and how to keep well. Dansville: A. Jackson & Co., 1868. 21p. DNLM **60-0958**

JACKSON, James Caleb (1811-1895)
Flesh as food for man. Dansville, N.Y.: Austin, Jackson & Co., 1868. 18p. DNLM **60-0959**

JACKSON, James Caleb (1811-1895)
The weak backs of American women. Dansville, N.Y.: Austin, Jackson & Co., 1868. 17p. DNLM **60-0960**

JACKSON, James Caleb (1811-1895)
Piles, and their treatment. Dansville, N.Y.: Austin, Jackson & Co., 1868. 14p. DNLM **60-0961**

JACKSON, James Caleb (1811-1895)
How to cure drunkards. Dansville, N.Y.: Austin, Jackson & Co., 1868. 20p. DNLM **60-0962**

JACKSON, James C[aleb] (1811-1895)
The four drunkards. Dansville, N.Y.: Austin, Jackson & Co., 1868. 10p. DNLM **60-0963**

JACKSON, James Caleb (1811-1895)
How to nurse the sick. Dansville, N.Y.: Austin, Jackson & Co., 1868. 19p. DNLM **60-0964**

JACKSON, James Caleb (1811-1895)
The philosophy of drunkenness and its cure. [1869?] 20p. DNLM **60-0965**

JACKSON, John Davies (1834-1875)
Trichiniasis. [Philadelphia, 1867.] 21p. DNLM; PPC **60-0966**

JACKSON, John Davies (1834-1875)
Address before the Boyle County Medical Society of the State of Kentucky. Louisville, Ky.: Bell & Co., 1869. 23p. DNLM **60-0967**

JACOBI, Abraham (1830-1919)
Report on the clinic for diseases of children, held in the New York Medical College, session 1860-1861. With essays on some of the more important points of infantile therapeutics. New York: Hall, Clayton & Co., 1861. 82p. DNLM; NNNAM; NNU-M **60-0968**

JACOBI, Abraham (1830-1919)
Dentition and its derangements. A course of lectures delivered in the New York Medical College. New York, London, Paris: Bailliere Bros., 1862. 172p. DNLM; NNNAM; NNU-M **60-0969**

JACQUES, D. H. (*c.* **1825-1877)**
The philosophy of human beauty; or, hints toward physical perfection: showing how to acquire and retain bodily symmetry, health, and vigor. . . . New York: Miller, Wood & Co., 1867. 244p. DNLM; NNNAM **60-0970**

JAEGER, Eduard (1818-1884)
Test-types for the determination of the acuteness of vision, myopia, range of accommodation, etc., corresponding to the Schrift-Scalen of Eduard Jaeger. New York: William Wood & Co., 1868. 10 l. DNLM; NNNAM **60-0971**

JAHR, Gottlieb Heinrich Georg (1800-1875)
Hull's Jahr; a new manual of homoeopathic practice. . . . Repertory. New York: William Radde, 1861. 804p. PPHa; PPC; PU **60-0972**

JAHR, Gottlieb Heinrich Georg (1800-1875)
Hull's Jahr: a new manual of homoeopathic practice. 4th American ed. Edited, with annotations and additions, by Frederick G. Snelling, M.D. Symptomatology. New York: W. Radde; Boston: O. Clapp; [etc., etc.], 1862. 1204p. DLC; MBM; NNNAM; PPC **60-0973**

JAHR, Gottlieb Heinrich Georg (1800-1875)
The venereal diseases; their pathological nature, correct diagnosis, and homoeopathic treatment. . . . Transl., with numerous and important additions from the works of other authors and from his own experience, by Charles J. Hempel, M.D. New York: W. Radde; Boston: O. Clapp; [etc., etc.], 1868. 428p. DLC; MBM; NNNAM; PPC **60-0974**

JAHR, Gottlieb Heinrich Georg (1800-1875)
The clinical guide; or, Pocket-repertory for the treatment of acute and chronic diseases. . . . Transl. by Charles J. Hempel, M.D. 2nd American rev. and enl. ed., from the 3rd German ed., enriched by the addition of the new remedies, by Samuel Lilienthal, M.D. New York: Boericke & Tafel; Philadelphia: F. E. Boericke & A. J. Tafel; [etc., etc.], 1869. 624p. DLC; MBM; NNNAM; PPC **60-0975**

JAHR, Gottlieb Heinrich Georg (1800-1875)
Therapeutic guide: the most important results of more than forty years' practice, with personal observations regarding the truly-reliable and practically-verified curative indications in actual cases of diseases. Transl. with notes and new remedies by Charles J. Hempel. Philadelphia: F. E. Boericke & A. F. Tafel, 1869. 364p. NNNAM; OCIM; PPC **60-0976**

JAMES, John
The American household book of medicine, or, Every one's guide in sickness: containing directions on the diseases of men, women, and children; on bathing, diet . . . adapted to popular use and ready reference . . . assisted by an eminent western physician. . . . Cincinnati: R. W. Carroll & Co., 1866. 810p. DLC; OCIM **60-0977**

JARVIS, Edward (1803-1884)
Memorial to the honorable the senate and house of representatives of Massachusetts. [Concerning sanitary legislation]. [Boston, 1861.] 31p. DNLM; MBM **60-0978**

JARVIS, Edward (1803-1884)
The sanitary condition of the Army of the United States. [1862.] 35p. DNLM **60-0979**

JARVIS, Edward (1803-1884)
Employment for patients in the British lunatic asylums. . . . [1862?] 17p. DLC **60-0980**

JARVIS, Edward (1803-1884)
Influence of distance from and nearness to an insane hospital on its use by the people. [1866?] 46p. DNLM **60-0981**

JARVIS, Edward (1803-1884)
Communications concerning the ninth census of the United States. [1869.] 16p. DNLM **60-0982**

JARVIS, Edward (1803-1884)
Mania transitoria. [1869.] 32p. DNLM **60-0983**

JARVIS, Edward (1803-1884)
Trial of Samuel M. Andrews for the murder of Cornelius Holmes. [1869.] 23p. DNLM **60-0984**

JEAFFRESON, John Cordy (1831-1901)
A book about doctors. . . . Reprinted from the English ed. New York: Carleton, 1864. 488p. DLC; MH; NN; NNC **60-0985**

JEFFERSON MEDICAL COLLEGE. PHILADELPHIA
Catalogue of graduates of the Jefferson Medical College from its organization. Philadelphia: Ledger Job Printing Office, 1869. 48p. DLC; DNLM; PPJ **60-0986**

JEFFERSON, R.
The family doctor. A dictionary of domestic medicine and surgery, especially adapted for family use. 15th ed. Philadelphia: G. Gebbie, 1869. 750p. DNLM; PPC; PPHa; PU **60-0987**

JEFFRIES, Benjamin Joy (1833-1915)
I. Enucleation of the eyeball. II. Section of the ciliary nerves and optic nerve. III. Some unnecessary causes of impaired vision. Boston: D. Clapp & Son, 1868. 22, 17p. DNLM; MBM **60-0988**

JENKINS, J[ohn] Foster (1826-1882)
Relations of the war to medical science. Annual address before the Westchester County [N.Y.] Medical Society. New York: Bailliere Bros., 1863. 16p. DNLM; NNNAM **60-0989**

JENNINGS, Isaac
The tree of life; or, human degeneracy; its nature and remedy, as based on the elevating principle of orthopathy. New York: Miller, Wood & Co., 1867. 279p. DNLM; NNNAM **60-0990**

JEWELL, Wilson (1800-1867)
Mortality of Philadelphia for 1859. Report on meteorology and epidemics. Read before the College of Physicians of Philadelphia. Philadelphia: Collins, 1860. 22p. DNLM; PPC **60-0991**

JEWELL, Wilson (1800-1867)
Mortality of Philadelphia for 1861. Report on meteorology and epidemics. Philadelphia: Collins, 1862. 61p. DNLM; PPC; PU **60-0992**

JEWELL, Wilson (1800-1867)
Address before the American Medical Association. Philadelphia: Collins, 1863. 22p. DNLM; PPC; PU **60-0993**

JEWELL, Wilson (1800-1867)
Mortality of Philadelphia for 1862. Report on meteorology and epidemics. Philadelphia: Collins, 1863. 40p. DNLM; PPC
60-0994

JEWELL, Wilson (1800-1867)
Address delivered before the Medical Society of the State of Pennsylvania. Philadelphia: Collins, 1864. 23p. DNLM; PPC
60-0995

JEWELL, Wilson (1800-1867)
Mortality of Philadelphia for 1863. Report on meteorology and epidemics. Read before the College of Physicians of Philadelphia, February 3, 1864. Philadelphia: Collins, 1864. 27p. DNLM; PPC **60-0996**

JEWETT'S PATENT ARTIFICIAL LEG COMPANY, Washington, D.C. Washington, D.C.: McGill & Witherow, 1865. 8p. DNLM
60-0997

JOHNS, Montgomery (1830?-1871)
Valedictory, delivered at the commencement of the Medical Department of Georgetown College.... Washington, D.C.: W. H. Moore, printer, 1862. 23p. DLC
60-0998

JOHNSON, Charles Earl (1812-1876)
The question of insanity and its medico-legal relations considered upon general principles. Raleigh, N.C.: T. M. Hughes, 1869. 250p. DNLM; NcD; NcU; PPC
60-0999

JOHNSON, Isaac D. (1827-1911)
An address delivered at the third annual meeting of the Homoeopathic Medical Society of Chester County, Pa., October 3, 1860. West Chester, Pa.: James, Printer, 1860. 16p. PPHa **60-1000**

JOHNSTON, Christopher (1822-1891)
History of the discovery of the circulation of the blood. A lecture. Baltimore: Published by the Medical Class, 1867. 15p. DNLM **60-1001**

JONES, C. Handfield (1819-1890)
Clinical observations on functional nervous disorders. Philadelphia: Henry C. Lea, 1867. 348p. NNNAM; LNT-M; PPC; PU
60-1002

JONES, Joseph (1833-1896)
Suggestions on medical education. Introductory lecture to the course of 1859-1860, in the Medical College of Georgia. . . . Augusta, Ga.: Printed at the Constitutionalist Book and Job Office, 1860. 26p. DLC **60-1003**

JONES, Joseph (1833-1896)
Inquiries upon hospital gangrene. Richmond, Va., 1864. 8p. DNLM **60-1004**

JONES, Joseph (1833-1896)
Quinine as a prophylactic against malarial fever: being an appendix to the third report on typhoid and malarial fevers delivered to the surgeon general of the late C.S.A., August, 1864. . . . Nashville, Tenn.: University Medical Press, 1867. 34p. DLC **60-1005**

JONES, Joseph (1833-1896)
Researches upon "spurious vaccination," or the abnormal phenomena accompanying and following vaccination in the Confederate army during the recent American civil war, 1861-1865. . . . Nashville, Tenn.: University Medical Press, 1867. 164p. DLC; DNLM; GU; PPC **60-1006**

JONES, Joseph (1833-1896)
Observations on malarial fever: . . . [Augusta, Ga., 1868.] 182p. DLC; GU **60-1007**

JONES, Joseph (1833-1896)
Observations and researches on albinism in the Negro race. . . . Philadelphia: Collins, printer, 1869. 46p. DLC; PPC; PU
60-1008

JONES, Joseph (1833-1896)
Mollities ossium. Philadelphia: Collins, 1869. 72p. DNLM
60-1009

JONES, Joseph (1833-1896)
Outline of observations on hospital gangrene as it manifested itself in the Confederate armies, during the American civil war, 1861-1865. . . . New Orleans: Printed at the "Bronze Pen" Book and Job Office, 1869. 60p. DLC; LNT-M
60-1010

JONES, Joseph E. (*d.* 1899)
Homoeopathy and its practitioners in Chester County, Pennsylvania. Published by the Homoeopathic Medical Society of Chester and Delaware Counties, Pa. West Chester: American Republican Print., 1869. 15p. DNLM; PPHa
60-1011

JONES, Joseph H[untington] (1797-1868)
Man, moral and physical; or, the influence of health and disease on religious experience. Philadelphia: W. S. & A. Martien, 1861. 324p. DNLM; NN; NNC; PPC
60-1012

JONES, Marie M.
Woman's dress; its moral and physical relations, being an essay delivered before the World's Health Convention, New York City. New York: Miller, Wood & Co., 1865. 29p. DNLM; NN; NNC; NNNAM **60-1013**

JONES, Thomas Wharton (1808-1891)
The principles and practice of ophthalmic medicine and surgery. . . . 3rd and rev. American ed., with additions, from the 2nd London ed. Philadelphia: Blanchard & Lea, 1863. 455p. DLC; DNLM; MBM; PPC **60-1014**

JORDAN, R. M.
Jordan White Sulphur Springs, Frederick County, Va., containing a description of the springs and surrounding country, the analysis of its waters, the history and use of mineral waters, and letters from professional and other gentlemen, etc., with some account of the diseases to which the waters are specially applicable. Baltimore: Guggenheimer, Weil & Co., [1867?]. 21p. DNLM **60-1015**

JOSELIN, Benjamin Franklin (1796-1861)
Potencies in connection with crudities, showing why small doses can supply great deficiencies, and operate where there is no lack of material, and without interference from matter less attenuated. New York: J. T. Smith & Sons, 1860. 11p. DNLM; NNNAM **60-1016**

JUDD, Homer
Valedictory address, delivered at the first commencement of the Missouri Dental College, St. Louis, February 22, 1867. St. Louis, Mo.: R. P. Studley, 1867. 12p. DNLM
60-1017

KAMMERER, Joseph (1822-1875)
On the treatment of uterine catarrh. New York: Townsend & Adams, 1869. 23p. DNLM; NNNAM **60-1018**

KAMMERER, Joseph (1822-1875)
On the pathological conditions causing sterility in the female; founded on clinical observations. New York, 1869. 10p. DNLM; NNNAM **60-1019**

KECKELER, T. Hartman
Thaleia: women: her physiology and pathology, in connection with maternity, with hygienic and medical directions. . . . Cincinnati: A. T. & T. H. Keckeler, 1869. 357p. DLC; OCIM
60-1020

KEEP, N. C.
The aims and duties of the dental profession. Boston: T. R. Marvin & Son, 1865. 15p. DNLM; MBM
60-1021

KEEP, N. C.
Aluminum as a basis for artificial teeth. [Boston, 1866.] 2p. DNLM **60-1022**

KEITH, B., & Co.
Manual of the active principles of indigenous and foreign medicinal plants, as prepared at the laboratory of B. Keith & Co. New York: W. H. Trafton & Co., 1863. 38p. DNLM; NNNAM **60-1023**

KELLOGG, John L[eonard] (1811-1893)
Disease, it intricacies. Introductory lecture to the course in the Hahnemann Medical College of Chicago, October 20, 1860. Chicago: Cowdery, Printer, 1860. 16p. IU-M; PPHa
60-1024

KELLOGG, John L[eonard] (1811-1893)
Valedictory address to the graduating class of Hahnemann Medical College, February 26, 1863. Chicago: Beach & Barnard, 1863. 22p. PPHa **60-1025**

KEMBLE, George S[howers] (1827-1884)
The medical profession and the community. Their mutual duties, relations, and inerests. An address by . . . February — 1860. Before the Westmoreland County Medical Association. And biographical sketch of the late Dr. Samuel P. Brown, of Greensburg. Greensburg, [Pa.]: J. Keenan & Co., printers, 1860. 29p. DLC **60-1026**

KENNEDY, Duncan (1809-1887)
A sermon on occasion of the death of Thomas W. Blatchford, M.D. Troy, N.Y.: A. W. Schribner, 1866. 58p. DNLM
60-1027

KEYSER, Peter Dirck (1835-1897)
Glaucoma: its symptoms, diagnosis, and treatment. . . . Philadelphia: Lindsay & Blakiston, 1864. 88p. DLC; DNLM; NNNAM; PPC **60-1028**

KING, Albert Freeman Africanus (1841-1914)
An essay on the ligation and management of the umbilical cord at childbirth; . . . Washington, D.C.: Printed by W. H. Moore, 1867. 37p. DLC; DNLM **60-1029**

KING, Dan (1791-1864)
Tobacco; what it is, and what it does. New York: S. S. & W. Wood, 1861. 171p. DNLM; NN; NNC; NNNAM
60-1030

KING, James (1816-1880)
Annual address, delivered before the Medical Society of Pennsylvania, at the meeting held in Pittsburgh June 12, 1867. Philadelphia: Collins, 1867. 20p. DNLM; PPC; PU
60-1031

KING, John (1813-1893)
The American family physician; or, Domestic guide to health. Prepared expressly for the use of families, in language adapted to the understanding of the people. Arranged in two divisions. . . . Indianapolis, Ind.: A. D. Streight, 1860. 794, 333p. DLC; OCIM; NNNAM **60-1032**

KING, John (1813-1893)
Medical chart, for the use of all persons afflicted with chronic disease, whether males or females. . . . Cincinnati, O., [1863]. 16p. DLC **60-1033**

KING, John (1813-1893)
The American dispensatory. . . . 6th ed., rev. and enl. . . . Cincinnati: Moore, Wilstach & Baldwin, 1864. 1509p. DLC; OCIM; OCLloyd **60-1034**

KING, John (1813-1893)
American eclectic obstetrics. . . . 2nd ed., rev. and enl. . . . Cincinnati: Moore, Wilstach & Baldwin, 1866. 768p. DLC; OCIM **60-1035**

KINGSBURY, C[harles] A.
Valedictory address delivered before the first graduating class of the Philadelphia Dental College, session 1863-1864, Feb. 29, 1864. Philadelphia: H. B. Ashmead, 1864. 20p. DNLM; PPC **60-1036**

KINGSLEY, Norman W[illiam] (1829-1913)
Congenital cleft palate. New York: New York Printing Company, 1860. 15p. DNLM; NNNAM **60-1037**

KINNE, William W.
. . . A treatise on hernia, trusses, and rupture pads, with illustrations. . . . [New York]: B. Urner, Steam Book and Job Printer, [1860]. 16p. DLC; NNNAM **60-1038**

[KINNE, William W.]
Introductory remarks on trusses, as a curative agent. [New York? 1860?] 16p. DLC **60-1039**

KIRBY, Stephen R[eynolds] (1801-1876)
The introduction and progress of homoeopathy in the United States. An inaugural address before the Homoeopathic Medical Society of the County of New York, delivered April 11, 1864. New York: By the Society, 1864. 21p. NNNAM; PPHa
60-1040

KIRKES, William Senhouse (1823-1864)
Manual of physiology. . . . 7th ed., edited by W. Morrant Baker. Philadelphia: Lindsay & Blakiston, 1869. 838p. DNLM; NNNAM; PPC; PU **60-1041**

KLOB, Julius M. (1831-1879)
Pathological anatomy of the female sexual organs. . . . Transl. from the German by Joseph Kammerer . . . and Benjamin F. Dawson. . . . [Vol. I. Affections of the uterus] New York: Moorhead, Simpson & Bond, 1868. 299p. DLC; DNLM; NNNAM **60-1042**

KNAPP, Frederick N[ewman] (1821-1889)
Report concerning the aid and comfort given by the Sanitary Commission to sick soldiers found at the railroad station. Sept. 23, 1861. [1861.] 13p. DNLM [No. 29. U.S. San. Com. Documents, 1861-1865.] **60-1043**

KNAPP, Frederick N[ewman] (1821-1889)
Two reports concerning the aid and comfort given by the Sanitary Commission to sick soldiers passing through Washington. 1. report made September 23, 1861; 2., October 21, 1861. [1861.] 23p. DNLM [No. 35, U.S. San. Com. Documents, 1861-1865; 1st report published separately as No. 29; 3rd report, March 21, 1862, 29p.; 4th report, December 15, 1862, 16p.; Supplement to 4th report, 14p.; 5th report, October 1st, 1863, 63p.] **60-1044**

KNAPP, Frederick N[ewman] (1821-1889)
"Sanitaria": or, homes for discharged disabled soldiers. [Suggestions how to provide permanently for disabled soldiers. Washington, May 5, 1865.] [Washington, 1865.] Broadside folio. DNLM **60-1045**

KNAPP, J[akob] H[ermann] (1832-1911)
Embolic diseases of the eye. [New York, 1869.] 16p. DNLM; NNNAM **60-1046**

KNAPP, J[akob] Hermann (1832-1911)
New York Ophthalmic and Aural Institute. [Announcement of the opening of the . . . Sept., 1869.] New York, 1869. 2 l. DNLM; NNNAM **60-1047**

KNAPP, J[akob] Hermann (1832-1911)
Report and remarks on a third series of one hundred cases of cataract extraction by the peripheric-linear method. New York: William Wood & Co., 1869. 29p. DNLM; NNNAM **60-1048**

KNAPP, J[akob] Hermann (1832-1911)
A treatise on intraocular tumors, from original clinical observations and anatomical investigations. Transl. by S. Cole. New York: William Wood & Co., 1869. 323p. 16 plates. DNLM; MBM; NNNAM; PPC **60-1049**

KNIGHT, James (1810-1887)
The improvement of the health of enfeebled children and adults by natural means, including a history of food and a consideration of its substantial qualities. . . . New York: Sackett & Mackay, 1868. 406p. CtY-M; DLC; NNNAM; PU **60-1050**

KOCH, Richard
General introductory address to the first session of the Hahnemann Medical College of Philadelphia. Philadelphia: King & Baird, 1867. 13p. PPHa **60-1051**

KOLBÉ, D. W., & SON
Orthopaedic apparatus and description of the mechanical applicances employed in the treatment of deformities and deficiencies of the body, with directions for taking measurements for their application. Philadelphia: Collins, 1868. 37p. DNLM; PP; PPF; PPC **60-1052**

KOST, John (1819-1904)
Domestic medicine, a treatise on the practice of medicine, adapted to the reformed system, comprising a materia medica. . . . Cincinnati: Melick & Bunn, 1868. 624p. DLC; OCIM **60-1053**

LALLEMAND, Claude François (1790-1854)
A practical treatise on the causes, symptoms, and treatment of spermatorrhoea. Transl. and edited by Henry J. McDougall. 4th American ed. To which is added, on diseases of the vesiculae seminales and their associated organs, by Marris Wilson. Philadelphia: Blanchard & Lea, 1861. 380p. DNLM; MBM; NNNAM; PPC **60-1054**

LAMBERT, Thomas Scott (1819-1897)
A description of the newly invented elastic tourniquet for the use of armies and employment in civil life. New York, 1862. 31p. DNLM; NNNAM **60-1055**

LAMBERT, Thomas Scott (1819-1897)
Systematic human physiology, anatomy, and hygiene: being an analysis and synthesis of the human system, with practical conclusions. . . . New York: William Wood & Co., 1865. 420p. plates. DLC; NNNAM; PPC; PU **60-1056**

LAMBERT, Thomas Scott (1819-1897)
Systematic human physiology, anatomy, and hygiene: being an analysis and synthesis of the human system, with practical conclusions. . . . 2nd ed. New York: William Wood & Co., 1866. 420p. plates CtY-M; DLC; NNNAM; PPC **60-1057**

LAMBERT, T[homas] S[cott] (1819-1897)
Primary systematic human physiology, anatomy, and hygiene: a new and improved method of analysis and classification, both simple and complete, practical and interesting. . . . New York: William Wood & Co., 1867. 177p. DLC; MBM; NNNAM; PPC **60-1058**

LAMBERT, Thomas Scott (1819-1897)
Longevity. Part I. Biometry (the measure or span of life). A new philosophy, answering the questions: Am I probably long or short lived? Can I myself know the indications? An exposition of the laws of life or life-time, exhibited in family inheritance and personal indications of longevity. Followed by two ($500) prize essays on the physical indications of longevity, by J. V. C. Smith and John Griscom. To which is added a "Brief application of the exposition and essays," including extracts, "Striking pen-pictures of indications of impending incipient diseases," from a paper by C. L. Hubbell. New York: William Wood & Co., 1869. 98p. DNLM; NNNAM **60-1059**

LANE, Levi Cooper (1830-1902)
Introductory address delivered at the opening of the course on physiology for the session of 1861-1862, in the medical department of the University of the Pacific, at San Francisco, Cal. San Francisco: Painter & Co., 1861. 14p. DNLM **60-1060**

LANE, Levi Cooper (1830-1902)
Valedictory address delivered at the closing exercises of Toland Medical College, November 4th, 1869. San Francisco: Spear & Co., [1869?] 18p. DNLM **60-1061**

LANSING, John V. (1824-1880)
Frogs, and contributions to science. Albany, N.Y. J. Munsell, 1869. 18p. DNLM **60-1062**

LANSING, John V. (1824-1880)
Therapeutical skepticism; an address introductory to the course of 1869. (Albany Medical College.) Albany: J. Munsell, 1869. 12p. DNLM **60-1063**

LAPHAM, Ephraim
Cause and effect cure. Cause, philosophy, and cure of typhoid and typhus fever, including typhoid enteritis, & other complications, also the philosophy of fevers in general, and how to break any fever in 1 to 5 days. . . . Adrian, Mich.: Steam Publishing House of S. P. Jermain & Co., 1864. 32p. DLC
60-1064

LA ROCHE, René (1795-1872)
Annual address delivered before the Philadelphia Medical Society, at its meeting held on the 26th March, 1860. . . . Published by order of the Society. Philadelphia: Collins, printer, 1860. 61p. DLC; PPC; PPJ **60-1065**

[LA ROCHE, René] (1795-1872)
. . . Catalogue of an extensive and valuable medical and scientific library: being part of the collection of R. La Roche, M.D., of Philadelphia . . . to be sold . . . October 24th, 1865, and following days . . . at the auction rooms of the subscribers, M. Thomas & Sons, auctioneers. . . . Philadelphia: Collins, printer, 1865. 100p. DLC; PPJ; PU **60-1066**

LAURENCE, John Z[achariah] (1830-1874)
A handy-book of ophthalmic surgery for the use of practitioners. Assisted by Robert C. Moon. Philadelphia: Henry C. Lea, 1866. 191p. MBM; PPJ; PPC; PU **60-1067**

LAURENCE, John Z[achariah] (1830-1874)
A handy-book of ophthalmic surgery for the use of practitioners. Assisted by Robert C. Moon. 2nd ed., rev. and enl. Philadelphia: Henry C. Lea, 1869. 227p. CtY-M; MBM; NNNAM; PPC **60-1068**

LAWSON, George (1831-1903)
Injuries of the eye, orbit and eyelids. From the last English ed. Philadelphia: Henry C. Lea, 1867. 404p. CtY-M; PPHa; PPJ; PU **60-1068A**

LAWSON, Leonidas Merion (1812-1864)
Remarks on the treatment of inflammation, with special reference to pneumonia. Philadelphia: Collins, 1860. 28p. DNLM; PPC **60-1069**

LAWSON, Leonidas Merion (1812-1864)
A practical treatise on phthisis pulmonalis; embracing its pathology, causes, symptoms, and treatment. Cincinnati: Rickey, Mallory & Co., 1861. 557p. DNLM; OCIM
60-1070

LAYCOCK, Thomas (1812-1876)
Mind and brain, or the correlations of consciousness and organization systematically investigated and applied to philosophy, mental science, and practice. With a preliminary dissertation on method, and illustrations of the text. 2nd ed. New York: D. Appleton & Co., 1869. 2 v. DNLM; NN; NNC; NNNAM **60-1071**

LEA, HENRY C. PHILADELPHIA
Illustrated catalogue of medical, surgical, and scientific publications. Philadelphia, 1866. 64p. DNLM; PPC; PPJ
60-1072

LEAMING, J[ames] R[oseburgh] (1820-1892)
Cardiac murmurs. New York: Moorhead, Bond & Co., 1868. 37p. DNLM; NNNAM **60-1073**

LEE, Benjamin (1833-1913)
A protest and appeal; or the brief consideration of certain errors in regard to the pathology and treatment of ulcerative inflammation of the spine, commonly called "Pott's disease." Philadelphia, 1865. 23p. DNLM; PPC; PU
60-1074

LEE, Benjamin (1833-1913)
Contributions to the pathology, diagnosis, and treatment of angular curvature of the spine. . . . Philadelphia: J. B. Lippincott & Co., 1867. 129p. DLC; DNLM; MBM; PPC
60-1075

LEE, Charles Alfred (1801-1872)
Hospital construction, with notices of foreign military hospitals. Albany: C. Van Benthuysen, 1863. 32p. 6 plates. DNLM **60-1076**

LEE, Charles Alfred (1801-1872)
On provision for the insane poor of the State of New York, and the adaptation of the "asylum and cottage plan" to their wants; as illustrated by the history of the colony of Fitz James at Clermont, France. . . . Albnay: Van Benthuysen's Steam Printing House, 1866. 32p. DLC; DNLM
60-1077

LEE, Charles Alfred (1801-1872)
Report on insanity. . . . Philadelphia: Collins, printer, 1868. 32p. DLC; DNLM; PPC; PU **60-1078**

LEE, Charles Alfred (1801-1872)
Lecture introductory to the course on materia medica and hygiene, delivered before the medical class of the University of Buffalo. Buffalo, 1869. 16p. DNLM
60-1079

LEE, John K[idd] (1824-1887)
Valedictory address to the graduating class of the Homoeopathic Medical College of Pennsylvania, at its 14th annual commencement, March 3, 1862. Philadelphia: Collins, 1862. 20p. PPHa **60-1080**

LEEDS, Lewis W.
Lectures on ventilation: being a coure delivered in the Franklin Institute of Philadelphia, during the winter of 1866-1867. New York: J. Wiley, 1868. 60p. NN; NNC; NNNAM
60-1081

LEIDY, Joseph (1823-1891)
An elementary treatise on human anatomy. Philadelphia: J. B. Lippincott & Co., 1861. 663p. CtY-M; DNLM; PPC; PU
60-1082

LENTE, Frederick Divoux (1823-1883)
Sulphuric ether and chloroform as anaesthetics, considered with reference to their relative safety and efficiency. Philadelphia: Collins, 1861. 16p. DNLM; PPC
60-1083

LENTE, Frederick Divoux (1823-1883)
Medical notes on the island of Jamaica. New York, [1868]. 35p. DNLM; NNNAM **60-1084**

LENTE, Frederick Divoux (1823-1883)
A new method for securing divided vessels, and on the use of carbolic acid in surgical operations, for facilitating union by first intention. 1869. 12p. DNLM **60-1085**

LETTERMAN, Jonathan (1824-1872)
Medical recollections of the Army of the Potomac. . . . New York: D. Appleton & Co., 1866. 194p. DLC; NN; NNC; NNNAM **60-1086**

LEVICK, James J[ones] (1824-1893)
A historical sketch of the dance of St. Vitus, with notices of some kindred disorders. [Philadelphia, 1862?] 13p. DNLM **60-1087**

LEWES, George Henry (1817-1878)
The physiology of common life. New York: D. Appleton & Co., 1867. 2 v. DNLM; MH; NN; NNC **60-1088**

LEWIS, Dioclesian (1823-1886)
Weak lungs and how to make them strong; or diseases of the organs of the chest, with their home treatment by the movement cure. Boston: Ticknor & Fields, 1863. 360p. DNLM; MH-M; NNNAM; PPC **60-1089**

LEWIS, Dioclesian (1823-1886)
The new gymnastics for men, women, and children. 10th ed. Boston: Ticknor & Fields, 1868. 286p. DNLM; MBM; MH; MWA **60-1090**

LEWIS, John B[enjamin] (1832-1914)
Hereditary predisposition. The annual dissertation delivered before the convention of the Connecticut Medical Society. Hartford: Case, Lockwood & Co., 1861. 20p. CtY-M; DNLM **60-1091**

LEWIS, William Beale (*d.* 1874)
The pathology of Bright's disease. . . . New York: Turner & Mignard, Steam Book and Job Printers, 1869. 29p. DLC; NNNAM **60-1092**

LIDELL, John A. (1823-1883)
A case of neuroma of the optic nerve, with remarks and illustrations. . . . 2nd ed. New York: Holman, printer, 1863. 15p. DLC; NNNAM **60-1093**

LIDELL, John A. (1823-1883)
On gunshot wounds of arteries, traumatic hemorrhage and traumatic aneurism. . . . Washington, D.C. McGill & Witherow, printers, 1863. 24p. DLC **60-1094**

LIDELL, John A. (1823-1883)
A memoir on osteomyelitis. Read before the New York Academy of Medicine. New York, 1866. 33p. DNLM; NNNAM **60-1095**

LIGHTHILL, August P.
A popular treatise on deafness: its causes and prevention. By Drs. Lighthill. Ed. by E. Bunford Lighthill. . . . New York: Carleton, 1862. 133p. plates. DLC; NNNAM **60-1096**

LIGHTHILL, Edward Bunford
Nephotherapy: the new system for the treatment of diseases of the throat, catarrh, asthma, affections of the voice, laryngeal, bronchial, pulmonary complaints, and inflammation of the eyes, and all diseases of the respiratory organs. . . . New York: Carleton, 1865. 44p. DLC; NNNAM **60-1097**

LINCOLN, Marvin
Lincoln's patent artificial arm. Boston, 1865. 12p. DNLM [*also*: Boston, 1866, 14p.] **60-1098**

LINES, Leverett H.
Thirty years of female life. A treatise on the diseases of females, incident to this period, with their causes, symptoms and treatment; including the theory of conception, and the symptoms of pregnancy. . . . New York: Printed by W. E. Hilton, 1862. 336p. DLC; NNNAM **60-1099**

LINES, Leverett H.
From fifteen to forty-five: or, Thirty years of female life. A treatise on the diseases of females, incident to this period, with their causes, symptoms and treatment, including the theory of conception, and the symptoms of pregnancy. . . . New York: Printed by F. Somers, 1863. 336p. DLC; NNNAM **60-1100**

LINTON, Moses L. (1808-1872)
Medicine for the million; a lecture introductory to the session 1860-1861 of the St. Louis Medical College. St. Louis: G. Knapp & Co., 1860. 24p. DNLM **60-1101**

LIPPE, Adolph (1812-1888)
Who is a homoeopathician? A lecture delivered before the Hahnemann Institute, Philadelphia, February 17, 1865. Published by order of the Hahnemannian Institute. Philadelphia: King & Baird, 1865. 26p. PPHa **60-1102**

LIPPE, Adolph (1812-1888)
Valedictory address delivered at the 18th annual commencement of the Homoeopathic Medical College of Pennsylvania. Also lists of matriculants and graduates, session of 1865-1866. Philadelphia: King & Baird, 1866. 30p. DLC **60-1103**

LIPPE, Adolph (1812-1888)
Text-book of materia medica. Philadelphia: A. J. Tafel, 1866. 714p. DLC; DNLM **60-1104**

LIPPE, Adolph (1812-1888)
Cholera. Lecture delivered at the Homoeopathic Medical College of Pennsylvania, December 8, 1865. Published by the Class. Philadelphia: Collins, 1866. 24p. PPHa **60-1105**

LITTELL, Squire, Jr. (1803-1886)
Memoir of Isaac Remington. Read before the College of Physicians. [Philadelphia, 1861.] 10p. DNLM **60-1106**

LITTELL, Squire, Jr. (1803-1886)
On the relations which electricity sustains to the causes of disease. Philadelphia, 1866. 54p. DNLM; PPC; PU **60-1107**

LITTLE, James Laurence (1836-1885)
A report on the use of plaster of Paris in surgery. . . . Philadelphia: Collins, printer, 1867. 12p. DLC; PPC **60-1108**

LODGE, Edwin A.
Asiatic cholera: history, description, causes, prevention, treatment,—allopathic, homoeopathic,—comparisons, results, etc. Detroit: E. A. Lodge, 1866. 32p. PPHa **60-1109**

LOGAN, Cornelius Ambrose (1836-1899)
An essay on the remote and proximate causes of miasmatic fever. . . . Leavenworth: Printed at the Daily Conservative Book & Job Office, 1861. 19p. DLC **60-1110**

LOGAN, Cornelius Ambrose (1836-1899)
Report on the sanitary relations of the State of Kansas. Lawrence: J. Speer, 1866. 50p. DNLM **60-1111**

LOGAN, Samuel (1831-1893) and A. S. GATES
Valedictory addresses delivered at the commencement exercises of the New Orleans School of Medicine, March 14, 1869. New Orleans: Bronze Office, 1868. 24p. DNLM; LNT-M **60-1112**

LOGAN, Thomas Muldrup (1808-1876)
Report on the medical topography and epidemics of California. . . . Philadelphia: Collins, printer, 1865. 75p. CU-M; DLC; DNLM **60-1113**

LOGAN, Thomas Muldrup (1808-1876)
Medical history of the year 1868, in California. A paper read before the "Sacramento Society for Medical Improvement," February 16th, 1869, and pub. by order of the Society. . . . San Francisco, Cal.: Printed by F. Clarke, 1869. 24p. CU-M; DLC; DNLM **60-1114**

LONGMORE, T. (1816-1895)
A treatise on gunshot wounds. Authorized and adopted by the Surgeon-General of the United States Army for the use of surgeons in the field and general hospitals. Philadelphia: J. B. Lippincott & Co., 1863. 132p. DNLM; PPC; PU **60-1115**

LONGSHORE, Joseph Skelton (1809-1879)
Introductory lecture delivered in the female department of the Penn Medical University of Philadelphia, Oct. 1, 1860. Being a review of the action of the Pennsylvania State Medical Society in relation to female physicians and female medical colleges. Philadelphia: Harbach & Bro., 1861. 18p. DNLM; PPC; PU **60-1116**

LONGSHORE, Joseph Skelton (1809-1879)
The Philadelphia system of obstetrics. . . . Designed for a text-book for students, and as reference for the practitioner. . . . Philadelphia: University Publication Society, 1868. 800p. DLC; PPC; PPJ; PU **60-1117**

LOOMIS, Alfred Lebbeus (1831-1895)
Lessons in physical diagnosis. . . . New York: R. M. De Witt, [1868]. 159p. DLC; MBM; NNNAM; PPC **60-1118**

LOOMIS, Justin R[udolph] (1810-1898)
Elements of the anatomy, physiology, and hygiene of the human system. New York: Sheldon & Co., 1860. 221p. DNLM; NNNAM **60-1119**

LOOMIS, Lafayette C[harles] (1824-1905)
Howard University Medical College, Washington, D.C. Address of . . . delivered at the opening of the first course of lectures, November 5, 1868. Washington: Government Printing Office, 1869. 10p. DNLM **60-1120**

LOOMIS, Silas Lawrence (1822-1896)
Introductory address to the course of medical lectures at Georgetown College. Washington: McGill & Witherow, 1862. 19p. DNLM **60-1121**

LOOMIS, Silas Lawrence (1822-1896)
Valedictory address at the fifteenth annual commencement of the medical department of the Georgetown College. Washington: McGill & Witherow, 1865. 14p. DNLM **60-1122**

LOOMIS, Silas Lawrence (1822-1896)
Address delivered at the opening of the nineteenth annual course of lectures of the medical department of Georgetown College. Washington, D.C.: L. Towers, 1867. 12p. DNLM **60-1123**

LORING, Edward Greely (1837-1888)
The causes of exudation in inflammation. An essay to which was awarded one of the prizes of the Boylston Medical Society in 1864. Boston: D. Clapp, 1864. 9p. DNLM; MH-M **60-1124**

LORING, Edward Greely (1837-1888)
Remarks on strabismus. 1869. 27p. DNLM **60-1125**

LORING, Edward Greely (1837-1888)
Relative accommodation. 1869. 16p. DNLM **60-1126**

LUDLAM, Reuben (1831-1899)
An essay on stomatitis materna; presented at the American Institute of Homoeopathy, Philadelphia, June, 1860. New York: J. T. S. Smith & Sons, 1860. 16p. NN **60-1127**

LUDLAM, Reuben (1831-1899)
Introductory lecture to the course upon physiology and pathology in the Hahnemann Medical College, delivered October 16, 1860. Chicago: Halsey & King, 1860. 16p. DLC **60-1127A**

LUDLAM, Reuben (1831-1899)
The relations of morbid anatomy to practical medicine. (A lecture before the Hahnemann Medical College, Chicago.) New York: H. Ludwig, 1861. 16p. PPHa **60-1128**

LUDLAM, Reuben (1831-1899)
Valedictory address to the graduating class of Hahnemann Medical College, delivered February 27, 1862. Chicago: Hyatt & Calhoun, 1862. 22p. PPHa **60-1129**

LUDLAM, Reuben (1831-1899)
A lecture on some minor superiorities of the homoeopathic treatment. Introductory to the course of clinical medicine in Hahnemann Medical College, October 17, 1861. Chicago: H. L. Chapin, 1862. 24p. PPHa **60-1130**

LUDLAM, Reuben (1831-1899)
A plea for physiology. An introductory lecture to the course in physiology in the Hahnemann Medical College, Chicago. New York: H. Ludwig, 1863. 16p. PPHa **60-1131**

LUDLAM, Reuben (1831-1899)
A course of clinical lectures on diphtheria; delivered before the class of Hahnemann Medical College, Chicago, session of 1862-1863. Chicago: C. S. Halsey, 1863. 126p. DNLM **60-1132**

LUDLAM, Reuben (1831-1899)
The ups and downs of a doctor's life. Chicago: C. S. Halsey, 1864. 16p. DNLM **60-1133**

LUDLAM, Reuben (1831-1899)
The methodical physician; being the closing lecture of the course in Hahnemann Medical College, session 1864-1865. Chicago: C. S. Halsey, 1865. 24p. PPHa **60-1134**

LUDLAM, Reuben (1831-1899)
The nurse; her natural history, duties, and responsibilities, as an aid to the physician. A lecture introductory to the course delivered in Hahnemann Medical College for the session 1866-1867. Published for the Class. Chicago: C. S. Halsey, 1866. 28p. PPHa **60-1135**

LUDLAM, Reuben (1831-1899)
A lecture on criminal abortion. Delivered in Hahnemann Medical College, Chicago, February 4th, 1867. Chicago: C. S. Halsey, 1867. 17p. NN **60-1135A**

LUDLOW, John Livingston (1819-1888)
Address delivered at the opening of the new clinical lecture room of the Philadelphia Hospital. Philadelphia: H. Bryson, 1861. 26p. DNLM; PPC **60-1136**

LUDLOW, John Livingston (1819-1888)
A manual of examinations upon anatomy, physiology, surgery, practice of medicine, chemistry, obstetrics, materia medica, pharmacy, and therapeutics. Especially designed for students of medicine. To which is added a medical formulary. A new ed. Philadelphia: Henry C. Lea, 1865. 816p. DNLM; MBM; NNNAM; PPC **60-1137**

LUTZE, Arthur (1813-1870)
Manual of homoeopathic theory and practice. Designed for the use of physicians and families. Transl. from the German, with additions, by C. J. Hempel, M.D. . . . New York: William Radde, 1862. 750p. NNNAM; PPHa **60-1138**

LYELL, Charles (1797-1875)
The geological evidences of the antiquity of man, with remarks on theories of the origin of species by variation. 2nd American from the latest London ed. Philadelphia: G. W. Childs, 1863. 526p. 2 plates. DNLM; MH; NN; NNC **60-1139**

LYMAN, A. S.
The purification and disinfection of the system by a proper use of fresh-burned charcoal and pure air better than poisoning it for the prevention and cure of the great majority of diseases. New York: E. O. Jenkins, 1863. 31p. DNLM; NNNAM **60-1140**

LYONS, Robert Spencer Dyer (1826-1886)
A handbook of hospital practice; or, An introduction to the practical study of medicine at the bedside. . . . New York: S. S. & W. Wood, 1861. 185p. forms. CtY-M; DLC; NNNAM; PPC **60-1141**

LYONS, Robert Spencer Dyer (1826-1886)
A treatise on fever: or Selections from a course of lectures on fever. Being part of a course of theory and practice of medicine delivered by. . . . Philadelphia: Blanchard & Lea, 1861. 362p. DLC; MBM; NNNAM; PPC **60-1142**

McBRIDE, Alexander (1822-1876)
The cause, treatment, and cure of cholera. Cincinnati: A. Moore, 1866. 16p. DNLM **60-1143**

McCLINTOCK, James (1809-1881)
Introductory lecture to session of 1860 and '61 in the Eclectic Medical College of Philadelphia. Philadelphia: W. S. Young, 1860. 20p. DNLM; PPC **60-1144**

McCONAUGHY, James (*b.* 1810)
True medical science, versus quacks and quackeries: an address, delivered in the Court House, Greensburg, on Tuesday evening, Nov. 12, 1861 . . . before the Westmoreland County Medical Association. Greensburg, [Pa.]: Printed by J. Keenan & Co., 1862. 25p. DLC **60-1145**

McCOY, Amasa
Development of the vocal organs; statements of results to the singing and speaking voice; also, to the health. Chicago, 1868. 34p. DNLM **60-1146**

McDERMONT, Clarke (*b.* 1823)
Report on inebriate asylums. Philadelphia, 1861. 14p. DNLM **60-1147**

McDOWELL, Joseph Nash (1803-1868)
A report on the improvements in the art and science of surgery in the last fifty years. Saint Louis: Herald Office, 1860. 38p. DNLM; OCIM **60-1148**

McELROY, Z. Collins
On the dynamics, principles and philosophy of organic life; an effort to obtain definite conceptions of how do medicines produce their effects. Valedictory address delivered to the Muskingum County Medical Society, May 6th, 1868. Saint Louis, 1869. 40p. DNLM **60-1149**

McGILL, George M. (1838-1867)
Observation book. Ante mortems and post mortems. Ante mortems by medical officers of wards; post mortems by the surgeon in charge. National and Hicks United States Army General Hospitals, Baltimore, Maryland. Baltimore: J. S. Clarke & W. Beck, National & Hicks' Gen'l. Hospitals, 1865-1866. 213p. DNLM; MdU-D **60-1150**

McGUIER, Henry
A concise history of High Rock Spring. Albany: C. Van Benthuysen & Sons, 1868. 42p. DNLM **60-1151**

McILVAINE, R. R. (*d.* 1881)
A synoptical history of the intellectual powers of man and what he has accomplished by them. Demonstrating by comparison his superiority over all other animals. A lecture introductory to a course on physiology. Reported by J. A. Thacker, M.D. Cincinnati: W. Doyle, 1861. 15p. DNLM; OC **60-1152**

MACKALL, Louis (1802-1876)
Essays on muscular action, written in 1843 and 1844, by. . . . Washington: T. McGill, printer, 1860. 24p. DLC **60-1153**

MACKALL, Louis (1802-1876)
Extract from an unpublished essay on physical force. Washington: H. Polkinhorn & Son, 1865. 34p. DNLM **60-1154**

MACKALL, Louis (1802-1876)
An essay on the law of muscular action. . . . 2nd ed., cor. and enl. Washington: McGill & Witherow, Printers and Stereotypers, 1865. 34p. DLC **60-1155**

MACKENZIE, Morell (1837-1892)
The use of the laryngoscope in diseases of the throat; with an appendix on rhinoscopy. Philadelphia: Lindsay & Blakiston, 1865. 160p. DNLM; NNNAM; PPC; PU **60-1156**

MACKENZIE, Morell (1837-1892)
The use of the laryngoscope in diseases of the throat with an essay on hoarseness, loss of voice, and stridulous breathing, in relation to nervo-muscular affections of the larynx. . . . 2nd ed. With additions, and a chapter on the examination of the nasal passages, by J. Solis Cohen. Philadelphia: Lindsay & Blakiston, 1869. 289p. DLC; MBM; NNNAM; PPC
60-1157

McLAIN, Andrew Ferdinand
Causes of decay in the human teeth. New Orleans: L. Graham, 1867. 13p. DNLM **60-1158**

McLAIN, Andrew Ferdinand
Prophylaxis, or prevention to dental decay. July 12, 1869. [New Orleans, 1869.] 8p. DNLM **60-1159**

MacLEOD, George H. B. (1828-1892)
Notes on the surgery of the war in the Crimea, with remarks on the treatment of gunshot wounds. Philadelphia: J. B. Lippincott & Co., 1862. 403p. MH-M; NNNAM; PPC; PU
60-1160

McMANUS, Felix R. (1807-1835)
An address delivered at the seventeenth annual meeting of the American Institute of Homoeopathy, held in the City of Philadelphia, June 6, 1860. Published by order of the Institute. New York: American Homoeopathic Review Press, 1860. 24p. NNNAM; PPHa **60-1161**

MACNAMARA, Nottidge C[harles] (1832-1918)
A manual of diseases of the eye. Philadelphia: Lindsay & Blakiston, [1869?] 620p. 7 plates. CtY-M; DNLM; MBM; NNNAM [2nd ed., Philadelphia: Lindsay & Blakiston, 1872. 620p.; 3rd ed., Philadelphia: Lindsay & Blakiston, 1876. 614p; 4th ed., Philadelphia: P. Blakiston, Son & Co., 1882. 520p.] **60-1162**

McNAUGHTON, James (1796-1874), James P. BOYD, and James H. ARMSBY
The last illness of Dr. Alden March. [1869.] 11p. DNLM
60-1163

McQUILLEN, John Hugh (1826-1879)
The anatomy and physiology of expression, and the human teeth in their relation to mastication, speech, appearance. Two addresses. Philadelphia: J. B. Lippincott & Co., 1864. 34p. DNLM; PPC **60-1164**

McQUILLEN, John Hugh (1826-1879)
Valedictory address delivered before the graduating class of the Philadelphia Dental College, March 1, 1865. Philadelphia: J. B. Lippincott & Co., 1865. 16p. DNLM; PU
60-1165

McQUILLEN, John Hugh (1826-1879)
Microscopy of the dental tissues. An address before the Connecticut State Dental Association. [1865.] 12p. DNLM
60-1166

McQUILLEN, John Hugh (1826-1879)
Pain; its beneficient uses, and means of alleviation. Synopsis of an address delivered before the Hartford Society of Dentists. [1866.] 4p. DNLM **60-1167**

McQUILLEN, John Hugh (1826-1879)
Dental education. An address. [1866.] 6p. DNLM
60-1168

McQUILLEN, John Hugh (1826-1879)
Cuvierian classification of animated nature. An address. [1866.] 16p. DNLM **60-1169**

McQUILLEN, John Hugh (1826-1879)
Action of anaesthetics on the blood corpuscles. [1869.] 7p. DNLM **60-1170**

McSHERRY, Richard (1817-1885)
Valedictory address to the graduating class of the Medical Department of the University of Maryland. . . . Delivered at the Holliday Street Theatre, March 7, 1863. Published by the class. Baltimore: Printed by W. M. Innes, 1863. 19p. DLC
60-1171

McSHERRY, Richard (1817-1885)
Essays and lectures on: 1. The early history of Maryland. 2. Mexico and Mexican affairs. 3. A Mexican campaign. 4. Homoeopathy. 5. Elements of hygiene. 6. Health and happiness. Baltimore: Kelly, Piet & Co., 1869. 125p. DNLM; MdU-D **60-1172**

MAISCH, John M. (1831-1903)
Report on legislation regulating the practice of pharmacy in the United States. Philadelphia: Merrihew & Son, 1868. 48p. DNLM; PU **60-1173**

MANSFIELD, Edward D[eering] (1801-1880)
Memoirs of the life and services of Daniel Drake, M.D. Cincinnati: Applegate & Company, 1860. 408p. OC; OCIM
60-1174

MARCET, William
On a new process for preparing meat for weak stomachs. With an inquiry into the influence of the abuse of alcohol as a predisposing cause of disease. 1st American from 2nd English ed. New York: Moorhead, Simpson & Bond, 1868. 178p. DNLM; NNNAM **60-1175**

MARCH, Alden (1795-1869)
Compound, comminuted, and complicated fracture of the upper end of the tibia. Albany: C. Van Benthuysen, 1861. 12p. DNLM **60-1176**

MARCH, Alden (1795-1869)
Address delivered before the American Medical Association. Philadelphia: Collins, 1864. 14p. DNLM; PPC
60-1177

MARCH, Alden (1795-1869)
An unusual place of lodgment and exit of a biliary calculus. Albany: C. Van Benthuysen & Sons, 1867. 8p. 1 plate. DNLM
60-1178

MARCH, Alden (1795-1869)
A new method employed for removing a urinary calculus from the urethra. Albany: C. Van Benthuysen & Sons, 1867. 6p. DNLM **60-1179**

MARCH, Alden (1795-1869)
Scirrhus or malignant disease of the rectum. Albany: C. Van Benthuysen & Sons, 1868. 11p. DNLM
60-1180

MARCH, Alden (1795-1869)
Spontaneous lithotomy. [New York, 1869.] 4p. DNLM
60-1181

MARCY, Erastus Edgerton (1815-1900) and Franklin W. HUNT
The homoeopathic theory and practice of medicine. New York: William Radde, 1864. 2 v. NNNAM; PPHa; PU
60-1182

MARIX, Martin Mayer (1832?-1877)
Homoeopathy; its theory and practice. A lecture delivered before the students and faculty of Lawrence University, Kansas. Leavenworth, Kansas: Bulletin Print., 1866. 16p. PPHa **60-1183**

MARKOE, Thomas Masters (1819-1901)
Median lithotomy. [New York, 1866.] 35p. DNLM; NNNAM
60-1184

MARKS, [A. A.]
Patent artificial limbs with india-rubber hands and feet. New York: W. B. Smyth, 1865. 24p. DNLM; NNNAM [*also*: New York: W. B. Smyth, 1867. 36p; New York: W. B. Smyth, 1869. 44p.] **60-1185**

MARSH, Seymour N.
A plain and popular explanation of the nature, varieties, treatment and cure of hernia, or rupture . . . with an appendix on mechanical surgery, and the application of the various instruments for prolapsus, varicocele, piles, curved spine, bow legs, club-feet, and other deformities. . . . [New York: Electrotyped and printed by Hall, Clayton & Co., 1860]. 71p. DLC; NNNAM **60-1186**

MARSHALL, John (1818-1891)
Outlines of physiology, human and comparative. . . . With additions, by Francis G. Smith. . . . Philadelphia: Henry C. Lea, 1868. 1026p. DLC; NIC; NN; NNC
60-1187

MARSHALL, N. B.
Introductory lecture before the medical class of the Kentucky School of Medicine, on the truth of medicine, as evinced by its origin, progress, and present condition. Louisville: Courier Office, 1860. 19p. DNLM **60-1188**

MARTIN, Henry Noah (1829-1889)
Valedictory address delivered at the fifteenth annual commencement of the Hahnemannian Institute of Philadelphia, March 1, 1865. Published by request of the Institute. Buffalo: Franklin Printing House, 1865. 15p. PPHa
60-1189

MARTIN, Henry Noah (1829-1889)
Valedictory address delivered at the annual commencement of the Homoeopathic Medical College of Philadelphia, at the Academy of Music, March 3, 1869. Philadelphia: W. P. Kildare, 1869. 14p. PPHa **60-1190**

MARWEG, Gustav
Das Kranken-Büchel für meine Patienten. 4. Aufl. New York: J. Weber, 1867. 24p. DNLM; NNNAM **60-1191**

MASON, Augustus (1822-1882)
The cholera. Brief hints for the prevention of cholera, with a plain account of its symptoms, the proper preventive measures, and the management of its early stages. Sanctioned by the Medical Faculty of Lowell. 14th ed., revised, with an appendix. Boston: Walker, Fuller & Co., 1866. 12p. DNLM; MH-M **60-1192**

MASON, John Thomson (1815-1873)
The country physician. An address upon the life and character of the late Dr. Frederick Dorsey, of Washington County, Maryland, delivered in the Lutheran Church, at Hagerstown. . . . 2nd ed. Baltimore: Printed by William K. Boyle, 1867. 50p. DLC; DNLM; MdU-D **60-1193**

MASTIN, Claudius H[enry] (1826-1898)
Inguinal aneurism; successful ligation of external iliac artery by means of silver wire. New Orleans: L. Graham, 1866. 8p. DNLM **60-1194**

MATHEWS, Charles
On fumigation of the lungs, throat, etc. With formulas, authorities, directions, and forms of prescription. New York: Livesey Bros., 1861. 10p. DNLM; NNNAM **60-1195**

MATTSON, Morris
Manual of directions for the employment of injections in various diseases, with remarks upon the nature and treatment of habitual constipation; preceded by a treatise on the intestinal canal, its structure, functions, etc.; with a description of the digestive process. Boston, 1862. 164p. 5 plates. DNLM; MH-M **60-1196**

MAUDSLEY, Henry (1835-1918)
Physiology and pathology of the mind. . . . New York: D. Appleton & Co., 1867. 442p. CtY-M; DLC; MBM; NNNAM
60-1197

MAUGHS, G. M. B. (*d.* 1901)
Menstruation; or the menstrual flow: an epiphenomenon of ovulation. An argumental treatise. . . . Saint Louis, 1867. 59p. DNLM **60-1198**

MAUL, W. C.
Address of . . . and valedictory of Prof. Lunsford P. Yandell, Jr., at the commencement of the University of Louisville Medical Department. Louisville: Bradley & Gilbert, 1869. 24p. DNLM; OCIM **60-1199**

MAURAN, Joseph (1796-1873)
An address delivered before the Alumni Association of the College of Physicians and Surgeons, Medical Department of Columbia College, N.Y. (Personal reminiscences of "Old New York," 1817.) Providence: A. C. Green, [1864.] 24p. DNLM; NNC **60-1200**

MAURAN, Joseph (1796-1873)
An address delivered before the Alumni Association of the College of Physicians and Surgeons, Medical Department of Columbia College, New York, at the spring commencement, March 10, 1864. . . . New York: F. Hart & Co., Printers, 1864. 25p. DLC; NNNAM **60-1201**

MAURAN, Joseph (1796-1873)
Anniversary address delivered before the Alumni Association of the College of Physicians and Surgeons, Medical Department of Columbia College, New York City, March 2, 1869. Providence: Hammond, Angell & Co., 1869. 24p. DNLM; NNNAM **60-1202**

MAXSON, Edwin R.
A treatise on the practice of medicine. . . . Philadelphia: Lindsay & Blakiston, 1861. 705p. CU-M; DLC; PPC; PU
60-1203

MAXSON, Edwin R.
Hospitals, British, French, and American. To which is appended, a glance at the British Islands, France, and America. Ethnological, climatic, and general. . . . Philadelphia: Pub. for the Author, 1868. 122p. DLC; NN; PPC; PU
60-1204

MAXWELL, W. H. (1813-1889)
A female physician to the ladies of the United States; being a familiar and practical treatise on matters of utmost importance peculiar to women. Adapted for every woman's own private use. New York: W. H. Maxwell, 1860. 111p. NN; NNC; NNNAM; PU **60-1205**

MAYBURRY, William (1816-1873)
Address before the Philadelphia County Medical Society. Philadelphia, 1867. 37p. DNLM; PPC **60-1206**

MEADER, L. P.
The people's physician; designed as a manual of medicine, expressly for the use of families and individuals. . . . To which is added a list of synonyms of many common medical plants. . . . Cincinnati: Pub. by the Author, 1860. 450p. plates. DLC; OCLloyd; OCIM **60-1207**

MEADER, L. P.
The people's medical companion and family guide, in the preparation of medicine for the sick and afflicted. . . . Cincinnati: Pub. by the Author, 1861. 239p. plates. DLC; OCLloyd; OCIM **60-1208**

THE MEDICAL register of New York, New Jersey, and Connecticut. . . . Pub. under the supervision of the New York Medico-Historical Society. . . . New York, 1865-. DLC; MB; NcD; NNNAM [Title varies: 1865-1866, Medical register of the City of New York; 1873-1874, Medical register of the City of New York and vicinity; 1874-1875, Medical register of New York and vicinity; 1875-, Medical register of New York, New Jersey, and Connecticut.] **60-1208A**

MEDICAL SCHOOL OF MAINE. THE MEDICAL DEPARTMENT OF BOWDOIN COLLEGE, BRUNSWICK
Annual announcements for the session of 1866 (46.); 1867 (47.); 1881-1883 (61.-63.); 1885 to 1904-1905 (65.-85.). Brunswick, 1865-1904. DNLM **60-1209**

MEIGS, Charles Delucena (1792-1869)
A farewell address to his class, Feb. 27, 1861. Philadelphia: Collins, 1861. 16p. DNLM; PPJ **60-1210**

MEIGS, Charles D[elucena] (1792-1869)
Obstetrics; the science and the art. . . . 4th ed. Philadelphia: Blanchard & Lea, 1863. 730p. DNLM; IEN-M; NNNAM; PPC
60-1211

MEIGS, James Aitken (1829-1879)
Observations upon the cranial forms of the American aborigines, based upon specimens contained in the collection of the Academy of Natural Sciences of Philadelphia. Philadelphia, [1866]. 39p. DNLM; PU **60-1212**

MEIGS, James Aitken (1829-1879)
Correlation of the physical and vital forces. An inaugural address introductory to the course on institutes of medicine in the Jefferson Medical College. Delivered October 12, 1868. . . . Published by the class. Philadelphia: Office of Medical and Surgical Reporter, 1868. 32p. DLC; PPJ
60-1213

MENDENHALL, George (1814-1874)
Introductory address at the opening of the sixth session of the Miami Medical College of Cincinnati, Nov. 1st, 1865, on: Professional success. Cincinnati: A. Moore, 1865. 24p. DNLM
60-1214

MENEES, Thomas (1823-1905) and John W. MORTON
Addresses, delivered at the public commencement, Feb. 28th, 1868, Medical Department, University of Nashville. Nashville: W. H. F. Ligon, 1867. 30p. DNLM **60-1215**

MERRILL, A. P[hillips] (1793-1873)
Lectures on fever. Delivered in the Memphis Medical College, 1853-1856. New York: Harper & Brothers, 1865. 235p. DNLM; IU-M; NNNAM; PPC **60-1216**

MERRILL, A. P[hillips] (1793-1873)
The cholera pestilence. New York, 1865. 27p. DNLM; NNNAM **60-1217**

METCALFE, Joseph
Memoir of the Rev. Wm. Metcalfe, M.D. Philadelphia: J. L. Capen, 1866. 38p. DNLM; PU **60-1218**

METZ, A[bram] (1828-1876)
The anatomy and histology of the human eye. . . . Philadelphia: Office of the Medical and Surgical Reporter, 1868. 184p. DLC; PPC; PU **60-1219**

MEYER, Georg Hermann (1815-1892)
Procrustes ante portas. Why the shoe pinches; a contribution to applied anatomy. Transl. from the German, by John Stirling Craig. Boston: J. C. Plumer, 1861. 24, 14, 4p. 4 plates. DNLM; MBM **60-1220**

MICHEL, Middleton (1822-1894)
Monograph on the pathology of the pituitary body. Charleston, S.C.: James & Williams, 1860. DNLM
60-1221

MICHEL, R. Fraser (1827-1907)
Monograph on haemorrhagic malarial fever. Montgomery, Ala., 1869. 19p. DNLM **60-1222**

MILLARD, Henry B. (1832-1893)
The climate and statistics of consumption. A paper read before the American Geographical and Statistical Society. . . . With extensive additions by the author. New York, Philadelphia: W. Radde; [etc., etc.], 1861. 108p. DLC; NNNAM; PPC; PPHa **60-1223**

MILLARD, Henry B. (1832-1893)
A guide for emergencies; containing the homoeopathic treatment of such diseases as require immediate attention, and of such as may be treated without the assistance of a physician; and also containing the treatment of cases of poisoning and of every common variety of accidents. For the use of families. New York: C. T. Hurlburt, 1863. 124p. NNNAM; PPHa
60-1224

MILLER, Eli P[eck]
A treatise on the cause of exhausted vitality; or abuses of the sexual function. New York: Gray & Green, 1867. 131p. DNLM; NNNAM **60-1225**

MILLER, Eli P[eck]
How to bathe; a family guide for the use of water in preserving health and treating disease. New York: American News Co., 1869. 72p. DNLM; NNNAM **60-1226**

MILLER, Henry (1800-1874)
An address delivered before the American Medical Association, at its thirteenth annual meeting, held in the city of New Haven, Conn., on the 5th of June, 1860. . . . president of the association. . . . Philadelphia: Collins, printer, 1860. 28p. DLC; PPC **60-1227**

MILLER, Henry (1800-1874)
Brief notes of four additional cases of ovariotomy. [Philadelphia, 1869.] 7p. DNLM **60-1228**

MINTON, Henry B[rewster] (1831-1895)
A practical homoeopathic treatise on the diseases of women and children. Intended for intelligent heads of families and students in medicine. New York: W. Radde, [1866]. 461p. DNLM; NNNAM; PPC **60-1229**

MITCHELL, J. H.
Introductory lecture delivered before the class of medical students at Willamette University for the session of 1867. Salem, Oregon, 1867. 8p. DNLM **60-1230**

MITCHELL, Joseph Sidney (*d.* 1898)
Introductory address delivered before the students of Hahnemann Medical College of Chicago, October 26, 1866. Published by the Class. Chicago, 1866. 14p. PPHa **60-1231**

MITCHELL, Silas Weir (1829-1914)
On the treatment of rattlesnake bites, with experimental criticisms upon the various remedies now in use. Philadelphia: J. B. Lippincott & Co., 1861. 45p. DNLM; PPC; PP; PU **60-1232**

MITCHELL, Silas Weir (1829-1914)
Paralysis from peripheral irritation. New York: J. Medole, 1866. 67p. DNLM: NNNAM **60-1233**

[MITCHELL, Silas Weir] (1829-1914)
A list of the original memoirs of S. Weir Mitchell. Philadelphia: J. B. Lippincott & Co., 1868. 8p. DNLM; PPJ; PU **60-1234**

MITCHELL, Thomas Duché (1791-1865)
Professor Mitchell's farewell to the graduating class of Jefferson Medical College. (With a list of the graduates.) Philadelphia: Collins, 1861. 12, 4p. DNLM; PPJ **60-1235**

MITCHELL, Thomas Duché (1791-1865)
The professor and the pupil; a general introductory lecture, delivered October 13th in Jefferson Medical College. Philadelphia: H. B. Ashmead, 1862. 23p. DNLM; PPJ **60-1236**

MOORE & GARDINER's imperishable raw hide artificial limbs. New York: H. Croker, 1866. DNLM; NNNAM **60-1237**

MOORE, George (1803-1880)
The desire for intoxicating liquors a disease; its causes, its effects, and its cure, with the danger of a relapse, together with illustrative sketches: The good salesman: The would-be politician, etc. Baltimore: Sherwood & Co., 1864. 216p. DNLM; MdU-D **60-1238**

MOORE, Levi (1827-1880)
Address delivered before the Medical Society of the County of Albany, November 3, 1866. Albany: C. Van Benthuysen & Sons, 1867. 11p. DNLM **60-1239**

MOORE, Thomas (1827-1882)
Valedictory address to the graduating class of the Homoeopathic Medical College of Pennsylvania. Philadelphia: King & Baird, 1861. 16p. DNLM; PPHa **60-1240**

MOORMAN, John J. (*d.* 1885)
The mineral waters of the United States and Canada. With a map and [4] plates, and general directions for reaching mineral springs. Baltimore: Kelly & Piet, 1867. 507p. DNLM **60-1241**

MOORMAN, John J. (*d.* 1885)
Virginia White Sulphur Springs, with the analysis of its waters, the diseases to which they are applicable, etc. Baltimore: Kelly, Piet & Co., 1869. 27p. 1 map. DNLM **60-1242**

[MORGAN & ALLEN, Druggists]
Observations on tubercular or scrofulous diseases, and the use of the perchloride of gold with iodine, with sketches of cases. [New York, 1868.] 40p. DLC; NNNAM **60-1243**

MORGAN, Alonzo Richardson (*b.* 1830)
Valedictory address delivered at the twentieth annual commencement of the Homoeopathic Medical College of Pennsylvania, February 28, 1868, with names of matriculants and graduates. Philadelphia: King & Baird, 1868. 32p. DNLM; PPHa **60-1244**

MORGAN, Charles E. (1833-1867)
Electrophysiology and therapeutics; being a study of the electrical and other physical phenomena of the muscular and other systems during health and disease, including the phenomena of the electrical fishes. New York: William Wood & Co., 1868. 714p. DNLM; NNNAM; PU **60-1245**

MORGAN, James Ethelbert (1822-1889)
Valedictory delivered at the commencement of the Medical Department of Georgetown College, March 19, 1863. Washington, D.C.: Gibson Bros., 1863. 11p. DNLM **60-1246**

MORGAN, James Ethelbert (1822-1889) and Frank COWAN
Addresses delivered at the annual commencement of the Medical Department of Georgetown College, March 2, 1869, with a catalogue of the faculty and students. Washington, 1869. 15p. DNLM **60-1247**

MORGAN, John Coleman (1831-1899)
Introductory lecture delivered at the Hahnemann Medical College of Philadelphia. Published by the Class of 1867-1868. Wilmington, Del.: H. & E. F. James, 1867. 18p. PPHa **60-1248**

MORGAN, John Coleman (1831-1899)
Homoeopathic Medical College of Pennsylvania. Professor Morgan's valedictory; delivered at Musical Fund Hall, Philadelphia, March 2, 1867; with catalogue of matriculants and graduates, session of 1866-1867. Philadelphia: A. J. Tafel, 1867. 24p. PPHa **60-1249**

MORGAN, John Coleman (1831-1899)
The action and classification of medicines in connection with the anatomy of temperaments. Albany: C. Van Benthuysen & Sons, 1868. 48p. PPHa **60-1250**

MORGAN, Samuel
The text-book for domestic practice; being plain and concise directions for the administration of homoeopathic medicines in simple ailments. New York, [1869?] 191p. DNLM; NNNAM **60-1251**

MORLAND, William Wallace (1818-1876)
The morbid effects of the retention in the blood of the elements of the urinary secretions (Fiske fund prize essay). Philadelphia: Blanchard & Lea, 1861. 83p. DNLM; PPC; PU **60-1252**

MORLEY, John (*d.* 1776)
The thirty-first edition, revised, of an essay on the nature and cure of scrofulous disorders, commonly called the king's evil; deduced from long observation and practice, with additions, and above sixty cases; the remedies in them used, and occasional remarks. To which is prefixed a plate of the herb vervain, and its root. Published for the good of mankind. By the late John Morely. . . . New York: Reprinted from the London ed. of 1797, 1861. [1861]. 51p. CtY-M; DLC; MBM; NNNAM **60-1253**

MORRILL, C.
The physiology of woman and her diseases from infancy to old age. . . . 5th ed. Boston: Charles, 1868. 433p. MBM; MH; MWA **60-1254**

MORRILL, Frederic
The gentleman's medical adviser, and sure guide to health and long life. . . . Boston: The Author, 1869. 80p. DLC; MBM; NNNAM **60-1255**

MORRILL, Frederic
The ladies' new guide to health and long life. . . . Boston: The Author, 1869. 64p. DLC; MBM; MH **60-1256**

MORSE, Verranus (1818-1904)
The renewal of prescriptions. Proceedings of the East River and other medical societies, and a paper, with an appendix. New York: East River Medical Association, 1869. 16p. DNLM; NNNAM **60-1257**

MORTON TESTIMONIAL ASSOCIATION
A representation to Congress by the . . . covering a portion of the new and recently received petitions, memorials, resolutions, and letters from a large number of the American Medical Association, scientific societies, professors, and surgeons of the principal colleges and hospitals, surgeons, officers, and wounded soldiers of the Federal Army, etc., urging compensation for the use of anaesthetics in the Army and Navy. Submitted to the Thirty-eighth Congress and printed for the use of its members. [Washington, 1864?] 67p. DNLM **60-1258**

MOSES, Israel (*d.* 1870)
Surgical notes of cases of gun-shot injuries occurring during the advance of the Army of the Cumberland, 1863. [1864.] 20p. DNLM **60-1259**

MOTT, Alexander Brown (1826-1889)
Advantages of clinical teaching. An address introductory to the regular course of lectures at the Bellevue Hospital Medical College, N.Y. New York: C. A. Alvord, 1868. 30p. DNLM; NNNAM; NNU-M **60-1260**

MOTT, Valentine (1785-1865)
Address . . . before the graduates of 1860 of the University Medical College of New York. . . . New York: Miller, Mathews & Clasback, 1860. 25p. DLC; DNLM; NNNAM **60-1261**

MOTT, Valentine (1785-1865)
Eulogy on the late John W. Francis, M.D., LL.D., being a disclosure on his life and character. . . . Delivered before the New York Academy of Medicine, May 29, 1861. (Published by order of the Academy.) New York: S. S. & W. Wood, 1861. 33p. DLC; DNLM; NNNAM **60-1262**

MOTT, Valentine (1785-1865)
Pain and anaesthetics: an essay introductory to a series of surgical and medical monographs. . . . Washington: Government Printing Office, 1862. 16p. DLC **60-1263**

MOTT, Valentine (1785-1865)
Pain and anaesthetics: an introductory to a series of surgical and medical monographs. . . . 2nd ed. Washington: McGill & Witherow, printers, 1863. 16p. DLC; DNLM **60-1264**

MOTT, Valentine (1785-1865)
. . . On hemorrhage from wounds, and the best means of arresting it. . . . New York: A. D. F. Randolph, 1863. 16p. 4 diag. DLC [U.S. Sanitary Commission; Medical and Surgical Monographs, R] **60-1265**

THE MOUTH and its diseases. A manual of the best means of preserving the teeth. . . . New York: W. B. Hurd, 1862. 30p. DNLM; NNNAM **60-1266**

MUNROE, Henry (1818-1887)
The physiological action of alcohol. New York, [1865]. 24p. DNLM; NNNAM **60-1267**

MURCHISON, Charles (1830-1879)
Clinical lecture on diseases of the liver, jaundice and abdominal dropsy. . . . New York: William Wood & Co., 1868. 556p. 2 plates. DLC; IEN-M; NNNAM; PPC **60-1268**

MURRAY, William (1839-1920)
Treatise on emotional disorders of the sympathetic system of nerves. Philadelphia: J. B. Lippincott & Co., 1866. 118p. CtY-M; DNLM; PPC; PU **60-1269**

MURRAY, William (1839-1920)
Treatise on emotional disorders of the sympathetic system of nerves. New York: A. Simpson & Co., 1867. 95p. DNLM; MBM; NNNAM **60-1270**

MURRAY, William (1839-1920)
Treatise on emotional disorders of the sympathetic system of nerves. 2nd American ed. New York: Moorhead, Simpson & Bond, 1868. 92p. DNLM; MBM; NNNAM; PPC **60-1271**

MUSSEY, Reuben Dimond (1780-1866)
Anatomical cabinet belonging to. . . . Printed for the use of pupils. [Cincinnati, 1860?] 20p. DNLM **60-1272**

MUSSEY, Reuben Dimond (1870-1866)
Health; its friends and its foes. Boston: Gould & Lincoln, 1866. 380p. 1 plate. DNLM; MBM **60-1273**

MUSSEY, William Heberden (1818-1882)
A case of fraction of the os inominatum; and death in connection with the administration of sulphuric ether. Cincinnati, [1861]. 8p. DNLM; OCIM **60-1274**

MUSSEY, William Heberden (1818-1882)
Successful double ovariotomy. [1867.] 7p. DNLM **60-1275**

MUSSEY, William Heberden (1818-1882)
Report on surgery. A paper read before the Ohio State Medical Society, at the annual meeting, held at Delaware, June, 1868. Cincinnati: A. Abraham, 1868. 16p. DNLM; OCIM **60-1276**

NASH, James Addison
The southern family physician. . . . 2nd ed. Philadelphia: Pile & McElroy, printers, 1860. 52p. DLC; PPC; PU **60-1277**

NEBINGER, Andrew (1819-1886)
Biography of William Darrach, M.D. . . . Read before the Philadelphia County Medical Society, Jan. 23, 1867. Philadelphia: Collins, Printer, 1867. 24p. DLC; PPC; PU **60-1278**

NEIDHARD, Charles (1809-1895)
On the efficacy of Crotalus horridus in yellow fever; also in malignant, bilious, and remittent fevers. With an account of Humboldt's prophylactic inoculation of the venom of a serpent, at Havana, Cuba. New York: W. Radde, 1860. 82p. DNLM; NNNAM **60-1279**

NEIDHARD, Charles (1809-1895)
Crotalus horridus; its analogy to yellow fever, malignant, bilious, and remittent fevers, demonstrated by the action of the venom on man and animals. With an account of Humboldt's prophylactic inoculation [etc.]. 2nd ed. New York, 1868. 87p. DNLM; NNNAM **60-1280**

NEIDHARD, Charles (1809-1895)
Diphtheria, as it prevailed in the United States from 1860 to 1866, preceded by an historical account of its phenomena, its nature and homoeopathic treatment. New York: W. Radde, 1867. 176p. DNLM; NNNAM **60-1281**

NEIDHARD, Charles (1809-1895)
Homoeopathy in France, Germany and England in the year 1869. Read before the Philadelphia County Homoeopathic Medical Society, Philadelphia. [1869.] 19p. PPHa **60-1282**

NEILL, Edward D.
Biographical sketch of Doctor Jonathan Potts, with extracts from his correspondence. Albany: J. Munsell, 1863. 18p. DNLM **60-1283**

NEILL, John (1819-1880) and Francis Gurney SMITH
Analytical compendium of the various branches of medical science. A new ed., revised and improved. Philadelphia: Blanchard & Lea, 1864. 974p. DNLM; PPC; PU **60-1284**

NELIGAN, John Moore (1815-1863)
A practical treatise on diseases of the skin. 4th American ed. Philadelphia: Blanchard & Lea, 1864. 333p. DNLM; MBM; NNNAM; PPC **60-1285**

NELIGAN, John Moore (1815-1863)
A practical treatise on diseases of the skin. 5th American from the 2nd rev. and enl. Dublin ed., by T. W. Belcher. Philadelphia: Henry C. Lea, 1866. 462p. DNLM; IEN-M; NNNAM; PPC **60-1286**

NELSON, Robert (1794-1873)
Gastrotomy, for the removal of non-malignant tumors from the abdominal cavity. New York: J. H. Tobitt, 1864. 32p. DNLM; NNNAM **60-1287**

NELSON, Robert (1794-1873)
Asiatic cholera, its origin and spread in Asia, Africa, and Europe, introduction into America through Canada, remote and proximate causes, symptoms, and pathology, and the various modes of treatment analyzed. New York: W. A. Townsend, 1866. 206p. DNLM; NNNAM **60-1288**

NEWBERRY, John Strong (1822-1892)
Report on the sanitary condition of the U.S. troops in the Mississippi valley, during the month of Aug., 1861. [1861.] 11p. DNLM [U.S. Sanitary Commission, Documents, 1861-1865, No. 27] **60-1289**

NEWBERRY, John Strong (1822-1892)
Report on the condition of the troops, and the operations of the Sanitary Commission in the valley of the Mississippi, for the three months ending Nov. 30, 1861. Cleveland: Fairbanks, Benedict & Co., 1861. 48p. DNLM [U.S. Sanitary Commission, Documents, 1861-1865, No. 36] **60-1290**

NEWBERRY, John Strong (1822-1892)
A visit to Fort Donelson, Tenn., for the relief of the wounded of Feb. 15, 1862. A letter by. . . . [1862.] 10p. DNLM [U.S. Sanitary Commission, Documents, 1861-1865, No. 42] **60-1291**

NEWBERRY, John Strong (1822-1892)
What the U.S. Sanitary Commission is doing in the valley of the Mississippi. Letter from . . . to W. P. Sprague. 2nd ed. Louisville, Feb. 16, 1863. [Washington, 1863.] 31p. DNLM [U.S. Sanitary Commission, Documents, 1861-1865, No. 64] **60-1292**

NEWBERRY, John Strong (1822-1892)
Report on the operations of the U.S. Sanitary Commission in the valley of the Mississippi, made Sept. 1, 1863. [1863.] 24p. DNLM [U.S. Sanitary Commission, Documents, 1861-1865, No. 75] **60-1293**

NEWBERRY, John Strong (1822-1892)
Report on the operations of the U.S. Sanitary Commission in the valley of the Mississippi for the quarter ending Oct. 1, 1864, Louisville, Oct. 22, 1864. [New York, 1864.] 29p. DNLM [U.S. Sanitary Commission, Documents, 1861-1865, No. 84] **60-1294**

NEWBERRY, John Strong (1822-1892)
Circular from the sanitary reporter. A mistake corrected. [Being a true statement of the expenditures, to correct a false one circulated by enemies of the commission.] Louisville, Dec. 1, 1864. [Louisville, 1864.] 1 broadside. DNLM **60-1295**

NEWBERRY, John Strong (1822-1892)
Modern scientific investigation; its methods and tendencies; an address delivered before the American Association for the Advancement of Science, August, 1867. Salem, 1867. 23p. DNLM **60-1296**

NEWTON, Calvin (1800-1853)
Diseases of the lungs, heart and blood: scrofula, consumption, bronchitis, their causes, prevention and cure, by Marshall Calkins. . . . With the posthumous writings of Calvin Newton. . . . Philadelphia: H. Cowperthwait & Co., 1860. 546p. DLC; PPC; PU **60-1297**

NEWTON, Orin E.
An essay on Asiatic cholera, as it appeared in Cincinnati, O., in the years 1849, 1850, and 1866, with remarks upon its treatment, and a tabulated statement of one hundred and seventeen cases treated. . . . New York and Cincinnati: The Office of the American Eclectic Review, 1867. 30p. tables. DLC; DNLM; OCIM; NNNAM **60-1298**

NEWTON, Robert Safford (1818-1881)
An eclectic treatise on the practice of medicine, embracing the pathology of inflammation and fever, with its classification and treatment. Cincinnati, 1861. 144p. DNLM; OCIM **60-1299**

NEWTON, Robert Safford (1818-1881)
Ancient and modern eclecticism in medicine. An address delivered before the Eclectic Medical Society of the State of New York. Brooklyn: W. C. Wilton, 1864. 8p. DNLM; NNNAM **60-1300**

NEWTON, Robert Safford (1818-1881) and William Byrd POWELL
An eclectic treatise on diseases of children. New York: J. F. Trow & Co., 1867. 610p. DNLM; NNNAM **60-1301**

NEW YORK CITY
Hospital formulary of the Department of Public Charities and Correction of the City of New York. [New York, 1868.] 14p. NNNAM; OCLloyd **60-1302**

NEW YORK HOMOEOPATHIC MEDICAL COLLEGE AND HOSPITAL. NEW YORK CITY
Annual announcements for the sessions of 1868-1869 (9.9); 1876-1877 (17.); 1880-1881 (21.); 1887-1888 to 1901-1902 (28-.42.) New York, 1868-1901. DNLM **60-1303**

NEW YORK MEDICAL ASSOCIATION FOR THE SUPPLY OF LINT, BANDAGES, ETC. TO THE UNITED STATES ARMY
Final report of the New York Medical Association for the supply of lint, bandages, etc. to the United States Army. Presented July 25th, 1861. New York: The Association, 1861. 32p. DLC; NNNAM **60-1304**

NEW YORK MEDICAL COLLEGE AND CHARITY HOSPITAL. NEW YORK CITY
Annual announcement for the session of 1859-1860 (10.). New York, W. F. Kost, 1860. [1859.] 3 l. DNLM **60-1305**

NIEMEYER, Felix von (1820-1871)
. . . Clinical lectures on pulmonary phthisis. Transl. by permission of the author, from the 2nd German ed., by J. L. Parke. New York: Moorhead, Simpson & Bond, 1868. 116p. CtY-M; DLC; NNNAM; PPC **60-1306**

NIEMEYER, Felix von (1820-1871)
A text-book of practical medicine, with particular reference to physiology and pathological anatomy. . . . Transl. from the 7th German ed., by special permission of the author, by George H. Humphreys . . . and Charles E. Hackley. . . . New York: D. Appleton & Company, 1869. 2 v. CU-M; DLC; IU-M; NNNAM **60-1307**

NIGHTINGALE, Florence (1820-1910)
Notes on nursing: what it is, and what it is not. . . . New York: D. Appleton & Company, 1860. 140p. DLC; NN; NNC; NNNAM **60-1308**

NORTH, Nelson L[uther] (1830-1904)
On epidemic cholera, the phenomena, causes, prevention and treatment. With an appendix, relating to the Brooklyn city sewerage. Brooklyn: Daily Times Presses, 1865. 39p. DNLM; NNNAM **60-1309**

NORTH, Nelson L[uther] (1830-1904)
A theory of inflammation; its cause, course, and rationale of treatment. New York: William Wood & Co., 1867. 46p. DNLM; NNNAM **60-1310**

NORTON, Sidney A[ugustus] (1835-1918)
A lecture on measures and weights, delivered October 5, 1869, as introductory to the tenth annual course of lectures in the Miami [Medical] College of Cincinnati. Cincinnati: R. Clarke & Co., 1869. 21p. DNLM; OCIM **60-1311**

NORWOOD, Wesley C.
The authorship and therapeutical powers of *Veratrum viride* more fully examined. . . . Albany, N.Y.: C. Van Benthuysen & Sons, Printers and Stereotypers, 1868. 39p. DLC; DNLM **60-1312**

NOYES, Henry Drury (1832-1900)
Sclerotico-choroiditis posterior, with cases and illustrations. New York: T. Holman, 1860. 16p. DNLM; NNNAM **60-1313**

NOYES, Henry Drury (1832-1900)
Specialties in medicine. . . . Read before the American Ophthalmological Society, June, 1865. [New York]: J. Medole, printer, [1865]. 16p. DLC; DNLM; NNNAM **60-1314**

NOYES, Henry Drury (1832-1900)
Glaucoma: read before the New York State Medical Society, at the annual session, February, 1869. . . . Albany: Weed, Parsons & Co., printers, 1869. 13p. DLC; DNLM **60-1315**

NOYES, John Humphrey (1811-1886)
Male continence, or self-control in sexual intercourse. A letter of inquiry answered. [Oneida, N.Y., 1866.] 4p. DNLM **60-1316**

O'BYRNE, John (*d.* 1876)
Introductory lecture delivered before the under-graduates of the Philadelphia University of Medicine and Surgery, October 6, 1869. Philadelphia: University Publication Society's Print, 1869. 16p. DNLM **60-1317**

OLDSHUE, L.
Urino-pathology, or the uroscopian system of diagnosing diseases by ocular inspection, chemical analysis, and microscopic examination of the urine. Pittsburgh, 1864. 264p. DNLM **60-1318**

ORDRONAUX, John (1830-1908)
Hints on the preservation of health in armies. For the use of volunteer officers and soldiers. New York: D. Appleton & Co., 1861. 142p. DNLM; NNNAM **60-1319**

ORDRONAUX, John (1830-1908)
Hints on the preservation of health in armies. For the use of volunteer officers and soldiers. 2nd ed., with additions. New York: D. Van Nostrand, 1863. 142p. DNLM; NNNAM **60-1320**

ORDRONAUX, John (1830-1908)
Manual of instructions for military surgeons, on the examination of recruits and discharge of soldiers. With an appendix, containing the official regulations of the provost-marshal general's bureau and those for the formation of the invalid corps, etc. Prepared at the request of the United States Sanitary Commission. New York: D. Van Nostrand, 1863. 238p. DNLM; NNNAM; PU **60-1321**

ORDRONAUX, John (1830-1908)
Proposed scheme for the relief of disabled soldiers. New York: W. C. Bryant & Co., 1863. 8p. DNLM [U.S. Sanitary Commission, Documents, 1861-1865, No. 58] **60-1322**

ORDRONAUX, John (1830-1908)
On a system for the economical relief of disabled soldiers, and on certain proposed amendments to our present pension laws. New York: Sanford, Harroun & Co., 1864. 163p. DNLM; NNNAM **60-1323**

ORDRONAUX, John (1830-1908)
A valedictory address delivered before the medical class of the University of Vermont, May 31st, 1865. New York: Baker & Godwin, 1865. 32p. DNLM **60-1324**

ORDRONAUX, John (1830-1908)
Valedictory address delivered before the graduating class, National Medical College. Washington: McGill & Witherow, 1867. 20p. DNLM **60-1325**

ORDRONAUX, John (1830-1908)
Prophylaxis, an anniversary oration delivered before the New York Academy of Medicine, Wednesday, Dec. 19th, 1866. . . . New York: Bailliere Brothers; London: H. Bailliere; [etc., etc.], 1867. 70p. DLC; DNLM; NNNAM **60-1326**

ORDRONAUX, John (1830-1908)
On hallucinations consistent with reason. A lecture delivered before the students of Columbia College, New York. [New York, 1868?] 23p. DNLM; NNC **60-1327**

ORDRONAUX, John (1830-1908)
The jurisprudence of medicine in its relations to the law of contracts, torts, and evidence, with a supplement on the liabilities of vendors of drugs. . . . Philadelphia: T. & J. W. Johnson & Co., 1869. 310p. DLC; DNLM; PPC; PU **60-1328**

ORDRONAUX, John (1830-1908)
On suicide. A lecture delivered before the students of Columbia College. [New York, 1869?] 35p. DNLM; NNC **60-1329**

O'REILLY, John (1813-1868)
The anatomy and physiology of the placenta. The connection of the nervous centres of animal and organic life. . . . New York: Hall, Clayton & Co., 1860. 111p. DLC; NNNAM **60-1330**

O'REILLY, John (1813-1868)
On the placenta, and the phenomena connected with the animal and organic nervous system. New York: Hall, Clayton & Co., 1861. 46p. DNLM; NNNAM **60-1331**

O'REILLY, John (1813-1868)
The modus propagandi of the human species, physiologically explained. . . . New York: Hall, Clayton & Co., printers, 1861. 28p. DLC; NNNAM **60-1332**

O'REILLY, John (1813-1868)
Course of lectures on the physiology and pathology of the central nervous system. By C.-E. Brown-Séquard. [Review of.] New York, 1861. 3p. DNLM **60-1333**

O'REILLY, John (1813-1868)
The placenta, the organic nervous system, the blood, the oxygen, and the animal nervous system, physiologically examined. . . . [2nd ed.] New York: S. S. & W. Wood; [etc., etc.], 1861. 204p., 2 plates. DLC; NNNAM **60-1334**

O'REILLY, John (1813-1868)
The modus operandi of various kinds of baths, sea-bathing, heat and cold, physiologically explained. New York: Hall, Clayton & Co., 1861. 23p. DNLM; NNNAM **60-1335**

O'REILLY, John (1813-1868)
Is tracheotomy in true croup a justifiable operation? New York: Hall, Clayton & Medale, 1862. 23p. DNLM; NNNAM **60-1336**

O'REILLY, John (1813-1868)
Hints on the treatment of strangulated hernia. The properties of opium as antiphlogistic, anatomically and physiologically explained. . . . Read before the Academy of Medicine of New York. New York: William Wood & Co., 1863. 24p. DLC; DNLM; NNNAM **60-1337**

O'REILLY, John (1813-1868)
Gastrotomy. Large abdominal-uterine tumor, extirpated by. . . . New York: R. Craighead, 1863. 8p. DNLM **60-1338**

O'REILLY, John (1813-1868)
What is the modus operandi of medicine? Do they produce their effects by action on the blood, as taught by all modern physiologists? Or, do they produce their effects by their action on the organic nervous system, through the agency of the blood? The latter question considered and affirmatively answered. . . . New York: R. Craighead, printer, 1863. 11p. DLC; NNNAM **60-1339**

O'REILLY, John (1813-1868)
The nervous and vascular connection between the mother and foetus in utero. . . . New York: Printed by R. Craighead, 1864. 76p. DLC; NNNAM **60-1340**

O'REILLY, John (1813-1868)
The nervous and vascular connection between the mother and foetus in utero. . . . Rev. and enl. . . . New York: Printed by R. Craighead, 1864. 86p. DLC; DNLM **60-1341**

THE ORIGIN, history, cause, prevention, and cure of cholera, with an account of its progress and ravages through the world, and the latest and most successful treatment, endorsed and approved by the medical faculty. By a New York physician. New York: G. Munroe & Co., [1865]. 86p. DNLM; NNNAM **60-1342**

ORME, Francis Hodgson (1834-1913)
Homoeopathy; an explanation of what it is, with the design of correcting existing erroneous impressions concerning it, and of showing its claim to be regarded as the superior method of medical practice. Detroit, Mich.: E. A. Lodge Homoeopathic Pharmacy, 1868. 38p. PPHa **60-1343**

ORME, Francis Hodgson (1834-1913)
Homoeopathy; the superior method of medical practice. . . . Detroit, Mich.: E. A. Lodge, 1868. 7p. PPHa **60-1344**

ORME, Francis Hodgson (1834-1913)
Homoeopathy: is it quackery? Has it been shown fair play? Detroit: Lodge, 1868. 8p. PPHa **60-1345**

OSGOOD, Charles (1808-1881)
The causes, treatment, and cure of fever and ague, and other diseases of bilious climates. New York, 1865. 15p. DNLM; NNNAM **60-1346**

OTIS, George Alexander (1830-1881) and Joseph Janvier WOODWARD
Circular No. 6, Nov. 1, 1865. Reports on the extent and nature of the materials available for the preparation of a medical and surgical history of the rebellion. Philadelphia: J. B. Lippincott & Co., 1865. 166p. 5 plates. DNLM; PPC; PU **60-1347**

OTIS, George Alexander (1830-1881)
Histories of two hundred and ninety-six surgical photographs, prepared at the Army Medical Museum. Washington: Surgeon-General's Office, 1866-1871. 296 l. DNLM **60-1348**

OTIS, George Alexander (1830-1881)
Photographs of surgical cases and specimens: taken at the Army Medical Museum, Washington, D.C. Washington, 1866-1871. 5 v. DNLM **60-1349**

OTIS, George Alexander (1830-1881)
Circular No. 7, 1867. A report on amputations at the hip-joint in military surgery. Washington: Government Printing Office, 1867. 87p. 9 plates. DNLM **60-1350**

OTIS, George A[lexander] (1830-1881)
Drawings, photographs, and lithographs illustrating the histories of seven survivors of the operation of amputation at the hip-joint, during the war of the rebellion, together with abstract of these seven successful cases. Washington: Surgeon-General's Office, 1867. 16 sheets. folio. DNLM **60-1351**

OTIS, George Alexander (1830-1881)
Circular No. 2, Jan. 2, 1869. A report on exicisions of the head of the femur for gunshot injury. Washington: Government Printing Office, 1869. 141p. 3 plates. DNLM **60-1352**

OTTO & REYNDERS
Description of aspirators, surgical and orthopoedical instruments of every description, etc. New York: H. D. Gerdts & Co., [1869?] 17p. DNLM **60-1353**

[PACKARD, John Hooker] (1832-1907)
. . . Report of a committee of the associate medical members of the Sanitary Commission on the subject of the treatment of fractures in military surgery. Philadelphia: J. B. Lippincott & Co., 1862. 15p. DLC [U.S. Sanitary Commission, Medical and Surgical Monographs, O] **60-1354**

PACKARD, John Hooker (1832-1907)
A manual of minor surgery. . . . With 145 illustrations. Authorized and adopted by the Surgeon-General of the United States Army for the use of surgeons in the field and general hospitals. Philadelphia: J. B. Lippincott & Co., 1863. 288p. DLC; DNLM; PPC; PU **60-1355**

PACKARD, John Hooker (1832-1907)
Lectures on inflammation. . . . Delivered before the College of Philadelphia, under the bequest of Dr. Mütter. . . . Philadelphia: J. B. Lippincott & Co., 1865. 276p. DLC; DNLM; NNNAM; PPC **60-1356**

PACKARD, John Hooker (1832-1907)
On amputation at the hip-joint. Philadelphia, 1865. 8p. DNLM **60-1357**

PACKARD, John Hooker (1832-1907)
Notes on fractures of the upper extremity. New York: J. Medole, 1867. 58p. DNLM; NNNAM **60-1358**

PAGE, Calvin G[ates] (1830-1869)
Local anaesthesia by the artificial production of cold. [1866.] 7p. DNLM **60-1359**

PAGET, James (1814-1899)
Lectures on surgical pathology. . . . 3rd American ed. Philadelphia: Lindsay & Blakiston, 1865. 737p. CtY-M; DNLM; MBM; NNNAM **60-1360**

PAINE, Henry D.
Address before the Homoeopathic Medical Society of the State of New York. Albany: Van Benthuysen, 1865. 22p. DNLM; PPHa **60-1361**

PAINE, H[orace Marshfield] (1827-1903)
Uniformity of drug proving. Read before the semi-annual meeting of the Homoeopathic Medical Society of Oneida County, N.Y. [1861.] 4p. DNLM **60-1362**

PAINE, Horace Marshfield (1827-1903)
Manual of reference of epidemic cholera; its causes, prevention, symptoms and treatment. Albany: Weed, Parsons & Co., 1866. 16p. PPHa **60-1363**

PAINE, Martyn (1794-1877)
The institutes of medicine. . . . 6th ed. New York: Harper & Brothers, [etc., etc.], 1860. 1109p. DNLM; MBM; NNNAM **60-1364**

PAINE, Martyn (1794-1877)
The institutes of medicine. . . . 7th ed. New York: Harper & Brothers, [etc., etc.], 1861. 1130p. DNLM; MBM; PPC; PU **60-1365**

PAINE, Martyn (1794-1877)
The institutes of medicine. . . . 8th ed., rev. New York: Harper & Brothers, [etc., etc.], 1867. 1145p. CtY-M; DLC; DNLM; OCIM **60-1366**

PAINE, William (*b.* 1821)
Introductory lecture to the session of 1861 and 1862, delivered in the hall of the Eclectic Medical College of Philadelphia. Philadelphia: : W. S. Young, 1861. 14p. DNLM; PPC **60-1367**

PAINE, William (*b.* 1821)
History of the rise, progress, and principles of the American eclectic practice of medicine. [Philadelphia, 1862.] 34p. DNLM; PPC **60-1368**

PAINE, William (*b.* 1821)
An epitome of the American eclectic practice of medicine, surgery, obstetrics, diseases of women and children, materia medica, and pharmacy. . . . Designed as a text-book for physicians and students of medicine. 3rd ed. Philadelphia: W. Paine, 1863. 1203p. 1 plate. DNLM; PPC; PPJ; PU
60-1369

PAINE, William (*b.* 1821)
The medical properties and uses of concentrated medicines. Philadelphia: J. B. Rodgers, 1865. 184p. DNLM; PPC; PU
60-1370

PALLEN, Montrose Anderson (1836-1892)
Report of the various surgical operations for the relief of defective vision. Philadelphia: Collins, 1860. 63p. DNLM; PPC
60-1371

PALLEN, Montrose Anderson (1836-1892)
Prize essay. On the treatment of certain uterine abnormities. Philadelphia: Collins, 1867. 26p. 8 plates. DNLM; PPC
60-1372

PALLEN, Moses Montrose (1810-1876)
An address to the graduates of the St. Louis Medical College, delivered March 4, 1864. St. Louis: G. Knapp & Co., 1864. 19p. DNLM **60-1373**

PALMER, Alonzo Benjamin (1815-1887)
A report upon the epidemic occurring at Maplewood Young Ladies Institute, Pittsfield, Mass., in July and August, 1864: including a discussion of the causes of typhoid fever. By A. B. Palmer . . . C. L. Ford . . . and Pliny Earle. . . . Boston: D. Clapp & Son, printers, 1865. 36p. DLC; MBM
60-1374

PALMER, Alonzo Benjamin (1815-1887)
A lecture on sanitary science: its importance as a branch of general education. . . . Delivered to the medical class in the Department of Medicine and Surgery, as introductory to the course on pathology and practice of medicine for 1865-1866: with an appendix containing the outlines of a course of instruction on sanitary science established in the Literary Department of the university. Published by the class. Ann Arbor: Press of Dr. A. W. Chase, 1865. 32p. DLC **60-1375**

PALMER, Alonzo Benjamin (1815-1887)
Epidemic cholera; its pathology and treatment. Detroit: W. Graham, 1866. 33p. DNLM; OCIM
60-1376

PALMER, Alonzo Benjamin (1815-1887)
Four lectures on homoeopathy; delivered in Ann Arbor, Michigan on the 28th to the 31st of December, 1868. . . . Published by request. Ann Arbor, Mich.: Gilmore & Fiske, Booksellers, 1869. 100p. DLC; DNLM; OCIM
60-1377

PALMER, B. Frank (*fl.* 1845-1870)
The Palmer arm and leg. Correspondence with the Surgeon-General, U.S.A., and the Chief of Bureau of Medicine and Surgery, U.S.N., with letters of eminent surgeons and a communication from B. Frank Palmer to the board of surgeons, convened to decide on the best patent artifical limbs to be adopted for use by the Army and Navy of the United States. Philadelphia: C. Sherman & Son, 1862. 48p. DNLM
60-1378

PALMER, B. Frank (*fl.* 1845-1870)
The Palmer arm and leg. . . . Manufactured only under the direction of the investor and patentee, B. Frank Palmer. Philadelphia, 1865. 48p. DNLM **60-1379**

PALMER, B. Frank (*fl.* 1845-1870)
[Brief history of the great national benefaction (or gift of 7,000 arms and legs) to the mutilated heroes of the great war.] Philadelphia: Sherman & Co., 1868. 32p. DNLM
60-1380

PALMER, Edward R[ush] (1842-1895)
Introductory address to the medical class of the University of Louisville. Louisville, Ky.: Bradley & Gilbert, 1868. 16p. DNLM **60-1381**

PALMER, Henry (1827-1895)
On the application of localized galvanism in the treatment of nervous rheumatic and other affections. Chicago: R. P. P. Assn., 1866. 60p. DNLM **60-1382**

PANCOAST, Joseph (1805-1882)
Valedictory address to the graduating class of Jefferson Medical College of Philadelphia on the 10th day of March, 1865. Philadelphia: Collins, 1865. 20p. DNLM; PPJ
60-1383

PANCOAST, Joseph (1805-1882)
Lecture introductory to the course of Jefferson Medical College for the session of 1869-1870. Philadelphia: Collins, 1869. 27p. DNLM; PPJ **60-1384**

PARIGOT, Julius (*b.* 1806)
Moral insanity in relation to criminal acts. New York: Hall, Clayton & Medole, [1861]. 31p. DNLM; NNNAM
60-1385

PARIGOT, Julius (*b.* 1806)
Legislation on insanity; an address before the New York Academy of Medicine, Feb. 1, 1865. New York, 1865. 14p. DNLM; NNNAM **60-1386**

PARKER, H. C.
Some account of the yellow fever as it appeared in Galveston and Houston, Texas, in 1867, together with its symptoms, treatment, etc. Galveston: Daily Civilian and Gazette, 1868. 34p. DNLM **60-1387**

PARRISH, Edward (1822-1872)
A treatise on pharmacy. Designed as a text-book for the student, and as a guide for the physician and pharmaceutist. Containing the officinal and many unofficinal formulas and numerous examples of extemporaneous prescriptions. . . . 3rd ed., thoroughly rev. and improved with important additions. With two hundred and thirty-eight illustrations. Philadelphia: Henry C. Lea, 1867. 850p. DLC; PPC; PPJ; PU
60-1388

PARRISH, Edward (1822-1872)
Historical memoirs of the Philadelphia College of Pharmacy. A discourse read at the opening of the new College Hall, October 7, 1869. Philadelphia: Merrihew & Son, 1869. 29p. DNLM; PPC; PU **60-1389**

PARSONS, Charles W. (1823-1893)
Report on the medical topography and epidemic diseases of Rhode Island. Philadelphia: Collins, 1864. 27p. 1 map. DNLM; PPC **60-1390**

PARVIN, Theophilus (1829-1898)
Address delivered before the State Medical Society of Indiana, November 18th, 1862. Indianapolis: Elder, Harkness & Bingham, 1862. 20p. DNLM **60-1391**

PARVIN, Theophilus (1829-1898)
Introductory address delivered Oct. 31, 1864, at the Medical College of Ohio before the class, at the commencement of the regular course. Cincinnati, 1864. 15p. DNLM **60-1392**

PARVIN, Theophilus (1829-1898)
Introductory address delivered before the class of the Medical College of Ohio, Oct. 6th, 1868. Cincinnati: R. Clarke & Co., 1868. 32p. DNLM **60-1393**

PASTEUR, Louis (1822-1895)
Researches on the molecular dissymmetry of natural organic products. Transl. from "Leçons de chimie professées en 1860." By W. S. W. Ruschenberger. [Philadelphia], 1862. 32p. DNLM; PPC; PU **60-1394**

PATTON, William W. (1821-1889) and R. N. ISHAM
Report on the condition of camps and hospitals at Cairo and vicinity, Paducah, and St. Louis. By . . . of the Chicago Branch of the U.S. Sanitary Commission, Oct., 1861. Chicago: Dunlop, Sewell & Spalding, 1861. 11p. DNLM [U.S. Sanitary Commission, Documents, 1861-1865, No. 38] **60-1395**

PATTON, William W. (1821-1889)
The compensated agency of the U.S. Sanitary Commission explained and defended. Chicago, Ill.: Dunlop, Sewell & Spalding, 1864. 8p. DNLM **60-1396**

PAVY, Frederick W[illiam] (1829-1911)
A treatise on the function of digestion, its disorders and their treatment. From the second London ed. Philadelphia: Henry C. Lea, 1869. 238p. CtY-M; ICJ; PPC; PU **60-1396A**

PEALE, Franklin (1795-1870)
A memorial of the late Robley Dunglison, M.D., one of the vice-presidents of the Pennsylvania Institution for the Instruction of the Blind. Philadelphia: Collins, 1869. 19p. DNLM; PPJ; PPC **60-1397**

PEASLEE, E[dmund] R[andolph] (1814-1878)
Successful case of double ovariotomy. Philadelphia, 1864. 11p. DNLM; PU **60-1398**

PEASLEE, Edmund Randolph (1814-1878)
Ovarian tumors and their treatment (excepting ovariotomy). New York: R. Craighead, 1864. 18p. DNLM; NNNAM **60-1399**

PEASLEE, Edmund Randolph (1814-1878)
Retroflexion of the unimpregnated uterus. Albany: C. Van Benthuysen & Sons, 1866. 45p. 4 plates. DNLM **60-1400**

PEEBLES, H. E.
An address on dental education, before the Chicago Dental Society. Cincinnati: Wrightson & Co., 1867. 24p. DNLM **60-1401**

PENNSYLVANIA HOSPITAL. PHILADELPHIA
Reports. Philadelphia: Lindsay & Blakiston, 1868-1869. 2 v. [Ed. by J. M. Da Costa and Wm. Hunt] DNLM; PC; PU [No more published] **60-1402**

PENNSYLVANIA HOSPITAL. PHILADELPHIA
Descriptive catalogue of the pathological museum of the . . . by Wm. Pepper. Philadelphia: Collins, 1869. 119, 19p. DNLM; PU **60-1403**

PERCY, Samuel R[otton] (1816-1890)
An inquiry into the physiological and medicinal properties of the veratrium viride; together with some physiological and chemical observations upon the alkaloid veratria obtained from this and other species, being the prize essay to which the American Medical Association awarded the gold medal for 1863. Philadelphia: Collins, 1864. 87p. DNLM; PU **60-1404**

PERCY, Samuel R[otton] (1816-1890)
On the food of cities. Read before the Medical Society of the State of New York at its annual meeting, February, 1864. [New York, 1864.] 25p. DLC **60-1405**

PERCY, Samuel R[otton] (1816-1890)
What effect has the meat or milk from diseased animals upon the public health? (Prize essay of the Alumni Association of the Medical Department of Columbia College, 1866.) New York: J. Medole, 1866. 49p. DLC; NNC **60-1406**

PERCY, Samuel R[otton] (1816-1890)
Digitalin; its chemical, physiological, and therapeutic action. (An essay which was awarded a prize by the American Medical Association, May, 1866.) Philadelphia: Collins, 1866. 39p. DNLM; PPC **60-1407**

PERCY, Samuel R[otton] (1816-1890)
Atropia: its chemical, physiological, and therapeutic action; together with experiments instituted to ascertain its toxicological properties. (An essay, for which was awarded the prize for the years 1867 and 1868 of the Alumni Association of the Medical Department of Columbia College.) New York: D. Appleton & Co., 1868. 47p. DNLM; NNC **60-1408**

PEREIRA, Jonathan (1804-1853)
Physician's prescription book. . . . 14th ed. Philadelphia: Lindsay & Blakiston, 1865. 298p. DNLM; OCLloyd; PPC; PU **60-1409**

PEREIRA, Jonathan (1804-1853)
Manual of materia medica and therapeutics. Being an abridgement of the late Dr. Pereira's elements of materia medica. Arranged in conformity with the British Pharmacopoeia, and adapted to the use of medical practitioners, chemists and druggists, medical and pharmaceutical students, etc., by Frederick John Farre, assisted by Robert Bentley and Robert Warington. Edited with numerous references to the U.S. Pharmacopoeia, and many other additions, by Horatio C. Wood, Jr., Philadelphia: Henry C. Lea, 1866. 1030p. DNLM; PPC; PPJ; PU **60-1410**

PERKINS, Stephen H.
Report on the pension systems and invalid hospitals of France, Prussia, Austria, Russia, and Italy, with some suggestions upon the best means of disposing of our disabled soldiers. New York: W. C. Bryant & Co., 1863. 52p. DNLM; NNNAM [U.S. Sanitary Commission, Documents, 1861-1865, No. 67] **60-1411**

PERRY, Bela C.
The human hair, and the cutaneous diseases which affect it: together with essays on acne, syncosis, and cholasma. . . . New York: J. Miller, 1865. 402p. plates. DLC; DNLM; NNNAM **60-1412**

PETERS, George A[bsalom] (*d.* **1894)**
An essay on acupressure, with some reference to its application in the continuity of arteries. New York: D. Appleton & Co., 1869. 39p. DNLM; NNNAM **60-1413**

PETERS, John Charles (1819-1893)
A review of some of the late reforms in pathology and therapeutics. With an appendix on the illnesses of Washington Irving. New York: H. Ludwig, 1860. 76p. DNLM; PPHa **60-1414**

PETERS, John Charles (1819-1893) and F. G. SNELLING
Index raisonné to the new materia medica. [New York, 1861.] 88p. DNLM; NNNAM **60-1415**

PETERS, John Charles (1819-1893)
Hints toward the treatment of uraemia. [New York, 1865.] 8p. DNLM **60-1416**

PETERS, John Charles (1819-1893)
The elements of a new materia medica and therapeutics, based upon an entirely new collection of drug-provings and clinical experience. By E. E. Marcy, M.D., J. C. Peters, M.D., and Otto Füllgraff, M.D. [1866.] 856p. OCLoyd; PPHa **60-1417**

PETERS, John Charles (1819-1893)
A treatise on the origin, nature, prevention, and treatment of Asiatic cholera. . . . New York: D. Van Nostrand, 1866. 162p. DLC; DNLM; NNNAM **60-1418**

PETERS, John Charles (1819-1893)
Hints about the nature and treatment of the active congestive variety of Bright's disease. [New York, 1866.] 9p. DNLM **60-1419**

PETERS, John Charles (1819-1893)
On the conveyance of cholera from India through Persia, Armenia, and Georgia, to Russia and the rest of Europe. . . . [1866.] 14p. folding map. DLC; DNLM **60-1420**

PETERS, John Charles (1819-1893)
Notes on the origin, nature, prevention, and treatment of Asiatic cholera. . . . 2nd ed., with an appendix. New York: D. Van Nostrand, 1867. 200p. DLC; DNLM [The appendix, and press notices, contained in the preceding edition, with same title page.] **60-1421**

PETERS, John Charles (1819-1893)
. . . Conveyance of cholera from Ireland to Canada and the United States Indian territory, in 1832. . . . [Leavenworth? 1867.] 3p. DLC; DNLM **60-1422**

PETERS, John Charles (1819-1893)
On the origin of cholera in Hindostan, and its conveyance to Europe. . . . [Chicago, 1868.] 12p. DLC; DNLM **60-1423**

PETERS, John Charles (1819-1893)
. . . On the conveyance of Asiatic cholera from northern Hindostan to Central Asia. . . . [Leavenworth? 1868.] 4p. DLC; DNLM **60-1424**

PETERS, John Charles (1819-1893)
On the conveyance of Asiatic cholera from Hindostan, through Central Asia and Persia, to Russia and England, from 1817 to 1831. [1869?] 4p. DNLM **60-1425**

THE PHARMACOPOEIA of the United States of America. Fourth decennial revision. By authority of the national convention for revising the pharmacopoeia, held at Washington, A.D., 1860. Philadelphia: J. B. Lippincott & Co., 1863. 399p. DLC; OCLloyd: PPC; PU **60-1426**

PHILADELPHIA COUNTY MEDICAL SOCIETY
Discussions before the Philadelphia County Medical Society at the conversational meetings, from October, 1861, to March, 1862. Ed. and pub. by Wm. B. Atkinson, M.D. Philadelphia: King & Baird, printers, 1863. 46p. DLC; PU **60-1427**

PHILADELPHIA COUNTY MEDICAL SOCIETY
Report to the Philadelphia County Medical Society of the special committee on cholera. Read before the Society, approved and ordered to be published November 8, 1865. 6p. DLC **60-1428**

PHILLIPS, Henry, Jr.
Medicine and astrology. A paper read before the Numismatic and Antiquarian Society of Philadelphia, June 7, 1866. Philadelphia: H. B. Ashmead, 1867. 9p. DNLM **60-1429**

PHILLIPS, Henry John (1830-1879)
A practical treatise on diseases of the throat and lungs. . . . New York: Baldwin & Jones, printers, 1864. 70p. DLC; DNLM; NNNAM; PU **60-1430**

PHILLIPS, John
Ophthalmic surgery and treatment; with advice on the use and abuse of spectacles. Chicago: W. B. Keen & Co., 1869. 510p. 1 plate. DLC; DNLM; OCIM; PPC **60-1431**

PHILLIPS, John
Advice on the use and abuse of spectacles, briefly explaining the fabric of the eye and the nature of vision. . . . Chicago: J. Phillips, 1869. 90p. DLC **60-1432**

PINCKARD, F.
The sanitary brace, a simple mechanical invention intended to force the closure of the mouth during sleep, and thereby absolutely compel the nose to perform all that nature designed in the act of breathing. New Orleans, 1869. 23p. DNLM **60-1433**

POPE, Charles (1818-1870)
Valedictory address to the graduating class of the St. Louis Medical College. St. Louis: McKee & Fishback, 1860. 17p. DNLM **60-1434**

PORCHER, Francis Peyre (1825-1895)
Prize essay . . . February, 1860. Illustrations of disease with the microscope. Clinical investigations, aided by the microscope, and by chemical reagents; with microscopical observations of pathological specimens, medical and surgical, obtained in Charleston, S.C. A contribution intended to disclose the minute history of the diseases prevailing in this latitude, and to assist future students. Pt. 1. Charleston: Evans & Cogswell, 1861. 133p. 1 tab. DNLM **60-1435**

PORCHER, Francis Peyre (1825-1895)
Resources of the southern fields and forests, medical, economical, and agricultural. Being also a medical botany of the Confederate States; with practical information on the useful properties of the trees, plants, and shrubs. . . . Prepared and published by order of the Surgeon-General, Richmond, Va. Richmond: West & Johnston, 1863. 594p. DLC; ViRA
60-1436

PORCHER, Francis Peyre (1825-1895)
Resources of the southern fields and forests, medical, economical, and agricultural. Being also a medical botany of the Confederate States; with practical information on the useful properties of the trees, plants, and shrubs. . . . Prepared and published by order of the Surgeon-General, Richmond, Va. Charleston: Steampower Press of Evans & Cogswell, 1863. 601p. DLC; DNLM; ViRA **60-1437**

PORCHER, Francis Peyre (1825-1895)
Resources of the southern fields and forests, medical, economical, and agricultural; being also a medical botany of the southern states; with practical information on the useful properties of trees, plants and shrubs. . . . New ed., rev. and largely augm. Charleston: Walker, Evans & Cogswell, printers, 1869. 733p. DLC; DNLM; OCIM; NNNAM
60-1438

PORTER, Charles H. (1834-1903)
Medico-legal contributions on arsenic: containing reports of a number of cases of arsenical poisoning, together with an account of the methods employed in their chemical examination. Albany: C. Van Benthuysen, 1862. 58p. DNLM
60-1439

POST, Alfred Charles (1806-1866) and William H. VAN BUREN
Report of the committee on military surgery of the New York Academy of Medicine to the surgical section on military hygiene and therapeutics. Printed for circulation by the Sanitary Commission. [New York], 1861. 27p. DNLM; NNNAM [*also*: New York: S. S. & W. Wood, 1861, 31p.]
60-1440

POST, Alfred Charles (1806-1886)
Eulogy on the late Valentine Mott, M.D., LL.D. . . . Delivered before the New York Academy of Medicine, November 27, 1865. New York: Bailliere Brothers, 1866. 30p. DLC; DNLM; NNNAM **60-1441**

POST, Alfred Charles (1806-1886)
An address delivered before the Alumni Association of the College of Physicians and Surgeons in the city of New York, Medical Department of Columbia College. New York: Baker & Godwin, 1867. 13p. DNLM; NNC **60-1442**

POWELL, Thomas Spencer (1826-1895)
A colloquy on the duties and elements of a physician. Atlanta, Ga., 1860. 68p. DNLM **60-1443**

POWELL, Thomas Spencer (1826-1895)
Independent thought. An introductory lecture delivered at the opening of the session of the Atlanta Medical College of Georgia on the first Tuesday in November, 1865. Atlanta, 1865. 38p. DNLM **60-1444**

POWELL, William Byrd (1799-1866) and Robert Safford NEWTON
An eclectic treatise on diseases of children. New York: J. F. Trow & Co., 1867. 610p. DNLM; NNNAM
60-1445

POWELL, W[illiam] Byrd (1799-1866)
The natural history of the human temperaments; their laws in relation to marriage, and the fatal consequences of their violation to progeny, with the indications of vigorous life and longevity; followed by a fugitive essay on the protection of society against crime. 2nd ed. Cincinnati: A. T. & T. H. Keckler, 1869. 246p. 1 plate, 1 phot. DNLM
60-1446

POWER, John Hatch (1806-1863)
Anatomy of the arteries of the human body, descriptive and surgical, with the descriptive anatomy of the heart; with illustrations by B. Wills Richardson. . . . Philadelphia: J. B. Lippincott & Co., 1862. 401p. DNLM; ICRM; IU-M; PPC
60-1447

POWER, John Hatch (1806-1863)
Anatomy of the arteries of the human body, descriptive and surgical, with the descriptive anatomy of the heart. . . . Authorized and adopted by the Surgeon-General of the United States Army for use in field and general hospitals. Philadelphia: J. B. Lippincott & Co., 1863. 401p. DLC; DNLM; PPC; PU
60-1448

POWERS, Elvira J.
Hospital pencillings; being a diary while in Jefferson General Hospital, Jeffersonville, Indiana, and others at Nashville, Tennessee, as matron and visitor. Boston: Mitchell, 1866. 211p. MA; MH; NN; NNC **60-1449**

PRATT, L. (1819-1900) and J. Y. SHIRLEY
Annual address delivered before the Illinois State Homoeopathic Medical Association, at Bloomington, May 15, 1861. With a valedictory of J. Y. Shirley, retiring President. Mount Carroll, Ill.: Hollinger & Windle, 1861. 16p. PPHa
60-1450

PRATT, S. Clesson
Hydrokonion, or catarrh and its complications; comprising the causes, symptoms, and treatment by medical hydrokonia; with notes on diseases and treatment of the eye and ear; the cause and cure of stammering; the Atmisterian treatment of deafness; new theory on the electrical relations of mind and body, in health and disease, etc. Boston: the author, 1865. 127p. DNLM; MBM; MWA **60-1451**

PRESTON, Ann (1813-1872)
Nursing the sick and the training of nurses. An address delivered at the request of the board of managers of the Woman's Hospital, at Philadelphia. Philadelphia: King & Baird, 1863. 15p. DNLM; PPC **60-1452**

PRESTON, Ann (1813-1872)
Valedictory address to the graduating class of the Female Medical College of Pennsylvania. Philadelphia: W. S. Young, 1864. 16p. DNLM **60-1453**

PRESTON, Ann (1813-1872)
Women as physicians. [Philadelphia, 1867.] 4p. DNLM
60-1454

PRICE, James W.
An essay upon the practice of medicine. Atlanta, Ga.: Daily Intelligencer Print, 1862. 24p. DNLM
60-1455

PRINCE, David (1816-1890)
Report on orthopedic surgery made to the Illinois State Medical Society. Part I. Talipes. Chicago: G. H. Fergus, 1864. 50p. DNLM; IU-M **60-1456**

PRINCE, David (1816-1890)
Orthopedics; a systematic treatise upon the prevention and correction of deformities. . . . Philadelphia: Lindsay & Blakiston, 1866. 240p. DLC; DNLM; PPC; PU **60-1457**

PROCEEDINGS of the general meeting of the medical profession, in relation to the deaths of Charles Frick and Berwick B. Smith, March 29, 1860. Baltimore: J. Murphy & Co., 1860. 32p. DNLM **60-1458**

PULTE, Joseph Hippolyte (1811-1884)
Letters on diphtheria, by J. H. Pulte, M.D. and Egbert Guernsey, M.D. Saint Louis, Mo.: R. & H. Luyties, [1860]. 16p. DLC **60-1459**

PULTE, Joseph Hippolyte (1811-1884)
Homoeopathic domestic physician, containing the treatment of diseases; popular explanations of anatomy, physiology, hygiene, and hydropathy, a treatise on domestic surgery, and an abridged materia medica. 8th ed. Cincinnati: W. B. Smith & Co., 1863. 719p. DNLM; OCIM **60-1460**

PULTE, Joseph Hippolyte (1811-1884)
Asiatic cholera; its preventives and homoeopathic treatment; for travelers' and domestic use. St. Louis, Mo.: H. C. G. Luyties, [1866]. 24p. DNLM **60-1461**

PULTE, Joseph Hippolyte (1811-1884)
The spectroscope, and the law "Similia similibus curantur." Boston: G. C. Rand & Avery, 1867. 10p. DNLM **60-1462**

PURCELL, J. B.
Wilmington in health and disease. Wilmington, N.C., 1867. 51p. DNLM **60-1463**

QUACKENBUSH, John Van Pelt (1819-1876)
Pelvic presentation; its mechanism and treatment. Spontaneous evolution of the foetus; its mechanism and treatment. Papers submitted to the N.Y. State Medical Society. Albany: C. Benthuysen & Sons, 1868. 24p. 1 plate. DNLM **60-1464**

[QUININE]
Sanitary Commission. D. Report. . . . On the use of quinine as a prophylactic agent against malarious diseases. Washington: McGill, Witherow, 1862. 19p. DNLM [Committee chaired by William H. Van Buren] **60-1465**

RADCLIFFE, Charles Bland (1822-1889)
Lectures on epilepsy, pain, paralysis, and certain other disorders of the nervous system. . . . Philadelphia: Lindsay & Blakiston, 1866. 280p. DLC; PPC; PPJ; PU **60-1466**

RALPH, Joseph E.
Seminalia; or an enquiry into the symptoms, consequences, causes, signs, nature, and treatment of seminal diseases, whether arising from abuse, excess, or irregularity in either sex; including spermatorrhoea, stricture, impotence, seminal gleet; and intended to be a faithful and practical guide to all who in any way may be interested. New York: E. Warner, 1865. 7-210p. DLC; DNLM; NNNAM **60-1467**

RALPH, Joseph E.
. . . Stricture, the signs—nature and varieties—causes—consequences—remedies and cure; diseases resembling and liable to be mistaken for it. . . . [New York, 1866.] 21p. DLC; NNNAM **60-1468**

RALPH, Joseph E.
New practical medical tracts. Rheumatism: its nature. Its varieties; eight different kinds. Its causes; predisposing—exciting. Its treatment; preventive—curative. With an appendix. . . . New York: D. Taylor, book and commercial job printer, 1869. 24, 8p. DLC; NNNAM **60-1469**

RALPH, Joseph E.
. . . Stricture: its true nature and radical treatment. Its symptoms, causes, varieties, consequences, and the diseases resembling and mistaken for it. With an appendix. . . . 2nd ed. New York: D. Taylor, 1869. 19, 8p. DLC; NNNAM **60-1470**

RAND, Benjamin Howard (1827-1883)
Valedictory address to the graduates of the medical department of Pennsylvania College. Philadelphia: Collins, 1861. 13p. DNLM; PU **60-1471**

RAND, Benjamin Howard (1827-1883)
Introductory address delivered before the students of Jefferson Medical College. Philadelphia: H. B. Ashmead, 1864. 13p. DNLM; PPJ **60-1472**

RAND, Benjamin Howard (1827-1883)
Valedictory address to the graduates of the Jefferson Medical College. Philadelphia: Collins, 1866. 16p. DNLM; PPJ **60-1473**

RAND, Benjamin Howard (1827-1883)
Elements of medical chemistry. Philadelphia: T. E. Zell & Co., 1867. 399p. DNLM; NNNAM; PPC **60-1474**

RAUE, Charles Godlove (1820-1896)
Subjective and objective symptoms. A preliminary lecture delivered at the Hahnemann Medical College of Philadelphia. Philadelphia: Wm. P. Kildare, 1868. 16p. DNLM **60-1475**

RAUE, Charles Godlove (1820-1896)
Special pathology and diagnostics with therapeutic hints. Philadelphia: F. E. Boericke, 1868. 644p. DNLM; PPC; PPHa **60-1476**

RAUE, Charles Godlove (1820-1896)
Mental symptoms. [A preliminary lecture, delivered at the New York Homoeopathic Medical College.] [1869?] 14p. DNLM; NNNAM; PPHa **60-1477**

RAY, Isaac (1807-1881)
A treatise on the medical jurisprudence of insanity. Boston: Little, Brown & Co., 1860. 595p. DNLM; MH-M; NNNAM; PPC **60-1478**

RAY, Isaac (1807-1881)
A discourse on the life and character of Dr. Luther V. Bell, read to the Association of Superintendents of North American Institutions for the Insane, at its annual meeting, in Providence, R.I., June 10th, 1862. . . . Boston: J. H. Eastburn's Press, 1863. 52p. DLC; DNLM; MBM **60-1479**

RAY, Isaac (1807-1881)
Mental hygiene. . . . Boston: Ticknor & Fields, 1863. 338p. DLC; DNLM; MBM; NNNAM **60-1480**

RAY, Isaac (1807-1881)
Homicide; epilepsy. [Utica, 1867.] 20p. DNLM **60-1481**

RAY, Isaac (1807-1881)
Address delivered on the occasion of laying the corner stone of the State Hospital for the Insane, at Danville, Pennsylvania. . . . August 26th, 1869. Harrisburg: T. F. Scheffer, printer, 1869. 20p. DLC; DNLM **60-1482**

RAY, Robert, Jr. (1832-1860)
A catalogue of the pathological cabinet of the New York Hospital, classified and arranged by. . . . With a memoir of the author [by John Watson]. Edited by H. D. Bulkley. New York: S. S. & W. Wood, 1869. 364p. DNLM; NNNAM **60-1483**

RAYMOND, John C.
Essay on diphtheria. Read before the Homoeopathic Medical Society of Oneida County. New York: J. T. S. Smith, 1860. 7p. NNNAM; PPHa **60-1484**

READ, William (1820-1889)
Placenta praevia; its history and treatment. Philadelphia: J. B. Lippincott & Co., 1861. 340p. DNLM; PPC; PPJ; PU **60-1485**

READ, William (1820-1889)
Report of the city physician on the Asiatic cholera. To the mayor and aldermen of the city of Boston. Oct. 2, 1865. City Doc. No. 73. [Boston, 1865.] 17p. DNLM; MBM **60-1486**

READ, William (1820-1889)
A letter to the consulting physicians of Boston. [On cholera.] Boston: A. Mudge & Son, 1866. 29p. DNLM; MBM **60-1487**

READ, William (1820-1889)
The treatment of diseases of the air-passages by inhalation. [1866.] 6p. DNLM; MBM **60-1488**

READ, William (1820-1889)
A communication from the city physician on Asiatic cholera. Is it a contagious disease? City Doc. No. 21, 1866. [Boston, 1866.] 14p. DNLM; MBM **60-1489**

A **RECORD** of the Metropolitan Fair in aid of the United States Sanitary Commission, held at New York, in April, 1864. New York: Hurd & Houghton, 1867. 261p. 8 photo., 1 plan. DNLM; NNNAM **60-1490**

RECORDS of facts in relation to the dismissal of the faculty of the Medical Department of the University of Louisville. Published by the former faculty. Louisville: Bradley & Gilbert, 1866. 23p. DNLM **60-1491**

REDFIELD, J. W.
New views of the cause, prevention, and cure of yellow fever, and other diseases produced by miasma and mephitic vapors. Presented for the safety of the army of occupation in the Southern States. New York: J. A. Gray, 1863. 16p. DNLM; NNNAM **60-1492**

REED, William Howell (1837-1914)
Hospital life in the army of the Potomac. Boston: W. V. Spencer, 1866. 199p. DNLM; MBM; MH; NN **60-1493**

REESE, John James (1818-1892)
On the detection of strychnia as a poison, and the influence of morphia in disguising the usual colour-test. [Philadelphia: Collins, 1861.] 13p. DNLM; PPC **60-1494**

REIL, A.
A monograph upon aconite; its therapeutic and physiological effects, together with its uses; and accurate statments, derived from the various sources of medical literature. Transl. from the German of Dr. Reil, by H. B. Millard, M.D. Prize essay. New York: William Radde, 1860. 168p. NNNAM; PPHa **60-1495**

REMINGTON, Isaac (1804-1862)
Address before the Philadelphia County Medical Society, delivered January 30, 1861. Philadelphia: Collins, 1861. 21p. DNLM; PPC **60-1496**

REPORT of the committee on the drug market (for the fiscal year ending June 30, 1868); read before the American Pharmaceutical Association . . . Sept. 9, 1868, by Daniel C. Robbins, chairman of the committee. Philadelphia: Merrihew & Son, 1868. 43p. DNLM; PPC **60-1497**

A **REPORT** on excisions of the head of the femur for gunshot injury. Circular No. 2. War Department. Surgeon-General's Office. Washington, 1869. 141p. DNLM **60-1498**

REYBURN, Robert (1833-1899) and George M. WELLMAN
Addresses delivered at the 19th annual commencement of the Medical Department of Georgetown College, March 11, 1868. With a catalogue of the faculty and students. Washington: Cunningham, Lane & McIntosh, 1868. 20p. DNLM **60-1499**

RICHARDS, W.E.
The origin of homoeopathy, and reasons for preferring it to the common system of medical treatment; with the by-laws of the Worcester County Homoeopathic Medical Society. Worcester, Mass.: Goddard & Nye, [1867]. 12p. DNLM; MBM **60-1500**

RICHARDSON, B. F[ranklin] (1817?-1890)
Introductory address of the eighth regular session of the Miami Medical College of Cincinnati, Ohio. Cincinnati, O.: P. C. Browne, 1867. 17p. DNLM **60-1501**

RICHARDSON, Benjamin Ward (1828-1896)
On local anaesthesia by ether spray, as a means for the entire extinction of pain in operations on the inferior animals. New York: Bergen & Tripp, 1868. 12p. DNLM; NNNAM **60-1502**

RICHARDSON, Joseph (1824-1890)
A practical treatise on mechanical dentistry. . . . With one hundred and ten illustrations. Philadelphia: Lindsay & Blakiston, 1860. 427p. DLC: MdU-D; PPC; PU **60-1503**

RICHARDSON, Joseph (1824-1890)
A practical treatise on mechanical dentistry. . . . 2nd ed., very much enl., with one hundred and fifty-nine illustrations. Philadelphia: Lindsay & Blakiston, 1869. 442p. DLC; MdU-D; PPC; PU **60-1504**

RICHARDSON, T. G[ibson] (1827-1892)
Elements of human anatomy: general, descriptive, and practical. . . . 2nd ed. Carefully rev. and illustrated by nearly three hundred engravings. . . . Philadelphia: J. B. Lippincott & Co., 1867. 671p. DLC; DNLM; PPC; PU **60-1505**

RIGGS, J. W.
Hernia; causes of its frequency, means of prevention, and policy as regards its treatment. . . . New York, 1861. 8p. DNLM; NNNAM **60-1506**

RIGGS, J. W.
Hernia, and its treatment by trusses. New York: Hall, Clayton & Co., 1861. 16p. DNLM; NNNAM **60-1507**

ROBBINS, E. Y[oung]
Abstract of a lecture introductory to a course, on sanitary science, now in process of delivery at the Cooper Institute, New York, March 24, 1860. New York: B. F. Corlies, 1860. 15p. DNLM; NN; NNNAM **60-1508**

ROBERTS, William (1830-1899)
A practical treatise on urinary and renal disease including urinary deposits illus. by numerous cases and illustrations. Philadelphia: Henry C. Lea, 1866. 516p. CtY-M; PPC; PPJ; PU **60-1509**

ROBERTS, William Currie (1810-1873)
The eulogium of medical science. An anniversary discourse, delivered before the New York Academy of Medicine, November 2nd, 1859. . . . [Published by order of the Academy.] New York: Printed for the Academy by W. H. Tinson, 1860. 48p. DLC; DNLM; NNNAM **60-1510**

ROBERTS, William Currie (1810-1873)
A manual on extracting teeth. Founded on the anatomy of the parts involved in the operation; the kinds and proper construction of the instruments to be used; the accidents liable to occur from the operation, and the proper remedies to retrieve such accidents. Philadelphia: Lindsay & Blakiston, 1863. 209p. DNLM; PPC; PPJ; PU **60-1511**

ROBERTS, William Currie (1810-1873)
An address delivered before the Alumni Association of the College of Physicians and Surgeons, Medical Department of Columbia College, New York. New York: J. A. Gray & Green, 1864. 19p. DNLM; NNNAM **60-1512**

ROBERTS, William Currie (1810-1873)
Eulogium upon the life, professional labors and public services of Joseph Mather Smith, M.D., late professor of the theory and practice of physic, and of materia medica and clinical medicine, in the College of Physicians and Surgeons, New York . . . delivered before the New York Academy of Medicine, Wednesday evening, Feb. 6, 1867. . . . New York: A. D. F. Randolph, 1867. 79p. DLC; DNLM; NNNAM **60-1513**

ROBERTSON, Abraham
A manual on extracting teeth. . . . Philadelphia: Lindsay & Blakiston, 1863. 198p. DLC; MdU-D; PPC; PU **60-1514**

ROCHESTER, Thomas Fortescue (1823-1887)
Introductory address to the undergraduates of the Medical Department of the University of Buffalo. Buffalo: Commercial Advertiser Steam Press, 1860. 15p. DNLM **60-1515**

ROCHESTER, Thomas Fortescue (1823-1887)
The army surgeon: an address to the graduates of the Medical Department of the University of Buffalo. Buffalo: J. Warren & Co., 1863. 16p. DNLM **60-1516**

ROCKWELL, Alphonso David (1840-1925)
On the treatment of paralysis by electrization, with an explanation of a new galvanic apparatus. Being a paper read before the New York Academy of Medicine, Nov. 19th, 1868. . . . New York: Printed by the New York Printing Company, 1869. 14p. DLC; DNLM; NNNAM **60-1517**

ROCKWELL, Alphonso David (1840-1925)
Electricity as a means of diagnosis. With a tabulated statement of 500 cases of disease, treated mainly by the method of general electrization; being a paper read before the New York Medical Journal Association, Oct., 1869. . . . New York: The Trow & Smith Book Manufacturing Co., 1869. 20p. DLC; DNLM; NNNAM **60-1518**

RODGERS, Stephen (1826-1878)
Quinine as a prophylactic or protective from miasmatic poisoning, a preventive of paroxysms of miasmatic diseases, together with some remarks upon its use in the treatment of developed miasmatic diseases. Albany: C. Van Benthuysen, 1862. 24p. DNLM **60-1519**

RODGERS, Stephen (1826-1878)
An inquiry relative to the subject of the information and expectoration of fibrinous bronchial casts, accompanied by the history of an illustrative case. Albany: C. Van Benthuysen, 1866. 16p. DNLM **60-1520**

RODGERS, Stephen (1826-1878)
Extra-uterine foetation and gestation, and the early signs which characterize it; symptoms of the fatal hemorrhage into the peritoneal cavity, its usual termination; suggestions for the positive diagnosis of this fatal condition, and a plea for the treatment indicated in it, with the view of saving the life of the woman. Philadelphia: Collins, 1867. 61p. DNLM; PPC **60-1521**

RODGERS, Stephen (1826-1878)
Case of excision of the entire scapula, to which is added a history of the operations involving the removal of all or a considerable part of this bone; with a view of establishing the surgical character and prognosis of this class of operations. Philadelphia, 1868. 22p. DNLM; PPC **60-1522**

RODGERS, Stephen (1826-1878)
Summer mortality in the cities of the United States. [New York, 1869.] 18p. DNLM; NNNAM **60-1523**

RODMAN, William W[oodbridge] (1817-1900)
An address delivered at the 18th annual meeting of the American Institute of Homoeopathy, at Cincinnati, O., June 7, 1865. Chicago: Jameson & Morse, 1865. 20p. DNLM **60-1524**

RODMAN, William W[oodbridge] (1817-1900)
The materia medica in its scientific relations. New Haven, Conn.: Judd & White, 1868. 42p. CtY-M; DNLM **60-1525**

ROLETTE, Francis Xavier de
Lecture on the fever & ague, and other intermittent fevers. . . . Pittsburgh, Pa.: A. A. Anderson & Sons, printers, 1865. 16p. DLC **60-1526**

ROOSA, D[aniel] B[ennett] St. John (1858-1908)
A vest-pocket medical lexicon. Being a dictionary of the words, terms, and symbols of medical science. . . . With an appendix. . . . New York: William Wood & Co., 1865. 268p. DLC; NNNAM; PPC; PU **60-1527**

ROOSA, D[aniel] B[ennett] St. John (1858-1908)
Recent advances in the diagnosis and treatment of diseases of the ear. Albany: Van Benthuysen & Sons, 1868. 23p. 5 plates. DNLM **60-1528**

ROOSA, D[aniel] B[ennett] St. John (1858-1908)
Statistical report of five hundred cases of aural disease. New York: D. Appleton & Co., 1869. 20p. DNLM; NNNAM **60-1529**

ROSCOE, Henry E[nfield] (1833-1915)
Lessons in elementary chemistry, inorganic and organic. New York: William Wood & Co., 1868. 383p. DNLM; NN; NNNAM **60-1530**

ROSCOE, Henry E[nfield] (1833-1915)
Spectrum analysis. Six lectures, delivered in 1868, before the Society of Apothecaries of London. New York: D. Appleton & Co., 1869. 348p. 5 plates. DNLM; NNNAM; PPC; PU **60-1531**

ROSEBRUGH, A. M.
Chloroform, and a new method of administering it. New York: William Wood & Co., 1869. 31p. DNLM; NNNAM **60-1532**

ROSER, W.
Chirurgisch-Anatomisches Vade-Mecum für studiende und Artze. Amerikanische Original-Ausgable. Philadelphia: Schaefer & Koradi, 1867. 226p. PPC; PPHa; PP; PU **60-1533**

ROWSEY, Thomas
Prize essay on prairie itch. Chicago: Halsey, 1867. 17p. PPHa **60-1534**

RUBINI, Rocco
Cactus grandiflorus. Its pathogenesis; for observation on the healthy organism, and confirmed on the sick. . . . Philadelphia: Jas. B. Rodgers, 1865. 32p. 1 plate. PPHa **60-1535**

RUDDER, William
The complete physician. An address pronounced before the graduates of the Albany Medical College. Albany: F. H. Little, 1861. 30p. DNLM **60-1536**

RUDDOCK, E. Harris (1822-1875)
On consumption; its symptoms, signs, causes, and preventive and general treatment. Detroit, Mich.: E. A. Lodge, 1869. 78p. OCIM; PPHa **60-1537**

RUPPANER, Antoine (1825-1892)
On the treatment of neuralgia by subcutaneous injection, with cases. Boston: D. Clapp, 1860. 36p. DNLM; MBM **60-1538**

RUPPANER, Antoine (1825-1892)
Hypodermic injections in the treatment of neuralgia, rheumatism, gout, and other diseases. Boston: T. O. H. P. Burnham, 1865. 160p. DNLM; MH-M **60-1539**

RUPPANER, Antoine (1825-1892)
The principles and practice of laryngoscopy and rhinoscopy in diseases of the throat and nasal passages. New York: A. Simpson & Co., 1868. 153p. DNLM; NNNAM; PPC; PU **60-1540**

RUPPANER, Antoine (1825-1892)
On the removal of enlarged tonsils without cutting, with 123 cases. [Philadelphia, 1869.] 14p. DNLM; PPC **60-1541**

RUSCHENBERGER, W[illiam] S. W. (1807-1895)
A notice of the origin, progress, and present condition of the Academy of Natural Sciences of Philadelphia. (Read before the Society, February 10, 1852.) 2nd ed., revised and corrected up to January 1, 1860. by the author. Philadelphia: Collins, 1860. 102p. DNLM; PHi; PP; PPL **60-1542**

RUSCHENBERGER, W[illiam] S. W. (1807-1895)
Contributions to the statistics of human growth. [Philadelphia, 1867.] 4p. 3 tables. DNLM **60-1543**

RUSH, James (1786-1869)
The philosophy of the human voice, embracing its physiological history; together with a system of principles by which criticism in the art of elocution may be rendered intelligible, and instruction definite and comprehensive. To which is added a brief analysis of songs and recitative. 6th ed. Philadelphia: J. B. Lippincott & Co., 1867. 648p. DNLM; PPC; PPF; PPL **60-1544**

RUSH MEDICAL COLLEGE. MEDICAL DEPARTMENT OF THE UNIVERSITY OF CHICAGO
Announcement of the spring and summer course of lectures for the years 1869 (10.); 1872 (13.); 1875-1883) (16.-24.). Chicago, 1869-1879. DNLM; ICRM **60-1545**

SAGER, Abram (1810-1877)
Report on obstetrics. Read before the State Medical Society, session of 1868. Ann Arbor: E. B. Pond, 1869. 22p. DNLM **60-1546**

SALISBURY, James Henry (1823-1905)
Some experiments on poisoning with the vegetable alkaloids. [Philadelphia, 1862.] 28p. DNLM **60-1547**

SALISBURY, James Henry (1823-1905)
Inoculating the human system with straw fungi, to protect it against the contagion of measles, with some additional observations relating to the influence of fungoid growth in producing disease and in the fermentation and putrefaction of organic bodies. Philadelphia, 1862. 8p. DNLM **60-1548**

SALISBURY, James Henry (1823-1905)
Experiments connected with the discovery of cholesterine and seroline, as secretions, in health, of the salivary, tear, mammary, and sudorific glands; of the testis and ovary; of the kidneys in hepatic derangements; of mucous membranes, when congested and inflamed; and in the fluid of ascites and that of spina bifida. Philadelphia, 1863. 17p. 2 plates. DNLM **60-1549**

SALISBURY, James Henry (1823-1905)
Microscopic examinations of blood; and vegetations found in variola, vaccina, and typhoid fever. . . . New York: Moorhead, Bond & Co., printers, 1868. 65p. 3 plates. DLC; DNLM; NNNAM **60-1550**

SALISBURY, James Henry (1823-1905)
. . . On the parasitic forms developed in parent epithelial cells of the urinary and genital organs and in their secretions. . . . [Philadelphia, 1868.] 10p. DLC; DNLM; PPC
60-1551

SALISBURY, Stephen
An address delivered before the Norfolk District Medical Society at the annual meeting, May 8th, 1866. Boston: D. Clapp & Son, 1866. 12p. DNLM; MBM **60-1552**

SALTER, Henry Hyde (1823-1871)
On asthma; its pathology and treatment. . . . Philadelphia: Blanchard & Lea, 1864. 260p. DNLM; MH-M; OCIM; PPC
60-1553

SAMSON, George Whitefield (1819-1896)
Address at the opening of the hall presented by W. W. Corcoran to the Columbian College for the use of the National Medical College. Washington, D.C., Thursday, Nov. 1, 1866. 11p. Washington, D.C.: McGill & Witherow, 1866. DNLM
60-1554

SANBORN, Eben K. (1827-1862)
The silver wire in ununited fractures, with a case. [Philadelphia, 1860.] 4p. DNLM **60-1555**

SANDS, Henry Berton (1830-1888)
A case of sudden monocular amaurosis, presenting unusual difficulties in diagnosis. New York: J. Medole, 1866. 11p. DNLM; NNNAM **60-1556**

SANFORD, Leonard J[acob] (1833-1896)
Memorial of Prof. Charles Hooker, M.D. Inaugural address, in Yale College, delivered September 17, 1863. New Haven: T. H. Pease, 1863. 42p. CtY-M; DNLM **60-1557**

SANITARY COMMISSION. E. Report . . . on the value of vaccination in armies. 2nd edition. (Washington, 1861). 34p. DNLM [Committee chaired by Francis G. Smith, and including Alfred Stillé. Appendix contains articles by Gregor, Husband, Collins and Martin.] **60-1558**

SANITARY COMMISSION. F. Report . . . on the subject of amputations 2nd edition. (1861). 8p. DNLM [Prepared by D. D. Slade with the approval of the Boston Committee, Geo. Hayward, S. D. Townsend, John Ware, J. M. Warren, S. Cabot, Jr., and R. M. Hodges.] **60-1559**

SANITARY COMMISSION. No. 46. Preliminary report on the mortality and sickness of the volunteer forces of the United States Government, during the present war. New York: Bryant, 1862. 28p. DNLM [By E. B. Elliott.] **60-1560**

SANITARY COMMISSION. G. Report of a Committee of the Associate Medical Members of the Sanitary Commission on the subject of amputations through the foot, and at the ankle-joint. New York: Bailliere, 1862. 28p. DNLM
60-1561

SANITARY COMMISSION. J. Report . . . on the subject of pneumonia. Washington, McGill, Witherow, 1862. 24p. DNLM [Prepared by committee chaired by Austin Flint and including A. Clark, John T. Metcalfe, Benj. W. McCready.]
60-1562

SANITARY COMMISSION. K. Report . . . on the subject of continued fevers. Washington: Government Printing Office, 1862. 27p. DNLM [Reprot prepared by Drs. J. Baxter Upham and approved by Geo. Hayward, J. Mason Warren, S. Cabot, Jr., S. D. Townsend, John Ware and R. N. Hodges.]
60-1563

SANITARY COMMISSION. N. Report . . . on the subject of scurvy with special reference to practice in the army and navy. Washington: Government Printing Office, 1862. 29p. DNLM [Committee chaired by Wm. A. Hammond, and including Joseph Carson, Richard Hartshorne, Walter F. Atlee, S. Weir Mitchell.] **60-1564**

SANITARY COMMISSION. O. Report . . . on the subject of the treatment of fractures in military surgery. Philadelphia: J. B. Lippincott & Co., 1862. 15p. DNLM [Prepared by the Philadelphia Committee, John H. Packard, Chairman; including George W. Norris, Gurdon Buck, W. H. Van Buren, Wm. A. Hammond. Edw. Hartshorne.] **60-1565**

SANITARY COMMISSION. P. Report . . . on the subject of the nature and treatment of miasmatic fevers. Washington: McGill, Witherow, 1862. 23p. DNLM [Prepared by John T. Metcalfe.]
60-1566

SARATOGA: its mineral waters, and their use in preventing and eradicating disease, and as a refreshing beverage. New York: Russell Bros., 1868. 64p. DNLM **60-1567**

SARGENT, F[itzwilliam] W. (1820-1889)
On bandaging and other operations of minor surgery. New ed. With an additional chapter on military surgery, by W. F. Atlee. Philadelphia: Blanchard & Lea, 1862. 383p. DNLM; PPC; PJ PU **60-1568**

SATTERLEE, Richard Sherwood (1798-1880)
Statement of medical and hospital supplies furnished to the sick and wounded of the United States Army and moneys expended for the same, at New York, from April 15, 1861, to December 31, 1865. New York, 1866. 8p. DNLM; NNNAM
60-1569

SAYRE, Lewis Albert (1820-1900)
Report on morbus coxarius, or hip disease. Philadelphia: Collins, 1860. 94p. 1 plate. DNLM; PPC; PU
60-1570

SAYRE, Lewis Albert (1820-1900)
A new operation for artificial hip joint in bony anchylosis. Illustrated by two cases. Albany: C. Van Benthuysen, 1863. 19p. DNLM **60-1571**

SAYRE, Lewis Albert (1820-1900)
Morbus coxarius. Art. I. Clinical lecture. Art. II. Objections to its treatment in the advanced stages by extension, unless preceded by tenotomy. Illustrated by cases. New York: R. Craighead, 1863. 16, 8p. DNLM; NNNAM
60-1572

SAYRE, Lewis Albert (1820-1900)
Remarkable case of deception. A woman professing to secrete nothing but charcoal and stones for a number of years, all the natural functions being arrested. And the deception unmasked. Albany: C. Van Benthuysen, 1863. 7p. 1 plate. DNLM
60-1573

SAYRE, Lewis Albert (1820-1900)
Croup. Case of traumatic hemorrhage following tracheotomy, arising from the imperfect form of the tracheal tubes used, and some remarks on the treatment of croup by inhalating of steam. Illustrated by cases. Albany: C. Van Benthuysen, 1864. 11p. 1 plate. DNLM **60-1574**

SAYRE, Lewis Albert (1820-1900)
On the mechanical treatment of chronic inflammation of the joints of the lower extremities, with a description of some new apparatus for producing extension at the knee and ankle joints. Philadelphia: Collins, 1865. 25p. DNLM; PPC **60-1575**

SAYRE, Lewis Albert (1820-1900)
Case of luxation of femur into ischiatic notch, of nine months' standing, reduced by manipulation. Philadelphia: Collins, 1866. 9p. DNLM; PPC **60-1576**

SAYRE, Lewis Albert (1820-1900)
Lecture introductory to the course of orthopaedic surgery, delivered at Bellevue Hospital Medical College. New York: Moorhead, Simpson & Bond, 1868. 19p. DNLM; NNNAM; NNU-M **60-1577**

SAYRE, Lewis Albert (1820-1900)
Introductory lecture of 1868-1869 at Bellevue Hospital Medical College. New York: Sun Job Print., 1869. 18p. DNLM; NNNAM **60-1578**

SAYRE, Lewis Albert (1820-1900)
Introductory lecture of 1868-1869 at Bellevue Hospital Medical College. New York: J. Sarell, [1869]. 19p. DNLM **60-1579**

SAYRE, Lewis Albert (1820-1900)
Three cases of lead palsy from the use of a cosmetic called "Laird's bloom of youth." Philadelphia: Collins, 1869. 12p. DNLM **60-1580**

SAYRE, Lewis Albert (1820-1900)
A practical manual of the treatment of club foot. New York: D. Appleton & Co., 1869. 91p. DLC; DNLM; NNNAM; OCIM **60-1581**

SAYRE, Lewis Albert (1820-1900)
A new operation for artificial hip joint in bony anchylosis. With additional notes and letters from eminent medical gentlemen, who examined the subject, and have testified to its perfect success. New York: D. Appleton & Co., 1869. 39p. DNLM; NNNAM **60-1582**

SCANZONI, Friedrich Wilhelm von (1821-1891)
A practical treatise on the diseases of the sexual organs of woman. Transl. from the French of Drs. H. Dor and A. Socin, and annotated, with the approval of the author, by Augustus K. Gardner. 4th American ed. New York: R. M. De Witt, [1861]. 669p. DNLM; NNNAM; OCIM; PU **60-1583**

SCHIEFERDECKER, Christian Charles
Hints about the proper treatment of typhus; a letter to an inquiring friend. [New York, 1864.] 8p. DNLM **60-1584**

SCHIEFERDECKER, Christian Charles
The curability of consumption demonstrated, and the applicability of the celebrated remedies of Julius Lobethal, M.D., of Breslau, Prussia, fully established, and particularly elucidated to physicians. New York: W. C. Bryant & Co., 1864. 32p. DNLM; NNNAM **60-1585**

SCHIEFERDECKER, Christian Charles
Nature, prevention and cure of cholera. . . . New York: American News Company, 1866. 40p. DLC; DNLM; NNNAM **60-1586**

SCHMIDT, Henry D. (1823-1888)
Microscopical anatomy of the human liver. [New Orleans, 1869.] 59p. 2 plates. DNLM; LNT-M **60-1587**

SCHROEDER van der KOLK, Jacobus L. C. (1797-1862)
Pathology and therapeutics of insanity. Transl. by J. Workman. [Utica, N.Y., 1864.] 91p. DNLM **60-1588**

SCHULTZ, Carl
Schultz and Warker's mineral spring waters, their chemical composition, physiological action and therapeutical use; with a short review of the history of mineral waters. . . . New York: Baker & Godwin, printers, 1865. 70p. DLC; DNLM; NNNAM **60-1589**

SCHUPPERT, Moritz (1818-1887)
A treatise on gunshot wounds. Written for and dedicated to the surgeons of the Confederate States army. New Orleans, 1861. 47p. DNLM; LNT-M; ViRA **60-1590**

SCHUPPERT, Moritz (1818-1887)
A treatise on vesico-vaginal fistula. . . . New Orleans: Daily Commercial Bulletin Print., 1866. 46p. DLC; DNLM **60-1591**

SCOTT, J. Walter
The University guide to health; explaining the causes, symptoms, and treatment of various diseases, hygiene, and the administration of the University medicines. New York, [1869]. 116p. DNLM; NNNAM **60-1592**

SCUDDER, John Milton (1829-1894)
The eclectic practice of medicine. . . . Cincinnati: Moore, Wilstach, Keys, & Co., printers, 1864. 578p. DLC; DNLM; OCIM **60-1593**

SCUDDER, John Milton (1829-1894)
Domestic medicine: or, Home book of health, a popular treatise on anatomy, physiology, hygiene, materia medica, surgery, practice of medicine, and nursing. . . . Volume I, complete in itself. Cincinnati: J. R. Hawley & Co., 1865. 595p. DLC; OCIM **60-1594**

SCUDDER, John Milton (1829-1894)
On the use of medicated inhalations, in the treatment of diseases of the respiratory organs. . . . With an introduction to the subject, by W. Abbots Smith. . . . Cincinnati: Moore, Wilstach & Baldwin, printers, 1866. 94p. DLC; OCIM **60-1595**

SCUDDER, John Milton (1829-1894)
A familiar treatise on medicine. 10th ed. 2 v. in 1. Cincinnati: Moore, Wilstach & Moore, 1869. 595, 242p. DNLM; OCIM **60-1596**

SCUDDER, John Milton (1829-1894)
The eclectic practice in diseases of children. . . . Cincinnati: American Publishing Company, 1869. 456p. DLC; DNLM; OCIM **60-1597**

SEDGWICK, Parker
Scarlet fever, diphtheria, cholera infantum, typhoid and typhus fever, and how to cure them. By Drs. P. and S. P. Sedgwick, Wheaton, DuPage County, Ill.[Wheaton? Ill., 1868]. 8p. DLC **60-1598**

SEDGWICK, Parker
The house we live in: how to keep it in order; or, The experience of seventy years' successful practice of the medical profession, east and west, in plain English for the people. By Drs. Parker Sedgwick and S. P. Sedgwick. . . . Chicago: Church, Goodman & Donnelly, 1869. 428p. DLC **60-1599**

SEGUIN, Edouard (1812-1880)
Idiocy: and its treatment by the physiological method. . . . New York: William Wood & Co., 1866. 457p. DLC; DNLM; NNNAM; PPC **60-1600**

SEMPLE, Matthew
Valedictory address delivered at the twelfth annual commencement of the Homoeopathic Medical College of Pennsylvania, March 1, 1860. Philadelphia, 1860. 24p. DNLM; PPHa **60-1601**

SEWARDSON, Seward
The Russian medical adviser; or, Treatise on private diseases. . . . [New York, 1866.] 23p. DLC; NNNAM **60-1602**

SHADOAN, W. H.
A treatise on alveolar abscess. Cincinnati: Wrightson & Co., 1868. 31p. DNLM; OCIM **60-1603**

SHARP, William (1805-1896)
What is homoeopathy? Revised with additions and published for gratuitous circulation by William Q. Mansfield. Philadelphia: May Bros., 1867. 20p. DNLM; PPC; PPHa; PU **60-1604**

SHARPLES, A.
Introductory address on the commencement of the session of the medical department of the Willamette University for the year 1867. Salem, Oregon, 1867. 16p. DNLM **60-1605**

SHATTUCK, George Cheyne, Jr. (1813-1893)
An address delivered at the annual commencement of the Medical School of Harvard University. Boston: D. Clapp, 1861. 15p. DNLM; MH-M **60-1606**

SHATTUCK, George Cheyne, Jr. (1813-1893)
The medical profession and society. The annual discourse before the Massachusetts Medical Society, May 30, 1866. Boston: D. Clapp & Son, 1866. 34p. DLC; MBM **60-1607**

SHAW, S. Parsons
Odontalgia, commonly called toothache; its causes, prevention, and cure. Philadelphia: J. B. Lippincott & Co., 1868. 258p. DNLM; PPC; PPJ; PU **60-1608**

SHERMAN, Julian S. (*d.* 1876)
Treatment of inflammation of joints, talipes, and similar deformities, with description of new apparatus. Chicago: R. Fergus' Sons, 1867. 16p. DNLM; ICRM; IEN-M **60-1609**

SHERRILL, Hunting (1773-1866)
Family physician, or homoeopathic practice of medicine. 4th ed. New York, 1860. 445p. NNNAM; PPHa **60-1610**

SHERRILL, Hunting (1773-1866)
A lecture on the epidemic sore throat sometimes called diphtheria. An appendix containing important remarks on remittent and typhoid fevers, also directions for nursing. New York: S. Tousey, 1863. 32p. DNLM; NNNAM; PPHa **60-1611**

SHEW, Joel (1816-1855)
The cholera, its causes, prevention, and cure, showing the inefficacy of drug-treatment, and the superiority of the water-cure, in this disease. . . . New York: Fowlers & Wells, [186-?]. 98p. DLC; NNNAM **60-1612**

SHIPMAN, George Elias (1820-1893)
The homoeopathic family guide. For the use of twenty-eight principal remedies in the treatment of the more simple forms of disease. . . . Together with directions for the treatment of dengue and yellow fever, by W. H. Holcombe, M.D., of New Orleans, La. Chicago: C. S. Halsey, 1865. 91p. OCIM; PPHa **60-1613**

SHIPMAN, George Elias (1820-1893)
The homoeopathic family guide, for the use of twenty-five principal remedies in the treatment of the more simple forms of disease. . . . Together with directions for the treatment of dengue and yellow fever, by W. H. Holcombe. . . . 2nd ed. Chicago: C. S. Halsey, 1865. 247p. DLC; PPHa **60-1614**

SHIPMAN, George Elias (1820-1893)
Cholera; its prevention and cure. Chicago: C. S. Halsey, 1866. 22p. PPHa **60-1615**

SHIRLEY, T. W.
The therapeutic agency of the mind. Read before the Illinois State Homoeopathic Medical Association at the 5th annual meeting, November 2, 1859. Jacksonville, Ill.: Young America Print., 1860. 12p. PPHa **60-1616**

SHIRLEY, T. W.
Valedictory address before the Illinois Homoeopathic Association. Mt. Carroll, 1861. 5p. PPHa **60-1617**

SHORB, J. Campbell (1837-1889) and René La ROCHE
Addresses. On the occasion of the presentation of the portrait of George B. Wood, to the Wistar and Horner Museum, on his retirement from the chair, March 15, 1860, by J. Campbell Shorb, on the part of the class of 1859-1860, and R. La Roche in reply on behalf of the board of trustees. Philadelphia: Collins, 1860. 17p. DNLM; PPC **60-1618**

SHORB, J. Campbell (1837-1889)
Benevolence in medicine. An introductory address at the sixth session of lectures at the Toland Medical College. July 1, 1869. San Francisco: A. Roman & Co., 1869. 21p. DNLM **60-1619**

SHUBERT, William Augustus
Yellow fever; its origin, improper treatment, prevention, and cure; with remarks regarding alive burials in times of the epidemic, and an interesting narrative of facts. Savannah: J. M. Cooper, 1860. 50p. DNLM; GU **60-1620**

SIMPSON, James Young (1811-1870)
Clinical lectures on diseases of women. Philadelphia: Blanchard & Lea, 1863. 510p. CtY-M; DNLM; ICRM; PPC **60-1621**

SIMS, James Marion (1813-1883)
Amputation of the cervix uteri. New York: "Home" Book & Job. Print. Office, 1861. 16p. DNLM; NNNAM **60-1622**

SIMS, James Marion (1813-1883)
Clinical notes on uterine surgery; with special reference to the management of the sterile condition. New York: William Wood & Co., 1866. 401p. CtY-M; DNLM; NNNAM; PPC **60-1623**

SIMS, James Marion (1813-1883)
The Woman's Hospital. Anniversary address. New York: Baker & Godwin, 1868. 11p. DNLM; NNNAM **60-1624**

SIMS, James Marion (1813-1883)
On the microscope in the diagnosis and treatment of sterility. New York: D. Appleton & Co., 1869. 25p. DNLM; NNNAM **60-1625**

SINGLETON, James William (1829-1881)
Dr. Isaac Casselberry and his writings. Nashville: J. T. S. Fall, 1860. 22p. DNLM **60-1626**

SKEY, Frederic Carpenter (1798-1872)
Hysteria: Remote causes of disease in general; treatment of disease by tonic agency; local or surgical forms of hysteria. . . . Six lectures delivered to the students of St. Bartholomew's Hospital, 1866. 2nd American ed. New York: Moorhead, Simpson, & Bond, 1868. 110p. DNLM; NNNAM; PPC; PU **60-1627**

SLADE & BROTHER
Practical hints on dentistry; designed for friends and patrons. New York: P. Eckler, 1860. 24p. DNLM; NNNAM **60-1628**

[SLADE, Daniel Denison] (1823-1896)
. . . Report of a committee of the associate medical members of the Sanitary Commission on the subject of amputations. Boston: D. Clapp, Printer, 1861. 10p. DNLM [U.S. Sanitary Commission, Medical and Surgical Monographs, F] **60-1629**

SLADE, Daniel Denison (1823-1896)
. . . Diphtheria; its nature and treatment, with an account of the history of its prevalence in various countries. . . . Being the dissertation to which the Fiske fund prize was awarded July 11, 1860. Philadelphia: Blanchard & Lea, 1861. 85p. DLC; DNLM; PPC; PU **60-1630**

[SLADE, Daniel Denison] (1823-1896)
. . . Report of a committee of the associate medical members of the Sanitary Commission on the subject of amputations. 2nd ed. [Washington? 1861.] 8p. DNLM [U.S. Sanitary Commission, Medical and Surgical Monographs, F] **60-1631**

SLADE, Daniel Denison (1823-1896)
Diphtheria: its nature and treatment. With an account of the history of its prevalence in various countries. . . . Being a 2nd and rev. ed. of an essay to which was awarded the Fiske fund prize of 1860. Philadelphia: Blanchard & Lea, 1864. 166p. DLC; DNLM; NNNAM; PPC **60-1632**

SMALL, Alvan Edmond (1811-1886)
Hahnemann and his doctrines. An address, introductory to the first course of lectures in Hahnemann Medical College, delivered Oct. 15, 1860. Chicago: Beebe Brothers, 1861. 30p. DNLM **60-1633**

SMALL, Alvan Edmond (1811-1886)
Valedictory address. Hahnemann Medical College, Chicago, February 14, 1861. Chicago: Scott & Co., 1861. 12p. PPHa **60-1634**

SMALL, Alvan Edmond (1811-1886)
The pocket manual of homoeopathic practice, arranged from the manual of homoeopathic practice of . . . by Jacob F. Sheek. 5th ed. Philadelphia: F. A. Boericke, 1863. 126p. DNLM; PPHa; PPC; PU **60-1635**

SMALL, Alvan Edmond (1811-1886)
Manual of homoeopathic practice for the use of families and private individuals. 10th enlarged ed. New York: W. Radde; Philadelphia: F. A. Boericke, 1864. 831p. DNLM; NNNAM; PPC **60-1636**

SMALL, Alvan Edmond (1811-1886)
The pocket manual of homoeopathic practice. Abridged from the manual of homoeopathic practice, by Jacob F. Sheek. 6th ed. New York: W. Radde, 1864. 126p. DNLM; NNNAM; PPHa **60-1637**

SMALL, Alvan Edmond (1811-1886)
The past and present; an introductory lecture. Chicago: C. S. Halsey, 1865. 19p. DNLM **60-1638**

SMALL, Alvan Edmond (1811-1886)
Valedictory address to the graduating class of Hahnemann Medical College. Chicago, 1868. 19p. DNLM **60-1639**

SMALL, Alvan Edmond (1811-1886)
Manual of homoeopathic practice for the use of families and private individuals. 13th enlarged ed. New York: W. Radde; Philadelphia: F. A. Boericke, 1869. 831p. DNLM; NNNAM PPHa; PPC **60-1640**

SMALL, E.
Anatomy and physiology rendered attractive, and the laws of health made plain, in conversations between a physician and his children. Designed for schools and families, and for general reading. Boston: Degen & Estes, 1864. 441p. CtY-M; DNLM; MBM; MWA **60-1641**

SMITH, Albert Holmes (1835-1885)
Description of a new utero-vaginal speculum. Lancaster, 1869. 2 l. DNLM **60-1642**

SMITH, Daniel Drowne
Introductory lecture to the course of the Homoeopathic Medical College of New York City, October 14, 1861. New York: American Homoeopathic Review Print., 1861. 31p. NNNAM; PPHa **60-1643**

SMITH, Edward (1819-1874)
Consumption: its early and remediable stages. Philadelphia: Blanchard & Lea, 1865. 253p. DNLM; NNNAM; PPC; PU
60-1644

[SMITH, Francis Gurney] (1818-1878)
. . . Report of a committee appointed by the Sanitary Commission to prepare a paper on the value of vaccination in armies. Philadelphia: Collins, printer, 1861. 32p. DNLM [U.S. Sanitary Commission, Medical and Surgical Monographs, E]
60-1645

[SMITH, Francis Gurney] (1818-1878)
. . . Report of a committee appointed by the Sanitary Commission to prepare a paper on the value of vaccination in armies. 2nd ed. [Washington? 1861.] 34p. DNLM [U.S. Sanitary Commission, Medical and Surgical Monographs, E]
60-1646

SMITH, George K.
The insertion of the capsular ligament of the hip-joint, and its relation to intra-capsular fracture. New York: S. S. & W. Wood, 1862. 44p. DNLM; NNNAM **60-1647**

SMITH, Gouverneur Mather (*d.* 1898)
On vegetable assimilation. [New York, 1868.] 8p. DNLM
60-1648

SMITH, Gouverneur Mather (*d.* 1898)
On the etiology of Bright's disease, with remarks on the prophylaxis. New York, 1869. 34p. DNLM; NNNAM
60-1649

SMITH, Henry Hollingsworth (1815-1890)
The principles and practice of surgery, embracing minor and operative surgery; with a bibliographical index of American surgical writers from the year 1783 to 1860. Arranged for the use of students. . . . Philadelphia: J. B. Lippincott & Co., 1863. 3 v. 80 plates. DLC; DNLM; PPC; PU [Embraces the substance of three treatises, on "Minor Surgery," "Operative Surgery," and "The Practice of Surgery."] **60-1650**

SMITH, J. Heber (1842-1898)
Valedictory address delivered at the 16th annual commencement of the Hahnemannian Institute of Philadelphia, February 27, 1866. Boston: C. C. P. Moody, 1866. 16p. PPHa
60-1651

SMITH, J[ob] Lewis (1827-1897)
A treatise on the diseases of infancy and childhood. Philadelphia: H. C. Lea, 1869. 620p. DNLM; MBM; NNNAM; PPC
60-1652

SMITH, Joseph Mather (1789-1866)
Report on the medical topography and epidemics of the State of New York. Submitted to the American Medical Association at its annual meeting at New Haven in June, 1860. . . . Philadelphia: Collins, printer, 1860. 189p. tables; fold. map. DLC; NNNAM; PPC; PU **60-1653**

SMITH, Nathan Ryno (1797-1877)
Treatment of fractures of the lower extremity by the use of the anterior suspensory apparatus. . . . Baltimore: Kelly & Piet, 1867. 70p. DLC; DNLM; MdU-D; PPC
60-1654

SMITH, Southwood (1788-1861)
The common nature of epidemics, and their relation to climate and civilization. Also remarks on contagion and quarantine. From writings and official reports by Southwood Smith. . . . Edited by T. Baker, Esq. . . . Philadelphia: J. B. Lippincott & Co., 1866. 130p. DLC; DNLM; PPC; PU
60-1655

[SMITH, Stephen] (1823-1922)
. . . Report of a committee of the associate medical members of the Sanitary Commission, on the subject of amputations through the foot, and at the ankle-joint. New York: Bailliere Brothers, 1862. 28p. DLC; DNLM [U.S. Sanitary Commission, Medical and Surgical Monographs, G]
60-1656

SMITH, Stephen (1823-1922)
Hand-book of surgical operations. . . . New York: Bailliere Brothers; [etc., etc.], 1862. 279p. DLC; DNLM; NNNAM; PU
60-1657

SMITH, Stephen (1823-1922)
Hand-book of surgical operations. 2nd ed. New York: Bailliere Brothers, 1862. 274p. CtY-M; DNLM; NNNAM; PPC
60-1658

SMITH, Stephen (1823-1922)
Hand-book of surgical operations. 3rd ed. New York: Bailliere Brothers, 1862. 274p. CtY-M; DNLM; NNNAM; ViRA
60-1659

SMITH, Stephen (1823-1922)
Hand-book of surgical operations. 4th ed. New York: Bailliere Brothers, 1863. 274p. DNLM; MBM; NNNAM; OCIM
60-1660

SMITH, Stephen (1823-1922)
Hand-book of surgical operations. 5th ed. New York: Bailliere Brothers, 1863. 274p. DNLM; NNNAM; PPC; PPJ
60-1661

SMITH, Stephen (1823-1922)
Principles of hospital construction being an abstract of a report on hospitical construction made to the trustees of the Roosevelt Hospital. New York: Holman, 1866. 52p. 6 plates. DNLM; NNNAM; PPC; PU **60-1662**

SMITH, Truman (1791-1884)
Anaesthesia. Who is entitled to the credit of making the great discovery? Wm. T. G. Morton and his designs on the U.S. Treasury. His letters patent null and void. New York: R. Larter, 1864. 16p. DNLM: NNNAM
60-1663

SMITH, Truman (1791-1884)
An inquriy into the origin of modern anaesthesia. Hartford: Brown & Gross, 1867. 165p. port. DNLM; MBM; NNNAM; PPC **60-1664**

SMITH, William Manlius (1824?-1900)
An attempt to answer the question: Which part of the plant Conium maculatum is the best for medicinal use? Albany: C. Van Benthuysen & Sons, 1867. 8p. DNLM
60-1665

SMYTH, Andrew W[oods] (1833-1916)
Report of a successful operation in a case of subclavian aneurism. New Orleans: True Delta Steam Job Office, 1864. 15p. DNLM **60-1666**

SMYTH, Andrew W[oods] (1833-1916)
A case of successful ligature of the innominate artery. [New Orleans, 1869.] 6p. DNLM **60-1667**

SNELLING, Frederick Greenwood (1831-1878)
The homoeopathic treatment of diphtheria. New York: W. Radde, 1861. 16p. DNLM; NNNAM **60-1668**

SNELLING, Frederick Greenwood (1831-1878)
Nocturnal enuresis and incontinence of urine. New York: Turner & Mignard, 1869. 18p. DNLM; NNNAM **60-1669**

SNOW, Edwin Miller (1820-1888)
Report on registration, presented to the quarantine and sanitary convention at its fourth annual meeting, held in the city of Boston, June 14, 1860. [Boston, 1860.] 23p. DNLM; MBM **60-1670**

SNOW, Edwin Miller (1820-1888)
Measures proposed for the prevention of Asiatic cholera, in the city of Providence; a report to the board of aldermen. City doc. no. 8. Providence, 1865. 15p. DNL; MBM **60-1671**

SNOW, Edwin Miller (1820-1888)
A report upon sundry documents relating to Asiatic cholera, transmitted by the governor of Rhode Island to the board of health of the city of Providence. City doc. No. 5. Providence: H. H. Thomas & Co., 1865. 13p. DNLM; RPM **60-1672**

SNOW, Edwin Miller (1820-1888)
Report upon the prevention of diseases in the city of Providence, R.I., in 1866 and 1867. Presented to the board of aldermen, May 2, 1869. Providence, 1867. 15p. DNLM **60-1673**

SNOW, Edwin Miller (1820-1888)
Small-pox and the protective power of vaccination in the city of Providence. A report to the board of aldermen, April 26, 1869. City doc. no. 44. Providence: Angell & Co., 1869. 9p. DNLM **60-1674**

SOME general considerations with regard to the treatment of yellow fever. Galveston, 1868. 29p. DNLM **60-1675**

SOME practical observations on yellow fever. Published for the use of surgeons of the volunteer forces in the Department of the Gulf. New Orleans, 1862. 20p. DNLM **60-1676**

SOME suggestions concerning the nature and treatment of the teeth. Baltimore: J. Murphy & Co., 1866. 45p. DNLM; MdU-D **60-1677**

SOUCHON, Edmund (1841-1924)
An essay on the history of aneurisms of the arch of the aorta. New Orleans: L. Graham, 1867. 72p. DNLM; LNT-M **60-1678**

SPRING, Charles H[arrison] (1831-1887)
Curvatures of the spine and spinal diseases. Boston: C. C. P. Moody, 1864. 14p. DNLM; MBM **60-1679**

SPRING, Charles H[arrison] (1831-1887)
Curvatures of the spine and spinal diseases. [With additions.] Boston: H. W. Harrington & Co., 1867. 15p. DNLM; MBM **60-1680**

SPURZHEIM, Joh. Gaspar (1776-1832)
The natural laws of man; a philosophical catechism. 6th ed. New York: Fowler & Wells, [1863?]. 171p. DNLM; MBM; MWA; NNNAM **60-1681**

SQUIBB, Edward Robinson (1819-1900)
Notes upon new remedies. Albany: C. Van Benthuysen, 1860. 22p. DNLM **60-1682**

SQUIBB, Edward Robinson (1819-1900)
Remarks upon the practical working of the U.S. drug law. Philadelphia: Collins, 1864. 12p. DNLM **60-1683**

SQUIBB, Edward Robinson (1819-1900)
Advice upon epidemic cholera. New York, 1866. 4p. DNLM **60-1684**

SQUIBB, Edward Robinson (1819-1900)
An appeal for the materia medica. [Albany, 1866.] 8p. DNLM **60-1685**

SQUIBB, Edward Robinson (1819-1900)
Disinfectants. New York, 1866. 43p. DNLM **60-1686**

SQUIBB, Edward Robinson (1819-1900)
Pharmacy of the cinchonas and of podophyllum, with suggestions upon their therapeutic uses, modes of application, and tests of quality. Philadelphia: Merrihew & Son, 1868. 72p. DNLM **60-1687**

SQUIBB, Edward Robinson (1819-1900)
Notes on the alcohols from coal tar (the so-called carbolic acid), and on rhubarb. Philadelphia: Merrihew & Son, 1869. 30p. DNLM **60-1688**

SQUIBB, Edward Robinson (1819-1900)
Notes on the phenols from coal-tar (the so-called carbolic acid), and on rhubarb. Revised by the author, with additions and corrections. Philadelphia: Merrihew & Son, 1869. 32p. DNLM **60-1689**

STAFFORD, Edward
Medical directions written for Governor Winthrop by Edward Stafford, of London, in 1643. (With notes by O. W. Holmes, M.D.). . . . Boston: John Wilson & Son, 1862. 23p. MH-M **60-1690**

STANDARD LIFE INSURANCE COMPANY OF NEW YORK
Instructions to the medical examiners of the. . . . New York: Peck & Winchell, 1868. 28p. DNLM; NN; NNC; NNNAM **60-1691**

STARKEY, George R. (1823-1896)
An introductory to the fifteenth annual course of lectures in the Homoeopathic Medical College of Pennsylvania. Philadelphia: A. M. Spangler, 1862. 21p. DNLM; PPHa **60-1692**

STARKEY, George R. (1823-1896)
Valedictory address delivered before the Homoeopathic Medical College of Pennsylvania. Philadelphia: Spangler & Davis, 1865. 21p. DNLM; PPHa **60-1693**

STARLING MEDICAL COLLEGE. COLUMBUS, OHIO
Announcement for the summer session of 1865 (1.). [Columbus, 1864.] DNLM **60-1694**

STEARNS, Charles W. (1818-1887)
Palatine fissure: its remedy by artificial means considered. New York: E. O. Jenkins, 1860. 23p. DNLM; NNNAM **60-1695**

STEARNS, Charles W. (1818-1887)
Shakespeare's medical knowledge. New York: D. Appleton & Co., 1865. 78p. DNLM; NNNAM **60-1696**

STEINER, Lewis Henry (1827-1892)
Animal magnetism and hypnotism. Chambersburg, Pa.: M. Kieffer & Co., 1861. 16p. DNLM **60-1697**

STEINER, Lewis H[enry] (1827-1892)
Valedictory address delivered at the fifth annual commencement of the Maryland College of Pharmacy, March 1, 1861. . . . Baltimore: Printed by F. A. Hanzsche, 1861. 22p. DLC; DNLM **60-1698**

STEINER, Lewis Henry (1827-1892)
Report of Lewis H. Steiner, M.D., inspector of the Sanitary Commission, containing a diary kept during the Rebel occupation of Frederick, Md., and an account of the operations of the U.S. Sanitary Commission during the campaign in Maryland, September, 1862. Pub. by permission of the Sanitary Commission. New York: A. D. F. Randolph, 1862. 43p. DLC; NNNAM **60-1699**

STEINER, Lewis Henry (1827-1892)
Account of the field relief corps, of the United States Sanitary Commission, in the Army of the Potomac. New York: W. C. Bryant & Co., 1863. 12p. DNLM; NNNAM **60-1700**

STEINER, Lewis Henry (1827-1892)
A sketch of the history, plan of organization, and operations of the United States Sanitary Commission. Philadelphia: J. B. Rodgers, 1866. 13p. DLC; DNLM; PPC; PU **60-1701**

STELLWAG VON CARION, Carl (1823-1904)
Treatise on the diseases of the eye, including the anatomy of the organ. Transl. from the 3rd German ed., and edited by Charles E. Hackley and D. B. St. John Roosa. With an appendix by the editors. New York: William Wood & Co., 1868. 774p. 3 col. plates. CtY-M; DNLM; NNNAM; PPC **60-1702**

STEPHENS, Lemuel
Inaugural address delivered at the Hahnemann Medical College of Philadelphia, at the opening of the session of 1869-1870. Published by the faculty. Philadelphia: William P. Kildare, 1869. 16p. DNLM; PPHa **60-1703**

STEVENS, Alexander Hodgdon (1789-1869)
Electropathy. A new and complete system of medical electricity, by. . . . Philadelphia: [T. Simax, printer, 1863?] 16p. DLC; PPC **60-1704**

STEVENS, Edward B[ruce] (1823-1896)
Introductory address to the ninth annual course of lectures in the Miami Medical College of Cincinnati. Cincinnati: A. Abraham, 1868. 20p. DNLM **60-1705**

STEVENS, Edward B[ruce] (1823-1896)
Ohio State Medical Society. Annual address of the retiring president. Cincinnati: A. Abraham, 1868. 15p. DNLM **60-1706**

STEVENS, George T[homas] (1832-1921)
On excisions in cases of gunshot wounds. Albany, 1866. 13p. 2 plates. DNLM **60-1707**

STEVENS, John (*d.* 1840?)
Man-midwifery exposed; or, The danger and immorality of employing men in midwifery proved; and the remedy for the evil found. Addressed to the Society for the Suppression of Vice. . . . 3rd ed., enl. . . . 80p. New York [1866.] DLC; DNLM **60-1708**

STEVENSON, William B.
Thirteen months in the Rebel Army. Being a narrative of personal adventures in the infantry, ordnance, cavalry, courier, and hospital services; with an exhibition of the power, purposes, earnestness, military despotism, and demoralization of the South. By an impressed New Yorker. New York: Barnes & Burr, 1862. 232p. MH; NN; NNC **60-1709**

STEWART, Thomas Grainger (1837-1900)
A practical treatise on Bright's disease of the kidneys. New York: William Wood & Co., 1868. 188p. 7 plates. DNLM; NNNAM; OCIM; PPC **60-1710**

STILES, R. Cresson (1830-1873)
A valedictory address delivered before the medical class of the University of Vermont. Burlington: Free Press Print, 1860. 25p. DNLM; VtHi **60-1711**

STILES, R. Cresson (1830-1873)
On the direct influence of medicinal and morbific agents upon the muscular tissue of the blood-vessels. New York: C. A. Alvord, 1865. 18p. DNLM; NNNAM **60-1712**

STILES, R. Cresson (1830-1873)
On the direct influence of medicinal and morbific agents upon the muscular tissue of the blood-vessels. Action of medicines on the blood-vessels. Buffalo: J. Warren & Co., 1865. 30p. DNLM **60-1713**

STILES, R. Cresson (1830-1873)
An introductory lecture to a course of demonstrative instruction in histology and pathological anatomy. New York: C. A. Alvord, 1866. 14p. DNLM; NNNAM **60-1714**

STILES, R. Cresson (1830-1873)
The life and doctrines of Haller. An anniversary address before the Kings County Medical Society. New York: C. A. Alvord, 1867. 24p. DNLM; NBM; NNNAM **60-1715**

STILLÉ, Alfred (1813-1900)
Therapeutics and materia medica. A systematic treatise on the action and uses of medicinal agents, including their description and history. Philadelphia: Blanchard & Lea, 1860. 2 v. DLC; DNLM; MdBM; PPC **60-1716**

STILLÉ, Alfred (1813-1900)
. . . Report of a committee of the associate members of the Sanitary Commission on dysentery. Philadelphia: Collins, printer, 1862. 40p. DLC; DNLM [U.S. Sanitary Commission, Medical and Surgical Monographs, M] **60-1717**

STILLÉ, Alfred (1813-1900)
Address before the Philadelphia County Medical Society. Delivered February 11, 1863. . . . Philadelphia: Collins, printer, 1863. 20p. DLC; DNLM; PU **60-1718**

STILLÉ, Alfred (1813-1900)
Therapeutics and materia medica. A systematic treatise on the action and uses of medicinal agents, including their description and history. 2nd ed. Philadelphia: Blanchard & Lea, 1864. 2 v. DNLM; PPC; PPJ; PU **60-1719**

STILLÉ, Alfred (1813-1900)
Epidemic meningitis; or, cerebro-spinal meningitis. . . . Philadelphia: Lindsay & Blakiston, 1867. 178p. DLC; DNLM; PPC; PU **60-1720**

STILLÉ, Alfred (1813-1900)
Therapeutics and materia medica. A systematic treatise on the action and uses of medicinal agents, including their description and history. . . . 3rd ed., rev. and enl. . . . Philadelphia: Henry C. Lea, 1868. 2 v. DLC; OCIM; PPC; PU **60-1721**

STILLÉ, Charles Janeway (1819-1899)
Memorial of the great central fair for the U.S. Sanitary Commission, held at Philadelphia, June, 1864. Philadelphia: U.S. Sanitary Commission, 1864. 211p. 3 plates. DNLM; PPC; PPJ; PU **60-1722**

STILLÉ, Charles Janeway (1819-1899)
History of the United States Sanitary Commission, being the general report of its work during the war of the rebellion. . . . Philadelphia: J. B. Lippincott & Co., 1866. 553p. DNLM; NNNAM; PPC; PU **60-1723**

STILLÉ, Charles Janeway (1819-1899)
History of the United States Sanitary Commission, being the general report of its work during the war of the rebellion. . . . New York: Hurd & Houghton, 1868. 553p. DNLM; NNC; NNNAM; OCIM **60-1724**

STILWELL, T. H[unt]
A treatise on deafness, catarrh, and scrofula. With a description of his great invention of the organic vibrator. [New York, 1869.] 36p. DNLM; NNNAM **60-1725**

STOCKTON-HOUGH, John
Description of a new vaginal speculum. [Philadelphia, 1869.] 4p. DNLM **60-1726**

STOCKTON-HOUGH, John
Description of a new self-retaining vaginal, uterine, and anal speculum combined, for examinations and operations. [Philadelphia, 1869.] 3p. DNLM **60-1727**

STONE, Alexander J. (1845-1910)
A new property of the bromide of potassium. Its power in checking the reflex nausea induced by the administration of anaesthetics. Boston: D. Clapp & Son, 1868. 23p. DNLM; MBM **60-1728**

STONE, Andrew
Pulmonary consumption, that fatal destroyer of man! Its curability demonstrated on natural principles alone. Combining medicated air, medicated inhalation, and natural hygiene. . . . Troy, N.Y.: Troy Lung and Hygienic Institute, 1863. 309p. DLC **60-1729**

STORER, David Humphreys (1804-1891)
Address. Philadelphia: Collins, 1866. 13p. DNLM **60-1730**

STORER, Horatio Robinson (1830-1922)
On criminal abortion in America. . . . Philadelphia: J. B. Lippincott & Co., 1860. 107p. DLC; DNLM **60-1731**

STORER, Horatio Robinson (1830-1922)
Studies of abortion. [Boston, 1863.] 7p. DNLM **60-1732**

STORER, Horatio Robinson (1830-1922)
On artificial dilatation of the os and cervix uteri by fluid pressure from above; a reply to Drs. Keiller, of Edinburgh, and Arnott and Barnes, of London. Boston: D. Clapp, 1863. 11p. DNLM **60-1733**

STORER, Horatio Robinson (1830-1922)
Eutokia: a word to physicians and to women upon the employment of anaesthetics in childbirth. Boston: A. Williams & Co., 1863. 30p. DNLM **60-1734**

STORER, Horatio Robinson (1830-1922)
On chloroform inhalation during labor; with especial reference to a later paper by Dr. Johns, of Dublin. Boston: D. Clapp, 1863. 8p. DNLM **60-1735**

STORER, Horatio Robinson (1830-1922)
The surgical treatment of amenorrhoea. [Philadelphia, 1864.] 10p. DNLM **60-1736**

STORER, Horatio Robinson (1830-1922)
The relations of female patients to hospitals for the insane; the necessity on their account of a board of consulting physicians to every hospital. Philadelphia: Collins, 1864. 11p. DNLM **60-1737**

STORER, Horatio Robinson (1830-1922)
The medical management of insane women. [Boston, 1865.] 10p. DNLM; MBM **60-1738**

STORER, Horatio Robinson (1830-1922)
Report of the delegate to the Association of Superintendents of Asylums for the Insane, for 1865-1866. Philadelphia: Collins, 1866. 14p. DNLM; MBM **60-1739**

STORER, Horatio Robinson (1830-1922)
Successful removal of the uterus and both ovaries by abdominal section, the tumor, fibrocystic, weighing thirty-seven pounds. Boston: D. Clapp & Son, 1866. 32p. DNLM; MBM **60-1740**

STORER, Horatio Robinson (1830-1922)
Why not? A book for every woman. The prize essay to which the American Medical Association awarded the gold medal for 1865. Boston: Lee & Shepard, 1866. 91p. DNLM; MBM **60-1741**

STORER, Horatio Robinson (1830-1922)
Is it I? A book for every man. A companion to Why not? A book for every woman. Boston: Lee & Shepard, 1867. 154p. DNLM; MBM **60-1742**

STORER, Horatio Robinson (1830-1922)
On the decrease of the rate of increase of population now obtaining in Europe and America. [New Haven, 1867.] 15p. DNLM; MBM **60-1743**

STORER, Horatio Robinson (1830-1922) and Franklin Fiske HEARD
Criminal abortion: its nature, its evidence, and its law. Boston: Little, Brown & Co., 1868. 215p. DNLM; MBM; NNNAM **60-1744**

STORER, Horatio Robinson (1830-1922)
On nurses and nursing; with especial reference to the management of sick women. . . . Boston: Lee & Shepard, 1868. 80p. DLC; DNLM; MBM **60-1745**

STORER, Horatio Robinson (1830-1922)
Pocketing the pedicle: a new and successful method of treating the ovarian stump after excision. Philadelphia, 1868. 11p. DNLM; PPC **60-1746**

[STORER, Horatio Robinson] (1830-1922)
Fiat justitia, ruat coelum. To the fellows of the Massachusetts Medical Society, Boston, Oct. 1, 1869. [Boston, 1869.] 14p. DNLM; MBM **60-1747**

THE STORY of a stomach; an egotism. By a reformed dyspeptic. 3rd ed. New York: Fowler & Wells, 1867. 60p. DNLM; NNNAM **60-1748**

STOUT, Arthur B.
Amputation at the hip joint; hip disease—epilepsy. [San Francisco, 1862.] 4p. DNLM **60-1749**

STOUT, Arthur B.
Carbolization in small-pox. [San Francisco, 1868.] 1 l. fol. DNLM **60-1750**

STOUT, S[amuel] H[ollingsworth] (1822-1903)
An address, introductory to the eighth regular summer course of lectures in the Atlanta Medical College. Atlanta, Ga.: J. J. Toon, 1866. 19p. DNLM **60-1751**

STRICKLAND, A.
Cholera, its symptoms and treatment. Cincinnati, 1866. 24p. DNLM **60-1752**

STROMEYER, Georg Friedrich Louis (1804-1876)
Gunshot fractures. By Louis Stromeyer. Resection in gunshot injuries. By Friedrich Esmarch. Transl. by S. F. Statham. Philadelphia: J. B. Lippincott & Co., 1862. 68, 120p. DNLM; PPC; PU **60-1753**

STURGIS, D. B.
The vademecum of valuable medical information, for the people. . . . Goshen, Ind.: Copeland & Smith, printers, 1864. 35p. DLC **60-1754**

STURGIS, Frederic Russell (1844-1919)
Human cestoids: an essay to which was awarded the second prize of the Boylston Medical Society for 1867. Cambridge: J. Wilson & Son, 1867. 81p. 3 plates. DNLM; MH-M **60-1755**

SUTTON, George (1812-1886)
Report on cholera, to the Indiana State Medical Society. [Indianapolis, 1868.] 16p. DNLM **60-1756**

SWEETSER, William (1797-1875)
Human life; considered in its present condition and future developments, especially with reference to its duration. . . . New York: G. B. Putnam & Son, 1867. 322p. DLC; NN; NNC **60-1757**

SWINBURNE, John (1820-1889)
Report of two cases of extra uterine pregnancy. Albany: C. Van Benthuysen, 1860. 5p. DNLM **60-1758**

SWINBURNE, John (1820-1889)
Treatment of fractures of long bones by simple extension. Albany: C. Van Benthuysen, 1861. 50p. 3 plates. DNLM **60-1759**

SWINBURNE, John (1820-1889)
A new method for the treatment of fractures and dislocations, with fractures in and near the elbow-joint. [Philadelphia, 1861.] 4p. DNLM **60-1760**

SWINBURNE, John (1820-1889)
Poisoning by aconite. Synopsis of the trial of Hendrickson for the murder of his wife. Philadelphia, 1862. 16p. DNLM **60-1761**

SWINBURNE, John (1820-1889)
Report of Dr. . . . giving an account of his services on the peninsula. [n.p., 1862.] 11p. DNLM **60-1762**

SWINBURNE, John (1820-1889)
Reports on the peninsular campaign, surgical experiences, etc. Albany: C. Van Benthuysen, 1863. 67p. DNLM **60-1763**

SWINBURNE, John (1820-1889)
Compound and comminuted gun-shot fractures of the thigh, and means for their transportation, etc. Albany: C. Van Benthuysen, 1864. 16p. 1 plate. DNLM **60-1764**

SYME, James (1799-1870)
The principles of surgery. By John Syme. . . . To which are appended his treatises on "The diseases of the rectum," "Stricture of the urethra and fistula in perineo," "The excision of diseased joints," and numerous additional contributions to the pathology and practice of surgery. Ed. by . . . Donald Maclean. . . . Philadelphia: J. B. Lippincott & Co., 1866. 880p. DLC; NNNAM; OCIM; PPC **60-1765**

SYME, James (1799-1870)
Principles and practice of surgery. . . . Ed. with notes and illustrations. By Robert S. Newton. . . . 5th American, from the last Edinburgh ed. New York: J. F. Trow & Co., printers, 1866. 908p. DLC; NNNAM; PPC; PU **60-1766**

TAFT, Jonathan (1820-1903)
A practical treatise on operative dentistry. . . . 2nd ed. with eighty-six illustrations. Philadelphia: Lindsay & Blakiston, 1868. 430p. DLC; MBM; MdU-D; PPC **60-1767**

TALBOT, I. T[isdale] (1829-1899)
"The common sense of homoeopathy." Annual address, delivered before the Massachusetts Homoeopathic Medical Society, April 10, 1861. Boston: J. Wilson & Son, 1862. 26p. DNLM; MBM; PPHa **60-1768**

TALBOT, I. T[isdale] (1829-1899)
Tracheotomy in croup. Boston: J. Wilson & Son, 1866. 25p. DNLM; MBM **60-1769**

TANNER, Thomas Hawkes (1824-1871)
A practical treatise on the diseases of infancy and childhood. Philadelphia: Lindsay & Blakiston, 1861. 464p. DNLM; ICRM; NNNAM; PPC **60-1770**

TANNER, Thomas Hawkes (1824-1871)
Memoranda on poisons. From the last London ed. Philadelphia: Lindsay & Blakiston, 1864. 112p. IEN-M; MBM; NNNAM; PPC **60-1771**

TANNER, Thomas Hawkes (1824-1871)
A manual of the practice of medicine. 3rd ed., revised and improved. From the last London ed., enlarged and improved. Philadelphia, 1864. 699p. DNLM; MBM; NNNAM; PU **60-1772**

TANNER, Thomas Hawkes (1824-1871)
The practice of medicine. . . . From the 5th London ed.: enl. and improved. Philadelphia: Lindsay & Blakiston, 1866. 835p. DLC; MH-M; PPC; PU **60-1773**

TANNER, Thomas Hawkes (1824-1871)
A practical treatise on the diseases of infancy and childhood. 2nd American ed. Philadelphia: Lindsay & Blakiston, 1866. 464p. DNLM; MdU-D; OCIM; PPC **60-1774**

TANNER, Thomas Hawkes (1824-1871)
The practice of medicine. 4th American from the 5th London ed. Philadelphia: Lindsay & Blakiston, 1867. 839p. CtY-M; MBM; NNNAM; PPC **60-1775**

TANNER, Thomas Hawkes (1824-1871)
An index of diseases and their treatment. 4th ed., revised by Percy Boulton. Philadelphia: Lindsay & Blakiston, 1867. 397p. DNLM; MBM; NNNAM; PPC **60-1776**

TANNER, Thomas Hawkes (1824-1871)
On the signs and diseases of pregnancy. From the 2nd and enlarged London ed. Philadelphia: Henry C. Lea, 1868. 490p. 4 plates. DNLM; OCIM; PPC; PU **60-1777**

TARBELL, John Adams (1810-1864)
Homoeopathy simplified; or, Domestic practice made easy. Containing explicit directions for the treatment of disease, the management of accidents, and the preservation of health. . . . Rev. ed. Boston: O. Clapp. 1863. 372p. DLC; MBM; PPHa; PU **60-1778**

TAYLOR, Alfred B[ower] (1824-1898)
Weights of the pharmacopoeia. [Philadelphia, 1860.] 8p. DNLM; PPC **60-1779**

TAYLOR, Alfred Swaine (1806-1880)
Medical jurisprudence. . . . 5th American from the 7th and rev. London ed. Ed., with additions, by Edward Hartshorne. . . . Philadelphia: Blanchard & Lea, 1861. 714p. DLC; OCIM; NNNAM; PPC **60-1780**

TAYLOR, Alfred Swaine (1806-1880)
A manual of medical jurisprudence. . . . 6th American from the 8th and rev. London ed., with notes and references to American decisions. By Clement B. Penrose. . . . Philadelphia: Henry C. Lea, 1866. 776p. DLC; DNLM; NNNAM; PPC **60-1781**

TAYLOR, Charles Fayette (1827-1899)
Pathology of paralysis of motion, with its treatment by specific exercises. New York: Dodge & Grattan, 1860. 32p. DNLM; NNNAM **60-1782**

TAYLOR, Charles Fayette (1827-1899)
Theory and practice of the movement-cure; or, the treatment of lateral curvature of the spine, paralysis, indigestion, constipation, consumption, angular curvatures and other deformities, diseases incident to women, derangements of the nervous system and other chronic affections by the Swedish system of localized movements. Philadelphia: Lindsay & Blakiston, 1861. 295p. DNLM; MBM; NNNAM; PPC **60-1783**

TAYLOR, Charles Fayette (1827-1899)
The mechanical treatment of angular curvature, or Pott's disease of the spine. . . . New York: Bailliere Brothers, 1863. 48p. DLC; NNNAM **60-1784**

TAYLOR, Charles Fayette (1827-1899)
"Spinal irritation"; or, The causes of back-ache among American women. . . . New York: William Wood & Co., 1864. 32p. 15 plates. DLC; NNNAM **60-1785**

TAYLOR, Charles Fayette (1827-1899)
Theory and practice of the movement-cure; or, The treatment of lateral curvature of the spine; paralysis; indigestion; constipation, consumption; angular curvatures, and other deformities, disease incident to women; derangements of the nervous system; and other chronic affections, by the Swedish system of localized movements. . . . 2nd ed. Philadelphia: Lindsay & Blakiston, 1864. 295p. DLC; NNNAM; PPC; PU **60-1786**

TAYLOR, Charles Fayette (1827-1899)
The pathology of the lateral curvature of the spine. Philadelphia: Collins, 1865. 8p. DNLM **60-1787**

TAYLOR, Charles Fayette (1827-1899)
Infantile paralysis, and its attendant deformities. . . . Philadelphia: J. B. Lippincott & Co., 1864. 119p. DLC; PPC; PPF; PU **60-1788**

TAYLOR, Charles Fayette (1827-1899)
The pathology and treatment of lateral curvature of the spine. New York: N.Y. Printing Co., 1868. 18p. DNLM; NNNAM **60-1789**

TAYLOR, Charles Fayette (1827-1899)
Differential diagnosis in diseases of the spine. New York: D. Appleton & Co., 1869. 16p. DNLM; NNNAM **60-1790**

TAYLOR, George Henry (1821-1896)
An exposition of the Swedish movement-cure . . . together with a summary of the principles of general hygiene. . . . New York: Fowler & Wells, 1860. 396p. DLC; NNNAM **60-1791**

TAYLOR, George H. (1821-1896)
A sketch of the movement-cure, with illustrative cases. New York, 1860. 24p. DNLM; NNNAM **60-1792**

TAYLOR, George H. (1821-1896)
The movement-cure in every chronic disease; a summary of its principles, processes, and results. New York: R. Larter, 1861. 64p. DNLM; NNNAM **60-1793**

TAYLOR, George Henry (1821-1896)
An illustrated sketch of the movement-cure; its principles, methods and effects. . . . New York: Published at the Institute, 1868. 60, 12p. DLC; NNNAM **60-1794**

TAYLOR, Henry S.
The family doctor: a counsellor in sickness, pain, and distress, for childhood, manhood, and old age, [etc.]. 21st ed. Philadelphia: J. E. Potter, 1863. 308p. DNLM; NNNAM; PPC; PU
60-1795

TAYLOR, Isaac Ebenezer (1812-1889)
Facts in relation to placenta praevia, with a review of the various opinions respecting its anatomy, physiology, pathology, and treatment. Albany: C. Van Benthuysen, 1865. 37p. DNLM **60-1796**

TAYLOR, Isaac Ebenezer (1812-1889)
Recto-vaginal and recto-labial fistula, a new method of operating for. Albany: C. Van Benthuysen, 1866. 5p. DNLM
60-1797

TAYLOR, Isaac Ebenezer (1812-1889)
On amputation of the cervix uteri in certain forms of procidentia and on complete eversion of the cervix uteri. New York: D. Appleton & Co., 1869. 66p. 1 plate. DNLM; NNNAM
60-1798

TAYLOR, Isaac Ebenezer (1812-1889)
On the spontaneous and artificial delivery of the child in face presentations, with the chin posteriorly. New York: D. Appleton & Co., 1869. 26p. DNLM; NNNAM
60-1799

TAYLOR, Othniel Hart (1803-1869)
[Medical topography of Camden County, New Jersey.] [New York, 1862.] 12p. DNLM; NjR **60-1800**

TEMPLE, John Taylor (1803-1877)
Valedictory address to the graduating class of the Homoeopathic Medical College of Missouri, February 27, 1867. By the Dean of the Faculty. St. Louis, Mo.: Ustick, 1867. 11p. PPHa
60-1801

TESTE, Alphonse (*b.* 1814)
A homoeopathic treatise on the diseases of children. Translated from the French by Emma H. Coté. 3rd ed. Revised by J. H. Pulte, M.D. Cincinnati: Moore, Wilstach, Keys & Co., 1860. 342p. OCIM; PPHa **60-1802**

TESTIMONIAL of members of the medical profession of Philadelphia, New York, and Boston, in behalf of Wm. T. G. Morton, M.D. Philadelphia: Collins, printer, 1860. 32p. CtY-M; DLC; MA; MBM **60-1803**

TETER, H[enry]
A book for every family: the science of medicine made known in a plain, comprehensive and practical manner. The guide to health and married woman's companion. . . . Columbus, O.: Osgood & Pearce, printers, 1860. 740p. DLC; OCIM
60-1804

THACHER, James (1754-1844)
Military journal of the American revolution, from the commencement to the disbanding of the American army. . . . To which is added the life of Washington. . . . Hartford, Conn.: Hurlbut, Williams & Co., 1862. MA; MB; NN; NNC
60-1805

THAYER, William Henry (1822-1897)
Diphtheria: its history, nature, and treatment. Pittsfield, Mass., 1861. 38p. DNLM **60-1806**

THOMAS, Amos Russell (1826-1892)
Inaugural address delivered at the Hahnemann Medical College of Philadelphia, at the opening of the session of 1868-1869. Published by the Faculty. Philadelphia: W. P. Kildare, 1868. 21p. DNLM; PPHa **60-1807**

THOMAS, Charles Monroe
Catalogue of the Museum and Library of the Hahnemann Medical College of Philadelphia, No. 1105 Filbert Street, Philadelphia. Wm. P. Kildare, 1869. 45p. DNLM; PPHa
60-1808

THOMAS, Joseph (1811-1891)
A comprehensive medical dictionary. . . . With an appendix, comprising a complete list of all the more important articles of the materia medica . . . with the necessary directions for writing Latin prescriptions, etc., etc. . . . Philadelphia: J. B. Lippincott & Co., 1864. 704p. DLC; MBM; NNNAM; PPC
60-1809

THOMAS, T[heodore] Gaillard (1832-1903)
Introductory address delivered at the College of Physicians and Surgeons, New York. New York: W. H. Trafton & Co., 1864. 31p. DNLM; NNNAM **60-1810**

THOMAS, T[heodore] Gaillard (1832-1903)
A practical treatise on the diseases of women. . . . With two hundred and nineteen illustrations. Philadelphia: Henry C. Lea, 1868. 625p. DLC; DNLM; NNNAM; PPC
60-1811

THOMAS, T[heodore] Gaillard (1832-1903)
A practical treatise on the diseases of women. . . . With two hundred and twenty-five illustrations. 2nd ed., rev. and improved. Philadelphia: Henry C. Lea, 1869. 647p. DLC: MBM; NNNAM; PPC **60-1812**

THOMAS, T[heodore] Gaillard (1832-1903)
The history of four cases of chronic inversion of the uterus, with the account of an operation designed as a substitute for amputation. [New York, 1869.] 47p. DNLM; NNNAM
60-1813

THOMAS, T[heodore] Gaillard (1832-1903)
The history of nine cases of ovariotomy. New York: D. Appleton & Co., 1869. 27p. DNLM; NNNAM
60-1814

THOMPSON, Augustine
Valedictory address delivered at the 17th annual commencement of the Hahnemannian Medical Institute of Philadelphia, February 26, 1867. Published by request of the graduating class. Rockland, Maine: Democrat Office Print., 1867. 17p. DNLM; PPHa **60-1815**

THOMPSON, Henry (1820-1904)
Clinical lectures on diseases of the urinary organs. Delivered at University College Hospital. Philadelphia: Henry C. Lea, 1869. 204p. DNLM; NNNAM; OCIM; PPC
60-1816

THOMPSON, Rezin
A treatise on fever: its cause, phenomena, and treatment, with an appendix, containing views on some female diseases, some diseases of children. . . . Memphis, 1869. 448p. DNLM; OCIM
60-1817

THOMS, Wm. Faulds
Health in country and cities. Illustrated by tables of the death-rates, sickness-rates, etc., etc., in country and cities. Philadelphia: Collins, 1866. 16p. DNLM **60-1818**

THOMS, Wm. Faulds
Tenant houses: their ground area, cubic feet of air space, and ventilation. Albany: C. Van Benthuysen & Sons, 1866. 18p. DNLM **60-1819**

THOMS, Wm. Faulds
Weather chart, showing the effects of the meteorological influences on mortality in the city of New York. Aug., 1868. [New York: Endicott & Co., 1868.] Broadside fol. DNLM **60-1820**

THOMSON, Anthony Todd (1778-1849)
A conspectus of the pharmacopoeias of the London, Edinburgh, and Dublin colleges of physicians, and of the United States Pharmacopoeia; being a practical compendium of materia medica and pharmacy. 7th American ed. Edited by Charles A. Lee (from the 13th English ed.). New York: William Wood & Co., 1862. 322p. DNLM; NNNAM; OCLloyd; PU **60-1821**

THOMSON, M. S.
Reply to Dr. J. Dickson Smith's pamphlet on "Lobeliaism." Macon, Ga.: Telegraph Steam Printing House, 1860. 16p. DNLM **60-1822**

THOMSON, William (1833-1907)
Report of cases of hospital gangrene treated in Douglas Hospital, Washington, D.C. [Philadelphia, 1864.] 18p. DNLM **60-1823**

THORN, James (1802-1876)
Memorial of the late Thomas M. Blatchford, read at a meeting of the governors of the Marshall Infirmary, Troy, N.Y., January 29, 1866. Troy, N.Y.: Daily & Weekly Times, 1866. 7p. DNLM **60-1824**

THRAILKILL, John W. (*d.* 1883)
An essay on the causes of infant mortality. . . . St. Louis: S. W. Book & Publishing Co., 1869. 62p. DLC; DNLM; OCIM **60-1825**

[TIEMANN, George & Co.]
Catalogue of surgical instruments, apparatus for deformities and fractures, bandages, trusses, spine braces, &c. manufactured and sold by George Tiemann & Co., No. 67 Chatham St., New York. 1869. 80p. NNNAM **60-1826**

TILDEN & CO. NEW LEBANON, N.Y.
Formulae for making tinctures, infusions, syrups, wines, mixtures, pills, etc., simple and compound, from the fluid and solid extracts, prepared at the laboratory of Tilden & Co. [New York], 1861. 162p. NNNAM **60-1827**

TILDEN & CO. NEW LEBANON, N.Y.
The therapeutical powers and properties of wild cherry, and its preparations, with a synopsis of the properties of other valuable remedies. New York, [1867]. 16p. DNLM; NNNAM **60-1828**

TILDEN & CO. NEW LEBANON, N.Y.
Prices current of medicinal preparations, prepared in vacuo, at a temperature not exceeding 100°F. New York, [1867]. 17p. DNLM **60-1829**

TILDEN & CO. NEW LEBANON, N.Y.
Formulae for making tinctures, infusions, syrups, wines, mixtures, pills, etc., simple and compound, from the fluid and solid extracts prepared at the laboratory of Tilden & Co., New Lebanon, N.Y. Established in 1848. New Lebanon, N.Y.: Tilden & Co., 1868, 162, 32p. DNLM; NNNAM **60-1830**

TILT, Edward [John] (1815-1893)
A handbook of uterine therapeutics, and of diseases of women. 3rd ed. New York: William Wood & Co., 1864. 2 v. DNLM; MH-M; NNNAM; PU **60-1831**

TIRRELL, N.D.
Valedictory address to the members of the graduating class of the seventh annual session of the Homoeopathic Medical College of Missouri, February 25, 1869. St. Louis, Mo.: Clayton & Babington, 1869. 20p. PPHa **60-1832**

TOBOLD, Adelbert (1827-1907)
Chronic diseases of the larynx, with special reference to laryngoscopic diagnosis and local therapeutics. . . . Transl. from the German and ed. by George M. Beard. . . . With an introduction on the history and art of laryngoscopy and rhinoscopy . . . by the editor. . . . New York: William Wood & Co., 1868. 279p. DLC; NNNAM; PPC; PU **60-1833**

TODD, Robert Bentley (1809-1860)
Clinical lectures on certain acute diseases. . . . Philadelphia: Blanchard & Lea, 1860. 308p. DLC; MBM; NNNAM; PPC **60-1834**

TOLAND, Hugh Hughes (1806-1880)
Valedictory address delivered before the graduating class of Toland Medical College, March 8th, 1865. [San Francisco, 1865.] 7p. DNLM **60-1835**

TONER, Joseph Meredith (1825-1896)
Maternal instinct, or love. Baltimore: Murphy & Co., 1864. 152p. DNLM; MdU-D; PPC; PU **60-1836**

TONER, Joseph Meredith (1825-1896)
. . . Inoculation in Pennsylvania. . . . [Philadelphia, 1865] 20p. DLC; DNLM; PPC; PU **60-1837**

TONER, Joseph Meredith (1825-1896)
A paper on the propriety and necessity of compulsory vaccination. . . . Philadelphia: Collins, printer, 1865. 26p. DLC; DNLM; PPC **60-1838**

[TONER, Joseph Meredith] (1825-1896)
A catalogue of medical works on cholera, in the library of J. M. Toner, M.D. [Washington, D.C., 1865.] 4 p. DLC; DNLM **60-1839**

TONER, Joseph Meredith (1825-1896)
Medical register of the District of Columbia, 1867. Embracing notices of the medical, benevolent and public institutions of Washington. . . . Washington, D.C.: Blanchard & Mohun, 1867. 102p. DLC; DNLM **60-1840**

TONER, Joseph Meredith (1825-1896)
Anniversary oration delivered before the Medical Society of the District of Columbia, September 26, 1866. . . . Washington, D.C.: Cunningham & McIntosh, printers, 1869. 80p. DLC; DNLM **60-1841**

TOWNSEND, Howard (1823-1867)
Glycogenic function of the liver. Albany: C. Van Benthuysen, 1864. 10p. DNLM **60-1842**

TOWSEND, Stephen (1804-1881)
Sermon to the medical students of Jefferson Medical College. Philadelphia: Perkinpino & Higgins, 1863. 24p. DNLM; PPJ **60-1843**

TOYNBEE, Joseph (1815-1866)
The diseases of the ear; their nature, diagnosis, and treatment. 2nd American ed. Philadelphia: Blanchard & Lea, 1865. 440p. DNLM; NNNAM; OCIM; PPC **60-1844**

TRALL, Russell Thacher (1812-1877)
Water-cure for the million. The processes of water-cure explained. Popular errors exposed. Hygienic and drug-medication contrasted; rules for bathing, dieting, exercising, etc.; recipes for cooking; directions for home-treatment; remarkable cases to illustrate, etc. . . . New York: Fowler & Wells, 1860. 72p. DLC; DNLM; NNNAM **60-1845**

TRALL, Russell Thacher (1812-1877)
Diseases of the throat and lungs. . . . New York: Fowler & Wells, 1861. 39p. DLC; NNNAM **60-1846**

TRALL, Russell Thacher (1812-1877)
Diphtheria: its nature, history, causes, prevention, and treatment on hygienic principles; with a resumé of the various theories and practices of the medical profession. . . . New York: Fowler & Wells, 1862. 276p. DLC; NNNAM; PU **60-1847**

TRALL, Russell Thacher (1812-1877)
The true healing art; or hygienic vs. drug medicaton. An address delivered in the Smithsonian Institute, Washington, D.C., February 12, 1862. New York: R. T. Trall & Co., [1862]. 83p. 1 plate. DNLM; NNNAM **60-1848**

TRALL, Russell Thacher (1812-1877)
Drug-medicines; their nature, consequences, and modus operandi; with an exposition of the false doctrines on which their employment is predicated. . . . New York: [Davies & Kent], 1862. 30p. DLC; NNNAM **60-1849**

TRALL, Russell Thacher (1812-1877)
The health and diseases of woman. . . . New York: Fowler & Wells, 1862. 31p. DLC; DNLM; NNNAM **60-1850**

TRALL, Russell Thacher (1812-1877)
Pathology of the reproductive organs; embracing all forms of sexual disorders. Boston: B. L. Emerson, 1862. 242p. DNLM; MBM **60-1851**

TRALL, Russell Thacher (1812-1877)
Hand-book of hygienic practice; intended as a practical guide for the sick room, arranged alphabetically. . . . With an appendix illustrative of the hygeio-therapeutic movements. New York: Miller & Wood, 1864. 300p. DLC; DNLM; NNNAM **60-1852**

TRALL, Russell Thacher (1812-1877)
The true temperance platform; or an exposition of the fallacy of alcoholic medication; being the substance of addresses delivered in the Queen's Concert Rooms, Hannover Square, and in Exeter Hall, London, during the session of the International Temperance Convention, September 2, 3 and 4, 1862. To which is added a discussion between Dr. Trall and Rev. J. C. Hurd, on the modus operandi of alcohol. New York: R. T. Trall & Co., 1864. 162p. DNLM; NNNAM **60-1853**

TRALL, Russell Thacher (1812-1877)
Alcoholic medication. . . . New York: Miller, Wood & Co.; [etc., etc.], 1866. 48p. DLC; NNNAM **60-1854**

TRIPLER, Charles Stuart (1806-1866) and George C. BLACKMAN
Handbook for the military surgeon: being a compendium of the duties of the medical officer in the field, the sanitary management of the camp, the preparation of food, etc.; with forms for the requisitions for supplies, returns, etc.; the diagnosis and treatment of camp dysentery; and all the important points in war surgery, including gun-shot wounds, amputation, wounds of the chest, abdomen, arteries and head, and the use of choloroform. Cincinnati: R. Clarke & Co., 1861. 121, 42p. DNLM; OCIM **60-1855**

TRIPLER, Charles Stuart (1806-1866)
Manual of the medical officer of the Army of the United States. Part I. Recruiting and the inspection of recruits. Washington: Government Printing Office, 1866. 100p. DNLM; NNNAM; PU **60-1856**

TRÖLTSCH, Anton Friedrich (1829-1890)
The diseases of the ear, their diagnosis and treatmnet. A text-book of . . . academical lectures. . . . Transl. from the German, and ed. by D. B. St. John Roosa. . . . From the 2nd and last German ed. New York: William Wood & Co., 1864. 254p. DLC; DNLM; NNNAM; PPC **60-1857**

TRÖLTSCH, Anton Friedrich (1829-1890)
Treatise on the diseases of the ear, including the anatomy of the organ. . . . Transl. and ed. by D. B. St. John Roosa. . . . 2nd American from the 4th German ed. New York: William Wood & Co., 1869. 565p. DLC; DNLM; NNNAM; PU **60-1858**

TROUSSEAU, Armand (1801-1867)
Lectures on clinical medicine, delivered at the Hôtel-Dieu, Paris. Transl. from the ed. of 1868 by John Rose Cormack. Philadelphia: Lindsay & Blakiston, 1867-1871. 4 v. DNLM; NNNAM; OCIM; PPC **60-1859**

TUCKER, Henry H. (1819-1890)
The true physician: an address delivered before the graduating class of the Medical College of Georgia. Augusta, Ga.: E. H. Pughe, 1867. 15p. DNLM; GU **60-1860**

TURNBULL, Laurence (1821-1900)
Hints and observations on military hygiene; with the best means of treating the medical and surgical diseases of the Army. Philadelphia, 1862. 62p. DNLM; PPC **60-1861**

TURNBULL, Laurence (1821-1900)
Defective and impaired vision, with the clinical use of the ophthalmoscope in their diagnosis and treatment. Philadelphia: Lindsay & Blakiston, 1865. 36p. DNLM; PPC; PU **60-1862**

TURNBULL, Laurence (1821-1900)
On foreign bodies in the ear; with a bibliography and a condensed statement of the present condition of aural surgery. Philadelphia: Collins, 1865. 23p. DNLM; PPC **60-1683**

TURNER, Henry McNeal
Health, and the best means of preserving it. A prize essay. Baltimore: Bull & Tuttle, [1860]. 20p. DNLM; MdU-D **60-1864**

TYRRELL, Walter
On the use of strychnine in epilepsy. New York: C. O. Jones, 1866. 16p. DNLM; NNNAM **60-1865**

UNITED STATES MEDICAL MUSEUM
Catalogue of the medical and microscopical sections of the United States Army Medical Museum. Prepared under the direction of the Surgeon-General, U.S. Army. Washington: Government Printing Office, 1867. 136, 161p. plates. DNLM [Medical section: By J. J. Woodward] **60-1866**

UNITED STATES SANITARY COMMISSION
Western Sanitary Commission; a sketch of its origin, history, labors for the sick and wounded of the Western armies, and aid given to freedmen and Union refugees, with incidents of hospital life. St. Louis: R. P. Studley & Co., 1864. 144p. DNLM; OCIM **60-1867**

UNITED STATES SANITARY COMMISSION
The Sanitary Commission of the United States Army; a succinct narrative of its works and purposes. New York: Pub. for the benefit of the United States Sanitary Commission, 1864. 318p. plates. DLC; DNLM; NNNAM **60-1868**

UNITED STATES SANITARY COMMISSION
Narrative of privations and sufferings of United States officers and soldiers while prisoners of war in the hands of the Rebel authorities. Being the report of a Commission of Inquiry, appointed by the United States Sanitary Commission. With an appendix, containing the testimony, printed for the U.S. Sanitary Commission by King & Baird, 1864. 283p. 4 plates. DNLM [Members of the Commission included: Valentine Mott, M.D., Edward Delafield, M.D., Gov. Morris Wilkins, Ellerslie Wallace, M.D., Hon. J. I. Clark Hare, Rev. T. Walden.] **60-1869**

UNITED STATES SANITARY COMMISSION
Military, medical and surgical essays prepared for the United States Sanitary Commission. 1862-1864. Washington, D.C., 1865. 448p. plates. DLC; DNLM [A collection of reports with separate t.-p. and paging. Contents—Introductory—Pain and anaesthetics [by] Valentine Mott—A. Military hygiene and therapeutics [by] A. C. Post [and] W. H. Van Buren—B. Directions to surgeons on the field of battle [by] G. J. Guthrie—C. Rules for preserving the health of the soldier [by] W. H. Van Buren—D. Quinine as a prophylactic [by] W. H. Van Buren—E. Vaccination in armies [by] F. G. Smith [and] Alfred Stillé—F. Amputations [by] D. D. Slade—G. Amputations, foot and ankle joint [by] Stephen Smith—H. Venereal diseases [by] F. J. Bumstead—J. Pneumonia [by] Austin Flint—K. Continued fevers [by] J. B. Upham—L. Excision of joints [by] R. M. Hodges—M. Dysentery [by] Alfred Stillé—N. Scurvy [by] W. A. Hammond—O. Fractures in military surgery [by] J. H. Packard—P. Miasmatic fevers [by] J. T. Metcalfe—Q. Yellow fever [by] J. T. Metcalfe—R. Hemorrhage from wounds [by] Valentine Mott—S. Infectious diseases [by] Elisha Harris—T. Plaster of paris splints [by] J. L. Little.] **60-1870**

UNITED STATES SANITARY COMMISSION
History of the United States Sanitary Commission, being the general report of its work during the war of the rebellion. By Charles J. Stillé. Philadelphia: J. B. Lippincott & Co., 1866. 553p. DLC; DNLM; PPC; PU **60-1871**

UNITED STATES SANITARY COMMISSION
Documents of the U.S. Sanitary Commission, vol. I-[III], numbers 1-96. [1861-1866]. New York, [etc.], 1866-1871. 3 v. DLC; DNLM [The collection includes in part the original documents and in part reprints of the originals. Contents of the documents (nos. 1-95) are given in the "Index-catalogue of the library of the Surgeon-General's Office, U.S. Army" under the heading "U.S. Sanitary Commission." Vol. [3] (Document no. 96) has title: . . . The U.S. Sanitary Commission in the valley of the Mississippi, during the war of the rebellion, 1861-1866. Final report of Dr. J. S. Newberry, secretary Western Department, Cleveland, Fairbanks, Benedict & Co., printers, 1871.] **60-1872**

UNITED STATES SANITARY COMMISSION
Sanitary memoirs of the war of the rebellion. Collected and published by the United States Sanitary Commission. [New York, U.S. Sanitary Commission; Cambridge: Riverside Press, 1867-1869]. 2 v. DLC; DNLM; MBM; NNNAM [Lettered on back "Medical" and "Statistical" respectively. Contents—[v. 1] Contributions related to the causation and prevention of disease, and to camp diseases; together with a report of the diseases, etc., among the prisoners at Andersonville, Ga. Ed. by Austin Flint, M.D., 1867.—[v. 2] Investigations in the military and anthropological statistics of American soldiers. By Benjamin Apthorp Gould. 1869] **60-1873**

UNITED STATES SANITARY COMMISSION
History of the United States Sanitary Commission, being the general report of its work during the war of the rebellion. By Charles J. Stillé. New York: Hurd & Houghton, 1868. 553p. DLC; DNLM; NNNAM **60-1874**

U.S. SURGEON-GENERAL'S OFFICE
Statistical report of the sickness and mortality in the Army of the United States, comp. from the records of the Surgeon-General's Office; embracing a period of five years from January 1855 to January 1860. Prepared under the direction of Brevet Brigadier General Thomas Lawson. Washington: George W. Bowman, 1860. 515p. map, charts. DNLM **60-1875**

U.S. SURGEON-GENERAL'S OFFICE
Catalogue of the Surgeon-General's Office library. May 10, 1864. [Washington, D.C., 1864.] 54p. DLC; DNLM **60-1876**

U.S. SURGEON-GENERAL'S OFFICE
Catalogue of the Surgeon-General's Office library. October 23, 1865. [Washington, 1865.] 32 l. DLC; DNLM **60-1877**

U.S. SURGEON-GENERAL'S OFFICE
. . . Report on epidemic cholera in the Army of the United States, during the year 1866. Washington: Government Printing Office, 1867. 65p. tables. DLC; DNLM [Circular No. 5, May 4, 1867] **60-1878**

U.S. SURGEON-GENERAL'S OFFICE
Catalogue of books in the library of the Surgeon-General's Office, Washington, D.C. Alphabetically arranged—with an appendix. [Washington], 1868. 147p. DLC; DNLM **60-1879**

U.S. SURGEON-GENERAL'S OFFICE
. . . Report on epidemic cholera and yellow fever in the Army of the United States, during the year 1867. Washington: Government Printing Office, 1868. 156p. DLC; DNLM [Circular No. 1, June 10, 1868] **60-1880**

U.S. SURGEON-GENERAL'S OFFICE
List of works on yellow fever in the library of the Surgeon-General's Office . . . August 20, 1869. [Washington, 1869.] 10p. DLC; DNLM **60-1881**

UPHAM, J. Baxter (1820?-1902)
Sanitary Commission. K. Report of a committee of the associated medical members of the Sanitary Commission, on the subject of continued fevers. Washington: Government Printing Office, 1862. 27p. DNLM **60-1882**

UPHAM, J. Baxter (1820?-1902)
Sanitary Commission. K. Report of a committee of the associated medical members of the Sanitary Commission, on the subject of continued fevers. 23p. Boston: J. E. Farwell & Co., 1862. DNLM **60-1883**

UPHAM, J. Baxter (1820?-1902)
Sanitary Commission. K. Report of a committee of the associated medical members of the Sanitary Commission, on the subject of continued fevers. 2nd ed. Printed for circulation by the Sanitary Commission. [Washington, D.C.], 1863. 23p. DNLM **60-1884**

UPHAM, J. Baxter (1820?-1902)
Hospital notes and memoranda; in illustration of the congestive fever (so-called), or epidemic cerebro-spinal meningitis, as it occurred in the winter and spring of 1862-1863 in the camps in and around the town of Newbern; with some account of its origin, nature, and treatment. Boston: D. Clapp, 1863. 38p. DNLM; MBM **60-1885**

VALERI, Gaetano (1818-1882)
An introduction to the study of clinical medicine; an introductory lecture to the medical class in the University of Rome, Italy. Transl. from the Italian by the author. Boston: D. Clapp & Sons, 1866. 45p. DNLM; MBM
60-1886

VAN BIBBER, W[ashington] C[hew] (1824-1892)
An analysis of a few cases of abdominal disease. Baltimore: Innes & Co., 1867. 14p. DNLM; MdU-D
60-1887

VAN BUREN, William Holme (1819-1883)
Contributions to practical surgery. . . . Philadelphia: J. B. Lippincott & Co., 1865. 208p. DLC; DNLM; NNNAM; NNU-M
60-1888

VAN BUREN, William Holme (1819-1883)
Medical study, A.D. 1869. Introductory address, annual session of Bellevue Hospital Medical College. New York: D. Appleton & Co., 1869. 20p. DNLM; NNNAM; NNU-M
60-1889

VANDER POEL, Samuel Oakley (1824-1886)
Suggestions relative to the pathology of pneumonia. Albany, N.Y.: C. Van Benthuysen, 1865. 7p. DNLM; NNNAM
60-1890

VANDER POEL, Samuel Oakley (1824-1886)
Progressive locomotor ataxy. Albany: C. Van Benthuysen, 1865. 7p. DNLM; NNNAM **60-1891**

VANDER POEL, Samuel Oakley (1824-1886)
Albany Medical College. Lecture, introductory to the course of 1867. Albany: Weed, Parsons & Co., 1867. 13p. DNLM
60-1892

VAN DEUSEN, E. H. (1829-1909)
Observations on a form of nervous prostration (neurasthenia), culminating in insanity. [A supplement to report of the Michigan Asylum for the Insane, for the years 1867-1868.] Lansing: W. S. George & Co., 1869. 19p. DNLM
60-1893

VAN GIESON, Ransford E.
The application of photography to medical science, including a process for photographing the microscopic field. New York: T. Holman, 1860. 16p. DNLM; NNNAM
60-1894

VELPEAU, [Alfred Armand Louis Marie] (1795-1867)
Surgical clinic at La Charité. Lessons upon the diagnosis and treatment of surgical diseases. Delivered in the month of August, 1865, by Professor Velpeau. . . . Collected and ed. by A. Regnard. . . . Transl. by W. C. B. Fifield. Boston: J. Campbell, 1866. 103p. DLC; DNLM; MBM; NNNAM
60-1895

[VENEREAL DISEASE]
Sanitary Commission. H. Report . . . on the subject of venereal diseases, with special reference to practice in the army and navy. Washington: McGill, Witherow, 1862. 19p. DNLM [Committee chaired by F. J. Bumstead and including J. Mason Warren, R. M. Hodges, Edward Hartshorne, J. H. Packard, William Parker, Wm. H. Van Buren.] **60-1896**

VIRCHOW, Rudolf Ludwig Karl (1821-1902)
Cellular pathology as based upon physiological and pathological histology. Twenty lectures delivered in the Pathological Institute of Berlin during the months of February, March and April, 1858. . . . Transl. from the 2nd ed. of the original. By Frank Chance . . . with notes and numerous emendations, principally from ms. notes of the author, and illustrated by 144 engravings on wood. New York: R. M. De Witt [1860?] 554p. DLC; DNLM; NNNAM; PU **60-1897**

VIRCHOW, Rudolf Ludwig Karl (1821-1902)
Cellular pathology as based upon physiological and pathological histology. Transl. from the 2nd ed. of the original by Frank Chance. . . . Philadelphia: J. B. Lippincott & Co., 1863..554p. DNLM; ICRM; NNNAM; PPC **60-1898**

VIRCHOW, Rudolf Ludwig Karl (1821-1902)
Cellular pathology as based upon physiological and pathological histology. Twenty lectures delivered in the Pathological Institute of Berlin during the months of February, March, and April, 1858. Transl. from the German by Frank Chance, with notes and numerous emendations, principally from MS. notes of the author. 8th Americn ed. Philadelphia: P. Blakiston, Son & Co., [1868?]. 554p. DNLM; MBM; NNNAM; PPC [An edition by Blakiston & Co. (1887) is simply the edition of 1860, New York, by R. M. De Witt, with title-page pasted in.]
60-1899

VON NIEMEYER, Felix (1820-1871)
Clinical lectures on pulmonary phthisis. Transl., by permission of the author, from the 2nd German ed., by J. L. Parke. New York: Moorhead, Simpson & Bond, 1868. 116p. DNLM; NNNAM; PPC; PU **60-1900**

VON NIEMEYER, Felix (1820-1871)
A textbook of practical medicine. . . . New York: D. Appleton & Co., 1869. 2 v. MBM; NNNAM; PPC; PU
60-1901

WAGNER, Clinton (1837-1914)
Report of interesting surgical operations performed at the United States Army General Hospital, Beverly, New Jersey. [1865.] 16p. 1 plate. DNLM; NjR **60-1902**

WALES, Philip Skinner (1837-1906)
Mechanical therapeutics. A practical treatise on surgical apparatus, appliances, and elementary operations; embracing bandaging, minor surgery, orthopraxy, and the treatment of fractures and dislocations. Philadelphia: Henry C. Lea, 1867. 685p. CtY-M; DNLM; PPC; PU **60-1903**

WALKER, George S. (*b.* 1820)
Epidemic cholera; its history and homoeopathic treatment. St. Louis: H. C. C. Luyties, 1866. 39p. DNLM **60-1904**

WALLACE, Ellerslie (1819-1885)
Charge to the graduating class of Jefferson Medical College, of Philadelphia. Philadelphia: Collins, 1863. 16, 3p. DNLM; PPJ **60-1905**

WALLACE, Ellerslie (1819-1885)
General introductory lecture delivered before the class of Jefferson Medical College. Philadelphia: T. Hamilton, 1866. 15p. DNLM; PPJ **60-1906**

WALLIS, Severn Teackle (1816-1894)
Valedictory address to the graduating class of the School of Medicine of the University of Maryland. Baltimore: Kelly, Piet & Co., 1869. 27p. DNLM; MdBM; MdU-D **60-1907**

WALSHE, Walter Hayle (1812-1892)
A practical treatise on the diseases of the lungs: including the principles of physical diagnosis. . . . A new American from the 3rd rev. and much enl. English ed. Philadelphia: Blanchard & Lea, 1860. 468p. DLC; DNLM; NNNAM; PPC **60-1908**

WALSHE, Walter Hayle (1812-1892)
A practical treatise on the diseases of the heart and great vessels, including the principles of physical diagnosis. A new American from the 3rd London ed. Philadelphia: Blanchard & Lea, 1862. 420p. CtY-M; DNLM; LNT-M; MdU-D **60-1909**

WALTER, Albert G. (1811-1876)
Conservative surgery in its general and successful adaptation in cases of severe traumatic injuries of the limbs; with a report of cases. Pittsburgh: W. G. Johnston & Co., 1867. 213p. DNLM **60-1910**

WARD, Isaac Moreau (1806-1895)
Valedictory address delivered at the 2nd annual commencement of the Homoeopathic Medical College of New York. New York: Francis Hart & Co., 1862. 24p. DNLM; NNNAM **60-1911**

WARD-JACKSON, E.
Ward-Jackson's gymnastics for the fingers and wrist, being a system of gymnastics, based on anatomical principles, for developing and strengthening the muscles of the hand, for musical, mechanical, and medical purposes. New edition, intended for schools. New York: G. Schirmer, 1865. 72p. DNLM; NNNAM **60-1912**

WARE, John (1795-1864)
On hemoptysis as a symptom. Boston: D. Clapp, 1860. 31p. DNLM; MBM **60-1913**

WARING, Edward John (1819-1891)
Practical therapeutics. From 2nd London ed. Philadelphia: Lindsay & Blakiston, 1866. 815p. DNLM; NNNAM; OCIM; PPC **60-1914**

WARING, James J[ohnston] (1830-1888)
Natural laws vs. political issues. A lecture delivered to the graduating class of the National Medical College, Feb. 21, 1861. Washington: H. Polkinhorn, 1861. 14p. DNLM **60-1915**

WARK, David
Of the Swedish movement-cure in consumption. Albany: C. Van Benthuysen & Sons, 1868. 16p. DNLM; NNNAM **60-1916**

WARREN, Edward (1804-1878)
The life of John Collins Warren, M.D., comp. chiefly from his autobiography and journals. . . . Boston: Ticknor & Fields, 1860. 2 v. plates. DLC; DNLM; MH; NN **60-1917**

WARREN, Edward (1828-1893)
An introductory lecture delivered in the University of Maryland, Oct. 15th, 1860. Baltimore: Kelly, Hedian & Piet, 1860. 22p. DNLM; MdU-D **60-1918**

WARREN, Edward (1828-1893)
An epitome of practical surgery for field and hospital. . . . 1st ed. Richmond, Va.: West & Johnston, 1863. 401p. tables. DLC; ViRA **60-1919**

[WARREN, John Collins] (1778-1856)
Memoir of John Collins Warren. [Boston, 1865.] 14p. port. DNLM; MH-M **60-1920**

WARREN, Jonathan Mason (1811-1867)
Cases in surgery. Gun-shot wounds. Plural births. . . . Boston: D. Clapp, printer, 1862. 28p. DLC; DNLM; MBM [*also*: Boston: D. Clapp, 1862. 26p.] **60-1921**

WARREN, Jonathan Mason (1811-1867)
On operations for cleft palate. Philadelphia, 1863. 8p. DNLM **60-1922**

WARREN, Jonathan Mason (1811-1867)
Hypertrophic elongation of the cervix uteri of twenty-six years' standing, with projection of the enlarged os beyond external organs; ulceration; hemorrhage; operation, followed by complete cure. [Philadelphia, 1864.] 6p. DNLM; PPC **60-1923**

WARREN, Jonathan Mason (1811-1867)
On neuralgic affections following injuries of nerves. Boston, 1864. 8p. DNLM **60-1924**

WARREN, Jonathan Mason (1811-1867)
Recent progress in surgery. The annual address delivered before the Massachusetts Medical Society, May 25, 1864. Boston: D. Clapp, 1864. 84p. DNLM; MBM **60-1925**

WARREN, Jonathan Mason (1811-1867)
Recent progress in surgery. The annual address delivered before the Massachusetts Medical Society, May 25, 1864. Boston: J. Wilson & Son, 1864. 70p. DNLM; MBM **60-1926**

WARREN, Jonathan Mason (1811-1867)
Fissures of the soft and hard palate. Philadelphia: Collins, 1865. 26p. DNLM **60-1927**

WARREN, Jonathan Mason (1811-1867)
Cystic tumors of the jaw. Read before the annual meeting of the Massachusetts Medical Society, May 29, 1866. [Boston, 1866.] 7p. DNLM; MBM **60-1928**

WARREN, Jonathan Mason (1811-1867)
Surgical observations, with cases and operations. . . . Boston: Ticknor & Fields, 1867. 630p. 5 plates. DLC; DNLM; MBM **60-1929**

WATERMAN, S[igismund] (1819-1899)
Practical remarks on scarlatina. New York: Turner & Mignard, 1869. 10p. DNLM; NNNAM **60-1930**

WATERMAN, Thomas (1842-1901)
Dislocation of the elbow; a new method of reduction. [Boston, 1869.] 1 l. DNLM **60-1931**

WATSON, John (1807-1863)
Memoir of Robert Jay, Jr. New York: S. S. & W. Wood, 1860. 11p. DNLM; NNNAM **60-1932**

WATSON, John (1807-1863)
The true physician. An anniversary discourse delivered before the New York Academy of Medicine. New York: S. S. & W. Wood, 1860. 44p. DNLM; NNNAM **60-1933**

WATSON, John (1807-1863)
Catalogue of the private library of medical and miscellaneous books of the late. . . . New York: C. C. Shelly, 1867. 58p. DNLM; NNNAM **60-1934**

WATSON, John McClaran (1796-1866)
Influence of the mother's mind on the foetus in utero: a lecture. Nashville: J. T. S. Fall, printer, 1860. 16p. DNLM **60-1935**

WATSON, Thomas (1792-1882)
Watson abridged; a synopsis of the lectures on the principles and practice of physic, delivered at King's College, London. (Abridged from the last English edition.) With a concise but complete account of the properties, use, preparations, doses, etc. (taken from the U.S. Dispensatory), of all the medicines mentioned in these lectures, and with other valuable additions, by J. J. Meylor. Philadelphia: [J. J. Meylor], 1867. 277p. DNLM; MBM; PPC; PU **60-1936**

WATSON, William Argyle (1828-1901)
On the history and uses of cod-liver oil in pulmonary consumption and other diseases. . . . with opinions thereon from the most eminent physicians of Europe and America. Also, notes on the value of pyrophosphate of iron in anaemia, chlorosis, debility, etc., etc. By E. N. Chapman. . . . New York: Caswell, Hazard & Co., [1868]. 42p. DLC; DNLM **60-1937**

WATSON, William Henry (*b.* 1829)
Address on the past and present position of homoeopathy, and the duties of its practitioners, delivered at the inauguration of the Homoeopathic Medical Society of the State of New York, held in Albany, February 28, 1861. Published by request of the Society. New York: Henry Ludwig, 1861. 15p. DNLM; NNNAM **60-1938**

WATSON, William Henry
The inaugural and annual addresses before the Homoeopathic Medical Society of the State of New York. Albany, N.Y.: Argus Co., 1869. 20p. DNLM **60-1939**

WATTERS, J. H.
Doctrines of life. [Reply to the letter of W. B. Carpenter. Controversy on the priority of the doctrine of the "Correlation and conservation of forces."] [St. Louis, 1868.] 28p. DNLM **60-1940**

WATTERS, J. H.
Dr. Watters' doctrines of life. Reply to London Lancet, and closing remarks. St. Louis, 1869. 10p. DNLM **60-1941**

WEBBER, Samuel G[ilbert] (1838-1926)
Cerebro-spinal meningitis. The Boylston prize essay for 1866. Boston: D. Clapp & Son, 1866. 104p. DNLM; MBM **60-1942**

WEBBER, Samuel G[ilbert] (1838-1926)
Progressive locomotor ataxy. (Read before the Boston Society for Medical Observation.) [Boston, 1868.] 6p. DNLM **60-1943**

WEBER, Leonard
A short treatise on the Kissingen Rakoczy and bitter water. Kurze Abbhandlung über Kissingen's Rakoczy und Bitterwasser. New York: N.Y. Staatszeitung, 1861. 20p. DNLM; NNNAM [English and German text.] **60-1944**

WEBSTER, J. G.
Epidemic cholera; its phenomena, causes, and mode of communication; together with its prevention and proper treatment. Being the substance of two popular lectures. New York: Miller, Wood & Co., 1866. 48p. DNLM; NNNAM **60-1945**

WEBSTER, Warren (1835-1896)
Regulations for the government of the De Camp General Hospital, U.S.A., at David's Island, New York Harbor. New York: De Camp Hospital Press, 1864. 31p. DNLM **60-1946**

WEBSTER, Warren (1835-1896)
The army medical staff. An address delivered at the inauguration of the Dale General Hospital, U.S.A., Worcester, Massachusetts, February 22, 1865. Boston: Wright & Potter, 1865. 56p. DNLM **60-1947**

WEBSTER, Warren (1835-1896)
Quarantine regulations for the fifth military district (State of Texas). Austin, Texas, [1869]. 8p. DNLM **60-1948**

WELCH, Benjamin (1798-1873)
Surgeons' splints and improved apparatus for fractures. New York: J. Russell, 1861. 43p. 2 plates. DNLM; NNNAM **60-1949**

WELCH, R.
Chemical commerce and its commodities. A valedictory address at commencement of Hahnemann Medical College, 1866. Chicago: C. S. Halsey, 1866. 14p. DNLM **60-1950**

WELLS, John Sollberg (1834-1879)
On a long, short, and weak sight, and their treatment by the scientific use of spectacles. 3rd ed. Philadelphia: Lindsay & Blakiston, 1869. 248p. 1 plate. DNLM; PPC; PU
60-1951

WELLS, Phineas P[arkhurst] (1808-1891)
The homoeopathic treatment of diarrhoea and dysentery. New York, 1862. 40p. DNLM; NNNAM
60-1952

WELLS, S. M.
The elctropathic guide: prepared with particular reference to home practice; containing hints on the care of the sick, the treatment of disease, and the use of electricity; with full directions for treating over 100 cases. . . . Chicago: Horton & Leonard, Book & Job Printers, 1867. 90p. DLC; IEN-M; IU-M **60-1953**

WELLS, W. R.
A new theory of disease; based upon the principle that man is a compound electrical magnet; also a new method of cure, by means of the various qualities of electricity. Revised and enlarged ed. Rochester: Tracy & Rew, 1869. 178p. DNLM
60-1954

WELLS, Walter S[cott] (*d.* 1897)
An epitome of Braithwaite's retrospect of practical medicine and surgery: containing a condensed summary of the most important cases; their treatment, and all the remedies and other useful matters embraced in the 40 volumes. New York: Dick & Fitzgerald, 1860. 2 v. DNLM; NNNAM
60-1955

WEST, Charles (1816-1898)
Lectures on the diseases of infancy and childhood. 3rd American from the 4th London ed. Philadelphia: Blanchard & Lea, 1860. 630p. DNLM; NNNAM; PPC; PU
60-1956

WEST, Charles (1816-1898)
Lectures on the disease of infancy and childhood. 4th American from the 5th English ed. Philadelphia: Henry C. Lea, 1866. 653p. DNLM; MBM; PPC; PPJ
60-1957

WEST, Charles (1816-1898)
Lectures on the diseases of women. . . . 3rd American from the 3rd English ed. Philadelphia: Henry C. Lea, 1867. 543p. DNLM; NNNAM; PPC; PU **60-1958**

WESTERN SANITARY COMMISSION ON HOSPITALS
Report to the Western Sanitary Commission, on the general military hospitals of St. Louis, Missouri. St. Louis: Studley, 1862. 75p. DNLM **60-1959**

WESTMORELAND, John G. (1816-1887)
Address introductory to the sixth course of lectures in the Atlanta Medical College. Atlanta, Ga.: Intelligencer Press, 1860. 16p. DNLM; GU **60-1960**

WETHERBEE, Isaac J.
The past and future of the dental profession. Address before the Massachusetts Dental Society at its second annual meeting, May 24, 1866. Boston: T. R. Marvin & Son, 1866. 16p. DNLM; MBM **60-1961**

WESTMORE, Edmund (1838-1918)
Statutory law of New York regarding the insane. Utica, N.Y.: Roberts, 1867. 35p. DNLM **60-1962**

WEY, William C. (1829-1897)
The late Alden March. A paper read at a meeting of the Elmira Academy of Medicine, August 3rd, 1869. 20p. DNLM
60-1963

WHARTON, Francis (1820-1889)
Involuntary confessions. A monograph. Philadelphia: Kay & Bro., 1860. 36p. DNLM; PPC; PU **60-1964**

WHARTON, Francis (1820-1889) and Moreton STILLÉ
A treatise on medical jurisprudence. The medical part revised and corrected, with numerous additions, by Alfred Stillé. 2nd and revised ed. Philadelphia: Kay & Bro., 1860. 1031p. CU-M; DNLM; NNNAM; PPC **60-1965**

WHITALL, Samuel (1840-1882)
A case of elephantiasis arabum, successfully operated on by J. S. Theband. New York: Bradstreet Press, 1867. 19p. 2 plates. DNLM; NNNAM **60-1966**

WHITE, George A.
A practical monograph on the treatment of local complaints of the feet. Washington: J. L. Pearson, 1869. 26p. 3 plates. DNLM **60-1967**

WHITE, James C[larke] (1833-1916)
Scabies. Boston, 1864. 11p. DNLM **60-1968**

WHITE, James Platt (1811-1881)
Charge to the graduating class, delivered at the commencement in the Medical Department of the University of Buffalo. [Buffalo]: J. Warren & Co., 1867. 19p. DNLM
60-1969

WHITE, James William (1826-1891)
Dental materia medica. . . . Philadelphia: S. S. White, 1868. 108p. DLC; DNLM; PPC; PPF **60-1970**

WHITE, SAMUEL S. DENTAL MANUFACTURERS, PHILADELPHIA
Catalogue of dental materials, furniture, instruments, etc. for sale by Samuel S. White. . . . [Philadelphia: Lippincott's Press], 1867. 226p. plates. DLC; DNLM; PPC; PPF
60-1971

WHITE, SAMUEL S. DENTAL MANUFACTURERS, PHILADELPHIA
Catalogue of dental materials, furniture, instruments, etc. Philadelphia: Lippincott's Press, 1867. 226p. DNLM; PPC
60-1972

WHITE, SAMUEL S. DENTAL MANUFACTURERS, PHILADELPHIA
Physicians' microscope for medical investigations and appratus for producing local anaesthesia by narcotic spray. Philadelphia, 1867. 16p. DNLM; PPC **60-1973**

WHITE, William
The student's manual of medical electricity. Showing its most scientific and rational application to all forms of acute and chronic disease. . . . Boston: Pub. by the author, 1869. 191p. DLC; MBM **60-1974**

WHITEHEAD, William Riddick (1831-1902)
On excision of the superior maxilla: report of a case, with remarks on certain tumors of this bone. New York: J. Medole, 1866. 28p. DNLM; NNNAM **60-1975**

WHITEHEAD, William Riddick (1831-1902)
Perineal urethrotomy; relation of a case suggestive of remarks on the treatment of stricture of the urethra. New York: New York Printing Co., 1867. 15p. DNLM; NNNAM **60-1976**

WHITEHEAD, William Riddick (1831-1902)
Report on the best methods of treatment for different forms of cleft palate. Philadelphia: Collins, 1869. 12p. 8 plates. DNLM; PPC **60-1977**

WHITEHEAD, William Riddick (1831-1902)
Surgical treatment of cleft of the hard palate; with an illustrated case. New York: D. Appleton & Co., 1869. 16p. 1 plate. DNLM; NNNAM **60-1978**

WHITNEY, E[lijah] and A. B. WHITNEY
Asiatic cholera: a treatise on its origin, pathology, treatment, and cure. New York: M. W. Dodd, 1866. 214p. DNLM; NNNAM **60-1979**

WHO, which, what, and wherefore; or, a few facts for the homoeopathic profession. Philadelphia, 1860. 8p. DNLM; PPHa **60-1980**

WILBUR, H[ervey] B[ackus] (1820-1883)
Aphasia. [Philadelphia, 1867.] 30p. DNLM; PPC; PU **60-1981**

WILDER, Alexander (1823-1908)
An address delivered before the Eclectic Medical Society of the State of New York. Albany, N.Y.: Weed, Parsons & Co., 1869. 13p. DNLM **60-1982**

WILDER, Alexander (1823-1908)
New Platonism and alchemy; a sketch of the doctrines and principal teachers of the eclectic or Alexandrian school; also, an outline of the interior doctrines of the alchemists of the Middle Ages. Albany, N.Y.: Weed, Parsons & Co., 1869. 30p. DNLM **60-1983**

WILKINSON, James John Garth (1812-1899)
On social health. A discourse delivered before the London "Ladies' Sanitary Association," February 28, 1865. Boston: S. W. Cone, 1865. 38p. DNLM **60-1984**

WILLAMETTE UNIVERSITY. MEDICAL DEPARTMENT, PORTLAND, ORE.
Annual announcements for the sessions of 1868-1869 (3.); 1870-1871 to 1872-1873 (5.-7.); 1878-1879 to 1886-1887 (13.-21.); 1888-1889 to 1893-1894 (23.-28.). Salem & Portland, 1868-1893. DNLM **60-1985**

WILLARD, Emma (1787-1870)
Theory of circulation by respiration. Synopsis of its principles and history. New York: F. Hart & Co., 1861. 20p. DNLM; NNNAM **60-1986**

WILLARD, Sylvester David (1825-1865)
Biographical memoir of Casper Van Wie Burton, of Laningsburg. Troy, N.Y.: Troy Daily Times Print., 1861. 13p. DNLM **60-1987**

WILLARD, Sylvester David (1825-1865)
Conservative surgery, with a list of the medical and surgical force of New York in the war of the rebellion, 1861-1862. To which is added a brief notice of the hospitals at Fortress Monroe and White House, Virginia. Albany: C. Van Benthuysen, 1862. 41p. DNLM; NNNAM **60-1988**

WILLARD, Sylvester David (1825-1865)
Regimental surgeons of the State of New York, in the war of the rebellion, 1861-1863. [Albany, 1863.] 33p. DNLM; N **60-1989**

WILLARD, Sylvester David (1825-1865)
Report on the condition of the insane poor in the county poorhouses of New York [to the legislature, Jan. 12, 1865]. Albany: C. Van Benthuysen, 1865. 70p. DNLM **60-1990**

WILLIAMS, Charles James Blasius (1805-1889)
Principles of medicine: comprising general pathology and therapeutics, and a brief general view of etiology, nosology, semeiology, diagnosis, and prognosis. . . . With brief remarks on hygienics, or the preservation of health. From the last revised London ed. Philadelphia: Blanchard & Lea, 1864. 486p. DNLM; NNNAM; PPC; PU **60-1991**

WILLIAMS, E[lkannah] (1822-1888)
Practical observations in ophthalmology. Philadelphia: Collins, 1865. 14p. DNLM; PPC **60-1992**

WILLIAMS, Henry Willard (1821-1895)
A practical guide to the study of the diseases of the eye; their medical and surgical treatment. Boston: Ticknor & Fields, 1862. 317p. CtY-M; DNLM; MBM; NNNAM **60-1993**

WILLIAMS, Henry Willard (1821-1895)
Recent advances in ophthalmic science. The Boylston prize essay for 1865. Boston: Ticknor & Fields, 1866. 166p. DNLM; MBM; MH **60-1994**

WILLIAMS, Henry Willard (1821-1895)
Practical guide to the study of the diseases of the eye; their medical and surgical treatment. Second edition, revised and enlarged. Boston: Ticknor & Fields, 1867. 422p. MBM; OCIM; PPC **60-1995**

WILLIAMS, Henry Willard (1821-1895)
Optical defects of school children. An address before the Massachusetts Teachers' Association. Boston: A. Mudge, 1869. 13p. DNLM; MB; MBM **60-1996**

WILLIAMS, Henry Willard (1821-1895)
A practical guide to the study of the diseases of the eye: their medical and surgical treatment. 3rd ed. Boston: Fields, Osgood & Co., 1869. 422p. CU-M; DNLM; MBM; PPC **60-1997**

WILLIAMSON, Walter (1811-1870)
Diseases of females and children, and their homoeopathic treatment. Containing a full description of the dose of each medicine. 3rd enlarged edition. New York: William Radde, 1860. 256p. NNNAM; PPHa **60-1998**

WILSON, Erasmus (1809-1884)
On diseases of the skin. 5th American from the 5th and revised London ed. Philadelphia: Blanchard & Lea, 1863. 694p. CtY-M; DNLM; MdBM; PPC **60-1999**

WILSON, Erasmus (1809-1884)
On diseases of the skin. . . . 6th American from the 5th and revised London ed. With illustrations on wood. Philadelphia: Lea & Blanchard, 1865. 694p. DLC; DNLM; PPC; PU
60-2000

WILSON, Erasmus (1809-1884)
The student's book of cutaneous medicine and diseases of the skin. New York: William Wood & Co., 1865. 445p. CtY-M; DLC; ICJ; NN **60-2000A**

WILSON, Erasmus (1809-1884)
On diseases of the skin: A system of cutaneous medicine. 7th American edition. Philadelphia: Henry C. Lea, 1868. 808p. DNLM; OCIM; PPC; PU **60-2001**

WILSON, Erasmus (1809-1884)
Plates illustrative of Wilson on diseases of the skin. 7th edition. Philadelphia: Henry C. Lea, 1868. 32p. DLC; PPC; PPJ; PU
60-2002

WINSLOW, Forbes Benignus (1810-1874)
On obscure diseases of the brain, and disorders of the mind. Philadelphia: Blanchard & Lea, 1860. 576p. CtY-M; DNLM; PPC; PU **60-2003**

WINSLOW, Forbes Benignus (1810-1874)
On obscure diseases of the brain, and disorders of the mind. 2nd American from the 3rd and rev. London ed. Philadelphia: Henry C. Lea, 1866. 483p. DNLM; ICRM; LNT-M; PPC
60-2004

WINSLOW, Forbes Benignus (1810-1874)
Light: its influence on life and health. New York: Moorhead, Simpson & Bond, 1868. 200p. DNLM; NNNAM; OCIM; PU
60-2005

WOLFE, N[apoleon] B.
An historical essay on medicated inhalation, and letters on consumption, asthma, [etc.]. 2nd ed. Cincinnati, O.: H. Watkin, 1862. 64p. DNLM; OCIM **60-2006**

WOLFE, Napoleon B.
Essay and letters on the treatment of consumption, bronchitis, asthma, and other diseases of the nose, throat, and lungs by medicated inhalation. 1st revised, 9th regular ed. Cincinnati: Moore, Wilstach & Baldwin, 1866. 96p. 1 plate. DNLM
60-2007

WOLFE, Napoleon B.
Common sense book on the new treatment of consumption, asthma, bronchitis, and all diseases of the nose, throat, and lungs by medicated inhalations. Cincinnati, 1869. 96p. 1 plate. DNLM; OCIM **60-2008**

WOOD, George Bacon (1797-1879)
A treatise on therapeutics, and pharmacology or materia medica. . . . 2nd ed. . . . Philadelphia: J. B. Lippincott & Co.; London: Trübner & Co., 1860. 2 v. DLC; OCLloyd; PPC; PU
60-2009

WOOD, George Bacon (1797-1879)
Annual address of the president of the American Philosophical Society. [Philadelphia, 1860.] 6p. DNLM
60-2010

WOOD, George Bacon (1797-1879)
Biographical memoir of the late Franklin Bache, prepared at the request of the American Philosophical Society, and read before the Society June 16, 1865. Philadelphia: Sherman & Co., 1865. 18p. DNLM; PPF; PPL; PU **60-2011**

WOOD, George B[acon] (1797-1879)
Biographical memoir of Franklin Bache, M.D., prepared at the request of the College of Physicians of Philadelphia, and read before the College, May 3rd and June 7th, 1865. . . . Philadelphia: J. B Lippincott & Co., 1865. 66p. DLC; PP; PPC; PU
60-2012

WOOD, George Bacon (1797-1879) and Franklin BACHE
The dispensatory of the United States of America. . . . 12th ed., carefully rev. Philadelphia: J. B. Lippincott & Co., 1865. 1704p. DLC: OCLloyd; PPC; PU **60-2013**

WOOD, George Bacon (1797-1879)
A treatise on the practice of medicine. . . . 6th ed. . . . Philadelphia: J. B. Lippincott & Co., 1866. 2 v. DLC; NNNAM; OCIM; PPC **60-2014**

WOOD, George Bacon (1797-1879)
A treatise on therapeutics, and pharmacology, or materia medica. . . . 3rd ed. . . . Philadelphia: J. B. Lippincott & Co., 1868. 2 v. DLC; OCLloyd; NNNAM; PPC
60-2015

WOOD, Jacob A. (1810-1879)
Beneficial results from the use of mechanical appliances in Pott's disease of the spine, illustrated with cases. New York, 1862. 22p. DNLM; NNNAM **60-2016**

WOOD, Luther Hodges
Researches on the influence of mental activity upon the excretion of phosphoric acid by the kidneys. [New Haven, 1869.] 18p. 4 plates. CtY-M; DNLM **60-2017**

WOOD, William Maxwell (1809-1880)
Report upon the rank of the naval medical staff. Philadelphia: Collins, 1868. 13p. DNLM; PU **60-2018**

WOOD, William Maxwell (1809-1880)
Special report of the Chief of Bureau of Medicine and Surgery, on the difficulty of officering the medical corps of the Navy; its causes and the remedy. [Washington, 1869?] 8p. DNLM
60-2019

WOOD, William & Co.
Archives of ophthalmology and otology, edited and published simultaneously in English and German by H. Knapp and S. Moos. [Prospectus] New York: William Wood & Co., 1869. 8p. NNNAM **60-2020**

WOODHULL, Alfred A[lexander] (1837-1921)
Catalogue of the surgical section of the United States Army Medical Museum. Prepared under the direction of the Surgeon-General, U.S. Army. Washington: Government Printing Office, 1866. 664p. 1 plate. DNLM **60-2021**

WOODHULL, Alfred A[lexander] (1837-1921)
A medical report upon the uniform and clothing of the soldiers of the United States Army. Washington: Surgeon-General's Office, 1868. 26p. DNLM **60-2022**

WOODS, Leonard
An address delivered on the opening of the new hall of the Medical School of Maine, February 21, 1862. Brunswick: A. G. Tenny, 1862. 24p. DNLM **60-2023**

WOODVINE, D[enton] G[eorge] (1834-1894)
Taenia solium. Albany: C. Van Benthuysen & Sons, 1868. 8p. 3 plates. DNLM **60-2024**

WOODWARD, Ashbel (1804-1885)
Medical ethics. The annual address delivered before the convention of the Connecticut Medical Society, at Hartford, May 23rd, 1860. Hartford: Case, Lockwood & Co., 1860. 35p. CtY-M; DNLM **60-2025**

WOODWARD, Ashbel (1804-1885)
Life. The annual address delivered before the convention of the Connecticut Medical Society at New Haven, May 22, 1861. Hartford: Case, Lockwood & Co., 1861. 15p. CtY-M; DNLM **60-2026**

WOODWARD, Ashbel (1804-1885)
Specialism in medicine. New Haven: Tuttle, Morehouse & Taylor, 1866. 7p. CtY-M; DNLM **60-2027**

WOODWARD, Joseph Janvier (1833-1884)
The hospital steward's manual: for the instruction of hospital stewards, ward-masters, and attendants, in their several duties. Prepared in strict accordance with existing regulations and the customs of service in the armies of the United States of America, and rendered authoritative by order of the Surgeon-General. . . . Philadelphia: J. B. Lippincott & Co., 1862. 324p. DLC; DNLM; PPF; PPC **60-2028**

WOODWARD, Joseph Janvier (1833-1884)
Outlines of the chief camp diseases of the United States armies, as observed during the present war. A practical contribution to military medicine. Philadelphia: J. B. Lippincott & Co., 1863. 364p. DNLM; PPC; PU; ScCM **60-2029**

WOODWARD, Joseph Janvier (1833-1884)
Report on the causes and pathology of pyaemia (septaemia). Philadelphia: Collins, 1866. 37p. DNLM; PPC **60-2030**

WOODWARD, Joseph Janvier (1833-1884)
On photo-micrography with the highest powers, as practiced in the Army Medical Museum. [New Haven, 1866.] 7p. DNLM **60-2031**

WOODWARD, Joseph Janvier (1833-1884)
Circular No. 5, May 4, 1867. Report on epidemic cholera in the Army of the United States, during the year 1866. Washington: Government Printing Office, 1867. 65p. DNLM **60-2032**

WOODWARD, Joseph Janvier (1833-1884)
Catalogue of the medical section of the United States Army Medical Museum. Prepared under the direction of the Surgeon-General, U.S. Army. Washington: Government Printing Office, 1867. 136p. 5 plates. DNLM **60-2033**

WOODWARD, Joseph Janvier (1833-1884)
Circular No. 1, June 10, 1868. Report on epidemic cholera and yellow fever in the Army of the United States during the year 1867. Washington: Government Printing Office, 1868. 156p. DNLM **60-2034**

WOODWORTH, B[enjamin] S[tudley] (1816-1891)
An address, read before the Indiana State Medical Society, May 21, 1861. Fort Wayne: D. W. Jones & Son, 1866. 10p. DNLM **60-2035**

WOOSTER, David (*b.* 1827)
Diseases of the heart: their diagnosis and treatment. San Francisco: H. H. Bancroft & Co., 1867. 209p. 1 plate. CU-M; DNLM; NNNAM **60-2036**

WORCESTER DISTRICT MEDICAL SOCIETY, WORCESTER, MASS. LIBRARY
Catalogue of the library of the Worcester District Medical Society. Worcester: E. R. Fiske, 1865. 144p. DLC **60-2037**

WORMLEY, Theodore George (1826-1897)
Micro-chemistry of poisons, including their physiological, pathological, and legal relations. New York: Bailliere Bros., 1867. 668p. 13 plates. 1 tab. DNLM; NN; NNNAM [Also: New York: W. Wood, 1869, 702p.] **60-2038**

WORMLEY, Theodore G[eorge] (1826-1897)
A contribution to our knowledge of the chemical composition of Gelsemium sempervirens. Case of fatal poisoning by three drachms of the fluid extract, and recovery of the poison some months after death. [Philadelphia], 1869. 16p. 1 plate. DNLM; PPL; PU **60-2039**

WORSTER, Joseph
A case of reduction of a completely inverted uterus of four years' standing, by means of pressure and a peculiar mode of manipulation. New York: Bergen & Tripp, 1867. 8p. DNLM; NNNAM **60-2040**

WORSTER, Joseph
A case of fibrous tumor of the uterus, successfully treated by incisions into its substance, the os and cervix being previously dilated by means of slips of the laminaria digitata, and subsequent extraction; and a case of vaginismus, treated after the method of Sims, by exsection of the hymen and meatus urinarius, etc. New York: A. Henderson, 1868. 8p. DNLM; NNNAM **60-2041**

WRAGG, William T.
Memoir of Dr. James Moultrie, late professor of physiology in the Medical College of South Carolina. Report of committee. Charleston, S.C.: W. G. Mazyck, 1869. 22p. DNLM; ScCM **60-2042**

WRIGHT, Henry C.
The empire of the mother over the character and destiny of the race. Boston: B. Marsh, 1863. 132p. DNLM; MA; MB; MH **60-2043**

WRIGHT, Henry Good (1828-1869)
Headaches, their cause and their cure. From the 4th London ed. Philadelphia: Lindsay & Blakiston, 1867. 154p. DNLM; ICRM; PPC; PU **60-2044**

WRIGHT, John W.
A treatise on medical psychology; or, the influence of the mind over the health of the body, and sketch of practice, designed both for use of practitioners of medicine and the people. 1st ed. Louisville: The author, 1866. 301p. DNLM **60-2045**

WRIGHT, Marmaduke Burr (1803-1879)
An introductory lecture delivered in the Medical College of Ohio, session 1860-1861. Cincinnati: Gazette Co., 1860. 23p. DNLM **60-2046**

WRIGHT, Thomas Lee (1825-1893)
Medico-legal: an inquiry concerning the value of testimony respecting facts as they appear to a mind partly conscious. Columbus: Follet, Foster & Co., 1860. 32p. DNLM
60-2047

WRIGHT, Thomas Lee (1825-1893)
Observations on some of the prominent traits of cholera. Cincinnati: A. Moore, 1866. 14p. DNLM
60-2048

WYMAN, Morrill (1812-1903)
The reality and certainty of medicine. An address delivered at the annual meeting of the Massachusetts Medical Society, June 17, 1863. Boston: D. Clapp, 1863. 52p. DNLM; MBM; MH **60-2049**

WYNNE, James (1814-1871)
A paper on diphtheria. New York: Bailliere Bros., 1861. 32p. DNLM; NNNAM **60-2050**

WYTHE, Joseph Henry (1822-1901)
The physician's dose and symptom book. . . . 4th ed. Philadelphia: Lindsay & Blakiston, 1864. 266p. DLC; PPC; PPJ; PU
60-2051

YANDELL, David Wendell (1826-1898)
The progress of medicine: an introductory lecture. Louisville, Ky.: Bradley & Gilbert, 1869. 20p. DNLM
60-2052

YANDELL, Lunsford Pitts, Jr. (1837-1884)
Letters from London. [Nashville, 1867.] 8, 8p. DNLM
60-2053

[YELLOW FEVER]
Sanitary Commission Q. Report . . . on the subject of the nature and treatment of yellow fever. New York: Bryant, 1862. 25p. DNLM [Committee chaired by John T. Metcalfe.]
60-2054

YELLOW fever and its treatment homoepathically; together with some general reflections upon its allopathic medication and non-local origin. By an allopathist and a homoeopathist. Galveston: Daily Civilian & Gazette, 1868. 21p. DNLM
60-2055

YOULIN, J[ohn] Juvenal (1821-1881)
An address delivered before the Homoeopathic Medical Society at its first annual meeting, April 15, 1869, in Newark. [With directory of homoeopathic physicians in the State of New Jersey.] New York: Charles Harvey, 1869. 30p. DNLM; NNNAM **60-2056**

YOUNG, James
The true physician! Heat, moisture, electricity, the vital principles of life, health, and growth, combined in Young's electro-thermal baths without medicine. The universal remedy, invented by. . . . Cleveland, O.: Nonpareil Steam Printing House, 1864. 40p. DNLM; OCIM **60-2057**

YOUNG, Noble (1808-1883)
Valedictory address to graduating class of the Medical Department of Georgetown College. Washington: H. Polkinhorn, 1860. 16p. DNLM **60-2058**

YOUNG, Noble (1808-1883)
Valedictory delivered at the annual commencement of the Medical Department of Georgetown College, March 6, 1866. Washington: H. Polkinhorn, 1866. 14p. DNLM
60-2059

YOUNG, Noble (1808-1883) and J. H. THOMPSON
Introductory addresses to the 20th session, 1869-1870, of the Medical Department of Georgetown College. Washington: W. H. Moore, 1869. DNLM **60-2060**

ZENDER, J. D. L.
Anthroponomy, or magneto-physiognomico-craniology. A new system . . . improved from the systems of . . . Lavater, Spurzheim, etc. New York, 1863. 99p. DNLM; NNNAM
60-2061

VI. AMERICAN MEDICAL IMPRINTS, 1870-1879

The meaning of *Conservative Surgery* is well understood. This phrase has been sufficiently common of late years. The conservative surgeon aims to preserve the integrity of the body. He spares diseased or wounded members whenever there are good grounds for believing that by skilful management they may be saved. He resorts to mutilations only when they are clearly necessary. He weighs carefully the dangers of operations, so as not to incur too much risk of shortening life by resorting to the scapel. By conservative medicine, I mean an analogous line of conduct in the management of maladies which are not surgical. The conservative physician shrinks from employing potential remedies whenever there are good grounds for believing that diseases will pursue a favorable course without active interference. He resorts to therapeutical measures which must be hurtful if not useful, only when they are clearly indicated. He appreciates injurious medication, and hence does not run a risk of shortening life by adding dangers of treatment to those of disease.

Austin Flint, *Essays on Conservative Medicine and Kindred Topics* (1874)

AN ACCOUNT of the medicinal properties of the Healing Springs, Bath Co., Va. To which is added a few certificates of cure (out of a large number) of scrofula, diseases of the skin, rheumatism, dyspepsia, chronic diarrhoea and dysentery, scrofulous ophthalmia, aptha, spinal irritation, etc. Richmond, Va.: J. D. Hammersley, 1870. 36p. DNLM **70-0001**

AN ACCOUNT of the Alleghany Springs in Montgomery County, Va., with an elaborate analysis of the water, and well authenticated cases establishing their efficacy in the treatment of a large class of prevalent and obstinate chronic complaints. Lynchburg: C. H. Bryant, 1871. 43p. DNLM **70-0002**

AN ACCOUNT of the medicinal properties of the Healing Springs, Bath Co., Va. . . . B. M. Quarles, agent. . . . Richmond: Clemmitt & Jones, printers, 1873. 24p. DNLM **70-0003**

ADAMS, John Glover (1807-1884)
Discourse commemorative of the life and character of Alex. Hodgdon Stevens, delivered by appointment of the N.Y. Academy of Medicine, May 25, 1871. New York: A. D. F. Randolph & Co., [1871]. 42p. DNLM; NNNAM **70-0004**

AN ADDRESS to the alumni of Hahnemann Medical College and Hospital of Chicago, Illinois, by the faculty of the College. Chicago: Culver, Page, Hoyne & Co., 1879. 24p. DNLM; OCIM **70-0005**

AGNEW, Cornelius Rea (1830-1888)
A contribution to the surgery of divergent squint. [New York, 1871.] 5p. DNLM **70-0006**

AGNEW, Cornelius Rea (1830-1888)
Ophthalmic notes. 1. Trephining the cornea to remove a foreign body deeply embedded in its substance. 2. A case of double, extremely minute and apparently congenital lachrymal fistula. 3. A contribution to the statistics of cataract extraction of one hundred and eighteen recent cases. New York: William Wood & Co., 1874. 30p. DNLM; NNNAM **70-0007**

AGNEW, Cornelius Rea (1830-1888)
Otitis. New York. G. P. Putnam's Sons, 1875. 22p. DNLM; NNNAM **70-0008**

AGNEW, Cornelius Rea (1830-1888)
Cantho-plasty as a remedy in certain diseases of the eye. New York: G. P. Putnam's Sons, 1875. 10p. DNLM **70-0009**

AGNEW, Cornelius Rea (1830-1888)
A preliminary analysis of ten hundred and sixty cases of asthenopia. New York: D. Appleton & Co., 1877. 12p. DNLM; NNNAM **70-0010**

AGNEW, Cornelius Rea (1830-1888)
A case of myxofibroma of the auricle. [Boston, 1878.] 2p. 1 plate. DNLM **70-0011**

AGNEW Cornelius Rea (1830-1888)
Clinical contribution to otology. Reported by David Webster. [New York, 1879.] 16p. DNLM **70-0012**

AGNEW, D[avid] Hayes (1818-1892)
Lecture introductory to the one hundred and fifth course of instruction in the Medical Department of the University of Pennsylvania, delivered Monday, October 10, 1870. Published by the class. Philadelphia: R. P. King's Sons, Printers, 1870. 33p. DNLM; PPC; PU **70-0013**

AGNEW, D[avid] Hayes (1818-1892)
Lacerations of the female perineum; and vesico-vaginal fistula; their history and treatment. Philadelphia: Lindsay & Blakiston, 1873. 141p. MBM; OCIM; PPC; PU **70-0014**

AGNEW, D[avid] Hayes (1818-1892)
Address delivered before the Philadelphia County Medical Society, January 5, 1875. (Published by order of the Society.) Philadelphia: Collins, 1875. 19p. DNLM; PPC; PU **70-0015**

AGNEW, D[avid] Hayes (1818-1892)
Hydrocele. New York: G. P. Putnam's Sons, 1877. 14p. DNLM **70-0016**

AGNEW, D[avid] Hayes (1818-1892)
Principles and practice of surgery, being a treatise on surgical diseases and injuries. Philadelphia: J. B. Lippincott & Co., 1878-1883. 3 v. MH-M; NNNAM; PPC; PU **70-0017**

AGNEW, D[avid] Hayes (1818-1892)
Biographical sketch of Dr. John Rhea Barton. Philadelphia: J. B. Lippincott & Co., 1879. 16p. PPC **70-0018**

AITKEN, William (1825-1892)
The science and practice of medicine. 3rd American from the 6th London ed., greatly enl., remodelled, carefully rev., and many portions rewritten . . . with additions by Meredith Clymer. Philadelphia: Lindsay & Blakiston, 1872. 2 v. DNLM; NNNAM; PPC; PU **70-0019**

ALCOTT, Louisa May (1832-1888)
Hospital sketches, and camp and fireside stories. Boston: Roberts Brothers, 1872. 379p. MA; MB; MH; NN **70-0020**

ALLEGHANY Springs, Montgomery Co., Va. Philadelphia: Merrihew & Sons, 1874. 60p. DNLM; PU **70-0021**

ALLEKTON. The antiseptic. A work of wonder. Middleton & Warner. New York: Rodgers Allekton Co., 1879. 16 l. DNLM **70-0022**

ALLEN, Harrison (1841-1897)
A description of the anatomy of the fifth pair of nerves. . . . Plate by Henry A. Daniels, M.D. Philadelphia: S. S. White, 1874. 41p. plate. DLC; PPC **70-0023**

ALLEN, Harrison (1841-1897)
Report of an autopsy on the bodies of Chang and Eng Bunker, commonly known as the Siamese twins. . . . Philadelphia: Collins, printer, 1875. 46p. DLC; DNLM **70-0024**

ALLEN, Harrison (1841-1897)
Studies in the facial region. [Philadelphia]: J. B. Lippincott & Co., 1875. 117p. DLNM; PPC; PU **70-0025**

ALLEN, Harrison (1841-1897)
Introductory lecture to the winter course of the Philadelphia Dental College, session 1876-1877. Delivered November 6th, 1876. New York: Johnston Bros., 1877. 12p. DLC; DNLM; NNNAM **70-0026**

ALLEN, Harrison (1841-1897)
The localization of diseases action in the oesophagus. . . . Philadelphia: J. B. Lippincott & Co., 1877. 8p. DLC **70-0027**

ALLEN, Henry C. (1836-1909)
The homoeopathic therapeutics of intermittent fever. . . . Detroit, Mich.: Drake's Homoeopathic Pharmacy, [1879]. 232p. DLC; PPHa **70-0028**

ALLEN, Jonathan Adams (1825-1890)
Medical examinations for life insurance. . . . Rev. and enl. ed., with new introductory chapter and an extensive appendix. New York: J. H. & C. M. Goodsell, 1870. 181p. DLC; DNLM; NNNAM **70-0029**

ALLEN, Nathan (1813-1889)
Medical problems of the day. The annual discourse before the Massachusetts Medical Society, June 3, 1874. . . . Boston: A. Williams & Co., 1874. 92p. DLC; DNLM; MH-M **70-0030**

ALLEN, Nathan (1813-1889)
The law of longevity, with special reference to life insurance. New York, 1874. 15p. DNLM **70-0031**

ALLEN, Nathan (1813-1889)
State medicine in its relations to insanity. Read at the meeting of the American Social Science Association, Detroit, May 13, 1875. Boston: Tolman & White, 1875. 31p. DNLM **70-0032**

ALLEN, Nathan (1813-1889)
The treatment of the insane. Read at the meeting of the American Social Science Association, Saratoga, September 6, 1876. Albany: Joel Munsell, 1876. 20p. DNLM; NNNAM **70-0033**

ALLEN, Nathan (1813-1889)
The normal standard of woman for propagation. New York: William Wood & Co., 1876. 39p. DNLM; MBM; NNNAM **70-0034**

ALLEN, Nathan (1813-1889)
Claims of the sick poor; paper read before the Middlesex North District Medical Society, January 31, 1877. Lowell: Marden & Rowell, 1877. 8p. DNLM **70-0035**

ALLEN, Nathan (1813-1889)
Changes in New England population. Read at the meeting of the American Social Science Association, Saratoga, September 6, 1877. Lowell, Mass.: Stone, Huse & Co., 1877. 16p. DNLM **70-0036**

ALLEN, Nathan (1813-1889)
The prevention of disease, insanity, crime, and pauperism. A paper read before the conference of charities, at Cincinnati, May 22, 1878. Boston: Rand, Avery & Co., 1878. 25p. DNLM; MBM **70-0037**

ALLEN, Nathan (1813-1889)
Changes in medical practice. [Boston, 1879.] Galley sheet. DNLM **70-0038**

ALLEN, Peter (1826-1874)
Lectures on aural catarrh; or the commonest forms of deafness and their cure (mostly delivered at St. Mary's Hospital). New York: William Wood & Co., 1872. 277p. 4 plates. DNLM; NNNAM; OCIM; PPC **70-0039**

ALLEN, Timothy Field, ed. (1837-1902)
The encyclopedia of pure materia medica. A record of the positive effects of drugs upon the healthy human organism. . . . With contributions from Dr. Richard Hughes . . . and others. New York, Philadelphia: Boericke & Tafel, [1874]-79. 10v. DNLM; DLC; PPHa; PU [*also*: Index, New York & Philadelphia: Boericke & Tafel . . . , 1880, 1331p.] **70-0040**

ALLEN, Timothy Field (1837-1902) and George S. NORTON
Ophthalmic therapeutics. . . . New York and Philadelphia: Boericke & Tafel, 1876. 269p. NNNAM; PPHa; PPC; PU **70-0041**

ALLINGHAM, William (1829-1908)
Fistula, haemorrhoids, painful ulcer, stricture, prolapsus, and other diseases of the rectum: their diagnosis and treatment. Philadelphia: Lindsay & Blakiston, 1872. 239p. NNNAM; PPC; PU [2nd ed. (1873), 265p.; 3rd ed. (1879), 325p.] **70-0041A**

ALLIS, Oscar H. (1836-1921)
Strangulated hernia, with cases and remarks upon early operative procedure in cases of doubtful diagnosis. Philadelphia: J. B. Lippincott & Co., 1877. 27p. DNLM **70-0042**

ALLIS, Oscar H. (1836-1921)
A brief account of the mechanism of the hip-joint, with diagnostic points upon dislocation and fracture of the neck of the femur. [Philadelphia, 1877.] 7p. DNLM **70-0043**

ALLIS, Oscar H. (1836-1921)
An examination of the usual signs of dislocation of the hip; also, an inquiry into the proper mode of procedure when dislocation of the hip is accompanied with fracture of the femur. Philadelphia: Collins, 1879. 23p. DNLM **70-0044**

ALLPORT, W. W[ebb] (1824-1893)
Address delivered before the American Academy of Dental Science, at their seventh annual meeting. Boston: Harris & Co., 1874. 16p. DNLM; MBM **70-0045**

AMERICAN ACADEMY OF DENTAL SCIENCE, BOSTON
A history of dental and oral science in America. Prepared under direction of the American Academy of Dental Science. Philadelphia: S. S. White, 1876. 271p. DLC; DNLM; PPC [Edited by James E. Dexter.] **70-0046**

AMERICAN DENTAL CONVENTION
Transactions, 1855-1873. New York: Sears & Cole, 1874. 356p. DNLM; NNNAM **70-0047**

AMERICAN ECLECTIC MEDICAL COLLEGE OF OHIO, AT CINCINNATI
Private circular to the graduates [soliciting their cooperation in securing a large class for the next session, offering ten dollars cash for every student they may induce to attend the lectures in this college. Signed W. Nicely, M.D.] [Cincinnati, 1879.] 1 sheet. DNLM **70-0048**

AMERICAN ECLECTIC MEDICAL COLLEGE OF OHIO, AT CINCINNATI

Annual announcements and catalogues for the sessions of 1879-1880 (4.); 1880-1881 (5.), 1882-1883 to 1892-1893 (7.-17.) Cincinnati, 1879-1892. DNLM [Organized in 1879 under the name of "Physio-Eclectic Medical College." In 1879, obtained a new charter as above, and in 1883 it was reorganized under the same name, but the control of the college passed to a new management. List of students and graduates for the years 1876-1877 to 1881-1882, in announcement for 1882-1883; for the years 1883-1884 to 1885-1886, in announcement for 1886-1887. List of students and graduates for 1886-1887 to 1888-1889, 1890-1891, 1891-1892, in announcements for subsequent years. In announcement for 1883-1884 and subsequent years title reads: American Eclectic Medical College of Ohio, at Cincinnati.] **70-0049**

AMERICAN GYNECOLOGICAL SOCIETY

Organized 1876. Constitution and by-laws, with a list of officers and fellows. Boston: Riverside Press, 1876. 12p. DNLM; MBM **70-0050**

AMERICAN HEALTH PRIMERS. EDITED BY W. W. KEEN

No. 1. Hearing, and how to keep it, by C. H. Burnett. Philadelphia: Lindsay & Blakiston, 1879-1880. 152p. DNLM; No. 2. Long life and how to reach it, by Joseph G. Richardson. Philadelphia, 1879. 160p. DNLM; No. 3. The summer and its diseases, by James C. Wilson. Philadelphia, 1879. 160p. DNLM; No. 4. Eyesight, and how to care for it, by George C. Harlan. Philadelphia, 1880. 139p. DNLM; No. 5. The throat and the voice, by Solis Cohen. Philadelphia, 1880. 159p. DNLM; No. 6. Winter and its dangers, by Hamilton Osgood. Philadelphia, 1879. 160p. DNLM; No. 7. The mouth and the teeth, by J. W. White. Philadelphia, 1880. 150p. DNLM; No. 8. Our homes, by Henry Hartshorne. Philadelphia, 1880. 149p. DNLM; No. 9. The skin in health and disease, by L. Duncan Bulkley. Philadelphia, 1880. 148p. DNLM; No. 10. Brain-work and overwork, by H. C. Wood. Philadelphia, 1880. 126p. DNLM; No. 11. Sea-air and sea-bathing, by John H. Packard. Philadelphia, 1880. 124p. DNLM; No. 12. School and industrial hygiene, by D. F. Lincoln. Philadelphia, 1880. 152p. DNLM **70-0051**

AMERICAN INSTITUTE OF HOMOEOPATHY

Record of the World's Homoeopathic Convention, to be held in Philadelphia, June 26, 1876. Philadelphia: Jackson Bros., 1875. 11p. DNLM; PPHa **70-0052**

AMERICAN INSTITUTE OF HOMOEOPATHY

Special report of the Homoeopathic Yellow Fever Commission, ordered by . . . for presentation to Congress. New York & Philadelphia: Boericke & Tafel, [1879.] 32p. DNLM; PPHa **70-0053**

AMERICAN INSTITUTE OF HOMOEOPATHY

Special report of the Homoeopathic Yellow Fever Commission, ordered by the . . . for presentation to Congress. New Orleans, La.: A. H. Nelson, 1879. 56p. DNLM **70-0054**

AMERICAN INSTRUCTORS OF THE DEAF AND DUMB

Proceedings of the convention held August, 1878 (9.) Columbus: Nevins & Myers, 1879. 317p. DNLM **70-0055**

AMERICAN MEDICAL ASSOCIATION

Plan of organization and code of ethics. Philadelphia: Collins, 1871. 30p. DNLM **70-0056**

AMERICAN MEDICAL ASSOCIATION

Report of the committee on criminal abortion. Philadelphia: Collins, 1871. 22p. DNLM **70-0057**

AMERICAN MEDICAL ASSOCIATION

Handbook for the use of the members of the American Medical Association, Philadelphia, 1872. Philadelphia: Collins, 1872. 82p. 2 maps. DNLM; PPC; PU **70-0058**

AMERICAN MEDICAL ASSOCIATION

Memorial to the senate and house of delegates of the State of West Virginia [for the establishment of a State board of health. By the special committee of the American Medical Association for the State of West Virginia. Appointed at the annual meeting, held at Philadelphia, June, 1876]. [Wheeling, 1876.] 2 l. DNLM **70-0059**

AMERICAN MEDICAL COLLEGE OF SAINT LOUIS (ECLECTIC)

Annual announcements for the sessions of 1875-1876 (3.); 1878-1879 (6.); 1879-1880 (7.); 1881-1882 to 1885-1886 (9.-13.); 1889-1890 (17.); 1890-1891 (18.); 1892-1893 (20.); 1893-1894 (21.). St. Louis, 1875-1893. DNLM [List of students and graduates for the years 1874-1875; 1877-1878; 1878-1879; 1880-1881; 1881-1882 to 1884-1885; 1888-1889; 1889-1890; 1891-1892; 1892-1893, in announcements for subsequent years. List of graduates from 1874 to 1890, in announcement for 1890-1891.] **70-0060**

AMIDON, R[oyal] W[ells] (*b.* **1853)**

Some new points on the pathological anatomy of tetanus. [New York, 1879.] 18p. 1 plate. DNLM **70-0061**

AMORY, Robert (1842-1910)

Physiological action of nitrous oxide, as shown by experiments on man and lower animals. Boston: J. Campbell, 1870. 31p. DNLM; MBM **70-0062**

AMORY, Robert (1842-1910)

Recent progress in therapeutics. [Boston, 1876.] 16p. DNLM **70-0063**

AMORY, Robert (1842-1910)

A contribution to the haematinic properties of dialized iron, being extracts from communications read before the Boston Society of the Medical Sciences and the Boston Society for Medical Observation. . . . Philadelphia: Lehman & Bolton, lithographers, engravers and printers, 1879. 16p. 5 plates. DLC; MBM; MWA **70-0064**

THE ANATOMICAL remembrancer, or complete pocket anatomist. . . . 3rd ed. With corrections and additions by C. E. Isaacs. . . . New York: William Wood & Co., 1871. 265p. DLC; NNNAM **70-0065**

ANDERSON, R. S.

Valedictory address to the class of graduates of the Missouri Medical College . . . , March 6, 1872. St. Louis: Printed by Missouri Democrat, 1872. 17p. DNLM; KU **70-066**

ANDERSON, T. McCall (1836-1908)

On the treatment of diseases of the skin: with an analysis of eleven thousand consecutive cases. Philadelphia: Henry C. Lea, 1873. 84p. DNLM; PPC; PPJ; PU **70-0067**

ANDERSON, W. C.
Curiosities of medical experience on Staten Island. A paper read before the Richmond County Medical Society, April, 1877. Stapleton, 1877. 12p. DNLM **70-0068**

ANDERSON, William H[enry] (1820-1887)
The climate of Alabama and its adaptation to health and comfort. Mobile: H. Farrow & Co., 1879. 11p. DNLM **70-0069**

ANDREWS, Edmund (1824-1904)
The relative dangers of anaesthesia by chloroform and ether, from statistics of 209,893 cases. Chicago: R. Fergus' Sons, 1870. 12p. DNLM; OCIM **70-0070**

ANDREWS, Edmund (1824-1904)
Prostitution and its sanitary management. Chicago, 1871. 33p. DNLM **70-0071**

ANDREWS, Edmund (1824-1904)
The unity or duality of the syphilitic virus. Chicago, 1871. 8p. DNLM **70-0072**

ANDREWS, Edmund (1824-1904)
Improved methods of treatment in joint and spinal diseases. [1872?] 16p. 8 fig. DNLM **70-0073**

ANDREWS, Edmund (1824-1904)
The mortality of surgical operations in the Upper Lake States, compared with that of other regions. By . . . assisted by Thomas B. Lacey. Chicago: Hazlitt & Reed, 1877. 123p. DNLM; ICRM; IEN-M **70-0074**

ANDREWS, Judson B. (1834-1894)
Exophthalmic goitre with insanity. [Utica, N.Y., 1870.] 15p. DNLM **70-0075**

ANDREWS, Judson B. (1834-1894)
The physiological action and therapeutic use of chloral. Utica, N.Y.: Roberts, 1871. 24p. DNLM **70-0076**

ANGELL, Henry Clay (1829-1911)
A treatise on diseases of the eye. For the use of general practitioners. . . . 2nd ed. Boston: James Campbell, 1871. 343p. MBA; PPHa **70-0078**

ANGELL, Henry Clay (1829-1911)
A treatise on diseases of the eye. For the use of general practitioners. . . . 2nd ed. James Campbell, 1871. 343p. MBA; PPHa **70-0078**

ANGELL, Henry Clay (1829-1911)
A treatise on diseases of the eye. For the use of general practitioners. . . . 3rd ed. Boston: James Campbell, 1870. 343p. MBA; PPHa **70-0079**

ANGELL, Henry Clay (1829-1911)
A treatise on diseases of the eye; for the use of students and general practitioners. To which is added, a series of test types for determining the exact state of vision. . . . 4th ed., enl. and illustrated. New York and Philadelphia: Boericke & Tafel, [etc., etc.], 1876. 343p. 3 plates. DLC; NNNAM; PPHa; PPC **70-0080**

ANGELL, Henry Clay (1829-1911)
A treatise on diseases of the eye. For the use of general practitioners. . . . 5th ed. Philadelphia: Boericke & Tafel, 1878. 344p. NNNAM; PPC; PPHa; PU **70-0081**

ANGELL, John
Elements of animal physiology, chiefly human. New York: G. P. Putnam's Sons, [1873]. 184p. DNLM; NN; NNNAM; NNC **70-0082**

ANSTIE, Francis Edmund (1833-1874)
On the uses of wines in health and disease. . . . New York: J. S. Redfield, 1870. 34p. DLC; NNNAM **70-0083**

ANSTIE, Francis Edmund (1833-1874)
Neuralgia and the diseases that resemble it. New York: D. Appleton & Co., 1872. 362p. NNNAM; OCIM; PPC; PU **70-0084**

ARLT, Ferdinand (1812-1887)
Injuries of the eye and their medico-legal aspect. . . . Transl. with the permission of the author, by Chas. S. Turnbull. . . . Philadelphia: Claxton, Remsen & Haffelfinger, 1878. 198p. DLC; NNNAM; PPC **70-0085**

ARMOR, Samuel Glasgow (1819-1885)
Catarrhal and croupous inflammation of mucous membranes. 1871. 12p. DNLM **70-0086**

ARMSTRONG, M. F.
Preventable diseases. New York: G. P. Putnam's Sons, 1879. 14p. DNLM; NNNAM [Hampton Tracts for the People, Sanitary Series, No. 3] **70-0087**

ARNOTT, Neil (1788-1874)
Elements of physics, or natural philosophy, general and medical, explained independently of technical mathematics, and containing new disquisitions and practical suggestions. . . . 7th ed., edited by Alexander Bain and Alfred Swaine Taylor. New York: D. Appleton & Co., 1877. 873p. CtY-M; DNLM; MBM; PPC **70-0088**

ARTHUIS, Arthur (*b.* 1842)
Treatment of nervous and rheumatic affections by static electricity. . . . Transl. from the French by J. H. Etheridge. . . . Chicago: W. B. Keen, Cooke & Co., 1874. 144p. DLC **70-0089**

ARTHUR, Robert (1819-1880)
Treatment and prevention of decay of the teeth. . . . Philadelphia: J. B. Lippincott & Co., 1871. 256p. DLC; DNLM; MdU-D; PPC **70-0090**

ARTHUR, Robert (1819-1880)
Treatment and prevention of decay of the teeth. . . . 2nd ed. . . . Philadelphia: J. B. Lippincott & Co., 1879. 216p. DLC; MdU-D; PPC **70-0091**

ASHHURST, John (1839-1900)
The principles and practice of surgery. . . . Illustrated with five hundred and thirty-three engravings. Philadelphia: Henry C. Lea, 1871. 1011p. DLC; MH-M; OCIM; PPC **70-0092**

ASHHURST, John (1839-1900)
The principles and practice of surgery. . . . 2nd ed. enl. and thoroughly rev. with five hundred and forty-two illustrations. Philadelphia: Henry C. Lea, 1878. 1040p. DLC; IU-M; LNT-M; PU **70-0093**

ASHHURST, John (1839-1900)
Valedictory address. University of Pennsylvania [Medical Department]. March 14, 1879. Philadelphia, 1879. 22p. DNLM; PU **70-0094**

ATKINSON, Isaac Edmondson (1846-1906)
The etiology of congenital syphilis, histologically considered. New York: D. Appleton & Co., 1875. 16p. DNLM
70-0095

ATKINSON, Isaac Edmondson (1846-1906)
Early syphilis in the Negro. Baltimore: J. H. Foster, [1877]. 12p. DNLM **70-0096**

ATKINSON, Isaac Edmondson (1846-1906)
An account of a case of syphilis inherited through two generations. New York: G. P. Putnam's Sons, 1877. 5p. DNLM
70-0097

ATKINSON, Isaac Edmondson (1846-1906)
The botanical relations of Tricophyton tonsurans. New York: D. Appleton & Co., 1878. 17p. DNLM
70-0098

ATKINSON, Isaac Edmondson (1846-1906)
The pigmentary syphiloderm. Chicago: Bulletin Print. Co., 1878. 8p. DNLM **70-0099**

ATKINSON, Isaac Edmondson (1846-1906)
Some phases of cerebral syphilis. Richmond: J. W. Ferguson & Son, 1879. 15p. DNLM **70-0100**

ATKINSON, William Biddle (1832-1909)
Evidence of life in the newly-delivered child. [1873.] 3p. DNLM **70-0101**

ATKINSON, William Biddle (1832-1909)
Hints in the obstetric procedure. The annual address before the Philadelphia County Medical Society. By. . . . Delivered May 8, 1874. Published by order of the Society. Philadelphia: Collins, printer, 1874. 28p. DLC; PPC
70-0102

ATKINSON, William Biddle (1832-1909)
The address in obstetrics. Delivered before the Medical Society of the State of Pennsylvania, May, 1874. . . . Philadelphia: Collins, printer, 1874. 48p. DLC; DNLM; PPC
70-0103

ATKINSON, William Biddle (1832-1909)
Hints in the obstetric procedure. . . . Philadelphia: Collins, printer, 1875. 89p. DLC; DNLM; PPC; PU
70-0104

ATKINSON, William Biddle (1832-1909)
Medical organizations and their value; an address delivered before the Alumni Association of Jefferson Medical College, March 9, 1877. Philadelphia: Collins, 1877. 20p. DNLM; PPJ **70-0105**

ATKINSON, William Biddle, ed. (1832-1909)
The physicians and surgeons of the United States. . . . Philadelphia: Charles Robson, 1878. 788p. DLC; DNLM; PPC; PU
70-0106

ATKINSON, William Biddle (1832-1909)
Hints in the obstetric procedure. . . . [2nd ed.] Philadelphia: D. G. Brinton, 1879. 121p. DLC; NNNAM; PPC; PU
70-0107

ATKINSON, William H.
Dental histology. Remarks before the Brooklyn Dental Society, reported by John C. Wyman. Philadelphia, 1872. 8p. DNLM **70-0108**

ATKINSON, William H.
Histology and microscopy. An essay. [Chicago, 1873.] 19p. DNLM **70-0109**

ATLEE, Washington Lemuel (1808-1878)
General and differential diagnosis of ovarian tumors, with specific reference to the operation of ovariotomy; and occasional pathological and therapeutical considerations. Philadelphia: J. B. Lippincott & Co., 1873. 482p. CtY-M; DNLM; PPC; PU **70-0110**

ATLEE, Washington Lemuel (1808-1878)
Reminiscences of the earliest days of Jefferson Medical College. An address delivered before the Alumni Association of the Jefferson Medical College of Philadelphia at its third anniversary, March 11, 1873. Philadelphia: P. Madeira, 1873. 16p. DNLM; PPJ **70-0111**

ATLEE, Washington Lemuel (1808-1878)
Old physic and young physic; some of the changes of the past half century contrasted and compared and their advantages estimated; the annual address before the Medical Society of the State of Pennsylvania. Philadelphia: Collins, 1875. 24p. DNLM; PPC **70-0112**

ATLEE, Washington Lemuel (1808-1878)
A retrospect of the struggles and triumph of ovariotomy in Philadelphia, with some additional remarks on allied subjects. The annual address before the Philadelphia County Medical Society, delivered Feb. 1, 1875. Philadelphia: Collins, 1875. 26p. DNLM; PPC **70-0113**

ATLEE, Washington Lemuel (1808-1878)
The treatment of fibroid tumors of the uterus. Philadelphia: Collins, 1877. 18p. DNLM; PPC; PPJ
70-0114

ATLEE, Washington Lemuel (1808-1878)
On sarcoma of the ovaries. [Philadelphia, 1878.] 20p. DNLM; PPC; PPJ **70-0115**

ATTFIELD, John (1835-1911)
Chemistry: general, medical, and pharmaceutical, including the chemistry of the U.S. pharmacopoeia. A manual on the general principles of the science, and their applications in medicine and pharmacy. . . . 7th ed. Rev. from the 6th (English) ed. by the author. Philadelphia: Henry C. Lea, 1876. 668p. tables. DLC; OCLloyd; PPC; PU **70-0116**

ATTFIELD, John (1835-1911)
Chemistry: general, medical, and pharmaceutical, including the chemistry of the U.S. pharmacopoeia. A manual on the general principles of the science, and their applications in medicine and pharmacy. . . . 8th ed., rev. by the author. Philadelphia: Henry C. Lea, 1879. 668p. tables. DLC; MBM; OCIM; OCLloyd
70-0117

AUSTEN, Philip H. (1822-1878)
Address delivered before the American Academy of Dental Science, at their sixth annual meeting, held in Boston, September 29, 1873. Boston: J. Harris & Co., 1874. 15p. DNLM; MBM **70-0118**

AUSTIN, Harriet N.
Baths and how to take them. [1875?] 11p. DNLM
70-0119

AYERS, J. Hamilton
. . . Ayers' Every man his own doctor. A family medical adviser; containing knowledge that will promote health, cure disease and prolong life, describing all diseases, and teaching how to cure them by the simplest medicines. . . . New ed., rev. and enl. . . . New York: G. W. Carleton & Co., [etc., etc.], 1879. 598p. DLC; NNNAM **70-0120**

AYRES, S[tephen] C.
Five cases of sympathetic ophthalmia. [New York, 1876.] 9p. DNLM **70-0121**

AYRES, Stephen C.
A comparison between the results of the treatment in one hundred cases of ophthalmia neonatorum in private and one hundred cases in hospital practice. [1876?] 8p. DNLM **70-0122**

AYRES, Stephen C.
Paracentesis of the cornea. [1877.] 15p. DNLM **70-0123**

AYRES, Stephen C.
Glaucoma. Columbus, O.: Cott & Hann, 1879. 10p. DNLM **70-0124**

BABBITT, E[dwin] D[wight] (1828-1905)
The health guide; aiming at a higher science of life and the life forces; giving nature's simple and beautiful laws of cure; the science of magnetic manipulation, bathing, electricity, food, sleep, exercise, marriage, and the treatment for one hundred diseases; thus constituting a home doctor far superior to drugs. New York: E. D. Babbitt, [1874]. 164p. DNLM; NNNAM **70-0125**

BABBITT, E[dwin] D[wight] (1828-1905)
Vital magnetism the life-fountain. Being an answer to Dr. Brown-Séquard's lectures on nerve force. The magnetic theory defended and a better philosophy of cure explained. Including also numerous quotations from "Babbitt's health guide," embracing the subjects of food, sleep, clothing, baths, rules for magnetizing, rules for the family, courtship, marriage, etc. New York: E. D. Babbitt, [1874]. 31p. DNLM; NNNAM **70-0126**

BABBITT, E[dwin] D[wight] (1828-1905)
The principles of light and color, including, among other things, the harmonic laws of the universe, the etherio-atomic philosophy of force, chromo-chemistry, chromo-therapeutics, and general philosophy of the fine forces, together with numerous discoveries and practical applications. New York: Babbitt & Co., 1878. 560p. 4 plates col. DNLM; NNNAM **70-0127**

BABBITT, E[dwin] D[wight] (1828-1905)
The wonders of light and color, including cromopathy, or the new science of color healing. New York: Babbitt & Co., 1879. 40p. DNLM; NNNAM **70-0128**

BACON, Francis (1831-1912)
Civilization and health. Cambridge, Mass., 1870. 20p. DNLM **70-0129**

BACON, Francis, (1831-1912), Wm. A. HAMMOND, and David F. LINCOLN
Vaccination. A report read before the American Social Science Association, at New York, October 27, 1869. New York: Nation Press, 1870. 19p. DNLM; NNNAM **70-0130**

BACON, Greenville
Tapeworms, their cause and treatment. Carefully collated from reliable data. . . . With the formulae for their total expulsion in every case as successfully used by J. B. Cherry, M.D. Printed for the author. . . . Boston: S. Woodberry & Co., printers, 1878. 56p. DLC **70-0131**

BACON, James G.
On the medicinal character of Hathorn spring water; the diseases in which it is useful, and the method of using the same. Also, a lecture by S. A. Fisk. Buffalo: Haas, Nauert & Co., 1876. 32p. DNLM **70-0132**

BACON, James G.
On the medicinal character of Hathorn spring water of Saratoga, N.Y.; the diseases in which it is useful and the method of using the same; also, a lecture by S. A. Fisk. Albany: C. Van Benthuysen, 1878. 30p. DNLM **70-0133**

BAILEY, Wm. (1833-1911)
Albuminuria. Read before the Kentucky State Medical Society, 1874. Louisville: J. P. Morton & Co., 1874. 14p. DNLM; KyLoJM **70-0134**

BAILHACHE, P[reston] H.
Syphilis and chancroid. Brief history, differential diagnosis, prophylaxis, and treatment. [Washington, D.C.], 1875. 30p. DNLM **70-0135**

BAKER, Henry B[rooks] (1837-1920)
The cause of chorea. [Detroit, 1876.] 7p. DNLM **70-0136**

BAKER, Louise S[outhard] (1846-1896)
A paper written for the Women's Christian Temperance Union of Mass., and read before the Suffolk County Medical Society in Boston, Feb. 22, 1879. [Boston, 1879.] 6p. DNLM; MH-M **70-0137**

BAKER, Rufus (1815-1891)
Management of our indigent insane. Read before the committee on humane institutions, in session February 11, 1879. Middletown, Conn., [1879]. 15p. DNLM **70-0138**

BAKER, William H[enry] (1845-1914)
Cases of amenorrhoea resulting from undeveloped uteri. New York, 1873. 7p. DNLM **70-0139**

BAKER, William H[enry] (1845-1914)
Malpositions of the uterers. New York: D. Appleton & Co., 1878. 17p. DNLM; NNNAM **70-0140**

BALCH, G[alusha] B.
Cancer of the bladder and prostate. Columbus: Nevins & Myers, 1877. 3p. DNLM **70-0141**

BALDWIN, Henry N.
Hahnemann Medical College and Hospital, Chicago. Seventeenth annual commencement, February 22, 1877. The class valedictory. . . . The class poem. By Jackson B. Whittier, M.D., of Wisconsin, and the list of graduates for the session of 1876-1877. Chicago: Culver, Page, Hoyne & Co., 1877. 12p. PPHa **70-0142**

BALL, John (1818-1890)
Forcible and rapid dilatation of the cervix uteri, for the relief of stricture, chronic endo-cervicitis, conical cervix, flexions, sterility, etc. New York: T. B. Sidebotham, 1877. 9p. DNLM; NNNAM **70-0143**

BANNING, Edmund Prior (*b.* 1810)
A peep into the house you live in; an essay on the causes of some of the ailments to which flesh is heir, and on the value of mechanical appliances in their treatment. New York, 1872. 64p. DNLM; NNNAM **70-0144**

BANNING, Edmund Prior (*b.* 1810)
The pathology and therapeutics of uterine displacements. [Read in brief before the Academy of Medicine, New York]. . . . [Boston, 1879.] 24p. DLC; DNLM; NNNAM **70-0145**

BANNISTER, H. M[artyn] (*b.* 1844)
Moral insanity. [Chicago, 1877.] 24p. DNLM **70-0146**

BANTING, William (1797-1878)
Letter on corpulence, addressed to the public. . . . 12th ed. Philadelphia: J. B. Lippincott & Co., [187?]. 51p. DLC; PPC **70-0147**

BARKER, [Benjamin] Fordyce (1818-1891)
Some clinical observations on the malignant diseases of the uterus. [New York, 1870.] 32p. DNLM; NNNAM **70-0148**

BARKER, [Benjamin] Fordyce (1818-1891)
On the treatment of croup. A letter to Prof. A. Jacobi, M.D. [New York, 1870.] 16p. DNLM; NNNAM **70-0149**

BARKER, [Benjamin] Fordyce [(1818-1891)
On sea-sickness. . . . New York: D. Appleton & Co.; [etc., etc.], 1870. 36p. DLC; DNLM; NNNAM **70-0150**

BARKER, [Benjamin] Fordyce (1818-1891)
Bloodletting as a therapeutic resource in obstetric medicine. . . . New York: D. Appleton & Co., 1871. 14p. DLC; DNLM; NNNAM **70-0151**

BARKER, [Benjamin] Fordyce (1818-1891)
The age of women when the capacity for child-bearing ceases. [Philadelphia, 1874.] 14p. DNLM **70-0152**

BARKER, [Benjamin] Fordyce (1818-1891)
The puerperal diseases. Clinical lectures delivered at Bellevue Hospital. . . . New York: D. Appleton & Co., 1874. 526p. DNLM; NNNAM; OCIM **70-0153**

BARKER, [Benjamin] Fordyce (1818-1891)
Vaginal hernia, or vaginal enterocele. Remarks before the New York Obstetrical Society, on a case communicated by B. A. Clements. [New York, 1876.] 16p. DNLM **70-0154**

BARKER, [Benjamin] Fordyce (1818-1891)
Annual address by the president. [Boston, 1876.] 17p. DNLM **70-0155**

BARKER, [Benjamin] Fordyce (1818-1891)
Annual address by the president. Medical gynecology. [Boston, 1877.] 18p. DNLM **70-0156**

BARKER, [Benjamin] Fordyce (1818-1891)
Biographical tribute, read before the New York Academy of Medicine, by vote of the council, February 7th, 1878. . . . Remarks by Drs. T. Gaillard Thomas, Austin Flint and R. J. O'Sullivan. New York: G. P. Putnam's Sons, 1878. 42p. DLC; DNLM; NNNAM [On cover: In memoriam Edmund Randolph Peaslee. Transactions of the Academy of Medicine.] **70-0157**

BARKER, [Benjamin] Fordyce (1818-1891)
On the induction of premature labor in the albuminuria of pregnancy. New York: William Wood & Co., 1878. 13p. DNLM; NNNAM **70-0158**

BARKER, [Benjamin] Fordyce (1818-1891)
Remarks on the obstetric forceps, with a description and demonstration of Tarnier's new instrument. New York: William Wood & Co., 1878. 13p. DNLM; NNNAM **70-0159**

BARKER, [Benjamin] Fordyce (1818-1891)
An inaugural address delivered before the New York Academy of Medicine, January 16, 1879. . . . New York: Printed for the Academy, 1879. 30p. DLC; NNNAM **70-0160**

BARKER, George T. (1836-1878)
An essay on the abuse of nitrous oxide; with discussions upon the same, before the Pennsylvania Association of Dental Surgeons, Feb. 13, 1877. Philadelphia: S. S. White, 1877. 16p. DNLM; PPC **70-0161**

BARNARD, Horace
Experts as witnesses. A lecture delivered before the New York Medico-Legal Society, February 26, 1874. New York: Russell Bros., 1874. 28p. DNLM; NNNAM **70-0162**

BARNES, Fancourt (1849-1908)
A manual for midwifery for midwives and medical students. Philadelphia: Henry C. Lea, 1879. 201p. DNLM; NNNAM; PPC **70-0163**

BARNES, John D.
Ancient and modern secrets of animal magnetism, clairvoyancy, mind reading and mesmerism; or, how to develop the magnetic power. Compiled from ancient and modern philosophers. Buffalo, N.Y.: Webster, [1870?] 61p. NN; NNNAM **70-0164**

BARNES, Robert (1817-1907)
Obstetric operations, including the treatment of hemorrhage. . . . With additions, by Benjamin F. Dawson, M.D. New York: D. Appleton & Co., 1870. 483p. DLC; MBM; NNNAM; PPC **70-0165**

BARNES, Robert (1817-1907)
Lectures on obstetric operations, including the treatment of hemorrhage, and forming a guide to the management of difficult labour. With additions by Benjamin F. Dawson. 2nd American ed. New York: D. Appleton & Co., 1871. 503p. DNLM; NNNAM; OCIM; PPC **70-0166**

BARNES, Robert (1817-1907)
A clinical history of the medical and surgical diseases of women. Philadelphia: Henry C. Lea, 1874. 791p. CtY-M; DNLM; PPC; PU **70-0167**

BARNES, Robert (1817-1907)
On the relations of pregnancy to general pathology. Boston, 1876. 27p. DNLM **70-0168**

BARNES, Robert (1817-1907)
A clinical history of the medical and surgical diseases of women. 2nd American from 2nd London ed. Philadelphia: Henry C. Lea, 1878. 784p. DNLM; PPC; PPJ; PU **70-0169**

BARRETT, W[illiam] C[ary] (1834-1903)
New principles in dental pathology. A review of the so-called new departure. [New York, 1878.] 8p. DNLM **70-0170**

BARTHOLOW, Roberts (1831-1904)
Fiske fund prize essay. Bromides: their physiological effects, and therapeutical uses. Providence: S. S. Rider & Bro., 1871. 47p. DNLM **70-0171**

BARTHOLOW, Roberts (1831-1904)
Spermatorrhoea: its causes, symptoms, results, and treatment. . . . 3rd ed., rev. New York: William Wood & Co., 1871. 120p. DLC; NNNAM; OCIM; PU **70-0172**

BARTHOLOW, Roberts (1831-1904)
Manual of hypodermic medication. . . . 2nd ed., rev. and enl. Philadelphia: J. B. Lippincott & Co., 1873. 170p. diags. (3 fold.). DLC; NNNAM; PPC; PU **70-0173**

BARTHOLOW, Roberts (1831-1904)
Cui bono? and what nature and what art does in the cure of disease. Two introductory lectures delivered in the Medical College of Ohio, sessions of 1872-1873 and 1873-1874. And, the doctor of the modern novel, read before the Cincinnati Literary Club, November 22, 1873. Cincinnati: Robert Clarke & Co., 1874. 66p. OCIM **70-0174**

BARTHOLOW, Roberts (1831-1904)
Annual oration on the degree of certainty in therapeutics, delivered before the Medical and Chirurgical Faculty at its seventy-eighth annual session, held at Baltimore, April, 1876. [Baltimore, 1876.] 18p. DNLM **70-0175**

BARTHOLOW, Roberts (1831-1904)
The principle of physiological antagonism as applied to the treatment of the febrile state. New York: G. P. Putnam's Sons, 1876. 21p. DNLM; NNNAM **70-0176**

BARTHOLOW, Roberts (1831-1904)
A practical treatise on materia medica and therapeutics. New York: D. Appleton & Co., 1876. 537p. CU-M; DNLM; IU-M; NNNAM **70-0177**

BARTHOLOW, Roberts (1831-1904)
Typho-malarial fever, and the opinions of Dr. Woodward, U.S.A., in 1863 and in 1877. . . . Cincinnati: R. Clarke & Co., 1877. 23p. DLC; DNLM **70-0178**

BARTHOLOW, Roberts (1831-1904)
The opinions, past and present, of Col. J. Woodward, M.D., U.S.A., in respect to typho-malarial fever and some other subjects. Cincinnati, 1878. 12p. DNLM; OCIM **70-0179**

BARTHOLOW, Roberts (1831-1904)
A practical treatise on materia medica and therapeutics. . . . New and enlarged ed. New York: D. Appleton & Co., 1878. 505p. DLC; ICJ; OCLloyd; PPC **70-0180**

BARTHOLOW, Roberts (1831-1904)
A practical treatise on materia medica and therapeutics. . . . 3rd ed., rev. New York: D. Appleton & Co., 1878. 595p. DLC; NNNAM; OCIM; PPC **70-0181**

BARTHOLOW, Roberts (1831-1904)
A case of human vivisection. Experimental investigations into the functions of the human brain. Washington, 1879. 10p. DNLM **70-0182**

BARTHOLOW, Roberts (1831-1904)
On spermatorrhoea. 4th ed. revised. New York: William Wood & Co., 1879. 128p. 1 plate. DNLM; IEN-M; LNT-M; NNNAM **70-0183**

BARTHOLOW, Roberts (1831-1904)
The hygiene of suburban life. A lecture delivered at Clifton Hall, suburb of Cincinnati, Friday evening, March 29th, 1879. . . . Philadelphia: Collins, printer, 1879. 22p. DLC; PPC **70-0184**

BARTHOLOW, Roberts (1831-1904)
The treatment of diseases by the hypodermic method: a manual of hypodermic medication. . . . 3rd ed., enl. Philadelphia [etc.]: J. B. Lippincott & Co., 1879. 249p. diags. (3 fold.). DLC; NNNAM; NNU-M; PPC **70-0185**

[BARTLETT, Elisha] (1804-1855)
A brief memoir of Dr. Elisha Bartlett, with selections from his writings and a bibliography of the same. Providence: S. S. Rider, 1878. 71p. DLC; MB; MH; MWA **70-0186**

BATES, W. H.
On the necessity of sufficiently extended urethral incisions for the permanent cure of strictures of the urethra. New York: D. Appleton & Co., 1877. 11p. DNLM; NNNAM **70-0187**

BATTEY, Robert (1828-1895)
Fibro-cystic tumor of the neck. [New York, 1877.] 7p. DNLM; NNNAM **70-0188**

BAUDUY, Jerome K[eating] (1842-1914)
Lectures on diseases of the nervous system. . . . Reported by V. Biart, M.D., rev. and ed. by the author. Philadelphia: J. B. Lippincott & Co., 1876. 484p. DLC; NNNAM; PPC; PU **70-0189**

BAUDUY, J[erome] K[eating] (1842-1914)
Emotional insanity. St. Louis: G. O. Rumbold & Co., 1879. 24p. DNLM **70-0190**

BAUER, Louis (1814-1898)
On the dressing of stumps. Old method; Lister's antiseptic plan; the Bordeaux treatment of stumps; Burow's plan, modified by the author; comparative statistics. [St. Louis, 1877.] 15p. DNLM **70-0191**

BAUER, Louis (1814-1898)
Original lecture on eucalyptol. The etherial oil of the leaves of Eucalyptus globulus. Its uses in medicine and surgery. [St. Louis, 1879?] 4p. DNLM **70-0192**

BAYLES, George (1836-1901)
Scarlet fever: suggestions concerning its treatment. . . . New York: D. Appleton & Co., 1873. 18p. DLC; DNLM **70-0193**

BAYLES, George (1836-1901)
Clinical study of diphtheria; treatment with elixir iodo-bromide of calcium comp., and bromo-chloralum. Read before the State Medical Society of New York, June, 1876. New York: Tilden & Co., 1877. 15 l. DNLM; NNNAM
70-0194

BEADLE, Hiram
The new medical era. A popular medical treatise on cholera, cholera morbus, cholera infantum, yellow fever, and cerebro-spinal meningitis, or spotted fever. St. Louis, 1874. 215p. OCIM; PPHa **70-0195**

BEADLE, Hiram
A popular treatise on yellow fever; being an original scientific and practical exposition of its nature and causes; also prevention and cure. Based on philosophical principles supported by facts, proving also its non-contagious character. . . . St. Louis: C. R. Burns, printer, 1878. 64p. DLC
70-0196

BEALE, Lionel Smith (1828-1906)
The mystery of life: an essay in reply to Dr. Gull's attack on the theory of vitality in his Harveian oration for 1870. . . . Philadelphia: Lindsay & Blakiston, 1871. 71p. 11 col. plates. DLC; NNNAM; PPC **70-0197**

BEALE, Lionel Smith (1828-1906)
Bioplasm: an introduction to the study of physiology and medicine. . . . Philadelphia: Lindsay & Blakiston, 1872. 345p. plates. DLC; PPC; PU **70-0198**

BEALE, Lionel Smith (1828-1906)
The machinery of life. A lecture. . . . Philadelphia: Lindsay & Blakiston, [1875]. 47p. DLC; PPC
70-0199

BEALE, Lionel Smith (1828-1906)
The microscope in medicine. 4th ed., much enlarged. . . . Philadelphia: Lindsay & Blakiston, 1878. 539p. CtY-M; DNLM; PPC; PU **70-0200**

BEARD, George Miller (1839-1883)
. . . Eating and drinking; a popular manual of food and diet in health and disease. . . . New York: G. P. Putnam & Sons, 1871. 180p. DLC; DNLM; NNNAM; PPC **70-0201**

BEARD, George Miller (1839-1883)
A practical treatise on the medical and surgical uses of electricity, including localized and general electrization. By George M. Beard . . . and A. D. Rockwell. . . . New York: William Wood & Co., 1871. 694p. plates. DLC; NNNAM; OCIM; PPC
70-0202

BEARD, George Miller (1839-1883)
. . . Stimulants and narcotics; medically, philosophically, and morally considered. . . . New York: G. P. Putnam & Sons, 1871. 155p. DLC; NNNAM; NNU-M
70-0203

BEARD, George Miller (1839-1883)
The cosmic law of intemperance. A contribution to the scientific study of the temperance question. [Ann Arbor, 1872.] 16p. DNLM **70-0204**

BEARD, George Miller (1839-1883)
Certain queries in electro-physiology and electro-therapeutics. [New York, 1872.] 13p. DNLM
70-0205

BEARD, George Miller (1839-1883)
A plea for scientific reform: a letter to Rev. Theodore L. Cuyler, D.D., on the attitude of physicians and scientists towards the temperance cause. New York, 1872. 23p. DNLM
70-0206

BEARD, George Miller (1839-1883)
Dr. George M. Beard's lecture before the Long Island Historical Society, on the decline of the moral faculties in old age. [Abstr.] [n.p., 1873(?).] 4p. DNLM **70-0207**

BEARD, George Miller (1839-1883)
Representative cases of nervous disease. [New York, 1874.] 8p. DNLM **70-0208**

BEARD, George Miller (1839-1883)
A practical treatise on the medical and surgical uses of electricity. Including localized and general faradization; localized and central galvanization: electrolysis and galvano-cautery. By George M. Beard . . . and A. D. Rockwell. . . . 2nd ed., rev., enl., and mostly re-written. . . . New York: William Wood & Co., 1875. 794p. DLC; NNNAM; OCIM; PPC
70-0209

BEARD, George Miller (1839-1883)
Hay-fever: or, summer catarrh: its nature and treatment. Including the early form, or "rose cold"; the later form, or "autumnal catarrh": and a middle form, or July cold, hitherto undescribed. . . . New York: Harper & Brothers, 1876. 266p. DLC; NNNAM; OCIM; PPC **70-0210**

BEARD, George Miller (1839-1883)
The scientific basis of delusions; a new theory of trance, and its bearings on human testimony. [Read before the New York Medico-Legal Society, November 1st, 1876.] New York: G. P. Putnam's Sons, 1877. 47p. DNLM **70-0211**

BEARD, George Miller (1839-1883)
Certain symptoms of nervous exhaustion. [Richmond, 1878.] 24p. DNLM **70-0212**

BEARD, George Miller (1839-1883)
Are inebriates automatons? [Hartford, 1878.] 12p. DNLM
70-0213

BEARD, George Miller (1839-1883)
The nature and diagnosis of neurasthenia (nervous exhaustion). New York: D. Appleton & Co., 1879. 29p. DNLM
70-0214

BEARD, George Miller (1839-1883)
Conclusions from the study of one hundred and twenty-five cases of writers' cramp and allied affections. New York, [1879]. 4p. DNLM **70-0215**

BEARD, George Miller (1839-1883)
Experiments with living human beings. [New York, 1879.] 18p. DNLM **70-0216**

BEARD, George Miller (1839-1883)
Other symptoms of nervous exhaustion (neurasthenia). Chicago: J. J. Spaulding & Co., 1879. 16p. DNLM
70-0217

BEARD, George Miller (1839-1883)
American nervousness: its philosophy and treatment. Richmond: J. W. Ferguson & Son, 1879. 24p. DNLM
70-0218

BEARD, George Miller (1839-1883)
Neurasthenia (nervous exhaustion) as a cause of inebriety. [Hartford, 1879.] 9p. DNLM **70-0219**

BECKWITH, David H[errick] (1825-1909)
Address delivered before the American Institute of Homoeopathy, by the president of the Association, at the twenty-eighth annual session, held in the hall of the Mercantile Library Association, Philadelphia, Pa., June 6, 7, 8, and 9, 1871. Cleveland: G. S. Newcomb & Co., 1871. 8p. PPHa **70-0220**

BECKWITH, Simeon W.
. . . Treatment of chronic diseases by means of electricity. . . . Philadelphia: Enterprise Print, 1871. 16p. DLC; DNLM **70-0221**

BEDELL, Gregory T[hurston] (1817-1892)
The therapeutical influence of high character in a physician: an address delivered before the graduating class of the Medical Department of the University of Wooster, Cleveland, February 24th, 1876. Published by request of the faculty of the Medical College. Cleveland, O.: Standard of the Cross, 1876. 15p. DNLM **70-0222**

BEDFORD, Gunning S. (1806-1870)
The principles and practice of obstetrics. [8th thousand] New York: William Wood & Co., 1873. 763p. DNLM; NNNAM; PPC; PU **70-0223**

BEEBE, Gaylord Dewitt (1835-1877)
Strangulated umbilical hernia. Removal of fifty-eight inches of mortified intestine during pregnancy—recovery. . . . [Chicago, 1870?] 7p. DLC **70-0224**

BEEBE, Gaylord Dewitt (1835-1877)
Ovariotomy; a clinical report of eight cases, giving a new and improved method of treating the pedicle, with brief remarks upon the natural history, diagnosis and treatment of ovarian tumors. . . . Chicago: Dr. G. D. Beebe, 1871. 35p. DLC **70-0225**

BEER, Robert Karl
Pharmacological dictionary. A lexicon of pharmaceutical terminology, containing all the terms of the pharmacopoeias of the United States and Germany, in English, German and Latin. . . . Baltimore, Md.: Beer & Sadler, 1876. 80p. DLC; DNLM; MdU-D **70-0226**

BELL, Agrippa Nelson (1820-1911)
Medical progress. An oration on the forty-seventh anniversary of the Medical Society of the County of Kings. . . . Brooklyn, April 27th, 1870. [Brooklyn, 1870.] 33p. DLC **70-0227**

BELL, A[grippa] N[elson] (1820-1911)
Sanitary work. [1875.] 1 l. DNLM **70-0228**

BELL, A[grippa] N[elson] (1820-1911)
Report on the bearing of the sanitary conditions of towns, and the crowding of population into filthy, ill-ventilated and badly drained tenement houses, upon the increase of pauperism. Albany: Weed, Parsons & Co., 1876. 22p. DNLM **70-0229**

BELL, Alexander Graham (1847-1922)
On the nature and uses of visible speech. Boston: Rand, Avery, & Co., 1872. 8p. DNLM **70-0230**

BELL, John (1796-1872)
Obituary notice of Charles D. Meigs. [Philadelphia, 1873.] 10p. DNLM; PPJ **70-0231**

BELLAMY, Edward (1842-1891)
The student's guide to surgical anatomy. . . . Philadelphia: Henry C. Lea, 1874. 300p. DNLM; ICU; OCIM; PPC **70-0231A**

BELLEVUE HOSPITAL MEDICAL COLLEGE, NEW YORK CITY
Annual circular and catalogue of the Bellevue Hospital Medical College, City of New York, 1870-1871. New York: Baker & Godwin, 1870. 16p. NNU-M **70-0232**

BELLEVUE HOSPITAL MEDICAL COLLEGE, NEW YORK CITY
First decennial catalogue of the trustees, faculty, officers, and of the alumni of the . . . of the city of New York, from 1861 to 1871. Compiled by Frederick A. Castle. Preceded by a history of the college from its organization to 1872. by Leroy Milton Yale. New York: D. Appleton & Co., 1873. 60p. DNLM; NNU-M **70-0233**

BELLOWS, Albert J[ones] (1804-1869)
The philosophy of eating. Boston: Houghton Mifflin Co., 1870. 426p. MBM [Homoeopathy] **70-0234**

BEMISS, S. M[errifield] (1821-1884)
Report to the faculty of the Medical Department of the University of Louisiana, in regard to the convention of medical teachers, lately held in Washington City. Published by order of the faculty. New Orleans: Bronze Pen Book Office, 1870. 7p. DNLM; LNT-M **70-0235**

BEMISS, S. M[errifield] (1821-1884)
Sanitary legislation in New Orleans. [New Orleans, 1870.] 33p. DNLM; LNT-M **70-0236**

BEMISS, S. M[errifield] (1821-1884)
Sudden death of an applicant for life insurance. Louisville: J. P. Morton & Co., 1871. 8p. DNLM **70-0237**

BENNETT, John Hughes (1812-1875)
Clinical lectures on the principles and practice of medicine. 5th American from the 4th London ed. New York: William Wood & Co., 1870. 1022p. DNLM; NNNAM; OCIM; PPC **70-0238**

BERNARDY, Eugene Prosper
The recurrence of puerperal fever. [New York, 1879.] 6p. DNLM **70-0239**

BERRY, J[ohn] C[utting] (1847-1936)
Climate and diseases of Japan. Portland: S. Berry, 1879. 14p. DNLM **70-0240**

BERRY, William and F. C. WILSON
A history of cholera in Lancaster, Ky., in 1873. Louisville: J. P. Morton & Co., 1873. 14p. 1 map. DNLM; KyLoJM **70-0241**

BERTOLET, R. M[orris] (*d.* 1882)
On the guaiacum process for the detection of blood as a valuable aid in distinguishing nucleated from non-nucleated red blood disks. [Philadelphia, 1871.] 4p. DNLM **70-0242**

BIDDLE, John Barclay (1815-1879)
Materia medica, for the use of students. . . . 4th ed., rev. and enl. . . . Philadelphia: Lindsay & Blakiston, 1871. 385p. DLC; MBM; OCLloyd; PPC **70-0243**

BIDDLE, John Barclay (1815-1879)
Lecture introductory to the course of Jefferson Medical College for the session of 1873-1874. Delivered October 6, 1873. Philadelphia: P. Madeira, 1873. 16p. DNLM; PPJ **70-0244**

BIDDLE, John Barclay (1815-1879)
Materia medica, for the use of students. . . . 5th ed., rev. and enl. . . . Philadelphia: Lindsay & Blakiston, 1873. 404p. DLC; NNNAM; OCIM; OCLloyd **70-0245**

BIDDLE, John Barclay (1815-1879)
Materia medica, for the use of students. . . . 6th ed., rev. and enl. . . . Philadelphia: Lindsay & Blakiston, 1874. 435p. DLC; NNNAM; OCLloyd; PPC **70-0246**

BIDDLE, John Barclay (1815-1879)
Materia medica, for the use of students. . . . 7th ed., rev. and enl. . . . Philadelphia: Lindsay & Blakiston, 1876. 454p. DLC; MBM; OCIM; OCLloyd **70-0247**

BIDDLE, John Barclay (1815-1879)
Materia medica, for the use of students. . . . 8th ed., rev. and enl. . . . Philadelphia: Lindsay & Blakiston, 1878. 462p. DLC; DNLM; PPC; PU **70-0248**

BIGELOW, C.
Sexual pathology; a practical and popular review of the principal diseases of the reproductive organs. Chicago: Ottaway & Colbert, 1875. 194p. DNLM; OCIM **70-0249**

BIGELOW, Henry Jacob (1818-1890)
Medical education in America: being the annual address read before the Massachusetts Medical Society, June 7, 1871. Cambridge: Welch, Bigelow & Co., 1871. 83p. DLC; MH-M; NNNAM; PU **70-0250**

BIGELOW, Henry Jacob (1818-1890)
Litholapaxy or rapid lithotrity with evacuation. Boston & New York, 1878. 42p. DNLM; MBM; NNNAM **70-0250A**

[BILLINGS, John Shaw] (1838-1913)
. . . A report on barracks and hospitals, with descriptions of military posts. Washington: Government Printing Office, 1870. 494p. DLC [U.S. Surgeon-General's Office, Circular, No. 4] **70-0251**

BILLINGS, John Shaw, comp. (1838-1913)
A report on the hygiene of the United States Army, with descriptions of military posts. Washington: Government Printing Office, 1875. 567p. fold. map, plates. DNLM; NNNAM; PPC; PU **70-0252**

[BILLINGS, John Shaw] (1838-1913)
Johns Hopkins Hospital. Reports and papers relating to construction and organization. No. 2—with plates. [Baltimore, 1876.] 18p. 14 plates. MdBJ-W **70-0253**

BILLINGS, John Shaw (1838-1913)
Medical education. Extracts from lectures delivered before the Johns Hopkins University. Baltimore, 1877-1878. . . . Baltimore: W. K. Boyle & Son, 1878. 42p. DLC; MdBJ-W **70-0254**

BILLINGTON, C[ornelius] E[varts] (1844?-1904)
Diphtheria and its treatment, with statistics of one hundred and seventy-nine cases. New York: D. Appleton & Co., 1876. 31p. DNLM; NNNAM **70-0255**

BILLROTH, Theodor (1829-1894)
General surgical pathology and therapeutics, in fifty lectures. A text book for students and physicians. . . . Transl. from the 4th German ed., with the special permission of the author, by Charles E. Hackley. . . . New York: D. Appleton & Co., 1871. 676p. DLC; NNNAM; OCIM; PPC **70-0256**

BILLROTH, Theodor (1829-1894)
General surgical pathology and therapeutics in fifty lectures. New York: 1874. (Transl. from 4th German ed., revised from 6th ed. by Chas. E. Hackley). New York: D. Appleton & Co., 1874. 697p. NNNAM **70-0257**

BILLROTH, Theodor (1829-1894)
General surgical pathology and therapeutics, in fifty-one lectures. . . . Transl from the 4th German ed. . . . and rev. from the 8th ed., by Charles E. Hackley. . . . New York: D. Appleton & Co., 1879. 773p. DLC; NNNAM; OCIM; PU **70-0258**

BIRD, O. B.
Progress and result of homoeopathy. Compiled by O. B. Bird, Secretary of the Oregon State Homoeopathic Medical Society. Portland, Oregon: Publishing House of Himes, 1879. 14p. PPHa **70-0259**

BISHOP, W. B.
An account of the medicinal properties of the Healing Springs, Bath County, Va. Richmond, 1876. 24p. DNLM **70-0260**

BIXBY, George H[olmes] (1837-1901)
A new instrument for the ready and effective use of the double current in the treatment of suppurating cavities and pelvic drainage. Cambridge: Riverside Press, 1875. 15p. DNLM; MBM **70-0261**

BLACK, D[onald] Campbell (1841-1898)
On the functional diseases of the renal, urinary, and reproductive organs, with a general review of urinary pathology. Philadelphia: Lindsay & Blakiston, 1872. 300p. CtY-M; DNLM; NNNAM; PPC **70-0262**

[BLACK, James Rush]
Alcohol as medicine, and how its use affects the temperance cause. A discussion between an M.D. of Newark, Ohio, and Thos. F. Hicks, M.D. Syracuse, N.Y.: Wesleyan Methodist Publishing House, 1870. 32p. DLC **70-0263**

BLACK, James Rush
The ten laws of health; or, How disease is produced and can be prevented. . . . Philadelphia: J. B. Lippincott & Co., 1872. 322p. DLC; PPC; PPHa; PPJ **70-0264**

BLACK, John Janvier (1837-1909)
Delaware State Medical Society. Session at Dover, Delaware, June, 1877, address of the president, ... Wilmington, Del.: James & Webb, printers, 1877. 28p. DLC; DNLM **70-0265**

BLACKMAN, George C[urtis] (1819-1871)
Catalogue of the library of the late. . . . Cincinnati, Ohio, [1871]. 12p. DNLM **70-0266**

BLAKE, Clarence J[ohn] (1843-1919)
Manometric cicatrix of the membrana tympani. New York, 1876. 15p. DNLM **70-0267**

BLAKE, Clarence J[ohn] (1843-1919)
Application of paper dressings in treatment of perforations of the membrana tympani. New York, 1877. 10p. DNLM **70-0268**

BLAKE, Clarence J[ohn] (1843-1919)
On the best mode of testing the hearing of school children, and of providing for the instruction of partially deaf children. Philadelphia, 1877. 10p. DNLM **70-0269**

BLAKE, Clarence J[ohn] (1843-1919)
Report of the progress of otology. Part II. Pathology and therapeutics. New York: D. Appleton & Co., 1877. 33p. DNLM **70-0270**

BLAKE, Clarence J[ohn] (1843-1919)
The use of membrana tympani as a phonautograph and logograph. New York: William Wood & Co., 1879. 10p. DNLM **70-0271**

BLAKE, John Ellis (1831-1880)
A case of grapeshot-wound of the chest. New York: D. Appleton & Co., 1872. 12p. DNLM **70-0272**

BLAKE, John Ellis (1831-1880)
Premature ossification of the fetal cranium as a cause of dystocia, and of impairment of intellect in children. New York: William Wood & Co., 1879. 12p. DNLM **70-0273**

BLANCHARD, Virgil W.
The Blanchard system of physical culture; embodied in the scientific application of food for the prevention and cure of physical and mental disease, intemperance, etc. [New York, 1877.] 23p. DNLM; NNNAM **70-0274**

BLANDFORD, G[eorge] Fielding (1829-1911)
Insanity and its treatment: lectures on the treatment, medical and legal, of insane patients. . . . With a summary of the laws in force in the United States on the confinement of the insane by Isaac Ray. Philadelphia: Henry C. Lea, 1871. 471p. CtY-M; NNNAM; PPC; PU **70-0275**

BLANE, John (1802-1885)
History of the District Medical Society for the County of Hunterdon, from its organization in 1821 to the annual meeting in 1871; together with the medical history of the county, as its boundaries now exist, from its first settlement to the present time, 1872. Newark, N.J.: Jennings & Hardham, 1872. 125p. DNLM; NjR **70-0276**

BLODGETT, F[rank] M.
A synopsis of dermatology. For the use of physicians and students. Boston: Rockwell & Churchill, 1876. 1 broadside. DNLM **70-0277**

BÖDECKER, C. F. W.
Necrosis. [New York, 1878.] 8p. DNLM **70-0278**

BODENHAMER, William (1808-1905)
The physical exploration of the rectum: with an appendix on the ligation of haemorrhoidal tumors. . . . New York: William Wood & Co., 1870. 34p. DLC; NNNAM **70-0279**

BODENHAMER, William (1808-1905)
An essay on rectal medication. . . . New York: William Wood & Co., 1878. 58p. DLC; NNNAM **70-0280**

BODINE, J[ames] M[orrison] (*b.* 1831)
The physician as a public educator: introductory address delivered at the opening of the session of the Medical Department of the University of Louisville, October 7, 1872. . . . [Louisville, Ky., 1872.] 19p. DLC **70-0281**

BODINE, J[ames] M[orrison] (*b.* 1831)
"What am I?" A valedictory address to the graduates delivered at the close of the forty-first session of the Medical Department of the University of Louisville, February 28, 1878. . . . Louisville, Ky.: Printed by J. P. Morton & Co., 1878. 28p. DLC; DNLM **70-0282**

BODLEY, Rachel L. (1831-1888)
Introductory lecture, Women's Medical College of Pennsylvania. Philadelphia: Grant, Faires & Rodgers, 1875. 16p. DNLM; PU **70-0283**

BOENNINGHAUSEN, Clemens Maria Franz von (1785-1864)
The homoeopathic treatment of hooping cough. Transl. with additions, by Carroll Dunham, M.D. New York: Henry M. Smith & Brother, 1870. 199p. DLC; NNNAM; PPHa **70-0284**

BOENNINGHAUSEN, Clemens Maria Franz von (1785-1864)
Boenninghausen's homoeopathic therapia of intermittent and other fevers. Transl., with the addition of new remedies, by A. Korndoerfer, M.D. New York and Philadelphia: Boericke & Tafel, 1873. 243p. NNNAM; PPHa **70-0285**

BOERICKE, Francis E[dmund] (1826-1901)
Three lectures on homoeopathic pharmaceutics. . . . New York, Philadelphia: Boericke & Tafel, [1878]. 50p. DLC; NNNAM **70-0286**

[BOERICKE & TAFEL]
The homoeopathic treatment of catarrh, or cold in the head. By eight remedies. New York: Boericke & Tafel, 1871. 8p. DLC **70-0287**

[BOERICKE & TAFEL]
The homoeopathic treatment of sea sickness, by eight remedies. New York: Boericke & Tafel, 1871. 22p. DLC **70-0288**

[BOERICKE & TAFEL]
The homoeopathic treatment of dyspepsia, or indigestion. By eight remedies. New York: Boericke & Tafel, 1871. 12p. DLC **70-0289**

[BOERICKE & TAFEL]
Toothache: useful hints upon, and how to treat it, by eight homoeopathic remedies. New York: Boericke & Tafel, 1871. 11p. DLC **70-0290**

[BOERICKE & TAFEL]
Medical index and key to the treatment of all common complaints, and list of medicines from the Homoeopathic Pharmacy of Boericke & Tafel, 145 Grand Street, New York, 1874. 32p. PPHa **70-0291**

[BOERICKE & TAFEL]
Homoopathischer wegweiser, oder schlussel zur Behandling gewohnlicher krankheiten. Boericke & Tafel's Homoopatischer Apotheken. New York, Philadelphia, Baltimore, Washington, Pittsburgh, Chicago, 1878. 32p. PPHa
70-0292

BOERICKE & TAFEL
Descriptive catalogue of homoeopathic publications. [Philadelphia, 1879?] 32p. DNLM; PPHa **70-0293**

BOGUE, R[oswell] G[riswold] (1832-1893)
A report of fifteen cases of tracheotomy in diphtheritic group, six of them successful. Chicago, 1878. 24p. DNLM
70-0294

BOLLES, J. A[ugustus] (1809-1878)
Address delivered at the fiftieth annual commencement of the National Medical College (Medical Department of the Columbian College), March 7, 1872. Washington, D.C.: Judd & Detweiler, 1872. 13p. DNLM **70-0295**

THE BOOK of travels of a doctor of physic, containing his observations made in certain portions of the two continents. Philadelphia: J. B. Lippincott & Co., 1871. 373p. DNLM; NN; NNC; PU **70-0296**

BORCK, [Mathias Adolph] Edward (1834-1912)
On fracture of the femur. . . . St. Louis: G. O. Rumbold & Co., 1879. 52p. DLC **70-0297**

BORLAND, J[ohn] Nelson (1828-1890)
First medical and surgical report of the Boston City Hospital. By J. Nelson Borland and David Cheever. Boston: By the Board of Trustees, 1870. 688p. 9 plates. DLC; DNLM; MBM; MH **70-0297A**

BOSTON CITY HOSPITAL
Medical formulary of the City Hospital. Boston: Rockwell & Churchill, 1873. 16p. MBM **70-0298**

BOSTON TRAINING SCHOOL FOR NURSES, MASSACHUSETTS GENERAL HOSPITAL
Circular [of the committee to physicians, calling their attention to the establishment of the school]. Aug. 11, 1873. [Boston, 1873.] 1 sheet. DNLM **70-0299**

BOSTON UNIVERSITY. SCHOOL OF MEDICINE (HOMOEOPATHIC)
Annual announcements for the sessions of 1876-1877 to 1895-1896 (4.-23.). Boston, 1876-1895. DNLM [List of the students and graduates for the sessions of 1873-1874 to 1894-1895 in announcements for subsequent years. Alumni from 1874 to 1895 in announcement for 1895-1896.]
70-0300

BOTH, Carl
Dr. C. Both's method for the radical arrest of tuberculosis of the lungs by artifical calcification. Transl. by the author. . . . [1872.] 2 l. DNLM **70-0301**

BOTH, Carl
Small-pox: the predisposing conditions and their prevention. Boston: A. Moore, 1872. 50p. DNLM; MBM
70-0302

BOTH, Carl
Small-pox: the predisposing conditions and their prevention. With a scientific exposition of vaccination. 2nd ed. Boston: A. Moore, 1872. 82p. DNLM; MBM **70-0303**

BOTH, Carl
On the treatment of severe case of lignitudo capitis. Rochester, N.Y., 1873. 4p. DNLM **70-0304**

BOTH, Carl
Consumption and its treatment in all its forms. Boston: A. Moore, 1873. 157p. 1 plate. DNLM; MH-M; NNNAM
70-0305

BOWDITCH, Henry Ingersoll (1808-1892)
Letter from the chairman of the State Board of Health, concerning houses for the people, convalescent homes, and the sewage question. [Boston, 1870.] 64p. DNLM; MBM
70-0306

BOWDITCH, Henry Ingersoll (1808-1892)
Thoracentesis, and its general results during twenty years of professional life. New York: William Wood & Co., 1870. 16p. DNLM; NNNAM **70-0307**

BOWDITCH, Henry Ingersoll (1808-1892)
Intemperance in New England. How shall we treat it? Boston, 1872. 4p. DNLM; MWA **70-0308**

BOWDITCH, Henry Ingersoll (1808-1892)
Venesection, its abuse formerly, its neglect at the present day. Boston: D. Clapp & Son, 1872. 23p. DNLM; MWA
70-0309

BOWDITCH, Henry Ingersoll (1808-1892)
Analysis of the correspondence on the use and abuse of intoxicating drinks throughout the globe, which was presented to the legislature in 1871; or, intemperance as seen in the light of cosmic law. Boston: Wright & Potter, 1872. 59p. 1 chart. DNLM; MBM; MHi **70-0310**

BOWDITCH, Henry Ingersoll (1808-1892)
Brief memories of Louis and some of his contemporaries in the Parisian school of medicine of forty years ago. Boston: J. Wilson & Son, 1872. 37p. DNLM; MH-M
70-0311

BOWDITCH, Henry Ingersoll (1808-1892)
Analysis of a correspondence on some of the causes or antecedents of consumption. [Boston, 1873.] 82p. DNLM; MBM; PPC **70-312**

BOWDITCH, Henry Ingersoll (1808-1892)
Massachusetts State Board of Health. Circular, being the address on the life and services of the late secretary of the Board, Dr. George Derby. July 1, 1874. [Boston, 1874.] 3p. DNLM; MH **70-0313**

BOWDITCH, Henry Ingersoll (1808-1892)
Address at a meeting of the Massachusetts State Board of Health, announcing the death and services of Dr. George Derby. Boston, July 1, 1874. [1874.] 3p. DNLM
70-0314

BOWDITCH, Henry Ingersoll (1808-1892)
Electrolysis in thoracic aneurism. Read at a meeting of the Suffolk District Medical Society, March 27, 1875. [1875.] 11p. DNLM **70-0315**

BOWDITCH, Henry Ingersoll (1808-1892)
Address on hygiene and preventive medicine, delivered before the International Medical Congress, at Philadelphia, September 5, 1876. Philadelphia, 1876. 32p. DNLM; PPC
70-0316

BOWDITCH, Henry Ingersoll (1808-1892)
Public hygiene in America: being the centennial discourse delivered before the International Medical Congress, Philadelphia, September, 1876. . . . With extracts from correspondence from the various states. Together with a digest of American sanitary law, by Henry G. Pickering, Esq. Boston: Little, Brown, & Co.; [etc., etc.], 1877. 498p. DLC; MH; NN; NNNAM **70-0317**

BOWDITCH, Henry Ingersoll (1808-1892)
Studies of an epidemic of diphtheria, which prevailed at Ferrisburg (adjacent to Vergennes), Vt. during the summer of 1877. Philadelphia: Collins, 1878. 15p. 1 map. DNLM
70-0318

BOWDITCH, H[enry] P[ickering] (1840-1911)
The school of physiology at Leipzig. Boston: D. Clapp & Son, 1870. 11p. DNLM; MH-M **70-0319**

BOWDITCH, Henry Pickering (1840-1911)
The lymph spaces in fasciae; a new method of injection. Boston: D. Clapp & Son, 1873. 2 l. 1 plate. DNLM
70-0320

BOWDITCH, Henry Pickering (1804-1911) and Charles Sedgwick MINOT
The influence of anaesthetics on the vaso-motor centres. Boston: D. Clapp & Son, 1874. 8p. 3 plates. DNLM
70-0321

BOWDITCH, Henry Pickering (1840-1911)
Recent progress in physiology. [Reports.] Course of nerve fibres in the spinal cord. [Boston, 1875.] 12p. DNLM; MH-M
70-0322

BOWDITCH, Henry Pickering (1840-1911)
Recent progress in physiology [Reports.] Functions of the cortex cerebri. Boston, 1876. 11p. DNLM; MH-M
70-0323

BOWDITCH, Henry Pickering (1840-1911)
Recent progress in physiology. [Reports.] Transfusion. [Boston, 1876.] 11p. DNLM; MH-M **70-0324**

BOWDITCH, Henry Pickering (1840-1911)
Force of ciliary motion. Cambridge, 1876. 5p. DNLM
70-0325

BOWDITCH, Henry Pickering (1840-1911)
The growth of children. Boston: A. J. Wright, 1877. 51p. 15 plates, 15 tab. DNLM; MBM **70-0326**

BOWDITCH, Henry Pickering (1840-1911)
Recent progress in physiology. [Reports.] Vaso-motor mechanism. Boston, 1877. 8p. DNLM; MH-M
70-0327

BOWDITCH, Henry Pickering (1840-1911)
Recent progress in physiology. [Reports.] Air in the circulatory system, etc. [Boston, 1878.] 10p. DNLM; MH-M
70-0328

BOWDITCH, Henry Pickering (1840-1911)
Contributions from the physiological laboratory of the Harvard Medical School. A new form of plethysmograph. [Salem, 1879.] 2 l. DNLM **70-0329**

BOWDITCH, Nathaniel Ingersoll (1805-1861)
History of the Massachusetts General Hospital. (To August 5, 1851). 2nd ed., with a continuation to 1872. Boston: Printed by the Trustees from the Bowditch Fund, 1872. 734p. DNLM; MBM; MWA; NNNAM **70-0330**

BOWDITCH, Nathaniel Ingersoll (1805-1861)
Extracts from a history of the Massachusetts General Hospital, 1810-1851 . . . with a continuation, 1851-1872, by George E. Ellis. Boston, [1872]. 98p. MBM **70-0331**

BOWDOIN COLLEGE AND THE MEDICAL SCHOOL OF MAINE
Catalogues of the officers and students of Bowdoin College and the Medical School of Maine, at Brunswick, for the sessions of 1823, 1826, 1828, 1835-1838, 1840, 1846-1849, 1853, 1855-1858, 1860. 1863-1864, 1866-1867 to 1875-1876. Brunswick, 1823-1876. DNLM **70-0332**

BOWLING, William K. (1808-1885)
An account of the cholera, as it appeared at Nashville, in the year 1873. Nashville, Tenn.: Union & American Co., 1873. 63p. 1 map. DNLM **70-0333**

BOWLING, William K. (1808-1885)
An inquiry concerning priority in the ligation of the internal carotid artery. Nashville, Tenn.: Union & American Co., 1874. 20p. DNLM **70-0334**

BOYLAND, George Halstead (1845-1919)
Six months under the Red Cross, with the French army. Cincinnati: R. Clarke & Co., 1873. 232p. DNLM; ICU; NN; NNC **70-0335**

BOYLAND, George Halstead (1845-1919)
On the treatment of venereal disease by salicyclic acid, with eight illustrative cases. [1875.] 3p. DNLM
70-0336

BOZEMAN, Nathan (1825-1905)
Vesico-vaginal fistules: comparative analysis of different surgical methods; results, American and European. [Philadelphia, 1870.] 13p. DNLM **70-0337**

BOZEMAN, Nathan (1825-1905)
On urethrocele, catarrh, and ulceration of the bladder in females. New York: W. Baldwin & Co., 1871. 27p. DNLM
70-0338

BOZEMAN, Nathan (1825-1905)
On urethrocele, catarrh, and ulceration of the bladder in females. Albany: Argus Co., 1872. 19p. DNLM
70-0339

BOZEMAN, Nathan (1825-1905)
Kolpokleisis as a means of treating vesico-vaginal fistule; is the procedure ever necessary? Philadelphia: Collins, 1877. 13p. DNLM **70-0340**

BOZEMAN, Nathan (1825-1905)
Retroversion in relation to lacerations of the cervix uteri, etc. [Boston, 1879.] 18p. DNLM **70-0341**

BOZEMAN, Nathan (1825-1905)
Remarks on ovariotomy, with relation of cases and peculiarities in treatment. New York: William Wood & Co., 1879. 60p. DLC; DNLM; NNNAM **70-0342**

BRADFORD, Edward H. (1848-1926)
Reflex symptoms in hip disease. Read at the annual meeting of the Massachusetts Medical Society, June 11, 1878. [Boston, 1878.] 18p. DNLM **70-0343**

BRADLEY, W[illiam] Lockwood (1837-1903)
The treatment of puerperal convulsions. New Haven: Tuttle, Morehouse & Taylor, 1872. 13p. DNLM **70-0344**

BRADNER, N. Roe
Sanity and insanity. Philadelphia: J. B. Lippincott & Co., 1874. 8p. DNLM **70-0345**

BRANDRETH, Benjamin (1807-1880)
The doctrine of purgation. . . . 2nd ed. New York: Baker & Godwin, printers, 1871. 224p. NNNAM **70-0346**

BRANDRETH, Benjamin (1807-1880)
The doctrine of purgation. . . . 3rd ed. New York: Baker & Godwin, printers, 1873. 246p. NNNAM **70-0347**

BREYFOGLE, William L. (*b.* 1845)
A lecture on homoeopathy. Louisville: Sherrill, Wilson & Co., 1873. 28p. PPHa **70-0348**

BREYFOGLE, William L. (*b.* 1845)
Treatise on the effects of coffee, by S. Hahnemann. Transl. by W. L. Breyfogle, M.D. Louisville, Ky.: Bradley & Gilbert, 1875. 36p. PPHa **70-0349**

BRICKELL, Daniel Warren (1824-1881)
Rupture of the perineum. With a description of a new operation. Philadelphia, 1875. 9p. DNLM **70-0350**

BRIDGMAN, M[arcus] F[ayette] (1824-1899)
Laceration of the soft parturient passages, including one unreported case, and some details of ten others reported in various publications illustrative of the subject. A monograph. Boston: J. Adams, 1875. 33p. DNLM; MBM **70-0351**

BRIGGS, Robert
On the relation of moisture in air to health and comfort. [Philadelphia, 1878.] 5p. DNLM **70-0352**

BRIGGS, Wm. T[hompson] (1828-1894)
Extract from a report on the history of surgery of Tennessee, comprising the subjects of stone in bladder, ovarian tumours, vesico-vaginal fistula, made to the Tennessee State Medical Society, April 3, 1872. Nashville, 1874. 98p. 1 plate. DNLM **70-0353**

BRIGGS, Wm. T[hompson] (1828-1894)
An address delivered before the McDowell Medical Society of Kentucky. Nashville, Tenn.: Wheeler, Marshall & Bonce, 1874. 15p. DNLM **70-0354**

BRIGGS, Wm. T[hompson] (1828-1894)
An address delivered before the McDowell Medical Society of Kentucky, at its semi-annual meeting, in Madisonville, Ky., Nov. 4, 1874. Nashville: Wheeler, Marshall & Bonce, 1874. 15p. DNLM **70-0355**

BRIGHAM, Amariah (1798-1849)
Influence of mental cultivation in producing of dyspepsia. 3rd ed. New York: M. L. Holbrook & Co., 1878. 95-145p. DNLM [Separate title-page. In: M. L. Holbrook, Liver Complaint. . . . (1878)] **70-0356**

BRIGHAM, Charles B[rooks] (1845-1903)
Valedictory address in behalf of the faculty of the Medical Department of the University of California to the graduating class of 1873. [1873.] 17p. DNLM **70-0357**

BRIGHAM, Charles B[rooks] (1845-1903)
Surgical cases, with illustrations. [Cambridge: H. O. Houghton & Co.], 1876. 110p. 23 plates. DNLM; MH-M **70-0358**

BRIGHT, J. W.
Cancer: its classification and remedies. . . . Philadelphia: S. W. Butler, 1871. 190p. DNLM; DLC; PPC; PU **70-0359**

BRISTOWE, John Syer (1827-1895)
A treatise on the theory and practice of medicine. . . . Ed., with notes, by James H. Hutchinson. Philadelphia: Henry C. Lea, 1876. 1089p. DLC; CtY-M; ICJ; MB **70-0360**

BRISTOWE, John Syer (1827-1895)
A treatise on the theory and practice of medicine. . . . 2nd American ed., rev. by the author. With notes and additions by James H. Hutchinson. Philadelphia: Henry C. Lea, 1879. 1081p. diags. DLC; NNNAM; PPC; PU **70-0360A**

BRISTOWE, John Syer (1827-1895)
Diseases of the intestines and peritoneum. By John Syer Bristowe, M.D., J. R. Wardell, M.D., J. W. Begbie, M.D., S. O. Habershon, M.D., T. B. Curling, F.R.S., and W. H. Ransom, M.D. New York: William Wood & Co., 1879. 243p. DLC; MBM; OCIM; NNNAM **70-0361**

BROCKLESBY, John (1811-1889)
The amateur microscopist: or views of the microscopic world. A handbook of microscopic manipulation and microscopic objects. New York: William Wood & Co., 1871. 144p. 9 plates. DNLM; NNNAM; OCIM; PU **70-0362**

BRODIE, Wm. (1823-1890)
Address of the president [of the] Michigan State Medical Society. Delivered at Ann Arbor, May 10, 1876. [1876?] 16p. DNLM **70-0363**

BRONSON, Henry (1804-1893)
History of intermittent fever in the New Haven region, with an attempt to distinguish known from unknown causes. [New Haven, 1875.] 52p. CtY-M; DNLM **70-0364**

BRONSON, Henry (1804-1893)
Medical history and biography. [Read at different dates, between Dec. 9, 1872, and Oct. 16, 1876.] [1876?] 150p. CtY-M; DNLM **70-0365**

BRONSON, J. R[ichardson] (1829-1900)
A review of medicine; its work and its worth. The annual address delivered before the Massachusetts Medical Society. Boston: D.C. Clapp & Son, 1877. 38p. DNLM; MH-M **70-0366**

BROOMALL, Anna E. (1847-1931)
The operation of epistotomy as a prevention of perineal ruptures during labor. New York: William Wood & Co., 1878. 13p. DNLM; NNNAM **70-0367**

BROWN, Buckminster (1819-1891)
Femoral aneurism cured by direct compression, while the patient was taking active exercise; death from peritonitis six years afterwards; with an account of the post-mortem appearances by Henry H. A. Beech. Cambridge: Riverside Press, 1875. 8p. 1 plate. DNLM; MBM **70-0368**

BROWN, Buckminster (1819-1891)
Spinal disease and spinal curvature. Their treatment by suspension and by the use of the plaster of Paris bandage. A review. Cambridge: Riverside Press, 1878. 4p. DNLM **70-0369**

BROWN, Buckminster (1819-1891)
Hints on the diagnosis and treatment of club-foot. Cambridge, [1879]. 12p. DNLM **70-0370**

BROWN, Buckminster (1819-1891)
Influence of the prevailing methods of education on the production of deformity in young persons of both sexes. Cambridge, 1879. 8p. 2 plates. DNLM **70-0371**

BROWN, C. W.
Analysis of one hundred and nine cases of rheumatism treated with salicylic acid and salicine. Cambridge: Riverside Press, 1877. 12p. DNLM; MBM **70-0372**

BROWN, E. O.
Official report of the yellow fever hospital, Louisville, Ky., 1878. Louisville, Ky., 1878. 12p. 2 tab. DNLM **70-0373**

BROWN, Francis Henry (1835-1917)
The medical register for New England. Boston: H. O. Houghton, 1877. 413p. DNLM; MBM; MH; MWA **70-0374**

BROWN, Francis Henry (1835-1917)
The medical register of the cities of Boston, Cambridge, Charlestown, and Chelsea. Boston: J. Wilson & Son, 1873. 170p. DNLM; MBM **70-0375**

BROWN, Francis Henry (1835-1917)
The medical register of the cities of Boston, Cambridge, Charlestown, and Chelsea. For the State of Massachusetts. Boston: W. P. Lunt, 1875. 296p. DNLM; MBM **70-0376**

BROWN, Francis Henry (1835-1917)
Arsenical paper hangings. [Boston, 1876.] 7p. DNLM **70-0377**

BROWN, George William
Address to the medical graduates of the University of Maryland. [Baltimore, 1872.] 14p. DNLM **70-0378**

BROWN, Harvey E. (1840-1889)
Report on a "more efficient system of quarantine on the southern and gulf coasts." [Transmitted by the Secretary of War, with communication from the Surgeon-General, U.S.A., in regard to the same.] Senate, 42nd Congress, 3rd session, Ex. Doc. 9, pts. 1 and 2. Washington: Government Printing Office, 1872. 117p. DNLM **70-0379**

BROWN, Harvey E. (1840-1889)
The Medical Department of the United States Army from 1775 to 1873. Compiled under the direction of the Surgeon-General. Washington: Surgeon-General's Office, 1873. 314p. DNLM **70-0380**

BROWN, Henry James
An opium cure: based upon science, skill and matured experience. . . . 2nd ed. New York: F. M. Brown & Co., 1872. 48p. DLC; NNNAM **70-0381**

BROWN, M. G.
Metaphysical pamphlet. A synopsis of metaphysics. Cause, cure, and prevention of disease. Life lengthened, disease kept at bay. New York: Metaphysical University, [1871?]. 48, 10, 6p. DNLM; NNNAM **70-0382**

BROWN, O. Phelps
The complete herbalist; or the people their own physicians, by the use of nature's remedies. Jersey City, N.J.: the author, 1872. 504p. DNLM; NjR **70-0383**

BROWN, R. T.
Annual address to the students of the Indiana Medical College. Indianapolis, 1871. 15p. DNLM **70-0384**

BROWN, R. T.
Elements of physiology and hygiene. Cincinnati & New York: Wilson, Hinkle & Co., [1872]. 286p. DNLM; OCIM; NNNAM **70-0385**

BROWN, Thomas Richardson (1846-1879)
Urethral stricture. Baltimore: Innes & Co., 1878. 16p. DNLM **70-0386**

BROWN, Thomas Richardson (1846-1879)
Urethral fever. New York: D. Appleton & Co., 1878. 16p. DNLM; NNNAM **70-0387**

BROWN-SÉQUARD, Charles Edouard (1817-1894)
Dual character of the brain. Delivered April 22, 1874. Washington: Smithsonian Institution, 1877. 21p. DLC; DNLM **70-0388**

BROWN-SÉQUARD, Charles Edouard (1817-1894)
Two lectures on convulsions and paralysis as effects of disease of the base of the brain. Philadelphia: Collins, 1878. 32p. DNLM; PPC **70-0389**

BROWNE, B. B. (1842-1922)
A paper on subinvolution of the uterus. Louisville, 1877. 7p. DNLM; KyLoJM **70-0390**

BROWNE, B. B. (1842-1922)
A case of fibroid tumor of the uterus, causing eclampsia; with remarks on uterine fibroids in general, and on the causes of puerperal and non-pueperal eclampsia. New York: W. Wood & Co., 1877. 10p. DNLM; NNNAM **70-0391**

BROWNE, Edgar A.
How to use the ophthalmoscope. Being elementary instructions in ophthalmoscopy. Arranged for the use of students. Philadelphia: Henry C. Lea, 1877. 120p. CtY-M; DNLM; MBM; PPC **70-0392**

BROWNE, John Hutton Balfour (1845-1921)
The medical jurisprudence of insanity. . . . 2nd ed. With references to the Scotch and American decisions. San Francisco: S. Whitney & Co., 1875. 713p. DLC **70-0393**

BRUCE, W. T.
Annual directory of the homoeopathic physicians residing in New York, Pennsylvania, New Jersey, Maryland, Delaware, District of Columbia, 1878. 4th ed. Quakertown, [1878]. 24p. DNLM **70-0394**

BRUEN, Edward Tunis (1851-1889)
Anasarca as a symptom of deficient vaso-motor tonus. [Philadelphia, 1879.] 12p. DNLM **70-0395**

BRYAN, L. H.
Great medical discovery. The blood poison, its origin and nature; and how it acts upon the system to cause the many and varied diseases that afflict mankind. Philadelphia: J. Moore & Sons, 1872. 119p. DNLM; PPC **70-0396**

BRYANT, Thomas (1828-1914)
The practice of surgery. A manual. Philadelphia: Henry C. Lea, 1873. 984p. DNLM; OCIM; PPC; PU **70-0397**

BRYANT, Thomas (1828-1914)
The practice of surgery. A manual. 2nd American from the 3rd English ed. Philadelphia: Henry C. Lea, 1879. 945p. CtY-M; DNLM; IU-M; PPC **70-0398**

BRYCE, Peter (1834-1893)
Annual message of [the] president of the Medical Association of the State of Alabama. Montgomery, Ala.: Barrett & Brown, 1878. 55p. DNLM **70-0399**

BUCHANAN, John
The physiological and therapeutic uses of our new remedies. 2nd ed. Philadelphia: J. Buchanan, 1873. 152p. DNLM; PPC; PU **70-0400**

BUCHANAN, John
The centennial practice of medicine. Philadelphia: J. Buchanan, 1876. 456p. DNLM; NNNAM; PPC; PU **70-0401**

BUCHANAN, John and John F. SIGGINS
Dispensatory and pharmacopoeia of North America and Great Britain. Philadelphia: John Buchanan, 1878. 630p. OCLloyd; PPC; PU **70-0402**

BUCHANAN, Joseph Rodes (1814-1899)
Triumphs of medicine. Address. New York: Trow's Print. Co., 1878. 24p. DNLM **70-0403**

BUCK, Albert Henry (1842-1922)
Case of angioma cavernosum, situated in the external auditory canal, and attached by a slender pedicle to the manubrium mallei. [1870?] 7p. 1 plate. DNLM **70-0404**

BUCK, Albert Henry (1842-1922)
An essay on the mechanism of the ossicles of the ear. New York: William Wood & Co., 1870. 18p. 2 plates. DNLM; NNNAM **70-0405**

BUCK, Albert Henry (1842-1922)
Report on the progress of otology. [Boston, 1871.] 10p. DNLM **70-0406**

BUCK, Albert Henry (1842-1922)
A report of three cases of acute diseases of the ear. [1873?] 12p. DNLM **70-0407**

BUCK, Albert Henry (1842-1922)
On the mechanism of hearing. New York: D. Appleton & Co., 1874. 21p. DNLM **70-0408**

BUCK, Albert Henry (1842-1922)
Ultimate forms of granulation tissue in the ear. [1874?] 5p. DNLM **70-0409**

BUCK, Albert Henry (1842-1922)
Cyclopedia of the practice of medicine. Edited by H. von Ziemssen. Transl. by R. H. Fitz, C. P. Putnam, and others. . . . New York: William Wood & Co., 1874-1880. 20 v. DNLM; NNNAM; OCIM; PU [Of this v. 1-17 are translations of v. 2-16 of: Handbuch der speciellen Pathologie und Therapie. Bearbeitet von Drs. Geigel, Hirt, Merkel, [*et al.*] Hrsg. von H. v. Ziemssen. Leipzig, 1874-1878. CONTENTS. v. 1-2. Acute infectious diseases; v. 3. Chronic infectious diseases; v. 4-5. Diseases of the respiratory organs; v. 6. Diseases of the circulatory system; v. 7. Diseases of the chylopoetic system. Together with the chapter on diseases of the naso-pharyngeal cavity and pharynx. Laryngitis phlegmonosa, perichondritis laryngea, ulcerations and tumors, and nerves of the larynx; v. 8. Diseases of the chylopoetic system, with chapters relating to diseases of the bladder and urethra; and functional affections of the male genital organs; v. 9. Diseases of the liver and portal vein. With a chapter relating to interstitial pneumonia; v. 10. Diseases of the female sexual organs; v. 11. Diseases of the peripheral cerebro-spinal nerves; v. 12. Diseases of the brain and its membranes; v. 13. Diseases of the spinal cord and medulla oblongata; v. 14. Diseases of the nervous system, and disturbances of speech; v. 15. Diseases of the kidney, by Carl Bartels and Wilhelm Ebstein; v. 16. Diseases of the locomotive apparatus, and general anomalies of nutrition; v. 17. General anomalies of nutrition, and poisons; v. 18-19. Supplementary volumes. On hygiene and public health; v. 20. General index. Supplement to Ziemssen's Cyclopedia. Edited by Geo. L. Peabody. 1881.] **70-0410**

BUCK, Albert Henry (1842-1922)
A method of using medicated Eustachian bougies. Boston: A. Mudge & Sons, 1875. 12p. DNLM; MBM **70-0411**

BUCK, Albert Henry (1842-1922)
Diseases of the mastoid process; their diagnosis, pathology, and treatment. New York: William Wood & Co., [1876?] 47p. DNLM; NNNAM **70-0412**

BUCK, Albert Henry (1842-1922)
The importance of treatment of aural diseases in their early stages, especially when arising from the exanthemata. Philadelphia: Collins, 1877. 13p. DNLM **70-0413**

BUCK, Albert Henry (1842-1922)
Complete occlusion of the external auditory canal by a dermoid membrane: as evidence of horizontal motion outward in the epidermis of the canal. [Boston, 1878.] 3p. DNLM **70-0414**

BUCK, Albert Henry (1842-1922)
Syphilitic affections of the ear. [New York, 1879.] 16p. DNLM **70-0415**

BUCK, Albert Henry, ed. (1842-1922)
A treatise on hygiene and public health. . . . New York: William Wood & Co., 1879. 2 v. DLC; MBM; NNNAM; PPC **70-0416**

BUCK, Gurdon (1807-1877)
A contribution to plastic surgery. A case of destruction of the right half of the upper lip, neighboring portion of the cheek, and ala nasi. Repaired by a series of autoplastic operations. Philadelphia: Collins, 1870. 8p. 4 plates. DNLM; PPC
70-0417

BUCK, Gurdon (1807-1877)
A contribution to surgical therapeutics of the air passages; illustrated by two cases. [1870.] 23p. 1 plate. DNLM
70-0418

BUCK, Gurdon (1807-1877)
Case of cicatricial contractions after burns, involving the chin and neck, successfully treated. [1871.] 7p. 4 figs. DNLM
70-0419

BUCK, Gurdon (1807-1877)
Observations on the operation for harelip, with cases and illustrations. [New York, 1872.] 5p. DNLM
70-0420

BUCK, Gurdon (1807-1877)
Lithotomy and lithotrity. Illustrated by cases. New York: William Wood & Co., 1872. 59p. DNLM; NNNAM
70-0421

BUCK, Gurdon (1807-1877)
A case of rhinoplastic operation, performed for the restoration of the apex of the nose after it has been bitten off. [New York, 1872.] 4p. DNLM **70-0422**

BUCK, Gurdon (1807-1877)
Report of a case of congenital hypertrophy of the under lip successfully treated by surgical operations. Albany: Argus Co., 1873. 5p. 1 plate. DNLM **70-0423**

BUCK, Gurdon (1807-1877)
Reconstruction of the mouth after loss of the under lip by a new operation. Louisville: J. P. Morton & Co., 1873. 13p. DNLM **70-0424**

BUCK, Gurdon (1807-1877)
Abscesses originating in the right iliac fossa. New York: D. Appleton & Co., 1874. 16p. DNLM **70-0425**

BUCK, Gurdon (1807-1877)
On abscesses in the lower abdominal cavity and its parietes. New York: J. F. Trow & Son, 1876. 11, 19, 19p. DNLM; NNNAM **70-0426**

BUCK, Gurdon (1807-1877)
Contributions to reparative surgery; showing its application to the treatment of deformities produced by destructive disease or injury; congenital defects from arrest or excess of development; and cicatricial contractions from burns. New York: D. Appleton & Co., 1876. 237p. DNLM; NNNAM; OCIM; PPC
70-0427

BUCK, Jirah D[ewey] (1839-1916)
Annual address delivered before the Cleveland Homoeopathic Hospital College, February 14, 1872. [1872.] 14p. PPHa
70-0428

BUCK, Jirah D[ewey] (1839-1916)
The office of the true physician. An address delivered at Hopkins Hall, February 12, 1874, at the graduating exercises of Pulte Medical College. [1874.] 8p. PPHa
70-0429

BUCKINGHAM, Charles Edward (1821-1877)
Correspondence concerning a fatal case of placenta praevia. Boston: A. Mudge & Son, 1870. 29p. DLC; DNLM; MBM
70-0430

BUCKINGHAM, Charles Edward (1821-1877)
Correspondence concerning a fatal case of placenta praevia. Republished with an appendix by D. Barnard. Boston: Nation Press, 1870. 37p. DLC; DNLM; MBM **70-0431**

BUCKINGHAM, Charles Edward (1821-1877)
The proper treatment of children, medical or medicinal, being the annual discourse before the Massachusetts Medical Society, June 4, 1873. Boston: D. Clapp & Son, 1873. 48p. DNLM; MBM **70-0432**

BUCKINGHAM, Charles Edward (1821-1877)
The mutual relations of druggists and physicians. An address before the graduating class of the Massachusetts College of Pharmacy, April 22, 1874. . . . Boston: Printed by D. Clapp & Son, 1874. 15p. DLC; MBM **70-0433**

BUCKNER, J. H.
Report on ophthalmology. A paper read before the Ohio State Medical Society. Dayton, O.: United Brethren Pub. House, 1873. 16p. DNLM **70-0434**

BUCKNER, J. H.
Astigmatism. Illustrative cases from clinical memoranda. Cincinnati: R. Clarke & Co., 1875. 15p. DNLM; OCIM
70-0435

BUCKNER, J. H.
The preservation of good eyesight. Columbus: Cott & Hahn, 1879. 10p. DNLM **70-0436**

BUFFALO SPRINGS, MECKLENBURG CO., VA.
Analysis, letters of eminent men, with cases illustrative of the effects of the waters in the various forms of disease. Baltimore: King Bros., 1874. 44p. DNLM **70-0437**

BULKLEY, Lucius Duncan (1845-1928)
The relations of the nervous system to diseases of the skin. New York: G. P. Putnam's Sons, 1874. 45p. DNLM; NNNAM
70-0438

BULKLEY, Lucius Duncan (1845-1928)
A new antipuritic remedy. [Philadelphia, 1874.] 4p. DNLM
70-0439

BULKLEY, Lucius Duncan (1845-1928)
Rare cases of congenital syphilis. New York: D. Appleton & Co., 1874. 19p. DLC; DNLM; NNNAM
70-0440

BULKLEY, Lucius Duncan (1845-1928)
Herpes gestationis: a rare affection of the skin peculiar to pregnancy. New York: William Wood & Co., 1874. 32p. DNLM; NNNAM **70-0441**

BULKLEY, Lucius Duncan (1845-1928)
The relations of the urine to diseases of the skin. New York: G. P. Putnam's Sons, 1875. 33p. DLC; DNLM; NNNAM
70-0442

BULKLEY, Lucius Duncan (1845-1928)
Analysis of one thousand cases of skin-disease, with cases and remarks on treatment. Louisville: J. P. Morton & Co., 1875. 29p. DNLM; KyLoJM **70-0443**

BULKLEY, L[ucius] D[uncan] (1845-1928)
Two cases of exophthalmic goitre, associated with chronic urticaria; illustrative of the relations of the nervous system to diseases of the skin. New York: G. P. Putnam's Sons, 1875. 10p. DNLM **70-0444**

BULKLEY, L[ucius] D[uncan] (1845-1928)
A clinical study on herpes zoster. [Philadelphia, 1876.] 10p. DNLM **70-0445**

BULKLEY, Lucius Duncan (1845-1928)
Analysis of six hundred and seventeen cases of skin-disease, with cases and remarks on treatment. Being a study on the cases of disease of the skin treated at Demilt Dispensary during the year 1875. New York: G. P. Putnam's Sons, 1876. 41p. DNLM; NNNAM **70-0446**

BULKLEY, L[ucius] D[uncan] (1845-1928)
Diseases of the skin. [New York, 1877.] 8p. DNLM **70-0447**

BULKLEY, L[ucius] D[uncan] (1845-1928)
Two cases of morphoea, with remarks on the disease and its differential diagnosis. New York: G. P. Putnam's Sons, 1877. 6p. DNLM **70-0448**

BULKLEY, Lucius Duncan (1845-1928)
On the nomenclature and classification of diseases of the skin. New York: G. P. Putnam's Sons, 1877. 10p. DNLM; NNNAM **70-0449**

BULKLEY, Lucius Duncan (1845-1928)
Analysis of seven hundred and seventy-four cases of skin-disease, treated at the Demilt Dispensary during the year 1876, with cases and remarks on treatment. New York: D. Appleton & Co., 1877. 48p. DLC; DNLM; NNNAM **70-0450**

BULKLEY, Lucius Duncan (1845-1928)
Are eczema and psoriasis local diseases of the skin, or are they manifestations of constitutional disorders? Philadelphia, 1877. 19p. DNLM; PPC **70-0451**

BULKLEY, Lucius Duncan (1845-1928)
On the recognition and management of the gouty state in diseases of the skin. New York: G. P. Putnam's Sons, 1877. 25p. DLC; DNLM; NNNAM **70-0452**

BULKLEY, Lucius Duncan (1845-1928)
On the so-called eczema marginatum of Hebra (tinea circinata cruris), as observed in America. New York: G. P. Putnam's Sons, 1877. 28p. DNLM; NNNAM **70-0453**

BULKLEY, Lucius Duncan (1845-1928)
On diet and hygiene in diseases of the skin. New York: G. P. Putnam's Sons, 1878. 18p. DNLM; NNNAM **70-0454**

BULKLEY, Lucius Duncan (1845-1928)
On the use of the solid rubber bandage in the treatment of eczema and ulcers of the leg. New York: G. P. Putnam's Sons, 1878. 21p. DNLM; NNNAM **70-0455**

BULKLEY, Lucius Duncan (1845-1928)
New method of permanently removing superfluous hairs. New York: G. P. Putnam's Sons, 1878. 7p. DNLM; NNNAM **70-0456**

BULKLEY, Lucius Duncan (1845-1928)
On the nomenclature and classification of diseases of the skin; with remarks upon that recently adopted by the American Dermatological Association. [New York, 1879.] 15p. DNLM; NNNAM **70-0457**

BULL, Charles Stedman (1844-1911)
On the treatment of various forms of amblyopia and amaurosis. [Philadelphia, 1873.] 19p. DNLM **70-0458**

BULL, Charles Stedman (1844-1911)
Retinal hemorrhage and its connection with cerebral, cardiac, and renal lesions. [1874?] 12p. DNLM **70-0459**

BULL, Charles Stedman (1844-1911)
On some forms of kerato-iritis and their effect in hindering the osmotic action of the cornea and conjunctiva. New York: D. Appleton & Co., 1874. 10p. DNLM **70-0460**

BULL, Charles Stedman (1844-1911)
Cases illustrating two rare diseases of the eyelids. Syphilitic gummata of the conjunctiva. [New York, 1878.] 15p. DNLM **70-0461**

BULL, Charles Stedman (1844-1911)
Observations on infiltration of the retina in lardaceous disease of the kidneys due to chronic suppuration from bone disease. [Philadelphia, 1879.] 7p. DNLM **70-0462**

BULL, William T. (1849-1909)
Perityphlitis. New York: D. Appleton & Co., 1873. 27p. DNLM; NNNAM **70-0463**

BULLARD, W[illiam] E.
A successful case of intra-venous injection of milk. New York: D. Appleton & Co., 1878. 8p. 1 tab. DNLM; NNNAM **70-0464**

BULLOCK & CRENSHAW
Catalogue of chemicals, chemical and pharmaceutical apparatus. Philadelphia, 1875. 140p. DNLM; PU **70-0465**

BUMSTEAD, Freeman Josiah (1826-1879)
The pathology and treatment of the venereal diseases. 3rd ed. Philadelphia: Henry C. Lea, 1870. 704p. CtY-M; DNLM; NNNAM; PPC **70-0466**

BUMSTEAD, Freeman J[osiah] (1826-1879)
Hints on the treatment of syphilis. Louisville: J. P. Morton & Co., 1871. 12p. DNLM **70-0467**

BUMSTEAD, Freeman J[osiah] (1826-1879)
The virus of venereal sores; its unity or duality. Philadelphia, 1877. 10p. DLC; DNLM **70-0468**

BUMSTEAD, Freeman Josiah (1826-1879)
The pathology and treatment of the venereal diseases. 4th ed., revised, enlarged, and in great part rewritten by the author and by Robert W. Taylor. Philadelphia: Henry C. Lea, 1879. 855p. CtY-M; DLC; DNLM; PPC **70-0469**

BURGE, J. H. Hobart (1823-1901)
The relations subsisting between physicians and apothecaries, and also between these and their respective patients and patrons. New York: D. Appleton & Co., 1870. 15p. DNLM; NNNAM **70-0470**

BURGE, J. H. Hobart (1823-1901)
Practical reflections on the nature and treatment of croup. New York: D. Appleton & Co., 1870. 23p. DNLM; NNNAM
70-0471

BURGE, J. H. Hobart (1823-1901)
An address delivered before the medical Society of the County of Kings, on its forty-seventh anniversary, A.D. 1868. New York: F. Hart & Co., 1871. 27p. DNLM; NNNAM
70-0472

BURGHER, John C. (1822-1901)
The year's progress. Address delivered before the American Institute of Homoeopathy, by the president, J. C. Burgher . . . at the opening of its thirty-first annual session at Put-in-Bay, June 18th, 1878. Philadelphia: Sherman & Co., printers, 1878. 13p. DLC; PPC **70-0473**

BURNETT, Charles Henry (1842-1902)
An investigation concerning the mechanism of the ossicles of hearing, and the membrane of the round window. . . . New York: William Wood & Co., 1872. 13p. DLC; DNLM; NNNAM
70-0474

BURNETT, Charles Henry (1842-1902)
A contribution to the comparative distribution of bloodvessels in the membrana tympani. Philadelphia: Collins, 1873. 11p. DNLM; PPC **70-0475**

BURNETT, Charles Henry (1842-1902)
Report on the progress of otology. Read before the American Otological Society, at the annual meeting, July 16, 1873. Boston: A. Mudge & Son, 1873. 57p. DNLM; MBM
70-0476

BURNETT, Charles H[enry] (1842-1902) and Clarence J. BLAKE
Report on the progress of otology. Boston: A. Mudge & Son, 1874. 73p. DNLM; MH-M **70-0477**

BURNETT, Charles H[enry] (1842-1902)
Three cases of tinnitus aurium and deafness, accompanied by very distinct flushing of the cutaneous surface adjacent to the ear. [New York, 1875.] 3p. DNLM **70-0478**

BURNETT, Charles Henry (1842-1902)
The ear; its anatomy, physiology, and diseases. A practical treatise for the use of medical students and practitioners. . . . Philadelphia: Henry C. Lea, 1877. 615p. DLC; DNLM; NNNAM; PPC **70-0479**

BURNETT, Charles H[enry] (1842-1902)
The growth of the fungus aspergillus in the human ear. Philadelphia, 1878. 17p. DNLM **70-0480**

BURNETT, Charles H[enry] (1842-1902)
Twenty cases of the growth of aspergillus in the living human ear. New York, 1879. 36p. DNLM **70-0481**

BURNETT, Charles Henry (1842-1902)
. . . Hearing and how to keep it. . . . Philadelphia: Lindsay & Blakiston, 1879. 152p. DLC; DNLM; OCIM; PPC
70-0482

BURNETT, Swan M[oses] (1847-1906)
A case of diplacusis binauralis, with remarks. A case of restricted range of audition. . . . New York: William Wood & Co., 1877. 10p. DLC; DNLM **70-0483**

BURNETT, Swan Moses (1847-1906)
A case of choroiditis exaudativa, accompanied with partial micropsia, metamorphopsia, and chromatopsic scotomata of singularly regular forms. . . . New York: William Wood & Co., 1878. 11p. DLC; DNLM **70-0484**

BURNETT, Swan Moses (1847-1906)
Double optic neuritis (choked disc) and sloughing of the right cornea accompanying a sarcomatous tumor on the right side of the brain. . . . New York: William Wood & Co., 1878. 10p. DLC; DNLM **70-0485**

BURNETT, Swan M[oses] (1847-1906)
Objective aural sounds produced by voluntary contraction of the tubal muscles. [New York, 1879.] 3p. DLC; DNLM
70-0486

BURNETT, Swan Moses (1847-1906)
A systematic method for the education of the color-sense in children. [Washington, 1879.] 4p. DNLM
70-0487

BURNETT, Swan Moses (1847-1906)
Results of an examination of the color-sense of 3,040 children in the colored schools of the District of Columbia. [New York, 1879.] 9p. DNLM **70-0488**

BURRALL, F[rederick] A[ugustus]
Nitrate of amyl as an antidote to chloroform. New York: D. Appleton & Co., 1876. 17p. DNLM **70-0489**

BURROUGH BROS. formulary and descriptive catalogue of their fluid and solid extracts, with a complete botanical index. Prepared by Burrough Bros. Philadelphia: [Collins], 1871. 180p. DNLM; OCLloyd; PPHa **70-0490**

BURROWS, C. H.
Dyspepsia, or: What shall we eat, and how shall we eat it. A lecture on the health and diseases of the stomach, liver, kidneys and bowels. . . . Atlanta, Ill.: C. H. Burrows, 1875. 16p. DLC **70-0491**

BURT, W[illiam] H. (1836-1897)
Cinchona officinalis and its alkaloid, the sulphate of quinine. St. Louis: John W. Munson's Homoeopathic Pharmacy, 1871. 33p. DNLM; PPHa **70-0492**

BURT, William H. (1836-1897)
Characteristic materia medica. . . . 2nd ed. New York and Philadelphia: Boericke & Tafel, 1873. 542p. OCLloyd; PPHa
70-0493

BURT, William H. (1836-1897)
Therpeutics of tuberculosis, or pulmonary consumption. . . . New York and Philadelphia: Boericke & Tafel; [etc., etc.], 1876. 230p. DLC; PPHa **70-0494**

BUSEY, Samuel Clagett (1828-1901)
Artificial induction of labor in uremia. . . . Washington, D.C.: National Medical Journal Office, [1871]. 62p. DLC; DNLM
70-0495

BUSEY, Samuel Clagett (1828-1901)
An inquiry into the nature of the uterine supports and of the causes of displacements. New York, 1872. 39p. DNLM
70-0496

BUSEY, Samuel Clagett (1828-1901)
Address in obstetrics and diseases of women and children. Delivered before the American Medical Association, June 8, 1876. Philadelphia: Collins, 1876. 33p. DLC; DNLM; PPC **70-0497**

BUSEY, Samuel Clagett (1828-1901)
Occlusion and dilatation of lymph channels. New Orleans, 1877. 84p. DNLM; LNT-M; PPC **70-0498**

[BUSEY, Samuel Clagett] (1828-1901)
The Columbia Hospital and Lying-in Asylum, a government institution. Its past and present management. By a citizen of Washington, D.C. Louisville, Ky., 1877. 18p. DNLM **70-0499**

BUSEY, Samuel Clagett (1828-1901) and Frank J. O'CONNOR
Addresses delivered at the twenty-eighth annual commencement of the Medical Department of the University of Georgetown . . . March 19, 1877. Washington, D.C. H. I. Rose, 1877. 21p. DNLM **70-0500**

[BUSEY, Samuel Clagett] (1828-1901)
The truth admitted. The Columbia Hospital for Women and Lying-in Asylum. By a citizen of Washington, D.C. Louisville, Ky., 1878. 16p. DNLM **70-0501**

BUSEY, Samuel Clagett (1828-1901)
Congenital occlusion and dilatation of lymph channels. New York: William Wood & Co., 1878. 187p. DLC; DNLM; NNNAM; PPC **70-0502**

BUSEY, Samuel Clagett (1828-1901)
Narrowing, occlusion, and dilatation of lymph channels, acquired forms. . . . [New Orleans, 1878]. 195p. DLC **70-0503**

BUSEY, Samuel Clagett (1828-1901)
The potassium bromide and suspension of the action of the stomach in the treatment of uncontrollable vomiting of pregnancy. [1879.] 6p. DNLM **70-0504**

BUSEY, Samuel Clagett (1828-1901)
Alternating anterior and posterior version of the uterus. [Boston, 1879.] 12p. DLC; DNLM **70-0505**

BUSH, L. P[otter] (1812-1892)
Some vital statistics of the city of Wilmington; read before the Delaware State Medical Society, June, 1877. Wilmington: Glatts & Eckel, 1877. 12p. DNLM **70-0506**

BUTLER, John (1844-1885)
Experiences in galvano-surgery. Brooklyn, N.Y.: J. O. Noxon, 1875. 25p. DNLM; NNNAM **70-0507**

BUTLER, John (1844-1885)
Paper on clinical electrolysis. [New York, 1877.] 7p. DNLM **70-0508**

BUTLER, John (1844-1885)
A text-book of electro-therapeutics and electro-surgery. New York & Philadelphia: Boericke & Tafel, 1878. 271p. DNLM; PPHa **70-0509**

BUTLER, John (1844-1885)
A text-book of electro-therapeutics and electro-surgery, for the use of students and general practitioners. 2nd ed. New York & Philadelphia: Boericke & Tafel, 1879. 323p. PPHa **70-0510**

BUTLER, John (1844-1885)
A paper on the uses of electricity in gynaecology. Read before the New York Medico-Chirurgical Society. New York & Philadelphia: Boericke & Tafel, 1879. 24p. PPHa **70-0511**

BUTLER, John S[impkins] (1803-1890)
State preventive medicine. The first annual address to the State Board of Health of Connecticut. Hartford, Conn.: Lockwood & Bromard Co., 1879. 31p. DNLM **70-0512**

BUTLER, Samuel Worcester (1823-1874)
The physician's daily pocket record. Philadelphia: Med. & Surg. Reporter, 1871. 232p. DNLM; PPC; PU **70-0513**

BUTLER, Samuel Worcester (1823-1874)
The medical register and directory of the United States . . . comprising names . . . of more than fifty thousand physicians; with lists of medical societies, colleges, hospitals and other medical institutions, with abstracts of medical laws of each state, notices of mineral springs, etc. . . . Philadelphia: Office of the Medical and Surgical Reporter; [etc., etc.], 1874. 854p. DLC; PPC; PU **70-0514**

BUTLER, Samuel Worcester (1823-1874)
The medical register and directory of the United States . . . comprising names . . . of more than fifty thousand physicians; with lists of medical societies, colleges, hospitals and other medical institutions, with abstracts of medical laws of each state, notices of mineral springs, etc. . . . 2nd ed., rev. and cor. Philadelphia: Office of the Medical and Surgical Reporter; [etc., etc.], 1877. 874p. DLC; PPC; PPJ; PU **70-0515**

BYFORD, William Heath (1817-1890)
A treatise on the theory and practice of obstetrics. New York: William Wood & Co., 1870. 457p. DLC; DNLM; NNNAM; PPC **70-0516**

BYFORD, William Heath (1817-1890)
An address introductory to the course of instruction in the Woman's Hospital Medical College, session of 1870-1871. Chicago: R. Fergus' Sons, [1870?]. 16p. DNLM **70-0517**

BYFORD, William Heath (1817-1890)
A treatise on the chronic inflammation and displacements of the unimpregnated uterus. 2nd ed. Philadelphia: Lindsay & Blakiston, 1871. 248p. DNLM; MBM; NNNAM; PPC **70-0518**

BYFORD, William Heath (1817-1890)
A treatise on the theory and practice of obstetrics. 2nd ed., thoroughly revised. New York: William Wood & Co., 1873. 469p. DLC; DNLM; NNNAM; PPC **70-0519**

BYFORD, William Heath (1817-1890)
The address in obstetrics and diseases of women and children. Philadelphia: Collins, 1875. 24p. DNLM; PPC **70-0520**

BYFORD, William Heath (1817-1890)
Fibrous tumors of the uterus. New York: G. P. Putnam's Sons, 1878. 41p. DNLM; NNNAM **70-0521**

BYFORD, William Heath (1817-1890)
Dermoid ovarian tumors. [Boston, 1879.] 14p. DNLM **70-0522**

BYRD, William A. (1843-1887)
On the wire ligature in the treatment of ununited fractures, and in resections of bones for deformity. New York: D. Appleton & Co., 1876. 19p. DNLM; NNNAM
70-0523

BYRD, William A. (1843-1887)
Strangulated hernia, with fecal fistula, treated by a new and simple enterotome and an anaplastic operation. [1879?] 3p. DNLM **70-0524**

BYRD, William A. (1843-1887)
Tracheotomy with the galvano-cautery. [Quincy, 1879.] 7p. DNLM **70-0525**

BYRN, Marcus Lafayette
How to live a hundred years, or The art of preserving health, curing disease and prolonging life. With plain instructions for improving the memory. . . . New York: Hurst & Co., [1876]. 107p. DLC; NNNAM **70-0526**

BYRNE, John (1825-1902)
Clinical notes on the electric cautery in uterine surgery. New York: William Wood & Co., 1873. 68p. DNLM; IU-M; NNNAM; PPC **70-0527**

BYRNE, John (1825-1902)
Amputations and excisions of the cervix uteri; their indications and methods. Boston, 1878. 48p. 1 plate. DNLM; MH-M
70-0528

BYRNE, John (1825-1902)
A case of acute puerperal inversion of the uterus. A clinical description of a new instrument successfully employed. With remarks on the mechanism of restoration. New York: D. Appleton & Co., 1878. 16p. DNLM; NNNAM
70-0529

CABELL, James L. (1813-1889)
Etiology of enteric fever. Philadelphia: Collins, 1877. 51p. DNLM; PPC **70-0530**

CABELL, James L. (1813-1889)
Address in state medicine and public hygiene, before the American Medical Association, June 6, 1878. Philadelphia: Collins, 1878. 35p. DNLM; PPC **70-0531**

CALDWELL, John J[abez] (*b.* 1836)
Report of cases treated by electricity, and addenda: Electro-medicine and electro-surgery. Baltimore: W. K. Boyle & Son, 1873. 23p. DNLM **70-0532**

CALDWELL, John J[abez] (*b.* 1836)
The connection between excessive nerve and brain worry and bodily disease, with pathology and treatment of cancers, tumors, etc. [Baltimore, 1874.] 7p. DNLM
70-0533

CALDWELL, John J[abez] (*b.* 1836)
A review of the recent researches in the pathology and treatment of cancer. Baltimore: Hammond & Jones, 1874. 8p. DNLM **70-0534**

CALDWELL, John J[abez] (*b.* 1836)
The pathology of club-foot and electro-massage and mechanical treatment of the same. Read before the Baltimore Medical Association, regular meeting, Jan. 26, 1874. [Baltimore, 1874?] 2p. DNLM **70-0535**

CALDWELL, John J[abez] (*b.* 1836)
Electricity in medicine and surgery, with cases to illustrate. Baltimore, [1874?]. 32p. DNLM **70-0536**

CALDWELL, John J[abez] (*b.* 1836)
Electricity as a restorative agent in narcosis and asphyxia. Baltimore, 1874? 8p. DNLM **70-0537**

CALDWELL, John J[abez] (*b.* 1836)
Involuntary action of the nervous system. Cincinnati, 1877. 19p. DNLM **70-0538**

CALDWELL, John J[abez] (*b.* 1836)
The treatment of the genito-urinary organs, the use of electricity, damiana, ... St. Louis, 1878, 8p. DNLM
70-0539

CALHOUN, Abner W. (1846-1910)
Résumé of cataract operations. Atlanta, Ga.: Dunlop, Wynne & Co., 1874. 7p. DNLM; GU **70-0540**

CALHOUN, Abner W. (1846-1910)
Iridotomy, and its applicability as a remedy for certain defects of the eye. With four illustrative cases. Atlanta, Ga.: Southern Publishing Co., 1875. 8p. DNLM; GU **70-0541**

CALHOUN, Abner W. (1846-1910)
Defects of hearing and other evils, the result of enlarged or hypertrophied tonsils, and the urgent necessity of immediate and proper treatment in order to restore the ear and other neighboring organs to their accustomed functions. Read before the Medical Association of Georgia. Atlanta, Ga.: H. H. Dickson, 1877. 12p. DNLM **70-0542**

CALHOUN, Abner W. (1846-1910)
Is modern education exerting an evil influence upon the eyesight of our children? Read before the Georgia Teachers' Association and the Atlanta Academy of Medicine. Atlanta, Ga.: H. H. Dickson, 1878. 18p. DNLM; GU
70-0543

CALHOUN, Abner W. (1846-1910)
Tobacco poisoning and its effects upon the eyesight. Atlanta, Ga.: J. P. Harrison & Co., [1879]. 8p. DNLM
70-0544

CALKINS, Alonzo (1804-1878)
Opium and the opium appetite; with notices of alcoholic beverages, cannabis indica, tobacco and coca, and tea and coffee, in their hygienic aspects and pathologic relations. Philadelphia: J. B. Lippincott & Co., 1871. 390p. DNLM; PPC; PU **70-0545**

CALKINS, Alonzo (1804-1878)
Felonious homicide; its penalty, and the execution thereof judicially. Read before the Medico-Legal Society of the City of New York. New York: Russell Brothers, 1873. 21p. DNLM; NNNAM **70-0546**

CALKINS, Marshall (1828-1922)
An introductory address delivered before the medical class of the University of Vermont, Thursday, March 8th, 1877. Burlington, 1877. 23p. DNLM **70-0547**

CALLAN, Peter A.
Examination of colored school children's eyes. New York: Wood & Reilly, 1875. 11p. DNLM; NNNAM
70-0548

CAMPBELL, Alexander James
How to be healthy. A collection from the writings and experience of many eminent physicians, on preventing disease, preserving youth and beauty, prolonging life, and producing a cheerful, happy old age. . . . Cleveland, O.: A. J. Campbell, 1878. 800p. DLC; OCIM **70-0549**

CAMPBELL, A. Sibley (*b.* 1849)
Full-term extra-uterine gestation of the tubo-ovarian form; with special examination of the sac, uterus, and appendages. New York: William Wood & Co., 1876. 20p. DNLM; NNNAM **70-0550**

CAMPBELL, A. Sibley (*b.* 1849)
Penumatic pressure and the genu-pectoral posture in the reduction of the uterine luxations. New York: William Wood & Co., 1877. 14p. DNLM; NNNAM **70-0551**

CAMPBELL, Henry Fraser (1824-1891)
Résumé of a report on position, pneumatic pressure and mechanical appliance in uterine displacements. Read before the Georgia Medical Association at Savannah, April 23, 1875. Atlanta, Ga.: Dunlop & Dickson, 1875. 18p. 1 plate. DNLM **70-0552**

CAMPBELL, Henry Fraser (1824-1891)
Résumé of a report on position, pneumatic pressure and mechanical appliance in uterine displacements. Read before the Georgia Medical Association at Savannah, April 23, 1875. Augusta, Ga.: J. L. Gow, [1875]. 18p. 1 plate. DNLM; GU **70-0553**

CAMPBELL, Henry Fraser (1824-1891)
Blood-letting in puerperal eclampsia. Pathology and therapeutics: The old and the new. New York: William Wood & Co., 1876. 48p. DNLM; NNNAM **70-0554**

CAMPBELL, Henry Fraser (1824-1891)
The yellow fever germ on coast and inland. A discussion of ship and railroad quarantine, before the Medical Association of Georgia, Rome, April 18, 1879. Atlanta: J. P. Harrison & Co., 1879. 26p. DLC; DNLM; GU **70-0555**

CAMPBELL, Henry Fraser (1824-1891)
Rectal alimentation in the nausea of pregnancy. Intestinal inhaustion, the rationale of its efficiency. [Boston, 1879.] 31p. DNLM; MH-M **70-0556**

CAMPBELL, Henry Fraser (1824-1891)
The soft rubber spring-stem pessary, in the treatment of uterine flexions. "Dangers avoided, benefits secured." Atlanta: J. P. Harrison, 1879. 10p. DNLM; GU **70-0557**

CAMPBELL, Howard S.
Homoeopathy; is there any truth in is? "Prove all things and hold fast to that which is good." Philadelphia: King & Baird, 1870. 4p. PPHa **70-0558**

CAMPBELL, James
List of new works and new editions in every department of medical literature. Contents: List of medical journals, visiting lists for 1873, sets of medical journals, new books and editions, James Campbell's publications, old and valuable medical works. Boston, 1875. 14p. 17 l. DNLM; MH; MHi **70-0559**

CAMPBELL, Robert
The relations existing between eczema and psoriasis. New York: G. P. Putnam's Sons, 1877. 9p. DNLM **70-0560**

CAMPBELL, Robert
Clinical reports of the Demilt Dispensary. Department for diseases of the skin. [New York, 1878.] 12p. DNLM; NNNAM **70-0561**

CAPELLMANN, Carl Franz Nicolaus (1841-1898)
Pastoral medicine, by. . . . Transl. with the author's sanction, by Rev. Wm. Dassell. . . . New York and Cincinnati: F. Pustet, 1879. 262p. DLC; NN; NNNAM; PPC **70-0562**

CARNOCHAN, J[ohn] M[urray] (1817-1887)
Contributions to operative surgery and surgical pathology. . . . New York: Harper & Brothers, 1877[-87]. 424p. 16 col. plates. DLC; NNNAM; OCIM; PU [Issued in parts, 1877-1887] **70-0563**

CARPENTER, H. W.
Annual address delivered before the Madison County Medical Society, July 8, 1873. [Oneida, N.Y., 1873.] 2 l. DNLM **70-0564**

CARPENTER, William Benjamin (1813-1885)
Principles of mental physiology, with their applications to the training and discipline of the mind, and the study of its morbid conditions. New York: D. Appleton & Co., 1874. 737p. MH; NN; NNC; NNNAM **70-0565**

CARPENTER, William Benjamin (1813-1885)
The microscope and its revelations. 5th ed. prepared with the assistance of H. J. Slack. Philadelphia: Lindsay & Blakiston, 1875. 848p. MBM; NNNAM; PPC; PU **70-0566**

CARPENTER, William Benjamin (1813-1885)
Principles of human physiology. . . . Ed. by Henry Power. . . . A new American from the 8th rev. and enl. English ed., with notes and additions, by Francis G. Smith. . . . Philadelphia: Henry C. Lea, 1876. 1083p. 2 plates. DLC; NN; NNNAM; PPC **70-0567**

CARROLL, Alfred Ludlow (1833-1893)
The question of quarantine: the nature and prevention of communicable zymotic diseases. New York: Leypoldt, 1872. 21p. DNLM; NNNAM **70-0568**

CARROLL, Alfred Ludlow (1833-1893)
Management of the gouty temperament; read before the New York Medical-Journal Association, November 19, 1875. . . . Louisville: Printed by J. P. Morton & Co., 1876. 8p. DLC **70-0569**

CARSON, Joseph (1808-1876)
A discourse commemorative of the life and character of Samuel Jackson, M.D., late professor of the institutes of medicine in the University of Pennsylvania. . . . Delivered October 7, 1872, before the trustees, professors, and students of the University of Pennsylvania. Philadelphia: Collins, printer, 1872. 32p. DLC; PPC; PU **70-0570**

CARTER, Robert Brudenell (1828-1918)
A practical treatise on diseases of the eye. Edited, with additions and test-types, by John Green. Philadelphia: Henry C. Lea, 1876. 505p. 1 plate. CU-M; DNLM; NNNAM; PPC **70-0571**

CASTLE, F[ranklin] D[ick]
. . . Hygiene of the eye. . . . Philadelphia, 1875. 12p. DLC; DNLM **70-0572**

CASTLE, Frederick Albert, comp. (1842-1902)
First decennial catalogue of the trustees, faculty, officers, and of the alumni of the Bellevue Hospital Medical College, of the City of New York, from 1861 to 1871. . . . Preceded by a history of the college, from its organization to 1872, by Leroy Milton Yale. . . . New York: D. Appleton & Co., 1873. 66p. DLC; NNNAM; NNU-M **70-0573**

CASWELL, Edward T[homas] (1833-1887)
Medical education. Annual address delivered before the Rhode Island Medical Society. Providence, 1875. 20p. DNLM **70-0574**

CASWELL, HAZARD & CO., NEW YORK
Illustrated catalogue of surgical instruments and appliances. . . . W. F. Ford, manufacturer. . . . New York, [1874]. 129p. DLC; NNNAM **70-0575**

CERNA, David (*b.* 1857)
Thevetia iccotli and its glucoside. [Philadelphia, 1879.] 6p. DNLM **70-0576**

CERNA, David (*b.* 1857)
Phenol (carbolic acid), its poisonous effects, and the soluble sulphates as antidotes. [Philadelphia, 1879.] 5p. DNLM **70-0577**

CHACE, George I.
Memorial of Thomas Perkins Shepard, M.D. Read before the trustees of the Rhode Island Hospital, September 19, 1877. Providence: S. S. Rider, 1877. 35p. port. DNLM **70-0578**

CHADWICK, James Read (1844-1905)
Amputations at the Massachusetts General Hospital. Compiled by James R. Chadwick, late surgical house officer, May 1, 1871. Boston: D. Clapp & Son, [1871?]. 22p. DNLM; MBM **70-0579**

CHADWICK, James Read (1844-1905)
Palpation in obstetrics as practiced in Germany. [Boston, 1872.] 14p. DNLM **70-0580**

CHADWICK, James Read (1844-1905)
Transfusion. Read at the annual meeting of the Mass. Medical Society, June 3, 1874. [1874.] DNLM **70-0581**

CHADWICK, James Read (1844-1905)
Report on obstetrics and diseases of women. [Boston, 1874.] 10p. DNLM **70-0582**

CHADWICK, James Read (1844-1905)
The injection of fluids through the abdominal walls into the large intestine by means of the trocar. Read before the N.Y. Obstetrical Society, Nov. 2, 1875. [New York, 1875.] 5p. DNLM **70-0583**

CHADWICK, James Read (1844-1905)
Ovariotomy. Read before the Suffolk District Medical Society, Jan. 30, 1875. [Boston, 1875.] 8p. DNLM **70-0584**

CHADWICK, James Read (1844-1905)
Extirpation of the uterus by abdominal section. [1875.] 4p. DNLM **70-0585**

CHADWICK, James Read (1844-1905)
Clinical lecture on the diagnostic value of abdominal palpation in pregnancy. Indianapolis, 1876. 22p. DNLM **70-0586**

CHADWICK, James Read (1844-1905)
The medical libraries of Boston; a report read at the first annual meeting of the Boston Medical Library Association, held on Oct. 3, 1876. . . . Cambridge: Riverside Press, 1876. 11p. DLC; MBM **70-0587**

CHADWICK, James Read (1844-1905)
Labor complicated with uterine fibroids and placenta previa. [Boston, 1876.] 13p. DNLM **70-0588**

CHADWICK, James Read (1844-1905)
Rare forms of umbilical hernia, in the fetus. [Boston, 1876.] 19p. 5 plates. DNLM **70-0589**

CHADWICK, James Read (1844-1905)
Cases of double uterus and vagina. Read before the Obstetrical Society of Boston. [1877.] 7p. DNLM **70-0590**

CHADWICK, James Read (1844-1905)
Pus in ovarian fluids. Boston: Rockwell & Churchill, 1877. 7p. DNLM **70-0591**

CHADWICK, James Read (1844-1905)
Cases of vaginismus traced to spasmodic turgescence of clitoris. [Boston, 1877.] 4p. DNLM **70-0592**

CHADWICK, James Read (1844-1905)
The functions of the anal sphincters, so-called, and the act of defecation. [1877.] 14p. 2 plates. DNLM **70-0593**

CHADWICK, James Read (1844-1905)
Expedients in gynaecological practice. [1877.] 3p. DNLM **70-0594**

CHAILLÉ, Stanford Emerson (1830-1911)
The yellow fever, sanitary commission, and vital statistics of New Orleans, during its military occupation, the four years 1862-1865. New Orleans, 1870. 36p. DNLM; LNT-M **70-0595**

CHAILLÉ, Stanford Emerson (1830-1911)
The vital statistics of New Orleans, from 1769 to 1874. New Orleans: J. A. Gresham, [1874.] 37p. DNLM; LNT-M **70-0596**

CHAILLÉ, Stanford Emerson (1830-1911)
Vital statistics applied to the "military-reconstruction" politics of Louisiana, 1868-1874. [1875.] 20p. DNLM; LNT-M **70-0597**

CHAILLÉ, Stanford Emerson (1830-1911)
Origin and progress of medical jurisprudence. 1776-1876. A centennial address. . . . A reprint from the "Transactions of the International Medical Congress," Philadelphia, September, 1876. Philadelphia: Collins, printer, 1876. 40p. DLC; DNLM; PPC; PU **70-0598**

CHAILLÉ, Stanford Emerson (1830-1911)
The climatotherapy of, and the American mountain sanitarium for consumption. Baltimore: Sherwood & Co., 1876. 15p. DNLM; MdU-D **70-0599**

CHAILLÉ, Stanford Emerson (1830-1911)
The American mountain sanitarium for consumption at Asheville, North Carolina. [New Orleans]: T. H. Thomason, 1878. 16p. DNLM; LNT-M **70-0600**

CHAILLÉ, Stanford Emerson (1830-1911)
Address on state medicine and medical organization. With the recommendations in reference to state medicine of the Louisiana State Medical Society and of the Orleans Parish Medical Society to the Louisiana Constitutional Convention of 1879. New Orleans, 1879. 15p. DNLM; LNT-M
70-0601

CHAILLÉ, Stanford Emerson (1830-1911)
Evolution and human anatomy. New York: Trow's Co., 1879. 21p. DNLM; NNNAM **70-0602**

CHAILLÉ, Stanford Emerson (1830-1911)
State medicine and State medical societies. Philadelphia: Collins, 1879. 59p. DNLM; PPC **70-0603**

CHAILLÉ, Stanford Emerson (1830-1911) and George Miller STERNBERG
The Havana Commission. Preliminary report of the Havana Yellow-Fever Commission of the National Board of Health, submitted Nov. 18, 1879. [Washington, 1879.] 19p. DNLM
70-0604

CHAMBERLAIN, William Mellen (1826-1887)
Rupture of an atheromatous aorta, and embolism of the left iliac artery. New York: D. Appleton & Co., 1874. 8p. DNLM; NNNAM **70-0605**

CHAMBERLAIN, William Mellen (1826-1887)
The relation of the urinary organs to puerperal diseases. New York: William Wood & Co., 1877. 31p. DNLM; NNNAM
70-0606

CHAMBERLAIN, William Mellen (1826-1887)
The germ theory of disease. Columbus: Nevins & Myers, 1877. 29p. 1877. DNLM **70-0607**

CHAMBERS, Thomas King (1818-1889)
Restorative medicine; an Harveian annual oration, delivered at the Royal College of Physicians, London, on June 21, 1871 (the 210th anniversary); with two sequels. Philadelphia: Henry C. Lea, 1871. 85p. DNLM; MBM; OCIM; PPC
70-0608

CHAMBERS, Thomas King (1818-1889)
A manual of diet in health and disease. Philadelphia: Henry C. Lea, 1875. 310p. DNLM; MBM; NNNAM; PPC
70-0609

CHANCELLOR, Charles Williams (1831-1915)
Vindication of the report of C. W. Chancellor, M.D., secretary of the State Board of Health, upon the public charities, etc. of the State of Maryland. March, 1878. Baltimore: Printed by J. Cox, 1878. 55p. DLC **70-0610**

CHANCELLOR, Charles Williams (1831-1915)
Contagious and epidemic diseases considered with reference to quarantine and sanitary laws. Is yellow fever contagious? . . . . Baltimore: Printed by J. Cox, 1878. 22p. DLC **70-0611**

CHANCELLOR, Charles Williams (1831-1915)
An inquiry into the history and etiology of plague, considered with reference to quarantine and sanitary laws. Should a national quarantine be established? Baltimore: J. Cox, 1879. 16p. DNLM **70-0612**

CHANNING, Walter (1849-1921)
A case of feigned insanity. Cambridge: Riverside Press, 1878. 7p. DNLM **70-0613**

CHANNING, Walter (1849-1921)
Case of Helen Miller; self-mutilation; tracheotomy. [New York, 1878.] 11p. DNLM; NNNAM
70-0614

CHANNING, Walter (1849-1921)
Buildings for insane criminals. Boston: Rand, Avery & Co., 1879. 18p. DNLM; MBM **70-0615**

CHAPIN, John B[assett] (1829-1918)
Report on insanity. Read before the conference of public charities, Saratoga, N.Y., September 5, 1877. Boston: A. J. Wright, 1877. 18p. DNLM **70-0616**

CHAPMAN, Edwin Nesbit (1819-1888)
Hysterology; a treatise, descriptive and clinical, on the diseases and the displacements of the uterus. New York: William Wood & Co., 1872. 504p. DLC; DNLM; NNNAM; PPC
70-0617

CHAPMAN, Edwin Nesbit (1819-1888)
The true uterine mucous membrane; its structure, function and morbid states. Buffalo: Baker, Jones & Co., 1875. 21p. DNLM **70-0618**

CHAPMAN, Edwin Nesbit (1819-1888)
Treatment of diphtheria. Buffalo: Baker, Jones & Co., 1877. 13p. DNLM **70-0619**

CHAPMAN, Edwin Nesbit (1819-1888)
Antagonism of alcohol and diphtheria. . . . Brooklyn, Union-Argus Steam Printing Establishment, 1878. 98p. DLC; NNNAM **70-0620**

CHAPMAN, Henry C[adwalader] (1845-1909)
Evolution of life. Philadelphia: J. B. Lippincott & Co., 1873. 193p. 32 plates. DNLM; ICU; MH; NNC
70-0621

CHARCOT, Jean Martin (1825-1893)
Lectures on Bright's disease of the kidneys, delivered at the School of Medicine of Paris . . . collected and published by Drs. Bourneville and Sevestre . . . and transl., with permission of the author, by Henry B. Millard. New York: William Wood & Co., 1878. 100p. 11 col. plates. CtY-M; ICJ; PPC; PU
70-0621A

CHARCOT, Jean Martin (1825-1893)
Lectures on localization in diseases of the brain, delivered at the Faculté de Médecine, Paris, 1875. . . . Ed. by Bourneville. Transl. by Edward P. Fowler. . . . New York: William Wood & Co., 1878. 133p. DLC; NNNAM; OCIM; PPC
70-0622

CHARCOT, Jean Martin (1825-1893)
Lectures on the diseases of the nervous system. Delivered at La Salpêtrière. Transl. from the 2nd ed. by George Sigerson. Philadelphia: Henry C. Lea, 1879. 271p. DNLM; MBM; NNNAM; PU **70-0623**

CHASE, Alvin Wood (1817-1885)
Dr. Chase's recipes; or, Information for everybody: an invaluable collection of about eight hundred practical recipes. . . . [53rd ed., four hundred and fifth thousand, English and German]. Stereotyped, carefully rev., illustrated, and much enl., with remarks and full explanations. . . . Ann Arbor, Mich.: R. A. Beal, 1870. 384p. DLC; OCIM; NNNAM
70-0624

CHASE, Alvin Wood (1817-1885)
Dr. Chase's recipes; or, Information for everybody; an invaluable collection of about eight hundred practical recipes. . . . New [61st] ed. [five hundred and tenth thousand]. Ann Arbor, Mich.: R. A. Beal, 1872. 400p. DLC; OCIM
70-0625

CHASE, Alvin Wood (1817-1885)
. . . Dr. Chase's family physician, farrier, bee-keeper, and second receipt book, being an entirely new and complete treatise. . . . Ann Arbor, Mich.: Ann Arbor Printing and Publishing Co., 1873. 644p. DLC; NNNAM; OCIM
70-0626

CHASE, Alvin Wood (1817-1885)
Dr. Chase's recipes; or, Information for everybody: an invaluable collection of about eight hundred practical recipes. . . . Greatly enl. and improved by the publisher . . . [1st enl. ed. Tenth thousand. Five hundred and ninetieth thousand of old ed.] Ann Arbor, Mic.: R. A. Beal, 1874. 648p. DLC; NNNAM; PP; PU **70-0627**

CHAVASSE, Pye Henry (1810-1879)
Woman as a wife and mother. . . . Philadelphia: W. B. Evans & Co., [1871]. 2 v. in 1. plates. DLC; PPC; PPHa; PU
70-0628

CHAVASSE, Pye Henry (1810-1879)
The physical training of children . . . with a preliminary dissertation by F. H. Getchell. Philadelphia: New World Publishing Co., 1873. 364p. OCIM; PPC; ScCM **70-0629**

CHEEVER, David W[illiams] (1831-1915)
Spontaneous fracture. . . . Boston: Printed by D. Clapp & Son, 1871. 8p. DLC; DNLM **70-0630**

CHEEVER, David Williams (1831-1915)
How to study medicine. An introductory lecture. Oct. 2, 1871. [1871.] 10p. DNLM **70-0631**

CHEEVER, David W[illiams] (1831-1915)
Three cases of ovariotomy, of which two were successful. Boston: D. Clapp & Son, 1873. 8p. DNLM **70-0632**

CHENERY, Elisha (1830?-1900)
Relation of alcoholism to other forms of disease. [Hartford], 1879. 11p. DNLM **70-0633**

CHENEY & MYRICK
Druggist's hand-book of American and foreign drugs; their common English and botanical names, arranged in alphabetical order. Boston: J. E. Farwell & Co., 1878. 110p. DNLM; MH-M; OCLloyd **70-0634**

CHEW, Samuel Claggett (1837-1915)
Introductory address delivered before the medical class of the University of Maryland. Baltimore: Sherwood & Co., 1871. 17p. DNLM **70-0635**

CHEW, Samuel Claggett (1837-1915)
A medical survey of the trial of Mrs. E. G. Wharton on the charge of poisoning Gen. W. S. Ketchum. [1872?] 23p. DNLM
70-0636

CHEW, Samuel Claggett (1837-1915)
An examination of the medical evidence in the trial of Mrs. E. G. Wharton, on the charge of attempting to poison Eugene Van Ness, esq. New York: William Wood & Co., 1873. 28p. DNLM; NNNAM **70-0637**

CHEW, Samuel Claggett (1837-1915)
Notes on thoracentesis. Read before the Medical and Chirurgical Faculty of Maryland, April 15, 1873. [Baltimore, 1873.] 9p. DNLM; MdBM **70-0638**

CHEW, Samuel Claggett (1837-1915)
Thoracentesis; with illustrative cases. New York: D. Appleton & Co., 1876. 15p. DNLM; NNNAM **70-0639**

CHEW, Samuel Claggett (1837-1915)
Notes on pneumonia, with cases. Baltimore: J. H. Foster, [1877?] 6 l. DNLM **70-0640**

CHEW, Samuel Claggett (1837-1915)
An address commemorative of Nathan Ryno Smith. Baltimore: J. H. Foster & Co., 1878. 20p. DNLM
70-0641

CHILD, Duff [pseud.?]
Diagnosis. A story for amateur physicians as well as for regular practitioners. . . . Louisville: A. A. Gosnell, 1872. 102p. DLC; DNLM **70-0642**

CHISOLM, Julian John (1830-1903)
Ophthalmic and aural surgery reports. Louisville: Med. Jour. print, 1873. 24p. DNLM **70-0643**

CHISOLM, Julian John (1830-1903)
Intra-ocular enchondroma of twenty-two years' growth removed at the Baltimore Eye and Ear Infirmary. With a description of the microscopic condition of the tumor, by H. Knapp. [New York, 1873.] 16p. 2 plates. DNLM; NNNAM
70-0644

CHISOLM, Julian John (1830-1903)
Making of both lids to the left eye from contiguous skin. A keloid growth of twenty-seven years, involving the entire lower lid and two-thirds of the upper lid, including the skin of the left side of the nose. Growth removed and deformity corrected by a blepharo-plastic operation, manufacturing the two lids from contiguous skin surfaces. [Baltimore, 1873.] 9p. 1 phot. DNLM **70-0645**

CHISOLM, Julian John (1830-1903)
Intra-ocular enchondroma of twenty-two years' growth. With a description of the microscopic condition of the tumor, by H. Knapp. New York: William Wood & Co., [1873?]. 16p. 2 plates. DNLM; NNNAM **70-0646**

CHISOLM, Julian John (1830-1903)
Misapplication of remedies in the treatment of eye diseases. Louisville, Ky.: Med. J. print, 1873. 8p. DNLM
70-0647

CHISOLM, Julian John (1830-1903)
Ophthalmic and aural surgery reports. Baltimore, 1873. 22p. DNLM **70-0648**

CHISOLM, Julian John (1830-1903)
Blepharoplasty; making lids to the left eye, after the removal of a keloid growth [of twenty-seven years], which involved both lids. [1873?] 9p. 1 phot. DNLM **70-0649**

CHISOLM, Julian John (1830-1903)
What course should be pursued with an eye lost through an accident? Baltimore: Kelly, Piet & Co., 1875. 8p. DNLM; MdU-D **70-0650**

CHISOLM, Julian John (1830-1903)
What anaesthetic shall we use? Baltimore, 1877. 23p. DNLM; MdU-D **70-0651**

CHISOLM, Julian John (1830-1903)
Treatment of chronic aural discharges. Baltimore: J. H. Foster & Co., 1878. 10p. DNLM; MdU-D **70-0652**

CHISOLM, Julian John (1830-1903)
Neurotomy: a substitute for enucleation. A new operation in ophthalmic surgery. Richmond: J. W. Fergusson & Son, 1879. 16p. DNLM **70-0653**

CHISOLM, Julian John (1830-1903)
A few well established facts in connection with squint. Baltimore, 1879. 15p. DNLM **70-0654**

CLAIBORNE, John Herbert (1828-1905)
Clinical reports from private practice. . . . Petersburg, Va.: J. van H. Nash, 1873. 424p. DLC **70-0655**

CLAPP, Herbert Codman (1846-1929)
A tabular handbook of auscultation and percussion. For students and physicians. . . . Boston: Houghton, Osgood & Co., 1879. 97p. 4 plates. DLC; MBM; NNNAM **70-0656**

CLAPP, Otis
Prevention as a means of reducing the material, social, and moral burdens and devastations of intemperance. Boston: Wright & Potter, 1872. 11p. DNLM; MB **70-0657**

CLAPP, Otis
The Washingtonian Home and its sixteen years' work. An address delivered at the dedication of its new building, Dec. 21, 1873. South Framingham: J. C. Clark, 1874. 16p. DNLM **70-0658**

Dr. CLARK's new illustrated marriage guide. A treatise on the anatomy and physiology of the generative organs of both sexes, and their organic and functional diseases. . . . Newark, N.J.: J. W. Stephens, 1873. 384p. DLC; PPC **70-0659**

CLARK, Anson L.
A treatise on the medical and surgical diseases of women. . . . Chicago: Jansen, McClurg & Co., 1879. 410p. DLC; IEN-M; OCIM **70-0660**

CLARK, Daniel (1835-1912)
A newly discovered system of electrical medication. Cincinnati: Hitchcock & Walden, 1875. 142p. DNLM; OCIM **70-0661**

CLARK, E. A. (1836?-1871)
A report on the progress of surgery, made to the St. Louis Medical Society. St. Louis: Levison & Blythe, 1871. 101p. DNLM **70-0662**

CLARK, E. A. (1836?-1871)
Effects of increased atmospheric pressure upon the human body; with a report of 35 cases brought to city hospital from the caisson of the St. Louis and Illinois bridge. [St. Louis, 1874.] 30p. DNLM **70-0663**

CLARK, James (1788-1870)
The management of infancy, physiological and moral. Intended chiefly for the use of parents. 1st American from the 10th London ed. New York: D. Appleton & Co., 1871. 301p. DNLM; NNNAM; PPC; PU **70-0664**

CLARK, T. Edwards
Notes on the pathology of the sympathetic nervous system. Chicago: J. J. Spalding & Co., 1876. 15p. DNLM **70-0665**

CLARKE, Edward Hammond (1820-1877)
Classification of medicines employed in the lectures of Dr. Edward H. Clarke. . . . Boston: Rockwell & Churchill, printers, 1870. 12p. DLC **70-0666**

CLARKE, Edward Hammond (1820-1877) and Robert AMORY
The physiological and therapeutical action of the bromide of potassium and bromide of ammonium. In 2 pts. Boston: J. Campbell, 1872. 178p. DLC; DNLM **70-0667**

CLARKE, Edward Hammond (1820-1877)
Sex in education; or, a fair chance for the girls. Boston: J. R. Osgood & Co., 1873. 181p. DNLM; MB; NN **70-0668**

CLARKE, Edward Hammond (1820-1877)
The building of a brain. Boston: J. R. Osgood & Co., 1874. 153p. DNLM; MH-M; NNNAM; PPC **70-0669**

CLARKE, Edward Hammond, ed. (1820-1877)
A century of American medicine, 1776-1876. Philadelphia: Henry C. Lea, 1876. 366p. DNLM; NNNAM; PPC; PU **70-0670**

CLARKE, Edward Hammond (1820-1877)
Visions: a study of false sight (pseudopia). . . . With an introduction and memorial sketch by Oliver Wendell Holmes, M.D. Boston: Houghton, Osgood & Co., 1878. 315p. DLC: DNLM; MBM; NNNAM **70-0671**

CLARKE, Robert & Co.
Bibliotheca medica. A catalogue of American and British books, periodicals, transactions, etc., relating to medicine, surgery, dentistry, pharmacy, chemistry, and kindred subjects, classified by subjects, with an index by authors. Cincinnati, 1878. 244p. AU; DNLM; MH; NN **70-0672**

CLARKE, W. Fairlie (1833-1884)
A manual of the practice of surgery. From the last London edition. New York: William Wood & Co., 1879. 316p. CtY-M; NNNAM; OCIM; PPC **70-0673**

CLEAVE, E.
Cleave's biographical cyclopaedia of homoeopathic physicians and surgeons. Philadelphia: Galaxy Publishing Co., 1873. 512p. PPHa; PU **70-0674**

CLEAVELAND, Charles Harley (1820-1863)
Pronouncing medical lexicon, containing the correct pronunciation and definition of terms used in medicine and the collateral sciences. 14th ed. Philadelphia: Lindsay & Blakiston, 1872. 302p. DNLM; PPC; PPJ; PU **70-0675**

CLEAVELAND, Charles Harley (1820-1863)
Pronouncing medical lexicon. . . . With addenda containing abbreviations used in prescriptions, and lists of poisons and their antidotes. [16th ed.] Philadelphia: Lindsay & Blakiston, 1875. 302p. DNLM; PP; PPC; PU **70-0676**

CLELAND, John (1835-1925)
. . . Animal physiology: the structure and function of the human body. . . . New York: G. P. Putnam's Sons, [1873]. 335p. DLC; NN; NNC; PU **70-0677**

CLELAND, John (1835-1925)
A directory for the dissection of the human body. Philadelphia: Henry C. Lea, 1877. 182p. DNLM; OCIM; PPC: PU **70-0678**

CLENDINEN, Alexander (1841-1891)
Artificial feeding of infants, and description of instruments and apparatus of the author, [etc.]. Newark, N.J.: L. F. Hardham, 1878. 17p. 1 plate. DNLM; PPC **70-0679**

CLENDINEN, Alexander (1841-1891)
. . . Résumé of yellow fever (quarantine and home sanitation) being abstract of report by A. Clendinen, M.D., as chairman of Committee of Intelligence, District Society of Bergen County. Read before the Medical Society of New Jersey, May 28, 1879. . . . [Newark, N.J., 1879]. 39p. DLC **70-0680**

CLEVELAND MEDICAL COLLEGE. MEDICAL DEPARTMENT OF WESTERN RESERVE COLLEGE, AT HUDSON
Annual announcement for the session of 1875-1876 (33.). Cleveland, 1875. 10p. DNLM [Organized in 1843 as the Cleveland Medical College. In 1844 it became the Medical Department of Western Reserve College, at Hudson. Reorganized in July, 1881, by a union of the faculty of the Cleveland Medical College and a majority of the faculty of the Medical Department of Wooster University, as the Medical Department of Western Reserve University. In March, 1882, the board of trustees of Western Reserve University conferred the *ad enudem* degree of Doctor of Medicine upon all graduates of the Cleveland Medical College, and upon such graduates of the Wooster Medical Department prior to 1881, as desired it.] **70-0681**

CLEVENGER, S. Vail (1843-1920)
Neurility: correlated, converted physical forces. [Chicago, 1879.] 24p. DNLM **70-0682**

CLINICAL charts of temperature, vital signs, and septenaries to register three weeks' observations made with the fever and surface thermometer. Analytical records of excreta, ingesta, and physiological symptoms, corresponding day for day with the clinical charts, for hospital and private practice. [New York, 1872.] 2 l. fol. DNLM **70-0683**

CLOUSTON, T. S. (1840-1915)
An asylum, or "hospital-home," for two hundred patients: . . . . [January, 1879.] 32p. DLC **70-0684**

CLYMER, Meredith (1817-1902)
Notes on the physiology and pathology of the nervous system, with reference to clinical medicine. a. Disseminated sclerosis of the brain and spinal cord. b. Annular or cortical sclerosis of the spinal cord. New York: D. Appleton & Co., 1870. 53p. DNLM; NNNAM **70-0685**

CLYMER, Meredith (1817-1902)
Hereditary genius: an analytical review. New York: D. Appleton & Co., 1870. 19p. DNLM **70-0686**

CLYMER, Meredith (1817-1902)
Epidemic cerebro-spinal meningitis. With an appendix on some points on the causes of the disease as shown by the history of the present epidemic in the city of New York. . . . Philadelphia: Lindsay & Blakiston, 1872. 59p. fold. front. (map). DLC; PPC **70-0687**

CLYMER, Meredith (1817-1902)
Dr. Benjamin Rush. The annual oration delivered before the Society of the Alumni of the Medical Department of the University of Pennsylvania. 34p. Philadelphia, 1876. DNLM; PU **70-0688**

CLYMER, Meredith (1817-1902)
Annual address before the alumni of the Medical Department of the University of Pennsylvania. [Life of Dr. Benjamin Rush.] With the proceedings of the alumni meeting of 1876. Philadelphia: Collins, 1876. 50p. DNLM; PU **70-0689**

COBBOLD, T. Spencer (1826-1886)
Worms. A series of lectures on practical helminthology. Delivered at the Medical College of the Middlesex Hospital. Philadelphia: Lindsay & Blakiston, 1872. 178p. DLC; PU **70-0690**

COCHRAN, Jerome (1831-1896)
The general principles of organization, and the evolution of organic forms. First annual address before the Alumni Society of the Medical Department of the University of Nashville. Delivered in the hall of the Medical College, February 28, 1870. . . . Nashville, Tenn.: W. C. Collier & Co., 1871. 53p. DLC; DNLM **70-0691**

COCHRAN, Jerome (1831-1896)
The endemic and epidemic diseases of Mobile: their causes and prevention. Mobile: Daily Register print, 1871. 48p. DNLM **70-0692**

COCHRAN, Jerome (1831-1896)
Contributions to the Transactions of the Medical Association of the State of Alabama, session of 1874. I. The yellow-fever epidemic of 1873. II. The white blood-corpuscle. Montgomery, Ala.: Barrett & Brown, 1874. 115p. DNLM **70-0693**

COCHRAN, Jerome (1831-1896)
History of the small-pox epidemic in the city of Mobile, 1874-1875: with mortuary & meteorological tables. Also, notes and reflections upon diphtheria and typho-malarial fever; together with an ordinance to secure the public health. . . . Montgomery, Ala.: Barrett & Brown, 1873. 122p. DLC; DNLM **70-0694**

CODMAN, Benjamin S. (1816?-1894) and Ashahel M. SHURTLEFF
Supplementary dental catalogue. Boston, 1874. 36p. DNLM **70-0695**

CODMAN, Benjamin S. (1816?-1894) and Ashahel M. SHURTLEFF
Surgical and dental instruments and kindred articles. Boston, 1875. 88p. DNLM **70-0696**

CODMAN, Benjamin S. (1816?-1894) and Ashahel M. SHURTLEFF
Illustrated catalogue of surgical instruments and appliances. Boston: T. W. Ripley, 1875. 88p. DNLM **70-0697**

CODMAN, Benjamin S. (1816?-1894) and Ashahel M. SHURTLEFF
Illustrated catalogue of surgical instruments and appliances. Boston: J. Wilson & Son, [1877]. 128p. DNLM; MBM **70-0698**

CODMAN, Benjamin S. (1816?-1894) and Ashahel M. SHURTLEFF
Illustrated catalogue of surgical instruments and appliances. Boston, [1878]. 132p. DNLM; MBM
70-0699

CODMAN, Benjamin S. (1816?-1894) and Ashahel M. SHURTLEFF
Illustrated catalogue of surgical instruments and appliances. Boston, Mass., [1879]. 136p. DNLM
70-0700

CODMAN, Benjamin S. (1816?-1894) and Ashahel M. SHURTLEFF
Manufacturers and importers of surgical instruments and appliances, trusses, apparatus for deformities and deficiencies, electro-medical apparatus, elastic hose, [etc.]. Boston: Rand, Avery & Co., 1879. 95-133p. DNLM; MH-M
70-0701

CODMAN, John T[homas]
Foul breath. St. Louis, 1879. 14p. DNLM
70-0702

COE, Grover (1825-1860)
Concentrated organic medicines; being a practical exposition of the therapeutic properties and clinical employment of the combined proximate medicinal constituents of indigenous and foreign plants, etc. 11th ed. New York: R. Keith & Co., 1870. 448p. DNLM; NNNAM; OCLloyd **70-0703**

COHEN, Jacob [da Silva] Solis (1838-1927)
A brief exposition of the management of the laryngoscope. Atlanta, Ga., 1871. 19p. DNLM **70-0704**

COHEN, Jacob [da Silva] Solis (1838-1927)
Diseases of the throat: a guide to the diagnosis and treatment of affections of the pharynx, aesophagus, trachea, larynx, and nares. . . . New York: William Wood & Co., 1872. 582p. DNLM; NNNAM; OCIM; PPC **70-0705**

COHEN, Jacob [da Silva] Solis (1838-1927)
Sore throat; two lectures delivered Sept. 24 and Oct. 1, 1874, in Jefferson Medical College. Philadelphia: J. A. Moore, 1874. 11p. DNLM; PPJ **70-0706**

COHEN, Jacob [da Silva] Solis (1838-1927)
Fetid coryza. Philadelphia: J. B. Lippincott & Co., 1874. 16p. DNLM **70-0707**

COHEN, Jacob [da Silva] Solis (1838-1927)
Croup, in its relations to tracheotomy. Philadelphia: Lindsay & Blakiston, 1874. 78p. DNLM; PPC; PPJ
70-0708

COHEN, Jacob [da Silva] Solis (1838-1927)
Apsithuria. [Philadelphia, 1875.] 4p. DNLM
70-0709

COHEN, Jacob [da Silva] Solis (1838-1927)
Inhalation in the treatment of disease: its therapeutics and practice. A treatise on the inhalation of gases, vapors, fumes, compressed and rarefied air, nebulized fluids, and powders. . . . 2nd ed., rev. and enl. with many new illustrations. Philadelphia: Lindsay & Blakiston, 1876. 392p. DNLM; ICRM; NNNAM; PPC **70-0710**

COHEN, Jacob [da Silva] Solis (1838-1927)
. . . The throat and the voice. . . . Philadelphia: Lindsay & Blakiston, 1879. 159p. DLC; MH-M; PPC; PPJ
70-0711

COHEN, J[acob da Silva] Solis (1838-1927)
Diseases of the throat and nasal passages; a guide to the diagnosis and treatment of affections of the pharynx, aesophagus, trachea, larynx, and nares. . . . 2nd ed. New York: William Wood & Co., 1879. 742p. DLC; DNLM; PPC; PPJ
70-0712

COLEMAN, John Scott (1837-1892)
Cephalic version by the external bi-polar method; arrest of profuse post-partum hemorrhage with tincture of iodine. New York: William Wood & Co., 1877. 6p. DNLM; NNNAM
70-0713

COLES, Walter (1839-1892)
Anaesthetics. . . . Wheeling, [W. Va.]: Frew, Hagans & Hall, Steam Job Printers, 1871. 14p. DLC; DNLM
70-0714

COLES, Walter (1839-1892)
Hepatic abscess; with some remarks on Dr. Hammond's paper. St. Louis: G. O. Rumbold & Co., 1878. 16p. DNLM
70-0715

COLLEGE OF THE NEW YORK OPHTHALMIC HOSPITAL, NEW YORK CITY
Annual announcements for the sessions of 1879-1880 to 1885-1886 (1.-7.). New York, 1879-1885. DNLM [List of graduates from 1880 to 1884, in announcement for 1884-1885. First to third announcements, in Reports N.Y. Ophthalmic Hospital for the preceding years. The third announcement of the college is in the thirtieth annual course held at the hospital.]
70-0716

COLLEGE OF OBSTETRICS AND GYNAECOLOGY, WASHINGTON, D.C.
[Announcement of a course of clinical lectures in Columbia Hospital for Women and Lying-in Asylum. April to June, 1873.] [Washington, 1873.] 1 sheet. DNLM
70-0717

COLLEGE OF PHYSICIANS AND SURGEONS, BALTIMORE
Annual announcements for the sessions of 1873-1874 (2.); 1875-1876 to 1897-1898 (4.-26.). Baltimore, 1873-1897. DNLM [List of students and graduates for 1872-1873; 1874-1875 to 1896-1897, in announcements for subsequent years. List of graduates from 1873 to 1879, in announcement for 1879-1880. Organized and incorporated in 1872. The Washington University School of Medicine was established in 1872. By act of the legislature the two schools were consolidated in 1878.] **70-0718**

COLLEGE OF PHYSICIANS AND SURGEONS, KEOKUK
Annual announcements for the sessions of 1874-1875 (30.); 1875-1876 (32.); 1876-1877 (34.); 1877-1878 (36.); 1879-1880 to 1883-1884 (38.-43.); 1890-1891 (50.); 1893-1894 to 1896-1897 (53.-56.). Keokuk, 1874-1896. DNLM [List of students and graduates for 1873-1874 to 1876-1877; 1878-1879 to 1882-1883; 1889-1890; 1892-1893 to 1895-1896, in announcements for subsequent years. Alumni since the organization of the institution in 1849 to 1896, in announcement for 1896-1897.] **70-0719**

COLLEGE OF PHYSICIANS AND SURGEONS, SAINT JOSEPH, MO.
Annual announcements for the sessions of 1879-1880 to 1881-1882 (1.-3.). St. Joseph, 1879-1881. DNLM [Ceased to exist in 1882, by uniting with the Saint Joseph Medical College, forming the Saint Joseph Medical College.]
70-0720

COLLINS, Samuel B.
Theriaki and their last dose. Letters of Fitz Hugh Ludlow and others, to Dr. Samuel B. Collins, relating to the most wonderful medical discovery of the age. Chicago: Evening Journal Print, 1870. 109p. DLC **70-0721**

COLTON, J. J.
The physiological action of nitrous oxide gas, as shown by experiments upon man and the lower animals. Together with experiments as to its safety, uses and abuses. . . . Philadelphia: S. S. White, 1871. 32p. DNLM; PPC
70-0722

COLUMBIA COLLEGE. NEW YORK CITY
Catalogue embracing the names of its trustees, officers, and graduates. . . . From 1754 to 1870 [including graduates in medicine]. New York: D. Van Nostrand, 1871. 163p. DNLM; NNC **70-0723**

COLUMBIA COLLEGE. NEW YORK CITY
Catalogues of the officers and students [including the medical department] for the years 1856-1857 (103.), 1858-1859 (105.), 1860-1861 (107.), 1862-1863 (109.). 1865-1866 (112.), 1869-1870 to 1871-1872 (116.-118.). New York, 1857-1872. DNLM; NNC **70-0724**

COLUMBIA HOSPITAL FOR WOMEN AND LYING-IN ASYLUM. WASHINGTON, D.C.
[Refutation of the anonymous accusations of mismanagement which appeared in the October number, 1877, of the Richmond and Louisville Medical Journal, by a citizen of Washington. J. K. Barnes, M.D., Chas. H. Cargin, J. T. Mitchell, committee on expenditures. Dec. 1, 1877.] Washington, 1877. 15p. DNLM. [Bound with: Annual report for 1876-1877.]
70-0725

COMBE, Andrew (1797-1847)
The management of infancy, physiological and moral. Intended chiefly for the use of parents. . . . Revised and edited by Sir James Clark, bart. . . . 1st American from the 10th London ed. New York: D. Appleton & Co., 1871. 302p. DLC; NNNAM; OCIM; PPC **70-0726**

COMBE, Andrew (1797-1847)
The mother's guide for the care of her children; or, The management of infancy. . . . Rev. and ed. by Sir James Clark, bart. . . . New York: Continental Publishing Company, [1872]. 303p. DLC; NNNAM; PPC; PU **70-0727**

COMBE, George (1788-1858)
Lectures on phrenology; . . . including its application to the present and prospective condition of the United States. With notes, an introductory essay and an historical sketch: by Andrew Boardman, M.D. 3rd ed., with corrections and additions. . . . New York: S. R. Wells, 1871. 391p. DLC; NN; NNNAM; PU **70-0728**

COMPTON, J. W[illiam] (1825-1905)
Sulphate of chinchonidia; a substitute for sulphate of quinine. Paducah, Ky.: Martin & Co., 1876. 7p. DNLM
70-0729

COMPTON, J. W[illiam] (1825-1905)
Solution and absorption of medicines, or the best means of securing the good effects of medicines in the cure of disease. [Evansville? 1876.] 7p. DNLM **70-0730**

COMPTON, J. W[illiam] (1825-1905)
Medicine, the present and future. An address delivered to the graduates of Evansville Medical College, February 27, 1878. St. Louis, 1878. 12p. DNLM **70-0731**

COMPTON, J. W[illiam] (1825-1905)
The therapeutic value of ergot. [1879.] 8p. DNLM
70-0732

COMPTON, J. W[illiam] (1825-1905)
Precautions requisite in the administration of ergot. Detroit: G. S. Davis, 1879. 7p. DNLM **70-0733**

CONKLIN, W. J[udkins] (1844-1916)
Report of the temperature of certain nervous diseases. Columbus, O.: Nevins & Myers, 1870. 24p. DNLM; OCIM
70-0734

CONKLIN, W. J[udkins] (1844-1916)
The relations of epilepsy to insanity and jurisprudence. [1871.] 43p. DNLM **70-0735**

CONKLIN, W. J[udkins] (1844-1916)
History of the discovery of the circulation of the blood. Columbus: Nevins & Myers, 1877. 14p. DNLM
70-0736

CONKLIN, W. J[udkins] (1844-1916)
The medical expert. Columbus: Nevins & Myers, 1878. 20p. DNLM **70-0737**

CONKLING, F. A[ugustus] (1816-1891)
Cottage hospitals. Remarks upon the report of the committee on a village of cottage hospitals, delivered at a meeting of the governors of the Society of the New York Hospital. [New York, 1876.] 23p. DNLM; NNNAM **70-0738**

COOK, A. B[rown] (1828-1895)
Reply to the action of the College of Physicians and Surgeons of Louisville, Ky. Louisville: Terrell, Hays & Co., 1871. 15p. DNLM **70-0739**

COOK, A. B[rown] (1828-1895)
Carbolic acid injections in the treatment of piles; radical cures. Louisville, 1878. 8p. DNLM **70-0740**

COOK, A. B[rown] (1828-1895)
How to elevate the standard of medical education and medical teaching. Louisville, Ky., 1879. 4p. DNLM
70-0741

COOK, Joseph
Heredity, with preludes on current events. Boston: Houghton, Osgood & Co., 1879. 268p. DNLM; MH; NN; NNC
70-0742

COOK, William H[enry] (1832-1899)
Physiomedical dispensatory. . . . Cincinnati, 1870. [1869.] 832p. OCLloyd **70-0743**

COOKE, Nicholas Francis (1829-1885)
Licensed foeticide. Detroit: Am. Observer Off., [1878]. 15p. DNLM **70-0744**

COOKE, Thomas (1841-1899)
Tablets of anatomy and physiology. Bones of upper limb. New York: William Wood & Co., 1874. 5 l. DNLM
70-0745

COOKE, Thomas (1841-1899)
Tables of anatomy and physiology. Bones and cavities of face; under surface of base and lateral region of skull. New York: William Wood & Co., 1874. 5 l. DNLM; NNNAM
70-0746

COOKE, Thomas (1841-1899)
Tablets of anatomy and physiology. Arteries of the head and neck. New York: William Wood & Co., 1874. 4 l. DNLM; NNNAM **70-0747**

COOKE, Thomas (1841-1899)
Tablets of anatomy and physiology. Arteries of the limbs. New York: William Wood & Co., 1874. 6 l. DNLM
70-0748

COOKE, Thomas (1841-1899)
Tablets of anatomy and physiology. Cranial nerves. (Third thousand, enlarged.) New York: William Wood & Co., 1874. 9 l. DNLM; NNNAM **70-0749**

COOKE, Thomas (1841-1899)
Tablets of anatomy and physiology. Physiology: General development of the embryo. New York: William Wood & Co., 1874. 5 l. DNLM **70-0750**

COOKE, Thomas (1841-1899)
Tablets of anatomy and physiology . . . being a synopsis of demonstrations given in the Westminster Hospital Medical School in the years 1871.-1872.-1873.-1874. and -1875. With an appendix containing most of the new discoveries of importance made known up to the date of publication. Anatomy complete. 2nd ed. . . . New York: William Wood & Co.; [etc., etc.], 1878. 385p. DLC; NNNAM; OCIM; PPC
70-0751

COOMES, Martin F. (*b.* 1847)
Catarrhal affections of the eye, nose, and ear. Louisville, Ky.: L. H. Bell, 1876. 18p. DNLM **70-0752**

COOMES, Martin F. (*b.* 1847)
Remarks on naso-pharyngeal catarrh. Louisville, Ky., 1878. 8p. DNLM **70-0753**

COOPER, J. F[awcett] (1822-1899)
A proving of arsenite of soda (hydro-disodic arseniate). By the Homoeopathic Materia Medica Club of Allegheny County, Pa. The prover's record arranged by J. F. Cooper, M.D. Contributed to the proceedings of the Homoeopathic Medical Society of Pennsylvania at the session of 1875. Printed by the Hahnemannian Monthly, 1876. 56p. PPHa
70-0754

CORNWELL, Henry G[ilbert]
A clinical report of eleven cases of dislocation of the crystalline lens. Read before the Union Medical Association of North Eastern Ohio, in session at Akron. Youngstown, Ohio: Woodrow, [1878]. 8p. DNLM **70-0755**

CORNWELL, Henry G[ilbert]
Observations on the treatment of blepharospasm. Youngstown, Ohio, 1879. 6p. DNLM **70-0756**

CORNWELL, Henry G[ilbert]
An analytical report of 407 cases of eye and ear diseases. Youngstown, 1879. 7p. DNLM **70-0757**

CORR, Lucinda H.
Obstetrics, reduced to questions and answers. . . . Chicago: D. B. Cooke & Co., 1878. 336p. DLC **70-0758**

CORSON, John W. (1816-1882)
On the treatment of pleurisy; with an appendix of cases, showing the value of combinations of croton oil, ether, and iodine, as counter-irritants in other diseases. New York: William Wood & Co., 1874. 31p. 1 plate. DLC; DNLM; NNNAM **70-0759**

COTTING, Benjamin Eddy (1812-1897)
Medical addresses. . . . Boston: D. Clapp & Son, 1875. 123p. DLC; DNLM; MBM **70-0760**

COUES, S. F.
Possibilities of organism. Stat nominis pro umbra. An address. Washington, D.C.: Mohun Bros., 1878. 37p. DNLM
70-0761

COURTRIGHT, Geo. S.
Dislocations of the shoulder-joint, and some of the accidents resulting therefrom. With history of a case, and post-mortem examination of the same. [Cincinnati, 1871?] 8p. DNLM
70-0762

COWDIN, Robert
Remarks . . . on the subject of admitting female students to clinical lectures at the City Hospital. City Doc. No. 37. May 8, 1871. [Boston, 1871.] 11p. DNLM; MBM
70-0763

COWLING, Richard Oswald (1839-1881)
The relations of medicine to modern unbelief. A valedictory address . . . commencement of the University of Louisville, March 1, 1876. Louisville: J. P. Morton & Co., 1876. 11p. DNLM **70-0764**

COWLING, Richard O[swald] (1839-1881)
Pathology and treatment of sprains. A paper read before the Kentucky State Medical Society. Louisville, Ky.: J. P. Morton & Co., 1877. 11p. DNLM **70-0765**

COWLING, Richard O[swald] (1839-1881)
An address upon the life and character of Lunsford Pitts Yandell, M.D. Louisville, Ky.: J. P. Morton & Co., 1879. 10p. DNLM **70-0766**

COWPERTHWAITE, Allen Corson (*b.* 1848)
Insanity in its medico-legal relations. Philadelphia: J. M. Stoddart & Co., 1876. 85p. DLC; DNLM
70-0767

COWPERTHWAITE, Allen Corson (*b.* 1848)
Science in therapeutics. The annual address delivered before the Nebraska Homoeopathic Medical Association by the President, at Omaha, May 15, 1877. Omaha: Redfield Bros., 1877. 18p. PPHa **70-0768**

CRABTRE, Addison Darre
The funny side of physic; or, the mysteries of medicine, presenting the humorous and serious sides of medical practice. An exposé of medical humbugs, quacks, and charlatans in all ages and all countries. Hartford: J. B. Burr & Hyde, 1872. 816p. 36 plates. DLC; DNLM; MH **70-0769**

CRANK, Charles Dake
Valedictory address delivered at the 21st annual commencement of the Hahnemannian Medical Institute, March 9, 1871. Published by the Institute. Philadelphia: A. Hull & Co., 1871. 15p. PPHa **70-0770**

CRAWFORD, John B. (*d.* 1894)
An essay on malpractice; read before the Luzerne County Medical Society, at Wilkes-Barre. [n.p.], R. Baur, 1879. 20p. DNLM **70-0771**

CROSBY, Alpheus Benning (1832-1877)
A contribution to the medical history of New Hampshire. Nashua: Moore & Langley, 1870. 32p. DNLM **70-0772**

CROSBY, Alpheus Benning (1832-1877)
Enthusiasm the condition of professional success. A valedictory address. Ann Arbor, Mich.: Courier Steam Ptg. House, 1872. 19p. DNLM **70-0773**

CROSBY, Alpheus Benning (1832-1877)
A lost art in surgery; read before the New York County Medical Society, New Hampshire State Medical Society, and the White Mountain Medical Society. New York: Rutledge & Co., 1877. 24p. DNLM; NNNAM **70-0774**

CROSBY, Dixi (1801-1873)
The first operation on record for the removal of the entire arm, scapula, and three-fourths of the clavicle. Reported with comments by his son, A. B. Crosby. Concord, N.H.: Republican Press Assoc., 1875. 13p. DNLM; MH-M **70-0775**

CROSBY, Howard (1826-1891)
The ethics of medical men. An introductory lecture to the medical course of the University of the City of New York, September 28th, 1875. New York: J. F. Trow & Son, 1875. 15p. DNLM; NNNAM **70-0776**

CROSBY, Nathan
Inebriate asylums. Remarks in opposition to them before the committee on charitable institutions. Boston: Nation Press, 1871. 12p. DNLM **70-0777**

CROSS, T. M. B.
Amnesic and ataxic aphasia with agraphia and temporary right hemiplegia, the result of embolism of the left middle cerebral artery. Louisville: J. P. Morton & Co., 1872. 13p. DNLM **70-0778**

CROWE, J. E.
An introductory lecture delivered in the University of Louisville, on the evening of October 3, 1870. Louisville: J. P. Morton & Co., 1870. 14p. DNLM **70-0779**

CULBERTSON, Howard (1828-1890)
Excision of the larger joints of the extremities. Prize essay. Philadelphia: Collins, 1876. 672p. 15 plates. DNLM; NNNAM; PPC; PU **70-0780**

CULBERTSON, Howard (1828-1890)
Are there one or two syphilitic poisons? [Cincinnati, 1877.] 12p. DNLM **70-0781**

CULBERTSON, H[oward] (1828-1890)
On a modified mode of detecting paralysis of the ocular muscles. [Philadelphia, 1877.] 9p. DNLM **70-0782**

CULBERTSON, H[oward] (1828-1890)
Waste and repair; a few thoughts upon the doctrine of waste and repair of organized bodies, considered in relation to the subject of zymotic and parasitoid diseases. Cincinnati, 1879. 9p. DNLM **70-0783**

CULBERTSON, Howard (1828-1890)
On a modified form of canula eye forceps. Cincinnati, 1879. 8p. DNLM **70-0784**

CULBERTSON, Howard (1828-1890)
Closing address to the class of the Columbus Medical College. [1879?] 14p. DNLM **70-0785**

CURTIS, Alva (1797-1881)
The provocation and the reply; or, Allopathy versus physiomedicalism in a review of Prof. M. B. Wright's remarks at the dedication of the Cincinnati new hospital, January 8th, 1869. . . . Cincinnati: Pub. by the proprietor, 1870. 162p. DLC **70-0786**

CURTIS, Alva (1797-1881)
A fair examination and criticism of all the medical systems in vogue. 4th ed. Cincinnati, 1872. 205p. 1 phot. DNLM **70-0787**

CURTIS, Alva (1797-1881)
A synopsis of lectures on medical science; embracing the principles of medicine, or physiology, pathology, and therapeutics, as discovered in nature; and the practice according to those principles, as applied by art. . . . 7th ed. Carefully rev., and much enl. . . . New York: A. J. Graham, 1877. 411, 16, 413-428p. DLC; NNNAM; PPC **70-0788**

CURTIS, Edward M. (1840-1874)
Asthenopia, or weak sight. Oswego, N.Y.: Morrison & Co., 1870. 14p. DNLM **70-0789**

CURTIS, Edward M. (1840-1874)
Why do we wear spectacles? [1871.] 15p. DNLM **70-0790**

CURTIS, Edward (1838-1912)
The protoplasm theory: an introductory lecture delivered at the opening of the winter session of the College of Physicians and Surgeons, New York, October 1, 1873. . . . Published by the medical class. New York: C. E. Wilbour, printer and bookbinder, 1873. 23p. DLC; NNNAM **70-0791**

CURTIS, Edward (1838-1912) and Thomas E. SATTERWAITE
Report of investigations into the pathogeny of diphtheria. [New York, 1876.] 56p. DNLM; NNNAM **70-0792**

CURTIS, T[homas] B. (1842-1881)
Recent progress in genito-urinary surgery. Cambridge, 1878. 14p. DNLM **70-0793**

CURTIS, T[homas] B. (1842-1881)
A new apparatus for fractures of the leg. Cambridge, 1878. 4p. DNLM **70-0794**

CURWEN, John (1821-1901)
Report on the proper treatment of the insane. Philadelphia: Collins, 1870. 17p. DNLM **70-0795**

CURWEN, John (1821-1901)
Report on mental disorders. Philadelphia: Collins, 1875. 12p. DNLM **70-0796**

CURWEN, John (1821-1901)
History of the Association of Medical Superintendents of American Institutions for the Insane, from 1844 to 1874, inclusive; with a list of the different hospitals for the insane, and the names and dates of appointment and resignation of the medical superintendents. Harrisburg: T. F. Scheffer, 1875. 121p. DNLM; PPC **70-0797**

CURWEN, John (1821-1901)
An appeal for the insane poor in the county poor-houses in Pennsylvania. [Harrisburg, 1876.] 11p. DNLM **70-0798**

CURWEN, John (1821-1901)
Address in mental disorders. Philadelphia: Collins, 1877. 28p. DNLM **70-0799**

CURWEN, John (1821-1901)
Report on the care of the insane. Philadelphia: Collins, 1878. 20p. DNLM **70-0800**

CUSHING, Alvin Matthew (*b.* 1829)
Leucorrhoea, its concomitant symptoms, and its homoeopathic treatment. . . . Lynn, Mass.: T. P. Nichols, printer, 1872. 70p. DLC; MBM **70-0801**

CUTTER, Calvin (1807-1872)
Second book on analytic anatomy, physiology and hygiene, human and comparative. . . . With numerous illustrations. Philadelphia: J. B. Lippincott & Co., 1871. 310p. DLC; NN; NNC; PU **70-0802**

CUTTER, [Calvin] (1807-1872)
Questions, diagrams and illustrations for analytic study and recitation. Also for unific and synthetic review of Cutter's new analytic anatomy, physiology and hygiene, human and comparative. Philadelphia: J. B. Lippincott & Co., [1871]. 66p. DLC; MB; PP; PU **70-0803**

CUTTER, Calvin (1807-1872)
New analytic anatomy, physiology and hygiene, human and comparative. . . . With numerous engravings. Philadelphia: J. B. Lippincott & Co., 1871. 322p. DLC; PPC; PU **70-0804**

CUTTER, Calvin (1807-1872)
First book on analytic anatomy, physiology and hygiene, human and comparative. . . . with numerous engravings. Philadelphia: J. B. Lippincott & Co., 1872. 197p. DLC; PPC; PU **70-0805**

CUTTER, Calvin (1807-1872)
Second book on analytic anatomy, physiology and hygiene, human and comparative. For academies, grammar schools, and families. Philadelphia: J. B. Lippincott & Co., 1872. 310p. DNLM; PU **70-0806**

CUTTER, Calvin (1807-1872)
A treatise on anatomy, physiology, and hygiene. . . . With one hundred and fifty engravings. Rev. stereotype ed., Philadelphia: J. B. Lippincott & Co., 1874. 466p. DLC; MB; NN; PU **70-0807**

CUTTER, Ephraim (1832-1917)
Thyrotomy for the removal of laryngeal growths. Boston: J. Campbell, 1871. 30p. DLC; DNLM; MH-M **70-0808**

CUTTER, Ephraim (1832-1917)
A contribution to the treatment of the versions and flexions of the unimpregnated uterus. Boston: J. Campbell, 1871. 44p. DNLM; MBM **70-0809**

CUTTER, Ephraim (1832-1917)
Partial report on the production of vaccine virus in the United States. Philadelphia: Collins, 1872. 39p. DLC; DNLM; PPC **70-0810**

CUTTER, Ephraim (1832-1917)
Is flour our proper food? With some remarks upon the effect of animal food in consumption. . . . A lecture delivered before the N.H. State Medical Society, June 16, 1875. Concord, N.H.: Printed by the Republican Press Association, 175. 36p. DLC; DNLM; NNNAM **70-0811**

CUTTER, Ephraim (1832-1917)
New electrodes and battery for electrolysis of uterine fibroids. [Boston, 1876.] 8p. DNLM **70-0812**

CUTTER, Ephraim (1832-1917)
A contribution to the treatment of uterine versions and flexions. . . . 2nd ed., entirely rewritten. Boston: J. Campbell, 1876. 216p. DLC; DNLM; MBM **70-0813**

CUTTER, Ephraim (1832-1917)
Salisbury's new physical sign of syphilis. [Baltimore, 1879.] 12p. DNLM **70-0814**

CUTTER, Ephraim (1832-1917)
Primer of the clinical microscope. Boston optical works. . . . Boston: C. Stodder, 1879. 24p. DLC; DNLM; MH-M **70-0815**

CUTTER, George Rogers (1840-1891)
A dictionary of the German terms used in medicine. New York: G. P. Putnam's Sons, 1879. 304p. DLC; DNLM; NN; RPB **70-0816**

DABNEY, Wm. C[ecil] (1849-1894)
The value of chemistry to the medical practitioner. Charlottesville: Chronicle Printing House,] 1873] . 57p. DNLM **70-0817**

DA COSTA, Jacob Mendes (1833-1900)
Medical diagnosis; with special reference to practical medicine. . . . 3rd ed. Philadelphia: J. B. Lippincott & Co., 1870. 844p. CtY-M; DNLM; NNNAM; PPC **70-0818**

DA COSTA, J[acob] Mendes (1833-1900)
Modern medicine: a lecture delivered October 7th, 1872. Introductory to the course at the Jefferson Medical College. . . . Philadelphia: J. B. Lippincott & Co., 1872. 38p. DLC; DNLM; PPJ **70-0819**

DA COSTA, Jacob Mendes (1833-1900)
. . . On strain and over-action of the heart. . . . Washington: Smithsonian Institution, 1874. 28p. DLC; DNLM **70-0820**

DA COSTA, Jacob Mendes (1833-1900)
Valedictory address to the graduating class of Jefferson Medical College, Philadelphia. Delivered March 11, 1874, at the Academy of Music. . . . Published by the class. Philadelphia: P. Madeira, 1874. 20, 4p. DLC; DNLM; PPJ
70-0821

DA COSTA, Jacob Mendes (1833-1900)
Respiratory percussion. [Philadelphia, 1875.] 10p. DNLM
70-0822

DA COSTA, Jacob Mendes (1833-1900)
Medical diagnosis, with special reference to practical medicine. A guide to the knowledge and discrimination of diseases. . . . Illustrated with engravings on wood. 4th ed., rev. Philadelphia: J. B. Lippincott & Co., 1876. 835p. DLC; NNNAM; OCIM; PPC **70-0823**

DA COSTA, Jacob Mendes (1833-1900)
Harvey and his discovery: a lecture delivered October 1st, 1878, introductory to the course at the Jefferson Medical College, by. . . . Philadelphia: J. B. Lippincott & Co., 1878. 45p. DLC; DNLM; PPJ **70-0824**

DA COSTA, Jacob Mendes (1833-1900)
Harvey and his discovery. . . . Philadelphia: J. B. Lippincott & Co., 1879. 57p. DLC; DNLM; PPJ **70-0825**

DAKE, Jabez Philander (1827-1894)
Acute diseases and their homoeopathic treatment; also directions for the treatment of injuries received by accident and from poisons. 2nd family ed., carefully rev. and enl. Nashville: William Gamble & Co., 1871. 130p. PPHa
70-0826

DAKE, Jabez Philander (1827-1894)
Medical legislation. No state medicine and no sectarian health boards. Report of the committee on legislation to the American Institute of Homoeopathy at its twenty-eighth session, held at Put-in-Bay, O., June 15, 16, 17, 18, 1875. Philadelphia: Sherman & Co., 1876. 14p. DNLM
70-0827

DAKE, J[abez] Philander (1827-1894)
Medicinal forces, as a distinct class in nature. A paper presented at the late meeting of the American Association for the Advancement of Science, at Nashville, and declined by the publishing committee, as "not appropriate." . . . Philadelphia: Sherman & Co., [1877]. 9p. DLC **70-0828**

DAKE, Jabez Philander (1827-1894)
The science of therapeutics in outline; a systematic arrangement of principles concerned in the care of human health, showing their several departments. Nashville: Tavel, Eastman & Howell, 1878. 46p. DNLM; OCIM **70-0829**

DAKE, Jabez Philander (1827-1894)
The yellow fever and the American Public Health Association. What shall we expect from the investigation? [Nashville, Tenn.: Mayfield, Patton & Truett, 1878.] 8p. DNLM
70-0830

DAKE, William Church
Diphtheria: its pathology and treatment; a report of one hundred and seventy-six cases, treated, during a period of eleven months. Nashville: Wheeler Bros., 1877. 55p. DNLM; PPHa **70-0831**

DALTON, John Call (1825-1889)
Trichina spiralis; a lecture. New York: William Wood & Co., [1870]. 4p. 1 plate. DNLM **70-0832**

DALTON, John Call (1825-1889)
A treatise on human physiology. . . . 5th ed., rev. and enl. . . . Philadelphia: Henry C. Lea, 1871. 728p. DLC; NN; NcD; PPC
70-0833

DALTON, John Call (1825-1889)
Sugar formation in the liver. [Read before the New York Academy of Medicine.] [New York, 1871.] 19p. DNLM; NNNAM **70-0834**

DALTON, John Call (1825-1889)
Memorial of Edward B. Dalton, M.D. . . . New York, 1872. 49p. DLC; NNNAM **70-0835**

DALTON, John Call (1825-1889)
Spontaneous generation. The substance of two lectures delivered in the College of Physicians and Surgeons, New York, January 12 and 13. New York: D. Appleton & Co., 1872. 42p. DNLM; NNNAM **70-0836**

DALTON, John Call (1825-1889)
Galen and Paracelsus. . . . New York: D. Appleton & Co., 1873. 29p. DLC; NNNAM **70-0837**

DALTON, John Call (1825-1889)
On the spectrum of bile. New York: D. Appleton & Co., 1874. 22p. DNLM; NNNAM **70-0838**

DALTON, John C[all] (1825-1889)
The origin and propagation of disease. An anniversary discourse, delivered before the New York Academy of Medicine, November 20, 1873. . . . New York: D. Appleton & Co., 1874. 30p. DLC; DNLM; NNNAM **70-0839**

DALTON, John Call (1825-1889)
Experimentation on animals, as a means of knowledge in physiology, pathology, and practical medicine. New York: F. W. Christern, 1875. 71p. DNLM; NNNAM; NNU-M
70-0840

DALTON, John Call (1825-1889)
A treatise on physiology and hygiene. . . . With illustrations. New York: Harper & Bros., 1875. 424p. DLC; MA; MWA; PPC **70-0841**

DALTON, John Call (1825-1889)
A treatise on human physiology. . . . 6th ed. . . . Philadelphia: Henry C. Lea, 1875. 830p. MBM; NNNAM; PPC; PU
70-0842

DALTON, John Call (1825-1889)
Experimental production of anesthesia by cerebral compression. New York: D. Appleton & Co., 1876. 10p. DNLM
70-0843

DALTON, John Call (1825-1889)
Report on the corpus luteum. Boston: Houghton, Osgood & Co., 1878. 50p. 4 plates. DNLM; MBM
70-0844

DALTON, John Call (1825-1889)
A treatise on physiology and hygiene; for schools, families, and colleges. . . . New York: Harper Brothers, 1878. 424p. DLC; NN; NNC; PP **70-0845**

DAMON, Howard F. (1833-1884)
Photographs of skin diseases, taken from life. Boston: J. Campbell, 1870. 26p. DNLM; MBM **70-0846**

DANA, Israel Thorndike (1827-1904)
History of the Portland School for Medical Instruction. An address at the dedication of the new school rooms. With the remarks of Hon. Israel Washburn, Jr., Hon. W. W. Thomas, Jr., Dr. Alfred Mitchell, Rev. E. Y. Hincks. Portland: S. Berry, 1874. 33p. DNLM **70-0847**

DANFORTH, I. N. (1835-1911)
The lesions of cholera. A report founded on two cases. Chicago, 1874. 14p. DNLM **70-0848**

DANIELS, Henry A.
Surgical tracts for the people; anal and rectal diseases; diseases of the genito-urinary organs; deformities of the eyes, nose, and face. New York, 1870. 52p. DNLM; NNNAM **70-0849**

DANIELS, Henry A.
Books on stricture, fistula, piles, impotence; diseases of the genito-urinary organs; deformity of the eyes, nose, and face. New York, 1873. 52p. DNLM **70-0850**

DANIELS, Henry A.
Curious marriages and instances of longevity. New York: Lange, Little & Hillman, 1873. 150p. DNLM; NN **70-0851**

DARBY, John Thompson (1836-1879)
Hair as a suture and ligature. Louisville, Ky.: Bell & Co., 1870. 20p. DNLM **70-0852**

DAVIES, Thomas
The preparation and mounting of microscopic objects. New York: William Wood & Co., 1870. 144p. DNLM; NNNAM; PPC **70-0853**

DAVIES, Thomas
The preparation and mounting of microscopic objects. Ed. by John Matthews. 2nd ed. New York: William Wood & Co., 1874. 214p. MBM; NNNAM; PPC; PU **70-0854**

[DAVIS, Andrew Jackson] (1826-1910)
Mental disorders; or, Diseases of the brain and nerves, developing the origin and philosophy of mania, insanity, and crime, with full directions for their treatment and cure. By the author of "The physician," [etc.]. Special edition. New York: American News Company; Philadelphia, Pa.: The Central News Company; [etc., etc.], 1871. 487p. DLC; DNLM; PP; PPC **70-0855**

DAVIS, C[harles] H[enry] S[tanley]
Clergyman's sore throat. (Chronic follicular pharyngitis.) Buffalo: Baker, Jones & Co., 1879. 7p. DNLM **70-0856**

DAVIS, C[harles] H[enry] S[tanley]
Is consumption a preventable disease? [Richmond, 1879.] 7p. DNLM **70-0857**

DAVIS, F[rank] H[oward] (1848-1880)
Liebig's extract of malt and its chemical composition, manufacture, and therapeutical uses. Philadelphia: Collins, 1876. 8p. DNLM **70-0858**

DAVIS, F[rank] H[oward] (1848-1880)
A study of nine hundred and sixty-five cases of chronic pulmonary disease. Philadelphia: Collins, 1877. 10p. DNLM; PPC **70-0859**

DAVIS, George S.
An explanation by the publisher . . . of the nature, scope, form, and method of preparation of the Index Medicus. Editors: Dr. John S. Billings and Dr. Robert Fletcher. Detroit, Mich., [1879]. 24p. DNLM **70-0860**

DAVIS, J. C.
Microscopical studies on abscess of the liver. New York: G. P. Putnam's Sons, 1879. 12p. 1 plate. DNLM **70-0861**

DAVIS, Nathan Smith (1817-1904)
Clinical lectures on various important diseases; being a collection of the clinical lectures delivered in the medical wards of Mercy Hospital, Chicago. Edited by Frank H. Davis. Chicago: J. J. Spalding, 1873. 262p. DLC; DNLM; ICRM; IU-M **70-0862**

DAVIS, Nathan Smith (1817-1904)
Clinical lectures on various important diseases; being a collection of the clinical lectures delivered in the medical wards of Mercy Hospital, Chicago. Edited by Frank H. Davis. 2nd ed. Philadelphia: Henry C. Lea, 1874. 283p. DNLM; NNNAM; PPC; PU **70-0863**

DAVIS, Nathan Smith (1817-1904)
Address on the progress of medical education in the United States of America, during the century commencing in 1776. Delivered before the International Medical Congress, at Philadelphia. September 9, 1876. . . . Philadelphia: [Collins, printer], 1876. 23p. DLC; PPC **70-0864**

DAVIS, Nathan Smith (1817-1904)
Contributions to the history of medical education and medical institutions in the United States of America. 1776-1876. Special report. Prepared for the United States Bureau of Education. . . . Washington: Government Printing Office, 1877. 60p. DLC; DNLM; NNNAM; PPC **70-0865**

DAVIS, Nathan Smith (1817-1904)
Some thoughts concerning the origin and spread of yellow fever, and the means of preventing it. . . . Baltimore: J. H. Foster & Co., 1878. 15p. DLC; MdU-D **70-0866**

DAVIS, R.
Address in obstetrics. Philadelphia: Collins, 1876. 22p. DNLM **70-0867**

DAVIS, William Bramwell (1832-1893)
Report on vaccination [to] Ohio State Medical Society. [Cleveland, 1870.] 36p. DNLM **70-0868**

DAVIS, William Bramwell (1832-1893)
An inquiry into the mortality from consumption in life insurance. Cincinnati, 1875. 17p. DNLM **70-0869**

DAVIS, William Bramwell (1832-1893)
Report on vaccination, read before the Ohio State Medical Society . . . being an inquiry concerning human vaccine, vaccino-syphilis and animal vaccine, with an appendix. Cincinnati: A. H. Pounsford & Co., 1876. 32p. DNLM **70-0870**

DAWSON, B[enjamin] F[rederick] (1847-1888)
A new ovariotomy clamp. Also applicable for other surgical purposes. [New York, 1871.] 6p. 1 fig. DNLM
70-0871

DAWSON, B[enjamin] F[rederick] (1847-1888)
On vascular naevi and their treatment by the actual cautery. [New York, 1871.] 20p. DNLM **70-0872**

DAWSON, B[enjamin] F[rederick] (1847-1888)
The treatment of whooping-cough with quinine. New York: William Wood & Co., 1873. 14p. DNLM; NNNAM
70-0873

DAWSON, B[enjamin] F[rederick] (1847-1888)
Report of a case of inversio uteri of two years' standing, reduced by taxis; with remarks. New York: D. Appleton & Co., 1875. 8p. DNLM; NNNAM **70-0874**

DAWSON, B[enjamin] F[rederick] (1847-1888)
Alimentation and its gastro-intestinal disorders of infants and young children. New York: William Wood & Co., 1875. 22p. DNLM; NNNAM **70-0875**

DAWSON, William Wirt (1828-1893)
Chloroform deaths. Twelve unpublished cases. Comparison between chloroform and other anaesthetics. Cincinnati: R. Clark & Co., [1871?]. 34p. DNLM; OCIM
70-0876

DAWSON, William Wirt (1828-1893)
State Medical Society of Ohio. Annual address of the retiring president. Cincinnati, 1872. 20p. DNLM; OCIM
70-0877

DAY, Albert (*d.* 1894)
The disease of inebriety. [Circular announcing the establishment of Greenwood Institute, Feb. 22, 1872.] [Boston, 1872.] 2 l. DNLM **70-0878**

DAY, Albert (*d.* 1894)
Washingtonian Home, Boston. [Circular announcing the opening of the new building.] [Boston, 1875.] 2 l. DNLM
70-0879

DAY, Albert (*d.* 1894)
Inebriety and its cure. Boston: C. W. Calkins & Co., 1877. 18p. DNLM; MB **70-0880**

DAY, Albert (*d.* 1894)
The curability of inebriety. Hartford, Conn.: Lockwood & Brainard Co., 1878. 24p. DNLM **70-0881**

DEAN, Amos (1803-1868)
Principles of medical jurisprudence: designed for the professions of law and medicine. . . . New York, Albany: Banks & Brothers, 1877. 664p. DLC; MBM; NNNAM
70-0882

DEAN, Richard C.
Naval medical schools of France and England, with observations on the naval hospitals of Toulon. Washington: Government Printing Office, 1876. 94p. 9 plates. DNLM
70-0883

DEANE, C. F.
Valedictory delivered at Toland Medical College. San Francisco: E. Bosqui & Co., 1871. 17p. DNLM
70-0884

[DEBILITY]
The causes, prevention and cure of debility, including consumption, dyspepsia, nervous disorders, &c. giving sure and simple methods of self treatment, by means within reach of all at no expense. Showing how to build up vigorous constitutions and overcome tendencies to disease. . . . New York: J. Haney & Co., [1870]. 158p. DLC; NNNAM **70-0885**

DEECKE, Theodore (1836-1905)
On the treatment of chronic catarrh of the bladder and of some forms of acute cystitis. Buffalo: Baker, Jones & Co., 1879. 7p. DNLM **70-0886**

DEECKE, Theodore (1836-1905)
Urea and phosphoric acid in the urine in anaemia. [Utica, N.Y., 1879.] 24p. DNLM **70-0887**

DEECKE, Theodore (1836-1905)
The structure of the vessels of the nervous centers in health, and their changes in disease. Pts. 1-6. [Utica, 1879-81.] 82p. DNLM; NNNAM **70-0888**

DE HART, J[ohn] N.
Practical hygiene, as it relates to a proper water supply, and the defective sewerage of cities and towns, hospitals, and asylums. Chicago: Bull. Print. Co., 1879. 13p. DNLM
70-0889

DELAFIELD, Francis (1841-1915)
Tumors of the retina. New York: William Wood & Co., 1871. 13p. 2 plates. DNLM; NNNAM **70-0890**

DELAFIELD, Francis (1841-1915)
A hand-book of post-mortem examinations and of morbid anatomy. . . . New York: William Wood & Co., 172. 376p. DLC; DNLM; NNNAM; PPC **70-0891**

DELAFIELD, Francis (1841-1915)
Some forms of dyspepsia. New York: G. P. Putnam's Sons, 1876. 14p. DNLM; NNNAM **70-0892**

DELAFIELD, Francis (1841-1915) and Charles F. STILLMAN
A manual of physical diagnosis. New York: William Wood & Co., 1878. 30p. [interleaved]. 3 plates. DNLM; NNNAM; OCIM; PU **70-0893**

DELAFIELD, Francis (1841-1915)
Studies in pathological anatomy. New York: William Wood & Co., 1878-1891. 2 v. [v. 1; v. 2, pts. 1-4; 126p., 93 plates; 90+ p., 133 plates]. DNLM; MH-M; NNNAM; PPC
70-0894

DE MARMON, Paluel
Report of three cases of poisoning by whiskey in children, with remarks on alcoholism. New York: D. Appleton & Co., 1870. 23p. DNLM; NNNAM **70-0895**

DE MARMON, Paluel
Medico-legal considerations upon alcoholism, and the moral and criminal responsibility of inebriates. . . . New York: W. Baldwin & Co., 1872. 24p. DLC; DNLM; NNNAM
70-0896

DENISON, Charles (1845-1909)
The best welfare of invalids seeking the benefits of climate, with suggestions for the co-operation of physicians, life insurance officials, etc. [Denver, Col., 1875.] 11p. DNLM
70-0897

DENISON, Charles (1845-1909)
The extension windlass, an extension and adjusting apparatus, a device especially adapted for treatment of fracture of the patella, for making extension of joints, for use in the treatment of certain difficult fractures, and as a tourniquet. Boston: Codman & Shurtleff, 1875. 10p. DNLM **70-0898**

DENISON, Charles (1845-1909)
The extension windlass, an extension and adjusting apparatus, a device especially adapted for treatment of fracture of the patella, for making extension of joints, for use in the treatment of certain difficult fractures, and as a tourniquet. Presented to the American Medical Association, May, 1975. New York: D. Appleton & Co., 1875. 11p. DNLM; NNNAM **70-0899**

DENISON, Charles (1845-1909)
The influence of the climate of Colorado on the nervous system. . . . Denver, Col.: Richards, 1875. 16p. DLC **70-0900**

DENISON, Charles (1845-1909)
Report on the climate of Colorado, and its relation to pulmonary diseases. Philadelphia: Collins, 1876. 21p. DNLM **70-0901**

DENISON, Charles (1845-1909)
The influence of high altitudes on the progress of phthisis. . . . Philadelphia, 1877. 39p. DLC **70-0902**

DENNIS, Frederic S[hepard] (1850-1934)
On the treatment of amputations by the open method. New York: D. Appleton & Co., 1876. 21p. DNLM; NNNAM **70-0903**

D'EPISY, Gilbert
A medical declaration of war: one against many, for the sake and benefit of all; addressed to the empirical members of all the medical faculties of the world. St. Louis: C. H. Lamoreaux, 1871. 7p. DNLM **70-0904**

DERBY, Hasket (1835-1914)
The modern operation for cataract. A lecture delivered at the Harvard Medical School, April 5, 1871. With an analysis of sixty-one operations. Boston, 1871. 23p. 2 plates. DNLM; MH-M **70-0905**

DERBY, Hasket (1835-1914)
Near-sighted—treated by atropia. New York, 1875. 8p. 8 tab. DNLM **70-0906**

DERBY, Hasket (1835-1914)
I. A report on the percentage of near-sight found to exist in the class of 1880 at Harvard College, with some account of similar investigations. II. An account of the phakometer of Snellen. Cambridge, 1877. 9p. 1 plate. DNLM; MH-M **70-0907**

DERBY, Richard H[enry] (1844-1907)
Color-blindness, and its acquisition through the abuse of alcohol and tobacco. New York: D. Appleton & Co., 1871. 9p. DNLM **70-0908**

DERBY, Richard H[enry] (1844-1907)
Progressive myopia and its operative cure. New York: D. Appleton & Co., 1873. 18p. DNLM **70-0909**

DESICCATED blood for rectal alimentation, and other literature on the subject of alimentation per rectum. Detroit, Mich.: Parke, Davis & Co., [1879]. 57p. 1 plate DNLM **70-0910**

DETMOLD, William Ludwig (1808-1894)
Facial paralysis treated by a new method. New York: D. Appleton & Co., 1873. 7p. DNLM **70-0911**

DEWEES, William B[ushy] (1854-1912)
An essay on means of lessening the sufferings of parturition. [Salina, Kansas, 1877.] 26p. DNLM **70-0912**

DEWEY, B. M.
Special hygienic and medical information for parents, embracing health and diseases of the reproductive organs, urinary apparatus, recum, diseases of childhood, everyday emergencies, household recipes, and common disorders and what to do. With copious index and glossary. . . . Chicago: Knight & Leonard, printers, 1878. 319p. DLC **70-0913**

DICKSON, Samuel Henry (1798-1872)
Lecture introductory to the course of Jefferson Medical College for the session, 1870-1871. Philadelphia, 1870. 27p. DNLM; PPJ **70-0914**

DIDAMA, Henry D.
The model physician. A valedictory address. Syracuse, N.Y.: Truair, Smith & Co., 1875. 16p. DNLM **70-0915**

DIXON, Edward H. (1808-1880)
The kidney; its structure, functions, and diseases; Bright's disease; the urine. . . . New York: J. S. Redfield, 1871. 45p. DLC; DNLM; NNNAM **70-0916**

DOANE, Charles Russell (1840-1884)
Our valedictory. College of Physicians and Surgeons, Medical Department of Columbia College. Class of 1872. [New York, 1872.] 2 l. DNLM **70-0917**

DOANE, William C.
Annual address before the Homoeopathic Medical Society of Pennsylvania. Philadelphia: Senseman & Son, 1871. 32p. DNLM; PPHa **70-0918**

DOBELL, Horace (1828-1917)
On coughs, consumption, and diet in disease. . . . Philadelphia: D. G. Brinton, 1877. 222p. DLC; DNLM; PPC; PU **70-0919**

DOE, O[rlando] W[itherspoon] (1843-1890)
The efficacy of cold-water treatment in typhoid fever. [Boston, 1876.] 6p. DNLM; MBM **70-0920**

DOLE, John (1838-1872)
The practical aspects of medical science. Boston, 1871. 20p. DNLM **70-0921**

DOLLEY, Sarah R. A.
Closing lecture to the class of 1873-1874, delivered at the Woman's Medical College of Pennsylvania, March 5th, 1874. [Philadelphia, 1874.] 8p. DNLM **70-0922**

DONALDSON, Francis (1823-1891)
Thirty-seven operations of thoracentesis by pneumatic aspiration. Baltimore: Innes & Co., 1876. 8p. DNLM **70-0923**

DONALDSON, Francis (1823-1891)
The influence of city life and occupations in developing pulmonary consumption. A discourse delivered before the American Health Association, October, 1875. Cambridge: Riverside Press, 1876. 20p. DNLM; MH-M
70-0924

DONALDSON, F[rancis] (1823-1891)
House-air the cause and promoter of disease. Baltimore: Innes & Co., 1878. 23p. DNLM **70-0925**

DOUGHERTY, Alexander N. (1820-1883)
Observations (historical and clinical) on glycosuria. Newark, N.J.: L. J. Hardham, 1878. 70p. DNLM
70-0926

DOUGHTY, William H[enry] (1836-1905)
The primary conversion of occipito-posterior into occipito-anterior positions of the vertex; with cases illustrating the practice. New York: William Wood & Co., 1878. 14p. DNLM; NNNAM **70-0927**

DOWELL, Greensville (1822-1881)
Original contributions to surgery, with inventions of instruments, and new operative procedures. . . . [Galveston? 187-] 12p. DLC; DNLM **70-0928**

DOWELL, Greensville (1822-1881)
Yellow fever and malarial diseases embracing a history of the epidemics of yellow fever in Texas: new views on its diagnosis, treatment, propagation and control. . . . Philadelphia: Medical Publication Office, 1876. 244p. tables, 2 plates. DLC; DNLM; PPC; PU **70-0929**

DOWELL, Greensville (1822-1881)
A treatise on hernia: with a new process for its radical cure, and original contributions to operative surgery, and new surgical instruments. . . . Philadelphia: D. G. Brinton, 1876. 206p. DLC; DNLM; PPC; PPJ **70-0930**

DOWLING, J[ohn] W[illiam] (1837-1892)
Annual address before the New York State Homoeopathic Medical Society, delivered in the assembly chamber at Albany, Feb. 11, 1873. New York: Carle & Grener, 1873. 19p. DNLM **70-0931**

DOWSE, Thomas Stretch
The brain and its diseases. Pt. I. Syphilis of the brain and spinal cord, showing the part which this agent plays in the production of paralysis, epilepsy, insanity, headache, neuralgia, hysteria, hypochondriasis, and other mental and nervous derangements. New York: G. P. Putnam's Sons, 1879. 144p. 5 plates. DNLM; NNNAM; PU **70-0932**

DRAKE, Daniel (1785-1852)
Pioneer life in Kentucky. A series of reminiscential letters from Daniel Drake . . . to his children. Edited with notes and a biographical sketch by his son, Charles D. Drake. Cincinnati: R. Clarke & Co., 1870. 263p. DLC; DNLM; OCIM; PPC
70-0933

DRAPER, John C[hristopher] (1835-1885)
The heat produced in the body, and the effects of exposure to cold. [New Haven, 1872.] 5p. DNLM
70-0934

DRAPER, John William (1811-1882)
Human physiology, statistical and dynamical; or, the conditions and course of the life of man. New York: Harper & Brothers, 1870. 649, 4p. 294 fig. DNLM; NN; NNC; NNNAM
70-0935

DRAPER, John William (1811-1882)
History of the conflict between religion and science. New York: D. Appleton & Co., 1875. 373p. DNLM; MB; NIC; NN
70-0936

DRAPER, John William (1811-1882)
Scientific memoirs, being experimental contributions to a knowledge of radiant energy. New York: Harper & Brothers, 1878. 473p. 1 plate. DNLM; ICU; MB; NN
70-0937

DRAPER, Joseph (1824-1892)
The responsibility of the insane in asylums. Utia, 1879. 17p. DNLM **70-0938**

DRAPER, William Henry (1830-1901)
On the nature of the gouty vice. New York: G. P. Putnam's Sons, 1875. 32p. DNLM; NNNAM **70-0939**

DRAPER, William Henry (1830-1901)
Memorial of Foster Swift, read before the New York Medical and Surgical Society. New York, 1875. 5p. DNLM
70-0940

DRESS and care of the feet. . . . New York: Samuel R. Wells, 1871. 202p. NNNAM **70-0941**

DREWRY, George Overend
Common-sense management of the stomach. New York: Dodd & Mead, [1875]. 138p. DNLM; NNNAM
70-0942

DROMGOOLE, John Parham
Dr. Dromgoole's yellow fever heroes, honors, and horrors of 1878. A list of over ten thousand victims, martyr death-roll of volunteer physicians, nurses, etc. . . . Thomas D. Osborne, assistant. With ninety-six resident correspondents. Louisville, [Ky.]: Printed by J. P. Morton & Co., 1879. 176p. DLC
70-0943

DRUMMOND, William Hamilton (1778-1865)
Love of science perverted. Vivisection. Philadelphia: W. Kildare, 1870. 22p. DNLM **70-0944**

DUDLEY, J. G.
Alcohol; its combinations, adulterations and physical effects. New York: G. P. Putnam's Sons, 1874. 68p. DNLM
70-0945

DUDLEY, Pemberton (1837-1907)
Directory of the homoeopathic physicians of the State of Pennsylvania. . . . Presented by the Mutual Life Insurance Company, of New York. Philadelphia: Jackson, 1874. 16p. DNLM; PPHa **70-0946**

DUDLEY, Pemberton (1837-1907)
Directory of homoeopathic physicians residing in New Jersey, Pennsylvania, Delaware, Maryland, and District of Columbia. 2nd ed. Philadelphia, 1875. 13p. DNLM; PPHa
70-0947

DUHRING, Louis Adolphus (1845-1913)
Pathology of alopecia areata. [Philadelphia, 1870.] 4p. DNLM
70-0948

DUHRING, Louis Adolphus (1845-1913)
On the study of dermatology. New York: F. W. Christern, 1871. 6 l. DNLM **70-0949**

DUHRING, Louis Adolphus (1845-1913)
Case of painful neuroma of the skin. Philadelphia: Collins, 1873. 11p. DNLM **70-0950**

DUHRING, Louis Adolphus (1845-1913)
Pruritus hiemalis; an undescribed form of pruritus. Philadelphia: J. B. Lippincott & Co., 1874. 20p. DNLM; PPC
70-0951

DUHRING, Louis Adolphus (1845-1913)
Atlas of skin diseases. . . . Philadelphia: J. B Lippincott & Co., 1876[-81]. 76p. 30 col. plates. DLC; DNLM; NNNAM; PPC
70-0952

DUHRING, Louis Adolphus (1845-1913)
Case of a bearded woman. New York: G. P. Putnam's Sons, 1877. 10p. DNLM **70-0953**

DUHRING, Louis Adolphus (1845-1913)
A practical treatise on diseases of the skin. . . . Philadelphia: J. B. Lippincott & Co., 1877. 618p. DLC; DNLM; NNNAM; PPC **70-0954**

DUHRING, Louis Adolphus (1845-1913)
A case of tinea tricophytina unguium. [Philadelphia, 1878.] 4p. DNLM **70-0955**

DUHRING, Louis Adolphus (1845-1913)
Case of an undescribed form of atrophy of the hair of the beard. [Philadelphia, 1878.] 5p. DNLM **70-0956**

DUHRING, Louis Adolphus (1845-1913)
A case of the so-called xeroderma (or parchment skin) of Hebra. [Philadelphia, 1878.] 7p. DNLM
70-0957

DUHRING, Louis Adolphus (1845-1913)
A case of inflammatory fungoid neoplasm. Philadelphia: J. B. Lippincott & Co., 1879. 28p. 3 plates. DNLM; PPC; PPJ
70-0958

DULLES, Charles Winslow (1850-1921)
Supra-pubic lithotomy. New York: D. Appleton & Co., 1878. 9p. DNLM **70-0959**

DULLES, Charles Winslow (1850-1921)
What is a chancre? [Philadelphia, 1879.] 5p. DNLM
70-0960

DUNCAN, Thomas Cation
How to be plump: or Talks on physiological feeding. . . . Chicago: Duncan Brothers, 1878. 60p. DLC
70-0961

DUNCAN, Thomas Cation, ed.
Diseases of infants and children, with their homoeopathic treatment. . . . Chicago: Duncan Bros., 1878-1880. 2 v. PPHa; OCIM **70-0962**

DUNGLISON, Richard James (1834-1901)
The public medical libraries of Philadelphia. . . . Philadelphia: J. B. Lippincott & Co., 1871. 46p. DLC; DNLM; PPC; PU
70-0963

DUNGLISON, Richard James (1834-1901)
The ready reference list for physicians. Philadelphia, 1876. 54p. DNLM; PPC; PPJ; PU **70-0964**

DUNGLISON, Richard James (1834-1901)
The practitioner's reference book. Adapted to the use of the physician, the pharmacist, and the student. . . . Philadelphia: Lindsay & Blakiston, 1877. 341p. DLC; DNLM; NNNAM; PPC
70-0965

DUNGLISON, Robley (1798-1869)
History of medicine from the earliest ages to the commencement of the nineteenth century. Arranged and ed. by Richard J. Dunglison, M.D. Philadelphia: Lindsay & Blakiston, 1872. 287p. DLC; DNLM; NNNAM; PU
70-0966

DUNGLISON, Robley (1798-1869)
. . . Catalogue of valuable medical library of the late Prof. Robley Dunglison . . . to be sold at public sale . . . October 31st and November 1st, 1872 . . . Davis & Harvey, auct'rs. . . . [Philadelphia: Selheimer, printer, 1872]. 38p. DLC; DNLM; PPC; PU **70-0967**

DUNGLISON, Robley (1798-1869)
Medical lexicon; a dictionary of medical science. Containing a concise explanation of the various subjects and terms of anatomy, physiology, pathology, hygiene, therapeutics, pharmacology, pharmacy, surgery, obstetrics, medical jurisprudence and dentistry; notices of climate and of mineral waters; formulae for officinal, empirical and dietetic preparations; with the accentuation and etymology of the terms, and the French and other synonyms, so as to constitute a French as well as an English medical lexicon. A new edition. Thoroughly revised and very greatly modified and augmented by Richard J. Dunglison, M.D. Philadelphia: Henry C. Lea, 1874. 1139p. DLC; MBM; OCIM; PPC
70-0968

DUNHAM, Carroll (1828-1877)
Valedictory address to the graduating class of the New York Homoeopathic Medical College, delivered in Association Hall, New York, February 29, 1872. New York: Francis Hart & Co., 1872. 15p. NNNAM; PPHa **70-0969**

DUNHAM, Carroll (1828-1877)
Address before the World's Homoeopathic Convention of 1876. Delivered at Philadelphia, Monday, June 26, 1876. Philadelphia: Sherman & Co., 1876. 15p. PPHa
70-0970

DUNHAM, Carroll (1828-1877)
Homoeopathy the science of therapeutics. A collection of papers elucidating and illustrating the principles of homoeopathy. New York: Francis Hart & Co., 1877. 529p. DLC; PPHa **70-0971**

DUNHAM, Carroll (1828-1877)
Lectures on materia medica. New York: F. Hart & Co., 1878. 2 v. DLC; PPHa **70-0972**

DUNHAM, William Russell (*b.* 1833)
Theory of medical science. The doctrine of an inherent power in medicine a fallacy. The ultimate special properties of vitality and the laws of vital force constitute the fundamental basis of medical philosophy and science. . . . Boston: J. Campbell, 1876. 150p. DLC; MBM; NNNAM **70-0973**

DUNMAN, Thomas (1849-1882)
A glossary of biological, anatomical, and physiological terms. . . . New York: D. Appleton & Co., 1879. 161p. DLC; NNNAM; PU **70-0974**

DUNN, James B. (1822?-1895)
A memorial sermon upon the life and character of Sir James Y. Simpson, the Christian physician. Boston: J. Campbell, 1870. 27p. DNLM; MH; MBM **70-0975**

DUNSTER, Edward Swift (1834-1888)
The relations of the medical profession to modern education. An address delivered at the commencement of the medical department of the University of Vermont, June 16, 1869. New York: D. Appleton & Co., 1870. 25p. DNLM; NNNAM **70-0976**

DUNSTER, Edward Swift (1834-1888)
The logic of medicine. An address delivered on the occasion of the twenty-fifth anniversary of the New York Academy of Medicine, December 30, 1872. . . . New York: D. Appleton & Co., 1873. 31p. DLC; DNLM; NNNAM **70-0977**

DUNSTER, Edward Swift (1834-1888)
Remarks on double monsters. [Ann Arbor, 1874.] 13p. DNLM **70-0978**

DUNSTER, Edward Swift (1834-1888)
The history of anaesthesia. Ann Arbor: Fiske & Douglas, 1875. 20p. DNLM **70-0979**

DUNSTER, Edward Swift (1834-1888)
The history of spontaneous generation. Ann Arbor, 1876. 30p. DNLM **70-0980**

DUNSTER, Edward Swift (1834-1888)
The use of obstetric forceps in abbreviating the second stage of labor. Lansing: W. S. George & Co., 1877. 33p. DNLM; OCIM **70-0981**

DUNSTER, Edward Swift (1834-1888)
The prophylaxis of puerperal convulsions. Toledo, 1878. 16p. DNLM **70-0982**

DUNSTER, Edward Swift (1834-1888)
A case of fracture of the humerus; death on the eighteenth day from fatty degeneration of the heart; with remarks on osteogenesis. [1879.] 6p. DNLM **70-0983**

DUNSTER, Edward Swift (1834-1888)
An argument made before the American Medical Association . . . against the proposed amendment to the code of ethics, restricting the teaching of students of irregular or exclusive systems of medicine. Ann Arbor, Mich.: Ann Arbor Printing & Publishing Co., 1879. 28p. DNLM **70-0984**

DURANT, Ghislani
Hygiene of the voice. Its physiology and anatomy. . . . A new and rev. ed. New York: Cassell, Petter, Galpin & Co., 1879. 188p. plates. DLC; NNNAM **70-0985**

DURKEE, Silas
Contributions to dermatology; eczema, impetigo, scabies, ecthyma, rupia, lupus. Boston: J. Campbell, 1870. 76p. DNLM; MH-M **70-0986**

DUTCHER, Addison Porter (1818-1884)
Pulmonary tuberculosis: its pathology, nature, symptoms, diagnosis, prognosis, causes, hygiene, and medical treatment. . . . Philadelphia: J. B. Lippincott & Co., 1875. 380p. DLC; NNNAM; PPC; PPJ **70-0987**

DWIGHT, Thomas, Jr. (1843-1911)
The action of the intercostal muscles. [Boston, 1873.] 8p. DNLM **70-0988**

DWIGHT, Thomas, Jr. (1843-1911)
The structure and action of striated muscular fibre. [Boston, 1873.] 10p. 1 plate. DNLM **70-0989**

DWIGHT, Thomas, Jr. (1843-1911)
The anatomy of the head, with plates representing frozen sections. Boston: H. G. Houghton & Co., 1876. 136p. 4 plates. DNLM; MH-M; NNNAM; PPC **70-0990**

DWIGHT, Thomas, Jr. (1843-1911)
The identification of the human skeleton. A medico-legal study. To which was awarded the prize of the Massachusetts Medical Society for 1878. Boston: D. Clapp & Sons, 1878. 54p. MH-M; MWA **70-0991**

EARLE, Charles Warrington (1845-1893)
Scarlatina in Chicago, particularly the epidemic of 1876-1877. Chicago: A. S. Kissell & Co., [1877]. 22p. DNLM; ICRM **70-0992**

EARLE, Charles Warrington (1845-1893)
The demand for a woman's medical college in the West. Waukegan, Ill., 1879. 13p. DNLM **70-0993**

EARLE, Pliny (1809-1892)
The curability of insanity. . . . Utica, N.Y.: E. H. Roberts & Co., printers, 1877. 52p. DLC; DNLM **70-0994**

EARLE, Pliny (1809-1892)
A glance at insanity and the management of the insane in the American states. . . . Read before the Conference of Charities, held at Chicago, Ill., June 10, 1879. Boston: Franklin Press, Rand, Avery & Co., 1879. 19p. DLC; DNLM **70-0995**

EASLEY, Edward Tandy (1842-1878)
Argument in favor of a contagious diseases act. Its present state. Louisville, Ky., 1876. 32p. DNLM **70-0996**

EASLEY, Edward Tandy (1842-1878)
A paper on surgery of the hand. Louisville, Ky., 1877. 25p. DNLM **70-0997**

EASSIE, William
Healthy houses. A handbook to the history, defects, and remedies of drainage, ventilation, warming, and kindred subjects. New York: D. Appleton & Co., 1872. 228p. DNLM; NN; PP; PU **70-0998**

EATON, Dorman B[ridgman] (1823-1899)
Sanitary regulations in England and New York: New York: J. W. Amerman, 1872. 46p. DNLM; NNNAM **70-0999**

EATON, Dorman B[ridgman] (1823-1899)
The essential conditions of good sanitary administration. Cambridge: Riverside Press, 1876. 17p. DNLM; MH-M
70-1000

EATON, Hosea Ballou (1822-1887)
Inaugural address read before the Maine Homoeopathic Medical Society. . . . Portland: B. Thurston & Co., 1870. 22p. 1 plate. DNLM; PPHa **70-1001**

ECKER, Alexander (1816-1887)
The cerebral convolutions of man, represented according to original observations, especially upon their development in the foetus. Intended for the use of physicians. . . . Transl. by Robert T. Edes, M.D. New York: D. Appleton & Co., 1873. 87p. DLC; NNNAM **70-1002**

EDES, Robert T[haxter] (1838-1923)
The treatment of typhoid fever by cold baths. [Boston, 1875.] 14p. DNLM **70-1003**

EDES, Robert T[haxter] (1838-1923)
A case of anterior spinal paralysis with formation of vacuoles in the ganglion cells of the spinal cord. Cambridge: Riverside Press, 1879. 5p. 1 plate. DNLM **70-1004**

EDGERTON, Joseph K[etchum] (1818-1893)
Education and the medical profession in Indiana. Address at the annual commencement of Fort Wayne Medical College. Fort Wayne, 1879. 12p. DNLM **70-1005**

AN EDITORIAL chameleon. [Addressed to physicians whose names appear in the medical register for 1872. A controversy occasioned by the advertisement of a graduate of the medical department of the University of the City of New York.] [New York, 1872.] 6p. DNLM
70-1006

EDMONDSON, George D.
Treatise on the art of fitting spectacles by test card, or grade of letters, for presbyopic or myopic vision; with mathematical tables of distances. . . . Detroit: O. S. Gulley, 1874. 4p. DLC
70-1007

EDMUNDS, James
The medical use of alcohol; and stimulants for women. . . . New York: National Temperance Society and Publication House, 1874. 96p. DLC; DNLM **70-1008**

EDWARDS, Arthur Mead
Notes on diatomaceae. Boston: A. A. Kingman, 1870. 14p. DNLM **70-1009**

EDWARDS, Arthur Mead
The microscope in gynaecology. Newark, N.J.: Jennings & Hardham, 1875. 23p. DNLM **70-1010**

EGGERT, William
Therapeutics of ovarian diseases. Chicago: Duncan Bros., 1878. 29p. DNLM **70-1011**

EGGERT, William
The homoeopathic treatment of prolapsus uteri. Chicago: Duncan Bros., 1878. 39p. DNLM **70-1012**

EGGERT, William
The homoeopathic therapeutics of uterine and vaginal discharges. . . . New York, Philadelphia: Boericke & Tafel, 1878. 543p. DLC; PPC; PPHa **70-1013**

ELA, Walter (*b.* 1848)
Fractures of the elbow joint. [Boylston prize essay.] Cambridge: Welch, Bigelow & Co., 1873. 57p. 1 plate. DNLM; MBM; MWA **70-1014**

ELDRIDGE, Stuart (1841?-1901)
On so-called hernia of the trachea, with a case of incomplete internal fistula of the trachea (or larynx), accompanied by the development of air sacs. [Philadelphia, 1879.] 9p. 1 plate. DNLM **70-1015**

ELIOT, Charles W. (1834-1926)
Address delivered before the American Academy of Dental Science. Cambridge: J. Wilson & Son, 1879. 30p. DNLM; MH
70-1016

ELIOT, Johnson (1815-1888), Herbert BOARDMAN and R. De L. FRENCH
Addresses delivered at the 23rd annual commencement of the medical department of Georgetown College. Washington: J. S. Tomlinson, 1872. 34p. DNLM **70-1017**

ELIOT, Johnson (1815-1888)
Simultaneous ligation of the carotid and subclavian arteries for aneurism of the arteria innominata. [Philadelphia, 1877.] 6p. DNLM **70-1018**

ELIOT, Johnson (1815-1888)
Palato-pharyngeal tumor. [Philadelphia, 1879.] 3p. DNLM
70-1019

ELLIOTT, [E.] H.
Dr. Elliott's pamphlet guide for mothers, or, A few diseases peculiar to women, with their treatment, being an auxiliary and appendix to the author's household guide map, or, what to use in illness or accident. Hartland, N.Y., 1870. 20p. DLC
70-1020

ELLIOTT, John B[arnwell] (1841-1921)
Prevention of disease; prophylaxis in person. New Orleans: L. Graham, 1879. 15p. DNLM; LNT-M
70-1021

ELLIS, Barnard
Generalized vaso-motor paralysis of the superior extremities. Transl. from the French. Columbus: Nevins & Myers, 1877. 17p. DNLM **70-1022**

ELLIS, Calvin (1826-1883)
Capillary bronchitis of adults. New York: G. P. Putnam's Sons, 1875. 36p. DNLM; NNNAM **70-1023**

ELLIS, Calvin (1826-1883)
Ulcerative endocarditis; embolism of the arteries of the left leg. [Boston, 1877.] 6p. DNLM **70-1024**

ELLIS, Edward
A practical manual of the diseases of children, with a formulary. 3rd ed. New York: William Wood & Co., 1879. 213p. DNLM; NNNAM; OCIM; PPC **70-1025**

ELLIS, George Viner (1812-1900)
Demonstrations of anatomy; being a guide to the knowledge of the human body by dissection. From the 8th and rev. English ed. Philadelphia: Henry C. Lea, 1879. 716p. DNLM; MBM; NNNAM; PPC **70-1026**

ELLIS, John (1815-1896)
The avoidable causes of disease, insanity, and deformity. 6th ed. New York: Boericke & Tafel, 1876. 348, 48p. DNLM; NNNAM; PPC; PPHa **70-1027**

ELLIS, John (1815-1896)
Family homoeopathy. 9th ed. Cleveland, Ohio: L. W. Witte, 1872. 404p. DNLM **70-1028**

ELWELL, John J. (1820-1900)
A medico-legal treatise on malpractice and medical evidence, comprising the elements of medical jurisprudence. 3rd ed. New York: Baker, Voorhis & Co., 1871. 600p. DNLM; NNNAM; PPC; PU **70-1029**

ELY, Edward T[albot] (1850-1885)
Note on the treatment of acute suppuration of the middle ear. [New York, 1879.] 5p. DNLM **70-1030**

ELY, William S.
An address ["the philosophy of disease"] as retiring president of the Medical Association of Central New York. [1876.] 12p. DNLM **70-1031**

EMERSON, Edward Waldo (1844-1930)
Some points in the pathology and treatment of cholera infantum. [Boston, 1876.] 17p. DNLM; MH-M **70-1032**

EMERSON, George Barrell (1797-1881)
What we owe to Louis Agassiz, as a teacher; an address before the Boston Society of Natural History, Boston, 1874. 14p. DNLM **70-1033**

EMERSON, N. B.
A clinical study of tetany. [New York, 1877.] 17p. DNLM **70-1034**

EMMET, Thomas Addis (1828-1919)
Prolapsus uteri, its chief causes and treatment. New York, 1871. 34p. DNLM; NNNAM **70-1035**

EMMET, Thomas Addis (1828-1919)
Chronic cystitis in the female, and mode of treatment. Louisville: J. P. Morton & Co., 1872. 30p. DNLM; OCIM **70-1036**

EMMET, Thomas Addis (1828-1919)
The philosophy of uterine disease, with the treatment applicable to displacements and flexures. New York: D. Appleton & Co., 1874. 26p. DNLM; NNNAM **70-1037**

EMMET, Thomas Addis (1828-1919)
Laceration of the cervix uteri, as a frequent and unrecognized cause of disease. New York: William Wood & Co., 1874. 15p. DNLM; NNNAM **70-1038**

EMMET, Thomas Addis (1828-1919)
The etiology of uterine flexures, with the proper mode of treatment indicated. [Boston, 1877.] 34p. DNLM; MBM **70-1039**

EMMET, Thomas Addis (1828-1919)
Proper treatment for lacerations of the cervix uteri. Indianapolis, 1877. 15p. DNLM **70-1040**

EMMET, Thomas Addis (1828-1919)
Congenital absence and accidental atresia of the vagina. Mode of operating to establish the canal and evacuate retained menstrual blood. [Boston, 1878.] 42p. DNLM; MBM **70-1041**

EMMET, Thomas Addis (1828-1919)
The principles and practice of gynaecology. . . . With one hundred and thirty illustrations. Philadelphia: Henry C. Lea, 1879. 855p. DLC; NNNAM; PPC; PU **70-1042**

EMMONS, F. A.
Annual medical directory of regular physicians in the State of Illinois for the year 1877. Chicago: R. R. McCabe & Co., 1877. 109p. DNLM; ICU; IEN-M **70-1043**

EMMONS, F. A.
Annual medical directory of regular physicians in the State of Illinois for the year 1878. Chicago: R. R. McCabe & Co., 1878. 112p. DNLM; OCIM; IU-M **70-1044**

ENGELMANN, George Julius (1847-1903)
On prolapse of the umbilical cord, its causes and treatment. New York: William Wood & Co., 1874. 76p. 2 tab. DNLM; NNNAM **70-1045**

ENGELMANN, George Julius (1847-1903)
The mucous membrane of the uterus, with special reference to the development and structure of the deciduae. New York: William Wood & Co., 1875. 65p. 1 plate. DNLM; NNNAM **70-1046**

ENGELMANN, George Julius (1847-1903)
Early pregnancy, simulating acute uterine and circumuterine inflammation. St. Louis: W. P. Kremer, 1877. 7p. DNLM **70-1047**

ENGELMANN, George Julius (1847-1903)
Battey's operation; three fatal cases, with some remarks upon the indications for the operation. New York: William Wood & Co., 1878. 25p. DNLM; NNNAM **70-1048**

ENGELMANN, George Julius (1847-1903)
The difficulties and dangers of Battey's operation. Philadelphia: Collins, 1878. 13p. DNLM; PPC **70-1049**

ENGELMANN, George Julius (1847-1903)
The hystero-neuroses, with especial reference to the menstrual hystero-neurosis of the stomach. [St. Louis, 1878.] 38p. DNLM **70-1050**

ENGELMANN, George Julius (1847-1903)
A hystero-psychosis. Epilepsy dependent upon erosions of the cervix uteri. St. Louis, 1878. 5p. DNLM **70-1051**

ENGELMANN, George Julius (1847-1903)
The obstetric forceps; when and how to use it. Cairo, Ill.: Cairo Printing Co., 1878. 9p. DNLM **70-1052**

ERB, Wilhelm Heinrich (1840-1921)
Diseases of the peripheral cerebro-spinal nerves. Transl. by Henry Power. New York: William Wood & Co., 1876. 623p. DNLM; OCIM; PPC; PU **70-1053**

ERB, Wilhelm Heinrich (1840-1921)
Diseases of the spinal cord and medulla oblongata. Transl. by Edward G. Geoghegan, Edward W. Schauffler, David F. Lincoln, and John A. McCreery. New York: William Wood & Co., 1878. 975p. DNLM; MBM; NNNAM; PPC
70-1054

ERICHSEN, John Eric (1818-1896)
The science and art of surgery. Being a treatise on surgical injuries, diseases, and operations. . . . A new ed., enlarged and carefully rev. by the author. Philadelphia: Henry C. Lea, 1873. 2 v. DNLM; OCIM; PPC; PU **70-1055**

ERICHSEN, John Eric (1818-1896)
On concussion of the spine, nervous shock, and other obscure injuries of the nervous system, in their clinical and medico-legal aspects. New York: William Wood & Co., 1875. 340p. DNLM; LNT-M; NNNAM; PPC **70-1056**

ERICHSEN, John Eric (1818-1896)
The science and art of surgery. Being a treatise on surgical injuries, diseases, and operations. . . . Rev. by the author from the 7th and enlarged English ed. Philadelphia: Henry C. Lea, 1878. 2 v. DNLM; MBM; NNNAM; PPC
70-1057

ESMARCH, Friedrich von (1823-1908)
The surgeon's handbook on the treatment of the wounded in war. . . . Transl. by H. H. Clutton. New York: L. W. Schmidt, 1878. 31p. DLC; OCIM; PP; PPC **70-1058**

EVANS, Elizabeth Edson
The abuse of maternity. Philadelphia: J. B. Lippincott & Co., 1875. 129p. DNLM; NN; NNNAM; PU
70-1059

EVANS, G[eorge] G.
What shall we drink? or alcohol, its uses and abuses. Philadelphia: G. G. Evans, 1877. 96p. DNLM; PP; PU
70-1060

EVANS, John Wesley
A new treatise on assimilation and digestion, showing the different solvent juices and fluids, their origin and their uses in the human system, the glands from which they are secreted and their relation to each other. . . . Quincy, Ill.: Daily Whig Book and Job Printing House, 1878. 112p. DLC
70-1061

EVANS, Warren Felt (1817-1889)
Mental medicine: a theoretical and practical treatise on medical psychology. Boston: W. White & Co., [1872]. 216p. DNLM
70-1062

EVANS, Warren Felt (1817-1889)
Mental medicine: a theoretical and practical treatise on medical psychology. 15th ed. Boston: H. H. Carter, 1872. 216p. DNLM
70-1063

EVANS, Warren Felt (1817-1889)
Soul and body; or, the spiritual science of health and disease. Boston: H. H. Carter & Co., 1876. 147p. DNLM
70-1064

EVE, Paul Fitzsimmons (1806-1877)
Contributions to surgery, for 1869. Nashville, Tenn.: N. Chammings, 1870. 12p. DNLM
70-1065

EVE, Paul Fitzsimmons (1806-1877)
A synsopsis and analysis of one hundred cases of lithotomy, lithotrity, etc. Philadelphia: Collins, 1871. 10p. DNLM; PPC
70-1066

EVE, Paul Fitzsimmons (1806-1877)
Amputation at the hip-joint, complicated by complete ankylosis; death in twenty-five hours. Nashville, Tenn., [1871]. 7p. DNLM **70-1067**

EVE, Paul Fitzsimmons (1806-1877)
Lithotomy. Removal of a calculous mass, deposited on a piece of bougie, by lithotomy, being the ninetieth bilateral operation, with only two deaths in the last forty-five cases, and these independent of it; and, moreover, without ever having refused a single applicant of the one hundred and three, for relief. Nashville: Roberts & Purvis, 1873. 7p. DNLM
70-1068

EVERETT, J. T.
Removal of a calcified fibroid of the uterus by laparo-elytrotomy. [New York, 1879.] 10p. 1 plate. DNLM; NNNAM
70-1069

EVERY MAN his own doctor! A medical hand book, containing a brief summary of the symptoms and cure of every disease. Also, a variety of popular prescriptions, and a very full chapter upon the efficacy of plants and herbs; and some remarks on physiology. Hinsdale, N.H.: Hunter & Co., 1870. 134p. DLC
70-1070

FAIRCHILD, Maria Augusta (*b.* 1834)
How to be well; or, Common-sense medical hygiene. A book for the people. . . . New York: S. H. Wells & Co., 1879. 180p. DLC; NNNAM **70-1071**

FALLIGANT, Louis A[lexander] (1836-1903)
Yellow fever. A paper read before the Homoeopathic Yellow Fever Commission, at New Orleans. [1878.] 1 broadside sheet. DNLM **70-1072**

FARQUHARSON, Robert (1836-1918)
A guide to therapeutics and materia medica. . . . Enl. and adapted to the U.S. pharmacopoeia by Frank Woodbury. . . . Philadelphia: Henry C. Lea, 1877. 410p. DLC; DNLM; OCLloyd; PU **70-1073**

FARQUHARSON, Robert (1836-1918)
A guide to therapeutics and materia medica. . . . 2nd American ed., rev. by the author. Enl. and adapted to the U.S. pharmacopoeia, by Frank Woodbury. . . . Philadelphia: Henry C. Lea, 1879. 498p. DLC; DNLM; OCLloyd; PPC
70-1074

FARRAR, I.
Medical advice, or A book for you, on the cause, symptoms, and treatment of chronic, or long-standing diseases. . . . Hartford: Case, Lockwood & Brainard, printers, 1870. 42p. DLC
70-1075

FAULKNER, Thomas
The book of nature, a full and explicit explanation of all that can or ought to be known of the structure and uses of the organs of life and generation. . . . To which is added a complete medical treatise upon all diseases of the generative organs. . . . New York: Hurst & Co., [1875]. 143p. DLC; NNNAM
70-1076

FENN, A[rtemas] I.
The medical and surgical companion. For the use of families, seamen, travellers, miners, &c. Giving a brief description, in plain language, of the diseases of men, women, and children. With the most approved methods of treating them. . . . Boston: Pub. by the author, 1870. 384p. DLC; MBM
70-1077

FENNER, Byron (*b.* **1844)**
Formulary, containing formulae for the preparation of all the elixirs, emulsions, essences, flavoring extracts, glycerites, solutions, syrups, wines, etc., known as elegant preparations, now in use. As well as formulae for such miscellaneous preparations as are in use in the drug business that are not officinal, and general directions for making fluid extracts. 5th ed. New York: B. Fenner, 1879. 402p. DNLM; NNNAM; OCLloyd
70-1078

FENNER, Christopher Smith (1823-1879)
A treatise on the diseases of refraction and accommodation. Louisville, Ky.: Richmond & Louisville Med. J. print., 1873. 29p. DNLM **70-1079**

FENNER, Christopher Smith (1823-1879)
Résumé of the modern views of the pathology and treatment of glaucoma. Louisville: J. P. Morton & Co., 1874. 13p. DNLM **70-1080**

FENNER, Christopher Smith (1823-1879)
Visions; its optical defects, and the adaptation of spectacles. Embracing, first, physical optics; second, physiological optics; third, errors of refraction and defects of accommodation, or optical defects of the eye, with selections from the test types of Jaeger and Suellen. Philadelphia: Lindsay & Blakiston, 1875. 299p. DNLM; NNNAM; OCIM; PPC **70-1081**

FIELD, A. G. (1829-1924)
Annual address delivered at the twentieth annual meeting of the Iowa State Medical Society. Des Moines: Carter, Hussey & Curl, 1873. 14p. DNLM **70-1082**

FIELD, A. G. (1829-1924)
Public health. An address before the Workingmen's Institute, Des Moines, Iowa. [Des Moines, 1877.] 8p. DNLM
70-1083

FIELD, David Dudley (1805-1894)
Emotional insanity. Read before the Medico-Legal Society of the city of New York. New York: Russell Bros., 1873. 16p. DNLM **70-1084**

FIELD, Henry M[artyn] (1822-1907)
A memorial of Dr. Peaslee. Newton, Mass.: Newton Republican Co., 1879. 12p. DNLM **70-1085**

FIELD, Henry M[artyn] (1822-1907)
Monograph of cinchona; its action and applications. (Neutral bromide of quinia and the hypodermic method of use.). St. Albans, 1879. 38p. DNLM **70-1086**

FINLAYSON, James (1840-1906)
Clinical diagnosis; a handbook for students and practitioners of medicine. Philadelphia: Henry C. Lea, 1878. 546p. CtY-M; DNLM; NNNAM; PPC **70-1087**

FISHBLATT, Edward N.
Lecture on the causes and treatment of syphilis. New York: Randel & Bruno, 1879. 36p. DNLM; NNNAM
70-1088

FISHER, G. C., comp.
Homoeopathic treatment of yellow fever by the physicians of the Homoeopathic Relief Association of New Orleans, La. A. guide for diagnosing, medicating and nursing yellow fever; by the most experienced and successful homoeopathic physicians of New Orleans. A. H. Nelson Print., 1879. 15p. LNT-M; PPHa **70-1089**

FISHER, George Jackson (1825-1893)
Are malformations or monstrosities of the foetus in utero ever produced by the power of maternal mental emotions? Utica, N.Y.: Roberts, 1870. 57p. DNLM **70-1090**

FISHER, George Jackson (1825-1893)
Inaugural and anniversary addresses delivered before the Medical Society of the State of New York, at its sixty-ninth session, held at the city of Albany, February 2nd, 3rd, and 4th, 1875. . . . New York: G. P. Putnam's Sons, 1875. 12, 57p. DLC; DNLM; NNNAM **70-1091**

FISHER, George Jackson (1825-1893)
A brief historical sketch of the discovery of the circulation of the blood. New York: D. Appleton & Co., 1877. 14p. DNLM; NNNAM **70-1092**

FISHER, L. C.
Yellow fever's origin. The disease not endemic in this country. [Galveston, 1878.] 14p. DNLM **70-1093**

[FISHER, L. C.]
Absolute quarantine. Non-intercourse with certain foreign ports in summer. [Galveston, 1878.] 20p. DNLM
70-1094

FISHER, T. W[illis] (*b.* **1837)**
Plain talk about insanity; its causes, forms, symptoms, and the treatment of mental diseases. With remarks on hospitals and asylums, and the medico-legal aspect of insanity. Boston: A. Moore, 1872. 97p. DNLM; MB; MH-M
70-1095

FITCH, Samuel Sheldon
Six lectures on the functions of the lungs, and causes, prevention, and cure of pulmonary consumption, asthma and diseases of the heart; on the laws of life and on the mode of preserving male and female health to a hundred years. Also, a treatise on medicated inhalation. 30th ed. New York, 1870. 351p. DNLM; NNNAM **70-1096**

FITCH, S[amuel] S[heldon]
Family physician, teaching how to prevent and cure disease, and prolong life and health for one hundred years. New York: S. S. Fitch & Son, 1876. 89p. NNNAM; MH-M
70-1097

FITCH, Simon (1820-1905)
Peculiarities in the operations of the great ovariotomists: Wells of London, Atlee of Philadelphia, and Thomas Keith of Edinburgh. Philadelphia: J. B. Lippincott & Co., 1872. 16p. DNLM; PPC; PU **70-1098**

FITCH, Simon (1820-1905)
The dome-trocar: its application to ovariotomy, aspiration, and transfusion. New York: D. Appleton & Co., 1875. 12p. DNLM; NNNAM **70-1099**

FITZ, Reginald Heber (1843-1913)
The theory of tuberculosis. A brief account of some of its more important features. (Read at the annual meeting of the Massachusetts Medical Society, June 6, 1871.) [Boston, 1871.] 30p. DNLM; MH-M **70-1100**

FITZ, Reginald [Heber] (1843-1913)
Reports on pathology and pathological anatomy. [Boston, 1873-1875.] 8, 10, 7, 12, 12p. DNLM; MBM **70-1101**

FITZ, Reginald H[eber] (1843-1913)
Report on pathology and pathological anatomy. [Boston, 1874.] 10p. DNLM **70-1102**

FITZ, Reginald H[eber] (1843-1913)
Tubo-uterine or interstitial pregnancy. Philadelphia, 1875. 8p. DNLM **70-1103**

FITZ, Reginald Heber (1843-1913)
Anatomy of the Fasciola Jacksoni. New York: D. Appleton & Co., 1876. 8p. DNLM **70-1104**

FLEMING, Andrew
Address in medicine. Emotional fever. Philadelphia: Collins, 1879. 15p. DNLM; PPC **70-1105**

FLINT, Austin (1812-1886)
A practical treatise on the diagnosis, pathology, and treatment of diseases of the heart. . . . 2nd ed. thoroughly rev. and enl. Philadelphia: Henry C. Lea, 1870. 550p. DLC; DNLM; NNNAM; PPC **70-1106**

FLINT, Austin (1812-1886)
A treatise on the principles and practice of medicine; designed for the use of practitioners and students of medicine. . . . 4th ed., carefully rev. Philadelphia: Henry C. Lea, 1873. 1070p. DLC; DNLM; OCIM; PPC **70-1107**

FLINT, Austin (1812-1886)
Essays on conservative medicine and kindred topics. . . . Philadelphia: Henry C. Lea, 1874. 214p. DLC; DNLM; ICRM; PPC **70-1108**

FLINT, Austin (1812-1886)
Pneumothorax. New York: G. P. Putnam's Sons, 1875. 19p. port. DNLM; NNNAM **70-1109**

FLINT, Austin (1812-1886)
Phthisis: its morbid anatomy, etiology, symptomatic events and complications, fatality and prognosis, treatment and physical diagnosis. In a series of clinical studies. . . . Philadelphia: Henry C. Lea, 1875. 446p. DLC; DNLM; MBM; NNNAM **70-1110**

FLINT, Austin (1812-1886)
Objects and work; a valedictory address delivered before the New York Academy of Medicine. New York: D. Appleton & Co., 1875. 9p. DNLM; NNNAM **70-1111**

FLINT, Austin (1812-1886)
A manual of percussion and auscultation; of the physical diagnosis of diseases of the lungs and heart, and of thoracic aneurism. . . . Philadelphia: Henry C. Lea, 1876. 255p. DLC; IU-M; NNNAM; PPC **70-1112**

FLINT, Austin (1812-1886)
Clinical medicine: a systematic treatise on the diagnosis and treatment of diseases. Designed for the use of students and practitioners of medicine. . . . Philadelphia: Henry C. Lea, 1879. 795p. DLC; DNLM; MdBJ-W; PPC **70-1113**

FLINT, Austin, Jr. (1836-1915)
The physiology of man. . . . Secretion; excretion; ductless glands; nutrition; animal heat; movements; voice and speech. New York: D. Appleton & Co., 1870. 526p. DNLM; NNNAM; NcD; PPC **70-1114**

FLINT, Austin, Jr. (1836-1915)
Manual of chemical examination of the urine in diesase; with brief directions for the examination of the most common varieties of urinary calculi. . . . New York: D. Appleton & Co., 1870. 76p. fold. tab. DLC; DNLM; IU-M; NNNAM **70-1115**

FLINT, Austin, Jr. (1836-1915)
On the physiological effects of severe and protracted muscular exercise; with special reference to its influence upon the excretion of nitrogen. . . . New York: D. Appleton & Co., 1871. 91p. DLC; DNLM; NNNAM; PU **70-1116**

FLINT, Austin, Jr. (1836-1915)
Manual of chemical examination of the urine in disease. . . . 2nd ed. New York: D. Appleton & Co., 1871. 76p. fold. plate. NNNAM; OCIM; PPC; PU **70-1117**

FLINT, Austin, Jr. (1836-1915)
The physiology of man. . . . vol. 4. Nervous system. New York: D. Appleton & Co., 1872. 470p. DNLM; NNNAM; PPC; PU **70-1118**

FLINT, Austin, Jr. (1836-1915)
Manual of chemical examination of the urine in disease. . . . 3rd ed., revised and corrected. New York: D. Appleton & Co., 1872. 76p. fold. tab. NNNAM; NNU-M; NcU; PPC **70-1119**

FLINT, Austin, Jr. (1836-1915)
Mechanism of reflex nervous action in normal respiration. An address delivered before the New York Society of Neurology and Electrology. Chicago: J. J. Spalding & Co., 1874. 12p. DNLM; NNNAM **70-1120**

FLINT, Austin, Jr. (1836-1915)
The physiology of man. . . . vol. 5. (With a general index to the five volumes.) Contents: Special senses; generation. New York: D. Appleton & Co., 1874. 517p. DNLM; NNNAM; OCIM; PPC **70-1121**

FLINT, Austin, Jr. (1836-1915)
Directions for the examination of urine of applicants for life insurance. . . . New York: D. Appleton & Co., 1874. 10p. DLC; DNLM; NNNAM **70-1122**

FLINT, Austin, Jr. (1836-1915)
Manual of chemical examination of the urine in disease; with brief directions for the examination of the most common varieties of urinary calculi. . . . 4th ed., revised and corrected. New York: D. Appleton & Co., 1875. 76p. fold. tab. DLC; NNNAM; OCIM; ScCM **70-1123**

FLINT, Austin, Jr. (1836-1915)
A text-book of human physiology. New York: D. Appleton & Co., 1876. 978p. 3 plates. DNLM; NN; NNNAM; OCIM
70-1124

FLINT, Austin, Jr. (1836-1915)
The excretory function of the liver. Philadelphia: Collins, 1877. 15p. DNLM **70-1125**

FLINT, Austin, Jr. (1836-1915)
On the source of muscular power. Arguments and conclusions drawn from observations upon the human subject, under conditions of rest and of muscular exercise. . . . New York: D. Appleton & Co., 1878. 103p. DLC; DNLM; NNNAM; PPC
70-1126

FLINT, Austin, Jr. (1836-1915)
A text-book of human physiology; designed for the use of practitioners and students of medicine. . . . 2nd ed., rev. and cor. New York: D. Appleton & Co., 1879. 978p. 3 plates. DLC; NNNAM; OCIM; ScCM **70-1127**

FLOWER, William Henry (1831-1899)
Diagrams of the nerves of the human body; exhibiting their origin, divisions, and connections. . . . 2nd American from the 2nd English ed. Ed., with additions, by William W. Keen. . . . Philadelphia: T. Hamilton, 1874. 12p. 6 plates. DLC; PPC; PPJ **70-1128**

FOLSOM, Charles Follen (1842-1907)
The treatment of insanity in England and America. [Boston, 1875.] 7p. DNLM **70-1129**

FOLSOM, Charles Follen (1842-1907)
The treatment of insanity. [Boston, 1876?] 2p. DNLM
70-1130

FOLSOM, Charles Follen (1842-1907)
Registration of deaths and of diseases. Boston: A. J. Wright, 1877. 43p. DNLM; MBM **70-1131**

FOLSOM, Charles Follen (1842-1907)
Disease of the mind. Boston: A. J. Wright, 1877. 109p. 1 plate. DNLM; MH-M; NNNAM; PU **70-1132**

FOLSOM, N. L.
Contributions to medicine and surgery. Portsmouth, N.H.: O. M. Knight, 1876. 26p. DNLM **70-1133**

FONSSAGRIVES, Jean Baptiste (1823-1884)
. . . The mother's work with sick children. . . . Transl. from the 4th Paris ed. By F. P. Foster. . . . New York: G. P. Putnam & Sons, [1872]. 244p. DLC; NN; NNNAM; PU
70-1134

FONSSAGRIVES, J[ean] B[aptiste] (1823-1884)
The mother's register; current notes on the health of children. . . . The mother records for the physician to interpret. From the French. . . . New York: G. P. Putnam & Sons, 1873. 97p. DLC; NN; OCIM; PPC **70-1135**

FOOTE, Edward B[liss] (1829-1906)
Medical common sense applied to the causes, prevention, and cure of chronic diseases; and plain home talk about the sexual organs; the natural relation of the sexes; society, civilization; and marriage. . . . 3rd rev. and enl. ed. New York: Pub. by the author, 1870. 912p. DLC; NNNAM; PPC; PPJ
70-1136

FOOTE, Edward B[liss] (1829-1906)
Plain home talk about the human system; the habits of men and women; the causes and prevention of disease; our sexual relations and social natures, [etc.]. New York: Wells & Coffin, 1870. 912p. 2 plates, port. DNLM; NNNAM
70-1137

FOOTE, Edward B[liss] (1829-1906)
The allopathic crusade; an essay, exhibiting the aggressive spirit of the allopathic school of medicine, and presenting views in opposition to proposed legislation, for the pretended purpose of promoting medical reform. New York: Wells & Co., 1872. 39p. DNLM; NNNAM **70-1138**

FOOTE, Edward Bliss (1829-1906)
Physiological marriage. An essay designed to set the people thinking. . . . New York: Murray Hill Publishing Company, 1876. 13p. DLC **70-1139**

FOOTE, Edward B[liss] (1829-1906)
Health in the sunbeam; or, the blueglass cure; containing practical observations on the remedial value of sunshine. New York: Murray Hill Publishing Company, 1877. 63p. DNLM; NNNAM **70-1140**

FOOTE, George F[ranklin] (1817-1889)
State Homoeopathic Asylum for the Insane, at Middletown, N.Y. [Circular of information relating to the proposed institution, with an address.] [1870.] 16p. DNLM **70-1141**

FOOTE, George F[ranklin] (1817-1889)
Inebriety and opium eating, in both cases a disease. Method of treatment and conditions of success. Portland, Me.: Tucker, 1877. 19p. DNLM **70-1142**

FORBES, W[illiam] S[mith] (1831-1905)
Harvey and the transit of the blood from the arteries to the veins "per porositates." Philadelphia, 1878. 7p. DNLM
70-1143

FORCHHEIMER, Frederick (1853-1913)
In memoriam Dr. Landon R. Longworth. An address read at the commencement of the Medical College of Ohio, Feb. 28, 1879. [Cincinnati: R. Clarke & Co., 1879.] 12p. DNLM
70-1144

FORD, Corydon La (1813-1894)
Questions on anatomy, for the use of students. 2nd ed., enlarged. Ann Arbor, Mich.: Ann Arbor Ptg. & Publishing Co., 1873. 136p. DNLM **70-1145**

FORD, C[orydon] La (1813-1894)
Questions on the structure and development of the teeth, for the use of dental students. . . . Ann Arbor: Fiske & Douglas, 1876. 16p. DLC; DNLM **70-1146**

FORD, Corydon La (1813-1894)
Questions on anatomy, histology and physiology for the use of students. . . . Ann Arbor: Courier Steam Printing House, 1878. 152p. DLC; DNLM **70-1147**

FORD, Samuel Payne, ed.
The American cyclopaedia of domestic medicine and household surgery. A reliable guide for every family. Containing, in the plainest language, full descriptions of the various parts of the human body; accounts of the numerous diseases to which man is subject—their causes, symptoms, treatment and prevention. . . . Chicago: E. P. Kingsley, 1879. 1215p. DLC; ICJ; ICRM **70-1148**

FORD, W. Hutson
A case of urinary suppression in yellow fever; treated by superoxygenated air and jaborandi. [St. Louis, 1878.] 8p. DNLM
70-1149

FORD, W. Hutson
A reply to the card of Doctors Dorsett and Outley. [On yellow fever.] [St. Louis, 1879.] 2 l. DNLM
70-1150

FORD, W. Hutson
Reports to the St. Louis Medical Society on yellow fever; consisting of the report of the committee appointed to inquire into the relations of the epidemic of 1878 to the city of St. Louis, and a report on the meteorological conditions and etiology of yellow fever, and of certain other diseases associated with a higher temperature, and on the treatment of yellow fever. St. Louis: G. O. Rumbold & Co., 1879. 320p. DNLM; OCIM **70-1151**

FORMAD, H[enry] (1847-1892)
Classification and condensed description of tumors, on Virchow's histogenetic basis, as taught by Prof. James Tyson. Edited and dedicated to the medical class of the University of Pennsylvania. [Philadelphia], 1879. 1 broadside eleph. fol. DNLM; PU **70-1152**

FORMULAS for some elixirs and medicated wines, adopted by the Louisville College of Pharmacy, Jan. 16, 1872. Chicago: J. J. Spalding & Co., 1872. 9p. DNLM
70-1153

FORSTER, Edward Jacob (1846-1896)
A manual for medical officers of the militia of the United States. . . . New York: Hurd & Houghton; Boston: H. O. Houghton & Co., 1877. 102p. DLC; DNLM; MBM; NNNAM
70-1154

FORSTER, Edward Jacob (1846-1896)
A case of third dentition. [1877.] 1 l. DNLM
70-1155

FOSTER, Frank Pierce (1841-1911)
Practical remarks on vaccination. New York: D. Appleton & Co., 1872. 4p. DNLM **70-1156**

FOSTER, Frank Pierce (1841-1911)
Report of the vaccine department, for the year 1873. New York: J. W. Amerman, 1874. 23p. DNLM; NNNAM
70-1157

FOSTER, Frank Pierce (1841-1911)
Report of the vaccine department of the New York Dispensary, for the years 1873; 1874. New York: J. W. Amerman, 1874-1875. 23p. 15p. DNLM; NNNAM
70-1158

FOSTER, Frank Pierce (1841-1911)
On prolapse of the arm in transverse presentation. New York: William Wood & Co., 1876. 25p. DNLM; NNNAM
70-1159

FOSTER, Harriet McI. (*b.* 1844)
The education of idiots and imbeciles. A paper read before the Social Science Association of Indiana. Indianapolis, 1879. 14p. DNLM **70-1160**

FOSTER, J. H.
Address delivered before the American Academy of Dental Science at their third annual meeting. Boston: Rockwell & Churchill, 1871. 31p. DNLM, MH-M
70-1161

FOSTER, James A.
Illustrations and a brief description of James A. Foster's patent union artificial limbs. With testimonials of surgeons, the press, and those wearing them. [Philadelphia], 1870. 80p. DNLM; PPC **70-1162**

FOSTER, Michael (1836-1907)
. . . Physiology. . . . New York: D. Appleton & Co., 1874. 132p. DLC; MH; ICU; NIC **70-1163**

FOSTER, Michael (1836-1907)
. . . Nociones de fisiologia. . . . Con láminas. Nueva York: D. Appleton y compañia, 1879. 159p. DLC
70-1164

FOSTER, Richard Norman
Valedictory address to the graduating class of Hahnemann Medical College of Chicago, February 22, 1871, with catalogue of students and graduates. Chicago, 1871. 24p. PPHa
70-1165

FOTHERGILL, John Milner (1841-1888)
The maintenance of health. A medical work for lay readers. New York: G. P. Putnam's Sons, 1875. 366p. DLC; NN; NNNAM; PU **70-1166**

FOTHERGILL, John Milner (1841-1888)
The practitioner's handbook of treatment; or, the principles of therapeutics. Philadelphia: Henry C. Lea, 1877. 575p. DNLM; MBM; NNNAM; PPC **70-1167**

FOTHERGILL, J[ohn] Milner (1841-1888)
The antagonism of therapeutic agents: and what it teaches. The essay to which was awarded the Fothergillian Gold Medal of the Medical Society of London for 1878. Philadelphia: Henry C. Lea, 1878. 157p. MBM; NNNAM; OCIM; PPC
70-1168

FOTHERGILL, J[ohn] Milner (1841-1888)
The heart and its diseases, with their treatment; including the gouty heart. 2nd ed. Philadelphia: Lindsay & Blakiston, 1879. 476p. 3 plates. DNLM; NNNAM; PPC; PU
70-1169

FOUGERA, F. & CO.
Descriptive catalogue of standard medicinal preparations, and new remedies. New York: J. L. Black, 1875. 105p. DNLM; NNNAM; OCLloyd **70-1170**

FOURNIER, [Jean] A[lfred] (1832-1914)
On the treatment of syphilis. Transl. by R. W. Taylor. New York: D. Appleton & Co., 1872. 16p. DNLM; NNNAM
70-1171

FOWLER, Edward Payson (1833-1914)
Medical science against exclusive homoeopathy. A reply to Dr. Edward Bayard's "Plea for Pure Homoeopathy against Electric Homoepathy." New York: John Polhemus, April, 1878. 12p. DNLM; NNC **70-1172**

FOWLER, George B[ingham] (1847-1907)
Examination of the urine. New York: D. Appleton & Co., 1874. 80p. DNLM; NNNAM **70-1173**

FOWLER, George B[ingham] (1847-1907)
The spectroscope; its value in medical science. New York: D. Appleton & Co., 1876. 29p. 2 plates. DNLM; NNNAM **70-1174**

FOWLER, George B[ingham] (1847-1907)
Chemical and microscopical analysis of the urine in health and disease. 2nd ed. New York: G. P. Putnam's Sons, 1876. 97p. DNLM; NNNAM **70-1175**

FOWLER, George B[ingham] (1847-1907)
On a new and simple method for the quantitative estimation of urea. New York: D. Appleton & Co., 1877. 11p. DNLM **70-1176**

FOWLER, George B[ingham] (1847-1907)
Chemical and microscopical analysis of the urine in health and disease. 3rd ed. New York: G. P. Putnam's Sons, 1879. 103p. DNLM; NNNAM **70-1177**

FOWLER, George B[ingham] (1847-1907)
Intra-vascular alimentation; the nutritive value of peptones. New York: D. Appleton & Co., 1879. 18p. DNLM **70-1178**

FOWLER, Harriet P.
Vegetarianism the radical cure for intemperance. New York: M. L. Holbrook & Co., 1879. 79p. DNLM; NNNAM **70-1179**

FOWLER, Orson Squire (1809-1887)
Maternity; or, Bearing, confinement, and the treatment of infants: including the analysis, preservation, and restoration of the female health and beauty; the causes and cures of feminine ailments . . . as taught by phrenology and physiology. . . . Boston: O. S. Fowler, 1870. 236p. DLC; MBM; NNNAM **70-1180**

FOWLER, Orson Squire (1809-1887)
Creative and sexual science: or manhood, womanhood and their mutual interrelations, as taught by phrenology and physiology. Philadelphia: National Pub. Co., 1875. 1065p. NNNAM; PPC; PPU **70-1181**

FOWNES, George (1815-1849)
Elementary chemistry. . . . From the 10th English ed. Edited by R. Bridges. Philadelphia: Henry C. Lea, 1870. 857p. DNLM; NNNAM; OCIM; PU **70-1182**

FOWNES, George (1815-1849)
Fownes' Manual of Chemistry. . . . Philadelphia: Henry C. Lea, 1878. 1027p. CtY-M; PPC; PPJ; PU **70-1183**

FOX, George Henry (1846-1937)
On the so-called pigmentary syphilide. [Philadelphia, 1875.] 6p. DNLM **70-1184**

FOX, George Henry (1846-1937)
A clinical study of molluscum contagiosum. Chicago, 1878. 10p. DNLM **70-1185**

FOX, George Henry (1846-1937)
On the permanent removal of hair by electrolysis. New York: Trow & Co., 1879. 4p. DNLM **70-1186**

FOX, George Henry (1846-1937)
Photographic illustrations of skin diseases. . . . Forty-eight plates from life. Colored by hand. New York: E. B. Treat, [1879-]80. 102p. 48 col. plates. DLC; NNNAM; PPC; PU [Issued in 12 parts] **70-1187**

FOX, William Tilbury (1836-1879)
Skin diseases; their description, pathology, diagnosis, and treatment. 1st American from the last London ed. Edited by M. H. Henry. New York: William Wood & Co., 1871. 313p. DNLM; NNNAM; PPC; PU **70-1188**

FOX, [William] Tilbury (1836-1879)
Skin diseases: their description, pathology, diagnosis, and treatment. . . . 2nd American from 3rd London ed., rewritten and enl. With a cutaneous pharmacopoeia, a glossarial index. . . . New York: William Wood & Co., 1873. 532p. DLC; DNLM; MBM; PPC **70-1189**

FOX, William Tilbury (1836-1879) and Thomas Colcott FOX
Epitome of skin diseases, with formulae. Philadelphia: Henry C. Lea, 1876. 120p. DNLM; NNNAM; OCIM; PPC **70-1190**

FOX, William Tilbury (1836-1879) and Thomas Colcott FOX
Epitome of skin diseases, with formulae, for students and practitioners. . . . 2nd American ed., enl. and rev. by the authors. Philadelphia: Henry C. Lea, 1879. 216p. DLC; DNLM; MBM; PPC **70-1191**

FOX, Wilson (1831-1887)
The diseases of the stomach. Being the third edition of the "Diagnosis and treatment of the varieties of dyspepsia." Philadelphia: Henry C. Lea, 1875. 283p. DNLM; NNNAM; OCIM; PPC **70-1192**

FRANCIS, Samuel W[ard] (1835-1886)
Novel device for heating and ventilating railroad cars. Newport, R.I., [1874]. Broadside. DNLM **70-1193**

FRANCIS, Samuel Ward (1835-1886)
Curious facts, concerning man and nature; with a few practical suggestions on other subjects. [Medical series No. 3.] Newport, R.I.: C. E. Hammett, Jr., 1874. 15p. DNLM **70-1194**

FRANCIS, Samuel Ward (1835-1886)
Curious facts, concerning man and nature; part second. [Medical series No. 4.] Newport, R.I.: C. E. Hammett, Jr., 1875. 28p. DNLM **70-1195**

FRANKLAND, A. E.
Report on the yellow fever epidemic in Memphis, Tenn., 1873. Memphis: Price, Jones & Co., 1873. 14p. DNLM **70-1196**

FRANKLIN, E[dward] C. (1822-1885)
Homoeopathic therapeutics in gunshot wounds, and the sequelae of operations. Philadelphia, 1876. 32p. DNLM; PPHa **70-1197**

FRANKLIN, E[dward] C. (1822-1885)
Address before the American Institute of Homoeopathy, at the thirtieth session held at Lake Chautauqua, N.Y., June 26, 1877. Philadelphia: Sherman & Co., 1877. 16p. DNLM **70-1198**

FRANKLIN, Edward C. (1822-1885)
The homoeopathic treatment of spinal curvatures according to the new principle. . . . 1st ed. St. Louis: H. C. G. Luyties, 1878. 80p. OCIM; PPHa **70-1199**

FRASER, John
A Scotch insane asylum. [Boston, 1875.] 7p. DNLM **70-1200**

FREEDLEY, S.
Catalogue of rare botanical, medical, and miscellaneous books. Philadelphia, [1887]. 12p. DNLM **70-1201**

FRELIGH, Martin (1813-1889)
Homoeopathic practice of medicine: embracing the history, diagnosis and treatment of diseases in general, including those peculiar to females and the management of children. 12th ed., rev. and enl. . . . New York: C. T. Hurlburt; Boston: O. Clapp; [etc., etc.], 1870. 864p. DLC; MBM; PPHa; PPC **70-1202**

FRELIGH, Martin (1813-1889)
Homoepathic materia medica: being a summary of the curative action of the principal remedial agents employed in the homoeopathic practice. Comp. from Hahnemann, Jahr . . . and other distinguished members of the profession, together with additions, references, and notes. . . . New York: C. T. Hurlburt; Boston: O. Clapp; [etc., etc.], 1870. [629]-841p. DLC; NNNAM; OCLloyd; PPHa **70-1203**

FRELIGH, Martin (1813-1889)
Homoeopathic practice of medicine. . . . 13th ed., rev. and enl. New York: C. T. Hurlburt; Boston: O. Clapp; [etc., etc.], 1873. 864p. MH-M; NNNAM; PPHa; PPC **70-1204**

FRENCH, Elizabeth J.
A new path in electrical therapeutics: an account of Prof. Elizabeth J. French's great discovery of electrical cranial diagnosis, and the scientific application of nine different currents of electricity to the cure of disease. A complete manual of anatomy and physiology. . . . Philadelphia: Pub. by the author, 1873. 251p. DLC; DNLM; NNNAM; PU **70-1205**

FRENCH, Elizabeth J.
Alcohol an enemy to health, morals, and happiness. Philadelphia: J. B. Lippincott & Co., 1873. 24p. DNLM; PPC; PU **70-1206**

FRENCH, Elizabeth J.
A new manual of electro-therapeutics, and a brief treatise on anatomy and physiology. . . . Ed. by M. L. French. Chicago: W. B. Keen, Cooke & Co., 1875. 242p. DLC; OCIM **70-1207**

FRENCH, Elizabeth J.
Family guide for the application of electricity, in some of the common ailments of life, by the use of the combination battery. . . . Cincinnati: Spencer & Craig, 1877. 16p. DLC **70-1208**

FRENCH, Elizabeth J.
A new path in electrical therapeutics: an account of Prof. Elizabeth J. French's great discovery of electrical cranial diagnosis and the scientific application of nine different currents of electricity to the cure of disease; a complete manual of anatomy and physiology, [etc.]. 4th ed. Philadelphia, 1877. 259p. DNLM; PU **70-1209**

FRENCH, George F[ranklin] (1837-1897)
The respiratory brace; a new appliance devised for the relief of orthopnoea. Cambridge, 1877. 5p. DNLM **70-1210**

FRENCH, George F[ranklin] (1837-1897)
The eradication of syphilis and crime by the extirpation, in that class, of the procreative power. Portland: S. Berry, 1878. 8p. DNLM **70-1211**

FREUND, Wilhelm Alexander (1833-1918) and James R. CHADWICK
Four cases of echinococci in the female pelvis. [New York, 1875.] 12p. DNLM; NNNAM **70-1212**

FREY, Heinrich (1822-1890)
The microscope and microscopical technology. Transl. by George R. Cutter. From the 4th German ed. New York: William Wood & Co., 1872. 658p. CtY-M; DNLM; MBM; NNNAM **70-1213**

FREY, Heinrich (1822-1890)
The histology and histochemistry of man. Transl. from the 4th German ed., by Arthur E. J. Barker. New York: D. Appleton & Co., 1875. 683p. DNLM; NNNAM; PPC; PU **70-1214**

FREY, Heinrich (1822-1890)
Compendium of histology. Twenty-four lectures by Heinrich Frey. . . . Transl. from the German, by permission of the author, by George R. Cutter. . . . Illustrated by 208 engravings on wood. New York: G. P. Putnam's Sons, 1876. 274p. DLC; DNLM; NNNAM; PU **70-1215**

FROST, J. H. P[aine] (1825-1875)
Introductory address at the opening of the third session of the Detroit Homoeopathic Medical College. Detroit: Daily Post. Ptg. Establishment, 1873. 24p. DNLM **70-1216**

FROTHINGHAM, George E[dward] (1836-1900)
Sympathetic ophthalmia. [Lansing, 1876.] 28p. DNLM **70-1217**

FROTHINGHAM, Richard (1812-1880)
Memoir of the Hon. Josiah Bartlett, M.D. Cambridge: J. Wilson & Son, 1879. 10p. DNLM; MH **70-1218**

FULLERTON, R. E.
An American Italy for invalids. A dissertation, showing the advantages, incidents, etc., of a journey on the plains, in the Rocky Mountains and Mexico, for the cure of all chronic diseases. Chicago: H. D. Chapin & Co., [1871?] 64p. DNLM **70-1219**

FULTON COUNTY MEDICAL SOCIETY, ATLANTA, GEORGIA
Report of the delegate of the Fulton County Medical Society, with the report of its committee. Also, a history of the controversy between the old board of trustees and the faculty of the Atlanta Medical College and the Fulton County Medical Society to the time of its introduction into the Georgia Medical Association. Also, Dr. Geo. G. Crawford's reply to an article styled "A statement of facts" . . . . Also, Dr. E. J. Roach's statements. Atlanta, Ga.: Franklin Steam Printing-House, 1871. 107p. DNLM **70-1220**

FULTON COUNTY MEDICAL SOCIETY, ATLANTA, GEORGIA
Proceedings of a meeting of the Fulton County Medical Society. Embracing the report of Dr. T. S. Powell, as a delegate to the late annual meeting of the American Medical Association; together with the report of the committee to whom was referred the action of the Georgia Medical Association. Atlanta, [1871?]. 1 broadside. DNLM **70-1221**

FULTON, J.
A text book of physiology. . . . 2nd ed., rev. and enl. . . . Philadelphia: Lindsay & Blakiston, [etc.], 1879. 416p. DLC; PP; PPC; PU **70-1222**

GAILLARD, Edwin Samuel (1827-1885)
Medical and general science as vindicators of the Mosaic record, and as repudiators of the modern doctrines of development and selection. Louisville: Medical Journal Office, 1872. 52p. DNLM **70-1223**

GALTON, Francis (1822-1911)
Hereditary genius: an inquiry into its laws and consequences. . . . New York: D. Appleton & Co., 1870. 390p. diagr., tables. DLC; DNLM; NN; PU **70-1224**

GALTON, Francis (1822-1911)
Hereditary genius: an inquiry into its laws and consequences. . . . New and rev. ed., with an American preface. New York: D. Appleton & Co., 1871. 390p. diagr., tables. DLC; ICU; NIC; NNC **70-1225**

GAMGEE, John (1831-1894)
Yellow fever, a nautical disease. Its origin and prevention. . . . New York: D. Appleton & Co., 1879. 207p. DLC; NNNAM; OCIM; PPC **70-1226**

GANT, Frederick James (1825-1905)
The irritable bladder, its causes and treatment; including a practical view of urinary pathology, deposits, and calculi. 3rd ed., revised and enlarged. Philadelphia: Lindsay & Blakiston, 1872. 221p. DNLM; NNNAM; PPC; PPJ **70-1227**

GANTILLON, H. E.
Diseases of the womb. Uterine catarrh frequently the cause of sterility. New treatment. [Transl. by the author.] Boston: J. Campbell, 1871. 54p. DNLM; MBM **70-1228**

GARDETTE, Emile B[laise] (1803-1887)
Memoir of John Barclay Biddle. Read before the College of Physicians of Philadelphia, June 4, 1879. Philadelphia: Collins, 1879. 22p. DNLM; PPC **70-1229**

GARDNER, Augustus Kinsley (1821-1876)
Conjugal sins against the laws of life and health and their effects upon the father, mother, and child. New York: J. S. Redfield, 1870. 240p. DLC; DNLM; NN; NNNAM **70-1230**

GARDNER, Augustus Kinsley (1821-1876)
Our children: their physical and mental development. Hartford: Belknap & Bliss, 1872. 340p. 6 plates. DNLM; MB; MH; NN **70-1231**

GARDNER, Augustus Kinsley (1821-1876)
Rupture of the perinaeum; its causes and cure. New York, 1872. 12p. DNLM **70-1232**

GARDNER, James T.
Relation between topographical surveys and the study of public health. An address delivered before the American Public Health Association, at Boston, Oct. 6, 1876. Albany: Argus Co., 1876. 10p. DNLM **70-1233**

GARDNER, John (1804-1880)
Longevity; the means of prolonging life after middle age. 3rd ed., revised and enlarged. Boston: W. F. Gill & Co., 1875. 191p. DNLM; MB; MH **70-1234**

[GARRETSON, James Edmund] (1828-1895)
Odd hours of a physician, by John Darby [pseud.]. Philadelphia: J. B. Lippincott & Co., 1871. 256p. DNLM; PU **70-1235**

GARRETSON, James Edmund (1828-1895)
A system of oral surgery; being a consideration of the diseases and surgery of the mouth, jaws, and associate parts. 2nd ed. Philadelphia: J. B. Lippincott & Co., 1873. 1091p. 17 plates. DNLM; NNNAM; PPC; PU **70-1236**

GARRIGUES, Henry Jacques (1831-1913)
Apparatus for transfusion. Asphyxia in new-born children considered from a medical and a legal stand-point. New York: William Wood & Co., 1878. 14p. DNLM; NNNAM **70-1237**

GARRIGUES, Henry Jacques (1831-1913)
On gastro-elytrotomy. New York: D. Appleton & Co., 1878. 78p. DNLM; NNNAM **70-1238**

GARRIGUES, Henry Jacques (1831-1913)
On lying-in institutions, especially those of New York. [Boston, 1878.] 58p. DNLM; MH-M **70-1239**

GARRIGUES, Henry Jacques (1831-1913)
Danger of stem pessaries. New York: William Wood & Co., 1879. 7p. DNLM **70-1240**

GAUSE, Owen B[everly] (1825-1895)
Valedictory address delivered at the annual commencement of the Hahnemann Medical College of Philadelphia, March 10, 1875. Philadelphia: Hering, Pope & Co., 1875. 14p. PPHa **70-1241**

GAY, Charles Curtis Fenn (1821-1886)
Defense of taxis in strangulated hernia. [Buffalo, 1872.] 8p. DNLM **70-1242**

GAY, Charles Curtis Fenn (1821-1886)
Preventive medicine. An address delivered June 8, 1875, before the Medical Society of Erie County. Buffalo: Baker, Jones & Co., 1875. 12p. DNLM **70-1243**

GAY, Charles Curtis Fenn (1821-1886)
Injuries of the skull; their relation to medical evidence, with reports of cases, and remarks upon the employment of the trephine. [Buffalo, 1875.] 11p. DNLM **70-1244**

GAZZO, John B. C.
Yellow fever facts, as to its nature, prevention, and treatment. New Orleans: M. F. Dunn & Bro., 1878. 35p. DNLM; LNT-M **70-1245**

GEDDINGS, William H. (1838-1892)
Aiken as a health station. Charleston, S.C.: Walker, Evans & Cogswell, 1877. 31p. DNLM; ScCM **70-1246**

GEDDINGS, William H. (1838-1892)
A case of sarcoma of the kidney in a Negro child. [1878.] 3p. 1 plate. DNLM **70-1247**

GEDDINGS, William H. (1838-1892)
Report of the results in thirty-one cases of phthisis treated at Aiken, S.C., during the season 1878-1879. New York: William Wood & Co., 1879. 24p. DNLM; NNNAM; ScCM **70-1248**

GEDDINGS, William H. (1838-1892)
Hints for invalids visiting southern health resorts. . . . New York: G. P. Putnam's Sons, 1879. 17p. DLC; DNLM; NNNAM; ScU **70-1249**

GEMRIG, J. H.
Illustrated catalogue of surgical instruments, appliances, bandages, apparatus for deformities, dislocations, and fractures, trusses, etc. Philadelphia, [1879?]. 128p. DNLM; PPC; PU **70-1250**

GENTRY, William D. (*b.* **1836)**
An answer to the question, what is homoeopathy? and how it differs from the old system of treating diseases. Memphis: Baptist Publishing House, 1875. 16p. PPHa **70-1251**

GERMAN MEDICAL INSTITUTE. ST. LOUIS, MO.
The book on gout and rheumatism. Safe and certain cure of gout and rheumatism, or instructions regarding the only easy, absolutely certain and expedient treatment in cases of gout and rheumatism, by the application of cheap natural remedies of never failing effect; written in the interest of all such sufferers, and as a caution against useless and injurious medicines and preparations, by a philanthropist, published by the German Medical Institute. St. Louis, Mo.: M. Olshausen, [1879?]. 43p. DNLM **70-1252**

GERRISH, Frederic Henry (1845-1920)
Prescription writing. Designed for the use of medical students who have never studied Latin. . . . Portland, Me.: Loring, Short & Harmon; Philadelphia: J. B. Lippincott & Co., 1878. 51p. DLC; NNNAM; PPC **70-1253**

GERRISH, Frederic Henry (1845-1920)
The duties of the medical profession concerning prostitution and its allied vices. Being the oration before the Maine Medical Association at its annual meeting, 12th of June, 1878. . . . 2nd ed. Portland, [Me.]: Loring, Short & Harmon, 1879. 31p. DLC **70-1254**

THE GETTYSBURG katalysine waters, its source, history of its discovery and wonderful cures. Testimony of invalids, physicians, medical journals, and others. Philadelphia: Haddock & Son, 1872. 63p. DNLM **70-1255**

GIBBONS, Abby Hopper
Compulsory medication of prostitutes by the State. . . . New York: Burton & Covey, [1876]. 23p. DLC; NNNAM **70-1256**

GIBBONS, Henry, Sr. (1808-1884)
Introductory lecture to the eighth session of the medical department of the University of the Pacific. San Francisco: J. H. Carmany & Co., 1870. 14p. DNLM **70-1257**

GIBBONS, Henry, Sr. (1808-1884)
Letheomania; the result of the hypodermic injection of morphia. San Francisco: F. Clarke, [1870]. 15p. DNLM **70-1258**

GIBBONS, Henry, Sr. (1808-1884)
Introductory lecture to the eighth session of the medical department of the University of the Pacific: delivered July 5, 1870. . . . [San Francisco: J. H. Carmany & Co., 1870.] 14p. DLC **70-1259**

GIBBONS, Henry, Sr. (1808-1884)
Illustrations of the literature of quackery. [San Francisco, 1874.] 20p. DNLM **70-1260**

GIBBONS, Henry, Sr. (1808-1884)
Modern spiritism; annual address before the San Francisco Medical Society. San Francisco: Woman's Publishing Co., 1875. 21p. DNLM **70-1261**

GIBBONS, Henry, Sr. (1808-1884)
Fifty years ago. An address to the graduating class of the Medical College of the Pacific for 1878. [San Francisco]: A. L. Bancroft & Co., [1878]. 21p. DNLM **70-1262**

GIBBONS, Henry, Sr. (1808-1884)
On feticide. [Sacramento, 1878.] 16p. DNLM **70-1263**

GIBBONS, Henry, Sr. (1808-1884)
A protest against meddlesome midwifery. (Read . . . before the San Francisco County Medical Society.) S[an] F[rancisco]: W. M. Hinton & Co., printers, [1879]. 11p. DLC **70-1264**

GIBBONS, Henry, Sr. (1808-1884)
Notes of hospital and private practice. San Francisco: A. L. Bancroft & Co., [1879]. 14p. DNLM **70-1265**

GIBERSON, Charles H. (1838-1879)
Medical practice modified. A semi-centennial address. Brooklyn: W. C. Wilton, 1873. 29p. DNLM **70-1266**

GIBNEY, Virgil P[endleton] (1847-1927)
Peri-nephritic abscess in children, with a report of nine cases. New York: William Wood & Co., 1876. 20p. DNLM; NNNAM **70-1267**

GIBNEY, Virgil P[endleton] (1847-1927)
The strumous element in the etiology of joint-disease, from an analysis of eight hundred and sixty cases. New York: D. Appleton & Co., 1877. 46p. DNLM; NNNAM **70-1268**

GIBNEY, Virgil P[endleton] (1847-1927)
Spinal irritation in children as related to true and false arthropathies. New York: G. P. Putnam's Sons, 1877. 23p. DNLM; NNNAM **70-1269**

GIBNEY, Virgil P[endleton] (1847-1927)
The paralyses of Pott's diseases; being a clinical study of fifty-eight cases. Chicago: J. Spalding & Co., 1878. 23p. DNLM **70-1270**

GIBNEY, Virgil P[endleton] (1847-1927)
Galvanism in the treatment of sciatica. Indianapolis, 1879. 26p. DNLM **70-1271**

GIBNEY, Virgil P[endleton] (1847-1927)
A case of scleroderma vel morphoea, with hemiatrophia facialis, alopecia areata, and canities. [With case of morphoea, by P. A. Morrow.] [New York, 1879.] 6p. DNLM **70-1272**

GIHON, Albert Leary (1833-1901)
Practical suggestions in naval hygiene. . . . Washington: Government Printing Office, 1871. 151p. DLC **70-1273**

GIHON, Albert Leary (1833-1901)
Practical suggestions in naval hygiene. . . . (3rd ed.) Published by order of the Navy Department. Washington: Government Printing Office, 1873. 151p. DLC **70-1274**

GIHON, Albert Leary (1833-1901)
Sanitary commonplaces applied to the Navy; an address. Claremont, N.H., 1877. 32p. DNLM **70-1275**

GIHON, Albert Leary (1833-1901)
The need of sanitary reform in ship life. Cambridge, 1877. 14p. DNLM **70-1276**

GILCHRIST, James Grant (1842-1906)
The homoeopathic treatment of surgical diseases. . . . Chicago: C. S. Halsey; New York: Boericke & Tafel, 1873. 421p. DLC; DNLM; NNNAM; PPC **70-1277**

GILCHRIST, J[ames] Grant (1842-1906)
Tumors, their etiology and curability. Detroit, Mich.: [W. A. Scripps, 1877.] 42p. DNLM **70-1278**

GILL, H. Z.
Intra-ocular tumors. [St. Louis, 1872.] 24p. DNLM **70-1279**

GILL, H. Z.
Abstract of the report of the special committee on croup of the Illinois State Medical Society, with a list of eighty-three cases of tracheotomy, for croup and diphtheria, performed in the State of Illinois. Chicago: H. Wilson & Co., 1878. 44p. DNLM; ICJ; ICU **70-1280**

GILLETTE, Walter R[oberts] (*b.* 1840)
The narcotic effect of morphia on the new-born child, when administered to the mother in labor. New York: William Wood & Co., 1877. 13p. DNLM **70-1281**

GILLETTE, Walter R[oberts] (*b.* 1840)
A new operation for the cure of rectocele and cystocele. New York: William Wood & Co., 1877. 6p. DNLM **70-1282**

GLASGOW, William Carr (1845-1907)
A few suggestions on anaesthesia of the larynx. [St. Louis, 1879.] 3p. DNLM **70-1283**

GLEASON, C[loye] W. (1822-1902)
How to acquire and preserve good health. [Philadelphia, 1872.] 54p. DNLM; PPC **70-1284**

GLEASON, C[loye] W. (1822-1902)
Everybody's own physician; or, How to acquire and preserve health. . . . 3rd thousand. Philadelphia: H. N. McKinney & Co., [1873]. 472p. DLC; PPC; PU **70-1285**

GLEASON, C[loye] W. (1822-1902)
Everybody's own physician; or, How to acquire and preserve health. Seventh thousand. Philadelphia: H. N. McKinney & Co., [1874]. 472p. DNLM; PPJ; PU **70-1286**

GLEASON, C[loye] W. (1822-1902)
Everybody's own physician, or, How to acquire and preserve health. 9th thousand. Philadelphia: H. N. McKinney & Co.; Boston, Mass.: I. N. Richardon & Co.; [etc., etc., 1875]. 488p. DLC; NNNAM; PPC **70-1287**

GLEITSMANN, [Joseph] William (1841-1914)
On the nature and curability of pulmonary phthisis. Baltimore: Hanzsche & Co., 1874. 19p. DNLM **70-1288**

GLEITSMANN, [Joseph] William (1841-1914)
On altitude and climate in the treatment of pulmonary phthisis. Baltimore: Innes & Co., 1875. 10p. DNLM **70-1289**

GLEITSMANN, [Joseph] William (1841-1914)
Statistics of mortality from pulmonary phthisis in the United States and in Europe. Baltimore: Turnbull Bros., 1875. 53p. DNLM **70-1290**

GLEITSMANN, [Joseph] William (1841-1914)
Mountain Sanitarium for Pulmonary Diseases, Asheville, N.C. [Circular letter announcing the establishment of.] [1875.] 2 l. DNLM **70-1291**

GLEITSMANN, [Joseph] William (1841-1914)
Western North Carolina as a health resort. Baltimore: Sherwood & Co., 1876. 8p. DNLM **70-1292**

GLEITSMANN, [Joseph] William (1841-1914)
Biennial report of the Mountain Sanitarium for Pulmonary Diseases, Asheville, N.C. Baltimore: Sherwood & Co., 1877. 8p. DNLM **70-1293**

GLEITSMANN, [Joseph] William (1841-1914)
Contributions to the treatment of pulmonary phthisis. [New Orleans, 1877.] 13p. DNLM **70-1294**

GOODELL, William (1829-1894)
The report on the progress of obstetrics and of gynaecology; read before the Medical Society of the State of Pennsylvania. Philadelphia: Collins, 1873. 32p. DNLM; PPC **70-1295**

GOODELL, William (1829-1894)
Prolapse of the womb. Philadelphia: J. B. Lippincott & Co., 1873. 36p. DNLM; PU **70-1296**

GOODELL, William (1829-1894)
The report of the progress of obstetrics and of gynaecology. Philadelphia: Collins, 1873. 32p. DNLM; PPC; PU **70-1297**

GOODELL, William (1829-1894)
In memory of George Pepper, M.D. An obituary read before the Obstetrical Society of Philadelphia. New York: William Wood, 1873. 7p. DNLM; PPC **70-1298**

GOODELL, William (1829-1894)
Some practical hints for the treatment and the prevention of diseases of women. Philadelphia: J. A. Moore, 1874. 33p. DNLM; PPC **70-1299**

GOODELL, William (1829-1894)
On means employed at the Preston Retreat for the prevention and treatment of puerperal diseases. Philadelphia: Collins, 1874. 15p. DNLM **70-1300**

GOODELL, William (1829-1894)
Biographical memoir of Hugh L. Hodge. Philadelphia: Collins, 1874. 19p. DNLM; PPJ; PU **70-1301**

GOODELL, William (1829-1894)
Clinical memoir on turning in pelves narrowed in the conjugate diameter. Philadelphia: Collins, 1875. 22p. DNLM; PPC **70-1302**

GOODELL, William (1829-1894)
A sketch of the life and writings of Louyse Bourgeois, midwife to Marie de Medici, the queen of Henry IV, of France. Philadelphia: Collins, 1876. 52p. port. DNLM; PU
70-1303

GOODELL, William (1829-1894)
When and why were male physicians employed as accoucheurs? [New York, 1876.] 10p. DNLM **70-1304**

GOODELL, William (1829-1894)
The mechanism of natural and of artificial labor in narrow pelves. Philadelphia, 1876. 18p. DNLM
70-1305

GOODELL, William (1829-1894)
The valedictory address to the graduating class of the medical department of the University of Pennsylvania. Philadelphia: Collins, 1878. 12p. DNLM; PU **70-1306**

GOODELL, William (1829-1894)
A case of vaginal ovariotomy. Boston, 1878. 18p. DNLM
70-1307

GOODELL, William (1829-1894)
Laceration of the cervix uteri. The address in obstetrics, delivered before the Society of the State of Pennsylvania, at its annual meeting held at Pittsburgh, May, 1878. Philadelphia: Collins, 1878. 16p. DNLM; PPC **70-1308**

GOODELL, William (1829-1894)
A case of spaying for fibroid tumor of the womb. [Philadelphia, 1878.] 14p. DNLM **70-1309**

GOODELL, William (1829-1894)
Annual address on the relation of neurasthenia to diseases of the womb. [Boston, 1879.] 20p. DNLM
70-1310

GOODELL, William (1829-1894)
The extirpation of the ovaries for some of the disorders of menstrual life. Philadelphia: Collins, 1879. 15p. DNLM
70-1311

GOODELL, William (1829-1894)
Clinical observations upon the treatment of uterine fibroids; with a case illustrating the operation of enucleation. Philadelphia: Henry C. Lea, [1879]. 16p. DNLM; PPC
70-1312

GOODELL, William (1829-1894)
Lessons in gynecology. . . . With eighty illustrations. Philadelphia, Pa.: D. G. Brinton, 1879. 380p. DLC; DNLM; NNNAM; PPC **70-1313**

GOODMAN, J[ohn] (1837-1912)
Menstruation and the law of monthly periodicity. Louisville, 1875. 16p. DNLM **70-1314**

GOODMAN, J[ohn] (1837-1912)
The cyclical theory of menstruation. New York: William Wood & Co., 1878. 24p. DNLM **70-1315**

GOODWILLIE, D[avid] H[enderson] (*b.* 1834)
Resections of the maxillary bones without external incision, illustrated by cases, and a description of instruments. New York: D. Appleton & Co., 1872. 19p. 12 fig. DNLM; NNNAM
70-1316

GOODWILLIE, D[avid] H[enderson] (*b.* 1834)
Anchylosis of the temporo-maxillary articulation of long standing; fracture of the right condyle; atrophy of the depressors and contraction of the elevator muscle of the inferior maxillary. New York: D. Appleton & Co., 1875. 12p. DNLM; NNNAM **70-1317**

GOODWILLIE, D[avid] H[enderson] (*b.* 1834)
Lesions of the trifacial (especially facial neuralgia), resulting from diseases of the dental organs and adjacent parts. [Chicago: A. S. Kissell & Co., 1876.] 20p. DNLM
70-1318

GOODWILLIE, D[avid] H[enderson] (*b.* 1834)
Extirpation of the bones of the nose and mouth by the use of the surgical engine. New York: William Wood & Co., 1879. 16p. DNLM; NNNAM **70-1319**

GOODWIN, E. J.
The family's medical guide. . . . Louisville, Ky.: J. C. Webb & Co., printers and binders, 1871. 102p. DLC
70-1320

GORDON, S[eth] C[hase] (*b.* 1830)
The mechanical treatment of sterility; with a report of cases. Portland: S. Berry, 1878. 10p. DNLM **70-1321**

GORTON, David Allyn (1832-1916)
Medicine a learned and liberal profession. An essay read before the Homoeopathic Medical Society of the County of Kings, August 6, 1872. Albany: The Argus Co., 1872. 20p. PPHa **70-1322**

GORTON, David Allyn (1832-1916)
An essay on the principles of mental hygiene. Philadelphia: J. B. Lippincott & Co., 1873. 242p. DLC; DNLM
70-1323

GORTON, David Allyn (1832-1916)
The drift of medical philosophy; an essay. Philadelphia: J. B. Lippincott & Co., 1875. 70p. DLC; DNLM
70-1324

GOSS, Francis W.
The dressing of wounds. [Boston, 1874.] 8p. DNLM
70-1325

GOSS, I[sham] J[abez] M[arshall]
New medicines, and their special therapeutics. St. Louis, 1877. 111p. DNLM; OCIM; OCLloyd **70-1326**

GOSS, I[sham] J[abez] M[arshall]
The new materia medica and therapeutics. . . . A compend of materia medica written with especial reference to the more direct or positive action of medicines, and the introduction of new ones. St. Louis, Mo.: G. H. Field, 1877. 437p. ICJ; IU-M; NjR; PPJ **70-1326A**

GOULEY, John William Severin (1832-1920)
Diseases of the urinary organs: including stricture of the urethra, affections of the prostate, and stone in the bladder. . . . New York: William Wood & Co., 1873. 368p. DLC; DNLM; NNNAM; PPC **70-1327**

GOULEY, John William Severin (1832-1920)
Perityphlitic abscess due to perforation of the appendix vermiformis, with remarks upon the surgical treatment thereof. . . . New York: G. P. Putnam's Sons, 1875. 9p. DLC; DNLM
70-1328

GOULEY, John William Severin (1832-1920)
Urethroplastic operations to remedy hypospadias, epispadias, and also incurvation of the penis. New York: William Wood & Co., 1876. 15p. DNLM **70-1329**

GOULEY, John William Severin (1832-1920)
Report of a case of sub-periosteal excision and disarticulation of the entire inferior maxillary bone for phosphorus necrosis. . . . Philadelphia: [Collins, printer], 1877. 4p. DLC **70-1330**

GOULEY, John William Severin (1832-1920)
Internal urethrotomy and lithotripsy at the same sitting, in a patient seventy-nine years of age; with remarks on rapid lithotripsy, and on the evacuation of detritus from the bladder. . . . New York: Trow's Printing & Bookbinding Company, 1879. 16p. DLC; DNLM; NNNAM **70-1331**

GOULLON, Heinrich (1801-1883)
Scrofulous affections and the advantages of their treatment according to the principles and experiences of homoeopathy; described and demonstrated by numerous examples of successful cures. . . . New York and Philadelphia: Boericke & Tafel, 1872. 255p. NNNAM; PPC; PPHa **70-1332**

GRAHAM, Douglas (*b.* 1848)
Massage in amenorrhoea and dysmenorrhoea. [Boston, 1876.] 7p. DNLM **70-1333**

GRAHAM, Douglas (*b.* 1848)
The history of massage. New York: William Wood & Co., 1879. 30p. DNLM; NNNAM **70-1334**

GRANT, Thomas P[age]
Diagnosis of spinal disease, and observations on hip disease. [Louisville, 1876.] 6p. DNLM **70-1335**

GRANVOGL, Eduard von
Text book of homoeopathy. . . . Transl. by Geo. E. Shipman, at the request of the author. Chicago: C. S. Halsey; New York: Boericke & Tafel; [etc., etc.], 1870. 341, 438p. fold. chart. DLC; NNNAM; PPC; PPHa **70-1336**

GRANVOGL, Eduard von
The homoeopathic law of similarity. An open letter to Professor Justus baron v. Liebig. . . . Transl. from the German by Geo. E. Shipman. Chicago: Foundlings' Home Print, 1879. 85p. DLC; PPHa **70-1337**

GRAY, Henry (1825-1861)
Anatomy descriptive and surgical. . . . The drawings by H. V. Carter . . . , the dissections jointly by the author and Dr. Carter. . . . A new American from the 5th and enlarged English ed. Philadelphia: Henry C. Lea, 1870. 876p. MBM; OCIM; NNNAM; PPC **70-1338**

GRAY, Henry (1825-1861)
Anatomy descriptive and surgical. . . . With five hundred and twenty-two engravings on wood. The drawings by H. V. Carter, M.D., and Dr. Westmacott. The dissections jointly by the author and Dr. Carter. With an introduction on general anatomy and development. By T. Holmes. . . . A new American from the 8th and enl. English ed. To which is added Landmarks, medical and surgical. By Luther Holden. . . . Philadelphia: Henry C. Lea, 1878. 983p. DLC; DNLM; NNNAM; PPC **70-1339**

GRAY, John Franklin (1804-1882)
American medical education. Annual address before the Homoeopathic Medical Society of the State of New York. Albany: The Argus Co., 1872. 14p. PPHa **70-1340**

GRAY, John P[erdue] (1825-1886)
Insanity; its dependence on physical disease. Utica, N.Y.: Roberts, 1871. 36p. DNLM **70-1341**

GRAY, John P[erdue] (1825-1886)
Thoughts on the causation of insantiy. [Utica, N.Y., 1872.] 22p. DNLM **70-1342**

GRAY, John P[erdue] (1825-1886)
Pathology of insanity. [Utica? 1874.] 30p. 6 plates. DNLM **70-1343**

GRAY, John P[erdue] (1825-1886)
Responsibility of the insane; homicide in insanity. [Utica, N.Y., 1875.] 57p. 1 tab. DNLM **70-1344**

GRAY, John P[erdue] (1825-1886)
Pathological researches. [Utica, N.Y., 1876.] 21p. DNLM **70-1345**

GRAY, John P[erdue] (1825-1886)
Mental hygiene. [Utica, N.Y., 1878.] 35p. DNLM **70-1346**

GRAY, John P[erdue] (1825-1886)
An abstract of the laws of the State of New York, in regard to the commitment of insane to asylums, their detention and discharge, and comparisons of the same, with the statutory provisions of England. [Utica, N.Y., 1879.] 16p. DNLM **70-1347**

GRAY, John P[erdue] (1825-1886)
Suicide. [Utica, N.Y., 1879.] 37p. DNLM **70-1348**

GRAY, Landon Carter (1850-1900)
Chorcic and choreiform movements in hysterical children. New York: G. P. Putnam's Sons, 1879. 8p. DNLM **70-1349**

GREEN, Ezra (1746-1847)
Diary of . . . surgeon on board the continental ship-of-war "Ranger," under John Paul Jones, from November 1, 1777, to September 27, 1778. With historical notes and a biography by Com. Geo. Henry Preble and Walter. C. Green. . . . Boston, 1875. 31p. DNLM; MB; MBAt **70-1350**

GREEN, Horace (1802-1866)
Selections from favorite prescriptions of living American practitioners. New York: J. Wiley & Son, 1872. 214p. DNLM; MBM; NNNAM; PPC **70-1351**

GREEN, J[ohn] Orne, Jr. (1841-1922)
Report on the progress of otology for 1869-1870. New York: D. Appleton & Co., 1870. 23p. DNLM; NNNAM **70-1352**

GREEN, J[ohn] Orne, Jr. (1841-1922)
Five cases of fatal otorrhoea, with remarks on the course by which such cases lead to death. [New York, 1870.] 21p. DNLM; NNNAM **70-1353**

GREEN, J[ohn] Orne, Jr. (1841-1922)
Report on otology. [Boston, 1873.] 11p. DNLM
70-1354

GREEN, J[ohn] Orne, Jr. (1841-1922)
Neuralgia in and about the ear. Boston: A. Mudge & Son, 1874. 11p. DNLM **70-1355**

GREEN, J[ohn] Orne, Jr. (1841-1922)
Disease of the brain in its relation to inflammations of the ear. Boston: Rockwell & Churchill, 1877. 26p. DNLM; MH-M
70-1356

GREEN, J[ohn] Orne, Jr. (1841-1922)
Phlebitis of the venae emissariae mastoideae. New York: William Wood & Co., 1879. 16p. DNLM; NNNAM
70-1357

GREEN, T. Henry (1841-1923)
An introduction to pathology and morbid anatomy. Philadelphia: Henry C. Lea, 1871. 252p. CtY-M; DNLM; OCIM; PPC
70-1358

GREEN, T. Henry (1841-1923)
An introduction to pathology and morbid anatomy. 2nd American from 3rd English ed. Philadelphia: Henry C. Lea, 1876. 316p. DNLM; MBM; NNNAM; PU
70-1359

GREEN, Traill (1813-1897)
First annual address delivered before the American Academy of Medicine. Also, the constitution and by-laws, etc. Carlisle, Pa., 1877. 30, 11p. DNLM **70-1360**

GREEN, Wm. A.
The cause and cure of yellow fever, and the Bedford (Va.) iron and alum mass as a remedial agent. [Atlanta, 1878.] 8p. DNLM **70-1361**

GREENE, Francis V[inton] (1850-1921)
Jaborandi. Communicated to the Bureau of Medicine and Surgery, Navy Department. [Philadelphia, 1875.] 8p. DNLM
70-1362

GREENE, James S[umner]
An unusual case of cancer. [Philadelphia, 1876.] 10p. DNLM
70-1363

GREENE, W[illiam] A[lexander] (*b.* 1834)
Haemorrhagic malarial fever, and its treatment with seven springs iron and alum mass. [Abingdon, Va., 1878.] 10p. DNLM **70-1364**

GREENE, William Warren (1831-1881)
Reduction of dislocations. [Boston, 1870.] 11p. DNLM
70-1365

GREENE, William Warren (1831-1881)
Report on ovariotomy. [Portland, 1870.] 23p. DNLM
70-1366

GREENFIELD, W. S.
Health primers. No. 2. Alcohol; its use and abuse. New York: D. Appleton & Co., 1879. 95p. DNLM; NN; NNC
70-1367

GREGG, Rollin Robinson (1828-1886)
The "febrinous crasis," its cause a loss of albumen from the blood. Buffalo, N.Y., 1870. 23p. DNLM **70-1368**

GREGG, Rollin Robinson (1828-1886)
An illustrated repertory of pains in chest, sides, and back; their direction and character, confirmed by clinical cases. 2nd ed. Chicago: Duncan Brothers, 1879. 97p. 5 plates. DNLM; OCIM; PPC **70-1369**

GREGG, Rollin Robinson (1828-1886)
The cause of consumption, a loss of albumen from the blood through irritated and abraded mucous membranes. [Buffalo, N.Y., 1879.] 4p. DNLM **70-1370**

GREGG, Rollin Robinson (1828-1886)
Consumption; the Academy of Medicine, Paris, in error on a most vital question. [Buffalo, N.Y., 1879.] 8p. DNLM
70-1371

GREGORY, T. A.
An essay written and published by . . . , dentist, New Albany, Ind. New Albany, Ind., 1872. 30p. DNLM
70-1372

GRIFFIN, E. L[eonard] (1821-1892)
Vaccination. A report. 22p. Milwaukee: Frayser, Williams & Walters, 1874. 22p. DNLM **70-1373**

GRIFFIN, E. L[eonard] (1821-1892)
Diphtheria; its relation to filth causes. Madison. D. Atwood, [1879]. 21p. DNLM **70-1374**

GRIFFITH, M[atthew] M[ilton]
Corpulence treated without starvation, or how to get lean. 2nd ed. Wilkes-Barre: E. B. Yordy, 1877. 79p. DNLM
70-1375

GRIFFITH, Robert Eglesfeld (1798-1850)
A universal formulary: containing the methods of preparing and administering officinal and other medicines. The whole adapted to physicians and pharmaceutists. By. . . . 3rd ed., carefully rev. and much enl., by John M. Maisch. . . . Philadelphia: Henry C. Lea, 1874. 779p. DLC; DNLM; OCLloyd; PPC
70-1376

GRISSOM, Eugene (1831-1902)
Mania transitoria. Raleigh, N.C.: Edwards, Broughton & Co., 1876. 48p. DNLM **70-1377**

GRISSOM, Eugene (1831-1902)
The border-land of insanity. Illustrated by examples selected from among the illustrious insane. [Richmond, 1876.] 37p. DNLM **70-1378**

GRISSOM, Eugene (1831-1902)
The border-land of insanity. Illustrated by examples selected from among the illustrious insane. Raleigh: J. Nichols, 1877. 44p. DNLM **70-1379**

GRISSOM, Eugene (1831-1902)
Mental hygiene for pupil and teacher. A lecture. Raleigh: J. Nichols, 1877. 36p. DNLM **70-1380**

GRISSOM, Eugene (1831-1902)
Mechanical protection for the violent insane. [Utica, 1878.] 32p. DNLM **70-1381**

GRISSOM, Eugene (1831-1902)
True and false experts. [Utica, 1878.] 36p. DNLM
70-1382

GRISSOM, Eugene (1831-1902)
True and false experts. To which is appended a rejoinder to Dr. Hammond's "Open letter." Raleigh, N.C.: J. Nichols, [1878]. 48p. DNLM **70-1383**

GRISSOM, Eugene (1831-1902)
Ture and false experts. To which is appended a rejoinder to Dr. Hammond's "Open letter." With a postscript. Raleigh: J. Nichols. [1878]. 51p. DNLM **70-1384**

GROSS, Samuel David (1805-1884)
Address before the Medical Society of the State of Pennsylvania at its twenty-second annual session, June 1871. Philadelphia: Collins, 1871. 28p. DNLM; PPJ **70-1385**

GROSS, Samuel David (1805-1884)
An address delivered before the Alumni Association of the Jefferson Medical College of Philadelphia, at its first anniversary, March 11, 1871. Philadelphia: Collins, 1871. 29p. DNLM; PPJ **70-1386**

GROSS, Samuel David (1805-1884)
A system of surgery; pathological, diagnostic, therapeutic, and operative. . . . Illustrated by upward of fourteen hundred engravings. 5th ed., greatly enl. and thoroughly rev. . . . Philadelphia: Henry C. Lea, 1872. 2 v. DLC; OCIM; PPC; PU **70-1387**

GROSS, Samuel David (1805-1884)
Discourse upon the life, character, and services of Ambrose Paré; delivered before the class of the Jefferson Medical College of Philadelphia, Feb. 12, 1873. Philadelphia: P. Madeira, 1873. 32p. PPJ **70-1388**

GROSS, Samuel David (1805-1884)
Syphilis in its relation to the national health; being the address in surgery. Philadelphia: Collins, 1874. 48p. DNLM; PPJ **70-1389**

GROSS, Samuel David (1805-1884)
A discourse on bloodletting considered as a therapeutic agent. Philadelphia: Collins, 1875. 19p. DNLM; PPJ **70-1390**

GROSS, Samuel David (1805-1884)
The glory and the hardships of the medical life; being the valedictory address delivered at the Philadelphia Academy of Music, March 11, 1875, before the trustees, faculty, and students of the Jefferson Medical College, at its 49th annual commencement. Philadelphia: P. Madeira, 1875. 31, 4p. DNLM; PPJ **70-1391**

GROSS, Samuel David (1805-1884)
A practical treatise on the diseases, injuries, and malformations of the urinary bladder, the prostate gland, and the urethra. . . . 3rd ed., rev. and ed. by Samuel W. Gross. . . . Philadelphia: Henry C. Lea, 1876. 574p. DLC; DNLM; NNNAM; PPC **70-1392**

GROSS, Samuel David (1805-1884)
History of American medical literature, from 1776 to the present time. . . . Philadelphia: Collins, printer, 1876. 85p. DLC; DNLM; NN; PPC **70-1393**

GROSS, Samuel David (1805-1884)
Obituary notice of Isaac Hays, M.D. . . . Philadelphia: Collins, printer, 1879. 14p. DLC; DNLM; PPJ **70-1394**

GROSS, Samuel David (1805-1884)
Memorial oration in honor of Ephraim McDowell, "The father of ovariotomy." . . . delivered at Danville, Ky., at the dedication of the monument erected to the memory of Dr. Ephraim McDowell by the Kentucky State Medical Society, May 14, 1879. Pub. by the Society. Louisville, Ky.: Printed by J. P. Morton & Co., 1879. 77p. DLC; DNLM; PPJ **70-1395**

[GROSS, Samuel David] (1805-1884)
Complimentary dinner given to Professor S. D. Gross by his medical friends in commemoration of his fifty-first year in the profession, April 10, 1879. Philadelphia: Lindsay & Blakiston, 1879. 42p. port. DNLM; PPJ **70-1396**

GROSS, Samuel Weissell (1837-1889)
Observations on ulceration of the jugular veins, communicating with an abscess or an open sore. Philadelphia: Collins, 1871. 18p. DNLM; PPJ **70-1397**

GROSS, Samuel Weissell (1837-1889)
On sexual debility and impotence, resulting from stricture and inflammation of the curved portion of the urethra, with special reference to masturbation as an exciting cause of stricture. [Philadelphia, 1877.] 9p. DNLM; PPJ **70-1398**

GUERNSEY, Henry Newell (1817-1885)
Before, during and after parturition. Prepared by special request for the Cumberland Valley Homoeopathic Medical Society and read before that body, May 3, 1870. New York: Boericke & Tafel, 1870. 16p. PPHa **70-1399**

GUERNSEY, Henry Newell (1817-1885)
Uterine haemorrhage. Philadelphia, 1870. 16p. PPHa **70-1400**

GUERNSEY, Henry Newell (1817-1885)
The homoeopathic treatment of disordered dentition. Philadelphia: Sherman & Co., 1870. 16p. PPHa **70-1401**

GUERNSEY, Henry Newell (1817-1885)
The homoeopathic materia medica. Read before the Pennsylvania State Homoeopathic Society, June, 1870. Philadelphia: Sherman & Co., 1870. 7p. PPHa **70-1402**

GUERNSEY, Henry Newell (1817-1885)
Notes of lectures on materia medica, delivered in the Hahnemann Medical College of Philadelphia. Reported by Joseph C. Guernsey, M.D. Philadelphia: W. P. Kildare, 1873. 234p. DNLM **70-1403**

GUERNSEY, Henry Newell (1817-1885)
The application of the principles and practice of homoeopathy to obstetrics and the disorders peculiar to women and young children. 2nd ed., revised, enlarged, and greatly improved. With numerous illustrations. Philadelphia: Boericke & Tafel, 1873. 986p. PPC; PPHa; PU **70-1404**

GUERNSEY, Henry Newell (1817-1885)
Ovarian tumors. Philadelphia, [1877]. 8p. DNLM **70-1405**

GUERNSEY, Henry Newell (1817-1885)
The application of the principles and practice of homoeopathy to obstetrics and the disorders peculiar to women and young children. 3rd ed. New York and Philadelphia: Boericke & Tafel, 1878. 1004p. PPC; PPHa; PU **70-1406**

GUERNSEY, Henry Newell (1817-1885)
Annual address to the Homoeopathic Medical Society of Pennsylvania. [1878.] 8p. DNLM; PPHa **70-1407**

GUERNSEY, Henry Newell (1817-1885)
A treatise. Death-rates in childbed. [New York, 1879.] 12p. DNLM **70-1408**

GUERNSEY, R. S.
Juries and physicians on questions of insanity. New York: J. R. McDivitt & Co., [1872]. 11p. DNLM **70-1409**

GUERNSEY, William Jefferson
Menstruation. . . . [Philadelphia, 1878.] 17p. DLC **70-1410**

GUERNSEY, William Jefferson
The traveller's medical repertory and family adviser, for the homoeopathic treatment of acute diseases. New York: Boericke & Tafel, 1879. 36p. DNLM; PPHa **70-1411**

GUILD, J. H.
A practical treatise on spasmodic asthma, with the various methods of its treatment. . . . Rutland: Tuttle & Co., 1873. 48p. DNLM **70-1412**

GUNN, John C. (1800-1863)
Domestic medicine. . . . New family physician; or, home-book of health. 100th ed. Cincinnati, O.: C. F. Wilstach & Co., 1870. 1218p. 4 plates. DNLM; OCIM **70-1413**

GUNN, John C. (1800-1863)
. . . Gunn's newer family physician; or, Home-book of health: an approved household guide for avoiding disease and prolonging life . . . assisted by Johnson H. Jordan. . . . Louisville: Moore Publishing Co., 1871. 1190p. plates. DLC; OCIM **70-1414**

GUNN, John C. (1800-1863)
. . . Gunn's new family physician: or Home-book of health; forming a complete household guide. . . . With supplementary treatises on anatomy, physiology and hygiene, on domestic and sanitary economy, and on physical culture and development. . . . Cincinnati: Wilstach, Baldwin & Co., 1873. 1230p. DLC; OCIM **70-1415**

GUNN, John C. (1800-1863)
. . . Gunn's newest family physician; or, Home-book of health; an approved household guide . . . assisted by Johnson H. Jordan, M.D., and several scientific writers of the highest eminence. Cincinnati, Philadelphia [etc.]; W. H. Moore & Co., 1876. 1190p. plates. DLC; OCIM; PPC **70-1416**

GUNN, Moses (1822-1887)
Valedictory address. Rush Medical College, 1870-1871. Chicago: Rand, McNally & Co., 1871. 15p. DNLM **70-1417**

GUNN, Robert A[lexander] (*b.* 1844)
The nature and treatment of venereal diseases; with numerous cases, formulae, and clinical observations. New York: A. K. Butts & Co., 1874. 182p. DNLM; NNNAM **70-1418**

GUNN, Robert A[lexander] (*b.* 1844)
Medical intolerance. A lecture delivered before the New York Liberal Club, November 2, 1877. New York: Monroe & Metz, 1877. 23p. DNLM **70-1419**

GUNNING, Robert Brian
The larynx the source of the vowel sounds. Baltimore, 1874. 29p. DNLM **70-1420**

GUNNING, Robert Brian
Hard rubber appliance for congenital cleft palate. New York: D. Appleton & Co., 1878. 11p. DNLM **70-1421**

GUNNING, Thomas Brian
A protest against the surrender to non-members of the dental profession of the right and duty of deciding upon the fitness of the faculties of dental colleges. [Baltimore, 1874.] 12p. DNLM **70-1422**

HABERSHON, Samuel Osborne (1825-1889)
Lettsomian lectures on the pathology and treatment of some diseases of the liver. Philadelphia: Lindsay & Blakiston, 1872. 91p. MBM; NNNAM; PPC; PPJ **70-1423**

HABERSHON, Samuel Osborne (1825-1889)
Pathological and practical observations on diseases of the abdomen, comprising those of the stomach, and other parts of the alimentary canal, oesophagus, caecum, intestines, and peritoneum. . . . 3rd ed. Considerably enlarged and revised. Philadelphia: Lindsay & Blakiston, 1878. 706p. tables. MH-M; NNNAM; PPC; PU **70-1424**

HABERSHON, Samuel Osborne (1825-1889)
On diseases of the stomach, the varieties of dyspepsia, their diagnosis and treatment. 3rd ed. Philadelphia: Lindsay & Blakiston, 1879. 324p. CtY-M; ICRM; NNNAM; PPC **70-1425**

HABERSHON, Samuel Osborne (1825-1889)
Diseases of the abdomen, comprising those of the stomach, and other parts of the alimentary canal, oesophagus, caecum, intestines, and peritoneum. . . . 2nd American from the 3rd enl. and rev. English ed. Philadelphia: Henry C. Lea, 1879. 554p. LNT-M; MdBJ-W; NNNAM; PPC **70-1426**

HABERSHON, Samuel Osborne (1825-1889)
Pathological and practical observations on diseases of the alimentary canal, oesophagus, stomach, caecum and intestines. 2nd American from the 3rd London ed. Philadelphia: Henry C. Lea, 1879. 554p. CU-M; IEN-M; NNNAM; PPC **70-1427**

HAHNEMANN MEDICAL COLLEGE AND HOSPITAL. CHICAGO
An address to the alumni by the faculty of the College. Chicago: Culver, Page, Hoyne & Co., 1879. 24p. DNLM; ICRM **70-1428**

HAHNEMANN MEDICAL COLLEGE AND HOSPITAL OF PHILADELPHIA
Annual announcements [of the College] for the sessions of 1879-1880 to 1901-1902 (13.-34., or 53., by consolidation). Philadelphia, 1879-1900. DNLM [List of students and graduates for the years 1867-1868 to 1899-1900, in announcements for subsequent years.] **70-1429**

HAHNEMANN, Samuel Christian Friedrich (1755-1843)
A treatise on the effects of coffee. Transl. by Wm. L. Breyfogle. Louisville: Bradley & Gilbert, 1875. 35p. DNLM; OCIM **70-1430**

HAHNEMANN, Samuel Christian Friedrich (1755-1843)
Organon of the art of healing. . . . 5th American ed., transl. from the 5th German ed., by C. Wesselhoeft, M.D. New York, Philadelphia: Boericke & Tafel; [etc., etc.], 1876. 244p. DLC; DNLM; PPHa; PPJ **70-1431**

HAHNEMANN, Samuel Christian Friedrich (1755-1843)
The genius of the homoeopathic healing art. Transl. by A. Lippe. Preface to the second volume of the materia medica pura. Philadelphia: J. A. Moore, 1878. 16p. DNLM; PPHa **70-1432**

HAILES, William Jr.
Sections and section cutting. With a description of a new poly-microtome for freezing. [Utica, 1879.] 12p. DNLM **70-1433**

HALE, Edwin Moses (1829-1899)
The bromides; their pathogenetic and therapeutic action. Published by the author, Chicago, 1871. 41p. OCLloyd; PPHa **70-1434**

HALE, Edwin Moses (1829-1899)
Lectures on diseases of the heart. . . . New York, [etc.]; Boericke & Tafel; [etc., etc.], 1871. 206p. DLC; DNLM; PPHa **70-1435**

HALE, Edwin Moses (1829-1899)
Lectures on diseases of the heart. . . . 2nd ed. New York: Boericke & Tafel, 1872. 248p. DLC; DNLM; PPHa **70-1436**

HALE, Edwin Moses (1829-1899)
The characteristics of the new remedies. . . . 3rd ed., remodeled and rewritten. Detroit, Mich.: Lodge's Homoeopathic Pharmacy; New York: Boericke & Tafel; [etc., etc.], 1873. 544p. DLC **70-1437**

HALE, Edwin Moses (1829-1899)
Materia medica and special therapeutics of the new remedies. . . . 4th ed., rev. and enl. New York and Philadelphia: Boericke & Tafel; [etc., etc.], 1875. 2 v. DLC; DNLM; PPHa **70-1438**

HALE, Edwin Moses (1829-1899)
Repertory to the new remedies. Based upon, and designed to accompany Hale's special symptomatology and therapeutics. By C. P. Hart. . . . New York, Philadelphia: Boericke & Tafel, 1876. 199p. DLC; OCLloyd; PPHa **70-1439**

HALE Edwin Moses (1829-1899)
A critical period for homoeopathy. [Chicago, 1877.] 2 l. DNLM **70-1440**

HALE, Edwin Moses (1829-1899)
An open letter to the medical profession; being a history and defense of Dr. Hale's pamphlet, entitled: "On the homoeopathic treatment of abortion, its causes and consequences, with some suggestions and indications for the use of the new remedies." Also an exposure of the animus of the attacks upon its author by Dr. G. D. Beebe and others. To which is added the republication of a fac-simile of the original pamphlet. Chicago: J. Millikan, 1877. 22, 22p. DNLM **70-1441**

HALE, Edwin Moses (1829-1899)
The medical, surgical, and hygienic treatment of diseases of women, especially those causing sterility, the disorders and accidents of pregnancy, and painful and difficult labor. New York & Philadelphia: Boericke & Tafel, 1878. 298p. DNLM; NNNAM; PPC; PPHa **70-1442**

[HALE, George S.] (1825-1897)
Medical charities; a paper read at the meeting of the Social Science Association, held at Detroit in May, 1875. Boston: Tolman & White, 1875. 17p. DNLM **70-1443**

HALL, Edward D.
The metric dose book. Boston: A. T. Bliss & Co., 1879. 28p. DNLM; MBM **70-1444**

HALL, F[rancis de Havilland] (1847-1929)
Differential diagnosis; a manual of the comparative semeiology of the more important diseases. American ed., with extensive additions. Philadelphia: D. G. Brinton, 1879. 205p. DNLM; NNNAM; OCIM; PPC [2nd American ed. Edited by Frank Woodbury. Philadelphia: D. G. Brinton, 1881. 223p.; 3rd ed., thoroughly rev. and greatly enl. Edited by Frank Woodbury. Philadelphia: D. G. Brinton, 1887. 255p.] **70-1445**

HALL, George A.
Valedictory address to the graduating class of Hahnemann Medical College and Hospital of Chicago, February 22, 1877, with the President's address, the report of the Dean, and catalogue of students and graduates. Chicago: George W. Blair, 1877. 18p. PPHa **70-1446**

HALL, George Emmet
Hints to medical examiners. . . . Presented by the Hahnemann Life Insurance Company. . . . Cleveland: Printed at the Office of the Hahnemannian, 1871. 70p. DLC; DNLM; OCIM **70-1447**

HALL, William Whitty (1810-1876)
Bronchitis, and kindred diseases. . . . New York: Hurd & Houghton, 1870. 400p. DLC; NNNAM **70-1448**

HALL, William Whitty (1810-1876)
Health and disease as affected by constipation. New York: Hurd & Houghton, 1870. 298p. NNNAM **70-1149**

HALL, William Whitty (1810-1876)
Health by good living. . . . 6th thousand. New York: Hurd & Houghton, 1870. 277p. DLC; NNNAM **70-1450**

HALL, William Whitty (1810-1876)
The guide-board to health, peace and competence; or, The road to happy old age. . . . Springfield, Mass.: D. E. Fisk & Company; Philadelphia: Crittenden & McKinney, [1870]. 752p. DLC; PPHa **70-1451**

HALL, William Whitty (1810-1876)
Sleep; or the hygiene of the night. New York: Hurd & Houghton, 1870. 352p. DNLM; NNNAM **70-1452**

[HALL, William Whitty] (1810-1876)
Coughs and colds; or, The prevention, cause, and cure of various affections of the throat; with cases, illustrating the remarkable efficacy of out-door activity and horseback exercise, in permanently arresting the progress of diseases of the chest. New York: Hurd & Houghton, 1871. 362p. DLC; DNLM; NNNAM **70-1453**

HALL, William Whitty (1810-1876)
Fun better than physic: or everybody's life-preserver. Springfield, Mass.: D. E. Fisk, 1871. 333p. MBM; MWA; PP **70-1454**

HALL, William Whitty (1810-1876)
The guide-board to health, peace and competence; or, The road to happy old age. . . . Springfield, Mass.: D. E. Fisk & Company; Philadelphia: H. N. McKinney & Co., [1872]. 752p. DLC; NNNAM; PPC **70-1455**

HALL, William Whitty (1810-1876)
Health by good living. New York: Hurd & Houghton, 1872. 285p. DNLM **70-1456**

HALL, William Whitty (1810-1876)
Health at home, or Hall's family doctor. . . . Hartford, Conn., and Cincinnati, O.: S. M. Betts & Company, 1873. 799p. plates. DLC; OCIM **70-1457**

HALL, William Whitty (1810-1876)
How to live long; or, Health maxima, physical, mental, and moral. . . . New York: Hurd & Houghton; Cambridge: The Riverside Press, 1875. 316p. DLC; MWA; NNNAM **70-1458**

HALL, William Whitty (1810-1876)
Dyspepsia, and its kindred diseases. . . . New York: R. Worthington, 1877. 272p. DLC; NNNAM **70-1459**

[HALSEY, Clinton S.]
Medical hints for the people. . . . Galesburg, Ill.: C. S. Halsey, 1879. 72p. DLC **70-1460**

HAM, John Randolph
The Dover (N.H.) physicians. Read before the N.H. Medical Society, June 17, 1879. . . . Concord: Printed by Evans, Sleeper & Evans, 1879. 22p. DLC **70-1461**

HAMILTON, Allan McLane (1848-1919)
Galvano-puncture applied to the treatment of aneurisms. Poughkeepsie, N.Y.: I. Platt & Sons, 1870. 28p. 1 plate. DNLM **70-1462**

HAMILTON, Allan McLane (1848-1919)
Clinical electro-therapeutics, medical and surgical: a handbook for physicians in the treatment of nervous and other diseases. . . . New York: D. Appleton & Co., 1873. 184p. DLC; DNLM; NNNAM; PU **70-1463**

HAMILTON, Allan McLane (1848-1919)
A consideration of certain symptoms associated with morbid changes in the medulla oblongata. New York: D. Appleton & Co., 1875. 15p. DNLM; NNNAM **70-1464**

HAMILTON, Allan McLane (1848-1919)
The therapeutics of epilepsy. [Chicago, 1876.] 15p. DNLM **70-1465**

HAMILTON, Allan McLane (1848-1919)
Nervous diseases: their description and treatment. . . . Philadelphia: Henry C. Lea, 1878. 512p. DLC; DNLM; NNNAM; PPC **70-1466**

HAMILTON, Allan McLane (1848-1919)
The value of absent "tendon reflex" as a diagnostic sign in locomotor ataxia. With an analysis of eight cases. Cambridge: Riverside Press, 1879. 8p. DNLM **70-1467**

HAMILTON, Frank Hastings (1813-1886)
A practical treatise on fractures and dislocations. . . . 4th ed., rev. and improved. Illustrated with three hundred and twenty-two wood-cuts. Philadelphia: Henry C. Lea, 1871. 789p. DLC; NNNAM; PPC; PU **70-1468**

HAMILTON, Frank Hastings (1813-1886)
The principles and practice of surgery. . . . New York: William Wood & Co., 1872. 943p. DLC; DNLM; OCIM; PPC **70-1469**

HAMILTON, Frank Hastings (1813-1886)
A practical treatise on fractures and dislocations. . . . 5th ed., rev. and improved. Illustrated with three hundred and forty-four woodcuts. Philadelphia: Henry C. Lea, 1875. 831p. DLC; DNLM; NNNAM; PPC **70-1470**

HAMILTON, Frank Hastings (1813-1886)
Address delivered at the third annual meeting of the association of alumni and officers of the medical department of the University of Buffalo. Buffalo: Hansman & Burow, 1877. 10p. DNLM **70-1471**

HAMILTON, Frank Hastings (1813-1886)
Annual address delivered before the American Academy of Medicine, at Easton, Pa. [n.p., 1878.] 16p. DNLM **70-1472**

HAMILTON, Frank Hastings (1813-1886) and George H. YEAMAN
The Medico-Legal Society of the City of New York; its status, purposes, and scientific aspects. Annual meeting, November 7, 1877. [New York, 1878.] 13p. DNLM; NNNAM **70-1473**

HAMILTON, Frank Hastings (1813-1886)
Alimentation in surgical accidents and diseases, and its general value as contrasted with the value of medicine. New York, 1878. 12p. DNLM; NNNAM **70-1474**

HAMILTON, Frank Hastings (1813-1886)
Posture as a means of relief in strangulated and incarcerated hernia, with general consideration of the mechanism of reduction. [New York, 1879.] 20p. DNLM; NNNAM **70-1475**

HAMILTON, Frank Hastings (1813-1886)
Posture in the treatment of intestinal colic and ileus, with a consideration of the pathology of spasmodic colic; being the supplement to a paper read before the New York Academy of Medicine, May 1, 1879. [New York, 1879.] 8p. DNLM; NNNAM **70-1476**

HAMILTON, George (1808-1885)
Obituary notice of Doctor Lewis P. Gebhard. Philadelphia: Collins, 1874. 8p. DNLM **70-1477**

HAMILTON, John B[rown] (1847-1898)
A report on the treatment of fractures. Chicago: Fergus Printing Co., 1873. 20p. 1 plate. DNLM **70-1478**

HAMILTON, J. W. (1826?-1898) and J. F. BALDWIN
"The physicians and surgeons of the United States." A review editorial. Columbus, O.: Cott & Hann, 1878. 8p. DNLM **70-1479**

HAMILTON, R. Leonidas
The discoveries and unparalleled experience of Prof. R. Leonidas Hamilton, M.D., with regard to the nature and treatment of diseases of the liver, lungs, blood, and other chronic diseases; containing, also a biographical sketch of his life . . . with his common sense theory of diseases and the evidence of his wonderful cures. . . . [New York, 1870.] 112p. DLC; NNNAM **70-1480**

HAMLIN, Augustus C[hoate] (1829-1905)
Transmission of diseases. First paper. Consumption. [1876?] 9p. DNLM **70-1481**

HAMLIN, Augustus C[hoate] (1829-1905)
Transfusion. [1876?] 14p. DNLM **70-1482**

HAMMOND, William Alexander (1828-1900)
Spinal irritation. New York: D. Appleton & Co., 1870. 42p. DNLM; NNNAM **70-1483**

HAMMOND, William Alexander (1828-1900)
A medico-legal study of the case of Daniel McFarland. New York: D. Appleton & Co., 1870. 35p. DNLM; NNNAM **70-1484**

HAMMOND, William Alexander (1828-1900)
A treatise on diseases of the nervous system. . . . New York: D. Appleton & Co., 1871. 754p. DLC; DNLM; NNNAM; PU **70-1485**

HAMMOND, William Alexander (1828-1900)
The physics and physiology of spiritualism. New York: D. Appleton & Co., 1871. 86p. DNLM; NNNAM **70-1486**

HAMMOND, William Alexander (1828-1900)
A treatise on diseases of the nervous system. . . . 2nd ed. New York: D. Appleton & Co., 1872. 754p. NNNAM; MH-M; PPC; PU **70-1487**

HAMMOND, William Alexander (1828-1900)
A treatise on the diseases of the nervous system. 3rd ed., enl. New York: D. Appleton & Co., 1872. 754p. CtY-M; ICRM; MBM; NNNAM **70-1488**

HAMMOND, William Alexander (1828-1900)
Insanity in its relations to crime. A text and a commentary. . . . New York: D. Appleton & Co., 1873. 77p. DLC; DNLM; NNNAM **70-1489**

HAMMOND, William Alexander (1828-1900)
A treatise on diseases of the nervous system. . . . 4th ed. New York: D. Appleton & Co., 1873. 754p. CU-M; NNNAM; MBM; PPC **70-1490**

HAMMOND, William Alexander (1828-1900)
Clinical lectures on diseases of the nervous system. . . . Reported, ed., and the histories of the cases prepared, with notes, by T. M. B. Cross. . . . New York: D. Appleton & Co., 1874. 291p. DLC; DNLM; NNNAM; PPC **70-1491**

HAMMOND, William Alexander (1828-1900)
A treatise on diseases of the nervous system. . . . 5th ed. New York: D. Appleton & Co., [1875?]. [No locations found] **70-1492**

HAMMOND, William Alexander (1828-1900)
On pigmentary deposits in the brain, resulting from malarial poisoning. . . . New York: S. W. Green, printer and electrotyper, [1875]. 15p. DLC; DNLM; NNNAM **70-1493**

HAMMOND, William Alexander (1828-1900)
On the cause of Vice-President Wilson's death. . . . Cambridge: Printed at the Riverside Press, 1875. 14p. DLC; DNLM; MH-M **70-1494**

HAMMOND, William Alexander (1828-1900)
Spinal irritation; its pathology and treatment. New York: G. P. Putnam's Sons, 1876. 20p. DNLM; NNNAM **70-1495**

HAMMOND, William Alexander (1828-1900)
A treatise on the diseases of the nervous system. . . . 6th ed., rewritten, enl. and improved. New York: D. Appleton & Co., 1876. 883p. col. plate. CLM; DLC; DNLM; MdBJ-W **70-1496**

HAMMOND, William Alexander (1828-1900)
Spiritualism and allied causes and conditions of nervous derangement. . . . New York: G. P. Putnam's Sons, 1876. 366p. DLC; NNNAM; MH-M **70-1497**

HAMMOND, William Alexander (1828-1900)
Neurological contributions. I. The odor of the human body as developed by certain affections of the nervous system. II. On a hitherto undescribed form of muscular incoordination. New York: G. P. Putnam's Sons, 1877. 15p. DNLM; NNNAM **70-1498**

HAMMOND, William Alexander (1828-1900)
Cerebral hyperaemia the result of mental strain or emotional disturbance. . . . Read before the New York Neurological Society (in outline) Nov. 5th, 1877. New York: G. P. Putnam's Sons, 1878. 106p. DLC; DNLM; NNNAM **70-1499**

HAMMOND, William Alexander (1828-1900)
An open letter to Eugene Grissom. New York: Trow, 1878. 13p. DNLM **70-1500**

HAMMOND, William Alexander (1828-1900)
A second open letter to Dr. Eugene Grissom. New York: Trow's Print. Co., 1878. 18p. DNLM **70-1501**

HAMMOND, William Alexander (1828-1900)
An open letter to Eugene Grissom. 2nd ed., with a preface and a postscript. New York, 1878. 16p. DNLM **70-1502**

HAMMOND, William Alexander (1828-1900)
Insane asylum reform. I. The non-asylum treatment of the insane. . . . New York: G. P. Putnam's Sons, 1879. 24p. DLC; DNLM; NNNAM **70-1503**

HAMMOND, William Alexander (1828-1900)
Fasting girls; their physiology and pathology. New York: G. P. Putnam's Sons, 1879. 76p. DNLM; NNNAM **70-1504**

HAMMOND, William Alexander (1828-1900)
To the medical profession. Jan. 15, 1879. [Being the third communication in his controversy with Eugene Grissom.] [New York, 1879.] 4p. DNLM **70-1505**

HAND, H. C[lay] (1848-1876)
Malformation of pulmonic valves; two instead of three. [St. Paul, 1873.] 1 l. 1 plate. DNLM **70-1506**

A HAND-BOOK of nursing for family and general use. Published under the direction of the Connecticut Training-School for Nurses. Philadelphia: J. B. Lippincott & Co., 1879. 266p. DNLM; NNNAM; PU **70-1507**

HANKS, H[orace] T[racy] (1837-1900)
A contribution to the study of dysmenorrhoea, when occasioned by anteflexion of the uterus or cervix. With a tabulated report of thirty-seven cases treated. Albany, N.Y.: Van Benthuysen, 1877. 16p. 1 tab. DNLM **70-1508**

HARDENSTEIN, Ernest
The epidemic of 1878 and its homoeopathic treatment; a general history of the origin, progress, and end of the plague in the Mississippi Valley. . . . To this is added a treatise on the disease by A. O. H. Hardenstein, and other valuable papers and statistics from the most reliable sources. New Orleans: J. S. Rivers, 1879. 105p. DNLM; LNT-M **70-1509**

HARLAN, George C[uvier] (1835-1909)
Retinitis albuminurica. Philadelphia, 1877. 7p. DNLM **70-1510**

HARLEY, George (1829-1896)
The urine and its derangements. With the application of physiological chemistry to the diagnosis and treatment of constitutional as well as local diseases. Philadelphia: Lindsay & Blakiston, 1872. 334p. DNLM; NNNAM; PPC; PPJ **70-1511**

HARRIS, Chapin Aaron (1806-1860)
The principles and practice of dentistry, including anatomy, physiology, pathology, therapeutics, dental surgery and mechanism. . . . 10th ed. Rev. and ed. by Philip H. Austen. . . . Philadelphia: Lindsay & Blakiston, 1871. 794p. col. plates. DLC; MdU-D; PU **70-1512**

HARRIS, Charles T[aylor] (1818-1890)
The nurse; or hints on the care of the sick; including mothers and infants, and a digest of domestic medicine. Chicago: Duncan Bros., 1879. 120p. PPHa **70-1513**

HARRIS, Elisha (1824-1884)
General health laws and local ordinances, considered with reference to State and local sanitary organization. Cambridge: Riverside Press, 1874. 13p. DNLM; MWA **70-1514**

HARRIS, Elisha (1824-1884)
Conclusions concerning cholera. Causes and preventive measures. Cambridge: Riverside Press, 1874. 16p. DNLM; MBM **70-1515**

HARRIS, Elisha (1824-1884)
A report on laws, provisions, and methods for securing general vaccination throughout the country. . . . Cambridge, [Mass.]: Printed at the Riverside Press, 1877. 16p. DLC; DNLM; MH-M; MWA **70-1516**

HARRIS, Elisha (1824-1884)
Report on plans for securing complete and authentic records of the deaths and the causes of death in the United States. Cambridge: Riverside Press, 1878. 15p. DNLM; MBM **70-1517**

HARRIS, James C.
An essay on the climate and fevers of the South-Western, South Atlantic, and Gulf States, embracing a brief exposition and defense of the existence and essential nature of malaria; accompanied and illustrated with a medico-topographical and meteorological account of the Dead Sea region. Charleston: Walker, Evans & Cogswell, 1872. 103p. DNLM; ScMS; ScU **70-1518**

HARRIS, R. Duncan
Abstract of the principal laws of the State of New York relating to the medical profession. New York: G. P. Putnam's Sons, 1875. 25p. DNLM; NNNAM **70-1519**

HARRIS, Robert Patterson (1822-1899)
Lessons from a study of the Caesarean operation in the City and State of New York, and their bearing upon the true position of gastro-elytrotomy. New York: William Wood & Co., 1879. 12p. DNLM; NNNAM **70-1520**

HARRIS, Robert Patterson (1822-1899)
A study and analysis of one hundred Caesarean operations performed in the United States during the present century, and prior to the year 1878. [Philadelphia, 1879.] 22p. DNLM; PPC **70-1521**

HARRIS, Robert Patterson (1822-1899)
Foot-binding in China. An account of the process and its effects; and a correction of many erroneous statements which have been made, chiefly by travellers, in regard to it. [Philadelphia, 1879.] 17p. DNLM **70-1522**

HARRISBURG HOSPITAL
Report of the managers of the Harrisburg Hospital, to the contributors, of the facts connected with the resignation of the first medical staff. Harrisburg: T. F. Scheffer, 1877. 16p. DNLM **70-1523**

HARRISBURG HOSPITAL
To the medical profession. Statement from the staff of the Harrisburg Hospital, denying the assertions of the Dauphin County Medical Scoeity, which accuse them and the institution of being in homoeopathic affiliation. March 12, 1877. [Harrisburg, 1877.] 8p. DNLM **70-1524**

HARRISON, J. S.
Valedictory address to the graduating class of the New Orleans Dental College. New Orleans, 1870. 14p. DNLM **70-1525**

HARRISS, Juriah (1825-1876)
Annual address delivered before the Georgia Medical Association. Savannah, Ga.: E. J. Purse, 1870. 20p. DNLM; GU **70-1526**

HART, Charles A. (1842-1885)
A case of hydrocele of the round ligament, mistaken for and operated upon as a strangulated hernia, with remarks. New York: D. Appleton & Co., 1872. 7p. DNLM **70-1527**

HART, Charles A. (1842-1885)
Successful applications of Dr. S. Fleet Spier's artery constrictor. New York: D. Appleton & Co., 1872. 11p. DNLM
70-1528

HART, Charles Porter (*b.* 1827)
Repertory of the new remedies. . . . New York and Philadelphia: Boericke & Tafel, 1876. 199p. NNNAM; PPHa
70-1529

HART, Charles Porter (*b.* 1827)
A systematic treatise on diseases of the eye, for general practitioners and students. Detroit, Mich.: E. A. Lodge, 1877. 336p. DLC; OCIM; PPHa **70-1530**

HART, Charles Porter (*b.* 1827)
Homoeopathic medical practice: a systematic treatise on diseases of the brain and eye. For the use of general practitioners and students. Detroit. E. A. Lodge, 1877. 428p. DLC; OCIM; PPHa **70-1531**

HARTMAN, J[acob] H.
Eight cases of intralaryngeal growths removed through the natural passages. [Richmond, 1878.] 11p. DNLM
70-1532

HARTMAN, J[acob] H.
Laryngeal hemorrhage. St. Louis: G. O. Rumbold & Co., 1879. 4p. DNLM **70-1533**

HARTSHORNE, Henry (1823-1897)
Essentials of the principles and practice of medicine. A handbook for students and practitioners. 2nd ed. . . . Philadelphia: Henry C. Lea, 1871. 487p. CtY-M; NNNAM; PPC; PU
70-1534

HARTSHORNE, Henry (1823-1897)
Valedictory address to the twentieth graduating class of the Woman's Medical College of Pennsylvania. . . . Philadelphia: J. B. Rodgers Co., printers, 1872. 14p. DLC; DNLM
70-1535

HARTSHORNE, Henry (1823-1897)
On organic physics. Philadelphia, 1872. 6p. DNLM
70-1536

HARTSHORNE, Henry (1823-1897)
On the present condition of vaso-motor physiology. Philadelphia: Collins, 1872. 10p. DNLM **70-1537**

HARTSHORNE, Henry (1823-1897)
Essentials of the principles and practice of medicine. A handbook for students and practitioners. 3rd ed., revised and enlarged. Philadelphia: Henry C. Lea, 1874. 324p. DNLM; NNNAM; PPC; PPJ **70-1538**

HARTSHORNE, Henry (1823-1897)
Essentials of the principles and practice of medicine. A handbook for students and practitioners. . . . 4th ed., thoroughly rev.; with one hundred illustrations. Philadelphia: Henry C. Lea, 1874. 548p. DLC; DNLM; NNNAM; PPC
70-1539

HARTSHORNE, Henry (1823-1897)
Conspectus of the medical sciences comprising manuals of anatomy, physiology, materia medica, etc. 2nd ed. Philadelphia: Henry C. Lea, 1874. 1024p. DNLM; MBM; NNNAM; PU **70-1540**

HARTSHORNE, Henry (1823-1897)
On some disputed points in physiological optics. . . . I. On the theory of erect vision, with inverted retinal images. II. On extuition, as a new term in psychology. III. On ocular color spectra, and their causation. [Philadelphia, 1877.] 12p. DLC; DNLM **70-1541**

HARTSHORNE, Henry (1823-1897)
. . . A commonly accepted theory in ophthalmic physiology disproved by a crucial experiment. . . . [New York, 1878.] 2p. DLC **70-1542**

HARVARD UNIVERSITY. DENTAL SCHOOL. BOSTON
Annual announcements for the sessions of 1878-1879 (11.); 1880-1881 to 1897-1898 (13.-30.). Boston & Cambridge, 1878-1897. DNLM; MH-M [List of students and graduates for the years 1897-1898; 1879-1880 to 1896-1897, in announcements for subsequent years.] **70-1543**

HARVARD UNIVERSITY. MEDICAL SCHOOL. BOSTON
A descriptive catalogue of the Warren Anatomical Museum of Harvard University, by J. B. S. Jackson. Boston: A. Williams & Co., 1870. 759p. 1 plate. DNLM; MH
70-1544

HARVARD UNIVERSITY. MEDICAL SCHOOL. BOSTON
[Notice of a meeting to be held Oct. 22, 1874, in favor of erecting a new building for the Harvard Medical School.] [Boston, 1874.] 1 sheet. DNLM; MH
70-1545

HARVARD UNIVERSITY. MEDICAL SCHOOL. BOSTON
Subscriptions in aid of the Harvard Medical School building fund. To date, Dec. 24, 1874. [Boston, 1874.] 2 l. DNLM; MH **70-1546**

HARVARD UNIVERSITY. MEDICAL SCHOOL. BOSTON
Medical education. [Extracts from addresses of President Eliot and Dr. O. W. Holmes. Being an appeal to the public to subscribe towards the erection of a new building, on a new site, to meet the requirements of the new system of medical instruction, now in successful operation.] [Boston, 1874.] 2 l. DNLM; MH **70-1547**

HARVARD UNIVERSITY. MEDICAL SCHOOL. BOSTON
Photo-autographs of the faculty of the Medical School of Harvard University. [Boston, 1876.] 16 port. DNLM; MH
70-1548

HARWOOD, Edward C[oke] (1838-1891)
Clinical observations on inflammation of the mastoid cells. Richmond: J. W. Fergusson & Son, 1877. 8p. DNLM
70-1549

HATCH, F. W[inslow] (1822-1885)
Report on climatology and diseases of California. Philadelphia: Collins, 1872. 35p. 1 map. DNLM **70-1550**

HATCH, F. W[inslow] (1822-1885)
Climatology and epidemics. [Scaramento, 1872.] 35p. DNLM
70-1551

HATCH, F. W[inslow] (1822-1885)
Address on the reciprocal relations existing between physicians and the public. Sacramento: T. A. Springer, 1873. 15p. DNLM
70-1552

HATFIELD, Nathan L[ewis] (1804-1887)
Address delivered before the Alumni Association of Jefferson Medical College, March 10, 1875, on the close of his official term as president. Philadelphia: Collins, 1876. 16p. DNLM; PPJ **70-1553**

HAWLEY, J[ames] S.
Note on the value of wheat phosphates in therapeusis. Greenpoint, N.Y., [1870]. 4 l. DNLM **70-1554**

HAWLEY, J[ames] S.
The use of pepsine in the diarrhoea of infants. [1871, *vel subseq.*] 16p. DNLM **70-1555**

HAWLEY, J[ames] S.
Dr. Hawley's restorative and nutritive agents. [Brooklyn, N.Y., 1872.] 2 l. DNLM **70-1556**

HAWLEY, J[ames] S.
Some thoughts on the nutrition of the sick. Brooklyn, N.Y., 1872.] 2 l. DNLM **70-1557**

HAWLEY, J[ames] S.
Pepsin; its physiological and therapeutical actions. New York: G. F. Nesbitt & Co., [1876?]. 20p. DNLM **70-1558**

HAWLEY, J[ames] S.
Liebig's food for infants. [1879?] 12p. DNLM **70-1559**

HAY, Thomas
History of a case of recurring sarcomatous tumor of the orbit in a child, extirpated for the third time, and ultimately causing the death of the patient. Philadelphia: Lindsay & Blakiston, 1877. 14p. 3 plates. DNLM; PPC **70-1560**

HAYDEN, W. R.
Hayden's cold concentrated saturates, for physicians' prescriptions. Cambridge, Mass.: J. Ford & Son, 1870. 48p. 1 l. DNLM **70-1561**

HAYDEN, W[illiam] R.
Physicians' hand book of cold concentrated saturates, embracing brief treatises on the especial value of many valuable plants. Bedford Springs, 1872. 66p. DNLM; OCLloyd **70-1562**

HAYES, Albert H[amilton]
A medical treatise on nervous affections. The result of an extensive experience in the treatment of nervous disorders. . . . Boston: Peabody Medical Institute, [1870]. 137p. DLC; DNLM; MBM; NNNAM **70-1563**

HAYES, J. J.
Yellow fever; a treatise on its cause, nature, prevention, and cure; a synopsis of the pamphlet published and copyrighted in 1858 on the same subject and by the same author; and embraced in an appeal to four of the most learned physicians of the city of New Orleans, for perusal and consideration, and for their decision on its merits, on its truth. The fever as an epidemic, checked in a few days; as a complaint, cured in a few hours. New Orleans: T. H. Thomasson, 1879. 16p. DNLM; LNT-M **70-1564**

HAYES, Justin
Therapeutic use of faradic and galvanic currents in the electro-thermal bath, with history of cases. Chicago: Jansen, McClurg & Co., 1877. 112p. DNLM; OCIM **70-1565**

[HAYWARD, Aaron S.]
Vital magnetic cure: an exposition of vital magnetism, and its application to the treatment of mental and physical disease. By a magnetic physician. Boston: W. White & Co.; New York: The American News Co., 1871. 216p. DLC; MBM; NNNAM **70-1566**

[HAYWARD, Aaron S.]
Vital magnetic cure: an exposition of vital magnetism, its application to the treatment of mental and physical disease. By a magnetic physician. Boston: W. White & Co., 1873. 216p. DLC; MBM **70-1567**

HAZARD, Thomas Robinson (1797-1886)
A family medical instructor. Civil and religious persecution in the state of New York. . . . Boston: Colby & Rich, 1876. 124p. DLC; MBM **70-1568**

HEALTH REFORM INSTITUTE, BATTLE CREEK, MICH.
The proper diet for man: a summary of the principal evidences which prove the natural and proper diet of man to be composed wholly of fruits, grains, and other vegetable food. . . . Battle Creek, Mich.: The Office of the Health Reformer, 1874. 48, 16p. DLC **70-1569**

HEALY, P. F., F. A. ASHFORD, and Patrick J. TIMMENS
Addresses delivered at the twenty-ninth annual commencement of the medical department of the University of Georgetown. Washington, D.C.: H. L. Rose, 1878. 18p. DNLM **70-1570**

HEARING on the appointment of a medical inspector for the public schools, November 23, 1876. Boston: Rand, Avery & Co., 1877. 15p. DNLM; MWA **70-1571**

HEATH, Asahel Hawley (1824-1899)
Chronic diseases of the renal, urinary, reproductive organs, throat, lungs, stomach, liver, heart and bowels. . . . New York, 1874. 60p. DLC; NNNAM **70-1572**

HEATH, Christopher (1835-1905)
Practical anatomy; a manual of dissections. . . . 1st American from the 2nd English ed. Edited with additions, by William W. Keen. . . . Philadelphia: Henry C. Lea, 1870. 572p. DLC; NNNAM; PPC; PU **70-1573**

HEATH, Christopher (1835-1905)
A manual of minor surgery and bandaging, for the use of house-surgeons, dressers, and junior practitioners. 1st American from the 2nd English ed. Edited, with additions, by William W. Keen. Philadelphia: Henry C. Lea, 1870. 572p. CtY-M; DNLM; PPC; PU **70-1574**

HEATH, Christopher (1835-1905)
A manual of minor surgery and bandaging. . . . 5th ed. Philadelphia: Lindsay & Blakiston, 1875. 308p. MH-M; NNNAM; PPC; PPJ **70-1575**

HEATH, Christopher (1835-1905)
A course of operative surgery with plates drawn from nature by M. Sévillé and colored by hand under his direction. Philadelphia: Lindsay & Blakiston, 1878. 130p. 20 col. plates. NNNAM **70-1576**

HEATH, Christopher (1835-1905)
A guide to surgical diagnosis. Philadelphia: Lindsay & Blakiston, 1879. 214p. NNNAM **70-1577**

HEINTZELMAN, R. B.
Treatise on the value of resolvent herbal vapor inhalations for diseases of the nasal organs, throat, and lungs, with original views, showing the causes which produce consumption, and the true method of cure. . . . New York, [1873]. 48p. DLC; NNNAM **70-1578**

HELMUTH, William Tod (1833-1902)
Ten cases in surgery. Albany: The Argus Company, 1870. 28p. PPHa **70-1579**

HELMUTH, William Tod (1833-1902)
A system of surgery. Illustrated with 571 engravings on wood. New York: Carle & Grener, 1873. 1228p. DLC; NNNAM; PPC [2nd ed. New York, 1874. 1228p. DLC; DNLM] **70-1580**

HELMUTH, William Tod (1833-1902)
A dozen cases of clinical surgery. Albany: Weed, Parsons & Co., 1876. 36p. 7 plates. DNLM **70-1581**

HELMUTH, William Tod (1833-1902)
A system of surgery. Illustrated with 568 engravings on wood. 3rd ed. New York and Philadelphia: Boericke & Tafel, 1878. 1000p. DLC; NNNAM; PPJ; PU **70-1582**

HELMUTH, William Tod (1833-1902)
A system of surgery. Illustrated by 568 engravings on wood. 4th ed. New York and Philadelphia: Boericke & Tafel, 1879. 1000p. DLC; NNNAM; PPC; PU **70-1583**

HELMUTH, William Tod (1833-1902)
Scratches of a surgeon. Chicago: W. A. Chatterton & Co., 1879. 120p. PPHa **70-1584**

HELMUTH, William Tod (1833-1902)
Nerve stretching; with a short history of the operation, and illustrative cases. Boston: Otis Clapp & Son, 1879. 23p. DNLM **70-1585**

HEMPEL, Charles Julius (1811-1879)
The science of homoeopathy; or, a critical and synthetical exposition of the doctrines of the homoeopathic school. New York: Boericke & Tafel, 1874. 177p. NNNAM; PPHa **70-1586**

HEMPEL, Charles Julius (1811-1879)
The science of homoeopathy; or, a critical and synthetical exposition of the doctrines of the homoeopathic school. 2nd ed. Revised and enlarged. New York: Boericke & Tafel, 1876. 200p. NNNAM; PPC; PPHa **70-1587**

HENRY, Frederick Porteous (1844-1919) and Charles B. NANCREDE
Blood-cell counting; a series of observations with the hématimètre of MM. Hayem and Nachet, and the harmacytometer of Dr. Gowers. Cambridge, 1879. 11p. DNLM **70-1588**

HENRY, Morris Henry (1835-1895)
On amputation of redundant scrotum in the treatment of varicocele. New York: F. W. Christern, 1871. 10p. DNLM **70-1589**

HENRY, Morris Henry (1835-1895)
The treatment of venereal diseases; a monograph on the method pursued in the Vienna Hospital under the direction of Prof. von Sigmund; including all the formulae. Adapted and arranged from the German. New York: William Wood & Co., 1872. 49p. DNLM; NNNAM **70-1590**

HENRY, Morris Henry (1835-1895)
Clinical observations on the dementia and the hemiplegia of syphilis. New York: F. W. Christern, 1872. 15p. DNLM; NNNAM **70-1591**

HENRY, Morris Henry (1835-1895)
Clinical contributions. Three cases of induration of the os and cervix uteri, the result of syphilis. Two cases of syphilitic insanity. Four cases of anomalous localities of chancres, extra-genital. New York: F. W. Christern, 1874. 16p. DNLM; NNNAM **70-1592**

HENRY, Morris Henry (1835-1895)
Specialists and specialties in medicine. Address delivered before the Alumni Association of the medical department of the University of Vermont. New York: William Wood & Co., 1876. 22p. DNLM; NNNAM **70-1593**

HERING, Constantine (1800-1880)
The homoeopathic domestic physician. The only authorized English edition. By the author himself thoroughly revised and reformed from the latest German edition. New York: Boericke & Tafel, 1870. 399p. NNNAM; PPHa **70-1594**

HERING, Constantine (1800-1880)
The treatment of typhoid fevers, with a few additions. A part of the analytical therapeutics. New York and Philadelphia: Boericke & Tafel, 1873. 24p. DLC; PPHa **70-1595**

HERING, Constantine (1800-1880)
C. Hering's materia medica, with a pathological index. [Vol. 1.] Containing 16 remedies. New York and Philadelphia: Boericke & Tafel, 1873. 706p. PPHa; OCLloyd **70-1596**

HERING, Constantine (1800-1880)
The twelve tissue remedies and their use in trituration of Dr. Schuessler, recommended for investigation by Dr. C. Hering. New York: Boericke & Tafel, 1874. 44p. PPHa **70-1597**

HERING, Constantine (1800-1880)
The twelve tissue remedies and their use in trituration of Dr. Schuessler, recommended for investigation by Dr. C. Hering. 2nd ed. Much enlarged by Schuessler's and other additions. New York and Philadelphia: Boericke & Tafel, 1874. 88p. PPHa **70-1598**

HERING, Constantine (1800-1880)
The twelve tissue remedies and their use in trituration of Dr. Schuessler, recommended for investigation by Dr. C. Hering. 3rd ed. Much improved. Boericke & Tafel, 1875. 93p. DLC **70-1599**

HERING, Constantine (1800-1880)
Analytical therapeutics. [Vol. 1.] New York and Philadelphia: Boericke & Tafel, 1875. 352p. PPHa; OCLloyd **70-1600**

HERING, Constantine (1800-1880)
Condensed materia medica. . . . Compiled with the assistance of Drs. A. Korndoerfer and E. A. Farrington. New York and Philadelphia: Boericke & Tafel, 1877. 870p. DLC **70-1601**

HERING, Constantine (1800-1880)
The guiding symptoms of the materia medica. Philadelphia: The American Publishing Co., J. M. Stoddart & Co., 1878-1891. 10 v. PPHa ["This work was edited by Drs. C. G. Raue, C. B. Knerr, and C. Mohr. It was issued by the American Homoeopathic Publishing Society (J. M. Stoddart & Co.) The price to members of this Society was about the actual cost of publication. To non-subscribers, the price was $5 per volume. After volume 4 the Publishing Society was obliged to relinquish this work, and F. A. Davis, Esq., Medical Publisher and Bookseller, of 1231 Filbert Street, Philadelphia, became its publisher. He republished vols. 1, 2, 3 and 4 in 1889; and as the original plates had been destroyed, the matter had to be entirely reset." (Bradford, p. 153)] **70-1602**

HERING, Constantine (1800-1880)
Condensed material medica. . . . Compiled with the assistance of Drs. A. Korndoerfer and E. A. Farrington. 2nd revised and improved ed. New York and Philadelphia: Boericke & Tafel, 1879. 886p. PPHa **70-1603**

HERRICK, H. J. (1833-1901)
Annual address of the retiring president of the Ohio Medical Society, June, 1874. Piqua: Helmet Steam Print, 1874. 16p. DNLM **70-1604**

HEWITT, Charles N.
Report on the climatology and epidemics of Minnesota. Philadelphia: Collins, 1871. 19p. DNLM [*also*: Philadelphia: Collins, 1872. 15p.] **70-1605**

HEWITT, Charles N.
Doctors and drunkards. 1874. 9p. DNLM **70-1606**

HEWITT, Charles N.
The relations of scholastic methods to the health of pupils in the public schools. Minneapolis: Johnson, Smith & Harrison, 1879. 14p. DNLM **70-1607**

HEWSEN, Addinell (1828-1889)
Earth as a topical application in surgery. Being a full exposition of its use in all the cases requiring topical applications admitted in the men's and women's surgical wards of the Pennsylvania Hospital during a period of six months in 1869. Philadelphia: Lindsay & Blakiston, 1872. 309p. 4 plates. DNLM; PPC; PU **70-1608**

HEWSEN, Addinell (1828-1889)
On various purposes to which earth may be applied in medicine and surgery. An address before the Delaware County Medical Society. Philadelphia: Lindsay & Blakiston, 1874. 28p. DNLM; PU **70-1609**

HEYL, Albert G.
Coloboma lentis. Philadelphia: Collins, 1877. 12p. DNLM **70-1610**

HIBLER, J. Phelps
Pathology and therapeutics of dentistry: with miscellaneous essays on dental subjects. St. Louis: J. Hogan, Printer, 1874. 285p. DNLM; OCIM **70-1611**

HICKS, J. L.
A case of acute inflammation of the middle ear, with symptoms of meningitis; paraceutesis of the membrana typani; complete recovery. New York: William Wood & Co., 1879. 6p. DNLM **70-1612**

HICKS, Thomas F.
The difference in men, or how to keep well and live long. A dialogue. [Wilmington, Del.: Wayside Book-Store, 1878. 4p.] DNLM **70-1613**

HICKS, Thomas F.
Nature in disease. A lecture. [Wilmington, Del.: Wayside Book-Store, 1878.] 12p. DNLM **70-1614**

HIGGINS, S. B.
Ophidians; zoological arrangement of the different genera, including varieties known in North and South America, the East Indies, South Africa, and Australia; their poisons and all that is known of their nature; their galls as antidotes to the snake venom; pathological, toxicological, and microscopical facts; together with much interesting matter hitherto not published. 1st American ed. New York and Philadelphia: Boericke & Tafel, 1873. 239p. NNNAM; PPHa **70-1615**

HILDEBRANDT, H[ugo] (1833-1882)
Catarrh of the female sexual organs. Transl. by S. Lilienthal. New York: Boericke & Tafel, 1873. 40p. NNNAM; PPHa **70-1616**

HILDRETH, Eugenius Augustus (1821-1885)
Second report on the climatology and epidemic diseases of West Virginia. Philadelphia: Collins, 1872. 32p. 1 map. DNLM **70-1617**

HILDRETH, Eugenius Augustus (1821-1885)
President's address, delivered before the Medical Society of the State of West Virginia. Wheeling, 1877. 19p. DNLM **70-1618**

HILDRETH, Eugenius Augustus (1821-1885)
Synopsis of observations on some of the relations of meteorology and disease. Wheeling, 1879. 15p. DNLM **70-1619**

HILL, Benjamin L[ord] (1813-1871)
Lectures on the American eclectic system of surgery. Edited, with notes and additions, and a treatise on the venereal disease, by John M. Scudder. Cincinnati: Medical Publishing Co., 1870. 795p. DNLM; OCIM **70-1620**

HILLER, Frederick (*b.* 1820)
Allopathy and homoeopathy before the judgment of common sense. San Francisco: Bruce, printer, 1871. 32p. PPHa **70-1621**

HILLER, Frederick (*b.* 1820)
Diphtheria. Read before the California State Homoeopathic Medical Society. San Francisco: G. H. Floto, 1877. 8p. PPHa **70-1622**

HILLER, Frederick (*b.* 1820)
Hip-joint disease, and its homoeopathic treatment. San Francisco, Cal., 1878. 30p. PPHa **70-1623**

HILLER, Frederick (*b.* 1820)
A monograph on morbus coxarius; its pathology, diagnosis, and homoeopathic treatment. Philadelphia: Globe Printing House, 1878. 30p. PPHa **70-1624**

HILLS, Alfred K.
Instructions to patients for communicating with physicians. New York: H. M. Smith & Co., [1870]. 8p. DNLM **70-1625**

HILTON, John (1804-1878)
On rest and pain: a course of lectures on the influence of mechanical and physiological rest in the treatment of accidents and surgical diseases and the diagnostic value of pain. Delivered at the Royal College of Surgeons of England in the years 1860, 1861, and 1862. Edited by W. H. A. Jacobson. 2nd ed. New York: William Wood & Co., 1879. 299p. DNLM; NNNAM; OCIM; PPC **70-1626**

HINTON, James (1822-1875)
Physiology for practical use. With an introduction by E. L. Youmans. New York: D. Appleton & Co., 1874. 507p. DNLM; MH; NN; PU **70-1627**

HISTORY, character, and medicinal properties of Orkney Springs, Virginia. Season of 1878. Woodbridge, N.J.: Independent Hour Book Office, 1878. 16p. DNLM **70-1628**

HITCHCOCK, H. O[wen] (1827-1882)
Fertility of the native Americans of the present generation, as compared with that of previous generations and that of other nationalities among us; with certain inquiries, inferences, and remarks, based upon some statistics of the population of Kalamazoo, Michigan. Ann Arbor, 1871. 14 l. DNLM **70-1629**

HITCHCOCK, H. O[wen] (1827-1882)
The entailments of alcohol. Lansing: W. S. George & Co., 1874. 32p. DNLM **70-1630**

HITCHCOCK, Thomas B. (1839-1874)
Report on dental histology and microscopy. [Chicago, 1873.] 8p. 9 plates. DNLM **70-1631**

HITCHCOCK, Thomas B. (1839-1874)
The physical properties of dental amalgams. . . . The physical properties and pathological action of dental amalgams, by E. A. Bogue. [New York], 1875. 42p. DNLM; NNNAM **70-1632**

HODGE, Hugh L[enox] (1796-1873)
On the "synclitism" of the fetal head in natural labour. [Philadelphia, 1870.] 12p. DNLM **70-1633**

HODGE, Hugh L[enox] (1796-1873)
On compression of the foetal head by the forceps and cephalotribe. New York: William Wood & Co., 1875. 29p. DNLM; NNNAM **70-1634**

HODGE, Hugh Lenox, Jr. (1836-1881)
Note book for cases of ovarian tumors, and other abdominal enlargements. Philadelphia: Lindsay & Blakiston, 1875. 35p. DNLM; PPC; PU **70-1635**

HODGE, Hugh Lenox, Jr. (1836-1881)
Anatomical rooms; plan for their construction, ventilation, and hygienic management. Richmond: J. W. Fergusson & Son, 1875. 10p. DNLM **70-1636**

HODGE, Hugh Lenox, Jr. (1836-1881)
Address in surgery; delivered before the Medical Society of the State of Pennsylvania. Philadelphia: Collins, 1877. 26p. DNLM; PPC **70-1637**

[HODGE, Hugh Lenox, Jr.] (1836-1881)
[Memorial to the trustees of the University of Pennsylvania, recommending the appointment of Dr. H. Lenox Hodge as a professor of clinical surgery. Philadelphia, May 26, 1877.] [Philadelphia, 1877.] 1 sheet. DNLM **70-1638**

HODGE, H[ugh] Lenox, Jr. (1836-1881)
Subcutaneous osteotomy, illustrated by a case in which the femur was sawn through the neck, and also through the shaft. Philadelphia: J. A. Moore, 1878. 15p. DNLM; PPC; PU **70-1639**

HODGEN, John Thompson (1826-1882)
Double-acting elastic stomach-pump. [St. Louis, 1870.] 1 l. DNLM **70-1640**

HODGEN, John Thompson (1826-1882)
On fractures. [St. Louis], 1870. 4p. DNLM **70-1641**

HODGEN, John Thompson (1826-1882)
Indications for treatment of fractures. [St. Louis], 1870. 5p. DNLM **70-1642**

HODGEN, John Thompson (1826-1882)
Remarks on shock. [St. Louis], 1870. 7p. DNLM **70-1643**

HODGEN, John Thompson (1826-1882)
Union of fractures. [St. Louis], 1870. 5p. DNLM **70-1644**

HODGEN, John Thompson (1826-1882)
Treatment of oblique and compound fractures of the leg. [St. Louis], 1871. 14p. DNLM **70-1645**

HODGEN, John Thompson (1826-1882)
Cell or skin grafting. [St. Louis], 1871. 8p. DNLM **70-1646**

HODGEN, John Thompson (1826-1882)
On the treatment of fractures of the femur. [St. Louis, 1871.] 12p. DNLM **70-1647**

HODGEN, John Thompson (1826-1882)
Apparatus for suspension of inferior extremities, in case of fractures or other injuries. [1874?]. 1 l. DNLM **70-1648**

HODGEN, John Thompson (1826-1882)
Surgeon's reel and artery forceps. [1874?]. 2p. DNLM **70-1649**

HODGEN, John Thompson (1826-1882)
A modification of the usual operation for "lacerated perineum." [1876?]. 4p. DNLM **70-1650**

[HODGEN, John Thompson] (1826-1882)
Hodgen's wire suspension splint, made by A. M. Leslie & Co. [St. Louis, 1878?]. 2 l. DNLM **70-1651**

HOFF, Oliver
On haematuria as a symptom of diseases of the genito-urinary organs. . . . Philadelphia: Lindsay & Blakiston, 1878. 50p. DLC; DNLM; PPC; PU **70-1652**

HOFFMANN, Frederick (1832-1904)
Pharmacy in Prussia and in the German Empire. Philadelphia: Merrihew & Son, 1871. 15p. DNLM **70-1653**

HOFFMANN, Frederick (1832-1904)
Manual of chemical analysis as applied to the examination of medicinal chemicals. New York: D. Appleton & Co., 1873. 393p. DNLM; NNNAM; PU **70-1654**

HOFFMANN, Frederick (1832-1904)
The problems and future of pharmacy in Germany. Philadelphia: Merrihew & Son, 1874. 12p. DNLM
70-1655

HOLBROOK, Arthur
Practical information about the teeth. . . . Milwaukee, Wis.: State Dental Society, 1879. 200p. plates. DLC
70-1656

HOLBROOK, Martin Luther (1831-1902)
Parturition without pain; a code of directions for escaping from the primal curse. New York: Wood & Holbrook, 1871. 113p. DNLM; NNNAM **70-1657**

HOLBROOK, Martin Luther (1831-1902)
Liver complaint, nervous dyspepsia, and headache; their causes, prevention, and cure. . . . New York: M. L. Holbrook & Co., [1877]. 141p. DLC; NNNAM [*Vel. subseq.*]
70-1658

HOLBROOK, Martin Luther (1831-1902)
Hygiene of the brain and nerves and the cure of nervousness. With twenty-eight original letters from leading thinkers and writers concerning their physical and intellectual habits. New York: M. L. Holbrook & Co., 1878. 279p. DNLM; NN; NNNAM **70-1659**

HOLBROOK, Martin Luther (1831-1902)
Parturition without pain: a code of directions for escaping from the primal curse. New York: M. L. Holbrook & Co., 1878. 159p. DNLM; NNNAM **70-1660**

HOLCOMBE, William Henry (1825-1893)
Why are not all physicians homoeopathists? Chicago: Halsey Bros., 1874. 20p. DNLM **70-1661**

HOLCOMBE, William Henry (1825-1893)
How I became a homoeopath. New York and Philadelphia: Boericke & Tafel, 1874. 28p. DNLM; NNNAM
70-1662

HOLCOMBE, William Henry (1825-1893)
Why is homoeopathy more curative than other systems of medicine? An address delivered before the Hahnemann Medical Society of Cincinnati. Cincinnati: R. Clarke & Co., 1875. 24p. PPHa **70-1663**

HOLCOMBE, William Henry (1825-1893)
Historical significance of homoeopathy. An address delivered by the president, before the American Institute of Homoeopathy, at its twenty-eighth annual session, held at Put-in-Bay, O., June 15-18, 1875. Philadelphia: Sherman & Co., 1875. 15p. PPHa **70-1664**

HOLCOMBE, William Henry (1825-1893)
Special report of the Homoeopathic Yellow Fever Commission. Ordered by the American Institute of Homoeopathy for presentation to Congress, 1879. New Orleans: A. H. Nelson, Printer, 1879. 56p. PPHa **70-1665**

HOLDEN, Edgar (1838-1909)
The sphygmograph and the physiology of the circulation. New York: William Wood & Co., 1871. 29p. 1 plate. DNLM; NNNAM **70-1666**

HOLDEN, Edgar (1838-1909)
Banishment from home in the treatment of consumption. Remarks based upon personal observations at the principal resorts for consumptives, both of this country and of Europe. Newark, N.J.: Jennings & Hardman, 1872. 19p. DNLM
70-1667

HOLDEN, Edgar (1838-1909)
The sphygmograph: its physiological and pathological indications. The essay to which was awarded the Stevens triennial prize, by the College of Physicians and Surgeons, New York, April, 1873. . . . Philadelphia: Lindsay & Blakiston, 1874. 169p. plates. DLC; MBM; NNNAM; PPC **70-1668**

HOLDEN, Edgar (1838-1909)
Is consumption contagious? Newark, N.J., 1879. 22p. DNLM
70-1669

HOLDEN, Luther (1815-1905)
Landmarks, medical and surgical. . . . From the 2nd English ed. . . . Philadelphia: Henry C. Lea, 1878. 128p. CtY-M; MH-M; NNNAM; PPC **70-1670**

HOLLICK, Frederick (*b.* 1818)
The male generative organs in health and disease, from infancy to old age. 120th ed., much enlarged and improved. New York: Strong, [1873?]. 461p. NNNAM **70-1671**

HOLLICK, Frederick (*b.* 1818)
The nerves and the nervous. A practical treatise on the anatomy and physiology of the nervous system. . . . Including also, an explanation of the new practice of neuropathy. . . . New York: The American News Company, [1873]. 432p. DLC; NNNAM **70-1672**

HOLLICK, Frederick (*b.* 1818)
Diseases of women, their causes and cure familiarly explained; with practical hints for their prevention, and for the preservation of female health. . . . 63rd ed., much enl. and improved. New York: The American News Company, [1876]. 466p. DLC; NNNAM **70-1673**

HOLLICK, Frederick (*b.* 1818)
The male generative organs in health and disease. . . . 200th ed., much enl. and improved. New York: The American News Company, [1877]. 466p. 2 col. plates. DLC; NNNAM
70-1674

HOLLISTER, F. H.
A public address delivered at the twenty-fifth anniversary of the Illinois State Medical Society, Chicago, 1875. 16p. DNLM; ICRM; IU-M **70-1675**

HOLMES, Oliver Wendell (1809-1894)
Valedictory address delivered to the graduating class of the Bellevue Hospital College, March 2, 1871. New York: D. Appleton & Co., 1871. 23p. MH; MH-M; NNNAM
70-1676

HOLMES, Oliver Wendell (1809-1894)
The claims of dentistry. An address delivered at the commencement exercises of the dental department in Harvard University, February 14, 1872. . . . Boston: Printed by Rand, Avery & Co., 1872. 35p. DLC; DNLM; MH **70-1676A**

HOLMES, Oliver Wendell (1809-1894)
Dedicatory address at the opening of the new building and hall of the Boston Medical Library Association. Cambridge, 1879. 14p. DNLM; MH **70-1677**

HOLMES, Timothy, ed. (1825-1907)
A system of surgery, theoretical and practical, in treatises by various authors. 2nd ed. New York: William Wood & Co., 1870[1869]-1871. 5 v. DNLM; NNNAM; PPC; PU
70-1678

HOLMES, Timothy (1825-1907)
A treatise on surgery, its principles and practice. Philadelphia: Henry C. Lea, 1876. 960p. CtY-M; DNLM; NNNAM; PPC
70-1679

HOLT, Daniel (1810-1883)
Medicine as an art and as a science. An address before the Massachusetts Homoeopathic Medical Society. Taunton, Mass.: C. A. Hack & Son, 1871. 39p. DNLM; MBM
70-1680

HOLT, E. E[ugene] (1849-1931)
Report on otology. A paper read before the Maine Medical Association, June 12, 1877. Portland: S. Berry, 1877. 25p. DNLM **70-1681**

HOLT, E. E[ugene] (1849-1931)
Strabismus convergens. A paper read before the Maine Medical Association, June 11, 1879. Portland: Berry, 1879. 19p. DLC
70-1682

HOLT, Joseph (1839-1922)
Analysis of the record of yellow fever in New Orleans in 1876. [New Orleans, 1876?] 16p. DNLM **70-1683**

HOLT, Joseph (1839-1922)
Analysis of the record of yellow fever in New Orleans in 1876. [New Orleans, 1878.] 15p. DNLM **70-1684**

HOLT, Joseph (1839-1922)
Yellow fever in New Orleans during the year 1879. New Orleans: L. Graham, 1879. 11p. DNLM; LNT-M
70-1685

HOLT, Joseph (1839-1922)
History of the yellow fever epidemic in the fourth district. New Orleans: J. S. Rivers, 1879. 14p. DNLM
70-1686

HOLT, Joseph (1839-1922)
The chain of circumstances connected with the appearance of yellow fever in New Orleans during the summer of 1879. New Orleans: L. Graham, 1879. 10p. DNLM **70-1687**

HOMANS, John (1836-1903)
Cases of antiseptic ovariotomy. Cambridge, 1879. 7p. DNLM
70-1688

HOMES and hospitals: or two phases of woman's work as exhibited in the labors of Amy Dutton and Agnes E. Jones. Boston: American Tract Society, 1873. 326p. DLC; MH
70-1689

HOMOEOPATHIC MEDICAL COLLEGE OF THE UNIVERSITY OF MICHIGAN, ANN ARBOR
Annual announcements for the sessions of 1875-1876 to 1880-1881 (1.-6.); 1884-1885 (10.); 1885-1886 (11.); 1888-1889 (14.); 1890-1891 (15.); 1891-1892 to 1891-1895 (17.-20.); 1896-1897 to 1898-1899 (22.-24.); 1900-1901 (26.). Ann Arbor, 1875-1900. DNLM [List of students and graduates for the sessions of 1875-1876 to 1879-1880; 1883-1884; 1884-1885; 1887-1888; 1888-1889; 1890-1891 to 1893-1894, in announcements for subsequent years.] **70-1690**

HOMOEOPATHIC MEDICAL SOCIETY OF THE COUNTY OF NEW YORK
List of active members. [New York, 1878.] 7p. DNLM
70-1691

HOMOEOPATHIC RELIEF ASSOCIATION, NEW ORLEANS
Report of the Homoeopathic Relief Association, with valuable papers on yellow fever by the leading homoeopathic physicians of New Orleans, La., 1878. New Orleans: A. H. Nelson, 1878. 89p. LNT-M; PPHa **70-1692**

HOMOEOPATHIC YELLOW FEVER COMMISSION
Special report of the Homoeopathic Yellow Fever Commission, ordered by the American Institute of Homoeopathy. For presentation to Congress. New Orleans, La.: A. H. Nelson, print, 1879. 56p. DLC; LNT-M **70-1693**

HOMOEOPATHY
Trial of William Bushnell, M.D. and others. . . , all of Boston, for practicing homoeopathy, while they were members of the Massachusetts Medical Society. . . . Printed for the examination and consideration of the Fellows of the Massachusetts Medical Society, Boston, May, 1873. 60p. MBM; MH; MWA
70-1694

HOMOEOPATHY in Michigan University. Further facts and opinions. [Detroit, 1876.] 16p. DNLM
70-1695

HOOPER, Joseph
The match of medical science: past, present and future. By Jos. Hooper, M.D. and C. S. Eldridge, M.D. Cleveland, O.: L. H. White, 1871. 40p. DLC **70-1696**

HOOPER, Joseph
Cholera. Its causes, its prevention, and its cure. A brief monogram for the use of families. . . . Bay City, Mich.: C. C. Gustin; Cleveland, O.: L. H. Witte, 1873. 26p. DLC
70-1697

HOPKINS, Johns (1795-1873)
Letter to the trustees of "The Johns Hopkins Hospital." Baltimore: W. K. Boyle & Son, 1873. 9p. DNLM; MdBJ-W
70-1698

HORNBY, John
On alcoholic liquors predisposing the system to the generation of syphilis and gonorrhoea. Albany, 1870. 12p. DNLM
70-1699

HORTON, Henry L. (1826-1885)
On the effect of atropine in diminishing the pains and shortening the duration of the first stage of labor. New York: William Wood & Co., 1878. 20p. DNLM; NNNAM
70-1700

HOSMER, George H.
How to get well, keep well, and live long. The everyday doctor. A household book of practical medicine, containing a full account of the diseases of the human system, with appropriate remedies and a collection of valuable receipts. . . . New York: D. Appleton & Co., 1876. 467p. DLC; NNNAM; PPJ; PU
70-1701

HOTZ, F[erdinand] C[arl] (1843-1909)
The relation of ametropia to blepharitis ciliaris. [Chicago, 1878.] 10p. DNLM **70-1702**

HOTZ, F[erdinand] C[arl] (1843-1909)
Two cases of clonic blepharospasmus as traumatic reflex neurosis. [Philadelphia, 1879.] 5p. DNLM
70-1703

HOTZ, F[erdinand] C[arl] (1843-1909)
Notes on intra-ocular lesions produced by sunstroke. [Philadelphia, 1879.] 8p. DNLM **70-1704**

HOUGHMAN, C. E.
Lecture on otology. Milwaukee, 1874. 19p. DNLM
70-1705

HOVEY, Bleeker Lansing
Annual address delivered before the Medical Association of Central New York, and an essay on Asiatic cholera, by W. S. Ely. Rochester: E. Darrow, 1872. 12p. DNLM
70-1706

HOVEY, B[leeker] L[ansing] and W. C. WEY
Addresses delivered June 13, 1878, before the alumni and before the graduating class of the College of Medicine of the Syracuse University. Syracuse, N.Y.: Standard Publ. Co., 1878. 32p. DNLM **70-1707**

HOW to prevent chills and fevers, and all other miasmatic diseases. Baltimore: T. A. Hansche, 1875. 12p. DNLM
70-1708

HOW to read character: New illustrated hand-book of phrenology and physiognomy, for students and examiners; with a descriptive chart. New York: Wells, 1877. 191p. NN; NNNAM
70-1709

HOWARD ASSOCIATION OF CHARLESTON, S.C.
Transactions, during the epidemic of 1871. Charleston, S.C.: Walker, Evans & Cogswell, [1871]. 41p. DNLM; ScMS
70-1710

HOWARD ASSOCIATION OF NEW ORLEANS
Report of receipts, expenditures, and their work in the epidemic of 1878, with names of contributors, etc. New Orleans: A. W. Hyatt, 1878. 59p. DNLM; LNT-M
70-1711

HOWARD, Benjamin (*d.* 1900)
Address delivered at the annual commencement before the graduating class of the medical department, University of Vermont. New York: D. Appleton & Co., 1874. 23p. DNLM; NNNAM **70-1712**

HOWARD, Edward Lloyd (1837-1881)
The legal relations of emotional insanity. Philadelphia: Collins, 1874. 12p. DNLM **70-1713**

HOWARD, Flodoardo (1811-1888), William WARD, and R. S. L. WALSH
Addresses delivered at the 22nd annual commencement of the medical department of Georgetown College. Washington: R. Beresford, 1871. 29p. DNLM **70-1714**

HOWARD, Horton
Supplement to Howard's domestic medicine; being a practical treatise on midwifery and the diseases peculiar to women . . . to which is added illustrations and descriptions of medicinal plants recommended in this work. Philadelphia, Pa.: Hubbard Brothers, [1879]. 175p. DNLM; PP; PPC; PPF
70-1715

HOWE, Andrew Jackson (1825-1892)
A practical and systematic treatise on fractures and dislocations. . . . Cincinnati: C. F. Wilstach & Co., 1870. 424p. DNLM; OCIM **70-1716**

HOWE, Andrew Jackson (1825-1892)
A practical and systematic treatise on fractures and dislocations. 2nd ed. Cincinnati: J. M. Scudder, 1873. 424p. DNLM; OCIM **70-1717**

HOWE, Andrew Jackson (1825-1892)
Manual of eye surgery. . . . Cincinnati: Printed by Wilstach, Baldwin & Co., 1874. 204p. DLC; DNLM; OCIM
70-1718

HOWE, Andrew Jackson (1825-1892)
Hunterian oration; addressed to the Cincinnati Society of Natural History. [1874.] 7p. DNLM
70-1719

HOWE, Andrew Jackson (1825-1892)
The art and science of surgery. . . . Cincinnati: Wilstach, Baldwin & Co., printers, 1876. 886p. DLC; OCIM
70-1720

HOWE, Joseph William (1843-1890)
Emergencies and how to treat them. The etiology, pathology, and treatment of the accidents, diseases, and cases of poisoning, which demand prompt action. . . . New York: D. Appleton & Co., 1871. 265p. DLC; NNNAM; PPC; PU
70-1721

HOWE, Joseph William (1843-1890)
The breath, and the diseases which give it a fetid odor. With directions for treatment. . . . New York: D. Appleton & Co., 1874. 108p. DLC; DNLM; NNNAM [*Vel. subseq.*]
70-1722

HOWE, Joseph William (1843-1890)
Winter homes for invalids, an account of the various localities in Europe and America, suitable for consumptives and other invalids during the winter months. . . . New York: G. P. Putnam's Sons, 1875. 205p. DLC; DNLM; NNNAM
70-1723

HOWE, Julia Ward (1819-1910)
Memoir of Dr. Samuel Gridley Howe; with other memorial tributes. Boston: A. J. Wright, 1876. 127p. DNLM; MH; MWA
70-1724

HOWE, Samuel (*d.* 1879)
Milk fever. A treatise to show the relation which exists between the rise in temperature on the third or fifth day, and the beginning of the milk secretion. [Harvard Medical School.] New York: William Wood & Co., 1876. 24p. 4 plates. DNLM; NNNAM **70-1725**

HOWE, Samuel Gridley (1801-1876)
Laura Bridgman [the deaf, dumb, and blind girl]. Extracts from the report for 1840. Boston: South Boston Inquirer Office, 1873. 11p. DNLM **70-1726**

HOY, P[hilo] R. (1816-1892)
Cases of injury of the brain, involving speech. [Chicago, 1877.] 3p. DNLM **70-1727**

HOYNE, Temple S. (1841-1899)
Valedictory address to the graduating class of Hahnemann Medical College of Chicago. With the president's address, the report of the dean, and catalogue of students and graduates. Chicago: Sinclair & Blair, 1873. 19p. DNLM
70-1728

HOYNE, Temple S. (1841-1899)
Hoyne's annual directory of homoeopathic physicians of the Western States, containing a lsit of homoeopathic physicians residing in the States of Illinois, Indiana, Iowa, Missouri, Nebraska, Kansas, and Wisconsin. For the years 1873-1884 (1.-12.). Chicago, 1873-1884. DNLM [1873-1882 bound in 1 v.; 1873 for Illinois only; Indiana added in 1874, Missouri in 1877, Kansas in 1879, Wisconsin in 1881, Iowa and Nebraska in 1884.] **70-1729**

HOYNE, Temple S. (1841-1899)
Clinical therapeutics. Chicago: Duncan Brothers, 1878-1880. 2 v. DLC; DNLM; PPHa **70-1730**

HOYNE, Temple S. (1841-1899)
Valedictory address to the graduating class of Hahnemann Medical College of Chicago, February 27, 1879. With the president's address, the report of the dean, and catalogue of students and graduates. Chicago: Dunn & Heggie, 1879. 24p. DNLM **70-1731**

HOYT, W. D.
Malarial intestinal obstructions. [Atlanta, 1875.] 5p. DNLM
70-1732

HOYT, W. D.
A contribution to the study of puerperal convulsions. [Louisville, 1877.] 7p. DNLM **70-1733**

HOYT, W. D.
Account of a peculiar form of malarial pneumonia, with a suggested plan of treatment. [Atlanta, 1879?] 3p. DNLM
70-1734

HUBBARD, Oliver P. (1809-1900)
A lecture introductory to the eighty-third course of the New Hampshire Medical Institution at Dartmouth College. Concord: Evans, Sleeper & Evans, 1879. 36p. DNLM
70-1735

HUBBARD, S. G. (1816-1905)
Observations, ante-mortem and post-mortem, upon the case of the late President Jeremiah Day. [1871?] 11p. 1 plate. DNLM
70-1736

HUDSON, Erasmus Darwin (1805-1880)
Mechanical surgery. New York, 1871. 47p. DNLM
70-1737

HUDSON, Erasmus Darwin (1805-1880)
Mechanical surgery. Artificial limbs; apparatus for resections; apparatus for united fractures; feet for limbs shortened by hip-disease. New York, 1871. 43p. DNLM; NNNAM
70-1738

HUDSON, Erasmus Darwin (1805-1880)
The pathology and etiology of pulmonary phthisis, in relation to its prevention and early arrest. New York: D. Appleton & Co., 1875. 24p. DNLM; NNNAM **70-1739**

HUDSON, Erasmus Darwin (1805-1880)
Doctors, hygiene, and therapeutics; an anniversary discourse delivered before the New York Academy of Medicine. New York: D. Appleton & Co., 1876. 20p. DNLM; NNNAM
70-1740

HUDSON, E[rasmus] D[arwin] (1805-1880)
Mechanical surgery. Prothetic appliances and apparatus for amputations, resections, ununited fractures, diseases of joints, deformities, curvatures of spine, and paralysis. New York: E. D. Hudson, [1878]. 48p. DNLM; NNNAM
70-1741

HUGHES, Charles Hamilton (1839-1916)
The hereditary insane neuroses, or neuroses spasmodica, with illustrative cases. [St. Louis, 1874.] 17p. DNLM
70-1742

HUGHES, C[harles] H[amilton] (1839-1916)
On the vicarious function of the cerebral hemispheres and convolutions, considered in relation to unilateral wounds of the head and insanity. [Utica, N.Y., 1875.] 14p. DNLM
70-1743

HUGHES, Charles Hamilton (1839-1916)
Case of unilateral cerebellar abscess and tumors without persistence of symptoms. [1877.] 11p. DNLM
70-1744

HUGHES, C[harles] H[amilton] (1839-1916)
An address on insanity. [St. Louis, 1879.] 18p. DNLM
70-1745

HUGHES, Charles Hamilton (1839-1916)
Aphasia, or aphasic insanity, which? A medico-legal inquiry. [1879.] 12p. DNLM **70-1746**

HUGHES, Charles Hamilton (1839-1916)
Reflex cerebral hyperaemia [and] a medical brief on reserve force. [St. Louis, 1879.] 8p. DNLM **70-1747**

HUGHES, Charles Hamilton (1839-1916)
A remarkable case of semi-conscious epileptic automatism. St. Louis, 1879. broadside. DNLM **70-1748**

HULL, A. G. (1810-1859)
Hull's Jahr: a new manual of homoeopathic practice. Edited with annotations by Frederick G. Snelling. 6th American ed. With an appendix of the new remedies by Dr. C. J. Hempel. Repertory. New York: Boericke & Tafel, 1870. 804p. NNNAM; PPG; PPHa **70-1749**

HULL, A. G. (1810-1859)
Hull's Jahr: a new manual of homoeopathic practice. Edited, with annotations by Frederick G. Snelling. 6th American ed. With an appendix of the new remedies, by Dr. C. J. Hempel. Symptomatology. New York: Boericke & Tafel, 1870. 1200p. NNNAM; PPHa **70-1750**

HUMPHREYS, Frederick (1816-1900)
Plantago major, its pathogenesis or proving and therapeutic indications. New York: S. W. Green, 1871. 58p. DNLM; NNNAM **70-1751**

HUMPHREYS, Frederick (1816-1900)
Humphreys' homoeopathic mentor, or Family adviser in the use of specific homoeopathic medicine. . . . New York: Humphreys' Specific Homoeopathic Medicine Co., 1872. 364p. DLC; NNNAM; PPC; PPJ **70-1752**

HUNT, David (*b.* 1845)
A comparative sketch of the early development of the ear and eye in the pig, together with a new account of the development of the meatus externus, drum, and Eustachian tube. New York: D. Appleton & Co., 1877. 11p. DNLM
70-1753

HUNT, David (*b.* 1845)
On the development of the external ear passages. [Boston, 1877.] 5p. DNLM **70-1754**

HUNT, David (*b.* 1845)
Some general ideas concerning medical reform. Boston: A. Williams & Co., 1877. 50p. DNLM; MBM
70-1755

HUNT, David (*b.* 1845)
The obstetric forceps. [Suffolk, 1877.] 4p. DNLM
70-1756

HUNT, David (*b.* 1845)
Some recent opinions concerning the development of the external ear passages. New York: Trow, 1879. 11p. DNLM; NNNAM **70-1757**

HUNT, Ezra Mundy (1830-1894)
The lights and shadows of medical science. An address. New York: Bradstreet Press, 1872. 27p. DNLM; NNNAM
70-1758

HUNT, Ezra Mundy (1830-1894)
Professional ethics. An essay read before the Medical Society of New Jersey. Newark, N.J.: Jennings & Hardham, 1873. 17p. DNLM **70-1759**

HUNT, Ezra Mundy (1830-1894)
The deeds and the needs of hygiene. Philadelphia: Collins, 1877. 27p. DNLM **70-1760**

HUNT, Ezra Mundy (1830-1894)
Alcohol; as a food and medicine. A paper from the Transactions of the International Medical Congress, at Philadelphia, September, 1876. . . . New York: National Temperance Society and Publication House, 1877. 137p. DLC: DNLM; NN; NNNAM **70-1761**

HUNT, Thomas Sterry (1826-1892)
An address delivered before the Massachusetts College of Pharmacy, at the ninth annual commencement, on the relations of chemistry to pharmacy and therapeutics. With the valedictory to the graduating class of 1875, by Prof. William P. Bolles. Boston, May 20, 1875. Boston: A. Mudge & Son, 1875 27p. DNLM; MBM **70-1762**

HUNT, William (1825-1896)
Memoir of Dr. George W. Norris. Read Oct. 6, 1875. [Philadelphia, 1876.] 20p. DNLM **70-1763**

HUNTER, James A.
Selections from James A. Hunter's letters upon diseases of the air passages of the head, throat and lungs, and affections of the heart, and their auxiliary treatment by medicated inhalation, and other methods of local medication, with numerous illustrations; and a supplement, containing miscellaneous papers on kindred subjects. New York, 1872. 51p. DLC; NNNAM **70-1764**

HUNTER, James A.
Letters upon some of the more common and important diseases of the head, throat and chest . . . and their auxiliary treatment by medicated inhalation, and other methods of local medication. . . . San Francisco: Bacon & Company, book and job printers, 1877. 2 v. [paged continuously]. plates. DLC
70-1765

HUNTER, James A.
Health tracts: comprising papers upon affections of the nasal cavities, lungs and ears and their treatment by medicated inhalation. . . . San Francisco: Bacon & Company, book and job printers, 1878. 32p. DLC **70-1766**

HUNTER, James B[radbridge] (1837-1889)
A review of Darwin's theory of the origin and development of man. New York: D. Appleton & Co., 1871. 19p. DNLM; NNNAM **70-1767**

HUNTER, Robert (*b.* 1826)
A popular treatise on bronchitis, embracing bronchial consumption, hooping-cough, and asthma; their nature, causes, and treatment. Revised from 6th London ed. New York: J. Miller, 1871. 179p. DNLM; NNNAM
70-1768

HUPP, John C[ox] (1819-1909)
Vaccination and its protective power in the State of West Virginia; a report to the governor. Wheeling: J. Frew, 1871. 12p. DNLM **70-1769**

HUPP, John C[ox] (1819-1909)
Report of cases of phymosis and adherent prepuce. Wheeling, 1877. 10p. DNLM **70-1770**

HUPP, John C[ox] (1819-1909)
The diagnostic importance of symptoms. Wheeling, 1878. 8p. DNLM **70-1771**

HURLBURT, E. T. M.
Homoeopathy, hygiene and opium. An address delivered at Omaha, before the Nebraska State Homoeopathic Medical Association. Lincoln, Nebraska: Journal Co., 1874. 18p. PPHa
70-1772

HURLBUT, J. Searle
Address delivered before the Massachusetts Dental Society at its fourteenth annual meeting, held in Boston, December 12, 1878. Boston: A. T. Bliss & Co., 1879. 22p. DNLM; MBM
70-1773

HUTCHINS, Alexander (1835?-1906)
The physiological reasons why. An essay on school hygiene, with reference to the physiological relations of age and sex to mental and physical education, to which the Medical Society of the State of New York awarded the prize for 1875. Brooklyn: W. W. Swayne, 1875. 50p. DNLM
70-1774

HUTCHINSON, Edwin (1840-1887)
Hospital construction. [Utica], 1875. 10p. 1 plate. DNLM
70-1775

HUTCHINSON, James H[owell] (1834-1889)
On intracranial aneurism, with the report of a case observed, and a table containing 33 cases. [1874.] 25p. DNLM
70-1776

HUTCHINSON, James H[owell] (1834-1889)
The inflammatory origin of phthisis. New York: G. P. Putnam's Sons, 1875. 21p. DNLM; NNNAM
70-1777

HUTCHINSON, William F[rancis] (1838-1893)
The present status of electricity in medicine, being the semi-annual address before the Rhode Island Medical Society. Providence, 1875. 29p. DNLM **70-1778**

HUTCHISON, Joseph C[hrisman] (1827-1887)
A treatise on physiology and hygiene for educational institutions and general readers; fully illustrated. New York: Clark & Maynard, 1870. 276p. 2 plates. DNLM; NN; NNC
70-1779

HUTTON, T. J.
The emergency medicine chest hand book. . . . Minneapolis: Johnson, Smith & Harrison, 1879. 31p. DLC
70-1780

HYDE, James Nevins (1840-1910)
Early medical Chicago; an historical sketch of the first practitioners of medicine in the city. Chicago: W. B. Keen; Cooke & Co., 1876. 47p. 2 plates. DNLM; IEN-M; OCIM
70-1781

HYDE, James Nevins (1840-1910)
Early medical Chicago; an historical sketch of the first practitioners of medicine, with the present faculties, and graduates since their organization, of the medical college of Chicago. . . . Chicago: Fergus Printing Company, 1879. 78p. DLC
70-1782

HYDE, James Nevins (1840-1910)
A clinical lecture on tubercular leprosy, delivered at the dermatological and venereal clinic, Rush Medical College, Sept. 28, 1879. Chicago, 1879. 15p. DNLM; ICRM
70-1783

HYDE, James Nevins (1840-1910)
A contribution to the study of the bullous eruption inducted by the ingestion of the iodide of potassium. Philadelphia, 1879. 10p. DNLM **70-1784**

INGALS, Ephraim Fletcher (1848-1918)
How shall the degree of doctor of medicine be conferred? Chicago, 1879. 8p. DNLM **70-1785**

INGALS, Ephraim Fletcher (1848-1918)
Laryngeal tumors and tuberculous laryngitis. Chicago, 1879. 12p. DNLM **70-1786**

INGALS, Ephraim Fletcher (1848-1918)
Report of special committee on medical education. [Lincoln, 1879.] 13p. DNLM **70-1787**

INGALLS, William (1813-1903)
A case of progressive muscular sclerosis, with a paper on the same. Boston, 1870. 6p. 2 tab. DNLM
70-1788

INGALLS, William (1813-1903)
A synopsis of private obstetrical practice for forty-two years previous to January 1, 1876. Cambridge: Riverside Press, 1877. 14p. DNLM; MH-M **70-1789**

INTERNATIONAL MEDICAL CONGRESS. PHILADELPHIA, 1876
Transactions of the International Medical Congress of Philadelphia. 1876. Ed. for the Congress by John Ashhurst, Jr. . . . Philadelphia: Printed for the Congress, 1877. 1153p. DLC; PPC; PPJ; PU **70-1790**

IRWIN, B[ernard] J. D[owling] (1830-1917)
Case of osteophytic inflammation of the right radius; resection; preservation of a useful hand. [Philadelphia, 1874.] 4p. DNLM
70-1791

IRWIN, B[ernard] J. D[owling] (1830-1917)
Extensive laceration of the hand, caused by the explosion of a bottle of "white gunpowder" while held in the hand. [Philadelphia, 1875.] 5p. DNLM **70-1792**

IRWIN, B[ernard] J. D[owling] (1830-1917)
Concussion of the brain, with cases illustrative of different degrees of severity. [Philadelphia, 1876.] 7p. DNLM
70-1793

IRWIN, B[ernard] J. D[owling] (1830-1917)
Catalogue of the library pertaining to the Cadets' Hospital, United States Military Academy, West Point, N.Y., 1877. [1877.] 7p. DNLM **70-1794**

ISAACS, Charles Edward (1811-1860)
The anatomical remembrancer, or complete pocket anatomist; containing a concise description of the structure of the human body. 3rd ed. New York: William Wood & Co., 1871. 265p. DNLM; NNNAM; PPC; PU **70-1795**

ISHAM, A. B[rainerd] (*b.* (1844)
Recent contributions to sphygmographic science. New York: G. P. Putnam's Sons, 1879. 8p. DNLM
70-1796

IVES, John
Electricity as a medicine, and its mode of application. New York: John Ives, 1879. 123p. NNNAM
70-1797

IZARD, Ant.-Alphonse
New treatment of venereal diseases and of ulcerative syphilitic affections by iodoform. Transl. from the French, by Howard F. Damon. Boston: J. Campbell, 1872. 73p. DNLM; MBM
70-1798

JACK, Louis
The conservative treatment of the dental pulp. Philadelphia, 1873. 16p. DNLM **70-1799**

JACKSON, A[braham] Reeves (1827-1892)
Remarks on intra-uterine polypi with special reference to their diagnosis and surgical treatment. Chicago: W. B. Keen, Cooke & Co., 1876. 20p. DNLM **70-1800**

JACKSON, A[braham] Reeves (1827-1892)
The ovulation theory of menstruation: will it stand? New York: William Wood & Co., 1876. 34p. DNLM
70-1801

JACKSON, A[braham] Reeves (1827-1892)
Vascular tumors of the female urethra, with the description of a speculum devised to facilitate their removal. Boston, 1878. 9p. DNLM **70-1802**

JACKSON, A[braham] Reeves (1827-1892)
Laceration of the cervix uteri. Chicago, 1879. 25p. DNLM
70-1803

JACKSON, A[braham] Reeves (1827-1892)
On some points in connection with the treatment of sterility. [Boston, 1879.] 16p. DNLM **70-1804**

JACKSON, James C[aleb] (1811-1895)
The gluttony plague; or how persons kill themselves by eating. Dansville, N.Y.: A. Jackson & Co., 1870. 25p. DNLM
70-1805

JACKSON, James C[aleb] (1811-1895)
Dyspepsia and its treatment. Dansville, N.Y.: Austin, Jackson & Co., 1871. 16p. DNLM **70-1806**

JACKSON, James C[aleb] (1811-1895)
"The curse" lifted; or, maternity made easy. Dansville, N.Y.: Astin, Jackson & Co., 1871. 24p. DNLM
70-1807

JACKSON, James C[aleb] (1811-1895)
Consumption; how to prevent it and how to cure it. New York: B. L. Emerson, 1879. 400p. DNLM; NNNAM; OCIM; PU
70-1808

JACKSON, John Davies (1834-1875)
The black arts in medicine. Read before the members of the Boyle County, Lincoln County, and Mercer County Medical Societies. . . . Danville, Ky., Tuesday, Sept. 13, 1870. . . . Cincinnati: R. Clarke & Co., 1870. 28p. DLC; DNLM
70-1809

JACKSON, John Davies (1834-1875)
Medical office pupilage. . . . Read before the Kentucky State Medical Society, at its annual meeting, held in Covington, in 1871. Louisville: Davidson Bros. & Co., printers, 1871. 13p. DLC; DNLM **70-1810**

JACKSON, John Davies (1834-1875)
Biographical sketch of Dr. Ephraim McDowell. Louisville, Ky., 1873. 19p. DNLM **70-1811**

JACOBI, Abraham (1830-1919)
[Letter from . . . a member of the medical staff of the Nursery and Child's Hospital, in the city of New York, to Mrs. R. H. Lemist, secretary of the board of lady managers, on his forced removal or resignation as a member of the medical board. Oct., 1870.] [New York, 1870.] 25p. DNLM; NNNAM
70-1812

JACOBI, Abraham (1830-1919)
The raising and education of abandoned children in Europe, with statistics and general remarks on that subject. New York: Bellevue Hospital Printing Office, 1870. 43p. DNLM; NNNAM; NNU-M **70-1813**

JACOBI, Abraham (1830-1919)
Inaugural address, including a paper on infant asylums. New York: D. Appleton & Co., 1872. 46p. DNLM; NNNAM
70-1814

JACOBI, Abraham (1830-1919)
Infant diet. A paper read before the Public Health Association of New York. New York: G. P. Putnam's Sons, 1873. 50p. DNLM; NNNAM **70-1815**

JACOBI, Abraham (1830-1919)
Infant diet. . . . Revised, enlarged, and adapted to popular use, by Mary Putnam Jacobi. New York: G. P. Putnam's Sons, 1874. 119p. DNLM; NNNAM; NNU-M; PU
70-1816

JACOBI, Abraham (1830-1919)
Gastrotomy in stricture of the oesophagus. New York: D. Appleton & Co., 1874. 25p. DNLM; NNNAM
70-1817

JACOBI, Abraham (1830-1919)
Contributions to the pathology and therapeutics of diphtheria. New York: William Wood & Co., 1875. 40p. DNLM; NNNAM
70-1818

JACOBI, Abraham (1830-1919)
Acute rheumatism in infancy and childhood. New York: G. P. Putnam's Sons, 1875. 38p. DNLM; NNNAM
70-1819

JACOBI, Abraham (1830-1919)
On masturbation and hysteria in young children. New York: William Wood & Co., 1876. 32p. DNLM; NNNAM
70-1820

JACOBI, Abraham (1830-1919)
Treatment of infant diarrhea and dysentery. New York: William Wood & Co., 1879. 33p. DNLM; NNNAM
70-1821

JACOBI, Mary Putnam (1842-1906)
The question of rest for women during menstruation. Boylston prize essay for 1876. New York: G. P. Putnam's Sons, 1877. 232p. 14 plates. DNLM; NNNAM; NNU-M
70-1822

JACOBI, Mary Putnam (1842-1906)
Acute fatty degneration of new-born. New York: William Wood & Co., 1878. 16p. DNLM; NNNAM
70-1823

JACQUES, D. H. (*c.* 1825-1877)
The temperaments; or, the varieties of physical constitution in man, considered in their relations to mental character and the practical affairs of life, etc. With an introduction by H. S. Drayton. New York: S. R. Wells & Co., 1878. 239p. 55 plates. DNLM; NN; NNC **70-1824**

JACQUES, J.
The science of life. A treatise on the cause, symptoms and treatment of nervous and physical debility, spermatorrhoea, and the secret infirmities of youth. . . . [Baltimore, 1874.] 125p. DLC **70-1825**

JAHR, Gottlieb Heinrich Georg (1800-1875)
A new manual of homoeopathic practice. Edited, with annotations and additions, by F. G. Snelling. 6th American ed. With an appendix of the new remedies, by C. J. Hempel. New York: Boericke & Tafel, 1870. 1200, 72p. DNLM; NNNAM; PPHa; PU **70-1826**

JAHR, Gottlieb Heinrich Georg (1800-1875)
Therapeutic guide; the most important results of more than 40 years' practice. . . . Transl. by C. J. Hempel. New York: Boericke & Tafel, 1873. 364p. NNNAM; OCIM; PPHa; PU
70-1827

JAMES, Bushrod W[ashington] (1836-1903)
Rules for the treatment of Asiatic cholera homoeopathically; intended for the people. 2nd ed. Philadelphia, 1872. 28p. DNLM; PPHa **70-1828**

JAMES, Bushrod W[ashington] (1836-1903)
Report of the Bureau of General Sanitary Science, Climatology and Hygiene, to the American Institute of Homoeopathy, session of 1879. Philadelphia: Sherman & Co., 1879. 88p. PPC; PPHa; PU **70-1829**

JAMES, Martin L. (1829-1907)
Heart clots. A report of three cases (two long existing), and the etiology, diagnosis, prognosis, and treatment of cardiac thrombosis, based on an analysis of sixty-eight cases and physiological experiments. [Richmond, 1877.] 25p. DNLM **70-1830**

JAMES, Martin L. (1829-1907)
Observations on amphoric respiration and amphoric respiratory echo. [Richmond, 1879.] 2 l. DNLM **70-1831**

JAMINET, A[lphonse]
Physical effects of compressed air, and of the causes of pathological symptoms produced on man by increased atmospheric pressure employed for the sinking of piers, in the construction of the Illinois and St. Louis bridge, over the Mississippi River at St. Louis, Missouri. St. Louis: R. & T. A. Ennis, 1871. 135p. DNLM **70-1832**

JARVIS, Edward (1803-1884)
Proper provision for the insane. [Boston?], 1870. 20p. DNLM; MBM **70-1833**

JARVIS, Edward (1803-1884)
Relation of education to insanity. Washington: Government Printing Office, 1872. 11p. DNLM **70-1834**

JARVIS, Edward (1803-1884)
The increase of human life. Read before the American Statistical Society. Boston: D. Clapp & Sons, 1872. 55p. DNLM; MBM; MH **70-1835**

JARVIS, Edward (1803-1884)
Proper provision for the insane. . . . Boston: Wright & Potter, State Printers, 1872. 23p. DLC; DNLM; MBM **70-1836**

JARVIS, Edward (1803-1884)
Infant mortality. . . . Boston: Wright & Potter, printers, 1873. 41p. DLC; DNLM; MH-M **70-1837**

JARVIS, Edward (1803-1884)
History of the progress of population of the United States. From 1790 to 1870. Boston: D. Clapp & Son, 1877. 16p. DNLM; MH; NN; NNC **70-1838**

JEFFERSON MEDICAL COLLEGE. PHILADELPHIA
List of graduates for the years 1870 to 1875; 1877. [Philadelphia, 1870-77.] DNLM; PPJ **70-1839**

JEFFERSON MEDICAL COLLEGE. PHILADELPHIA
An interlineal, literal, and free translation of the diploma of the Jefferson Medical College. By Thomas J. Mullen, M.D. Philadelphia: T. Hamilton, 1874. 8p. DLC; PPJ **70-1840**

JEFFERSON MEDICAL COLLEGE. PHILADELPHIA
Catalogue of graduates from its organization. 1826-1879. Philadelphia: Collins, 1879. 64p. DNLM; PPJ **70-1841**

JEFFRIES, Benjamin Joy (1833-1915)
Report on the progress of ophthalmology. New York: J. Medole, 1871. 51p. DNLM; NNNAM **70-1842**

JEFFRIES, Benjamin Joy (1833-1915)
Report on the progress of ophthalmology. [New York, 1871.] 59p. DNLM; NNNAM **70-1843**

JEFFRIES, Benjamin Joy (1833-1915)
The eye in health and disease: being a series of articles on the anatomy and physiology of the human eye, and its surgical and medical treatment. . . . Boston: A Moore, 1871. 119p. plates. DLC; DNLM; NNNAM; PPC **70-1844**

JEFFRIES, Benjamin Joy (1833-1915)
. . . Diseases of the skin: the recent advances in their pathology and treatment. . . . Boston: A. Moore, 1871. 79p. DLC; DNLM; NNNAM; PU **70-1845**

JEFFRIES, Benjamin Joy (1833-1915)
Re-introduction of ether into England. [Boston, 1872.] 7p. DNLM **70-1846**

JEFFRIES, Benjamin Joy (1833-1915)
Animal and vegetable parasites of the human skin and hair. . . . Boston: A. Moore, 1872. 102p. DLC; DNLM; MBM; NNNAM **70-1847**

JEFFRIES, B[enjamin] Joy (1833-1915)
Report on the progress of ophthalmology, 1872. [Prepared for the American Ophthalmological Society.] [New York, 1872.] 60p. DNLM; NNNAM **70-1848**

JEFFRIES, Benjamin Joy (1833-1915)
Report on the progress of ophthalmology, 1872. Prepared for the American Ophthalmological Society. [Boston, 1873.] 60p. DNLM **70-1849**

JEFFRIES, Benjamin Joy (1833-1915)
[Miscellaneous papers.] (1) White sarcomatous intra-ocular tumor; enucleation. Intra-ocular tumor; white fusiformed-cell sarcoma; enucleation; (2) Two cases of herpes zoster ophthalmicus, destroying the eye; (3) Traumatic rupture of the choroid, without direct injury to the eye. [1873.] 11p. DNLM **70-1850**

JEFFRIES, Benjamin Joy (1833-1915)
Records of one hundred and five cases of operations for cataract. [Boston, 1874.] 15p. DNLM **70-1851**

JEFFRIES, B[enjamin] Joy (1833-1915)
Reports of sixteen cases of cataract operations. [Boston, 1875.] 7p. DNLM **70-1852**

JEFFRIES, Benjamin Joy (1833-1915)
A lecture on color-blindness and its practical relations. [1878.] 4p. DNLM **70-1853**

JEFFRIES, Benjamin Joy (1833-1915)
Relative frequency of color-blindness in males and females. Cambridge, 1878. 7p. DNLM **70-1854**

JEFFRIES, Benjamin Joy (1833-1915)
. . . Incurability of congenital color-blindness. . . . [Boston, 1878?] 8p. DLC; DNLM **70-1855**

JEFFRIES, Benjamin Joy (1833-1915)
. . . Dangers from color-blindness in railroad employees and pilots. . . . Boston: Rand, Avery & Co., printers, 1878. 40p. DLC; DNLM **70-1856**

JEFFRIES, Benjamin Joy (1833-1915)
Color-blindness. Dr. B. Joy Jeffries before the Society of Arts. A lecture on color-blindness and its practical relations, delivered April 11, 1878, at the Institute of Technology. . . . [Boston, 1878?] 4p. DLC; DNLM **70-1857**

JEFFRIES, Benjamin Joy (1833-1915)
Color-blindness: its dangers and its detection. . . . Boston: Houghton, Osgood & Co., 1879. 312p. col. front; diags. DLC; DNLM; OCIM; PPC **70-1858**

JENKINS, J[ohn] Foster (1826-1882)
Tent hospitals. [Am. Soc. Sc. Ass.] Cambridge, Mass.: Riverside Press, 1874. 26p. DNLM; MBM **70-1859**

JENKINS, Walworth
Prostitution and its management. Consideration of the license system in Europe and in St. Louis, Missouri. Special report to board of health of Louisville, Ky. Louisville: Bradley & Gilbert, 1873. 14p. DNLM **70-1860**

JENKS, Edward Watrous (1833-1903)
Coccyodynia. Lansing: W. S. George & Co., 1873. 13p. DNLM **70-1861**

JENKS, Edward Watrous (1833-1903)
President's address before the Michigan State Medical Society. Lansing: W. S. George & Co., 1874. 15p. DNLM **70-1862**

JENKS, Edward Watrous (1833-1903)
Viburnum prunifolium (black haw); its uses in the treatment of the diseases of women. [Boston, 1876.] DNLM **70-1863**

JENKS, Edward Watrous (1833-1903)
Two cases of elephantiasis arabum. Detroit, 1876. 5p. 1 plate. DNLM **70-1864**

JENKS, Edward Watrous (1833-1903)
Report upon obstetrics. A paper read before the Detroit Medical and Library Association. Detroit: W. A. Scripps, 1877. 16p. DNLM **70-1865**

JENKS, Edward Watrous (1833-1903)
The relations of ancient medicine to gynaecology. Detroit: W. A. Scripps, 1877. 22p. DNLM **70-1866**

JENKS, Edward Watrous (1833-1903)
Report of a successful case of caesarean section after seven days' labor. New York: William Wood & Co., 1877. 9p. DNLM **70-1867**

JENKS, Edward Watrous (1833-1903)
On the postural treatment of tympanites intestinalis following ovariotomy. New York: William Wood & Co., 1878. 6p. DNLM **70-1868**

JENKS, Edward Watrous (1833-1903)
The causes of sudden death of puerperal women. An address. Philadelphia: Collins, 1878. 21p. DNLM; PPC **70-1869**

JENKS, Edward Watrous (1833-1903)
Perineorrhaphy, with special reference to its benefits in slight lacerations, and a description of a new mode of operating. New York: William Wood & Co., 1879. 20p. DNLM; NNNAM **70-1870**

JENKS, William Furness (1842-1881)
On sarcomatous growths of the uterus. Philadelphia: Collins, 1873. 15p. DNLM **70-1871**

JENNEY, William H.
Address delivered before the Missouri Institute and How Valley Homoeopathic Society. . . . Published by resolution of the Missouri State Institute of Homoeopathy. Kansas City, Mo.: Ramsey, Millett & Hudson, 1878. 11p. PPHa **70-1872**

JESSEN, H. C.
The pathology and treatment of hereditary syphilis. A monograph in six letters. Chicago: W. A. Chatterton, 1879. 24p. PPHa **70-1873**

JEWELL, J. S[tewart] (1837-1887)
On certain forms of morbid nervous sensibility. New York: G. P. Putnam's Sons, 1876. 18p. DNLM **70-1874**

JEWETT, Charles (1839-1910)
Report upon the case of the late Dr. E. A. Groux, to the Brooklyn Anatomical and Surgical Club, November 18, 1878. [Brooklyn, 1878.] 10p. 1 plate. DNLM **70-1875**

JEWETT, Milo P[arker] (1808-1882)
Relation of boards of health to intemperance. A paper read before the National Convention of Health Boards assembled in Washington City, Jan. 21-23, 1874. Milwaukee: Milwaukee News Company, 1874. 11p. DNLM **70-1876**

JEWETT, Pliny Adams (1816-1884)
Semi-centennial history of the General Hospital Society of Connecticut, with a history of the Hartford Hospital, being the annual address read before the State Medical Society at its session, May, 1876. New Haven: Tuttle, Morehouse & Taylor, 1876. 93p. CtY-M; DNLM **70-1877**

JEWISH HOSPITAL ASSOCIATION. PHILADELPHIA
Ceremonies on laying the corner-stone of the Jewish Hospital, on the Olney Road, Oct. 9, 1872. Philadelphia: Jones & Potsdamer, 1872. 24p. DNLM; PPC **70-1878**

JOHNS HOPKINS HOSPITAL, BALTIMORE
Letter of Johns Hopkins to the trustees of "The Johns Hopkins Hospital." [Baltimore: W. R. Boyle & Son], 1873. 9p. DNLM; MdBJ-W **70-1879**

JOHNS HOPKINS HOSPITAL. BALTIMORE
Hospital plans. Five essays, relating to the construction, organization, and management of hospitals, contributed by the authors for the use of the Johns Hopkins Hospital of Baltimore. By John S. Billings, Norton Folsom, Joseph Jones, Caspar Morris, and Stephen Smith. appendices i and ii, by John R. Niernsée. New York: William Wood & Co., 1875. 353p. 48 plates. DLC; DNLM; MdBJ-W **70-1880**

JOHNS HOPKINS HOSPITAL. BALTIMORE
Review of "Hospital plans" by John R. Niernsée. [With description of wards.] [Baltimore, 1876.] 44, 5p. DNLM; MdBJ-W **70-1881**

JOHNS HOPKINS HOSPITAL. BALTIMORE
"Hospital plans" condensed for the use only of the trustees of the Johns Hopkins Hospital, 1875. Baltimore: W. R. Boyle & Son, [1876]. 51p. DNLM; MdBJ-W **70-1882**

JOHNS HOPKINS HOSPITAL. BALTIMORE
Reports and papers relating to construction and organization. Nos. 1-5, 7, 10-13. [Baltimore, 1876-1885]. MdBJ-W **70-1883**

JOHNS HOPKINS UNIVERSITY. BALTIMORE
Preliminary medical course. For the session of 1878-1879. Baltimore, 1878. 12p. DNLM; MdBJ-W **70-1884**

JOHNSON, Hosmer Allen (1822-1891)
History of the Chicago Medical College. An introductory lecture to the college session of 1870-1871. Chicago: R. Fergus' Sons, 1870. 20p. DNLM; ICRM **70-1885**

JOHNSON, Hosmer Allen (1822-1891)
Thyrotomy; with reports of four operations. [Chicago, 1877.] 13p. DNLM **70-1886**

JOHNSON, Hosmer Allen (1822-1891)
The regulation of medical practice by State boards of health, as exemplified by the execution of the law of Illinois. Philadelphia: Collins, 1879. 8p. DNLM **70-1887**

JOHNSON, Isaac D. (1827-1911)
Therapeutic key; or, Practical guide for the homoeopathic treatment of acute diseases. . . . Philadelphia: F. E. Boericke; New York: Boericke & Tafel, 1872. 179p. DLC; DNLM; PPHa; PU **70-1888**

JOHNSON, Isaac D. (1827-1911)
Therapeutic key; or, Practical guide for the homoeopathic treatment of acute diseases. . . . [2nd ed.] Philadelphia: Boericke & Tafel, 1874. 179p. PPHa **70-1889**

JOHNSON, Isaac D. (1827-1911)
Therapeutic key; or, Practical guide for the homoeopathic treatment of acute diseases. 3rd ed., rev. and improved. . . . Philadelphia: F. E. Boericke; New York: Boericke & Tafel, 1877. 312p. DLC; PPC; PPHa **70-1890**

JOHNSON, Isaac D. (1827-1911)
A guide to homoeopathic practice. Designed for the use of families and private individuals. New York and Philadelphia: Boericke & Tafel, 1879. 494p. NNNAM; PPHa; PU **70-1891**

JOHNSON, John M[ilton] (1812-1886)
Dysmenorrhoea. [Read before Atlanta Academy of Medicine, Jan. 12, 1875.] Atlanta, Ga.: Dunlop, Wynne & Co., 1875. 18p. DNLM **70-1892**

JOHNSON, Joseph Taber (1845-1921)
An address delivered before the Academy of Medicine, Washington, D.C. Washington, D.C.: Judd & Detweiler, 1871. 22p. DNLM **70-1893**

JOHNSON, John Taber (1845-1921)
Angina pectoris, illustrated by the case of Charles Sumner. [Boston, 1874.] 12p. DNLM **70-1894**

JOHNSON, John Taber (1845-1921)
On some of the apparent peculiarities of parturition in the Negro race, with remarks on race pelves in general. New York: William Wood & Co., 1875. 36p. DNLM; NNNAM **70-1895**

JOHNSON, John Taber (1845-1921)
On the treatment of placenta praevia. Washington, D.C., 1878. 11p. DNLM **70-1896**

JOHNSON, John Taber (1845-1921)
Address delivered at the thirtieth annual commencement of the medical department of the University of Georgetown. Washington: H. L. Rose, 1879. 18p. DNLM **70-1897**

JOHNSON, John Taber (1845-1921)
A case of head and foot presentation; fracture of the spine in utero. . . . [Boston, 1879?] 5p. DLC; DNLM **70-1898**

JOHNSON, William O[tis] (1825?-1873)
Modern medicine. Boston: J. R. Osgood & Co., 1873. 39p. DNLM; MH-M **70-1899**

JOHNSTON, Christopher (1822-1891)
Report on surgery [to the Medical and Chirurgical Faculty of Maryland]. [Baltimore, 1874.] 13p. DNLM; MdBM **70-1900**

JOHNSTON, Christopher (1822-1891)
Report on surgery. Baltimore: Innes & Co., 1876. 12p. DNLM **70-1901**

JOHNSTON, Christopher (1822-1891)
Epithelioma penis. Baltimore: J. H. Foster, [1877]. 3p. DNLM **70-1902**

JOHNSTON, Christopher (1822-1891)
The microscopy of the blood. Philadelphia, 1877. 22p. DNLM **70-1903**

JOHNSTON, Christopher (1822-1891)
The opening address before the Medical and Chirurgical Faculty of Maryland, 1877. Baltimore: Innes & Co., 1877. 14p. DNLM; MdBM **70-1904**

JOHNSTON, Samuel
Removal of a toy locomotive from subglottic cavity by tracheotomy and thyrotomy; recovery. New York: Rutledge & Co., 1876. 6p. DNLM **70-1905**

JONES, Alexander H.
Remarks on sulphate of quinia. [Philadelphia: Collins], 1877. 16p. DNLM **70-1906**

JONES, James (1807-1873)
Obstetric report of the Charity Hospital to the medical faculty of the University of Louisiana, to the surgeon and board of administrators of the hospital, from October 23, 1870, to March 7, 1871. New Orleans: G. Ellis & Bro., 1871. 3 l. DNLM; LNT-M **70-1907**

JONES, James (1807-1873)
Grand catalogue sale of the complete medical library of standard modern and miscellaneous books accumulated through a series of over forty years' practice by the late James Jones. New Orleans: A. W. Hyatt, 1877. 45p. DNLM; LNT-M
70-1908

JONES, John (1729-1791)
Plain, concise, practical remarks on the treatment of wounds and fractures; to which is added a short appendix on camp and military hospitals, principally assigned for the use of young military surgeons in North America. New York: J. Holt, 1775 [1871]. 18p. DNLM [A reprint of the original, issued with centenary address by J. W. Beekman in 1871.]
70-1909

JONES, Joseph (1833-1896)
Memoranda of medical clinic at Charity Hospital, New Orleans, La., 1869-1870. New Orleans, La., 1871. 156p. DNLM; LNT-M **70-1910**

JONES, Joseph (1833-1896)
Observations upon the treatment of yellow fever. Louisville: J. P. Morton & Co., 1873. 11p. DNLM
70-1911

JONES, Joseph (1833-1896)
General conclusions as to the nature of yellow fever; drawn from original investigations. New York: D. Appleton & Co., 1873. 11p. DNLM **70-1912**

JONES, Joseph (1833-1896)
Changes of temperature and pulse in yellow fever. Louisville: J. P. Morton & Co., 1873. 19p. DNLM
70-1913

JONES, Joseph (1833-1896)
Temperature in yellow fever. [1873.] 6p. DNLM
70-1914

JONES, Joseph (1833-1896)
Spontaneous combustion. New Orleans, [1874]. 6p. DNLM
70-1915

JONES, Joseph (1833-1896)
Explorations of the aboriginal remains of Tennessee. Washington, 1876. 171p. DNLM **70-1916**

JONES, Joseph (1833-1896)
Medical and surgical memoirs: containing investigations on the geographical distribution, causes, nature, relations and treatment of various diseases. . . . New Orleans: Printed for the author, by Clark & Hofeline, 1876-1890. 3 v. in 4 v. plates, maps. DLC; DNLM; LNT-M; NNNAM **70-1917**

JONES, Joseph (1833-1896)
Compulsory vaccination. The establishment of a uniform system of vaccination for all citizens and inhabitants of the State of Louisiana, by legislative enactment. New Orleans: T. H. Thomason, 1878. 17p. DNLM **70-1918**

JONES, Joseph (1833-1896)
Medico-legal evidence relating to the detection of human blood presenting the alterations characteristic of malarial fever, on the clothing of a man accused of murder, [etc.]. New Orleans: L. Graham, 1878. 18p. DNLM; LNT-M
70-1919

JONES, Lorenzo E.
Exposition! Scudder's school. Is it eclectic? The doctrine of specifics examined. Cincinnati: Miami Printing Co., 1872. 24p. DNLM; OCIM **70-1920**

JONES, Samuel A[rthur] (1834-1912)
Homoeopathy; its nature, purpose, and place. A lecture delivered at the opening of the Homoeopathic Medical College of the University of Michigan, October 1, 1875. Detroit, Mich.: American Observer Office, 1875. 16p. DNLM
70-1921

JONES, Samuel A[rthur] (1834-1912)
Woman's sphere in medicine. An introductory to the woman's class of 1879-1880, University of Michigan. Detroit: American Observer Office, 1879. 18p. OCIM **70-1922**

JONES, Samuel J. (1836-1901)
Report on otology. [Chicago, 1870.] 8p. DNLM
70-1923

JONES, Talbot
A plea for cold climates, in the treatment of pulmonary consumption. Minnesota as a health resort. New York, 1879. 32p. DNLM; NNNAM **70-1924**

JONES, W[illiam] W. (1819-1892)
President's annual address before the Ohio State Medical Society, at Put-in-Bay, June, 1875. Toledo: [Spear, Johnson & Co.], 1875. 12p. DNLM **70-1925**

JORDAN, H. J., *et al.*
Practical observations on nervous debility and physical exhaustion; to which is added an essay on marriage, with important chapters on disorders on the reproductive organs, [etc.]. Philadelphia, [1871]. 164p. DNLM; PPC; PU
70-1926

JORDAN, H. J.
The philosophy of marriage. Being eight important lectures on the functions and disorders on the nervous system, reproductive organs, and special diseases, as delivered at the New York Museum of Anatomy. New York, [1872?]. 176p. DNLM; NN; NNNAM **70-1927**

JORDAN, L. J.
Man's mission on earth! A treatise on nervous debility and physical exhaustion. New York, [1871]. 181p. DNLM; NN
70-1928

THE JORDAN Rockbridge Alum Springs, in Rockbridge County Va., with an analysis of the waters, and their medicinal properties, [etc.]. Richmond: Whittel & Shepperson, 1875. 18p. DNLM **70-1929**

JOSELIN, Benjamin Franklin (1796-1861)
Inaugural address, delivered before the Homoeopathic Medical Society of the County of New York. Englewood, N.J., 1875. 18p. DNLM **70-1930**

JOYNES, Levin Smith (1819-1881)
Curiosities of medical history. The Paris pharmacopoeia of 1758 and its treasures. [Richmond, 1875.] 20p. DNLM
70-1931

JOYNES, Levin Smith (1819-1881)
Yellow fever. Liability of Richmond to the disease and the need of preventive measures. [Richmond, 1878.] 23p. DNLM
70-1932

JUDSON, Adoniram Brown (1837-1916)
The cause of rotation in lateral curvature of the spine. New York: D. Appleton & Co., 1876. 18p. 1 plate. DNLM
70-1933

JUDSON, Eliza E. (*d.* 1880)
Address in memory of Ann Preston, M.D., delivered by request of the corporation and faculty of the Woman's College of Pennsylvania. [1873.] 29p. DNLM; PPC; PPJ; PU
70-1934

KAHN, L. J.
Nervous exhaustion; its cause and cure. A series of lectures on debility and disease, with practical information on marriage, its obligations and impediments; illustrated with cases. To which is added pictures from real life, or photographic life studies, addressed to the young, the old, the grave, the gay. New York, [1870]. 198p. DNLM; NN; NNC
70-1935

KAMPF, [H.]
The causes and prevention of near-sightedness. Transl. from the "Winer Zeitung" by Henry W. Williams. Boston: D. Clapp & Son, 1871. 22p. DNLM; MH-M **70-1936**

KANE, H[arry] H[ubbell] (*b.* 1854)
The sick-room; a practical manual on nursing, with a chapter on the dietary of the sick. . . . New York: National Printing Co., 1879. 88p. DLC; NNNAM **70-1937**

KEAN, John
Domestic medical lectures, embracing a thorough treatise on the cause, prevention, treatment and cure of the most prevalent diseases. . . . Chicago, Ill., 1879. 536p. DLC; OCIM
70-1938

KEATING, John McLeod (1830-1906)
A history of the yellow fever. The yellow fever epidemic of 1878, in Memphis, Tenn., embracing a complete list of the dead, the names of the doctors and nurses employed, names of all who contributed money or means, and the names and history of the Howards, together with other data, and lists of the dead elsewhere. . . . Memphis, Tenn.: Printed for the Howard Association, 1879. 454p. DLC; DNLM; LNT-M
70-1939

KEDZIE, Robert Clark (1823-1902)
Shadows from the walls of death; facts and inferences prefacing a book of specimens of arsenical wall papers. Lansing: W. S. George & Co., 1874. 8p. DNLM
70-1940

KEDZIE, Robert Clark (1823-1902)
Circular to the members of the section on state medicine and public hygiene of the American Medical Association. [The water supply as related to public health.] Lansing, 1875. broadside. DNLM **70-1941**

KEEN, William W[illiams] (1837-1932)
A sketch of the early history of practical anatomy. Philadelphia: Madeira, 1870. 31p. DNLM; PPJ
70-1942

KEEN, William Williams (1837-1932)
A sketch of the early history of practical anatomy. Philadelphia: J. B. Lippincott & Co., 1874. 43p. DLC; DNLM; PPJ; PPC **70-1943**

KEEN, William Williams (1837-1932)
The anatomical, pathological, and surgical uses of chloral. Philadelphia: J. B. Lippincott & Co., 1874. 19p. DNLM; PPJ; PPC **70-1944**

KEEN, William Williams (1837-1932)
. . . The anatomical, pathological, and surgical uses of chloral. . . . [Philadelphia, 1875.] 11p. DLC
70-1945

KEEN, William Williams (1837-1932)
The history of the Philadelphia School of Anatomy, and its relation to medical teaching. With photograph of the building; and blank diploma, fol. Philadelphia: J. B. Lippincott & Co., 1875. 32p. DNLM; PPC **70-1946**

KEEN, William Williams (1837-1932)
Directions to accompany the clinical charts. Philadelphia: T. Hamilton, 1875. 4p. and charts folded. DNLM
70-1947

KEEN, William Williams (1837-1932)
. . . On the surgical complications and sequels of the continued fevers. . . . Washington: Smithsonian Institution, 1877. 68p. DLC; DNLM; PPC; PU **70-1948**

KEITH, B., & CO.
Hand-book of practice; employing concentrated medicines. Jersey City: Pangborn, Dunning & Dear, 1874. 143p. DNLM
70-1949

KELLER, J. M.
The hot springs of Arkansas as a health resort; their waters as remedial agents. St. Louis: G. O. Rumbold & Co., 1879. 12p. DNLM **70-1950**

KELLOGG, A. O[tis] (1818-1888)
Notes of a visit to some of the principal hospitals for the insane in Great Britain, France, and Germany, with observations on the use of mechanical restraint in the treatment of the insane. [1871?] 28p. DNLM **70-1951**

KELLOGG, John Harvey (1852-1943)
The uses of water in health and disease. A practical treatise on the bath, its history and uses. . . . Battle Creek, Mich.: The Office of the Health Reformer, 1876. 154p. DLC
70-1952

KELLOGG, John Harvey (1852-1943)
The uses of water in health and disease, comprising an account of the physical properties, hygienic relations, physiological effects and remedial properties of water, together with a history of water-cure, an exposure of errors in water-cure and a description of the various baths and other water appliances. Battle Creek, Mich., 1877. 133p. DNLM; OCIM
70-1953

KELLOGG, John Havey (1852-1943)
Diphtheria: its causes, prevention, and proper treatment. . . . Battle Creek, Mich.: Good Health Publishing Co., [1879]. 64p. DLC **70-1954**

KELLOGG, M. G.
The bath; its use and application. Battle Creek, Mich., 1873. 64p. DNLM **70-1955**

KELLOGG, M. G.
The hygienic family physician: a complete guide for the preservation of health, and the treatment of the sick without medicine. . . . Battle Creek, Mich., Office of the Health Reformer, 1873. 380p. DLC; DNLM
70-1956

KELLOGG, M. G.
The treatment of disease by hygienic agencies. A guide for treating the sick without medicine. . . . Battle Creek, Mich.: The Office of the Health Reformer, 1873 [1874]. 160p. DLC **70-1957**

KELLOGG, M. G.
Disease and drugs: a brief treatise on the nature and cause of disease, and the so-called action of drugs. . . . Battle Creek, Mich.: The Office of the Health Reformer, 1874. 48p. DLC
70-1958

KELLOGG, Ulysses H. (1850-1917)
Magnum Dei donum, the cure of opium habit, neuralgia, nervous affections, delirium tremens, etc. . . . Jamestown, N.Y., [1872]. 44p. DLC **70-1959**

KELSEY, Charles B. (1850-1917)
Functional heart troubles. [New York, 1879.] 11p. DNLM
70-1960

KEMPER, Andrew C[arr] (1832-1905)
The annual address before the Cincinnati Medical Society by the retiring president. Cincinnati: R. Clarke & Co., [1875]. 12p. DNLM **70-1961**

KEMPER, G. William Harrison (1839-1927)
Retention in utero of the dead fetus. Considered particularly with regard to its effect on the mother. . . . Indianapolis: Baker, Schmidlap & Co., [1875]. 11p. DLC; DNLM
70-1962

KEMPER, G. William Harrison (1839-1927)
Affections of the gall-bladder, tending to result in cutaneous biliary fistula. Indianapolis: Baker & Randolph, 1879. 16p. DNLM **70-1963**

KEMPSTER, Walter (1841-1918)
Some of the preventable causes of insanity. Madison: D. Atwood, [1879]. 19p. DNLM **70-1964**

KENNEDY, Donald
On diseases of the skin, 2nd ed. Roxbury, Mass.: D. Kennedy, [1871]. 128p. 3 plates. DNLM; MH-M
70-1965

KENNEDY, Stiles
The magnetic and mineral springs of Michigan, to which is prefixed an essay on the climate of Michigan. Wilmington, Del.: James & Webb, 1872. 115p. 6 plates. DNLM
70-1966

KENNEDY, Stiles
Iodoform (ter iodide of formyl C_2HI_3); its therapeutical effects. [Philadelphia, 1872.] 16p. DNLM
70-1967

KENNEDY, Stiles
Record of new remedies and their therapeutical effects. Iodoform. Philadelphia, [1873]. 16p. DNLM
70-1968

KENNEDY, W. F.
Hints to mothers about their children. Wilmington, Del.: Glatts & Eckel, 1875. 41p. PPHa **70-1969**

KENTUCKY SCHOOL OF MEDICINE. LOUISVILLE
Letter to Medical School Convention. [The reply of the medical faculty of the . . . to Dr. J. Biddle, stating their reasons why they could not be present, by delegation, at the convention to be held at Philadelphia, June 2, 1876, "To consider all matters relating to reform in medical college work." May 20, 1876.] Louisville, 1876. 1 l. DNLM **70-1970**

KENTUCKY SCHOOL OF MEDICINE. LOUISVILLE
Response of the . . . to charge and specification preferred by Drs. Gross, Flint, and Davis against it and the Louisville Medical College, before the American Medical College Association, at its session held at Atlanta, Ga., 3rd of May, 1879. Louisville: Brewer, 1879. 13p. DNLM; PPJ
70-1971

KENTUCKY SCHOOL OF MEDICINE AND HOSPITAL IN THE CITY OF LOUISVILLE
Register of students, and circulars of information for the sessions of 1879 (23.); 1881 (25.); 1883 (27.); 1884 (28.); 1886-1896 (30.-40.); 1898-1903 (42.-47.). Louisville, 1878-1902. DNLM [Prior to 1893, called Annual announcements. In 1894, the words "and Hospital" were added to the title.]
70-1972

KENTUCKY STATE DENTAL ASSOCIATION
Transactions for the year 1878. Cincinnati: J. P. Geppert, 1878. 92p. DNLM **70-1973**

KERLIN, Isaac Newton (1834-1893)
Juvenile insanity. Philadelphia: J. B. Lippincott & Co., 1879. 11p. DNLM **70-1974**

KERN, Horatio G.
Catalogue of surgical and dental instruments, elastic trusses, etc. Philadelphia, 1877. 61p. DNLM
70-1975

KERR, J. G[lasgow] (1824-1901)
Medical missions at home and abroad. San Francisco: A. L. Bancroft & Co., 1878. 34p. DNLM **70-1976**

KERSHAW, James Martine
Diseases of the brain and nervous system. . . . Issued in eight parts. Facial neuralgia and the visceralgiae. Their diagnosis and treatment. pt. I. St. Louis: Schroback & Co., printers, 1878. 66p. DLC; DNLM **70-1977**

KERSHAW, James Martine
Femoro-popliteal neuralgia. Neuralgia ischiadica, sciatica. Cincinnati: J. P. Geppert, 1878. 23p. DNLM
70-1978

KETCHUM, George A. (1825-1906)
Address before the Medical Association of the State of Alabama. . . . With Board of Health bill. Montgomery, Ala.: Barrett & Brown, printers, 1874. 32p. DLC **70-1979**

KEYES, Edward Lawrence (1843-1924)
Syphilis of the nervous system. A clinical study chiefly in regard to diagnosis and treatment, founded on the cases of Prof. Wm. H. Van Buren, M.D., and those of the author. . . . New York: D. Appleton & Co., 1870. 44p. DLC; DNLM; NNNAM **70-1980**

KEYES, Edward Lawrence (1843-1924)
The effects of small doses of mercury in modifying the number of the red blood corpuscles in syphilis; a study of blood-counting with the hématimètre. Philadelphia, 1876. 23p. DNLM **70-1981**

KEYES, Edward Lawrence (1843-1924)
The tonic treatment of syphilis. . . . New York: D. Appleton & Co., 1877. 83p. DLC; DNLM; NNNAM **70-1982**

KEYES, Edward Lawrence (1843-1924)
The treatment of syphilis, with special reference to the constitutional remedies appropriate to its various stages, the duration of their use, and the question of their continuous or intermittent employment. Philadelphia: Collins, 1877. 15p. DNLM; PPC; PU **70-1983**

KEYSER, Peter Dirk (1835-1897)
Clinical contributions to ophthalmology. [Philadelphia, 1874.] 7, 3p. DNLM **70-1984**

KEYSER, Peter Dirk (1835-1897)
Supplemental report of cataract extractions. Philadelphia: Collins, 1875. 13p. DNLM **70-1985**

KEYSER, Peter Dirk (1835-1897)
Blepharitis and ametropia. [Philadelphia, 1877.] 3p. DNLM **70-1986**

KEYSER, Peter Dirk (1835-1897)
On some forms of inflammatory diseases of the eye, being caused by defects in refraction and accommodation. Philadelphia: Collins, 1877. 21p. DNLM; PPC **70-1987**

KEYSER, Peter Dirk (1835-1897)
The physiological action of belladonna and its alkaloid, atropia, on the eye. Philadelphia, 1878. 16p. DNLM **70-1988**

KIDD, Joseph (1824-1918)
The laws of therapeutics; or the science and art of medicine. Philadelphia: Lindsay & Blakiston, 1879. 196p. DNLM; MBM; PPC; PU **70-1989**

KIDDER, Jerome
Extra appliances for electro-therapeutic uses. [1871?] 2 l. DNLM **70-1990**

KIDDER, Jerome
Electro-allotropic-physiology. Uses of different qualities of electricity to cure disease. New York, 1873. 14p. DNLM **70-1991**

KIDDER, Jerome
Researches in electro-allotropic physiology. Uses of different qualities of electricity to cure disease. New York, [1877]. 18p. DLC; DNLM **70-1992**

KING, A[lfred] F[reeman] A[fricanus] (1841-1914)
On the etiology and pathology of areolar hyperplasia of the uterus. [New York, 1875.] 14p. DNLM **70-1993**

KING, A[lfred] F[reeman] A[fricanus] (1841-1914)
A new basis for uterine pathology. . . . New York: William Wood & Co., 1875. 20p. DLC; NNNAM **70-1994**

KING, John (1813-1893)
The causes, symptoms, diagnosis, pathology, and treatment of chronic diseases. Cincinnati: Med. Publ. Co., 1870. 1607p. DNLM; OCIM **70-1995**

KING, John (1813-1893)
American eclectic dispensatory. . . . 7th ed. Cincinnati: Wilstach, Baldwin & Co., 1870. 1509p. DNLM; OCLloyd **70-1996**

KING, John (1813-1893)
The American dispensatory. . . . 8th ed., rev. and enl. . . . Cincinnati: Wilstach, Baldwin & Co., 1870. 1439p. DLC; OCLloyd **70-1997**

KING, John (1813-1893)
Woman; her diseases and their treatment. 3rd ed. Cincinnati: J. M. Scudder, 1870. 366p. DNLM; OCIM **70-1998**

KING, John (1813-1893)
American eclectic obstetrics. 2nd ed. Cincinnati: Moore, Wilstach, Keys & Co., 1871. 768p. DNLM; OCIM **70-1999**

KING, John (1813-1893)
American eclectic dispensary. . . . 8th ed. Cincinnati: Wilstach, Baldwin & Co., 1876. 1440p. DNLM; OCLloyd **70-2000**

KING, John (1813-1893)
Urological dictionary: containing an explanation of numerous technical terms; the qualitative and quantitative methods employed in urinary investigations. . . . Cincinnati: Wilstach, Baldwin & Co., 1878. 266p. tables. DLC; DNLM; OCIM **70-2001**

KING, John C.
Headaches and their concomitant symptoms. With a complete and concise repertory-analysis. . . . Chicago: W. A. Chatterton & Co., 1879. 235, 62p. DLC; DNLM **70-2002**

KING's patent splints and limb straighteners. Washington, D.C.: Powell, Ginck & Co., 1870. 15p. DNLM **70-2003**

KINGSLEY, Charles (1819-1874)
Health and education. New York: D. Appleton & Co., 1874. 411p. DNLM; MH; NN; NNC **70-2004**

KINGSLEY, Norman W[illiam] (1829-1913)
An inquiry into the causes of irregularities in the development of the teeth. [New York], 1875. 42p. DNLM **70-2005**

KINGSLEY, Norman W[illiam] (1829-1913)
Mechanism of speech. New York: D. Appleton & Co., 1879. 42p. DNLM **70-2006**

KINLOCH, R[obert] A[lexander] (1826-1891)
A new form of intra-uterine stem pessary, with remarks upon the general use of intra-uterine stems. [Charleston, 1875.] 10p. 1 plate. DNLM **70-2007**

KINNEY, J. R.
Valedictory address delivered at the eleventh commencement of the Bellevue Hospital Medical College. New York: Baker & Godwin, 1873. 11p. DNLM; NNU-M **70-2008**

KIPP, Charles John (1835-1911)
Affections of the eye from small-pox. Newark, N.J.: Jennings & Hardham, 1874. 12p. DNLM **70-2009**

KIPP, Charles John (1835-1911)
A case of primary sarcoma of the iris cured by excision of the tumor. New York: William Wood & Co., 1876. 8p. 1 plate. DNLM **70-2010**

KIRKBY, Edmund A[dolphus]
On the administration of phosphorus, as a remedy for loss of nerve power, neuralgia, hysteria, melancholia, and other atonic conditions of the cerebro-spinal system. With formulae for its combination with iron, quinine, and nux vomica. With formulae for its administration and general directions for regimen and diet. 2nd ed. Philadelphia: Lindsay & Blakiston, [1876?] 63p. DNLM; PPC; PU **70-2011**

KIRBY, Edmund A[dolphus] and J. A. THOMPSON
Functional disorders of the brain and nervous system, induced by overwork and other influences incidental to modern life, with the formulae and treatment by the use of phosphorus. Philadelphia: W. R. Warner & Co., 1879. 47p. DNLM; PU **70-2012**

KIRKBRIDE, Thomas Story (1809-1883)
Resolutions offered and unanimously adopted by the Association of Medical Superintendents of American Institutes for the Insane at the meeting in Toronto June 7, 1871. [On the construction and organization of hospitals for the insane.] [1871.] 2 l. DNLM **70-2013**

KIRKES, William Senhouse (1823-1864)
Manual of physiology. . . . A new American from the 8th enlarged English ed. Philadelphia: Henry C. Lea, 1873. 656p. DNLM; MH-M; NNNAM; PU **70-2014**

KITCHEN, Daniel H[ixon] (*b.* 1847)
Conium in the treatment of insanity. [1873.] 24p. DNLM **70-2015**

KITCHEN, Daniel H[ixon] (*b.* 1847)
Nitrite of amyl in the treatment of spasmodic asthma and acute bronchitis. [1873.] 8p. DNLM **70-2016**

KITCHEN, Daniel H[ixon] (*b.* 1847)
Ergot in the treatment of nervous diseases. Utica, N.Y., 1873. 16p. DNLM **70-2017**

KITCHEN, Daniel H[ixon] (*b.* 1847)
Lectures on insanity and hysteria. [New York], Bellevue Press, 1876. 104p. DNLM; NNNAM **70-2018**

KITTRELL, B[enjamin] F[ranklin] (1836-1897)
Address before the State Medical Association, at its twelfth annual session, held at Aberdeen, Miss., April 1st, 2nd, and 3rd, 1879. Jackson, Miss., 1879. 16p. DNLM **70-2019**

KNAPP, J[akob] H[ermann] (1832-1911)
Remarks on some practical points concerning cataract extraction. [New York, 1870]. 2 l. DNLM **70-2020**

KNAPP, J[akob] H[ermann] (1832-1911)
I. Purulent otitis media, caused by the nasal douche, and accompanied by double hearing. II. The influence of spectacles on the optical constants and visual acuteness of the eye. III. Large cyst of the iris, cured by operation. IV. A case of extirpation of a cancroid growth of the inner canthus and upper eyelid. Blepharoplasty by sliding flaps. New York: William Wood & Co., 1870. 66p. DNLM **70-2021**

KNAPP, J[akob] H[ermann] (1832-1911)
A clinical analysis of the inflammatory affections of the inner ear. New York: William Wood & Co., 1871. 80p. DNLM **70-2022**

KNAPP, J[akob] H[ermann] (1832-1911)
Blindness from ischaemia retinae in hooping-cough. [New York, 1875.] 4p. DNLM **70-2023**

KNAPP, J[akob] H[ermann] (1832-1911)
Ophthalmological contributions. New York: William Wood & Co., 1875. 15p. 1 plate. DNLM **70-2024**

KNAPP, J[akob] H[ermann] (1832-1911)
A case of carcinoma of the outer sheath of the optic nerve, removed with preservation of the eyeball. New York: William Wood & Co., 1875. 32p. 4 plates. DNLM **70-2025**

KNAPP, J[akob] H[ermann] (1832-1911)
On the diagnosis of one-sided deafness. On fibroma of the lobule of the ear. New York: William Wood & Co., 1875. 12p. DNLM **70-2026**

KNAPP, J[akob] H[ermann] (1832-1911)
On the operations for traumatic colobomata of the eyelids. New York: William Wood & Co., 1876. 10p. DNLM **70-2027**

KNAPP, J[akob] H[ermann] (1832-1911)
Large orbital sarcoma, removed with preservation of the eyeball; death from acute nephritis; autopsy. New York: William Wood & Co., 1876. 16p. DNLM **70-2028**

KNAPP, J[akob] H[ermann] (1832-1911)
On the operative treatment of vascular tumors of the eyelids and anterior part of the orbit. New York: William Wood & Co., 1877. 13p. DNLM **70-2029**

KNAPP, J[akob] H[ermann] (1832-1911)
Report and remarks on a fourth and a fifth hundred of cataract extractions, according to von Graefe's method. New York: William Wood & Co., 1877. 134p. DNLM **70-2030**

KNAPP, J[akob] H[ermann] (1832-1911)
A case of parotidean and intra-tympanic malignant tumor. New York, 1879. 11p. DNLM **70-2031**

KNAPP, J[akob] H[ermann] (1832-1911)
I. Case of trephining the mastoid in acute suppurative otitis media. II. Case of supernumerary auricle of rudimentary development. New Bedford: Mercury Publ. Co., 1879. 6p. DNLM **70-2032**

KNAPP, J[akob] H[ermann] (1832-1911)
On disease of the mastoid process. Philadelphia: Collins, 1879. 10p. DNLM **70-2033**

KNAPP, J[akob] H[ermann] (1832-1911)
The removal of foreign bodies from the interior of the eye. New York: William Wood & Co., 1879. 38p. DNLM
70-2034

KNAPP, J[akob] H[ermann] (1832-1911)
Report and remarks on a sixth hundred of cataract extractions, performed according to von Graefe's method. New York: G. P. Putnam's Sons, 1879. 24p. DNLM **70-2035**

KNERR, Calvin B.
"Coup de soleil"; sunstroke and its homoeopathic treatment. Chicago: Duncan Brothers, 1878. 15p. PPHa
70-2036

KNIGHT, Frederick Irving (1841-1909)
Report on diseases of the throat. [Boston, 1872]. 10p. DNLM
70-2037

KNIGHT, Frederick Irving (1841-1909)
A brief sketch of the methods of removing growths from the larynx with the aid of the laryngoscope; with a case in which a fibrocellular growth was removed from the right vocal cord. [Boston, 1873.] 7p. DNLM **70-2038**

KINGHT, Frederick Irving (1841-1909)
Report on diseases of the throat. [Boston, 1873.] 15p. DNLM
70-2039

KNIGHT, Frederick Irving (1841-1909)
The action of the soft palate in speaking and swallowing, as seen through the nose in certain cases. [Boston, 1874.] 1 l. DNLM **70-2040**

KNIGHT, Frederick Irving (1841-1909)
Retro-pharyngeal sarcoma. St. Louis: G. O. Rumbold & Co., 1879. 16p. 1 plate. DNLM **70-2041**

KNIGHT, James (1810-1887)
Orthopaedia or a practical treatise on the aberrations of the human form. New York: G. P. Putnam's Sons, 1874. 364p. NNNAM; OCIM; PPC; PU **70-2042**

KNIGHT, J[ames] (1810-1887)
The improvement of the health of children and adults by natural means. Including a history of food and a consideration of its substantial qualities. 2nd ed. New York: G. P. Putnam's Sons, 1875. 406p. 6 plates. DNLM; NNNAM
70-2043

KNIGHT, William L[ambdin] (1811-1877)
The powers and undeveloped resources of the Philadelphia County Medical Society. An address delivered December 24, 1873. Published by the Society. Philadelphia: Collins, 1874. 25p. DNLM; PPC; PU **70-2044**

KNIGHT, William Lambdin (1811-1877)
Catalogue of the medical library of . . . . To be sold Friday, October 12, 1877. Philadelphia: Selheimer & Moore, [1877]. 18p. DNLM; PU **70-2045**

KNIGHT, William Lambdin (1811-1877)
Catalogue of the medical library of . . . . Also, engravings and paintings of distinguished physicians. [Philadelphia, 1877.] 11p. DNLM **70-2046**

KOBER, George Martin (1850-1931)
Uronology and its practical applications; a guide to the examination of urine and its diagnostic value, [etc.]. Louisville, Ky., 1875. 107 pp. 3 plates. DNLM; OCIM **70-2047**

KOCH, Richard
Valedictory address delivered at the annual commencement of the Hahnemann Medical College of Philadelphia, March 10, 1871, at the Academy of Music. Philadelphia: W. P. Kildare, 1871. 17p. DNLM; PPHa **70-2048**

KOLBÉ, D. W., & SON. PHILADELPHIA
Artificial legs, arms, and apparatus for disabilities and deformities, invented and manufactured by . . . . Philadelphia, Pa.: Philadelphia: Collins, 1870. 15p. DNLM
70-2049

KOLBÉ, D. W., & SON. PHILADELPHIA
Orthopaedic apparatus. . . . 2nd ed. Philadelphia: Collins, 1870. 57p. DNLM **70-2050**

KOLBÉ, D. W. & SON. PHILADELPHIA
Orthopaedic apparatus. . . . 3rd ed. Philadelphia: Collins, 1874. 60p. DNLM; PU **70-2051**

KOLBÉ, D. W., & SON. PHILADELPHIA
Orthopaedic apparatus. . . . 4th ed. Philadelphia: Collins, 1876. 60p. DNLM **70-2052**

KOLBÉ, D. W. & SON. PHILADELPHIA
Description of the orthopaedic apparatus employed in the treatment of deformities and deficiencies of the human body, with directions for taking measurements for their application. 6th ed. Philadelphia: Collins, 1879. 62p. DLC; DNLM
70-2053

KOLBÉ, D. W., & SON. PHILADELPHIA
Illustrated catalogue of surgical instruments manufactured by. . . . Philadelphia: W. P. Kildare, printer, 1879. 202p. DLC; DNLM **70-2054**

KOLBÉ, D. W., & SON. PHILADELPHIA
Illustrated catalogue of surgical instruments. Philadelphia: Sherman & Co., [1879]. 218p. DNLM
70-2055

KREUTZBERG, Charles
Guide to the European anatomical, pathological, and ethnological museum of . . . . Buffalo: Haas, Nauert & Co., 1875. 36p. DNLM **70-2056**

KÜSS, ÉMILE (1851-1871)
A course of lectures on physiology; as delivered by Professor Küss. . . . Ed. by Mathias Duval. . . . Transl. from the second and rev. ed. by Robert Amory. . . . Boston: J. Campbell, 1875. 531p. DLC; MH-M; NNNAM; PU **70-2057**

LAGENBECK, Bern. Rud. Conrad
Bone-formation after resection of the lower jaw. New York: D. Appleton & Co., 1878. 6p. DNLM **70-2058**

LA GRANGE, Robert J.
What to eat, drink and avoid. With a chapter on dyspepsia. . . . Philadelphia, 1879. 72p. DLC **70-2059**

LAMBERT, John (*b.* 1828)
Tubercular nephritis, resulting in abscess of both kidneys. Boston: J. Campbell, 1871. 13p. DNLM
70-2060

LAMBERT, John (*b.* 1828)
The treatment of uterine displacements, from the standpoint of a country gynaecological practice; especially regarding the employment of pessaries. Salem, N.Y., [1872]. 2 l. DNLM
70-2061

LAMBERT, John (*b.* 1828)
Notes on the relations of uterine disease to insanity. Read before a meeting of the County Medical Society, held at Salem, N.Y., Jan. 20, 1877. [1877.] 8p. DNLM
70-2062

LAMBERT, John (*b.* 1828)
Sanitary reform and preventive medicine; annual address delivered before the Medical Society of the county of Washington, on the occasion of its seventy-third anniversary, at Cambridge, June 24, 1879. [1879.] 8p. DNLM
70-2063

LAMBERT, Thomas Scott (1819-1897)
Systematic human physiology, anatomy, and hygiene; being an analysis and synthesis of the human system, with practical conclusions. 2nd ed. New York: William Wood & Co., 1873. 420p. 31 plates. DNLM; NNNAM; PPC; PU
70-2064

LAMBERT, Thomas Scott (1819-1897)
They are not dead. Restoration by the "heat method," of those drowned, or otherwise suffocated. . . . New York: Wright & Schondelmeier, 1879. 120p. 4 plates. DLC; DNLM; NNNAM **70-2065**

LAMBORN, L.
Non-medicinal therapeutics; the treatment of disease without medicine. A new dispensation in the healing art. . . . [no. 1] [n.p., 1876.] 54p. DLC **70-2066**

LANDOLT, Edmund (1846-1926)
A manual of examination of the eyes. A course of lectures delivered at the "École pratique." Transl. by Swan M. Burnett. Revised ed. Philadelphia: D. G. Brinton, 1879. 312p. 1 ch., 1 tab. DNLM; NNNAM; PPC; PPJ **70-2067**

LANOIX, Gustave (*b.* 1837)
Essay on vaccinal syphilis. Extract from Dr. Lanoix's conference in the ampitheatre of the Sorbonne at Paris. On the 26th of July, 1869. Transl. from the "La Tribune Medical." New York: Milhaus, 1872. 8p. NNNAM **70-2068**

LA ROCHE, René (1795-1872)
Remarks on the origin and mode of progression of yellow fever in Philadelphia, based on the occurrence of the disease in that city and at the lazaretto in the months of July, August, and September, 1870. Philadelphia: [E. C. Markley & Son, Printers], 1871. 86p. DLC; DNLM; PPC
70-2069

LATIMER, Thomas Sargent (1839-1906)
Annual oration before the Medical and Chirurgical Faculty of the State of Maryland. Anaesthetics in midwifery. [Baltimore, 1872.] 18p. DNLM; MdBM **70-2070**

LATTIMORE, S. A.
The relations of typhoid fever to contaminated well-water. Report on the chemical analysis of water from forty suspected wells. Why well-water is liable to contamination. Published for general circulation, by order of the board of health of the city of Rochester, [Sept. 29, 1877.] [Rochester, 1877.] 2 l. DNLM
70-2071

LAURIE, Joseph (*d.* 1865)
The homoeopathic domestic medicine. . . . 1st American from the 21st English ed. Edited and revised, with numerous important additions, and the introduction of the new remedies and a repertory and a glossary, by Robert J. McClatchey. New York: Boericke & Tafel, 1871. 1044p. NNNAM; PPHa; PU
70-2072

LAWRENCE, William Richards
Medical relief to the poor. Boston: Rockwell & Churchill, 1877. 54p. DNLM; MBM **70-2073**

LAYTON, Thomas
History of a phosphatic calculus spontaneously expelled through the vagina from a cyst of the anterior vaginal wall. [New Orleans, 1878.] 23p. DNLM **70-2074**

LEA, HENRY C. PHILADELPHIA
Illustrated catalogue of medical, surgical, and scientific publications. Philadelphia, 1873. 64p. DNLM; PPC; PPJ; PU
70-2075

LEALE, Charles Augustus (*b.* 1842)
Observations on thoracentesis. . . . New York: D. Appleton & Co., 1874. 26p. DLC; DNLM **70-2076**

LEALE, Charles Augustus (*b.* 1842)
Degenerations of the placenta as a cause of the death of the child. New York: D. Appleton & Co., 1876. 20p. DNLM; NNNAM **70-2077**

LEAMING, J[ames] R[oseburgh] (1820-1892)
Annual address before the Alumni Association of the University of the City of New York Medical Department. New York: G. W. Carleton, 1870. 20p. DNLM; NNNAM
70-2078

LEAMING, J[ames] R[oseburgh] (1820-1892)
Respiratory murmurs. New York: D. Appleton & Co., 1872. 19p. DNLM; NNNAM **70-2079**

LEAMING, J[ames] R[oseburgh] (1820-1892)
Significance of disturbed action and functional murmurs of the heart. New York: D. Appleton & Co., 1875. 27p. DNLM; NNNAM **20-2080**

LEAMING, J[ames] R[oseburgh] (1820-1892)
Physical signs of inter-pleural pathological processes. New York: Trow's Printing Company, 1878. 24p. DNLM; NNNAM
70-2081

LEBER, Theodor (1840-1917)
Dental caries and its causes. An investigation into the influence of fungi in the destruction of the teeth. By Drs. Leber and Rottenstein. Transl. by Thomas H. Chandler. . . . Philadelphia: Lindsay & Blakiston, 1873. 103p. 2 plates. DLC; DNLM; MdU-D; PU **70-2082**

LEE, Benjamin (1833-1913)
Report of the special committee on meteorology and epidemics of the Philadelphia County Medical Society, for the year 1870. Philadelphia: Collins, 1871. 38p. DNLM
70-2083

LEE, Benjamin (1833-1913)
The correct principles of treatment for angular curvature of the spine. . . . Philadelphia: J. B. Lippincott & Co., 1872. 77p. DLC; DNLM; PPC **70-2084**

LEE, Benjamin (1833-1913)
. . . Address in hygiene. Proposed act to create a state board of health. Report of Philadelphia County Medical Society. Diagnosis of psoas abscess. . . . Philadelphia: Collins, printer, 1877. 51p. DLC; DNLM **70-2085**

LEE, Benjamin (1833-1913)
Suspension as a means of treating spinal distortions. Philadelphia: Collins, 1877. 23p. 7 plates. DNLM **70-2086**

LEE, Benjamin (1833-1913)
A plea for a State Board of Health; read before the Philadelphia Social Science Association, March 7, 1878. Philadelphia: Philadelphia Social Science Association, [1878]. 16p. DNLM **70-2087**

LEE, Benjamin (1833-1913)
Medical Society of the State of Pennsylvania, session of 1878. The address in hygiene. Report of the Philadelphia County Medical Society on meteorology and epidemics. Philadelphia: Collins, 1878. 29p. 1 map. DNLM **70-2088**

LEE, Benjamin (1833-1913)
Remarks on the horizontal extension for the purpose of applying the porous felt jacket for curvatures of the spine. Philadelphia, 1879. 9p. 6 plates. DNLM **70-2089**

LEE, Charles Alfred (1801-1872)
Medical opinion of . . . in the matter of Carlton Gates, deceased. New York: W. J. Read, 1870. 30p. DNLM **70-2090**

LEE, Charles Alfred (1801-1872)
Remarks on wines and alcohol. New Lebanon, N.Y.: Tilden & Co., 1871. 22p. DNLM **70-2091**

LEE, Charles Alfred (1801-1872)
The late Dr. John Conolly, of Hanwell, England. Louisville: J. P. Morton & Co., 1871. 14p. DNLM **70-2092**

LEE, Charles Carroll (1838-1893)
Remarks upon the diagnosis of ovarian tumors from fibrocystic tumors of the uterus. New York: D. Appleton & Co., 1871. 33p. DNLM; NNNAM **70-2093**

LEE, Henry (1817-1898)
Lectures on syphilis and on some forms of local disease affecting principally the organs of generation. Philadelphia: Henry C. Lea, 1875. 246p. CtY-M; DNLM; NNNAM; OCIM **70-2094**

LEEDS, Albert R[ipley] (1843-1902)
Upon the presence of nitric acid in healthy urine, with a method for its accurate determination. [1879.] 5p. DNLM **70-2095**

LEFFERTS, George Morewood (1846-1920)
A brass ring lodged in the larynx for four years; removal by subhyoidean laryngotomy; cure. New York: J. McGee, 1875. 16p. DNLM **70-2096**

LEFFERTS, George Morewood (1846-1920)
The modern methods of examining the upper air passages. New York: G. P. Putnam's Sons, 1876. 39p. DNLM; NNNAM **70-2097**

LEFFERTS, George M[orewood] (1846-1920)
A unique case of prolapse of both ventricles of the larynx; their removal by the operation of thyrotomy; cure. New York: J. F. Trow & Son, 1876. 16p. DNLM **70-0298**

LEFFERTS, George M[orewood] (1846-1920)
Lupus of the larynx, a clinical study. [Philadelphia, 1878.] 8p. DNLM **70-2099**

LEFFERTS, George Morewood (1846-1920)
A clinical account of some cases of intra-laryngeal growths. New York: Trow, 1878. 20p. DNLM **70-2100**

LEFFERTS, George Morewood (1846-1920)
Two cases of bilateral paralysis of the dilator muscles of the glottis (musculi crico-arytaenoidei postici); cure. New York: D. Appleton & Co., 1878. 11p. DNLM **70-2101**

LEFFERTS, George Morewood (1846-1920)
Some of the commoner affections of the tonsils, from a diagnostic and therapeutic standpoint. New York: J. F. Trow & Son, 1879. 30p. DNLM **70-2102**

LEFFMANN, Henry (1847-1930)
First step in chemical principles, an introduction to modern chemistry, intended especially for beginners. Philadelphia: E. Stern & Co., 1879. 51p. DNLM; PP; PPL; PU **70-2103**

LEGG, John Wickham (1843-1921)
A guide to the examination of the urine, designed chiefly for the use of clinical clerks and students. 3rd ed. Philadelphia: Lindsay & Blakiston, 1872. 96p. DNLM; PPC; PU **70-2104**

LE HARDY, Julius Caesar (*b.* 1831)
Quarantine. Its sanitary and political aspect in relation to the spread of epidemic diseases. . . . Atlanta, Ga.: J. P. Harrison & Co., [1879]. 45p. DLC **70-2105**

LEISHMAN, William (1834-1894)
A system of midwifery, including the diseases of pregnancy and the puerperal state. Philadelphia: Henry C. Lea, 1873. 715p. DNLM; NNNAM; OCIM; PPC **70-2106**

LEISHMAN, William (1834-1894)
A system of midwifery, including the diseases of pregnancy and the puerperal state. . . . 2nd American from the 2nd and rev. English ed. With additions by John S. Parry. . . . Philadelphia: Henry C. Lea, 1875. 766p. CtY-M; DLC; DNLM; MH-M **70-2107**

LEISHMAN, William (1834-1894)
A system of midwifery, including the diseases of pregnancy and the puerperal state. . . . 3rd American ed., rev. by the author. With additions by John S. Parry. . . . Philadelphia: Henry C. Lea, 1879. 732p. DLC; DNLM; MBM; NNNAM **70-2108**

LE MONNIER, Y. R.
Are carbolic acid disinfections useful in yellow fever? [New Orleans, 1875.] 6p. DNLM **70-2109**

LE MONNIER, Y. R.
A case of resection of elbow-joint. [New Orleans, 1876.] 7p. DNLM **70-2110**

LENTE, Frederick Divoux (1823-1883)
The mineral waters of Saratoga. [New York, 1870.] 4p. DNLM
70-2111

LENTE, Frederick Divoux (1823-1883)
On the "sedative" action of calomel in disease. New York: D. Appleton & Co., 1870. 24p. DNLM
70-2112

LENTE, Frederick Divoux (1823-1883)
Intra-uterine medication. New York: D. Appleton & Co., 1870. 31p. DNLM **70-2113**

LENTE, Frederick Divoux (1823-1883)
The objects and aims of medical science, and the relations existing between the medical profession and the public. (The anniversary oration before the Alumni Association of the Medical Department of the University of the City of New York.) New York: D. Appleton & Co., 1871. 38p. DNLM; NNU-M **70-2114**

LENTE, Frederick Divoux (1823-1883)
Treatment of vomiting by electricity. New York: T. L. Clacher, 1874. 15p. DNLM **70-2115**

LENTE, Frederick Divoux (1823-1883)
On the treatment of intermittent fever by the hypodermic injection of quinine. New York: D. Appleton & Co., 1874. 27p. DNLM **70-2116**

LENTE, Frederick Divoux (1823-1883)
The value of transfusion of blood. Louisville, Ky., 1874. 27p. DNLM **70-2117**

LENTE, Frederick Divoux (1823-1883)
Superficial lacerations of the perineum. New York: J. F. Trow & Son, 1875. 20p. DNLM **70-2118**

LENTE, Frederick Divoux (1823-1883)
Neuralgia and other neuroses arising from cicatrices of the scalp, and their surgical treatment. New York: S. W. Green, 1875. 19p. DNLM **70-2119**

LENTE, Frederick Divoux (1823-1883)
The neurotic origin of disease, and the action of remedies on the nervous system. New York: McDivitt, Campbell & Co., 1875. 107p. DNLM **70-2120**

LENTE, Frederick Divoux (1823-1883)
Cases illustrating the direct action of remedies on the nervous system. Louisville, Ky., 1875. 36p. DNLM
70-2121

LENTE, Frederick Divoux (1823-1883)
Florida as a health resort. New York: D. Appleton & Co., 1876. 34p. DNLM; NNNAM **70-2122**

LENTE, Frederick Divoux (1823-1883)
The constituents of climate with special reference to the climate of Florida. Louisville, Ky., 1878. 56p. DNLM
70-2123

LEONARD, Charles Henri (1850-1925)
The pocket case reference and dose book. . . . Chagrin Falls, O.: Stranahan & Hohler, 1874. 28p. DLC
70-2124

LEONARD, Charles Henri (1850-1925)
The multum in parvo reference and dose book. . . . 2nd ed., rev. and enl. Fifth thousand. Detroit: Detroit Post Book & Job Printing Establishment, 1875. 77p. DLC; OCIM
70-2125

LEONARD, C[harles] Henri (1850-1925)
The vest-pocket anatomist. (Founded upon "Gray."). . . . Enl. ed. Detroit: Detroit Post Book & Job Printing Establishment, 1875. 56p. DLC; OCIM **70-2126**

LEONARD, Charles Henri (1850-1925)
. . . The codes of medical ethics. (American Medical Association, American Institute of Homoeopathy, National Eclectic Society) and Advertiser, arranged and comp. by . . . . Detroit, Mich., 1876. 31p. DLC **70-2127**

LEONARD, Charles Henri (1850-1925)
A manual of bandaging. Adapted for self-instruction. . . . With over one hundred illustrations. Detroit: Daily Post Book Printing Establishment, 1876. 132p. DLC; DNLM; OCIM; PPC
70-2128

LEONARD, C[harles] Henri (1850-1925)
The physician's dose and day-book . . . . 3rd ed., rev. and enl. Thirteenth thousand. . . . Detroit: [Printed by W. A. Scripps], 1878 [1877]. 99p. DLC **70-2129**

LEONARD, C[harles] Henri (1850-1925)
The vest-pocket anatomist (founded upon "Gray"). Enlarged ed. Detroit, 1877. 56p. DNLM; OCIM
70-2130

LEONARD, C[harles] Henri (1850-1925)
The vest-pocket anatomist. (Founded upon "Gray."). . . . 2nd enl. ed. VIth thousand. . . . Detroit, 1878. 60p. DLC; DNLM; OCIM **70-2131**

LEONARD, C[harles] Henri (1850-1925)
The codes of medical ethics: American Medical Association, American Institute of Homoeopathy, National Eclectic Society, and Advertiser. Detroit, Mich., 1878. 29p. DNLM
70-2132

LEONARD, Charles Henri (1850-1925)
The multum in parvo reference and dose book. . . . 3rd ed. Rev. and enl. 23rd thousand. . . . Detroit, 1879. 99p. DLC; DNLM; NNNAM **70-2133**

LESLIE, A. M. & CO.
Illustrated catalogue of surgical instruments and appliances, bandages, trusses, supporters, orthopedic apparatus, elastic hose, etc. St. Louis: A. M. Leslie & Co., [1874]. 104p. DNLM; OCIM **70-2134**

LETHEBY, H[enry] (1816-1876)
On food; its varieties, chemical composition, nutritive value, comparative digestibility, physiological functions and uses, preparation, culinary treatment, preservation, adulteration, etc., being the substance of four Cantor lectures. 2nd ed. New York: William Wood & Co., 1872. 255p. DNLM; NNNAM; PU
70-2135

[LETTER] to all true Hahnemaniacs, who are interested in securing the establishment of Hahnemann's dogmas, [and against] the Milwaukee test. [Philadelphia, 1879.] 4 l. DNLM; PPHa **70-2136**

LEVIS, R[ichard] J. (1827-1890)
The treatment of aneurism of large arterial trunks by complete compression; with a report of its successful application to a case of aneurism of the external iliac artery. [Philadelphia, 1871.] 4p. DNLM **70-2137**

LEVIS, R[ichard] J. (1827-1890)
The new operation for coloring corneal opacities. [Philadelphia, 1872.] 3p. DNLM **70-2138**

LEVIS, R[ichard] J. (1827-1890)
Skin grafting. Philadelphia: Sherman & Co., [1873]. 8p. DNLM **70-2139**

LEVIS, R[ichard] J. (1827-1890)
The treatment of fracture of the lower end of the radius. [Philadelphia, 1879.] 2 l. DNLM **70-2140**

LEWES, George Henry (1817-1878)
The physiology of common life. New York: D. Appleton & Co., 1871. 2 v. DNLM; NN; NNC; NNNAM **70-2141**

LEWES, George Henry (1817-1878)
The physical basis of mind. Being the second series of problems of life and mind. Boston: J. R. Osgood & Co., 1877. 556p. DNLM; ICU; KU; MH **70-2142**

LEWI, Joseph (1820-1897)
Annual address delivered before the Medical Society of the County of Albany, Nov. 12, 1872. Albany: J. Munsell, 1873. 13p. DNLM **70-2143**

LEWIN, Georg Richard (1820-1896)
The treatment of syphilis with subcutaneous sublimate injections. Transl. by Carl Proegler and E. H. Gale. Philadelphia: Lindsay & Blakiston, 1872. 249p. 1 plate. DNLM; NNNAM; PPC; PU **70-2144**

LEWIS, Albert
The medical companion and guide to health, by . . . . A treatise on the anatomy and physiology of the organs of generation and their diseases, with observations on onanism and its baneful results, including an essay on spermatorrhoea, mental and sexual incapacity, and impotence, and the venereal and syphilitic maladies, with plain and clear directions for the removal of secondary symptoms, gonorrhoea, gleets, strictures, and all diseases of the skin, such as scurvy, scrofula, ulcers, boils, blotches and pimples, on the face and body. . . . New York: The author, 1870. 256p. DLC; NNNAM **70-2145**

LEWIS, Albert
The medical companion and guide to health. A treatise on the anatomy and physiology of the organs of generation and their diseases. 6th ed. New York, 1876. 252p. DNLM; NNNAM; PU **70-2146**

LEWIS, Charlton T[homas] (1834-1904)
Address to the graduating class of the College of Physicians and Surgeons at their annual commencement, March 1, 1871. New York, 1871. 13p. DNLM **70-2147**

LEWIS, Daniel (1846-1919)
Cancer and its treatment. New York: A. C. Maclauchlan, 1875. 16p. DNLM **70-2148**

LEWIS, Dio (1823-1886)
Our digestion; or, my jolly friend's secret. Philadelphia: G. MacLean, 1872. 407p. port. DNLM; PPC; PP; PU **70-2149**

LEWIS, Edwin W.
Dr. Lewis' family guide and medical manual. . . . Rochester, N.Y.: M. H. Smith, book and job printer, 1872. 66p. DLC **70-2150**

LEWIS, Emlen
Maternity made easy; or Fruit diet during pregnancy and its effects upon gestation and labor. . . . Oskaloosa, Ia.: F. M. Roberts, job printer, 1877. 29p. DLC **70-2151**

LEWIS, Winslow (1799-1875)
The Boston Gynaecological Society, and its work during 1870. The annual address for 1871. Boston: J. Campbell, 1870. 25p. DNLM; MH-M **70-2152**

LIDELL, John A. (1823-1883)
I. On the wounds of blood-vessels, traumatic hemorrhage, traumatic aneurism, and traumatic gangrene. II. On the secondary traumatic lesions of bone: namely, osteo-myelitis, periostitis, ostitis, osteo-porosis, caries, and necrosis. III. On pyaemia. . . . Ed. by Prof. Frank Hastings Hamilton. New York: U.S. Sanitary Commission, 1870. 586p. DLC [U.S. Sanitary Commission. Surgical Memoirs of the War of the Rebellion] **70-2153**

LIDELL, John A. (1823-1883)
A treatise on apoplexy, cerebral hemorrhage, cerebral embolism, cerebral gout, cerebral rhematism, and epidemic cerebrospinal meningitis. New York: William Wood & Co., 1873. 395p. DLC; DNLM; NNNAM **70-2154**

LIEBREICH, Richard (1830-1917)
On a new method for extraction of cataract. Philadelphia: Claxton, Remsen & Haffelfinger, 1873. 20p. DNLM **70-2155**

LILIENTHAL, Samuel (1815-1891)
Valedictory address at the commencement exercises, March 4, 1875. Published by request of the graduating class of the New York Homoeopathic Medical College. [1875.] 7p. PPHa **70-2156**

LILIENTHAL, Samuel (1815-1891)
A treatise on diseases of the skin. New York and Philadelphia: Boericke & Tafel, 1876. 495p. DLC; DNLM **70-2157**

LILIENTHAL, Samuel (1815-1891)
Homoeopathic therapeutics. New York and Philadelphia: Boericke & Tafel, 1878. 710p. DLC; PPHa **70-2158**

LILIENTHAL, Samuel (1815-1891)
Homoeopathic therapeutics. 2nd ed. Philadelphia: Boericke & Tafel, 1879. 835p. DNLM; PPHa **70-2159**

LINCOLN, David Francis (1841-1916)
Vienna medical education. Boston, 1871. 6p. DNLM **70-2160**

LINCOLN, David Francis (1841-1916)
Report of 211 cases at the Boston Dispensary for Diseases of the nervous system. Boston: D. Clapp & Son, 1873. 7p. DNLM **70-2161**

LINCOLN, David Francis (1841-1916)
A report on school hygiene. Cambridge, Mass.: Ptd. for the American Social Science Association, 1874. 11p. DNLM
70-2162

LINCOLN, David Francis (1841-1916)
Electro-therapeutics: a condensed manual of medical electricity. . . . Philadelphia: Henry C. Lea, 1874. 186p. DLC; DNLM; NNNAM; PU **70-2163**

LINCOLN, David Francis (1841-1916)
A case of spinal paralysis in an adult, resembling the so-called infantile paralysis. [Boston, 1875.] 7p. DNLM
70-2164

LINCOLN, David Francis (1841-1916)
Notes on the climate of the Isles of Shoals and of Nantucket. [Boston, 1875.] 7p. DNLM **70-2165**

LINCOLN, David Francis (1841-1916)
Hygiene of public schools in Massachusetts. Boston: Rand, Avery & Co., 1879. 69p. DNLM **70-2166**

LINCOLN, Rufus P[ratt] (1841-1900)
Laryngeal phthisis. New York: William Wood & Co., 1874. 41p. DNLM; NNNAM **70-2167**

LINCOLN, R[ufus] P[ratt] (1841-1900)
Selected cases of diseases in the nasal and post-nasal region treated with the galvano-cautery; together with remarks and description of an instrument. New York: William Wood & Co., 1877. 8p. DNLM **70-2168**

LINCOLN, R[ufus] P[ratt] (1841-1900)
Naso-pharyngeal polypi, with illustration of cases. St. Louis: G. O. Rumbold & Co., 1879. 8p. 1 plate. DNLM
70-2169

LINDEN, John
Manual of the exanthematic method of cure, also known as Baunscheidtism. . . . Cleveland, Evangelical Association, 1878. 380p. OCIM **70-2170**

LINDSAY, W[illiam] Lauder (1829-1880)
Mechanical restraint in English asylums. Utica, N.Y., 1879. 13p. DNLM **70-2171**

LINDSAY, W[illiam] Lauder (1829-1880)
Rib-fracture in English asylums. [Utica, 1879.] 22p. DNLM
70-2172

LINDSLEY, C. A. (1826-1906)
Precautions respecting diphtheria and scarlet fever. Special report. Issued by order of the board of health of New Haven. [New Haven, 1878.] 2 l. DNLM **70-2173**

LINDSLEY, S. van (1840-1885)
Orthopedic surgery. Deformities of the lower extremities. [Nashville], 1876. 8p. DNLM **70-2174**

LIPPE, Adolph (1812-1888)
Liberty of medical opinion and action. Philadelphia, 1870. 11p. DNLM **70-2175**

LIPPE, Adolph (1812-1888)
A reply to Prof. William Pepper's insult to the homoeopathic school of medicine, in his opening address, delivered at the University of Pennsylvania, October 1, 1877. [Philadelphia]: Sherman & Co., 1877. 6p. DNLM **70-2176**

LITTELL, Squire, Jr. (1803-1886)
Memoir of John Rodman Paul. Philadelphia, 1878. 21p. DNLM
70-2177

LITTLE, James L[aurence] (1836-1885)
A paper on median lithotomy. . . . Philadelphia: Collins, printer, 1870. 20p. DLC; DNLM **70-2178**

LITTLE, James Laurence (1836-1885)
Puncture of the bladder by Dieulafoy's aspirator; with a description of the instrument. . . . New York: D. Appleton & Co., 1872. 12p. DLC; DNLM **70-2179**

LITTLE, James Laurence (1836-1885)
A case of anchylosis of the temporo-maxillary articulation; successfully treated by excision of the right condyle. Albany: C. Van Benthuysen & Sons, 1874. 11p. 2 plates. DLC; DNLM
70-2180

LITTLE, James Laurence (1836-1885)
A case of naso-pharyngeal tumor; removed by the galvano-cautery; excision of the greater portion of the superior maxillary to reach the tumor; operation preceded by the introduction of Trendelberg's tampon tracheotomy tube; ether administered through tube. New York: Rutledge & Co., 1876. 6p. DNLM **70-2181**

LITTLE, James Laurence (1836-1885)
A remarkable case of morphine tolerance by an infant. . . . New York: William Wood & Co., 1878. 6p. DLC; DNLM
70-2182

LITTLE, James L[aurence] (1836-1885)
Two lectures on Lister's antiseptic method of treating surgical injuries, delivered at the College of Physicians and Surgeons, New York. . . . Reprint from the Hospital Gazette, May 9th and 16th, 1878. [New York, 1878.] 15p. DLC; DNLM [*also*: New York: G. P. Putnam's Sons, 1878, 32p.]
70-2183

LIVEING, Robert (1834-1919)
Notes on the treatment of skin diseases. 4th ed. New York: William Wood & Co., 1878. 197p. CtY-M; DNLM; NNNAM
70-2184

LIVEING, Robert (1834-1919)
A handbook on the diagnosis of skin diseases. New York: William Wood & Co., 1879. 266p. DNLM; MBM; NNNAM; PPC **70-2185**

LIVINGSTON, J.
The cause of, and remedy for, yellow fever, as explained in a few articles published in the Daily City Item. New Orleans: A. W. Hyatt, 1879. 16p. DNLM; LNT-M
70-2186

LOCHMAN, C. L.
Dose and price labeles of the principal articles of the materia medica and preparations used in the United States; with some useful hints and formulas, and with prominent marks, calling attention to all active and poisonous articles. Allentown, Pa.: C. L. Lochman & Haines & Worman, 1877. 96 l. DNLM; PU
70-2187

LOCKE, Joseph Morris
Report on the analysis of three specimens of milk, made at the request of the health officer of the city of Cincinnati. Cincinnati: Bloch & Co., 1870. 19p. 2 tab. DNLM
70-2188

LOGAN, Cornelius Ambrose (1836-1899)
Physics of the infectious diseases. Comprehending a discussion of certain physical phenomena in connection with the acute infectious diseases. Chicago: Jansen, McClurg & Co., 1878. 212p. 1 map. DLC; DNLM **70-2189**

LOGAN, R. F.
How to prevent cholera. Shelbyville: A. C. Ellis, 1873. 25p. DNLM **70-2190**

LOGAN, R. F.
Report on surgery. Before the Kentucky State Medical Society, 1874. Louisville: J. P. Morton & Co., 1874. 14p. DNLM **70-2191**

LOGAN, Thomas Muldrup (1808-1876)
Report on the annual museum for the exhibition of the American Medical Association, in Philadelphia, and the contributions from California. Sacramento: T. A. Springer, 1872. 22p. DNLM **70-2192**

LOGAN, Thomas Muldrup (1808-1876)
Address delivered in St. Louis (Mo.), May 6, 1873, before the American Medical Association. [St. Louis, 1873.] 25p. DNLM **70-2193**

LOGAN, Thomas Muldrup (1808-1876)
Valedictory address at the commencement exercises of the Medical Department of the University of California, Oct. 29, 1874. [Sacramento, 1874.] 17p. DNLM **70-2194**

LOGAN, Wade Minor
Consumption; its pathology and treatment; to which is appended an essay on the use of alcohol in the treatment of consumption. Philadelphia: S. W. Butler, 1871. 90p. DNLM; PPC **70-2195**

LONGSHORE, Joseph Skelton (1809-1879)
Woman and her maladies: the little book of forbidden knowledge. . . . Philadelphia: Grant, Faires & Rodgers, 1878. 55p. DLC **70-2196**

LONGSTRETH, Morris (1846-1914)
Pathological anatomy; its growth, its use, and its methods. An address, introductory to the summer course of lectures in the Jefferson Medical College. Philadelphia: J. H. Gemrig, 1877. 20p. DLC; DNLM; PPJ; PU **70-2197**

LOOMIS, Alfred Lebbeus (1831-1895)
Lecture introductory to the course of 1871-1872 in the medical department of the University of New York: New York: J. C. Saxton, 1871. 17p. DNLM; NNNU-M **70-2198**

LOOMIS, Alfred L[ebbeus] (1831-1895)
Lessons in physical diagnosis. . . . 3rd ed.—rev. and enl. New York: William Wood & Co., 1872. 240p. DLC; DNLM; NNNAM; PU **70-2199**

LOOMIS, Alfred Lebbeus (1831-1895)
Lectures on diseases of the respiratory organs, heart, and kidneys. New York: William Wood & Co., 1875. 549p. DLC; DNLM; OCIM; PU **70-2200**

LOOMIS, Alfred Lebbeus (1831-1895)
Peritonitis. New York: G. P. Putnam's Sons, 1875. 30p. DNLM; NNNAM **70-2201**

LOOMIS, Afred Lebbeus (1831-1895)
Lectures on fevers. . . . New York: William Wood & Co., 1877. 403p. DLC; DNLM; NNNAM; PPC **70-2202**

LOOMIS, Alfred Lebbeus (1831-1895)
The Adirondack region as a therapeutical agent in the treatment of pulmonary phthisis. New York: William Wood & Co., 1879. 29p. DNLM **70-2203**

LOOMIS, Justin R[udolph] (1810-1898)
Elements of the anatomy, physiology, and hygiene of the human system. Revised ed. New York: Sheldon & Co., 1872. 254p. DNLM; NN; NNC **70-2204**

LORD, Fred A.
Valedictory address to the graduating class of Hahnemann Medical College of Chicago, February 23, 1872 . . . with the president's address, the report of the dean, and catalogue of students and graduates. Chicago: R. R. Donnelley, [1872]. 23p. DLC **70-2205**

LORD, Israel Shipman Pelton
On intermittent fever, and other malarious diseases. New York: Boericke & Tafel, 1871. 341p. NNNAM; PPHa **70-2206**

LORING, Edward Greely (1837-1888)
Some remarks on cataract. [1871.] 5p. DNLM [*also*: New York, 10p. (1871)] **70-2207**

LORING, Edward Greely (1837-1888)
Determination of the refraction of the eye by means of the ophthalmoscope. From advanced sheets on the ophthalmoscope. New York: William Wood & Co., 1876. 61p. 1 l. DNLM; NNNAM **70-2208**

LORING, Edward Greely (1837-1888)
Is the human eye changing its form under the influence of modern education? New York, 1878. 26p. DNLM **70-2209**

LORING, Edward Greely (1837-1888)
The light streak seen in the centre of the retinal vessels with the ophthalmoscope. [New York, 1879.] 7p. DNLM **70-2210**

LORING, Francis B.
Modification of the artificial leech. [Washington, D.C., 1879.] 3p. DNLM **70-2211**

LOTHROP, Charles Henry (1831-1890)
The Medical and Surgical Directory of the State of Iowa. Containing the names, post-office address, and professional status of the physicians; the various medical societies, with names and residence of the officers and members; a list of members of the American Medical Association from Iowa; a roster of United States examining surgeons for pensions for the State. Lyons, Iowa: J. C. Hopkins, Jr., 1876. 246p. DNLM **70-2212**

LOTHROP, Charles Henry (1831-1890)
The Medical and Surgical Directory of the State of Iowa. Containing the names, post-office address, and professional status of the physicians; the various medical societies, with names and residence of the officers and members; a list of members of the American Medical Association from Iowa; a roster of United States examining surgeons for pensions for the State. For 1878 and 1879. [Containing] also, medical colleges, State charitable institutions, hospitals, medical laws, fee bills of medical societies in different parts of the State. Clinton, Iowa: L. P. Allen, 1878. DNLM **70-2213**

LOUISVILLE MEDICAL COLLEGE
Annual announcements for the sessions of 1878-1879 (10.); 1889-1890 (21.); 1892-1893 to 1896-1897 (24.-28.); 1898-1899 (30.); 1900-1901 (31.). Louisville, 1878-1898. DNLM [List of students and graduates for the sessions of 1877-1878; 1888-1889; 1891-1892 to 1895-1896; 1897-1898; 1898-1899, in announcements for subsequent years.]
70-2214

LOUISVILLE MEDICAL COLLEGE
Response of the Louisville Medical College to charge and specification preferred before the American Medical College Association, at the third annual meeting, held at Atlanta, Ga., 3rd of May, 1879, by Drs. Flint, Gross, and Davis, committee. Louisville: Brewer's [1879]. 13p. PPJ
70-2215

LOUISVILLE MEDICAL COLLEGE FREE DISPENSARY
[Announcement of the faculty of the college of the opening of the . . . .]. [Louisville, 1879.] 1 sheet. DNLM
70-2216

LOVE, William Abram (1824-1898)
A plea for principles and conservatism in the treatment of diseases peculiar to females, embracing the report of a case of superinduced pseudo-cyesis, with results. Atlanta: Dunlop & Dickson, 1876. 18p. DNLM **70-2217**

LOVE, William Abram (1824-1898)
The soft palate. Its value in diagnosis as compared with the tongue in derangements of the liver, malarial diseases, and exanthematous fevers. Atlanta: J. P. Harrison & Co., 1878. 9p. DNLM **70-2218**

LOVING, Starling (1827-1911)
Clinical lectures. Locomotor ataxia. [Columbus, O., 1874?] 12p. DNLM **70-2219**

LOVING, Starling (1827-1911)
A lecture. Exophthalmic goitre. Columbus: Nevins & Meyers, 1877. 11p. DNLM **70-2220**

LUDLAM, Reuben (1831-1899)
Lectures, clinical and didactic, on the diseases of women. Pt. 1. Chicago: C. S. Halsey, 1870. 112p. DNLM; PPHa
70-2221

LUDLAM, Reuben (1831-1899)
Woman and homoeopathy. Annual address, delivered before the American Institute of Homoeopathy. Boston: A. Mudge & Son, 1870. 16p. DNLM **70-2222**

LUDLAM, Reuben (1831-1899)
Lectures, clinical and didactic, on the diseases of women. . . . 2nd ed. . . . Chicago: C. S. Halsey; Philadelphia: F. E. Boericke; [etc., etc.], 1872. 612p. DLC; OCIM; PPHa [3rd ed., 1877. 612p.] **70-2223**

LUDLAM, R[euben] (1831-1899)
. . . Valedictory address to the graduating class of Hahnemann Medical College and Hospital, of Chicago, March 19th, 1874 . . . with the report of the registrar, the president's address, and catalogue of the students and graduates. Chicago: Sinclair & Blair, printers, 1874. 19p. DLC **70-2224**

LUDLAM, R[euben] (1831-1899)
Ovariotomy by enucleation, being an extract from a clinical lecture. Chicago, 1874. 8p. DNLM
70-2225

LUDLAM, R[euben] (1831-1899)
Three months in the old hospitals of Paris. A lecture delivered before the Hahnemannian Institute, in the Hahnemann Medical College and Hospital of Chicago, November 12, 1875. Philadelphia: Sherman & Co., 1875. 16p. PPHa
70-2226

LUDLAM, Reuben (1831-1899)
Stomatitis materna. [Chicago, 1877?] 16p. DNLM
70-2227

LUDLAM, Reuben (1831-1899)
Lectures, clinical and didactic on the diseases of women. 4th ed. Chicago: Duncan Brothers, 1879. 648p. PPHa; OCIM
70-2228

LUDLUM, William S. (1830?-1890)
Dispensaries, their origin, progress and efficiency. . . . New York: G. P. Putnam's Sons, [1876]. 30p. DLC; DNLM
70-2229

LUNDY, Charles J. (1846-1892)
Optic neuritis, with notes of three cases. Detroit, 1878. 17p. DNLM **70-2230**

LUSE, J. P.
Agassiz; the lessons of his life. Lecture. [Louisville, 1874.] 38p. DNLM **70-2231**

LUSK, William T[hompson] (1838-1897)
On the origin of diabetes, with some new experiments regarding the glycogenic function of the liver. New York: D. Appleton & Co., 1870. 19p. DNLM **70-2232**

LUSK, William T[hompson] (1838-1897)
The etiology and indications for treatment of irregular uterine action during labor. New York: D. Appleton & Co., 1873. 19p. DNLM; NNNAM **70-2233**

LUSK, William T[hompson] (1838-1897)
Clinical report of the lying-in service at Bellevue Hospital for the year 1873. New York: D. Appleton & Co., 1874. 9p. DNLM **70-2234**

LUSK, William T[hompson] (1838-1897)
The genesis of an epidemic of puerperal fever. New York: William Wood & Co., 1875. 31p. DNLM
70-2235

LUSK, William T[hompson] (1838-1897)
On the nature, origin, and prevention of puerperal fever. Philadelphia, 1877. 29p. DNLM **70-2236**

LUTZ, Frank J. (1855-1916)
Diastasis of the sternum by the violent action of the diaphragm during coughing. St. Louis, [1877]. 6p. DNLM
70-2237

LYMAN, George H. (1819-1891)
The interests of the public and the medical profession. The annual discourse before the Massachusetts Medical Society. Boston: D. Clapp & Son, 1875. 46p. DNLM; MBM
70-2238

LYMAN, George H. (1819-1891)
In memoriam; Charles Edward Buckingham. [1878.] 3p. port. DNLM **70-2239**

LYMAN, Henry Munson (1835-1904)
Cervico-dorsal paralysis of peripheral origin. New York: G. P. Putnam's Sons, 1878. 18p. DNLM; NNNAM
70-2240

LYNCH, John S. (1828-1888)
A reply to Dr. John Van Bibber on "The future influence of the Johns Hopkins Hospital on the medical profession of Baltimore." Richmond: Whittet & Shepperson, 1879. 11p. DNLM **70-2241**

LYONS, Albert Brown (1841-1926)
Medicinal plants indigenous in Michigan. . . . Read before the Detroit Academy of Medicine, Nov. 27th, 1877. . . . [Detroit, 1878.] 25p. DLC; DNLM **70-2242**

LYONS, Frederick A.
Address delivered at the commencement of the College of Physicians and Surgeons, Medical Department of Columbia College, New York. New York, [1876]. 18p. DNLM
70-2243

McALLISTER, T. H.
Illustrated price list of microscopes, microscopic apparatus, lenses. . . . 3rd ed. New York: T. H. McAllister, 1877. 64p. DNLM; NNNAM **70-2244**

McARTHUR, J. A[mbrose] (1831-1887)
Notes on the treatment of consumption with the syrup of the hypophosphites. Boston: A. Mudge & Son, 1878. 32p. DNLM; MH-M **70-2245**

McBRIDE, James H.
Experimental and clinical observations on the use of nitrite of amyl in epilepsy. Chicago: J. J. Spalding & Co., 1875. 15p. DNLM **70-2246**

McBRIDE, Thomas Alexander (1844-1886)
The utility of the sphygmograph in medicine. New York: G. P. Putnam's Sons, 1879. 15p. DNLM; NNNAM
70-2247

McCLELLAN, Ely (1834-1893)
Obstetric procedures among the aborigines of North America. Louisville: J. P. Morton, 1873. 15p. DNLM
70-2248

McCLELLAN, Ely (1834-1893)
Cholera hygiene. Louisville: J. P. Morton & Co., 1874. 24, 22p. DNLM **70-2249**

McCELLLAN, Ely (1834-1893)
Fibroid tumors of the uterus. Louisville: J. P. Morton, 1874. 28p. DNLM **70-2250**

McCLELLAN, Ely (1834-1893)
Common carriers as the porters of disease. Part I. Louisville: J. P. Morton & Co., 1874. 11p. DNLM
70-2251

McCLELLAN, Ely (1834-1893)
An account of the epidemic of cholera, during the summer of 1873, in eighteen counties of the State of Kentucky. Cambridge: Riverside Press, 1874. 24p. DNLM
70-2252

McCLELLAN, Ely (1834-1893)
A note of warning. Lessons to be learned from the cholera facts of the past year, and from recent cholera literature. Louisville, Ky., 1876. 45p. DNLM **70-2253**

McCLELLAN, Ely (1834-1893)
Public health papers. No. 1. On the relations of health boards and other sanitary organizations with civic authorities. Atlanta: J. P. Harrison, 1876. 36p. DNLM **70-2254**

McCLELLAN, Ely (1834-1893)
A review of the latest work of Dr. Max von Pettenkofer: "An outbreak of cholera among convicts." Louisville, 1877. 43p. DNLM **70-2255**

McCLELLAN, E. S[pencer] (1824-1911)
Infant feeding and its relation to infant mortality. New York, N.Y.: Medical Review Office, [1873]. 16p. DNLM
70-2256

McCLELLAND, James H[enderson] (1849-1913)
The mind. The annual address delivered before the Homoeopathic Medical Society of Pennsylvania, October 15, 1875, at Library Hall, and in a modified form before the Legislature of Pennsylvania, March, 1876. Pittsburgh: William G. Johnson & Co., 1876. 45p. PPHa **70-2257**

McCLELLAND, Milo Adams (*b.* 1837)
Civil malpractice. A report presented to the Military Tract Medical Society at its fifteenth semi-annual meeting, Jan. 14, 1873. Chicago: Keen, Cooke & Co., 1873. 74p. DNLM; ICRM
70-2258

McCLELLAND, Milo Adams (*b.* 1837)
Civil malpractice: a treatise on surgical jurisprudence. With chapters on skill in diagnosis and treatment, prognosis in fractures and on negligence. . . . New York: Hurd & Houghton; Boston: H. O. Houghton & Co., 1877. 554p. DLC; DNLM; NNNAM **70-2259**

McCLINTOCK, James (1809-1881)
Medical lectures to gentlemen. . . . Philadelphia, Pa.: J. McClintock, [1872]. 144p. DLC; PPC; PU
70-2260

McCOMBER, Joel
An address delivered before the polytechnic branch of the American Institute of the City of New York, May 20, 1875, on the human foot; its use, abuse, and preservation. New York, 1875. 60p. DNLM; NNNAM **70-2261**

McCOMBER, Joel
McComber's tracks; an appeal to fathers and mothers to save their children's feet from deformity. New York, 1876. 17p. DNLM **70-2262**

MacDONALD, A. E. (*b.* 1845)
A lecture delivered before the pupils of the School for Nurses, Charity Hospital, New York, October 6, 1875, on the nursing of the insane. New York: Bellevue Press, 1875. 24p. DNLM
70-2263

MacDONALD, A. E. (*b.* 1845)
Feigned insanity. New York: Campbell & Co., 1876. 11 l. DNLM **70-2264**

MacDONALD, A. E. (*b.* 1845)
General paresis. Utica, 1877. 32p. DNLM
70-2265

MacDONALD, Carlos F.
Feigned insanity, homicide, suicide. Case of William Barr, alias Ball. [1879.] 22p. DNLM **70-2266**

McDONNELL, Robert (1828-1889)
On the torsion of blood-vessels. New York: G. P. Putnam's Sons, 1874. 6p. DNLM **70-2267**

McELROY, Z. Collins
The bromides; their physiological effects and therapeutic uses. New York: D. Appleton & Co., 1870. 26p. DNLM **70-2268**

McELROY, Z. Collins
The clinical thermometer; its lessons and teachings tentatively expressed in numbers. New York: W. Baldwin & Co., [1871]. 17p. DNLM **70-2269**

McELROY, Z. Collins
The essential nature and purpose of the fever process in living human bodies. Delivered before the Muskingum County Medical Society. Columbus: Nevins & Myers, 1876. 14p. DNLM **70-2270**

McELROY, Z. Collins
Hydroadipsia and the water supply of living bodies clinically illustrated. Cincinnati, 1876. 9p. DNLM **70-2271**

McELROY, Z. Collins
What is the nature and purpose of the fever process in human bodies? [Cincinnati, 1876.] 7p. DNLM **70-2272**

McELROY, Z. Collins
On artificially produced fever processes in the human body. Columbus: Nevins & Myers, 1877. 13p. DNLM **70-2273**

McELROY, Z. Collins
Curative relation of measles to whooping-cough, with some observations on the epidemics of measles and whooping-cough in the city of Zanesville, Ohio. Columbus: Nevins & Myers, 1877. 9p. DNLM **70-2274**

McELROY, Z. Collins
Clinical cases of hydroadipsia, with some facts concerning the water supply of living bodies. [Cincinnati, 1877.] 9p. DNLM **70-2275**

McELROY, Z. Collins
What medicine offers for the relief of common drunkenness. A clinical report and study of it. [Cincinnati, 1877.] 13p. DNLM **70-2276**

MacFARLAN, Malcolm (*b.* 1841)
Valedictory address to the graduates of the Hahnemann Medical College of Philadelphia, delivered at the twenty-fifth annual commencmeent, held at the Academy of Music, March 10, 1873. Philadelphia: W. P. Kildare, 1873. 18p. DNLM; PPHa **70-2277**

McFARLAND, Andrew (1817-1891)
The better way; or, considerations upon the natural system of providing for the treatment of the insane. [St. Louis, 1872.] 40p. DNLM; OCIM **70-2278**

McFARLAND, Andrew (1817-1891)
Commitments to institutions for the insane. A letter to Hon. Thos. P. Rogers. Carrollton, Ill.: Patriot Printing Establishment, 1879. 17p. DNLM **70-2279**

McILVAINE, Robert R. (*d.* 1881)
Remarks before the Ohio Medical Society, 1871, on the special report of the committee on sanitary science. Reported by J. W. Haddock, M.D. [1871.] 4p. DNLM **70-2280**

McINTOSH NATURAL UTERINE SUPPORTER CO.
Some practical facts about displacement of the womb, with suggestions for treatment. Chicago, [1870?]. 15p. DNLM **70-2281**

MACKALL, Louis (1802-1876)
Critique on Prof. Tyndall's course of lectures on light. In three essays. Washington, D.C.: McGill & Witherow, 1873. 29p. DNLM **70-2282**

MACKALL, Louis (1802-1876)
Darwinism reproved and refuted. Washington: McGill & Witherow, 1873. 25p. DNLM **70-2283**

MACKALL, Louis (1802-1876), Edward CRANCH, and Charles ALLEN
Addresses delivered at the twenty-fourth annual commencement of the Medical Department of the University of Georgetown, March 6, 1873. Washington, D.C.: D. McIntosh, 1873. 30p. DNLM **70-2284**

McKAY, Lawrence
Aima Tomaton; or new cupping and puncturing apparatus. Rochester, N.Y.: Express Printing House, 1870. 11p. DNLM **70-2285**

McKAY, Read J[ennings]
Some of the practical relations of ophthalmology and otology to the general practice of medicine. Wilmington, Del., 1879. 8p. DNLM **70-2286**

MACKENZIE, Morell (1837-1892)
Essay on growths in the larynx; with reports and an analysis of one hundred consecutive cases treated by the author, and a tabular statement of all published cases treated by other practitioners since the invention of the laryngoscope. Philadelphia: Lindsay & Blakiston, 1871. 263p. 5 plates. DNLM; MBM; NNNAM; PPC **70-2287**

McKESSON & ROBBINS. NEW YORK CITY
Prices current of drugs and druggists' articles, chemical and pharmaceutical preparations. . . . New York: Thitchener & Glastaeter, 1872. 128p. NNNAM **70-2288**

MACLAY, J. W.
Prize essay on the relations of the different professions and vocations to longevity. New York: F. Hart & Co., 1873. 58p. DNLM; NNNAM **70-2289**

McLEAN, Le Roy (1831-1897)
Two cases of oesophagotomy. West Roy, N.Y.: J. Treanor, 1877. 10p. 1 tab. DNLM **70-2290**

McMURRAY, Robert (1844-1896)
Medical education; annual address delivered before the Homoeopathic Medical Society of the State of New York, [1871]. 12p. DNLM; PPHa **70-2291**

McMURTRIE, Henry (1793-1865)
The woman's medical companion, and nursery adviser: containing rules for preserving the health of unmarried females; directions to pregnant and lying-in women; and an account of their diseases. . . . Philadelphia: T. E. Zell, 1871. 299p. plates. DLC; PPC; PU **70-2292**

McMURTRY, Lewis Samuel (1850-1924)
Memoir of John D. Jackson. [1876?] 12p. DNLM **70-2293**

McNAUGHTON, James (1796-1874)
Reply to Dr. C. A. Robertson's review of the report concerning the last illness of Dr. Alden March. New York: D. Appleton & Co., 1870. 16p. DNLM **70-2294**

McNAUGHTON, James (1796-1874)
A brief sketch of the life of the late Dr. Alden March, of Albany. [1871.] 6p. DNLM **70-2295**

McNUTT, W. F[letcher] (*b.* **1839)**
Valedictory address to the graduating class of the Medical Department of the University of California. [1879.] 8p. DNLM **70-2296**

McQUILLEN, John Hugh (1826-1879)
Remarks on dental education. [1873.] 4p. DNLM **70-2297**

McQUILLEN, John Hugh (1826-1879)
A case of oral surgery. [1875.] 4p. DNLM **70-2298**

McQUILLEN, John Hugh (1826-1879)
Oral organisms. [1875.] 7p. DNLM **70-2299**

McQUILLEN, John Hugh (1826-1879)
Introductory lecture to the winter course of the Philadelphia Dental College, session 1875-1876. New York: Johnston Bros., 1876. 15p. DNLM **70-2300**

McSHERRY, H. Clinton
Laryngeal stenosis. Baltimore: J. H. Foster, 1877. 12p. DNLM **70-2301**

McSHERRY, Richard (1817-1885)
Health, and how to promote it. New York: D. Appleton & Co., 1879. 185p. DNLM; NNNAM **70-2302**

MADDEN, Thomas More (1838-1902)
The principal health resorts of Europe and Africa for the treatment of chronic diseases. . . . Philadelphia: Lindsay & Blakiston, 1876. 276p. DLC; NNNAM; PPC **70-2303**

MAGITOT, Emile (1833-1897)
Treatise on dental caries. Experimental and therapeutic investigations. Transl. by Thomas H. Chandler. Boston: Houghton, Osgood & Co., 1878. 275p. 2 plates. DNLM; MH-M; NNNAM; PU **70-2304**

MAISCH, John M. (1831-1903)
Valedictory address delivered before the graduating class of the Philadelphia College of Pharmacy, March 16, 1875. [Philadelphia, 1875.] 11p. DNLM; PPC; PPHa **70-2305**

MANN, Edward Cox (1850-1908)
Insanity in the Middle States. [1873.] 12p. DNLM **70-2306**

MANN, Edward Cox (1850-1908)
Insanity; its nature, pathology, and treatment. New York: D. Appleton & Co., 1874. 20p. DNLM; NNNAM **70-2307**

MANN, Edward Cox (1850-1908)
Insanity; its etiology, diagnosis, pathology, and treatment, with cases illustrating pathology, morbid histology, and treatment. New York: G P. Putnam, 1875. 50p. DNLM; NNNAM **70-2308**

MANN, Edward Cox (1850-1908)
The nature and treatment of inebriety. Also the opium habit and its treatment. New York: C. A. Coffin, 1878. 86p. DNLM; NNNAM **70-2309**

MANN, M[atthew] D[arbyshire] (1845-1921)
The immediate treatment of superficial ruptures of the perineum. New York: William Wood & Co., 1874. 10p. DNLM **70-2310**

MANN, Matthew Darbyshire (1845-1921)
A manual of prescription writing with a full explanation of the methods of correctly writing prescriptions, a table of doses expressed in both the apothecaries' and metric systems; rules for avoiding incompatibilities and for combining medicines. . . . New York: G. P. Putnam's Sons, 1878. 155p. DLC; NNNAM; PPJ; PU **70-2311**

MANN, William B.
How to care for the teeth: being practical advice and valuable suggestions, designed for popular distribution, Baltimore, Md., 1877. 80p. DLC; MdU-D **70-2312**

MANNING, J. M[errill] (1824-1882)
An address delivered before the Massachusetts College of Pharmacy, at the third annual commencement. An outside view of pharmacy. Boston: A. A. Blair, [1871]. 16p. DNLM; MH-M; MSaE **70-2313**

MANSILL, Richard
Cholera and planetary epidemics. Cholera waves or periods—the rise and fall of the scourge. Epidemics and other pestilences. Cattle plagues and other diseases. Periodical maladies of slow fevers and agues. Sun-strokes, etc. Crop blighting years. Unseasonable hot and cold weather. . . . Rock Island, Ill.: Daily Union Steam Printing House, 1874. 28p. DLC; DNLM **70-2314**

A MANUAL of nursing. Prepared for the training school for nurses attached to Bellevue Hospital. New York: G. P. Putnam's Sons, 1878. 142p. DNLM; NNNAM; NNU-M **70-2315**

MARCY, Henry Orlando (1837-1924)
Fracture of the patella, and treatment by a new method. Cambridge: Riverside Press, 1876. 6p. DNLM **70-2316**

MARCY, Henry Orlando (1837-1924)
Plastic splints in surgery. Cambridge: Riverside Press, 1877. 9p. DNLM **70-2317**

MARCY, Henry Orlando (1837-1924)
The radical cure of hernia by the antiseptic use of the carbolized catgut ligature. Cambridge, Mass., 1879. 23p. DNLM
70-2318

MARKOE, Thomas Masters (1819-1901)
A treatise on diseases of the bones. New York: D. Appleton & Co., 1872. 416p. DNLM; MBM; NNNAM **70-2319**

MARKS, A. A., & CO.
Patent artificial limbs with India-rubber hands and feet. New York: N. F. Turner, 1876. 112p. DNLM; NNNAM
70-2320

MARKS, A. A., & CO.
Patent artificial limbs with India-rubber hands and feet. New York: N. F. Turner, 1876. 85p. 1 phot. DNLM; NNNAM
70-2321

MARSDEN, John Hatton (1803-1883)
Hand-book of practical midwifery, including full instruction for the homoeopathic treatment of the disorders of pregnancy, and the accidents and diseases incident to labor and the puerperal state. New York: Boericke & Tafel, 1879. 315p. DNLM; NNNAM; PPC; PPHa **70-2322**

MARSH, Elias J. (*b.* 1835)
Hay fever, or pollen poisoning. Newark, N.J.: L. J. Hardham, 1877. 26p. DNLM **70-2323**

MARTIN, Henry A[ustin] (1824-1884)
The American Medical Association vs. Henry A. Martin, M.D., member of said association, and late chairman of its committee on vaccination. Boston: Rand, Avery & Frye, 1871. 16p. DNLM **70-2324**

MARTIN, Henry A[ustin] (1824-1884)
Dr. Martin on vaccination. Erie, Pa., 1873. 6p. DNLM
70-2325

MARTIN, Henry A[ustin] (1824-1884)
Colles's fracture and Dr. Carr's splint. [Boston, 1876?] 7p. DNLM **70-2326**

MARTIN, Henry A[ustin] (1824-1884)
A few words on "unfortunate results of vaccination." Cambridge, 1877. 7p. DNLM **70-2327**

MARTIN, Henry A[ustin] (1824-1884)
A new adhesive plaster, especially adapted to the requirements of modern surgery. [Boston, 1877.] 4p. DNLM
70-2328

MARTIN, Henry A[ustin] (1824-1884)
Remarks on the treatment of fistula in ano by caustics. [Boston, 1877.] 4p. DNLM **70-2329**

MARTIN, Henry A[ustin] (1824-1884)
Tracheotomy without tubes. Philadelphia: Collins, 1878. 19p. DNLM **70-2330**

MARTIN, Henry A[ustin] (1824-1884)
On animal vaccination. Boston: J. Campbell, 1878. 62p. 2 plates. DNLM **70-2331**

MARTIN, Henry A[ustin] (1824-1884)
Surgical uses other than haemostatic of the strong elastic bandage. Boston: J. Campbell, 1878. 27p. DNLM
70-2332

MARTIN, Henry A[ustin] (1824-1884)
Surgical uses other than haemostatic of the strong elastic bandage. 2nd ed. Boston: Leach & Green, 1879. 26p. DNLM
70-2333

MARTIN, Henry A[ustin] (1824-1884)
Surgical uses other than haemostatic of the strong elastic bandage. 2nd ed., with some additions. Boston: Wright & Potter; London: Krohne & Seseman, 1879. 26p. DNLM
70-2334

MARTIN, Henry A[ustin] (1824-1884)
Toe nail ulcer; what it is and its treatment, ancient and modern. Toledo, [1879]. 16p. DNLM **70-2335**

MARTIN, Henry A[ustin] (1824-1884)
On miscarriage, and especially on the use of Loomis's forceps in its management. Chicago, 1879. 16p. DNLM
70-2336

MARTIN, H[enry] Newell (1818-1896)
The physiology of secretion. Baltimore, 1879. 27p. DNLM
70-2337

MARVIN, Frederick R. (1847-1918)
Epidemic delusions; a lecture read before the New York Liberal Club. New York: A. K. Butts & Co., 1874. 28p. DNLM; NNNAM **70-2338**

MARVIN, Frederick R. (1847-1918)
The philosophy of spiritualism and the pathology and treatment of mediomania. New York: A. K. Butts & Co., 1874. 68p. DNLM; NNNAM **70-2339**

MARVIN, Frederick R. (1847-1918)
The literature of the insane. Truth seeker tracts. Scientific series, No. 4. [New York, 1875.] 25p. DNLM; NNNAM
70-2340

MARVIN, Joseph Benson (1852-1913)
A history of the diagnosis, pathology, and treatment of yellow fever. Louisville, Ky., 1878. 15p. DNLM
70-2341

MARYLAND EYE AND EAR INSTITUTE. BALTIMORE
Bericht über die fünfjährige Wirksamkeit der ersten deutschen Augen- und Ohren-Klinik in den Vereinigten Staaten. Von George Reuling. Baltimore: Guggenheimer & Weil, 1875. 16p. DNLM **70-2342**

MASON, Erskine (1837-1882)
A case of strangulated oblique inguinal hernia, reduced en masse; together with strangulated ventral hernia; operation; recovery; and remarks upon the accident of reduction en masse. New York: D. Appleton & Co., 1870. 15p. DNLM
70-2343

MASON, Erskine (1837-1882)
A case of rupture of the urinary bladder, with remarks upon the treatment of this accident. New York: D. Appleton & Co., 1872. 22p. DNLM **70-2344**

MASON, Erskine (1837-1882)
Two successful cases of amputation at the hip-joint, with remarks upon the operation. New York: D. Appleton & Co., 1876. 26p. 1 plate. DNLM **70-2345**

MASON, John J[ames]
On the pathogeny of the infractions or congested patches which follow embolism. New York: D. Appleton & Co., 1872. 8p. DNLM **70-2346**

MASON, John J[ames]
Experiments on the tonicity of the arterioles. New York: D. Appleton & Co., 1872. 7p. DNLM **70-2347**

MASON, John J[ames]
Peristaltic arterial action; objections to this theory. New York: D. Appleton & Co., 1873. 10p. DNLM **70-2348**

MASON, John J[ames]
The polar action of electricity in physiology. New York: D. Appleton & Co., 1874. 15p. 2 plates. DNLM **70-2349**

MASON, John J[ames]
The polar action of electricity in physiology. Second article. [1874?] 4p. DNLM **70-2350**

MASON, Lewis D[uncan] (*b.* 1843)
The rubber air-cushion in the treatment of complicated fractures and other serious injuries of the lower extremities; with illustrated cases. New York: D. Appleton & Co., 1870. 12p. DNLM **70-2351**

MASSACHUSETTS MEDICAL SOCIETY
Fellows of the Massachusetts Medical Society, 1781-1870. Alphabetically arranged. Boston: Printed by D. Clapp & Son, 1870. 52p. DLC; MH; MWA **70-2352**

MASSEY, Thomas E.
Relations of Colorado to pulmonary consumption. Denver (Col.): Daily & Smart, 1874. 26p. DNLM **70-2353**

MASTIN, Claudius Henry (1826-1898)
Internal urethrotomy as a cure of urethral stricture. Mobile: Tribune Office, 1871. 34p. DNLM **70-2354**

MASTIN, Claudius Henry (1826-1898)
Chronic urethral discharges. Louisville, 1872. 32p. DNLM **70-2355**

MASTIN, Claudius Henry (1826-1898)
A new method of treating strictures of the urethra, after external sections. Louisville: Med. Jour. Print, 1873. 39p. DNLM **70-2356**

MASTIN, Claudius Henry (1826-1898)
The causes and geographical distribution of calculous diseases. Philadelphia: [Collins], 1877. 17p. DNLM **70-2357**

MATHEWS, J. McDowell (*b.* 1847)
Objections to the use of carbolic acid in the treatment of piles. Louisville, 1878. 8p. DNLM **70-2358**

MATHEWSON, Arthur (1837-1920)
A case of exostosis of the external auditory meatus drilled out by the "dental engine." New York: D. Appleton & Co., 1877. 12p. DNLM **70-2359**

MATTISON, J. B[eemer] (*b.* 1845)
Chloral inebriety; read before the Kings County Medical Society April 15, 1879. New York: H. T. Cornett, 1879. 13p. DNLM **70-2360**

MAUDSLEY, Henry (1835-1918)
Body and mind: an inquiry into their connection and mutual influence, specially in reference to mental disorders. Being the Gulstonian lectures for 1870, delivered before the Royal College of Physicians. With appendix. . . . New York: D. Appleton & Co., 1871. 155p. DLC; DNLM; NNNAM; PPC **70-2361**

MAUDSLEY, Henry (1835-1918)
Body and mind: an inquiry into their connection and mutual influence, specially in reference to mental disorders: an enl. and rev. ed. To which are added psychological essays. . . . New York: D. Appleton & Co., 1874. 275p. DLC; NNNAM; OCIM; PU **70-2362**

MAUDSLEY, Henry (1835-1918)
. . . Responsibility in mental disease. . . . New York: D. Appleton & Co., 1875. 313p. DLC; DNLM; NNNAM; PU **70-2363**

MAUGHS, G. M. B. (*d.* 1901)
Placenta praevia. St. Louis: C. R. Barns & Co., 1879. 24p. DNLM **70-2364**

MAURY, Francis Fontaine (1840-1879)
Case of stricture of the oesophagus in which gastrotomy was performed. Philadelphia: J. B. Chandler, 1870. 8p. DNLM **70-2365**

MAURY, Francis Fontaine (1840-1879) and Louis A. DUHRING
Case of exsection of the brachial plexus of nerves for the relief of painful neuroma of the skin. Philadelphia: Collins, 1874. 13p. DNLM **70-2366**

MAURY, Francis Fontaine (1840-1879) and C. W. DULLES
Tattooing as a means of communicating syphilis; an investigation of twenty-two cases exposed to inoculation with the virus of mucous patches, in fifteen of which syphilis followed. [Philadelphia, 1878.] 19p. DNLM **70-2367**

MAURY, Francis Fontaine (1840-1879)
Catalogue of the valuable medical library of the late Dr. . . . Philadelphia: W. B. Selheimer, 1879. 11p. DNLM **70-2368**

MAURY, Richard Brooke (1834-1919)
The treatment of chronic dysentery by topical medication. New York: D. Appleton & Co., 1876. 12p. DNLM **70-2369**

MAYS, Thomas Jefferson (1846-1918)
On the therapeutic forces: an effort to consider the action of medicines in the light of the modern doctrine of the conservation of force. . . . Philadelphia: Lindsay & Blakiston, 1878. 143p. DLC; DNLM; NNNAM; PPC **70-2370**

MAYS, Thomas Jefferson (1846-1918)
An improved method of applying heat to the chest. New York: D. Appleton & Co., 1879. 7p. DNLM **70-2371**

MAYS, Thomas Jefferson (1846-1918)
On the elective action and small doses of medicines. With illustrative cases. New York: D. Appleton & Co., 1879. 19p. DNLM; NNNAM **70-2372**

MAYS, Thomas Jefferson (1846-1918)
Consumption and how to prevent it. . . . New York: G. P. Putnam's Sons, 1879. 89p. DLC; DNLM; NNNAM; PU
70-2373

MEAD, Edward (1819-1883)
Announcement of the Psychopathic Retreat, an institution for the treatment of mental and nervous diseases under the superintendence of . . . . Boston: W. F. Brown & Co., 1874. 5 l. DNLM **70-2374**

MEADOWS, Alfred (1823-1887)
A manual of midwifery, including the signs and symptoms of pregnancy, obstetric operations, diseases of the puerperal state, etc. 1st American from 2nd London ed. Philadelphia: Lindsay & Blakiston, 1871. 487p. CtY-M; DNLM; NNNAM; PPC **70-2375**

MEARS, George Washington (1803-1879)
Address on the etiology and treatment of unavoidable hemorrhage. Indianapolis: Indianapolis Journal Co., 1878. 9p. DNLM **70-2376**

MEARS, James Ewing (1838-1918)
Description of the anomalous origin of the right subclavian artery associated with anomalies of origin of the branches of both subclavian arteries. Philadelphia, 1871. 14p. DNLM **70-2377**

MEARS, James Ewing (1838-1918)
Ligation of the femoral artery for large aneurism of the popliteal artery; recovery. Philadelphia, 1873. 1p. DNLM **70-2378**

MEARS, James Ewing (1838-1918)
Report of two cases of amputation in which a modification of the Esmarch apparatus was employed. Philadelphia, 1874. 2p. DNLM **70-2379**

MEARS, James Ewing (1838-1918)
Practical surgery: including surgical dressings, bandaging, ligations and amputations. . . . Philadelphia: Lindsay & Blakiston, 1878. 279p. DLC; MBM; OCIM; PPC **70-2380**

MEDICAL handbook of Philadelphia, 1876. Designed for the use of the International Medical Congress, American Medical Association, and Medical Society of the State of Pennsylvania. Philadelphia: Collins, 1876. 26p. DLC; DNLM; PPC; PU **70-2381**

MEDICAL SOCIETY OF SOUTH CAROLINA
Prof. Eli Geddings. The tribute of the Medical Society to his memory. [Charleston, 1878.] 8p. DNLM; ScCM
70-2382

MEDICO-LEGAL SOCIETY OF THE CITY OF NEW YORK
Report of the committee on criminal abortion. New York: D. Appleton & Co., 1872. 15p. DNLM; NNNAM
70-2383

MEDICO-LEGAL SOCIETY OF THE CITY OF NEW YORK
First annual dinner, March 19, 1873. New York: H. E. Thomson & Co., 1873. 45p. 1 phot. DNLM; NNNAM
70-2384

MEDICO-LEGAL SOCIETY OF THE CITY OF NEW YORK
[Organization, objects, and plans.] List of papers read and of officers for 1872-1873. [1873.] 5p. DNLM; NNNAM
70-2385

MEDICO-LEGAL SOCIETY OF THE CITY OF NEW YORK
Constitution, by-laws, and list of officers, members, library contributions, etc. New York: C. Levey & Co., 1874. 28p. DNLM; NNNAM **70-2386**

MEDICO-LEGAL SOCIETY OF THE CITY OF NEW YORK
Proceedings, March 26, 1874. Care and safe keeping of lunatics. Medical jurisprudence of the Stokes case. New York: Sanitarian Publ. Office, 1874. 15p. DNLM; NNNAM
70-2387

MEDICO-LEGAL SOCIETY OF THE CITY OF NEW YORK
Proceedings, April 23, 1874. Discussion of Prof. W. A. Hammond's paper on morbid impulse. New York: Sanitarian Publ. Office, 1874. 9p. DNLM; NNNAM
70-2388

MEDICO-LEGAL SOCIETY OF THE CITY OF NEW YORK
Papers read before the Medico-Legal Society of New York, from its organization. First series. Revised edition. New York: McDivitt, Campbell & Co., 1874. 552p. DNLM; NNNAM **70-2389**

MEDICO-LEGAL SOCIETY OF THE CITY OF NEW YORK
Report of special committee upon school hygiene. New York: Terwilliger & Peck, 1876. 12p. DNLM; NNNAM
70-2390

MEDICO-LEGAL SOCIETY OF THE CITY OF NEW YORK
Charter, constitution, by-laws, and list of officers and members. 5th ed. New York: Terwilliger & Peck, 1877. 20p. DNLM; NNNAM **70-2391**

MEIGS, James Aitken (1829-1879)
Valedictory address to the graduating class of Jefferson Medical College. Philadelphia: Collins, 1870. 29p. DNLM; PPJ **70-2392**

MEIGS, James Aitken (1829-1879)
Valedictory address to the graduating class of Jefferson Medical College. Philadelphia: Collins, 1879. 20p. DLC; DNLM; PPJ **70-2393**

MEIGS, John Forsyth (1818-1882)
A practical treatise on the diseases of children. By J. Forsyth Meigs . . . and William Pepper. . . . 4th ed. (of Meigs on diseases of children) rev. and greatly enl. . . . Philadelphia: Lindsay & Blakiston, 1870. 921p. DLC; DNLM; NNNAM; PPC
70-2394

MEIGS, J[ohn] Forsyth (1818-1882)
Address delivered before the managers, medical staff, and students of the Pennsylvania Hospital, on the occasion of the opening of the new lecture and operating room, Jan. 9th, 1869. . . . Philadelphia: Lindsay & Blakiston, 1871. 35p. DLC; DNLM; PU **70-2395**

MEIGS, John Forsyth (1818-1882)
A practical treatise on the diseases of children. By J. Forsyth Meigs . . . and William Pepper. . . . 5th ed., rev. and enl. Philadelphia: Lindsay & Blakiston, 1874. 1008p. DLC; DNLM; NNNAM; PU **70-2396**

MEIGS, John Forsyth (1818-1882)
A practical treatise on the diseases of children. By J. Forsyth Meigs . . . and William Pepper. . . . 6th ed., rev. and enl. Philadelphia: Lindsay & Blakiston, 1877. 1012p. DLC; DNLM; NNNAM; PPC **70-2397**

MEIGS, John Forsyth (1818-1882)
A history of the first quarter of the second century of the Pennsylvania Hospital. Read before the Board of Managers at their stated meeting held 9th mo. 25th, 1876. . . . Published by the Board of Managers. Philadelphia: Collins, printer, 1877. 145p. DLC; DNLM; PPC; PU **70-2398**

MEIGS, J[ohn] Forsyth (1818-1882)
An address on the occasion of the one hundred and twenty-fifth celebration of the founding of the Pennsylvania Hospital, delivered Sept. 25, 1876. Philadelphia: Collins, 1877. 87p. DNLM; PU **70-2399**

MEIGS, J[ohn] Forsyth (1818-1882)
Case of collapse of the lung and cyanosis in a young infant, produced by violent crying, in which the symptoms were such as to cause a suspicion of opium-poisoning; with remarks on the nature and treatment of temporary cyanosis from post-natal collapse of the lung. New York: William Wood & Co., 1879. 16p. DNLM **70-2400**

MEMOIR of Élie-Magloire Durand. [Philadelphia, 1873.] 10p. DNLM **70-2401**

MEMOIR of William Proctor, Jr., late professor of pharmacy in the Philadelphia College of Pharmacy. Philadelphia: Merrihew & Sons, 1874. 27p. DNLM; PPC **70-2402**

MENDENHALL, George (1814-1874)
Address delivered before the American Medical Association at its twenty-first annual meeting. Philadelphia: Collins, 1870. 21p. DNLM; PPC **70-2403**

MENDENHALL, George (1814-1874)
The medical student's vade mecum. A compendium of anatomy, physiology, chemistry, poisons, materia medica, pharmacy, surgery, obstetrics, practice of medicine, diseases of the skin, etc. 10th ed. Philadelphia: Lindsay & Blakiston, 1871. 692p. DNLM; MBM; NNNAM; PPC **70-2404**

[MENDENHALL, George] (1814-1874)
Catalogue of the medical library, and surgical instruments, etc., of the late. . . . Cincinnati: J. Barclay, [1877]. 17p. DNLM **70-2405**

MERCER, Alfred (1820-1914)
The relations of general (scientific medicine) to special and specific modes of medication. Buffalo: Baker, Jones & Co., 1874. 18p. DNLM **70-2406**

MERCER, Alfred (1820-1914)
An address, presenting the claims of the medical department, read before a council in the interest of Syracuse University, held at Syracuse, N.Y., December 18, 19, 1878. Syracuse, N.Y.: Masters & Stone, 1979. 19p. DNLM **70-2407**

MERCER, Samuel David
Spinal curvatures, and treatment of spinal diseases by plaster of Paris jacket (Sayre's method). . . . Omaha, Neb.: Republican Steam Book and Job Print, 1878. 12p. OCIM **70-2408**

MEREDITH, L. P.
The teeth and how to save them. . . . Philadelphia: J. B. Lippincott & Co., 1871. 271p. DLC; DNLM; PPC; PU **70-2409**

MEREDITH, L. P.
Examination, appreciation, and fees. A lecture delivered at the Cincinnati College of Medicine and Surgery, Feb. 12, 1874. [Cincinnati], 1874. 20p. DNLM **70-2410**

MEREDITH, L. P.
Our teeth and their preservation. . . . Popular lecture. Cincinnati: Hitchcock & Walden, 1875. 43p. DNLM **70-2411**

MEREDITH, L. P.
The teeth and how to save them. . . . Philadelphia: J. B. Lippincott & Co., 1877. 274p. DLC; MdU-D; PU **70-2412**

MERRICK, William Matthews (1818-1889)
Address to the medical graduates of the University of Maryland . . . at the commencement held in the Academy of Music, Baltimore, Md., March 1, 1875. Published by the Faculty of Physic. Baltimore: Kelly, Piet & Co., 1875. 11p. DLC **70-2413**

MERRILL, A. P[hillips] (1793-1873)
Observations on the use of mercury. Louisville: J. P. Morton, 1871. 8p. DNLM **70-2414**

MERRILL, A. P[hillips] (1793-1873)
Uterine diseases. Pneumonia. Louisville: J. P. Morton & Co., 1871. 16p. DNLM **70-2415**

MERRILL, A. P[hillips] (1793-1873)
Puerperal fever. Chloroform as an internal remedy. Louisville: J. P. Morton & Co., 1871. 16p. DNLM **70-2416**

MERRILL, A. P[hillips] (1793-1873)
The necessity of dentists in the army and navy. New York: J. J. Pusey, 1875. 8p. DNLM **70-2417**

[MESMERISM]
Library of mesmerism and psychology. New York: Wells, [1876]. 2 v. in 1. NN; NNC; NNNAM; PU [Includes: William Fishbough, The macrocosm and microcosm. . . . 1876; John B. Newman, Fascination, or the philosophy of charming. . . . 1875; John Bovee Dods, The philosophy of electrical psychology; in a course of twelve lectures, 1876; John Bovee Dods, Six lectures on the philosophy of mesmerism. . . . 1876; Joseph Haddock, Psychology; or the science of the soul, considered psychologically and philosophically, 1876.] **70-2418**

METCALF, THEODORE, & CO.
Notes on new remedies, collated from medical and pharmaceutical periodicals, etc. Boston, 1877. 32p. DNLM **70-2419**

MEYER, Georg Hermann (1815-1892)
Procrustes ante portas. Why the shoe pinches; a contribution to applied anatomy. Transl. from the German by John Stirling Craig. New York: G. F. Nesbitt & Co., 1877. 29p. 1 plate. DNLM; NNNAM **70-2420**

MICHEL, Carl
Diseases of the nasal cavity and the vault of the pharynx. Transl. from the German. With an introduction by E. L. Shurly and C. C. Yemans. 1st American ed. Detroit: C. Jung, 1877. 109p. DNLM; OCIM **70-2421**

MICHEL, Middleton (1822-1894)
Cases of cataract extracted by the corneal-flap, with comments on Graefe's operation. Charleston: Walker, Evans & Cogswell, 1871. 20p. DNLM; ScCM **70-2422**

MICHEL, Middleton (1822-1894)
Effects consequent upon the section of the posterior muscles of the neck, with a short history of the cerebro-spinal fluid. [1874?] 12p. DNLM **70-2423**

MICHEL, Middleton (1822-1894)
Cancroid or epithelioma of the lower lip modified operation for its removal; cure. [Charleston, 1875.] 6p. DNLM **70-2424**

MICHEL, Middleton (1822-1894)
Anatomy of the bullet-track, and cicatrices of the wounds of entrance and exit. [Charleston, 1875.] 14p. DNLM **70-2425**

MICHEL, R. Fraser (1827-1907)
Objections to the term "purpuraemia" being applied to the disease known as "hemorrhagic malarial fever." Montgomery, Ala., 1870. 10p. DNLM **70-2426**

MICHEL, R. Fraser (1827-1907)
Reflections on the anatomy and physiology of some parts of the eye. Mobile, 1871. 11p. DNLM **70-2427**

MICHEL, R. Fraser (1827-1907)
Epidemic yellow fever in Montgomery, Ala., during the summer of 1873. Charleston, 1874. 17p. DNLM **70-2428**

MICHEL, R. Fraser (1827-1907)
Epidemic yellow fever in Montgomery, Ala., during the summer of 1873. Montgomery: Barrett & Brown, 1874. 25p. DNLM **70-2429**

MICHEL, R. Fraser (1827-1907)
A history of break-bone-fever, as it prevailed in the city of Montgomery, Alabama, during the summer of 1866. Charleston, 1874. 12p. DNLM **70-2430**

MICHIGAN. UNIVERSITY OF MICHIGAN, ANN ARBOR. HOMOEOPATHIC MEDICAL COLLEGE
Annual announcements for the sessions of 1876-1877 to 1880-1881 (2.-6.); 1884-1885 (10.); 1885-1886 (11.); 1888-1889 (14.); 1889-1890 (15.); 1891-1892 to 1894-1895 (17.-20.); 1896-1897 to 1900-1901 (22.-26.); 1904-1905 (30.). Ann Arbor, 1876-1904. DNLM [List of students and graduates for the years 1875-1876 to 1879-1880; 1883-1884; 1884-1885; 1887-1888; 1888-1889; 1890-1891 to 1893-1894; 1895-1896 to 1899-1900; 1903-1904, in: Announcements for subsequent years.] **70-2431**

MICHIGAN. UNIVERSITY OF MICHIGAN, ANN ARBOR. SCHOOL OF PHARMACY
Index to the contributions of original work done by the alumni, 1870-1876. [Ann Arbor: Register Print. House, 1876.] 8p. DNLM **70-2432**

MILES, A[bijah] J.
The forceps in breech deliveries; with description of a new instrument. Cincinnati, 1876. 8p. DNLM **70-2433**

MILES, C. Richardson
Address to the graduates of the Medical College of the State of South Carolina at the annual commencement, held at Hibernian Hall, Charleston, S.C., March 5, 1878. Charleston, S.C., 1878. 7p. DNLM; ScCM **70-2434**

MILES, Francis Turquand (1827-1903)
Peripheral paralysis. New York: G. P. Putnam's Sons, 1876. 16p. DNLM **70-2435**

MILES, Francis Turquand (1827-1903)
A contribution to regional diagnosis in brain lesion. New York: G. P. Putnam's Sons, 1877. 7p. DNLM **70-2436**

MILES, Francis Turquand (1827-1903)
Electricity in medicine. Baltimore: J. H. Foster & Co., 1878. 17p. DNLM **70-2437**

MILLARD, Henry Benton (1832-1893)
A guide for emergencies, containing the homoeopathic treatment. . . . 3rd ed. . . . New York: C. T. Hurlbutt, 1871. 136p. DLC; NNNAM **70-2438**

MILLARD, Henry Benton (1832-1893)
On diphtheria. Illustrated by cases. Read before the New York Medico-Chirurgical Society. . . . New York and Philadelphia: Boericke & Tafel, 1879. 32p. DNLM; PPHa **70-2439**

MILLARD, Henry Benton (1832-1893)
Lectures on Bright's disease of the kidneys. Delivered at the School of Medicine in Paris, by J. M. Charcot. Collected and published by Drs. Bourneville and Levestre. Transl. by Henry B. Millard. New York: William Wood & Co., 1879. 100p. NNNAM; PPHa **70-2440**

MILLER, Eli Peck
Dyspepsia: its varieties, causes, symptoms, and treatment by hydropathy and hygiene. . . . New York: Miller, Haynes & Co., 1870. 94p. DLC; NNNAM **70-2441**

MILLER, Eli Peck
The improved Turkish bath; what is it, who should take it, why, when, how, and where? New York: Miller, Haynes & Co., 1871. 27p. DNLM **70-2442**

MILLER, Eli Peck
Vital force: how wasted and how preserved. 3rd ed. New York: E. P. Miller, 1874. 131p. DNLM; NNNAM **70-2443**

MILLER, Henry (1800-1874)
Thoughts on chronic inversion of the uterus; specially with reference to gastrotomy as a substitute for amputation of the uterus. Louisville, Ky.: Bell & Co., 1870. 42p. DNLM **70-2444**

MILLER, Henry (1800-1874)
Retrospect of uterine pathology and therapeutics in the United States, specially in regard to intra-uterine medication in chronic internal metritis. [Louisville, 1870.] 37p. DNLM **70-2445**

MILLER, Henry (1800-1874)
Retrospect of uterine pathology and therapeutics in the United States; specially in regard to intra-uterine medication in chronic internal metritis. New York: W. Baldwin & Co., 1871. 37p. DNLM; NNNAM **70-2446**

MILLER, James (1812-1864) and John LIZARS
Alcohol and tobacco. Alcohol: its place and power. The use and abuse of tobacco. Philadelphia: Lindsay & Blakiston, 1870. 179, 138p. DNLM; NNNAM; PU
70-2447

MILLER, J. P.
The hydatiform mole. The report of a case, together with a disquisition upon its history, pathology, etiology, diagnosis, prognosis, and treatment. Wheeling, 1879. 34p. DNLM
70-2448

MILLER, Samuel M.
Notes of hospital practice. Philadelphia, 1879-1882. 3 v. DNLM; PPJ; PU [Pt i. Philadelphia hospitals; Pts. ii-iv. New York and Philadelphia hospitals.] **70-2449**

MILLER, T. Clarke
A contribution to the etiology, pathology, and therapeutics of cholera infantum. New York: William Wood & Co., 1879. 18p. DNLM **70-2450**

MILLS, George A.
How to keep teeth clean and healthful. [Philadelphia, 1879.] 7p. DNLM **70-2451**

MILLS, George A.
Strengthening weak teeth by heavy gold and screws. The use of smooth convex-face fillers. [Philadelphia, 1879.] 4p. DNLM
70-2452

MINNESOTA. UNIVERSITY OF MINNESOTA, MINNEAPOLIS
Catalogues and calendars for the years 1876-1877; 1880-1881; 1882-1883 to 1884-1885; 1887-1888 to 1894-1895; 1896-1897 to 1903-1904, and announcements for the years 1877-1878; 1881-1882; 1883-1884 to 1885-1886; 1888-1889 to 1895-1896; 1897-1898 to 1904-1905. Minneapolis, 1877-1904. DNLM [Contains announcements of the College of Medicine and Surgery, the College of Homoeopathic Medicine and Surgery, the College of Dentistry, and the College of Pharmacy. The years 1876-1877; 1880-1881; 1882-1883 to 1884-1885, are called calendars.] **70-2453**

MINOR, Thomas Chalmers (1846-1912)
Erysipelas and child-bed fever. Cincinnati: R. Clarke & Co., 1874. 131p. 2 tab. DNLM; OCIM **70-2454**

MINOR, Thomas Chalmers (1846-1912)
Scarlatina statistics of the United States. Cincinnati: R. Clarke & Co., 1875. 55p. DNLM; OCIM **70-2455**

MINOR, Thomas Chalmers (1846-1912)
Notes on the epidemiology of Ohio. [Cincinnati, 1877.] 103p. DNLM; OCIM **70-2456**

MINOR, Thomas Chalmers (1846-1912)
Report on yellow fever in Ohio, as it appeared during the summer of 1878. Cincinnati, 1878. 122p. DNLM; OCIM
70-2457

MINOT, C[harles] S[edgwick] (1852-1914)
Transfusion and auto-transfusion. Cambridge, 1876. 3p. DNLM **70-2458**

MINOT, Francis (1821-1899)
Hints in ethics and hygiene. The annual discourse delivered in Boston, before the Massachusetts Medical Society, June 12, 1878. Boston: D. Clapp & Son, 1878. 30p. DNLM; MH-M
70-2459

MINTON, Henry (1831-1895)
Uterine fibroid tumors. A lecture delivered at the Hahnemann Medical College of Philadelphia. Albany: The Argus Co., 1870. 19p. DNLM; PPHa **70-2460**

MITCHELL, Clifford (1854-1939)
Students' manual of urinary analysis, chemical and microscopical. Comp., transl. and abridged from the most recent French authorities. . . . With a preface by Chas. Adams. . . . Chicago: Jansen, McClurg & Co., 1879. 24p. DLC
70-2461

MITCHELL, Joseph Sidney (*d.* 1898)
Valedictory address to the graduating class of Hahnemann Medical College, February 24, 1870, with inaugural address by A. E. Small. Chicago: Horton & Leonard, 1870. 23p. OCIM; PPHa **70-2462**

MITCHELL, J. W.
The compound oxygen treatment; its mode of action and results. New York: Kelly, Rorty & Gibson, 1871. 28p. DNLM; NNNAM **70-2463**

MITCHELL, J. W.
Hygienic hints to health seekers, while using the compound oxygen treatment. Philadelphia: Collins, 1872. 15p. DNLM
70-2464

MITCHELL, Robert Wood (1831-1903)
Yellow fever in Memphis in 1873. Louisville, 1874. 11p. DNLM **70-2465**

MITCHELL, Silas Weir (1829-1914)
Researches upon the venom of the rattlesnake. [Washington: Smithsonian Inst.], 1870. 145p. DNLM
70-2466

MITCHELL, S[ilas] Weir (1829-1914)
Wear and tear, or hints for the overworked. Philadelphia: J. B. Lippincott & Co., 1871. 59p. DNLM; NNNAM; PPC; PU
70-2467

MITCHELL, S[ilas] Weir (1829-1914)
Wear and tear, or hints for the overworked. [2nd ed.] Philadelphia: J. B. Lippincott & Co., 1871. 59p. PPJ; PU
70-2468

MITCHELL, S[ilas] Weir (1829-1914)
Wear and tear, or hints for the overworked. [3rd ed.] Philadelphia: J. B. Lippincott & Co., 1871. 59p. NNNAM; PU
70-2469

MITCHELL, Silas Weir (1829-1914)
Injuries of nerves, and their consequences. Philadelphia: J. B. Lippincott & Co., 1872. 377p. DNLM; MBM; NNNAM; PPC
70-2470

MITCHELL, S[ilas] Weir (1829-1914)
The rate of growth of the nails as a means of diagnosing certain forms of paralysis. [Philadelphia, 1872.] 2 l. DNLM
70-2471

MITCHELL, Silas Weir (1829-1914)
Wear and tear, or hints for the overworked. 4th ed. Philadelphia: J. B. Lippincott & Co., 1874. 59p. DNLM; NNNAM; PPJ; PPC **70-2472**

MITCHELL, Silas Weir (1829-1914)
On some of the disorders of sleep. Richmond, 1875. 13p. DNLM **70-2473**

MITCHELL, Silas Weir (1829-1914)
On rest in the treatment of nervous disease. New York: G. P. Putnam's Sons, 1875. 20p. DNLM; NNNAM **70-2474**

MITCHELL, Silas Weir (1829-1914)
Neurotomy. With an examination of three [re] generated nerves, and notes upon neural repair, by R. M. Bertolet. [Philadelphia, 1876.] 14p. DNLM **70-2475**

MITCHELL, Silas Weir (1829-1914)
The annual oration before the Medical and Chirurgical Faculty of Maryland, 1877. Baltimore: Jones & Co., 1877. 18p. DNLM; MdBM **70-2476**

MITCHELL, Silas Weir (1829-1914)
Nurse and patient, and Camp cure. . . . Philadelphia: J. B. Lippincott & Co., 1877. 73p. DLC; DNLM; PPC; PU **70-2477**

MITCHELL, Silas Weir (1829-1914)
Fat and blood, and how to make them. Philadelphia: J. B. Lippincott & Co., 1877. 101p. DNLM; MH-M; NNNAM; PU **70-2478**

MITCHELL, Silas Weir (1829-1914)
Fat and blood: and how to make them. . . . 2nd ed., rev. Philadelphia, [etc.]: J. B. Lippincott & Co., 1878. 109p. DLC; DNLM; PPJ; PU **70-2479**

MITCHELL, Silas Weir (1829-1914)
Address dedicatory of the new buildings erected by the University of Pennsylvania for its dental school and medical laboratories. Philadelphia: J. B. Lippincott & Co., 1878. 16p. DNLM; PU **70-2480**

MOHR, Charles (1844-1907)
The incompatible remedies of the homoeopathic materia medica. A paper read before the Homoeopathic Medical Society of the County of Philadelphia. New York & Philadelphia: Boericke & Tafel, [1879]. 9p. DNLM; PPHa **70-2481**

MONTGOMERY, Edward (1816-1883)
A plea for the antiphlogistic treatment of disease. St. Louis, 1872. 20p. DNLM **70-2482**

MONTGOMERY, Joseph Fauntleroy (1812-1883)
The ethics of the medical profession. [Read before the Sacramento Society for Medical Improvement.] San Francisco: J. H. Carmany & Co., 1871. 14p. DNLM **70-2483**

MONTGOMERY, Joseph Fauntleroy (1812-1883)
Burns and scalds; their treatment, with cases. San Francisco: J. F. Brown, 1872. 24p. DNLM **70-2484**

MONTGOMERY, Joseph Fauntleroy (1812-1883)
The treatment of typhoid fever. Sacramento: F. A. Springer, 1873. 28p. DNLM **70-2485**

MONTGOMERY, Joseph Fauntleroy (1812-1883)
Fracture of the inferior maxillary bone. Sacramento, Cal.: H. S. Crocker & Co., 1875. 17p. DNLM **70-2486**

MONTGOMERY, Joseph Fauntleroy (1812-1883)
Annual address delivered before the Sacramento Society for Medical Improvement. March 23, 1875. San Francisco: Woman's Publishing Co., 1875. 8p. DNLM **70-2487**

MONTGOMERY, Joseph Fauntleroy (1812-1833)
Report of the committee on medical education, made by the Medical Society of the State of California. Sacramento: Sacramento Leader Printing Office, 1876. 20p. DNLM **70-2488**

MOORE, E[dward] M[ott] (1814-1902)
Treatment of the clavicle when fractured or dislocated. [Rochester, N.Y., 1870.] 2p. 1 plate. DNLM **70-2489**

MOORE, E[dward] M[ott] (1814-1902)
A luxation of the ulna not hitherto described, with a plan of reduction and mode of after treatment; including the management of Colles' fracture. Albany: Weed, Parsons & Co., 1872. 12p. 4 plates. DNLM **70-2490**

MOORE, George (1803-1880)
Scarlatina; its prevention by belladonna and carbolic acid; their success and mode of use. American revised ed., by Edwin A. Lodge. . . . Detroit, Mich.: Lodge's Homoeopathic Pharmacy, 1870. 23p. DNLM **70-2491**

MOORE, James
The knowledge and cure of diseases. . . . Philadelphia: Allen, Lane & Scott's Printing House, 1873. 15p. DLC **70-2492**

MOORE, Thomas (1827-1882)
Homoeopathy, the science of therapeutics; its natural law and the essential conditions of that law. Annual address before the Homoeopathic Medical Society of the State of Pennsylvania. Germantown: W. H. Bonsall, 1873. 42p. DNLM; PPHa **70-2493**

MOORE, Thomas (1827-1882)
Dietetics in relation to infants and young children. Philadelphia: Sherman & Co., 1877. 14p. DNLM; PPHa **70-2494**

MOORMAN, John J. (*d.* 1885)
Mineral springs of North America; how to reach and how to use them. Philadelphia: J. B. Lippincott & Co., 1873. 294p. DNLM; PU **70-2495**

MORGAN, Ethelbert Carroll (1856-1891)
Diphthonia paralytica. Washington, D.C., 1879. 6p. DNLM **70-2496**

MORGAN, Ethelbert Carroll (1856-1891)
A contribution to the study of laryngeal syphilis. [Richmond, 1879.] 17p. DNLM **70-2497**

MORGAN, John Coleman (1831-1899)
Introductory address delivered at the opening of the course of lectures for 1870-1871 at the Hahnemann Medical College, October 10, 1870. Philadelphia: W. P. Kildare, 1870. 35p. DNLM; PPHa **70-2498**

MORGAN, John Coleman (1831-1899)
Diet of infants and young children. Philadelphia: W. P. Kildare, 1873. 22p. DNLM **70-2499**

MORGAN, John C[oleman] (1831-1899)
Valedictory address delivered at the annual commencement of the Hahnemann Medical College of Philadelphia, March 10, 1874. Philadelphia: W. P. Kildare, 1874. 26p. DNLM; PPHa **70-2500**

MORGAN, John C[oleman] (1831-1899)
The claim of homoeopathy to a place among the sciences. A lecture introductory to the course in the Homoeopathic Medical College of the University of Michigan. Detroit, 1875. 11p. DNLM **70-2501**

[MORGAN, Samuel]
Popular guide to homoeopathy, for family and private use; comp. from the standard works of Pulte, Hering, Hempel, and Ruddock. For the use of twenty-seven homoeopathic remedies. Cincinnati: Smith & Worthington, 1871. 191p. DLC; OCIM; OCLloyd **70-2502**

MORGAN, Samuel
Text book for domestic practice: being plain and concise directions for the administration of homoeopathic medicines in common forms of disease. 2nd ed., thoroughly rev. and enl. . . . Cincinnati: Smith & Worthington, 1871. 191p. DLC **70-2503**

MORLAND, William Wallace (1818-1876)
Florida and South Carolina as health resorts. Boston: J. Campbell, 1873. 20p. DNLM **70-2504**

MORRILL, Frederic
The medical adviser and guide to health, designed to illustrate the author's new system of practice, in the cure of all sexual diseases incident to exposure, early indiscretions, etc. . . . A new and rev. ed. Boston: The author, 1870. 127p. DLC: MH-M **70-2505**

MORRILL, Frederic
The medical adviser and guide to health. . . . Rev. and enl. ed. Boston: Morrill Medical Institute, 1871. 575p. DLC: MBM; MWA **70-2506**

MORRILL, Frederic
The pocket medical adviser and guide to health. . . . A new and rev. ed. Boston, Mass.: The author, 1871. 127p. DLC; MBM **70-2507**

MORRILL, F. Gordon
A case of typhlitis, with some statistics of the disease. Cambridge: Riverside Press, 1875. 5p. DNLM **70-2508**

MORRIS, F. Baldwin (1829-1894)
The panorama of a life, and experience in associating and battling with opium and alcoholic stimulants. A treatise for the cure of opium and alcoholic inebriacy. Philadelphia: G. W. Ward, 1878. 107p. DNLM; PPC; PPJ; PU **70-2509**

MORRIS, Moreau (1825-1904)
Epidemic cerebro-spinal meningitis. New York: Tower, Gildersleeve & Co., 1873. 26p. 1 map. DNLM; NNNAM **70-2510**

MORRIS, Moreau (1825-1904)
Medical supervision in distinction from medical selection in life insurance. Quarterly report. Appendix. Confirmatory evidence of the value of medical supervision by T. S. Lambert. Remarks upon biometry incidental to Dr. Morris's report by W. H. Dwinelle. New York, [1874]. 17, 15p. DNLM; NNNAM **70-2511**

MORRIS, Moreau (1825-1904)
Biometry; its relation to the practice of medicine. [1875.] 30p. DNLM; NNNAM **70-2512**

MORRIS, Moreau (1825-1904)
Biometry; its relation to the practice of medicine. New York: J. F. Trow & Son, 1875. 16p. DNLM **70-2513**

MORSE, David Appleton (*b.* 1840)
Report on dipsomania and drunkenness. [Dayton, Ohio, 1873.] 52p. DNLM **70-2514**

MORSE, David Appleton (*b.* 1840)
Report on monomania. [1874.] 46p. DNLM **70-2515**

MORSE, David Appleton (*b.* 1840)
Report on general paralysis. [1874.] 120p. DNLM **70-2516**

MORSE, David Appleton (*b.* 1840)
The mind; an introductory lecture. Cincinnati, 1875. 28p. DNLM **70-2517**

MORSE, David Appleton (*b.* 1840)
Mental and nervous disorders. Review of nervous disorders, insanity, and medical jurisprudence. [1876.] 8p. DNLM **70-2518**

MORSE, David Appleton (*b.* 1840)
A review of the literature of nervous disorders and insanity for the year 1878. [Cincinnati, 1878.] 4p. DNLM **70-2519**

MORSE, David Appleton (*b.* 1840)
Cerebral circulation. The duties of the medical witness and his privileges. The mind; lectures delivered. Dayton, 1879. 72p. DNLM **70-2520**

MORSE, E. Malcolm
A treatise on the hot sulphate springs of El Paso de Robles. . . . With a description of its natural beauties and improvements, and how to get there. Edited by W. W. Messer, Jr. San Francisco: H. S. Crocker & Co., 1875. 38p. DNLM **70-2521**

MORSE, Lucius D.
Homoeopathy. What it is, and what it is not. Nashville, Tenn.: Wheeler, Marshall & Berne, 1874. 24p. OCIM; PPHa **70-2522**

MORSE, Lucius D.
On nasal catarrh; its symptoms, causes, complications, prevention, treatment, etc., with illustrative cases. Memphis: A. F. Dod & Co., 1876. 72p. DNLM **70-2523**

MORSE, Lucius D.
Popular exposition of homoeopathy. 6th ed. St. Louis: H. C. G. Luyties, 1878. 24p. DNLM **70-2524**

MORTON, Henry (1836-1902)
Carbonic oxide; is it a harmless anaesthetic or a virulent poison? New York, 1978. 12p. DNLM **70-2525**

MORTON, Thomas George (1835-1903)
A peculiar and painful affection of the fourth metatarso-phalangeal articulation. [Philadelphia, 1876.] 10p. DNLM **70-2526**

MORTON, Thomas George (1835-1903)
Transfusion of blood and its practical application. New York: G. P. Putnam, 1877. 35p. DNLM **70-2527**

MORTON, William James (1846-1920)
Mount Desert and typhoid fever during the summer of 1873. [Boston, 1873.] 8p. DNLM **70-2528**

MORTON, William James (1846-1920)
South African diamond fields and the journey to the mines. New York, 1877. 28p. DNLM **70-2529**

MORTON, William James (1846-1920)
Anaesthetic inhalation. Rival claimants to the discovery. Dr. Long's claim criticized; the priority of Dr. Morton's announcement maintained. [New York, 1879.] 3 l. DNLM **70-2530**

[MOSHER, Jacob Simmons] (1834-1883)
Catalogue of the medical and scientific portion of the library of . . . comprising many scarce books on insanity, yellow fever, sanitation, medical journals, reports, etc., etc. Albany, [1879]. 21 l. DNLM **70-2531**

MOTT, J. Varnum (1851-1904)
A paper on medicated ice. New York: Mucklow & Simon, 1877. 7p. DNLM **70-2532**

MOUNT SINAI HOSPITAL. NEW YORK CITY
Ceremonies attending the laying the corner-stone of the new building, May 25, 1870. New York: D. Taylor, 1870. 24p. DNLM; NNNAM **70-2533**

MOUNT SINAI HOSPITAL. NEW YORK CITY
Proceedings attending the ceremonies of laying the corner-stone of the new building, May 25, 1870. [New York, 1870.] 22p. DNLM; NNNAM **70-2534**

MOWRIS, James A.
Reform; medicine and morals. No. 3. An address delivered before the Onondaga Medical Society, at Syracuse, N.Y., June 14, 1870. [Syracuse: Durston's Book, Store, 1870.] 2 l. DNLM **70-2535**

MOWRIS, James A.
An expose of surgical seduction! As practiced by physicians who specialize on female diseases. . . . Medicine and morals—No. 5. . . . The uterine specialty. [Syracuse, N.Y., 1871.] 4p. DLC **70-2536**

MUNDÉ, Paul F[ortunatus] (1846-1902)
Report on diseases of women for the year 1874. New York, 1875. 31p. DNLM **70-2537**

MUNDÉ, Paul F[ortunatus] (1846-1902)
The reposition of retro-displacement of the gravid uterus by posture and atmospheric pressure. New York: William Wood & Co., 1876. 10p. DNLM **70-2538**

MUNDÉ, Paul F[ortunatus] (1846-1902)
The value of electrolysis in the treatment of ovarian tumors. [Boston, 1878.] 89p. DNLM **70-2539**

MUNDÉ, Paul Fortunatus (1846-1902)
The indications for hystero-trachelorrhaphy, or the operation for laceration of the cervix uteri. New York: William Wood & Co., 1879. 20p. 2 col. plates. DNLM; NNNAM **70-2540**

MUNROE COUNTY BOARD OF HEALTH, MISSISSIPPI
Quarantine notice! [In consequence of the prevalence of yellow fever in Memphis, Tenn.] July 21, 1879. [Aberdeen, 1879.] broadside. DNLM **70-2541**

MUNROE, William H.
Munroe's philosophy of cure. Originated at Chelsea, Mass., in the year 1856. Cambridge: Printed for the Author, 1874. 134p. MBM **70-2542**

MUNSON, Franklin Avery (1852-1878)
The errors of refraction demonstrated by a new and original model. Albany, N.Y.: G. C. Riggs, 1877. 11p. DNLM **70-2543**

MURCHISON, Charles (1830-1879)
Clinical lectures on diseases of the liver, jaundice, and abdominal dropsy, including the Croonian lectures on functional derangements of the liver; delivered at the Royal College of Physicians in 1874. 2nd ed. New York: William Wood & Co., 1877. 644p. DNLM; NNNAM; PPC; PU **70-2544**

MURPHY, Edward A.
Notes on electro-surgery, with cases and operations. Chicago: Lakeside Press, 1874. 15p. DNLM **70-2545**

MURPHY, Edward A.
Yellow fever; its treatment and prevention. [Homoeopathic.] [1876.] 25p. DNLM **70-2546**

MURRAY, John
Observations on the pathology and treatment of cholera, the result of forty years' experience. . . . New York: G. P. Putnam's Sons, 1874. 58p. DLC; NNNAM **70-2547**

MURRAY, William (1839-1920)
A treatise on emotional disorders of the sympathetic system of nerves. New York: William Wood & Co., 1872. 92p. IU-M **70-2547A**

MURRELL, William J. (1832-1890)
A chapter on yellow fever. Originally prepared in a concise form for Dr. Adam Miller's "Plain talk to the sick, with directions for homoeopathic treatment." Opportunely enlarged to the present essay, by request of friends of homoeopathy in Mobile. Mobile: Henry Farrow & Co., 1879. 41p. AU; PPHa **70-2548**

MURTOUGH, Peter
Condensed history of the great yellow fever epidemic of 1878. Personal sketches and incidents, full particulars of the Father Mathew Camp, list of cities and towns visited by the scourge, and names of the victims of the fever in Memphis. Memphis: S. C. Toof & Co., 1879. 103p. DLC; DNLM; OCIM **70-2549**

MUSSEY, William Heberden (1818-1882)
Death from inhalation of chloroform. [Cincinnati, 1873.] 3p. DNLM **70-2550**

NAPHEYS, George Henry (1842-1876)
Modern therapeutics: a compendium of recent formulae and specific therapeutical directions. . . . Philadelphia: S. W. Butler, 1870. 309p. DLC; DNLM; PPC; PU **70-2551**

NAPHEYS, George Henry (1842-1876)
Modern therapeutics; a compendium of recent formulae and specific therapeutical directions. 2nd ed. Philadelphia: S. W. Butler, 1871. 412p. DNLM; OCIM; PPC; PU
70-2552

NAPHEYS, George Henry (1842-1876)
Modern medical therapeutics: a compendium of recent formulae, and specific therapeutical directions. . . . 3rd ed., rev. and improved. Philadelphia: S. W. Butler, 1871. 496p. DLC; DNLM; NNNAM; PPC **70-2553**

NAPHEYS, George Henry (1842-1876)
The transmission of life. Counsels on the nature and hygiene of the masculine function. 9th ed. Philadelphia: J. G. Fergus & Co., 1871. 346p. DNLM; NN; PU **70-2554**

NAPHEYS, George H[enry] (1842-1876)
The prevention and cure of disease: a practical treatise on the nursing and home treatment of the sick. . . . Springfield, [Mass.]: W. J. Holland & Co., 1872. 1151p. plates. DLC; MH-M **70-2555**

NAPHEYS, George Henry (1842-1876)
The prevention and cure of disease: a practical treatise on the nursing and home treatment of the sick. . . . Springfield, [Mass.]: W. J. Holland & Co., 1872. 1110p. plates. DLC; MBM **70-2556**

NAPHEYS, George Henry (1842-1876)
The physical life of woman: advice to the maiden, wife, and mother. . . . New stereotype ed., entirely rewritten, enl. and rev. Philadelphia: J. F. Fergus & Co.; Cincinnati: E. Hannaford & Co.; [etc., etc.], 1873. 436p. DLC; OCIM; PPC; PU
70-2557

NAPHEYS, George Henry (1842-1876)
The body and its ailments: a handbook of familiar directions for care and medical aid in the more usual complaints and injuries. . . . Philadelphia: H. C. Watts & Co., 1876. 438p. DLC; PPC; PPJ; PU **70-2558**

NAPHEYS, George Henry (1842-1876)
Modern therapeutics: a compendium of recent formulae, approved treatment, and specific methods in medicine and surgery, with an appendix on hypodermic medication, inhalation, aeration, and other remedial agents and therapeutic methods, of recent introduction. . . . 4th ed., rewritten and enl. Philadelphia: D. G. Brinton, 1877. 609p. DLC; DNLM; NNNAM; PPC **70-2559**

NAPHEYS, George Henry (1842-1876)
Handbook of popular medicine, embracing the anatomy and physiology of the human body . . . etc. With over 300 choice dietetic and remedial recipes. . . . Rev. to the latest date. Philadelphia: H. C. Watts Co., 1878. 438p. DLC; NNNAM; PPC; PU **70-2560**

NAPHEYS, George Henry (1842-1876)
Modern medical therapeutics: a compendium of recent formulae and specific therapeutical directions, from the practice of eminent contemporary physicians, American and foreign. . . . 5th ed., enl. and rev. Philadelphia: D. G. Brinton, 1878. 598p. DLC; DNLM; NNNAM; PPC **70-2561**

NAPHEYS, George Henry (1842-1876)
Modern surgical therapeutics: a compendium of current formulae, approved dressings and specific methods for the treatment of surgical diseases and injuries. . . . Rev. to the most recent date. Philadelphia: D. G. Brinton, 1878. 587p. DLC; DNLM; PPC; PU **70-2562**

NAPHEYS, George Henry (1842-1876)
Modern surgical therapeutics: a compendium of current formulae, approved dressings and specific methods for the treatment of surgical diseases and injuries. . . . 6th ed., rev. to the most recent date. Philadelphia: D. G. Brinton, 1879. 605p. DLC; DNLM; NNNAM; PPC **70-2563**

NAPHEYS, George Henry (1842-1876)
Modern medical therapeutics: a compendium of recent formulae and specific therapeutical directions, from the practice of eminent contemporary physicians, American and foreign. . . . 6th ed., enl. and rev. Philadelphia: D. G. Brinton, 1879. 607p. DLC; DNLM; NNNAM; PU **70-2564**

NASH, Eugene Beauharnais (*b.* 1838)
Directions for the domestic use of important homoeopathic remedies. . . . [Cortland? N.Y., 1874]. 22p. DLC
70-2565

NASH, James Addison
The third edition of Dr. Nash's practice, containing all the practical matter of the two former editions of the "Southern family physician." Rev. and improved. Dallas, Tex.: Texas Baptist Publishing House, 1878. 220p. DLC
70-2566

NATIONAL COLLEGE OF PHARMACY, WASHINGTON, D.C.
Review of Dr. Squibb's proposed plan for the future revision of the U.S. Pharmacopoeia, being a special report upon this subject by the committee of National College of Pharmacy on the U.S. Pharmacopoeia, and resolutions adopted by the National College of Pharmacy, Washington, D.C., at a special meeting held May 28, 1877. [Washington]: Judd & Detweiler, 1877. 8p. DNLM **70-2567**

NEBINGER, Andrew (1819-1886)
Criminal abortion; its extent and prevention. Philadelphia: Collins, 1876. 24p. DNLM **70-2568**

NEFTEL, William Basil (1830-1906)
Galvano-therapeutics. The physiological and therapeutical action of the galvanic current upon the acoustic, optic, sympathetic, and pneumogastric nerves. . . . New York: D. Appleton & Co., 1871. 161p. DLC; NNNAM **70-2569**

NEFTEL, William Basil (1830-1906)
The electrolytic treatment of malignant tumors. New York: J. F. Trow & Son, 1876. 8p. DNLM **70-2570**

NEFTEL, William Basil (1830-1906)
The treatment of some forms of dyspepsia (chronic catarrh of the stomach). New York: J. F. Trow & Son, 1878. 29p. DNLM
70-2571

NEIDHARD, Charles (1809-1895)
On the universality of the homoeopathic law of cure. 2nd ed. New York and Philadelphia: Boericke & Tafel, 1874. 34p. DNLM; PPHa **70-2572**

NEIDHARD, Charles (1809-1895)
On the universality of the homoeopathic law of cure. . . . New York and Philadelphia: Boericke & Tafel, 1875. 60p. PPHa
70-2573

NEIDHARD, Charles (1809-1895)
Homoeopathy in Europe, 1878. Germ theories of disease. Read before the Homoeopathic Medical Society of the County of Philadelphia. [1878.] 14p. PPHa **70-2574**

NELSON, R. W.
A clinical assistant; being reliable gleanings from practice. Chicago: Duncan Bros., 1879. 134p. PPHa
70-2575

NEUBAUER, Carl (1830-1879) and Julius VOGEL
A guide to the qualitative and quantitative analysis of the urine. Designed for physicians, chemists, and pharmacists. With a preface by R. Fresenius. Transl. from the 7th enlarged and revised German ed. by Elbridge G. Cutler, revised by Edward S. Wood. New York: William Wood & Co., 1879. 55p. 4 plates. DNLM; NNNAM; PU **70-2576**

NEUMANN, Isidor (1832-1906)
Handbook of skin diseases. . . . Transl. from the 2nd German ed., with notes by Lucius D. Bulkley. New York: D. Appleton & Co., 1872. 467p. DLC; MB; NcD; PU
70-2576A

NEWBERRY, John Strong (1822-1892)
[Sanitary Commission No. 96.] The U.S. Sanitary Commission in the valley of the Mississippi during the war of the rebellion, 1861-1866. (Final report.) Cleveland: Fairbanks, Benedict & Co., 1871. 543p. DNLM; OCIM **70-2577**

NEWCOMB, Daniel
When and how; or, a collection of the more recent facts and ideas upon raising healthy children. Chicago: A. W. Penny & Co., 1872. 324p. 1 plate. DNLM **70-2578**

NEWELL, Charles M.
Pneumatic therapia: the cure of chronic diseases by rarefied air. . . . [Boston: W. Y. Brown & Co., printers], 1879. 40p. DLC **70-2579**

NEW JERSEY. DISTRICT MEDICAL SOCIETY FOR THE COUNTY OF HUDSON
A documentary history of recent dissensions in the District Medical Society for the County of Hudson, N.J. Compiled by J. E. Culver. New York, 1873. 39p. DNLM
70-2580

NEWMAN, Robert (*d.* 1903)
Treatment of strictures of the urethra by Laminaria digitata and galvanism. . . . New York, [1871]. 5p. DNLM
70-2581

NEWMAN, Robert (*d.* 1903)
The endoscope in granular urethritis in the male. Louisville: J. P. Morton & Co., 1871. 16p. DNLM
70-2582

NEWMAN, Robert (*d.* 1903)
The endoscope; considered particularly in reference to diseases of the female bladder and urethra. Albany: Weed, Parsons & Co., 1872. 17p. 6 plates. DNLM
70-2583

NEWMAN, Robert (*d.* 1903)
Electrolysis in the treatment of stricture of the urethra. Albany: C. Van Benthuysen & Sons, 1874. 29p. DNLM
70-2584

NEWMAN, Robert (*d.* 1903)
Electrolysis in the treatment of stricture of the urethra. New York: T. L. Clacher, 1874. 32p. DNLM; NNNAM
70-2585

NEWMAN, Robert (*d.* 1903)
Stricture of the urethra in the female, and its treatment by electrolysis. [New York, 1875.] 11p. DNLM
70-2586

NEWMAN, W. H.
On rupture of the cervix uteri occurring at the time of parturition; its remote consequences. The power of the perineum in preventing prolapsus uteri; abstract of four cases. Louisville: J. P. Morton & Co., 1871. 16p. DNLM
70-2587

NEWPHER, Henry A.
. . . A treatise on chronic diseases. . . . New York, 1874. 32p. DLC **70-2588**

NEWTON, A. E. (1822-1889)
Pre-natal culture; being suggestions to parents relative to systematic methods of moulding the tendencies of offspring before birth. Washington, D.C. R. H. Darby, 1879. 67p. DNLM
70-2589

NEWTON, A. E. (1822-1889)
The modern Bethesda, or the gift of healing restored; being some account of the life and labors of Dr. J. R. Newton, healer; with observations on the nature and sources of the healing power, and the conditions of its exercise. Notes of valuable auxiliary remedies. Health maxims, etc. New York: Newton Pub. Co., 1879. 322p. DNLM; NNNAM; PU
70-2590

NEWTON, Orin E.
Asiatic cholera: as it appeared in Cincinnati in 1849-1850 and in 1866. . . . [Cincinnati, O., 1871.] 12p. DLC
70-2591

NEWTON, Robert Safford (1818-1881)
Explorations in cell-pathology; or, observations in regard to the causes, character, and treatment of cancer; made from 1843 till the present time. New York: Logan & Forbes, 1877. 20p. DNLM; NNNAM **70-2592**

NEW YORK (CITY). DEPARTMENT OF PUBLIC CHARITIES. BELLEVUE HOSPITAL
Catalogue of house staff from 1850 to 1873. New York: Bellevue Press, 1873. 34p. DNLM; NNNAM; NNU-M
70-2593

NEW YORK (CITY). DEPARTMENT OF PUBLIC CHARITIES
Hospital formulary for the use of the . . . . New York: Department Press, 1878. 168p. DNLM; NNU-M **70-2594**

NICHOLS, C. F[essenden]
Home made treatment. Boston: W. F. Towns, 1879. 46p. DNLM **70-2595**

NICHOLS, C. F[essenden]
Multum in parvo. Boston: Walter F. Towns, 1879. 24p. MBM
70-2596

NIEMEYER, Felix von (1820-1871)
A text-book of practical medicine, with particular reference to physiology and pathological anatomy. . . . Transl. from the 7th German ed., by special permission of the author. By George H. Humphreys . . . and Charles E. Hackley. . . . 3rd American ed. New York: D. Appleton & Co., 1870. 2 v. DLC; NNNAM; PPC; PU **70-2597**

NIEMEYER, Felix von (1820-1871)
A text-book of practical medicine, with particular reference to physiology and pathological anatomy. . . . Transl. from the 8th German edition by special permission of the author. By George H. Humphreys . . . and Charles E. Hackley. . . . Rev. ed. New York: D. Appleton & Co., 1873. 2 v. DLC; MH-M; OCIM; PPC **70-2598**

NIEMEYER, Felix von (1820-1871)
A text-book of practical medicine, with particular reference to physiology and pathological anatomy. . . . Transl. from the 8th German edition, by special permission of the author. By George H. Humphreys . . . and Charles E. Hackley. . . . Rev. ed. New York: D. Appleton & Co., 1878. 2 v. CtY-M; DLC; NNNAM; PU **70-2599**

NIERNSÉE, John R[udolph]
Review of "Hospital plans" of the Johns Hopkins Hospital [with description of wards]. [Baltimore, 1876.] 41, 5p. DNLM; MdBJ-W **70-2600**

NOEGERRATH, Emil Jacob (1827-1895)
The vesico-vaginal and vesico-rectal touch; a new method of examining the uterus and appendages. New York, 1875. 16p. DNLM; NNNAM **70-2601**

NOMENCLATURE of diseases prepared for the use of the medical officers of the United States Marine Hospital Service, by the supervising surgeon, J. M. Woodworth. (Being the classification and English-Latin terminology of the provisional nomenclature of the Royal College of Physicians, London.) Washington: Government Printing Office, 1874. 210p. DNLM **70-2602**

NORCOM, William A. B. (1836-1881)
Haemorrhagic malarial fever, an address delivered before the Medical Society of North Carolina, at its 21st annual meeting, held in Charlotte in May, 1874. . . . Raleigh, N.C.: Edwards, Broughton & Co., Book & Job printers, 1874. 30p. DLC **70-2603**

NORRIS, George W. (1808-1872)
Contributions to practical surgery. Philadelphia: Lindsay & Blakiston, 1873. 318p. DNLM; NNNAM; PPC; PU **70-2604**

NORRIS, William Fisher (1839-1901)
Cases of optic neuritis. [Philadelpia, 1874.] 7p. 4 plates. DNLM **70-2605**

NORRIS, William Fisher (1839-1901)
Three cases of intraocular tumor. Philadelphia: J. B. Lippincott & Co., 1874. 8p. DNLM **70-2606**

NORRIS, William Fisher (1839-1901)
Duboisia as a mydriatic, with remarks on its physiological and toxic effects. Philadelphia, 1879. 8p. DNLM **70-2607**

THE NORTH American Homoeopathic Directory for 1877-1878, compiled and publised by J. Pettel. . . . Cleveland: Robinson, Savage & Co., 1878. 117p. DNLM; OCIM; PPHa **70-2608**

NORTON, Jane C.
An interior view of Bloomingdale Asylum, also reply to Dr. Ordronaux's report. [Brooklyn, 1877.] 38p. DNLM; NNNAM **70-2609**

NORTON, Sidney A[ugustus] (1835-1918)
A valedictory address delivered before the class graduating Feb. 29, 1872. from the Miami Medical College of Cincinnati. Cincinnati: Bradley & Power, [1872]. 16p. DNLM **70-2610**

NOTES on new remedies, collated from medical and pharmaceutical periodicals, etc. Infants' food. 3rd ed. Boston: T. Metcalf & Co., 1878. 64p. DNLM; MBM **70-2611**

NOTTINGHAM, Custis Bell (1818-1876)
An address delivered before the Georgia Medical Association at its 21st meeting. Savannah, Ga.: E. J. Purse, 1870. 20p. DNLM; GU **70-2612**

NOXON, J. O.
Noxon's directory of the homoeopathic physicians of Brooklyn, May 1, 1876. United States Homoeopathic Pharmacy, [1876.] 8p. PPHa **70-2613**

NOYES, Henry Drury (1832-1900)
Ectropium, exophthalmus, extirpation, plastic operation. [1871.] 8p. 3 plates. DNLM **70-2614**

NOYES, Henry Drury (1832-1900)
Report on ophthalmology for 1870. New York: D. Appleton & Co., 1871. 37p. DNLM; NNNAM **70-2615**

NOYES, Henry Drury (1832-1900)
Ophthalmoscopic examination of sixty insane patients in the State Asylum at Utica. [New York, 1872.] 23p. DNLM **70-2616**

NOYES, Henry Drury (1832-1900)
Report on ophthalmology for 1871. New York: D. Appleton & Co., 1872. 21p. DNLM; NNNAM **70-2617**

NOYES, Henry D[rury] (1832-1900)
Selections from recent ophthalmic literature. New York: D. Appleton & Co., 1873. 15p. DNLM; NNNAM **70-2618**

NOYES, Henry Drury (1832-1900)
Syphilis of the eye. Being chapter 8 [pt. 2] of a "Practical treatise on the surgical diseases of the genito-urinary organs, including syphilis," by W. H. Van Buren and E. L. Keyes. New York: D. Appleton & Co., 1874. 22p. DLC; DNLM; NNNAM **70-2619**

NOYES, Henry Drury (1832-1900)
A case of irritation of the chorda tympani. Boston: A. Mudge & Sons, 1874. 5p. DNLM **70-2620**

NOYES, Henry Drury (1832-1900)
Cases of disease in the orbit. . . . New York: G. P. Putnam's Sons, 1875. 20p. DLC; DNLM; NNNAM **70-2621**

NOYES, Henry Drury (1832-1900)
Diagnosis of those diseases of the eye which can be seen without the ophthalmoscope. New York: G. P. Putnam's Sons, 1876. 61p. DNLM; NNNAM **70-2622**

NOYES, Henry Drury (1832-1900)
Papers presented to the Fifth International Congress of Ophthalmology. On the use of a naso-buccal flap for blepharoplasty, with two cases and illustrations. On additional means for relieving pressure on the eyelids in diseases of the cornea, with an illustration. On the optical error of conical cornea, and report of two cases treated by operation. New York: D. Appleton & Co., 1877. 25p. DNLM; NNNAM; PU **70-2623**

NOYES, Henry Drury (1832-1900)
Eye troubles in general practice. New York: William Wood & Co., 1879. 24p. DNLM; NNNAM **70-2624**

NOYES, Henry Drury (1832-1900)
Ophthalmology in the last quarter century. An address before the Medical Society of the State of New York. . . . February 1879. Syracuse, N.Y.: Truair, Smith & Bruce, printers and binders, 1879. 19p. DLC; DNLM **70-2625**

NOYES, Isaac Pitman (*b.* 1840)
Hospital construction; suggestion for the combination of the pavilion and corridor plan. Washington, 1877. 4p. DNLM **70-2626**

NOYES, T. R.
Report on the health of children in the Oneida Community. Oneida, N.Y., 1878. 8p. DNLM **70-2627**

NUTE, Timothy Riker
A new remedy of great promise. OEnothera biennis; its history and therapeutic power over diseases and functional derangements of the mucous surface. . . . Chicago: Inter-ocean (Beach & Barnard) print, 1873. 30p. DLC **70-2628**

OBSERVATIONS on the dietetic and hygienic treatment of tuberculous consumption. Philadelphia: The Leisenring Printing House, 1870. 45p. DNLM; PPJ; PPC **70-2629**

OBSTETRICAL SOCIETY OF PHILADELPHIA
Special rules for the management of infants during the hot season, recommended by the Obstetrical Society of Philadelphia to the thoughtful attention of the mothers in Philadelphia. Philadelphia: Collins, printer, 1873. 8p. DLC; DNLM; PPJ; PU **70-2630**

OBSTETRICAL SOCIETY OF PHILADELPHIA
Special rules for the management of infants during the hot season, recommended by the . . . to the thoughtful attention of the mothers in Philadelphia. Philadelphia: E. C. Markley & Son, 1875. 6p. DNLM; PU **70-2631**

OCTERLONY, John Arvid (1838-1905)
A case of molluscum simplex, with illustrations. New York: G. P. Putnam's Sons, 1875. 9p. 2 plates. DNLM **70-2632**

OCTERLONY, John Arvid (1838-1905)
A paper on chole-lithiasis. Louisville, Ky.: J. P. Morton & Co., 1877. 22p. DNLM **70-2633**

O'DANIEL, W.
Address delivered at the twenty-ninth annual meeting, Medical Association, Georgia. [Macon: J. W. Burke & Co., 1878.] 8p. DNLM **70-2634**

O'DEA, James J. (*b.* 1837)
The sphere, rights, and obligations of medical experts. New York: D. Appleton & Co., 1871. 41p. DNLM; NNNAM **70-2635**

O'DEA, James J. (*b.* 1837)
The physiology and psychology of dreams. New York: D. Appleton & Co., 1873. 31p. DNLM **70-2636**

OEHME, Ferdinand Gustave (*b.* 1826)
Therapeutics of diphtheritis. A compilation and critical review of the German and American homoeopathic literature. New York and Philadelphia: Boericke & Tafel, 1876. 68p. NNNAM; PPHa; PPC **70-2637**

OESTERREICHER, Johann Heinrich (1805-1843)
Atlas of human anatomy, containing 197 large plates taken from the original designs from nature by Drs. Oesterreicher & Erdl and many other of the greatest anatomists of modern times; with explanatory text by J. A. Jeancon. Cincinnati: A. E. Wilde & Co., [1879-1885]. 4p. 197 plates. DLC; OCIM; PU [*also*: Explanatory text to the Atlas of human anatomy, by Drs. Oesterreicher and Erdl. Cincinnati: A. Bicker, (1885). 173p.] **70-2638**

OGSTON, Francis (1803-1887)
Lectures on medical jurisprudence. Edited by Francis Ogston, Jr. Philadelphia: Lindsay & Blakiston, 1878. 663p. 12 plates. DNLM; PPC; PPJ; PU **70-2639**

OLDBERG, Oscar (1846-1913)
Inaugural address delivered at the opening of lectures in the National College of Pharmacy, City of Washington. Washington, D.C.: Judd & Detweiler, 1873. 8p. DNLM **70-2640**

OLIVER, Joseph P. (1845-1903)
On the treatment of diarrhoea in young children; read before the Boston Society for Medical Observation. [Boston, 1879?] 7p. DNLM; MH-M **70-2641**

O'NEAL, J. W. C.
Contribution to the history and use of the Katalysine spring water, at Gettysburg, Pa., and a comparison of its powers with waters of foreign springs. Gettysburg, Pa.: H. J. Stahle, 1876. 7p. DNLM **70-2642**

O'NEAL, J. W. C.
Report of the Adams County Medical Society. Philadelphia: Collins, 1879. 19p. 1 map. DNLM; PPC **70-2643**

OPIUM eating. An autobiographical sketch. By an habituate. Philadelphia: Claxton, Remsen & Haffelfinger, 1876. 154p. DNLM; PU **70-2644**

ORDRONAUX, John (1830-1908)
Valedictory address delivered before the graduating class of the National Medical College. Washington, D.C.: Judd & Detweiler, 1870. 22p. DNLM **70-2645**

ORDRONAUX, John (1830-1908)
Questions relating to poorhouses, hospitals, and insane asylums, prepared for the use of the visiting committees, Feb. 1, 1874. New York: Cushing & Bardua, 1874. 11p. DNLM; NNNAM **70-2646**

O'REILLY, John
On cholera infantum. Louisville, Ky.: J. P. Morton & Co., 1872. 8p. DNLM **70-2647**

O'REILLY, John
On the art of prescribing. An introductory address. Louisville: J. P. Morton & Co., 1872. 8p. DNLM **70-2648**

ORTH, Johannes (1847-1923)
A compend of diagnosis in pathological anatomy, with directions for making post-mortem examinations. . . . Transl. by Frederick Cheever Shattuck and George Krans Sabine. Rev. by Reginald Heber Fitz. . . . With numerous additions from ms. prepared by the author. Sole authorized English ed. New York: Hurd & Houghton; Boston: H. O. Houghton & Co.; [etc., etc.], 1878. 440p. DLC; MBM; NNNAM; PPC **70-2649**

OSBORN, Thomas Crutcher (1818-1902)
Annual address, delivered before the Medical Association of the State of Alabama. [1872.] 14p. DNLM **70-2650**

OSGOOD, Charles (1808-1881)
The causes, treatment, and cure of fever and ague, and other diseases of bilious climates. . . . New York, 1874. 15p. DLC **70-2651**

OSGOOD, Samuel
Health and the higher culture. A discourse delivered before the American Public Health Association in Philadelphia. New York: E. P. Dutton & Co., 1876. 10p. DNLM; NNNAM **70-2652**

OSTROM, Homer I[rvin] (*b.* 1852)
A treatise on the breast and its surgical diseases. Philadelphia: J. M. Stoddart & Co., 1877. 180p. DNLM; NNNAM; PU **70-2653**

OTIS, Fessenden Nott (1825-1900)
On chronic urethral discharges. Article 1. New York: D. Appleton & Co., 1870. 25p. DNLM **70-2654**

OTIS, Fessenden Nott (1825-1900)
On the physiology of syphilitic infection. New York: F. Leypoldt, 1872. 29p. DNLM **70-2655**

OTIS, Fessenden Nott (1825-1900)
On the physiology of syphilitic infection, as applied to the successive manifestations of the disease. Pt. 2. New York: D. Appleton & Co., 1872. 28p. DNLM **70-2656**

OTIS, Fessenden Nott (1825-1900)
Remarks on strictures of the urethra of extreme calibre, with cases, and a description of new instruments for their treatment. New York: D. Appleton & Co., 1872. 25p. DNLM **70-2657**

OTIS, Fessenden Nott (1825-1900)
On strictures on the urethra. Results of operation with the dilating urethrotome, with cases. New York: D. Appleton & Co., 1873. 20p. DNLM **70-2658**

OTIS, Fessenden Nott (1825-1900)
Urethrotomy, external and internal combined, in cases of multiple and difficult stricture; with remarks on the urethral calibre. New York: D. Appleton & Co., 1874. 24p. DNLM **70-2659**

OTIS, Fessenden Nott (1825-1900)
On reflex irritations throughout the genito-urinary tract, resulting from contraction of the urethra, at or near the meatus urinarius, congenital or acquired. Charleston, S.C., 1874. 16p. DNLM **70-2660**

OTIS, Fessenden Nott (1825-1900)
On reflex irritations throughout the genito-urinary tract, resulting from contraction of the urethra, at or near the meatus urinarius, congenital or acquired. New York: McDivitt, Campbell & Co., 1875. 37p. DLC; DNLM **70-2661**

OTIS, Fessenden Nott (1825-1900)
A case of reflex neuralgia, associated with urethral contractions and a rare form of urinary sinus. With a description of the cold-water coil. New York: D. Appleton & Co., 1875. 12p. 1 plate. DNLM **70-2662**

OTIS, Fessenden Nott (1825-1900)
On spasmodic urethral stricture. New York: G. P. Putnam's Sons, 1875. 15p. DLC; DNLM **70-2663**

OTIS, Fessenden Nott (1825-1900)
On stricture of the male urethra, its radical cure. . . . New York: G. P. Putnam's Sons, 1875. 36p. DLC; DNLM **70-2664**

OTIS, Fessenden Nott (1825-1900)
Gleet and its relations to urethral stricture. New York: G. P. Putnam's Sons, 1875. 24p. DNLM **70-2665**

OTIS, Fessenden Nott (1825-1900)
A description of the instruments and apparatus of the author, with directions for their use in operations on the genito-urinary organs. New York: G. P. Putnam's Sons, 1875. 17p. DNLM **70-2666**

OTIS, Fessenden Nott (1825-1900)
A lecture delivered before the ladies of the School for Nurses. [New York]: Bellevue Press, 1876. 15p. DNLM **70-2667**

OTIS, Fessenden Nott (1825-1900)
A lecture delivered before the School for Nurses, at Charity Hospital. Columbus: Nevins & Myers, 1876. 23p. DNLM **70-2668**

OTIS, Fessenden Nott (1825-1900)
On stricture as the initial cause of gleet, with remarks on the urethral calibre. Being a reply to the paper of Dr. H. B. Sands on the same subject. New York: D. Appleton & Co., 1876. 30p. DLC; DNLM **70-2669**

OTIS, Fessenden Nott (1825-1900)
On reflex irritations throughout the genito-urinary tract, resulting from contraction of the urethra, at or near the meatus urinarius, cogenital or acquired. Columbus, 1877. 38p. DNLM **70-2670**

OTIS, Fessenden Nott (1825-1900)
A description of the intruments and apparatus of the author, with directions for their use in operations on the genito-urinary organs. Columbus: Nevins & Myers, 1877. 13p. DNLM **70-2671**

OTIS, Fessenden Nott (1825-1900)
Report of a case of spasmodic urethral stricture, of seventeen years' duration, simulating organic stricture. [1877.] 9p. DNLM **70-2672**

OTIS, Fessenden Nott (1825-1900)
Stricture of the male urethra, its radical cure. . . . New York: G. P. Putnam's Sons, 1878. 352p. DLC; DNLM; NNNAM; PPC **70-2673**

OTIS, F[essenden] N[ott] (1825-1900)
Classroom lessons on syphilis and the genito-urinary diseases. First fasciculus. Initiatory period of syphilis. Nos. 1 to 8. [New York, 1878.] 33p. DNLM; NNNAM **70-2674**

OTIS, F[essenden] N[ott] (1825-1900)
Classroom lessons on syphilis and the genito-urinary diseases. First fasciculus. Initiatory period of syphilis. 2nd ed. [New York, 1878.] 18p. DNLM; NNNAM **70-2675**

OTIS, Fessenden Nott (1825-1900)
Urethrismus, or chronic spasmodic stricture. [New York, 1879.] 22p. DNLM **70-2676**

OTIS, Fessenden Nott (1825-1900)
Chronic spasmodic stricture, or urethrismus. Second paper in reply to Dr. H. B. Sands. New York, 1879. 22p. DNLM **70-2677**

OTIS, Fessenden Nott (1825-1900)
Addendum to the controversy on chronic spasmodic structure or urethrismus. [New York?], 1879. 4p. DNLM **70-2678**

OTIS, George Alexander (1830-1881)
Circular No. 3, Aug. 17, 1871. A report of surgical cases treated in the army of the United States from 1865 to 1871. Washington: Government Printing Office, 1871. 296p. 3 plates. DNLM **70-2679**

OTIS, George Alexander (1830-1881)
A report on a plan for transporting wounded soldiers by railway in time of war; with descriptions of various methods employed for this purpose on different occasions. Washington: Surgeon-General's Office, 1875. 56p. DNLM **70-2680**

OTIS, George Alexander (1830-1881)
Description of selected specimens from the surgical section of the Army Medical Museum at Washington. Philadelphia, 1876. 28p. DNLM [No. 7 of U.S. Army Med. Dept. Exhibits, International Exhibition of 1876.] **70-2681**

OTIS, George Alexander (1830-1881)
Check list of preparations and objects in the section of human anatomy of the United States Army Medical Museum for use during the International Exhibition of 1876. Washington, D.C., 1876. 135p. DNLM [No. 8 of U.S. Army Med. Dept. Exhibits, International Exhibition, 1876.] **70-2682**

OTIS, George Alexander (1830-1881)
A report to the Surgeon-General on the transport of sick and wounded by pack animals. Circular No. 9. War Department, Surgeon-General's Office. Washington, March 1, 1877. Washington: Government Printing Office, 1877. 32p. DNLM **70-2683**

OTT, Isaac (1847-1916)
Cocain, veratria and gelsemium. Toxicological studies. Philadelphia: Lindsay & Blakiston, 1874. 66p. 2 plates. DNLM; PPC PU **70-2684**

OTT, Isaac (1847-1916)
Note on the action of lobelina on the circulation. [Boston, 1875.] 7p. DNLM **70-2685**

OTT, Isaac (1847-1916)
The physiological action of thebain. [Boston, 1875.] 12p. DNLM **70-2686**

OTT, Isaac (1847-1916)
Physiological action of gelsemia. [Philadelphia, 1875.] 17p. DNLM **70-2687**

OTT, Isaac (1847-1916)
Poisonous mushrooms. [Chicago, 1877.] 6p. DNLM **70-2688**

OTT, Isaac (1847-1916)
The action of medicines. Philadelphia: Lindsay & Blakiston, 1878. 168p. DNLM; OCIM; OCLloyd; PU **70-2689**

OTT, Isaac (1847-1916)
Contributions to the physiology and pathology of the nervous system. Pts. 1-3; 5; 7-9; 11-16. Easton, Pa., 1879-1905. DNLM **70-2690**

OTT, Isaac (1847-1916)
The paths of conduction of sensory and motor impulses in the cervical segment of the spinal cord. [Philadelphia, 1879.] 8p. DNLM **70-2691**

OTT, Isaac (1847-1916) and Robert Meade SMITH
The inhibitory fibres in the spinal cord. [New York, 1879.] 3p. DNLM **70-2692**

OTTO, F. G., & SONS
Catalogue and price-list of surgical and orthopedical instruments, trusses, bandages, etc. New York, [1875]. 64p. DNLM; NNNAM **70-2693**

OTTO, F. G., & SONS
Price-list of orthopedic appliances. [1876?] 47p. DNLM; NNNAM **70-2694**

PACIFIC HOMOEOPATHIC MEDICAL SOCIETY OF THE STATE OF CALIFORNIA
Transactions of the . . . from 1874 to 1876, with constitution and by-laws. San Francisco. Cubery & Co., 1876. 208p. 6 plates. DNLM **70-2695**

PACKARD, John Hooker (1832-1907)
A hand-book of operative surgery. . . . Philadelphia: J. B. Lippincott & Co., 1870. 211p. 54 plates. DLC; DNLM; NNNAM; PPC **70-2696**

PACKARD, John Hooker (1832-1907)
. . . Training of nurses for the sick. Read before the [Social Science] Association January 20, 1876. . . . Philadelphia, Pa. [1876]. 12p. DLC; DNLM **70-2697**

PACKARD, John Hooker (1832-1907)
Urethral fistula, treated by means of the elastic ligature. [n.p., 1877.] 3p. DNLM **70-2698**

PAGET, James (1814-1899)
Clinical lectures and essays. Edited by Howard Marsh. New York: D. Appleton & Co., 1875. 428p. DNLM; MBM; NNNAM; PPC **70-2699**

PAINE, Horace Marchfield (1827-1903)
Registration of prevailing acute diseases, in connection with meteorological conditions of the atmosphere. [1878.] 22p. DNLM **70-2700**

PAINE, Martyn (1794-1877)
The institutes of medicine. . . . 9th ed. New York: Harper & Brothers; [etc., etc.], 1870. 1151p. DLC; NNNAM; OCIM; PU **70-2701**

PAINE, Martyn (1794-1877)
Physiology of the soul and instinct, as distinguished from materialism; with supplementary demonstrations of the divine communication of the narratives of creation and the flood. New York: Harper & Brothers, 1872. 707p. port. DNLM; NNNAM; PPC; PPJ **70-2702**

PAINE, William (*b.* 1821)
An epitome of the American eclectic practice of medicine. . . . New school remedies and their application to the cure of diseases, including those of women, children, and surgery; designed for physicians, surgeons, students of medicine, and families. Philadelphia: Claxton, Remsen & Haffelfinger, 1874. 633p. 1 plate. DNLM; OCIM; PPC; PPJ **70-2703**

PAINE, William (*b.* 1821)
New school treatment reduced to a science, with rules and directions so plain that all who can read understandingly may treat disease with far better success than physicians of the sectarian schools of physic. Philadelphia, 1875. 40p. DNLM; PPC; PU **70-2704**

PALLEN, Montrose Anderson (1836-1892)
Absence of the vagina; three operations; establishment of the menstrual flow. [1870.] 10p. DNLM **70-2705**

PALLEN, Montrose Anderson (1836-1892)
On some of the accidents of parturition requiring surgical treatment. Louisville, 1874. 28p. DNLM **70-2706**

PALLEN, Montrose Anderson (1836-1892)
Vagino-cerviplasty in lieu of amputation of the cervix uteri, in certain forms of intravaginal elongation. New York: William Wood & Co., 1875. 10p. DNLM; NNNAM **70-2707**

PALLEN, Montrose Anderson (1836-1892)
The philosophy of menstruation, conception, and sterility. New York: G. P. Putnam's Sons, 1877. 25p. DNLM; NNNAM **70-2708**

PALLEN, Montrose Anderson (1836-1892)
Kolpo-cystotomy, or artificial vesico-vaginal fistula. New York: William Wood & Co., 1878. 11p. DNLM **70-2709**

PALLEN, Montrose Anderson (1836-1892)
On the management of pregnant women. Louisville, Ky., 1878. 29p. DNLM **70-2710**

PALLEN, Montrose A[nderson] (1836-1892)
Case of abdominal pregnancy treated by laparotomy. With remarks concerning the etiology of extrauterine fetation. 1879. 11p. DNLM **70-2711**

PALMER, A[lonzo] B[enjamin] (1815-1887)
Dry earth as a means of disposing of excreta. [Ann Arbor, 1871.] 16p. DNLM **70-2712**

PALMER, Alonzo Benjamin (1815-1887)
Law and intelligence in nature; and the improvement of the race in accordance with the law. President's address: Lansing: W. S. George & Co., 1873. 31p. DNLM **70-2713**

PALMER, Alonzo Benjamin (1815-1887)
A statement of the relations of the faculty of medicine and surgery in the University of Michigan to homoeopathy. Detroit: W. A. Scripps, 1875. 12p. DNLM **70-2714**

PALMER, Alonzo Benjamin (1815-1887)
Letter on the homoeopathic complication in the University of Michigan. [1876.] 7p. DNLM **70-2715**

PALMER, Alonzo Benjamin (1815-1887)
The new departure in medical teaching. A lecture delivered at the beginning of the course on pathology and practice of medicine in the University of Michigan, October 1st, 1877. . . . [Ann Arbor, Mich.]: The Senior Lyceum of the Department, [1877]. 24p. DLC; DNLM **70-2716**

PALMER, Alonzo Benjamin (1815-1887)
Homoeopathy; its status in public institutions of learning. [1879.] 4p. DNLM; PPHa **70-2717**

PALMER, Alonzo Benjamin (1815-1887)
Quinine in acute pneumonia. Ann Arbor, Mich., 1879. 14p. DNLM **70-2718**

PALMER, Edward R[ush] (1842-1895)
Intellectual culture. A valedictory address delivered to the graduating class of the medical department of the University of Louisville, 1874. Louisville: J. P. Morton & Co., 1874. 20p. DNLM **70-2719**

PALMER, O. H.
Suicide not evidence of insanity. Utica, 1878. 37p. DNLM [*also*: New York (1878), 40p.] **70-2720**

PANCOAST, Joseph (1805-1882)
Valedictory address to the graduating class of Jefferson Medical College. Philadelphia: P. Madeira, 1872. 19, 4p. DNLM; PPJ **70-2721**

PANCOAST, Seth (1823-1889)
The cholera; its history, cause, symptoms, and treatment, with an appendix. Philadelphia: H. N. McKinney & Co, 1873. 48p. DNLM; PPC **70-2722**

PANCOAST, Seth (1823-1889)
The ladies' medical guide; a complete instructor and counsellor; embracing a full and exhaustive account of the structure and functions of the reproductive organs, the diseases of females and children, with their causes, symptoms and treatment: the toilet considered in reference to female health, beauty and longevity, with an appendix containing startling facts in plain words for mothers and the young. With more than 100 illustrated engravings. Chicago: W. H. Harrison, Jr., 1875. 612p. IEN-M; OCIM; PP; PU **70-2723**

PANCOAST, Seth (1823-1889)
Blue and red light: or, Light and its rays as medicine; showing that light is the original and sole source of life, as it is the source of all the physical and vital forces in nature; and that light is nature's own and only remedy for disease . . . together with a chapter on light in the vegetable kingdom. . . . Philadelphia: J. M. Stoddart & Son, [1877]. 312p. col. plates. DLC; PPC; PU **70-2724**

PANCOAST, Seth (1823-1889)
The Kabbala: or, The true science of light; an introduction to the philosophy and theosophy of the ancient sages. Together with a chapter on light in the vegetable kingdom. . . . Philadelphia: J. M. Stoddart & Co., [1877]. 312p. plates. DLC; NNNAM; PPC; PU **70-2725**

PANCOAST, William H. (1835-1897)
Lecture introductory to the course of Jefferson Medical College for the session of 1874-1875. Philadelphia, 1874. 24p. DNLM; PPJ **70-2726**

PANCOAST, William H. (1835-1897)
Valedictory address to the graduating class of Jefferson Medical College. Philadelphia: P. Madeira, 1876. 16, 4p. DNLM; PPJ **70-2727**

PANELLI, Francesco
A treatise on typhoid fever and its homoeopathic treatment. Transl., with notes by G. E. Shipman, with a chapter by Dr. Hering. Chicago: Duncan Bros., 1878. 297p. NNNAM; OCIM; PPHa; PU **70-2728**

PARK, Roswell (1852-1914)
A conspectus of the different forms of phthisis, intended as an aid to differential diagnosis. Chicago: Bulletin Ptg. Co., 1878. 19p. DNLM **70-2729**

PARK, Roswell (1852-1914)
On a new modification of the anterior splint. [1878.] 4p. DNLM **70-2730**

PARK, Roswell (1852-1914)
A conspectus of three different forms of acute inflammatory cardiac disorder. Chicago: Bulletin Ptg. Co., 1879. 17p. DNLM **70-2731**

PARK, Roswell (1852-1914)
Maternal impressions: mother's marks. An exposé of a popular fallacy. Richmond: Whittel & Shepperson, 1879. 13p. DNLM **70-2732**

PARKER, Edward Hazen (1823-1896)
Heredity as a factor in pauperism and crime. [Poughkeepsie, 1877.] 12p. DNLM **70-2733**

PARKER, Langston (1805?-1871)
The treatment of the syphilitic diseases by the mercurial vapour bath; comprising the treatment of constitutional and confirmed syphilis by this safe and successful method; with numerous cases and clinical observations. . . . Comp, from the 5th London ed. by John W. Foye. . . . [Boston]: A. Williams & Co., 1874. 17, 40, 23, 92p. DLC; MH-M; NNNAM **70-2734**

PARKES, Edmund Alexander (1819-1876)
A manual of practical hygiene, prepared especially for use in the medical service of the army. Intended especially for medical officers of the army, and for civil medical officers of health. 4th ed. Philadelphia: Lindsay & Blakiston, 1873. 672p. DNLM; NNNAM; PPC; PU **70-2735**

PARKES, Edmund Alexander (1819-1876)
A manual of practical hygiene, prepared especially for use in the medical service of the army. Intended especially for medical officers of the army, and for civil medical officers of health. Edited by F. S. B. François de Chaumont. 5th ed. Philadelphia: Lindsay & Blakiston, 1878. 733p. CtY-M; DNLM; OCIM; PPC **70-2736**

PARRISH, Edward (1822-1872)
A treatise on pharmacy; designed as a text-book for the student, and as a guide for the physician and pharmacist, containing the officinal and many unofficinal formulas, and numerous examples of extemporaneous prescriptions. . . . 4th ed., enl. and thoroughly rev. by Thos. S. Wiegand. . . . With two hundred and eighty illustrations. Philadelphia: Henry C. Lea, 1874. 977p. DLC; OCLloyd; PP; PU **70-2737**

PARRISH, Joseph (1818-1891)
The classification and treatment of inebriates. [New York, 1871.] 16p. DNLM **70-2738**

PARRISH, Joseph (1818-1891)
The pathology of inebriety. A lecture before the Medical and Chirurgical Faculty of Maryland. Baltimore: Innes & Co., 1874. 17p. DNLM **70-2739**

PARRISH, Joseph (1818-1891)
An open letter to John Charles Bucknill, M.D., of London, England. "Habitual drunkenness." Burlington, 1877. 13p. DNLM **70-2740**

PARROT, Jules (1829-1883)
The urine of the new-born, consisting of practical studies of the urine of the new-born with applications to physiology and the clinique, and clinical studies of the urine of the new-born in athrepsin. By J. Parrot . . . and Albert Robin. . . . Transl. from the Archives Générales de Médecine, 1878, by Geo. E. Shipman, M.D. Chicago: Foundlings' Home Press, 1878. 66p. DLC; IU-M; OCIM **70-2741**

PARRY, John S. (1843-1876)
Infant mortality and the necessity of a foundling hospital in Philadelphia. Read May 5, 1871. [Philadelphia, 1871.] 28p. DNLM **70-2742**

PARRY, John S. (1843-1876)
Vaccination; its uses and alleged dangers. Lancaster: Wylie & Griest, 1872. 24p. DNLM **70-2743**

PARRY, John S. (1843-1876)
Two lectures on inherited syphilis. Philadelphia: J. B. Lippincott & Co., 1872. 35p. DNLM; PPC **70-2744**

PARRY, John S. (1843-1876)
The comparative merits of craniotomy and the Caesarean section in small pelvis with conjugate diameter of two and a half inches or less. New York: William Wood & Co., 1873. 43p. DNLM; NNNAM **70-2745**

PARRY, John S. (1843-1876)
Abscess of the larynx in young children. Philadelphia: J. B. Lippincott & Co., 1873. 8p. DNLM **70-2746**

PARRY, John S. (1843-1876)
Extra-uterine pregnancy; its causes, species, pathological anatomy, clinical history, diagnosis, prognosis and treatment. Philadelphia: Henry C. Lea, 1876. 276p. DNLM; NNNAM; OCIM; PPC **70-2747**

PARSON, Frederick T.
Vital magnetism in the treatment of disease. New York: C. P. Thore & Co., 1875. 8p. DNLM **70-2748**

PARSON, Frederick T.
Vital magnetism; its power over disease. A statement of the facts developed by men who have employed this agent under various names, as animal magnetism, mesmerism, hypnotism, etc., from the earliest times down to the present. New York: Adams, Victor & Co., 1877. 235p. DLC; NN; PP
70-2749

PARSONS, Charles William (1823-1893)
. . . Memoir of Usher Parsons, M.D., of Providence, R.I., By his son, Charles W. Parsons. Providence: Hammond, Angell & Co., printers, 1870. 72p. DLC; DNLM
70-2750

PARSONS, Charles William (1823-1893)
Hydrate of chloral. Providence: Hammond, Angell & Co., 1872. 23p. DNLM **70-2751**

PARSONS, Charles William (1823-1893)
Outline of lectures. [Providence], 1877. 12p. DNLM
70-2752

PARSONS, E.
Conversations on the teeth, illustrating the judicious management of these important organs and the proper treatment of the ordinary diseases of the mouth. . . . Savannah, Ga.: Printed at the Office of the Evening Recorder, 1879. 42p. DLC
70-2753

PARSONS, Scott B.
An index to the titles of the most important surgical papers, including lectures, and orginal communications, together with clinical reports in surgery, published in the homoeopathic journals during the year 1877. St. Louis: Slawson & Pierrot, 1878. 8p. OCIM; PPHa **70-2754**

PARTRIDGE, Edward L.
Remarks on the history and treatment of two cases of face-presentation. New York: D. Appleton & Co., 1877. 11p. DNLM **70-2755**

PARVIN, Theophilus (1829-1898)
Woman and her physician: a lecture delivered in the Medical Department of the University of Louisville. . . . Louisville, Ky.: Printed by J. P. Morton & Co., 1870. 21p. DLC; DNLM
70-2756

PARVIN, Theophilus (1829-1898)
Galenism; an address before the graduating class of the College of Physicians and Surgeons of Indiana. Louisville: J. P. Morton & Co., 1875. 15p. DNLM **70-2757**

PARVIN, Theophilus (1829-1898)
Address on obstetrics, delivered before the International Medical Congress, at Philadelphia, September 7, 1876. Philadelphia, 1876. 31p. DNLM; PPC **70-2758**

PARVIN, Theophilus (1829-1898)
Three cases of rupture of the uterus. [Boston, 1879.] 8p. DNLM **70-2759**

PARVIN, Theophilus (1829-1898)
Philosophical problems in medicine. Presidential address before the American Medical Association. Indianapolis: Cathcart & Cleland, 1879. 34p. DNLM **70-2760**

PARVIN, Theophilus (1829-1898)
Philosophical problems in medicine. Presidential address before the American Medical Association at its thirtieth annual session, Atlanta, Ga., May 6th, 1879. Philadelphia: Collins, 1879. 33p. DNLM; PPC **70-2761**

PATRICK, John J. R. (1828-1895)
Dental fallacies. St. Louis: G. O. Rumbold & Co., 1879. 9p. DNLM **70-2762**

PAUL, Josias and Constantin PAUL
Notes on hydrophobia. Transl. from the French, by Bernard Ellis. Columbus: Nevins & Myers, 1877. 14p. DNLM
70-2763

PAVY, Frederick William (1829-1911)
A treatise on food and dietetics, physiologically and therapeutically considered. Philadelphia: Henry C. Lea, 1874. 574p. DNLM; IEN-M; NNNAM; PPC **70-2764**

PAYNE, Robert Lee (1834-1895)
North Carolina Board of Health. Limitation and prevention of diphtheria. Raleigh: P. M. Hale [*et al.*], 1879. 10p. DNLM
70-2765

PAYNE, William Elisha (1815-1877)
Boston University School of Medicine. Opening exercises and address. Boston, 1874. 28p. DNLM **70-2766**

PEABODY, Andrew P[reston] (1811-1893)
What the physician should be. An address delivered at the commencemet of the medical school of Harvard University, March 9, 1870. Cambridge: Welch, Bigelow & Co., 1870. 23p. DNLM; MBM; MH **70-2767**

PEASE, Roger William (1828-1886)
Address to the graduates of the College of Physicians and Surgeons of the Syracuse University; delivered February 12, 1873. [Syracuse, 1873.] 14p. DNLM
70-2768

PEASE, Roger William (1828-1886)
Improved methods of diagnosis and treatment of strictures of the urethra; with a tabulated report of forty-five cases. Syracuse, 1878. 22p. DNLM **70-2769**

PEASLEE, Edmund Randolph (1814-1878)
Injections into the peritoneal cavity after ovariotomy. New York, 1870. 19p. DNLM; NNNAM **70-2770**

PEASLEE, Edmund Randolph (1814-1878)
Intra-uterine medication; its uses, limitations, and methods. New York: D. Appleton & Co., 1870. 23p. DNLM; NNNAM
70-2771

PEASLEE, Edmund Randolph (1814-1878)
Note on the intra-uterine medicaton. [New York, 1871.] 2p. DNLM **70-2772**

PEASLEE, Edmund Randolph (1814-1878)
Ovarian tumors; their pathology, diagnosis, and treatment, especially by ovariotomy. New York: D. Appleton & Co., 1872. 551p. DNLM; MH-M; NNNAM; PPC
70-2773

PEASLEE, Edmund Randolph (1814-1878)
A case of solid uterus bipartitus. Both ovaries removed for the relief of epileptic seizures ascribed to ovarian irritation. [Philadelphia], 1876. 12p. DNLM **70-2774**

PEASLEE, Edmund Randolph (1814-1878)
Incision and discission of the cervix uteri. New York: D. Appleton & Co., 1876. 32p. DNLM; NNNAM
70-2775

PEASLEE, Edmund Randolph (1814-1878), Thomas Addis EMMET, and T. Gaillard THOMAS
Reply to Dr. J. Marion Sims' pamphlet, entitled "The Woman's Hospital in 1874," by his former colleagues. New York: Trow's Co., 1877. 24p. DNLM; NNNAM
70-2776

PEASLEE, Edmund Randolph (1814-1878), Thomas Addis EMMET, and T. Gaillard THOMAS
To the medical profession. Statements respecting the separation of Dr. J. Marion Sims from the Woman's Hospital, New York. [New York, 1877.] 1 l. DNLM; NNNAM
70-2777

PECK, Washington F. (1841-1891)
Address of . . . president of the Iowa State Medical Society at its annual meeting, held at Des Moines January 26, 1876. Davenport Iowa, 1876. 8p. DNLM **70-2778**

PEEDEN, James T.
President's address: delivered before the Jefferson County Medical Society at the annual meeting, January 3, 1871. Watertown, N.Y., 1870. 7p. DNLM **70-2779**

PENDLETON, Lewis Warrington (1844-1898)
Involuntary action. Annual address delivered before the Maine Medical Association. Portland: S. Berry, 1876. 22p. DNLM
70-2780

PENFIELD, E. C. & CO.
Illustrated catalogue of trusses, abdominal supporters, shoulder braces, elastic stockings, etc. Philadelphia: E. Stern & Co., [1877]. 38p. DNLM [*also*: Philadelphia, 1878. 40p.]
70-2781

PENNSYLVANIA HOSPITAL. PHILADELPHIA
A history of the first quarter of the second century of the . . . read before the board of managers at their stated meeting, held 9th Mo. 25, 1876. Published by the board of managers. Philadelphia: Collins, 1877. 145p. DNLM; PPPH; PU
70-2782

PENROSE, Richard Alexander F[ullerton] (1827-1908)
A discourse commemorative of the life and character of Hugh L. Hodge. Philadelphia: Collins, 1873. 31p. DNLM; PP
70-2783

PENROSE, R[ichard] A[lexander] F[ullerton] (1827-1908)
The treatment of face presentations. Philadelphia, 1876. 11p. DNLM **70-2784**

PENROSE, Richard Alexander F[ullerton] (1827-1908)
Medical education in the United States. [1879?] 8p. DNLM
70-2785

PENROSE, Richard Alexander F[ullerton] (1827-1908)
Treatment of post-partum hemorrhage. [Boston, 1879.] 12p. DNLM **70-2786**

PEPPER, William (1843-1898)
Clinical lecture on a case of progressive muscular sclerosis. Delivered May 13, 1871. Philadelphia: J. B. Lippincott & Co., 1871. 24p. 2 plates. DNLM
70-2787

PEPPER, William (1843-1898)
Cases of abdominal tumor attended with profuse sweating; with remarks on the influence of the abdominal sympathetic nerve over the state of the skin and intestinal mucous membrane. [Philadelphia, 1871.] 12p. DNLM
70-2788

PEPPER, William (1843-1898)
Obituary of Edward Rhoads. Philadelphia, 1872. 13p. DNLM
70-2789

PEPPER, William (1843-1898)
The sanitary relations of hospitals. Nov. 10, 1874. [Philadelphia, 1874.] 10p. DNLM **70-2790**

PEPPER, William (1843-1898)
On the local treatment of pulmonary cavities by injections through the chest-wall. [Philadelphia, 1874.] 30p. DNLM
70-2791

PEPPER, William (1843-1898)
International Exhibition, 1876, Philadelphia. Bureau of medical service. [Table showing the relative mortality of Philadelphia and some of the larger American and European cities.] [Philadelphia, 1876.] 1 broadside. DNLM
70-2792

PEPPER, William (1843-1898)
Higher medical education the true interest of the public and of the profession. An address. Philadelphia: Collins, 1877. 46p. DLC; DNLM **70-2793**

PEPPER, William (1843-1898)
A contribution to the clinical study of catarrhal inflammation of the bile-ducts, with remarks on the use of nitrate of silver in its treatment. [Philadelphia, 1878.] 24p. DNLM
70-2794

PEPPER, William (1843-1898)
Koumiss; its mode of preparation and its remedial value. [Philadelphia, 1878.] 11p. DNLM **70-2795**

PEPPER, William (1843-1898)
A contribution to the clinical study of exophthalmic goitre. [Philadelphia, 1879.] 17p. DNLM **70-2796**

PERCY, Samuel Rotton (1816-1890)
What physiological value has phosphorus as an organismal element? An essay to which was awarded the prize of the American Medical Association for the year 1872. Philadelphia: Collins, 1872. 56p. DNLM; PPC; PU
70-2797

PERCY, Samuel Rotton (1816-1890)
What is the comparative physiological and therapeutic action of free phosphorus and the hypophosphites. An essay to which the Merrit H. Cash prize was awarded by the New York State Medical Society, 1876. New York: E. P. Coby & Co., 1877. 23p. DNLM; NNNAM **70-2798**

PEREIRA, Jonathan (1804-1853)
The physician's prescription book; containing list of terms, phrases, contractions, and abbreviations used in prescriptions, with explanatory notes; also, the grammatical construction of prescriptions, etc. To which is added a key, containing the prescriptions in an unabbreviated form, with a literal translation, intended for the use of medical and pharmaceutical students. Philadelphia: Lindsay & Blakiston, 1871, *vel. subseq.* 286p. DNLM; NNNAM; PPC; PU **70-2799**

PEREIRA, Jonathan (1804-1853)
The physician's prescription book. . . . [16th ed.] Philadelphia: Lindsay & Blakiston, 1877. 286p. CtY-M; DNLM; MH-M; PPC **70-2800**

PETERS, George Absalom (*d.*, 1894)
An address delivered before the Alumni Association of the College of Physicians and Surgeons, in the city of New York, February 28, 1871. New York, 1872. 22p. DNLM; NNC **70-2801**

PETERS, John Charles (1819-1893)
On the origin and travels of Asiatic cholera. . . . New York: D. Appleton & Co., 1871. 31p. 2 fold. maps. DLC; DNLM; NNNAM **70-2802**

PETERS, John Charles (1819-1893)
On phosphoric acid. [1871?] 1 double galley sheet. DNLM **70-2803**

PETERS, John Charles (1819-1893)
The southwestern cholera, 1873. [New York, 1873.] 6p. DNLM **70-2804**

PETERS, John Charles (1819-1893)
On sects in medicine. . . . New York: J. R. McDivitt, 1874. 24p. DLC; DNLM **70-2805**

PETERS, John Charles (1819-1893)
On neurotics. [Read before the New York Neurological Society, Nov. 2, 1874.] New York: F. W. Christern, 1874. 22p. DNLM **70-2806**

PETERS, John Charles (1819-1893)
The Asiatic or Bengal cholera, of 1867 to 1873. . . . Cambridge, [Mass.] : Printed at the Riverside Press, 1874. 7p. DLC; DNLM **70-2807**

PETERS, John Charles (1819-1893)
An historical sketch of the origin and progress of the Medical Library and Journal Association of New York. [Abstract.] [1875.] 11p. DNLM **70-2808**

PETERS, John Charles (1819-1893)
On the origin and spread of the Asiatic cholera which reached the United States in 1873. Washington: Government Printing Office, 1875. 16p. DNLM **70-2809**

PETERS, John Charles (1819-1893)
Notes on the history of diphtheria in the United States. [Wheeling, 1876.] 8, 3p. DNLM **70-2810**

PETERS, John Charles (1819-1893)
Memoir of the late John Osgood Stone; read before the New York Academy of Medicine on Thursday evening, Dec. 21st, 1876. New York: G. P. Putnam's Sons, 1877. 36p. DNLM; NNNAM **70-2811**

PETTET, J.
Annual directory of the homoeopathic physicians residing in Ohio. Revised and greatly enlarged by the addition of a list of homoeopathic physicians residing in Alabama, Alaska, Arizona, Arkansas, California, Colorado, Connecticut, Dakota, District of Columbia, Florida, Georgia, Idaho, Indian Territory, Kentucky, Louisiana, Mississippi, Montana, Nebraska, New Mexico, North Carolina, South Carolina, Texas, Virginia, Washington Territory, West Virginia, and Wyoming Territory. Cleveland, Ohio, 1876. 40p. DNLM; OCIM; PPHa **70-2812**

PETTET, J.
The North American homoeopathic directory for 1877-1878. Cleveland, Ohio: Robison, Savage & Co., 1878. 117p. DNLM; OCIM; PPHa **70-2813**

PEUGNET, Eugène (1836-1879)
Medico-legal toxicology. Read by invitation before the Medico-Legal Society of the City of New York, February 27, 1873. New York: H. E. Thomson & Co., [1873]. 20p. DNLM; NNNAM **70-2814**

PEUGNET, Eugène (1836-1879)
The nature of gunshot wounds of the abdomen, and their treatment; based on a review of the case of the late James Fisk, Jr., in its medico-legal aspects. New York: William Wood & Co., 1874. 96p. DNLM; NNNAM **70-2815**

PEUGNET, Eugène (1836-1879)
Clinical notes in obstetrics and gynaecology. Read before the Yonkers Medical Association at its stated meeting, March 15, 1878. Columbus: Nevins & Myers, 1878. 3 pts., 27, 22, 34p. DNLM; OCIM **70-2816**

THE PHARMACOPOEIA of the United States of America. Fifth decennial revision. By authority of the national convention for revising the pharmacopoeia, held at Washington, A.D. 1870. Philadelphiia: J. B. Lippincott & Co., 1873. 383p. DLC; OCLloyd; PPC; PU [*also*: 5th decennial revision. . . . Philadelphia: J. B. Lippincott & Co., 1876. 383p.] **70-2817**

PHILADELPHIA COUNTY MEDICAL SOCIETY
Officers of the . . . since its organization. Philadelphia: Collins, 1874. 16p. DNLM; PPC **70-2818**

PHILLIPS, Charles Douglas Fergusson (1830-1904)
Materia medica and therapeutics. . . . New York: William Wood & Co., 1879-1882. 3 v. DLC; NNNAM; PPC; PU **70-2819**

THE PHYSICIAN'S annual for 1872. A complete calendar for the city and country practitioner: comprising a monthly calendar; hospital calendar of the principal cities of the United States. . . . Ed. by S. W. Butler, M.D., and Geo. H. Napheys, M.D. Philadelphia: S. W. Butler, 1872. 83p. DLC; PPC; PPJ; PPL **70-2820**

PHYSIO-MEDICAL COLLEGE OF INDIANA, INDIANAPOLIS
Annual announcements for the sessions of 1874-1875 (2.); 1889-1890 to 1904-1905 (17.-32.). Indianapolis, 1874-1904. DNLM **70-2821**

PIERCE, George Augustus (1828-1885)
Case of ovarian tumor treated by electricity. Reported by A. Van Derveer. [New York, 1878.] 3p. DNLM **70-2822**

PIERCE, Ray Vaughn (*b.* 1840)
. . . Chronic diseases of the generative and urinary organs, their rational treatment and positive cure. . . . Buffalo, N.Y., 1871. 23p. DLC **70-2823**

PIERCE, Ray Vaughn (*b.* 1840)
. . . Chronic diseases of the generative and urinary organs, their rational treatment and positive cure. 2nd ed. Buffalo, N.Y., 1871. 31p. NNNAM **70-2824**

PIERCE, Ray Vaughn (*b.* **1840)**
. . . Chronic diseases of the generative and urinary organs of males, their nature, rational treatment and positive cure. . . . Buffalo, N.Y., 1874. 23p. DLC **70-2825**

PIERCE, Ray Vaughn (*b.* **1840)**
Chronic diseases peculiar to women; their nature, rational treatment and positive cure. . . . Buffalo, N.Y., 1874. 23p. DLC **70-2826**

PIERCE, Ray Vaughn (*b.* **1840)**
The people's common sense medical adviser in plain English, or Medicine simplified. . . . Buffalo, N.Y.: World Dispensary Printing Office & Bindery, 1875. 885p. DLC; NNNAM; PU **70-2827**

PIERCE, Ray Vaughn (*b.* **1840)**
The people's common sense medical adviser in plain English, or Medicine simplified. . . . 2nd ed.–Rev. Buffalo, N.Y.: World's Dispensary Printing Office & Bindery, 1875. 888p. 5 col. plates. DLC; NNNAM; PPJ **70-2828**

PIERCE, Ray Vaughn (*b.* **1840)**
The people's common sense medical adviser in plain English; or Medicine simplified. . . . 3rd ed.–Rev. Buffalo, N.Y.: World's Dispensary Printing Office & Bindery, 1876. 912p. 5 col. plates. DLC; NNNAM; OCIM **70-2829**

PIERCE, Ray Vaughn (*b.* **1840)**
The people's common sense medical adviser in plain English; or, Medicine simplified. . . . 4th ed.–Rev. Buffalo, N.Y.: World Dispensary Printing Office & Bindery, 1876. 912p. 5 col. plates. DLC; NNNAM; OCIM **70-2830**

PIFFARD, Henry Granger (1842-1910)
A guide to urinary analysis, for the use of physicians and students. . . . New York: William Wood & Co., 1873. 88p. tables. DLC; DNLM; NNNAM; OCIM **70-2831**

PIFFARD, Henry Granger (1842-1910)
Clinical ureametry. New York: D. Appleton & Co., 1874. 7p. DNLM **70-2832**

PIFFARD, Henry Granger (1842-1910)
The compound microscope as an aid to the study of the skin and skin lesions in situ. New York: G. P. Putnam's Sons, 1875. 5p. DNLM **70-2833**

PIFFARD, Henry Granger (1842-1910)
The proper construction, care, and uses of the galvano-cautery apparatus. New York: D. Appleton & Co., 1876. 15p. DNLM **70-2834**

PIFFARD, Henry Granger (1842-1910)
The rheumic diathesis in dermatology. New York: D. Appleton & Co., 1876. 18p. DNLM **70-2835**

PIFFARD, Henry Granger (1842-1910)
The treatment of the scrofulides (lupus). New York: Macmillan & Co., 1876. 11p. DNLM **70-2836**

PIFFARD, Henry Granger (1842-1910)
The actual cautery and its employment in cutaneous surgery. Charleston, S.C., 1876. 8p. DNLM **70-2837**

PIFFARD, Henry Granger (1842-1910)
On certain points relating to the nature and treatment of lupus. Albany, N.Y., 1877. 10p. DNLM **70-2838**

PIFFARD, Henry Granger (1842-1910)
The local treatment of eczema. New York: Trow's Co., 1878. 8p. DNLM **70-2839**

PIFFARD, Henry Granger (1842-1910)
Bibliotheca dermatologica. Catalogue of cutaneous literature in the library of . . . . New York: Bradstreet, 1879. 37p. DNLM **70-2840**

PIFFARD, Henry Granger (1842-1910)
Further contributions to the treatment of lupus. New York: Trow's Co., 1879. 10p. DNLM **70-2841**

PIFFARD, Henry Granger (1842-1910)
On the treatment of strictures of the fossa navicularis. New York: E. O'Keefe, 1879. 7p. DNLM **70-2842**

PILCHER, Lewis S[tephen] (1845-1934)
Croup and tracheotomy in the city of Brooklyn, State of New York; a study of local conditions and local experience, with map showing location of croup areas in that city. A report made to the Medical Society of the County of Kings, N.Y., April 17, 1877. [Brooklyn, 1877.] 29p. 1 map. DNLM; NNNAM; NNU-M **70-2843**

PINKHAM, Lydia E. (1819-1883)
Private test-book. Revised ed. Lynn, Mass.: Lydia E. Pinkham Medicine Co., [1878?]. 61p. MA; MB; NN **70-2844**

PLAIN directions for accidents, emergencies, and poisons. By a fellow of the College of Physicians of Philadelphia. Distributed to its policy holders by the Mutual Life Insurance Company of New York. [New York: S. W. Green, 1875.] 126p. DNLM; NNNAM **70-2845**

PLAIN directions for accidents, emergencies, and poisons. By a fellow of the College of Physicians of Philadelphia. 80th thousand. Distributed to its policy holders by the Mutual Life Insurance Company of New York. [New York: S. W. Green, 1875.] 126p. DNLM; NNNAM [*also*: New York: S. W. Green, n.d., 144p.] **70-2846**

PLAIN directions for the care of the sick, and recipes for sick people. By a fellow of the College of Physicians of Philadelphia, and physician to several of the charitable institutions of the same city. New York: S. W. Green, [1875.] 64p. DNLM; NNNAM **70-2847**

PLAIN directions for the care of the sick, and recipes for sick people. By a fellow of the College of Physicians of Philadelphia, and physician to several of the charitable institutions of the same city. 60th thousand. New York: S. W. Green, [1875]. 64p. DNLM; NNNAM [*also*: enlarged ed. (New York: S. W. Green, 1875), 72p.] **70-2848**

PLAIN words on health in homes, or how we daily invite headache, loss of appetite, paleness, unpleasant odors, languor, malaria, zymotic diseases, etc., by imperfect house drainage. New York: The Germicide Co., [1879]. 17p. 3 plates. DNLM **70-2849**

PLAYFAIR, William S[moult] (1836-1903)
A treatise on the science and practice of midwifery. Philadelphia: Henry C. Lea, 1876. 576p. CtY-M; MB; NcU; PPC **70-2850**

PLAYFAIR, William S[moult] (1836-1903)
A treatise on the science and practice of midwifery. . . . With notes and additions by Robert P. Harris, M.D. 2nd American from the 2nd and rev. London ed. . . . Philadelphia: Henry C. Lea, 1878. 639p. DLC; DNLM; NNNAM; PPC **70-2850A**

PLEASONTON, Augustus James (1808-1894) and others
The influence of the blue ray of the sunlight and of the blue color of the sky in developing animal and vegetable life: in arresting disease, and in restoring health in acute and chronic disorders to human and domestic animals. . . . Philadelphia: Claxton, Remsen, 1877, 185p. DLC; PP; PPL **70-2851**

POLLAK, S[imon] (*b.* 1814)
Simultaneous intra- and extra-uterine pregnancy to full term. St. Louis, 1871. 8p. DNLM **70-2852**

POLLOCK, Allan
A botanical index to all the medicinal plants, barks, roots, seeds and flowers usually kept by druggists. . . . New York: A. Pollock, 1872. 137p. DLC; DNLM; NNNAM; OCLloyd **70-2853**

POLLOCK, Allan
A botanical index to all the medicinal plants, barks, roots, seeds and flowers usually kept by druggists, arranged in alphabetical order, with their officinal and common names. New ed., revised and enlarged. New York: A. Pollock, 1873. 137p. DNLM; NNNAM; OCLloyd **70-2854**

POMEROY, John M.
The New York State Inebriate Asylum; its objects, its system, and its results. . . . [New York: Pub. by direction of the Superintendent, 1870.] 16p. DLC **70-2855**

POMEROY, Thomas Fuller (1816-1892)
The elementary principles of medicine. [Philadelphia, 1875.] 12p. DNLM; PU **70-2856**

POOLEY, James Henry (1839-1897)
Three cases of imperforate anus. New York, 1870. 20p. DNLM; NNNAM **70-2857**

POOLEY, James Henry (1839-1897)
Report of the surgical cases treated in the St. John's Riverside Hospital, Yonkers, New York, during the year 1870. New York: D. Appleton & Co., 1871. 19p. DNLM; NNNAM **70-2858**

POOLEY, James Henry (1839-1897)
Report of the surgical cases treated in the St. John's Riverside Hospital, Yonkers, New York, during the year 1871. (2nd year.) New York: D. Appleton & Co., 1872. 20p. DNLM; NNNAM **70-2859**

POOLEY, James Henry (1839-1897)
On imperforate anus; the rectum communicating with the vagina. New York: William Wood & Co., 1872. 34p. DNLM; NNNAM **70-2860**

POOLEY, James Henry (1839-1897)
Some general remarks on the surgery of childhood. Albany, 1872. 14p. DNLM; NNNAM **70-2861**

POOLEY, James Henry (1839-1897)
Two cases of rare disease of the tongue. [Philadelphia, 1872.] 4p. DNLM; NNNAM **70-2862**

POOLEY, James Henry (1839-1897)
Report of the surgical cases treated in the St. John's Riverside Hospital, Yonkers, New York, during the year 1872. (3rd year.) New York: D. Appleton & Co., 1873. 30p. DNLM; NNNAM **70-2863**

POOLEY, James Henry (1839-1897)
Case of epithelioma of the cheek and the lower eyelid. Removal; blepharoplasty. New York: William Wood & Co., [1873]. 8p. DNLM; NNNAM **70-2864**

POOLEY, James Henry (1839-1897)
Naevus. New York: D. Appleton & Co., 1873. 28p. DNLM; NNNAM **70-2865**

POOLEY, James Henry (1839-1897)
Cases in surgery, lumbar colotomy, etc. New York: D. Appleton & Co., 1874. 11p. DNLM; NNNAM **70-2866**

POOLEY, James Henry (1839-1897)
Report of the surgical cases treated in the St. John's Riverside Hospital, Yonkers, New York, during the year 1873. (4th year.) New York: D. Appleton & Co., 1875. 29p. DNLM; NNNAM **70-2867**

POOLEY, James Henry (1839-1897)
Enuresis nocturna, incontentia urinae, mictio involuntaria, incontinence of childhood, etc. [Cincinnati]: R. Clarke & Co., [1875]. 10p. DNLM; NNNAM **70-2868**

POOLEY, James Henry (1839-1897)
On the surgical treatment of perityphlitic abscess. [New York, 1875.] 15p. DNLM; NNNAM **70-2869**

POOLEY, James Henry (1839-1897)
A surgical study; gastrotomy and gastrostomy. Columbus: Nevins & Meyers, 1876. 27p. 1 tab. DNLM; NNNAM **70-2870**

POOLEY, James Henry (1839-1897)
Points in the surgery of childhood. New York: G. P. Putnam's Sons, 1876. 26p. DNLM; NNNAM **70-2871**

POOLEY, James Henry (1839-1897)
Median lithotomy. [Cincinnati, 1876.] 11p. DNLM; NNNAM **70-2872**

POOLEY, James Henry (1839-1897)
A case of intra-thoracic cancer. Columbus: Nevins & Meyers, 1877. 8p. DNLM; NNNAM **70-2873**

POOLEY, James Henry (1839-1897)
Tracheotomy in diphtheria. Louisville, 1877. 22p. DNLM; NNNAM **70-2874**

POOLEY, James Henry (1839-1897)
Clinical lectures on surgery, delivered at Starling Medical College, Columbus, Ohio. Lecture I. [1. Cancer of the breast; 2. Chronic periostitis, with ulceration; 3. Fracture of clavicle, produced by muscular contraction; 4. Depressed and adherent cicatrix of the face.] Columbus: Nevins & Meyers, 1877. 25p. DNLM; NNNAM **70-2875**

POOLEY, James Henry (1839-1897)
Clinical lectures on surgery, delivered at Starling Medical College, Columbus, Ohio. Lecture II. [Hydrocele.] Columbus: Nevins & Meyers, 1878. 20p. DNLM; NNNAM **70-2876**

POOLEY, James Henry (1839-1897)
Clinical lectures on surgery, delivered at Starling Medical College, Columbus, Ohio. Lecture III. [Tumor of the male breast and cyst of the neck.] Columbus: Nevins & Meyers, 1878. 15p. DNLM; NNNAM **70-2877**

POOLEY, James Henry (1839-1897)
Memoir of Samuel D. Turney, M.D., of Circleville, Ohio. Cincinnati: R. Clarke & Co., 1878. 36p. DNLM; NNNAM **70-2878**

POOLEY, Thomas Rickett (1841-1926)
Sympathetic ophthalmia. New York: D. Appleton & Co., 1870. 18p. DNLM **70-2879**

POOLEY, Thomas Rickett (1841-1926)
A case of wound of the sclera treated by suture, with remarks. [New York, 1873.] 7p. DNLM **70-2880**

POOLEY, Thomas Rickett (1841-1926)
Three cases of ear disease. New York: D. Appleton & Co., 1874. 10p. DNLM **70-2881**

POOLEY, Thomas Rickett (1841-1926)
An ordinary strabismus operation followed by tendinitis, perforation of the sclerotic, detachment of the retina, recovery. [New York, 1875.] 4p. DNLM **70-2882**

POOLEY, Thomas Rickett (1841-1926)
Three cases of foreign bodies in the eye. New York: G. P. Putnam's Sons, 1875. 10p. DNLM **70-2883**

POOLEY, Thomas Rickett (1841-1926)
Convergent strabismus. New York: G. P. Putnam's Sons, 1877. 29p. DNLM **70-2884**

POOLEY, Thomas Rickett (1841-1926)
Irido-choroiditis in the puerperal state. Albany: Van Benthuysen, 1877. 9p. DNLM **70-2885**

POOLEY, Thomas Rickett (1841-1926)
Ischaemia of the retina. [Syracuse, 1878.] 8p. DNLM **70-2886**

POOLEY, Thomas Rickett (1841-1926)
Contribution to the pathology of the temporal bone. New Bedford, 1879. 7p. DNLM **70-2887**

POOLEY, Thomas Rickett (1841-1926)
Sulphate of eserine in the treatment of acute glaucoma. New York: G. P. Putnam's Sons, 1879. 5p. DNLM **70-2888**

POORE, Charles T[albot] (1846-1911)
Disease of the sacro-iliac synchondrosis. [Philadelphia, 1878.] 12p. DNLM **70-2889**

POPE, Bolling A. (1825?-1894)
Opium as a tonic and alterative; with remarks upon the hypodermic use of the sulphate of morphia and its use in the debility and amaurosis consequent upon onanism. [New Orleans, 1879.] 14p. DNLM; LNT-M **70-2890**

PORCHER, Francis Peyre (1825-1895)
Yellow fever in Charleston, 1871, with remarks upon its treatment. President's address before South Carolina Medical Association. Charleston, S.C.: Walker, Evans & Cogswell, 1872. 30p. DNLM; ScCM **70-2891**

PORCHER, Francis Peyre (1825-1895)
President's address: before South Carolina Medical Association, meeting held in Columbia, April, 1872. Yellow fever in Charleston, 1871, with remarks upon its treatment. . . . Charleston, S.C.: Walker, Evans & Cogswell, printers and stationers, 1872. 30p. DLC; ScCM **70-2892**

[PORCHER, Francis Peyre] (1825-1895)
Suggestion of a plan of treatment for yellow fever, to be used by those who are unable to procure medical aid without delay. Letter from a physician. [Charleston, S.C., 1878.] 1 l. DLC **70-2893**

PORTER, P. Brynberg (1845-1915)
Report of two thousand cases of disease in children treated at the Demilt Dispensary, New York. New York: William Wood & Co., 1878. 30p. DNLM; NNNAM **70-2894**

PORTER, William (1852-1921)
Aphonia; its causes and treatment. [St. Louis], 1876. 16p. DNLM **70-2895**

PORTER, William (1852-1921)
Syphilitic phthisis. [St. Louis, 1877.] 7p. DNLM **70-2896**

PORTER, William (1852-1921)
Life and its forces; health and disease correctly defined. A reliable guide to health without the use of mineral or vegetable poisons or irritants, the conclusions from forty years' practice of medicine. Hartford, Conn.: Case, Lockwood & Brainard Co., 1878. 133p. DLC; DNLM **70-2897**

PORTER, William (1852-1921)
Tubercular-laryngitis. [St. Louis, 1878.] 8p. DNLM **70-2898**

PORTER, William (1852-1921)
Excision of the epiglottis. [Philadelphia, 1879.] 4p. DNLM **70-2899**

POST, Alfred Charles (1806-1886)
On contraction of the palmar fascia, and of the sheaths of the flexor tendons. New York: Rutledge & Co., 1876. 16p. DNLM; NNNAM **70-2900**

POST, Alfred Charles (1806-1886)
Exsection of the articular extremities of the phalanges of the fingers and toes for the relief of deformity of those members. Also blepharoplastic operations. Philadelphia: Collins, 1878. 6 plates. DNLM; PPC **70-2901**

POST, Alfred Charles (1806-1886)
Cicatricial contraction from burns; deformity of face and both hands; reparative operations. Philadelphia: Collins, 1879. 14p. DNLM; PPC **70-2902**

POTTER, Alonzo (*b.* 1800)
The drinking usages of society. An address. New York, 1871. 24p. DNLM; NN **79-2903**

POTTER, Samuel O. Lewis (1846-1914)
The logical basis of the high potency questions. Abstr. of a paper read before the Milwaukee Academy of Medicine, April, 1879. [Philadelphia, 1879.] 25p. DNLM **70-2904**

POTTER, Samuel O. Lewis (1846-1914)
High potency criticism. [Philadelphia, 1879.] 7p. DNLM **70-2905**

POTTER, Samuel O. Lewis (1846-1914)
Munchausen microscopy. Comments of the work of a microcrith. [n. p., 1879?] 7p. DNLM **70-2906**

POTTER, Samuel O. Lewis (1846-1914)
The Milwaukee test. [New York, 1879.] 8p. DNLM **70-2907**

POTTER, Stephen H.
A compendium of the principles and practice of medicine, for the use of students and practitioners. Nos. 1-6, January-June, 1878. 2nd ed. Hamilton, O.: J. H. Long, 1878. 240p. DNLM; OCIM **70-2908**

POTTER, Stephen H.
A compendium of the principles and practice of medicine, for the use of students and practitioners. . . . 2nd ed., rev. and enl. Hamilton, O.: Butler County Democrat Print, 1879. 500p. DLC **70-2909**

POTTER, William Warren (1838-1911)
Umbilical hernia in the adult. Buffalo: Baker, Jones & Co., 1879. 19p. DNLM **70-2910**

POTTER, William Warren (1838-1911)
On the induction of premature labor in puerperal eclampsia. New York: William Wood & Co., 1879. 8p. DNLM **70-2911**

POWELL, Thomas Spencer (1826-1895)
Reply to the strictures of E. S. Gaillard contained in the Richmond and Louisville Medical Journal. [Atlanta, 1872.] 12p. DNLM **70-2912**

POWER, J. L[ogan] (1834-1901)
The epidemic of 1878, in Mississippi. Report of the yellow fever relief work through . . . grand secretary of Masons and grand treasurer of Odd Fellows. . . . Jackson, 1879. 216p. DNLM **70-2913**

PRATT, Edwin Hartley (1849-1930)
Introductory lecture to the sixteenth session of Hahnemann Medical College, Chicago. Given on the evening of October 6, 1875. Published by the class. Chicago: Culver, Page, Hoyne & Co., 1875. 16p. DNLM **70-2914**

PRATT, Edwin Hartley (1849-1930)
Introductory lecture to the fourth course of lectures of the Chicago Homoeopathic College, on the evening of September 30, 1879. Published by the class. Chicago: Binney, Hand & Co., 1879. 16p. PPHa **70-2915**

PRATT, Foster (1823-1898)
Legal relations of insane patients. Lansing: W. S. George & Co., 1878. 36p. DNLM **70-2916**

PRAY, T[homas] J[efferson] W[orcester] (1819-1888)
The reasons for modern alcoholic stimulation examined. Concord, 1878. 15p. DNLM **70-2917**

PREMATURE death; its promotion or prevention. New York: D. Appleton & Co., 1879. 94p. DNLM; NN; NNNAM **70-2918**

PRENTISS, Daniel Webster (1843-1899)
A contribution to the clinical history of croupous pneumonia. A report of eleven cases of croupous pneumonia occurring in private practice between the dates of February and June, 1878. [Washington, 1879.] 29p. DNLM **70-2919**

PRESTON, Ann (1813-1872)
Valedictory address to the graduating class of the Woman's Medical College of Pennsylvania, at the eighteenth annual commencement, March 12th, 1870. . . . Philadelphia: Loag, printer, 1870. 15p. DLC; DNLM **70-2920**

PRINCE, David (1816-1890)
Plastics and orthopedics: a report republished from the Transactions of the Illinois State Medical Society for 1871. Jacksonville, Ill., [1871]. 16p. DNLM **70-2921**

PRINCE, David (1816-1890)
Plastics and orthopedics; . . . being editions of three reports made to the Illinois State Medical Society, in the years, respectively, 1864, 1867, and 1871, upon plastic and orthopedic surgery. Philadelphia: Lindsay & Blakiston, 1871. 96, 240p. DLC; PPC; PU **70-2922**

PRINCE, David (1816-1890)
Galvano-therapeutics. A revised reprint of a report made to the Illinois State Medical Society, 1873. Philadelphia: Lindsay & Blakiston, 1873. 63p. DNLM **70-2923**

PRINCE, David (1816-1890)
Palatoplasty; the substance of a report made to the St. Louis Medical Society, Nov. 28, 1874. St. Louis: E. F. Hobart & Co., 1875. 8p. DNLM **70-2924**

PRINCE, David (1816-1890)
Diphtheria. A paper read before the St. Louis Medical Society, Dec. 18, 1875, in which a weak solution of iodine in perpetual spray is advocated. [n. p., 1876.] 8p. DNLM **70-2925**

PRINCE, David (1816-1890)
A case of ovariotomy. [n. p., 1876.] 12p. DNLM **70-2926**

PRINCE, David (1816-1890)
Considerations in relation to diseases of the joints. [Louisville, 1877.] 8p. DNLM **70-2927**

PRINCE, David (1816-1890)
Sprague's galvanometer arranged for therapeutic uses. 1878. 4p. DNLM **70-2928**

PRINCE, David (1816-1890)
Lithotomy. A tabulated statement of cases, with considerations in relation to the operation, the treatment, and the preventives most promising of success. [St. Louis, 1878.] 7p. DNLM **70-2929**

PRINCE, David (1816-1890)
Bathing, cupping, electricity, massage. A comparison of the therapeutic effects of bathing, of cupping or atmospheric exhaustion, of electricity in the form of galvanism and faradism, and of massage, in the treatment of debilities, deformities, and chronic diseases. [Louisville, 1878.] 8p. DNLM **70-2930**

PRINCE, David (1816-1890)
Bathing, cupping, electricity, massage. A comparison of the therapeutic effects of bathing, of cupping or atmospheric exhaustion, of electricity in the form of galvanism and faradism, and of massage, in the treatment of debilities, deformities, and chronic diseases. With additions. [Louisville, 1878. 16p. DNLM **70-2931**

PRINCE, David (1816-1890)
The sanitation of small cities. Soil, drainage, sewerage, and the disposal of sewage. [1879.] 8p. DNLM
70-2932

PRINCE, David (1816-1890)
Partial forward dislocation of the head of the humerus, or backward displacement of the tendon of the long head of the biceps flexor cubiti; replaced after the lapse of one month. [St. Louis, 1879.] 4p. DNLM **70-2933**

PRITCHETT, J. W.
Address before the McDowell Medical Society, at its meeting in Henderson, Ky., May 8, 1878. Madisonville, 1878. 12p. DNLM **70-2934**

PROCTER, John R.
Notes on the yellow fever epidemic at Hickman, Ky., 1878. [Frankfort, 1878.] 42p. 3 plates. DNLM
70-2935

[PROCTOR, William] (1817-1874)
Memoir of William Proctor, Jr., late professor of pharmacy in the Philadelpia College of Pharmacy. Philadelphia: Merrihew & Son, 1874. 27p. DNLM; PLF **70-2936**

PROCTOR, William, Jr. (1817-1874)
A memorial of Elias Durand. Philadelphia: Merrihew & Son, 1873. 10p. DNLM **70-2937**

PRUDDEN, Theophil Mitchell (1849-1921)
Notes on the practical course in normal histology given in the laboratory of the Alumni Association of the College of Physicians and Surgeons, New York City. New York: Trow, 1879. 128p. DNLM; NNNAM **70-2938**

PULTE, Joseph Hippolyt (1811-1884)
Homoeopathic domestic physician containing the treatment of diseases. . . . Treatise on domestic surgery and an abridged materia medica. Cincinnati: Smith & Worthington, 1871, *vel subseq.* 719p. OCIM; PPHa **70-2939**

PULTE, Joseph Hippolyt (1811-1884)
. . . Homoeopathic domestic physician, containing the treatment of diseases; popular explanations of physiology, hygiene, hydropathy, anatomy and surgery, with illustrations, and an abridged materia medica. . . . With full explanations as to the use of the new remedies. [12th ed. enl. and rev.] Fiftieth thousand. Cincinnati: Smith & Worthington; New York: Boericke & Tafel; [etc., etc.], 1872. 743p. DLC; OCIM; PPHa
70-2940

PULTE MEDICAL COLLEGE. CINCINNATI (HOMOEOPATHIC)
Prospectus. May, 1872. Cincinnati: Bradley & Power, 1872. 1 sheet. DNLM **70-2941**

PULTE MEDICAL COLLEGE. CINCINNATI (HOMOEOPATHIC)
Annual announcements for the sessions of 1872-1873 to 1881-1882 (1.-10.); 1885-1886 (4.) Cincinnati, 1872-1885. DNLM [List of students for the years 1875-1876 to 1880-1881, in announcement for subsequent years. List of alumni from 1873-1881, in announcement for 1881-1882.]
70-2942

PULTE MEDICAL COLLEGE. CINCINNATI (HOMOEOPATHIC)
Annual catalogue for the session of 1873-1874. Cincinnati: E. W. Fish, 1873. 18p. DNLM **70-2943**

PULTE MEDICAL COLLEGE. CINCINNATI (HOMOEOPATHIC)
Special announcement for session of 1873-1874. Cincinnati, 1873. 2 l. DNLM **70-2944**

PULTE MEDICAL COLLEGE. CINCINNATI (HOMOEOPATHIC)
Announcement of the spring session of 1876. Cincinnati: J. P. Geppert, 1875. 13p. DNLM **70-2945**

PURPLE, Samuel Smith (1822-1900)
Objects and purposes: an inaugural address delivered before the New York Academy of Medicine, January 21, 1875, at the College of Physicians and Surgeons. New York: D. Appleton & Co., 1875. 8p. DNLM; NNNAM **70-2946**

PURPLE, Samuel Smith (1822-1900)
Medical libraries; an address delivered before the New York Academy of Medicine, January 18, 1877, on taking the chair as president a second term. New York, 1877. 26p. DNLM; NNNAM **70-2947**

PURPLE, Samuel Smith (1822-1900)
A valedictory address delivered before the New York Academy of Medicine, January 16, 1879. . . . New York: Printed for the Academy, 1879. 13p. DLC; DNLM; NNNAM
70-2948

PUTNAM, James Jackson (1846-1919)
Report on electro-therapeutics (containging some final alterations). [Boston, 1873.] 6p. DNLM **70-2949**

PUTNAM, James Jackson (1846-1919)
Rare form of rhythmical irregularity in the action of the heart. New York: D. Appleton & Co., 1874. 8p. DNLM
70-2950

PUTNAM, James Jackson (1846-1919)
Contribution to the physiology of the cortex cerebri. [Boston, 1874.] 4p. DNLM **70-2951**

PUTNAM, James Jackson (1846-1919)
Case of circumscribed analgesia. New York: S. W. Green, 1875. 24p. DNLM; NNNAM **70-2952**

PUTNAM, James Jackson (1846-1919)
Pathology of the nervous system. Second report. [Boston, 1875.] 8p. DNLM **70-2953**

PUTNAM, James Jackson (1846-1919)
Wernecke on the theory of aphasia. An abstract. [Boston, 1875.] 7p. DNLM **70-2954**

PUTNAM, James Jackson (1846-1919)
To members of the Massachusetts Medical Society. [Circular requesting answers to a series of questions in connection with the recent epidemic of diphtheria, especially in regard to post-diphtheritic paralysis, that the facts may be collated and properly classified. 1875.] [1875.] 1 sheet. DNLM
70-2955

PUTNAM, James Jackson (1846-1919)
Case of cutaneous disease, confined to the palmar surface of the thumb, successfully treated by nerve-section. Boston, [1878]. 4p. DNLM **70-2956**

PYBURN, George (*b.* 1831)
An exposition and defense of homoeopathy, or The treatment of diseases by similarly-perturbing specifics. . . . Georgetown, Col.: J. S. Randall, book and job printer, 1876. 36p. DLC
70-2957

QUEEN, JAMES W., & CO. PHILADELPHIA
Priced and illustrated catalogue of optical instruments. Pt. 2. 25th ed. Philadelphia: [H. B. Ashmead], 1872. 107p. DNLM
70-2958

QUEEN, JAMES W., & CO. PHILADELPHIA
Priced and illustrated catalogue of optical instruments. 31st ed. Philadelphia, 1872. 156p. DNLM
70-2959

QUEEN, JAMES W., & CO. PHILADELPHIA
Priced and illustrated catalogue of optical instruments. 38th ed. Philadelphia, 1875, 84p. DNLM
70-2960

QUEEN, JAMES W., & CO. PHILADELPHIA
Priced and illustrated catalogue of optical instruments. Pt. 2. 39th ed. Philadelphia, 1876. 120p. DNLM
70-2961

QUEEN, JAMES W., & CO. PHILADELPHIA
Perfect sight, how to retain it. Imperfect sight, how to restore it. Philadelphia: J. W. Queen & Co., [1876]. 16p. DNLM
70-2962

QUIMBY, Isaac Newton (1831-1898)
A new mode of treatment of congenital talipes; also a new mode of amputation at the ankle-joint. Jersey City: Pangborn, Dunning & Dear, 1875. 12p. DNLM
70-2963

QUINQUINIA. A natural combination of the alkaloids of cinchona bark. Manufactured by the Charles T. White Co. [New York, 1879.] 15p. DNLM; NNNAM **70-2964**

RAE, Julius H.
On the application of electricity as a therapeutic agent. New York and Philadelphia: Published for the Author by Boericke & Tafel, 1877. 132p. DNLM; PPHa **70-2965**

RAINS, George W.
Strange forces in nature; and their relation to the healing art. An introductory lecture. Augusta, Ga.: E. H. Pughe, 1874. 16p. DNLM **70-2966**

RALFE, Charles Henry
Health primers. No. 1. Exercise and training. New York: D. Appleton & Co., 1879. 96p. DNLM; NN; NNNAM
70-2967

RAND, Benjamin Howard (1827-1883)
Elements of medical chemistry. 2nd ed. Philadelphia: J. B. Lippincott & Co., 1871. 420p. CtY-M; DNLM; ICRM; PPC
70-2968

RAND, Benjamin Howard (1827-1883)
Charge to the graduating class of Jefferson Medical College, Philadelphia, delivered March 12, 1873, at the Academy of Music. Philadelphia: P. Madeira, 1873. 15, 4p. DNLM; PPJ
70-2969

RAND, Benjamin Howard (1827-1883)
Catalogue of valuable medical and miscellaneous books from the library of . . . . To be sold Friday, February 1, 1878. Philadelphia: Selheimer & Moore, [1878]. 16p. DNLM; PPC; PPL; PU **70-2970**

RANNEY, Ambrose Loomis (1848-1905)
A practical treatise on surgical diagnosis, designed as a manual for practitioners and students. New York: William Wood & Co., 1879. 386p. DLC; DNLM; NNNAM; PPC
70-2971

RANNEY, Ambrose Loomis (1848-1905)
Causes of death in surgical operations. New York: William Wood & Co., 1879. 24p. DNLM; NNNAM
70-2972

RANNEY, George E.
Achievements in medicine. Incentives to its scientific study. [Detroit, 1876.] 14p. DNLM **70-2973**

RAUE, Charles Godlove (1820-1896)
Valedictory address delivered at the annual commencement of the Hahnemann Medical College of Philadelphia, March 9, 1870, at the Academy of Music. Philadelphia: Wm. P. Kildare, 1870. 15p. PPHa **70-2974**

RAUE, Charles Godlove (1820-1896)
Annual record of homoeopathic literature. 1870. Edited by C. G. Raue, M.D., assisted by Drs. T. F. Allen, T. Bacmeister, G. W. Barnes, J. B. Bell, J. W. Blakely, H. B. Fellows, O. B. Gause, E. M. Hale, A. H. Hull, C. Hering, F. G. Houard, T. S. Hoyne, R. Koch, S. Lilienthal, F. A. Lord, R. J. McClatchey, M. Macfarlan, H. Minton, W. E. Payne, H. Ring, G. R. Starkey, C. Wesselhoeft. New York, San Francisco: Boericke & Tafel, 1870. 416p. PPHa **70-2975**

RAUE, Charles Godlove (1820-1896)
Annual record of homoeopathic literature. 1871. Assisted by Drs. T. F. Allen, T. Bacmeister, J. W. Blakely, Chas. Cropper, H. B. Fellows, E. A. Farrington, C. Hering, W. C. Goodno, T. S. Hoyne, A. Korndoerfer, F. A. Lord, R. J. McClatchey, M. Macfarlan, H. Minton, H. Ring, E. Tietze, C. Wesselhoeft. New York, San Francisco: Boericke & Tafel, 1871. 255p. PPHa
70-2976

RAUE, Charles Godlove (1820-1896)
Annual record of homoeopathic literature. 1872. Assisted by Drs. T. Bacmeister, Charles Cropper, E. A. Farrington, C. Hering, T. S. Hoyne, E. U. Jones, A. Korndoerfer, S. Lilienthal, R. J. McClatchey, M. Macfarlan, E. Mussina, J. Pettet, A. R. Thomas, C. Wesselhoeft. New York and Philadelphia: Boericke & Tafel, 1872. 338p. PPHa **70-2977**

RAUE, Charles Godlove (1820-1896)
Annual record of homoeopathic literature 1873. Assistants: Drs. T. Bacmeister, C. Cropper, E. A. Farrington, C. Hering, A. K. Hills, T. S. Hoyne, J. R. Kippax, A. Korndoerfer, S. Lilienthal, R. J. McClatchey, M. Macfarlan, W. S. Searle, A. R. Thomas, Charles Von Tagen, C. Wesselhoeft. New York and Philadelphia: Boericke & Tafel, 1873. 332p. PPHa
70-2978

RAUE, Charles Godlove (1820-1896)
Annual record of homoeopathic literature. 1874. Assistants: Drs. T. Bacmeister, C. M. Conant, C. Cropper, E. A. Farrington, C. Hering, T. S. Hoyne, J. R. Kippax, A. Korndoerfer, S. Lilienthal, O. W. Lounsbury, R. J. McClatchey, M. Macfarlan, J. N. Mitchell, C. F. Nichols, W. S. Searle, C. Von Tagen, C. Wesselhoeft. New York and Philadelphia: Boericke & Tafel, 1874. 376p. PPHa **70-2979**

RAUE, Charles Godlove (1820-1896)
Annual record of homoeopathic literature. 1875. Assistants: Drs. T. Bacmeister, C. Cropper, C. Hering, S. B. Higgins, J. R. Kippax, A. Korndoerfer, S. Lilienthal, O. W. Lounsbury, R. J. McClatchey, M. Macfarlan, J. N. Mitchell, Thos. Nichol, C. F. Nichols, W. S. Searle, C. M. Thomas, C. H. Von Tagen, C. Wesselhoeft. New York and Philadelphia: Boericke & Tafel, 1875. 376p. PPHa **70-2980**

RAWLEY Springs, in Rockingham Co., Va., with an analysis of the waters, and letters of skilful and eminent physicians and certificates of cure, showing the great remedial effects of these waters in many diseases. Philadelphia, 1878. 19p. DNLM **70-2981**

RAWSON, Charles Hamilton (1828-1884)
Puerperal convulsions. Treatment of, etc. Des Moines: Carter, Hussey & Curl, 1878. 11p. DNLM **70-2982**

RAY, Isaac (1807-1881)
A treatise on the medical jurisprudence of insanity. . . . 5th ed., with additions. Boston: Little, Brown & Co., 1871. 658p. DLC; DNLM; NNNAM; PPC **70-2983**

RAY, Isaac (1807-1881)
Contributions to mental pathology. . . . Little, Brown & Co., 1873. 558p. DLC; DNLM; MH-M; NNNAM **70-2984**

RAY, Isaac (1807-1881)
Ideal characters of the officers of a hospital for the insane. . . . Read to the Association of Superintendents of North American Hospitals for the Insane, at its annual meeting in Baltimore, May 29, 1873, and ordered to be printed. Philadelphia: [J. B. Chandler, printer], 1878. 45p. DLC; DNLM; NNNAM; PU **70-2985**

RAY, Isaac (1807-1881)
What shall Philadelphia do for its paupers? [Philadelphia, 1872.] 23p. DNLM **70-2986**

RAYMOND, Rossiter W[orthington] (1840-1918)
The hygiene of mines. [New York, 1879.] 24p. DNLM **70-2987**

READ, Henry N., and Jerome WALKER
Tabulated notes on children and some of their diseases, for the use of students. Brooklyn: Rome Brothers, 1878. 36p. [interleaved copy]. DNLM; NNNAM **70-2988**

READ, William (1820?-1889)
Cases of cerebro-spinal meningitis, in 1873 and 1874. [Philadelphia, 1874.] 16p. DNLM; PPC **70-2989**

REED, Joseph Allison (1823-1884), David D. RICHARDSON, and G. COOK
To the legislature. In the matter of the insane in the prisons and poorhouses of Pennsylvania. Letter of . . . . Philadelphia: A. C. Bryson & Co., 1874. 8p. DNLM **70-2990**

REESE, C. Girard
Second edition on consumption of the lungs, or decline; and the only successful treatment. Showing that formidable disease to be curable in all its stages. . . . New York: The Author, [1870]. 24p. DLC **70-2991**

REESE, John James (1818-1892)
A manual of toxicology, including the consideration of the nature, properties, effects, and means of detection of poisons, more especially in their medico-legal relations. Philadelphia: J. B. Lippincott, 1874. 507p. DLC; DNLM; PPC; PU **70-2992**

REEVE, John Charles (1826-1920)
The brain and nervous system, in their relations to teaching and learning; a lecture delivered before the Teachers' Institute of Dayton, Ohio. Dayton, 1878. 32p. DNLM **70-2993**

REEVE, John Charles (1826-1920)
An office table for surgical and gynecological purposes. New York: William Wood & Co., 1878. 5p. DNLM; NNNAM **70-2994**

REEVES, James Edmund (1829-1896)
The physical and medical topography, including vital, manufacturing, and other statistics of the city of Wheeling. Wheeling, 1870. 50p. DNLM **70-2995**

REEVES, James Edmund (1829-1896)
The health and wealth of the city of Wheeling, including its physical and medical topography; also, general remarks on the natural resources of West Virginia. 2nd ed. Baltimore: Sun Office, 1871. 158p. DNLM **70-2996**

REEVES, James Edmund (1829-1896)
The physical and moral causes of bad health in American women. Read before the American Public Health Association. Wheeling, 1875. 43p. DNLM **70-2997**

REITER, William C. (1817-1882)
A monograph on the treatment of diphtheria, based upon a new etiology and pathology. Philadelphia: J. B. Lippincott, 1878. 47p. NNNAM; PPC; PPJ; PU **70-2998**

REPORT of the autopsy of the Siamese twins, together with other interesting information concerning their life. Philadelphia: J. B. Lippincott & Co., 1874. 39p. DNLM; PPC **70-2999**

A REPORT of the origin and cause of the late epidemic (yellow fever) in Augusta. Submitted to a meeting of the physicians of Augusta, on the 10th Dec., 1839. Reprinted by order of council, Nov., 1877. Augusta: Chronicle & Constitutionalist Print, 1877. 16p. DNLM; GU **70-3000**

REYBURN, Robert (1833-1889), Oliver O. HOWARD and Charles S. SHADD
Addresses delivered at the third annual commencement of the medical department of Howard University, Washington, D.C. With a catalogue of the faculty and students. Washington, D.C.: Reed & Woodward, 1873. 35p. DNLM **70-3001**

REYNDERS, JOHN & CO.
Illustrated catalogue and price-list of surgical instruments, orthopaedical apparatus, trusses, etc. New York: J. Reynders & Co., [1875]. 184p. DNLM; NNNAM **70-3002**

REYNDERS, JOHN & CO.
Illustrated catalogue and price-list of surgical instruments, orthopaedical apparatus, trusses, etc. New York: Cherouny & Kieule, [1879]. 184p. DNLM; NNNAM **70-3003**

REYNDERS, JOHN & CO.
Illustrated catalogue and price-list of surgical instruments, orthopaedical apparatus, trusses, etc. 2nd ed. New York, [1879]. 194p. DNLM; NNNAM **70-3004**

REYNOLDS, Dudley Sharpe (1842-1915)
Granular lids. Louisville: J. P. Morton & Co., 1872. 8p. DNLM **70-3005**

REYNOLDS, Dudley Sharpe (1842-1915)
Accommodation and refraction: a review of Dr. Fenner's pamphlet. Louisville: J. P. Morton & Co., 1873. 12p. DNLM **70-3006**

REYNOLDS, Dudley Sharpe (1842-1915)
Recent improvements in ophthalmic surgery. Louisville: J. P. Morton & Co., 1873. 15p. DNLM **70-3007**

REYNOLDS, Dudley Sharpe (1842-1915)
Diseases of the conjunctiva. Louisville: J. P. Morton & Co., 1874. 13p. DNLM **70-3008**

REYNOLDS, J[ohn] Russell (1828-1896)
Lectures on the clinical uses of electricity delivered in University College Hospital. 2nd ed. Philadelphia: Lindsay & Baikiston, 1874. 118p. DNLM; NNNAM; PPC; PU **70-3009**

REYNOLDS, John Russell, ed. (1828-1896)
A system of medicine. . . . With numerous additions and illustrations, by Henry Hartshorne. . . . Philadelphia: Henry C. Lea, 1879-1880. 3 v. DLC; OCIM; PPC; PU **70-3010**

REYNOLDS, Thomas Noble (1843-1885)
Medical education of the people their best safeguard against imposition in the practice of medicine. Detroit, 1878. 7p. DNLM **70-3011**

RIBOT, Théodule (1839-1916)
Heredity: a psychological study of its phenomena, laws, causes, and consequences. New York: D. Appleton & Co., 1875. 393p. CtY-M; DNLM; NN; MH **70-3012**

RICE, Charles (1841-1901)
Posological table, including all the officinal and the most frequently employed unofficinal preparations. New York: William Wood & Co., 1879. 95p. DNLM; NNNAM; PPJ; PU **70-3013**

RICHARDSON, Benjamin Franklin (1817-1890)
Address, introductory to the twelfth regular session of the Miami Medical College of Cincinnati, O. Cincinnati: Bradely & Power, 1871. 25p. DNLM **70-3014**

RICHARDSON, Benjamin Ward (1828-1896)
The action of alcohol on the body and on the mind. New York: J. N. Stearns, 1878. 58p. DNLM; NNNAM **70-3015**

RICHARDSON, Benjamin Ward (1828-1896)
Moderate drinking, for and against, from scientific points of view. New York: J. N. Stearns, 1879. 47p. DNLM; NN **70-3016**

RICHARDSON, Benjamin Ward (1828-1896)
The medical profession and alcohol. An inaugural address. New York, 1879. 33p. DNLM **70-3017**

RICHARDSON, John W. (1809-1872)
Puerperal convulsions. A general view of two hundred and ninety-seven cases. Nashville, Tenn.: "Union & American" Book and Job Office, 1872. 44p. DNLM **70-3018**

RICHARDSON, Joseph Gibbons (1836-1886)
On the cellular structure of the red blood corpuscle. Philadelphia: Collins, 1870. 12p. 1 plate. DNLM **70-3019**

RICHARDSON, Joseph Gibbons (1836-1886)
On the identity of the white corpuscles of the blood with the salivary, pus, and mucous corpuscles. [1870, *vel subseq.*] 6p. DNLM **70-3020**

RICHARDSON, Joseph Gibbons (1836-1886)
On the diagnostic value of the corpuscular blood-elements in the urine of Bright's diease. [Philadelphia, 1870.] 15p. DNLM **70-3021**

RICHARDSON, Joseph Gibbons (1836-1886)
A handbook of medical microscopy. Philadelphia: J. B. Lippincott & Co., 1871. 333p. DNLM **70-3022**

RICHARDSON, Joseph Gibbons (1836-1886)
Detection of pulmonary elastic tissue in the sputum of phthisis. Albany: Argus Co., 1871. 8p. DNLM **70-3023**

RICHARDSON, Joseph Gibbons (1836-1886)
Introductory lecture to the course on pathological anatomy at the University of Pennsylvania. Philadelphia: J. B. Lippincott & Co., 1871. 16p. DNLM **70-3024**

RICHARDSON, Joseph Gibbons (1836-1886)
Report on the structure of the white blood corpuscle. Philadelphia: Collins, 1872. 22p. DNLM **70-3025**

RICHARDSON, Joseph Gibbons (1836-1886)
On certain human parasitic fungi, and their relation to disease. Philadelphia: J. B. Lippincott & Co., 1872. 16p. DNLM **70-3026**

RICHARDSON, Joseph Gibbons (1836-1886)
New method of preserving tumors and certain urinary deposits during transportation. Philadelphia: J. B. Lippincott & Co., 1873. 8p. DNLM **70-3027**

RICHARDSON, Joseph Gibbons (1836-1886)
A lecture on the true nature and origin of the salivary globules, and their identity with the white corpuscles of the blood. Philadelphia: S. S. White, 1874. 16p. DNLM **70-3028**

RICHARDSON, Joseph Gibbons (1836-1886)
Improved method of applying the microspectroscopic test for blood-stains. [Philadelphia, 1876.] 2p. 1 broadside. DNLM **70-3029**

RICHARDSON, Joseph Gibbons (1836-1886)
On fungous growths in solutions for hypodermic medication, and their prevention by salicyclic acid. Philadelphia, 1877. 7p. DNLM **70-3030**

RICHARDSON, Joseph Gibbons (1836-1886)
On the identity of the red blood corpuscles in different races of mankind. [Philadelphia, 1877.] 3p. DNLM
70-3031

RICHARDSON, Joseph Gibbons (1836-1886)
The germ theory of disease, and its present bearing upon public and personal hygiene. Read before the Philadelphia Social Science Association Oct. 17, 1878. Philadelphia: E. Stern & Co., [1878]. 14p. DNLM **70-3032**

RICHARDSON, Joseph Gibbons (1836-1886)
Report of the Philadelphia County Medical Society on meteorology and epidemics, for the year 1878. Philadelphia: Collins, 1879. 19p. DNLM **70-3033**

RICHARDSON, Joseph Gibbons (1836-1886)
Long life, and how to reach it. Philadelphia: Lindsay & Blakiston, 1879. 160p. DNLM; PPC; PU
70-3034

RICHARDSON, T[obias] Gibson (1827-1892)
Address delivered before the American Medical Association, at its twenty-ninth annual session, held at Buffalo, N.Y., June 4th to 7th, 1878. . . . Philadelphia: Collins, printer, 1878. 21p. DLC; DNLM **70-3035**

RICHARDSON, William C. (*b.* 1849)
Cholera infantum and its sequelae—convulsions, diarrhoea and dysentery. Detroit, Mich.: Lodge's Homoeopathic Pharmacy, 1874. 52p. OCIM; PPHa **70-3036**

RICHARDSON, William C. (*b.* 1849)
A system of obstetrics on homoeopathic principles. St. Louis: Schroback & Co., 1877. 458p. 11 plates. DLC; DNLM; OCIM; PU **70-3037**

RICHARDSON, William Lambert (1842-1932)
External manipulation in obstetric practice. [1871.] 18p. 1 l. DNLM **70-3038**

RICHARDSON, William Lambert (1842-1932) and Thomas DWIGHT
A rare form of monstrosity. Two cases of apparently true hermaphroditism. Cambridge, 1875. 10p. 3 plates. DNLM
70-3039

RICHARDSON, William Lambert (1842-1932)
Summary of seven years' work on the State Board of Health of Massachusetts. Boston: Wright & Potter, 1876. 61p. DNLM; MH **70-3040**

RICHARDSON, William Lambert (1842-1932)
Subacute cystitis following parturition. [Boston, 1876.] 8p. 1 ch. DNLM **70-3041**

RICHARDSON, William Lambert (1842-1932)
Hydrate of chloral in obstetric practice. [Boston, 1877.] 9p. DNLM **70-3042**

RICHARDSON, William Lambert (1842-1932)
A contribution to the study of the treatment of the acute parenchymatous nephritis of pregnancy. [Boston, 1879.] 18p. DNLM **70-3043**

RICHARDSON, William Lambert (1842-1932)
The recurrence of nausea and vomiting during the latter months of pregnancy. New York: William Wood & Co., 1879. 7p. DNLM **70-3044**

RICHET, Charles (1850-1935)
Physiology and histology of the cerebral convolutions. Also poisons of the intellect. Transl. by Edward P. Fowler. New York: William Wood & Co., 1879. 170p. 1 plate. CtY-M; DNLM; NNNAM; PPC **70-3045**

RICHET, Louis-Alfred (1816-1891)
Notes on salivary calculus; with an appendix by Sirus Pirondi. Transl. from the French by Barnard Ellis. Columbus: Nevins & Myers, 1877. 22p. DNLM **70-3046**

RICHEY, S. O.
Restoration of the membrane tympani. Chicago: H. Willson & Co., 1878. 6p. DNLM **70-3047**

RICHEY, S. O.
Exfoliation of the cochlea. [Chicago, 1878.] 7p. DNLM
70-3048

RICHFIELD SPRINGS, OTSEGO COUNTY, NEW YORK
. . . Its attractions as a summer resort; its scenery, mountains, valleys . . . and the medicinal virtues of its waters. [1876.] 15p. DNLM **70-3049**

RICHFIELD SPRINGS, OTSEGO COUNTY, NEW YORK
Richfield Springs, N.Y. Visitors' list, spring house, June 16th to August 1st, 1877. Utica, N.Y.: White & Floyd, [1877]. 8p. DNLM **70-3050**

RINDFLEISCH, Edward (1836-1908)
A text-book of pathological histology: an introduction to the study of pathological anatomy. Transl. from the second German edition, with permission of the author, by William C. Kloman, assisted by F. T. Miles. Philadelphia: Lindsay & Blakiston, 1872. 695p. CtY-M; NNNAM; OCIM; PPJ
70-3051

RINGER, Sydney (1835-1910)
A handbook of therapeutics. . . . New York: William Wood & Co., 1870. 485p. CtY-M; MBM; NNNAM; PPC
70-3052

RINGER, Sydney (1835-1910)
A handbook of therapeutics. . . . 2nd ed. New York: William Wood & Co., 1871. 483p. LNT-M; OCLloyd; PPC; PU
70-3053

RINGER, Sydney (1835-1910)
A handbook of therapeutics. . . . 3rd ed. New York: William Wood & Co., 1873. 576p. MBM; OCIM; PPC; PU
70-3054

RINGER, Sydney (1835-1910)
A handbook of therapeutics. . . . 4th ed. New York: William Wood & Co., 1875. 632p. MBM; OCIM; PPC; PU
70-3055

RINGER, Sydney (1835-1910)
A handbook of therapeutics. . . . 5th ed. New York: William Wood & Co., 1876. 597p. MBM; OCIM; PPC; PU
70-3056

RINGER, Sydney (1835-1910)
A handbook of therapeutics. . . . 6th ed. New York: William Wood & Co., 1879. 665p. MBM; OCIM; PPC; PU
70-3057

RINGER, Sydney (1835-1910)
A handbook of therapeutics. . . . 7th ed. New York: William Wood & Co., 1879. 647p. DLC; DNLM; NNNAM; PPC
70-3058

RISLEY, S[amuel] D[oty] (1845-1920)
A clinical study of the more frequently occurring forms of conjunctival disease. [Philadelphia, 1877.] 6p. DNLM
70-3059

RITTER, Thomas
A medical manual and medicine chest companion, for popular use in families and on ship-board, for the treatment of the ordinary diseases of the human system. . . . 38th thousand, rev. and enl. New York: S. W. Green, printer and stereotyper, 1878 [1877]. 364p. DLC; NNNAM; PU **70-3060**

ROBB, R. L.
Robb & Co.'s family physician. A work on domestic medicines, designed to show how to have health, which is equivalent to time and money, by R. L. Robb, M.D., homoeopathic, J. V. Bean, M.D., allopathic [and] S. Lucretia Robb. . . . Burlington, Ia.: Robb & Co., [1879]. 854p. DLC; MH-M
70-3061

ROBBINS, Daniel C.
Remarks upon the last meeting of the American Pharmaceutical Association, which was held in Philadelphia, in September, and the Centennial Exposition in connection with pharmacy in the United States. New York: Thitchener & Glastaeter, 1876. 14p. DNLM **70-3062**

ROBBINS, Daniel C.
Annual review of the drug trade of New York, for the year 1878, prepared for the twenty-first annual report of the Chamber of Commerce of the State of New York. New York: H. Bessey, 1879. 10p. DNLM **70-3063**

ROBERTS, Frederick Thomas (1838-1919)
A handbook of the theory and practice of medicine. Philadelphia: Lindsay & Blakiston, 1874. 1052p. DNLM; NNNAM; OCIM; PU **70-3064**

ROBERTS, Frederick Thomas (1838-1919)
The theory and practice of medicine. 2nd American from the last London ed. Philadelphia: Lindsay & Blakiston, 1876. 920p. CtY-M; DNLM; OCIM; PU **70-3065**

ROBERTS, John Bingham (1852-1924)
Paracentesis of the pericardium, with an analysis of forty-one cases. New York: D. Appleton & Co., 1876. 16p. DNLM
70-3066

ROBERTS, John Bingham (1852-1924)
Acute bronchocele with cardiac hypertrophy occurring during pregnancy, and producing fatal dyspnoea. Philadelphia: Collins, 1876. 14p. DNLM **70-3067**

ROBERTS, John Bingham (1852-1924)
Excision of the lower end of the rectum in cases of cancer. Philadelphia: Sherman & Co., 1877. 16p. DNLM; PU
70-3068

ROBERTS, William (1830-1899)
A practical treatise on urinary and renal diseases, including urinary deposits. 2nd American from the 2nd revised and considerably enlarged London ed. Philadelphia: Henry C. Lea, 1872, 616p. 1 col. plate. DNLM; LNT-M; MH-M; NNNAM
70-3069

ROBERTS, William (1830-1899)
A practical treatise on urinary and renal diseases, including urinary deposits. Illustrated by numerous cases and engravings. 3rd ed. Philadelphia: Henry C. Lea, 1879. 625p. DNLM; IU-M; MH-M; NNNAM **70-3070**

ROBERTSON, Charles Archibald (1829-1880)
General nervous commotion, caused by a wounded eye. . . . A case reported to the American Ophthalmological Society. New York: J. Medole, 1870. 7p. DNLM
70-3071

ROBERTSON, Charles Archibald (1829-1880)
"Lo, the cranes of Ibycus!" A review of the report concerning the last illness of Dr. Alden March, with critical comments on the improper medical treatment of the case, and strictures on pitiful devices for concealment. New York: D. Appleton & Co., 1870. 28p. DNLM **70-3072**

ROBERTSON, Charles Archibald (1829-1880)
The strange defense of Dr. James H. Armsby against the criticism of his report. Albany: Argus Co., 1870. 16p. DNLM
70-3073

ROBERTSON, Charles Archibald (1829-1880)
Medical ethics; with remarks concerning the present state of the medical profession in Albany. Published from the records of the Albany County Medical Society. Albany: Argus Company, 1871. 97p. DNLM **70-3074**

ROBERTSON, Charles Archibald (1829-1880)
An eye case in the courts. Albany: Argus Co., 1873. 21p. DNLM **70-3075**

ROBERTSON, Charles Archibald (1829-1880)
Diagnosis of diseases of the eye. Albany: C. Van Benthuysen & Sons, 1874. 15p. DNLM **70-3076**

ROBERTSON, Charles Archibald (1829-1880)
Obituary of John Van Peet Quackenbush. Albany, N.Y.: Van Benthuysen, 1876. 12p. DNLM **70-3077**

ROBERTSON, Charles Archibald (1829-1880)
Intra-ocular disease: an interesting case in diagnosis. 1878. 4 l. DNLM **70-3078**

ROBERTSON, Francis Marion (1807-1892)
Modification of the obstetrical forceps, with practical observations on their application. New York: J. Ross & Co., 1872. 24p. DNLM; NNNAM **70-3079**

ROBINSON, [Andrew] R[ose] (1845-1924)
Pompholyx [cheiro-pompholyx (Hutchinson); dysidrosis (Tilbury Fox)]. A study on this disease with special reference to its nature and pathological history. New York: G. P. Putnam's Sons, 1877. 17p. 5 plates. DNLM; NNNAM
70-3080

ROBINSON, [Andrew] R[ose] (1845-1924)
Sycosis: prize essay for 1877 of the Bellevue Hospital Medical College Alumni Association. New York: D. Appleton & Co., 1877. 48p. DNLM; NNU-M **70-3081**

ROBINSON, [Andrew] R[ose] (1845-1924)
On the nature and pathological histology of psoriasis. New York: D. Appleton & Co., 1878. 32p. DNLM
70-3082

ROBINSON, Beverley (1844-1924)
A contribution to the study of post-nasal catarrh. New York: J. F. Trow & Son, 1875. 29p. DNLM **70-3083**

ROBINSON, Beverley (1844-1924)
On the sequelae and prophylaxis of simple tonsillar hypertrophy in children. New York: William Wood & Co., 1875. 8p. DNLM **70-3084**

ROBINSON, Beverley (1844-1924)
Case of chronic laryngitis, serving to illustrate how the mucous membrane of the vocal cords may be in an objective morbid condition, though their physiological functions be restored. [New York, 1875.] 4p. DNLM **70-3085**

ROBINSON, Beverley (1844-1924)
On certain morbid alterations of mucous membrane; their influence on speech, and their apparent relations with diseased nerve-structure. New York: D. Appleton & Co., 1875. 13p. DNLM **70-3086**

ROBINSON, Beverley (1844-1924)
Case of intra-laryngeal tumour (showing under the microscope mixed characters, principally, however, those of small-cell sarcoma), in a syphilitic subject. Partial evulsion, perichondritis, abscess pointing exteriorly, fistula of larynx, necrosis of thyroid cartilage; tracheotomy; death, examination post-mortem; remarks. [New York, 1875.] 13p. DNLM **70-3087**

ROBINSON, Beverley (1844-1924)
On the pathogenetic physiology of follicular disease of the throat and air-passages. [Philadelphia, 1876.] 7p. DNLM **70-3088**

ROBINSON, E. T.
The hygienic system: or The principles of hygienic medication briefly explained. . . . Pomfret, Conn.: E. T. Robinson, 1870. 15p. DLC **70-3089**

ROCHESTER, Thomas Fortescue (1823-1887)
Medical men and medical matters of 1776. Anniversary address before the Medical Society of the State of New York. Albany, N.Y., Van Benthuysen, 1876. 30p. DNLM **70-3090**

ROCKWELL, Alphonso David (1840-1925) and George M. BEARD
Observations on the physiological and therapeutical effects of galvanization of the sympathetic. New York: N.Y. Print Co., 1870. 16p. 1 plate. DLC; DNLM **70-3091**

ROCKWELL, Alphonso David (1840-1925)
Electrization in the treatment of the diseases of the organs of digestion. New York, 1871. 20p. DNLM **70-3092**

ROCKWELL, Alphonso David (1840-1925)
Electrolysis and its application to the treatment of disease. New York: D. Appleton & Co., 1871. 16p. DNLM **70-3093**

ROCKWELL, Alphonso David (1840-1925)
Faradization and galvanization in the treatment of amenorrhoea. [New York, 1872.] 10p. DNLM **70-3094**

ROCKWELL, Alphonso David (1840-1925)
Present state of electro-therapeutics. Louisville: J. P. Morton & Co., 1872. 22p. DNLM **70-3095**

ROCKWELL, Alphonso David (1840-1925) and George M. BEARD
Clinical researches in electro-surgery. New York: William Wood & Co., 1873. 72p. 2 plates. DNLM **70-3096**

ROCKWELL, Alphonso David (1840-1925)
On the application of electricity to the central nervous system. (Central galvanization.) [New York, 1873.] 20p. DNLM **70-3097**

ROCKWELL, Alphonso David (1840-1925)
On the application of electricity to the central nervous system. A reply to the objections of Anstie, Brown-Séquard, Cyon, and others. New York: D. Appleton & Co., 1873. 12p. DNLM **70-3098**

ROCKWELL, Alphonso David (1840-1925)
Observations in electro-therapeutics. Buffalo: Baker, Jones & Co., 1874. 9p. DNLM **70-3099**

ROCKWELL Alphonso David (1840-1925)
The electrolytic treatment of cancer. [New York, 1874.] 12p. DNLM **70-3100**

ROCKWELL, Alphonso David (1840-1925)
Electro-therapeutics of the male genital organs. New York: William Wood & Co., 1874. 12p. DNLM **70-3101**

ROCKWELL, Alphonso David (1840-1925)
A brief résumé of the indications for the use of electricity in disease. New York: William Wood & Co., 1875. 4p. DNLM **70-3102**

ROCKWELL, Alphonso David (1840-1925)
Aphasia. Chicago: J. J. Spalding & Co., 1875. 8p. DNLM **70-3103**

ROCKWELL, Alphonso David (1840-1925)
The relation of electro-therapeutics to electro-physiology. New York: William Wood & Co., 1875. 11p. DNLM **70-3104**

ROCKWELL, Alphonso David (1840-1925)
The physiological and therapeutical relations of electricity to the nervous system. New York: William Wood & Co., 1875. 12p. DNLM **70-3105**

ROCKWELL, Alphonso David (1840-1925)
On the differential indications for the use of the faradic and galvanic currents. New York: D. Appleton & Co., 1877. 10p. DNLM **70-3106**

ROCKWELL, Alphonso David (1840-1925)
Intermittent hemiplegia, with results of a post-mortem examination. [New York, 1877.] 4p. DNLM **70-3107**

ROCKWELL, Alphonso David (1840-1925)
On the use of electricity in the treatment of epilepsy. New York: Trow's Printing Co., 1878. 11p. DNLM **70-3108**

ROCKWELL, Alphonso David (1840-1925)
Lectures on electricity in its relations to medicine and surgery. New York: William Wood & Co., 1879. 99p. DNLM **70-3109**

ROCKWITH, Frank A.
General introductory discourse upon the therapeutics of midwifery and the sexual diseases of women. Delivered at the annual opening of the second course of lectures before the Homoeopathic Medical College, Department of the University of Michigan, October 2, 1876. East Saginaw, Mich.: E. W. Lyon, Book and Job Pr., 1876. 29p. OCIM
70-3110

RODENSTEIN, Charles Frederick (1826-1876)
A contribution to the natural history of tubercles. New York: D. Appleton & Co., 1871. 20p. DNLM
70-3111

RODENSTEIN, Charles Frederick (1826-1876)
The origin of Caesarean section; an historical sketch. New York: D. Appleton & Co., 1872. 19p. DNLM
70-3112

RODENSTEIN, Louis A.
A report on sewers, drainage, and public health. New York, 1873. 8p. DNLM **70-3113**

RODENSTEIN, Louis A.
A case of enormous polycystic ovarian tumor. New York: William Wood & Co., 1879. 5p. DNLM
70-3114

RODGERS, Stephen (1826-1878)
Inaugural address on assuming the presidency of the New York Medico-Legal Society. [New York, 1870?] 12p. DNLM
70-3115

RODGERS, Stephen (1826-1878)
Can chloroform be used to facilitate robbery? New York: D. Appleton & Co., 1871. 21p. DNLM **70-3116**

RODGERS, Stephen (1826-1878)
Professorial infamy. To the medical profession. [1872.] 2 l. DNLM **70-3117**

RODGERS, Stephen (1826-1878)
Intussusception. Albany, 1873. 38p. DNLM
70-3118

RODGERS, Stephen (1826-1878)
The true object of medical legislation. Albany, 1873. 15p. DNLM **70-3119**

RODGERS, Stephen (1826-1878)
The influence of uraemic and alcoholic poisoning on testamentary capacity. New York: D. Appleton & Co., 1873. 16p. DNLM **70-3120**

RODGERS, Stephen (1826-1878)
The hypodermic use of quinine: a dangerous experimental medication, and rarely justifiable. New York: D. Appleton & Co., 1874. 15p. DNLM **70-3121**

ROE, John Orlando (1848-1915)
Adenoid growths in the vault of the pharynx, their removal by the galvano-cautery. New York: William Wood & Co., 1879. 23p. DNLM; NNNAM **70-3122**

ROGERS, Lewis (1812-1875)
Facts and reminiscences of the medical history of Kentucky: an address before the Kentucky State Medical Society. Louisville: J. P. Morton, 1873. 32p. DNLM
70-3123

ROGERS, Lewis (1812-1875)
Climate in pulmonary consumption, and California as a health resort. Louisville: J. P. Morton & Co., 1874. 16p. DNLM
70-3124

ROHÉ, George H. (1851-1899)
The prevention of syphilis. [1876.] 3p. DNLM
70-3125

ROHLAND, Robert
Od, or odo-magnetic, force: and explanation of its influence on homoeopathic medicines, from the odic stand point, with opinions of medical homoeopathic authorities on the sanative effect of od-preparations, together with several sketches of interesting cases of disease. Appendix: "The conscientious, educated physician at the sick-bed, according to the odic laws. Magnetizing and odic touch." From the German, after the best sources. Transl. by . . . . New York, 1871. 39p. DNLM; NN; NNNAM **70-3126**

ROKENBAUGH, Henry S.
Testamentary capacity and the mental conditions affecting it. A paper read before the Medico-Legal Society of New York, May 1, 1878. New York: D. C. Gardner, 1878. 31p. DNLM; NN **70-3127**

ROOSA, Daniel Bennett St. John (1838-1908)
Statistical report of 494 cases of diseases of the ear. Albany: Argus Company, 1872. 10p. DNLM
70-3128

ROOSA, Daniel Bennett St. John (1838-1908)
A vest-pocket medical lexicon, being a dictionary of the words, terms, and symbols of medical science, collated from the best authorities, with the addition of new words not before introduced into a lexicon. With an appendix. 2nd ed. New York: William Wood & Co., 1872. 280p. CtY-M; DNLM; NNNAM; OCIM **70-3129**

ROOSA, Daniel Bennett St. John (1838-1908)
Anniversary address delivered before the alumni of the medical department of the city of New York, March 4, 1872. New York: D. Appleton & Co., 1872. 23p. DNLM; NNNAM
70-3130

ROOSA, Daniel Bennett St. John (1838-1908)
The nasal douche in aural disease. New York, 1872. 15p. DNLM **70-3131**

ROOSA, Daniel Bennett St. John (1838-1908)
A practical treatise on the diseases of the ear, including the anatomy of the organ. . . . New York: William Wood & Company, 1873. 535p. DLC; DNLM; NNNAM; PPC
70-3132

ROOSA, Daniel Bennett St. John (1838-1908)
The coming medical man: an anniversary discourse delivered before the New York Academy of Medicine, December 8, 1874. New York: D. Appleton & Co., 1874. 26p. DNLM
70-3133

ROOSA, Daniel Bennett St. John (1838-1908)
A practical treatise on the diseases of the ear, including the anatomy of the organ. . . . 2nd ed. New York: William Wood & Co., 1874. 535p. CtY-M; NNNAM; OCIM; PU
70-3134

ROOSA, Daniel Bennett St. John (1838-1908)
The coming medical man: an anniversary discourse delivered before the New York Academy of Medicine, December 8, 1874. New York: D. Appleton & Co., 1875. 24p. DNLM **70-3135**

ROOSA, Daniel Bennett St. John (1838-1908)
Ophthalmic and optic memoranda. By D. B. St. John Roosa . . . and Edward T. Ely. . . . New York: William Wood & Co., 1876. 264p. DLC; DNLM; NNNAM; PPC **70-3136**

ROOSA, Daniel Bennett St. John (1838-1908)
A practical treatise on the diseases of the ear, including the anatomy of the organ. . . . 3rd ed. New York: William Wood & Co., 1876. 535p. MH-M; NNNAM; PPJ; PU **70-3137**

ROOSA, Daniel Bennett St. John (1838-1908)
The relations of blepharitis ciliaris to ametropia. [New York, 1878.] 10p. DNLM **70-3138**

ROOSA, Daniel Bennett St. John (1838-1908)
An examination under atropine of the refractive state of eyes with normal vision (20/20), and which had never been affected with asthenopia or inflammation. [New York, 1878(?).] 5p. DNLM **70-3139**

ROOSA, Daniel Bennett St. John (1838-1908)
A case of acute inflammation of the middle ear, with inflammation of the muscles of the neck, and facial paralysis of the same side. Recovery. With some remarks upon the indications for Wilde's incision and trephining the mastoid process. [1879.] 14p. DNLM **70-3140**

ROOSA, Daniel Bennett St. John (1838-1908)
A case of poisoning from the use of the compound tincture of cinchona, producing permanent contraction of the visual fields and temporary impairment of sight and hearing. [New York, 1879.] 4p. DNLM **70-3141**

ROOSA, Daniel Bennett St. John (1838-1908)
The relations of the medical profession to the state. Being the anniversary discourse delivered before the Medical Society of the State of New York. New York, 1879. 24p. DNLM **70-3142**

ROSCOE, Henry E[nfield] (1833-1915)
Lessons in elementary chemistry; inorganic and organic. New York: William Wood & Co., 1871. 383p. 1 plate. DNLM; NN; NNC; PU **70-3143**

ROSENTHAL, Moritz (1833-1889)
A clinical treatise on the diseases of the nervous system, by M. Rosenthal. . . . With a preface by Professor Charcot; transl. from the author's rev. and enl. ed. by L. Putzel. New York: William Wood & Co., 1879. 2 v. DLC; NNNAM; OCIM; PU **70-3144**

ROSENTHAL, Moritz (1833-1889)
A clinical treatise on the diseases of the nervous system. New York: William Wood & Co., 1879. 555p. NNNAM; MBM; PPJ; PU **70-3145**

ROTCH, Thomas Morgan (1849-1914)
The emigration of the white corpuscle in inflammation. An essay to which was awarded the first prize of the Boylston Medical Society for 1873. Cambridge: Welch, Bigelow & Co., 1873. 37p. 1 plate. DNLM; MH-M **70-3146**

ROTCH, Thomas Morgan (1849-1914)
Absence of resonance in the fifth right intercostal space, diagnostic of pericardial effusion. Boston: D. Clapp & Son, 1878. 21p. 6 plates. DNLM [*also*: Boston: D. Clapp & Son, 1878, 27p.] **70-3147**

THE ROWE Truss Company's illustrated catalogue of trusses, supporters, elastic stockings, and deformity instruments. New York: Watson's Press, 1874. 17p. DNLM; NNNAM **70-3148**

RUDDOCK, E. Harris (1822-1875)
The stepping stone to homoeopathy and health. 1st American ed., from the 6th London ed., with notes by the American editor: Chicago: C. S. Halsey, 1870. 241p. OCIM; PPHa **70-3149**

RUDDOCK, E. Harris (1822-1875)
The lady's manual of homoeopathic treatment in the various derangements incident to her sex, with a chapter on the management of infants. 1st American, from the 3rd London ed., with notes and additions by R. Ludlam. Chicago: C. S. Halsey, 1870. 231p. OCIM **70-3150**

RUDDOCK, E. Harris (1822-1875)
The stepping stone to homoeopathy and health. 2nd American, from the 7th London ed. 60th thousand, with alterations and additions, adapting it to the climate. diseases and customs of Americans. By the American editor. Chicago: Halsey Bros., 1872. 259p. OCIM **70-3151**

RUDDOCK, E. Harris (1822-1875) and E. B. SHULDHAM
Essentials of diet; or, hints on food, in health and disease. New York & Philadelphia: Boericke & Tafel, Homoeopathic Pharmacies, 1876. 252p. NNNAM; PPHa; PPJ **70-3152**

RUMBOLD, Thomas F[razier] (1830-1901)
The function of the Eustachian tube, in its relation to the renewal and density of the air in the tympanic cavity, and to the concavity of the membrana tympani. St. Louis: Southwestern Book & Publishing Co., 1873. 40p. DLC; DNLM **70-3153**

RUMBOLD, Thomas F[razier] (1830-1901)
A description of new instruments for making examinations and applications to the cavities of the nose, throat, and ear, and a few remarks about the remedies that may be administered by means of them. St. Louis: Southwestern Book & Publishing Co., 1873. 16p. DNLM **70-3154**

RUMBOLD, Thomas F[razier] (1830-1901)
Direct local medication in the treatment of chronic catarrhal inflammation of the nasal and pharyngo-nasal cavities. Kansas City, Mo.: Ramsey, Millett & Hudson, 1874. 8p. DNLM **70-3155**

RUMBOLD, Thomas F[razier] (1830-1901)
A description of new instruments for making examinations and applications to the cavities of the nose, throat, and ear, and a few remarks about the remedies that may be administered by means of them. 3rd ed. St. Louis: A. M. Leslie & Co., [1875]. 24p. 1 tab. **70-3156**

RUMBOLD, Thomas F[razier] (1830-1901)
The function of the uvula and the prominence formed by the azygos uvulae muscles. [1876.] 8p. DLC; DNLM **70-3157**

RUMBOLD, Thomas F[razier] (1830-1901)
A simple mode of cleansing the nasal and pharyngo-nasal passages. [1877.] 7p. DNLM **70-3158**

RUPPANER, Antoine (1825-1892)
Contributions to practical laryngoscopy. Four cases of morbid growths within the larynx. New York: D. Appleton & Co., 1870. 20p. 1 plate. DNLM; NNNAM **70-3159**

RUPPANER, Antoine (1825-1892)
Reply to Dr. Lewis A. Sayre's review of Dr. Ruppaner's case of laryngo-tracheotomy, to which is added a full account of the great poisoning case by partridges at the Fifth Avenue Hotel. New York: D. Appleton & Co., 1870. 29p. DLC; NNNAM **70-3160**

RUPPANER, Antoine (1825-1892)
Contributions to practical laryngoscopy. . . . Second series. Large fibrous polypus (fibro-sarcoma-polyposum), in the larynx, removed by thyrotomy, preceded by laryngo-tracheotomy. New York: Bradstreet Press, 1871. 16p. 1 col. plate. DNLM; NNNAM **70-3161**

RUPPANER, Antoine (1825-1892)
Statement of the "Sayre-Ruppaner case," and opinion of the Supreme Court. New York: Bradstreet Press, 1871. 36p. DNLM; NNNAM **70-3162**

RUPPANER, Antoine (1825-1892)
. . . Report on medicine and surgery. . . . Washington: Government Printing Office, 1876. 15p. DLC [U.S. Commission to the Vienna Exhibition, 1876] **70-3163**

RUSCHENBERGER, W[illiam] S. W. (1807-1895)
A report on the origin and therapeutic properties of cundurango. (Published by order of the Navy Department.) Washington: Government Printing Office, 1873. 25p. DNLM [*also*: Washington Government Printing Office, 1873. 28p.] **70-3164**

RUSH, Benjamin (1745-1813)
An account of the causes and indications of longevity and of the state of the body and mind in old age: with observations on its diseases, and their remedies. (First printed at Philadelphia, an. 1793.) New York: Poole & Maclauchlan, 1872. 12p. DLC; DNLM; NN; NNNAM **70-3165**

RUSH MEDICAL COLLEGE. MEDICAL DEPARTMENT OF THE UNIVERSITY OF CHICAGO
Dedicatory exercises of the new building of Rush Medical College. Introductory lecture to the thirty-fourth annual session, Oct. 4, 1876. [By J. Adams Allen.] With an appendix, containing a historical sketch of the college; proceedings at the laying of the corner stone, Nov. 20, 1875, etc., etc. Chicago: C. H. Blakely & Co., 1876. 48p. DLC; DNLM; ICRM **70-3166**

RUSH MEDICAL COLLEGE. MEDICAL DEPARTMENT OF THE UNIVERSITY OF CHICAGO
Triennials. Containing annual announcements for the sessions of 1877-1878 and 1880-1881. With a list of graduates from its organization, 1843-1844 to 1880. Chicago, 1877-1880. DNLM; ICRM **70-3167**

RUSH MEDICAL COLLEGE. MEDICAL DEPARTMENT OF THE UNIVERSITY OF CHICAGO
Post graduate course. Announcement for the session of 1880. Chicago: Bulletin Print. Co., 1879. 12p. DNLM; ICRM **70-3168**

RYDER, John Adam (1852-1895)
Addenda to etiological views expressed in a paper on the mechanical genesis of tooth-forms. Philadelphia, 1878. 3p. DNLM **70-3169**

SAGER, Abram (1810-1877)
A reply to Prof. Dunster's letter on "homoeopathy in the University" [of Michigan], Aug. 17, 1875. [Also, an explanation from Prof. A. B. Palmer, called for by one of his old students, Henry A. Cleland, Aug., 1875.] [Ann Arbor, 1875.] 2 l. DNLM **70-3170**

SAGER, Abram (1810-1877)
Review of Prof. Palmer's statement respecting the relations of himself and colleagues to homoeopathy in the University [of Michigan]. Also, further facts and opinions respecting the situation at the Michigan University Medical School. [Detroit, 1875.] 12p. DNLM **70-3171**

SAINT LOUIS HOMOEOPATHIC COLLEGE OF MEDICINE AND SURGERY
Thirteenth annual announcement; being the second of the St. Louis Homoeopathic College of Medicine and Surgery; the tenth of the Homoeopathic Medical College of Missouri; and the third of the St. Louis College of Homoeopathic Physicians and Surgeons; comprising a catalogue of the corporators, fellows, professors, lecturers, alumni and students of the united colleges, from the date of the act of incorporation in 1875. Session of 1872-1873. St. Louis: Musick, Harris & Co., 1872. 20p. DNLM **70-3172**

SAINT LOUIS MEDICAL SOCIETY OF MISSOURI
Reports to the St. Louis Medical Society on yellow fever; consisting of the report of the Committee appointed to inquire into the relations of the epidemic of 1878 to the city of St. Louis, and a report on the meteorological conditions and etiology of yellow fever, and of certain other diseases associated with a high temperature, and on the treatment of yellow fever, by W. Hutson Ford. . . . Rev. by the Committee on publication: Thos. Kennard, M.D., chairman, Walter Coles, M.D., John Bryson, M.D. St. Louis: G. O. Rumbold & Co., 1879. 320p. 5 plates. DLC **70-3173**

SALTER, Samuel James Augustus (1825-1897)
Dental pathology and surgery. New York: William Wood & Co., 1875. 399p. DNLM; NNNAM; PPC; PU **70-3174**

SALTER, Seaborn Freeman
Woman: and her diseases, from infancy to old age. Wtih the diseases of children. . . . Atlanta, Ga.: Economical Book & Job Printing House, 1872. 128p. DLC **70-3175**

SALTER, S[eaborn] F[reeman]
The American practice of domestic medicine. . . . Atlanta, Ga.: J. P. Harrison & Co., 1877. 347p. DLC **70-3176**

SANDS, Henry Berton (1830-1888)
On the use of the plaster-of-Paris bandage in the treatment of fracture, especially fracture of the femur. New York: D. Appleton & Co., 1871. 23p. DNLM; NNNAM **70-3177**

SANDS, Henry Berton (1830-1888)
A case of bony anchylosis of the hip-joint, successfully treated by subcutaneous division of the neck of the femur. New York: D. Appleton & Co., 1873. 8p. DNLM **70-3178**

SANDS, Henry Berton (1830-1888) and E. C. SEGUIN
A case of traumatic brachial neuralgia, treated by excision of the cords of the brachial plexus. Philadelphia: J. B. Lippincott & Co., [1873]. 18p. 1 plate. DNLM; PPC
70-3179

SANDS, Henry Berton (1830-1888)
A case of haemorrhage from the internal carotid artery, treated successfully by the ligature. New York: D. Appleton & Co., 1874. 9p. DNLM **70-3180**

SANDS, Henry Berton (1830-1888)
Esmarch's bloodless method. New York: D. Appleton & Co., 1875. 21p. DNLM **70-3181**

SANDS, Henry Berton (1830-1888)
On the causes of gleet and on the calibre of the male urethra. New York: D. Appleton & Co., 1876. 23p. DNLM
70-3182

SANDS, Henry Berton (1830-1888)
On tracheotomy and laryngotomy. New York: G. P. Putnam's Sons, 1876. 40p. DNLM **70-3183**

SANDS, Henry Berton (1830-1888)
On the treatment of intussusception by abdominal section, with the report of a case in which the operation proved successful. New York: D. Appleton & Co., 1877. 24p. DNLM
70-3184

SANDS, Henry Berton (1830-1888)
On spasmodic stricture of the urethra. A reply to Dr. F. N. Otis. [New York: W. L. Mershon, 1869.] 12p. DNLM
70-3185

SANDS, Henry Berton (1830-1888)
A clinical lecture on inflammatory and on spasmodic stricture of the urethra. [New York, 1879.] 10p. DNLM
70-3186

SANDS, Henry Berton (1830-1888)
Chronic spasmodic stricture of the urethra. [New York, 1879.] 4p. DNLM **70-3187**

SANGER, Eugene Francis (1829-1897)
Report on malpractice. A paper read before the Maine Medical Association, June 12, 1878. Portland: S. Berry, 1878. 25p. DNLM **70-3188**

SANGER, Eugene Francis (1829-1897)
Review of malpractice suit, Bowley *vs.* Sanger, January term, 1878. [Bangor, Me., 1878.] 20p. DNLM
70-3189

SANGER, Eugene Francis (1829-1897)
Report of the committee on suits for malpractice. Bangor: S. S. Smith, 1879. 22p. DNLM **70-3190**

SATCHWELL, Solomon Sampson (1821-1892)
Treatment of fever and inflammation. An essay on the topography and prevailing diseases of New Hanover County, N.C., read before the North Carolina Medical Society. Wilmington, N.C.: Engelhard & Price, 1870. 69p. DNLM
70-3191

SATTERLEE, F. Le Roy (1847-1917)
Psoriasis; its etiology, relation to rheumatic disease, and the rationale of a cognate treatment. New York: Poole & Maclauchlan, 1873. 8p. DNLM **70-3192**

SATTERLEE, F. Le Roy (1847-1917)
Erysipelas; its etiology, pathology, and abortive treatment by quinine and opium. New York: D. Appleton & Co., 1874. 16p. DNLM **70-3193**

SATTERTHWAITE, Thomas Edward (*b.* 1843)
On the structure and development of connective substances. New York: D. Appleton & Co., 1876. 28p. 1 plate. DNLM
70-3194

SATTERTHWAITE, Thomas Edward (*b.* 1843)
The present condition of the evidence concerning disease germs. Philadelphia, 1877. 20p. DNLM
70-3195

SATTERTHWAITE, Thomas Edward (*b.* 1843)
Notes and practical studies on the minute elements of the nervous system. New York: D. Appleton & Co., 1878. 21p. 2 plates. DNLM **70-3196**

SATTERTHWAITE, Thomas Edward (*b.* 1843) and W. H. PORTER
Observations in one hundred cases of carcinoma. New York: D. Appleton & Co., 1879. 101p. DNLM; NNNAM
70-3197

SAWYER, Edward Warren (1840-1897)
Affections of the nipple and breast incident to early lactation; a lecture delivered at Rush Medical College, Chicago. Chicago: A. S. Kissell & Co., 1877. 22p. DNLM
70-3198

SAWYER, Edward Warren (1840-1897)
How to save the perineum. A new use of the obstetric forceps. An improved instrument. [Chicago, 1878.] 6p. DNLM
70-3199

SAYRE, Lewis Albert (1820-1900)
Partial paralysis from reflex irritation, caused by congenital phimosis and adherent prepuce. Philadelphia: Collins, 1870. 9p. DNLM **70-3200**

SAYRE, Lewis Albert (1820-1900)
Review of Dr. Ruppaner's case of laryngo-tracheotomy. New York: D. Appleton & Co., 1870. 8p. DNLM
70-3201

SAYRE, Lewis Albert (1820-1900)
Answer to Dr. A. Ruppaner, with a review and criticism on his recent report of a case of laryngo-tracheotomy, including all the attested facts regarding the recent partridge poisoning case at the Fifth Avenue Hotel. . . . New York: D. Appleton & Co., 1870. 38p. DLC; DNLM **70-3202**

SAYRE, Lewis Albert (1820-1900)
A simple dressing for fracture of the clavicle. Louisville: J. P. Morton & Co., 1871. 8p. DNLM **70-3203**

SAYRE, Lewis Albert (1820-1900)
Cases of luxation of the elbow. Albany: The Argus Co., 1871. 7p. DNLM **70-3204**

SAYRE, Lewis Albert (1820-1900)
Cases of luxation of the elbow. Report of two cases of luxation of the elbow, also a description of a new vertebrated probe and catheter. Albany: The Argus Co., 1871. 10p. 1 plate DNLM
70-3205

SAYRE, Lewis Albert (1820-1900)
Report on fractures. Philadelphia: Collins, 1874. 30p. DNLM; PPC **70-3206**

SAYRE, Lewis Albert (1820-1900)
On anchylosis. New York: D. Appleton & Co., 1874. 20p. DNLM **70-3207**

SAYRE, Lewis Albert (1820-1900)
A practical manual of the treatment of club-foot. . . . 2nd ed., enl. and cor. New York: D. Appleton & Co., 1874. 117p. DLC; DNLM; NNNAM; PU **70-3208**

SAYRE, Lewis Albert (1820-1900)
A practical manual of the treatment of club-foot. 3rd ed. New York: D. Appleton & Co., 1875. 129p. DNLM; NNNAM; NNU-M **70-3209**

SAYRE, Lewis Albert (1820-1900)
On disease of the hip-joint. New York: G. P. Putnam's Sons, 1875. 24p. DNLM; NNNAM **70-3210**

SAYRE, Lewis Albert (1820-1900)
Spinal anaemia with partial paralysis and want of co-operation, from irritation of the genital organs. Philadelphia: Collins, 1875. 29p. DNLM **70-3211**

SAYRE, Lewis Albert (1820-1900)
Lectures on orthopedic surgery and diseases of the joints, delivered at Bellevue Hospital Medical College, during the winter session of 1874-1875. . . . Illustrated by 274 wood-engravings. New York: D. Appleton & Co., 1876. 476p. DLC; NNNAM; NNU-M; PU **70-3212**

SAYRE, Lewis Albert (1820-1900)
Report on Pott's disease, or caries of the spine, treated by extension and the plaster of Paris bandage. Philadelphia: Collins, 1877. 68p. DNLM; PPC; PPJ **70-3213**

SAYRE, Lewis Albert (1820-1900)
Spinal disease and spinal curvature, their treatment by suspension and the use of the plaster of Paris bandage. Philadelphia: J. B. Lippincott & Co., 1877. 121p. 19 phot. plates. CtY-M; DNLM; IU-M; PPC **70-3214**

SAYRE, Lewis Albert (1820-1900)
A succinct history of the plan of treatment of Pott's disease by suspension and the use of plaster of Paris bandage. Louisville, Ky., 1878. 22p. DNLM **70-3215**

SAYRE, Lucius E[lmer] (1847-1925)
Conspectus of organic materia medica and pharmacal botany, comprising the vegetable and animal drugs: their physical character, geographical origin, classification, constituents, doses, adulterations, &c. Table of the tests and solubilities of the alkaloids appended. . . . Philadelphia: D. G. Brinton, 1879 [1878]. 220p. fold. tab. DLC; OCLloyd; PU **70-3216**

SCHÄFER, Edward Albert (1850-1935)
A course of practical histology. Being an introduction to the use of the microscope. Philadelphia: Henry C. Lea, 1877. 304p. 1 plate. CU-M; DNLM; MBM; NNNAM **70-3217**

SCHAFER, GEORGE H., & CO., FORT MADISON, IA.
Descriptive catalogue of pharmaceuticals with quantitative composition, dose and price list. Fort Madison, Ia.: G. H. Schafer & Co., [1872]. 24p. DLC **70-3218**

SCHIEFERDECKER, Christian Charles
Horrors of vaccination. New York: American News Co., 1870. 48p. DNLM; NNNAM **70-3219**

SCHMIDT, Henry D. (1823-1888)
On the origin and development of the bacillus tuberculosis in the human lung, liver, spleen, etc. Chicago: The Clark & Longley Co., [1879?]. 125p. 3 plates. DNLM; OCIM **70-3220**

SCHÖPF, Johann David (1752-1800)
The climate and diseases of America. . . . Transl. by James Read Chadwick. . . . Boston: H. O. Houghton & Co.; New York: Hurd & Houghton; [etc., etc.], 1875. 31p. DLC; MH; MBM; MWA **70-3221**

SCHROEDER, Carl Ludwig Ernst (1838-1887)
A manual of midwifery, including the pathology of pregnancy and the puerperal state. Transl. into English from the 3rd German ed. by Charles H. Carter. New York: D. Appleton & Co., 1873. 388p. DNLM; ICRM; NNNAM; PPC **70-3222**

SCHROEDER, Carl Ludwig Ernst (1838-1887)
Diseases of the female sexual organs. Transl. by E. W. Schauffler, L. Wheeler, W. L. Richardson, E. B. Bronson, J. H. Emerson, and P. F. Mundé. New York: William Wood & Co., 1875. 575p. DNLM; IEN-M; MBM; NNNAM **70-3223**

SCHULTZ, Carl H.
Mineral spring waters, their chemical composition, physiological action, therapeutic and general use. New York: W. Wallach, 1876. 36p. DNLM **70-3224**

SCHUPPERT, Moritz (1818-1887)
Excision of the entire scapula with preservation of a useful arm. [New Orleans], 1870. 4p. DNLM **70-3225**

SCHÜSSLER, Wilhelm Heinrich (1821-1898)
Abridged therapeutics founded upon histology & cellular pathology . . . with an appendix: special indications for the application of the inorganic tissue-formers. . . . Authorized transl. by M. Docetti Walker. . . . [5th ed.] New York: G. Houston, 1879. 91p. DLC; NNNAM; MH-M; PU **70-3226**

SCHWABE, Willmar
Pharmacopoea homoeopathica polyglottica. . . . New York, 1872. 251p. OCLloyd **70-3227**

SCHWEIG, George M.
On some of the uses of galvanic and faradic baths. New York: J. F. Trow & Sons, 1874. 12p. DNLM **70-3228**

SCHWEIG, George M.
Cerebral exhaustion with special reference to its galvano-balneological treatment. New York, [1876]. 15p. DNLM **70-3229**

SCHWEIG, George M.
The electric bath; its medical uses, effects, and applicance. New York: G. P. Putnam's Sons, 1877. 134p. DNLM **70-3230**

SCHWEIGGER, Karl Ernst Theodor (1830-1905)
Handbook of ophthalmology. . . . Transl. from the 3rd German ed. by Porter Farley. . . . Philadelphia: J. B. Lippincott & Co., 1878. 555p. DLC; DNLM; NNNAM; PPC **70-3231**

SCOTT, J. Walter
History of the cancer-plant. New York: University Publishing Society, [1870]. 16 l. DNLM **70-3232**

SCOTT, M. J.
On hysteria. [St. Louis, 1870.] 8p. DNLM
70-3233

SCOVELL, J[osiah] T[homas] (*b.* 1841)
Lessons in physiology. . . . Terre Haute: Moore & Langen, printers, 1879. 80p. DLC **70-3234**

SCUDDER, John Milton (1829-1894)
The eclectic practice of medicine. . . . 5th thousand. Rev. ed. Cincinnati: Medical Publishing Company, 1870. 743p. DLC; DNLM; OCIM; NNNAM **70-3235**

SCUDDER, John Milton (1829-1894)
Specific medication and specific medicine. . . . Cincinnati: Wilstach, Baldwin & Co., printers, 1870. 253p. DLC; DNLM; OCIM **70-3236**

SCUDDER, John Milton (1829-1894)
Specific medication and specific medicines. Revised, with an appendix containing the articles published on the subject since the 1st ed. And a report of cases illustrating specific medication. 4th ed. Cincinnati: Wilstach, Baldwin & Co., 1873. 377p. DNLM; ICRM; OCIM; NNNAM **70-3237**

SCUDDER, John Milton (1829-1894)
Specific medication and specific medicines. Rev., with an appendix containing the articles published on the subject since the first edition. And a report of cases illustrating specific medication. . . . 5th ed. Cincinnati: Wilstach, Baldwin & Co., printers, 1874. 393p. DLC; DNLM; OCIM; PU
70-3238

SCUDDER, John Milton (1829-1894)
On the reproductive organs, and the venereal. . . . Cincinnati: Wilstach, Baldwin & Co., printers, 1874. 393p. col. plates. DLC; IU-M; OCIM; PPC **70-3239**

SCUDDER, John M[ilton] (1829-1894)
Specific diagnosis: a study of diseases with special reference to the administration of remedies. . . . Cincinnati: Wilstach, Baldwin & Co., printers, 1874. 387p. DLC; OCIM; NNNAM; PU **70-3240**

SCUDDER, John Milton (1829-1894)
The eclectic practice of medicine for families. . . . 17th ed. Cincinnati: Wilstach, Baldwin & Co., printers, 1876. 884p. DLC; IEN-M; OCIM; NNNAM **70-3241**

SEARLE, William S. (*b.* 1833)
The status of the medical profession in America. Annual address before the New York State Homoeopathic Medical Society, February 8, 1870. Albany: The Argus Co., 1870. 24p. NNNAM; PPHa **70-3242**

SEARLE, William S. (*b.* 1833)
A new form of nervous disease. Thesis for fellowship in the Medico-Chirurgical Society of New York, January, 1879. Philadelphia: Globe Printing House, 1879. 33p. NNNAM; PPHa **70-3243**

SEGUIN, Edouard (1812-1880)
New facts and remarks concerning idiocy, being a lecture delivered before the New York Medical Journal Association, October 15, 1869. . . . New York: William Wood & Co., 1870. 44p. DLC; DNLM; NNNAM **70-3244**

SEGUIN, Edouard (1812-1880)
Family thermometry; a manual of thermometry, for mothers, nurses, hospitalers, etc., and all who have charge of the sick and of the young. . . . New York: G. P. Putnam & Sons, 1873. 72p. DLC; DNLM; NNNAM **70-3245**

[SEGUIN, Edouard] (1812-1880)
Clinical thermometers and thermography. [New York: J. F. Trow & Son, 1875.] 8p. DLC **70-3246**

[SEGUIN, Edouard] (1812-1880)
The clinical thermoscope and uniformity of means of observation. Two notes. New York: G. P. Putnam's Sons, 1875. 8p. DNLM **70-3247**

SEGUIN, Edouard (1812-1880)
Medical thermometry and human temperature. . . . New York: William Wood & Co., 1876. 446p. DLC; DNLM; NNNAM; PPC
70-3248

SEGUIN, Edouard (1812-1880)
International uniformity in the practice and records of physic. New York: J. F. Trow & Son, 1876. 12p. DNLM
70-3249

SEGUIN, Edouard (1812-1880)
Psycho-physiological training of an idiotic hand. New York: G. P. Putnam's Sons, 1879. 8p. 1 plate. DNLM
70-3250

SEGUIN, Edward C[onstant] (1843-1898)
Spinal paralysis of the adult; acute, subacute, and chronic. (Inflammation of the motor tract of the spinal cord.) New York: D. Appleton & Co., 1874. 39p. 1 phot. plate. DNLM
70-3251

SEGUIN, Edward C[onstant] (1843-1898)
An outline of the physiology of the nervous system. New York: William Wood & Co., 1874. 18p. DNLM
70-3252

SEGUIN, Edward C[onstant] (1843-1898)
Infantile spinal paralysis. A clinical lecture. New York: D. Appleton & Co., 1875. 18p. DNLM **70-3253**

SEGUIN, Edward C[onstant] (1843-1898)
Hysterical symptoms in organic nervous affections. New York: J. F. Trow & Son, 1875. 16p. DNLM **70-3254**

SEGUIN, Edward C[onstant] (1843-1898)
The treatment of mild cases of melancholia at home. New York: G. P. Putnam's Sons, 1876. 25p. DNLM
70-3255

SEGUIN, Edward C[onstant] (1843-1898)
I. A clinical contribution to the study of post-paralytic chorea. II. A contribution to the study of localized cerebral lesions. New York: G. P. Putnam's Sons, 1877. 39p. DNLM
70-3256

SEGUIN, Edward C[onstant] (1843-1898)
Myelitis of the anterior horns, or spinal paralysis of the adult and child. . . . New York: G. P. Putnam's Sons, 1877. 120p. DLC; NNNAM; MBM **70-3257**

SEGUIN, Edward C[onstant] (1843-1898)
The diagnosis of progressive locomotor ataxia. New York: G. P. Putnam's Sons, 1878. 17p. DNLM **70-3258**

SEGUIN, Edward C[onstant] (1843-1898)
A contribution to the therapeutics of migraine. (Read before the section on practice of medicine in the New York Academy of Medicine, Nov. 20, 1877.) . . . New York: Trow's Printing & Bookbinding Company, 1878. 8p. DLC **70-3259**

SEGUIN, Edward C[onstant] (1843-1898)
Clinical lecture on syphilitic brain-lesions. [New York, 1878.] 8p. DNLM **70-3260**

SEGUIN, Edward C[onstant] (1843-1898), J. C. SHAW and A. VANDER VEER
A contribution to the pathological anatomy of disseminated cerebro-spinal sclerosis. Chicago: J. J. Spalding & Co., 1878. 13p. 1 plate. DNLM **70-3261**

SEGUIN, Edward C[onstant] (1843-1898)
Report on aconitia in trigeminal neuralgia. New York: D. Appleton & Co., 1878. 10p. DNLM **70-3262**

SEGUIN, Edward C[onstant] (1843-1898)
Lectures on the localization of spinal and cerebral diseases. Delivered at the College of Physicians and Surgeons. New York, 1878. 82p. DNLM **70-3263**

SEGUIN, Edward C[onstant] (1843-1898)
A contribution to the medicinal treatment of chronic trigeminal neuralgia. New York: J. F. Trow & Son, 1879. 13p. DNLM **70-3264**

SEGUIN, Edward C[onstant] (1843-1898)
Lunacy reform. Historical considerations. New York: G. P. Putnam's Sons, 1879. 15p. DNLM **70-3265**

SEGUIN, Edward C[onstant] (1843-1898)
Lunacy reform. II. Insufficiency of the medical staff of asylums. New York: G. P. Putnam's Sons, 1879. 9p. DNLM **70-3266**

SEGUIN, Edward C[onstant] (1843-1898)
A series of American clinical lectures. . . . New York: G. P. Putnam's Sons, 1879. 341p. DLC; NNNAM; PPC; PU [Issued in monthly numbers, January 1875 - December 1879] **70-3267**

SEILER, Carl (1849-1905)
Handbook of diagnosis and treatment of diseases of the throat and nasal cavities. . . . With thirty-five illustrations. Philadelphia: Henry C. Lea, 1879. 156p. DLC; MH-M; NNNAM; PPC **70-3268**

SEILER, EMMA
The voice in speaking. Transl. from the German by W. H. Furness. Philadelphia: J. B. Lippincott & Co., 1875. 164p. DNLM; MH; NN; NNC **70-3269**

SENN, Nicholas (1844-1908)
Medical legislation: being the annual address before the State Medical Society. Milwaukee, 1879. 24p. DNLM **70-3270**

SEYMOUR, William Pierce (1825-1893)
An introductory address to the medical class of 1873, of the Albany Medical College, Union University, delivered October 2, 1873. Albany: Van Benthuysen, 1873. 31p. DNLM **70-3271**

SHAFFER, Newton M[elman] (*b.* 1846)
The etiology and pathology of chronic joint disease. New York: G. P. Putnam's Sons, 1877. 41p. DNLM; NNNAM **70-3272**

SHAFFER, Newton M[elman] (*b.* 1846)
On reflex muscular contraction and atrophy in joint disease. With remarks on mechanical extension and a description of new apparatus. New York: Rutledge Co., 1877. 15p. DNLM **70-3273**

SHAFFER, Newton M[elman] (*b.* 1846)
Pott's disease, its pathology and mechanical treatment, with remarks on rotary lateral curvature. New York: G. P. Putnam's Sons, 1879. 82p. DLC; DNLM; NNNAM; PU **70-3274**

SHAKESPEARE, Edward O[ram] (1846-1900)
The Toner lectures. Lecture VII. The nature of reparatory inflammation in arteries after ligature, acupressure, and torsion. Washington: Smithsonian Institution, 1879. 70p. 7 plates. DLC; DNLM **70-3275**

SHARPLES, Stephen P[aschall] (*b.* 1842)
Milk analysis. Philadelphia, 1876. 7p. DNLM **70-3276**

SHATTUCK, Frederick Cheever (1847-1929)
Floating spleen. [Boston, 1878.] 6p. DNLM; MH-M **70-3277**

SHAW, Henry L.
The injurious effects of the nasal douche and other appliances for flooding the nasal cavity; with eighteen cases. Cambridge: Riverside Press, 1876. 8p. DNLM **70-3278**

SHAW, John Cargill (1845-1900)
Hysterical trismus. New York: G. P. Putnam's Sons, 1877. 14p. DNLM **70-3279**

SHAW, John Cargill (1845-1900)
Some peculiarities in the myeline of peripheral nerves after treatment by osmic acid. [Chicago, 1878.] 3p. DNLM **70-3280**

SHAW, John Cargill (1845-1900)
A case of progressive muscular atrophy with sclerosis of the lateral columns. [Chicago, 1879.] 9p. 1 plate. DNLM **70-3281**

SHEPARD, Charles U[pham], Jr. (1842-1915)
Foreign phosphates, being a lecture delivered before the Young Men's Christian Association, April 21, 1879, at the laboratory of the Medical College, Charleston, S.C. Charleston, S.C., 1879. 32p. DNLM **70-3282**

SHEPARD & DUDLEY's descriptive catalogue of apparatus for deformities and deficiencies, elastic stockings, galvanic batteries, inhalation apparatus, etc., etc. 150 William Street, New York, May, 1873. 121p. NNNAM **70-3283**

SHEPARD & DUDLEY. NEW YORK CITY
Catalogue of surgical instruments. New York: E. J. Kerr & Co., [1878?] 40p. DNLM; NNNAM **70-3284**

SHEPARD & DUDLEY. NEW YORK CITY
Illustrated catalogue of surgical instruments. Pt. 2. New York: Styles & Cash, 1878. 501-926p. DNLM; NNNAM **70-3285**

SHEPARD & DUDLEY. NEW YORK CITY
Descriptive catalogue of apparatus for deformities and deficiencies, elastic stockings, galvanic batteries, inhalation apparatus, etc. New York, 1879. 133p. DNLM; NNNAM **70-3286**

SHEPARD & DUDLEY. NEW YORK CITY
Catalogue of surgical instruments. New York: E. J. Kerr & Co., [1879?] 40p. DNLM; NNNAM **70-3287**

SHERMAN, Lewis
Directory of the homoeopathic physicians in the State of Wisconsin, containing a list of homoeopathic physicians in the State of Minnesota for the year 1874. Milwaukee: Godfrey & Crandall, 1874. 24p. DNLM **70-3288**

SHERMAN, Lewis
A test of the efficacy of the high dilutions. Published by the Milwaukee Academy of Medicine, December, 1878. Milwaukee, Wis.: Cramer, Aikens & Cramer, 1878. 7p. PPHa **70-3289**

SHERMAN, Lewis
Therapeutics and materia medica for the use of families and physicians. Milwaukee: Cramer, Aikens & Cramer, 1878. 203p. OCIM; PPHa **70-3290**

SHERMAN, Lewis
The potency question; or, the doctrine of transubstantiation. [Philadelphia, 1879.] 7p. DNLM **70-3291**

SHEW, Abram Marvin (1841-1886)
History and description of the Connecticut Hospital for the Insane. Middletown, Conn.: Pelton & King, 1876. 17p. 1 plate. **70-3292**

SHEW, Abram Marvin (1841-1886)
Mechanical restraint. [Utica, N.Y., 1879.] 7p. DNLM **70-3293**

SHEW, Joel (1816-1855)
The hydropathic family physician; a ready prescriber and hygienic adviser [etc.]. New York: S. R. Wells, 1873. 816p. DNLM; NNNAM **70-3294**

SHIPMAN, George Elias (1820-1893)
The homoeopathic family guide, for the use of twenty-eight principal remedies in the treatment of the more simple forms of disease. . . . Together with directions for the treatment of dengue and yellow fever. By W. H. Holcombe. . . . 8th ed. Chicago: The Western News Company, 1873. 311p. DLC; ICRM; IU-M; OCIM **70-3295**

SHOEMAKER, C. E. (*d.* 1891)
The ear: its diseases and injuries and their treatment. Reading, Pa.: Press of B. F. Owen, 1879. 375p. DLC; PPC; PPJ; PU **70-3296**

SHOEMAKER, John Veitch (1852-1910)
Valedictory address to the class on diseases of the skin at the Philadelphia School of Anatomy and Surgery, January 12, 1877. Philadelphia: Castle & King, 1877. 10p. DNLM; PPC **70-3297**

SHOEMAKER, John Veitch (1852-1910)
Baths, and their uses in the treatment of diseases of the skin. Valedictory address. January 16, 1878. Philadelphia: Collins, 1878. 31p. DNLM **70-3298**

SHOEMAKER, John Veitch (1852-1910)
Ringworm in public institutions. Rosacea. Philadelphia: Collins, 1878. 16p. DNLM **70-3299**

SHREVEPORT MEDICAL SOCIETY
Report of the committee on the yellow fever epidemic of 1873, at Shreveport, Louisiana. [Signed A. B. Snell, D. P. Fenner, J. F. Davis.] Shreveport: Simmons & Co., 1874. 23p. DNLM; LNT-M **70-3300**

SHURLY, Ernest Lorenzo (1845-1913)
On albumen in the treatment of pulmonary consumption. Buffalo: Baker, Jones & Co, 1877. 19p. DNLM **70-3301**

SHURTLEFF, George Augustus (1819-1902)
Address delivered before the Medical Society of the State of California at its annual session, April, 1873. Sacramento: T. A. Springer, 1873. 22p. CLM; CU-M; DNLM **70-3302**

SIBBET, R. Lowry (1826-1898)
An address read at the first meeting of the American Academy of Medicine in Philadelphia, September 6, 1876, on the necessity of an organization which shall encourage a higher standard of qualifications in the medical profession in the United States. Carlisle, Pa., 1877. 11p. DNLM **70-3303**

SICHEL, Arthur, *fils*
Lecture upon granulations of the conjunctiva. From the Archives générales de médecine. Transl. by Miss A. V. Culbertson. Cin[cinnati]: R. Clarke & Co., [1875]. 24p. DNLM; OCIM **70-3304**

SIEVEKING, Edward Henry (1816-1904)
The medical adviser in life assurance. Hartford, Conn.: N. P. Fletcher & Co., 1878. 183p. CtY-M; DNLM; MH-M **70-3305**

SILLIMAN, Benjamin (1816-1885)
A century of medicine and chemistry. A lecture introductory to the course of lectures to the medical class in Yale College. New Haven: C. C. Chatfield & Co., 1871. 65p. CtY-M; DNLM **70-3306**

SILLIMAN, Benjamin (1816-1885)
A fatal case of poisoning by arseniate of sodium. New York: Vanden Houten & Co., [1876]. 10p. DNLM **70-3307**

SIMMONS, Thomas Warfield (1836-1905)
Description of a splint for combined suspension and extension in the treatment of fracture of the lower extremity. Philadelphia, 1875. 5p. DNLM **70-3308**

SIMON, Christoph. Jakob F. L. (1824-1876)
Methods of rendering the female urinary bladder accessible, and on probing the ureter in women. A clinical lecture. Transl. expressly for the New York Medical Journal, with the consent and under the supervision of the author, by Augustus C. Bernays. New York: D. Appleton & Co., 1875. 33p. DNLM; NNNAM; NNU-M **70-3309**

SIMON, John (1816-1904)
Filth-diseases and their prevention. 1st American ed. Boston: J. Campbell, 1876. 96p. DNLM; MBM; MH-M; MdBJ-W **70-3310**

SIMONS, Manning (*b.* 1846)
Report on the climatology and epidemics of South Carolina. Philadelphia: Collins, 1872. 59p. DNLM **70-3311**

SIMONS, Manning (*b.* 1846)
Report of the committee on state medicine and public hygiene. [Charleston, 1877.] 77p. DNLM **70-3312**

SIMPSON, James Young (1811-1870)
A reply to Dr. Jacob Bigelow's second letter. [Anaesthetics.] [Boston, 1870.] 19p. DNLM **70-3313**

SIMPSON, James Young (1811-1870)
Anaesthesia, hospitalism, hermaphroditism, and a proposal to stamp out small-pox and other contagious diseases. . . . Ed. by Sir W. G. Simpson. . . . New York: D. Appleton & Co., 1872. 562p. DLC; NNNAM; PPC; PPJ **70-3314**

SIMPSON, James Young (1811-1870)
Clinical lectures on the diseases of women. Edited by Alexander R. Simpson. New York: D. Appleton & Co., 1872. 789p. CtY-M; DNLM; NNNAM; PPC **70-3315**

SIMS, James Marion (1813-1883)
On ovariotomy. New York: D. Appleton & Co., 1873. 85p. DNLM; NNNAM **70-3316**

SIMS, James Marion (1813-1883)
Legislation and "contagious diseases." An extract [etc.]. Philadelphia: Collins, 1876. 14p. DNLM **70-3317**

SIMS, James Marion (1813-1883)
Obituary. Gustav Simon. New York, 1877. 7p. DNLM **70-3318**

SIMS, James Marion (1813-1883)
The Woman's Hospital in 1874. A reply to the printed circular of Drs. E. R. Peaslee, T. A. Emmet, and T. Gaillard Thomas, addressed "To the medical profession," "May 5th, 1877." . . . New York: Kent & Co., printers, 1877. 24p. DLC; DNLM; NNNAM **70-3319**

SIMS, James Marion (1813-1883)
. . . The discovery of anaesthesia. . . . Richmond, [Va.] : J. W. Fergusson & Son, 1877. 20p. DLC; DNLM **70-3320**

SIMS, James Marion (1813-1883)
The treatment of epithelioma of the cervix uteri. New York: William Wood & Co., 1879. 41p. DNLM; NNNAM **70-3321**

SIMS, James Marion (1813-1883)
History of the discovery of anaesthesia. Richmond, 1877; New York, 1879. 14p. DNLM; NNNAM; ViRA **70-3322**

SIMS, James Marion (1813-1883)
Remarks on abscess of the liver. [Richmond], 1879. 6p. DNLM **70-3323**

SINGLETON, James William (1829-1881)
Medical heroism of 1878. St. Louis: G. O. Rumbold & Co., 1879. 11p. DNLM **70-3324**

SIZER, Nelson B.
A case of puerperal peritonitis complicated with acute yellow atrophy of the liver, with remarks. New York: William Wood & Co., 1874. 14p. DNLM **70-3325**

SKENE, Alexander Johnston Chalmers (1837-1900)
The relation of medical societies to progress in science. Inaugural address delivered before the Medical Society of the County of Kings, New York. Brooklyn: Rome Bros., 1874. 27p. DNLM; NBM; NNNAM **70-3326**

SKENE, Alexander Johnston Chalmers (1837-1900)
Diseases of the bladder and urethra in women. New York: William Wood & Co, 1878. 374p. DLC; DNLM; NNNAM; NNU-M **70-3327**

SKINNER, Thomas
Homoeopathy in its relation to the diseases of women. Philadelphia: Porter & Coates, 1876. 74p. DNLM **70-3328**

SKINNER, Thomas
Essay on the all-sufficiency of constitutional treatment in the special diseases of women. Read before the Hahnemann Academy of Medicine of New York, June 21, 1876. Printed for the Academy. Chicago: Duncan Brothers, 1876. 14p. DNLM **70-3329**

SKINNER, Thomas
Homoeopathy in its relation to the diseases of women. Philadelphia: Globe Printing House, 1879. 84p. PPHa **70-3330**

SMALL, Alvan Edmond (1811-1886)
The pocket manual of homoeopathic practice, arranged from the manual of homoeopathic practice of . . . by Jacob F. Sheek. New York: Boericke & Tafel; Philadelphia: F. E. Boericke, 1870. 126p. DNLM; NNNAM; PPC; PPHa **70-3331**

SMALL, Alvan Edmond (1811-1886)
Handbuch der Homoöpathie für Familien und das Publikum in Allgemeinen. In's Deutsche übersetzt von Karl Julius Hempel. 11. Aufl. New York: Boericke & Tafel, 1871. 643p. DNLM; NNNAM; PPG **70-3332**

SMALL, Alvan Edmond (1811-1886)
Annual address to the students and friends of Hahnemann Medical College, delivered October 3, 1876. Published by universal request. Chicago: S. H. Oakley, 1876. 12p. OCIM **70-3333**

SMALL, Alvan Edmond (1811-1886) and H. P. COLE
Address introductory to the 18th course of lectures of the Hahnemann Medical College and Hospital of Chicago, Ill. Delivered at the College October 2, 1877. Chicago: The United States Medical Investigator Print, 1877. 14p. OCIM
70-3334

SMART, Charles (1841-1905)
On mountain fever and malarious waters. [Philadelphia, 1878.] 27p. DNLM **70-3335**

SMEE, Alfred (1818-1877)
Accidents and emergencies: a guide containing directions for treatment in bleeding, cuts, stabs, bruises, sprains, ruptures. . . . With alterations, corrections, and appendix, by Dr. R. T. Trall. . . . New and rev. ed. New York: S. R. Wells & Co, 1876. 43p. DLC; NNNAM; PPJ **70-3336**

SMITH, Albert Holmes (1835-1885)
Clinical observations on the use of pessaries in the early months of pregnancy. [Philadelphia: Henry C. Lea, 1875.] 16p. 1 l. DNLM **70-3337**

SMITH, Albert Holmes (1835-1885)
Retarded dilatation of the os uteri in labor. Philadelphia: J. A. Moore, 1877. 46p. DNLM; PPC **70-3338**

SMITH, Albert Holmes (1835-1885)
Pendulum leverage of the obstetric forceps. [Boston, 1879.] 26p. DNLM **70-3339**

SMITH, Andrew Heermance (1837-1910)
. . . Oxygen gas as a remedy in disease. 2nd ed. . . . New York: D. Appleton & Company, 1870. 56p. DLC; DNLM; NNNAM
70-3340

SMITH, Andrew Heermance (1837-1910)
. . . The effects of high atmospheric pressure, including the caisson disease. . . . Brooklyn: Eagle Print, 1873. 53p. DLC; DNLM; NNNAM **70-3341**

SMITH, Andrew Heermance (1837-1910)
Supplementary rectal alimentation, and especially by defibrinated blood, as applicable to a large range of cases in which nutritive enemata have not heretofore been employed. New York: G. P. Putnam's Sons, 1879. 25p. DNLM; NNNAM
70-3342

SMITH, Andrew Heermance (1837-1910)
The first year of the Therapeutical Society of New York. New York: G. P. Putnam's Sons, 1879. 5p. DNLM
70-3343

SMITH, D[avid] D.
Combination and therapeutic action of some filling-materials. Philadelphia, 1878. 5p. DNLM **70-3344**

SMITH, Edward (1819-1874)
Foods. New York: D. Appleton & Co., 1873. 485p. 2 plates. DNLM; NN; NNC **70-3345**

SMITH, Edward (1819-1874)
Health: a handbook for households and schools. New York: D. Appleton & Co., 1875. 198p. DNLM; NN; NNNAM
70-3346

SMITH, Eugene R.
Homoeopathy in Tennessee; a brief sketch of its progress in the State, giving the number of societies and their respective officers, alphabetical list of the homoeopathic physicians, statistics, etc. Nashville: Tavel, Eastman & Howell, 1875. 23p. DNLM; OCIM; PPHa **70-3347**

SMITH, Eustace (1835-1914)
On the wasting diseases of infants and children. Philadelphia: Henry C. Lea, 1870. 195p. CtY-M; DNLM; NNNAM; PPC
70-3348

SMITH, Eustace (1835-1914)
On the wasting diseases of infants and children. 2nd American from the 2nd rev. and enl. English ed. Philadelphia: Henry C. Lea, 1871. 266p. ICRM; MBM; NNNAM; PU
70-3349

SMITH, Gouverneur Mather (*d.* 1898)
Discourse delivered on the occasion of the twenty-second anniversary of the New York Academy of Medicine, November 11, 1869. New York: William Wood & Co, 1870. 76p. DNLM; NNNAM **70-3350**

SMITH, Gouverneur Mather (*d.* 1898)
On diabetes. New York: William Wood & Co., 1871. 47p. DNLM **70-3351**

SMITH, Gouverneur Mather (*d.* 1898)
On the uses and derangements of the glycogenic function of the liver. Being remarks before the New York Academy of Medicine, June 15, 1871, in the discussion of Dr. J. C. Dalton's paper on "Sugar-formation in the liver." [New York, 1871.] 11p. DNLM **70-3352**

SMITH, Gouverneur Mather (*d.* 1898)
Memoir of the late William C. Roberts. Read before the New York Academy of Medicine, Thursday evening, April 2, 1874. New York: A. D. F. Randolph & Co., 1874. 30p. DNLM; NNNAM **70-3353**

SMITH, Gouverneur Mather (*d.* 1898)
Epidemics of the century, and lessons derived from them. New York: D. Appleton & Co., 1876. 34p. DNLM; NNNAM
70-3354

SMITH, Gouverneur Mather (*d.* 1898)
Derangement of the glycogenic function of the liver as a cause of Bright's disease. Philadelphia: Collins, 1878. 8p. DNLM
70-3355

SMITH, Henry
Report of the yellow fever epidemic of 1873, Shreveport, La. New Orleans: L. Graham & Co., 1874. 12p. DNLM; LNT-M
70-3356

SMITH, Henry Hollinsworth (1815-1890)
Biographical sketch of William L. Knight, ex-president of the Society, read before the Philadelphia County Medical Society. Philadelphia: Collins, 1878. 18p. DNLM; PPC
70-3357

SMITH, Henry Hollinsworth (1815-1890)
Address on certain points in the pathology of bones, especially tubercle. Philadelphia: Collins, 1878. 39p. 6 plates. DNLM; PU **70-3358**

SMITH, Henry Mitchell (*d.* 1901)
Smith's homoeopathic directory of New York and vicinity, 1872-1873. New York: Henry M. Smith. Smith's Homoeopathic Pharmacy, 1872. 32p. DNLM; NNNAM
70-3359

SMITH, Henry Mitchell (*d.* 1901)
List of medicines mentioned in homoeopathic literature. New York: Smith, 1879. 160p. DNLM; NNNAM; PPHa
70-3360

SMITH, J. Heber (1842-1898)
Thoughts for the times. An address delivered before the Homoeopathic Medical Society of Massachusetts. Boston: O. Clapp & Son, [1872]. 13p. DNLM; PPHa
70-3361

SMITH, J[ob] Lewis (1827-1897)
A treatise on the diseases of infancy and childhood. 2nd ed., enl. and thoroughly rev. . . . Philadelphia: Henry C. Lea, 1872. 741p. DLC; IU-M; NNNAM; PU
70-3362

SMITH, J[ob] Lewis (1827-1897)
A treatise on the diseases of infancy and childhood. . . . 3rd ed., enl. and thoroughly rev. . . . Philadelphia: Henry C. Lea, 1876. 724p. DLC; MdU-D; NNNAM; PPC
70-3363

SMITH, J[ob] Lewis (1827-1897)
Are diphtheritic and pseudo-membranous croup identical or distinct affections? Philadelphia: [Collins], 1877. 27p. DNLM; PPJ **70-3364**

SMITH, J[ob] Lewis (1827-1897)
A treatise on the diseases of infancy and childhood. . . . 4th ed., thoroughly rev. . . . Philadelphia: Henry C. Lea, 1879. 758p. DLC; MdBJ-W; PPC; PU **70-3365**

SMITH, Joel Washington (1824-1897)
Medical schools and their relations to the profession. Charles City [Iowa]: "Intelligencer," 1876. 6p. DNLM
70-3366

SMITH, Nathan Ryno (1797-1877)
Address concerning the late Dr. John H. O'Donovan, before the Medical and Chirurgical Faculty of Maryland. Baltimore: Kelly, Piet & Co., 1870. 16p. DNLM; MdBM
70-3367

SMITH, Nathan Ryno (1797-1877)
Semi-annual address before the Medical and Chirurgical Faculty of Maryland. Baltimore, 1872. 14p. DNLM; MdBM
70-3368

SMITH, Stephen (1823-1922)
Analysis of four hundred and thirty-nine recovered amputations in the continuity of the lower extremity. New York, 1871. 141p. DNLM; NNNAM **70-3369**

SMITH, Stephen (1823-1922)
Doctor in medicine, and other papers on professional subjects. New York: William Wood & Co., 1872. 308p. DNLM; ICU; NIC; NNNAM **70-3370**

SMITH, Stephen (1823-1922)
On the effects of high temperature upon the public health, and on measures of prevention. New York: T. L. Clacher, 1873. 25p. DNLM; NNNAM **70-3371**

SMITH, Stephen (1823-1922)
On the reciprocal relations of an efficient public health service and the highest educational qualifications of the medical profession. Cambridge, 1876. 16p. DNLM; MBM
70-3372

SMITH, Stephen (1823-1922)
Manual of the principles and practice of operative surgery. . . . Boston: Houghton, Osgood & Co.; Cambridge: The Riverside Press, 1879. 689p. DLC; DNLM; MH-M; NNNAM
70-3373

SMITH, W. H.
Practical mode of studying the heart. [Ann Arbor, 1879.] 15p. DNLM **70-3374**

SMYTH, Andrew W[oods] (1833-1916)
The collateral circulation in aneurism. Report of the successful ligation of the innominate, the common carotid, the vertebral, and the internal mammary arteries, in a case of right subclavian aneurism. New Orleans, La.: [L. Graham & Co.], 1876. 25p. DNLM; LNT-M **70-3375**

SMYTH, Andrew W[oods] (1833-1916)
The collateral circulation in aneurism. Report of the successful ligation of the innominate, the common carotid, the vertebral, and the internal mammary arteries, in a case of right subclavian aneurism. New Orleans: [German Gazette Job Office], 1877. 17p. DNLM; LNT-M **70-3376**

SNELLING, Frederick Greenwood (1831-1878)
Relaxation of the pelvic symphyses during pregnancy and parturition. New York: W. A. Townsend & Adams, 1870. 36p. DNLM; NNNAM **70-3377**

SNOW, C. W. & CO.
Illustrated catalogue of surgical instruments and appliances, galvanic batteries, elastic stockings, trusses, etc. Syracuse, N.Y.: C. M. Cornwell, 1878. 251p. DNLM **70-3378**

SNOW, Norman Leslie (1839-1885)
Some practical facts in fractures of the thigh, verified by the treatment of twenty-five cases occurring in private practice. New York: D. Appleton & Co., 1879. 13p. DNLM; NNNAM
70-3379

SOLLY, Samuel Edwin (1845-1906)
Manitou, Colorado, U.S.A., its mineral waters and climate. Saint Louis: J. McKittrick & Co., 1875. 39p. DNLM
70-3380

SPALDING, F. A.
A classification of the arterial, venous, and nervous systems of the human body. . . . Ann Arbor: Ann Arbor Printing & Publishing Co., 1873. 28p. DLC **70-3381**

SPENCER, Horatio N. (*b.* 1842)
Statistical report of 166 cases of diseases of the ear. [St. Louis, 1872.] 8p. DNLM **70-3382**

SPENCER, H[oratio] N. (*b.* 1842)
Statistical report of two hundred and fifty-five cases of diseases of the ear. St. Louis: The R. P. Studley Co., 1873. 16p. DNLM **70-3383**

SPENCER, H[oratio] N. (*b.* 1842)
Chronic suppuration of the middle ear in its relation to the brain. St. Louis: The R. P. Studley Co., 1875. 12p. 1 plate. DNLM **70-3384**

SPENCER, H[oratio] N. (*b.* **1842)**
The ear in the exanthemata. [St. Louis: L. C. Lavat & Co., 1878.] 12p. DNLM **70-3385**

SPINZIG, Carl
Epidemic diseases as dependent upon meteorological influences. St. Louis: Abner, Menning & Co., 1874. 58p. DNLM **70-3386**

SPINZIG, Carl
Cholera. The laws of its occurrence, non-occurrence and its nature. St. Louis, Mo.: Abner, Menning & Co., 1877. 52p. DNLM **70-3387**

SPINZIG, Carl
Variola: its causes, nature, and prophylaxis, and the dangers of vaccination. St. Louis: Buxton & Skinner, 1878. 86p. DNLM; OCIM **70-3388**

SPITZKA, Edward C[harles] (1852-1914)
Contributions to encephalic anatomy. [Chicago, 1877.] 11p. DNLM **70-3389**

SPITZKA, Edward C[harles] (1852-1914)
Reform in the scientific study of psychiatry. An address. Chicago, [1878]. 29p. DNLM **70-3390**

SQUIBB, Edward Robinson (1819-1900)
Liquor opii compositus, or compound solution of opium. Philadelphia: Merrihew & Son, 1870. 28p. DNLM **70-3391**

SQUIBB, Edward Robinson (1819-1900)
Report on the U.S. pharmacopoeia. Note on rhubarb, for 1869. Note on collodion by F. C. Mussgiller. Liquor opii compositus. Philadelphia: Merrihew & Son, 1870. 96p. DNLM **70-3392**

SQUIBB, Edward Robinson (1819-1900)
Anaesthetics. Read before the Medical Society of the State of New York, February 8, 1871. New York, 1871. 30p. DNLM **70-3393**

SQUIBB, Edward Robinson (1819-1900)
Notes on fluid extract of senega, cantharides and a blistering liquid, officinal extract of jalap, rhubarb, pareira, litmus paper, commercial bicarbonate of soda, and chloral. Philadelphia: Sherman & Co., 1872. 36p. DNLM **70-3394**

SQUIBB, Edward Robinson (1819-1900)
Notes, on a new form of percolator. The triplex pill. Rhubarb. Aconite root. Citrate of bismuth and ammonia. Aloes. Philadelphia: Sherman & Co., 1873. 30p. DNLM **70-3395**

SQUIBB, Edward Robinson (1819-1900)
Report on the new or fifth decennial revision of the United States Pharmacopoeia, to the Medical Society of the State of New York. New York: D. Appleton & Co., 1873. 25p. DNLM **70-3396**

SQUIBB, Edward Robinson (1819-1900)
Medical and pharmaceutical notes. On the preservation of hypodermic solutions. On ergot and its preparations. On rhubarb. On physician's pocket cases. On buying alcohol and distilled spirits. On a general apparatus stand, upright condenser, pinchcock, and burette stand. Philadelphia: Sherman & Co., 1874. 66p. DNLM **70-3397**

SQUIBB, Edward Robinson (1819-1900)
Note on salicyclic acid. Brooklyn, 1875. 10p. DNLM **70-3398**

SQUIBB, Edward R[obinson] (1819-1900)
Note on salicyclic acid. Brooklyn Eagle Print, 1875. 10p. DNLM **70-3399**

SQUIBB, Edward R[obinson] (1819-1900)
The American Medical Association and United States Pharmacopoeia. A reprint of the pamphelts of H. C. Wood, Alfred B. Taylor, the Philadelphia Medical Society, and the National College of Pharmacy, with a rejoinder addressed to the professions of medicine and pharmacy of the United States. Brooklyn, 1877. 157p. DLC; DNLM **70-3400**

SQUIBB, Edward Robinson (1819-1900)
The American Medical Association and the Pharmacopoeia of the United States of America. . . . Brooklyn: Eagle Print, 1877. 59p. DLC; DNLM **70-3401**

SQUIBB, Edward Robinson (1819-1900)
A universal pharmacopoeia. Philadelphia, 1877. 5p. DNLM **70-3402**

SQUIBB, Edward Robinson (1819-1900)
Note on the administration of phosphorus. Philadelphia: Sherman & Co., 1877. 15p. DNLM **70-3403**

SQUIBB, Edward Robinson (1819-1900)
Fluid extracts by repercolation. Philadelphia: Merrihew & Son, 1878. 43p. DNLM **70-3404**

SQUIBB, Edward Robinson (1819-1900)
Note on hydrobromic acid. Brooklyn, 1878. 11p. DNLM **70-3405**

SQUIBB, Edward Robinson (1819-1900)
Notes on the estimation of urea; and on the revision of the United States Pharmacopoeia in 1880. Syracuse: Truair, Smith & Bruce, 1879. 4p. DNLM **70-3406**

SQUIBB, Edward Robinson (1819-1900)
Proposed legislation on the adulteration of food and medicine. Rough draft of a proposed law to prevent the adulteration of food and medicine, and to create a State Board of Health, with explanations and illustrations of the principle points of the law. Notes in reply to criticisms by the press. The British "sales of food and drugs act of 1875," with notices of some rulings of the British court. New York: G. P. Putnam's Sons, 1879. 57p. DNLM **70-3407**

[STAMMERING]
The causes, prevention and treatment of stammering and stuttering, with the most approved and successful methods of self cure. Carefully compiled from the best authorities. New York: Haney & Co., [1870]. 42p. DLC; NNNAM **70-3408**

STAPLES, Franklin (1833-1904)
Report on the influence of climate on pulmonary diseases in Minnesota. Philadelphia: Collins, 1876. 41p. DNLM **70-3409**

STAPLES, Franklin (1833-1904)
Treatment of fracture of the shaft of the femur, the "American method." St. Paul: H. M. Smyth & Co., 1878. 22p. DNLM **70-3410**

STARKEY, George R. (1823-1896)
The compound oxygen treatment: its mode of action and results. Enlarged ed. Philadelphia: G. R. Starkey, [1870]. 144p. port. DNLM; PU **70-3411**

STARKEY, George R. (1823-1896)
The compound oxygen treatment: its mode of action and results. Enlarged ed. Philadelphia: G. R. Starkey, 1872. 144p. DNLM; PU **70-3412**

STARKEY, George R. (1823-1896)
The compound oxygen treatment: its mode of action and results. 3rd ed. Philadelphia: Starkey & Palen, 1877. 202p. DNLM; PU **70-3413**

STARKEY, George R. (1823-1896)
The compound oxygen treatment: its mode of action and results. 5th ed. Philadelphia: Starkey & Palen, 1879. 218p. DNLM; PU **70-3414**

STARR, Louis (1849-1925) and James B. WAKER
Chart of the physiological action of medicines. Philadelphia: Collins, 1877. 1 broadside. DNLM **70-3415**

STARTLING facts for the people regarding vaccination, for everybody who has any intention of being vaccinated; giving good reasons why caution should be taken; showing how thousands are being poisoned outright by impure virus, and giving in plain language such advice, from physicians eminent in the profession as will enable the public to take advantage of Jenner's discovery without imperilling life and health. New York: G. P. Sykes & Co., 1872. 53p. DNLM; NNNAM **70-3416**

STEARNS, Henry Putnam (1828-1905)
On medical examinations for life insurance. Hartford: Hutchings, 1873. 41p. CtY-M; DNLM **70-3417**

STEARNS, Henry Putnam (1828-1905)
The discovery of modern anaesthesia; a critique. . . . Hartford: Press of the Case, Lockwood & Brainard Co., 1876. 15p. DLC; DNLM **70-3418**

STEARNS, Henry Putnam (1828-1905)
An address: delivered to the graduating class in the medical department of Yale College. New Haven: Tuttle [and others], 1876. 15p. CtY-M; DNLM **70-3419**

STEARNS, Henry Putnam (1828-1905)
Statistics of insanity relative to readmissions to the Retreat. Hartford: The Lockwood & Brainard Co., 1876. 18p. DNLM; MBM **70-3420**

STEARNS, Henry Putnam (1828-1905)
The relations of insanity to modern civilization. Hartford, Conn.: The Case, Lockwood & Brainard Co., 1879. 14p. DNLM **70-3421**

STEELE, A. John (1835-1917)
Theory and practice of electrical therapeutics, or electricity as a curative agent. New York: Am. News Co., 1871. 192p. 5 plates. DNLM; NNNAM; PU **70-3422**

STEELE, Joel Dorman (1836-1886)
Fourteen weeks in human physiology. New York & Chicago: A. S. Barnes & Co., 1874. 238p. DNLM; MH; NN **70-3423**

STEIN, Alexander W. (1841-1897)
Pathology and treatment of urethritis. New York: D. Appleton & Co., 1870. 26p. DNLM **70-3424**

STEIN, Alexander W. (1841-1897)
Retention of urine depending on stricture. New York: R. J. Johnston, 1870. 16p. DNLM **70-3425**

STEIN, Alexander W. (1841-1897)
The histology and physiology of the penis. New York: D. Appleton & Co., 1872. 14p. 1 plate. DNLM **70-3426**

STEIN, Alexander W. (1841-1897)
Retention of urine. New York: D. Appleton & Co., 1874. 30p. DNLM **70-3427**

STEINER, Johann (1832-1876)
Compendium of children's diseases. A handbook for practitioners and students. Transl. from the 2nd German ed. by Lawson Tait. New York: D. Appleton & Co., 1875. 408p. CtY-M; DNLM; NNNAM; PPC **70-3428**

STEINER, Lewis H[enry] (1827-1892)
Annual oration before the Medical and Chirurgical Faculty of the State of Maryland, April 1874. . . . Baltimore: Innes & Co., printers, 1874. 18p. DLC; DNLM **70-3429**

STEINER, Lewis Henry (1827-1892)
Am I my brother's keeper? A discourse delivered before the American Public Health Association. Cambridge, 1876. 11p. DNLM **70-3430**

STEINER, Lewis Henry (1827-1892)
Health a prerequisite to national success in peace and war. Annapolis: G. Colton, 1878. 16p. DNLM **70-3431**

STEINER, Lewis Henry (1827-1892)
Annual address before the American Academy of Medicine, at New York, September 16th, 1879. . . . New York: C. L. Bermingham & Co., 1879. 16p. DLC; DNLM; NNNAM **70-3432**

STEINER, Lewis H[enry] (1827-1892)
Some changes required by the present status of medicine. Annual address delivered before the Society of the alumni of the Medical Department of the University of Pennsylvania, March 13, 1879. . . . Philadelphia: Collins, printer, 1879. 40p. DLC; DNLM; PPC **70-3433**

STELLWAG VON CARION, Carl (1823-1904)
Treatise on the diseases of the eye, including the anatomy of the organ. Transl. from the 3rd German ed. and edited by Charles E. Hackley and D. B. St. John Roosa. 2nd American ed. New York: William Wood & Co, 1870. 774p. 4 plates. DNLM; MdBJ-W; NNNAM; PU **70-3434**

STELLWAG VON CARION, Carl (1823-1904)
Treatise on the diseases of the eye, including the anatomy of the organ. Transl. from the 4th German ed., and edited by D. B. St. John Roosa, Charles S. Bull, and Charles E. Hackley. 4th ed. New York: William Wood & Co., 1873. 915p. 3 plates. CtY-M; DNLM; ICRM; NNNAM **70-3435**

STEPHENS, Charles R.
Inebriety, or vini morbus; a disease, and to be treated as such; modes of treatment, etc. Salem, Mass.: T. J. Hutchinson & Son, 1877. 61p. DNLM **70-3436**

STEPHENS, Philetus J.
A record of the surgical clinics of Wm. Tod Helmuth, M.D., held at the N.Y. Homoeopathic Medical College during the session of 1874-1875. To which is added a synopsis of the clinics of 1873-1874. New York, 1875. 207p. DNLM; NNNAM; PPHa; PU **70-3437**

STERNBERG, George M. (1838-1915)
An inquiry into the modus operandi of the yellow fever poison. [New Orleans, 1875.] 23p. DNLM **70-3438**

STERNBERG, George M. (1838-1915)
A study of the natural history of yellow fever and some remarks upon the treatment based upon the same; with cases and tables of observations upon the temperature and urine. [New Orleans, 1877.] 36p. DNLM **70-3439**

STERNBERG, George M. (1838-1915)
Photo micrographs. Washington, 1879. 69 plates. fol. DNLM **70-3440**

STEUDENER, Fridericus [Guilelmus Ernestus] (1839-1880)
Vegetable organisms as causes of disease. Transl. from the German by Conrad Georg. Ann Arbor, Mich.: J. R. Webster & Co., 1872. 41p. DNLM; OCIM **70-3441**

STEVENS, Edward B.
Pregnancy with albuminuric amaurosis. New York: William Wood & Co, 1878. 14p. DNLM; NNNAM **70-3442**

STEVENS, George T[homas] (1832-1921)
Method of study in medicine. Introductory lecture, Albany Medical College. Albany: Van Benthuysen, 1872. 15p. DNLM **70-3443**

STEVENS, George T[homas] (1832-1921)
Chorea: its cause and treatment. June 15, 1876. New York: D. Appleton & Co., 1876. 19p. DNLM; NNNAM **70-3444**

STEVENS, George T[homas] (1832-1921)
On light in some of its relations to disease. New York: D. Appleton & Co, 1877. 12p. DNLM **70-3445**

STEVENS, Thaddeus M. (1829-1885)
Medico-legal sciences. Indianapolis: Wright, Baker & Co., 1872. 10p. DNLM **70-3446**

STEVENS, Thaddeus M. (1829-1885)
Medico-legal investigations. [Indianapolis: Wright, Baker & Co., 1872.] 2p. DNLM **70-3447**

STEVENS, Thaddeus M. (1829-1885)
Expert testimony. [Indianapolis, 1873.] 11p. DNLM **70-3448**

STEVENS, Thaddeus M. (1829-1885)
Malpractice: responsibilities of surgeons and physicians. [Indianapolis, 1875.] 8p. DNLM **70-3449**

STEVENS, Thaddeus M. (1829-1885)
State boards of health. [Indianapolis, 1875.] 9p. DNLM **70-3450**

STEVENS, Thaddeus M. (1829-1885)
The psychology of Kathrina. [Cincinnati, 1877.] 8p. DNLM **70-3451**

STEVENS, Thaddeus M. (1829-1885)
Report of certain medico-legal cases. St. Louis: G. O. Rumbold & Co., 1879. 15p. DNLM **70-3452**

STEVENS, Thaddeus M. (1829-1885)
Address on state medicine. Cincinnati, 1879. 8p. DNLM **70-3453**

STEWARDSON, Thomas (1807-1878)
Biographical memoir of William W. Gerhard. Read before the College of Physicians of Philadelphia. Philadelphia: Collins, 1874. 13p. DNLM; PPC **70-3454**

STEWART, James Logan (1825-1890)
An address delivered before the Medical Society of the State of Pennsylvania. Philadelphia: Collins, 1879. 20p. DNLM **70-3455**

STEWART, Morse (1818-1906)
Pocket therapeutics and dose book: with classification and explanation of the action of medicines; index of diseases with appropriate remedies, classification of symptoms; poisons and their antidotes. . . . Detroit, Mich.: E. Schober, printer and binder, 1878. 101p. DLC; DNLM **70-3456**

STEWART, Morse (1818-1906)
Pocket therapeutics and dose book; with classification and explanation of the action of medicines . . . index and definition of diseases, with appropriate remedies . . . classification of symptoms. . . . By Morse Stewart, Jr. . . . 2nd ed. Rev. and enl. Detroit: G. D. Stewart, 1878. 263p. DLC; OCIM **70-3457**

STEWART, R[enel]
Comparative merits of cephalic and podalic (or vertex-first and vertex-last) deliveries through pelves narrowed in the conjugate diameter. Philadelphia: E. C. Markley & Son, 1875. 14p. 1 plate. DNLM; PPC **70-3458**

STEWART, Thomas Grainger (1837-1900)
A practical treatise on Bright's disease of the kidneys. 2nd ed. New York: William Wood & Co, 1871. 334p. 9 plates. CtY-M; DNLM; NNNAM; PPC **70-3459**

STILLÉ, Alfred (1813-1900)
Annual address, with the proceedings of the Society of the Alumni of the Medical Department of the University of Pennsylvania, at the anniversary meeting for 1873. Philadelphia: Collins, 1873. 52p. DNLM **70-3460**

STILLÉ, Alfred (1813-1900)
Epidemic or malignant cholera. Philadelphia: J. P. Lippincott & Co., 1873. 45p. DNLM **70-3461**

STILLÉ, Alfred (1813-1900)
Medical education; what it is, and what it might be made. An address. Philadelphia: Collins, 1873. 34p. DNLM **70-3462**

STILLÉ, Alfred (1813-1900)
Introductory lecture of the one hundred and ninth session of the Medical Department of the University of Pennsylvania. Philadelphia: Collins, 1874. 19p. DNLM
70-3463

STILLÉ, Alfred (1813-1900)
Therapeutics and materia medica. A systematic treatise on the action and uses of medicinal agents, including their description and history. . . . 4th ed., thoroughly rev. and enl. . . . Philadelphia: Henry C. Lea, 1874. 2 v. DLC; NNNAM; PPC; PU
70-3464

STILLÉ, Alfred (1813-1900)
The national dispensatory. Containing the natural history, chemistry, pharmacy, actions and uses of medicines, including those recognized in the pharmacopoeias of the United States and Great Britain. By Alfred Stillé . . . and John M. Maisch. . . . With two hundred and one illustrations. Philadelphia: Henry C. Lea, 1879. 1628p. DLC; OCLloyd; PPC; PU
70-3465

STILLÉ, Alfred (1813-1900)
The national dispensatory. Containing the natural history, chemistry, pharmacy, actions and uses of medicines. Including those recognized in the pharmacopoeias of the United States, Great Britain, and Germany, with numerous references to the French codex. Alfred Stillé . . . and John M. Maisch. . . . 2nd ed., thoroughly rev., with numerous additions. With two hundred and thirty-nine illustrations. Philadelphia: Henry C. Lea, 1879. 1680p. DLC; OCLloyd; PPJ; PU
70-3466

STILLÉ, Alfred (1813-1900)
The origin, nature, symptoms, and treatment of yellow fever. Philadelphia: S. M. Miller, [1879]. 20p. DNLM
70-3467

STIMSON, Lewis Atterbury (1844-1917)
Bacteria and their influence upon the origin and development of septic complications of wounds. Wood prize essay, 1875. New York: D. Appleton & Co., 1875. 34p. 1 plate. DNLM; NNNAM **70-3468**

STIMSON, Lewis Atterbury (1844-1917)
A manual of operative surgery. . . . With three hundred and thirty-two illustrations. Philadelphia: Henry C. Lea, 1878. 477p. DLC; IEN-M; NNNAM; PPC **70-3469**

STIMSON, Lewis Atterbury (1844-1917)
A contribution to the study of cancer of the rectum. New York: G. P. Putnam's Sons, 1879. 33p. DNLM
70-3470

STOCKTON-HOUGH, John
Description of an improved speculum. [Philadelphia, 1870.] 2p. DNLM **70-3471**

STOCKTON-HOUGH, John
Longevity, or, the relative viability of the sexes: particularly with regard to the relative liability to the inheritance of certain transmitted diseases, considered in relation to the selection of life insurance risks, with a view of exhibiting the unjustness of the practice of charging higher rates for women. Illustrated, in part, by the statistics of Philadelphia, for the eleven years ending 1871. [New York, 1873.] 9p. DNLM
70-3472

STOCKTON-HOUGH, John
Statistics relating to the births, deaths, marriages, and movements of population in the city of Philadelphia, from January 1, 1861, to January 1, 1872. [Philadelphia, 1873.] 24p. DNLM **70-3473**

STOCKTON-HOUGH, John
The laws of transmission of resemblance from parents to their children. [New York, 1873.] 16p. DNLM
70-3474

STOCKTON-HOUGH, John
On the relative influence of city and country life, on morality, health, fecundity, longevity, and mortality; read before the Social Science Association of Philadelphia. [Philadelphia, 1874.] 38p. DNLM **70-3475**

STOCKWELL, Cyrus M. (1823-1899)
Puerperal convulsions. A paper read before the St. Clair, Sanilac and Lapeer Medical Society. [Detroit, 1876.] 20p. DNLM **70-3476**

STOKES, William (1804-1878)
Lectures on fever, delivered in the theatre of the Meath Hospital and County of Dublin Infirmary. Ed. by John W. Moore. Philadelphia: Henry C. Lea, 1876. 264p. DLC; DNLM; NNNAM; PPC **70-3477**

STONE, Andrew
The new gospel of health, an effort to teach people the principles of vital magnetism; or how to replenish the springs of life without drugs or stimulants. Troy, N.Y.: Lung and Hygienic Institute, 1875. 519p. DLC; DNLM **70-3478**

STONE, John Osgood (1813-1876)
Clinical cases, medical and surgical. By the late . . . . New York: G. P. Putnam's Sons, 1878. 230p. 1 diag. DNLM; NNNAM; NNU-M **70-3479**

STONE, Warren (1843-1883)
A case of traumatic aneurism of the left subclavian artery treated successfully by distal compression. [New Orleans, 1875.] 5p. DNLM **70-3480**

STORER, David Humphreys (1804-1891)
Two frequent causes of uterine disease. Boston: J. Campbell, 1872. 11p. DNLM; MBM **70-3481**

STORER, Horatio Robinson (1830-1922)
The causation, course, and treatment of reflex insanity in women. . . . Boston: Lee & Shepard; New York: Lee, Shepard & Dillingham, 1871. 236p. DLC; DNLM; MBM; NNNAM
70-3482

STORER, Horatio [Robinson] (1830-1922)
The mutal relations of the medical profession, its press, and the community. . . . Boston: J. Campbell, 1872. 23p. DLC; DNLM; MBM **70-3483**

STORER, Horatio [Robinson] (1830-1922)
Female hygiene: a lecture delivered at Sacramento and San Francisco, by request of the State Board of Health of California. Boston: J. Campbell, 1872. 20p. DNLM
70-3484

STORER, Horatio [Robinson] (1830-1922)
Upon the treatment of strumous disease by what may be called the Solfatara method. Cambridge: Riverside Press, 1878. 10p. DNLM **70-3485**

STORER, Horatio [Robinson] (1830-1922)
The frequently gynaecological origin of inherited forms of strumous disease. Philadelphia: Collins, 1878. 14p. DNLM
70-3486

STORER, Horatio [Robinson] (1830-1922)
New or unappreciated aids in the treatment of strumous disease. [Richmond, 1879.] 7p. DNLM
70-3487

STOUT, Arthur B.
Report on medical education to the Medical Society of the State of California, April 18th, 1877. . . . Read by Jas. M. Browne, chairman of the standard committee on medical education, as a supplement to his report. San Francisco: E. Bosqui & Co., printers, 1877. 11p. DLC
70-3488

STOUT, Arthur B.
Report on mental diseases, to the Medical Society of the State of California, April, 1879. . . . [Sacramento? 1879?] 7p. DLC **70-3489**

STOWELL, T. B[lanchard] (*b.* 1846)
Syllabus of lectures in anatomy and physiology, for students of the State Normal and Training School, at Cortland, N.Y. Syracuse, N.Y.: David, Bardeen & Co., 1877. 80p. DNLM
70-3490

STRAWBRIDGE, George (1844-1914)
Ophthalmic contributions. I. Dermoid tumor of the cornea. II. An additional method for the determination of astigmatism. With an abstract from a paper on "Ophthalmometrical measurements of the cornea and cyrstalline lens." [By Woinow.] Repr. from: Tr. German Ophth. Soc. Heidelberg, Sept., 1869. III. Cyst of the iris, removed by operation. Philadelphia: Lindsay & Blakiston, 1873. 26p. 3 plates. DNLM; PPC; PPJ; PU **70-3491**

STRAWBRIDGE, George (1844-1914)
Report of forty recent cases of cataract extractions. Philadelphia, 1876. 8p. DNLM **70-3492**

STRICKER, Salomon (1834-1898)
A manual of histology . . . in cooperation with Th. Meynert, F. von Recklinghausen, Max Schultze, W. Waldeyer, and others. Transl. by Henry Power . . . James J. Putnam . . . J. Orme Green . . . Henry C. Eno, Thomas E. Satterthwaite, Edward C. Seguin, Lucius D. Bulkley, Edward L. Keyes and Francis E. Delafield. . . . American translation ed. by Albert H. Buck . . . with 431 illustrations. New York: William Wood & Co., 1879. 1106p. DLC; NNNAM; OCIM; PU
70-3493

STURGES, Edward B[aker] (*b.* 1845)
The durggist's legal directory. Philadelphia: Evans, Stoddart & Co., [1870]. 366p. DNLM; PPC; PPL
70-3494

STURGES, Octavius (1833-1894)
An introduction to the study of clinical medicine, being a guide to the investigation of disease for the use of students. Philadelphia: Henry C. Lea, 1873. 127p. DNLM; PPC; PPJ; PU **70-3495**

STURGIS, Frederic Russell (1844-1919)
On the etiology of hereditary syphilis. New York: D. Appleton & Co., 1873. 38p. DNLM **70-3496**

STURGIS, Frederic Russell (1844-1919)
On the prognosis of syphilis. Philadelphia, 1873. 8p. DNLM
70-3497

STURGIS, Frederic Russell (1844-1919)
What effect does syphilis have upon the duration of life? [New York, 1874.] 12p. DNLM **70-3498**

STURGIS, Frederic Russell (1844-1919)
Scleritis syphilitica; its pathology, course and treatment. New York: G. P. Putnam's Sons, 1875. 11p. DNLM
70-3499

STURGIS, Frederic Russell (1844-1919)
Upon some points in the etiology of hereditary syphilis. Chicago, 1876. 16p. DNLM **70-3500**

STURGIS, Frederic Russell (1844-1919)
Relations of syphilis to the public health. New York: H. Truss, Jr., 1877. 40p. DNLM **70-3501**

STURGIS, Frederic Russell (1844-1919)
Responsibility of the medical profession for the abuses of free medical services. [New York, 1879.] 8p. DNLM
70-3502

SUMMERS, Thomas Osmond (1852-1899)
Yellow fever. Nashville, Tenn.: Wheeler Bros., 1879. 72p. DNLM **70-3503**

SUSSDORFF, G. E.
A contribution to the differential diagnosis between hollow uterine polypus and complete inversion of the uterus. New York: William Wood & Co., 1877. 16p. DNLM; NNNAM
70-3504

SUTTON, George (1812-1886)
Man's power over nature, and medicines as means by which he aids and controls the laws of life. An address. Indianapolis: J. G. Doughty, 1870. 24p. DNLM **70-3505**

SUTTON, George (1812-1886)
Report on the diseases of Indiana for the year 1872; with a brief outline of the medical topography and climatology of different localities. Indianapolis, 1873. 33p. DNLM
70-3506

SUTTON, George (1812-1886)
A report on trichinosis, as observed in Dearborn Co., Ind., in 1874. Indianapolis: Baker, Schmidlap & Co., [1875]. 23p. DNLM **70-3507**

SUTTON, George (1812-1886)
Placenta previa, and its treatment. Aurora, Ind., 1878. 16p. DNLM **70-3508**

SWAYNE, Joseph Griffiths (1819-1903)
Obstetric aphorisms; for the use of students commencing midwifery practice. From the 4th revised English ed., with additions by Edward R. Hutchins. Philadelphia: Henry C. Lea, 1870. 177p. CtY-M; DNLM; NNNAM; PPC
70-3509

SWAYNE, Joseph Griffiths (1819-1903)
Obstetric aphorisms: for the use of students commencing midwifery practice. 2nd American from the 5th rev. English ed., with additions by Edward R. Hutchins. Philadelphia: Henry C. Lea, 1873. 189p. NNNAM; OCIM; PPJ; PU
70-3510

SWERINGEN, H. V.
Pharmaceutical lexicon; a dictionary of pharmaceutical science, [etc.]. Philadelphia: Lindsay & Blakiston, 1873. 576p. DNLM; OCLloyd; PPC; PU **70-3511**

SYDENHAM MEDICAL ASSOCIATION OF VINELAND, N.J.
Health influences of the climate of Vineland, New Jersey. Vineland, N.J.: F. P. Crocker, 1874. 41p. DNLM **70-3512**

TAFT, Jonathan (1820-1903)
A practical treatise on operative dentistry. . . . 3rd ed., with one hundred and twenty-eight illustrations. Philadelphia: Lindsay & Blakiston, 1877. 521p. DLC; ICRM; NNNAM; PPC **70-3513**

TAIT, [Robert] Lawson (1845-1899)
Hermaphroditism. Boston, 1876. 8p. DNLM **70-3514**

TAIT, [Robert] Lawson (1845-1899)
Diseases of women. New York: William Wood & Co., 1879. 192p. DNLM; MBM; NNNAM; PU **70-3515**

TALCOTT, Selden Haines (*d.* 1902)
Prognosis in insanity. New York, 1878. 20p. DNLM **70-3516**

TALCOTT, Selden Haines (*d.* 1902)
Medical notes on the treatment of mental and nervous diseases. New York, [1879]. 8p. DNLM **70-3517**

TALIAFERRO, Valentine Ham (1831-1887)
Observations upon medication by the use of uterine cloth tents, in diseases of the body and cavity of the uterus. Atlanta, Ga., 1871. 15p. DNLM **70-3518**

TALIAFERRO, Valentine Ham (1831-1887)
The corset in its relations to uterine diseases. Atlanta, Ga.: Herald Publishing Co., 1873. 13p. DNLM **70-3519**

TALIAFERRO, Valentine Ham (1831-1887)
New intra-uterine pessary, secured and steadied in position by silver suture. Atlanta, Ga.: H. H. Dickson, 1877. 6p. DNLM **70-3520**

TALIAFERRO, Valentine Ham (1831-1887)
The application of pressure in diseases of the uterus. Atlanta, Ga.: J. F. Harrison & Co., [1878]. 26p. DNLM **70-3521**

TALLEY, A[lexander] N[icholas] (1827-1897)
An address delivered before the South Carolina Medical Association. Columbia, S.C.: Presbyterian Publishing House, 1870. 16p. DNLM; ScMS **70-3522**

TANNER, Thomas Hawkes (1824-1871)
A manual of the practice of medicine. . . . 5th American from the 6th London ed. Philadelphia: Lindsay & Blakiston, 1870. 1200p. DNLM; MH-M; NNNAM; PPC **70-3523**

TANNER, Thomas Hawkes (1824-1871)
A practical treatise on the diseases of infancy and childhood. 3rd American ed., from the last London ed., revised and enlarged by Alfred Meadows. Philadelphia: Lindsay & Blakiston, 1871. 559p. CtY-M; DNLM; MH-M; NNNAM **70-3524**

TANNER, Thomas Hawkes (1824-1871)
Memoranda of poisons. 3rd American ed. from the last London enlarged ed. Philadelphia: Lindsay & Blakiston, 1875. 155p. CtY-M; DNLM; MBM; PU **70-3525**

TANNER, Thomas Hawkes (1824-1871)
A manual of clinical medicine and physical diagnosis. 3rd American from the 2nd English ed. Rev. and enl. by Tilbury Fox. Philadelphia: Henry C. Lea, 1876. 366p. ICRM; MdU-D; NNNAM; PU **70-3526**

TANNER, Thomas Hawkes (1824-1871)
Memoranda on poisons. 4th American from the last London enlarged and revised ed. Philadelphia: Lindsay & Blakiston, 1879. 201p. DNLM; MdBJ-W; NNNAM; PPJ **70-3527**

TAYLOR, Alfred B[ower] (1824-1898)
The pharmacopoeia of the United States and the American Medical Association. A review of a plan of revision proposed by Edward R. Squibb. Philadelphia: Merrihew & Son, [1877]. 18p. DNLM; PPC **70-3528**

TAYLOR, Alfred B[ower] (1824-1898)
Proposed changes in the U.S. pharmacopoeia. [Philadelphia, 1877.] 28p. DNLM **70-3529**

TAYLOR, Alfred Swaine (1806-1880)
A manual of medical jurisprudence. . . . 7th American ed., rev. from the author's latest notes and ed. with additional notes and references, by John J. Reese. . . . Philadelphia: Henry C. Lea, 1873. 879p. DLC; LNT-M; OCIM; NNNAM **70-3530**

TAYLOR, Alfred Swaine (1806-1880)
On poisons in relation to medical jurisprudence and medicine. 3rd American from the 3rd English ed. Philadelphia: Henry C. Lea, 1875. 788p. CU-M; DNLM; MBM; NNNAM **70-3531**

TAYLOR, Charles Bell (1830-1909)
On vivisection. [Philadelphia, 1879?] 2p. DNLM **70-3532**

TAYLOR, Charles Fayette (1827-1899)
On the management of lumbar and psoas abscess. New York: Turner & Mignard, 1870. 16p. DNLM **70-3533**

TAYLOR, Charles Fayette (1827-1899) and William R. FISHER
Papers on the therapeutic value of localized movements. Philadelphia: J. B. Lippincott & Co., 1871. 39p. DLC; DNLM **70-3534**

TAYLOR, Charles Fayette (1827-1899)
On the mechanical treatment of synovitis of the knee-joint. New York: D. Appleton & Co., 1873. 14p. DNLM **70-3535**

TAYLOR, Charles Fayette (1827-1899)
On the mechanical treatment of disease of the hip-joint. New York: William Wood & Co., 1873. 62p. DLC; DNLM **70-3536**

TAYLOR, Charles Fayette (1827-1899)
Observations on the mechanical treatment of disease of the hip-joint. [Boston, 1879.] 8p. DNLM **70-3537**

TAYLOR, Charles Fayette (1827-1899)
Emotional prodigality. Philadelphia: S. S. White, 1879. 16p. DNLM **70-3538**

TAYLOR, Edward R.
Stanzas written for the Sacramento Society for Medical Improvement and addressed to Thomas M. Logan. [Sacramento]: Carr, Dunn & Newhoff, [1872]. 11 l. DNLM **70-3539**

TAYLOR, George H. (1821-1896)
An illustrated sketch of the movement-cure: its principles, methods and effects. . . . New York: Pub. at the Institute, 1870. 48, 12p. DLC; NNNAM **70-3540**

TAYLOR, George H. (1821-1896)
Paralysis and other affections of the nerves; their cure by vibratory and special movements. New York: S. R. Wells, 1871. 149p. DNLM; OCIM; NNNAM; PU **70-3541**

TAYLOR, George H. (1821-1896)
Diseases of women: their causes, prevention, and radical cure. . . . Philadelphia, New York, [etc.]: G. Maclean, 1871. 318p. DLC; MdU-D; MBM; NNNAM **70-3542**

TAYLOR, George H. (1821-1896)
The cure of deformities by progressive divulsion and the development. New York: S. R. Wells, 1874. 28p. DNLM; NNNAM **70-3543**

TAYLOR, Isaac Ebenezer (1812-1889)
On the mechanism of spontaneous active uterine inversion, and the reduction of a case of complete inversion by the combined rectal and vaginal taxis. New York: D. Appleton & Co., 1872. 43p. 2 plates. DNLM; NNNAM **70-3544**

TAYLOR, Isaac Ebenezer (1812-1889)
What is the best treatment in contracted pelves? New York: D. Appleton & Co., 1876. 64p. 3 plates. DNLM; NNNAM; PPC **70-3545**

TAYLOR, Isaac Ebenezer (1812-1889)
On the early delivery of the placenta when previa. [Boston, 1879.] 27p. 3 plates. DNLM; MH-M **70-3546**

TAYLOR, Morse K. (1823-1889)
Poisoning by bin-iodide of mercury. Report of a case of poisoning by bin-iodide of mercury, occurring at Fort Gratiot, Michigan, June 27, 1869. Port Huron, Mich.: Port Huron Times Co., 1870. 3 l. DNLM **70-3547**

TAYLOR, Robert William (1842-1908)
On dactylitis syphilitica, with observations on syphilitic lesions of the joints. New York: F. W. Christern, 1871. 30p. DNLM **70-3548**

TAYLOR, Robert William (1842-1908)
On chronic hypertrophy of the lips. New York: W. Baldwin & Co., 1871. 8p. DNLM **70-3549**

TAYLOR, Robert William (1842-1908)
Clinical observations on contagious impetigo. [New York, 1872.] 4p. DNLM **70-3550**

TAYLOR, Robert William (1842-1908)
On some practical points in the treatment of the phimosis produced by chancroidal ulcers. New York: F. W. Christern, 1872. 19p. DNLM **70-3551**

TAYLOR, Robert William (1842-1908)
On the question of the transmission of syphilitic contagion in the rite of circumcision. New York: D. Appleton & Co., 1873. 24p. DNLM **70-3552**

TAYLOR, Robert William (1842-1908)
The dangers of the transmission of syphilis between nursing children and nurses in infant asylums and in private practice. New York: William Wood & Co., 1875. 18p. DNLM **70-3553**

TAYLOR, Robert William (1842-1908)
Syphilitic lesions of the osseous system in infants and young children. New York: William Wood & Co., 1875. 179p. DLC; NNNAM; PU **70-3554**

TAYLOR, Robert William (1842-1908)
Etiology of infantile eczema. Louisville: I. P. Morton & Co., 1875. 20p. DNLM **70-3555**

TAYLOR, Robert William (1842-1908)
On a rare form of idiopathic localized or partial atrophy of the skin. New York: G. P. Putnam's Sons, 1876. 8p. DNLM **70-3556**

TAYLOR, Robert William (1842-1908)
On the treatment of eczema. New York: G. P. Putnam's Sons, 1876. 28p. DNLM **70-3557**

TAYLOR, Robert William (1842-1908)
A case in which syphilitic contagion was conveyed in the operation of vaccination, with remarks upon the means of prevention. New York: G. P. Putnam's Sons, 1876. 9p. DNLM **70-3558**

TAYLOR, Robert William (1842-1908)
A contribution to the study of syphilis of the nervous system. Chicago: J. J. Spalding & Co., 1876. 23p. DNLM; NNNAM **70-3559**

TAYLOR, Robert William (1842-1908)
A contribution to the study of the transmission of syphilis. New York: Rutledge & Co., 1876. 15p. DNLM **70-3560**

TAYLOR, Robert William (1842-1908)
On the various forms of pruritus cutaneus, and their treatment. New York: Rutledge & Co., 1877. 18p. DNLM **70-3561**

TAYLOR, Robert William (1842-1908)
On the treatment of the various forms of acne and of rosacca. New York: G. P. Putnam's Sons, 1878. 32p. DNLM; NNNAM **70-3562**

TAYLOR, Walter C.
A physician's counsels to woman, in health and disease. . . . Springfield, [Mass.]: W. J. Holland & Co., 1871. 403p. DLC; MH; MH-M **70-3563**

TAYLOR, Walter C.
A physician's counsels to man, in health and disease. . . . Springfield, [Mass.]: W. J. Holland & Co., 1872. 399p. DLC; MH-M **70-3564**

TEWKSBURY, Samuel Henry (1819-1880)
Vesico-vaginal lithotomy in a child seven years old. Portland: S. Berry, 1871. 8p. DNLM **70-3565**

THACHER, L. K.
Kansas City College of Physicians and Surgeons. Second annual commencement, March 7th, 1871. Address by. . . . Valedictory by T. B. Lester. Kansas City, Mo., 1871. 14p. DNLM **70-3566**

THACKER, John Adams (1833-1891)
Psychology of vice and crime. Valedictory address. [Cincinnati] : H. Watkin, 1873. 17p. DNLM **70-3567**

THAYER, B. B.
Thayer's elixir of chloral hydrate; remarks upon and details of cases treated with chloral hydrate. San Francisco: E. Bosqui & Co., [1870?] . 20p. DNLM **70-3568**

THAYER, Charles P.
The Vermont Medical Register, for the year 1877, containing a complete list of the regular physicians, dentists, and druggists of the State, with their residences, post-office address, dates and source of degrees, laws of the State affecting these professions, and a mass of other useful information concerning them. Burlington, 1877. 12p. CtY-M; DNLM; MBM **70-3569**

THAYER, David (1813-1893)
"The coming doctor." Annual address before the Massachusetts Homoeopathic Medical Society, 1870. Taunton: C. A. Hack & Son, 1875. 26p. DNLM; MH-M **70-3570**

THAYER, HENRY & CO.
Descriptive catalogue of fluid and solid extracts in vacuo, also concentrations and officinal pills, prepared by Henry Thayer & Co. with formulas and receipts. Cambridgeport, Mass., 1876. 218p. MH; MWA; OCLloyd **70-3571**

THAYER, William Henry (1822-1897)
Obligations and duties of a county medical society. Inaugural address of the president of the Medical Society of the County of Kings, New York. Brooklyn: J. Keller, 1872. 10p. DNLM **70-3572**

THEOBOLD, Samuel (1846-1930)
An endeavor to show that insufficiency of the internal recti muscles and myopia have been erroneously associated; and that the muscular asthenopia of myopia is not the result of such insufficiency, but of the anomaly of refraction. [Philadelphia, 1874.] 13p. DNLM **70-3573**

THEOBOLD, Samuel (1846-1930)
Tinnitus aurium; a consideration of the causes upon which it depends, and an attempt to explain its production in accordance with physical principles. Baltimore: Innes & Co., 1875. 13p. DNLM **70-3574**

THEOBOLD, Samuel (1846-1930)
Notes on the progress of ophthalmology. [Baltimore, 1876.] 11p. DNLM **70-3575**

THEOBOLD, Samuel (1846-1930)
Remarks on the nature and treatment of convergent strabismus. Baltimore: J. H. Foster, 1877. 10p. DNLM **70-3576**

THEOBOLD, Samuel (1846-1930)
On the use of large probes in the treatment of strictures of the nasal duct. Baltimore: Innes & Co., 1877. 22p. DNLM **70-3577**

THEOBOLD, Samuel (1846-1930)
Further testimony in favor of the use of large probes in the treatment of strictures of the nasal duct. New York: William Wood & Co., 1878. 6p. DNLM **70-3578**

THEOBOLD, Samuel (1846-1930)
Some cases of traumatic lesions of the eye of unusual character. [Richmond, 1878.] 8p. DNLM **70-3579**

THEOBOLD, Samuel (1846-1930)
The scepticism prevalent regarding the efficacy of aural therapeutics. To what extent is it justifiable? [Baltimore, 1879.] 10p. DNLM **70-3580**

THEOBOLD, Samuel (1846-1930)
The value of atropia in the treatment of acute inflammation of the middle ear. New York: William Wood & Co., 1879. 6p. DNLM **70-3581**

THOMAS, Amos Russell (1826-1892)
Valedictory address to the graduates of the Hahnemann Medical College of Philadelphia, delivered at the 24th annual commencement, held at the Academy of Music, March 11, 1872. Philadelphia: William P. Kildare, 1872. 16p. DNLM; PPHa **70-3582**

THOMAS, Amos Russell (1826-1892)
A practical guide for making post-mortem examinations, and for the study of morbid anatomy, with directions for embalming the dead, and for the preservation of specimens of morbid anatomy. New York and Philadelphia: Boericke & Tafel, 1873. 337p. DNLM; PPHa; PU **70-3583**

THOMAS, Charles Hermon (*b.* 1839)
A general system of measurements for urethral, uterine, rectal and other instruments; and an adaptable metric gauge. [Philadelphia, 1879.] 2 l. DNLM **70-3584**

THOMAS, Charles Monroe
On the importance of correcting optical defects in the eye, in the treatment of certain neuralgic pains in the head, with other sympathetic affections. Philadelphia: W. P. Kildare, 1876. 14p. PPHa **70-3585**

THOMAS, Charles Monroe
Laceration of the female perineum. Philadelphia: Sherman & Co., 1877. 11p. PPHa **70-3586**

THOMAS, Charles Monroe
Glaucoma; the importance of its early recognition and proper treatment. Philadelphia: Sherman & Co., 1877. 8p. PPHa **70-3587**

THOMAS, Daniel Golden (1806-1880)
History of the Medical Society of Oneida County, from its organization, July, 1806, to July, 1878. Utica, N.Y.: T. J. Griffiths, 1878. 40p. DNLM **70-3588**

THOMAS, F[rederick] R.
Manual of the discovery, manufacture, and administration of nitrous oxide, or laughing gas, in its relations to dental or minor surgical operations, and particularly for the painless extraction of teeth. Philadelphia: S. S. White, 1870. 122p. DNLM; MWA; PU **70-3589**

THOMAS, James Gray (1835-1884)
The use of baths in typhoid fever. Charleston, S.C.: News & Courier Job Presses, 1876. 8p. 1 ch. DNLM; ScCM
70-3590

THOMAS, Joseph (1811-1891)
A comprehensive medical dictionary: containing the pronunciation, etymology, and signification of the terms made use of in medicine and the kindred sciences. With an appendix, comprising a complete list of all the more important articles of the materia medica, arranged according to their medicinal properties. Philadelphia: J. B. Lippincott & Co., 1872. 704p. DNLM; NNNAM; PPC; PU **70-3591**

THOMAS, T[heodore] Gaillard (1832-1903)
Gastro-elytrotomy: a substitute for the Caesarean section. New York: W. A. Townsend & Adams, [1870]. 15p. DNLM
70-3592

THOMAS, T[heodore] Gaillard (1832-1903)
A practical treatise on the diseases of women. . . . 3rd ed., enl. and thoroughly rev., with two hundred and forty-six illustrations on wood. Philadelphia: Henry C. Lea, 1872. 784p. DLC; OCIM; PPC; PU **70-3593**

THOMAS, T[heodore] Gaillard (1832-1903)
A practical treatise on the diseases of women. . . . 4th ed. Philadelphia: Henry C. Lea, 1874. 801p. DNLM; NNNAM; PPC; PU **70-3594**

THOMAS, T[heodore] Gaillard (1832-1903)
A clinical contribution to the treatment of tubal pregnancy. New York: D. Appleton & Co., 1875. 11p. DNLM
70-3595

THOMAS, T[heodore] Gaillard (1832-1903)
Remarks on chronic dysentery; with the history of a case of five years' standing cured within five weeks by topical treatment. New York: D. Appleton & Co., 1876. 10p. DNLM
70-3596

THOMAS, T[heodore] Gaillard (1832-1903)
Remarks upon the enucleation of uterine fibroids, with illustrative cases. New York: Rutledge & Co., 1876. 14p. DNLM
70-3597

THOMAS, T[heodore] Gaillard (1832-1903)
Double ovariotomy performed for the removal of solid ovarian tumors. Transfusion of milk four days after operation. Philadelphia: Collins, 1876. 8p. DNLM **70-3598**

THOMAS, T[heodore] Gaillard (1832-1903)
A case of abdominal pregnancy treated by laparatomy. [Boston, 1877.] 9p. DNLM **70-3599**

THOMAS, T[heodore] Gaillard (1832-1903)
The prophylactic treatment of placenta praevia. Indianapolis, Ind., 1877. 16p. DNLM **70-3600**

THOMAS, T[heodore] Gaillard (1832-1903)
The influences which are elevating medicine to the position of a science; an anniversary discourse delivered before the New York Academy of Medicine. New York, 1877. 24p. DNLM
70-3601

THOMAS, T[heodore] Gaillard (1832-1903)
Laparo-elytrotomy; a substitute for the Caesarean section. New York: William Wood & Co., 1878. 25p. DNLM
70-3602

THOMAS, T[heodore] Gaillard (1832-1903)
The intra-venous injection of milk as a substitute for the transfusion of blood. Illustrated by seven operations. New York: D. Appleton & Co., 1878. 19p. DNLM
70-3603

THOMAS, T[heodore] Gaillard (1832-1903)
Comparison of the results of the Caesarean section and laparo-elytrotomy in New York. [New York, 1878.] 3p. DNLM
70-3604

THOMAS, T[heodore] Gaillard (1832-1903)
The most effectual method for controlling the high temperature occurring after ovariotomy. New York: D. Appleton & Co., 1878. 21p. DNLM **70-3605**

THOMAS, T[heodore] Gaillard (1832-1903)
Notes from lectures on obstetrics. New York: J. J. O'Brien, 1878. 81p. DNLM **70-3606**

THOMAS, T[heodore] Gaillard (1832-1903)
A new method of removing interstitial and submucous fibroids of the uterus; illustrated by cases. New York: G. P. Putnam's Sons, 1879. 32p. DNLM **70-3607**

THE THOMAS WILSON SANITARIUM FOR CHILDREN OF BALTIMORE CITY
[Circular of the trustees to persons of experience, requesting their views on the treatment and care of children, and the best method of establishing a sanitarium, or summer retreat.] Dec. 8, 1879. [Baltimore, 1879.] 3 sheets. DNLM [Incorporated July 2, 1875; opened June 16, 1884.]
70-3608

THOMPSON, Henry (1820-1904)
The diseases of the prostate: their pathology and treatment; comprising the Jacksonian prize essay for the year 1860. 4th ed. Philadelphia: Henry C. Lea, 1873. 364p. NNNAM; MBM; PPC; PU **70-3609**

THOMPSON, Henry (1820-1904)
Clinical lectures on the diseases of the urinary organs. Delivered at the University College Hospital. 2nd American from the 3rd and revised English ed. Philadelphia: Henry C. Lea, 1874. 195p. CtY-M; DNLM; NNNAM; PPC
70-3610

THOMPSON, J. Harry
Operations for the radical cure of lacerated or ruptured perineum. [Washington, 1870.] 32p. DNLM
70-3611

THOMPSON, J. Harry and P. T. KEENE
Addresses delivered at the 21st commencement of the Medical Department of Georgetown College. Washington, D.C.: Judd & Detweiler, 1870. 27p. DNLM **70-3612**

THOMPSON, J. Harry
Report of the Columbia Hospital for Women and Lying-in Asylum, Washington, with appendix. Washington: Government Printing Office, 1873. 430p. 1 l. DNLM
70-3613

THOMPSON, Joseph W. (1838-1886)
Tri-States Medical Society. Address of the president. Paducah, Ky.: Martin & Co., 1877. 19p. DNLM
70-3614

THOMPSON, Rezin
Specimen pages [of] The medical adviser: a full and plain treatise on the theory and practice of medicine, especially adapted to family use. Cincinnati: Nat. Pub. Co.; Chicago: Jones, Junkin & Co., 1870. 23 l. 8 plates. DNLM
70-3615

THOMSON, Spencer (1848-1883)
A dictionary of domestic medicine and household surgery. . . . 10th American, from the last London ed. Rev. with additions, by Henry H. Smith. . . . Philadelphia: Claxton, Remsen & Haffelfinger, 1877. 582p. DLC; NNNAM; PPC; PU
70-3616

THOMSON, William (1833-1907)
An additional test for the diagnosis and correction of the optical defects of the eye. [Philadelphia, 1870.] 4p. DLC; DNLM **70-3617**

THOMSON, William (1833-1907)
An additional method to determine the degree of ametropia. [New York, 1871.] 8p. DLC; DNLM **70-3618**

THOMSON, William (1833-1907)
An additional test for the diagnosis of ametropia, with a method to determine its various degrees. New York: William Wood & Co., 1872. 14p. DNLM **70-3619**

THOMSON, William (1833-1907)
Relation of ophthalmology to practical medicine. An introductory to the summer course of lectures of the Jefferson Medical College. Philadelphia: J. B. Lippincott & Co., 1875. 27p. DLC; DNLM **70-3620**

THOMSON, William (1833-1907)
A practical and rapid method, with an instrument, for the diagnosis of the refraction. [New York, 1878.] 7p. DNLM
70-3621

THOMSON, William Henry (*d.* 1893)
Lectureships for physicians. An anniversary discourse delivered before the New York Academy of Medicine. New York, 1878. 21p. DNLM; NNNAM **70-3622**

THRESHER, Leonard
The ladies' private medical guide; an essay giving the causes, symptoms, and treatment of all diseases peculiar to women, infants, and older children, with an appendix giving recipes for the preparation of medicines and their uses; followed by an address and advice to young females. Montpelier, 1875. 104p. DNLM **70-3623**

THUDICHUM, Joh. Ludwig. Wilh. (1829-1901)
A manual of chemical physiology, including its points of contact with pathology. New York: William Wood & Co., 1872. 195p. DNLM; NNNAM; PPJ; PU
70-3624

TIEMANN, GEORGE, & CO., NEW YORK
Catalogue of surgical instruments, manufactured and sold by Geo. Tiemann & Co. . . . New York: H. Ludwig, printer (1872-1875] . 4 v. DLC; NNNAM **70-3625**

TIEMANN, GEORGE, & CO., NEW YORK
The American armamentarium chirurgicum. A representation of modern, chiefly American, patterns of surgical instruments. . . . New York: Carle & Grener, printers, 1872. 17p. 41 plates. DLC; NNNAM **70-3626**

TIEMANN, GEORGE & CO.
Catalogue of surgical instruments for 1872; 1874. New York, [1872-1874] . 114p. DNLM; NNNAM **70-3627**

TIEMANN, GEORGE & CO.
Illustrated catalogue of surgical instruments. Index and price-list to Part I. New York: H. Ludwig, [1874] . 64p. DNLM; NNNAM **70-3628**

TIEMANN, GEORGE & CO.
Illustrated catalogue of surgical instruments. Index and price-list to Part II. New York, [1874] . 114p. DNLM; NNNAM
70-3629

TIEMANN, GEORGE & CO.
Illustrated catalogue of surgical instruments. Index and price-list to Part IV. New York: Carle & Grener, 1874. 88p. DNLM; NNNAM **70-3630**

TIEMANN, GEORGE & CO.
Catalogue of surgical instruments. New York, [1876] . 64p. DNLM; NNNAM **70-3631**

TIEMANN, GEORGE & CO.
The American armamentarium chirurgicum. New York. [C. H. Ludwig, 1879] . 33, 134, 102, 126, 136, 14, 32, 36p. DNLM; NNNAM **70-3632**

TIFFANY, Louis McLane (1844-1916)
Removal of naso-pharyngeal polypus by temporary depression of both upper jaws. Baltimore: Innes & Co., 1878. 8p. DNLM
70-3633

TILDEN & CO. NEW LEBANON, N.Y.
Catalogue of pure medicinal preparations. [New York, 1874, *vel subseq.*] 16 l. DNLM; NNNAM **70-3634**

TILDEN & CO. NEW LEBANON, N.Y.
Formulae for making tinctures, infusions, syrups, wines, mixtures, pills. . . . New Lebanon, N.Y., 1874. 230p. DNLM; NNNAM **70-3635**

TILT, [John] Edward (1815-1893)
The change of life, [etc.] . On the preservation of the health of women at the critical periods of life. From 3rd London ed. Philadelphia: Lindsay & Blakiston, 1871. 292p. DNLM; NNNAM; PPC; PU **70-3636**

TODD, S[imeon] S[eymour] (1826-1899)
Anesthetics in labor. [Kansas City, Mo., 1875.] 25p. DNLM
70-3637

TODD, S[imeon] S[eymour] (1826-1899)
Report of two cases of ovariotomy. St. Louis, Mo.: W. P. Kremer, [1877] . 13p. DNLM **70-3638**

TOLAND, Hugh Hughes (1806-1880)
Lectures on practical surgery. 2nd ed. Philadelphia: Lindsay & Blakiston, 1879. 520p. DNLM; LNT-M; NNNAM; PPC [1st ed. 1877] **70-3639**

TOMES, Charles S[issmore] (1846-1928)
An address delivered at the commencement exercises of the dental department in Harvard University, February 12, 1873. Saint Louis: Missouri Dental Journal, 1873. 12p. DNLM; MH-M **70-3640**

TONER, Joseph Meredith (1825-1896)
Facts of vital statistics in the United States; with tables and diagrams. Extracts from an address. [Washington, 1872.] 9p. 7 tables. DNLM **70-3641**

TONER, Joseph Meredith (1825-1896)
The late Charles A. Lee, M.D. Obituary notice. [New York, 1872.] 12p. DNLM **70-3642**

TONER, Joseph Meredith (1825-1896)
Free parks and camping grounds; or sanitariums for the sick and debilitated children of large cities during the summer months. By J. M. Toner. Infant mortality, by H. C. Hand. Minneapolis: Johnson & Smith, [1872]. 16p. DNLM **70-3643**

TONER, Joseph Meredith (1825-1896)
Address of . . . , President of the American Medical Association. Extracted from the Transactions of the American Medical Association. Philadelphia: Collins, 1874. 20p. DNLM **70-3644**

TONER, Joseph Meredith (1825-1896)
Contributions to the study of yellow fever, a paper read before the American Public Health Association, New York, November 12, 1873, on the natural history and distribution of yellow fever in the United States. . . . [Washington, 1874.] 36p. tables, fold. map. DLC; DNLM; PU **70-3645**

TONER, Joseph Meredith (1825-1896)
. . . Contributions to the study of yellow fever. A. —The distribution and natural history of yellow fever in the United States. . . . by J. M. Toner, M.D. B — The yellow-fever epidemic of 1873; reports from medical officers, U.S. marine-hospital service, with note by the supervising surgeon, John M. Woodworth, M.D. Washington, 1874. 51p. tables, fold. map. DLC; DNLM **70-3646**

TONER, Joseph Meredith (1825-1896)
Contributions to the annals of medical progress and medical education in the United States before and during the war of independence. . . . Washington: Government Printing Office, 1874. 118p. DLC; DNLM; NNNAM; PPC **70-3647**

TONER, Joseph Meredith (1825-1896)
Annual oration before the Medical and Chirurgical Faculty of Maryland, April 14, 1875. Contribution to the medical history and physical geography of Maryland. . . . Baltimore: Innes & Co., printers and binders, 1875. 31p. DLC; DNLM; MdBM **70-3648**

TONER, Joseph Meredith (1825-1896)
The medical men of the revolution, with a brief history of the medical department of the Continental Army. Containing the names of nearly twelve hundred physicians. An address before the Alumni Association of Jefferson Medical College, March 11, 1876. . . . Philadelphia: Collins, printer, 1876. 140p. DLC; DNLM; PPJ; PU **70-3649**

TONER, Joseph Meredith (1825-1896) and L. S. McMURTRY
A biographical sketch of John D. Jackson, M.D., of Danville, Ky. Louisville, Ky., 1876. 11p. port. DNLM **70-3650**

TONER, Joseph Meredith (1825-1896)
An address on some of the leading public health questions; with remarks on the extent of swamp lands in the United States, and their reclamation as a sanitary and economic measure. Delivered at the opening of the third annual meeting of the American Public Health Association, Baltimore, Md., November 9, 1875. . . . Cambridge: Printed at the Riverside Press, 1876. 40p. DLC; DNLM; MH-M **70-3651**

TONER, Joseph Meredith (1825-1896)
An address on medical biography. (Delivered before the International Medical Congress at Philadelphia, September 5, 1876.) Philadelphia, 1876. 49p. DNLM **70-3652**

TONER, Joseph Meredith (1825-1896)
Address before the Rocky Mountain Medical Association, June 6, 1877, containing some observations on the geological age of the world, the appearance of animal life upon the globe, the antiquity of man, and the archeological remains of extinct races found on the American continent, with views of the origin and practice of medicine among uncivilized races, more especially the North American Indians. . . . Washington: Pub. for the Association, 1877. 112p. DLC; DNLM **70-3653**

TONER, Joseph Meredith (1825-1896)
Address before the Rocky Mountain Medical Association, June 6, 1877, containing some observations on the geological age of the world, the appearance of animal life upon the globe, the antiquity of man, and the archeological remains of extinct races found on the American continent, with views of the origin and practice of medicine among uncivilized races, more especially the North American Indians; to which is appended a synopsis of the previous addresses and also biographies of the members of the Association. . . . Washington, D.C.: Pub. for the Association, 1877. 414p. DLC; DNLM; NN **70-3654**

TONER, Joseph Meredith (1825-1896)
A sketch of the life of Horatio R. Storer, M.D. Washington, D.C., 1878. 14p. DNLM **70-3655**

TONER, Joseph Meredith (1825-1896)
Biographical sketch of Washington L. Atlee, M.D., of Philadelphia. Lancaster, Pa., 1878. 11p. DNLM **70-3656**

THE TONER LECTURES
The Toner lectures, instituted to encourage the discovery of new truths for the advancement of medicine. Washington: Smithsonian Institution, 1873-1885. DNLM [Contents: Lecture I. On the structure of cancerous tumors and the mode in which adjacent parts are invaded. By J. J. Woodward. Delivered March 28, 1873. 40p. 74 plates; Lecture II. Dual character of the brain. By C. E. Brown-Séquard. Delivered April 22, 1874. 21p.; Lecture III. On strain and over action of the heart. By J. M. Da Costa. Delivered May 14, 1874. 28p.; Lecture IV. A study of the nature and mechanism of fever. By Horatio C. Wood. Delivered Jan. 20, 1875. 45p.; Lecture V. On the surgical complications and sequels of the continued fevers. By Wm. Keen. Delivered Feb. 17, 1876. 68p.; Lecture VI. Subcutaneous surgery: its principles, and its recent extension in practice. By Wm. Adams. Delivered Sept. 13, 1876. 15p.; Lecture VII. The nature of reparatory inflammation in arteries after ligature, acupressure, and torsion. By Edward O. Shakespeare. Delivered June 27, 1878. 57p. 7 plates; Lecture VIII. Suggestions for the sanitary drainage of Washington. By George E. Waring, Jr. Delivered May 26, 1880. 23p.; Lecture IX. Mental over-work and premature disease among public and professional men. By Charles K. Mills. Delivered March 19, 1884. 34p.] **70-3657**

TOWNSEND, Ralph M[ilbourne] (*d.* 1877)
Student's chart of the sympathetic nerve. Philadelphia: T. Hamilton, 1871. 1 chart [in frame 10 by 12 inches]. DNLM
70-3658

TOWNSEND, Ralph M[ilbourne] (*d.* 1877)
Some medical pilgrimages abroad. An introductory to the summer course of lectures of the Jefferson Medical College, delivered March 30, 1874. Philadelphia: P. Madeira, 1874. 23p. 1 plate. DLC; DNLM; PPJ **70-3659**

TRADER, John W.
A case of skin grafting. Saint Louis, Mo.: Levison & Blythe, 1871. 7p. DNLM **70-3660**

TRADER, John W.
Anaesthesia and anaesthetics. [Kansas City, Mo., 1875.] 16p. DNLM **70-3661**

TRADER, John W.
President's annual address to the Medical Association of the State of Missouri, April 17, 1877. [St. Louis, Mo., 1877.] 12p. DNLM **70-3662**

TRALL, Russell Thacher (1812-1877)
The hygienic system. . . . Battle Creek, Mich.: The Office of the Health Reformer, 1872. 83p. DLC; DNLM
70-3663

TRALL, Russell Thacher (1812-1877)
An essay on tobacco-using, being a philosophical explanation of the effects of tobacco on the human system. Battle Creek, Mich., 1872. 62p. DNLM **70-3664**

TRALL, Russell Thacher (1812-1877)
The hygienic hand-book intended as a practical guide for the sick room. Arranged alphabetically. With an appendix, illustrative of the hygeio-therapeutic movements. . . . Rev. ed. New York: S. R. Wells, 1873. 300p. DLC; DNLM; NNNAM
70-3665

TRALL, R[ussell] T[hacher] (1812-1877)
The health and diseases of woman. Battle Creek, Mich.: Office of the Health Reformer, 1873. 60p. DLC; OCIM
70-3666

TRALL, R[ussell] T[hacher] (1812-1877)
The bath; its history and uses in health and disease. New York: S. R. Wells, 1873. 70p. DNLM; NNNAM
70-3667

TRALL, R[ussell] T[hacher] (1812-1877)
Diseases of the throat and lungs. New York: S. R. Wells, 1873. 39p. DNLM; NNNAM **70-3668**

TRALL, Russell Thacher (1812-1877)
Digestion and dyspepsia; a complete explanation of the physiology of the digestive processes, with the symptoms and treatment of dyspepsia and other disorders of the digestive organs. . . . New York: S. R. Wells & Co., 1875. 160p. DLC; DNLM; NNNAM **70-3669**

TRALL, Russell Thacher (1812-1877)
The human voice: its anatomy, physiology, pathology, therapeutics, and training; with rules of order for lyceums. . . . New York: S. R. Wells & Co., 1876. 111p. DLC; NNNAM
70-3670

TRANSACTIONS of the Howard Association, of Charleston, South Carolina during the epidemic of 1871. Charleston, S.C.: Evans & Cogswell, [c. 1871]. 41p. ScMS; ScU
70-3671

A TREATISE on the hair. Nashua, N.H.: R. P. Hall & Co., [1876]. 24p. DNLM **70-3672**

TREATISE on the immediate cause and the specific treatment of pulmonary consumption, nervous and general debility, with notes of cases, reports of physicians, embracing many wonderful and remarkable cures. New York, 1870. 32p. DNLM
70-3673

TRESCOT, George E[dward]
The study and value of therapeutics. [Charleston, 1871.] 16p. DNLM **70-3674**

TROUSSEAU, Armand (1801-1867)
Trousseau condensed, by Dr. L. Hale. Albany, N.Y.: L. H. Burdick, [1872]. 35p. DLC **70-3675**

TROUSSEAU, Armand (1801-1867)
Lectures on clinical medicine, delivered at the Hôtel Dieu, Paris. Transl. from the 3rd and revised ed. by John Rose Cormack and P. Victor Bazire. Philadelphia: Lindsay & Blakiston, 1873. 2 v. DNLM; IEN-M; NNNAM; PPC
70-3676

TUCKER, James Ioannes (1840?-1899)
Herpes zoster frontalia. Chicago: A. S. Kissell & Co., [1876]. 15p. DNLM **70-3677**

TUCKER, Willis G[aylord] (1849-1922)
Organic chemistry and therapeutics. [Introductory lecture.] Albany: Van Benthuysen, 1875. 19p. DNLM
70-3678

TUCKER, Willis G[aylord] (1849-1922)
Alcohol: is it a food? Albany, N.Y.: J. Munsell, 1877. 22p. DNLM **70-3679**

TUKE, Daniel Hack (1827-1895)
Illustrations of the influence of the mind upon the body in health and disease, designed to elucidate the action of the imagination. Philadelphia: Henry C. Lea, 1873. 415p. DNLM; NN; NNNAM; PU **70-3680**

TURNBULL, Charles S[mith] (1847-1918)
Filaria in the eye. [Philadelphia, 1878.] 8p. DNLM
70-3681

TURNBULL, Charles S[mith] (1847-1918)
Filaria in the eye. [Philadelphia, 1878.] 7p. DNLM
70-3682

TURNBULL, Charles S[mith] (1847-1918)
The audiphone and dentaphone. New York: G. P. Putnam's Sons, 1879. 8p. DNLM **70-3683**

TURNBULL, Charles S[mith] (1847-1918)
A clinical lecture on perforating wounds and injuries of the membrana tympani, with a case of fracture of the handle of the malleus. Philadelphia: Dickson & Gilling, 1879. 8p. DNLM
70-3684

TURNBULL, Charles S[mith] (1847-1918)
On cysticercus cellulose. [Philadelphia, 1879.] 8p. DNLM
70-3685

TURNBULL, Laurence (1821-1900)
Report of six hundred cases of diseases of the ear. [Philadelphia, 1871.] 7p. DNLM **70-3686**

TURNBULL, Laurence (1821-1900)
A clinical manual of the diseases of the ear. Philadelphia: J. B. Lippincott & Co., 1872. 486p. 1 col. plate. DLC; DNLM; NNNAM; PPC **70-3687**

TURNBULL, Laurence (1821-1900)
Observations on Bell's system of "visible speech" for the deaf mute. Philadelphia: S. W. Butler, 1873. 12p. DNLM **70-3688**

TURNBULL, Laurence (1821-1900)
On deaf-mutism and the method of educating the deaf and dumb. [Philadelphia, 1874.] 7p. DNLM **70-3689**

TURNBULL, Laurence (1821-1900)
Tinnitus aurium, or noises in the ears. Philadelphia: J. B. Lippincott & Co., 1874. 16p. DNLM **70-3690**

TURNBULL, Laurence (1821-1900)
Tinnitus aurium, or noises in the ears. 2nd ed., with cases. Philadelphia: J. B. Lippincott & Co., 1875. 39p. DNLM **70-3691**

TURNBULL, Laurence (1821-1900)
On the several methods of educating, and on the selection of proper schools for the deaf and dumb. On bathing, swimming, and diving, as causes of aural disease. Philadelphia: Collins, 1877. 8p. DNLM **70-3692**

TURNBULL, Laurence (1821-1900)
Artificial perforation of the membrana tympani. Philadelphia: J. A. Moore, 1877. 7p. DNLM **70-3693**

TURNBULL, Laurence (1821-1900)
The advantages and accidents of artificial anaesthesia. Being a manual of anaesthetic agents, and their modes of administration, considering their relative risk, tests of purity, treatment of asphyxia, spasm of the glottis, syncope, etc. . . . Philadelphia: Lindsay & Blakiston, 1878. 210p. DLC; DNLM; PPC; PU **70-3694**

TURNBULL, Laurence (1821-1900)
The advantages and accidents of artificial anaesthesia: a manual of anaesthetic agents, and their employment in the treatment of disease. . . . 2nd ed., rev. and enl. . . . Philadelphia: Lindsay & Blakiston, 1879. 322p. DLC; DNLM; NNNAM; PPC **70-3695**

TURNER, William Mason (1835-1877)
Phosphorus: its claims as a therapeutic agent. Philadelphia, 1875. 16p. DNLM **70-3696**

TURNEY, Samuel Denny (1824-1878)
Solid food in typhoid fever. Columbus: Nevins & Myers, 1877. 8p. DNLM **70-3697**

TYNDALE, J. Hilgard (*b.* 1843)
The present status of the pathology of consumption and tuberculosis. New York: Trow, 1878. 93p. DNLM; NNNAM **70-3698**

TYNDALE, J. Hilgard (*b.* 1843)
Influence of altitudes on consumptives. St. Louis: C. R. Barns, 1879. 29p. DNLM **70-3699**

TYNDALE, J. Hilgard (*b.* 1843)
Summar sanitarium at Manitou Park, Colorado. [Circular to the profession announcing the opening about July 1, 1879.] [1879.] 2 l. 1 chart. DNLM **70-3700**

TYNDALE, Theodore H.
The law of coroners. [Boston, 1877.] 16p. DNLM; MH **70-3701**

TYSON, James (1841-1919)
The cell doctrine: its history and present state. For the use of students in medicine and dentistry. Also, a copious bibliography of the subject. . . . Philadelphia: Lindsay & Blakiston, 1870. 150p. col. front. DLC; DNLM; PPJ; PPC **70-3702**

TYSON, James (1841-1919)
The glykogenic function of the liver. [Philadelphia, 1870.] 6p. DNLM **70-3703**

TYSON, James (1841-1919)
An introduction to the study of practical histology. For beginners in microscopy. Philadelphia: J. B. Lippincott & Co., 1873. 50p. 1 plate. DNLM; PPC; PU **70-3704**

TYSON, James (1841-1919)
Practical histology in Vienna, and the microscopical study of blood and epithelium. Philadelphia: J. B. Lippincott & Co., 1873. 34p. DNLM; PPC **70-3705**

TYSON, James (1841-1919) and R. M. BERTOLET
Catalogue of the specimens in the pathological museum of the Philadelphia Hospital. Philadelphia: Collins, 1874. 21p. DNLM; PPC; PU **70-3706**

TYSON, James (1841-1919)
A guide to the practical examination of urine. For the use of physicians and students. . . . Philadelphia: Lindsay & Blakiston, 1875. 182p. plates, tables. DLC; NNNAM; OCIM; PPC **70-3707**

TYSON, James (1841-1919)
A guide to the practical examination of urine. For the use of physicians and students. 2nd ed., rev. and improved. . . . Philadelphia: Lindsay & Blakiston, 1878. 172p. plates, tables. DLC; MBM; NNNAM; PU **70-3708**

TYSON, James (1841-1919)
The cell doctrine: its history and present state. For the use of students in medicine and dentistry. Also, a copious bibliography of the subject. . . . 2nd rev., cor. and enl. . . . Philadelphia: Lindsay & Blakiston, 1878. 202p. col. fronts, fold. plate. DLC; NNNAM; OCIM; PU **70-3709**

TYSON, James (1841-1919)
The causal lesions of puerperal convulsions. Philadelphia: J. B. Lippincott, 1879. 56p. DNLM; PPC **70-3710**

UNDERHILL, Alfred (1809-1873)
Symptoms and signs of pregnancy in their diagnostic relations. New York: William Wood & Co., 1870. 14p. DNLM; NNNAM **70-3711**

UNDERHILL, J[oshua] W.
The hydatidiform mole; its causes, pathology, medico-legal relations, diagnosis and treatment. Cincinnati, 1879. 20p. DNLM **70-3712**

U.S. BUREAU OF MEDICINE AND SURGERY
Medical essays: compiled from reports to the Bureau of Medicine and Surgery, by medical officers of the U.S. Navy. Pub. by order of the Navy Department. Washington: Government Printing Office, 1872. 367p. DLC
70-3713

U.S. BUREAU OF MEDICINE AND SURGERY
. . . Naval medical schools of France and England, with observations on the naval hospitals of Toulon. Reported to the Bureau of Medicine and Surgery, by Richard C. Dean. . . . Washington: Government Printing Office, 1876. 94p. 9 fold. plans. DLC **70-3714**

UNITED States homoeopathic pharmacopoeia. . . . Chicago, 1878. 281p. OCLloyd; PPHa; PU **70-3715**

UNITED STATES. NAVY DEPARTMENT.
BUREAU OF MEDICINE AND SURGERY
Catalogue of the library of the . . . Washington, 1877. 28p. DNLM **70-3716**

UNITED STATES SANITARY COMMISSION
Surgical memoirs of the war of the rebellion. Collected and published by the United States Sanitary Commission. [New York: U.S. Sanitary Commission; Cambridge: Riverside Press, 1870-1871.] 2 v. col. plates. DLC [Contents — [v. 1] I. On the wounds of blood-vessels, traumatic hemorrhage, traumatic aneurism, and traumatic gangrene. II. On the secondary traumatic lesions of bone: namely, osteo-myelitis, periostitis, ostitis, osteoporosis, caries, and necrosis. III. On pyaemia. By John A. Lidell . . . Ed. by Prof. Frank Hastings Hamilton, 1870. [v. 2] I. Analysis of four hundred and thirty-nine recorded amputations in the contiguity of the lower extremity. By Stephen Smith, M.D. II. Investigations upon the nature, causes, and treatment of hospital gangrene, as it prevailed in the Confederate armies, 1861-1865. By Joseph Jones, M.D. . . . Ed. by Prof. Frank Hastings Hamilton, 1871.]
70-3717

U.S. SURGEON-GENERAL'S OFFICE
The medical and surgical history of the war of the rebellion. (1861-1865). Prepared, in accordance with the acts of Congress, under the direction of Surgeon-General Joseph K. Barnes, United States Army. Washington: Government Printing Office, 1870-1888, 3 v. in 6 v. plates [part col. and mounted], maps, diags. DLC; NN; NNNAM; PU [Of the medical history v. 1 and 2 were prepared by J. J. Woodward, 1870-1879; v. 3 by Charles Smart, 1888. v. 1 contains also an appendix with reports of medical directors and other documents by J. J. Woodward and George A. Otis, with separate t.-p. and pagination. Of the surgical history v. 1 and 2 were prepared by George A. Otis, 1870-1876; v. 3, by G. A. Otis and D. L. Huntington, 1883. Vol. 3 of the surgical history is first issued. There is also a "second issue" of the same date.]
70-3718

U.S. SURGEON-GENERAL'S OFFICE. LIBRARY
Catalogue of the library of the Surgeon-General's Office, United States Army. With an alphabetical index of subjects. Washington: Government Printing Office, 1872. 454p. DLC
70-3719

U.S. SURGEON-GENERAL'S OFFICE. LIBRARY
. . . Supplement to Catalogue. No. I. List of American medical journals. Washington: Government Printing Office, 1872. 26p. DLC **70-3720**

U.S. SURGEON-GENERAL'S OFFICE. LIBRARY
Catalogue of the library of the Surgeon-General's Office, United States Army. . . . Washington: Government Printing Office, 1873-1874. 3 v. DLC **70-3721**

U.S. SURGEON-GENERAL'S OFFICE
The Medical Department of the United States Army from 1775 to 1873. Comp. under the direction of the Surgeon-General by Harvey E. Brown. . . . Washington, D.C.: Surgeon-General's Office, 1873. 314p. DLC **70-3722**

U.S. SURGEON-GENERAL'S OFFICE
. . . The cholera epidemic of 1873 in the United States. Washington: Government Printing Office, 1875. 1025p. plates, maps (part fold.). DLC ["Bibliography of Cholera" by John S. Billings, pp. 707-1025] **70-3723**

U.S. SURGEON-GENERAL'S OFFICE. LIBRARY
Specimen fasciculus of a catalogue of the national medical library, under the direction of the Surgeon-General, United States Army, at Washington, D.C. Washington: Government Printing Office, 1876. 72p. DLC **70-3724**

U.S. SURGEON-GENERAL'S OFFICE. LIBRARY
Abbreviation of titles of medical periodicals to be used in the subject-catalogue of the library of the Surgeon-General's Office. Washington: Government Printing Office, 1878. 96p. DLC **70-3725**

UNMASKED, or the science of immorality. To gentlemen. By a woman physician and surgeon [Mary Walker]. Philadelphia: W. H. Boyd, 1878. 146p. 7 plates. DNLM; PPC; PU
70-3726

UPHAM, J[abez] Baxter (1820?-1902)
A tabular history and analysis of all the undoubted cases of typhoid and typhus fever treated at the Boston City Hospital, from the date of its opening, June 1, 1864, to June 1, 1869. Boston, 1870. 93p. DNLM **70-3727**

UPHAM, J[abez] Baxter (1820?-1902)
Some additional reflections upon the late epidemic of cerebro-spinal meningitis. [Boston, 1874.] 8p. DNLM
70-3728

UPHAM, J[abez] Baxter (1820?-1902)
Cerebro-spinal meningitis in Massachusetts; being a succinct history of the epidemic of 1873, with an analysis of upwards of 500 cases, collected from every part of the State. Boston: Wright & Potter, 1874. 52p. DNLM **70-3729**

UPHAM, W. R.
Report of surgical cases of St. John's Riverside Hospital, Yonkers, N.Y. Ninth year, ending May 1, 1879. Yonkers, 12p. DNLM **70-3730**

THE USE of sulphate of cinchonidia in parts of the States of Illinois, Indiana, Missouri, Kentucky, and in the Mississippi Valley, in 1875. From medical journals, societies, and individual physicians. Philadelphia: J. A. Moore, 1876. 24p. DNLM
70-3731

THE USE of sulphate of cinchonidia in parts of the States of Illinois, Indiana, Missouri, Kentucky, and in the Mississippi Valley, in 1875. From medical journals, societies, and individual physicians. [With additions.] Philadelphia: J. A. Moore, 1876. 36p. DNLM **70-3732**

VAN BIBBER, John P. (1850-1892)
A new apparatus for extensor paralysis. New York: D. Appleton & Co., 1874. 6p. DNLM **70-3733**

VAN BIBBER, John P. (1850-1892)
Treatment of paralyzed muscles by elastic relaxation. Baltimore: Innes & Co., 1875. 8p. DNLM **70-3734**

VAN BIBBER, John P. (1850-1892)
On the successful treatment of some forms of peripheral paralysis. Baltimore: Innes & Co., 1876. 7p. DNLM; MdU-D **70-3735**

VAN BIBBER, John P. (1850-1892)
The new treatment for chorea. Baltimore: Innes & Co., 1878. 8p. DNLM; MdU-D **70-3736**

VAN BIBBER, John P. (1850-1892)
The future influence of the Johns Hopkins Hospital on the medical profession of Baltimore. Baltimore: Innes & Co., 1879. 22p. DNLM; MdBJ-W; MdU-D **70-3737**

VAN BIBBER, Washington Chew (1824-1892)
Supplemental report upon therapeutics. Baltimore: Innes & Co., 1877. 12p. DNLM; MdU-D **70-3738**

VAN BIBBER, Washington Chew (1824-1892)
Ventilation. Written for the Maryland State Board of Health. Annapolis: G. Colton, 1878. 36p. 1 plate. DNLM; MdU-D **70-3739**

VAN BUREN, William Holme (1819-1883)
Lectures upon diseases of the rectum, delivered at the Bellevue Hospital Medical College, session 1869-1870. . . . New York: D. Appleton & Co., 1870. 164p. DLC; DNLM; NNNAM; PU **70-3740**

VAN BUREN, William Holme (1819-1883)
A practical treatise on the surgical diseases of the genito-urinary organs, including syphilis. Designed as a manual for students and practitioners. . . . By W. H. Van Buren . . . and E. L. Keyes. . . . New York: D. Appleton & Co., 1874. 672p. DLC; DNLM; NNNAM; PPC **70-3741**

VAN BUREN, William Holme (1819-1883) and E. L. KEYES
Self-injection of the bladder, in the treatment of the consequences of obstructing enlargement of the prostate, and the best means of accomplishing it; together with two cases illustrating another method of removing foreign bodies from the urethra. New York: D. Appleton & Co., 1875. 33p. DNLM; NNNAM **70-3742**

VAN BUREN, William Holme (1819-1883)
Ulcer of the rectum. New York: G. P. Putnam's Sons, 1879. 29p. DNLM; NNNAM **70-3743**

VANCE, Ap Morgan (1854-1915)
A new removable paper brace for the treatment of caries of the spine and of lateral curvature by the insertion of a rubber band to exert continuous pressure over the deformity. [New York, 1879.] 14p. DNLM **70-3744**

VANCE, Reuben A[leshire] (1845-1894)
The treatment of paralysis by hypodermic injections of strychnia. New York: D. Appleton & Co., 1870. 34p. DNLM; NNNAM **70-3745**

VANCE, Reuben A[leshire] (1845-1894)
On syphilitic epilepsy. New York: F. W. Christern, 1871. 15p. DNLM; NNNAM **70-3746**

VANCE, Reuben A[leshire] (1845-1894)
The prevention of abscesses in hypodermic medication; with a description of an instrument for the injection of strychnia. New York: W. Baldwin & Co., 1871. 8p. DNLM; NNNAM **70-3747**

VANCE, Reuben A[leshire] (1845-1894)
The physical diagnosis of brain disease. New York: W. Baldwin & Co., 1871. 8p. DNLM; NNNAM **70-3748**

VANCE, Reuben A[leshire] (1845-1894)
The ophthalmoscope in the treatment of epilepsy. New York: D. Appleton & Co., 1871. 10p. DNLM; NNNAM **70-3749**

VANCE, Reuben A[leshire] (1845-1894)
Clinical examination of urine. With a description of a convenient apparatus for its speedy analysis. New York: W. Baldwin & Co., [1871]. 12p. DNLM; NNNAM **70-3750**

VANCE, Reuben A[leshire] (1845-1894)
A case of Bright's disease of the kidneys, in which there was no albuminuria, the only evidence of renal disease being the characteristic alterations of the intra-ocular structures as determined by the ophthalmoscope. [Boston, 1872.] 4p. DNLM; MBM **70-3751**

VANCE, Reuben A[leshire] (1845-1894)
Writer's cramp, or scrivener's palsy. Boston: D. Clapp & Son, 1873. 12p. DNLM; MBM **70-3752**

VANCE, Reuben A[leshire] (1845-1894)
Lithotrity. Cincinnati, 1877. 20p. DNLM **70-3753**

VANDER POEL, Samuel Oakley (1824-1886)
Pathological anatomy: the necessity for its study, and its influence upon medicine as a positive science. Anniversary address delivered before the Medical Society of the State of New York. Utica, N.Y.: Roberts, 1871. 36p. DNLM **70-3754**

VANDER POEL, Samuel Oakley (1824-1886)
Inaugural address at the sixty-fifth meeting of the Medical Society of the State of New York. [Albany, 1872.] 9p. DNLM **70-3755**

VANDER POEL, Samuel Oakley (1824-1886)
General principles affecting the organization of quarantine. A paper read before the New York Academy of Medicine. [Also:] On the transmissibility of yellow fever and cholera in their relations to quarantine. Albany: C. Van Benthuysen & Sons, 1874. 43p. 2 plates. DNLM; NNNAM **70-3756**

VANDER POEL, Samuel Oakley (1824-1886)
General principles affecting the organization of quarantine. A paper read before the New York Academy of Medicine. [Also:] On the transmissibility of yellow fever and cholera in their relations to quarantine. New York: D. Appleton & Co., 1874. 36p. 2 plates. DNLM; NNNAM **70-3757**

VANDER POEL, Samuel Oakley (1824-1886)
Quarantine. (With reference solely to sea-port towns.) [n.p., 1874?] 25p. DNLM **70-3758**

VANDER VEER, Albert (1841-1929)
Stricture of the male urethra, with report of twenty-seven cases. Annual address delivered before the Medical Society of the County of Albany, November 11, 1873. Albany: "The Argus Company," 1874. 35p. DNLM **70-3759**

VANDER VEER, Albert (1841-1929)
The operation for stone as observed in some of the London hospitals, together with a report of cases from private practice. New York: Rutledge & Co., 1876. 20p. DNLM **70-3760**

VANDER VEER, Albert (1841-1929)
Operation for closure of cleft of the hard and soft palate. [New York: G. P. Putnam's Sons, 1878.] 15p. DNLM; NNNAM **70-3761**

VANDER VEER, Albert (1841-1929)
Report of two cases of excision of the rectum. New York: William Wood & Co., 1879. 10p. DNLM **70-3762**

VANDER VEER, Albert (1841-1929)
Report of eight cases of uterine fibroids. Cambridge: Riverside Press, 1879. 11p. DNLM; MBM **70-3763**

VANDER VEER, Albert (1841-1929)
Facts in relation to the history of the Albany Medical College Museum, together with a comparative review of the museums of Great Britain. Albany: J. Munsell, 1879. 17p. DNLM; N **70-3764**

VAN DE WARKER, Ely (1841-1910)
Sunstroke and its theory. New York: D. Appleton & Co., 1870. New York: D. Appleton & Co., 1870. 24p. DNLM; NNNAM **70-3765**

VAN DE WARKER, Ely (1841-1910)
The detection of criminal abortion. Boston: J. Campbell, 1871. 16p. DNLM; MBM **70-3766**

VAN DE WARKER, Ely (1841-1910)
The detection of criminal abortion and a study of foeticidal drugs. Boston: J. Campbell, 1872. 88p. DNLM; MBM **70-3767**

VAN DE WARKER, Ely (1841-1910)
The use of the seton in the treatment of some cases of chronic affections of the womb. New York: J. Ross & Co., 1872. 16p. DNLM; NNNAM **70-3768**

VAN DE WARKER, Ely (1841-1910)
The criminal use of proprietary or advertised nostrums. New York: D. Appleton & Co., 1873. 15p. DNLM; NNNAM **70-3769**

VAN DE WARKER, Ely (1841-1910)
The treatment of uterine flexions. Buffalo: Baker, Jones & Co., 1874. 13p. DNLM **70-3770**

VAN DE WARKER, Ely (1841-1910)
A study of the normal movements of the unimpregnated uterus. New York: D. Appleton & Co., 1875. 26p. DNLM; NNNAM **70-3771**

VAN DE WARKER, Ely (1841-1910)
The treatment of anteflexions of the uterus. New York: D. Appleton & Co., 1876. 14p. DNLM; NNNAM **70-3772**

VAN DE WARKER, Ely (1841-1910)
Normal position and movements of the unimpregnated uterus. New York: William Wood & Co., 1878. 38p. DNLM; NNNAM **70-3773**

VAN DE WARKER, Ely (1841-1910)
Impotency in women. New York: William Wood & Co., 1878. 14p. DNLM; NNNAM **70-3774**

VAN HARLINGEN, Arthur (1845-1936)
On scleroderma. New York: F. W. Christern, 1873. 19p. DNLM; NNNAM **70-3775**

VANSANT, John (*d.* 1902)
On the physiological action of magnetism. New York: D. Appleton & Co., 1870. 30p. DNLM **70-3776**

VARICK, Theodore Romeyn (1825-1887)
The causes of death after operations and grave injuries. New York: D. Appleton & Co., 1875. 15p. DNLM; NNNAM **70-3777**

VARICK, Theodore Romeyn (1825-1887)
Cases of subperiosteal resection. New York: D. Appleton & Co., 1878. 14p. DNLM **70-3778**

VARICK, Theodore Romeyn (1825-1887)
A case of femoral aneurism successfully treated by intermittent pressure. New York: D. Appleton & Co., 1878. 6p. DNLM **70-3779**

VAUGHAN, R. A.
Public health. An address. [Columbus, Miss., 1878.] 10p. DNLM **70-3780**

VAUGHAN, Victor C[larence] (1851-1929)
Lecture notes on chemical physiology and pathology. 2nd ed. Ann Arbor, 1879. 315p. DNLM; OCIM **70-3781**

VERDI, Tullio Suzzara (1829-1902)
Maternity: a popular treatise for young wives and mothers. New York: J. B. Ford & Co., 1873. 451p. CtY-M; DNLM; NNNAM; PU **70-3782**

VERDI, Tullio Suzzara (1829-1902)
Report as special sanitary commissioner to European cities. Washington: Gibson Bros., 1873. 48p. DNLM **70-3783**

VERRILL, A[ddison] E[mory] (1839-1926)
The external and internal parasites of man and domestic animals. Hartford, Conn.: Case, Lockwood & Brainard, [1870?]. 140p. DNLM **70-3784**

VILAS, Charles H[arrison] (*b.* 1846)
The Eustachian catheter. Read before the Chicago Academy of Homoeopathic Physicians and Surgeons. Chicago: Duncan Brothers, 1876. 12p. OCIM **70-3785**

VILAS, Charles H[arrison] (*b.* 1846)
Valedictory address to the graduating class of Hahnemann Medical College and Hospital of Chicago, February 21, 1878; with the President's address, the report of the Dean, and catalogue of students and graduates. Chicago: Culver, Page, Hoyne & Co., 1878. 23p. OCIM **70-3786**

VILAS, Charles H[arrison] (*b.* **1846)**
Eye notes. [Chicago, 1878.] 23 cards. DNLM
70-3787

VILAS, Charles H[arrison] (*b.* **1846)**
Medical observations abroad; an address delivered at the Hahnemann Medical College and Hospital of Chicago, on invitation of the Hahnemannian Medical Institute, December 19, 1878. Printed by request. Chicago: The United States Medical Investigator Print, 1879. 15p. DNLM; PPHa
70-3788

VOGEL, Alfred (1829-1890)
A practical treatise on the diseases of children. Transl. and edited by H. Raphael. From the 4th German ed. New York: D. Appleton & Co., 1870. 603p. 6 plates. CU-M; DNLM; IU-M; NNNAM [2nd American ed., 1871; 3rd American ed., 1885] **70-3789**

WADDEL, Thomas (1843-1879)
Maternal impressions. Report of the obstetric section of the Toledo Medical Association. [Toledo], 1876. 32p. DNLM; OCIM **70-3790**

WADSWORTH, Oliver Fairfield (1838-1911)
Report on ophthalmology. [Boston, 1874.] 8p. DNLM
70-3791

WADSWORTH, Oliver Fairfield (1838-1911)
Recent progress in ophthalmology. [Boston, 1875.] 12p. DNLM; MBM **70-3792**

WADSWORTH, Oliver Fairfield (1838-1911)
A modification of the ophthalmoscope. Read before the Boston Society of Medical Science, December 25, 1876. [Boston, 1876.] 1 long sheet. DNLM; MBM **70-3793**

WADSWORTH, Oliver Fairfield (1838-1911)
A case of ectropion treated by transplantation of large flap without predicle. Cambridge: Riverside Press, 1877. 4p. DNLM **70-3794**

WADSWORTH, Oliver Fairfield (1838-1911) and James J. PUTNAM
Intra-ocular circulation; rhythmical changes in the venous pulse of the optic disk. Chicago, 1878. 4p. DNLM
70-3795

WAGNER, Clinton (1837-1914)
Certain nervous affections of the throat. New York: F. W. Christern, 1874. 18p. DNLM; NNNAM **70-3796**

WAGNER, Clinton (1837-1914)
Case of acne rosacea, or hypertrophica. Outgrowths removed by operation. New York: Rutledge & Co., 1876. 6p. DNLM
70-3797

WAGNER, Clinton (1837-1914)
Hoarseness and its causes. A lecture delivered at the Grand Conservatory of Music, New York, March 29, 1876. New York: G. P. Putnam's Sons, 1876. 15p. DNLM; NNNAM
70-3798

WAGNER, Clinton (1837-1914)
Syphilis of the nose and larynx. Columbus, O.: Nevins & Myers, 1876. 15p. DNLM **70-3799**

WAGNER, Clinton (1837-1914)
I. Case of sub-lingual follicular cyst, with sebaceoid contents. II. Case of nasal vascular myxoma: removal, alarming hemorrhage, recovery. New York: Rutledge & Co., 1877. 5p. DNLM
70-3800

WAGNER, Clinton (1837-1914)
A case of synovial bursa of the hyoid bone. Pharyngeal tumor treated by incisions and injections through the mouth. Columbus: Nevins & Myers, 1877. 5p. DNLM
70-3801

WAGNER, Clinton (1837-1914)
A paper on intra-laryngeal growths. Columbus: Nevins & Myers, 1878. 15p. DNLM **70-3802**

WAGNER, Ernst (1829-1888)
A manual of general pathology for the use of students and practitioners of medicine. Transl. from the 6th German ed. by John Van Duyn and E. C. Seguin. New York: William Wood & Co., 1877. 728p. CtY-M; ICRM; NNNAM; PU
70-3803

WAGNER, Henry
The young man's pocket companion: a digest on venereal diseases! . . . Virginia, Nev.: Brown & Mahanny, printers, 1877. 76p. DLC **70-3804**

WAGNER, [Joh.] Rudolf (1822-1880)
A handbook of chemical technology. Transl. and edited from 8th German ed., with extensive additions by William Crookes. New York: D. Appleton & Co., 1872. 745p. DNLM; MH; NN; PU **70-3805**

WALES, Philip Skinner (1837-1906)
A new rectal dilator and explorer, with two cases illustrating their use. Washington: Columbian Press, 1877. 9p. 1 plate. DNLM **70-3806**

WALES, Philip Skinner (1837-1906)
A new method of rhinoscopic exploration. Washington: Columbian Press, 1877. 10p. 1 plate. DNLM
70-3807

WALKER, George Brinton (1807-1887)
The medical profession. . . . What it is not, and what it is. Introductory lecture delivered at the opening of the session of 1875-1876 of the Medical College of Evansville, Oct. 4th, 1875. 25p. DNLM; IU-M **70-3808**

WALKER, George Brinton (1807-1887)
Observations in practice, surgery, gynecology and especially obstetrics. Chicago: Chicago Med. Press Ass., 1878. 33p. DNLM; ICRM; IEN-M; OCIM **70-3809**

WALKER, Jerome (*b.* **1845)**
The digestion and dilution of cow's milk, in the artificial feeding of children. [Brooklyn, 1877.] 10p. DNLM
70-3810

WALKER, M[ahlon] M. (1845-1896)
Teratology, or the science of monsters; a lecture delivered before the class of the Hahnemann Medical College of Philadelphia, January 1878. Philadelphia: Sherman & Co., 1878. 15p. DNLM; PPHa **70-3811**

[WALKER, Mary E.] (1832-1919)
Unmasked, or the science of immorality. To gentlemen. By a woman physician and surgeon. Philadelphia: W. H. Boyd, 1878. 146p. 7 plates. DNLM; PPC; PU **70-3812**

WALL, John P. (1836-1895)
The climate and diseases of the Gulf coast of the Florida peninsula, with remarks on the former in relation to pulmonary tuberculosis. Charleston, S.C.: H. P. Cooke & Co., 1874. 16p. DNLM; ScCM **70-3813**

WALL, John P. (1836-1895)
Climatological and sanitary report of Florida. Philadelphia: Collins, 1875. 30p. DNLM; PPC **70-3814**

WALLACE BROS.
Centennial Exhibition, 1876, of . . . . Catalogue of 562 materia medica pressed plants, giving their habitat and officinal qualities. [Philadelphia, 1876.] 64p. DNLM; OCLloyd **70-3815**

WALLACE, D[avid] Richard (*b.* 1825)
An address before the Waco Medical Association, delivered January 2, 1872. Waco: Golledge & Tomlinson, 1879. 15p. DNLM **70-3816**

WALLACE, Ellerslie (1819-1885)
Valedictory address. . . . Jefferson Medical College. . . . [With list of graduates.] Philadelphia: P. Medina, 1878. 11, 6p. DNLM; PPJ **70-3817**

WALSH, Ralph S. L. (*b.* 1841), J. Llewellin ELIOT and Wm. H. ROSS
Address delivered at the twenty-fifth annual commencement of the Medical Department of Georgetown University, March 10, 1874. Washington, D.C.: J. S. Tomlinson, 1874. 31p. DNLM **70-3818**

[WALSH, W. M.]
Correspondence between the Georgia Medical Society and W. M. Walsh.] [Savannah, Ga., 1870.] 13p. DNLM **70-3819**

WALTER, Albert G. (1811-1876)
Arthroplastic operation upon both femurs, below the great trochanters. New York: Rutledge & Co., 1876. 13p. DNLM; NNNAM **70-3820**

WALTON, George E[dward] (*b.* 1839)
The mineral springs of the United States and Canada, with analyses and notes on the prominent spas of Europe, and a list of seaside resorts. New York: D. Appleton & Co., 1873. 390p. 1 map. DLC; DNLM; NN **70-3821**

WALTON, George E[dward] (*b.* 1839)
The mineral springs of the United States and Canada, with analyses and notes on the prominent spas of Europe, and a list of seaside resorts. 2nd ed., revised and enlarged. New York: D. Appleton & Co., 1874. 414p. DLC; DNLM; NNNAM **70-3822**

WARD, Electus B.
Physiological antagonism the therapeutic law of cure. [Detroit, 1879.] 7p. DNLM **70-3823**

WARD, Henry A[ugustus] (1834-1906)
Catalogue of cabinet of comparative osteology. Rochester, N.Y.: E. R. Andrews, 1873. 39p. DNLM **70-3824**

WARD, Henry A[ugustus] (1834-1906)
Catalogue of specimens of comparative osteology. Rochester, N.Y.: E. R. Andrews, 1875. 43p. DNLM **70-3825**

WARD, Henry A[ugustus] (1834-1906)
Catalogue of specimens of comparative osteology. Rochester, N.Y.: E. R. Andrews, 1877. 63p. DNLM **70-3826**

WARD, Samuel B[aldwin] (*b.* 1842)
Embolism of the arteries of the extremities. New York: D. Appleton & Co., 1874. 18p. DNLM; NNNAM **70-3827**

WARD, Samuel Baldwin (*b.* 1842)
Progress in surgery. New York: D. Appleton & Co., 1875. 13p. DNLM; NNNAM **70-3828**

WARD, Samuel Baldwin (*b.* 1842)
The introductory lecture to the course of 1878-1879 at the Albany Medical College. Albany: Weed, Parsons & Co., 1878. 18p. DNLM **70-3829**

WARING, Edward John (1819-1891)
Practical therapeutics, considered chiefly with reference to articles of the materia medica. 2nd American ed. from 3rd London ed. Philadelphia: Lindsay & Blakiston, 1871. 765p. CU-M; DNLM; OCIM; PPC **70-3830**

WARING, Edward John (1819-1891)
A manual of practical therapeutics, considered chiefly with reference to articles of the materia medica. 3rd American from the last London ed. Philadelphia: Lindsay & Blakiston, 1874. 765p. DNLM; MH-M; MdBJ-W; NNNAM **70-3831**

WARING, George E[dwin], Jr. (1833-1898)
The causation of typhoid fever. Fiske Fund prize essay. Cambridge: Riverside Press, 1878. 16p. DNLM; MBM **70-3832**

WARING, George E[dwin], Jr. (1833-1898)
Excremental diseases: their causation and their prevention by hygienic means. [Newport, R.I., 1879.] 17p. DNLM **70-3833**

WARNER, Levi Farr (1822-1889)
On the connection of the hepatic functions with uterine hyperaemias, fluxions, congestions, and inflammations; with appendix. Cambridge, 1879. 37p. DNLM; MBM **70-3834**

WARNER, Lucien Calvin (1841-1925)
A popular treatise on the functions and diseases of woman. . . . Cortland, N.Y., 1873. 345p. DLC **70-3835**

WARNER, Oliver
Instructions concerning the registration of births, marriages, and deaths in Massachusetts; designed for town clerks and physicians. Boston: Wright & Potter, 1873. 32p. DNLM; MH; MHi; MWA **70-3836**

WARREN ANATOMICAL MUSEUM
A descriptive catalogue of the Warren Anatomical Museum, Harvard University. By J. B. S. Jackson, Boston: A. Williams, 1870. 759p. MH; MH-M; MWA **70-3837**

WARREN, Edward (1804-1878)
The life of John Warren, M.D., Surgeon-general during the war of the revolution; first professor of anatomy and surgery in Harvard College; president of the Massachusetts Medical Society, etc. . . . Boston: Noyes, Holmes & Co., 1874. 568p. front. (port.). DLC; MH; MH-M; NN **70-3838**

WARREN, Ira (1806-1864)
The household physician; for the use of families, planters, seamen, and travellers. Being a brief description, in plain language, of all the diseases of men, women, and children. . . . By Ira Warren . . . and A. E. Small. . . . Boston: I. Bradley & Co.; New York City: J. Taylor; [etc., etc.], 1870. 898p. col. plates. DLC; MH-M; NNNAM; NNU-M **70-3839**

WARREN, Ira (1806-1864)
The household physician; for the use of families, planters, seamen, and travellers. Being a brief description, in plain language, of all the diseases of men, women, and children, with the newest and most approved methods of curing them. By Ira Warren . . . and A. E. Small. . . . Illustrated by thirty-six figures on eight splendid colored lithograph plates, and three hundred and thirty-six engravings. . . . One hundred and fifth thousand. Boston: I. Bradley & Co.; New York City: J. Taylor; [etc., etc.], 1877. 893p. 8 col. plates. DLC; MBM; NNNAM; PPC **70-3840**

WARREN, John Collins (1842-1927)
The anatomy and development of rodent ulcer. A Boylston medical prize essay for 1872. Boston: Little, Brown & Co., 1872. 66p. 2 plates. DNLM; MBM **70-3841**

WARREN, John Collins (1842-1927)
Recent progress in surgery. [Cambridge, 1875.] 6, 8p. DNLM **70-3842**

WARREN, John Collins (1842-1927)
Vaginal lithotomy. Cambridge: Riverside Press, 1876. 11p. DNLM **70-3843**

WARREN, John Collins (1846-1927)
Note on the anatomy and pathology of the skin. Cambridge: Riverside Press, 1877. 8p. DNLM **70-3844**

WARREN, John S.
Two cases of intussusception successfully treated by fluid injections. New York: D. Appleton & Co., 1875. 10p. DNLM **70-3845**

WARREN, Samuel (1807-1877)
Passages from the diary of a late physician. From the 5th London ed. New York: Harper & Bros., 1875. 3 v. NN; NNC; MH; PP **70-3846**

WATERS, [Alderman] Thomas Houghton (1826-1912)
On diseases of the chest; being contributions to their clinical history, pathology, and treatment. 2nd ed. Philadelphia: Lindsay & Blakiston, 1874. 431p. CtY-M; DNLM; NNNAM; PPC **70-3847**

WATHEN, William H[udson] (1846-1913)
Sterility and its treatment. Louisville: J. P. Morton & Co., 1877. 11p. DNLM **70-3848**

WATHEN, William H[udson] (1846-1913)
Amputation of cervix uteri. Louisville, 1878. 12p. DNLM **70-3849**

WATHEN, William H[udson] (1846-1913)
Clinical gynecology. Louisville, 1878. 13p. DNLM **70-3850**

WATSON, Beriah André (1836-1892)
The pathology and treatment of chronic ulcers. New York: D. Appleton & Co., 1875. 17p. DNLM; NNNAM **70-3851**

WATSON, Beriah André (1836-1892)
Pyaemia and septicaemia. New York: D. Appleton & Co., 1877. 52p. DNLM; NNNAM **70-3852**

WATSON, Beriah André (1836-1892)
Disease germs: their origin, nature, and relation to wounds. Philadelphia: Collins, 1878. 22p. DNLM; PPC **70-3853**

WATSON, Thomas (1792-1882)
Lectures on the principles and practice of physic. Delivered at King's College, London. . . . From the 5th rev. and enl. English ed. Ed. with additions and numerous illustrations, by Henry Hartshorne. . . . Philadelphia: Henry C. Lea, 1872. 2 v. DLC; LNT-M; MBM; NNNAM **70-3854**

WATSON, William H[enry] (*b.* 1829)
Allopathic bigotry, popular opinion in reference to it as evidenced by the public press and the reflex action of popular opinion upon the New York Academy of Medicine. Albany: Argus Co., 1870. 19p. DNLM; NNNAM **70-3855**

WATTS, Henry (1815-1884)
A dictionary of chemistry and the allied branches of other sciences. Supplement. New York: William Wood & Co., 1872. 1136p. CU-M; MH; NN; NNNAM **70-3856**

WEATHERLY, J[ob] S[obieski] (1828-1892)
Addresses and reports read before the Medical Association of the State of Alabama, at the annual meetings of 1869 and 1870. Mobile: Tribune Job Office, 1870. 10p. DNLM **70-3857**

WEBB, M[elville] E[merson]
On the smallpox epidemic in Boston in 1872-1873. Read before the Massachusetts Medical Society, June 3, 1873. [Boston, 1873.] 13p. DNLM; MBM; MHi **70-3858**

WEBB, W[illiam] H. (1839?-1903)
Is Phthisis pulmonalis contagious, and does it belong to the zymotic group? Philadelphia: J. B. Chandler, 1878. 38p. DNLM; PPJ; PU **70-3859**

WEBBER, Samuel G[ilbert] (1838-1926)
A contribution to the study of myelitis. New York: S. W. Green, [1875]. 16p. 2 plates. DNLM; NNNAM **70-3860**

WEBER, Leonard
The therapeutic value of the hot mustard-bath in pneumonia in children. New York: William Wood & Co., 1878. 10p. DNLM; NNNAM **70-3861**

WEBSTER, David (*b.* 1842)
Is glaucoma ever of sympathetic origin? New York: G. P. Putnam's Sons, 1879. 9p. DNLM **70-3862**

WEIR, Robert F[ulton] (1838-1927)
Photographs of surgical specimens from United States General Hospital, Frederick, Maryland. [1873?] 49p. DNLM
70-3863

WEIR, Robert F[ulton] (1838-1927)
Elephantiasis of the penis from stricture of the urethra; amputation. New York: G. P. Putnam's Sons, 1874. 8p. DNLM **70-3864**

WEIR, Robert F[ulton] (1838-1927)
Two cases of congenital curvature of the penis, with hypospadias and adhesion to the scrotum; successfully relieved by operation. New York: D. Appleton & Co., 1874. 7p. 1 plate. DNLM **70-3865**

WEIR, Robert F[ulton] (1838-1927)
Ichthyosis of the tongue and vulva. New York: D. Appleton & Co., 1875. 19p. DNLM **70-3866**

WEIR, Robert F[ulton] (1838-1927)
The hypertrophied prostate. New York: G. P. Putnam's Sons, 1876. 28p. DNLM **70-3867**

WEIR, Robert F[ulton] (1838-1927)
On the normal urethra and its construction in relation to strictures of large calibre. New York: D. Appleton & Co., 1876. 21p. DNLM **70-3868**

WEIR, Robert F[ulton] (1838-1927)
On the antiseptic treatment of wounds, and its results. New York: D. Appleton & Co., 1878. 42p. DNLM
70-3869

WEIR, Robert F[ulton] (1838-1927)
Gritti's supra-condyloid amputation of the thigh. Syracuse, N.Y.: Truair, Smith & Bruce, 1879. 20p. DNLM
70-3870

WEIR, Robert F[ulton] (1838-1927)
Notes on practice in the New York Hospital. New York: D. Appleton & Co., 1879. 10p. DNLM
70-3871

WEIR, Robert F[ulton] (1838-1927)
Two cases of intratympanic vascular tumor, with a pulsating intact drum membrane. New York: Trow, 1879. 8p. DNLM
70-3872

WEISSE, Faneuil Dunkin (1842-1915)
Address before the graduating class of 1871 of the New York College of Dentistry. New York: Thitchener & Glastaeter, 1871. 14p. DNLM; NNNAM **70-3873**

WEISSE, Faneuil Dunkin (1842-1915)
Nitrous oxide gas. New York: Sanitarian Publ. Off., 1874. 11p. DNLM **70-3874**

WELCH, William M[iller] (*b.* 1837)
Report of the Municipal Hospital [for 1871] (comprising statistics of 1,227 cases of smallpox). Philadelphia: E. C. Markley & Son, 1872. 35p. DNLM; PPC
70-3875

WELCH, William M[iller] (*b.* 1837)
Report of the Municipal Hospital [for 1872] (comprising statistics of 2,377 cases of smallpox). Philadelphia: E. C. Markley & Son, 1873. 81p. 1 diag., 1 plate. DNLM; PPC
70-3876

WELLING, James Clarke (1825-1894), J. A. BOLLES, and James M. GASSAWAY
Addresses delivered at the fiftieth annual commencement of the National Medical College (Medical Department of the Columbian College), March 7, 1872. Washington, D.C.: Judd & Detweiler, 1872. 28p. DNLM **70-3877**

WELLING, James Clarke (1825-1894), W. PINKNEY, and S. L. CRISSEY
Addresses delivered at the fifty-first annual commencement of the National Medical College, March 8, 1873. Washington: J. C. Parker, 1873. 36p. DNLM **70-3878**

WELLING, James Clarke (1825-1894). A. F. A. KING, and L. T. BREMERMAN
Addresses delivered at the fifty-second annual commencement of the National Medical College, March 4, 1874. Washington, D.C.: R. Beresford, 1874. 32p. DNLM
70-3879

WELLING, James Clarke (1825-1894), Edward T. FRISTOE, and Charles L. DANA
Addresses delivered at the fifty-fourth annual commencement of the National Medical College, March 9, 1876. Washington, D.C.: W. H. Moore, 1876. 24p. DNLM
70-3880

WELLING, James Clarke (1825-1894), William LEE, and C. T. LEWIS
Addresses delivered at the fifty-sixth annual commencement of the National Medical College, March 21, 1878. Washington, D.C.: Darby & Duvall, 1878. 30p. DNLM
70-3881

WELLINGTON, William W[illiamson] (1814-1896)
Modern medicine, its needs and its tendency. The annual discourse before the Massachusetts Medical Society, May 25, 1870. Boston: D. Clapp & Son, 1870. 44p. DNLM; MH; MHi
70-3882

WELLS, Edward F[ranklin] (*b.* 1853)
Cholera infantum. Treatment of the cold stage. Cincinnati, 1877. 5p. DNLM **70-3883**

WELLS, Frank
Filth in its relation to disease. A report made to the board of police commissioners of the city of Cleveland. [Cleveland, Ohio, 1876.] 163p. 4 plates. DNLM; OCIM
70-3884

WELLS, John Soelberg (1834-1879)
A treatise on the diseases of the eye. 2nd ed. Philadelphia: Lindsay & Blakiston, 1870. 797p. 6 plates. DNLM; NNNAM; PPC; PPJ **70-3885**

WELLS, John Solberg (1834-1879)
A treatise on disease of the eye. 2nd American from the 3rd English ed., with additions. [Edited by I. M. Hays.] Philadelphia: Henry C. Lea, 1873. 836p. 6 col. plates, 4 plates [test types]. CtY-M; DNLM; PPC; PU **70-3886**

WELLS, P[hineas] Parkhurst (1808-1891)
Eruptive fevers. Philadelphia, 1876. 7 plates
70-3887

[WELLS, Phineas Parkhurst] (1808-1891)
What is homoeopathy, and what the possibilities and duties of its practice? Syracuse, N.Y.: Masters & Stone, 1878. 12p. DLC; DNLM; PPHa **70-3888**

WELLS, Thomas Spencer (1818-1897)
Diseases of the ovaries: their diagnosis and treatment. New York: D. Appleton & Co., 1873. 478p. DNLM; NNNAM; PPC; PU **70-3889**

WENZEL, Henry T. (1848-1897)
Protrusion of the stump of the pedicle through the cicatrix more than three years after ovariotomy. Deligation of the protruding part, and complete recovery. [Richmond, 1879.] 4p. DNLM **70-3890**

WENZEL, Henry T. (1848-1897)
New remedies. Report to the Wisconsin State Medical Society. Milwaukee: Sentinel Company. 1879. 15p. DNLM **70-3891**

WESSELHOEFT, Conrad (1834-1904)
The cause of contention between old and new. An address delivered before the Massachusetts Homoeopathic Medical Society, April 10, 1872. Philadelphia: Hering & Co., 1872. 8p. PPHa **70-3892**

WEST, Charles (1816-1898)
On some disorders of the nervous system in childhood: being the Lumleian lectures delivered at the Royal College of Physicians of London in March, 1871. Philadelphia: Henry C. Lea, 1871. 131p. DNLM; ICJ; NNNAM; PPC **70-3893**

WEST, Charles (1816-1898)
Lectures on the diseases of infancy and childhood. . . . 5th American from the 6th rev. and enl. English ed. Philadelphia: Henry C. Lea, 1874. 678p. DLC; DNLM; LNT-M; PPC **70-3894**

WEST, N[athaniel] (1840-1906)
The medical science and profession. Commencement address. Cincinnati, 1877. 14p. DNLM; OCIM **70-3895**

WEST PHILADELPHIA MEDICAL INSTITUTE
Announcement for the session of 1874-1875. [Philadelphia, 1874.] DNLM **70-3896**

WESTCOTT, Amos (1815-1873)
Adhesive gold foil: its discovery, history, and use. Philadelphia: S. White, 1870. 10p. DNLM; PPC; PU **70-3897**

WESTMORELAND, John Gray (1816-1887)
A treatise on acology and therapeutics, with some of the most prominent principles and rules of chemical and mechanical pharmacy. Atlanta, Ga., 1873. 391p. DNLM; GU **70-3898**

WETMORE, S[amuel] W[illiam] (*b.* 1832)
What is modern homoeopathy? Detroit, Mich.: E. A. Lodge, [1877]. 16p. DNLM; PPHa **70-3899**

WETMORE, Samuel William (*b.* 1832)
A therapeutical inquiry into rational medicine. Buffalo, N.Y.: Hutchinson & Gatchell, 1878. 35p. DNLM **70-3900**

WEY, William C. (1829-1897)
Medical responsibility and malpractice: an address. Albany: Argus Co., 1872. 35p. DNLM **70-3901**

WEY, William C. (1829-1897)
A medical aspect of drunkenness. Elmira, N.Y.: Advertiser Ass., 1877. 16p. DNLM **70-3902**

WEY, William C. (1829-1897)
A medical aspect of drunkenness. Syracuse: Masters & Stone, 1877. 16p. DNLM **70-3903**

WHARTON, Francis (1820-1889) and Moreton STILLÉ
A treatise on medical jurisprudence. . . . 3rd ed. Philadelphia: Kay & Bro., 1873. 2 v. in 3. CtY-M; DNLM; IU-M; PPC **70-3904**

WHARTON, George M. (*d.* 1853)
A Southern medical student's portfolio. . . . With illustrations by Croome. Philadelphia: Claxton, Remsen & Haffelfinger, 1872. 186p. plates. DLC **70-3905**

WHEELER, C. Gilbert (1836-1912)
Medical chemistry, including the outlines of organic and physiological chemistry. Based in part upon Riche's "Manuel de chimie." Philadelphia: Lindsay & Blakiston; Chicago: S. J. Wheeler, 1879. 424p. DNLM; NNNAM; NcD; PPL **70-3906**

WHITE, Charles Brainon (1826-1882)
Remarks on the proceedings of the meeting of physicians to discuss carbolic acid disinfection, published in the New Orleans Medical and Surgical Journal, November, 1875. New Orleans: Seymour & Stevens, 1876. 9p. DNLM; LNT-M **70-3907**

WHITE, Charles Brainon (1826-1882)
Disinfection in yellow fever, as practiced at New Orleans, in the years 1870 to 1875 inclusive. . . . Submitted to the American Public Health Association at Boston, October, 1876. New Orleans: J. W. Madden, printer, 1876. 16p. DLC; DNLM **70-3908**

WHITE DENTAL MANUFACTURERS, PHILADELPHIA
. . . List of changes in price necessarily made since publication of catalogue of 1867. With additions. Philadelphia: S. S. White, [1873]. 80p. DLC **70-3909**

WHITE DENTAL MANUFACTURERS, PHILADELPHIA
Catalogue of dental materials. Furniture, instruments, etc., for sale by Samuel S. White. . . . [Philadelphia: Press of J. B. Lippincott & Co., 1876.] 406p. DLC **70-3910**

WHITE, George A.
A practical monograph on the treatment of local complaints of the feet. Washington, D.C.: Judd & Detweiler, 1877. 48p. 4 plates. DNLM **70-3911**

WHITE, James C[larke] (1833-1916)
An introductory lecture delivered before the medical and dental schools of Harvard University, November 2, 1870. Boston: D. Clapp & Son, 1870. 30p. DNLM; MH; MH-M **70-3912**

WHITE, James C[larke] (1833-1916)
Review on modern dermatology. [Philadelphia, 1871.] 24p. DNLM; PPC **70-3913**

WHITE, James Clarke (1833-1916)
Vegetable parasites, and the diseases caused by their growth upon man. Boston: Wright & Potter, 1872. 50p. DNLM; MBM **70-3914**

WHITE, James Clarke (1833-1916)
On the action of Rhus venenata and Rhus toxicodendron upon the human skin. New York: D. Appleton & Co., 1873. 27p. DNLM; NNNAM **70-3915**

WHITE, James Clarke (1833-1916)
Four cases of scleroderma. [New York, 1875.] 8p. DNLM **70-3916**

WHITE, James Clarke (1833-1916)
An analysis of five thousand cases of skin disease, with remarks upon some of the principal groups and cases. Cambridge: Riverside Press, 1876. 32p. DNLM; MBM **70-3917**

WHITE, James Clarke (1833-1916)
Variations in type and in prevalence of diseases of the skin in different countries of equal civilization. Philadelphia, 1877. 20p. DNLM; PPC **70-3918**

WHITE, James Clarke (1833-1916)
Dermatology in America; being the president's address before the first meeting of the American Dermatological Association, New York: G. P. Putnam's Sons, 1878. 14p. DNLM; NNNAM **70-3919**

WHITE, James Clarke (1833-1916)
A contribution to the study of the aetiology of skin diseases. Cambridge 1879. 12p. DNLM; MH-M **70-3920**

WHITE, James Platt (1811-1881)
Progress in medicine. Annual address before the Medical Society of the State of New York: Buffalo: Sage, Sons & Co., 1870. 32p. DNLM **70-3921**

WHITE, James Platt (1811-1881)
Inaugural address before the Medical Society of the State of New York. Buffalo: Baker, Jones & Smith, 1870. 8p. DNLM **70-3922**

WHITE, James Platt (1811-1881)
A report of the reduction of two cases of chronic inversion of the uterus. Being cases X and XI of his series. Albany: C. Van Benthuysen & Sons, 1874. 13p. DNLM **70-3923**

WHITE, James Platt (1811-1881)
Address. Chronic inversion of the uterus. [Philadelphia, 1877.] 17p. DNLM; PPC **70-3924**

WHITE, James Platt (1811-1881)
Address in obstetrics and diseases of women and children. Philadelphia: Collins, 1877. 28p. DNLM; PPC **70-3925**

WHITE, James Platt (1811-1881)
Progress and prospect of the Buffalo Medical College. [Buffalo, 1877?] 7p. DNLM **70-3926**

WHITE, James William (1826-1891)
Taking impressions of the mouth. To which is appended a chapter on "porcelain teeth," from the new ed. of Harris's Principles and Practice of Dentistry. Philadelphia: S. S. White, 1871. 96p. DNLM; MdU-D; PPC; PU **70-3927**

WHITE, James W[illiam] (1826-1891)
The teeth; natural and artificial. Philadelphia, 1872. 31p. DNLM **70-3928**

WHITE, James William (1826-1891)
The teeth; natural and artificial. Philadelphia: S. S. White, 1873. 31p. DLC; DNLM; PPC **70-3929**

WHITE, James William (1826-1891)
Pathological dentition. Philadelphia: Collins, 1878. 10p. DNLM **70-3930**

WHITE, James William (1826-1891)
The mouth and the teeth. Philadelphia: Lindsay & Blakiston, 1879. 150p. CtY-M; MBM; NNNAM; PU **70-3931**

WHITE, J[ames] William (1850-1916)
On the diagnosis of urethral stricture by bulbous bougies, with illustrative cases. Philadelphia: J. B. Lippincott & Co., 1877. 25p. DNLM; PPC; PPJ **70-3932**

WHITE, Joseph A.
The ophthalmoscope as a diagnostic means in various forms of disease. Louisville, Ky., 1878. 25p. DNLM **70-3933**

WHITE, Octavius Augustus (1826-1903)
Varicocele and its radical cure. New York: D. Appleton & Co., 1873. 13p. DNLM; NNNAM **70-3934**

WHITE, Octavius Augustus (1826-1903)
Report upon yellow fever as it appeared in Savannah in 1876. New York: D. Appleton & Co., 1877. 27p. 1 map. DNLM; NNNAM **70-3935**

WHITE, Octavius Augustus (1826-1903)
The haemarumascope. [Philadelphia, 1877.] 4p. DNLM; PPC **70-3936**

WHITE, Octavius Augustus (1826-1903)
A normal pulse in the veins. [Louisville, 1878.] 7p. DNLM **70-3937**

WHITE, William
Medical electricity. A manual for students. Showing its most scientific and rational application to all forms of acute and chronic disease, by the different combinations of electricity, galvanism, electro-magnetism, magneto-electricity, and human magnetism. New York: S. R. Wells, 1872. 203p. DLC; DNLM; NNNAM; PU **70-3938**

WHITE, Wlliam T[homas] (1829-1893)
An anniversary discourse, delivered before the New York Academy of Medicine, Nov. 16, 1876. New York: D. Appleton & Co., 1876. 36p. DNLM; NNNAM **70-3939**

WHITEHEAD, William Riddick (1831-1902)
Remarks on the management of the intermaxillary bone in the double hair-lip. Denver, Col.: Tribune Printing House, 1874. 4p. DNLM **70-3940**

WHITENEY, William Fiske (1850-1921)
On empysema; an analysis of the cases in which pus has occurred in the pleural cavity, which have been treated at the Massachusetts General Hospital. [Boston, 1875.] 6p. DNLM; MH-M **70-3941**

WHITTAKER, James Thomas (1843-1900)
The morbid anatomy of the placenta. New York: W. A. Townsend & Adams, 1870. 108p. DNLM; NNNAM **70-3942**

WHITTAKER, James Thomas (1843-1900)
Physiology; preliminary course lectures on the influence of physiology upon practice; on the conservation of force; on the origin of life and the evolution of its forms, and on protoplasm, bone, muscle, nerve, and blood. Cincinnati: C. R. Murry, 1879. 288p. plates. DLC; DNLM; OCIM
70-3943

WICKES, Stephen (1813-1889)
History of medicine in New Jersey, and of its medical men, from the settlement of the province in A.D. 1800. . . . Newark, N.J.: M. R. Dennis & Co., 1879. 449p. DLC; DNLM; NNNAM; NjR **70-3944**

WIGGIN, Oliver Chase (1839-1903)
Artificial feeding of infants. [And:] Cholera infantum; its causes, nature and treatment. Charles Edward Banks Fiske Fund Prize essays, 1879. Providence: E. L. Freeman & Co., 1879. 66p. DNLM; RPJCB **70-3945**

WIGGLESWORTH, Edward (1840-1896)
Alopecia. [Boston, 1871.] 28p. DNLM
70-3946

WIGGLESWORTH, Edward (1840-1896)
Affections of the sebaceous glands. [Boston, 1875.] 11p. DNLM **70-3947**

WIGGLESWORTH, Edward (1840-1896)
Fibromata of the skin and subjacent tissues. [Fibroma molluscum, cutis pendula, "fibro-cellular" tumors.] New York: G. P. Putnam's Sons, 1876. 12p. 1 plate. DNLM; NNNAM
70-3948

WIGGLESWORTH, Edward (1840-1896)
A case of idiopathic multiple medullary round-celled sarcoma of the skin, with a retrospect of all recorded similar cases. New York: G. P. Putnam's Sons, 1876. 10p. DNLM; NNNAM
70-3949

WIGGLESWORTH, Edward (1840-1896)
Auto-inoculation of vegetable parasites of the skin, and the clinical testimony for their identity or non-identity. New York: G. P. Putnam's Sons, 1878. 9p. DNLM
70-3950

WIGGLESWORTH, Edward (1840-1896)
Faulty innervation as a factor in skin diseases. [New York, 1878.] 7p. DNLM **70-3951**

WIGGLESWORTH, Edward (1840-1896)
The metric system in a nut-shell. [Boston, 1878.] 2 l. DNLM
70-3952

WIGGLESWORTH, Edward (1840-1896)
New formations. [New York, 1878.] 16p. DNLM
70-3953

WILBUR, H[ervey] B[ackus] (1820-1883)
Materialism in its relations to the causes, conditions, and treatment of insanity. New York: D. Appleton & Co., 1872. 35p. DNLM; NNNAM **70-3954**

WILBUR, H[ervey] B[ackus] (1820-1883)
Management of the insane. A series of articles published in the Northern Christian Advocate, Syracuse, N.Y., Feb. 19, 26, and March 5 and 12, 1874. [Syracuse, 1874.] 12p. DNLM
70-3955

WILBUR, H[ervey] B[ackus] (1820-1883)
Government supervision of the insane. [n.p., 1876.] 20p. DNLM **70-3956**

WILBUR, H[ervey] B[ackus] (1820-1883)
Governmental supervision in the management of the insane. [Syracuse? 1876.] 45p. DNLM **70-3957**

WILBUR, H[ervey] B[ackus] (1820-1883)
Buildings for the insane. A report read at the Saratoga Conference of Charities, Sept. 6, 1877. Boston: A. J. Wright, 1877. 24p. DNLM; MH-M **70-3958**

WILBUR, H[ervey] B[ackus] (1820-1883)
Report on the management of the insane in Great Britain. Albany: Weed, Parsons & Co., 1877. 74p. DLC; DNLM
70-3959

WILDER, Alexander (1823-1908)
Plea for collegiate education of women. Address delivered before the Eclectic Medical Society of the State of New York, at Cooper Institute, New York, October 21, 1874. . . . [New York? 1874.] 15p. DLC **70-3960**

WILDER, Alexander (1823-1908)
Vaccination a medical fallacy. [n.p., 1875.] 39p. DNLM; PPC
70-3961

WILDER, Alexander (1823-1908)
Intermarriage of kindred. Consanguineous marriages not forbidden by moral or physiological law. Evils of connubial alliances between persons of diverse race. Annual address delivered before the Eclectic Medical Society of the State of New York. New York: Trow & Smith. 1870. 32p. DNLM; NN; NNNAM **70-3962**

WILDER, Burt Green (1841-1925)
The Cornell University. Lectures on human physiology and hygiene. Fall trimester, 1872-1873. [Syllabus.] [Ithaca, N.Y., 1872.] unpag. DNLM **70-3963**

WILDER, Burt Green (1841-1925)
Questions upon a course of forty lectures in human physiology, for the use of the candidates for graduation at the Medical School of Maine, session of 1875. [1875.] 4p. DNLM
70-3964

WILEY, Harvey Washington (1844-1930)
The relation of the physician to the education of the people. Indianapolis: J. G. Doughty, 1873. 17p. DNLM
70-3965

WILKINS, E. T. (1824-1890)
Insanity and insane asylums. Report of E. T. Wilkins, commissioner in lunacy for the State of California, made to the governor of the State, Dec. 2, 1871. Sacramento: T. A. Springer, 1872. 345, 15p. CLM; CU-M; DNLM
70-3966

WILLARD, Frances E[lizabeth] (1839-1898)
Hints and help in our temperance work. New York: Nat. Temperance Soc. & Pub. House, 1875. 72p. DNLM; NN
70-3967

WILLIAMS, A. D.
Diseases of the ear, including the necessary anatomy of the organ. Cincinnati: R. Clarke & Co., 1873. 209p. 1 lith. plate. DNLM; OCIM **70-3968**

WILLIAMS, BROWN & EARLE
A condensed list of a few of the most desirable microscopes, . . . accessories, mounting implements and materials, spectacles, eyeglasses, photographic outfits, etc. Philadelphia, [1878?]. [unp.] DNLM; PPC; PPJ; PU **70-3969**

WILLIAMS, Charles Herbert (1850-1918)
The prize essay of the Boylston Medical Society, for 1874. I. Experiments on the action of bile in promoting the absorption of fats [by Charles Herbert Williams]. II. On intestinal digestion [by George Minot Garland]. Boston: Printed by D. Clapp & Son, 1874. 26p. 2 plates. DLC; DNLM; MH-M **70-3970**

WILLIAMS, Harold
A comparison between the Caesarean section and the high forceps operation. New York: William Wood & Co., 1879. 11p. DNLM; NNNAM **70-3971**

WILLIAMS, Henry Willard (1821-1895)
A practical guide to the study of the diseases of the eye: their medical and surgical treatment. 4th ed. Boston: J. R. Osgood & Co., 1873. 422p. CtY-M; DNLM; MBM; NNNAM **70-3972**

WILLIAMS, Henry Willard (1821-1895)
On the comparative value of caustics and astringents in the treatment of diseases of the conjunctiva, and on the best mode of applying these remedies. Philadelphia, 1877. 12p. DNLM; PPC **70-3973**

WILLIAMS, Henry Willard (1821-1895)
Eserine and pilocarpine in the treatment of eye disease. Cambridge, 1878. 5p. DNLM; MBM **70-3974**

WILLIAMS, Philip Croudson (1828-1896)
An examination of Prof. Reese's "Review of the trial of Mrs. Wharton for the murder of General Ketchum." Baltimore: Turnbull Brothers, 1872. 31p. DNLM; MdU-D **70-3975**

WILLIAMS, Philip Croudson (1828-1896)
A reply to Dr. H. C. Wood's "Review of the medical testimony for the alleged attempt to poison Mr. Van Ness." Louisville, Ky., 1873. 31p. DNLM **70-3976**

WILLIAMS, Philip Croudson (1828-1896)
Hypodermic injection of ergot in post-partum hemorrhage. Baltimore, 1874. 4p. DNLM **70-3977**

[WILLIAMS, Thaddeus Warsaw]
The vade-mecum of nature: being a practical treatise on the medical and surgical diseases of the urinary and generative organs of both sexes; and their treatment upon improved principles. . . . Milwaukee, Wis.: Milwaukee Medical and Surgical Institute, [1872]. 194, 16p. plates. DLC **70-3978**

[WILLIAMS, Thaddeus Warsaw]
The people's medical guide, and family vade-mecum. . . . St. Louis, Mo.: The Butts Dispensary, [1877]. DLC **70-3979**

[WILLIAMS, Thaddeus Warsaw]
The people's marriage guide. Sexual & chronic diseases, reproduction, and the diseases of women. . . . Vol. 1. Milwaukee, Wis.: M. & S. Institute, [1878]. 301p. plates. DLC **70-3980**

WILLIAMSON, Allan N[eale]
Observations on the principal diagnostic points in diseases of the liver. New York: D. Appleton & Co., 1872. 14p. DNLM; NNNAM **70-3981**

WILLIAMSON, Allan N[eale]
Observations on nasal catarrh and catarrhal deafness. . . . [New York]: New York Throat and Ear Institute, 1877. 14p. DLC; DNLM **70-3982**

WILSON, Erasmus (1809-1884)
The anatomist's vade mecum, a system of human anatomy. Edited by George Buchanan, assisted by Henry E. Clark. 9th ed. Philadelphia: Lindsay & Blakiston, 1873. 743p. CtY-M; IEN-M; NNNAM; PPC **70-3983**

WILSON, Frank C[aruther] (*b.* 1841)
Fetal physical diagnosis. With an analysis of the physical examination of one hundred and twenty-six cases. Louisville: J. P. Morton, [1873]. 19p. DNLM; OCIM **70-3984**

WILSON, F[red] M[orse] (*b.* 1851)
Astringents in chronic conjunctivitis. [Hartford, 1879.] 4p. DNLM **70-3985**

WILSON, George (1811-1897)
A handbook of hygiene and sanitary science. 3rd ed. Philadelphia: Lindsay & Blakiston, 1877. 490p. DNLM; NNNAM; PPJ; PPC **70-3986**

WILSON, H[enry] P[arke] C[ustis] (1827-1898)
A fatty tumor; with some remarkable points in the case. [Baltimore, 1877.] 4p. DNLM **70-3987**

WILSON, H[enry] P[arke] C[ustis] (1827-1898)
Epithelioma of the cervix uteri, amputation with Paquelin's thermo-cautery. Baltimore: J. H. Foster & Co., 1878. 8p. DNLM **70-3988**

WILSON, H[enry] P[arke] C[ustis] (1827-1898)
Sub-sulphate of iron as an atiseptic in the surgery of the pelvis. [Boston, 1878.] 11p. DNLM **70-3989**

WILSON, H[enry] P[arke] C[ustis] (1827-1898)
The hand as a curette in post-partum hemorrhage. [Boston, 1879.] 5p. DNLM **70-3990**

WILSON, H[enry] P[arke] C[ustis] (1827-1898)
Inversion of the uterus. New York: D. Appleton & Co., 1879. 11p. DNLM **70-3991**

WILSON, H[enry] P[arke] C[ustis] (1827-1898)
Paquelin's thermo-cautery with Wilson's antithermic shield in epithelioma of the cervix uteri. [Richmond, 1879.] 16p. DNLM **70-3992**

WILSON, H[enry] P[arke] C[ustis] (1827-1898)
The thermantidote. An instrument for preventing the evil effects of heat from Paquelin's thermo-cautery when operating in deep cavities. Baltimore, Md.: M. J. Printing House, 1879. 12p. DNLM **70-3993**

WILSON, James Cornelius (1847-1934)
. . . The summer and its diseases. . . . Philadelphia: Lindsay & Blakiston, 1879. 160p. DLC; DNLM; PPC; PU [American Health Primers, vol. 3]. **70-3994**

WILSON, Joseph (1816-1887)
Naval hygiene . . . with an appendix: Moving wounded men on shipboard, by Albert C. Gorgas. . . . Reported to the Bureau of Medicine and Surgery. Pub. by order of the Navy Department. Washington: Government Printing Office, 1870. 234p. col. plates. DLC; DNLM; MBM; NNNAM
70-3995

WILSON, Joseph (1816-1887)
Naval hygiene. Human health and the means of preventing disease, with illustrative incidents principally derived from naval experience. . . . 2nd ed. Philadelphia: Lindsay & Blakiston, 1879. 274p. col. plates. DLC; DNLM; PPC; PU
70-3996

WILSON, Joseph M[iller] (1838-1902)
The new pavilion ward of the Presbyterian Hospital of Philadelphia. Philadelphia: W. Kildare, 1875. 3p. 2 plates. DNLM; PPPrHi **70-3997**

WILSON, T[homas] Pardon (1832-1909)
The rejected address. Man's true relation to nature: his origin, character, and destiny. Delivered in Philadelphia, June 6, 1871. Cleveland: L.H. Witte, 1871. 26p. DNLM; OCIM
70-3998

WILSON, T[homas] Pardon (1832-1909)
Graduation address of the Homoeopathic Hospital College, at Cleveland, session 1870-1871, 1871-1872. Cleveland, O.: S. H. Witte, 1872. 13p. DNLM; OCIM
70-3999

WILSON, T[homas] Pardon (1832-1909)
Ophthalmology and other modern sciences. Together with the first annual report of the Cincinnati Eye and Ear Institute. Cincinnati: J. P. Geppert, 1874. 20p. DLC; DNLM
70-4000

WINCKEL, Franz Karl Ludwig Wilhelm von (1837-1911)
The pathology and treatment of childbed: a treatise for physicians and students. From the 2nd German ed., with many additional notes by the author. Transl. by James R. Chadwick. Philadelphia: Henry C. Lea, 1876. 484p. CtY-M; DNLM; MH-M; NNNAM **70-4001**

WING, Clifton Ellis (1848-1911)
Poisoning by nitro-benzole. [Boston, 1872.] 7p. DNLM; MBM
70-4002

WING, Clifton Ellis (1848-1911)
On so-called "ulcerations" of the os uteri. Cambridge: Riverside Press, 1876. 8p. DNLM; MBM **70-4003**

WING, Clifton Ellis (1848-1911)
Vaginal ovariotomy. Cambridge, 1876. 7p. DNLM; MBM
70-4004

WING, Clifton Ellis (1848-1911)
The use of uterine supporters. [Boston, 1877.] 8p. DNLM; MBM **70-4005**

WING, Clifton Ellis (1848-1911)
The specialty of diseases of women. [Boston, 1877.] 8p. DNLM; MBM **70-4006**

WING, Clifton Ellis (1848-1911)
Some hints regarding uterine supporters. [Boston: D. Clapp & Son, 1877.] 7p. DNLM; MBM
70-4007

WING, Clifton Ellis (1848-1911)
A case of complete inversion of the uterus; reposition 14 months after the confinement by means of continued moderate pressure, without the aid of anesthesia; remarks upon the modern treatment of chronic inversion. [Boston, 1879.] 12p. DNLM; MBM **70-4008**

WING, Clifton Ellis (1848-1911)
. . . The aid of anaesthesia; remarks upon the modern treatment of chronic inversion. [Boston, 1879.] 12p. DNLM; MBM
70-4009

WINSTON, Gustavus Storrs (1833-1899) and E. M. MARSH
Preliminary report of the mortality experience of the Mutual Life Insurance Company of New York. From 1843 to 1874. v. 1. New York: Printed by order of the Board of Trustees, 1875. 46p. 3 diag. DNLM; NNNAM **70-4010**

WINSTON, Gustavus Storrs (1833-1899), *et al.*
Mortuary experience of the Mutual Life Insurance Company of New York, with tabulated reports, and an analysis of the causes of death. v. 2. New York: Printed by order of the Board of Trustees, 1877. 225p. DNLM; NNNAM
70-4011

WINSTON, Gustavus Storrs (1833-1899) and W. R. GILLETTE
On the examination of the urine of applicants for life insurance. New York, 1879. 15p. DNLM; NNNAM
70-4012

WITTHAUS, Rudolph August (1846-1915)
Essentials of chemistry, inorganic and organic, for the use of students in medicine. . . . New York: William Wood & Co., 1879. 257p. DLC; DNLM; NNNAM; PU
70-4013

WAOKES, Edward (1837-1912)
Throat deafness associated with paresis of the palato-tubal muscles. New York: Trow's, 1879. 10p. DNLM; NNNAM
70-4014

WOLFE, N[apoleon] B.
Common sense book on the new treatment of consumption, asthma, bronchitis, and all diseases of the nose, throat, and lungs by medicated inhalations. Cincinnati, 1872. 93p. DNLM; OCIM **70-4015**

WOLFE, N[apoleon] B.
The guide-book. A sequel to medical common sense, for the use and benefit of patients employing medicated inhalations under the direction of . . . Cincinnati, 1872. 60p. 1 plate. DNLM; OCIM **70-4016**

WOLFE, N[apoleon] B.
Inhalation: or, how to cure catarrh, asthma, and consumption. Cincinnati, 1875. 72p. 1 plate. DNLM; OCIM
70-4017

WOLFF, Lawrence (1845?-1901)
Supposed toxic effect of artificial vanillin. [Philadelphia, 1879.] 1 l. DNLM **70-4018**

WOOD, Edward S[tickney] (1846-1905)
Recent progress in medical chemistry. Boston, 1877. 8p. DNLM **70-4019**

WOOD, Edward S[tickney] (1846-1905)
Illuminating gas in its relation to health. Cambridge: Riverside Press, 1877. 7p. DNLM **70-4020**

WOOD, George Bacon (1797-1879)
The dispensatory of the United States of America. By George B. Wood . . . and Franklin Bache. . . . 13th ed., carefully rev. Philadelphia: J. B. Lippincott & Co., 1870. 1810p. DLC; DNLM; OCLloyd; PPC **70-4021**

WOOD, George Bacon (1797-1879)
Introductory lectures and addresses, on medical subjects, delivered chiefly before the medical classes of the University of Pennsylvania. . . . 2nd ed. Philadelphia: J. B. Lippincott & Co., 1872. 476p. DLC; NNNAM; PPC; PU **70-4022**

WOOD, George Bacon (1797-1879)
Historical and biographical memoirs, essays, addresses, etc., written at various times during the last fifty years, and now first published in collected form. Philadelphia: J. B. Lippincott & Co., 1872. 576p. DNLM; NNNAM; PPC; PU **70-4023**

WOOD, George Bacon (1797-1879)
The dispensatory of the United States of America. 14th ed. Carefully rev. by Dr. George B. Wood. Assisted by Dr. H. C. Wood. Philadelphia: J. B. Lippincott & Co., 1877. 1879p. DLC; OCIM; OCLloyd; NNNAM **70-4024**

WOOD, George Bacon (1797-1879)
The last will and codicils of . . . , deceased. [Philadelphia, privately printed, not published, 1879.] 41p. DNLM; PU **70-4025**

WOOD, Horatio C. (1841-1920)
A contribution to the knowledge of the physiological action of the alkaloids, viridia, veratroidia, and veratria of commerce, and of the resin of Veratrum viride. [Philadelphia, 1870.] 18p. DNLM **70-4026**

WOOD, Horatio C. (1841-1920)
On the influence of section of the cervical pneumogastrics upon the action of emetics and cathartics. [Philadelphia, 1870.] 25p. DNLM; PU **70-4027**

WOOD, Horatio C. (1841-1920)
On a case of splenic and lymphatic hypertrophy without leucocythaemia (Hodgkins' disease, pseudo-leucaemia). [Philadelphia, 1870.] 9p. DNLM **70-4028**

WOOD, Horatio C. (1841-1920)
Experimental researches on the physiological action of nitrite of amyl. (Memoir to which was awarded the Warren prize, for 1871, of the Massachusetts General Hospital.) [Philadelphia, 1871.] 27p. DNLM; MBM **70-4029**

WOOD, Horatio C. (1841-1920)
Contribution to the knowledge of the physiological action of atropia. No. 1. Its influence on pigeons. [Philadelphia, 1871.] 5p. DNLM **70-4030**

WOOD, Horatio C., ed. (1841-1920)
A year-book of therapeutics, pharmacy and allied sciences. . . . New York: William Wood & Co., 1872. 360p. DLC; NNNAM; PPJ; PU **70-4031**

WOOD, Horatio C. (1841-1920)
Thermic fever, or sunstroke. Boylston prize essay. Philadelphia: J. B. Lippincott & Co., 1872. 128p. DNLM; MBM; MH; PPC **70-4032**

WOOD, Horatio C. (1841-1920)
A treatise on therapeutics, comprising materia medica and toxicology, with special reference to the application of the physiological action of drugs to clinical medicine. . . . Philadelphia: J. B. Lippincott & Co., 1874. 578p. DLC; DNLM; OCLloyd; PPC **70-4033**

WOOD, Horatio C. (1841-1920) and Joseph BERENS
An investigation into the action of Veratrum viride upon the circulation. [Philadelphia, 1874.] 51p. DNLM **70-4034**

WOOD, Horatio C. (1841-1920)
A study of the nature and mechanism of fever. Toner lectures. Washington, 1875. 45p. DNLM; PPJ; PPC; PU **70-4035**

WOOD, Horatio C. (1841-1920)
On the diagnosis of diseases accompanied with real or apparent paraplegia without marked muscular degeneration. New York: G. P. Putnam's Sons, 1875. 27p. CtY-M; DNLM; NNNAM; PPC **70-4036**

WOOD, Horatio C. (1841-1920)
A treatise on therapeutics, comprising materia medica and toxiciology, with especial reference to the application of the physiological action of drugs to clinical medicine. . . . 2nd ed., rev. and enl. Philadelphia: J. B. Lippincott & Co., 1876. 674p. DLC; DNLM; OCLloyd; PPC **70-4037**

WOOD, Horatio C. (1841-1920)
The United States Pharmacopoeia and the American Medical Association. [Philadelphia, 1877.] 11p. DNLM; PPC **70-4038**

WOOD, Horatio C. (1841-1920)
Preliminary note on a new medicinal plant and its alkaloid. [Philadelphia, 1877.] 4p. DNLM **70-4039**

WOOD, Jacob A. (1810-1879)
Beneficial results from the use of mechanical appliances in Pott's disease of the spine. New York: Steam Printing House, 1873. 41p. NNNAM **70-4040**

WOOD, James Rushmore (1816-1883)
Report of four cases of neurotomy of the superior maxillary nerve, with extirpation of Meckel's ganglion for the cure of tic-douloureux. New York: D. Appleton & Co., 1879. 10p. DNLM; NNNAM **70-4041**

WOOD, WILLIAM, & CO.
Code of medical ethics of the American Medical Association. With illustrated catalogue of the medical publications of William Wood & Co. New York, 1878. NNNAM [12p. (the Code of Ethics); 42p. (1878 catalog); 58p. (prospectus for Cyclopedia of Medicine by Ziemssen); 31p. (list of more 1878 publications by title only)] **70-4042**

WOODBURY, Frank (1848-1927)
Cases called hysterical. Philadelphia: J. A. Moore, 1877. 8p. DNLM **70-4043**

WOODHULL, Alfred Alexander (1837-1921)
Clinical studies with large non-emetic doses of ipecacuanha. [With a contribution to the therapeusis of cholera.] Atlanta, Ga.: Dunlop, Wynne & Co., 1875. 63p. DNLM; GU **70-4044**

WOODHULL, Alfred Alexander (1837-1921)
Clinical studies with the non-nauseating use of ipecacuanha, chiefly in intermittents. Atlanta, Ga.: Dunlop & Dickson, 1875. 23p. DNLM; GU **70-4045**

WOODHULL, Alfred Alexander (1837-1921)
Studies, chiefly clinical, in the non-emetic use of ipecacuanha: with a contribution to the therapeusis of cholera. . . . Philadelphia: J. B. Lippincott & Co., 1876. 155p. DLC; NNNAM; PPC; PU **70-4046**

WOODS, J[oseph] T.
Woods' hammock splint, for all fractures of the leg and thigh. Toledo, 1874. 12p. DNLM **70-4047**

WOODWARD, A[lfred] W. (1839-1902)
Modifying influence of epidemics on therapeutics. Philadelphia, 1876. 18p. DNLM; PPC; PU **70-4048**

WOODWARD, Ashbel (1804-1885)
Small-pox at South Windham, Conn. [New Haven, 1874.] 4p. CtY-M; DNLM **70-4049**

WOODWARD, Joseph Janvier (1833-1884)
. . . Report to the Surgeon-General of the United States Army on certain points connected with the histology of minute blood-vessels. . . . Washington, 1870. 8p. 11 photo. DLC; DNLM **70-4050**

WOODWARD, Joseph Janvier (1833-1884)
Report to the Surgeon-General of the United States Army, on the magnesium and electric lights, as applied to photo-micrography. Washington, 1870. 3 l. 11 photo. DLC; DNLM **70-4051**

WOODWARD, Joseph Janvier (1833-1884)
Report to the Surgeon-General of the United States Army, on the oxy-calcium light, as applied to photo-micrography. Washington, 1870. 2 l. 2 photo. DLC; DNLM **70-4052**

WOODWARD, Joseph Janvier (1833-1884)
Memorandum on the Amphipleura pellucida. Washington, 1871. 1p. 2 photo. DLC; DNLM **70-4053**

WOODWARD, Joseph Janvier (1833-1884)
Memorandum on Pleurosigma angulatum and Pleurosigma formosum. Washington, 1871. 4p. 8 photo. DLC; DNLM **70-4054**

WOODWARD, Joseph Janvier (1833-1884)
Memorandum on the Surirella gemma. Washington, 1871. 1p. 2 photo. DLC; DNLM **70-4055**

WOODWARD, Joseph Janvier (1833-1884)
Memorandum on the test Podura. Washington, 1871. 3p. 5 photo. DLC; DNLM **70-4056**

WOODWARD, Joseph Janvier (1833-1884)
Photographs of Surirella gemma, Amphipleura pellucida and test Podura. Washington: Surgeon-General's Office, 1871. 9 photo. DLC; DNLM **70-4057**

WOODWARD, Joseph Janvier (1833-1884)
Photo-micrographs of the Pleurosigma angulatum, Pleurosigma formosum, and Nobert's plate. Washington: Surgeon-General's Office, 1871. 20 photo. DLC; DNLM **70-4058**

WOODWARD, Joseph Janvier (1833-1884)
Report to the Surgeon-General of the United States Army, on an improved method of photographing histological preparations by sunlight. Washington, 1871. 10p. 10 photo. DLC: DNLM **70-4059**

WOODWARD, Joseph Janvier (1833-1884)
Report to the Surgeon-General of the United States Army, on an improved method of photographing histological preparations by sunlight. Washington, 1871. 10p. 9 photo. DLC; DNLM **70-4060**

WOODWARD, Joseph Janvier (1833-1884)
. . . Report to the Surgeon-General of the United States Army on the minute anatomy of two cases of cancer. . . . Washington, D.C., 1872. 10p. DLC; DNLM **70-4061**

WOODWARD, Joseph Janvier (1833-1884)
Photo-micrographs of certain parasites. [Washington, 1872.] DLC; DNLM **70-4062**

WOODWARD, Joseph Janvier (1833-1884)
Remarks on the nomenclature of achromatic objectives for the compound microscope. [New Haven, 1872.] 9p. DLC; DNLM **70-4063**

WOODWARD, Joseph Janvier (1833-1884)
Letter to the Surgeon-General of the Army, accompanying seven photographs of some of the external appearances of the mosquito. [Washington, 1872.] 2p. 7 photo. DLC; DNLM **70-4064**

WOODWARD, Joseph Janvier (1833-1884)
Letter to the Surgeon-General of the Army, accompanying eleven miscellaneous photographs of insects and parts of insects. [Washington], 1872. 2p. 11 photo. DLC; DNLM **70-4065**

WOODWARD, Joseph Janvier (1833-1884)
Letter to the Surgeon-General of the Army, accompanying ten photographs of certain parasites. [Washington], 1872. 2p. 10 photo. DLC; DNLM **70-4066**

WOODWARD, Joseph Janvier (1833-1884)
Letter to the Surgeon-General of the Army, accompanying seven photographs of the proboscides of certain flies. [Washington], 1872. 2p. 7 photo. DLC; DNLM **70-4067**

WOODWARD, Joseph Janvier (1833-1884)
Memorandum on the nineteen-band test-plate of Nobert. [Washington, 1872.] 2 l. 9 photo. DLC; DNLM **70-4068**

WOODWARD, Joseph Janvier (1833-1884)
On the structure of cancerous tumors and the mode in which adjacent parts are invaded. Toner Lectures, No. I. Washington, 1872. 40p. DNLM **70-4069**

WOODWARD, Joseph Janvier (1833-1884)
The application of photography to micrometry, with special reference to the micrometry of blood in criminal cases. . . . Philadelphia: Press of J. B. Lippincott & Co., 1876. 13p. DLC; DNLM **70-4070**

WOODWARD, Joseph Janvier (1833-1884)
International Exhibition of 1876. Hospital of Medical Department, United States Army, No. 2. Description of the models of hospital cars exhibited in Room No. 2. [Washington: Gibson Bros.], 1876. 10p. 1 plate. DLC; DNLM
70-4071

WOODWARD, Joseph Janvier (1833-1884)
International Exhibition of 1876. Hospital of Medical Department, United States Army. No. 3. Description of the models of hospitals. [Washington: Gibson Bros.], 1876. 23p. 3 plates. DLC; DNLM **70-4072**

WOODWARD, Joseph Janvier (1833-1884)
International Exhibition of 1876. Hospital of Medical Department, United States Army. No. 4. Description of the models of hospital steam vessels exhibited in Room No. 2. [Washington: Gibson Bros.], 1876. 12p. 1 plate. DLC; DNLM
70-4073

WOODWARD, Joseph Janvier (1833-1884)
Photo-micrograph, 1876. Blood corpuscles of man, dog, etc. Philadelphia, 1876. Washington, 1876. 45 photo. DLC; DNLM
70-4074

WOODWARD, Joseph Janvier (1833-1884)
Photo-micrographs, 1870-1871. Cancer. Philadelphia, 1876. Washington: Surgeon-General's Office, 1876. 74 photo. DLC; DNLM **70-4075**

WOODWARD, Joseph Janvier (1833-1884)
Photo-micrographs. Fibers of wool, calf-hair, etc. Washington: Surgeon-General's Office, 1876. 26 photo. DLC; DNLM
70-4076

WOODWARD, Joseph Janvier (1833-1884)
Photo-micrographs. Histology of minute blood vessels and other histological photo-micrographs. Philadelphia, 1876. Washington: Surgeon-General's Office, 1876. 45 photo. DLC; DNLM **70-4077**

WOODWARD, Joseph Janvier (1833-1884)
Photo-micrographs of Nobert's nineteen-band plate, Webb's test, Nobert's wave-plate, Amphipleura pellucida, etc. [Washington: Surgeon-General's Office, 1876.] 24 photo. DLC; DNLM **70-4078**

WOODWARD, Joseph Janvier (1833-1884)
Photo-micrographs of Pleurosigma angulatum and formosum, Surirella gemma and Podura scales. Washington: Surgeon-General's Office, 1876. 20 photo. DLC; DNLM
70-4079

WOODWARD, Joseph Janvier (1833-1884)
The medical staff of the United State Army and its scientific work. An address delivered to the International Medical Congress, at Philadelphia, September 6, 1876. [Washington: Gibson Bros.], 1876. 28p. DLC; DNLM
70-4080

WOODWARD, Joseph Janvier (1833-1884)
Typho-malarial fever. Is it a special type of fever? Being remarks introductory to the discussion of the question in the section of medicine, International Medical Congress. [Washington: Gibson Bros.], 1876. 44p. DLC; DNLM
70-4081

WOODWARD, Joseph Janvier (1833-1884)
Dysentery and bacteria. An address delivered before the Society of the Alumni of the Medical Department of the University of Pennsylvania, March 10, 1877. With the proceedings of the alumni meeting of 1877. Philadelphia: Collins, 1878. 66p. DLC; DNLM **70-4082**

WOODWORTH, John M[aynard] (1837-1879)
Report on the immigration service, to the Secretary of the Treasury, Nov. 1, 1873. [Washington, 1873.] 46p. DNLM
70-4083

WOODWORTH, John M[aynard] (1837-1879)
Hospitals and hospital construction. Washington, 1874. 13p. 8 plates. DLC; DNLM **70-4084**

WOODWORTH, John M[aynard] (1837-1879) and Heber SMITH
Migrants and sailors, considered in their relation to the public health. Cambridge, 1875. 21p. DNLM **70-4085**

WOODWORTH, John M[aynard] (1837-1879)
Cholera epidemic of 1873 in the United States. The introduction of epidemic cholera through the agency of the mercantile marine: suggestions of measures of prevention. Washington: Government Printing Office, 1875. 28p. DNLM
70-4086

WOODWORTH, John M[aynard] (1837-1879)
The safety of ships, and of those who travel in them. Cambridge, 1877. 8p. DNLM **70-4087**

WOODWORTH, John M[aynard] (1837-1879)
The general subject of quarantine, with particular reference to cholera and yellow fever. Philadelphia, 1877. 13p. DLC; DNLM **70-4088**

WOOLLEY, B[asil] M.
The opium habit and its cure. And what others say of his cures. Atlanta, 1879. 62p. DNLM; GU; NNNAM; PU
70-4089

WOOLMAN, G. S.
Priced and illustrated catalogue of microscopes and optical instruments. New York, 1879. 13p. DNLM; NNNAM
70-4090

[WOOLSEY, Abby Howland] (1828-1893)
Handbook for hospital visitors. State Charities Aid Association. No. 13. New York: G. P. Putnam's Sons, 1877. 151p. DNLM; NN; MH; PU **70-4091**

WOOLWORTH, Isaac
Our children's teeth, or the dentist to mothers; a manual of dentistry for the household; embracing many practical and useful suggestions relating to our teeth, addressed to every person, through mothers. New Haven: Punderson, Crisand & Co., 1871. 158p. CtY-M; DNLM; MBM; NNNAM
70-4092

WORMLEY, Theodore G[eorge] (1826-1897)
The alkaloids of Veratrum viride and album. History, preparation, and recovery from complex mixtures and the blood. Philadelphia: Merrihew & Son, 1876. 12p. DNLM; PPC
70-4093

WORMLEY, Theodore G[eorge] (1826-1897)
Medical chemistry and toxicology. An address delivered before the International Medical Congress, at Philadelphia. Philadelphia: Collins, 1876. 26p. DNLM; PPC **70-4094**

WRIGHT, Charles Edward (1843-1893)
Address to the graduating class of Indiana Medical College. [On opium habit.] Indianapolis: Weekly Herald, 1879. 1p. DNLM 70-4095

WRIGHT, Thomas Lee (1825-1893)
Some points connected with the question of responsibility as it relates to the partially insane. [Cincinnati, 1879.] 15p. DNLM; OCIM 70-4096

WRIGHT, Thomas Lee (1825-1893)
Responsibility restricted by insane delusions. [Cincinnati, 1879.] 16p. DNLM; OCIM 70-4097

WYETH, John Allan (1845-1922)
A hand-book of medical and surgical reference. . . . New York: William Wood & Co., 1873. 279p. DLC; NNNAM; PPC; PU 70-4098

WYETH, John A[llan] (1845-1922)
A chapter in minor surgery. . . . New York: [J. F. Trow & Son], 1875. 30p. DLC; DNLM; NNNAM 70-4099

WYETH, John Allan (1845-1922)
. . . A prize essay upon the surgical anatomy of the tibio-tarsal articulation, with special regard to amputations at this joint. . . . [Philadelphia? 1876.] 12p. DLC; DNLM 70-4100

WYETH, John Allan (1845-1922)
The surgical anatomy of the carotid arteries, as deduced from one hundred and three consecutive dissections. New York: J. F. Trow & Son, 1876. 33p. DNLM; NNNAM 70-4101

WYETH, John Allan (1845-1922)
Prize essay.—Essays upon the surgical anatomy and history of the common, external, and internal carotid arteries, and the surgical anatomy and history of the innominate and subclavian arteries. . . . [Philadelphia, 1878.] 245p. plates. DLC; PPC; PPJ; PU 70-4102

WYETH, John Allan (1845-1922)
Essays in surgical anatomy and surgery. . . . New York: William Wood & Co., 1879. 262p. 12 plates. DLC; DNLM; MBM; NNNAM 70-4103

WYETH, JOHN & BRO.
Papoma. A farinaceous food for infants and invalids. [Philadelphia, 1872?] 2 l. DNLM 70-4104

WYETH, JOHN & BRO.
Dialyzed iron (ferrum dialysatum). A neurtral solution of oxide of iron in the colloid form. The result of endosmosis and diffusion with distilled water. [Philadelphia, 1877.] 16p. DNLM 70-4105

WYLIE, Walker Gill (1848-1923)
Hospitals: history of their origin and development: their progress during the century of the American republic. . . . New York: D. Appleton & Co., 1876. 37p. DLC; NNNAM 70-4106

WYLIE, Walker Gill (1848-1923)
Hospitals: their history, organization, and construction. Boylston prize essay of Harvard University for 1876. . . . New York: D. Appleton & Co., 1877. 240p. 2 fold. plates. DLC; DNLM; MH-M; NNNAM 70-4107

WYMAN, Morrill (1812-1903)
Autumnal catarrh (hay fever). New York: Hurd & Houghton, 1872. 173p. 3 maps. DLC; DNLM; MBM; NNNAM 70-4108

WYMAN, Morrill (1812-1903)
Autumnal catarrh (hay fever). . . . New York: Hurd & Houghton, 1876. 221p. 4 maps. DLC; NNNAM; PU 70-4109

WYMAN, Morrill (1812-1903)
The early history of the McLean Asylum for the Insane. A criticism of the report of the Massachusetts State Board of Health for 1877. Cambridge: Riverside Press, 1877. 15p. 5 plates. DNLM; MBAt; MBM; MWA 70-4110

WYTHE, Joseph Henry (1822-1901)
The physician's dose and symptom book, containing the doses and uses of all the principal articles of the materia medica and officinal preparations. . . . 10th ed. Philadelphia: Lindsay & Blakiston, 1871. 277p. DLC; DNLM; PPC; PPJ 70-4111

WYTHE, Joseph Henry (1822-1901)
The physician's dose and symptom book, containing the doses and uses of all the principal articles of the materia medica and officinal preparations. . . . 11th ed., rev. Philadelphia: Lindsay & Blakiston, 1874. 236p. DLC; PPC; PPJ; PU 70-4112

WYTHE, J[oseph] H[enry] (1822-1901)
The microscopist: a manual of microscopy and compendium of the microscopic sciences. . . . 3rd ed. Rewritten and greatly enl. . . . Philadelphia: Lindsay & Blakiston, 1877. 259p. 27 col. plates. DLC; OCIM; PPC; PPJ 70-4113

WYTHE, Joseph Henry (1822-1901)
Disease-germs. An address delivered at the anniversary meeting of the San Francisco Medical Society, November, 1879. 10p. [San Francisco: W. M. Hinton & Co., 1879.] 10p. DNLM 70-4114

YALE, Leroy Milton (1841-1906)
The argument for the antipyretic treatment of fever. New York: D. Appleton & Co., 1874. 20p. DNLM; NNNAM 70-4115

YALE, Leroy Milton (1841-1906)
Phimosis; a report from the surgical section to the New York Academy of Medicine. New York: D. Appleton & Co., 1877. 15p. DNLM; NNNAM 70-4116

YALE, Leroy Milton (1841-1906)
Certain general considerations respecting the mechanical treatment of chronic diseases of the joints. With especial reference to the use of traction. New York: Trow, 1878. 16p. DNLM; NNNAM 70-4117

YALE, Leroy Milton (1841-1906)
The Academy as a teacher. An anniversary discourse delivered before the New York Academy of Medicine, December 11, 1879. New York, 1879. 19p. DNLM; NNNAM 70-4118

YALE UNIVERSITY. MEDICAL DEPARTMENT. NEW HAVEN
Announcements for the spring terms of 1873-1876. New Haven, 1873-1876. CtY-M 70-4119

YALE UNIVERSITY. MEDICAL DEPARTMENT. NEW HAVEN
Alumni of the medical institution of Yale College [from 1814 to 1874]. [New Haven, 1875?] 11p. CtY-M; DNLM
70-4120

YANDELL, David Wendell (1826-1898)
Reply to the attack of Dr. E. S. Gaillard. Louisville: J. P. Morton & Co., 1871. 20p. DNLM **70-4121**

YANDELL, David Wendell (1826-1898)
Address before the American Medical Association. Philadelphia, May 7, 1872. Louisville: J. P. Morton & Co., 1872. 29p. DLC; DNLM; PPC **70-4122**

YANDELL, David Wendell (1826-1898)
Valedictory address to the medical graduates of the University of Louisville, March 1st, 1875. Louisville: J. P. Morton & Co., 1875. 21p. DNLM **70-4123**

YANDELL, David Wendell (1826-1898) and Ely McCLELLAN
Battey's operation. Louisville: J. P. Morton & Co., 1875. 16p. DNLM **70-4124**

YANDELL, David W[endell] (1826-1898)
A clinical lecture on the use of plastic dressing in fractures of lower extremity. Indianapolis, 1876. 10p. DNLM
70-4125

YANDELL, Lunsford Pitts (1805-1878)
A memoir of Dr. Benjamin W. Dudley. Louisville, Ky.: J. P. Morton & Co., 1870. 16p. DNLM; KyLoJM
70-4126

YANDELL, Lunsford Pitts (1805-1878)
Biographical sketch of Dr. B. F. Shumard. Indianapolis, 1870. 16p. DNLM **70-4127**

YANDELL, Lunsford Pitts (1805-1878)
On puerperal convulsions.. Louisville: J. P. Morton & Co., 1871. 16p. DNLM; KyLoJM **70-4128**

YANDELL, Lunsford Pitts (1805-1878)
Epidemic cholera: its origin and treatment. Louisville: J. P. Morton & Co., 1871. 16p. DNLM; KyLoJM
70-4129

YANDELL, Lunsford Pitts (1805-1878)
Recollections of the Medical Society of Tennessee. . . . Pub. by permission from Lindsley's Medical Annals of Tennessee. [Louisville, Ky., 1872.] 28p. DLC; DNLM
70-4130

YANDELL, Lunsford Pitts (1805-1878)
A biographical sketch of the late Amasa Converse, D.D. Louisville: Webb & Breeding, 1873. 15p. DNLM; KyLoJM
70-4131

YANDELL, Lunsford Pitts (1805-1878)
Medical literature of Kentucky. . . . Read before the Kentucky State Medical Society, 1874. Louisville: Printed by J. P. Morton & Co., 1874. 52p. DLC; DNLM
70-4132

YANDELL, Lunsford Pitts (1805-1878)
Address on American medical literature. Philadelphia, 1876. 44p. DNLM; PPC **70-4133**

YANDELL, Lunsford Pitts (1805-1878)
Notes on the life and writings of Dr. Benjamin Rush. Indianapolis: Journal Co., 1876. 16p. DNLM
70-4134

YANDELL, Lunsford Pitts (1805-1878)
Old age; its diseases and its hygiene. Louisville, 1878. 14p. DNLM **70-4135**

YANDELL, Lunsford Pitts, Jr. (1837-1884)
A report on dermatology, read before the Kentucky State Medical Society. Indianapolis, 1876. 7p. DNLM
70-4136

YANDELL, Lunsford Pitts, Jr. (1837-1884)
A case of syphilitic aphasia. [Philadelphia, 1877.] 8p. DNLM
70-4137

YANDELL, Lunsford Pitts, Jr. (1837-1884)
Report on dermatology; syphilis and other exanthemata. Louisville, Ky.: J. P. Morton & Co., 1877. 8p. DNLM
70-4138

YANDELL, Lunsford Pitts, Jr. (1837-1884)
Report on dermatology; syphilis and other exanthemata. [Louisville, 1877.] 8p. DNLM
70-4139

YANDELL, Lunsford Pitts, Jr. (1837-1884)
Malaria and struma; their relation to the etiology of skin diseases. Louisville, 1878. 15p. DNLM
70-4140

YELLOW FEVER COMMISSION
Circular letter of the . . . [to physicians, requesting replies to queries]. S. M. Bemiss, M.D., chairman; Jerome Cochran, M.D.; E. Lloyd Howard, M.D. Oct. 7, 1878. [New Orleans, 1878.] 2 l. DNLM; LNT-M **70-4141**

YELLOW FEVER NATIONAL RELIEF COMMISSION
Report of the executive committee, organized at Washington, D.C., Sept. 11, 1878, with accompanying reports of the operations of the relief boat "John M. Chambers," receipts, expenditures, etc. Washington, 1879. 76p. DNLM
70-4142

YOULIN, John Juvenal (1821-1881)
Address before the American Institute of Homoeopathy, twenty-seventh annual session, held at Niagara Falls, N.Y., June, 1874. Philadelphia: Sherman & Co., 1875. 15p. PPHa
70-4143

YOUNG, D[elos] W. (1829-1874)
Bloodletting not necessary in the treatment of pneumonia. A contribution to the report on practical medicine. Chicago: R. Fergus & Son, 1870. 25p. DNLM **70-4144**

YOUNG, Delos W. (1829-1874)
Cholera infantum; its cause, pathology, and treatment. Chicago: R. Fergus' Sons, 1871. 28p. DNLM
70-4145

YOUNG, Noble (1808-1883)
Address delivered on the occasion of laying the corner stone of the building for the College of Physicians and Surgeons, of Wilmington, N.C., Dec. 27, 1871. Wilmington, N.C.: J. A. Engelhard, 1872. 20p. DNLM; NcD; NcU
70-4146

YOUNG, Noble (1808-1883), John Edwin MASON, and Thomas ROBINSON
Addresses delivered at the twenty-seventh annual commencement of the Medical Department of Georgetown University, March 10, 1876. Washington: R. O. Polkinhorn, 1876. 31p. DNLM **70-4147**

ZIEMSSEN, Hugo Wilhelm von (1829-1902), ed.
Cyclopaedia of the practice of medicine. . . . Albert H. Buck . . . , editor of American ed. New York: William Wood & Co., 1874-1881. 20 v. DLC; NNNAM; PPC; PPJ [and *Supplement* (1881), ed. by George L. Peabody] **70-4148**

VII. AMERICAN MEDICAL IMPRINTS, 1880-1889

As it is now seven years since I first published a formal statement of this method, it seems to me that the time has come when I should say in what respect my opinions have been altered or confirmed, and what changes I would desire to suggest. I shall, therefore, give here a condensed statement of the treatment in question, and referring to my former publications for minute details, shall criticize it in the light of what, without want of modest statement, I may venture to call an enormous experience.

The treatment to which in these pages I so many times refer, consists in an effort to lift the health of patients to a higher plane by the use of seclusion, which cuts off excitement and foolish sympathy; by rest, so complete as to exclude all causes of tire; by massage, which substitutes passive exercise for exertion; and by electrical muscular excitation, which acts in a somewhat similar manner to massage, and with it by depriving rest in bed of its essential evils, leaves only its good. These means enable us to over-feed our patients, and to enable them to digest with ease large amounts of food.

S. Weir Mitchell, *Lectures on Diseases of the Nervous System, Especially in Women* (1881)

ABBE, Robert (1851-1928)
On Dupuytren's finger-contraction, its nervous origin. New York: D. Appleton & Co., 1884. 25p. DNLM
80-0001

ABBE, Robert (1851-1928)
Intestinal anastomosis. Philadelphia: W. J. Dornan, 1889. 18p. DNLM **80-0002**

ABBE, Robert (1851-1928)
The surgical treatment of inveterate tic douloureux. New York, 1889, 8p. DNLM **80-0003**

ABBOTT, Frank (1836-1897)
Address delivered before the American Academy of Dental Science, at their fifteenth annual meeting. Boston: T. Todd, 1882. 18p. DNLM **80-0004**

ABBOTT, Frank (1836-1897)
Microscopical studies upon absorption of the roots of temporary teeth. New York, [1884]. 10p. DNLM
80-0005

ABBOTT, Frank (1836-1897)
Studies of the pathology of enamel of human teeth, with special reference to the etiology of caries. [Minneapolis, 1885.] 13p. DNLM **80-0006**

ABBOTT, Frank (1836-1897)
Hyperostosis of roots of teeth. Philadelphia, 1886. 19p. DNLM
80-0007

ABBOTT, Frank (1836-1897)
A contribution to the study of the minute anatomy of enamel. Philadelphia, 1887. 7p. DNLM **80-0008**

ABBOTT, Frank (1836-1897)
Teeth of rabbits. Philadelphia, 1887. 11p. DNLM
80-0009

ABBOTT, Frank (1836-1897)
Odontoblasts in their relation to developing dentine. Philadelphia, 1888. 11p. DNLM **80-0010**

ABBOTT, Frank (1836-1897)
Diseases of the antrum due to dental complications, and its treatment. Philadelphia, 1888. 8p. DNLM
80-0011

ABBOTT, Frank (1836-1897)
Growth of enamel. Philadelphia, 1889. 14p. DNLM
80-0012

ABEL-MUSGRAVE, Curt
The cholera in San Francisco: a contribution to the history of corruption in California. San Francisco: San Francisco News Co., 1885. 28p. CU-M **80-0013**

ACTON, William (1813-1875)
The functions and disorders of the reproductive organs in childhood, youth, adult age, and advanced life, considered in their physiological, social and moral relations. 6th ed. Philadelphia: P. Blakiston, Son & Co., 1883. 267p. CtY-M; IU-M; PPC; PPJ **80-0014**

ADAMS, A. Wellington
The electric laryngoscope. [New York: G. P. Putnam's Sons, 1880.] 5p. DNLM **80-0015**

ADAMS, A. Wellington
Flagrant abuses requiring correction; proprietary vs. legitimate pharmacy. [Kansas City, 1889.] 4p. DNLM
80-0016

ADAMS, George F.
Turkish bath hand book. St. Louis: Little & Becker, 1881. 242p. OCIM **80-0017**

ADAMS, J[ames] F[orster] Alleyne (1844-1914)
Malaria in New England. Cambridge: Riverside Press, 1882. 6p. DNLM; MH-M **80-0018**

ADAMS, J[ames] F[orster] Alleyne (1844-1914)
The New Lenox malaria case. Cambridge: Riverside Press, 1883. 16p. DNLM; MH-M **80-0019**

ADAMS, J[ames] F[orster] Alleyne (1844-1914)
Substitutes for opium in chronic disease. Philadelphia: W. J. Dornan, 1889. 17p. DNLM **80-0020**

ADAMS, J. Howe (1866-1919)
The use of carbolic acid in diarrhoea. [Philadelphia, 1889.] 2p. DNLM **80-0021**

ADAMS, Samuel S[hugert] (1853-1928)
Incontinence of urine in children. New York: William Wood & Co., 1884. 14p. DNLM; NNNAM **80-0022**

ADAMS, Samuel S[hugert] (1853-1928)
Sudden death in diphtheria. New York: William Wood & Co., 1884. 26p. DNLM; NNNAM **80-0023**

ADAMS, Samuel S[hugert] (1853-1928)
Strabismus convergence unaccompanied by paralysis of accommodation as a sequela of diphtheria. Philadelphia: J. E. Potter & Co., 1884. 5 l. DNLM **80-0024**

ADAMS, Samuel S[hugert] (1853-1928)
The systematic training of nursery-maids. Chicago, 1887. 11p. DNLM **80-0025**

ADAMS, Samuel S[hugert] (1853-1928)
The relation of dentition to diseases of the alimentary tract. [Philadelphia, 1889.] 16p. DNLM **80-0026**

ADAMS, Wellington
Dawn of a new era in ontological surgery. [St. Louis, 1881.] 8p. MB **80-0026A**

ADDRESSES at the inauguration of William Pepper as provost of the University of Pennsylvania, Feb. 22, 1881. Philadelphia: Collins, 1881. 62p. DNLM; PPC; PHi; PU
80-0027

ADLER, Lewis H., Jr.
The technique of ovariotomy as practiced at the University Hospital by Prof. Wm. Goodell. Philadelphia, 1888. 12p. DNLM **80-0028**

ADLER, Lewis H., Jr.
A case of Hodgkin's disease accompanied with a possible resulting paraplegia. Philadelphia, 1889. 6p. DNLM
80-0029

ADLER, Lewis H., Jr.
Report of a case of hysteria simulating laryngismus stridulus. Philadelphia, 1889. 2p. DNLM **80-0030**

ADLER, Lewis H., Jr.
Report of a case of hystero-epilepsy in a man. Philadelphia, 1889. 7p. DNLM **80-0031**

ADLER, Lewis H., Jr.
Lacerated cervix uteri as treated at the University Hospital by Professor William Goodell. New York, 1889. 9p. DNLM **80-0032**

ADLER, Lewis H., Jr.
Report of amputations performed at the hospital of the University of Pennsylvania, from September 30, 1874, to December 31, 1888. [Philadelphia, 1889.] 9p. DNLM **80-0033**

ADLER, Lewis H., Jr.
Report of a case of stricture of the rectum, the probable result of a specific vaginitis. [Philadelphia, 1889.] 5p. DNLM **80-0034**

ADLER, Lewis H., Jr.
Prolapse of the womb, with especial reference to the (so-called) hypertrophic elongation of the supra-vaginal portion of the cervix, with report of a case. [Philadelphia, 1889.] 12p. DNLM **80-0035**

ADLER, Lewis H., Jr.
A case of cerebral syphilis following an attack of thermic fever. [Boston, 1889.] 5p. DNLM **80-0036**

ADLER, Lewis H., Jr.
Diphtheritic paralysis. [Detroit, 1889.] 8p. DNLM **80-0037**

AGNEW, Cornelius Rea (1830-1888)
Contributions to ophthalmology. [I. The insufficiency of the ophthalmoscope as the sole test of errors of refraction. II. Three cases of persistent pupillary membrane.] [New York, 1880.] 15p. DNLM; NNNAM **80-0038**

AGNEW, Cornelius Rea (1830-1888)
The limits of medical ethics. [New York, 1882.] 8p. DNLM **80-0039**

AGNEW, Cornelius Rea (1830-1888)
Notes on contagious diseases of the eyes in schools and asylums. State Board of Health of New York. [Albany, 1882.] 9p. DNLM **80-0040**

AGNEW, Cornelius Rea (1830-1888)
An operation with a double needle or bident, for the removal of a crystalline lens dislocated into the vitreous chamber. [Philadelphia, 1885.] 12p. DNLM; PPC **80-0041**

AGNEW, D[avid] Hayes (1818-1892)
Lacerations of the female perineum and vesico-vaginal fistula, their history and treatment with an account of the methods of performing the operations and the instruments used illustrated by cases. Philadelphia: P. Blakiston, Son & Co., 1882. 141p. PPC **80-0042**

AGNEW, D[avid] Hayes (1818-1892)
Memoir of John Light Atlee, M.D., LL.D. Philadelphia: W. J. Doran, 1886. 11p. PPC **80-0043**

AGNEW, D[avid] Hayes (1818-1892)
University of Pennsylvania. Medical Department of, Philadelphia. [Circular of the committee representing the three undergraduate classes, the hospital staff, and the faculty of the medical department of the university, requesting the co-operation of the alumni in the celebration of the fiftieth anniversary of Professor D. Hayes Agnew's graduation.] March 1, 1888. Philadelphia, 1888. DNLM; PU **80-0044**

AGNEW, D[avid] Hayes (1818-1892)
The principles and practice of surgery, being a treatise on surgical diseases and injuries. 2nd ed., thoroughly rev., with additions. Philadelphia: J. B. Lippincott & Co., 1889. 3 v. MBM; NNNAM; PPC; PU **80-0045**

AITKEN, William (1825-1892)
A complete handbook of treatment, arranged as an alphabetical index of diseases to facilitate reference and containing nearly one thousand formulae. New York: Bermingham & Co., 1882. 444p. DNLM; NNNAM; PPC; PPJ [Bermingham's Medical Library] **80-0046**

AITKEN, William (1825-1892)
A complete handbook of treatment, arranged as an alphabetical index of diseases to facilitate reference and containing nearly one thousand formulae. . . . Edited with notes and additions by A. D. Rockwell. New York: E. B. Treat, 1887. 444p. CU-M; ICRM; NNNAM; PU [Medical Classics] **80-0047**

AITKEN, William (1825-1892)
On the animal alkaloids, the ptomaines, leucomaines, and extractives in their pathological relations; being a short summary of recent researches as to the origin of some diseases by or through the physiological processes going on during life. Philadelphia: P. Blakiston, Son & Co., 1887, 61p. CtY-M; MH-M; NNNAM; PPC **80-0048**

AITKEN, William (1825-1892)
On the animal alkaloids, the ptomaines, leucomaines, and extractives in their pathological relations; being a short summary of recent researches as to the origin of some diseases by or through the physiological processes going on during life. 2nd ed. Philadelphia: P. Blakiston, Son & Co., 1889. 112p. NNNAM; NNU-M; PPC; PU **80-0049**

ALLBUTT, Thomas Clifford (1836-1925)
On visceral neuroses, being the Gulstonian lectures on neuralgia of the stomach and allied disorders, delivered at the Royal College of Physicians in March, 1884. Philadelphia: P. Blakiston, Son & Co., 1884. 103p. DNLM; NNNAM; PPC; PPJ **80-0050**

THE ALLEGHANY Springs, Montgomery County, Va. An elaborate analysis of the water. Lynchburg, Va.: J. P. Bell & Co., 1884. 60p. DNLM **80-0051**

ALLEMAN, L. A. W[elles]
An ophthalmo-dynamometer. [Brooklyn, 1889.] 7p. DNLM **80-0052**

ALLEN, Charles W[arrene] (1854-1906)
Cholera in America. How to meet it. How to treat it. . . . [Hartford, Conn.: The Case, Lockwood & Brainard Co., print], 1885. 15p. DLC **80-0053**

ALLEN, Charles W[arrene] (1854-1906)
Molluscum contagiosum; an analysis of fifty cases. New York: William Wood & Co., 1886. 7p. 1 plate. DNLM
80-0054

ALLEN, Charles W[arrene] (1854-1906)
Practical observations on the gonococcus and Roux's method of confirming its identity. [New York, 1887.] 11p. DNLM
80-0055

ALLEN, Harrison (1841-1897)
A system of human anatomy, including its medical and surgical relations. . . . with a section on histology. By E. O. Shakespeare. . . . Illustrated with . . . one hundred and nine full-page lithographic plates. . . . The drawings by Hermann Faber. . . . Also two hundred and forty-one woodcuts in the text. Philadelphia: Henry C. Lea's Son & Co., 1884. 812p. 109 plates. DLC; DNLM; PPC; PU **80-0056**

ALLEN, Harrison (1841-1897)
On a new method of recording the motions of the soft palate. . . . Philadelphia: P. Blakiston, Son & Co., 1884. 34p. DLC; DNLM **80-0057**

ALLEN, Harrison (1841-1897)
Electricity in medicine. Philadelphia: J. S. Smith, 1885. 10p. DNLM **80-0058**

ALLEN, Harrison (1841-1897)
On the methods of study on the crowns of the human teeth, including their variations. [Philadelphia, 1888.] 4p. DNLM
80-0059

ALLEN, Harrison (1841-1897)
The palatal rugae in man. Philadelphia, 1888. 19p. DNLM
80-0060

ALLEN, Harrison (1841-1897)
The anatomy of the nasal chambers. New York, 1889. 11p. DNLM **80-0061**

ALLEN, Henry C. (1836-1909)
The therapeutics of intermittent fever. Philadelphia: F. E. Boericke, 1884. 342p. DNLM; PPHa
80-0062

ALLEN, Henry C. (1836-1909)
Secale cornutum. A fragmentary proving. By H. C. Allen, M.D., and the students of the University of Michigan. Pittsburgh: Stevenson & Foster, 1885. 18p. 1 plate. DNLM; PPHa
80-0063

ALLEN, Henry C. (1836-1909)
Consumption: its cause and nature by Rollin R. Gregg, M.D. to which is added the Therapeutics of Tuberculosis Affections. Ann Arbor, [Mich.], 1889. 477p. OCIM; PPHa
80-0064

ALLEN, John Adams
Hints to physicians concerning water drinking. By J. Adams Allen, M.D., William T. Belfield, M.D., Oscar C. De Wolf, M.D., and Walter S. Haines, M.D. Chicago: F. H. Revell, 1884. 55p. DLC **80-0065**

ALLEN, Jonathan Adams (1825-1890)
Medical examinations for life insurance. . . . 7th ed., rev. and enl. . . . New York and Chicago: The Spectator Company, 1880. 181p. DLC; NNNAM; OCIM
80-0066

ALLEN, Jonathan Adams (1825-1890)
Progress in medical education, being the doctorate address at the thirty-ninth annual commencemnt of the Rush Medical College; Feb. 22, 1881. [With secretary's report for the session of 1880-1881.] Chicago: Chicago Legal News Co., 1881. 20p. DNLM; ICRM **80-0067**

ALLEN, Joseph Eve
A case of puerperal eclampsia, with remarks; read before the Augusta Medical Society. [Atlanta, 1880.] 9p. DNLM
80-0068

ALLEN, Joseph Eve
The uses of tar-water in obstetrical and gynaecological practice; read before the Doctors' Society of Augusta, Ga. [Atlanta, 1880.] 9p. DNLM **80-0069**

ALLEN, Joseph Eve
The treatment of delay in the first stage of natural labor, with special reference to the early use of the forceps. [Atlanta, 1882.] 9p. DNLM **80-0070**

ALLEN, J[oshua] G[ibbons] (1832-1903)
Orthopaedic notes; with report of interesting cases treated at the Surgical Institute, corner of Broad and Arch Streets, Philadelphia. Philadelphia, 1887. 24p. DNLM; PPC
80-0071

ALLEN, Nathan (1813-1889)
Supervision of lunatic hospitals; a paper read at Cleveland, Ohio, July 2, 1880. before the National Conference of Charities. Boston: Tolman & White, 1880. 16p. DNLM
80-0072

ALLEN, Nathan (1813-1889)
Influence of medical men. Read before the American Academy of Medicine at its annual meeting in Philadelphia, Oct. 26, 1882. [Bridgeport, Conn., 1882.] 5p. DNLM
80-0073

ALLEN, Nathan (1813-1889)
The law of human increase. [New York, 1882.] 10p. DNLM
80-0074

ALLEN, Nathan (1813-1889)
Insanity in its relations to the medical profession and lunatic hospitals. Read at the annual meeting of the American Association for the Protection of the Insane in New York. January 29, 1882. [1882.] 1 broadside. DNLM **80-0075**

ALLEN, Nathan (1813-1889)
The prevention of insanity. Boston: Wright & Potter, 1883. 23p. DNLM **80-0076**

ALLEN, Nathan (1813-1889)
Changes in New England population. [With explanation and defense of the preceding paper.] [New York, 1883.] 16p. DNLM **80-0077**

ALLEN, Nathan (1813-1889)
Laws of heredity. [New York, 1883.] 1 broadside. DNLM
80-0078

ALLEN, Nathan (1813-1889)
Normal standard of physiology. [Sandy Hook, Conn., 1885.] 5p. DNLM **80-0079**

ALLEN, Nathan (1813-1889)
Normal standard of physiology. Lowell, 1885. 1 broadside. DNLM **80-0080**

ALLEN, Nathan (1813-1889)
Physiology in its more public relations. [1885.] 1 broadside. DNLM **80-0081**

ALLEN, Nathan (1813-1889)
Laws of maternity. [Sandy Hook, Conn., 1885.] 7p. DNLM **80-0082**

ALLEN, Nathan (1813-1889)
Laws of inheritance. [Bridgeport, Conn., 1886.] 5p. DNLM **80-0083**

ALLEN, Nathan (1813-1889)
Physical culture in Amherst College. Read at the tenth annual meeting of the American Academy of Medicine at Pittsburgh, Penn., Oct. 12, 1886. [1886.] 16p. DNLM **80-0084**

ALLEN, Nathan (1813-1889)
The relations between sanitary science and the medical profession. [Concord, N.H., 1887.] 14p. DNLM **80-0085**

ALLEN, Nathan (1813-1889)
The relations between sanitary science and the medical profession. [1886.] 1 broadside. DNLM **80-0086**

ALLEN, Nathan (1813-1889)
Physical development, or the laws governing the human system. Boston: Lee & Shepard; New York: C. T. Dillingham, 1888. 34p. port. DNLM; NNNAM **80-0087**

ALLEN, Timothy Field (1837-1902)
A general symptom register of the homoeopathic materia medica. . . . New York & Philadelphia: Boericke & Tafel, 1880. 1331p. OCLloyd; PPHa; PPJ **80-0088**

ALLEN, Timothy Field (1837-1902)
A critical examination of our materia medica. [New York, 1880-1881.] 64+ p. DNLM; PPHa **80-0089**

ALLEN, Timothy Field (1837-1902)
A critical revision of the encyclopedia of pure materia medica. [1886?] 16+ p. DNLM; PPHa **80-0090**

ALLEN, Timothy Field (1837-1902)
A handbook of materia medica, and homoeopathic therapeutics. . . . Philadelphia: F. E. Boericke, 1889. 1165p. DLC; DNLM; OCLloyd; PPHa **80-0091**

ALLEN, William A.
Repertory to the symptoms of intermittent fever. Philadelphia: F. E. Boericke, 1883. 107p. DNLM; PPHa **80-0092**

ALLINGHAM, William (1829-1908)
Fistula, haemorrhoids, painful ulcer, stricture, prolapsus, and other diseases of the rectum: their diagnosis and treatment. 4th ed. New York: Bermingham & Co., 1882. 252p. CtY-M; DNLM; IU-M; NNNAM **80-0093**

ALLINGHAM, William (1829-1908)
Fistula, hemorrhoids, painful ulcer, stricture, prolapsus, and other diseases of the rectum: their diagnosis and treatment. . . . 4th rev. and enl. ed. . . . Philadelphia: P. Blakiston, Son & Co., 1883. 88p. DLC; INE-M; PPC; PU **80-0094**

ALLIS, Oscar H. (1836-1921)
Deformity from fractures at the lower end of the humerus, and how it may be avoided. New York: G. P. Putnam's Sons, 1880. 20p. DNLM; NNNAM **80-0095**

ALLIS, Oscar H. (1836-1921)
Upon the danger from fractures in close proximity to the knee-joint. Philadelphia: Collins, 1881. 15p. DNLM **80-0096**

ALLIS, Oscar H. (1836-1921)
The formation of the tunica vaginalis; the descent of the testes and their relation to oblique inguinal hernia and hydrocele. Brooklyn, 1883. 15p. DNLM; NNNAM **80-0097**

ALLISON, Henry Edward (1851-1904)
The moral and industrial management of the insane. [St. Louis, 1886.] 12p. DNLM **80-0098**

ALLISON, Henry Edward (1851-1904)
On a general system of reporting autopsies in American asylums for the insane. [With form for post-mortem records.] [Utica, N.Y., 1889.] 8p. DNLM **80-0099**

ALLPORT, Walter Webb (1824-1893)
The relation of dentistry to medicine. [Toledo], 1882. 8p. DNLM **80-0100**

ALTHAUS, Julius (1833-1900)
On sclerosis of the spinal cord. . . . New York: G. P. Putnam's Sons, 1885. 394p. NNNAM **80-0101**

AMERICAN homoeopathic pharmacopoeia. . . . New York & Philadelphia: Boericke & Tafel, 1882. 523p. DLC; NNNAM; OCLloyd; PPHa **80-0102**

THE AMERICAN homoeopathic pharmacopoeia. 2nd ed., thoroughly rev. and augm. by Joseph T. O'Connor. . . . New York, Philadelphia and Chicago: Boericke & Tafel, 1883. 511p. DLC; MBM; OCLloyd. PPHa **80-0103**

THE AMERICAN homoeopathic pharmacopoeia. 3rd ed., thoroughly rev. and augm. by Joseph T. O'Connor. New York & Philadelphia: Boericke & Tafel, 1885. 521p. OCIM; OCLloyd; PPHa **80-0104**

AMERICAN INSTITUTE OF HOMOEOPATHY
Report of the bureau of organization, registration, and statistics to the American Institute of Homoeopathy, at its session held in Milwaukee, June 15, 1880. Boston: A. Mudge & Son, 1880. 22p. DNLM; OCIM; PPHa **80-0105**

AMERICAN INSTITUTE OF HOMOEOPATHY
Transactions of the World's Homoeopathic Convention, held at Philadelphia, under the auspices of the American Institute of Homoeopathy, at its 29th session, June 26th to July 1st, 1876. History of homoeopathy. Philadelphia: Sherman & Co., 1880-1881. 2 v. DNLM; PPC; PPHa; PPJ **80-0106**

AMERICAN INSTITUTE OF HOMOEOPATHY
Circular letter to the honorable the members of the Senate and House of Representatives of the United States [asking that physicians of the homoeopathic schools be made eligible to positions in the medical departments of the United States]. [Philadelphia, 1883.] 18p. DNLM; PPHa
80-0107

AMERICAN MEDICAL ASSOCIATION
General programme . . . thirty-second annual meeting, Richmond, Va., May, 1881. Richmond: J. W. Fergusson & Son, [1881]. 4 l. DNLM **80-0108**

AMERICAN MEDICAL ASSOCIATION
Index to the transactions of the . . . . 1-33. Prepared by William B. Atkinson. Philadelphia: W. F. Fell & Co., 1883. 130p. DNLM; MBM; NNNAM; PU **80-0109**

AMERICAN MEDICAL ASSOCIATION
Programme of proceedings of the thirty-fifth annual session of the . . . held at Washington, D.C., May 6, 7, 8, and 9, 1884. Washington, D.C.: Gray & Clarkson, 1884. 4, 8p. DNLM
80-0110

AMERICAN MEDICAL ASSOCIATION
Proceedings of the thirty-fifth annual meeting, held in Washington, May 6-9, inclusive, 1884. Together with the plan of organization, by-laws, and code of ethics of the association, and the list of members in attendance at the recent meeting. Chicago: A. G. Newell, 1884. 38p. DNLM; IEN-M
80-0111

AMERICAN MEDICAL ASSOCIATION
Memorial to the Senate and House of Representatives of the Untied States [with accompanying] documents with reference to the proposed building for the Army Medical Museum and library of the Surgeon-General's Office. [n.p., 1884?] 14p. DNLM **80-0112**

AMERICAN MEDICAL ASSOCIATION
Programme of proceedings of the thirty-sixth annual session of the . . . held at New Orleans, La., April 28, 29, 30, and May 1, 1885. New Orleans: L. Graham & Son, 1885. 10p. DNLM; LNT-M **80-0113**

AMERICAN MEDICAL ASSOCIATION
Memorial of committee of the American Medical Association in relation to the prevention of yellow fever, June 14, 1886. 49th Congress, 1st session. Mis. Doc. No. 129. In S., June 18, 1886. Presented by Mr. Butler. [Washington, 1886.] 8p. DNLM **80-0114**

AMERICAN MEDICAL ASSOCIATION
Memorial of the American Medical Association, praying certain legislation for the better protection of the health and lives of immigrants on board passenger vessels. Report of the committee on memorializing Congress relative to medical sanitary service on board immigrant passenger vessels. 50th Congress, 1st session. S. Mis. Doc. No. 57. Feb. 14, 1888. Presented by Mr. Frye. [Washington, 1888.] 3p. DNLM
80-0115

AMERICAN ORTHOPEDIC ASSOCIATION
Constitution and by-laws. New York: M. J. Rooney, 1887. 8p. DNLM; NNNAM **80-0116**

AMERICAN PEDIATRIC SOCIETY
The constitution and by-laws, with the officers and members for 1888-1889. Philadelphia: J. B. Lippincott Co., 1888. 9p. DNLM; PPC [Organized in Washington, D.C., Sept. 18, 1888.]
80-0117

AMERICAN PHYSIOLOGICAL SOCIETY
Constitution and list of members. [Baltimore: I. Friedenwald, 1887.] 11p. DNLM; MdU-D [Founded December 30, 1887.]
80-0118

AMERICAN POPULAR HEALTH ASSOCIATION
Prospectus. Chicago, 1888. 8p. DNLM **80-0119**

AMERICAN SOCIETY FOR THE RESTRICTION OF VIVISECTION
A reply to certain charges against the Society for the Restriction of Vivisection, contained in a report made to the College of Physicians of this city, by Drs. Mitchell and Wood. [Philadelphia, 1885?] 7p. DNLM; PPC **80-0120**

AMERICAN SURGICAL ASSOCIATION
Constitution and by-laws adopted May 31, 1882, and names of officers and fellows. [n.p.]: M. Cullaton & Co., 1883. 11p. DNLM; NNNAM; PPC **80-0121**

AMERICAN SURGICAL ASSOCIATION
Transactions, history of the organization, abstract of the proceedings of the meetings held from the organization, June 1, 1880, to April 30, 1884, constitution and by-laws, and names of fellows of the Association. Richmond, Ind.: M. Cullaton & Co., 1884. 63p. DNLM; PPC; PU **80-0122**

AMERLING, H. Wharton
Address upon the formation of the American Society for the Prevention of Adulteration of Food, Drugs, etc., at Philadelphia, Pa. Philadelphia, 1885. 24p. DNLM
80-0123

AMICK, M[arion] L. (*b.* 1843)
Cranial nerves as taught by Prof. . . . Cincinnati, Ohio. Cincinnati, 1883. 1 sheet. DNLM **80-0124**

AMIDON, Royal W[ells] (*b.* 1853)
A new study of cerebral cortical localization. The effect of willed muscular movements on the temperature of the head. The essay to which was awarded the prize of the Alumni Association of the College of Physicians and Surgeons, New York, March 12, 1880. New York: G. P. Putnam's Sons, 1880. 57p. 1 plate. DNLM; NNNAM **80-0125**

AMIDON, Royal W., ed. (*b.* 1853)
. . . A year-book of therapeutics for 1883. . . . New York, London: G. P. Putnam's Sons, 1884. 250p. DLC; NNNAM; OCIM **80-0126**

AMIDON, Royal W[ells] (*b.* 1853)
Student's manual of electro-therapeutics, embodying lectures delivered in the course on therapeutics at the Women's Medical College of the New York Infirmary. New York [etc.]: G. P. Putnam's Sons, 1884. 93p. CtY-M; DNLM; NNNAM; PU
80-0127

AMIDON, Royal W[ells] (*b.* 1853)
A plea for more heroic surgical interference in affections of the brain. [Philadelphia, 1884.] 23p. DNLM; PPC
80-0128

AMMERMAN, Coleman R.
The medical surgical directory of the State of Missouri for 1884 and 1885. . . . Quincy: Volk & Jones, 1885. 223p. DNLM; IU-M; OCIM **80-0129**

AMORY, Robert (1842-1910)
A contribution to the haematinic properties of dialyzed iron; being extracts from communications read before the Boston Society of the Medical Sciences, and the Boston Society for Medical Observation. Philadelphia: G. F. Lasher, 1882. 20p. 5 plates. DNLM; MBM; MWA **80-0130**

AMORY, Robert (1842-1910)
A treatise on electrolysis and its applications to therapeutics and surgical treatment in disease. New York: William Wood & Co., 1886. 307p. DLC; DNLM; NNNAM; PU **80-0131**

ANDERS, James M[eschter] (1854-1936)
Sanitary influences of forest growth. Philadelphia, 1885. 15p. DNLM **80-0132**

ANDERS, James M[eschter] (1854-1936)
House-plants as sanitary agents; or, the relation of growing vegetation to health and disease. Comprising also a consideration of the subject of practical floriculture, and of the sanitary influences of forests and plantations. Philadelphia: J. B. Lippincott & Co., 1887. 334p. DNLM; NN; MH; PU **80-0133**

ANDERSON, J. C.
Trophic surgery. A paper read before the post-graduate class, New York City, January, 1888. [n.p.], 1888. 8p. DNLM **80-0134**

ANDERSON, Thomas McCall (1836-1908)
A treatise on diseases of the skin, with special reference to their diagnosis and treatment, including an analysis of 11,000 consecutive cases. Philadelphia: P. Blakiston, Son & Co., 1887. 662p. 4 plates. CU-M; DNLM; ICRM; PPC **80-0135**

ANDERSON, William Henry (1820-1887)
Medical Association of the State of Alabama. The annual message of the president. Montgomery, Ala.: Barrett & Brown, 1881. 27p. DNLM; AU **80-0136**

ANDERSON, William Henry (1820-1887)
The city of Mobile and the contiguous country about the Gulf coast as a winter resort for health and pleasure of invalids and others from the North and Northwest. Mobile, 1881. 16p. DNLM; AU **80-0137**

ANDREWS, Edmund (1824-1904)
Rectal and anal surgery, with a description of the secret methods of the itinerants, by Edmund Andrews . . . and E. Wyllys Andrews. . . . With original illustrations. Chicago: W. T. Keener, 1888. 111p. DLC; DNLM; IEN-M; NNNAM **80-0138**

ANDREWS, Edmund (1824-1904)
Rectal and anal surgery, with a description of the secret methods of the itinerants, by Edmund Andrews . . . and E. Wyllys Andrews. . . . 2nd ed. rev. and enl., with illustrations and formulary. Chicago: W. T. Keener, 1889. 140p. DLC; DNLM; ICRM; PPC **80-0139**

ANDREWS, Joseph A[lfred]
Trachoma and the etiology of jequirity ophthalmia. [New York, 1884.] 40p. DNLM **80-0140**

ANDREWS, Joseph A[lfred]
Contagious conjunctivitis; its causes, prevention, and treatment. [New York, 1885.] 24p. DNLM **80-0141**

ANDREWS, Joseph A[lfred]
Contagious eye-disease. [New York, 1886.] 20p. DNLM **80-0142**

ANDREWS, Joseph A[lfred]
The electric light as an illuminator. The effect of strong light on the eye. [New York, 1886.] 15p. DNLM **80-0143**

ANDREWS, Joseph A[lfred]
Successful removal of two osteomata of the orbit: one originating in the frontal, the other in the ethmoidal cells. With a history of osteomata of the neighboring pneumatic cavities of the orbit. New York: Trow's Co., 1887. 56p. DNLM **80-0144**

ANDREWS, Joseph A[lfred]
Enucleation of the eyeball during purulent panophthalmitis. Twelve consecutive enucleations of the eyeball during purulent panophthalmitis, in all of which the course of healing was uninterrupted by unfavorable symptoms. [New York, 1888.] 11p. 1 table. **80-0145**

ANDREWS, Judson B[oardman] (1834-1894)
Urethran. Utica, N.Y., [1886]. 9p. DNLM **80-0146**

ANGELL, Henry C[lay] (1829-1911)
A treatise on diseases of the eye. For the use of general practitioners. 6th ed. Boston and Providence: Otis Clapp & Son, 1884. 404p. MBM; NNNAM; PPC; PU **80-0147**

ANSTIE, Francis Edmund (1833-1874)
Neuralgia and the diseases that resemble it. . . . New York: Bermingham & Co., 1882. 233p. DLC; MBM; NNNAM; PU **80-1048**

ARLT, [Carl] Ferdinand von (1812-1887)
Clinical studies on diseases of the eye, including those of the conjunctiva, cornea, sclerotic, iris, and ciliary body. Transl. by Lyman Ware. Philadelphia: P. Blakiston, Son & Co., 1885. 325p. 1 plate. CLM; DNLM; IU-M; NNNAM **80-0149**

[ARMOR, Samuel Glasgow] (1819-1885)
The beloved physician: a tribute to the memory of the late Samuel G. Armor. New York: New York Acad. Anthrop., [1885]. 16p. DNLM; NNNAM **80-0150**

ARMSTRONG, W. P.
A hand-book of the diseases of the heart, and their homoeopathic treatment. Chicago: Duncan Bros., 1882. 271p. IEN-M; OCIM; PPHa **80-0151**

ARMY Medical Museum catalogs of exhibits at the World Industrial and Cotton Centennial Exposition, New Orleans, 1884-1885. Description of selected specimens from the Medical and Surgical Section of the Army Medical Museum. Exhibit-Class 4, No. 5. 20p. DNLM **80-0152**

ARMY Medical Museum catalogs of exhibits at the World Industrial and Cotton Centennial Exposition, New Orleans, 1884-1885. Description of the microscopes and microscopical preparations from the Army Medical Museum, Exhibit-Class 4, No. 6. 15p. DNLM **80-0153**

ARNDT, Hugo R., ed. (*b.* **1848)**
A system of medicine based upon the law of homoeopathy. Philadelphia: Hahnemann Publishing House. F. E. Boericke, 1885-1886. 3 v. OCLloyd; PPHa **80-0154**

ARNOLD, Abraham Blumenthal (1820-1904)
Manual of nervous diseases and an introduction to medical electricity. New York: J. H. Vail & Co., 1885. 170p. 9 plates. DLC; DNLM; NNNAM; PPC **80-0155**

ARNOLD, Abraham Blumenthal (1820-1904)
Circumcision. New York, 1886. 22p. DNLM; NNNAM **80-0156**

ARNOLD, Howard Payson (1831-1900)
Memoir of John Collins Warren, M.D. Prepared at the request of the New England Historic Genealogical Society, and privately reprinted from their volume of memoirs. Cambridge: J. Wilson & Son, 1882. 74p. DNLM; MH; MWA; MWiW **80-0157**

ARNOLD, Howard Payson (1831-1900)
Memoirs of Jonathan Mason Warren. Boston, 1886. 329p. DNLM; MBM; MH **80-0158**

ARNOLD, J[ohn] W[illiam] S[chmidt] (1846-1888)
Catalogue of the medical and scientific library of Dr. . . . sold by M. Thomas & Sons. Philadelphia, 1889. 22p. DNLM; PU **80-0159**

ASHBY, Henry (1846-1908)
Memoranda of physiology. . . . 3rd ed., thoroughly revised, with additions and corrections by an American editor. New York: William Wood & Co., 1882. 319p. DLC; ICRM; NNNAM; PU **80-0160**

ASHBY, Thomas Almond (1846-1916)
On some of the uses of antiseptics in obstetrics and gynecology. Baltimore, 1880. 13p. DNLM **80-0161**

ASHBY, Thomas Almond (1846-1916)
Observations on the part the obstetrical forceps plays in the induction and prevention of perineal lacerations. [Baltimore, 1882.] 6p. DNLM **80-0162**

ASHBY, Thomas Almond (1846-1916)
A contribution to the study of neglected lacerations of the cervix uteri and perineum. [Baltimore], 1883. 11p. DNLM **80-0163**

ASHBY, Thomas Almond (1846-1916)
Observations and suggestions in regard to the method of operating during the same anesthetization for lacerations of the cervix uteri and ruptured perineum. Baltimore: Journal Publ. Co., 1886. 10p. DNLM **80-0164**

ASHBY, Thomas Almond (1846-1916)
A contribution to the study of the operation of shortening the round ligaments: Alexander's operation. Baltimore: Journal Publ. Co., 1887. 20p. DNLM **80-0165**

ASHBY, Thomas Almond (1846-1916)
Note on the treatment of amenorrhoea with permanganate of potash. Baltimore, [1887]. 12p. DNLM **80-0166**

ASHBY, Thomas Almond (1846-1916)
Syphilis of the endometrium. Baltimore, 1887. 16p. DNLM **80-0167**

ASHBY, Thomas Almond (1846-1916)
The animal suture in intravaginal plastic surgery. Baltimore: Journal Publ. Co., 1889. 16p. DNLM **80-0168**

ASHBY, Thomas Almond (1846-1916)
Laparotomy for ascites. Baltimore, 1889. 11p. DNLM **80-0169**

ASHBY, Thomas Almond (1846-1916)
The origin and treatment of pus accumulations in the female pelvis. Baltimore: Journal Publ. Co., 1889. 23p. DNLM **80-0170**

ASHBY, Thomas Almond (1846-1916)
The value of laparotomy in the diagnosis and treatment of minor forms of intra-abdominal and intra-pelvic diseases. Philadelphia: W. J. Dornan, 1889. 26p. DNLM **80-0171**

ASHFORD, Francis Asbury (1841-1882)
Catalogue sale of the medical library and instruments of the late . . . . Washington, 1883. 14p. DNLM **80-0172**

ASHHURST, John, ed. (1839-1900)
The international encyclopedia of surgery; a systematic treatise on the theory and practice of surgery by authors of various nations. . . . New York: William Wood & Co., 1881-1886. 6 v. 35 part. col. plates. DLC; DNLM; NNNAM; PU **80-0173**

ASHHURST, John (1839-1900)
The principles and practice of surgery. . . . 3rd ed., enl. and thoroughly rev. . . . Philadelphia: Henry C. Lea's Sons & Co., 1882. 1064p. DLC; DNLM; OCIM; PPC **80-0174**

ASHHURST, John (1839-1900)
The principles and practice of surgery. . . . 4th ed., enl. and thoroughly rev. . . . Philadelphia: Lea Bros. & Co., 1885. 1118p. DLC; DNLM; IU-M; NNNAM **80-0175**

ASHHURST, John (1839-1900)
Biographical notice of George Hamilton. Philadelphia: W. J. Dornan, 1886. 11p. DNLM **80-0176**

ASHHURST, John (1839-1900)
Valedictory address delivered at the annual commencement of the departments of medicine and dentistry of the University of Pennsylvania, May 1, 1888. Philadelphia, 1888. 14p. DNLM; PU **80-0177**

ASHHURST, John (1839-1900)
The principles and practice of surgery. . . . 5th ed., enl. and thoroughly rev. With six hundred and forty-two illustrations. Philadelphia: Lea Bros. & Co., 1889. 1148p. DLC; DNLM; ICRM; PU **80-0178**

ASHTON, William Easterly (1859-1933)
Questions and answers on the essentials of obstetrics, prepared especially for students of medicine. . . . Philadelphia: W. B. Saunders, 1888. 230p. DLC; MH-M; NNNAM; PU
80-0179

ATKINS, Edward Babcock
The relation of homoeopathy to natural science. New York: A. L. Chatterton & Co., 1889. 195p. NNNAM; PPHa
80-0180

ATKINSON, Archer
Clinical studies on hyosciamia. [Bridgeport, 1886.] 5p. DNLM
80-0181

ATKINSON, Isaac Edmondson (1846-1906)
A clinical lecture upon cutaneous epithelioma. [Richmond, 1880.] 16p. DNLM **80-0182**

ATKINSON, Isaac Edmondson (1846-1906)
May iodide of potassium excite Bright's disease? [Philadelphia, 1881.] 14p. DNLM **80-0183**

ATKINSON, Isaac Edmondson (1846-1906)
On "kerion Celsi," a variety of tinea tonsurans. [New York, 1881.] 20p. DNLM **80-0184**

ATKINSON, Isaac Edmondson (1846-1906)
Notes on a case of erythematous lupus, complicated by the tubercular syphiloderm. [Baltimore, 1883.] 6p. DNLM
80-0185

ATKINSON, Isaac Edmondson (1846-1906)
Bright's disease of malarial origin. [Philadelphia, 1884.] 18p. DNLM **80-0186**

ATKINSON, Isaac Edmondson (1846-1906)
Carcinoma of the peritoneum. [New York, 1884.] 14p. DNLM
80-0187

ATKINSON, Isaac Edmondson (1846-1906)
Scarlatina and scarlatiniform eruptions, following injuries and operations. [Baltimore, 1886.] 6p. DNLM **80-0188**

ATKINSON, Isaac Edmondson (1846-1906)
Rubella (Rötheln). [Philadelphia, 1887.] 18p. DNLM
80-0189

ATKINSON, Isaac Edmondson (1846-1906)
President's address delivered before the American Dermatological Association at its twelfth annual meeting. [Boston], 1888. 7p. DNLM **80-0190**

ATKINSON, Isaac Edmondson (1846-1906)
Some of the graver and rarer forms of cinchonism. Chicago, 1889. 16p. DNLM **80-0191**

ATKINSON, William Biddle, ed. (1832-1909)
A biographical dictionary of contemporary American physicians and surgeons. . . . 2nd ed., enl. and rev. Philadelphia: D. G. Brinton, 1880. 747p. DLC; MH; NN; PU
80-0192

ATKINSON, William Biddle, ed. (1832-1909)
The therapeutics of gynecology and obstetrics, comprising the medical, dietetic, and hygienic treatment of diseases of women, as set forth by distinguished contemporary specialists. . . . Philadelphia: D. G. Brinton, 1880. 365p. DLC; DNLM; NNNAM; PPC **80-0193**

ATKINSON, William Biddle, ed. (1832-1909)
The therapeutics of gynecology and obstetrics, comprising the medical, dietetic, and hygienic treatment of diseases of women. 2nd ed., thoroughly rev. and greatly enl. . . . Philadelphia: D. G. Brinton, 1881. 571p. CtY-M; DLC; NNNAM; PU
80-0194

ATKINSON, William H.
Report on nomenclature and terminology. [Chicago, 1880.] 5p. DNLM **80-0195**

ATKINSON, William H.
Disease. Paper read at the May (1883) meeting of the Dental Society of the State of New York. [Buffalo, 1883.] 8p. DNLM
80-0196

ATKINSON, William H.
Ripening and ripeness. [Philadelphia, 1885.] 4p. DNLM
80-0197

ATKINSON, William H.
Reproduction of tissue by sponge-grafting. (Whitney memorial prize essay.) Correspondence. [Rochester], 1885. 8p. DNLM
80-0198

ATLEE, John Light (1799-1885)
A case of strangulated hernia, complicated by a very extraordinary diseased spermatic cord. A case of ovariotomy, in which the expanded bladder was wounded, with recovery, by Walter F. Atlee. A case of congenital cyst of the back of the head, with serous contents, its cavity unconnected with that of the skull, by Louis W. Atlee. [Philadelphia, 1883.] 12p. DNLM
80-0199

ATLEE, Walter Franklin (1828-1910)
On vaccination. [Philadelphia, 1880.] 2p. DNLM
80-0200

ATLEE, Walter Franklin (1828-1910)
Report of a case where mother and child died during labor from difficulties attributed to shortness of the pedicle secured by a clamp in ovariotomy. [Philadelphia, 1880.] 3p. DNLM
80-0201

ATLEE, Walter Franklin (1828-1910)
A case of ovariotomy in which phlegmasia dolens followed the operation. [Philadelphia, 1880.] 3p. DNLM
80-0202

ATTFIELD, John (1835-1911)
Chemistry: general, medical, and pharmaceutical, including the chemistry of the U.S. pharmacopoeia. A manual on the general principles of the science, and their applications in medicine and pharmacy. . . . 12th ed. Philadelphia: Lea Bros. & Co., 1889. 770p. tables. DLC; OCLloyd; PPC; PU
80-0203

AUSTIN, G. Lowell (1849-1893)
The physicians' pocket manual and year-book. Boston: The Author, 1880. 176p. DNLM; MBM; NNNAM; PPC
80-0204

AUSTIN, G. Lowell (1849-1893)
Perils of American women, or a doctor's talk with maiden, wife, and mother. Boston: Lee & Shepard, 1883. 240p. MH; NN; PU **80-0205**

AYRES, Mortimer
Some of the diseases of the rectum and their homoeopathic and surgical treatment. Chicago: Duncan Bros., 1884. 78p. OCIM; PPHa **80-0206**

AYRES, William C.
The development of the eye. New York, 1881. 18p. DNLM; NNNAM **80-0207**

BAAS, Johann Hermann (1838-1909)
Outlines of the history of medicine and the medical profession. Transl., and in conjunction with the author revised and enlarged, by H. E. Handerson. New York: J. H. Vail & Co., 1889. 1173p. CtY-M; DNLM; NNNAM; PPC **80-0208**

BABCOCK, Cyrus M.
Odds and ends of practical pharmacology, for the use of students and practitioners of homoeopathic medicine. Practical elucidation of the thousand and one ever recurring problems connected with the pharmacology of our school, etc. Chicago: Halsey Bros., 1887. 48p. OCIM; PPHa **80-0209**

BABER, E[dward] Cresswell (1851-1910)
A guide to the examination of the nose; with remarks on the diagnosis of diseases of the nasal cavities. New York: J. H. Vail & Co., 1886. 163p. DNLM; LNT-M; NNNAM; PPC **80-0210**

BACON, Francis (1831-1912)
Some account of the medical profession in New Haven, as written by . . . for "A history of the city of New Haven to the present time, by an association of writers." New York: W. W. Munsell & Co., 1887. 44p. CtY-M; DNLM; NNNAM **80-0211**

BACON, Gorham (*b.* 1855)
Calcium sulphide in aural diseases. [New York, 1883.] 2p. DNLM **80-0212**

BACON, Gorham (*b.* 1855)
A report of twenty-one cases of traumatic lesions of the ear; with remarks. [New York, 1887.] 14p. DNLM **80-0213**

BACON, Gorham (*b.* 1855)
On the use of the wet-cup in place of the leech in certain acute diseases of the ear. [New York, 1888.] 5p. DNLM **80-0214**

BAER, B[enjamin] F[ranklin] (1846-1920)
An analysis of twenty-seven operations for the restoration of the lacerated cervix uteri, with special reference to the effect of the operation on fertility and labor. Philadelphia, 1883. 12p. DNLM **80-0215**

BAER, B[enjamin] F[ranklin] (1846-1920)
A case of suppurating cyst of the broad ligament, rupture into the bladder; laparotomy and removal; death. New York: William Wood & Co., 1883. 10p. DNLM **80-0216**

BAER, B[enjamin] F[ranklin] (1846-1920)
The significance of metrorrhagia recurring about and after the menopause. Read before the Obstetrical Society of Philadelphia, March 6, 1884. New York: William Wood & Co., 1884. 16p. DNLM **80-0217**

BAER, B[enjamin] F[ranklin] (1846-1920)
Recurrent pelvic peritonitis. A clinical lecture. Philadelphia, 1888. 8p. DNLM **80-0218**

BAER, B[enjamin] F[ranklin] (1846-1920)
Report of a case of pregnancy in the right horn of a uterus bicornis, treated successfully by a modified Caesarean operation, twelve months after the death of the child at the full term of gestation; so-called "missed labor." [Philadelphia, 1888.] 16p. DNLM **80-0219**

BAER, B[enjamin] F[ranklin] (1846-1920)
Report of some recent cases of abdominal section for the removal of tumors, of unusual interest regarding the character of the tumors and the method of operating. [Philadelphia, 1889.] 10p. DNLM **80-0220**

BAKER, Albert Rufus (*b.* 1858)
Consequences of acute suppuration of the middle ear, with special reference to opening the mastoid. Cleveland, O., [1888]. 20p. DNLM **80-0221**

BAKER, Albert Rufus (*b.* 1858)
A few observations on the etiology, prognosis, and cure of incipient cataract without operative interference. Cleveland, O., [1889]. 7p. DNLM **80-0222**

BAKER, Albert Rufus (*b.* 1858)
Address at the opening of the medical department of Wooster University, Cleveland, Ohio, Wednesday, Feb. 27, 1889. Cleveland, 1889. 16p. DNLM **80-0223**

BAKER, Albert Rufus (*b.* 1858)
Impaired vision as the result of sunstroke. Chicago, 1889. 7p. DNLM **80-0224**

BAKER, Frank (1841-1918)
President Garfield's case. A diagnosis made two days after the injury. Washington: Judd & Detweiler, 1882. 8p. DNLM **80-0225**

BAKER, Frank (1841-1918)
The rational method of teaching anatomy. New York: Trow, 1884. 20p. DNLM **80-0226**

BAKER, Frank (1841-1918)
What is anatomy? A lecture delivered October 5, 1887, at the opening of the anatomical course at the medical department, University of Georgetown, Washington, D.C. [Washington, 1887.] 22p. DNLM **80-0227**

BAKER, Henry A.
An appliance for congenital cleft palate. Read before the Massachusetts Dental Society. Philadelphia: Trustees of S. S. White, 1881. 12p. DNLM **80-0228**

BAKER, Henry A.
An improved appliance in the physiological treatment of cleft palate. Cambridge: Riverside Press, 1884. 16p. DNLM **80-0229**

BAKER, Henry B[rooks] (1837-1920)
Regulation of medical practice. [Ann Arbor, 1880.] 10p. DNLM **80-0230**

BAKER, Henry B[rooks] (1837-1920)
Diagrams illustrating a paper on the systematic study of the causes of sickness and deaths, read at the sanitary convention at Battle Creek, Mich., March 29, 1881. 1881. 15p. DNLM **80-0231**

BAKER, Henry B[rooks] (1837-1920)
General sanitation; its importance to the public welfare, and a plea for better methods. [Lansing, 1881.] 16p. DNLM
80-0232

BAKER, Henry B[rooks] (1837-1920)
The relations of schools to diphtheria and to similar diseases. Boston: Rand, Avery & Co., 1881. 19p. 4 charts. DNLM
80-0233

BAKER, Henry B[rooks] (1837-1920)
The Michigan plan for general boards of health. [Detroit, 1882.] 1 l. DNLM **80-0234**

BAKER, Henry B[rooks] (1837-1920)
A proposed bill to regulate the practice of medicine in Michigan. [Detroit, 1882.] 3p. DNLM
80-0235

BAKER, Henry B[rooks] (1837-1920)
Climate and health in Michigan. 1884. 1 l. DNLM
80-0236

[BAKER, Henry B[rooks] (1837-1920) and J. N. McCORMACK
Concerted action by state boards of health. [Committee call for meeting of State boards of health, at Washington, in May, 1884.] [1884.] 3p. DNLM **80-0237**

BAKER, Henry B[rooks] (1837-1920)
Climate and health in Michigan. [Lansing], 1885. 1 diag. DNLM **80-0238**

BAKER, Henry B[rooks] (1837-1920)
Diagrams exhibiting the relation between sickness, and deaths, from pneumonia and the average relation to humidity, etc. 1878-1884. [Lansing, 1885.] 30 sheets. DNLM
80-0239

BAKER, Henry B[rooks] (1837-1920)
Preparation in Michigan against cholera. Statement of the status of the public health work in Michigan. [Detroit, 1885.] 8p. DNLM **80-0240**

BAKER, Henry B[rooks] (1837-1920)
Time of greatest danger from typhoid fever. Diagram A. Exhibiting for a period of five years (1878-1882) the average monthly oscillations of ground-water in Michigan, the deaths reported from typhoid fever, and what per cent of the weekly reports of sickness received stated the presence of typhoid fever. [Lansing, 1885.] 1 diag. DNLM
80-0241

BAKER, Henry B[rooks] (1837-1920)
Diagrams to illustrate a paper on the relations of certain meteorological conditions to diseases of the lungs and air-passages. Lansing: Thorp & Godfrey, [1887]. 11 l. DNLM
80-0242

BAKER, Henry B[rooks] (1837-1920)
Scientific collective investigation of disease. Chicago, 1887. 11p. 1 diag. DNLM **80-0243**

BAKER, Henry B[rooks] (1837-1920)
Diphtheria in Michigan in 1886, exhibiting the average numbers of cases and deaths per outbreak. [Lansing, 1888.] 1 diag. DNLM **80-0244**

BAKER, Henry B[rooks] (1837-1920)
Address in state medicine. Recent advance in state medicine. Chicago, 1888. 27p. DNLM **80-0245**

BAKER, Henry B[rooks] (1837-1920)
The prevention of the communicable diseases, from the standpoint of the State board of health. Reprint No. 277. [Lansing, 1888.] 7p. DNLM **80-0246**

BAKER, Henry B[rooks] (1837-1920)
Malaria; and the causation of periodic fever. Chicago, 1888. 30p. DNLM **80-0247**

BAKER, Lucius Willard (1862-1902)
Cottage hospitals. Read before the Massachusetts Medical Society, June 13, 1882. West Gardner, 1882. 10p. DNLM
80-0248

BAKER, Lucius Willard (1862-1902)
Mental epilepsy. [New York, 1886.] 22p. DNLM
80-0249

BAKER, Lucius Willard (1862-1902)
The alcohol habit. [St. Louis, 1888.] 10p. DNLM
80-0250

BAKER, Lucius Willard (1862-1902)
The continuous use of the bromides. Philadelphia: Records, McMullin & Co., 1888. 10p. DNLM **80-0251**

BAKER, Luicus Willard (1862-1902)
How shall we deal with the inebriate? [Hartford, Conn., 1889.] 7p. DNLM **80-0252**

BAKER, Rufus (1815-1891)
Specialties in medicine. [Hartford, 1882.] 8p. DNLM
80-0253

BAKER, William H[enry] (1845-1914)
Drainage in the removal of submucous fibroids. New York: G. P. Putnam's Sons, 1882. 23p. DNLM
80-0254

BAKER, William H[enry] (1845-1914)
The treatment of cancer of the uterus. New York: William Wood & Co., 1882. 25p. DNLM **80-0255**

BAKER, William H[enry] (1845-1914)
Vaginal ovariotomy. [New York, 1882.] 6p. DNLM
80-0256

BAKER, William H[enry] (1845-1914)
Hyperemia of the vesico-urethral membrane. [1883.] 23p. 1 plate. DNLM **80-0257**

BAKER, William H[enry] (1845-1914)
Unusual cases of vesico-vaginal and vesico-uterine fistula. Boston: Stanley & Usher, 1885. 15p. DNLM
80-0258

BAKER, William H[enry] (1845-1914)
The use and abuse of Battey's and Tait's operations. Boston: Stanley & Usher, 1885. 15p. DNLM **80-0259**

BAKER, William H[enry] (1845-1914)
Cancer of the uterus; its treatment by high amputation compared with total extirpation. [New York: D. Appleton & Co., 1886.] 18p. DNLM **80-0260**

BAKER, William H[enry] (1845-1914)
Electrolysis in gynecological surgery. [New York, 1886.] 14p. DNLM **80-0261**

BALDWIN, David A.
The family pocket homoeopathist. A concise manual of homoeopathic practice for families and travellers. 2nd ed. Rochester: E. Darrow & Co., 1886. 158p. LNT-M; NNNAM; OCIM **80-0262**

BALDWIN, J[ames] F[airchild] (1850-1936)
The Columbus Medical College imbroglio. A reply to certain widely-circulated misstatements and slanders. To the medical profession. [Columbus, 1882.] 16p. DNLM **80-0263**

BALDWIN, J[ames] F[airchild] (1850-1936)
"The Columbus Medical College imbroglio." Our vindication. The voice of the medical press. [Columbus, 1882.] 8p. DNLM **80-0264**

BALDWIN, W[illiam] O[wen] (1818-1886)
On the poisonous properties of quinine; with remarks by J. Marion Sims. New York: Bermingham & Co., [1881]. 8p. DNLM; NNNAM **80-0265**

BALDWIN, W[illiam] O[wen] (1818-1886)
Tribute to the late James Marion Sims. Montgomery, Ala.: W. D. Brown & Co., 1884. 31p. DLC; DNLM **80-0266**

BALDY, J[ohn] M[ontgomery] (1860-1934)
The relation of pyosalpinx to puerperal fever. Philadelphia: W. J. Dornan, 1887. 7p. DNLM **80-0267**

BALDY, J[ohn] M[ontgomery] (1860-1934)
Exploratory laparotomy. [Philadelphia, 1888.] 16p. DNLM **80-0268**

BALDY, J[ohn] M[ontgomery] (1860-1934)
The early diagnosis of extra-uterine pregnancy. [New York, 1889.] 8p. DNLM **80-0269**

BALDY, J[ohn] M[ontomgery] (1860-1934)
A plea for prompt interference in abdominal diseases. [Philadelphia, 1889.] 13p. DNLM **80-0270**

BALDY, J[ohn] M[ontgomery] (1860-1934)
Three cases of appendicitis; operation; recovery. [Philadelphia, 1889.] 7p. DNLM **80-0271**

BALDY, J[ohn] M[ontgomery] (1860-1934)
Twenty consecutive cases of abdominal section, with one death. [Philadelphia, 1889.] 12p. 1 tab. DNLM **80-0272**

BALL, A[lonzo] B[rayton]
A contribution to the study of aphasia, with special reference to "word-deafness" and "word-blindness." New York: G. P. Putnam's Sons, 1881. 26p. DNLM; NNNAM **80-0273**

BALL, Benjamin (1834-1893)
The morphine habit (morphinomania). With four lectures on the borderland of insanity; cerebral dualism; prolonged dreams, insanity in twins. Translated from the French for the Humboldt Library. New York: J. Fitzgerald, 1887. 43p. DNLM; NNNAM **80-0274**

BALL, Charles B[ent] (1851-1916)
The rectum and anus; their diseases and treatment. Philadelphia: Lea Bros. & Co., [1887]. 410p. 4 plates. DNLM; MBM; PPC; PU **80-0275**

BALL, John (1818-1890)
Rapid dilatation of the cervix uteri, for the relief of chronic cervical endo-metritis, conical cervix, flexions, stricture, sterility, etc. [n.p., 1883.] 12p. DNLM **80-0276**

BANGS, L[emuel] Bolton (1842-1914)
A contribution to the study of neuroses of the genito-urinary system. New York: De Leeuw, Oppenheimer & Myers, 1886. 12p. DNLM **80-0277**

BANGS, L[emuel] Bolton (1842-1914)
On the diagnosis of hypertrophied prostate, and the treatment of its effects. New York, [1887]. 12p. DNLM **80-0278**

BANGS, L[emuel] Bolton (1842-1914)
External urethrotomy. A plea for its early performance in minor traumatisms of the urethra. New York: Trow, 1887. 8p. DNLM **80-0279**

BANGS, L[emuel] Bolton (1842-1914)
On some of the indications for external urethrotomy, with a case of unusual difficulty. [Danbury, Conn., 1887.] 6p. DNLM **80-0280**

BANGS, L[emuel] Bolton (1842-1914)
Clinical observation of diseases of the testicle. New York, 1888. 11p. DNLM **80-0281**

BANGS, L[emuel] Bolton (1842-1914)
Cases of suprapubic cystotomy. [New York, 1889.] 15p. DNLM **80-0282**

BANGS, L[emule] Bolton (1842-1914)
On spasmodic urethral stricture from anal fissure. New York: Trow, 1889. 7p. DNLM **80-0283**

BANISTER, J. M.
Lateral lithotomy, with the successful removal of a calculus and seven pieces of necrosed bone from the bladder of an Indian scout, nineteen months after the reception of a gunshot wound. [Philadelphia, 1880.] 6p. DNLM **80-0284**

BANNING, E[dumund] P[rior] (*b.* 1810)
The human spine. An analysis of the comparative merits of the gypsum jacket and compound adjustable supports in the physical treatment of spinal irritation, caries, curvature. . . . Boston: A Mudge & Sons, 1881. 32p. DLC **80-0285**

BANNING, E[dmund] P[rior] (*b.* 1810)
. . . Vital mechanics. . . . [Boston, 1881?] 68p. DLC; MH-M **80-0286**

BANNING, Edmund Prior (*b.* 1810)
Two monographs. 1. The comparative merits of the gypsum jacket and adjustable supports in the treatment of spinal affections. 2. The pathology and therapeutics of uterine displacements. New York: A. G. Sherwood & Co., 1882. 32p. DNLM; NNNAM **80-0287**

BANNING, Edmund Prior (*b.* 1810)
Two monographs. 1. The comparative merits of the gypsum jacket and adjustable supports in the treatment of spinal affections. 2. The pathology and therapeutics of uterine displacements. New York: J. J. Little & Co., 1884. 32p. DNLM; NNNAM **80-0288**

BANNING, Edmund Prior (*b.* 1810)
On spinal deformities. From Banning's mechanical pathology and therapeutics. New York: Banning & Co., [1885?] 12p. DNLM **80-0289**

BANNING, E[dmund] P[rior] (*b.* 1810)
Spinal diseases, weakness and deformity with a rational method of cure. A monograph. . . . 35th ed. New York: Press of G. F. Isley, 1886. 12, [4] p. DLC **80-0290**

BANNISTER, Henry Martyn (1844-1920)
On some points in regard to color blindness. [New York], 1881. 15p. DNLM **80-0291**

BANNISTER, Henry Martyn (1844-1920) and Ludwig HEKTOEN
Race and insanity. [Utica,, 1888.] 16p. 1 tab. DNLM **80-0292**

BANTON, J[ohn] F[loyd]
Vaccination refuted. Cleveland, O., 1882. 15p. DNLM; OCIM **80-0293**

BANTON, J[ohn] Floyd
Physicians a scourge. . . . Showing the vagueness of practical medicine of today. . . . Chicago, 1883. 24p. DLC **80-0294**

BANTON, John Floyd
Revolution in the practice of medicine. . . . 2nd ed. . . . Chicago, Ill.: [Review Printing & Publishing Co.], 1885. 55p. DLC; DNLM **80-0295**

BAR, Paul (*b.* 1853)
The principles of antiseptic methods applied to obstetric practice. . . . Transl. by Henry D. Fry. Philadelphia: P. Blakiston, Son & Co., 1887. 175p. fold. chart. DLC; NNNAM; OCIM; PPC **80-0296**

BARBOUR, Alexander Hugh Freeland (1856-1927)
The diagnosis of advanced extra-uterine gestation after the death of the foetus, with a frozen section. New York, 1882. 8p. DNLM **80-0297**

BARBOUR, Alexander Hugh Freeland (1856-1927)
Spinal deformity in relation to obstetrics. Being a thesis for graduation in medicine at the University of Edinburgh, for which a gold medal was awarded in 1883. New York: J. H. Vail & Co., [1885]. 35p. 39 plates. DNLM; NNNAM **80-0298**

BARKAN, A[dolph] (1845-1935)
Does cocaine improve the changes of success in operations for cataract? San Francisco: W. A. Woodward & Co., [1887]. 5p. DNLM **80-0299**

BARKAN, Adolph (1845-1935)
Expert medical report on one hundred and fifty-eight inmates of the Institution for the Deaf and Dumb and the Blind, at Berkeley, Cal. [San Francisco]: W. B. Bancroft & Co., [1887]. 44p. 2 tab. CU-M; DNLM **80-0300**

BARKER, Benjamin Fordyce (1818-1891)
Puerperal malarial fever. New York: William Wood & Co., 1880. 10p. DNLM **80-0301**

BARKER, Benjamin Fordyce (1818-1891)
New York Academy of Medicine, 1881. Second inaugural address. New York, 1881. 20p. DNLM; NNNAM **80-0302**

BARKER, Benjamin Fordyce (1818-1891)
Leucorrhea considered in relation to its constitutional causes and treatment. [New York, 1882.] 11p. DNLM **80-0303**

BARKER, Benjamin Fordyce (1818-1891)
The prevention and treatment of puerperal fever. New York: D. Appleton & Co., 1884. 21p. DNLM; NNNAM **80-0304**

BARKER, Benjamin Fordyce (1818-1891)
Valedictory address by the retiring president, delivered before the New York Academy of Medicine, Feb. 5th, 1885. New York, 1885. 17p. DNLM; NNNAM **80-0305**

BARKER, Benjamin Fordyce (1818-1891)
The influence of maternal impressions of the fetus. [New York, 1886.] 24p. DNLM **80-0306**

BARKER, Benjamin Fordyce (1818-1891)
Is the danger from post-partum hemorrhage increased by the use of anaesthetics during parturition? [Philadelphia, 1887.] 11p. DNLM **80-0307**

BARLOW, Thomas W.
Philadelphia Social Science Association. A plea for a new city hospital. Read at a meeting of the Association, February 15th, 1883. Philadelphia: Phila. Soc. Sc. Ass., 1883. 16p. DNLM; PU **80-0308**

BARNES, J[oseph] Deane (1845-1882)
Catalogue of the medical and miscellaneous library of the late . . . also of other medical books, to be sold June 26 and 27, 1882. Washington, 1882. 18p. DNLM **80-0309**

BARNES, Robert (1817-1907)
On antiseptic midwifery and septicemia in midwifery. New York: William Wood & Co., 1882. 17p. DNLM; NNNAM **80-0310**

BARNES, Robert (1817-1907) and Robert Sydenham Fancourt BARNES
A system of obstetric medicine and surgery, theoretical and clinical, for the student and practitioner. Philadelphia: Lea Bros. & Co., 1885. 884p. CtY-M; DNLM; MBM; NNNAM **80-0311**

BARNES, Robert (1817-1907)
Lectures on obstetric operations, including the treatment of haemorrhage, and forming a guide to the management of difficult labour. 4th ed. Philadelphia: P. Blakiston, Son & Co., 1886. 503p. DNLM; ICRM; LNT-M; PPC **80-0312**

BARRET, William L.
New method of performing the primary operation for laceration of the perineum. St. Louis, Mo.: Commercial Print. Comp., 1883. 8p. DNLM **80-0313**

BARRETT, Ashley W[illiam]
Dental surgery for general practitioners and students of medicine. Philadelphia: P. Blakiston, Son & Co., 1885. 83p. DNLM; MdU-D; PPC; PPJ **80-0314**

BARRETT, John A.
Chloride of silver, complete and perfected medical batteries. Invented and patented by . . . . [New York: Beeken & Geery, 1887.] 16p. DNLM **80-0315**

BARRETT, William Cary (1834-1903)
Anaesthesia. Philadelphia: Trustees of S. S. White, 1881. 16p. DNLM **80-0316**

BARRETT, William Cary (1834-1903)
Nervous force: its origin and physiology. Read before the American Dental Association at its twenty-second annual meeting, held in Cincinnati, August 1-5, 1882. [Toledo, Ohio, 1882.] 15p. DNLM **80-0317**

BARRETT, William Cary (1834-1903)
Diseases of the period of dentition. Address delivered before the American Academy of Dental Science at its 18th annual meeting, held in Boston, Nov. 4, 1885. Buffalo: Independ. Pract. Print, 1885. 18p. DNLM **80-0318**

BARROW, David
How the refinements of abdominal surgery have influenced general surgery. Philadelphia: W. J. Dornan, 1889. 10p. DNLM; PPC **80-0319**

BARROWS, C. M.
Bread-pills; a study of mind-cure. What it is, and how to do it. 2nd ed. Boston: Deland & Barton, 1885. 88p. DNLM; MH; NNNAM; PU **80-0320**

BARTHOLOW, Roberts (1831-1904)
A treatise on the practice of medicine, for the use of students and practitioners. . . . New York: D. Appleton & Co., 1880. 853p. plates, diags. DLC; MBM; MdU-D; PPC **80-0321**

BARTHOLOW, Roberts (1831-1904)
A practical treatise on materia medica and therapeutics. 3rd ed. New York: D. Appleton & Co., 1880. 595p. DNLM; OCLloyd; NNNAM; PU **80-0322**

BARTHOLOW, Roberts (1831-1904)
On the antagonism between medicines and between remedies and diseases. Being the Cartwright lectures for the year 1880. . . . New York: D. Appleton & Co., 1881. 122p. DLC; DNLM; NNNAM; PU **80-0323**

BARTHOLOW, Roberts (1831-1904)
A treatise on the practice of medicine, for the use of students and practitioners. . . . 2nd ed., rev. and enl. New York: D. Appleton & Co., 1881. 872p. plates, diags. DLC; IU-M; NNNAM; PPC **80-0324**

BARTHOLOW, Roberts (1831-1904)
A practical treatise on materia medica and therapeutics. . . . 4th ed. rev. and enl. New York: D. Appleton & Co., 1881. 662p. DLC; OCLloyd; OCIM; PPC **80-0325**

BARTHOLOW, Roberts (1831-1904)
Medical electricity; a practical treatise on the applications of electricity to medicine and surgery. Philadelphia: Henry C. Lea's Sons & Co., 1881. 262p. CtY-M; DNLM; MBM; PPC **80-0326**

BARTHOLOW, Roberts (1831-1904)
Medical electricity; a practical treatise on the applications of electricity to medicine and surgery. 2nd ed. Philadelphia: Henry C. Lea's Son & Co., 1882. 291p. DNLM; MH-M; NNNAM; PPC **80-0327**

BARTHOLOW, Roberts (1831-1904)
A treatise on the practice of medicine, for the use of students and practitioners. . . . 3rd ed., rev. and enl. New York: D. Appleton & Co., 1882. 918p. plates. diags. DLC; MdU-D; NNNAM; PU **80-0328**

BARTHOLOW, Roberts (1831-1904)
A manual of hypodermatic medication. The treatment of diseases by the hypodermatic method. . . . 4th ed., rev. and enl. Philadelphia: J. B. Lippincott & Co., 1882. 365p. DLC; DNLM; LNT-M; PPC **80-0329**

BARTHOLOW, Roberts (1831-1904)
A treatise on the practice of medicine, for the use of students and practitioners. . . . 4th ed. [5th ed.], rev. and enl. New York: D. Appleton & Co., 1883. 936p. plates. diags. DLC; DNLM; MBM; NNNAM **80-0330**

BARTHOLOW, Roberts (1831-1904)
A practical treatise on materia medica and therapeutics. . . . 5th ed., rev. and enl. New York: D. Appleton & Co., 1884. 738p. DLC; DNLM; NNNAM; PU **80-0331**

BARTHOLOW, Roberts (1831-1904)
Permanganate of potassium; its action and uses. [Philadelphia, 1884.] 15p. DNLM **80-0332**

BARTHOLOW, Roberts (1831-1904)
The physiological effects and therapeutical uses of hydrastis. Cincinnati, 1885. 6p. 1 diag. DNLM **80-0333**

BARTHOLOW, Roberts (1831-1904)
Note on the use of cocaine in hay fever. [Philadelphia, 1885.] 5 l. DNLM **80-0334**

BARTHOLOW, Roberts (1831-1904)
Medical education and the Jefferson Medical College of Philadelphia; an open letter to the Secretary of the Illinois State Board of Health. Philadelphia: W. F. Fell & Co., 1886. 17p. PPJ **80-335**

BARTHOLOW, Roberts (1831-1904)
A treatise on the practice of medicine, for the use of students and practitioners of medicine. . . . 6th ed., rev. and enl. New York: D. Appleton & Co., 1886. 990p. diags. DLC; DNLM; MBM; PPC **80-0336**

BARTHOLOW, Roberts (1831-1904)
Medical electricity; a practical treatise on the application of electricity to medicine and surgery. 3rd ed. Philadelphia: Lea Bros. & Co., 1887. 304p. DNLM; IEN-M; OCIM; PU **80-0337**

BARTHOLOW, Roberts (1831-1904)
A treatise on the practice of medicine, for the use of students and practitioners of medicine; . . . 7th ed., rev. and enl. New York: D. Appleton & Co., 1889. 1003p. diags. DLC; DNLM; MBM; PPC **80-0338**

BARTHOLOW, Roberts (1831-1904)
A practical treatise on materia medica and therapeutics, by.... 7th ed., rev. and enl. New York: D. Appleton & Co., 1889. 802p. DLC; DNLM; OCLloyd; PU **80-0339**

BARTLETT, Ezra A.
... Cholera; its history, cause and prevention.... Albany, N.Y.: H. H. Bender, 1885. 105p. DLC; DNLM; MBM; NNNAM **80-0340**

BARTLETT, G[eorge] T.
Congenital hydrocephalus. A case in practice. Read before the Southeast Missouri Medical Association, at Marble Hill, Nov. 1, 1887. Poplar Bluff, Mo., 1887. 3p. DNLM **80-0341**

BARTLEY, Elias Hudson (1849-1937)
A text-book of medical chemistry. For medical and pharmaceutical students and practitioners.... With forty illustrations. Philadelphia: Blakiston, Son & Co., 1885. 376p. DLC; MBM; NNNAM; PU **80-0342**

BARTON, James M[orrie] (*b.* 1846)
A report of some cases of abdominal surgery. [Philadelphia, 1888.] 16p. DNLM **80-0343**

BARUCH, Simon (1840-1921)
Causes and prevention of "liver complaint" among the rural and laboring population of South Carolina. [Charleston, 1881.] 15p. DNLM **80-0344**

BARUCH, Simon (1840-1921)
Malaria as an etiological factor in New York City. New York: Trow's Printing and Bookbinding Co., 1883. 22p. DNLM **80-0345**

BARUCH, Simon (1840-1921)
The prevention of puerperal infection. A study of antiseptic practice in the maternity hospitals of Paris, Prague, Berlin, Parma, Glasgow, Copenhagen, and New York. New York: D. Appleton & Co., 1884. 23p. DNLM **80-0346**

BARUCH, Simon (1840-1921)
The management of the third stage of labor. New York: William Wood & Co., 1885. 34p. DNLM **80-0347**

BARUCH, Simon (1840-1921)
The therapeutic significance of the cervical follicles. [New York, 1885.] 31p. DNLM **80-0348**

BARUCH, Simon (1840-1921)
A clinical study of the etiology and treatment of summer diarrhoea of infants. [Philadelphia, 1888.] 32p. DNLM **80-0349**

BARUCH, Simon (1840-1921)
The treatment of typhoid fever. Philadelphia: W. J. Dornan, 1889. 15p. DNLM **80-0350**

BARWELL, Richard (1827-1916)
A treatise on diseases of the joints. 2nd ed. New York: William Wood & Co., 1881. 463p. CtY-M; NNNAM; OCIM; PPC **80-0351**

BASTIAN, Henry Charlton (1837-1915)
The brain as an organ of mind. New York: D. Appleton & Co., 1880. 708p. DNLM; LNT-M; OCIM; PPC **80-0352**

BASTIAN, Henry Charlton (1837-1915)
Paralyses, cerebral, bulbar, and spinal. A manual of diagnosis for students and practitioners. New York: D. Appleton & Co., 1886. 671p. 1 tab. DNLM; ICRM; MH-M; NNNAM **80-0353**

BATES, N[ewton] L.
Intestinal concretions resembling sand, and originating in cells from the banana. [Philadelphia, 1887.] 4p. DNLM **80-0354**

BATES, William H[oratio] (1860-1931)
A new operation for the alleviation of persistent deafness. New York: Trow, 1886. 8p. DNLM **80-0355**

BATTEY, Robert (1828-1895)
Antisepsis in ovariotomy and Battey's operation; eighteen consecutive cases; all successful. Richmond: J. W. Fergusson & Son, 1883. 16p. DNLM; ViRA **80-0356**

BATTEY, Robert (1828-1895)
Antisepsis in ovariotomy and Battey's operation; seventy consecutive cases with sixty-eight recoveries and two deaths. [Atlanta, 1886.] 41p. DNLM; GU; PPC **80-0357**

BATTEY, Robert (1828-1895)
The president's annual address [Am. Gynec. Soc.]. Philadelphia: W. J. Dornan, 1888. 15p. DNLM; PPC **80-0358**

BAUMGARTEN, G[ustav] (1837-1911)
Disturbances of the heart rhythm with reference to their causation and their value in diagnosis. Philadelphia: W. J. Dornan, 1888. 13p. DNLM **80-0359**

BEACH, H[enry] H[arris] A[ubrey]
Styrone: a consideration of its value as an antiseptic. Copaiba in surgery. Boston: Damrell & Upham, 1889. 18p. DNLM; MBM **80-0360**

BEADLE, H[iram]
Synopsis of Dr. Beadle's theory of disease, and practice of medicine, having special relation to pestilential and epidemic diseases.... St. Louis, Mo., 1881. 13p. DLC **80-0361**

BEALE, James Sheilds (1841-1884)
Address to the graduates in medicine, delivered at Lincoln Hall, Washington, D.C., on Thursday evening, April 27, 1882. Washington, D.C.: Judd & Detweiler, [1882]. 10p. DNLM **80-0362**

BEALE, James Sheilds (1841-1884)
Report of case of Hodgkin's disease. Read before the Medical Society of the District of Columbia. [Washington]: Judd & Detweiler, [1883]. 8p. DNLM **80-0363**

BEALE, Lionel Smith (1828-1906)
On slight ailments: their nature and treatment.... Philadelphia: P. Blakiston, 1880. 353p. DLC; NNNAM; PPC; PU **80-0364**

BEALE, Lionel Smith (1828-1906)
. . . One hundred urinary deposits: in eight sheets. With brief directions for the clinical examination of urine. . . . 2nd ed. Philadelphia: P. Blakiston, Son, & Co., 1883. 3p. 8 plates. DLC; MH-M; NNNAM; PPC **80-0365**

BEALE, Lionel Smith (1828-1906)
Urinary and renal derangements and calculous disorders: hints on diagnosis and treatment. Philadelphia: P. Blakiston, Son & Co., 1885. 356p. CtY-M; DNLM; NNNAM; PPC **80-0366**

BEALL, Elias James (*b.* 1835)
Hernia cerebri. [Fort Worth, Texas, 1885.] 7p. DNLM **80-0367**

BEALL, Elias James (*b.* 1835)
A reprint of the report on surgery. Read before the Texas State Medical Association at its seventeenth annual convocation, held at Houston, Texas, April 21, 22, and 23, 1885. Austin, Tex.: Draughton & Lambert, [1885]. 48p. DNLM **80-0368**

BEALL, Elias James (*b.* 1835)
Impetigo contagiosa. [Austin, 1886.] 12p. DNLM **80-0369**

BEALL, Elias James (*b.* 1835)
Interstitial fibro-myoma of the uterus, complicating parturition; tumor enucleated; child living; complete recovery of mother. Fort Worth, Tex. 1887. 1 sheet. DNLM **80-0370**

BEALL, Elias James (*b.* 1835)
Dermoid cysts of the coccygeal region. [Austin, 1888.] 7p. DNLM **80-0371**

BEALL, Elias James (*b.* 1835)
Fibro-cystic tumor of the uterus; unusual treatment; cure. Philadelphia, 1889. 10p. DNLM **80-0372**

BEANE, Frank Dudley (1851-1894)
Uncommon aural cases. [New York, 1888.] 6p. DNLM **80-0373**

BEARD, George Miller (1839-1883)
The symptoms of sexual exhaustion (sexual neurasthenia). Baltimore, 1880. 19p. DNLM **80-0374**

BEARD, George Miller (1839-1883)
Why we need a national association for the protection of the insane. A paper read at Cleveland, Ohio, July 1st, 1880, before the Conference of Charities. Boston: Tolman & White, 1880. 11p. DNLM **80-0375**

BEARD, George Miller (1839-1883)
What constitutes a discovery in science? New York, 1880. 7p. DNLM **80-0376**

BEARD, George Miller (1839-1883)
The dosage of electricity. [Chicago, 1880.] 19p. DNLM **80-0377**

BEARD, George Miller (1839-1883)
The problems of insanity; a paper read before the N.Y. Medico-Legal Society, March 3rd, 1880. [New York, 1880.] 24p. DNLM **80-0378**

BEARD, George Miller (1839-1883)
Notes on sexual neurasthenia. [Detroit: G. S. Davis, 1880.] 6p. DNLM **80-0379**

BEARD, George Miller (1839-1883)
A reply to criticisms on "The problems of insanity," with remarks on the Gosling case. Delivered before the New York Medico-Legal Society, April 16, 1880. New York, 1880. 34p. DNLM **80-0380**

BEARD, George Miller (1839-1883)
A practical treatise on nervous exhaustion (neurasthenia), its symptoms, nature, sequences, treatment. . . . New York: William Wood & Co., 1880. 198p. DLC; NNNAM; PPC; PU **80-0381**

BEARD, George Miller (1839-1883)
A practical treatise on sea-sickness: its symptoms, nature and treatment. . . . New York: E. B. Treat, 1880. 74p. DLC; MBM; PPC; PU **80-0382**

BEARD, George Miller (1839-1883)
The asylums of Europe. Cambridge: Riverside Press, 1881. 12p. DNLM **80-0383**

BEARD, George Miller (1839-1883)
Nature and phenomena of trance. ("Hypnotism," or "somnambulism.") New York: G. P. Putnam's Sons, 1881. 31p. DNLM **80-0384**

BEARD, George Miller (1839-1883)
Trance and trancoidal states in the lower animals. New York: W. L. Hyde & Co., 1881. 17p. DNLM **80-0385**

BEARD, George Miller (1839-1883)
How to use the bromides. . . . Read before the American Neurological Association, June, 1881. . . . [New York: G. P. Putnam's Sons, printers, 1881.] 15p. DLC **80-0386**

BEARD, George Miller (1839-1883)
American nervousness, its causes and consequences, a supplement to nervous exhaustion (neurasthenia). . . . New York: G. P. Putnam's Sons, 1881. 352p. DLC; IEN-M; NNNAM; PPC **80-0387**

BEARD, George Miller (1839-1883)
A practical treatise on the medical and surgical uses of electricity. Including localized and general faradization; localized and central galvanization; electrolysis and galvano-cautery. By Geo. M. Beard . . . [and] A. D. Rockwell. . . . 3rd ed. Rev. by A. D. Rockwell. . . . New York: William Wood & Co., 1881. 758p. DLC; IU-M; MH-M; NNNAM **80-0388**

BEARD, George Miller (1839-1883)
A practical treatise on sea-sickness; its symptoms, nature and treatment; . . . Enlarged edition. 4th thousand. New York: E. B. Treat, 1881. 108p. DLC; MdBJ-W; NNNAM; PPC **80-0389**

BEARD, George Miller (1839-1883)
The new cyclopaedia of family medicine. Our home physician: a popular guide to the art of preserving health and treating disease; with plain advice for all the medical and surgical emergencies of the family. . . . Rev. and enl. New York: E. B. Treat, 1881. 2 v. in 1. plates. DLC; MdU-D; NNNAM; PPC **80-0390**

BEARD, George Miller (1839-1883)
The case of Guiteau—a psychological study. [New York, 1882.] 36p. DNLM **80-0391**

BEARD, George Miller (1839-1883)
Current delusions relating to hypnotism (artificial trance). [St. Louis, 1882?]. 9p. DNLM **80-0392**

BEARD, George Miller (1839-1883)
The study of trance, muscle-reading and allied nervous phenomena in Europe and America, with a letter on the moral character of trance subjects, and a defense of Dr. Charcot. New York, 1882. 40p. 1 plate. DNLM **80-0393**

BEARD, George Miller (1839-1883)
The psychology of the Salem witchcraft excitement of 1692 and its practical application to our own time. New York: G. P. Putnam's Sons, 1882. 112p. 1 plate. DNLM **80-0394**

BEARD, George Miller (1839-1883)
Herbert Spencer on American nervousness. A scientific coincidence. New York: G. P. Putnam's Sons, 1883. 17p. DNLM **80-0395**

BEARD, George Miller (1839-1883) and A. D. ROCKWELL
A practical treatise on the medical and surgical uses of electricity, including localized and general faradization; localized and central galvanization; franklinization; electrolysis and galvano-cautery. 4th ed., revised by A. D. Rockwell. New York: William Wood & Co., 1883. 758p. CtY-M; DNLM; MH-M; NNNAM **80-0396**

BEARD, George Miller (1839-1883)
Sexual neurasthenia (nervous exhaustion). Its hygiene, causes, symptoms, and treatment, with a chapter on diet for the nervous. [. . . .] (Posthumous manuscript.) Ed. by A. D. Rockwell. . . . New York: E. B. Treat, 1884. 270p. DLC; MBM; NNNAM; PPC **80-0397**

BEARD, George Miller (1839-1883)
Sexual neurasthenia [nervous exhaustion]; its hygiene, causes, symptoms, and treatment, with a chapter on diet for the nervous. [Posthumous manuscript.] Edited by A. D. Rockwell. 2nd ed., with formulas. New York: E. B. Treat, 1886. 274p. DNLM; NNNAM; PPJ; PU **80-0398**

BEARD, George Miller (1839-1883)
A practical treatise on nervous exhaustion (neurasthenia), its symptoms, nature, sequences, treatment. Edited, with notes and additions, by A. D. Rockwell. New York: E. B. Treat, 1888. 254p. DNLM **80-0399**

BEARD, Richard O[lding] (*b.* 1856)
Elementary lessons in hygiene. The action and uses of alcohol in the human body. . . . Chicago: Beard Brothers, 1882. 66p. DLC; OCIM **80-0400**

BEASLEY, Henry
The pocket formulary and synopsis of the British and foreign pharmacopoeias, comprising standard, approved, and most recent formulae for the preparations and compounds employed in medical practice. 11th ed. Philadelphia: P. Blakiston, Son & Co., 1886. 517p. DNLM; OCLloyd; MBM; NNNAM **80-0401**

BEASLEY, Henry
The druggist's general receipt book, comprising a copious veterinary formulary, numerous recipes in patent and proprietary medicines, druggists' nostrums, etc., perfumery and cosmetics, beverages, dietetic articles, and condiments, photographic chemicals and formulae, trade chemicals, scientific processes, and an appendix of useful tables. 9th ed. Philadelphia: P. Blakiston, Son & Co., 1886. 507p. DNLM; OCLloyd; NNNAM; PPC **80-0402**

BECK, Richard and Joseph BECK
A condensed list of a few of the most desirable microscopes, of moderate cost, and accessories, mounting implements and materials, clinical thermometers, telescopes, barometers, etc., made, imported, and for sale by . . . manufacturing opticians, Philadelphia. [Philadelphia, 1883?] 32p. DNLM; PPC; PU **80-0403**

BECK, Theodoric Romeyn (1791-1855)
Elements of medical jurisprudence. By Theodoric Romeyn Beck . . . and John B. Beck . . . 11th ed., with notes by an association of the friends of Drs. Beck. The whole revised by C. R. Gilman. . . . Philadelphia: J. B. Lippincott & Co., 1880. 2 v. DLC; MH-M; NNNAM; PPC **80-0404**

BECKWITH, F[rank] E. (1847-1906)
On the treatment of laceration of the cervix uteri, with histories of twenty-six original cases. Hartford: The Case, Lockwood & Brainard Co., 1886. 21p. DNLM **80-0405**

BECKWITH, F[rank] E. (1847-1906)
Remarks on the recent outbreak of typhoid or enteric fever at Southampton, L.I. New Haven: O. A. Dorman, 1887. 18p. CtY-M; DNLM **80-0406**

BEDELL, Leila G.
The abdominal brain. . . . Chicago: Gross & Delbridge, 1885. 45p. OCIM; PPHa **80-0407**

BEEBE, E. W.
Annual address, delivered before the Homoeopathic Medical Society of the State of Wisconsin, by the President; at its twenty-fifth annual session, held at Racine, May 29 and 30, 1889. Chicago: W. A. Chatterton, 1889. 16p. OCIM; PPHa **80-0408**

BEECHER, [Maximillian P.]
Beecher's manual and dental directory of the United States. M. P. Beecher, editor and compiler. New York: Beecher & Co., 1884. 70, 163p. DLC; NNNAM **80-0409**

BEECHER, [Maximillian P.]
A revised and corrected list of the dentists of Ohio, from Beecher's dental directory of the United States. . . . New York: Beecher & Co., 1886. 16 [20] p. DLC **80-0410**

BEECHER, [Maximillian P.]
A revised and corrected list of the dentists of New York, and New Jersey, from Beecher's dental directory of the United States. . . . New York: Beecher & Co., 1886. 41p. DLC **80-0411**

BEECHER, [Maximillian P.]
A supplement to Beecher's Dental Directory of the United States. New York, 1889. 13p. DNLM; NNNAM **80-0412**

BELFIELD, William Thomas (1856-1929)
On the relations of microorganisms to disease. The Cartwright lectures delivered before the Alumni Association of the College of Physicians and Surgeons, New York, February 19, 21, 24, and 27, 1883. New York: Trow, 1883. 131p. DLC; DNLM; NNNAM; NNU-M **80-0413**

BELFIELD, William Thomas (1856-1929)
. . . Diseases of the urinary and male sexual organs. . . . New York: William Wood & Co., 1884. 351p. DLC; DNLM; NNNAM; PPJ **80-0414**

BELL, Agrippa Nelson (1820-1911)
. . . Climatology and mineral waters of the United States. . . . New York: William Wood & Co., 1885. 386p. maps. DLC; DNLM; NNNAM; OCIM **80-0415**

BELL, A[grippa] N[elson] (1820-1911)
Merritt H. Cash prize essay: The physiological conditions and sanitary requirements of school-houses and school-life. [Syracuse, 1887.] 83p. DNLM **80-0416**

BELL, Alexander Graham (1847-1922)
Upon the electrical experiments to determine the location of the bullet in the body of the late President Garfield; and upon a successful form of induction balance for the painless detection of metallic masses in the human body. With an appendix. Washington, D.C.: Gibson Brothers, 1882. 58p. DNLM
80-0417

BELL, Alexander Graham (1847-1922)
Upon a method of teaching language to a very young congenitally deaf child. Washington: Gibson Brothers, 1883. 16p. DNLM **80-0418**

BELL, Alexander Graham (1847-1922)
Memoir upon the formation of a deaf variety of the human race. [Washington, 1885.] 86p. 1 chart. DNLM
80-0419

BELL, Alonzo
Report on the Hot Springs of Arkansas, made to the Secretary of the Interior, 1882. Washington: Government Printing Office, 1882. 27p. DNLM **80-0420**

BELL, Clark (1832-1918)
The coroner's office: should it be abolished? New York: T. B. Mead, 1881. 32p. DNLM; NNNAM **80-0421**

BELL, Clark (1832-1918)
Proposed reforms in the coroner's office. [New York, 1881.] 30p. DNLM; NNNAM **80-0422**

BELL, Clark, (1832-1918)
The Medico-Legal Society of New York. Fifth inaugural address. [New York, 1883.] 24p. DNLM; NNNAM
80-0423

BELL, Clark (1832-1918)
The Medico-Legal Society of New York. Sixth inaugural address. [New York], 1884. 15p. DNLM; NNNAM
80-0424

BELL, Clark (1832-1918)
The Medico-Legal Society of New York. Seventh inaugural address. New York: Vanden Houten & Co., 1884. 24p. DNLM; NNNAM **80-0425**

BELL, Clark (1832-1918)
Report on classification of mental diseases as a basis of international statistics of the insane, made to the Belgian Society of Mental Medicine. [New York, 1886.] 14p. DNLM; NNNAM
80-0426

BELL, Clark (1832-1918)
The Medico-Legal Society of New York. [New York, 1887.] 13p. DNLM; NNNAM **80-0427**

BELL, Clark (1832-1918)
Insanity and the care of the insane. [New York, 1887.] 43p. DNLM; NNNAM **80-0428**

BELL, Clark (1832-1918)
The medical jurisprudence of inebriety. [New York, 1887.] 11p. DNLM; NNNAM **80-0429**

BELL, Clark (1832-1918)
The Medico-Legal Society of New York. Eighth inaugural address. New York, 1888. 20p. DNLM; NNNAM
80-0430

BELL, Clark (1832-1918)
The Medico-Legal Society of New York. Ninth inaugural address. New York, 1889. 15p. DNLM; NNNAM
80-0431

BELL, Clark (1832-1918)
Monomania. [New York, 1889.] 17p. DNLM; NNNAM
80-0432

BELL, F[rancis] Jeffrey (1855-1924)
Comparative anatomy and physiology. Philadelphia: Lea Brothers & Co., 1885. 555p. CtY-M; DNLM; MBM; NNNAM
80-0433

BELL'S HOMOEOPATHIC PHARMACY
. . . Bell's family guide to homoeopathy and health. [New rev. ed. New York, 1888.] 64p. DLC; NNNAM
80-0434

BELL, James Bachelder (1838-1914)
The homoeopathic therapeutics of diarrhoea, dysentery, cholera, cholera morbus, cholera infantum and all other loose evacuations of the bowels. . . . 2nd ed. By Drs. Bell and Laird. . . . New York, Philadelphia: Boericke & Tafel; [etc., etc.], 1881. 275p. DLC; DNLM; NNNAM; PPHa **80-0435**

BELL, James Bachelder (1838-1914)
The homoeopathic therapeutics of diarrhoea, dysentery, cholera, cholera morbus, cholera infantum, and all other loose evacuations of the bowels. . . . 3rd ed. Philadelphia: F. E. Boericke, 1888. 191p. DLC; DNLM; NNNAM; PPHa
80-0436

BELLEVUE HOSPITAL MEDICAL COLLEGE. NEW YORK
Second decennial catalogue of the trustees, faculty, officers, and of the alumni of the Bellevue Hospital Medical College of the City of New York, 1861-1881; together with a history of the College, directory to alumni, and an appendix containing graduates of 1882, 1883, and 1884; the officers, constitution, and by-laws of the Alumni Association of the Bellevue Hospital [Medical] College . . . by Frederick Castle. New York: The Association, 1884. 255p. NNNAM; NNU-M
80-0437

BELT, E[dward] Oliver (1861-1906)
Report of one hundred cataract extractions at the Presbyterian Eye, Ear, and Throat Charity. [New York: G. P. Putnam's Sons, 1888.] 8p. DNLM; NNNAM **80-0438**

BEMISS, J[ohn] Harrison (1856-1891)
A few cases of leprosy. New Orleans: L. Graham, 1880. 16p. 12 plates. DNLM **80-0439**

BEMISS, Samuel Merrifield (1821-1884)
Dengue. Clinical lecture. [New Orleans, 1880.] 12p. DNLM; LNT-M **80-0440**

BEMISS, Samuel Merrifield (1821-1884)
Report upon yellow fever in Louisiana in 1878, and subsequently. New Orleans: L. Graham & Son, 1883. 55p. 4 charts. DNLM; LNT-M **80-0441**

[BEMISS, Samuel Merrifield (1821-1884)]
Biographical sketch of Dr. Samuel Merrifield Bemiss. Late professor of the theory and practice of medicine and clinical medicine, University of Louisiana; member of the National Board of Health, etc., etc. . . . [New Orleans, 1885.] 8p. port. DLC; LNT-M **80-0442**

BENDER, Prosper (1844-1917)
The pathology and physiology of diabetes. [Boston, 1887.] 19p. DNLM; MH-M **80-0443**

BENDER, Prosper (1844-1917)
Address on hospital and dispensary clinics, and the art of prescribing. [Boston, 1888.] 12p. DNLM **80-0444**

BENNETT, Alice (*b.* 1851)
Periodic insanity as illustrated in the case of Sarah J. Whiteling and others. [New York, 1888.] 36p. DNLM **80-0445**

BERMANN, I[sidor] (1845-1918)
The fungus of syphilis. New York: G. P. Putnam's Sons, 1880. 7p. DNLM **80-0446**

BERMANN, I[sidor] (1845-1918)
Some points on staining in toto and dry section cutting. New York: G. P. Putnam's Sons, 1881. 6p. DNLM **80-0447**

BERMANN, I[sidor] (1845-1918)
The Bacillus leprae. New York: G. P. Putnam's Sons, 1882. 5p. DNLM **80-0448**

BERMINGHAM & COMPANY. NEW YORK CITY
Descriptive catalogue of Bermingham's medical library. 2nd ed. New York & London, [1883]. 9 l. DNLM; NNNAM **80-0449**

BERMINGHAM & COMPANY. NEW YORK CITY
Descriptive catalogue of the medical and surgical publications of . . . . New York & London, [1884]. 15p. DNLM; NNNAM **80-0450**

BERMINGHAM, Edward John (*b.* 1853)
The disposal of the dead, a plea for cremation. New York: Bermingham & Co., 1881. 89p. DNLM; NN; NNNAM **80-0451**

BERMINGHAM, Edward John, ed. (*b.* 1853)
An encyclopaedic index of medicine and surgery. . . . New York: Bermingham & Co., 1882. 934p. DNLM; NNNAM; PPJ; PU **80-0452**

BERMINGHAM, Edward John (*b.* 1853)
Practical therapeutics: a compendium of selected formulae and practical hints on treatment. Systematically arranged, interleaved, and copiously indexed. . . . New York: J. R. Bermingham, 1885. 420p. DLC; MH-M; NNNAM; PPC **80-0453**

BERNARD, Henry (1874-1906)
The homoeopathic treatment of constipation. Transl. and revised from the 2nd Belgian ed. by T. M. Strong. Chicago: W. A. Chatterton; New York: A. L. Chatterton Pub. Co., 1882. 192p. DNLM; NNNAM; PPHa **80-0454**

BERNARDY, Eugene Prosper
Biniodide of mercury as a disinfectant in obstetrics, and the value of biniodide of mercury as an antiseptic in obstetrics. [Philadelphia, 1886.] 20p. DNLM **80-0455**

BERNARDY, Eugene Prosper
Ten attacks of appendicitis within eleven months; operation; cure. [Philadelphia, 1889.] 3p. DNLM **80-0456**

BERNARDY, Eugene Prosper
Biniodide of mercury; its antiseptic use. Philadelphia: W. J. Dornan, 1889. 14p. DNLM **80-0457**

BERNAYS, Augustus Charles (1854-1907)
Contribution to the physiology of parturition, illustrated by the history of a case of labor during paralysis. St. Louis, 1883. 4p. DNLM **80-0458**

BERNAYS, Augustus Charles (1854-1907)
Chip No. VII. Kolpohysterectomy. Successful cases of total extirpation of the uterus through the vagina, with epicritical remarks and a description of the author's method of operating. [*Also*: The uterotractor.] St. Louis, Mo.: J. Bucchel, 1885. 14p. DNLM **80-0459**

BERNAYS, Augustus Charles (1854-1907)
Ideal cholecystotomy, a successful case; with critical remarks on the pathology and the different operative procedures practiced on the system of gall vessels. St. Louis: J. H. Chambers, [1885]. 23p. DNLM **80-0460**

BERNAYS, Augustus Charles (1854-1907)
Chip No. VIII. A case of cystic tumor of the jaw in a Negro, and some new observations on the pathological histology of this disease. St. Louis, Mo.: Nixon-Jones Print. Co., 1885. 22p. DNLM **80-0461**

BERNAYS, Augustus Charles (1854-1907)
On the relations between cells and micro-organisms. Chicago, 1886. 11p. DNLM **80-0462**

BERNAYS, Augustus Charles (1854-1907)
Clinical report of surgical cases operated upon by . . . . Reported by Dr. W. V. Kingsbury. St. Louis: Nixon-Jones Print. Co., 1887. 8p. DNLM **80-0463**

BERNHEIM, Hippolyte M[arie] (1840-1919)
Suggestive therapeutics; a treatise on the nature and uses of hypnotism. Transl. from the 2nd French ed. by Christian A. Herter. New York & London: G. P. Putnam's Sons, 1889. 420p. DNLM; IU-M; NNNAM; PPC **80-0464**

BERRY, George A[ndreas] (*b.* 1853)
Diseases of the eye. A practical treatise for students of ophthalmology. Philadelphia: Lea Bros. & Co., 1889. 670p. CtY-M; DNLM; IEN-M; NNNAM **80-0465**

BEUERMANN, John Augustus
The "cell-theory"; can the cell-theory be maintained in the light of recent investigations? New York, 1888. 13p. DNLM
80-0466

BEYER, Henry Gustav (1850-1918)
The influence of cocaine, atropine, and caffeine on the heart and blood-vessels. [Philadelphia, 1885.] 31p. DNLM
80-0467

BEYER, Henry Gustav (1850-1918)
The direct action of calcium, sodium, potassium, and ammonium salts on the blood-vessels. [Philadelphia: Lea Bros. & Co., 1886.] 19p. DNLM **80-0468**

BIDDLE, John Barclay (1815-1879)
Materia medica, for physicians and students. . . . 9th ed. rev., rewritten and enl. in accordance with the 6th revision of the U.S. pharmacopoeia, by Clement Biddle. . . . Philadelphia: P. Blakiston, Son & Co., 1883. 537p. DLC; OCLloyd. PPC; PU
80-0469

BIDDLE, John Barclay (1815-1879)
Materia medica and therapeutics for physicians and students. . . . 10th ed. rev. and enl. with special reference to therapeutics and to the physiological action of medicines. By Clement Biddle . . . and Henry Morris. . . . Philadelphia: P. Blakiston, Son & Co., 1886. 524p. DLC; DNLM; OCLloyd; NNNAM
80-0470

BIDDLE, John Barclay (1815-1879)
Materia medica and therapeutics, for physicians and students. . . . 11th ed., rev. and enl., with special reference to therapeutics and to the physiological action of medicines. By Clement Biddle . . . and Henry Morris. . . . Philadelphia: P. Blakiston, Son & Co., 1889. 607p. DLC; OCLloyd; NNNAM; PPC **80-0471**

BIEGLER, Joseph A.
Domestic guide to homoeopathic treatment, also the hygienic measures required in the management of epidemic cholera. Rochester: Schlicht & Field, 1885. 56p. PPHa
80-0472

BIGELOW, Henry Jacob (1818-1890)
Fees in hospitals. [Boston, 1889.] 8p. DNLM
80-0473

BIGELOW, Horatio Ripley
Hydrophobia. . . . Philadelphia: D. G. Brinton, 1881. 154p. DLC; MH-M; PPC; PPJ **80-0474**

BIGELOW, Horatio Ripley
The rest treatment in gynaecology. [Baltimore, 1881.] 4p. DNLM **80-0475**

BIGELOW, Horatio Ripley
American ovariotomies. New York: William Wood & Co., 1882. 31p. DNLM; NNNAM **80-0476**

BIGELOW, Horatio Ripley
American ovariotomies. [With additions.] New York: William Wood & Co., 1882. 52p. DLC; DNLM; NNNAM
80-0477

BIGELOW, Horatio Ripley
Physicians, pharmacists, and the Therapeutic Gazette. Bridgeport, Conn.: Gould & Stiles, 1882. 8p. DNLM
80-0478

BIGELOW, Horatio Ripley
The surgical treatment of prolapsus uteri. [Cincinnati, 1883.] 10p. DNLM **80-0479**

BIGELOW, Horatio Ripley
The moral significance of sterility. [Cincinnati], 1883. 24p. DNLM **80-0480**

BIGELOW, Horatio Ripley
Some points connected with the pathology, histology, etiology, and diagnosis of myofibromata of the uterus. (Read before the Med. Society of the District of Columbia.) [Baltimore], 1884. 11p. DNLM **80-0481**

BIGELOW, Horatio Ripley
Berlin as a medical center. A guide for American practitioners and students. . . . Sandy Hook, Conn.: New England Publishing Co., 1885. 117p. fold. map. DLC **80-0482**

BIGELOW, Horatio Ripley
Conservative gynaecology. [Washington: McQueen & Wallace, 1887.] 16p. DNLM **80-0483**

[BIGELOW, Jacob] (1787-1879)
Memoir of Jacob Bigelow by George E. Ellis. Cambridge: John Wilson & Son, 1880. 105p. MBM; MH **80-0484**

BIGGS, Hermann Michael (1859-1923)
The aetiology of rabies and the method of M. Pasteur for its prevention. [New York, 1886.] 34p. DNLM
80-0485

BIGGS, Hermann Michael (1859-1923)
Pasteur's prophylactic treatment of rabies. [New York, 1887.] 19p. 1 tab. DNLM **80-0486**

BIGGS, Hermann Michael (1859-1923)
The accidents incidental to the use of the exploring needle for diagnosis. [New York, 1888.] 12p. DNLM
80-0487

BIGGS, T. J.
Haematherapy: present status and technique of the new treatment. New York, [1888]. 111p. 6 plates. DNLM; NNNAM **80-0488**

BILLINGS, John Shaw (1838-1913)
The National Board of Health and national quarantine. Philadelphia: Collins, 1880. 23p. DNLM **80-0489**

BILLINGS, John S[haw] (1838-1913)
Medical bibliography. . . . Baltimore: I. Friedenwald, 1883. 23p. DLC **80-0490**

BILLINGS, John Shaw (1838-1913)
The principles of ventilation and heating and their practical application. New York: The Sanitary Engineer, 1884. 216p. DNLM **80-0491**

BILLINGS, John Shaw (1838-1913)
The World's Industrial and Cotton Centennial Exposition, New Orleans, La., 1884-1885. Medical Department, United States Army. Exhibit Class 4, No. 5. Description of selected specimens from the medical and surgical section of the Army Medical Museum, at Washington, D.C. New Orleans, 1884. 20p. DNLM **80-0492**

BILLINGS, John Shaw (1838-1913)
The World's Industrial and Cotton Centennial Exposition, New Orleans, La., 1884-1885. Medical Department. United States Army. Exhibit Class 4, No. 6. Description of the microscopes and microscopical preparations from the Army Medical Museum, Washington, D.C. New Orleans, 1884. 15p. DNLM
80-0493

BILLINGS, John Shaw (1838-1913)
The World's Industrial and Cotton Centennial Exposition, New Orleans, La., 1884-1885. Medical Department, United States Army. Exhibit Class 4, No. 7, Description of the composite photographs of crania, and of crania from the Army Medical Museum, Washington, D.C. New Orleans, 1884. 15p. DNLM
80-0494

BILLINGS, John Shaw (1838-1913)
Memoir of Joseph Janvier Woodward. Washington, D.C.: Judd & Detweiler, 1885. 7p. DNLM **80-0495**

BILLINGS, John Shaw (1838-1913)
Report on the mortality and vital statistics of the United States as returned at the Tenth Census (June 1, 1880). Washington: Government Print. Office, 1885-1886. 2 v. 19 plates, 20 maps, 38 diags. DNLM **80-0496**

BILLINGS, John Shaw (1838-1913)
Medicine in the United States, and its relations to cooperative investigation; the annual address in medicine, delivered before the British Medical Associations, August 11, 1886. [Philadelphia, 1886.] 30p. DNLM **80-0497**

BILLINGS, John Shaw (1838-1913)
Methods of research in medical literature. [Boston, 1887.] 13p. DNLM **80-0498**

BILLINGS, John Shaw (1838-1913)
Forms of tables of vital statistics, with special reference to the needs of the health department of a city. Concord, N.H., 1888. 21p. DNLM **80-0499**

BILLINGS, John Shaw (1838-1913)
Medical museums, with special reference to the Army Medical Museum at Washington, Philadelphia, 1888. 43p. DNLM
80-0500

BILLINGS, John Shaw (1838-1913)
Memoir of Spencer Fullerton Baird. Washington: Judd & Detweiler, 1889. 9 l. DNLM **80-0501**

BILLINGS, John Shaw (1838-1913)
The plans and purposes of the Johns Hopkins Hospital. [Philadelphia, 1889.] 20p. DNLM **80-0502**

BILLINGS, John Shaw (1838-1913)
On vital and medical statistics. The Cartwright lectures, 1889. New York: Trow, 1889. 37p. DNLM; NNNAM
80-0503

BILLINGTON, C[ornelius] Evarts (1844?-1904)
Diphtheria, its nature and treatment; and intubation in croup and other acute and chronic forms of stenosis of the larynx, by Joseph O'Dwyer. New York: William Wood & Co., 1889. 326p. CtY-M; DNLM; MBM; NNNAM
80-0504

BILLROTH, Theodor (1829-1894)
General surgical pathology and therapeutics, in fifty-one lectures. . . . With additions by Dr. Alexander von Winiwarter. . . . Transl. from the 4th German ed. . . . and rev. from the 10th ed., by Charles E. Hackley. . . . New York: D. Appleton & Co., 1883. 835p. DLC; IEN-M; MBM; NNNAM
80-0505

BILLROTH, Theodor (1829-1894)
Diseases of the female mammary glands. . . . New growths of the uterus by A. Gusserow . . . New York: William Wood & Co., 1887. 426p. MH-M; NNNAM; PPJ; PU
80-0506

BIRD, Francis William (1809-1894)
Physiological reform. An address, delivered before the American Physiological Society at their first annual meeting, June 1, 1837. . . . Published by the request of the Society. Boston: Marsh, Capen & Lyon, 1887. 48p. DLC; MBM
80-0507

BISHOP, Seth Scott (1852-1923)
Cocaine in hay fever. Chicago, 1886. 13p. DNLM
80-0508

BISHOP, Seth Scott (1852-1923)
Operations on the drum-head for impaired hearing; with fourteen cases. Chicago, 1886. 13p. DNLM
80-0509

BISHOP, Seth Scott (1852-1923)
Hay fever. The first prize essay of the United States Hay Fever Association for 1887. Chicago, 1887. 11p. DNLM
80-0510

BISHOP, Seth Scott (1852-1923)
Novel methods of treating diseases of the middle ear. Chicago, 1887. 8p. DNLM **80-0511**

BISHOP, Seth Scott (1852-1923)
Operations for mastoid disease. Chicago, 1887. 8p. DNLM
80-0512

BISHOP, Seth Scott (1852-1923)
Statistical report of 5,700 cases of ear diseases, classified by age, sex, occupation, and disease; causation. Chicago, 1887. 7p. **80-0513**

BISHOP, Seth Scott (1852-1923)
Treatment of chronic suppurative otitis . . . . Chicago, 1887. 4p. DNLM **80-0514**

BISHOP, Seth Scott (1852-1923)
A new adjustable lamp bracket. [Chicago, 1888.] 1p. DNLM
80-0515

BISHOP, Seth Scott (1852-1923)
The pathology of hay fever. Chicago, 1888. 11p. DNLM
80-0516

BISHOP, Seth Scott (1852-1923)
Report of the committee on ophthalmology and otology. [Chicago, 1888.] 11p. DNLM **80-0517**

BISSELL, J[oseph] Bidlemann (1859-1918)
The morbid anatomy of congenital talipes equino-varus. Philadelphia: J. B. Lippincott & Co., 1888. 14p. DNLM
80-0518

BIXBY, George H[olmes] (1837-1901)
A case of shot wound of the bladder. [Boston, 1880.] 4p. DNLM **80-0519**

BIXBY, George H[olmes] (1837-1901)
A case of hystero-neurosis. Cambridge: Riverside Press, 1881. 8p. DNLM **80-0520**

BIXBY, George H[olmes] (1837-1901)
The histories of six cases of ovariotomy. New York: D. Appleton & Co., 1884. 19p. DNLM **80-0521**

BLACK, Greene Vardiman (1836-1915)
The formation of poisons by micro-organisms. A biological study of the germ theory of disease. Philadelphia: P. Blakiston, Son & Co., 1884. 178p. DLC; DNLM; MH **80-0522**

BLACK, Greene Vardiman (1836-1915)
A study of the histological characters of the periosteum and peridental membrane. Chicago: W. T. Keener, 1887. 138p. 15 plates. DNLM **80-0523**

BLACK, John J[anvier] (1837-1909)
A Porro-Caesarean section rendered necessary by a deformed pelvis and a uterus enormously enlarged by fibroid growths; together with a cyst of the right broad ligament. [Philadelphia, 1889.] 8p. DNLM **80-0524**

BLACKWOOD, W[illiam] R[obert] D[ouglas] (1839-1922)
[Report of the "committee on the abuse of medical charities."] [Philadelphia, 1880.] 10p. DNLM **80-0525**

BLAKE, Clarence J[ohn] (1843-1919)
On the occurrence of exostoses within the external auditory canal in prehistoric man. New York: Trow, 1880. 12p. DNLM **80-0526**

BLAKE, Clarence J[ohn] (1843-1919)
Intra-tympanic pressure during phonation. [Boston, 1881]. 5p. DNLM **80-0527**

BLAKE, Clarence J[ohn] (1843-1919)
Acute congestion of the upper portion of the tympanic cavity and membrana tympani. [New York, 1882.] 4p. DNLM **80-0528**

BLAKE, Clarence J[ohn] (1843-1919)
Aural polypus snare. [New York, 1882.] 1 l. DNLM **80-0529**

BLAKE, Clarence J[ohn] (1843-1919)
The progressive growth of the dermoid coat of the membrana tympani. [n.p., 1882.] 3p. DNLM **80-0530**

BLANDFORD, G[eorge] Fielding (1829-1911)
Insanity and its treatment; lectures on the treatment, medical and legal, of insane patients. 3rd ed., together with, types of insanity, an illustrated guide in the physical diagnosis of mental disease, by Allan McLane Hamilton. New York: William Wood & Co., 1886. 379p. CtY-M; DNLM; LNT-M; NNNAM **80-0531**

BLEE, Charles G.
A modern treatise on the most rational treatment of cancer, tumors and other important diseases. . . . Cincinnati: Issued by the author, C. T. Woodrow & Co., print., [1883]. 28p. DLC **80-0532**

BLEYER, J[ulius] Mount (1859-1915)
Apparatus for the administration of ozonized vapor, and inhaler for the special use of Ch. Marchand's peroxide of hydrogen in pulmonary, bronchial, throat, and nasal affections. [New York, 1887.] 36p. DNLM; NNNAM **80-0533**

BLEYER, J[ulius] Mount (1859-1915)
Scientific methods of capital punishment. New York: J. Fitzgerald, 1887. 9p. DNLM **80-0534**

BLEYER, J[ulius] Mount (1859-1915)
Some practical hints in connection with intubation of the larynx, and a résumé of 206 cases operated on from 1886 to 1888. [New York, 1889.] 12p. DNLM **80-0535**

BLISS, D. W[illard] (1825-1889)
Feeding per rectum, as illustrated in the case of the late President Garfield, and others. [Washington, 1882.] 16p. DNLM **80-0536**

BLODGETT, A[lbert] N[ovatus] (1843-1923)
The treatment of strains and sprains by collodion. Cambridge: Riverside Press, 1881. 14p. DNLM; MH-M **80-0537**

BLODGETT, A[lbert] N[ovatus] (1843-1923)
The management of chronic inebriates and insane drunkards. Boston: G. H. Ellis, 1882. 24p. DNLM; MBM **80-0538**

BLODGETT, A[lbert] N[ovatus] (1843-1923)
A case of subscapular abscess, with remarks. [Philadelphia, 1884.] 8p. DNLM **80-0539**

BLODGETT, A[lbert] N[ovatus] (1843-1923)
A handbook of dental pathology. For students and practitioners. Philadelphia: P. Blakiston, Son & Co., 1888. 279p. DLC; DNLM; MdU-D; PPC **80-0540**

BLUMER, G. Adler
A case of perverted sexual instinct. (Conträre Sexualempfindung.) [Utica, N.Y., 1882.] 14p. DNLM **80-0541**

BLYTH, Alexander Wynter (1844-1921)
Poisons, their effects and detection; a manual for the use of analytical chemists and experts, with an introductory essay on the growth of modern toxicology. . . . New York: William Wood & Co., 1885. 2 v. fold. tab. DLC; NNNAM **80-0542**

BOARDMAN, William E[lbridge]
The management of cases of rigidity of the os uteri in labor. [Boston, 1886.] 17p. DNLM; MBM **80-0543**

BOARDMAN, William E[lbridge]
Aseptic obstetrics. [Boston, 1889.] 18p. DNLM **80-0544**

BÖDECKER, C. F. W.
The Herbst method of filling teeth. New York, [1884]. 10p. DNLM **80-0545**

BÖDECKER, C. F. W.
Iodoform in dental surgery. Buffalo, N.Y., [1884]. 12p. DNLM **80-0546**

BODENHAMER, William (1808-1905)
A theoretical and practical treatise on the hemorrhoidal disease, giving its history, nature, causes, pathology, diagnosis, and treatment. . . . New York: William Wood & Co., 1884. 297p. col. plates. DLC; NNNAM; NNU-M; PPC
80-0547

BODLEY, Rachel L. (1831-1888)
Valedictory address to the twenty-ninth graduating class of the Woman's Medical College of Pennsylvania. . . . March 17th, 1881. . . . Philadelphia: Grant, Faires & Rogers, printers, 1881. 16p. DLC; DNLM **80-0548**

BOERICKE & TAFEL
Drug prices current. Philadelphia, 1889. 140p. PPHa; PU
80-0549

BOERICKE, William (1849-1929)
The twelve tissue remedies of Schüssler, comprising the theory, therapeutical appliction, materia medica, and a complete repertory of these remedies. Arranged and comp. by William Boericke . . . and Willis A. Dewey. . . . Philadelphia: F. E. Boericke, Hahnemann Publishing House, 1888. 303p. DLC; NNNAM; PPHa; PPJ **80-0550**

BOHNE, William
Hand-book for young and old opticians. A concise and comprehensive treatise on the theory of the optical trade and of its mechanical manipulations. New Orleans: Published by the Author, 1888. 108p. LNT-M; OCIM; PPC
80-0551

BOLDT, H[ermann] J[ohn] (*b.* 1856)
Interstitial salpingitis. New York: William Wood & Co., 1888. 14p. DNLM **80-0552**

BOLDT, H[ermann] J[ohn] (*b.* 1856)
Suppurative exfoliative cystitis. New York: William Wood & Co., 1888. 21p. DNLM; NNNAM
80-0553

BOLDT, H[ermann] J[ohn] (*b.* 1856)
The manual treatment in gynecology. New York: William Wood & Co., 1889. 22p. DNLM; NNNAM
80-0554

BOLDT, H[ermann] J[ohn] (*b.* 1856)
The treatment of suppurative disease of the uterine appendages. New York: William Wood & Co., 1889. 16p. DNLM; NNNAM **80-0555**

BOLLES, William P[almer] (1845-1916)
New surgical apparatus. Boston: Rockwell & Churchill, 1882. 16p. 2 plates. DNLM; MBM **80-0556**

BONWILL, W. G. A[rlington]
Rapid breathing as a pain obtunder in minor surgery, obstetrics, the general practice of medicine and of dentistry. [New York, 1881.] 16p. DNLM **80-0557**

BONWILL, W. G. A[rlington]
The geometrical and mechanical laws of the articulation of the human teeth; the anatomical articulator. [Philadelphia, 1889.] 16p. DNLM **80-0558**

BONWILL, W. G. A[rlington]
The philosophy of eating and drinking from a dental and medical standpoint with personal experiences. Read before the Odontological Society of Pennsylvania, April 7th, 1888. Philadelphia, 1889. 21p. PPC **80-0559**

BOOKER, William D[avid] (1844-1921)
A study of some of the bacteria found in the dejecta of infants afflicted with summer diarrhoea. Philadelphia: W. F. Fell & Co., [1888]. 10 l. DNLM **80-0560**

BORCK, [Mathias Adolph] Edward (1834-1912)
Simple methods to stanch accidental hemorrhage. St. Louis, Mo., 1881. 4p. 1 plate. DNLM **80-0561**

BORCK, [Mathias Adolph] Edward (1834-1912)
Observations on surgery in children. St. Louis: Med. J. Pub. Co., 1882. 13p. DLC; DNLM **80-0562**

BORCK, [Mathias Adolph] Edward (1834-1912).
Spinal deformities. Fracture of the femur. Orthopaedics and injuries. Extracts of clinical lectures. [St. Louis, Mo.], 1882[-3]. 14p. DNLM **80-0563**

BORCK, [Mathias Adolph] Edward (1834-1912)
Diagnosis of ovarian tumors. St. Louis, Mo.: C. M. Curtman, 1883. 16p. DNLM **80-0564**

BORCK, [Mathias Adolph] Edward (1834-1912)
Memorandum of contributions towards medical and surgical literature, up to date. St. Louis, 1884. 4p. DNLM
80-0565

BORCK, [Mathias Adolph] Edward (1834-1912)
Home again! A synopsis of a tour abroad, by . . . one of the delegates . . . [to] the International Medical Congress, held at Copenhagen, Denmark, from August 10-16, 1884. [St. Louis]: J. H. Chambers & Co., 1884. 24p. DNLM **80-0566**

BORCK, [Mathias Adolph] Edward (1834-1912)
Abnormal positions of the head. What do they indicate? A Clinical lecture delivered before his private class of medical practitioners, with a case of dislocation of the cervical vertebrae. St. Louis, Mo.: Weiss & Maccallum, 1885. 14p. DNLM **80-0567**

BORCK, [Mathias Adolph] Edward (1834-1912)
Ovarian tumors, and remarks on abdominal surgery, with the result of 50 cases. 2nd revised reprint ed. St. Louis: Weiss & Maccallum, 1887. 22p. DNLM **80-0568**

BORCK, [Mathias Adolph] Edward (1834-1912)
Short notes on the surgical diseases of children. [Philadelphia, 1889.] 9p. DNLM **80-0569**

BOSTON MEDICAL LIBRARY ASSOCIATION
Address delivered at the dedication of the hall of the Boston Library Association, on Dec. 3, 1878, by Oliver Wendell Holmes, pres. Report of C. P. Putnam, Remarks of J. S. Billings, Justin Winsor, G. H. Lyman, C. W. Elliot, D. P. Smith, D. C. Ellis, and H. I. Bowditch. Exhibition of medical portraits. Report of the librarian James R. Chadwick, read at the 6th annual meeting, held on Oct. 4, 1881. Report of F. C. Shattuck on the Directory for Nurses. Cambridge: Riverside Press, 1881. 39p. 18p. DNLM; MB **80-0570**

BOSTON POLYCLINIC
Clinical courses of medical instruction. Bulletins, etc. Boston, 1885-1895. DNLM; MBM [Includes bulletins for Sept. to Dec., 1885; June to Oct., 1888; Jan. to May, 1889; Jan. to Feb., 1890. Summer courses for 1885-1887; 1890-1892; 1894. Autumn courses for 1886; 1887; 1891-1893. Winter courses for 1887; 1892; 1893; 1895. Spring courses for 1894; 1895. Commenced in 1880, and regularly organized in the summer of 1881 as the Summer School for Clinical Instruction. Summer courses only from 1880 to 1884. Winter courses commenced in 1885.] **80-0571**

BOSTON POLYCLINIC
Its faculty and history. [Boston, 1886.] 22p. DNLM; MBM **80-0572**

BOSTON UNIVERSITY. SCHOOL OF MEDICINE (HOMOEOPATHIC)
What it is doing and what it needs. March 1, 1887. [Boston: A. Mudge & Son, 1887.] 16p. DNLM; MBM **80-0573**

BOSWORTH, Francke H[untington] (1845-1925)
Some of the unsettled questions concerning nasal catarrh. New York: Trow, 1880. 30p. DNLM; NNNAM **80-0574**

BOSWORTH, Francke H[untington] (1845-1925)
A manual of diseases of the throat and nose. New York: William Wood & Co., 1881. 427p. DLC; DNLM; NNNAM; PPC **80-0575**

BOSWORTH, Francke H[untington] (1845-1925)
Jarvis' operation; its relation to nasal catarrh. New York: Trow, 1881. 12p. DNLM **80-0576**

BOSWORTH, Francke H[untington] (1845-1925)
Adenoma at the vault of the pharynx. Cambridge: Riverside Press, 1882. 8p. DNLM **80-0577**

BOSWORTH, Francke H[untington] (1845-1925)
A study of nasal catarrh, based on pathological investigation. New York: Trow, 1882. 24p. DNLM; NNNAM **80-0578**

BOSWORTH, Francke H[untington] (1845-1925)
Growths in the nasal passages. New York: Trow, 1883. 27p. DNLM; NNNAM **80-0579**

BOSWORTH, Francke H[untington] (1845-1925)
The relation of laryngeal to pulmonary diseases. New York, 1884. 7p. DNLM **80-0580**

BOSWORTH, Francke H[untington] (1845-1925)
The three tonsils; some practical suggestions in regard to their structure, function, and diseases. New York: Trow, 1884. 20p. DNLM; NNNAM **80-0581**

BOSWORTH, Francke H[untington] (1845-1925)
Hay fever, asthma, and allied affections. [New York, 1886.] 20p. DNLM **80-0582**

BOSWORTH, Francke H[untington] (1845-1925)
The use of caustics in the nasal cavities. New York, 1888. 9p. DNLM **80-0583**

BOSWORTH, Francke H[untington] (1845-1925)
A treatise on diseases of the nose and throat. . . . New York: William Wood & Co., 1889-1892. 2 v. col. plates. DLC; ICRM; NNNAM; PU **80-0584**

BOVEE, J. W[esley] (1861-1927)
A few interesting clinical cases. Cincinnati, 1888. 8p. DNLM **80-0585**

BOWDITCH, Henry Ingersoll (1808-1892)
Sanitary organization of nations. . . . Cambridge, [Mass.]: Printed at the Riverside Press, 1880. 24p. DLC; DNLM **80-0586**

BOWDITCH, Henry Ingersoll (1808-1892)
The medical education of women. The present hostile position of Harvard University and the Massachusetts Medical Society. What remedies therefor can be suggested? [Boston, 1881.] 4p. DNLM; MH-M **80-0587**

BOWDITCH, Henry Ingersoll (1808-1892)
The past, present, and future treatment of homoeopathy, eclecticism, and kindred delusions which may hereafter arise in the medical profession, as viewed from the history of medicine and of personal experience. Boston: Cupples, Upham & Co., 1887. 20p. DNLM; MH-M; PPHa **80-0588**

BOWDITCH, Henry Ingersoll (1808-1892)
Yellow fever epidemic. What should be done; imperative need of national sanitary board. To the editor of the Post. Sept. 14, 1888. Boston, 1888. 1 sheet. fol. DNLM; MBM **80-0589**

BOWDITCH, Henry Ingersoll (1808-1892)
Open-air travel as a curer and preventer of consumption, as seen in the history of a New England family. Philadelphia: W. J. Dornan, 1889. 10p. DNLM **80-0590**

BOWDITCH, Henry Pickering (1840-1911)
[Cards for registering the growth of children], single and successive observations. [Boston, 1880.] 4 cards, 3 by 4 inches. DNLM; MBM **80-0591**

BOWDITCH, Henry Pickering (1840-1911)
The relation between growth and disease. Philadelphia: Collins, 1881. 9p. DNLM **80-0592**

BOWDITCH, Henry Pickering (1840-1911)
On the collection of data at autopsies. [Cambridge, 1882.] 4p. DNLM **80-0593**

BOWDITCH, Henry Pickering (1840-1911)
Vaso-motor nerves of the limbs. [Abstr.] [Salem, 1886.] 1 l. DNLM **80-0594**

BOWDITCH, Henry Pickering (1840-1911)
What is nerve force? Salem, 1886. 12p. DNLM **80-0595**

BOWDITCH, Henry Pickering (1840-1911)
Remarks made at a meeting of the academic council of Harvard University, held on Wednesday, Dec. 22, 1886. Boston: D. Clapp & Son, 1887. 19p. DNLM; MH **80-0596**

BOWDITCH, Henry Pickering (1840-1911)
The action of sulphuric ether on the peripheral nervous system. From experiments performed in the physiological laboratory of the Harvard Medical School, by Dr. F. H. Hooper, Dr. F. W. Ellis, and Mr. J. W. Perkins. [Philadelphia, 1887.] 11p. DNLM; MH-M **80-0597**

BOWDITCH, Henry Pickering (1840-1911)
The reinforcement and inhibition of the knee-jerk. Boston: Cupples & Hard, 1888. 6p. DNLM **80-0598**

BOWDITCH, Henry Pickering (1840-1911)
. . . Hints for teachers of physiology. . . . Boston: D. C. Heath & Co., 1889. 58p. DLC; ICU; MBM; MH **80-0599**

BOWDITCH, Vincent Y[ardley] (1852-1929)
A case of traumatic linear atrophy. Boston: Cupples, Upham & Co., 1885. 8p. DNLM **80-0600**

BOWDITCH, Vincent Y[ardley] (1852-1929)
The treatment of pulmonary diseases by means of "pneumatic differentiation." [Boston: Cupples, Upham & Co., 1885.] 11p. DNLM **80-0601**

BOWDITCH, Vincent Y[ardley] (1852-1929)
A case of phthisis with numerous bacilli; complete arrest of the disease. [Boston: Cupples, Upham & Co., 1885.] 8p. DNLM **80-0602**

BOWDITCH, Vincent Y[ardley] (1852-1929)
Ten months' experience with pneumatic differentiation. New York, 1886. 40p. DNLM **80-0603**

BOWDITCH, Vincent Y[ardley] (1852-1929)
Homoeopathy as viewed by a member of the Massachusetts Medical Society. An address delivered April 15, 1886, before the Hahnemannian Society of the Boston University School of Medicine. Boston: Cupples, Upham & Co., 1886. 29p. DNLM; MBM **80-0604**

BOWDITCH, Vincent Y[ardley] (1852-1929)
The use of strophanthus hispidus in heart disease. [Boston, 1887.] 11p. DNLM **80-0605**

BOWDITCH, Vincent Y[ardley] (1852-1929)
The comparative importance of different climatic attributes in the treatment of pulmonary consumption. [Philadelphia, 1888.] 10p. DNLM **80-0606**

BOWDITCH, Vincent Y[ardley] (1852-1929)
Comparative results in ninety cases of pleurisy, with special reference to the development of phthisis pulmonalis. Philadelphia: W. J. Dornan, 1889. 13p. 1 tab. DNLM; PPC **80-0607**

BOWDITCH, Vincent Y[ardley] (1852-1929) and William N. BULLARD
Two cases of phthisis treated by intra-pulmonary injections. [Boston, 1889.] 14p. DNLM **80-0608**

BOWEN, Cuthbert
Hand-book of materia medica, pharmacy, and therapeutics. Compiled for the use of students preparing for examination. Philadelphia: F. A. Davis, 1888. 366p. DLC; DNLM; OCLloyd; NNNAM **80-0609**

BOWEN, John George (1855?-1886)
Cholera: its preventive and curative treatment, simplified for domestic use. [New Orleans], 1885. 80p. DNLM; LNT-M **80-0610**

BOWEN, John T[empleton] (*b.* 1857)
On the occurrence of small-pox lesions in the internal organs, with some studies of the skin eruptions. Boston: Rockwell & Churchill, 1888. 16p. 1 plate. DNLM; MBM **80-0611**

BOWLBY, Anthony Alfred (1855-1929)
Surgical pathology and morbid anatomy. Philadelphia: P. Blakiston, Son & Co., 1887. 543p. DNLM; IEN-M; NNNAM; PPC **80-0612**

BOWLING, William K. (1808-1885)
Life of John M. Briggs, M.D., of Bowling Green, Ky. Nashville, 1882. 20p. DNLM **80-0613**

BOWMAN, John E[ddowes] (1819-1854)
An introduction to practical chemistry, including analysis. Edited by Charles L. Bloxam. 8th ed. Philadelphia: P. Blakiston, Son & Co., 1885. 248p. DNLM; ICU; NN; NNC **80-0614**

BOWMAN, Winthrop H.
Lecture delivered at Tremont Temple, May 11, 1882, introducing his system of respiration for the development and treatment of the vital organs of the body. Boston: A. Mudge & Son, 1883. 30p. DNLM; MBM **80-0615**

BOWMAN, Winthrop H.
A system of respiration for the development and treatment of the vital organs of the body. Boston: A Mudge & Sons, 1888. 19p. DNLM; MBM **80-0616**

BOYCE, C. W. (1822-1900)
Electricity; its nature and forms, with a study on electro-therapeutics. Chicago. W. A. Chatteron, 1880. 85p. DNLM; OCIM **80-0617**

[BOYD, J. C.]
"The blood is the life." An astonishing discovery; accomplished at last, the efficacy of electricity. Nearly all diseases effectually cured by Boyd's miniature galvanic battery. [New York, 1880.] 842p. DNLM; NNNAM **80-0618**

BOYD, James P., [Jr.]
A contribution to the study of placenta praevia. [Albany, 1883.] 11p. DNLM **80-0619**

BOYLAND, G. Halsted (1845-1919)
The Buffalo lithia waters in the treatment of the diseases of the nervous system. New York: D. Appleton & Co., 1887. 11p. DNLM **80-0620**

BOZEMAN, Nathan (1825-1905)
Removal of a cyst of the pancreas weighing twenty and one-half pounds. [New York, 1882.] 4p. DNLM **80-0621**

BOZEMAN, Nathan (1825-1905)
On genital renovation by kolpostenotomy and kolpoecpetasis in urinary and fecal fistules. [Philadelphia, 1882.] 43p. DNLM; PU **80-0622**

BOZEMAN, Nathan (1825-1905)
The value of graduated pressure in the treatment of diseases of the vagina, uterus, ovaries, and other appendages. [Atlanta, 1883.] 62p. DNLM **80-0623**

BOZEMAN, Nathan (1825-1905)
History of the clamp suture of the late Dr. J. Marion Sims, and why it was abandoned by the profession. [Philadelphia, 1884.] 59p. DNLM; PPC **80-0624**

BOZEMAN, Nathan (1825-1905)
The gradual preparatory treatment of the complications of urinary and faecal fistulae in women, including a special consideration of the treatment of pyelitis by a new method, and the prevention of the evils of incontinence of urine by a new system of drainage. [New York, 1887.] 13p. DNLM
80-0625

BOZEMAN, Nathan (1825-1905)
The gradual preparatory treatment of the complications of urinary and faecal fistulae in women, including a special consideration of the treatment of pyelitis by a new method, and the prevention of the evils of incontinence of urine by a new system of drainage. [Philadelphia: W. F. Fell & Co., 1887.] 23 l. DNLM **80-0626**

BOZEMAN, Nathan (1825-1905)
Chronic pyelitis; successfully treated by kolpo-uretero-cystotomy; irrigation of the pelvis of the kidney, and intra-vaginal drainage. [Philadelphia, 1888.] 19p. DNLM
80-0627

BOZEMAN, Nathan (1825-1905)
Renal tenesmus. New York: Trow's Co., 1888. 36p. DNLM; NNNAM **80-0628**

BOZEMAN, Nathan G.
The after-treatment of kolpo-uretero-cystotomy and other similar operations, by a new system of continuous irrigation and drainage. [New York, 1889.] 12p. DNLM
80-0629

BRACKETT, C. A[lbert] (1850-1927)
Some of the opportunities, responsibilities, and encouragements of life. An address delivered before the Massachusetts Dental Society at its eighteenth annual meeting in Boston, December 14, 1882. Boston, Mass.: Wright & Potter, 1883. 19p. DNLM; MBM **80-0630**

BRADBURY, Robert
Bradbury's unofficial formulary and memory work of pharmacy. . . . Chicago, Ill.: Bradbury Publishing Co., 1889. 356, [18] p. DLC; OCIM; OCLloyd; PU **80-0631**

BRADFORD, Edward Hickley (1848-1926)
The treatment of hip disease. Read before the Boston Society for Medical Improvement, June 28, 1880. Cambridge, 1880. 21p. DNLM **80-0632**

BRADFORD, Edward Hickley (1848-1926)
On the use of force in the treatment of resistant club-foot. Cambridge: Riverside Press, 1881. 15p. DNLM
80-0633

BRADFORD, Henry W.
The electro-magnet in ophthalmology, with a description of a new magnet. Cambridge, 1881. 8p. 1 plate. DNLM
80-0634

BRADFORD, Henry W.
Rapid cocainization. Cambridge: Riverside Press, 1884. 12p. DNLM **80-0635**

BRADFORD, Henry W.
A case of enucleation with replacement of the human globe by that of a rabbit. [Boston, 1885.] 4p. DNLM
80-0636

BRADFORD, Thomas Lindsley (1847-1918)
A monograph on croup; its pathology, diagnosis, and treatment. Philadelphia: Sherman & Co., 1880. 24p. DNLM; PPHa
80-0637

BRADFORD, Thomas Lindsley (1847-1918)
Complete list of homoeopathic medical journals published in the United States, between the years 1835 and 1888. Philadelphia, [1889]. 9p. DNLM; PPHa
80-0638

BRADFORD, W. Ellis
Physiological law governing the production of the human sex. Dix, Ill., 1889. 9p. DNLM **80-0639**

BRADLEY, John E[dwin] (*b.* 1839)
Science and industry; the relation of science to material prosperity. An address to the graduating class of the Albany college of Pharmacy, March 1, 1886. Albany, N.Y.: Burdick & Taylor, 1886. 12p. DNLM **80-0640**

BRAMBLE, D[avid] D. (*b.* 1839)
Antiseptics in the treatment of certain forms of bone disease, especially necrosis and its consequences. . . . Cincinnati: Aldine Printing Works, 1881. 16p. DLC **80-0641**

BRAMWELL, Byrom (1847-1931)
The diseases of the spinal cord. New York: William Wood & Co., 1882. 300p. 40 plates. DNLM; IU-M; NNNAM; PPC
80-0642

BRAMWELL, Byrom (1847-1931)
Diseases of the heart and thoracic aorta. New York: D. Appleton & Co., 1884. 783p. 36 plates. DNLM; NNNAM; PPC; PU **80-0643**

BRAMWELL, Byrom (1847-1931)
The diseases of the spinal cord. 2nd ed. New York: William Wood & Co., 1886. 298p. 53 plates. CtY-M; DNLM; NNNAM; PU **80-0644**

BRAMWELL, Byrom (1847-1931)
Practical medicine and medical diagnosis. Methods of diagnosis. Case-taking and case-recording. Medical thermometry. New York: J. H. Vail & Co., 1887. 149p. DNLM; OCIM; NNNAM; PPC **80-0645**

BRAMWELL, Byrom (1847-1931)
Intracranial tumours. Philadelphia: J. B. Lippincott Co., 1888. 270p. CtY-M; DNLM; NNNAM; PPC
80-0646

BRASTED, Horace Kimball
Facts on homoeopathy. . . . Lima, N.Y.: A. T. Norton, printer, 1883. 92p. DLC **80-0647**

BREWER, George E[merson] (1861-1939)
Some observations upon the modern treatment of urethritis. New York: William Wood & Co., 1887. 23p. DNLM; NNNAM
80-0648

BREWER, George E[merson] (1861-1939)
Typical cases illustrating the advantages of the use of nitrate of silver in the deep urethra. [New York, 1889.] 8p. DNLM
80-0649

BRIDGER, Adolphus E[dward]
Man and his maladies; or the way to health. A popular handbook of physiology and domestic medicine in accord with the advance in medical science. New York: Harper & Bros., 1889. 593p. DNLM; NN; NNC **80-0650**

BRIEF description of the Swedish movement, massage, and mechanical vibration for the treatment of diseases, as used by Prof. Hartvig Nissen, of Stockholm, Sweden, and Profs. S. Weir Mitchell, Hammond, Graham, Taylor, Schreibert, and others. Compiled by J. A. Stucky and Mrs. A. Bealert. Lexington, Ky., 1889. 41p. DNLM **80-0651**

BRIGGS, F[rederic] M[elancthon]
A case of papillomatous urethritis. Boston: Damrell & Upham, 1889. 9p. DNLM **80-0652**

BRIGGS, James Edwin
Nervous diseases and magnetic therapeutics. . . . New York: G. W. Wheat, printer, 1881. 60p. DLC; NNNAM **80-0653**

BRIGGS, William Ellery
Notes on the electro-magnetic in ophthalmology, with a report of nine cases. Sacramento, 1889. 6p. DNLM **80-0654**

BRIGGS, W[illiam] T[hompson] (1828-1894)
The surgical treatment of intestinal obstruction. Nashville, 1880. 25p. DNLM; OCIM **80-0655**

BRIGGS, W[illiam] T[hompson] (1828-1894)
The antiseptic treatment of wounds after operations and injuries. Nashville, Tenn., 1882. 19p. DNLM; OCIM **80-0656**

BRIGGS, W[illiam] T[hompson] (1828-1894)
The surgical treatment of epilepsy arising from injuries of the head, with special reference to the use of the trephine. Louisville: J. P. Morton & Co., 1884. 24p. DNLM; OCIM **80-0657**

BRIGHAM, Gershom N[elson] (1820-1886)
Catarrhal diseases of the nasal and respiratory organs. New York: A. L. Chatterton Publishing Co., 1881. 112p. DNLM; PPHa **80-0658**

BRIGHAM, Gershom N[elson] (1820-1886)
Catarrhal diseases of the nasal and respiratory organs. 2nd ed. New York: A. L. Chatterton Publishing Co., 1884. 112p. DNLM; PPHa **80-0659**

BRIGHAM, Gershom N[elson] (1820-1886)
Phthisis pulmonalis; or, tubercular consumption. New York and Philadelphia: Boericke & Tafel. 1882. 241p. DNLM; PPHa **80-0660**

BRILL, Nathan E[dwin] (1860-1925)
Lyssa and the Pasteur fiasco. [Philadelphia, 1888.] 23p. DNLM **80-0661**

BRINKERHOFF, Alexander W. (*d.* 1887)
Diseases of the rectum and new method of rectal treatment. . . . Columbus, O.: The author, 1881. 266p. DLC; OCIM **80-0662**

BRINTON, John Hill (1832-1907)
The faculty of 1841. A lecture delivered before the Alumni Association of the Jefferson Medical College, March 11th, 1880. Philadelphia: Collins, 1880. 14p. DNLM; PPJ **80-0663**

BRINTON, John Hill (1832-1907)
The march of surgery. An address. Philadelphia: W. F. Fell & Co., 1882. 13p. DNLM; PPJ **80-0664**

BROKOW, A[ugustus] V. L. (1836-1907)
An experimental study of intestinal anastomosis. With some practical suggestions as to a modified technique. [St. Louis, 1889.] 2 l. DNLM **80-0665**

BROKAW, A[ugustus] V. L. (1836-1907)
The use of segmented rubber ring in intestinal anastomotic and other operations. New York: E. P. Coby & Co., [1889]. 18p. DNLM **80-0666**

BRONSON, Edward Bennet
The objects of dermatological classification, with especial reference to Auspitz's system. New York: William Wood & Co., 1884. 21p. DNLM; NNNAM **80-0667**

BRONSON, Edward Bennet
A study of the considerations relating to the classification of skin diseases, with an attempt to construct a logical system in accordance with fundamental principles of etiology. New York: William Wood & Co., 1887. 19p. 1 tab. DNLM; NNNAM **80-0668**

BRONSON, Edward Bennet
On preventive treatment in primary syphilis. [New York, 1888.] 21p. DNLM **80-0669**

BROOKLYN VACUUM CURE CO.
Illustrated catalogue of vacuum apparatus, pneumatic equalizer, . . . with nature of treatment. . . . Brooklyn, 1888. 23p. NNNAM **80-0670**

BROWN, A. P.
President's annual address before the Texas State Medical Association, at Belton, Tex., April 23rd, 1884. Jefferson, 1884. 14p. DNLM **80-0671**

BROWN, Bedford (1825-1897)
Report on the advances in the practice of medicine, submitted to the Medical Society of Virginia at its annual meeting, October 21, 1881. Alexandria, Va.: Ramey & Son, 1881. 13p. DNLM **80-0672**

BROWN, Bedford (1825-1897)
Observations on the treatment of scarlet fever. [New York, 1885.] 9p. DNLM **80-0673**

BROWN, Bedford (1825-1897)
The medical treatment of fibroid tumors of the uterus. [New York, 1888.] 14p. DNLM **80-0674**

BROWN, Buckminster (1819-1891)
Description of an apparatus for the treatment of contraction and false anchylosis of the hip-joint. Cambridge, 1881. 6p. DNLM **80-0675**

BROWN, Buckminster (1819-1891)
Extension in the treatment of diseased vertebrae. Cambridge: Riverside Press, 1884. 8p. DNLM **80-0676**

BROWN, Buckminster (1819-1891)
Double congenital displacement of the hip. Description of a case with treatment resulting in cure. Boston: Cupples, Upham & Co., 1885. 24p. 4 plates. DNLM; MBM
80-0677

BROWN, C[harles] W.
In memoriam Hervey Backus Wilbur, M.D. New York: G. P. Putnam's Sons, 1883. 3p. DNLM **80-0678**

BROWN, C[harles] W.
The treatment and cure of rheumatism, gout, lumbago, etc. Philadelphia, [1885?]. 3 l. DNLM **80-0679**

BORWN, C[harles] W.
The treatment and cure of rheumatism, gout, lumbago, etc. [Philadelphia: W. R. Warner & Co., [1885]]. 11p. DNLM **80-0680**

BROWN, C[harles] W.
Railway injuries. [New York, 1888.] 16p. DNLM
80-0681

BROWN, Dillon
Intubation of the larynx in diphtheritic croup. Analysis of two hundred cases operated upon. [New York, 1889.] 15p. 1 tab. DNLM; NNNAM **80-0682**

BROWN, Francis Henry (1835-1917)
The medical register for New England. Boston: Houghton, Osgood & Co., 1880. 45p. DNLM; MBM; MH; MWA
80-0683

BROWN, Francis Henry (1835-1917)
Impacted foreign bodies in the external auditory meatus. New York: Trow, 1881. 8p. DNLM **80-0684**

BROWN, Francis Henry (1835-1917)
Indexes to medical literature. Cambridge: Riverside Press, 1881. 8p. DNLM **80-0685**

BROWN, Francis Henry (1835-1917)
The first medical school in America; an historical item. [Boston, 1882?] 1 galley sheet. DNLM
80-0686

BROWN, F. Tilden (1853-1910)
A new universal syringe and aspirator. [New York, 1886.] 5p. DNLM; NNNAM **80-0687**

BROWN, F. Tilden (1853-1910)
The meto-urethrotome. [New York, 1887.] 1 broadside. DNLM; NNNAM **80-0688**

BROWN, F. Tilden (1853-1910)
The limitations of electrolysis as a therapeutic agent in organic and spasmodic stricture of the urethra, with cases. New York: William Wood & Co., 1888. 31p. DNLM; NNNAM
80-0689

BROWN, Harvey Ellicott (*d.* 1889)
The influence of the commercial prosperity of the county on epidemics. [New Orleans: L. Graham & Son, 1884.] 14p. DNLM **80-0690**

BROWN, J[ohn James] Graham (1853-1925)
Medical diagnosis; a manual of clinical methods. 2nd ed. New York & London: Bermingham & Co., 1884. 285p. CtY-M; DNLM; MBM; NNNAM **80-0691**

BROWN, William Symington
A clinical hand-book on the diseases of women. . . . New York: William Wood & Co., 1882. 247p. DLC; DNLM; NNNAM; PPC
80-0692

BROWNE, B[ennet] Bernard (1842-1922)
Address of . . . , delivered at the celebration of the Medical and Chirurgical Faculty of the State of Maryland, held in honor of the sesqui-centennial anniversary of the founding of Baltimore, at the hall of the faculty. . . . Baltimore, Md., on the evening of Wednesday, October 13, 1880. [Baltimore: J. W. Borst & Co., 1881.] 20p. DLC **80-0693**

BROWNE, B[ennet] Bernard (1842-1922)
The surgeons of Baltimore and their achievements. Baltimore: J. W. Borst & Co., 1881. 20p. DNLM; MdU-D
80-0694

BROWNE, B[ennet] Bernard (1842-1922)
On the use of the curette as a therapeutic agent in gynecological practice. Cincinnati, 1882. 4p. DNLM
80-0695

BROWNE, B[ennet] Bernard (1842-1922)
A contribution to the history of combined intra-uterine and extra-uterine twin pregnancy. With an analysis of twenty-four cases, and full extracts from the most important cases. [Philadelphia, 1882.] 19p. DNLM **80-0696**

BROWNE, B[ennet] Bernard (1842-1922)
A new operation for the reduction of chronic inversion of the uterus. New York, 1883. 2 l. DNLM **80-0697**

BROWNE, B[ennet] Bernard (1842-1922)
Malformation of the female sexual organs resulting from arrest of development. Chicago: Review Print. Co., 1884. 16p. DNLM **80-0698**

BROWNE, B[ennet] Bernard (1842-1922)
The curette as a diagnostic and therapeutic agent in gynecology and obstetrics. Baltimore: Guggenheimer, Weil & Co., 1886. 6p. DNLM **80-0699**

BROWNE, [Isaac] Lennox (1841-1902) and Emil BEHNKE
Voice, song, and speech; a practical guide for singers and speakers, from the combined view of vocal surgeon and voice trainer. New York: G. P. Putnam's Sons, 1884. 322p. 2 plates. DNLM; ICU; NN; MH **80-0700**

BROWNE, [Isaac] Lennox (1841-1902)
The throat and its diseases. 2nd ed. Philadelphia: Lea Bros. & Co., 1887. 614p. 15 plates. CU-M; DNLM; IEN-M; PPC
80-0701

BROWNING, William (1855-1941)
The veins of the brain and its envelopes. Their anatomy and bearing on the intracranial circulation. Brooklyn: F. B. O'Connor, 1884. 79p. 2 plates. DNLM; NNU-M
80-0702

BROWNING, William (1855-1941)
The occurrence of coma in sudden spontaneous brain lesions. Philadelphia, 1888. 12p. 1 tab. DNLM
80-0703

BROWNING, William (1855-1941)
Severe continuous cephalalgia as an early secondary in syphilis. [Brooklyn, 1889.] 5p. DNLM **80-0704**

BROWNSON, W[illiam] G[reen] (1830-1899)
The country doctor. Bridgeport, Conn.: Gould & Stiles, [1883]. 19p. DNLM **80-0705**

BRUBAKER, Albert P. (1852-1943)
. . . A compend of human physiology. . . . Philadelphia: P. Blakiston, Son & Co., 1883. 133p. DLC; IU-M; NNNAM; PU **80-0706**

BRUBAKER, Albert P. (1852-1943)
. . . A compend of human physiology. . . . 2nd ed., rev. and enl. With a table of physiological constants. Philadelphia: P. Blakiston, Son & Co., 1884. 154p. DLC; NNNAM; PPJ; PU **80-0707**

BRUBAKER, Albert P. (1852-1943)
. . . A compend of human physiology. . . . 3rd ed., rev. and enl. With illustrations, and a table of physiological constants. Philadelphia: P. Blakiston, Son & Co., 1886. 166p. DLC; MH-M; NNNAM; PPC **80-0708**

BRUBAKER, Albert P. (1852-1943)
. . . A compend of human physiology. . . . 4th ed., rev. and enl. With illustrations and a table of physiological constants. Philadelphia: P. Blakiston, Son & Co., 1888. 174p. DLC; DNLM; PPC; PU **80-0709**

BRUBAKER, Albert P. (1852-1943)
. . . A compend of human physiology. . . . 5th ed., rev. and enl. With new illustrations and a table of physiological constants. Philadelphia: P. Blakiston, Son & Co., 1889. 188p. DLC; DNLM; NNNAM; PPC **80-0710**

BRUCE, John Mitchell (1846-1929)
Materia medica and therapeutics: an introduction to the rational treatment of disease. Philadelphia: Henry C. Lea's Son & Co., 1884. 547p. CU-M; DNLM; OCLloyd; PU **80-0711**

BRUEN, Edward Tunis (1851-1889)
A pocket book of physical diagnosis, for the student and physician. . . . Philadelphia: P. Blakiston, 1881. 256p. 4 plates. DLC; OCIM; NNNAM; PPC **80-0712**

BRUEN, Edward Tunis (1851-1889)
A pocket book of physical diagnosis, of the diseases of the heart and lungs. For the student and physician. . . . 2nd ed. Rev., with additional illustrations. Philadelphia: P. Blakiston, Son & Co., 1883. 228p. plates. DLC; IEN-M; NNNAM; PPC **80-0713**

BRUEN, Edward Tunis (1851-1889)
. . . Outlines for the management of diet; or, The regulation of food to the requirements of health and the treatment of diseases. . . . Philadelphia, [etc.]: J. B. Lippincott Co., 1887. 138p. DLC; MBM; NNNAM; PU **80-0714**

BRUEN, Edward Tunis (1851-1889)
The relative importance of different climatic elements in the treatment of phthisis. [Philadelphia, 1888.] 14p. DNLM **80-0715**

BRUNTON, Thomas Lauder (1844-1916)
A text-book of pharmacology, therapeutics, and materia medica. Adapted to the United States Pharmacopoeia, by Francis H. Williams. Philadelphia: Lea Bros. & Co., 1885. 1035p. CtY-M; DNLM; OCLloyd; PU **80-0716**

BRUNTON, Thomas Lauder (1844-1916)
A text-book of pharmacology, therapeutics, and materia medica. Adapted to the United States Pharmacopoeia, by Francis H. Williams. 3rd ed. Philadelphia: Lea Bros. & Co., 1888. 1261p. DNLM; OCIM; OCLloyd; NNNAM **80-0717**

BRUSH, Edward N[athaniel] (1852-1933)
Notes on some clinical experiences with insomnia. [Utica, N.Y., 1889.] 9p. DNLM **80-0718**

BRYAN, James (1810-1881)
A treatise on nervous diseases. . . . [New York, 1882.] 51p. DLC; NNNAM **80-0719**

BRYAN, Joseph Hammond (1856-1935)
Diagnosis and treatment of abscess of the antrum. Chicago, 1889. 16p. DNLM **80-0720**

BRYANT, Joseph Decatur (1845-1914)
Manual of operative surgery. . . . New York, [etc.]: Bermingham & Co., 1884. 2 v. DLC; DNLM; NNNAM; NNU-M **80-0721**

BRYANT, Joseph Decatur (1845-1914)
Manual of operative surgery. . . . With about eight hundred illustrations. New York: D. Appleton & Co., 1887 [1886]. 530p. DLC; DNLM; NNNAM; PPC **80-0722**

BRYANT, Joseph Decatur (1845-1914)
Treatment of penetrating gun-shot wounds of the cranium. New York, 1888. 21p. DNLM **80-0723**

BRYANT, Joseph Decatur (1845-1914)
Malignant neoplasmata. Read in the discussion before the New York State Medical Association, October 10, 1888. [New York, 1888.] 12p. DNLM **80-0724**

BRYANT, Thomas (1828-1914)
A manual for the practice of surgery. 3rd American from 3rd English ed. Edited and enlarged for the use of the American student and practitioner, by John B. Roberts. Philadelphia: Henry C. Lea's Son & Co., 1881. 1005p. CtY-M; DNLM; NNNAM; PPC **80-0725**

BRYANT, Thomas (1828-1914)
A manual for the practice of surgery. 4th ed. Philadelphia: Henry C. Lea's Son & Co. 1885. 1039p. CU-M; DNLM; OCIM; NNNAM **80-0726**

BRYANT, W[illiam] S[ohier] (*b.* 1861)
Valves in the veins of the human intestines. Boston: Cupples & Hurd, 1888. 9p. DNLM **80-0727**

BRYCE, Peter (1834-1893)
Moral and criminal responsibility. [St. Louis, 1888.] 22p. DNLM **80-0728**

BUCHANAN, John
The family physician, and domestic practice of medicine. . . . Philadelphia: R. Russell, 1884. 903p. DLC; MdU-D; PPC; PPJ **80-0729**

BUCHANAN, Joseph Rodes (1814-1899)
The American system of medicine. Address delivered by Prof. Joseph Rodes Buchanan, at the opening of the twentieth session of the Eclectic Medical College, of New York, Friday, October 1, 1880. New York: Russell Brothers, Printers, 1880. 24p. DLC **80-0730**

BUCHANAN, Joseph Rodes (1814-1899)
. . . Moral education: its laws and methods. . . . New York: Printed for the Author by S. W. Green's Son, [1882]. 395p. DLC; NNNAM; OCIM; PU **80-0731**

BUCHANAN, Joseph Rodes (1814-1899)
Therapeutic sarcognomy, a scientific exposition of the mysterious union of soul, brain and body, and a new system of therapeutic practice without medicine, by the vital nervaura, electricity and external applications, giving the only scientific basis for therapeutic magnetism and electro-therapeutics. . . . Volume 1st—Nervauric and electric. Boston: The Author, [1884]. 269p. fold. plate. DLC; DNLM; MBM; NNNAM **80-0732**

BUCK, Albert Henry (1842-1922)
Diagnosis and treatment of ear diseases. . . . New York: William Wood & Co., 1880. 411p. DLC; DNLM; NNNAM; PPC **80-0733**

BUCK. Albert Henry (1842-1922)
Vascular tumors of the membrana tympani. [Boston, 1881.] 2p. DNLM **80-0734**

BUCK, Albert Henry (1842-1922)
Microphotograph of a peculiar pear-shaped body found in the middle ear. Cambridge, 1882. 1 l. 1 plate. DNLM **80-0735**

BUCK, Albert Henry (1842-1922)
The value of counter-irritation in the treatment of certain affections of the middle ear. [New York, 1882.] 3p. DNLM **80-0736**

BUCK, Albert Henry (1842-1922)
Two papers on topics relating to aural pathology and treatment. [New Bedford, 1886.] 55p. DNLM **80-0737**

BUCK, Albert Henry, ed. (1842-1922)
A reference hand-book of the medical sciences, embracing the entire range of scientific and practical medicine and allied science by various writers; illustrated by chromolithographs and fine wood engravings. . . . New York: William Wood & Co., 1886-1893. 9 v. CtY-M; DNLM; NNNAM; PPC [vol. 9 has title: Supplement to the Reference Handbook. . . .] **80-0738**

BUCK, Albert Henry (1842-1922)
A case of rapid and almost total loss of hearing in a child, seven years of age; inherited syphilis apparently the cause; marked improvement following the use of iodide of potassium. New Bedford: Mercury Pub. Co., 1887. 9p. DNLM **80-0739**

BUCK, Albert Henry (1842-1922)
A contribution to the anatomy of the elephant's ear. [New Bedford, 1888.] 15p. DNLM **80-0740**

BUCK, Albert Henry (1842-1922)
A manual of diseases of the ear, for the use of students and practitioners of medicine, by . . . . New York: William Wood & Co., 1889. 420p. DLC; DNLM; NNNAM; OCIM **80-0741**

BUCKHAM, M. H[enry] (1832-1910)
Medical education. An address. Burlington: Free Press Assoc., 1881. 16p. DNLM **80-0742**

BUCKHAM, T[homas] R.
Insanity considered in its medico-legal relations. Philadelphia: J. B. Lippincott & Co, 1883. 265p. CtY-M; DNLM; MBM; PPC **80-0743**

BUCKLER, Thomas Hepburn (1812-1901)
Notes on the anatomical relations of uterine structures; with surgical remarks and therapeutical suggestions. Cambridge, 1880. 34p. DNLM; MBM **80-0744**

BUCKLER, Thomas Hepburn (1812-1901)
Strangulated veins of the uterus, and other papers, gynaecological and surgical. Cambridge, 1881. 72p. DNLM; MH-M; NNNAM **80-0745**

BUCKLEY, C. F.
Cerebral hyperaemia; does it exist? A consideration of some views of Dr. William A. Hammond. . . . New York: G. P. Putnam's Sons, 1882. 129p. DLC; NNNAM **80-0746**

BUCKLIN, C[harles] A.
Practical hints about sympathetic diseases of the eye. [New York, 1886.] 8p. DNLM **80-0747**

BUCKLIN, Charles A.
Practical contributions to special surgery for the use of practitioners and students. Nasal stenosis, its effects on the eye, ear, pharynx, larynx, voice, and brain. Report and remarks on a series of two hundred cataract extractions. Practical hints on sympathetic diseases of the eye. [New York: G. Lauter, 1887.] 16p. DNLM; NNNAM **80-0748**

BUCKMASTER, A[ugustus] H[arper] (*b.* 1859)
Pregnancy, together with artificial impregnation, as a substitute for removal of the uterine appendages in a certain class of cases. [New York, 1887.] 14p. DNLM **80-0749**

BUCKMASTER, A[ugustus] H[arper] (*b.* 1859)
A review of twenty-two cottage cases occurring in the Women's Hospital, in the service of Dr. T. Gaillard Thomas. Brooklyn: G. Tremlett, 1887. 14p. DNLM; NNU-M **80-0750**

BUCKMASTER, A[ugustus] H[arper] (*b.* 1859)
The galvanic treatment of fibro-myomata. Prize essay of the Alumni Association of the Long Island College Hospital for 1888. New York: M. J. Rooney & Co., 1888. 27p. DNLM; NNU-M **80-0751**

BUCKMASTER, A[ugustus] H[arper] (*b.* 1859)
A case of extrauterine pregnancy; embryo destroyed by a twenty-milliampere current without interruptions; together with remarks on the best manner of using electricity for this purpose. [Philadelphia, 1888.] 12p. DNLM **80-0752**

BUFFUM, Joseph Howard (*b.* 1849)
Diseases and injuries of the eye. A practical treatise on the medical and surgical treatment of the diseases and injuries of the eye. Chicago: Gross & Delbridge, 1883. 428p. ICRM; OCIM **80-0753**

BUFFUM, Joseph Howard (*b.* 1849)
Clinical papers on ophthalmology and otology. Chicago: Gross & Delbridge, 1883. 22p. ICRM; OCIM **80-0754**

BUFFUM, Joseph Howard (*b.* **1849)**
The diseases of eye: their medical and surgical treatment. . . . Chicago: Gross & Delbridge, 1884. 428p. 5 col. plates. diags. DLC; OCIM **80-0755**

BULKLEY, L[ucius] Duncan (1845-1928)
The skin in health and disease. American Health Primers, edited by W. W. Keen. Philadelphia: P. Blakiston, 1880. 148p. CU-M; DLC; DNLM; PPC **80-0756**

BULKLEY, L[ucius] Duncan (1845-1928)
On the use of sulphur and its compounds in diseases of the skin. [New York, 1880.] 10p. DNLM; NNNAM **80-0757**

BULKLEY, L[ucius] Duncan (1845-1928)
On the management of infantile eczema. New York: G. P. Putnam's Sons, 1880. 15p. DNLM; NNNAM **80-0758**

BULKLEY, L[ucius] Duncan (1845-1928)
On the use of water in the treatment of diseases of the skin. New York, 1880. 14p. DNLM **80-0759**

BULKLEY, L[ucius] Duncan (1845-1928)
Eczema and its management; a practical treatise based on the study of two thousand five hundred cases of the disease. New York: G. P. Putnam's Sons, 1881. 344p. DNLM; NNNAM; PPC **80-0760**

BULKLEY, L[ucius] Duncan (1845-1928)
On the nomenclature and classification of diseases of the skin. [New York, 1881.] 17p. DNLM; NNNAM; PPC **80-0761**

BULKLEY, L[ucius] Duncan (1845-1928)
Clinical illustrations of favus and its treatment by a new method of depilation. . . . New York: G. P. Putnam's Sons, 1881. 14p. DLC; DNLM **80-0762**

BULKLEY, L[ucius] Duncan (1845-1928)
Analysis of eight thousand cases of skin disease. New York: G. P. Putnam's Sons, 1882. 30p. DNLM; NNNAM; PPC **80-0763**

BULKLEY, L[ucius] Duncan (1845-1928)
The malignity of syphilis, with an analysis of 450 cases of the disease. New York: G. P. Putnam's Sons, 1882. 27p. DNLM; NNNAM; PPC **80-0764**

BULKLEY, L[ucius] Duncan (1845-1928)
Manual of diseases of the skin, with an analysis of eight thousand consecutive cases and a formulary. . . . New York: G. P. Putnam's Sons, 1882. 312p. DLC; DNLM; NNNAM; PPC **80-0765**

BULKLEY, L[ucius] Duncan (1845-1928)
Eczema and its management; a practical treatise based on the study of three thousand cases of the disease. 2nd ed. New York: G. P. Putnam's Sons, [1884]. 344p. DNLM; NNNAM; PPC **80-0766**

BULKLEY, L[ucius] Duncan (1845-1928)
Acne; its etiology, pathology, and treatment. A practical treatise based on the study of one thousand five hundred cases of sebaceous disease. New York & London: G. P. Putnam's Sons, 1885. 280p. DNLM; NNNAM; PPC **80-0767**

BULKLEY, L[ucius] Duncan (1845-1928)
Specialties and their relation to the medical profession. Chicago, 1885. 16p. DNLM; NNNAM; PPC **80-0768**

BULKLEY, L[ucius] Duncan (1845-1928)
On the existence of "dermatitis herpetiformis" (of Duhring) as a distinct disease. . . . New York: William Wood & Co., 1886. 12p. DLC; DNLM **80-0769**

BULKLEY, L[ucius] Duncan (1845-1928)
Clinical notes on pruritus. New York: William Wood & Co., 1887. 14p. DNLM; NNNAM; PPC **80-0770**

BULKLEY, L[ucius] Duncan (1845-1928)
Infant feeding, especially with reference to subjects with infantile eczema. Chicago, 1887. 12p. DNLM; NNNAM; PPC **80-0771**

BULKLEY, L[ucius] Duncan (1845-1928)
On the treatment of felon without incision. Chicago: Office Am. Med. Ass., 1887. 8p. DNLM; NNNAM; PPC **80-0772**

BULKLEY, L[ucius] Duncan (1845-1928)
A clinical study on alopecia areata and its treatment. New York: Trow's Co., 1889. 12p. DNLM; NNNAM; PPC **80-0773**

BULKLEY, L[ucius] Duncan (1845-1928)
On the relation between the general practitioner and the consultant or specialist. Chicago, 1889. 12p. DNLM; NNNAM; PPC **80-0774**

BULKLEY, L[ucius] Duncan (1845-1928)
On unusual methods of acquiring syphilis. With report of cases. [Philadelphia, 1889.] 32p. DNLM; NNNAM; PPC **80-0775**

BULKLEY, L[ucius] Duncan (1845-1928)
On the value of frequently repeated doses of arsenic in the treatment of bullous diseases of the skin, especially in children. New York: D. Appleton & Co., 1889. 17p. DNLM; NNNAM; PPC **80-0776**

BULL, Charles Stedman (1844-1911)
A contribution to the pathology and treatment of vascular tumors of the eyelids and vicinity. New York: D. Appleton & Co., 1880. 11p. DNLM; NNNAM **80-0777**

BULL, Charles Stedman (1844-1911)
On the removal of foreign bodies from the eye; with four cases. [New York, 1880.] 9p. DNLM; NNNAM **80-0778**

BULL, Charles Stedman (1844-1911)
Syphilitic diseases of the lachrymal apparatus. [New York, 1882.] 12p. DNLM; NNNAM **80-0779**

BULL, Charles Stedman (1844-1911)
The treatment of scars of the face involving the eyelids, directly or indirectly. New York: Trow, 1882. 7p. DNLM; NNNAM **80-0780**

BULL, Charles Stedman (1844-1911)
Analysis of one hundred and three cases of exudative neuro-retinitis, associated with chronic Bright's disease. [Boston, 1886.] 10p. DNLM; NNNAM **80-0781**

BULL, Charles Stedman (1844-1911)
A consideration of some unusual forms of intra-ocular hemorrhage, with special reference to etiology and prognosis. New York: Trow, 1886. 19p. DNLM; NNNAM **80-0782**

BULL, Charles Stedman (1844-1911)
Passive motion in the treatment of paralysis of the ocular muscles. [Boston, 1887.] 12p. DNLM; NNNAM **80-0783**

BULL, Charles Stedman (1844-1911)
A contribution to the surgical treatment of membranous opacities in the vitreous. Hartford, Conn., 1888. 16p. DNLM; NNNAM **80-0784**

BULL, Charles Stedman (1844-1911)
An analysis of ninety cases of simple chronic glaucoma, with special reference to the effects of iridectomy on the acuity of vision and the visual field. [New York, 1889.] 11p. DNLM; NNNAM **80-0785**

BULL, Charles Stedman (1844-1911)
Contributions to the subject of tumours of the orbit and neighboring cavities. New York: Trow's Co., 1889. 11p. DNLM; NNNAM **80-0786**

BULL, Charles Stedman (1844-1911)
Extraction of cataract without iridectomy. Report of one hundred cases, with remarks. [New York, 1889.] 16p. 1 tab. DNLM; NNNAM **80-0787**

BULLARD, William N[orton] (*b.* 1853)
Chronic tea poisoning. Boston: Cupples, Upham & Co., 1886. 16p. DNLM; MBM **80-0788**

BULLARD, William N[orton] (*b.* 1853)
A case of cerebral localization, with double trephining. (Acquired spastic hemiplegia; porencephalus.) Boston: Cupples & Hurd, 1888. 8p. DNLM; MBM **80-0789**

BULLARD, William N[orton] (*b.* 1853)
Cases of febrile delirium tremens. Boston: Cupples & Hurd, 1888. 18p. DNLM; MBM **80-0790**

BULLARD, William N[orton] (*b.* 1853) and E. G. BRACKETT
Observations on steadiness of the hand and on static equilibrium. Boston: Cupples & Hurd, 1889. 21p. DNLM; MBM **80-0791**

BULLARD, William N[orton] (*b.* 1853) and Herbert L. BURRELL
Surgical operations for the relief of pressure paralysis in caries of the spine. Boston: Damrell & Upham, 1889. 11p. DNLM; MBM **80-0792**

BULLOCK & CRENSHAW
Prices current for wholesale druggists and manufacturing pharmacists. Philadelphia, [*c.*] 1880. 104p. PPC; PU **80-0793**

BULLOCK & CRENSHAW
Illustrated catalogue of drugs and sundries. Philadelphia, 1880. 152p. DNLM **80-0794**

BUMSTEAD, Freeman Josiah (1826-1879)
The pathology and treatment of venereal diseases. By Freeman J. Bumstead . . . and Robert W. Taylor. . . . 5th ed., rev. and rewritten, with many additions by Dr. Taylor. . . . Philadelphia: Henry C. Lea's Son & Co., 1883. 906p. 11 col. plates. DLC; DNLM; NNNAM; PPJ **80-0795**

BURDON-SANDERSON, John Scott (ed) (1828-1905)
A handbook for the physiological laboratory. . . . Histology: parts I and II. By E. Klein. . . . Physiology: part I. Blood circulation, respiration and animal heat. By . . . . Part II. The functions of the muscles and nerves. By Michael Foster. . . . Part III. Digestion and secretion. By T. Lauder Brunton. . . . Ed. by . . . . With one hundred and thirty-three full-page plates. . . . Philadelphia: P. Blakiston, Son & Co., 1884. 2 v. 133 plates. DLC; LNT-M; OCIM; PPC **80-0796**

BURGGRAEVE, Adolphe Pierre (1806-1902)
New manual of alkaloidal therapeutics. From the French of Dr. Ad. Burggraeve. Transl. by C. C. P. Silva . . . and W. T. Thackeray. . . . Chicago: [Press of G. T. Halla], 1888. **80-0797**

BURGGRAEVE, Adolphe Pierre (1806-1902)
Dyspepsia and its dosimetric treatment. Transl. from the French by T. L. Phipson. 2nd ed. New York: Morrison & Titus, 1888. 34p. DNLM; NNNAM **80-0798**

BURGHER, J[ohn] C. (1822-1901)
The year's progress. Address delivered before the American Institute of Homoeopathy. Philadelphia: Sherman & Co., 1880 [1878]. 13p. DNLM; PPHa **80-0799**

BURGHER, John C., ed. (1822-1901)
Semi-centennial celebration of the introduction of homoeopathy west of the Allegheny Mountains, held at Pittsburgh, Pa., September 20, 1887, under the auspices of the Homoeopathic Medical Society of Allegheny County, Pa. Published by the Society. Pittsburgh: Stevenson & Foster, 1888. 72p. PPHa **80-0800**

BURNETT, Charles H[enry] (1842-1902)
A case of probable syphilitic deafness in one ear. New York: Trow & Co., 1881. 4p. DNLM **80-0801**

BURNETT, Charles H[enry] (1842-1902)
Aural vertigo. Philadelphia, 1882. 8p. DNLM **80-0802**

BURNETT, Charles H[enry] (1842-1902)
Chronic otitis media purulenta: its treatment in the Presbyterian Hospital, Philadelphia. Reported by Thomas A. Downes. Further observations on the usefulness of chinoline salicylate in otorrhoea. Cambridge: Riverside Press, 1882. 5p. DNLM **80-0803**

BURNETT, Charles H[enry] (1842-1902) and Charles A. OLIVER
Clinical history of a case of recurrent dropsy of the left middle ear, complicated after eight years' duration, by an acute attack of monocular optic neuritis (choked disk) on the same side, follwed by general tabetic symptoms. With remarks. [Philadelphia, 1884.] 26p. DNLM; PU **80-0804**

BURNETT, Charles H[enry] (1842-1902)
The ear: its anatomy, physiology, and diseases. . . . 2nd ed., rev. and rewritten. Philadelphia: Henry C. Lea's Son & Co., 1884. 585p. DLC; DNLM; NNNAM; PPC **80-0805**

BURNETT, Charles H[enry] (1842-1902)
The frequent dependence of disease of the ear upon catarrhal disease of the nose. [Philadelphia, 1886.] 24p. DNLM **80-0806**

BURNETT, Charles H[enry] (1842-1902)
. . . Diseases and injuries of the ear: their prevention and cure. . . . Philadelphia: J. B. Lippincott Co., 1889. 154p. DLC; DNLM; MBM; PPC **80-0807**

BURNETT, J. Compton (1840-1901)
The prevention of congenital malformations, defects, and diseases, by the medicinal and nutritional treatment of the mother during pregnancy. Edited, with notes from Grauvogl, by T. C. Duncan, M.D. Chicago: Duncan Bros., 1881. 26p. OCIM; PPHa **80-0808**

BURNETT, J. Compton (1840-1901)
Dr. Burnett's essays. Ecce medicus; natrum muriaticum; gold; the causes of cataract; curability of cataract; diseases of the veins; supersalinity of the blood. New York and Philadelphia: Boericke & Tafel, 1882. 296p. DNLM; PPHa **80-0809**

BURNETT, Swan Moses (1847-1906)
A case of acute chemosis. [New York, 1880.] 3p. DNLM **80-0810**

BURNETT, Swan Moses (1847-1906)
A case of primary external inflammation of the mastoid. [New York, 1880.] 1 l. DNLM **80-0811**

BURNETT, Swan M[oses] (1847-1906)
Color-perception and color-blindness. [New York, 1881.] 7p. DNLM **80-0812**

BURNETT, Swan M[oses] (1847-1906)
Refraction in the principal meridians of a triaxial ellipsoid, with remarks on the correction of astigmatism by cylindrical glasses; and an historical note on corneal astigmatism. With a communication on the monochromatic aberration of the human eye in aphakia, by Prof. Wm. Harkness. [New York, 1883.] 21p. DNLM **80-0813**

BURNETT, Swan M[oses] (1847-1906)
Are there separate centres for light, form, and color perception? New York: G. P. Putnam's Sons, 1884. 17p. DNLM **80-0814**

BURNETT, Swan M[oses] (1847-1906)
A nomenclature of ophthalmology. St. Louis: J. H. Chambers & Co., [1884]. 19p. DNLM **80-0815**

BURNETT, Swan M[oses] (1847-1906)
Theories of colour perception. [Philadelphia, 1884.] 25p. DNLM **80-0816**

BURNETT, Swan M[oses] (1847-1906)
The dioptry again. [New York, 1886.] 5p. DNLM **80-0817**

BURNETT, Swan M[oses] (1847-1906)
The metre-lens: its English name and equivalent. [New York, 1886.] 6p. DNLM **80-0818**

BURNETT, Swan M[oses] (1847-1906)
Clinical contributions to the study of ringscotoma. [Boston, 1887.] 15p. DNLM **80-0819**

BURNETT, Swan M[oses] (1847-1906)
Remarks on cataract extraction. Chicago, 1887. 12p. DLC; DNLM **80-0820**

BURNETT, Swan Moses (1847-1906)
A theoretical and practical treatise on astigmatism. . . . With fifty-nine diagrams and illustrations. St. Louis, Mo.: J. H. Chambers & Co., 1887. 245p. tables, diags. DLC; DNLM; OCIM; PU **80-0821**

BURNETT, Swan M[oses] (1847-1906)
An analysis of the refraction of 576 healthy human corneae examined with the ophthalmometer of Javal and Schiötz. [Hartford, 1888.] 12p. DNLM **80-0822**

BURNETT, Swan M[oses] (1847-1906)
Models, demonstrative of cylindrical refraction. 1888. 1 phot. plate. DNLM **80-0823**

BURNETT, Swan M[oses] (1847-1906)
Skiascopy; or the "shadow" test for the determination of the refraction of the eye. Philadelphia, 1888. 20p. DNLM **80-0824**

BURR, C[olonel] B. (1856-1931)
Cocculus indicus in epilepsy. [Lansing, 1881.] 8p. DNLM **80-0825**

BURR, C[olonel] B. (1856-1931)
The insanity of masturbation. [Ann Arbor, Mich., 1882.] 8p. DNLM **80-0826**

BURR, C[olonel] B. (1856-1931)
A case of primary monomania (primäre Verrücktheit). [Philadelphia, 1883.] 8p. DNLM **80-0827**

BURR, C[olonel] B. (1856-1931)
Amelioration of paretic dementia after extensive sloughs. New York: Indust. Print. Co., 1884. 17p. DNLM **80-0828**

BURR, C[olonel] B. (1856-1931)
The insanity of pubescence. [Utica, N.Y., 1887.] 12p. DNLM **80-0829**

BURR, C[olonel] B. (1856-1931)
Muscular action a cause of fracture among paretics. [Utica, N.Y., 1889.] 5p. DNLM **80-0830**

BURR, George (1813-1882)
The New York State Inebriate Asylum. A defense of its management and operations. Syracuse: Truair, Smith & Bruce, 1881. 22p. DNLM **80-0831**

BURRELL, Herbert Leslie (1856-1910)
Fracture of the spine: its immediate treatment by rectification of the deformity and fixation by plaster of Paris jacket. [Boston, 1887.] 27p. 7 tabs., 2 plates. DNLM; MBM **80-0832**

BURRELL, Herbert Leslie (1856-1910)
The reimplantation of a trephine button of bone. Boston: Cupples & Hurd, 1888. 4p. DNLM; MBM **80-0833**

BURRELL, Herbert Leslie (1856-1910) and Greenleaf R. TUCKER
Some practical experiments in the details of aseptic surgery. [Boston, 1889.] 20p. DNLM; MBM **80-0834**

BURT, F[rank] L[eslie]
The animal suture. Concerning its preparation and uses. [Boston, 1888.] 4 l. DNLM **80-0835**

BURT, Stephen Smith (*b.* 1850)
A clinic on phthisis pulmonalis, acute and chronic; acute miliary tuberculosis; mitral and tricuspid insufficiency, mitral stenosis; hydro-thorax, hydro-pericardium, and chronic pneumonia; emphysema. [New York, 1883.] 7p. DNLM
80-0836

BURT, Stephen Smith (*b.* 1850)
A clinical lecture on diseases of the heart and lungs, with special reference to physical diagnosis. [New York, 1885.] 8p. DNLM **80-0837**

BURT, Stephen Smith (*b.* 1850)
Remarks on Bright's disease. [New York, 1885.] 4p. DNLM
80-0838

BURT, Stephen Smith (*b.* 1850)
A clinic on heart disease. New York: Pusey & Co., 1887. 7p. DNLM **80-0839**

BURT, Stephen Smith (*b.* 1850)
Pleurisy. New York: Pusey & Co., 1887. 17p. DNLM
80-0840

BURT, Stephen Smith (*b.* 1850)
Exploration of the chest in health and disease. New York: D. Appleton & Co., 1889. 206p. 6 plates. DNLM
80-0841

BURT, Stephen Smith (*b.* 1850)
Some of the limitations of medicine. [New York, 1889.] 5p. DNLM **80-0842**

BURT, Stephen Smtih (*b.* 1850)
Views on the prevention and treatment of typhoid fever. New York: Pusey & Co., 1889. 11p. DNLM
80-0843

BURT, W[illiam] H. (1836-1897)
Clinical companion to "physiological materia medica"; a compendium of diseases, their homoeopathic and accessory treatment, with valuable tables and practical hints on aetiology, pathology, hygiene, etc. Chicago: Gross & Delbridge, 1883. 251p. DLC; DNLM; OCIM; PPHa **80-0844**

BURT, W[illiam] H. (1836-1897)
Physiological materia medica, containing all that is known of the physiological action of our remedies; together with their characteristics, indications, and pharmacology. Chicago: Gross & Delbridge, 1883. 992p. DLC; DNLM; OCIM; PPHa
80-0845

BURT, W[illiam] H. (1836-1897)
Physiological materia medica, containing all that is known of the physiological action of our remedies; together with their characteristics, indications, and pharmacology. [4th ed.] Chicago: Gross & Delbridge, 1888. 1109p. OCIM; PPHa [Contains a clinical index of diseases]
80-0846

BUSEY, Samuel Clagett (1828-1901)
Thrombosis of the sinuses of the dura mater in fatal cases of dysentery in young children. New York: William Wood & Co., 1880. 8p. DNLM; NNNAM **80-0847**

BUSEY, Samuel Clagett (1828-1901)
A contribution to the pathology of the cicatrices of pregnancy. Boston, [1880]. 22p. DLC; DNLM
80-0848

BUSEY, Samuel Clagett (1828-1901)
Chronic Bright's disease in children caused by malaria. Philadelphia: Collins, 1880. 14p. DNLM; PPC
80-0849

BUSEY, Samuel Clagett (1828-1901)
A case of tuberculosis of the peritoneum, with the formation of a sac simulating an ovarian cyst. [Washington, D.C., 1880.] 12p. DNLM **80-0850**

BUSEY, Samuel Clagett (1828-1901)
Washington malaria and the "catching of cold." [Washington, D.C., 1882.] 8p. DNLM **80-0851**

BUSEY, Samuel Clagett (1828-1901)
The influence of the constant use of high-heeled French shoes upon the health and form of the female, and upon the relation of the pelvic organs, [Philadelphia, 1883.] 19p. DNLM
80-0852

BUSEY, Samuel Clagett (1828-1901)
First annual address of the president . . . delivered before the Washington Obstetrical and Gynecological Society, October 5, 1883. [Craniotomy upon the living foetus is not justifiable.] New York: William Wood & Co., 1884. 19p. DLC
80-0853

BUSEY, Samuel Clagett (1828-1901)
Scarlatina puerperalis. Philadelphia, 1884. 15p. DNLM
80-0854

BUSEY, Samuel Clagett (1828-1901)
The causal relation of obstructed cardiac circulation to lymph stasis. Philadelphia, 1885. 8p. DNLM **80-0855**

BUSEY, Samuel Clagett (1828-1901)
A reply to Dr. A. Y. P. Garnett, Sr. [Washington, 1885.] 28p. DNLM **80-0856**

BUSEY, Samuel Clagett (1828-1901)
Washington Obstetrical and Gynecological Society. Third annual address of the president, Samuel C. Busey, M.D. The hygiene of pregnancy. . . . New York: William Wood & Co., 1885. 15p. DLC; DNLM **80-0857**

BUSEY, Samuel Clagett (1828-1901)
A reply to Dr. A. Y. P. Garnett, Sr. [Washington, 1885.] 33p. DNLM **80-0858**

BUSEY, Samuel Clagett (1828-1901)
The hygiene of pregnancy. New York: William Wood & Co., 1886. 15p. DNLM **80-0859**

BUSEY, Samuel Clagett (1828-1901)
The natural hygiene of childbearing life. [New York, 1886.] 14p. DNLM **80-0860**

BUSEY, Samuel Clagett (1828-1901)
Maternal impressions. Discussion on Dr. Barker's essay. [New York, 1887.] 19p. DNLM **80-0861**

BUSEY, Samuel Clagett (1828-1901)
Persistent vomiting during labor relieved by anaesthesia. Chicago, 1887. 11p. DNLM **80-0862**

BUSEY, Samuel Clagett (1828-1901)
Some rare clinical observations in obstetric practice. New York: William Wood & Co., 1887. 14p. DNLM
80-0863

BUSEY, Samuel Clagett (1828-1901)
Cystocolpocele complicating pregnancy and labor. [New York, 1888.] 44p. DNLM **80-0864**

BUSEY, Samuel Clagett (1828-1901)
First annual address of the president . . . delivered before the Washington Obstetrical and Gynecological Society, October 5, 1883. [Craniotomy upon the living foetus is not justifiable.] Reprinted under the auspices of St. Mary's Seminary. Washington: W. H. Lepley, 1888. 19p. DNLM **80-0865**

BUSEY, Samuel Clagett (1828-1901)
The effusion of chyle and of chyle-like, milky, fatty, and oily fluids into the serous cavities. Philadelphia, 1889. 23p. DNLM **80-0866**

BUSEY, Samuel Clagett (1828-1901)
The wrong of craniotomy upon the living fetus. New York: William Wood & Co., 1889. 21p. DLC **80-0867**

BUSH, Lewis P[otter] (1812-1892)
The Delaware State Medical Society and its founders in the eighteenth century. New York, 1886. 16p. DNLM **80-0868**

BUTLER, F. W. P.
Gangrene following continued fever; double amputation; recovery. [Charleston, S.C., 1889.] 3p. DNLM **80-0869**

BUTLER, Glentworth Reeve (1855-1926)
Emergency notes. What to do in accidents and sudden illness until the doctor comes. . . . New York: Funk & Wagnalls, 1889. 102p. DLC; NNNAM **80-0870**

BUTLER, John (1844-1885)
A text-book of electro-therapeutics and electro-surgery. 2nd ed. New York & Philadelphia: Boericke & Tafel, 1880. 323p. DNLM; NNNAM; PPHa; PU **80-0871**

BUTLER, John (1844-1885)
Electro-massage. Philadelphia, 1880. 16p. DNLM **80-0872**

BUTLER, John (1844-1885)
Three cases of stricture of the urethra cured by electrolysis after all other methods of treatment had failed. New York, 1882. 4p. DNLM **80-0873**

BUTLER, John (1844-1885)
Electricity in surgery. New York & Philadelphia: Boericke & Tafel, 1882. 111p. DNLM; NNNAM; PPHa **80-0874**

BUTLER, John Simpkins (1803-1890)
The curability of insanity and the individualized treatment of the insane. . . . New York and London: G. P. Putnam's Sons, 1887. 59p. DLC; NNNAM **80-0875**

BUTLIN, Henry Trentham (1845-1912)
Diseases of the tongue. Philadelphia: Lea Brothers & Co., 1885. 451p. 7 plates. DNLM; NNNAM; PPC; PU **80-0876**

BUTLIN, Henry Trentham (1845-1912)
On the operative surgery of malignant disease. Philadelphia: P. Blakiston, Son & Co., 1887. 408p. CtY-M; DNLM; MBM PPC **80-0877**

BUXTON, Dudley Wilmot (1855-1931)
Anaesthetics, their uses and administration. Philadelphia: P. Blakiston, Son & Co., 1888. 164p. DNLM; MBM; NNNAM; PU **80-0878**

BUZZARD, Thomas (1831-1919)
Clinical lectures on diseases of the nervous system. Philadelphia: P. Blakiston, Son & Co., 1882. 466p. CU-M; ICRM; NNNAM; PPC **80-0879**

BYERS, J. Wellington
Fracture of the coracoid process. Charlotte, N.C.: Hirst Print. Co., 1885. 10p. DNLM **80-0880**

BYFORD, Henry [Turman] (*b.* 1853)
Functions of the membranes in labor. Chicago, 1885. 11p. DNLM **80-0881**

BYFORD, Henry T[urman] (*b.* 1853)
Observations on the cause and treatment of infantile eczema and allied eruptions. Chicago, 1885. 7p. DNLM **80-0882**

BYFORD, Henry T[urman] (*b.* 1853)
Mechanical treatment of retroversion of the uterus. Chicago, 1886. 24p. DNLM **80-0883**

BYFORD, Henry T[urman] (*b.* 1853)
The production and prevention of perineal lacerations during labor, with description of an unrecognized form. Chicago, 1886. 16p. DNLM **80-0884**

BYFORD, Henry T[urman] (*b.* 1853)
Report of a case of pelvic abscess, with autopsy. Chicago: Clark & Longley, 1886. 15p. DNLM **80-0885**

BYFORD, Henry T[urman] (*b.* 1853)
A study of the causation and treatment of pelvic hematocele. New York: William Wood & Co., 1886. 18p. DNLM **80-0886**

BYFORD, Henry T[urman] (*b.* 1853)
Lecture on the operative treatment of retroversion. Alexander's operation. Chicago, 1888. 12p. DNLM **80-0887**

BYFORD, Henry T[urman] (*b.* 1853)
Removal of the uterine appendages and small ovarian tumors by vaginal section, with a report of twelve successful cases. [New York, 1888.] 13p. DNLM **80-0888**

BYFORD, Henry T[urman] (*b.* 1853)
The so-called physiological argument in obstetrics. [New York, 1888.] 7p. DNLM **80-0889**

BYFORD, Henry T[urman] (*b.* 1853)
Twelve months of abdominal and vaginal section. [Chicago, 1888.] 13p. DNLM **80-0890**

BYFORD, Henry T[urman] (*b.* 1853)
Vaginal hysterectomy. [Chicago, 1889.] 8p. DNLM **80-0891**

BYFORD, William Heath (1817-1890)
The practice of medicine and surgery, applied to the diseases and accidents incident to women. . . . 3rd ed. Thoroughly rev. and rewritten. With one hundred and sixty-four illustrations. Philadelphia: Lindsay & Blakiston, 1881. 682p. DLC; OCIM; NNNAM; PPC **80-0892**

BYFORD, William Heath (1817-1890)
The practice of medicine and surgery, applied to the diseases and accidents incident to women. By W. H. Byford . . . and Henry T. Byford. . . . 4th ed. Rev., rewritten and very much enl. with three hundred and six illustrations. Philadelphia: P. Blakiston, Son & Co., 1888. 820p. DLC; DNLM; NNNAM; PU **80-0893**

BYRD, William A[ndrew] (1843-1887)
Extirpation of rectum, without destroying the sphincter and muscle. Philadelphia, 1880. 4p. DNLM **80-0894**

BYRD, William A[ndrew] (1843-1887)
Clinical notes upon the use of the galvano-cautery. Baltimore: Practitioner Publishing Co., 1880. 8p. DNLM; MdU-D **80-0895**

BYRD, William A[ndrew] (1843-1887)
Lumbo-colotomy in the new-born for relief of imperforate rectum. [St. Louis, 1881.] 8p. DNLM **80-0896**

BYRD, William A[ndrew] (1843-1887)
Abdominal section in the treatment of ulceration and perforation of the caecum and the appendix vermiformis. Philadelphia: Collins, 1881. 7p. DNLM **80-0897**

BYRD, William A[ndrew] (1843-1887)
Address in surgery. Excisions of portions of the alimentary canal covered by peritoneum. Philadelphia: Times Print. House, [1882]. 11p. DNLM **80-0898**

BYRD, William A[ndrew] (1843-1887)
Report of a case of successful amputation of the hip-joint; being the third amputation at the hip-joint within a year. [St. Louis, 1886.] 7p. DNLM **80-0899**

BYRN, M[arcus] Lafayette
The best family physician and household companion. (The mystery of medicine explained!) Prepared for the use of families, farmers, mechanics, travelers, everybody. . . . New York: The Coast City Publishing Co., 1889. 509p. col. front. DLC; NNNAM **80-0900**

BYRNE, John (1825-1902)
Kolpo-cystotomy by electro-cautery; with remarks on other methods of operating. [Boston, 1880.] 8p. DNLM **80-0901**

BYRNE, John (1825-1902)
Contributions to gynaecology, No. 10. 1. Fibro-sarcomatous tumor of the uterus; operation; recovery. 2. Cancer of the rectum; excision; recovery. New York: G. P. Putnam's Sons, 1880. 13p. DNLM; NNNAM **80-0902**

BYRNE, John (1825-1902)
A digest of twenty years' experience in the treatment of uterine cancer, including 367 operations by galvano-cautery. Philadelphia: W. J. Dornan, 1889. 25p. DNLM; PPC **80-0903**

CABELL, James Lawrence (1813-1889)
The National Board of Health and the International Sanitary Conference of Washington. Philadelphia: Collins, 1881. 21p. DNLM **80-0904**

CABELL, James Lawrence (1813-1889)
A brief historical notice of the origin and progress of international hygiene. A paper presented at the ninth annual meeting of the American Public Health Association, Savannah, Ga., Nov. 29 to Dec. 3, 1881. Boston: Rand, Avery & Co., 1882. 18p. DNLM; MBM **80-0905**

CABELL, James Lawrence (1813-1889)
On sanitary conditions in relation to the treatment of surgical operations and injuries. [Richmond], 1882. 41p. DNLM **80-0906**

CABELL, James Lawrence (1813-1889)
Remarks before the committee on public health of the House of Representatives, in support of House Bill 2785, 48th Cong., 1st sess., for the protection of the public health. Washington: Gibson Bros., 1884. 20p. DNLM **80-0907**

CABOT, Arthur Tracy (1852-1912)
A contribution to the treatment of empyema. Cambridge: Riverside Press, 1883. 13p. DNLM; MBM **80-0908**

CABOT, Arthur Tracy (1852-1912)
Papers upon genito-urinary surgery. I. Nephrotomy for hydronephrosis; recovery. II. The constrictor urethrae muscle; its relation to urethral pathology and treatment. III. Case of multiple calculi in the bladder. IV. The application of antiseptic principles to genito-urinary surgery. Boston: D. Clapp & Son, 1886. 39p. DNLM; MBM **80-0909**

CABOT, Arthur Tracy (1852-1912)
Papers upon genito-urinary surgery. V. Notes on the treatment of stone in the bladder [etc.]. VI. A case of suprapubic lithotomy. VII. A case of hysterectomy for the relief of pyelitis from obstruction. Boston: D. Clapp & Son, 1887. 26p. DNLM; MBM **80-0910**

CABOT, Arthur Tracy (1852-1912)
A case of atresia and urethralis; operation with relief. [Philadelphia, 1888.] 7p. DNLM **80-0911**

CABOT, Arthur Tracy (1852-1912)
The choice of operation for stone in the bladder. Chicago, 1889. 16p. DNLM **80-0912**

CABOT, Arthur Tracy (1852-1912)
Bony anchylosis of the temporo-maxillary joint relieved by osteotomy of the neck of the inferior maxilla. St. Louis, 1889. 7p. DNLM **80-0913**

CAILLÉ, Augustus (1854-1935)
Acute Carbol-Vergiftung. New York, 1886. 7p. DNLM **80-0914**

CAILLÉ, Augustus (1854-1935)
Permanent drainage for ascites. [New York, 1886.] 10p. DNLM **80-0915**

CAILLÉ, Augustus (1854-1935)
Sterilized milk. A report of some experiments made to determine the proper manner of boiling and preserving milk for the use of infants. New York, 1888. 2 l. DNLM **80-0916**

CAILLÉ, Augustus (1854-1935)
A method of prophylaxis in diphtheria. New York: Trow's Co., 1888. 11p. DNLM **80-0917**

CAILLÉ, Augustus (1854-1935)
Prolapse of the inverted lower portion of the right ureter through the urethra in a child two weeks old. Philadelphia, 1888. 6p. DNLM **80-0918**

CAILLÉ, Augustus (1854-1935)
Our present knowledge concerning the aetiology of typhoid fever. New York, 1889. 11p. DNLM **80-0919**

CALDWELL, John J[abez] (1836-1888?)
Genius resistless: a Pindaric ode, a tribute to Jenner and Pasteur. Baltimore, Md.: W. K. Boyle, 1882. 12p. DNLM **80-0920**

CALDWELL, John J[abez] (1836-1888?)
Some interesting reflex neuroses, with treatment and comments. [Richmond, 1885.] 12p. DNLM **80-0921**

CALHOUN, Abner W. (1846-1910)
School hygiene in relation to its influence upon the vision of children, or school sanitation. An address delivered before the Medical Association of Georgia, 1884. Atlanta, Ga.: J. P. Harrison & Co., 1884. 15p. DNLM **80-0922**

CALLENDER, John H[ill] (1832-1896)
Address before the Association of Medical Superintendents of American Institutions for the Insane, Newport, R.I., June 26, 1883. Utica, N.Y.: E. H. Roberts & Co., 1883. 32p. DNLM **80-0923**

CAMPBELL, Amory Sibley (*b.* 1849)
Ophthalmic operations, with remarks on after-treatment. The ophthalmic use of quinine, and its therapeutic action. . . . [Atlanta, Ga.: J. P. Harrison & Co., state printers, 1880.] 35p. DLC; DNLM **80-0924**

CAMPBELL, Amory Sibley (*b.* 1849)
Gun-shot wound of the abdomen; fecal fistula—spontaneous closure; recovery; with remarks on treatment; including a further consideration of the action and application of quinine. Augusta: J. Loveday, 1881. 16p. DNLM **80-0925**

CAMPBELL, Frederick Ransom (1860-1888)
The relation of meteorology to disease. Buffalo: The Times Co., 1885. 23p. DNLM **80-0926**

CAMPBELL, Frederick Ransom (1860-1888)
The causes and prevention of infantile diarrhoeal diseases. Buffalo, 1887. 23p. DNLM **80-0927**

CAMPBELL, Frederick Ransom (1860-1888)
The language of medicine; a manual giving the origin, etymology, pronunciation, and meaning of the technical terms found in medical literature. . . . New York: D. Appleton & Co., 1888. 318p. DLC; DNLM; NNNAM; PU **80-0928**

CAMPBELL, Henry Fraser (1824-1891)
Premature senile obliteration of the uterine cervical canal. [Boston, 1880.] 10p. DNLM **80-0929**

CAMPBELL, Henry Fraser (1824-1891)
The widespread influence of the cerebro-spinal centres over the ganglionic plexuses. Richmond, 1880. 11p. DNLM; PU **80-0930**

CAMPBELL, Henry Fraser (1824-1891)
The yellow fever quarantine of the future, based upon the portability of atmospheric germs, and the non-contagiousness of the disease. Read at the seventh annual meeting of the American Public Health Association, at Nashville, Tenn., November 20, 1879. . . . Cambridge, [Mass.]: Printed at the Riverside Press, 1880. 16p. DLC; DNLM; MBM **80-0931**

CAMPBELL, Henry Fraser (1824-1891)
Registration and sanitation; their value; a preliminary report read before the board of health of the State of Georgia. Augusta, 1881. 23p. DNLM **80-0932**

CAMPBELL, Henry Fraser (1824-1891)
The prophylactic and therapeutic value of quinine in gynecic and obstetric practice. Boston, 1881. 45p. DNLM **80-0933**

CAMPBELL, Henry Fraser (1824-1891)
Strictures of the oesophagus. Their nature and treatment, with cases. Philadelphia: Collins, 1883. 35p. 1 plate. DNLM **80-0934**

CAMPBELL, Henry Fraser (1824-1891)
Arrest and deficient lactation, and the neuro-dynamic influence controlling the secretion of milk. Atlanta: J. P. Harrison & Co., 1885. 8p. DNLM **80-0935**

CAMPBELL, Henry Fraser (1824-1891)
The genu-pectoral posture; its value in impeded uterine reduction and in the prolonged nausea and vomiting of pregnancy. [New York, 1886.] 76p. DNLM **80-0936**

CAMPBELL, Henry Fraser (1824-1891)
Uterine fibroids and other pelvic tumors: their therapeutic treatment and conduct to the menopause. New Orleans: L. Graham & Sons, 1887. 16p. DNLM **80-0937**

CAMPBELL, Henry Fraser (1824-1891)
The infertility of women. The nervous system in sterility. Some of the requirements of treatment. Philadelphia, 1888. 32p. DNLM **80-0938**

CANFIELD, Ralph M., and James J. PUTNAM
A case of acute hemiplegic chorea. With autopsy and remarks. Cambridge: Riverside Press, 1884. 13p. DNLM **80-0939**

CANFIELD, William B[uckingham] (1857-1899)
Cyclic albuminuria. [Philadelphia, 1887.] 8p. DNLM **80-0940**

CANFIELD, William B[uckingham] (1857-1899)
Practical notes on urinary analysis. Baltimore, 1887. 38p. DNLM **80-0941**

CANFIELD, William B[uckingham] (1857-1899)
On the study of normal histology. [Baltimore, 1887.] 3p. DNLM **80-0942**

CANFIELD, William B[uckingham] (1857-1899)
The gonococcus. [Detroit, 1888.] 4p. DNLM **80-0943**

CANFIELD, William B[uckingham] (1857-1899)
Report of section on microscopy, microchemistry, and spectral analysis. On the microscopical examination of urinary sediment. [Baltimore, 1888.] 4p. DNLM
80-0944

CANFIELD, William B[uckingham] (1857-1899)
Report of the section on practice of medicine. I. The relation of dusty occupations to pulmonary phthisis. II. The present aspect of the question as to the etiology of pneumonia. III. The more recent treatment of pulmonary phthisis. [Baltimore, 1889.] 10p. DNLM **80-0945**

CANFIELD, William B[uckingham] (1857-1899)
Some complications of chronic endarteritis. Baltimore: Jour. Pub. Co., 1889. 10p. DNLM **80-0946**

CAPEN, Nahum (1804-1886)
Reminiscences of Dr. Spurzheim and George Combe. New York: Fowler & Wells, 1881. 262p. NN; NNNAM
80-0946A

CARMALT, William H. (1836-1929)
Some limits in the use of the ophthalmoscope. [Hartford, 1880.] 16p. DNLM **80-0947**

CARMALT, William H. (1836-1929)
Cases of interest. Hartford: Lockwood & Brainard Co., 1884. 16p. 1 plate. DNLM **80-0948**

CARNOCHAN, John Murray (1817-1887)
Cerebral localization in relation to insanity, with cases. New York: J. H. Vail & Co., 1884. 48p. DNLM; NNNAM
80-0949

CARPENTER, J[ames] G[iven]
Sequels of naso-pharyngeal and aural catarrh, illustrated by cases from private practice. [New York, 1884.] 6p. DNLM
80-0950

CARPENTER, J[ames] G[iven]
Treatment of neoplasms of the naso-pharyngeal cavity. Chicago, 1885. 7p. DNLM **80-0951**

CARPENTER, Julia W.
Hygiene versus surgery in gynecology. New York: William Wood & Co., 1889. 9p. DNLM **80-0952**

CARPENTER, William Benjamin (1813-1885)
The microscope and its revelations. 6th ed. New York: William Wood & Co., 1883. 2 v. CtY-M; NNNAM; OCIM; PPC
80-0953

CARPENTER, William Benjamin (1813-1885)
Principles of mental physiology, with their applications to the training and discipline of the mind, and the study of its morbid conditions. . . . New York: D. Appleton & Co., 1888. 737p. DLC; MH-M; NNNAM; PU **80-0954**

CARSON, William (1827-1893)
Cincinnati Hospital. Clinical lecture series, 1885-1886. No. 1. Broncho-pneumonia. Cincinnati: A. Bicker, [1885]. 2 l. DNLM **80-0955**

CARTER, Alfred Henry (1849-1918)
Elements of practical medicine. 3rd ed. New York: D. Appleton & Co., 1885. 447p. DNLM; NNNAM; OCIM; PPC
80-0956

CARTER, James Madison Gore
A synopsis of the medical botany of Illinois. . . . Chicago: Cowdrey, Clark & Co, printers, 1884. 45p. DLC
80-0957

CARTER, J[ames] M[adison] G[ore]
A synopsis of the medical botany of the United States. St. Louis: G. H. Field, 1888. 176p. DNLM; OCLloyd
80-0958

CARTER, Robert Brudenell (1828-1918) and William Adams FROST
Ophthalmic surgery. Philadelphia: Lea Bros. & Co., [1888]. 554p. 2 plates. CtY-M; DNLM; NNNAM; PPC
80-0959

CARTWRIGHT, Sarah
Magnetism clairvoyantly discerned. Lessons from nature. Inherited characteristics explained. New light on the treatment of diseases, medicine and how to take it. With treatises on various subjects of general interest. . . . Detroit, Mich.: O. S. Gulley, Bornman & Co., 1884. 269p. DLC; NN; MH; PU
80-0960

CASSELBERRY, W[illiam] Evans (1858-1916)
A new method of feeding in cases of intubation of the larynx, by position, head downward, on an inclined plane. [Chicago, 1888.] 5p. DNLM **80-0961**

CASTLE, Frederick Albert, ed. (1842-1902)
Wood's household practice of medicine, hygiene and surgery, a practical treatise for the use of families, travelers, seamen, miners, and others. . . . New York: William Wood & Co., 1880. 2 v. DLC; NNNAM; PPC; PU **80-0962**

CASTLE, Frederick A[lbert] (1842-1902)
Design for an isolating pavilion for the use in connection with a hospital, or as one of a series of cottage hospitals. [New York, 1886.] 6p. 1 plate. DNLM **80-0963**

CASTRO, D'Oliveira
Elements of therapeutics and practice according to the dosimetric system. New York: D. Appleton & Co., 1888. 448p. NNNAM; OCIM; PPC; PU **80-0964**

CASWELL, Edward T[hompson] (1833-1887)
Fractures at the Rhode Island Hospital, 1868-1878. Cambridge, 1880. 10p. DNLM **80-0965**

CASWELL, Edward T[hompson] (1833-1887)
Address delivered at the annual meeting of the Rhode Island Medical Society, June 11, 1879, by the president. Providence: E. L. Freeman & Co., 1880. 26p. DNLM **80-0966**

CASWELL, Edward T[hompson] (1833-1887)
Annual address delivered before the alumni of Jefferson Medical College, Philadelphia, March 11, 1879. Providence: E. L. Freeman & Co., 1880. 25p. DNLM; PPJ
80-0967

CASWELL, Edward T[hompson] (1833-1887)
Public health. An address. [Providence, 1881.] 2p. DNLM
80-0968

CASWELL, Edward T[hompson] (1833-1887)
Reform in medical education the aim of the academy. The annual address delivered before the American Academy of Medicine, New York, Sept. 20, 1881. Philadelphia: W. F. Fell & Co., 1881. 16p. DLC; DNLM; NNNAM **80-0969**

CASWELL, HAZARD & CO., NEW YORK
Illustrated catalogue of surgical instruments and appliances. Caswell, Hazard & Co. . . . W. F. Ford, manufacturer. . . . New York, [1880]. 227p. NNNAM **80-0970**

CASWELL, HAZARD & CO., NEW YORK
Registered physicians in the county of New York. Compiled and alphabetically arranged from the official list in the office of the county clerk, to Jan. 1, 1881. [New York, 1881.] 40p. DNLM; NNNAM **80-0971**

CASWELL, HAZARD & CO., NEW YORK
Registered physicians in the county of New York. Compiled and alphabetically arranged from the official list in the office of the county clerk. . . . Revised to Jan. 1, 1883. [New York, 1883.] 53p. DNLM; NNNAM **80-0972**

CASWELL, HAZARD & CO., NEW YORK
Illustrated catalogue of surgical instruments and appliances. W. F. Ford, manufacturerer. New York, [1884]. 129p. DNLM; NNNAM **80-0973**

CATE, S[hadrach] M.
A treatise on some diseases of the bones and ligaments of the spine. . . . Washington: J. F. Sheiry, printer, 1886. 24p. DLC; DNLM **80-0974**

CATE, William Mellen (*b.* 1851)
The child of promise or the Isaac of medicine, and Ishamel the half-brother, being a comprehensive glance at the instincts and predilections of the rival schools of medicines. Washington, D.C.: H. B. Burnham & Co., 1882. 280p. PPHa **80-0975**

CATHELL, Daniel Webster (1839-1925)
The physician himself and what he should add to the strictly scientific. . . . Baltimore: Cushings & Bailey, 1882. 194p. DNLM; NcD; NNNAM; PU **80-0976**

CATHELL, Daniel Webster (1839-1925)
The physician himself and what he should add to his scientific acquirements. . . . 2nd ed., carefully rev. Baltimore: Cushing & Bailey, 1882. 208p. DNLM; ICRM; MBM; NNNAM **80-0977**

CATHELL Daniel Webster (1839-1925)
The physician himself and what he should add to his scientific acquirements. . . . 3rd ed. Baltimore: Cushings & Bailey, 1883. 208p. DNLM; MdBJ-W; MdU-D; PPC **80-0978**

CATHELL, Daniel Webster (1839-1925)
The physician himself and what he should add to his scientific acquirements in order to secure success. . . . 4th ed. Enlarged by the addition of nearly three hundred new suggestions. Baltimore: Cushings & Bailey, 1885. 284p. DNLM; IEN-M; MH-M; ScCM **80-0979**

CATHELL, Daniel Webster (1839-1925)
The physician himself and what he should add to his scientific acquirements in order to secure success. . . . 5th ed., thoroughly rev. Baltimore: Cushings & Bailey, 1885. 284p. DLC; NNNAM; PPJ; PU [Reprinted as 6th ed. (1886), 7th ed. (1887), 8th ed. (1888); Baltimore; Gessings & Bailey, 284p.] **80-0980**

CATHELL, Daniel Webster (1839-1925)
Rectal medication, Baltimore, 1885. 12p. DNLM **80-0981**

CATHELL, Daniel Webster (1839-1925)
A case of pregnancy complicated with uterine fibroids and measles. Baltimore: Guggenheimer, Weil & Co., 1886. 8p. DNLM **80-0982**

CATHELL, Daniel Webster (1839-1925)
Book on the physician himself and things that concern his reputation and success. . . . 9th ed., rev. and enl. Philadelphia and London: F. A. Davis, 1889. 298p. DLC; NNNAM; OCIM; PPC **80-0983**

CATLETT, G[eorge] C[almes] (1830-1886)
Report on the asylum treatment of the insane. St. Louis, 1885. 28p. DNLM **80-0984**

CATLIN, R[obert]
The relations of pain to weather, studied during eleven years of a case of traumatic neuralgia. With notes by S. Weir Mitchell. Philadelphia: Collins, 1883. 19p. 2 charts. DNLM; PPC **80-0985**

CAZEAUX, Pierre (1808-1862)
. . . Obstetrics: the theory and practice; including the diseases of pregnancy and parturition, obstetrical operations, etc. . . . Remodelled and rearranged, with additions and revisions, by S. Tarnier. . . . The 7th American ed. Edited and rev., based in part upon the 8th French and a recent Italian ed., with additions from other recent authorities, a new chapter upon lacerations of the perineum and an article on puerperal insanity, by Robert J. Hess. . . . With twelve full-page plates, five being colored, and one hundred and sixty-five wood engravings. Philadelphia: P. Blakiston, Son & Co., 1884. 1081p. 12 plates. DLC; MBM; NNNAM; PPC **80-0986**

CAZEAUX, Pierre (1808-1862)
. . . The theory and practice of obstetrics; including diseases of pregnancy and parturition, obstetrical operations, etc. . . . Remodelled and rearranged, with additions and revisions, by S. Tarnier. . . . The 8th American ed. Edited and rev. by Robert J. Hess. . . . With an appendix by Paul F. Mundé. . . . Philadelphia: P. Blakiston, Son & Co., 1886. 2 v. DLC; DNLM; MH-M; NNNAM **80-0987**

CHADBOURNE, E. R.
Observations upon an epidemic of measles at the New York Foundling Asylum, with cases illustrating complications and sequelae. New York: William Wood & Co., 1880. 14p. DNLM; NNNAM **80-0988**

CHADWICK, James Read (1844-1905)
Cases of sporadic septicemia in gynecological practice. [Boston, 1880.] 12p. DNLM **80-0989**

CHADWICK, James Read (1844-1905)
Obstetric and gynaecological literature, 1876-1880. . . . Cambridge: Riverside Press, 1881. 17p. DLC; DNLM **80-0990**

CHADWICK, James Read (1844-1905)
The hot rectal douche. [Boston, 1881.] 9p. DNLM **80-0991**

CHADWICK, James Read (1844-1905)
Admission of women to the Massachusetts Medical Society. Boston, 1882. 11p. DNLM **80-0992**

CHADWICK, James Read (1844-1905)
Extirpation of a retro-renal sarcoma by abdominal section. Cambridge: Riverside Press, 1884. 8p. DNLM
80-0993

CHADWICK, James Read (1844-1905)
Ten cases of pregnancy and labor, complicated with fibroids, with remarks. Read at the meeting of the Massachusetts Medical Society, June 9, 1885. [Boston, 1885.] 19p. DNLM
80-0994

CHADWICK, James Read (1844-1905)
Peristalsis of the genital tract, and a new theory to explain relaxation of the vaginal outlet during labor. [New York, 1885.] 8p. DNLM **80-0995**

CHADWICK, James Read (1844-1905)
Cases of stenosis and atresia of the female genital canal. Boston: Cupples, Upham & Co., 1886. 19p. DNLM; MBM
80-0996

CHADWICK, James Read (1844-1905)
The value of the bluish coloration of the vaginal entrance as a sign of pregnancy. [New York, 1886.] 17p. 1 plate. DNLM
80-0997

CHADWICK, James Read (1844-1905)
Ventral hernia after laparotomy, and its surgical treatment. [New York, 1887.] 16p. 1 plate. DNLM
80-0998

CHADWICK, James Read (1844-1905)
Discussion to treatment of uterine fibromata. [Philadelphia, 1889.] 4p. DNLM **80-0999**

CHAILLÉ, Stanford Emerson (1830-1911)
Extramicroscopic organisms. [New Orleans, 1880.] 3p. DNLM
80-1000

CHAILLÉ, Stanford Emerson (1830-1911)
Eadsport, Ship Island quarantine and the National Board of Health. June 9, 1881. 3p. New Orleans: Democrat Print, 1881. 3p. DNLM **80-1001**

CHAILLÉ, Stanford Emerson (1830-1911)
The vital statistics of New Orleans as taught by the U.S. census, 1880. [New Orleans, 1881.] 13p. 4 tabs. DNLM
80-1002

CHAILLÉ, Stanford Emerson (1830-1911)
The Louisiana State Board of Health in its annual report for 1881, versus the National Board of Health. Reply in behalf of the latter. New Orleans: L. Graham & Son, 1882. 14p. DNLM
80-1003

CHAILLÉ, Stanford Emerson (1830-1911)
The prevention of yellow fever. Report of the flushing committee, New Orleans Auxiliary Sanitary Association, June 24, 1882, submitted by Edward Fenner. New Orleans: L. Graham & Son, 1882. 22p. DNLM; LNT-M **80-1004**

CHAILLÉ, Stanford Emerson (1830-1911)
Yellow fever, or yellow jaundice in New Orleans in 1882; disputed case of Louis (or Ludwig) Deschler. New Orleans: Graham & Son, 1882. 12p. DNLM; LNT-M
80-1005

CHAILLÉ, Stanford Emerson (1830-1911)
The importance of introducing the study of hygiene into the public and other schools; address on the forty-eighth commencement day, March 29th, 1882, of the Medical Department of the University of Louisiana. New Orleans: L. Graham & Son, 1882. 19p. DNLM; LNT-M **80-1006**

CHAILLÉ, Stanford Emerson (1830-1911)
Inundations of New Orleans and their influence on its health. [New Orleans, 1882.] 18p. DNLM; LNT-M
80-1007

CHAILLÉ, Stanford Emerson (1830-1911)
Inundations in Louisiana; their influence on health. [New Orleans, 1883.] 27p. DNLM **80-1008**

CHAILLÉ, Stanford Emerson (1830-1911)
The New Orleans Auxiliary Sanitary Association publishes for the benefit of the public the following information as to samll-pox and vaccination, written at the request of the Association by . . . New Orleans, June, 1883. New Orleans: W. B. Stansbury & Co., 1883. 28p. DNLM
80-1009

CHAILLÉ, Stanford Emerson (1830-1911)
Yellow fever in Vera Cruz and Colon in 1882, and the Louisiana State Board of Health thereon in 1882 and in 1883. [New Orleans, 1884.] 10p. DNLM **80-1010**

CHAILLÉ, Stanford Emerson (1830-1911)
[Medical science] on the abuse of alcoholics by the healthy. Concord, N.H., 1886. 36p. DNLM **80-1011**

CHAILLÉ, Stanford Emerson (1830-1911)
Infants, their chronological progress. [New Orleans, 1887.] 20p. DNLM **80-1012**

CHAILLÉ, Stanford Emerson (1830-1911)
Life and death-rates. New Orleans and other cities compared. New Orleans, 1888. 16p. DNLM **80-1013**

CHAMBERLAIN, William Mellen (1826-1887)
Notes on the sanitary and climatic conditions of Southern California. New York: Trow's, 1886. 19p. DNLM; NNNAM
80-1014

CHAMBERLAIN, William Mellen (1826-1887)
Pasadena as a sanitarium. New York: D. Appleton & Co., 1888. 15p. 1 plate. DNLM **80-1015**

CHANCELLOR, Charles Williams (1831-1915)
Report to the State Board of Health, on the epidemic of diphtheria in Frederick City, Maryland. And the small-pox in Charles County, Md. . . . Baltimore: The Sun Book & Job Printing Office, 1882. 63p. fold. plan. DLC; DNLM; MdU-D
80-1016

CHANCELLOR, Charles Williams (1831-1915)
The Liernur system of sewerage. A refutation of the criticisms of Colonel Waring and Dr. Billings. [Baltimore, 1883.] 14p. DNLM **80-1017**

CHANCELLOR, Charles Williams (1831-1915)
A treatise on mineral waters and sea-side resorts, descriptive and medical. . . . Baltimore: J. H. Piet & Co., 1883. 160p. DLC; DNLM; MdU-D **80-1018**

CHANCELLOR, Charles Williams (1831-1915)
Sewerage of cities. A reply to the paper of Col. George E. Waring, C.E., of Newport, R.I., on "The Liernur system of sewerage for Baltimore." An important question involving the interests of health, commerce, and agriculture. Baltimore: J. Young, [1884]. 24p. DNLM; MdU-D
80-1019

CHANCELLOR, Charles Williams (1831-1915)
The climate of the eastern shore of Maryland, considered with reference to its sanative and curative influence in pulmonary consumption and other diseases. . . . Baltimore: Walworth & Co., 1889. 107p. DLC; MdU-D **80-1020**

CHANNING, Walter (1849-1921)
Note on the construction of hospitals for insane paupers, read at the Conference of Charities, Cleveland, Ohio, June, 1880. 6p. DNLM **80-1021**

CHANNING, Walter (1849-1921)
The mental status of Guiteau, the assassin of President Garfield. Cambridge: Riverside Press, 1882. 22p. DNLM
80-1022

CHANNING, Walter (1849-1921)
A consideration of the causes of insanity. Boston: Wright & Potter Ptg. Co., 1884. 31p. DNLM **80-1023**

CHANNING, Walter (1849-1921)
The connection between insanity and crime. Read at the meeting of the Association of Medical Superintendents of American Institutions for the Insane, at Saratoga, N.Y., June 17, 1885. [Utica, N.Y., 1886.] 21p. DNLM
80-1024

CHANNING, Walter (1849-1921)
Report of a case of epilepsy of forty-five years' duration, with autopsy. (Read March 18, 1886, before the Boston Medico-Psychological Society.) [Boston, 1886.] 20p. DNLM
80-1025

CHANNING, Walter (1849-1921)
An international classification of mental diseases. Utica, 1888. 20p. DNLM **80-1026**

CHANNING, Walter (1849-1921)
The Codman will case. [Utica, N.Y., 1888.] 11p. DNLM
80-1027

CHANNING, Walter (1849-1921)
Physical training of the insane, with remarks by Miss A. W. Adams. Utica, N.Y. 1889. 11p. DNLM
80-1028

CHAPIN, Charles V[alue] (1856-1941)
The origin and progress of the malarial fever now prevalent in New England. Providence: Kellogg Print. Co., 1884. 41p. DNLM **80-1029**

CHAPIN, Charles V[alue] (1856-1941)
The present state of the germ theory of disease. Providence: Kellogg Print. Co., 1885. 47p. DNLM
80-1030

CHAPIN, Charles V[aule] (1856-1941)
The original Jennerian vaccine virus as preserved and used in the public vaccinations in the city of Providence, Rhode Island. [With notes by C. H. Leonard.] [Providence, 1886.] 11p. DNLM **80-1031**

CHAPIN, Charles V[alue] (1856-1941)
What changes has the acceptance of the germ theory made in measures for the prevention and treatment of consumption? Providence, 1888. 47p. DNLM
80-1032

CHAPIN, Charles V[alue] (1856-1941)
Methods for the prevention of scarlet fever. An address delivered at the annual meeting of the R.I. Medical Society, June 9, 1888. [1889.] 25p. DNLM **80-1033**

CHAPIN, Charles V[alue] (1856-1941)
Edwin Miller Snow, M.D. [Biography.] [Providence, 1889.] 6p. DNLM **80-1034**

CHAPIN, Charles V[alue] (1856-1941)
Some points in the etiology of typhoid fever. [Boston, 1889.] 14p. DNLM **80-1035**

CHAPIN, Henry Dwight (1857-1942)
Typhoid fever in young children. New York: William Wood & Co., 1883. 10p. DNLM; NNNAM **80-1036**

CHAPIN, Henry Dwight (1857-1942)
Two cases of branchial cyst. New York: W. R. Jenkins, [1885]. 7p. DNLM; NNNAM **80-1037**

CHAPIN, Henry Dwight (1857-1942)
Rheumatism in early life. New York: Trow, 1886. 23p. DNLM; NNNAM **80-1038**

CHAPIN, Henry Dwight (1857-1942)
Septic poisoning in early life. [New York, 1889.] 11p. DNLM; NNNAM **80-1039**

CHAPIN, John B[assett] (1829-1918)
Experts and expert testimony. Read before the Association of Superintendents of American Asylums for the Insane, May, 1880. [n.p.], 1880. 29p. DNLM **80-1040**

CHAPIN, John B[assett] (1829-1918)
Public complaints against asylums for the insane, and the commitment of the insane. [Utica, N.Y. 1883.] 17p. DNLM
80-1041

CHAPIN, John B[assett] (1829-1918)
On mental capacity in certain states of typhoid fever. [Utica, N.Y., 1884.] 7p. DNLM **80-1042**

CHAPIN, John B[assett] (1829-1918)
Address delivered at the forty-third annual meeting of the Association of Medical Superintendents of American Institutions for the Insane, Newport, R.I., June 18, 1889. [Newport, 1889.] 35p. DNLM **80-1043**

CHAPMAN, GREEN & CO.
Desc. dose and price list of drugs. . . . Chicago, 1882. 140p. DLC **80-1044**

CHAPMAN, Henry Cadwalader (1845-1909)
History of the discovery of the circulation of the blood. . . . Philadelphia: P. Blakiston, Son & Co., 1884. 56p. DLC; NNNAM; PPC; PPJ **80-1045**

CHAPMAN, Henry Cadwalader (1845-1909)
Treatise on human physiology. . . . Philadelphia: Lea Bros. & Co., 1887. 945p. DLC; OCIM; PPC; PU
80-1046

CHAPMAN, Henry Cadwalader (1845-1909) and Albert P. BRUBACKER
Researches on general nerve muscle physiology, made in the laboratory of the Jefferson Medical College. Philadelphia, 1888. 7p. DNLM; PPJ **80-1047**

CHAPMAN, Norman H.
Extensive scalding from prolonged exposure to steam at high temperature. [Philadelphia, 1881.] 12p. DNLM **80-1048**

CHARCOT, Jean Martin (1825-1893)
Clinical lectures on the diseases of old age. . . . Transl. by Leigh H. Hunt. . . . With additional lectures by Alfred L. Loomis. . . . New York: William Wood & Co., 1881. 280p. 3 plates. DLC; DNLM; NNNAM; PPC **80-1049**

CHARCOT, Jean Martin (1825-1893)
Lectures on the pathological anatomy of the nervous system. Diseases of the spinal cord. . . . Transl. from the reports by Dr. E. Brissaud, in the Progrés médicale, by Cornelius G. Comegys. . . . Cincinnati: P. G. Thomson, 1881. 165p. DLC; DNLM; NNNAM; OCIM **80-1050**

CHARCOT, Jean Martin (1825-1893)
Clinical lectures on certain diseases of the nervous system. . . . Transl. by E. P. Hurd. . . . Detroit, Mich.: G. S. Davis, 1888. 155p. DLC; OCIM; PPC; PU **80-1051**

CHARPENTIER, Louis Arthur Alphonse (1836-1899)
A practical treatise on obstetrics. Transl. under the supervision of, and with notes and additions by, Egbert H. Grandin. New York: William Wood & Co., 1887. 4 v. CtY-M; DNLM; NNNAM; PPC **80-1052**

CHARTIER, M[elite] E[lysée]
Alkaloïdo-therapy: an introduction to a treatise on alkaloïdo-therapy. . . . St. Louis: American Alkaloïdo-Therapic Society, 1885. 27p. DLC **80-1053**

CHASE, Alvin Wood (1817-1885)
. . . Dr. Chase's family physician, farrier, bee-keeper, and second receipt book, being an entirely new and complete treatise. . . . Rev. and enl. by the author. . . . Toledo, O.: Chase Publishing Co., 1881. 652p. DLC; OCIM **80-1054**

CHASE, Alvin Wood (1817-1885)
. . . Dr. Chase's third, last and complete receipt book and household physician; or, Practical knowledge for the people. . . . [Memorial ed.] Detroit, Mich.: F. B. Dickerson & Co., 1887. 808p. DLC; OCIM **80-1055**

CHASE, Walter B[ennaiah]
Mechanical support in uterine displacements, with reference to the management of certain complications. [New York, 1886.] 12p. DNLM **80-1056**

CHAVANNES, Albert
Heredity, cross-breeding, and pre-natal influences. New York: Murray Hill Pub. Co., 1885. 19p. DNLM; NNNAM **80-1057**

CHAVANNES, Albert
Vital force and magnetic exchange; their relation to each other and to life and happiness. Followed by a brief study of their agency upon conduct and the phenomena of mind reading and magnetic cures. Knoxville: T. Haws, 1888. 45p. DNLM **80-1058**

CHAVASSE, Pye Henry (1810-1879)
Man's strength and woman's beauty; or, The royal road to life, love, and longevity. A treatise on the physical laws of being, embracing an outline of how human life begins; its growth and expansion in youth; its perfection under the laws of love; and the general discipline by which its happiness is fostered and matured. . . . With notes and additions by an eminent American author. . . . Cincinnati, Philadelphia, [etc.]: Jones Brothers & Co.; San Francisco: A. L. Bancroft & Co., 1880. 515p. plates. DLC; NNNAM; PPC; PPJ **80-1059**

CHAVASSE, Pye Henry (1810-1879)
. . . The mental culture and training of children. . . . Philadelphia: Lindsay & Blakiston, 1881. 286p. DLC; DNLM; PPC; PU **80-1060**

CHAVASSE, Pye Henry (1810-1879)
Gynecology: the ladies' guide and counsellor. . . . With an introduction by Sarah Hackett Stevenson. . . . Together with chapters on the sacred rights of offspring, the physiology of marriage, and happiness in wedlock, by N. F. Cooke. . . . Chicago: Park City Publishing House, 1886. 614p. DLC; OCIM; PU **80-1061**

CHAVASSE, Pye Henry (1810-1879)
Wife and mother; or, Information for every woman. Adapted from the writings of . . . . Together with an introduction by Sarah Hackett Stevenson. . . . Chicago: Smith & Miller, 1886. 526p. DLC; NNNAM; OCIM; PPC **80-1062**

CHAVASSE, Pye Henry (1810-1879)
Ladies family physician. . . . New York: Butler Bros., 1888. 273p. NNNAM **80-1063**

CHAVASSE, Pye Henry (1810-1879)
Wife and mother; or, Information for every woman. Adapted from the writings of . . . . Together with an introduction by Sarah Hackett Stevenson. . . . Rev. and enl. . . . 30th ed. Philadelphia, Chicago, [etc.]: H. J. Smith & Co., 1888. 575p. DLC; MBM; OCIM; PU **80-1064**

CHEATHAM, W[illiam]
Intubation of larynx for true and diphtheritic croup. Louisville: J. P. Morton & Co., 1886. 11p. DNLM **80-1065**

CHEATHAM, W[illiam]
Nasal reflexes as a cause of diseases of the eye. Louisville: J. P. Morton & Co., 1887. 8p. DNLM **80-1066**

CHEATHAM, W[illiam]
Diseases of the nose and pharynx, and their treatment. [Richmond, 1888.] 80p. DNLM **80-1067**

CHEATHAM, W[illiam]
Granular conjunctivitis with and without pannus. [Atlanta, 1888.] 5p. DNLM **80-1068**

CHEATHAM, W[illiam]
Points of interest to the general practitioner, deducted from 5,409 cases of diseases of the eye, ear, throat, and nose, seen in private practice, 1887-1888. Louisville: J. P. Morton & Co., 1889. 21p. DNLM **80-1069**

CHEEVER, C[larence] A[lonzo]
A case of multiple sarcoma of the skin. Boston: Cupples, Upham & Co., 1886. 7p. DNLM **80-1070**

CHEEVER, David W[illiams] (1831-1915)
Shock. Boston: Cupples & Hurd, 1888. 7p. DNLM
80-1071

CHEEVER, David W[illiams] (1831-1915)
The future of surgery without limit. Boston: Damrell & Upham, 1889. 10p. DNLM **80-1072**

CHEW, Samuel Claggett (1837-1915)
Medicine in the past and in the future; an inaugural address delivered before the Medical and Chirurgical Faculty of Maryland. Baltimore: W. Borst & Co., 1880. 21p. DNLM; MdBM **80-1073**

CHEW, S[amuel] C[laggett] (1837-1915)
The use of strophanthus in dilatation of the heart. New York: Trow, 1887. 7p. DNLM **80-1074**

CHILDS, William Riddle (1838-1888)
Address delivered before the Homoeopathic Medical Society of Pennsylvania, by the President, at the opening of its twentieth annual session, held at Pittsburgh, Pa., September 17, 18, 1884. Pittsburgh: J. H. Barrows & Co., 1884. 8p. PPHa **80-1075**

CHIPLEY, W[illiam] S. (1810-1880)
Catalogue of medical and miscellaneous books from the library of the late Dr. . . . Cincinnati, O.: J. Barclay, [1880]. 10p. DNLM **80-1076**

CHIPMAN, M[arshall] M[ead] (1822-1899)
Report of the committee on medical topography, meteorology, endemics and epidemics. Subject: Mining débris deposits. San Francisco: W. M. Hinton & Co., 1884. 21p. DNLM
80-1077

CHIPMAN, M[arshall] M[ead] (1822-1899)
Report of the committee on medical topography, meteorology, endemics, etc. Importance of forest preservation and timber cultivation. San Francisco, 1883. 31p. DNLM
80-1078

CHISOLM, Julian John (1830-1903)
Myopia in its various phases. Richmond, 1880. 32p. DNLM
80-1079

CHISOLM, Julian John (1830-1903)
Optico-ciliary neurotomy, the proposed substitute for extirpation of a lost and painful eye ball. Baltimore: J. W. Borst & Co., 1880. 13p. DNLM; MdU-D **80-1080**

CHISOLM, Julian John (1830-1903)
Salicylate of sodium in the treatment of iritis. [New York, 1880.] 4p. DNLM **80-1081**

CHISOLM, Julian John (1830-1903)
Myopia (commonly called near-sightedness) in its various phases. [Baltimore, 1880.] 32p. DNLM
80-1082

CHISOLM, Julian John (1830-1903)
Spasm of the intra-ocular eye muscles; a frequent cause of annoying and serious eye defects. Baltimore: Thomas & Evans, 1881. 10p. DNLM **80-1083**

CHISOLM, Julian John (1830-1903)
Report on ophthalmology, made to the Medical and Chirurgical Faculty of Maryland, at the eighty-fourth session, April, 1882. [Baltimore, 1882.] 15p. DNLM **80-1084**

CHISOLM, Julian John (1830-1903)
Bromide of ethyl, the most perfect anaesthetic for short, painful surgical operations. [Baltimore], 1883. 8p. DNLM
80-1085

CHISOLM, Julian John (1830-1903)
Address on ophthalmology. Chicago: A. G. Newell, 1884. 19p. DNLM **80-1086**

CHISOLM, Julian John (1830-1903)
Removal of a piece of iron from the vitreous chamber by means of the magnetic needle. Baltimore, 1884. 8p. DNLM
80-1087

CHISOLM, Julian John (1830-1903)
The after-treatment of cataract cases, to the exclusion of compresses, bandages, dark rooms, and restraint. Chicago, 1887. 21p. DNLM **80-1088**

CHISOLM, Julian John (1830-1903)
Report of the section on ophthalmology, otology, and laryngology. A simple and valuable optometer. [Baltimore, 1887.] 13p. DNLM **80-1089**

CHISOLM, Julian John (1830-1903)
Rest for painful eyes; is this advice always good? Baltimore, 1887. 23p. DNLM **80-1090**

CHISOLM, Julian John (1830-1903)
Cataract extractions, with only the eye operated upon closed by adhesive strips; the other eye left open for the guidance of the patient. Chicago, 1888. 11p. DNLM
80-1091

CHISOLM, Julian John (1830-1903)
Chloroform, the best of anaesthetics. Baltimore, 1888. 26p. DNLM **80-1092**

CHISOLM, Julian John (1830-1903)
The great value of a 0.25 D. cylinder in the relief of headache and eye pains. Chicago, 1888. 12p. DNLM
80-1093

CHISOLM, Julian John (1830-1903)
A very valuable lesson for those who use anaesthetics. [Baltimore: Guggenheimer, Weil & Co., 1888.] 15p. DNLM
80-1094

CHITTENDEN, R[ussell] H[enry] (1856-1943)
Observations on the digestive ferments. Philadelphia, 1889. 15p. DNLM **80-1095**

CHOATE, Clara E.
True Christianity; the basis of healing with mind. Boston: H. H. Carter & Karrick, 1886. 27p. DNLM; MH
80-1096

CHOATE, Clara E.
Mental healing. Boston: H. H. Carter & Karrick, 1886. 21p. DNLM; MH **80-1097**

CHOATE, Clara E.
The unfolding; or mind understood the healing power. Boston: H. H. Carter & Co., 1886. 21p. DNLM; MH
80-1098

CHRISTIAN, E[dmund] A.
A case of general paralysis apparently of traumatic origin. [Utica, N.Y., 1888.] 5p. DNLM **80-1099**

CHRISTIAN, Walter Shield (1859-1905)
Chemical experiments for medical students. Arranged after Beilstein. . . . Cincinnati: R. Clarke & Co., 1888. 84p. DLC; OCIM **80-1100**

CHURCHILL, Frederick (1843-1916)
Face and foot deformities. With illustrations of new appliances for the cure of birth-mark, club-foot, etc. . . . Philadelphia: P. Blakiston, Son & Co., 1885. 195p. NNNAM; OCIM; PPC; PU **80-1101**

CLAIBORNE, John Herbert (1861-1922)
The theory and practice of the ophthalmoscope. A handbook for students. . . . Detroit, Mich.: G. S. Davis, 1888. 77p. diags. DLC; DNLM; OCIM; PU **80-1102**

CLAPP, Dwight M.
Address before the 24th annual meeting of the Massachusetts Dental Society, December 13th, 1888. Salem, 1889. 13p. DNLM **80-1103**

CLAPP, Herbert Codman (1846-1929)
Is consumption contagious? And can it be transmitted by means of food? . . . Boston and Providence: O. Clapp & Son, 1881. 178p. DLC; DNLM; MBM **80-1104**

CLAPP, Herbert C[odman] (1846-1929)
Empyema. Twenty-four cases of the radical operation. Read at the annual meeting of the Boston Homoeopathic Medical Society. Boston: Rand, Avery & Co., 1886. 20p. MBM; PPHa **80-1105**

[DR. CLARK]
The physician and druggist, a description of disease and its treatment with eighteen medical prescriptions made plain for general use. . . . [2nd ed.] New York and Philadelphia: F. H. Reynolds & Co., [1882]. 262p. DLC; PPC; PU **80-1106**

CLARK, Alonzo (1807-1887)
Lectures on diseases of the heart, delivered at the College of Physicians and Surgeons, New York. . . . New York, London: Bermingham & Co., 1884. 251p. DLC; DNLM; NNNAM; PPC **80-1107**

CLARK, Alonzo (1807-1887)
Lectures on diseases of the heart, delivered at the College of Physicians and Surgeons, New York. . . . New York: E. B. Treat, 1887. 251p. DLC; NNNAM; OCIM; PU **80-1108**

CLARK, Daniel (1835-1912)
A psycho-medical history of Louis Riel. [Utica, N.Y., 1887.] 19p. DNLM **80-1109**

CLARK, [Daniel] (1835-1912)
A revised and enlarged edition of Clark's new system of electrical medication. By A. W. Tipton. . . . Chicago: C. J. Johnson, printer, 1882. 259p. DLC; OCIM **80-1110**

CLARK, Daniel (1835-1912)
A revised and enlarged edition of Clark's new system of electrical medication. By A. W. Tipton. . . . Chicago: C. J. Johnson, printer, 1885. 264p. DLC; DNLM; OCIM **80-1111**

CLARKE, Augustus P[eck] (1833-1912)
Vascular growths of the female meatus urinarius. Cambridge, Mass., 1888. 4 l. 1 plate. DNLM **80-1112**

CLARKE, Augustus P[eck] (1833-1912)
Faradism in the practice of gynaecology. [Boston, 1889.] 16p. DNLM **80-1113**

CLARKE, John Henry (1852-1931)
The prescriber: a dictionary of the new therapeutics. . . . New York: Boericke & Tafel, 1885. 187p. DLC; NNNAM; PPHa **80-1114**

CLARKE, ROBERT, & CO.
Bibliotheca medica. Supplement, November, 1880. Cincinnati, 1880. 26p. [New books and new editions issued in America and Great Britain from August, 1878 to November, 1880] DNLM; ICU; MH; NNC **80-1115**

CLARKE, ROBERT, & CO.
Bibliotheca medica. A catalogue of American and British books relating to medicine, surgery, dentistry, pharmacy, chemistry, and kindred subjects, with an index by authors. 6th ed. Cincinnati, 1883. 282p. DNLM; OCIM; PPC; PU **80-1116**

CLARKE, W[illiam] Bruce (1850-1914) and Charles Barrett LOCKWOOD
The dissector's manual. Philadelphia, Pa., [1883]. 390p. 1 plate. DNLM; NNNAM; PPC; PPJ **80-1117**

CLARKE, William Bruce (1850-1914)
An oxygen exposé. [Indianapolis, 1885.] 4 l. DNLM **80-1118**

CLARKE, William Bruce (1850-1914)
Hydrogen peroxide. [Chicago, 1886.] 36p. DNLM **80-1119**

CLAYPOOL, Albert
Annual address read before the Homoeopathic Medical Society of Ohio. Toledo, O.: B. F. Wade & Co., 1887. 9p. OCIM; PPHa **80-1120**

CLEAVELAND, D[aniel] A.
A notable defect in medical education. [Hartford], 1880. 9p. DNLM **80-1121**

CLEMMER, John W.
Medical education and legislation. President's address delivered before the Central Ohio Homoeopathic Medical Society, September 4, 1884. [1884.] 14p. OCIM; PPHa **80-1122**

CLEVELAND, Charles Luther (*d.* 1890)
An introduction to the study of the homoeopathic materia medica. A lecture delivered in the Homoeopathic Hospital College of Cleveland, Ohio, January 3, 1887. (Published by the Class.) [1887.] 6p. PPHa **80-1123**

CLEVELAND, Charles Luther (*d.* 1890)
Salient materia medica and therapeutics. Philadelphia: F. E. Boericke, Hahnemann Publishing House, 1888. 171p. DLC; PPHa **80-1124**

CLEVELAND, Clement (*b.* 1843)
A case of interstitial pregnancy. New York: William Wood & Co., 1880. 6p. 1 plate. DNLM **80-1125**

CLEVELAND, Clement (*b.* 1843)
Model of a gynecological examining table invented by Dr. Samuel W. Francis; with remarks. [New York, 1880.] 1 l. DNLM **80-1126**

CLEVENGER, S[hobal] Vail (1843-1920)
Therapeutic action of mercury. Inaugural thesis read before the Chicago Biological Society, Feb. 4, 1880. Chicago: Knight & Leonard, 1880. 27p. DNLM **80-1127**

CLEVENGER, S[hobal] Vail (1843-1920)
Traumatic insanity and other effects of head injuries. [St. Louis, 1888.] 27p. DNLM **80-1128**

CLEVENGER, S[hobal] Vail (1843-1920)
Spinal concussion surgically considered as a cause of spinal injury, and neurologically restricted to a certain symptom group, for which is suggested the designation Erichsen's disease, as one form of traumatic neuroses. Philadelphia & London: F. A. Davis, 1889. 359p. 12 plates. DLC; DNLM; NNNAM; PPC **80-1129**

CLOUSTON, Thomas Smith (1840-1915)
Clinical lectures on mental diseases. . . . To which is added, an abstract of the statutes of the United States and of several states and territories relating to the custody of the insane. By Charles F. Folsom. . . . Philadelphia: Henry C. Lea's Son, & Co., 1884. 550p. 8 plates. DLC; DNLM; NNNAM; PPC **80-1130**

CLOUSTON, Thomas Smith (1840-1915)
Reprint of Dr. T. S. Clouston's review of Dr. Kirkbride's work on the construction, etc., of insane hospitals. With a brief introduction. [Syracuse, N.Y., 188?]. 16p. DLC **80-1131**

CLUM, Franklin D.
Men and women; their structure and function, and how to supply their wants, direct their powers, avoid their afflictions, and sustain their lives. Boston: D. Lothrop & Co., [1882]. 400p. DNLM; MB; MH; NN **80-1132**

CLUM, Franklin D.
Inebriety; its causes, its results, its remedy. Philadelphia: J. B. Lippincott Co., 1888. 252p. DNLM; MH; NN; PU **80-1133**

COATS, Joseph (1846-1899)
A manual of pathology. Philadelphia: Henry C. Lea's Son & Co., 1883. 818p. CtY-M; DNLM; MBM; NNNAM **80-1134**

COCHRAN, Jerome (1831-1896)
Sketches of yellow fever on the Gulf Coast of Florida. [Montgomery, 1881.] 39p. DNLM **80-1135**

COCHRAN, Jerome (1831-1896)
Problems in regard to yellow fever and the prevention of yellow fever epidemics. Concord, N.H., 1888. 12p. DNLM **80-1136**

CODMAN, Benjamin S. (1816?-1894) and Ashahel M. SHURTLEFF
Surgical instruments and appliances. Boston, [1881, *vel. subseq.*]. 12 l. DNLM; MBM **80-1137**

CODMAN, Benjamin S. (1816?-1894) and Ashahel M. SHURTLEFF
Illustrated catalogue of surgical instruments and appliances. Boston: Stanley & Usher, [1883?]. 24p. DNLM; MBM **80-1138**

CODMAN, John T[homas]
Inflamed and sensitive teeth. [Philadelphia, 1885.] 7p. DNLM **80-1139**

CODMAN, John T[homas]
Enforced climate and diet as affecting the teeth. [New York, 1888.] 10p. DNLM **80-1140**

COE, Henry C[larke] (1856-1940)
The exaggerated importance of minor pelvic inflammations. [New York, 1886.] 22p. DNLM; NNNAM **80-1141**

COE, Henry C[larke] (1856-1940)
Malarial manifestations due to traumatism. New York, 1886. 20p. DNLM; NNNAM **80-1142**

COE, Henry C[larke] (1856-1940)
Is disease of the uterine appendages as frequent as it has been represented? New York: William Wood & Co., 1886. 17p. DNLM; NNNAM **80-1143**

COE, Henry C[larke] (1856-1940)
The clinical versus the microscopical evidences of malignant disease. [New York, 1887.] 11p. DNLM **80-1144**

COE, Henry C[larke] (1856-1940)
Post-graduate instruction in gynaecology. [New York, 1887.] 12p. DNLM **80-1145**

COE, Henry C[larke] (1856-1940)
The significance and localization of pain in pelvic disease. New York: Judson Co., 1888. 10p. DNLM **80-1146**

COE, Henry C[larke] (1856-1940)
The use of the curette for the relief of hemorrhage due to uterine fibroids. New York: Trow's Print. & Bookbinding Co., 1888. 12p. DNLM **80-1147**

COE, Henry C[larke] (1856-1940)
So-called "varicocele" in the female. New York: William Wood & Co., 1889. 11p. DNLM **80-1148**

COE, Henry C[larke] (1856-1940)
Death from visceral affections after ovariotomy. Philadelphia: W. J. Dornan, 1889. 24p. DNLM **80-1149**

COE, Henry C[larke] (1856-1940)
In memoriam, James Bradbridge Hunter, M.D. [Philadelphia, 1889.] 4p. DNLM **80-1150**

COE, Henry C[larke] (1856-1940)
A successful case of laparotomy and supra-vaginal amputation of the uterus for rupture. New York: Trow's, 1889. 7p. 1 tab. DNLM **80-1151**

COE, Henry C[larke] (1856-1940)
The early recognition of cancer of the cervix uteri. Philadelphia, 1889. 16p. DNLM **80-1152**

COE, Henry C[larke] (1856-1940)
The immediate application of forceps to the after-coming head in cases of version with partial dilatation of the cervix. New York: Trow's, 1889. 7p. DNLM **80-1153**

COGSHALL, Bela
Is tubercular consumption a contagious and parasitic disease? [Boston, 1882.] 12p. DNLM **80-1154**

COHEN, Jacob [da Silva] Solis (1838-1927)
Case of cystic adenoma of base of tongue with retropharyngeal and cervical adenoma. [Philadelphia, 1880.] 2p. DNLM **80-1155**

COHEN, Jacob [da Silva] Solis (1838-1927)
The throat and the voice. Philadelphia: P. Blakiston, 1880. 159p. CtY-M; DNLM; NNNAM; PPC **80-1156**

COHEN, Jacob [da Silva] Solis (1838-1927)
Hyper-distention of the pulmonary alveoli as a therapeutic agent in chronic disease of the respiratory mucous membrane. [Philadelphia, 1880.] 4p. DNLM **80-1157**

COHEN, Jacob [da Silva] Solis (1838-1927)
Some clinical considerations on access to benign intralaryngeal neoplasms through external incisions; as illustrated in a small group of personal observations heretofore unreported. [Philadelphia, 1880.] 10p. DNLM **80-1158**

COHEN, Jacob [da Silva] Solis (1838-1927)
Some remarks on tuberculous laryngitis, as viewed laryngoscopically. [Philadelphia, 1880.] 2 l. DNLM **80-1159**

COHEN, Jacob [da Silva] Solis (1838-1927)
Hyper-distension of the air cells as a therapeutic measure. [Philadelphia, 1880.] 3p. DNLM **80-1160**

COHEN, Jacob [da Silva] Solis (1838-1927)
A case of primary tuberculosis of the larynx. Read before the American Laryngological Association, session 1880. [Philadelphia, 1881.] 7p. DNLM **80-1161**

COHEN, Jacob [da Silva] Solis (1838-1927)
Address in medicine, delivered before the Medical Society of the State of Pennsylvania, at its annual meeting held at Lancaster, May, 1881. Philadelphia: Collins, 1881. 9p. DNLM **80-1162**

COHEN, Jacob [da Silva] Solis (1838-1927)
A case of prolapse of the laryngeal sac. New York: G. P. Putnam's Sons, 1882. 2p. DNLM **80-1163**

COHEN, Jacob [da Silva] Solis (1838-1927)
Tuberculosis as manifested in the larynx. Philadelphia, 1883. 20p. DNLM **80-1164**

COHEN, Jacob [da Silva] Solis (1838-1927)
Does excision of the larynx tend to the prolongation of life? Philadelphia: Collins, 1883. 19p. DNLM **80-1165**

COHEN, Jacob [da Silva] Solis (1838-1927)
A case of thyrotomy for mobid growth, with subsequent development of epithelioma in the cutaneous cicatrix, but without involvement of the interior of the larynx. [New York, 1883.] 5p. DNLM **80-1166**

COHEN, Jacob [da Silva] Solis (1838-1927)
On the elements of prognosis and of therapeusis in tuberculosis of the larynx. [Chicago, 1883.] 11p. DNLM **80-1167**

COHEN, Jacob [da Silva] Solis (1838-1927)
Apsithyria. [Philadelphia, 1883.] 4p. DNLM **80-1168**

COHEN, Jacob [da Silva] Solis (1838-1927)
A case of paralysis of the left vocal band in extreme abduction, following an incised wound in the neck. New York. D. Appleton & Co., 1884. 4p. DNLM **80-1169**

COHEN, Jacob [da Silva] Solis (1838-1927)
The use of compressed and rarefied air, as a substitute for change of climate, in the treatment of pulmonary diseases. New York, 1884. 6p. DNLM **80-1170**

COHEN, Jacob [da Silva] Solis (1838-1927)
Three cases of pressure upon the recurrent laryngeal nerve from different causes, with fixation of the left vocal band in phonatory position. Philadelphia: W. J. Dornan, 1886. 16p. DNLM **80-1171**

COHEN, Jacob [da Silva] Solis (1838-1927)
Further history of the case of paralysis of the posterior crico-arytenoid muscles, presented at the first meeting of the association in 1879. With report of autopsy and exhibition of specimen and microscopic preparations. [New York: D. Appleton & Co., 1886.] 10p. DNLM **80-1172**

COHEN, Jacob [da Silva] Solis (1838-1927)
The appearance of larynx nearly twenty years after the extirpation of an epithelioma by external access. [Philadelphia, 1887.] 4p. DNLM **80-1173**

COHEN, Jacob [da Silva] Solis (1838-1927)
Phonatory pneumatic distention, or hernia of the laryngeal sac. [Philadelphia, 1887.] 1 l. DNLM **80-1174**

COHEN, Jacob [da Silva] Solis (1838-1927)
The treatment of affections of the respiratory passages and of blood-poisoning by gaseous enemata. A clinical demonstration before the members of the Philadelphia County Medical Society, at the German Hospital of Philadelphia, March 30, 1887. [Philadelphia, 1887.] 11p. DNLM **80-1175**

COHEN, Jacob [da Silva] Solis (1838-1927)
The treatment of affections of the respiratory passages and of blood-poisoning by gaseous enemata. A clinical demonstration before the members of the Philadelphia County Medical Society, at the German Hospital of Philadelphia, March 30, 1887. [*Also*:] The treatment of pulmonary diseases by gaseous enemata. A preliminary report by Edward T. Bruen. [Philadelphia, 1887.] 15p. DNLM **80-1176**

COHEN, Jacob [da Silva] Solis (1838-1927)
Extracts from an address on the treatment of affections of the respiratory passages and of blood poisonings by gaseous enemata. Boston: Codman & Shurtleff, [1887]. 2 l. DNLM **80-1177**

COHEN, Jacob [da Silva] Solis (1838-1927)
Description of a modified laryngectomy. [New York, 1887.] 4p. DNLM **80-1178**

COHEN, Jacob [da Silva] Solis (1838-1927)
Presidential address delivered before the Philadelphia County Medical Society, Jan. 18, 1888. Philadelphia: W. J. Dornan, 1888. 11p. DNLM **80-1179**

COHEN, Jacob [da Silva] Solis (1838-1927)
Syphilis of the larynx, trachea, and bronchi. Philadelphia: W. J. Dornan, 1888. 24p. DNLM **80-1180**

COHEN, Jacob [da Silva] Solis (1838-1927)
Cantatory paresis. [Philadelphia, 1888.] 4p. DNLM **80-1181**

COHEN, Jacob [da Silva] Solis (1838-1927)
Stricture of the larynx; with extensive cicatrization, from ulcerative tuberculosis. [Philadelphia, 1888.] 4p. DNLM **80-1182**

COHEN, Jacob [da Silva] Solis (1838-1927)
Common membranous sore throat. [New York, 1889.] 6p. DNLM **80-1183**

COHEN, Jacob (da Silva) Solis (1838-1927)
A case of sarcoma of the thyroid gland. [New York, 1889.] 6p. DNLM **80-1184**

COHEN, Solomon Solis (1857-1948)
Pneumato-therapy. A paper read before the Philadelphia County Medical Society, Dec. 8, 1886. Detroit. G. S. Davis, 1887. 31p. DNLM **80-1185**

COHEN, Solomon Solis (1857-1948)
Recent advances in the treatment of pulmonary consumption. A paper read before the Medical Society of the State of Pennsylvania at Bedford Springs, Pa., June 30, 1887. Philadelphia, 1887. 14p. DNLM **80-1186**

COHEN, Solomon Solis (1857-1948)
A case of chyluria, with exhibition of patient and specimens. [Philadelphia, 1889.] 2p. DNLM **80-1187**

COHEN, Solomon Solis (1857-1948)
A design for an apparatus for pneumatic treatment in hospitals. [New York, 1889.] 6p. DNLM **80-1188**

COHEN, Solomon Solis (1857-1948)
Therapeutics of the gouty diathesis. [Philadelphia], 1889. 13p. DNLM **80-1189**

COHEN, Solomon Solis (1857-1948)
Exhibition of an improved apparatus for the therapeutic use of compressed and rarefied air, with remarks on the home-treatment of pulmonary affections. [New York, 1889.] 18p. DNLM **80-1190**

COLE, Palmer Cook (1835-1906)
Tests for diabetes mellitus. Read before the Northwestern Medical and Surgical Society of New York, June 29, 1888. New York: Trow's, 1888. 8p. DNLM **80-1191**

COLEMAN, Alfred (1828-1902)
Manual of dental surgery and pathology. . . . Thoroughly rev. and adapted to the use of American students and practitioners. By Thomas C. Stellwagen. . . . Philadelphia: H. C. Lea's Son & Co., 1882. 408p. DLC; DNLM; MdU-D; PPC **80-1192**

COLEMAN, John Scott (1837-1892)
The multiple wedge principle in the treatment of organic strictures of the urethra. Philadelphia: Collins, 1884. 12p. DNLM **80-1193**

COLEMAN, John Scott (1837-1892)
Combined rectal and intra-uterine irrigator. [Chicago, 1885.] 1 l. DNLM **80-1194**

COLEMAN, John Scott (1837-1892)
Division of the funis during forceps delivery. [New York, 1888.] 2 l. DNLM **80-1195**

COLEMAN, John Scott (1837-1892)
Caesarean section, necessitated and justified by hypertrophic elongation of the cervix; removal of a living female child of seven pounds weight. New York: William Wood & Co., 1888. 17p. DNLM **80-1196**

COLEMAN, John Scott (1837-1892)
Mercuric bi-chloride in diphtheria. Chicago, 1889. 8p. DNLM **80-1197**

COLEMAN, W[illiam] Franklin (1838-1917)
Does tobacco produce amblyopia? [Baltimore, 1885.] 16p. DNLM **80-1198**

COLES, Walter (1839-1892)
On the relations of the placenta to post-partum hemorrhage. [St. Louis, 1880.] 12p. DNLM **80-1199**

COLES, Walter (1839-1892)
The nurse and mother. A manual for the guidance of monthly nurses and mothers. . . . Chicago, Ill., St. Louis, Mo. [etc.]: J. H. Chambers & Co., 1881. 153p. DLC; OCIM; NNNAM; PU **80-1200**

COLES, Walter (1839-1892)
Post-partum atrophy of the uterus. . . . Read before the St. Louis Obstetrical and Gynecological Society, May 19, 1881. . . . St. Louis, Mo.: Chambers' Publishing House, 1881. 12p. DLC **80-1201**

COLES, Walter (1839-1892)
Remarks on syphilis. [St. Louis, 1881.] 16p. DNLM **80-1202**

COLES, Walter (1839-1892)
Post-partum atrophy of the uterus. St. Louis: J. H. Chambers & Co., 1881. 12p. DNLM **80-1203**

COLES, Walter (1839-1892)
A large fibro-cyst of the uterus and ovarian cystoma, co-existing with pregnancy; operation; recovery. [St. Louis, 1882.] 16p. DNLM **80-1204**

COLES, Walter (1839-1892)
Coca; its physiological properties. [Chicago & St. Louis, 1883.] 8p. DNLM **80-1205**

COLES, Walter (1839-1892)
The induction of premature labor in certain cases. St. Louis, 1885. 16p. DNLM **80-1206**

COLLEGE OF DENTISTRY OF THE UNIVERSITY OF CALIFORNIA
Annual announcements for the sessions of 1882-1884 (1.-3.); 1891 to 1897-1898 (10.-16.). San Francisco, 1882-1897. DNLM [List of students and graduates for 1882, 1883, 1890 to 1896-1897, in announcements for subsequent years. List of graduates from 1882 to 1896-1897, in announcement for 1897-1898. Organized in 1882, under the title of the Dental Department of the University of California.] **80-1207**

COLLEGE FOR MEDICAL PRACTITIONERS OF SAINT LOUIS, MO.
Preliminary notice of the . . . March 21, 1882. [St. Louis, 1882.] 1 sheet. DNLM **80-1208**

COLLEGE FOR MEDICAL PRACTITIONERS OF SAINT LOUIS, MO.
Articles of agreement or constitution and the rules of the . . . , in the State of Missouri. [Inaugurated March 21, 1882. Incorporated April 11, 1882.] St. Louis: Med. J. Pub. Co., 1882. 19p. DNLM **80-1209**

COLLEGE FOR MEDICAL PRACTITIONERS OF SAINT LOUIS, MO.
Announcements for the sessions of 1882-1883; 1883-1884. St. Louis, 1882-1883. DNLM [Inaugurated March 21, and incorporated April 11, 1882. Three announcements covering six sessions, commencing Nov. 6, 1882, and ending April 15, 1884. The third session called annual announcement.] **80-1210**

COLLEGE OF MEDICINE OF SYRACUSE UNIVERSITY
Annual announcements for the sessions of 1881-1882 to 1897-1898 (10.-26.). Syracuse, 1881-1897. DNLM [List of students and graduates for 1880-1881 to 1896-1897, in announcements for subsequent years. Graduates from 1873 to 1894, in announcement for 1894-1895.] **80-1211**

COLLEGE OF MEDICINE OF THE UNIVERSITY OF SOUTHERN CALIFORNIA, LOS ANGELES
Annual announcements for the sessions of 1885-1886 (1.); 1892-1893 (8.); 1893-1894 (9.); 1896-1897 (12.). Los Angeles, 1885-1896. DNLM [Established November 1884.] **80-1212**

COLLEGE OF PHYSICIANS OF PHILADELPHIA
Transactions of the College of Physicians of Philadelphia. Centennial volume. Philadelphia, 1887. 391p. DNLM; PPC; PU **80-1213**

COLLEGE OF PHYSICIANS OF PHILADELPHIA
Centennial celebration. Catalogue of loan collection of portraits. 1887. [Philadelphia, 1887.] 23p. PPC **80-1214**

COLLEGE OF PHYSICIANS OF PHILADELPHIA
Catalogue of duplicates in the library of the College of Physicians of Philadelphia. For sale. Philadelphia: W. M. Christy's Sons, 1887. 103p. PPC **80-1215**

COLLEGE OF PHYSICIANS OF PHILADELPHIA
I. An address from a special committee of . . . to the medical societies of the United States, concerning the dangers to which the country is exposed by the ineffectual methods of quarantine at its ports, and in regard to the necessity of national control of maritime quarantine. II. Report of the committee of the College of Physicians of Philadelphia, appointed to investigate the efficiency of our quarantine arrangements for the exclusion of cholera and other epidemic diseases. Philadelphia, 1888. 45p. DLC; DNLM; PPC **80-1216**

COLLEGE OF PHYSICIANS AND SURGEONS. BOSTON
Annual announcements for the sessions of 1880-1881 to 1894-1895 (1.-15.). Boston, 1880-1894. DNLM [List of students and graduates for 1880-1881 to 1893-1894, in announcements for subsequent years. No announcement issued for 1885-1886, temporarily suspended during that year. Organized in 1880, for the co-education of the sexes.] **80-1217**

COLLEGE OF PHYSICIANS AND SURGEONS, BUFFALO [HOMOEOPATHIC]
Annual announcement for the session of 1883 (3.). Buffalo: Haas & Klein, [1882?]. 8p. DNLM [Organized in 1879. No session held in 1881-1882. Ceased to exist after the third session.] **80-1218**

COLLEGE OF PHYSICIANS AND SURGEONS OF CHICAGO
Annual announcements for the sessions of 1882-1883 to 1895-1896 (1.-14.); 1897-1898 (16.). Chicago, 1882-1897. DNLM [List of students and graduates for 1882-1883 to 1894-1895; 1896-1897, in announcements for subseequent years. Announcement for 1892-1893 contains the first decennial catalogue, 1881-1891. Organized in 1882. In 1897 it became the Medical Department of the University of Illinois.] **80-1219**

COLLEGE OF PHYSICIANS AND SURGEONS OF CHICAGO
Announcement of the spring session of lectures and practitioners course for 1883. Chicago: A. G. Newell, 1883. 8p. DNLM **80-1220**

COLLEGE OF PHYSICIANS AND SURGEONS IN THE CITY OF NEW YORK. MEDICAL DEPARTMENT OF COLUMBIA UNIVERSITY
Syllabus of Cartwright lectures. 1886. Lecture II. Degeneration and regeneration. [New York, 1886.] 2 l. DNLM; NNC **80-1221**

COLLEGE OF PHYSICIANS AND SURGEONS IN THE CITY OF NEW YORK. MEDICAL DEPARTMENT OF COLUMBIA UNIVERSITY
Addresses at the inauguration of the new college building, Sept. 29, 1887; and of the Sloane Maternity Hospital and Vanderbilt Clinic, Dec. 29, 1887. New York: By the College, 1888. 56p. DNLM; NNC **80-1222**

COLLEGE OF THERAPEUTICS. THE MEDICAL DEPARTMENT OF THE AMERICAN UNIVESITY, BOSTON
Announcement for the session of 1883-1884 (1.). [Boston, 1883.] 1 l. DNLM; MBM **80-1223**

COLLINS, James (1831-1895) and Charles K. MILLS
Cases with hydrophobic symptoms; with microscopical reports by Carl Seiler. [Philadelphia, 1880.] 11p. DNLM **80-1224**

COLLINS, Samuel B.
Theriaki: a treatise on the habitual use of narcotic poison. How the habit is formed, its consequences and cure. Laporte, Ind., [1887]. 64p. DLC; DNLM **80-1225**

COLLINS, Samuel B.
Theriaki: a treatise on the habitual use of narcotic poison. How the habit is formed, its consequences and cure. [La Porte, Ind., 1888.] 76p. 1 l. DNLM **80-1226**

COLLINS, Samuel H.
Yellow fever; a brief sketch of its natural and clinical history, together with some practical suggestions relating to the sanitary control of yellow fever outbreaks. [Indianapolis: W. B. Burford, 1889.] 7p. DNLM **80-1227**

COMBE, George (1877-1858)
Essay on the constitution of man, and its relations to external objects. With an additional chapter on the harmony between phrenology and revelation, by Joseph A. Warne. Only authorized American ed. New ed. New York: S. R. Wells & Co., 1880. 436p. DNLM; NNNAM; PPC; PU **80-1228**

CONANT, Clarence M.
An obstetric mentor. A hand-book of homoeopathic treatment required during pregnancy, parturition, and the puerperal season. New York: A. L. Chatterton Pub. Co., 1884. 212p. DNLM; NNNAM; PPHa; PU **80-1229**

CONKLIN, W. Judkins (1844-1916)
A report upon the sanitary condition of the public schools of Dayton, with special reference to the eyesight of the pupils. Dayton, O., 1880. 32p. DNLM **80-1230**

CONKLIN, William Judkins (1844-1916)
Impacted fracture of the neck of the femur, with inversion of the foot. [Columbus, O., 1882.] 8p. DNLM **80-1231**

CONN, Granville Priest (1832-1916)
State medicine. Concord: Evans & Sleeper, 1881. 20p. DNLM **80-1232**

CONN, Granville Priest (1832-1916)
Observations upon the importance and means of ventilation. Concord: P. B. Cogswell, 1882. 28p. DNLM **80-1233**

CONN, Granville Priest (1832-1916)
Disposal of garbage. Remarks upon the necessity of some advancement in the conditions now existing in New Hampshire. Concord: Repub. Press Ass., 1889. 13p. DNLM **80-1234**

CONNER, Phineas Sanborn (1839-1909)
Hospitals for the sick; their construction and management. [Boston, 1886.] 14p. DNLM **80-1235**

CONNOR, Leartus (1843-1911)
Glaucoma caused by mental worry, illustrated by the report of a case. Detroit: Post & Tribune Co., 1881. 6p. DNLM **80-1236**

CONNOR, Leartus (1843-1911)
The use of hot water in the local treatment of diseases of the eye. [Philadelphia, 1881.] 7p. DNLM **80-1237**

CONNOR, Leartus (1843-1911)
A clinical study of syphilis of the eye and its appendages. [Philadelphia, 1883.] 12p. DNLM **80-1238**

CONNOR, Leartus (1843-1911)
Notes on the treatment of trachoma by jequirity. [Detroit, 1884.] 16p. DNLM **80-1239**

CONNOR, Leartus (1843-1911)
Mumps as a cause of sudden deafness. [Philadelphia, 1884.] 9p. DNLM **80-1240**

CONNOR, Leartus (1843-1911)
Hot water in the management of eye diseases. Some suggestions. Detroit: D. O. Haynes & Co., 1887. 16p. DNLM **80-1241**

CONNOR, Leartus (1843-1911)
The American Academy of Medicine; its objects, its signs of promise, and its obstacles, its field of work, and some suggestions looking to an increase of its efficiency. The president's address, delivered . . . Chicago, Nov. 13, 1889. Detroit, 1889. 43p. DNLM **80-1242**

CONRAD, J[ohn] S[ummerfield] (1839-1896)
A paper on small-pox. Baltimore: Innes & Co., 1884. 26p. 3 tabs. DNLM; MdU-D **80-1243**

CONRAD, J[ohn] S[ummerfield] (1839-1896)
Hallucination, and its allied states. Baltimore: I. Friedenwald, 1888. 13p. DNLM **80-1244**

COOK, A. B[rown] (1828-1895)
Elixir paraldehyde; the coming remedy, as a substitute for opiates and anodynes. Louisville, 1888. 2 l. DNLM **80-1245**

COOK, Charles H.
Pyaemia of doubtful origin; apparently "spontaneous." [Boston, 1880.] 15p. DNLM **80-1246**

COOK, George Wythe
Is dentition a cause of disease? Washington; Taylor & Bart, 1887. 9p. DNLM **80-1247**

COOK, Marc (1854-1822)
The wilderness cure. New York: William Wood & Co., 1881. 153p. CtY-M; DNLM; NNNAM; PU **80-1248**

COOK, W. C.
Entero-colitis (summer diarrhoea of children). Read before the Nashville Academy of Medicine and Surgery. Nashville, Tenn.: Brandon Print. Co., 1886. 14p. DNLM **80-1249**

COOK, W. C.
Necessity for teaching hygiene in schools. Read before and unanimously adopted by the Ninth International Medical Congress, Washington, D.C., September 5-10, 1887. Nashville: Brandon Print. Co., 1887. 14p. DNLM **80-1250**

COOKE, Nicholas Francis (1829-1885)
A treatise on antiseptic medication, or Déclat's method. . . . Chicago: Gross & Delbridge, 1882. 120p. DLC; DNLM; OCIM; NNNAM **80-1251**

COOKE, Nicholas Francis (1829-1885)
The pocket doctor. . . . Chicago, Ill.: Park City Publishing House, 1886. 34p. DLC; OCIM **80-1252**

COOMES, Martin F. (*b.* 1847)
Naso-pharyngeal catarrh. Louisville, Ky.: Bradley & Gilbert, 1880. 105p. DNLM; OCIM **80-1253**

COOMES, Martin F. (*b.* 1847)
Observations on strabismus. [Louisville, 1882.] 2 l. DNLM **80-1254**

COOMES, M[artin] F. (*b.* 1847)
Some thoughts on phthisis, with special reference to the value of laryngeal symptoms in diagnosis. [New York, 1882.] 7p. DNLM **80-1255**

COOMES, M[artin] F. (*b.* 1847)
Menstrual amblyopia. [Louisville, 1882.] 4p. DNLM **80-1256**

COOMES, M[artin] F. (*b.* 1847)
Florida as a health resort. [Louisville, 1883.] 10p. DNLM **80-1257**

COOMES, M[artin] F. (*b.* **1847)**
Inflammations of the iris, with report of cases. [Louisville, 1885.] 8p. DNLM **80-1258**

COOMES, M[artin] F. (*b.* **1847)**
A description of the improved sonometer. Opium eating. [Louisville, 1885.] 8p. DNLM **80-1259**

COOPER, Alfred (1838-1908)
Syphilis and pseudo-syphilis. Philadelphia: P. Blakiston, Son & Co., 1884. 339p. CtY-M; DNLM; NNNAM; PPC **80-1260**

COOPER, Hunter P[ope] (1860-1906)
The early diagnosis of spinal caries, with remarks on treatment. Atlanta, [1887]. 10p. DNLM **80-1261**

COOPER, Hunter P[ope] (1860-1906)
The treatment of hemorrhoids. [Atlanta], 1888. 9p. DNLM **80-1262**

CORDELL, Eugene F[auntleroy] (1843-1913)
On the continuous inhalation of the vapor of slacking lime in the treatment of membranous laryngitis. [Baltimore, 1882.] 4p. DNLM **80-1263**

CORDELL, Eugene F[auntleroy] (1843-1913)
Woman as a physician; illustrious examples drawn from history; the advantages of the female medical student of to-day compared with those of her predecessors, with suggestions as to their proper utilization. [Baltimore, 1883.] 4p. DNLM **80-1264**

CORNIL, Victor (1837-1908)
A manual of pathological histology. By V. Cornil . . . and L. Ranvier. . . . Transl. with notes and additions, by E. O. Shakespeare and J. Henry C. Simes. . . . Philadelphia: Henry C. Lea, 1880. 784p. DLC; DNLM; NNNAM; PPC **80-1265**

CORNIL, Victor (1837-1908)
Syphilis. . . . Transl., with notes and additions, by J. Henry C. Simes . . . and J. William White. With eighty-four illustrations. Philadelphia: Henry C. Lea's Son & Co., 1882. 461p. DLC; DNLM; MBM; PPC **80-1266**

CORNING, James Leonard (1853-1923)
Carotid compression and brain rest. . . . New York: A. D. F. Randolph & Co., [1882]. 39p. DLC; DNLM; NNNAM **80-1267**

CORNING, James Leonard (1853-1923)
Brain-rest. . . . New York: G. P. Putnam's Sons, 1883. 103p. DLC; DNLM; NNNAM; PU **80-1268**

CORNING, James Leonard (1853-1923)
Brain exhaustion, with some preliminary considerations on cerebral dynamics. . . . New York: D. Appleton & Co., 1884. 234p. DLC; DNLM; MBM; NNNAM **80-1269**

CORNING, James Leonard (1853-1923)
Brain exhaustion and its treatment. New York: D. Appleton & Co., 1884. 13p. DNLM **80-1270**

CORNING, James Leonard (1853-1923)
Electrization of the sympathetic and pneumogastric nerves, with simultaneous bilateral compression of the carotids. New York: D. Appleton & Co., 1884. 11p. DNLM **80-1271**

CORNING, James Leonard (1853-1923)
On the prolongation of the anesthetic effects of the hydrochlorate of cocaine when subcutaneously injected. An experimental study. [New York, 1885.] 6p. DNLM **80-1272**

CORNING, James Leonard (1853-1923)
Local anaesthesia in general medicine and surgery, being the practical application of the author's recent discoveries. . . . New York: D. Appleton & Co., 1886. 103p. DLC; DNLM; MH-M; NNNAM **80-1273**

CORNING, James Leonard (1853-1923)
A treatise on headache and neuralgia, including spinal irritation and a disquisition on normal and morbid sleep. . . . New York: E. B. Treat, 1888. 231p. DLC; DNLM; OCIM; NNNAM **80-1274**

CORNING, James Leonard (1853-1923)
A treatise on hysteria and epilepsy, with some concluding observations on epileptic insomnia. . . . Detroit, Mich.: G. S. Davis, 1888. 176p. DLC; DNLM; OCIM; PPC **80-1275**

CORNWELL, Henry G.
The origin and prevalence of myopia among school children. Youngstown, O., 1880. 11p. DNLM **80-1276**

CORNWELL, Henry G.
A case of Basedow's disease, terminating in total loss of sight from [neuro-paralytic] inflammation of the cornea. Youngstown, O., 1881. 8p. DNLM **80-1277**

CORNWELL, Henry G.
A compound dermoid cyst of the orbit. Columbus, 1882. 7p. 1 plate. DNLM **80-1278**

CORNWELL, Henry G.
The first quarterly report of the Eye and Ear Dispensary of Starling Medical College, July 1, 1882. Cincinnati: Cincinnati Lancet Press Print, 1882. 8p. DNLM **80-1279**

CORNWELL, Henry G.
Consultation chart of the eye-symptoms and eye-complications of general diseases, arranged after Foerster and others. Columbus: H. C. McClelland & Co., [1883?]. Broadside. DNLM; OCIM **80-1280**

CORR, Lucinda H.
Hygiene and heredity, with anatomy and physiology in outline lessons for blackboard instruction. . . . Carlinville, Ill.: Macoupin Printing Co., 1883. 26p. DLC **80-1281**

CORSON, Eugene R[ollin] (*b.* **1855)**
The future of the colored race in the United States from an ethnic and medical standpoint. New York, 1887. 32p. DNLM; NN **80-1282**

CORSON, Hiram (1804-1896)
Notes on the treatment of cholera during the epidemic of 1832. Philadelphia, 1884. 9p. DNLM; PPC **80-1283**

CORSON, Hiram (1804-1896)
Reminiscences of the cholera epidemic of 1832. Philadelphia, 1884. 6p. DNLM **80-1284**

CORSON, Hiram (1804-1896)
Our hospitals for the insane poor. A plea to the legislature for a reorganization of the acts of assembly regulating the State hospitals. [n.p., 1885, *vel subseq.*] 13p. DNLM
80-1285

CORSON, Hiram (1804-1896)
Chorea and its treatment by cimicifuga racemosa. [Philadelphia, 1886.] 7p. DNLM **80-1286**

CORSON, Hiram (1804-1896)
On the statistics of three thousand and thirty-six cases of labor. [New York, 1886.] 39p. DNLM
80-1287

CORSON, Hiram (1804-1896)
The rhus glabrum. A remedy for stomatitis. [Philadelphia, 1887.] 4p. DNLM **80-1288**

CORSON, Hiram (1804-1896)
An almost unrecognized cause of disease in young children. Philadelphia, 1888. 5p. DNLM **80-1289**

CORSON, Hiram (1804-1896)
Our hospitals for the insane. Philadelphia, 1888. 8p. DNLM
80-1290

CORSON, Hiram (1804-1896)
A brief history of the proceedings in the Medical Society of Pennsylvania, in the years 1859, 1860, 1866-1868, 1870, 1871, to procure the recognition of women physicians by the medical profession of the State; to which is added an account of the measures adopted by the society at its annual meetings, in, 1877-1879 to procure a law to authorize trustees of hospitals for the insane-poor, under the control of the State, to appoint women physicians to have entire medical control of the insane of their sex. Philadelphia: J. B. Rodgers, 1888. 40p. DNLM; PPC; PU **80-1291**

CORSON, Hiram (1804-1896)
State hospitals for the insane poor. New York, 1889. 5p. DNLM **80-1292**

CORSON, John W. (1816-1882)
Essay on a healthy impulse of the heart as a valuable sign of comparative safety in the use of anaesthetics. Newark, N.J.: L. J. Hardham, 1880 [1879]. DNLM **80-1293**

COTTELL, H[enry] A.
Esthetics of medicine. Louisville, Ky.: J. P. Morton & Co., 1886. 26p. DNLM **80-1294**

COTTING, B[enjamin] E[ddy] (1812-1898)
Historical sketch of the Obstetrical Society of Boston. [*Also*:] Biographical sketches of deceased members of the Obstetrical Society of Boston; with an outline of the earlier obstetrical history of Boston and vicinity. By William W. Wellington. Boston: D. Clapp & Son, 1881. 73p. CtY-M; DNLM; MBM
80-1295

COTTING, B[enjamin] E[ddy] (1812-1898)
A few fragmentary remarks on the radical relief of infleshed toe-nail. [Boston, 1887. 4p. DNLM **80-1296**

COTTING, B[enjamin] E[ddy] (1812-1898)
Professional reminiscences. Prepared for the Norfolk District Medical Society. Boston: D. Clapp & Son, 1888. 112p. DNLM; MA; MBM; MWA **80-1297**

COTTING, B[enjamin] E[ddy] (1812-1898)
The life of the foetus. [Boston, 1889.] 8p. DNLM
80-1298

COTTING, B[enjamin] E[ddy] (1812-1898)
A murderer's dying confession disproved by surgical and anatomical facts. Boston, 1889. 16p. DNLM; MH-M
80-1299

COUES, Elliott (1842-1899)
The nature of the human temporal bone. Cambridge, 1882. 36p. DNLM; MBM **80-1300**

COUES, Elliott (1842-1899) and Leonard K. GRAVES
Addresses delivered at the sixty-third annual commencement of the Medical College (Medical Department of the Columbian University), March 18, 1885. Washington, D.C.: W. H. Moore, 1885. 16p. DNLM **80-1301**

COUES, Elliott (1842-1899) and D. K. SHUTE
Neuro-myology; classification of the muscles of the human body with reference to their innervation, and new nomenclature of the muscles. New York: Trow's Co., 1887. 48p. DNLM; NNNAM **80-1302**

COUES, Elliott (1842-1899)
"A woman in the case." An address, delivered at the annual commencement of the National Medical College, in the Congregational Church of Washington, March 16, 1887. . . . Washington, D.C. [etc.]: Brentano's (A. S. Witherbee & Co., proprietors), [1887]. 32p. DLC **80-1303**

COULSON, William (1802-1877)
. . . Coulson on the diseases of the bladder and prostate gland. 6th ed., rev. by Walter J. Coulson. . . . New York: William Wood & Co., 1881. 393p. DLC; NNNAM; OCIM; PPC
80-1304

COUNCILMAN, William Thomas (1854-1933)
A contribution to the study of inflammation as illustrated by induced keratitis. Prize essay of the Baltimore Academy of Medicine. Baltimore: J. Murphy & Co., 1880. 28p. 1 plate. DNLM; MdU-D **80-1305**

COWAN, Frank (1844-1906)
The principles and practice of medicine in Corea. . . . Greenesburgh, Pa.: The Oliver Publishing House, 1888. 24p. DLC
80-1306

COWL, Walter Y.
A brief history of the definition of disease, with a consideration of the pathological concepts of Hahnemann. The definition of an homoeopathist. New York, 1883. 22p. DNLM; PPHa **80-1307**

COWL, Walter Y. and LEAL
A brief résumé of the clinical examination of urine, chemical and microscopical. New York: Anderson, Stanley & Brown, 1883. 40p. hectograph. DNLM; NNNAM
80-1308

COWL, Walter Y.
Inaugural address on the work of the New York Society for Medico-Scientific Investigation. New York: M. J. Rooney, 1887. 7p. DNLM **80-1309**

COWLES, Edward (1837-1919)
Nursing-reform for the insane. [Utica, N.Y., 1887.] 16p. 1 plate. DNLM **80-1310**

COWLES, Edward (1837-1919)
Insistent and fixed ideas. [Baltimore, 1888.] 48p. DNLM
80-1311

COWLING, Richard O[swald] (1839-1881)
Aphorisms in fractures. Louisville: J. P. Morton & Co., 1881. 70p. DNLM; OCIM **80-1312**

COWPERTHWAITE, Allen Corson (*b.* 1848)
An elementary text-book of the materia medica. Characteristic, analytical, and comparative. Chicago: Duncan Bros., 1880. 339p. OCIM; PPHa **80-1313**

COWPERTHWAITE, Allen Corson (*b.* 1848)
Text-book of materia medica. Characteristic, analytical, and comparative. Second edition, revised and enlarged. Chicago: Duncan Bros., 1882. 576p. OCLloyd; PPHa
80-1314

COWPERTHWAITE, Allen Corson (*b.* 1848)
Text-book of materia medica. Characteristic, analytical, and comparative. Third edition. Chicago: Gross & Delbridge, 1885. 697p. DLC; PPHa **80-1315**

COWPERTHWAITE, Allen Corson (*b.* 1848)
Text-book of materia medica. Characteristic, analytical, and comparative. Fourth edition. Revised and enlarged, with clinical index. Chicago: Gross & Delbridge, 1887. 722p. OCIM; PPHa **80-1316**

COWPERTHWAITE, Allen Corson (*b.* 1848)
A text-book of gynecology. . . . Chicago: Gross & Delbridge, 1888. 533p. DLC; DNLM; NNNAM; PPHa
80-1317

CRANDALL, Charles R.
Diagnosis of consumption during the first stage. [New York, 1886.] 10p. DNLM **80-1318**

CRANE, James (1818-1888)
The prevention of certain contagious diseases, by local boards of health. Boston: Rand, Avery & Co., 1881. 3 l. DNLM
80-1319

CRAWFORD, John B. (*d.* 1894)
An essay on the indigenous malarial diseases of Wyoming Valley. Wilke-Barre, Pa., 1881. 21p. DNLM
80-1320

CRAWFORD, John B. (*d.* 1894)
Wounds of the brain. Read by appointment before the Luzerne County Medical Society at Wilkes-Barre, Jan. 14, 1885. Wilkes-Barre, Pa., 1885. 21p. DNLM **80-1321**

CROCKER, Henry Radcliffe (1845-1909)
Diseases of the skin; their description, pathology, diagnosis, and treatment. . . . Philadelphia: P. Blakiston, Son & Co., 1888. 746p. DNLM; IEN-M; NNNAM; PPC
80-1322

CROCKER, SAM'L A. & CO.
Illustrated catalogue of surgical instruments and appliances. Cincinnati, O.: Spencer & Craig, 1886. 216p. DNLM; OCIM
80-1323

CROOKSHANK, Edgar M[arch] (1858-1928)
Manual of bacteriology. 2nd ed. New York: J. H. Vail & Co., 1887. 439p. 29 plates. DNLM; NN; NNNAM; PU
80-1324

CROTHERS, Thomas Davison (1842-1918)
What shall we do with the inebriate? St. Louis, 1881. 24p. DNLM **80-1325**

CROTHERS, Thomas Davison (1842-1918)
A clinical study of the disease, and curability of inebriety. Philadelphia, 1882. 9p. DNLM **80-1326**

CROTHERS, Thomas Davison (1842-1918)
The trance state in inebriety; its medico-legal relations. With an introduction on the nature and character of the trance state, by Geo. M. Beard. Hartford: Lockwood & Brainard Co., 1882. 39p. DNLM **80-1327**

CROTHERS, Thomas Davison (1842-1918)
The disease of inebriety and its social science relations, read before the American Social Science Association, at Saratoga, New York, September 5, 1884. Boston, 1884. 14p. DNLM
80-1328

CROTHERS, Thomas Davison (1842-1918)
Neuratrophia. The cause of inebriety; a clinical study. St. Louis, 1883. 9p. DNLM **80-1329**

CROTHERS, Thomas Davison (1842-1918)
Inebriate automatism. [Chicago, 1884.] 9p. DNLM
80-1330

CROTHERS, Thomas Davison (1842-1918)
Certain hereditary and psychical phenomena in inebriety. St. Louis, 1886. 15p. DNLM **80-1331**

CROTHERS, Thomas Davison (1842-1918)
Editorial reprints from the Journal of Inebriety. [Inebriety.] [Hartford, 1886.] 20p. DNLM **80-1332**

CROTHERS, Thomas Davison (1842-1918)
Inebriety and heredity. Read before the Temperance Institute of the Presbyterian churches of New York City, February 7, 1886. Hartford, Conn., 1886. 16p. DNLM
80-1333

CROTHERS, Thomas Davison (1842-1918)
Inebriate. Maniacs. [New York, 1886.] 8p. DNLM
80-1334

CROTHERS, Thomas Davison (1842-1918)
The Otto case; a medico-legal study. [Hartford, 1886.] 9p. DNLM **80-1335**

CROTHERS, Thomas Davison (1842-1918)
States of delirium in inebriety. [St. Louis, 1886.] 7p. DNLM
80-1336

CROTHERS, Thomas Davison (1842-1918)
The alcoholic question medically considered. [Hartford, 1887.] 5p. DNLM **80-1337**

CROTHERS, Thomas Davison (1842-1918)
An address delivered before the corporation of the Washingtonian Home, Boston, Mass., on its thirtieth anniversary, February 20, 1888. [Boston], 1888. 18p. DNLM
80-1338

CROTHERS, Thomas Davison (1842-1918)
Alcoholic trance in criminal cases. Hartford, Conn.: The Case, Lockwood & Brainard Comp., 1889. 12p. DNLM
80-1339

CROTHERS, Thomas Davison (1842-1918)
Inebriate asylums and their work. Part of a lecture delivered before the Young Men's Christian Association, at Toronto, Canada, Oct. 2, 1888. [Hartford, 1888.] 16p. DNLM **80-1340**

CROTHERS, Thomas Davison (1842-1918)
Should inebriates be punished by death for crime? [New York, 1888.] 8p. DNLM **80-1341**

CROTHERS, Thomas Davison (1842-1918)
Medico-legal problems of inebriety. Illustrated by the Swift case. Hartford, Conn.: The Case, Lockwood & Brainard Comp., 1889. 15p. DNLM **80-1342**

CROTHERS, Thomas Davison (1842-1918)
Sketch of the late Dr. Edward Turner, the founder of inebriate asylums. Hartford, Conn.: Case, Lockwood & Brainard, 1889. 25p. 2 plates. DNLM **80-1343**

CROWLEY, C. George
Dental bibliography: a standard reference list of books on dentistry published throughout the world from 1536 to 1885. Arranged chronologically, and supplemented with a complete cross-reference to authors. . . . Philadelphia: The S. S. White Dental Mfg. Co., 1885. 180p. DLC; DNLM; PPC; PU **80-1344**

CRUMPLER, Rebecca
A book of medical discourses, in two parts. Part 1: treating of the cause, prevention, and cure of infantile bowel complaints. . . . Part 2: containing miscellaneous information concerning the life and growth of beings; the beginning of womanhood; also, the cause, prevention, and cure of many . . . complaints of women, and youth of both sexes. . . . Boston: Cashman, Keating & Co., printers, 1883. 144p. DLC; MBM **80-1345**

CULBERTSON, H[oward] (1828-1890)
Several cases of cataract, illustrating the importance of Prof. H. Knapp's method of extraction. [Zanesville, O., 1880.] 15p. DNLM **80-1346**

CULBERTSON, H[oward] (1828-1890)
Report of a case of glycosuric retinitis. [Detroit] : G. S. Davis, [1880]. 12p. DNLM **80-1347**

CULBERTSON, H[oward] (1828-1890)
Medical doses and therapeutic effects. [Detroit] : G. S. Davis, [1880]. 16p. DNLM **80-1348**

CULBERTSON, H[oward] (1828-1890)
Refraction of the eye, as distinguished from accommodation and estimated as an equivalent, from the index of refraction. [Cincinnati, 1882.] 6p. DNLM **80-1349**

CULBERTSON, H[oward] (1828-1890)
A form of spectacle frames in lieu of nose pieces. [Chicago, 1883.] 7p. DNLM **80-1350**

CULBERTSON, H[oward] (1828-1890)
A comparison of total and manifest hypermetropia, as determined by the prisoptometer, with and without the use of mydriatics. New York: D. Appleton & Co., 1884. 8p. 1 tab. DNLM **80-1351**

CULBERTSON, H[oward] (1828-1890)
On the value of the prisoptometer in determining the degree of myopia. [St. Louis, 1884.] 8p. 1 tab. DNLM **80-1352**

CULBERTSON, H[oward] (1828-1890)
An alleged defect of the prisoptometer. St. Louis: J. H. Chambers & Co., 1888. 6p. DNLM **80-1353**

CULBERTSON, H[oward] (1828-1890)
Binocular astigmatism. Chicago, 1888. 8p. DNLM **80-1354**

CULBERTSON, H[oward] (1828-1890)
In memoriam. The life and character of C. C. Hildreth. A memorial sketch read before the Zanesville Medical Society, September 5, 1889. [Cincinnati, 1889.] 2 l. DNLM **80-1355**

CULBERTSON, H[oward] (1828-1890)
Personal reminiscences of the subject of anaesthesia. Cleveland, O.: Williams Publishing Co., [1889]. 12p. DNLM **80-1356**

CULIN, Stewart (1858-1929)
Chinese drug stores in America. [Philadelphia, 1887.] 6p. DNLM **80-1357**

CULIN, Stewart (1858-1929)
The practice of medicine by the Chinese in Ámerica. [Philadelphia, 1887.] 3p. DNLM **80-1358**

CURRIER, Andrew F[ay] (*b.* 1851)
Eucalyptus globulus in gynaecological practice, together with an account of several cases in which it was used. [Philadelphia, 1882.] 4p. DNLM **80-1359**

CURRIER, Andrew F[ay] (*b.* 1851)
Gonorrhoea in the female. New York, 1885. 21p. DNLM **80-1360**

CURRIER, Andrew F[ay] (*b.* 1851)
Local vs. general treatment in gynaecology. [New York, 1886.] 14p. DNLM **80-1361**

CURRIER, Andrew F[ay] (*b.* 1851)
Some considerations concerning cancer of the uterus, especially its palliative treatment in its later stages. [New York, 1887.] 17p. DNLM **80-1362**

CURRIER, Andrew F[ay] (*b.* 1851)
The disorders of menstruation. [Philadelphia, 1889.] 26p. DNLM **80-1363**

CURRIER, Charles G[ilman]
The efficacy of filters and other means employed to purify drinking-water. A bacteriological study. [Philadelphia], 1889. 42p. DNLM **80-1364**

CURRIER, Charles S.
Chronic nasal catarrh. San Francisco: Crocker & Co., 1884. 9p. CU-M **80-1365**

CURRIER, Charles S.
A few words about oxygen. San Francisco: Murdock & Co., 1888. 18p. CU-M **80-1366**

CURTIN, Roland G[ideon] (1839-1913)
The influence of sea air on syphilitic phthisis. Philadelphia: W. J. Dornan, 1887. 7p. DNLM **80-1367**

CURTIN, Roland G[ideon] (1839-1913)
Rocky Mountain fever. [New York, 1887.] 11p. DNLM **80-1368**

CURTIN, Roland G[ideon] (1839-1913)
Climate as an etiological factor in Graves's disease. Philadelphia: W. J. Dornan, 1889. 7p. DNLM
80-1369

CURTIN, Roland G[ideon] (1839-1913)
The climatology of hemoptysis in chronic lung disease from an etiological and therapeutic standpoint. Philadelphia: W. J. Dornan, 1889. 13p. DNLM **80-1370**

CURTIS, B. Farquhar (1857-1924)
The results of laparotomy for acute intestinal obstruction. [New York, 1888.] 24p. DNLM **80-1371**

CURTIS, Edward (1838-1912)
Manual of general medical technology including prescription-writing. . . . New York: William Wood & Co., 1883. 234p. DLC; NNNAM; OCIM; PPC **80-1372**

CURTIS, F[rederic] C[olton] (*b.* 1843)
Report on sudden outbreak of enteric fever, at Port Jervis, during the fall of 1883. [Albany, 1884.] 23p. 1 map, 1 plan. DNLM **80-1373**

CURTIS, F[rederic] C[olton] (*b.* 1843)
Glimpses of early medicine in Albany. The introductory address of the course of 1886-1887 at the Albany Medical College, delivered September 21, 1886. Albany: Burdick & Taylor, 1886. 14p. DNLM **80-1374**

CURTIS, H[enry] Holbrook (1856-1920)
The nasal trephine and its advantages. With a consideration of batteries and electrical apparatus used in nasal surgery. With practical demonstrations. [New York, 1887.] 10p. DNLM
80-1375

CURTISS, Romaine J.
Clinical cases of surgical diseases of women. [Philadelphia, 1882.] 7p. DNLM **80-1376**

CURTISS, Romaine J.
Nervous shock as a therapeutical agent. St. Louis, 1882. 13p. DNLM **80-1377**

CURWEN, John (1821-1901)
On the propositions of the Association of Superintendents of American Hospitals for the Insane. [Harrisburg, 1880.] 16p. DNLM **80-1378**

CURWEN, John (1821-1901)
The original thirteen members of the Association of Medical Superintendents, of American Institutions for the Insane. Warren, Pa.: E. Cowan & Co., 1885. 49p. 13 port. DNLM
80-1379

CURWEN, John (1821-1901)
History of the Association of Medical Superintendents of American Institutions for the Insane, from 1844 to 1884, inclusive; with a list of the different hospitals for the insane, and the names and dates of appointment and resignation of the medical superintendent, compiled from the records of the Association. Warren, Pa.: E. Cowan & Co., 1885. 210p. DNLM; NNNAM; PPC **80-1380**

CURWEN, John (1821-1901)
Memoir of Thomas S. Kirkbirde, M.D., LL.D., prepared by direction of the Association of Medical Superintendents of American Institutions for the Insane, by John Curwen, M.D., Charles H. Nichols, M.D., John H. Callender, M.D.; read at the meeting of the Association at Saratoga, New York, June 16, 1885. Warren, Pa.: E. Cowan & Co., printers, 1885. 38p. DLC **80-1381**

CUSHIER, Elizabeth M.
A case of myxoedema. New York: G. P. Putnam's Sons, 1882. 16p. DNLM **80-1382**

CUSHING, Alvin Matthew (*b.* 1829)
Leucorrhoea. Its concomitant symptoms and its homoeopathic treatment. Rev. and enl. 2nd ed. Boston: Alfred Mudge & Son, 1882. 163p. DLC; DNLM; MBM; NNNAM
80-1383

CUSHING, Clinton (1840-1904)
A year's work in abdominal surgery. [San Francisco, 1889.] 13p. 1 tab. DNLM **80-1384**

CUSHING, E[rnest] W[atson] (1847-1916)
The specific and infectious character of tuberculosis, with exhibition of the bacilli of tuberculosis, and those of malignant pustule (anthrax). Read before the section for clinical medicine, pathology, and hygiene of the Suffolk District Medical Society, Nov. 11, 1885. Boston: Cupples, Upham & Co., 1885. 20p. DNLM; MBM **80-1385**

CUSHING, E[rnest] W[atson] (1847-1916)
On the examination of sputa for tubercle bacilli, with cases. Boston: Cupples, Upham & Co., 1886. 15p. DNLM
80-1386

CUSHING, E[rnest] W[atson] (1847-1916)
History and value of antiseptics; together with remarks on antiseptic dressings. Boston: Grosvenor & Richards, 1886. 23p. DNLM **80-1387**

CUSHING, E[rnest] W[atson] (1847-1916)
Relations of certain bacteria to puerperal inflammations. [Philadelphia], 1886. 22p. DNLM **80-1388**

CUSHING, E[rnest] W[atson] (1847-1916)
On erosions of the cervix uteri; their pathology and treatment. [Hartford, 1887.] 18p. DNLM **80-1389**

CUSHING, E[rnest] W[atson] (1847-1916)
"Septic bacteria" and antiseptic dressings. . . . Boston: Grosvenor & Richards, [1887]. 24p. DNLM
80-1390

CUSHING, E[rnest] W[atson] (1847-1916)
Tubal pregnancy; rupture; recovery. Boston, 1888. 9 l. 1 sheet with 8 plates. DNLM **80-1391**

CUSHING, H[ayworth] W[arren]
An improved method for the radical cure of femoral hernia. Boston: Cupples & Hurd, 1889. 6p. DNLM
80-1392

CUSHING, H[ayworth] W[arren]
The "right angle" continuous intestinal suture. Boston: Rockwell & Churchill, 1889. 9p. 7 plates. DNLM
80-1393

CUTLER, Condict W[alker] (1859-1930)
The medical student's essentials of physics. . . . New York: J. H. Vail & Co., 1884. 123p. DLC; DNLM; NNNAM; PPJ
80-1394

CUTLER, Condict W[alker] (1859-1930)
Student's essentials of chemistry, theoretical and inorganic. New York, 1885. 192p. DNLM; NN; PU
80-1395

CUTLER, Condict W[alker] (1859-1930)
Manual of differential medical diagnosis. . . . New York: G. P. Putnam's Sons, 1886. 161p. DLC; DNLM; NNNAM; PPC
80-1396

CUTLER, Condict W[alker] (1859-1930)
Introductory lessons in organic chemistry. New York: J. H. Vail & Co., 1886. 121p. DNLM; MH; NNNAM; PU
80-1397

CUTLER, Condict W[alker] (1859-1930)
Differential diagnosis of the diseases of the skin. . . . New York: G. P. Putnam's Sons, 1887. 139p. DLC; DNLM; NNNAM; PPC **80-1398**

CUTLER, Condict W[alker] (1859-1930)
The medical student's essentials of physics and chemistry. . . . [2nd ed.] New York: J. H. Vail & Co., 1887. 140p. DLC; NNNAM; PPC; PU **80-1399**

CUTLER, Condict W[alker] (1859-1930)
Essentials of physics and chemistry written especially for the use of students in medicine. 3rd ed. New York & London: G. P. Putnam's Sons, 1889. 296p. DNLM; OCIM; NNNAM; PPC **80-1400**

CUTLER, Elbridge G[erry] (*b.* 1846) and G. M. GARLAND
Percussion outlines. Boston: Houghton Mifflin, 1882. 65p. MBM **80-1401**

CUTLER, Elbridge G[erry] (*b.* 1846)
Iodoform poisoning. Read before the Boston Society for Medical Improvement, May 10, 1886. Boston: Cupples, Upham & Co., 1886. 31p. DNLM **80-1402**

CUTTER, Calvin (1807-1872)
A treatise on anatomy, physiology, and hygiene. . . . With one hundred and fifty engravings. Rev. stereotype ed. Philadelphia: J. B. Lippincott & Co., [1880]. 466p. DLC; OCIM; PPC; PU
80-1403

CUTTER, Calvin (1807-1872)
Intermediate anatomy, physiology, and hygiene, including scientific instruction upon the effects of narcotics and stimulants upon the human body. A revision of Calvin Cutter's First book on anatomy, etc. By John C. Cutter. . . . Illustrated. Philadelphia: J. B. Lippincott Co., [1887]. 221p. DLC; NNNAM; PPJ; PU **80-1404**

CUTTER, Ephraim (1832-1917)
Nervousness, divorce, food. Detroit, 1880. 2p. DNLM
80-1405

CUTTER, Ephraim (1832-1917)
Food, Open letter to J. Marion Sims. [New York], 1881. 10p. DNLM **80-1406**

CUTTER, Ephraim (1832-1917)
List of food stuffs examined. Prepared for the "Medical News." New York, [1881]. 4p. DNLM
80-1407

CUTTER, Ephraim (1832-1917)
A contribution to the treatment of uterine lesions, by iodoform, cotton, and mechanics. Detroit, 1882. 8p. DNLM
80-1408

CUTTER, Ephraim (1832-1917)
Infants' and invalids' cereal foods under the microscope. New York: E. S. Gaillard, 1882. 14p. DNLM
80-1409

CUTTER, Ephraim (1832-1917)
Uterine disease, sometimes called consumption. . . . Atlanta, Ga.: J. P. Harrison & Co., printers, [1883]. 24p. DLC
80-1410

CUTTER, Ephraim (1832-1917)
The therapeutical drinking of hot water: its origin and use. . . . Boston: A. Mudge & Sons, printers, 1883. 9p. DLC
80-1411

CUTTER, Ephraim (1832-1917)
The therapeutical drinking of hot water; its origin and use. New York: W. A. Kellogg, 1883. 9p. DNLM
80-1412

CUTTER, Ephraim (1832-1917)
A porcelain stem pessary. New York: H. A. Vonneid-Hutz, 1884. 8p. DNLM **80-1413**

CUTTER, Ephraim (1832-1917)
Diagnosis of consumption by means of the microscope, with reference to life insurance. New York: W. A. Kellogg, [1886]. 17p. DNLM; NNNAM **80-1414**

CUTTER, Ephraim (1832-1917)
Baked beans; a serio-humorous medical paper. Albany, N.Y.: Burdick & Taylor, 1887. 20p. DNLM
80-1415

CUTTER, Ephraim (1832-1917)
Contributions to gynecology, fasciculus I. The galvanic treatment of uterine fibroids; full text of first fifty cases. . . . New York: W. A. Kellogg, 1887. 73p. DLC; DNLM; NNNAM
80-1416

CUTTER, Ephraim (1832-1917)
Galvanism of uterine fibroids. . . . Philadelphia, Pa.: Press of W. F. Fell & Co., [1887]. 14p. DLC; DNLM
80-1417

CUTTER, Ephraim (1832-1917)
Feeding patients against the appetite. New York: W. A. Kellogg, 1887. 44p. DNLM; NNNAM
80-1418

CUTTER, Ephraim (1832-1917)
Diet in cancer. I. Full text of nine cases. II. Theoretical considerations. New York: W. A. Kellogg, 1887. 33p. DNLM; NNNAM **80-1419**

CUTTER, Ephraim (1832-1917)
The contras and pros of the Cutter stem pessary, with a description of a new platina-plated sound. New York, 1888. 9p. DNLM **80-1420**

CUTTER, Ephraim (1832-1917)
Partial syllabic lists of the clinical morphologies of the blood, sputum, feces, skin, urine, vomitus, foods, including potable waters, ice and the air, and the clothing (after Salisbury). . . . New York: The Ariston, 1888. 81p. DLC; DNLM; NNNAM
80-1421

CUTTER, Ephraim (1832-1917)
Food versus bacilli in consumption (opus 286). An open letter from . . . to his son, John Ashburton Cutter, with answer. New York: Published by the Author, 1888. 22p. DNLM; NNNAM
80-1422

CUTTER, Ephraim (1832-1917) and John Ashburton CUTTER
Vinegar and vinegar yeasts. Philadelphia: Med. Press Co., 1889. 4p. DNLM **80-1423**

CUTTER, George R[ogers] (1840-1891)
A dictionary of the German terms used in medicine. New York: G. P. Putnam's Sons, 1882. 304p. CtY-M; DNLM; NN; MH **80-1424**

CUTTER, John Ashburton (1867-1944)
Some facts regarding medical missions and the International Medical Missionary Society. [Albany, 1887.] 4p. DNLM
80-1425

CUTTER, John Ashburton (1867-1944)
The thirty-third annual meeting of the Kentucky State Medical Society, held at Crab Orchard Springs, July 11-13, 1888. [n.p., 1888.] 3p. DNLM **80-1426**

CUTTER, John Ashburton (1867-1944)
Clinical morphology versus bacteriology, with some therapeutic deductions. [New York, 1889.] 2 l. 1 plate. DNLM
80-1427

CUTTER, John C[larence] (*b.* 1851)
Comprehensive anatomy, physiology, and hygiene . . . containing brief directions for illustrative dissections of mammals, for elementary work with the microscope, for physiological demonstrations of the human body, and for the management of emergent cases. . . . With one hundred and forty illustrations. Philadelphia: J. B. Lippincott & Co., 1885. 376p. DLC; MH; NN; PU **80-1428**

CUTTER, John Clarence (*b.* 1851)
Lessons in hygiene: an elementary text-book on the maintenance of health, with the rudiments of anatomy and physiology. . . . Philadelphia: J. B. Lippincott Co., 1885. 180p. DLC; ICU; MH; NN **80-1429**

CUTTER, John Clarence (*b.* 1851)
Beginner's anatomy, physiology, and hygiene, including scientific instruction on the effects of stimulants and narcotics on the growing body. . . . Philadelphia: J. B. Lippincott & Co., [1887]. 144p. DLC; MH; NN; PU
80-1430

CUTTER, John Clarence (*b.* 1851)
Comprehensive anatomy, physiology, and hygiene . . . with instruction on the effects of stimulants and narcotics, and brief directions for illustrative dissections of mammals, for elementary work with the microscope, for physiological demonstrations on the human body, and for the management of emergent cases. . . . With one hundred and forty illustrations. 2nd ed. Philadelphia: J. B. Lippicott Co., [1888]. 376p. DLC; ICU; MA; MB **80-1431**

CYCLOPAEDIA of obstetrics and gynecology. New York: William Wood & Co., 1887. 12 v. DNLM; OCIM; NNNAM; PPC
80-1432

DABNEY, William Cecil (1849-1894)
The atopical forms of typhoid fever. [Richmond, 1888.] 9p. DNLM **80-1433**

DA COSTA, JACOB MENDES (1833-1900) and Morris LONGSTRETH
Researches on the state of the ganglionic centers in Bright's disease. [Philadelphia, 1880.] 35p. DNLM
80-1434

DA COSTA, Jacob Mendes (1833-1900)
The fluorides in medicine. New York: G. P. Putnam's Sons, 1881. 6p. DNLM **80-1435**

DA COSTA, Jacob Mendes (1833-1900)
The nervous symptoms of lithaemia. [Philadelphia: Henry C. Lea's Son & Co., 1881.] 18p. DNLM
80-1436

DA COSTA, Jacob Mendes (1833-1900)
Medical diagnosis, with special reference to practical medicine. A guide to the knowledge and discrimination of diseases. . . . Illustrated with engravings on wood. 5th ed., rev. Philadelphia [etc.]: J. B. Lippincott & Co., 1881. 924p. DLC; NNNAM; OCIM; PPC **80-1437**

DA COSTA, Jacob Mendes (1833-1900)
Some points in the pathology of tubercle. Philadelphia: Collins, 1882. 16p. DNLM **80-1438**

DA COSTA, Jacob Mendes (1833-1900)
Observations on the salts of nickel, especially the bromide of nickel. [Philadelphia, 1883.] 7p. DNLM
80-1439

DA COSTA, Jacob Mendes (1833-1900)
The higher professional life. Valedictory address to the graduating class of Jefferson Medical College, Philadelphia, delivered April 2, 1883. Philadelphia: J. B. Lippincott & Co., 1883. 18p. DNLM **80-1440**

DA COSTA, Jacob Mendes (1833-1900)
Speech delivered at the dinner given to Prof. Alfred Stillé, by the medical profession of Philadelphia, Thursday, June 5, 1884. [Philadelphia], 1884. 4p. DNLM
80-1441

DA COSTA, Jacob Mendes (1833-1900)
Medical diagnosis, with special reference to practical medicine. A guide to the knowledge and discrimination of diseases. . . . Illustrated with engravings on wood. 6th ed., rev. Philadelphia [etc.]: J. B. Lippincott & Co., 1884. 967p. diags. DLC; NNNAM; PPC; PU **80-1442**

DA COSTA, Jacob Mendes (1833-1900)
Biographical sketch of Professor Samuel D. Gross. . . . [Philadelphia: Times Printing House, 1884.] 16p. DLC; DNLM; PPJ **80-1443**

DA COSTA, Jacob Mendes (1833-1900)
Address before the College of Physicians of Philadelphia. Delivered Feb. 4, 1885. Philadelphia: Time Print. House, 1885. 8p. DNLM **80-1444**

DA COSTA, Jacob Mendes (1833-1900)
Address of welcome to the newly-elected associate fellows. Delivered Jan. 4, 1887, at the centennial celebration of the College of Physicians of Philadelphia. [Philadelphia, 1887.] 4 l. DNLM **80-1445**

DA COSTA, Jacob Mendes (1833-1900)
The methods in medicine in the near present. An introductory lecture to the course at the Jefferson Medical College for the session of 1887. Philadelphia: [Times Print. House], 1887. 31p. PPJ **80-1446**

DA COSTA, Jacob Mendes (1833-1900)
Relation of the diseases of the kidney, especially the Bright's diseases, to the diseases of the heart. The Middleton Goldsmith lecture, delivered before the New York Pathological Society, April 18, 1888. [Philadelphia], 1888. 37p. DNLM **80-1447**

DA COSTA, Jacob Mendes (1833-1900)
The treatment of valvular diseases of the heart. Philadelphia: W. J. Dornan, 1888. 16p. DNLM **80-1448**

DA COSTA, Jacob Mendes (1833-1900)
The treatment of valvular diseases of the heart. Philadelphia: W. J. Dornan, 1888. 16p. DNLM **80-1449**

DA COSTA, Jacob Mendes (1833-1900)
Address at the dinner given Friday, April 6, 1888, to Dr. D. Hayes Agnew by the medical profession, in honor of the fiftieth anniversary of his entrance into the profession. Philadelphia, 1888. 3 l. DNLM **80-1450**

DA COSTA, Jacob Mendes (1833-1900)
Relation of the diseases of the kidney, especially the Bright's diseases, to the diseases of the heart. The Middleton Goldsmith lecture, delivered before the New York Pathological Society, April 18, 1888. [New York, 1889.] 27p. DNLM **80-1451**

DA COSTA, Jacob Mendes (1833-1900) and E. P. HERSHEY
The use of oxygen in the treatment of leukaemia and grave anaemias. [Philadelphia, 1889.] 10p. DNLM **80-1452**

DA COSTA, John Chalmers (1834-1910)
An easy method of repairing the perinaeum. [Boston: Rockwell & Churchill], 1889. 6p. DNLM **80-1453**

DAGGETT, William G.
The treatment of typhoid fever. Bridgeport, Conn.: Gould & Stiles, 1889. 12p. DNLM **80-1454**

DAKE, Jabez Philander (1827-1894)
Drug attenuation, its objects, modes, means, and limits, in homoeopathic pharmacy and posology. By the Bureau of Materia Medica, Pharmacy and Provings in the American Institute of Homoeopathy, 1879 and 1880, J. B. Dake, Chairman. Philadelphia: Sherman & Co., 1880. 189p. DNLM **80-1455**

DAKE, Jabez Philander (1827-1894)
Materia medica as a science. A discussion at the World's Homoeopathic Convention, under the auspices of the American Institute of Homoeopathy, Philadelphia, June, 1876. Philadelphia: Sherman & Co., 1881. 25p. PPHa **80-1456**

DAKE, Jabez Philander (1827-1894)
Quarantine; when and by what authority, and for what purpose maintained. Answers to the leading questions submitted by the State Board of Health of Louisiana to the Quarantine Convention at New Orleans, December 8, 1880. Philadelphia: Sherman & Co., 1881. 6p. DNLM; PPHa **80-1457**

DAKE, Jabez Philander (1827-1894)
Fermentation as a process in the disinfection of rooms after small-pox. Philadelphia: Sherman & Co., 1881. 4p. PPHa **80-1458**

DAKE, Jabez Philander (1827-1894)
Drug attenuation; its influence upon drug matter and drug power. Nashville: Haynes & Camp., 1881. 35p. DNLM **80-1459**

DAKE, Jabez Philander (1827-1894)
Susceptibility to malaria; or, personal predisposition to malarial fevers. A paper read at Niagara Falls during the thirty-sixth annual session of the American Institute of Homoeopathy. Pittsburgh: Stevenson & Foster, 1883. 9p. PPHa **80-1460**

DAKE, Jabez Philander (1827-1894)
Introductory to the report of the bureau of materia medica, with synopses of the papers presented at the 36th annual session of the American Institute of Homoeopathy. Pittsburgh: Stevenson & Foster, 1883. 20p. DNLM **80-1461**

DAKE, Jabez Philander (1827-1894)
Medical legislation in the United States. A discussion of the principles involved in American laws regulating the practice of medicine, showing their characters and results. Philadelphia: Sherman & Co., 1884. 14p. DNLM **80-1462**

DAKE, Jabez Philander (1827-1894)
Therapeutic methods. An outline of principles observed in the art of healing. Boston and Providence: Otis Clapp & Son, 1886. 195p. DLC **80-1463**

DALAND, Judson
A case of pyopneumothorax of nine months' duration. Philadelphia: W. J. Dornan, 1887. 5p. DNLM **80-1464**

DALAND, Judson
Dilatation of ureter and hypertrophy of the bladder. [*Also*:] Chronic interstitial nephritis, with enormous dilatation of the right pelvis, without apparent cause. [Philadelphia, 1887.] 3p. DNLM **80-1465**

DALTON, John C[all] (1825-1889)
Mr. Bergh as a commentator. A criticism of quotations. New York: Trow's, 1880. 15p. DNLM **80-1466**

DALTON, John Call (1825-1889)
A treatise on human physiology. . . . 7th ed. Philadelphia: Henry C. Lea's Son & Co., 1882. 722p. DLC; LNT-M; NNNAM; PPC **80-1467**

DALTON, John C[all] (1825-1889)
The experimental method in medical science; second course of the Cartwright lectures of the Alumni Association, College of Physicians and Surgeons, New York, delivered January 24, January 31, and February 7, 1882. New York: G. P. Putnam's Sons, 1882. 108p. DNLM; NNNAM; NNU-M; PPC **80-1468**

DALTON, John Call (1825-1889)
Doctrines of the circulation; a history of physiological opinion and discovery, in regard to the circulation of the blood. . . . Philadelphia: Henry C. Lea's Son & Co., 1884. 296p. DLC; DNLM; NNNAM; PPC **80-1469**

DALTON, John Call (1825-1889)
Topographical anatomy of the brain. . . . Philadelphia: Lea Bros. & Co., 1885. 3 v. 48 plates. DLC; DNLM; NNNAM; PPC **80-1470**

DALTON, John C[all] (1825-1889)
History of the College of Physicians and Surgeons in the City of New York. Medical Department of Columbia College. New York: Columbia College, 1888. 208p. DNLM; NN; NNC; NNNAM **80-1471**

DALY, W[illiam] H[udson] (1842-1901)
Stenosis of the larynx, with fibrous adhesive bands of the true vocal cords; tracheotomy, rupture of the bands, and cure of stenosis by general and local treatment. Some remarks concerning the value of the galvano-cautery in treatment of diseases and growths of the naso-pharynx. [New York: G. P. Putnam's Sons, 1880.] 12p. DNLM; NNNAM **80-1472**

DALY, W[illiam] H[udson] (1842-1901)
Elongating hypertrophy of the femur and tibia of opposite sides (the osteitis deformans of Paget). New York: Trow, 1880. 12p. DNLM **80-1473**

DALY, W[illiam] H[udson] (1842-1901)
Nasal polyps. [New York, 1881.] 12p. DNLM **80-1474**

DALY, W[illiam] H[udson] (1842-1901)
Naso-antral catarrh and its treatment. New York, 1882. 6p. DNLM **80-1475**

DALY, W[illiam] H[udson] (1842-1901)
A peculiar injury of the hip-joint, followed by tetanus and death; post-mortem examination of the parts. Philadelphia, 1882. 11p. DNLM **80-1476**

DALY, W[illiam] H[udson] (1842-1901)
On the relation of hay asthma and chronic naso-pharyngeal catarrh. [New York, 1882.] 5p. DNLM **80-1477**

DALY, W[illiam] H[udson] (1842-1901)
A discussion of some questions relating to tonsillotomy; and clinical remarks upon deflections of the nasal septum, with a presentation of two cases. [Philadelphia, 1883.] 14p. DNLM **80-1478**

DALY, W[illiam] H[udson] (1842-1901)
Address in medicine, delivered before the Medical Society of the State of Pennsylvania, at its annual meeting held at Philadelphia, May, 1884. Philadelphia: Collins, 1884. 12p. DNLM **80-1479**

DALY, W[illiam] H[udson] (1842-1901)
Gunshot wounds of the larynx, with the report of a case in which the vocal bands were involved. New York: D. Appleton & Co. [1884]. 11p. DNLM **80-1480**

DALY, W[illiam] H[udson] (1842-1901)
Two papers. 1. Laryngology and its cognate branches in America. 2. The simplest and most efficient treatment of diphtheria. 1886. 8p. DNLM **80-1481**

DALY, W[illiam] H[udson] (1842-1901)
On some mild measures in the treatment of intra-nasal hypertrophies and inflammations. [Philadelphia, 1888.] 6p. DNLM **80-1482**

DANA, C[harles] L[oomis] (1852-1935)
The asylum superintendents on the needs of the insane, with statistics of insanity in the United States. [New York: G. P. Putnam's Sons, 1882.] 17p. DNLM **80-1483**

DANA, C[harles] L[oomis] (1852-1935)
The digestive power of commercial pepsin in artificial digesters and in the stomach. [Philadelphia, 1882.] 11p. DNLM **80-1484**

DANA, C[harles] L[oomis] (1852-1935)
A study of some points in the physiology of digestion. Cambridge, 1882. 12p. DNLM **80-1485**

DANA, C[harles] L[oomis] (1852-1935)
On the pathology and treatment of certain forms of nerve-weakness. New York: Trow, 1883. 28p. DNLM **80-1486**

DANA, C[harles] L[oomis] (1852-1935)
On morbid drowsiness and somnolence. A contribution to the pathology of sleep. [Chicago], 1884. 27p. DNLM **80-1487**

DANA, C[harles] L[oomis] (1852-1935)
Some certainties in the therapeutics of epilepsy. [New York, 1886.] 13p. DNLM **80-1488**

DANA, C[harles] L[oomis] (1852-1935)
A clinical study of neuralgias and of the origin of reflex or transferred pains. [New York, 1887.] 31p. 1 plate. DNLM **80-1489**

DANA, Israel T[horndike] (1827-1904)
The pathology of pulmonary phthisis. Portland, Me.: S. Berry, 1880. 16p. DNLM **80-1490**

DANELSON, J. Edwin
Dr. Danelson's counselor with recipes: a practical and trusty guide for the family, and a suggestive hand-book for the physician. . . . New York: Nickles Publishing Co., 1880. 720p. DLC; NNNAM **80-1491**

DANELSON, J. Edwin
The family medical guide. Comprising chapters on physiology, hygiene, marriage, and medical practice; giving descriptions of diseases, with directions and prescriptions for their cure. . . . Springfield, Mass.: The Phelps Publishing Co., [1889]. 720p. DLC; MBM; NNNAM **80-1492**

DANELSON, J. Edwin
The model home physician. With recipes. A practical and trusty guide for the family, and a suggestive hand-book for the physician. . . . Rev. and enl. Springifeld, O.: Mast, Crowell & Kirkpatrick, [1889]. 720p. DLC **80-1493**

DANIEL, Ferdinand Eugene (1839-1914)
On the necessity of organization of the medical profession. Philadelphia, 1886. 8p. DNLM **80-1494**

DARBY, Edwin T[yler] (1845-1927)
Professional services and professional fees. [Baltimore, 1884.] 8p. DNLM **80-1495**

DARBY, John Custis
Science and the healing art, or A new book on old facts. . . . Louisville, Ky.: J. P. Morton & Co., 1880. 403p. DLC; OCIM **80-1496**

DARLING, William (1802-1884)
The essentials of anatomy, designed as a text-book for students and as a book of easy reference for the practitioner; by William Darling . . . and Ambrose L. Ranney. . . . New York: G. P. Putnam's Sons, 1880. 629p. 4 fold. tab., diags. DLC; DNLM; NNNAM; PPC **80-1497**

DAVENPORT, Francis Henry (*b.* 1851)
Uterine displacements and their influence on the general nervous system. Boston, 1888. 16p. DNLM **80-1498**

DAVENPORT, Francis Henry (*b.* 1851)
Diseases of women: a manual of non-surgical gynecology, designed especially for the use of students and general practitioners. . . . Philadelphia: Lea Bros. & Co., 1889. 317p. DLC; DNLM; NNNAM; PPC **80-1499**

DAVENPORT, Isaac B.
Harmony and discord, health and disease, healing and hindering. Philadelphia: W. P. Fell & Co., [1887]. 4 l. DNLM **80-1500**

DAVENPORT, Isaac B.
Non-cohesive half-cylinder and loop filling. Philadelphia, 1889. 6p. DNLM **80-1501**

DAVIES, Nathaniel Edward (*b.* 1844)
Foods for the fat. A treatise on corpulency, with dietary for its cure. American ed., edited by Charles W. Greene. Philadelphia: J. B. Lippincott & Co., 1889. 138p. DNLM; MBM; NNNAM; PPC **80-1502**

DAVIS, A[lexander] H.
Improved theory and practice of medicine, deduced from forty years successful practice. . . . Chicago: Pub. by the Author, 1880. 383p. DLC; OCIM **80-1503**

DAVIS, C[harles] G[ilbert] (1848-1928)
Five cases of ovariotomy. Chicago: Clark & Longley, 1885. 16p. DNLM **80-1504**

DAVIS, C[harles] H[enry] S[tanley] (1840-1917)
Idiocy and its treatment. [Richmond, 1882.] 4p. DNLM **80-1505**

DAVIS, C[harles] H[enry] S[tanley] (1840-1917)
Psycho-physiological training of an idiot. [Newtown, Conn., 1882.] 2 l. DNLM **80-1506**

DAVIS, C[harles] H[enry] S[tanley] (1840-1917)
The classification, training and education of the feeble-minded, imbecile and idiotic. New York: E. Steiger & Co., 1883. 46p. DNLM; NNNAM **80-1507**

DAVIS, C[harles] H[enry] S[tanley] (1840-1917)
Diagnosis of female diseases. [Meriden, Conn., [1883]]. 10p. DNLM **80-1508**

DAVIS, Irenaeus P.
Hygiene for girls. New York: D. Appleton & Co., 1883. 210p. DNLM; NN; MB; MH **80-1509**

DAVIS, John D[aniel] S[inkler] (*b.* 1859)
Epicystic surgical fistula for cystoscopic exploration; intravesical treatment and drainage. [Birmingham, Ala., 1889.] 1 galley sheet. DNLM **80-1510**

DAVIS, Nathan S[mith] (1817-1904)
An address on the nature of the science and art of medicine and their relations to the various important interests of the people. Chicago, 1880. 13p. DNLM **80-1511**

DAVIS, Nathan S[mith] (1817-1904)
Lecture: Alcoholic liquids as therapeutic agents. Chicago. [1884]. 12p. DNLM **80-1512**

DAVIS, Nathan Smith (1817-1904)
Lectures on the principles and practice of medicine. Delivered in Chicago Medical College, Medical Department of the Northwestern University. . . . Chicago: Jansen, McClurg & Co., 1884. 896p. DLC; IEN-M; OCIM; NNNAM **80-1513**

DAVIS, N[athan] S[mith], Jr. (1858-1920)
Arsenite of bromine in diabetes mellitus. Chicago, 1886. 7p. DNLM **80-1514**

DAVIS, N[athan] S[mith], Jr. (1858-1920)
Antipyrin in rheumatism; its value and mode of action. Chicago, 1887. 8p. DNLM **80-1515**

DAVIS, N[athan] S[mith], Jr. (1858-1920)
Cellular digestion; its utility in pathological processes. [Philadelphia: W. Fell & Co., 1887.] 4 l. DNLM **80-1516**

DAVIS, T[homas] D[avis] (*b.* 1846)
Gradual dilatation of oesophageal strictures. Chicago, 1888. 12p. DNLM **80-1517**

DAWBARN, Robert Hugh Mackay (1860-1915)
An aid to materia medica. . . . New York: J. H. Vail & Co., 1884. 86p. DLC; NNNAM; OCLloyd; PU **80-1518**

DAWBARN, Robert Hugh Mackay (1860-1915)
An aid to materia medica. 2nd ed. New York: J. H. Vail & Co., 1886. 86p. DNLM; NNNAM; PU **80-1519**

DAWBARN, Robert Hugh Mackay (1860-1915)
Doctors and politicians. New York: M. J. Rooney & Co., [1889]. 14p. DNLM; NNNAM **80-1520**

DAWBARN, Robert Hugh Mackay (1860-1915)
A successful case of spinal resection. With neurological notes by Landon Carter Gray. New York: M. J. Rooney & Co., [1889]. 15p. DNLM; NNNAM **80-1521**

DAWSON, W[illiam] W[irt] (1828-1893)
Address before the American Medical Association, delivered at Newport, R.I., June 25, 1889. Cincinnati: Wrightson Print. Co., 1889. 26p. DNLM; OCIM **80-1522**

DAY, R[ichard] H[ance] (1813-1892)
Malarial haematuria. [New Orleans, 1886.] 12p. DNLM
80-1523

DAY, R[ichard] H[ance] (1813-1892)
Remarks in regard to the nature and treatment of yellow fever. [New Orleans, 1888.] 16p. DNLM
80-1524

DAY, W[illiam] H[enry] (1830-1907)
Headaches, their nature, causes, and treatment. 3rd ed. New York: Bermingham & Co. 1880? 104p. NNNAM; PPC; PPJ; PU **80-1525**

DAY, W[illiam] H[enry] (1830-1907)
Headaches, their nature, causes, and treatment. 3rd ed. Philadelphia: Lindsay & Blakiston, 1880. 322p. CtY-M; MH-M; NNNAM; PPC **80-1526**

DAY, W[illiam] H[enry] (1830-1907)
Headaches, their nature, causes, and treatment; 4th ed. Philadelphia: P. Blakiston, Son & Co., 1883. 149p. CtY-M; DNLM; PPC; PU [This is a reprint of the third London edition (1880).] **80-1527**

DAYFOOT, Herbert M. (1846-1894)
Homoeopathy; its principles, practice and achievements. An address delivered before the Rochester Academy of Science, March 14, 1887. Rochester, N.Y.: Rochester Democrat & Chronicle Print, 1887. 20p. PPHa
80-1528

DAYTON MEDICAL UNIVERSITY
Annual announcements for the sessions of 1886-1887 (1).; 1887-1888 (2.). [Dayton, 1886-1887.] 14, 15p. DNLM
80-1529

DEAN, M. S.
Address delivered at the commencement of the Ohio College of Dental Surgery, Cincinnati. March 6th, 1880. Cincinnati: Spencer & Craig, 1880. 15p. DNLM
80-1530

DE BECK, David
Acetate of lead in ocular therapeutics. Cincinnati: R. Clarke & Co., 1884. 11p. DNLM; OCIM **80-1531**

DE BECK, David
A rare family history of congenital coloboma of the iris, etc. [New York, 1886.] 16p. DNLM **80-1532**

DE BECK, David
Hard chancre of the eyelids and conjuctiva. Cincinnati: R. Clarke & Co., 1886. 51p. 1 plate. DNLM; OCIM
80-1533

DE BECK, David
Diagnosis and after-treatment of cataract cases. [Cincinnati, 1888.] 9p. DNLM **80-1534**

DE DERKEY, Francis Foeldvar
Gynaecology; a treatise on the diseases of women, their prevention and cure. Chicago: W. A. Chatteron, 1889. 32p. OCIM; PPHa **80-1535**

DE ECKE, Theodore (*d.* 1905)
The condition of the brain in insanity. [Utica, N.Y., 1881.] 32p. DNLM **80-1536**

DE ECKE, Theodore (*d.* 1905)
On some changes in the ganglion cells of the grey cortex of the brain in acute delirium, and their relation to those in acute insanity and in dementia. Pt. I. [Utica, N.Y. 1881.] 10p. 1 plate. DNLM **80-1537**

DE ECKE, Theodore (*d.* 1905) and John P. GRAY
Medulla oblongata. Case of general paralysis. [Utica, 1882?] 25 plates. DNLM **80-1538**

DEEMS, Frank M[elville] (1846-1918)
Handbook of systematic urinary analysis, chemical and microscopical. For the use of physicians, medical students, and clinical assistants. New York: Industrial Publ. Co., 1880. 30p. 1 plate. CtY-M; DNLM; NNNAM; PU
80-1539

DELAFIELD, Francis (1841-1915)
Lectures on the practice of medicine. Phonographically reported, arranged and pub. by M. Josiah Roberts, M.D. New York, 1881. 315p. DLC; NNNAM; MBM; PPC
80-1540

DELAFIELD, Francis (1841-1915)
Studies in pathological anatomy. . . . New York: William Wood & Co., 1882-1891. 2 v. DLC; NNNAM; OCIM; PU
80-1541

DELAFIELD, Francis (1841-1915)
A handbook of pathological anatomy and histology, with an introductory section on post-mortem examinations and the methods of preserving and examining diseased tissues, by Francis Delafield . . . and T. Mitchell Prudden. . . . [2nd ed.]. New York: William Wood & Co., 1885. 575p. DLC; OCIM; NNNAM; PPC **80-1542**

DELAFIELD, Francis (1841-1915)
A handbook of pathological anatomy and histology, with an introductory section on post-mortem examinations and the methods of preserving and examining diseased tissues, by Francis Delafield . . . and T. Mitchell Prudden. . . . 3rd ed., illustrated by 224 wood engravings printed in black and colors. New York: William Wood & Co., 1889. 600p. illus. (part col.). DLC; ICRM; NNNAM; PPC **80-1543**

DELAVAN, D. Bryson (1850-1942)
The tonsils; their general, surgical, and minute anatomy. [New York, 1880.] 5p. DNLM **80-1544**

DELAVAN, D. Bryson (1850-1942)
Primary epithelioma of larynx below vocal cords; unique case; bilateral paralysis of laryngeal abductus; death. [New York, 1881.] 4p. DNLM **80-1545**

DELAVAN, D. Bryson (1850-1942)
Nine cases of tumor of the nasal septum, anteriorly. [New York, 1882.] 5p. DNLM **80-1546**

DELAVAN, D. Bryson (1850-1942)
Otalgia from reflex dental irritation. Cambridge: Riverside Press, 1882. 2p. DNLM **80-1547**

DELAVAN, D. Bryson (1850-1942)
Primary epithelioma of the tonsil. [New York, 1882.] 6p. DNLM **80-1548**

DELAVAN, D. Bryson (1850-1942)
On the question of hypertrophy of the osseous structure of the turbinated bodies, practically considered. [New York: G. P. Putnam's Sons, 1882.] 10p. DNLM
80-1549

DELAVAN, D. Bryson (1850-1942)
Case of acute idiopathic perichondritis and abscess of the nasal septum. [New York: G. P. Putnam's Sons, 1883.] 2p. DNLM **80-1550**

DELAVAN, D. Bryson (1850-1942)
On the "lacunae tonsillarum." New York: G. P. Putnam's Sons, 1883. 4p. DNLM **80-1551**

DELAVAN, D. Bryson (1850-1942)
Practical suggestions upon the alimentation of patients suffering from dysphagia. [Philadelphia, 1884.] 11p. DNLM
80-1552

DELAVAN, D. Byson (1850-1942)
A case of primary epithelioma of the larynx; tracheotomy; death ten months later; autopsy; remarks. New York; Trow, 1885. 8p. DNLM **80-1553**

DELAVAN, D. Bryson (1850-1942)
Erysipelas of the larynx and pharynx. New York: D. Appleton & Co., 1885. 10p. DNLM **80-1554**

DELAVAN, D. Bryson (1850-1942)
On the localization of the cortical motor center of the human larynx. New York: Trow, 1885. 8p. DNLM
80-1555

DELAVAN, D. Bryson (1850-1942)
The social history of the Eighth International Medical Congress, held in Copenhagen, August, 1884. New York: D. Appleton & Co., 1885. 36p. DNLM
80-1556

DELAVAN, D. Bryson (1850-1942)
The social history of the Eighth International Medical Congress, held in Copenhagen, Augsut, 1884. 2nd ed. New York & London: G. P. Putnam's Sons, 1885. 36p. DNLM
80-1557

DELAVAN, D. Bryson (1850-1942)
Foreign bodies in the nose. [New York, 1886.] 4p. DNLM
80-1558

DELAVAN, D. Bryson (1850-1942)
On the etiology of deflections of the nasal septum. [New York, 1887.] 12p. DNLM **80-1559**

DELAVAN, D. Bryson (1850-1942)
Seven cases of buccal tuberculosis; with remarks upon tubercular ulceration of the tongue. New York: D. Appleton & Co., 1887. 14p. DNLM **80-1560**

DELAVAN, D. Bryson (1850-1942)
On the etiology, surgical pathology, and treatment of haemorrhage after tonsillotomy. New York: Trow, 1889. 11p. DNLM
80-1561

DELAVAN, D. Bryson (1850-1942)
Further investigations as to the existence of a cortical motor center for the human larynx. [New York, 1889.] 9p. DNLM
80-1562

[DE MARMON, PALUEL]
Catalogue of the valuable medical library of . . . New York: D. Taylor, [1880]. 21p. DNLM; NNNAM
80-1563

DEMARQUAY, Jean Nicolas (1814-1875)
Essay on medical pneumatology: a physiological, clinical, and therapeutic investigation of the gases. . . . Transl., with notes, additions, and omissions, by Samuel S. Wallian. . . . Philadelphia and London: F. A. Davis, 1889. 300p. DLC; MBM; NNNAM; PU **80-1564**

DENISON, Charles (1845-1909)
Rocky Mountain health resorts. An analytical study of high altitudes in relation to the arrest of chronic pulmonary disease. . . . Boston: Houghton, Osgood & Co., 1880. 192p. fold. map, chart. DLC; DNLM; MBM; NNNAM
80-1565

DENISON, Charles (1845-1909)
Rocky Mountain health resorts. An analytical study of high altitudes in relation to the arrest of chronic pulmonary disease. . . . 2nd ed. . . . Boston: Houghton, Mifflin & Co., 1881. 192p., fold. map. DLC; DNLM; MBM; NNNAM
80-1566

DENISON, Charles (1845-1909)
The infectiousness of phthisis. Denver. E. Price & Co., 1882. 15p. DLC **80-1567**

DENISON, Charles (1845-1909)
The climatic treatment of pulmonary consumption. . . . [Denver, 1883.] 7p. DLC **80-1568**

DENISON, Charles (1845-1909)
The preferable climate for phthisis; or, the comparative importance of different climatic attributes in the arrest of chronic pulmonary diseases. Chicago: Rand, McNally & Co., [1887]. 15p. 1 map. DLC; DNLM **80-1569**

DENISON, Charles (1845-1909)
The preferable climate for phthisis; or, the comparative importance of different climatic attributes in the arrest of chronic pulmonary diseases. [Denver: Collier & Cleaveland, 1887.] 15p. 1 map. DLC; DNLM **80-1570**

DENISON, Charles (1845-1909)
The extension-windlass method of treating fracture of long bones; especially illustrated with reference to fracture in upper third of femur. New York, 1888. 16p. DNLM
80-1571

DENNIS, Frederick S[hepard] (1850-1934)
Head injuries accompanied by paralysis. A clinical lecture. [Philadelphia, 1884.] 12p. DNLM **80-1572**

DENNIS, Frederick S[hepard] (1850-1934)
A memoir of James R. Wood, M.D. New York: D. Appleton & Co., 1884. 31p. port. DNLM **80-1573**

DENNIS, Frederick S[hepard] (1850-1934)
A memoir of James R. Wood, M.D. New York: D. Appleton & Co., 1884. 24p. port. DNLM **80-1574**

DENNIS, Frederick S[hepard] (1850-1934)
The action of micro-organisms upon surgical wounds, with demonstrations. New York, 1885. 38p. DNLM
80-1575

DENNIS, Frederick S[hepard] (1850-1934)
Laparotomy in the treatment of penetrating wounds and visceral injuries of the abdomen. [Philadelphia, 1886.] 55p. DNLM **80-1576**

DENNIS, Frederick S[hepard] (1850-1934)
The treatment of fracture of the patella by the metallic suture. New York: D. Appleton & Co., 1886. 33p. 1 tab. DNLM **80-1577**

DENNIS, Frederick S[hepard] (1850-1934)
Some practical hints upon the technique of an aseptic surgical operation. A clinical lecture delivered in the Carnegie Laboratory. [Reported by Dr. H. Seymour Houghton.] Chicago, 1886. 22p. DNLM **80-1578**

DENNIS, Frederick S[hepard] (1850-1934)
Some points of special interest in the treatment of compound fractures, including a report of five hundred and sixteen cases. [Philadelphia], 1886. 29p. DNLM **80-1579**

DENNIS, Frederick S[hepard] (1850-1934)
Laparotomy in the treatment of spontaneous gluteal and sciatic aneurisms. [Philadelphia], 1886. 21p. DNLM **80-1580**

DENNIS, Frederick S[hepard] (1850-1934)
Selected cases from the surgical clinic of . . . . [Pittsburgh], 1887. 8p. DNLM **80-1581**

DENNIS, Frederick S[hepard] (1850-1934)
Rickets, its treatment by osteotomy. [New York], 1887. 10p. DNLM **80-1582**

DENNIS, Frederick S[hepard] (1850-1934)
Clinical lecture on the general principles involved in amputation, with a consideration of some points in the technique. Chicago, 1887. 18p. DNLM **80-1583**

DENNIS, Frederick S[hepard] (1850-1934)
Suprapubic cystotomy, its technique illustrated by anatomical preparations. [Philadelphia], 1887. 21p. DNLM **80-1584**

DERBY, Hasket (1835-1914)
The prevention of near-sight in the young. Boston, 1880. 11p. DNLM **80-1585**

DERBY, Hasket (1835-1914)
Anaesthesia and non-anaesthesia in the extraction of cataract. With some practical suggestions regarding the performance of this operation, and comparative statistics of two hundred cases. Cambridge: Riverside Press, 1882. 32p. DNLM; MH-M **80-1586**

DERBY, Hasket (1835-1914)
Anaesthesia and non-anaesthesia in the extraction of cataract; with some practical suggestions regarding the performance of this operation, and comparative statistics of two hundred cases. Cambridge, 1882. 32p. DNLM; MBM **80-1587**

DERBY, Richard H[enry] (1844-1907)
Contagious ophthalmia in asylums and residential schools. [New York, 1885.] 11p. DNLM **80-1588**

DERCUM, Francis X[avier] (1856-1931)
A brief synopsis of the various points involved in the coarse examination of the brain and spinal cord. Norristown, Pa., 1886. 11p. DNLM **80-1589**

DERCUM, Francis X[avier] (1856-1931)
Description of the brain of John M. Wilson, recently hanged at Norristown. Philadelphia, 1887. 4p. 1 plate. DNLM **80-1590**

DERCUM, Francis X[avier] (1856-1931)
Remarks on spinal injuries, more especially "railway spine"; with hints on expert testimony. Detroit: G. S. Davis, 1889. 31p. DNLM **80-1591**

DERCUM, Francis X[avier] (1856-1931)
Some thoughts on surgical shock, with special reference to brain and spinal operations. [Philadelphia, 1889.] 8p. DNLM **80-1592**

DERCUM, Francis X[avier] (1856-1931)
Railway shock and its treatment. Detroit: G. S. Davis, 1889. 35p. DNLM **80-1593**

DERCUM, Francis X[avier] (1856-1931) and J[ohn] William WHITE
Two cases of spinal surgery. [St. Louis, 1889.] 15p. DNLM **80-1594**

DESSAU, S. Henry
Hysteria in boys; with the report of a case. New York: William Wood & Co., 1880. 10p. DNLM **80-1595**

DESSAU, S. Henry
Observations on pertussis; based upon an analysis of 361 cases. New York: William Wood & Co., 1881. 16p. DNLM **80-1596**

DESSAU, S. Henry
Convulsive affections in children and their treatment. New York: Trow, 1883. 20p. DNLM **80-1597**

DESSAU, S. Henry
The treatment of diphtheria. New York: Trow, 1886. 11p. DNLM **80-1598**

DEUTSCH, Solomon (1816-1897)
Medical German; a manual designed to aid physicians in their intercourse with German patients and in reading medical works and publications in the German language. . . . New York: [Baltimore, Press of I. Friedenwald], 1884. 336p. DLC; MdU-MdU-D; NNNAM; OCIM **80-1599**

DEWEES, William Bushy (1854-1912)
Impure sexual intercourse the primitive cause of syphilis, scrofula, and phthisis. Philadelphia: Record, McMullin & Co., 1888. 30p. DNLM; PPC; PU **80-1600**

DEWEY, B. M.
Special hygienic and medical information for parents, embracing health and diseases of the reproductive organs, urinary apparatus, rectum, diseases of childhood, everyday emergencies, household recipes, and common disorders and what to do. With copious index and glossary. . . . Chicago: Knight & Leonard, printers, 1880 [1879]. 398p. DLC; OCIM **80-1601**

DEWEY, J. H.
The new departure in healing and physical culture. Based upon the discovery of means for the more direct conservation of physical energy and its transformation into nerve-force and recuperative power. A discovery which renders complete physical reconstruction not only possible but practicable. Chicago: W. A. Chatterton, 1880. 48p. OCIM; PPHa
80-1602

DICKEY, John L.
The errors of refraction. Wheeling, 1885. 7p. DNLM
80-1603

DICKEY, John L.
Report of committee on necrology. Wheeling, 1886. 7p. DNLM **80-1604**

DICKINSON, Robert L[atou] (1861-1950)
The corset: questions of pressure and displacement. New York, 1887. 33p. DNLM; NNNAM **80-1605**

DICKINSON, Robert L[atou] (1861-1950)
Studies of the levator and muscle. New York, 1889. 24p. DNLM **80-1606**

DICKINSON, William
Hemiopia. Mechanism of its caustion on the theory of total decussation of the optic nerve fibres in the optic tracts at the chiasma (optic commissure). [St. Louis, 1881.] 11p. DNLM
80-1607

DICKINSON, W[illiam] H[owship] (1832-1913)
A treatise on albuminuria. 2nd ed. New York: William Wood & Co., 1881. 300p. 11 plates. CtY-M; DNLM; NNNAM; OCIM
80-1608

DICKINSON, W[illiam] H[owship] (1832-1913)
On renal and urinary affections. In three parts. Part III. Miscellaneous affections of the kidneys and urine. New York: William Wood & Co., 1885. 343p. DNLM; OCIM; PPC; PU [This edition differs from the original in that detailed reports of cases are omitted.] (London, 1885)
80-1609

DICKINSON, Wilmot Horton (*b.* 1829)
Homoeopathic principles and practice of medicine. Des Moines: Mills & Co., 1883. 730p. IEN-M; OCIM
80-1610

DIDAY, Paul (1812-1894)
A treatise on syphilis in new-born children and infants at the breast. . . . Transl. by G. Whitley, M.D. With notes and an appendix by F. R. Sturgis. . . . New York: William Wood & Co., 1883. 310p. col. front plate. DLC; NNNAM; OCIM; PPC
80-1611

DILLER, Theodore (*b.* 1863)
Antifebrin in the treatment of epilepsy. Detroit: G. S. Davis, 1889. 7p. DNLM **80-1612**

DILLER, Theodore (*b.* 1863)
Case of large cerebellar and several smaller cerebral hemorrhages. [Philadelphia, 1889.] 8p. DNLM
80-1613

DILLER, Theodore (*b.* 1863)
Some observations on the hereditary form of chorea, with the report of a case. [Philadelphia, 1889.] 9p. DNLM
80-1614

DILLOW, George M[orris]
Inaugural address delivered before the Homoeopathic Medical Society of the County of New York, January 14, 1885. New York: Martin B. Brown, 1885. 12p. NNNAM; PPHa
80-1615

DIX, Tandy L.
The healthy infant; a treatise on the healthy procreation of the human race, embracing the obligations to offspring, the management of the pregnant female, the management of the newly born, the management of the infant, and the infant in sickness. Cincinnati: P. G. Thomson, 1880. 134p. DNLM; OCIM **80-1616**

DIXON, Edward H. (1808-1880)
Back-bone; photographed from "The Scalpel." . . . New York: R. M. De Witt, [1886]. 396p. DLC; NNNAM; PPJ; PU
80-1617

DIXON, Robert B[rewer]
Is craniotomy upon the living fetus ever justifiable? Boston: Cupples, Upham & Co., 1885. 24p. DNLM; MBM
80-1618

DIXON, Samuel Gibson (1851-1918)
Possibility of establishing tolerance for the tubercle bacillus. Philadelphia, 1889. 2 l. DNLM **80-1619**

DIXON, Samuel Gibson (1851-1918)
A bacteriological manipulating chamber. Detroit, Mich.: G. S. Davis, 1889. 6p. DNLM **80-1620**

DOCK, George (*b.* 1860)
Aneurism of the aorta simulating cardiac valvular disease. [Philadelphia, 1889.] 7p. DNLM **80-1621**

DOCK, George (*b.* 1860)
The examination of sputum in the diagnosis of tuberculosis. [Dallas, 1889.] 5p. DNLM **80-1622**

DOCK, George (*b.* 1860)
Leprosy, with a report on two cases. [San Antonio, 1889.] 6p. DNLM **80-1623**

DODS, John Bovee (1795-1872)
The philosophy of electrical psychology; in a course of twelve lectures. Stereotype ed. New York: S. R. Wells & Co., 1880. 252p. DNLM; NN; NNNAM **80-1624**

DOERING, Edmund J.
The overcrowding of the profession. Extracts from an address delivered March 23, 1885, before the Alumni Association of the Chicago Medical College. Chicago, 1885. 8p. DNLM
80-1625

DOERING, Edmund J.
Some remarks on the value of permanganate of potassium in amenorrhea. Chicago: Clark & Longley, 1885. 5p. DNLM
80-1626

DOERING, Edmund J.
Report of a case of hydatiform pregnancy. Chicago, 1886. 5p. DNLM **80-1627**

DOLLEY, Charles S[umner] (*b.* 1856)
Bacteria as beneficial and noxious agents. Read before the Rochester Society of Natural Sciences. [Rochester, 1885?] 16p. DNLM **80-1628**

DOLLEY, Charles S[umner] (*b.* 1856)
The technology of bacteria investigation, explicit directions for the study of bacteria, their culture, staining, mounting, etc., according to the methods employed by the most eminent investigators. Boston: S. E. Cassino & Co., 1885. 263p. CtY-M; DNLM; MH-M; NNNAM **80-1629**

DOMVILLE, Edward J[ames] (1849-1925)
A manual for hospital nurses and others engaged in attending on the sick. 5th ed. Philadelphia: P. Blakiston, Son & Co., 1885. 96p. DNLM; NNNAM; PPC; PU **80-1630**

DOMVILLE, Edward J[ames] (1849-1925)
A manual for hospital nurses and others engaged in attending on the sick. 6th ed. Philadelphia: P. Blakiston, Son & Co., 1888. 100p. DNLM; OCIM; PPJ; PU **80-1631**

DONALDSON, Francis (1823-1891)
Domestic hygiene. A lecture before the St. Peter's Brotherhood. Baltimore: Sun Book & Job Print. Office, 1881. 40p. DNLM **80-1632**

DONALDSON, Francis (1823-1891)
The influence of lung retractility in pleurisy and pneumothorax. Baltimore, 1884. 15p. DNLM **80-1633**

DONALDSON, Francis (1823-1891)
Personal observations on the value of cocaine in nose and throat surgery. [Baltimore, 1885.] 8p. DNLM **80-1634**

DONALDSON, Francis (1823-1891)
A case of primary epithelioma of the tonsil. [New York, 1885.] 8p. DNLM **80-1635**

DONALDSON, Francis (1823-1891)
Hard chancre of the tonsil. [Philadelphia, 1885.] 15p. DNLM **80-1636**

DONALDSON, Francis (1823-1891)
A case of congenital defect of the epiglottis, illustrating its function in deglutition. [New York: D. Appleton, 1886.] 16p. DNLM **80-1637**

DONALDSON, Francis (1823-1891)
On the causes of dyspnoea and cardiac failure in high altitudes. [Philadelphia, 1886.] 12p. DNLM **80-1638**

DONALDSON, Francis (1823-1891)
The function of the recurrent laryngeal nerve. From experimental studies in the Biological Laboratory of the Johns Hopkins University [Philadelphia, 1886.] 11p. DNLM **80-1639**

DONALDSON, Francis (1823-1891)
The pneumatic cabinet and pneumatic differentiation. [Baltimore, 1886.] 7p. DNLM **80-1640**

DONALDSON, Francis (1823-1891)
A study of diaphragmatic pleurisy. [Philadelphia: Lea Bros. & Co.], 1886. 14p. DNLM **80-1641**

DONALDSON, Francis (1823-1891)
Treatment of nasal growths and hypertrophies. [Richmond, 1886.] 11p. DNLM **80-1642**

DONALDSON, Francis (1823-1891)
Heredity in tuberculosis. President's address at the meeting of the American Climatological Association, May 31st, 1887. [Baltimore, 1887.] 22p. DNLM **80-1643**

DONALDSON, Francis (1823-1891)
On the causes of cardiac failure in high altitudes. Buffalo: Bigelow Bros., [1887]. 4p. DNLM **80-1644**

DONALDSON, Francis (1823-1891)
Further researches upon the physiology of the recurrent laryngeal nerve. [New York, 1887.] 24p. DNLM **80-1645**

DONALDSON, Francis (1823-1891)
Paralysis of the lateral adductor muscle of the larynx, with unique case. [New York, 1887.] 6p. DNLM **80-1646**

DONALDSON, Francis (1823-1891)
The prognosis of certain heart murmurs with special reference to the selection of risks for life insurance. [Philadelphia, 1887.] 18p. DNLM **80-1647**

DONALDSON, Francis (1823-1891)
Note on the physiology of the recurrent laryngeal nerves. [New York, 1888.] 1 l. DNLM **80-1648**

DONALDSON, Francis (1823-1891)
The diagnostic significance of the mitral presystolic murmur. Philadelphia, 1888. 24p. DNLM **80-1649**

DONALDSON, S[amuel] James
Contributions to practical gynecology. Pt. I. Practical observations upon uterine deflections. Pt. II. Practical observations upon dysmenorrhoea. New York: Trow's Print. & Bookbind. Co., 1882. 134p. DNLM; NNNAM **80-1650**

DONALDSON, S[amuel] James
Thoughts regarding the treatment of uterine displacements. New York: Trow's Print. & Bookbind. Co., 1882. 24p. DNLM; NNNAM **80-1651**

DONALDSON, S[amuel] James
A treatise on uterine displacements. 2nd ed. Boston, 1883. 83p. DNLM; MBM **80-1652**

DONALDSON, S[amuel] James
A treatise on dysmenorrhoea. Boston: A. Mudge & Co., 1884. 32p. DNLM; MBM **80-1653**

DONALDSON, S[amuel] James
An essay on habitual constipation. New York: E. P. Coby & Co., [1885]. 72p. DNLM; NNNAM **80-1654**

DONALDSON, S[amuel] James
Bodily posture in gynecology. New York: William Wood & Co., 1885. 24p. DNLM; NNNAM **80-1655**

DONALDSON, S[amuel] James
A contribution to the treatment of displacements of the uterus. New York: William Wood & Co., 1885. 16p. DNLM; NNNAM **80-1656**

DORCHESTER, Daniel (1827-1907)
The liquor problem in all ages. New York and Cincinnati: Phillips & Hunt, 1884. 478p. ICU; NN; NNC; MB **80-1657**

DOTY, Alvah Hunt (*b.* **1854**)
A manual of instruction in the principles of prompt aid to the injured; designed for military and civic use. . . . New York [etc.]: D. Appleton & Co., 1889. 224p. col. front. DLC; NNNAM; PPC; PU **80-1658**

DOUGHTY, F[rancis] E. (*b.* **1847**)
Inaugural address, delivered before the Homoeopathic Medical Society of the County of New York, January 10, 1883. [New York], 1883. 17p. DNLM; PPHa **80-1659**

DOUGHTY, William Henry (1836-1905)
Yellow fever. An open letter to E. S. Gaillard. Aug. 25, 1883. [New York, 1883.] 2 l. DNLM **80-1660**

DOUGLAS, Richard (1860-1908)
Hysterectomy; report of a case, with remarks. [New York, 1889.] 10p. DNLM **80-1661**

DOWD, Daniel Lawrence (*b.* **1854**)
Physical culture for home and school, scientific and practical. New York: the Author, 1889. 300p. NN; NNC; MB; MH **80-1662**

DOWLING, J[ohn] W[illiam] (1837-1892)
The sphygmograph, what it tells us, and its value as an aid to the diagnosis of disease. Havana, N.Y.: L. E. Keyser, 1881. 14p. DNLM **80-1663**

DOWLING, J[ohn] W[illiam] (1837-1892)
American Institute of Homoeopathy, 1881. Meeting held at Brighton Beach, June 14-17. Address. Pittsburgh: J. Eichbaum, 1881. 16p. DNLM **80-1664**

DOWLING, J[ohn] W[illiam] (1837-1892)
Old-school medicine and homoeopathy . . . , being a reply to Prof. Palmer's article . . . entitled "The fallacies of homoeopathy." New York: C. T. Hurlburt, 1882. 26p. DLC; DNLM; NNNAM **80-1665**

DOWLING, J[ohn] W[illiam] (1837-1892)
Nature of malaria, and its peculiarities of origin as to place. Pittsburgh: Stevenson & Foster, 1883. 16p. DNLM **80-1666**

DOWLING, J[ohn] W[illiam] (1837-1892)
The effects of the abuse of alcohol on the circulatory and respiratory organs. Pittsburgh: Stevenson & Foster, 1884. 16p. DNLM **80-1667**

DOWLING, J[ohn] W[illiam] (1837-1892)
Functional disturbances and organic diseases arising from lithaemia. Written by special request for the Pennsylvania State Homoeopathic Medical Society, session of 1886. New York: J. C. Rankin, Printer, 1886. 23p. PPHa **80-1668**

DOWLING, J[ohn] W[illiam] (1837-1892)
Is the American heart wearing out? New York, 1888. 18p. DNLM **80-1669**

DOWNES, Andrew J.
A cyst of the spleen; splenotomy (splenectomy?); recovery. Philadelphia: W. J. Dornan, 1888. 7p. DNLM **80-1670**

DOWSE, Thomas Stretch
The brain and the nerves; their ailments and their exhaustion. New York: G. P. Putnam's Sons, 1884. 150p. 1 tab. CtY-M; DNLM; MBM; NNNAM **80-1671**

DOWSLEY, Thomas M.
Plain and important information concerning the teeth, natural and artificial. . . . Boston, 1889. 24p. DLC **80-1672**

DRAPER, F[rank] W[inthrop] (1843-1909)
Medical expert testimony. [Boston, 1880.] 16p. DNLM; MBM **80-1673**

DRAPER, F[rank] W[inthrop] (1843-1909)
On sudden death by the entrance of air into the uterine veins. Boston, 1883. 24p. DNLM; MBM **80-1674**

DRAPER, John Christopher (1835-1885)
A text-book on anatomy, physiology, and hygiene. . . . 6th ed., rev. New York: Harper & Bros., 1883. 200p. plates. DLC; NNNAM; MBM; PPC **80-1675**

DRAPER, John C[hristopher] (1835-1885)
A text-book of medical physics. For the use of students and practitioners of medicine. Philadelphia: Lea Bros. & Co., 1885. 733p. DNLM; IU-M; NNNAM; PPC **80-1676**

DRAPER, Joseph (1824-1892)
Insanity in Great Britain and upon the continent of Europe. Its different phases and modes of treatment compared with those prevailing in the United States. St. Louis, 1882. 37p. DNLM; OCIM **80-1677**

DRAPER, Joseph (1824-1892)
The responsibility of the insane outside of asylums. Utica, 1883. 14p. DNLM **80-1678**

DRAPER, W[illiam] H[enry] (1830-1901)
A memorial of Dr. Henry Berton Sands. Read at a meeting of the Medical and Surgical Society, November 23, 1889. [New York, 1889.] 20p. DNLM; NNNAM **80-1679**

DRAYTON, H. S[hipman] (1840-1923)
Two cases of epilepsy. [New York, 1889.] 1 galley sheet. DNLM **80-1680**

DRURY, W. V[allancey]
Teething and croup. . . . Enriched with notes and additions, by T. C. Duncan, M.D. Chicago: Duncan Bros., 1881. 58p. OCIM; PPHa **80-1681**

DUANE, Alexander (1858-1926)
The corpuscular elements of the blood; their anatomy and physiology, normal and pathological. [New York, 1881-1882.] 108p. DNLM; NNNAM **80-1682**

DUANE, Alexander (1858-1926)
Some new tests for insufficiencies of the ocular muscles, together with a system of abbreviations suitable for note-taking. [New York, 1889.] 21p. DNLM; NNNAM **80-1683**

DUCKWORTH, Dyce (1840-1928)
A treatise on gout. Philadelphia: Blakiston, Son & Co., [1889]. 476p. 1 plate. DNLM; PPC; PPJ; PU **80-1684**

DUDLEY, A[ugustus] Palmer (1835-1905) and H. C. COE
A case of ovarian tumor with rare complications. [New York, 1882.] 10p. DNLM **80-1685**

DUDLEY, A[ugustus] Palmer (1835-1905)
Vaginal hysterectomy in America, with report of two cases. [New York, 1887.] 20p. DNLM; NNNAM **80-1686**

DUDLEY, A[ugustus] Palmer (1835-1905)
Two cases of ovariotomy; with remarks on the importance of position in this operation, and on the simultaneous and rapid development of pelvic abscess and ovarian cyst in immediate proximity. [New York, 1887.] 7p. DNLM **80-1687**

DUDLEY, A[ugustus] Palmer (1835-1905)
Varicocele in the female. What is its influence upon the ovary? [New York, 1888.] 19p. DNLM; NNNAM **80-1688**

DUDLEY, E. C. (1850-1928)
Pressure forceps versus the ligature and the suture in vaginal hysterectomy. Philadelphia: W. J. Dornan, 1888. 16p. DNLM **80-1689**

DUDLEY, William H[enry] (1811-1886)
Address at the alumni dinner, May 20, 1884. [Sketch of the origin of clinical teaching in the Long Island College Hospital.] [Brooklyn, 1884.] 8p. DNLM **80-1690**

DUDLEY, William L[ofland] (1859-1914)
A chart for the chemical examination of urine; also tables of the metric weights and measures, and rules for converting the apothecaries' weights and measures into metric terms. For the use of the students. [Cincinnati], 1880. 2 l. DNLM **80-1691**

DUDLEY, William L[ofland] (1859-1914)
Chemical examination of the urine, compiled and arranged for the use of the students of the Miami Medical College of Cincinnati, Ohio. [Cincinnati, 1880.] Broadside. DNLM **80-1692**

DUHRING, Louis Adolphus (1845-1913)
The rise of American dermatology, being the president's address . . . American Dermatological Association. New York: A. G. Sherwood & Co., 1880. 39p. DNLM; NNNAM **80-1693**

DUHRING, Louis Adolphus (1845-1913)
Supplement to a case of inflammatory fungoid neoplasm. Philadelphia: J. B. Lippincott & Co., 1880. 17p. DNLM; PPC **80-1694**

DUHRING, Louis Adolphus (1845-1913)
Pityriasis maculata et circinata. [Philadelphia, 1880.] 19p. DNLM **80-1695**

DUHRING, Louis Adolphus (1845-1913)
A practical treatise on diseases of the skin. 2nd ed. Philadelphia: J. B. Lippincott, 1881. 644p. DLC; DNLM; NNNAM; PPC **80-1696**

DUHRING, Louis Adolphus (1845-1913)
The foundation of American dermatology: being the president's address . . . American Dermatological Association. Philadelphia: J. B. Lippincott & Co., 1881. 29p. DNLM; PPC **80-1697**

DUHRING, Louis Adolphus (1845-1913)
Supplement to a case of painful neuroma of the skin. [Philadelphia, 1881.] 7p. DNLM **80-1698**

DUHRING, Louis Adolphus (1845-1913)
A practical treatise on diseases of the skin. . . . 3rd ed., rev. and enl. Philadelphia [etc.]: J. B. Lippincott & Co., 1882. 685p. DLC; OCIM; PPC; PU **80-1699**

DUHRING, Louis Adolphus (1845-1913)
A case of sarcomatous inflammatory neoplasm. [Philadelphia, 1883.] 4p. DNLM **80-1700**

DUHRING, Louis Adolphus (1845-1913)
Case of impetigo herpetiformis; recovery. [Philadelphia]: W. J. Dornan, [1883]. 8p. DNLM **80-1701**

DUHRING, Louis Adolphus (1845-1913)
On the value of a lotion of sulphide of zinc in the treatment of superficial lupus erythematosus. [Philadelphia]: W. J. Dornan, [1883]. 8p. DNLM **80-1702**

DUHRING, Louis Adolphus (1845-1913)
Two cases of Paget's disease of the nipple [Philadelphia, 1883]. 6p. DNLM **80-1703**

DUHRING, Louis Adolphus (1845-1913)
Notes on a case of dermatitis herpetiformis, extending over eleven years illustrating the several varieties of the disease. [Philadelphia, 1884.] 3p. DNLM **80-1704**

DUHRING, Louis Adolphus (1845-1913)
Dermatitis herpetiformis. Chicago: A. G. Newell, 1884. 16p. DNLM **80-1705**

DUHRING, Louis Adolphus (1845-1913)
A case of ainhum. With microscopic examination by Henry Wile. [Philadelphia, 1884.] 5p. DNLM **80-1706**

DUHRING, Louis Adolphus (1845-1913)
Epitome of diseases of the skin. Being an abstract of a course of lectures delivered in the University of Pennsylvania during the session of 1883 and 1884. . . . Reported by Henry Wile. . . . Philadelphia: J. B. Lippincott & Co., 1886 [1885]. 130p. DLC; DNLM; NNNAM; PPC **80-1707**

DUHRING, Louis Adolphus (1845-1913)
Case of dermatitis herpetiformis of the pustular variety. [Philadelphia], 1887. 7p. DNLM **80-1708**

DUHRING, Louis Adolphus (1845-1913)
Two cases of typical dermatitis herpetiformis. [New York, 1887.] 7p. DNLM **80-1709**

DUHRING, Louis Adolphus (1845-1913)
Case of dermatitis herpetiformis resembling erythema multiforme. New York: William Wood & Co., 1887. 6p. DNLM **80-1710**

DUJARDIN-BEAUMETZ, Georges Octave (1833-1895)
Clinical therapeutics. Lectures in practical medicine, delivered in the Hospital St. Antoine, Paris, France. The treatment of nervous diseases, of general diseases, and of fevers. Transl. by E. P. Hurd. Detroit: G. S. Davis, 1885. 491p. DLC; DNLM; OCIM; PU **80-1711**

DUJARDIN-BEAUMETZ, Georges Octave (1833-1895)
Diseases of the stomach and intestines; a manual of clinical therapeutics, for the student and practitioner. Transl. from the 4th French ed. by E. P. Hurd. New York: William Wood & Co., 1886. 389p. 1 chart. DLC; DNLM; NNNAM; PPC
80-1712

DUJARDIN-BEAUMETZ, Georges Octave (1833-1895)
The modern treatment of diseases of the heart. A manual of clinical therapeutics. Transl. from the 4th French ed. by E. P. Hurd. Detroit: G. S. Davis, 1887. 316p. DLC; DNLM; OCIM
80-1713

DUJARDIN-BEAUMETZ, Georges Octave (1833-1895)
The modern treatment of diseases of the liver. Transl. from the 5th French ed. by E. P. Hurd. Detroit: G. S. Davis, 1888. 185p. DLC; DNLM; OCIM **80-1714**

DUJARDIN-BEAUMETZ, Georges Octave (1833-1895)
The modern treatment of diseases of the kidney. Transl. from the 5th French ed. by E. P. Hurd. Detroit: G. S. Davis, 1888. 169p. DLC; DNLM; OCIM **80-1715**

DULLES, Charles Winslow (1850-1921)
What to do first, in accidents or poisoning. Philadelphia: P. Blakiston, 1880. 64p. DNLM; IU-M; NNNAM; PPC
80-1716

DULLES, Charles Winslow (1850-1921)
Remarks on hydrophobia. [Philadelphia, 1883.] 12p. DNLM
80-1717

DULLES, Charles Winslow (1850-1921)
What to do first in accidents and emergencies; a manual explaining the treatment of surgical and other injuries in the absence of the physician. 2nd ed. Philadelphia: P. Blakiston, Son & Co., 1883. 119p. 1 plate. DLC; DNLM
80-1718

DULLES, Charles Winslow (1850-1921)
Criticisms on the specific theory of hydrophobia. Philadelphia, 1884. 35p. DLC; PU **80-1719**

DULLES, Charles Winslow (1850-1921)
Disorders mistaken for hydrophobia. Philadelphia: Collins, 1884. 37p. DLC; PPC **80-1720**

DULLES, Charles Winslow (1850-1921)
A new bandage for fixation of the humerus and shoulder-blade. [Philadelphia], 1885. 8p. DNLM **80-1721**

DULLES, Charles Winslow (1850-1921)
Comments on Pasteur's method of treating hydrophobia. New York, 1886. 20p. DNLM; NNNAM
80-1722

DULLES, Charles Winslow (1850-1921)
The mechanism of indirect fractures of the skull. Philadelphia: W. J. Dornan, 1886. 55p. 14 plates. DNLM; PPC
80-1723

DULLES, Charles Winslow (1850-1921)
Supra-public lithotomy; a historical sketch. Philadelphia, 1887. 8p. DNLM **80-1724**

DULLES, Charles Winslow (1850-1921)
Report on hydrophobia. Philadelphia: W. J. Dornan, 1888. 8p. DNLM **80-1725**

DULLES, Charles Winslow (1850-1921)
Accidents and emergencies. A manual of the treatment of surgical and other injuries in the absence of a physician. 3rd ed. Philadelphia: P. Blakiston, Son & Co., 1888. 123p. 1 plate. DLC; DNLM **80-1726**

DUNCAN, J[ames] Matthews (1826-1890)
Clinical lectures on the diseases of women, delivered in Saint Bartholomew's Hospital. Philadelphia: Henry C. Lea, 1880. 175p. CtY-M; DNLM; NNNAM; PPC **80-1727**

DUNCAN, J[ames] Matthews (1826-1890)
Clinical lectures on the diseases of women, delivered in Saint Bartholomew's Hospital. Philadelphia: Henry C. Lea's Son & Co., 1881. 100p. DNLM; ICRM; MBM; PU
80-1728

DUNCAN, J[ames] Matthews (1826-1890)
Clinical lectures on the diseases of women, delivered in Saint Bartholomew's Hospital. New York: Bermingham & Co., 1881. 67p. DNLM; MBM; NNNAM; PU **80-1729**

DUNCAN, Thomas Cation
The feeding and management of infants and children, and the home treatment of their diseases. . . . Chicago: Duncan Bros., 1880. 426p. DLC; OCIM; PPHa **80-1730**

DUNCAN, Thomas Cation, ed.
Diseases of infants and children, with their homoeopathic treatment. . . . 2nd ed. Chicago: Duncan Bros., 1880. 2 v. DLC; IEN-M; OCIM; PPHa **80-1731**

DUNCAN, Thomas Cation
Diseases of children and their homoeopathic treatment. . . . 3rd ed. Chicago: Duncan Bros., 1882. 1006p. IEN-M; OCIM; PPHa
80-1732

DUNGLISON, Richard James (1834-1901)
A new school physiology. . . . Illustrated with one hundred and seventeen engravings. Philadelphia: Porter & Coates, [1880]. 114p. DLC; ICU; NN; MB **80-1733**

DUNGLISON, Richard James (1834-1901)
The practitioner's reference book. . . . 2nd ed., rev. and enl. Philadelphia: Lindsay & Blakiston, 1880. 476p. DLC; MBM; NNNAM; PPC **80-1734**

DUNGLISON, Richard James (1834-1901)
The practitioner's ready reference book. A handy guide in office and bedside practice. . . . 3rd ed., thoroughly rev. and enl. Philadelphia: P. Blakiston, Son & Co., 1883. 529p. DLC; DNLM; NNNAM; PPC **80-1735**

DUNGLISON, Richard James (1834-1901)
The present treatment of disease. An outline of the medical practice of the day. Based upon recent clinical cases. . . . Philadelphia: Press of W. F. Fell & Co., 1886. 308p. DLC; MH-M; NNNAM; PPC **80-1736**

DUNHAM, Carroll (1828-1877)
Lectures on materia medica. Philadelphia: F. E. Boericke, 1884. 419p. DNLM; OCLloyd; PPC; PPHa
80-1737

DUNHAM, Carroll (1828-1877)
Homoeopathy the science of therapeutics; a collection of papers elucidating and illustrating the principles of homoeopathy. Philadelphia: F. E. Boericke, 1885. 529p. DNLM; OCLloyd; PPHa; PPJ **80-1738**

DUNN, William A.
The therapeutics of venesection. Cambridge: Riverside Press, 1882. 20p. DNLM; MH-M **80-1739**

DUTTON, George (*b.* 1830)
Anatomy scientific and popular. . . . Boston: Cynosure Publishing Co., 1886. 443p. 2 col. plates. DLC; MBM; NNNAM **80-1740**

DWIGHT, Theodore W.
The opinion of . . . concerning the New York Ophthalmic and Aural Institute. New York: E. O. Jenkins, 1882. 12p. DNLM; NNNAM **80-1741**

DWIGHT, Thomas, Jr. (1843-1911)
Frozen sections of a child. Fifteen drawings from nature by H. P. Quincy. New York: William Wood & Co., 1881. 66p. 15 plates. CtY-M; DNLM; NNNAM; PPC **80-1742**

DWIGHT, Thomas, Jr. (1843-1911)
The significance of bone structure. Boston, 1886. 15p. 3 plates. DNLM; MBM **80-1743**

DWIGHT, Thomas, Jr. (1843-1911)
The bones of the leg considered as one apparatus. Boston: Cupples & Hurd, 1888. 18p. DNLM; MBM **80-1744**

DYE, John H.
Painless childbirth. A book for women; containing practical rules how the pains and perils, the difficulties and dangers of childbirth may be effectually avoided. . . . Silver Creek, N.Y.: The Local Printing House, 1880. 200p. DLC **80-1745**

DYE, John H.
Painless childbirth; or Healthy mothers and healthy children. A book for women. . . . 2nd ed., rev. and enl. Silver Creek, N.Y.: The Local Printing House, 1882. 294p. DLC **80-1746**

DYE, John H.
Painless childbirth; or Healthy mothers and healthy children. A book for all women. . . . 3rd ed., rev. and enl. Silver Creek, N.Y.: Brown, Elliott & Spears, 1884. 451p. DLC **80-1747**

DYE, John H.
Painless childbirth; or Healthy mothers, and healthy children. A book for all women. . . . 7th ed., rev. and enl. Buffalo, N.Y.: Baker, Jones & Co., 1888. 451p. DLC **80-1748**

EARLE, Charles Warrington (1845-1893)
The cinchona cure for intemperance. Chicago, 1880. 19p. DNLM **80-1749**

EARLE, Charles Warrington (1845-1893)
The opium habit. A clinical lecture. Chicago: Chandler & Engelhard, 1880. 31p. DNLM; OCIM **80-1750**

EARLE, Charles Warrington (1845-1893)
Cephalhaematoma of the new-born. Chicago, 1883. 7p. DNLM **80-1751**

EARLE, Charles Warrington (1845-1893)
Cirrhosis of the pancreas, or pancreatic anaemia. [Chicago, 1884.] 11p. DNLM **80-1752**

EARLE, Charles Warrington (1845-1893)
Observations in Chiara's clinic and the Hospital St. Maria Nuova, Florence, Italy. Chicago, 1887. 7p. DNLM **80-1753**

EARLE, Charles Warrington (1845-1893)
Retained débris as one of the causes of puerperal fever; the intra-uterine douche and curette. Chicago, [1887]. 3 l. DNLM **80-1754**

EARLE, Charles Warrington (1845-1893)
Antiseptic obstetrics. [Chicago, 1888.] 12p. DNLM **80-1755**

EARLE, Charles Warrington (1845-1893)
Infant feeding. Chicago, 1888. 15p. DNLM **80-1756**

EARLE, Charles Warrington (1845-1893)
The influence of sewerage and water pollution on the prevalence and severity of diphtheria. [Philadelphia, 1888.] 9p. DNLM **80-1757**

EARLE, Charles Warrington (1845-1893)
Observations in Vienna; the General Hospital, Billroth, Carl Braun, Bandl, and others. [Chicago, 1888.] 18p. DNLM **80-1758**

EARLE, Charles Warrington (1845-1893)
The responsibilities and duties of the medical profession regarding alcoholic and opium inebriety. [Chicago, 1889.] 19p. DNLM **80-1759**

EARLE, Charles Warrington (1845-1893)
The treatment (not preventive) of puerperal fever. [Chicago, 1889.] 8p. DNLM **80-1760**

EARLE, Pliny (1809-1892)
The curability of insanity. A statistical study. [Utica, N.Y., 1885.] 31p. DNLM **80-1761**

EARLE, Pliny (1809-1892)
The curability of insanity: a series of studies. . . . Philadelphia: J. B. Lippincott Co., 1887. 23p. DLC; DNLM; NNNAM; PPC **80-1762**

EASTMAN, Joseph (1842-1902)
The evolution of surgery. [n.p., 1886.] 16p. DNLM **80-1763**

EASTMAN, Joseph (1842-1902)
Four cases of abdominal surgery, with remarks. [Indianapolis, 1886.] 15p. DNLM **80-1764**

EASTMAN, Joseph (1842-1902)
A case of hysterectomy, with practical comments on laparotomy. Indianapolis: A. R. Baker, [1887]. 10p. DNLM **80-1765**

EASTMAN, Joseph (1842-1902)
Intraligamentous tubal pregnancy; successful removal by abdominal section of a four-pound living child with all its appendages; mother and child still living and in good health January 15, 1889. [Remarks on pelvic peritonitis, and on my year's work in abdominal surgery (forty cases).] [New York, 1889.] 7p. DNLM **80-1766**

EATON, Morton Monroe (1839-1889)
A treatise on the medical and surgical diseases of women, with their homoeopathic treatment. . . . New York, Philadelphia: Boericke & Tafel, [etc., etc.], 1880. 782p. 31 plates. DLC; DNLM; NNNAM; PPHa **80-1767**

EATON, Morton M[onroe] (1839-1889)
Eaton's domestic practice for parents and nurses. . . . Cincinnati: M. M. Eaton, Jr., & Co., 1882. 703p. DLC; OCIM; PPHa **80-1768**

EATON, Morton M[onroe] (1839-1889)
Eaton's illustrated domestic practice for married people and nurses. Cincinnati, O.: M. M. Eaton, Jr. & Co., 1882. 730p. OCIM; PPHa **80-1769**

ECCLES, Robert G[ibson] (1848-1934)
Drugs and digestion. [New York, 1886.] 26p. DNLM **80-1770**

ECCLES, Robert G[ibson] (1848-1934)
Descent and disease. Brooklyn: M. J. Rogers & Co., 1889. 21p. DNLM **80-1771**

ECLECTIC MEDICAL COLLEGE OF THE CITY OF NEW YORK
Annual announcements for the sessions of 1883-1884 to 1895-1896 (23.-35.); 1897-1898 (37.); 1898-1899 (38.). New York, 1883-1898. DNLM; NNNAM **80-1772**

ECLECTIC MEDICAL COLLEGE OF MAINE IN THE CITY OF LEWISTON
Annual announcements for the sessions of 1881-1882 (1.); 1883-1884 (3.). Lewiston, 1881-1883. 7, 15p. [Ceased to exist in 1887.] DLC **80-1773**

ECLECTIC MEDICAL INSTITUTE, CINCINNATI
Catalogue of graduates, 1845 to 1881. With the graduates of the Medical College, Worthington, 1834 to 1838. [Cincinnati, 1882.] 20p. DNLM; OCIM **80-1774**

ECLECTIC MEDICAL INSTITUTE, CINCINNATI
Annual announcements for the sessions of 1882-1883 to 1893-1894 (38.-49.); 1895-1896 to 1898-1899 (51.-54.). Cincinnati, 1882-1898. DNLM; OCIM; [List of students and graduates for the sessions of 1881-1882 to 1892-1893, 1894-1895 to 1897-1898, in announcements for subsequent years.] **80-1775**

THE ECLECTIC physiology, or guide to health. With special reference to the nature of alcoholic drinks and narcotics and their effects upon the human system. New York, Cincinnati, Chicago: Am. Book Comp., [1888]. 189p. 5 plates. DNLM; OCIM; NN; NNNAM **80-1776**

EDDY, Mary Morse Baker (1821-1910)
Defense of Christian science against Rev. Joseph Cook and Dr. A. J. Gordon's religious ban. Boston, 1885. 15p. DNLM; MH **80-1777**

EDDY, Mary Morse Baker (1821-1910)
Science and health, with key to the Scriptures. 24th ed. Boston, 1886, *vel subseq.* DNLM; ICU; MH; NN [1st ed., 1875] **80-1778**

EDDY, Mary Morse Baker (1821-1910)
The people's idea of God; its effects on health and Christianity. 2nd ed. Cambridge: J. Wilson & Son, 1886. 14p. DNLM; MH **80-1779**

EDDY, Mary Morse Baker (1821-1910)
Christian healing. A lecture delivered at Boston. 2nd ed. Cambridge: J. Wilson & Son, 1886. 17p. DNLM; MH **80-1780**

EDES, Robert T[haxter] (1838-1923)
Connection of cardiac and renal disease. Cambridge: Riverside Press, 1881. 22p. DNLM **80-1781**

EDES, Robert T[haxter] (1838-1923)
High-pressure education: its effects. Boston: Rockwell & Churchill, 1882. 13p. DNLM **80-1782**

EDES, Robert T[haxter] (1838-1923)
The excretion of phosphoric acid by the kidneys as affected by mental labor. [New York, 1883.] 7p. DNLM **80-1783**

EDES, Robert Thaxter (1838-1923)
Therapeutic handbook of the United States pharmacopoeia, being a condensed statement of the physiological and toxic action, medicinal value, methods of adminsitration and doses of the drugs and preparations in the latest ed. of the United States pharmacopoeia (apothecaries' and metric system) with some remaks on unofficinal preparations. . . . New York: William Wood & Co., 1883. 397p. DLC; NNNAM; OCLloyd; PU **80-1784**

EDES, Robert T[haxter] (1838-1923)
Text-book of therapeutics and materia medica, intended for the use of students and practitioners. Philadelphia: Lea Bros. & Co., 1887. 178, 552p. DLC; DNLM; OCLloyd; PU **80-1785**

EDES, Robert T[haxter] (1838-1923)
On the absolute and relative value of albumen and casts, and of renal inadequacy, in the diagnosis and prognosis of diseases of the kidney. Philadelphia: W. J. Dornan, 1888. 24p. DNLM **80-1786**

EDES, Robert T[haxter] (1838-1923)
Cases of idiopathic anaemia; large-celled sarcoma of the lumbar vertebrae. Chicago, 1888. 20p. DNLM **80-1787**

EDES, Robert T[haxter] (1838-1923)
A new clinical sphygmograph. Chicago, 1888. 7p. DNLM **80-1788**

EDES, Robert T[haxter] (1838-1923)
The relation of renal diseases to diseases of the nervous system. New York: M. J. Rooney & Co., 1888. 28. DNLM **80-1789**

EDES, Robert T[haxter] (1838-1923)
Tumor of the choroid plexus in the neighborhood of the foramen of Monro. [Philadelphia, 1888.] 10p. DNLM **80-1790**

EDES, Robert T[haxter] (1838-1923)
Hydronephrosis and renal atrophy, especially as resulting from functional disturbances of micturition. [Philadelphia, 1889.] 18p. DNLM **80-1791**

EDIS, Arthur W[ellesley] (1840-1893)
Diseases of women: including their pathology, causation, symptoms, diagnosis, and treatment. A manual for students and practitioners. Philadelphia: Henry C. Lea's Son & Co., 1882. 576p. CU-M; IU-M; PPJ; PPC **80-1792**

EDMONDS, William D.
A treatise on diseases peculiar to infants and children. New York and Philadelphia: Boericke & Tafel, 1881. 300p. MH-M; NNNAM; PPHa **80-1793**

[EDWARDS, Arthur Mead]
Catalogue of the libraries of Arthur Mead Edwards and S. S. Haldeman, forming a valuable collection of works relating to natural history, astronomy, chemistry, entomology, medicine and surgery, etc. To be sold Thursday, June 2, 1881. New York, 1881. 50p. DNLM; NN **80-1794**

EDWARDS, D. M.
A short memoir of Dr. Ariel Ballou. Providence, R.I.: E. L. Freeman & Son, 1889. 12p. DNLM **80-1795**

EDWARDS, Joseph F. (1853-1897)
Malaria; what it means and how avoided. Philadelphia: P. Blakiston, 1881. 81p. DLC; DNLM; NNNAM; PPC **80-1796**

EDWARDS, Joseph F. (1853-1897)
Dyspepsia. How to avoid it. Philadelphia: P. Blakiston, 1881. 87p. DLC; DNLM; NNNAM; PPC **80-1797**

EDWARDS, Joseph F. (1853-1897)
Constipation, plainly treated, and relieved without the use of drugs. . . . Philadelphia: P. Blakiston, 1881. 72p. DLC; NNNAM; PPC; PU **80-1798**

EDWARDS, Joseph F. (1853-1897)
Constipation, plainly treated, and relieved without the use of drugs. . . . 2nd ed., with additions. Philadelphia: P. Blakiston, 1881. 88p. DLC; OCIM; PPC; PU **80-1799**

EDWARDS, Joseph F. (1853-1897)
How a person threatened or afflicted with Bright's disease ought to live. . . . Philadelphia: P. Blakiston, 1881. 87p. DLC; MBM; NNNAM; PPC **80-1800**

EDWARDS, Joseph F. (1853-1897)
How we ought to live; a practical guide, written in plain, intelligible language, for the preservation of health, and the attainment of longevity; designed to enable all so to live that they may reach old age in health and comfort. . . . Philadelphia: H. C. Watts Co., 1882. 636p. DLC; DNLM; NNNAM; PPC **80-1801**

EDWARDS, Joseph F. (1853-1897)
Vaccination; arguments pro and con; with a chapter on the hygiene of small-pox. Philadelphia: P. Blakiston, Son & Co., 1882. 80p. DLC; DNLM; NNNAM; PPC **80-1802**

EDWARDS, Joseph F. (1853-1897)
Edwards' health books, containing: Constipation plainly treated. Bright's disease; how to live with it. Malaria; what it means. Vaccination; pro and con. Philadelphia: P. Blakiston, Son & Co., 1884. 4 pts. in 1 v. DNLM; NNNAM; OCIM; PPC **80-1803**

EDWARDS, Joseph F. (1853-1897)
Modern therapeutics of the diseases of children, with observations on the hygiene of infancy. . . . Philadelphia: D. G. Brinton, 1885. 346p. DLC; NNNAM; PPJ; PU **80-1804**

EDWARDS, Joseph F. (1853-1897)
The brittle thread of life; unfolding the true rules of life and action by which to nurture and strengthen, to guard and lengthen this vital cord, this brittle thread. [Philadelphia]: Edgewood Publishing Co., [Hubbard Bros., 1888]. 548p. 8 plates. DNLM; ICU; MB; NN **80-1805**

EDWARDS, N[athan] B[rown] (1820?-1893)
Historical address delivered before the Middlesex North District Medical Society, July 28, 1880. Lowell, Mass.: Stone, Bacheller & Livingston, 1880. 8p. DNLM **80-1806**

EDWARDS, W[illiam] A[loysius] (*b.* 1860)
Is the ovarian cell pathognomonic? [Philadelphia, 1882.] 6p. DNLM **80-1807**

EDWARDS, W[illiam] A[loysius] (*b.* 1860)
Peculiar cases of typhoid fever. Philadelphia, 1883. 4p. DNLM **80-1808**

EDWARDS, W[illiam] A[loysius] (*b.* 1860)
A contribution to the clinical study of Rötheln or German measles. Philadelphia: Henry C. Lea's Son & Co., 1884. 10p. DNLM **80-1809**

EDWARDS, W[illiam] A[loysius] (*b.* 1860)
An anomalous human lung, having four lobes on the right side. [Philadelphia, 1885.] 5p. DNLM **80-1810**

EDWARDS, W[illiam] A[loysius] (*b.* 1860)
Deductions from ninety-one (91) cases of rheumatism; being a consideration of the report of the committee on the collective investigation of disease of the Medical Society of the State of Pennsylvania. Philadelphia, [1886]. 3p. DNLM **80-1811**

EDWARDS, W[illiam] A[loysius] (*b.* 1860)
Intestinal casts; with the report of a case. [Philadelphia, 1886.] 11p. DNLM **80-1812**

EDWARDS, W[illiam] A[loysius] (*b.* 1860)
Southern Florida; a winter sanitarium. [Philadelphia, 1886.] 12p. DNLM **80-1813**

EDWARDS, W[illiam] A[loysius] (*b.* 1860)
Supernumerary mammary glands and nipples; three cases. [Philadelphia, 1886.] 8p. DNLM **80-1814**

EDWARDS, W[illiam] A[loysius] (*b.* 1860)
Notes on some forms of purpura rheumatica. [Philadelphia, 1889.] 3p. DNLM **80-1815**

EGGERT, William
The treatment of uterine displacements, including prolapsus, anteversion, retroversion, and retroflexion. 2nd ed. Chicago: Duncan Bros., 1884. 136p. DNLM; OCIM **80-1816**

EGGLESTON, E[ugene] R.
The dynamics of sanitary science, or the relations of the natural forces to the etiology of epidemics. [Ann Arbor], 1882. 21p. DNLM **80-1817**

EGGLESTON, E[ugene] R.
Natural law applied to etiology. [Cleveland, 1884.] 10p. DNLM **80-1818**

EHINGER, Clyde E.
Oxygen in therapeutics; a treatise explaining the apparatus, the materials, the chemicals and processes used in the preparation of oxygen and other gases with which it may be combined; also, its administration and effects, illustrated by clinical experience of the author and of others. Chicago: Chatterton & Co., 1886. 157p. IU-M; OCIM **80-1819**

EICHHORST, Hermann Ludwig (1849-1921)
Handbook of practical medicine. . . . New York: William Wood & Co., 1886. 4 v. DLC; MBM; NNNAM; PPC **80-1820**

ELA, Walter (*b.* 1848)
Some observations on the surgical treatment of rectal affections. [Boston, 1881.] 8p. DNLM **80-1821**

ELDRIDGE, Stuart (1841?-1901)
On beri-beri, the kak'ke of Japan. [San Francisco, 1881.] 18p. DNLM **80-1822**

ELDRIDGE, Stuart (1841?-1901)
Echinococci in the female bladder; cystitis; excessive dilatation of urethra; cure. New York: William Wood & Co., 1881. 3p. DNLM **80-1823**

ELDRIDGE, Stuart (1841?-1901)
The "pathfinder," a new instrument for facilitating the diagnosis and treatment of strictures of small calibre. [Philadelphia, 1881.] 3p. DNLM **80-1824**

ELIOT, Gustavus (1857-1932)
Poliomyelitis anterior in adults. Philadelphia, 1885. 9p. DNLM **80-1825**

ELIOT, Gustavus (1857-1932)
The prevention of insanity. Hartford, Conn.: Lockwood & Brainard, 1886. 8p. DNLM **80-1826**

ELIOT, Gustavus (1857-1932)
The treatment of neuralgia in general practice. Buffalo: J. Laughlin & Co., 1887. 8p. DNLM **80-1827**

ELIOT, Llewellyn (*b.* 1853)
Case of poisoning resulting from chloroform taken internally; recovery; supplemented with a table of reported cases. New York: Trow, 1885. 22p. 1 tab. DNLM **80-1828**

ELIOT, Llewellyn (*b.* 1853)
The metric system in medicine. [New York, 1885.] 3p. DNLM **80-1829**

ELIOT, Llewellyn (*b.* 1853)
Permanent drainage for ascites. [New York, 1886.] 3p. DNLM **80-1830**

ELIOT, Llewellyn (*b.* 1853)
Persistent vomiting of labor arrested by tincture of iodine. New York: Trow, 1887. 8p. DNLM **80-1831**

ELIOT, Llewellyn (*b.* 1853)
The prophylaxis of diphtheria. [Philadelphia, 1887.] 3p. DNLM **80-1832**

ELIOT, Llewellyn (*b.* 1853)
A case of poisoning by sulphate of atropia; recovery. [Chicago, 1888.] 8p. DNLM **80-1833**

ELIOT, Llewellyn (*b.* 1853)
On the diagnosis of pregnancy in the early months. Chicago, 1889. 8p. DNLM **80-1834**

ELIOT, Llewellyn (*b.* 1853)
Four narrow escapes from death from hyperanaesthesia at surgical operations. [Philadelphia, 1889.] 4p. DNLM **80-1835**

ELIOT, Llewellyn (*b.* 1853)
The resuscitation of asphyxiated newborn infants by the suspension method. Philadelphia: W. J. Dornan, 1889. 7p. DNLM **80-1836**

ELLINGWOOD, Finley (1852-1920)
A synopsis of medical chemistry. A brief suggestive consideration of the practical facts in theoretical, inorganic and organic chemistry. . . . Chicago: The J. M. W. Jones Stationery & Printing Co., 1889. 84p. DLC; ICU **80-1837**

ELLIOT, George T[homas]
A contribution to the histology and pathology of herpetiform hydroa. [New York, 1887.] 24p. 1 plate. DNLM; NNNAM **80-1838**

ELLIOT, J[ohn] W[heelock] (1852-1925)
The treatment of retroversion of the uterus with adhesions. Cambridge: Riverside Press, 1884. 16p. DNLM; MBM **80-1839**

ELLIOT, J[ohn] W[heelock] (1852-1925)
Five cases of ovariotomy. [Boston, 1885.] 8p. DNLM **80-1840**

ELLIOT, J[ohn] W[heelock] (1852-1925)
Three cases of suppurating ovarian tumor treated by drainage. [Boston, 1886.] 10p. DNLM **80-1841**

ELLIOT, J[ohn] W[heelock] (1852-1925)
A case of chronic salpingitis; tubo-ovarian cyst, acutely inflamed; hemorrhage into the cyst; operation; recovery. New York, 1887. 6p. DNLM **80-1842**

ELLIOT, J[ohn] W[heelock] (1852-1925)
Papers on abdominal surgery. Bsoton: Cupples & Hurd, 1889. 26p. DNLM; MBM **80-1843**

ELLIOTT, George R.
The pressure paralysis of Pott's disease. [New York, 1888.] 27p. DNLM **80-1844**

ELLIOTT, John B[arnwell] (1841-1921)
A rational explanation of fever and its phenomena. [New Orleans, 1882.] 14p. DNLM; LNT-M **80-1845**

ELLIOTT, John B[arnwell] (1841-1921)
Exercise as a physiological necessity. New Orleans: L. Graham & Son, [1883]. 11p. DNLM **80-1846**

ELLIS, Edward
What every mother should know. Philadelphia: P. Blakiston, Son & Co., [1880]. 132p. DNLM; NNNAM; PPC; PU **80-1847**

ELLIS, Edward
A practical manual of the diseases of children, with a formulary. 4th ed., revised and enlarged. New York: Bermingham & Co., 1882. 218p. CtY-M; DNLM; MBM; NNNAM
80-1848

ELLIS, Erastus R[anney] (1832-1914)
Homoeopathic family guide, and information for the people. . . . 2nd ed. [Detroit: O. S. Gulley, Book and Job Printer, 1882.] 244p. OCIM; PPHa **80-1849**

ELLIS, Fred W[arren]
The circulation of the blood in the orbit studied by means of the plethysmograph. Boston: Cupples & Co., 1887. 6p. DNLM
80-1850

ELLIS, Fred W[arren]
Oxaluria. [Boston, 1888.] 19p. DNLM
80-1851

ELLIS, George E[dward] (1814-1894)
Memoir of Jacob Bigelow, M.D. Cambridge: J. Wilson & Son, 1880. 105p. 1 plate. DNLM; MH; MH-M; NN
80-1852

ELLIS, George Viner (1812-1900) and G. H. FORD
Illustrations of dissections in a series of original colored plates the size of life, representing the dissection of the human body. 2nd ed. New York: William Wood & Co., 1882. 2 v. DNLM; NNNAM; PPC; PU **80-1853**

ELSBERG, Louis (1836-1885)
The throat and its functions in swallowing, breathing, and the production of the voice. New York: G. P. Putnam's Sons, 1880. 60p. DNLM; NNNAM **80-1854**

ELSBERG, Louis (1836-1885)
The galvanic accumulator for storing dynamical electricity for cautery and illuminating purposes. New York: Trow, 1881. 13p. DNLM **80-1855**

ELSBERG, Louis (1836-1885)
Laryngological instruction. Address. [New York, 1881.] 7p. DNLM **80-1856**

ELSBERG, Louis (1836-1885)
The throat and its functions in swallowing, breathing, and the production of the voice. 2nd ed. Albany, N.Y.: E. S. Werner, 1882. 60p. DNLM; NNNAM **80-1857**

ELSBERG, Louis (1836-1885)
Case of eversion and prolapse of both sacculi laryngis; successful intralaryngeal extirpation of one and almost complete reduction of the other. [New York, 1882.] 4p. DNLM
80-1858

ELSBERG, Louis (1836-1885)
Case of unilateral acute inflammation of the crico-arytenoid joint. [New York, 1882.] 1 l. DNLM **80-1859**

ELSBERG, Louis (1836-1885)
Changes in biological doctrines during the past twenty-five years. Philadelphia, 1882. 16p. DNLM
80-1860

ELSBERG, Louis (1836-1885)
Neuroses of sensation of the pharynx and larynx, or sensory neuroses of the throat. New York: G. P. Putnam's Sons, 1882. 30p. DNLM **80-1861**

ELSBERG, Louis (1836-1885)
Paralysis of muscles of the larynx. [New York, 1882.] 9p. DNLM **80-1862**

ELSBERG, Louis (1836-1885)
The structure of hyaline cartilage. With deductions regarding the cell doctrine and the bioplasson doctrine, being the first chapter of contributions to the histology of the cartilages of the larynx. [New York, 1882.] 36p. 1 plate. DNLM
80-1863

ELSBERG, Louis (1836-1885)
Lecture, introductory to the eighty-seventh course of instruction in the Medical Department of Dartmouth College, delivered August 1, 1883. [Hanover, N.H.: Dartmouth Press], 1883. 23p. DNLM **80-1864**

ELSBERG, Louis (1836-1885)
Reflex and other phenomena due to nasal disease. [New York: G. P. Putnam's Sons, 1883]. 3p. DNLM
80-1865

ELSBERG, Louis (1836-1885)
Two cases of successful internal oesophagotomy. [New York, 1883.] 5p. DNLM **80-1866**

ELSBERG, Louis (1836-1885)
On angioma of the larynx. [New York, 1884.] 18p. DNLM
80-1867

ELSBERG, Louis (1836-1885)
Hereditary transmission; illustrations of its occurrence, explanation of its phenomena by the plastidule theory, and modification of the evolution doctrine. [New York, 1884.] 32p. DNLM **80-1868**

ELSNER, H[enry] Leopold (1857-1916)
Typhoid fever as we see it in central New York. New York, 1885. 13p. DNLM; NNNAM **80-1869**

ELSNER, H[enry] Leopold (1857-1916)
Early diagnosis of tubercular meningitis in children. Buffalo: Times Print. House, 1888. 8p. DNLM
80-1870

ELY, Edward T[albot] (1850-1885)
Refraction of the eyes of newly-born children. [New York, 1880.] 12p. DNLM; NNNAM **80-1871**

EMERSON, Edward Waldo (1844-1930)
The man as doctor. An oration delivered at the annual meeting of the Middlesex South District Medical Society. Cambridge: Riverside Press, 1882. 27p. DNLM; MBM
80-1872

EMERY, Z. T.
Report of thirty-two cases of poisoning by locust bark. [New York, 1887.] 3p. DNLM **80-1873**

EMMET, John Duncan
Impressions of German and English gynaecology, from the standpoint of a woman's hospital alumnus. [New York, 1886.] 12p. DNLM; NNNAM **80-1874**

EMMET, Thomas Addis (1828-1919)
The principles and practice of gynaecology. . . . 2nd ed., thoroughly rev. With one hundred and thirty-three illustrations. Philadelphia: Henry C. Lea, 1880. 875p. DLC; MBM; NNNAM; PPC **80-1875**

EMMET, Thomas Addis (1828-1919)
A new method of exploration with the pathology and treatment of certain lesions of the female urethra. [Philadelphia, 1883.] 27p. DNLM; PPC **80-1876**

EMMET, Thomas Addis (1828-1919)
The principles and practice of gynaecology. . . . 3rd ed., thoroughly rev. With one hundred and fifty illustrations. Philadelphia: Henry C. Lea's Son & Co., 1884. 876p. DLC; DNLM; NNNAM; PPC **80-1877**

EMMET, Thomas Addis (1828-1919)
A study of the etiology of perineal laceration, with a new method for its proper repair. [New York, 1884.] 12p. DNLM **80-1878**

EMMET, Thomas Addis (1828-1919)
A memoir of James Marion Sims, M.D., LL.D. . . . New York: D. Appleton & Co., 1884. 19p. DLC; DNLM; NN; NNNAM **80-1879**

EMMET, Thomas Addis (1828-1919)
Pelvic inflammations; or, cellulitis versus peritonitis. [New York, 1887.] 11p. DNLM **80-1880**

EMMET, Thomas Addis (1828-1919)
Tracheotomy without the cannula. [New York, 1888.] 5p. DNLM **80-1881**

EMMET, Thomas Addis (1828-1919)
On the use of the vaginal tampon in the treatment of certain effects following pelvic inflammations. [New York, 1888.] 16p. DNLM **80-1882**

EMMET, Thomas Addis (1828-1919)
A study of the causes and treatment of uterine displacements. [New York, 1888.] 14p. DNLM; NNNAM **80-1883**

ENGELMANN, George J[ulius] (1847-1903)
The treatment of post-partum hemorrhage. St. Louis: G. O. Rumbold & Co., 1880. 26p. DNLM; OCIM **80-1884**

ENGELMANN, George J[ulius] (1847-1903)
Time of conception and duration of pregnancy. St. Louis: McCormick, Nixon & Co., 1880. 7p. DNLM **80-1885**

ENGELMANN, George J[ulius] (1847-1903)
The danger incident to the simplest uterine manipulations and operations. St. Louis: Davis & Freegard, 1880. 35p. DNLM; OCIM **80-1886**

ENGELMANN, George J[ulius] (1847-1903)
Time of conception and duration of pregnancy; supplementary. [St. Louis, 1880.] 6p. DNLM **80-1887**

ENGELMANN, George J[ulius] (1847-1903)
Two cases of anterior displacement of the ovary, simulating inguinal hernia; Battey's operation. [Boston, 1881.] 17p. DNLM **80-1888**

ENGELMANN, George J[ulius] (1847-1903)
Primary cancer of the corpus uteri; diagnosis and treatment; Freund's operation and the scoop. [St. Louis, 1881.] 12p. DNLM **80-1889**

ENGELMANN, George J[ulius] (1847-1903)
Posture in labor. [Boston, 1881.] 95p. DNLM; MBM; NNNAM **80-1890**

ENGELMANN, George J[ulius] (1847-1903)
Pregnancy, parturition, and childbed among primitive people. New York, 1881. 16+ p. DNLM **80-1891**

ENGELMANN, George J[ulius] (1847-1903)
Ovariotomy; difficulties, diagnostic and operative; continued menstruation after double ovariotomy. [Philadelphia, 1882.] 16p. DNLM **80-1892**

ENGELMANN, George J[ulius] (1847-1903)
Massage and expression or external manipulations in the obstetric practice of primitive people. [New York, 1882.] 25p. DNLM; NNNAM **80-1893**

ENGELMANN, George J[ulius] (1847-1903)
Clitoridectomy. Louisville: J. P. Morton & Co., 1882. 12p. DNLM **80-1894**

ENGELMANN, George J[ulius] (1847-1903)
Labor among primitive peoples. St. Louis: J. H. Chambers & Co., 1882. 203p. 1 plate. DNLM; ICU; MBM; NNNAM **80-1895**

ENGELMANN, George J[ulius] (1847-1903)
Insidious septicemia. A rare, deceptive, and fatal form of the disease. Boston, 1884. 17p. DNLM; MBM **80-1896**

ENGELMANN, George J[ulius] (1847-1903)
Labor among primitive peoples showing the development of the obstetric science of today, from the natural and instinctive customs of all races. . . . 3rd ed., rev. and enl. St. Louis: J. H. Chambers & Co., 1884. 227p. ICU; OCIM; PU **80-1897**

ENGELMANN, George J[ulius] (1847-1903)
A new departure in uterine therapeutics; the dry treatment. [St. Louis, 1886.] 11p. DNLM **80-1898**

ENGELMANN, George J[ulius] (1847-1903)
The use of electricity in gynecological practice. [New York, 1887.] 149p. CtY-M; DNLM; MBM; NNNAM **80-1899**

ENGELMANN, George J[ulius] (1847-1903)
The polar method of electrotherapy in gynecology. Application, dosage, and medication. [Philadelphia], 1887. 39p. DNLM; PPC; PU **80-1900**

ENGELMANN, George J[ulius] (1847-1903)
Galvanic and faradic electricity in the treatment of uterine displacements. St. Louis: J. H. Chambers & Co., [1887]. 30p. DNLM; OCIM **80-1901**

ENGELMANN, George J[ulius] (1847-1903)
Electro-therapy and surgery in gynecology. Philadelphia: W. J. Dornan, 1888. 21p. DNLM **80-1902**

ENGELMANN, George J[ulius] (1847-1903)
Renal disease following utero-ovarian lesions. Philadelphia: W. J. Dornan, 1889. 24p. DNLM; PPC **80-1903**

AN EPITOME of the newer materia medica, standard medicinal products, and fine pharmaceutical specialties introduced and manufactured by Parke Davis & Company, to which is added a complete property and dose list of all the fluid, solid, and powdered extracts, German tinctures, normal liquids, and concentrations prepared by them, together with a complete formula list of their sugar and gelatin coated pills. Designed for the special convenience of the busy physician. 4th ed. Detroit: Parke Davis & Co., 1886. 76p. DNLM; OCIM; OCLloyd **80-1904**

AN EPITOME of the newer materia medica, standard medicinal products, and fine pharmaceutical specialties introduced and manufactured by Parke Davis & Company, to which is added a complete property and dose list of all the fluid, solid, and powdered extracts, German tinctures, normal liquids, and concentrations prepared by them, together with a complete formula list of their sugar and gelatin coated pills. Designed for the special convenience of the busy physician. 5th ed. Detroit: Parke Davis & Co., 1889. 88p. DNLM; OCLloyd **80-1905**

AN EPITOME of medicine, surgery, obstetrics and pathology, consisting of revised stenographic reports of the lectures of Alfred Stillé . . . D. Hayes Agnew . . . R. A. F. Penrose . . . and James Tyson . . . 3rd ed. Philadelphia: Samuel M. Miller, 1886. 552p. DLC; ICJ; NNNAM; PU [1st ed., 188-?, 451p.; 2nd ed., 1883, 478p.] **80-1905A**

ERB, Wilhelm H[einrich] (1840-1921)
Spinal myosis and reflex pupillary immobility. New York: G. P. Putnam's Sons, 1880. 15p. DNLM; NNNAM **80-1906**

ERB, Wilhelm H[einrich] (1840-1921)
Handbook of electro-therapeutics. Transl. by L. Putzel. New York: William Wood & Co., 1883. 366p. IEN-M; LNT-M; NNNAM; PPC **80-1907**

ERCOLANI, Giovanni Battista (1819-1883)
The utricular glands of the uterus, and the glandular organ of new formation which is developed during pregnancy in the uterus of the *Mammalia*, including the human species. . . . To which is appended his monograph upon the unity of the anatomical type of the placenta in all the *Mammalia*, and the physiological unity of the nutrition of the foetus in all the vertebrates. Also, a general summary and classification, written expressly for this edition. With a quarto atlas of fifteen plates, engraved by Bettini, and reproduced by the heliotype process. Transl. from the Italian under the direction of Henry O. Marcy. . . . Boston: Houghton, Osgood & Co., 1880. 305p. atlas, 16 plates. DLC; NNNAM; PPC; PU **80-1908**

ERCOLANI, Giovanni Battista (1819-1883)
The reproductive process: its history, physiology, and pathology. Demonstrating the unity of the anatomical type of the placenta in all the *Mammalia*, and the physiological unity of the nutrition of the foetus in all the vertebrates. In two volumes: one a quarto atlas of illustrations, engraved by Bettini, and reproduced by the heliotype process. Transl. by Henry O. Marcy. . . . Boston, New York: Houghton, Mifflin & Co., 1884. 435p. DLC; NNC; OCIM; PU **80-1909**

ERICH, Augustus Frederick (1837-1886)
Seven cases of retroflexion of the uterus with peritoneal adhesions of the fundus in the hollow of the sacrum, treated by forcible separation of adhesions. New York: William Wood & Co., 1880. 12p. DNLM; NNNAM **80-1910**

ERICH, Augustus Frederick (1837-1886)
A case of encysted ascites stimulating ovarian dropsy; operation; death; autopsy. [Boston, 1880.] 7p. DNLM **80-1911**

ERICH, Augustus Frederick (1837-1886)
Atresia of the vagina and uterus. Atlanta: H. H. Dickson, 1881. 9p. DNLM **80-1912**

ERICH, Augustus Frederick (1837-1886)
A device to facilitate the removal of deep wire sutures in the operation for ruptured peritoneum. Baltimore: J. W. Borst & Co., [1881]. 7p. DNLM **80-1913**

ERICH, Augustus Frederick (1837-1886)
An improved self-retaining rectal and vaginal speculum. Cincinnati: Lancet Press Print, 1881. 8p. DNLM **80-1914**

ERICH, Augustus Frederick (1837-1886)
Chronic pelvic abscess. A contribution to the differential diagnosis of abdominal tumors. [Baltimore, 1882.] 6p. DNLM **80-1915**

ERICHSEN, Hugo (1860-1944)
The London medical student and other comicalities. Selected and compiled by . . . . Detroit, Mich.: Detroit Free Press, 1885. 207p. DNLM **80-1916**

ERICHSEN, Hugo (1860-1944)
The cremation of the dead considered from an aesthetic, sanitary, religious, historical, medico-legal, and economical standpoint. With an introductory note by Sir T. Spencer Wells. Detroit: D. O. Haynes & Co., 1887. 264p. 1 plate. DNLM; OCIM **80-1917**

ERICHSEN, John Eric (1818-1896)
On concussion of the spine, nervous shock, and other obscure injuries of the nervous system, in their clinical and medico-legal aspects. New and rev. ed. New York: Bermingham & Co., 1882. 300p. MdBJ-W; NNNAM; NNU-M; PU **80-1918**

ERICHSEN, John Eric (1818-1896)
On concussion of the spine, nervous shock and other obscure injuries to the nervous system in their clinical and medico-legal aspects. . . . A new and rev. ed. New York: William Wood & Co., 1883. 163p. DLC; DNLM; NNNAM; PPC **80-1919**

ERICHSEN, John Eric (1818-1896)
The science and art of surgery. Being a treatise on surgical injuries, diseases, and operations. 8th ed., revised and edited by Marcus Beck. Philadelphia: Henry C. Lea's Son & Co., 1884. 1124p. CU-M; DNLM; IU-M; PPC **80-1920**

ERLENMEYER, [Friedrich] Albrecht (1822-1877)
On the treatment of the morphine habit. . . . Transl. from the German [by E. P. Hurd]. Detroit, Mich.: G. S. Davis, 1889. 113p. DLC; NNNAM; OCIM; PU **80-1921**

ESHNER, Augustus A[dolph] (*b.* 1862)
Exophthalmic goitre. Prize essay, Jefferson Medical College, 1888. Philadelphia, 1888. 8p. DNLM; PPJ **80-1922**

ESHNER, Augustus A[dolph] (*b.* 1862)
Large doses of iodide of potassium. [Philadelphia, 1889.] 3p. DNLM **80-1923**

ESKRIDGE, Jeremiah Thomas (1848-1902)
Tubercular cerebro-spinal meningitis. [New York, 1883.] 29p. DNLM **80-1924**

ESKRIDGE, Jeremiah Thomas (1848-1902)
Abscess of the brain; operation; death on the ninth day. New York: M. J. Rooney & Co., 1889. 7p. DNLM **80-1925**

ESKRIDGE, Jeremiah Thomas (1848-1902)
Cases of syphilis of the brain. St. Louis, 1889. 20p. DNLM **80-1926**

ESKRIDGE, Jeremiah Thomas (1848-1902)
Spinal irritation, and some points in the diagnosis of affections that may be mistaken for it. [St. Louis, 1889.] 21p. DNLM **80-1927**

von ESMARCH, Friedrich (1823-1908)
Early aid in injuries and accidents. . . . Transl. by H. R. H. Princess Christian. Philadelphia: Henry C. Lea's Son & Co., 1883. 117p. NNNAM; OCIM; PPC; PU **80-1928**

ESSIG, Charles James (1841-1901)
Dental metallurgy: a manual for the use of dental students. . . . Philadelphia: The S. S. White Dental Mfg. Co., 1882. 253p. DLC; MdU-D; NNNAM; PPC **80-1929**

ESSIG, Charles James (1841-1901)
Dental metallurgy: a manual for the use of dental students. . . . 2nd ed., rev. Philadelphia: The S. S. White Dental Mfg. Co., 1888. 268p. DLC; MdU-D; OCIM; PPC **80-1930**

EVANS, D[aniel] W.
An address to the members of the general assembly of Pennsylvania, supporting "An act to establish a State board of medical examiners and licensers and to define the duties and powers of such board." By the Cambria County Medical Society. [Johnstown, Pa., 1889.] 4p. DNLM **80-1931**

EVANS, E[van] W.
The antipyretic action of antifebrin. [Philadelphia, 1887.] 8, 9p. DNLM **80-1932**

EVANS, George (1844-1942)
A practical treatise on artificial crown- and bridge-work. . . . With 500 illustrations. Philadelphia: The S. S. White Dental Mfg. Co., 1888. 263p. plates. DLC; MdU-D; NNNAM; PU **80-1933**

EVANS, George (1844-1942)
A practical treatise on artificial crown- and bridge-work. . . . 2nd ed., rev. and enl. With 547 illustrations. Philadelphia: The S. S. White Dental Mfg. Co., 1889. 296p. plates. DLC; MBM; MdU-D; PPC **80-1934**

EVANS, George A. (1850-1925)
Handbook of historical and geographical phthisiology, with special reference to the distribution of consumption in the United States. New York: D. Appleton & Co., 1888. 295p. DNLM; NNNAM; OCIM; PPC **80-1935**

EVANS, Thomas B[enjamin] (1832-1891)
Oration, delivered by request, before the Medical and Surgical Society of Baltimore, Md., commemorate of Dr. Augustus Frederick Erich. Baltimore: I. Friedenwald, 1887. 15p. DNLM; MdU-D **80-1936**

EVANS, W[arren] Felt (1817-1889)
The divine law of cure. Boston: H. H. Carter & Co., 1881. 302p. DNLM; MB; MBM **80-1937**

EVANS, W[arren] Felt (1817-1889)
The primitive mind-cure. The nature and power of faith; or, elementary lessons in Christian philosophy and transcendental medicine. Boston: H. H. Carter & Co., 1885. 215p. DNLM; MB **80-1938**

EVANS, W[arren] Felt (1817-1889)
The mental-cure, illustrating the influence of the mind on the body, both in health and disease, and the psychological method of treatment. . . . 7th ed. Boston: Colby & Rich, 1885. 364p. DLC; MH **80-1939**

EVANS, W[arren] Felt (1817-1889)
Mental medicine: a theoretical and practical treatise on medical psychology. . . . 15th ed. Boston: H. H. Carter, 1885. 216p. DLC; NN; MH **80-1940**

EVANS, W[arren] Felt (1817-1889)
The primitive mind-cure. The nature and power of faith; or, elementary lessons in Christian philosophy and transcendental medicine. 5th ed. Boston: H. H. Carter & Karrick, 1886. 215p. DNLM; MH **80-1941**

EVANS, W[arren] Felt (1817-1889)
Esoteric Christianity and mental therapeutics. Boston: H. H. Carter & Karrick, 1886. 174p. DNLM; MH **80-1942**

EVE, Duncan (*b.* 1852)
The prophecy of science; an address to the graduating class of the Medical Department of the University of Tennessee, Nashville, Feb. 27, 1883. [n.p., 1883.] 8p. DNLM **80-1943**

EWALD, C[arl] A[nton] (1845-1915)
Lectures on digestion; an introduction to the clinical study of diseases of the digestive organs. Twelve lectures, delivered to the practitioners and advanced students of medicine during the winter session 1878-1879. Transl. by Robert Saundby. New York: William Wood & Co., 1881. 149p. CtY-M; DNLM; NNNAM; PPC **80-1944**

EXCERPTS from opinions of distinguished medical men in this and other countries justifying the treatment of the late President Garfield, together with a letter in reply to the resolution of the special committee of the House of Representatives referring to the expenses consequent upon his illness and death. Washington: D. C. Gibson Bros., 1882. 24p. DNLM **80-1945**

EXPLANATORY index to accompany "White's physiological manikin, medical edition"; prepared under the supervision of Frank H. Hamilton, illustrating the effects of alcohol and narcotics by colored plates, and by a series of microscopical sections prepared under the authority of the State of New York by Francis Delafield and T. Mitchell Prudden. New York: J. T. White & Co., [1889]. 41p. DNLM; NNNAM **80-1946**

FAGGE, [Charles] Hilton (1838-1883)
The principles and practice of medicine. Including a section of cutaneous diseases, by P. H. Pye-Smith; chapters on cardiac diseases, by Samuel Wilkes; and complete indexes, by Robert Edmund Carrington. Philadelphia: P. Blakiston, Son & Co., 1886. 2 v. DNLM; NNNAM; OCIM; PPC **80-1947**

FAIRCHILD, D. W.
Something I have yearned for. [Circular of "Phosphatine," and Rowe's improved rupture appliances.] New York: Russell Bros., 1880. 24p. DNLM; NNNAM **80-1948**

FALLIGANT, Louis A[lexander] (1836-1903)
The dengue fever of 1880 in Savannah, Georgia. Philadelphia, 1881. 32p. DNLM; LNT-M **80-1949**

FALLIGANT, Louis A[lexander] (1836-1903)
A monograph on the yellow fever of 1876 in Savannah, Ga. Savannah, Ga.: The Morning News Print, September, 1888. 4pp. LNT-M; PPHa **80-1950**

THE FAMILY physician. A manual of domestic medicine, by physicians and surgeons of the principal London hospitals. American ed. Ed. by Ghislani Durant. . . . New York: Cassell, Petter, Galpin & Co., [1880]. 1030p. DLC; NNNAM; PPC; PU **80-1951**

FARLOW, J[ohn] W[oodford] (1853-1937)
Five cases of large, visible, pulsating artery on the posterior wall of the pharynx. [Boston, 1887.] 7p. DNLM **80-1952**

FARLOW, J[ohn] W[oodford] (1853-1937)
On examination of the throat, with especial reference to the manner of using the tongue-depressor. [Boston, 1887.] 5p. DNLM **80-1953**

FARLOW, J[ohn] W[oodford] (1853-1937)
An analysis of one hundred and forty-one cases of pregnancy, with reference to the blue color of the vagina. Boston: Cupples & Hurd, 1887. 9p. DNLM **80-1954**

FARLOW, J[ohn] W[oodford] (1853-1937)
Cascara sagrada, and its use in the treatment of constipation. Boston: Cupples & Hurd, 1887. 8p. DNLM **80-1955**

FARLOW, J[ohn] W[oodford] (1853-1937)
Hypertrophy of the glandular tissue at the base of the tongue; with report of cases. Boston: Cupples & Hurd, 1888. 5p. DNLM **80-1956**

FARLOW, J[ohn] W[oodford] (1853-1937)
A case of suppression of urine for twelve days, from compression of both ureters; autopsy. [Boston, 1889.] 16p. DNLM **80-1957**

FARNHAM, A. B[radford]
When to operate in the nasal passages; and a nasal cutting-forceps. [New York, 1887.] 7p. DNLM **80-1958**

FARNSWORTH, P[hilo] J[udson] (*b.* 1830)
Abstract of a course of lectures on materia medica and therapeutics. Clinton, Iowa, 1882. 55p. DNLM; OCLloyd **80-1959**

FARNSWORTH, W. A.
Annual directory of homoeopathic physicians and surgeons of the state of Michigan. East Saginaw, [1885]. 35p. DNLM; OCIM **80-1960**

FARQUHARSON, Robert (1836-1918)
A guide to therapeutics and materia medica. Enlarged and adapted to the U.S. Pharmacopoeia. . . . 3rd American ed. Philadelphia: Henry C. Lea's Son & Co., 1882. 526p. DLC; DNLM; OCLloyd; PPC **80-1961**

FARQUHARSON, Robert (1836-1918)
A guide to therapeutics and materia medica. 4th American from 4th English ed. Enlarged so as to include all preparations officinal in the U.S. Pharmacopoeia, by Frank Woodbury. Philadelphia: Lea Bros. & Co., 1889. 598p. DLC; DNLM; OCLloyd; PU **80-1962**

[FARQUHARSON, Robert James] (1824-1884)
Hospitals for contagious diseases, and their proper location. A paper prepared by request for the State Medical Society, and printed by order of the State Board of Health. [Des Moines, 1883.] 12p. DLC; DNLM **80-1963**

FARRAND TRAINING SCHOOL FOR NURSES, DETROIT
Rules for nurses in Harper Hospital. Detroit: Winn & Hammond, 1884. 12p. DNLM **80-1964**

FARRAND TRAINING SCHOOL FOR NURSES, DETROIT
Announcement for the year 1886. Detroit: O. S. Gulley, Bornman & Co., [1885]. 11p. DNLM **80-1965**

FARRAND TRAINING SCHOOL FOR NURSES, DETROIT
Annual reports of the training school committee to the board of trustees of Harper Hospital. 1., 1884-1886. Detroit: Winn & Hammond, 1887. 32p. DNLM [Established in memory of David Osburn Farrand in connection with Harper Hospital. Organized in the fall of 1883 and opened April, 1884. First report from organization to April, 1886.] **80-1966**

FARRAND TRAINING SCHOOL FOR NURSES, DETROIT
[Circular of information for candidates and probationers.] [Detroit, 1889?] 1 sheet. DNLM **80-1967**

FARRAND TRAINING SCHOOL FOR NURSES, DETROIT
[Rules, course of instruction, with list of questions to be filled out in the candidate's own handwriting.] [Detroit: R. & B. Co., 1889?] 2 l. DNLM **80-1968**

FARRAR, J. N[utting]
Importance of direct sunlight in the work-room; usefulness in art, and its bearings upon the general health. New York, [1880?] 19p. DNLM **80-1969**

FARRAR, J. N[utting]
Courtesy among dentists at professional meetings. Annual oration delivered before the American Academy of Dental Science, Boston, Mass., Nov. 10th, 1886. Buffalo, 1887. 8p. DNLM **80-1970**

FARRINGTON, Ernest Albert (1847-1885)
A clinical materia medica. Being a course of lectures delivered at the Hahnemann Medical College, of Philadelphia. . . . Reported phonographically and ed. with the assistance of the lecturer's manuscript, by Clarence Bartlett, M.D., and rev. by S. Lilienthal, M.D. With a memorial sketch of the author, by Aug. Korndoerfer, M.D. Philadelphia: Sherman & Co., 1887. 752p. DLC; MdU-D; PPC; PPHa **80-1971**

FAULKNER, Richard B[iddle] (*b.* 1853)
Some remarks on the treatment of spasmodic asthma. [New York, 1880.] 4p. DNLM **80-1972**

FAULKNER, Richard B[iddle] (*b.* 1853)
The rational treatment of spasmodic asthma. New York, 1883. 5p. DNLM **80-1973**

FAULKNER, Thomas
Each person his own physician! The doctor at home; or, The unfailing medical instructor, filled with the proven facts of medical science, and family experience. . . . New York: Hurst & Co., [1881]. 510p. DLC; DNLM; NNNAM
80-1974

FAULKNER, Thomas
The cottage physician, proven facts of medical science and family experience. . . . By Thomas Faulkner . . . J. H. Carmichael. . . . Springfield, Mass., Des Moines, Ia., [etc.]: W. C. King & Co., 1885. 640p. DLC; DNLM; MBM; OCIM
80-1975

FENGER, Christian (1840-1902) and J[ohn] H. HOLLISTER
Opening and drainage of cavities in the lungs. [Philadelphia, 1881.] 23p. DNLM; PPC **80-1976**

FENGER, Christian (1840-1902)
Total extirpation of the uterus through the vagina. [Philadelphia, 1882.] 31p. DNLM; PPC **80-1977**

FENGER, Christian (1840-1902)
Chronic peri-uterine abscess, and its treatment by laparotomy. St. Louis, Mo.: J. H. Chambers & Co., 1885. 31p. DNLM
80-1978

FENGER, Christian (1840-1902)
Vaginal hysterectomy; the actual status of the operation, and report of four cases. Chicago, 1887. 13p. DNLM
80-1979

FENGER, Christian (1840-1902)
A new kolpoplastic operation for atresia or defect of the vagina. Philadelphia: W. J. Dornan, 1887. 11p. DNLM
80-1980

FENGER, Christian (1840-1902)
Living and dead osteomas of the nasal and its accessory cavities. Chicago, 1888. 16p. DNLM **80-1981**

FENNEL, Adolphus
Principles of general pharmacy, with special reference to systems of weights and measures, specific gravity and its uses, pharmaceutical manipulations. Pursuant to a course of Adolphus Fennel . . . . Comp. by Charles T. P. Fennel. . . . Cincinnati: McDonald & Eick, 1886. 124p. DLC; DNLM; OCLloyd; PU **80-1982**

FENNER, B[yron] (*b.* 1844)
Working formulae. A handbook of the old and the new pharmacopoeias, containing weight and measure standards, working processes, working formulae, the medicinal properties and doses of drugs and their preparations, and being a comparison of the 1870 with the 1880 pharmacopoeia; with remarks, suggestions, original processes and formulae, and other matter of interest and value to druggists and physicians. Westfield, N.Y.: B. Fenner, 1884. 528p. DNLM; NNNAM; OCLloyd
80-1983

FENNER, Edward
Annual address of . . . vice-president, with remarks by C. A. Whitney, president, C. Bussey, chairman executive committee, and A. Baldwin, chairman finance committee, at regular meeting of the New Orleans Auxiliary Sanitary Association, Nov. 23, 1880. New Orleans, 1880. 20p. DNLM
80-1984

FENNER, Edward
Annual address, New Orleans Auxiliary Sanitary Association. What has been done and what remains to be accomplished to render New Orleans healthy and prosperous. Delivered Feb. 15, 1883. New Orleans: W. B. Stansbury & Co., 1883. 18p. DNLM **80-1985**

FENWICK, Samuel (1821-1902)
Outlines of the practice of medicine, with special reference to the prognosis and treatment of disease with appropriate formulae and illustrations. Philadelphia: Lindsay & Blakiston, 1880. 387p. NNNAM; OCIM; PPC; PU **80-1986**

FERNALD, F[rank] C[linton] (*d.* 1889)
Pleurotomy for empysema; recovery. Chicago, 1886. 8p. DNLM **80-1987**

FERNALD, F[rank] C[linton] (*d.* 1889)
Three unusual cases of diphtheria. [Philadelphia, 1887.] 11p. DNLM **80-1988**

FERNANDEZ [DE IBARRA], Augustin M.
Contributions to the diagnosis of yellow fever. [Philadelphia, 1887.] 8p. DNLM **80-1989**

FERRIER, David (1843-1928)
The function of the brain. 2nd ed., rewritten and enlarged. New York: G. P. Putnam's Sons, 1886. 498p. DNLM; MBM; NNNAM; OCIM **80-1990**

FERRY, A. L.
Phrenology made easy; a new system of mental science. . . . (2nd ed., rev.). Cincinnati: R. Clarke & Co., 1886. 60p. DLC
80-1991

FIELD, George Washington (*d.* 1889)
Field's medico-legal guide for doctors and lawyers. . . . Albany, New York: Banks & Bros., 1887. 291p. DLC; NN
80-1992

FIELD, Henry M[artyn] (1822-1907)
Some of the present phases of therapeutics. Hanover, N.H., 1881. 18p. DNLM **80-1993**

FIELD, Henry M[artyn] (1822-1907)
The balsamics. Concord, N.H.: Evans, Sleeper & Woodbury, 1882. 20p. DNLM **80-1994**

FIELD, Henry M[artyn] (1822-1907)
Modifications in the action of remedies occasioned by six generic conditions. Cambridge, 1884. 30p. DNLM
80-1995

FIELD, Henry M[artyn] (1822-1907)
Evacuant medication (cathartics and emetics). . . . Philadelphia: P. Blakiston, Son & Co., 1887. 288p. DLC
80-1996

FIELD, Henry M[artyn] (1822-1907)
Sulphonal. Detroit: G. S. Davis, 1889. 28p. DNLM
80-1997

FIELD, James B[rainerd] (1859-1915)
Membranous enteritis. Fiske fund prize dissertation. Providence: Kellogg Print. Co., 1887. 57p. 5 tabs. DNLM
80-1998

FIELD, Mathew D[ickinson] (1853-1895)
Is belief in spiritualism ever evidence of insanity *per se*? New York: M. J. Rooney & Co, 1888. 7p. DNLM
80-1999

FILLEBROWN, Thomas (1836-1908)
The relations of the teeth and palate to vocalism. Buffalo, 1888. 10p. DNLM **80-2000**

FILLEBROWN, Thomas (1836-1908)
A text book of operative dentistry. Written by invitation of the National Association of Dental Faculties. Philadelphia: P. Blakiston, Son & Co., 1889. 273p. DNLM; MdU-D; NNNAM; PPC **80-2001**

FINGER, Ernst A[nton] F[ranz] (1856-1939)
Blenorrhoea of the sexual organs and its complications. New York: William Wood & Co., 1889. [33-] 304p. DLC; ICJ; LNT-M; MH-M [Printed out of Wood's Medical and Surgical Monographs, vol. 2, No. 1 (1889), pp. 33-304]
80-2001A

FINLAYSON, James, ed. (1840-1906)
Clinical manual for the study of medical cases. 2nd ed., rev. and enl. Philadelphia: Lea Bros. & Co., 1886. 683p. CtY-M; MBM; NNNAM; PPC **80-2002**

FIRST district Dental Society of the State of New York: Souvenir. Seventeeth anniversary of the .... Dec. 9, 1885. Philadelphia, 1885. 73p. DNLM **80-2003**

FIRST lessons on health. Adapted from the works of Huxley, Carpenter, Oding, and E. Smith. 1st American from the 5th London ed.: rev. and improved. New York: T. A. Wright, 1882. 59p. DLC **80-2004**

[FISHER, C[harles] H[arris]] (1822-1893)
Consumption in Rhode Island. [Providence, 1882.] 11p. DNLM **80-2005**

FISHER, C[hester] Irving (*b.* 1847)
The other infectious disease; a plea for a new hospital. Boston, 1889. 7p. DNLM **80-2006**

FISHER, E[dward] D.
Clinical report of cases of epilepsy following cerebral hemiplegia. New York: M. J. Rooney & Co., 1888. 12p. DNLM
80-2007

FISHER, E[dward] D. and Frederick PETERSON
Cranial measurements in twenty cases of infantile cerebral hemiplegia. [New York, 1889.] 9p. DNLM
80-2008

FISHER, Frank
Hints to wife and mother; hand-book for women. . . . By Frank Fisher, M.D., and J. Aubrey Davis, M.D. Philadelphia: Weston & Bryan, 1889. 142p. DLC; PPC; PU
80-2009

FISHER, George Jackson (1825-1893)
Historical and bibliographical notes. A series of sketches of the lives, times, and works of some of the old masters of anatomy, surgery, and medicine. Brooklyn, N.Y., 1883. 27p. DNLM
80-2010

FISHER, George Jackson (1825-1893)
A memorial sketch of the life and character of the late John Foster Jenkins, A.M., M.D., of Yonkers, N.Y. . . . Syracuse: Smith & Bruce, printers and book binders, 1884. 21p. DLC
80-2011

FISHER, George Jackson (1825-1893)
The famous historic masters of the healing art were men of classical education. [Detroit, 1889.] 23p. DNLM
80-2012

FISHER, Theodore W[illis] (1837-1914)
A case of tumor of the brain. [Utica, 1885.] 14p. DNLM
80-2013

FISHER, Theodore W[illis] (1837-1914)
Two unique cases of insanity; possibly epileptic. [Utica, 1887.] 21p. DNLM **80-2014**

FISK, Samuel A[ugustus], Jr.
The cottage plan of treating consumption in Colorado. [Philadelphia, 1889.] 13p. DNLM **80-2015**

FISK, Samuel A[ugustus], Jr.
The effects of the climate of Colorado upon phthisis pulmonalis, as shown by the analysis of one hundred recorded cases. Boston: Damrell & Upham, 1889. 16p. DNLM
80-2016

FISK, Samuel A[ugustus], Jr.
A study of the climate of Colorado as applied to the arrest and cure of pulmonary disease. [Philadelphia, 1889.] 20p. DNLM **80-2017**

FITZ, Reginald H[eber] (1843-1913)
Persistent omphalo-mesenteric remains, their importance in the causation of intestinal duplication, cyst-formation and obstruction. [Philadelpia, 1884.] 28p. DNLM; PPC
80-2018

FITZ, Reginald H[eber] (1843-1913)
Perforating inflammation of the vermiform appendix; with special reference to its early diagnosis and treatment. Philadelphia: W. J. Dornan, 1886. 31p. DNLM; PPC
80-2019

FITZ, Reginald H[eber] (1843-1913)
Acute pancreatitis: a consideration of pancreatic hemorrhage, hemorrhagic, suppurative, and gangrenous pancreatitis, and of desseminated fat-necrosis. The Middleton-Goldsmith lecture for 1889. Boston: Cupples & Hurd, 1889. 91p. DNLM; MBM
80-2020

FITZ, Reginald H[eber] (1843-1913)
The diagnosis and medical treatment of acute intestinal obstruction. Boston: Cupples & Hurd, 1889. 64p. DNLM; MBM **80-2021**

FLAGG, J[osiah] Foster (1789-1853)
Plastics and plastic filling; as pertaining to the filling of all cavities of decay in teeth below medium in structure, and to difficult and inaccessible cavities in teeth of all grades of structure. . . . Philadelphia: P. Blakiston, 1881. 207p. plates. DLC; MBM; NNNAM; PPC **80-2022**

FLAGG, J[osiah] Foster (1789-1853)
The amalgam question. Philadelphia, 1882. 25p. DNLM
80-2023

FLAGG, J[osiah] Foster (1789-1853)
Quiz questions, course on dental pathology and therapeutics, Philadelphia Dental College. . . . Answered by William C. Foulks. . . . Philadelphia: G. A. Fowler & Co., 1882. 98p. DLC; DNLM; PPJ; PU **80-2024**

FLAGG, J[osiah] Foster (1789-1853)
Quiz questions: course on dental pathology and therapeutics. Philadelphia Dental College. . . . Answered by William C. Foulks. . . . 2nd ed., rev. and enl. Philadelphia: S. S. White Dental Manufacturing Co., [1882]. 122p. DLC; OCIM; PPC; PU **80-2025**

FLAGG, J[osiah] Foster (1789-1853)
Quiz questions: course on dental pathology and therapeutics, Philadelphia Dental College. . . . Answered by William C. Foulks. . . . 3rd ed., rev. and enl. Philadelphia: S. S. White Dental Manufacturing Co., [1885]. 122p. DLC; NNNAM; PPC; PU **80-2026**

FLETCHER, Moore Russell
Our home doctor. Domestic and botanical remedies simplified and explained for family treatment. With a treatise upon suspended animation, the danger of burying alive, and directions for restoration. . . . Boston: Pub. by the author, 1883. 332, 70p. DLC; MBM **80-2027**

FLICK, Lawrence F[rancis] (1856-1938)
The contagiousness of phthisis (tubercular pulmonitis). Philadelphia: W. J. Dornan, 1888. 21p. 2 maps. DNLM **80-2028**

FLICK, Lawrence F[rancis] (1856-1938)
The hygiene of phthisis. Philadelphia: W. J. Dornan, 1888. 14p. DNLM **80-2029**

FLICK, Lawrence F[rancis] (1856-1938)
How to take care of the lungs. Philadelphia: Buck & McFetridge, 1889. 14p. DNLM **80-2030**

FLICK, Lawrence F[rancis] (1856-1938)
The mode of entrance of the bacillus tuberculosis into the system. Philadelphia, 1889. 9p. DNLM **80-2031**

FLICK, Lawrence F[rancis] (1856-1938)
A review of the cases of tuberculosis which terminated in death in the fifth ward of the city of Philadelphia during the year 1888. [Philadelphia, 1889.] 7p. DNLM **80-2032**

FLINT, Austin (1812-1886)
A manual of auscultation and percussion; embracing the physicial diagnosis of diseases of the lungs and heart, and of thoracic aneurism. . . . 2nd ed., rev. Philadelphia: Henry C. Lea, 1880. 240p. DLC; DNLM; NNNAM; PPC **80-2033**

FLINT, Austin (1812-1886)
The treatment of pneumonic fever (acute lobar pneumonia) by the employment of the wet-sheet. [New York, 1881.] 7p. DNLM **80-2034**

FLINT, Austin (1812-1886)
A treatise on the principles and practice of medicine; designed for the use of practitioners and students of medicine. . . . 5th ed., rev. and largely re-written. Philadelphia: Henry C. Lea's Son & Co., 1881. 1150p. DLC; ICRM; IU-M; PPC **80-2035**

FLINT, Austin (1812-1886)
. . . Physical exploration of the lungs by means of auscultation and percussion. A course of three lectures delivered by invitation before the Philadelphia County Medical Society. . . . Philadelphia: Henry C. Lea's Son & Co., 1882. 83p. DLC; DNLM; PPC; PU **80-2036**

FLINT, Austin (1812-1886)
Medical ethics and etiquette. The code of ethics adopted by the American Medical Association, with commentaries. . . . New York: D. Appleton & Co., 1883. 97p. DLC; DNLM; NNNAM; PPC **80-2037**

FLINT, Austin (1812-1886)
A manual of auscultation and percussion; embracing the physical diagnosis of diseases of the lungs and heart, and of thoracic aneurism. . . . 3rd ed., rev. Philadelphia: Henry C. Lea's Son & Co., 1883. 242p. DLC; NNNAM; OCIM; PPC **80-2038**

FLINT, Austin (1812-1886)
On the pathological and practical relations of the doctrine of the bacillus tuberculosis. [Philadelphia, 1884.] 16p. DNLM; PPC **80-2039**

FLINT, Austin (1812-1886)
A treatise on the principles and practice of medicine; designed for the use of practitioners and students of medicine. . . . 5th ed., rev. and largely re-written. With an appendix on the researches of Koch. . . . Philadelphia: Henry C. Lea's Son & Co., 1884. 1160p. DLC; NNNAM; PPC; PU [2nd issue of 5th edition; 1st issue, without appenix: 1881.] **80-2040**

FLINT, Austin (1812-1886)
A manual of auscultation and percussion; embracing the physical diagnosis of diseases of the lungs and heart, and of thoracic aneurism. . . . 4th ed., thoroughly rev. and enl. Illustrated with fourteen woodcuts. Philadelphia: Lea Bros. & Co.,1885. 280p. DLC; MBM; NNNAM; PU **80-2041**

FLINT, Austin (1812-1886)
Medicine of the future: an address prepared for the annual meeting of the British Medical Association in 1886. . . . New York: D. Appleton & Co., 1886. 37p. DLC; DNLM; PPC: PU **80-2042**

FLINT, Austin (1812-1886)
A treatise on the principles and practice of medicine; designed for the use of practitioners and students of medicine. . . . 6th ed., rev. and largely re-written by the author. Assisted by William H. Welch . . . and Austin Flint. . . . Philadelphia: Lea Bros. & Co., 1886. 1160p. CtY-M; DLC; NNNAM; PPC **80-2043**

FLINT, Austin (1836-1915)
A text-book of human physiology; designed for the use of practitioners and students of medicine. . . . 3rd ed., rev. and cor. New York: D. Appleton & Co., 1881. 978p. 3 plates. DLC; NNNAM; PPC; PU **80-2044**

[FLINT, Austin] (1836-1915)
Catalogue of a portion of the medical library of . . . . New York, 1883. 38p. DNLM; NNNAM **80-2045**

FLINT, Austin (1836-1915)
Manual of chemical examination of the urine in disease; with brief directions for the examination of the most common varieties of urinary calculi, and an appendix, containing a diet-table for diabetes. . . . 6th ed., rev. and cor. New York: D. Appleton & Co., 1884. 87p. fold. tab. DLC; MH-M; NNNAM; PPC **80-2046**

FLINT, Austin (1836-1915)
The treatment of diabetes mellitus. Chicago: A. G. Newell, 1884. 35p. DNLM; OCIM **80-2047**

FLINT, Austin (1836-1915)
A text-book of human physiology. . . . 4th ed., entirely rewritten. New York: D. Appleton & Co., 1888. 872p. 2 plates. DLC; NNNAM; OCIM; PU **80-2048**

FLINT, Austin (1836-1915)
A tonic formula. New York, 1889. 2 l. DNLM **80-2049**

FLINT, James Milton (1838-1919)
. . . Reports on the pharmacopoeias of all nations. . . . Washington: Government Printing Office, 1883. 28p. DLC; DNLM; OCLloyd; PU **80-2050**

FLOWER, Richard C.
The allopathic czar. A lecture delivered by Dr. R. C. Flower, of Boston, in Foster's Opera House, Des Moines, December ninth. A severe indictment of the allopathic school of practice. . . . Rev. and cor. [5th ed.] Only authorized ed. Boston, Mass.: Massachusetts Medical Liberty League, 1888. 43p. DLC; DNLM; MBM **80-2051**

FOLSOM, Charles F[ollen] (1842-1907)
Observations on the births, marriages, and deaths in Massachusetts in 1879. Prepared for the thirty-eighth Massachusetts registration report. Boston: Rand, Avery & Co., 1880. 91p. DNLM; MB; MBM **80-2052**

FOLSOM, Charles F[ollen] (1842-1907)
Four introductory lectures on insanity. A portion of a course delivered before the graduation class of the Harvard Medical School. Cambridge, 1880. 44p. DNLM; MBM **80-2053**

FOLSOM, Charles F[ollen] (1842-1907)
Abstract of the statutes of the United States, and of the several states and territories, relating to the custody of the insane. With the assistance of Hollis R. Bailey. Philadelphia: Henry C. Lea's Son & Co., 1884. 111p. DNLM; NNNAM; OCIM; PPC **80-2054**

FOOTE, Edward Bliss (1829-1906)
. . . Dr. Foote's hand-book of health-hints and ready recipes; comprising information of the utmost importance to everybody, concerning their daily habits of eating, drinking, sleeping, dressing, bathing, working, etc., together with many useful suggestions on the management of various diseases. . . . New York: Murray Hill Publishing Co., 1881. 128p. DLC; NNNAM; PPJ; PU **80-2055**

FOOTE, Edward Bliss (1829-1906)
Reply to the Alphites, giving some cogent reasons for believing that sexual continence is not conducive to health. New York: Murray Hill Publishing Co., 1882. 39p. DNLM; NNNAM **80-2056**

FOOTE, Edward Bond
. . . An illustrated treatise on gynecology or diseases of women. . . . New York: Murray Hill Publishing Co., 1887. 48p. DLC; NNNAM **80-2057**

FORBES, W[illiam] Smith (1831-1905)
The diaphragm; a protector of the heart and cardiac vessels; its influence on the organs of circulation. [Philadelphia, 1880.] 9p. DNLM **80-2058**

FORBES, W[illiam] Smith (1831-1904)
The liberating of the ring finger, in musicians, by dividing the accessory tendons of the extensor communis digitorum muscle. [Philadelphia, 1884.] 6p. DNLM **80-2059**

FORD, Corydon La (1813-1894)
Syllabus of lectures and questions on odontology, human and comparative, for the use of students in the dental college, of the University of Michigan. . . . Ann Arbor: Register Printing House, 1884. 44p. DLC; OCIM **80-2060**

FORD, C[orydon] La (1813-1894)
Questions on the structure and development of the human teeth, and some closely related subjects, for the use of dental students. Ann Arbor: Andrews & Witherby, 1884. 46p. DNLM; OCIM **80-2061**

FORD, Samuel Payne, ed.
The American cyclopaedia of domestic medicine and household surgery. A reliable guide for every family. Containing full descriptions of the various parts of the human body; accounts of the numerous diseases to which man is subject—their causes, symptoms, treatment and prevention. . . . With an appendix by N. H. Paaren. . . .Chicago, Ill.: E. P. Kingsley & Co.; Cincinnati: O. J. Hugill; [etc., etc.], 1880. 1215p. col. plates. DLC; OCIM **80-2062**

FORD, Samuel Payne, ed.
The American cyclopaedia of domestic medicine and household surgery. A reliable guide for every family. . . . With an appendix by N. H. Paaren. . . . Chicago: E. P. Kingsley & Co.; Cincinnati: O. J. Hugill; [etc., etc.], 1880. 3 v. col. plates. DLC; OCIM **80-2063**

FORD, Samuel Payne, ed.
The American cyclopaedia of domestic medicine and household surgery. . . . With an appendix by N. H. Paaren. . . . Chicago: E. P. Kingsley; Little Rock, Ark.: A. J. Lappeus; [etc., etc.], 1882. 3 v. col. plates. DLC **80-2064**

FORD, William H[enry] (1839-1897)
Principles of sanitary inspection; reprinted, with additions for the use of the Philadelphia Board of Health, from "The reference handbook of the medical sciences." Philadelphia: Dunlap & Clarke, 1889. 59p. DNLM; PU **80-2065**

FORD, Willis E.
Some of the limitations of galvanism in gynecology. Philadelphia: W. J. Dornan, 1889. 18p. DNLM; PPC **80-2066**

FORDYCE, John Addison (1858-1925)
Fatal peritonitis following ovarian apoplexy of the menstrual period. New York, 1889. 5p. DNLM **80-2067**

FOREST, W[illiam] E.
Intussusception in children. New York: William Wood & Co., 1886. 27p. DNLM; NNNAM **80-2068**

FORMAD, H[enry] F. (1847-1892)
Some comments and discussion on the paper: "The etiology of tumors." Philadelphia, 1881. 13p. DNLM **80-2069**

FORMAD, H[enry] F. (1847-1892)
The etiology of tumors. Philadelphia: Globe Printing House, 1881. 53p. DNLM; PPC **80-2070**

FORMAD, H[enry] F. (1847-1892)
The inflammatory origin of tumors. New York: G. P. Putnam's Sons, 1881. 28p. DNLM **80-2071**

FORMAD, H[enry] F. (1847-1892)
The bacillus tuberculosis and some anatomical points which suggest the refutation of its etiological relation with tuberculosis. Philadelphia, 1882. 12p. DNLM **80-2072**

FORMAD, H[enry] F. (1847-1892)
Special edition of seventy-four plates, illustrating the histology of tumors, extracted from A manual of microscopic diagnosis. . . . Illustrated with two hundred original engravings by I. W. Blackburn, M.D. Philadelphia: J. B. Lippincott & Co., 1883. 4p. 74 plates. DLC; DNLM; PPC; PU **80-2073**

FORMAD, H[enry] F. (1847-1892)
The bacillus tuberculosis and the etiology of tuberculosis. Is consumption contagious? Second communication read before the Philadelphia County Medical Society, November 14, 1883. [Philadelphia, 1883.] 9 galley sheets. DNLM **80-2074**

FORMAD, H[enry] F. (1847-1892)
The bacillus tuberculosis and the etiology of tuberculosis. Is consumption contagious? Second communication read before the Philadelphia County Medical Society, November 14, 1883. Philadelphia, 1884. 36p. DNLM **80-2075**

FORMAD, H[enry] F. (1847-1892)
Fatal cases of intracranial hemorrhage. Philadelphia, 1886. 12p. DNLM **80-2076**

FORMAD, H[enry] F. (1847-1892)
The "pig-backed" or alcoholic kidney of drunkards. A contribution to the post-mortem diagnosis of alcoholism. [Philadelphia, 1886.] 16p. DNLM **80-2077**

FORMAD, H[enry] F. (1847-1892)
Comparative studies of mammalian blood, with special reference to the microscopical diagnosis of blood stains in criminal cases. Philadelphia: A. L. Hummel, 1888. 61p. 5 plates. DNLM **80-2078**

FORMAD, H[enry] F. (1847-1892)
Anatomical relations of lesions of the heart and the kidneys in Bright's disease. From the study of three hundred autopsies. Philadelphia: W. J. Dornan, 1889. 36p. DNLM; PPC **80-2079**

FORSTER, Edward Jacob (1846-1896)
Improved and new powder insufflators. An improved ear spout. Cambridge: Riverside Press, 1881. 4p. DNLM **80-2080**

FORSTER, Edward Jacob (1846-1896)
The necessity of using the long nozzle in making intra-uterine injections after confinement. Cambridge: Riverside Press, 1881. 8p. DNLM **80-2081**

FORT, George Franklin (1809-1872)
Medical economy during the middle ages; a contribution to the history of European morals, from the time of the Roman Empire to the close of the fourteenth century. New York: J. W. Bouton, 1883. 488p. DNLM; ICU; MH; NN **80-2082**

FOSTER, Eugene (1850-1903)
Prevention and control of small-pox. Atlanta: H. H. Dickson, [1881?]. 21p. DNLM **80-2083**

FOSTER, Eugene (1850-1903)
The relative merits of humanized and bovine vaccine virus. [Augusta, Ga., Chronicle, 1882.] 45p. DNLM **80-2084**

FOSTER, Eugene (1850-1903)
Vaccination, its control, efficiency, and safety. Concord, N.H.: P. B. Cogswell, 1884. 54p. DNLM **80-2085**

FOSTER, Frank Pierce (1841-1911)
An illustrated encyclopaedic medical dictionary. Being a dictionary of the technical terms used by writers on medicine and the collateral sciences, in the Latin English, French and German languages. . . . New York: D. Appleton & Co., 1888-1894. 4 v. DLC; DNLM; NNNAM; PU **80-2086**

FOSTER, Michael (1836-1907)
A textbook of physiology. 3rd ed., rev. New York: Macmillan & Co., 1880. 804p. CtY-M; NNNAM; OCIM; PPC **80-2087**

FOSTER, Michael (1836-1907)
A text-book of physiology. . . . From the 3rd and rev. English ed., with notes and additions, by Edward T. Reichert. . . . Philadelphia: Henry C. Lea's Son & Co., 1880. 1030p. DLC; DNLM; NNNAM; PPC **80-2088**

FOSTER, Michael (1836-1907)
A text-book of physiology. . . . 2nd American from the 3rd and rev. English ed. With extensive notes and additions, by Edward T. Reichert. . . . With two hundred and fifty-nine illustrations. Philadelphia: Henry C. Lea's Son & Co., 1881. 987p. DLC; NNNAM; OCIM; PU **80-2089**

FOSTER, Michael (1836-1907)
. . . Physiology. By M. Foster. . . . Hygiene. By R. S. Tracy. . . . New York: D. Appleton & Co., 1883. 170p. DLC: ICU; MB; NN **80-2090**

FOSTER, Michael (1836-1907)
A text-book of physiology. . . . 3rd American from the 4th and rev. English ed. With extensive notes and additions, by Edward T. Reichert. . . . Philadelphia: Lea Bros. & Co., 1885. 911p. DLC; DNLM; NNNAM; OCIM **80-2091**

FOSTER, M. Whilldin
Abnormal conditions of the antrum, and restorative treatment. Philadelphia, 1886. 14p. DNLM **80-2092**

FOSTER, R[ichard] N.
The therapeutics of food. Chicago, 1886. 16p. DNLM **80-2093**

FOSTER, R[ichard] N.
Modern medicine. Chicago, 1887. 24p. DNLM
80-2094

FOSTER, Simeon A. (1843-1885)
Remarks on chronic inflammation of the knee joint, with description of a new apparatus. Brooklyn, 1882. 7p. DNLM
80-2095

FOSTER, William D[avis] (*b.* 1841)
History of trephining; fracture of the inner table of the cranium; depressed bone; compression of the brain; a case; strabismus; recovery. Kansas City, 1884. 22p. DNLM
80-2096

FOSTER, William D[avis] (*b.* 1841)
Rules for the treatment of Asiatic cholera homoeopathically; intended for the people. [St. Louis, 1884.] 11p. DNLM
80-2097

FOTHERGILL, J[ohn] Milner (1841-1888)
The practitioner's handbook of treatment; or the principles of therapeutics. 2nd American from 2nd English ed. Philadelphia: Henry C. Lea's Son & Co., 1880. 641p. CtY-M; DNLM; NNNAM; PPC **80-2098**

FOTHERGILL, J[ohn] Milner (1841-1888)
Food for the invalid; the convalescent; the dyspeptic; and the gouty. By J. Milner Fothergill . . . and Horatio C. Wood. . . . New York: Macmillan & Co., 1880. 157p. DLC; NNNAM; OCIM; PPC **80-2099**

FOTHERGILL, J[ohn] Milner (1841-1888)
Indigestion, biliousness, and gout in its protean aspects. Part I: Indigestion and biliousness. New York: William Wood & Co., 1881. 320p. NNNAM; OCIM; PPC; PU [Part II, on gout, was never published.] **80-2100**

FOTHERGILL, J[ohn] Milner (1841-1888)
Indigestion and biliousness. New York: Bermingham & Co., 1881. 89p. DNLM; MBM; NNNAM; PU
80-2101

FOTHERGILL, J[ohn] Milner (1841-1888)
Some practical points in digestion. [New York: D. D. Comes, 1881.] 16p. DNLM **80-2102**

FOTHERGILL, J[ohn] Milner (1841-1888)
Chronic bronchitis; its forms and treatment. New York: G. P. Putnam's Sons, 1882. 160p. 1 plate. DNLM; IEN-M; NNNAM; PU **80-2103**

FOTHERGILL, J[ohn] Milner (1841-1888)
Aids to diagnosis. Pt. III: What to ask. New York: G. P. Putnam's Sons, 1882. 66p. DNLM; NNNAM; PPC; PU
80-2104

FOTHERGILL, J[ohn] Milner (1841-1888)
The physiological factor in diagnosis. A work for young practitioners. New York: William Wood & Co., 1883. 256p. DNLM; MBM; NNNAM; OCIM **80-2105**

FOTHERGILL, J[ohn] Milner (1841-1888)
Gout in its protean aspects. Detroit: G. S. Davis, 1883. 303p. DNLM; OCIM **80-2106**

FOTHERGILL, J[ohn] Milner (1841-1888)
Aids to rational therapeutics. New York: G. P. Putnam's Sons, 1883. 121p. CtY-M; DNLM; NNNAM; PPC **80-2107**

FOTHERGILL, J[ohn] Milner (1841-1888)
A brief treatise on therapeutics. . . . Ed. for the U.S. pharmacopoeia by Wm. H. Rouse . . . with the addition of chapters on diet for the sick, by Mrs. Emma Drant. . . . Detroit: The Illustrated Medical Journal Co., 1884. 140p. DLC; OCLloyd; OCIM; PU **80-2108**

FOTHERGILL, J[ohn] Milner (1841-1888)
The diseases of sedentary and advanced life. A work for medical and lay readers. New York: D. Appleton & Co., 1885. 295p. CtY-M; DNLM; NNNAM; PU **80-2109**

FOTHERGILL, J[ohn] Milner (1841-1888)
A manual of dietetics. . . . New York: William Wood & Co., 1886. 255p. DLC; NNNAM; PPC; PU
80-2110

FOTHERGILL, J[ohn] Milner (1841-1888)
The practitioner's handbook of treatment, or the principles of therapeutics. 3rd American from the 3rd English ed. Philadelphia: Lea Bros. & Co., 1887. 660p. CtY-M; DNLM; NNNAM; PPC **80-2111**

FOTHERGILL, J[ohn] Milner (1841-1888)
Vaso-renal change versus Bright's disease. New York: G. P. Putnam's Sons, 1887. 219p. 6 plates. DNLM; NNNAM; PPJ; PPC **80-2112**

FOULKS, William C.
Practical information concerning the care of the mouth and teeth in adults and children. . . . 2nd ed. Philadelphia, 1888. 13p. DLC **80-2113**

FOURNIER, [Jean] A[lfred] (1832-1914)
Syphilis and marriage. Lectures delivered at the St. Louis Hospital, Paris. Transl. by P. Albert Morrow. New York: D. Appleton & Co., 1881. 251p. DLC; DNLM; NNNAM; PPC **80-2114**

FOURNIER, [Jean] A[lfred] (1832-1914)
Syphilitic teeth. Transl. by J. William White. Philadelphia, 1884. 37p. DNLM; MdU-D **80-2115**

FOWLER, C. H. and W. H. DE PUY
Home and health and home economics; a cyclopedia of facts and hints for all departments of home life, health, and domestic economy. New York: Phillips & Hunt, 1880. 352p. DNLM; MH; NN; NNNAM **80-2116**

FOWLER, Edward Payson (1833-1914)
Are brains of criminals anatomical perversions? [New York, 1880.] 32p. DNLM; NNNAM **80-2117**

FOWLER, Edward Payson (1833-1914)
Suppression of urine; clinical descriptions and analysis of symptoms. . . . Ninety-three clinical cases, with illustrations, tables, and diagrams. Paper presented to the New York Medico-Chirurgical Society, 14th December, 1880. New York: William Wood & Co., 1881. 86p. col. front. plate, diags. DLC; DNLM; NNNAM; PU **80-2118**

FOWLER, Edward Payson (1833-1914)
Annual address before the New York Medico-Chirurgical Society by the president. New York, 1883. 34p. DNLM; NNNAM **80-2119**

FOWLER, George B[ingham] (1847-1907)
Chemical and microscopical analysis of the urine in health and disease, designed for physicians and students. 3rd ed. New York: G. P. Putnam's Sons, 1881. 103p. DNLM
80-2120

FOWLER, George B[ingham] (1847-1907)
Farinaceous infant foods. New York: William Wood & Co., 1882. 19p. DNLM **80-2121**

FOWLER, George B[ingham] (1847-1907)
Incontinence of feces in children. New York: William Wood & Co., 1882. 7p. DNLM **80-2122**

FOWLER, George B[ingham] (1847-1907)
The dietetic value of water. [New York, 1886.] 8p. DNLM
80-2123

FOWLER, George B[ingham] (1847-1907)
Digestion and diet; their relation to disease. Brooklyn, 1888. 15p. DNLM **80-2124**

FOWLER, George B[ingahm] (1847-1907)
The significance and detection of sugar in the urine, with some reference to life-insurance. New York, 1888. 16p. DNLM
80-2125

FOWLER, George R[yerson] (1848-1906)
On elbow-joint fractures; being a clinical study of twenty cases of fracture at the lower end of the humerus involving or approximating the elbow-joint. New York: G. P. Putnam's Sons, 1880. 12p. DNLM; NNNAM **80-2126**

FOWLER, George R[yerson] (1848-1906)
Hydronaphthol; a new antiseptic. New York: D. Appleton & Co., 1885. 31p. DNLM; NNNAM **80-2127**

FOWLER, George R[yerson] (1848-1906)
A review of the new antiseptic hydronaphthol, in surgery. New York, 1885. 23p. DNLM; NNNAM **80-2128**

FOWLER, George R[yerson] (1848-1906)
Explorative laparotomy. New York, 1886. 13p. DNLM; NNNAM **80-2129**

FOWLER, George R[yerson] (1848-1906)
Surgical infection; is it a chimera? New York, 1886. 8p. DNLM; NNNAM **80-2130**

FOWLER, George R[yerson] (1848-1906)
Syllabus of a course of lectures on first aids to the injured, arranged for the medical officers of the second brigade, N. G. S. N. Y. New York: A. Coffin & Rogers, 1887. 57p. DNLM; NNNAM **80-2131**

FOWLER, George R[yerson] (1848-1906)
A case of modified laryngectomy for epithelioma of the larynx; recovery. [Philadelphia], 1889. 6p. DNLM; NNNAM
80-2132

FOWLER, Orson Squire (1809-1887)
The practical phrenologist; and records and delineator of the character and talents . . . a compendium of phreno-organic science. . . . Boston: O. S. Fowler, [1880]. 174p. DLC; MH; MWA; NNNAM **80-2133**

FOWNES, George (1815-1849)
Manual of chemistry, theoretical and practical. A new American from the 12th English ed., embodying Watts' "Physical and inorganic chemistry." Philadelphia: Lea Bros. & Co., 1885. 1056p. 1 plate. CtY-M; DNLM; NNNAM; PU
80-2134

FOX, Cornelius B[enjamin] (*b.* 1839)
Sanitary examinations of water, air, and food. A vade-mecum for the medical officer of health. Philadelphia: P. Blakiston, Son & Co., 1887. 563p. DNLM; MBM; NN; PU
80-2135

FOX, George Henry (1846-1937)
Photographic illustrations of skin diseases. New York: E. B. Treat, 1880. 51 l. 48 plates. DNLM; NNNAM; PPC; PU
80-2136

FOX, George Henry (1846-1937)
Photographic illustations of cutaneous syphilis. Forty-eight plates from life. Colored by hand. New York: E. B. Treat, 1881. 106p. 48 col. plates. DLC; NNNAM; OCIM; PPC [Issued in 12 numbers, 1880-1881.] **80-2137**

FOX, George Henry (1846-1937)
Photographic illustrations of skin diseases. . . . 2nd ed. New York: E. B. Treat, 1885. 208p. 48 col. plates. DLC; NNNAM; PPC; PU **80-2138**

FOX, George Henry (1846-1937)
Photographic illustrations of cutaneous syphilis. New York: E. B. Treat, 1885. 106p. 48 plates. DNLM; NNNAM; OCIM; PPJ **80-2139**

FOX, George Henry (1846-1937)
The use of electricity in the removal of superfluous hair and the treatment of various facial blemishes. . . . Detroit, Mich.: G. S. Davis, 1886. 67p. DLC; DNLM; OCIM; PU
80-2140

FOX, George Henry (1846-1937)
Photographic illustrations of skin diseases. 2nd ed. New York: E. B. Treat, 1887. 208p. 85 plates. CtY-M; DNLM; NNNAM; PPC **80-2141**

FOX, L[awrance] Webster (1853-1931)
The ointment of boroglyceride (unguentum boroglyceridi). [Philadelphia: Lea Bros. & Co., 1884.] 7p. DNLM
80-2142

FOX, L[awrance] Webster (1853-1931)
An improved refraction ophthalmoscope. [Philadelphia: Lea Bros. & Co., 1885.] 4p. DNLM **80-2143**

FOX, L[awrance] Webster (1853-1931) and George M. GOULD
Retinal insensibility to ultra-violet and infra-red rays. [St. Louis, 1886.] 20p. 1 plate. DNLM **80-2144**

FOX, L[awrance] Webster (1853-1931) and George M. GOULD
The oculist, the optician, and the public. [Philadelphia, 1886.] 1 l. DNLM **80-2145**

FOX, L[awrance] Webster (1853-1931) and George M. GOULD
The human color-sense considered as the organic response to natural stimuli. [St. Louis, 1886.] 20p. DNLM
80-2146

FOX, L[awrance] Webster (1853-1931) and George M. GOULD
On heat considered as the retinal intermediate of light and color sensation. [St. Louis: J. H. Chambers & Co., 1886.] 23p. DNLM **80-2147**

FOX, L[awrance] Webster (1853-1931)
. . . A compend of the diseases of the eye, including refraction and surgical operations. By L[awrance] Webster Fox . . . and Geo. M. Gould. Philadelphia: P. Blakiston, Son & Co., 1887. 148p. diag. DLC; NNNAM; PPC; PU **80-2148**

FOX, L[awrance] Webster (1853-1931)
Ophthalmology. [Philadelphia, 1887.] 11p. DNLM **80-2149**

FOX, L[awrance] Webster (1853-1931)
. . . A compend of the diseases of the eye; including refraction and surgical operations. By L[awrance] Webster Fox . . . and Geo. M. Gould, M.D. 2nd ed., rev. and enl. With 71 illustrations. Philadelphia: P. Blakiston, Son & Co., 1888. 164p. diag. DLC; LNT-M; NNNAM; PPC **80-2150**

FOX, L[awrance] Webster (1853-1931)
Blindness and the blind. Philadelphia, 1889. 30p. DNLM **80-2151**

FOX, Sidney Allan (1856-1890)
A report of three interesting cases, viz.: Case 1. Adenoid of the vault of the pharynx. Case 2. Strumous ozoena. Case 3. Tubercular phthisis; secondary tubercular ulcer of the tongue. [New York, 1889.] 6p. DNLM **80-2152**

FOX, Tilbury (1836-1870)
Epitome of skin diseases, with formulae, for students and practitioners. By the late Tilbury Fox . . . and by T. Colcott Fox. . . . 3rd American ed., rev. and with additions. By T. Colcott Fox. . . . Philadelphia: Henry C. Lea's Son & Co., 1883. 240p. DLC; DNLM; NNNAM; PPC **80-2153**

FRAKER, George Wilhelm
Health and disease. The people's book, being a treatise on clothing, exercise, sleep, bathing, air, sunshine, food and drink. . . . Excelsior Springs, Mo.: Sentinel of Truth Job Print, 1886. 47p. DLC **80-2154**

FRANCIS, Joseph (1801-1893)
Appendix to History of life-saving appliances and military and naval constructions. Washington: Judd & Detweiler, 1885. 34p. DNLM **80-2155**

FRANCIS, Samuel W[ard] (1835-1886)
Interesting medical and surgical cases. Probable epithelioma, cured by astringent washes. Newport, R.I.: Davis & Pitman, 1883. 9p. DNLM **80-2156**

FRANKLAND, Edward (1825-1899)
Water analysis for sanitary purposes; with hints for the interpretation of results. Philadelphia: P. Blakiston, 1880. 149p. DNLM **80-2157**

FRANKLIN, Edward Carroll (1822-1885)
A complete minor surgery. The physician's vade mecum. Including a treatise on venereal diseases. . . . Illustrated with 260 wood cuts. Chicago: Gross & Delbridge, 1882. 423p. OCIM; PPHa **80-2158**

FRANKLIN, Edward Carroll (1822-1885)
The practitioner's and student's manual of the science of surgery. Being a compendium of the course of lectures delivered in the Homoeopathic College, University of Michigan. Ann Arbor: S. C. Andrews, Publisher, 1882. 187p. OCIM; PPHa **80-2159**

FRANKLIN, Edward Carroll (1822-1885)
The science and art of surgery, or The semeiology, pathology, therapeutics and operations of surgery. . . . . 2nd ed., rev., abridged and illustrated. Ann Arbor: S. C. Andrews, 1882. 187, 865p. DLC; IEN-M; OCIM **80-2160**

FRANKLIN, Edward Carroll (1822-1885)
A manual of venereal diseases; being a condensed description of those affections and their homoeopathic treatment. Chicago: Gross & Delbridge, 1883. 111p. DLC; DNLM; IU-M; OCIM **80-2161**

FRANKLIN, Emmanuel Zeus
Illustrated domestic medical counsellor. Laws and science of life, health, and self-preservation. Materia medica and pharmacy, [etc.]. Boston, 1884. unp. DNLM; MBM; MWA **80-2162**

FRANKLIN, Emmanuel Zeus
Cosmical science of creation; divinity and destiny of mind; universal laws of the mental constitution; redemption and perfection of man; a new mental, moral, and social world, [etc.]. Boston, 1884. unp. DNLM; ICU; MH; NN **80-2163**

FREELAND, J. T.
Phymosis in children. Indianapolis: Baker & Randolph, 1888. 7p. DNLM **80-2164**

FREES, C. A. INVENTOR & MFG.
Illustrated catalog of artificial limbs and apparatus. New York, 1887. 83p. NNNAM **80-2165**

FRELIGH, Martin (1813-1889)
Homoeopathic practice of medicine. . . . 14th ed., rev. and enl. New York: C. T. Hurlburt, 1884. 705p. NNNAM; PPHa; PU **80-2166**

FRENCH, Elizabeth J.
. . . A complete manual of electro-therapeutics, and a brief treatise on anatomy and physiology. . . . [3rd ed. rev. and cor.] Philadelphia: J. B. Lippincott Co., 1886. 262p. DLC; NNNAM; PPC; PU **80-2167**

FRENCH, Elizabeth J.
. . . A new path in electrical therapeutics: an account of the author's great discovery of electrical cranial diagnosis. . . . [5th ed. rev. and cor.] . . . . Philadelphia: J. B. Lippincott Co., 1886. 269p. DLC; NNNAM; OCIM; PPC **80-2168**

FRENCH, M[orris] S.
Report of the physical examination of men upon the police force of Philadelphia, and those who were applicants for appointment; also, of the sanitary condition of the station houses, and facts relating to the medical service of the police department. Philadelphia: Schall & Bro., 1885. 16p. DNLM; PU **80-2169**

FRENCH, M[orris] S. and Edward O[ram] SHAKESPEARE
The lesson taught by the epidemic at Plymouth concerning typhoid fever. [New York, 1885.] 6p. DNLM **80-2170**

FRENCH, M[orris] S. and Edward O[ram] SHAKESPEARE
Report upon the epidemic of typhoid fever at Plymouth, Luzerne County, Pa. Philadelphia, 1885. 20p. 1 map. DNLM
80-2171

FRENCH, Thomas R[ushmore] (1849-1929)
A case of double epiglottis and double voice. [Brooklyn, N.Y., 1880.] 2 l. DNLM **80-2172**

FRENCH, Thomas R[ushmore] (1849-1929)
A case of hypertrophy of the larynx. [Brooklyn, N.Y., 1880.] 2 l. DNLM **80-2173**

FRENCH, Thomas R[ushmore] (1849-1929)
Mouth breathing; its causes, effects, and treatment. [Brooklyn, 1882.] 10p. DNLM **80-2174**

FRENCH, Thomas R[ushmore] (1849-1929)
On photographing the larynx. New York: G. P. Putnam's Sons, 1882. 2p. 1 phot. DNLM **80-2175**

FRENCH, Thomas R[ushmore] (1849-1929)
On photographing the larynx. [New York: G. P. Putnam's Sons, 1883.] 9p. 1 plate. DNLM; NNNAM
80-2176

FRENCH, Thomas R[ushmore] (1849-1929)
On a perfected method of photographing the larynx. [New York, 1884.] 10p. 1 plate. DNLM; NNNAM
80-2177

FRENCH, Thomas R[ushmore] (1849-1929)
A photographic study of the laryngeal image during the formation of the registers in the singing voice. New York, 1889. 8p. DNLM **80-2178**

FREUDENTHAL, W[olff] (1858-1929)
Zur Aetiologie der Unterleibsbrüche. [New York, 1888.] 11p. DNLM **80-2179**

FREY, Heinrich (1822-1890)
The microscope and microscopical technology; a text-book for physicians and students. . . . Transl. and ed. by George R. Cutter. . . . Illustrated by three hundred and eighty-eight engravings on wood. 2nd ed. New York: William Wood & Co., 1880. 660p. DLC; NNNAM; OCIM; PPC
80-2180

FRIEDENWALD, A[aron] (1836-1902)
Optic neuritis. Baltimore, [1881]. 10p. DNLM; MdU-D
80-2181

FRIEDENWALD, A[ron] (1836-1902)
Relation of eye and spinal diseases. [Baltimore, 1883.] 13p. DNLM; MdU-D **80-2182**

FRIEDLAENDER, Carl (1847-1887)
A manual of microscopical technology for use in the investigations of medicine and pathological anatomy, by . . . . Transl. from the 2nd enl. and cor. ed. by Stephen Yates Howell. New York & London: G. P. Putnam's Sons, 1885. 249p. DLC: IEN-M; NNNAM; PPC **80-2183**

FRIEDLAENDER, Carl (1847-1887)
The use of the microscope in clinical and pathological examinations. . . . 2nd ed., enl. and improved, with a chromo-lithograph. Transl. by Henry C. Coe. . . . New York: D. Appleton & Co., 1885. 195p. col. front. DLC; MH-M; NNNAM; PPC
80-2184

FROTHINGHAM, George E[dward] (1836-1900)
Report on ophthalmology. Detroit: J. F. Eby & Co., [1886]. 25p. DNLM **80-2185**

FROTHINGHAM, George E[dward] (1836-1900)
A lecture on the code of medical ethics. Tecumseh, Mich., 1886. 44p. DNLM **80-2186**

FROTHINGHAM, George E[dward] (1836-1900)
Some cases illustrating the safety of cocaine as an anesthetic in cataract extractions. Chicago. Office Am. M. Ass., 1886. 12p. DNLM **80-2187**

FRUITNIGHT, J[ohn] Henry (1851-1900)
Pudendal hematocele. New York: William Wood & Co., 1884. 12p. DNLM **80-2188**

FRUITNIGHT, J[ohn] Henry (1851-1900)
Local treatment in diphtheria. [Philadelphia, 1888.] 3p. DNLM **80-2189**

FRUITNIGHT, J[ohn] Henry (1851-1900)
Urinary concretions in children. New York, 1889. 16p. DNLM
80-2190

FRUITNIGHT, J[ohn] Henry (1851-1900)
Treatment of scarlet fever and its complications. [New York, 1889.] 14p. DNLM **80-2191**

FRY, Henry D[avidson] (1853-1919)
Some observations on the diagnosis of pregnancy in its early stage, with special reference to temperature of the genital canal. New York: William Wood & Co., 1884. 12p. DNLM
80-2192

FRY, Henry D[avidson] (1853-1919)
The value of the antiseptic system in private obstetric practice; conclusions based on a study of the puerperal temperature. New York: William Wood & Co., 1886. 19p. DNLM
80-2193

FRY, Henry D[avidson] (1853-1919)
Electricity as a substitute for the curette in the treatment of retained secundines after abortion. New York: William Wood & Co., 1888. 11p. DNLM **80-2194**

FRY, Henry D[avidson] (1853-1919)
Observations on child-bearing complicated by organic disease of the heart. New York: William Wood & Co., 1888. 24p. DNLM **80-2195**

FRY, Henry D[avidson] (1853-1919)
The application of forceps to transverse and oblique positions of the head. Description of a new forceps. Chicago, 1889. 24p. DNLM **80-2196**

FRY, Henry D[avidson] (1853-1919)
The function of the coccyx in the mechanism of labor. New York: William Wood & Co., 1889. 11p. DNLM
80-2197

FRY, Henry D[avidson] (1853-1919)
A new obstetric forceps. [New York, 1889.] 4p. DNLM
80-2198

FRYE, George C.
Illustrated catalogue of surgical instruments and appliances. Portland, Me., [1880]. 226p. DNLM
80-2199

FRYE, George C.
Bulletin of surgical instruments. Portland, Me., [1883?]. 1 sheet, printed on both sides. eleph. fol. DNLM
80-2200

FRYE, George C.
Illustrated catalogue and price-list of surgical instruments, electric batteries, orthopedic appliances, etc. Portland, Me., 1883. 111 l. DNLM **80-2201**

FRYER, B. E.
Recent advances in ophthalmology. Atchison, Kansas: E. W. Beall, 1882. 17p. DNLM **80-2202**

FÜLLGRAFF, Otto (1819-1893)
Spray in the trachea. [New York, 1885.] 8p. DNLM
80-2203

FÜLLGRAFF, Otto (1819-1893)
The importance of proper respiration in the treatment of non-surgical diseases of the larynx, trachea, and bronchial tubes with medicated spray, and some explanations and suggestions as to the achievement of beneficial results. [New York, 1887.] 8p. DNLM **80-2204**

FULTON, John F.
The influence of climate on the treatment of chronic catarrh of the middle ear. Chicago: A. G. Newell, 1884. 8p. DNLM
80-2205

GAGE, Simon Henry (1851-1944)
Notes on microscopical methods. For the use of laboratory students in the anatomical department of the Cornell University. . . . Ithaca, N.Y.: Andrus & Church, 1886-1887. 32p. DLC **80-2206**

GALABIN, Alfred Lewis (1843-1913)
A manual of midwifery. Philadelphia: P. Blakiston, Son & Co., 1886. 753p. DNLM; NNNAM; PPC; PU
88-2207

GALENTIN, Christopher B.
Diphtheria, croup, etc.; or, The membranous diseases; their nature, history, causes, and treatment. . . . Cleveland, O.: Printed at the Publishing House of the Evangelical Association, 1884. 174p. DLC; OCIM **80-2208**

GALTON, Francis (1822-1911)
Hereditary genius: an inquiry into its laws and consequences. New and revised ed., with American preface. New York: D. Appleton & Co., 1883. 390p. ICU; MH; NN; NNC
80-2209

GAMA LOBO, Manoel da
The swamps and the yellow fever, with medium, minimum, and maximum thermometric, barometric and hygrometric and direction of winds of the city of Rio de Janeiro during 26 years. . . . New York, 1881. 28p. tables, 3 plates. DLC; NNNAM **80-2210**

GARBIT, Frederick J.
The woman's medical companion and guide to health. A practical treatise on the diseases of women and children, with full and definite directions for their treatment, giving the causes, symptoms, and means of prevention or cure, with the latest and most approved methods of treatment, adopted by all schools of medicine; their doses and modes of administration carefully prescribed. 2nd ed. Boston: J. P. Dale & Co., 1880. 512p. 1 plate. DNLM; MBM; NNNAM **80-2211**

GARBIT, Frederick J.
Diseases of the skin and blood, and how to cure them. Boston: A Mudge & Son, 1882. 64p. DNLM; MH-M
80-2212

GARBIT, Frederick J.
Diseases of the skin and blood, and how to cure them. Boston: Forbes Lith. Co., 1883. 64p. DNLM; MBM **80-2213**

GARDENIER, A., & CO.
Physiology and hygiene. A manual to accompany Gardenier's movable atlas. Albany: A. Gardenier & Co., 1887. 47p. DLC
80-2214

GARDENIER, Adelbert
A manual of physiology, anatomy, and hygiene. To accompany the "Man wonderful" manikin, a chart of the human body. Devised and arranged by Adelbert Gardinier. New York and Chicago: E. L. Kellogg & Co., [1889]. 33p. DLC; NNNAM; OCIM **80-2215**

GARDINER, James T[erry] (1842-1912)
Report to the State Board of Health on the methods of sewerage for cities and villages, in the State of New York. [Albany, 1881.] 15p. DNLM **80-2216**

GARDINER, James T[erry] (1842-1912)
Report to the State Board of Health on the methods of sewerage for cities and large villages in the State of New York. Albany: Weed, Parsons & Co., 1882. 15p. DNLM
80-2217

GARDINER, James T[erry] (1842-1912)
Report on a law for the sanitary protection of water supplies. [Albany, 1885.] 8p. DNLM **80-2218**

GARDINER, James T[erry] (1842-1912)
Report of the State Board of Health on the sanitary qualities of water supplies proposed for the city of Syracuse. Syracuse: Journal Co., 1887. 79p. DNLM **80-2219**

GARDINER, Thomas
Illustrated catalogue of surgical instruments and appliances. Minneapolis, [1880]. 226p. DNLM; OCIM
80-2220

GARDNER, JOHN H., & SONS
Introduction of the most approved European methods of using sulphur water at Sharon Springs, N.Y., for treatment of nasal catarrh and diseases of the respiratory organs, with translations from the notes of French physicians on these methods and the results as observed in France. New York: T. L. De Vinne & Co., 1885. 32p. DNLM; NNNAM **80-2221**

GARDNER, JOHN H., & SONS
Introduction of the most approved European methods of using sulphur water at Sharon Springs, N.Y., for treatment of nasal catarrh and diseases of the respiratory organs, with translations from the notes of French physicians on these methods and the results as observed in France. New York: T. L. De Vinne & Co., 1888. 42p. DNLM; NNNAM **80-2222**

GARDNER, R[obert] W[inslow] (1835-1911)
Hydriodic acid; its chemical character, history, incompatibles, condition, doses, etc., hypophosphites and phosphates chemically compared. History of three selected typical cases of phthisis, first stage, intermediate, second stage, cured by hypophosphites. [New York, 1880.] 16p. DNLM
80-2223

GARDNER, R[obert] W[inslow] (1835-1911)
Hydriodic acid. Additional notes in the treatment of acute inflammatory rheumatism, asthma, chronic bronchitis, adenitis, etc. Dr. Churchill's method of using the hypophosphites in phthisis, with detailed history of four cases, in the cavernous state successfully treated by him. Physiogenic and pathogenic effects of the hypophosphites, and conditions claimed by him to be necessary to their successful use in phthisis. 2nd ed. [New York, 1883.] 40p. DNLM; NNNAM [*also*: 3rd ed., New York, 1884. 63p. DNLM] **80-2224**

GARDNER, R[obert] W[inslow] (1835-1911)
Hydriodic acid; hypophosphites in phthisis. 5th ed. [New York, 1887.] 15p. DNLM; NNNAM **80-2225**

GARDNER, R[obert] W[inslow] (1835-1911)
Hydriodic acid, hypophospites in phthisis. 6th ed. [New York], 1888. 47p. DNLM; NNNAM **80-2226**

[GARFIELD, James Abram] (1831-1881)
Complete medical record of President Garfield's case, containing all of the official bulletins, from the day of the shooting to the day of his death, together with the official autopsy, made September 20, 1881, and a diagram showing the course taken by the ball. Compiled from the records of the Executive Mansion. Washington: C. A. Wimer, 1881. 106p. 1 plate. DNLM **80-2227**

GARLAND, George Minott
The modern treatment of pleurisy and pneumonia. Detroit: G. S. Davis, 1887. 108p. DNLM; OCIM; PPC; PU **80-2228**

GARMANY, Jasper Jewett (1859-1947)
Operative surgery in the cadaver. . . . New York: D. Appleton & Co., 1887. 150p. 2 col. plates. DLC; NNNAM; PPC; PU **80-2229**

GARRATT, Alfred C[harles] (1813?-1891)
Atmospheric electricity as a remedy. Cambridge, 1883. 20p. DNLM; MH-M **80-2230**

GARRATT, Alfred C[harles] (1813?-1891)
Myths in medicine and old-time doctors. New York & London: G. P. Putnam's Sons, 1884. 242p. CtY-M; DNLM; NNNAM; PU **80-2231**

GARRETSON, James E[dmund] (1828-1895)
A system of oral surgery; being a treatise on the diseases and surgery of the mouth, jaws, and associate parts. 3rd ed. Philadelphia: J. B. Lippincott & Co., 1881. 916p. DNLM; MdU-D; NNNAM; PPC [4th ed., 1884; 1037p.] **80-2232**

GARRIGUES, Henry Jacques (1831-1913)
Rest after delivery. New York: William Wood & Co., 1880. 21p. DNLM; NNNAM **80-2233**

GARRIGUES, Henry Jacques (1831-1913)
The obstetric treatment of the perineum. New York: William Wood & Co., 1880. 36p. DNLM; NNNAM **80-2234**

GARRIGUES, Henry Jacques (1831-1913)
Laceration of the cervix uteri. New York: G. P. Putnam's Sons, 1881. 5p. DNLM **80-2235**

GARRIGUES, Henry Jacques (1831-1913)
Dissecting metritis. [New York, 1882.] 9p. DNLM **80-2236**

GARRIGUES, Henry Jacques (1831-1913)
Diagnosis of ovarian cysts by means of the examination of their contents. New York: William Wood & Co., 1882. 112p. CtY-M; DNLM; NNNAM; PPC **80-2237**

GARRIGUES, Henry Jacques (1831-1913)
Obstetrical tetanus and tetanoid contractions. New York: William Wood & Co., 1882. 46p. DNLM; NNNAM **80-2238**

GARRIGUES, Henry Jacques (1831-1913)
The improved Caesarean section; containing the description of a kyphotic pelvis. New York: William Wood & Co., 1883. 55p. DNLM; NNNAM **80-2239**

GARRIGUES, Henry Jacques (1831-1913)
On lying-in institutions, especially those in New York. [New York, 1883.] 58p. DNLM; NNNAM **80-2240**

GARRIGUES, Henry Jacques (1831-1913)
Electricity in extra-uterine pregnancy. Boston, 1883. 35p. DNLM; MH-M **80-2241**

GARRIGUES, Henry Jacques (1831-1913)
Additional remarks on gastro-elytrotomy, with special reference to Porro's operation. New York: William Wood & Co., 1883. 20p. DNLM; NNNAM **80-2242**

GARRIGUES, Henry Jacques (1831-1913)
Prevention of ophthalmia neonatorum. [Philadelphia, 1884.] 4p. DNLM **80-2243**

GARRIGUES, Henry Jacques (1831-1913)
Prevention of puerperal infection. New York: Trow, 1884. 15p. DNLM **80-2244**

GARRIGUES, Henry Jacques (1831-1913)
The removal of the after-birth. New York: William Wood & Co., 1884. 14p. DNLM **80-2245**

GARRIGUES, Henry Jacques (1831-1913)
Extra-uterine pregnancy changed to intra-uterine, by means of faradization. [Philadelphia, 1885.] 14p. DNLM **80-2246**

GARRIGUES, Henry Jacques (1831-1913)
Practical guide in antiseptic midwifery in hospital and private practice. . . . Detroit: G. S. Davis, 1886. 128p. DLC; DNLM; OCIM; NNNAM **80-2247**

GARRIGUES, Henry Jacques (1831-1913)
Puerperal diphtheria. New York, 1886. 16p. DNLM **80-2248**

GARRIGUES, Henry Jacques (1831-1913)
The improved Caesarean section. Philadelphia: W. J. Dornan, 1888. 20p. DNLM **80-2249**

GARRIGUES, Henry Jacques (1831-1913)
Der Scheintod. Vortrag gehalten im Deutschen gesellig-wissenschaftlichen Verein von New York am 15. December 1886. New York: H. Bartsch, 1889. 28p. DNLM **80-2250**

GATCHELL, Charles (1851-1910)
"Doctor, what shall I eat?" A handbook of diet in disease. For the profession and the people. . . . Milwaukee: Cramer, Aikens & Cramer, printers, 1880. 147p. DLC; OCIM **80-2251**

GATCHELL, Charles (1851-1910)
. . . How to feed the sick, or, Diet in disease. For the profession and the people. . . . 2nd ed., rev. and enl. Chicago: Gross & Delbridge, 1882. 150p. DLC; OCIM **80-2252**

GATCHELL, Charles (1851-1910)
The key notes of medical practice. Chicago: Gross & Delbridge, 1883. 217p. OCIM; PPHa **80-2253**

GATCHELL, Charles (1851-1910)
The treatment of cholera as practiced by the leading homoeopathic physicians of the world. . . . Chicago: Gross & Delbridge, 1884. 32p. DLC; DNLM; OCIM **80-2254**

GATCHELL, Charles (1851-1910)
The key notes of medical practice. . . . Chicago: Gross & Delbridge, 1884. 172p. DLC; OCIM **80-2255**

GATCHELL, Charles (1851-1910)
The key notes of medical practice. 2nd ed. Chicago: Gross & Delbridge, 1885. 217p. DNLM; OCIM **80-2256**

GATCHELL, Charles (1851-1910)
How to feed the sick. A hand-book of diet in disease. 3rd ed. Chicago: Gross & Delbridge, 1885. 162p. OCIM; PPHa **80-2257**

GAY, George W[ashington] (1842-1931)
The management of patients during captial operations. Cambridge: Riverside Press, 1883. 8p. DNLM **80-2258**

GAY, George W[ashington] (1842-1931)
Tracheotomy in croup. [Philadelphia, 1884.] 12p. DNLM **80-2259**

GAY, George W[ashington] (1842-1931)
The plaster-posterior splint in the treatment of fractures of the leg. [Boston], 1884. 9p. DNLM **80-2260**

GAY, George W[ashington] (1842-1931)
The comparative merits of tracheotomy and intubation in the treatment of croup. Boston: Cupples & Hurd, 1888. 21p. DNLM; MBM **80-2261**

GEHRUNG, Eugene C[harles] (1841-1924)
Improved plaster of Paris jacket, or "cuirasse," for posterior spinal curvature in the middle and upper dorsal regions. St. Louis: Nixon & Penn, 1880. 8p. DNLM **80-2262**

GEHRUNG, Eugene C[harles] (1841-1924)
The mechanical treatment of cystocele and procidentia uteri. New York: William Wood & Co., 1880. 23p. DNLM **80-2263**

GEHRUNG, Eugene C[harles] (1841-1924)
The effects of ante-displacements of the uterus on pregnancy and labor. New York: William Wood & Co., 1882. 8p. DNLM **80-2264**

GEHRUNG, Eugene C[harles] (1841-1924)
Are uterine displacements curable by position, reposition, electricity, therapeutic means, pregnancy, surgical operations, or pessaries? [St. Louis, 1882.] 13p. DNLM **80-2265**

GEHRUNG, Eugene C[harles] (1841-1924)
Peculiar displacement of the arm in utero at birth. St. Louis, 1885. 7p. DNLM **80-2266**

GEHRUNG, Eugene C[harles] (1841-1924)
A new instrument for intra-uterine medication. New York, 1886. 4p. DNLM **80-2267**

GEHRUNG, Eugene C[harles] (1841-1924)
A new system of uterine medication. New York, 1886. 13p. DNLM **80-2268**

GEHRUNG, Eugene C[harles] (1841-1924)
Electrolysis; its value in diagnosis as well as in treatment of intra-abdominal and intra-pelvic tumors by the aid of a new instrument. New York: William Wood & Co., 1888. 12p. DNLM **80-2269**

GEHRUNG, Eugene C[harles] (1841-1924)
Repression of menstruation as a curative agent in gynecology. New York: William Wood & Co., 1888. 12p. DNLM **80-2270**

GEMRIG, J. H.
Illustrated catalogue of surgical instruments, appliances. . . . Philadelphia: [J. H. Gemrig, 1880?]. 139p. DNLM; PPC **80-2271**

GEMRIG, J. H.
Illustrated catalogue of surgical instruments, appliances. . . . Philadelphia: [J. H. Gemrig, 1881?] 188p. DNLM; PU **80-2272**

GEMRIG, J. H.
Illustrated catalogue of surgical instrumens, appliances. . . . [5th ed.] Philadelphia, 1882. 216p. DNLM; PPC **80-2273**

GEMRIG, J. H.
Illustrated catalogue of the apparatus required for the treatment of deformities, contractions, debilities, and paralysis of the human frame, and diseases of the joints. Philadelphia: J. H. Gemrig, [1884?] 12 l. DNLM **80-2274**

GEORGIA COLLECE OF ELECTIC MEDICINE AND SURGERY, ATLANTA
Annual announcements for the sessions 1880-1881 to 1895-1896 (41.-56.); 1897-1898 to 1899-1900 (58.-60.). Atlanta, 1880-1899. DNLM [The original charter of this school was granted in 1839 to the Southern Botanico-Medical College at Forsyth, which removed to Macon in 1846, and was succeeded by the Reform Medical College of Georgia in 1854. Suspended during the civil war. Reorganized in 1867, and in 1874 changed title to the College of American Medicine and Surgery. Removed to Atlanta in 1880. In 1884, united with the Georgia Eclectic Medical College (organized in 1877). In 1886, the present title was adopted. In 1887, the announcements were numbered from the original charter of 1839. Lists of graduates from 1878 to 1898, in announcement for 1898-1899.] **80-2275**

GEROULD, H[enry]
A practical and successful mode of disinfecting the room in case of cancer. Cleveland, 1887. 1 galley sheet. DNLM **80-2276**

GERRISH, Frederic Henry (1845-1920)
Prescription writing. Designed for the use of medical students who have never studied Latin. . . . 3rd ed., with an appendix on the metric system in prescriptions. Portland, Me.: Loring, Short, & Harmon; Philadelphia: J. B. Lippincott & Co., 1880. 53p. DLC; PPC; PPJ; PU **80-2277**

GERRISH, Frederic Henry (1845-1920)
The best equipment for medical study. Portland, Me.: W. M. Marks, 1887. 33p. DNLM **80-2278**

GERRISH, Frederic Henry (1845-1920)
Prescription writing. Designed for the use of medical students who have never studied Latin. . . . 7th and rev. ed. Portland, Me.: Loring, Short, & Harmon; Philadelphia: J. B. Lippincott & Co., 1888. 55p. DLC; PU **80-2279**

GERRISH, Frederic Henry (1845-1920)
The special function of the American Academy of Medicine. Address of the president, 13th November, 1888. Philadelphia, 1889. 27p. DNLM; PPC **80-2280**

GERSTER, Arpad G. (1848-1923)
The rules of aseptic and antiseptic surgery. A practical treatise for the use of students and the general practitioner. New York: D. Appleton & Co., 1888. 332p. CtY-M; DNLM; NNNAM; OCIM **80-2281**

GETCHELL, F. H[orace] (1836-1907)
An illustrated encyclopedia of the science and practice of obstetrics. Philadelphia: Gebbie & Co., 1885. 276p. IEN-M; NNNAM; PPC; PU **80-2282**

GIBBES, Heneage (*d.* 1912)
Practical histology and pathology. Philadelphia: P. Blakiston, 1881. 107p. CtY-M; DNLM; NNNAM; PPC **80-2283**

GIBBES, Heneage (*d.* 1912)
Practical histology and pathology. 2nd ed. Philadelphia: P. Blakiston & Co., 1883. 154p. DNLM; LNT-M; NNNAM; PU **80-2284**

GIBBES, Heneage (*d.* 1912)
Practical histology and pathology. 3rd ed. Philadelphia: P. Blakiston, Son & Co., 1885. 196p. DNLM; MBM; NNNAM; PU **80-2285**

GIBBES, Heneage (*d.* 1912)
Fistula in ano in phthisis and actinomycosis bovis. [Chicago, 1889.] 8p. DNLM **80-2286**

GIBBONS, Henry, Sr. (1808-1884)
A protest against meddlesome midwifery. [San Francisco]: W. M. Hinton & Co., [1880?]. 11p. DNLM **80-2287**

GIBIER, Paul (1851-1900)
Etiology and treatment of yellow fever. Transl. by Joseph A. Pacetti. Spec. sess. S. Mis. Doc. No. 13, March 30, 1889. Presented by Mr. Call. [Washington, 1889.] 8p. DNLM **80-2288**

GIBNEY, V[irgil] P[endleton] (1847-1927)
The strong galvanic current in the treatment of sciatica. The results in thirty-two cases. Philadelphia: Collins, 1880. 11p. DNLM **80-2289**

GIBNEY, V[irgil] P[endleton] (1847-1927)
Notes on the management of orthopedic cases. Louisville: J. P. Morton & Co., 1880. 9p. DNLM **80-2290**

GIBNEY, V[irgil] P[endleton] (1847-1927)
Perinephritis; fifteen additional cases in children, completing a total of twenty-eight. Chicago, 1880. 30p. DNLM **80-2291**

GIBNEY, V[irgil] P[endleton] (1847-1927)
Caries of the ankle in children. The results of expectant treatment from a study of thirty cases. New York: William Wood & Co., 1880. 26p. DNLM; NNNAM **80-2292**

GIBNEY, V[irgil] P[endleton] (1847-1927)
Periarthritis; a study of forty-seven cases. New York: D. Appleton & Co., 1880. 16p. DNLM **80-2293**

GIBNEY, V[irgil] P[endleton] (1847-1927)
Perityphlitis in children. Illustrating points in the differential diagnosis of hip-disease. A report of six cases. Philadelphia: Collins, 1881. 11p. DNLM **80-2294**

GIBNEY, V[irgil] P[endleton] (1847-1927)
Intermittent spinal paralysis of malarial origin. New York: B. Westermann & Co., 1882. 20p. DNLM **80-2295**

GIBNEY, V[irgil] P[endleton] (1847-1927)
A case of slow and one of swift compression of the spinal cord from dislocation of the odontoid process. New York, 1882. 11p. 1 plate. DNLM **80-2296**

GIBNEY, V[irgil] P[endleton] (1847-1927)
The diagnosis of Pott's disease of the spine before the stage of deformity. Cambridge: Riverside Press, 1882. 30p. DNLM **80-2297**

GIBNEY, V[irgil] P[endleton] (1847-1927)
The hip and its diseases. New York: Bermingham & Co., 1884. 412p. DNLM **80-2298**

GIBNEY, V[irgil] P[endleton] (1847-1927)
The surgical management of rhachitic deformities of the lower extremities. [New York, 1884.] 19p. DNLM **80-2299**

GIBNEY, V[irgil] P[endleton] (1847-1927)
The treatment of sciatica. New York: Trow's, 1884. 16p. DNLM **80-2300**

GIBNEY, V[irgil] P[endleton] (1847-1927)
Excision of the accessory tendons of the extensor communis digitorum of the ring-finger in a pianist. [New York, 1886.] 4p. DNLM **80-2301**

GIBNEY, V[irgil] P[endleton] (1847-1927)
The limitation of therapeutics in infantile paralysis. [New York, 1886.] 12p. DNLM **80-2302**

GIBNEY, V[irgil] P[endleton] (1847-1927)
The management of abscesses in connection with the bone-diseases of childhood. [Philadelphia, 1887.] 16p. DNLM **80-2303**

GIBNEY, V[irgil] P[endleton] (1847-1927)
The "boat-belly" of tubercular meningitis. A clinical report. [Philadelphia, 1889.] 3p. 1 plate. DNLM **80-2304**

GIBNEY, V[irgil] P[endleton] (1847-1927)
The immediate correction of deformities resulting from disease of the hip. New York, 1889. 17p. DNLM
80-2305

GIHON, Albert Leary (1833-1901)
The prevention of venereal disease by legislation. New York, 1882. 23p. DNLM; NNNAM **80-2306**

GIHON, Albert Leary (1833-1901)
The domain of climatology and demography as dependencies of medicine. . . . [Philadelphia: W. F. Fell & Co., prs., 1887.] 15p. DLC **80-2307**

GILBERT, Luther M.
The home physician; a summary of practical medicine and surgery for the use of travellers, and of families at a distance from physicians. . . . New York: G. P. Putnam's Sons, 1883. 131p. DLC; NNNAM; PPC; PU **80-2308**

[GILBERT, William Kent] (1827-1880)
Catalogue of the library of the late Wm. Kent Gilbert, M.D., of Philadelphia: Containing many early American imprints, both in medicine and history. The whole to be sold by auction Monday, May 16, 1881. Philadelphia, 1881. 16p. DNLM; PPC
80-2309

GILCHRIST, J[ames] Grant (1842-1906)
Surgical diseases and their homoeopathic treatment. 3rd ed. Rewritten, revised and enlarged. Chicago: Duncan Bros., 1880. 464p. OCIM; PPHa **80-2310**

GILCHRIST, J[ames] Grant (1842-1906)
Surgical principles and minor surgery. Chicago: Duncan Bros., 1881. 205p. DNLM **80-2311**

GILCHRIST, J[ames] Grant (1842-1906)
Surgical emergencies and accidents. Chicago: Duncan Bros., 1881. 599p. DNLM; OCIM **80-2312**

GILES, Alfred E[llenwood]
Civil and medical liberty in the healing art, including the practice of therapeutics by clairvoyants, spirit mediums, healing and magnetic mediums and magnetizers. With corroborative letters from Eugene Crowell and Joseph R. Buchanan. Boston: Colby & Rich, 1880. 34p. DNLM; MBM
80-2313

GILES, Alfred E[llenwood]
The iniquity of compulsory vaccination and the unconstitutionality of its statues. A reply to Dr. W. S. Everett's "Utility of vaccination." Hyde Park, Mass., 1881. 7p. DNLM
80-2314

GILL, H. Z.
Eclampsia. Puerperal convulsions. [Chicago, 1881.] 16p. DNLM **80-2315**

GILLETTE, W[alter] R[oberts] (*b.* 1840)
A postural method of copulation for the cure of some forms of sterility in the female. [New York, 1880.] 8p. DNLM
80-2316

GILLETTE, W[alter] R[oberts] (*b.* 1840)
A successful case of laparo-elytrotomy, with remarks on the indications, dangers, and results of the operation. New York: William Wood & Co., 1880. 10p. DNLM
80-2317

GILLETTE, W[alter] R[oberts] (*b.* 1840)
A point in the management of the first stage of labor. [Boston, 1882.] 11p. DNLM **80-2318**

GILLIAM, David Tod (1844-1923)
The essentials of pathology. . . . Philadelphia: P. Blakiston, Son & Co., 1883. 296p. DLC; DNLM; NNNAM; PPC
80-2319

GLASGOW, William Carr (1845-1907)
Varicose aneurism of the aorta; a report of a case of aneurism of the aorta communicating with the superior vena cava. St. Louis: H. Chambers & Co., [1885]. 7p. 2 plates. DNLM
80-2320

GLASGOW, William Carr (1845-1907)
On certain measures for the relief of congestive headaches. [New York, 1887.] 5p. DNLM **80-2321**

GLEITSMANN, [Joseph] William (1841-1914)
Deviation of the nasal septum. [Philadelphia, 1885.] 11p. DNLM **80-2322**

GLEITSMANN, [Joseph] William (1841-1914)
Mundathmung, ihre Ursachen, practische Bedentung und Behandlung. [New York, 1886.] 5p. DNLM
80-2323

GLEITSMANN, [Joseph] William (1841-1914)
Hypertrophy of the tonsil of the tongue, with history of cases. New York: Trow's Co., 1887. 11p. DNLM
80-2324

GLEITSMANN, [Joseph] William (1841-1914)
Traumatic haematoma of the larynx. [New York, 1887.] 4p. DNLM **80-2325**

GLEITSMANN, [Joseph] William (1841-1914)
Zweiter Jahresbericht der Halsabtheilung des Deutschen Dispensary in New York. [New York, 1887.] 9p. DNLM
80-2326

GLEITSMANN, [Joseph] William (1841-1914)
Nasal instruments. [New York, 1889.] 1 sheet. DNLM
80-2327

GLISAN, Rodney (1827-1890)
Text book of modern midwifery. Philadelphia: P. Blakiston, 1881. 639p. CtY-M; DNLM; NNNAM; PPC
80-2328

GODDING, William Whitney (1831-1899)
Progress in provision for the insane, 1844-1884. Utica, N.Y., 1884. 22p. DNLM **80-2329**

GODDING, William Whitney (1831-1899)
The rights of the insane in hospitals. Philadelphia, 1884. 24p. DNLM **80-2330**

GODDING, William Whitney (1831-1899)
Our insane neighbor; his rights and ours. Pt. 1. [Philadelphia, 1884.] 4p. DNLM **80-2331**

GODDING, William Whitney (1831-1899)
Our insane neighbor: his rights and ours. Pt. 2. [Philadelphia, 1884.] 22p. DNLM **80-2332**

GODDING, William Whitney (1831-1899)
The recognition of classes of the insane in asylum construction. St. Louis, 1885. 9p. DNLM **80-2333**

GODDING, William Whitney (1831-1899)
A vindication of history, by the author of Two hard cases. St. Louis, 1885. 19p. DNLM **80-2334**

GODDING, William Whitney (1831-1899) and W. W. L. CISSEL
Addresses delivered at the sixty-fourth annual commencement of the National Medical College (Medical Department of the Columbian University) March 17, 1886. Washington, D.C.: W. H. Moore, 1886. 15p. DNLM **80-2335**

GODDING, William Whitney (1831-1899)
Sketch of Charles H. Nichols, M.D., LL.D. Utica, N.Y, 1889. 7p. port. DNLM **80-2336**

GODFREY, E. L. B.
Dr. Edward Jenner's discovery of vaccination. Philadelphia: Hoeflich & Senseman, 1881. 16p. DNLM **80-2337**

GODFREY, John
Medicine and medicine men. Anniversary address, before the New Orleans Medical and Surgical Association, Dec. 20, 1882. New Orleans: L. Graham & Son, 1883. 17p. DNLM; LNT-M **80-2338**

GODLEE, Rickman John (1849-1925)
An atlas of human anatomy; illustrating most of the ordinary dissections and many not usually practiced by the student. With explanatory text. Philadelphia: P. Blakiston, 1880. 459p. 48 plates. DNLM; NNNAM; OCIM; PPC **80-2339**

GOELET, Augustin H. (1854-1910)
Electrolysis in gynaecology. Wilmington, 1888. 7p. DNLM **80-2340**

GOELET, Augustin H. (1854-1910)
The use of the dilator and intra-uterine stem in the treatment of dysmenorrhoea and sterility (rapid dilatation). New York, 1888. 19p. DNLM **80-2341**

GOELET, Augustin H. (1854-1910)
A new suture-fastener for silver wire, especially adapted for operations upon the cervix and perinaeum. [New York, 1888.] 5p. DNLM **80-2342**

GOELET, Augustin H. (1854-1910)
A perineal retractor for the dorsal position, with elevator for the anterior vaginal wall, especially adapted for applications of electricity to the uterus and vagina. [New York, 1889.] 8p. DNLM **80-2343**

GOELET, Augustin H. (1854-1910)
The value of electricity as a substitute for laparotomy in diseases of the uterine appendages. [New York, 1889.] 24p. DNLM **80-2344**

GOLDSMITH, W[illiam] B[enjamin] (1854-1888)
A case of moral insanity [with removal of ovaries and recovery]. [Utica, N.Y., 1883.] 16p. DNLM **80-2345**

GOLDSMITH, W[illiam] B[enjamin] (1854-1888)
The early symptoms of general paralysis of the insane. [New York, 1883.] 12p. DNLM **80-2346**

GOLDTHWAIT, Joel E[rnest] (*b.* 1866)
Ultimate results of osteotomy and osteoclasis. [Boston, 1889.] 12p. DNLM **80-2347**

GOODELL, William (1829-1894)
Lessons in gynecology. . . . With ninety-two illustrations. [2nd ed.] Philadelphia, Pa.: D. G. Brinton, 1880. 454p. DLC; DNLM; NNNAM; PPC **80-2348**

GOODELL, William (1829-1894)
Clinical notes on the elongation of the cervix uteri. [Boston, 1880.] 25p. DNLM; MH-M **80-2349**

GOODELL, William (1829-1894)
Clinical observations on the radical treatment of fibroid tumors of the womb. Philadelphia: Collins, 1880. 12p. DNLM **80-2350**

GOODELL, William (1829-1894)
The dangers and the duty of the hour. Baltimore: J. W. Borst & Co., 1881. 17p. DNLM; MdU-D **80-2351**

GOODELL, William (1829-1894)
Statistics of ovariotomies. New York: William Wood & Co., 1882. 10p. DNLM **80-2352**

GOODELL, William (1829-1894)
A year's work in ovariotomy. [Philadelphia, 1883.] 15p. DNLM **80-2353**

GOODELL, William (1829-1894)
On the treatment of painful menstruation and sterility from flexion. Philadelphia, 1885. 15p. DNLM **80-2354**

GOODELL, William (1829-1894)
A year's work in laparotomy. [Philadelphia, 1886.] 8p. 1 tab. DNLM **80-2355**

GOODELL, William (1829-1894)
Lessons in gynecology. . . . 3rd ed., thoroughly rev. and greatly enl. With one hundred and twelve illustrations. Philadelphia, Pa.: D. G. Brinton, 1887. 579p. CtY-M; DLC; NNNAM; PPC **80-2356**

GOODELL, William (1829-1894)
The abuse of uterine treatment through mistaken diagnosis. Philadelphia, 1889. 16p. DNLM **80-2357**

GOODELL, William (1829-1894)
Mechanical dysmenorrhoea. Philadelphia, 1889. 7p. DNLM **80-2358**

GOODHART, James Frederic (1845-1916)
A guide to the diseases of children. . . . Rev. and ed. by Louis Starr. . . . With formulae. Philadelphia: P. Blakiston, Son & Co., 1885. 738p. DLC: DNLM; MBM; PU **80-2359**

GOODHART, James Frederic (1845-1916)
A guide to the diseases of children. . . . Rearranged, rev. and ed. by Louis Starr. . . . 2nd American from the 3rd English ed., with numerous formulae. . . . Philadelphia: P. Blakiston, Son & Co., 1889. 772p. diags. DLC; DNLM; NNNAM; PPC **80-2360**

GOODMAN, J[ohn] (1837-1912)
Reprints of papers upon gynecological subjects. Louisville, 1880. 78p. DNLM; OCIM **80-2361**

GOODNO, William C[olby]
Valedictory address delivered at the Academy of Music upon the 38th annual commencement of the Hahnemann Medical College of Philadelphia. [Philadelphia, 1886.] 14p. DNLM; PPHa **80-2362**

GOODWILLIE, D[avid] H[enderson] (*b.* 1834)
Surgical treatment of naso-pharyngeal catarrh. 1st ed. New York, 1880. 8p. DNLM **80-2363**

GOODWILLIE, D[avid] H[enderson] (*b.* 1834)
Surgical treatment of naso-pharyngeal catarrh. Philadelphia: Collins, 1880. 13p. DNLM **80-2364**

GOODWILLIE, D[avid] H[enderson] (*b.* 1834)
Thumb sucking. [New York, 1881.] 2p. DNLM **80-2365**

GOODWILLIE, D[avid] H[enderson] (*b.* 1834)
Treatment of arthritis of the temporo-maxillary articulation. New York: G. P. Putnam's Sons, 1881. 5p. DNLM **80-2366**

GOODWILLIE, D[avid] H[enderson] (*b.* 1834)
An address on oral surgery. Philadelphia, 1882. 16p. DNLM **80-2367**

GOODWILLIE, D[avid] H[enderson] (*b.* 1834)
The application by insufflation of medicated powders to the upper air-passages for the relief of catarrhal conditions. New York: G. P. Putnam's Sons, 1882. 5p. DNLM **80-2368**

GOODWIN, Charles H.
The hospital treatment of diseases of the heart and lungs, with over three hundred and fifty formulae and prescriptions. . . . New York: C. H. Goodwin, 1883. 196p. DLC; NNNAM **80-2369**

GOODWIN, Charles H.
Treatment of diseases of infancy and childhood, with over four hundred formulae and prescriptions, as exemplified in the services of Drs. A. Jacobi et al. 2nd ed. New York: C. H. Goodwin, 1883. 284p. DLC; DNLM **80-2370**

GOODWIN, Charles H.
Treatment of diseases of women, puerperal and non-puerperal. Being the latest contributions to this important branch of medical science, based upon the most recent practical experiences and investigations of the present day, by the following eminent gynaecologists and specialists: Drs. T. Gaillard Thomas, et al. 2nd ed. New York: C. H. Goodwin, 1884. 436p. DLC; DNLM **80-2371**

GOODWIN, GEORGE & CO.
Catalog of drugs and sundries. Boston, 1880. 268p. MBM **80-2372**

GOODWIN, GEORGE & CO.
Catalog of drugs and sundries. . . . Boston, 1885. 384p. MH-M **80-2373**

GORDINIER, H[ermon] C. (*b.* 1864)
A case of sclerodactyle with diffuse scleroderma. [Philadelphia, 1889.] 10p. DNLM **80-2374**

GORDON, Joseph C[laybaugh] (1842-1903)
Practical hints to parents of young deaf children concerning preliminary home training. Washington: Gibson Bros., 1886. 45p. DNLM **80-2375**

GORDON, S[eth] C[hase] (*b.* 1830)
President's address to the Maine Medical Association. Portland: S. Berry, 1880. 13p. DNLM **80-2376**

GORDON, S[eth] C[hase] (*b.* 1830)
Results of treatment of injuries occurring at parturition. Portland: S. Berry, 1883. 11p. DNLM **80-2377**

GORDON, S[eth] C[hase] (*b.* 1830)
The operative treatment of hyperplasia of the uterus and vagina, with special reference to the cure of displacements. [New York, 1884.] 5p. DNLM **80-2378**

GORDON, S[eth] C[hase] (*b.* 1830)
A new surgical dressing for wounds. [Boston, 1885.] 6p. DNLM **80-2379**

GORDON, S[eth] C[hase] (*b.* 1830)
Hysteria and its relation to diseases of the uterine appendages. Chicago, 1886. 24p. DNLM **80-2380**

GORDON, S[eth] C[hase] (*b.* 1830)
A case of extra-uterine (tubal) pregnancy; rupture at three months; laparotomy; recovery. [New York, 1888.] 7p. DNLM **80-2381**

GORGAS, Ferdinand James Samuel (1835-1914)
Dental medicine; a manual of dental materia medica and therapeutics, for practitioners and students. . . . Philadelphia: P. Blakiston, Son & Co., 1884. 311p. DLC; MdU-D; PPC; PU **80-2382**

GORGAS, Ferdinand James Samuel (1835-1914)
A series of questions pertaining to the curriculum of the dental student. . . . Baltimore, Md.: W. K. Boyle & Son, 1885. 133p. DLC; MdU-D **80-2383**

GORGAS, Ferdinand James Samuel (1835-1914)
Dental medicine. A manual of dental materia medica and therapeutics, for practitioners and students. . . . 2nd ed. Rev. and enl. Philadelphia: P. Blakiston, Son & Co., 1885. 379p. DLC; DNLM; MdU-D; PPC **80-2384**

GORGAS, Ferdinand James Samuel (1835-1914)
Dental medicine; a manual of dental materia medica and therapeutics. . . . 3rd ed. Rev. and enl. Philadelphia: P. Blakiston, Son & Co., 1889. 446p. DLC; MdU-D; NNNAM; PU **80-2385**

GOSS, Francis W.
A membrane-like affection of the bowels. Cambridge: Riverside Press, 1881. 12p. DNLM **80-2386**

GOSS, I[sham] J[abez] M[arshall]
The American practice of medicine. Including the diseases of women and children. Based upon the pathological indication of the remedies advised. 2nd ed. Philadelphia: Miller, 1885. 336p. DNLM; IU-M; OCIWHi; PU [1st ed. (1882), 641p.] **80-2387**

GOSS, I[sham] J[abez] M[arshall]
The practice of medicine, or, The specific art of healing. . . . Chicago: W. T. Keener, 1888. 569p. DLC; DNLM; OCIM **80-2387A**

GOSS, I[sham] J[abez] M[arshall]
A text book of materia medica, pharmacology, and special therapeutics, with many new remedies of late introduction. Designed as a text book for the student and as a ready reference for the practitioner. A compend of materia medica, written with especial reference to the more direct or positive action of medicines and the introduction of new ones. 2nd ed. Chicago: W. T. Keener, 1889. 586p. DLC; OCIM
80-2388

GOULD, George M[ilbry] (1848-1922)
The homing instinct. An explanation suggested. Louisville, 1888. 12 l. DNLM **80-2389**

GOULD, George M[ilbry] (1848-1922)
Is the electric light injurious to the eyes? [Philadelphia, 1888.] 23p. DNLM **80-2390**

GOULD, George M[ilbry] (1848-1922)
Mixed astigmatism, the result of severe inflammation of an eye. [Philadelphia, 1888.] 1 sheet. DNLM
80-2391

GOULD, George M[ilbry] (1848-1922)
A new style of bi-focal lenses. [Philadelphia, 1888.] 7p. DNLM **80-2392**

GOULD, George M[ilbry] (1848-1922)
A peculiar case of herpes zoster ophthalmicus, serous iritis, or "ophthalmo-neuritis." [Philadelphia, 1888.] 6p. DNLM
80-2393

GOULD, George M[ilbry] (1848-1922)
The psychological influence of errors of refraction and of their correction. [Philadelphia, 1888.] 6p. DNLM
80-2394

GOULD, George M[ilbry] (1848-1922)
Concerning reflex neuroses due to eye-strain. I. Three remarkable cases of reflex neuroses due to eye-strain. II. The influence of sexualism in reflex ocular neuroses. [Philadelphia, 1889.] 14p., 11p. DNLM **80-2395**

GOULD, George M[ilbry] (1848-1922)
Dreams, sleep, consciousness. A psychological study. Chicago, 1889. 24p. DNLM **80-2396**

GOULD, George M[ilbry] (1848-1922)
The modern Frankenstein. Chicago, [1889]. 25p. DNLM
80-2397

GOULEY, John William Severin (1832-1920)
Note on cystorrhagia from retention of urine. . . . Syracuse, N.Y.: Standard Steam Book & Job Printing House, 1880. 15p. DLC **80-2398**

GOULEY, John William Severin (1832-1920)
Sacculation and perforation of the bladder as consequences of chronic retention of urine. . . . [New York, 1886.] 14p. DLC
80-2399

GOULEY, John William Severin (1832-1920)
Diseases of man: data of their nomenclature, classification & genesis. . . . New York: J. H. Vail & Co., [etc., etc.], 1888. 412p. DLC; DNLM; NNNAM; PU
80-2400

GOULEY, John William Severin (1832-1920)
A general consideration of tumors from a surgical point of view. New York, 1888. 32p. DNLM; NNNAM
80-2401

GOULEY, John William Severin (1832-1920)
Abstract of a paper on the choice of treatment of urinary concretions. . . . Chicago: Printed at the Office of the Association, 1889. 23p. DLC; DNLM **80-2402**

GOWERS, William R[ichard] (1845-1915)
A manual and atlas of medical ophthalmoscopy. Philadelphia: P. Blakiston, 1882. 384p. 16 plates. CtY-M; DNLM; NNNAM; PPC **80-2403**

GOWERS, William R[ichard] (1845-1915)
Lectures on the diagnosis of diseases of the brain, delivered at University College Hospital. Philadelphia: P. Blakiston, Son & Co., 1885. 246p. DNLM; NNNAM; OCIM; PU
80-2404

GOWERS, William R[ichard] (1845-1915)
Diagnosis of diseases of the brain and of the spinal cord. New York: William Wood & Co., 1885. 293p. DNLM; IEN-M; NNNAM; PU **80-2405**

GOWERS, William R[ichard] (1845-1915)
Epilepsy and other chronic convulsive diseases; their causes, symptoms, and treatment. New York: William Wood & Co., 1885. 255p. DNLM; IU-M; NNNAM; PPC
80-2406

GOWERS, William R[ichard] (1845-1915)
A manual of diseases of the nervous system. Philadelphia: P. Blakiston, Son & Co., 1886. v. 1. 463p. CtY-M; DNLM; PPC; PU **80-2407**

GOWERS, William R[ichard] (1845-1915)
Lectures on the diagnosis of diseases of the brain, delivered at University College Hospital. 2nd ed. Philadelphia: P. Blakiston, Son & Co., 1887. 254p. CU-M; DNLM; PPC; PU
80-2408

GOWERS, William R[ichard] (1845-1915)
A manual of diseases of the nervous system. American ed., under the supervision of the author, and containing all the material of the two-volume English edition, with some additions and revisions. Philadelphia: P. Blakiston, Son & Co., 1888. 25, 1357p. DNLM; MBM; NNNAM; PPC
80-2409

GRADLE, Henry (1855-1911)
Bacteria and the germ theory of disease. Eight lectures delivered at the Chicago Medical College. . . . Chicago: W. T. Keener, 1883. 219p. DLC; DNLM; OCIM
80-2410

GRADY, Richard
Dental jurisprudence. Baltimore: Snowden & Cowman, 1884. 21p. DNLM; MdU-D **80-2411**

GRADY, Richard
A case of closure of the jaws. [Philadelphia, 1888.] 1 galley sheet. DNLM **80-2412**

GRAHAM, D[avid] W[ilson]
The demand for medically-educated women. Chicago, 1886. 14p. DNLM **80-2413**

GRAHAM, D[avid] W[ilson] and J. Suydam KNOX
Practitioner's handbook, designed to accompany Physician's anatomical aid [Knox, Graham, and Owens]. Chicago: Western Publishing House, [1889]. 93p. DNLM
80-2414

GRAHAM, Douglas (1848-1928)
A practical treatise on massage, its history, mode of application, and effects. . . . New York: William Wood & Co., 1884. 286p. DLC; DNLM; NNNAM; OCIM
80-2415

GRANDIN, Egbert H[enry] (*b.* 1855)
Certain causes of sterility in the female, and their treatment. Nashville: Brandon Printing Co., [1887]. 8p. DNLM
80-2416

GRANDIN, Egbert H[enry] (*b.* 1855)
Electrolysis in uterine flexions. [New York, 1888.] 5p. DNLM
80-2417

GRANDIN, Egbert H[enry] (*b.* 1855)
A plea for the active treatment of puerperal endometritis by means of the curette. New York, 1889. 15p. DNLM
80-2418

GRAY, Harry C.
A condensed compendium of pharmaceutical knowledge. A quiz book, by H. C. Gray, Ph.G., and C. H. Bryan, M.D. . . . [2nd ed.] Springfield, O.: C. H. Bryan, 1888. 72p. DLC; OCIM; OCLloyd
80-2419

GRAY, Harry C.
A condensed compendium of pharmaceutical knowledge. A quiz book by H. C. Gray and C. H. Bryan. 3rd ed. Springfield, O.: C. H. Bryan, 1888. 178p. OCIM; OCLloyd
80-2420

GRAY, Harry C.
A condensed compendium of pharmaceutical knowledge. A quiz book by H. C. Gray and C. H. Bryan. 4th ed. Chicago: Gray & Bryan, 1888. 90p. IU-M; OCIM; OCLloyd
80-2421

GRAY, H[arry] C.
A condensed compendium of pharmaceutical knowledge. A quiz book by H. C. Gray, Ph.G., and C. H. Bryan, M.D. 5th ed. . . . Chicago, Ill.: Gray & Bryan, 1889. 96p. DLC; IU-M; OCIM; OCLloyd
80-2422

GRAY, Harry C.
Gray's elements of pharmacy, a treatise on elementary pharmacy, chemistry, and botany. . . . By H. C. Gray . . . and C. H. Bryan. . . . Chicago, Ill.: Gray & Bryan, 1889. 98p. DLC; IU-M; OCIM; OCLloyd
80-2423

GRAY, Henry (1827-1861)
Anatomy, descriptive and surgical. . . . With an introduction on general anatomy and development. By T. Holmes. The drawings by H. V. Carter. . . . With additional drawings in later editions. Ed. by T. Pickering Pick. A new American from the 10th English ed. To which is added Landmarks, medical and surgical. By Luther Holden. . . . With additions by William W. Keen. . . . Philadelphia: Henry C. Lea's Son & Co., 1883. 1023p. DLC; IU-M; NNNAM; PPC
80-2424

GRAY, Henry (1827-1861)
Anatomy, descriptive and surgical. . . . The drawings by H. V. Carter. . . . With additional drawings in later editions. Ed. by T. Pickering Pick. . . . A new American from the 11th English ed. Thoroughly rev. and re-ed. with additions, by William W. Keen. . . . To which is added Landmarks, medical and surgical. By Luther Holden. . . . With additions by William W. Keen, M.D. Philadelphia: Lea Bros. & Co., 1887. 1100p. DLC; DNLM; NNNAM; PPC
80-2425

GRAY, John P[erdue] (1825-1886)
The United States *vs.* Charles J. Guiteau, indicted for the murder of James A. Garfield, twentieth President of the United States. Opinion of . . . . on the sanity of the prisoner. Washington, 1882. 34p. DNLM
80-2426

GRAY, John P[erdue] (1825-1886)
Introductory address of the course of 1883-1884, at the Albany Medical College, delivered Sept. 11, 1883. Albany: Weed, Parsons & Co., 1883. 20p. DNLM
80-2427

GRAY, John P[erdue] (1825-1886)
Heredity. [Utica, N.Y., 1884.] 21p. DNLM
80-2428

GRAY, John P[erdue] (1825-1886)
Review of Dr. Godding's paper on progress in provision for the insane. [Utica, N.Y., 1884.] 32p. DNLM
80-2429

GRAY, John P[erdue] (1825-1886)
Insanity; some of its preventable causes. A lecture in the regular course of the Utica Mechanics' Association, delivered March 18, 1885. Utica, N.Y.: E. H. Roberts, 1885. 47p. DNLM
80-2430

GRAY, John P[erdue] (1825-1886)
Insanity; its frequency, and some of its preventable causes. [Utica, N.Y., 1886.] 26p. DNLM
80-2431

GRAY, J[oseph] L.
Ligation of the vertebral arteries for the relief or cure of epilepsy. Chicago: Rand, McNally & Co., 1886. 12p. DNLM
80-2432

GRAY, Landon Carter (1850-1900)
The use of quinine with nervous sedatives. New York: G. P. Putnam's Sons, 1880. 6p. DNLM
80-2433

GRAY, Landon Carter (1850-1900)
The effect of genital irritation in the production of nervous disorders. Brooklyn, N.Y., 1882. 30p. DNLM
80-2434

GRAY, Landon Carter (1850-1900)
The treatment of epilepsy. New York: D. Appleton & Co., 1884. 28p. DNLM
80-2435

GRAY, Landon Carter (1850-1900)
The nervous symptoms of so-called lithaemia. [New York, 1886.] 29p. DNLM
80-2436

GRAY, Landon Carter (1850-1900)
The present state of our knowledge regarding localization in the cortex cerebri. [New York, 1887.] 22p. DNLM
80-2437

GRAY, Landon Carter (1850-1900)
Syphilis of the nervous system, and its treatment. [Philadelphia, 1887.] 18p. DNLM **80-2438**

GRAY, Landon Carter (1850-1900)
Syphilis of the nervous system, and its treatment. Philadelphia, 1887. 2 galley sheets. DNLM **80-2439**

GRAY, Landon Carter (1850-1900)
Our present knowledge regarding muscular atrophies and hypertrophies. [New York, 1888.] 29p. DNLM **80-2440**

GRAY, Landon Carter (1850-1900)
The curability of locomotor ataxia, with an account of our present knowledge of its pathological anatomy. [New York, 1889.] 33p. DNLM **80-2441**

GRAY, William B[rooks] (*b.* 1833)
Diagnositc value of the phosphates in pregnancy. [Richmond, 1887.] 7p. DNLM **80-2442**

GRAY, William Merrick (*b.* 1868)
Alveolar sarcoma of tonsil. [Philadelphia, 1889.] 4p. DNLM **80-2443**

GRAYDON, Andrew W. (*d.* 1900)
Electricity in gynecological practice. [Philadelphia, 1887.] 12p. DNLM **80-2444**

GREEN, Adolphus
Asiatic cholera; its etiology and treatment. [St. Louis, 1885.] 12p. DNLM **80-2445**

GREEN, Charles M[ontraville] (1850-1928)
The delivery of the second fetus in labor with twins. New York: William Wood & Co., 1884. 9p. DNLM **80-2446**

GREEN, Charles M[ontraville] (1850-1928)
The etiology and treatment of occipito-posterior positions. [Boston, 1886.] 8p. DNLM **80-2447**

GREEN, Charles M[ontraville] (1850-1928)
The treatment of prolapse of the uterus and vagina, especially in the aged, with illustrative cases. Boston: Cupples, Upham & Co., 1887. 14p. DNLM **80-2448**

GREEN, Charles M[ontraville] (1850-1928)
A case of rupture of the uterus in labor at term, the child being born alive; recovery of the mother, and subsequent delivery of a full-term child in normal labor. Philadelphia: W. J. Dornan, 1888. 8p. DNLM **80-2449**

GREEN, Edgar Moore
On the value of Brücke's method for the removal of interfering substances from urine in testing for glucose. [Baltimore, 1886.] 14p. DNLM; MdU-D **80-2450**

GREEN, Frank B[ertangue] (1849?-1887)
A history of the medical profession in the county of Kings and the city of Brooklyn, New York, including the hospitals, dispensaries, and semi-medical institutions. . . . New York: W. W. Munsell & Co., 1884. 68p. NNNAM; NNU-M **80-2451**

GREEN, James S[proat] (1829-1892)
Chronic club-foot successfully treated without tenotomy, by continuous extension and stretching. [New York, 1881.] 9p. DNLM **80-2452**

GREEN, James S[proat] (1829-1892)
A review of the surgery of the knee joint for the last fifty years. Newark: L. F. Hardham, 1888. 22p. DNLM; NjR **80-2453**

GREEN, John (1835-1913)
Die Operation des Entropium. Historische Studie. St. Louis, Mo., 1886. 26p. DNLM **80-2454**

GREEN, John Orne (1799-1885)
The importance of early recognition of ear disease. Boston: D. Clapp & Son, 1880. 15p. DNLM; MBM **80-2455**

GREEN, John Orne (1799-1885)
Phlebitis of the mastoid emissary vein, from phlebitis of the lateral sinus; death from pyaemia; autopsy. New York: Trow, 1880. 10p. DNLM **80-2456**

GREEN, Milbrey
A sketch of obstetrics and gynaecology in America; the annual address before the Massachusetts Eclectic Medical Society. Boston: A Mudge & Son, 1880. 66p. DNLM; MH-M **80-2457**

GREEN, Milbrey
Qualifications, duties, and responsibilities of the medical profession; the annual address before the National Eclectic Medical Association. New York: A. Metz & Co., 1881. 33p. DNLM; NNNAM **80-2458**

GREEN, Samuel Abbott (1830-1918)
History of medicine in Massachusetts. A centennial address delivered before the Massachusetts Medical Society at Cambridge, June 7, 1881. Boston: A. Williams & Co., 1881. 131p. DLC; DNLM; MH-M; MWA **80-2459**

GREEN, Samuel Abbott (1830-1918)
A centennial address delivered in the Sanders Theatre, at Cambridge, June 7, 1881, before the Massachusetts Medical Society. Groton, 1881. 112p. DNLM; MBM **80-2460**

GREEN, Samuel Abbott (1830-1918)
Notes on a copy of Dr. Wm. Douglass's almanack for 1743, touching on the subject of medicine in Massachusetts before his time. Cambridge: J. Wilson & Son, 1884. 8p. DNLM **80-2461**

GREEN, T[homas] Henry (1841-1923)
An introduction to pathology and morbid anatomy. 5th American ed. from 6th English ed. Philadelphia: Henry C. Lea's Son & Co., 1884. 481p. DNLM; NNNAM; PPC; PU **80-2462**

GREEN, T[homas] Henry (1841-1923)
An introduction to pathology and morbid anatomy. 6th American from the 7th English ed., revised and enlarged by Stanley Boyd. Philadelphia: Lea Bros. & Co., 1889. 539p. DNLM; NNNAM; OCIM; PU **80-2463**

GREEN, Traill (1813-1897)
Proceedings of the Alumni Society of the Medical Department of the University of Pennsylvania for 1879, with the annual address by . . . . Words of encouragement to the medical profession. Delivered March 13, 1880. Philadelphia: Collins, 1880. 38p. DNLM; PPC; PU **80-2464**

GREEN, Traill (1813-1897)
The annual address delivered before the American Academy of Medicine, at its seventh annual meeting in Philadelphia, Oct. 26th, 1882. A retrospective glance at the origin and progress of the Academy. Philadelphia, 1883. 16p. DNLM; PPC **80-2465**

GREEN, Walter D[avenport] (*d.* 1914)
On a source of error in the estimation of urea by the hypobromate method, with apparatus of the Russell and West type. [Baltimore, 1886.] 4p. DNLM **80-2466**

GREENE, C. A.
Medical compendium, containing his sanitary platform and a brief history of the reformatory code or omnipathy, [etc.]. Harrisburg, Pa., 1882. 40p. DNLM **80-2467**

GREENE, Charles Lyman (*b.* 1862) and J. L. ROTHROCK
A case of concentric displacement of the heart to the right, presenting some unusual features. Philadelphia, 1889. 4p. DNLM **80-2468**

GREENE, James S[umner]
Neurasthenia; its causes and its home treatment. Cambridge, 1883. 14p. DNLM; MBM **80-2469**

GREENE, James S[umner]
Some uses of the vaginal tampon in obstetric art. Boston: Cupples & Hurd, 1889. 13p. DNLM; MBM **80-2470**

GREENE, R[euben] (*b.* 1817)
Alcoholic stimulants as medicines. Boston: J. E. Farwell & Co., 1881. 11p. DNLM **80-2471**

GREENE, William H[ouston] (1853-1918)
A practical handbook of medical chemistry applied to clinical research and the detection of poisons. Philadelphia: Henry C. Lea's Son & Co., 1880. 310p. DNLM; NNNAM; PPC; PU **80-2472**

GREENE, William Warren (1831-1881)
Contributions to clinical surgery; ten cases of litholapaxy. Cambridge, 1880. 12p. DNLM **80-2473**

GREENLEES, T[homas] Duncan
Cases illustrating cortical paralysis with loss of speech. [Utica, N.Y., 1887.] 13p. DNLM **80-2474**

GREENOUGH, F[rancis] B[oott] (1837-1904)
Herpes progenitalis. Read at the fourth annual meeting of the American Dermatological Assoc., Newport, R.I., September 1, 1880. [1880.] 29p. DNLM **80-2475**

GREENOUGH, F[rancis] B[oott] (1837-1904)
The routine treatment of venereal diseases. Cambridge: Riverside Press, [1882]. 24p. DNLM; MH-M **80-2476**

GREENOUGH, F[rancis] B[oott] (1837-1904)
Clinical notes on psoriasis. Boston: Cupples, Upham & Co., 1885. 16p. DNLM; MH-M **80-2477**

GREENOUGH, F[rancis] B[oott] (1837-1904)
Five cases of cerebral symptoms in early (secondary) syphilis. Boston: Cupples, Upham & Co., 1885. 27p. DNLM; MBM **80-2478**

GREENOUGH, F[rancis] B[oott] (1837-1904)
Clinical notes on scabies. Boston, 1886. 13p. DNLM **80-2479**

GREENOUGH, F[rancis] B[oott] (1837-1904)
Some additional clinical notes on psoriasis. Boston: Cupples, Upham & Co., 1886. 7p. DNLM **80-2480**

GREGG, Rollin R[obinson] (1828-1886)
Diphtheria; its cause, nature, and treatment. Buffalo: Matthews Bros. & Bryant, 1880. 133p. DLC; DNLM; PPHa **80-2481**

GREGG, Rollin R[obinson] (1828-1886)
Diphtheria and bacteria. [Buffalo, 1880.] 8p. DNLM **80-2482**

GREGG, Rollin R[obinson] (1828-1886)
Prof. Pasteur's experiments. Bacteria in various diseases. [Buffalo, 1881.] 10p. DNLM **80-2483**

GREGG, Rollin R[obinson] (1828-1886)
A simple solution of the mystery of tubercle. Chyle-corpuscles, red blood-corpuscles, and tubercular corpuscles, shown to be all one and the same under different conditions. [Buffalo, 1882.] 1 l. DNLM **80-2484**

GREGG, Rollin R[obinson] (1828-1886)
A simple solution of the mystery of tubercles, and other important questions. Buffalo: Haas & Klein, 1883. 19p. 1 plate. DLC; DNLM **80-2485**

GREGG, Rollin R[obinson] (1828-1886)
Constituents of tubercles, and explanation regarding them. [Buffalo, 1883.] 8p. DNLM **80-2486**

GREGG, Rollin R[obinson] (1828-1886)
The revelations of fibrin. Unexpected proof of the immortality of life. [Buffalo, 1884.] 7p. DNLM **80-2487**

GREGG, Rollin R[obinson] (1828-1886)
Consumption: its cause and nature, by . . . , to which is added, The therapeutics of tuberculous affections, by H. C. Allen, M.D. Ann Arbor, Mich.: Ann Arbor Register Printing & Publishing Co., 1889. 477p. col. plate. DLC; IEN-M; IU-M; OCIM **80-2488**

GREGORY, Elisha Hall (1824-1906)
Neoplasms from a practical point of view. Philadelphia: Collins, 1885. 11p. DNLM; PPC **80-2489**

GRIESINGER, Wilhelm (1817-1868)
Mental pathology and therapeutics. Transl. from the German (2nd ed.) by C. Lochart Robertson and J. Rutherford. New York: William Wood & Co., 1882. 375p. DNLM; NNNAM; PPC; PU **80-2490**

GRIFFITH, J[ohn] P. Crozer (1856-1941)
On the employment of thallin in febrile affections. [Philadelphia, 1886.] 8p. DNLM **80-2491**

GRIFFITH, J[ohn] P. Crozer (1856-1941)
Rubella (Rötheln, German measles); with a report of 150 cases. New York: Trow, 1887. 36p. DNLM **80-2492**

GRIFFITH, J[ohn] P. Crozer (1856-1941)
Glycerine enemata and suppositories in constipation, based on a trial of them in 234 cases. Philadelphia, 1888. 19p. DNLM
80-2493

GRIFFITH, J[ohn] P. Crozer (1856-1941)
Notes on the treatment of whooping cough with antipyrine. Philadelphia: W. J. Dornan, 1888. 14p. DNLM
80-2494

GRIFFITH, J[ohn] P. Crozer (1856-1941) and Elwood R. KIRBY
Notes on the employment of urethan and of amyl hydrate in insomnia. [Philadelphia, 1888.] 18p. DNLM
80-2495

GRIFFITH, J[ohn] P. Crozer (1856-1941)
A contribution to the study of Friedreich's ataxia; with exhibition of cases. Philadelphia: W. J. Dornan, 1889. 80p. 1 tab. DNLM **80-2496**

GRIFFITH, J[ohn] P. Crozer (1856-1941)
The graphic clinical chart. Philadelphia: P. Blakiston, Son & Co., [1889]. 50 sheets. roy. DNLM **80-2497**

GRIFFITH, J[ohn] P. Crozer (1856-1941)
Remarks on the unpleasant effects of sulphonal. Detroit, Mich.: G. S. Davis, 1889. 18p. DNLM **80-2498**

GRISSOM, Eugene (1831-1902)
Medical science in conflict with materialism. Wilmington, N.C.: Jackson & Bell, 1880. 31p. DNLM **80-2499**

GRISSOM, Eugene (1831-1902)
Report of the trial of James Thomas De Jarnette for homicide, with an appendix. Wilmington, N.C., 1881. 66p. DNLM
80-2500

GROFF, George G. (1851-1910)
A manual of accidents and emergencies, or How to avoid accidents and what to do when they occur. With notes on the preservation of health. . . . Lewisburg, Pa.: Printed for the Author, 1881. 92p. DLC **80-2501**

GROSS, James E.
. . . Homoeopathic guide to domestic practice, by Gross & Delbridge. . . . Chicago: N. W. Homoeopathic Pharmacy, 1883. 64p. DLC; IU-M; OCIM; PPHa **80-2502**

GROSS, James E.
Home guide in the use of forty-eight homoeopathic remedies. . . . 2nd ed. Chicago: Gross & Delbridge, 1884. 53p. DLC; IU-M; OCIM; PPHa **80-2503**

GROSS MEDICAL COLLEGE, DENVER. MEDICAL DEPARTMENT OF THE ROCKY MOUNTAIN UNIVERSITY
Circulars of information and register of students for the sessions of 1887-1888 to 1889-1890 (1.-3.); 1891-1892 (5.); 1892-1893 (6.); 1894-1895 to 1900-1901 (8.-14.). Denver, 1887-1900. DNLM [Incorporated May 7, and opened Sept. 21, 1887. Prior to 1895-1896 were called announcements. List of students and graduates for the sessions of 1887-1888 to 1889-1890; 1891-1892; 1892-1893; 1894-1895 to 1899-1900, in announcements and circulars for subsequent years. Alumni from 1888 to 1899, in circular for 1899-1900.]
80-2504

GROSS, Samuel D[avid] (1805-1884)
John Hunter and his pupils. . . . Philadelphia: P. Blakiston, 1881. 106p. DLC; DNLM; PPC; PPJ **80-2505**

GROSS, Samuel D[avid] (1805-1884)
A system of surgery; pathological, diagnostic, therapeutic, and operative. . . . Illustrated by upwards of sixteen hundred engravings. 6th ed., thoroughly rev. and greatly improved. . . . Philadelphia: Henry C. Lea's Son & Co., 1882. 2 v. DLC; IU-M; NNNAM; PPC **80-2506**

GROSS, Samuel D[avid] (1805-1884)
Remarks on the importance of having trained nurses. [Philadelphia], 1883. 11p. PPJ **80-2507**

GROSS, Samuel D[avid] (1805-1884)
Autobiography of Samuel D. Gross, M.D. . . . emeritus professor of surgery in the Jefferson Medical College of Philadelphia. With sketches of his contemporaries. Ed. by his sons. . . . Philadelphia: G. Barrie, 1887. 2 v. DLC; NNNAM; PPJ; PU
80-2508

GROSS, Samuel Weissell (1837-1889)
A practical treatise on tumors of the mammary glands, embracing their histology, pathology, diagnosis, and treatment. . . . New York: D. Appleton & Co., 1880. 246p. DLC; DNLM; NNNAM; PPC **80-2509**

GROSS, Samuel Weissell (1837-1889)
A practical treatise on impotence, sterility, and allied disorders of the male sexual organs. . . . Philadelphia: Henry C. Lea's Son & Co., 1881. 174p. DLC; DNLM; NNNAM; PPJ
80-2510

GROSS, Samuel Weissell (1837-1889)
A practical treatise on impotence, sterility and allied disorders of the male sexual organs. . . . 2nd ed., thoroughly rev. . . . Philadelphia: Henry C. Lea's Son & Co., 1883. 176p. DLC; NNNAM; PPC; PPJ **80-2511**

GROSS, Samuel Weissell (1837-1889)
The impress of American surgery upon surgical practice. Philadelphia, 1884. 35p. DNLM; PPC; PPJ
80-2512

GROSS, Samuel Weissell (1837-1889)
A practical treatise on impotence, sterility, and allied disorders of the male sexual organs. . . . 3rd ed., thoroughly rev. . . . Philadelphia: Lea Bros. & Co., 1887. 172p. DLC; DNLM; MBM; PPJ **80-2513**

GROSSMAN, Paul
A modified Porro-Caesarean operation; the pedicle dropped in. Philadelphia, 1883. 3p. DNLM **80-2514**

GUERNSEY, Henry Newell (1817-1885)
Plain talks on avoided subjects. Philadelphia: F. A. Davis, 1882. 126p. DNLM; PPHa **80-2515**

GUERNSEY, Henry Newell (1817-1885)
Key-notes to the materia medica, as taught by Henry N. Guernsey. . . . Ed. by Joseph C. Guernsey. . . . Philadelphia: F. E. Boericke, 1887 [1886]. 267p. DLC; PPHa
80-2516

GUERNSEY, R[ocellus] S.
Medico-Legal sciences; the analyses and classification of them. New York, 1882. 7p. DNLM **80-2517**

GUITERAS, John and J. William WHITE
A contribution to the history of influenza. A study of a series of cases. Philadelphia: J. B. Lippincott & Co., 1880. 31p. DNLM; PPC; PU **80-2518**

GUNN, J. A.
Memorial sketches of Doctor Moses Gunn, by his wife. . . . Chicago: W. T. Keener, 1889. 380p. DNLM; IU-M; OCIM
80-2519

GUNN, John C. (1800-1863)
. . . Gunn's newest family physician; or, Home-book of health. . . . By John C. Gunn . . . assisted by Johnson H. Jordan, M.D., and several scientific writers of the highest eminence. Chicago, [etc.]: W. H. Moore & Co.; New York: J. S. Ogilvie & Co., 1884. 1190p. plates. DLC; IEN-M; NNNAM; PU
80-2520

GUNN, John C. (1800-1863)
Gunn's neuer hausarzt, oder Handbuch der gesundheit. . . . Nach der 17. steretyp-aufl. des englischen originals für das deutsche publikum bearbeitet von Dr. C. A. Rodin, unter mitwirkung von Johann Eggers. 35. aufgabe, verb. Chicago: W. H. Moore & Co., 1884. 1038p. illus., plates. DLC; IU-M; OCIM; PPG **80-2521**

GUNN, John C. (1800-1863)
. . . Gunn's newest family physician; or, Home-book of health: an approved household guide. . . . By John C. Gunn . . . assisted by Johnson H. Jordan, M.D. and several scientific writers of the highest eminence. Chicago, [etc.]: W. H. Moore & Co.; New York: J. S. Ogilvie & Co., 1885. 1190p. plates. DLC; IEN-M; OCIM **80-2522**

GUNN, John C. (1800-1863)
. . . Gunn and Jordan's newest revised physician; being the first New domestic physician, or, Home book of health; by John C. Gunn, M.D., as originally enl. and now issued with renewed copyright to the author who prepared the large additions . . . Johnson H. Jordan. . . . Cincinnati; Philadelphia: J. E. Moore & Co., 1887. 1190p. plates. DLC; OCIM
80-2523

GUNN, John C. (1800-1863)
. . . Gunn's new domestic physician: or, Home book of health. A complete guide for families. . . . With an appendix on anatomy, physiology, etc., etc. Cincinnati: J. E. Moore & Co., 1888. 1030p. plates. DLC; IEN-M; OCIM
80-2524

GUNN, John C. (1800-1863)
Gunn & Jordan's neuer hausarzt, oder Handbuch der gesundheit. . . . Von John C. Gunn, M.D., und Johnson H. Jordan, M.D. . . . Nach der 17. stereotyp-aufl. des englischen originals für das deutsche publikum bearbeitet von Dr. C. A. Rodin, unter mitwirkung von Johann Eggers. 36. verb. aufl. Chicago und Cincinnati: J. G. Moore & Co., 1889 [1888]. 1038p. plates. DLC; IU-M; OCIM; PPG **80-2525**

GUNN, Moses (1822-1887)
The doctorate address . . . Rush Medical College, Chicago. Chicago: A. G. Newell, 1883. 17p. DNLM; ICRM
80-2526

GUNN, Moses (1822-1887)
The philosophy of manipulation in the reduction of hip and shoulder dislocations. Chicago: A. G. Newell, 1884. 22p. DNLM; ICRM; IEN-M **80-2527**

GUNN, Robert A[lexander] (*b.* 1844)
Diseases and deformities of the spine. [New York, 1880.] 19p. DNLM **80-2528**

GUNN, Robert A[lexander] (*b.* 1844)
Vaccination; its fallacies and evils. New York: Munroe & Metz, [1880]. 20p. DNLM; NNNAM **80-2529**

GUNN, Robert A[lexander] (*b.* 1844)
Vaccination; its fallacies and evils. 3rd ed., revised and enlarged. New York: Nickles Publ. Co., 1882. 38p. DNLM; NNNAM **80-2530**

GUNN, Robert A[lexander] (*b.* 1844)
Everybody's doctor, a new and improved hand-book of hygiene and domestic medicine. . . . 1st ed. New York: The Dennis Manufacturing Co. (Limited), 1885. 692p. DLC; NNNAM **80-2531**

GUNN, Robert Alexander (*b.* 1844)
Medical and literary reference manual, comprising a complete "family physician" . . . and also a select bibliography of American and European authors, by F. T. Jones . . . and other eminent bibliographers. New York and Chicago: Home Knowledge Association, [1887]. 74p. plates. DLC; IU-M; NNNAM
80-2532

GUNNING, Thomas Brian
Treatment of fracture of the jaw, with critical remarks as sent to Prof. D. Hayes Agnew. Baltimore: Snowden & Cowman, 1884. 21p. DNLM; MdU-D **80-2533**

GUNNING, Thomas Brian
Critical remarks upon the misstatements as to interdental splints in the surgical treatise of D. Hayes Agnew. [Springfield, 1884.] 12p. DNLM **80-2534**

GUTHRIE, George W.
. . . An essay on antiseptic surgery; read by appointment before the Luzerne County Medical Society, November 10th, 1880. . . . Published by request of the Society. [Wilkes Barre, Pa.]: R. Lambert, 1881. 35p. DLC **80-2535**

GUTMANN, Edward
The watering places and mineral springs of Germany, Austria, and Switzerland; with notes on climatic resorts and consumption, sanitariums, peat, mud, and sand baths, whey and grape cures, &c. A popular medical guide. . . . New York: D. Appleton & Co., 1880. 331p. plates, fold. map. DLC; DNLM; NNNAM; PU **80-2536**

GUTTMANN, Oskar
Gymnastics of the voice; a system of correct breathing in singing and speaking, based upon physiological laws; a self-instructor in the training and use of the singing and speaking voice. Albany: E. S. Werner, 1882. 138p. 1 diag. DNLM
80-2537

GUTTMANN, Paul (1834-1893)
A handbook of physical diagnosis, comprising the throat, thorax, and abdomen. Transl. from the 3rd German ed. by Alex. Napier. New York: William Wood & Co., 1880. 344p. 1 col. plate. CtY-M; DNLM; NNNAM; PPC
80-2538

GWYN, Charles L.
Reflex irritation from hypertrophy of labia minora. Galveston: W. A. Shaw & Co, 1886. 7p. DNLM
80-2539

GWYN, Charles L.
Babies and their troubles. [Austin, 1886.] 8p. DNLM
80-2540

GWYN, Charles L.
Elongated nyphae a sign of sterility. Galveston: C. P. Marye, 1887. 5p. DNLM **80-2541**

HABERSON, Samuel Osborne (1825-1889)
The Lettsomian lectures delivered at the Medical Society of London, 1872, on the pathology and treatment of some diseases of the liver. 2nd ed. Philadelphia: P. Blakiston, Son & Co., 1885. 111p. IEN-M; NNNAM; PPC; PU **80-2542**

HADDON, Alfred C[ort] (1855-1940)
An introduction to the study of embryology. Philadelphia: P. Blakiston, Son & Co., 1887. 336p. CtY-M; DNLM; MBM; PPC **80-2543**

HADRA, Berthold Ernest (1842-1908)
Lesions of the vagina and pelvic floor, with special reference to the uterine and vaginal prolapse; . . . with 88 illustrations. Philadelphia: Records, McMullin & Co, 1888. 329p. DLC; NNNAM; PPC; PU **80-2544**

HAGEN, Richard
A guide to the clinical examination of patients and the diagnosis of disease. . . . Transl. from the second revised and enlarged edition, by G. E. Gramm. New York and Philadelphia: Boericke & Tafel, 1881. 223p. NNNAM; OCIM; PPHa **80-2545**

HAHNEMANN HOSPITAL COLLEGE OF SAN FRANCISCO
Annual announcements for the sessions of 1884-1885 to 1894 (1.-11.); 1895-1896 to 1899-1900 (13.-17.). San Francisco, 1884-1899. DNLM [Organized in 1884. In 1888 the word "Hospital" was substituted in lieu of the word "Medical." In 1895 the session was changed from summer to fall and winter. The summer session was again adopted in 1899. Alumni from 1884 to 1898, in announcement for 1899-1900.] **80-2546**

HAHNEMANN MEDICAL COLLEGE AND HOSPITAL OF CHICAGO
Closing exercises of the practitioner's course of lectures, delivered in the spring of 1883. [Chicago, 1883.] 24p. DNLM; IU-M **80-2547**

HAHNEMANN MEDICAL COLLEGE AND HOSPITAL OF CHICAGO
A prospectus of an extra course of twenty lectures on puerperal diseases. To be given in the Hahnemann Hospital during the winter term of 1883-1884, by Prof. R. Ludlam. [Chicago, 1883.] 8p. DNLM; IU-M **80-2548**

HAHNEMANN MEDICAL COLLEGE AND HOSPTIAL, PHILADELPHIA
Programme of Masonic ceremonies of the laying of the corner stone, Nov. 6, 1884. Philadelphia: W. P. Kilder, [1884]. 8p. DNLM; PPHa **80-2549**

HAHNEMANN MEDICAL COLLEGE AND HOSPITAL, PHILADELPHIA
Description with ground plans and elevations of the Hahnemann College and Hospital of Philadelphia. Philadelphia, 1884. 8p. plates, plan (1 fold.). DLC; PPHa **80-2550**

HAHNEMANN MEDICAL COLLEGE AND HOSPITAL, PHILADELPHIA
Dedication week. Hahnemann Medical College and Hospital of Philadelphia. Monday to Saturday, September 20-25, 1886. . . . [Philadelphia? 1886?] 18p. DLC; PPHa **80-2551**

HAILES, William Jr.
The introductory address of the course of 1880-1881 at the Albany Medical College. Albany, N.Y.: Burdick & Taylor, 1881. 20p. DNLM **80-2552**

HALE, Amie M.
The management of children in sickness and in health. A book for mothers. . . . Philadelphia: P. Blakiston, 1880. 110p. DLC; DNLM; NNNAM; PPC **80-2553**

HALE, Amie M.
The management of children in sickness and in health. A book for mothers. 2nd ed. Philadelphia: P. Blakiston, 1881. 110p. DNLM; MBM; NNNAM; PU **80-2554**

HALE, Edwin M[oses] (1829-1899)
Materia medica and special therapeutics of the new remedies. 5th ed. With appendix. Philadelphia: F. E. Boericke, Hahnemann Publishing House, 1880-1886. 2 v. DNLM; OCIM; OCLloyd **80-2555**

HALE, Edwin M[oses] (1829-1899)
The medical, surgical and hygienic treatment of diseases of women; especially those causing sterility: the disorders and accidents of pregnancy; and painful and difficult labor. 2nd ed. New York and Philadelphia: Boericke & Tafel, 1880. 378p. NNNAM; OCIM; PPHa **80-2556**

HALE, Edwin M[oses] (1829-1899)
The heart, and how to take care of it. Chicago: A. L. Chatterton Publishing Co., 1881. 94p. DLC; OCIM **80-2557**

HALE, Edwin M[oses] (1829-1899)
The heart; how to take care of it. Chicago: Gross & Delbridge, 1884. 100p. IU-M; OCIM; PPHa **80-2558**

HALE, Edwin M[oses] (1829-1899) and Charles A. WILLIAMS
The compendium of health; pertaining to the physical life of man and the animals which serve him. Chicago: The American Book Co., 1884. 945p. IU-M; OCIM; NNNAM **80-2559**

HALE, Edwin M[oses] (1829-1899)
Lectures on diseases of the heart. With a repertory of heart symptoms. 3rd ed. Philadelphia: Boericke & Tafel, 1889. 478p. NNNAM; PPC; PPHa **80-2560**

HALE, Lorenzo
The medical annals; official register, 1881, of medical societies, giving officers, members, delegates, etc., with addresses and office hours. Albany: Burdick & Taylor, 1881. 13p. DNLM **80-2561**

HALL, C. Lester
Diphtheria and diphtheroid. [St. Louis, 1889.] 11p. DNLM **80-2562**

HALL, Henry Clay (*d.* 1887)
Medical journal directory. Cincinnati, 1883, 12p. DNLM **80-2563**

HALL & RUCKEL
8th annual catalogue. Prices current. [Drugs, druggists' supplies.] New York, 1880. 365p. NNNAM **80-2564**

HALL, William Whitty (1810-1876)
Fun better than physic; or, Everybody's life-preserver. . . . Chicago, Ill.: Rand, McNally & Co., 1882. 333p. DLC; IU-M; NNNAM; PU **80-2565**

HALSEY, Clinton S.
Halsey's homoeopathic guide. For families, travelers, missionaries, pioneers, miners, farmers, stock raisers, horse owners, dog fanciers, poultry keepers. . . . Chicago: C. S. & G. E. Halsey, 1885. 262, 84p. DLC; IU-M; PPHa **80-2566**

HALSTED, William S[tewart] (1852-1922)
The effects of adduction and abduction on the length of the limb in fractures of the neck of the femur. [New York, 1884.] 13p. DNLM; NNNAM **80-2567**

HAM, John Randolph
A contribution to the study of fractures and dislocations. . . . Concord: Evans & Sleeper, printers, 1881. 9p. DLC **80-2568**

HAMILTON, Allan McLane (1848-1919)
Nervous diseases: their description and treatment. A manual for students and practitioners of medicine. . . . 2nd ed.—rev. and enl. . . . Philadelphia: Henry C. Lea's Son & Co., 1881. 598p. DLC; IU-M; NNNAM; PU **80-2569**

HAMILTON, Allan McLane (1848-1919)
The use of nitrous oxide gas in certain nervous affections. [Baltimore, 1881.] 8p. DNLM **80-2570**

HAMILTON, Allan McLane (1848-1919)
On cortical sensory discharging lesions. [Sensory epilepsy.] New York: Appleton & Co., 1882. 12p. DNLM **80-2571**

HAMILTON, Allan McLane (1848-1919)
The case of Guiteau. Cambridge: Riverside Press, 1882. 11p. DNLM **80-2572**

HAMILTON, Allan McLane (1848-1919)
Upon transferred patellar tendon-reflex. [Chicago, 1883.] 5p. DNLM **80-2573**

HAMILTON, Allan McLane (1848-1919)
A manual of medical jurisprudence, with special reference to diseases and injuries of the nervous system. . . . New York, [etc.]: Bermingham & Co., 1883. 380p. DLC; NNNAM; PPC; PU **80-2574**

HAMILTON, Allan McLane (1848-1919)
Types of insanity: an illustrated guide in the physical diagnosis of mental disease. . . . New York: William Wood & Co., 1883. 36p. DLC; NNNAM **80-2575**

HAMILTON, Allan McLane (1848-1919)
A case of word-blindness with impairment of the faculty of space association. [Philadelphia, 1884.] 8p. DNLM **80-2576**

HAMILTON, Allan McLane (1848-1919)
A manual of medical jurisprudence, with special reference to diseases and injuries of the nervous system. New York: J. R. Bermingham, 1885. 386p. DNLM; MBM; NNNAM; PU **80-2577**

HAMILTON, Allan McLane (1848-1919)
A manual of medical jurisprudence, with special reference to diseases and injuries of the nervous system. . . . New York: E. B. Treat, 1887. 390p. DLC; MBM; NNNAM; OCIM **80-2578**

HAMILTON, Allan McLane (1848-1919)
The modern treatment of headaches. . . . Detroit, Mich.: G. S. Davis, 1888. 124p. DLC; DNLM; IU-M; OCIM **80-2579**

HAMILTON, Frank Hastings (1813-1886)
A practical treatise on fractures and dislocations. . . . 6th American ed., rev. and improved. Illustrated with three hundred and fifty-two wood-cuts. Philadelphia: Henry C. Lea's Son & Co, 1880. 909p. DLC; MBM; NNNAM; PPC **80-2580**

HAMILTON, Frank Hastings (1813-1886)
Fracture of the patella; a study of one hundred and twenty-seven cases. New York: L. Bermingham & Co, 1880. 106p. DNLM; NNNAM **80-2581**

HAMILTON, Frank Hastings (1813-1886)
. . . Health aphorisms, and an essay on the struggle for life against civilization, luxury, and aestheticism. . . . New York: Bermingham & Co., 1882. 64p. DLC; DNLM; NNNAM **80-2582**

HAMILTON, Frank Hastings (1813-1886)
A practical treatise on fractures and dislocations. . . . 7th American ed., revised and improved. Illustrated with three hundred and seventy-nine wood-cuts. Philadelphia: Henry C. Lea's Son & Co., 1884. 1005p. DLC; IU-M; NNNAM; PPC **80-2583**

HAMILTON, Frank Hastings (1813-1886)
Conversations between Drs. Warren and Putnam on the subject of medical ethics, with an account of the medical empiricisms of Europe and America. . . . New York, etc.: Bermingham & Co., 1884. 129p. DLC: DNLM; NNNAM **80-2584**

HAMILTON, Frank Hastings (1813-1886)
The army surgeons. Buffalo, 1886. 10p. DNLM; NNNAM **80-2585**

HAMILTON, Frank Hastings (1813-1886)
The art of primary union or union by adhesion in large incised wounds. New York: Trow, 1886. 22p. DNLM; NNNAM **80-2586**

HAMILTON, Frank Hastings (1813-1886)
Cremation of human bodies not a necessary sanitary measure. New York: Judson Print. Co., [1886]. 11p. DNLM; NNNAM **80-2587**

HAMILTON, Frank Hastings (1813-1886)
The essentials of physiology and hygiene, a text-book to accompany White's physiological manikin. Prepared under the supervision of . . . illustrating the effects of alcohol and narcotics by colored plates and by a series of microscopical sections, prepared under the authority of the State of New York, by Francis Delafield and T. Mitchell Prudden. New York: J. T. White & Co., 1886. 47p. DNLM; NNNAM **80-2588**

HAMILTON, Frank Hastings (1813-1886)
The principles and practice of surgery. . . . Illustrated with 472 engravings on wood. 3rd ed., rev. and cor. New York: William Wood & Co., 1886. 989p. DLC; MH-M; NNNAM; PU
80-2589

[HAMILTON, Frank Hastings] (1813-1886)
Catalogue of the library of the late Frank H. Hamilton, A.M., M.D., LL.D. New York: M. J. Rooney, Steam Printer & Stationer, 1886. 36p. DLC; DNLM; NNNAM
80-2590

HAMILTON, George (1808-1885)
Biographical sketch of James Aitken Meigs, M.D. Philadelphia: Collins, 1880. 22p. DNLM; PPC **80-2591**

HAMILTON, G[eorge] (1808-1885)
The status of professional opinion and popular sentiment regarding sewer-gas and contaminated water as causes of typhoid fever; with allusions to a paper by Dr. Alfred L. Carroll upon this subject. [New York, 1883.] 10p. DNLM
80-2592

HAMILTON, G[eorge] (1808-1885)
The question of vivisection. Was the act of the British Parliament in restricting vivisection inconsiderate and unnecessary? [Philadelphia, 1883?] 12p. DNLM
80-2593

HAMILTON, G[eorge] (1808-1885)
The Hamilton library. Part I. Bibliotheca medica, anatomica et chirurgica, or catalogue of rare and curious medical books; an extraordinary collection, forming the medical library of the late Dr. . . . to be sold Thursday and Friday afternoons, March 25th and 26th, 1886. Philadelphia: S. V. Henkels & Co., 1886. 44p. DNLM; PPC **80-2594**

HAMILTON, Hugh (*b.* 1847)
Artificial infant alimentation. Philadelphia: Collins, 1883. 12p. DNLM **80-2595**

HAMILTON, Hugh (*b.* 1847)
The relation dairy products bear to disease. Harrisburg: L. S. Hart, 1884. 6p. DNLM **80-2596**

HAMILTON, Hugh (*b.* 1847)
The sanitary condition of Harrisburg (Pennsylvania). Harrisburg: E. K. Meyers, 1886. 12p. 10 maps, 2 plans, 6 diag. DNLM **80-2597**

HAMILTON, John B. (1847-1898)
Lessons in longevity. Paragraphs on home hygiene and the art of prolonging life. Washington: W. H. Morrison, 1884. 77p. DNLM **80-2598**

HAMILTON, John B. (1847-1898)
Penetrating pistol-shot wound of abdomen; laparatomy; suture of intestines; pelvic hematoma; recovery. [Washington, D.C., 1885.] 7p. DNLM **80-2599**

HAMILTON, John B. (1847-1898)
On the radical cure of inguinal hernia; a review of the existing status of the operation, with remarks on its past history. Chicago, 1886. 16p. DNLM **80-2600**

HAMILTON, John B. (1847-1898)
College addresses. [1887.] 32p. DNLM
80-2601

HAMILTON, John B. (1847-1898)
Annual oration before the Alumni Association of the Medical Chirurgical College of Philadelphia, 1888. "Our alumnus and his medical environment." Philadelphia, 1888. 12p. DNLM
80-2602

HAMILTON, John B. (1847-1898)
Remarks made at the Medical Society of the District of Columbia on the death of Dr. A. Y. P. Garnett. [Washington, 1888.] 2 l. DNLM **80-2603**

HAMILTON, John B. (1847-1898)
International comity in state medicine. Chicago, 1889. 7p. DNLM **80-2604**

HAMILTON, John W[aterman] (1826?-1898)
The examinations of A. M. Dent, by the Columbus Medical College. A firm of congenial spirits in affectionate embrace. [Reply to charges made in J. F. Baldwin's pamphlet, Sept. 5, 1882.] [Columbia, 1882.] 8p. DNLM
80-2605

HAMILTON, W[eston] G.
A compend of domestic medicine and household remedies. . . . Greensboro, N.C.: Phillips & Stout Bros., printers, 1887. 250p. DLC; NcD; NcU **80-2606**

HAMILTON, W[illiam] D.
Disarticulation of the right half of the lower jaw for enchondroma. [New York, 1887.] 5p. DNLM
80-2607

HAMMOND, Graeme M[onroe]
A new cortical centre. New York: Trow, 1881. 10p. DNLM
80-2608

HAMMOND, William Alexander (1828-1900)
A treatise on the diseases of the nervous system. . . . 7th ed., rewritten, enl. and improved. New York: D. Appleton & Co., 1881. 929p. col. plate. DLC; DNLM; NNNAM; PPC
80-2609

HAMMOND, William Alexander (1828-1900)
On certain conditions of nervous derangement, somnambulism—hypnotism—hysteria—hysteroid affections, etc. . . . New York: G. P. Putnam's Sons, 1881. 256p. DLC; MBM; NNNAM; PPC **80-2610**

HAMMOND, William Alexander (1828-1900)
The official correspondence between Surgeon-General Wm. A. Hammond, U.S.A., and the adjutant-general of the Army relative to the founding of the Army Medical Museum, and the inauguration of the Medical and Surgical History of the War. New York: D. Appleton & Co., 1883. 8p. DNLM; NNNAM
80-2611

HAMMOND, William Alexander (1828-1900)
A treatise on insanity in its medical relations. . . . New York: D. Appleton & Co., 1883. 767p. DLC: DNLM; NNNAM; PPC
80-2612

HAMMOND, William Alexander (1828-1900)
Sexual impotence in the male. . . . New York: Bermingham & Co., 1883. 274p. DLC; DNLM; NNNAM; PU
80-2613

HAMMOND, William Alexander (1828-1900)
A treatise on the diseases of the nervous system. . . . 8th ed., with corrections and additions. . . . New York: D. Appleton & Co., 1886. 945p. col. plate. DLC; DNLM; IU-M; NNNAM
80-2614

HAMMOND, William Alexander (1828-1900)
Spinal irritation. (Posterior spinal anaemia). . . . Detroit, Mich.: G. S. Davis, 1886. 80p. DLC; DNLM; OCIM
80-2615

HAMMOND, William Alexander (1828-1900) and Clara LANZA
Tales of eccentric life. New York: D. Appleton & Co., 1886. 209p. DNLM; ICU; MH; NN **80-2616**

HAMMOND, William Alexander (1828-1900)
Sexual impotence in the male and female. . . . Detroit: G. S. Davis, 1887. 305p. DLC; DNLM; IU-M; NNNAM
80-2617

HAMMOND, William Alexander (1828-1900)
Coca; its preparations and their therapeutical qualities, with some remarks on the so-called cocaine habit. [Richmond, 1887.] 2 l. DNLM **80-2618**

HANAFORD, J. H.
The Plowman manual of health; a practical treatise on the conditions conducive to good health, and the sources of disease. . . . Moline, Ill.: Plowman Publishing Co., printers, 1888. 46p. DLC **80-2619**

HANCHETT, Henry G[ranger] (1853-1918)
The elements of modern domestic medicine. A plain and practical hand-book, describing simple diseases. . . . The whole issued after careful revision by A. H. Laidlaw. . . . New York: C. T. Hurlburt, 1887. 377p. DLC; DNLM; NNNAM
80-2620

HANCHETT, Henry G[ranger] (1853-1918)
Sexual health. A companion to "Modern domestic medicine." A plain and practical guide for the people in all matters concerning the organs of reproduction in both sexes and all ages. . . . Issued after careful revision by A. H. Laidlaw. . . . New York: C. T. Hurlburt, 1887. 86p. DLC; NNNAM
80-2621

HANCHETT, H[enry] G[ranger] (1853-1918)
The prophylactic and therapeutic resources of mankind. [New York], 1888. 15p. DNLM; NNNAM
80-2622

HAND-BOOK of eclampsia; or notes and cases of puerperal convulsions, comprising all the cases which have occurred during the present century, within a radius of several miles around Avondale, Chester Co., Penn'a., so far as can be ascertained by E. Michener, J. H. Stubbs, B. Thompson, R. B. Ewing, S. Stebbins. Philadelphia: F. A. Davis, 1883. 68p. DNLM; PPC; PU **80-2623**

HANDERSON, Henry E[benezer] (1837-1918)
The school of Salernum. An historical sketch of mediaeval medicine. New York, 1883. 60p. DNLM; ICU; MH; NN
80-2624

HANKS, H[orace] T[racy] (1837-1900)
The operations necessary for restoring complete lacerations of the female perineum involving the sphincter ani and the subsequent management without constipating the bowels. New York: Trow, 1882. 24p. DNLM; NNNAM **80-2625**

HANKS, H[orace] T[racy] (1837-1900)
Remarks upon peri-uterine cellulitis and peri-uterine peritonitis. Albany: Burdick & Taylor, 1885. 16p. DNLM
80-2626

HARDAWAY, William A[ugustus] (1850-1923)
Essentials of vaccination; a compilation of facts relating to vaccine inoculation and its influence in the prevention of smallpox. . . . Chicago: Jansen, McClurg & Co., 1882. 146p. DLC; DNLM; IU-M; NNNAM **80-2627**

HARDAWAY, W[illiam] A[ugustus] (1850-1923)
The lymphatic theory of syphilitic infection; with a new view of the relation between the chancre and chancroid, and suggestions for the treatment of syphilis. New York: D. Appleton & Co., [1882?]. 26p. DNLM **80-2628**

HARDAWAY, W[illiam] A[ugustus] (1850-1923)
A case of multiple xanthoma, exhibiting the plane, tubercular, and tuberose varieties of the disease. St. Louis: J. H. Chambers & Co., [1884]. 10p. DNLM **80-2629**

HARDAWAY, W[illiam] A[ugustus] (1850-1923)
Essentials of vaccination: a compilation of facts relating to vaccine inoculation and its influence in the prevention of smallpox. St. Louis: J. H. Chambers & Co., 1886. 146p. DNLM; IU-M; OCIM **80-2630**

HARDAWAY, W[illiam] A[ugustus] (1850-1923)
Note on the treatment of port-wine mark by electrolysis. [St. Louis, 1886.] 6p. DNLM **80-2631**

HARDAWAY, W[illiam] A[ugustus] (1850-1923)
Observations on feigned and artificial eruptions of the skin. [St. Louis, 1886.] 6p. DNLM **80-2632**

HARDAWAY, W[illiam] A[ugustus] (1850-1923)
Report of a case of multiple myomata of the skin, accompanied by severe pain. Philadelphia, 1886. 6p. DNLM
80-2633

HARDON, Virgil O.
Vesical irritation in women. [Atlanta, 1887.] 13p. DNLM
80-2634

HARDON, Virgil O.
The treatment of uterine flexions. [Atlanta, 1887.] 13p. DNLM **80-2635**

HARDON, Virgil O.
Some observations upon pelvic cellulitis. [Atlanta, 1888.] 14p. DNLM **80-2636**

HARDON, Virgil O.
Superinvolution of the uterus following trachelorraphy. [Atlanta, 1888.] 4p. DNLM **80-2637**

HARE, Hobart Amory (1862-1931)
. . . The physiological and pathological effects of the use of tobacco. . . . Philadelphia: P. Blakiston, Son & Co., 1885. 86p. plate, diag. DLC; DNLM; PPC; PU
80-2638

HARE, Hobart Amory (1862-1931)
. . . New and altered forms of disease, due to the advance of civilization in the last half century. . . . Philadelphia: P. Blakiston, Son & Co., 1886. 17p. DLC; DNLM; NNNAM; PPC
80-2639

HARE, Hobart Amory (1862-1931)
The physiological action of the heavy oil of wine. [Philadelphia, 1886.] 11p. DNLM **80-2640**

HARE, Hobart Amory (1862-1931)
The influence of antifebrin, salicyclic acid, and carbolic acid on normal and abnormal bodily temperature. Detroit: G. S. Davis, 1887. 21p. DNLM; OCIM **80-2641**

HARE, Hobart Amory (1862-1931)
Experiments to determine the influence of etherization on the normal bodily temperature with reference to the use of external heat. Detroit, Mich.: G. S. Davis, 1888. 5p. DNLM **80-2642**

HARE, Hobart Amory (1862-1931)
Questions and answers on the essentials of physiology, prepared especially for students of medicine. . . . Philadelphia: W. B. Saunders, 1888. 170p. DLC; NNNAM; PPC; PPJ **80-2643**

HARE, Hobart Amory (1862-1931)
The fatality of cardiac injuries. [Philadelphia, 1889.] 6p. DNLM **80-2644**

HARE, Hobart Amory (1862-1931)
The fatality of heart wounds. Pt. 2. [Philadelphia, 1889.] 10p. DNLM **80-2645**

HARE, Hobart Amory (1862-1931)
The effect of the entrance of air into the circulation. Detroit: G. S. Davis, 1889. 5p. DNLM **80-2646**

HARE, Hobart Amory (1862-1931)
. . . Essentials of physiology arranged in the form of questions and answers. Prepared especially for students of medicine. . . . 2nd ed., thoroughly rev. and enl. Philadelphia: W. B. Saunders; [etc., etc.], 1889. 193p. DLC; MBM; NNNAM; PPC **80-2647**

HARE, Hobart Amory (1862-1931)
The pathology, clinical history, and diagnosis of affections of the mediastinum other than those of the heart and aorta. With tables giving the clinical history of five hundred and twenty cases. Being an essay to which was awarded the Fothergillian medal of the Medical Society of London, March, 1888. . . . Philadelphia: P. Blakiston, Son & Co., 1889. 150p. tables. DLC; DNLM; NNNAM; PPC **80-2648**

HARE, Hobart Amory (1862-1931) and Edward MARTIN
The value of the electrical methods employed for the resuscitation of persons who have ceased breathing. [Philadelphia, 1889.] 5p. 1 diag. DNLM **80-2649**

HARGIS, Robert Bell Smith (1818-1893)
Practical hints relating to yellow fever prevention. Baltimore, 1880. 9p. DNLM **80-2650**

HARGIS, Robert Bell Smith (1818-1893)
The ship origin of yellow fever, with comments on the preliminary report of the Havana Yellow Fever Commission. . . . Pensacola: Gazette Book & Job Office, 1880. 19p. DLC; DNLM **80-2651**

HARGIS, Robert Bell Smith (1818-1893)
Yellow fever: its ship origin and prevention. . . . Philadelphia: D. G. Brinton, [1880]. 76p. DLC; DNLM; PPC; PU **80-2652**

HARGIS, Robert Bell Smith (1818-1893)
The genius of medicine. Annual address presented to the Florida State Medical Association, 1882. New Orleans: L. Graham & Son, [1882]. 19p. 1 l. DNLM **80-2653**

HARLAN, George C[uvier] (1835-1909)
Eyesignt, and how to care for it. Philadelphia: P. Blakiston, 1880. 139p. DNLM; NNNAM; PPC; PU **80-2654**

HARRINGTON, A[rthur] H[udson] (*b.* 1856)
Clinical case. Hereditary cases of progressive muscular atrophy. [Utica, N.Y., 1887.] 4p. DNLM **80-2655**

HARRINGTON, Charles (1856-1908)
Proper and improper methods of disinfection. Boston: Cupples & Hurd, 1888. 15p. DNLM; MBM **80-2656**

HARRINGTON, Charles (1856-1908)
The value of so-called diabetic foods. Boston: Cupples & Hurd, 1888. 8p. DNLM **80-2657**

HARRINGTON, F[rancis] B[ishop] (1854-1914)
Ante-partum haemorrhage, with the infusion of sixty-six ounces of salt solution. Boston: Cupples, Upham & Co., 1886. 8p. DNLM **80-2658**

HARRINGTON, F[rancis] B[ishop] (1854-1914)
The operation of shortening the round ligaments; with two cases. Boston: Cupples, Upham & Co., 1886. 7p. DNLM **80-2659**

HARRINGTON, F[rancis] B[ishop] (1854-1914)
Apparatus for the intra-venous injection of salt solution in cases of haemorrhage. [Boston, 1886.] 1 l. DNLM **80-2660**

HARRIS, Chapin Aaron (1806-1860)
A dictionary of medical terminology, dental surgery, and the collateral sciences. 4th ed., carefully revised and enlarged, by Ferdinand J. S. Gorgas. Philadelphia: P. Blakiston, Son & Co., 1882. 754p. DNLM; MdU-D; NNNAM; PPC **80-2661**

HARRIS, Chapin Aaron (1806-1860)
The principles and practice of dentistry, including anatomy, physiology, pathology, therapeutics, dental surgery and mechanism. . . . 11th ed. Rev. and ed. by Ferdinand J. S. Gorgas. . . . Philadelphia: P. Blakiston, Son & Co., 1885. 994p. col. plate. DLC; DNLM; NNNAM; PPC **80-2662**

HARRIS, Chapin Aaron (1806-1860)
The principles and practice of dentistry including anatomy, physiology, pathology, therapeutics, dental surgery and mechanism. . . . 12th ed. Rev. and ed. by Ferdinand J. S. Gorgas. . . . With one full page plate and one thousand and twenty-eight illustrations. Philadelphia: P. Blakiston, Son & Co., 1889. 1222p. DLC; DNLM; MdU-D; PPC **80-2663**

HARRIS, Edward N.
Address delivered before the American Academy of Dental Science at their seventeenth annual meeting, held in Boston, November 5, 1884. Boston: T. Todd, 1885. 29p. DNLM **80-2664**

HARRIS, Philander A. (*b.* 1852)
The treatment of mastitis by bandaging and rest. New York: William Wood & Co., 1885. 47p. DNLM; NNNAM
80-2665

HARRIS, Robert Patterson (1822-1899)
If a woman has ruptured her uterus during labor, what should be done in order to save her life? New York: William Wood & Co., 1880. 22p. DNLM: NNNAM **80-2666**

HARRIS, Robert Patterson (1822-1899)
The practice of obstetrics among the Chinese. New York: William Wood & Co., 1881. 14p. DNLM; NNNAM
80-2667

HARRIS, Robert Patterson (1822-1899)
The revival of symphysiotomy in Italy, with comparative tables of the early and later cases, showing that the operation has been more frequently performed in that country in the last seventeen years than in all Europe in the previous eighty, and with far better results. The whole subject examined historically and clinically. Philadelphia, 1883. 16p. DNLM
80-2668

HARRIS, Robert P[atterson] (1822-1899)
The operation of primary laparotomy in cases of extrauterine pregnancy; with a tabular record, showing the results in twenty-seven women under twenty-six operators. New York: William Wood & Co., 1887. 16p. DNLM; NNNAM
80-2669

HARRIS, Robert P[atterson] (1822-1899)
Extrauterine pregnancy treated by cystectomy, or cystotomy without exsection, with special reference to cases in which the foetus is living and viable. Philadelphia, 1888. 13p. DNLM
80-2670

HARRIS, Thomas
Post-mortem handbook, or how to conduct post-mortem examinations for clinical and for medico-legal purposes. New York: J. H. Vail & Co., 1887. 78p. 8 plates. CtY-M; DNLM; NNNAM; PU **80-2671**

HARRISON, George L[eib] (1811-1885)
Legislation on insanity; a collection of all the lunacy laws of the States and Territories of the United States to the year 1883, inclusive; also, the laws of England on insanity, legislation in Canada on private houses, and important portions of the lunacy laws of Germany, France, etc. Philadelphia: Privately Printed, 1884. 1119p. DNLM; NNNAM; PPC; PU
80-2672

HARRISON, George T[ucker] (1835-1925)
The natural mechanism of the expulsion of the placenta and the proper management of the placental period. New York: Judson Co., 1888. 7p. DNLM **80-2673**

HART, Charles Porter (*b.* 1827)
Diseases of the nervous system; being a treatise on spasmodic, paralytic, neuralgic, and mental affections. New York: Trübner & Co., 1881. 409p. DNLM; NNNAM; PPHa
80-2674

HART, Charles Porter (*b.* 1827)
Diseases of the nervous system; being a treatise on spasmodic, paralytic, neuralgic, and mental affections. For the use of students and practitioners of medicine. New York and Philadelphia: Boericke & Tafel, 1881. 409p. DNLM; PPHa
80-2675

HART, Charles Porter (*b.* 1827)
A treatise on the diseases of the respiratory passages, for the use of students and general practitioners. Detroit, Mich.: E. A. Lodge, 1882. 336p. OCIM; PPHa **80-2676**

HART, Charles Porter (*b.* 1827)
A treatise on intracranial diseases, inflammatory, organic, and symptomatic. Philadelphia: F. E. Boericke, Hahnemann Publishing House, 1884. 312p. DLC; DNLM
80-2677

HART, Charles Porter (*b.* 1827)
Diseases of the nervous system; being a treatise on spasmodic, paralytic, neuralgic and mental affections. For the use of students and practitioners of medicine; to which is added a supplement on intracranial diseases. Philadelphia: F. E. Boericke, Hahnemann Publishing House, 1884. 720p. DLC; PPC; PPHa **80-2678**

HART, Charles Porter (*b.* 1827)
Therapeutics of nervous diseases, including also their diagnosis and pathology. Philadelphia: F. E. Boericke, Hahnemann Publishing House, 1889. 268p. DLC; DNLM; PPHa
80-2679

HART, David Berry (1851-1920) and A. H. BARBOUR
Manual of gynecology. New York: William Wood & Co., 1883. 2 v. DNLM; MH-M; NNNAM; PU **80-2680**

HART, David Berry (1851-1920)
Atlas of female pelvic anatomy. New York: D. Appleton & Co., 1884. 89p. 37 plates. CtY-M; DNLM; NNNAM; PPC
80-2681

HART, John I.
Diseases of the antrum. [n. p., 1880.] 5p. DNLM
80-2682

HARTFORD MEDICAL SOCIETY
History of the presentation of the loving cup by the Hartford City Medical Society to Gurdon W. Russell, M.D., and of the complimentary dinner given to him in honor of his fifty years of actual service in the profession, November 21, 1887. [Hartford, Conn.: The Case, Lockwood & Brainard Co., printers, 1887.] 94p. front. (port.) plate. CtY-M; DLC
80-2683

HARTIGAN, J[ames] French (1843-1894)
The lockjaw of infants (trismus nascentium), or nine day fits, crying spasms, etc. Its history, cause, prevention, and cure. New York: Bermingham & Co., 1884. 123p. 1 plate. DLC; DNLM; NNNAM **80-2684**

HARTIGAN, James French (1843-1894)
Trismus nascentium; or, The lockjaw of infants. Its history, cause, prevention, and cure. . . . [Philadelphia: Henry C. Lea's Son & Co., 1884.] 39p. DLC; PPC; PU
80-2685

HARTIGAN, J[ames] French (1843-1894)
Left laparotomy, followed (a week later) by right laparotomy, for suppurative peritonitis. Consequent upon bulimia, foecal impaction, perityphlitis, and septicaemia. Recovery. Also on the use of arsenic in septicaemia. Chicago, 1888. 12p. DNLM
80-2686

HARTMAN, J[acob] H.
Some results in the treatment of atrophic rhinitis, with the galvanic current. [New York, 1889.] 4p. DNLM
80-2687

HARTMANN, Arthur (1849-1931)
The diseases of the ear and their treatment. Transl. from the German by J. Erskine. New York: G. P. Putnam's Sons, 1887. 283p. CtY-M; MBM; NNNAM; PPC **80-2688**

HARTRIDGE, Gustavus (1849-1923)
The refraction of the eye. A manual for students. 2nd ed. Philadelphia: P. Blakiston, Son & Co., 1886. 228p. 1 test type plate. CtY-M; DNLM; NNNAM; PPC
80-2689

HARTRIDGE, Gustavus (1849-1923)
The refraction of the eye. A manual for students. 3rd ed. Philadelphia: P. Blakiston, Son & Co., 1888. 240p. 1 test-type plate. DNLM; MBM; NNNAM; PU
80-2690

HARTSHORNE, Henry (1823-1897)
Our homes. Philadelphia: P. Blakiston, 1880. 149. DNLM; NNNAM; PPC; PU **80-2691**

HARTSHORNE, Henry (1823-1897)
Memoir of George B. Wood. Philadelphia, 1880. 35p. DNLM; PPC; PPJ; PU **80-2692**

HARTSHORNE, Henry (1823-1897)
Essentials of the principles and practice of medicine. A handbook for students and practitioners. . . . 5th ed., thoroughly rev. and improved. With one hundred and forty-four illustrations. Philadelphia: Henry C. Lea's Son & Co., 1881. 669p. DLC; NNNAM; OCIM; PPC **80-2693**

HARTSHORNE, Henry (1823-1897)
A household manual of medicine, surgery, nursing, and hygiene; for daily use in the preservation of health and care of the sick and injured. . . . Philadelphia: Lea Bros. & Co., 1886. 953p. col. plates. DLC; MBM; NNNAM; PPC
80-2694

HARTSHORNE, Henry (1823-1897)
Pneumonia; its mortality and treatment. A statistical and rational inquiry. Philadelphia: W. J. Dornan, 1888. 35p. DNLM; PPC **80-2695**

HARTSHORNE, Henry (1823-1897)
The practical household physician. A cyclopedia of family medicine, surgery, nursing and hygiene. . . . Philadelphia, Pa., Chicago, Ill.: J. C. Winston & Co., 1889. 971p. col. plates. DLC; IU-M; NNNAM; PPC **80-2696**

HARVARD UNIVERSITY. MEDICAL SCHOOL (BOSTON)
Annual circulars and announcements for the sessions of 1811-1812 (29.); (1838-1839 (56.); 1840-1841 (58.); 1841-1842 (59.); 1843-1844 to 1846-1847 (61.-64.); 1849-1850 (67.); 1855-1856 to 1859-1860 (73.-77.); 1863-1864 (81.); 1865-1866 to 1881-1882 (83.-99.); 1883-1884 (101.). Boston, 1811-1883. DNLM; MH [Since 1872-1873 the announcements are contained in the annual catalogues for the preceding years.] **80-2697**

HARVARD UNIVERSITY. MEDICAL SCHOOL (BOSTON)
Programme of the celebration of the one hundredth annivarsary, 1783-1883, of the foundation of the Medical School of Harvard University, and dedication of its new building, Oct. 7, 1883. [Boston, 1883.] 1 sheet. DNLM; MH
80-2698

HARVARD UNIVERSITY. MEDICAL SCHOOL (BOSTON)
The new century and the new building of the Harvard Medical School. 1783-1883. Addresses and exercises at the one hundredth anniversary of the foundation of the Medical School of Harvard University, October 17, 1883. Cambridge: J. Wilson & Son, 1884. 55p. 3 plates. DLC; DNLM; MH
80-2699

HARVEY, T[homas] B. (1827-1889)
The advance in medicine. An address. Indianapolis: Carlon & Hollenbeck, 1881. 16p. DNLM **80-2700**

HARVEY, T[homas] B. (1827-1889)
A report on laceration of the cervix uteri. Stenographically reported. Indianapolis: Baker & Randolph, [1883]. 15p. DNLM **80-2701**

HARVEY, T[homas] B. (1827-1889)
Conditions rendering diagnosis difficult in pelvic and abdominal diseases. With illustrative cases. Including an oral report on an ovarian tumor, with discussions. Indianapolis: Baker & Randolph, 1888. 14p. DNLM **80-2702**

HARWOOD, Edward C[oke] (1838-1891)
Statement of facts in connection with the quarterly report of the treasurer of the Medico-Legal Society of New York, prepared for presentation at the meeting of September 6th, 1882. New York: W. R. Jenkins, 1882. 32p. DNLM; NNNAM
80-2703

HARWOOD, Edward C[oke] (1838-1891)
Report of a case of pistol shot wound of the second and third cervical vertebrae. Considered in its medico-legal aspects; attempted suicide; death. New York: T. B. Mead, 1881. 12p. DNLM; NNNAM **80-2704**

HASBROUCK, Everitt (*d.* 1906)
Annual address before the Homoeopathic Medical Society of the State of New York, February 12, 1884. By the President. New York: J. F. Baker, printer, 1884. 26p. NNNAM; PPHa **80-2705**

HATCH, F. W[inslow] (1822-1885)
Report on small-pox in California, 1880 and 1881. Sacramento: J. D. Young, 1882. 16p. DNLM
80-2706

HATFIELD, Marcus P[atten] (1849-1909) and Roswell PARK
The abuses of medical charities. Chicago: Knight & Leonard, 1880. 22p. DNLM; IU-M **80-2707**

HATFIELD, Marcus P[atten] (1849-1909) and Roswell PARK
The physiology and hygiene of the house in which we live. New York: Chautauqua Press, 1888. 283p. DNLM; NN; NNNAM **80-2708**

HAVENS, H[enry] C[ecil]
The etiology and treatment of the summer diarrhea of infants. Philadelphia: J. E. Potter & Co., 1886. 26p. DNLM; PPC
80-2709

HAWES, Jesse (1843-1901)
Charlatanism in Colorado. [Denver, 1883.] 23p. DNLM
80-2710

HAWKES, W[illiam] J.
Characteristic indications of prominent remedies for the use of students of materia medica and therapeutics. 2nd ed. Chicago: Halsey Bros., 1884. 131p. DNLM; IU-M; OCIM
80-2711

HAWLEY, J. S.
Remarks on pepsine. Brooklyn, 1880. 40p. DNLM
80-2712

HAWTHORNE, R. M.
How every fat person may become lean without medicine, starvation, suffering or discomfort. The result of one month's actual experience. New York, 1880. 16p. DNLM; NNNAM
80-2713

HAY, C[harles] M.
Unusual epileptic phenomena. New York: J. Rooney & Co., 1889. 11p. DNLM **80-2714**

HAY, C[harles] M.
A clinical study of paraldehyde and sulphonal. [Philadelphia, 1889.] 10p. DNLM **80-2715**

HAYDEN, W[illiam] R.
The viburnum compound. The formula of . . . . [New York, 1880.] 18p. 1 plate. DNLM **80-2716**

HAYDEN, W[illiam] R.
The viburnum compound, the formula of . . . . [1881.] 24p. DNLM [*also*: New York, 1884, 43p.; New York (1884?), 27p. 1 plate] **80-2717**

HAYES, Albert H[amilton]
The science of life, or self-preservation. A medical treatise on nervous and physical debility, spermatorrhoea, [etc.]. Boston, [1881]. 276p. 2 plates. DNLM; MH-M; NNNAM
80-2718

HAYES, Harriet E., ed.
The home nurse and nursery. A practical treatise on the management of the sick-room . . . with . . . special department on the management and care of infants. . . . New York, Portland, Me.: Union Publishing House, 1888. 363p. DLC; NNNAM **80-2719**

HAYES, Plymmon S[anford] (1850-1894)
Electricity and the methods of its employment in removing superfluous hair and other facial blemishes. Chicago: Keener, 1889. 128p. IU-M; OCIM **80-2720**

HAYMOND, William S[ummerville] (1823-1885)
Concussion of the brain, and its mechanism. Indianapolis: Carlon & Hollenbeck, 1882. 14p. DNLM
80-2721

HAYNES, Celia M.
Elementary principles of electrotherapeutics for the use of physicians and students. . . . Chicago, Ill.: The McIntosh Galvanic & Faradic Battery Co., [1884]. 426p. plates. DLC; IU-M; OCIM **80-2722**

HAYNES, Celia M.
Elementary principles of electrotherapeutics for the use of physicians and students. . . . 2nd ed. Chicago, Ill.: McIntosh Galvanic & Faradic Battery Co., [1884]. 426p. DNLM; IU-M; OCIM **80-2723**

HAYNES, Celia M.
Elementary principles of electrotherapeutics for the use of physicians and students. . . . 3rd ed. Chicago: McIntosh Galvanic & Faradic Battery Co., [1884]. 426p. DNLM; IU-M; OCIM **80-2724**

[HAYNES, Celia M.]
A book for men, by a woman physician, Mrs. Barbara C. Morgan [*pseud.*] . . . . Chicago, Ill.: Dr. Haynes Publishing Co., [1888]. 408p. DLC; IEN-M; IU-M; OCIM
80-2725

HAYNES, Celia M.
Conditions of healthy manhood. . . . Chicago, Ill.: Dr. Haynes Publishing Co., [1888]. 408p. DLC **80-2726**

HAYNES, Francis L. (1850-1898)
Cocaine spray in epistaxis, and in nasal surgery generally. Detroit, 1886. 1 l. DNLM **80-2727**

HAYNES, Francis L. (1850-1898)
An easy method of plugging the posterior nares. Detroit, 1886. 1 l. DNLM **80-2728**

HAYNES, Francis L. (1850-1898) and John R. HAYNES
Hyoscine hydrobromate as a hypnotic in private practice. Detroit, 1886. 8p. DNLM **80-2729**

HAYNES, Francis L. (1850-1898)
On the treatment of piles by injection of carbolic acid. Los Angeles, [1887]. 6p. DNLM **80-2730**

HAYNES, Francis L. (1850-1898)
Suppurating ovarian cyst; ovariotomy; recovery. Los Angeles, [1888]. 4p. DNLM **80-2731**

HAYNES, Francis L. (1850-1898)
Suprapubic lithotomy; history of one operation. Los Angeles, [1889]. 4p. DNLM **80-2732**

HAYNES, Francis L. (1850-1898) and John R. HAYNES
Irrigation of the puerperal uterus; its uses and dangers. With especial reference to the treatment of puerperal fever. [New York, 1889.] 14p. DNLM **80-2733**

HAYNES, W[illiam] H[enry] (1856?-1902)
A case of left inguinal colotomy for imperforate rectum; recovery. [Philadelphia, 1884.] 5p. DNLM
80-2734

HAYS, Benjamin Frank
The life-work of Carl Wilhelm Scheele, the Swedish apothecary. New York: P. W. Bedford, 1884. 14p. DNLM; NNNAM
80-2735

HAYS, I[saac] Minis (1847-1925)
Memoir of Samuel D. Gross. Philadelphia: Collins, 1884. 29p. DNLM; PPJ **80-2736**

HAYS, I[saac] Minis (1847-1925)
A memoir of Samuel D. Gross. [Philadelphia: Henry C. Lea's Son & Co.], 1884. 16p. port. DNLM; PPJ
80-2737

HAYWARD, George G[riswold]
A case of labor at eight months; shoulder presentation; version; adherent placenta; child with imperforate rectum; operation; recovery. Boston: Cupples & Hurd, 1887. 12p. DNLM
80-2738

HAYWARD, George G[riswold]
A complicated case of labor at eight months. Boston: Cupples & Hurd, 1887. 12p. DNLM **80-2739**

HAZARD, Alexander
Pocket medical formulary, arranged therapeutically. By Alexander Hazard, M.D., and Bernard M. Goldberg, M.D. Rev. and enl. by Abraham S. Gerhard. . . . With an appendix. . . . Philadelphia, Pa.: Collins, printer, 1886. 333p. DLC; DNLM; PPC; PU **80-2740**

HAZARD, Alexander
Pocket medical formulary, arranged therapeutically. . . . Rev. and enl. by Abraham S. Gerhard. . . . With an appendix. . . . 2nd ed. Phialdelphia, Pa.: A. L. Hummel, 1888. 334p. DLC; NNNAM; PPC; PU **80-2741**

HAZARD, HAZARD & CO.
Illustrated catalogue of surgical instruments. . . , mfg. by W. F. Ford. New York, 1880. 179p. NNNAM **80-2742**

HAZARD, W[illiam] B. (1843-1888)
The bromides; their physiological action, therapeutical and toxic effects, alone and in combination. [New York, 1886.] 19p. DNLM; NNNAM **80-2743**

HEALTH influences of the climate of Vineland, New Jersey, better than Florida or the Far West. A series of papers prepared by the Sydenham Medical Association of Vineland, N.J. New York: C. H. Jones & Co., 1880. 47p. DNLM; NNNAM
80-2744

HEATH, Christopher (1835-1905)
A manual of minor surgery and bandaging for the use of house-surgeons, dressers, and junior practitioners. 6th ed. Philadelphia: Lindsay & Blakiston, 1880. 342p. NNNAM; OCIM; PPC; PU **80-2745**

HEATH, Christopher (1835-1905)
The student's guide to surgical diagnosis. New York: Bermingham & Co., 1881. 58p. NNNAM; OCIM; PPJ; PU
80-2746

HEATH, Christopher (1835-1905)
Practical anatomy: a manual of dissections. 5th ed. Philadelphia: P. Blakiston, Son & Co., 1881. 549p. CtY-M; NNNAM; PPC; PU **80-2747**

HEATH, Christopher (1835-1905)
Handbook of surgical diagnosis for physicians and students. Philadelphia: P. Blakiston, Son & Co., 1882. 214p. CtY-M; NNNAM; OCIM; PPC **80-2748**

HEATH, Christopher (1835-1905)
A guide to surgical diagnosis. Philadelphia: P. Blakiston & Son, 1882. 36p. DNLM; NNNAM; PPC; PU
80-2749

HEATH, Christopher (1835-1905)
Injuries and diseases of the jaws; the Jacksonian prize essay of the Royal College of Surgeons of England, 1867. . . . Philadelphia: P. Blakiston, Son & Co., 1884. 480p. IEN-M; NNNAM; PPC; PU **80-2750**

HEATH, Christopher (1835-1905)
A course of operative surgery, with plates drawn from nature by J. B. Léveillé. 2nd ed. Philadelphia: P. Blakiston, Son & Co., 1884. 128p. 20 plates. CtY-M; NNNAM; OCIM; PPC
80-2751

HEATH, Christopher (1835-1905)
Practical anatomy: a manual of dissections. 6th ed., revised by Rickman J. Godlee. Philadelphia: P. Blakiston, Son & Co., 1885. 567p. 24 plates. DNLM; NNNAM; OCIM; PPC
80-2752

HEATH, Christopher (1835-1905)
Dictionary of practical surgery by various British hospital surgeons. Philadelphia: J. B. Lippincott Co., 1886. 2 v. in 1. DNLM; NNNAM; OCIM; PPC **80-2753**

HEATH, Christopher (1835-1905)
A manual of minor surgery and bandaging for the use of house-surgeons, dressers, and junior practitioners. 8th ed. Philadelphia: P. Blakiston, Son & Co., [1886]. 360p. CtY-M; DNLM; NNNAM; PPC **80-2754**

HEATH, Christopher (1835-1905)
Lectures on certain diseases of the jaws, delivered at the Royal College of England, 1867. Philadelphia: P. Blakiston, Son & Co., 1888. 128p. CtY-M; DNLM; MBM; NNNAM
80-2755

HEATH, Christopher (1835-1905)
Practical anatomy: a manual of dissections. 7th ed., revised by Richman J. Godlee. Philadelphia: P. Blakiston, Son & Co., 1888. 598p. 24 col. plates. DNLM; NNNAM; PPJ; PPC
80-2756

HEATH, Christopher (1835-1905)
A manual of minor surgery and bandaging for the use of house-surgeons, dressers, and junior practitioners. 9th ed. Philadelphia: P. Blakiston, Son & Co., 1889. 361p. DNLM; IU-M; NNNAM; PU **80-2757**

HECKER, J[ustus] F[riedrich] C[arl] (1795-1850)
The black death; an account of the deadly pestilence of the fourteenth century. Transl. for the Sydenham Society of London by B. G. Babington. New York: J. Fitzgerald, 1885. 47p. DNLM; ICU; MH; NN
80-2758

HECKER, J[ustus] F[riedrich] C[arl] (1795-1850)
The dancing mania of the middle ages. Transl. by B. G. Babington. New York: J. Fitzgerald, 1885. 53p. DNLM; MB; MH; NN **80-2759**

HEFFENGER, Arthur C.
The pavilion in hospital construction. [Boston, 1886.] 19p. DNLM **80-2760**

HEFFLEFINGER, M. L.
Dysentery. [Dallas, 1889.] 3p. DNLM
80-2761

HEGAR, Alfred (1830-1914) and R[udolph] KALTENBACH
A hand-book of general and operative gynecology. New York: William Wood & Co., 1887. 2 v. DNLM; NNNAM; OCIM; PPC [Forms v. 7 and 8 of: Cyclopaedia of obstetrics and gynecology.] **80-2762**

HEINIGKE, Carl
Pathogenetic outlines of homoeopathic drugs. . . . Transl. from the German by Emil Tietze, M.D. . . . New York and Philadelphia: Boericke & Tafel, 1880. 576p. OCLloyd; PPHa; PU **80-2763**

HEITZMANN, C[arl] (1836-1896)
The minute anatomy of the teeth in the light of the bioplasson theory, and the minute anatomy, physiology, pathology, and therapeutics of the dental pulp, by C. F. W. Bödecker. Philadelphia, 1882. 45p. DNLM; MdU-D; PPC **80-2764**

HEITZMANN, C[arl] (1836-1896)
The intimate nature of tuberculosis; its transmissibility, and its parasitic origin. New York: G. P. Putnam's Sons, 1883. 25p. DNLM; NNNAM **80-2765**

HEITZMANN, C[arl] (1836-1896)
Anatomy, descriptive and topographical, in 625 illustrations. English ed., by Louis Heitzmann. New York: J. H. Vail & Co., 1887. 238, 270, 36p. DNLM; MBM; NNNAM; PPC **80-2766**

HEITZMANN, C[arl] (1836-1896) and Frank ABBOTT
Contributions to the knowledge of tumors of the jaws. Philadelphia, 1888. 32p. DNLM; PPC **80-2767**

HEITZMANN, C[arl] (1836-1896) and C. F. W. BÖDECKER
Contributions to the history of development of the teeth. [New York, 1888.] 98p. DNLM; MdU-D **80-2768**

HELMUTH, William Tod (1833-1902)
Epicystotomy; hypogastric lithotomy; supra-pubic lithotomy; the high operation for stone. Detroit: B. F. Saunders, 1880. 13p. DNLM **80-2769**

HELMUTH, William Tod (1833-1902)
The influence of homoeopathy upon surgery. [Philadelphia, 1881.] 41p. DNLM; PPHa **80-2770**

HELMUTH, William Tod (1833-1902)
Supra-pubic lithotomy; the high operation for stone; epicystotomy; hypogastric lithotomy; "The high apparatus." With lithographic plates. New York and Philadelphia: Boericke & Tafel, 1882. 93p. DNLM; NNNAM; PPHa **80-2771**

HELMUTH, William Tod (1833-1902)
The present status of antiseptic surgery. Pittsburgh: Stevenson & Foster, 1883. 22p. DNLM **80-2772**

HELMUTH, William Tod (1833-1902)
Fourteen consecutive completed ovariotomies. [New York]: E. P. Coby & Co., 1884. 9p. DNLM; NNNAM **80-2773**

HELMUTH, William Tod (1833-1902)
Ovarian tumors and ovariotomy. New York: A. L. Chatterton & Co., 1885. 43p. NNNAM; PPHa **80-2774**

HELMUTH, William Tod (1833-1902)
American Institute of Homoeopathy: Bureau of Surgery. Inguinal and femoral hernia. Synopsis of a paper on hernia. Boston: Alfred Mudge & Son, 1886. 12p. MH-M; PPHa **80-2775**

HELMUTH, William Tod (1833-1902)
A system of surgery. Illustrated with 718 engravings on wood. 5th ed. Enlarged, rearranged, revised. Many parts rewritten and much new matter added. Philadelphia: F. E. Boericke, Hahnemann Publishing House, 1887. 1111p. DLC; NNNAM; PPC; PPHa **80-2776**

HELMUTH, William Tod (1833-1902)
Sectarianism in medicine. Presidential address delivered before the Homoeopathic Medical Society of the State of New York, February 12, 1889. . . . New York: J. C. Rankin, Jr., 1889. 20p. NNNAM; PPHa **80-2777**

HEMPEL, Charles Julius (1811-1879)
Materia medica and therapeutics, arranged upon a physiological and pathological basis. . . . 3rd ed. Rev. by the author and greatly enl. by the addition of many new and valuable remedies, personal observations, and numerous clinical contributions from public and private sources, by H. R. Arndt. Chicago: W. A. Chatterton, 1880. 2 v. DLC; OCLloyd; PPHa; PU **80-2778**

HENKE, [Philipp Jakob] Wilhelm (1834-1896)
Henke's atlas of surgical anatomy; a series of plates illustrating the application of anatomy to medicine and surgery. Transl. and ed. by W. A. Rothacker. . . . Cincinnati: A. E. Wilde & Co., [1884]. 20p. 81 plates. DLC: IU-M; NNNAM; PPC **80-2779**

HENOCH, Eduard Heinrich (1820-1900)
. . . Lectures on diseases of children: a handbook for physicians and students. . . . New York: William Wood & Co., 1882. 357p. DLC; NNNAM; OCIM; PPC **80-2780**

HENRY, Frederick P[orteous] (1844-1919)
Cartwright prize essay. Observations with the haemacytometer upon the globular composition of the blood and milk. [Philadelphia, Pa., 1880?] 37p. DNLM; PPC **80-2781**

HENRY, Frederick P[orteous] (1844-1919)
A case of asynchronous contraction of the cardiac ventricles, with remarks upon reduplication of heart sounds. New York: G. P. Putnam's Sons, 1881. 8p. DNLM **80-2782**

HENRY, Frederick P[orteous] (1844-1919)
Cartwright prize essay. Observations with the haemacytometer upon the globular compositions of the blood and milk. Philadelphia: F. A. Davis, 1881. 37p. DNLM; PPC **80-2783**

HENRY, Frederick P[orteous] (1844-1919)
A contribution to the study of anaemia. New York: G. P. Putnam's Sons, 1882. 5p. DNLM **80-2784**

HENRY, Frederick P[orteous] (1844-1919)
A contribution to the study of icterus neonatorum. New York, 1883. 10p. DNLM **80-2785**

HENRY, Frederick P[orteous] (1844-1919)
The coagulation of the blood. [New York, 1884.] 8p. DNLM **80-2786**

HENRY, Frederick P[orteous] (1844-1919) and William OSLER
Atrophy of the stomach, with the clinical features of progressive pernicious anaemia. [Philadelphia, 1886.] 14p. DNLM; PPC **80-2787**

HENRY, Frederick P[orteous] (1844-1919)
Anaemia. Philadelphia: P. Blakiston, Son & Co., 1887. 136p. DNLM; NNNAM; PPC; PU **80-2788**

HENRY, Frederick P[orteous] (1844-1919)
The relations between chlorosis, simple anaemia, and pernicious anaemia, including leucocythaemia and Hodgkin's disease. [Philadelphia, 1889.] 22p. DNLM; PPC **80-2789**

HENRY, M[orris] H[enry] (1835-1895)
Treatment of varicocele by excision of redundant scrotum, illustrated by new instruments and an account of fifteen successful cases. New York: J. H. Vail & Co., 1881. 27p. DNLM; NNNAM **80-2790**

HENRY, M[orris] H[enry] (1835-1895)
A higher standard of medical education. Speech of . . . before the American Medical Association at the meeting in Washington, D.C., May 7, 1884. [n. p., 1884.] 3p. DNLM **80-2791**

HENRY, M[orris] H[enry] (1835-1895)
The radical cure of varicocele attended with redundancy of scrotum, demonstrated by time. [Chicago, 1888.] 12p. DNLM **80-2792**

HENRY, M[orris] H[enry] (1835-1895)
Suggestions on the treatment and influence of diet in the management of rheumatic diseases. New York, 1889. 7p. DNLM **80-2793**

HERDMAN, William James (1848-1896)
A guide to the dissection of the human body. . . . Ann Arbor, Mich.: G. Osius & Co., 1883. 30p. DLC **80-2794**

HERING, Constantin (1800-1880)
Catalogue of a very rare and curious collection of the different editions of the works of Theophrastus Bombastus Paracelsus; together with several hundred commentaries and translations, collected during fifty years. Philadelphia: The Globe Printing House, 1881. 20p. PPHa ["This is the most complete library of the works of Paracelsus in existence. The catalogue embraces 189 titles of books, with 18 bound pamphlets, and a number of manuscripts about Paracelsus, by Dr. Hering. There are 30 pictures of Paracelsus, his residence, his study, and a photograph of his skull. After Dr. Hering's death, it was offered for sale, collectively; after some competition, it was purchased by the Hahnemann Medical College of Philadelphia, and now occupies a very handsome case in its Library." Bradford, p. 154.] **80-2795**

HERING, Constantin (1800-1880)
Analytical repertory of the symptoms of the mind. 2nd ed. Philadelphia: American Homoeopathic Publishing Society. J. M. Stoddart & Co., 1881. 361p. PPHa **80-2796**

HERING, Constantin (1800-1880)
The homoeopathic domestic physician. 7th American ed. Philadelphia: F. E. Boericke. Hahnemann Publishing House, 1883. 458p. PPHa **80-2797**

HERING, Constantin (1800-1880)
The homoeopathic domestic physician. 9th American ed. Philadelphia: Hahnemann Publishing House, [1883]. 458p. DNLM; PPHa **80-2798**

HERING, Constantin (1800-1880)
Condensed materia medica. 3rd ed. More condensed, revised, enlarged and improved. Edited by Dr. E. A. Farrington. Philadelphia: F. E. Boericke, 1884. 968p. OCLloyd; PPHa **80-2799**

[HERING, Constantin] (1800-1880)
. . . Catalogue of the miscellaneous portion of the library of the late Constantin Hering, M.D., of Philadelphia, Pa. . . . To be sold . . . April 24 & 25, 1884. . . . Stan V. Henkles & Co., auctioneers. . . . Philadelphia, 1884. 31p. DLC; DNLM; PPHa **80-2800**

HERING, Constantin (1800-1880)
Repertory to Hering's condensed materia medica. Published by the Homoeopathic Medical Society of Pennsylvania. Philadelphia: Globe Printing House, 1889. 432p. OCLloyd; PPHa **80-2801**

HERON-ALLEN, Edward (1861-1945)
A manual of cheirosophy; being a complete practical hand book of the twin sciences of cheirognomy and cheiromancy, [etc.]. New York: G. P. Putnam's Sons, [1885]. 319p. DNLM; MH; NN; NNNAM **80-2802**

HERRICK, H[enry] J[ustus] (1833-1901)
The radical cure of hernia. [Columbus, 1887.] 4p. DNLM **80-2803**

HERRICK, O. E.
Abortion and its lesson. Detroit, 1882. 8p. DNLM **80-2804**

HERRICK, O. E.
An operation for closing Douglas' cul-de-sac. [Cincinnati, 1883.] 4p. DNLM **80-2805**

HESS, Oliver
Diphtheria, its causes, symptoms, treatment and cure. . . . Lowell, Mich.: Journal Steam Printing Office, 1880. 10p. DLC **80-2806**

HEUBNER, Otto (1843-1926)
. . . Experimental diphtheria. . . . Transl. by H. G. Beyer. . . . Detroit: G. S. Davis, 1885. 56p. col. plate. DLC; IUM; OCIM **80-2807**

HEWITT, [William Morse] Graily (1828-1893)
The pathology, diagnosis, and treatment of the diseases of women. . . . A new American from the 4th rev. and enl. London ed. . . . Ed. with notes and additions, by Harry Marion Sims. New York: Bermingham & Co., 1883. 2 v. DLC; DNLM; NNNAM; PPC **80-2808**

HEWITT, [William Morse] Graily (1828-1893)
The pathology, diagnosis, and treatment of the diseases of women. . . . A new American from the 4th rev. and enl. London ed. With 236 illustrations. Edited with notes and additions by H. Marion Sims. . . . New York: E. B. Treat, 1887-1893. 3 v. DLC; DNLM; NNNAM; PU **80-2809**

HEWSON, Addinell (1828-1889)
On the treatment of fibroids of the uterus by means of dry earth. With outline tracings of three cases so treated, in their various stages of progress. Philadelphia: Collins, 1880. 22p. DNLM; PPC **80-2810**

HEWSON, Addinell (1828-1889)
Electric light as an aid to diagnosis in surgery, or externally affected parts. Philadelphia, 1885. 9p. DNLM
80-2811

HEWSON, Addinell (1828-1889)
Earth as a topical application in surgery. Being a full exposition of its use in all the cases requiring topical applications admitted in the men's and women's surgical wards of the Pennsylvania Hospital during a period of six months in 1869. 2nd ed. Philadelphia: Medical Register Co., 1887. 309p. 4 plates. CtY-M; DNLM; MBM; PPC **80-2812**

HEWSON, Addinell (1828-1889)
Some results of excessive conservatism in the treatment of disease in large joints. Chicago, 1889. 25p. 1 plate. DNLM
80-2813

HEWSON, Addinell (1828-1889)
Medical and scientific library of Dr. . . . Philadelphia, [1889]. 42p. DNLM; PPC **80-2814**

HEYL, Albert G.
Intra-ocular lipaemia. Philadelphia: Collins, 1881. 16p. DNLM
80-2815

HEYL, Albert G.
The new constants of the Helmholtz diagrammatic eye. Philadelphia: Collins, 1881. 6p. DNLM
80-2816

HIGBEE, Edwin W.
A treatise on domestic medicine. The standard homoeopathic remedies, and how to use them. Dr. Higbee's complete family medicine case. . . . [Northampton, Mass., 1883.] 39p. DLC
80-2817

HIGGENS, Charles
Handbook of ophthalmic practice. 2nd ed. Philadelphia: P. Blakiston, Son & Co., 1882. 116p. DNLM; NNNAM; PPC; PU **80-2818**

HIGGENS, Charles
A manual of ophthalmic practice. Philadelphia: P. Blakiston, Son & Co., 1888. 314p. DNLM; MH-M; NNNAM; PPC
80-2819

HILDRETH, Eugenius A[ugustus] (1821-1885)
Synopsis of observations on some of the relations of meteorology and disease. Wheeling, W. Va., 1882. 10p. DNLM
80-2820

HILL, Hampton E[ugene] (1850-1894)
Reasons for drainage in ovariotomy. Philadelphia: W. J. Dornan, 1889. 7p. DNLM **80-2821**

[HILL, Hiram H.] (1810-1889)
Complimentary banquet to H. H. Hill, M.D., given at the Augusta House, Tuesday, June 15, 1886, it being the 50th anniversary of his continuous practice of the medical profession. Augusta, Maine. 1887. 48p. 1 table. DNLM
80-2822

HILL, [Matthew] Berkeley (1834-1892)
A manual of venereal diseases, for students and practitioners, being a concise description of those affections and of their treatment, by Berkeley Hill . . . and by Arthur Cooper. New York: Bermingham & Co., 1881. 25p. DNLM; NNNAM
80-2823

HILL, [Matthew] Berkeley (1834-1892)
The student's manual of venereal diseases, being a concise description of those affections and their treatment, by Berkeley Hill . . . and by Arthur Cooper. . . . 2nd ed. New York: William Wood & Co., 1881. 62p. DLC; DNLM; NNNAM
80-2824

HILL, [Matthew] Berkeley (1834-1892)
The essentials of bandaging; with directions for managing fractures and dislocations, for administering ether and chloroform, and for using other surgical apparatus. With a chapter on surgical landmarks. [5th ed.] New York: J. H. Vail & Co., 1887. 341p. 136 engr. DNLM; NNNAM; PPC; PU
80-2825

HILL, [Matthew] Berkeley (1834-1892) and Arthur COOPER
The student's manual of venereal diseases; being a concise description of those affections and of their treatment. 4th ed., revised. Philadelphia: P. Blakiston, Son & Co., 1887. 132p. DNLM; IU-M; NNNAM; PPC **80-2826**

HILLS, Alfred K.
Some observations on the therapeutic use of alcohol. [New York, 1882.] 27p. DNLM; NNNAM
80-2827

HILSMAN, P. L.
Double ovariotomy; operation; death from tetanus. Atlanta: J. P. Harrison & Co., [1880]. 6p. DNLM
80-2828

HINTS on digestion. A brief résumé of the latest physiological investigations. From various English, American, French, and German physiological writings. New York, [1882]. 23p. DNLM; NNNAM **80-2829**

HIRST, Barton Cooke (1861-1935)
The death-rate of lying-in hospitals in the United States. [Philadelphia, 1887.] 12p. DNLM; PPC
80-2930

HIRST, Barton Cooke, ed. (1861-1935)
A system of obstetrics. By American authors. . . . Philadelphia: Lea Bros. & Co., 1888-1889. 2 v. col. plates. DLC; DNLM; NNNAM; PPC **80-2831**

HITZ, Gertrude
The importance of knowledge concerning the sexual nature. [Washington]: Brentano Bros., 1884. 32p. DNLM
80-2832

HODENPYL, Eugene (1863-1910)
A case of adeno-sarcoma of the dura-mater spinalis. [Philadelphia, 1888.] 4p. DNLM **80-2833**

HODGE, C[lifton] F[remont] (*b.* 1859)
Some effects of electrically stimulating ganglion cells. [Baltimore, 1889.] 27p. 1 plate. DNLM; MdU-D
80-2834

HODGES, Richard Manning (1827-1896)
So-called concussion of the spinal cord. Cambridge: Riverside Press, 1881. 27p. DNLM; MH-M **80-2835**

HODGES, Richard Manning (1827-1896)
Undercurrents of modern medicine. The annual discourse. Boston: D. Clapp & Son, 1886. 59p. DNLM; MBM; NNNAM [*also*: Boston, 1886, 45p.] **80-2836**

HODGES, William D[ennison] (1854-1893)
Massachusetts General Hospital surgical cases. Antiseptic treatment. Services of Drs. Bigelow, Hodges, and Beach. [Philadelphia, 1886.] 4p. 1 tab. DNLM
80-2837

HOFF, John Van Rensselaer (1848-1920)
Notes on bearer drill with hand-litter, ambulance-wagon, etc., supplementary to a provisional manual of instruction for the Hospital Corps, U.S. Army, and company bearers. [Fort Reno, I. T., 1889.] 53p. DNLM **80-2838**

HOFFMAN, Frederick (1832-1904) and Frederick B. POWER
A manual of chemical analysis as applied to the examination of medicinal chemicals. 3rd ed. Philadelphia: Henry C. Lea's Son & Co., 1883. 624p. DNLM; ICU; NNC; PU
80-2839

HOLBROOK, Arthur
Practical suggestions on personal care of the teeth. . . . Milwaukee, Wis., 1889. 18p. DLC **80-2840**

HOLBROOK, Martin Luther, ed. (1831-1902)
Parturition without pain; a code of directions for escaping from the primal curse. New York: M. L. Holbrook, 1885. 159p. NNNAM **80-2841**

HOLBROOK, M[artin] L[uther] (1831-1902)
How to strengthen the memory; or, natural and scientific methods of never forgetting. New York: M. L. Holbrook & Co., 1886. 152p. DNLM; NNNAM **80-2842**

HOLBROOK, M[artin] L[uther] (1831-1902)
Eating for strength; or, food and diet in their relation to health and work, together with several hundred recipes for wholesome foods and drinks. New York: M. L. Holbrook & Co., [1888]. 246p. DNLM; NNNAM **80-2843**

HOLDEN, Edgar (1838-1909)
Mortality and sanitary record of Newark, N.J., [during the past twenty years]. A report presented to the president and directors of the Mutual Benefit Life Insurance Co., January, 1880. [Newark, 1880.] 25p. 4 maps, 9 diag., 1 tab. DNLM
80-2844

HOLDEN, Edgar (1838-1909)
A contribution to the study of chorea laryngis. [New York, 1885.] 8p. DNLM **80-2845**

HOLDEN, Luther (1815-1905)
Landmarks, medical and surgical. . . . 3rd ed. Assisted by James Shuter. Philadelphia: P. Blakiston, 1881. 73p. CtY-M; DNLM; IU-M; PPC **80-2846**

HOLDEN, Luther (1815-1905)
Landmarks, medical and surgical. . . . Assisted by James Shuter. . . . From the 3rd English ed., with additions, by William W. Keen. . . . Philadelphia: Henry C. Lea's Son & Co., 1881. 148p. DLC; NNNAM; PPJ; PU **80-2847**

HOLDEN, Luther (1815-1905)
Holden's anatomy. . . . A manual of dissection of the human body. 5th ed. Philadelphia: P. Blakiston, 1885. 886p. CU-M; IEN-M; MBM; PU **80-2848**

HOLDEN, Luther (1815-1905)
Human osteology comprising a description of the bones with delineations of the attachments of the muscles, the general and microscopic structure of bone and its development. . . . Assisted by James Shuter. . . . 6th ed. New York: William Wood & Co., 1885. 276p. DLC; NNNAM; PPC; PU
80-2849

HOLDEN, Luther (1815-1905)
Human osteology; comprising a description of the bones, with delineations of the attachments of the muscles, the general and microscopic structure of bone, and its development. To which is added a brief notice of the unity of type in the construction of the vertebrate skeleton. Edited by Charles Stewart and R. W. Reid. 7th ed. Philadelphia: P. Blakiston, Son & Co., 1887. 356p. 58 plates. CU-M; DNLM; MH-M; PPC
80-2850

HOLDEN, Luther (1815-1905)
Landmarks, medical and surgical. . . . 4th ed. Philadelphia: P. Blakiston, Son & Co., 1888. 79p. DNLM; MdBJ-W; PPC; PPJ **80-2851**

HOLLAND, James William (1849-1922)
Diet for the sick; notes medical and culinary. Louisville: J. P. Morton & Co., 1880. 68p. DLC; DNLM; IU-M; OCIM
80-2852

HOLLAND, James William (1849-1922)
Our thirtieth year; annual address before the Kentucky State Medical Society. Louisville: J. P. Morton & Co., 1882. 22p. DNLM **80-2853**

HOLLAND, James William (1849-1922)
The urine. Memoranda, chemical and microscopical, for laboratory use. . . . Philadelphia: P. Blakiston, Son & Co., 1887. 43p. DLC; NNNAM; PPC; PU
80-2854

HOLLAND, James William (1849-1922)
The urine and the common poisons. Memoranda, chemical and microscopical, for laboratory use. . . . Illustrated. 2nd ed., rev. and much enl. Philadelphia: P. Blakiston, Son & Co., 1888. 65p. DLC; MH-M; NNNAM; PU **80-2855**

HOLLAND, James William (1849-1922)
The urine, the common poisons, and the milk. Memoranda, chemical and microscopical, for laboratory use. . . . 3rd ed., rev. and much enl. Philadelphia: P. Blakiston, Son & Co., 1889. 84p. DLC; MH-M; NNNAM; PPC
80-2856

HOLLETT, Arthur P. (*b.* 1847)
Annual directory of homoeopathic physicians, societies, and institutions, in the State of New York. May, 1881. [Havana, N.Y., 1881.] 33p. DNLM **80-2857**

HOLLICK, Frederick (*b.* 1818)
The marriage guide, or Physiological and hygienic instructor, for the married, or those intending to marry, both male and female. . . . 500th ed., rev., and with new matter and illustrations. New York: The American News Co., [1883]. 414p. col. plates. DLC; NNNAM; PPJ; PU **80-2858**

HOLLICK, Frederick (*b.* 1818)
The male generative organs in health and disease. . . . 300th ed., rev., and with additions, New York: Excelsior Publishing House, [1886]. 377p. col. plates. DLC; IU-M; NNNAM; OCIM
80-2859

HOLMES, Bayard Taylor (1852-1924)
Secondary mixed infection in typhoid fever. [Chicago, 1888.] 11p. DNLM **80-2860**

HOLMES, Bayard Taylor (1852-1924)
Secondary mixed infection in typhoid fever. Chicago, 1888. 16p. DNLM **80-2861**

HOLMES, Bayard Taylor (1852-1924)
Secondary mixed infection in some of the acute infectious diseases of children. [Chicago, 1889.] 28p. DNLM **80-2862**

HOLMES, J. P. and W. R. HOLMES
Some remarks on diseases of the gums and mouth, with numerous testimonials of the virtues of Holmes' sure cure mouth wash and dentifrice. Macon: J. W. Burke & Co., [1884]. 30p. DNLM **80-2863**

HOLMES, Oliver Wendell (1809-1894)
Address delivered at the dedication of the Boston Medical Library Association, on December 3, 1878. Cambridge: Riverside Press, 1881. 39p. DNLM; MBM **80-2864**

HOLMES, Oliver Wendell (1809-1894)
Farewell address of Dr. Oliver Wendell Holmes, Parkman professor of anatomy in the medical school of Harvard University, delivered Nov. 28, 1882. Boston: Heliotype Printing Co., [1882]. 1 photog. plate. DNLM; MBM **80-2865**

HOLMES, Oliver Wendell (1809-1894)
Medical essays, 1842-1882. . . . Boston, [etc.]: Houghton, Mifflin & Co., 1883. 445p. DLC; MBM; MH; NN **80-2866**

[HOLMES, Oliver Wendell] (1809-1894)
Proceedings at the dinner given by the medical profession of the city of New York, April 12, 1883, to Oliver Wendell Holmes. New York: G. P. Putnam's Sons, 1883. 61p. MBM; NNNAM [Ed. by Wesley M. Carpenter] **80-2867**

[HOLMES, Oliver Wendell] (1809-1894)
Complimentary dinner to Professor Oliver Wendell Holmes, M.D., LL.D., by the medical profession of New York City. Delmonico's, April 12th, 1883. New York: Dempsey & Carroll, [1883]. 6 l. DNLM; MBM; NNNAM **80-2868**

HOLMES, Timothy, ed. (1825-1907)
A system of surgery, theoretical and practical. In treatises by various authors. . . . 1st American, from the 2nd English ed., thoroughly rev. and much enl. by John H. Packard. . . . Assisted by a large corps of the most eminent American surgeons. . . . Philadelphia: Henry C. Lea's Son & Co., 1881-1882. 3 v. col. plates. DLC; DNLM; NNNAM; PPC **80-2869**

HOLMES, Timothy (1825-1907)
A treatise on surgery, its principles and practice. 5th ed., edited by T. Pickering Pick. Philadelphia: Lea Bros. & Co., 1889. 1008p. CtY-M; DNLM; IU-M; NNNAM **80-2870**

[HOLT, Joseph] (1839-1922)
Discussion on the Memphis system of sewerage. A defense of the principle of organized effort in the sanitation of New Orleans. New Orleans, 1881. 8p. DNLM **80-2871**

HOLT, Joseph (1839-1922)
The ethical problem as demonstrated by the history of medical societies in New Orleans. An address before the New Orleans Medical and Surgical Association. New Orleans: Graham & Son, 1883. 11p. DNLM **80-2872**

HOLT, Joseph (1839-1922)
Board of Health of the State of Louisiana; its policy declared in the resolutions adopted at the reorganization, April 12th, 1884; inaugural address of the president. New Orleans, 1884. 9p. DNLM **80-2873**

HOLT, Joseph (1839-1922)
Quarantine and commerce. Their antagonism destructive to the prosperity of city and state. A reconciliation an imperative necessity. . . . Remarks of the president of the board of health of the State of Louisiana. . . . New Orleans: L. Graham & Son, 1884. 24p. DNLM; LNT-M [*also*: New Orleans, 1884, 19p.] **80-2874**

HOLT, Joseph (1839-1922)
The new quarantine system. New Orleans: L. Graham & Son, 1885. 12p. DNLM **80-2875**

HOLT, Joseph (1839-1922)
Prevention of yellow fever. [A letter to George M. Sternberg.] [New Orleans, 1885.] 3p. DNLM **80-2876**

HOLT, Joseph (1839-1922)
A reply to a letter entitled "Dr. Joseph Holt and steam as a disinfectant." Commercial relations with Brazil as affected by quarantine regulations. New Orleans, 1885. 15p. DNLM **80-2877**

HOLT, Joseph (1839-1922)
The sanitary relief of New Orleans. New Orleans: L. Graham & Son, 1885. 15p. DNLM **80-2878**

HOLT, Joseph (1839-1922)
Some quarantine reflections. [New Orleans, 1885.] 7p. DNLM **80-2879**

HOLT, Joseph (1839-1922)
Excerpta from the biennial report of the board of health to the general assembly of the State of Louisiana, 1884-1885. New Orleans: E. A. Brandao & Co., 1886. 44p. DNLM **80-2880**

HOLT, Joseph (1839-1922)
The National Board of Health in its relations to the Mississippi Valley and States of the Gulf. New Orleans: E. A. Brandao & Co., 1886. 10p. DNLM **80-2881**

HOLT, Joseph (1839-1922)
Prevention of yellow fever. Commercial relations with Brazil, as affected by quarantine regulations. Brazil and New Orleans. New Orleans: L. Graham & Son, [1886]. 12p. DNLM **80-2882**

HOLT, Joseph (1839-1922)
The proposed yellow fever commission and the National Board of Health. [Atlanta, 1886.] 6p. DNLM **80-2883**

HOLT, Joseph (1839-1922)
The sanitary protection of New Orleans, municipal and maritime. [New York, 1886.] 15p. DNLM **80-2884**

HOLT, Joseph (1839-1922)
"In shipping all industries unite." Conference of the American Shipping and Industrial League, held at Pensacola, Fla., Nov. 10-12, 1886. Address on relation of quarantine to shipping interests. [Pensacola, 1886.] 15p. DNLM
80-2885

HOLT, Joseph (1839-1922)
The quarantine system of Louisiana. Methods of disinfection practiced. An addendum to the report of the committee of the American Public Health Association. New Orleans. L. Graham & Son, 1887. 20p. 9 plates. DNLM **80-2886**

HOLT, Joseph (1839-1922)
A letter upon the causes of the introduction of yellow fever into Florida, and advice as to disinfection and sanitation. [New Orleans, 1888.] 8p. DNLM **80-2887**

HOLT, [Luther] Emmett (1855-1924)
True aneurism of the brachial artery at its upper third; cured by compression maintained for ten hours by means of a conical pad; with a résumé of the literature of the subject. [n.p., 1882.] 13p. DNLM **80-2888**

HOLT, [Luther] Emmett (1855-1924)
The symptoms and diagnosis of malaria in children. New York: William Wood & Co., 1883. 34p. DNLM; NNNAM
80-2889

HOLT, L[uther] Emmett (1855-1924)
A successful case of tetanus neonatorum treated with bromide of potassium. Cambridge: Riverside Press, 1883. 8p. DNLM
80-2890

HOLT, L[uther] Emmett (1855-1924)
Pneumonia in young children. New York: Trow's Print. & Bookbind. Co., 1885. 29p. DNLM
80-2891

HOLT, L[uther] Emmett (1855-1924)
Does quinine abort pneumonia? New York, 1885. 7p. DNLM
80-2892

HOLT, L[uther] Emmett (1855-1924)
The non-identity of croupous tonsillitis with diphtheria. [New York, 1886.] 9p. DNLM **80-2893**

HOLT, L[uther] Emmett (1855-1924)
The antiseptic treatment of summer diarrhea. [New York, 1887.] 31p. DNLM **80-2894**

HOLT, L[uther] Emmett (1855-1924)
Cerebral symptoms in the pneumonia of children. New York: Trow's Print. & Bookbind. Co., 1888. 12p. DNLM
80-2895

HOLT, L[uther] Emmett (1855-1924)
The prevention of summer diarrhoea among infants, viewed in the light of the lesions. [Philadelphia, 1889.] 8p. DNLM
80-2896

HOLT, L[uther] Emmett (1855-1924)
The relation of bacteria to diarrhoeal diseases in infancy. [New York, 1889.] 10p. DNLM **80-2897**

HOMAN, George (*b.* 1849)
Railway sanitation and quarantine. Read before the Beaumont Medical Club, Dec. 18, 1879. St. Louis: McCormick, Nixon & Co., 1880. 10p. DNLM **80-2898**

HOMAN, George (*b.* 1849)
On some salient points of likeness in the lives and characters of John Hunter and John Hodgen. [St. Louis], 1882. 8p. DNLM
80-2899

HOMAN, George (*b.* 1849)
On some points in regard to outbreaks of Asiatic cholera. [Read before the St. Louis Medical Society, May 19th, 1883.] [St. Louis, 1883?] 7p. DNLM **80-2900**

HOMAN, George (*b.* 1849)
On the rise and progress of epidemics. Read before the St. Louis Medico-Chirurgical Society, July 22, 1884. St. Louis: J. H. Chambert & Co., 1884. 7p. DNLM
80-2901

HOMAN, George (*b.* 1849)
On the course and destiny of population infections. [St. Louis, 1885.] 11p. DNLM **80-2902**

HOMAN, George (*b.* 1849)
Observations on police service and physique in Saint Louis. Essential individual hygiene of a municipal police force for the prevention of pulmonary diseases. St. Louis: Nixon-Jones Print. Co., 1887. 20p. DNLM **80-2903**

HOMAN, George (*b.* 1849)
Reports on the physical condition of the police force of St. Louis, made to the board of police commissioners. [St. Louis, 1888.] 14p. 2 diag. DNLM **80-2904**

HOMANS, John (1836-1903)
Twenty-five consecutive cases of ovariotomy. Cambridge, 1881. 22p. DNLM; MH-M **80-2905**

HOMANS, John (1836-1903)
One hundred cases of antiseptic ovariotomy. [Boston, 1882.] 4p. DNLM **80-2906**

HOMANS, John (1836-1903)
Three hundred and eighty-four laparotomies for various diseases, with tables showing the results of the operations and the subsequent history of the patients. A résumé of the writer's experience in abdominal surgery during the last fifteen years. . . . Boston: N. Sawyer & Son, printers, 1887. 56p. 26 fold. tables. DLC; DNLM; MBM **80-2907**

[HOMERGUE, Louis C.]
Valuable medical prescriptions; or, Get well and keep so. . . . New York: F. Harrison & Co., [1880]. 57p. DLC
80-2908

HOMOEOPATHIC MEDICAL SOCIETY OF ALLEGHENY COUNTY, PA.
Semi-centennial celebration of the introduction of homoeopathy west of the Allegheny mountains, held at Pittsburgh, Pa., September 20th, 1887, under the auspices of the Homoeopathic Medical Society of Allegheny County, Pa. Pub. by the Society. Ed. by J. C. Burgher, M.D. Pittsburgh: From the Press of Stevenson & Foster, 1888. 72p. DLC
80-2909

HOMOEOPATHIC MEDICAL SOCIETY OF THE COUNTY OF NEW YORK
List of active members. May, 1886. New York: M. J. Rooney, [1886]. 11p. DNLM; NNNAM
80-2910

HOMOEOPATHIC MEDICAL SOCIETY OF THE COUNTY OF PHILADELPHIA
Sanitary hints for the summer; published for distribution by the . . . . June, 1885. [Philadelphia, 1885.] 8p. DNLM; PPHa **80-2911**

HOOD & REYNOLDS
Illustrated catalogue of dentists' furniture, tools, instruments and supplies. Boston, 1881. 302p. MH-M **80-2912**

HOOPER, Franklin Henry (1850-1892)
On the treatment and recurrence of papilloma of the larynx. [New York, 1882.] 10p. DNLM **80-2913**

HOOPER, Franklin Henry (1850-1892)
Experimental researches on the tension of the vocal bands. (a) The action of the thyrocricoid muscle. (b) The action of the expiratory blast of air. [New York: G. P. Putnam's Sons, 1883.] 20p. DNLM; NNNAM **80-2914**

HOOPER, Franklin Henry (1850-1892)
A case of cavernous papilloma of the vocal band. [New York, 1884.] 3p. DNLM **80-2915**

HOOPER, Franklin Henry (1850-1892)
The respiratory function of the human larynx. From experimental studies in the physiological laboratory of Harvard University. [New York, 1885.] 20p. DNLM; NNNAM **80-2916**

HOOPER, Franklin Henry (1850-1892)
Adenoid vegetations in the naso-pharyngeal cavity. [Boston, 1886.] 16p. DNLM **80-2917**

HOOPER, Franklin Henry (1850-1892)
Concerning the positions of paralyzed vocal bands. [New York, 1886.] 16p. DNLM **80-2918**

HOOPER, Franklin Henry (1850-1892)
Concerning the positions of paralyzed vocal bands. [New York, 1886.] 11p. DNLM **80-2919**

HOOPER, Franklin Henry (1850-1892)
The anatomy and physiology of the recurrent laryngeal nerves. [Boston, 1887.] 40p. DNLM **80-2920**

HOOPER, Franklin Henry (1850-1892)
Effects of varying rates of stimulation on the action of the recurrent laryngeal nerves. [New York, 1887.] 1 l. DNLM **80-2921**

HOOPER, Franklin Henry (1850-1892)
Adenoid vegetations in children: their diagnosis and treatment. Boston: Cupples & Hurd, 1888. 19p. DNLM **80-2922**

HOOPER, Franklin Henry (1885-1892)
Effects of varying rates of stimulation on the action of the recurrent laryngeal nerves. [New York, 1888.] 8p. DNLM **80-2923**

HOOPER, Franklin Hnery (1850-1892)
A combined nasal snare and écraseur. Boston, 1889. 6p. DNLM **80-2924**

HOOPER, Franklin Henry (1850-1892)
The mechanical effects of adenoid vegetations in children. Boston: Rockwell & Churchill, 1889. 15p. DNLM **80-2925**

HOPKIN, H[enry] R[eed]
Sphygmograms; with notes on autopsies. Philadelphia: Collins, 1880. 10p. DNLM **80-2926**

HOPKINS, H[enry] R[eed]
An improved sphygmograph and its work. [Buffalo, 1886.] 10p. DNLM **80-2927**

HOPKINS, H[enry] R[eed]
The relations of mind and body. [Buffalo, 1887.] 7p. DNLM **80-2928**

HOPKINS, William Barton (1853-1904)
The roller bandage . . . with seventy-three illustrations. Philadelphia: J. B. Lippincott & Co., 1883. 95p. DLC; DNLM; NNNAM; PPC **80-2929**

HOPKINS, William Barton (1853-1904)
Report of a case of Wladimiroff-Mikulicz osteoplastic resection of the foot. [Philadelphia, 1887.] 7p. 1 tab. DNLM [*also*: Philadelphia: W. J. Dornan, 1888. 9p.] **80-2930**

HORWITZ, Orville (1859-1913)
. . . A compend of surgery. For students and physicians. . . . With fifty illustrations. Philadelphia: P. Blakiston, Son & Co., 1883. 133p. DLC; NNNAM; PPJ; PU **80-2931**

HORWITZ, Orville (1859-1913)
. . . A compend of surgery. For students and physicians. . . . 2nd ed., rev. and enl. With sixty-two illustrations. Philadelphia: P. Blakiston, Son & Co., 1885. 156p. DLC; IU-M; NNNAM; PPC **80-2932**

HORWITZ, Orville (1859-1913)
. . . A compend of surgery. For students and physicians. . . . 3rd ed., thoroughly rev., enl., and improved. With ninety-one illustrations. Philadelphia: P. Blakiston, Son & Co., 1887. 210p. DLC; DNLM; NNNAM; PPC **80-2933**

HOTZ, F. C. (1843-1909)
A clinical lecture upon the operation for inversion of the lower eyelid. Chicago, 1880. 11p. DNLM **80-2934**

HOUGHTON, Alfred S. and P. C. JENSEN
Pneumatic therapeutics. With editorial comments. Chicago, 1885. 28p. DNLM; IU-M; OCIM **80-2935**

HOUGHTON, Henry C[larke] (1837-1901)
Lectures on clinical otology, delivered before the senior class in the New York Homoeopathic Medical College; to which are added, cases from practice, and summaries of remedies. Boston: O. Clapp & Son, 1885. 260p. 2 plates. DNLM; MH-M; NNNAM; PU **80-2936**

HOVEY, E.
An address to the members of "the Southwest Dental Society." [Columbus, Kans.: J. W. McCullah & Co., 1881.] 4p. DNLM **80-2937**

HOW fevers are bred. New York, 1885. 1 sheet. DNLM **80-2938**

HOW, Lyman B[artlett] (1838-1893)
Ligation of the common carotid. Exsection of the inferior dental nerve. Concord, N.H.: Evans & Sleeper, 1880. 9p. DNLM; MH-M **80-2939**

HOW not to have the small-pox. Some advice on vaccination. [Lansing, 1881.] galley sheet. DNLM
80-2940

HOW, W. Storer
Mode of mounting the new Richmond tooth-crown. Philadelphia, 1887. 4p. DNLM **80-2941**

HOW, W. Storer
Professional patents. 1888. 8p. DNLM
80-2942

HOW, W. Storer
Flasking dentures for vulcanization. Philadelphia, 1889. 7p. DNLM **80-2943**

HOWARD, Erving Melville (*b.* 1848)
List of vegetable substances used in medicine, arranged under their proper botanical orders, for the use of the students of the Hahnemann Medical College of Philadelphia. Camden, N.J.: Senseman's Printing House. 58p. OCLloyd; PPC; PPHa; PU
80-2944

HOWARD UNIVERSITY. MEDICAL DEPARTMENT
Annual announcements, including the medical, dental, and pharmaceutical colleges, for the sessions of 1883-1884 to 1898-1899 (16.-31.). Washington, 1883-1898. DNLM [List of students for the sessions of 1882-1883 to 1897-1898, in announcements for subsequent years. Graduates in medicine, dentistry, and pharmacy, in announcement for 1898-1899.]
80-2945

HOWARD UNIVERSITY. MEDICAL DEPARTMENT
Addresses delivered at the eighteenth annual commencement of the Medical Department, including the medical, dental, and pharmaceutical colleges, at Congregational Church, March 9, 1887. Washington: R. Beresford, 1887. 29p. DNLM
80-2946

HOWARD UNIVERSITY. MEDICAL DEPARTMENT
Post graduate course, April and May, 1889. [Programme of lectures.] [Washington, 1889.] 1 sheet. DNLM
80-2947

HOWARD, W[illiam] T[ravis] (1821-1907)
Report of the section on obstetrics and gynaecology. Baltimore: I. Friedenwald, [1883]. 39p. DNLM; MdBM
80-2948

HOWARD, W[illiam] T[ravis] (1821-1907)
The president's address. Two rare cases in abdominal surgery. [New York, 1886.] 35p. DNLM; MdBM [M. & Chir. Fac. Maryland, Balt.] **80-2949**

HOWE, J. Morgan
Difficult dentition, reflex actions, and the use of the gum lancet. Buffalo, N.Y.: Baker, Jones & Co., [1883]. 9p. DNLM
80-2950

HOWE, Joseph William (1843-1890)
Emergencies, and how to treat them. The etiology, pathology, and treatment of the accidents, diseases, and cases of poisoning which demand prompt action. 3rd ed. New York: D. Appleton & Co., 1881. 265p. CtY-M; DNLM; NNNAM; PPC
80-2951

HOWE, Joseph William (1843-1890)
Excessive venery, masturbation and continence. The etiology, pathology and treatment of the diseases resulting from venereal excesses, masturbation and continence. . . . New York, [etc.]: Bermingham & Co., 1883. 291p. DLC; DNLM; NNNAM; PU
80-2952

HOWE, Joseph William (1843-1890)
Emergencies. The etiology, pathology, and treatment of the accidents, diseases, and cases of poisoning which demand prompt action. Designed for students and practitioners of medicine. . . . 4th ed. New York: D. Appleton & Co., 1884. 267p. DLC; NNNAM; PPC; PU **80-2953**

HOWE, Joseph William (1843-1890)
Excessive venery, masturbation, and continence; the etiology, pathology and treatment of the diseases resulting from venereal excesses, masturbation and continence. . . . New York, London: Bermingham & Co., 1884. 299p. DLC; NNNAM; PPJ; PU **80-2954**

HOWE, Lucien (1848-1928)
A protective shield for the eye. Buffalo, 1885. 1 l. DNLM
80-2955

HOWE, Lucien (1848-1928)
Effect of cocaine upon the healing of wounds. New York, [1885]. 7p. DNLM **80-2956**

HOWE, Lucien (1848-1928)
The purulent conjunctivitis of infants, and blindness in New York State. Philadelphia: W. J. Dornan, 1889. 8p. DNLM
80-2957

HOWE, Lucien (1848-1928), E. V. STODDARD and H. D. NOYES
Report of the committee of New York State Medical Society on the causes and prevention of blindness. [New York, 1889.] 9p. DNLM **80-2958**

HOWE, Sarah
Nature the best physician. A new method of treating female diseases, without the use of injurious or expensive instruments, on a principle hitherto unknown. . . . Wellington, Kans.: Press Steam Book and Job Printing House, 1880. 16p. DLC; DNLM **80-2959**

HOYNE, Temple S[toughton] (1841-1899)
Venereal and urinary diseases. . . . Chicago and Detroit: Halsey Bros., [1883]. 125p. DLC; DNLM; IU-M; OCIM
80-2960

HOYT, E[ugene] F. (*b.* 1846)
Observations and experiences involving rectal diseases. Philadelphia: Med. Print. Co., 1889. 16p. DNLM; PPC
80-2961

HUBBARD, Frederick Heman
The opium habit and alcoholism; a treatise on the habits of opium and its compounds; alcohol; chloral hydrate; chloroform; bromide of potassium; and Cannabis indica; including their therapeutical indications; with suggestions for treating various painful complications. New York: A. S. Barnes & Co., [1881]. 259p. DNLM; MBM; NNNAM; PU
80-2962

HUBBARD, Frederick Heman
Diphtheria. A constitutional disease. Its local manifestations, clinical history, and treatment. New York: Wynkoop & Hallenbeck, [1881]. 16p. DNLM; NNNAM
80-2963

HUBBARD, Oliver P[ayson] (1809-1900)
The early history of the New Hampshire Medical Institution, with a sketch of its founder, Nathan Smith. Washington, D.C.: Globe Ptg. & Publ. House, 1880. 41p. DNLM; MBM
80-2964

HUBBARD, S[tephen] G[rosvenor] (1816-1905)
Centennial observations on the past, present, and future of the Connecticut Medical Society. Hartford: Case, Lockwood & Brainard Co., 1885. 19p. CtY-M; DNLM
80-2965

HUBBELL, Alvin A[llace] (1846-1911)
Congenital occlusion of the posterior nares. Buffalo: Times Print. House, 1886. 16p. 1 l. DNLM
80-2966

HUBBELL, Alvin A[llace] (1846-1911)
The electro-magnet in removal of steel from the interior of the eye. [Buffalo, 1888.] 8p. DNLM
80-2967

HUBBELL, Alvin A[llace] (1846-1911)
Exudative conjunctivitis. [Concord, N.H., 1888.] 13p. DNLM
80-2968

HUBBELL, Alvin A[llace] (1846-1911)
Cases of ocular paralysis. [Buffalo, 1889.] 7p. DNLM
80-2969

HUDSON, E[rasmus] Darwin, Jr. (1843-1887)
Johnson's family physician, from the ablest medical authorities. Giving numerous and dangerous diseases to which the human race is subject, the symptoms and treatment . . . with articles from the most eminent physicians. . . . New York: A. J. Johnson & Son, 1880. 127p. DLC; NNNAM
80-2970

HUDSON, E[rasmus] Darwin, Jr. (1843-1887)
Essentials of the physical diagnosis of thoracic diseases. New York: Styles & Cash, 1885. 63p. DLC; DNLM; NNNAM
80-2971

HUDSON, E[rasmus] Darwin, Jr. (1843-1887)
The limitations of the diagnosis of malaria. New York, 1885. 15p. DLC; DNLM; NNNAM **80-2972**

HUDSON, E[rasmus] Darwin, Jr. (1843-1887)
The physical examination of weak chests and differential diagnosis of the several forms of early phthisis. New York: Styles & Cash, 1885. 24p. DNLM; NNNAM
80-2973

HUDSON, E[rasmus] Darwin, Jr. (1843-1887)
Some of the diagnostic relations of the indigestions. New York: Styles & Cash, 1885. 19p. DNLM
80-2974

HUDSON, E[rasmus] Darwin, Jr. (1843-1887)
The results of the home treatment of phthisis contrasted with those of changed residence and travel. [New York, 1886.] 27p. DNLM; NNNAM **80-2975**

HUDSON, E[rasmus] Darwin, Jr. (1843-1887)
A manual of the physical diagnosis of thoracic diseases. New York: William Wood & Co., 1887. 150p. DLC; DNLM; NNNAM; PPC **80-2976**

HUDSON, William H.
Sea-sickness; its cause, nature, and prevention without medicine or change in diet. A scientific and practical solution of the problem. Boston: S. E. Cassino & Co., 1883. 147p. DNLM; MBM **80-2977**

HUEPPE, Ferdinand Adolph Theophil (1852-1938)
The methods of bacteriological investigation. . . . Transl. by Herman M. Biggs. . . . Illustrated by thirty-one wood-cuts. New York: D. Appleton & Co., 1886. 218p. DLC; NNNAM; PPC; PPJ **80-2978**

HUESTED, Alfred Birch
Albany College of Pharmacy. Introductory address delivered at the opening of the seventh course of lectures. October 1, 1887. . . . Albany, N.Y.: Burdick & Taylor, Printers, 1887. 13p. DLC
80-2979

HUGHES, Charles Hamilton (1839-1916)
Illusion, hallucination, and delusion; a differential study for forensic purposes. [St. Louis, 1881.] 9p. DNLM
80-2980

HUGHES, C[harles] H[amilton] (1839-1916)
Clinical notes illustrative of consciousness in epilepsia. [St. Louis, 1881.] 4p. DNLM **80-2981**

HUGHES, Charles Hamilton (1839-1916)
Note on the essential psychic signs of general functional neuratrophia or neurasthenia. [St. Louis, 1882.] 8p. DNLM
80-2982

HUGHES, Charles Hamilton (1839-1916)
Moral (affective) insanity. A plea for its retention in medical nomenclature. [St. Louis, 1882.] 14p. DNLM **80-2983**

HUGHES, C[harles] H[amilton] (1839-1916)
Acute dementia occurring in an old man; recovery after two and one-half months of treatment. [St. Louis, 1882.] 6p. DNLM **80-2984**

HUGHES, C[harles] H[amilton] (1839-1916)
Report on bibliography. Presented to the thirty-ninth annual meeting of superintendents of American hospitals for the insane, at Newport, Rhode Island, June, 1883. [St. Louis, 1883.] 20p. DNLM **80-2985**

HUGHES, Charles Hamilton (1839-1916)
Glycosuria and melancholia. [Chicago? 1883.] 3p. DNLM
80-2986

HUGHES, Charles Hamilton (1839-1916)
The therapeutic value of cephalic and spinal electrizations. [St. Louis, 1883.] 11p. DNLM **80-2987**

HUGHES, C[harles] H[amilton] (1839-1916)
Borderland psychiatric records. Prodromal symptoms of psychical impairment. [St. Louis, 1884.] 7p. DNLM
80-2988

HUGHES, C[harles] H[amilton] (1839-1916)
The curability of locomotor ataxia and simulations of posterior spinal sclerosis. [St. Louis, 1884.] 12p. DNLM
80-2989

HUGHES, C[harles] H[amilton] (1839-1916)
Migraine. [St. Louis, 1884.] 12p. DNLM
80-2990

HUGHES, C[harles] H[amilton] (1839-1916)
Moral (affective) insanity; psycho-sensory insanity. [St. Louis, 1884.] 18p. DNLM **80-2991**

HUGHES, C[harles] H[amilton] (1839-1916)
The opium psycho-neurosis; chronic meconism or papaverism. [St. Louis, 1884.] 23p. DNLM **80-2992**

HUGHES, C[harles] H[amilton] (1839-1916)
Psycho-senory insanity; moral (affective) insanity. [St. Louis, 1884.] 18p. DNLM **80-2993**

HUGHES, C[harles] H[amilton] (1839-1916)
A short case record in psychiatry, with a moral. A morbidly sensitive moral sense. [St. Louis, 1884.] 18p. DNLM
80-2994

HUGHES, C[harles] H[amilton] (1839-1916)
Borderland psychiatric records, continued. Psychical concussion and perversion of self-sense; aberrations of sensation associated with probable lesion of the sympathetic system. [St. Louis, 1885.] 3p. DNLM **80-2995**

HUGHES, C[harles] H[amilton] (1839-1916)
A case of psycho-sensory (affective or moral) insanity. [St. Louis, 1885.] 7p. DNLM **80-2996**

HUGHES, C[harles] H[amilton] (1839-1916)
Editorials: General Grant. Apropos of the threatened invasion of cholera. "Dangerous physicians." Ferran and his inoculations. A melancholic attempt to commit suicide while under the influence of cocaine. St. Louis, 1885. 9p. DNLM
80-2997

HUGHES, C[harles] H[amilton] (1839-1916)
The hygiene of the nervous system and the mind. The relation of the nervous system to cholera and its prophylaxis and neurotherapy. The cure and prevention of dyspepsia as a nervous disease. The neuropathic diathesis; its quarantine and treatment. [St. Louis, 1885.] 22p. DNLM
80-2998

HUGHES, C[harles] H[amilton] (1839-1916)
Insanity and divorce. The neuropathic conditions and treatment of cancer. Mysomania. [St. Louis, 1885.] 9p. DNLM
80-2999

HUGHES, C[harles] H[amilton] (1839-1916)
Note on a form of post-neuralgic encelphalatrophic or cerebrasthenic insanity. [St. Louis, 1885.] 6p. DNLM
80-3000

HUGHES, C[harles] H[amilton] (1839-1916)
State provision for the insane. [St. Louis, 1885.] 8p. DNLM
80-3001

HUGHES, C[harles] H[amilton] (1839-1916)
Meconeuropathia. [St. Louis, 1886.] 15p. DNLM
80-3002

HUGHES, C[harles] H[amilton] (1939-1916)
An outline brief in the management of melancholia, designed chiefly for the home physician. St. Louis, 1886. 20p. DNLM
80-3003

HUGHES, C[harles] H[amilton] (1839-1916)
The curability of epilepsy and epileptoid affections by galvanism and the phosphated and arseniated bromides. [St. Louis, 1887.] 7p. DNLM **80-3004**

HUGHES, C[harles] H[amilton] (1839-1916)
The relation of the nervous system to haemophilia, malarial haematuria, etc. Second paper. [St. Louis, 1887.] 11p. DNLM
80-3005

HUGHES, C[harles] H[amilton] (1839-1916)
The scientific rationale of electrotherapy. A revised paper on the therapeutic applications of electricity. [St. Louis, 1887.] 11p. DNLM **80-3006**

HUGHES, C[harles] H[amilton] (1839-1916)
The true nature and definition of insanity. [St. Louis, 1887.] 30p. DNLM **80-3007**

HUGHES, C[harles] H[amilton] (1839-1916)
A unique case of bi-lateral athetosis. [St. Louis,1887.] 7p. DNLM **80-3008**

HUGHES, C[harles] H[amilton] (1839-1916)
My first case of cocainophobia and cocainomania. What will become of it? [St. Louis, 1888.] 4p. DNLM
80-3009

HUGHES, C[harles] H[amilton] (1839-1916)
The neural and psycho-neural factor in gynaeciac disease. [St. Louis, 1888.] 16p. DNLM **80-3010**

HUGHES, C[harles] H[amilton] (1839-1916)
Overstrain and under-power of brain. [St. Louis, 1889.] 22p. DNLM **80-3011**

HUGHES, Daniel E. (1851-1902)
. . . A compend of the practice of medicine. Especially adapted for the use of medical students. . . . Philadelphia: P. Blakiston, Son & Co., 1882-1883. 2 v. DLC; DNLM; NNNAM; PPC
80-3012

HUGHES, Daniel E. (1851-1902)
. . . A compend of the practice of medicine. . . . 2nd ed., rev. and enl. . . . Philadelphia: P. Blakiston, Son & Co., 1885. 2 v. DLC; MBM; NNNAM; PU **80-3013**

HUGHES, Daniel E. (1851-1902)
A compend of the practice of medicine. . . . Physicians' ed. Based on the revision of the quiz-compend ed., and including a very complete section on skin diseases. Philadelphia: P. Blakiston, Son & Co., 1886 [1885]. 399p. DLC; IU-M; NNNAM; PPC **80-3014**

HUGHES, Daniel E. (1851-1902)
A compend of the practice of medicine. Physicians' ed. Thorougly rev. and enl. Based on the 3rd revision of the quiz-compend ed., and including a very complete section on skin diseases. Philadelphia: P. Blakiston, Son & Co, 1887. 408p. DLC; IEN-M; PPC; PU **80-3015**

HUGHES, Daniel E. (1851-1902)
A compend of the practice of medicine. . . . Physicians' ed. Thoroughly rev. and enl. Based on the 4th revision of the quiz-compend ed. and including a very complete section on skin diseases. Philadelphia: P. Blakiston, Son & Co., 1889. 462p. CtY-M; DLC; MBM; PPC
80-3016

HUGHES, Daniel E. (1851-1902)
A compend of the practice of medicine. . . . 4th ed. Philadelphia: P. Blakiston, Son & Co., 1889. 174p. DNLM; NNNAM; PPC; PU **80-3017**

HUGHES, Richard
The knowledge of the physician; a course of lectures delivered at the Boston University School of Medicine, May, 1884. Boston: O. Clapp & Son, 1884. 292p. DLC; DNLM; MH-M; NNNAM **80-3018**

HUMPHREYS' SPECIFIC HOMEOPATHIC MEDICINE COMPANY
Catalogue and price current. New York, 1882. 97p. NNNAM **80-3019**

HUMPHREYS, Frederick (1816-1900)
Humphreys' homeopathic mentor, or Family adviser in the use of specific homeopathic medicine. By F. Humphreys. . . . Rev. and enl. ed. New York: Humphreys' Specific Homoeopathic Medicine Co., 1882. 508p. DLC; NNNAM **80-3020**

HUMPHREYS, Frederick (1816-1900)
Humphreys Homeopathischer Mentor odor familien Rathgeger. N.Y.: Humphreys' Specific Homeopathic Medicine Co., 1884. 542p. NNNAM **80-3021**

HUMPHREYS, Frederick (1816-1900)
. . . Mentor homeopathico, on Conselheiro da familia para uso da medicina specifica homeopathica. . . . Ed., corr. e. augm. New York: Humphreys' Specific Homeopathic Medicine Co., 1885. 435p. DLC; NNNAM **80-3022**

HUMPHREYS, Frederick (1816-1900)
Mentor homeopatico de Humphreys, o Guia de las familias en el uso de la medicina específica homeopática. . . . Ed., corr. y aum. Nueva York: Humphreys' Specific Homeopathic Medicine Co., 1886. 448p. DLC; NNNAM **80-3023**

HUMPHREYS, Frederick (1816-1900)
. . . Humphreys' manual of specific homeopathy for the administration of medicine and cure of disease. . . . [Rev. ed.] New York: Humphreys' Homeopathic Medicine Co., 1887. 144p. DLC; NNNAM **80-3024**

HUMPHREYS, Frederick (1816-1900)
Humphreys' homoeopathic mentor, or family adviser in the use of specific homoeopathic medicine. Revised and enlarged ed. New York: Humphreys' Specific Homeopathic Medicine Co., 1889. 533p. NNNAM; PPHa **80-3025**

HUN, Henry (1854-1924)
A guide to American medical students in Europe. . . . New York: William Wood & Co., 1883. 151p. DLC; MBM; NNNAM; PPC **80-3026**

HUN, Henry (1854-1924)
Alcoholic paralysis. Philadelphia, 1885. 17p. DNLM **80-3027**

HUN, Henry (1854-1924)
Differential diagnosis between locomotor ataxia and spasmodic spinal paralysis. Albany: Burdick & Taylor, 1885. 16p. DNLM **80-3028**

HUN, Henry (1854-1924)
Reduction of temperature by cold baths. Albany: Burdick & Taylor, 1885. 12p. DNLM **80-3029**

HUN, Henry (1854-1924)
Some cases of delirium tremens, treated with half-ounce doses of tincture of digitalis. Albany: Burdick & Taylor, 1885. 10p. DNLM **80-3030**

HUN, Henry (1854-1924)
The bacteria of disease. Albany: Burdick & Taylor, 1886. 11p. 1 plate. DNLM **80-3031**

HUN, Henry (1854-1924)
A clinical study of cerebral localization, illustrated by seven cases. [Philadelphia, 1887.] 29p. DNLM **80-3032**

HUN, Henry (1854-1924)
Gliomatous hypertrophy of the pons. Albany: Burdick & Taylor, 1887. 8p. DNLM **80-3033**

HUN, Henry (1854-1924)
The introductory lecture of the course of 1887-1888 at the Albany Medical College, delivered September 20, 1887. Published by the class. Albany: Burdick & Taylor, 1887. 8p. DNLM **80-3034**

HUN, Henry (1854-1924)
Sewer-gas poisoning. [Philadelphia, 1887.] 24p. DNLM **80-3035**

HUN, Henry (1854-1924)
A case of Pott's disease, presenting in the arms symptoms resembling those of locomotor ataxia, and in the legs those of spinal spasmodic paralysis. [Philadelphia, 1888.] 7p. DNLM **80-3036**

HUN, Henry (1854-1924)
Cases of tetany, hysterical contraction, and reflex contraction; illustrating varieties of chronic functional tonic spasm. [Philadelphia], 1888. 12p. DNLM **80-3037**

HUN, Henry (1854-1924)
Clinical reports. I. Two cases of tumor of the cerebellum. [Albany, 1888.] 17p. DNLM **80-3038**

HUN, Henry (1854-1924)
Clinical reports. II. Traumatic rupture of the valves of the heart. [Albany, 1888.] 8p. DNLM **80-3039**

HUN, Henry (1854-1924)
Clinical reports. III. Treatment of the pressure paralysis of Pott's disease by the plaster-of-Paris jacket. [Albany, 1888.] 9p. DNLM **80-3040**

HUN, Henry (1854-1924)
Clinical reports. IV. A case illustrating the relationship between cerebro-spinal meningitis and pneumonia. [Albany, 1888.] 11p. DNLM **80-3041**

HUN, Henry (1854-1924)
Myxoedema; four cases with two autopsies. With a report of the microscopical examination by T. Mitchell Prudden. Philadelphia, 1888. 40p. 3 plates. DNLM **80-3042**

HUNT, De Forest
Homeopathic treatment of diphtheria. . . . comprising a general history of the disease; and a manual of ready reference for the use of students and practitioners. Grand Rapids, Mich.: Eaton, Lyon & Co., 1880. 102p. DLC; PPHa
80-3043

HUNT, Ezra [Mundy] (1830-1894)
Hygiene; its scope, its progress and its leading aims. [n. p., 1883.] 22p. DNLM **80-3044**

HUNT, Ezra M[undy] (1830-1894)
Principals of hygiene for the school and the house, together with so much of anatomy and physiology as is necessary to the correct teaching of the subject. New York & Chicago: Ivison, Blakeman, Taylor & Co., 1886. 382p. DNLM; IU-M; OCIM; NN **80-3045**

HUNT, Lucy B.
Hand-book of light gymnastics. Boston: Lee & Shepard, 1882 [1881]. 87p. ICU; MH; NN **80-3046**

HUNT, William (1825-1896)
On injuries of the spine; a clinical lecture. [Philadelphia, 1881]. 14p. DNLM **80-3047**

HUNT, William (1825-1896)
Esmarch, antisepsis and bacillus. The annual address delivered before the Philadelphia Academy of Surgery. [Philadelphia], 1883. 22p. DNLM; PPC **80-3048**

HUNT, William (1825-1896)
Proceedings of the Alumni Society of the medical department of the University of Pennsylvania for 1884. With the annual address, by . . . . Philadelphia, 1884. 31p. DNLM; PU
80-3049

HUNT, William (1825-1896)
Health gymnastics at Baden-Baden. Philadelphia: Med. Bull. Print. House, 1888. 15p. DNLM **80-3050**

HUNT, William (1825-1896)
The rights of a consultant in compensation. [Philadelphia, 1888.] 5p. DNLM **80-3051**

HUNT, William (1825-1896)
Diabetic gangrene. Philadelphia: W. J. Dornan, 1889. 19p. DNLM **80-3052**

HUNTER, James B[radbridge] (1837-1889)
Ovariotomy. [New York, 1884.] 18p. DNLM
80-3053

HUNTER, James B[radbridge] (1837-1889)
Endometritis fungosa; its pathologic diagnosis and treatment. New York: Trow, 1885. 16p. **80-3054**

HUNTER, James B[radbridge] (1837-1889)
Fifty cases of abdominal section; with remarks on laparotomy. [New York, 1885.] 18p. DNLM **80-3055**

HUNTER, James B[radbridge] (1837-1889)
Fifty cases of abdominal section. (Second series.) [New York, 1886.] 16p. 1 tab. DNLM **80-3056**

HUNTER, James B[radbridge] (1837-1889)
Introductory remarks made at the first meeting of the Alumni Association of the Woman's Hospital in the State of New York. [New York, 1886.] 5p. DNLM **80-3057**

HUNTER, James B[radbridge] (1837-1889)
Persistent pain after abdominal section. [New York, 1887.] 10p. DNLM **80-3058**

HUNTER, James B[radbridge] (1837-1889)
The influence of the Woman's Hospital. [New York, 1887.] 9p. DNLM **80-3059**

HURD, Anson (1824-1910)
A paper on the close relation and probable identity existing between scarlatina and diphtheria. [n. p., 1883.] 8p. DNLM
80-3060

HURD, Henry M[ills] (1843-1927)
A plea for systematic therapeutical, clinical and statistical study. Read before the Association of Medical Superintendents of American Institutions for the Insane, at the annual meeting in Toronto, June, 1881. [Utica, 1881.] 16p. DNLM
80-3061

HURD, Henry M[ills] (1843-1927)
Future provision for the Insane in Michigan. [n. p., 1883.] 9p. DNLM **80-3062**

HURD, Henry M[ills] (1843-1927)
The data of recovery from insanity. [Utica, N.Y., 1886.] 13p. DNLM **80-3063**

HURD, Henry M[ills] (1843-1927)
Gastric, secretory, and other crises in general paresis. [Utica, N.Y., 1887.] 6p. DNLM **80-3064**

HURD, Henry M[ills] (1843-1927)
Imbecility with insanity. [Utica, N.Y., 1888.] 9p. DNLM
80-3065

HURD, Henry M[ills] (1843-1927)
The religious delusions of the insane. [Utica, N.Y., 1888.] 17p. DNLM **80-3066**

HURD, Henry M[ills] (1843-1927)
A case of inebriety with insantiy. Utica, N.Y., 1889. 10p. DNLM **80-3067**

HUTCHINS, Alexander (1835?-1906)
The reciprocal attitude of the medical profession and the community. The anniversary address before the Medical Society of the State of New York. [n. p.], 1884. 25p. DNLM; NNNAM **80-3068**

HUTCHINSON, Jonathan (1828-1913)
The pedigree of disease. Being six lectures on temperament, idiosyncrasy and diathesis. Delivered in the theatre of the Royal College of Surgeons in the session of 1881. New York: William Wood & Co., 1885. 113p. IU-M; NNNAM; OCIM; PPC **80-3069**

HUTCHINSON, Jonathan (1828-1913)
Syphilis. . . . Philadelphia: Lea Bros. & Co., [1887]. 532p. 8 plates. CtY-M; DNLM; NNNAM; PPC **80-3070**

HUTCHISON, Joseph Chrisman (1827-1887)
Contributions to orthopedic surgery; including observations on the treatment of chronic inflammation of the hip, knee, and ankle joints, by a new and simple method of extension, the physiological method; and lectures on club-foot, delivered at the College of Physicians and Surgeons, New York (special course). New York: G. P. Putnam's Sons, 1880. 121p. DNLM; NNNAM; OCIM; PPC **80-3071**

HUTCHISON, Joseph Chrisman (1827-1887)
The laws of health. Physiology, hygiene, stimulants, narcotics, for educational institutions and general readers. New York: Clark & Maynard, [1884]. 223p. 2 plates. DNLM; NNNAM; PPC; PU **80-3072**

HUTCHINSON, William F[rancis] (1838-1893)
Practical electro-therapeutics in children's diseases. Bridgeport, Conn.: Gould & Stiles, 1884. 7p. CtY-M; DNLM **80-3073**

HUTTON, Terry J.
The family emergency medicine chest hand-book, by . . . . [2nd ed.] Chicago: R. R. McCabe & Co., printers, 1886. 87p. DLC; OCIM [1st ed. published 1879 under title: The Emergency Medicine Chest Hand Book.] **80-3074**

HUTTON, Terry J.
The family emergency medicine chest hand-book. . . . [3rd ed.] Chicago: R. R. McCabe & Co., printers, 1889. 96p. DLC; IU-M **80-3075**

HYDE, James Nevins (1840-1910)
A practical treatise on diseases of the skin, for the use of students and practitioners. . . . Philadelphia: Henry C. Lea's Son & Co., 1883. 572p. DLC; DNLM; NNNAM; PPC **80-3076**

HYDE, James Nevins (1840-1910)
A clinical study of lupus erythematosus as it affects the hands. New York, [1884]. 15p. DNLM **80-3077**

HYDE, James Nevins (1840-1910)
On the affections of the skin induced by temperature variations in cold weather. Chicago: Clark & Longley, 1885. 24p. DNLM **80-3078**

HYDE, James Nevins (1840-1910)
On the affections of the skin induced by temperature variations in cold weather. With incidental reference to so-called prairie itch, Ohio scratches, Michigan itch, Texas mange, camp itch, prairie digs, lumbermen's itch, swamp itch, etc. Chicago: Clark & Longley, 1886. 51p. DNLM **80-3079**

HYDE, James Nevins (1840-1910)
Observations on three cases of symmetrical hand and foot disease. Philadelphia, 1887. 16p. DNLM **80-3080**

HYDE, James Nevins (1840-1910)
A practical treatise on diseases of the skin, for the use of students and practitioners. 2nd ed., thoroughly rev. and enl. . . . Philadelphia: Lea Bros. & Co., 1888. 676p. col. front. and plates. DLC; DNLM; NNNAM; PPC **80-3081**

HYDE, Joel W[ilson] (*b.* 1839)
Four cases of Tait's operation. New York, 1885. 12p. DNLM; NNNAM **80-3082**

INGALS, Ephraim Fletcher (1848-1918)
Cases of tracheotomy for croup and diphtheria. [Chicago, 1880.] 3p. DNLM **80-3083**

INGALS, Ephraim Fletcher (1848-1918)
Lectures on the diagnosis and treatment of diseases of the chest, throat, and nasal cavities. . . . New York: William Wood & Co., 1881. 437p. DLC; DNLM; NNNAM; PPC **80-3084**

INGALS, Ephraim Fletcher (1848-1918)
Report to the Illinois State Medical Society on laryngeal tumors. Chicago: Johnson, Olds & Co., 1881. 24p. DNLM; IU-M **80-3085**

INGALS, Ephraim Fletcher (1848-1918)
Report to the Illinois State Medical Society on laryngeal tumors. Chicago: Tucker, Newell & Co., 1881. 23p. DNLM; IU-M **80-3086**

INGALS, Ephraim Fletcher (1848-1918)
Deflection of the septum narium. [New York, 1882.] 9p. DNLM **80-3087**

INGALS, Ephraim Fletcher (1848-1918)
Obstructions in the larynx and trachea. Chicago: C. J. Johnson, 1882. 8p. DNLM **80-3088**

INGALS, Ephraim Fletcher (1848-1918)
Treatment of empyema. Chicago: A. G. Newell, 1883. 11p. DNLM **80-3089**

INGALS, Ephraim Fletcher (1848-1918)
Hay-fever; its cause and cure. Chicago: Clark & Longley, 1885. 14p. DNLM **80-3090**

INGALS, Ephraim Fletcher (1848-1918)
Leukoplakia buccalis et lingualis, or ichthyosis linguae; successful treatment with the galvanocautery. [New York, 1885.] 18p. DNLM **80-3091**

INGALS, Ephraim Fletcher (1848-1918)
Recurrent laryngitis and obstruction of the nares, or ordinary catarrh. Chicago, 1885. 16p. DNLM **80-3092**

INGALS, Ephraim Fletcher (1848-1918)
Intubation of the larynx for diphtheritic croup. Chicago, 1886. 7p. DNLM **80-3093**

INGALS, Ephraim Fletcher (1848-1918)
Intubation of the larynx. [New York, 1887.] 25p. DNLM **80-3094**

INGALS, Ephraim Fletcher (1848-1918)
Suppurative inflammation of the antrum. Chicago, 1887. 8p. DNLM **80-3095**

INGALS, Ephraim Fletcher (1848-1918)
Chronic rheumatic laryngitis. Chicago, 1888. 8p. DNLM **80-3096**

INGALS, Ephraim Fletcher (1848-1918)
Naso-pharyngeal fibromata. Chicago, 1888. 8p. DNLM **80-3097**

INGALS, Ephraim Fletcher (1848-1918)
Subglottic laryngeal tumor. [Philadelphia, 1888.] 5p. DNLM **80-3098**

INGALLS, P[hineas] H[enry]
The non-surgical treatment of anteflexion. [New York, 1886.] 11p. DNLM **80-3099**

INGLIS, David (*b.* 1850)
The future of therapeutics. Chicago, 1886. 8p. DNLM **80-3100**

INGLIS, David (*b.* **1850)**
A contribution to the pathology of trophic diseases of the muscular system. [New York, 1888.] 12p. DNLM
80-3101

INGLIS, Otto E[dward] (*b.* **1864)**
Dental pathology and therapeutics in the form of questions and answers. Carefully revised and approved by J. Foster Flagg. Philadelphia, 1887. 105p., interleaved. DNLM; MdU-D; PPC; PU **80-3102**

INSTRUCTIONS for L. A. Berteling's compound optometer for correcting errors of refraction. San Francisco: G. Spaulding & Co., 1885. 18p. DNLM **80-3103**

INTERNATIONAL MEDICAL CONGRESS. 9th, WASHINGTON, D.C., 1887.
International Medical Congress, ninth session, to be held in Washington, D.C., in 1887. Rules and preliminary organization. Washington, D.C., 1885. 31p. DLC
80-3104

INTERNATIONAL SANITARY CONFERENCE. 5th, WASHINGTON, D.C., 1881.
Proceedings of the International Sanitary Conference provided for by joint resolutions of the Senate and House of Representatives in the early part of 1881. Washington: Government Printing Office, 1881. 449p. DLC **80-3105**

IOWA. STATE UNIVERSITY OF IOWA. COLLEGE OF HOMOEOPATHIC MEDICINE
Annual announcements for the sessions 1886-1887 to 1897-1898 (10.-21.); 1899-1900 to 1902-1903 (23.-26). Des Moines & Iowa City, 1886-1902. DNLM [List of students and graduates for the years 1885-1886 to 1896-1897; 1898-1899 to 1901-1902 in announcements for subsequent years. Prior to 1901-1902 called Homoeopathic Medical Department.]
80-3106

IRWIN, B[ernard] J. D[owling] (1830-1917)
Fracture of the sternum, with dislocation of the fragments, treatment and result. Philadelphia, 1888. 3p. DNLM
80-3107

IRWIN, J[ohn] A[rthur] (1853-1912)
The influence of sea-voyaging upon the genito-uterine functions. New York: Trow, 1885. 30p. DNLM; NNNAM
80-3108

ISHAM, A. B[rainerd] (*b.* **1844)**
Inebriate reform. Annual address to the society of the alumni of the Medical College of Ohio. [Cincinnati, 1881.] 3p. DNLM
80-3109

IVINS, Horace F[remont] (1856-1899)
A case of bilateral paralysis of the abductor muscles of the larynx; tracheotomy; cure. Philadelphia, 1884. 8p. DNLM
80-3110

IVINS, Horace F[remont] (1856-1899)
Intubation of the larynx in a case of pharyngo-laryngeal diphtheria. Philadelphia, 1886. 8p. DNLM
80-3111

IVINS, Horace F[remont] (1856-1899)
Three cases of papillomata of the larynx. Philadelphia, 1888. 6p. DNLM **80-3112**

JACCOUD, Sigismond (1830-1913)
The curability and treatment of pulmonary phthisis. Transl. and edited by Montagu Lubbock. New York: D. Appleton & Co., 1885. 407p. CtY-M; DNLM; NNNAM; PPC
80-3113

JACK, Frederick L[afayette]
A case of necrosis of the temporal bone; removal of the labyrinth; recovery. Boston: Damrell & Upham, [1888]. 6p. DNLM **80-3114**

JACKSON, A[braham] Reeves (1827-1892)
Laceration of the neck of the uterus. Louisville, Ky.: J. P. Morton & Co., 1880. 22p. DNLM **80-3115**

JACKSON, A[braham] Reeves (1827-1892)
Uterine massage as a means of treating certain forms of enlargement of the womb. [Boston, 1881.] 15p. DNLM
80-3116

JACKSON, A[braham] Reeves (1827-1892)
A contribution to the relations of ovulation and menstruation. Chicago: Review Printing Co., 1884. 19p. DNLM
80-3117

JACKSON, A[braham] Reeves (1827-1892)
Is the extirpation of the cancerous uterus a justifiable operation? [New York, 1884.] 17p. DNLM
80-3118

JACKSON, A[braham] Reeves (1827-1892)
The ethics of female sterility. [Philadelphia, 1885.] 10p. DNLM **80-3119**

JACKSON, A[braham] Reeves (1827-1892)
Vaginal hysterectomy for cancer. Chicago, 1885. 12p. DNLM
80-3120

JACKSON, A[braham] Reeves (1827-1892)
The intra-uterine stem in the treatment of flexions. [Philadelphia, 1887.] 9p. DNLM **80-3121**

JACKSON, A[braham] Reeves (1827-1892)
Conservatism in gynaecology. Chicago, [1888]. 7p. DNLM
80-3122

JACKSON COUNTY MEDICAL SOCIETY
List of officers and members of the Jackson County Medical Society, together with the constitution and by-laws and fee-bill of the society. Kansas City: Argo Print, 1889. 30p. DNLM; IU-M **80-3123**

JACKSON, Edward (1856-1942)
Alarming and dangerous doses of the mydriatics. [Philadelphia, 1884.] 8p. DNLM **80-3124**

JACKSON, Edward (1856-1942)
The measurement of refraction by the shadow-test, or retinoscopy. [Philadelphia, 1885.] 8p. DNLM
80-3125

JACKSON, Edward (1856-1942)
The best form and practical value of the shadow test in the measurement of refraction. Chicago, 1886. 7p. DNLM
80-3126

JACKSON, Edward (1856-1942)
The relation of eye-strain to headache. [Philadelphia, 1886.] 8p. DNLM **80-3127**

JACKSON, George Thomas (1852-1916)
Iodide of potassium. New York, 1882. 10p. DNLM
80-3128

JACKSON, George Thomas (1852-1916)
Dandruff; what it is, and how to cure it. New York: Trow's Printing & Bookbinding Co., 1884. 11p. DNLM
80-3129

JACKSON, George Thomas (1852-1916)
Atrophia pilorum propria. New York, [1884]. 6p. DNLM
80-3130

JACKSON, George Thomas (1852-1916)
Lecture on general dermatological diagnosis. Detroit, 1884. 11p. DNLM **80-3131**

JACKSON, George Thomas (1852-1916)
Canities. New York, [1885]. 5 plates. DNLM
80-3132

JACKSON, George Thomas (1852-1916)
Superfluous hair. The Russian dog-faced boy, and facial hirsuties in women. New York, 1885. 15p. DNLM
80-3133

JACKSON, George Thomas (1852-1916)
Alopecia areata; its etiology, diagnosis, and tratment. [New York, 1886.] 12p. DNLM **80-3134**

JACKSON, George Thomas (1852-1916)
Baldness; what can we do for it? New York: Trow, 1887. 20p. DNLM **80-3135**

JACKSON, George Thomas (1852-1916)
Ichthyol and resorcin. A clinical study of their effects. [New York, 1887.] 11p. DNLM **80-3136**

JACKSON, George Thomas (1852-1916)
Impetigo contagiosa. New York, 1887. 8p. DNLM
80-3137

JACKSON, George Thomas (1852-1916)
A practical treatise on the diseases of the hair and scalp. . . . New York: E. B. Treat, 1887. 356p. DLC; NNNAM; PPC; PU
80-3138

JACKSON, George Thomas (1852-1916)
Sycosis; a clinical study. New York, 1889. 19p. DNLM
80-3139

JACKSON, James Caleb (1811-1895)
How to treat the sick without medicine. New York: Baker, Pratt & Co., 1881. 537p. DNLM; NNNAM
80-3140

JACKSON, James Caleb (1811-1895)
"The curse" lifted, or maternity made easy. Dansville, N.Y., 1885. 24p. DNLM **80-3141**

JACKSON, John Davies (1834-1875)
The black arts in medicine, with Anniversary address. . . . Ed. by L. S. McMurtry. . . . [2nd ed.] Cincinnati: R. Clarke & Co., 1880. 74p. DLC; DNLM; OCIM **80-3142**

JACOBI, Abraham (1830-1919)
A treatise on diphtheria. . . . New York: William Wood & Co., 1880. 252p. DLC; DNLM; NNNAM; PC
80-3143

JACOBI, Abraham (1830-1919)
Die Johns Hopkins Universität. Vortrag gehalten vor dem Deutschen-Gesellig-Wissenschaftlichen Vereine von New York. New York: E. Steiger & Co., 1881. 33p. DNLM; MdBJ-W; NNNAM **80-3144**

JACOBI, Abraham (1830-1919)
Anaemia in infancy and early childhood. New York: G. P. Putnam's Sons, 1881. 27p. DNLM; NNNAM
80-3145

JACOBI, Abraham (1830-1919)
Rudolph Virchow; an address, introductory to the course of lectures of the term, 1881-1882. New York: Trow & Co., 1881. 35p. DNLM; NNNAM **80-3146**

JACOBI, Abraham (1830-1919)
Festrede zur Feier des fünfundzwanzigjährigen Jubilaums des Deutschen Dispensary der Stadt New York, und der Einweihung des Ottendorfer-Pavilions im Deutschen Hospital am 27. Mai 1882. New York: E. Steiger & Co., 1882. 23p. DNLM; NNNAM **80-3147**

JACOBI, Abraham (1830-1919)
Infant feeding and infant foods. The anniversary address, delivered before the New York State Medical Society. Philadelphia, 1882. 24p. DNLM; PU **80-3148**

JACOBI, Abraham (1830-1919)
The historical development of modern nursing. [New York, 1883.] 15p. DNLM **80-3149**

JACOBI, Abraham (1830-1919)
Diphtheria spread by adults. Part of a paper read before the Medical Society of the County of New York. New York, 1884. 12p. DNLM; NNNAM **80-3150**

JACOBI, Abraham (1830-1919)
Congenital lipoma. Jersey City, [1884]. 21p. DNLM
80-3151

JACOBI, Abraham (1830-1919)
Inaugural address, delivered before the New York Academy of Medicine. New York: Trow's Ptg. Co., 1885. 24p. DNLM; NNNAM **80-3152**

JACOBI, Abraham (1830-1919)
Catalepsy in a child three years old. [n. p., 1885.] 3p. DNLM
80-3153

JACOBI, Abraham (1830-1919)
Volksmedicin. Vortrag gehalten vor dem deutschen gesellig-wissenschaftlichen Verein von New York am 11. März 1885. New York: Cherouny Print. & Publ. Co., 1885. 38p. DNLM; NNNAM **80-3154**

JACOBI, Abraham (1830-1919)
Follicular amygdalitis. New York: Trow, 1886. 16p. DNLM; NNNAM **80-3155**

JACOBI, Abraham (1830-1919)
Memoir of Austin Flint. New York: Trow, 1886. 11p. DNLM; NNNAM **80-3156**

JACOBI, Abraham (1830-1919)
The intestinal diseases of infancy and childhood. Physiology, hygiene, pathology, and therapeutics. Detroit: G. S. Davis, 1887. 301p. DNLM; NNNAM; OCIM
80-3157

JACOBI, Abraham (1830-1919)
Contributions to the anatomy and pathology of the thymus gland. Philadelphia: W. J. Dornan, 1888. 23p. 14 plates. DNLM; PPC **80-3158**

JACOBI, Abraham (1830-1919)
Heart and blood vessels in the young. New York: M. J. Rooney & Co., 1888. 19p. DNLM; NNNAM **80-3159**

JACOBI, Abraham (1830-1919)
The therapeutics of diphtheria. Philadelphia: W. J. Dornan, 1888. 23p. DNLM; PPC; PU **80-3160**

JACOBI, Mary Putnam (1842-1906)
Case of tubercular meningitis, with measurements of cranial temperatures. [Chicago, 1880.] 6p. DNLM **80-3161**

JACOBI, Mary Putnam (1842-1906)
On the use of the cold pack followed by massage in the treatment of anaemia, by Mary Putnam Jacobi and Victoria A. White. New York: G. P. Putnam's Sons, 1880. 76p. NNNAM; PPC; PU **80-3162**

JACOBI, Mary Putnam (1842-1906)
Case of uterine fibroid treated by ergotine injections, and finally removed by means of Thomas's scoop. [Philadelphia, 1880.] 5p. DNLM **80-3163**

JACOBI, Mary Putnam (1842-1906)
The prophylaxis of insanity. New York: G. P. Putnam's Sons, 1881. 16p. DNLM; NNNAM **80-3164**

JACOBI, Mary Putnam (1842-1906)
Review of: Fever; a study in morbid and normal in physiology, by H. C. Wood. New York: G. P. Putnam's Sons, 1881. 17p. DNLM; NNNAM **80-3165**

JACOBSON, Nathan (1857-1913)
The early diagnosis and treatment of tumors of the jaw. Philadelphia, 1889. 10p. DNLM **80-3166**

JACOBSON, W[alter] H[amilton] A[cland] (1847-1924)
The operations of surgery. . . . A systematic handbook for practitioners, students, and hospital surgeons. Philadelphia: P. Blakiston, Son & Co., 1889. 1006p. DNLM; IU-M; NNNAM; PPC **80-3167**

JACOBUS, Arthur M.
Inflammation and abscess of the breast during lactation. New York, 1883. 15p. DNLM **80-3168**

JACOBUS, Arthur M.
A case of congenital hernia of the abdominal viscera and left lung. Presentation of the hernia sac, left arm, and shoulder. Podalic version. [New York, 1887.] 4p. DNLM **80-3169**

JACOBUS, Arthur M.
A case of perforation of the veriform appendix, general peritonitis, laparotomy, accident, and recovery. New York, 1889. 22p. DNLM **80-3170**

JACOBY, George W. (1856-1940)
The neurotic disturbances after joint affections. [New York, 1884.] 22p. DNLM **80-3171**

JACOBY, George W. (1856-1940)
The use of osmic acid in peripheral neuralgias. New York: Trow, 1885. 12p. DNLM **80-3172**

JACOBY, George W. (1856-1940)
Massage in nervous diseases. [New York, 1885.] 28p. DNLM; NNNAM **80-3173**

JACOBY, George W. (1856-1940)
Trigger finger (doigt à ressort). [New York, 1886.] 12p. DNLM **80-3174**

JACOBY, George W. (1856-1940)
Massage in nervous diseases. [New York, 1886.] 21p. DNLM **80-3175**

JACOBY, George W. (1856-1940)
Microscopical studies in a case of pseudo-hypertrophic paralysis. New York, 1887. 13p. DNLM **80-3176**

JAEGER, Gustav (1832-1917)
Selections from essays on health culture and the sanitary woolen system. . . . (Transl. from the German.) New York: Dr. Jaeger's Sanitary Woolen System Co., 1886. 199p. DLC; NNNAM **80-3177**

JAHR, Gottlieb Heinrich Georg (1800-1875)
Therapeutic guide; the most important results of more than forty years' practice with personal observations regarding the truly-reliable and practically-verified curative indications in actual cases of disease. . . . Transl., with notes and new remedies, by Charles J. Hempel. . . . Philadelphia: F. E. Boericke, 1887. 364p. DLC; NNNAM; PPC; PPHa **80-3178**

JAMES, Bushrod W[ashington] (1836-1903)
American resorts, with notes upon their climate . . . with translations from the German by Mr. S. Kauffmann. Intended for invalids and those who desire to preserve good health in a suitable climate. Philadelphia: F. A. Davis, 1889. 285p. DNLM; NNNAM; PPHa **80-3179**

JAMES, Martin L. (1829-1907)
Treatment of consumption indicated by the discoveries of Koch and others of its parasitic origin. [Richmond, 1882.] 4p. DNLM **80-3180**

JAMES, Prosser
Sore throat, its nature, varieties, and treatment; including the use of the laryngoscope as an aid to diagnosis. Including the connection between affections of the throat and other diseases. 4th ed. Philadelphia: P. Blakiston, Son & Co., 1882. 318p. 2 plates. DNLM; NNNAM; OCIM; PPC **80-3181**

JAMES, Prosser
The therapeutics of the respiratory passages. New York: William Wood & Co., 1884. 316p. CtY-M; DNLM; NNNAM; PPC **80-3182**

JARVIS, O. A.
The dentist. A popular treatise on the care of the teeth. 2nd ed. . . . New York: Press of S. W. Green's Son, 1880. 56p. DLC; NNNAM **80-3183**

JARVIS, William C[hapman] (1855-1895)
The pathology and surgical treatment of hypertrophic nasal catarrh. Description of a new operation for the radical cure of nasal catarrh. New York: G. Putnam's Sons, 1881. 12p. DNLM **80-3184**

JARVIS, William C[hapman] (1855-1895)
Chronic irritative hyperaemia of the larynx. [New York, 1882.] 5p. DNLM **80-3185**

JARVIS, William C[hapman] (1855-1895)
Removal of hypertrophied turbinated tissues by écrasement with the cold wire. [New York, 1882.] 7p. DNLM **80-3186**

JARVIS, William C[hapman] (1855-1895)
The healing of ulcers in laryngeal phthisis. [New York, 1883.] 6p. DNLM **80-3187**

JARVIS, William C[hapman] (1855-1895)
A new method for the removal of laryngeal growths, with illustrative case. New York: Trow, 1884. 12p. DNLM **80-3188**

JARVIS, William C[hapman] (1855-1895)
Catarrhal affections of the nasal passages as a cause of pulmonary phthisis, with special reference to the question of heredity. New York: D. Appleton & Co., 1885. 35p. DNLM; NNNAM **80-3189**

JARVIS, William C[hapman] (1855-1895)
A new electric light, for the diagnosis and treatment of diseases of the nose and throat, with a practical demonstration. Syracuse, N.Y.: Smith & Bruce, 1885. 4p. DNLM **80-3190**

JARVIS, William C[hapman] (1855-1895)
A novel procedure for the removal of subglottic laryngeal growths, with the report of an illustrative case. New York: D. Appleton & Co., 1886. 12p. DNLM **80-3191**

JARVIS, William C[hapman] (1855-1895)
A novel system of operating for the correction of the deflected septum by means of an electric motor, nasal drills, and an original spray-producing device, with illustrative cases. New York: Trow, 1887. 12p. DNLM **80-3192**

JARVIS, William C[hapman] (1855-1895)
Two unique cases of congenital occlusion of the anterior nares. New York, 1887. 12p. DNLM **80-3193**

JARVIS, William C[hapman] (1855-1895)
Notes on a case of nasal caries complicated with meningitis, successfully treated by means of the surgical drill. Philadelphia: Records, McMullen & Co., 1888. 12p. DNLM **80-3194**

JEANÇON, John A.
Pathological anatomy, pathology and physical diagnosis. A series of clinical reports comprising the principal diseases of the human body. Systematically arranged in one hundred full-page illustrations and one hundred pages text. . . . Cincinnati, O.: Progress Publishing Co., [1883]-85. 100p. 98 plates (part col., part fold.). DLC; ICJ; NN **80-3194A**

JEANÇON, John A.
Diseases of the sexual organs. Anatomy, normal and morbid; pathology, physical diagnosis and treatment of the diseases of those organs. Arranged in eighty full-page colored illustrations and one hundred and sixty-two pages text, royal folio. . . . Cincinnati: Progress Publishing Co., 1886. 2 v. in 1. 80 plates (part col.). ICJ **80-3194B**

JEFFERSON MEDICAL COLLEGE. PHILADELPHIA
Annual announcements for the sessions of 1881-1882 to 1900-1901 (57.-76.); 1902-1903 (78.). Philadelphia, 1881-1902. DNLM; PPJ **80-3195**

JEFFERSON MEDICAL COLLEGE. PHILADELPHIA
Announcement for the spring session of 1887 (55.). [Philadelphia, 1887.] 2 l. DNLM; PPJ **80-3196**

JEFFERSON MEDICAL COLLEGE. PHILADELPHIA
Colegio de medicina. El curso del Colegio de medicina de Jefferson, Filadelfia, de 1887-1888 (63.). [Filadelfia? 1887.] 1 sheet. DNLM; PPJ **80-3197**

JEFFERSON MEDICAL COLLEGE. PHILADELPHIA
Catalogue of graduates from 1880-1889. Philadelphia: W. F. Fell & Co., 1889. 20p. DNLM; PPJ **80-3198**

JEFFERSON MEDICAL COLLEGE. PHILADELPHIA
Directory of the class of 1888 of the . . . and report of the class reunion held April 3, 1889. [Philadelphia, 1889.] 29p. DNLM; PPJ **80-3199**

JEFFERSON MEDICAL COLLEGE HOSPITAL. PHILADELPHIA
Report of the trustees of the Jefferson Medical College of Philadelphia . . . exhibiting the operations of the hospital from its foundation to the end of the third fiscal year, Sept. 30, 1880. Philadelphia: McLaughlin Bros., 1881. 48p. DNLM; PPJ **80-3200**

JEFFRIES, Benjamin Joy (1833-1915)
. . . Report of the examination of 27,927 school children for color-blindness. . . . Boston: Rockwell & Churchill, City Printers, 1880. 9p. DLC; DNLM **80-3201**

JEFFRIES, Benjamin Joy (1833-1915)
Synopsis of a lecture on color-blindness and its dangers on the sea. Claremont, N.H., 1880. 4p. DNLM **80-3202**

JEFFRIES, Benjamin Joy (1833-1915)
Color-names, color-blindness, and the education of the color-sense in our schools. Boston: L. Prang & Co., 1882. 11p. DNLM **80-3203**

JEFFRIES, Benjamin Joy (1833-1915)
Color-blindness: its dangers and its detection. . . . Rev. and enl. ed. Boston, New York: Houghton, Mifflin & Co., 1883. 334p. col. front., diags. DLC; MBM; NNNAM; PPC **80-3204**

JEFFRIES, B[enjamin] (1833-1915)
Our eyes and our industries. Boston: Rand, Avery & Co., 1883. 31p. DNLM; MH **80-3205**

JEFFRIES, B[enjamin] Joy (1833-1915)
Some medico-legal cases under state and national laws. [Boston, 1886.] 11p. DNLM **80-3206**

JEFFRIES, B[enjamin] Joy (1833-1915)
Physical examination of candidates for the United States Naval and Military Academies. Boston, 1886. galley sheet. DNLM **80-3207**

JEFFRIES, B[enjamin] Joy (1833-1915)
Re-establishment of the medical profession. Boston: D. Clapp & Son, 1888. 39p. DNLM; MH-M **80-3208**

JEFFRIES, John Amory (1859-1892)
The anti-bacterial action of iodoform. [Philadelphia, 1888.] 7p. DNLM **80-3209**

JEFFRIES, John Amory (1859-1892)
The bacteria of the alimentary canal, especially in the diarrhoeas of infancy. Boston: Cupples & Hurd, 1888. 24p. DNLM; MBM **80-3210**

JEFFRIES, John Amory (1859-1892)
On the sterilization of milk and foods for infants. [Philadelphia, 1888.] 11p. DNLM **80-3211**

JEFFRIES, John Amory (1859-1892)
The reaction of the blood. [Boston, 1889.] 17p. DNLM **80-3212**

JELKS, James T[homas] (1849-1902)
Papers read before the State Medical Society of Arkansas. Little Rock: Mitchell & Bettis, 1889. 8p. DNLM **80-3213**

[JENKINS, J[ohn] Foster] (1826-1882)
Catalogue of the medical library of the late . . . a large and valuable collection: comprising many old, very curious and rare works, illustrating the growth of anatomical and physiological knowledge, and the science and practice of medicine and surgery from early times, to be sold at auction, Feb. 12 and following days, 1883, by Bangs & Co. New York: D. Taylor, 1883. 109p. DNLM; NNNAM **80-3214**

JENKS, Edward W[atrous] (1833-1903)
The treatment of puerperal septicemia by intra-uterine injections. Boston, 1880. 24p. DNLM; MBM **80-3215**

JENKS, Edward W[atrous] (1833-1903)
On coccygodynia; a lecture. Chicago, 1880. 15p. DNLM **80-3216**

JENKS, Edward W[atrous] (1833-1903)
Artresia of the genital passages of women. [Chicago, 1880.] 24p. DNLM **80-3217**

JENKS, Edward W[atrous] (1833-1903)
The relations of goitre to pregnancy and derangements of the generative organs of women. New York: William Wood & Co., 1881. 39p. DNLM; NNNAM **80-3218**

JENKS, Edward W[atrous] (1833-1903)
Contribution to surgical gynecology. Chicago: C. J. Johnson, 1882. 21p. DNLM **80-3219**

JENKS, Edward W[atrous] (1833-1903)
The practice of gynecology in ancient times. [Philadelphia], 1882. 46p. 3 plates. DNLM; PPC; PU **80-3220**

JENKS, Edward W[atrous] (8133-1903)
Modified Listerism in ovariotomy, with a report of five recent operations. [Detroit, 1882.] 7p. DNLM **80-3221**

JENKS, Edward W[atrous] (1833-1903)
On a new mode of operating for fistula in ano. [Boston, 1883.] 9p. DNLM **80-3222**

JENKS, Edward W[atrous] (1833-1903)
Open letter to Dr. N. S. Davis [in regard to controversy with Dr. Geo. E. Ranney as to performance of an ovariotomy]. [Detroit, Mich., 1885.] 8p. DNLM **80-3223**

JENKS, Edward W[atrous] (1833-1903)
Report of a case of Caesarean operation, with some comments. [New York, 1886.] 11p. DNLM **80-3224**

JENKS, Edward W[atrous] (1833-1903)
Disorders of menstruation. Detroit: G. S. Davis, 1887. 120p. DNLM; IU-M; OCIM; NNNAM **80-3225**

JENKS, Edward W[atrous] (1833-1903)
The education of girls from a medical standpoint. [Lansing, 1889.] 11p. DNLM **80-3226**

JENNINGS, Charles Goodwin (1857-1936)
Practical urine testing; a guide to office and bedside urine analysis, for physicians and students. Detroit: D. O. Haynes & Co., 1887. 124p. DLC; DNLM; OCIM **80-3227**

JENNINGS, Charles Goodwin (1857-1936)
The technique of tracheotomy and intubation of the larynx. [Detroit, 1887.] 9p. DNLM **80-3228**

JESSEN, H. C.
Therapeutic materia medica, containing the chief symptoms and clinical uses of 216 remedies, arranged upon a new and available plan for practice. Chicago: Halsey Bros., 1880. 219p. IU-M; PPHa **80-3229**

JEWETT, Charles (1839-1910)
Outline of a course of lectures on obstetrics. . . . Long Island College Hospital, 1886-1887. [n. p., 1887.] 41p. DLC **80-3230**

JEWETT, Charles (1839-1910)
Note on the treatment of puerperal eclampsia. [New York, 1888.] 7p. DNLM **80-3231**

JEWETT, Charles (1839-1910)
Manual of rules for child-bed nursing. . . . Brooklyn, N.Y.: [Press of Brooklyn Eagle], 1889. 23p. DLC **80-3232**

JOHNSON, H[osmer] A[llen] (1822-1891)
Pneumatic differentiation and medication. [Chicago, 1887.] 4p. DNLM **80-3233**

JOHNSON, H[osmer] A[llen] (1822-1891)
Report of a case of chronic pseudo-membranous bronchitis. [Chicago, 1887.] 11p. DNLM **80-3234**

JOHNSON, Isaac D. (1827-1911)
Therapeutic key; or, Practical guide for the homoeopathic treatment of diseases in general. . . . 10th ed., rev., improved, and enl. New York, Philadelphia: Boericke & Tafel, 1881. 347p. DLC; NNNAM; PPC; PPHa **80-3235**

JOHNSON, Isaac D. (1827-1911)
Guide du Traietment Homeopathique pour l'usage des Families. Traduit de l'Anglais, annoté et vorrigé par le Dr. Charles Lopez, New Orleans. New York and Philadelphia: Boericke & Tafel, 1884. 484p. LNT-M; PPHa **80-3236**

JOHNSON, Isaac D. (1827-1911)
Therapeutic key: or, A practical guide for the homoeopathic treatment of disease. . . . 15th ed., rev., improved and enl. Philadelphia: F. E. Boericke, 1886. 306p. DLC; OCLloyd: PPHa **80-3237**

JOHNSON, Isaac D. (1827-1911)
Anleitung zur Ausubung der Homoopatischen Heilkunst, fur Familien und Privat-Gerbrauch. Aus dem Englisch übertragen. Philadelphia, 1888. 463 seiten. Geschmachvoll gebunden. PPG; PPHa **80-3238**

JOHNSON, Isaac D. (1827-1911)
Counsel to parents, and how to save the baby. Kennett Square, Pa. Published by the Author, 1889. 224p. PPC; PPHa; PU **80-3239**

JOHNSON, Isaac D. (1827-1911)
Johnson's therapeutic key. . . . 16th ed. Rev., improved and enl. Philadelphia: F. E. Boericke, 1889. 400p. DLC; PPHa **80-3240**

JOHNSON, John G.
Anaesthetics medico-legally considered. New York: T. B. Mead. 1881. 23p. DNLM; NNNAM **80-3241**

JOHNSON, John G.
Vaccination medico-legally considered: New York: T. B. Mead, 1881. 27p. DNLM; NNNAM **80-3242**

JOHNSON, John G.
Concussion of the spine in railway injuries. New York: Vanden Houten & Co., 1883. 31p. DNLM; NNNAM **80-3243**

JOHNSON, John G.
Concussion of the spine in railway injuries. New York, [1884]. 25p. DNLM; NNNAM **80-3244**

JOHNSON, John G.
Poisoning by canned goods. New York: Vanden Houten & Co., [1884]. 21p. DNLM; NNNAM **80-3245**

JOHNSON, Joseph Taber (1845-1921)
Mismanaged labor the source of much of the gynecological practice of the present day. [Boston, 1880.] 15p. DNLM **80-3246**

JOHNSON, Joseph Taber (1845-1921)
Introductory address, delivered at the opening of the second course of lectures of the Washington Training School for Nurses. Washington: H. A. Gibbs, 1880. 22p. DNLM **80-3247**

JOHNSON, Joseph Taber (1845-1921)
On the management of the third stage of abortion, with retention of membranes. Philadelphia: Collins, 1880. 11p. DNLM **80-3248**

JOHNSON, Joseph Taber (1845-1921)
Can we make a positive diagnosis of pregnancy previous to the occurrence of the audible sounds of the foetal heart and the direction of the foetal movements? Philadelphia: Collins, 1881. 9p. DNLM **80-3249**

JOHNSON, Joseph Taber (1845-1921)
Superinvolution of the uterus. [New York, 1883.] 11p. DNLM **80-3250**

JOHNSON, Joseph Taber (1845-1921)
A case of Battey's operation. [Baltimore, 1883.] 15p. 1 plate. DNLM **80-3251**

JOHNSON, Joseph Taber (1845-1921)
The proper use of ergot in obstetrics. [Philadelphia, 1883.] 25p. DNLM **80-3252**

JOHNSON, Joseph Taber (1845-1921)
On the importance of trachelorraphy, with cases and remarks. Chicago: A. G. Newell, 1884. 19p. DNLM; IU-M **80-3253**

JOHNSON, Joseph Taber (1845-1921)
On the immediate and remote effect of Emmet's operation. Read before the American Medical Association. Chicago: A. G. Newell, 1884. 12p. DNLM; IU-M **80-3254**

JOHNSON, Joseph Taber (1845-1921)
Four cases of oöphorectomy. [New York, 1886.] 12p. DNLM **80-3255**

JOHNSON, Joseph Taber (1845-1921)
The mechanical treatment of the vomiting of pregnancy. Chicago, 1886. 15p. DNLM **80-3256**

JOHNSON, Joseph Taber (1845-1921)
History of fifteen cases of abdominal section, with remarks upon the methods of foreign operators. [Richmond, 1887.] 34p. DNLM **80-3257**

JOHNSON, Joseph Taber (1845-1921)
Introductory address delivered at the opening of the thirty-ninth session of the Medical Department of Georgetown University, on the recent advances in abdominal surgery . . . October 3, 1887. Published by request of the students of the college. [Washington: W. H. Moore, print, 1887.] 21p. DLC **80-3258**

JOHNSON, Joseph Taber (1845-1921)
Can the Caesarean section be safely substituted for craniotomy in the United States at the present time? Chicago, 1887. 19p. DNLM **80-3259**

JOHNSON, Joseph Taber (1845-1921)
Introductory address delivered at the opening of the thirty-ninth session of the Medical Department of the Georgetown University, on the recent advances in abdominal surgery, October 3, 1887. [Washington: W. H. Moore, 1887.] 21p. DNLM **80-3260**

JOHNSON, Joseph Taber (1845-1921)
Three bad cases of ovariotomy; two double, one single. Chicago, 1888. 8p. DNLM **80-3261**

JOHNSON, Joseph Taber (1845-1921)
Brief remarks on a number of surgical operations performed in his private hospital. [Richmond, 1889.] 10p. DNLM **80-3262**

JOHNSON, Laurence (1845-1893)
A medical formulary based on the United States and British pharmacopoeias, together with numerous French, German and unofficinal preparations. . . . New York: William Wood & Co., 1881. 402p. DLC; DNLM; NNNAM; OCLloyd **80-3263**

JOHNSON, Laurence (1845-1893)
. . . A manual of the medical botany of North America. . . . New York: William Wood & Co., 1884. 292p. 9 col. plates. DLC; DNLM; NNNAM; OCLloyd **80-3264**

JOHNSON & LUND. PHILADELPHIA
Illustrated catalogue of instruments. . . . Philadelphia, 1888. 250p. PU **80-3265**

JOHNSON, Robert W.
Cryptorchidism, with an illustrative case. Baltimore, 1884. 11p. DNLM **80-3266**

JOHNSTON BROTHERS
Illustrated catalogue of new improved cone socket instruments. New York and Brooklyn, [1880]. 32p. NNNAM **80-3267**

JOHNSTON BROTHERS
Preliminary illustrated dental catalogue of materials and supplies. New York and Brooklyn, 1881. 220p. NNNAM **80-3268**

JOHNSTON, Edwin S.
The Philadelphia Institute for the Permanent Cure of Stammering. [Account of the foundation of the institute in 1884. With testimonials.] [Philadelphia, 1888.] 54p. DNLM; PPC **80-3269**

JOHNSTON, George Woodruff
A contribution to the study of cysts of the vagina; with the report of a case. New York: William Wood & Co., 1887. 49p. DNLM; NNNAM **80-3270**

JOHNSTON, George Woodruff
Certain facts, regarding fertility, utero-gestation, parturition, and the puerperium in the so-called "lower" or "laboring" classes. Observations made in the Woman's Clinic of the Central Dispensary and Emergency Hospital, Washington, D.C. New York: William Wood & Co., 1888. 19p. DNLM; NNNAM **80-3271**

JOHNSTON, George Woodruff
Occurrence of the mammary secretion, accompanied by certain rational signs of pregnancy in two non-pregnant women. [New York, 1888.] 6p. DNLM **80-3272**

JOHNSTON, Samuel
A case of primary nasal diphtheria. [New York: G. P. Putnam's Sons, 1882.] 3p. DNLM **80-3273**

JOHNSTON, William W[aring] (1843-1902) and T. N. McLAUGHLIN
Addresses delivered at the sixtieth annual commencement of the National Medical College (medical department of the Columbian University). Washington, D.C.: W. H. Moore, 1882. 14p. DNLM **80-3274**

JOHNSTON, William W[aring] (1843-1902)
The Eureka Springs, Arkansas. St. Louis, Mo.: Woodward & Tiernan, 1885. 48p. DNLM **80-3275**

JOHNSTONE, A[rthur] W[eir] (1853-1905)
Experimental and microscopical studies on the origin of the blood globules. New York: G. P. Putnam's Sons, 1881. 10p. DNLM **80-3276**

JOHNSTONE'S improved adaptable porous felt splints, with directions for their employment in fractures and other surgical lesions. Philadelphia: Lehman & Bolton, [1881?]. 30p. DNLM **80-3277**

JOHNSTONE'S improved Ahl's adaptable porous splints [etc.]. Philadelphia: Lehman & Bolton, [1882?]. 40p. DNLM **80-3278**

JONES, Charles N. Dixon
Acute suppurative inflammation of the middle ear; septic meningitis; pyaemia; marked pyrexia; death in eight days. [New York, 1886.] 8p. DNLM **80-3279**

JONES, Charles N. Dixon
The radical cure of hernia. New York: D. Appleton & Co., 1887. 20p. DNLM; NNNAM **80-3280**

JONES, Charles N. Dixon
Congenital club foot; its treatment by open incision and immediate rectification. Philadelphia, 1888. 16p. DNLM **80-3281**

JONES, Charles N. Dixon
The preparation of surgical dressings by sterilization with heat. Antiseptics as used in the Woman's Hospital, Brooklyn, N.Y. New York, 1888. 16p. DNLM; NNNAM **80-3282**

JONES, H. MacNaughton (1844-1918)
Practical manual of diseases of women and uterine therapeutics. New York: D. Appleton & Co., 1884. 410p. CtY-M; DNLM; NNNAM; PPC **80-3283**

JONES, J[ohn] Harris (*b.* 1851)
A report of cases (surgical and medical). Wilkes-Barre, 1887. 15p. DNLM **80-3284**

JONES, Joseph (1833-1896)
Acts of the legislature of Louisiana, establishing and regulating quarantine for the protection of the state; organizing and defining the powers of the Board of Health, and regulating the practice of medicine, midwifery, dentistry, and pharmacy; also, rules and regulations of the Board of Health of the State of Louisiana and health ordinances of the city of New Orleans, collected and classified in accordance with resolution of the Board of Health of the State of Louisiana, September 2, 1880. New Orleans: J. S. Rivers, 1880. 97p. DNLM; LNT-M **80-3285**

JONES, Joseph (1833-1896)
Outline of the history, theory, and practice of quarantine. Relation of quarantine to constitutional and international law and to commerce. New Orleans: E. A. Brandao & Co., 1883. 30p. DNLM; LNT-M **80-3286**

JONES, Joseph (1833-1896)
Contagious and infectious diseases, measures for their prevention and arrest. Small-pox (variola); modified small-pox (varioloid); chicken-pox (varicella); cow-pox (variolae vaccinae); vaccination; spurious vaccination. Circular No. 2, prepared for the guidance of the quarantine officers and sanitary inspectors of the Board of Health of the State of Louisiana. Baton Rouge: L. Jastremski, 1884. 410p. 8 col. plates. DNLM; LNT-M **80-3287**

JONES, Joseph (1833-1896)
Quarantine and sanitary operations of the Board of Health of the State of Louisiana during 1880, 1881, 1882, and 1883. Introduction to the annual report of the Board of Health to the General Assembly of the State of Louisiana, 1883-1884. Baton Rouge: L. Jastremski, 1884. ccclxciii p. DNLM; LNT-M **80-3288**

JONES, Joseph (1833-1896)
Observations and practical results of medical service, in the Charity Hospital of New Orleans, La., 1869-1886. New Orleans: L. Graham & Son, [1886]. 45p. DNLM; LNT-M **80-3289**

JONES, Joseph (1833-1896)
Philosophical principles of education and their scientific application to the development and perfection of medical science. [New Orleans], 1888. 114p. DNLM; LNT-M **80-3290**

JONES, Joseph (1833-1896)
Contribution to teratology. Definition of teratology; giants and dwarfs; classification of monstrosities; four-legged child, J. Myrtle Corban; Siamese twins; Hungarian sisters; Carolina twins; Millie and Christine; John Allen; hermaphroditism; Miss Emily Landry, the bearded girl. [New Orleans], 1888. 41p. DNLM; LNT-M **80-3291**

JONES, Joseph (1833-1896)
Vital capacity of the lungs in health and disease, vacuum pneumatic spirometer. [New Orleans], 1888. 8p. DNLM **80-3292**

JONES, Joseph (1833-1896)
The relations of quarantine to commerce in the valley of the Mississippi River, during a period of eight years, 1880-1887 inclusive, with observations upon the general mortality of New Orleans, 1880-1889. . . . New Orleans: L. Graham & Sons, 1889. 47p. DLC; LNT-M **80-3293**

JONES, Joseph (1833-1896)
A new method of testing germicidal and antiseptic powers of certain mineral and vegetable substances employed externally and internally in the treatment of wounds, tumors, enlarged glands, ulcers and syphilis. . . . New Orleans: Joseph Jones, 1889. 27p. LNT-M **80-3294**

[JONES, Lorenzo E.]
The American eclectic materia medica and therapeutics. By John M. Scudder. . . . 10th ed., rev. and rewritten. Cincinnati: Pub. by the Author, 1883. 748p. DLC; OCLloyd **80-3295**

JONES, Mary A[manda] Dixon (1828-1908)
Removal of the uterine appendages. Nine consecutive cases. New York: Trow, 1886. 39p. DNLM; NNNAM **80-3296**

JONES, Mary A[manda] Dixon (1828-1908)
Removal of the uterine appendages (five cases). New York: William Wood & Co., 1888. 20p. DNLM; NNNAM **80-3297**

JONES, Mary A[manda] Dixon (1828-1908)
Two cases of removal of uterine myoma; one, suprapubic hysterectomy; the other, complete hysterectomy. A new method of disposing of the stump. Microscopical examination of the appendages. Remarks on the treatment of uterine myoma by electricity. [New York, 1888.] 44p. DNLM; NNNAM **80-3298**

JONES, Mary A[manda] Dixon (1828-1908)
Misplacement of the uterus. History of cases showing how in many instances they are produced; the accompanying conditions; microscopical examinations. [Pittsburgh,1889.] 32p. DNLM **80-3299**

JONES, Mary A[manda] Dixon (1828-1908)
A hitherto undescribed disease of the ovary; endothelioma changing to angeioma and haematoma. [New York, 1889.] 29p. DNLM; NNNAM **80-3300**

JONES, Paul Barrington
Pearls of wisdom, gems of knowledge for all. Common-sense prescriptions and practical information; a systematic treatment in the domestic practice of medicine. Kansas City: I. P. Moore, 1880. 150p. DNLM; OCIM **80-3301**

JONES, Roland Davis
Rheumatism, neuralgia and gout. . . . [Philadelphia, 1886.] 30p. DLC **80-3302**

JONES, Samuel A[rthur] (1834-1912)
The grounds of a homoeopath's faith. Three lectures, delivered at the request of matriculates of the Department of Medicine and Surgery (old school) of the University of Michigan. . . . New York and Philadelphia: Boericke & Tafel, 1880. 92p. DNLM; PPHa **80-3303**

JONES, Samuel A[rthur] (1834-1912)
Our indigenous remedies. [n. p., 1883.] 8p. DNLM **80-3304**

JONES, Stacy (1828-1905)
The medical genius; a guide to the cure. . . . Philadelphia: J. C. Winston & Co., 1887. 320p. DLC; DNLM; PPC; PU **80-3305**

JONES, Talbot
A case of intra-ovarian pregnancy, with post-mortem examination. Philadelphia, 1880. 11p. DNLM **80-3306**

JONES, Talbot
Some recent progress in diseases of the nervous system. [St. Louis, 1884.] 11p. DNLM **80-3307**

JORDAN, Henry J.
A practical treatise on the skin and its complicated diseases, blood poisoning and impurities. . . . New York: Pub. by the Author, 1888. 103p. DLC; NNNAM **80-3308**

JORDAN, J. Eugene
The histogenetic system: the entire revolution of medicine: the story of its discovery and of its trial; together with an arraignment of the so-called medical science of today. 2nd ed. Chicago: Hanscom Printing Co., [1888]. 189p. IEN-M; IU-M; OCIM **80-3309**

JORDAN, Johnson H.
. . . "Anatomy, physiology and laws of health"; . . . [and] "Additional diseases" [described and treated]. . . . Chicago: W. H. Moore & Co., 1885. 88p. DLC **80-3310**

JOSELIN, Benjamin Franklin (1796-1861)
The homoeopathic treatment of epidemic cholera. Therapeutics and repertory. With notes and additions by P. P. Wells. [Philadelphia], 1885. 96p. DNLM; PPHa **80-3311**

JOUSSET, Pierre (1818-1910)
Lectures on clinical medicine, delivered in the Hospital Saint-Jacques, of Paris. . . . Transl., with copious notes and additions, by R. Ludlam. . . . Chicago: S. C. Griggs & Co., 1880. 510p. DLC; IU-M; OCIM; NNNAM **80-3312**

JOYE, Thomas A.
The treatment of chronic dacryo-cystitis. [New York], 1885. 9p. DNLM **80-3313**

[JOYNES, Levin Smith] (1819-1881)
Catalogue of the valuable medical library of the late Levin S. Joynes. Richmond, Va., 1883. 10p. DNLM **80-3314**

JUDSON, Adoniram Brown (1837-1916)
Coup de fouet, or rupture of the plantaris muscle. [New York, 1881.] 6p. DNLM **80-3315**

JUDSON, Adoniram Brown (1837-1916)
The question of axillary or ischiatic support in the treatment of joint diseases of the lower extremity. New York: Trow & Co., 1881. 12p. DNLM **80-3316**

JUDSON, Adoniram Brown (1837-1916)
A practical point in the mechanical therapeutics of hip-disease. Read before the Medical Society of the County of New York, November 28, 1881. New York, 1881. 4p. DNLM **80-3317**

JUDSON, Adoniram Brown (1837-1916)
Considerations respecting the mechanical treatment of hip disease, with especial reference to the value of traction. [St. Louis, 1881.] 6p. DNLM **80-3318**

JUDSON, Adoniram Brown (1837-1916)
Some practical inferences from the pathology of hip disease. [New York, 1882.] 19p. DNLM **80-3319**

JUDSON, Adoniram Brown (1837-1916)
The history of three cases of hip-disease in the third stage. New York: E. B. Treat, 1882. 4 l. fol. DNLM **80-3320**

JUDSON, Adoniram Brown (1837-1916)
Mr. Shaw's view of the cause of rotation in lateral curvature of the spine. New York: Trow, 1882. 9p. DNLM **80-3321**

JUDSON, Adoniram Brown (1837-1916)
The fixative power of traction in the treatment of hip disease. New York: Trow, 1883. 17p. DNLM **80-3322**

JUDSON, Adoniram Brown (1837-1916)
What is the rationale of traction and counter-traction in the treatment of hip-disease? New York: Trow, 1883. 12p. DNLM **80-3323**

JUDSON, A[doniram] B[rown] (1837-1916)
Mr. Brodhurst's view of the cause of rotation in lateral curvature of the spine. New York: Trow, 1884. 7p. DNLM **80-3324**

JUDSON, Adoniram Brown (1837-1916)
The management of the abscesses of hip-disease. Read before the New York Orthopaedic Society, January 29, 1885. New York, 1885. 19p. DNLM **80-3325**

JUDSON, Adoniram Brown (1837-1916)
The mechanical treatment of talipes calcaneus. New York: Trow, 1885. 10p. DNLM **80-3326**

JUDSON, A[doniram] B[rown] (1837-1916)
The treatment of white swelling of the knee. [New York, 1886.] 17p. DNLM; NNNAM **80-3327**

JUDSON, A[doniram] B[rown] (1837-1916)
Points in the therapeutics of diseases of the joints. [New York, 1886.] 4p. DNLM **80-3328**

JUDSON, A[doniram] B[rown] (1837-1916)
The ischiatic crutch. New York: Trow, 1887. 8p. DNLM **80-3329**

JUDSON, A[doniram] B[rown] (1837-1916)
The uses of adhesive plaster in orthopaedic surgery. [New York, 1887.] 12p. DNLM **80-3330**

JUDSON, A[doniram] B[rown] (1837-1916)
The orthopedic treatment of paralysis of the anterior muscles of the thigh. New York: Trow, 1888. 8p. DNLM **80-3331**

JUDSON, A[doniram] B[rown] (1837-1916)
The American hip-splint. Philadelphia: W. F. Fell & Co., [1888]. 2 l. DNLM **80-3332**

JUDSON, A[doniram] B[rown] (1837-1916)
A practical point in the treatment of Pott's disease of the spine. [New York, 1888.] 3p. DNLM **80-3333**

JUDSON, A[doniram] B[rown] (1837-1916)
Is more conservatism desirable in the treatment of the joint diseases of children? New York: Trow, 1889. 8p. DNLM **80-3334**

JUDSON, A[doniram] B[rown] (1837-1916)
The question of interfering with the abscesses of hip diseases. [New York, 1889.] 8p. DNLM **80-3335**

JULER, Henry E[dward] (1866-1921)
A handbook of ophthalmic science and practice. Philadelphia: Henry C. Lea's Son & Co., 1884. 467p. 31 plates. 4 tab. CtY-M; DNLM; NNNAM; PPC **80-3336**

JUSTI, H. D., & CO.
Illustrated price list of dental materials. Philadelphia, 1888. 239p. PU **80-3337**

KANE, Harry Hubbell (*b.* 1854)
The hypodermic injection of morphia. Its history, advantages and dangers. (Based on the experience of 360 physicians.) . . . New York: C. L. Bermingham & Co., 1880. 354p. DLC; DNLM; NNNAM; PU **80-3338**

KANE, Harry Hubbell (*b.* 1854)
Drugs that enslave. The opium, morphine, chloral and hashisch habits. . . . Philadelphia: P. Blakiston, 1881. 224p. DLC; DNLM; PPC; PU **80-3339**

KANE, Harry Hubbell (*b.* 1854)
Opium smoking in America and China; a study of its prevalence, and effects, immediate and remote, on the individual and the nation. . . . New York: G. P. Putnam's Sons, 1882. 156p. DLC; DNLM; NNNAM; PU **80-3340**

KANE, Harry Hubbell (*b.* **1854)**
The De Quincy home method by means of which any individual can cure himself promptly, painlessly, and permanently of the opium, morphine, or chloral habit and alcoholic inebriety. New York, [1882]. 30p. DNLM; NNNAM
80-3341

KANSAS CITY HOMEOPATHIC MEDICAL COLLEGE
Annual announcements for the sessions of 1888-1889 to 1895-1896 (1.-8.); 1898-1899 to 1900-1901 (11.-13.). Kansas City, 1888-1900. DNLM [Alumni from 1889 to 1900 in announcement for 1900-1901.] **80-3342**

KANSAS CITY HOSPITAL COLLEGE OF MEDICINE
Annual announcement for the session of 1885-1886 (4). Kansas City: Wimbush-Powell Co., 1885. DNLM. [Organized in 1882; ceased to exist in 1888.] **80-3343**

KANSAS CITY MEDICAL COLLEGE
Annual announcements for the sessions of 1888-1889 to 1898-1899 (20.-30.). Kansas City, 1888-1898. DNLM [List of students and graduates for the years 1884-1885; 1887-1888 to 1897-1898, in announcements for subsequent years. List of the graduates of the Kansas City City College of Physicians and Surgeons and the Kansas City Medical College, from 1870 to 1892, in announcement for 1892-1893.]
80-3344

KANSAS ECLECTIC MEDICAL ASSOCIATION
Transactions of the meeting held February 14 and 15, 1882, at Topeka, Kansas. Topeka: Daily Capital Publ. Co., 1882. 73p. DNLM **80-3345**

KAY, Thomas W[iles] (*b.* **1858)**
The blunt curette in uterine hemorrhage. [New York, 1889.] 7p. DNLM **80-3346**

KAY, Thomas W[iles] (*b.* **1858)**
Varicocele. Cleveland, 1889. 5p. DNLM
80-3347

KAY, Thomas W[iles] (*b.* **1858)**
Urinary calculus and lithotomy. Baltimore, 1889. 8p. DNLM
80-3348

KAY, Thomas W[iles] (*b.* **1858)**
Cerebral abscess following injury of the skull. [Chicago, 1889.] 2p. DNLM **80-3349**

KAY, Thomas W[iles] (*b.* **1858)**
The radical cure of hernia. Baltimore, 1889. 8p. DNLM
80-3350

KAY, Thomas W[iles] (*b.* **1858)**
Enucleation of tuberculous glands. Baltimore: Journal Publ. Co., 1889. 11p. DNLM **80-3351**

KEATING, John Marie (1852-1893)
The mother's guide in the management and feeding of infants. . . . Philadelphia: Henry C. Lea's Son & Co., 1881. 118p. DLC; DNLM; NNNAM; PPC **80-3352**

KEATING, John Marie (1852-1893)
Weak spines in young girls, and their treatment. [Philadelphia, 1881.] 3p. DNLM **80-3353**

KEATING, John Marie (1852-1893)
The presence of the micrococcus in the blood of malignant measles; its importance in treatment. Philadelphia, 1882. 7p. DNLM **80-3354**

KEATING, John Marie (1852-1893)
How to feed the baby. A lecture delivered before the Philadelphia Hospital Training School for Nurses; with some remarks on the practical methods of preparing foods, by B. T. Fairchild. Philadelphia: W. H. Morrison, 1885. 20p. DLC; DNLM; PPC
80-3355

KEATING, John Marie (1852-1893)
The artificial feeding of infants. [Philadelphia, 1886.] 10p. DNLM **80-3356**

KEATING, John Marie (1852-1893)
The climate of south central Florida, especially for the pulmonary diseases of women and children. [New York, 1886.] 12p. DNLM **80-3357**

KEATING, John Marie (1852-1893)
A few suggestions for the preparation of milk for infants. Philadelphia, 1886. 4p. DNLM **80-3358**

KEATING, John Marie (1852-1893)
Practical lessons in nursing. Maternity, infancy, childhood. Hygiene of pregnancy; nursing and weaning of infants; the care of children in health and disease, adapted especially to the use of mothers or those intrusted with the bringing up of infants and children, and training schools for nurses, as an aid to the teachng of the nursing of women and children. Philadelphia: J. P. Lippincott Co., 1887. 221p. DLC; DNLM; NNNAM; PU **80-3359**

KEATING, John Marie (1852-1893)
Announcement. Cyclopaedia of the diseases of children, medical and surgical. By American, British, and Canadian authors. Edited by . . . . Philadelphia: J. B. Lippincott & Co., 1889. 16p. DNLM; PPC **80-3360**

KEATING, John Marie (1852-1893) and William A. EDWARDS
Diseases of the heart and circulation in infancy and adolescence. Philadelphia: P. Blakiston, Son & Co., 1888. 215p. DLC; DNLM; NNNAM; PPC **80-3361**

KEATING, John Marie (1852-1893) and William A. EDWARDS
Clinical studies on the pulse in childhood. [New York, 1888.] 15p. DNLM; NNNAM **80-3362**

KEATING, John Marie, ed. (1852-1893)
Cyclopaedia of the diseases of children, medical and surgical. These articles written especially for the work by American, British, and Canadian authors. . . . Philadelphia: J. B. Lippincott & Co., [1889-1899]. 5 v. plates. DLC; NNNAM; OCIM; PPC
80-3363

KEELEY, Leslie E. (1832?-1900)
The opium habit; its proper method of treatment and cure without suffering or inconvenience. Dwight, Ill., 1880. 15p. DNLM **80-3364**

KEELEY, Leslie E. (1832?-1900)
The morphine eater; or, from bondage to freedom; the opium, morphine, and kindred habits, [etc.]. Dwight, Ill.: C. L. Palmer & Co., 1881. 200p. DLC; DNLM; ICU; OCIM
80-3365

KEELEY, Leslie E. (1832?-1900)
An essay upon the morphine and opium habit; its proper method of treatment and cure with the double chloride of gold. . . . Dwight, Ill., [1882]. 16p. DLC **80-3366**

KEEN, William W[illiams] (1837-1932)
A lecture on the clinical anatomy of the lower extremity and especially of the knee and ankle joints. Brooklyn, 1881. 20p. DNLM **80-3367**

KEEN, William Williams (1837-1932)
Our recent debts to vivisection. The address to the graduates at the thirty-third commencement of the Woman's Medical College of Pennsylvania, March 11, 1885. . . . Philadelphia: Porter & Coates, 1885. 17p. DLC; DNLM; PPJ **80-3368**

KEEN, William Williams (1837-1932)
Pistol-shot wound of the abdomen, involving the liver, stomach, superior mesenteric artery and vein, small intestine, and kidney; laparotomy; nephrectomy; death on the fifteenth day; autopsy. [Philadelphia], 1887. 19p. DNLM **80-3369**

KEEN, William Williams (1837-1932)
Exploratory trephining and puncture of the brain almost to the lateral ventricle, for intracranial pressure supposed to be due to an abscess in the temporo-sphenoidal lobe; temporary improvement; death on the fifth day; autopsy; meningitis with effusion into the ventricles; with a description of a proposed operation to tap and drain the ventricles as a definite surgical procedure. [Philadelphia, 1888.] 23p. DNLM **80-3370**

KEEN, William Williams (1837-1932)
Three successful cases of cerebral surgery, including (1) the removal of a large intracranial fibroma; (2) exsection of damaged brain tissue; and (3) exsection of the cerebral centre for the left hand; with remarks on the general technique of such operation. Philadelphia, 1888. 43p. DNLM **80-3371**

KEEN, William Williams (1837-1932)
Deformity from prominent ears cured by a new method of operating. Philadelphia: W. J. Dornan, 1889. 4p. 1 plate. DNLM **80-3372**

KEEN, William Williams (1837-1932)
Dupuytren's finger contraction; operation of removal of the contracting band by open wound; immediate cure without reaction or pain. Philadelphia: W. J. Dornan, 1889. 5p. DNLM **80-3373**

KEETLEY, C[harles] R[obert] B[ell] (1848-1909)
An index of surgery, being a concise classification of the main facts and theories of surgery for the use of senior students and others. New York: Bermingham & Co., 1882. 208p. CtY-M; DNLM; NNNAM; PPC **80-3374**

KEETLEY, C[harles] R[obert] B[ell] (1848-1909)
An index of surgery; being a concise classification of the main facts and theories of surgery, for the use of senior students and others. . . . New York: William Wood & Co., 1882. 320p. DLC; DNLM; NNNAM; PPC **80-3375**

KEITH, B., & CO.
Manual of the active principles of indigenous and foreign medicinal plants, as prepared at the laboratory of B. Keith & Co. New York: B. Keith & Co., 1881. 65p. DNLM; NNNAM **80-3376**

KEITH, B., & CO.
Revised and enlarged manual of the active principles of indigenous and foreign medicinal plants, as prepared at the laboratory of . . . . Jersey City: Evening Journal Print, 1882. 67p. DNLM; NNNAM; OCLloyd **80-3377**

KEITH, Thomas
On ovariotomy. Louisville, Ky.: J. P. Morton & Co., 1881. 19p. DNLM **80-3378**

KELCH, A. H.
Quinquinia. Proceedings of the Academy of Medicine and Surgery, in the Polytechnic Society of Kentucky, Jan. 6, 1881. [Louisville, 1881.] 12p. DNLM **80-3379**

KELLOGG, John H[arvey] (1852-1943)
The home hand-book of domestic hygiene and rational medicine. . . . Battle Creek, Mich.: Good Health Publishing Co., 1880. 1624p. col. plates. DLC; OCIM **80-3380**

KELLOGG, John H[arvey] (1852-1943)
A new form of suture pin for use in perineorrhaphy. [Chicago, 1887.] 4p. DNLM **80-3381**

KELLOGG, John H[arvey] (1852-1943)
Oxygen enemata. [Detroit, 1887.] 9p. DNLM **80-3382**

KELLOGG, John H[arvey] (1852-1943)
The radical cure of retro-displacements of the uterus and procidentia by Alexander's operation and median colporrhaphy. [Detroit, 1887.] 20p. 3 plates. DNLM **80-3383**

KELLOGG, John H[arvey] (1852-1943)
Experimental researches respecting the relation of dress to pelvic diseases in women. [Detroit], 1888. 22p. 5 plates. DNLM **80-3384**

KELLOGG, John H[arvey] (1852-1943)
New form of posterior colporrhaphy. [Boston, 1888.] 6p. DNLM **80-3385**

KELLOGG, John H[arvey] (1852-1943)
Plain facts for old and young; embracing the natural history and hygiene of organic life. New ed. Burlington, Iowa: I. F. Segner & Co., 1888. 644p. DNLM; OCIM **80-3386**

KELLOGG, John H[arvey] (1852-1943)
Report of forty-eight cases of Alexander's operation. Chicago, 1888. 33p. DNLM **80-3387**

KELLY, Howard A[twood] (1858-1943)
Removal of an ovarian cyst weighing one hundred and sixteen pounds; recovery. New York: William Wood & Co., 1885. 6p. DNLM **80-3388**

KELLY, Howard A[twood] (1858-1943)
A contribution to hepato-phlebotomy. Philadelphia, 1887. 8p. DNLM **80-3389**

KELLY, Howard A[twood] (1858-1943)
Hysterorrhaphy. New York: William Wood & Co., 1887. 16p. DNLM **80-3390**

KELLY, Howard A[twood] (1858-1943)
Results of some general work in abdominal surgery performed during seven and one-half months of 1886. Philadelphia: W. J. Dornan, 1887. 8p. DNLM **80-3391**

KELLY, Howard A[twood] (1858-1943)
A case of Caesarean section. Philadelphia, 1888. 7p. DNLM **80-3392**

KELLY, Howard A[twood] (1858-1943)
Discussion on the new Caesarean section. Philadelphia: W. J. Dornan, 1888. 8p. DNLM **80-3393**

KELLY, Howard A[twood] (1858-1943)
Hysterorrhaphy. [Philadelphia, 1888.] 14p. DNLM **80-3394**

KELLY, Howard A[twood] (1858-1943)
Palpation of the ureters in the female. Philadelphia: W. J. Dornan, 1888. 14p. DNLM **80-3395**

KELSEY, Charles B[oyd] (1850-1917)
The surgical treatment of cancer of the rectum. [Philadelphia, 1880.] 4 l. DNLM **80-3396**

KELSEY, Charles B[oyd] (1850-1917)
External rectotomy as a substitute for lumbar colotomy in the treatment of stricture of the rectum. New York: D. Appleton & Co., 1880. 12p. DNLM **80-3397**

KELSEY, Charles B[oyd] (1850-1917)
On division of the sphincter and muscle as a therapeutic measure. New York: D. Appleton & Co., 1880. 8p. DNLM **80-3398**

KELSEY, Charles B[oyd] (1850-1917)
An analysis of one hundred and forty cases of excision of cancer of the rectum. [New York, 1880.] 14p. DNLM **80-3399**

KELSEY, Charles B[oyd] (1850-1917)
The diagnosis of cancer of the rectum. [New York: D. Appleton & Co., 1881.] 20p. DNLM **80-3400**

KELSEY, Charles B[oyd] (1850-1917)
On rectal exploration and diagnosis. [New York: D. Appleton & Co., 1881.] 15p. DNLM **80-3401**

KELSEY, Charles Boyd (1850-1917)
Stricture of the rectum: a study of one hundred and thirty-eight cases. . . . 2nd ed., enl. [New York? 1881?] 15p. DNLM **80-3402**

KELSEY, Charles Boyd (1850-1917)
Diseases of the rectum and anus. . . . New York: William Wood & Co., 1882. 299p. DLC; DNLM; NNNAM; PPC **80-3403**

KELSEY, Charles Boyd (1850-1917)
The pathology, diagnosis and treatment of diseases of the rectum and anus. . . . New York: William Wood & Co., 1884. 416p. col. plates. DLC; DNLM; NNNAM; PU **80-3404**

KELSEY, Charles B[oyd] (1850-1917)
How to treat haemorrhoids by injections of carbolic acid. New York, 1885. 8p. DNLM **80-3405**

KELSEY, Charles B[oyd] (1850-1917)
The cure of fissure of the anus without operation. New York, 1886. 7p. DNLM **80-3406**

KELSEY, Charles B[oyd] (1850-1917)
The diagnosis and treatment of haemorrhoids; with general rules as to the examination of rectal diseases. Detroit: G. S. Davis, 1887. 78p. DNLM; NNNAM; OCIM **80-3407**

KEMP, William M[iller] (1814-1886)
What Baltimore did in a sanitary way during the yellow fever in Norfolk and Portsmouth in 1855. Baltimore, 1882. 13p. DNLM; MdU-D **80-3408**

KEMPER, W[illiam] H[arrison] (1839-1927)
Practical thoughts for physicians. [Indianapolis, 1887.] 12p. DNLM **80-3409**

KEMPF, E. J.
Fifty aphorisms in pregnancy. Louisville, 1888. 16p. DNLM **80-3410**

KEMPF, E. J.
Should the state take care of its inebriates? Read to the Mitchell District Medical Society, at Seymour, Indiana, December 28, 1888. [n. p., 1888.] 24p. DNLM **80-3411**

KENDALL, B. J., & CO.
The doctor at home, illustrated, treating the diseases of man and the horse. Enosburgh Falls, Vt., 1887. 96p. DNLM **80-3412**

KENISTON, J[ames] M[ortimer] (*b.* 1848)
Paraldehyde. [Utica, N.Y., 1888.] 5p. DNLM **80-3413**

KENNEDY, J. C.
The medical magician. Part I. How to preserve health and cure disease. An exposition of the progress of medical knowledge as exemplified in the successful treatment of obstinate and long-standing maladies by the new method cure. . . . Cincinnati, Detroit, Louisville, 1887. 224p. IU-M; OCIM **80-3414**

KENNEDY, J[osiah] F[orrest] (*b.* 1834)
Typhoid fever, its cause and prevention. [With appendix on disinfection and disinfectants.] Des Moines, Iowa: Carter & Hussey, 1886. 14p. DNLM **80-3415**

KENNEDY, Stiles
Iodoform. A powerful alterative and general tonic, valuable as a remedy in scrofula, anaemia, neuralgia, chlorosis, and rheumatism. Philadelphia, 1880. 14p. DNLM **80-3416**

KENNEDY, William Sloane (1850-1929)
Oliver Wendell Holmes; poet, littérateur, scientist. Boston: S. E. Cassino & Co., 1883. 356p. ICU; MB; MH; NN **80-3417**

KENNER, Robert C. (*b.* 1859)
The treatment of intermittent fever. Louisville: J. P. Morton & Co., 1888. 36p. DNLM; OCIM **80-3418**

KENSINGTON HOSPITAL FOR WOMEN, PHILADELPHIA
Annual reports of the board of directors and officers to the contributors. 5.-19., 1887-1888 to 1901-1902. Philadelphia, 1889-1903. DNLM [Organized in 1884, and incorporated June 11, 1887. No reports were issued until 1889. In 1890 began to number reports from the year of organization.]
80-3419

KENT, J[ames] Tyler (1849-1916)
An address before the Central New York Homoeopathic Society at Rochester, N.Y., Dec. 17, 1885. [n. p., 1885.] 2 l. DNLM **80-3420**

KENT, J[ames] Tyler (1849-1916)
Address before the International Hahnemannian Association, at its seventh annual meeting, held at Long Branch, New Jersey, June 21st and 24th, 1887. [Philadelphia, 1887.] 9p. DNLM; PPHa **80-3421**

KERLIN, Isaac N[ewton] (1834-1893)
Enumeration, classification, and causation of idiocy. Philadelphia: Collins, 1880. 30p. DNLM **80-3422**

KERLIN, Isaac N[ewton] (1834-1893)
The epileptic change, and its appearance among feeble-minded children. [1882.] 13p. DNLM **80-3423**

KERLIN, Isaac N[ewton] (1834-1893) and H. M. GREENE
Idiotic and feeble-minded children. Report of standing committee to the Eleventh National Conference of Charities and Reforms, St. Louis, 1884. Boston: G. H. Ellis, 1884. 28p. DNLM; MH **80-3424**

KERLIN, Isaac N[ewton] (1834-1893)
Provision for idiotic and feeble-minded children. . . . [*Also*:] The state's duty toward epileptics. By George H. Knight. [Boston, 1886.] 18p. DNLM; MBM **80-3425**

KERLIN, Isaac N[ewton] (1834-1893) and John M. BROOMALL
Moral imbecility; two papers read before the Association of Medical Officers of American Institutions for Idiotic and Feeble-Minded Persons. Philadelphia: J. B. Lippincott Co., 1889. 12p. DNLM **80-3426**

KERN, Horatio G.
Illustrated catalogue of surgical and dental instruments, orthopedical appliances, trusses, etc. Philadelphia: H. L. Butler, 1885. 110p. DNLM; PPC **80-3427**

KERR, Norman S[hanks] (1834-1899)
Inebriety. Philadelphia: P. Blakiston, Son & Co., 1888. 415p. DNLM; !EN-M; PPC; PU **80-3428**

KERSHAW, J. Martine
Care of mother and child in the lying-in room. St. Louis, 1886. 8p. DNLM **80-3429**

KESSLER, Adolph
A contribution to the hypodermic ergot treatment of uterine myomata. Large interstitial myoma; complete disappearance after ergot hypodermically; speedy pregnancy; return of tumor; abortion; septicemia; death; remarks. New York: William Wood & Co., 1880. 17p. DNLM; NNNAM
80-3430

KESSLER, Adolph
Fatal poisoning by mushrooms. [Philadelphia, 1880.] 6p. DNLM **80-3431**

KETCH, Samuel (1855?-1899)
Remarks on lateral curvature, with special reference to its occurrence in children. New York: Lehmaier & Bro., 1886. 13p. NNNAM **80-3432**

KEYES, E[dward] L[awrence] (1843-1924)
The venereal diseases, including stricture of the male urethra. . . . New York: William Wood & Co., 1880. 348p. DLC; DNLM; NNNAM; PPC **80-3433**

KEYES, E[dward] L[awrence] (1843-1924)
Litholapaxy. New York: G. P. Putnam's Sons, 1880. 18p. DNLM; NNNAM **80-3434**

KEYES, E[dward] L[awrence] (1843-1924)
Rapid lithotrity with evacuation. [New York, 1880.] 26p. DNLM; NNNAM **80-3435**

KEYES, E[dward] L[awrence] (1843-1924)
Arterio-venous aneurism. [Richmond, 1881.] 15p. DNLM
80-3436

KEYES, E[dward] L[awrence] (1843-1924)
The curability of urethral stricture by electricity. New York, 1888. 24p. 1 tab. DNLM; NNNAM
80-3437

KEYES, E[dward] L[awrence] (1843-1924)
The surgical diseases of the genito-urinary organs, including syphilis. A revision of Van Buren and Keyes's text-book upon the same subjects. New York: D. Appleton & Co., 1888. 704p. DLC; DNLM; NNNAM; PU **80-3438**

KEYSER, P[eter] D[irch] (1835-1897)
Some ophthalmological observations during ten years' service in Wills' Eye Hospital. Philadelphia: Collins, 1883. 46p. DNLM; PPC **80-3439**

KEYSER, P[eter] D[irch] (1835-1897)
Neoplasm of the lachrymal gland. Chicago: Review Printing Co., 1884. 8p. DNLM **80-3440**

KEYSER, P[eter] D[irch] (1835-1897)
The relation of medical colleges to preliminary education. [n. p., 1884.] 3p. DNLM **80-3441**

KEYSER, P[eter] D[irch] (1835-1897)
An instrument for measuring the face and eyes for the proper adjustment of spectacle-frames; also, a diagram for recording cases of refraction and accommodation, and for the prescribing of spectacles. [1884.] 2p. DNLM **80-3442**

KEYSER, P[eter] D[irch] (1835-1897)
Cocaine in ophthalmic surgery. [Detroit, 1885.] 8p. DNLM
80-3443

KEYT, Alonzo T[hrasher] (1827-1885)
A contribution to the cardio-sphygmography of tricuspid lesions. New York: G. P. Putnam's Sons, 1882. 6p. 2 diag. DNLM **80-3444**

KEYT, Alonzo T[hrasher] (1827-1885)
The claims of the graphic method. [Cincinnati, 1882.] 12p. DNLM **80-3445**

KEYT, Alonzo T[hrasher] (1827-1885)
An experiment in cardio-sphygmography, in which the heart, carotid, femoral, radial, and posterior tibial arteries, and the corresponding time, were traced simultaneously, with reproduction of the inscriptions obtained. New York: G. P. Putnam's Sons, 1882. 5p. 1 diag. DNLM
80-3446

KEYT, Alonzo T[hrasher] (1827-1885)
An experimental inquiry into the causes of the variations of pulse-wave velocity and duration of the cardio-aortic or presphygmic interval observed in man, etc. Chicago: A. G. Newell, 1883. 28p. DNLM **80-3447**

KEYT, Alonzo T[hrasher] (1827-1885)
Instructions relating to the use and management of Keyt's compound sphygmograph. [1884.] 8p. DNLM
80-3448

KEYT, Alonzo T[hrasher] (1827-1885)
Sphygmography and cardiography, physiological and clinical. Edited by Asa B. Isham and M. H. Keyt. New York & London: G. P. Putnam's Sons, 1887. 229p. DNLM; NNNAM; OCIM; PPC **80-3449**

KIDDER, Jerome Henry (1842-1889)
Note on the microscopic appearances presented by the blood of scarlatina and typhoid fever. Washington, 1882. 4p. 1 phot. plate. DNLM **80-3450**

KILMER, Fred. B[arnett] (*b.* 1851)
Review of the new drugs introduced during the past ten years. [n. p., 1882.] 19p. DNLM **80-3451**

KILNER, Walter B.
A compendium of modern pharmacy and druggists' formulary. . . . Springfield, Ill.: H. W. Rokker, printer, 1880. 478p. DLC; OCLloyd; PU **80-3452**

KILNER, Walter B.
A compendium of modern pharmacy and druggists' formulary. . . . 2nd ed. . . . Springfield, Ill.: H. W. Rokker, printer, 1881. 686p. DLC; OCLloyd; NNNAM; PPC **80-3453**

KIMBALL, Samuel A[yer]
A repertory of gonorrhoea, with the concomitant symptoms of the genital and urinary organs. Boston & Providence: O. Clapp & Son, 1888. 53p. DNLM; MH-M; NNNAM; PPHa
80-3454

KING, Albert F[reeman] A[fricanus] (1841-1914)
A manual of obstetrics. . . . Philadelphia: Henry C. Lea's Son & Co., 1882. 325p. DLC; DNLM; NNNAM; PPC
80-3455

KING, Albert F[reeman] A[fricanus] (1841-1914) and Philip G. WALES
Addresses delivered at the sixty-first annual commencement of the National Medical College (medical department of the Columbian University), March 15, 1883. Washington, D.C.: W. H. Moore, 1883. 17p. DNLM **80-3456**

KING, Albert F[reeman] A[fricanus] (1841-1914)
A manual of obstetrics. . . . 2nd ed. Philadelphia: Henry C. Lea's Son & Co., 1884. 338p. DLC; DNLM; NNNAM; PPC
80-3457

KING, Albert F[reeman] A[fricanus] (1841-1914)
On obstructed labor from short or coiled funis, and its treatment by change of position from recumbency to sitting. [Washington, 1885.] 7p. DNLM **80-3458**

KING, Albert F[reeman] A[fricanus] (1841-1914)
A manual of obstetrics. 3rd ed. Philadelphia: Lea Bros. & Co., 1886. 379p. DLC; DNLM; NNNAM; OCIM
80-3459

KING, Albert F[reeman] A[fricanus] (1841-1914)
Dystocia from short or coiled funis, and its treatment. Chicago, 1887. 15p. DNLM **80-3460**

KING, Albert F[reeman] A[fricanus] (1841-1914)
A new explanation of the renal troubles, eclampsia, and other pathological phenomena of pregnancy and labor. New York: William Wood & Co., 1887. 44p. DNLM; NNNAM
80-3461

KING, Albert F[reeman] A[fricanus] (1841-1914)
The physiological argument in obstetric studies and practice. New York: William Wood & Co., 1888. 18p. DLC; DNLM; NNNAM **80-3462**

KING, Albert F[reeman] A[fricanus] (1841-1914)
The natural rectification of malpresentations, and its imitation by art. New York: William Wood & Co., 1889. 21p. 2 plates. DNLM; NNNAM **80-3463**

KING, Albert F[reeman] A[fricanus] (1841-1914)
What is the normal posture for a parturient woman? New York: William Wood & Co., 1889. 23p. DNLM; NNNAM
80-3464

KING, Albert F[reeman] A[fricanus] (1841-1914)
A manual of obstetrics. 4th ed. Philadelphia: Lea Bros. & Co., 1889. 431p. DLC; DNLM; IU-M; PPC
80-3465

KING, Charles
Puerperal mania. Columbus, O., 1883. 8p. DNLM
80-3466

[KING, David] (1812-1882)
David King, M.D. By Wm. Dehon King. . . . [Providence]: Providence Press, 1882. 11p. RHi; RPM
80-3467

[KING, David] (1812-1882)
Catalogue of the library of the late David King, of Newport, R.I. Pt. 2. New York, 1884. 252p. DNLM; NNNAM
80-3468

KING, Ernest F.
Hysteria of a grave form in three successive pregnancies. Case. Chicago, 1888. 4p. DNLM **80-3469**

KING, E. H.
Treatment of the umbilicus in the new-born. Why should we use the belly-band on the infant? Davenport, Iowa, 1885. 25p. DNLM **80-3470**

KING, Enoch W[ood] (1846-1882)
Statistics of placenta previa. Collected from the practice of physicians in the State of Indiana. [New York, 1880.] 50p. DNLM **80-3471**

KING, John (1813-1893)
Supplement to the American dispensatory. By John King . . . and John U. Lloyd. . . . Cincinnati: Wilstach, Baldwin & Co., 1880. 202p. plates. DLC; OCLloyd; PU
80-3472

KING, John (1813-1893)
The American eclectic dispensatory. . . . 10th ed., rev. and enl. Cincinnati: Wilstach, Baldwin & Co., 1886. 1439p. + Supp., 202p. OCLoyd; PU **80-3473**

KING, Julius [Optical Co.]
Synopsis of lectures on the eye and the correction of defects of vision. . . . [Cleveland, O.: Brooks & Co., printers], 1888. 31p. diags. DLC **80-3474**

KING, William Harvey (*b.* 1861)
Electro-therapeutics, or electricity in its relation to medicine and surgery. New York: A. L. Chatterton & Co., 1889. 153p. NNNAM; PPHa **80-3475**

KING, Willis P[ercival] (1839-1909)
Quacks and quackery in Missouri. [St. Louis, 1882.] 35p. DNLM **80-3476**

KINGSLEY, George L[yle] (1864-1890)
A method of determining the angle of flexion of the diseased leg in hip disease. [Boston, 1888.] 3p. DNLM
80-3477

KINGSLEY, Norman W[illiam] (1829-1913)
A treatise on oral deformities as a branch of mechanical surgery. New York: D. Appleton & Co., 1880. 541p. DNLM; MdU-D; NNNAM; PU **80-3478**

KINGSLEY, Norman W[illiam] (1829-1913)
Civilization in its relation to the decay of the teeth. New York: D. Appleton & Co., [1881]. 10p. DNLM
80-3479

KINGSLEY, Norman W[illiam] (1829-1913)
Woman; an oration delivered before the American Academy of Dental Science. Boston: T. Todd, 1883. 20p. DNLM
80-3480

KINGSLEY, Norman W[illiam] (1829-1913)
Dentistry not a specialty in medicine. [Buffalo, 1887.] 15p. DNLM **80-3481**

KINGSLEY, Norman W[illiam] (1829-1913)
Dentistry not a specialty in medicine. Nashville, 1887. 15p. DNLM **80-3482**

KINLOCH, Robert Alexander (1826-1891)
Education the means for unifying the medical profession and strengthening the State Medical Association. Charleston: E. Perry, 1884. 26p. DNLM; ScCM **80-3483**

KINLOCH, R[obert] A[lexander] (1826-1891)
Two laparotomies on same patient; removal of both ovaries for cystic disease, and also a large tumor of the mesentery; silk ligature passes into the bladder and serves as the nucleus of a calculus. [Charleston, 1887.] 3p. DNLM
80-3484

KINNEAR, B[everley] O.
Explanatory remarks upon neurodynamic medicine, with cases. Cambridge: Riverside Press, 1883. 24p. DNLM; MBM
80-3485

KINNEAR, B[everley] O.
The dangers of an unskilful or careless application of heat and cold to the spine. New York: Trow, 1884. 14p. DNLM
80-3486

KINNEAR, B[everley] O.
Cholera, and its treatment by John Chapman's method, and twelve cases, with some answers to the microbe theory of the disease, and a full report of the discussion. Boston: D. Clapp & Son, 1885. 19p. DNLM; MBM **80-3487**

KINNEAR, B[everley] O.
Uterine diseases treated by heat and cold over the spinal cord and sympathetic ganglia. Boston, 1888. 4 l. DNLM
80-3488

KINNICUTT, Francis P[arker] (1846-1913)
Transient albuminuria as it occurs, particularly in children and adolescents, in apparent health. New York: G. P. Putnam's Sons, 1882. 19p. DNLM; NNNAM **80-3489**

KINNICUTT, Francis P[arker] (1846-1913)
Nitro-glycerine in the treatment of chronic nephritis. New York, 1886. 19p. DNLM; NNNAM **80-3490**

KIPP, Charles J[ohn] (1835-1911)
On gonorrhoic irido-choroiditis. New York: Trow's Co., 1880. 10p. DNLM **80-3491**

KIPP, Charles J[ohn] (1835-1911)
On eye affections from malarial poisoning. Newark, N.J.: L. J. Hardham, 1881. 12p. DNLM **80-3492**

KIPP, Charles J[ohn] (1835-1911)
Clinical notes on cases of foreign bodies lodged in or on the iris, and in the anterior chamber. St. Louis, Mo.: J. H. Chambers & Co., [1884]. 11p. DNLM
80-3493

KIPP, Charles J[ohn] (1835-1911)
Cases of disease of the frontal sinus. [New Bedford, 1884.] 8p. DNLM **80-3494**

KIPP, Charles J[ohn] (1835-1911)
A case of fatal ear disease. beginning as a circumscribed inflammation in the outer half of the external auditory canal. New Bedford, 1885, 8p. DNLM **80-3495**

KIPP, Charles J[ohn] (1835-1911)
On the significance of the development of optic neuritis in cases of purulent inflammation of the middle ear. New York, 1885. 5p. DNLM **80-3496**

KIPP, Charles J[ohn] (1835-1911)
A case of double vascular exophthalmos; recovery under intermittent compression of the right carotid artery and the internal use of the iodide of potassium; cocaine conjunctivitis. [Hartford, 1888.] 8p. DNLM **80-3497**

KIPP, Charles J[ohn] (1835-1911)
Three cases of transient bilaterial horizontal nystagmus occurring in connection with purulent inflammation of the middle ear. [New Bedford, 1888.] 18p. DNLM
80-3498

KIPPAX, John R[obert] (*b.* 1849)
A hand book of skin diseases and their homoeopathic treatment. Chicago: Duncan Bros., 1880. 208p. DNLM; PPHa
80-3499

KIPPAX, John R[obert] (*b.* **1849**)
A hand book of skin diseases and their homoeopathic treatment. 2nd ed. Chicago: Duncan Bros., 1882. 212p. OCIM; PPHa **80-3500**

KIPPAX, John R[obert] (*b.* **1849**)
Lectures on fevers. Delivered at the Chicago Homoeopathic Medical College; with a few additional lectures. Chicago: Gross & Delbridge, 1883. 400p. DLC; DNLM; IU-M; OCIM **80-3501**

KIPPAX, John R[obert] (*b.* **1849**)
A hand book of skin diseases and their homoeopathic treatment. 3rd ed. Revised, enlarged and illustrated. Chicago: Duncan Bros., 1884. 292p. DLC; PPHa **80-3502**

KIPPAX, John R[obert] (*b.* **1849**)
A hand book of skin diseases and their homoeopathic treatment. 4th ed. Chicago: Gross & Delbridge, 1885. 294p. DNLM; OCIM; PPHa **80-3503**

KIRBY, Edmund A.
On the value of phosphorus, as a remedy for loss of nerve power and functional disorders of the nervous system, induced by over-work and the exigencies of modern life. With formulae and directions for treatment. 5th ed. Philadelphia: P. Blakiston, 1881. 105p. DNLM; NNNAM; PPC; PU **80-3504**

KIRK, Edward C[ameron] (1856-1933)
A contribution to the etiology of erosion. Philadelphia, 1887. 9p. DNLM **80-3505**

KIRKBRIDE, Thomas Story (1809-1883)
On the construction, organization, and general arrangements of hospitals for the insane. With some remarks on insanity and its treatment. . . . 2nd ed. With revisions, additions, and new illustrations. Philadelphia, London: J. B. Lippincott & Co., 1880. 320p. 22 plates. DLC; DNLM; NNNAM; PU **80-3506**

KIRKBRIDE, Thomas Story (1809-1883)
Memoir of Isaac Ray, M.D., LL.D. Philadelphia, 1881. 19p. DNLM; PPC **80-3507**

[KIRKBRIDE, Thomas Story (1809-1883)]
Memoir of Thomas S. Kirkbride, prepared by direction of the Association of Medical Superintendents of American Institutions for the Insane. By John Curwen, Charles H. Nichols, John H. Callender. Read at the meeting of the Association at Saratoga, New York, June 16, 1885. Warren, Pa.: Cowan, 1885. 38p. NNNAM; PPC; PU **80-3508**

KIRKES, William Senhouse (1823-1864)
Manual of physiology. . . . Edited by W. Morrant Baker and Vincent Dormer Harris. 11th ed. New York: William Wood & Co., 1885. 2 v. 1 plate. DNLM; NNNAM; OCIM; PU **80-3509**

KIRKES, William Senhouse (1823-1864)
Manual of physiology. . . . By W. Morrant Baker and Vincent Dormer Harris. 12th ed. Philadelphia: P. Blakiston, Son & Co., 1889. 880p. 3 plates. CtY-M; DNLM; PPC; PU **80-3510**

KIRWAN, G[eorge] H[enry] (1856-1895)
Hemorrhoids and their treatment. [Philadelphia, 1888.] 19p. DNLM; PPC **80-3511**

KITCHEN, J[oseph] M[oses] W[ard] (1846-1931)
Students' manual of diseases of the nose and throat; a digest, descriptive of the more commonly seen diseases of the upper air-tract, with the methods of their treatment. . . . New York: G. P. Putnam's Sons, 1883. 127p. DLC; NNNAM; OCIM; PPC **80-3512**

KITCHEN, Joseph Moses Ward (1846-1931)
Catarrh, sore-throat and hoarseness; a description of the construction, action, and use of the nasal passages and throat. . . . New York, [etc.]: G. P. Putnam's Sons, 1884. 80p. DLC; DNLM; NNNAM; PPC **80-3513**

KITCHEN, Joseph Moses Ward (1846-1931)
Consumption; its nature, causes, prevention and cure. . . . New York, London: G. P. Putnam's Sons, 1885. 223p. DLC; DNLM; NNNAM; PU **80-3514**

KLEIN, Carl H. von
A manual of medical jurisprudence, instructing how to conduct inquests and post-mortems, and how to give official and expert testimony before courts of law, in cases of homicide. Hamilton, O., 1882. 35p. DNLM **80-3515**

KLEIN, Carl H. von
Tabulae anatomicae osteologiae. Cincinnati: Lithographic Co., 1883. 3 p. l. 32 plates. DNLM; OCIM **80-3516**

KLEIN, Carl H. von
Jewish hygiene and diet, the Talmud and various other Jewish writings, heretofore untranslated. [Chicago, 1884.] 22p. DNLM **80-3517**

KLEIN, Carl H. von
Tabulae anatomicae osteologiae. Editio emendata. Cincinnati: Cincinnati Lithographic Co., 1885. 2 p. l. 32 plates. DNLM; OCIM **80-3518**

KLEIN, Carl H. von
Medical jurisprudence in divorce. Dayton, O., [1885]. 8p. DNLM **80-3519**

KLEIN, Carl H. von
Voice in singers. Columbus, O.: Harn & Adair, 1885. 8p. DNLM **80-3520**

KLEIN, Carl H. von
Rhinology in the past and of the future. Chicago, 1886. 15p. DNLM **80-3521**

KLEIN, Carl H. von
Address on rhinology. The president's address before the American Rhinological Association. Chicago, 1888. 12p. DNLM **80-3522**

KLEIN, Carl H. von
New and illustrative points in examination of the nose and throat. Philadelphia: Records, Mullin & Co., 1888. 7p. DNLM **80-3523**

KLEIN, [Edward] Emanuel (1844-1925)
Elements of histology. Philadelphia: Henry C. Lea's son & Co., 1883. 352p. CtY-M; DNLM; NNNAM; PPC **80-3524**

KLINE, Robert H.
Woman. Her diseases and their treatment. . . . [Philadelphia, 1889.] 67p. DLC; PPC; PU **80-3525**

KLINGENSMITH, I[srael] P[utnam] (1850?-1904)
Hay asthma. Greensburg, Pa., 1887. 8p. DNLM
80-3526

KLOPHEL, C. G. Buchanan
Tuberculosis; with remarks on some of its manifestations and treatment. Memphis: E. Whitmore, [1886]. 40p. DNLM
80-3527

KLOPHEL, C. G. Buchanan
Gun-shot, stab, and other penetrating wounds of the abdomen. [Memphis, 1888.] 4p. DNLM **80-3528**

KLOPHEL, C. G. Buchanan
Xeroderma pigmentosum. [Memphis, 1888.] 8p. 1 plate. DNLM **80-3529**

KLOTZ, Herman G[ustav] (*b.* 1844)
Clinical observations on endoscopy of the male urethra. [New York, 1886.] 30p. DNLM; NNNAM
80-3530

KLOTZ, Herman G[ustav] (*b.* 1844)
On the advantages of a compound salicylated plaster in dermatological and surgical practice. [New York, 1887.] 11p. DNLM
80-3531

KLOTZ, Herman G[ustav] (*b.* 1844)
On the occurrence of ulcers resulting from spontaneous gangrene of the skin during the later stages of syphilis, and their relation to syphilis. [New York, 1887.] 12p. DNLM
80-3532

KLOTZ, Herman G[ustav] (*b.* 1844)
A case of syphilis in which several fingers of both hands became cold and livid; suspected arteritis. [Philadelphia, 1889.] 5p. DNLM **80-3533**

KNAPP, J[akob] Hermann (1832-1911)
Some observations concerning the value of the audiphone. [New York, 1880.] 9p. DNLM **80-3534**

KNAPP, J[akob] Hermann (1832-1911)
Methods of medical instruction. Introductory address delivered to the students of the medical department of the University of the City of New York, October 2, 1883. New York: Trow's Printing Co., 1883. 23p. DNLM; NNNAM
80-3535

KNAPP, J[akob] Hermann (1832-1911)
Cocaine and its use in ophthalmic and general surgery. With supplementary contributions by Drs. F. H. Bosworth, R. J. Hall, E. L. Keyes, H. Knapp, and Wm. M. Polk. New York & London: G. P. Putnam's Sons, 1885. 1 p. l. 87 plates. DNLM; NNNAM; PPC; PU **80-3536**

KNAPP, J[akob] H[ermann] (1832-1911)
Dioptry or dioptric? [New York, 1886.] 1 galley sheet. DNLM
80-3537

KNAPP, J[akob] H[ermann] (1832-1911)
Fermentation, putrefaction, and suppuration, with demonstrations and experiments. New York, 1886. 22p. DNLM; NNNAM
80-3538

KNAPP, J[akob] H[ermann] (1832-1911)
Report on a second series of one hundred successive cataract extractions without iridectomy. [New York, 1889.] 11p. DNLM **80-3539**

KNAPP, Philip Coombs (1858-1920)
A case of professional neurosis of coordination of unusual origin. [New York, 1887.] 5p. DNLM **80-3540**

KNAPP, Philip Coombs (1858-1920)
Hemiplegia in childhood. [New York, 1887.] 23p. DNLM; NNNAM **80-3541**

KNAPP, Philip Coombs (1858-1920)
Nervous affections following injury. "Concussion of the spine," "railway spine," and "railway brain." Boston: Cupples & Hurd, 1888. 35p. DNLM; MBM **80-3542**

KNAPP, Philip Coombs (1858-1920)
Some post-hemiplegic disturbances of motion in children. Boston: Cupples & Hurd, 1888. 12p. DNLM; MBM
80-3543

KNAPP, Philip Coombs (1858-1920)
Methods of examination in medico-legal cases involving suits for damages for real or supposed injuries to the brain and spinal cord. Boston: Damrell & Upham, 1889. 24p. DNLM; MBM **80-3544**

KNAPP, Philip Coombs (1858-1920) and E. H. BRADFORD
A case of tumor of the brain; removal; death. [Boston, 1889.] 43p. DNLM; MBM **80-3545**

KNIGHT, Charles Huntoon, ed. (1849-1913)
. . . A year-book of surgery for 1883; . . . New York, [etc.]: G. P. Putnam's Sons, 1884. 197p. DLC; DNLM; NNNAM
80-3546

KNIGHT, Charles Huntoon (1849-1913)
Abscess of the tongue, with report of a case. [New York, 1885.] 8p. DNLM **80-3547**

KNIGHT, Charles Huntoon (1849-1913)
Paralysis of the velum palati in acute naso-pharyngitis. [New York, 1886.] 8p. DNLM **80-3548**

KNIGHT, Charles Huntoon (1849-1913)
A case of perichondritis of the larynx; necrosis of the cricoid. [New York, 1887.] 6p. DNLM **80-3549**

KNIGHT, Charles Huntoon (1849-1913)
The galvano-cautery in the treatment of hypertrophied tonsils. [New York, 1887.] 9p. DNLM **80-3550**

KNIGHT, Charles Huntoon (1849-1913)
Congenital bony occlusion of the posterior nares. Philadelphia, 1888. 12p. DNLM **80-3551**

KNIGHT, Charles Huntoon (1849-1913)
The diagnosis and treatment of certain forms of rhinitis. [New York, 1889.] 11p. DNLM **80-3552**

KNIGHT, Charles Huntoon (1849-1913)
Note on the galvano-cautery in the treatment of hypertrophied tonsils. [New York, 1889.] 10p. DNLM
80-3553

KNIGHT, Frederick Irving (1841-1909)
Chorea laryngis. [New York: G. P. Putnam's Son, 1883.] 7p. DNLM **80-3554**

KNIGHT, Frederick Irving (1841-1909)
Laryngeal vertigo. New York, 1886. 12p. DNLM
80-3555

KNIGHT, Frederick Irving (1841-1909)
Indications and contra-indications for altitude in the treatment of pulmonary tuberculosis. [Philadelphia, 1888.] 8p. DNLM **80-3556**

KNIGHT, Frederick Irving (1841-1909)
On the selection of a climate for patients with pulmonary tuberculosis. Boston: Cupples & Hurd, 1888. 12p. DNLM **80-3557**

KNIGHT, Frederick Irving (1841-1909)
The climatic treatment of bronchial asthma. Philadelphia: W. J. Dornan, 1889. 8p. DNLM **80-3558**

KNIGHT, James (1810-1887)
A paper read before the Academy of Medicine, June 15th, 1882. . . . New York: E. W. Sackett & Rankin, printers and stationers, 1882. 15p. DLC; DNLM; NNNAM **80-3559**

KNIGHT, James (1810-1887)
Orthopaedia, or a practical treatise on the aberrations of the human form. 2nd ed. New York: J. H. Vail & Co., 1884. 388p. 5 plates. DLC; DNLM; NNNAM **80-3560**

KNIGHT, James (1810-1887)
Results of observations in the treatment of 2,072 cases of lateral curvature of the spine during a period of twenty-three years in the Hospital of the New York Society for the Relief of the Ruptured and Crippled. [New York, 1885.] 2 l. DNLM **80-3561**

KNIGHT, L. A.
Asthma, its cause and cure. Hay fever, rose cold, and catarrh. [Cincinnati, 1882.] 30p. DNLM; OCIM **80-3562**

KOBER, George M[artin] (1850-1931)
Report on the topography, botany, climatology, and diseases of Surprise and Goose Lake valleys. Sacramento: J. J. Ayers, 1886. 31p. CU-M; DNLM **80-3563**

KOLBÉ, D. W., & SON. PHILADELPHIA
Description of orthopaedic apparatus employed in the treatment of deformities. . . . 7th ed. Philadelphia: Collins, 1880. 62p. DNLM; PU **80-3564**

KOLBÉ, D. W., & SON. PHILADELPHIA
Illustrated catalogue of surgical instruments. Philadelphia: Sherman & Co., 1881. 202p. DNLM; PU **80-3565**

KOLBÉ, D. W., & CO. PHILADELPHIA
Suggestions on the treatment of club-foot. . . . Presented by D. W. Kolbé & Son. . . . Philadelphia: Globe Printing House, 1882. 23p. DLC; DNLM; PU **80-3566**

KOLBÉ, D. W., & SON. PHILADELPHIA
Illustrated catalogue of surgical instruments. Philadelphia: Sherman & Co., [1884]. 213p. DNLM; PU **80-3567**

KOLBÉ, D. W., & SON. PHILADELPHIA
Description of orthopaedic apparatus employed in the treatment of deformities. . . . 9th ed. Philadelphia: Collins, 1886. 62p. DNLM; PU **80-3568**

KOLBÉ, D. W., & SON. PHILADELPHIA
Description of orthopaedic apparatus employed in the treatment of deformities. . . . 10th ed. Philadelphia: Collins, 1887. 62p. DNLM; PU **80-3569**

KOLIPINSKI, Louis
Preliminary notes on some of the properties of sodium fluoride. [Philadelphia, 1886.] 12p. DNLM **80-3570**

KOPLIK, Henry (1858-1927)
Acute articular rheumatism in the nursing infant. [New York, 1888.] 12p. DNLM **80-3571**

KOST, John (1819-1904)
A text-book on medical jurisprudence; for medical and law colleges: . . . Cincinnati: Wilstach, Baldwin & Co., 1885. 360p. DLC; IU-M; OCIM; PU **80-3572**

KREIDER, George N[oble] (*b.* 1856)
How micro-organisms enter the body. St. Louis, 1888. 8p. DNLM **80-3573**

KREIDER, George N[oble] (*b.* 1856)
The treatment of pneumonia by tepid baths. [New York, 1889.] 6p. DNLM **80-3574**

KRETZSCHMAR, Paul H. (1847-1891)
Dilatation of the gall-bladder; its treatment by aspiration. Report of a case. [New York: Jenkins & Thomas, 1881.] 12p. DNLM; NNNAM **80-3575**

KRETZSCHMAR, Paul H. (1847-1891)
Dr. Dettweiler's method of treating pulmonary consumption; an appeal for the establishment of an institution for the rational treatment of pulmonary consumption. [New York, 1888.] 20p. DNLM; NNNAM **80-3576**

KRETZSCHMAR, Paul H. (1847-1891)
Public health reports vs. institutions for the treatment of bacillary phthisis. Philadelphia: Records, McMullin & Co., 1888. 22p. DNLM; PU **80-3577**

KRETZSCHMAR, Paul H. (1847-1891)
Institutions for the treatment of pulmonary consumption in the United States. Philadelphia: W. J. Dornan, 1889. 17p. DNLM; PPC **80-3578**

KRETZSCHMAR, Paul H. (1847-1891)
Notes on the prevention of pulmonary consumption. Concord, N.H.: Republican Press Assoc., 1889. 10p. DNLM **80-3579**

LA GRANGE, Robert J.
Useful information for the people. On the modern tretment of syphilis and hereditary disease. . . . [Philadelphia? 1886.] 32p. DLC; PPC; PU **80-3580**

LAIDLEY, L[eonidas] H. (1844-1881)
Papillomatous cystic tumor of ovary, with a hernial pouch developed in the cicatrix of the abdominal wound from a former ovariotomy. Chicago, 1888. 8p. DNLM **80-3581**

LAMB, Daniel Smith (1843-1929)
Introductory address to the fourteenth session of the medical department of Howard University. Washington, D.C.: R. Beresford, 1881. 12p. DNLM **80-3582**

LAMB, Daniel Smith (1843-1929)
Report of the post-mortem examination of the body of Chas. J. Giteau. [With report of the microscopical examination.] Philadelphia, 1882. 22p. DNLM **80-3383**

LAMB, Daniel Smith (1843-1929)
Address to the graduates of medical department of Howard University. Washington, D.C.: R. Beresford, 1885. 19p. DNLM **80-3584**

LAMB, Daniel Smith (1843-1929)
In clouds of smoke. Washington, D.C.: R. H. Darby, 1885. 20p. DNLM **80-3585**

LAMB, Daniel Smith (1843-1929)
Anomalous lobation of the human lung. [Philadelphia, 1886.] 3p. DNLM **80-3586**

LAMBERT, John (*b.* 1828)
Albuminuria in pregnancy. Read before the Union Medical Association of Bennington Co., Vt., July 14, 1880. [n. p., 1880.] 8p. DNLM **80-3587**

LAMBERT, John (*b.* 1828)
Medical expert witnesses. Salem, N.Y., [1881]. 15p. DNLM **80-3588**

LAMBERT, John (*b.* 1828)
Two cases of insanity before ecclesiastical courts. New York: Vanden Houten & Co., 1885. 13p. DNLM **80-3589**

LAMSON, Daniel L[owell] (1834-1894)
Report to the Maine Medical Association of the visitors to the Portland School for Medical Instruction, 1880. Portland: S. Berry, 1880. 3p. DNLM **80-3590**

LAMSON, Mary Swift
Life and education of Laura Dewey Bridgman, the deaf, dumb, and blind girl. Boston: Houghton, Mifflin, 1881. 373p. ICU; MB; MH; NN **80-3591**

LAND, Charles Henry (1847-1922)
The scientific adaptation of artificial dentures. . . . Detroit, Mich.: C. H. Land, 1885. 44p. DLC **80-3592**

LAND, C[harles] Henry (1847-1922)
Porcelain dental art. The new process of restoring decayed and defective teeth. . . . Detroit, Mich.: O. S. Gulley, Bornman & Co., 1888. 40p. DLC **80-3593**

LANDIS, Henry Gardner (1848-1886)
Vicarious menstruation. [Cincinnati, 1880.] 8p. DNLM **80-3594**

LANDIS, Henry Gardner (1848-1886)
How to use the forceps. With an introductory account of the female pelvis and of the mechanism of delivery. New York: E. B. Treat, 1880. 168p. 1 plate. DNLM; NNNAM; OCIM; PU **80-3595**

LANDIS, Henry Gardner (1848-1886)
. . . A compend of obstetrics. Especially adapted to the use of medical students and physicians. . . . Philadelphia: P. Blakiston, Son & Co., 1883. 107p. DLC; MBM; NNNAM; PPC **80-3596**

LANDIS, Henry Gardner (1848-1886)
. . . A compend of obstetrics. Especially adapted to the use of medical students and physicians. . . . 2nd ed. rev. and enl. . . . Philadelphia: P. Blakiston, Son & Co., 1885. 120p. DLC; IU-M; NNNAM; PU **80-3597**

LANDIS, Henry Gardner (1848-1886)
The management of labor and of the lying-in period. A guide for the young practitioner. . . . Philadelphia: Lea Bros. & Co., 1885. 334p. DLC; DNLM; PPC; PU **80-3598**

LANDIS, Henry Gardner (1848-1886)
. . . A compend of obstetrics. Especially adapted to the use of medical students and physicians. . . . 3rd ed., thoroughly rev. . . . Philadelphia: P. Blakiston, Son & Co., 1887. 118p. DLC; LNT-M; PPC; PU **80-3599**

LANDOIS, Leonard (1837-1902)
A text-book of human physiology, including histology and microscopical anatomy; with special reference to the requirements of practical medicine. Transl. from 4th German ed. With additions by William Stirling. Philadelphia: P. Blakiston, Son & Co., 1885. 2 v. DNLM; MH-M; NNNAM; PPC **80-3600**

LANDOIS, Leonard (1837-1902)
A text-book of human physiology, including histology and microscopical anatomy; with special reference to the requirements of practical medicine. Transl. from the 5th German ed., with additions by William Stirling. Philadelphia: P. Blakiston's Son & Co., 1886. 922p. DNLM; IU-M; PPC; PU **80-3601**

LANDOIS, Leonard (1837-1902)
A text-book of human physiology, including histology and microscopical anatomy; with special reference to the requirements of practical medicine. 3rd American, translated from the 6th German ed., with additions by William Stirling. Philadelphia: P. Blakiston's Son & Co., 1889. 974p. CtY-M; DNLM; NNNAM; PPC **80-3602**

LANE, Irvin J.
Convallaria majalis. [New York, 1883.] 18p. DNLM **80-3603**

LANE, Levi Cooper (1830-1902) and Edward R. TAYLOR
Addresses delivered on the occasion of the dedication of Cooper Medical College Building. San Francisco: A. L. Bancroft & Co., 1882. 42p. DLC; DNLM **80-3604**

LANE, L[evi] C[ooper] (1830-1902)
Ligations for the cure of aneurism. [San Francisco: Stanley & Davis, 1884.] 11p. DNLM **80-3605**

LANE, Levi Cooper (1830-1902)
Dr. Henry Gibbons. In memoriam. San Francisco: Howard & Pariser, 1885. 22p. DNLM **80-3606**

LANE, Levi Cooper (1830-1902)
Shadows in the ethics of the Internatioal Medical Congress. San Francisco: A. L. Brancroft, 1885. 12p. DNLM **80-3607**

LANE, L[evi] C[ooper] (1830-1902)
Memorial wreath for the prosecution in the Graves malpractice suit. San Francisco: W. A. Woodward & Co., [1886]. 6p. DNLM **80-3608**

LANE, L[evi] C[ooper] (1830-1902)
Dr. Augustus J. Bowie; in memoriam. [San Francisco, 1887.] 6p. DNLM **80-3609**

LANGDON, F[rank] W[arren] (1851-1933)
The germ theory of disease; its present status and practical applications. Cincinnati, 1885. 8p. DNLM **80-3610**

LANGLEY, John Williams (1841-1908)
Notes on a course of lectures on general chemistry. electro-therapeutics and chemical physics delivered by J. W. Langley. . . . Ed. by Orion J. Fay. . . . Ann Arbor, [Mich.]: S. C. Andrews, 1882. 102, 12p. DLC **80-3611**

LANGLEY, John Williams (1841-1908)
. . . Electro-therapeutics, a synopsis of lectures and laboratory work in applied electro-therapeutics. . . . Ann Arbor, Mich.: G. Osius & Co., 1884. 39p. DLC **80-3612**

LANKESTER, Edwin, ed. (1814-1874)
The family medical guide: a complete popular dictionary of medicine and hygiene. Comprising all possible self-aids in the treatment of diseases, accidents, emergencies, etc., with articles on general physiology; on diet and food . . . assisted by distinguished members of the Royal Colleges of Physicians and Surgeons, London. American ed. Carefully rev., with additions and amendments by competent authorities. New York: E. R. Pelton & Co., 1881. 496p. DLC; NNNAM; OCIM; PU **80-3613**

LANKESTER, Edwin, ed. (1814-1874)
A dictionary of popular medicine and hygiene. American domestic medicine and household physician. A companion for the traveler, emigrant, clergyman, and miner. . . . Augusta, Me.: True & Co., [1882]. 1008p. plates. DLC; MBM **80-3614**

LATIMER, Thomas S[argent] (1839-1906)
President's address on the origin and diffusion of cholera. [Baltimore, 1885.] 21p. DNLM; MdU-D **80-3615**

LATIMER, Thomas S[argent] (1839-1906)
Deep reflexes in health and in disease. Report of the section on anatomy, physiology and pathology. Baltimore, 1888. 12p. DNLM **80-3616**

LAURIE, Joseph (*d.* 1865)
The homoeopathic domestic medicine. Edited and revised, with numerous important additions and the introduction of the new remedies, a repertory, and a glossary, by Robert J. McClatchey. 10th American ed. Philadelphia: F. E. Boericke, [1887]. 1044p. DNLM; NNNAM; PPHa; PU **80-3617**

LAUTENBACH, Louis J. (*b.* 1860)
Ophthalmoscopic examinations of the insane at the State Hospital, Norristown, and the insane department of the Philadelphia Hospital. [Philadelphia, 1886.] 4p. DNLM **80-3618**

LAUTENBACH, Louis J. (*b.* 1860), and Alice BENNETT
Ophthalmoscopic studies of acute mania, with notes of cases. Histories of patients. [New York, 1886.] 16p. DNLM **80-3619**

LAUTENBACH, Louis J. (*b.* 1860)
The value of nitroglycerine in tinnitus aurium. [Washington, 1887.] 3p. DNLM **80-3620**

LAUTENBACH, Louis J. (*b.* 1860)
The prevention of ear-disease by care in childhood. [Philadelphia, 1888.] 10p. DNLM **80-3621**

LAWRENCE, Joseph B.
What to do in cases of accidents and emergencies; describing the symptoms in each case, and how to treat them on the moment. With a list of the principal poisons, which, if taken, require prompt treatment; their remedies and antidotes. Designed for family and general use. New York: J. H. Vail & Co., 1888. 139p. DNLM; NNNAM **80-3622**

LAWSON, John H.
Adjudged cases in insanity as a defense to crime. San Francisco: Bancroft-Whitney Co., 1887. 953p. CLM; DNLM; NNNAM **80-3623**

LAWTON, C[harles H.] (1832-1894)
Therapeutic force; or, proofs of medicinal power beyond the limit of drug attenuation, as furnished by analogy from natural philosophy and physical science. Philadelphia: Globe Pr. House, 1881. 8p. DNLM **80-3624**

LAWVER, Winfield Peter (1848-1891)
Tables for the practical examination of urine, urinary deposits and calculi, prepared for the use of students of the National Medical College, Columbian University. . . . Washington, D.C.: R. Beresford, printer, 1885. 7p. DLC; DNLM **80-3625**

[LEA BROTHERS & CO.]
One hundred years of publishing, 1785-1885. [Philadelphia, 1885.] 20p. DNLM; PPC; PU [The preeminent 19th century medical publisher, founded by Mathew Carey in 1785. Chronology of firm: Mathew Carey, 1785-1817; M. Carey & Son, 1817-1821; M. Carey & Sons, 1821; H. C. Carey & I. Lea, 1822-1827; Carey, Lea & Carey, 1827-1829; Carey & Lea, 1829-1832; Carey, Lea & Blanchard, 1833-1838; Lea & Blanchard, 1838-1851; Blanchard & Lea, 1851-1865; Lea & Blanchard, 1865; Henry C. Lea, 1865-1880; Henry C. Lea's Son & Co., 1880-1885; Lea Brothers & Co., 1885-1907; Lea & Febiger, 1907 to date.] **80-3626**

LEA BROTHERS & CO. PHILADELPHIA
Illustrated catalogue of medical works and periodicals. Philadelphia, [1888]. 48p. DNLM; PPC; PU **80-3627**

LEACH & GREENE
Illustrated catalogue of surgical instruments, etc. Boston: J. S. Adams, [1884]. 126p. DNLM; MBAt; MH-M **80-3628**

LEALE, Charles Augustus (*b.* 1842)
Eulogy delivered before the New York State Medical Association on Prof. Frank Hastings Hamilton, New York, November, 1886. . . . Concord, N.H.: Republican Press Association, 1887. 16p. DLC; DNLM **80-3629**

LEALE, Charles A[ugustus] (*b.* 1842)
. . . The prevention of chronic disease among the children of New York City. . . . Read before the New York County Medical Association, June 20, 1887. [New York? 1887.] 22p. DLC; DNLM; NNNAM **80-3630**

LEAMING, J[ames] R[oseburgh] (1820-1892)
Contributions to the study of diseases of the heart and lungs. New York & London: Bermingham & Co., 1884. 276p. DNLM; NNNAM; OCIM; PU 80-3631

LEAMING, J[ames] R[oseburgh] (1820-1892)
Acoustics applied to the human chest in physical diagnosis. Philadelphia: W. J. Dornan, 1889. 26p. DNLM; PPC; PU 80-3632

LEAVITT, Sheldon (1848-1933)
Homoeopathic therapeutics as applied to obstetrics. Chicago: Duncan Bros., 1881. 121p. DNLM; OCIM 80-3633

LEAVITT, Sheldon (1848-1933)
The science and art of obstetrics. With an introduction by Professor R. Ludlam. With 263 illustrations. Chicago: Gross & Delbridge, 1883. 659p. DLC; OCIM; PPHa 80-3634

LE CONTE, Joseph (1823-1901)
Sight; an exposition of the principles of monocular and binocular vision. New York: D. Appleton & Co., 1881. 275p. CtY-M; DNLM; MBM; NNNAM 80-3635

LEE, Arthur Bolles (1849-1927)
The microtomist's vade-mecum. A handbook of the methods of microscopic anatomy. Philadelphia: P. Blakiston, Son & Co., 1885. 424p. DNLM; IU-M; NNNAM; PU 80-3636

LEE, Benjamin (1833-1913)
Note on the alkaloids of cinchona. [Philadelphia, 1880.] 20p. DNLM 80-3637

LEE, Benjamin (1833-1913)
Massage; the latest handmaid of medicine. . . . Philadelphia: Collins, printer, 1884. 12p. DLC; DNLM; PPC 80-3638

LEE, Benjamin (1833-1913)
Differentiation the test of civilization. The education of the specialist. Annual address delivered before the American Academy of Medicine. Philadelphia: W. F. Fell & Co., 1884. 20p. DNLM; PPC 80-3639

LEE, Benjamin (1833-1913)
A clinical illustration of the value of combining motion with extension in the treatment of disease of the hip-joint. . . . Philadelphia: Collins, printer, 1884. 3p. DLC; DNLM 80-3640

LEE, Benjamin (1833-1913)
. . . The organization of local boards of health in Pennsylvania. Read at a meeting of the Association, January 28th, 1886. . . . Philadelphia: Philadelphia Social Science Association, [1886]. 16p. DLC; DNLM 80-3641

LEE, Benjamin (1833-1913)
Do the sanitary interests of the United States demand the annexation of Cuba? Concord, N.H., 1889. 8p. DNLM 80-3642

LEE, Charles Carroll (1838-1893)
The proper limitations of Emmet's operation for lacerations of the cervix uteri. New York, 1881. 19p. DNLM; NNNAM 80-3643

LEE, Charles Carroll (1838-1893)
The treatment of chronic perimetritis by puncture and iodine injections. [New York, 1882.] 8p. DNLM 80-3644

LEE, Charles Carroll (1838-1893)
The management of accidental puncture and other injuries of the gravid uterus, as complications of laparatomy. [1883.] 15p. DNLM 80-3645

LEE, Charles Carroll (1838-1893)
The future influence of surgery upon obstetrical art. New York: Trow, 1886. 22p. DNLM; NNNAM 80-3646

LEE, E[dmund] Jennings
Characteristic conditions of aggravation and amelioration. After Bönninghausen. Edited by . . . . The homoeopathic physician. Suppl. No. 4. [n. p.], 1884. 82p. DNLM; PPHa 80-3647

LEE, Edmund Jennings and George H. CLARK
Cough and expectoration. A repertorial index of their symptoms. New York: A. L. Chatterton & Co., 1884. 201p. NNNAM; PPHa 80-3648

LEE, John G.
Hand-book for coroners, containing a digest of all the laws in the thirty-eight States of the Union, together with a historical résumé from the earliest period to the present time, a guide to the physician in post-mortem examinations, and valuable miscellaneous matter never before collated. Philadelphia: W. Brotherhead, 1881. 288p. DNLM; ICU; MH; NN 80-3649

LEE, John G.
Homicide and suicide, in the city and county of Philadelphia, Pa., during a decade, 1871 to 1881 inclusive. Philadelphia: Times Printing House, 1883. 32p. DNLM 80-3650

LEE, William (1841-1893) and Henry S. T. HARRIS
Addresses delivered at the sixty-second annual commencement of the National Medical College (medical department of the Columbian University), March 20, 1884. Washington, D.C.: W. H. Moore, 1884. 16p. DNLM 80-3651

LEEDS, Albert R[ipley] (1843-1902)
On infant foods; a lecture. Boston: Doliber, Goodale & Co., 1883. 31p. DNLM 80-3652

LEETE, James M[adison] (1833-1897) and Robert MOORE
The sanitary condition of St. Louis, with special reference to Asiatic cholera. Reports to the Commercial Club, of St. Louis, Jan. 10, 1885. St. Louis, 1885. 16p. DNLM 80-3653

LEFFERTS, George M[orewood] (1846-1920)
Chorea of the laryngeal muscles (chorea laryngealis). St. Louis: G. O. Rumbold & Co., 1880. 8p. DNLM 80-3654

LEFFERTS, George M[orewood] (1846-1920)
Some practical suggestions in connection with the use of the laryngoscope in children. [New York, 1880.] 11p. DNLM 80-3655

LEFFERTS, George M[orewood] (1846-1920)
The question of hemorrhage after tonsillotomy. [New York, 1882.] 11p. DNLM **80-3656**

LEFFERTS, George M[orewood] (1846-1920)
Fistulae colli congenitae. A clinical lecture. [New York, Dornan], 1883. 12p. DNLM **80-3657**

LEFFERTS, George M[orewood] (1846-1920)
The diagnosis and treatment of chronic nasal catarrh. Three clinical lectures. St. Louis: Lambert & Co., 1884. 49p. DNLM; OCIM **80-3658**

LEFFERTS, George M[orewood] (1846-1920)
A pharmacopoeia for the treatment of diseases of the larynx, pharynx, and nasal passages, with remarks on the selection of remedies and choice of instruments and on the methods of making local applications. 2nd ed. New York & London: G. P. Putnam's Sons, 1884. 101p. DNLM; NNNAM; OCLloyd **80-3659**

LEFFERTS, George M[orewood] (1846-1920)
The diagnosis and treatment of chronic nasal catarrh. Three clinical lectures delivered at the College of Physicians and Surgeons, New York. 2nd ed. St. Louis: Lambert & Co., 1886. 57p. DNLM; IU-M; OCIM **80-3660**

LEFFINGWELL, Albert [Tracy] (1845-1916)
Vivisection. [Philadelphia, 1884.] 13p. DNLM **80-3661**

LEFFINGWELL, Albert [Tracy] (1845-1916)
On vivisection. Tract No. 1. [Boston: W. B. Clarke & Carruth, 1884.] 16p. DNLM; MdBM **80-3662**

LEFFINGWELL, Albert [Tracy] (1845-1916)
Vivisection. New York: J. W. Lovell Co., [1889]. 95p. DNLM; NNNAM **80-3663**

LEFFMANN, Henry (1847-1930)
The compend of chemistry. With which is included a 2nd and rev. ed. of the "First step in chemical principles." . . . Philadelphia: C. C. Roberts & Co., 1881. 160p. DLC; DNLM; PPJ; PU **80-3664**

LEFFMANN, Henry (1847-1930)
Elements of chemistry. Philadelphia: E. H. Butler & Co., [1882]. 227p. CtY-M; DNLM; NN; PU **80-3665**

LEFFMANN, Henry (1847-1930)
Medical relations of the prevailing forms of food adulterations. Philadelphia, 1882. 5p. DNLM **80-3666**

LEFFMANN, Henry (1847-1930)
The hygiene of exposure. [Philadelphia, 1883.] 6p. DNLM **80-3667**

LEFFMANN, Henry (1847-1930)
. . . A compend of organic and medical chemistry; including urinary analysis and the examination of water and food. . . . Philadelphia: P. Blakiston, Son & Co., 1884. 124p. DLC; DNLM; PPC; PU **80-3668**

LEFFMANN, Henry (1847-1930)
Typhoid fever in Philadelphia. [Philadelphia, 1885.] 8p. DNLM **80-3669**

LEFFMANN, Henry (1847-1930)
. . . A compend of chemistry, inorganic and organic; including urinary analysis, and the sanitary examination of water. . . . Rewritten and adapted to students in medicine and dentistry. Philadelphia: P. Blakiston, Son & Co., 1888. 190p. DLC; DNLM; NNNAM; PU **80-3670**

LEFFMANN, Henry (1847-1930)
Food laws. A paper read before the Medical Jurisprudence Society of Philadelphia, March 13, 1888. Philadelphia, [1888]. 7 p. DNLM **80-3671**

LEFFMANN, Henry (1847-1930) and William BEAM
Effects of food preservatives on the action of diastase, pancreatic extract, and pepsin. [Philadelphia: W. Fell & Co., 1888.] 9p. DNLM **80-3672**

LEFFMANN, Henry (1847-1930) and William BEAM
Examination of water for sanitary and technical purposes. Philadelphia: P. Blakiston, Son & Co., 1889. 106p. DNLM; PPC; PPJ; PU [2nd ed., rev. and enl., 1891, 130p.] **80-3673**

LEGARÉ, Thomas
. . . Observations on epidemic of scarlet fever at Charleston, S.C., in the spring of 1881. . . . Charleston, S.C.: E. Perry, printer [1881]. 8p. DLC; ScCM **80-3674**

LEGG, John Wickham (1843-1921)
A guide to the examination of the urine, designed chiefly for the use of clinical clerks and students. 6th ed. Philadelphia: P. Blakiston, Son & Co., [1885]. 120p. CtY-M; DNLM; NNNAM; PPC **80-3675**

LE HARDY, J[ulius] C[aesar] (*b.* 1831)
Annual address delivered before the Medical Association of Georgia, Thomasville, April 20th, 1881, by the president. . . . Augusta, Ga.: J. Loveday, 1881. 11p. DLC **80-3676**

LE HARDY, J[ulius] C[aesar] (*b.* 1831)
Syphilis; the importance of a thorough diagnosis and long-continued treatment. Atlanta, 1885. 20p. DNLM **80-3677**

LE HARDY, J[ulius] C[aesar] (*b.* 1831)
The yellow-fever panic. [Savannah]: Townsend, [1888]. 14p. DNLM **80-3678**

LE HARDY, J[ulius] C[aesar] (*b.* 1831)
The rational method of preventing yellow fever on the South Atlantic coast. Augusta, Ga.: J. M. Richards, 1889. 22p. DNLM **80-3679**

LEHLBACH, Charles F. J. (1835-1896)
State protection against quackery. Newark, N.J., 1888. 19p. DNLM **80-3680**

LEHLBACH, Charles F. J. (1835-1896)
What treatment will most effectually and promptly curtail the course of acute rheumatism? Newark, N.J.: J. L. Hardham, 1888. 9p. DNLM **80-3681**

LEIDY, Joseph (1823-1891)
An address on evolution and the pathological importance of lower forms of life. Detroit: G. S. Davis, 1886. 21p. DNLM **80-3682**

LEIDY, Joseph (1823-1891)
Experiments to determine the influence of digitalis on normal temperatures, and its action as an antipyretic in typhoid fever. Detroit: G. S. Davis, 1888. 5p. DNLM
80-3683

LEIDY, Joseph (1823-1891)
An elementary treatise on human anatomy. . . . 2nd ed., rewritten. With four hundred and ninety-five illustrations. Philadelphia: J. B. Lippincott Co., 1889. 950p. DLC; DNLM; NNNAM; PPC **80-3684**

LEIDY, Philip (1838-1891)
Medical and vital statistics; are they reliable? Philadelphia, 1883. 8p. DNLM **80-3685**

LEIGHTON, Alton W.
Laparotomy for ovarian cyst. [n. p., 1885.] 4p. DNLM
80-3686

LENTE, Frederick D[ivoux] (1823-1883)
Higher education of medical men, and its influence on the profession and the public. New York: C. T. Bermingham & Co., 1880. 16p. DNLM; NNNAM **80-3687**

LENTE, Frederick D[ivoux] (1823-1883)
A hitherto undescribed lesion of the knee-joint; a paper read before the New York Academy of Medicine. New York: Bermingham & Co., 1882. 15p. DNLM; NNNAM
80-3688

LEONARD, Charles Henri (1850-1925)
The hair: its growth, care, diseases and treatment. . . . Detroit: C. H. Leonard, 1880. 316p. DLC; IU-M; OCIM
80-3689

LEONARD, C[harles] Henri (1850-1925)
. . . The vest-pocket anatomist (founded upon "Gray.") . . . 11th rev. ed. . . . Detroit: The Illustrated Medical Journal Co., 1882. 82p. DLC; IU-M **80-3690**

LEONARD, C[harles] Henri (1850-1925)
The multum in parvo reference and dose book. Detroit, 1882. 32nd thousand. Detroit, 1882. 99p. DNLM; OCIM
80-3691

LEONARD, Charles Henri, ed. (1850-1925)
Auscultation, percussion, and urinalysis. An epitome of the physical signs of the heart, lung, liver, kidney and spleen in health and disease. . . . Detroit, Mich.: The Illustrated Medical Journal Co., [1883]. 166p. DLC; IEN-M; OCIM
80-3692

LEONARD, Charles Henri (1850-1925)
A manual of bandaging. Adapted for self-instruction. . . . With one hundred and thirty-nine engravings. 2nd ed., rev. and enl. Detroit: The Illustrated Medical Journal Co., [1884]. 159p. DLC; OCIM; NNNAM **80-3693**

LEONARD, Charles Henri (1850-1925)
. . . The vest-pocket anatomist (founded upon "Gray.") . . . 14th rev. ed. Containing dissection hints and visceral anatomy. Detroit: The Ilustrated Medical Journal Co., [1888]. 297p. DLC; IU-M; OCIM **80-3694**

LEONARD MEDICAL SCHOOL, SHAW UNIVERSITY, RALEIGH, N.C.
Annual announcements for the sessions of 1885-1886 (5.), 1886-1887 (6.). Raleigh, 1885-1886. DNLM [List of students and graduates for the sessions of 1884-1885; 1885-1886. Organized in 1882, for the eduction of Negro students.]
80-3695

LEONARD MEDICAL SCHOOL, SHAW UNIVERSITY, RALEIGH, N.C.
Annual announcements and catalogues for the sessions of 1885-1886 to 1891-1892 (5.-11.). Raleigh, 1885-1891. DNLM [List of students and graduates for the sessions of 1884-1885 to 1890-1891 in announcements for subsequent years. Organized in 1882 for the education of Negro students.]
80-3696

LEONARD, William E[dwin] (1855-1935)
Allopathic progress in the therapeutics of paedology. [Minneapolis], 1882. 5p. DNLM **80-3697**

LEONARD, W. T.
Rupture and its radical cure by J. A. Sherman's method, with an extract from an article on the radical cure of inguinal hernia. New York: McBride Bros., 1880. 85p. port. DNLM; NNNAM **80-3698**

LESZYNSKY, William M.
Leucorrhoea as the cause of a recent epidemic of purulent ophthalmia in one of our city charitable institutions. [New York, 1886.] 10p. DNLM **80-3699**

LESZYNSKY, William M.
Insanity and oophorectomy. [New York, 1887.] 7p. DNLM
80-3700

LESZYNSKY, William M.
An abstract of a lecture on the significance and value of pupillary phenomena in nervous disease. [New York], 1888. 7p. DNLM **80-3701**

LEUF, A. H. P. (*b.* 1867)
Additional factors concerned in fractures of the humerus in the vicinity of the elbow-joint. Brooklyn, N.Y., 1881. 9p. DNLM **80-3702**

LEUF, A. H. P. (*b.* 1867)
A report of anatomical anomalies. New York: G. P. Putnam's Sons, 1882. 8p. DNLM **80-3703**

LEUF, A. H. P. (*b.* 1867)
The treatment of scarlatina. Philadelphia: J. E. Potter & Co., 1885. 30p. DNLM **80-3704**

LEUF, A. H. P. (*b.* 1867)
Note on a peculiar form of pulmonary congestion not generally known and terminating in sudden death; together with a plea for cardiac aspiration. Philadelphia, 1885. 15p. DNLM
80-3705

LEVIS, R[ichard] J. (1827-1890)
Ethylization, the anaesthetic use of the bromide of ethyl. [Philadelphia: Sherman & Co., 1880.] 8p. DNLM
80-3706

LEVIS, R[ichard] J. (1827-1890)
The new anaesthetic, the bromide of ethyl. [Philadelphia, 1880.] 4p. DNLM **80-3707**

LEVIS, R[ichard] J. (1827-1890)
Priority in the anaesthetic use of the bromide of ethyl. [Philadelphia, 1880.] 4p. DNLM **80-3708**

LEVIS, R[ichard] J. (1827-1890)
The treatment of varicocele by excision of redundant scrotum. Philadelphia, 1881. 4p. DNLM **80-3709**

LEVIS, R[ichard] J. (1827-1890)
The treatment of hydrocele and serous cysts in general by the injection of carbolic acid. [Philadelphia, 1881.] 4p. DNLM **80-3710**

LEVIS, R[ichard] J. (1827-1890)
A winter climate for invalids. The Gulf coast of Florida. [n. p., 1882.] 11p. 1 map. DNLM **87-3711**

LEVIS, R[ichard] J. (1827-1890)
Extension apparatus. [Philadelphia, 1883.] 1 sheet. DNLM **80-3712**

LEWERS, Arthur [Hamilton Nicholson]
A practical text-book of the diseases of women. Philadelphia: P. Blakiston, Son & Co., 1888. 400p. DNLM; MBM; NNNAM; PPC **80-3713**

LEWIN, Louis (1850-1929)
The untoward effect of drugs. A pharmacological and clinical manual. . . . 2nd ed., rev. and enl. Transl. by J. J. Mulheron. . . . The only English translation having the author's endorsement. Detroit, Mich.: G. S. Davis, 1883. 216p. DLC; IU-M; NNNAM; OCIM **80-3714**

LEWIS, Daniel (1846-1919)
The development of cancer from non-malignant diseases. New York: D. Appleton & Co., 1883. 12p. DNLM **80-3715**

LEWIS, Daniel (1846-1919)
The Chian turpentine treatment of cancer. [New York, 1888.] 3p. DNLM **80-3716**

LEWIS, Daniel (1846-1919)
The treatment of epithelioma with mild caustics. New York, [1888]. 8p. DNLM **80-3717**

LEWIS, Dio (1823-1886)
Our digestion, or my jolly friend's secret. New York: H. C. Lewis & Co., 1885. 407p. DNLM; NNNAM **80-3718**

LEWIS, Dio (1823-1886)
Weak lungs and the remedy, or troubles of the chest, with their home treatment. New York: D. Lewis Co., 1885. 358p. DNLM; NNNAM **80-3719**

LEWIS, F. Park (1855-1940)
The eye as a factor in functional nervous diseases. [Philadelphia], 1888. 8p. DNLM **80-3720**

LEWIS, George W., Jr.
The comma bacillus of Asiatic cholera. Some observations of its life history. New York, [1885]. 7p. DNLM **80-3721**

LEWIS, George W., Jr.
Ten days in the laboratory with Dr. Robert Koch, of Berlin. The methods to be employed in the cultivation and detection of the comma bacillus of Asiatic cholera. Buffalo, 1885. 15p. DNLM **80-3722**

LEWIS, John B[enjamin] (1832-1914)
Intracranial hemorrhage in its medico-legal aspects. Hartford: Case, Lockwood & Brainard, 1886. 23p. CtY-M; DNLM **80-3723**

LEWIS, Louis (1839-1902)
The urine in disease. Philadelphia, 1884. broadside fol. DNLM; PPC **80-3724**

LEWIS, Morris J[ames] (*b.* 1852)
A partial study of the seasonal relations of chorea and rheumatism. [Philadelphia, 1886.] 8p. 1 tab. DNLM **80-3725**

LEWIS, Morris J[ames] (*b.* 1852) and G. E. DE SCHWEINITZ
A preliminary note on the use of eucalyptus in headache. [Philadelphia, 1889.] 6p. DNLM **80-3726**

LEWIS, Richard H[enry]
Higher medical education and how to secure it. The annual address before the Alumni Association of the University of Maryland [delivered April 8, 1889]. [Baltimore, 1889.] 20p. DNLM; MdU-D **80-3727**

LEWIS, William J.
Hair microscopically examined and medico-legally considered. Buffalo: Bigelow Bros., 1884. 10p. 2 plates. DNLM **80-3728**

LIGGINS, John
Opium: England's coercive policy and its disastrous results in China and India: the spread of opium-smoking in America. New York: Funk & Wagnalls, Publishers, 1882. 48p. NN **80-3729**

LILLARD, Benjamin (*b.* 1847)
Practical hints and formulas for busy druggists. Original, contributed, and compiled. New York: J. H. Vail & Co., 1884. 80p. NNNAM **80-3730**

LILLY'S hand book of pharmacy and therapeutics. 3rd ed. Indianapolis: E. Lilly & Co., 1888. 248p. DNLM; OCLloyd **80-3731**

LINCOLN, David Francis (1841-1916)
School and industrial hygiene. Philadelphia: P. Blakiston, 1880. 152p. DNLM; NNNAM; PPC **80-3732**

LINCOLN, David Francis (1841-1916)
American Public Health Association. Lomb prize essay. The sanitary conditions and necessities of school-houses and school life. Concord, N.H.: Republican Press Ass'n., 1886. 38p. DNLM; MBM **80-3733**

LINCOLN, R[ufus] P[ratt] (1841-1900)
On the results of the treatment of naso-pharyngeal fibromata, with demonstration of successful cases, together with a table of seventy-four operations by different surgeons. [New York, 1883.] 24p. DNLM; NNNAM **80-3734**

LINCOLN, R[ufus] P[ratt] (1841-1900)
A case of melano-sarcoma of the nose cured by galvano-cauterization. [New York, 1885.] 3p. DNLM **80-3735**

LINCOLN, R[ufus] P[ratt] (1841-1900)
Recurrent naso-pharyngeal tumor, cured by electrolysis; exhibition of the patinet. New York, 1887. 3p. DNLM **80-3736**

LINDEN, John
Manual of the exanthematic method of cure, also known as Baunscheidtism. First issue of the fifteenth edition, with an appendix on "The Eye" and "The Ear," their diseases and treatment by means of the exanthematic method of cure, for the practical use of everyone. . . . Cleveland, O.: Publishing House of the Evangelical Association, 1883. 332p. OCIM
80-3737

LINDSAY & BLAKISTON
Catalogue of medical, dental and scientific books. Philadelphia, 1880. 32p. DNLM; PPC; PPJ; PU **80-3738**

LINDSLEY, C[harles] A[ugustus] (1826-1906)
The prescription of proprietary medicines for the sick; its demoralizing effects on the medical profession. An essay read before the Connecticut Medical Society. [New Haven, 1882.] 16p. CtY-M; DNLM **80-3739**

LINDSLEY, C[harles] A[ugustus] (1826-1906)
Vaccination. From the report of the Secretary of State Board of Health. Hartford, Conn.: Lockwood & Brainard Co., 1882. 29p. CtY-M; DNLM **80-3740**

LINDSLEY, J[ohn] Berrien (1822-1897)
The medical profession and the public-health movement. Memphis: S. C. Toof & Co., 1887. 8p. DNLM
80-3741

LINDSLEY, J[ohn] Berrien (1822-1897)
Practitioners of medicine as students of science. Nashville: Hasslock & Ambrose, 1887. 3p. DNLM
80-3742

LIPPE, Adolph (1812-1888)
Cholera: its treatment by homoeopathy. Philadelphia, 1885. 6p. DNLM; PPHa **80-3743**

LIPPE, Adolph (1812-1888)
What is homoeopathy? A lecture delivered May 10, 1886, before the Women's Homoeopathic Association of Pennsylvania, at the Medical, Surgical and Maternity Hospital. . . . Philadelphia: Wm. F. Fell & Co., 1886. 23p. DNLM; PPHa
80-3744

LIPPINCOTT, E[ldridge]
Hay fever, or rhinitis vasomotoria periodica, and its radical cure. Chicago: Gross & Delbridge, 1888. 76p. DNLM; IU-M; OCIM **80-3745**

LIPPINCOTT, J. A[udrey] (*b.* 1847)
On the binocular metamorphopsia produced by correcting glasses. [New York, 1889.] 30p. DNLM; NNNAM
80-3746

[LISTER, Joseph] (1827-1912)
Macte Lister trimphator: a moist-Merry, humid-hilarious antiseptic vade-mecum of internal surgery, for the ambitious modern physician, by Dr. Risorius Santorini [pseud. of Charles Everett Warren]. Boston: Cupples & Hurd, 1888. 42p. MBM; NNNAM **80-3747**

LITCH, Wilbur F., ed. (1840-1912)
The American system of dentistry. In treatises by various authors. . . . Philadelphia: Lea Bros. & Co., 1886-1887. 3 v. plates. DLC; DNLM; MdU-D; PPC
80-3748

LITTLE, James Lawrence (1836-1885)
A lecture on median lithotomy. New York: G. P. Putnam's Sons, 1880. 24p. DNLM; NNNAM **80-3749**

LITTLE, James Lawrence (1836-1885)
A modification of Lister's antiseptic dressing. [New York: D. Appleton & Co., 1881.] 7p. DNLM
80-3750

LITTLE, James Lawrence (1836-1885)
Spurious hermaphroditism. A case of hypospadias, where the patient, mistaken for a female at birth, has passed as such to the present time. New York: E. B. Treat, 1882. 1 l. 1 plate. DNLM **80-3751**

LITTLE, James Lawrence (1836-1885)
The treatment of fractures of the patella by the plaster-of-Paris splint. Philadelphia: W. J. Dornan, 1884. 8p. DNLM
80-3752

LITTLE, William S[eely] (1849?-1887)
A case of persistent hyaloid artery. [Boston, 1881.] 3p. 1 plate. DNLM **80-3753**

LITTLE, William S[eely] (1849?-1887)
Subjective traumatism of the eye; its importance when the question of sympathetic irritation or sympathetic ophthalmia arises. Philadelphia, 1882. 12p. DNLM
80-3754

LITTLE, William S[eely] (1849?-1887)
The possibility of abnormal ocular conditions through the sympathetic system impairing the function of the uterus. [Philadelphia, 1883.] 4p. DNLM **80-3755**

LITTLE, William S[eely] (1849?-1887)
Address in ophthalmology. Philadelphia: Collins, 1884. 20p. DNLM **80-3756**

LITTLE, William S[eely] (1849?-1887)
A combined visual and astigmatic test-card of words made up of letters confusing to the astigmatic eye. Remarks on astigmatism, characteristic mannerisms. Chicago: A. G. Newell, 1884. 8p. DNLM **80-3757**

LITTLE, William S[eely] (1849?-1887)
The care of eyes in institutions for children; fourteen years' experience in hospitals and homes for children. With discussion. [Philadelphia, 1886.] 8p. DNLM
80-3758

LIVERMORE, Mary A. (1820-1905)
My story of the war: a woman's narrative of four years' personal experience as nurse in the Union Army, and in relief work at home, in hospitals, camps, and at the front, during the War of the Rebellion. . . . Hartford, Conn.: A. D. Worthington & Co., 1889. 700p. 18 plates. MA; MB; MH; NN
80-3759

LLOYD, James Hendrie (*b.* 1853)
Hysteria; a study in psychology. [New York: G. P. Putnam's Sons, 1883.] 21p. DNLM; NNNAM
80-3760

LLOYD, James Hendrie (*b.* 1853)
Faith-cures. New York: Trow, 1886. 12p. DNLM
80-3761

LLOYD, James Hendrie (*b.* **1853)**
Moral insanity; a plea for a more exact cerebral pathology. A thesis for admission into the American Neurological Association. [New York, 1886.] 17p. DNLM
80-3762

LLOYD, James Hendrie (*b.* **1853)**
A preliminary report on electrolysis, with special reference to its trial in inflammatory products in the female pelvis. Philadelphia, 1886. 4p. DNLM **80-3763**

LLOYD, James Hendrie (*b.* **1853)**
The claim of moral insanity in its medico-legal aspects. New York: Trow's, 1887. 16p. DNLM **80-3764**

LLOYD, James Hendrie (*b.* **1853)**
The insanity of Oscar Hugo Webber. Philadelphia, 1888. 5p. DNLM **80-3765**

LLOYD, James Hendrie (*b.* **1853) and John B. DEAVER**
A case of tumor of the cervical region of the spine; operation and death. [Philadelphia, 1888.] 7p. DNLM
80-3766

LLOYD, John Uri (1849-1936)
The chemistry of medicines, practical. A text and reference book for the use of students, physicians, and pharmacists, embodying the principles of chemical philosophy and their application to those chemicals that are used in medicine and in pharmacy, including all those that are officinal in the pharmacopoeia of the United States. . . . Cincinnati: The Author, 1881. 451p. DLC; OCIM; OCLloyd
80-3767

LLOYD, John Uri (1849-1936)
The chemistry of medicines, practical. A text and reference book for the use of students, physicians, and pharmacists, embodying the principles of chemical philosophy and their application to those chemicals that are used in medicine and in pharmacy, including all those that are officinal in the pharmacopoeia of the United States. 2nd e.d Cincinnati: R. Clarke & Co., 1881. 451p. DNLM; OCIM; OCLloyd [3rd ed.-8th ed., 1882-1897] **80-3768**

LLOYD, John Uri (1849-1936)
Pharmaceutical preparations. Elixirs: their history, formulae, and methods of preparation . . . with a résumé of unofficial elixirs from the days of Paracelsus; . . . Cincinnati: R. Clarke & Co., 1883. 187p. DLC; OCIM; OCLloyd
80-3769

LLOYD, John Uri (1849-1936)
Pharmaceutical preparations. Elixirs: their history, formulae, and methods of preparation . . . with a résumé of unofficial elixirs from the days of Paracelsus; . . . 2nd ed. Cincinnati: R. Clarke & Co., 1883. 187p. OCLloyd
80-3770

LLOYD, John Uri (1849-1936)
Pharmaceutical preparations. Elixirs: their history, formulae, and methods of preparation . . . with a résumé of unofficial elixirs from the days of Paracelsus; . . . 3rd ed. Cincinnati: R. Clarke & Co., 1885. 187p. OCLloyd
80-3771

LLOYD, John Uri (1849-1936)
Bright's disease as a complication of surgical procedures. [New York, 1887.] 11p. DNLM
80-3772

LLOYD, T[homas] Mortimer
Some evidence relating to Asheville and the mountains of North Carolina in the climatic treatment of phthisis. [New York, 1887.] 17p. DNLM **80-3773**

LOCKWOOD, Hilliard L.
Homoeopathic hints. A simplified arrangement of the principal remedies, with definite instructions for their selection and administration adapted to the treatment of those more ordinary ills in which professional advice is not always necessary. With especial reference to the diseases of infancy and childhood. . . . New York: J. Medole & Sons, 1887. 71p. DLC; NNNAM; PPHa; PU **80-3774**

LOGAN, Henry C.
. . . The hygienic curative treatment; a rational and advanced method for curing, without the aid of drugs, nauseous medicines or electric belts. . . . Philadelphia, Pa.: The Author, 1888. 20p. DLC **80-3775**

LOGAN, P. W.
Catarrhal mucous membrane. [n. p., 1885.] 10p. DNLM
80-3776

LOMBARD, Warren P[limpton] (1855-1939)
Is the "knee-kick" a reflex act? A research made at the physiological laboratory of the College of Physicians and Surgeons, New York. [New York, 1887.] 14p. DNLM
80-3777

LOMBARD, Warren P[limpton] (1855-1939)
A new method of testing the "knee-kick." [New York, 1887.] 1 broadside. DNLM **80-3778**

LOMBARD, Warren P[limpton] (1855-1939)
The variations of the normal knee-jerk, and their relation to the activity of the central nervous system. Baltimore, 1887. 67p. 2 plates. DNLM; MdU-D **80-3779**

LONG ISLAND COLLEGE HOSPITAL, BROOKLYN
Polhemus Memorial Clinic and Hoagland Laboratory. Annual announcements and circulars for the sessions of 1886-1887 to 1895-1896 (28.-37.); 1897-1898 (39.); 1898-1899 (40.); 1900-1901 to 1903-1904 (42.-45.). Brooklyn, 1886-1903. DNLM [List of students and graduates for the sessions of 1885-1886 to 1894-1895; 1896-1897; 1897-1898; 1899-1900 to 1902-1903, *in*: Announcements for subsequent years. The Polhemus Memorial Clinic and Hoagland Laboratory was added in 1897, by the gift of Mrs. Caroline H. Polhemus.]
80-3780

LONG, J[ohn] W[esley] (1859-1926)
Uterine irrigation. [New York, 1885.] 1 l. DNLM
80-3781

LONGSTRETH, Morris (1846-1914)
Rheumatism, gout, and some allied disorders. New York: William Wood & Co., 1882. 280p. DNLM; MH-M; NNNAM; PU **80-3782**

LOOMIS, Alfred L[ebbeus] (1831-1895)
Lessons in physical diagnosis. New York: William Wood & Co., 1881. 240p. IU-M; NNNAM; PPC
80-3783

LOOMIS, Alfred L[ebbeus] (1831-1895)
A text-book of practical medicine, designed for the use of students and practitioners of medicine. . . . New York: William Wood & Co., 1884. 1102p. diags. DLC; DNLM; NNNAM; PPC
80-3784

LOOMIS, Alfred L[ebbeus] (1831-1895)
Bright's disease of the kidney. . . . Detroit, Mich.: G. S. Davis, 1888. 117p. DLC; DNLM; OCIM; PPC
80-3785

LOOMIS, Alfred L[ebbeus] (1831-1895)
A text-book of practical medicine, designed for the use of students and practitioners of medicine. . . . 8th ed., rev. and enl. . . . New York: William Wood & Co., 1889. 1147p. col. plate, diags. DLC; DNLM; NNNAM; PPC
80-3786

LORD, STOUTENBURGH & CO.
Illustrated catalogue. [Drugs, druggists' sundries and supplies.] Chicago, 1881. 427p. IU-M; OCIM **80-3787**

LORENZ, P. C.
Illustrated catalogue of surgical instruments, physicians' supplies. . . . New York, 1887. 32p. NNNAM
80-3788

LORING, Edward G[reely] (1837-1888)
Text-book of ophthalmoscopy. Part I. The normal eye, determination of refraction, diseases of the media, physiological optics, and theory of the ophthalmoscope. New York: D. Appleton & Co., 1886. 274p. 4 plates. DNLM; IU-M; NNNAM; PU **80-3789**

LORING, Edward G[reely] (1837-1888)
Text-book of ophthalmoscopy. Edited by Francis B. Loring. New York: D. Appleton & Co., 1886-1891. 2 v. 7 plates. DNLM; NNNAM; OCIM; PU **80-3790**

LORING, Francis B[oott]
Peculiar anatomical development of one of the central arteries of the retina. [n. p., 1880.] 3p. DNLM
80-3791

LOTHROP, Charles H[enry] (1831-1890)
Malaria. [Clinton, Iowa]: Allen, 1880. 12. DNLM
80-3792

LOTHROP, Charles H[enry] (1831-1890)
The Medical and Surgical Directory of the State of Iowa. Containing the names, post-office address, and professional status of the physicians; the various medical societies, with names and residence of the officers and members; a list of members of the American Medical Association from Iowa; a roster of the United States examining surgeons for pensions for the State. . . . For 1880 and 1881. Clinton: Allen, 1880. 172p. DNLM; OCIM **80-3793**

LOTHROP, Charles H[enry] (1831-1890)
The remedial properties of the Hot Springs, Ark.; also, a brief consideration of the locality as a resort for phthisical invalids. St. Louis: Times Printing House, 1881. 28p. DNLM
80-3794

LOTHROP, Charles H[enry] (1831-1890)
The medical and surgical directory of the State of Iowa for 1886 and 1887, containing the names, post-office address, and professional status of the physicians; the various medical societies, with names and residence of the officers and members; a list of members of the American Medical Association from Iowa; rosters of the U.S. examining surgeons for pensions for the State, officers and members of the State Board of Health, and medical officers of the Iowa National Guard; also medical colleges, State charitable institutions, hospitals, medical laws, [etc.]. Clinton, Iowa: Allen, 1886. 218p. DNLM; OCIM **80-3795**

LOUISVILLE COLLEGE OF DENTISTRY, DENTAL DEPARTMENT OF THE CENTRAL UNIVERSITY OF KENTUCKY
Annual announcements for the sessions of 1888-1895 (2.-9.); 1898 to 1903-1904 (14.-18.). Louisville, 1887-1903. DNLM [List of graduates from 1887 to 1894 in Announcement for 1895.] **80-3796**

LOUISVILLE COLLEGE OF PHARMACY
Annual announcements for the sessions of 1886-1887 to 1893-1894 (16.-23.); 1898-1899 to 1902-1903 (28.-32.). Louisville, 1886-1902. DNLM [List of students and graduates for the years 1885-1886 to 1892-1893; 1897-1898 to 1901-1902, in Announcements for subsequent years. Class roll of graduates from 1873 to 1901 in Announcement for 1902-1903.]
80-3797

LOUISVILLE SCHOOL OF PHARMACY FOR WOMEN
Annual announcements for the sessions of 1888-1889 (6.); 1890-1891 (8.); 1891-1892 (9.). Louisville, 1888-1891. 16p. DNLM [Organized in 1883, and incorporated March 11, 1884.] **80-3798**

LOVE, I[saac] N[ewton] (1848-1903)
Address of the president. At Mississippi Valley Medical Association, thirteenth annual meeting, Crab Orchard Springs, Ky., July 13, 1887. [Chicago & St. Louis, 1887.] 3 l. DNLM
80-3799

LOVE, I[saac] N[ewton] (1848-1903)
One year of acetanilide in pediatric practice. [Philadelphia, 1889.] 10p. DNLM **80-3800**

LOVE, I[saac] N[ewton] (1848-1903)
The scrofulous diathesis. Danbury, Conn.: Danbury Med. Print. Co., 1889. 8p. DNLM **80-3801**

LOVETT, Robert W[illiamson] (1859-1924)
A clinical consideration of sixty cases of cerebral paralysis in children. Boston: Cupples & Hurd, 1888. 20p. DNLM; MBM
80-3802

LOVETT, Robert W[illiamson] (1859-1924)
A method of estimating adduction and abduction of the leg in hip disease. Boston: Cupples & Hurd, 1888. 10p. DNLM
80-3803

LOVETT, Robert W[illiamson] (1859-1924)
The use of salicylic acid in chronic tuberculous joint disease. Boston, 1889. 7p. DNLM **80-3804**

LOVETT, Robert W[illiamson] (1859-1924) and John C. MUNRO
A consideration of the results in 327 cases of tracheotomy, performed at the Boston City Hospital from 1864 to 1887. [Philadelphia, 1887.] 11p. 2 tab. DNLM; PPC
80-3805

LUCAS-CHAMPIONNIÈRE, Just Marie Marcelin (1843-1913)
Antiseptic surgery. The principles, modes of application, and results of the Lister dressing. . . . Transl. from the 2nd and completely rev. ed. with the special sanction of the author, and ed. by Frederic Henry Gerrish. . . . Portland, [Me.]: Loring, Short & Harmon; [Cambridge, Mass.: J. Wilson & Son], 1881. 239p. DLC; MBM **80-3806**

LUCE, Charles E[lmer]
The movements of the lower jaw. Boston: Damrell & Upham, [1889]. 8p. DNLM **80-3807**

LÜCKES, Eva C. E.
Hospital sisters and their duties. Philadelphia: P. Blakiston, Son & Co., 1886. 164p. DNLM; MB; NN; PU **80-3808**

LUDLAM, R[euben] (1831-1899)
Membraneous dysmenorrhoea from repelled eruptions. [Philadelphia, 1881.] 9p. DNLM **80-3809**

LUDLAM, R[euben] (1831-1899)
Lectures, clinical and didactic, on the diseases of women. 5th ed. Revised, enlarged and illustrated. Chicago: Duncan Bros., 1881. 1029p. DNLM; IU-M; PPHa **80-3810**

LUDLAM, R[euben] (1831-1899)
Hahnemann Medical College and Hospital of Chicago. A prospectus of an extra course of twenty lectures on the puerperal diseases. To be given in the Hahnemann Hospital during the winter term of 1883-1884. [Chicago, 1883.] 8p. DNLM; IU-M **80-3811**

LUDLAM, R[euben] (1831-1899)
The thorough physician. A lecture introductory to the twenty-sixth annual course of instruction in the Hahnemann Medical College and Hospital of Chicago, delivered September 22, 1885. [Chicago, 1885.] 12p. IU-M; PPHa **80-3812**

LUDLAM, R[euben] (1831-1899)
Medical and surgical lectures on the diseases of women, a clinical and systematic treatise. . . . Lectures delivered from 1870 to 1887. 6th ed., rev., enl. and illustrated. Chicago: Halsey Bros., 1888. 1093p. DLC; IU-M; PPHa **80-3813**

LUDLOW, William (1843-1901)
Water supply in relation to sanitation. An address to the County Medical Society of Philadelphia. Philadelphia: Dunlap & Clarke, 1885. 17p. DNLM; PU **80-3814**

LUECKE, Georg (1829-1894)
Surgical diagnosis of tumors. [Transl. by A. T. Cabot.] Boston: A. Williams & Co., 1880. 43p. DNLM; MH-M **80-3815**

LUNDY, Charles J. (1846-1892)
Light in the public schools, and school-life in relation to vision; a paper read before the Sanitary Convention at Detroit, January, 1880. Lansing. W. S. George & Co., 1880. 12p. DNLM **80-3816**

LUNDY, Charles J. (1846-1892)
Diabetic cataract, iritis, etc.; a clinical lecture. [Detroit, 1880.] 11p. DNLM **80-3817**

LUNDY, Charles J. (1846-1892)
Sympathetic affections of the eye. [Detroit, 1880.] 12p. DNLM **80-3818**

LUNDY, Charles J. (1846-1892)
Tubercular laryngitis, or laryngeal phthisis. Ann Arbor, Mich., 1881. 11p. DNLM **80-3819**

LUNDY, Charles J. (1846-1892)
Gonorrhoeal ophthalmia, its complications and results; iridectomy for artificial pupil; a clinical lecture. [Detroit, 1882.] 8p. DNLM **80-3820**

LUNDY, Charles J. (1846-1892)
Hygiene, in relation to the eye. [Detroit, 1882.] 8p. DNLM **80-3821**

LUNDY, Charles J. (1846-1892)
School hygiene. [Detroit, 1883.] 16p. DNLM **80-3822**

LUNDY, Charles J. (1846-1892)
Muriate of cocaine in ophthalmic surgery. Ann Arbor, 1884. 4p. DNLM **80-3823**

LUNDY, Charles J. (1846-1892)
The dry treatment of chronic suppurative inflammation of the middle ear. 1884. 8p. DNLM **80-3824**

LUNDY, Charles J. (1846-1892)
Iritis; its relation to the rheumatic diathesis, and its treatment. Ann Arbor, Mich., 1885. 10p. DNLM **80-3825**

LUNDY, Charles J. (1846-1892)
The relations of the State and the medical profession. An address delivered June 30, 1886, before the Alumni Association of the Department of Medicine and Surgery of the University of Michigan. Ann Arbor: F. E. Beeman, 1886. 12p. DNLM **80-3826**

LUSK, William [Thompson] (1838-1897)
The prognosis of Caesarean operations. New York: William Wood & Co., 1880. 8p. DNLM **80-3827**

LUSK, William [Thompson] (1838-1897)
The justo-minor pelvis, with presentation of specimen. [New York, 1880.] 14p. 1 plate. DNLM **80-3828**

LUSK, William [Thompson] (1838-1897)
On the necessity of caution in the use of chloroform during labor. [New York, 1881.] 11p. DNLM **80-3829**

LUSK, William [Thompson] (1838-1897)
The science and art of midwifery. . . . New York: D. Appleton & Co., 1882. 687p. DLC; IC-U; NNNAM; PPC **80-3830**

LUSK, William [Thompson] (1838-1897)
The science and art of midwifery. 2nd ed. New York: D. Appleton & Co., 1884. 697p. CtY-M; NNNAM; PPC; PU **80-3831**

LUSK, William [Thompson] (1838-1897)
The science and art of midwifery. . . . New [3rd] ed., rev. and enl. . . . New York: D. Appleton & Co., 1885. 763p. plates. DLC; MH-M; NNNAM; PPC **80-3832**

LUSK, William [Thompson] (1838-1897)
The new Caesarean section, with reports of three successful cases. [Philadelphia]: W. J. Dornan, 1888. 22p. DNLM; PU
80-3833

LUTZ, Frank J[oseph] (1855-1916)
Remarks on abdominal surgery. Cyst of broad ligament; laparotomy; recovery. St. Louis: Davis & Freegard, 1880. 9p. DNLM **80-3834**

LUTZ, Frank J[oseph] (1855-1916)
Adenoid of the rectum; extirpation; recovery. St. Louis: Medical Journal Pub. Comp., 1881. 8p. DNLM
80-3835

LUTZ, Frank J[oseph] (1855-1916)
Gastrostomy; establishment of a gastric fistula in a case of stricture of the oesophagus. St. Louis, 1881. 11p. DNLM
80-3836

LUTZ, Frank J[oseph] (1855-1916)
Excision of the rectum for the cure of malignant growths, St. Louis: Medical Journal Pub. Com., 1884. 7p. DNLM
80-3837

LUTZ, Frank J[oseph] (1855-1916)
Cases illustrating diseases and treatment of cicatrices, scar, ulcer, epithelioma, fastening of arm to thorax after burn; operation; recovery. St. Louis, 1885. 4p. DNLM
80-3838

LUTZ, Frank J[oseph] (1855-1916)
Excision of the os calcis. St. Louis, 1886. 4p. DNLM
80-3839

LUTZ, Frank J[oseph] (1855-1916)
A contribution to the literature of the rarer forms of abdominal tumors. [St. Louis, 1887.] 7p. DNLM
80-3840

LYDSTON, G[eorge] Frank (1858-1923)
The prophylaxis and treatment of puerperal septaemia and the puerperal inflammations. Chicago: A. M. Wood & Co., 1884. 30p. DNLM; OCIM **80-3841**

LYDSTON, G[eorge] Frank (1858-1923)
Lectures on syphilis. Delivered at the Chicago College of Physicians and Surgeons. . . . Reported by Wm. A. Walker. . . . Chicago: A. M. Wood & Co., 1885. 184p. DLC: IU-M; OCIM **80-3842**

LYDSTON, G[eorge] Frank (1858-1923)
Apparent cancerous transformation of syphiloma of the tongue; excision of the tongue by the galvanic-cautery. New York, 1889. 16p. DNLM; NNNAM **80-3843**

LYDSTON, G[eorge] Frank (1858-1923)
A lecture on sexual perversion, satyriasis and nymphomania. Chicago, [1889]. 22p. DNLM: IU-M
80-3844

LYDSTON, G[eorge] Frank (1858-1923)
Remarks on hypertrophy and atrophy of tissue. New Orleans, [1889]. 8p. DNLM **80-3845**

LYMAN, Albert J[osiah] (1845-1915)
The modern physician the mediator of science. An address delivered at the Academy of Music, Brooklyn, May 21, 1884, before the graduating class of the Long Island College Hospital. New York: D. Appleton & Co., 1884. 18p. DNLM; NNNAM
80-3846

LYMAN, Charles P[arker] (1846-1918)
Special report No. 31. Contagious pleuro-pneumonia. Third report of . . . . Washington: Government Printing Office, 1881. 20p. 7 plates. DNLM **80-3847**

LYMAN, G[eorge] H[inckley] (1819-1890)
Pelvic effusions, and the importance of their early recognition with reference to treatment. Report of eleven cases. Cambridge, 1882. [unp.] DNLM **80-3848**

LYMAN, G[eorge] H[inckley] (1819-1890)
Synopsis of gynecological cases treated in the Boston City Hospital for five years preceding January 1, 1881. Boston: Rockwell & Churchill, 1882. 20p. DNLM; MBM
80-3849

LYMAN, G[eorge] H[inckley] (1819-1890)
Notes on cases of pelvic effusion resulting in abscess. [Boston, 1882.] 44p. DNLM; MH-M **80-3850**

LYMAN, G[eorge] H[inckley] (1819-1890)
Tinnitus aurium and vertigo as prominent symptoms of lithaemia. Chicago: A. G. Newell, 1884. 16p. DNLM
80-3851

LYMAN, G[eorge] H[inckley] (1819-1890)
Tinnitus aurium and vertigo as prominent symptoms of lithaemia. Cambridge, 1884. 14p. DNLM; MBM
80-3852

LYMAN, G[eorge] H[inckley] (1819-1890)
Historical sketch of the Obstetrical Society of Boston in the War of the Rebellion. Boston: D. Clapp & Son, 1887. 62p. DNLM; MBM **80-3853**

LYMAN, Henry M[unson] (1835-1904)
. . . Artificial anaesthesia and anaesthetics. . . . New York: William Wood & Co., 1881. 338p. DLC; NNNAM; PPC; PU
80-3854

LYMAN, Henry M[unson] (1835-1904)
The practical home physician; a popular guide for the household management of disease. . . . Written by Henry M. Lyman . . . Christian Fenger . . . H. Webster Jones . . . W. T. Belfield. . . . Chicago, Ill.: Western Publishing House, 1884. 1115p. col. plates. DLC; IU-M; OCIM **80-3855**

LYMAN, Henry M[unson] (1835-1904)
Insomnia, and other disorders of sleep. . . . Chicago: W. T. Keener, 1885. 239p. DLC; DNLM; IU-M; OCIM
80-3856

LYONS, Albert B[rown] (1841-1926)
Manual of practical pharmaceutical assaying, including details of the simplest and best methods of determining the strength of crude drugs and galenical preparations. . . . Detroit: D. O. Haynes & Co., 1886. 151p. DLC; OCIM
80-3857

MABON, William
Clinical observations on the action of sulfonal in insanity. [Utica, 1889.] 7p. DNLM **80-3858**

MABON, William, William H. FLINT and Elon H. CARPENTER
Clinical observations on the action of Sulfonal-Bayer. New York: W. H. Schieffelin & Co., 1889. 16p. DNLM; NNNAM
80-3859

McALLISTER, William G.
A complete and profusely illustrated catalogue of spectacles, microscopes, thermometers, and other scientific instruments. Philadelphia, 1881. 132p. DNLM; PU
80-3860

McARDLE, Thomas E[ugene] (*b.* 1852)
Remarks on pyo- and hydro-salpinx. [Washington, 1885.] 5p. DNLM **80-3861**

McARDLE, Thomas E. (*b.* 1852) and Louis KOLIPINSKI
Hydrocele of the hernial sac. [Philadelphia, 1886.] 16p. DNLM **80-3862**

McARTHUR, John A[mbrose] (1831-1887)
Consumption and tuberculosis. Notes on their treatment by the hypophosphites. 2nd ed. Boston, 1880. 64p. DNLM; MBM
80-3863

McARTHUR, John A[mbrose] (1831-1887)
Consumption and tuberculosis. Notes on their treatment by hypophosphites. 3rd ed. Boston: Mills, Knight & Co., 1881. 64p. DNLM; MBM **80-3864**

MACAULAY, James (1817-1902)
Vivisection; is it scientifically useful or morally justifiable? An essay addressed specifically to the medical profession. From the London ed. Philadelphia: American Anti-Vivisect. Soc., 1884. 70p. DNLM; PPC; PU **80-3865**

McBRIDE, J[ames] H.
Circulatory and sensory disorders of neurasthenia. [St. Louis, 1889.] 8p. DNLM **80-3866**

McBRIDE, P[eter] (1854-1946)
Clinical notes on ear disease. Oedema of the drum membrane simulating polypus; deafness improved by electricity and phosphorus. [New York: G. P. Putnam's Sons, 1883.] 7p. DNLM **80-3867**

McBRIDE, T[homas] A[lexander] (1844-1886)
Auscultatory percussion. New York: G. P. Putnam's Sons, 1880. 10p. DNLM **80-3868**

McBRIDE, T[homas] A[lexander] (1844-1886)
The early diagnosis of chronic Bright's disease. New York: Trow's Printing Co., 1882. 51p. DNLM; NNNAM
80-3869

McBRIDE, T[homas] A[lexander] (1844-1886)
Coma in chronic Bright's disease; the differential diagnosis of coma due to uraemia and to cerebral hemorrhage. New York, 1883. 14p. DNLM **80-3870**

McCASKEY, G[eorge] W[ashington] (1853-1935)
Geographical pathology of consumption. Chicago, 1885. 28p. DNLM **80-3871**

McCLELLAN, Ely (1834-1893)
On the use of vaseline by atomization in diseases of the upper air passages. Jefferson Barracks, Mo.: Kittson & Waller, 1888. 4 l. DNLM **80-3872**

McCLELLAN, Ely (1834-1893)
Note on Rumbold's method of treatment of catarrhal inflammations of the upper air passages. Chicago, 1889. 16p. DNLM
80-3873

McCLELLAN, George (1849-1913)
An introductory lecture delivered at the opening of the Pennsylvania School of Anatomy and Surgery, October 4, 1881, including a study of the effects of shock. Philadelphia: W. H. Hoskins, 1881. 24p. DNLM; PPC; PU
80-3874

McCLELLAND, J[ames] H[enderson] (1849-1913)
Nephrectomy. Philadelphia: Sherman & Co., 1880. 7p. DNLM
80-3875

McCLELLAND, J[ames] H[enderson] (1849-1913)
Homoeopathic treatment of syphilis. [Philadelphia, 1881.] 9p. DNLM **80-3876**

McCLELLAND, J[ames] H[enderson] (1849-1913)
Address delivered before the Homoeopathic Medical Society of Pennsylvania. Pittsburgh: J. Eickbaum & Co., 1881. 15p. DNLM **80-3877**

McCLELLAND, Milo A[dams] (*b.* 1837)
Report of the special committee on medical legislation before the Illinois State Medical Society at its thirty-first anniversary meeting. Chicago: Johnson, Olds & Co., 1881. 31p. DNLM
80-3878

McCLELLAND, Milo A[dams] (*b.* 1837)
Teaching in medicine and licensing to practice. Report on the desirability and practicability of separating the work. Chicago: Brown, Pettibone & Kelly, 1883. 10p. DLC; DNLM
80-3879

McCONNELL, James
Commencement address, delivered at the commencement of Tulane University, June 17, 1886. Tulane University of Louisiana; the wisdom of its benefactor. [New Orleans, 1886.] 11p. DNLM; LNT-M **80-3880**

McCORKLE, John A.
Certain foods in relation to treatment. New York: M. J. Rooney & Co., 1888. 12p. DNLM **80-3881**

McCOWEN, Jennie
Insanity in women. Davenport, Iowa, 1886. 15p. DNLM
80-3882

McCOY, Alexander W.
Idiopathic retro-pharyngeal abscess. [Philadelphia, 1882.] 4p. DNLM **80-3883**

McCOY, Alexander W.
Notes on a case of idiopathic retro-pharyngeal abscess, with some observations on diagnosis and treatment. [Philadelphia, 1882.] 8p. DNLM **80-3884**

McCOY, Alexander W.
Observations on occlusion of the posterior nares as a result of nasal catarrh. [Philadelphia, 1883.] 15p. DNLM
80-3885

McCOY, J. Cresap
Healthy digestion. A popular treatise on indigestion, dyspepsia, and biliousness. Being the substance of a course of lectures on the physiology of digestion, delivered before popular audiences in the city of Harrisburg, during the month of September, 1882. . . . Harrisburg: L. S. Hart, printer and binder, 1883. 76p. plates. DLC **80-3886**

McDADE, George W.
Monographia syphilitica. Indianapolis: E. Lilly & Co., 1885. 32p. 1 plate. DNLM; OCIM **80-3887**

MacDONALD, Carlos F. (*b.* 1845)
Report of a case of insanity following gunshot injury to the head; cerebral cyst; aspiration; recovery. [Philadelphia, 1886.] 8p. DNLM **80-3888**

MacDONALD, Carlos F. (*b.* 1845)
Report of two successful cases of trephining for traumatic epilepsy. [New York, 1886.] 8p. DNLM **80-3889**

McELROY, Z. Collins
On some points in the pathological histology of so-called phthisis pulmonalis, or consumption. St. Louis, 1880. 7p. DNLM **80-3890**

McFARLAND, T. Fletcher
General paralysis of the insane. Jacksonville, [Ill.], [1882]. 12p. DNLM **80-3891**

McGILLICUDDY, T[imothy] J. (1857-1899)
Dilation for stenosis and flexions of the uterus, with new instruments. [New York, 1888.] 10p. DNLM **80-3892**

McGILLICUDDY, T[imothy] J. (1857-1899)
Some points on the perineum and forceps; with a description of a new method of assisting the perineum, and a new combined axis traction forceps to be used as an alternative for craniotomy. [New York, 1889.] 11p. DNLM **80-3893**

McGRAW, Theodore A[ndrews] (1839-1921)
Abscesses of the abdomen. Detroit: G. S. Daris, 1880. 12p. DNLM **80-3894**

McGRAW, Theodore A[ndrews] (1839-1921)
Fracture of the humeral epiphysis in old dislocations of the elbow. New York, 1880. 8p. DNLM **80-3895**

McGRAW, Theodore A[ndrews] (1839-1921)
A case of traumatic aneurism of the sub-scapular artery. [n. p., 1885.] 10p. DNLM **80-3896**

McGRAW, Theodore A[ndrews] (1839-1921)
A contribution to the history of gunshot wounds of the intestines. Philadelphia: W. J. Dornan, 1889. 25p. DNLM; PPC **80-3897**

McGUIRE, Hunter Holmes (1835-1900)
Operative interference in gun-shot wounds of the peritoneum. Philadelphia: Collins, 1881. 11p. DNLM **80-3898**

McGUIRE, Hunter Holmes (1835-1900)
Clinical remarks on cancer of the breast. Richmond: J. W. Fergusson & Son, 1882. 16p. DNLM **80-3899**

McGUIRE, Hunter [Holmes] (1835-1900)
Progress and development of medical science. [Richmond, 1887.] 27p. DNLM **80-3900**

McGUIRE, J[ames] Clark
The care of the skin. A lecture before the Y.M.C.A. Lyceum. Louisville: J. P. Morton & Co., 1887. 19p. DNLM **80-3901**

McGUIRE, J[ames] Clark
Dermatological notes. Arsenic. Syphilis. Acne. Treatment of warts. Ichthyol and resorcin. Resorcin. Ointment basis. Lanolin. Iodide potash eruptions. [Louisville, 1887.] 4p. DNLM **80-3902**

McGUIRE, J[ames] Clark
Dermatological notes. Washington: Gibson Bros., 1888. 70p. 1 plate. DNLM; MdU-D **80-3903**

McHATTON, H[enry]
Malarial haemoglobinuria. [Atlanta, 1886.] 13p. DNLM **80-3904**

McILHANY, James Stuart
The therapy of oxygen. Washington: R. Beresford, 1887. 24p. DNLM **80-3905**

McINTIRE, Charles (*b.* 1847)
The percentage of college-bred men in the medical profession. A paper read before the American Academy of Medicine, at its annual meeting in Philadelphia, October 27, 1882. . . . Philadelphia, 1883. 13p. DLC; DNLM **80-3906**

McINTYRE, John H[oge] (*b.* 1833)
Bichloride of methylene used in a Junkers inhaler. St. Louis, 1883. 8p. DNLM **80-3907**

MACK, Charles S[amuel]
Similia similibus curantur? Addressed to the medical profession. Boston & Providence: Otis, Clapp & Son, 1888. 31p. DNLM; MBM **80-3908**

McKAY, Read Jennings
Some practical remarks upon the anomalies of refraction and accommodation of the eye and their complications. Milford, Del.: Scott & Townsend, 1880. 9p. DNLM **80-3909**

McKEE, E. S.
Irregular contraction of the uterus. [n. p., 1884.] 16p. DNLM **80-3910**

McKEE, E. S.
Membrana virginatatis. [Nashville, 1884.] 12p. DNLM **80-3911**

McKEE, E. S.
The early diagnosis of pregnancy. Chicago, 1886. 12p. DNLM **80-3912**

McKEE, E. S.
Consanguinity in marriage. [Cincinnati, 1886.] 16p. DNLM **80-3913**

McKELWAY, George I.
[Circular] to the physicians of Philadelphia [soliciting their vindication of himself from the unfavorable verdict of the coroner's inquest upon the body of Annie Carrol]. Philadelphia, 1884. 2 l. DNLM **80-3914**

MACKENZIE, John N[oland] (1853-1925)
Congenital syphilis of the throat; based upon the study of one hundred and fifty cases. [Philadelphia, 1880.] 32p. DNLM
80-3915

MACKENZIE, John N[oland] (1853-1925)
Diphtheritic ulceration of the air-passages and its relations to pulmonary phthisis. [Baltimore, 1882.] 8p. DNLM
80-3916

MACKENZIE, John N[oland] (1853-1925)
Transfixion of the left arytenoid cartilage by a fish-bone; loss of motion in the corresponding half of the larynx; abscess; recovery. [Baltimore, 1882.] 3p. DNLM
80-3917

MACKENZIE, John N[oland] (1853-1925)
Tubercular tumors of the windpipe, tuberculosis of the laryngeal muscles. A contribution to the pathological histology of laryngo-tracheal phthisis. New York: G. P. Putnam's Sons, 1882. 8p. DNLM **80-3918**

MACKENZIE, John N[oland] (1853-1925)
Abstract of a paper on deflection of the nasal septum. Baltimore, 1883. 2p. DNLM **80-3919**

MACKENZIE, John N[oland] (1853-1925)
Abstract of a paper "on nose cough and the existence of a sensitive reflex area in the nasal mucous membrane." Baltimore, 1883. 4p. DNLM **80-3920**

MACKENZIE, John N[oland] (1853-1925)
Deflection of the nasal septum and its treatment. [Richmond, 1883.] 16p. DNLM **80-3921**

MACKENZIE, John N[oland] (1853-1925)
On a hitherto undescribed malformation of the naso-pharynx. [New York, 1883.] 4p. DNLM **80-3922**

MACKENZIE, John N[oland] (1853-1925)
The local use of the bichloride of mercury in diseases of the nose and throat. [Baltimore, 1883.] 3p. DNLM
80-3923

MACKENZIE, John N[oland] (1853-1925)
On nasal cough, and the existence of a sensitive reflex area in the nose. [Philadelphia], 1883. 11p. DNLM
80-3924

MACKENZIE, John N[oland] (1853-1925)
Some remarks on naso-aural catarrh and its rational treatment. [Baltimore], 1883. 22p. DNLM
80-3925

MACKENZIE, John N[oland] (1853-1925)
Cases of reflex cough due to nasal polypi; with remarks. Baltimore, 1884. 8p. DNLM **80-3926**

MACKENZIE, John N[oland] (1853-1925)
Some observations on the toxic effects of chrome on the nose, throat, and ear. (Read in the section of ophthalmology, otology, and laryngology of the American Medical Association, May, 1884.) Chicago, 1884. 7p. DNLM
80-3927

MACKENZIE, John N[oland] (1853-1925)
A contribution to the study of congenital syphilis. [New York, 1884.] 8p. DNLM **80-3928**

MACKENZIE, John N[oland] (1853-1925)
Coryza vasomotoria periodica (hay asthma) in the Negro. With some remarks upon the etiology of the disease. [New York, 1884.] 6p. DNLM **80-3929**

MACKENZIE, John N[oland] (1853-1925)
A contribution to the study of coryza vasomotoria periodica, or so-called "hay fever." [New York], 1884. 16p. DNLM
80-3930

MACKENZIE, John N[oland] (1853-1925)
Some notes on the pathology of intranasal inflammation. [Philadelphia], 1884. 12p. DNLM **80-3931**

MACKENZIE, John N[oland] (1853-1925)
An improved self-retaining nasal speculum. [n. p., 1884.] 1 l. **80-3932**

MACKENZIE, John N[oland] (1853-1925)
Irritation of the sexual apparatus as an etiological factor in the production of nasal disease. [Philadelphia], 1884. 7p. DNLM
80-3933

MACKENZIE, John N[oland] (1853-1925)
On removal of the inferior turbinated body of the obstructed side as a substitute for operation on the deflected nasal septum in certain cases. [n. p., 1885.] 3p. DNLM
80-3934

MACKENZIE, John N[oland] (1853-1925)
Review [of hay fever; its etiology and treatment; with an appendix on rose cold. By Morell Mackenzie, London, 1885]. Philadelphia, 1885. 17p. DNLM **80-3935**

MACKENZIE, John N[oland] (1853-1925)
Historical notes on the discovery of the nasal erectile tissue. [n. p., 1885.] 6p. DNLM **80-3936**

MACKENZIE, John N[oland] (1853-1925)
A contribution to the pathological histology of acute and chronic coryza. [New York, 1885.] 8p. DNLM
80-3937

MACKENZIE, John N[oland] (1853-1925)
Notes on the classification, diagnosis, and treatment of the stages of chronic nasal inflammation. [Philadelphia, 1885.] 11p. DNLM **80-3938**

MACKENZIE, John N[oland] (1853-1925)
Observations on the origin and cure of the disease called "hay asthma" (coryza vasomotoria periodica). Baltimore, 1885. 6p. DNLM **80-3939**

MACKENZIE, John N[oland] (1853-1925)
Reflections on the aetiology of the simple inflammatory affections of the upper air-passages. [New York, 1885.] 16p. DNLM **80-3940**

MACKENZIE, John N[oland] (1853-1925)
On removal of the inferior turbinated body of the obstructed side as a substitute for operation on the deflected nasal septum in certain cases. [Bridgeport, Conn., 1885.] 3p. DNLM
80-3941

MACKENZIE, John N[oland] (1853-1925)
The production of the so-called "rose cold" by means of an artificial rose; with remarks and historical notes. [Philadelphia, 1886]. 13p. DNLM **80-3942**

MACKENZIE, John N[oland] (1853-1925)
The relation of certain states of the atmosphere to the prevalence of catarrhal affections of the upper air-passages. Baltimore, 1886. 5p. DNLM **80-3943**

MACKENZIE, John N[oland] (1853-1925)
A contribution to the pathology and treatment of the respiratory vaso-motor neuroses. [New York, 1887.] 22p. DNLM **80-3944**

MACKENZIE, John N[oland] (1853-1925)
The pathological nasal reflex. An historical study. [New York, 1887.] 22p. DNLM **80-3945**

MACKENZIE, Morell (1837-1892)
A manual of diseases of the throat, and nose, including the pharynx, larynx, trachea, oesophagus, nose, and naso-pharynx. Philadelphia: P. Blakiston, 1880. 570p. [vol. 2: P. Blakiston, Son & Co., 1884. 550p.] DNLM; IU-M; PPC; PU **80-3946**

MACKENZIE, Morell (1837-1892)
Malformations of the oesophagus. New York, 1880. 15p. DNLM **80-3947**

MACKENZIE, Morell (1837-1892)
A manual of diseases of the throat and nose, including the pharynx, larynx, trachea, oesophagus, nose, and naso-pharynx. New York: William Wood & Co., 1880. 440p. [vol. 2: William Wood & Co., 1884. 400p.] DLC; DNLM; NNNAM; PPC **80-3948**

MACKENZIE, Morell (1837-1892)
Diphtheria; its nature and treatment, varieties and local expressions. Philadelphia: P. Blakiston, 1881. 32p. DNLM; PPC; PU **80-3949**

McKESSON & ROBBINS
Prices current of druggists' articles, flint and green glassware, implements, fancy moulds, cases, perfumes. . . . New York, 1880. 226p. NNNAM **80-3950**

McKESSON & ROBBINS
Illustrated catalog with prices current. New York, 1883. 244p. NNNAM **80-3951**

McKESSON & ROBBINS
Catalogo general y precios corrientes de las drogas. New York, 1884. 472p. NNNAM **80-3952**

McKESSON & ROBBINS
Illustrated catalog. New York, 1888. 218p. NNNAM **80-3953**

McKIM, W. Duncan (1855-1935)
The present status of laparo-clytrotomy, with report of a successful case. [New York, 1887.] 21p. 1 tab. DNLM; NNNAM **80-3954**

MACLAGAN, Thomas John (1838-1903)
Rheumatism; its nature, its pathology, and its successful treatment. New York: William Wood & Co., 1886. 277p. CtY-M; DNLM; NNNAM; PPC **80-3955**

McLAUGHLIN, J[ames] W[harton] (1840-1909)
Researches into the etiology of dengue. Chicago, 1886. 23p. 1 plate. DNLM **80-3956**

McLAUGHLIN, J[ames] W[harton] (1840-1909)
The nature of contagion. [Austin, 1887.] 8p. DNLM **80-3957**

McLAURY, William M[uir] (*d.* 1896)
A paper [The senses—five or seven?] read at a meeting of the Northwestern Medical and Surgical Society. New York, 1884. 14p. DNLM **80-3958**

McLAURY, William M[uir] (*d.* 1896)
Remarks on the relation of menstruation to the sexual functions. [New York, 1887.] 7p. DNLM **80-3959**

McLAURY, William M[uir] (*d.* 1896)
The senses, five or seven. [New York, 1889.] 12p. DNLM **80-3960**

MACLEAN, Donald (1839-1903)
Observations upon the mutual relations of the medical profession and the state. Lansing: W. S. George & Co., 1885. 18p. DNLM **80-3961**

MACLEAN, Donald (1839-1903)
Amputation at the hip joint for morbus coxae; with a case and a specimen. [Chicago, 1886.] 3p. DNLM **80-3962**

McLEAN, Leroy (1831-1897)
Successful esophagotomy for the removal of foreign bodies. Troy, N.Y.: Stowell, 1884. 29p. 1 tab. DNLM **80-3963**

McMUNN, Charles A[lexander] (1852-1911)
Outlines of the clinical chemistry of urine. Philadelphia: P. Blakiston, Son & Co., 1889. 254p. 1 plate. DNLM; NNNAM; PPC; PU **80-3964**

McMURTRY, Lewis S[amuel] (1852-1924)
A case of traumatic aneurism of the axillary artery; ligation of the subclavian; subsequent incision of the sac, followed by recovery. Chicago, 1885. 8p. DNLM **80-3965**

McMURTRY, Lewis S[amuel] (1852-1924)
A case of ovariotomy. [Louisville, 1886.] 8p. DNLM **80-3966**

McMURTRY, Lewis S[amuel] (1852-1924)
A cae of intra-ligamentous ovarian cyst; general peritonitis; universal adhesions; ovariotomy; recovery. Chicago, 1887. 7p. DNLM **80-3967**

McMURTRY, Lewis S[amuel] (1852-1924)
A case of typhlitis, with double perforation of the caecum, and peritonitis, in which laparotomy and suture of the gut were followed by recovery. Chicago: Office of the Association, 1888. 8p. DNLM **80-3968**

McMURTRY, Lewis S[amuel] (1852-1924)
The treatment of peritonitis by abdominal section. Some illustrative cases. Boston: Rockwell & Churchill, 1888. 16p. DNLM **80-3969**

McMURTRY, Lewis S[amuel] (1852-1924)
A case of extra-uterine pregnancy; operation; recovery. Philadelphia: W. J. Dornan, 1889. 5p. DNLM **80-3970**

McMURTRY, Lewis S[amuel] (1852-1924)
A study of the pathology and treatment of intra-pelvic inflammations. Philadelphia: W. J. Dornan, 1889. 9p. DNLM
80-3971

McNEIL, A.
A treatise on diphtheria; its history, etiology, varieties, pathology, sequelae, diagnosis, and homoeopathic therapeutics. A prize essay. Chicago: Duncan Bros., 1881. 145p. DNLM; OCIM; PPHa 80-3972

MacNEILL, J. E[dward]
Reformation in the practice of medicine by the dosimetric method of practice, or the method of small doses of the active principles of plants, mathematically measured and scientifically adapted to the varied abnormal conditions; with biographical sketch of Ad. Burggraeve. [Revised.] New York: W. J. Morrison, 1889. 11p. DNLM; NNNAM
80-3973

McNUTT, Sarah J.
Apoplexia neonatorum. New York: William Wood & Co., 1885. 11p. DNLM; NNNAM 80-3974

McNUTT, Sarah J.
The babies' hospital. A summer's work. New York: Trow, 1889. 23p. DNLM; NNNAM 80-3975

McNUTT, W[illiam] F[letcher] (*b.* 1839)
Malignant disease of intestine at sigmoid flexure; diagnosis by physical examination impossible; post-mortem. San Francisco, 1880. 4p. DNLM 80-3976

McNUTT, W[illiam] F[letcher] (*b.* 1839)
Ovariotomy. [San Francisco, 1880.] 7p. DNLM
80-3977

McNUTT, W[illiam] F[letcher] (*b.* 1839)
Treatment of pneumonitis or croupous pneumonia. [n. p., 1880.] 4p. DNLM 80-3978

McNUTT, W[illiam] F[letcher] (*b.* 1839)
Report on medical education. [n. p., 1884.] 13p. DNLM
80-3979

McNUTT, W[illiam] F[letcher] (*b.* 1839)
Essentials of physiology; a manual to accompany White's physiological manikin. Prepared under the supervision of Wm. F. McNutt. . . . San Francisco: J. T. White & Co., [1885]. 16p. DLC 80-3980

McNUTT, W[illiam] F[letcher] (*b.* 1839)
Report on the etiology of leprosy, to the California State Medical Society. San Francisco, 1887. 27p. DNLM
80-3981

McNUTT, W[illiam] F[letcher] (*b.* 1839)
Mineral and thermal springs of California. San Francisco, Cal., 1888. 5 l. DNLM 80-3982

McNUTT, W[illiam] F[letcher] (*b.* 1839)
Treatment of hydrocele by incision of the tunica vaginalis and by a new procedure. [Philadelphia, 1888.] 4p. DNLM
80-3983

McSHERRY, H. Clinton
Some remarks on growths in the larynx. Baltimore: J. W. Borst & Co., 1881. 7p. DNLM 80-3984

McSHERRY, H. Clinton
Laryngeal stenosis; report of cases, with remarks on the history and treatment. [Baltimore, 1883.] 16p. DNLM
80-3985

McSHERRY, H. Clinton
Conservatism in throat practice. [Baltimore, 1884.] 10p. DNLM 80-3986

McSHERRY, Richard (1817-1885)
Health, and how to promote it. From infancy to advanced age. 2nd ed. New York: D. Appleton & Co., 1884. 185p. DNLM; NNNAM 80-3987

MADDEN, Thomas More (1838-1902)
On the prevention and treatment of post-partum hemorrhage. [n. p., 1882.] 12p. DNLM 80-3988

MAGRUDER, George L[loyd] (1848-1914)
Some practrical observations made at the Department for the diseases of children at the Central Dispensary, Washington, D.C. . . . [Richmond? 1880.] 8p. DLC; DNLM
80-3989

MAGRUDER, George L[loyd] (1848-1914)
Pertussis treated by the chloride of gold and sodium. Washington: Gibson Bros., 1885. 5p. DNLM 80-3990

MAGRUDER, George L[loyd] (1848-1914)
Operations for phimosis as a means of cure or relief of some nervous and other symptoms. . . . Read before the Washington Obstetrical and Gynecological Society, June 15, 1883. Chicago: Printed at the Office of the Association, 1887. 14p. DLC; DNLM 80-3991

MAISCH, Henry Charles Christian (1865-1901)
Illicium Floridanum, Ellis; histological and chemical examination. [Philadelphia College of Pharmacy.] Philadelphia: J. S. Smith, [1885]. 11p. 4 plates. DNLM
80-3992

MAISCH, John Michael (1831-1903)
A manual of organic materia medica. Being a guide to materia medica of the vegetable and animal kingdoms for the use of students, druggists, pharmacists, and physicians. . . . Philadelphia: Henry C. Lea's Son & Co., 1882. 459p. DLC; DNLM; OCLloyd; NNNAM 80-3993

MAISCH, John Michael (1831-1903)
A manual of organic materia medica. Being a guide to materia medica of the vegetable and animal kingdoms for the use of students, druggists, pharmacists, and physicians. . . . 2nd ed. With two hundred and forty-two illustrations. Philadelphia: Lea Bros. & Co., 1882. 511p. DLC; DNLM; OCLloyd; PU
80-3994

MAISCH, John Michael (1831-1903)
A manual of organic materia medica. Being a guide to materia medica of the vegetable and animal kingdoms for the use of students, druggists, pharmacists, and physicians. . . . 3rd ed. With two hundred and fifty-seven illustrations. Philadelphia: Lea Bros. & Co., 1887. 532p. DLC; DNLM; NNNAM; OCLloyd
80-3995

MAJOR, George W.
Phonation on inspiration a cause of hysterical aphonia. [New York: G. P. Putnam's Sons, 1882.] 3p. DNLM
80-3996

MAJOR, George W.
Affections of the crico-arytenoid articulation. [New York, 1887.] 10p. DNLM **80-3997**

MAJOR, George W.
Prolapse of the laryngeal ventricles. [New York, 1887.] 5p. DNLM **80-3998**

MALLET, John William
The claims of science for its own sake upon the medical profession; address delivered before the Medical and Chirurgical Faculty of Maryland, April 14, 1880. Baltimore: J. W. Borst & Co., 1880. 28p. DNLM; MdBM **80-3999**

MANHATTAN EYE AND EAR HOSPITAL, NEW YORK CITY
Annual reports of the board of directors to the contributors. 18.-34., 1886-1887 to 1902-1903. New York, 1887-1903. DNLM; NNNAM **80-4000**

MANHATTAN EYE AND EAR HOSPITAL, NEW YORK CITY
Nomenclature and pharmacopoeia of the throat department. New York, 1888. 38p. DNLM; NNNAM **80-4001**

MANHATTAN EYE AND EAR HOSPITAL, NEW YORK CITY
Dr. C. R. Agnew Memorial Fund. [Circular letter of committee soliciting contributions, March 27, 1889.] [New York, 1889.] 1 l. port. DNLM; NNNAM **80-4002**

MANHATTAN SURGEONS' SUPPLY CO.
Illustrated catalogue of medical articles including ear trumpet canes. New York, [*c.* 1880]. 48p. plates. NNNAM **80-4003**

MANLEY, Thomas H[enry] (1851-1905)
Injuries to the skull, with some observations on one hundred and eighteen cases. New York: M. J. Rooney & Co., 1889. 18p. DNLM; NNNAM **80-4004**

MANN, Edward Cox (1850-1908)
The brain in health and disease. Richmond, 1880. 16p. DNLM **80-4005**

MANN, Edward Cox (1850-1908)
The brain in health and disease. On the importance of the early recognition and the repression of mental diseases in its incipient stages, including the consideration of modern nervous diseases. [Philadelphia, 1881.] 7p. DNLM **80-4006**

MANN, Edward Cox (1850-1908)
On the importance of the early recognition and the repression of mental disease in its incipient stages. [Philadelphia, 1881.] 4p. DNLM **80-4007**

MANN, Edward Cox (1850-1908)
Some considerations on insanity and its therapeutics. [New York], 1881. 7p. DNLM **80-4008**

MANN, Edward Cox (1850-1908)
Contribution to mental pathology. Codification of the common law as to insanity. [St. Louis, 1881.] 11p. DNLM **80-4009**

MANN, Edward Cox (1850-1908)
Hystero-epilepsy, relieved by central galvanization, etc., after failure of oophorectomy. New York, 1881. 8p. DNLM **80-4010**

MANN, Edward Cox (1850-1908)
General considerations on the development of the nervous system by evolution, and its condition in health and disease. [St. Louis, 1882.] 12p. DNLM **80-4011**

MANN, Edward Cox (1850-1908)
A manual of psychological medicine and allied nervous diseases . . . with especial reference to the clinical features of mental diseases, and the allied neuroses, and its medico-legal aspects, with a carefully prepared digest of the lunacy laws in the various states. . . . Designed for the geneal practitioner of medicine. . . . Philadelphia: P. Blakiston, Son & Co., 1883. 699p. plate, 2 facsim. DLC; DNLM; NNNAM; PPC **80-4012**

MANN, Edward Cox (1850-1908)
On the use of cocaine in the opium habit. With a few preliminary remarks on its physiological properties. [St. Louis, 1886.] 7p. DNLM **80-4013**

MANN, Edward Cox (1850-1908)
On the relations existing between the digestive system and the brain. [St. Louis, 1886.] 6p. DNLM **80-4014**

MANN, Edward Cox (1850-1908)
Sunnyside. A private medical home for the treatment of inebriety, the morphine habit, and mild, curable mental cases. Brooklyn: T. F. Larkin, 1887. 16p. DNLM **80-4015**

MANN, Edward Cox (1850-1908)
Sunnyside. A private medical home for the treatment of inebriety, the morphine habit, and mild, curable mental cases. Brooklyn, 1889. 20p. DNLM **80-4016**

MANN, M[atthew] D[arbyshire] (1845-1921)
A manual of prescription writing, with a full explanation of the methods of correctly writing prescriptions; a table of doses expressed in both the apothecaries' and metric systems; rules for avoiding incompatibilities and for combining medicines. 3rd ed. New York: G. P. Putnam's Sons, 1881. 157p. DNLM; NNNAM; OCLloyd; PU **80-4017**

MANN, M[atthew] D[abryshire] (1845-1921)
A case of fatal primary hemorrhage after excision of the cervix uteri for epithelioma, and a case of fatal secondary hemorrhage after removal of the cervix uteri for epithelioma with the galvano-cautery wire, followed by the Sharp curette and thermo-cautery, by Paul F. Mundé, with discussion. New York: William Wood & Co., 1882. 10p. DNLM **80-4018**

MANN, M[atthew] D[arbyshire] (1845-1921)
Surgical operations on the pelvic organs of pregnant women. Philadelphia, 1883. 42p. DNLM; PPC **80-4019**

MANN, M[atthew] D[arbyshire] (1845-1921)
A series of twenty-five laparotomies. Buffalo, [1887]. 11p. 1 tab. DNLM **80-4020**

MANN, M[atthew] D[arbyshire] (1845-1921)
Removal of solid uterine and ovarian tumors by laparotomy. With a report of nine cases. New York: William Wood & Co., 1887. 21p. DNLM; NNNAM **80-4021**

MANN, M[atthew] D[arbyshire] (1845-1921)
A system of gynecology. By American authors. . . . Philadelphia: Lea Bros. & Co., 1887-1888. 2 v. 7 col. plates. DLC; DNLM; NNNAM; PPC **80-4022**

MANSON, Otis F[rederick] (1822-1888)
Pneumonia cut short. [Richmond, 1880.] 7p. DNLM **80-4023**

MANSON, Otis F[rederick] (1822-1888)
Remittent fever. [Richmond, 1881.] 21p. DNLM **80-4024**

MANSON, Otis F[rederick] (1822-1888)
A treatise on the physiological and therapeutic action of the sulphate of quinine. Philadelphia: J. B. Lippincott & Co., 1882. 164p. DLC; DNLM **80-4025**

MANSON, Otis F[rederick] (1822-1888)
A treatise on the physiological and therapeutic action of the sulphate of quinine. . . . Richmond, Va.: J. W. Fergusson & Son, 1882. 164p. DLC; DNLM; ViRA **80-4026**

MANSON, Otis F[rederick] (1822-1888)
A treatise om malarial haemorrhage, embracing epistaxis, odontorrhagia, stomatorrhagia, haemoptysis, haematemesis, enterrorrhagia, metrorrhagia, and haematuria. Richmond: J. W. Fergusson & Son, 1886. 118p. DNLM; PCC; PPJ; ViRA **80-4027**

MANTON, Walter P[orter] (1858-1925)
Beginnings with the microscope; a working handbook, containing simple [in]structions in the art and method of using the microscope and preparing objects for examination. . . . Boston: Lee & Shepard; New York: C. T. Dillingham, 1884. 73p. DLC; ICU; NN **80-4028**

MANTON, Walter P[orter] (1858-1925)
Report on ophthalmia neonatorum. [Boston, 1885.] 8p. DNLM **80-4029**

MANTON, Walter P[orter] (1858-1925)
A plea for episotomy. New York, 1885. 13p. DNLM **80-4030**

MANTON, Walter P[orter] (1858-1925)
On the use and abuse of the pessary. [n. p., 1885.] 10p. DNLM **80-4031**

MANTON, Walter P[orter] (1858-1925)
On the treatment of the perineum in the second stage of labor and post partum. [Detroit, 1885.] 19p. DNLM **80-4032**

MANTON, Walter P[orter] (1858-1925)
Ovariotomy; with the report of a case. [Detroit, 1885.] 11p. DNLM **80-4033**

MANTON, Walter P[orter] (1858-1925)
Antiseptic midwifery. [St. Paul, 1888.] 16p. DNLM **80-4034**

MANTON, Walter P[orter] (1858-1925)
Shall the forceps be applied to the aftercoming head? [Detroit, 1888.] 7p. DNLM **80-4035**

MANTON, Walter P[orter] (1858-1925)
A contribution to the history of ovariotomy on the insane. Philadelphia: W. J. Dornan, 1889. 6p. DNLM **80-4036**

MANTON, Walter P[orter] (1858-1925)
Intra-uterine stems; their history, abuse and use. [Detroit, 1889.] 8p. DNLM **80-4037**

MANTON, Walter P[orter] (1858-1925)
Skin eruptions during the climacteric. Boston: Rockwell & Churchill, [1889]. 2 l. DNLM **80-4038**

MANTON, Walter P[orter] (1858-1925)
Vaginal tamponnement in the treatment of prolapsed ovaries. Philadelphia: W. J. Dornan, 1889. 7p. DNLM **80-4039**

MARBLE, John O[liver]
Cremation in its sanitary aspects. Boston, [1885]. 35p. DNLM; MB **80-4040**

MARCHAND, Charles
On bacterine. [New York, 1884.] 10p. DNLM **80-4041**

MARCHAND, Charles
The use of peroxide of hydrogen and glycozone in therapeutics. Diphtheria. [New York, 1888.] 6p. DNLM **80-4042**

MARCHAND, Charles
The therapeutical applications of peroxide of hydrogen and glycozone for the treatment of chronic and contagious diseases. Revised ed. New York: N. Thompson, 1889. 18p. DNLM; NNNAM **80-4043**

MARCY, Henry Orlando (1837-1924)
Aspiration of the knee-joint. Cambridge: Riverside Press, 1880. 32p. DNLM; MBM **80-4044**

MARCY, Henry Orlando (1837-1924)
The development of the osseous callus in fractures of the bones of man and animals. Philadelphia: Collins, 1880. 20p. DNLM **80-4045**

MARCY, Henry Orlando (1837-1924)
A lecture on the development of the osseous callus in fractures of the bones of man and animals. Brooklyn, N.Y., 1881. 22p. DLC; DNLM; NNNAM **80-4046**

MARCY, Henry Orlando (1837-1924)
The best methods of treating operative wounds. [New York], 1882. 16p. DNLM **80-4047**

MARCY, Henry Orlando (1837-1924)
The best methods of treating operative wounds. New York: Bermingham & Co., 1882. 16p. DNLM **80-4048**

MARCY, Henry Orlando (1837-1924)
The placental development in mammals; a unity of anatomical and physiological modality in all vertebrates. Brooklyn, 1882. 11p. DNLM **80-4049**

MARCY, Henry Orlando (1837-1924)
The recent advances of sanitary science. The relations of micro-organisms to disease. Annual address delivered before the American Academy of Medicine. Philadelphia, 1883. 23p. DNLM; PPC **80-4050**

MARCY, Henry Orlando (1837-1924)
The recent advances of sanitary science. The relation of micro-organisms to disease. Philadelphia, 1883. 23p. DNLM **80-4051**

MARCY, Henry Orlando (1837-1924)
The restoration of the perinaeum by a new method. Chicago: A. G. Newell, 1884. 7p. DNLM **80-4052**

MARCY, Henry Orlando (1837-1924)
The role of bacteria in infectious diseases. Chicago: Review Printing Co., 1884. 31p. DNLM **80-4053**

MARCY, Henry Orlando (1837-1924)
The relation of micro-organisms to surgical lesions. Chicago: Review Printing Co., 1884. 16p. DNLM **80-4054**

MARCY, Henry Orlando (1837-1924)
Medical legislation. The annual address delivered before the Association of American Medical Editors. Chicago, 1885. 21p. DNLM; OCIM **80-4055**

MARCY, Henry Orlando (1837-1924)
The role of bacteria in parturition. Chicago, 1885. 12p. DNLM **80-4056**

MARCY, Henry Orlando (1837-1924)
The climatic treatment of disease; Western North Carolina as a health resort. Chicago, 1886. 24p. DNLM **80-4057**

MARCY, Henry Orlando (1837-1924)
The climate of the southern Appalachians. Washington, 1887. 5 l. 2 tab. **80-4058**

MARCY, Henry Orlando (1837-1924)
The cure of hernia. Chicago, 1887. 11p. DNLM **80-4059**

MARCY, Henry Orlando (1837-1924)
The histology and surgical treatment of uterine myoma. Philadelphia: W. Fell & Co., 1887. 7 l. DNLM **80-4060**

MARCY, Henry Orlando (1837-1924)
Placental development. Philadelphia: W. F. Fell & Co., [1887]. 4 l. DNLM **80-4061**

MARCY, Henry Orlando (1837-1924)
Recent advances in abdominal surgery. [Philadelphia, 1887.] 18p. DNLM **80-4062**

MARCY, Henry Orlando (1837-1924)
Cystitis in the female. Chicago, 1888. 8p. DNLM **80-4063**

MARCY, Henry Orlando (1837-1924)
The surgical advantages of the buried animal suture, and its adaptability to special purposes. Chicago, 1888. 11p. DNLM **80-4064**

MARCY, Henry Orlando (1837-1924)
The animal suture; its place in surgery. Philadelphia: W. J. Dornan, 1889. 24p. DNLM **80-4065**

MARCY, Henry Orlando (1837-1924)
Chronic inversion of the uterus; reduction by a new method. Chicago, 1889. 16p. DNLM **80-4066**

MARCY, Henry Orlando (1837-1924)
The cure of hemorrhoids by excision and closure with the buried animal suture. [St. Louis, 1889.] 14p. DNLM **80-4067**

MARCY, Henry Orlando (1837-1924)
The cure of hernia by the use of buried antispetic animal suture. Chicago, 1889. 28p. 1 plate. DNLM **80-4068**

MARCY, Henry Orlando (1837-1924)
Exploratory laparotomy. Chicago, 1889. 8p. DNLM **80-4069**

MARCY, Henry Orlando (1837-1924)
The perineum; its anatomy, physiology, and methods of restoration after injury. Philadelphia: W. J. Dornan, 1889. 31p. 11 plates. DNLM **80-4070**

MARCY, Henry Orlando (1837-1924)
A treatise on hernia. The radical cure by the use of the buried antiseptic animal suture. Detroit: G. S. Davis, 1889. 251p. DLC; DNLM; NNNAM; OCIM **80-4071**

MARKOE, Thomas Masters (1819-1901)
Oesophagotomy for foreign bodies lodged in the tube. [New York, 1886.] 15p. DNLM; NNNAM **80-4072**

MARKS, A. A. & CO.
Patent artificial limbs with india-rubber hands and feet. New York: W. L. Mershon & Co., 1884. 158p. 1 phot. DNLM; NNNAM **80-4073**

MARKS, A. A. & CO.
Formula for measurements and drafts for artificial arms and legs. New York, [1885]. broadside fol. DNLM; NNNAM **80-4074**

MARKS, A. A. & CO.
Abstract (No. 21). Marks' patent artificial limbs. New York, 1886. 32p. DNLM; NNNAM **80-4075**

MARKS, George E[dwin] (1853-1932)
A treatise on Marks' patent artificial limbs with rubber hands and feet. New York: A. A. Marks, 1888. 397p. DLC; DNLM; NNNAM **80-4076**

MARKS, George E[dwin] (1853-1932)
A treatise on Marks' patent artificial limbs with rubber hands and feet. New York: A. A. Marks, 1889. 410p. DLC; DNLM; NNNAM **80-4077**

MARSH, F. H. (1839-1915)
The law of heredity. New York: Murray Hill Publ. Co., 1882. 34p. DNLM; NN; NNNAM **80-4078**

MARSH, Howard
Diseases of the joints. Philadelphia: Lea Bros. & Co., 1886. 461p. 1 plate. DNLM; MBM; NNNAM; PPC **80-4079**

MARSH, Luther R[awson] (1813-1902)
Discourse before the College of Physicians and Surgeons of New York, to its graduating class of students. New York, 1882. 32p. DNLM; NNNAM **80-4080**

MARSHALL BROS.
Green Spring Sanitarium and Water Cure. [Circular of the proprietors.] Detroit: J. F. Eby & Co., [1884]. 2 l. DNLM
80-4081

MARSHALL, Clara (1848-1931)
Two cases of congenital imperforate anus with fecal fistula in the adult female. [New York, 1885.] 7p. DNLM
80-4082

MARSHALL, Clara (1848-1931)
Valedictory address to the graduating class of the Woman's Medical College of Pennsylvania, delivered March 11, 1886. [Philadelphia, 1886.] 9p. DNLM
80-4083

MARSHALL, John (1855-1925)
Notes on the chemical lectures in the Medical Department of the University of Pennsylvania, for first-year students. Published by authority of Prof. Theo. G. Wormley. . . . Philadelphia: Press of W. F. Fell & Co., 1889. 166p. DLC; PU
80-4084

MARSHALL, John (1855-1925)
Notes on the chemical lectures in the Medical Department of the University of Pennsylvania, for second-year students. Pub. by authority of Prof. Theo. G. Wormley. . . . Philadelphia: Printed by J. B. Lippincott Co., 1889. 107p. DLC; PU
80-4085

MARSHALL, John S[ayre] (1846-1922)
Fracture and diastasis of the superior maxillae and upper bones of the face, treated by the aid of the interdental splint; with two cases. Chicago, 1888. 20p. DNLM; IU-M
80-4086

MARTIN, Eduard Arnold (1809-1875)
Martin's atlas of obstetrics and gynaecology, ed. by A[ugust] Edward Martin. 2nd ed. Transl. and ed. with additions by Fancourt Barnes. Philadelphia: P. Blakiston, 1881. 98 l. 98 plates. DLC; IU-M; NNNAM; PPC [98 lithographic plates facing text explanation; 12 col. plates; 4 plates are of instruments.] **80-4087**

MARTIN, Edward (1859-1938)
Questions and answers of the essentials of surgery: together with a full description of the handerchief and roller bandages. . . . With ninety illustrations. Philadelphia: W. B. Saunders, 1888. 314p. DLC; MH-M; NNNAM; PPJ
80-4088

MARTIN, Francis C[offin]
Martin's method of treatment of synovitis, especially of the knee-joint. New York, 1885. 4p. DNLM
80-4089

MARTIN, Franklin H[enry] (1857-1935)
Electrolysis in gynecology, with a report of three cases of fibroid tumor successfully treated by the method. With discussion. . . . Also, supplementary paper, citing two cases of fibroid tumor treated by electrolysis, by J. N. Freeman. Chicago: By the Association, 1886. 47p. DNLM; IU-M
80-4090

MARTIN, Henry A[ustin] (1824-1884)
Rubber bandage. Philadelphia, 1880. 3p. DNLM
80-4091

MARTIN, Henry Austin (1824-1884)
Jefferson as a vaccinator. [Wilmington, 1881.] 34p. DNLM; MdU-D **80-4092**

MARTIN, H[enry] Newell (1848-1896)
The human body. An account of its structure and activities, and the conditions of its healthy working. New York: H. Holt & Co., 1881. 621, 34p. DNLM; ICU; MB; NN
80-4093

MARTIN, H[enry] Newell (1848-1896)
Annual address. The study of the physiological action of drugs. [Baltimore, 1885.] 14p. DNLM
80-4094

MARTIN, H[enry] Noah (1829-1889)
Constipation. [Philadelphia, 1885.] 7p. DNLM .
80-4095

MARTIN, H[enry] Noah (1829-1889)
Prescribing by mail. Philadelphia, 1886. 1 sheet. fol. DNLM
80-4096

MARTIN, Solomon C[laiborne] (1837-1906)
The inoculation, propagation, and preservation of the virus of animal vaccine. Boston: Cupples, Upham & Co., 1885. 16p. DNLM; MBM **80-4097**

MARVIN, C. A.
Address delivered before the American Academy of Dental Science, at their twelfth annual meeting. Boston: I. G. Gates, 1880. 32p. DNLM; MBM **80-4098**

MARVIN, J[oseph] B[enson] (1852-1913)
Primary lateral spinal sclerosis. [Louisville, 1885.] 8p. DNLM
80-4099

MARVIN, J[oseph] B[enson] (1852-1913)
Progressive muscular atrophy, beginning in the legs. Louisville: J. P. Morton & Co., 1886. 11p. DNLM
80-4100

MARVIN, J[oseph] B[enson] (1852-1913)
The aim and purpose of the medical man. Louisville: J. P. Morton & Co., [1886]. 15p. DNLM
80-4101

MARVIN, J[oseph] B[enson] (1852-1913)
"Renal colic, parasitic and calculus." A criticism. Louisville: Bradley & Gilbert Co., [1887]. 28p. DNLM; OCIM
80-4102

MARYLAND COLLEGE OF PHARMACY. BALTIMORE
Annual circulars, announcements, and catalogues for the sessions of 1882-1883 (33.); 1889-1890 (40.); 1891-1892 (42.); 1893-1894 to 1898-1899 (44.-49.); Baltimore, 1882-1898. DNLM; MdU-D **80-4103**

MARYLAND EYE AND EAR INSTITUTE. BALTIMORE
[Circular of the surgeon in charge, stating the conditions of treatment for indoor and out-door patient.] [Baltimore, 1888.] 1 sheet. DNLM; MdU-D **80-4104**

MARYLAND. MEDICAL AND CHIRURGICAL FACULTY
Report of committee on lunacy commission, with the new lunacy law enacted by the Maryland legislature, January session, 1886. [Baltimore: Weil & Co., 1886.] 13p. DNLM; MdBM **80-4105**

MASON, Charles F[ield] (1864-1922)
A compend of electricity and its medical and surgical uses. With an introduction by Charles H. May. Philadelphia: P. Blakiston, Son & Co., 1887. 108p. DLC; DNLM; NNNAM; PPC **80-4106**

MASON, George W[ilcoxson] (1850-1887)
Sarcoma of the spermatic cord, with hernia of the vermiform appendix. [Philadelphia: W. J. Dornan, 1883.] 8p. DNLM **80-4107**

MASON, Lewis D[uncan] (*b.* 1843)
An improved method of treating depressed fractures of the nasal bones. [Brooklyn, 1880.] 5p. DNLM **80-4108**

MASON, Lewis D[uncan] (*b.* 1843)
A case of fracture of nasal bones treated by an improved method. [New York, 1880.] 2p. DNLM **80-4109**

MASON, Lewis D[uncan] (*b.* 1843)
A statistical report of two hundred and fifty-two cases of inebriety, treated at the Inebriates' Home, Fort Hamilton, L.I., from Nov. 1, 1879, to Sept. 10, 1880. [1881.] 25p. DNLM **80-4110**

MASON, Lewis D[uncan] (*b.* 1843)
Report of cases of extensive fracture of nasal bones treated by a new method. [Brooklyn, 1881.] 4p. DNLM **80-4111**

MASON, Lewis D[uncan] (*b.* 1843)
Alcoholic anaesthesia. Hartford: Case, Lockwood & Brainard Co., 1882. 8p. DNLM **80-4112**

MASON, Lewis D[uncan] (*b.* 1843)
Alcoholic insanity. [New York], 1883. 33p. DNLM **80-4113**

MASON, Lewis D[uncan] (*b.* 1843)
Alcohol in the treatment of acute and chronic forms of alcoholic mania. New York, 1885. 8p. DNLM **80-4114**

MASON, Lewis D[uncan] (*b.* 1843)
Modified lithotomy-staff. [1885.] 3p. DNLM **80-4115**

MASON, Lewis D[uncan] (*b.* 1843)
The relation which disease bears to alcoholic inebriety. [Hartford, 1887.] 15p. DNLM **80-4116**

MASON, Lewis D[uncan] (*b.* 1843)
The etiology of dipsomania and heredity of "alcoholic inebriety." Hartford: Case, Lockwood & Brainard Co., 1888. 21p. DNLM **80-4117**

MASON, Lewis D[uncan] (*b.* 1843)
The control and care of pauper inebriates of towns and cities. [Hartford, 1889.] 11p. DNLM **80-4118**

MASON, Lewis D[uncan] (*b.* 1843)
Pathological changes in chronic alcoholism. [Brooklyn, 1889.] 8p. DNLM **80-4119**

MASSEY, G[eorge] Betton (1856-1927)
Electricity in the diseases of women, with special reference to the application of strong currents. Philadelphia & London: F. A. Davis, 1889. 210p. DNLM; NNNAM; PPC **80-4120**

MASTIN, Claudius H[enry] (1826-1898)
Circumcision a cause of reflex irritation of the genito-urinary organs. Mobile, 1885. 8p. DNLM **80-4121**

MASTIN, Claudius H[enry] (1826-1898)
Subcutaneous division of urethral stricture. Philadelphia: W. J. Dornan, 1886. 32p. DNLM; PPC **80-4122**

MASTIN, Claudius H[enry] (1826-1898)
Hernia. A comparison of the various methods adopted for its cure; inviting discussion of their respective merits. Philadelphia: W. J. Dornan, 1889. 34p. DNLM; PPC; PU **80-4123**

MASTIN, William M.
Tracheotomy for croup in the United States; analysis of 863 operations. [New York, 1880.] 35p. DNLM; NNNAM **80-4124**

MATAS, Rudolph (1860-1957)
Morbid somnolence. [New Orleans, 1884.] 16p. DNLM; LNT-M **80-4125**

MATAS, Rudolph (1860-1957)
The peritoneal relations of the caecum. Rectification of an historical error. [New Orleans, 1887.] 10p. DNLM; LNT-M **80-4126**

MATAS, Rudolph (1860-1957)
Report of the case of a patient from whose subcutaneous tissue three larvae of a species of Dermatobia were removed. New Orleans: L. Graham & Son, [1887]. 19p. DNLM; LNT-M **80-4127**

MATAS, Rudolph (1860-1957)
Report of a case of thyroidectomy for malignant disease, with a synoptical consideration of the present status of the operation. [New Orleans, 1888.] 32p. 2 plates. DNLM; LNT-M **80-4128**

MATAS, Rudolph (1860-1957)
Multiple subperiosteal sarcoma of the skull, associated with necrosis of vertical plate of frontal. Extirpation of necrotic vertical plate and tumors; recovery. [New Orleans, 1889.] 10p. 1 plate. DNLM; LNT-M **80-4129**

MATHEWS, Joseph M[cDowell] (*b.* 1847)
Report on diseases of the rectum. Louisville: The Bradley & Gilbert Co., 1886. 7p. DNLM **80-4130**

MATTEI, Cesare
The principles of electro-homoeopathy. A new science discovered by Count Cesar Mattei, of Bologna. American ed. Milwaukee, Wis.: P. Kaindl, 1883. 229p. DLC **80-4131**

MATTISON, J[ansen] B[eemer] (*b.* **1845)**
Clinical notes on opium addiction. A paper read before the Kings County Medical Society. Cincinnati, 1883. 12p. DNLM
80-4132

MATTISON, J[ansen] B[eemer] (*b.* **1845)**
The curability of opium addiction. [Brooklyn, 1883.] 15p. DNLM **80-4133**

MATTISON, J[ansen] B[eemer] (*b.* **1845)**
Neurotic pyrexia, with special reference to opium addiction. [1883.] 8p. DNLM **80-4134**

MATTISON, J[ansen] B[eemer] (*b.* **1845)**
Neurotic pyrexia, with special reference to opium addiction. Bridgeport, 1883. 11p. DNLM **80-4135**

MATTISON, J[ansen] B[eemer] (*b.* **1845)**
Opium addiction among medical men. New York: Trow, 1883. 9p. DNLM **80-4136**

MATTISON, J[ansen] B[eemer] (*b.* **1845)**
A personal narrative of opium addiction. [New York, 1883.] 10p. DNLM **80-4137**

MATTISON, J[ansen] B[eemer] (*b.* **1845)**
The treatment of opium addiction. St. Louis: J. H. Chambers & Co., 1883. 15p. DNLM **80-4138**

MATTISON, J[ansen] B[eemer] (*b.* **1845)**
A somewhat unusual case of opium addiction. [New York, 1883.] 3 l. DNLM **80-4139**

MATTISON, J[ansen] B[eemer] (*b.* **1845)**
The genesis of opium addiction. [Brooklyn, 1884.] 8p. DNLM
80-4140

MATTISON, J[ansen] B[eemer] (*b.* **1845)**
A curious case of opium addiction. [Brooklyn, 1884.] 8p. DNLM **80-4141**

MATTISON, J[ansen] B[eemer] (*b.* **1845)**
The prevention of opium addiction, with special reference to the value of electricity in the treatment of neuralgic headaches. [Brooklyn, 1884.] 8p. DNLM **80-4142**

MATTISON, J[ansen] B[eemer] (*b.* **1845)**
Avena sativa in the treatment of opium addiction. A therapeutical fraud, a delusion, and a snare. [Philadelphia, 1885.] 16p. DNLM **80-4143**

MATTISON, J[ansen] B[eemer] (*b.* **1845)**
The treatment of opium addiction. New York & London: G. P. Putnam's Sons, 1885. 3 p. 1., 49 p. DNLM **80-4144**

MATTISON, J[ansen] B[eemer] (*b.* **1845)**
Opium antidotes and their vendors. [Chicago, 1886.] 10p. DNLM **80-4145**

MATTISON, J[ansen] B[eemer] (*b.* **1845)**
1. Cocaine dosage and cocaine addiction. 2. Cocaine toxaemia. [Brooklyn, 1888.] 44p. DNLM **80-4146**

MAUDSLEY, Henry (1835-1918)
The pathology of mind. Being the third edition of the second part of the "Physiology and pathology of mind," recast, enlarged, and rewritten. . . . New York: D. Appleton & Co., 1880. 580p. DLC; DNLM; NNNAM; PPC
80-4147

MAUDSLEY, Henry (1835-1918)
Body and will; being an essay concerning will in its metaphysical, physiological, and pathological aspect. New York: D. Appleton & Co., 1884. 333p. DNLM; ICU; MB; NN
80-4148

MAUDSLEY, Henry (1835-1918)
The physiology of mind. Being the first part of a 3rd ed., rev., enl., and in great part rewritten, of "The physiology and pathology of mind." . . . New York: D. Appleton & Co., 1887. 547p. DLC; NNNAM; OCIM; PU **80-4149**

MAUGHS, G. M. B. (*d.* **1901)**
Constitutional syphilis. A critic criticized. St. Louis, 1881. 27p. DNLM; OCIM **80-4150**

MAURY, Richard B[rooke] (1834-1919)
A clinical contribution to the study of the fevers of the Mississippi Valley. [Philadelphia, 1881.] 21p. DNLM; PPC; PU
80-4151

MAY, Charles H[enry] (1861-1943)
Statistics of four hundred cases of rheumatism, with especial reference to treatment, treated at the Roosevelt Hospital. New York: Trow, 1884. 12 l. DNLM **80-4152**

MAY, Charles H[enry] (1861-1943)
Manual of the diseases of women, being a concise and systematic exposition of the theory and practice of gynaecology. Philadelphia: Lea Bros. & Co., 1885. 357p. DLC; DNLM; PPC **80-4153**

MAY, Charles H[enry] (1861-1943)
Method in medical study. [New York, 1886.] 8p. DNLM
80-4154

MAY, Charles H[enry] (1861-1943)
Enucleation with transplantation and reimplantation of eyes. New York: Trow, 1886. 32p. DNLM **80-4155**

MAY, Charles H[enry] (1861-1943)
Method in medical study. [New York, 1886.] 7p. DNLM
80-4156

MAY, Charles H[enry] (1861-1943)
Practical examples in prescription writing. [New York, 1887.] 16p. DNLM; NNNAM **80-4157**

MAY, Charles H[enry] (1861-1943) and Charles F. MASON
An index of materia medica; with prescription writing, including practical exercises. New York: William Wood & Co., 1887. 267p. DLC; DNLM; NNNAM; OCLloyd
80-4158

MAY, Charles H[enry] (1861-1943)
A résumé of experience at the aural clinic of Hermann Schwartze, in Halle, Germany. [New York, 1889.] 18p. DNLM; NNNAM **80-4159**

MAY, Charles H[enry] (1861-1943)
Scarlatinous otitis. [New York], 1889. 12p. DNLM; NNNAM
80-4160

MAYO, U. K.
Mayo's compound vegetable anaesthetic. A safe and pleasant substitute for ether, chloroform, nitrous oxide, and all dangerous substances used to destroy pain in dentistry and surgery. Boston: Cochran & Sampson, 1883. 24p. DNLM; MBM
80-4161

MAYO, U. K.
The vegetable anaesthetic. A safe and pleasant substitute for ether, chloroform, nitrous oxide, and all dangerous substances used to destroy pain in dentistry and surgery. 2nd ed. Boston, [1883]. 32p. DNLM; MBM; MWA **80-4162**

MAYS, Thomas Jefferson (1846-1918)
The external therapeutics of pulmonary consumption. [Philadelphia: Lea Bros. & Co., 1884.] 20p. DNLM; PPC **80-4163**

MAYS, Thomas Jefferson (1846-1918)
The external therapeutics and the dietetics of pulmonary consumption. Detroit: G. S. Davis, 1885. 18p. DNLM **80-4164**

MAYS, Thomas Jefferson (1846-1918)
The external therapeutics of pulmonary consumption. A retrospect of twenty cases treated by this method. Fourth paper. Philadelphia, 1885. 20p. DNLM; PPC **80-4165**

MAYS, Thomas Jefferson (1846-1918)
The physiological action of cocaine and of its analogue, brucine. Detroit: G. S. Davis, 1885. 6p. DNLM **80-4166**

MAYS, Thomas Jefferson (1846-1918)
The therapeutic action of aconite in croupous pneumonia. [Detroit, 1885.] 4p. DNLM **80-4167**

MAYS, Thomas Jefferson (1846-1918)
The therapeutic action of theine; a new analgesic. [Philadelphia, 1885.] 6p. DNLM **80-4168**

MAYS, Thomas Jefferson (1846-1918)
The external therapeutics of pulmonary consumption. Third paper. [Philadelphia, 1885.] 15p. DNLM **80-4169**

MAYS, Thomas Jefferson (1846-1918)
Study of pulmonary consumption in the city of Philadelphia. Philadelphia: W. J. Dornan, 1886. 26p. DNLM; PPC **80-4170**

MAYS, Thomas Jefferson (1846-1918)
Theine in the treatment of neuralgia: being a physiological contribution to the therapeutics of pain. . . . Philadelphia: P. Blakiston, Son & Co., 1888. 84p. DLC **80-4171**

MEADOWS, Alfred (1823-1887)
Manual of midwifery. 3rd American, with additions from the 4th London ed. Philadelphia: P. Blakiston, Son & Co., 1882. 494p. DNLM; MBM; NNNAM; PPC **80-4172**

MEADOWS, Alfred (1823-1887)
Manual of midwifery. 4th ed., revised and enlarged by Albert J. Venn. New York: G. P. Putnam's Sons, 1882. 498p. CtY-M; DNLM; NNNAM; PU **80-4173**

MEARS, J[ames] Ewing (1838-1919)
Closure of the jaws and its treatment, with the report of a case in which complete occlusion followed a gunshot wound of the left superior maxilla, received at two-and-a-half years of age, and which was relieved eighteen years subsequently by operation according to a new method. Philadelphia: Collins, 1883. 16p. DNLM; PPJ **80-4174**

MEARS, J[ames] Ewing (1838-1919)
Practical surgery: including surgical dressing, bandaging, fractures, dislocations, ligature of arteries, amputations, and excisions of bones and joints. . . . [2nd ed.]. Philadelphia: P. Blakiston, Son & Co., 1885. 794p. DLC; DNLM; PPC; PU **80-4175**

MEARS, J[ames] Ewing (1838-1919)
A sketch of the life of Professor Samuel D. Gross, M.D. Read before the Philadelphia County Medical Society, May 13, 1885. Philadelphia: Wm. J. Dornan, printer, 1885. 18p. DNLM; PPJ **80-4176**

MEARS, J[ames] Ewing (1838-1919)
Study of the pathological changes occurring in trifacial neuralgia. With the report of a case in which three inches of the inferior dental nerve were excised. Philadelphia: Collins, 1885. 17p. DNLM; PPJ **80-4177**

MEARS, J[ames] Ewing (1838-1919)
Phosphorus-necrosis of the jaws. Philadelphia, 1885. 31p. DNLM; PPJ **80-4178**

MEARS, J[ames] Ewing (1838-1919)
Closure of the jaws, and its treatment. Philadelphia: W. J. Dornan, 1887. 15p. DNLM; PPJ **80-4179**

MEARS, J[ames] Ewing (1838-1919)
The propriety of surgical interference in perforating typhoid ulcer. Philadelphia: W. J. Dornan, 1888. 14p. DNLM; PPJ **80-4180**

MEARS, J[ames] Ewing (1838-1919)
The progress and limitations of operations upon the abdominal cavity. Philadelphia, 1887. 20p. DNLM; PPJ **80-4181**

MEARS, J[ames] Ewing (1838-1919)
Distended gall-bladder simulating floating kidney, cholecystotomy by the lumbar incision. Philadelphia: W. J. Dornan, 1889. 7p. DNLM **80-4182**

MEDICAL COLLEGE OF ALABAMA, MOBILE
Annual announcements for the sessions of 1884-1885 to 1894-1895 (20.-30.); 1898-1899 (34.); 1899-1900 (35.). Mobile, 1884-1899. DNLM [List of students and graduates for the years 1883-1884 to 1893-1894; 1897-1898; 1898-1899 in: Announcements for subsequent years. List of graduates from 1860 to 1891 in: Announcement for 1891-1892.] **80-4183**

MEDICAL COLLEGE OF GEORGIA, AUGUSTA
Medical Department of the University of Georgia. Annual announcements for the sessions of 1885-1886 (54.); 1887-1888 to 1891-1892 (56.-60.); 1893-1894 (62.). Augusta, 1885-1893. DNLM [List of graduates from 1829 to 1891 in: Announcement for 1891-1892.] **80-4184**

MEDICAL COLLEGE OF INDIANA, UNIVERSITY OF INDIANAPOLIS
Annual announcements for the sessions of 1887-1888 (18.); 1889-1890 (20.); 1891-1892 to 1893-1894 (22.-24); 1897-1898 (28.); 1898-1899 (29.). Indianapolis, 1887-1898. DNLM [Prior to 1883, was Medical Department of Butler University. Alumni from 1870 to 1897 in: Announcement for 1897-1898.] **80-4185**

MEDICAL COLLEGE OF OHIO, DEPARTMENT OF MEDICINE OF THE UNIVERSITY OF CINCINNATI
Annual announcements and circulars for the sessions of 1883-1884 to 1904-1905 (65.-86.). Cincinnati, 1883-1904. DNLM
80-4186

MEDICAL COLLEGE OF OHIO, DEPARTMENT OF MEDICINE OF THE UNIVERSITY OF CINCINNATI
Announcement for the regular spring course of 1889. [Cincinnati, 1889.] 8p. DNLM **80-4187**

MEDICAL COLLEGE OF THE STATE OF SOUTH CAROLINA AND DEPARTMENT OF PHARMACY, CHARLESTON
Annual announcements and circulars for the sessions of 1886-1887 to 1893-1894 (58.-65.); 1895-1896 to 1898-1899 (67.-70.); 1900-1901 (72.); 1902-1903 (74.); 1903-1904 (75.). Charleston, 1886-1903. DNLM; ScCM [List of students and graduates for the years 1885-1886 to 1892-1893; 1894-1895 to 1897-1898; 1899-1900; 1901-1902; 1903-1904 in: Announcements for subsequent years. The department of pharmacy was added in 1896.] **80-4188**

THE MEDICAL directory and register for Baltimore, Washington, Maryland, and District of Columbia. Containing full and complete list of physicians, dentists, and druggists; also descriptions and details relating to colleges, hospitals, dispensaries, homes, reformatories, and complete list of medical colleges in the United States and Canadas. Compiled and arranged by B. R. Sheriff, manager, 1888. Baltimore: R. L. Polk & Co., 1888. 407p. DNLM; MdU-D; PPC; PU **80-4189**

THE MEDICAL directory of the City of New York. Published by the Medical Society of the County of New York, for the years 1887-1889; 1891-1894; 1896-1901; 1903. New York, 1887-1903. 14 v. DNLM; NNNAM **80-4190**

THE MEDICAL directory of Philadelphia for 1884. Edited by Samuel B. Hoppin. Philadelphia: P. Blakiston, Son & Co., 1884. 205p. DNLM; PPC; PPJ; PU **80-4191**

THE MEDICAL directory of Philadelphia, Pennsylvania, Delaware, and the southern half of New Jersey, 1885. Philadelphia: P. Blakiston, Son & Co., 1885. 307p. DNLM; PPC; PU
80-4192

THE MEDICAL directory of Philadelphia, Pennsylvania, Delaware, and the southern half of New Jersey for 1887. 3rd issue. Philadelphia: P. Blakiston, Son & Co., 1887. 232, 161p. 1 map. DNLM; PPC; PU **80-4193**

THE MEDICAL directory of Philadelphia, comprising lists of physicians, dentists, druggists, and veterinarians in Philadelphia and Camden for 1889. 4th issue. Philadelphia: P. Blakiston, Son & Co., 1889. 318p. DNLM; PPC; PU
80-4194

MEDICAL facts concerning Colorado Springs. Colorado Springs, 1889. 32p. DNLM **80-4195**

MEDICAL SOCIETY OF THE DISTRICT OF COLUMBIA
Catalogue of members of the Medical Society of the District of Columbia, from its organization in 1817 to 1885. Washington, D.C.: Printed by W. H. Moore, 1885. 26p. DLC
80-4196

MEDICAL SOCIETY OF SOUTH CAROLINA
In memoriam. George Granby Kinloch. [Charleston]: Walker, Evans & Cogswell Co., [1886]. 16p. DNLM; ScC
80-4197

THE MEDICAL student, his qualifications, course of study, expenses, and business opportunities. Issued by the Hahnemann Medical College and Hospital, Philadelphia. Philadelphia, [1884]. 8p. DNLM; PPHa **80-4198**

MEDICO-CHIRURGICAL COLLEGE OF PHILADELPHIA
Annual announcements for the sessions of 1881-1882 (1.); 1882-1883 (2.); 1885-1886 (5.). Philadelphia, 1881-1885. DNLM [Opened April 4, 1881] **80-4199**

MEDICO-CHIRURGICAL COLLEGE OF PHILADELPHIA. DEPARTMENT OF MEDICINE
Annual announcements for the sessions of 1887-1888 to 1903-1904 (7.-23.). Philadelphia, 1887-1903. DNLM [List of students and graduates for the sessions of 1886-1887 to 1902-1903 in: Announcements for subsequent years.]
80-4200

MEDICO-LEGAL SOCIETY OF THE CITY OF NEW YORK
Charter, constitution, by-laws, and resolution establishing permanent commission. 6th ed. New York: T. B. Mead, 1881. [unp.] DNLM; NNNAM **80-4201**

MEDICO-LEGAL SOCIETY OF THE CITY OF NEW YORK
Constitution and by-laws, officers, committees, and members, and list of donors and contributors to the library to December 31, 1882. [New York, 1882.] 40p. DNLM; NNNAM
80-4202

MEDICAL-LEGAL SOCIETY OF THE CITY OF NEW YORK
Report of the permanent commission of the . . . in answer to the senate resolutions of January 4, 1882, in reply to the letter of the attorney-general and State commissioner in lunacy of the State of New York. [New York, 1882.] 16p. DNLM; NNNAM **80-4203**

MEDICO-LEGAL SOCIETY OF THE CITY OF NEW YORK
Papers read before the Medico-Legal Society of New York, from its organization. Second Series. Rev. ed. New York: W. F. Vanden Houten, 1882. 528p. 1 diag. DNLM; NNNAM
80-4204

MEDICO-LEGAL SOCIETY OF THE CITY OF NEW YORK
Papers read before the Medico-Legal Society of New York, from its organization. Third Series. Rev. ed. New York: Medical-Legal Society, 1886. 550p. DNLM; NNNAM
80-4205

MEDICO-LEGAL SOCIETY OF THE CITY OF NEW YORK
The medical jurisprudence of inebriety. Being the papers read before the . . . , the discussion thereon. New York, 1888. 183p. DLC; DNLM; NNNAM **80-4206**

MEDICO-LEGAL SOCIETY OF PHILADELPHIA
An act [proposed] to establish a State board of medical examiners and licensers, and to define the duties and power of such board. Philadelphia: Siddall Bros., [1884] 4 l. DNLM; PPC **80-4207**

MEHARRY MEDICAL COLLEGE. NASHVILLE, TENN.
College for Colored Medical Students in the South. [Resolutions adopted at a meeting of medical teachers and practitioners, held at the Hall of the College of Physicians, of Philadelphia, May 8, 1882, to promote the thorough training of colored physicians, and recommending the Meharry Medical Department of the Central College of Tennessee to the profession and the public for encouragement and liberal support.] [Philadelphia, 1882.] 2 l. DNLM **80-4208**

MEIGS, Arthur V[incent] (1850-1912)
Milk analysis. Philadelphia, 1882. 4p. DNLM **80-4209**

MEIGS, Arthur V[incent] (1850-1912)
Memoir of J. Forsyth Meigs. Read before the College of Physicians of Philadelphia, March 5, 1884. Philadelphia, 1884. 25p. DNLM; PPC **80-4210**

MEIGS, Arthur V[incent] (1850-1912)
Milk analysis and infant feeding. A practical treatise on the examination of human and cows' milk, cream, condensed milk, etc., and directions as to the diet of young infants. Philadelphia: P. Blakiston, Son & Co., 1885. 102p. DLC; DNLM; PPC; PPJ **80-4211**

MEIGS, Arthur V[incent] (1850-1912)
Report of a case of brain and spinal-cord syphilis, showing extensive disease of the blood-vessels. With an account of the autopsy and microscopic examination by Geo. E. de Schweinitz. [Chicago, 1887.] 12p. DNLM **80-4212**

MEIGS, Arthur V[incent] (1850-1912)
A study of the arteries and veins in Bright's disease. New York: Trow, 1888. 31p. DNLM **80-4213**

MEIGS, Arthur V[incent] (1850-1912)
The artificial feeding of infants. [Philadelphia, 1889.] 12p. DNLM **80-4214**

MEIGS, Arthur V[incent] (1850-1912)
The treatment of spasmodic croup with opium. [Philadelphia, 1889.] 13p. DNLM **80-4215**

MEIGS, Arthur V[incent] (1850-1912) and J. A. SCOTT
Experiments in weighing before and after feeding as a means of determining the amount of food taken. [Philadelphia, 1889.] 4p. DNLM **80-4216**

MEIGS, John Forsyth (1818-1882)
On the internal use of water for the sick, and on thirst. A clinical lecture at the Pennsylvania Hospital, October 25, 1879. . . . Philadelphia: Lindsay & Blakiston, 1880. 54p. DLC; DNLM; PPC **80-4217**

MEIGS, John Forsyth (1818-1882)
Proceedings of the Alumni Society of the Medical Department of the University of Pennsylvania for 1880. With the annual address by . . . . Philadelphia: Collins, 1881. 31p. 1 plate. DNLM; PU **80-4218**

MEIGS, John Forsyth (1818-1882)
Annual address before the Alumni Society of the Medical Department of the University of Pennsylvania, delivered Feb. 10, 1881. Philadelphia: Collins, 1881. 23p. DNLM; PU **80-4219**

MEIGS, John Forsyth (1818-1882)
A practical treatise on the diseases of children. By J. Forsyth Meigs . . . and William Pepper. . . . 7th ed., rev. and enl. Philadelphia: P. Blakiston, Son & Co., 1882. 1055p. DLC; NNNAM; OCIM; PU **80-4220**

MELTZER, S[amuel] J[ames] (1851-1920)
Intubation in cases of foreign bodies in the air-passages; with remarks concerning feeding after intubation. New York: Trow's Print. & Bookbind. Co., 1889. 8p. DNLM **80-4221**

MELTZER, S[amuel] J[ames] (1851-1920)
Ueber die mechanischen Verhältnisse bei der Entstehung der Pneumonie. [New York, 1889.] 4p. DNLM **80-4222**

MELTZER, S[amuel] J[ames] (1851-1920)
Carbolsänrevergiftung bei einem Kinde. [New York, 1889.] 1 l. DNLM **80-4223**

A **MEMOIR** of Charles Hilton Fagge. [Philadelphia: P. Blakiston, Son & Co., 1886.] 7p. DNLM; PPC **80-4224**

IN **MEMORY** of Édouard Séguin. Being remarks made by some of his friends at the lay funeral service held October 31, 1880. [1880.] 51p. port. DNLM; NNNAM **80-4225**

MEMPHIS HOSPITAL MEDICAL COLLEGE
Annual announcements and catalogues for the sessions of 1887-1888 to 1893-1894 (8.-14.); 1897-1898 to 1902-1903 (18.-23.). Memphis, 1887-1902. DNLM [List of students and graduates for the sessions of 1886-1887 to 1892-1893, 1896-1897 to 1901-1902, in: Announcements for years. Alumni from 1881-1902 in: Announcements for 1902-1903.] **80-4226**

MERCER, A. Clifford (*b.* 1855)
Myxoedema. New York: Trow, 1881. 16p. DNLM **80-4227**

. . . **MERCK'S** index of fine chemicals and drugs for the materia medica and the arts. . . . A guide for the physician, apothecary, chemist, and dealer. [1st American ed.] By E. Merck. [New York: Cherouny Printing & Publishing Co.], 1889. 168p. DLC; NNNAM **80-4228**

MERGIER, Marie-J[oséphine] (1851-1901)
Etiology and treatment of salpingitis, with report of a case of pyometra, followed by purulent salpingitis. [Chicago, 1888.] 6p. DNLM **80-4229**

MERIAM, Horatio C.
Footprints of a profession, or ethics in materials and methods. Address delivered before the Maine Dental Society, at their twenty-second annual meeting. St. Louis: J. H. Chambers & Co., 1887. 21p. DNLM **80-4230**

MERIAM, Horatio C.
Footprints of a profession, or ethics in materials and methods. Address delivered before the Maine Dental Society, at their twenty-second annual meeting. 2nd ed. St. Louis, 1888. 30p. DNLM **80-4231**

MERIAM, Horatio C.
Professional atmosphere and morals; or, patents and secrets vs. liberal profession. [Philadelphia, 1889.] 23p. DNLM **80-4232**

MERKEL, G. Hermann
Microscopy in medical practice; its necessity demonstrated in the investigation of disease. New York: A. Metz & Co., 1881. 22p. DNLM; NNNAM **80-4233**

MERKEL, G. Hermann
Ozone, its merits as a disinfectant, antiseptic and anti-zymotic. Boston: Rand & Avery, 1884. 19p. DNLM; MBM **80-4234**

MERRELL, WILLIAM S. & CO.
Revised current price list of drugs and pharmaceuticals for manufacturing druggists. Cincinnati, 1880. 2p. OC; OCIM **80-4235**

MERRELL, WILLIAM S. & CO.
Catalogue of drugs. . . . Cincinnati, 1881. 52p. OC; OCIM **80-4236**

MERRELL, WILLIAM S. & CO.
Catalogue of drugs. . . . Cincinnati, 1883. 48p. OC; OCIM **80-4237**

MERRILL, Cyrus S[trong] (*b.* 1847)
The introductory address of the course of 1882-1883 at the Albany Medical College. Albany: J. Munsell, 1882. 12p. DNLM **80-4238**

METTLER, Lee Harrison (*b.* 1863)
The biological cell. An argument. Philadelphia: Records, McMullin & Co., limited, 1888. 64p. DNLM; PPC; PU **80-4239**

MEYER, Eduard (1838-1902)
A practical treatise on diseases of the eye. Transl., with the assistance of the author, from the 3rd French ed., with additions as contained in the 4th German ed., by Freeland Fergus. Philadelphia: P. Blakiston, Son & Co., 1887. 647p. 3 plates. CtY-M; DNLM; NNNAM; PPC **80-4240**

MEYER, Georg Hermann (1815-1892)
The organs of speech, and their application in the formation of articulate sounds. New York: D. Appleton & Co., 1884. 349p. DNLM; MB; MH; NN **80-4241**

MEYER, Leo Theodor
Guide to the study of anatomy, based upon notes of the lectures of Prof. William Darling. . . . 2nd ed. New York: J. Batchelar, printer, 1880. 474p. DLC; NNNAM **80-4242**

MEYER, Willy (*b.* 1858)
On cystoscopy, and the new cystoscope of Nitze and Leiter, with a demonstration of the same. [New York], 1888. 22p. DNLM; NNNAM **80-4243**

MEYER, Willy (*b.* 1858)
A contribution to the surgery of the bladder. [New York, 1889.] 25p. DNLM; NNNAM **80-4244**

MEYLERT, Asa P. (*d.* 1893)
Notes on the opium habit. New York: G. P. Putnam's Sons, 1884. 36p. DNLM; NNNAM **80-4245**

MEYLERT, Asa P. (*d.* 1893)
Notes on the opium habit. 3rd ed., rev. and enl. New York: G. P. Putnam's Sons, 1885. 47p. NNNAM **80-4246**

MEYLERT, Asa P. (*d.* 1893)
Notes on the opium habit. 4th ed. New York: G. P. Putnam's Sons, 1885. 49p. DNLM; NNNAM **80-4247**

MEYNERT, Theodor H[ermann] (1833-1892)
Psychiatry; a clinical treatise on diseases of the fore-brain, based upon a study of its structure, functions, and nutrition. Transl. by B. Sachs. Pt. 1. The anatomy, physiology, and chemistry of the brain. New York: G. P. Putnam's Sons, 1885. 285p. DNLM; IU-M; NNNAM; PU **80-4248**

MIAMI MEDICAL COLLEGE, CINCINNATI
Annual announcements for the sessions of 1883-1884 to 1886-1887 (24.-27.); 1889-1890 to 1904-1905 (30.-45.). Cincinnati, 1883-1904. DNLM [List of students and graduates for the years 1882-1883 to 1885-1886; 1888-1889 to 1903-1904, in announcements for subsequent years.] **80-4249**

MIAMI MEDICAL COLLEGE, CINCINNATI
Annual reports of the eye and ear clinic held at the Miami Medical College. 5., 1883; 6., 1884; 8., 1886. Cincinnati, 1884-1887. DNLM **80-4250**

MICHAEL, J. Edwin (1843-1895)
A critical historical and clinical study of Smith's anterior splint. Brooklyn, N.Y.: Annals of Anatomy & Surgery, 1882. 26p. DNLM; NNNAM; NNU-M **80-4251**

MICHAELIS, Gustavus
The gradual development of pharmacy. [Introductory address, Albany College of Pharmacy.] Albany, N.Y.: Burdick & Taylor, 1886. 17p. DNLM **80-4252**

MICHEL, Middleton (1822-1894)
In memoriam. J. Lawrence Smith. Charlston, S.C., 1884. 11p. **80-4253**

MICHELL, Charles L.
Fixed adhesive dressings in the treatment of skin diseases. Philadelphia, [1885]. 12p. DNLM **80-4254**

MICHENER, Ezra (1794-1887), et al.
Hand-book of eclampsia, or notes and cases of puerperal convulsions, comprising all the cases which have occurred during the present century within a radius of several miles around Avondale, Chester County, Pa., so far as can be ascertained. Philadelphia: F. A. Davis, 1883. 68p. DNLM; PPC; PU **80-4255**

MICHIGAN. UNIVERSITY OF MICHIGAN, ANN ARBOR. COLLEGE OF DENTAL SURGERY
Annual announcements for the sessions of 1887-1888 to 1903-1904 (13.-29.). Ann Arbor, 1887-1903. DNLM [Register of graduates in: Announcements for 1903-1904.] **80-4256**

MICHIGAN. UNIVERSITY OF MICHIGAN, ANN ARBOR. DEPARTMENT OF MEDICINE AND SURGERY
Annual announcements for the sessions of 1883-1884 (34.); 1884-1885 (35.); 1886-1887 to 1896-1897 (37.-47.); 1898-1899 (49.). Detroit & Ann Arbor, 1883-1898. DNLM [List of students and graduates for the years 1882-1883; 1883-1884; 1885-1886 to 1895-1896; 1897-1898, in: Announcements for subsequent years.] **80-4257**

MICHIGAN. UNIVERSITY OF MICHIGAN, ANN ARBOR. SCHOOL OF PHARMACY
Annual announcements and registers of alumni for the sessions of 1880-1881 (13.); 1882-1883 to 1900-1901 (15.-37.). Ann Arbor, 1880-1904. DNLM [List of students and graduates for the years 1879-1880; 1881-1882 to 1903-1904, in: Announcements for subsequent years.] **80-4258**

MILES, Francis T[urquand] (1827-1903)
Effect of spinal concussion on the reflexes. Philadelphia, 1888. 6p. DNLM **80-4259**

MILES, T. Wesley
The influence of the nervous system on cell life (metabolism). New York, 1888. 10p. DNLM **80-4260**

MILLARD, Henry B[enton] (*d.* 1893)
Researches in the minute anatomy of the epithelia of the kidney. [New York, 1882.] 15p. DNLM; NNNAM **80-4261**

MILLARD, Henry B[enton] (*d.* 1893)
A treatise on Bright's disease of the kidneys; its pathology, diagnosis, and treatment. . . . New York: William Wood & Co., 1884. 246p. DLC; NNNAM; PPJ; PU **80-4262**

MILLEN, Charles W[atson]
Address . . . delivered at the 25th commencement of the Eclectic Medical College of the City of New York, Chickering Hall, March 25, 1886. New York: The Day Star, 1886. 8p. DLC **80-4263**

MILLER, B. Curtis
A year's record of seventy-five successful cases of abdominal section. New York: William Wood & Co., 1889. 14p. DNLM; NNNAM **80-4264**

MILLER, Eli P[eck]
A father's advice; a book for every boy. New York: E. P. Miller, 1881. 29p. DNLM; NN **80-4265**

MILLER, Eli P[eck]
A new treatment for piles or hemorrhoids, painful fissure, rectal ulcer, fistula, and other diseases of the rectum, without the use of the knife, ligature, clamp, écraseur, caustics, hot iron, etc., and by a process sure, safe, and painless. New York: Miller, Haynes & Co., 1883. 32p. DLC; DNLM **80-4266**

MILLER, John S.
A case of extensive recurrent sarcomatous disease. [Philadelphia, 1885.] 3p. DNLM **80-4267**

MILLER, John S.
A contribution to the study of bone repair. Philadelphia: W. J. Dornan, 1888. 7p. DNLM **80-4268**

MILLER, Maurice Norton (1838-1888)
Practical microscopy: a course of normal histology for students and practitioners of medicine. . . . Illustrated with one hundred and twenty-six photographical reproductions of the author's pen drawings. New York: William Wood & Co., 1887. 217p. DLC; DNLM; NNNAM; PPC **80-4269**

MILLER, Samuel M., ed.
Notes of hospital practice. I. Philadelphia hospitals, II. New York hospitals, III. New York & Philadelphia hospitals. Philadelphia: The author, 1881. 141, 110, 108p. NNNAM; PPC; PPJ; PU **80-4270**

MILLER, Wesley
The germ-theory of Pasteur, and new discoveries of Dr. Wesley Miller to prevent diseases in domestic animals and mankind generally by vaccination. [n. p., 1881.] 2 l. DNLM **80-4271**

MILLER, Wesley
Prevention of tubercular and other diseases, in man and domestic animals, by vaccination. [New York, 1882.] 8p. DNLM **80-4272**

MILLER, Wesley
New York Vaccine Co. Animal vaccine virus. New discoveries in the treatment of contagious or infectious diseases by vaccination or hypodermic injections. [New York, 1882.] 2 l. DNLM **80-4273**

MILLER, W[illoughby] D[ayton] (1838-1907)
Fermentation in the human mouth; its relation to caries of the teeth. The influence of antiseptics, filling materials, etc., upon the fungi of dental caries. The fungi of dental caries; their pure cultivation and effect upon lower animals. New York, 1884. 41p. DNLM; NNNAM **80-4274**

MILLER, W[illoughby] D[ayton] (1835-1907)
Biological studies of the fungi on the human mouth. New York: Dental J. Ass., [1885]. 11p. DNLM **80-4275**

MILLER, W[illoughby] D[ayton] (1835-1907)
On the antiseptic action of filling-materials. Philadelphia, 1889. 8p. DNLM **80-4276**

MILLS, Charles K[arsner] (1845-1931)
Tumor of the pons Varolii, with conjugate deviation of the eyes and rotation of the head. [New York, 1881.] 12p. DNLM **80-4277**

MILLS, Charles K[arsner] (1845-1931)
Reflections on criminal lunacy, with remarks on the case of Guiteau. Philadelphia, 1882. 26p. DNLM **80-4278**

MILLS, Charles K[arsner] (1845-1931)
Mental over-work and premature disease among public and professional men. Washington: Smithsonian Institution, 1885. 34p. DNLM **80-4279**

MILLS, Charles K[arsner] (1845-1931)
Benjamin Rush and American psychiatry. [New York, 1886.] 36p. DNLM **80-4280**

MILLS, Charles K[arsner] (1845-1931)
Arrested and aberrant development of fissures and gyres in the brains of paranoiacs, criminals, idiots, and Negroes. Preliminary study of a Chinese brain. [New York: G. P. Putnam's Sons, 1886.] 37p. 2 plates. DNLM **80-4281**

MILLS, Charles K[arsner] (1845-1931)
Practical lessons in nursing. The nursing and care of the nervous and the insane. Philadelphia: J. B. Lippincott & Co., 1887. 147p. DLC; DNLM; NNNAM; PPC **80-4282**

MILLS, Charles K[arsner] (1845-1931) and George A. BODAMER
Glioma of the right temporal lobe, with intercurrent hemorrhage. A case in which the questioning of trephining was considered and decided against. [New York, 1887.] 5p. DNLM **80-4283**

MILLS, Charles K[arsner] (1845-1931)
The treatment of nervous and mental disease by systematized active exercises. Philadelphia: W. J. Dornan, 1888. 20p. DNLM **80-4284**

MILLS, Charles K[arsner] (1845-1931)
Brain specimens chiefly illustrating localization. [Philadelphia, 1889.] 11p. DLC; DNLM **80-4285**

MILLS, Charles K[arsner] (1845-1931)
Lesions of the sacral and lumbar plexuses. [Philadelphia, 1889.] 22p. DLC; DNLM **80-4286**

MILLS, Charles K[arsner] (1845-1931)
Spinal localization in its practical relations. Detroit: G. S. Davis, 1889. 61p. DNLM **80-4287**

MILLS, George A.
Specialties and their advantages. New York: Jenkins & Thomas, [1882]. 14p. DNLM **80-4288**

MILLS, George A.
Pericementitis; its manifestations in the oral cavity, and its serious effects upon the general health. New York: Jenkins & Thomas, [1882]. 8p. DNLM **80-4289**

MILLS, George A.
Riggs' disease (pericementitis, pyorrhea, alveolaris, diseased gums, loose teeth, etc.). New York: Jenkins & McCowan, [1885]. 8p. DNLM **80-4290**

MILLS, George A.
Dental specialists of medicine and surgery, in the care and treatment of the disorders of the teeth and mouth. St. Louis: J. H. Chambers & Co., 1886. 10p. DNLM **80-4291**

MILLS, T. Wesley (1847-1915)
A physiological basis for an improved cardiac pathology. New York: Trow's 1887. 23p. DNLM **80-4292**

MILLS, T. Wesley (1847-1915)
Surgical puncture of the heart. A warning. [Philadelphia, 1887.] 4p. DNLM **80-4293**

MILLSPAUGH, Charles Frederick (1854-1923)
American medicinal plants; an illustrated and descriptive guide to the American plants used as homoeopathic remedies: their history, preparation, chemistry and physiological effects. . . . New York, Philadelphia: Boericke & Tafel, 1887. 2 v. 180 plates. DLC; DNLM; OCLloyd; PPHa [Originally, in 6 parts, 1884-1887] **80-4294**

MILLSPAUGH, Charles Frederick (1854-1923)
Reportory to eczema. New York: A. L. Chatterton Publishing Co., 1885. 43p. NNNAM; PPHa **80-4295**

MILNE, Alexander
The principles and practice of midwifery, with some of the diseases of women. 2nd ed. New York & London: Bermingham & Co., 1884. 371p. DNLM; MBM; NNNAM; PPC **80-4296**

MILNER, U. R.
Yellow fever not imported, nor contagious, but indigenous, and intrinsically identical with our paludal fevers. Preventable by well determined and wisely executed local sanitary measures. Quarantine a wide-spread calamity, and should not longer be tolerated. A lecture. New Orleans: M. J. Scott, 1880. 39p. DNLM; LNT-M **80-4297**

MILROY, W[illiam] F.
Typhoid fever and water supply in Omaha. [Omaha, 1889.] 11p. DNLM **80-4298**

MILTENBERGER, George W[arner] (1819-1905)
Puerperal eclampsia. [Baltimore: Guggenheimer, Weil & Co., 1886.] 29p. DNLM; MdBM **80-4299**

MILTENBERGER, George W[arner] (1819-1905)
President's address. [Baltimore, 1887.] 9p. DNLM; MdBM [M. & Chir. Fac. Maryland, Balt.] **80-4300**

MILTENBERGER, George W[arner] (1819-1905)
The etiology of puerperal fever; its direct causative factor. Baltimore: I. Friedenwald, 1889. 15p. DNLM; MdU-D **80-4301**

MILTON, John Laws (1820-1898)
On the pathology and treatment of gonorrhoea. 5th ed. New York: William Wood & Co., 1884. 306p. DNLM; IU-M; NNNAM; PPC **80-4302**

MILTON, John Laws (1820-1898)
On the pathology and treatment of gonorrhoea and spermatorrhoea. New York: William Wood & Co., 1887. 474p. DNLM; MH-M; NNNAM; PPC **80-4303**

MINNESOTA COLLEGE OF PHARMACY, MINNEAPOLIS
Annual announcements for the sessions of 1885-1886 to 1891-1892 (1.-7.); 1893-1894 to 1895-1896 (9.-11.). Minneapolis, 1885-1895. DNLM [In: Annual announcements of Minnesota College of Physicians and Surgeons, for the same years.] **80-4304**

MINNESOTA HOMOEOPATHIC MEDICAL COLLEGE, MINNEAPOLIS
Annual announcements for the sessions of 1886-1887 (1.); 1887-1888 (2.). Minneapolis: Tribune Print. Co., 1886-1887. 14p., 16p. DNLM **80-4305**

MINNESOTA HOSPITAL COLLEGE, MINNEAPOLIS
Announcement for the spring session of 1886. [Minneapolis, 1886.] 1 sheet. DNLM **80-4306**

MINNESOTA. UNIVERSITY OF MINNESOTA. COLLEGE OF HOMOEOPATHIC MEDICINE AND SURGERY, MINNEAPOLIS
Annual announcements for the sessions of 1888-1889 to 1895-1896 (1.-8.); 1897-1898 to 1905-1906 (10.-18.). Minneapolis, 1888-1905. DNLM **80-4307**

MINNESOTA. UNIVERSITY OF MINNESOTA. COLLEGE OF MEDICINE
Special announcement, May, 1884. Minneapolis: Johnson, Smith & Harrison, 1884. 57p. DNLM **80-4308**

MINNESOTA. UNIVERSITY OF MINNESOTA. STATE BOARD OF MEDICAL EXAMINERS
Explanatory announcement. [Minneapolis, 1883.] 3p. DNLM **80-4309**

MINOR, James L.
Experimental keratitis; its bearing upon Stricker's theory of inflammation. [Philadelphia, 1883.] 6p. DNLM
80-4310

MINOR, James L.
The field of vision. [Philadelphia, 1883.] 8p. DNLM
80-4311

MINOR, John C.
The relation of the law to medical education. New York: W. R. Jenkins, 1882. 19p. DNL; NNNAM **80-4312**

MINOR, John C.
Ethics and education. The annual address delivered November 14, 1883, before the New York Medico-Chirurgical Society. New York, 1884. 36p. DNLM; NNNAM
80-4313

MINOR, Thomas C[halmer] (1846-1912)
Athothis; a satire on modern medicine. Cincinnati: R. Clarke & Co., 1887. 194p. DNLM; OCIM
80-4314

MINTON, Henry B[rewster] (1831-1895)
Uterine therapeutics. New York: A. L. Chatterton Publishing Co., 1884. 710p. DNLM; NNNAM; OCIM; PPC
80-4315

MISSOURI DENTAL COLLEGE, ST. LOUIS
Annual announcements for the sessions of 1889-1890 (24.); 1891-1892 (26.). St. Louis: Continental Ptg. Co., 1889-1891. 16p; 16p. DNLM **80-4316**

MISSOURI MEDICAL COLLEGE, ST. LOUIS
Annual announcements and catalogues for the sessions of 1884-1885 to 1898-1899 (44.-58.). St. Louis, 1884-1898. DNLM [List of students and graduates for the years 1883-1884 to 1897-1898, in: Announcements for subsequent years. In 1899 it united with the St. Louis Medical College, forming the Medical Department of Washington University.]
80-4317

MITCHELL, Charles (*d.* 1900)
Condensed statement of mortality in the city of Nashville, Tenn., for the years 1879-1884. Nashville: J. B. Tavel, 1885. 44p. DNLM; OCIM **80-4318**

MITCHELL, Charles L.
Strictures of the urethra situated at or near the meatus; their causes, nature, and treatment, together with a description of a new meatome. [Philadelphia, 1883.] 7p. DNLM; PPC
80-4319

MITCHELL, Charles L.
Fixed adhesive dressings in the treatment of skin diseases. Philadelphia, [1884]. 12p. DNLM
80-4320

MITCHELL, Charles L.
The treatment of gonorrhoea and its sequelae. [Philadelphia, 1886, *vel subseq.*] 24p. DNLM; PPC
80-4321

MITCHELL, Charles L.
Illustrated catalogue of soluble medicated gelatin and other pharmaceutical preparations manufactured by . . . . [Philadelphia, 1887.] 24p. DNLM; PPC **80-4322**

MITCHELL, Charles L.
Should physicians be pharmacists? [Philadelphia, 1887.] 17p. DNLM; PPC **80-4323**

MITCHELL, Charles L.
The rational treatment of urethritis. [1887.] 32p. DNLM; PPC
80-4324

MITCHELL, C[harles] Pittfield
An evolution aspect of the healing of wounds. New York, 1882. 13p. DNLM **80-4325**

MITCHELL, C[harles] Pittfield
The treatment of wounds as based on evolutionary laws. New York: J. H. Vail & Co., 1883. 29p. DNLM; NNNAM
80-4326

MITCHELL, Clifford (1854-1939)
The practitioner's guide in urinalysis. . . . Chicago: Gross & Delbridge, 1882. 205p. DLC; IU-M; OCIM
80-4327

MITCHELL, Clifford (1854-1939)
A condensed chemistry for medical students and practitioners. Chicago: Gross & Delbridge, 1885. 200p. IU-M; PPHa
80-4328

MITCHELL, Clifford (1854-1939)
The physician's chemistry. . . . Chicago: Gross & Delbridge, 1886. 301p. DLC; NNNAM **80-4329**

MITCHELL, Clifford (1854-1939)
The physician's manual of simple chemical tests. Pt. I. Poisons. Pt. II. Constituents of urine. . . . Chicago: Gale & Blocki, 1886. 18p. DLC **80-4330**

MITCHELL, Clifford (1854-1939)
The dentist's manual of special chemistry. . . . Chicago: Pub. by the author, 1887. 259p. DLC; DNLM
80-4331

MITCHELL, Clifford (1854-1939)
The practitioner's guide in urinalysis. 2nd ed. Chicago: Gross & Delbridge, 1888. 188p. IU-M; OCIM **80-4332**

MITCHELL, C. L., M.D. & CO.
8th annual catalogue. Physicians' handbook and illustrated catalogue of soluble medicated gelatin preparations. Philadelphia, 1885. 48p. NNNAM; PPC **80-4333**

MITCHELL, Hubbard Winslow (*d.* 1913)
The operation for stellate and bilateral laceration of the cervix uteri. New York: T. A. Wright, 1888. 12p. DNLM
80-4334

MITCHELL, John Kearsley, Jr. (1859-1917)
The general and local effects of paraffin oil upon those working in it. Philadelphia, 1888. 11p. 3 phot. DNLM
80-4335

MITCHELL, John Kearsley, Jr. (1859-1917), and G. E. de SCHWEINITZ
Hysterical anaesthesia, with a study of the fields of vision. [Philadelphia, 1889.] 16p. DNLM
80-4336

MITCHELL, Joseph Sidney (*d.* 1898)
Homoeopathy in its relation to malignant diseases. A lecture delivered under the auspices of the Alumni Association of the New York Homoeopathic Medical College. New York, 1888. 17p. NNNAM **80-4337**

MITCHELL, S[ilas] Weir (1829-1914)
Lectures on diseases of the nervous system, especially in women. Philadelphia: Henry C. Lea's Son & Co., 1881. 238p. 5 plates. DNLM; NNNAM; OCIM; PPC **80-4338**

MITCHELL, S[ilas] Weir (1829-1914) and Edward T. REICHERT
A partial study of the poison of Heloderma suspectum Cope, the Gila monster. Philadelphia: Dornan, 1883. 16p. DNLM **80-4339**

MITCHELL, S[ilas] Weir (1829-1914) and Edward T. REICHERT
Preliminary report on the venoms of serpents. [Philadelphia, 1883.] 14p. DNLM **80-4340**

MITCHELL, S[ilas] Weir (1829-1914)
Fat and blood: an essay on the treatment of certain forms of neurasthenia and hysteria. . . . 3rd ed., rev., with additions. Philadelphia: J. B. Lippincott & Co., 1884. 164p. DLC; ICRM; NNNAM; PPC **80-4341**

MITCHELL, S[ilas] Weir (1829-1914)
Fat and blood: an essay on the treatment of certain forms of neurasthenia and hysteria. . . . 4th ed., rev., with additions. Philadelphia, [etc.]: J. B. Lippincott & Co., 1885. 166p. DLC; DNLM; PPC; PU **80-4342**

MITCHELL, S[ilas] Weir (1829-1914) and H. C. WOOD
A report made to the College of Physicians of Philadelphia: [Philadelphia, 1885.] 1 l. DNLM; PPC **80-4343**

MITCHELL, S[ilas] Weir (1829-1914)
Lectures on diseases of the nervous system, especially in women. 2nd ed. Philadelphia: Lea Bros. & Co., 1885. 287p. DNLM; NNNAM; PPC; PU **80-4344**

MITCHELL, S[ilas] Weir (1829-1914) and Edward T. REICHERT
Researches upon the venoms of poisonous serpents. Washington: Smithsonian Inst., 1886. 186p. 5 plates. DNLM **80-4345**

MITCHELL, S[ilas] Weir (1829-1914) and Morris J. LEWIS
Physiological studies of the knee-jerk, and of the reactions of muscles under mechanical and other excitants. [Philadelphia: Lea Bros. & Co., 1886.] 35p. DNLM; PPC **80-4346**

MITCHELL, S[ilas] Weir (1829-1914)
A doctor's century. [Philadelphia, 1887.] 4 l. DNLM **80-4347**

MITCHELL, S[ilas] Weir (1829-1914)
Celebration of the centennial anniversary of the institution of the College of Physicians of Philadelphia. Commemorative address. Delivered January 3, 1887. [Philadelphia, 1887.] 40p. DNLM; PPC **80-4348**

MITCHELL, S[ilas] Weir (1829-1914)
Wear and tear, or hints for the overworked. 5th ed. Philadelphia: J. B. Lippincott & Co., 1887. 76p. DNLM; NNNAM; PPC; PPJ **80-4349**

MITCHELL, S[ilas] Weir (1829-1914)
Fat and blood; an essay on the treatment of certain forms of neurasthenia and hysteria. . . . 5th ed. Philadelphia, [etc.]: J. B. Lippincott & Co., 1888. 166p. DLC; NNNAM; PPC; PU **80-4350**

MITCHELL, S[ilas] Weir (1829-1914)
[Minerva medica.] Read at the dinner commemorative of the fiftieth year of the doctorate of D. Hayes Agnew, M.D., April 6, 1888. [Philadelphia, 1888.] 6 l. DNLM **80-4351**

MITCHELL, S[ilas] Weir (1829-1914)
Doctor and patient. . . . Philadelphia, [etc.]: J. B. Lippincott & Co., 1888. 177p. DLC; DNLM; NNNAM; PPC **80-4352**

MITCHELL, Thomas Duché (1791-1865)
Materia medica and therapeutics: with . . . copious notes of toxicology. . . . New ed., rev. and enl. . . . Philadelphia: J. B. Lippincott & Co., 1880 [org. 1857]. 820p. DLC; OCLloyd; PPC; PU **80-4353**

MITTENDORF, William F.
A manual on diseases of the eye and ear, for the use of students and practitioners. New York: G. P. Putnam's Sons, [1881]. 445p. CtY-M; NNNAM; PU **80-4354**

MIXTER, S[amuel] J[ason] (1855-1926)
A case of Porro's operation performed on account of multiple myomata, saving both mother and child. Boston: Cupples & Hurd, 1888. 7p. DNLM **80-4355**

MOHR, Charles (1844-1907)
Directory of the homoeopathic physicians of the County of Philadelphia, 1880. Compiled and published for gratuitous circulation. Philadelphia: Globe Printing House, 1880. 8p. PPC; PPHa **80-4356**

MOHR, Charles (1844-1907)
Sanitary precautions in measles. [Philadelphia, 1880.] 5p. DNLM **80-4357**

MOHR, Charles (1844-1907)
Care of the mouth and teeth in infancy and childhood. [Philadelphia, 1880.] 10p. DNLM **80-4358**

MOHR, Charles (1844-1907)
General treatment of epilepsy. [Philadelphia, 1881.] 5p. DNLM **80-4359**

MOHR, Charles (1844-1907)
Verifications of unverified symptoms in Allen's Encyclopaedia. [Philadelphia, 1881.] 16p. DNLM **80-4360**

MOHR, Charles (1844-1907)
Homoeopathic register and directory for the use of the members of the Homoeopathic Medical Society of the County of Philadelphia, 1881-1882. Philadelphia, 1882. 4, 144p. DNLM; PPC; PU **80-4361**

MOHR, Charles (1844-1907)
Hydrastis canadensis. Philadelphia, 1886. 14p. DNLM
80-4362

MOHR, Charles (1844-1907)
Notes of interesting clinical cases. [Philadelphia, 1886.] 7p. DNLM **80-4363**

MOHR, Charles (1844-1907)
A case of carcinoma of the breast vs. erysipelas and arsenic. [Philadelphia, 1888.] 3p. DNLM **80-4364**

MOHR, Charles (1844-1907)
Introductory lecture on the occasion of the opening of the forty-first annual session of lectures at the Hahnemann Medical College of Philadelphia. [Philadelphia, 1888.] 6p. DNLM
80-4365

MOHR, Charles (1844-1907)
Provings of zincum picricum. [Philadelphia, 1888.] 7p. DNLM
80-4366

MOHR, Charles (1844-1907)
Two cases of ovarian tumor. [Philadelphia, 1889, *vel subseq.*] 4p. DNLM **80-4367**

MOIR, Henry C.
A manual of the practice of medicine. Designed for the use of students and the general practitioner. . . . New York: Steam Press of the Industrial School, H. O. A., 1881. 455p. DLC; NNNAM [2nd ed., New York: J. H. Bilding, 1883, 455p.]
80-4368

MOIR, Henry C.
A manual of the practice of medicine. Designed for the use of students and the general practitioner. . . . 3rd ed. New York: J. H. Vail & Co., 1884. 455p. col. plate. DLC; NNNAM [4th ed., 1886] **80-4369**

MONEY, Angel (1856-1904)
Treatment of disease in children, including the outlines of diagnosis and the chief pathological differences between children and adults. Philadelphia: P. Blakiston, Son & Co., 1887. 560p. NNNAM; PPC; PU **80-4370**

MONROE, Andrew L[eight]
Method of memorizing the materia medica. Louisville: J. P. Morton & Co., 1882. 44p. DNLM **80-4371**

MONTGOMERY, Edward E[mmet] (1849-1927)
Procidentia and its relief; with a case. Philadelphia, 1882. 9p. DNLM **80-4372**

MONTGOMERY, Edward E[mmet] (1849-1927)
Is craniotomy justified? [Philadelphia, 1883.] 8p. DNLM
80-4373

MONTGOMERY, Edward E[mmet] (1849-1927)
Abdominal surgery; seven cases. Philadelphia: F. A. Davis, 1885. 14p. DNLM **80-4374**

MONTGOMERY, Edward E[mmet] (1849-1927)
The bromide of ethyl as an anesthetic in labor. New York: William Wood & Co., 1886. 12p. DNLM
80-4375

MONTGOMERY, Edward E[mmet] (1849-1927)
Ovarian tumor complicating pregnancy. [Philadelphia, 1887.] 6p. DNLM **80-4376**

MONTGOMERY, Edward E[mmet] (1849-1927)
Tracheotomy and intubation in diphtheria. [Philadelphia, 1887.] 10p. DNLM **80-4377**

MOODY, G. W.
Veratrum viride. Nashville: Harslock & Ambrose, [1887]. 8p. DNLM **80-4378**

MOORE, Chas. W.
A review of the most important advances in surgery, medicine, and pharmacy in the last forty years. [San Francisco, 1887.] 16p. CU-M; DNLM **80-4379**

MOORE, Frederick F.
Old-school and new-school therapeutics; read before the Cambridge Society for Medical Improvement, December 22, 1879. Revised and enlarged. Boston: A. Mudge & Son, 1880. 59p. DNLM; MBM **80-4380**

MOORE, William Oliver (*b.* 1852)
A clinical lecture on herpes zoster. [New York, 1886.] 12p. DNLM **80-4381**

MOORE, William Oliver (*b.* 1852)
Diseases of the eye occurring in affections of the kidney. [New York, 1886.] 16p. DNLM **80-4382**

MOORE, William Oliver (*b.* 1852)
The ophthalmoscope in general medicine. Montpelier, Vt.: Argus & Patriot Printing House, 1887. 13p. DNLM
80-4383

MOORE, William Oliver (*b.* 1852)
Diabetic affections of the eye. [New York], 1888. 31p. DNLM
80-4384

MOORE, William Oliver (*b.* 1852)
Ocular symptoms in diseases of the spinal cord. [New York], 1888. 12p. DNLM **80-4385**

MOORE, William Oliver (*b.* 1852)
Lecture on vision and its defects. New York: M. J. Rooney & Co., [1889]. 8 l. DNLM **80-4386**

MORGAN, Ethelbert Carroll (1856-1891)
Cystic tumor of the epiglottis. [New York, 1882.] 4p. DNLM
80-4387

MORGAN, Ethelbert Carroll (1856-1891)
Diphthonia, or double voice. New York, 1882. 10p. DNLM
80-4388

MORGAN, Ethelbert Carroll (1856-1891)
Clinical lecture. [Laryngeal fibroma; relaxed pharynx.] [Baltimore, 1883.] 11p. DNLM **80-4389**

MORGAN, Ethelbert Carroll (1856-1891)
Aphonia due to chronic alcoholism. Paralysis of the lateral crico-arytenoids. Chicago, 1884. 8p. DNLM
80-4390

MORGAN, Ethelbert Carroll (1856-1891)
Extraction of a glosso-epiglottic myxo-sarcoma by means of the fingers; to which are added two cases of palato-pharyngeal tumor and a bibliography of pharyngeal growths. New York: G. P. Putnam's Sons, 1884. 15p. DNLM
80-4391

MORGAN, Ethelbert Carroll (1856-1891)
Submucous laryngeal hemorrhage. New York, 1885. 3p. DNLM **80-4392**

MORGAN, Ethelbert Carroll (1856-1891)
The value of the snare in performing uvulotomy. [Baltimore, 1885.] 3p. DNLM **80-4393**

MORGAN, Ethelbert Carroll (1856-1891)
The question of haemorrhage following uvulotomy. Report of twenty-three cases of obstinate uvular haemorrhage; description of a uvular clamp; bibliography. New York: D. Appleton & Co., 1886. 27p. DNLM; NNNAM **80-4394**

MORGAN, Ethelbert Carroll (1856-1891)
The administration of the hypophosphites in powder. [Baltimore, 1886.] 3p. DNLM **80-4395**

MORGAN, Ethelbert Carroll (1856-1891)
The bursa pharyngea and its relation to naso-pharyngeal diseases. Baltimore, 1887. 16p. DNLM **80-4396**

MORGAN, Ethelbert Carroll (1856-1891)
Universal scoop powder-blower and a uvular haemostatic clamp. New York: D. Appleton & Co., 1888. 4p. DNLM **80-4397**

MORGAN, James E[thelbert] (1822-1889)
A defense of medicine and of the medical profession. Annual address to the Medical Society of the District of Columbia, delivered Jan. 9, 1884. Washington: R. O. Polkinhorn, 1884. 15p. DNLM **80-4398**

MORGAN, John C[oleman] (1831-1899)
Diet of infants and young children. . . . 2nd ed. Philadelphia: J. Hogan, printer, 1882. 50p. DLC; DNLM **80-4399**

MORGAN, John C[oleman] (1831-1899)
Address delivered by the president of the Homoeopathic Medical Society of Pennsylvania, at the eighteenth annual session. Pittsburgh: Stevenson & Foster, 1882. 13p. DNLM **80-4400**

MORISON, Robert B.
Bacteria and their presence in syphilitic secretions. [Baltimore, 1883.] 4p. 1 plate. DNLM **80-4401**

MORRILL, S. E.
A treatise of practical instructions in the medical and surgical uses of electricity, including instructions in electrical diagnosing and a new method of general and local electrization. Also clinical experiences of fifteen years. [Prospectus.] Kalamazoo, Mich., 1882. [25p.] DNLM **80-4402**

MORRILL, S. E.
A treatise of practical instructions in the medical and surgical uses of electricity, including instructions in electrical diagnosing and a new method of general and local electrization. Also clinical experiences of fifteen years. Kalamazoo, 1882. 249p. DNLM **80-4403**

MORRIS, Henry (1844-1926)
. . . Essentials of materia medica, therapeutics, and prescription writing, arranged in the form of questions and answers, prepared especially for students of medicine. . . . Philadelphia: W. B. Saunders; London: H. Renshaw; [etc., etc.], 1889. 250p. DLC; NNNAM; PPC; PU **80-4404**

MORRIS, J[ames] Cheston (1831-1923)
Biographical sketch of Caspar Norris. Philadelphia: W. J. Dornan, 1888. 31p. 1 plate. DNLM; PPC **80-4405**

MORRIS, John (1824-1903)
Prison physicians, their duties and influence. Baltimore, 1886. 19p. DNLM **80-4406**

MORRIS, John (1824-1903)
Crime, its physiology and pathogenesis. How far can medical men aid in its prevention? [Baltimore, 1889.] 12p. DNLM **80-4407**

MORRIS, Malcolm (1849-1924)
Skin diseases, including their definition, symptoms, diagnosis, prognosis, morbid anatomy, and treatment. A manual for students and practitioners. Philadelphia: Henry C. Lea, 1880. 320p. DNLM; NNNAM; OCIM; PPC **80-4408**

MORRIS, Robert Tuttle (1857-1945)
How we treat wounds today; a treatise on the subject of antiseptic surgery which can be understood by beginners. . . . New York & London: G. P. Putnam's Sons, 1886. 162p. DLC; DNLM; NNNAM **80-4409**

MORRIS, Robert Tuttle (1857-1945)
How we treat wounds today; a treatise on the subject of antiseptic surgery which can be understood by beginners. . . . 2nd ed. New York & London: G. P. Putnam's Sons, 1886. 162p. DLC **80-4410**

MORRIS, Robert Tuttle (1857-1945)
How we treat wounds today; a treatise on the subject of antiseptic surgery which can be understood by beginners. . . . 3rd and rev. ed. New York & London: G. P. Putnam's Sons, 1887. 164p. DLC; NNNAM **80-4411**

MORRIS, Robert Tuttle (1857-1945)
A second series of one hundred consecutive operations showing the results of antiseptic methods of work. New York, 1889. 9p. 1 tab. DNLM **80-4412**

MORRISON, PLUMMER & CO.
Druggists' ready reference with illustrations and prices of sundries. . . . Chicago, 1880. 334p. DLC; OCIM **80-4413**

MORRIS, PLUMMER & CO.
Illustrated catalogue. . . . Chicago, 1887. 736p. IU-M; OCIM **80-4414**

MORROW, Prince Albert (1846-1913)
Venereal memoranda; a manual for the student and practitioner. . . . New York: William Wood & Co., 1885. 332p. DLC; NNNAM; OCIM; PPC **80-4415**

MORROW, Prince Albert (1846-1913)
Drug eruptions: a clinical study of the irritant effects of drugs upon the skin. . . . New York: William Wood & Co., 1887. 199p. col. front. DLC; DNLM; NNNAM; PU **80-4416**

MORROW, Prince Albert (1846-1913)
Atlas of skin and venereal diseases; comprising original illustrations and selections from the plates of Prof. M. Kaposi . . . J. Hutchinson . . . I. Neumann . . . and others. With original text by Prince A. Morrow. . . . New York: William Wood & Co., [1888-1889]. 120, 121-318p. 75 col. plates. DLC; DNLM; NNNAM; PPC **80-4417**

MORROW, Prince Albert (1846-1913)
Case of tuberculosis papillomatosa cutis, with remarks on the relation of papilloma to syphilis, lupus, etc. New York: William Wood & Co., 1888. 16p. 1 plate. DNLM **80-4418**

MORROW, Prince Albert (1846-1913)
Personal observations of leprosy in Mexico and the Sandwich Islands. [New York, 1889.] 15p. 1 plate. DNLM **80-4419**

MORSE, Willard H.
New therapeutical agents. Detroit: G. S. Davis, 1882. 208p. DNLM; IU-M; OCIM; NNNAM **80-4420**

MORSE, Willard H.
A contribution to the study of the therapeutics of pulmonary tuberculosis. [Louisville, 1887.] 19p. DNLM **80-4421**

MORTON, A. Stanford (1847-1925)
Refraction of the eye; its diagnosis and the correction of its errors, with chapter on keratoscopy. 3rd ed. Philadelphia: P. Blakiston, Son & Co., 1886. 67p. 2 plates. DNLM; PPC [1st ed., 1881. 57p.; 2nd ed., 1882. 60p.] **80-4422**

MORTON, Bowditch (1857-1909)
Handbook of first aid to the injured; prepared at the request of the Society for Instruction in First Aid to the Injured. 2nd ed. New York: M. B. Brown, [1884]. Frontispiece, 90p. DNLM; NNNAM [3rd ed., 1885] **80-4423**

MORTON, Henry H[oldich] (*b.* 1861)
Obstetric methods in Prague. [New York, 1888.] 6p. DNLM **80-4424**

MORTON, Thomas George (1835-1903) and William HUNT
Surgery in the Pennsylvania Hospital, being an epitome of the practice of the hospital since 1756; including collations from the surgical notes, and an account of the more interesting cases from 1873 to 1878; with some statistical tables; with papers by John B. Roberts and Frank Woodbury. Philadelphia: J. B. Lippincott & Co., 1880. 348p. 2 plates. DNLM; PPC; PU **80-4425**

MORTON, Thomas George (1835-1903)
On the antiseptic treatment of wounds. Clinical lectures. [Philadelphia, 1886.] 35p. DNLM **80-4426**

MORTON, Thomas George (1835-1903)
On asymmetry of the lower limbs as a cause of lateral spinal curvature, with a description of a new method for readily and accurately determining any variation in the lengths of the lower extremities. [Philadelphia, 1886.] 28p. DNLM **80-4427**

MORTON, Thomas George (1835-1903)
Clinical lecture on cases of painful affection of the foot. [Philadelphia, 1886.] 22p. DNLM **80-4428**

MORTON, Thomas George (1835-1903)
The duty of the State and the obligations of directors of the poor, with the policy of the State committee on lunacy, with regard to the management and care of the insane in the State of Pennsylvania. Read at the annual meeting of the association of directors of the poor at Gettysburg, Oct. 18, 1887. Harrisburg: E. K. Meyers, 1887. 27p. DNLM **80-4429**

MORTON, Thomas George (1835-1903)
On the antiseptic treatment of wounds. Clinical lectures. [Philadelpiha, 1887.] 31p. DNLM **80-4430**

MORTON, Thomas George (1835-1903)
Clinical lectures on the antiseptic treatment of wounds. [Philadelphia, 1887.] 35p. DNLM **80-4431**

MORTON, Thomas George (1835-1903)
Abdominal section for perforated typhoid ulcer. Philadelphia, 1887. 8p. DNLM **80-4432**

MORTON, Thomas S. K.
Hospital operating-table and ward dressing-carriage. [Extracts.] [Philadelphia, 1887.] 3p. DNLM **80-4433**

MORTON, Thomas S. K.
Surgical considerations of the abdominal complications of typhoid fever. [Philadelphia, 1887.] 12p. DNLM **80-4434**

MORTON, William J[ames] (1846-1920)
The invention of anaesthetic inhalation; or, discovery of anaesthesia. New York: D. Appleton & Co., 1880. 48p. DLC; DNLM **80-4435**

MORTON, William J[ames] (1846-1920)
A contribution to the subject of nerve-stretching. In 1. Lateral sclerosis; 2. Paralysis agitans; 3. Athetosis; 4. Chronic transverse myelitis; 5. Sciatica; 6. Reflex epilepsy. New York, 1882. 31p. DNLM; NNNAM **80-4436**

MORTON, William J[ames] (1846-1920)
Neurological specialism. Presidential address delivered at the annual meeting of the New York Neurological Society, May 1, 1883. [n. p., 1883.] 12p. DNLM **80-4437**

MOSELEY, William E.
The influence from a clinical standpoint, of cicatricial tissue in the angles of the lacerated cervix. [New York, 1886.] 12p. DNLM **80-4438**

MOSES, G. A[she]
Hysterectomy, in malignant disease. [St. Louis, 1882.] 7p. **80-4439**

[MOSHER, Jacob Simmons] (1834-1883)
Catalogue of the medical and scientific portion of the library of the late J. S. Mosher, comprising many scarce books on insanity, yellow fever, sanitation, medical journals, reports, etc. [Albany, 1884.] 21 l. DNLM **80-4440**

MOTT-RING, Allan
The treatment of uterine diseases by means of the hot-air bath and hot-vaginal douche. Boston: A. Williams & Co., 1882. 22p. DNLM; MBM **80-4441**

MUDD, Henry H[odgen] (1844-1899)
Rapid lithotrity. Chicago & St. Louis: J. H. Chambers & Co., [1883]. 11p. DNLM **80-4442**

MUDD, Henry H[odgen] (1844-1899)
A new method of incision of the intestine. Chicago, 1888. 7p. DNLM **80-4443**

MUDD, Henry H[odgen] (1844-1899)
Lacerations of the kidney, with a nephrectomy. [Philadelphia, 1889.] 6p. DNLM **80-4444**

MUNDÉ, Paul F[ortunatus] (1846-1902)
Minor surgical gynecology: a manual of uterine diagnosis and the lesser technicalities of a gynecological practice; for the use of the advanced student and general practitioner. . . . New York: William Wood & Co., 1880. 381p. DLC; DNLM; NNNAM; PPC **80-4445**

MUNDÉ, Paul F[ortunatus] (1846-1902)
The diagnosis and treatment of obscure pelvic abscess in women, with remarks on the differential diagnosis between pelvic peritonitis and pelvic cellulitis. New York: G. P. Putnam's Sons, 1880. 29p. DNLM; NNNAM **80-4446**

MUNDÉ, Paul F[ortunatus] (1846-1902)
Prolapse of the ovaries. [Boston, 1880.] 47p. DNLM **80-4447**

MUNDÉ, Paul F[ortunatus] (1846-1902)
The diagnosis and treatment of obstetric cases by external (abdominal) examination and manipulation. New York: William Wood & Co., 1880. 114p. DNLM; NNNAM **80-4448**

MUNDÉ, Paul F[ortunatus] (1846-1902)
The curability of uterine displacements. New York: William Wood & Co., 1881. 24p. DNLM **80-4449**

MUNDÉ, Paul F[ortunatus] (1846-1902)
Minor surgical gynecology; a treatise of uterine diagnosis and the lesser technicalities of gynecological practice. . . . 2nd ed., rev. and enl. New York: William Wood & Co., 1885. 552p. DLC; DNLM; NNNAM; OCIM **80-4450**

MUNDÉ, Paul F[ortunatus] (1846-1902)
Four cases of Alexander's operation of shortening the round ligaments of the uterus for retroversion. [Sandy Hook, Conn., 1885.] 5p. DNLM **80-4451**

MUNDÉ, Paul F[ortunatus] (1846-1902)
Clinical observations on reflex genital neuroses in the female. [Chicago, 1886.] 11p. DNLM **80-4452**

MUNDÉ, Paul F[ortunatus] (1846-1902)
The value of antipyrine in puerperal fever. [New York, 1886.] 6p. DNLM **80-4453**

MUNDÉ, Paul F[ortunatus] (1846-1902)
A plea for intra-uterine medication. [New York, 1887.] 13p. DNLM **80-4454**

MUNDÉ, Paul F[ortunatus] (1846-1902)
Three cases of pregnancy complicated by ovarian tumors. Ovariotomy; recovery. [New York, 1887.] 11p. DNLM **80-4455**

MUNDÉ, Paul F[ortunatus] (1846-1902)
A sketch of the management of pregnancy, parturition and the puerperal state, normal and abnormal. . . . Detroit, Mich.: G. S. Davis, 1887. 110p. DLC; DNLM; OCIM **80-4456**

MUNDÉ, Paul F[ortunatus] (1846-1902)
Drainage after laparotomy. [New York, 1887.] 18p. DNLM **80-4457**

MUNDÉ, Paul F[ortunatus] (1846-1902)
Intrapelvic kidney mistaken for diseased uterine appendages; abdominal nephrectomy; recovery. [New York, 1888.] 9p. DNLM **80-4458**

MUNDÉ, Paul F[ortunatus] (1846-1902)
Laparatomy for reduction of an inverted uterus. New York, 1888. 6p. DNLM **80-4459**

MUNDÉ, Paul F[ortunatus] (1846-1902)
A year's work in laparotomy. (Forty-five operations.) New York: William Wood & Co., 1888. 47p. 4 plates. DNLM **80-4460**

MUNDÉ, Paul F[ortunatus] (1846-1902)
Chronic endometritis and chronic vaginitis. A clinical lecture. Boston, 1889. 7p. DNLM **80-4461**

MUNDÉ, Paul F[ortunatus] (1846-1902)
The methods and limitation of treatment for uterine fibroids. Philadelphia: W. J. Dornan, 1889. 10p. DNLM **80-4462**

MUNDÉ, Paul F[ortunatus] (1846-1902)
A rare case of adeno-myxosarcoma of the cervix uteri. New York: William Wood & Co., 1889. 9p. DNLM **80-4463**

MUNSON, George S.
A case of chronic suppurative otitis, with exostosis of the auditory canal, abscess of the brain; autopsy. Albany: Burdick & Taylor, 1882. 17p. DNLM **80-4464**

MURDOCH, J[ames] B[issett] (1830-1896)
Surgical clinics at the Western Pennsylvania Hospital before the students of the Western Pennsylvania Medical College. Chicago: Office Am. Medical Ass., 1889. 59p. DNLM; OCIM **80-4465**

MURDOCH, Russell (1839-1905)
Ear instruments. New York, 1888. 1 l. DNLM **80-4466**

MURFREE, J[ames] B.
A case of abdominal pregnancy (extra-uterine) of fifty-five years' duration. [Nashville, 1886.] 8p. DNLM **80-4467**

MURPHY, P[atrick] J[oseph] (1844-1891)
Chylous ascites. Washington, [1887]. 49p. DNLM **80-4468**

MURPHY, P[atrick] J[oseph] (1844-1891)
Report of the Columbia Hospital for Women and Lying-in Asylum. Cincinnati, 1888. 22p. DNLM **80-4469**

MURPHY, P[atrick] J[oseph] (1844-1891)
Caesarean section vs. embryotomy. [Cincinnati, 1889.] 7p. DNLM **80-4470**

MURRAY, David (1830-1905)
Eulogy upon Jacob P. Mosher, [Albany, 1884.] 4p. DNLM **80-4471**

MURRAY, David (1830-1905)
Semi-centennial anniversary of the Albany Medical College, March 21, 1889. Historical address. Albany: Burdick & Taylor, 1889. 29p. DNLM **80-4472**

MURRAY, Francis W.
Anthrax maligna. New York, 1889. 10p. DNLM **80-4473**

MURRELL, William (1853-1912)
What to do in cases of poisoning. 2nd ed. Detroit: G. S. Davis, 1882. 96p. DNLM; OCIM [Also: 2nd ed. New York: C. H. Goodwin, 1884. 108p. ICJ; ICU] **80-4474**

MURRELL, William (1853-1912)
Massage as a mode of treatment. Philadelphia: P. Blakiston, Son & Co., 1886. 78p. DNLM; PPC; PU **80-4475**

MURRELL, William (1853-1912)
Massage as a mode of treatment. 2nd ed. Philadelphia: P. Blakiston, Son & Co., 1887. 100p. DNLM; PPC; PPJ; PU **80-4476**

MURRELL, William (1853-1912)
Massage as a mode of treatment. 3rd ed. Philadelphia: P. Blakiston, Son & Co., 1887. 143p. DNLM; NNNAM; PPC; PU **80-4477**

MURRELL, William (1853-1912)
What to do in cases of poisoning. . . . 1st American from the 5th English ed. Ed. by Frank Woodbury. . . . Philadelphia: Medical Register Co., 1887. 158p. DLC; NNNAM; PPC **80-4478**

MURRELL, William (1853-1912)
Massage as a mode of treatment. 4th ed. Philadelphia: P. Blakiston, Son & Co., 1889. 236p. DNLM; NNNAM; OCIM; PPC **80-4479**

MURSICK, Geo. A[ndrew] (1834-1895)
A case of complete intestinal occlusion by pressure of an ovarian tumor; ovariotomy; death. [New York, 1882.] 4p. DNLM **80-4480**

MUSSER, John H[err] (1856-1912) and W. W. KEEN
Cholecystotomy; with a report of two cases, a table of all the hitherto reported cases, and remarks. [n. p., 1884.] 59p. DNLM **80-4481**

MUSSER, John H[err] (1856-1912)
A modification of the sphygmograph, being a change in the base of the instrument of Pond. [Philadelphia, 1884.] 4p. DNLM **80-4482**

MUSSER, John H[err] (1856-1912)
[Collection of 30 monographs.] [Philadelphia, 1884-1898.] DNLM **80-4483**

MUSSER, John H[err] (1856-1912) and George A. PIERSOL
Notes of a case of infectious, so-called ulcerative, endocarditis and of a case of acute pericarditis. Philadelphia: W. J. Dornan, 1885. 15p. [8 photographic plates]. DNLM **80-4484**

MUSSER, John H[err] (1856-1912)
On idiopathic anaemia. A report of three cases, with remarks; and an analysis of the cases hitherto published in America. Philadelphia, 1885. 31p. DNLM **80-4485**

MUSSER, John H[err] (1856-1912)
Some statistics of hepatic diseases. An analysis of cases presented to the Pathological Society of Philadelphia from 1837 to 1881, inclusive; with a detailed study of the fatty, the cancerous, and the cirrhotic liver. [n. p., 1885.] 14p. DNLM **80-4486**

MUSSER, John H[err] (1856-1912)
Three cases of idiopathic anaemia, with remarks; and an analysis of the cases hitherto published in America. [Philadelphia, 1885.] 15p. DNLM **80-4487**

MUSSER, John H[err] (1856-1912)
Some remarks on the treatment of the summer gastro-intestinal diseases of childhood. Detroit: G. S. Davis, 1886. 10p. DNLM **80-4488**

MUSSER, John H[err] (1856-1912)
Notes on thirteen cases of tubercular meningitis. [Philadelphia, 1886.] 8p. DNLM **80-4489**

MUSSER, John H[err] (1856-1912)
Abscess of the pancreas and thrombosis of the portal vein. [Philadelphia, 1886.] 6p. DNLM **80-4490**

MUSSER, John H[err] (1856-1912)
Notes of a case of (1) Raynaud's disease, and (2) of gangrene complicating diabetes mellitus. Philadelphia: W. J. Dornan, 1886. 19p. DNLM **80-4491**

MUSSER, John H[err] (1856-1912)
On the influence of age on the dosage of nux vomica, with some remarks on its therapeutics. Detroit, Mich.: G. S. Davis, 1886. 7p. DNLM **80-4492**

MUSSER, John H[err] (1856-1912)
Two cases of malignant or ulcerative endocarditis. A clinical lecture. Boston, 1886. 16p. DNLM **80-4493**

MUSSER, John H[err] (1856-1912)
On the value of the oil of eucalyptus in some malarial affections. [Detroit, 1886.] 4p. DNLM **80-4494**

MUSSER, John H[err] (1856-1912)
Remarks on vomiting, physiological and clinical. Philadelphia, 1887. 8p. DNLM **80-4495**

MUSSER, John H[err] (1856-1912)
Some cases of purpura haemorrhagica, and leucocythaemia, from private practice. Philadelphia: W. J. Dornan, 1887. 8p. DNLM **80-4496**

MUSSER, John H[err] (1856-1912)
The treatment of the final stages of phthisis. Philadelphia: W. J. Dornan, 1887. 8p. DNLM **80-4497**

MUSSER, John H[err] (1856-1912)
Case of tubercular pericarditis; unusual amount of effusion; accidental paracentesis pericardii. Notes of the treatment of peritonitis. Philadelphia, 1888. 14p. DNLM **80-4498**

MUSSER, John H[err] (1856-1912)
Memoranda of the life and works of Benjamin Rush. Philadelphia: W. J. Dornan, 1888. 7p. DNLM **80-4499**

MUSSER, John H[err] (1856-1912)
The oil of eucalyptus in some forms of malaria. Philadelphia, 1889. 8p. DNLM **80-4500**

MUSSER, John H[err] (1856-1912)
Primary cancer of the gall-bladder and bile-ducts. Philadelphia: W. J. Dornan, 1889. 45p. DNLM **80-4501**

MYNTER, Herman (1845-1903)
Stricture of the trachea. [Buffalo, 1881.] 7p. DNLM **80-4502**

NANCREDE, Charles Beylard [Guerard de] (1847-1921)
Some points in the anatomy of the shoulder-joint examined with reference to its luxations. Philadelphia, [1880]. 2p. DNLM **80-4503**

NANCREDE, Charles Beylard [Guerard de] (1847-1921)
An analysis of the principles on which depends the success of the modern methods of treating wounds. New York: G. P. Putnam's Sons, 1881. 16p. DNLM; NNNAM **80-4504**

NANCREDE, Charles Beylard [Guerard de] (1847-1921)
Have we any therapeutic means, as proven by experiment, which directly affect the local processes of inflammation? Read before the Am. Surg. Ass., Cincinnati, May 31, 1883. [Philadelphia, 1883.] 16p. DNLM **80-4505**

NANCREDE, Charles Beylard [Guerard de] (1847-1921)
Two successful cases of brain surgery. [Philadelphia, 1888.] 14p. DNLM **80-4506**

NANCREDE, Charles Beylard [Guerard de] (1847-1921)
Recent advances in the surgery of the brain and its coverings. Philadelphia, 1888. 28p. DNLM; PPC **80-4507**

NANCREDE, Charles Beylard [Guerard de] (1847-1921)
. . . Essentials of anatomy including the anatomy of the viscera, arranged in the form of questions and answers. . . . 2nd ed., based upon the last edition of Gray's anatomy. . . . Philadelphia: W. B. Saunders; [etc., etc.], 1889. 352p. DLC; MBM; NNNAM; PPC **80-4508**

NAPHEYS, George H[enry] (1842-1876)
Modern medical therapeutics: a compendium of recent formulae and specific therapeutical directions, from the practice of eminent contemporary physicians, American and foreign. . . . 7th ed., enl. and rev. Philadelphia: D. G. Brinton, 1880. 612p. DLC; DNLM; PPC; PU **80-4509**

NAPHEYS, George H[enry] (1842-1876)
Modern surgical therapeutics: a compendium of current formulae, approved dressings and specific methods for the treatment of surgical diseases and injuries. . . . 7th ed., rev. to the most recent date. Philadelphia: D. G. Brinton, 1881. 612p. DLC; PPC **80-4510**

NAPHEYS, George H[enry] (1842-1876)
Handbook of popular medicine, embracing the anatomy and physiology of the human body; illustrations of home gymnastics; instructions for nursing the sick; the domestic treatment of the ordinary diseases and accidents of children and adults; plan for a family health record, etc. With over 300 choice dietetic and remedial recipes, and more than 100 engravings on wood. Especially adapted for general and family instruction and reference. Philadelphia: H. C. Watts Co., 1882. 408p. DNLM; PPC; PU **80-4511**

NAPHEYS, George H[enry] (1842-1876)
Modern medical therapeutics: a compendium of recent formulae and specific therapeutical directions, from the practice of eminent contemporary physicians, American and foreign. . . . Ed. by Joseph F. Edwards, M.D., and D. G. Brinton, M.D. 8th ed., enl. and rev. Philadelphia: D. G. Brinton, 1885. 629p. DLC; DNLM; PPC **80-4512**

NATIONAL COLLEGE OF PHARMACY. WASHINGTON, D.C.
Annual circulars for the sessions of 1885-1886 to 1905-1906 (14.-34.). Chicago, 1885-1905. DNLM [List of students and graduates for the sessions of 1884-1885 to 1904-1905 in announcements for subsequent years. List of alumni, 1873-1905, in announcement for 1905-1906.] **80-4513**

NATIONAL DENTAL ASSOCIATION (LATE SOUTHERN)
Proceedings of the . . . in connections with the Georgia State Dental Society and the North Carolina and South Carolina Dental Associations, 1879. Athens, Ga.: Yancey & Cranford, 1881. 96p. DNLM; GU; ScMS **80-4514**

THE NATIONAL formulary of unofficial preparations. [Baltimore]: American Pharm. Association, 1888. 176p. OCLloyd **80-4515**

NATIONAL INSTITUTE OF PHARMACY, CHICAGO
Special announcement. October, 1888. [Chicago: G. P. Engelhard & Co., 1888.] 1 l. DNLM **80-4516**

NATIONAL MEDICAL COLLEGE. MEDICAL DEPARTMENT OF COLUMBIAN UNIVERSITY
Annual announcements and catalogues for the sessions of 1888-1889 to 1893-1894 (67.-72.). Washington, 1888-1893. DNLM [List of students for the sessions of 1887-1888 to 1892-1893, in announcements for subsequent years.] **80-4517**

NATIONAL MEDICAL COLLEGE, WASHINGTON
Addresses delivered at the sixty-fourth annual commencement of the National Medical College (medical department of Columbian University) by W. W. Godding and W. L. Cissel, March 17, 1886. Washington: W. H. Moore, 1886. 15p. DNLM **80-4518**

NATIONAL UNIVERSITY, WASHINGTON. MEDICAL AND DENTAL DEPARTMENTS
Annual announcements for the sessions of 1888-1889 to 1898-1899 (5.-15.); 1900-1901 to 1902-1903 (17.-19.). Washington, 1888-1902. DNLM [List of graduates from 1885 to 1895, in announcement for 1895-1896.] **80-4519**

NEALE, L. E.
Placenta praevia, with report of case. Baltimore, 1887. 9p. DNLM **80-4520**

NEIDHARD, Charles (1809-1895)
Pathogenetic and clinical repertory of the most prominent symptoms of the head, with their concomitants and conditions. Philadelphia: F. E. Boericke, Hahnemann Publishing House, 1888. 188p. PPC; PPHa **80-4521**

NELSON, A. W.
Veratrum viride in typhoid fever; its lowering of the pulse and temperature; twenty-eight successive cases in private practice, all recovering, 1873-1882. [New York, 1883.] 17p. DNLM; NNNAM **80-4522**

NELSON, Daniel T[hurber] (*b.* 1839)
Clinical lecture delivered before the senior class at Rush Medical College. Bridgeport, Conn., 1885. 3p. DNLM
80-4523

NELSON, Daniel T[hurber] (*b.* 1839)
Uterine fibroids treated by ergot. Philadelphia: W. F. Pell & Co., [1887]. 30 l. DNLM **80-4524**

NELSON, Samuel N[ewell] (1857?-1893)
The etiology of diphtheria. Boston: Cupples & Hurd, [1889]. 9p. DNLM **80-4525**

[NELSON, Wolfred] (1846-1913)
Yellow fever. Absolute protection secured by scientific quarantine. New York, 1889. 50p. DNLM; NNNAM
80-4526

[NELSON, Wolfred] (1846-1913)
Yellow fever. A new treatment. A forecast for 1889, Panama, Colon, and Havana; its hot-beds and distributors. New York, 1889. 40p. DNLM; NNNAM **80-4527**

NETTLESHIP, Edward (1845-1913)
The student's guide to diseases of the eye. Philadelphia: Henry C. Lea, 1880. 369p. DNLM; MBM; OCIM; PPC
80-4528

NETTLESHIP, Edward (1845-1913)
Student's guide to diseases of the eye. . . . 2nd American from the 2nd rev. and enl. English ed. With a chapter on examination for color perception, by William Thomson. . . . Philadelphia: Henry C. Lea's Son & Co., 1883. 416p. diags. DLC; NNNAM; PPC; PPJ **80-4529**

NETTLESHIP, Edward (1845-1913)
Diseases of the eye. . . . 3rd American from the 4th English ed. with a chapter on examination for color-perception. By William Thomson. Philadelphia: Henry C. Lea's Son & Co., 1887. 475p. CtY-M; MH-M; NNNAM; PPC
80-4530

NEWELL, Otis K[imball]
The intestinal suture. Boston: Cupples, Upham & Co., 1887. 23p. DNLM **80-4531**

NEWELL, Otis K[imball]
The endoscopic instruments of Joseph Leiter, of Vienna, and the present development of endoscopy. Boston: Cupples & Hurd, 1887. 9p. DNLM **80-4532**

NEWELL, Otis K[imball]
The best surgical dressing; how to prepare it and how to use it. With a consideration of Beach's principle of bullet-wound treatment. Boston: Cupples & Hurd, 1888. 179p. DNLM
80-4533

NEWELL, Otis K[imball]
A new principle in the surgery of the bladder. Boston: Cupples & Hurd, 1888. 20p. DNLM **80-4534**

NEWELL, Otis K[imball]
Diagnosis of tumors of the bladder and stone with the cystoscope. Boston: Cupples & Hurd, [1889]. 6p. DNLM
80-4535

NEWMAN, Robert (*d.* 1903)
Urethrocele in the female. New York: William Wood & Co., 1880. 16p. DNLM; NNNAM **80-4536**

NEWMAN, Robert (*d.* 1903)
A successful ovariotomy in 1866. Galvano-caustic to pedicle, antiseptic dressing, drainage, silver wire ligatures left in abdominal cavity. [n. p.], 1882. 6p. DNLM
80-4537

NEWMAN, Robert (*d.* 1903)
Stricture of the rectum treated by electrolysis. Bridgeport, Conn.: Gould & Stiles, 1882. 7p. DNLM
80-4538

NEWMAN, Robert (*d.* 1903)
Ten years' experience in the treatment of stricture of the urethra by electrolysis. New York: Trow, 1882. 44p. DNLM; NNNAM **80-4539**

NEWMAN, Robert (*d.* 1903)
The treatment of urethritis and leucorrhoea. Richmond: The Southern Clinic Print, 1883. 15p. DNLM
80-4540

NEWMAN, Robert (*d.* 1903)
Additional answers to correspondents about the electrolytic treatment of urethral strictures; with a few select cases. [Bridgeport, Conn.: Gould & Stiles], 1883. 5p. DNLM
80-4541

NEWMAN, Robert (*d.* 1903)
Does the character of pus diagnosticate gonorrhoea as a specific infection from a simple (benign) urethritis? A medico-legal sketch. Richmond: Whittet & Shepperson, 1883. 8p. DNLM **80-4542**

NEWMAN, Robert (*d.* 1903)
Progress of electrolysis in surgery. Read at the first annual meeting of the Fifth District Branch of the New York State Medical Association, held at Brooklyn, October 13, 1885. New York, 1885. 8p. DNLM **80-4543**

NEWMAN, Robert (*d.* 1903)
Tabular statistics of one hundred cases of urethral stricture treated by electrolysis, without relapse. Bridgeport, Conn.: Gould & Stiles, 1885. 15p. DNLM **80-4544**

NEWMAN, Robert (*d.* 1903)
Is electrolysis a failure in the treatment of urethral strictures? New York: Trow's Printing Co., 1886. 12p. DNLM
80-4545

NEWMAN, Robert (*d.* 1903)
Galvano-cautery in diseases of the prostate, bladder, and urethra. Chicago, 1886. 13p. DNLM **80-4546**

NEWMAN, Robert (*d.* 1903)
Causes of failure in the treatment of urethral strictures by electrolysis. New York, 1886. 13p. DNLM
80-4547

NEWMAN, Robert (*d.* 1903)
The galvano-cautery sound and its application, especially in hypertrophy of the prostate; with reports of cases. Bridgeport, Conn.: Gould & Stiles, 1887. 53p. DNLM
80-4548

NEWMAN, Robert (*d.* 1903)
Synopsis of the second hundred cases of urethral stricture treated by electrolysis; with cases. Chicago, 1887. 15p. DNLM
80-4549

NEWMAN, Robert (*d.* **1903)**
A defense of electrolysis in urethral strictures, with documentary evidence. Philadelphia, 1888. 20p. DNLM
80-4550

NEWMAN, Robert (*d.* **1903)**
The failure of J. B. Thomas's treatment of urethral stricture by electrolysis. Chicago, 1888. 15p. DNLM
80-4551

NEWMAN, Robert (*d.* **1903)**
Success and failure of electrolysis in urethral strictures, especially Dr. Keyes' method reviewed. Philadelphia, 1888. 36p. DNLM **80-4552**

NEWMAN, Robert (*d.* **1903)**
Accumulators and their medical use. [Philadelphia], 1889. 24p. DNLM **80-4553**

NEWTH, Alfred Henry
Post-mortems; what to look for and how to make them with sections on infanticide, poisons, malformations, etc. . . . Ed., with numerous notes and additions, by F. W. Owen. Detroit, Mich.: The Illustrated Medical Journal Co., 1885. 136p. DLC
80-4554

NEWTON, A. E. (1822-1889)
The better way: an appeal to men in behalf of human culture through a wise parentage. New York: Wood & Holbrook, 1880. 48p. DNLM; NN **80-4555**

NEWTON, A. E. (1822-1889)
The better way; an appeal to men in behalf of human culture through a wise parentage. New York: M. L. Holbrook & Co., 1884. 48p. DNLM; NN **80-4556**

NEWTON, William K. (*b.* **1850)**
Some facts about the New Jersey milk adulteration act and the results of its enforcement. Notes on milk analysis, giving the results of 112 analyses and a brief account of methods. [Paterson, N.J., 1884.] 15p. DNLM
80-4557

NEWTON, William K. (*b.* **1850)**
Sanitary control of the food supply. Concord, N.H.: Republican Press Association, 1884. 25p. DNLM
80-4558

NEWTON, William K. (*b.* **1850)**
The sanitary survey of a house. Concord, N.H., 1885. 8p. DNLM **80-4559**

NEWTON, William K. (*b.* **1850)**
Report of the milk inspector. [Trenton, 1886?] 17p. DNLM
80-4560

NEW YORK ACADEMY OF MEDICINE
List of officers and resident fellows, October, 1887. New York, 1887. 7p. DNLM; NNNAM **80-4561**

NEW YORK (CITY). DEPARTMENT OF PUBLIC CHARITIES
Hospital formulary of. . . . 3rd ed. rev. . . . New York: Printing Bureau, 1886. 127p. DNLM; OCLloyd
80-4562

NEW YORK (CITY). DEPARTMENT OF PUBLIC CHARITIES
Hospital formulary of. . . . 4th ed., revised. New York: Printing Bureau, 1889. 143p. DNLM; NNNAM; OCLloyd
80-4563

NEW YORK CITY. GERMAN HOSPITAL AND DISPENSARY
Catalogue of the library of physicians to the . . . by Hermann G. Klotz, M.D., librarian. Mount Vernon, N.Y., 1880. 19p. DNLM **80-4564**

NEW YORK COLLEGE OF DENTISTRY, NEW YORK CITY
Annual announcements for the sessions of 1887-1888 to 1895-1896 (22.-30.); 1902-1903 (37.). New York, 1887-1902. DNLM; NNNAM **80-4565**

NICHOL, Thomas
Diseases of the nares, larynx, and trachea, in childhood. New York: A. L. Chatterton Publishing Co., 1885. 308p. NNNAM; PPHa **80-4566**

NICHOLS, C. F[essenden]
Quantum sufficit. A summary of cases chiefly treated by the higher homoeopathic attenuations, with comments. . . . Boston: Walter F. Towns, 1881. 26p. MBM; PPHa
80-4567

NICHOLS, Charles H[enry] (1820-1889)
Memoir of William B. Goldsmith. [Utica, 1888.] 14p. DNLM
80-4568

NICHOLS, Charles L.
On medical restrictions in Massachusetts. Annual address before the Massachusetts Homoeopathic Medical Society, April 15, 1886. Boston: Rand, Avery & Co., 1886. 12p. MBM
80-4569

NICHOLS, Thomas L[ow] (1815-1901)
Eating to live. The diet cure. An essay on the relations of food and drink to health, disease, and cure. New York: M. L. Holbrook & Co., 1881. 88p. DNLM; NNNAM
80-4570

NICHOLS, W. T.
Mind cure; its truths and fallacies from a common sense standpoint. Chicago, 1886. 76p. DNLM **80-4571**

NIEMEYER, Felix von (1820-1871)
A text-book of practical medicine, with particular reference to physiology and pathological anatomy. . . . Transl. from the 8th German ed., by special permission of the author. By George H. Humphreys . . . and Charles E. Hackley. . . . Rev. ed. . . . New York: D. Appleton & Co., 1880. 2 v. DLC: NNNAM; PPC; PU **80-4572**

NILES, Edward S.
Dental phosphorénèses, or caries. [Buffalo, 1886.] 8p. DNLM
80-4573

NOBLE, George Henry (1860-1932)
Abortive treatment of mammary abscesses, and the cure of fissured nipples by means of a new and effectual compress. Atlanta, 1882. 8p. DNLM **80-4574**

NOEGGERATH, Emile Jacob (1827-1895)
The diseases of blood-vessels of the ovary in relation to the genesis of ovarian cysts. New York: William Wood & Co., 1880. 19p. 2 plates. DNLM; NNNAM
80-4575

NORRIS, Basil (1828-1895)
A paper on dislocations of the astragalus. Read before the American Surgical Association, Cincinnati, 1883. Washington: Judd & Detweiler, 1883. 23p. DNLM
80-4576

NORRIS, George W[ashington] (1808-1875)
The early history of medicine in Philadelphia. . . . Philadelphia, 1886. 232p. NNNAM; PPC; PU [A limited edition of 125 copies for private distribution. The manuscript of Dr. Norris, surgeon of Philadelphia, was found among his papers after his death in 1875. It was written for the most part in 1845, and was published by his son, Dr. William F. Norris, who served as a surgeon in the Civil War and was a noted ophthalmologist. "Believing that the picture which its pages present of our early medical men and institutions, as well as of the customs and manners of our colonists, and the concise but vivid description of the privations of our Revolutionary Army, and of the struggles and necessities of its Medical Department, would be interesting to all antiquarians as well as to the Medical Professions, I have decided to print it. . . . "—Preface.] **80-4577**

NORRIS, William Fisher (1839-1901)
Retinitis in Bright's disease. Philadelphia: Sherman & Co., 1881. 10p. DNLM **80-4578**

NORRIS, William Fisher (1839-1901)
Case of embolism of the upper temporal division of the left central retinal artery. Philadelphia, 1882. 7p. DNLM **80-4579**

NORRIS, William Fisher (1839-1901)
Hereditary atrophy of the optic nerves. New York: Trow, 1883. 7p. DNLM **80-4580**

NORRIS, William Fisher (1839-1901)
Contributions to ophthalmology. New York: Trow, 1883. 7p. DNLM **80-4581**

NORRIS, William Fisher (1839-1901)
Medical ophthalmology. [Philadelphia, 1886.] 68p. DNLM; PPC **80-4582**

NORRIS, William Fisher (1839-1901)
Some remarks of asthenopia and the changes in refraction in adolescent and adult eyes. [Boston, 1886.] 13p. DNLM **80-4583**

NORRIS, William Fisher (1839-1901)
Cases of primary acute glaucoma, of hemorrhagic glaucoma, and of secondary glaucoma, with remarks and photomicrographs. [Philadelphia, 1887.] 11p. 3 plates. DNLM **80-4584**

NORTHRUP, William P[erry]
Extensive interlobular emphysema and abscess of the lung, after whooping cough in a child of two months; unique case. Philadelphia, 1883. 3p. DNLM **80-4585**

NORTON, Arthur B[righam] (1856-1919)
Advantages of systematic exercise over tenotomy in the treatment of heterophoria. Read before the American Institute of Homoeopathy, June 1889. New York: A. L. Chatterton & Co., 1889. 6p. NNNAM **80-4586**

NORTON, George S[almon] (1851-1891)
Ophthalmic therapeutics. With an introduction by Prof. T. F. Allen. 2nd ed. New York & Philadelphia: Boericke & Tafel, 1882. 242p. DNLM; NNNAM; PPC **80-4587**

NORTON, George S[almon] (1851-1891)
The eye as an agent in causing headaches and other nervous disturbances. Read before the New York Medico-Chirurgical Society, December 9, 1884. Philadelphia, 1885. 24p. DNLM **80-4588**

NORTON, George S[almon] (1851-1891)
Malignant tumors of the eyelids and orbit. New York: J. C. Rankin, 1886. 12p. DNLM **80-4589**

NOTHNAGEL, Hermann (1841-1905)
A treatise on materia medica (including therapeutics and toxicology) by Dr. H. Nothnagel . . . and Dr. M. J. Rossbach. . . . Transl. from the 4th enl. ed. by Dr. H. N. Heineman . . . and Dr. H. W. Berg. . . . New York, [etc.]: Bermingham & Co., 1883-1884. 3 v. DLC; NNNAM; OCLloyd **80-4590**

NOYES, Charles J[ohnson] (*b.* 1841)
Argument before the committee on the judiciary of the house of representatives of Massachusetts against a bill to regulate the practice of medicine. Delivered at the State House, Feb. 18, 1889. Boston: L. Barta & Co., 1889. 19p. DNLM **80-4591**

NOYES, Henry Drury (1832-1900)
. . . A treatise [on] diseases of the eye. . . . New York: William Wood & Co., 1881. 360p. 2 col. plates, diags. DLC; DNLM; NNNAM; PPC **80-4592**

NOYES, Henry D[rury] (1832-1900)
Pathfinding in medicine, being the anniversary address delivered before the New York Academy of Medicine, November 19, 1885. New York: William Wood & Co., 1885. 24p. DNLM; NNNAM **80-4593**

NOYES, P. J. MFG. PHARMACIST
Price list of gelatine coated pills and granules, tablets, extracts, tinctures. Lancaster, N.H., 1888. 76p. Nh **80-4594**

NOYES, Robt. F.
Perityphlitis. Providence, 1883. 47p. DNLM **80-4595**

NOYES, R. K[ing] (*b.* 1853)
The history of medicine for the last 4000 years. Lynn, Mass.: Leech & Lewis, 1880. 79p. DNLM; MBM; MH **80-4596**

NOYES, William (1845-1915)
Composite portrait of eight cases of melancholia (all men). Boston: Notman Co., 1887. 1 phot., 4¼ x 6½. DNLM **80-4597**

NOYES, William (1845-1915)
Composite portrait of eight cases of general paresis (five men and three women). Boston: Notman Co., 1887. 1 phot., 4¼ x 6½. DNLM **80-4598**

NOYES, William (1845-1915)
Paranoia. A study of the evolution of systematized delusions of grandeur. Baltimore, 1888. 19p. 6 plates. DNLM **80-4599**

NOYES, William (1845-1915)
Paranoia. A study of the evolution of systematized delusions of grandeur. [Baltimore, 1889.] 27p. 6 plates. DNLM **80-4600**

NOYES, William (1845-1915)
Clinical history and autopsy of a case of general paresis of nine years' duration. New York: M. J. Rooney & Co., 1889. 6p. DNLM **80-4601**

NUNN, R[ichard] J. (1831-1910)
Some practical suggestions in the treatment of diphtheria. Baltimore: Thomas & Evans, 1880. 7p. DNLM
80-4602

NUNN, R[ichard] J. (1831-1910)
Peptonized milk as food for infants and invalids. New York: William Wood & Co., 1880. 20p. DNLM
80-4603

NUNN, R[ichard] J. (1831-1910)
Female diseases; the result of errors in habit and hygiene during childhood and puberty; with remarks on the treatment of rachi-algia with igni-puncture (Paquelin's cautery). Augusta, Ga.: J. Loveday, 1881. 45p. DNLM; GU
80-4604

NUNN, R[ichard] J. (1831-1910)
Report on diseases of women from the First Congresssional district. Atlanta: J. P. Harrison & Co., [1883]. 32p. DNLM
80-4605

NUNN, R[ichard] J. (1831-1910)
Diet in consumption and other morbid states and processes in diseases of the genito-urinary system, to which is added several recipes for the preparation of animal food. Atlanta: J. P. Harrison & Co., [1884]. 54p. DNLM
80-4606

NUNN, R[ichard] J. (1831-1910)
A national and international medical degree. Atlanta, 1886. 19p. DNLM **80-4607**

[OBSTETRICAL SOCIETY OF BOSTON]
Historical and biographical sketches by Cutting and Wellington. [Boston: D. Clapp & Son, 1881.] 73p. DLC
80-4608

OCHSNER, A[lbert] J[ohn] (1858-1925)
The preparation of specimens for chemical microscopy. . . . Chicago: W. T. Keener, 1888. 19p. DLC
80-4609

OCKFORD, George M.
A hand-book of homoeopathic practice. Chicago: Duncan Bros., 1882. 435p. IU-M; PPHa **80-4610**

OCTERLONY, John Arvid (1838-1905)
Eulogy on the life and character of Lunsford Pitts Yandell. Louisville: J. P. Morton & Co., 1885. 16p. DNLM
80-4611

O'DANIEL, W.
Malaria and its toxic influences; malarial haematuria. Atlanta, Ga.: J. P. Harrison & Co., [1885]. 8p. DNLM
80-4612

O'DEA, James J. (*b.* 1837)
Suicide; studies on its philosophy, causes, and prevention. New York: G. P. Putnam's Sons, 1882. 322p. DNLM; ICU; MH; NN **80-4613**

O'DWYER, Joseph (1841-1898)
Analysis of fifty cases of croup treated by intubation of the larynx. New York, 1888. 11p. 1 tab. DNLM
80-4614

O'DWYER, Joseph (1841-1898)
Intubation in chronic stenosis of the larynx, with a report of five cases. [New York, 1888.] 23p. DNLM
80-4615

OFFICIAL formulae of American hospitals. Collected and arranged by C. F. Taylor. 2nd ed. Philadelphia: Medical World, [1886]. 256p. DNLM; OCLloyd; PPC; PU
80-4616

OFFICIAL record of the post-mortem examination of the body of President J. A. Garfield, made Sept. 20, 1881, commencing at 4:30 p.m., eighteen hours after death, at Francklyn Cottage, Elberon, New Jersey. [Philadelphia, 1881.] 8p. DNLM
80-4617

OFFICIAL register of physicians and midwives now in practice to whom certificates have been issued by the State Board of Health of Illinois, 1877-1886. Springfield, Ill.: Rokker, 1886. 314p. IU-M **80-4618**

O'HARA, Michael (1832-1905)
Case of recovery from occlusion of one or more of the cerebral sinuses. Philadelphia, 1880. 8p. DNLM
80-4619

O'HARA, Michael (1832-1905)
Case of recovery from occlusion of one or more of the cerebral sinuses. Philadelphia, 1888. 8p. DNLM
80-4620

OHMANN-DUMESNIL, A[mant] H[enry] (*b.* 1857)
A case of giant (?) urticaria. Read before the Linton District Medical Society, Nov. 15, 1882. [n. p.], 1882. 2p. DNLM
80-4621

OHMANN-DUMESNIL, A[mant] H[enry] (*b.* 1857)
A case of universal psoriasis. St. Louis: Med. J. Pub. Co., 1884. 7p. DNLM **80-4622**

OHMANN-DUMESNIL, A[mant] H[enry] (*b.* 1857)
A case of symmetrical vitiligo. St. Louis, 1884. 3p. DNLM
80-4623

OHMANN-DUMESNIL, A[mant] H[enry] (*b.* 1857)
The importance of local mercurial treatment in syphilis. St. Louis: Med. J. Pub. Co., 1885. 7p. DNLM
80-4624

OHMANN-DUMESNIL, A[mant] H[enry] (*b.* 1857)
The relations of skin diseases to marriage. St. Louis: Med. J. Pub. Co., 1885. 7p. DNLM **80-4625**

OHMANN-DUMESNIL, A[mant] H[enry] (*b.* 1857)
When is the proper time to institute specific treatment in syphilis? St. Louis: Med. J. Pub. Co., 1885. 6p. DNLM
80-4626

OHMANN-DUMESNIL, A[mant] H[enry] (*b.* 1857)
An unusual case of syphilis. St. Louis, 1886. 4p. DNLM
80-4627

OHMANN-DUMESNIL, A[mant] H[enry] (*b.* 1857)
Syphilis is a constitutional disease from its inception. St. Louis: Med. J. Pub. Co., 1886. 7p. DNLM
80-4628

OHMANN-DUMESNIL, A[mant] H[enry] (*b.* 1857)
The role of the nervous system in the causation of vitiligo. St. Louis, 1886. 7p. DNLM **80-4629**

OHMANN-DUMESNIL, A[mant] H[enry] (*b.* 1857)
Hypertrichosis due to general disease of the nervous system. St. Louis, 1887. 5p. DNLM **80-4630**

OHMANN-DUMESNIL, A[mant] H[enry] (*b.* 1857)
Double comedo. St. Louis, 1888. 17p. DNLM **80-4631**

OHMANN-DUMESNIL, A[mant] H[enry] (*b.* 1857)
A case of indigenous leprosy. Paper read before the Missouri State Medical Association, April, 1888. [St. Louis, 1888.] 6p. DNLM **80-4632**

OHMANN-DUMESNIL, A[mant] H[enry] (*b.* 1857)
Circumscribed hypertrichosis (acquired) in the lumbar region. The report of a case. New York: [Gillis Bros. & Turnure, 1888.] 4p. DNLM **80-4633**

OHMANN-DUMESNIL, A[mant] H[enry] (*b.* 1857)
A case of hereditary syphilis simulating leprosy. St. Louis, Mo., 1888. 4p. DNLM **80-4634**

OHMANN-DUMESNIL, A[mant] H[enry] (*b.* 1857)
A hand book of dermatology. For the use of students. . . . St. Louis: St. Louis Medical and Surgical Journal Publishing Co., [1889]. 167p. DLC; PPC **80-4635**

OLDBERG, Oscar (1846-1913)
The pharmacopoeial nomenclature. New York, 1880. 19p. DNLM; NNNAM **80-4636**

OLDBERG, Oscar (1846-1913)
The metric system in medicine, containing an account of the metric system of weights and measures, Americanized and simplified, a comprehensive dose table, and three hundred practical illustrations of metric prescription writing, selected from recipes in actual use in hospital and out-door practice. Philadelphia: P. Blakiston, 1881. 182p. DNLM; PU **80-4637**

OLDBERG, Oscar (1846-1913)
A companion to the United States Pharmacopoeia, being a commentary on the latest edition of the Pharmacopoeia, and containing the descriptions, properties, uses, and doses of all official and numerous unofficial drugs and preparations in current use in the United States, together with practical hints, working formulas, etc., designed as a ready reference book for pharmacists, physicians, and students, with over 650 original illustrations. New York: William Wood & Co., 1884. 1216p. DNLM; OCLloyd **80-4638**

OLDBERG, Oscar (1846-1913)
A manual of weights, measures, and specific gravity, including principles of metrology; the weights and measures now in use; weight and volume, and their reciprocal relations; weighing and measuring; balances (scales) and weights; measures of capacity; specific weight and specific volume, and their determination, and practical applications with rules and tables. Chicago, 1885. 238p. DNLM; IU-M **80-4639**

OLDBERG, Oscar (1846-1913)
An outline of a course of study in practical pharmacy. Chicago, 1885. 104p. DNLM; IU-M **80-4640**

OLDBERG, Oscar (1846-1913)
Pharmaceutical problems and exercises in metrology, chemistry, pharmacy, and pharmaceutical nomenclature. Chicago: W. T. Keener, 1887. 75p. DNLM **80-4641**

OLIVER, Charles A[ugustus] (1853-1911)
Iritis; diagnosis and treatment. [Philadelphia, 1880.] 5p. DNLM; PPC **80-4642**

OLIVER, Charles A[ugustus] (1853-1911)
The comparative action of hydrobromate of homatropine and of sulphate of atropia upon the iris and ciliary muscle. [Philadelphia, 1881.] 6p. DNLM **80-4643**

OLIVER, Charles A[ugustus] (1853-1911)
The hygiene of the eye; an address to physicians. Philadelphia, [1881]. 9p. DNLM **80-4644**

OLIVER, Charles A[ugustus] (1853-1911)
The comparative action of sulphate of daturia and of sulphate of hyoscyamia upon the iris and ciliary muscle. [Philadelphia], 1882. 7p. DNLM **80-4645**

OLIVER, Charles A[ugustus] (1853-1911)
Description of a revolving astigmatic disk. [Philadelphia], 1883.] 7p. DNLM **80-4646**

OLIVER, Charle A[ugustus] (1853-1911)
A new series of metric test-letters for determining the acuity of direct vision for form. Boston, 1885. 4p. DNLM **80-4647**

OLIVER, Charles A[ugustus] (1853-1911)
New series of metric test-letters and words for determining the amount and range of accommodation. Philadelphia, 1886. 1 p. l. 3 p. DNLM **80-4648**

OLIVER, Charles A[ugustus] (1853-1911)
A new series of Berlin wools for the scientific detection of subnormal color-perception (color-blindness). [Philadelphia, 1886.] 4p. DNLM **80-4649**

OLIVER, Charles A[ugustus] (1853-1911)
A new series of metric test-letters and words for determining the amount and range of accommodation. [Philadelphia, 1886.] 1 galley sheet. DNLM **80-4650**

OLIVER, Charles A[ugustus] (1853-1911)
The eye of the adult imbecile. [Philadelphia, 1887.] 4p. DNLM **80-4651**

OLIVER, Charles A[ugustus] (1853-1911)
An analysis of the ocular symptoms obtainable in epilepsy in the male adult. Philadelphia: J. B. Lippincott Co., 1887. 8p. DNLM **80-4652**

OLIVER, Charles A[ugustus] (1853-1911)
Description of a case of coloboma of the iris, lens, and choroid, with a study of the visual fields. [Hartford, 1887.] 6p. 1 plate. DNLM **80-4653**

OLIVER, Charles A[ugustus] (1853-1911)
Double chorio-retinitis, with partial degeneration of the optic nerve, associated with curious lymph extravasation into the retina and vitreous. [Hartford, 1887.] 6p. 2 col. plates. DNLM **80-4654**

OLIVER, Charles A[ugustus] (1853-1911)
The eye of the adult imbecile. [Hartford, 1887.] 6p. DNLM
80-4655

OLIVER, Charles A[ugustus] (1853-1911)
Description of a series of tests for the detection and determination of sub-normal color-perception (color-blindness), designed for use in railway service. [Hartford, Conn., 1888.] 8p. DNLM
80-4656

OLIVER, Charles A[ugustus] (1853-1911)
An analysis of some of the ocular symptoms observed in so-called general paresis. [Hartford, 1889.] 6p. DNLM
80-4657

OLIVER, Charles A[ugustus] (1853-1911)
Description of a case of embolism of the left central retinal artery. Hartford, Conn.: Case, Lockwood & Brainard Co., 1889. 5p. DNLM
80-4658

OLIVER, George (1841-1915)
Instruction for the use of the urinary test papers introduced for the clinical examination of the urine at the bedside. Detroit & New York: Parke, Davis & Co., [1888]. 16p. 1 tab. DNLM; NNNAM
80-4659

OLIVER, George P[owell] (1824-1884)
Opening address of the Medico-Chirurgical College of Philadelphia. Philadelphia: G. F. Lasher, 1881. 8p. DNLM; PPC
80-4660

OLIVER WENDELL HOLMES HOSPITAL. HUDSON, WIS.
Announcement [of its organization on the first day of May, 1887]. Minneapolis: Tribune Job Printing Co., 1887. 16p. DNLM
80-4661

OLIVER WENDELL HOLMES HOSPITAL. HUDSON, WIS.
Description of the . . . . Addresses delivered by the founder of the institution and others. Ceremonies attending the exercises. [Minneapolis, 1887.] [unp.] DNLM
80-4662

OMAHA MEDICAL COLLEGE, MEDICAL DEPARTMENT. UNIVERSITY OF OMAHA
Annual announcements for the sessions of 1887-1888 (7.); 1889-1890 (9.); 1891-1892 (11.); 1892-1893 (12.); 1897-1898 (17.); 1898-1899 (18.); 1900-1901 (20.). Omaha, 1887-1900. DNLM [List of students and graduates for the years 1885-1886; 1886-1887; 1888-1889; 1890-1891; 1891-1892; 1896-1897; 1897-1898; 1899-1900, in announcements for subsequent years.]
80-4663

OREGON. UNIVERSITY OF OREGON. MEDICAL DEPARTMENT, PORTLAND
Annual announcements for the sessions of 1887-1888 to 1906-1907 (1-20). Portland, 1887-1906. DNLM [List of students and graduates for the years 1887-1888 to 1905-1906 in announcements for subsequent years. Alumni from 1888 to 1902 in announcement for 1902-1903.]
80-4664

ORIGIN of yellow fever. [Letter of Sanford E. Chaillé, dated New Orleans, March 19, 1880, to the editor of the Pensacola Advance, with reply of Dr. Robt. B. S. Hargis.] [Pensacola, 1880.] 1 sheet. DNLM
80-4665

ORME, Francis Hodgson (1834-1913)
The charge of exclusivism as applied to homoeopathists. New York, 1883. 8p. DNLM
80-4666

ORME, Francis Hodgson (1834-1913)
Address delivered by the president of the American Institute of Homoeopathy, at the session on its forty-eighth anniversary, held at Saratoga Springs, June 27 to July 1, 1887. Atlanta: W. H. Scott, 1887. 30p. DNLM
80-4667

ORME, H. S[ayre] (*b.* 1837)
The climatology and diseases of southern California. Sacramento: State Office, 1886. 17p. DNLM
80-4668

OSBALDESTON, E. T.
Massage with rational home gymnastics. New York: G. P. Putnam's Sons, 1884. 27p. DNLM; NNNAM
80-4669

OSGOOD, Hamilton (*b.* 1839)
The need of a radical change in the training and education of the American girl, and the physician's duty therein. [Philadelphia, 1881.] 11p. DNLM
80-4670

OSGOOD, Hamilton (*b.* 1839)
A peculiar form of oesophagismus. Boston: Cupples & Hurd, [1880]. 16p. DNLM
80-4671

OSLER, William (1849-1919)
On the systolic brain murmur of children. Cambridge: Riverside Press, 1880. 8p. DNLM
80-4672

OSLER, William (1849-1919)
Notes on intestinal diverticula. Brooklyn, 1881. 6p. DNLM
80-4673

OSLER, William (1849-1919)
Infectious (so-called ulcerative) endocarditis. New York: G. P. Putnam's Sons, 1881. 25p. DNLM
80-4674

OSLER, William (1849-1919)
A clinical lecture on empyema and its antiseptic treatment. Philadelphia, 1882. 8p. DNLM
80-4675

OSLER, William (1849-1919)
Preataxic tabes dorsalis. A clinical lecture. Philadelphia, 1883. 12p. DNLM
80-4676

OSLER, William (1849-1919)
The third corpuscle of the blood. Philadelphia, 1883. 8p. DNLM
80-4677

OSLER, William (1849-1919)
On some natural modes of cure in empyema. A clinical lecture delivered during the summer session of the McGill Medical Faculty, June 20th, 1883. [New York, 1883.] 13p. DNLM
80-4678

OSLER, William (1849-1919)
Cartwright lectures. On certain problems of the blood corpuscles. Delivered before the Association of Alumni of the College of Physicians and Surgeons, New York, March 23, 27, and 30, 1886. 1. The blood plaque or third corpuscle. 2. Degneration and regeneration of the corpuscles. 3. The relation of the corpuscles to coagulation. Philadelphia, 1886. 55p. DNLM; KU
80-4679

OSLER, William (1849-1919)
The biscuspid condition of the aortic valves. Philadelphia: W. J. Dornan, 1886, 8p. DNLM
80-4680

OSLER, William (1849-1919)
On the use of arsenic in certain forms of anaemia. Detroit: G. S. Davis, 1886. 14p. DNLM **80-4681**

OSLER, William (1849-1919)
Antifebrin. Detroit: G. S. Davis, 1887. 5p. DNLM **80-4682**

OSLER, William (1849-1919)
Case of cholesteatoma of floor of third ventricle and of the infundibulum. New York, 1887. 19p. DNLM **80-4683**

OSLER, William (1849-1919)
Hereditary angio-neurotic oedema. Philadelphia, 1888. 6p. DNLM **80-4684**

OSLER, William (1849-1919)
Glioma of the medulla oblongata. [New York, 1888.] 5p. DNLM **80-4685**

OSLER, William (1849-1919)
Puerperal anaemia, and its treatment with arsenic. Boston, 1888. 7p. DNLM **80-4686**

OSLER, William (1849-1919)
On the diagnosis of duodenal ulcer. New York, 1888. 7p. DNLM **80-4687**

OSLER, William (1849-1919)
On lesions of the conus medullaris and cauda equina, and on the situation of the ano-vesical centre in man. Philadelphia, 1888. 7p. DNLM **80-4688**

OSLER, William (1849-1919)
On a form of purpura associated with articular, gastro-intestinal, and renal symptoms. New York, 1888. 5p. DNLM **80-4689**

OSLER, William (1849-1919)
The mortality of pneumonia. Philadelphia, 1889. 7p. DNLM **80-4690**

OSLER, William (1849-1919)
On phagocytes. [Philadelphia: Lea Bros. & Co., 1889.] 27p. DNLM **80-4691**

OSLER, William (1849-1919)
Pulsating pleurisy. Philadelphia, 1889. 8p. DNLM **80-4692**

OSLER, William (1849-1919)
Annual address. The license to practice. Baltimore, 1889. 13p. DNLM **80-4693**

OSLER, William (1849-1919)
Aequanimitas. Valedictory remarks to the graduates in medicine of the University of Pennsylvania, May 1, 1889. Philadelphia: W. F. Fell & Co., 1889. 10p. DNLM **80-4694**

OSLER, William (1849-1919)
The cerebral palsies of children; a clinical study from the Infirmary for Nervous Diseases, Philadelphia. Philadelphia: P. Blakiston, Son & Co., 1889. 103p. DNLM; IU-M; KU; NcD **80-4695**

OSLER, William (1849-1919)
Notes on intra-thoracic growths developing from the thyroid gland. Philadelphia, 1889. 3p. DNLM **80-4996**

OSLER, William (1849-1919)
On a case of simple idiopathic muscular atrophy, involving the face and the scapulo-humeral muscles. Philadelphia, 1889. 5p. DNLM **80-4697**

OSLER, William (1849-1919)
Case of syphiloma of the cord of the cauda equina; death from diffuse central myelitis. [New York, 1889.] 9p. DNLM **80-4698**

OSLER, William (1849-1919)
On the value of Laveran's organisms in the diagnosis of malaria. Baltimore, 1889. 2 l. DNLM **80-4699**

OSTROM, Homer I. (*b.* 1852)
A treatise on the breast and its surgical diseases. 2nd ed. New York: A. L. Chatterton & Co., 1885. 377p. NNNAM; PPC **80-4700**

OSTROM, Homer I. (*b.* 1852)
Epithelioma of the mouth. New York: A. L. Chatterton & Co., 1885. 120p. DLC; NNNAM **80-4701**

OSWALD, Felix L[eopold] (1845-1906)
Physical education, or the health-laws of nature. New York: D. Appleton & Co., 1882. 257p. DNLM; ICU; MH; NN **80-4702**

OSWALD, Felix L[eopold] (1845-1906)
The poison problem, or the cause and cure of intemperance. New York: D. Appleton & Co., 1887. 138p. DNLM; NN **80-4703**

OTIS, Edward O[sgood] (1848-1933)
Report on surgery. Manchester: J. B. Clarke, 1884. 20p. DNLM **80-4704**

OTIS, Edward O[sgood] (1848-1933)
Backward dislocation of the fingers upon the metacarpus. Boston: Cupples, Upham & Co., 1886. 11p. DNLM **80-4705**

OTIS, Edward O[sgood] (1848-1933)
Some observations on health resorts. Boston: Cupples, Upham & Co., 1886. 12p. DNLM **80-4706**

OTIS, Edward O[sgood] (1848-1933)
Notes on minor surgery. [Wilmington, 1887.] 11p. 1 plate. DNLM **80-4707**

OTIS, Edward O[sgood] (1848-1933)
Injuries of and operations upon the kidney. Boston: Cupples & Hurd, 1887. 26p. 1 tab. DNLM; MBM **80-4708**

OTIS, Edward O[sgood] (1848-1933)
Creolin. Boston: Damrell & Upham, [1889]. 19p. DNLM **80-4709**

OTIS, Edward O[sgood] (1848-1933)
The psychological factor in selecting a climate for invalids. Philadelphia: W. J. Dornan, 1889. 8p. DNLM **80-4710**

OTIS, Fessenden Nott (1825-1900)
Stricture of the male urethra, its radical cure. [2nd ed.] New York: G. P. Putnam's Sons, 1880. 360p. 2 plates. DNLM; NNNAM; PPC **80-4711**

OTIS, Fessenden Nott (1825-1900)
Prefatory remarks to the second edition of stricture of the male urethra. New York: G. P. Putnam's Sons, 1880. 24p. DNLM; NNNAM **80-4712**

OTIS, Fessenden Nott (1825-1900)
Clinical lectures on the physiological pathology and treatment of syphilis; together with a fasciculus of classroom lessons covering the initiatory period. . . . New York: G. P. Putnam's Sons, 1881. 116p. DLC; DNLM; NNNAM; PPC **80-4713**

OTIS, Fessenden Nott (1825-1900)
Practical clinical lessons on syphilis and the genito-urinary diseases. . . . New York: Bermingham & Co., 1883. 2 v. DLC; DNLM; NNNAM **80-4714**

OTIS, Fessenden Nott (1825-1900)
A simplified evacuator for the removal of débris from the bladder after lithotrity. New York: Trow, 1883. 19p. DNLM **80-4715**

OTIS, Fessenden Nott (1825-1900)
Practical clinical lessons on syphilis and the genito-urinary diseases. . . . New York: Bermingham & Co., 1883. 2 v in 1. DLC; NNNAM **80-4716**

OTIS, Fessenden Nott (1825-1900)
On the limitation of the contagious stage of syphilis, especially in its relation to marriage. New York: William Wood & Co., 1886. 16p. DNLM **80-4717**

OTIS, Fessenden Nott (1825-1900)
On the limitation of the contagious stage of syphilis, especially in its relations to marriage. Syracuse: Journal Co., 1886. 19p. DNLM **80-4718**

OTIS, Fessenden Nott (1825-1900)
On some important points in the treatment of deep urethral stricture. New York: D. Appleton & Co., 1887. 10p. DNLM **80-4719**

OTIS, Fessenden Nott (1825-1900)
On temporary overstrain of the bladder, producing localized stony and chronic retention of urine. New York: Trow's Co., 1887. 14p. DNLM **80-4720**

OTIS, Fessenden Nott (1825-1900)
The male urethra, its diseases and reflexes. . . . Detroit, Mich.: G. S. Davis, 1888. 86p. DLC; DNLM; OCIM **80-4721**

OTIS, Fessenden Nott (1825-1900)
Papillomatous tumor of the bladder demonstrated by means of the electro-cystoscope of Josef Leiter, of Vienna. Diagnosis confirmed by subsequent inspection through supra-pubic opening of the bladder. Successful removal. [New York, 1888.] 4p. DNLM **80-4722**

OTIS, Fessenden Nott (1825-1900)
Résumé of the experience of seventeen years in the operation of dilating urethrotomy. New York: Trow, 1889. 21p. DNLM **80-4723**

OTIS, Fessenden Nott (1825-1900)
The "perfected evacuator." New York: D. Appleton & Co., 1889. 16p. DNLM **80-4724**

OTIS, George Alexander (1830-1881)
List of the specimens in the anatomical section of the United States Army Medical Museum. Washington, D.C., 1880. 194p. DNLM **80-4725**

OTT, I[saac] (1847-1916)
The decussation of the spinal inhibitory fibres. [Chicago, 1880.] 5p. DNLM **80-4726**

OTT, I[saac] (1847-1916) and Michael T. PRENDERGRAST
The rapidity of perception of colored lights. [Chicago, 1880.] 4p. DNLM **80-4727**

OTT, I[saac] (1847-1916)
Bromide of ethyl; its toxicological action. [Detroit, 1880.] 8p. DNLM **80-4728**

OTT, I[saac] (1847-1916)
The decussation of the motor fibres in the medulla oblongata. [Detroit, 1880.] 8p. DNLM **80-4729**

OTT, I[saac] (1847-1916)
A new narcotic, Placidia erythrina; Jamaica dogwood; its physiological and toxicological action. [Detroit, 1880.] 12p. DNLM **80-4730**

OTT, I[saac] (1847-1916)
Paralysis and anaesthesia. [New York, 1880.] 4p. DNLM **80-4731**

OTT, I[saac] (1847-1916)
On the path of the inhibitory and sensory fibres in the medulla oblongata. [New York, 1880.] 4p. DNLM **80-4732**

OTT, I[saac] (1847-1916)
The path of sensory nerves in the spinal cord; the path of sensory and inhibitory nerves in the pons Varolii. [Detroit, 1880.] 8p. DNLM **80-4733**

OTT, I[saac] (1847-1916)
The physiological action of Urechites suberecta. [Detroit, 1880.] 15p. DNLM **80-4734**

OTT, I[saac] (1847-1916)
Bromide of ethyl; its physiological action. [Detroit, 1880.] 16p. DNLM **80-4735**

OTT, I[saac] (1847-1916)
The inhibition of sensibility and motion. [New York, 1881.] 7p. DNLM **80-4736**

OTT, I[saac] (1847-1916)
Urechites suberecta and digitalis. [Detroit, 1881.] 4p. DNLM **80-4737**

OTT, I[saac] (1847-1916)
The path of the vasomotor, sudorific, and sensory nerves in the spinal cord. [New York, 1881.] 6p. DNLM **80-4738**

OTT, I[saac] (1847-1916)
Effect of sections of the spinal cord upon the excretion of carbonic acid. [1885.] 5p. DNLM **80-4739**

OTT, I[saac] (1847-1916)
The heat-centre in the brain [1887.] 11p. DNLM
80-4740

OTT, I[saac] (1847-1916) and William S. CARTER
The four cerebral heat-centres. [Detroit, 1887.] 12p. DNLM
80-4741

OTT, I[saac] (1847-1916) and Charles COLLMAR
The thermo-inhibitory apparatus. [Chicago, 1887.] 11p. DNLM **80-4742**

OTT, I[saac] (1847-1916) and Charles COLLMAR
The thermogenetic apparatus; its relation to atropine. [Detroit, 1887.] 19p. DNLM **80-4743**

OTT, I[saac] (1847-1916)
The antipyretics, acetphenetidin and antithermin. [New York, 1888.] 11p. DNLM **80-4744**

OTT, I[saac] (1847-1916)
The heat centres of the cortex cerebri and pons Varolii. [New York, 1888.] 20p. DNLM **80-4745**

OTT, I[saac] (1847-1916)
Fever, thermotaxis, and calorimetry of malarial fever. [New York]: M. J. Rooney & Co., 1889. 1 p. l. 42, 54, 8p., 2 ch. DNLM **80-4746**

OTT, I[saac] (1847-1916)
Human calorimetry. [New York, 1889.] 13p. DNLM
80-4747

OTT, I[saac] (1847-1916)
Human calorimetry. Second contribution. [New York, 1889.] 11p. DNLM **80-4748**

OTTO, F. G. & SONS
Illustrated catalogue of surgical instruments, electric batteries, orthopaedic appliances. . . . New York, 1884. 244, 46p. NNNAM **80-4749**

OWEN, Edmund B[lackett] (1847-1915)
The surgical diseases of children. Philadelphia: Lea Bros. & Co., [1885]. 518p. 4 plates. DNLM; NNNAM; PPC; PU
80-4750

OWENS, William (1823-1897)
Introductory lecture delivered before the class of Pulte Medical College, September 30, 1881. Cincinnati, O.: Advance Printing Co., 1881. 31p. DNLM **80-4751**

OWENS, William (1823-1897)
The vaso-motor nerves, their origin, functions, and relations to morbid processes. Presented to the American Institute of Homoeopahty, at its thirty-fifth annual session, Indianapolis, Ind., June, 1882. Pittsburgh: Stevenson & Foster, 1882. 16p. DNLM **80-4752**

PACKARD, John Hooker (1832-1907)
On some important advantages to be secured by oblique section of the skin in surgical operations. [New York, 1880.] 8p. DNLM **80-4753**

PACKARD, John Hooker (1832-1907)
. . . Sea-air and sea-bathing. . . . Philadelphia: P. Blakiston, 1880. 124p. DLC; DNLM; NNNAM; PPC
80-4754

PACKARD, John Hooker (1832-1907)
The great advances in surgery and how they have been made. Philadelphia: J. B. Lippincott & Co., 1885. 25p. DNLM; PPC
80-4755

PACKARD, John H[ooker] (1832-1907)
Suprapubic cystotomy for purposes other than the extraction of calculus. Philadelphia: W. J. Dornan, 1887. 51p. DNLM; PPC **80-4756**

PACKARD, John H[ooker] (1832-1907)
On the proposed board of State medical examiners. Philadelphia: W. J. Dornan, 1888. 8p. DNLM
80-4757

PACKARD, John H[ooker] (1832-1907)
Laparotomy for injury by a circular saw. Laparotomy for a wandering fibroid tumor. Ligation of carotid and subclavian arteries for innominate aneurism. [Philadelphia, 1888, *vel subseq.*] 7p. DNLM **80-4758**

PAGE, C. E. (*b.* 1840)
The natural cure of consumption, constipation, Bright's disease, neuralgia, rheumatism, "colds" (fevers), etc. How sickenss originates, and how to prevent it. A health manual for the people. New York: Fowler & Wells, 1883. 278p. DNLM; NNNAM **80-4759**

PAGE, Charles W.
How can we escape insanity? Hartford, Conn.: Case, Lockwood & Brainard Co., 1883. 22p. DNLM
80-4760

PAGE, Herbert W[illiam] (1845-1926)
Injuries of the spine and spinal cord without apparent mechanical lesion and nervous shock, in their surgical and medico-legal aspects. Philadelphia: P. Blakiston, Son & Co., 1883. 374p. DNLM; NNNAM; PPC; PU **80-4761**

PAGE, Herbert W[illiam] (1845-1926)
Injuries of the spine and spinal cord without apparent mechanical lesions, and nervous shock, in their surgical and medico-legal aspects. 2nd ed. Philadelphia: P. Blakiston, Son & Co., 1885. 397p. DNLM; IU-M; PPC; PU
80-4762

PAGE, R[ichard] C[hanning] M[oore] (1841-1898)
A chart on physical signs of diseases of the heart and respiratory organs. Compiled from the works of various authors, with original ideas and observations. New York: J. H. Vail & Co., 1886. 1 sheet folded. DNLM; NNNAM
80-4763

PAGE, R[ichard] C[hanning] M[oore] (1841-1898)
A handbook of physical diagnosis of diseases of the organs of respiration and heart, and of aortic aneurism. New York: J. H. Vail & Co., 1889. 291p. 7 plates. DNLM; NNNAM
80-4764

PALMER, Alonzo B[enjamin] (1815-1887)
Homoeopathy, what is it? A statement and review of its doctrines and practice. 2nd ed. Detroit, Mich.: G. S. Davis, 1881. 109p. DNLM; OCIM; PPHa **80-4765**

PALMER, Alonzo B[enjamin] (1815-1887)
A treatise on the science and practice of medicine, or the pathology and therapeutics of internal diseases. New York: G. P. Putnam's Sons, 1882. 2 v. DLC; DNLM; MdBM; NNNAM
80-4766

PALMER, Alonzo B[enjamin] (1815-1887)
A treatise on epidemic cholera and allied diseases. Ann Arbor, Mich., 1885. 224p. DNLM; OCIM **80-4767**

PALMER, Alonzo B[enjamin] (1815-1887)
A report on alcohol, its action and effects in health and disease. Lansing: W. S. George & Co., 1885. 28p. DNLM **80-4768**

PALMER, Alonzo B[enjamin] (1815-1887)
Suggestions on the causes and treatment of inflammation of internal organs. Ann Arbor, 1886. 13p. DNLM **80-4769**

PALMER, Alonzo B[enjamin] (1815-1887)
Diarrhoea and dysentery. Modern views of their pathology and treatment. Detroit: G. S. Davis, 1887. 128p. DNLM; OCIM; NNNAM **80-4770**

PALMER, Benjamin W[ood] (*d.* 1895)
Favorite prescriptions of distinguished practitioners, with notes on treatment, comp. from the published writings or unpublished records of Drs. Fordyce Barker, Roberts Bartholow [etc.]. . . . 2nd ed. rev. and enl. New York: Bermingham & Company, [etc.], 1884. 136p. DLC; NNNAM; OCLloyd; PPC **80-4771**

PALMER, Benjamin W[ood] (*d.* 1895)
A practical treatise on palatable prescribing, containing the favorite formulary of the most eminent medical and surgical authorities. . . . Detroit: G. S. Davis, 1884. 136p. DLC; IU-M; OCLloyd; PU **80-4772**

PALMER, Benjamin W[ood] (*d.* 1895)
A practical treatise on palatable prescribing, containing the favorite formulary of the most eminent medical and surgical authorities. . . . 2nd ed. Detroit: G. S. Davis, 1885. 138p. OCIM; OCLloyd **80-4773**

PALMER, Benjamin W[ood] (*d.* 1895)
Favorite prescriptions of distinguished practitioners, with notes on treatment; comp. from the published writings or unpublished records of Drs. Fordyce Barker, Roberts Bartholow [etc.]. . . . New York: E. B. Treat, 1887. 256p. DLC; DNLM; NNNAM; OCLloyd **80-4774**

PALMER, Edward R[ush] (1842-1895)
Report on the progress of genito-urinary surgery. Some points in the management of urethral stricture. The specific microbe of gonorrhoea. Louisville: J. P. Morton & Co., 1888. 37p. DNLM **80-4775**

PALMER, E[dward] R[ush] (1842-1895)
Retrojection in gonorrhoea. New York, 1888. 7p. DNLM **80-4776**

PALMER, E[dward] R[ush] (1842-1895)
Report on the treatment of gonorrhoea and gonorrhoeal cystitis. [New York, 1889.] 2p. DNLM **80-4777**

PANCOAST, Seth (1823-1889)
What is Bright's disease? Its curability. . . . Philadelphia: The author, 1882. 152p. DLC; DNLM; PPC **80-4778**

PANCOAST, Seth (1823-1889)
The ladies' medical guide. An instructor, counsellor and friend; indispensable to mothers and daughters, embracing a full and exhaustive description of the structure and functions of the reproductive organs; anatomy and physical perfection of females; with diseases of women and children; their causes, symptoms and treatment. The toilet, beauty and longevity of females; startling facts in plain words, etc. Illustrated by over 100 engravings. To which is added the hygiene and care of children and the aged; care of the teeth, eyes, ears, skin, hands, and feet; early rising, exercise, tabulated matter, etc. by C. C. Vanderbeck. Philadelphia: John E. Potter & Co., 1886. 692p. PP; PPC; PPJ **80-4779**

PARISH, William H[enry] (1845-1903)
Puerperal septicaemia chiefly as observed at the Philadelphia Hospital. Philadelphia, 1880. 9p. DNLM **80-4780**

PARISH, William H[enry] (1845-1903)
The treatment of post-partum hemorrhage. Philadelphia, 1882. 8p. DNLM **80-4781**

PARISH, William H[enry] (1845-1903)
Pelvic abscess in the female. [Philadelphia, 1885.] 17p. DNLM **80-4782**

PARISH, William H[enry] (1845-1903)
Removal of the uterine appendages. Philadelphia, 1886. 8p. DNLM **80-4783**

PARK, Augustus V[itelius] (1851?-1901)
A case of ante-partum haemorrhage at term; recovery. Chicago, 1887. 8p. DNLM **80-4784**

PARK, Augustus V[itelius] (8151?-1901)
A case of pyelitis of nineteen years' duration caused by a renal calculus; recovery. Chicago, 1887. 7p. DNLM **80-4785**

PARK, Roswell (1852-1914)
The electric light in surgical diagnosis. Brooklyn, 1883. 22p. 2 plates. DNLM **80-4786**

PARK, Roswell (1852-1914)
Total extirpation of the larynx. [Buffalo], 1885. 12p. DNLM **80-4787**

PARK, Roswell (1852-1914)
Surgery of the brain, based on the principles of cerebral localization. New York, 1888. 63p. 1 tab. DNLM; NNNAM **80-4788**

PARKE, DAVIS & CO.
Complete price list of drugs. Detroit, 1880. 176p. DLC **80-4789**

PARKE, DAVIS & CO.
Descriptive circulars on new remedies presented to the members of the Ohio State Allopathic Association, 1881. Detroit, [1881]. 41 l. DNLM; OCLloyd **80-4790**

PARKE, DAVIS & CO.
Scientific pharmacy. Detroit, 1882. 8p. DNLM; OCLloyd **80-4791**

PARKE, DAVIS & CO.
Working bulletin for the collective investigation of Grindelia robusta. Detroit & New York, [1883]. 27p. DNLM; OCLloyd
80-4792

PARKE, DAVIS & CO.
Working bulletins for the scientific investigation of the newer materia medica. A plan to promote progress in the science of pharmacology, and consisting of a collection of all procurable information as it has appeared in contributions to medical literature, bearing on the botanical origin, history, chemical constituents, pharmaceutical preparations, adulterations and therapeutic properties of the several drugs considered. Detroit, 1883. 207p. 3 plates. DNLM; OCLloyd
80-4793

PARKE, DAVIS & CO.
Working bulletins for the scientific investigation of manaca (Franciscea uniflora) [etc.]. Detroit & New York, 1884. 35p. DNLM; OCLloyd **80-4794**

PARKE, DAVIS & CO.
Pharmacal facts, presented to the members of the American Medical Convention, Washington, D.C. Detroit & New York City, 1884. 18 l. DNLM; OCLloyd
80-4795

PARKE, DAVIS & CO.
An epitome of the newer materia medica, standard medicinal products, and fine pharmaceutical specialties, introduced and manufactured by . . . to which is added a complete property and dose list of all the fluid, solid and powdered extracts, German tinctures, normal liquids and concentrations prepared by them, together with a complete formula list of their sugar and gelatin pills. Designed for the special convenience of the busy physician. 4th ed. Detroit, Mich.: Parke, Davis & Co., 1886. 76p. DNLM; OCLloyd **80-4796**

PARKE, DAVIS & CO.
Cascara sagrada. (Rhamnus purshiana, D. C.) Its botanical origin. . . . With appendix of clinical reports of its use in private and hospital practice. Comp. from medical and pharmacal literature, and issued by the scientific department of Parke, Davis & Co. . . . [Detroit, Mich., 1889.] 71p. DLC; OCLloyd
80-4797

PARKE, DAVIS & CO.
Notes on alteratives with special reference to syrup trifolium compound. With appendix of clinical reports of its use in private and hospital practice. Detroit and New York City: Parke, Davis & Co., [1889]. 47p. DLC; NNNAM; OCLloyd
80-4798

PARKER, Andrew H.
The rational treatment of rupture. A study of the causation, pathology, and varieties of hernia; the application of improved modern trusses, elastic stockings, etc. Chicago: Shea, Smith & Co., 1885. 62p. DLC; DNLM **80-4799**

PARKER, Andrew H.
The rational treatment of rupture. A study of the causation, pathology, and varieties of hernia; the application of improved modern trusses, elastic stockings, etc. 3rd ed. Chicago: Shea, Smith & Co., 1887. 62p. DNLM; IU-M
80-4800

PARKER, Moses Greely (*b.* 1842)
Photo-micrography. The best means of illustrating and teaching pathology. Boston: Rockwell & Churchill, 1888. 23p. DNLM; MBM **80-4801**

PARKER, Willard (1800-1884)
Cancer: a study of three hundred and ninety-seven cases of cancer of the female breast, with clinical observations. [Compiled by his son, Willard Parker, Jr.] New York & London: G. P. Putnam's Sons, 1885. 61p. DNLM; NNNAM
80-4802

PARKER, William H[arwar] (1826-1896)
The science of life; or, self preservation. A medical treatise on nervous and physical debility, spermatorrhoea, impotence, and sterility, with practical observations on the treatment of diseases of the generative organs. Boston: Published by authority of the Peabody Medical Institute. Latest ed., 1881. 333p. MBM **80-4803**

PARKER, William Thornton (1849-1925)
Ventnor, Isle of Wight, and its peculiar advantages for the invalid. New York, 1881. 10p. DNLM
80-4804

PARKER, William Thornton (1849-1925)
Concerning the climate of New Mexico. [n. p., 1884.] 27p. DNLM **80-4805**

PARKER, William Thornton (1849-1925)
A new clothing case for the soldier. Chicago, 1886. 4p. DNLM
80-4806

PARKER, William Thornton (1849-1925)
A new clothing case for the soldier. Newport: Davis & Pitman, 1887. 15p. DNLM **80-4807**

PARKER, William Thornton (1849-1925)
The Burton case. Chicago, 1887. 19p. DNLM
80-4808

PARKER, William Thornton (1849-1925)
The genealogy of Wm. Thornton Parker, A.M., M.D., of Boston, Mass. Newport, R.I.: J. P. Sanborn, 1888. 10p. DNLM
80-4809

PARKER, William Thornton (1849-1925)
The military red cross corps. Philadelphia, 1888. 30p. DNLM
80-4810

PARKES, Charles T[heodore] (1842-1891)
A case of uterine cancer. Chicago, Bulletin Print, 1880. 8p. DNLM **80-4811**

PARKES, Charles T[heodore] (1842-1891)
Gun-shot wounds of the small intestines. Chicago: Cowdrey, Clarke & Co., 1884. 67p. DNLM **80-4812**

PARKES, Charles T[heodore] (1842-1891)
A review of some facts connected with gunshot wounds of the abdomen, and practical deductions thereform. [St. Louis, 1887.] 21p. DNLM **80-4813**

PARKES, Edmund Alexander (1819-1876)
A manual of practical hygiene. . . . Ed. by F. S. B. François de Chaumont. . . . 6th ed. Philadelphia: P. Blakiston, Son & Co., 1883. 731p. 9 plates. DLC; PPC; PU
80-4814

PARKES, Edmund Alexander (1819-1876)
A manual of practical hygiene. . . . Ed. by F. S. B. François de Chaumont. . . . From the last [6th] London ed. With an appendix giving the American practice in matters relating to hygiene, prepared by and under the supervision of Frederick N. Owen. New York: William Wood & Co., 1884. 2 v. in 1. 9 plates, maps, diags. DLC; NNNAM; PPC; PU
80-4815

PARKES, Edmund Alexander (1819-1876)
A manual of practical hygiene. . . . Ed. by F. S. B. François de Chaumont. . . . 7th ed. Philadelphia: P. Blakiston, Son & Co., 1887. 766p. 15 plates. DNLM; NNNAM; PPC
80-4816

PARKES, Louis C[oltman]
Hygiene and public health. Philadelphia: P. Blakiston, Son & Co., 1889. 471p. DNLM; NNNAM; PPC; PU
80-4817

PARREIDT, Julius (*b.* 1849)
A compendium of dentistry, for the use of students and practitioners. Authorized translation by Louis Ottofy; with notes and additions by G. V. Black. Chicago: W. T. Keener, 1889. 229p. 1 plate. DNLM; IU-M; MdU-D
80-4818

PARRISH, Edward (1822-1872)
A treatise on pharmacy: designed as a text-book for the student, and as a guide for the physician and pharmacist, containing the officinal and many unofficinal formulas, and numerous examples for extemporaneous prescriptions. . . . 5th ed. enl. and thoroughly revised. By Thos. S. Wiegand. . . . With two hundred and fifty-six illustrations. Philadelphia: Henry C. Lea's Son & Co., 1884. 1090p. DLC; NNNAM; OCLloyd; PPC **80-4819**

PARRISH, Joseph (1818-1891)
Alcoholic inebriety; from a medical standpoint. With cases from clinical records. . . . Philadelphia: P. Blakiston, Son & Co., 1883. 185p. DLC; DNLM; NNNAM; PPC
80-4820

PARRISH, Joseph (1818-1891)
Insanity and its problems. [Philadelphia, 1883.] 8p. DNLM
80-4821

PARRISH, Joseph (1818-1891)
The geography of malaria. An address. Newark, N.J.: L. J. Hardham, 1886. 10p. DNLM **80-4822**

PARRISH, Joseph (1818-1891)
Climate and malaria. Burlington, 1888. 4p. DNLM
80-4823

PARRISH, Joseph (1818-1891)
The medical jurisprudence of inebriety. [1888.] 7p. DNLM
80-4824

PARRISH, Joseph (1818-1891)
The legal responsibility of inebriates. [*Also*:] The unalterability of strychnia in the body after death, by Alfred H. Allen. Philadelphia, 1889. 5p. DNLM **80-4825**

PARSONS, Charles William (1823-1893)
The medical school formerly existing in Brown University, its professors and graduates. . . . Providence, R.I.: S. S. Rider, 1881. 59p. DLC; RHi: RPB **80-4826**

PARSONS, Ralph L[yman] (1828-1914)
On the private care of the insane. Greenmont, [1883]. 26p. DNLM **80-4827**

PARSONS, Ralph L[yman] (1828-1914)
Reciprocal insanity. [n. p., 1883.] 17p. DNLM
80-4828

PARSONS, Ralph L[yman] (1828-1914)
Detention in asylums. [n. p., 1884.] 17p. DNLM
80-4829

PARSONS, Ralph L[yman] (1828-1914)
On the classification of mental diseases. New York: D. Appleton & Co., 1887. 13p. 1 tab. DNLM
80-4830

PARSONS, Ralph L[yman] (1828-1914)
Nomenclature in psychiatry. Monomania or oligomania, which? Paranoia, what? Greenmont-on-the-Hudson, [1887]. 11p. DNLM **80-4831**

PARTRIDGE, Edward L.
Accidental ante-partum haemorrhage. New York, 1881. 13p. DNLM **80-4832**

PARTRIDGE, Edward L.
The histories of some unusual cases of labor, taken from the obstetric records of [the author]. New York: Trow's Co., 1882. 14p. DNLM **80-4833**

PARTRIDGE, Edward L.
A manual of obstetrics. New York: William Wood & Co., 1884. 295p. DNLM; NNNAM; PPC; PU **80-4834**

PARVIN, Theophilus (1829-1898)
In memoriam M. B. Wright. Boston, 1880. 5p. port. DNLM
80-4835

PARVIN, Theophilus (1829-1898)
Introductory address to the annual course of lectures, Jefferson Medical College, session 1883-1884. Philadelphia, 1883. 8p. DNLM; PPJ **80-4836**

PARVIN, Theophilus (1829-1898)
The physician is a good man, skilled in healing. The doctorate address in the medical department of the University of Louisville, 1883. Louisville, Ky.: J. P. Morton & Co., 1883. 23p. DNLM [*also*: Louisville: J. P. Morton & Co., 1883, 29p.]
80-4837

PARVIN, Theophilus (1829-1898)
The science and art of obstetrics. . . . Philadelphia: Lea Bros. & Co., 1886. 701p. col. plate. DLC; DNLM; PPC; PU
80-4838

PARVIN, Theophilus (1829-1898)
The necessity for practical obstetrics in the course of instruction given by medical schools. Philadelphia, 1888. 7p. DNLM
80-4839

PARVIN, Theophilus (1829-1898)
Annual address of the president of the Philadelphia Obstetrical Society. Boston: Rockwell & Churchill, [1889]. 8 l. DNLM
80-4840

PARVIN, Theophilus (1829-1898)
Lectures on obstetric nursing. Delivered at the training school for nurses of the Philadelphia Hospital. . . . Philadelphia: P. Blakiston, Son & Co., 1889. 104p. DLC; DNLM; PPC; PU
80-4841

PATCHEN, George H[enry] (*b.* 1845)
Clinical experience with vibratory and specialized motion. Ann Arbor Register Print, 1884. 18p. OCIM
80-4842

PATRICK, John J. R. (1828-1895)
Medical specialties. A paper read before the Illinois State Medical Society. Belleville, 1881. 10p. DNLM
80-4843

PATRICK, John J. R. (1828-1895)
"Oral electricity and the new departure." An essay read before the American Dental Association. Belleville, 1881. 20p. DNLM **80-4844**

PATRICK, John J. R. (1828-1895)
Civilization not the cause of tooth decay. An essay. [Chicago, 1882.] 37p. DNLM **80-4845**

PATRICK, John J. R. (1828-1895)
Closure of the jaws; and removal of a tumor. Two essays. Toledo, 1884. 24p. DNLM **80-4846**

PATRICK, John J. R. (1828-1895)
Irregularities in human teeth; or, dental teratology. An essay. [Chicago, 1884.] 20p. DNLM **80-4847**

PATRICK, John J. R. (1828-1895)
The progressive and retrogressive physiological metamorphosis of the jaws and teeth. [Philadelphia, 1886.] 19p. DNLM
80-4848

PATRICK, John J. R. (1828-1895)
The rationale of the construction of artificial crowns for the roots of natural teeth. [Philadelphia, 1888.] 14p. DNLM
80-4849

PATRICK, John J. R. (1828-1895)
"Professional atmosphere and morals; or, patents and secrets vs. a liberal profession." A reply. [St. Louis, 1889.] 24p. DNLM **80-4850**

PATTEE, Asa F[landers] (1835-1897)
Résumé of J. Mortimer Granville's book on nerve vibration and excitation, with notes of clinical experience with the percuteur. Chicago, 1885. 28p. DNLM **80-4851**

PATTERSON, J[ames] A.
Galvanism and bromide of quinine and the treatment of chronic catarrh of the middle ear. [Detroit, 1887.] 4p. DNLM
80-4852

PAUL, Constantin [Charles T.] (1833-1896)
. . . Diagnosis and treatment of diseases of the heart. . . . Transl. from the French. New York: William Wood & Co., 1884. 335p. diags. DLC; DNLM; NNNAM; PPC
80-4853

PAVY, Frederick William (1829-1911)
A treatise on food and dietetics physiologically and therapeutically considered. . . . 2nd ed. New York: William Wood & Co., 1881. 402p. DLC; DNLM; NNNAM; PU
80-4854

PAYNE, Joseph Frank (1840-1910)
A manual of general pathology designed as an introduction to the practice of medicine. Philadelphia: Lea Bros. & Co., 1888. 528p. 1 plate. DNLM; IEN-M; NNNAM; PPC
80-4855

PEABODY, George L., ed. (1850-1914)
Supplement to Ziemssen's Cyclopaedia of the practice of medicine. New York: William Wood & Co., 1881. 844p. NNNAM; NNU-M; PPC; PU **80-4856**

PEABODY, George L. (1850-1914)
The treatment of typhoid fever. [Philadelphia, 1884.] 30p. DNLM **80-4857**

PEARSON, Clement (1819-1886)
The present and future of homoeopathy. An address delivered before the International Hahnemannian Association at Niagara Falls, June 19, 1883. [Niagara Falls, 1883.] 11p. DNLM
80-4858

PEARSON, (R. I.) & CO.
Illustrated catalogue of surgical instruments. New York: Styles & Cash, 1889. Part 2. [501-] - 986p. DNLM; NNNAM
80-4859

PEASE, Edward Allen
Voluntary control of the heart. Boston: Damrell & Upham, [1889]. 12p. DNLM **80-4860**

PEASE, Giles M[oseley] (1838?-1891)
Gynaecological experiences. Read before the California State Homoeopathic Medical Society, San Francisco, November 8, 1882. C. A. Murdock & Co., 1883. 42p. CU-M
80-4861

PECK, Edward S[prague] (*b.* 1845)
An unique case of conjunctival lupus. New York: G. P. Putnam's Sons, 1880. 7p. DNLM **80-4862**

PECK, Edward S[prague] (*b.* 1845)
Foreign bodies in the nose and ear of children, with remarks on their removal. New York: William Wood & Co., 1881. 10p. DNLM **80-4863**

PECK, Edward S[prague] (*b.* 1845)
Inoculation of both eyes for complete pannus with gonorrhoeal pus. Recovery of sight after eleven years of blindness. New York: Trow's Print. & Bookbind. Co., 1881. 8p. DNLM
80-4864

PECK, Edward S[prague] (*b.* 1845)
Infusion of jequirity or licorice bean in invertebrate pannus, with a report of several successful cases. New York: Trow, 1883. 11p. DNLM **80-4865**

PECK, Edward S[prague] (*b.* 1845)
A case of severe purulent inflammation of the middle ear, with restoration of the drumhead; consecutive dentalgia without caries. New York, Buffalo, [1883]. 2 l. DNLM
80-4866

PECKHAM, Geo. W. (1845-1914)
The growth of children. [Milwaukee, 1882.] 40p. 12 charts. DNLM **80-4867**

PEIRCE, C[yrus] N[ewlin] (1829-1908)
Calcification and decalcification of the teeth. Philadelphia, 1884. 6p. DNLM **80-4868**

PEIRCE, C[yrus] N[ewlin] (1829-1908)
Function; its evolution and influence. Philadelphia, 1886. 7p. DNLM **80-4869**

PEIRCE, C[yrus] N[ewlin] (1829-1908)
The deciduous teeth; their eruption and removal. [Philadelphia], 1887. 6p. DNLM **80-4870**

PENFIELD, E. C. & CO.
Illustrated catalogue of trusses, abdominal supports, shoulder braces, elastic stockings, etc. [Philadelphia, 1882?] 17 l. DNLM [*also*: Philadelphia, n. d., 66p.] **80-4871**

PENNSYLVANIA HOSPITAL. PHILADELPHIA
Surgery in the . . . being an epitome of the practice of the hospital since 1756, including collations from the surgical notes, and an account of the more interesting cases from 1873 to 1878; with some statistical tables. By Thomas G. Morton and William Hunt, surgeons to the hospital. With papers by John B. Roberts and Frank Woodbury, late resident physicians in the hospital. Prepared by direction of the managers. Philadelphia: J. B. Lippincott & Co., 1880. 349p. DNLM; PPPH **80-4872**

PENROSE, Charles Bingham (1862-1925)
Antiseptic surgery in the Pennsylvania Hospital. [Philadelphia, 1886.] 10p. DNLM **80-4873**

PENROSE, Charles Bingham (1862-1925)
Intestinal obstruction in its surgical aspects. Chicago: Office Am. Medical Assoc., 1888. 19p. DNLM **80-4874**

PEPPER, Augustus J[oseph] (1849-1935)
Elements of surgical pathology. Philadelphia: Henry C. Lea's Son & Co., [1883]. 503p. CtY-M; DNLM; NNNAM; PPC **80-4875**

PEPPER, William (1843-1898)
A further contribution to the local treatment of pulmonary cavities. . . . Philadelphia: Collins, printer, 1880. 23p. DLC; DNLM; PU **80-4876**

PEPPER, William (1843-1898)
Address in medicine on some of the relations of catarrhal affections. Philadelphia: Collins, 1881. 18p. DNLM **80-4877**

PEPPER, William (1843-1898)
Remarks on some points in the treatment of typhoid fever. [Philadelphia, 1881.] 6p. DNLM **80-4878**

PEPPER, William (1843-1898)
Memoir of John Forsyth Meigs; read before the American Philosophical Society Oct. 19, 1883. [Philadelphia, 1883.] 14p. DNLM **80-4879**

PEPPER, William (1843-1898)
A contribution to the clinical study of typhlitis and perityphlitis. Philadelphia: Collins, 1883. 23p. DNLM **80-4880**

PEPPER, William (1843-1898)
Force vs. work; some practical remarks on dietetics in disease. Baltimore, 1884. 20p. DNLM **80-4881**

PEPPER, William (1843-1898)
Precautions suggested in the event of the existence of cholera as an epidemic. Philadelphia, 1885. 3 l. DNLM **80-4882**

PEPPER, William (1843-1898)
A system of practical medicine. By American authors. Ed. by William Pepper. . . . Assisted by Louis Starr. . . . Philadelphia: Lea Bros. & Co., 1885-1886. 5 v. DLC; DNLM; NNNAM; PPC **80-4883**

PEPPER, William (1843-1898)
Syllabus of notes from lectures on the theory and practice of medicine, delivered before the students of the University of Pennsylvania. . . . Prepared . . . by Cuthbert Bowen . . . '86-87. Philadelphia: Press of Burk & McFetridge, 1886. 178p. DLC; DNLM; PPC; PU **80-4884**

PEPPER, William (1843-1898)
A contribution to the climatological study of phthisis in Pennsylvania. Presidential address. . . . American Climatological Association. . . . New York: D. Appleton & Co., 1887. 77p. 1 map, 3 charts, 2 tabs. DNLM **80-4885**

PEPPER, William (1843-1898) and J. P. Crozer GRIFFITH
The treatment of phthisis by gaseous enemata. Philadelphia, 1887. 8p. DNLM **80-4886**

PERKINS, Daniel C[hastelar] (*b.* 1837)
The homoeopathic treatment of rheumatism and kindred diseases. With notes, suggestions and a complete repertory. Philadelphia: F. E. Boericke, Hahnemann Publishing House, 1888. 180p. DNLM; PPHa **80-4887**

PERRY, Safford G.
Concerning separators. Philadelphia, 1885. 11p. DNLM **80-4888**

PETERS, George A. (*d.* 1894)
In memory of Freeman J. Bumstead. Read before the New York Academy of Medicine, May 6, 1880. [New York, 1880.] 17p. DNLM; NNNAM **80-4889**

PETERS, George A. (*d.* 1894)
Excision of the superior maxilla, with remarks. [New York, 1885.] 14p. DNLM **80-4890**

PETERS, Hermann (1847-1920)
Pictorial history of ancient pharmacy; with sketches of medical practice. . . . Transl. and rev., with numerous additions, by Dr. William Netter. Chicago: G. P. Engelhard & Co., 1889. 184p. DLC; ICU **80-4891**

PETERS, John Charles (1819-1893)
A biographical sketch of the late Middleton Goldsmith. [New York, 1889.] 10p. DNLM **80-4892**

PETERSON, Frederick (1859-1938)
Remarks on some European asylums. [Utica, N.Y., 1887.] 20p. DNLM **80-4893**

PETERSON, Frederick (1859-1938)
The colonization of epileptics. New York: M. J. Rooney & Co., 1889. 11p. DNLM **80-4894**

PETERSON, Frederick (1859-1938)
A contribution to the study of muscular tremor. New York: M. J. Rooney & Co., [1889]. 13p. DNLM **80-4895**

PETERSON, Frederick (1859-1938)
The proposed new lunacy law. New York: Trow, 1889. 11p. DNLM **80-4896**

PETERSON, Frederick (1859-1938)
Electrothanasia. New York, 1889. 4p. DNLM **80-4897**

PETTIT, Elihu R.
Why teeth decay. Philadelphia, 1885. 15p. DNLM **80-4898**

PEUGNET, Eugène (1836-1879)
The nature of gunshot wounds of the abdomen, and their treatment: based on a review of the case of the late James Fisk, Jr., in its medico-legal aspects. . . . New York: William Wood & Co., 1874. 96p. DLC; NNNAM **80-4899**

The **PHARMACOPOEIA** of the United States of America. 6th decennial revision by authority of the national convention for revising the pharmacopoeia, held at Washington, 1880. New York: William Wood & Co., 1882. 488p. DLC; NNNAM; OCLloyd; PPC **80-4900**

The **PHARMACOPOEIA** of the United States of America. Digest of criticisms on the United States Pharmacopoeia, sixth decennial revision (1880). Published by the committee of revision and publication (1880-1890). Pts. 1-3. New York, 1889-1890. 335p. DNLM; NNNAM; OCLloyd; PU **80-4901**

PHELPS, A[bel] M[ix] (1851-1902)
The treatment of empyema by valvular drainage. Syracuse, N.Y., 1880. 14p. DNLM **80-4902**

PHELPS, A[bel] M[ix] (1851-1902)
A case of double talipes equino-varus, treated by open incision and fixed extension. Syracuse: Truair, Smith & Bruce, 1881. 8p. DNLM **80-4903**

PHELPS, A[bel] M[ix] (1851-1902)
The discussion which followed the paper read before the New York State Medical Society, in February, 1885, by Dr. A. Vanderveer, upon "Some personal observations on the work of Mr. Lawson Tait"; together with report of five cases of abdominal section by the writer. [Syracuse, 1885.] 14p. DNLM **80-4904**

PHELPS, A[bel] M[ix] (1851-1902)
An improved method of operation for harelip. Syracuse, N.Y.: Syracuse Jour. Comp., 1885. 6p. DNLM **80-4905**

PHELPS, A[bel] M[ix] (1851-1902)
Excision of the knee-joint, together with a report of three hundred and twenty-nine cases treated according to modern antiseptic methods, and four cases of resection of the hamstring tendon to prevent relapse in children. New York: Trow, 1886. 15p. 1 tab. DNLM **80-4906**

PHELPS, E[dward] J[ohn] (1822-1900)
Lectures on topics connected with medical jurisprudence, delivered before the Medical Department of the University of Vermont. Burlington, 1881. 100p. DNLM; VtHi **80-4907**

PHILADELPHIA DENTAL COLLEGE AND HOSPITAL OF ORAL SURGERY
Annual announcements for the sessions of 1885-1886 (23.); 1890-1891 (28.); 1892-1893 to 1897-1900 (30.-35.). Philadelphia, 1885-1897. DNLM [List of officers and students for 1890-1891 to 1895-1896, in announcements for subsequent years.] **80-4908**

PHILADELPHIA. PENNSYLVANIA HOSPITAL
Surgery in the Pennsylvania Hospital, being an epitome of the practice of the hospital since 1756; including collations from the surgical notes, and an account of the more interesting cases from 1873 to 1878; with some statistical tables. By Thomas G. Morton, M.D., and William Hunt, M.D. . . . With papers by John B. Roberts, M.D., and Frank Woodbury, M.D. . . . Prepared by direction of the managers of the hospital. Philadelphia, London: J. B. Lippincott & Co., 1880. 349p. DLC; PPPH; PU **80-4909**

PHILADELPHIA. PENNSYLVANIA HOSPITAL
. . . Addresses delivered by Dr. Thomas G. Morton and John B. Garrett, on the unveiling of West's picture, "Christ Healing the Sick." Eleventh month 10th, 1884. [Philadelphia: By order of the Board of Managers, 1884.] 30p. DLC; PPPH; PU **80-4910**

PHILADELPHIA POLYCLINIC AND COLLEGE FOR GRADUATES IN MEDICINE
Announcement of a special systematic course in ophthalmology. Sessions of 1889. [Philadelphia, 1889.] 2 l. DNLM **80-4911**

[PHILANTHROPOS]
Physiological cruelty: or, fact v. fancy. An inquiry into the vivisection question. New York: J. Wiley, 1883. 156p. NN; NNNAM **80-4912**

PHILLIPS, Charles D. F. (1830-1904)
Materia medica and therapeutics . . . inorganic substances. Edited and adapted to the U.S. Pharmacopoeia, by Laurence Johnson. New York: William Wood & Co., 1882. 2 v. DNLM; NNNAM; OCLloyd; PU **80-4913**

PHILLIPS, Walter P[olk] (1846-1920)
A mild corrective. New York, 1883. 22p. DNLM **80-4914**

The **PHYSICIANS** protective register, containing the names of physicians of the city of Philadelphia, regularly graduated from medical colleges of good standing, also their addresses, office hours, names of colleges from which they graduated, and years of graduation; together with a directory of the benevolent, charitable, and humane institutions in said city, presenting in addition a statement of the objects and workings of the most prominent of them. April, 1881. Philadelphia: A. W. Selden, 1881. 70p. DNLM; PPC; PU **80-4915**

PHYSICO-MEDICAL COLLEGE OF INDIANA. INDIANAPOLIS
Announcement of the practitioners' course, session of 1884. Indianapolis: J. Ratti, [1884]. 5p. DNLM **80-4916**

PHYSICO-MEDICAL INSTITUTE, CINCINNATI
Annual circulars for the sessions of 1883-1884 (25.); 1884-1885 (26.). Cincinnati: The College, 1883-1884. 14p., 14p. DNLM; OC [Opened Oct. 17 and chartered Dec. 5, 1859. List of graduates from 1860 to 1883 in announcement for 1883-1884.] **80-4917**

PIERCE, Franklin Duane
Tumors of the uterus and ovaries; their successful treatment by electrolysis. . . . [n. p., 1887.] 20p. DLC **80-4918**

PIERCE, Franklin D[uane]
Tumors, their curability by new methods. . . . 2nd ed. rev. [Union Springs, N.Y.], 1888. 22p. DLC **80-4919**

PIERCE, Ray V[aughn] (*b.* 1840)
The people's common sense medical adviser in plain English; or, medicine simplified. . . . 8th rev. ed. 140th thousand. Buffalo, N.Y.: World's Dispensary Printing-Office and Bindery, 1880. 922p. DLC **80-4920**

PIERCE, Ray V[aughn] (*b.* 1840)
The people's common sense medical adviser in plain English; or medicine simplified. 11th ed. Buffalo, 1883. 922p. 5 plates. DNLM **80-4921**

PIERCE, Ray V[aughn] (*b.* 1840)
The people's common sense medical adviser in plain English; or, medicine simplified. . . . 12th rev. ed. 240th thousand. Buffalo, N.Y.: World's Dispensary Printing-Office and Bindery, 1883. 1018p. col. plates. DLC **80-4922**

PIERCE, Ray V[aughn] (*b.* 1840)
Asthma or phthisic. A new, rational, and successful treatment. Pt. 14. Buffalo, N.Y., [1884]. 71p. DNLM **80-4923**

PIERCE, Ray V[aughn] (*b.* 1840)
The people's common sense medical adviser in plain English; or, medicine simplified. . . . 13th ed. 260th thousand. . . . Buffalo, N.Y.: World's Dispensary Printing-Office and Bindery, 1886. 1008p. col. plates. DLC **80-4924**

PIERCE & SON
Dr. Pierce's patent magnetic elastic truss, a new and valuable invention for the relief and radical cure of hernia or rupture. Illustrated [4th] ed. Magnetic Elastic Truss Co. . . . San Francisco [etc.], 1884. 32p. DLC **80-4925**

PIERSOL, George A[rthur] (1856-1924)
An illustrated synopsis of normal histology: adapted to the course of practical instruction in the University of Pennsylvania. . . . Illus. with forty plates. Philadelphia: P. Blakiston, Son & Co., 1885. 3p. 11 photos. DLC; PPC **80-4926**

PIERSOL, George A[rthur] (1856-1924)
Carmine staining for nervous tissues. [New York, 1889.] 8p. DNLM **80-4927**

PIFFARD, Henry Granger (1842-1910)
. . . A treatise on the materia medica and therapeutics of the skin. . . . New York: William Wood & Co., 1881. 351p. DLC; DNLM; NNNAM; OCLloyd **80-4928**

PIFFARD, Henry Granger (1842-1910)
On the Viola tricolor (L.) and its use in eczema. New York: Trow's Co., 1882. 20p. DNLM **80-4929**

PIFFARD, Henry Granger (1842-1910)
The status of the medical profession in the State of New York. New York: D. Appleton & Co., 1884. 64p. DLC; DNLM; NNNAM **80-4930**

PIFFARD, Henry Granger (1842-1910)
Cutaneous memoranda. . . . 3rd ed. New York: William Wood & Co., 1885. 268p. DLC; NNNAM **80-4931**

PIFFARD, Henry Granger (1842-1910)
The modern treatment of eczema. Detroit, Mich.: G. S. Davis, 1886. 54p. DNLM **80-4932**

PIFFARD, Henry Granger (1842-1910)
Salt in dermal hygiene and therapeutics. New York: William Wood & Co., 1887. 8p. DNLM **80-4933**

PILCHER, Lewis Stephen (1845-1934)
. . . The treatment of wounds: its principles and practice, general and special. . . . With one hundred and sixteen wood engravings. New York: William Wood & Co., 1883. 391p. DLC; NNNAM; PPC; PPJ **80-4934**

PILCHER, Lewis Stephen (1845-1934)
Some recent advances in methods of wound treatment. [New York, 1884.] 14p. DNLM **80-4935**

PILE, J. M.
Outlines of anatomy and physiology. . . . Dixon, Ill.: W. M. Kennedy, printer, 1882. 50p. DLC **80-4936**

PITTSBURGH COLLEGE OF PHARMACY. DEPARTMENT OF PHARMACY OF THE WESTERN UNIVERSITY OF PENNSYLVANIA
Prospectuses for the sessions of 1880-1881 to 1897-1898 (3.-20.); 1900-1901 to 1906-1907 (23.-29.). Pittsburgh, 1880-1906. DNLM [List of graduates from 1800 to 1906, in announcement for 1906-1907.] **80-4937**

A PLAIN exposition of the only practical and sure system for the prevention of disease ever offered to the public. Prospectus of the Manhattan Anti-Sewer Gas Company. New York: P. F. McBreen, 1883. 15p. DNLM; NNNAM **80-4938**

PLAYFAIR, William Smoult (1836-1903)
A treatise on the science and practice of midwifery. . . . 3rd American ed., rev. and cor. by the author. With notes and additions by Robert P. Harris. . . . Philadelphia: Henry C. Lea, 1880. 655p. plates. DLC; DNLM; NNNAM; PPC **80-4939**

PLAYFAIR, William Smoult (1836-1903)
The puerperal state. Being part the fifth from a treatise on the science and practice of midwifery. With notes and additions by Robert P. Harris. Philadelphia: Henry C. Lea's Son & Co., 1882. 67p. DNLM; PPC; PU **80-4940**

PLAYFAIR, William Smoult (1836-1903)
The systematic treatment of nerve prostration and hysteria. Philadelphia: Henry C. Lea's Son & Co., 1883. 111p. DNLM; PPC **80-4941**

PLAYFAIR, William Smoult (1836-1903)
A treatise on the science and practice of midwifery. . . . 4th American from the 5th English ed. With notes and additions by Robert P. Harris. . . . Philadelphia: Lea Bros. & Co., 1885. 663p. col. plates. DLC; DNLM; PPC; PU **80-4942**

PLAYFAIR, William Smoult (1836-1903)
A treatise on the science and practice of midwifery. . . . 5th American from the 7th English ed. With notes and additions by Robert P. Harris. . . . Philadelphia: Lea Bros. & Co., 1889. 671p. col. plates. DLC; MBM; NNNAM; PPC **80-4943**

PLUMMER, R[ichard] H. (1840-1899)
Address delivered at the opening of the 18th annual meeting of the Medical Society of the State of California. [San Francisco, 1888.] 15p. DLC **80-4944**

PLUMMER, R[ichard] H. (1840-1899)
Address delivered at the opening of the 18th annual meeting of the Medical Scoiety of the State of California. San Francisco: The Bancroft Co., 1888. 15p. DNLM **80-4945**

PLUNKETT, H. M. (*b.* 1826)
Women, plumbers, and doctors; or, Household sanitation, "Showing that if women and plumbers do their whole sanitary duty, there will be comparatively little occasion for the services of doctors." New York: D. Appleton & Co., 1885. 248p. ICU; NN **80-4946**

POLK, R. L. & CO.
Medical and surgical directory of the United States. Detroit, Mich.: R. L. Polk & Co., 1886. 1451p. DNLM; IU-M; NNNAM; PU **80-4947**

POLLAK, S[imon] (*b.* 1814)
Jequirity ophthalmia. St. Louis: Med. Jour. Pub. Co., 1883. 11p. DNLM **80-4948**

POMEROY, Harlan (*b.* 1853)
Medical electricity. A lecture delivered before the Hahnemannian Society, on the evening of January 19, 1886. Published by request of the Society. Cleveland, O.: Buel & Roberts, Printers, 1886. 23p. OCIM **80-4949**

POMEROY, Oren Day (1834-1902)
On some points in the management of asthenopic symptoms in emmetropic and ametropic eyes. New York: Trow, 1880. 24p. DNLM; NNNAM **80-4950**

POMEROY, Oren Day (1834-1902)
A case of intracranial myxosarcoma, destroying the whole of the organ of hearing, bursting through the external parts, and forming a large tumor which depended from the ear. New York: Trow, 1881. 23p. 2 plates. DNLM; NNNAM **80-4951**

POMEROY, Oren Day (1834-1902)
The diagnosis and treatment of diseases of the ear. . . . New York: Bermingham & Co., 1883. 392p. DLC; NNNAM **80-4952**

POMEROY, Oren Day (1834-1902)
The diagnosis and treatment of diseases of the ear. . . . With one hundred illustrations. 2nd ed. rev., with additions. New York: D. Appleton & Co., 1886. 413p. DLC; NNNAM **80-4953**

POOLEY, James Henry (1839-1897)
Clinical notes on nerve injuries. [Columbus, O., 1880.] 14p. DNLM **80-4954**

POOLEY, James Henry (1839-1897)
Anomalies of perspiration. Columbus: Cott & Hann, 1881. 81p. DNLM **80-4955**

POOLEY, James Henry (1839-1897)
Cases of tetanus. [Columbus: Cott & Hann, 1881.] 16p. DNLM **80-4956**

POOLEY, James Henry (1839-1897)
Re-amputation for neuralgic stump. [Attica, 1885.] 5p. DNLM **80-4957**

POOLEY, James Henry (1839-1897)
The physical or immediate cause of the death of Christ. [Yonkers, N.Y., 1885.] 8p. DNLM **80-4958**

POOLEY, Thoms Rickett (1841-1926)
Cases of rupture of the choroid. Syracuse: Truair, Smith & Bruce, 1883. 13p. DNLM **80-4959**

POORE, Charles Talbot (1846-1911)
Osteotomy and osteoclasis for deformities of the lower extremities. New York: D. Appleton & Co., 1884. 187p. NNNAM **80-4960**

POPE, John Hunter (1845-1915)
President's annual address before the Texas State Medical Association. Marshall, Tex.: Jennings Bros., 1880. 24p. DNLM **80-4961**

PORCHER, Francis Peyre (1825-1895)
Explanation of a simple method for the diagnosis of organic valvular diseases of the heart. [Philadelphia, 1880.] 6p. DNLM **80-4962**

PORCHER, Francis Peyre (1825-1895)
Report of nine cases (second series) of pleuritic effusion, with removal of nine hundred and six ounces of fluid. Also one of paracentesis in abscess of the liver; a pint and a half of pus evacuated, with recovery. Philadelphia, 1885. 7p. DNLM **80-4963**

PORCHER, Francis Peyre (1825-1895)
Report of ten cases of pleuritic effusion with aspiration of the chest. Fourth series. With a case of injection of carbolized iodine into a lung cavity. [Charleston, 1888.] 5p. DNLM **80-4964**

PORCHER, Francis Peyre (1825-1895)
Fifteen cases of hydrothorax (sixth series). [Charleston, 1889.] 6p. DNLM **80-4965**

PORCHER, W. Peyre
Cases from practice in diseases of the throat and nose. Read before the South Carolina Medical Association. [Charleston, 1888.] 8p. DNLM **80-4966**

PORTER, Dwight (1855-1935)
Report upon a sanitary inspection of certain tenement-house districts of Boston. Boston: Rockwell & Churchill, 1889. 76p. 2 plates, 8 plans, 2 diags. DNLM; MB; MH **80-4967**

PORTER, George L.
A xanthic oxide calculus from the kidney. [Newtown, Conn., 1881.] 11p. DNLM **80-4968**

PORTER, George L.
Sickness a factor of political economy. Cost of sickness to the individual and the state. Annual address delivered before the Connecticut Medical Society. [Danbury, Conn., 1889.] 28p. DNLM **80-4969**

PORTER, Horace P.
The common nervous trouble of old soldiers. Oneida, Kans., 1888. 1 broadside. DNLM **80-4970**

PORTER, Joshua Henry (*d.* 1880)
The surgeon's pocket-book: being an essay on the best treatment of the wounded in war, for which a prize was awarded by Her Majesty the Queen of Prussia and Empress of Germany in the year 1874. Specially adapted for the public medical services. . . . Philadelphia: P. Blakiston, Son & Co., 1887. 257p. 1 plate. DNLM; PPC; PU **80-4971**

PORTER, Noah (1811-1892)
Professor David Paige Smith. A memorial discourse. [New York, 1881.] 24p. port. MB; MH; NN **80-4972**

PORTER, P. Brynberg (1845-1915)
A complicated case: Remittent fever with jaundice and probable hepatitis, convulsions, hemiplegia, typhoid fever, occurring in a rachitical child. New York, [1881]. 12p. DNLM **80-4973**

PORTER, William (1852-1921)
Erysipelas of the larynx. New York, 1880. 5p. DNLM **80-4974**

PORTER, William (1852-1921)
The prognosis of laryngeal phthisis. New York, 1881. 12p. DNLM **80-4975**

POST-GRADUATE MEDICAL SCHOOL OF CHICAGO
Annual announcement for the session of 1887. Chicago: Jameson & Morse Co., 1887. 15p. DNLM; IU-M **80-4976**

POTTER, Frank Hamilton (1860-1891)
Report of a case of congenital bony occlusion of the posterior nares. [Buffalo, 1888.] 3p. DNLM **80-4977**

POTTER, George E.
My experinece with the Ninth International Medical Congress; its peculiar ways and methods illustrated. Johnstown, Penn., 1888. 19p. DNLM **80-4978**

POTTER, Samuel Otway Lewis (1846-1914)
An index of comparative therapeutics with tables of differential diagnosis, a pronouncing dose-list in the genitive case, a list of medicines used in homoeopathic practice, memoranda concerning clinical thermometry. . . . Chicago: Duncan Bros., 1880. 280p. DLC; DNLM; OCIM **80-4979**

POTTER, Samuel Otway Lewis (1846-1914)
Signs of the times. Read before the Wisconsin State Homoeopathic Medical Society, June 14, 1880. [n. p., 1880.] 5p. DNLM **80-4980**

POTTER, Samuel Otway Lewis (1846-1914) and Lewis SHERMAN
Papers on the Milwaukee test of the thirtieth dilution; with the reports of the Milwaukee Academy of Medicine on the result. [Milwaukee], 1880. 7, 6, 4 (2 l.), 25, 7, 8 (4 l.), 4, 7 (4 l.), 7, 5p. DNLM **80-4981**

POTTER, Samuel Otway Lewis (1846-1914)
An index of comparative therapeutics with tables of differential diagnosis, a pronouncing dose-list in the genitive case, a list of medicines used in homoeopathic practice, memoranda concerning clinical thermometry. . . . 2nd ed. Chicago: Duncan Bros., 1882. 279p. DNLM; OCIM **80-4982**

POTTER, Samuel Otway Lewis (1846-1914)
Speech and its defects: considered physiologically, pathologically, historically, and remedially. Lea prize thesis of Jefferson Medical College. Philadelphia: P. Blakiston, Son & Co., 1882. 117p. DNLM; PPJ **80-4983**

POTTER, Samuel Otway Lewis (1846-1914)
Questions on human anatomy. Philadelphia: P. Blakiston, Son & Co., 1883. 139p. DNLM; PPC; PU **80-4984**

POTTER, Samuel Otway Lewis (1846-1914)
. . . A compend of visceral anatomy especially adapted to the use of medical students. . . . With forty-one illustrations. Philadelphia: P. Blakiston, Son & Co., 1883. 101p. DLC; PPC; PPJ **80-4985**

POTTER, Samuel Otway Lewis (1846-1914)
. . . A compend on materia medica and therapeutics, with especial reference to the physiological actions of drugs. . . . Based on the sixth decennial revision of the U.S. pharmacopoeia, and including unofficial remedies. . . . Philadelphia: P. Blakiston, Son & Co., 1883. 141p. DLC; DNLM; OCLloyd; PPC **80-4986**

POTTER, Samuel Otway Lewis (1846-1914)
. . . A compend of human anatomy. . . . 3rd ed., rev. With sixty-three illustrations. Philadelphia: P. Blakiston, Son & Co., 1884. 139p. DLC; PPC **80-4987**

POTTER, Samuel Otway Lewis (1846-1914)
. . . A compend of visceral anatomy, especially adapted to the use of medical students. . . . 2nd ed., rev. With forty-one illustrations. Philadelphia: P. Blakiston, Son & Co., 1885. 104p. DLC; PPC **80-4988**

POTTER, Samuel Otway Lewis (1846-1914)
Handbook of materia medica, pharmacy, and therapeutics, including the physiological action of drugs, the special therapeutics of disease, official and extemporaneous pharmacy, and minute directions for prescription writing. . . . Philadelphia: P. Blakiston, Son & Co., 1887. 828p. DLC; DNLM; OCLloyd; PPC **80-4989**

POTTER, Samuel Otway Lewis (1846-1914)
. . . A compend of human anatomy, including the anatomy of the viscera. . . . 4th ed., rev. and enl. With one hundred and seventeen illustrations. Philadelphia: P. Blakiston, Son & Co., 1887. 223p. DLC; PPJ; PU **80-4990**

POTTER, Samuel Otway Lewis (1846-1914)
. . . A compend of materia medica, therapeutics, and prescription writing. . . . 4th ed., rev. and enl. Philadelphia: P. Blakiston, Son & Co., 1887. 160p. DLC; OCLloyd; PPC; PU **80-4991**

POTTER, Samuel Otway Lewis (1846-1914)
. . . A compend of materia medica, therapeutics, and prescription writing. . . . 5th ed., entirely rewritten and enl. Philadelphia: P. Blakiston, Son & Co., 1888. 248p. DLC; DNLM; PPC **80-4992**

POTTER, Samuel Otway Lewis (1846-1914)
The progress of medicine measured by the progress of therapeutics. The report on medicine. San Francisco: The Bancroft Co., 1888. 76p. DNLM **80-4993**

POTTER, Samuel Otway Lewis (1846-1914)
Professional success; a valedictory address delivered to the graduating class at Cooper Medical College, San Francisco, November 12th, 1889. San Francisco, Cal.: Woodward & Co., [1889]. 16p. DNLM **80-4994**

POTTER, Samuel Otway Lewis (1846-1914)
Modern homoeopathy viewed homoeopathically; the grounds of a homoeopath's loss of faith. [n. p., 1889.] 70p. DNLM **80-4995**

POTTER, Samuel Otway Lewis (1846-1914)
Periostitis of the ribs after typhoid fever, and its probable dependence on medication. [San Francisco, 1889.] 7p. DNLM **80-4996**

POTTER, William Warren (1838-1911)
On rectal alimentation and the induction of abortion for the relief of the obstinate vomiting of pregnancy. New York: William Wood & Co., 1880. 16p. DNLM **80-4997**

POTTER, William Warren (1838-1911)
On rectal alimentation and the induction of abortion for the relief of the obstinate vomiting of pregnancy. [1880.] 14p. DNLM **80-4998**

POTTER, William Warren (1838-1911)
Remarks on rectal feeding in disease. New York: Trow, 1880. 12p. DNLM **80-4999**

POTTER, William Warren (1838-1911)
The genu-pectoral posture in uterine and ovarian displacements. Syracuse: Truair, Smith & Bruce, 1882. 18p. DNLM **80-5000**

POTTER, William Warren (1838-1911)
Dysmenorrhoea, its treatment by dilatation. New York: Trow's Co., 1884. 12p. DNLM **80-5001**

POTTER, William Warren (1838-1911)
Remarks on pelvic inflammations and the management of their residues. Buffalo, 1888. 16p. DNLM **80-5002**

POTTER, William Warren (1838-1911)
Double ovariotomy during pregnancy; subsequent delivery at term. New York, 1888. 4p. DNLM **80-5003**

POTTER, William Warren (1838-1911)
Remarks on pelvic inflammations and the management of their residues. [Buffalo, 1888.] 16p. DNLM **80-5004**

POTTER, William Warren (1838-1911)
Reminiscences of field-hospital service with the Army of the Potomac. [Buffalo, 1889.] 27p. 4 plates. DNLM; MH; NN **80-5005**

POTTER, William Warren (1838-1911)
A dermoid cyst of the left ovary, with a pathological demonstration by William C. Krauss. Buffalo, 1889. 8p. DNLM **80-5006**

POULET, Alfred (*b.* 1849)
A treatise on foreign bodies in surgical practice. New York: William Wood & Co., 1880. 2 v. IU-M; KyLoJM; NNNAM; PU **80-5007**

POULSEN, Viggo Albert (1855-1919)
Botanical micro-chemistry; an introduction to the study of vegetable histology, prepared for the use of students. . . . Transl. with the assistance of the author and considerably enlarged by William Trelease. . . . Boston: S. E. Cassino & Co., 1884. 118p. DLC; MBM; MH; NN **80-5008**

POWELL, Richard Douglas (1842-1925)
On diseases of the lungs and pleurae, including consumption. 3rd ed. New York: William Wood & Co., 1886. 347p. 2 plates. DNLM; NNNAM; PPC; PU **80-5009**

POWER, Henry (1829-1911)
Elements of human physiology. Philadelphia: Henry C. Lea's Son & Co., 1884. 389p. DNLM; NN; PPC; PU **80-5010**

POWERS, Charles A.
A contribution to the treatment of fractures at the lower end of the humerus, based on the analysis of fifty consecutive cases. New York, 1888. 19p. 1 tab. DNLM **80-5011**

POWERS, Charles A.
Kocher's method of reducing subcoracoid dislocations of the humerus. A plea for its employment in every recent case. New York: Trow, 1889. 15p. DNLM; NN **80-5012**

POWERS, Geo. Hermon (*b.* 1840)
Cataract extraction without iridectomy. San Francisco: W. S. Duncombe & Co., 1886. 2 l. DNLM **80-5013**

PRACTICAL guide to homoeopathy, for family and private use, compiled from the standard works of Pulte, Laurie, Hempel, Ruddock, Burt, Verdi, and others, for the use of twenty-eight homoeopathic remedies. St. Louis, Mo., and Cincinnati: A. F. Worthington & Co., 1883. 180p. DNLM; NNNAM; OCIM; PPHa **80-5014**

A PRACTICAL treatise on how to preserve perfect nutrition in health and disease by natural means. [New York: The Bovinine Company, 1888.] 110p. DNLM; NNNAM **80-5015**

PRATT, Edwin Hartley (1849-1930)
Orificial surgery and its application to the treatment of chronic diseases. . . . Chicago: W. T. Keener, 1887. 139p. DLC; DNLM; IU-M **80-5016**

PRATT, Edwin Hartley (1849-1930)
Orificial surgery. [Chicago, 1888.] 3p. DNLM **80-5017**

PRATT, Foster (1823-1898)
A study of the 10th census. The increase of insanity in the United States, it causes and sources. Kalamazoo, Mich.: H. H. Everard & Co., 1883. 18p. DNLM **80-5018**

PRAY, T[homas] J[efferson] W[orcester] (1819-1888)
The etiology or nature, causes, etc., of diphtheria, an address delivered before the N.H. Medical Society. Concord: Evans & Sleeper, 1880. 49p. DNLM **80-5019**

PRENTICE, Chas. F[rederick] (*b.* **1854**)
A treatise on simple and compound ophthalmic lenses, their refraction and dioptric formulae, including tables of crossed cylinders and their sphero-cylindrical equivalents. New York: J. Prentice & Son, [1886]. 40p. 2 tab. DLC; DNLM
80-5020

PRENTICE, Chas. F[rederick] (*b.* **1854**)
Dioptric formulae for combined cylindrical lenses applicable for all angular deviations of their axes. New York: J. Prentice & Son, 1888. 48p. 1 phot., 2 plates. DNLM; NNNAM
80-5021

PRENTISS, D[aniel] W[ebster] (1843-1899)
National Medical College (Medical Department of the Columbian University), Washington, D.C. On the revision of the U.S. Pharmacopoeia. Addressed to the Pharmacopoeial Convention of 1880. Washington, D.C.: H. A. Gibbs, 1880. 14p. DNLM **80-5022**

PRENTISS, D[aniel] W[ebster] (1843-1899)
Death from diphtheritic paralysis. [Philadelphia, 1880.] 2p. DNLM **80-5023**

PRENTISS, D[aniel] W[ebster] (1843-1899)
1. Remarkable change in the color of the hair from light blonde to black in a patient while under treatment by pilocarpin. Report of a case of pyelo-nephritis, with unusually prolonged anuria. 2. Case of membranous croup treated successfully by pilocarpin. Philadelphia: J. B. Lippincott & Co., 1881. 15p. 1 plate. DNLM **80-5024**

PRENTISS, D[aniel] W[ebster] (1843-1899)
Croupous pneumonia; is it a zymotic disease? Philadelphia: Collins, 1881. 11p. DNLM **80-5025**

PRENTISS, D[aniel] W[ebster] (1843-1899)
A review of the sixth decennial revision of the Pharmacopoeia of the United States of America. New York, 1882. 12p. DNLM
80-5026

PRENTISS, D[aniel] W[ebster] (1843-1899)
An address delivered before the graduating class of the Washington Training School for Nurses. [n. p., 1883.] 3p. DNLM **80-5027**

PRENTISS, D[aniel] W[ebster] (1843-1899)
Case of double hydronephrosis with dilatation of the bladder and ureters due to disease of the prostate gland. [Baltimore, 1883.] 4p. DNLM **80-5028**

PRENTISS, D[aniel] W[ebster] (1843-1899)
An answer to a protest against the use of the metric system in prescribing. [Philadelphia], 1883. 10p. DNLM
80-5029

PRENTISS, D[aniel] W[ebster] (1843-1899)
Gall-stones or soap? Olive or cotton-seed oil in the treatment of gall-stones. [With a] Note on the action of the digestive fluids on oil, by H. W. Wiley. [Philadelphia, 1888.] 6p. DNLM
80-5030

PRENTISS, D[aniel] W[ebster] (1843-1899)
A report of five hundred consecutive cases of labor in private practice, in the District of Columbia, between the years 1864 and 1888. [Washington]: H. I. Rothrock, [1889]. 22p. DNLM
80-5031

PRENTISS, D[aniel] W[ebster] (1843-1899)
Change in the color of the hair, from the white hair of old age to black, produced by jaborandi. Detroit, Mich.: G. S. Davis, 1889. 6p. DNLM **80-5032**

PRENTISS, D[aniel] W[ebster] (1843-1899)
Cases of poisoning by Japanese lacquer, by administration of homoeopathic pellets labelled "Rhus," and by the cashew-nut, Anacardium occidentale. Detroit, Mich.: G. S. Davis, 1889. 7p. DNLM **80-5033**

PRENTISS, D[aniel] W[ebster] (1843-1899)
Cases of uterine fibroids from private practice, and their treatment. New York: William Wood & Co., 1889. 12p. DNLM
80-5034

PRENTISS, D[aniel] W[ebster] (1843-1899)
Change of color in the hair from the internal use of pilocarpin. Exhibition of specimens. Chicago, 1889. 19p. DNLM
80-5035

THE PRESCRIBER'S memoranda. New York: William Wood & Co., 1881. 301p. DLC; NNNAM; OCLloyd
80-5036

THE PRESENT relation of dentistry to medicine, by Norman W. Kingsley; and dentistry more than a specialty in medicine, by J. Foster Flagg. Discussion thereon by C. S. Stockton, W. H. Dwinelle [*et al.*] before the Central Dental Association of Northern New Jersey, March 21, 1887. Chicago, 1887. 28p. DNLM **80-5037**

PRESIDENTIAL and other addresses, by Ed. C. Harwood, together with addresses by George T. Elliot, Lewis A. Sayre, Frank H. Hamilton, A. B. Crosby, etc. New York: W. R. Jenkins, 1883. 81p. DNLM; NNNAM **80-5038**

THE PREVENTION of insanity, and the early and proper treatment of the insane. By Dr. Putnam Jacobi, Prof. Harris, Dr. Cleaves, and others. Boston: Tolman & White, 1882. 29p. DNLM; MBM **80-5039**

PREVENTION of yellow fever. Commercial relations with Brazil, as affected by quarantine regulations. Brazil and New Orleans. New Orleans, 1886. 12p. DNLM **80-5040**

PRICE and dose labels of drugs and preparations generally kept in a retail pharmacy, including, besides those officinal in the last revision of the United States Pharmacopoeia, many other new and rare drugs and chemicals, with the Latin, French, and German synonyms. Edited by Hans M. Wilder. New York: J. H. Vail & Co., 1888. 230p. DNLM; NNNAM; OCLloyd
80-5041

PRICE, Eldridge C. (*b.* **1854**)
Medical progress. A revision of the paper read at the sixth annual meeting of the Maryland Homoeopathic Medical Society, November 10, 1880. Philadelphia: Globe Printing House, 1881. 28p. DNLM **80-5042**

PRICE, Eldridge C. (*b.* **1854**)
The mind cure; or, the mental method of healing. New York: N.Y. Times Printing Co., 1886. 32p. DNLM
80-5043

PRICE, Joseph (1853-1911)
A consideration of some of the recent work in abdominal surgery. [Buffalo, 1888.] 15p. DNLM
80-5044

PRICE, Joseph (1853-1911)
Gonorrhoeal disease of the uterine appendages. [Philadelphia, 1889.] 12p. DNLM 80-5045

PRICE, Joseph (1853-1911)
A plea for early ovariotomy. Richmond, 1889. 7p. DNLM 80-5046

PRICE, Joseph (1853-1911)
A report of two cases of extra-uterine pregnancy. [Richmond, 1889.] 7p. DNLM 80-5047

PRICE, William H[enry]
Baby's guide to health, or, How to promote and preserve the health of babies from the time of birth to the age of two years or more in all seasons and climates. . . . New York: Pub. by the author, 1880. 47p. DLC 80-5048

PRINCE, A[rthur] E. (*b.* 1853)
Contribution to the correction of strabismus by the advancement of the rectus. St. Louis: Med. J. Pub. Co., 1881. 8p. DNLM 80-5049

PRINCE, A[rthur] E. (*b.* 1853)
Observations on the use of bromide and ethyl as an anaesthetic for short operations and as a precursor to the administration of ether. St. Louis, 1883. 8p. DNLM 80-5050

PRINCE, A[rthur] E. (*b.* 1853)
Report on ophthalmology and otology, delivered before the Illinois State Medical Society. Chicago, 1883. 21p. DNLM 80-5051

PRINCE, A[rthur] E. (*b.* 1853)
Peroxide of hydrogen in suppurative conjunctivitis and mastoid abscesses, with a report of two cases. St. Louis, Mo., 1884. 7p. DNLM 80-5052

PRINCE, A[rthur] E. (*b.* 1853)
An accidental divulsion of a pterygium leading to an improvement in the regular operation. New York: G. P. Putnam's Sons, 1885. 5p. DNLM 80-5053

PRINCE, A[rthur] E. (*b.* 1853)
The pulley modification of his limiting tenotomy and advancement of the rectus operation, with a report of a case of section and one of execution of the rectus. [1885.] 8p. DNLM 80-5054

PRINCE, A[rthur] E. (*b.* 1853)
The radical treatment of trachoma. [St. Louis, 1886.] 7p. DNLM 80-5055

PRINCE, A[rthur] E. (*b.* 1853)
The extraction of cataract as influenced by mycological development. [Jacksonville, Ill., 1888.] 4p. DNLM 80-5056

PRINCE, A[rthur] E. (*b.* 1853)
The pulley method of advancing the rectus, with indications for its employment. [St. Louis, 1888.] 8p. DNLM 80-5057

PRINCE, A[rthur] E. (*b.* 1853)
Section or exsection of the rectus in the treatment of paralytic strabismus, and that due to extreme overcorrection with loss of motion. Chicago, 1888. 16p. DNLM 80-5058

PRINCE, A[rthur] E. (*b.* 1853)
Expression in the treatment of trachoma. Read at the meeting of the Illinois State Medical Society, at Jacksonville, May 23-25, 1889. [1889.] 2 l. DNLM 80-5059

PRINCE, A[rthur] E. (*b.* 1853)
Evisceration. Chicago, 1889. 7p. DNLM 80-5060

PRINCE, A[rthur] E. (*b.* 1853)
Expression in the treatment of trachoma. Chicago, 1889. 4p. DNLM 80-5061

PRINCE, David (1816-1890)
The treatment of extrophy of the bladder, with some historical notes and general considerations, and an account of a case. St. Louis, 1881. 13p. DNLM 80-5062

PRINCE, David (1816-1890)
The management of wounds. Philadelphia: Lindsay & Blakiston, 1881. 54p. DNLM 80-5063

PRINCE, David (1816-1890)
A rectal obturator. St. Louis, 1881. 16p. DNLM 80-5064

PRINCE, David (1816-1890)
Lithotomy; a tabulated statement of cases, with considerations in relation to the operation, the treatment, and the preventives most promising of success. St. Louis, [1881]. 8p. DNLM 80-5065

PRINCE, David (1816-1890)
Palato-plasty. [St. Louis, 1881.] 20p. DNLM 80-5066

PRINCE, David (1816-1890)
Iodoform in surgery. [St. Louis], 1882. 3p. DNLM 80-5067

PRINCE, David (1816-1890)
The bead suture, a modification of the quilled suture for palatoplasty and for use in other situations in which the suture line requires to be supported for several days. Brooklyn, 1883. 5p. DNLM 80-5068

PRINCE, David (1816-1890)
Alcohol in some of its immediate surgical relations and in some of its remote effects. [1884.] 4p. DNLM 80-5069

PRINCE, David (1816-1890)
Floating minute organic matter in the air and its management to prevent disease and to mitigate or control it, with a new device for atmospheric purification, with an original illustration. [St. Louis, 1885.] 16p. DNLM 80-5070

PRINCE, David (1816-1890)
Erysipelas and other septic and infectious diseases incident to injuries and surgical operations prevented by a method of atmospheric purification. (Second presentation.) 2nd ed. [Louisville, 1886.] 20p. DNLM 80-5071

PRINCE, David (1816-1890)
An experimental study in relation to the removal from the air of the dust or particulate material supposed to produce yellow fever, small-pox, and other infectious diseases. [n. p., 1886.] 8p. DNLM 80-5072

PRINCE, David (1816-1890)
The action of the constant galvanic current, especially in the treatment of stricture of the urethra. [St. Louis, 1887.] 4p. DNLM **80-5073**

PRINCE, David (1816-1890)
Wounds; their aseptic and antiseptic management. [Philadelphia, 1887.] 15p. DNLM **80-5074**

PRINCE, David (1816-1890)
Pelvic and abdominal drainage. [Philadelphia, 1888.] 16p. DNLM **80-5075**

PRINCE, David (1816-1890)
An aseptic atmosphere. Club foot. A rectal obturator. Palatoplasty. St. Louis, 1888. 30p. DNLM **80-5076**

PRINCE, Morton (1854-1929)
How a lesion of the brain results in that disturbance of consciousness known as sensory aphasia. [Boston, 1885.] 17p. DNLM [*also*: New York, 1885. 14p.] **80-5077**

PRINCE, Morton (1854-1929)
The nautre of mind and human automatism. Philadelphia: J. B. Lippincott Co., 1885. 173p. DNLM; ICU; NN; NIC **80-5078**

PRINCE, Morton (1854-1929)
The exact measurement of the electric current, and other practical points in the destruction of hair by electrolysis, with especial reference to the use of the absolute galvanometer. Boston: Cupples, Upham & Co., 1886. 12p. DNLM **80-5079**

PRINCE, Morton (1854-1929)
Thought transference. A résumé of the evidence. Boston: Cupples, Upham & Co., 1887. 22p. DNLM; MBM **80-5080**

PRINCE, Morton (1854-1929)
Electrolysis. Proper and improper methods of using it in the removal of hair and kindred operations. [Philadelphia: Lea Bros. & Co., 1889.] 6p. DNLM **80-5081**

PRITCHARD, Urban (*b.* 1845)
A case of foreign body in the ear producing severe cerebral symptoms; removal and recovery. New York: Trow, 1880. 7p. DNLM **80-5082**

PRITCHARD, Urban (*b.* 1845)
Handbook of diseases of the ear for the use of students and practitioners. Philadelphia: P. Blakiston, Son & Co., 1886. 207p. 1 plate. DNLM; MH-M; NNNAM; PPC **80-5083**

PRUDDEN, T[heophil] Mitchell (1849-1924)
Contributions to the structure and clinical history of the multiple neuroma; from the pathological laboratory of the Alumni Association of the College of Physicians and Surgeons, New York City. [Philadelphia: Henry C. Lea's Son & Co., 1880.] 24p. DNLM **80-5084**

PRUDDEN, T[heophil] Mitchell (1849-1924)
On the action of carbolic acid upon ciliated cells and white blood cells. [Philadelphia, 1881.] 17p. DNLM **80-5085**

PRUDDEN, T[heophil] Mitchell (1849-1924)
A manual of practical normal histology. . . . New York: G. P. Putnam's Sons, 1882. 265p. DLC; DNLM; NNNAM; PU **80-5086**

PRUDDEN, T[heophil] Mitchell (1849-1924)
Cell life and animal life. An address. [New York, 1882.] 16p. DNLM **80-5087**

PRUDDEN, T[heophil] Mitchell (1849-1924)
An experimental study on the action of salicyclic acid upon blood-cells and upon amoeboid movements and emigration. Philadelphia, [1882]. 6p. DNLM **80-5088**

PRUDDEN, T[heophil] Mitchell (1849-1924)
Rhabdomyoma of the parotid gland. [Philadelphia, 1883.] 5p. DNLM **80-5089**

PRUDDEN, T[heophil] Mitchell (1849-1924)
On the occurrence of the bacillus tuberculosis in tuberculous lesions. New York: Trow's Printing Co., 1883. 20p. DNLM **80-5090**

PRUDDEN, T[heophil] Mitchell (1849-1924)
The description of an adenoma of the caruncle. New York, 1886. 3p. DNLM **80-5091**

PRUDDEN, T[heophil] Mitchell (1849-1924)
On bacteria in ice, and their relations to disease, with special reference to the ice supply of New York City. An experimental study. New York: Trow, 1887. 61p. DNLM **80-5092**

PRUDDEN, T[heophil] Mitchell (1849-1924)
An experimental study of mycotic or malignant ulcerative endocarditis. [New York], 1887. 21p. DNLM **80-5093**

PRUDDEN, T[heophil] Mitchell (1849-1924)
On the etiology of diphtheria. An experimental study. [Philadelphia, 1889.] 50p. DNLM **80-5094**

PRUDDEN, T[heophil] Mitchell (1849-1924) and William S. NORTHRUP
Studies on the etiology of the pneumonia complicating diphtheria in children. [Philadelphia, 1889.] 18p. DNLM **80-5095**

PRUDDEN, T[heophil] Mitchell (1849-1924)
The story of the bacteria and their relations to health and disease. . . . New York & London: G. P. Putnam's Sons, 1889. 143p. DLC; DNLM; NNNAM; PPC **80-5096**

PULTE, [Mrs.] Joseph Hippolyte
Domestic cook book. A companion to Pulte's Domestic Physician. Cincinnati: G. W. Smith, 1888. 370p. OCIM **80-5097**

PURDUE UNIVERSITY. SCHOOL OF PHARMACY, LAFAYETTE
Annual announcements. 1.-3., 1884-1885 to 1886-1887. Lafayette, 1884-1886. DNLM **80-5098**

PURDUE UNIVERSITY. SCHOOL OF PHARMACY, LAFAYETTE
Bulletin, No. 1. [Lafayette, 1886.] 22p. DNLM **80-5099**

PURDUE UNIVERSITY. SCHOOL OF PHARMACY, LAFAYETTE, INDIANA
Annual announcements. 4, 1887-1888; 6., 1889-1890; 8., 1891-1892; 9., 1892-1893. Lafayette, 1887-1892. DNLM
80-5100

PURDY, Charles W[esley] (1846-1901)
Suggestions on some symptoms of renal disease and their management. Chicago, 1885. 15p. DNLM
80-5101

PURDY, Charles W[esley] (1846-1901)
The pre-albuminuric stage of chronic Bright's disease. (Read before the Chicago Medical Society, May 18, 1885.) Chicago: Clark & Longley, 1885. 35p. DNLM
80-5102

PURDY, Charles W[esley] (1846-1901)
Bright's disease and allied affections of the kidneys. Philadelphia: Lea Bros. & Co., 1886. 295p. DLC; DNLM; PPC; PU
80-5103

PURDY, Charles W[esley] (1846-1901)
The specific gravity of the urine and its relations to structural diseases of the kidneys. Read before the Chicago Medical Society, September 5, 1887. Chicago, 1887. 19p. DNLM
80-5104

PURDY, Charles W[esley] (1846-1901)
Treatment of glycosuria. Chicago, 1889. 19p. DNLM
80-5105

PUTNAM, James Jackson (1846-1919)
A series of cases of paraesthesia, mainly of the hands, of periodical recurrence, and possibly of vaso-motor origin. New York: G. P. Putnam's Sons, 1880. 16p. DNLM
80-5106

PUTNAM, James Jackson (1846-1919)
A case of rapid and wide-spread muscular wasting without disease of the spinal cord. [Chicago, 1881.] 10p. DNLM
80-5107

PUTNAM, James Jackson (1846-1919)
Case of clonic facial spasm successfully treated by stretching the seventh nerve. New York: G. P. Putnam's Sons, 1881. 4p. DNLM
80-5108

PUTNAM, James Jackson (1846-1919)
Examination of the spinal cord in a case of poliomyelitis of the adult, of two months' standing. [Chicago, 1883.] 12p. DNLM
80-5109

PUTNAM, James Jackson (1846-1919)
Lead-poisoning: on certain unrecognized forms of lead-poisoning; and on the possibility of mistaking lead for bismuth in urine analyses. Read at the meeting of the American Neurological Association, June, 1883. Cambridge, 1883. 11p. DNLM
80-5110

PUTNAM, James Jackson (1846-1919)
The medico-legal significance of hemi-anaesthesia after concussion accidents. New York, 1884. 10p. DNLM
80-5111

PUTNAM, James Jackson (1846-1919)
Clinical notes on chronic lead poisoning. [New York, 1887.] 17p. DNLM
80-5112

PUTNAM, James Jackson (1846-1919)
Lead-poisoning as a cause of muscular inco-ordination (pseudo-tabes). Boston: S. J. Parkhill & Co., 1887. 14p. DNLM
80-5113

PUTNAM, James Jackson (1846-1919)
Lead in the urine. The frequency with which it is found, and certain points in the symptomatology of chronic lead-poisoning. Boston: Cupples & Hurd, 1887. 23p. DNLM
80-5114

PUTNAM, James J[ackson] (1846-1919)
A case of acute fatal neuritis of infectious origin, with post-mortem examination. [New York, 1888.] 20p. DNLM
80-5115

PUTNAM, James J[ackson] (1846-1919)
On chronic arsenic poisoning, especially from wall-paper, based on the analyses of twenty-five cases in which arsenic was found in the urine. [Boston: Cupples & Hurd, 1889.] 23p. DNLM; MBM
80-5116

PUTZEL, Leopold (*b.* 1855)
A treatise on common forms of functional nervous diseases. . . . New York: William Wood & Co., 1880. 256p. DLC; DNLM; MBM; NNNAM
80-5117

PYBURN, George (*b.* 1831)
Nasal catarrh, and ozaena. An exposition of the principles involved in their rational treatment and cure. . . . [Sacramento: Day & Joy, printers, 1881.] 16p. DLC
80-5118

QUAIN, Jones (1796-1851)
Quain's elements of anatomy, ed. by Allen Thomson, Edward Albert Schaefer, and George Dancer Thane. 9th ed. New York: William Wood & Co., 1882. 2 v. NNNAM; NNU-M; PPC; PU
80-5119

QUAIN, Richard, ed. (1816-1898)
A dictionary of medicine including general pathology, general therapeutics, hygiene, and the diseases peculiar to women and children. By various writers. 4th ed. New York: D. Appleton & Co., 1883. 1816p. CU-M; ICRM; NNNAM; PU
80-5120

QUEEN, JAMES W., & CO. PHILADELPHIA
Abridged catalogue; medical batteries, [etc.]. [Philadelphia, 1882.] 52p. DNLM
80-5121

QUEEN, JAMES W., & CO. PHILADELPHIA
Illustrated catalogue of chemical glassware for druggists, chemists. . . . Philadelphia, 1883. 50p. PPC; PU
80-5122

QUEEN, JAMES W., & CO. PHILADELPHIA
Catalogue of instruments of precision, for use in physiology and medicine. Philadelphia, 1883. 51p. 1 plate. DNLM
80-5123

QUEEN, JAMES W., & CO. PHILADELPHIA
Priced and illustrated catalogue of optical instruments. 55th ed. Philadelphia, 1885. 205p. DNLM
80-5124

QUEEN, JAMES W., & CO. PHILADELPHIA
Priced and illustrated catalogue of ophthalmological instruments, spectacles, and eye-glasses, made, imported, and sold wholesale and retail. . . . [Philadelphia, 1885.] 140p. DLC
80-5125

QUEEN, JAMES W., & CO. PHILADELPHIA
Catalogue of anatomical models, charts, and osteological preparations. No. 221. Philadelphia, 1886. 19p. DNLM
80-5126

QUEEN, JAMES W., & CO. PHILADELPHIA
Priced and illustrated catalogue of ophthalmological instruments, spectacles, and eyeglasses. Philadelphia, 1886. 137p. DNLM **80-5127**

QUEEN, JAMES W., & CO. PHILADELPHIA
New apparatus for treating consumption by gaseous enemata. Philadelphia, [1887]. 16p. DNLM
80-5128

QUEEN, JAMES W., & CO. PHILADELPHIA
How to fit glasses. A manual for the use of opticians, jewelers, druggists, and others who sell spectacles and eye-glasses. Philadelphia: J. W. Queen & Co., 1888. 96p. DNLM
80-5129

QUEEN, JAMES W., & CO. PHILADELPHIA
Priced and illustrated catalogue of ophthalmological instruments, spectacles, and eye-glasses, made, imported, and sold, wholesale and retail. . . . [Philadelphia, 1889.] 175p. col. front. DLC **80-5130**

QUIMBY, Isaac N[ewton] (1831-1898)
The criminal use of chloroform. Jersey City, 1881. 7p. DNLM
80-5131

QUIMBY, Isaac N[ewton] (1831-1898)
Pathological action of alcoholic stimulants on health and in disease. Camden, N.J., 1883. 24p. DNLM
80-5132

QUINAN, John R[ussell] (1822-1890)
The introduction of inoculation and vaccination into Maryland, historically considered. Read before Baltimore Med. Association, May 14, 1883. [Baltimore, 1883.] 12p. DNLM; MdBM **80-5133**

QUINAN, John R[ussell] (1822-1890)
Medical annals of Baltimore from 1608 to 1880, including events, men and literature. To which is added a subject index and record of public services. . . . Prepared at the request of the Medical and Chirurgical Faculty of Maryland, as a memorial volume, in honor of the sesquicentennial of Baltimore, October, 1880. Publication committee: G. Lane Taneyhill . . . [and others]. Baltimore: Press of L. Friedenwald, 1884. 274p. DLC; MdBM; PPC; PU
80-5134

QUINAN, John R[ussell] (1822-1890)
The chartered right of the Medical and Chirurgical Faculty of Maryland to exact licenses to practice in the State. The president's address, delivered before the Medical and Chirurgical Faculty of the State of Maryland, at Baltimore, Md., April 27, 1886. Baltimore, 1886. 11p. DNLM; MdBM
80-5135

QUINBY, Henry Clay
Notes on dental practice. Philadelphia: S. S. White Dental Mfg. Co., 1884. 202p. DNLM; MdU-D; PU
80-5136

QUINQUINIA: A natural combination of the alkaloids of cinchona bark. Manufactured by the Charles T. White Co. Philadelphia: G. F. Lasher, 1882. 48p. DNLM; OCLloyd; PU
80-5137

RALFE, Charles H[enry] (1842-1896)
Clinical chemistry. An account of the analysis of blood, urine, morbid products, etc.; with an explanation of some of the chemical changes that occur in the body in disease. Philadelphia: Henry C. Lea's Son & Co., [1883]. 308p. DNLM; NNNAM; PPC; PU **80-5138**

RALFE, Charles H[enry] (1842-1896)
A practical treatise on diseases of the kidneys and urinary derangements. Philadelphia: P. Blakiston, Son & Co., 1885. 572p. CtY-M; DNLM; NNNAM; PPC
80-5139

RALPH, Joseph E.
A practical treatise on organic obstructions (commonly called stricture) of the intestinal and urinary passages, and allied diseases: designed to lead to their prevention or early detection. . . . New York: The Standard Printing & Publishing Co., 1883. 53p. DLC; DNLM; NNNAM **80-5140**

von RAMDOHR, C. A.
Considerations on anterior uterine displacements and a new method of treatment for the same. [New York, 1883.] 7p. DNLM **80-5141**

RAND, Benjamin H[oward] (1827-1883)
Two lectures on impure air and ventilation. [Abstr.] Philadelphia: Collins, 1880. 8p. DNLM **80-5142**

RANDALL, B[urton] Alexander] (1858-1932)
A study of the eyes of medical students. Philadelphia, [1885]. 18p. DNLM **80-5143**

RANDALL, B[urton] Alexander (1858-1932)
The refraction of the human eye. A critical study of the statistics obtained by examinations of the refraction, especially among school children. Philadelphia, 1885. 30p. DNLM; PPC
80-5144

RANDALL, B[urton] Alexander (1858-1932)
The "Hohlschnitt" of von Jaeger in the extraction of cataract; cilio-retinal or aberrant vessels; sarcoma of the eyelid, simulating a Meibomian cyst. [Boston, 1887.] 16p. 1 plate. DNLM
80-5145

RANDALL, B[urton] Alexander (1858-1932) and Henry Lee MORSE
Photographic illustrations of the anatomy of the human ear, together with pathological conditions of the drum membrane, and descriptive text. Philadelphia: P. Blakiston, Son & Co., 1887. 18p. 25 plates. DNLM; PPC; PU
80-5146

RANDALL, B[urton] Alexander (1858-1932) and Henry Lee MORSE
Photographic illustrations of the anatomy of the ear. New Bedford: Mercury Pub. Co., 1887. 7p. 1 plate. DNLM
80-5147

RANDOLPH, Nathaniel A[rcher] (1858-1887) and A. E. ROUSSEL
A study of the nutritive value of branny food. Philadelphia: Collins, 1884. 20p. DNLM **80-5148**

RANDOLPH, Nathaniel A[rcher] (1858-1887)
A note on the behavior of hydrobromic acid and of potassium iodide in the digestive tract. [Philadelphia, 1884.] 1 l. DNLM **80-5149**

RANDOLPH, Nathaniel A[rcher] (1858-1887) and Samuel G. DIXON
Notes from the physiological laboratory of the University of Pennsylvania. Philadelphia: J. B. Lippincott Co., 1885. 88p. DNLM; PU **80-5150**

RANDOLPH, Nathaniel A[rcher] (1858-1887)
Inorganic foods. A lecture. [Philadelphia, 1886.] 9p. DNLM **80-5151**

RANDOLPH, Nathaniel A[rcher] (1858-1887)
A note on the irradiation of motor impulses. Philadelphia: W. J. Dornan, 1887. 14p. DNLM **80-5152**

RANDOLPH, Robert L[ee] (1860-1919)
Congenital clouding of the cornea affecting two sisters. [Philadelphia, 1888.] 8p. DNLM **80-5153**

RANDOLPH, Robert L[ee] (1860-1919)
A clinical study of some antiseptics in the treatment of otorrhoea. New York: Trow, 1889. 12p. DNLM **80-5154**

RANKIN, David N[evin]
Nasal alimentation. [New York: G. P. Putnam's Sons, 1882.] 3p. DNLM **80-5155**

RANKIN, David N[evin]
Epistaxis. Pittsburgh: C. M. Rodgers & Co., 1884. 13p. DNLM **80-5156**

RANNEY, Ambrose L[oomis] (1848-1905)
Internal urethrotomy: are the benefits to be derived from it, as now advocated for the relief of stricture, commensurate with its dangers? New York: D. Appleton & Co., 1880. 27p. DNLM **80-5157**

RANNEY, Ambrose L[oomis] (1848-1905)
The human face; its modifications in health and disease, and its value as a guide in diagnosis. [New York, 1880.] 37p. DNLM **80-5158**

RANNEY, Ambrose L[oomis] (1848-1905)
The applied anatomy of the nervous system, being a study of this portion of the human body from a standpoint of its general interest and practical utility, designed for use as a text-book and a work of reference. New York: D. Appleton & Co., 1881. 500p. DLC; DNLM **80-5159**

RANNEY, Ambrose L[oomis] (1848-1905)
A practical treatise on surgical diagnosis. Designed as a manual for practitioners and students. 2nd ed., enlarged and revised. New York: William Wood & Co., 1881. 471p. DNLM; NNNAM; PPC; PU **80-5160**

RANNEY, Ambrose L[oomis] (1848-1905)
Pyaemia and septicaemia. Their causes, diagnosis, and methods of treatment. Brooklyn, 1881. 26p. DNLM; NNNAM **80-5161**

RANNEY, Ambrose L[oomis] (1848-1905)
Practical medical anatomy. A guide to the physician in the study of the relations of the viscera to each other in health and disease, and in the diagnosis of the medical and surgical conditions of the anatomical structures of the head and neck. New York: William Wood & Co., 1882. 339p. DLC; DNLM **80-5162**

RANNEY, Ambrose L[oomis] (1848-1905)
The internal capsule of the cerebrum and the diagnosis of lesions affecting it. New York: G. P. Putnam's Sons, 1883. 23p. DNLM **80-5163**

RANNEY, Ambrose L[oomis] (1848-1905)
The corpora quadrigemina; with remarks concerning the diagnosis and localization of lesions affecting sight. New York: Trow, 1883. 33p. DNLM **80-5164**

RANNEY, Ambrose L[oomis] (1848-1905)
The topographical relations of the female pelvic organs. New York: William Wood & Co., 1883. 121p. DNLM **80-5165**

RANNEY, Ambrose L[oomis] (1848-1905)
A practical treatise on surgical diagnosis, designed as a manual for practitiones and students in medicine; by . . . 3rd ed.—thoroughly rev., enl., and profusely illustrated. New York: William Wood & Co., 1884. 608p. plates. DLC; NNNAM; OCIM; PPC **80-5166**

RANNEY, Ambrose L[oomis] (1848-1905)
Practical suggestions respecting the varieties of electric currents and the uses of electricity in medicine. With hints relating to the selection and care of electrical apparatus. New York: D. Appleton & Co., 1885. 147p. 15 plates. DLC; DNLM **80-5167**

RANNEY, Ambrose L[oomis] (1848-1905)
The eye as a factor in the causation of some common nervous symptoms, with hints respecting the examination of that organ. [New York, 1886.] 27p. DNLM **80-5168**

RANNEY, Ambrose L[oomis] (1848-1905)
"Eye-strain" in its relation to neurology. [New York, 1887.] 8p. DNLM **80-5169**

RANNEY, Ambrose L[oomis] (1848-1905)
Does a relationship exist between anomalies of the visual apparatus and the so-called neuropathic predisposition? Philadelphia, 1887. 24p. DNLM; PPC **80-5170**

RANNEY, Ambrose L[oomis] (1848-1905)
Static electricity in medicine. An exposition of the different forms of generators which may be employed, and the various methods of application of this therapeutical agent; together with hints respecting the care and management of induction-machines and the selection of apparatus. Ann Arbor, 1887. 43p. DNLM **80-5171**

RANNEY, Ambrose L[oomis] (1848-1905)
Lectures on nervous diseases from the standpoint of cerebral and spinal localization, and the latter methods employed in the diagnosis and treatment of these affections. Philadelphia: F. A. Davis, 1888. 778p. 1 plate. DLC; DNLM **80-5172**

RANNEY, Ambrose L[oomis] (1848-1905)
The applied anatomy of the nervous system, being a study of this portion of the human body from a standpoint of its general interest and practical utility, designed for use as a text-book and a work of reference. 2nd ed. New York: D. Appleton & Co., 1888. 791p. DLC; DNLM; NNNAM
80-5173

RANNEY, Ambrose L[oomis] (1848-1905)
"Eye-strain." Its bearings upon the duration of human life. [New York, 1889.] 27p. DNLM **80-5174**

RANNEY, George E[mery] (1839-1915)
Unilocular ovarian cyst weighing ninety-five pounds successfully removed. Chicago, 1884. 11p. DNLM
80-5175

RANNEY, George E[mery] (1839-1915)
Inaugural address on obstetrics and gynecology. [Lansing], 1888. 14p. DNLM **80-5176**

RANNEY, George E[mery] (1839-1915)
The treatment of galactorrhoea and mastitis by pressure. [Lansing], 1888. 10p. DNLM **80-5177**

RANSOHOFF, Joseph (1853-1921)
Two ovariotomies in the same patient. [Philadelphia, 1885.] 12p. 1 tab. DNLM **80-5178**

RANSOHOFF, Joseph (1853-1921)
A case of aortic aneurism, treated by the insertion of wire. [Philadelphia, 1886.] 18p. DNLM **80-5179**

RANSOHOFF, Joseph (1853-1921)
Considerations on the anatomy, physiology, and pathology of the caecum and appendix. Chicago, 1888. 20p. DNLM
80-5180

RAUE, Charles Godlove (1820-1896)
Special pathology and diagnostics, with therapeutic hints. . . . 2nd ed. rewritten and enl. New York, Philadelphia: Boericke & Tafel; [etc., etc.], 1882. 1072p. DLC; NNNAM; PPHa; PU
80-5181

RAUE, Charles Godlove (1820-1896)
Special pathology and diagnostics, with therapeutic hints. . . . 3rd ed., rev. and augm. Philadelphia: F. E. Boericke, 1885. 1094p. DLC; PPC; PPHa; PU **80-5182**

RAVOGLI, A[ugusto] (*b.* 1851)
The endoscope in diseases of the male urethra. Cincinnati, 1883. 32p. DNLM **80-5183**

RAWLEY SPRINGS in Rockingham Co., Va., with an analysis of the waters, and letters of skillful and eminent physicians and certificates of cure, showing the great remedial effects of these waters in many diseases. Dayton, Va.: Ruebush, Kieffer & Co., 1880. 23p. DNLM **80-5184**

RAY, Dwârka Nâth
Cholera and its preventive and curative treatment. With an introduction by T. F. Allen. New York: A. L. Chatterton, 1884. 128p. DNLM; NNNAM **80-5185**

RAY, Isaac (1807-1881)
. . . Isolation of persons in hospitals for the insane. Read before the . . . Association, October 23rd, 1879. . . . Philadelphia: Philadelphia: Social Science Association, [1880]. 18p. DLC; DNLM **80-5186**

RAYMOND, Henry I. (*b.* 1857)
Primary anti-septic occlusion in military practice, with cases from the Big-Dry-Wash fight. [New York], 1882. 16p. DNLM
80-5187

RAYMOND, Henry I. (*b.* 1857)
Elephantiasis arabum of the labia majora. A case of successful operation by excision. Philadelphia, 1886. 4p. DNLM
80-5188

RAYMOND, Joseph H[oward] (1845-1915)
Measles not a trivial disease; a report on the present epidemic in Brooklyn, and its treatment by the board of health. Brooklyn, 1880. 7p. DNLM **80-5189**

RAYMOND, Joseph H[oward] (1845-1915)
Progress in the management of contagious diseases by the Brooklyn board of health. [Brooklyn, 1880.] 7p. DNLM
80-5190

RAYMOND, Joseph H[oward] (1845-1915)
Report on the prevention of cholera, to the conference of State and municipal boards of health, at Washington, D.C., December 10, 1884. [1884.] 17p. DNLM
80-5191

RAYMOND, Joseph H[oward] (1845-1915)
Disinfectants. Preliminary reports of the committee on disinfectants of the American Public Health Association. XII. Experiments with sulphurous acid gas. [Philadelphia, 1885.] 7p. DNLM **80-5192**

RED SULPHUR SPRINGS
A specialty for lung and throat diseases. Located in Monroe County, West Virginia. Washington, D.C.: R. O. Polkinhorn, 1880. 24p. DNLM **80-5193**

RED SULPHUR SPRINGS, Monroe County, W. Va.
A mineral water unequalled for catarrh and all diseases of the mucous membrane. . . . Buffalo: Mathews-Northrup Co., [1883]. 16p. 1 plate. DNLM **80-5194**

REDDING, J[acob]
An address delivered before the Physio-Medical Association of Indiana, May 3, 1882. Is medicine a science? [Indianapolis, 1882.] 20p. DNLM **80-5195**

REED, Boardman (1842-1917)
Winter health-resorts. The climate of Atlantic City, and its effects on pulmonary diseases. [Philadelphia, 1880.] 7p. DNLM **80-5196**

REED, Boardman (1842-1917)
Atlantic City as a winter health resort; embracing official reports, meteorological tables, etc., concerning the climate of Atlantic City, N.J., the testimony of eminent physicians as to its effects on various forms of disease, hygienic hints for invalids at the seashore, and information about the sanitary conditions of Atlantic City. 2nd ed. Philadelphia: Allen, Lane & Scott, 1881. 22p. DNLM **80-5197**

REED, Boardman (1842-1917)
The insufficiency of the laws governing commitments to asylums for the insane; with reports of cases. [Philadelphia, 1883.] 6p. DNLM **80-5198**

REED, Boardman (1842-1917)
Healthfulness of sea-shore resorts: some pertinent facts about malaria. Philadelphia, 1883. 4p. DLC; DNLM
80-5199

REED, Boardman (1842-1917)
The effects of sea air upon diseases of the respiratory organs. Including a study of the influence upon health of changes in the atmospheric pressure. Read before the American Climatological Association at its first annual congress, in Washington, D.C., May 5, 1884.] 1884.] 7p. DNLM
80-5200

REED, Boardman (1842-1917)
The restorative treatment of sleeplessness from brain exhaustion. Chicago, [1887]. 3p. DNLM **80-5201**

REED, Boardman (1842-1917)
Diseased conditions for which sea air is of doubtful benefit. [n. p., 1887.] 8p. DNLM **80-5202**

REED, Boardman (1842-1917)
The double action of medicines as illustrated by digitalis. [Philadelphia, 1888.] 10p. DNLM **80-5203**

REED, Carl H[empel]
The histogenesis and histology of carcinoma. Philadelphia, 1883. 11p. DNLM **80-5204**

REED, Charles A[lfred] L[ee] (1856-1928)
Intraperitoneal haematocele considered as a consequence of ruptured tube-pregnancy, with report of a case. New York: Trow, 1887. 16p. DNLM; NNNAM **80-5205**

REED, R. Harvey (1851-1907)
A periodical painful affection, believed to be located in the liver, its capsule, or both, or possibly an irritation of the capsule of Glisson. Chicago: A. G. Newell, 1884. 19p. DNLM
80-5206

REED, R. Harvey (1851-1907)
Irritation of the prostate. Abstr. of a paper read before the Ohio State Medical Society, June 14, 1884. [1884.] 7p. DNLM **80-5207**

REED, R. Harvey (1851-1907)
Hydatid tumors in the brain. Chicago, 1885. 16p. DNLM
80-5208

REED, R. Harvey (1851-1907)
Vitiligo. [1885.] 16p. DNLM **80-5209**

REED, R. Harvey (1851-1907)
An interesting case of buzz-saw injury to the head. [Columbus, 1886.] 7p. DNLM **80-5210**

REED, R. Harvey (1851-1907)
Sanitary condition of Ohio's capitol. [Report.] [Columbus? 1886.] 1 sheet. DNLM **80-5211**

REED, R. Harvey (1851-1907)
A report on the public water-supply of the city of Mansfield, O. [Mansfield, 1887.] 2 l. DNLM **80-5212**

REED, R. Harvey (1851-1907)
Some of the practical results of our criminal laws from a sanitary standpoint. St. Louis, 1887. 8p. DNLM
80-5213

REED, R. Harvey (1851-1907)
Of an experimental demonstration of the value of gaseous enemata in the diagnosis of perforations of the intestines, and their repair by the rubber ring and decalcified bone plate method. Cleveland, O.: The Williams Pub. Co., 1888. 10p. DNLM **80-5214**

REED, R. Harvey (1851-1907)
Some new operations in abdominal surgery, illustrated with a number of specimens. [Columbus, 1888.] 11p. DNLM
80-5215

REED, R. Harvey (1851-1907)
A report on the sanitary inspection of passenger coaches. Sept. 8, 1887. Chicago, 1888. 12p. 2 tab. DNLM
80-5216

REED, R. Harvey (1851-1907)
The heating and ventilation of passenger coaches. [New York?], 1888. 4p. DNLM **80-5217**

REED, R. Harvey (1851-1907)
Clinical observations on some of the effects of direct and indirect traumatisms of the brain. Philadelphia: Medical Press Co., 1889. 25p. DNLM **80-5218**

REED, R. Harvey (1851-1907)
The heating and ventilation of the Mansfield schools and churches. Chicago, 1889. 31p. DNLM
80-5219

REED, William Howell (1837-1914)
Hospital life in the army of the Potomac. 2nd ed. Boston, 1881. 199p. DNLM; MA: MB; NN
80-5220

REED, William Howell (1837-1914)
Hospital life in the army of the Potomac. Special ed. [2nd ed.] Boston, 1881. 199p. DNLM; MBM; MH; NIC
80-5221

REESE, John J[ames] (1818-1892)
Text-book of medical jurisprudence and toxicology. Philadelphia: P. Blakiston, Son & Co., 1884. 606p. CtY-M; DLC; DNLM; PPC **80-5222**

REESE, John J[ames] (1818-1892)
Live birth, in its medico-legal relations. Annual address, delivered before the Medical Jurisprudence Society of Philadelphia. [Philadelphia, 1887.] 6p. DNLM
80-5223

REESE, John J[ames] (1818-1892)
Suicide in its relation to insantiy. An address delivered before the Medical Jurisprudence Society of Philadelphia. [Philadelphia], 1888. 15p. DNLM **80-5224**

REESE, John J[ames] (1818-1892)
Text-book of medical jurisprudence and toxicology. 2nd ed. Philadelphia: P. Blakiston, Son & Co., 1889. 646p. CtY-M; DLC; DNLM; PPC **80-5225**

REEVE, J[ohn] C[harles] (1826-1920)
The latest systems in medicine. The presidential address delivered to the Ohio State Medical Society, June, 1883. Columbus, O.: Hann & Adair, 1883. 33p. DNLM; OC
80-5226

REEVE, J[ohn] C[harles] (1826-1920)
The treatment of puerperal fever. Columbus, [1883]. 8p. DNLM **80-5227**

REEVE, J[ohn] C[harles] (1826-1920)
Historical and clinical notes on the delivery of the placenta. Columbus, O., 1884. 10p. DNLM **80-5228**

REEVES, Henry A[lbert]
Bodily deformities and their treatment, a handbook of practical orthopaedics. Philadelphia: P. Blakiston, Son & Co., 1885. 460p. DNLM; NNNAM; PPC; PU **80-5229**

REEVES, James E[dmund] (1829-1896)
Annual address by the president of the Medical Society of the State of West Virginia. Wheeling: L. Baker & Co., 1882. 19p. DNLM **80-5230**

REEVES, James E[dmund] (1829-1896)
How to work with the Bausch & Lomb Optical Co.'s microtome, and a method of demonstrating the tubercle-bacillus. . . . Rochester, N.Y.: Bausch & Lomb Optical Co., 1886. 27p. DLC **80-5231**

REEVES, James E[dmund] (1829-1896)
The value of sanitation in its national aspect, as compared with other public interests. Concord, N.H.: Republican Press Association, 1886. 26p. DLC **80-5232**

REIBMAYR, Albert
The art of massage. Tracts on massage. No. 1. Transl. from the German, with notes, by Benjamin Lee. Philadelphia, 1885. 41p. DNLM; PPC **80-5233**

REIBMAYR, Albert
The art of massage. Tracts on massage. No. 2. The physiological effects of massage. Transl. from the German, with notes, by Benjamin Lee. Philadelphia, 1885. 46p. DNLM; PPC **80-5234**

REICHERT, Edward T[yson] (*b.* 1855)
Ethylene bichloride as an anaesthetic agent; with a consideration of ethylene methylethylate, ethylene ethylate, ethyl nitrate, and ethylidene bichloride. [Philadelphia, 1881.] 12p. DNLM **80-5235**

REICHERT, Edward T[yson] (*b.* 1855)
Convulsions due to depression of spinal reflex-inhibitory centres; with special reference to the convulsions of apomorphine, atropine, strychnine, and other poisons. [Philadelphia, 1881.] 5p. DNLM **80-5236**

REICHERT, Edward T[yson] (*b.* 1855)
Amyl nitrite, a powerful cardiac stimulant. New York, 1881. 11p. DNLM **80-5237**

REICHERT, Edward T[yson] (*b.* 1855)
Are all anaesthetics dangerous which contain chlorine, bromine, or iodine? Philadelphia, 1881. 16p. DNLM **80-5238**

REICHERT, Edward T[yson] (*b.* 1855)
Contributions to the study of the toxicology of cardiac depressants. I. Carbolic acid; a summary of fifty-six cases of poisoning, with a study of its physiological action. [Philadelphia, 1881.] 25p. DNLM **80-5239**

REICHERT, Edward T[yson] (*b.* 1855)
Observations on the regeneration of the vagus and hypoglossal nerves. Philadelphia, 1885. 14p. DNLM **80-5240**

REMINGTON, Joseph P[rice] (1847-1918)
The practice of pharmacy: a treatise on the modes of making and dispensing officinal, unofficinal, and extemporaneous preparations, with descriptions of their properties, uses, and doses. Intended as a hand-book for pharmacists and physicians and a text-book for students. . . . With nearly five hundred illustrations. Philadelphia, [etc.]: J. B. Lippincott Co., 1885. 1080p. diags. DLC; DNLM; OCLloyd; PU **80-5241**

REMINGTON, Joseph P[rice] (1847-1918)
The practice of pharmacy. A treatise on the modes of making and dispensing officinal, unofficinal and extemporaneous preparations, with descriptions of their properties, uses, and doses. Intended as a hand-book for pharmacists and physicians, and a text-book for students. 2nd ed. Enl. and thoroughly rev. . . . With over six hundred illustrations. Philadelphia, [etc.]: J. B. Lippincott Co., 1889. 1300p. diags. DLC; IU-M; NNNAM; OCLloyd **80-5242**

REPERTORY to Hering's condensed materia medica. Published by the Homoeopathic Medical Society of Pennsylvania. Philadelphia, 1889. 432p. DNLM; OCLloyd; PPHa **80-5243**

REPORT of the post-mortem examination of the body of Chas. J. Guiteau, who died by hanging, June 30, 1882, at the United States jail, Washington, D.C., in execution of judicial sentence. [By D. S. Lamb. With report of the microscopical examination.] Philadelphia, 1882. 22p. DNLM **80-5244**

REPORTS of the application of hydrochlorate of cocaine in ophthalmology, otology, laryngology, gynaecology, genito-urinary, nasal, dental, and general surgery. Compiled from medical literature. Detroit & New York: Parke, Davis & Co., 1885. 36p. DNLM; NNNAM **80-5245**

REYNDERS, JOHN, & CO. NEW YORK
Illustrated catalogue and price-list of surgical instruments, orthopaedical apparatus, trusses, etc. . . . 3rd ed. New York, [1880]. 262p. DNLM; NNNAM **80-5246**

REYNDERS, JOHN, & CO. NEW YORK
. . . illustrated descriptive catalogue of orthopaedical apparatuses, trusses, bandages, elastic stockings, crutches, etc., etc. New York: J. Reynders & Co., [1884]. [291]-376p. DLC; NNNAM **80-5247**

REYNDERS, JOHN, & CO. NEW YORK
. . . illustrated catalogue and price-list of surgical instruments, orthopaedical apparatus, trusses, etc. . . . 5th ed. New York: J. Reynders & Co., [1884]. 386p. DLC; NNNAM **80-5248**

REYNDERS, JOHN, & CO. NEW YORK
. . . illustrated catalogue and price list of surgical instruments. . . . 6th ed. New York: J. Reynders & Co., 1889. 398p. DLC; NNNAM **80-5249**

REYNOLDS, Dudley S[harpe] (1842-1915)
Otitis media purulenta. A clinical lecture. [n. p.], 1882. 8p. DNLM **80-5250**

REYNOLDS, Dudley S[harpe] (1842-1915)
Some of the causes of failure in operations for the correction of squint. [Philadelphia], 1885. 7p. DNLM
80-5251

REYNOLDS, Dudley S[harpe] (1842-1915)
Oration delivered before the Alumni Association of the Medico-Chirurgical College of Philadelphia, April 7, 1887. [Philadelphia, 1887.] 10p. DNLM; PPC **80-5252**

REYNOLDS, Edward (*b.* 1860)
A contribution to the mechanism of descent and flexion in vertex presentations. New York: William Wood & Co., 1887. 9p. DNLM **80-5253**

REYNOLDS, Edward (*b.* 1860)
Stricture of the urethra. Urethrotomy under cocaine anaesthesia. A clinical lecture. Chicago, 1888. 14p. DNLM; ICRM
80-5254

REYNOLDS, Henry J.
Treatment of eczema. Chicago: Clark & Longley, 1885. 8p. DNLM **80-5255**

REYNOLDS, Henry J.
Address on dermatology. Chicago, 1886. 8p. DNLM
80-5256

REYNOLDS, Henry J.
A new method in the treatment of the vegetable parasitic diseases of the skin. With extract from a corroborative article by E. Charn and G. Gevaert. [Chicago, 1888.] 8p. DNLM
80-5257

REYNOLDS, Henry J.
Stricture of the urethra. Urethrotomy under cocaine anaesthesia. A clinical lecture. Chicago, 1888. 14p. DNLM
80-5258

REYNOLDS, J[ohn] Russell, ed. (1828-1896)
A system of medicine. . . . With additions by Henry Hartshorne. Philadelphia: Henry C. Lea's Son, 1880. 3 v. NNNAM; MBM; ICU; PPC **80-5259**

RHEIN, M[eyer] L.
Studies of pyorrhea alveolaris. Philadelphia, 1888. 6p. DNLM
80-5260

RHEIN, M[eyer] L.
Chloride of methyl. [Chicago, 1889.] 8p. DNLM
80-5261

RIBOT, Theodule A[rmand] (1839-1916)
An essay in the positive psychology. Transl. from the French by William Huntington Smith. New York: D. Appleton & Co., 1882. 209p. MA; NIC; NN **80-5262**

RIBOT, Theodule A[rmand] (1839-1916)
The diseases of memory. Transl. from the French by J. Fitzgerald. New York: J. Fitzgerald, 1882. 48p. DNLM; NNNAM **80-5263**

RIBOT, Theodule A[rmand] (1839-1916)
The diseases of the will, transl. from the French by J. Fitzgerald. New York: J. Fitzgerald, 1884. 45p. DNLM; NNNAM **80-5264**

RIBOT, Theodule A[rmand] (1839-1916)
German psychology of today. The empirical school. Transl. from the 2nd French edition by James Mark Baldwin. New York: C. Scribner's Sons, 1886. 307p. ICU; MB; MH; NN
80-5265

RICE, Charles (1841-1901)
Report on the revision of the U.S. Pharmacopoeia preliminary to the convention of 1880. Being a rough draft of the general principles, titles, and working formulae proposed for the next pharmacopoeia. New York, 1880. 202p. DNLM; NNNAM; OCLloyd **80-5266**

RICE, Clarence C.
Adhesion of the soft palate to the walls of the pharynx. [New York, 1885.] 15p. DNLM **80-5267**

RICE, Clarence C.
Some points in regard to the etiology and surgical treatment of "colds in the head." New York, 1886. 8p. DNLM
80-5268

RICE, Clarence C.
How the therapeutic value of our mineral springs may be increased. [New York, 1886.] 15p. DNLM
80-5269

RICE, Clarence C.
Unusual causes of coughing. New York: M. J. Rooney, [1886]. 10p. DNLM **80-5270**

RICE, Clarence C.
Glandular and connective-tissue hypertrophies of the lateral walls of the pharynx. [New York, 1887.] 9p. DNLM
80-5271

RICE, Clarence C.
The relation of laryngeal to pulmonary phthisis and the importance of local treatment. New York: Trow, 1887. 12p. DNLM
80-5272

RICE, Clarence C.
What cases of nasal catarrh require surgical treatment. [New York, 1887.] 12p. DNLM **80-5273**

RICE, Clarence C.
Antiseptic nasal surgery. [New York, 1889.] 17p. DNLM
80-5274

RICHARDS, Huntington
Two noteworthy cases of traumatic rupture of the membrana tympani. [New Bedford, 1889.] 4p. DNLM
80-5275

RICHARDSON, Benjamin Ward (1828-1896)
A synopsis of the temperance lesson-book of . . . by C. R. Agnew. New York, 1880. 23p. DNLM; NNNAM
80-5276

RICHARDSON, Benjamin Ward (1828-1896)
Diseases of modern life. New York: Bermingham & Co., 1882. 288p. IU-M; NNNAM; PPC **80-5277**

RICHARDSON, Benjamin Ward (1828-1896)
Ten lectures on alcohol. New York, 1882. 190, 58, 47, 33, 12, 8, 24p. DNLM; NNNAM **80-5278**

RICHARDSON, Benjamin Ward (1828-1896)
Twenty-one historic landmarks. New York: Nat. Temp. Soc., 1882. 24p. DNLM; NNNAM **80-5279**

RICHARDSON, Benjamin Ward (1828-1896)
Diseases of modern life. New York: D. Appleton & Co., 1883. 520p. DNLM; MBM; NNNAM; PU **80-5280**

RICHARDSON, Benjamin Ward (1828-1896)
The field of disease: a book of preventive medicine. . . . Philadelphia: Henry C. Lea's Son & Co., 1884. 737p. DLC; MH-M; NNNAM; PPC **80-5281**

RICHARDSON, C. W[illiamson] (1861-1929)
A case of laryngeal growth. Chicago, 1888. 7p. DNLM **80-5282**

RICHARDSON, C. W[illiamson] (1861-1929)
A pathological change at the base of the tongue, possibly explaining certain so-called functional diseases of that organ. Chicago, 1889. 8p. DNLM **80-5283**

RICHARDSON, C. W[illiamson] (1861-1929)
A contribution to the study of nervous cough. [Baltimore, 1889.] 9p. DNLM **80-5284**

RICHARDSON, Elliott (*d.* 1887)
Caesarean section with removal of uterus and ovaries after the Porro-Müller method. [Philadelphia, 1881.] 11p. DNLM **80-5285**

RICHARDSON, Elliott (*d.* 1887)
Remarks on the use of obstetric forceps. Philadelphia, 1883. 7p. DNLM **80-5286**

RICHARDSON, Joseph (1824-1890)
A practical treatise on mechanical dentistry. . . . 3rd ed., rev. and enl., with one hundred and eighty-five illustrations. Philadelphia: Lindsay & Blakiston, 1880. 433p. DLC; DNLM; PPC; PU **80-5287**

RICHARDSON, Joseph (1824-1890)
A practical treatise on mechanical dentistry. . . . 4th ed., rev. and enl., with four hundred and fifty-eight illustrations. Philadelphia: P. Blakiston, Son & Co., 1886. 710p. DLC; DNLM; MdU-D; PPC **80-5288**

RICHARDSON, Joseph (1824-1890)
A practical treatise on mechanical dentistry. 5th ed. Philadelphia: P. Blakiston, Son & Co., 1888. 710p. CtY-M; DNLM; MdU-D; PPC **80-5289**

RICHARDSON, Joseph Gibbons (1836-1886)
Why sewer traps are unreliable, and how to apply the ounce of prevention against disease germs in sewer air. Philadelphia, [1882]. 8p. DNLM **80-5290**

RICHARDSON, Joseph Gibbons (1836-1886)
Address in hygiene. Philadelphia, 1885. 23p. DNLM **80-5291**

RICHARDSON, Joseph Gibbons (1836-1886)
The modern family physician and hygienic guide. . . . By Joseph G. Richardson . . . William H. Ford . . . C. C. Vanderbeck. . . . Philadelphia: J. E. Potter & Co., [1885]. 1140p. plates (partly col.). DLC; MdBM; MdBJ-W; PPC **80-5292**

RICHARDSON, Joseph Gibbons (1836-1886)
The modern family physician and hygienic guide. . . . Philadelphia: J. E. Potter & Co., 1889. 1314p. col. plates. DLC; IU-M; MBM; PU **80-5293**

RICHARDSON, Maurice H[owe] (1851-1912)
A case of nephrorraphy for movable kidney; complete relief of symptoms. Boston: Cupples & Hurd, 1888. 19p. DNLM; MBM **80-5294**

RICHARDSON, Maurice H[owe] (1851-1912)
Operations on nerves. Cases of nerve suture, nerve section, nerve stretching, and operations to relieve pressure upon nerve trunks. Boston: Cupples & Hurd, 1888. 46p. 1 plate. DNLM; MBM **80-5295**

RICHARDSON, Maurice H[owe] (1851-1912)
On the surgical treatment of gangrenous hernia, with report of four cases. Philadelphia: W. J. Dornan, 1889. 18p. DNLM; PPC **80-5296**

RICHARDSON, William L[ambert] (1842-1932)
A new method of performing decapitation. [Boston, 1880.] 5p. DNLM **80-5297**

RICHARDSON, William L[ambert] (1842-1932)
Manual dilatation of the os uteri as a means of inducing premature labor. [Boston, 1881.] 8p. DNLM **80-5298**

RICHARDSON, William L[ambert] (1842-1932)
Diagnosis and treatment of posterior positions of the occiput. Read at the annual meeting of the Massachusetts Medical Society, June 10, 1885. [Boston, 1885.] 16p. DNLM **80-5299**

RICHARDSON, William L[ambert] (1842-1932)
The use of antiseptics in obstetric practice. Boston: Cupples, Upham & Co., 1887. 21p. 1 plate. DNLM **80-5300**

RICHARDSON, William L[ambert] (1842-1932)
Address on the duties and conduct of nurses in private nursing. Delivered at the Boston Training School for Nurses, June 18, 1886. Boston: G. H. Ellis, 1887. 23p. DNLM **80-5301**

RICHEY, Stephen O[lin]
A case of reproduction of the membrana tympani. [Washington, 1880.] 5p. DNLM **80-5302**

RICHEY, Stephen O[lin]
General atrophy of the conducting apparatus of the ear as related to progressive arthritis deformans. Philadelphia: W. Fell & Co., [1881]. 4 l. DNLM **80-5303**

RICHEY, Stephen O[lin]
Deterioration of vision in school children. Concord, N.H.: Republican Press Association, 1885. 8p. DNLM **80-5304**

RICHEY, Stephen O[lin]
A case of chronic simple glaucoma treated with escrine. [Washington, D.C., 1886.] 7p. DNLM **80-5305**

RICHEY, Stephen O[lin]
Prophylaxis in rhinitis sympathetica. [Chicago, 1886.] 4p. DNLM **80-5306**

RICHEY, Stephen O[lin]
General atrophy of the conducting apparatus of the ear (proliferous inflammation). New York, 1886. 29p. DNLM **80-5307**

RICHEY, Stephen O[lin]
A contribution to the management of general atrophy (sclerosis?) of the conducting apparatus of the ear. [Philadelphia, 1887.] 10p. DNLM **80-5308**

RICHEY, Stephen O[lin]
Eczema simplex dependent upon ametropia, Chicago, [1888]. 1 l. DNLM **80-5309**

RICHEY, Stephen O[lin]
The primary physiological purpose of the membrana tympani. [New Bedford, Mass., 1888.] 23p. DNLM **80-5310**

RICHEY, Stephen O[lin]
Binocular astigmatism? Chicago, 1888. 3p. DNLM **80-5311**

RICHEY, Stephen O[lin]
The physiology of the intra-tympanic muscles. [Washington, 1888.] 4p. DNLM **80-5312**

RICHEY, Stephen O[lin]
General atrophy of the conducting apparatus of the ear as related to progressive arthritis deformans. Philadelphia: W. F. Fell & Co., [1888]. 4 l. DNLM **80-5313**

RICHEY, Stephen O[lin]
A contribution to the management of initial myopia acquisita. [Philadelphia, 1889.] 7p. DNLM **80-5314**

von RICHTER, Victor (1841-1891)
A text-book of inorganic chemistry. Transl. by Edgar F. Smith. 2nd American from the 4th German ed. Philadelphia: P. Blakiston, Son & Co., 1885. 432p. 1 lithog. plate. DNLM; ICU; MA **80-5315**

von RICHTER, Victor (1841-1891)
Chemistry of the carbon compounds; or, organic chemistry. Authorized translation by Edgar F. Smith. From the 4th German ed. Philadelphia: P. Blakiston, Son & Co., 1886. 710p. DNLM; KU; NIC; NN **80-5316**

RICKETTS, B. Merrill (*b.* 1858)
The negligence and result of vaccination. Ironton: Register Office, 1882. 14p. DNLM **80-5317**

RICKETTS, B. Merrill (*b.* 1858)
Epithelioma; its etiology, diagnosis and treatment. [Cincinnati, 1886.] 8p. DNLM **80-5318**

RICKETTS, B. Merrill (*b.* 1858)
The management of eczema infantile. [Cincinnati, 1887.] 4p. DNLM **80-5319**

RICKETTS, B. Merrill (*b.* 1858)
The treatment of acne. Philadelphia, [1888]. 8p. DNLM **80-5320**

RICKETTS, B. Merrill (*b.* 1858)
Plasto-cosmetics in surgery of the face. Cincinnati, 1889. 8p. DNLM **80-5321**

RICKETTS, Edwin
Cholecystotomy: report of a case. [Cincinnati, 1889.] 8p. DNLM **80-5322**

RIDLON, John (1852-1936)
Contributions to orthopaedic surgery. New York, 1888. 18p. DNLM **80-5323**

RIDLON, John (1852-1936)
Contributions to orthopaedic surgery. New York. Knickerbocker Press, 1888. 110 (i.e., 106)p. (mounted). illus. NcD [A collection of reprints; title from first publication] **80-5323A**

RIDLON, John (1852-1936)
Contributions to orthopaedic surgery. New York: Trow's, 1888-1890. 119p. DNLM; PPC [Drawn from various medical journals] **80-5323B**

RING, Allan M[ott]
The treatment of uterine diseases by means of the hot-air bath and hot-vaginal douche. Boston: A. Williams & Co., 1882. 22p. DNLM; MBM **80-5324**

RINGER, Sydney (1835-1910) and E. E. MORSHEAD
On the physiological action of the bulb of the Buphane toxicaria or Hemanthus toxicarius; Amaryllidaceae. New York: G. P. Putnam's Sons, 1880. 19p. DNLM; NNNAM **80-5325**

RINGER, Sydney (1835-1910)
A handbook of therapeutics. . . . 10th ed. New York: William Wood & Co., 1883. 688p. DNLM; NNNAM; OCIM; PU **80-5326**

RINGER, Sydney (1835-1910)
A handbook of therapeutics. . . . 11th ed. New York: William Wood & Co., 1886. 668p. CtY-M; NN; PPC; PU **80-5327**

RINGER, Sydney (1835-1910)
A handbook of therapeutics. . . . 12th ed. New York: William Wood & Co., 1889. 524p. CtY-M; NNNAM; OCIM; PU **80-5328**

RISLEY, S[amuel] D[oty] (1845-1920)
Weak eyes in the public schools of Philadelphia. The report of the committee on examination of the eyes of the children in the public schools of Philadelphia. Philadelphia: Collins, 1881. 38p. 1 plate, 1 tab. DNLM; PPC **80-5329**

RISLEY, S[amuel] D[oty] (1845-1920)
The comparative value of the mydriatics. [Boston, 1881.] 29p. DNLM **80-5330**

RISLEY, S[amuel] D[oty] (1845-1920)
Incipient cataract; its aetiology, treatment, and prognosis. [Philadelphia, 1889.] 10p. DNLM **80-5331**

RITCHIE, Fred G.
The rectum and its diseases. . . . Worcester, Mass.: Press of D. Seagrave, 1886. 28p. DLC **80-5332**

ROBB, R. L.
Robb & Co.'s family physician. A work on domestic medicines, designed to show the causes, symptoms and treatment of disease. For the use of the people. By R. L. Robb, M.D., homoeopathic, J. V. Bean, M.D., regular, or allopathic [and] S. Lucretia Robb. . . . 2nd ed. Carefully rev. and enl. . . . Burlington, Ia., and London, Can.: Robb & Co., 1880. 736, 155, [802]-910p. fol. col. plates. DLC
80-5333

ROBB, R. L.
Robb's family physician: being a concise and comprehensive treatise on diseases, as they occur in every-day life. Showing the causes, explaining the symptoms and treatment, and demonstrating the cure of the various ills humanity is subject to. By J. V. Bean, M.D., allopathic, R. L. Robb, M.D., homoeopathic [and] Sarah L. Robb. . . . Philadelphia, Chicago, [etc.]: The National Publishing Co., 1884. 760, 155, [916]-934p. plates. DLC **80-5334**

ROBBINS, Daniel C.
Annual review of the drug trade of New York, for the year 1880. New York: H. Bessey, 1881. 13p. DNLM; NNNAM
80-5335

ROBBINS, Daniel C.
Review of the drug trade of New York, for the year 1882. New York: H. Bessey, 1883. 12p. DNLM; NNNAM
80-5336

ROBBINS, Daniel C.
Review of the drug trade of New York for the year 1887. Prepared for the thirtieth annual report of the Chamber of Commerce of the State of New York: New York: H. Bessey, 1888. 19p. DNLM; NNNAM **80-5337**

ROBERTS, A[lgernon] Sydney (1855-1896)
The spinal arthropathies. (A clinical report of Charcot's joints.) Philadelphia: W. J. Dornan, 1885. 15p. DNLM
80-5338

ROBERTS, A[lgernon] Sydney (1855-1896)
Clinical lectures on orthopaedic surgery, delivered at the Philadelphia Hospital. Nos. I, II. The etiology, morbid anatomy, varieties, and treatment of club-foot. Philadelphia: P. Blakiston, Son & Co., 1886. 32p. DNLM; PPC
80-5339

ROBERTS, A[lgernon] Sydney (1855-1896)
Clinical lectures on orthopaedic surgery, delivered at the Philadelphia Hospital. Nos. III, IV. Knock-knee and bow-legs, with remarks upon rachitis. Philadelphia: P. Blakiston, Son & Co., 1888. 24p. DNLM; PPC **80-5340**

ROBERTS, Frederick Thomas (1838-1919)
The theory and practice of medicine. 3rd American from 4th London ed. 2 pts. Philadelphia: Lindsay & Blakiston, 1881. 509, 530p. DNLM; MBM; NNNAM; PPC
80-5341

ROBERTS, Frederick Thomas (1838-1919)
The theory and practice of medicine. 5th American ed. Philadelphia: P. Blakiston, Son & Co., 1884. 1008p. DNLM; IU-M; NNNAM; PU **80-5342**

ROBERTS, Frederick Thomas (1838-1919)
Notes on materia medica and pharmacy. Philadelphia: P. Blakiston, Son & Co., 1884. 380p. DNLM; NNNAM; OCLloyd; PU **80-5343**

ROBERTS, Frederick Thomas (1838-1919)
A handbook of the theory and practice of medicine. 7th ed. Philadelphia: P. Blakiston, Son & Co., 1888. 1044p. DNLM; MdBM; MH-M; PPC **80-5344**

ROBERTS, John B[ingham] (1852-1924)
Paracentesis of the pericardium. A consideration of the surgical treatment of pericardial effusions. Philadelphia: J. B. Lippincott & Co., 1880. 100p. DNLM
80-5345

ROBERTS, John B[ingham] (1852-1924)
Ether death; a personal experience in four cases of death from anaesthetics. Philadelphia, 1881. 12p. DNLM
80-5346

ROBERTS, John B[ingham] (1852-1924)
The compend of anatomy. For use in the dissecting room, and in preparing for examinations. Philadelphia: C. C. Roberts & Co., 1881. 191p. DNLM [2nd ed., 1881, 198p.; 3rd ed., Lea Bros., 1885, 198p.] **80-5347**

ROBERTS, John B[ingham] (1852-1924)
The surgery of the pericardium. Brooklyn, 1881. 6p. DNLM
80-5348

ROBERTS, John B[ingham] (1852-1924)
Excision of cartilage in nasal obstructions due to deviated septum. Philadelphia, 1882. 4p. DNLM
80-5349

ROBERTS, John B[ingham] (1852-1924)
The clinical history and exact localization of perinephric abscesses. [Philadelphia, 1883.] 19p. DNLM
80-5350

ROBERTS, John B[ingham] (1852-1924)
Heart-puncture and heart-suture as therapeutic procedures. [Philadelphia, 1883.] 5p. DNLM **80-5351**

ROBERTS, John B[ingham] (1852-1924)
The legal control of medical practice by a state examination. [Philadelphia, 1884.] 4p. DNLM **80-5352**

ROBERTS, John B[ingham] (1852-1924)
The policlinic never-leaking ether bottle. Philadelphia, 1884. 1 galley sheet. DNLM **80-5353**

ROBERTS, John B[ingham] (1852-1924)
Surgical delusions and follies. A revision of the address in surgery for 1884 of the Medical Society of the State of Pennsylvania. Philadelphia: P. Blakiston, Son & Co., 1884. 55p. DNLM **80-5354**

ROBERTS, John B[ingham] (1852-1924)
The field and limitation of the operative surgery of the human brain. Philadelphia: P. Blakiston, Son & Co., 1885. 80p. DNLM **80-5355**

ROBERTS, John B[ingham] (1852-1924)
Remarks on the bill proposed by the Medical Society of the State of Pennsylvania for the establishment of a state board of medical examiners and licensers. [Philadelphia, 1888.] 10p. DNLM **80-5356**

ROBERTS, John B[ingham] (1852-1924)
The segment trephine and an aseptic trephine. [Philadelphia, 1889.] 4p. DNLM **80-5357**

ROBERTS, John B[ingham] (1852-1924)
The cure of crooked and otherwise deformed noses. Philadelphia: P. Blakiston, Son & Co., 1889. 24p. DNLM
80-5358

ROBERTS, John B[ingham] (1852-1924)
The science of successful surgery. The annual address of the Philadelphia Academy of Surgery. Chicago, 1889. 24p. DNLM
80-5359

ROBERTS, John B[ingham] (1852-1924)
Delusions in eye surgery. Philadelphia: B. F. Adams, 1889. 8p. DNLM **80-5360**

ROBERTS, John B[ingham] (1852-1924)
Extraction of cataract, with cases showing results of operation. Philadelphia: W. J. Dornan, 1889. 10p. DNLM
80-5361

ROBERTS, J. D.
Report of the chairman of the section on medical jurisprudence. [Wilmington, 1886.] 23p. DNLM
80-5362

ROBERTS, Milton J[osiah] (1850-1893)
Elastic tension therapeutically utilized in adhesive and medicated plasters. New York, 1882. 4p. DNLM
80-5363

ROBERTS, Milton J[osiah] (1850-1893)
Elastic tension and articular motion in Pott's disease. [1882]. 12p. DNLM **80-5364**

ROBERTS, Milton J[osiah] (1850-1893)
Non-uniformity in the principles of treating Pott's disease, as taught by Professor Sayre; elastic tension and articular motion as therapeutic agents. [n. p., 1882.] 16p. DNLM
80-5365

ROBERTS, Milton J[osiah] (1850-1893)
The electro-osteotome. A new instrument for the performance of the operation of osteotomy. [New York: J. J. O'Brien, 1883.] 8p. DNLM **80-5366**

ROBERTS, Milton J[osiah] (1850-1893)
The fundamental principles of mechanico-therapy in hip disease. Based on a consideration of clinical, pathological, and physico-physiological data, with a description of new forms of elastic tension hip splints. New York, 1885. 56p. DNLM
80-5367

ROBERTS, Milton J[osiah] (1850-1893)
Presentation of two patients, illustrating the favorable progress of suppurative knee-joint disease, while wearing elastic tension splints permitting articular motion of affected joints. [New York, 1886.] 4 l. DNLM **80-5368**

ROBERTS, Milton J[osiah] (1850-1893)
The exploration, excavation, and illumination of the interior bones in any part of the body. [New York, 1885.] 4p. DNLM
80-5369

ROBERTS, Milton J[osiah] (1850-1893)
Anatomical geometry and toponymy. An introduction to the scientific study of deformities, with a description of new mathematical instruments. Syracuse, N.Y., 1885. 14p. DNLM
80-5370

ROBERTS, Milton J[osiah] (1850-1893)
Description and practical demonstration of the working of Roberts' improved electro-osteotome, new electrical illuminating apparatus, and a new form of portable storage battery. New York: De Leeuw et al., 1886. 15p. DNLM
80-5371

ROBERTS, Milton J[osiah] (1850-1893)
Cuneiform osteotomy for anterior curvature of both tibiae and both fibulae; illustrating the great practical value of the electro-osteotome as a bone cutting instrument, and the sphenometer as an instrument of precision in bone surgery; suturing of the bones with kangaroo tendons; hydro-naptholized surgical dressings; Bruce's bow-leg brace. Detroit: G. S. Davis, 1887. 12p. DNLM **80-5372**

ROBERTS, Milton J[osiah] (1850-1893)
Remarks on a new spinal corset woven out of wire to fit the contour of the body. [Richmond], 1887. 3p. DNLM
80-5373

ROBERTS, William (1830-1899)
A practical treatise on urinary and renal diseases, including urinary deposits. . . . 4th ed. Philadelphia: Lea Bros. & Co., 1885. 628p. DNLM; IU-M; NNNAM; PPC
80-5374

ROBERTS, W. O.
Report on surgery; read before the Kentucky State Medical Society, April 5, 1882. Louisville: J. P. Morton & Co., 1882. 16p. DNLM **80-5375**

ROBERTS, W. O.
Aneurism of the femoral artery and a knife wound of the intestines. Louisville, Ky.: J. P. Morton & Co., 1884. 11p. DNLM **80-5376**

ROBERTSON, Joseph McGregor (1858-1925)
The elements of physiological physics: an outline of the elementary facts, principles, and methods of physics; and their applications in physiology. . . . Illustrated with 219 engravings on wood. Philadelphia: Henry C. Lea's Son & Co., 1884. 528p. DLC; DNLM; NNNAM; PPC **80-5377**

ROBINSON, A[ndrew] R[ose] (1845-1924)
The anatomical seat of the fungus in tinea tonsuraus capillitii. New York, 1881. 10p. DNLM **80-5378**

ROBINSON, A[ndrew] R[ose] (1845-1924)
Lichen ruber and lichen planus. New York: G. P. Putnam's Sons, 1883. 28p. DNLM **80-5379**

ROBINSON, A[ndrew] R[ose] (1845-1924)
A manual of dermatology. New York: D. Appleton & Co., 1885. 647p. DNLM; NNNAM; PPC; PU
80-5380

ROBINSON, Beverley (1844-1924)
Suggestions as to the therapeutic value of rest in the treatment of laryngeal diseases. [New York, 1880.] 13p. DNLM
80-5381

ROBINSON, Beverley (1844-1924)
A practical treatise on nasal catarrh. New York: William Wood & Co., 1880. 182p. CtY-M; DNLM; NNNAM; PPC
80-5382

ROBINSON, Beverley (1844-1924)
The laryngeal affections of pulmonary phthisis. [New York, 1881.] 23p. DNLM **80-5383**

ROBINSON, Beverley (1844-1924)
A clinical study of the action and uses of caffeine and Convallaria majalis as cardiac tonics. Detroit: J. S. Davis, 1883. 30p. DNLM **80-5384**

ROBINSON, Beverley (1844-1924)
A practical treatise on nasal catarrh and allied diseases. . . . 2nd ed., rev. and enl. . . . New York: William Wood & Co., 1885. 276p. DLC; DNLM; NNNAM; PPC **80-5385**

ROBINSON, Beverley (1844-1924)
A contribution to the study of hay fever (so-called). [Philadelphia], 1886. 12p. DNLM **80-5386**

ROBINSON, Beverley (1844-1924)
A manual on inhalers, inhalations, and inhalants, and guide to their disciminating use in the treatment of common catarrhal diseases of the respiratory tract. Detroit: G. S. Davis, 1886. 72p. DNLM; IU-M; NNNAM **80-5387**

ROBINSON, Beverley (1844-1924)
Creosote as a remedy in phthisis pulmonalis. Philadelphia: W. J. Dornan, 1888. 32p. DNLM **80-5388**

ROBINSON, Beverley (1844-1924)
A manual on inhalers, inhalations and inhalants. . . . 2nd ed. Detroit, Mich.: G. S. Davis, 1888. 72p. DLC; OCIM; PU **80-5389**

ROBY, Henry W.
The treatment of disease from the homoeopathic standpoint. Topeka: Capital City Printing Co., 1886. 37p. DNLM **80-5390**

ROCKWELL, Alphonso David (1840-1933)
Locomotor ataxia differentiated from functional conditions which simulate it. New York, 1881. 9p. DNLM **80-5391**

ROCKWELL, Alphonso David (1840-1933)
Observations on hemiplegia, based on eighty-one recorded cases, with special reference to cerebral localization. New York: Trow, 1882. 12p. DNLM **80-5392**

ROCKWELL, Alphonso David (1840-1933)
The induction coil; its varieties and the differential indications for their use. New York: Trow, 1884. 12p. DNLM **80-5393**

ROCKWELL, Frank W[arren] (1843-1889)
Case of mutton bone impacted in trachea; successful tracheotomy for its removal. Brooklyn, N.Y., 1881. 5p. DNLM **80-5394**

ROE, John O[rlando] (1848-1915)
The relation of membranous croup to diphtheria. Buffalo: Haas, Nauert & Klein, 1880. 20p. DNLM **80-5395**

ROE, John O[rlando] (1848-1915)
Fracture of the larynx. [New York, 1881.] 7p. DNLM **80-5396**

ROE, John O[rlando] (1848-1915)
Nasal stenosis: its influence on olfaction, audition, vocalization, and respiration, and its treatment. New York: Trow, 1881. 32p. DNLM **80-5397**

ROE, John O[rlando] (1848-1915)
Laryngeal whistling. [New York, 1882.] 3p. DNLM **80-5398**

ROE, John O[rlando] (1848-1915)
Internal oesophagotomy. The division of membranous or cicatricial constrictions or obstructions in the oesophagus by internal section. New York: Trow, 1882. 36p. DNLM **80-5399**

ROE, John O[rlando] (1848-1915)
The comparative value of atomized fluids in the treatment of diseases of the larynx. [New York: G. P. Putnam's Sons, 1882.] 4p. DNLM **80-5400**

ROE, John O[rlando] (1848-1915)
The pathology and radical cure of hay fever, or hay asthma. Syracuse: Truair, Smith & Bruce, 1883. 16p. DNLM **80-5401**

ROE, John O[rlando] (1848-1915)
Discussion on "the utility or non-utility of local applications in chronic catarrhal laryngitis." [New York, 1883.] 5p. DNLM **80-5402**

ROE, John O[rlando] (1848-1915)
The pathology and radical cure of hay fever, or hay asthma. New York: D. Appleton & Co., 1883. 21p. DNLM **80-5403**

ROE, John O[rlando] (1848-1915)
Retro-pharyngeal abscess. New York: D. Appleton & Co., 1884. 23p. DNLM **80-5404**

ROE, John O[rlando] (1848-1915)
The pathology and radical cure of hay fever, or hay asthma. 2nd article. New York: D. Appleton & Co., 1884. 16p. DNLM **80-5405**

ROE, John O[rlando] (1848-1915)
Bronchiectasis. Buffalo, 1885. 11p. DNLM **80-5406**

ROE, John O[rlando] (1848-1915)
Angioma of the nose. New York: D. Appleton & Co., 1886. 9p. 1 tab. DNLM **80-5407**

ROE, John O[rlando] (1848-1915)
Hay fever. Analysis of forty-four cases treated by the writer, together with the result of treatment. New York: D. Appleton & Co., 1887. 17p. DNLM **80-5408**

ROE, John O[rlando] (1848-1915)
An electric nasal saw. [New York, 1888.] 5p. 1 plate. DNLM **80-5409**

ROE, John O[rlando] (1848-1915)
The frequent dependence of persistent and so-called congestive headaches upon abnormal conditions of the nasal passages. New York: Trow's Printing & Bookbinding Co., 1888. 17p. DNLM **80-5410**

ROE, John O[rlando] (1848-1915)
Sir Morell Mackenzie's book on "The fatal illness of Frederick the Noble." An interview with . . . . Rochester, 1888. 14p. DNLM **80-5411**

ROE, John O[rlando] (1848-1915)
The treatment of diseased tonsils when unattended with hypertrophy. New York: D. Appleton & Co., 1889. 11p. DNLM **80-5412**

ROGERS, Joseph G[oodwin] (1841-1908)
The state and its insane. Notes on the location, construction, and equipment of hospitals for the insane. Read before the Indiana Social Science Association, May 8, 1883. Indianapolis: Carlon & Hollenbeck, 1883. 25p. DNLM **80-5413**

ROGERS, Joseph G[oodwin] (1841-1908)
Report to the commission to construct additional hospitals for the insane on the construction of hospitals for the insane. No. 1. Indianapolis: W. B. Burford, 1883. 20p. DNLM **80-5414**

ROGERS, W[illiam] B[oddie] (*b.* 1856)
Rogers' urethrotome. A dilating bulbous urethrotome (and urethrometer), adapted to strictures of both large and small caliber. [New York, 1888.] 6p. DNLM **80-5415**

ROHÉ, George H. (1851-1899)
A probable cause of tardy, painful labor, not hitherto recognized. [New York, 1881.] 5p. DNLM **80-5416**

ROHÉ, George H. (1851-1899)
The treatment of the various forms of acne. Baltimore, 1883. 7p. DNLM **80-5417**

ROHÉ, George H. (1851-1899)
Pemphigus, and the diseases liable to be mistaken for it. Philadelphia, 1883. 11p. DNLM **80-5418**

ROHÉ, George H. (1851-1899)
Hints on the treatment of some parasitic skin diseases. New York: Trow, 1883. 11p. DNLM **80-5419**

ROHÉ, George H. (1851-1899)
The treatment of acute eczema. Baltimore, 1883. 7p. DNLM **80-5420**

ROHÉ, George H. (1851-1899)
Some points concerning anaesthetics and their administration. A lecture. Baltimore, [1883?]. 18p. DNLM **80-5421**

ROHÉ, George H. (1851-1899)
Practical notes on the treatment of skin diseases. I. Diseases of the perspiratory and sebaceous glands, including hyperidrosis, bromidrosis, prickly heat, seborrhoea, comedo, acne, acne rosacea, sycosis, and other disorders of the cutaneous glandular system. Baltimore: Thomas & Evans, 1885. 52p. DNLM **80-5422**

ROHÉ, George H. (1851-1899)
A text-book of hygiene; a comprehensive treatise on the principles and practice of preventive medicine from an American standpoint. . . . Baltimore: Thomas & Evans, 1885 [1884]. 324p. DLC; DNLM; MdU-D **80-5423**

ROHÉ, George H. (1851-1899)
Practical notes on the treatment of skin diseases. . . . Baltimore: Press of Thomas & Evans, 1885-1888. 4 v. DLC; MdU-D **80-5424**

ROHÉ, George H. (1851-1899)
Practical notes on the treatment of skin diseases. II. Eczema. Baltimore: Thomas & Evans, 1886. 46p. DNLM **80-5425**

ROHÉ, George H. (1851-1899)
Address in state medicine. Recent advances in preventive medicine. Chicago, 1887. 33p. DNLM **80-5426**

ROHÉ, George H. (1851-1899)
Keratosis senilis and its relations to epithelioma. [Baltimore], 1887. 2p. DNLM **80-5427**

ROHÉ, George H. (1851-1899)
Memorial address delivered before the faculty and students of the College of Physicians and Surgeons on the first anniversary of the death of Professor A. F. Erich. Baltimore: Thomas & Evans, 1888. 15p. MdU-D **80-5428**

ROHÉ, George H. (1851-1899)
The electrolytic decomposition of organic tissues. New York, 1888. 15p. DNLM **80-5429**

ROHÉ, George H. (1851-1899)
Electrolysis in dermatology and in some other departments of practical surgery. [1888.] 12p. DNLM **80-5430**

ROHÉ, George H. (1851-1899)
Value and proper use of arsenic in skin diseases. [1888.] 8p. DNLM **80-5431**

ROHÉ, George H. (1851-1899)
On corpulence, especially its treatment by a pure milk diet. [Baltimore, 1889.] 4p. DNLM **80-5432**

ROHÉ, George H. (1851-1899)
Diseases of the skin associated with disorders of the female sexual organs. [Buffalo, 1889.] 13p. DNLM **80-5433**

ROHÉ, George H. (1851-1899)
Discussion on craniotomy. Philadelphia: W. J. Dornan, 1889. 39p. DNLM **80-5434**

ROOSA, Daniel Bennett St. John (1838-1908)
A practical treatise on the diseases of the ear, including the anatomy of the organ. . . . 4th ed. New York: William Wood & Co., 1880. 569p. NNNAM; NNU-M; PU **80-5435**

ROOSA, Daniel Bennett St. John (1838-1908)
Ophthalmic and otic contributions, by Daniel B. St. John Roosa . . . and Edward T. Ely. . . . New York: G. P. Putnam's Sons, 1880. 109p. DLC; NNNAM **80-5436**

ROOSA, Daniel Bennett St. John (1838-1908)
A doctor's suggestions to the community; being a series of papers upon various subjects from a physician's standpoint. New York: G. P. Putnam's Sons, 1880. 234p. DLC; DNLM **80-5437**

ROOSA, Daniel Bennett St. John (1838-1908)
A practical treatise on the diseases of the ear, including the anatomy of the organ. . . . 5th ed. New York: William Wood & Co., 1881. 569p. CtY-M; NNNAM; PPC; PU
80-5438

ROOSA, Daniel Bennett St. John (1838-1908)
Universities in the United States. An address delivered at the commencement of the medical department of the University of Vermont, June 27, 1881. Burlington, Vt., 1881. 15p. DNLM
80-5439

ROOSA, Daniel Bennett St. John (1838-1908)
The tuning fork in the differential diagnosis of diseases of the middle and the internal ear. [New Bedford, 1881.] 7p. DNLM
80-5440

ROOSA, Daniel Bennett St. John (1838-1908)
A pocket medical lexicon; being a dictionary of the words, terms, and symbols of medical science. . . . 2nd ed. New York: William Wood & Co., 1882. 280p. DNLM; NNANM; PPC; PU
80-5441

ROOSA, Daniel Bennett St. John (1838-1908)
The next step for the medical profession of the United States. An address delivered before the graduating class of the College of Medicine, medical department of Syracuse University, June 14, 1883. [New York] : Trow's Co., 1883. 16p. DNLM
80-5442

ROOSA, Daniel Bennett St. John (1838-1908)
A pocket medical lexicon; being a dictionary of the words, terms, and symbols of medical science. . . . 3rd rev. and enl. ed. New York: William Wood & Co., [1884]. 320p. DLC; NNNAM; PPJ; PU
80-5443

ROOSA, Daniel Bennett St. John (1838-1908)
A practical treatise on the diseases of the ear, including a sketch of aural anatomy and physiology. . . . 6th ed., rev. and enl. New York: William Wood & Co., 1885. 718p. col. plate. DLC; DNLM; NNNAM; PU
80-5444

ROOSA, Daniel Bennett St. John (1838-1908)
Presbykousis. New York, 1885. 4p. DNLM
80-5445

ROOSA, Daniel Bennett St. John (1838-1908)
James Lawrence Little, M.D., a sketch of his life and times. Syracuse, 1886. 16p. DNLM
80-5446

ROOSA, Daniel Bennett St. John (1838-1908)
The determination of the necessity for wearing glasses. Detroit: G. S. Davis, 1887. 73p. [1 tab.] . DNLM; OCIM
80-5447

ROOSA, Daniel Bennett St. John (1838-1908)
The means of effecting the unity of the medical profession. Being the anniversary discourse delivered before the New York Academy of Medicine. New York: Trow's Co., 1888. 34p. DNLM; NNNAM
80-5448

ROOSA, Daniel Bennett St. John (1838-1908)
The old hospital, and other papers. . . . 2nd rev. and enl. ed. of "A doctor's suggestions." . . . New York: William Wood & Co., 1889. 320p. DLC; DNLM; NNNAM
80-5449

ROOSEVELT, J[ames] West (1858-1896)
Medical education and methods of instruction in medicine. [New York, 1889.] 10p. DNLM
80-5450

ROSE, A[chilles] (1839-1916)
Carbonic acid as a local application to chronically inflamed mucous surfaces. Brooklyn, N.Y., 1883. 8p. DNLM
80-5451

ROSS, James (1837-1892)
A treatise on the diseases of the nervous system. New York: William Wood & Co., 1882. 2 v. ICRM; IEN-M; NNNAM; PU
80-5452

ROSS, James (1837-1892)
Handbook of the diseases of the nervous system. Philadelphia: Lea Bros. & Co. 1885. 723p. CU-M; IU-M; NNNAM; PPC
80-5453

ROSSE, Irving C[ollins] (1847-1901)
Illustrations of error in the diagnosis of some nervous diseases. New York, 1887. 23p. DNLM; NNNAM
80-5454

ROSSE, Irving C[ollins] (1847-1901)
Reversive anomalies in the study of the neuroses. Chicago, 1888. 15p. DNLM; NNNAM
80-5455

ROSSE, Irving C[ollins] (1847-1901)
Notes concerning a few cases in which the electro-static remedy was used. New York: Stettiner, Lambert & Co., 1888. 12p. DNLM; NNNAM
80-5456

ROTCH, Thomas M[organ] (1849-1914)
The artificial feeding of infants. [Philadelphia, 1887.] 23p. DNLM
80-5457

ROTHER, Reinhold
The beginnings in pharmacy, an introductory treatise on the practical manipulation of drugs and the various processes employed in the preparation of medicines. . . . Detroit, Mich.: W. Graham Printing Co., 1888. 342p. DLC; OCIM; OCLloyd
80-5458

ROTHER, Reinhold
The chemistry of pharmacy, an exposition of chemical science in its relations to medicinal substances according to a practical and original plan. . . . Detroit, Mich.: W. Graham Printing Co., 1888. 71p. DLC
80-5459

ROTHER, Reinhold
The beginnings in pharmacy, an introductory treatise on the practical manipulation of drugs and the various processes employed in the preparation of medicines; together with an exposition of chemical science in its relations to medicinal substances according to a practical and original plan. . . . 4th ed., rev. and enl. Detroit, Mich.: W. Graham Printing Co., 1889. 421p. DLC; OCLloyd [2nd, 3rd eds., 1888]
80-5460

ROTHWELL, P. D.
Oxygen as a therapeutic agent. Its germicidal and healing qualities; its consequent adaptability to the treatment of consumption and pulmonary and throat troubles. Denver: W. W. Rea, [1886] . 73p. DNLM
80-5461

von RUCK, Karl (1849-1921)
The management of pulmonary phthisis. Asheville: Citizens Pub. Co., 1889. 44p. DNLM
80-5462

RUDDOCK, E. Harris (1822-1875)
The stepping stone to homoeopathy and health. With alterations adapting it to the climate, diseases and customs of Americans. Chicago: Halsey Bros., 1881. 259p. IU-M; OCIM; PPHa **80-5463**

RUDDOCK, E. Harris (1822-1875)
Ruddock's family doctor. Being a reprint of Dr. Ruddock's vade mecum, diseases of women, diseases of infants and children, and essentials of diet. With notes and additional chapters by James E. Gross. Illustrated. Chicago: Gross & Delbridge, 1884. 734p. IU-M; PPHa **80-5464**

RUDDOCK, E. Harris (1822-1875)
Ruddock's family doctor. Being a reprint of Dr. Ruddock's vade mecum, diseases of women, diseases of infants and children, and essentials of diet. With notes and additional chapters by James E. Gross. Illustrated. 3rd ed. Chicago: Gross & Delbridge, 1889. 772p. IEN-M; OCIM **80-5465**

RUMBOLD, Thomas F[razier] (1830-1901)
Hygiene and treatment of catarrh; hygienic and sanative measures for chronic catarrhal inflammation of the nose, throat, and ears. Part I. St. Louis: G. O. Rumbold & Co., 1880. 174p. DLC; DNLM; OCIM **80-5466**

RUMBOLD, Thomas F[razier] (1830-1901)
The hygiene and treatment of catarrh. Part 1. Hygienic and sanative measures. Part 2. Therapeutic measures. St. Louis: G. O. Rumbold & Co., 1881. 473p. DLC; DNLM; OCIM **80-5467**

RUMBOLD, Thomas F[razier] (1830-1901)
Hygienic and sanative measures for chronic catarrhal inflammation of the nose, throat and ears. . . . 2nd ed. . . . St. Louis: Medical Journal Publishing Co., 1882. 190p. DLC **80-5468**

RUMBOLD, Thomas F[razier] (1830-1901)
Pruritic rhinitis (hay-fever, autumnal catarrh, etc.). Its medical and surgical treatment. . . . St. Louis: Medical Journal Publishing Co., 1885. 167p. DLC **80-5469**

RUMBOLD, Thomas F[razier] (1830-1901)
A practical treatise on the medical, surgical and hygienic treatment of catarrhal diseases of the nose, throat, and ears; including anatomy, physiology, pathology, etiology, and symptomatology connected therewith . . . with 32 lith. plates, showing anatomical sections of the nasal and pharyngo-nasal cavities, and the cells and sinuses connected with them. 2nd ed. St. Louis: Medical Journal Publishing Co., 1888. 1054p. DLC; DNLM; OCIM **80-5470**

RUNNELS, Moses T[hurston] (1830-1902)
Drugs vs. public health. [Read at the 15th annual session of the Indiana Institute of Homoeopathy.] New York, [1881]. 16p. DNLM **80-5471**

RUNNELS, Moses T[hurston] (1830-1902)
Physical degeneracy of American women. [Chicago, 1886.] 16p. DNLM **80-5472**

RUSCHENBERGER, W[illiam] S[amuel] W[aithman] (1807-1895)
A sketch of the life of Thomas Stewardson, read before the College [of Physicians of Philadelphia], November 7, 1883. Philadelphia, 1883. 22p. DNLM; PPC **80-5473**

RUSCHENBERGER, W[illiam] S[amuel] W[aithman] (1807-1895)
A memory of Dr. George Fox, read before the College [of Physicians of Philadelphia], November 7, 1883. Philadelphia, 1883. 23p. DNLM; PPC **80-5474**

RUSCHENBERGER, W[illiam] S[amuel] W[aithman] (1807-1895)
A sketch of Robert Bridges. Philadelphia, 1884. 23p. DNLM; PPC **80-5475**

RUSCHENBERGER, W[illiam] S[amuel] W[aithman] (1807-1895)
A sketch of the life of Robert E. Rogers, with biographical notices of his father and brothers. Philadelphia: McCalla & Stavely, 1885. 45p. DNLM; PPC **80-5476**

RUSCHENBERGER, W[illiam] S[amuel] W[aithman] (1807-1895)
An account of the institution and progress of the College of Physicians of Philadelphia, during a hundred years, from January, 1787. Philadelphia: W. J. Dornan, 1887. 308p. DNLM; PPC **80-5477**

RUSH MEDICAL COLLEGE. MEDICAL DEPARTMENT OF LAKE FOREST UNIVERSITY
Annual announcements for the sessions of 1889-1890 to 1901-1902 (47.-59.); 1904-1905 (62.). Chicago, 1889-1904. DNLM; ICRM **80-5478**

RUSH MEDICAL COLLEGE. MEDICAL DEPARTMENT OF THE UNIVERSITY OF CHICAGO
Progress in medical education; being the doctorate address at the thirty-ninth annual commencement of . . . Feb. 22, 1881, by J. Adams Allen. [With secretary's report for the session of 1880-1881.] Chicago: Chicago Legal News Co., 1881. 20p. DNLM; ICRM **80-5479**

RUSH MEDICAL COLLEGE. MEDICAL DEPARTMENT OF THE UNIVERSITY OF CHICAGO
Annual announcements for the sessions of 1845-1846 (3.); 1848-1849 (6.); 1849-1850 (7.); 1856-1857 to 1869-1870 (14.-27.); 1871-1872 to 1873-1874 (29.-31.); 1875-1876 to 1887-1888 (33.-45.). Chicago, 1845-1887. DNLM; ICRM [Incorporated March 2, 1837. First session commenced Dec. 4, 1843. In 1875 it became the medical department of the University of Chicago. List of students and graduates for the sessions of 1844-1845, 1846-1847, 1849-1850, 1855-1856 to 1868-1869, 1870-1871 to 1872-1873, 1874-1875, 1876-1877 to 1886-1887, in announcements for subsequent years. List of graduates since its organization, 1844 to 1884, in announcement for 1884-1885, 33., in the catalogue of the University of Chicago, for 1874-1875.] **80-5480**

RUSSELL, George H.
A new discovery. The functions of the spleen. Containing an explanation of the functions of the spleen; its relations to the circulation of the blood and the stomach, with advanced philosophical views upon the creation of force and motion in the circulation of the blood, etc. Newburg, Pa.: Telephone Print, 1882. 11p. DNLM **80-5481**

RUSSELL, Ira (1815-1888)
A case of general paresis. [St. Louis, 1880.] 12p. DNLM **80-5482**

RUSSELL, Ira (1815-1888)
Mysophobia. Melancholia with filth dread; mania contaminations. [St. Louis, 1880.] 5p. DNLM **80-5483**

RUSSELL, Ira (1815-1888)
Insanity; a description of some of its forms, symptoms, and method of treatment. Winchendon, Mass.: F. W. Ward, 1883. 18p. DNLM **80-5484**

RUST BROTHERS & BIRD
Catalogue of drugs and druggists' articles. Boston, 1880. 164p. MBM **80-5485**

SACHS, Bernard (1858-1944)
On the use of the absolute galvanometer, with description of Hirschmann's new instrument. [New York, 1885.] 8p. DNLM **80-5486**

SACHS, Bernard (1858-1944)
A contribution to the study of tumors of the spinal cord. New York, 1886. 22p. DNLM **80-5487**

SACHS, Bernard (1858-1944)
Intracerebral hemorrhage in the young. [Chicago, 1887.] 7p. DNLM **80-5488**

SACHS, Bernard (1858-1944)
On arrested cerebral development, with special reference to its cortical pathology. New York, 1887. 15p. 1 plate. DNLM **80-5489**

SACHS, Bernard (1858-1944)
Notes on the cause and treatment of functional insomnia. [Philadelphia, 1887.] 16p. DNLM **80-5490**

SACHS, Bernard (1858-1944)
Progressive muscular dystrophies: the relation of the primary forms to one another and to typical progressive muscular atrophy. New York, 1888. 44p. DNLM **80-5491**

SACHS, Bernard (1858-1944)
Polioencephalitis superior (nuclear ophthalmoplegia) and poliomyelitis. Philadelphia, 1889. 7p. DNLM **80-5492**

SADTLER, Samuel Philip (1847-1923)
The debt of medical and sanitary science to synthetic chemistry. Philadelphia, 1889. 17p. DNLM **80-5493**

SAINT LOUIS COLLEGE OF HOMOEOPATHIC PHYSICIANS AND SURGEONS
Annual announcement and catalogue for the session of 1881-1882. St. Louis: C. Maynard, 1881. 23p. DNLM [Official list of the alumni from 1860 to 1880, in announcement for 1881-1882.] **80-5494**

SAINT LOUIS COLLEGE OF PHYSICIANS AND SURGEONS
Annual announcements for the sessions of 1885-1886 (7.); 1890-1891 to 1898-1899 (12.-20.); 1906-1907 (28.). Saint Louis, 1885-1906. DNLM **80-5495**

SAINT LOUIS MEDICAL COLLEGE
Announcement for the spring session of 1882. St. Louis, 1882. 3 l. DNLM **80-5496**

SAJOUS, Charles Euchariste de Medici (1852-1929)
Glacial acetic acid in nasal hypertrophy. [Philadelphia, 1881.] 14p. DNLM **80-5497**

SAJOUS, Charles Euchariste de Medici (1852-1929)
A case of abductor paralysis due to lead poisoning. [New York, 1882.] 1 l. DNLM **80-5498**

SAJOUS, Charles Euchariste de Medici (1852-1929)
Two cases of fracture of the thyroid cartilage. [New York: G. P. Putnam's Sons, 1882.] 2p. DNLM **80-5499**

SAJOUS, Charles Euchariste de Medici (1852-1929)
Inhalations in laryngeal and pulmonary affections. A new instrument. [Philadelphia, 1883.] 4p. DNLM **80-5500**

SAJOUS, Charles Euchariste de Medici (1852-1929)
A new wire snare écraseur. Philadelphia, 1883. 1 galley sheet. DNLM **80-5501**

SAJOUS, Charles Euchariste de Medici (1852-1929)
Notes on hay fever. [Philadelphia, 1883.] 13p. DNLM **80-5502**

SAJOUS, Charles Euchariste de Medici (1852-1929)
Hydrochlorate of cocaine in the treatment of nasal affections. [Philadelphia, 1884.] 8p. DNLM **80-5503**

SAJOUS, Charles Euchariste de Medici (1852-1929)
Modification of Cohen's laryngeal forceps, making them adaptable for post-nasal, pharyngeal, and laryngeal applications. Philadelphia, 1884. 1 sheet. DNLM **80-5504**

SAJOUS, Charles Euchariste de Medici (1852-1929)
Hay fever and its successful treatment by superficial organic alteration of the nasal mucous membrane. Philadelphia: F. A. Davis, 1885. 103p. DNLM **80-5505**

SAJOUS, Charles Euchariste de Medici (1852-1929)
Lectures on the diseases of the nose and throat, delivered during the spring session of Jefferson Medical College. Philadelphia: F. A. Davis, 1885. 439p. 8 plates. DNLM **80-5506**

SALISBURY, James Henry (1823-1905)
Malaria. . . . McNaughton prize essay, 1882. Awarded by the Albany Medical College Alumni Association. New York: W. A. Kellogg, 1885. 152p. DLC; NNNAM **80-5507**

SALISBURY, James Henry (1823-1905)
The relation of alimentation and diseases. . . . New York: J. H. Vail & Co., 1888. 332p. DLC; DNLM; NNNAM **80-5508**

SALTER, Henry H. (1823-1871)
Asthma, its pathology and treatment. New York: William Wood & Co., 1882. 284p. IU-M; MBM; NNNAM; PPC **80-5509**

SALTER, S[eaborn] F[reeman]
Principles and practice of American medicine and surgery. . . . Atlanta, Ga.: J. P. Harrison & Co., 1883. 621p. DLC; GU **80-5510**

SALZER, L.
Lectures on cholera, and its homoeopathic treatment. Chicago: Duncan Bros., 1884. 236p. IU-M; OCIM; PPHa **80-5511**

SANDS, Henry Berton (1830-1888)
On the rupture of veins, with the report of a case in which the rupture of a deep femoral vein was successfully treated by ligation of the ruptured vessel. New York: G. P. Putnam's Sons, 1885. 15p. DNLM; NNNAM **80-5512**

SANDS, Henry Berton (1830-1888)
An account of a case in which recovery took place after laparotomy had been performed for septic peritonitis due to a perforation of the vermiform appendix. [New York, 1888.] 30p. DNLM; NNNAM **80-5513**

THE SARAH BERNHARDT book of beauty; ladies' and gentlemen's toilet companion; how to become beautiful forever; no more ugly faces, and handsome ones made still more handsome; cures for all diseases affecting personal appearance; all the valuable recipes of the world; how to become fat and how to become thin. New York: E. G. Rideout, 1881. 90p. DNLM; NN **80-5514**

SARGENT INVALID FURNITURE CO.
Price list of beds, chairs, operating tables. . . . Boston, 1883. 16p. NNNAM **80-5515**

SARGENT INVALID FURNITURE CO.
Illustrated catalogue of invalid beds, chairs, tables. . . . Boston, 1888. 96p. NNNAM **80-5516**

SATCHWELL, S[olomon] S[ampson] (1821-1892)
Memorial of Prof. Otis Frederick Manson. (1822-1888). [1888.] 7p. port. DNLM **80-5517**

SATTERTHWAITE, Thomas Edward (*b.* 1843)
Suppurative disease of the ankle in children and young adults. A record of twenty-six cases. New York: Trow, 1880. 20p. DNLM **80-5518**

SATTERTHWAITE, Thomas Edward, ed. (*b.* 1843)
A manual of histology, ed. and prepared by Thomas E. Satterthwaite . . . in association with Drs. Thomas Dwight, J. Collins Warren, William F. Whitney, Clarence J. Blake [and others] . . . . With one hundred and ninety-eight illustrations. New York: William Wood & Co., 1881. 478p. DLC; DNLM; NNNAM; PU **80-5519**

SATTERTHWAITE, Thomas Edward (*b.* 1843)
The study of comparative pathology. Introductory lecture of a course delivered at the Columbia Veterinary College, 1881-1882. New York: W. L. Hyde & Co., 1882. 13p. DNLM **80-5520**

SATTERTHWAITE, Thomas Edward (*b.* 1843)
An introduction to practical bacteriology. A guide for students and general practitioners. Detroit: G. S. Davis, 1887. 85p. 1 plate. DLC; DNLM; OCIM **80-5521**

SATTLER, Eric E[ricson] (*b.* 1859)
A history of tuberculosis from the time of Sylvius to the present day, being in part a transl., with notes and additions, from the German of Dr. Arnold Spina, containing also an account of the researches and discoveries of Dr. Robert Koch and other recent investigators. Cincinnati: R. Clarke & Co., 1883. 191p. DNLM; OCHP **80-5522**

SATTLER, Robert
A case of one-sided transitory exophthalmos, with undisturbed function and muscular movements of the eye and the co-existence of enophthalmos or recession of the globe. [Philadelphia, 1885.] 4p. DNLM **80-5523**

SATTLER, Robert
Pulsating proptosis and elastic tumor of left orbit consequent upon a trauma of the skull; ligation of left common carotid. New York: Trow's Co., 1885. 24p. DNLM **80-5524**

SATURDAY lectures delivered in the lecture-room of the U.S. National Museum under the auspices of the Anthropological and Biological Societies of Washington in March and April, 1882. Washington, D.C.: Judd & Detweiler, 1882. 185p. DNLM **80-5525**

SAVAGE, George H. (1842-1921)
Insanity and allied neuroses: practical and clinical. Philadelphia: Henry C. Lea's Son & Co., 1884. 544p. CtY-M; NNNAM; PPC; PU **80-5526**

SAVAGE, Henry (*d.* 1900)
The surgery, surgical pathology, and surgical anatomy of the female pelvic organs, in a series of plates taken from nature with commentaries, notes and cases. 3rd ed., rev. and greatly enl. New York: William Wood & Co., 1880. 129p. + 32 plates. IU-M; NNNAM; OCIM; PPC **80-5527**

SAWYER, Edward Warren (*d.* 1897)
Mania lactea, with the report of two cases. [Philadelphia, 1882.] 6p. DNLM **80-5528**

SAWYER, Edward Warren (*d.* 1897)
Remarks on the occipito-posterior position in vertex labors, with an analysis of thirty-eight cases. [Chicago, 1884.] 12p. DNLM **80-5529**

SAYRE, Lewis A[lbert] (1820-1900)
Presidential address before the American Medical Association at its thirty-firt annual session, New York City, June 1, 1880. Philadelphia: Collins, 1880. 20p. DNLM; PPC **80-5530**

SAYRE, Lewis A[lbert] (1820-1900)
A clinical surgical lecture delivered in Bellevue Hospital amphitheatre, December 24, 1879. New York, 1880. 15p. DNLM; NNU-M **80-5531**

SAYRE, Lewis A[lbert] (1820-1900)
Shortening of limbs after fracture. New York: Trow, 1881. 16p. DNLM; NNNAM **80-5532**

SAYRE, Lewis A[lbert] (1820-1900)
A practical manual of the treatment of club-foot. . . . 4th ed., enl. and cor. New York: D. Appleton & Co., 1882. 143p. DLC; NNNAM **80-5533**

SAYRE, Lewis A[lbert] (1820-1900)
Clinical lecture. Fracture of the clavicle. Newtown, Conn., 1883. 2p. DNLM **80-5534**

SAYRE, Lewis A[lbert] (1820-1900)
Lectures on orthopedic surgery and diseases of the joints, delivered at Bellevue Hospital Medical College, during the winter session of 1874-1875. . . . 2nd ed., rev. and greatly enl., with 324 illustrations. New York: D. Appleton & Co., 1883. 589p. tables, col. front. DLC; DNLM; NNNAM; NNU-M **80-5535**

SAYRE, Lewis A[lbert] (1820-1900)
On disease of the knee-joint. [Philadelphia, 1884.] 16p. DNLM **80-5536**

SAYRE, Lewis A[lbert] (1820-1900)
Spondylitis and rotary lateral curvature of spine; their proper treatment practically demonstrated, with exhibition of cases. New York, 1885. 46p. DNLM; NNNAM **80-5537**

SAYRE, Lewis A[lbert] (1820-1900)
On the advantages of plaster-of-Paris dressings as a means of spinal support. [New York, 1888.] 20p. DNLM **80-5538**

SAYRE, Lewis A[lbert] (1820-1900)
On the deleterious results of a narrow prepuce and preputial adhesions. Philadelphia: W. F. Fell & Co., [1888]. 8 l. DNLM **80-5539**

SAYRE, Lewis A[lbert] (1820-1900)
Section of contractured tissues essential before mechanical treatment can be effectual. Philadelphia: W. F. Fell & Co., [1888]. 7 l. DNLM **80-5540**

SAYRE, L[ucius] E[lmer] (1847-1925)
Conspectus of organic materia medica and pharmacal botany, comprising the vegetable and animal drugs: their physical character, geographical origin, classification, constituents, doses, adulterations, etc. Table of the tests and solubilities of the alkaloids appended. Detroit: G. S. Davis, 1880. 220p. 1 table. DNLM; OCLloyd **80-5541**

SAYRE, Reginald H[all] (1859-1929)
The immediate restoration of parts to the normal position, after tenotomy. New York: Gilliss Bros. & Turnure, 1886. 18p. 1 l. DNLM; NNNAM **80-5542**

SAYRE, Reginald H[all] (1859-1929)
The result of antiseptic treatment of abscesses connected with disease of the hip joint. New York, 1888. 7p. DNLM **80-5543**

SAYRE, Reginald H[all] (1859-1929)
The treatment of rotary lateral curvature of the spine. New York, 1888. 21p. DNLM; NNU-M **80-5544**

SCHÄFER, Edward Albert (1850-1935)
The essentials of histology, descriptive and practical. For the use of students. Philadelphia: Lea Bros. & Co., 1885. 245p. CtY-M; DNLM; NNNAM; PPC **80-5545**

SCHAPRINGER, Alois
Ueber Extraktion des Altersstaars ohne Iridektomie. [New York, 1887.] 8p. DNLM **80-5546**

SCHAPRINGER, Alois
Ein Fall von metastatischem Carcinom der Chorioidea. New York, 1888. 8p. 2 plates. DNLM **80-5547**

SCHAPRINGER, Alois
A case of metastatic carcinoma of the choroid. [New York, 1888.] 13p. DNLM **80-5548**

SCHAPRINGER, Alois
Miliartuberkulose der Iris und der Choroidea bei einem fünfmonatlichen Kinde. Wissenschaftliche Zusammenkünfte deutscher Aerzte von New York. [New York, 1888.] 3p. DNLM **80-5549**

SCHAPRINGER, Alois
Ueber angeborene beiderseitige Pleuroplegie (Abducens) und Facialislähmung. [New York, 1889.] 12p. DNLM **80-5550**

SCHENK, Peter V. (1838-1885)
A successful case of ovariotomy and hysterectomy combined. New York, 1881. 2p. DNLM **80-5551**

SCHENK, Peter V. (1838-1885)
Uterine functions and disease, one hundred and ten cases of Emmet's operation. St. Louis, 1881. 49p. DNLM **80-5552**

SCHENK, W. L.
Preventive and state medicine. An address delivered before the State Sanitary Convention, at Topeka, Kans., December, 1887. [n. p., 1887.] 13p. DNLM **80-5553**

SCHIEFFELIN, W. H. & CO.
Pharmaceutical preparations. . . . New York, 1880. 52p. NNNAM **80-5554**

SCHIEFFELIN, W. H. & CO.
General prices current. . . . New York, 1881. 427p. NNNAM **80-5555**

SCHIEFFELIN, W. H. & CO.
General prices current. . . . New York, 1883. 479p. NNNAM **80-5556**

SCHIEFFELIN, W. H. & CO.
General prices current. . . . New York, 1885. 554p. NNNAM **80-5557**

SCHIEFFELIN, W. H. & CO.
A treatise on salol, the new remedy for rheumatism and rheumatic affections, diarrhoea, dysentery, typhoid fever, etc., and antiseptically as a surgical dressing. Manufactured by Dr. F. von Heyden's successors at Radebeul-Dresden. 2nd ed. New York: W. H. Schieffelin & Co., 1888. 22p. DNLM; NNNAM **80-5558**

SCHMIDT, Henry D. (1823-1888)
The pathology and treatment of yellow fever; with some remarks upon the nature of its cause and its prevention. . . . Chicago: The Chicago Medical Press Association, 1881. 240p. DLC; IU-M; OCIM **80-5559**

SCHREIBER, Joseph (1835-1908)
A manual of treatment by massage and methodical muscle exercise; transl., with the author's permission by Walter Mendelson. Philadelphia: Lea Bros. & Co., 1887. 285p. DNLM; MBM; NNNAM; PPC **80-5560**

SCHULTZ, Carl H.
Carl H. Schultz's mineral spring waters, their chemical composition, physiological action, therapeutic and general use. . . . New York: W. Wallach, stationer and printer, 1880. 36p. DLC; NNNAM **80-5561**

SCHULTZ, Carl H.
The mineral water controversy. Artificial or natural? Conflicting official opinions. The U.S. chemists and the Attorney-General overruled by the Secretary of the Treasury. His novel chemical theory that natural products can be manufactured. A review of the whole question on behalf of American mineral waters. New York: E. Wells Sackett & Rankin, 1882. 32p. DNLM; NNNAM **80-5562**

SCHÜSSLER, Wilhelm Heinrich (1821-1898)
Abridged therapeutics, founded upon histology and cellular pathology, with an appendix giving special directions for the application of the inorganic cell salts, and indications of the underlying conditions of morbid states of tissue. Biochemic method of successfully treating disease. Authorized transl. by M. Docetti Walker. New York: Gavin Houston, 1880. 199p. NNNAM; OCLloyd; PPHa **80-5563**

SCHÜSSLER, Wilhelm Heinrich (1821-1898)
The cure of diphtheria by biochemic treatment: a word to educated laymen. . . . Ed. and transl. by M. Docetti Walker. By special permission. . . . New York: G. Houston, 1881. 51p. DLC; NNNAM **80-5564**

SCHÜSSLER, Wilhelm Heinrich (1821-1898)
Abridged therapeutics founded upon histology and cellular pathology with an appendix: special indications for the application of the inorganic tissue-formers. . . . Authorized transl. by M. Docetti Walker. 8th ed. New York: G. Houston, 1884. 215p. DLC; NNNAM **80-5565**

SCHÜSSLER, Wilhelm Heinrich (1821-1898)
Abridged therapeutics founded upon histology and cellular pathology with an appendix; giving special directions for the application of the inorganic cell salts and indications of the underlying condition of morbid states of tissue. Biochemic method of successfully treating disease. Authorized transl. by M. Docetti Walker. 9th ed. New York: G. Houston, 1884. 226p. DLC; DNLM; NNNAM; OCLloyd
80-5566

SCHÜSSLER, Wilhelm Heinrich (1821-1898)
An abbreviated therapy; the biochemical treatment of disease. 12th ed., partly rewritten, with appendix containing clinical histories. Transl., with the addition of a repertory, by J. T. O'Connor. Philadelphia: F. E. Boericke, 1885. 94p. DLC; DNLM; PPC; PPHa **80-5567**

SCHÜSSLER, Wilhelm Heinrich (1821-1898)
Abridged therapeutics founded upon histology and cellular pathology, with an appendix giving special directions for the application of the inorganic cell salts, and indications of the underlying condition of morbid states of tissue. Biochemic method of successfully treating disease. Authorized transl. by M. Docetti Walker. 13th ed. New York: G. Houston, [1886]. 166p. DLC; DNLM; NNNAM; OCLloyd
80-5568

SCHÜSSLER, Wilhelm Heinrich (1821-1898)
Abridged therapeutics founded upon histology and cellular pathology with an appendix; giving special directions for the application of the inorganic cell salts and indications of the underlying condition of morbid states of tissue. Biochemic method of successfully treating disease. Authorized transl. by M. Docetti Walker. 15th ed., enlarged. New York: G. Houston, [1883]. 112p. DLC; DNLM; NNNAM
80-5569

SCHWABE, Willmar, ed.
Pharmacopoea homeopathica polyglotta. . . . Rendered into English by Lemuel Steffens. Leipzig: W. Schwabe; New York: Boericke & Tafel, 1880. 374p. OCLloyd
80-5570

de SCHWEINITZ, G[eorg] E[dmund] (1858-1938)
Notes of a case of optic atrophy and temporal hemianopsia; suspected tumor of the pituitary body. [Philadelphia, 1887.] 8p. DNLM **80-5571**

de SCHWEINITZ, G[eorg] E[dmund] (1858-1938)
Tuberculous tumors of the cerebellum in a child four years old; autopsy and microscopical examination. [Philadelphia, 1887.] 2p. DNLM **80-5572**

de SCHWEINITZ, G[eorg] E[dmund] (1858-1938)
Acute unilateral optic neuritis, with the report of a case. Philadelphia: W. J. Dornan, 1888. 7p. DNLM
80-5573

de SCHWEINITZ, G[eorg] E[dmund] (1858-1938)
A case of leukaemic retinitis. [St. Louis, 1888.] 4p. DNLM **80-5574**

de SCHWEINITZ, G[eorg] E[dmund] (1858-1938)
An examination of the eyes of fifty cases of chorea of childhood. [New York, 1888.] 13p. DNLM
80-5575

de SCHWEINITZ, G[eorg] E[dmund] (1858-1938)
Ophthalmic memoranda. [Philadelphia, 1889.] 2p. DNLM **80-5576**

de SCHWEINITZ, G[eorg] E[dmund] (1858-1938)
Massage of the cornea. [Philadelphia, 1889.] 3p. DNLM **80-5577**

de SCHWEINITZ, G[eorg] E[dmund] (1858-1938)
The use of ascending doses of nux vomica, as an aid in the treatment of insufficiences of the ocular muscles. [Philadelphia, 1889.] 11p. DNLM **80-5578**

de SCHWEINITZ, G[eorg] E[dmund] (1858-1938)
Spontaneous dislocation of both crystalline lenses into the anterior chambers. [Philadelphia, 1889.] 2p. DNLM
80-5579

SCUDDER, Charles D[avies] (1856-1892)
Mollities uteri. [New York, 1886.] 7p. DNLM
80-5580

SCUDDER, Charles Locke (1860-1949)
Congenital talipes equinovarus. Boston: Cupples & Hurd, 1887. 20p. DNLM **80-5581**

SCUDDER, John Milton (1829-1894)
The eclectic practice in diseases of children. . . . Rev. ed. Cincinnati: Pub. by the author, 1881. 486p. DLC; OCIM **80-5582**

SCUDDER, John Milton (1829-1894)
Specific medication and specific medicines. 4th revision. With an appendix containing the articles published on the subject since the first edition. And a report of cases illustrating specific medication. . . . 11th ed. Cincinnati: Wilstach, Baldwin & Co., printers, 1884. 432p. DLC; OCIM; OCLloyd
80-5583

SCUDDER, John Milton (1829-1894)
Eclecticism. What is it? [1885?]. 8p. DNLM; OCLloyd
80-5584

SCUDDER, John Milton (1829-1894)
The eclectic family physician. . . . 21st ed., 5th revision. . . . With appendix. Cincinnati: J. K. Scudder, 1887. 884p. DLC; OCIM; OCLloyd **80-5585**

SCUDDER, John Milton (1829-1894)
A brief history of eclectic medicine. [1887?] 12p. DNLM; OCLloyd **80-5586**

SCUDDER, John Milton (1829-1894)
A complete descriptive catalogue and price-list of medical books published and for sale by . . . . Cincinnati, 1889. 6 l. DNLM; OCLloyd **80-5587**

SEARLE, William S. (*b.* 1833)
A new form of nervous disease: together with an essay on erythroxylon coca. New York: Ford, Howard & Hurlburt, 1881. 133p. NNNAM; PPHa **80-5588**

SEE, Germain (1818-1896)
Diseases of the lungs (of a specific not tuberculous nature). Acute bronchites; infectious pneumonia; gangrene, syphilis, cancer and hydatid of the lungs. Transl. by E. P. Hurd, with appendices by Geo. M. Sternberg [and] Dujardin Beaumetz. New York: William Wood & Co., 1885. 398p. DNLM; NNNAM; PPC **80-5589**

SEGUIN, Edward C[onstant] (1843-1898)
Lunacy reform. III. Our asylums as seen by a competent foreign visitor. [New York, 1880.] 12p. DNLM **80-5590**

SEGUIN, Edward C[onstant] (1843-1898)
Lunacy reform. IV. The right of the insane to liberty. New York: G. P. Putnam's Son, 1880. 10p. DNLM **80-5591**

SEGUIN, Edward C[onstant] (1843-1898)
A lecture on the localization of diseases in the spinal cord. Brooklyn, 1880. 20p. DNLM **80-5592**

SEGUIN, Edward C[onstant] (1843-1898)
On occipital headache as a symptom of uraemia. [New York, 1880.] 5p. DNLM **80-5593**

SEGUIN, Edward C[onstant] (1843-1898)
The cultivation of specialties in medicine. New York: G. P. Putnam's Sons, 1880. 14p. DNLM **80-5594**

SEGUIN, Edward C[onstant] (1843-1898)
On the coincidence of optic neuritis and subacute transverse myelitis. [New York, 1880.] 12p. DNLM **80-5595**

SEGUIN, Edward C[onstant] (1843-1898)
A second contribution to the study of localized cerebral lesions. [Chicago, 1881.] 43p. DNLM **80-5596**

SEGUIN, Edward C[onstant] (1843-1898)
A case of abscess of the left frontal lobe of the cerebrum, with special reference to localization. [New York, 1881.] 5p. DNLM **80-5597**

SEGUIN, Edward C[onstant] (1843-1898)
On the early diagnosis of some organic diseases of the nervous system. New York: Trow, 1881. 19p. DNLM **80-5598**

SEGUIN, Edward C[onstant] (1843-1898)
Higher medical education in New York. I. Organization of the medical staff of hospitals. New York: G. P. Putnam's Sons, 1881. 10p. DNLM **80-5599**

SEGUIN, Edward C[onstant] (1843-1898)
Higher medical education in New York. II. Reorganization of the medical staff of hospitals. New York: G. P. Putnam's Sons, 1881. 11p. DNLM **80-5600**

SEGUIN, Edward C[onstant] (1843-1898)
Higher medical education in New York. III. The system of clinical teaching in colleges. New York, 1881. 9p. DNLM **80-5601**

SEGUIN, Edward C[onstant] (1843-1898)
Importance of the early recognition of epilepsy. New York: Trow's Ptg. & Bookbndg. Co., 1881. 26p. DNLM; NNNAM **80-5602**

SEGUIN, Edward C[onstant] (1843-1898)
The efficient dosage of certain remedies used in the treatment of nervous diseases. Syracuse, 1882. 20p. DNLM **80-5603**

SEGUIN, Edward C[onstant] (1843-1898)
On a peculiar cutaneous lesion (ulcus elevatum) occurring during the use of bromide of potassium. New York: G. P. Putnam's Sons, 1882. 9p. DNLM **80-5604**

SEGUIN, Edward C[onstant] (1843-1898)
Post-graduate instruction. New York: G. P. Putnam's Sons, 1882. 11p. DNLM **80-5605**

SEGUIN, Edward C[onstant] (1843-1898)
Hysterical convulsions and hemianaesthesia in an adult male; cure by metallo-therapy (gold). [New York, 1882.] 3p. DNLM **80-5606**

SEGUIN, Edward C[onstant] (1843-1898)
Myelitis following acute arsenical poisoning (by Paris or Schweinfurth green). [New York, 1882.] 16p. DNLM **80-5607**

SEGUIN, Edward C[onstant] (1843-1898)
Notes on Spanish asylums for the insane. Lancaster, Pa., 1883. 42p. DNLM; NNNAM **80-5608**

SEGUIN, Edward C[onstant] (1843-1898)
Illustrations of the anomalous course of posterior spinal sclerosis. [New York, 1884.] 11p. DNLM **80-5609**

SEGUIN, Edward C[onstant] (1843-1898)
The American method of giving potassium iodide in very large doses for the later lesions of syphilis; more especially syphilis of the nervous system. [New York, 1884.] 18p. DNLM **80-5610**

SEGUIN, Edward C[onstant] (1843-1898)
Opera minora. A collection of essays, articles, lectures, and addresses, from 1866 to 1882, inclusive. New York: G. P. Putnam's Sons, 1884. 687p. DLC; DNLM **80-5611**

SEGUIN, Edward C[onstant] (1843-1898)
A contribution to the pathology of hemianopsia of central origin (cortex-hemianopsia). New York: G. P. Putnam's Sons, [1886]. 38p. DNLM **80-5612**

SEGUIN, Edward C[onstant] (1843-1898)
A contribution to the pathology of the cerebellum. New York: J. H. Vail & Co., 1887. 19p. DNLM **80-5613**

SEGUIN, Edward C[onstant] (1843-1898)
A second clinical study of hemianopsia. Cases of chiasm-lesion. Demonstration of hemiopic pupillary inaction. New York, 1887. 19p. DNLM **80-5614**

SEGUIN, Edward C[onstant] (1843-1898)
A third contribution to the study of localized cerebral lesions. New York: J. H. Vail & Co., 1887. 10p. DNLM **80-5615**

SEGUIN, Edward C[onstant] (1843-1898)
The relation between trophic lesions and diseases of the nervous system. New York: M. J. Rooney & Co., 1888. 10p. DNLM **80-5616**

DR. SEGUIN'S metric prescription book. New York & London: G. P. Putnam's Sons, 1885. 52 l. DNLM; NNNAM **80-5617**

SEIBERT, August (1854-1926)
Stomach washing in infants, with a demonstration on the living subject. [New York, 1889.] 9p. DNLM **80-5618**

SEIBERT, August (1854-1926)
The surgical treatment of erysipelas in children. [New York, 1889.] 4p. DNLM **80-5619**

SEIFERT, Otto (1853-1933) and Friedrich MÜLLER
Manual of clinical diagnosis. 3rd ed., revised and corrected by Friedrich Müller. Transl., with the permission of the authors, by William Buckingham Canfield. New York & London: G. P. Putnam's Sons, 1887. 173p. DNLM; NNNAM; OCIM; PPC **80-5620**

SEILER, Burkhard Wilhelm
A case of papillary growth of the larynx. [New York, 1881.] 6p. DNLM **80-5621**

SEILER, Burkhard Wilhelm
Catching cold. [Philadelphia, 1881.] 3p. DNLM **80-5622**

SEILER, Burkhard Wilhelm
Jarvis' operation in hypertrophic nasal catarrh; with report of three cases. New York: Trow, 1881. 14p. DNLM **80-5623**

SEILER, Burkhard Wilhelm
Two cases of reflex laryngeal cough, due to irritation of the nasal mucous membrane. New York, 1882. 5p. DNLM **80-5624**

SEILER, Burkhard Wilhelm
On the pathology of phthisis pulmonaris and its laryngeal complications. [Chicago, 1883.] 7p. DNLM **80-5625**

SEILER, Burkhard Wilhelm
Ecchondroses of the septum narium and their removal. [New York, 1888.] 12p. DNLM **80-5626**

SEILER, Carl (1849-1905)
Some remarks on the diagnosis and treatment of incipient phthisis. Read before the Philadelphia County Medical Society, May 12, 1880. [Philadelphia], 1880, 2 l. DNLM **80-5627**

SEILER, Carl (1849-1905)
Jarvis' operation in hypertrophic nasal catarrh, with report of three cases. New York: Trow, 1881. 14p. DNLM **80-5628**

SEILER, Carl (1849-1905)
Compendium of microscopical technology. A guide to physicians and students in the use of the microscope and in the preparation of histological and pathological specimens. . . . Philadelphia: D. G. Brinton, 1881. 130p. DLC; DNLM; PPC; PU **80-5629**

SEILER, Carl (1849-1905)
Handbook of the diagnosis and treatment of the diseases of the throat, nose, and naso-pharynx. . . . 2nd ed., thoroughly rev. and greatly enl. With thirty-seven illustrations. Philadelphia: Henry C. Lea's Son & Co., 1883. 295p. tables. DLC; NNNAM; PPC; PPJ **80-5630**

SEILER, Carl (1849-1905)
Ecchondroses of the septum narium and their removal. New York: Trow, 1888. 12p. DNLM; NNNAM **80-5631**

SEILER, Carl (1849-1905)
Handbook of the diagnosis and treatment of diseases of the throat, nose and naso-pharynx. . . . 3rd ed., thoroughly rev. and greatly enl. Illustrated with two lithographic plates containing ten figures, and one hundred and one wood engravings. Philadelphia: Lea Bros. & Co., 1889. 373p. tables, col. plates. DLC; NcD; NNNAM; PPC **80-5632**

SELL, E. H. M[iller] (1832-1920)
The opium habit; its successful treatment by the avena sativa. A paper read before the New York State Medical Society, February 9, 1882. New York: Bermingham & Co., [1882]. 8p. NNNAM **80-5633**

SEMON, Felix (1849-1921)
Proceedings of the subsection—diseases of the throat—of the seventh International Medical Congress, held in London, Aug. 2nd-9th, 1881. New York, 1881. 35p. DNLM; NNNAM **80-5634**

SEMON, Felix (1849-1921)
Clinical remarks on the proclivity of the abductor fibres of the recurrent laryngeal nerve to become affected sooner than the abductor fibres, or even exclusively, in cases of undoubted central or peripheral injury or disease of the roots or trunks of the pneumogastric, spinal accessory, or recurrent nerves. New York: G. P. Putnam's Sons, 1881. 26p. DNLM; NNNAM **80-5635**

SEMPLE, C. E. Armand (1845-1895)
Aids to materia medica and therapeutics. Pt. 2 (double part): The vegetable and animal substances. New York: G. P. Putnam's Sons, 1880. 152p. DNLM; NNNAM **80-5636**

SEMPLE, C. E. Armand (1845-1895)
Aids to medicine. Pt. 1 (double part): The general diseases, diseases of the lungs, heart, blood-vessels, and liver. New York: G. P. Putnam's Sons, 1883. 120p. DNLM; NNNAM **80-5637**

SEMPLE, C. E. Armand (1845-1895)
The diseases of children. A handbook for practitioners and students. New York & London: G. P. Putnam's Sons, 1884. 352p. DNLM; NNNAM; OCIM **80-5638**

SENN, N[icholas] (1844-1908)
The pathology and treatment of epulis. Address delivered by invitation, before the Wisconsin Dental Society. Philadelphia: J. B. Lippincott & Co., 1880. 13p. DNLM
80-5639

SENN, N[icholas] (1844-1908)
A contribution to a knowledge of fracture of the rim of the acetabulum, based on the reports of twenty-seven cases and experiments on the cadaver. Milwaukee, 1880. 30p. DNLM
80-5640

SENN, N[icholas] (1844-1908)
Spontaneous osteo-myelitis of the long bones. Chicago, 1880. 44p. DNLM **80-5641**

SENN, N[icholas] (1844-1908)
Recent progress in surgery; report to the Wisconsin State Medical Society. Milwaukee, 1881. 44p. DNLM
80-5642

SENN, N[icholas] (1844-1908)
Excision of the rectum for malignant disease. New York: W. S. Fowler, 1881. 16p. DNLM **80-5643**

SENN, N[icholas] (1844-1908)
Delayed and non-union of fractures. St. Louis: J. H. Chambers & Co., [1883]. 21p. DNLM **80-5644**

SENN, N[icholas] (1844-1908)
Fractures of the neck and femur, with special reference to bony union after intracapsular fracture. Philadelphia: Collins, 1883. 113p. DNLM **80-5645**

SENN, N[icholas] (1844-1908)
The pathology and morbid anatomy of tubercle. Report to the Wisconsin State Medical Society. Milwaukee, 1883. 33p. DNLM **80-5646**

SENN, N[icholas] (1844-1908)
On brachial cysts of the neck. Chicago: A. G. Newell, 1884. 44p. DNLM **80-5647**

SENN, N[icholas] (1844-1908)
Experimental researches on cicatrization in bloodvessels after ligature. Philadelphia: Collins, 1885. 117p. DNLM
80-5648

SENN, N[icholas] (1844-1908)
An experimental and clinical study of air-embolism. Philadelphia: Collins, 1885. 121p. DNLM **80-5649**

SENN, N[icholas] (1844-1908)
Introductory lecture on tumors. [Philadelphia], 1885. 22p. DNLM **80-5650**

SENN, N[icholas] (1844-1908)
The surgical treatment of cysts of the pancreas. Chicago, 1885. 58p. DNLM **80-5651**

SENN, N[icholas] (1844-1908)
Tetanus. Milwaukee, 1886. 27p. DNLM
80-5652

SENN, N[icholas] (1844-1908)
The address in surgery. The present status of abdominal surgery. Delivered at the thirty-seventh annual meeting of the American Medical Association. Chicago, 1886. 64p. DNLM
80-5653

SENN, N[icholas] (1844-1908)
Periostitis. [Philadelphia, 1886.] 20p. DNLM
80-5654

SENN, N[icholas] (1844-1908)
Surgical lesions of the brain, and its envelopes. [Philadelphia, 1886.] 23p. DNLM **80-5655**

SENN, N[icholas] (1844-1908)
Biology of tumors. Philadelphia, 1887. 36p. DNLM
80-5656

SENN, N[icholas] (1844-1908)
Four months among the surgeons of Europe. Being a series of letters to Dr. Chr. Fenger. Chicago, 1887. 157p. DNLM
80-5657

SENN, N[icholas] (1844-1908)
Importance and value of experimental research. Chicago: C. F. Ansell & Co., [1887]. 11p. DNLM
80-5658

SENN, N[icholas] (1844-1908)
Inflation of the stomach with hydrogen gas in the diagnosis of wounds and perforations of this organ. With the report of a case. 1888. 11p. DNLM **80-5659**

SENN, N[icholas] (1844-1908)
Rectal insufflation of hydrogen gas an infallible test in the diagnosis of visceral injury of the gastro-intestinal canal in penetrating wounds of the abdomen. Chicago, 1888. 48p. DNLM **80-5660**

SENN, N[icholas] (1844-1908)
Two cases of gunshot wound of the abdomen, illustrating the use of rectal insufflation with hydrogen gas as a diagnostic measure. 1888. 9p. DNLM **80-5661**

SENN, N[icholas] (1844-1908)
An experimental contribution to intestinal surgery with special reference to the treatment of intestinal obstruction. St. Louis: J. H. Chambers, 1888. 84p. 1 plate. DLC; DNLM
80-5662

SENN, N[icholas] (1844-1908)
On the healing of aseptic bone cavities by implantation of antiseptic decalcified bone. [Philadelphia, 1889.] 26p. DNLM
80-5663

SENN, N[icholas] (1844-1908)
A plea in favor of early laparotomy for catarrhal and ulcerative appendicitis, with the report of two cases. Chicago, 1889. 20p. DNLM **80-5664**

SENN, N[icholas] (1844-1908)
Experimental surgery. Chicago: W. T. Keener, 1889. 522p. DLC; DNLM **80-5665**

SENN, N[icholas] (1844-1908)
Intestinal surgery. Chicago: W. T. Keener, 1889. 269p. DLC; DNLM **80-5666**

SENN, N[icholas] (1844-1908)
Surgical bacteriology. Philadelphia: Lea Bros. & Co., 1889. 270p. 12 plates. DLC; DNLM **80-5667**

SENN, N[icholas] (1844-1908)
The surgical treatment of volvulus. [Philadelphia, 1889.] 29p. DNLM **80-5668**

SENN, N[icholas] (1844-1908)
The treatment of fractures of the neck of the femur by immediate reduction and permanent fixation. Chicago, 1889. 32p. DNLM **80-5669**

THE SEVEN mineral waters of Soden in the Taunus, Germany, and the diseases which are cured by them. A synopsis of medical monographs about Soden in the Taunus and its springs. New York, [1888]. 30p. DNLM **80-5670**

SEXTON, Samuel (1833-1896)
Causes of deafness among school children and its influences on education with remarks on the instruction of pupils with impaired hearing and on aural hygiene in the schools. Washington: Government Printing Office, 1881. 47p. DLC; DNLM **80-5671**

SEXTON, Samuel (1833-1896)
Anomalies of the membrana tympani and ossicles from interruption of intratympanic air-supply. New York: Trow's Printing & Bookbinding Co., 1881. 7p. DNLM **80-5672**

SEXTON, Samuel (1833-1896)
Occlusion of the external auditory meatus. Cambridge, 1882. 6p. DNLM **80-5673**

SEXTON, Samuel (1833-1896)
Employment of calcium sulphide in the treatment of inflammatory and suppurative aural disease. Cambirdge: Riverside Press, 1882. 8p. DNLM **80-5674**

SEXTON, Samuel (1833-1896)
On the necessity of providing for the better education of children with defective hearing in the public schools. New York: Trow's Printing & Bookbinding Co., 1884. 16p. DNLM **80-5675**

SEXTON, Samuel (1833-1896)
Destructive adenoma of the petrous portion of the temporal bone, involving the organ of hearing. [New York, 1884.] 15p. DNLM **80-5676**

SEXTON, Samuel (1833-1896)
On inflammation of the attic of the tympanium, and two fatal cases of ear disease in infants. New Bedford: Mercury Publishing Co., 1885. 22p. DNLM **80-5677**

SEXTON, Samuel (1833-1896)
The classification and treatment of over two thousand consecutive cases of ear diseases at Dr. Sexton's aural clinic, New York Eye and Ear Infirmary. Detroit: G. S. Davis, 1886. 95p. DNLM **80-5678**

SEXTON, Samuel (1833-1896)
Catarrh of the upper air-track; especially its effects on the ear, with suggestions as to treatment—both hygienic and medical. New York: J. H. Vail & Co., 1886. 33p. DNLM **80-5679**

SEXTON, Samuel (1833-1896)
The care of the teeth, from a medical practitioner's standpoint. New York: Trow's Printing & Bookbinding Co., 1889. 20p. DNLM **80-5680**

SEXTON, Samuel (1833-1896)
The ear and its diseases; being practical contributions to the study of otology. . . . Ed. by Christopher J. Colles. . . . New York: William Wood & Co., 1888. 461p. DLC; NNNAM **80-5681**

SEYMOUR, William Wotkyns (1853-1904)
The delivery of the after-coming head by the occiput. New York: William Wood & Co., 1883. 11p. DNLM **80-5682**

SEYMOURS, William Wotkyns (1853-1904)
A successful case of nephro-lithotomy for calculus-pyelitis. New York: D. Appleton & Co., 1885. 6p. DNLM **80-5683**

SEYMOUR, William Wotkyns (1853-1904)
A successful case of excision of the rectum. New York: D. Appleton & Co., 1885. 5p. DNLM **80-5684**

SEYMOUR, William Wotkyns (1853-1904)
A case of pistol-shot wound of the abdomen; abdominal section, resection of the colon, and suture of the small intestine; autopsy. New York, 1886. 5p. DNLM **80-5685**

SHAFFER, Newton M[elman] (*b.* 1846)
The hysterical element in orthopaedic surgery. New York: G. P. Putnam's Sons, 1880. 2 p. l. 66p. DLC; DNLM **80-5686**

SHAFFER, Newton M[elman] (*b.* 1846)
On indiscriminate circumcision. Brooklyn, 1881. 6p. DNLM **80-5687**

SHAFFER, Newton M[elman] (*b.* 1846)
A lecture on knock-knee and bow-legs. New York: William Wood & Co., 1881. 21p. DNLM **80-5688**

SHAFFER, Newton M[elman] (*b.* 1846)
A lecture on the prognosis and treatment of ankle-joint disease. Brooklyn, N.Y., 1882. 21p. DNLM **80-5689**

SHAFFER, Newton M[elman] (*b.* 1846)
A lecture on the pathology, symptoms, and diagnosis of ankle-joint disease. Brooklyn, 1882. 21p. DNLM **80-5690**

SHAFFER, Newton M[elman] (*b.* 1846)
A case of hip-joint disease, complicated by a fracture of the femur. Adam's subcutaneous section of the neck of the femur. Brooklyn, 1883. 13p. DNLM **80-5691**

SHAFFER, Newton M[elman] (*b.* 1846)
A preliminary paper upon the causes of lateral curvature of the spine; with the report of a case of lateral deformity due to occupation. [New York, 1884.] 11p. DNLM **80-5692**

SHAFFER, Newton M[elman] (*b.* 1846)
Remarks on the treatment of club-foot by open incision. [New York, 1887.] 4p. DNLM **80-5693**

SHAFFER, Newton M[elman] (b. 1846)
The use of traction in the treatment of club-foot, with a consideration of some of the mechanical points involved, and a description of the antero-posterior and lateral traction apparatus. New York: D. Appleton & Co., 1887. 51p. DNLM **80-5694**

SHAFFER, Newton M[elman] (*b.* 1846) and Robert W. LOVETT
On the ultimate results of the mechanical treatment of hip-joint disease. An analysis of fifty-one cases occurring in the service of the New York Orthopaedic Dispensary and Hospital. New York: D. Appleton & Co., 1887. 21p. DNLM **80-5695**

SHAKESPEARE, Edward O[ram] (1846-1900)
. . . Histology. Philadelphia: Henry C. Lea's Son & Co., 1882. 17-96p. 12 col. plates [folio]. DLC; NNNAM; PPC; PU **80-5696**

SHAKESPEARE, Edward O[ram] (1846-1900)
A criticism of Dr. Formad's printed statements and conclusions concerning the aetiology of tuberculosis. New York, 1884. 36p. DNLM; NNNAM **80-5697**

SHAKESPEARE, Edward O[ram] (1846-1900) and M. S. FRENCH
Epidemic of typhoid fever at Plymouth, Pa. [Philadelphia, 1885.] 4p. DNLM **80-5698**

SHALL we have a profession of pharmacy? [Detroit, 1884.] 2 l. DNLM **80-5699**

SHARP & DOHME
A brief summary of hypodermic medication, compiled for the convenience of the medical practitioner. Baltimore, 1887. 19p. DNLM; MdU-D **80-5700**

SHATTUCK, Frederick C[heever] (1847-1929)
The diagnosis of the so-called "functional murmurs." [Boston, 1883.] 8p. DNLM **80-5701**

SHATTUCK, Frederick C[heever] (1847-1929)
The home treatment of phthisis. New York, 1885. 19p. DNLM **80-5702**

SHATTUCK, Frederick C[heever] (1847-1929)
Over-distension of the right ventrical, with a report of six cases treated by leeches. Boston: Cupples & Co., 1887. 11p. DNLM **80-5703**

SHATTUCK, Frederick C[heever] (1847-1929)
Some hospital cases of phthisis: marked improvement under general treatment, with special reference to alimentation. Philadelphia: W. J. Dornan, 1887. 14p. DNLM **80-5704**

SHAW, Alexander B. (1847?-1896)
Suspension in the treatment of affections of the spinal cord. St. Louis, 1889. 4 l. DNLM **80-5705**

SHAW, John C[argyll] (1845-1900)
The practicability and value of non-restraint in treating the insane. Boston: Tolman & White, 1880. 8p. DNLM **80-5706**

SHAW, John C[argyll] (1845-1900)
The tendon reflex in general paralysis of the insane. New York: G. P. Putnam's Sons, 1881. 8p. DNLM **80-5707**

SHAW, John C[argyll] (1845-1900)
A second year's experience with non-restraint in the treatment of the insane. New York: G. P. Putnam's Sons, 1882. 11p. DNLM **80-5708**

SHAW, John C[argyll] (1845-1900) and G. N. FERRIS
Perverted sexual instinct. (Conträre Sexualempfindung. Westphal.) New York, 1883. 20p. DNLM **80-5709**

SHAW, John C[argyll] (1845-1900)
Raynaud's disease. [New York, 1886.] 13p. DNLM **80-5710**

SHAW, John C[argyll] (1845-1900)
Apoplectiform, epileptiform, and hemiparetic attacks in locomotor ataxia. [New York, 1888.] 10p. DNLM **80-5711**

SHEDD, Philander
Electropathy and homoeopathy combined. A new and complete system of therapeutics of medical electricity, by Philander Shedd, M.D., and Clark Otis. . . . Chicago: Halsey Bros., [1882], 131p. DLC; DNLM; IU-M **80-5712**

SHEFFIELD, L[ucius] T.
Artificial teeth without plates, by the perfect crowning system. . . . [New York], 1883. 22p. DLC **80-5713**

[SHEFFIELD, Lucius T.]
A new system of prosthetic dentistry. [New York: J. J. Little & Co., printers, 1883.] 19p. DLC **80-5714**

SHEFFIELD, [Lucius T.]
Treatise on a new system of prosthetic dentistry. . . . [New York], 1885. 23p. DLC **80-5715**

SHEPARD & DUDLEY
Descriptive catalogue of apparatus for deformities and deficiencies; elastic stockings, galvanic batteries, inhalation apparatus. . . . New York: W. J. Pell, 1886. [501-]977p. DNLM; NNNAM **80-5716**

SHEPHERD, E. R.
True manhood, a manual for young men; also the White Cross; its origin and progress, by B. F. de Costa. Chicago: A. B. Stockham & Co., [1889]. 314p. DNLM; ICU; NN **80-5717**

SHEPHERD, Francis J[ohn] (1851-1924)
On some anatomical variations. Brooklyn, 1881. 5p. DNLM **80-5718**

SHEPHERD, Francis J[ohn] (1851-1924)
Report on some anatomical variations for 1882. Brooklyn, 1882. 10p. DNLM **80-5719**

SHEPHERD, Francis J[ohn] (1851-1924)
Cervical ribs. [Philadelphia, 1883.] 5p. DNLM **80-5720**

SHEPHERD, Francis J[ohn] (1851-1924)
A case of sarcoma of the skin and cellular tissue about the ankle. Philadelphia, 1884. 7p. DNLM **80-5721**

SHEPHERD, Francis J. (1851-1924), James OLMSTEAD and F. E. BECKWITH
Frequency of albuminuria in healthy people. Hartford: Case, Lockwood & Brainard Co., 1889. 15p. 1 tab. DNLM
80-5722

SHEPHERD, George R.
Essays on the value of raw food extracts, read before the American Medical Association, [etc.]. Boston, [1881]. 23p. DNLM **80-5723**

SHEPHERD, George R.
Climacteric glycosuria. [Hartford, 1887.] 8p. DNLM
80-5724

SHEPHERD, Peter (*d.* 1879)
First aid to the injured. Revised and added to at the request of the First Aid to the Injured Association of New York by Bowditch Morton. New York: G. P. Putnam's Sons, 1882. 88p. DNLM; NNNAM **80-5725**

SHERMAN, J. A.
Convincing testimony. A pamphlet full of interest to the ruptured. Unparalleled success in the treatment of hernia, [etc.]. New York: McBride Bros., 1881. 11, 32p. DNLM; NNNAM **80-5726**

SHERMAN, Lewis
Experiments made for the purpose of determining the limit of drug presence and power in attentuation. [Milwaukee, 1880.] 2 l. DNLM **80-5727**

SHERWELL, Samuel (1841-1927)
Some general suggestions in dermatological therapy. [New York, 1889.] 6p. DNLM **80-5728**

SHEW, Abram M[arvin] (1841-1886)
A glance at the past and present condition of the insane. Middletown, Conn.: Pelton & Kina, 1880. 8p. DNLM
80-5729

SHEW, Abram M[arvin] (1841-1886)
California as a health resort. Hartford: Case, Lockwood & Brainard Comp., 1884. 8p. DNLM **80-5730**

SHEW, Abram M[arvin] (1841-1886)
California as a health resort. Boston: J. S. Adams, 1885. 8p. DNLM **80-5731**

SHEW, Abram M[arvin] (1841-1886)
Progress in the treatment of the insane. Utica, N.Y., 1886. 23p. DNLM **80-5732**

SHICK, William F.
Physiological action of sulphonal. [New York, 1889.] 12p. DNLM; NNNAM **80-5733**

SHIPPEN, Edward (1827-1895)
Memoir of John Neill, M.D.; read before the College of Physicians of Philadelphia, Oct. 6, 1880. Philadelphia: [Collins], 1880. 18p. DNLM; PPC **80-5734**

SHIPPEN, Edward (1827-1895)
Some account of the origin of the Naval Asylum at Philadelphia. [Philadelphia]: Collins, [1883]. 13 l. 1 plate. DNLM
80-5735

SHOEMAKER, George Erety
Adirondacks as a health resort. [Philadelphia, 1886.] 10p. DNLM **80-5736**

SHOEMAKER, John V[ietch] (1852-1910)
A history of the origin and growth of the Jefferson Quiz Association, together with a condensed account of six years' experience in medical teaching. Valedictory address. Philadelphia: Collins, 1880. 27p. DNLM; PPJ
80-5737

SHOEMAKER, John V[ietch] (1852-1910)
The treatment of scrofulous diseases of the skin. [Philadelphia, 1880.] 8p. DNLM **80-5738**

SHOEMAKER, John V[ietch] (1852-1910)
Some new remedies in the local treatment of skin diseases. [Philadelphia, 1880.] 7p. DNLM
80-5739

SHOEMAKER, John V[ietch] (1852-1910)
The oleates and oleo palmitates in skin diseases. [Philadelphia, 1883.] 16p. DNLM **80-5740**

SHOEMAKER, John V[ietch] (1852-1910)
The oleates and oleo palmitates in skin diseases. Detroit: G. S. Davis, 1883. 13p. DNLM **80-5741**

SHOEMAKER, John V[ietch] (1852-1910)
Jequirity; its uses in diseases of the skin. Philadelphia: Collins, 1884. 11p. DNLM **80-5742**

SHOEMAKER, John V[ietch] (1852-1910)
The treatment of the diseases of the skin by novel means and methods. Philadelphia, 1884. 13p. DNLM
80-5743

SHOEMAKER, John V[ietch] (1852-1910)
Address on practical medicine, delivered before the American Medical Association. Philadelphia, 1884. 16p. DNLM
80-5744

SHOEMAKER, John V[ietch] (1852-1910)
The oleates. Further investigation into their nature and action. Philadelphia: F. A. Davis, 1885. 15p. DNLM
80-5745

SHOEMAKER, John V[ietch] (1852-1910)
A practical treatise on diseases of the skin. New York: D. Appleton & Co., 1888. 633p. 6 plates. DLC; DNLM; NNNAM; PPC **80-5746**

SHOEMAKER, John V[ietch] (1852-1910)
A treatise on materia medica, pharmacology, and therapeutics. By John V. Shoemaker . . . and John Aulde. . . . Philadelphia and London: F. A. Davis, 1889-1991. 2 v. DLC; MBM; NNNAM; PPC **80-5747**

SHURLY, Ernest L[orenzo] (1845-1913)
Atrophic pharyngitis or pharyngitis sicca. [New York: G. P. Putnam's Sons, 1880.] 4p. DNLM **80-5748**

SHURLY, Ernest L[orenzo] (1845-1913)
The galvano-cautery as a therapeutical measure in chronic nasal and naso-pharyngeal catarrh. St. Louis: G. Rumbold & Co., 1880. 7p. DNLM **80-5749**

SHURLY, Ernest L[orenzo] (1845-1913)
Lupoid ulceration of the nasal septum. [New York: G. P. Putnam's Sons, 1881.] 7p. DNLM **80-5750**

SHURLY, Ernest L[orenzo] (1845-1913)
Lectures on phthisis pulmonalis, delivered at the Detroit Medical College, Detroit. Detroit: G. S. Davis, 1885. 117p. DLC; DNLM; OCIM **80-5751**

SHURLY, Ernest L[orenzo] (1845-1913)
A report on the origin and geographical distribution of phthisis pulmonalis for the State of Michigan. New York, 1885. 15p. DNLM **80-5752**

SHURLY, Ernest L[orenzo] (1845-1913)
Observations on the use of some of the newer remedies in diseases of the upper air-passages. New YOrk, 1886. 15p. DNLM **80-5753**

SHURLY, Ernest L[orenzo] (1845-1913)
The analogy between acute idiopathic pleuritis and acute articular rheumatism. [Detroit, 1887.] 6p. DNLM **80-5754**

SIBBERT, R. Lowry (1826-1898)
Report on medical legislation, presented to the Medical Society of the State of Pennsylvania. Philadelphia: Collins, 1880. 14p. DNLM **80-5755**

SIBBERT, R. Lowry (1826-1898)
The study of medicine as a means of education. Read before the American Academy of Medicine at its ninth annual meeting, in New York, October 28, 1885. Carlisle, Pa., [1885]. 18p. DNLM **80-5756**

SIBLEY, GIDEON, MFG.
Abridged price list of artificial teeth and dental supplies. Philadelphia, 1887. 36p. PU **80-5757**

SIMMONS, Gustavus L[incoln] (*d.* 1910)
An address delivered at the opening of the twenty-fifth annual meeting of the Medical Society of the State of California, held in San Francisco, April, 1885. [San Francisco, 1885.] 12p. DNLM **80-5758**

SIMMONS, Gustavus L[incoln] (*d.* 1910)
Report on surgery. Sacramento, 1886. 12p. DNLM **80-5759**

SIMON, William (1844-1916)
Manual of chemistry. A guide to lectures and laboratory-work for students of pharmacy and medicine. . . . With sixteen illustrations on wood and seven colored plates, representing fifty-six chemical reactions. Philadelphia: Henry C. Lea's Son & Co., 1884. 411p. col. plates. DLC; DNLM; NNNAM; PU **80-5760**

SIMON, William (1844-1916)
Manual of chemistry. A guide to lectures and laboratory-work for beginners in chemistry. A text-book specially adapted for students of pharmacy and medicine. . . . 2nd ed., thoroughly rev. and greatly enl. With forty-four illustrations and seven colored plates, representing fifty-six chemical reactions. Philadelphia: Lea Bros. & Co., 1888. 479p. col. plates. DLC; DNLM; PPC; PU **80-5761**

SIMPSON, James Young
Organic materia medica and therapeutics. In accordance with the 6th revision of the United States Pharmacopoeia. New York: J. H. Vail & Co., 1885. 337p. DNLM; NNNAM; OCLloyd; PU **80-5762**

SIMS, James Marion (1813-1883)
Thomas Keith and ovariotomy. . . . New York: William Wood & Co., 1880. 16p. DLC; DNLM; PPC **80-5763**

SIMS, James Marion (1813-1883)
Pregnancy-vomiting. New York: G. P. Putnam's Sons, 1880. 8p. DNLM; NNNAM **80-5764**

SIMS, James Marion (1813-1883)
The bromide of ethyl as an anaesthetic. [New York, 1880.] 22p. DNLM **80-5765**

SIMS, James Marion (1813-1833)
The treatment of syphilis. Indianapolis, [1883]. 7p. DNLM **80-5766**

SIMS, James Marion (1813-1883)
The treatment of syphilis. 2nd ed. Indianapolis, [1883]. 7p. DNLM **80-5767**

SIMS, James Marion (1813-1883)
The story of my life. . . . Ed. by his son, H. Marion Sims, M.D. New York: D. Appleton & Co., 1884. 471p. DLC: DNLM; NNNAM; PPC **80-5768**

SINCLAIR, Alexander D[oull]
Measurements of the uterine cavity in childbed. [Boston, 1880.] 9p. DNLM **80-5769**

SINCLAIR, Alexander D[oull]
Measurements of the uterine cavity in childbed. Boston, 1882. 14p. DNLM **80-5770**

SINCLAIR, A[lexander] G[rant]
Iritis. Nashville: Hasslock & Ambrose, [1886]. 3p. DNLM; KyLoJM **80-5771**

SINCLAIR, A[lexander] G[rant]
Electro-magnetism in ophthalmic surgery. With illustrative cases. Memphis: S. C. Toof & Co., 1887. 8p. DNLM; KyLoJM **80-5772**

SINGLETON, James W[illiam] (1829-1881)
Suggestions on the management of natural labor. [St. Louis, 1880.] 16p. DNLM **80-5773**

SINKLER, Wharton (1845-1910)
Two additional cases of hereditary chorea. New York: M. J. Rooney & Co., [1889]. 23p. DNLM; NNNAM **80-5774**

SINKLER, Wharton (1845-1910) and Edward N. BUSH
A case of general paresis of fourteen years' standing. [Utica, N.Y., 1889.] 5p. DNLM **80-5775**

SKENE, Alexander Johnston Chalmers (1837-1900)
The anatomy and pathology of two important glands of the female urethra. New York, 1880. 8p. 1 plate. DNLM **80-5776**

SKENE, Alexander Johnston Chalmers (1837-1900)
Gynecology as related to insanity. New York: G. P. Putnam's Sons, 1880. 31p. DNLM; NNNAM **80-5777**

SKENE, Alexander Johnston Chalmers (1837-1900)
Membranous dysmenorrhoea. [New York, 1885.] 16p. DNLM **80-5778**

SKENE, Alexander Johnston Chalmers (1837-1900)
Treatise on the diseases of women, for the use of students and practitioners . . . with 251 engravings and 9 chromo-lithographs. New York: D. Appleton & Co., 1888. 966p. col. plates. DLC; NNNAM; OCIM; PPC **80-5779**

SKENE, Alexander Johnston Chalmers (1837-1900)
Education and culture as related to the health and diseases of women. . . . Detroit, Mich.: G. S. Davis, 1889. 127p. DLC; DNLM; OCIM **80-5780**

SLAVJANSKI, Kronid F.
Rupture of uterus during pregnancy. Porro's operation; cure. Transl. by Robert T. Wilson, M.D., and Cara S. Harvey. . . . [Richmond], 1886. 11p. DNLM **80-5781**

SMALL, Alvan Edmond (1811-1886)
A systematic treatise on the practice of medicine. Chicago: Duncan Bros., 1886. 900p. IU-M; NNNAM; OCIM; PPHa **80-5782**

SMALL, H[oratio] N[elson] (1840-1886)
How the obstetrical forceps should be used. Portland, Me.: Ford & Rich, 1882. 16p. DNLM **80-5783**

SMALL, H[oratio] N[elson] (1840-1886)
Extra-uterine pregnancy. Portland: S. Berry, 1883. 13p. DNLM **80-5784**

SMART, Charles (1841-1905)
Report of an investigation to determine the prevalence of adulteration of food supplies. [Washington, 1881.] 14p. DNLM **80-5785**

SMART, Charles (1841-1905)
Handbook for the Hospital Corps of the U.S. Army and state military forces. . . . Approved by the Surgeon General of the Army. New York: William Wood & Co., 1889. 577p. DLC; DNLM; NNNAM; PPC **80-5786**

SMITH, Albert H[olmes] (1835-1885)
A clinical lecture on the relation of cleanliness to the prevention of puerperal septicaemia. New York, 1881. 9p. DNLM **80-5787**

SMITH, Albert H[olmes] (1835-1885)
The relation of the County Medical Society to the profession and the community. [Philadelphia, 1882.] 6p. DNLM **80-5788**

SMITH, A. Lapthorn (*b.* 1855)
A year's experience with Apostoli's method, with reports of cases. [New York, 1889.] 20p. DNLM **80-5789**

SMITH, Alder
Ringworm; its diagnosis and treatment. Philadelphia: P. Blakiston, 1881. 81p. 1 plate. DNLM; PPC; PU **80-5790**

SMITH, Allen J[ohn] (1836-1926)
A new chromogenic bacillus; bacillus coeruleus. Philadelphia, 1887. 3p. DNLM **80-5791**

SMITH, Allen J[ohn] (1836-1926)
Reports of several cases of angio-neurotic oedma. Philadelphia, 1889. 10p. DNLM **80-5792**

SMITH, Andrew H[eermance] (1837-1910)
Neuroses of the throat. [New York, 1881.] 7p. DNLM **80-5793**

SMITH, Andrew H[eermance] (1837-1910)
The influence of barometric changes upon the body in health and disease. New York: G. P. Putnam's Sons, 1881. 10p. DNLM **80-5794**

SMITH, Andrew H[eermance] (1837-1910)
On adhesion of the velum to the walls of the pharynx. [New York, 1883.] 6p. DNLM **80-5795**

SMITH, Andrew H[eermance] (1837-1910)
The principles involved in the construction of spray-tubes. New York, 1885. 3p. DNLM **80-5796**

SMITH, Andrew H[eermance] (1837-1910)
The physiological, pathological and therapeutical effects of compressed air. . . . Detroit, Mich.: G. S. Davis, 1886. 112p. DLC; DNLM; OCIM **80-5797**

SMITH, Andrew H[eermance] (1837-1910)
Waking numbness; a heretofore undescribed neurosis. [Philadelphia, 1887.] 4p. DNLM **80-5798**

SMITH, Andrew H[eermance] (1837-1910)
Diabetes. Mellitus and insipidus. . . . Detroit, Mich.: G. S. Davis, 1889. 74p. DLC; DNLM **80-5799**

SMITH, Charles Gilman (1828-1894)
Address delivered before the Alumni Society of the Medical Department of the University of Pennsylvania, March 26, 1886. Philadelphia: Collins, 1887. 17p. DNLM; PU **80-5800**

SMITH, Edgar F[ahs] (1854-1928) and John MARSHALL
Chemical analysis of the urine, based in part on Casselmann's Analyse des Harns. Philadelphia: P. Blakiston, 1881. 104p. 1 plate. DNLM; NNNAM; PPC; PU **80-5801**

SMITH, Edwin Dudley (1833-1906)
The new method. An interesting thesis on general debility and nervous exhaustion; with a full description of the generative organs of man, and their peculiar diseases. Also, the new method of treating nervous exhaustion. . . . [New York, 1880.] 172p. DLC; NNNAM **80-5802**

SMITH, Edwin Dudley (1833-1906)
Woman: her diseases and treatment. With advice in the different periods of her life; from the maiden to the mother; consisting of a full description of the generative organs of woman, and their peculiar diseases, causes, and cure. Also, the new modes of treatment. . . . New York, [1880]. 191p. DLC; NNNAM **80-5803**

SMITH, Eugene
Blepharoplasty sine pedicle. [Philadelphia, 1881.] 3p. DNLM **80-5804**

SMITH, Eugene
Jequirity in granular lids. Chicago: A. G. Newell, [1883]. 7p. DNLM **80-5805**

SMITH, Eugene
Jequirity; its use in the treatment of phlyctenular keratitis, phlyctenular conjunctivitis, ulcers of the cornea and granular lids. [Detroit, 1883.] 7p. DNLM **80-5806**

SMITH, Eustace (1835-1914)
A practical treatise on disease in children. . . . New York: William Wood & Co., 1884. 844p. DLC; NNNAM; OCIM; PU **80-5807**

SMITH, Eustace (1835-1914)
On the wasting diseases of infants and children. 4th ed. New York: William Wood & Co., 1885. 278p. DNLM; NNNAM; PPC; PPJ **80-5808**

SMITH, Eustace (1835-1914)
Clinical studies of disease in children. 2nd ed. Philadelphia: P. Blakiston, Son & Co., 1887. 318p. CtY-M; DNLM; NNNAM; PPC **80-5809**

SMITH, Eustace (1835-1914)
On the wasting diseases of infants and children. 5th ed. Philadelphia: P. Blakiston, Son & Co., 1888. 380p. DNLM; IU-M; NNNAM; PPC **80-5810**

SMITH, Henry (1812-1901)
The surgery of the rectum. 1st American, from 4th English ed., with additions and illustrations. Philadelphia: Henry C. Lea's Son & Co., 1881. 71p. DNLM; NNNAM; PPC; PPJ **80-5811**

SMITH, Henry (1812-1901)
A practical manual of the treatment of diseases of the rectum. 1st American from 4th English ed. New York: Bermingham & Co., [1881]. 44p. DNLM; NNNAM **80-5812**

SMITH, Henry H[ollinsworth] (1815-1890)
An address delivered before the Medical Society of the State of Pennsylvania, at its annual meeting held at Philadelphia, May, 1884. Philadelphia: Collins, 1884. 33p. DNLM; PPC **80-5813**

SMITH, Henry H[ollinsworth] (1815-1890)
The appendix vermiformis, its function, pathology, and treatment. [Also:] The diagnosis of pericaecal abscess, and its treatment by removal of the appendix vermiformis, by Thomas G. Morton. Chicago, 1888. 44p. DNLM **80-5814**

SMITH, Henry H[ollinsworth] (1815-1890)
Concussion of the spine in its medico-legal aspects. [Also:] The medico-legal aspect of concussion of the spine, by Herbert Judd. Chicago, 1889. 39p. DNLM **80-5815**

SMITH, H. Ralls
A popular treatise on the medical uses of electricity for the cure of nervous and chronic diseases without drugs. With instructions for self-treatment. . . . 2nd ed. rev. and enl. . . . Milwaukee, Wis., and St. Louis, Mo.: Pub. for the Author, 1880. 68p. DLC **80-5816**

SMITH, J. Edwards
How to see with the microscope; being useful hints connected with the selection and use of the instrument; also some discussion of the claims and capacity of the modern high-angled objectives, as compared with those of medium aperture; with instructions as to the selection and use of American object-glasses of wide apertures. Chicago: Duncan Bros., 1880. 410p. 12 plates. DNLM; IU-M; OCIM **80-5817**

SMITH, J[ames] Greig (1834-1897)
Abdominal surgery. . . . Philadelphia: P. Blakiston, Son & Co., 1887. 606p. DNLM; PPC; PU **80-5818**

SMITH, J[ames] Greig (1834-1897)
Abdominal surgery. . . . 3rd ed. Philadelphia: P. Blakiston, Son & Co., 1889. 799p. DNLM; MBM; NNNAM; PPC **80-5819**

SMITH, J[ob] Lewis (1827-1897)
A treatise on the diseases of infancy and childhood. . . . 5th ed., thoroughly rev. . . . Philadelphia: Henry C. Lea's Son & Co., 1881. 836p. DLC; NNNAM; PPC; PPJ **80-5820**

SMITH, J[ob] Lewis (1827-1897)
A treatise on the diseases of infancy and childhood. . . . 6th ed., thoroughly rev. . . . Philadelphia: Lea Bros. & Co., 1886. 870p. DLC; IEN-M; NNNAM; PU **80-5821**

SMITH, John Telemachus
Plain facts about small-pox. Everybody's questions about small-pox and vaccination plainly answered. Three dollars' worth of medical advice for ten cents. . . . New York: Murray Hill Publishing Co., 1882. 19p. DLC; NNNAM **80-5822**

SMITH, Joseph R[owe] (1831-1911)
The best form of report of diseases and wounds, regarded from a statistical standpoint. Philadelphia: W. F. Fell & Co., [1888]. 5 l. DNLM **80-5823**

SMITH, Robert Meade (*b.* 1854) and Andrew J. PARKER
Dissection of a human otocephalic cyclops monstrosity. [Philadelphia, 1882.] 10p. DNLM **80-5824**

SMITH, Robert Meade (*b.* 1854)
Methods of studying the physiological action of drugs. Detroit: G. S. Davis, 1884. 20p. DNLM; ICRM; IEN-M **80-5825**

SMITH, Robert Meade (*b.* 1854)
The thermic phenomena in contraction of mammalian muscles. New York: G. P. Putnam's Sons, 1884. 50p. DNLM **80-5826**

SMITH, Robert Meade (*b.* 1854)
The absorption of sugar and albuminoids by the stomach. Cambridge, 1884. 92p. DNLM **80-5827**

SMITH, Samuel W.
Original deductions based on a study of one hundred cases of fractures of the upper extremities, excluding the hand. New York: Trow, 1885. 21p. DNLM; NNNAM **80-5828**

SMITH, Samuel W.
Diphtheria and its treatment. New York: Trow, 1886. 14p. DNLM; NNNAM **80-5829**

[SMITH, Stephen] (1823-1922)
The care of health and life in the State of New York: A statement transmitted to the legislature of New York, recommending that a State board of health be established. Prepared by the New York member of the advisory committee of the American Public Health Association, by request of citizens. [New York, 1880.] 8p. DNLM; NNNAM
80-5830

SMITH, Stephen (1823-1922)
A State board of health. A communication to a member of the legislature on sanitary organization and administration in the State of New York. [New York, 1880.] 1[illegible]p. DNLM
80-5831

SMITH, Stephen (1823-1922)
Handbook of the principles and practice of operative surgery. 5th ed. Philadelphia: Samuel M. Miller, 1884. 689p. NNNAM; OCIM; PPC; PU **80-5832**

SMITH, Stephen (1823-1922)
Manual of the principles and practice of operative surgery. [8th ed.] Boston: Houghton, Mifflin & Co., 1886. 689p. CtY-M; MH-M; NNNAM; PU **80-5833**

SMITH, Stephen (1823-1922)
The care of the insane in the State of New York, historically considered. [Utica, N.Y., 1886.] 23p. DNLM
80-5834

SMITH, Stephen (1823-1922)
The principles and practice of operative surgery. . . . New and thoroughly rev. ed. . . . Philadelphia: Lea Bros. & Co., 1887. 877p. DLC; DNLM; NNNAM; PPC **80-5835**

SMITH, Theobald (1859-1934)
Some recent investigations concerning bacteria in drinking water. [Philadelphia, 1886.] 8p. DNLM
80-5836

SMITH, Theobald (1859-1934)
The relative value of cultures in liquid and solid media in the diagnosis of bacteria. [n. p., 1886.] 8p. DNLM
80-5837

SMITH, Thomas C[roggon] (1842-1913)
Ante-partum hour-glass contraction of the uterus. New York: William Wood & Co., 1882. 31p. DNLM; NNNAM
80-5838

SMITH, Thomas C[roggon] (1842-1913)
Sarcoma and multiple mucous polypi of the uterus in a child. New York, 1883. 8p. DNLM **80-5839**

SMITH, Thomas C[roggon] (1842-1913)
Hydatidiform mole. Chicago, 1887. 8p. DNLM
80-5840

SMITH, Thomas C[roggon] (1842-1913)
Tetanus following abortion. New York, 1887. 12p. DNLM
80-5841

SMITH, Thomas C[roggon] (1842-1913)
Case of tubal gestation. Baltimore, 1889. 3p. DNLM
80-5842

SMITH, W[illard] Everett (*d.* 1890)
The rational treatment of pulmonary diseases by the pneumatic cabinet. Chicago, 1885. 7p. DNLM **80-5843**

SMITH, W[illard] Everett (*d.* 1890)
Hereditary or degenerative ataxia; six cases in one family; death of one case and autopsy. Boston: Cupples, Upham & Co., 1885. 31p. DNLM **80-5844**

SMITH, W[illard] Everett (*d.* 1890)
A case of poisoning from arsenical wallpaper. [Boston, 1887.] 12p. DNLM **80-5845**

SMITH, W[illard] Everett (*d.* 1890)
Postero-lateral spinal sclerosis (generic origin); or generic ataxia. A name suggested in place of hereditary ataxia or Friedreich's disease. [Boston, 1888.] 8p. DNLM
80-5846

SMITH, W[illard] Everett (*d.* 1890)
A study of phthisis and pneumonia in Massachusetts; statistical and climatological. [Boston, 1888.] 28p. 3 charts. DNLM **80-5847**

SMITH, William M[anlius] (1824?-1900)
Report on quarantine, external and internal. Albany: Weed, Parsons & Co., 1881. 26p. DNLM **80-5848**

SMITH, William M[anlius] (1824?-1900)
Report of the standing committee on quarantine, external and internal. Albany: Weed, Parsons & Co., 1882. 41p. DNLM
80-5849

SMITH, William R[obert] (1850-1932)
Assassination and insanity. Guiteau's case examined and compared with analogous cases from the earlier to the present times. Washington, D.C.: W. R. Smith, 1881. 96p. DNLM
80-5850

SMYTH, Andrew W[oods] (1833-1916)
Interpretations of the structure and function of the kidney. Reported by John Gamgee. New Orleans: Eureka Book & Job Office, 1880. 22p. DNLM; LNT-M **80-5851**

SMYTH, George A.
Hygienic institutes. The utility of their work of investigation, and the need of it in this country. [Hartford, 1884.] 27p. DNLM **80-5852**

SMYTHE, Gonzalvo C[ordova] (1836-1897)
Medical heresies, historically considered. A series of critical essays on the origin and evolution of sectarian medicine, embracing a special sketch and review of homoeopathy, past and present. Philadelphia: P. Blakiston, 1880. 228p. DNLM; PPC; PU **80-5853**

SMYTHE, Gonzalvo C[ordova] (1836-1897)
The antipyretic treatment of typhoid fever. Cincinnati, 1883. 24p. DNLM **80-5854**

SMYTHE, Gonzalvo C[ordova] (1836-1897)
The hydro-therapeutic treatment of typhoid fever. Indianapolis: W. B. Burford, [1889]. 11p. DNLM
80-5855

SNADER, Edward R.
Repertory of the heart symptoms. [n. p., 1888.] 112p. DNLM; PPHa **80-5856**

SNOW, Norman Leslie (1839-1885)
Syphilitic degeneration of arteries as a cause of aneurism; with a report of two cases. Albany: Burdick & Taylor, 1880. 11p. DNLM **80-5857**

SOLLY, Samuel Edwin (1845-1906)
Colorado for invalids. Colorado Springs, 1880. 28p. DNLM
80-5858

SOLLY, Samuel Edwin (1845-1906)
The health resorts of Colorado Springs and Manitou; also a prize article descriptive of scenery, resources, etc., by Mrs. Simeon J. Dunbar. [n. p., 1883, *vel subseq.*] 136p. DNLM
80-5859

SOLLY, Samuel Edwin (1845-1906)
An invalid's day in Colorado Springs. Philadelphia: W. J. Dornan, 1888. 14p. DNLM **80-5860**

SOLLY, Samuel Edwin (1845-1906)
The physician in Colorado; being the president's address to the Colorado State Medical Society. [Denver]: Whipple & Pierson, [1888]. 10p. DNLM **80-5861**

SOLLY, Samuel Edwin (1845-1906)
Invalids suited for treatment at Colorado Springs. Philadelphia: W. J. Dornan, 1889. 15p. DNLM
80-5862

SOUTHWICK, George R[inaldo] (1859-1930)
A practical manual of gynaecology. Boston and Providence: Otis Clapp & Son, 1888. 408p. MBM; PPHa
80-5863

SPALDING, James A[fred] (*b.* 1846)
Ophthalmology, ancient and modern. Annual address before the Maine Medical Association. Portland: S. Berry, 1881. 27p. DNLM **80-5864**

SPEAR, Edmund D[oe], Jr. (*b.* 1852)
Clinical observations. New York, 1880. 12p. DNLM
80-5865

SPENCER, John C.
Review and translation in part from the German of the recent article on the cycle of evolution of the malaria-parasite of tertian intermittent fever, by Camillo Golgi. [San Francisco, 1889.] 14p. DNLM **80-5866**

SPERRY, Lyman Beecher
Diseases of the rectum. . . . Chicago, 1884. 48p. DLC
80-5867

SPINA, Arnold
A history of tuberculosis from the time of Sylvius to the present day. Being in part a transl. with notes and additions from the German, containing also an account of the researches and discoveries of Robert Koch and other recent investigators, by Erie E. Sattler. Cincinnati: R. Clarke & Co., 1883. 191p. DNLM; OC **80-5868**

SPINKS, E. E.
Directory of the practicing dentists of the State of Mississippi. Meridian, Miss.: Shannon & Dement, 1881. 11p. DNLM
80-5869

SPINZIG, Carl
Yellow fever; nature and epidemic character caused by meteorlogical influences, verified by the epidemics of Shreveport and Memphis in 1873, by that of Savannah in 1876, by the great epidemic of the Mississippi Valley in 1878 and (in the appendix) by the one of Memphis in 1879. St. Louis: G. O. Rumbold & Co., 1880. 205p. DNLM
80-5870

SPINZIG, Carl
Failure of vaccination. Variolous infection an illusion; vaccination an injury to health and a danger to life, and, as a protection against small-pox, a vanity. [St. Louis, 1881.] 15p. DNLM **80-5871**

SPITZKA, Edward C[harles] (1852-1914)
What has been done by the Asylum Association in the interest of scientific psychiatry? Chicago: Chandler & Engelhard, 1880. 24p. DNLM; IU-M **80-5872**

SPITZKA, Edward C[harles] (1852-1914)
The evidences of insanity discoverable in the brains of criminals and others whose mental state has been questioned; with some remarks on expert testimony and the Grappotte case. [New York, 1882.] 31p. DNLM; NNNAM
80-5873

SPITZKA, Edward C[harles] (1852-1914)
Insanity, its classification, diagnosis and treatment; a manual for students and practitioners of medicine. . . . New York: Bermingham & Co., 1883. 415p. DLC; DNLM; NNNAM; PU
80-5874

SPITZKA, Edward C[harles] (1852-1914)
The intra-axial course of the auditory tract. [New York, 1886.] 8p. DNLM **80-5875**

SPITZKA, Edward C[harles] (1852-1914)
The comparative anatomy of the pyramid tract. New York: W. R. Jenkins, [1886]. 46p. 1 plate. DNLM; NNNAM
80-5876

SPITZKA, Edward C[harles] (1852-1914)
Insanity, its classification, diagnosis and treatment; a manual for students and practitioners of medicine. . . . [2nd ed.] New York: E. B. Treat, 1887. 423p. DLC; MBM; NNNAM; PPC
80-5877

SPRAGUE, W[illiam] B. (1836-1891)
Uterine massage. [Detroit, 1888.] 10p. DNLM
80-5878

SPRATLING, William P[hilip] (1863-1915)
Primary dementia, with description of two cases. New York: M. J. Rooney, 1889. 7p. DNLM
80-5879

SQUIBB, Edward R[obinson] (1819-1900)
On the relations of the medical profession to the trade interests of the materia medica, and a note on pepsin, followed by a reprint of a paper entitled: A ready method of testing pepsin [by J. Merritt]. New York: H. T. Cornett, [1880]. 18p. DNLM **80-5880**

SQUIBB, Edward R[obinson] (1819-1900)
Semi-annual price lists of standard pharmaceutical preparations and pharmacopoeial reagents manufactured by . . . Nos. 50, 51, 52, 53, and 54. Brooklyn, 1883-1885. DNLM; NNNAM
80-5881

SQUIBB, Edward R[obinson] (1819-1900)
Semi-annual price list of standard pharmaceutical preparations and pharmacopoeial reagents. No. 60. [Brooklyn, N.Y., 1888.] DNLM; NNNAM **80-5882**

SQUIER, A. O[rin]
Some observations on the treatment of diphtheria. Springfield, Mass.: [D. Clapp & Son], 1888. 14p. DNLM **80-5883**

STANDISH, Myles (*b.* 1851)
Report of twenty-four cases of granular lids treated by jequirity. Boston: A. Mudge & Son, 1884. 7p. 1 tab. DNLM
80-5884

STANDISH, Myles (*b.* 1851)
A case of tuberculosis of the iris. Boston: D. Clapp & Son, 1885. 6p. DNLM **80-5885**

STANDISH, Myles (*b.* 1851)
Celloidin; the new material for embedding specimens for microscopic section cutting; its method of use and its advantages. St. Louis, 1885. 5p. DNLM **80-5886**

STANDISH, Myles (*b.* 1851)
A case of retinitis pigmentosa treated electrically. Boston: D. Clapp & Son, 1887. 6p. DNLM **80-5887**

STANDISH, Myles (*b.* 1851)
Partial tenotomies in cases of neurasthenia, with insufficiencies of the ocular muscles. Boston: Damrell & Upham, 1889. 23p. DNLM **80-5888**

STAPLES, Allen
Suicide by blows against the head. A medico-legal study. Chicago, 1887. 15p. DNLM **80-5889**

STAPLES, Franklin (1833-1904)
Report on diphtheria. [1881.] 44p. DNLM
80-5890

STAPLES, George A.
Hydronephrosis. An essay based upon the comparative study of seventy-one cases of that lesion, of which one case came under the personal observation of the writer. Chicago: A. G. Newell, 1884. 20p. DNLM **80-5891**

STARKEY, George R. (1823-1896)
The compound oxygen treatment: its mode of action and results. New and revised ed. Philadelphia: Starkey & Palen, [1881]. 182p. 5 plates, 2 port. DNLM; PPC; PPJ; PU
80-5892

STARLING MEDICAL COLLEGE, COLUMBUS, O. [FORMERLY MEDICAL DEPARTMENT OF WILLOUGHBY UNIVERSITY]
Annual announcements for the sessions of 1848-1849 (2.); 1850-1851 (4.); 1851-1852 (5.); 1853-1854 to 1887-1888 (7.-41.). Columbus, 1848-1887. DNLM [List of students and graduates for the sessions of 1847-1848 to 1850-1851, 1852-1853 to 1882-1883, 1886-1887, in announcements for subsequent years. List of graduates from 1848 to 1883 in announcement for 1883-1884.] **80-5893**

STARLING MEDICAL COLLEGE, COLUMBUS, OHIO
Annual announcemnts for the sessions of 1888-1889 to 1898-1899 (42.-52.); 1902-1903 (56.); 1904-1905 to 1906-1907 (58.-60.). Columbus, 1888-1906. DNLM
80-5894

STARR, Louis (1849-1925) and James B. WALKER
A synopsis of the physiological action of medicines. "A chart of the physiological action of medicines." 2nd ed. Philadelphia: Collins, 1880. 30p. DNLM; PPC; PU
80-5895

STARR, Louis (1849-1925)
Diseases of the digestive organs in infancy and childhood, with chapters on the investigation of disease, and on the general management of children. . . . Philadelphia: P. Blakiston, Son & Co., 1886. 385p. DLC; DNLM; PPC; PU
80-5896

STARR, Louis (1849-1925)
A synopsis of the physiological action of medicines, prepared for the use of students of the medical department of the University of Pennsylvania. With the approval of the professor of materia medica. By Louis Starr . . . and James B. Walker . . . assisted by W. M. Powell. . . . 3rd ed.; enl. Philadelphia: P. Blakiston, Son & Co., 1888 [1887]. 72p. DLC; DNLM; NNNAM; PPC **80-5897**

STARR, Louis (1849-1925)
Hygiene of the nursery. . . . With twenty-one illustrations. Philadelphia: P. Blakiston, Son & Co., 1888. 212p. DLC; DNLM; PPC: PU **80-5898**

STARR, Louis (1849-1925)
Hygiene of the nursery. Including the general regimen and feeding of infants and children, and the domestic management of the ordinary emergencies of early life. . . . 2nd ed. With twenty-five illustrations. Philadelphia: P. Blakiston, Son & Co., 1889. 280p. DLC; DNLM; PPC; PPJ **80-5899**

STARR, M[oses] Allen (1854-1932)
The sensory tract in the central nervous system. [New York: G. P. Putnam's Sons, 1884.] 81p. 1 plate. DNLM; NNNAM
80-5900

STARR, M[oses] Allen (1854-1932)
Syringomyelia; its pathology and clinical features; with a study of a case, and remarks upon its diagnosis. New York, 1888. 13p. DNLM **80-5901**

STEARNS, FREDERICK & CO. DETROIT
Catalogue of popular non-secret medicines. . . . Detroit, 1883-1884. 66p. OCIM **80-5902**

STEARNS, FREDERICK & CO. DETROIT
Revised price list. . . . Detroit, 1885. 8p. IU-M; OCIM
80-5903

STEARNS, FREDERICK & CO. DETROIT
Revised catalogue. . . . Detroit, 1885. 16p. OCIM
80-5904

STEARNS, FREDERICK & CO. DETROIT
Desc. catalogue with article on positive medication. . . . Detroit, 1886. 32p. NNNAM **80-5905**

STEARNS, FREDERICK & CO. DETROIT
Retail druggists' diary and want book. . . . Detroit, 1886. 80p. OCIM **80-5906**

STEARNS, FREDERICK & CO. DETROIT
Positive medication. A pamphlet on alkatrits, alkametric granules, and alkadermic pellets. . . . Also upon alkassayed fluids. . . . Pub. by Frederick Stearns & Co. . . . . Detroit, Mich.: F. Stearns & Co., [1886]. 28p. DLC
80-5907

STEARNS, Henry Putnam (1828-1905)
Physiology vs. philosophy. A short study. Hartford: Case, Lockwood & Brainard Co., 1880. 18p. DNLM
80-5908

STEARNS, Henry Putnam (1828-1905)
The care of some classes of the chronic insane. Hartford: Case, Lockwood & Brainard Co., 1881. 16p. DNLM
80-5909

STEARNS, Henry Putnam (1828-1905)
Insanity: its causes and prevention. . . . New York: G. P. Putnam's Sons, 1883. 248p. DLC; DNLM; NNNAM
80-5910

STEARNS, Henry Putnam (1828-1905)
Progress in the treatment of the insane. [Utica, 1884.] 18p. DNLM **80-5911**

STEDMAN, Henry R[ust] (1849-1926)
The family system as an accessory provision for our insane poor. [Boston, 1884.] 29p. DNLM **80-5912**

STEDMAN, Henry R[ust] (1849-1926)
The family system in practice. A report of the condition of the "boarded-out" insane in Massachusetts. [Boston, 1889.] 21p. DNLM **80-5913**

STEDMAN, Henry R[ust] (1849-1926)
On medical advice regarding the marriage of subjects, with a personal or family history of insanity. New York: M. J. Rooney & Co., 1889. 11p. DNLM **80-5914**

STEELE, D. A. K.
The differential diagnosis of scrotal tumors. Chicago, 1886. 12p. DNLM **80-5915**

STEELE, Joel Dorman (1836-1886)
Hygienic physiology, with special reference to the use of alcoholic drinks and narcotics. Being a revised ed. of the "Fourteen weeks in human physiology." Edited for the use of schools, in accordance with the recent legislation upon temperance instruction. New York & Chicago: A. S. Barnes & Co., [1888]. 276p. 3 col. plates included in pagination. DNLM; ICU; MH; NN **80-5916**

STEIN, Alexander W. (1841-1897)
A study of the tumors of the bladder, with original contributions and drawings. New York: William Wood & Co., 1881. 94p. DLC; DNLM; NNNAM **80-5917**

STEIN, Alexander W. (1841-1897)
A study of rupture of the bladder, with some experiments bearing upon the closure of the vesical wound. Brooklyn, N.Y.: G. E. Stechert, 1882. 42p. DNLM; NNNAM
80-5918

STELLWAGEN, Thomas C[ook] (*b.* 1841)
Physical and mental inheritances. An address read before the American Academy of Dental Science, Boston, November 15, 1887. Newton, Mass., 1888. 17p. DNLM
80-5919

STELWAGON, Henry W[eightman] (1853-1919)
Psoriasis in child under four years of age. [Philadelphia, 1881.] 2 l. DNLM **80-5920**

STELWAGON, Henry W[eightman] (1853-1919)
A case of phthiriasis palpebrarum. [New York, 1881.] 2 l. DNLM **80-5921**

STELWAGON, Henry W[eightman] (1853-1919)
A case of feigned eruption. [New York, 1882.] 2 l. DNLM
80-5922

STELWAGON, Henry W[eightman] (1853-1919)
An interesting case of herpes iris. [Philadelphia, 1882.] 2 l. DNLM **80-5923**

STELWAGON, Henry W[eightman] (1853-1919)
A sebaceous cyst containing a coil of hair consisting of two hairs, each several inches in length. [Philadelphia, 1883.] 2 l. DNLM **80-5924**

STELWAGON, Henry W[eightman] (1853-1919)
Vieminckx's solution in acne rosacea. [Philadelphia, 1883.] 2 l. DNLM **80-5925**

STELWAGON, Henry W[eightman] (1853-1919)
An erythematous eruption from chlorate of potassium. [New York, 1883.] 2 l. DNLM **80-5926**

STELWAGON, Henry W[eightman] (1853-1919)
Impetigo contagiosa; its clinical features. [Philadelphia, 1883.] 6p. DNLM **80-5927**

STELWAGON, Henry W[eightman] (1853-1919)
Acne indurata; its treatment. [New York, 1884.] 7p. DNLM
80-5928

STELWAGON, Henry W[eightman] (1853-1919)
Impetigo contagiosa; its individuality and nature. Philadelphia: Lloyd & Porter, 1884. 8p. DNLM **80-5929**

STELWAGON, Henry W[eightman] (1853-1919)
The oleates in cutaneous diseases. [Philadelphia, 1884.] 10p. DNLM **80-5930**

STELWAGON, Henry W[eightman] (1853-1919)
Iodide of potassium in eczema. Philadelphia, 1885. 3p. DNLM
80-5931

STELWAGON, Henry W[eightman] (1853-1919)
A case of late cutaneous syphilis (acne-like syphiloderm of the nose) illustrating the occasional necessity of large doses of potassium iodide. Philadelphia, 1885. 4p. DNLM
80-5932

STELWAGON, Henry W[eightman] (1853-1919)
A case of vitiligo involving the whole surface. [Philadelphia, 1885.] 3p. DNLM **80-5933**

STELWAGON, Henry W[eightman] (1853-1919)
Observations on the oleates. [Philadelphia, 1885.] 4p. DNLM
80-5934

STELWAGON, Henry W[eightman] (1853-1919)
Clinical notes on the value of resorcinichthyol, and lanolin in cutaneous diseases. New York, 1886. 4p. DNLM
80-5935

STELWAGON, Henry W[eightman] (1853-1919)
A case of purpura with circinate lesions. New York, 1887. 1 l. 1 plate. DNLM **80-5936**

STELWAGON, Henry W[eightman] (1853-1919)
Notes on the use of medicated rubber plasters in certain cutaneous diseases. [Philadelphia, 1887.] 4p. DNLM
80-5937

STELWAGON, Henry W[eightman] (1853-1919)
Molluscum contagiosum; a preliminary report. Read before the American Dermatological Association, Washington, Sept. 19, 1888. [New York, 1889.] 3p. DNLM **80-5938**

STELWAGON, Henry W[eightman] (1853-1919)
Molluscum contagiosum; a preliminary report. Read before the American Dermatological Association, Washington, Sept. 19, 1888. [With discussion.] [New York, 1889.] 4p. DNLM **80-5939**

STELWAGON, Henry W[eightman] (1853-1919)
On the alleged tolerance of the iodides in late syphilis. Detroit, Mich.: G. S. Davis, 1889. 7p. DNLM **80-5940**

STELWAGON, Henry W[eightman] (1853-1919)
A case of urticaria pigmentosa. [Philadelphia, 1889.] 4p. DNLM **80-5941**

STEPHENSON, F. B[ache] (*b.* 1848)
Yellow fever at Norfolk and Portsmouth, Virginia, in 1855. [Washington], 1883. 19p. DNLM **80-5942**

STEPHENSON, F. B[ache] (*b.* 1848)
Reparative surgery. Brooklyn, 1884. 10p. DNLM **80-5943**

STEPHENSON, F. B[ache] (*b.* 1848)
Arabic and Hebrew in anatomy. [New York: D. Appleton & Co., 1886.] 10p. DNLM **80-5944**

STEPHENSON, F. B[ache] (*b.* 1848)
Sydenham and Hahnemann. [New York, 1886.] 6p. DNLM **80-5945**

STEPHENSON, F. B[ache] (*b.* 1848)
A summary of Holsti's views on arteriocapillary sclerosis. [New York, 1886.] 6p. DNLM **80-5946**

STEPHENSON, F. B[ache] (*b.* 1848)
Duty of the State in public health. [New York, 1887.] 11p. DNLM **80-5947**

STEPHENSON, F. B[ache] (*b.* 1848)
Scientific work by alienists. [Boston, 1889.] 10p. DNLM **80-5948**

STEPHENSON, William
On the menstrual wave. New York, 1882. 10p. DNLM **80-5949**

STERLING, Charles Frederick
The diseases of the ear and their homoeopathic treatment, with a brief outline of the anatomy, physiology, and pathology. New York: A. L. Chatterton Co., 1885. 167p. DNLM; NNNAM; PPHa **80-5950**

STERNBERG, George M[iller] (1838-1915), J. Dickson BRUNS and John Pintard DAVIDSON
[Reports in regard to a form of fever recently prevailing on the Lower Mississippi River.] [New Orleans, 1880.] 18p. DNLM **80-5951**

STERNBERG, George M[iller] (1838-1915)
The diagnosis of yellow fever. Yellow fever and quarantine. New Orleans: L. Graham & Son, 1880. 17p. DNLM **80-5952**

STERNBERG, George M[iller] (1838-1915)
The microscopical investigations of the Havana yellow fever commission. New Orleans: L. Graham, 1880. 7p. DNLM **80-5953**

STERNBERG, George M[iller] (1838-1915)
A fatal form of septicaemia in the rabbit, produced by the subcutaneous injection of human saliva. Baltimore: J. Murphy & Co., 1881. 22p. 1 plate. DNLM **80-5954**

STERNBERG, George M[iller] (1838-1915)
Bacillus anthracis. New York: Thompson & Moreau, 1881. 4p. 1 plate. DNLM **80-5955**

STERNBERG, George M[iller] (1838-1915)
Experimental investigations relating to the etiology of the malarial fevers. [n. p., n. d.] 11p. 4 plates. DNLM **80-5956**

STERNBERG, George M[iller] (1838-1915)
Photo-micrographs and how to make them. Boston: J. R. Osgood & Co., 1883. 204p. 20 plates. DNLM; MBM **80-5957**

STERNBERG, George M[iller] (1838-1915)
Malaria and malarial diseases. New York: William Wood & Co., 1884. 329p. DLC; DNLM; NNNAM **80-5958**

STERNBERG, George M[iller] (1838-1915)
American Public Health Association, Lomb prize essay. Disinfection and individual prophylaxis against infectious diseases. Concord, N.H., 1886. 40p. DLC; DNLM **80-5959**

STERNBERG, George M[iller] (1838-1915)
Recent researches relating to the etiology of yellow fever. Philadelphia: W. J. Dornan, 1888. 11p. 1 plate. DNLM; PPC **80-5960**

STERNBERG, George M[iller] (1838-1915)
Bacteria, and the germ theory of disease. Sacramento: Day & Joy, [1888]. 8p. DNLM **80-5961**

STEVENS, Charles Wistar (*d.* 1901)
Revelations of a Boston physician. Boston: A. Williams & Co., 1881. 252p. MB **80-5962**

STEVENS, Edward S[ommerville] (*b.* 1857)
The best preliminary education for the study of medicine. Boylston prize essay, 1885. Lebanon, O., [1885]. 45p. DNLM; MH-M **80-5963**

STEVENS, George T[homas] (1832-1921)
Functional nervous diseases, their causes and their treatment. Memoir for the concourse of 1881-1883. Académie royale de médecine de Belgique. With a supplement on the anomalies of refraction and accommodation of the eye and of the ocular muscles. New York: D. Appleton & Co., 1887. 217p. DLC; DNLM; NNNAM **80-5964**

STEVENS, George T[homas] (1832-1921)
A system of terms relating to the condition of the ocular muscles known as "insufficiencies." New York, 1886. 11p. DNLM **80-5965**

STEVENS, George T[homas] (1832-1921)
Ocular irritations and nervous disorders. With remarks by Ambrose L. Ranney. New York: D. Appleton & Co., 1887. 40p. DNLM; NNNAM **80-5966**

STEVENS, Thaddeus M. (1829-1895)
The "essentials" of a law to regulate the practice of medicine in Indiana. [New Albany, 1881.] 3p. DNLM **80-5967**

STEVENS, Thaddeus M. (1829-1895)
State medicine; what has been accomplished and what is needed in Indiana. [Indianapolis, 1881.] 15p. DNLM
80-5968

STEVENS, Thaddeus M. (1829-1895)
State boards of health, their object and use, etc. Extracts, showing the views of practical workers and eminent sanitarians. Indianapolis: W. B. Burford, 1882. 40p. DNLM
80-5969

STEVENS, Thaddeus M. (1829-1895)
A history of health-work in Indiana. Boston: Rockwell & Churchill, 1883. 7p. DNLM **80-5970**

STEVENS, Thaddeus M. (1829-1895)
Charges made by the Indiana State Board of Health against Thad M. Stevens, M.D., secretary of the board, together with answers to such charges; with an appendix, containing statements offered in proof, and other matter. Indianapolis, 1883. 27p. DNLM **80-5971**

STEVENS, Thaddeus M. (1829-1895)
Answer to charges of the Indiana State Board of Health, together with statements in proof and other matters. Indianapolis: Baker & Randolph, 1883. 31p. DNLM **80-5972**

STEVENS, Thaddeus M. (1829-1895)
The relative value of bovine and humanized vaccine virus practically considered. [Indianapolis, 1883.] 9p. DNLM
80-5973

STEVENS, Thaddeus M. (1829-1895)
Report of committee on state medicine. Indianapolis: W. B. Burford, 1884. 18p. DNLM **80-5974**

STEVENSON, John Rudderow (1834-1917)
The history of medicine and medical men of Camden County, New Jersey. . . . Philadelphia. L. J. Richards & Co., 1886. 39p. DLC **80-5975**

STEVENSON, ROBERT & CO.
Wholesale catalogue of drugs and druggists' sundries, pharmaceuticals, . . . Chicago, 1887. 522p. IU-M; OCIM
80-5976

STEVENSON, Sarah Hackett (1843-1909)
The physiology of woman, embracing girlhood, maternity and mature age, with essays on "Coeducation of the sexes in medicine," "The physiological basis of education" . . . [etc.] . . . . 3rd ed. Chicago: Fairbanks, Palmer & Co.; Boston: Alden & Hazen; [etc., etc.], 1882. 230p. plates. DLC; ICU; MH; NN
80-5977

STEWART, David Denison (1859-1905)
Notes on some obscure cases of poisoning by lead chromate, manifested chiefly by encephalopathy. [Philadelphia], 1887. 20p. DNLM **80-5978**

STEWART, David Denison (1859-1905)
A clinical analysis of sixty-four cases of poisoning by lead chromate (chrome yellow), used as a cake-dye. [Philadelphia], 1887. 21p. DNLM **80-5979**

STEWART, David Denison (1859-1905)
Poisoning by chrome yellow, used as a cake dye; the subsequent clinical history of the cases, including a case of paralysis agitans, and of chronic endocarditis. [Philadelphia, 1889.] 24p. DNLM **80-5980**

STEWART, David Denison (1859-1905)
Report on the treatment of fourteen cases of diseases of the spinal cord by the method of suspension. Philadelphia, 1889. 19p. DNLM **80-5981**

STEWART, David Denison (1859-1905)
A suggestion as to the action of olive or cotton-seed oil in gall-stone colic; observations on the use of the oils, and reports of cases. [Philadelphia, 1889.] 12p. DNLM
80-5982

STEWART, F[erdinand] Campbell (1815-1899)
Eminent French surgeons, with a historical and statistical account of hospitals of Paris; together with miscellaneous information and biographical notices of the most eminent of the living Parisian surgeons. Buffalo: A. Burke, [1886?]. 432p. NNNAM **80-5983**

STEWART, F[rancis] E[dward] (1853-1941)
A new method of rectal medication. New York: William Wood & Co., 1880. 8p. DNLM **80-5984**

STEWART, F[rancis] E[dward] (1853-1941)
A new method of rectal alimentation. New York: Trow, 1880. 8p. DNLM **80-5985**

STEWART, F[rancis] E[dward] (1853-1941)
An old system and a new science. Detroit: G. S. Davis, [1882]. 31p. DNLM **80-5986**

STEWART, F[rancis] E[dward] (1853-1941)
How can physicians aid in elevating the profession of pharmacy? [Philadelphia, 1884.] 22p. DNLM
80-5987

STEWART, F[rancis] E[dward] (1853-1941)
A compend of pharmacy; based upon Prof. Joseph P. Remington's "Text-book of pharmacy." Philadelphia: P. Blakiston, Son & Co., 1886. 196p. DLC; DNLM; NNNAM; PPC **80-5988**

STEWART, F[rancis] E[dward] (1853-1941)
A compend of pharmacy; based upon Prof. Joseph P. Remington's "Text-book of pharmacy." 2nd ed. Philadelphia: P. Blakiston, Son & Co., 1887. 184p. DNLM; PPC; PU
80-5989

STEWART, F[rancis] E[dward] (1853-1941)
The increased efficacy of massage in combination with the electro-vapor bath. [Philadelphia, 1887.] 20p. DNLM
80-5990

STEWART, John S.
Obstetric synopsis. Philadelphia: F. A. Davis, 1888. 202p. DNLM; PPC; PU **80-5991**

STEWART, Morse (1818-1906)
Pocket therapeutics and dose-book. . . . 3rd ed. Detroit: G. D. Stewart & Co., 1882. 240p. DNLM; ICJ; PPC
80-5992

STEWART, R[obert] W. (*b.* 1853)
The action and use of alcohol in fevers. Pittsburgh, 1889. 12p. DNLM **80-5993**

STEWART, Thomas G[rainger] (1837-1900)
Clinical lectures on important symptoms. On giddiness . . . . Fasciculus II. On albuminuria. New York: William Wood & Co., 1888. 250p. DNLM; NNNAM **80-5994**

STICKLER, Joseph W[illiam] (1854-1899)
Hatter's consumption. [New York, 1886.] 14p. DNLM
80-5995

STICKLER, Joseph W[illiam] (1854-1899)
The Adirondacks as a health resort, showing the benefit to be derived by a sojourn in the wilderness, in cases of pulmonary phthisis, acute and chronic bronchitis, asthma, "hay-fever," and various nervous affections. New York & London: G. P. Putnam's Sons, 1886. 198p. DNLM; NNNAM
80-5996

STICKLER, Joseph W[illiam] (1854-1899)
Foot-and-mouth disease as it affects man and animals, and its relation to human scarlatina as a prophylactic. Also, remarks upon the transmission of human scarlatina to the lower animals, and the use of virus thus cultivated as a preventive agent. New York: Trow's Co., 1887. 31p. DNLM; NNNAM
80-5997

STILLÉ, Alfred (1813-1900)
Memoir of Isaac Hays. Philadelphia: Collins, 1880. 36p. DNLM; PPC
80-5998

STILLÉ, Alfred (1813-1900)
General introductory lecture delivered at the opening of the one hundred and eighteenth course of lectures in the medical department of the University of Pennsylvania, October 1, 1883. Philadelphia: J. B. Lippincott & Co., 1883. 36p. DNLM; PU
80-5999

STILLÉ, Alfred (1813-1900)
An address delivered to the medical classes of the University of Pennsylvania, on withdrawing from his chair, April 10, 1884. [Philadelphia, 1884.] 20p. DNLM; PU
80-6000

STILLÉ, Alfred (1813-1900)
The national dispensatory. Containing the natural history, chemistry, pharmacy, actions, and uses of medicines. Including those recognized in the pharmacopoeias of the United States, Great Britain, and Germany, with numerous references to the French codex. By Alfred Stillé . . . and John M. Maisch. . . . 3rd ed., thoroughly rev., with numerous additions. With three hundred and eleven illustrations. Philadelphia: Henry C. Lea's Son & Co., 1884. 1755p. DLC; DNLM; OCLloyd; PU
80-6001

STILLÉ, Alfred (1813-1900)
Cholera: its origin, history, causation, symptoms, lesions, prevention, and treatment. . . . Philadelphia: Lea Bros. & Co., 1885. 164p. fold. map. DLC; DNLM; PPC; PU
80-6002

STILLÉ, Alfred (1813-1900)
The national dispensatory. Containing the natural history, chemistry, pharmacy, actions, and uses of medicines. Including those recognized in the pharmacopoeias of the United States, Great Britain, and Germany, with numerous references to the French codex. By Alfred Stillé . . . and John M. Maisch. . . . 4th ed. Philadelphia: Henry C. Lea's Son & Co., 1886. 1781p. DNLM; NNNAM; OCLloyd; PPC
80-6003

STILLMAN, Charles Frederick (1853-1892)
The life insurance examiner. A practical treatise upon medical examinations for life insurance. . . . New York: The Spectator Company, 1888. 181p. col. plate. DLC; NN; NNNAM
80-6004

STIMSON, Lewis A[tterbury] (1844-1917)
Mr. Lister's antiseptic method. New York: G. P. Putnam's Sons, 1880. 13p. DNLM; NNNAM
80-6005

STIMSON, Lewis A[tterbury] (1844-1917)
A treatise on fractures. . . . With three hundred and sixty illustrations on wood. Philadelphia: Henry C. Lea's Son & Co., 1883. 598p. DLC; ICRM; NNNAM; PPC
80-6006

STIMSON, Lewis A[tterbury] (1844-1917)
An inquiry into the origin of the use of the ligature in the treatment of aneurism. [New York, 1884.] 16p. DNLM
80-6007

STIMSON, Lewis A[tterbury] (1844-1917)
Arterio-venous aneurism of the common carotid artery and internal jugular vein, with a case. [Philadelphia, 1884.] 13p. DNLM
80-6008

STIMSON, Lewis A[tterbury] (1844-1917)
A manual of operative surgery. . . . [2nd ed.] With three hundred and forty-two illustrations. Philadelphia: Lea Bros. & Co., 1885. 506p. DLC; GU; NNNAM; PU
80-6009

STIMSON, Lewis A[tterbury] (1844-1917)
Injuries of the main blood-vessels in the axilla caused by efforts to reduce dislocations of the shoulder. [New York, 1885.] 20p. DNLM
80-6010

STIMSON, Lewis A[tterbury] (1844-1917)
A treatise on dislocations. . . . With one hundred and sixty-three illustrations. Philadelphia: Lea Bros. & Co., 1888. 539p. DLC; LNT-M; NNNAM; PPC
80-6011

STIMSON, Lewis A[tterbury] (1844-1917)
On gunshot wounds of the abdomen, with especial reference to wounds of the intestines. [New York, 1889.] 48p. DNLM; NNNAM
80-6012

STIMSON, Lewis A[tterbury] (1844-1917)
On some modifications in the technique of abdominal surgery, limiting the use of the ligature en masse. [Philadelphia, 1889.] 12p. DNLM
80-6013

STIRLING, William (1851-1932)
A manual of human physiology, [etc.]. Philadelphia, 1885. 2 v. DNLM; PU
80-6014

STIRLING, William (1851-1932)
Outlines of practical physiology, being a manual for the physiological laboratory, including chemical and experimental physiology, with reference to practical medicine. Philadelphia: P. Blakiston, Son & Co., 1888. 309p. DNLM; NNNAM; PPC; PU
80-6015

STOCKEN, James
Elements of dental materia medica and therapeutics, with pharmacopoeia. 3rd ed. Assisted by Thomas Gaddes. Philadelphia: P. Blakiston, Son & Co., 1882. 400p. DNLM; MdU-D; PPC; PU
80-6016

STOCKHAM, Alice B[unker] (1833-1912)
Tokology. A book for every woman. Revised ed. Chicago: Sanitary Publishing Co., 1886. 374p. DNLM; ICU
80-6017

STOCKHAM, Alice B[unker] (1833-1912)
Tokology. A book for every woman. Revised ed. Chicago: Alice B. Stockham & Co., 1889. 374p. DNLM **80-6018**

STOCKTON-HOUGH, John
An inquiry concerning the relative influence of the sex of the fetus in utero on the mental, physical, physiological, pathological, and developmental condition of the mother during gestation, lactation, and subsequently. New York: William Wood & Co., 1884. 70p. DNLM; NNNAM **80-6019**

STOCKTON-HOUGH, John
The influence of sex of fetus-in-utero on length of intergestation period immediately following its birth. Forming a supplement to a paper entitled: "An inquiry concerning the influence of the sex of the fetus-in-utero on the . . . condition of the mother during gestation, and of the infant during lactation, and subsequently. . . ." To which is added a list of the various papers published by the author. New York: William Wood & Co., 1886. 9p. 1 l. DNLM **80-6020**

STOCKTON-HOUGH, John
Incunabula medica [prodromus bibliographicus] directorium bibliothecarum cum nominibus et locis earumque viginiti vel plura medicorum librorum quinto decimo saeculo typis excusorum exemplaria continent, in alphabetico auctorum ordine dispositum. Trentonii, in Nuovo-Caesarea, 1880. 30 l. DNLM **80-6021**

STOCKWELL C. Twitchell (1841-1911)
The combination of metals for filling teeth. [Philadelphia, 1887.] 7p. DNLM **80-6022**

STOCKWELL, G. Archie
The physicians' perfect call-book and record. Detroit: G. S. Davis, [1887]. 24p. DNLM **80-6023**

STONE, Alexander J. (1845-1910)
President's annual address to the Minnesota State Medical Society, June 22, 1881. [St. Paul, 1881.] 8p. DNLM **80-6024**

STONE, I[saac] S[cott] (*b.* 1851)
Modern trachelorrhaphy—what is it? Report of six cases. [Richmond, 1887.] 10p. DNLM **80-6025**

STONE, I[saac] S[cott] (*b.* 1851)
The treatment of contracted bladder by hot-water dilatation. [Philadelphia, 1889.] 9p. DNLM **80-6026**

STONE, J. L.
Morbi aëre vitali curantur, or philosophy and application of condensed air as a curative agent. Rochester, 1881. 35p. DNLM **80-6027**

STONE, R[ichard] French (1844-1913)
Elements of modern medicine; including principles of pathology, and therapeutics. . . . New York: D. Appleton & Co., 1885. 368p. DLC; DNLM; NNNAM **80-6028**

STONE, R[ichard] French (1844-1913)
Zymotic diseases considered with reference to their cause, extent, and prevention. [Indianapolis]: W. B. Burford, [1886]. 22p. DNLM **80-6029**

STORER, Horatio Robinson (1830-1922)
The anticipatory treatment of local epidemics. [Providence, 1886.] 12p. DNLM **80-6030**

STORER, Horatio Robinson (1830-1922)
. . . The medals, jetons and tokens illustrative of obstetrics and gynaecology. . . . [Newtown? Conn.], 1887. 14p. DLC; DNLM **80-6031**

STORER, Horatio Robinson (1830-1922)
The importance and eradication of syphilis. Chicago, 1888. 11p. DNLM **80-6032**

STORER, Horatio Robinson (1830-1922)
The medals of Benjamin Rush, obstetrician. . . . Read at the fortieth annual meeting of the American Medical Association, held at Newport, R.I., June, 1889. . . . Chicago, 1889. 20p. IU-M **80-6033**

STORY, Charles A.
Alcohol; its nature and effects. Ten lectures. New York, 1883. 392p. 1 plate. DNLM; NN **80-6034**

STOUT, Henry R[ice] (*b.* 1843)
Our family physician. A plain, practical and reliable guide to the detection and treatment of diseases common to this country. Designed for people who want information stated in plain English. Peoria, Ill.: Smith & Hilman, 1889. 477p. IC-U; OCIM **80-6035**

STOWELL, Charles Henry (1850-1932)
The students' manual of histology, for the use of students, practitioners and microscopists. . . . Illus. by one hundred and ninety-two engravings. Detroit: G. S. Davis, 1881. 279p. DLC; OCIM **80-6036**

STOWELL, Charles Henry (1850-1932) and Louisa Reed STOWELL
Microscopical diagnosis. Detroit: G. S. Davis, 1882. 93, 118, 32p. 10 plates. DNLM **80-6037**

STOWELL, Charles Henry (1850-1932)
The students' manual of histology, for the use of students, practitioners and microscopists. 3rd ed. Entirely rewritten; greatly enl.; and newly illustrated. . . . Illustrated by 178 engravings. Ann Arbor, Mich.: C. H. Stowell, 1884. 368p. DLC **80-6038**

STOWELL, Charles Henry (1850-1932)
The microscopic structure of a human tooth, together with some unusual and irregular forms of teeth. 2nd ed. Ann Arbor, Mich.: C. H. Stowell, 1888. 20 l. 12 plates, fol. DNLM **80-6039**

STRAHAN, John (1852-1896)
The diagnosis and treatment of extra-uterine pregnancy. The Jenks prize essay of the College of Physicians of Philadelphia. [Philadelphia: P. Blakiston, Son & Co., 1889.] 128p. DNLM; PPC **80-6040**

STRAWBRIDGE, George (1844-1914)
Report of 261 cases of cataract extraction. Boston: D. Clapp & Son, 1887. 20p. DNLM **80-6041**

STRAWBRIDGE, George (1844-1914)
Preliminary report of an operation for the formation of an artificial pupil through the sclerotic coat of the eyeball. [Philadelphia, 1888.] 12p. DNLM **80-6042**

STRECKER, Adolph (1822-1871)
Short text-book of organic chemistry; by Johannes Wislicenus. Transl. and edited, with extensive additions, by W. H. Hodgkinson and A. J. Greenaway. New York: D. Appleton & Co., 1882. 789p. DNLM; ICU; MB; NN **80-6043**

STRONG, Charles P[ratt] (1855-1893)
Rectal disease of uterine origin. Boston: Cupples & Upham, 1886. 12p. DNLM **80-6044**

STRONG, Charles P[ratt] (1855-1893)
Dystocia caused by tonic annular contraction of the uterus. [Boston, 1887.] 7p. DNLM **80-6045**

STRONG, Charles P[ratt] (1855-1893)
Six cases of uterine displacements treated by shortening of the round ligaments, with remote results. Boston: Cupples & Hurd, 1888. 8p. DNLM **80-6046**

STRONG, Thomas Morris
The homoeopathic treatment of constipation. Transl. and revised from the second Belgian edition, with additions and clinical cases from American sources. New York: A. L. Chatterton Publishing Co., 1882. 189p. NNNAM **80-6047**

STRÜMPELL, Adolf von (1853-1925)
. . . A text-book of medicine, for students and practitioners. . . . Transl. by permission from the 2nd and 3rd German editions by Herman F. Vickery . . . and Philip Coombs Knapp. . . . With editorial notes by Frederick C. Shattuck. . . . New York: D. Appleton & Co., 1886. 474p. diags. DLC; NNNAM; OCIM; PU **80-6048**

STRÜMPELL, Adolf von (1853-1925)
A text-book of medicine, for students and practitioners. . . . Transl. by permission from the 2nd and 3rd German editions by Herman F. Vickery . . . and Philip Coombs Knapp. . . . With editorial notes by Frederick C. Shattuck. . . . New York: D. Appleton & Co., 1887. 981p. diags. DLC; IU-M; NNNAM; PPC **80-6049**

STUART, Francis H[art] (*b.* 1846)
The management of the perineum during labor, and the immediate treatment of lacerations and the obstetrics and gynaecology of William Harvey. New York: Jenkins & Thomas, 1881. 30p. DNLM; NNNAM **80-6050**

STUBBLEFIELD, D[avid] R.
A hand-book of materia medica and therapeutics for dentists and dental students. . . . Nashville, Tenn.: Printed at the Southern Methodist Publishing House, for the Author, 1882. 187p. DLC **80-6051**

STUCKY, Joseph Addison (*b.* 1858)
The treatment of chronic nasal catarrh. Louisville, Ky., [1883]. 10p. DNLM **80-6052**

STUCKY, Joseph Addison (*b.* 1858)
Muriate of cocaine as a local anaesthetic. [Louisville, 1884.] 4p. DNLM **80-6053**

STUCKY, Joseph Addison (*b.* 1858)
Pruritic catarrh or hay fever. Its treatment. St. Louis, 1885. 12p. DNLM **80-6054**

STUCKY, Joseph Addison (*b.* 1858)
Two rare cases of abdominal injury. New York: Trow, 1885. 8p. DNLM **80-6055**

STUCKY, Joseph Addison (*b.* 1858)
Report on rhinology: the treatment of nasal and pharyngo-nasal catarrh. Lexington: Acme Printing Co., 1886. 12p. DNLM **80-6056**

STUCKY, Joseph Addison (*b.* 1858)
Notes on catarrhal inflammation of the nasal cavities in the young. Treatment. Cincinnati, 1888. 7p. DNLM **80-6057**

STURGIS, Frederic R[ussell] (1844-1919)
The student's manual of venereal diseases, being the University lectures delivered at Charity Hospital, B. I., during the winter session of 1879-1880. New York: G. P. Putnam's Sons, 1880. 196p. DNLM; MH-M; NNNAM; PU **80-6058**

STURGIS, Frederic R[ussell] (1844-1919)
On the affections of the middle ear during the early stages of syphilis. [Boston, 1880.] 7p. DNLM; MBM **80-6059**

STURGIS, Frederic R[ussell] (1844-1919)
Hints and suggestions for reform in medical education. [New York: W. Wieser, 1882.] 13p. DNLM; NNNAM **80-6060**

STURGIS, Frederic R[ussell] (1844-1919)
The student's manual of venereal diseases, being the University lectures delivered at Charity Hospital, B. I., during the winter session of 1879-1880. 5th ed. New York: G. P. Putnam's Sons, 1884. 196p. DNLM; NNNAM; [Earlier printings in 1880. 1881, 1883 by Putnam] **80-6061**

STURGIS, Russell, Jr. (1856-1899)
The use of lanolin and boracic acid in certain diseases of the skin of children. [Boston, 1888.] 2 l. DNLM **80-6062**

SULLIVAN, T. J.
Observations on the administation of chloroform. Read before the Michigan State Medical Society, June 9, 1886. Ann Arbor, Mich., [1886]. 8p. DNLM **80-6063**

SUMMA, Hugo (*b.* 1859)
The pseudo-parasitism of Diptera in man, or mylosis. St. Louis: Weiss & Maccallum, 1889. 16p. DNLM **80-6064**

SUMMERS, J. E., Jr. (*b.* 1858)
Observations on some modern surgical procedures. [n. p., 1889.] 8p. DNLM **80-6065**

SUMMERS, J. E., Jr. (*b.* 1858)
Notes on surgical cases. [Omaha, 1889.] 8p. DNLM **80-6066**

SUTTON, Francis (1831-1917)
A systematic handbook of volumetric analysis. . . . 4th ed. Philadelphia: P. Blakiston, 1882. 471p. PPF; PPL; PU **80-6067**

SUTTON, Francis (1831-1917)
A systematic handbook of volumetric analysis. . . . 5th ed. Philadelphia: P. Blakiston, Son & Co., 1886. 491p. NNNAM; PPC; PPF; PU **80-6068**

SUTTON, John Bland (1855-1936)
An introduction to general pathology, founded on three lectures, delivered at the Royal College of Surgeons. Philadelphia: P. Blakiston, Son & Co., 1886. 390p. CtY-M; DNLM; NNNAM; PPC **80-6069**

SUTTON, R[hoades] Stansbury (1841-1906)
Laceration of the cervix uteri. Twenty-fifth lecture of the course of 1880, at Rush Medical College, Chicago. New York: Trow's, 1880. 14p. DNLM; ICRM; NNNAM **80-6070**

SUTTON, R[hoades] Stansbury (1841-1906)
A case of cataleptic convulsion cured by trachelorraphy. Boston, 1881. 3p. DNLM; MBM **80-6071**

SUTTON, R[hoades] Stansbury (1841-1906)
Some remarks on ovariotomy, with special reference to the treatment of the pedicle. [1882?] 12p. DNLM **80-6072**

SUTTON, R[hoades] Stansbury (1841-1906)
The importance of cleanliness in surgical operations. [New York, 1884.] 13p. DNLM; NNNAM **80-6073**

SUTTON, R[hoades] Stansbury (1841-1906)
Annual address delivered before the American Academy of Medicine. Medical education in the United States; its defects and the remedy. Philadelphia: W. F. Fell & Co., 1887. 13p. DNLM; PPC **80-6074**

SWAIN, William Paul (1834-1916)
Surgical emergencies, together with the emergencies attendant on parturition and the treatment of poisoning. A manual for the use of general practitioners. 4th ed. Philadelphia: P. Blakiston, Son & Co., 1887. 229p. DNLM; NNNAM; PPC; PU **80-6075**

SWAN, Samuel (1815-1893)
Catalogue of morbific products, nosodes, and other remedies, in high potencies. New York: Pusey & Co., 1886. 32p. NNNAM; OCLloyd **80-6076**

SWAN, Samuel (1815-1893)
A materia medica containing provings and clinical verifications of nosodes and morbific products. Collated, arranged, and prepared for publication by E. W. Burridge. New York: Pusey & Co., 1888. 121p. DNLM; NNNAM; OCLloyd **80-6077**

SWANZY, Henry R[osborough] (1843-1913)
A handbook of the diseases of the eye and their treatment. . . . New York: D. Appleton & Co., 1884. 437p. CtY-M; DNLM; NNNAM; PPC **80-6078**

SWASEY, Edward
Hernia in children; based on a study of five hundred cases under personal observation. New York: William Wood & Co., 1880. 28p. DNLM **80-6079**

SWASEY, Edward
An interesting case of malformation of the female sexual organs; representing either a rare variety of hermaphroditism or of double congenital ovarian hernia with absence of uterus. New York: William Wood & Co., 1881. 13p. DNLM **80-6080**

SWAYNE, Joseph Griffiths (1819-1903)
Obstetric aphorisms; for the use of students commencing midwifery practice. 8th ed. Philadelphia: P. Blakiston, Son & Co., 1884. 156p. DNLM; NNNAM; PPC; PU **80-6081**

SWAYNE, Joseph Griffiths (1819-1903)
Obstetric aphorisms; for the use of students commencing midwifery practice. 9th ed. Philadelphia: P. Blakiston, Son & Co., 1888. 159p. DNLM; MBM; OCIM; PU **80-6082**

SWAYZE, George B. H.
Quackery and regular medicine. [Detroit, 1881.] 8p. DNLM **80-6083**

SWAYZE, George B. H.
How are we sustaining the medical constitution as editors, doctors, and medicine makers? [Detroit, 1881.] 14p. DNLM **80-6084**

TAFT, Jonathan (1820-1903)
A practical treatise on operative dentistry. . . . 4th ed., rev. . . . Philadelphia: P. Blakiston, Son & Co., 1883. 509p. DLC; NNNAM; PPC; PU **80-6085**

TAFT, Jonathan (1820-1903)
Index to the periodical literature of dental science and art, as presented in the English language. . . . Philadelphia: P. Blakiston, Son & Co., 1856. 212p. DLC; DNLM; PPC; PU **80-6086**

TAGEN, C. H. von
Biliary calculi; perineorrhaphy; hospital gangrene and its kindred diseases; with their respective treatments. New York & Philadelphia: Boericke & Tafel, 1881. 154p. DNLM; NNNAM; PPHa **80-6087**

TAGLIABUE, Chas. J.
Illustrated catalogue of barometers, thermometers, pyrometers and hydrometers. New York: J. B. Stilwell & Co., 1885. 96p. DNLM; NNNAM **80-6088**

[TAIT, Robert Lawson] (1845-1899)
Extracts from addresses of Mr. Lawson Tait, the eminent surgeon, and others. At the annual meeting of the Victoria Street Society for the Total Prohibition of Vivisection, 1882. [Philadelphia, 1882.] 4p. DNLM **80-6089**

TAIT, [Robert] Lawson (1845-1899)
The pathology and treatment of diseases of the ovaries (being the Hastings essay for 1873). . . . 4th ed., rewritten and greatly enlarged. Birmingham: Cornish Bros.; New York: William Wood & Co., 1883. 357p. DLC; IU-M; NNNAM; PU **80-6090**

TAIT, [Robert Lawson] (1845-1899)
The uselessness of vivisection upon animals as a method of scientific research. Philadelphia: Am. Anti-Vivisection Soc., 1883. 34p. DNLM; PPC **80-6091**

TAIT, [Robert] Lawson (1845-1899)
Abdominal section in diseases of the uterus, or of the uterine appendages. Philadelphia: Henry C. Lea's Son & Co., 1884. 22p. DNLM **80-6092**

TAIT, [Robert Lawson] (1845-1899)
A discussion of the general principles involved in the operation of removal of the uterine appendages. [New York, 1886.] 20p. DNLM; PPC **80-6093**

TAIT, [Robert] Lawson (1845-1899)
Diseases of women and abdominal surgery. Philadelphia: Lea Bros. & Co., 1889. 547p. DNLM; NNNAM; OCIM; PPC **80-6094**

TALBOT, Eugene Solomon (1847-1924)
Irregularities of the teeth and their treatment. . . . With 152 illustrations. Philadelphia: P. Blakiston, Son & Co., 1888. 163p. DLC; DNLM; MdU-D; PPC **80-6095**

TALBOT, Eugene Solomon (1847-1924)
Classification of typical irregularities of the maxillae and teeth. [Philadelphia, 1889.] 7p. DNLM **80-6096**

TALCOTT, Selden H[aines] (*d.* 1902)
General paresis. New York, 1880. 26p. DNLM **80-6097**

TALCOTT, Selden H[aines] (*d.* 1902)
The insane diathesis. Middletown: Slauson & Boyd, 1881. 21p. DNLM **80-6098**

TALCOTT, Selden H[aines] (*d.* 1902)
Two addresses by . . . and a poem by Wm. Tod Helmuth. Havana, N.Y.: L. E. Keyser & Co., 1882. 32p. DNLM **80-6099**

TALCOTT, Selden H[aines] (*d.* 1902)
Sleep without narcotics. Middletown, N.Y.: Press Job Printing House, 1883. 28p. DNLM **80-6100**

TALCOTT, Selden H[aines] (*d.* 1902)
Application of "new remedies" in the treatment of mental and nervous diseases. New York: E. P. Coby & Co., 1884. 12p. DNLM **80-6101**

TALCOTT, Selden H[aines] (*d.* 1902)
Hahnemann and his influence upon modern medicine. An address delivered at the Homoeopathic festival, Boston, April 12, 1887. [n. p., 1887.] 12p. DNLM **80-6102**

TALIAFERRO, Valentine H. (1831-1887)
The application of pressure in diseases of the uterus, ovaries and peri-uterine structures. [Atlanta, 1882.] 20p. DNLM **80-6103**

TANCRET, Charles
Ergotinine and pelletiérine. New York: E. Fougera & Co., [1882]. 16p. DNLM; NNNAM **80-6104**

TANNER, Thomas Hawkes (1824-1871)
Memoranda on poisons. . . . 6th American from the last London ed. Rev. by Henry Leffmann, M.D. Philadelphia: P. Blakiston, Son & Co., 1888. 177p. DLC; DNLM; PPC; PU **80-6105**

TARRANT & CO. MFG. AND IMP.
General prices current of drugs, chemicals, pharmaceuticals and druggists' sundries. New York, 1880. 170p. NNNAM **80-6106**

TARRANT & CO. MFG. AND IMP.
General prices current. . . . New York, 1882. 192p. NNNAM **80-6107**

TAYLOR, Alfred Swaine (1806-1880)
A manual of medical jurisprudence. . . . 8th American ed., from the 10th London ed., containing the author's latest notes made expressly for this ed.; ed., with additional notes and references, by John J. Reese. . . . Philadelphia: Henry C. Lea's Son & Co., 1880. 933p. DLC; NNNAM; OCIM; PPC **80-6108**

TAYLOR, Alfred Swaine (1806-1880)
The principles and practice of medical jurisprudence. 3rd ed., edited by Thomas Stevenson. Philadelphia: Henry C. Lea's Son & Co., 1883. 2 v. DNLM; IU-M; NNNAM; PPC **80-6109**

TAYLOR, Charles Fayette (1827-1899)
Sensation and pain. A lecture. New York: G. P. Putnam's Sons, 1881. 77p. DLC; DNLM **80-6110**

TAYLOR, Charles Fayette (1827-1899)
Genital irritation. Brooklyn, N.Y., 1881. 7p. DNLM **80-6111**

TAYLOR, Charles Fayette (1827-1899)
Effect on women of imperfect hygiene of the sexual function. New York, 1882. 19p. DNLM **80-6112**

TAYLOR, Charles Fayette (1827-1899)
Official formulae of American hospitals. Collected and arranged by . . . . Philadelphia: "The Medical World," [1885]. 238p. DLC; OCLloyd; PPC; PU **80-6113**

TAYLOR, Charles Fayette (1827-1899)
A home-made spinal apparatus. [New York, 1886.] 8p. DNLM **80-6114**

TAYLOR, Charles Fayette (1827-1899)
Official formulae of American hospitals. Collected and arranged by . . . . 2nd ed., enl. Philadelphia: "The Medical World," [1886]. 256p. DLC; PPC **80-6115**

TAYLOR, Charles Fayette (1827-1899)
Official formulae of American hospitals. Collected and arranged by . . . . 2nd ed., enl. Philadelphia: "The Medical World," [1886]. 272p. DLC; PU **80-6116**

TAYLOR, Charles Fayette (1827-1899) and W[illiam] F. WAUGH
Manual of treatment. A concise presentation of the modern methods of treating disease, employed by the best authors, teachers, and practitioners, arranged with special reference to the needs of American practitioners. Philadelphia: Medical World, 1887. 532p. DLC; DNLM; PPC **80-6117**

TAYLOR, George H[erbert] (1821-1896)
Paralysis, and other affections of the nerves; their cure by transmitted energy and special movements. New York: American Book Exchange, [1880]. 179p. DNLM; NNNAM **80-6118**

TAYLOR, George H[erbert] (1821-1896)
Health by exercise. What exercises to take and how to take them, to remove special physical weakness. Embracing an account of the Swedish methods, and a summary of the principles of hygiene. . . . New York: American Book Exchange, 1880. 408p. DLC; NNNAM
80-6119

TAYLOR, George H[erbert] (1821-1896)
Health for women. Showing the causes of feebleness and the local diseases resulting therefrom; with full directions for self-treatment. . . . New York: J. B. Alden, 1883. 249p. DLC; NNNAM **80-6120**

TAYLOR, George H[erbert] (1821-1896)
An exposition of the Swedish movement-cure. . . . the processes of massage. . . . New York: Fowler & Wells, 1884. 462p. NNNAM **80-6121**

TAYLOR, George H[erbert] (1821-1896)
Health by exercise, showing what exercises to take and how to take them to remove special physical weakness; embracing the history and philosophy of medical treatment by this system, including the process of massage; also a summary of the general principles of hygiene. New York: J. B. Alden, 1884. 454p. NNNAM **80-6122**

TAYLOR, George H[erbert] (1821-1896)
Health by exercise. The movement cure, embracing the history and philosophy of this system of medical treatment, with examples of single movements, the processes of massage . . . together with a summary of the principles of general hygiene. . . . New and enl. ed. New York: Fowler & Wells, 1884. 462p. DLC; NNNAM **80-6123**

TAYLOR, George H[erbert] (1821-1896)
Massage. Principles and practice of remedial treatment by imparted motion. Description of manual processes. . . . New York: Fowler & Wells, 1884. 203p. DLC; NNNAM
80-6124

TAYLOR, George H[erbert] (1821-1896)
Pelvic and hernial therapeutics. Principles and methods for remedying chronic affections of the lower part of the trunk, including processes for self-cure. . . . New York: J. B. Alden, 1885. 282p. DLC; NNNAM **80-6125**

TAYLOR, George H[erbert] (1821-1896)
Massage. Principles and practice of remedial treatment by imparted motion. Mechanical processes. . . . New York: J. B. Alden, 1887. 173p. DLC; NNNAM **80-6126**

TAYLOR, George H[erbert] (1821-1896)
The delusion of tonics. New York: J. B. Alden, [1887]. 23p. DNLM; NNNAM **80-6127**

TAYLOR, H[enry] Genet (*b.* 1837)
Retrospection of the Medical Society of New Jersey, with some suggestions as to its improvement. President's address. Newark, N.J.: L. J. Hardham, 1889. 19p. DNLM
80-6128

TAYLOR, Henry Ling (1857-1923)
Primary crural asymmetry. New York: Trow's, 1884. 12p. DNLM **80-6129**

TAYLOR, Henry Ling (1857-1923) and Robert W. LOVETT
The paralysis of Pott's diseases and its behavior under protective treatment. New York: Trow Co., 1886. 12p. DNLM
80-6130

TAYLOR, Henry Long (1857-1923)
A new method of overcoming adduction at the hip joint. [New York, 1887.] 4p. DNLM **80-6131**

TAYLOR, Henry Ling (1857-1923)
A case of Pott's disease with an unusual deformity; description of improved spinal apparatus. New York: Trow, 1887. 88p. DNLM; NNNAM **80-6132**

TAYLOR, Henry Ling (1857-1923)
Hygiene of reflex action. New York, 1888. 23p. DNLM
80-6133

TAYLOR, Henry Ling (1857-1923)
The mechanical treatment of senile coxitis. [New York, 1888.] 5p. DNLM **80-6134**

TAYLOR, Henry Ling (1857-1923)
The therapeutic value of systematic passive respiratory movements. New York: Trow's, 1889. 12p. DNLM
80-6135

TAYLOR, Henry Ling (1857-1923)
The prevention and treatment of crural adduction. [New York, 1889.] 18p. DNLM **80-6136**

TAYLOR, Henry Ling (1857-1923)
Principles and methods of examination in orthopaedic practice. Baltimore: Jour. Publ. Co. Print., 1889. 29p. DNLM
80-6137

TAYLOR, Hugh M[cGuire] (*b.* 1856)
Nervous mimicry. Richmond, 1886. 15p. DNLM
80-6138

TAYLOR, Isaac E[benezer] (1812-1889)
Atresia of the vagina, congenital or accidental, in the pregnant or non-pregnant female. [Boston, 1880.] 19p. DNLM
80-6139

TAYLOR, Isaac E[benezer] (1812-1889)
The prevention of uterine hemorrhage. Baltimore, 1880. 20p. DNLM **80-6140**

TAYLOR, Isaac E[benezer] (1812-1889)
Gastro-hysterectomy, or the recent modification of the Caesarian section by Dr. Porro. Philadelphia, 1880. 15p. 1 plate. DNLM **80-6141**

TAYLOR, Isaac E[benezer] (1812-1889)
The early application of the forceps in the first stage of natural labor. Boston, 1880. 22p. DNLM **80-6142**

TAYLOR, Isaac E[benezer] (1812-1889)
Lupus, or esthiomène, of the vulvo-anal region. [Philadelphia, 1882.] 21p. 2 plates. DNLM **80-6143**

TAYLOR, Isaac E[benezer] (1812-1889)
Occipito-posterior presentations. Chicago, 1884. 31p. DNLM
80-6144

TAYLOR, Isaac E[benezer] (1812-1889)
Recto-labial and vulvar fistulae. [New York, 1885.] 20p. DNLM **80-6145**

TAYLOR, Isaac E[benezer] (1812-1889)
Eclampsia during pregnancy. [New York], 1886. 12p. DNLM **80-6146**

TAYLOR, Isaac E[benezer] (1812-1889)
Placenta praevia. New York, 1887. 12p. DNLM **80-6147**

TAYLOR, Isaac E[benezer] (1812-1889)
Lupus of the cervix uteri and female genitalia. New York: J. H. Vail & Co., 1888. 24p. 12 col. plates. DNLM; NNNAM **80-6148**

TAYLOR, Isaac E[benezer] (1812-1889)
Inversion of the uterus after somatic death. [New York], 1889. 10p. DNLM **80-6149**

TAYLOR, James R[idley] (1820-1895)
Paper on fractures of the long bones and their treatment. New York: Photo-Engr. Co., 1883. 19p. DNLM **80-6150**

TAYLOR, Lewis H. (*b.* 1850)
Report upon the epidemic of typhoid fever at Plymouth, Pa. Wilkes-Barre, Pa.: E. B. Yordy, 1885. 25p. 1 plan. DNLM **80-6151**

TAYLOR, Morse K. (1823-1889)
On the abortive treatment of buboes and lymphadenitis generally, by injections of carbolic acid. [Philadelphia, 1882.] 12p. DNLM **80-6152**

TAYLOR, Robert William (1842-1908)
The use of chrysophanic acid in the treatment of diseases of the skin. St. Louis: McCormick, Nixon & Co., 1880. 8p. DNLM **80-6153**

TAYLOR, Robert William (1842-1908)
Clinical notes on neuralgia of the sciatic nerve caused by syphilis. New York: D. Appleton & Co., 1880. 12p. DNLM **80-6154**

TAYLOR, Robert William (1842-1908)
On the mode of development and course of molluscum fibrosum, and on the question of its relation to acrochordon and other cutaneous outshoots. New York: William Wood & Co., 1887. 13p. DNLM **80-6155**

TAYLOR, Robert William (1842-1908)
A further contribution to the study of molluscum fibrosum; etiology; fibromatous infiltration and its relation to keloid. New York: William Wood & Co., 1887. 12p. DNLM **80-6156**

TAYLOR, Robert William (1842-1908)
Precocious gummata. [Philadelphia, 1887.] 17p. DNLM **80-6157**

TAYLOR, Robert William (1842-1908)
The toxic effects of iodoform, cutaneous and systematic. [New York, 1887.] 20p. DNLM **80-6158**

TAYLOR, Robert William (1842-1908)
An address delivered to the graduating class of the Charity Hospital Training School for Nurses, Oct. 12, 1887. [New York, 1887.] 10p. DNLM **80-6159**

TAYLOR, Robert William (1842-1908)
Tubercle of the testis. [Philadelphia, 1888.] 8p. DNLM **80-6160**

TAYLOR, Robert, William (1842-1908)
Lichen ruber as observed in America and its distinction from lichen planus. New York: D. Appleton & Co., 1889. 7p. 2 plates. **80-6161**

TAYLOR, Robert William (1842-1908)
Primary melano-sarcoma of the vulva. New York: D. Appleton & Co., 1889. 9p. 1 plate. DNLM **80-6162**

TAYLOR, Robert William (1842-1908)
Some practical points in the treatment of syphilis. [Philadelphia, 1889.] 23p. DNLM **80-6163**

TAYLOR, Robert William (1842-1908)
A clinical atlas of venereal & skin diseases, including diagnosis, prognosis & treatment. . . . Illustrated with two hundred and thirteen figures . . . on fifty-eight beautifully colored plates. . . . Philadelphia: Lea Bros. & Co., 1889. 427p. 58 col. plates. DLC; NNNAM; PPC; PU **80-6164**

TAYLOR, Thomas M.
A case of spinal hemianaesthesia and hemiparaplegia after fracture of the dorsal vertebra. New York, 1884. 7p. DNLM **80-6165**

TAYLOR, William H[enry] (1836-1910)
Report of a case of gastro-elytrotomy. [Chicago, 1883.] 12p. DNLM **80-6166**

TAYLOR, William L.
1. Fixed uteri. 2. Uterine hemorrhage. Philadelphia: Med. Print. Co., 1889. 14, 16p. DNLM **80-6167**

TERRY, Herbert (*b.* 1854)
The prevention of laceration of the perineum. Providence, 1886. 8p. DNLM **80-6168**

TERRY, Samuel Hough
Controlling sex in generation. The physical law influencing sex in the embryo of man and brute, and its direction to produce male or female offspring at will. New York: Fowler & Wells Co., 1885. 147p. DNLM; NNNAM **80-6169**

TERRY, Samuel Hough
Controlling sex in generation. The physical law influencing sex in the embryo of man and brute, and its direction to produce male or female offspring at will. 2nd ed., with an appendix of corroborative proofs. New York: Fowler & Wells Co., 1887. 209p. DNLM; NNNAM **80-6170**

TESTE, Alphonse (*b.* 1814)
A homoeopathic treatise on the diseases of children. Transl. from the French by Emma H. Coté. 4th ed. New York and Philadelphia: Boericke & Tafel, 1880. 345p. NNNAM; PPC; PPHa **80-6171**

THACHER, James K[ingsley] (1847-1891)
Galvanism in diphtheritic paralysis. [Philadelphia, 1885.] 3p. DNLM **80-6172**

THACHER, James K[ingsley] (1847-1891)
An elementary text-book of anatomy, physiology, and hygiene, including a special account of the effects of alcoholic liquors, stimulants, and narcotics upon the human system. By James K. Thacher, M.D. . . . and Arthur B. Morrill. . . . Hartford, Conn.: The Case, Lockwood & Brainard Co., 1887. 56p. DLC **80-6173**

THACHER, James K[ingsley] (1847-1891)
The relation of cardiac hypertrophy to nephritis. [Hartford, 1888.] 8p. DNLM **80-6174**

THACHER, James K[ingsley] (1847-1891)
The pulse-wave velocity and ventricular close-time in health. Philadelphia: W. J. Dornan, 1888. 21p. DNLM; PPC **80-6175**

THACHER, James K[ingsley] (1847-1891)
Note on the counting of white blood-cells. [Philadelphia, 1888.] 1 galley sheet. DNLM **80-6176**

THACKER, John A[dams] (1833-1891)
A new, simple, and safe method of preventing hemorrhage, treating aneurisms, and applicable for other surgical purposes. Cincinnati, [1887]. 2 l. DNLM **80-6177**

THAYER, William H[enry] (1822-1897)
Umbilical haemorrhage. New York, 1885. 7p. DNLM **80-6178**

THAYER, William H[enry] (1822-1897) and J. E. BAKER
Report on cholera to the Medical Society of the County of Kings. New York, 1885. 28p. DNLM **80-6179**

THAYER, William H[enry] (1822-1897)
History of malarial fever in Brooklyn. [New York, 1886.] 15p. DNLM **80-6180**

THAYER, William H[enry] (1822-1897)
Angina and pneumonia before 1857 and since; with the pathology of diphtheria in its various phases. [New York, 1889.] 22p. DNLM; NNNAM **80-6181**

THEOBALD, Samuel (1846-1930)
Boracic acid; a new remedy in eye diseases. [With supplementary note.] New York: Trow's Co., 1880. 15p. DNLM **80-6182**

THEOBALD, Samuel (1846-1930)
A new eye bandage. [New York, 1880.] 3p. DNLM **80-6183**

THEOBALD, Samuel (1846-1930)
Some of the errors in the diagnosis of eye diseases into which general practitioners are most apt to fall. Baltimore: J. W. Borst & Co., 1880. 6p. DNLM **80-6184**

THEOBALD, Samuel (1846-1930)
Four cases of otomycosis aspergillina successfully treated by the insufflation of oxide of zinc and boracic acid. New York: Trow, 1881. 8p. DNLM **80-6185**

THEOBALD, Samuel (1846-1930)
Report of section on ophthalmology and otology. Baltimore: J. W. Borst & Co., 1881. 10p. DNLM **80-6186**

THEOBALD, Samuel (1846-1930)
The use of constitutional remedies in the treatment of ear diseases. Philadelphia, 1882. 16p. DNLM **80-6187**

THEOBALD, Samuel (1846-1930)
Suggestions regarding the local treatment of some of the commoner affections of the ear. Baltimore, 1882. 6p. DNLM **80-6188**

THEOBALD, Samuel (1846-1930)
Preventable blindness. Baltimore, 1884. 8p. DNLM **80-6189**

THEOBALD, Samuel (1846-1930)
Some instructive cases of ametropia. [St. Louis: J. H. Chambers & Co.], 1884. 4p. DNLM **80-6190**

THEOBALD, Samuel (1846-1930)
The amblyopia of squinting eyes: is it a determining cause, or a consequence of the squint? [Philadelphia, 1886.] 10p. DNLM **80-6191**

THEOBALD, Samuel (1846-1930)
Notes of a series of cataract extractions by von Graefe's method. Baltimore, 1886. 15p. DNLM **80-6192**

THEOBALD, Samuel (1846-1930)
Is astigmatism a factor in the causation of glaucoma? [St. Louis, 1888.] 7p. DNLM **80-6193**

THEOBALD, Samuel (1846-1930)
The influence which the discovery of cocaine has exerted upon ophthalmic surgery. [Baltimore, 1888.] 3p. DNLM **80-6194**

THEOBALD, Samuel (1846-1930)
An unpleasant experience with the new local anaesthetic, hydrochlorate of erythrophleine. Philadelphia, 1888. 4p. DNLM **80-6195**

THEOBALD, Samuel (1846-1930)
The employment of oleate of veratria to facilitate the determination of errors of refraction. Hartford, Conn.: Case, Lockwood & Brainard Co., 1889. 7p. DNLM **80-6196**

THE THERMAL spring (spring No. 3) of Soden in the Taunus; chemical analysis by R. Fresenius; bacteriological examination by Grandhomme; medical communications by Koehler; supplement by the administration of the springs, Ph. Herm. Fay & Co., New York, [1889]. 31p. DNLM **80-6197**

THOMAS, Amos R[ussell] (1826-1895)
Diseases of the pancreas. By Professors A. R. Thomas, J. C. Morgan, A. Kordoerfer and E. A. Farrington. Chicago: Duncan Bros., 1882. 70p. IU-M; OCIM; PPHa **80-6198**

THOMAS, Charles Hermon (b. 1839)
Researches on hearing through the medium of the teeth and cranial bones. [Philadelphia, 1880.] 4p. DNLM **80-6199**

THOMAS, Charles Hermon (*b.* **1839)**
Graduated tenotomy in the treatment of insufficiencies of the ocular muscles. Philadelphia: W. J. Dornan, 1888. 12p. 1 plate. DNLM **80-6200**

THOMAS, Charles M.
Rapid lithotrity, with a report of two cases. Philadelphia: Sherman & Co., 1880. 7p. DNLM **80-6201**

THOMAS, Charles M.
Radical cure of hernia. Philadelphia, 1880. 11p. DNLM **80-6202**

THOMAS, Henry M. (*b.* **1861)**
An electric apparatus used in the diagnosis of diseases of the nervous system. Baltimore, [1889]. 2 l. DNLM **80-6203**

THOMAS, James Gray (1835-1884)
Dengue. Boston: Rand, Avery & Co., 1881. 20p. 1 chart. DNLM; MBM **80-6204**

THOMAS, James Gray (1835-1884)
Address in defense of the National Board of Health, against attacks in Congress, and on the importance of Sapelo quarantine station as a place of refuge for the dangerous and infected vessels for the South-Atlantic States. Savannah, Ga.: Morning New Printing House, 1883. 23p. DNLM; GU **80-6205**

THOMAS, Joseph (1811-1891)
A complete pronouncing medical dictionary: embracing the terminology of medicine and the kindred sciences, with their signification, etymology, and pronunciation. . . . On the basis of Thomas's comprehensive pronouncing medical dictionary. Philadelphia, London: J. B. Lippincott Co., 1886 [1885]. 844p. DLC; DNLM; NNNAM; PU **80-6206**

THOMAS, J[oseph] P[otts] (1830-1894)
The annual or inaugural address of the president of the Kentucky State Medical Society, June 23, 1886. Pembroke, Ky., 1886. 21p. DNLM **80-6207**

THOMAS, Richard Henry (1854-1904)
A contribution of the influence of season and weather on the death-rate from diphtheria in Baltimore (1861-1862). [Baltimore, 1883.] 17p. 6 diags. DNLM; MdBM **80-6208**

THOMAS, Richard Henry (1854-1904)
Report of a case of so-called hay fever, treated by the galvano-cautery. [Philadelphia, 1885.] 8p. DNLM **80-6209**

THOMAS, T[heodore] Gaillard (1832-1903)
Annual address by the president. The gynecology of the future, and its relations to surgery. [Philadelphia, 1880.] 20p. DNLM **80-6210**

THOMAS, T[heodore] Gaillard (1832-1903)
Clinical contribution to the subject of removal of the uterus in whole or in part for the extirpation of tumors connected with that organ. Philadelphia: Collins, 1880. 20p. DNLM **80-6211**

THOMAS, T[heodore] Gaillard (1832-1903)
A practical treatise on the diseases of women. . . . 5th ed., enl. and thoroughly rev. Containing two hundred and sixty-six engravings on wood. Philadelphia: Henry C. Lea's Son & Co., 1880. 806p. DLC; NNNAM; NNU-M; PPC **80-6212**

THOMAS, T[heodore] Gaillard (1832-1903)
Expansions of the bladder over the surface of abdominal tumors, and its attachment to them or to the abdominal walls as a complication of laparotomy. [Philadelphia, 1882.] 12p. DNLM **80-6213**

THOMAS, T[heodore] Gaillard (1832-1903)
The prevention and treatment of puerperal fever. New York, 1883. 32p. DNLM; NNNAM **80-6214**

THOMAS, T[heodore] Gaillard (1832-1903)
The prevention and treatment of puerperal fever. New York: D. Appleton & Co., 1884. 14p. DNLM **80-6215**

THOMAS, T[heodore] Gaillard (1832-1903)
Vulvar and vaginal enterocele. [New York, 1885.] 23p. DNLM **80-6216**

THOMAS, T[heodore] Gaillard (1832-1903)
A eulogy upon Cornelius Rea Agnew, read before the New York Academy of Medicine. . . . By appointment of the council, June 7th, 1888. [New York, 1888.] 26p. DLC; DNLM; NNNAM **80-6217**

THOMAS, T[heodore] Gaillard (1832-1903)
Acute mania and melancholia as sequelae of gynecological operations. [Philadelphia, 1889.] 12p. DNLM **80-6218**

THE THOMAS WILSON SANITARIUM. BALTIMORE
The sanitary care and treatment of children and their diseases, being a series of five essays by Drs. Elizabeth Garrett-Anderson, Samuel C. Busey, A. Jacobi, J. Forsyth Meigs, and J. Lewis Smith. Prepared by request of the trustees of The Thomas Wilson Sanitarium of Baltimore, Md. Boston: Houghton, Mifflin & Co., 1881. 309p. 3 plates. DNLM; MBM; PPC; PU **80-6219**

THOMPSON'S bromine-arsenic water. Springs in Ashe County, N.C. [Prospectus.] [Saltville, Va., 1888.] 24p. DNLM **80-6220**

THOMPSON, Henry (1820-1904)
Clinical lectures on diseases of the urinary organs. Delivered at University College Hospital. 6th ed. Philadelphia: P. Blakiston, Son & Co., 1882. 175p. CtY-M; DNLM; NNNAM; PU **80-6221**

THOMPSON, Henry (1820-1904)
Clinical lectures on diseases of the urinary organs. Delivered at University College Hospital. 7th ed. Philadelphia: P. Blakiston, Son & Co., 1883. 190p. MBM; NNNAM; OCIM; PPC **80-6222**

THOMPSON, Henry (1820-1904)
The diseases of the prostate. . . . 5th ed. Philadelphia: P. Blakiston, Son & Co., 1883. 157p. MBM; NNNAM; PPC; PPJ **80-6223**

THOMPSON, Henry (1820-1904)
On tumours of the bladder, their nature, symptoms and surgical treatment. . . . Philadelphia: Blakiston, Son & Co., 1884. 111p. 6 plates. CtY-M; DNLM; PPC; PU **80-6224**

THOMPSON, Henry (1820-1904)
Lectures on some important points connected with the surgery of the urinary organs, delivered in the Royal College of Surgeons. Philadelphia: P. Blakiston, Son & Co., 1884. 147p. DNLM; NNNAM; PU **80-6225**

THOMPSON, Henry (1820-1904)
The pathology and treatment of stricture of the urethra, and urinary fistulae. Philadelphia: P. Blakiston, Son & Co., 1885. 254p. DNLM; PPC; PU [1st American from 3rd & rev. London ed. Philadelphia: H. C. Lea, 1869. 359p.] **80-6226**

THOMPSON, Henry (1820-1904)
The diseases of the prostate. . . . 6th ed. Philadelphia: P. Blakiston, Son & Co., 1886. 237p. DNLM; NNNAM; OCIM; PPC **80-6227**

THOMPSON, Henry (1820-1904)
Clinical lectures on diseases of the urinary organs. Delivered at University College Hospital. 8th ed. Philadelphia: P. Blakiston, Son & Co., 1888. 470p. DNLM; IU-M; PPC; PU **80-6228**

THOMPSON, Mary H[arris] (1829-1895)
Salpingitis; its diagnosis and treatment. [Chicago, 1889.] 16p. DNLM **80-6229**

THOMPSON, Pinckney
Public health. Henderson, Ky.: C. H. Johnson & Bro., 1881. 18p. DNLM **80-6230**

THOMPSON, William Gilman (1856-1927)
Training schools for nurses, with notes on twenty-two schools. . . . New York: G. P. Putnam's Sons, 1883. 57p. DLC; DNLM; NNNAM **80-6231**

THOMSON, William (1833-1907)
The practical examination of railway employees, as to color-blindness, acuteness of vision, and hearing. [Philadelphia: Lea Bros. & Co., 1882.] 18p. DNLM; PPC **80-6232**

THOMSON, William H[anna] (1833-1918)
Notes on materia medica and therapeutics, taken from the lectures delivered by. . . . New York: Trow, 1880?]. 379p. DNLM **80-6233**

THOMSON, William H[anna] (1833-1918)
Notes on materia medica and therapeutics, taken from the lectures delivered by. . . . [2nd ed.] [New York:] E. LeFevre, 1882. 379p. NN; NNNAM **80-6234**

THOMSON, William H[anna] (1833-1918)
Notes on materia medica and therapeutics, taken from the lectures delivered by. . . . 3rd ed., rev. and enl. New York: Press of Stettiner, Lambert & Co., 1886. 264p. NNNAM **80-6235**

THOMSON, William H[anna] (1833-1918)
Notes on materia medica and therapeutics, taken from lectures delivered by. . . . Edited by W. M. H. McEnroe. . . . 4th ed. completely rev. and enl. New York: Press of Stettiner, Lambert & Co., 1889. 303p. DLC; NNNAM; OCLloyd **80-6236**

[THORNE, Robert]
Asiatic cholera. A brief sketch of its nature and history, together with simple and practical measures of prevention and immediate treatment. . . . Published by G. E. Beers. . . . Hartford, Conn.: Clark & Smith, job and pamphlet printers, 1885. 14p. DLC **80-6237**

THORNER, Max (1859?-1899)
The removal of foreign bodies from the larynx: a cockleburr removed from the larynx by Voltolini's sponge method. Cincinnati, 1886. 8p. DNLM **80-6238**

THORNER, Max (1859?-1899)
Salol: with report on the use of salol in affections of the throat, ear, and eye. Cincinnati, 1887. 7p. DNLM **80-6239**

THORNER, Max (1859?-1899)
A new galvano-cautery handle. [New York, 1888.] 1 l. DNLM **80-6240**

THORNER, Max (1859?-1899)
Haematoma of the septum narium. [Philadelphia, 1889.] 4p. DNLM **80-6241**

THORNER, Max (1859?-1899)
A case of persistent tinnitus aurium relieved by the removal of a nasal obstruction. [Cincinnati, 1889.] 8p. DNLM **80-6242**

THORNER, Max (1859?-1899)
Chronic throat affections of rheumatic origin. Cleveland: Williams Publ. Co., 1889. 8p. DNLM **80-6243**

THORNTON, Gustavus B. (*b.* 1835)
Memphis sanitation and quarantine, 1879 and 1880. Boston: Rand, Avery & Co., 1881. 8 l. DNLM **80-6244**

THORNTON, Gustavus B. (*b.* 1835)
The death-rate of Memphis. To which is appended a circular on the Waring sewer system, by J. H. Humphreys. Memphis: Tracy & Co., 1881. 10p. DNLM **80-6245**

THORNTON, Gustavus B. (*b.* 1835)
Gulf coast quarantine. Report to the Tennessee State Board of Health, on the quarantine conference held at New Orleans, June 2nd, 3rd, and 4th, 1884. Nashville: Hasslock & Ambrose, 1884. 16p. DNLM **80-6246**

THORNTON, Gustavus B. (*b.* 1835)
Sanitation of the Mississippi Valley. Concord, N.H., 1885. 8p. DNLM **80-6247**

THORNTON, Gustavus B. (*b.* 1835)
Report to the Tennessee State Board of Health, on the conference of the State boards of health, held in St. Louis, Oct. 13th and 15th, and in Washington, Dec. 10th and 11th, 1884, Jan. 6, 1885. Nashville, 1885. 7p. DNLM **80-6248**

THORNTON, Gustavus B. (*b.* 1835)
The present improved sanitary condition of Memphis. Nashville: Hasslock & Ambrose, [1887]. 14p. DNLM **80-6249**

THORNTON, William (*b.* 1846)
Rationalism in medical treatment, or the restoration of chemism, the system of the future. Boston, 1885. 46p. DNLM
80-6250

THOROWGOOD, John C[harles] (1833-1913)
Aids to diagnosis. Part II. Physical. New York: G. P. Putnam's Sons, 1881. 61p. DNLM; NNNAM **80-6251**

THE THREE ethical codes. The code of ethics of the American Medical Association, its constitution and by-laws. The code of ethics of the American Institute of Homoeopathy. The code of ethics of the National Eclectic Medical Society. Detroit, [1888]. 54p. DNLM **80-6252**

THURBER, WHYLAND & CO.
General prices current. [Drugs, sundries.] New York, 1888. 208p. NNNAM **80-6253**

TIDY, Charles Meymott (1843-1892)
Legal medicine. Philadelphia: Henry C. Lea's Son & Co., 1882-1884. 2 v. DNLM; NNNAM; PPC; PU
80-6254

TIDY, Charles Meymott (1843-1892)
Legal medicine. New York: William Wood & Co., 1882-1884. 3 v. DNLM; NNNAM **80-6255**

TIDY, Charles Meymott (1843-1892)
Handbook of modern chemistry inorganic and organic. For the use of students. 2nd ed. Philadelphia: P. Blakiston, Son & Co., 1887. 894p. DNLM; IU-M; NNNAM; PU
80-6256

TIEMANN, GEO., & CO.
The American armamentarium chirurgicum. New York: [C. H. Ludwig, 1889.] 846p. DLC; NNNAM
80-6257

TIFFANY, Flavel B[enjamin] (1846-1918)
Skin grafting for malignancy of the orbit. [St. Louis, 1882.] 8p. DNLM **80-6258**

TIFFANY, Flavel B[enjamin] (1846-1918)
Glaucoma. St. Louis, 1883. 16p. DNLM
80-6259

TIFFANY, Louis McLane (1844-1916)
Diagnosis of malignant tumors of the upper jaw in youth. Baltimore: J. W. Borst & Co., 1880. 8p. DNLM
80-6260

TIFFANY, Louis McLane (1844-1916)
Treatment of irreducible epiplocele. Baltimore: J. W. Borst & Co., 1882. 7p. DNLM **80-6261**

TIFFANY, Louis McLane (1844-1916)
Treatment of cancer of the rectum. A case of amputation at the hip joint; recovery. [Baltimore, 1882.] 8p. DNLM
80-6262

TIFFANY, Louis McLane (1844-1916)
Observations upon mammary tumors, based on an analysis of thirty cases in practice. [Baltimore, 1883.] 5p. DNLM
80-6263

TIFFANY, Louis McLane (1844-1916)
The prone position during operations upon the jaws. Baltimore, Md., 1883. 3p. DNLM **80-6264**

TIFFANY, Louis McLane (1844-1916)
Plastic surgery of the face. [Richmond, 1883.] 6p. DNLM
80-6265

TIFFANY, Louis McLane (1844-1916)
Left lumbar colotomy and the position of the descending colon. [Baltimore, Md., 1883.] 1 l. DNLM
80-6266

TIFFANY, Louis McLane (1844-1916)
Intussusception in an infant; laparotomy; death; suggestions for treatment. [Baltimore, 1883.] 2p. DNLM
80-6267

TIFFANY, Louis McLane (1844-1916)
Sub-spinous dislocation of the right femur, occurring twice in the same person, with deformity of knee of long standing; reduction. [Baltimore, 1883.] 2p. DNLM
80-6268

TIFFANY, Louis McLane (1844-1916)
Division of the crucial ligaments for the relief of knee-joint ankylosis. [Baltimore, 1884.] 2p. DNLM
80-6269

TIFFANY, Louis McLane (1844-1916)
A contribution to the history of ligation of the common femoral artery. [Philadelphia, 1884.] 12p. DNLM
80-6270

TIFFANY, Louis McLane (1844-1916)
Results of operative measures for rectal cancer. [Baltimore, 1884.] 4p. DNLM **80-6271**

TIFFANY, Louis McLane (1844-1916)
Nephrolithotomy. Philadelphia: Collins, 1885. 13p. DNLM
80-6272

TIFFANY, Louis McLane (1844-1916)
A case of nephrolithotomy during the fifth month of pregnancy. [Philadelphia, 1887.] 4p. DNLM
80-6273

TIFFANY, Louis McLane (1844-1916)
Comparison between the surgical diseases of the white and colored races. Philadelphia: W. J. Dornan, 1887. 4p. 1 plate. DNLM **80-6274**

TIFFANY, Louis McLane (1844-1916)
A contribution to hepatic surgery, with a suggestion for rendering a portion of the liver extraperitoneal. [Philadelphia, 1888.] 6p. DNLM **80-6275**

TIFFANY, Louis McLane (1844-1916)
Pregnancy and operative surgery. Their mutual relations. Philadelphia: W. J. Dornan, 1889. 19p. DNLM
80-6276

TIFFANY, Louis McLane (1844-1916)
Free division of the capsule of the kidney for the relief of nephralgia. Philadelphia: W. J. Dornan, 1889. 17p. DNLM
80-6277

TILDEN & CO. NEW YORK CITY
Formulae for making tinctures, infusions, syrups . . . mixtures, pills. . . . [New York]: Tilden & Co., 1886. 315, 16p. NNNAM
80-6278

TILDEN, George H[orton] and F. S. WATSON
Nineteen cases of internal urethrotomy by Otis's method. Cambridge: Riverside Press, 1883. 16p. DNLM; MBM
80-6279

TILDEN, George H[orton]
The pathogenesis of certain affections of the skin. [Boston, 1885.] 13p. DNLM **80-6280**

TILDEN, George H[orton]
So-called mycosis fongoïde. Boston: Cupples, Upham & Co., 1885. 23p. DNLM **80-6281**

TILDEN, George H[orton]
Some points in the treatment of syphilis. [Boston, 1886.] 11p. DNLM **80-6282**

TILDEN, George H[orton]
Trophoneurosis of the skin caused by injury to the median nerve. New York: William Wood & Co., 1886. 6p. DNLM
80-6283

TILT, Edward [John] (1815-1893)
A hand-book of uterine therapeutics. New York: William Wood & Co., 1881. 328p. NNNAM; OCIM; PU
80-6284

TILT, Edward [John] (1815-1893)
The change of life in health and disease. A clinical treatise on the diseases of the ganglionic nervous system incidental to women at the decline of life. New York: Bermingham & Co., 1882. 250p. NNNAM; PU **80-6285**

TIPTON, A. W.
A revised and enlarged edition of Clark's new system of electrical medication. Chicago: C. J. Johnson, 1882. 264p. port. DNLM; IU-M; OCIM **80-6286**

TIPTON, F.
What the general practitioner should know of the throat and nose. Selma: The Times Job Print, 1883. 15p. DNLM
80-6287

TIPTON, F.
The Negro problem from a medical standpoint. [New York, 1886.] 11p. DNLM [*Also*: New York, 1886 (with additions). 12p.] **80-6288**

TITUS, E. C.
A few clinical cases showing the value of oxygen combined with nitrogen monoxide in the treatment of pulmonary and other troubles. [New York: Lehmaier & Bro., 1889.] 8p. DNLM **80-6289**

TODD, S[imeon] S[eymour] (1826-1899)
Treatment of hemorrhoids. [St. Louis, 1881.] 5p. DNLM
80-6290

TODD, S[imeon] S[eymour] (1826-1899)
Ovariotomy. [Fort Scott, Kans., 1881.] 8p. DNLM
80-6291

TOMES, John (1815-1895)
A system of dental surgery. 3rd ed. Philadelphia: P. Blakiston, Son & Co., 1887. 772p. DNLM; MdU-D; NNNAM; PPC
80-6292

TOOKER, Robert N[ewton] (1841-1902)
Homoeopathy and its relation to the germ-theory. Being the President's address delivered before the Illinois Homoeopathic Medical Association at its thirtieth annual session held at Peoria, Ill., May 20, 1885. Chicago: Gross & Delbridge, 1885. 21p. IU-M; OCIM; PPHa **80-6293**

TOWLES, William B[everly] (1847-1893)
Notes on anatomy. Lithographed by Anderson Bros. Charlottesville: University of Virginia, 1888. 413 l. DNLM
80-6294

TOWNSEND, Charles W[endell] (*b.* 1859)
The so-called physiological loss in infants. [Boton, 1887.] 10p. DNLM **80-6295**

TOWNSEND, Charles W[endell] (*b.* 1859)
Incontinence of urine in children. [Philadelphia, 1887.] 10p. DNLM **80-6296**

TOWNSEND, Charles W[endell] (*b.* 1859)
Endemic cerebro-spinal meningitis. Boston: Cupples & Hurd, 1888. 17p. 1 diag. DNLM **80-6297**

TOWNSEND, Charles W[endell] (*b.* 1859)
Two difficult cases of breech presentation. Boston: Cupples & Hurd, 1889. 7p. DNLM **80-6298**

TOWNSEND, Charles W[endell] (*b.* 1859)
Acute lobar pneumonia in children. [Philadelphia, 1889.] 23p. DNLM **80-6299**

TOWNSEND, Charles W[endell] (*b.* 1859) and A. COOLIDGE, Jr.
The mortality of acute lobar pneumonia, from a study of all the cases of this disease treated at the Massachusetts General Hospital from the first case, in 1822, up to the present day. Philadelphia: W. J. Dornan, 1889. 27p. DNLM
80-6300

TOWNSEND, M. M.
Hay fever, asthma, and chronic catarrh. Testimonials regarding cure, and special directions for treatment. Grinnell, Iowa: Cravath & Shaw, 1882. 19p. DNLM **80-6301**

TRACY, Roger S[herman] (1841-1926)
Hand-book of sanitary information for householders, containing facts and suggestions about ventilation, drainage, care of contagious diseases, disinfection, food and water; with appendices on disinfectants and plumbers' materials. New York: D. Appleton & Co., 1884. 110p. DNLM; NNNAM
80-6302

TRACY, Roger S[herman] (1841-1926)
The essentials of anatomy, physiology, and hygiene. A textbook for schools and academies. New York: D. Appleton & Co., 1884. 299p. 1 plate. DNLM; MH; NIC; NN
80-6303

TRACY, Roger S[herman] (1841-1926)
The outlines of anatomy, physiology, and hygiene. Being an edition of the essentials of anatomy, physiology and hygiene. New York, Cincinnati & Chicago, [1889]. 383p. 1 plate. DNLM; NN **80-6304**

TRALL, Russell Thacher (1812-1877)
Uterine diseases and displacements; a practical treatise on the various diseases, malpositions and structural derangements of the uterus and its appendages. New York: Fowler & Wells, 1881. 167p. 53 plates. DNLM; NNNAM
80-6305

TRALL, Russell Thacher (1812-1877)
The human voice: its anatomy, physiology, pathology, therapeutics, and training; with rules of order for lyceums. New York: Fowler & Wells, 1882. 107p. DNLM: NNNAM
80-6306

TRALL, Russell Thacher (1812-1877)
Popular physiology; a familiar exposition of the structures, functions, and relations of the human system. New York: Fowler & Wells, 1884. 223p. DNLM; NNNAM
80-6307

TRALL, Russell Thacher (1812-1877)
Digestion and dyspepsia; a complete explanation of the physiology of the digestive processes, with the symptoms and treatment of dyspepsia and other disorders of the digestive organs. New York: Fowler & Wells Co., 1884. 160p. DNLM; NNNAM **80-6308**

TRALL, Russell Thacher (1812-1877)
Sexual physiology and hygiene; or the mysteries of man. Rev. ed. New York: M. L. Holbrook, 1885. 344p. NNNAM
80-6309

TREAT, Charles R. (*d.* 1901)
Sanitary entombment; the ideal disposition of the dead. [New York, 1889.] 22p. DNLM **80-6310**

A TREATISE on the Greenbrier White Sulphur Springs and its waters. Baltimore, 1882. 48p. DNLM
80-6311

A TREATISE on the Greenbrier White Sulphur Springs and its waters. Richmond, Va.: Everett, Waddey & Co., 1886. 30p. DNLM **80-6312**

A TREATISE on trichina spiralis, the worm in the pig, the cause of sickness and death and serious loss to the national wealth. Referring to experiments by Virchow, Blasius, Leukert, Griepenkerl, Kuehn Engelbrecht, and others. Compiled and augmented by a German expert and microscopist. Transl. by Siegfried Sydow. New York: H. Cherouny, 1883. 32p. DNLM; NNNAM **80-6313**

TREATMENT of constipation. New York: McKesson & Robbins [1888, *vel subseq.*] 16p. DNLM; NNNAM **80-6314**

THE TREATMENT and cure of rheumatism, gout, lumbago, etc. By Chas. W. Brown, M.D., [*et al.*]. [Philadelphia: W. R. Warner & Co., 1889.] 3 l. DNLM **80-6315**

ON THE TREATMENT of diphtheria and dyspepsia by "papoid." Being a résumé of our present knowledge of the drug, compiled from the published writings of the most eminent English, continental, and United States authorities upon the subject. New York: Johnson & Johnson, [1886, *vel subseq.*]. 31p. DNLM; NNNAM **80-6316**

TREMAINE, William S[cott] (1838-1898)
Suprapubic lithotomy. Buffalo, N.Y.: Ulbrich & Kingsley, [1884]. 11p. DNLM **80-6317**

TREMAINE, William S[cott] (1838-1898)
Cyst of the pancreas successfully removed. [Philadelphia, 1888.] 3p. DNLM **80-6318**

TREVES, Frederick (1853-1923)
Scrofula and its gland diseases. An introduction to the general pathology of scrofula, with an account of the histology, diagnosis, and treatment of its glandular affections. New York: Bermingham & Co., 1882. 181p. DNLM; NNNAM; PU
80-6319

TREVES, Frederick (1853-1923)
Scrofula and its gland diseases. An introduction to the general pathology of scrofula, with an account of the histology, diagnosis, and treatment of its glandular affections. Philadelphia: Henry C. Lea's Son & Co., 1883. 77p. DNLM; NNNAM; PPC; PPJ **80-6320**

TREVES, Frederick (1853-1923)
Surgical applied anatomy. Philadelphia, Pa.: Henry C. Lea's Son & Co., [1883]. 531p. CtY-M; DNLM; NNNAM; PPC
80-6321

TREVES, Frederick (1853-1923)
Surgical applied anatomy. [2nd ed.] Philadelphia: Henry C. Lea's Son & Co., 1883. 531p. DNLM; PPC; PU
80-6322

TREVES, Frederick (1853-1923)
Intestinal obstruction; its varieties, with their pathology, diagnosis, and treatment. The Jacksonian prize essay. . . . Philadelphia: Henry C. Lea's Son & Co., 1884. 515p. DNLM; NNNAM; PPC; PU **80-6323**

TREVES, Frederick, ed. (1853-1923)
A manual of surgery. In treatises by various authors. Philadelphia: Lea Bros. & Co., 1886. 3 v. DNLM; NNNAM; OCIM; PU
80-6324

TREVES, Frederick (1853-1923)
Surgical applied anatomy. [3rd ed.] Philadelphia: Lea Bros. & Co., [1888]. 566p. DNLM; MBM; OCIM; PPC
80-6325

TROUSSEAU, Armand (1801-1867)
Treatise on therapeutics, transl. by D. F. Lincoln, M.D., from the French of A. Trousseau . . . and H. Pidoux. . . . 9th ed., rev. and enl., with the assistance of Constantine Paul. . . . New York: William Wood & Co., 1880. 3 v. DLC; DNLM; NNNAM; PPC **80-6326**

TRUAX, Charles, & CO.
Price list of medical supplies. . . . Manufacturers and jobbers of pharmaceutical preparations, surgical instruments, and strictly pure drugs. 3rd ed. Chicago: Charles Truax & Co., [1885?] 400p. ICU; NNNAM **80-6327**

TUCKER, James L.
Case of herpes omo-brachialis. Chicago, Ill.: Clark & Longley Co., 1887. 4p. DNLM **80-6328**

TUCKER, James L.
Hydrophobia vera, with report of a case. Chicago: Clark & Longley Co., 1887. 6p. DNLM **80-6329**

TUCKER, Joshua (1800-1881)
Address delivered before the American Academy of Dental Science, at their thirteenth annual meeting. Boston: S. Woodberry & Co., 1881. 22p. DNLM; MBM
80-6330

TUCKER, Willis G[aylord] (1849-1922)
A memorial sketch of the life and character of the late Jacob Simmons Mosher, of Albany, N.Y. New York, 1885. 7p. DNLM **80-6331**

TUCKER, Willis G[aylord] (1849-1922)
Report on the chemical examination of the waters of the public wells of Albany, N.Y. Albany, N.Y.: Burdick & Taylor, 1885. 10p. DNLM **80-6332**

TUCKER, Willis G[aylord] (1849-1922)
The introductory address of the fifth lecture course at the Albany College of Pharmacy. Albany, N.Y.: Burdick & Taylor, 1885. 14p. DNLM **80-6333**

TUCKER, Willis G[aylord] (1849-1922)
The introductory address to the eighth lecture course at the Albany College of Pharmacy. Published by the class. Albany, 1888. 18p. DNLM **80-6334**

TUHOLSKE, Herman (*b.* 1848)
Iodoform in surgery. St. Louis, Mo.: J. H. Chambers & Co., 1883. 15p. DNLM **80-6335**

TURNBULL, Charles S[mith] (1847-1918)
Second annual abstract of ophthalmological literature for 1881-1882. [Philadelphia], 1882. 33p. DNLM; PPC
80-6336

TURNBULL, Charles S[mith] (1847-1918)
Powdered boracic acid in the treatment of chronic purulent inflammation of the middle ear ("otorrhoea"). Philadelphia, 1882. 15p. DNLM **80-6337**

TURNBULL, Charles S[mith] (1847-1918)
Does a chronic discharge from the ear make life insurance hazardous? [Philadelphia, 1884.] 3p. DNLM
80-6338

TURNBULL, Charles S[mith] (1847-1918)
Ophthalmological miscellanies. [Philadelphia, 1884.] 6p. DNLM **80-6339**

TURNBULL, Charles S[mith] (1847-1918)
Address in otology. [Philadelphia, 1885.] 7p. DNLM
80-6340

TURNBULL, Charles S[mith] (1847-1918)
Ophthalmology. [Philadelphia, 1885.] 8p. DNLM
80-6341

TURNBULL, Charles S[mith] (1847-1918)
Address on ophthalmology. Philadelphia, 1887. 13p. DNLM
80-6342

TURNBULL, Laurence (1821-1900)
Hydrobromic ether or bromide of ethyl as an anaesthetic. [Philadelphia, 1880.] 2 l. DNLM
80-6343

TURNBULL, Laurence (1821-1900)
Memoir of James Aitken Meigs. Philadelphia: P. Madeira, 1881. 18p. DNLM; PU **80-6344**

TURNBULL, Laurence (1821-1900)
Imperfect hearing and the hygiene of the ear. Including nervous symptoms, tinnitus aurium, aural vertigo, diseases of the naso-pharyngeal membrane, middle ear, and mastoid region. With home instruction of the deaf. 3rd ed. Philadelphia: J. B. Lippincott & Co., 1881. 147p. DNLM; PPC: PPJ; PU **80-6345**

TURNBULL, Laurence (1821-1900)
Diseases of the ear in locomotive and other engineers, firemen, and conductors, which may endanger the lives of the traveling public. [Philadelphia, 1881.] 6p. DNLM
80-6346

TURNBULL, Laurence (1821-1900)
Deafness as the result of the poison of syphilis. Philadelphia: W. F. Fell & Co., [1881]. 8p. DNLM
80-6347

TURNBULL, Laurence (1821-1900)
Progress of otology. [Philadelphia, 1884.] 8p. DNLM
80-6348

TURNBULL, Laurence (1821-1900)
Report on the diseases of the ear in locomotive and other engineers, firemen, and conductors, which may endanger the lives of the traveling public. [Chicago, 1884.] 12p. DNLM
80-6349

TURNBULL, Laurence (1821-1900)
Hydrobromic ether or bromide of ethyl as an anaesthetic. Chicago, 1885. 20p. DNLM **80-6350**

TURNBULL, Laurence (1821-1900)
The new local anaesthetic; hydrochlorate of cocaine (muriate of cocaine), and etherization by the rectum. Philadelphia: P. Blakiston, Son & Co., 1885. 76p. DNLM; PPC; PU
80-6351

TURNBULL, Laurence (1821-1900)
A clinical manual of the diseases of the ear. 2nd ed. Philadelphia: J. B. Lippincott & Co., 1887. 567p. tables, col. front. DLC; DNLM; NNNAM; PPC **80-6352**

TURNER, Dawson W[illiam] (1815-1885)
Hints and remedies for the treatment of common accidents and diseases and rules of simple hygiene. The two parts complete. Compiled by. . . . Revised, corrected, and enlarged by twelve eminent medical men belonging to different hospitals in London and by one Right Rev. Bishop of the Established Church, formerly surgeon to one of the London hospitals and F.R.C.S. From the 8th English ed. New York: Macmillan & Co., 1882. 106p. DNLM; NNNAM
80-6353

TURNER, George A.
One hundred and thirty-eight cases amputation of scrotum for elephantiasis Arabum. . . . [New York,1882.] 8p. DNLM
80-6354

TURNER, J. Edward (1822-1889)
The history of the first inebriate asylum in the world by its founder. An account of his indictment. Also a sketch of the Woman's National Hospital by its projector. New York: Published by the Author, 1888. 508p. ICU; NN
80-6355

TURNER, Thomas J. (*d.* **1901)**
The hygiene of emigrant ships; read before the American Public Health Association. Boston: Rand, Avery & Co., 1881. 71p. DNLM **80-6356**

TURNER, Thomas J. (*d.* **1901)**
Some remarks upon national and international sanitary jurisprudence. Boston: Rand, Avery & Co., 1882. 40p. DNLM **80-6357**

TURNER, Thomas J. (*d.* **1901)**
Some considerations upon the naval retiring board in medico-legal relations. Washington: Government Printing Office, 1885. 10p. DNLM **80-6358**

TWITCHELL, Herbert F. (*b.* **1859)**
Pleuritic effusion; its treatment. Portland: S. Berry, 1889. 15p. DNLM **80-6359**

TYNDALE, J. Hilgard (*b.* **1843)**
The localized and diffused connective tissue processes in the lungs, and their relations to pulmonary phthisis. [St. Louis, 1882.] 11p. DNLM **80-6360**

TYNDALE, J. Hilgard (*b.* **1843)**
Catarrhal pneumonia, and its relation to pulmonary phthisis. Richmond: Whittet & Shepperson, 1882. 8p. DNLM **80-6361**

TYNDALE, J. Hilgard (*b.* **1843)**
Home and climatic treatment of pulmonary consumption on the basis of modern doctrines. New York: Bermingham & Co., 1882. 174p. DNLM; NNNAM **80-6362**

TYNDALE, J. Hilgard (*b.* **1843)**
Home treatment of pulmonary consumption by systematic antisepsis and counter-irritation. Richmond, Va.: Old Dominion Print, [1883]. 13p. DNLM **80-6363**

TYNDALE, J. Hilgard (*b.* **1843)**
New Mexico: Its climatic advantages for consumptives. Cambridge: Riverside Press, 1883. 24p. DNLM **80-6364**

TYNDALL, John (1820-1893)
Essays on the floating-matter of the air in relation to putrefaction and infection. New York: D. Appleton & Co., 1882. 338p. ICU, MH; NIC; NN **80-6365**

TYNER, E. S.
A treatise on yellow fever; containing a synopsis of its causes, nature, symptoms, treatment, precautions to be used to prevent its spread, and being indigenous to the tropical Atlantic and defined as a nautical disease. Jacksonville, Fla.: Da Costa, 1889. 65p. DNLM **80-6366**

TYNG, Anita E[lizabeth] (1838-1913)
A case of removal of both ovaries by abdominal section for the relief of an exhausting menorrhagia and uterine fibroid. [Providence, 1888.] 11p. DNLM **80-6367**

TYRRELL, Gerrard George (1831-1895)
Annual address delivered before the Medical Society of the State of California. Sacramento: Day & Joy, 1882. 25p. CLM; CU-M; DNLM **80-6368**

TYSON, James (1841-1919)
A guide to the practical examination of urine. For the use of physicians and students. 3rd ed., rev. and cor. Philadelphia: Lindsay & Blakiston, 1880. 183p. col. plates. DLC; NNNAM; PPC; PU **80-6369**

TYSON, James (1841-1919)
A treatise on Bright's disease and diabetes. With especial reference to pathology and therapeutics. . . . Including a section on retinitis in Bright's disease. By William F. Norris. . . . Philadelphia: Lindsay & Blakiston, 1881. 312p. col. plates. DLC; DNLM; PPC; PU **80-6370**

TYSON, James (1841-1919)
Higher medical education. [Philadelphia, 1882.] 8p. DNLM **80-6371**

TYSON, James (1841-1919)
A guide to the practical examination of urine. For the use of physicians and students. 4th ed. Rev. and cor. Philadelphia: P. Blakiston, Son & Co., 1883. 196p. col. plates. DLC; OCIM; PU **80-6372**

TYSON, James (1841-1919)
A guide to the practical examination of urine. For the use of physicians and students. 5th ed. Rev. & cor. Philadelphia: P. Blakiston, Son & Co., 1886. 249p. col. plates. DLC; NNNAM; PPC; PPJ **80-6373**

TYSON, James (1841-1919)
Does the present state of knowledge justify a clinical and pathological correlation of rheumatism, gout, diabetes, and chronic Bright's disease? Philadelphia: W. J. Dornan, 1886. 16p. DNLM; PPC **80-6374**

TYSON, James (1841-1919)
A guide to the practical examination of urine. For the use of physicians and students. 6th ed. Rev. & cor. Philadelphia: P. Blakiston, Son & Co., 1888. 253p. col. frontis. DLC; IU-M; PPC; PU **80-6375**

TYSON, James (1841-1919)
Chronic interstitial nephritis, or chronically contracted kidney; renal cirrhosis. Philadelphia, 1888. 8p. DNLM **80-6376**

TYSON, James (1841-1919)
Treatment of acute pneumonia. [Philadelphia, 1889.] 11p. DNLM **80-6377**

ULTZMANN, Robert (1842-1889)
Pyuria; or, pus in the urine, and its treatment. Comprising the diagnosis and treatment of acute and chronic urethritis, prostatitis, cystitis, and pyelitis, with especial reference to their local treatment. Transl. by permission by Walter B. Platt. New York: D. Appleton & Co., 1884. 98p. DLC; DNLM; NNNAM **80-6378**

ULTZMANN, Robert (1842-1889)
The neuroses of the genito-urinary system in the male, with sterility and impotence. Transl. by Gardner W. Allen. Philadelphia & London: F. A. Davis, 1889. 160p. DNLM; PPC; PU **80-6379**

UNDERHILL, Joshua W.
Valedictory address to the Obstetrical Society of Cincinnati and inaugural address by Thad. A. Reamy. [Cincinnati, 1880.] 24p. DNLM; OC **80-6380**

UNDERWOOD, Benoni F. (1843-1932)
Rationale of infant mortality. New York: A. L. Chatterton & Co., 1881. 16p. NNNAM **80-6381**

UNDERWOOD, Benoni F. (1843-1932)
Diseases of children, with therapeutic indications. New York: A. L. Chatterton & Co., 1882. 216p. NNNAM **80-6382**

UNDERWOOD, Benoni F. (1843-1932)
A materia medica of differential potency. New York: A. L. Chatterton & Co., 1884. 215p. DNLM; NNNAM **80-6383**

UNDERWOOD, Benoni F. (1843-1932)
Phthisis pulmonalis. New York: A. L. Chatterton & Co., 12p. NNNAM **80-6384**

UNDERWOOD, Benoni F. (1843-1932)
Headache, and its materia medica. New York: A. L. Chatterton & Co., 1889. 212p. NNNAM **80-6385**

U.S. BUREAU OF MEDICINE AND SURGERY
. . . Report on yellow fever in the U.S.S. Plymouth in 1878-1879. Prepared under direction of Philip S. Wales, Surgeon-General U.S. Navy. Washington: Government Printing Office, 1880. 85p. 8 plates, fold. maps. DLC **80-6386**

U.S. NAVY DEPARTMENT. BUREAU OF MEDICINE AND SURGERY
Report of the Surgeon-General of the Navy for the year 1886. Washington: Government Printing Office, 1886. 126p. **80-6387**

U.S. SURGEON-GENERAL'S OFFICE. LIBRARY
Index-catalogue of the library of the Surgeon-General's Office, United States Army. Authors and subjects. . . . Washington: Government Printing Office, 1880-1895. 16 v. DNLM; NNNAM; PPC: PU **80-6388**

UNIVERSITY MEDICAL COLLEGE OF KANSAS CITY
Annual announcements for the sessions of 1881-1882 (1); 1883-1884 (3); 1886-1887 (6); 1888-1889 to 1891-1892 (8-11). Kansas City, 1881-1891. DNLM [Formerly, Medical Department of the University of Kansas City, Missouri] **80-6389**

UNNA, Paul Gerson (1850-1929)
On herpes progenitalis, especially in women. New York, 1883. 14p. DNLM **80-6390**

UPSHUR, John N[ottingham] (1848-1924)
The disorders of menstruation. A practical treatise. New York & London: G. P. Putnam's Sons, 1886. 200p. DLC; DNLM; NNNAM **80-6391**

UTLEY, M. Howell
Didactic remarks respecting electricity and its application for the treatment and cure of diseases. New York: M. J. Rooney, 1886. 8p. DNLM **80-6392**

VALENTINE, Ferdinand Charles (1851-1910)
600 medical don'ts; or, The physician's utility enhanced. . . . New York: G. W. Dillingham; [etc., etc.], 1887. 144p. DLC; NNNAM **80-6393**

VALK, Francis (1845-1919)
Report of four operations for the removal of cataract without an iridectomy, and by an entirely new method. New York: M. J. Rooney, [1887]. 12p. DNLM **80-6394**

VALK, Francis (1845-1919)
Lectures on the errors of refraction and their correction with glasses. New York & London: G. P. Putnam's Sons, 1889. 241p. 8 plates. DNLM; NNNAM **80-6395**

VALLERY-RADOT, René (1853-1933)
Louis Pasteur, his life and labors, by his son-in-law. Transl. from the French, by Lady Claud Hamilton. New York: D. Appleton & Co., 1885. 300p. DNLM; ICU; MB; NN **80-6396**

VAN ARSDALE, William Waldo (1856?-1899)
On subluxation of the head of the radius in children; with a résumé of one hundred consecutive cases. St. Louis, 1889. 23p. DNLM **80-6397**

VAN BAUN, William W.
Oxygen, an adjuvant to the homoeopathic treatment of diseases of the respiratory and circulatory systems. Philadelphia, 1889. 10p. DNLM **80-6398**

VAN BIBBER, John P. (1850-1892)
The prospective advantages of Baltimore as a medical centre. Baltimore: J. W. Borst & Co., 1880. 15p. DNLM; MdU-D **80-6399**

VAN BIBBER, John P. (1850-1892)
The rational treatment of chorea. New York: Stettiner, Lambert & Co., 1884. 8p. DNLM; NNNAM **80-6400**

VAN BIBBER, John P. (1850-1892)
Intermediate hospitals for the treatment of acute mental diseases. Philadelphia, 1885. 15p. DNLM; PPC **80-6401**

VAN BIBBER, W[ashington] C[hew] (1824-1892)
Malaria. Written for the Maryland State Board of Health. Baltimore: J. Young, 1884. 10p. DNLM **80-6402**

VAN BIBBER, W[ashington] C[hew] (1824-1892)
The Baltimore Academy of Medicine. Baltimore, 1887. 16p. DNLM; MdBM **80-6403**

VAN BIBBER, W[ashington] C[hew] (1824-1892)
Prevention of yellow fever in Florida and the South. Baltimore: Journal Publ. Co., 1889. 26p. DNLM; MdBM **80-6404**

VAN BUREN, William Holme (1819-1883)
Lectures upon diseases of the rectum. Delivered at the Bellevue Hospital Medical College, 1869-1870. [2nd ed.] New York: D. Appleton & Co., 1881. 412p. DLC; DNLM; NNNAM; PPC **80-6405**

VAN BUREN, William Holme (1819-1883)
Lectures on the principles of surgery. Delivered at Bellevue Hospital Medical College. Edited by Lewis A. Stimson. New York: D. Appleton & Co., 1884. 588p. DLC; DNLM; NNNAM; PPC **80-6406**

VANCE, Ap Morgan (1854-1915)
Tenotomy in the treatment of congenital club-foot; with a tabular report of fifty-two cases, and remarks illustrating the management of the deformity. New York: Trow, 1881. 22p. 1 tab. DNLM; NNNAM **80-6407**

VANCE, Ap Morgan (1854-1915)
Cases in orthopaedic surgery. [New York, 1885.] 17p. DNLM **80-6408**

VANCE, Ap Morgan (1854-1915)
Femoral osteotomy for the correction of deformity resulting from hip-joint disease. New York, 1888. 15p. DNLM **80-6409**

VANCE, Reuben A[leshire] (1845-1894)
Remarks on lithotrity; an outline of a series of lectures delivered before the class of 1880 of the Evansville Medical College, February 11th, 1880. [Evansville, 1880.] 12p. DNLM **80-6410**

VANCE, Reuben A[leshire] (1845-1894)
The nature and diagnosis of certain diseases of the testicles, the symptoms accompanying which are generally denominated "spermatorrhoea." . . . Cincinnati: Aldine Printing Works, 1881. 16p. DLC **80-6411**

VANCE, Reuben A[leshire] (1845-1894)
The radical cure of hip-joint disease. [Columbus, O., 1882.] 4p. DNLM **80-6412**

VANCE, Reuben A[leshire] (1845-1894)
Surgery of arteries. Columbus, 1882. 8p. DNLM **80-6413**

VANCE, Reuben A[leshire] (1845-1894)
Cancer of the intestinal tract; operations for the removal of malignant strictures of pylorus and intestines. Together with a brief review of the historical development of modern abdominal surgery. Columbus, O.: Hann & Adair, 1883. 15p. DNLM; OCIM; OCIWHi **80-6414**

VANCE, Reuben A[leshire] (1845-1894)
Vesico-vaginal fistula. Cleveland, 1888. 35p. DNLM; OCIM; OCIWHi **80-6415**

VANDER VEER, A[lbert] (1841-1929)
Report of ten cases of gastric ulcer, one case malignant ulcer of the stomach, and two cases perforating ulcer of the jejunum. Albany: Burdick & Taylor, 1880. 16p. DNLM **80-6416**

VANDER VEER, A[lbert] (1841-1929)
Case of subcutaneous section of femur above trochanter major. [Syracuse, 1882.] 4p. DNLM **80-6417**

VANDER VEER, A[lbert] (1841-1929)
Report of cases of trifacial neuralgia, treated by removal of Meckel's ganglion; also by the successful internal administration of aconitia. St. Louis: E. E. Carreras, 1883. 10p. DNLM **80-6418**

VANDER VEER, A[lbert] (1841-1929)
Defective drainage. New York: Jenkins & Thomas, [1883]. 21p. DNLM; NNNAM **80-6419**

VANDER VEER, A[lbert] (1841-1929)
Some personal observations on the work of Lawson Tait, together with report of five cases of abdominal section by the writer. New York: William Wood & Co., 1885. 18p. DNLM; NNNAM **80-6420**

VANDER VEER, A[lbert] (1841-1929)
To what extent can we classify vesical calculi for operation? With a report of cases, and remarks on the different methods employed. Philadelphia: W. J. Dornan, 1887. 48p. DNLM; PPC **80-6421**

VANDER VEER, A[lbert] (1841-1929)
The history of abdominal section in Albany, with a report of seventy-five cases. Albany: Burdick & Taylor, 1888. 35p. DNLM **80-6422**

VANDER VEER, A[lbert] (1841-1929)
Intestinal obstruction. When should operative measures be resorted to in intestinal obstruction? [Albany, 1888.] 4p. DNLM **80-6423**

VANDER VEER, A[lbert] (1841-1929)
The relation of the abdominal surgeon to the obstetrician and gynaecologist. New York: Judson Printing Co., [1888]. 8p. DNLM **80-6424**

VANDER VEER, A[lbert] (1841-1829)
The relation of the abdominal surgeon to the obstetrician and gynaecologist. Philadelphia: W. J. Dornan, 1889. 11p. DNLM **80-6425**

VANDER VEER, A[lbert] (1841-1929)
Concealed pregnancy: its relations to abdominal surgery. Chicago, 1889. 28p. 1 tab. DNLM **80-6426**

VANDER VEER, A[lbert] (1841-1929)
Concealed pregnancy: its relations to abdominal surgery. New York: William Wood & Co., 1889. 28p. DNLM; NNNAM **80-6427**

VAN DE WARKER, [Edward] Ely (1841-1910)
The etiology of laceration of the cervix uteri. New York: William Wood & Co., 1882. 20p. DNLM; NNNAM **80-6428**

VAN DE WARKER, [Edward] Ely (1841-1910)
Forcible elongation of pelvic adhesions. [Philadelphia], 1882. 7p. DNLM **80-6429**

VAN DE WARKER, [Edward] Ely (1841-1910)
Mechanical treatment of versions and flexions of the uterus. A theoretical and practical study of the pessary. [Philadelphia, 1883.] 46p. 14 plates. DNLM; PPC **80-6430**

VAN DE WARKER [Edward] Ely (1841-1910)
An analysis of thirty-one operations for repair of laceration of the cervix uteri. New York: William Wood & Co., 1883. 22p. DNLM **80-6431**

VAN DE WARKER, [Edwrd] Ely (1841-1910)
A new method of partial extirpation of the cancerous uterus. [New York, 1884.] 17p. DNLM **80-6432**

VAN DE WARKER, [Edward] Ely (1841-1910)
A successful case of laparo-hysterectomy for uterine fibroids. [New York, 1884.] 6p. DNLM **80-6433**

VAN DE WARKER, [Edward] Ely (1841-1910)
A gynecological study of the Oneida community. New York: William Wood & Co., 1884. 28p. DNLM; NNNAM
80-6434

VAN DE WARKER, [Edward] Ely (1841-1910)
Caesarean operation in a dwarf. Philadelphia, 1885. 7p. 1 tab. DNLM **80-6435**

VAN DE WARKER, [Edward] Ely (1841-1910)
Laparotomy as a cure for tuberculosis of the peritoneum. New York: William Wood & Co., 1887. 12p. DNLM
80-6436

VAN DE WARKER, [Edward] Ely (1841-1910)
Stricture of the urethra in women. Philadelphia, 1887. 10p. DNLM **80-6437**

VAN DE WARKER, [Edward] Ely (1841-1910)
The dangers of galvano-puncture in pelvic tumors. Philadelphia: W. J. Dornan, 1888. 15p. DNLM
80-6438

VAN DE WARKER, [Edward] Ely (1841-1910)
Extra-uterine pregnancy and its treatment by electricity. [New York, 1888.] 8p. DNLM **80-6439**

VAN DE WARKER, [Edward] Ely (1841-1910)
Address in gynecology. How gynecology is taught. Chicago, 1888. 15p. DNLM **80-6440**

VAN DE WARKER, [Edward] Ely (1841-1910)
An experience with sloughing intra-uterine fibroids. Philadelphia: W. J. Dornan, 1889. 15p. DNLM; PPC; PPJ
80-6441

VAN DE WARKER, [Edward] Ely (1841-1910)
Diseased tubes and ovaries. [Boston: Rockwell & Churchill, 1889.] 7p. 2 plates. DNLM; MBM
80-6442

VAN DE WARKER, [Edward] Ely (1841-1910)
The islands of the afternoon. Philadelphia: Lea Bros. & Co., 1889. 32p. DNLM; PU **80-6443**

VAN DUZER, S. R.
Prices current of drugs, chemicals, pharmaceuticals, paints, oils, . . . New York, 1883. 108, 40p. NNNAM
80-6444

VAN DYCK, J.
Treatise on personal beauty, the complexion, bearded belles, blessings for the bald, catarrh and skin diseases. Washington, D.C., [1884]. 48p. DNLM **80-6445**

VAN GIESON, Ira T. (1866-1913)
Laboratory notes of technical methods for the nervous system. [New York, 1889.] 14p. DNLM; NNNAM
80-6446

VAN HARLINGEN, Arthur (1845-1936)
Three cases of syphilitic muscular contraction. Philadelphia, 1880. 6p. DNLM **80-6447**

VAN HARLINGEN, Arthur (1845-1936)
Case of a chronic inflammatory tuberculo-vescular skin disease. [Philadelphia, 1880.] 5p. DNLM
80-6448

VAN HARLINGEN, Arthur (1845-1936)
Medicinal eruptions. [Philadelphia, 1880.] 31p. DNLM
80-6449

VAN HARLINGEN, Arthur (1845-1936)
Handbook of the diagnosis and treatment of skin diseases. . . . With two colored plates. Philadelphia: P. Blakiston, Son & Co., 1884. 282p. DLC; DNLM; NNNAM; PPC
80-6450

VAN HARLINGEN, Arthur (1845-1936)
Handbook of the diagnosis and treatment of skin diseases. . . . 2nd ed., enl. and rev. With eight full-page plates and other illustrations. Philadelphia: P. Blakiston, Son & Co., 1889. 410p. DLC; DNLM; IU-M; PU **80-6451**

VAN HOREN, Fred. D.
Physicians' and surgeons' supplies; the professional reference lists. [New York, 1886.] 19 l. DNLM; NNNAM
80-6452

VAN LENNEP, William B. (1853-1919)
A case of double genu valgum. Philadelphia, 1885. 10p. DNLM
80-6453

VAN LENNEP, William B. (1853-1919)
The use and abuse of instruments in the male urethra. Philadelphia, 1885. 10p. DNLM **80-6454**

VAN LENNEP, William B. (1853-1919)
Necrosis of the femur with implantation of decalcified bone chips. [Philadelphia, 1889.] 3p. DNLM
80-6455

VAN LENNEP, William B. (1853-1919)
Studies in intestinal surgery. [Philadelphia, 1889.] 15p. DNLM
80-6456

VAN LENNEP, William B. (1853-1919)
The radical cure of hernia, with the report of three rather unusual cases. New York: J. C. Rankin, Jr., 1889. 15p. DNLM
80-6457

VAN SCHAACK, PETER & SONS
Illustrated catalogue of drugs and pharmaceuticals, sundries, furniture, glassware. . . . Chicago, 1887. 739p. OCIM
80-6458

VAN VALZAH, W. W. (*b.* 1849)
Notes regarding the management of chronic gastro-intestinal catarrh. New York: Trow, 1889. 12p. DNLM
80-6459

VAN VALZAH, W. W. (*b.* 1849) and Charles R. CRANDALL
Nervous sysmptoms caused by functional gastro-intestinal disorders. [New York, 1889.] 13p. DNLM
80-6460

VARICK, Theodore R[omeyn] (1825-1887)
Statistics of amputations performed at St. Francis Hospital, Jersey City, N.J., from 1871 to 1881. Philadelphia, 1881. 7p. DNLM **80-6461**

VARICK, Theodore R[omeyn] (1825-1887)
Distal compression applied in a case of inguinal aneurism, with a successful result. [Philadelphia, 1881.] 2p. DNLM
80-6462

VARICK, Theodore R[omeyn] (1825-1887)
A case of amputation at the hip-joint, in which Prof. Trendelenburg's method of controlling hemorrhage was resorted to, with recovery of the patient. [Philadelphia, 1882.] 3p. DNLM **80-6463**

VARICK, Theodore R[omeyn] (1825-1887)
On railroad injuries of the extremities of the human body, with observations on the site of amputation and subsequent treatment of the stump. New York: Morgenthaler & Watson, 1884. 16p. DNLM **80-6464**

VARICK, Theodore R[omeyn] (1825-1887)
The protective treatment of open wounds. New York: Holt Bros., 1885. 11p. DNLM **80-6465**

VARICK, Theodore R[omeyn] (1825-1887)
The use of hot water in surgery. New York: D. Appleton & Co., 1887. 15p. DNLM **80-6466**

VAUGHAN, Victor C[larence] (1851-1929)
Hand-book of chemical physiology and pathology, with lectures upon normal and abnormal urine. . . . 3rd ed., rev. and enl. Ann Arbor: Ann Arbor Printing and Publishing Co., 1880. 351p. DLC **80-6467**

VAUGHAN, Victor C[larence] (1851-1929) and P. E. NAGLE
Contamination of drinking-water by filtration of organic matter through the soil. [Read at the sanitary convention in Detroit, Mich., January 7, 1880.] [Lansing, 1880.] 4p. DNLM **80-6468**

VAUGHAN, Victor C[larence] (1851-1929)
American Public Health Association. Lomb prize essay. Healthy homes and foods for the working classes. Concord, N.H.: Republican Press Ass'n., 1886. 62p. DNLM; MH; NN **80-6469**

VAUGHAN, Victor C[larence] (1851-1929)
The prevention of cholera infantum and kindred diseases, and of poisoning by cheese, milk, etc. Abstract of a paper on the chemistry of tyrotoxicon, its action upon lower animals, and its relation to the summer diarrheas of infancy. No. 123. [Lansing, 1887.] 4p. DNLM **80-6470**

VAUGHAN, Victor C[larence] (1851-1929) and Frederick G. NOVY
Ptomaines and leucomaines, or the putrefactive and physiological alkaloids. Philadelphia: Lea Bros. & Co., 1888. 314p. AU; DNLM; PPC; PU **80-6471**

VERDI, Ciro de Suzzara
Progressive medicine. A scientific and practical treatise on diseases of the digestive organs and the complications arising therefrom. Philadelphia: F. E. Boericke, 1885. 349p. DNLM; PPC; PPHa; PU **80-6472**

VERRIER, Eugène (1824-1910)
Practical manual of obstetrics. 4th ed., with the four obstetric tables of Prof. Pajot. 1st American ed., with revision and annotations by Edward L. Partridge. New York: William Wood & Co., 1884. 395p. CtY-M; DNLM; MBM; PPC **80-6473**

VILAS, Charles H[arrison] (*b.* 1846)
Spectacles; and how to choose them; an elementary monograph. Chicago: Duncan Bros., 1881. 160p. DNLM; OCIM **80-6474**

VILAS, Charles H[arrison] (*b.* 1846)
The ophthalmoscope; its theory and practical uses. Chicago: Duncan Bros., 1882. 150p. DNLM; ICU; IEN-M; NNNAM **80-6475**

VILAS, Charles H[arrison] (*b.* 1846)
Therapeutics of the eye and ear. An elementary manual. . . . Chicago: W. A. Chatterton; New York: A. L. Chatterton Pub. Co., 1883. 233p. DLC; DNLM; MH **80-6476**

VINEBERG, Hiram N.
The internal administration of bichloride of mercury as an adjunct to the local treatment of circumuterine inflammations. New York, 1888. 15p. DNLM **80-6477**

VIRCHOW, Rudolf Ludwig Karl (1821-1902)
Post-mortem examinations, with especial reference to medico-legal practice; transl. from the 2nd German ed. by T. P. Smith. Philadelphia: P. Blakiston, 1880. 145p. 4 plates. DNLM; MBM; NNNAM; PPC **80-6478**

VIRCHOW, Rudolf Ludwig Karl (1821-1902)
Post-mortem examinations, with especial reference to medico-legal practice; transl. from the 4th German ed. With additional notes and new plates. Philadelphia: P. Blakiston, Son & Co., 1885. 138p. 4 plates. DLC; DNLM; ICRM; PPC **80-6479**

VON TAGEN, Charles H.
Biliary calculi; perineorrhaphy; hospital gangrene and its kindred diseases, with their respective treatments. New York and Philadelphia: Boericke & Tafel, 1881. 154p. NNNAM; PPHa; PU **80-6480**

WADE, De Witt Clinton
Displacements of the uterus; together with formula for official dilute hydrobromic acid of the United States Pharmacopoeia. Philadelphia: W. F. Fell & Co., [1887]. 6p. DNLM **80-6481**

WADE, De Witt Clinton
A new antiseptic. [Detroit], 1888. 3p. DNLM **80-6482**

WADSWORTH, Oliver Fairfield (1838-1911)
Optico-ciliary neurotomy. Boston, 1882. 24p. DNLM **80-6483**

WADSWORTH, Oliver Fairfield (1838-1911)
Phlyctenular disease of the eyes. [Boston, 1883.] 15p. DNLM **80-6484**

WADSWORTH, Oliver Fairfield (1838-1911)
The amblyopia of squint. Boston: Cupples, Upham & Co., 1887. 14p. DNLM **80-6485**

WAGNER, Clinton (1837-1914)
Myxomata of the left laryngeal ventricle; spontaneous expulsion. [New York, 1880.] 5p. DNLM **80-6486**

WAGNER, Clinton (1837-1914)
Habitual mouth-breathing. Its causes, effects, and treatment. New York: G. P. Putnam's Sons, 1881. 52p. 3 plates. DNLM **80-6487**

WAGNER, Clinton (1837-1914)
Habitual mouth-breathing. Its causes, effects, and treatment. 2nd ed. Albany, N.Y.: E. S. Werner, 1884. 52p. 2 l. DNLM **80-6488**

WAGNER, Clinton (1837-1914)
Sub-hyoidean pharyngotomy for the removal of the epiglottis for epithelioma, with illustrative cases. New York: Trow, 1881. 12p. DNLM **80-6489**

WAGNER, Clinton (1837-1914)
Case of exsection of the right half of the larynx for epithelioma. [New York: G. P. Putnam's Sons, 1883.] 2p. DNLM **80-6490**

WAGNER, Clinton (1837-1914)
On intra-laryngeal growths. A clinical lecture. [Philadelphia]: Dornan, 1883. 15p. DNLM **80-6491**

WAGNER, Clinton (1837-1914)
Ossification of the right arytenoid cartilage; separation and expulsion following thyrotomy for the removal of a papilloma. New York: [G. P. Putnam's Sons, 1883.] 3p. DNLM **80-6492**

WAGNER, Clinton (1837-1914)
Diseases of the nose. New York: Bermingham & Co., 1884. 252p. DNLM **80-6493**

WAGNER, Clinton (1837-1914)
Three cases of thyreotomy; recovery in each case, with excellent voice. [New York, 1880.] 4p. DNLM **80-6494**

WAGNER, Clinton (1837-1914)
Colorado Springs and Davosplatz, as winter health resorts, compared. New York: Trow, 1887. 12p. DNLM **80-6495**

WAINWRIGHT, William A. M. (1844-1894)
The modern treatment of wounds. Hartford: Case, Lockwood & Brainard Co., 1887. 12p. DNLM **80-6496**

WAINWRIGHT, William A. M. (1844-1894)
. . . The medical history of Hartford County. . . . [Hartford? 1887?] 14p. DLC **80-6497**

WAITE & BARTLETT MFG. CO.
Illustrated price list of electro-medical and electro-surgical instruments. New York, 1889. 64p. NNNAM **80-6498**

WALES, Philip S[kinner] (1837-1906)
Rectal palpation and inspection as means of diagnosis. Washington: Judd & Detweiler, 1883. 44p. DNLM **80-6499**

WALKER, George S. (*b.* 1820)
Address delivered before the joint convention of the Western Academy and Minnesota Institute of Homoeopathy, at Minneapolis, Minn., June 10, 1880. [Minneapolis, Minn., 1880.] 15p. DNLM **80-6500**

WALKER, H[enry] O. (1843-1912)
Litholapaxy and lithotomy. A report of eight cases of removal of stone from the bladder by those methods. [Grand Rapids, 1880.] 16p. DNLM **80-6501**

WALKER, H[enry] O. (1843-1912)
Plaster-of-Paris as a surgical dressing. Detroit, Mich.: G. S. Davis, 1884. 16p. DNLM **80-6502**

WALKER, H[enry] O. (1843-1912)
Eighteen cases of external perineal urethrotomy. [Philadelphia, 1887.] 8p. DNLM **80-6503**

WALKER, H[enry] O. (1843-1912)
Report of four cases of trephining the skull. [Philadelphia], 1888. 15p. DNLM **80-6504**

WALKER, Jerome (*b.* 1845)
Anatomy, physiology, and hygiene; a manual for the use of colleges, schools, and general readers. New York: A. Lovell & Co., 1884. 415p. DNLM; ICU; MH; NN **80-6505**

WALL, John P. (1836-1895)
As to yellow fever. [Tampa, 1886.] 7p. DNLM **80-6506**

WALL, John P. (1836-1895)
Observations on yellow fever, with special reference to diagnosis, prognosis, and treatment. Jacksonville, Fla.: The Dacosta, 1888. 9p. DNLM **80-6507**

WALL, Otto A[ugustus] (1846-1922)
The prescription therapeutically, pharmaceutically, and grammatically considered. St. Louis: A. Gast Lith. Co., 1888. 184p. DLC; DNLM **80-6508**

WALLACE, James
An improved astigmatic chart. [Philadelphia, 1889.] 3p. DNLM **80-6509**

WALLIAN, Samuel S[pencer] (1836-1907)
On oxygen, as a remedial agent. New York: Trow, 1884. 52p. DNLM **80-6510**

WALLIAN, Samuel S[pencer] (1836-1907)
Oxygen; a rational study of its place in therapeutics; and further report on oxygen; with cases treated. Philadelphia: Foote & Swift, 1886. 30p. DNLM **80-6511**

WALLIAN, Samuel S[pencer] (1836-1907)
Oxygen treatment and oxygen charlatans. New York, 1886. 8p. DNLM **80-6512**

WALLIAN, Samuel S[pencer] (1836-1907)
Medical fetichism, and a suggested basis for a science of medicine. Read before the Section in Therapeutics and Materia Medica, International Medical Congress, at Washington, D.C., Sept. 6, 1887. New York: Clark & Zugalla, 1887. 11p. DNLM **80-6513**

WALLIAN, Samuel S[pencer] (1836-1907)
A further study of the therapeutic value of oxygen; with cases treated. [Chicago, 1887.] 8p. DNLM **80-6514**

WALLIAN, Samuel S[pencer] (1836-1907)
Suggestions toward a more rational procedure in wasting diseases. [New York, 1888.] 6p. DNLM **80-6515**

WALLIAN, Samuel S[pencer] (1836-1907)
An abused and neglected remedy. [Boston, 1888.] 8p. DNLM **80-6516**

WALLIS, Severn T[eackle] (1816-1894)
The Johns Hopkins University in its relations to Baltimore. An address delivered at the seventh anniversary of the Johns Hopkins University, 1883. Baltimore: J. Murphy & Co., 1883. 37p. DNLM; MdBM; MdU-D; MdBJ-W
80-6517

WALSHAM, William J[ohnson] (1847-1903)
Surgery: its theory and practice. Philadelphia: P. Blakiston, Son & Co., 1887. 655p. DNLM; MBM; NNNAM; PPC
80-6518

WALTER, Robert (*b.* 1841)
The standard series. The nutritive cure, a statement of its principles and methods; with introduction by Rev. Joel Swartz. New York: I. K. Funk & Co., 1881. 52p. DNLM
80-6519

WALTER, Robert (*b.* 1841)
The philosophy of the health-reform. Reading, Pa., 1884. 36p. DNLM **80-6520**

WALTER, Robert (*b.* 1841)
The best means of preserving and regaining health. Reading, Pa.: Health Publishing Co., 1885. 64p. DNLM
80-6521

WALTER, Robert (*b.* 1841)
Recent important discoveries in vital science, constituting a philosophical and practical basis for an exact science of human health. Reading. B. F. Owen, 1887. 64p. DNLM
80-6522

WALTON, Alfred
Oxygen and nitrogen as therapeutic agents in the treatment of pulmonary and other chronic diseases. [New York, 1880?] 16p. DNLM **80-6523**

WALTON, George E[dward] (*b.* 1839)
The mineral springs of the United States and Canada, with analyses and notes on the prominent spas of Europe, and a list of sea-side resorts. . . . 3rd ed., rev. and much enl. New York: D. Appleton & Co., 1883. 468p. fold. maps. DLC; NNNAM **80-6524**

WALTON, George E[dward] (*b.* 1839)
Monograph on sulphur waters of Sharon Springs, N.Y. New York: T. L. De Vinne & Co., 1883. 32p. DNLM; NNNAM
80-6525

WALTON, George L[incoln] (1854-1941)
Neglect of ear-symptoms in the diagnosis of diseases of the nervous system. [New York, 1883.] 11p. DNLM
80-6526

WALTON, George L[incoln] (1854-1941)
Possible cerebral origin of the symptoms usually classed under "railway spine." Cambridge: Riverside Press, 1883. 14p. DNLM **80-6527**

WALTON, George L[incoln] (1854-1941)
Two cases of hysteria. 1. Hysterical hemianaesthesia in a man, following injury; 2. hysterical anaesthesia of special sense, accompanying cutaneous hyperaesthesia. A paper presented at the meeting of the American Neurological Association, June 22, 1882. [New York], 1883. 7p. DNLM
80-6528

WALTON, George L[incoln] (1854-1941)
Spinal irritation; probable cerebral origin of the symptoms sometimes classed under this head. Cambridge: Riverside Press, 1884. 12p. DNLM **80-6529**

WALTON, George L[incoln] (1854-1941)
Case of hysterical hemianaesthesia, convulsions, and motor paralysis, brought on by a fall. Cambridge, 1884. 12p. DNLM
80-6530

WALTON, George L[incoln] (1854-1941)
A contribution to the study of hysteria, bearing on the question of oöphorectomy. New York, 1884. 11p. DNLM
80-6531

WALTON, George L[incoln] (1854-1941)
Katalytic action of electricity; its practical value in rheumatic affections. Boston, [1888]. 2 l. DNLM **80-6532**

WALTON, George L[incoln] (1854-1941)
Case of cerebral tumor involving the facial centre; autopsy. Boston: Cupples & Hurd, [1889]. 6p. DNLM
80-6533

WALTON, George L[incoln] (1854-1941)
Dislocation of cervical vertebrae. Five cases: recovery without operation. Boston: Damrell & Upham, 1889. 16p. 1 plate. DNLM **80-6534**

WALTON, George L[incoln] (1854-1941)
Latency of ataxic symptoms in cases of optic atrophy. Boston: Damrell & Upham, 1889. 10p. DNLM
80-6535

WARD, Elijah J. (1842-1892)
Some observations on the possibilities of preventive surgery. Austin, [1889]. 16p. DNLM **80-6536**

WARD, Henry A[ugustus] (1834-1906)
Catalogue of human skeletons and anatomical preparations. [Rochester, N.Y., 1884.] 25p. DNLM
80-6537

WARD, H. O. (1824-1899)
The first requisites in physician and nurse for the cure of insanity. . . . Philadelphia: Sherman & Co., 1881. 9p. DNLM
80-6538

WARD, Samuel B[aldwin] (*b.* 1842)
Carcinomatous papilloma of bladder. Occlusion of orifices of ureters. Death by uraemic coma. New York: G. P. Putnam's Sons, [1882]. 17p. DNLM; NNNAM
80-6539

WARD, Whitfield
Singers' throat troubles; their cause and cure; course of lectures delivered at the Grand Conservatory of Music, during the season 1883-1884. . . . New York: The Grand Conservatory Publishing Co., 1885. 37p. DLC **80-6540**

WARDER, Robert B.
Examination of commercial black antimony, tartar emetic, and glycerine. [Philadelphia, 1885.] 8p. DNLM
80-6541

WARDNER, Horace (1829-1905)
Care of the chronic insane. A paper read before the Tenth Annual Conference of Charities and Corrections, held at Louisville, Ky., September 24-30, 1883. Madison: Midland Publishing Co., 1884. 13p. DNLM **80-6542**

WARDNER, Horace (1829-1905)
Occupation in treatment of insanity. St. Louis, 1888. 10p. DNLM **80-6543**

WARING, Edward John (1819-1891)
Practical therapeutics. Edited by Dudley W. Buxton. 4th ed. Philadelphia: P. Blakiston, Son & Co., 1886. 666p. PPC; PPHa; PU **80-6544**

WARING, George E[dwin], Jr. (1833-1898)
The drainage question in Philadelphia. A public lecture delivered June 12, 1885, at the hall of the College of Physicians of Philadelphia, by invitation of the committee on hygiene of the County Medical Society. [Philadelphia, 1885.] 11p. DNLM; PPC **80-6545**

WARK, David
Prevention and cure of chronic consumption. New York, 1880. 103p. DNLM; NNNAM **80-6546**

WARK, David
The practical home doctor for women. New York: Gray Bros. & Co., [1882]. 420p. DNLM; NNNAM **80-6547**

THE WARM SULPHUR SPRINGS, Bath County, Virginia. Richmond, Va.: Baughman Bros., 1884. 24p. DNLM **80-6548**

WARNER, Francis (1847-1926)
The student's guide to medical casetaking. Philadelphia: P. Blakiston, Son & Co., 1881. 211p. NNNAM: PPC; PPJ; PU **80-6549**

WARNER, Francis (1847-1926)
The student's guide to clinical medicine and case-taking. 2nd ed. Philadelphia: P. Blakiston, Son & Co., 1885. 211p. DNLM; NNNAM; PPC; PU **80-6550**

WARNER, Francis (1847-1926)
Physical expression, its modes and principles. [Internat. Scient. Ser.] New York: D. Appleton & Co., 1886. 372p. DNLM; ICU; MH; NN **80-6551**

WARNER, Lucien Calvin (1841-1925)
Woman's hand-book in health and disease. A popular treatise on the functions and diseases of woman with the most approved hygienic and medical treatment. . . . Rev. and enl. by a member of the medical staff of the N.Y. State Woman's Hospital, New York City. . . . New York: E. B. Treat, 1886. 359p. DLC; NNNAM **80-6552**

WARNER, William R.
Ingluvin. To the medical profession only. Philadelphia, [1880]. 7 l. DNLM **80-6553**

WARNER, William R.
Coca, erythroxylon coca. Philadelphia, 1885. 28p. DNLM **80-6554**

WARNER, William R., & CO.
Therapeutic reference book. . . . Philadelphia, 1889. 119p. NNNAM; PPC **80-6555**

WARREN, Edward (1828-1893)
A doctor's experiences in three continents; in a series of letters addressed to John Morris. Baltimore: Cushing & Bailey, 1885. 613p. DLC; DNLM; MH; NN **80-6556**

WARREN, Ira (1806-1864)
Warren's household physician, enlarged and revised, for the use of physicians, families, mariners, and miners. . . . By Ira Warren . . . and A. E. Small. . . . Allopathic department revised by William Thorndike. . . . Homoeopathic department revised by Heber Smith. . . . Boston: I. Bradley & Co., 1885. 902p. col. plates. DLC; MBM; NNNAM **80-6557**

WARREN, John Collins (1842-1927)
Medical societies; their organization and the nature of their work. An address delivered at the centennial meeting of the Massachusetts Medical Society, June 8, 1881. Cambridge: Riverside Press, 1881. 68p. DLC; DNLM **80-6558**

WARREN, John Collins (1842-1927)
Columane adiposae. A newly-described structure of the cutis vera, with its pathological significance in carbuncle and other affections. Cambridge: Riverside Press, 1881. 28p. 4 plates. DNLM **80-6559**

WARREN, John Collins (1842-1927)
New operation for rupture of the perineum through the sphincter. [Philadelphia, 1883.] 9p. DNLM **80-6560**

WARREN, John Collins (1842-1927)
Provisional report on healing of arteries after ligature. Cambridge: Riverside Press, 1884. 8p. DNLM **80-6561**

WARREN, John Collins (1842-1927)
The healing of arteries after ligature in man and animals. New York: William Wood & Co., 1886. 3 p. l. 184p., 14 plates. DLC; DNLM **80-6562**

WARREN, John Collins (1842-1927)
Personal experience in the treatment of cancer. Boston: Cupples & Hurd, 1887. 14p. DNLM **80-6563**

WARREN, John Collins (1842-1927)
A case of gastrotomy for cancer of the oesophagus. New York: Trow's Co., 1887. 8p. DNLM **80-6564**

WARREN, John Collins (1842-1927)
The process of repair after resection of the intestine and intestinal suture. Philadelphia: W. J. Dornan, 1887. 16p. DNLM **80-6565**

WARREN, John Collins (1842-1927)
The diagnosis and treatment of cancer of the breast. Boston: Cupples & Hurd, [1889]. 16p. DNLM **80-6566**

WARREN, Joseph H[uckins] (1831-1891)
Hernia, strangulated and reducible. With cure by subcutaneous injections, together with sug[g]ested and improved methods for kelotomy. Also an appendix giving a short account of various new surgical instruments. . . . Boston: C. N. Thomas; [etc., etc.], 1881. 280p. DLC; MBM **80-6567**

WARREN, Joseph H[uckins] (1831-1891)
Report of chairman of committee of foreign delegates. Also essay on new surgical instruments. Philadelphia: Collins, 1881. 16p. DNLM **80-6568**

WARREN, Joseph H[uckins] (1831-1891)
A practical treatise on hernia. . . . 2nd and rev. ed. Boston: J. R. Osgood & Co.; [etc., etc.], 1882 [1881]. 428p. 3 plates. DLC; DNLM; MH-M **80-6569**

WARREN, Joseph H[uckins] (1831-1891)
Clinical report on cases of lacerated cervix and ovariotomy. From private practice. Cambridge: Riverside Press, 1883. 19p. DNLM **80-6570**

WARREN, Joseph H[uckins] (1831-1891)
Clinical report of interesting cases in private practice. Boston: J. R. Osgood & Co., 1883. 15p. DNLM **80-6571**

WARREN, Joseph H[uckins] (1831-1891)
Clinical report of interesting cases in private practice. Richmond, 1883. 15p. DNLM **80-6572**

WARREN, Joseph H[uckins] (1831-1891)
A plea for the cure of rupture; or, The pathology of the subcutaneous operation by injection for the cure of hernia. . . . Boston: J. R. Osgood & Co.; [etc., etc], 1884. 117p. plates. DLC; DNLM; MH-M **80-6573**

WARREN, Joseph W[eatherhead]
Alcohol again: a consideration of recent misstatements of its physiological action. Boston: Cupples & Hurd, 1887. 39p. DNLM **80-6574**

WARREN, Joseph W[eatherhead]
Notes on the digestion of "living" tissues. Boston: Cupples, Upham & Co., 1887. 14p. DNLM **80-6575**

WARREN, Stanley P[erkins] (*b.* 1846)
Cases of: 1. Rudimentary uterus and vagina. II. Cyst of Gärtner's canal. A paper read before the Maine Medical Association, June 12, 1883. Portland: S. Berry, 1883. 7p. DNLM **80-6576**

WARREN, Stanley P[erkins] (*b.* 1846)
Case of missed labor with Caesarean section. New York, 1885. 16p. DNLM **80-6577**

WARREN, Stanley P[erkins] (*b.* 1846)
A case of incomplete abortion in twin pregnancy. One fetus lost at third month, but its placenta retained to delivery at term of the other twin. [New York, 1887.] 7p. DNLM **80-6578**

WARREN, Stanley P[erkins] (*b.* 1846)
Accidental hemorrhage in labor. [New York, 1888.] 8p. DNLM **80-6579**

[WASHINGTON OBSTETRICAL AND GYNECOLOGICAL SOCIETY]
In memoriam. Francis Asbury Ashford, M.D. Born September 19, 1841. Died May 19, 1883. 20p. DLC **80-6580**

WATHEN, William H[udson] (1846-1913)
Sterility. Management of the secundines. [Louisville, 1887.] 8p. DNLM **80-6581**

WATHEN, William H[udson] (1846-1913)
A successful vaginal hysterectomy for carcinoma uteri. [Birmingham, 1888.] 2p. DNLM **80-6582**

WATHEN, William H[udson] (1846-1913)
1. Rapid dilatation of the cervix uteri. 2. Surgical treatment for lacerations of the perineum and pelvic floor. 3. A successful vaginal hysterectomy for carcinoma uteri. 4. The pathology of ectopic pregnancy and pelvic hematocele. Louisville: Courier-Journal, 1889. 20p. DNLM **80-6583**

WATSON, Beriah André (1836-1892)
The proper period for the performance of amputation in cases of traumatic injuries. [Jersey City, 1880.] 13p. DNLM **80-6584**

WATSON, Beriah André (1836-1892)
An experimental and clinical inquiry into the etiology and distinctive peculiarities of traumatic fever. Philadelphia: Collins, 1881. 17p. DNLM **80-6585**

WATSON, Beriah André (1836-1892)
Lister's system of aseptic wound treatment versus its modifications. Philadelphia: Collins, 1883. 17p. DNLM **80-6586**

WATSON, Beriah André (1836-1892)
A treatise on amputations of the extremities and their complications. Philadelphia: P. Blakiston & Sons, 1885. 762p. 2 plates. DNLM; NNNAM; PPC **80-6587**

WATSON, Beriah André (1836-1892)
Fibro- or spindle-celled sacromatous tumors, with the report of a case and presentation of the specimen. Chicago, 1886. 16p. DNLM **80-6588**

WATSON, Beriah André (1836-1892)
An experimental study of the effects of puncture of the heart in cases of chloroform narcosis. Philadelphia: W. J. Dornan, 1887. 37p. DNLM **80-6589**

WATSON, Beriah André (1836-1892)
Rational medicine versus empiricism. [n. p.], 1887. 15p. DNLM **80-6590**

WATSON, Francis S[edgwick] (1853-1942)
A case of successful removal of a papilloma from the male bladder, by the supra-pubic operation. Boston: Cupples & Hurd, 1887. 13p. DNLM **80-6591**

WATSON, Francis S[edgwick] (1853-1942)
The operative treatment of the hypertrophied prostate. . . . Boston: Cupples & Hurd, 1888. 167p. plates. DLC; MH-M **80-6592**

WATSON, Francis S[edgwick] (1853-1942)
Supra-pubic prostatectomy in a patient aged sixty-nine years, the subject of profuse haematuria from an unusual source; recovery. [Boston: Cupples & Hurd, 1889.] 6p. DNLM
80-6593

WATSON, Irving A[llison] (1849-1918)
Sanitary suggestions. Concord, N.H.: Evans, Sleeper & Woodbury, 1882. 17p. DNLM **80-6594**

WATSON, Irving A[[ison] (1849-1918)
Address to the graduating class of Dartmouth Medical College. Manchester, N.H.: J. B. Clarke, 1885. 12p. DNLM; Nh
80-6595

WATSON, Irving A[llison] (1849-1918)
Extent and distribution of consumption in New Hampshire. Concord, 1888. 14p. DNLM **80-6596**

WATSON, William H[enry] (*b.* 1829)
Medical education and medical licensure. An address. Albany: Weed, Parsons & Co., 1886. 13p. DNLM
80-6597

WATSON, William [Perry]
An address on cholera infantum. Philadelphia: J. E. Potter & Co., 1885. 21p. DNLM **80-6598**

WATSON, William P[erry]
The therapeutics of high temperatures in young children. Philadelphia: J. E. Potter & Co., 1885. 13p. DNLM
80-6599

WATSON, William P[erry]
Atropine in enuresis. [Philadelphia, 1887.] 7p. DNLM
80-6600

WATSON, William P[erry]
The value of creosote in fifty cases of diseases of the air passages. Richmond, 1889. 20p. DNLM
80-6601

WATTS, Henry (1815-1884)
Watts' manual of chemistry, theoretical and practical (based on Fownes' manual). Vol. II. Chemistry of carbon-compounds or organic chemistry. 2nd ed. (13th ed. of Fownes). By William A. Tilden. Philadelphia: P. Blakiston, Son & Co., 1886. 662p. DNLM; ICU; MH; NN **80-6602**

WAUGH, William F[rancis] (1849-1918)
A case of broncho-pulmonary mycosis. [Philadelphia, 1887.] 2p. DNLM **80-6603**

WAXHAM, F[rank] E. (1852-1911)
Intubation of the larynx, with history of cases. Chicago: Clark & Longley, 1885. 11p. DNLM **80-6604**

WAXHAM, F[rank] E. (1852-1911)
Intubation of the larynx, with history of cases. [Chicago, 1886.] 20p. DNLM **80-6605**

WAXHAM, F[rank] E. (1852-1911)
Intubation of the larynx, as a substitute for tracheotomy in the treatment of pseudo-membraneous laryngitis; with a report of eighty-three cases. [Chicago, 1886.] 15p. DNLM
80-6606

WAXHAM, F[rank] E. (1852-1911)
Clinical lecture on intubation of the larynx. [Chicago, 1889.] 9p. DNLM **80-6607**

WEAVER, Benjamin F[ranklin] (*b.* 1839)
Woman's guide to health. A treatise on the diseases of the female genital organs. . . . Bucyrus, O.: The Author, [1889]. 114p. DLC **80-6608**

WEBB, Marshall H.
Notes on operative dentistry . . . . Philadelphia: The S. S. White Dental Manufacturing Company, 1883. 175p. DLC
80-6609

WEBB, Marshall H.
Notes on operative dentistry . . . . 2nd ed. Philadelphia: The S. S. White Dental Manufacturing Co., 1883. 175p. DLC
80-6610

WEBB, R[obert] D[ickens] (1824-1894)
Typho-malarial or continued malarial fever. Philadelphia, 1883. 20p. DNLM; PPC **80-6611**

WEBB, W[illiam] H. (1839?-1903)
Reasons for believing in the contagiousness of phthisis. Philadelphia: W. P. Kildare, 1884. 16p. DNLM
80-6612

WEBB, W[illiam] H. (1839?-1903)
Facts serving to prove the contagiousness of tuberculosis. Philadelphia: W. F. Fell & Co., 1885. 28p. DNLM
80-6613

WEBBER, Samuel G[ilbert] (1838-1926)
The pathological history of the spinal cord with a short introduction of the normal histology. Boston, 1881. 33p. 3 plates. DNLM **80-6614**

WEBBER, Samuel G[ilbert] (1838-1926)
Ocular symptoms as localizing symptoms. Cambridge: Riverside Press, 1883. 29p. DNLM
80-6615

WEBBER, Samuel G[ilbert] (1838-1926)
A treatise on nervous diseases; their symptoms and treatment. New York: D. Appleton & Co., 1885. 410p. DNLM; NNNAM
80-6616

WEBBER, Samuel G[ilbert] (1838-1926)
A study of arterial tension in neurasthenia. Boston: Cupples & Hurd, 1888. 18p. DNLM
80-6617

WEBER, Theodor
The construction of Suersen's obturators. New York, [1885]. 11p. DNLM **80-6618**

WEBSTER, David (*b.* 1842)
Amblyopia from the abuse of tobacco and alcohol; a clinical paper based upon cases in the practice of C. R. Agnew and David Webster. New York: Trow, 1880. 24p. DNLM **80-6619**

WEBSTER, David (*b.* 1842)
Extraction of a splinter of wood from the cornea. [New York, 1880.] 3p. DNLM **80-6620**

WEBSTER, David (*b.* 1842)
A remarkable case of detachment of the retina, with hemorrhage into the vitreous simulating intra-ocular tumor. [New York, 1880.] 3p. DNLM **80-6621**

WEBSTER, David (*b.* 1842)
Sympathetic inflammation following operations for cataract. [New York, 1880.] 14p. DNLM **80-6622**

WEBSTER, David (*b.* 1842)
Calx sulphurata in diseases of the eye. New York: G. P. Putnam's Sons, 1883. 16p. DNLM **80-6623**

WEBSTER, David (*b.* 1842)
Two cases of quinine amaurosis, from the practice of Dr. C. R. Agnew and Dr. D. Webster. [New York, 1883.] 3p. DNLM **80-6624**

WEBSTER, David (*b.* 1842)
A new method of treating episcleritis. New York: E. P. Coby & Co., 1888. 8p. DNLM **80-6625**

WEBSTER, Frank P.
Allopathic opinions of homoeopathy. Norfolk, Va., [1883]. 20p. DNLM **80-6626**

WEEKS, Clara S[haw]
Science in the sick room. Cambridge: J. Wilson & Son, 1883. 12p. DNLM **80-6627**

WEEKS, Clara S[haw]
A text-book of nursing. For the use of training schools, families, and private students. . . . New York: D. Appleton & Co., 1885. 396p. col. plate, fold. diag. DLC; NNNAM; PPC; PU **80-6628**

WEEKS & POTTER
Illustrated catalogue of druggists' sundries. Revised prices. Boston, 1888. 300p. MBM **80-6629**

WEIGEL, Louis A. (1854?-1906)
State control of medicine. [Buffalo, 1887.] 11p. DNLM **80-6630**

WEIGEL, Louis A. (1854?-1906)
The value of elastic tension in the treatment of fibrous anklyosis: also the description of an apparatus for producing extension and at the same time rotation of the forearm. New York: D. Appleton & Co., 1888. 12p. DNLM **80-6631**

WEIGERT, Louis
Consumption and its cure. A popular treatise on the new method of treating consumption through inhalation of superheated dry air. . . . Transl. . . . by Robert Briscoe Earée. New York: J. H. Vail & Co., 1889. 15p. DNLM; NNNAM **80-6632**

WEIR, F[rank] Le Sieur
Oleate of copper; its employment in five hundred cases of parasitic disease of the skin. With analytical tables. [New York: D. Appleton & Co., 1884.] 24p. DNLM; NNNAM **80-6633**

WEIR, Robert F[ulton] (1838-1927)
Remarks on a fatal result from the use of elastic bandage in the treatment of a popliteal aneurism. A paper read before the New York Surgical Society, February 10, 1880. New York: G. P. Putnam's Sons, 1880. 9p. DNLM **80-6634**

WEIR, Robert F[ulton] (1838-1927)
On litholapaxy. [Philadelphia, 1880.] 8p. DNLM **80-6635**

WEIR, Robert F[ulton] (1838-1927)
Remarks on antiseptic dressings. [New York, 1880.] 3p. DNLM **80-6636**

WEIR, Robert F[ulton] (1838-1927) and E. C. SEGUIN
Contribution to the diagnosis and surgical treatment of tumors of the cerebrum. [Philadelphia, 1888.] 48p. DNLM **80-6637**

WEIR, Robert F[ulton] (1838-1927)
On the treatment of the so-called perityphlitic abscess. Philadelphia: W. J. Dornan, 1889. 20p. DNLM **80-6638**

WEISSE, Faneuil D[unkin] (1842-1915)
Practical human anatomy, a working guide for students of medicine and a ready-reference for surgeons and physicians. New York: William Wood & Co., 1886. 456p. 222 plates. CtY-M; DNLM; NNNAM; PPC **80-6639**

WEIST, J[acob] Rollin (1834-1900)
Problems in relation to the prevention of disease. Annual address of the president. Richmond, Ind., 1880. 25p. DNLM **80-6640**

WEIST, J[acob] Rollin (1834-1900)
Report on the water supply of Richmond, Indiana, made to the common council, Dec. 6th, 1880. Richmond, 1880. 14p. 1 map. DNLM **80-6641**

WEIST, J[acob] Rollin (1834-1900)
Foreign bodies in the air-passages. A study of one thousand cases to determine the propriety of bronchotomy in such cases. Louisville, Ky.: J. P. Morton & Co., 1882. 16p. 1 tab. DNLM **80-6642**

WEIST, J[acob] Rollin (1834-1900)
The evolution of a doctor. The annual address before the Alumni Association of Jefferson Medical College. Richmond, Ind.: M. Cullaton & Co., 1883. 30p. DNLM
80-6643

WEIST, J[acob] Rollin (1834-1900)
Civil malpractice suits: how can the physician protect himself against them? [Indianapolis, 1884.] 15p. DNLM
80-6644

WEIST, J[acob] Rollin (1834-1900)
A monument to the late Samuel David Gross. [1885?] 2 l. DNLM **80-6645**

WELCH, Francis H[enry] (1840-1910)
Enteric fever, its prevalence and modifications; aetiology; pathology and treatment: as illustrated by army data at home and abroad. Philadelphia: P. Blakiston, Son & Co., 1883. 190p. DNLM; NNNAM; PU **80-6646**

WELCH, Geo. T[heodore] (*b.* 1845)
Many drugs; few remedies. Paterson, N.J.: Guardian Printing Establishment, 1885. 12p. DNLM; NjR
80-6647

WELCH, Uriah
The new American, Richfield Springs. 7th season. New York, 1887. 16p. 2 maps. DNLM **80-6648**

WELCH, William Henry (1850-1934)
An experimental study of glomerulo-nephritis. Philadelphia: W. J. Dornan, 1886. 12p. 1 plate. DNLM; PPC; PU
80-6649

WELCH, William Henry (1850-1934)
Annual address. Modes of infection. Baltimore, 1887. 21p. DNLM **80-6650**

WELCH, William Henry (1850-1934)
The structure of white thrombi. Philadelphia: W. J. Dornan, 1888. 22p. DNLM; PU **80-6651**

WELCH, William Henry (1850-1934)
On the general pathology of fever. Lecture I. The nature of fever. Lecture II. The effects of increased temperature of the body. Lecture III. The etiology of fever. Philadelphia, 1888. 101p. DNLM; PPC; PU **80-6652**

WELCH, William Henry (1850-1934)
Some of the advantages of the union of medical school and university. An address delivered at Yale University, June 26th, 1888. [New Haven], 1888. 19p. DNLM
80-6653

WELCH, William Henry (1850-1934)
Preliminary report of investigations concerning the causation of hog cholera. [Baltimore, 1889.] 3 l. DNLM
80-6654

WELCH, William Henry (1850-1934)
Hydrophobia. Report of the section on anatomy, physiology, and pathology. [Baltimore, 1889.] 16p. DNLM
80-6655

WELCH, William Henry (1850-1934)
Considerations, concerning some external sources of infection in their bearing on preventive medicine. [Philadelphia, 1889.] 32p. DNLM **80-6656**

WELCH, William M[iller] (*b.* 1837)
The Jenner of America. An address delivered before the Philadelphia County Medical Society. Philadelphia: W. P. Kildare, 1885. 32p. DNLM; PU **80-6657**

WELLING, James Clarke (1825-1894), Elliott COUES, and T. J. C. MADDOX
Addresses delivered at the fifty-eighth annual commencement of the National Medical College, March 18, 1880. Washington: W. H. Moore, 1880. 29p. DNLM
80-6658

WELLNER, George C. (*b.* 1849)
The medical graduate and his needs. Detroit: G. S. Davis, 1884. 100p. DNLM **80-6659**

WELLS, John S[oelberg] (1834-1879)
A treatise on diseases of the eye. 3rd American from 3rd English ed., with copious additions, by Charles Stedman Bull . . . together with selections from the test-types of E. Jaeger and H. Snellen. Philadelphia: Henry C. Lea's Son & Co., 1880. 897p. 6 col. plates, 4 plates [test types]. DNLM; NNNAM; PPC; PPJ **80-6660**

WELLS, John S[oelberg] (1834-1879)
A treatise on the diseases of the eye. 4th American from 3rd English ed. Philadelphia: Henry C. Lea's Son & Co., 1883. 846p. 6 col. plates, 4 plates [test types]. DNLM; ICRM; PPPH; PPC **80-6661**

WELLS, Phineas P[arkhurst] (1808-1891)
The philosophy of homoeopathy. [Philadelphia, 1881.] 12p. DNLM **80-6662**

WELLS, Phineas P[arkhurst] (1808-1891)
Essays on the treatment of diarrhoea and dysentery, with repertory by E. J. Lee. Philadelphia: The Homoeopathic Physician, 1884. 68p. DNLM; NNNAM; PPHa
80-6663

WELLS, Thomas Spencer (1818-1897)
On ovarian and uterine tumours; their diagnosis and treatment. Philadelphia: P. Blakiston, Son & Co., 1882. 530p. DNLM; NNNAM; PPC **80-6664**

WELLS, Thomas Spencer (1818-1897)
Diagnosis and surgical treatment of abdominal tumours. Philadelphia: P. Blakiston, Son & Co., 1885. 216p. DNLM; PPC; PU **80-6665**

WENDT, Edmund C[harles] (1857-1903)
The biology of the blood-vessels. New York: D. Appleton & Co., 1880. 16p. DNLM **80-6666**

WENDT, Edmund C[harles] (1857-1903)
A contribution to the pathological histology of acute parotitis. New York: D. Appleton & Co., 1880. 16p. DNLM
80-6667

WENDT, Edmund C[harles] (1857-1903)
Histological contributions: 1. The blood vessels. 2. The alimentary canal. 3. The urinary excretory passages. 4. The suprarenal capsules. 5. The mammary gland. [New York, 1881.] 12p. DNLM **80-6668**

WENDT, Edmund C[harles] (1857-1903)
The histology of the salivary glands. [New York, 1882.] 10p. DNLM **80-6669**

WENDT, Edmund C[harles] (1857-1903)
A case of unilateral spasm of the tongue. [Philadelphia, 1885.] 2p. DNLM **80-6670**

WENDT, Edmund C[harles] (1857-1903)
A treatise on Asiatic cholera, edited and prepared by Edmund Charles Wendt . . . in association with Drs. John C. Peters . . . Ely McClellan . . . John B. Hamilton . . . and Geo. M. Sternberg. New York: William Wood & Co., 1885. 403p. maps. DLC; NNNAM; PU **80-6671**

WENDT, Edmund C[harles] (1857-1903)
Congenital haemophilia, with the history of a remarkable case. New York: Trow's Co., 1887. 12p. DNLM **80-6672**

WENDT, Edmund C[harles] (1857-1903)
Recent views regarding the pathology and treatment of pertussis. [Philadelphia, 1888.] 19p. DNLM **80-6673**

WENDT, Edmund C[harles] (1857-1903)
Sulfonal, a new hypnotic. New York: William Wood & Co., 1888. 7p. DNLM **80-6674**

WENDT, Edmund C[harles] (1857-1903)
Advanced pyelo-nephritis in an infant. New York: William Wood & Co., 1889. 6p. DNLM **80-6675**

WENZEL, Henry T. (1848-1897)
Is the obstetric binder necessary? Milwaukee: Sentinel Co., 1881. 4p. DNLM **80-6676**

WERUM, J. H.
A short description of hernia, or rupture. . . . [Toledo, O.]: Montgomery & Vrooman, printers, 1884. 31p. DLC **80-6677**

WESCOTT, Robert
President's address to the New Jersey Sanitary Association. [Duties of physicians as sanitarians.] [Elizabeth], 1886. 21p. DNLM **80-6678**

WESSELHOEFT, C[onrad] (1834-1904)
The effects of trituration, with observations on the limit of mechanical divisibility of metals and hard substances. [Boston, 1880.] 25p. DNLM; MBM **80-6679**

WESSELHOEFT, C[onrad] (1834-1904)
A plea for a standard limit of attenuated doses. [Boston, 1881.] 25p. DNLM **80-6680**

WESSELHOEFT, C[onrad] (1834-1904)
The law of similars. Its dosage and the action of attenuated medicines. Boston: Otis Clapp & Son, 1883. 71p. MBM **80-6681**

WESSELHOEFT, C[onrad] (1834-1904)
A lecture on homoeopathy before the members of the Boylston Medical Society (of Harvard Medical School). Boston: O. Clapp & Son, 1885. 46p. DNLM; MH-M **80-6682**

WESSELHOEFT, C[onrad] (1834-1904)
A lecture on homoeopathy before the members of the Boylston Medical Society (of Harvard Medical School). 2nd ed. Boston: O. Clapp & Son, 1886. 46p. DNLM; MH-M **80-6683**

WEST, W[ashington]
An essay on typho-malaria. Belleville, Ill.: Advocate Steam Printing House, 1881. 10p. DNLM **80-6684**

WESTBROOK, Benjamin F[ranklin] (1851-1895)
On abstraction of blood from the right heart, as a means of relieving intense pulmonary congestion. [New York, 1882.] 9p. DNLM **80-6685**

WESTBROOK, Benjamin F[ranklin] (1851-1895)
On the aetiology of pulmonary phthisis. [New York, 1884.] 23p. DNLM **80-6686**

WESTBROOK, Benjamin F[ranklin] (1851-1895)
On cough as a symptom of disease. New York: Stettiner, Lambert & Co., 1884. 25p. DNLM **80-6687**

WESTBROOK, Benjamin F[ranklin] (1851-1895)
Local treatment of diseases of the bronchial tubes and lungs. [Philadelphia, 1887.] 20p. DNLM **80-6688**

WESTBROOK, Benjamin F[ranklin] (1851-1895)
A method for the surgical treatment of sero-fibrinous pleurisy. [New York, 1887.] 6p. DNLM **80-6689**

WESTBROOK, Benjamin F[ranklin] (1851-1895)
Pleurisy as a predisposing cause of phthisis pulmonalis. [New York, 1888.] 10p. DNLM **80-6690**

WESTBROOK, Benjamin F[ranklin] (1851-1895)
Treatment of fever. New York, 1888. 21p. DNLM **80-6691**

WESTON, Edward B.
A new procedure in cases of anticipated complete rupture of the perineum. Read before the Chicago Gynaecological Society, Nov. 16, 1888. [Chicago, 1888.] 2 l. DNLM **80-6692**

WETHERILL, Henry M[ayer], Jr. (1852?-1904)
The modern hypnotics. [Utica, N.Y., 1889.] 20p. DNLM **80-6693**

WHARTON, Francis (1820-1889) and Moreton STILLÉ
A treatise on medical jurisprudence. . . . 4th ed. Philadelphia: Kay & Bro., 1882. 3 v. CU-M; DNLM; ICRM; PPC **80-6694**

WHARTON, Henry R[edwood] (1853-1925)
Charles T. Hunter, 1843-1884. [Philadelphia, 1884.] 3p. DNLM **80-6695**

WHARTON, Henry R[edwood] (1853-1925)
Osteotomy for the correction of deformities in the lower extremities. Philadelphia, [1885]. 15p. DNLM **80-6696**

WHEELER, H. A.
Abstracts of pharmacology. Prepared for the use of physicians and pharmacists, and especially for the use of students of medicine and pharmacy, [etc.]. Onawa, Iowa, 1889. 180p. DNLM **80-6697**

WHEELER, John B[rooks] (*b.* 1853)
Cocaine in general surgery. Montpelier, Vt., 1887. 6p. DNLM **80-6698**

WHEELER, John B[rooks] (*b.* **1853)**
Antiseptic surgery in the country. Philadelphia: Med. Press Co., 1889. 7p. DNLM **80-6699**

WHELPLEY, Henry Milton (1861-1926)
Chemical lecture notes. Taken from Prof. C. O. Curtman's lectures at the St. Louis College of Pharmacy. . . . St. Louis: The Author, 1886. 143p. diags. DLC **80-6700**

WHELPLEY, Henry Milton (1861-1926)
Chemical lecture notes. Taken from Prof. C. O. Curtman's lectures at the St. Louis College of Pharmacy. . . . 2nd ed., rev. and enl. by the addition of notes on the metals. St. Louis, Mo.: The Author, 1888. 211p. diags. DLC **80-6701**

WHITALL, TATUM & CO.
Illustrated catalogue. [Druggists' supplies.] Philadelphia & New York, 1880. 72p. NNNAM; PPC **80-6702**

WHITALL, TATUM & CO.
Illustrated catalogue. [Druggists' supplies.] Philadelphia & New York, 1881. 80p. NNNAM **80-6703**

WHITALL, TATUM & CO.
Illustrated catalogue. [Druggists' supplies.] Philadelphia & New York, 1882. 88p. PPC; PU **80-6704**

WHITALL, TATUM & CO.
Illustrated catalogue. [Druggists' supplies.] Philadelphia & New York, 1883. 88p. PPC **80-6705**

WHITALL, TATUM & CO.
Illustrated catalogue. [Druggists' supplies.] Philadelphia & New York, 1884. 104p. PPC; PU **80-6706**

WHITALL, TATUM & CO.
Illustrated catalogue. [Druggists' supplies.] Philadelphia & New York, 1885. 106p. NNNAM **80-6707**

WHITALL, TATUM & CO.
Illustrated catalogue. [Druggists' supplies.] Philadelphia & New York, 1886. 148p. NNNAM **80-6708**

WHITE, Caroline Earle (1833-1916)
An answer to Dr. Keen's address entitled "Our recent debts to vivisection." Philadelphia, 1886. 24p. DNLM **80-6709**

WHITE, Charles B[rainon] (1826-1882)
Remarks upon "disinfection," as found on pages 81 and 82 of a pamphlet prepared by Dr. Joseph Jones and published by the board of health; a pamphlet entitled, "Acts of the legislature of Louisiana, establishing and regulating quarantine, etc."; also, discussion of analyses of Dr. Jones, appearing in the same article, by Jos. Albrecht. [New Orleans, 1880.] 12p. DNLM; LNT-M **80-6710**

WHITE, Frances Emily (1832-1903)
Hygiene as a basis of morals. Address to graduates at the thirty-fifth annual commencement of the Woman's Medical College of Pennsylvania. New York: D. Appleton & Co., 1887. 16p. DNLM; NNNAM; PPC **80-6711**

WHITE, Horace C[arr] (1836-1903)
Annual address on the progressive and conservative spirit in medical science. Chicago: Office American Medical Association, 1888. 8p. DNLM; ICRM **80-6712**

WHITE, James Clarke (1833-1916)
Some of the causes of infantile eczema, and the importance of mechanical restraint in its treatment. Cambridge, 1881. 15p. DNLM **80-6713**

WHITE, James Clarke (1833-1916)
The limitations of internal therapeutics in skin diseases. New York: J. P. Putnam's Sons, [1882]. 10p. DNLM; NNNAM **80-6714**

WHITE, James Clarke (1833-1916)
The question of contagion in leprosy. [Philadelphia, 1882.] 22p. DNLM; PPC **80-6715**

WHITE, James Clarke (1833-1916)
A case of unilateral chromidrosis? New York: William Wood & Co., 1884. 7p. DNLM; NNNAM **80-6716**

WHITE, James Clarke (1833-1916)
Cases of arsenical dermatitis. Cambridge: Riverside Press, 1884. 11p. DNLM; MBM **80-6717**

WHITE, James Clarke (1833-1916)
Angioma pigmentosum et atrophicum. New York: William Wood & Co., 1885. 7p. 1 plate. DNLM; NNNAM **80-6718**

WHITE, James Clarke (1833-1916)
Psoriasis, verruca, epithelioma: a sequence. Philadelphia, 1885. 10p. DNLM **80-6719**

WHITE, James Clarke (1833-1916)
On the treatment of lupus by parasiticides. Boston: Cupples, Upham & Co., 1885. 20p. DNLM; MBM **80-6720**

WHITE, James Clarke (1833-1916)
An introduction to the study of the influence of diet in the production and treatment of skin diseases. New York: William Wood & Co., 1887. 16p. DNLM; NNNAM **80-6721**

WHITE, James Clarke (1833-1916)
Dermatitis venenata: an account of the action of external irritants upon the skin. . . . Boston: Cupples & Hurd, 1887. 216p. DLC; DNLM; MH-M **80-6722**

WHITE, James Clarke (1833-1916)
Dermatitis gestationis, the history of a recurrent dermatosis. Boston: Cupples & Hurd, [1889]. 12p. DNLM; MBM **80-6723**

WHITE, James Clarke (1833-1916)
A case of keratosis (ichthyosis) follicularis. [1889.] 8p. 1 plate. DNLM **80-6724**

WHITE, James Clarke (1833-1916)
On the increasing prevalence of scabies, with remarks upon treatment. Boston: Cupples & Hurd, 1889. 9p. DNLM; MBM **80-6725**

WHITE, James Platt (1811-1881)
Hints relative to intra-uterine medication. [n. p., 1880.] 10p. DNLM **80-6726**

WHITE, James W[illiam] (1826-1891)
The teeth; natural and artificial. Philadelphia: S. S. White, 1880. 32p. DNLM; PPC **80-6727**

WHITE, James W[illiam] (1826-1891)
. . . The mouth and the teeth. . . . Philadelphia: P. Blakiston, 1880. 150p. DLC; DNLM; MdU-D; PPC **80-6728**

WHITE, James W[illiam] (1826-1891)
A consideration of temperament in relation to teeth. Philadelphia, 1884. 8p. DNLM **80-6729**

WHITE, James W[illiam] (1826-1891)
Diseases incident to the first dentition. Philadelphia: S. S. White, 1887. 30p. DNLM **80-6730**

WHITE, J[ames] William (1850-1916)
The prevention of syphilis: an address. [Philadelphia, 1882.] 20p. DNLM **80-6731**

WHITE, J[ames] William (1850-1916)
A review of some of the more important surgical problems of President Garfield's case. Philadelphia, 1882. 24p. DNLM **80-6732**

WHITE, J[ames] William (1850-1916)
First aid to the injured. An abstract of lectures. [Philadelphia], 1883. 25p. DNLM **80-6733**

WHITE, J[ames] William (1850-1916)
A case of supposed dislocation of the tendon of the long head of the biceps muscle. Philadelphia: Collins, 1884. 41p. DNLM **80-6734**

WHITE, J[ames] William (1850-1916)
Elementary directions for personal hygiene and physical development. Philadelphia: Patterson & White, 1886. 19p. DNLM **80-6735**

WHITE, J[ames] William (1850-1916)
The abortive treatment of syphilis. [Philadelphia, 1888.] 16p. DNLM **80-6736**

WHITE, J[ames] William (1850-1916)
A case of rupture of the urethra, with some remarks upon the symptoms and treatment of that injury. Boston: Cupples & Hurd, 1888. 16p. DNLM **80-6737**

WHITE, J[ames] William (1850-1916)
A note on two cases illustrating some minor difficulties in the diagnosis of hernia. [Philadelphia, 1888.] 2 l. DNLM **80-6738**

WHITE, J[ames] William (1850-1916)
The surgical importance of strictures of large calibre. [Philadelphia, 1888.] 20p. DNLM **80-6739**

WHITE, J[ames] William (1850-1916)
Two cases of the radical cure of hernia. [Philadelphia, 1888.] 11p. DNLM **80-6740**

WHITE, J[ames] William (1850-1916)
Some glimpses of British surgery. Philadelphia, 1888. 15p. DNLM **80-6741**

WHITE, J[ames] William (1850-1916)
Record of one term of service in the surgical wards of the German Hospital of Philadelphia. Philadelphia, 1888. 24p. DNLM **80-6742**

WHITE, J[ames] William (1850-1916)
The aseptic use of Malgaigne's hooks in the transverse fracture of the patella. New York, 1888. 14p. DNLM **80-6743**

WHITE, J[ames] William (1850-1916) and Horatio C. WOOD
Iodide of potassium in syphilis. Detroit: G. S. Davis, 1888. 19p. DNLM **80-6744**

WHITE, J[ames] William (1850-1916)
Anaesthetics. [Philadelphia, 1889.] 34p. DNLM **80-6745**

WHITE, J[ames] William (1850-1916)
The aseptic theory and its practice. Philadelphia, 1889. 26p. DNLM **80-6746**

WHITE, J[ames] William (1850-1916) and H. C. WOOD
Contributions to the discussion on the diagnostic value of the tolerance of the iodides in syphilis. Detroit, Mich.: G. S. Davis, 1889. 14p. DNLM **80-6747**

WHITE, J[ames] William (1850-1916)
Notes of a case of cure of aneurism of the posterior tibial artery through position after failure of digital compression. [Philadelphia, 1889.] 4p. DNLM **80-6748**

WHITE, J[ames] William (1850-1916)
Notes from clinical lectures delivered during a term of service at the Philadelphia Hospital. [Philadelphia, 1889.] 11p. DNLM **80-6749**

WHITE, J[ames] William (1850-1916)
The radical cure of hernia: a report of four successful cases. [Philadelphia, 1889.] 8p. DNLM **80-6750**

WHITE, J[ames] William (1850-1916)
The relation of the prostate to chronic urethral discharge. [Philadelphia, 1889.] 7p. DNLM **80-6751**

WHITE, J[ames] William (1850-1916)
The surgery of the spine. [St. Louis, 1889.] 39p. 1 tab. DNLM **80-6752**

WHITE, J[ames] William (1850-1916)
The surgical aspects of Dr. Wood's case of brain tumor. [Philadelphia, 1889.] 3p. DNLM **80-6753**

WHITE, J[ames] William (1850-1916)
The toxic action of chromic acid used as a cauterant. [Philadelphia, 1889.] 4p. DNLM **80-6754**

WHITE, J[ames] William (1850-1916)
The transplantation of bone: with two illustrative cases. [Philadelphia, 1889.] 9p. DNLM **80-6755**

WHITE, J[ames] William (1850-1916)
Tumors of the female breast. A clinical lecture. [Philadelphia, 1889.] 15p. DNLM **80-6756**

WHITE, J[ames] William (1850-1916)
A note on the use of the bidet in surgery. New York, 1889. 11p. DNLM **80-6757**

WHITE, John Blake (*b.* 1850)
Eleven cases of phthisis treated by intra-pulmonary injections of carbolized iodine. New York: Trow, 1886. 16p. DNLM **80-6758**

WHITE, John Blake (*b.* 1850)
Some remarks on the diagnosis and treatment of spasmodic stricture. New York: William Wood & Co., 1886. 6p. DNLM **80-6759**

WHITE, John Blake (*b.* 1850)
The diagnosis and treatment of uterine flexions. New York: Judson Printing Co., 1887. 10p. DNLM **80-6760**

WHITE, John Blake (*b.* 1850)
A case of icterus infantum from congenital deficiency of the ductus communis choledochus. [New York, 1888.] 7p. DNLM **80-6761**

WHITE, John Blake (*b.* 1850)
Remarks on the vesico-urethral erethism peculiar to locomotive engineers. [New York, 1888.] 7p. DNLM **80-6762**

WHITE, Joseph A.
Otorrhoea. Richmond: J. W. Fergusson & Son, 1880. 10p. DNLM **80-6763**

WHITE, Joseph A.
Some remarks about a common functional eye trouble. Read before the Medical Society of Virginia, 1880. [Richmond, 1880.] 13p. DNLM **80-6764**

WHITE, Joseph A.
Report on advances in ophthalmology, otology and laryngology. [Richmond, 1882.] 10p. DNLM **80-6765**

WHITE, Joseph A.
Naso-pharyngeal catarrh. [Richmond, 1883.] 16p. DNLM **80-6766**

WHITE, Joseph A.
Influence of naso-pharyngeal growths, obstructions and hypertrophies upon the hearing, with a few cases in point. [Richmond, 1885.] 13p. DNLM **80-6767**

WHITE, Samuel S[tockton] (1822-1879)
Catalogue of gum sectional teeth. Philadelphia, 1887. 72p. DNLM; PPC **80-6768**

THE S. S. WHITE DENTAL MFG. CO.
Catalogue of procelain teeth manufactured by The S. S. White Dental Mfg. Co. . . . Philadelphia: The S. S. White Dental Mfg. Co., [1889]. 158p. fold. plate. DLC; PPC **80-6769**

WHITEHEAD, William R[iddick] (1831-1902)
Address delivered at the fourteenth annual convention of the Colorado Sate Medical Society (June 1884). [Denver, 1884.] 9p. DNLM **80-6770**

WHITEHEAD, William R[iddick] (1831-1902)
The "Medical Record's" position editorially, as to the value of exsection for hip disease. [Denver, 1886.] 6p. DNLM **80-6771**

WHITEHEAD, William R[iddick] (1831-1902)
1. A report on orthopedic surgery to the Colorado State Medical Society. 2. Remarks on stricture of the rectum. [Denver]: Whipple & Pierson, [1887]. 16p. DNLM **80-6772**

WHITEMAN, Charles Otis (1842-1910)
Methods of research in microscopical anatomy and embryology. Boston: Cassino, 1885. 255p. MBM; NNNAM **80-6773**

WHITMAN, Royal (1857-1946)
Some observations on bow-leg and in-knee, with especial reference to the question of outgrowth of these deformities. New York: Trow's Co., 1887. 7p. DNLM **80-6774**

WHITMAN, Royal (1857-1946)
Observations on forty-five cases of flat-foot, with particular reference to etiology and treatment. Boston: Cupples & Hurd, 1888. 24p. DNLM; MBM **80-6775**

WHITMAN, Royal (1857-1946)
Observations on seventy-five cases of flat-foot, with particular reference to treatment. Boston: L. P. Kellogg & Son, 1889. 24p. DNLM; MBM **80-6776**

WHITNEY, James O[rne] (1823-1895)
Diagnosis of the posture of the child in utero, by palpation. Pawtucket, R.I., 1880. 7p. DNLM **80-6777**

WHITNEY, N. D., & CO.
Testing for color-blindness. [Boston, 1880.] 1 l. DNLM **80-6778**

WHITTEMORE, Frank H.
The treatment of stricture of the urethra. New York, 1885. 12p. DNLM **80-6779**

WHITWELL, William S[collay] (1847-1903?)
Report of a case of successful transfusion in typhoid fever. San Francisco: W. S. Duncombe & Co., 1886. 6p. 1 diag. DNLM **80-6780**

WHITWELL, William S[collay] (1847-1903?)
The opium habit. [San Francisco, 1887.] 18p. DNLM **80-6781**

[WICKES, Edward Zeus Franklin]
Illustrated medical counsellor. A strictly private book for married people. . . . By the president of the Phreno-Medical College of Pa. . . . [New York, 1882.] 190p. DLC; NNNAM **80-6782**

WICKES, Edward Zeus Franklin
Domestic materia medica. The family doctor. . . . All rights reserved by the author. . . . In two volumes. . . . Boston, Mass.: The Author, 1884. 136p. DLC; MBM **80-6783**

WICKES, Edward Zeus Franklin
Illustrated domestic medical counsellor. Laws and science of life, health and self-preservation. Materia medica and pharmacy. Embracing all the latest discoveries in cosmic science. . . . Boston, Mass.: Mutual Benefit Publishing M'f'g. Co., 1884. 5 v. in 1. DLC; MH; MSaE **80-6784**

WICKES, Stephen (1813-1889)
Sepulture, its history, methods, and sanitary requisites. Philadelphia: P. Blakiston, Son & Co., 1884. 156p. DNLM; PPC; PU **80-6785**

WIGGLESWORTH, Edward (1840-1896) and E. W. CUSHING
Buccal ulcerations of constitutional origin. [New York, 1882.] 18p. DNLM **80-6786**

WIGGLESWORTH, Edward (1840-1896)
Address delivered before the American Dermatological Association, at the tenth annual meeting. Boston, 1886. 13p. DNLM **80-6787**

WIGHT, Jervis [Sherman] (1834-1901)
The fallacies of popular clinical medicine. An introductory lecture. New York: G. P. Putnam's Sons, 1880. 16p. DNLM **80-6788**

WIGHT, Jervis [Sherman] (1834-1901)
The principles of myodynamics. New York: Bermingham & Co., 1881. 162p. DNLM; NNNAM **80-6789**

WIGHT, Jervis [Sherman] (1834-1901)
A plea for the treatment of criminals. New York, 1884. 13p. DNLM **80-6790**

WIGHT, Jervis [Sherman] (1834-1901)
In memorium. Professor Frank Hastings Hamilton. [1886.] 39p. NNNAM **80-6791**

WIGHT, Orlando Williams (1824-1888)
How to combat small-pox. Detroit, 1882. 27p. DNLM **80-6792**

WIGHT, Orlando Williams (1824-1888)
Laws requiring medical men to report deaths and cases of infectious disease to the public authorities. Detroit: Post & Tribune Co., 1882. 8p. DNLM **80-6793**

WIGHT, Orlando Williams (1824-1888)
Report to the city council on the pavement question, by the health officer. [Detroit, 1882.] 2 l. DNLM **80-6794**

WIGHT, Orlando Williams (1824-1888)
Maxims of public health. New York: D. Appleton & Co., 1884. 176p. DNLM; NNNAM **80-6795**

WILBUR, H[ervey] B[ackus] (1820-1883)
"Chemical restraint" in the management of the insane. New York: G. P. Putnam's Sons, 1881. 22p. DNLM; NNNAM **80-6796**

WILBUR, H[ervey] B[ackus] (1820-1883)
A Scotch asylum for the insane. [n. p., 1881.] 2 l. DNLM **80-6797**

WILCOX, Reynold W[ebb] (1856-1931)
Is albuminuria a contra-indication to ovariotomy? St. Louis, 1884. 13p. DNLM **80-6798**

WILCOX, Reynold W[ebb] (1856-1931)
The mechanical treatment of hip-disease. [St. Louis, 1884.] 4p. DNLM **80-6799**

WILCOX, Reynold W[ebb] (1856-1931)
A successful case of hysterectomy. [St. Louis, 1885.] 4p. DNLM **80-6800**

WILCOX, Reynold W[ebb] (1856-1931)
The therapeutic and operative treatment of hip disease. [St. Louis, 1885.] 4p. DNLM **80-6801**

WILCOX, Sidney F[reeman]
President's address, read before the New York Society for Medico-Scientific Investigation, January 5th, 1886. [New York, 1886.] 3 l. DNLM **80-6802**

WILDER, A[braham] M. (1840-1886)
Old and new codes. [Sacramento], 1884. 20p. DNLM **80-6803**

WILDER, A[braham] M. (1840-1886)
Report on ophthalmology, read before the California State Medical Society, April, 1885. [San Francisco, 1885.] 19p. DNLM **80-6804**

WILDER, Alexander (1823-1908)
The ganglionic nervous system. . . . [Orange, N.J., 1884.] 29p. DLC; DNLM **80-6805**

WILDER, Alexander (1823-1908)
Eclectic medicine; its history and scientific basis. [1884?] 18p. DNLM **80-6806**

WILDER, Burt Green (1841-1925)
The names of the encephalic arteries. New York, 1885. 1 l. DNLM **80-6807**

WILDER, Hans M[atthias], ed.
Price and dose labels of drugs and preparations generally kept in a retail pharmacy, including besides those officinal in the last revision of the United States Pharmacopoeia, many other new and rare drugs and chemicals, with the Latin, French, and German synonyms. New York: J. H. Vail & Co., 1888. 230p. DNLM; NNNAM; OCLloyd **80-6808**

WILE, Henry (1859?-1887)
The pathogenesis of secondary tumors. Philadelphia, 1882. 1882. 16p. DNLM **80-6809**

WILE, Henry (1859?-1887)
Some notes on the histology of lupus vulgaris. [New York, 1882.] 6p. DNLM **80-6810**

WILE, William C[onrad] (1847-1913)
Hydrocele in the female. New York: William Wood & Co., 1881. 15p. DNLM **80-6811**

WILE, William C[onrad] (1847-1913)
Surgical notes from the case book of a general practitioner. [Bridgeport, Conn., 1885.] 22p. 2 plates. DNLM **80-6812**

WILE, William C[onrad] (1847-1913)
Surgical notes from the case book of a general practitioner. [Bridgeport, Conn. 1886.] 16p. DNLM **80-6813**

WILLARD, DeForest (1846-1910)
Hip-injuries, including hip-joint disease, and fractures of the femoral neck, splint for. [Philadelphia, 1880.] 4p. DNLM **80-6814**

WILLARD, DeForest (1846-1910)
Hip-joint disease: death in early stage from tubercular meningitis; microscopical appearances, by E. O. Shakespeare. Cambridge: Riverside Press, 1880. 77p. DNLM
80-6815

WILLARD, DeForest (1846-1910)
Adherent and contracted prepuce, commonly called congenital phimosis. [Philadelphia, 1883.] 7p. DNLM
80-6816

WILLARD, DeForest (1846-1910)
Ambulance service in Philadelphia, 1883. [Philadelphia, 1883.] 24p. DNLM **80-6817**

WILLARD, DeForest (1846-1910)
Club-foot; simple measures for its early relief. [Philadelphia, 1883.] 4p. DNLM **80-6818**

WILLARD, DeForest (1846-1910)
Club-foot. Is excision of the tarsus necessary in children? Philadelphia: Collins, 1884. 29p. DNLM
80-6819

WILLARD, DeForest (1846-1910)
Joint diseases; treatment by rest and fixation. [New York: D. Appleton & Co.], 1885. 15p. DNLM
80-6820

WILLARD, DeForest (1846-1910)
Surgical treatment of infants. [Philadelphia, 1885.] 12p. DNLM **80-6821**

WILLARD, DeForest (1846-1910)
Foreign bodies in the urethra and bladder; removal by the litholapaxy evacuator with large, straight, open-ended cannula. [Philadelphia, 1887.] 8p. DNLM **80-6822**

WILLARD, DeForest (1846-1910)
Nephrectomies for gunshot wound, and for tuberculous kidney. Philadelphia: W. J. Dornan, 1889. 20p. DNLM
80-6823

WILLARD, DeForest (1846-1910)
Osteotomy for anterior curves of the leg. [Philadelphia, 1889.] 20p. DNLM **80-6824**

WILLARD, DeForest (1846-1910)
Spinal caries: operative treatment; laminectomy, or so-called trephining of spine. Philadelphia: W. J. Dornan, 1889. 8p. DNLM **80-6825**

WILLIAMS, Charles (*d.* 1907)
Stone in the bladder in connexion with enlargement of the spleen. Norwich: Fletcher & Son, 1888. 11p. DNLM
80-6826

WILLIAMS, Charles J[ames] B[lasius] (1805-1889) and Charles Theodore WILLIAMS
Pulmonary consumption; its etiology, pathology, and treatment. With an analysis of 1,000 cases to exemplify its duration and modes of arrest. 2nd ed., enlarged and rewritten by C. Theodore Williams. Philadelphia: P. Blakiston, Son & Co., 1887. 446p. 4 plates. DNLM; NNNAM; PPC; PU
80-6827

WILLIAMS, Harold
The climatic treatment of phthisis. Boston: Cupples, Upham & Co., 1885. 19p. DNLM **80-6828**

WILLIAMS, Henry Smith (1863-1943)
The encephalic circulation and its relation to the mind. [Utica, N.Y., 1889.] 24p. DNLM **80-6829**

WILLIAMS, Henry Willard (1821-1895)
The diagnosis and treatment of the diseases of the eye. Boston: Houghton, Mifflin & Co., 1881. 464p. 7 plates. CtY-M; DNLM; MBM; NNNAM **80-6830**

WILLIAMS, Henry Willard (1821-1895)
A practical guide to the study of diseases of the eye: their medical and surgical treatment. 2nd ed. Boston: Cupples, 1886. 484p. 5 charts. MBM; NNNAM; PPC; PU
80-6831

WILLIAMS, Henry Willard (1821-1895)
Advances in our knowledge of some cerebral, ocular, and intra-orbital lesions which facilitate the diagnosis and treatment of important diseases. Chicago: Office of American Medical Association, 1889. 11p. DNLM **80-6832**

WILLIAMS, Herbert F. (*b.* 1850)
Antiseptic treatment of pulmonary disease by means of pneumatic differentiation. New York, 1885. 22p. DNLM; NNNAM
80-6833

WILLIAMS, Herbert F. (*b.* 1850)
A clinical report of cases treated by pneumatic differentiation. [New York, 1886.] 42p. DNLM; NNNAM
80-6834

WILLIAMS, J[ohn] L.
A consideration of the merits and claims of artificial crown- and bridge-work. Philadelphia, 1884. 16p. DNLM
80-6835

WILLIAMS, J[ohn] L.
Artificial teeth without plates; the merits and claims of crown- and bridge-work. Philadelphia: Patterson & White, 1885. 15p. DNLM **80-6836**

WILLIAMS, Philip C[roudson] (1828-1896)
Malarial fever in puerperal women. [Baltimore, 1883.] 6p. DNLM **80-6837**

WILLIAMS, Philip C[roudson] (1828-1896)
The use of ergot in obstetrics. Baltimore, 1884. 10p. DNLM
80-6838

WILLIAMS, R. E.
Cremation and other modes of sepulture. Philadelphia: J. B. Lippincott & Co., 1884. 82p. DNLM; PPC; PU
80-6839

WILLIAMS, Richard J. (1830-1915)
A view of the laws relating to physicians, druggists and dentists. Philadelphia: W. P. Kildare, 1884. 115p. DNLM; ICU; MH; NN **80-6840**

WILLIAMS, T. D.
The American Homoeopathic Dispensatory. Designed as a text-book for the physician, student and druggist. Chicago: Gross & Delbridge, 1884. 705p. OCLloyd
80-6841

WILLIS, A. E.
Illustrated physiognomy. Chicago, 1881. 51p. 19 plates. DNLM **80-6842**

WILSON, Charles Meigs (1860-1891)
Mechanical dilatation of the uterus. Philadelphia, 1885. 8p. DNLM **80-6843**

WILSON, George (1811-1897)
Health and healthy homes . . . with notes and additions by J. G. Richardson. Philadelphia: P. Blakiston, 1880. 307p. DNLM; PPC; PU **80-6844**

WILSON, George (1811-1897)
A handbook of hygiene and sanitary science. 4th ed. Philadelphia: Lindsay & Blakiston, 1880. 468p. DNLM; PPC; PPJ; PU **80-6845**

WILSON, George (1811-1897)
How to live, or health and healthy homes. Philadelphia: P. Blakiston, Son & Co., 1884. 314p. DNLM; NNNAM; PU **80-6846**

WILSON, George (1811-1897)
A handbook of hygiene and sanitary science. 5th ed., enl. and carefully rev. Philadelphia: P. Blakiston, Son & Co., 1884. 512p. MBM; NNNAM; PPC; PU **80-6847**

WILSON, George (1811-1897)
A text-book of hygiene. Domestic hygiene and sanitary information, including articles on the human body, digestion, and nutrition, the causes of disease, the effects of intemperance, food and diet, cleanliness and clothing, exercise, recreation and training, the home and its surroundings, the prevention of infectious diseases, etc. Edited with notes and additions by J. G. Richardson. Philadelphia: P. Blakiston, Son & Co., 1885. 314p. DNLM; NNNAM; PU **80-6848**

WILSON, George (1811-1897)
A handbook of hygiene and sanitary science. 6th ed. Philadelphia: P. Blakiston, Son & Co., 1886. 520p. DNLM; PPC; PU **80-6849**

WILSON, Grove H[errick] (*d.* 1902)
Epidemic intermittent fever; its annual progress in Connecticut and other parts of New England. Hartford: Case, Lockwood & Brainard Co., 1883. 8p. 1 map. DNLM **80-6850**

WILSON, Harold B.
Foreign sketches from Wiesbaden and the German universities, being chiefly upon ophthalmological subjects. [Detroit], 1888. 30p. DNLM **80-6851**

WILSON, Harry Augustus (1853-1919)
Anaesthesia by ethyl bromide. Philadelphia: W. F. Fell & Co., [1880]. 7p. DNLM **80-6852**

WILSON, Harry Augustus (1853-1919)
Soluble compressed pellets, a new form of remedies for hypodermic use. Philadelphia, 1880. 3p. DNLM **80-6853**

WILSON, Harry Augustus (1853-1919)
A brief consideration of twenty cases of foreign bodies in the eyes. [Philadelphia, 1881.] 3p. DNLM **80-6854**

WILSON, Harry Augustus (1853-1919)
The differential diagnosis of fractures, and dislocations of the femur at the hip joint. [Brooklyn, 1881.] 2 l. DNLM **80-6855**

WILSON, Harry Augustus (1853-1919)
Soluble compressed hypodermic tablets. [n. p., 1881, *vel subseq.*] 6p. DNLM **80-6856**

WILSON, Harry Augustus (1853-1919)
Soluble compressed pellets; a new form of remedies for hypodermic use, and applicable to ophthalmic and general medication. Philadelphia: Collins, 1881. 4p. DNLM **80-6857**

WILSON, Harry Augustus (1853-1919)
A study of transverse fracture of the patella. [Philadelphia, 1881.] 8p. DNLM **80-6858**

WILSON, H[enry] P[arke] C[ustis] (1827-1898)
A case of combined intrauterine and abdominal twin pregnancy; the first child born naturally at eight months; the second delivered alive at term by laparotomy. New York: William Wood & Co., 1880. 18p. DNLM **80-6859**

WILSON, H[enry] P[arke] C[ustis] (1827-1898)
Ovariotomy during pregnancy. [Baltimore, 1881.] 11p. DNLM **80-6860**

WILSON, H[enry] P[arke] C[ustis] (1827-1898)
Uterine dilatation with a new instrument. New York: William Wood & Co., 1881. 9p. DNLM **80-6861**

WILSON, H[enry] P[arke] C[ustis] (1827-1898)
A case of hysterectomy with a new clamp for the removal of large uterine tumors. New York: William Wood & Co., 1883. 12p. DNLM **80-6862**

WILSON, H[enry] P[arke] C[ustis] (1827-1898)
Foreign bodies left in the abdomen after laparotomy. [New York, 1884.] 15p. DNLM **80-6863**

WILSON, H[enry] P[arke] C[ustis] (1827-1898)
Circumscribed peritoneal dropsy simulating ovarian dropsy. Baltimore: Journal Pub. Co., 1886. 13p. DNLM **80-6864**

WILSON, H[enry] P[arke] C[ustis] (1827-1898)
Division of the cervix backward in some forms of anteflexion of the uterus, with dysmenorrhoea and sterility. [New York, 1886.] 13p. DNLM **80-6865**

WILSON, H[enry] P[arke] C[ustis] (1827-1898)
The president's annual address. [American Gynecological Society.] Philadelphia: W. J. Dornan, 1889. 11p. DNLM **80-6866**

WILSON, James Cornelius (1847-1934)
A treatise on the continued fevers. . . . With an introduction by J. M. Da Costa. . . . New York: William Wood & Co., 1881. 365p. diags. DLC; DNLM; NNNAM **80-6867**

WILSON, James Cornelius (1847-1934)
Observations on the management of enteric fever according to a plan based upon the so-called specific treatment. Philadelphia: Collins, 1883. 13p. DNLM **80-6868**

WILSON, James Cornelius (1847-1934)
Remarks upon the climate of Florida. New York: D. Appleton & Co., 1885. 12p. DNLM **80-6869**

WILSON, James Cornelius (1847-1934)
. . . Fever-nursing: designed for the use of professional and other nurses, and especially as a text-book for nurses in training. . . . Philadelphia, London: J. B. Lippincott Co., 1888. 210p. fold. charts. DNLM; PPC; PU
80-6870

WILSON, James Cornelius (1847-1934)
Casual therapeutics in the infectious diseases. [Detroit, 1888.] 16p. DNLM **80-6871**

WILSON, James Cornelius (1847-1934)
The causes and prevention of the opium habit and kindred affections. [Philadelphia, 1888.] 15p. DNLM
80-6872

WILSON, James Cornelius (1847-1934)
Climate and Bright's disease. [Philadelphia, 1888.] 7p. DNLM
80-6873

WILSON, James Cornelius (1847-1934)
Note on the treatment of syphilis by the hypodermatic injection of calomel. Philadelphia, 1888. 19p. DNLM
80-6874

WILSON, James Cornelius (1847-1934)
The etiology and prophylaxis of the tuberculous diseases. [Philadelphia, 1889.] 16p. DNLM **80-6875**

WILSON, James Cornelius (1847-1934)
Pulsating empyema; report of a case. [Philadelphia, 1889.] 8p. DNLM **80-6876**

WILSON, James Cornelius (1847-1934)
Remarks upon the treatment of the opium habit and kindred affections. [Philadelphia, 1889.] 18p. DNLM
80-6877

WILSON, John
Health and health resorts. Philadelphia: Porter & Coates, [1880]. 288p. DNLM; PU **80-6878**

WILSON, Joseph M[iller] (1838-1902)
Drainage for health, or easy lessons in sanitary science. Philadelphia: P. Blakiston, 1881. 68p. 1 plate. DNLM; PPC; PU
80-6879

WILSON, Joseph M[iller] (1838-1902)
Drainage for health, or easy lessons in sanitary science. 2nd ed., with important additions. Philadelphia: P. Blakiston, Son & Co., 1886. 74p. 1 plate. DNLM; MdBM; PU
80-6880

WILSON, L[ouis] D.
The plea of an aggrieved uterus. [Wheeling, 1886.] 13p. DNLM
80-6881

WILSON, O. S.
Report on the sanitary condition of Havana, [N.Y.]. [Albany, 1885.] 8p. DNLM **80-6882**

WILSON, Robert [Taylor]
Combined sponge and placental forceps, and curettes, etc. [Philadelphia, 1886.] Galley sheet. DNLM
80-6883

WILSON, Robert [Taylor]
Hysterectomy for removal of a fibro-cystic tumor. [Also] ovariotomy, with the history of a case. Baltimore: Journ. Publ. Co. print, 1886. 22p. DNLM **80-6884**

WILSON, Robert [Taylor]
Temporary clamp, to be used especially in "ovariotomy," "Battey's operation," and "Tait's operation," with remarks on these operations. Baltimore, 1886. 5p. DNLM
80-6885

WILSON, Robert [Taylor]
A contribution to the history of hydramnios. New York: William Wood & Co., 1887. 27p. DNLM
80-6886

WILSON, Thomas P[ardon] (1832-1909)
Special indications for twenty-five remedies in intermittent fever. Philadelphia: Boericke & Tafel, 1880. 53p. DLC; DNLM; PPHa **80-6887**

WILSON, W. R.
The right relation of the general public to state preventive medicine. The annual address delivered before the Medical Society of North Caorlina. (Published gratuitously by the North Carolina Board of Health.) Raleigh: Edwards, Broughton & Co., 1883. 15p. DNLM **80-6888**

WILTROUT, Irving D.
Brain and spinal surgery in Philadelphia. [St. Paul, 1889.] 15p. DNLM **80-6889**

WILTROUT, Irving D.
Multiple neuritis. Milwaukee: Corbitt & Skidmore Co., 1889. 9p. DNLM **80-6890**

WIMMER, Sebastian J.
Improprieties of dress an important etiological factor in many of the diseases peculiar to women. Philadelphia: Records, McMullin & Co., 1888. 10p. DNLM **80-6891**

WIMMER, Sebastian J.
Terebene: its medical uses and its value. [New York, 1889.] 5p. DNLM **80-6892**

WINANS, Henry C.
Prosposed medical legislation for Indiana. Muncie, 1880. 14p. DNLM **80-6893**

von WINCKEL, Franz Karl Ludw. Wilh. (1837-1911)
Diseases of women. A hand-book for physicians and students. Authorized transl. by J. H. Williamson. Under the supervision and with an introduction by Theophilus Parvin. Philadelphia: P. Blakiston, Son & Co., 1887. 774p. DNLM; MBM; NNNAM; PPC **80-6894**

von WINCKEL, Franz Karl Ludw. Wilh. (1837-1911)
Diseases of women. A hand-book for physicians and students. Authorized transl. by J. H. Williamson. Under the supervision and with an introduction by Theophilus Parvin. 2nd ed. Philadelphia: P. Blakiston, Son & Co., 1889. 766p. DNLM; OCIM; PPJ; PU **80-6895**

WING, Clifton Ellis (1848-1911)
Modern abuse of gynaecology. [Boston: D. Clapp & Son, 1880.] 8p. DNLM **80-6896**

WING, Clifton Ellis (1848-1911)
On certain uterine displacements. [Boston, 1880.] 3p. DNLM
80-6897

WING, Clifton Ellis (1848-1911)
The "abdominal method" of singing and breathing as a cause of "female weaknesses." [Boston: D. Clapp & Son, 1880.] 8p. DNLM **80-6898**

WING, Clifton Ellis (1848-1911)
On unnecessary surgical operations in the treatment of the diseases of women. [Boston, 1881.] 16p. DNLM
80-6899

WING, Clifton Ellis (1848-1911)
Some points regarding the diagnosis of uterine anteflexions and anteversions. [Boston, 1882.] 7p. DNLM
80-6900

WINSEY, Whitfield
Some thoughts on phthisis pulmonalis. Baltimore: Guggenheimer, Cox & Co., [1886]. 11p. DNLM
80-6901

WINSLOW, Randolph (*b.* 1852)
The surgical treatment of abscess of the liver. Brooklyn, 1881. 7p. DNLM **80-6902**

WINSLOW, Randolph (*b.* 1852)
External rectotomy in benign stricture of the rectum. [Baltimore, 1881.] 4p. DNLM **80-6903**

WINSLOW, Randolph (*b.* 1852)
A study of the malformations, variations, and anomalies of the circulatory apparatus in man. With a brief consideration of some of the principles governing their production. Brooklyn, N.Y., 1883. 40p. DNLM; NNNAM
80-6904

WINSLOW, William H.
The human ear and its diseases; a practical treatise upon the examination, recognition, and treatment of affections of the ear and associate parts, [etc.]. New York & Philadelphia: Boericke & Tafel, 1882. 526p. DLC; DNLM; NNNAM; PPC
80-6905

WINTER, John Thomas (1842-1902)
Croup. New York: William Wood & Co., 1888. 15p. DNLM
80-6906

WINTER, John Thomas (1842-1902)
A case of absence of the bladder. New York: William Wood & Co., 1889. 3p. 1 plate. DNLM **80-6907**

WINTERBURN, George William (1845-1911)
Purpura. . . . New York: A. L. Chatterton & Co., 1886. 240p. DLC; NNNAM **80-6908**

WINTERBURN, George William, ed. (1845-1911)
A repertory of the most characteristic symptoms of the materia medica. . . . New York: A. L. Chatterton & Co., 1886. 182p. DLC; DNLM; NNNAM; PU **80-6909**

WINTERBURN, George William (1845-1911)
The value of vaccination. A non-partisan review of its history and results. . . . Philadelphia: F. E. Boericke, 1886. 182p. tables. DLC; NNNAM; PPHa **80-6910**

WINTERS, Joseph Edeil (*d.* 1922)
Is the operation of tracheotomy in diphtheritic croup dangerous? When should the operation be performed? New York: Trow's, 1884. 33p. DNLM; NNNAM **80-6911**

WINTERS, Joseph Edeil (*d.* 1922)
Is the operation of tracheotomy in diphtheritic croup dangerous? When should the operation be performed? New York, [1885]. 8p. DNLM **80-6912**

WINTERS, Joseph Edeil (*d.* 1922)
Diphtheria and its management. Are membranous croup and diphtheria distinct diseases? New York: Trow's, 1885. 43p. DNLM; NNNAM **80-6913**

WINTERS, Joseph Edeil (*d.* 1922)
The relative influences of maternal and wet-nursing on mother and child. New York: Trow's, 1886. 39p. DNLM; NNNAM
80-6914

WISTAR, Thomas (1836-1913)
Ode to Prof. D. Hayes Agnew, M.D., LL.D., on the fiftieth anniversary of his graduation in medicine, April 6th, 1888. [Philadelphia, 1888.] 2 l. DNLM; PPC
80-6915

WITHERSTINE, C. Sumner (*b.* 1854)
International pocket medical formulary. With an appendix. Philadelphia & London: F. A. Davis, 1888. 269p. DNLM; MBM; NNNAM; PPC **80-6916**

WITHINGTON, Charles Francis (1852-1917)
Observations upon the apparent curve of the sagittal suture in vertex presentations. [New York, 1885.] 8p. DNLM
80-6917

WITHINGTON, Charles Francis (1852-1917)
Consanguineous marriages: their effect upon offspring. [Boston, 1885.] 32p. DNLM; MBM **80-6918**

WITHINGTON, Charles Francis (1852-1917)
The relation of hospitals to medical education. Boston: Cupples, Upham & Co., 1886. 47p. DNLM; MBM
80-6919

WITHINGTON, Charles Francis (1852-1917)
An inquiry into the transmission of infectious diseases through the medium of rags. [Boston, 1887.] 69p. 8 tabs. DNLM; MBM **80-6920**

WITTHAUS, R[udolph] A[ugust] (1846-1915)
. . . General medical chemistry for the use of practitioners of medicine. . . . New York: William Wood & Co., 1881. 443p. DLC; DNLM; NNNAM; PU **80-6921**

WITTHAUS, R[udolph] A[ugust] (1846-1915)
The medical student's manual of chemistry. . . . New York: William Wood & Co., 1883. 370p. DLC; DNLM; NNNAM; PU **80-6922**

WITTHAUS, R[udolph] A[ugust] (1846-1915)
A laboratory guide in urinalysis and toxicology. . . . New York: William Wood & Co., 1886. 75p. DLC; DNLM; NNNAM; PU
80-6923

WITTHAUS, R[udolph] A[ugust] (1846-1915)
The medical student's manual of chemistry. . . . 2nd ed. New York: William Wood & Co., [*c.* 1887]. 391p. DNLM; NNNAM; PPC; PU **80-6924**

WITTHAUS, R[udolph] A[ugust] (1846-1915)
Essentials of chemistry and toxicology, for the use of students in medicine. . . . 2nd ed. New York: William Wood & Co., 1888. 294p. DLC; DNLM; NNNAM; PPC [*vel subseq.*]
80-6925

WITTHAUS, R[udolph] A[ugust] (1846-1915)
A laboratory guide in urinalysis and toxicology. . . . 2nd ed. New York: William Wood & Co., 1889. 75p. DLC; MBM; NNNAM; PPC **80-6926**

WOAKES, Edward (1837-1912)
Post-nasal catarrh and diseases of the nose causing deafness. Being vol. I of the third edition of "Deafness, giddiness, and noises in the head." Philadelphia: P. Blakiston, Son & Co., 1884. 224p. DNLM; PPC; PU **80-6927**

WOAKES, Edward (1837-1912)
Nasal polypus with neuralgia, hay fever, and asthma in relation to ethmoiditis. Philadelphia: P. Blakiston, Son & Co, 1887. 140p. DNLM; NNNAM; PPC **80-6928**

WOLFE, John Reissberg (1824-1904)
. . . On diseases and injuries of the eye, a course of systematic and clinical lectures to students and medical practitioners. . . . With ten coloured plates and 157 wood engravings. Philadelphia: P. Blakiston, 1882. 452p. 10 col. plates. DLC; NNNAM; OCIM; PPC **80-6929**

WOLFE, Mary
Prize paper on physiology and histology. Cincinnati, 1882. 32p. 1 plate. DNLM **80-6930**

WOLFF, Lawrence (1845?-1901)
Ethyl bromide. [Philadelphia]: Merrihew & Son, [1880]. 8p. DNLM **80-6931**

WOLFF, Lawrence (1845?-1901)
Soluble compressed pellets for hypodermic medication. [Philadelphia, 1880.] 3p. DNLM **80-6932**

WOLFF, Lawrence (1845?-1901)
Oleates and oleo-palmitates. Formic acid as an atiseptic. Cascara sagrada. Philadelphia: Merrihew & Lippert, 1881. 13p. DNLM **80-6933**

WOLFF, Lawrence (1845?-1901)
Chlorinated oil and the chlorine substitution in fat oils. Pepo as a taenifuge. Philadelphia: J. S. Smith, 1882. 10p. DNLM
80-6934

WOLFF, Lawrence (8145?-1901)
A review of new drugs and remedies introduced during the last ten years. Harrisburg: L. S. Hart, 1883. 36p. DNLM
80-6935

WOLFF, Lawrence (1845?-1901)
Applied medical chemistry. A manual for students and practitioners of medicine. . . . Philadelphia: P. Blakiston, Son & Co., 1885. 174p. DLC; DNLM; NNNAM; PPC
80-6936

WOLFF, Lawrence (1845?-1901)
Die Behandlung der Harnröhrenstrikturen durch Elektrolyse. [New York, 1887.] 6p. DNLM
80-6937

WOLFF, Lawrence (1845?-1901)
Questions and answers on the essentials of medical chemistry. . . . Philadelphia: W. B. Saunders, 1888. 214p. DLC; NNNAM; PPC; PU **80-6938**

WOLFF, Lawrence (1845?-1901)
The ptomaines; their forensic and pathological importance. Detroit: G. S. Davis, 1888. 19p. DNLM
80-6939

WOLFF, Lawrence (1845?-1901)
The chemistry of gastric digestion. Philadelphia: W. J. Dornan, 1889. 10p. DNLM **80-6940**

WOLFF, Lawrence (1845?-1901)
The hypodermic use of mercurials in the treatment of syphilis. Detroit, Mich.: G. S. Davis, 1889. 14p. DNLM
80-6941

WOLFF, Lawrence (1845?-1901)
Recent advances in the diagnosis and treatment of some diseases of the stomach. [Philadelphia, 1889.] 32p. DNLM
80-6942

WOMAN'S MEDICAL COLLEGE OF BALTIMORE
List of students and graduates for the years 1882-1883; 1891-1892; 1893-1894 to 1901-1902. Baltimore, 1883-1902. DNLM
80-6943

WOMAN'S work in the field of medicine. New York: College of Midwifery, [1883]. 54p. DNLM; NNNAM **80-6944**

WOOD, A. L.
The medical and surgical uses of electricity. . . . By A. L. Wood, M.D., and B. C. Woodruff. . . . Brooklyn, N.Y.: A. L. Wood, 1885. 95p. DLC **80-6945**

WOOD, E[dward] A[ddison]
Heredity and education: their relation to each other, and to the human race. Pittsburg: Herald Printing Co., 1886. 12p. DNLM **80-6946**

WOOD, Edward Stickney (1846-1905)
Arsenic as a domestic poison. Boston: Wright & Potter, 1885. 57p. 6 tabs. DNLM; MBM **80-6947**

WOOD, E[ugene] Halsey
Gangliasthenia. [Detroit, 1881.] 7p. DNLM
80-6948

WOOD, George Bacon (1797-1879)
The dispensatory of the United States of America. . . . 14th ed., carefully rev. by Dr. George B. Wood, assisted by Dr. H. C. Wood. Philadelphia: J. B. Lippincott & Co., 1882. 1879p. DLC; NNNAM; OCLloyd; PU
80-6949

WOOD, George Bacon (1797-1879)
The dispensatory of the United States of America. . . . 15th ed. Rearranged, thoroughly rev., and largely rewritten. With illustrations. By H. C. Wood . . . Joseph P. Remington . . . and Samuel P. Sadtler. . . . Philadelphia: J. B. Lippincott & Co., 1883. 1923p. DLC; DNLM; OCLloyd; PU
80-6950

WOOD, George Bacon (1797-1879)
The dispensatory of the United States of America. By George B. Wood . . . and Franklin Bache. . . . 16th ed. Rearranged, thoroughly rev., and largely rewritten. . . . By H. C. Wood . . . Joseph P. Remington . . . and Samuel P. Sadtler. . . . Philadelphia: J. B. Lippincott & Co., 1888. 2091p. DLC; DNLM; OCLloyd; PPC **80-6951**

WOOD, Horatio C. (1841-1920) and Henry F. FORMAD
Research on the effects of inoculating the lower animals with diphtheritic exudation. [Washington, 1880.] 6p. DNLM **80-6952**

WOOD, Horatio C. (1841-1920)
A treatise on therapeutics, comprising materia medica and toxicology. . . . 3rd ed., rev. and enl. Philadelphia: J. B. Lippincott & Co., 1880. 720p. DLC; DNLM; NNNAM; PU **80-6953**

WOOD, Horatio C. (1841-1920)
Brain-work and overwork. Philadelphia: P. Blakiston, 1880. 126p. DNLM; NNNAM; PPC **80-6954**

WOOD, Horatio C. (1841-1920)
Fever: a study in morbid and normal physiology. Washington, [1880]. 258p. 5 plates. DNLM; MdU-D; PPC **80-6955**

WOOD, Horatio C. (1841-1920) and Henry F. FORMAD
Report on diphtheria. [Washington, 1882.] 18p. DNLM **80-6956**

WOOD, Horatio C. (1841-1920)
A treatise on therapeutics, comprising materia medica and toxicology, with especial reference to the application of the physiological action of drugs to clinical medicine. . . . 4th ed., rev. and enl. Philadelphia: J. B. Lippincott & Co., 1882. 736p. DLC; IU-M; NNNAM; PPC **80-6957**

WOOD, Horatio C. (1841-1920)
A treatise on therapeutics, comprising materia medica and toxicology, with especial reference to the application of the physiological action of drugs to clinical medicine. . . . 5th ed., rev. and enl. Philadelphia: J. B. Lippincott & Co., 1883. 740p. DLC; DNLM; IEN-M; PU **80-6958**

WOOD, Horatio C. (1841-1920)
Hyoscine; its physiological and therapeutic action. Detroit, Mich.: G. S. Davis, 1885. 10p. DNLM **80-6959**

WOOD, Horatio C. (1841-1920)
Clinical aspects of cerebral syphilis. [Philadelphia, 1884.] 37p. DNLM **80-6960**

WOOD, Horatio C. (1841-1920) and F. X. DERCUM
Cases of spinal diseases, with autopsies. [Detroit, 1885.] 28p. DNLM **80-6961**

WOOD, Horatio C. (1841-1920)
Chorea; a study in clinical pathology. Detroit, Mich.: G. S. Davis, 1885. 10p. DNLM **80-6962**

WOOD, Horatio C. (1841-1920), E. T. REICHERT, and Hobart A. HARE
A contribution to our knowledge of fever and of the agents which produce or arrest it. Detroit: G. S. Davis, 1886. 40p. DNLM **80-6963**

WOOD, Horatio C. (1841-1920)
The hygiene of old age. Detroit, Mich.: G. S. Davis, 1886. 8p. DNLM **80-6964**

WOOD, Horatio C. (1841-1920)
A treatise on therapeutics, comprising materia medica and toxicology, with especial reference to the application of the physiological action of drugs to clinical medicine. . . . 6th ed., rev. and enl. Philadelphia, [etc.]: J. B. Lippincott & Co., 1886. 779p. DLC; DNLM; ICRM; PPC **80-6965**

WOOD, Horatio C. (1841-1920)
Remarks upon chronic contracted kidney with normal urine; acute gouty dementia with a perforating recto-vaginal ulcer, and death from sudden pulmonic oedema. [Philadelphia, 1886.] 12p. DNLM **80-6966**

WOOD, Horatio C. (1841-1920)
Nervous diseases and their diagnosis: a treatise upon the phenomena produced by diseases of the nervous system, with especial reference to the recognition of their causes. Philadelphia: J. B. Lippincott & Co., 1887. 501p. DLC; DNLM; MBM; NNNAM **80-6967**

WOOD, Horatio C. (1841-1920)
The treatment of phthisis by sulphuretted hydrogen. Detroit: G. S. Davis, 1887. 13p. DNLM **80-6968**

WOOD, Horatio C. (1841-1920)
Therapeutics: its principles and practice. . . . The 7th ed. of a treatise on therapeutics, rearranged, rewritten, and enl. Philadelphia, [etc.]: J. B. Lippincott & Co., 1888. 908p. DLC; NNNAM; PPC; PPJ **80-6969**

WOOD, Horatio C. (1841-1920)
Insanity in its relation to law. An address delivered before the Medical Society of the State of Pennsylvania, June, 1888. . . . Philadelphia: W. J. Dornan, printer, 1888. 11p. DLC **80-6970**

WOOD, Horatio C. (1841-1920)
The medical profession; the medical sects; the law. The address in medicine, Yale University, 1889. [New Haven, 1889.] 19p. CtY-M; DNLM **80-6971**

WOOD, Horatio C. (1841-1920)
Syphilis of the nervous system. . . . Detroit, Mich.: G. S. Davis, 1889. 135p. DLC; DNLM; OCIM; PU **80-6972**

WOOD, Luther Hodges
Phthisis pulmonalis. How affected by the climate of Colorado, and what are the proper cases to be sent here. [Denver, 1884.] 19p. DNLM **80-6973**

WOOD MUSEUM OF BELLEVUE HOSPITAL, NEW YORK CITY
Catalogue, comprising a description and classified list of anatomical and pathological specimens. New York: Department Press, 1880. 256p. DNLM; NNNAM; NNU-M **80-6974**

WOOD, Robert W.
Memorial of Edward Jarvis. Boston: T. R. Marvin & Son, 1885. 24p. DNLM; MBM **80-6975**

WOOD, William B.
Report of a case of tubercular phthisis treated with the pneumatic cabinet. New York, 1887. 6p. DNLM **80-6976**

WOOD, WILLIAM, & CO. NEW YORK
Route of the steamer Grand Republic on the excursion given by Messrs. William Wood & Co., New York, in honor of the American Medical Association June 4th, 1880. 22p. NNNAM
80-6977

WOOD, WILLIAM, & CO. NEW YORK
Prospectus of Wood's Library of standard medical authors for 1880. [New York, 1880.] 16p. DNLM; NNNAM
80-6978

WOOD, WILLIAM, & CO. NEW YORK
Pictures for physicians' offices and libraries. New York, [1880?] 8 l. DNLM **80-6979**

WOOD, WILLIAM, & CO. NEW YORK
Medical publications. New York, [1881?] 40p. DNLM; NNNAM **80-6980**

WOOD, WILLIAM, & CO. NEW YORK
A catalogue of the medical publications. . . . New York, [1882]. 61p. DNLM; NNNAM **80-6981**

WOOD, WILLIAM, & CO. NEW YORK
Medical publications. New York, [1884?] 47p. DNLM; NNNAM **80-6982**

WOOD, WILLIAM, & CO. NEW YORK
Index to Wood's library of standard medical authors for the years 1879, 1880, 1881, 1882, 1883, 1884. New York: William Wood & Co., 1885. [unp.] DNLM; MB; PPC; PU
80-6983

WOOD, WILLIAM, & CO. NEW YORK
Index to Wood's libary of standard medical authors, complete in one hundred volumes. New York: William Wood & Co., 1887. 568p. NNNAM; PPC **80-6984**

WOOD's household practice of medicine, hygiene, and surgery. A practical treatise for the use of families, travelers, seamen, miners, and others. Edited by Frederick A. Castle. New York: William Wood & Co., 1880. 2 v. CtY-M; DNLM; MBM; NNNAM **80-6985**

WOOD's medical and surgical monographs, consisting of original treatises and of complete reproductions in English of books and monographs selected from the latest literature of foreign countries, with all illustrations, etc. New York: William Wood & Co., 1889-1892. 12 v. DNLM; NNNAM; PPC
80-6986

WOODBRIDGE, John Eliot (1846?-1901)
The duty of the Ohio Medical Society to consumptives. Cleveland: Williams Pub. Co., 1889. 9p. DNLM; OCIM
80-6987

WOODBRIDGE, L[uther] D[ana] (1850-1899)
Abortive treatment of typhoid fever. Chicago, 1888. 36p. DNLM **80-6988**

WOODBURY, Frank (1848-1927)
Remarks upon clinical phases of poisoning by alcohol. [Philadelphia, 1881.] 6p. DNLM **80-6989**

WOODBURY, Frank (1848-1927)
Guide to therapeutics and materia medica. Philadelphia: Henry C. Lea's Son, 1882. 526p. NNNAM; OCLloyd; PPC; PU
80-6990

WOODBURY, Frank (1848-1927)
On disordered digestion and dyspepsia. Detroit, Mich.: G. S. Davis, 1889. 82p. DNLM; OCIM **80-6991**

WOODFORD, H. T.
Venerology. The causes, treatment, and cure of venereal diseases. . . . Chicago: Hoke & Bros., 1886. 111p. DLC
80-6992

WOODHEAD, G[erman] Sims (1855-1921)
Practical pathology. Philadelphia: Henry C. Lea's Son, 1884. 484p. 136 color plates. NNNAM; PPC; PU
80-6993

WOODHULL, Alfred A[lexander] (1837-1921)
Provisional manual for exercise of company bearers and hospital corps. Fort Leavenworth, 1889. 34p. DNLM
80-6994

WOODRUFF, Elmer
The female medical counselor, being a domestic treatment on the diseases of females and children. . . . San Francisco: Printed for the Author, 1885. 383p. DLC **80-6995**

WOODWARD, A[lfred] W. (1839-1902)
A new similia. First principles of homoeopathic therapeutics. Chicago: Duncan Bros., 1881. 39p. DNLM; IU-M
80-6996

WOODWARD, Joseph J[anvier] (1833-1884)
Pathological histology of yellow fever. April 6, 1880. [Washington, 1880.] 8p. DNLM **80-6997**

WOODWARD, Joseph J[anvier] (1833-1884)
Report to the Secretary of War on the case of Capt. Jonathan G. Bigelow. Washington: J. L. Pearson, 1880. 4p. DNLM
80-6998

WOODWARD, Joseph J[anvier] (1833-1884)
Modern philosophical conceptions of life; an address delivered before the Philosophical Society of Washington, December 3, 1881. Washington: Judd & Detweiler, 1881. 38p. DNLM
80-6999

WOODWARD, Joseph J[anvier] (1833-1844)
Pseudo-polypi of the colon; an anomalous result of follicular ulceration. [Philadelphia, 1881.] 14p. DNLM
80-7000

WOODWARD, Joseph J[anvier] (1833-1884)
Photographs. Camp fever and camp dysentery. Washington, [1882?] 28 phot. DNLM **80-7001**

WOODY, Samuel E. (*b.* 1854)
The essentials of medical chemistry and urinalysis. 2nd ed. Louisville: J. P. Morton, 1888. 140p. DNLM; KyLoJM; OC; OCIM **80-7002**

WOOLLEY, B[asil] M.
The opium and whisky habits and their cure. Atlanta, [1888]. 32p. DNLM **80-7003**

WOOLSEY, Abbey H[owland] (1828-1893)
Handbook for hospitals. New York & London: G. P. Putnam's Sons, 1883. 263p. DLC; NN; NNNAM; PU
80-7004

WORCESTER, A[lfred] (1855-1951)
A new way of training nurses. Boston: Cupples & Hurd, 1888. 118p. DNLM; MBM **80-7005**

WORCESTER, Samuel (1847-1918)
Repertory to the modalities, in their relations to temperature, air, water, winds, weather, and seasons. Based mainly upon Hering's condensed materia medica, with additions from Allen, Lippe, and Hale. New York: Boericke & Tafel, 1880. 160p. DLC; DNLM; NNNAM; PPHa **80-7006**

WORCESTER, Samuel (1847-1918)
Insanity and its treatment. Lectures on the treatment of insanity and kindred nervous diseases. New York & Philadelphia: Boericke & Tafel, 1882. 262p. DLC; DNLM; NNNAM; PPHa **80-7007**

WORCESTER, William L. (1845-1901)
Clinical case. Cases illustrative of the localization of cerebral functions. [Utica, N.Y., 1887.] 8p. DNLM **80-7008**

WORCESTER, William L. (1845-1901)
Delirium. [Utica, N.Y., 1889.] 6p. DNLM **80-7009**

WORMLEY, Theodore G[eorge] (1826-1897)
Quantitative determination of urea by alkaline hypochlorites and hypobromites. [Philadelphia, 1881.] 3p. DNLM **80-7010**

WORMLEY, Theodore G[eorge] (1826-1897)
Is gelsemic acid identical with aesculin? With observations on the preparation, properties and recovery, when absorbed, of the important constituents of Gelsemium sempervirens, and gelsemium poisoning. Philadelphia: J. S. Smith, 1882. 8p. DNLM **80-7011**

WORMLEY, Theodore G[eorge] (1826-1897)
Micro-chemistry of poisons, including their physiological, pathological, and legal relations. With an appendix on the detection and microscopic discrimination of blood. 2nd ed. Philadelphia: J. B. Lippincott Co., 1885. 741p. 17 plates, 1 chart. DNLM; NNNAM; PPC; PU **80-7012**

WRIGHT, Jonathan (1860-1928)
Nasal bacteria in health. [New York, 1889.] 21p. DNLM **80-7013**

WRIGHT, Jonathan (1860-1928)
Two cases of laryngeal paralysis, with a consideration of the points involved. [New York, 1889.] 20p. DNLM **80-7014**

WRIGHT, J. Williston
Lectures on diseases of the rectum. Delivered at the Medical Department of the Univesity of the City of New York. . . . New York, [etc.]: Bermingham & Co., 1884. 170p. DLC; NNNAM **80-7015**

WRIGHT, Thomas Lee (1825-1893)
Observations on the origin, character, and treatment of cinomania. [St. Louis, 1881.] 18p. DNLM **80-7016**

WRIGHT, Thomas Lee (1825-1893)
Inebriety; a study upon alcohol in its relations to mind and conduct. [St. Louis: Carreras, 1882.] 23p. DNLM **80-7017**

WRIGHT, Thomas Lee (1825-1893)
Inebriism, a pathological and psychological study. Columbus, O.: W. G. Hubbard, 1885. 222p. DNLM; OCIM **80-7018**

WRIGHT, Thomas R.
Three cases of compound comminuted fracture of the leg; recovery without suppuration. Augusta: J. Loveday, 1881. 11p. DNLM; GU **80-7019**

WYETH, John Allan (1845-1922)
A text-book on surgery, general, operative, and mechanical. . . . New York: D. Appleton & Co., 1887. 777p. DLC; DNLM; NNNAM; PU **80-7020**

WYETH, John Allan (1845-1922)
Laparotomy and intestinal suture. Exsection of a portion of the ileum, with restoration of function of the alimentary canal by suture. A novel operation for the cure of urethro-rectal fistula. New York: Trow's Co., [1887]. 21p. DNLM; NNNAM **80-7021**

WYETH, JOHN, & BRO.
The two new cholagogues. Euonymus atropurpureus (wahoo) and Iris versicolor (blue flag). [Philadelphia, 1880?] 9p. DNLM **80-7022**

WYETH, JOHN, & BRO.
Purity, activity, and beauty. Elegant pharmaceutical preparations, compressed powders or pills, and medicinal fluid extracts. With formulary dose list, and quantitative composition. Philadelphia: G. F. Lasher, 1882. 47 l. DNLM **80-7023**

WYETH, JOHN, & BRO.
Catalogue of fluid extracts, standard formulae. . . . Philadelphia, 1883. 176p. PPC **80-7024**

WYETH, JOHN, & BRO.
The model vaccine propagating establishment of the United States. Bovine virus; its production and preservation; comparative value of bovine and humanized lymph. Philadelphia, 1885. 8p. DNLM **80-7025**

WYETH, JOHN, & BRO.
Price list of suppositories. . . . Philadelphia, 1886. 20p. DNC; PU **80-7026**

WYLIE, W[alker] Gill (1848-1923)
Observations on laceration of the cervix uteri; its etiology, pathology, prevention, and treatment. New York: William Wood & Co., 1882. 29p. DNLM **80-7027**

WYLIE, W[alker] Gill (1848-1923)
Anteflexion of the uterus: its etiology and associated pathological conditions. New York: William Wood & Co., 1884. 47p. DNLM **80-7028**

WYLIE, W[alker] Gill (1848-1923)
Memorial sketch of the life of J. Marion Sims. New York: D. Appleton & Co., 1884. 26p. DNLM **80-7029**

WYLIE, W[alker] Gill (1848-1923)
Disease of the Fallopian tubes, and histories of fourteen cases operated upon and reports on specimens. New York: Trow's Co., 1885. 43p. DNLM **80-7030**

WYLIE, W[alker] Gill (1848-1923)
The local use of antiseptics in gynaecology. [New York, 1885.] 9p. DNLM **80-7031**

WYLIE, W[alker] Gill (1848-1923)
Report of one hundred and twenty-five laparotomies, with observations on the use of hot water within the peritoneal cavity during and after laparotomy to prevent shock. New York, 1887. 8p. 2 charts. DNLM **80-7032**

WYLIE, W[alker] Gill (1848-1923)
One hundred and ten laparotomies for the removal of the uterine appendages. Sixty-one consecutive operations without a death. [Boston, 1888.] 5 l. 8 plates. DNLM **80-7033**

WYLIE, W[alker] Gill (1848-1923)
A year's work in abdominal surgery, with a report of 80 laparotomies done in 1887. [New York, 1888.] 8p. 1 tab. DNLM **80-7034**

WYMAN, Hal C. (1852-1908)
(A) A useful catheter for the operation for vesico-vaginal fistula. (B) The management of Potts' disease of the spine in young children. [Detroit, 1883.] 16p. DNLM **80-7035**

WYMAN, Hal C. (1852-1908)
Abdominal surgery. . . . Detroit, Mich.: G. S. Davis, 1888. 87p. DLC **80-7036**

WYMAN, Hal C. (1852-1908)
The training of nurses. Address. Philadelphia: Records, McMullin & Co., 1888 [1889]. 15p. DNLM **80-7037**

WYMAN, Hal C. (1852-1908)
Diastasic food in the treatment of chronic diseases and deformities of the bones of children. [Cincinnati, 1889.] 6p. DNLM **80-7038**

WYMAN, Hal C. (1852-1908)
The constitutional treatment of caries and necrosis. [New York, 1889.] 7p. DNLM **80-7039**

WYMAN, Walter (1848-1911)
Quarantine. Baltimore: J. Young, 1884. 17p. DNLM **80-7040**

WYMAN, Walter (1848-1911)
Treatment of cholera by Parisian physicians. [St. Louis: J. H. Chambers & Co., 1885.] 8p. DNLM **80-7041**

WYTHE, Joseph Henry (1822-1901)
The microscopist: a manual of microscopy and compendium of the microscopic sciences. . . . 4th ed.; greatly enl. . . . Philadelphia: Lindsay & Blakiston, 1880. 434p. col. plates. DLC; NNNAM; PPC; PU **80-7042**

WYTHE, Joseph Henry (1822-1901)
The physician's dose and symptom book, containing the doses and uses of all the principal articles of the materia medica and officinal preparations; also table of weights and measures, rules to proportion the doses of medicine, common abbreviations used in writing prescriptions, [etc.]. 17th ed. Philadelphia: P. Blakiston, Son & Co., 1887. 226p. DLC; DNLM; PPC; PU **80-7043**

YALE, Leroy Milton (1841-1906)
Remarks on excision of the hip. [New York, 1885.] 15p. DNLM **80-7044**

YANDELL, David W[endell] (1826-1898)
A discourse on the life and character of Richard Oswald Cowling. A valedictory address. Louisville: J. P. Morton & Co., 1882. 26p. DNLM **80-7045**

YANDELL, David W[endell] (1826-1898)
Supplement. A reply [to circular issued by the Louisville Medical College of this city]. [Louisville, 1884.] 19p. DNLM **80-7046**

YANDELL, David W[endell] (1826-1898)
The doctorate address delivered at the semi-centennial anniversary of the University of Louisville, medical department. [Reminiscences of the teachers of medicine in the University of Louisville.] March 2, 1887. Louisville: J. P. Morton & Co., 1887. 26p. DNLM **80-7047**

YARNALL, E. A., & CO.
Illustrated catalogue of surgical and orthopaedical appliances, acoustic apparatus. Philadelphia, 1889. 306p. DNLM; PPC **80-7048**

YARNALL, E. A., & CO.
Surgical instruments, orthopedical appliances, etc. Acoustic apparatus, and instruments to assist in hearing. [Philadelphia, 1889.] 8p. DNLM; PPC **80-7049**

YARROW, Henry C[récy] (1840-1929)
A tampon carrier and new vaginal speculum. [New York, 1883.] 3p. DNLM **80-7050**

YARROW, Henry C[récy] (1840-1929)
Chart of skin diseases as taught in the National Medical College, Columbian Univesity. [Washington, 1884.] 2 l. DNLM **80-7051**

[YELLOW FEVER]
Outbreak of yellow fever at Biloxi, Harrison County, Miss., and its relation to inter-State notification. New Orleans, 1886. 51p. DNLM **80-7052**

YEO, Gerald Francis (1845-1909)
Manual of physiology. A text-book for students of medicine. . . . Philadelphia: P. Blakiston, Son & Co., 1884. 749p. DLC; DNLM; OCLloyd; PU **80-7053**

YEO, Gerald Francis (1845-1909)
Manual of physiology. A textbook for students of medicine. 2nd American ed. Philadelphia: P. Blakiston, Son & Co., 1886. 743p. DLC; DNLM; NNNAM; PPC **80-7054**

YEO, Gerald Francis (1845-1909)
Manual of physiology. A textbook for students of medicine. 3rd English ed. Philadelphia: P. Blakiston, Son & Co., 1888. 758p. CtY-M; DNLM; PPC; PU **80-7055**

YEO, I[saac] Burney (1835-1914)
Food in health and disease. . . . Philadelphia: Lea Bros. & Co., [1889]. 583p. PPC **80-7056**

YOUNG, Edward J[ames] (1829-1906)
Subjects for master's degree in Harvard College [including questions relating to medicine]. 1655-1791. Boston: J. Wilson & Son, 1880. 38p. DNLM; MH **80-7057**

YOUNG, James Kelly (1862-1923)
. . . Synopsis of human anatomy, being a compend of anatomy, including the anatomy of the viscera and numerous tables. . . . Philadelphia and London: F. A. Davis, 1889. 393p. fold. table. DLC; DNLM; NNNAM; PPC **80-7058**

YOUNGE, J[ohn] W. (1841-1899)
Malaria and its effects. Fort Wayne, Ind.: Page, Taylor & Co., 1880. 22p. DNLM **80-7059**

YOUNGER, William J.
Implantation of teeth and cemental life. Individual report of the committee on pathology and surgery, read before the California State Dental Association, July 21, 1886. San Francisco: W. S. Duncombe & Co., 1886. 14p. DNLM **80-7060**

YOUNGER, William J.
Transplantation of teeth into artificial sockets. San Francisco, 1886. 20p. DNLM **80-7061**

YOUNGMAN, Maurice D.
Atlantic City, N.J., as a resort for invalids; comprising statistics, meteorological tables, etc., concerning the climate of Atlantic City, N.J., its sanitary regulations, and observations on its value as a resort in various diseased conditions. Atlantic City: W. W. Holdzkom, 1884. 16p. DNLM **80-7062**

YOUNGMAN, Maurice D.
Atlantic City as a resort for invalids. . . . Philadelphia: E. Patteson Press, 1889. 22p. DNLM **80-7063**

ZARTMAN, Joseph H., ***et al.***
Alumni record of Syracuse University, 1872-1886, including Genesee College, 1852-1871 and Geneva Medical College, 1835-1872. Syracuse: Master & Sons, 1887. 368p. N; NN **80-7064**

ZIEGLER, Ernst (1849-1905)
A text-book of pathological anatomy and pathogenesis. Transl. and edited for English students by Donald MacAlister. New York: William Wood & Co., 1883-1887. 2 pts. in 3 v. DNLM; NNNAM; PPC; PU **80-7065**

ZIEGLER, George Jacob (1821-1895)
The basic pathology and specific treatment of diphtheria, typhoid, zymotic, septic, scorbutic, and putrescent diseases generally. . . . Philadelphia: G. J. Ziegler, 1884. 225p. CtY-M; DLC; PPC; PU **80-7066**

ZIEMSSEN, Hugo Wilhelm von, ed. (1829-1902)
Handbook of diseases of the skin. . . . New York: William Wood & Co., 1885. 653p. col. illus., map. DLC; NNNAM; PPC; PU **80-7067**

ZIEMSSEN, Hugo Wilhelm von (1829-1902)
Pulmonary tuberculosis. Its etiology, symptomatology and therapeutics. . . . Transl. by David J. Doherty. . . . Detroit, Mich.: G. S. Davis, 1888. 118p. DLC; IU-M; OCIM; PPC **80-7068**

ZEISSL Hermann von (1817-1884)
Outlines of the pathology and treatment of syphilis and allied venereal diseases. . . . 2nd ed., rev. by Maximilian von Zeissl. . . . Authorized ed. transl. with notes, by H. Raphael. . . . New York: D. Appleton & Co., 1886. 402p. DLC; NNNAM; PPJ; PU **80-7069**

ZINKE, [Ernst] Gustav (*b.* 1846)
Emmet's operation. When shall it, and when shall it not, be performed? [Chicago, 1885.] 16p. 1 chart. DNLM **80-7070**

FRANCESCO CORDASCO

AMERICAN MEDICAL IMPRINTS, 1820-1910

A CHECKLIST OF PUBLICATIONS ILLUSTRATING THE HISTORY
AND PROGRESS OF MEDICAL SCIENCE,
MEDICAL EDUCATION, AND THE HEALING ARTS
IN THE UNITED STATES
A PRELIMINARY CONTRIBUTION

Foreword
by
James Tait Goodrich, M.D., Ph.D.

Volume II

1985

ROWMAN & LITTLEFIELD, PUBLISHERS
TOTOWA, NEW JERSEY

JUNIUS-VAUGHN PRESS, INC.
FAIRVIEW, N.J. & LONDON

Library of Congress Cataloging in Publication Data

Cordasco, Francesco, 1920-
American medical imprints, 1820-1910.

Bibliography: p.
Includes index.
1. Medicine—United States—Bibliography. 2. Medicine —Bibliography. 3. Medicine—United States—History—19th century—Sources—Bibliography. 4. United States—Imprints. I. Title. [DNLM: 1. Bibliography of Medicine—United States. ZWB 100 C794a 1820-1910]
Z6661.U5C67 1984 [R152] 016.61'0973 84-11829
ISBN 0-8476-7338-3 Set
ISBN 0-8476-7422-3 Vol. I
ISBN 0-8476-7423-1 Vol. II

First published in the United States 1985 by:

Rowman & Littlefield, Publishers
81 Adams Drive
Totowa, New Jersey 07512 USA
****
[Junius Vaughn Press, Inc.]
PO Box 85, Fairview, New Jersey 07022 USA
St. John's Road, London SW11 U.K.

Printed & bound in the United States of America

FOR MY WIFE
EDNA MAE VAUGHN CORDASCO
AND
IN MEMORY OF MY MOTHER
CARMELA MADORMA CORDASCO (1883–1962)

The theme which I have selected for my discourse is, "The Progress of American Medical Literature during the last Century;" a theme which, while it may, I think, incite your ambition, will afford us an opportunity of discharging a debt of gratitude to our predecessors and contemporaries; men who have advanced the interests of the profession and surrounded it with a halo of glory. I have undertaken this task, difficult as it is, the more willingly because my entrance into the profession fifty years ago was coeval with the birth of our medical literature. . . . We have medical literature, based upon a broad and solid foundation; a literature full of vigor and inspiration, honorable alike to the profession and to the nation. I have portrayed to you, perhaps too feebly, one of the noble legacies bequeathed to us by our forefathers. Let us, their heirs, cherish their memories, and strive to render ourselves worthy of our inheritance.

Samuel D. Gross,
History of American
Medical Literature
(1876)

FOREWORD

BY JAMES TAIT GOODRICH, M.D., Ph.D.

I

Bibliography is a noble and ancient art and only with its evolution has come systematic access to the literature: with its development the interested writer is able now to trace a theme, subject, or author. Anyone who has ever attempted even so simple a task as a bibliography for publication will appreciate the work, endurance and scholarship that go into a study such as this. Many a student, bibliophile, antiquarian, and librarian will thank Dr. Francesco Cordasco for providing this bibliography of American medical imprints. "Learning, as with water, is never more fair, pure and simple than at its source." (Naude)

Bibliography has an ancestral and honorable design. The subject of bibliography dates at least to the great library of Alexandria when listings were provided with references to authors and subjects. The great Pergamite, Galen (130-200 A.D.) compiled two classified bibliographies of his own writings, this in the 2nd century A.D. (*De libris propriis and De oridine librorum suorum ad Eugenianum*). In these works, Galen classified his writings into seventeen various categories. Fulton called this the ". . . first attempt at classified bibliography by a medical writer."[1] In recent history, the first systematization of the literature of medicine and science was the *Bibliotheca universalis* . . . (1545) by Conrad Gesner (1516-1565).[2] Gesner, while only in his twenties, compiled a "universal dictionary" which listed the writings of all authors, famous, obscure, ancient, and modern, each entry with a brief resume and all this done in three languages, Latin, Greek, and Hebrew. This work laid the foundation of modern medical bibliography and was listed as the first work of medical bibliography in Garrison-Morton.[3] The irony was that while twenty-one books were to be published, in actual

[1] Fulton, J. F. *The Great Medical Bibliographers*. Philadelphia: The University of Pennsylvania Press, 1951, p. 1.

[2] Gesner, Conrad. *Bibliotheca universalis . . . in tribus linguis. Tiguri*, apud C. Froschouerum, 1545-1555.

[3] Morton, T. *A Medical Bibliography* (Garrison-Morton) . . . Edinburgh: Deutsch 1970. See G. M. citation 6743.

fact only twenty were. The twenty-first book on medicine was never completed. This left the first systematic medical bibliography to Pascal Lecoq[4] (1567-1632) who published his *Bibliotheca medica* . . . in 1590, a listing of 1224 authors. Further significant works in medical bibliography were issued by Linden[5] (1609-1664) *De Scriptus medicis* . . . (1637) and by Lipen[6] (1630-1692) *Bibliotheca realis medica* . . . (1679). This last work contained an elaborate subject analysis, numerous cross references, author and subject indices. With the 18th century came the great father of medical bibliography, Albrecht von Haller (1708-1777), an extraordinary man, physician, scientist and man of letters who continued Gesner's great effort. Haller's intellectual powers and feats of memory are legend. Fulton[7] notes that at the age of four, Haller could repeat the Scriptures at great length to the family servants. At age eight, he succeeded in writing two thousand brief biographies of great historical figures. At age ten, he completed a Greek lexicon with supplements in Hebrew and Chaldee—certainly an awesome mind by any standard. Haller went on to complete four great bibliographies on botany, anatomy, surgery, and medicine. With a classified analysis of over 52,000 publications of all countries, this compendium formed the most complete reference work of its time. The bibliographies are still in use today.

The practice of medical bibliography continued, even though it could be ". . . dry, dusty, tedious, accursed, hateful"[8] as described by James Atkinson (1759-1839). Works by James Douglas (1675-1742), *Bibliographiae anatomicae* . . . (Londini: G. Sayes, 1715); Herman Boerhaave (1668-1738) *Methodus discendi medicinam* (London, 1726); J. F. Blumenbach (1752-1840) *Medicinische Bibliothek* (Göttingen, J. C. Dieterich, 1783-1788) were with others to round out the 18th century. The 19th century was to see a virtual explosion of works in medical bibliography by Hain, Choulant, Forbes, The Royal Society of London, Gross, and finally the spectacular work of Billings.

John Shaw Billings (1839-1913) provided a work unique in the history of medical bibliography, a work that William Henry Welch (1850-1934) proclaimed one of the four greatest contributions that the United States has made to medicine. The *Index-Catalogue,*[9] for the first time in a medical bibliography, provided author and subject indices in one alphabet. Titles of books and periodicals were included. William Osler (1849-1919) commented

[4] Lecoq, Pascal. *Bibliotheca medica. Sive catalogus illorum, qui ex professo artem medicam in hunc usque annum scriptis illustrarunt.* Basileae: C. Waldkirch, 1590.

[5] Linden, J. A. *De scriptis medicis, libri duo.* Amstelredami: J. Blaeu, 1637.

[6] Lipen, M. *Bibliotheca realis medica, omnium materiarum, rerum, et titulorum, in universa medicina occurrentium.* Francofurti ad Moenum, J. Friderici, 1679.

[7] Fulton, J. F. *The Great Medical Bibliographers.* Philadelphia: The University of Pennsylvania Press, 1951. p. 39.

[8] *Ibid.*, p. 52.

[9] Billings, J. S. *Index-Catalogue of the Library of the Surgeon-General's Office.* Washington: GPO, 1880-1961.

on this work: "No undertaking in bibliography of the same magnitude dealing with a special subject had ever been issued, and its extraordinary value was at once appreciated all over the world."[10] While this work was intended as a catalogue of the Surgeon-General's Library (SGL) holdings, in actual fact, because of Billings determined efforts to compile a "complete" medical library, it became a comprehensive index to the world literature as it existed then. The first series of sixteen volumes was completed in 1895. By the time of completion of the fourth series, some three million books, journal articles, and pamphlets had been catalogued.

Billings built this collection and bibliography from almost nothing. In 1860 the Surgeon-General's Library, the precursor to the present National Library of Medicine, had a total of 304 volumes in its collection. When Billings took charge in 1865, the collection had expanded to a grand sum of 2,253 books, journals, and pamphlets.[11] Billings determined that this country needed a medical library, central in location, to house the medical works of the world. We had no Bibliothèque Nationale, British Museum, or the like to turn to for medical information. In 1872 Billings issued a short-title catalogue of the holdings and, by this point, the SGL collection had grown to 13,300 volumes; by 1878 the card catalogue held over 400,000 subject cards. Billings, long a historian, realized the value of bibliography and approached Congress on the funding of a catalogue listing of the SGL collection. He was successful in obtaining support; and in 1880 the first volume of the *Index-Catalogue of the Library of the Surgeon-General* was published with over 50,000 volumes and 60,000 pamphlets listed. To put the size of the SGL collection in perspective, consider that the oldest library in the country, Pennsylvania Hospital, listed 1200 volumes in 1876.[12] The College of Physicians of Philadelphia listed 19,000 volumes; Harvard University had 7000 volumes. The Manchester Medical Library in England listed 130,000 volumes. Personal collections of physicians in the United States had varying numbers, *e.g.*, Samuel D. Gross (1805-1884)–4500; Robley Dunglison (1799-1869)–5000; David Hosack (1769-1835)–2500; Samuel Smith Purple (1822-1900)–6000. The enormity and rapidity at which the SGL collection evolved was such that by 1895, when Billings retired from the SGL, sixteen volumes of his first series of the *Index-Catalogue* had been published. The SGL collection now totaled some 116,847 books and 191,598 pamphlets. Today, the National Library of Medicine stands as the largest repository of biomedical literature in the world, attesting to this man's genius and foresight for gathering together these written dictates of medicine, both old and new. William Henry Welch

[10] Fulton, J. F. *The Great Medical Bibliographers*. Philadelphia: The University of Pennsylvania Press, 1951, p. 74.

[11] National Library of Medicine. *John Shaw Billings Centennial*. 1965. See page 2.

[12] Gross, S. D. *History of American Medical Literature, from 1776 to the Present Time*. Philadelphia: Collins, 1876. See p. 74.

considered the *Index-Catalogue* to be the "most important American contribution to medical science in the 19th century."[13]

II

A review of Professor Cordasco's bibliography shows that mediocrity was not necessarily a result of 19th century medical education. Imperfect as the system may have been, physicians of distinction were produced, eminent in the art of practicing medicine. Personalities are, by and large, self-made; the ability to persevere is a major key to success. It is a person's intrinsic drive and intellectual delights that subserve genius. An education, no matter what the design, cannot create talent nor compel taste: "You may, indeed, give it opportunity, but you cannot force it."[14]

A look at the early American medical literature, as cited in Guerra[15] and Austin[16] shows the earliest literature dealt with the local medical experience of our founders and contained mostly medical observations. Medicine, as practiced in this early period, was mostly an ancillary preoccupation, usually involving the clergy. Clergy received some medical education as part of their training; hence, it was they who provided the earliest medical writings. An example of a clergy-physician was Thomas Thacher (1620-1678) who provided the first known medical publication in a broadside: *A Brief Rule to Guide the Common People of New England on How to Order Themselves and Theirs in the Small-pox and Measles* (Boston: J. Foster, 1678).

With the rise of the first two medical schools in Philadelphia and New York City in the late 18th century, the rate at which medical literature appeared accelerated. Two influential papers by Samuel Bard[17] (1742-1821) and John Morgan[18] (1735-1789) signify the early influence American medicine was to have. Both the high standard of conduct, as outlined by Bard, and the course of education with topics in anatomy, materia medica, chemistry, and botany, as outlined by Morgan were discussed in these germinal works.

In the post-Revolutionary War era, a new development took place: the introduction of the American medical journal, long a familiar item in England and the Continent, but conspicuously lacking here. With this new medium the practitioner could now publish his observations for wide public distribution. Prior to this period the medical writer could only disseminate

---

[13] *John Shaw Billings Centennial*, p. v.

[14] Bigelow, H. J. *Medical Education in American* ... Cambridge: Welch, Bigelow, and Company, 1871. p. 14.

[15] Guerra, F. *American Medical Bibliography 1639-1783.* New York: Lathrop and Harper, 1962.

[16] Austin, R. *Early American Medical Imprints 1668-1820.* Washington: GPO, 1961.

[17] Bard, S. *A Discourse upon the Duties of a Physician.* New York: A. and J. Robertson, 1769.

[18] Morgan, J. *A Discourse upon the Institution of Medical Schools in America* ... Philadelphia: William Bradford, 1765.

his works by bearing the expense of publishing his own pamphlet or broadside. It is interesting to note that before 1800, only one journal was in print, but by 1850 there were over 117 journals. This number does not even begin to account for those that opened and failed.[19]

In discussing 19th century American medicine, many authors have shown this era as being essentially devoid of extensive research efforts, either applied or pure. This comparison is inevitable when one looks at the work of the British and the Continentals. While this may be true in pure numbers of original efforts, one only has to consult Professor Cordasco on American papers and realize that in actual fact there was a tremendous effort being undertaken, albeit by a few. While American physicians were "practical" in their outlook, this by the very design of the land and their pioneering heritage, they produced several significant and important original contributions, *e.g.*, works by Oliver Wendell Holmes (1809-1894) on puerperal fever,[20] Austin Flint (1812-1886) on cardiac disease,[21] William Beaumont (1785-1853) on physiology of digestion,[22], S. Weir Mitchell (1829-1914) on diseases of the nervous system, Samuel D. Gross (1805-1884) on surgery,[23] and John Shaw Billings in bibliography. Examination of Cordasco entries reflects a developmental theme: American physicians were making their major contributions in the field of differential diagnosis and clinical observation. Without the extensive didactic education of the Europeans, the Americans made their studies by doing what they could do best—observation of the patient. Journals of this era are replete with reports of diseases presented in the descriptive sense. From this, one sees that the American physician reflected upon his profession as an "art" versus a "science." This development was all a result of the style of education the American physician was exposed to here versus his European counterpart.

What was this "style" of education for the 19th century physician? Prior to 1800 American physicians were heavily dependent on European and English authors for their texts. After 1800 this was to change with the dominance of the early New York and Philadelphia schools. It was these sources along with a growing number of medical periodicals that were to influence 19th century American medical men. In the first half of the 19th century, Americans were under the influence of the French, German, and English schools. German medical sciences emerged from an *a priori* 18th century speculative science to 19th century Baconian reasoning. The Germans substituted rigorous deduction from ascertained

[19]Shaftel, N. "The Evolution of American Medical Literature." In *History of American Medicine. A Symposium.* Edited by Felix Marti-Ibañez. New York: MD Publication, 1959, pp. 95-118. See p. 103.

[20]Holmes, O. W. "The Contagiousness of Puerperal Fever." *New England Quarterly Journal of Medical Surgery,* 1842-43. 1:503-30.

[21]Flint, A. "On Cardiac Murmurs." *American Journal of Medical Science,* 1862, n.s. 44:29-54.

[22]Beaumont, W. *Experiments and Observations on the Gastric Juice, and the Physiology of Digestion.* Plattsburgh: F. P. Allen, 1833.

[23]Gross, S. D. *A System of Surgery.* Philadelphia: Blanchard & Lea, 1859.

facts for vain discussion and ignored in turn the earlier flatulent pedantry enunciated from the magisterial chairs.[24] With exact observation the German schools laid a foundation for a new style of science. Their neighbors, the French were, at the same time, providing the most prominent educational schools of the period for Americans. With personalities like Laennec (1781-1826), Magendie (1783-1855), Bouillard (1796-1881), Corvisart (1755-1821) and others, the physical diagnostic art was introduced on a firm ground. Across the channel in England great strides were being made by the works and investigations of Bright (1789-1858), Addison (1793-1860), Hodgkin (1798-1866), Watson (1792-1882) and others. Americans, at this time, were more involved with internal and external strife and with shifting transportation routes. As a result of this American medical schools developed along their separate themes.

How evident these various themes were can be seen by reviewing Professor Cordasco's bibliography: homeopathy, eclectic, Thomasonian, botanic, allopathic. In discussing the state of American medicine in the early 19th century, the president of the New York State Medical Society commented in 1818: "With a few, honorable exceptions . . . the practitioners were ignorant, degraded and contemptible."[25] Medical licensure at this time was in a ludicrous state. While there were medical societies in nearly all the states by 1830, few were compelled to give rigorous exams. Just the opposite was occurring in Europe and Great Britain where medical boards were being set up to establish and enforce uniform standards of medical practice.[26] In this American era there was a plethora of new and dubious schools opening (1810-1840, twenty-six new schools; 1840-1875, forty-seven new schools). These schools were mostly proprietary in style with loosely defined requirements where professors were supported by students' fees, hardly a pedantic playground. These schools for profit followed many a philosophy depending upon the mountebank character leading the forum. An enterprising student could study homeopathy, eclectic, botanic, Thomasonian, to name but a few; and, of course, these competed with the "regular" or allopathic schools of medicine.

By 1900 the ratio of doctors to patients in America had exceeded England by about two to one: In the United Kingdom the ratio was 1:1100 and in the United States it was 1:600.[27] Shryock did an analysis on the education of "practitioners" in eastern Tennessee in 1850 and found that there were 201 "physicians" serving a population of 164,000. In analyzing their educational achievements, it was noted, of these 35 (17%) were graduates of some sort of regular school; 42 (20%) said they had "taken

---

[24] Anderson, W. *British Journal of Medicine.* 2:351, 1895.

[25] Shryock, R. H. *Medical Licensing in America, 1650-1965.* Baltimore: Johns Hopkins Press, 1967. p. 4.

[26] *Ibid.*, p. 27.

[27] *Ibid.*, p. 30. See footnote #44.

one course of lectures," but had not graduated; and 27 (13%) were "botanic and steamers." The rest (some 50%) had received no other education other than some reading, most likely as apprentices.[28] To appreciate what some people thought of an average medical student, consider the following quote which appeared in an editorial in *The New York Sun* in 1861; when describing a Southern medical student one editor observed ". . . a long haired, lantern-jawed verdant youth afflicted with chronic salivation and inveterate profanity . . . deriving his ideas of morals, grammar, and behavior from his negro nurse . . . he becomes in New York a puzzle to professors, a terror to landladies, and a munificient patron of grog shops"[29] – not exactly flowery praise. But then one must also appreciate this was a Northerner writing about a Southerner in 1861. Nevertheless, this was probably not too far from an accurate description of medical students at some of the schools of this era.

William Henry Welch, educator, pathologist, and a founder of Johns Hopkins could only describe native medical education in the United States in 1878 as "simply horrible."[30] This unflattering view does unfortunately detract from the many good students and physicians in practice at this time. A study of Professor Cordasco's bibliography graphically illustrates the logarithmic increases in American medical literature as the 19th century progressed. A good deal of this came from physicians traveling abroad and returning with new information, which was then published locally (Shryock reports that some 15,000 American physicians traveled abroad between 1875 and 1914).[31] In the latter half of the 19th century, American physicians began to introduce their own "systems" of medicine, detailed in example by Pepper[32] and Osler.[33] In this period the American Medical Association and its president, Nathan S. Davis (1817-1904) were demanding educational reform with pre-clinical education requirements, minimum medical school and hospital clinical experience. Improved licensing examinations by state boards and improved medical schools were advocated.[34]

Out of this came the great Hopkins experiment and a paradigm for future medical education. Founded by a philanthropist, patterned after the German medical institutions, and led by the medical greats of this era, a revolution in medical education occurred with the Hopkins experience.

---

[28] Shryock, R. H. *Medical Licensing in America, 1650-1965.* Baltimore: Johns Hopkins Press, 1967. p. 4.

[29] *Ibid.*, p. 36.

[30] *Ibid.*, p. 43.

[31] *Ibid.*, p. 4.

[32] Pepper, W. *A System of Practical Medicine by American Authors.* Philadelphia: Lea Brothers, 1885-1886. 5 vols.

[33] Osler, W. and T. McCrae. *Modern Medicine, Its Theory and Practice. In Original Contributions by American and Foreign Authors.* Philadelphia and New York: Lea Brothers, 1907-1910. 7 vols.

[34] Shryock, R. H. *Medical Licensing in America, 1650-1965.* Baltimore: Johns Hopkins Press, 1967. p. 47.

For the first time there were strict pre-medical requirements; a four-year graded course, full-time pre-clinical professors, and emphasis on both teaching and research. In 1900 the United States Office of Education reported 151 active medical schools in the United States of which eight were eclectic and physiomedical and twenty-two homeopathic. In 1910 Flexner issued *Bulletin #4*, a now well-known and heavily cited work which devastated the medical profession at this time. The "Flexner Report"[35] was undertaken by Abraham Flexner on behalf of the Carnegie Foundation. In 1908 Henry Pritchett had read *The American College*, a criticism of the elective and lecture system.[36] Pritchett discussed with Flexner a study which would analyze American medical education from the perspective of educational theory and practice: the rest is history. After Flexner's work, many of the worst medical schools closed. By the end of the Great War the epoch of European research had slowed, and the Americans headed to the forefront.

From this brief foreword, it can be seen how appropriate it was for Dr. Cordasco to select a bibliographic period crucial to American medicine—a period embryonic for American physicians. No medical man can practice in a chronological vacuum for our methods today were developed yesterday. In this wonderful work of Professor Cordasco, we see a compendium of our past. The lapse of centuries has removed the amulet from the physician's sanctum, the bleeding lancets from our bags, and added anesthesia and antiseptics to our surgical techniques. Professor Cordasco has outlined it all here, a crucial period in our development of medical knowledge. Professor Cordasco's work will rank with the great studies of Billings, Evans, Sabin, Austin, and Guerra. Happy the student, be he physician, historian, librarian, or antiquarian dealer, who pulls this work from the shelf for he will now be able to locate, with ease and leisure, the works of this most important era in American medicine. This bibliographic repository will stand as an enduring tribute to Dr. Francesco Cordasco for his experience, erudition, and multitudinous talents. By returning to the original descriptions of diseases, clinical pictures are etched more deeply in the mind of the student, practitioner, and the researcher. Here, uninterrupted over a period of 90 years, lies our medical heritage. *Pigmei gigantum humeris imposit plusauam ipsi gigantes vident.*[37]

Acknowledgment: The author would like to express his sincere thanks to Karen Hall, Historical Librarian, Columbia University Health Science Library for her assistance and guidance.

[35] Flexner, A. *Medical Education in the United States and Canada. Bulletin Number Four*. The Carnegie Foundation for the Advancement of Learning, 1910.

[36] Kaufman, M. *American Medical Education. The Formative Years 1765-1910*. Westport: Greenwood Press, 1976. p. 167.

[37] "A Dwarfe standing on the shoulders of a giant may see farther than a giant himselfe." From: Burton, R. *The Anatomy of Melancholy* . . . Oxford: John Lichfield and James Short for Henry Cripps A°Dom, 1624. p. 7.

PREFACE

The genesis of this work lies in those expectant and exciting years in the 1930's when I was an undergraduate student in New York City's Columbia College, a formidable citadel of learning, and of social privilege in an America, at that time, wrenched by economic privation. For the most part excluded (by the lack of money, and by blatantly undisguised discrimination) from the round of social activities found in any collegial environment (and at the Columbia of my time predicated on the money and social privilege of its national and international student constituency), I turned to the wondrous resources of the city: to its libraries and museums, to the exploration of its ethnic communities, and the contemplation of its historic monuments; and, out of these contemplative wanderings, with a kind of fated inevitability, I discovered, fortuitously, a fabled antiquarian book market which extended from the John Wanamaker emporium off Astor Place north along Fourth Avenue to 14th Street and Union Square. Although, it is long since gone, part of a vanished era, it remains, for me, as real as yesterday.

The Fourth Avenue book bazaar (truly, a *bazaar* in seemingly inexhaustible stocks spilling out of its shops onto outside tables and shelving, disordered and overseen by idiosyncratic, impecunious entrepreneurs whose penury was exceeded only by their amiable arrogance) for me, was a vertiginous source of continuing excitement; it was here that I spent all of my free time; reading, browsing, talking to shopkeepers, and in day-dreaming reveries which magically provided me with all the money needed to buy any (and all) of the wares which had captured my fancy.

I did acquire a multitude of volumes (*belles-lettres*, history, social sciences) for nickels and dimes (and an occasional dollar), and as token payment for a wide range of chores for shopkeepers: and from the earliest sojourns my attention was drawn to the ubiquitously scattered 19th century medical textbooks, with few exceptions, disdained by both the shopkeepers and buyers. My preoccupation with the medical texts (more often than not enormously thick non-descripto, teutonic shape, tub-model tomes) was not altogether fortuitous: at Columbia, I was a pre-medical student, and a mentor at the University (whose influence I can only inadequately acknowledge) was the medical sociologist, Bernhard J. Stern, whose *Society and Medical Progress* (1941) and *American Medical Practice* (1945) have become prophetically classic statements.

Professor Stern was a tragic figure, denied promotion at a WASPish Columbia because he was a Jew and a reputed Marxist (it would appear); to me, Professor Stern was a source of sustained inspiration and encouragement who marvelled over the medical texts I brought him from Fourth Avenue for examination; it was Professor Stern who first explained to me the 19th century social contexts out of which Austin Flint, Sr., Samuel D. Gross, Charles D. Meigs, and J. Marion Sims (with a multitude of others) emerged, and *pari passu*, related them to the evolving history of American medicine and its social relationships.

The nucleus of the medical titles described in *American Medical Imprints, 1820-1910* is my collection of some 2500 19th century medical textbooks, some 1500 of which derive from my excursions to the Fourth Avenue enchanted book "bazaar" of the 1930's, and assembled with Professor Stern's encouragement. In a sense, then, *American Medical Imprints, 1820-1910* has been in progress for over forty years.

In the last ten years, I have worked steadily toward the work's completion. Using my collection as a core-base, I articulated a practicable framework, defined bibliographical descriptive canons, and established criteria for entry inclusion. It has been a one-man task, and however formidable, it has not been objectionable or onerous: painful, at times, to be sure, yet a continuing source of delight and wonder as it evolved, with little attention to mounting costs and little expectation of even modest remuneration. I am reminded of Samuel D. Gross's plaintive lamentation on the meagre financial gains from his monumental *System of Surgery* (1859; 6th ed., 1882): "What compensation does the reader think I obtained for this hard work, this excessive toil of my brain, including original composition, the correction and improvement of new editions, and the proof-reading, in itself a horrible task, death to brain and eyes, extending over a period certainly not less than fifteen years? Eighty-five cents a copy, all told, and no extra dividends! Two dollars and a half ought to have been the price, or, what would have been more equitable, an equal distribution of the profits from the sale of the work. No wonder authors are poor and publishers are rich!" (*Autobiography*, I, 141)

American Medical Imprints, 1820-1910 includes over 36,000 entries. Its subtitle calls it "a preliminary contribution," and, hopefully, critics will remain mindful of this caveat. I am not unaware of the carping criticisms which have purused Francisco Guerra's *American Medical Bibliography, 1639-1783* (1962) and Robert B. Austin's *Early American Medical Imprints . . . , 1668-1820* (1961), and I am resigned to the inevitable critical prattle which will greet *American Medical Imprints, 1820-1910* and dog its heels. Of the work's value, I have no doubt; and, given the bibliographical canons and inclusion-criteria, the work is honest to its task. Completeness is not proposed, and any such pretension would be palpably both presumptuous and ludicrous: anyone familiar with the byzantine bibliographical history of 19th century America (and for that matter, of the entire history of American book publishing) recognizes the virtue of modest affirmations.*

I welcome constructive criticism, and look forward to receiving notices of corrections, additions, and ancillary emendations. I have a special fondness for *American Medical Imprints, 1820-1910*: not only because, of its long gestation, or because, like a petulant offspring, it has made such heavy demands on my time: its titles gather together a multiplicity of themes which I have explored in other books, themes not incongruent with an expanding America and its evolving social institutions. It is only with reluctance (but with unconcealed glee) that an author recalls Samuel Johnson's caustic commentary on launching his *Dictionary*: "I have protracted my work till most of those whom I wished to please, have sunk into the grave, and success and miscarriage are empty sounds: I therefore dismiss it with frigid tranquillity, having little to fear or hope from censure or from praise." G. Thomas Tanselle, with a touching magnanimity, is closer to the mark in his *Guide to the Study of United State Imprints* (1971) with this plaintive observation: "Bibliographers traditionally end their introductory remarks with a reference to the inevitable omissions which will be discovered in their work, and sometimes their tone suggests a grudging acceptance of an unfortunate fact. They should rather feel pleased that their work is being used and that it is serving to stimulate the recording of additional relevant material. Margaret B. Stillwell, recalling the time when she took her 'first plunge into the study of Americana,' says in her preface to *Incunabula and Americana,* 'I felt often haunted by a questioning fear. Had I not overlooked the obvious?' If a checklist is to allay such fears on the part of its users, it must be constructed through a collaborative effort in which additional information can be gathered in a meaningful way; it provides a framework into which the community of workers in a field can place further references in an organized fashion. Not until the additions and corrections to this book begin to flow in, therefore, can it be thought of as fulfilling its true function." (I, iii)

There is, of course, a serious concern to be addressed. Of what value is retrospective bibliography? *American Medical Imprints, 1820-1910* is a retrospective bibliography consciously predicated on retrieval systems imbedded in and dependent on traditional deposit libraries with vast and continuously expanding holdings. In a new printing of her seminal *The*

*John Tebbel, in contemplating the fortunes of his *A History of Book Publishing in the United States* (1972-1981, 4v.) spoke to this issue: "Whatever their considerable virtues, none of these volumes offers a detailed view of publishing in America that even approaches the comprehensive. While I agree with Professor [G. Thomas] Tanselle that individual scholars will still confront the necessity of doing a host of small-scale studies before the pieces can be put together in a general publishing history of the kind he envisions, I disagree with him that what has been done to date is adequate as even a first step in synthesis and generalization. I intend the volumes on which I have embarked to be that first step, and make no more claims for them than that. (I, xv)

Development of Medical Bibliography (1954; rep. 1982), Estelle Brodman presciently observes that "The growth of automation from the first fumbling attempts to use punched cards and sorting and printing machines to the present on-line systems of bibliographical control has been a revolution all of whose effects have still not been understood." Of this there is no doubt; and it may well be that the traditional library, as we have known it, will be ineluctably changed with the continuing advance of a technology whose advocates predict the replacement of paper and print by electronic recording: all remains uncertain.

The new technology (with promise of protean videotext capabilities), and its multitudinous applications, has proven to be both blessing and bane. Medical bibliography presents special problems, and, in the main, the caution expressed by Scott Adams is judicious: "In the last analysis, there is only one thing which can be said with any degree of certainty about the future forms and content of biomedical bibliography; they will continue to be responsive to the socio-political-technological changes in the society they serve. Since such changes interact with each other, it would take a brave person to predict the results of three forces whose directions are only partially understood." (*Medical Bibliography In An Age of Discontinuity*, [1981], 186). And these sentiments are echoed in Frank B. Roger's prognostications in a centennial tribute to the *Index Medicus*, the companion to the *Index-Catalogue of the Library of the Surgeon-General's Office*: "I do not foresee the demise of a printed version of the *Index Medicus* store; I do, however, believe that inevitably we must see radical changes in the periodicity of publication, and at the same time marked changes in the shape and configuration and relationships of the *Index Medicus* family membership—the *Index Medicus* siblings and all the *Index Medicus* children, and the cousins, too. It is bound to happen that some of them are going to have their lease on printed life rescinded, and will remain only as ghosts within the machine." (*Centenary of Index Medicus 1879-1979* [1980], 59)

I remain confident that *American Medical Imprints, 1820-1910* will, for a long time, meet the needs I had in mind when I compiled it. Above all else, it adds to the corpus of systematic and enumerative bibliography which evolves into a national form: and this is adequate reason, alone, for its compilation.* It affords, also, easy access to a multifarious literature

---

*The *doyen* of bibliographers, Theodore Besterman (1904-1976), saw no need to justify *American Medical Imprints, 1820-1910* as anything more than systematic and enumerative bibliography, a part of an evolving national bibliographical register. In long discursive bibliothecal discussions with Dr. Besterman while preparing the publication of the *Supplement* (1977, 2v.) to his *World Bibliography of Bibliographies* (4th ed., 1965-1966, 5v.), Dr. Besterman applauded the design of the *American Medical Imprints, 1820-1910*, and encouraged its completion. He scoffed at the electronic threat to libraries, and predicted that the libraries would shape and adapt the new technology to *their* needs, not the other way around. Dr. Besterman's prediction is congruent with the historical patterns of societal and institutional change: libraries are not immune to axiomatic phenomenon.

integrally coincident with the age out of which it emerges and of which it is a dimensional representation. It incorporates the archives out of which the sociologist and cultural historian recreate a vanished era which explain both the genesis and transformation of contemporary reality; and for the medical historian and investigator, *American Medical Imprints, 1820-1910* affords limitless opportunities to explore, in its thousands of entries, the evolution and formation of the profession. The history of medicine and its archives, of course, go far beyond antiquarian pursuits and systematic bibliography. Owsei Temkin's *obiter dicta* are not inappropriate. "Indeed, why turn to new fields to study the moral nature of man? We can behold truth only in the form of samples, and if the historiography of medicine is to comprise 'all that is historical in medicine, as well as all that is medical in history,' it constitutes a sample of considerable size. It is also a good sample, I believe. Hippocrates, Galen, Avicenna, Averröes, Maimonides, Paracelsus, Rabelais, Haller, Virchow, Claude Bernard, and Freud were among the intellectual leaders of mankind. Physicians have been both praised and ridiculed in novels and on the stage. Health and disease have been subjects of religious and philosophical meditation, and as metaphors they are to be found in politics, science, and literature. The human body in the glory of health and in the wretchedness of sickness has been depicted in art. Man has speculated over the meaning of his disease for himself and for his community. Medicine is not only a science and an art; it is also a mode of looking at man with compassionate objectivity. Why turn elsewhere to contemplate man's moral nature?" (*The Double Face of Janus* [1977], 37)

In a centennial review of the state of American medical publishing, John S. Billings (1838-1913), the creator of the Surgeon General's library and architect of its *Index Catalogue*, proudly observed: "In the retrospective reviews, historical sketches, and centennial addresses which have, during the past year, been devoted to American medicine, our most important contributions to the healing art have been duly pointed out and, for the most part, sufficiently eulogized. That the United States has a medical literature, has been cumulatively demonstrated, even to the extent of raising a suspicion of the existence of a doubt upon this point; and that this literature contains many valuable original contributions to the art, if not to the science, of medicine may be considered and unanimously affirmed and admitted." (*A Century of American Medicine, 1776-1876* [1876], 291-292). *American Medical Imprints 1820-1910* documents Billings's proud affirmations.

FRANCESCO CORDASCO
West New York, New Jersey
December, 1983

ACKNOWLEDGMENTS

Over the years, I have incurred many obligations while preparing *American Medical Imprints, 1820-1910*. Many of these obligations cannot be acknowledged, lost as they are in the hundreds of fortuitous encounters in libraries and institutions where my questions were answered, and resources placed at my disposal by countless but nameless individuals always courteous and helpful. However anonomously, they figure in the history of this work. I salute and applaud this library phalanx and the institutions they serve: The Yale University School of Medicine; Library of Congress; National Library of Medicine; John Crerar Library; Health Sciences Library, University of Louisville; Rudolph Matas Medical Library, Tulane University; Boston Public Library; The Francis A. Countway Library of Medicine; William H. Welch Medical Library, Johns Hopkins University; New York Public Library; Health Sciences Library, Columbia University; New York Academy of Medicine; Lloyd Library and Museum; Cleveland Health Sciences Library, Case Western Reserve University; College of Physicians of Philadelphia; Hahnemann University of the Health Sciences; Scott Memorial Library, Jefferson Medical College; Library of the School of Medicine, University of Pennsylvania; Richmond Academy of Medicine.

I owe a special debt to Dr. James Tait Goodrich of the College of Physicians and Surgeons, Columbia University, who graciously prepared a foreword to the work; and to R. Kenneth Bussy, executive editor at Lea & Febiger of Philadelphia, who made available to me the rich resources of the 19th century premier medical publisher, now on the threshold of its third century. Special thanks are due: Stanly B. Burns, M.D.; Heidi E. Duda, Francis A. Countway Library of Medicine; Ellen G. Gartrell, College of Physicians of Philadelphia; John B. Griggs and Rebecca A. Perry, Lloyd Library and Museum; Miriam Mandelbaum and Anne M. Pascarelli, New York Academy of Medicine; Alice Kennedy, Library of the School of Medicine, University of Pennsylvania; Caroline Morris, Pennsylvania Hospital Medical Library; and Barbara Williams, Hahnemann University of the Health Sciences.

American Medical Imprints, 1820-1910 could not have been done without Mrs. Chalmers Morehead who brought to the task those bountiful skills which disciplined a project always on the verge of tumbling out of control; Mary Faith Daly attended to a constellation of needs which brought the work to completion and for these services, I am grateful; and special thanks are due Edna Cordasco, Carmela Cordasco, Michael Cordasco and Gaetana Cordasco for a multitude of tasks cheerfully performed. My bibliographical assistant, John M. Macagne, made his way back and forth through the formidable "Mansell" in his continuing pursuit of evasive and perplexing entries, and his tireless efforts contributed to the completion of this work.

TABLE OF CONTENTS

VIII. AMERICAN MEDICAL IMPRINTS, 1890-1899

The management of the present epidemic as compared with former ones manifests a distinct tendency toward germicide, or antiseptic remedies, and is characterized by the introduction and general use of expedients of a surgical kind—such as enteroclysis, intra-venous transfusion, hypodermatoclysis, and subcutaneous injection. Whether the results are as successful as the devices are ingenious, may admit of question in the light of the mortality statistics. Judged dispassionately and all deductions allowed, it must be admitted, I think, that some progress has been made, and although the number of deaths in some localities may be equal to those in former epidemics, it yet appears certain that our therapeutical measures are attended with a constantly increasing improvement in the proportion of cures.

Roberts Bartholow,
Cholera: Its Causes, Symptoms, Pathology and Treatment (1893)

ABBE, Robert (1851-1928)
Spinal surgery; a report of eight cases. New York: Trow, 1890. 31p. DNLM **90-0001**

ABBE, Robert (1851-1928)
A case of hemiplegic epilepsy, probably diabetic, simulating cerebral abscess. [New York, 1890.] 6p. DNLM **90-0002**

ABBE, Robert (1851-1928)
Paranephric cysts. [New York, 1890.] 11p. DNLM **90-0003**

ABBE, Robert (1851-1928)
Cases of gall-bladder surgery. [New York, 1892.] 10p. DNLM **90-0004**

ABBE, Robert (1851-1928)
Intestinal anastomosis and suturing. New York: Trow Directory, Printing & Bookbinding Co., 1892. 23p. DNLM **90-0005**

ABBE, Robert (1851-1928)
A new and safe method of cutting oesophageal strictures. New York: Trow's Co., 1893. 8p. DNLM **90-0006**

ABBE, Robert (1851-1928)
The surgery of gall-stone obstruction. New York: Trow Co., 1893. 16p. DNLM **90-0007**

ABBE, Robert (1851-1928)
The surgery of the hand, being the Carpenter lectureship address before the New York Academy of Medicine, November 20, 1893. [New York, 1893.] 24p. DNLM; NNNAM **90-0008**

ABBE, Robert (1851-1928)
The surgery of the hand, being the Carpenter lectureship address before the New York Academy of Medicine, November 20, 1893. [New York, 1894.] 27p. DNLM **90-0009**

ABBE, Robert (1851-1928)
Sarcoma of the kidney; its operative treatment. [Philadelphia, 1894.] 12p. 3 plates. DNLM **90-0010**

ABBOTT, Alexander C[rever] (1860-1935)
Further studies upon the relation of the pseudo-diphtheritic bacillus to the diphtheritic bacillus. [Baltimore, 1891.] 7 l. DNLM **90-0011**

ABBOTT, Alexander C[rever] (1860-1935)
The principles of bacteriology: a practical manual. . . . Philadelphia: Lea Bros. & Co., 1892. 263p. NNNAM; OCIM; PPC; PU **90-0012**

ABBOTT, Alexander C[rever] (1860-1935)
The etiology of membranous rhinitis (rhinitis fibrinosa). [Philadelphia: Lea Bros. & Co., 1893.] 15p. DNLM **90-0013**

ABBOTT, Alexander C[rever] (1860-1935)
Considerations concerning Asiatic cholera. Philadelphia, 1893. 14p. DNLM **90-0014**

ABBOTT, Alexander C[rever] (1860-1935)
The results of the inoculations of milch cows with cultures of the bacillus diphtheriae. [Philadelphia, 1893.] 21p. 2 plates. **90-0015**

ABBOTT, Alexander C[rever] (1860-1935)
A review of some of the disputed points in connection with diphtheria and conditions with which it has been confounded. Philadelphia: Lea Bros. & Co., 1894. 16p. DNLM **90-0016**

ABBOTT, Alexander C[rever] (1860-1935)
The principles of bacteriology: a practical manual. . . . 2nd ed. Philadelphia: Lea Bros. & Co., 1894. 471p. CtY-M; NNNAM; PPC; PPJ **90-0017**

ABBOTT, Alexander C[rever] (1860-1935)
The principles of bacteriology: a practical manual. . . . 3rd ed. Philadelphia: Lea Bros. & Co., 1895. 493p. ICRM; IU-M; NNNAM; PU **90-0018**

ABBOTT, Alexander C[rever] (1860-1935)
The principles of bacteriology: a practical manual. . . . 4th ed. Philadelphia: Lea Bros. & Co., 1897. 543p. NNNAM; NNU-M; PPC; PU **90-0019**

ABBOTT, Alexander C[rever] (1860-1935)
The principles of bacteriology: a practical manual. . . . 5th ed. Philadelphia: Lea Bros. & Co., 1899. 590p. MH-M; NNNAM; PPC; PPJ **90-0020**

ABBOTT, Alexander C[rever] (1860-1935)
The hygiene of transmissible diseases: their causation, modes of dissemination, and methods of prevention. Philadelphia: W. B. Saunders & Co., 1899. 311p. MBM; NNNAM; PPC; PU **90-0021**

ABBOTT, Frank (1836-1897)
Congenital defects in enamel. Philadelphia, 1891. 12p. DNLM **90-0022**

ABEL, William J.
School hygiene including simple directions respecting ventilation, eyesight, infectious diseases, and first aid in injuries for schools and families. New York: Longmans, Green & Co., 1890. 53p. ICU; MB; NIC; NN **90-0023**

ABRAMS, Albert (1863-1924)
Manual of clinical diagnosis. . . . San Francisco: The Bancroft Co., 1891. 207p. CU-M; NNNAM **90-0024**

ABRAMS, Albert (1863-1924)
Report of one hundred and sixty-three cases treated with the pneumatic cabinet. Read before the San Francisco County Medical Society, Aug. 11, 1891. San Francisco: W. A. Woodward & Co., [1891]. 11p. DNLM **90-0025**

ABRAMS, Albert (1863-1924)
Report of committee on pathological anatomy. Parenchymatous aspiration: a new method of diagnosis. Read before the Medical Society of the State of California, April 21, 1891. [San Francisco, 1891.] 5p. DNLM **90-0026**

ABRAMS, Albert (1863-1924)
Pulmonary atelectasis as a cause of anemia. [San Francisco, 1892.] 4p. DNLM **90-0027**

ABRAMS, Albert (1863-1924)
Manual of clinical diagnosis. . . . Rev. 2nd ed. San Francisco: The S. Carson Co., 1892. 207p. NNNAM
90-0028

ABRAMS, Albert (1863-1924)
Clinical diagnosis. . . . 3rd ed., rev. and enl. . . . New York: E. B. Treat, 1894. 273p. NNNAM **90-0029**

ABRAMS, Albert (1863-1924)
A case of gastroptosis and merycismus, with voluntary dislocation of the stomach and kidney. Philadelphia, 1895. 4p. DNLM **90-0030**

ABRAMS, Albert (1863-1924)
Transactions of the antiseptic club, reported by Albert Abrams. . . . New York: E. B. Treat & Co., 1895. 206p. NNNAM **90-0031**

ACHENBACH, J. G.
Regional symptomatology and therapeutics; or, help for the sick. A system to simplify the medical treatment for the people, arranged and compiled from the best authors. Weeping Water, Neb., 1890. 48p. OCIM; PPHa
90-0032

ACTON, William (1813-1875)
The functions and disorders of the reproductive organs in childhood, youth, adult age and advanced life, considered in their physiological, social and moral relations. 8th ed. Philadelphia: P. Blakiston, Son & Co., 1895. 263p. PPC; PPJ; PU **90-0033**

ADAMS, A. Wellington
Electricity: its applications in medicine and surgery. A brief and practical exposition of modern scientific electro-therapeutics. Detroit: G. S. Davis, 1891. 2 v. DNLM; OCIM
90-0034

ADAMS, Francis (1796-1861)
On the construction of the human placenta. An historical sketch. New York, [1891]. 42p. DNLM
90-0035

ADAMS, Frederick E.
Report on the health of Bolton during the year 1890. Bolton: Tillottson & Son, 1891. 47p. 16 diag., 1 tab. DNLM; MBM
90-0036

ADAMS, J[ames] F[orster] Alleyne (1844-1914)
A case of biliary calculus; cholecystotomy; duodenal fistula; recovery. Boston: Damrell & Upham, 1892. 9p. DNLM
90-0037

ADAMS, J[ames] F[orster] Alleyne (1844-1914)
The Shattuck lecture, 1892. The prevention of disease in Massachusetts. Boston: D. Clapp & Son, 1892. 30p. 1 diag. DNLM; MBM **90-0038**

ADAMS, Jedidiah Howe (1866-1919)
History of the life of D. Hayes Agnew. Philadelphia: F. A. Davis, 1892. 376p. DNLM; NNNAM; PPC; PU
90-0039

ADAMS, Jedidiah Howe (1866-1919)
An account of the influenza as it appeared in Philadelphia in the winters of 1889-1890 and 1891-1892. [Philadelphia: Univ. Penn. Press, 1892.] 24p. DNLM; PU
90-0040

ADAMS, Samuel S[hugert] (1853-1928)
The diploma of the nurse, and what she owes to it. Delivered on the part of the faculty to the graduating class of the Washington Training School for Nurses, June 11, 1891. Washington, D.C.: R. O. Polkinhorn, 1891. 6p. DNLM
90-0041

ADAMS, Samuel S[hugert] (1853-1928)
Typhoid fever in infants under two years of age. Etiology; pathology; symptomatology. New York: William Wood & Co., 1895. 7p. DNLM **90-0042**

ADDRESSES delivered at the dedication of the Training School for Nurses of the Newton Hospital, February 14, 1894. Newton, Mass., 1894. 32p. 1 plate. DNLM
90-0043

ADDRESSES delivered before the Mutual Aid Association of the Philadelphia County Medical Society for the relief of the widows and orphans of medical men, December 14, 1892. By Drs. Billings, Keen, and Willard, and George D. McCreary, esq. [Philadelphia], 1892. 11p. DNLM **90-0044**

ADDRESSES delivered at the opening of the Cincinnati Hospital Medical Library, May 11, 1892. [By C. G. Comegys, David Judkins, Hon. Wm. M. Ramsey, and Wm. Carson.] [Cincinnati, 1892.] 12p. DNLM; OC **90-0045**

ADDRESSES delivered at the opening of the Walter Garrett Memorial Building of the Pennsylvania Hospital, April 23, 1897. Philadelphia: Times Printing House, [1897]. 47p. PPPH; PU **90-0046**

ADLER, I[saac] (*b.* 1849)
A case of so-called laryngeal vertigo. New York: D. Appleton & Co., 1892.] 10p. DNLM **90-0047**

ADLER, Lewis H., Jr.
Normal liquid ergot in enuresis nocturna. [Detroit, 1890.] 8p. DNLM **90-0048**

ADLER, Lewis H., Jr.
Report of a case of a dissecting aneurism of the aorta; rupture and death. [Philadelphia, 1891.] 2p. DNLM
90-0049

ADLER, Lewis H., Jr.
Cocaine as a local anaesthetic in cases requiring amputation of the digits, with a report of fifty such operations in which the drug was employed. [Detroit, 1891.] 4p. DNLM
90-0050

ADLER, Lewis H., Jr.
The status of the hydrochlorate of cocaine in minor surgery, as based upon the experience of Philadelphia physicians. Detroit: G. S. Davis, 1891. 48p. DNLM
90-0051

ADLER, Lewis H., Jr.
A report of five cases of chronic mercurial poisoning. [Philadelphia, 1891.] 7p. DNLM **90-0052**

ADLER, Lewis H., Jr.
Two cases of fracture of the body of the scapula. [Detroit, 1891.] 2p. DNLM **90-0053**

ADLER, Lewis H., Jr.
Ligation of the internal jugular vein for profuse hemorrhage caused by a sloughing adenitis, which followed malignant scarlet fever. [Philadelphia, 1891.] 2p. DNLM **90-0054**

ADLER, Lewis H., Jr.
Anal fissure; its etiology, symptomatology, physical exploration, diagnosis, and prognosis. [Philadelphia, 1892.] 8p. DNLM **90-0055**

ADLER, Lewis H., Jr.
Fistula in ano; general considerations; etiology, symptomatology, diagnosis, prognosis. [Philadelphia, 1892.] 17p. DNLM **90-0056**

ADLER, Lewis H., Jr.
The operative treatment of fistula in ano. [Philadelphia, 1892.] 8p. DNLM **90-0057**

ADLER, Lewis H., Jr.
The treatment of anal fissure, or irritable ulcer of the rectum. [Philadelphia, 1892.] 7p. DNLM **90-0058**

ADLER, Lewis H., Jr.
Fissure of the anus and fistula in ano. Detroit, Mich.: G. S. Davis, 1892. 78p. DNLM **90-0059**

ADLER, Lewis H., Jr.
The treatment of anal fissure, or irritable ulcer of the rectum. [Detroit, 1893.] 12p. DNLM **90-0060**

ADLER, Lewis H., Jr.
The treatment of fistula in ano by Lange's method of immediate suture of the tract. Philadelphia, 1895. 4p. DNLM **90-0061**

ADLER, Lewis H., Jr.
Extirpation and colotomy in cases of carcinoma of the rectum. Philadelphia, 1895. 4p. DNLM **90-0062**

ADLER, Lewis H., Jr.
I. The etiology and symptomatology of pruritus ani. II. The constitutional treatment directed toward the relief of pruritus ani. III. The local treatment of pruritus ani. Philadelphia, 1895. 6p. DNLM **90-0063**

ADLER, Lewis H., Jr.
Excision of the coccyx for constant pain resulting from an ununited fracture. Philadelphia, 1895. 3p. DNLM **90-0064**

AGNEW, D[avid] Hayes, ed. (1818-1892)
History and reminiscences of the Philadelphia Almshouse and Philadelphia Hospital. Philadelphia: Deltre, 1890. 144p. PPC; PPPH **90-0065**

ALBANY MEDICAL COLLEGE. MEDICAL DEPARTMENT OF UNION UNIVERSITY (FORMERLY MEDICAL DEPARTMENT OF THE UNIVERSITY OF ALBANY)
Annual catalogues and announcements for the sessions of 1839-1840 (2.); 1853-1854 (17.); 1854 s. (18.); 1855s (20.); 1856 s. (22.); 1857 s. (24.); 1861 (31.); 1862 (31.); 1865 (35.); 1866 (36.); 1880-1881 to 1895-1896 (49.-65.). Albany, 1839-1895. DNLM [List of graduates from 1839 to 1890, in announcement for 1890-1891. Organized April 14, 1838. First course of lectures commenced Jan. 3, 1839. From 1839 to 1895, inclusive, there were 65 lecture terms and commencements; 57 fall and 8 spring. Summer sessions 1868. In 1873 it became the medical department of Union University. In 1877 the term was lengthened to 20 weeks.] **90-0066**

ALDEN, Charles H.
The special training of the medical officer, with brief notes on army medical schools abroad and at home. An address delivered before the Association of Military Surgeons of the United States, at Washington, D.C., May 3, 1894. Washington, 1894. 15p. DNLM **90-0067**

ALLAN, George S.
Address delivered before the American Academy of Dental Science, at its twenty-fourth annual meeting, held in Boston, November 11, 1891. Boston: Rockwell & Churchill, 1892. 12p. DNLM **90-0068**

ALLBUTT, Thomas Clifford, ed. (1836-1925)
A system of medicine, by many writers. . . . New York & London: Macmillan & Co., 1896-1898. 8 v. NNNAM; OCIM; PPC; PU **90-0069**

ALLBUTT, Thomas Clifford, ed. (1836-1925)
A system of gynaecology by many writers, ed. by Thomas Clifford Allbutt . . . and W. S. Playfair. . . . New York: The Macmillan Co.; London: Macmillan & Co., Ltd., 1897. 973p. DLC; NNNAM; PPC; PU **90-0070**

ALLEMAN, L. A. W[elles]
Galvanism in the treatment of corneal opacities. New York: M. J. Rooney, [1890]. 16p. DNLM **90-0071**

ALLEN, Alfred H. (1847-1904)
Chemistry of urine; a practical guide to the analytical examination of diabetic, albuminous, and gouty urine. Philadelphia: P. Blakiston, Son & Co., 1895. 212p. CtY-M; DNLM; NNNAM; PPC **90-0072**

ALLEN, Charles W[arrene] (1854-1906)
Pemphigus circinatus. [New York, 1890.] 6p. DNLM **90-0073**

ALLEN, Charles W[arrene] (1854-1906)
The treatment of erysipelas. A personal experience in fifty cases. [Philadelphia, 1891.] 15p. DNLM **90-0074**

ALLEN, Charles W[arrene] (1854-1906)
Clinical comments on cutaneous cases. New York: M. J. Rooney, 1891. 5p. DNLM **90-0075**

ALLEN, Charles W[arrene] (1854-1906)
Syphilis of the epididymis. Philadelphia, 1894. 11p. DNLM **90-0076**

ALLEN, Charles W[arrene] (1854-1906)
Handy book of medical progress; a lexicon of the recent advances in medical science, by Charles Warrene Allen . . . and Jacob Sobel. . . . New York: William Wood & Co., 1899. 184p. DLC; NNNAM **90-0077**

ALLEN, Charles W[arrene] (1854-1906)
The practitioner's manual: a condensed system of medical diagnosis and treatment. . . . New York: William Wood & Co., 1899. 851p. DLC; NNNAM **90-0078**

ALLEN, Dudley P[eter] (1852-1915)
Meckel's diverticulum as a cause of intestinal obstruction. Philadelphia, 1892. 10p. DNLM **90-0079**

ALLEN, Dudley P[eter] (1852-1915)
A résumé of surgical operations from April 1, 1892, to April 1, 1893, in the practice of . . . by William H. Nevison. Cleveland, 1893. 103p. DNLM; OCIM **90-0080**

ALLEN, Dudley P[eter] (1852-1915)
A résumé of surgical operations from April 26, 1893, to May 3, 1894, in the practice of . . . , by William H. Nevison. Cleveland, 1894. 87p. DNLM; OCIM
90-0081

ALLEN, Gardner W[eld] (1856-1901)
Some points in the treatment of gonorrhoea. Boston: Damrell & Upham, 1890. 20p. DNLM **90-0082**

ALLEN, Gardner W[eld] (1856-1901)
Cases of renal colic. Boston, 1891. 4p. DNLM
90-0083

ALLEN, Gardner W[eld] (1856-1901)
The etiology and pathology of impotence. New York, 1893. 15p. DNLM **90-0084**

ALLEN, Gardner W[eld] (1856-1901)
Two cases of litholapaxy. Boston, 1894. 7p. DNLM
90-0085

ALLEN, Gardner W[eld] (1856-1901)
Chronic inflammation of the seminal vesicles. Boston, 1894. 10p. DNLM **90-0086**

ALLEN, Gardner W[eld] (1856-1901)
Remarks on the treatment of cystitis. New York, 1895. 5p. DNLM **90-0087**

ALLEN, Harrison (1841-1897)
A description of the anatomy of the fifth pair of nerves. By Harrison Allen. . . . Plate by Henry A. Daniels, M.D. Philadelphia: The S. S. White Dental Mfg. Co., 1890. 40p. DLC; PPC
90-0088

ALLEN, Harrison (1841-1897)
Smithsonian miscellaneous collections. 708. The Toner lectures, instituted to encourage the discovery of new truths for the advancement of medicine. Lecture X. A clinical study of the skull, delivered May 29, 1889. Washington: Smithsonian Inst., 1890. 77p. 1 l. DNLM **90-0089**

ALLEN, Harrison (1841-1897)
Addresses on anatomy. I. Comparative anatomy as a part of the medical curriculum. II. On the teaching of anatomy to advanced medical students. Philadelphia, 1891. 19p. DNLM
90-0090

ALLEN, Harrison (1841-1897)
Clinical signs common to mouth, nose, throat, and ear. [Philadelphia, 1891.] 14p. DNLM **90-0091**

ALLEN, Harrison (1841-1897)
Defective conditions of the vocal organs studied, in connection with questions of the oral method of training the deaf; the tongue. Philadelphia, 1892. 22p. DNLM [Lectures delivered before the American Association to Promote the Teaching of Speech to the Deaf, at its second summer meeting, at Lake George, 1892.] **90-0092**

ALLEN, Harrison (1841-1897)
The tonsils in health and disease. Philadelphia, 1892. 17p. DNLM **90-0093**

ALLEN, Harrison, ed. (1841-1897)
A handbook of local therapeutics. General surgery, by Richard H. Harte. . . . Diseases of the skin, by Arthur Van Harlingen. . . . Diseases of the ear and air-passages, by Harrison Allen. . . . Diseases of the eye, by George C. Harlan. . . . Philadelphia: P. Blakiston, Son & Co., 1893. 505p. DLC; DNLM; NNNAM; PPC **90-0094**

ALLEN, Harrison (1841-1897)
The objects of the Wistar Institute. [Philadelphia, 1894.] 7p. DNLM **90-0095**

ALLEN, Harrison (1841-1897)
The etiology of fracture of the lower end of the radius. [Philadelphia, 1894.] 3p. DNLM **90-0096**

ALLEN, Harrison (1841-1897)
Rhinoliths. [Philadelphia, 1894.] 3p. DNLM
90-0097

ALLEN, Harrison (1841-1897)
On a new species of Ametrida. [Boston, 1894.] 7p. DNLM
90-0098

ALLEN, Harrison (1841-1897)
Morphology as a factor in skin disease. [New Haven, 1894.] 27p. DNLM **90-0099**

ALLEN, Harrison (1841-1897)
Speech without a larynx. [Philadelphia: Lea Bros. & Co., 1894.] 13p. DNLM **90-0100**

ALLEN, Harrison (1841-1897)
Another word on adenoid growths of the pharynx. Philadelphia, 1895. 5p. DNLM **90-0101**

ALLEN, Harrison (1841-1897)
Demonstration of skulls showing the effects of cretinism on the shape of the nasal chambers. [New York: D. Appleton & Co., 1895.] 5p. DNLM **90-0102**

ALLEN, Henry C. (1836-1909)
Keynotes and characteristics, with comparisons of some of the leading remedies of the materia medica. . . . Philadelphia and Chicago: Boericke & Tafel, 1898. 179p. DLC; IU-M; PPC; PPHa **90-0103**

ALLEN, Henry C. (1836-1909)
Keynotes and characteristics, with comparisons of some of the leading remedies of the materia medica. . . . 2nd ed., rev. and enl. Philadelphia and Chicago: Boericke & Tafel, 1899. 318p. DLC; OCLloyd; PPC; PPHa **90-0104**

ALLEN, Joseph Eve
The aseptic dressing of the umbilical stump. New York, 1894. 5p. DNLM **90-0105**

ALLEN, Samuel Ellsworth
The mastoid operation, including its history, anatomy, and pathology. Cincinnati: R. Clarke & Co., 1892. 111p. DLC; DNLM; OC **90-0106**

ALLEN, Timothy Field (1837-1902)
A primer of materia medical for practitioners of homoeopathy. . . . Philadelphia: Boericke & Tafel, 1892. 480p. DLC; NNNAM; OCLloyd; PPHa **90-0107**

ALLIS, Oscar H. (1836-1921)
Fracture in the upper third of the femur exclusive of the neck. [Philadelphia, 1891.] 21p. DNLM **90-0108**

ALLIS, Oscar H. (1836-1921)
Cramming in our medical schools. Philadelphia, 1894. 6p. DNLM **90-0109**

ALLIS, Oscar H. (1836-1921)
An inquiry into the difficulties encountered in the reduction of dislocations of the hip. The Samuel D. Gross Prize Essay. Philadelphia: W. Dornan, 1896. 171p. NNNAM; PPC; PPJ; PU **90-0110**

ALLISON, Charles C.
Some practical observations upon the origin, communications, and distributions of the cranial nerves. [Omaha, 1893.] 7p. DNLM **90-0111**

ALLISON, Charles C.
Causes and treatment of rectal fistulae. [Omaha, 1893.] 8p. DNLM **90-0112**

ALLISON, Henry E[dward] (1851-1904)
Insanity among criminals. Chicago: Rand, McNally & Co., 1894. 10p. DNLM **90-0113**

ALLISON, Henry E[dward] (1851-1904)
The care of the criminal insane in the State of New York. Middletown, N.Y., 1894. 16p. DNLM **90-0114**

ALLPORT, Frank (1856-1935)
Purulent brain deposits, and phlebitis and thrombosis of the cerebral veins and sinuses following ear disease. Chicago, 1892. 83p. 4 tabs., 1 plate. DNLM; IU-M **90-0115**

ALLPORT, Frank (1856-1935)
Refraction in schools. Chicago, 1895. 23p. DNLM **90-0116**

[ALLPORT, W[alter] W[ebb]] (1824-1893)
The death of Dr. W[alter] W[ebb] Allport. Obituary. Chicago, 1893. 3p. DNLM **90-0117**

ALLYN, Herman B[ryden]
Meningitis complicating influenza; autopsy. Philadelphia, 1894. 3p. DNLM **90-0118**

ALLYN, Herman B[ryden]
The reciprocal relations of mitral stenosis and pregnancy. Philadelphia, 1894. 19p. DNLM **90-0119**

ALOE, A. S., CO.
Catalogue of superior surgical instruments and physician's and surgeon's supplies. 6th ed. St. Louis, [1891]. 1068p. NNNAM **90-0120**

AMERICAN ASSOCIATION FOR THE STUDY AND CURE OF INEBRIETY
Proceedings of a complimentary dinner given to Dr. Joseph Parish, of Burlington, N.J., with a sketch of his life by Col. Shipman, etc. Hartford, Conn.: Case, Lockwood & Brainard, 1890. 86p. port. CtY-M; DNLM **90-0121**

AMERICAN ASSOCIATION FOR THE STUDY AND CURE OF INEBRIETY
The disease of inebriety from alcohol, opium and other narcotic drugs, its etiology, pathology, treatment and medico-legal relations. New York: E. B. Treat, 1893. 404p; NNNAM **90-0122**

AMERICAN DENTAL ASSOCIATION
Instructions, tables, and diagrams for the examination of human crania. Series A. [1891.] 101 l. DNLM **90-0123**

THE AMERICAN DENTAL FORCEPS CO.
. . . The manufacture and sale of an entirely new scientific and mechanical design of dental forceps. [1892?] 20p. DNLM **90-0124**

AMERICAN ELECTRO-THERAPEUTICAL ASSOCIATION
Proceedings of first annual meeting. September 24-26, 1891. [Philadelphia, 1891.] 63p. DNLM; PPC; PU **90-0125**

AMERICAN HOMOEOPATHIC BIOGRAPHICAL ASSOCIATION
Biographical cyclopaedia of homoeopathic physicians and surgeons. Chicago: American Homoeopathic Biographical Association, 1893. 172p. ports. DLC; ICU **90-0126**

AMERICAN homoeopathic pharmacopoeia. . . . 4th ed. Rev. and augm. by Joseph T. O'Connor. New York: Boericke & Tafel, 1890. 521p. NNNAM; OCLloyd **90-0127**

AMERICAN homoeopathic pharmacopoeia. . . . 5th ed. Rev. and augm. by Joseph T. O'Connor. New York: Boericke & Tafel, 1896. 521p. NNNAM; OCLloyd **90-0128**

AMERICAN homoeopathic pharmacopoeia. . . . 6th ed. Rev. and augm. by Joseph T. O'Connor. Philadelphia: Boericke & Tafel, 1899. 521p. OCLloyd; PPHa **90-0129**

AMERICAN INSTITUTE OF HOMOEOPATHY
Transactions of the World's Congress of Homoeopathic Physicians and Surgeons. Held under the auspices of the World's Congress Auxiliary of the World's Columbian Exposition in Chicago, 1893. Published by the American Institute of Homoeopathy. Philadelphia: Sherman & Co., 1894. 1109p. DNLM; PPC; PPHa; PU **90-0130**

AMERICAN INSTITUTE OF HOMOEOPATHY. COMMITTEE ON PHARMACOPOEIA
Pharmacopoeia of the American Institute of Homoeopathy. Pub. for the Committee on Pharmacopoeia of the American Institute of Homoeopathy. Boston: O. Clapp & Son, 1897. 674p. DLC; MBM; OCLloyd **90-0131**

THE AMERICAN Invalid Aid Society, its aims and purposes. [Boston, 1893.] 4p. DNLM; MB **90-0132**

AMERICAN INVALID AID SOCIETY, BOSTON
Constitution and by-laws. Boston: J. W. Calley & Sons, [1893]. 3 l. DNLM; MB **90-0133**

AMERICAN MEDICAL ASSOCIATION
List of officers and programme of the forty-first annual meeting, 1890. Nashville: Foster & Webb, 1890. 30p. DNLM **90-0134**

AMERICAN MEDICAL ASSOCIATION
Programme forty-first meeting, 1890. [New York, 1890.] 24p. DNLM **90-0135**

AMERICAN MEDICAL ASSOCIATION
Addresses, papers, and discussions in the section of the practice of medicine and physiology of the forty-second annual meeting of the . . . Washington, D.C., 1891. Chicago, 1891. 324p. DNLM; IU-M **90-0136**

AMERICAN MEDICAL ASSOCIATION
Addresses, papers, and discussions in the section of surgery and anatomy at the forty-second annual meeting of the . . . Washington, D.C., 1891. Chicago, 1891. 318p. 1 tab. DNLM **90-0137**

AMERICAN MEDICAL ASSOCIATION
Addresses, papers, and discussions in the section of obstetrics and diseases of women at the forty-second annual meeting of the . . . Washington, D.C., 1891. Chicago, 1891. 394p. 1 tab. DNLM **90-0138**

AMERICAN MEDICAL ASSOCIATION
Organization and regulations of the board of trustees of the . . . Chicago, 1892. 11p. DNLM **90-0139**

AMERICAN MEDICAL ASSOCIATION
Addresses, papers, and discussions in the section on surgery and anatomy at the forty-fifth annual meeting of the . . . , held at San Francisco, June 5-8, 1894. Chicago, 1894. 414p. DNLM **90-0140**

AMERICAN PEDIATRIC SOCIETY
Transactions. First session, Washington, D.C., Sept. 20, and Baltimore, Md., Sept. 21, 1889. Together with the proceedings of the meeting for organization, held in Washington, D.C., Sept. 18, 1888. Edited by Wm. Perry Watson. [Philadelphia]: J. B. Lippincott Co., 1890. 315p. DNLM; PPC; PU **90-0141**

AMERICAN PSYCHOLOGICAL ASSOCIATION
Proceedings. I. Preliminary meeting, 1892. II. First annual meeting, 1892. III. Second annual meeting, 1893. New York: Macmillan & Co., 1894. 29p. DNLM; NNNAM **90-0142**

AMERICAN SURGICAL ASSOCIATION
A complete list of the officers and fellows of the . . . together with an alphabetically arranged index of v. 1-10, 1880-1892. [1892.] 31p. DNLM; NNNAM; PPC **90-0143**

AMES, Delano (1868-1899)
A laboratory manual of pathological anatomy. . . . Baltimore, Md.: Printed by A. Haskell, 1895. 122p. DLC; MdBM **90-0144**

AMICK, W[illiam] R.
A treatise on lung diseases, giving the methods of diagnosis and treating these diseases as employed by . . . . Cincinnati, O., [1893]. 100p. DNLM; OC **90-0145**

ANDERS, Howard S[chultz] (*b.* 1866)
Public sanitary aid indispensable to the general health. [Philadelphia: Univ. Penn. Press], 1892. 7p. DNLM **90-0146**

ANDERS, Howard S[chultz] (*b.* 1866)
Present status of the sanitary movement for the adoption of the individual communion cup. Philadelphia, 1895. 2 l. DNLM **90-0147**

ANDERS, Howard S[chultz] (*b.* 1866)
Two cases of gastric cancer, with interesting clinical features. Philadelphia, 1895. 2 l. 2 plates. DNLM **90-0148**

ANDERS, Howard S[chultz] (*b.* 1866)
A case of uremic convulsions; venesection; recovery, remarks. Charlotte, 1895. 4p. DNLM **90-0149**

ANDERS, Howard S[chultz] (*b.* 1866)
A case of third attack of typhoid fever; with remarks on recrudescence, relapse, and recurrence in typhoid fever. Philadelphia, 1895. 2 l. DNLM **90-0150**

ANDERS, James M[eschter] (1854-1936)
The complicating conditions, associated disease, and mortality rate in erysipelas. Philadelphia: J. B. Lippincott & Co., 1893. 6p. DNLM **90-0151**

ANDERS, James M[eschter] (1854-1936)
Points in the etiology and clinical history of erysipelas. Chicago, 1893. 12p. DNLM **90-0152**

ANDERS, James M[eschter] (1854-1936)
Seasonal influences in erysipelas, with statistics. [Philadelphia], 1893. 12p. DNLM **90-0153**

ANDERS, James M[eschter] (1854-1936)
The treatment of erysipelas. Detroit, Mich.: G. S. Davis, 1894. 13p. DNLM **90-0154**

ANDERS, James M[eschter] (1854-1936)
Beriberi, with report of cases. Philadelphia, 1894. 13p. DNLM **90-0155**

ANDERS, James M[eschter] (1854-1936)
The external and internal use of guaiacol, with brief reports of cases. Detroit: G. S. Davis, 1895. 9p. DNLM **90-0156**

ANDERS, James M[eschter] (1854-1936)
A textbook of the practice of medicine. Philadelphia: W. B. Saunders & Co., 1897. 1287p. CtY-M; NNNAM; PPC; PU **90-0157**

ANDERS, James M[eschter] (1854-1936)
A textbook of the practice of medicine. 2nd ed. Philadelphia: W. B. Saunders & Co., 1898. 1287p. MBM; NNNAM; OCIM; PPC **90-0158**

ANDERS, James M[eschter] (1854-1936)
A textbook of the practice of medicine. 3rd ed. Philadelphia: W. B. Saunders & Co., 1899. 1292p. IU-M; OC; PPC; PU **90-0159**

ANDERSON MFG. CO.
Catalogue No. 2. Pharmaceutical apparatus, machinery and supplies. . . . Detroit, 1890. 32p. OCIM **90-0160**

ANDERSON, P. L.
Abnormities of the nasal septum and their treatment in the cure of catarrh. [New York: D. Appleton & Co., 1895.] 6p. DNLM **90-0161**

ANDERSON, Winslow (1860-1917)
Mineral springs and health resorts of California, with a complete chemical analysis of every important mineral water in the world. Illustrated. A prize essay; annual prize of the Medical Society of the State of California, awarded April 20, 1889. San Francisco: Bancroft Co., 1890. 384p. DNLM
80-0162

ANDREWS, Edmund (1824-1904)
Rectal and anal surgery, with a full description of the secret methods of itinerant specialists. By Edmund Andrews . . . and Edward Wyllis Andrews. . . . 3rd ed., rev. and enl., with illustrations and formulary. Chicago: W. T. Keener, 1892. 164p. DLC; NNNAM; OCIM **90-0163**

ANDREWS, Joseph A[lfred]
A new portable apparatus for sterilizing eye instruments by boiling in water. An aluminum shield for protecting the eye after cataract extraction. [New York; D. Appleton & Co., 1893.] 4p. DNLM **90-0164**

ANGELL, Henry Clay (1829-1911)
A treatise on diseases of the eye; for the use of students and practitioners. To which is added, a series of test types for determining the exact state of vision. . . . 7th ed., rewritten and illustrated. Boston: O. Clapp & Son, 1891. 357p. DLC; MBM; NNNAM **90-0165**

ANGELL, Henry C[lay] (1829-1911)
A treatise on diseases of the eye for the use of general practitioners. 7th ed. Rewritten and illustrated. Ed. by F. Park Lewis. Boston: Otis Clapp & Son, 1891. 404p. MBM; NNNAM; PPC **90-0166**

ANGLE, Edward Hartley (1855-1930)
The Angle system of regulation and retention of the teeth. 3rd ed., rev. and enl. . . . Philadelphia, Pa.: The Wilmington Dental Manufacturing Co., 1892. 51p. DLC
90-0167

ANGLE, Edward Hartley (1855-1930)
The Angle system of regulation and retention of the teeth, and treatment of fractures of the maxillae. 4th ed., rev. and enl. With one hundred and thirteen illustrations. . . . Philadelphia: The S. S. White Dental Mfg. Co., 1895. 112p. DLC; PPC; PU
90-0168

ANGLE, Edward Hartley (1855-1930)
The Angle system of regulation and retention of the teeth, and treatment of fractures of the maxillae. 5th ed., rev. With one hundred and fifteen illustrations. . . . Philadelphia: The S. S. White Dental Mfg. Co., 1897. 111p. DLC; PPC; PU
90-0169

[ANSHUTZ, Edward Pollock] (1846-1918)
Safety in cholera time. Homoeopathic treatment. Philadelphia: Boericke & Tafel, [1892]. 63p. DLC; PPHa
90-0170

[ANSHUTZ, Edward Pollock] (1846-1918)
Sexual ills and diseases. A popular manual, based on the best homoeopathic practice and the latest text book. Philadelphia: Boericke & Tafel, 1896. 160p. DLC; PPC; PPHa
90-0171

ARNOLD, Abraham B[lumenthal] (1820-1904)
Manual of nervous diseases. . . . 2nd ed. rev. and enl. San Francisco: The Bancroft Co., 1890. 332p. DLC
90-0172

ARNOLD, F. & SONS
Descriptive circular and price list of Howard A. Kelly's new instruments. Baltimore, 1894. 21p. NNNAM
90-0173

ASHBY, Henry (1846-1908)
The diseases of children. medical and surgical, by Henry Ashby . . . and G. A. Wright. . . . 2nd ed., edited for American students, by William Perry Northrup. . . . New York and London: Longmans, Green & Co., 1893. 773p. diags. DLC; NNNAM; PPC; PU **90-0174**

ASHBY, Henry (1846-1908)
The diseases of children, medical and surgical, by Henry Ashby . . . and G. A. Wright. . . . 3rd ed., edited for American students by William Perry Northrup. . . . New York, London and Bombay: Longmans, Green & Co., 1896. 840p. diags. DLC; NNNAM; OCIM; PU **90-0175**

ASHBY, Thomas A[lmond] (1848-1916)
Clinical observations on salpingitis. Baltimore, 1890. 21p. DNLM **90-0176**

ASHHURST, John (1839-1900)
Memoir of James H. Hutchinson, M.D. Philadelphia: W. J. Dornan, 1890. 16p. DNLM **90-0177**

ASHHURST, John (1839-1900)
On the surgery of the larger blood-vessels. [Charleston, 1891.] 23p. DNLM **90-0178**

ASHHURST, John (1839-1900)
The principles and practice of surgery. . . . 6th ed., enl. and thoroughly rev. with a colored plate and six hundred and fifty-six illustrations. . . . Philadelphia: Lea Bros. & Co., 1893. 1166p. DLC; NNNAM; PPC; PPJ **90-0179**

ASHMEAD, Albert S[idney] (1850-1911)
Christianity in Japan and the leper problem. An address. New York: Moore & Co., 1891. 8p. DNLM
90-0180

ASHMEAD, Albert S[idney] (1850-1911)
Pre-Columbian syphilis. [Philadelphia, 1891.] 4p. DNLM
90-0181

ASHMEAD, Albert S[idney] (1850-1911)
Some observations on kakké, the national disease of Japan. [Philadelphia, 1891.] 8p. DNLM **90-0182**

ASHMEAD, Albert S[idney] (1850-1911)
Migration of syphilis from East Asia into America by way of the Behring Sea. Chicago, 1894. 8p. DNLM
90-0183

ASHMEAD, Albert S[idney] (1850-1911)
Opinions of a noted Japanese specialist in matters of leprosy. [New York, 1894.] 11p. DNLM **90-0184**

ASHMEAD, Albert S[idney] (1850-1911)
Synopsis of a Chinese secret; manuscript on syphilis, reprinted in Japan, A.D. 1724, originally written by Chin-Shi-Sei, who lived under the dynasty of Ming (A.D. 1368-1644). Philadelphia, 1894. 5p. DNLM **90-0185**

ASHMEAD, Albert S[idney] (1850-1911)
Prof. Bandelier's views on Huacos pottery deformations and pre-Columbian syphilis. New York, 1896. 11p. DNLM
90-0186

ASHTON, Thomas G.
Angio-neurotic edema: a report of three cases showing some interesting manifestations. [Philadelphia, 1893.] 5p. DNLM
90-0187

ASHTON, Thomas G.
Chronic valvular disease of the heart. A study from clinical observations of 1024 cases, with especial reference to the causative influences and relative distribution of the lesions. Philadelphia, 1894. 13p. DNLM **90-0188**

ASHTON, Thomas G. and Alonzo H. STEWART
The employment of centrifugal force as an aid to the examination of sputum. Philadelphia: Lea Bros. & Co., 1894. 14p. DNLM **90-0189**

ASHTON, Thomas G. and Alonzo H. STEWART
Report of a case of tricuspid stenosis associated with mitral stenosis and aortic stenosis. Philadelphia, 1895. 11p. DNLM
90-0190

ASHTON, William Easterly (1859-1933)
. . . Essentials of obstetrics, arranged in the form of questions and answers, prepared especially for students of medicine. . . . 3rd ed., rev. and enl. Seventy-five illustrations. Philadelphia: W. B. Saunders, 1891. 252p. DLC; DNLM; NNNAM; PPC
90-0191

ASHTON, William Easterly (1859-1933)
The pathology of intestinal obstructions following abdominal and pelvic operations. Philadelphia, 1892. 18p. DNLM
90-0192

ASHTON, William Easterly (1859-1933)
A successful case of cholecystotomy for the removal of gall-stones obstructing the cystic duct. Detroit, Mich.: G. S. Davis, 1892. 5p. DNLM **90-0193**

ASHTON, William Easterly (1859-1933)
A successful case of lateral anastomosis of the ileum for malignant structure. Detroit: G. S. Davis, 1892. 15p. DNLM
90-0194

ASHTON, William Easterly (1859-1933)
The surgical treatment of appendicitis and its limits. Detroit: G. S. Davis, 1892. 13p. DNLM **90-0195**

ASHTON, William Easterly (1859-1933)
An outline of the technique of abdominal and pelvic operations as performed in the Medico-Chirurgical Hospital of Philadelphia. Philadelphia: Med. Bull. Print. House, 1893. 7 l. DNLM **90-0196**

ASHTON, William Easterly (1859-1933)
Ventral hernia following abdominal operations. Philadelphia, [1893]. 8p. DNLM **90-0197**

ASHTON, William Easterly (1859-1933)
A simple device for sterilizing in private houses. Philadelphia, [1894]. 1 l. 1 plate. DNLM **90-0198**

ASHTON, William Easterly (1859-1933)
The treatment of fibroid tumors of the uterus. New York, 1896. 12p. DNLM **90-0199**

ATKINS, Francis H.
The health of Las Vegas, New Mexico. . . . Also the death-rate of Las Vegas, New Mexico. . . . Manhattan, Kan., 1890. 8p. DNLM **90-0200**

ATKINSON, Edward (1827-1905)
The science of nutrition. Treatise upon the science of nutrition. The Aladdin oven, invented by Edward Atkinson. What it is, what it does, how it does it. Dietaries carefully computed under the direction of Mrs. Ellen H. Richards. Tests of the slow methods of cooking in the Aladdin oven, by Mrs. Mary H. Abel and Miss Maria Daniell; with instructions and recipes. Nutritive values of food materials, collated from the writings of Prof. W. O. Atwater. Appendix: letters and reports. Springfield, Mass.: C. W. Bryan & Co., 1892. 179p. DNLM; MB; MH; NN **90-0201**

ATKINSON, Edward (1827-1905)
The science of nutrition. Treatise upon the science of nutrition. The Aladdin oven, invented by Edward Atkinson. What it is, what it does, how it does it. Dietaries carefully computed under the direction of Mrs. Ellen H. Richards. Tests of the slow methods of cooking in the Aladdin oven, by Mrs. Mary H. Abel and Miss Maria Daniell; with instructions and recipes. Nutritive values of food materials, collated from the writings of Prof. W. O. Atwater. Appendix: letters and reports. Eighth thousand. Boston: Damrell & Upham, 1896. 246p. 1 plate. DNLM; MB; NN **90-0202**

ATTFIELD, John (1835-1911)
Chemistry; general, medical, and pharmaceutical, including the chemistry of the U.S. pharmacopoeia. A manual on the general principles of the science, and their applications in medicine and pharmacy. . . . 14th ed. Philadelphia: Lea Bros. & Co., 1894. 794p. tables, diags. DLC; NNNAM; OCLloyd: PU
90-0203

ATTFIELD, John (1835-1911)
Chemistry; general, medical, and pharmaceutical, including the chemistry of the U.S. pharmacopoeia. A manual on the science of chemistry, and its applications in medicine and pharmacy. . . . 16th ed. Philadelphia and New York: Lea Bros. & Co., 1899. 780p. tables. DLC: NNNAM; PPC; PU
90-0204

ATWATER, Wilbur Olin (1844-1907 and C. F. LANGWORTHY
A digest of metabolism experiments in which the balance of income and outgo was determined. Revised ed. Washington: Government Printing Office, 1898. 434p. DNLM
90-0205

AURAND, Samuel Herbert (*b.* 1854)
Botanical materia medica and pharmacology; drugs considered from a botanical, pharmaceutical, physiological, therapeutical and toxicological standpoint. . . . Chicago: P. H. Mallen Co., 1899. 406p. DLC; OCLloyd **90-0206**

AUSTIN, A. E[verett] (*b.* 1861)
Clinical value of renal casts. Philadelphia, 1894. 3p. DNLM
90-0207

AUVARD, Alfred (*b.* 1855)
A system of obstetrics. . . . Based upon a transl. from the French of Auvard. Rev. by Curtis M. Beebe. . . . New York: J. B. Flint & Co., 1892. 436p. DLC; NNNAM
90-0208

AYRES, Samuel
Address in mental disorders. Gastro-intestinal and hepatic disorders, especially chronic gastro-intestinal catarrh, in relation to the etiology of some cases of insanity. [Philadelphia, 1891.] 11p. DNLM **90-0209**

AYRES, Samuel
Ayres' hernia truss. Richmond, Va.: Gillis, [1892?]. 2 l. DNLM **90-0210**

AYRES, Stephen C.
Tumors of the optic nerve; with report of two original cases. Cincinnati: R. Clarke & Co., 1890. 38p. 2 plates. DNLM **90-0211**

AYRES, Stephen C.
Traumatic hemorrhages in the region of the macula lutea. [Cincinnati, 1891.] 11p. DNLM **90-0212**

AYRES, Stephen C.
The treatment of blepharitis marginalis by hydrogen dioxide. [Philadelphia, 1892.] 2p. DNLM **90-0213**

BABCOCK, Robert H[all] (*b.* 1851)
The remarkable effects of diuretin in removing dropsy. With report of cases. [New York, 1891.] 8p. DNLM **90-0214**

BABCOCK, Warren L[a Verne] (*d.* 1942)
On the morbid heredity and predisposition to insanity of the man of genius. New York, 1895. 23p. DNLM **90-0215**

[BACON, Charles A[ustin]] (1838-1892)
Catalogue sale of the valuable medical library of the late Dr. . . . ; also his miscellaneous books, including some very fine illustrated works [etc.]. Washington, D.C.: Judd & Detweiler, [1892]. 25p. DNLM **90-0216**

BACON, C. S.
The mortality from puerperal infection in Chicago. New York, 1896. 18p. DNLM **90-0217**

BACON, C. S.
Diagnosis of ectopic gestation. New York, 1896. 9p. DNLM **90-0218**

BACON, Gorham (*b.* 1855)
A case of mastoid disease following an operation for the removal of adenoid vegetations. [New Bedford, Mass., 1892.] 3p. DNLM **90-0219**

BACON, Gorham (*b.* 1855)
Middle-ear operations. New York, 1894. 8p. DNLM **90-0220**

BACON, Gorham (*b.* 1855)
A case of sarcoma of the neck involving the tonsil and causing deafness in a boy seven years of age. New York: D. Appleton & Co., 1895. 5p. DNLM **90-0221**

BACON, Gorham (*b.* 1855)
A case of brain abscess; secondary to chronic suppurative otitis media, and presenting unusual symptoms; operation; recovery. New York, 1896. 6p. DNLM **90-0222**

BACON, Gorham (*b.* 1855)
A manual of otology. . . . With an introductory chapter by Clarence John Blake. . . . With 110 illustrations and a colored plate. New York and Philadelphia: Lea Bros. & Co., 1898. 398p. DLC; NNNAM; PPC; PU **90-0223**

BAER, B[enjamin] F[ranklin] (1846-1920)
Clinical lecture. Dysmenorrhoea from haematoma of the ovary; double dermoid cyst of the ovary; two cases of fibro-sarcoma of the ovary; remarks on drainage and the after-treatment in laparotomy. [Delivered at the hospital of the Philadelphia Polyclinic.] [Philadelphia, 1890.] 12p. DNLM **90-0224**

BAER, B[enjamin] F[ranklin] (1846-1920)
A plea for early diagnosis in the pelvic diseases of women. [Philadelphia, 1892.] 13p. DNLM **90-0225**

BAER, B[enjamin] F[ranklin] (1846-1920)
Supra-vaginal hysterectomy without ligature of the cervix, in operation for uterine fibroids. A new method. Cases of chronic ovarian abscess illustrating the danger of delay in their proper management. Drainage in abdominal surgery. Its unnecessary and excessive use. [Philadelphia, 1893.] 20p. DNLM **90-0226**

BAER, B[enjamin] F[ranklin] (1846-1920)
A supplemental paper upon supra-vaginal hysterectomy by the new method, with report of additional cases. [Philadelphia, 1893.] 12p. DNLM **90-0227**

BAER, B[enjamin] F[ranklin] (1846-1920)
Report of cases, with presentation of specimens. New York, 1895. 7p. DNLM **90-0228**

BAILEY, Pearce (1865-1922)
Three cases of Brown-Séquard paralysis, with remarks, on the sensory tract in the human spinal cord. New York, 1895. 14p. DNLM **90-0229**

BAILEY, Pearce (1865-1922)
Valvular disease of the heart in tabes. [New York, 1895.] 4p. DNLM **90-0230**

BAILEY, Pearce (1865-1922)
Report upon two cases of tumor of the spinal cord, unaccompanied by severe pain. New York, 1896. 8p. DNLM **90-0231**

BAILEY, Pearce (1865-1922) and James EWING
A contribution to the study of acute ascending (Landry's) paralysis. New York: D. Appleton & Co., 1896. 38p. 1 plate. DNLM; NNNAM **90-0232**

BAILEY, Pearce (1865-1922)
Accident and injury; their relations to diseases of the nervous system. . . . New York: D. Appleton & Co., 1898. 430p. col. plates. DLC; NNNAM **90-0233**

BAKER, Albert Rufus (*b.* 1858)
Myopia. Cleveland, 1890. 11p. DNLM **90-0234**

BAKER, Albert Rufus (*b.* 1858)
Functional nervous diseases of reflex origin. Chicago, 1890. 16p. DNLM **90-0235**

BAKER, Albert Rufus (*b.* 1858)
Coughs, colds, and catarrh: how to avoid. Cleveland, 1891. 15p. DNLM **90-0236**

BAKER, Albert Rufus (*b.* 1858)
Infantile cataract. Chicago, 1892. 12p. DNLM **90-0237**

BAKER, Albert Rufus (*b.* 1858)
The use of the electro-magnet in removing foreign bodies from the eye. [Cincinnati, 1893.] 4p. DNLM
90-0238

BAKER, Albert Rufus (*b.* 1858)
Dermoid tumors of the cornea. Chicago, 1896. 4p. DNLM
90-0239

BAKER, Frank (1841-1918)
Recent discoveries in the nervous system. New York, 1893. 41p. DNLM **90-0240**

BAKER, Henry B[rooks] (1837-1920)
Scarlet fever in Michigan in 1886: the average number of cases and deaths per outbreak. [Lansing, 1890.] 1 diag. DNLM
90-0241

BAKER, Henry B[rooks] (1837-1920)
Small-pox. Now is a good time to be vaccinated. [Lansing, 1890.] 1 broadside. DNLM **90-0242**

BAKER, Henry B[rooks] (1837-1920)
The climatic causation of consumption, with tables and diagrams representing the same. Chicago: Office of the Association, 1890. 40p. port. DNLM **90-0243**

BAKER, Henry B[rooks] (1837-1920)
A plea for public health work in villages. Harrisburg: E. K. Myers, 1891. 10p. DNLM **90-0244**

BAKER, Henry B[rooks] (1837-1920)
Sanitation in 1890. 31p. Chicago: Office American M. Association, 1891. 31p. DNLM **90-0245**

BAKER, William H[enry] (1845-1914)
Cancer of the cervix uteri; result in its treatment by high amputation. Philadelphia: W. J. Dornan, 1891. 38p. DNLM; PPC **90-0246**

BAKODY, Theodor von (*b.* 1825)
Scientific medicine in its relation to homoeopathy. Transl. from the German by Rudolph F. Bauer. Philadelphia: Boericke & Tafel, 1891. 60p. DNLM; PPHa **90-0247**

BALCH, Franklin G[reen] (*b.* 1864)
Five cases of compound fracture of the ankle-joint. Boston: Damrell & Upham, 1894. 7p. DNLM **90-0248**

BALCH, Lewis (1847-1909)
A manual for boards of health and health officers. Albany & New York: Banks & Brothers, 1893. 242p. DNLM; NN
90-0249

BALDWIN, David A.
The family pocket homoeopathist, a concise manual of homoeopathic practice, for families and travelers. 2nd ed. Rochester: E. Darrow & Co., 1890. 158p. NNNAM
90-0250

BALDWIN, David A.
The family pocket homoeopathist, a concise manual of homoeopathic practice, for families and travelers. 3rd ed. Rochester: E. Darrow & Co., 1894. 148p. NNNAM
90-0251

BALDY, J[ohn] M[ontgomery] (1860-1934)
Uterine fibromata; removal of twenty-seven, with two deaths. Philadelphia, 1892. 6p. DNLM **90-0252**

BALDY, J[ohn] M[ontgomery] (1860-1934)
Hysterectomy, indications and technique. New York, 1893. 13p. DNLM **90-0253**

BALDY, J[ohn] M[ontgomery] (1860-1934)
Removal of the uterus and its appendages for pelvic inflammatory disease. [Philadelphia, 1893.] 4p. DNLM
90-0254

BALDY, J[ohn] M[ontgomery] (1860-1934)
Phlegmasia alba dolens complicating laparotomy. New York, 1894. 3p. DNLM **90-0255**

BALDY, J[ohn] M[ontgomery], ed. (1860-1934)
An American text-book of gynecology, medical and surgical, for practitioners and students. By Henry T. Byford, M.D., J. M. Baldy, M.D., Edwin B. Cragin, M.D. . . . [and others]. . . . Philadelphia: W. B. Saunders, 1894. 713p. 37 plates, part col. DLC; DNLM; NNNAM; PPC
90-0256

BALDY, J[ohn] M[ontgomery], ed. (1860-1934)
An American text-book of gynecology, medical and surgical, for practitioners and students. By Henry T. Byford, M.D., J. M. Baldy, M.D., Edwin B. Cragin, M.D. . . . [and others]. . . . 2nd ed., rev. With 341 illustrations in the text, and 38 colored and half-tone plates. Philadelphia: W. B. Saunders, 1898. 718p. DLC; NNNAM; OCIM; PPC
90-0257

BALL, Francis P.
Remarks on pseudo-membranous croup, and diphtheric croup, and the value of intubation. Philadelphia: Lea Bros. & Co., 1894. 20p. DNLM **90-0258**

BALL, James B[arry] (1849-1926)
A handbook of diseases of the nose and naso-pharynx. 2nd ed. New York: William Wood & Co., 1895. 364p. DNLM; NNNAM
90-0259

BALL, M[ichael] V[alentine] (*b.* 1868)
Essentials of bacteriology; being a concise and systematic introduction to the study of micro-organisms for the use of students and practitioners. Philadelphia: W. B. Saunders, 1891. 159p. DLC; DNLM; PPC; PU **90-0260**

BALL, M[ichael] V[alentine] (*b.* 1868)
Essentials of bacteriology; being a concise and systematic introduction to the study of micro-organisms for the use of students and practitioners. 2nd ed. Philadelphia: W. B. Saunders, 1893. 205p. 5 plates. DLC; DNLM; PPC
90-0261

BALL, M[ichael] V[alentine]. (*b.* 1868)
The opium habit. Sudden and complete withdrawal without other medication as a method of treatment. Philadelphia, 1895. 2p. DNLM **90-0262**

BALL, M[ichael] V[alentine] (*b.* 1868)
. . . Essentials of bacteriology: being a concise and systematic introduction to the study of micro-organisms. . . . 3rd ed., rev. With eighty-one illustrations . . . and five plates. Philadelphia: W. B. Saunders, 1897. 218p. DLC: PPC; PPJ; PU
90-0263

BANE, William C.
Headache due to eye-strain. [Philadelphia, 1892.] 4p. DNLM
90-0264

BANE, William C.
Practical points in the treatment of some common diseases of the eye. [New York, 1892.] 9p. DNLM
90-0265

BANE, William C.
Inflammation of the middle ear, with involvement of the mastoid. Report of cases. Denver, 1895. 8p. DNLM
90-0266

BANGS, L[emuel] Bolton (1842-1914)
A case of obscure disease of the bladder treated by suprapubic cystotomy and prolonged drainage. [New York, 1890.] 8p. DNLM **90-0267**

BANGS, L[emuel] Bolton (1842-1914)
Some clinical features of stone in the bladder. [New York, 1891.] 15p. DNLM **90-0268**

BANGS, L[emuel] Bolton (1842-1914)
On the choice of operation for the removal of stone from the bladder. [St. Louis, 1892.] 6p. DNLM
90-0269

BANGS, L[emuel] Bolton (1842-1914)
A peculiar accident during a litholapaxy. [Baltimore, 1892.] 2p. DNLM **90-0270**

BANGS, L[emuel] Bolton (1842-1914)
Blood in the urine; how to discover its source, and what to do for it. [New York, 1892.] 8p. DNLM
90-0271

BANGS, L[emuel] Bolton (1842-1914)
Some of the effects of withdrawal. [Richmond, 1892.] 7p. DNLM **90-0272**

BANGS, L[emuel] Bolton (1842-1914)
The relative value of operative and hygienic measures in the treatment of tuberculosis and neoplasms of the bladder. Philadelphia, 1895. 12p. DNLM **90-0273**

BANGS, L[emuel] Bolton (1842-1914)
An American text-book of genito-urinary diseases, syphilis and diseases of the skin. Ed. by L. Bolton Bangs . . . and W. A. Hardaway. . . . Illustrated with 300 engravings and 20 full-page colored plates. Philadelphia: W. B. Saunders, 1898. 1229p. DLC; MBM; NNNAM; PPC **90-0274**

BANTA, Francis M.
The prevention of sepsis in the practice of midwifery. [New York, 1893.] 10p. DNLM **90-0275**

[BARBER, Elmer De Vergne] (*b.* 1858)
Osteopathy; the new science of healing. Kansas City, Mo.: Press of Hudson-Kimberly Publishing Co., [1896]. 170p. plates. **90-0276**

BARBER, Elmer De Vergne (*b.* 1858)
Osteopathy complete. . . . [Kansas City, Mo.: Press of Hudson-Kimberly Publishing Co., 1898.] 566p. plates. DLC
90-0277

BARBOUR, John Ford (1861-1896)
The uric acid diathesis and its treatment. New York, 1894. 8p. DNLM **90-0278**

BARBOUR, L. P.
The hygienic and dietetic management of phthisis. Atlanta, 1894. 8p. DNLM **90-0279**

BARCUS, Paul J.
Sudden death from shock due to the intra-uterine injection of a solution of lead acetate to induce abortion. Philadelphia, 1895. 2p. DNLM **90-0280**

BARD, Cephas L[yttle] (1843-1902)
Case of supra-pubic cystotomy performed to secure continuous drainage of the bladder. [Los Angeles, 1893.] 4p. DNLM
90-0281

BARD, Cephas L[yttle] (1843-1902)
The advantages of extension of the head during anaesthesia and some other conditions. [Los Angeles, 1893.] 12p. DNLM
90-0282

BARD, Cephas L[yttle] (1843-1902)
A contribution to the history of medicine in southern California. Annual address of the retiring president of the Southern California Medical Society, delivered at San Diego, August 8, 1894. [Los Angeles, 1894.] 34p. DNLM
90-0283

BARKAN, Louis
How to preserve health. New York, 1890. 344p. DNLM; NNNAM **90-0284**

BARKER, H[oward] H[inos] (1848-1910)
An open letter to Dr. Samuel C. Busey in review of Dr. Swan M. Burnett's "Historical sketch" of the Central Dispensary and Emergency Hospital. Washington, D.C.: Gibson Bros., 1895. 32p. DNLM **90-0285**

BARKER, Lewellys F[ranklin] (1867-1943)
A case of circumscribed unilateral and elective sensory paralysis. New York: D. Appleton & Co., 1896. 13p. DNLM
90-0286

BARKER, Lewellys F[ranklin] (1867-1943)
The nervous system and its constituent neurones; designed for the use of practitioners of medicine and of students of medicine and psychology. . . . With two colored plates and six hundred and seventy-six illustrations. . . . New York: D. Appleton & Co., 1899. 1122p. 2 fold. col. plates. DLC; MBM; NNNAM; PPC **90-0287**

BARNES, Justin L.
On symptomatic heterophoria. New York: D. Appleton & Co., 1894. 11p. DNLM **90-0288**

BARNEY, George D.
Anemia, its cause and treatment with pepto-mangan (Dr. Gude's). [New York: D. Appleton & Co., 1895.] 13p. DNLM
90-0289

BARR, Martin W. (1860-1938)
Cerebral meningitis. Its history, diagnosis, prognosis, and treatment. Detroit, Mich.: G. S. Davis, 1892. 93p. DNLM; OCIM **90-0290**

BARRETT, A[shley] William
Dental surgery for general practitioners and students of medicine. 2nd ed. Philadelphia: P. Blakiston, Son & Co., 1890. 136p. DNLM; MdU-D; PPC; PU
90-0291

BARRETT, A[shley] William
Dental surgery for general practitioners and students of medicine and dentistry. . . . 3rd ed. Philadelphia: P. Blakiston, Son & Co., 1897. 152p. DNLM; MdU-D; PPC; PU
90-0292

BARRETT, W[illiam] C[ary] (1834-1903)
Oral pathology and practice. A text-book for the use of students in dental colleges, and a hand-book for dental practitioners. . . . Philadelphia: S. S. White Dental Mfg. Co., 1898. 239p. DLC; MdU-D; PPC; PU **90-0293**

BARRINGER, Paul B[randon] (1857-1941)
The venomous reptiles of the United States, with the treatment of wounds inflicted by them. [Philadelphia, 1891.] 18p. DNLM **90-0294**

BARRINGER, Paul B[randon] (1857-1941)
An abstract of physiology for medical students and practitioners. 2nd ed. [University of Virginia]. Charlottesville: Anderson Bros., 1899. 474p. GU; NNNAM
90-0295

BARROW, David
Gun-shot wounds of the abdomen; with cases. Chicago, 1890. 12p. DNLM **90-0296**

BARROW, David
Cases of intestinal obstruction; laparotomy; remarks. [Toledo, 1891.] 8p. DNLM **90-0297**

BARROWS, Charles Clifford
Puerperal eclampsia treated by Duehrssen's incisions and veratrum viride; gangrene of the appendix vermiformis. [New York: D. Appleton & Co., 1895.] 13p. DNLM
90-0298

BARROWS, Isabel Chapin (1845-1913)
Physical training; a full report of the papers and discussions of the conference held in Boston in November, 1889, rep. and ed. by Isabel C. Barrows. Boston: George H. Ellis, 1899. 135p. MB; MH; NN **90-0299**

BARTHOLOW, Roberts (1831-1904)
A manual of hypodermatic medication; the treatment of diseases by the hypodermatic or subcutaneous method. . . . 5th ed. Rev. and enl. Philadelphia, [etc.]: J. B. Lippincott Co., 1891. 540p. DLC; MBM; NNNAM; PPC
90-0300

BARTHOLOW, Roberts (1831-1904)
A practical treatise on materia medica and therapeutics. . . . 8th ed., rev. and enl. New York: D. Appleton & Co., 1893. 820p. DLC; NNNAM; OCLloyd; PU
90-0301

BARTHOLOW, Roberts (1831-1904)
Cholera: its causes, symptoms, pathology and treatment. . . . Philadelphia: Lea Bros. & Co., 1893. 132p. DLC: NNNAM; PPC **90-0302**

BARTHOLOW, Roberts (1831-1904)
A treatise on the practice of medicine, for the use of students and practitioners of medicine. . . . 8th ed., rev. and enl. New York: D. Appleton & Co., 1895. 1003p. diags. DLC: NNNAM; OCIM; PPC **90-0303**

BARTHOLOW, Roberts (1831-1904)
A practical treatise on materia medica and therapeutics. . . . 9th ed., rev. and enl. New York: D. Appleton & Co., 1896. 866p. DLC; NNNAM; OCLloyd; PU **90-0304**

BARTHOLOW, Roberts (1831-1904)
A practical treatise on materia medica and therapeutics by. . . . 10th ed., rev. and enl. New York: D. Appleton & Co., 1899. 866p. DLC; MBM; OCLloyd; PPC **90-0305**

BARTLETT, Clarence (1858-1935)
Five cases in cerebral surgery. [Philadelphia, 1890.] 22p. DNLM **90-0306**

BARTLETT, Clarence (1858-1935)
The diagnostic significance of the tendon reflexes. [Philadelphia, 1890.] 13p. DNLM **90-0307**

BARTLETT, Clarence (1858-1935)
The treatment of apoplexy. [Philadelphia, 1892.] 5p. DNLM
90-0308

BARTLETT, Clarence (1858-1935)
The treatment of epilepsy. [Philadelphia, 1892.] 14p. DNLM
90-0309

BARTLETT, Clarence (1858-1935) and W. B. VAN LENNEP
Two cases of brain tumor. A contribution to cerebral surgery. Philadelphia: Sherman & Co., 1894. 10p. 1 plate. DNLM
90-0310

BARTLETT, E[dwin] J[ulius] (1851-1932)
The doctor and the lawyer, or Expert testimony again. . . . with discussion by Mr. J. H. Albin. . . . Concord, N.H.: Printed by The Rumford Press, [1898]. 36p. DLC
90-0311

BARTLETT, Frank H.
The relation of eye-strain to certain functional nervous disturbances. [New York: D. Appleton & Co., 1894.] 14p. DNLM
90-0312

BARTLETT, James W.
A short biographical sketch, and in memoriam of Dr. Carl Herrmann Horsch, 1822-1891. Cambridge: Riverside Press, 1893. 27p. DNLM; MBM **90-0313**

BARTLEY, Elias Hudson (1849-1937)
Text-book of medical chemistry. For medical and pharmaceutical students and practitioners. . . . 2nd ed. Rev. and enl. With sixty-two illustrations. Philadelphia: P. Blakiston, Son & Co., 1890. 423p. DLC; PPC; PU **90-0314**

BARTLEY, Elias Hudson (1849-1937)
Text-book of medical chemistry for medical and pharmaceutical students and practitioners. . . . 3rd ed., rev. and enl. With eighty-four illustrations. Philadelphia: P. Blakiston, Son & Co., 1894. 684p. DLC; MH-M; NNNAM; PPC
90-0315

BARTLEY, Elias Hudson (1849-1937)
Text-book of medical and pharmaceutical chemistry. . . . 4th ed., rev. and enl. With ninety-two illustrations. Philadelphia: P. Blakiston, Son & Co., 1895. 711p. DLC; IU-M; PPC: PPJ
90-0316

BARTLEY, Elias Hudson (1849-1937)
Text-book of medical and pharmaceutical chemistry. . . . 5th ed., rev. and enlarged. Philadelphia: P. Blakiston, Son & Co., 1898. 738p. DLC; NNNAM; OCIM; PU
90-0317

BARTLEY, Elias Hudson (1849-1937)
Manual of clinical chemistry. . . . Thirty-three illustrations. Philadelphia: P. Blakiston, Son & Co., 1899. 150p. DLC; ICRM; PPC; PPJ **90-0318**

BARTON, Clara (1821-1912)
The Red Cross, a history. . . . Washington, D.C.: American National Red Cross, 1898. 684p. MB; NIC; NN; PP
90-0319

BARTON, Clara (1821-1912)
The Red Cross in peace and war. [Washington, D.C.]: American Historical Press, 1899. 703p. ICU; MB; MH; NN
90-0320

BARTON, James M[orrie] (*b.* 1846)
Intestinal obstruction. [Philadelphia: Lea Bros. & Co., 1892.] 12p. DNLM **90-0321**

BARUCH, Simon (1840-1921)
The relation of peripheral irritation to disease; considered from a therapeutic standpoint. [Philadelphia, 1890.] 17p. DNLM
90-0322

BARUCH, Simon (1840-1921)
A plea for public baths, together with an inexpensive method for their hygienic utilization. [New York, 1891.] 45p. DNLM
90-0323

BARUCH, Simon (1840-1921)
Conditions indicating change of air and baths in the summer diarrhoea of children. [Philadelphia, 1892.] 10p. DNLM
90-0324

BARUCH, Simon (1840-1921)
The successful treatment of chronic diseases. A plea for their more methodical management. . . . [New York], 1892. 63p. DLC; NNNAM **90-0325**

BARUCH, Simon (1840-1921)
The uses of water in modern medicine. . . . Detroit, Mich.: G. S. Davis, 1892. 2 v. DLC; OCIM **90-0326**

BARUCH, Simon (1840-1921)
Practical data on the application of water in some intractable diseases. Read before the New York County Medical Society. New York: Stettiner, Lambert & Co., 1893. 12p. DNLM
90-0327

BARUCH, Simon (1840-1921)
Therapeutic reflections; a plea for physiological remedies. New York: Stettiner, Lambert & Co., 1893. 11p. DNLM
90-0328

BARUCH, Simon (1840-1921)
The clinical aspect of dyspepsia. [Charleston, 1895.] 20p. DNLM **90-0329**

BARUCH, Simon (1840-1921)
The principles and practice of hydrotherapy: a guide to the applicaton of water in disease, for student and practitioners of medicine. . . . New York: William Wood & Co., 1898. 455p. DLC; NNNAM **90-0330**

BARUCH, Simon (1840-1921)
The evolution of modern therapy. An address read before the Society of the Alumni of the Medical College of Virginia. Detroit, Mich.: W. M. Warren, 1899. 46p. DLC
90-0331

BASE, Daniel (*b.* 1869)
Elements of vegetable microscopy. . . . Preparatory to the study of pharmacognosy. . . . Baltimore, 1897. 66p. plates. DLC **90-0332**

BASSETTE, M. Imogene
The paralyses in children which occur during and after infectious diseases. [Chicago, 1892.] 33p. DNLM
90-0333

BATES, Kinzie
Vivisection. [Detroit, Mich.], 1895. 12p. DNLM
90-0334

BATES, William H[oratio] (1860-1931)
Treatment of chronic inflammation of the mucous membrane of the eye, ear, and throat. [Richmond, 1892.] 11p. DNLM
90-0335

BATES, William H[oratio] (1860-1931)
Conjunctivitis as a cause of poor vision. New York: Stettiner, Lambert & Co., 1892. 12p. DNLM
90-0336

BATES, William H[oratio] (1860-1931)
Notes on cataract extraction. Richmond, 1893. 12p. DNLM
90-0337

BATES, William H[oratio] (1860-1931)
Report of a case of plastic operation for the repairs of the inner canthus. Kansas City, 1893. 4p. DNLM
90-0338

BATES, William H[oratio] (1860-1931)
Traumatic deafness. [New York, 1893.] 6p. DNLM
90-0339

BATES, William H[oratio] (1860-1931)
A suggestion of an operation to correct astigmatism. New York, 1894. 13p. DNLM **90-0340**

BATES, William H[oratio] (1860-1931)
Syringing in lachrymal disease. Danbury, Conn., 1896. 16p. DNLM **90-0341**

BATTLE, Samuel Westray
A review of the mountain health resorts of North Carolina, and their possibilities; suggesting the desirability of graduated sanitaria or health stations at different elevations on and about the Asheville plateau. Asheville: D. W. Furman, 1892. 23p. DNLM **90-0342**

BAUDUY, J[erome] K[eating] (1842-1914)
Diseases of the nervous system. 2nd ed. Philadelphia: J. B. Lippincott Co., 1892. 352p. DLC; DNLM; PPC; PPJ
90-0343

BAUDUY, J[erome] K[eating] (1842-1914)
Observations upon the treatment of some cases of neurasthenia. . . . St. Louis, Mo., [1898]. 8p. DLC
90-0344

BAUER, Joseph L.
Two cases of stricture of the urethra, with interesting features. New York, 1892. 7p. DNLM **90-0345**

BAUER, Joseph L.
The why and wherefore of nervous prostration and allied states; some typical illustrations of the exercise of positive individuality and change of habit. St. Louis, [1894]. 8p. DNLM **90-0346**

BAUER, Joseph L.
The analysis of a crime. St. Louis, 1895. 10p. DNLM **90-0347**

BAUMGARTEN, Gustav (1837-1911)
On a simple continued fever. [Philadelphia], 1893. 13p. DNLM **90-0348**

BAUMGARTEN, Gustav (1837-1911)
The St. Louis Medical College. An historical address. Delivered at the semi-centennial celebration of the college, in Memorial Hall, October 18, 1892. St. Louis: Nixon-Jones, 1893. 19p. DNLM **90-0349**

BAUMGARTEN, Gustav (1837-1911)
Renal affections following influenza. Philadelphia, 1895. 12p. DNLM **90-0350**

BEACH, Bennett S[heldon]
Histology, pathology, and bacteriology. A manual for students and practitioners. Philadelphia: Lea Bros. & Co., [1892]. 165p. DLC; DNLM; PPC; PU **90-0351**

BEACH, Henry Harris Aubrey
Cerebral surgery. Observations. I. Traumatic epilepsy; operation; recovery. II. Tumor of brain; operation; death. Boston, Mass., 1890. 18p. 1 plate. DNLM **90-0352**

BEACH, Henry Harris Aubrey
Compression in the treatment of aneurism, with the description of a new appliance. Boston: Damrell & Upham, 1891. 10p. DNLM **90-0353**

BEACH, Henry Harris Aubrey
Exploration and treatment of fissures from skull fractures. Chicago, 1896. 8p. DNLM **90-0354**

BEAL, James Hartley (*b.* 1861)
Notes on equation writing and chemical arithmetic. . . . Columbus, O.: Nitschke Bros., 1896. 94p. DLC **90-0355**

BEAL, James Hartley (*b.* 1861)
Pharmaceutical interrogations, a list of classified questions upon subjects pertaining to pharmacy. . . . Columbus, O.: Press of Nitschke Bros., 1896. 154p. DLC **90-0356**

BEALL, Elias James (*b.* 1835), Amos C. WALKER and Edgar D. CAPPS
The fitness of the climate of Texas for operative surgery demonstrated by results in recent capital cases. [St. Louis: Commercial Pr. Co., 1894.] 9, 12p. DNLM **90-0357**

BEARD, George M[iller] (1839-1883)
Our home physician: the new encyclopaedia of family medicine. A popular guide to the art of preserving health and treating disease; with plain advice for all the medical and surgical emergencies of the family. . . . With an appendix giving homoeopathic remedies. By Samuel Lilienthal. . . . Rev., enl. and illustrated. . . . New York, Chicago: E. B. Treat, 1890. 1239, 105, [1481]-1506p. col. plates. DLC: IU-M; NNNAM; PPC **90-0358**

BEARD, George M[iller] (1839-1883)
On the medical and surgical uses of electricity by Geo. M. Beard . . . and A. D. Rockwell. . . . 8th ed. With over two hundred illustrations. New York: William Wood & Co., 1891. 788p. DLC; NNNAM; PPC; PU **90-0359**

BEARD, George M[iller] (1839-1883)
A practical treatise on nervous exhaustion (neurasthenia), its symptoms, nature, sequences, treatment. . . . Ed., with notes and additions, by A. D. Rockwell. . . . 3rd ed.—enl. New York: E. B. Treat, 1894. 262p. DLC; NNNAM **90-0360**

BEASLEY, Henry
The book of prescriptions, containing upwards of 3,000 prescriptions. . . . 7th ed. Philadelphia: P. Blakiston, Son & Co., 1892. 599p. DNLM; OCLloyd; PPC; PU **90-0361**

BECK, Carl (1856-1911)
On surgical diseases of the neck. New York, 1893. 44p. DNLM; NNNAM **90-0362**

BECK, Carl (1856-1911)
Zur Ehrenrettung des Perinealschnitts. Vortrat, verbunden mit Krankenvorstellung, gehalten in der deutschen medicinischen Gesellschaft von New York, 5. Dec. 1892. New York: The Cherouny Print. & Publ. Co., 1893. 8p. DNLM **90-0363**

BECK, Carl (1856-1911)
The value of ethereal solution of iodoform in the treatment of haemorrhoids. New York: D. Appleton & Co., 1894. 4p. DNLM **90-0364**

BECK, Carl (1856-1911)
On tubercular and suppurative peritonitis. New York, 1894. 25p. DNLM; NNNAM **90-0365**

BECK, Carl (1856-1911)
Pyothorax and its treatment. New York: Trow, 1894. 31p. DNLM **90-0366**

BECK, Carl (1856-1911)
. . . A manual of the modern theory and technique of surgical asepsis. . . . Philadelphia: W. B. Saunders, 1895. 306p. DLC; DNLM; NNNAM; PPC **90-0367**

BECK, Carl (1856-1911)
Exploratory pleurotomy and resection of costal pleura. New York, 1895. 8p. DNLM **90-0368**

BECK, Carl (1856-1911)
On some points in regard to sterilization in private dwellings. With the demonstration of some new aseptic appliances. Chicago, 1895. 7p. DNLM **90-0369**

BECK, Carl (1856-1911)
Subphrenic abscess. New York, 1896. 40p. DNLM
90-0370

BECK, Carl (1856-1911)
On some difficulties in reference to the early surgical treatment of appendicitis. Chicago, 1896. 16p. 2 plates. DNLM
90-0371

BECKWITH, S. R.
A new therapeutics for the cure of disease by sending ozone, oxygen, and medicine into diseased tissues. . . . New York: Thermo-Ozone Co., [1899]. 286p. DLC; NNNAM
90-0372

BEECHER, Abraham C. W. (1959?-1893)
California as a winter resort for invalids. [Philadelphia, 1891.] 2 galley sheets. DNLM **90-0373**

BEECHER, Maximilian P.
Beecher's dental directory, of the United States. [5th ed.] Brooklyn, N.Y.: M. P. Beecher, 1893. 180p. DLC; NNNAM
90-0374

BEECHHAVEN SANATORIUM. NEW PARIS, OHIO
A private hospital. "Beechhaven," for the treatment of nervous and mental diseases, opium, morphine, and chloral habits. [Illustrated circular of the management.] Dayton: Groneweg Print. Co., 1892. 15p. DNLM **90-0375**

BEELY, F[lorian] (*b.* 1846)
On the scope of orthopaedics. [New York: D. Appleton & Co., 1892.] 7p. DNLM **90-0376**

BELL, Alexander Graham (1847-1922)
Address upon the condition of articulation teaching in American schools for the deaf. Boston: N. Sawyer & Sons, 1893. 72p. DNLM **90-0377**

BELL, Alexander Graham (1847-1922)
Utility of signs. Penna. Inst. Print, 1894. 23p. DNLM
90-0378

BELL, James
Two cases of syphilis having a bearing on the question of the period during which the disease is communicable. [New York, 1894.] 4p. DNLM **90-0379**

BELL, James Bachelder (1838-1914)
The homoeopathic therapeutics of diarrhoea, dysentery, cholera, cholera morbus, cholera infantum, and all other loose evacuations of the bowels. . . . Philadelphia: Boericke & Tafel, 1897. 316p. DLC: PPC; PPHa **90-0380**

BELL, James H.
The question of general medical culture in an expanding science and a contracting personal field. [New York: D. Appleton & Co., 1891.] 6p. DNLM **90-0381**

BELL, James H.
Medical ethics gone to seed. [Philadelphia, 1892.] 10p. DNLM
90-0382

BELL, Victor C[harles] (*b.* 1867)
Popular essays upon the care of the teeth and mouth. [Buffalo, N.Y.], 1894. 103p. DLC; DNLM; NNNAM: PU
90-0383

BELL, Victor C[harles] (*b.* 1867)
Popular essays upon the care of the teeth and mouth. . . . [2nd ed.] New York, [etc.]: V. C. Bell, 1896. 112p. DLC; NN; NNNAM **90-0384**

BELLEVUE HOSPITAL. NEW YORK CITY
An account of Bellevue Hospital, with a catalogue of the medical and surgical staff from 1736 to 1894. Ed. by Robert J. Carlisle. New York: Society of the Alumni of Bellevue Hospital, 1893. 381p. 8 plates, 14 port. DNLM; NNNAM; NNU-M **90-0385**

BELT, Edward Oliver (1861-1906)
Rat-tail sutures. Philadelphia, 1891. 8p. DNLM
90-0386

BELT, Edward Oliver (1861-1906)
Ocular signs as aids to diagnosis. [Philadelphia, 1891.] 8p. DNLM **90-0387**

BELT, Edward Oliver (1861-1906)
Otitis media; abscess of neck; death. Nashville, Tenn.: A. R. Gray & Son, 1892. 8p. DNLM **90-0388**

BELT, Edward Oliver (1861-1906)
Sulphuric-acid paste in the treatment of epithelioma of the face. Philadelphia, 1894. 3p. DNLM **90-0389**

BELT, Edward Oliver (1861-1906)
Consanguineous marriage as a factor in the cause of disease. Philadelphia, 1896. 10p. DNLM **90-0390**

BELT, Edward Oliver (1861-1906)
Sponge grafting in the orbit for support of artificial eye. Philadelphia, 1896. 3p. DNLM **90-0391**

BENEDICT, A[rthur] L[incoln] (1865-1950)
The use of methol through the stomach tube. [Philadelphia, 1892.] 6p. DNLM **90-0392**

BENEDICT, A[rthur] L[incoln] (1865-1950)
The tube stripper. Philadelphia, 1894. 3p. DNLM
90-0393

BENEDICT, A[rthur] Lincoln] (1865-1950)
Auscultatory percussion and allied methods of physical diagnosis. [Philadelphia, 1895.] 12p. DNLM
90-0394

BENNETT, Alice (*b.* 1851)
Insanity as a symptom of "Bright's disease." Philadelphia: W. J. Dornan, 1890. 32p. DNLM **90-0395**

BENSON, John Alfred (1859-1898)
Asiatic cholera: its genesis, etiological facors, clinical history, pathology, and treatment. . . . Chicago: The J. H. White Co., 1893. 248p. fold. plate. DLC **90-0396**

BENSON, John A[lfred] (1859-1898)
Synopsis of a course of lectures on the anatomy, physiology and histo-chemistry of the nervous system. . . . Chicago: E. H. Colegrove & Co., 1895. 28p. DLC **90-0397**

BERMINGHAM, Edward John (*b.* 1853)
Chronic nasal catarrh, and what the general practitioner can do for it. New York: Chambers Print. Co., 1893. 45p. DLC; DNLM; NNNAM **90-0398**

BERMINGHAM, Edward John (*b.* **1853)**
Hypertrophic rhinitis. New York, 1895. 15p. DNLM
90-0399

BERMINGHAM, Edward John (*b.* **1853)**
Rhinological don'ts. What not to do in nasal affections. [Austin, 1895.] 2 l. DNLM **90-0400**

BERNARDY, Eugene Prosper
Use and abuse of the obstetrical forceps. Philadelphia: W. J. Dornan, 1890. 15p. DNLM **90-0401**

BERNARDY, Eugene Prosper
Hysterectomy for cancer in a pregnant uterus. New York, 1895. 5p. DNLM **90-0402**

BERNAYS, Augustus Charles (1854-1907)
Chips from a surgeon's workshop; five consecutive cases of gun-shot wounds of the abdominal viscera treated by abdominal section; two deaths, three recoveries. [St. Louis, 1890.] 27p. 1 plate. DNLM **90-0403**

BERNAYS, Augustus Charles (1854-1907)
The principles which govern our treatment of wounds; a résumé of our knowledge up to the present time. [St. Louis, 1890.] 7p. DNLM **90-0404**

BERNAYS, Augustus Charles (1854-1907)
The complete method of operation in cases of cancer of the breast. [St. Louis, 1895.] 7p. DNLM
90-0405

BERNAYS, Augustus Charles (1854-1907)
Report of a surgical clinic (illustrated). Complimentary to the visiting members of the Mississippi Valley Medical Association. St. Louis: C. B. Woodward Co., 1895. 20p. DNLM
90-0406

BERNHEIM, Hippolyte (1840-1919)
Suggestive therapeutics; a treatise on the nature and uses of hypnotism. . . . Transl. from the 2nd and rev. French ed. by Christian A. Herter. . . . New York, [etc.]: G. P. Putnam's Sons, 1895. 420p. diags. DLC; NNNAM; OCIM; PPC
90-0407

BERRY, George A[ndreas] (*b.* **1853)**
Diseases of the eye. A practical treatise for students of ophthalmology. 2nd ed. Philadelphia: Lea Bros. & Co., 1893. 727p. CtY-M; DNLM; PPC; PPJ **90-0408**

BERRY, H. S. D.
Irrigation in diseases of the male urethra. Milwaukee: The R. Hyde Co., [1890]. 2 l. DNLM **90-0409**

BETTMAN, Boerne (1856-1906)
The relation between the eyes and disease of the female genital organs. New York: William Wood & Co., 1893. 6p. DNLM
90-0410

BETTMAN, Boerne (1856-1906)
Spastic senile entropion cured by canthotomy. [Chicago, 1893.] 4p. DNLM **90-0411**

BETTMAN, Boerne (1856-1906)
Ripening of immature cataracts by direct trituration. Chicago, 1893. 7p. DNLM **90-0412**

BETTMAN, Boerne (1856-1906)
The treatment of blennorrhoea neonatorum. Chicago, 1893. 7p. DNLM **90-0413**

BETTMAN, Boerne (1856-1906)
Subvolution: a new pterygium operation. Chicago, 1894. 7p. DNLM **90-0414**

BETTMAN, Boerne (1856-1906)
The spectacle treatment of hypermetropia. [Chicago, 1894.] 3p. DNLM **90-0415**

BETTMAN, Boerne (1856-1906)
Ripening of immature cataract by direct trituration. [St. Louis, 1895.] 5p. DNLM **90-0416**

BETTMANN, Henry W.
The present status of the diphtheria-question. Philadelphia, 1895. 16p. DNLM **90-0417**

BETTMANN, Henry W.
Diphtheria, its bacterial diagnosis and treatment with the antitoxin. Philadelphia, 1895. 16p. DNLM
90-0418

BETZ, Frank S.
Illustrated catalogue of ear trumpets, trusses, surgical instruments, apparatus, etc. offered after twenty years' experience and growth. Hammond, Ind., [*c.* 1890]. 16p. OCIM
90-0419

BEUERMANN, John Augustus
The differential diagnosis between benign lymphomyxoma and malignant lymphomyeloma. New York: D. Appleton & Co., 1896. 13p. DNLM **90-0420**

BEYER, Henry G[ustav] (1850-1918)
A lecture on physical training and gymnastic exercise, delivered to the naval cadets at Annapolis, Md. [Annapolis?], 1892. 15p. DNLM **90-0421**

BEYER, Henry G[ustav] (1850-1918)
The influence of exercise on growth. [New York]: D. Appleton & Co., 1896. 13p. DNLM
90-0422

BIDDLE, John Barclay (1815-1879)
Materia medica and therapeutics, for physicians and students. . . . 12th ed. rev., rearranged and enl., with special reference to therapeutics, toxicology, and to the physiological action of medicine. By Clement Biddle. . . . With numerous illustrations, many of which are new to this edition. Philadelphia: P. Blakiston, Son & Co., 1892. 639p. DLC; DNLM; OCLloyd; PPC **90-0423**

BIDDLE, John Barclay (1815-1879)
Materia medica and therapeutics for physicians and students. . . . 13th ed. rev., rearranged and enl., with special reference to therapeutics, toxicology, the physiological action of medicines, and containing all the preparations and remedies described in the U.S. pharmacopoeia of 1890, to which the work has been made to conform. By Clement Biddle. . . . Philadelphia: P. Blakiston, Son & Co., 1895. 714p. DLC: DNLM; OCLloyd; PU
90-0424

BIGELOW, Horatio Ripley
Plain talks on electricity and batteries with therapeutic index. . . . Philadelphia: P. Blakiston, Son & Co., 1891. 85p. DLC; PPC; PU **90-0425**

BIGELOW, Horatio Ripley
Plain talks on electricity and batteries with therapeutic index. . . . 2nd ed., rev. Philadelphia: P. Blakiston, Son & Co., 1892. 85p. DLC; NNNAM; PPC; PU **90-0426**

BIGELOW, Horatio Ripley, ed.
An international system of electro-therapeutics . . . [with] thirty-eight associate editors. . . . Philadelphia: The F. A. Davis Co.; [etc., etc.], 1894. 1179p. plates, diags. DLC; MBM; NNNAM; PPC **90-0427**

BIGGS, Hermann M. (1859-1923) and John Henry HUDDLESTON
The sanitary supervision of tuberculosis as practiced by the New York City Board of Health. Philadelphia: Lea Bros. & Co., 1895. 9p. DNLM **90-0428**

BIGLER, William H[oward] (1840-1904)
Syllabus of lectures on physiology. Philadelphia: The Morris Press, 1898. 191p. DLC; PU **90-0429**

BILLINGS, John Shaw (1838-1913)
Vital statistics of the Jews in the United States. Washington, D.C., [1890]. 19p. 4 diags. DNLM **90-0430**

BILLINGS, John Shaw (1838-1913)
. . . Description of the Johns Hopkins Hospital. . . . Baltimore: [Press of J. Friedenwald], 1890. 116p. 56 plates. DLC; DNLM; MdBJ-W **90-0431**

BILLINGS, John Shaw (1838-1913)
The national medical dictionary: including English, French, German, Italian, and Latin technical terms used in medicine and the collateral sciences, and a series of tables of useful data. . . . Philadelphia: Lea Bros. & Co., 1890. 2 v. DLC; DNLM; NNNAM; PPC **90-0432**

BILLINGS, John Shaw (1838-1913)
American inventions and discoveries in medicine, surgery, and practical sanitation. Boston: Damrell & Upham, 1891. 12p. DNLM **90-0433**

BILLINGS, John Shaw (1838-1913)
. . . Ideals of medical education. The address in medicine, Yale University, 1891. . . . [New Haven], 1891. 22p. CtY-M; DLC **90-0434**

BILLINGS, John Shaw (1838-1913)
. . . Public health and municipal government. . . . An address delivered . . . Jan. 14, 1891. Philadelphia, [1891]. 23p. DLC **90-0435**

BILLINGS, John Shaw (1838-1913)
The objects, plans, and needs of the Laboratory of Hygiene. [Philadelphia, 1892.] 17p. DNLM **90-0436**

BILLINGS, John Shaw (1838-1913)
St. Augustine: report upon her present sanitary condition. New York: Trow Directory, 1892. 7p. DNLM **90-0437**

BILLINGS, John Shaw (1838-1913)
St. Augustine: report upon her present sanitary condition. New York: J. B. Watkins, 1892. 7p. DNLM **90-0438**

BILLINGS, John Shaw (1838-1913) and A[lexander] C. ABBOTT
A syllabus of the lectures on hygiene, vital statistics, etc., at the University of Pennsylvania. 1891-1892. Edited by Seneca Egbert. Philadelphia: Collins, 1892. 29p. DNLM **90-0439**

BILLINGS, John Shaw (1838-1913)
A condensed statement of the requirements of the principal university medical schools in Europe with regard to candidates for the degree of doctor of medicine. Baltimore: Privately printed, 1893. 25p. [printed only on one side]. DNLM **90-0440**

BILLINGS, John Shaw (1838-1913)
Ventilation and heating. New York: The Engineering Record, 1893. 500p. DNLM **90-0441**

BILLINGS, John Shaw (1838-1913)
Vital statistics of the District of Columbia and Baltimore, covering a period of six years, ending May 31, 1890. 52. Cong., 1. sess. H. R. Misc. Doc. No. 340, part 8. Washington: Government Printing Office, 1893. 241p. 12 col. maps. DNLM **90-0442**

BILLINGS, John Shaw (1838-1913)
World's Columbian Exposition, Chicago, Ill., 1892-1893. War Department exhibit. Medical Department, United States Army, No. 5. Description of microscopes from the Army Medical Museum, Washington, D.C. Chicago, 1893. 6p. DNLM **90-0443**

BILLINGS, John Shaw (1838-1913)
World's Columbian Exposition, Chicago, Ill., 1892-1893. War Department exhibit. Medical Department, United States Army, No. 5. Description of selected specimens from the Army Medical Museum, Washington, D.C. Chicago, 1893. 14p. DNLM **90-0444**

BILLINGS, John Shaw (1838-1913) and W[illiam] M. GRAY
Photomicrographs of normal histology, human and comparative, prepared by direction of the Surgeon-General. Washington: Government Printing Office, 1893. 2p. 76 phot. DNLM **90-0445**

BILLINGS, John Shaw (1838-1913)
Hygiene in university education. Boston: Damrell & Upham, 1894. 24p. DNLM **90-0446**

BILLINGS, John Shaw (1838-1913)
Methods of teaching surgery. Boston: Damrell & Upham, 1894. 13p. DNLM **90-0447**

BILLINGS, John Shaw (1838-1913)
Vital statistics of New York and Brooklyn, covering a period of six years, ending May 31, 1890. 52. Cong., 1. sess. H. R. Misc. Doc. 340, part 13. Washington: Government Printing Office, 1894. 529p. 12 maps. DNLM **90-0448**

BILLINGS, John Shaw (1838-1913)
Bibliography (preliminary) of the literature on the physiological and pathological effects of alcohol and alcoholic drinks. Edited for "The committee of fifty for the investigation of the liquor problem." . . . Washington, D.C.: Judd & Detweiler, 1894. 28p. DNLM **90-0449**

BILLINGS, John Shaw (1838-1913)
Municipal mortality statistics. Philadelphia, 1895. 9p. DNLM
90-0450

BILLINGS, John Shaw (1838-1913)
Report on the social statistics of cities in the United States at the Eleventh Census, 1890. Washington: Government Printing Office, 1895. 137p. 1 cartog., 33 diags. DNLM
90-0451

BILLINGS, John Shaw (1838-1913)
Waste. Address on commencement day at Miami University, Oxford, Ohio. Oxford, 1895. 19p. DNLM
90-0452

BILLINGS, John Shaw (1838-1913)
Vital statistics of Boston and Philadelphia, covering a period of six years, ending May 31, 1890. Washington: Government Printing Office, 1895. 229p. 12 maps. DNLM
90-0453

BILLINGS, John Shaw (1838-1913)
The William Pepper Laboratory of Clinical Medicine. Address given at the opening of the laboratory, December 4, 1895. [Philadelphia, 1895.] 15p. DNLM
90-0454

BILLINGS, John Shaw (1838-1913)
The history and literature of surgery. New York, 1895. 144p. DNLM; NNNAM; PPC; PU [Rep. from Dennis, Syst. Surg. (New York, 1895), I] **90-0455**

[BILLINGS, John Shaw] (1838-1913)
Banquet and presentation in honor of John S. Billings. Philadelphia: Lea Bros. & Co., 1895. 24p. DNLM
90-0456

BILLINGS, John Shaw (1838-1913)
Suggestions to hospital and asylum visitors. By John S. Billings . . . and Henry M. Hurd. . . . With an introduction by S. Weir Mitchell, M.D. Philadelphia: J. B. Lippincott Co., 1895. 48p. DLC; DNLM; PPC; PU **90-0457**

BILLINGS, John S., Jr.
The leucocytes in croupous pneumonia. [Baltimore, 1894.] 22p. DNLM **90-0458**

BILLINGS, John S., Jr.
The leucocytes in malarial fever. [Baltimore, 1894.] 10p. DNLM **90-0459**

BILLINGS, John S., Jr.
Therapeutic use of extract of bone marrow. [Baltimore, 1894.] 6p. 3 charts. DNLM **90-0460**

BISHOP, Francis B[esant] (1853-1916)
Electricity versus old methods in female pelvic disorders. Richmond, 1895. 8p. DNLM **90-0461**

BISHOP, Louis Faugères (1864-1941)
A new measurement in the study of fever. Philadelphia, 1893. 5p. DLC; DNLM **90-0462**

BISHOP, Louis Faugères (1864-1941)
Paroxysmal hemoglobinuria due to cold. [Philadelphia, 1895.] 2p. DNLM **90-0463**

BISHOP, Louis Faugères (1864-1941)
The value of bimanual simultaneous examination of symmetric structures. Philadelphia, 1895. 3p. DNLM
90-0464

BISHOP, Louis Faugères (1864-1941)
The diagnosis and treatment of gout. Philadelphia, 1896. 14p. DLC; DNLM **90-0465**

BISHOP, Louis Faugères (1864-1941)
Medicine as a profession. New York: McAuliffe & Booth, 1896. 8p. DLC; DNLM **90-0466**

BISHOP, Louis Faugères (1864-1941)
The theory and treatment of rheumatism . . . with discussion by Wm. H. Draper, M.D., Beverly Robinson, M.D., Robert W. Taylor, M.D., and Wm. H. Thomson, M.D. . . . New York: The Publishers' Printing Co., 1896. 23p. DLC; NNNAM
90-0467

BISHOP, Louis Faugères (1864-1941)
The importance of the habit of prognosis in the development of the individual physician. . . . Chicago: American Medical Association Press, 1897. 4p. DLC **90-0468**

BISHOP, Louis Faugères (1864-1941)
A study of the symptomatology of the neurasthenia in women. . . . [New York, 1897.] 11p. DLC **90-0469**

BISHOP, Louis Faugères (1864-1941)
I. The scientific spirit in practical medicine. . . . II. The importance of the habit of prognosis in the development of the individual physician. . . . III. Some points, important for consideration, in the treatment of acute lobar pneumonia. . . . New York, 1897. 22p. DLC; NNNAM **90-0470**

BISHOP, Louis Faugères (1864-1941)
The debility of adolescence. . . . Chicago: American Medical Association Press, 1898. 8p. DLC **90-0471**

BISHOP, Louis Faugères (1864-1941)
The influence of sex on disease. Presented to the section of obstetrics and diseases of woman at the forty-ninth annual meeting of the American Medical Association held at Denver, Colo., June 7-10, 1898. . . . Chicago: American Medical Association Press, 1898. 4p. DLC **90-0472**

BISHOP, Louis Faugères (1864-1941)
The evolution of scientific medicine. . . . [New York, 1898.] 4p. DLC **90-0473**

BISHOP, Seth Scott (1852-1923)
Imperforate auditory canals. Chicago, 1890. 8p. DNLM
90-0474

BISHOP, Seth Scott (1852-1923)
Camphor-menthol in catarrhal diseases. Chicago, 1891. 3 l. DNLM **90-0475**

BISHOP, Seth Scott (1852-1923)
A new pathology and treatment of nervous catarrh. Chicago, 1893. 16p. DNLM **90-0476**

BISHOP, Seth Scott (1852-1923)
New instruments. Chicago, 1894. 3p. DNLM
90-0477

BISHOP, Seth Scott (1852-1923)
Address on the founding of the Illinois Hospital. Chicago, 1895. 4p. DNLM **90-0478**

BISHOP, Seth Scott (1852-1923)
Camphor-menthol; a supplementary report. Chicago, 1895. 4p. DNLM **90-0479**

BISHOP, Seth Scott (1852-1923)
The dilator in diseases of the air passages and the ear. [Chicago], 1895. 4p. DNLM **90-0480**

BISHOP, Seth Scott (1852-1923)
Grip, and its effects on the nose, throat, and ear. Detroit, 1895. 6p. DNLM **90-0481**

BISHOP, Seth Scott (1852-1923)
Improved double retractors. Chicago, 1895. 1 l. DNLM **90-0482**

BISHOP, Seth Scott (1852-1923)
Diseases of the ear, nose, and throat and their accessory cavities. A condensed text-book. . . . Philadelphia, New York, [etc.]: The F. A. Davis Co., 1897. 496p. col. plates. DLC; NNC; NNNAM; PPC **90-0483**

BISHOP, Seth Scott (1852-1923)
Diseases of the ear, nose, and throat, and their accessory cavities. . . . 2nd ed., thoroughly rev. and enl. Illustrated with ninety-four colored lithographs and sixteen additional illustrations. Philadelphia, New York, [etc.]: The F. A. Davis Co., 1898. 554p. col. plates. DLC; NNNAM; PPC; PU **90-0484**

BISS, Cecil Yates and A. Pierce GOULD
A case of intussusception treated by laparotomy, terminating in complete recovery. Philadelphia, 1892. 5p. DNLM **90-0485**

BISSEL, J. Dougal (*b.* 1864)
A trocar which both clamps and empties a cyst without permitting the escape of fluid into the abdominal cavity. New York, 1894. 4p. DNLM **90-0486**

BISSELL, Mary Taylor
Household hygiene. New York: N. D. C. Hodges, 1890. 83p. DNLM; NN **90-0487**

BISSELL, Mary Taylor
A manual of hygiene. New York, [1894]. 338p. DNLM; NNNAM **90-0488**

BISSELL, William G[rosvenor] (*b.* 1870)
Bacteriologic examination in the diagnosis of diphtheria. [Philadelphia, 1895.] 10p. DNLM **90-0489**

BLACK, D[onald] Campbell (1841-1898)
The urine in health and disease, and urinary analysis, physiologically and pathologically considered. Philadelphia: Lea Bros. & Co., 1895. 246p. ICJ; PPC; PPJ; PU **90-0490**

BLACK, G. Melville
Strychnine nitrate in toxic amblyopia from alcohol and tobacco. With report of cases. [New York: D. Appleton & Co., 1895.] 6p. DNLM **90-0491**

BLACK, G. Melville
Removal of the drum-head and ossicles in diseases of the middle ear. [Philadelphia, 1893.] 11p. DNLM **90-0492**

BLACK, G. Melville
A new instrument for vibratory massage of the nasal mucous membrane. New York, 1894. 5p. DNLM **90-0493**

BLACK, G. Melville
Nasal sarcoma cured by operation. New York, 1896. 6p. DNLM **90-0494**

BLACK, Greene Vardiman (1836-1915)
Descriptive anatomy of the human teeth. . . . Philadelphia: The Wilmington Dental Manufacturing Co., 1890. 153p. plates. DLC; PU **90-0495**

BLACK, Greene Vardiman (1836-1915)
Descriptive anatomy of the human teeth. 2nd ed. . . . Philadelphia: The Wilmington Dental Manufacturing Co., 1892. 161p. plates. DLC; PPC; PU **90-0496**

BLACK, Greene Vardiman (1836-1915)
Descriptive anatomy of the human teeth. 3rd ed. . . . Philadelphia: The Wilmington Dental Manufacturing Co., [1894]. 171p. plates. DLC; DNLM; PPC **90-0497**

BLACK, Greene Vardiman (1836-1915)
Descriptive anatomy of the human teeth. 4th ed. . . . Philadelphia: The S. S. White Manufacturing Co., 1897. 169p. plates. DLC; PPC; PU **90-0498**

BLACK, Greene Vardiman (1836-1915)
The technical procedure in filling teeth. . . . Chicago: The H. O. Shepard Co., printers, 1899. 156p. DLC **90-0499**

[BLACK, J[ames] M.]
Ectopic-gestation. A living foetus at twelve months; report of a case. New York, 1895. 2p. DNLM **90-0500**

BLACKBURN, Isaac W[right] (1851-1911)
A manual of autopsies, designed for the use of hospitals for the insane and other public institutions. . . . Philadelphia: P. Blakiston, Son & Co., 1892. 84p. plates. DLC; DNLM; PPC; PU **90-0501**

BLACKFORD, Charles Minor (1865-1924)
Medical education, as it was, as it is, and as it might be. [Richmond, 1891.] 18p. DLC; DNLM **90-0502**

BLACKFORD, Charles Minor (1865-1924)
Bacteria nd disease. Richmond, 1892. 11p. DNLM **90-0503**

BLACKFORD, Charles Minor (1865-1924)
Tetanus. The essay for which Dr. Hunter McGuire's prize of one hundred dollars was awarded. [Richmond, 1892.] 13p. DNLM **90-0504**

BLACKFORD, Charles Minor (1865-1924)
The pathology and treatment of gonorrhoea. Atlanta, 1894. 6p. DNLM **90-0505**

BLACKWELL, Elizabeth (1821-1910)
The influence of women in the profession of medicine. Address given at the opening of the winter session of the London School of Medicine for Women. [Baltimore], 1890. 32p. MdBM; MdU-D **90-0506**

BLACKWELL, Elizabeth (1821-1910)
Pioneer work in opening the medical profession to women; autobiographical sketches. . . . London and New York: Longmans, Green & Co., 1895. 265p. DLC; MB; MH; NN **90-0507**

BLACKWOOD, W[m.] R[obt.] D[oug.] (1839-1922)
A year's work in electro-therapeutics. Concerning the merits of differently made apparatus. Baltimore, 1894. 15p. DNLM **90-0508**

BLAIKIE, William (1843-1904)
How to get strong and how to stay so. With numerous portraits. New & enl. ed. from new plates. New York: Harper Bros., 1898. 510p. ICU; MB; NN; NIC **90-0509**

BLAKE, Clarence J[ohn] (1843-1919)
The Boston City Hospital. Boston: Damrell & Upham, 1890. 7p. DNLM **90-0510**

BLAKE, Clarence J[ohn] (1843-1919)
Boston hospitals. Boston: Damrell & Upham, 1891. 16p. 1 plate. DNLM **90-0511**

BLAKE, Clarence J[ohn] (1843-1919)
Mastoid cases. [New Bedford, Mass., 1893.] 43p. DNLM **90-0512**

BLAKE, Clarence J[ohn] (1843-1919)
Middle ear operations. [New Bedford, Mass., 1893.] 12p. DNLM **90-0513**

BLAKE, Edward T. (1842-1905)
Constipation and corpulency, etiologically considered. Philadelphia: F. J. Redman, 1893. 25p. DNLM **90-0514**

BLANC, Henry William (1861?-1896)
A review of five years of physiological practice in New Orleans. [New York, 1892.] 24p. DNLM **90-0515**

BLAND-SUTTON, John (1855-1936)
Tumours. Innocent and malignant. Their clinical features and appropriate treatment. Philadelphia: Lea Bros. & Co., 1893. 511p. CtY-M; NNNAM; PPC; PU **90-0516**

BLAND-SUTTON, John (1855-1936)
The diseases of women; a handbook for students and practitioners, by J. Bland Sutton . . . and Arthur E. Giles. . . . With 115 illustrations. Philadelphia: W. B. Saunders, 1897. 436p. DLC; MBM; PPC; PU **90-0517**

BLECH, Gustavus M[aximillian] (*b.* 1870)
Rational therapeutics. New York, 1895. 4p. DNLM **90-0518**

BLECH, Gustavus M[aximillian] (*b.* 1870)
What is asepsis? New York, 1895. 3p. DNLM **90-0519**

BLECH, Gustavus M[aximillian] (*b.* 1870)
Can antitoxin statistics be relied upon? Chicago, 1896. 2 l. DNLM **90-0520**

BLECH, Gustavus M[aximillian] (*b.* 1870)
Modern methods of treatment of typhoid fever critically reviewed, with suggestions for a rational therapeusis. Chicago, 1896. 12p. DNLM **90-0521**

BLEYER, J[ulius] Mount (1859-1915)
A new method of laryngeal and bronchial medication by means of a spray and tube during the act of deep inspiration. Chicago, 1890. 7p. DNLM **90-0522**

BLEYER, J[ulius] Mount (1859-1915)
A record of the results of five hundred and twelve cases of intubation of the larynx operated on between 1886 and the present year. [New York, 1891.] 14p. DNLM **90-0523**

BLEYER, J[ulius] Mount (1859-1915) and M. Milton WEILL
The primary action of the galvanic current; it increases the amount of ozone in the blood as shown by chemical test of the blood in the arteries; with our theory of animal electricity. [New York, 1893.] 16p. DNLM **90-0524**

BLEYER, J[ulius] Mount (1859-1915)
An abstract of a lecture on the new rays of Röntgen, the new photography, and the photo-fluoroscope, Their joint application in medicine. New York, 1896. 14p. DNLM **90-0525**

BLEYER, J[ulius] Mount (1859-1915)
Crookes's "X" and other light rays. A problem yet to be solved in therapeutics, etc. New York, 1896. 11p. DNLM **90-0526**

BLICKBAHN, W[alter] L.
A case of ankylostomiasis. [Philadelphia, 1893.] 4p. DNLM **90-0527**

BLISS, Arthur Ames (*d.* 1913)
Three cases of occlusion of the nares by deflection of the nasal septum; operation. [Philadelphia, 1890.] 3p. DNLM **90-0528**

BLISS, Arthur Ames (*d.* 1913)
General report of an examination of 415 young deaf-mutes, in regard to the nasal chambers, ears, and organs of phonation. [Philadelphia: Lea Bros. & Co., 1892.] 8p. DNLM **90-0529**

BLISS, Arthur Ames (*d.* 1913)
Abnormalities of the upper respiratory tract and ear, found commonly among deaf-mutes. Rochester, 1894. 41p. DNLM **90-0530**

BLISS, Arthur Ames (*d.* 1913)
Report of a case of epithelioma and of one of sarcoma of the larynx. New York: D. Appleton & Co., 1894. 6p. DNLM **90-0531**

BLISS, Arthur Ames (*d.* 1913)
A contribution to the study of deaf-mutism. Philadelphia, 1895. 12p. DNLM **90-0532**

BLODGETT, Albert Novatus (1848-1923)
The continuous inhalation of oxygen in cases of pneumonia otherwise fatal, and in other diseases. Boston: Damrell & Upham, 1890. 21p. DNLM; MBM **90-0533**

BLODGETT, Samuel
The scientific skeleton. . . . Grafton, N.D.: [S. Blodgett, 1897.] 105p. diags. DLC **90-0534**

BLUMER, George and Hugh H. YOUNG
A case of anthrax septicaemia in a human being associated with acute endocarditis and peritonitis. Baltimore, 1895. 16p. DNLM **90-0535**

BLYTH, Alexander Wynter (1844-1921)
A manual of public health. . . . New York: Macmillan & Co., 1890. 653p. col. plates. DLC: ICU; NNNAM; PU **90-0536**

BOARDMAN, William S.
The treatment of pulmonary tuberculosis by the subcutaneous use of the chloride of gold and sodium with the iodide of manganese. Boston, 1894. 6p. 2 tables. DNLM **90-0537**

BODINE, John A[lfred] (1865-1919)
New method of performing intestinal anastomosis with special reference to its adaptability to inguinal colostomy and subsequent restoration of the fecal current. New York, 1897. 15p. DNLM **90-0538**

BODINE, J[ames] M[orrison] (1831-1915)
The four commencements. Valedictory address. Louisville: J. P. Morton & Co., 1890. 19p. DNLM **90-0539**

BOECKEL, WILLIAM & CO.
Illustrated catalogue of surgical goods and chemical apparatus. Philadelphia, 1893. 54p. NNNAM; PU **90-0540**

BOENNING, Henry C.
A treatise on practical anatomy: for students of anatomy and surgery. . . . Illustrated with 198 wood engravings. Philadelphia and London: F. A. Davis, 1891. 481p. DLC; NNNAM; PPC; PU **90-0541**

BOENNINGHAUSEN, C. von (1785-1864)
Boenninghausen's therapeutic pocket-book for homoeopathic physicians; to use at the bedside, and in the study of the materia medica. A new American edition, by Timothy Field Allen. Philadelphia: The Hahnemann Publishing House, 1891. 484p. NNNAM; PPC; PPHa; PU **90-0542**

BOERICKE & RUNYON
Descriptive catalogue of homoeopathic pharmaceuticals. San Francisco, [*c.* 1895] . 87p. IU-M; OCLloyd **90-0543**

BOERICKE & TAFEL
Physicians' catalogue, medicines and books, sundries for physicians. New York, 1894. 184p. NNNAM; PPHa **90-0544**

BOERICKE, William (1849-1929)
The twelve tissue remedies of Schüssler, comprising the theory, therapeutical application, materia medica, and a complete repertory of these remedies. Homoeopathically and biochemically considered. By William Boericke . . . and Willis A. Dewey. . . . 3rd ed., rewritten and enl. Philadelphia: Boericke & Tafel, 1893. 384p. DLC; PPC; PPHa **90-0545**

BOERICKE, William (1849-1929)
A compend of the principles of homoeopathy as taught by Hahnemann, and verified by a century of clinical application. . . . San Francisco: Boericke & Runyon, 1896. 160p. DLC **90-0546**

BOERICKE, William (1849-1929)
The treatment of disease with the twelve tissue remedies being a treatise on biochemistry. . . . San Francisco, Cal.: Boericke & Runyon, 1897. 194p. DLC **90-0547**

BOERICKE, William (1849-1929)
The twelve tissue remedies of Schüssler, comprising the theory, therapeutic application, materia medica, and a complete repertory of these remedies. Homoeopathically and biochemically considered. By William Boericke . . . and Willis A. Dewey. . . . 4th ed., rewritten and enl. Philadelphia: Boericke & Tafel, 1899. 424p. DLC; OCIM; PPC; PPHa **90-0548**

BOISE, Eugene (*b.* 1846)
Opium and catharsis after abdominal section. [New York, 1894.] 10p. DNLM **90-0549**

BOISE, Eugene (*b.* 1846)
The pathology and treatment of shock. New York, 1896. 13p. DNLM **90-0550**

BOISLINIÈRE, Louis Charles C[herot] (1816-1896)
Obstetric accidents, emergencies, and operations. Philadelphia: W. B. Saunders, 1896. 381p. DNLM; MBM; NNNAM; PPC **90-0551**

BOLAND, Mary A. (*b.* 1852)
A handbook of invalid cooking, for the use of nurses in training schools, nurses in private practice, and others who care for the sick; containing explanatory lessons on the properties and value of different kinds of food, and recipes for the making of various dishes. New York: Century Co., 1893. 323p. DNLM; NN **90-0552**

BOLDT, H[ermann] John (*b.* 1856)
Contribution to the literature concerning the normal mucous membrane of the uterus. [Philadelphia, 1890.] 2 l. 2 plates. DNLM **90-0553**

BOLDT, H[ermann] John (*b.* 1856)
Peritonitis due to rupture of an ovarian haematoma; laparotomy; recovery. [Philadelphia, 1890.] 7p. DNLM **90-0554**

BOLDT, H[ermann] John (*b.* 1856)
Salpingo-oöphorectomy and its results. New York: Trow, 1890. 7p. DNLM **90-0555**

BOLDT, H[ermann] John (*b.* 1856)
The treatment of posterior displacements of the uterus. New York: William Wood & Co., 1890. 13p. DNLM **90-0556**

BOLDT, H[ermann] John (*b.* 1856)
The treatment of posterior displacements of the uterus with the utero-vaginal ligature. [Philadelphia: Lea Bros. & Co., 1891.] 6p. DNLM **90-0557**

BOLDT, H[ermann] John (*b.* 1856)
Suppurative oöphoritis. New York: M. J. Rooney, 1892. 17p. DNLM **90-0558**

BOLDT, H[ermann] John (*b.* 1856)
Vaginal hysterectomy in cancer of the uterus. New York: William Wood & Co., 1892. 30p. DNLM
90-0559

BOLDT, H[ermann] John (*b.* 1856)
The operative treatment for myo-fibroma of the uterus. New York, 1893. 23p. DNLM **90-0560**

BOLDT, H[ermann] John (*b.* 1856)
Pelvic elevation in abdominal surgery, with a new transportable table for obtaining this posture. New York, 1893. 2 l. DNLM
90-0561

BOLDT, H[ermann] John (*b.* 1856)
The effects of various metals on the growth of certain bacteria. Philadelphia, 1894. 10p. DNLM **90-0562**

BOLDT, H[ermann] John (*b.* 1856)
Ligation of the uterine arteries for the cure of a fibro-myomatous tumor of the uterus. [New York, 1894.] 3p. DNLM **90-0563**

BOND, C[harles] S.
Early diagnosis of chronic kidney lesions. [Philadelphia, 1890.] 14p. DNLM **90-0564**

BOND, Young H.
A knowledge or a time requirement. A plea for a more rational system of medical legislation. [St. Louis, 1891.] 12p. DNLM
90-0565

BONDURANT, E[ugene] D[u Bose]
Duplication of the spinal cord, as a result of post-mortem injury. Philadelphia, 1894. 10p. DNLM
90-0566

BONDURANT, Eugene D[u Bose]
"Horse-nettle" in the treatment of epilepsy. Philadelphia, 1895. 7p. DNLM **90-0567**

BONDURANT, Eugene D[u Bose]
Brief studies in tuberculosis among the insane. [New York: D. Appleton & Co., 1895.] 10p. DNLM
90-0568

BONDURANT, Eugene D[u Bose]
Report of thirteen cases of multiple neuritis occurring among insane patients. Philadelphia, 1896. 16p. DNLM
90-0569

BONDURANT, Eugene D[u Bose]
Arterio-sclerosis among the insane. Philadelphia, 1896. 12p. DNLM **90-0570**

BOOKER, William D[avid] (1844-1921)
The relation of pseudo-diphtheric angina to diphtheria, with special reference to scarlatinal pseudo-membranous angina. [Baltimore, 1892.] 10 l. DNLM **90-0571**

BOONE, H. W.
Disarticulation at the hip-joint. A new method of controlling hemorrhage during the operation. Philadelphia, 1892. 3p. DNLM **90-0572**

BOOTH, James Arthur (*b.* 1856)
Two cases of tumor of the cerebellum. [New York, 1890.] 9p. DNLM **90-0573**

BOOTH, James Arthur (*b.* 1856) and B. Farquhar CURTIS
Report of a case of tumor of the left frontal lobe of the cerebrum; operation; recovery. Philadelphia: Univ. Penn. Press, 1893. 13p. DNLM **90-0574**

BOOTH, James Arthur (*b.* 1856)
Some clinical notes on eight cases of exophthalmic goitre. New York, 1894. 12p. DNLM **90-0575**

BORCK, Mathias Adolph Edward (1834-1912)
Synopsis of one hundred ovariotomies. St. Louis: Weiss & Maccallum, 1895. 12p. DNLM **90-0576**

BORCK, Mathias Adolph Edward (1834-1912)
I. Sleeve bandage for fracture of the clavicle. II. Fractures and dislocations of radius and ulna. St. Louis: Weiss & Maccallum, 1896. 16p. DNLM **90-0577**

BOSTON vegetable vapor. A safe and pleasant substitute for ether, chloroform, nitrous oxide, and all dangerous substances used to destroy pain in dentistry and surgery. 7th ed. Boston, [1892]. 46p. DNLM; MBM **90-0578**

BOSWORTH, Francke H[untington] (1845-1925)
A treatise on diseases of the nose and throat. New York: William Wood & Co., 1890-1892. 2 v. plates. DNLM; NNNAM; OCIM; PU **90-0579**

BOSWORTH, Francke H[untington] (1845-1925)
Taking cold. Detroit: G. S. Davis, 1891. 69p. DLC; DNLM; NNNAM **90-0580**

BOSWORTH, Francke H[untington] (1845-1925)
A text-book of diseases of the nose and throat. New York: William Wood & Co., 1896. 814p. 7 plates. DLC; DNLM; NNNAM; PPC **90-0581**

BOSWORTH, Francke H[untington] (1845-1925)
. . . The doctor in old New York. . . . New York, [etc.]: G. P. Putnam's Sons, 1898. [277]-317p. DLC; NNNAM
90-0582

BOUCHARD, Charles (1837-1915)
Lectures on auto-intoxication in disease, or self-poisoning of the individual. Transl., with a preface, by Thomas Oliver. Philadelphia: F. A. Davis, 1894. 302p. NNNAM; PPC
90-0583

BOVEE, J. W[esley] (1861-1927)
An unusual case of pelvic enucleation per vaginam. Cancer of the cervix, fibroma of the fundus and tubo-ovarian abscess; recovery. Richmond, 1895. 4p. DNLM
90-0584

BOVEE, J. W[esley] (1861-1927)
Case of ruptured tubal pregnancy at seven weeks; laparotomy and recovery; remarks. Richmond, 1895. 3p. DNLM
90-0585

BOVEE, J. W[esley] (1861-1927)
A case of ruptured tubal pregnancy; attempted criminal abortion; septic infection; celiotomy and curettage; recovery. New York: William Wood & Co., 1895. 4p. DNLM
90-0586

BOVEE, J. W[esley] (1861-1927)
Treatment of pelvic pus cases by abdominal section; report of sixty-six cases, with remarks. Chicago, 1895. 16p. DNLM
90-0587

BOVEE, J. W[esley] (1861-1927)
Anterior colpotomy in pelvic disease. New York: William Wood & Co., 1896. 8p. DNLM **90-0588**

BOVEE, J. W[esley] (1861-1927)
Uretero-ureteral anastomosis. Philadelphia, 1897. 31p. DNLM **90-0589**

[BOWDITCH, Henry Ingersoll] (1808-1892)
Henry Ingersoll Bowditch; the memorial meeting of the section for clinical medicine, pathology and hygiene of the Massachusetts Medical Society, Suffolk district. Boston, 1892. 40p. DNLM; MBM **90-0590**

BOWDITCH, Henry Pickering (1840-1911)
Is Harvard a university? Cambridge, 1890. 8p. DNLM; MH **90-0591**

BOWDITCH, Henry Pickering (1840-1911)
The physique of women in Massachusetts. [Boston, 1890.] 20p. 1 table. DNLM; MBM **90-0592**

BOWDITCH, Henry Pickering (1840-1911)
. . . Hints for teachers of physiology. . . . Boston: D. C. Heath & Co., 1897. 58p. DLC; MB; MH; NN **90-0593**

BOWDITCH, Vincent Y[ardley] (1852-1929)
The effect of change of posture upon heart murmurs. Philadelphia: J. B. Lippincott Co., 1892. 3p. DNLM **90-0594**

BOWDITCH, Vincent Y[ardley] (1852-1929)
The establishment of sanitaria for pulmonary diseases in the vincinity of our great cities. Boston: Damrell & Upham, 1892. 12p. DNLM **90-0595**

BOWDITCH, Vincent Y[ardley] (1852-1929)
Three years' experience with sanitarium treatment of pulmonary diseases near Boston. Boston: Damrell & Upham, 1894. 21p. DNLM; MBM **90-0596**

BOWDOIN COLLEGE. BRUNSWICK, MAINE
General catalogue of Bowdoin College and the Medical School of Maine, 1794-1894. Including a historical sketch of the institution during its first century, prepared by George Thomas Little, the librarian. Brunswick: By the College, 1894. 216p. 7 plates. DNLM; MH; MWA **90-0597**

BOWEN, John T[empleton] (*b.* 1857)
Cases of cutaneous tuberculosis, with histological studies. [New York, 1890.] 10p. DNLM **90-0598**

BOWEN, John T[empleton] (*b.* 1857)
The association of purpura and acute circumscribed oedema. New York, 1892. 7p. DNLM **90-0599**

BOWEN, John T[empleton] (*b.* 1857)
The present position of electrolysis in the treatment of cutaneous affections. Boston: Damrell & Upham, 1892. 15p. DNLM **90-0600**

BOWEN, John T[empleton] (*b.* 1857)
The epitrichial layer of the epidermis and its relationship to ichthyosis congenita. [New York: D. Appleton & Co., 1895.] 7p. DNLM **90-0601**

BOWEN, John T[empleton] (*b.* 1857)
Keratosis follicularis (psorospermose folliculaire végétante, Darier), apropos of a new case. New York, 1896. 11p. DNLM **90-0602**

BOWES, W[illiam] W.
A new varicocele needle, and how to use it. New York, 1895. 2p. DNLM **90-0603**

BOWHILL, Thomas
Manual of bacteriological technique and special bacteriology . . . with one hundred original illustrations. New York: William Wood & Co., 1899. 284p. plates. DLC; NNNAM **90-0604**

BOWLBY, Anthony Alfred (1855-1929)
Injuries and diseases of nerves and their surgical treatment. Philadelphia: P. Blakiston, Son & Co., 1890. 510p. 20 plates. CtY-M; DNLM ; PPC; PU **90-0605**

BOWMAN, Winthrop H[eight]
New method for the cure of organic diseases and its results in sixty-three cases. [Boston, 1890?] 15p. DNLM **90-0606**

BOWMAN, Winthrop H[eight]
The treatment of organic diseases by the system of respiration and compatibilities. Boston: A Mudge & Son, 1891. 14p. DNLM **90-0607**

BOWMAN, Winthrop H[eight]
Respiration and compatibilities, their value in restoring health and prolonging life. Boston: A Mudge & Son, 1893. 8p. DNLM **90-0608**

BOWMAN, Winthrop H[eight]
Respiration and absorption in the treatment of disease and restoration of functional power. Boston: A Mudge & Son, 1894. 14p. DNLM **90-0609**

BOYCE, Rubert [William]
A textbook of morbid histology for students and practitioners. New York: D. Appleton & Co., 1892. 477p. 65 plates. DNLM; NNNAM; OCIM; PPC **90-0610**

BOYD, George M[elick]
A case of puerperal pelvic abscess, with some remarks on septic infection. New York, 1894. 3p. DNLM **90-0611**

BOYD, George M[elick]
Two cases of tubal pregnancy operated upon more than a month after rupture. New York, 1895. 7p. DNLM **90-0612**

BOYD, George M[elick]
Symphyseotomy. New York, 1896. 10p. DNLM **90-0613**

BOYLAN, J[oseph] E.
A simple and effective method of anesthetizing the pharyngeal tonsil. Cincinnati, 1890. 8p. DNLM **90-0614**

BOYLAND, G. Halsted (1845-1919)
The solvent properties of the Buffalo lithia waters of Virginia. New York, 1896. 14p. DNLM **90-0615**

BOZEMAN, Nathan G.
Accidental uretero-vaginal fistula following hysterectomy; cure by kolpo-uretero-cystotomy, gradual preparatory treatment and button-suture. New York: M. Rooney, 1892. 7p. DNLM **90-0616**

BOZEMAN, Nathan G.
An air and water irrigator and drain for prolonged douching in deep cavities. New York, 1893. 4p. DNLM **90-0617**

BOZEMAN, Nathan G.
A new vaginal douche with automatic outflow. New York: D. Appleton & Co., 1894. 3p. DNLM **90-0618**

BRACKEN, Henry M[artyn] (1854-1938)
Outlines of material medica and pharmacology. Philadelphia: P. Blakiston, Son & Co., 1895. 383p. DLC; NN; PPC; PU **90-0619**

BRADBURY, Robert
Bradbury's unofficinal formulary and memory work of pharmacy . . . 2nd ed. . . . Chicago, Ill.: Bradbury Publishing Co., 1891. 264 (*i.e.,* 432)p. [Paging irregular.] DLC; OCLloyd **90-0620**

BRADFORD, Edward H[ickling] (1848-1926)
A treatise on orthopedic surgery, by Edward H. Bradford . . . and Robert W. Lovett. . . . Illustrated with 789 wood engravings. New York: William Wood & Co., 1890. 783p. DLC; NNNAM; PPC; PPJ **90-0621**

BRADFORD, Edward H[ickling] (1848-1926)
Operative treatment of resistant club-foot. [Philadelphia, 1892.] 20p. DNLM **90-0622**

BRADFORD, Edward H[ickling] (1848-1926) and E. G. BRACKETT
Treatment of lateral curvature by means of pressure correction. [Boston: S. J. Parkhill & Co., 1893.] 5p. DNLM **90-0623**

BRADFORD, Edward H[ickling] (1848-1926)
Treatment of congenital dislocation of the hip. Philadelphia, 1894. 9p. 2 plates. DNLM **90-0624**

BRADFORD, Edward H[ickling] (1848-1926) and Robert W. LOVETT
Distraction in the treatment of hip disease. New York, 1894. 20p. 5 plates. DNLM; NNNAM **90-0625**

BRADFORD, Edward H[ickling] (1848-1926) and E. G. BRACKETT
The employment of mechanical force in the treatment of lateral curvature. Boston, 1895. 5p. DNLM **90-0626**

BRADFORD, Edward H[ickling] (1848-1926)
Treatise on orthopedic surgery, by Edward H. Bradford . . . and Robert W. Lovett. . . . Illustrated with six hundred and twenty-one engravings. 2nd rev. ed. New York: William Wood & Co., 1899. 655p. DLC; NNNAM; OCIM; PU **90-0627**

BRADFORD, E[noch] F[reeman]
Handbook of emergencies and common ailments. Explaining the latest approved treatment of injuries, sudden and painful attacks, poisoning, and many common diseases. Boston: B. B. Russell, 1892. 448p. MBM **90-0628**

BRADFORD, T. Hewson
Retroverted gravid uterus causing retention of urine. Philadelphia, 1891. 4p. DNLM **90-0629**

BRADFORD, Thomas Lindsley (1847-1918)
Catalogue of scientific and medical books in Latin, French, German, and English; works on homoeopathy, botany, etc., for sale by . . . . Philadelphia, 1890. 19p. DNLM; PPHa **90-0630**

BRADFORD, Thomas Lindsley (1847-1918)
Homoeopathic bibliography of the United States, from the year 1825 to the year 1891, inclusive. Part I. Alphabetical list of homoeopathic books and pamphlets; books against homoeopathy; magazines, directories; list of homoeopathic publishers; libraries, previous American homoeopathic bibliography. Part II. Condensed histories, data, and bibliography of the homoeopathic societies, colleges, hospitals, asylums, homes, sanitariums, asylums for the insane, dispensaries, pharmacies, life insurance, legislation, now or at any time existent in the United States. Philadelphia: Boericke & Tafel, 1892. 596p. 1 plate. DLC; DNLM; PPC; PPHa **90-0631**

BRADFORD, Thomas Lindsley (1847-1918)
The life and letters of Dr. Samuel Hahnemann. . . . Philadelphia: Boericke & Tafel, 1895. 513p. DLC; NNNAM; PPC; PPHa **90-0632**

BRADFORD, Thomas Lindsley (1847-1918)
The pioneers of homoeopathy. . . . Philadelphia: Boericke & Tafel, 1897. 677p. DLC; NNNAM; PPHa; PU **90-0633**

BRADFORD, Thomas Lindsley (1847-1918)
History of the Homoeopathic Medical College of Pennsylvania; the Hahnemann Medical College and Hospital of Philadelphia. . . . Philadelphia: Boericke & Tafel, 1898. 904p. plates. DLC; NNNAM; PPC; PPHa **90-0634**

BRADFUTE, C. S.
Some experimental and clinical observations on the therapeutical value of salicylbromide. Danbury, Conn.: Danbury Med. Print. Co., 1891. 13p. DNLM **90-0635**

BRADLEE, Caleb Davis (1831-1897)
A brief sketch of the life of Prof. George Cheyne Shattuck, H.U., 1831. Boston: Privately printed, 1894. 6p. port. DNLM; MBM **90-0636**

BRADLEY, George B.
La grippe epidemic, with treatment. New York: G. B. Bradley, 1892. 16p. DLC; DNLM **90-0637**

BRADLEY, W. I.
On hemorrhagic cysts of the thyroid gland. New York: D. Appleton & Co., 1896. 18p. 1 plate. DNLM **90-0638**

BRAMWELL, Byron (1847-1931)
The diseases of the spinal cord. 3rd ed. New York: William Wood & Co., 1896. 659p. DNLM; NNNAM **90-0639**

BRANNAN, John Winters (*b.* 1853)
The varying significance of intermittent albuminuria. Report of autopsy of a case. [New York, 1891.] 13p. DNLM
90-0640

BRANNAN, John Winters (*b.* 1853) and Timothy Matlack CHEESMAN
A study of typhus fever, clinical, pathological, and bacteriological. New York, 1892. 15p. DNLM
90-0641

BRANNAN, John Winters (*b.* 1853)
Observations on a case of recurrent amoebic dysentery with successive large hepatic abscesses. New York: D. Appleton & Co., 1893. 9p. DNLM **90-0642**

BRANNAN, John Winters (*b.* 1853)
Quinsy and its treatment by early incision. New York: Trow Directory, 1893. 16p. DNLM **90-0643**

BRANNAN, John Winters (*b.* 1853)
State and municipal control of infections and contagious diseases. New York: Trow Co., 1894. 8p. DNLM
90-0644

BRANNAN, John Winters (*b.* 1853)
The treatment of the pulmonary haemorrhage. New York, 1896. 10p. DNLM **90-0645**

BRANNAN, John Winters (*b.* 1853)
Sero-diagnosis of typhoid fever. A study of its practical clinical value, with a demonstration of the blood reactions. New York, 1897. 16p. DNLM **90-0646**

BREMER, L[udwig] (1844-1914) and N. B. CARSON
A case of brain tumor (angioma cavernosum), causing spastic paralysis and attacks of tonic spasms; operation. [Philadelphia], 1890. 24p. DNLM **90-0647**

BREMER, L[udwig] (1844-1914) and N. B. CARSON
Aphasia due to sub-dural hemorrhage without external signs of injury; operation; recovery. [Philadelphia, 1892.] 14p. DNLM **90-0648**

BREMER, L[udwig] (1844-1914)
Itching of central origin, or brain itch. [Milwaukee, 1892.] 14p. DNLM **90-0649**

BREMER, L[udwig] (1844-1914)
Tobacco insanity, and nervousness. St. Louis: M. Brothers, 1892. 16p. DNLM **90-0650**

BREMER, L[udwig] (1844-1914)
Typhoid fever in the light of modern research. Facts and doubts about cholera. St. Louis: Nixon-Jones, 1892. 28p. 1 plate. DNLM **90-0651**

BREMER, L[udwig] (1844-1914)
A case of hysterical astasia-abasia suing for damages, with remarks on the nature of this disease and the hysterical temperament. [New York: Raff & Co., 1893.] 16p. DNLM
90-0652

BREMER, L[udwig] (1844-1914)
Traumatic neuroses in court. [St. Louis, 1893.] 14p. DNLM
90-0653

BREMER, L[udwig] (1844-1914)
On certain morphologic and microchemic peculiarities of the blood in diabetes and glycosuria. [Philadelphia, 1894.] 8p. DNLM **90-0654**

BREMER, L[udwig] (1844-1914) and N. B. CARSON
Cylindroma endothelioides of the dura mater causing localizing symptoms and early musculary atrophy. [Philadelphia: Lea Bros. & Co., 1895.] 18p. DNLM **90-0655**

BREMER, L[udwig] (1844-1914)
An improved method of diagnosticating diabetes from a drop of blood. New York, 1896. 9p. DNLM **90-0656**

BREMER, L[udwig] (1844-1914)
On cyclone-neuroses and psychoses. St. Louis, 1896. 14p. DNLM **90-0657**

BREMER, L[udwig] (1844-1914)
On the chemical behavior of cosin and gentian violet toward normal and diabetic urines. New York, 1897. 8p. DNLM
90-0658

BREMER, L[udwig] (1844-1914)
Current fallacies about "nervous prostration." [St. Louis]: Nixon-Jones Co., [1897]. 30p. DNLM
90-0659

BRÈS, Madeline (*b.* 1842)
A clinical report on vin nourry iodotané. New York: E. Fougera & Co., 1893. 15p. DNLM
90-0660

BREWER, Edward P.
Six cases of diphtheria treated with the antitoxin. Philadelphia, 1895. 7p. DNLM **90-0661**

BREWER, George E[merson] (1861-1939)
Accidents, complications, and results following internal urethrotomy upon one hundred and twenty cases of stricture. New York: E. P. Coby & Co., 1890. 32p. DNLM; NNNAM
90-0662

BREWER, George E[merson] (1861-1939)
Operative surgery at the City Hospital, with a preliminary report on the study of wound infection. New York, 1896. 27p. DNLM; NNNAM **90-0663**

BREWER, George E[merson] (1861-1939) and Pearce BAILEY
Clinical and pathological report of a case of cerebral syphilis. New York, 1896. 6p. DNLM **90-0664**

BRIDGE, Norman
Tuberculosis. . . . Philadelphia: W. B. Saunders Co., 1894. 302p. DLC; ICRM; OCIM; PPC **90-0665**

BRIGGS, Charles S.
Phelp's operation for club-foot. Nashville, 1895. 6p. DNLM
90-0666

BRIGGS, Charles S.
Some points in the technique of kidney operations. Nashville, 1895. 8p. DNLM **90-0667**

BRIGGS, F[rederic] M[elancthon]
Torsion, with description of an automatic forceps for rapid torsion. Boston: Damrell & Upham, 1891. 8p. DNLM
90-0668

BRIGGS, F[rederic] M[elancthon]
A self-retaining drainage canula for preventing scar in cervical abscess. Boston: Damrell & Upham, 1895. 12p. DNLM
90-0669

BRIGGS, F[rederic] M[elancthon]
Two cases of cyst of the finger. Boston: Damrell & Upham, 1895. 7p. DNLM **90-0670**

BRIGGS, F[rederic] M[elancthon]
The treatment of cervical adenitis. Boston: Damrell & Upham, 1896. 12p. 1 plate. DNLM **90-0671**

BRIGGS, Wallace A.
Antiseptic cataphoresis in the treatment of diseases of the uterus and its appendages. [Philadelphia, 1893.] 12p. DNLM
90-0672

BRINKERHOFF, Alexander W. (*d.* 1887)
Haemorrhoids (piles), rectal ulcer, fistula in ano, fissure, pruritus, polypus recti, stricture, &c, &c. . . . Part 1st. Diseases of the rectum and their reflex results. Surgical operations for the cure of piles absolutely unnecessary. Dr. Alexander W. Brinkerhoff's system of rectal treatment. Part 2nd. Medical code of ethics. . . . Writings of the late Dr. A. W. Brinkerhoff, as revised by William C. Brinkerhoff. . . . Chicago: Thayer & Jackson, 1895, 80p. DLC **90-0673**

BRINTON, John Hill (1832-1907)
Valedictory address to the graduating class of the Army Medical School, Washington, D.C. Chicago, 1896. 16p. DNLM
90-0674

BRISTOWE, John S[yer] (1827-1895)
A treatise on the theory and practice of medicine. 7th ed. Philadelphia: Lea Bros. & Co., 1890. 1285p. DNLM; MBM; NNNAM; PPC **90-0675**

BROADBENT, William H[enry] (1835-1907)
The pulse. Philadelphia: Lea Bros. & Co., [1890]. 317p. AU; CtY-M; OCIM; PPHa **90-0676**

BROADBENT, William H[enry] (1835-1907)
Heart disease, with special reference to prognosis and treatment. By W. H. Broadbent . . . , and John F. H. Broadbent. New York: William Wood & Co., 1897. 331p. ICJ; OCIM; PPC; PU **90-0677**

BROCKWAY, Fred J[ohn] (1860-1901)
. . . Anatomy. A manual for students and practitioners. By Fred J. Brockway . . . and A. O'Malley. . . . Philadelphia: Lea Bros. & Co., [1892]. 376p. DLC; DNLM; NNNAM; PPC
90-0678

BROCKWAY, Fred J[ohn] (1860-1901)
Essentials of physics, arranged in the form of questions and answers, prepared especially for students of medicine. Philadelphia: W. B. Saunders, 1892. 330p. DNLM; PPC; PU
90-0679

BROCKWAY, Fred, J[ohn] (1860-1901)
. . . Anatomy. A manual for students and practitioners. By Fred J. Brockway . . . and A. O'Malley. . . . 2nd ed. . . . Philadelphia: Lea Bros. & Co., [1893]. 376p. plates. DLC; PPC; PPJ; PU **90-0680**

BROKAW, A[ugustus] V. L. (1863-1907)
Intestinal anastomotic operations with segmented rubber rings, with some practical surgical suggestions as to their use in other operations. Philadelphia: W. J. Dornan, 1890. 10p. DNLM
90-0681

BROKAW, A[ugustus] V. L. (1863-1907)
A new intestinal clamp. [St. Louis, 1890.] 2 l. DNLM
90-0682

BROKAW, A[ugustus] V. L. (1863-1907)
New methods of performing pylorectomy, with remarks upon intestinal anastomotic operations. St. Louis, 1890. 12p. DNLM
90-0683

BROKAW, A[ugustus] V. L. (1863-1907)
The direct treatment of diseased tubes and ovaries. [St. Louis, 1891.] 5p. DNLM **90-0684**

BROKAW, A[ugustus] V. L. (1863-1907)
Extirpation of the kidney for an enormous myxo-sarcoma in a child aged three years and eight months. [Philadelphia, 1891.] 4p. DNLM **90-0685**

BROKAW, A[ugustus] V. L. (1863-1907)
Some practical points in the technique of abdominal and pelvic surgery. [St. Louis, 1891.] 7p. DNLM
90-0686

BROKAW, A[ugustus] V. L. (1863-1907)
The technique and management of pelvic surgical cases. Philadelphia, 1891. 4p. DNLM **90-0687**

BROKAW, A[ugustus] V. L. (1863-1907)
Experiences in pelvic surgery. [Philadelphia, 1892.] 11p. DNLM **90-0688**

BROKAW, A[ugustus] V. L. (1863-1907)
Peritonitis from a surgical standpoint. St. Louis, 1892. 7p. DNLM **90-0689**

BROKAW, A[ugustus] V. L. (1863-1907)
A unique case of stab wound of thorax and abdomen; recovery. Detroit, 1892. 4p. DNLM **90-0690**

BROKAW, A[ugustus] V. L. (1863-1907)
Some conclusions drawn from experiences in pelvic surgery. St. Louis, 1896. 2 l. DNLM **90-0691**

BRONSON, Edward Bennet
The sensation of itching. New York, 1890. 22p. DNLM
90-0692

BRONSON, Edward Bennet
The etiology of itching. New York: Trow's Co., 1891. 20p. DNLM **90-0693**

BRONSON, Edward Bennet
On the origin of type in disease. New York: Trow's Co., 1892. 12p. DNLM **90-0694**

BRONSON, Edward Bennet
A case of symmetrical cutaneous atrophy of the extremities. New York, 1895. 10p. 1 plate. DNLM
90-0695

BRONSON, Edward Bennet
On the topical treatment of acne. New York, 1896. 14p. DNLM **90-0696**

[BRONSON, Henry] (1804-1893)
Biographical sketch of the life and writings of the late Professor Henry Bronson, M.D. (New Haven, 1895). New Haven, 1895. 117p. CtY-M; MBM **90-0697**

BROOKE, John (1830-1902)
Military hygiene. A lecture in the course on military hygiene, at the U.S. Infantry and Cavalry School, Fort Leavenworth, Kansas. Fort Leavenworth, 1893. 9p. DNLM **90-0698**

BROOKE, John B. (1833-1898)
An improved fracture-box for the repair of injuries of the lower extremities requiring extension and counter extension. Philadelphia, 1894. 5p. DNLM **90-0699**

BROOME, G. Wiley
Typical uterus-bicornis; living seven-months' child expelled from left horn; laparotomy for parovarian cyst; uterus-bicornis then discovered; recovery. [St. Louis, 1891.] 9p. 1 plate. DNLM **90-0700**

BROOME, G. Wiley
The technique of cerebral surgery. [St. Louis, 1891.] 11p. DNLM **90-0701**

BROOME, G. Wiley
Ideal surgery. Chicago, 1893. 15p. DNLM **90-0702**

BROOMELL, Isaac Norman (*b.* 1858)
Anatomy and histology of the mouth and teeth. . . . With 284 illustrations. Philadelphia: P. Blakiston's Son & Co., 1898. 428p. DLC; MdU-D; PPC **90-0703**

BROSIUS, Mariott (1843-1901)
The medical profession and the State. The alumni oration. Philadelphia, 1895. 14p. DNLM **90-0704**

BROTHERS, A[bram] (*b.* 1861)
Infantile mortality during child-birth and its prevention. [William Furness Jenks' prize essay of the College of Physicians of Philadelphia.] Philadelphia: P. Blakiston, Son & Co., 1896. 179p. DLC; DNLM; PPC **90-0705**

BROTHERS, Abram (*b.* 1861)
Intra-uterine vaporization. . . . [New York: D. Appleton & Co.], 1899. 13p. DLC **90-0706**

BROWER, Daniel R[oberts] (1839-1909)
Cerebral syphilis; some observations on its diagnosis and treatment. Peoria, 1896. 4p. DNLM **90-0707**

BROWN, Bedford (1825-1897)
Personal recollections of the late Dr. Benjamin W. Dudley, of Lexington, Ky., and of his surgical methods and work. [Philadelphia, 1892.] 18p. DNLM **90-0708**

BROWN, Bedford (1825-1897)
Observations on the action of chloroform on the functions of the human brain and spinal cord, as witnessed in extensive injuries of the cranium and brain. Detroit, Mich.: G. S. Davis, 1894. 25p. DNLM **90-0709**

BROWN, Christian Henry (1857-1933)
Opticians' record book of optometric examinations. . . . Philadelphia: The Author, 1896. 102p. DLC **90-0710**

BROWN, Christian Henry (1857-1933)
The optician's manual. Chapters 1-10, inclusive. A treatise on the science and practice of optics, comp. from the serial written by C. H. Brown. . . . 1st ed. Philadelphia: The Keystone, [1896]. 376p. diags. DLC; PPC **90-0711**

BROWN, Christian Henry (1857-1933)
The optician's manual. Chapters 1-10, inclusive. A treatise on the science and practice of optics, comp. from the serial written by C. H. Brown. . . . 2nd ed. Philadelphia: The Keystone, 1897. 417p. col. plates, diags. DLC **90-0712**

BROWN, C[hristian] H[enry] (1857-1933)
Supplement to The optician's manual. Chapters 11 and 12. A treatise on the science and practice of optics, comp. from the serial written by C. H. Brown. . . . Philadelphia: The Keystone, 1899. 203p. diag. DLC **90-0713**

BROWN, Dillon
The surgical treatment of erysipelas; a successful case in an infant. [Philadelphia, 1890.] 2p. DNLM **90-0714**

BROWN, Dillon
The construction of O'Dwyer tubes with a report of three hundred and fifty cases of intubation of the larynx. [Philadelphia, 1891.] 15p. DNLM **90-0715**

BROWN, Dillon
Some practical points in the treatment of diphtheria by calomel fumigations. Philadelphia, 1894. 10p. DNLM **90-0716**

BROWN, Dillon
A new extractor for the removal of intubation tubes from the larynx. Philadelphia, 1895. 4p. DNLM **90-0717**

BROWN, Francis Henry (1835-1917)
The medical register for New England. 8th ed. Boston: Damrell & Upham, 1895. 589p. DNLM; MH; MBM; MWA **90-0718**

BROWN, F[rederic] Tilden (1853-1910)
The ocular and tactile demonstration of urethral lesions by the aid of new instruments. Shown with cases. New York: D. Appleton & Co., 1891. 16p. DNLM **90-0719**

BROWN, F[rederic] Tilden (1853-1910)
A case of cystitis, pyelonephritis due to colon-bacillus infection. Presentation of two kidneys showing different stages of infective disease, the bacillus coli communis only being found. Presentation of one kidney in the early stage of cortical tuberculosis. New York, 1895. 10p. 2 plates. DNLM **90-0720**

BROWN, F[rederic] Tilden (1853-1910)
Case of double ligation of the vasa deferentia for hypertrophy of the prostate. New York, 1896. 4p. DNLM **90-0721**

BROWN, F[rederic] Tilden (1853-1910)
Report of two successful hip-joint amputations, the second of which was performed by a new method. St. Louis, 1896. 10p. 3 plates. **90-0722**

BROWN, F[rederick] K.
Poisoning by oil of cedar. Philadelphia, 1893. 2p. DNLM
90-0723

BROWN, George S.
Cholecystotomy necessitated by obstruction of the cystic duct. [Philadelphia, 1893.] 4p. DNLM **90-0724**

BROWN, George S.
A case of incarcerated hernia and its reduction by means of rectal taxis. Philadelphia, 1895. 3p. DNLM
90-0725

BROWN, George S.
The mental state as conducive to organic disease. Philadelphia, 1895. 14p. DNLM **90-0726**

BROWN, Moreau R.
Suppuration of the antrum of Highmore. [New York], 1890. 10p. DNLM **90-0727**

BROWN, Moreau R.
The relation of acute diseases of the nose and throat to disorders of digestion. New York, 1896. 10p. DNLM
90-0728

BROWN, Price
Organic stricture of the oesophagus. [New York, 1893.] 8p. DNLM **90-0729**

BROWN UNIVERSITY. MEDICAL DEPARTMENT
The Medical Department of Brown University. [n. p., 1898.] 59p. DNLM; RPB **90-0730**

BROWNE, [Isaac] Lennox (1841-1902)
The throat and nose and their diseases. 3rd ed. Philadelphia: Lea Bros. & Co., 1890. 716p. 15 plates. DNLM; NNNAM; OCIM; PPC **90-0731**

BROWNE, [Isaac] Lennox (1841-1902)
Koch's remedy in relation specially to throat consumption. Philadelphia: Lea Bros. & Co., 1891. 114p. DNLM; NNNAM; PPC; PPJ **90-0732**

BROWNE, [Isaac] Lennox (1841-1902)
The throat and nose and their diseases. 4th ed. Philadelphia: Lea Bros. & Co., 1893. 734p. 15 plates. CtY-M; DNLM; PPC; PU **90-0733**

BROWNE, [Isaac] Lennox (1841-1902)
Diphtheria and its associates. Philadelphia: J. B Lippincott Co., 1895. 272p. DNLM; NNNAM; PPC; PU
90-0734

BROWNING, William (1855-1941)
The arrangement of the supra-cerebral veins in man as bearing on Hill's theory of a developmental rotation of the brain. [New York, 1891.] 5p. DNLM **90-0735**

BROWNING, William (1855-1941)
The bilateral paresis and pseudoplegias of childhood, with special reference to a type of malarial origin. [Philadelphia, 1891.] 13p. DNLM **90-0736**

BROWNING, William (1855-1941)
Inequality of the pupils in epileptics, with a note on latent anisocoria. [New York, 1892.] 5p. DNLM
90-0737

BROWNING, William (1855-1941)
The epileptic interval; its phenomena and their importance as a guide to treatment. [New York: Raff & Co., 1893.] 68p. DNLM **90-0738**

BROWNING, William (1855-1941)
The nervous affections that may arise from malaria. New York: M. J. Rooney, 1893. 14p. DNLM **90-0739**

BROWNING, William (1855-1941)
Lumbar puncture for the removal of cerebro-spinal fluid. New York: Alliance Press, 1894. 8p. DNLM
90-0740

BROWNING, William (1855-1941)
Some etiological types of hysteria. [Brooklyn, 1894.] 7p. DNLM **90-0741**

BROWNING, William (1855-1941)
On the relation of sex to the prognosis of epilepsy. Chicago, 1895. 7p. DNLM **90-0742**

BROWNING, William (1855-1941)
Pitting about the hair-cups. A trophic change of the skin in certain nervous disorders of central origin. New York, 1896. 8p. DNLM **90-0743**

BROWNSON, J[ohn] J.
Vesico-vaginal fistula; suture of bladder with catgut. Philadelphia, 1895. 3p. DNLM **90-0744**

BROWNSON, J[ohn] J.
Chest drainage in empyema. St. Louis, 1896. 7p. DNLM
90-0745

BRUBAKER, Albert P. (1852-1943)
. . . A compend of human physiology. . . . 6th ed., rev. and improved. With new illustrations and a table of physiological constants. Philadelphia: P. Blakiston, Son & Co., 1891. 198p. DLC; DNLM; PPC; PU **90-0746**

BRUBAKER, Albert P. (1852-1943)
. . . A compend of human physiology. . . . 7th ed., rev. and enl. With new illustrations and a table of physiological constants. Philadelphia: P. Blakiston, Son & Co., 1893. 236p. DLC; NNNAM; PPC **90-0747**

BRUBAKER, Albert P. (1852-1943)
. . . A compend of human physiology. . . . 8th ed., rev. and enl. With new illustrations and table of physiological constants. Philadelphia: P. Blakiston, Son & Co., 1896. 250p. DLC; PPC; PPJ **90-0748**

BRUBAKER, Albert P. (1852-1943)
. . . A compend of human physiology. Especially adapted for the use of medical students. . . . 9th ed., rev. and enl. With new illustrations and a table of physiologic constants. Philadelphia: P. Blakiston, Son & Co., 1899. 266p. DLC; IU-M; PPC; PU
90-0749

BRUNTON, T[homas] Lauder (1844-1916)
Index of diseases and remedies reprinted from the "Pharmacology, Therapeutics and Materia Medica" with supplement. Detroit, Parke, Davis & Co., 1890. 264p. OCLloyd; PPC
90-0750

BRUSH, Arthur Conklin
The neurological causes of impotence. [New York, 1893.] 10p. DNLM **90-0751**

BRYAN, Joseph Hammond (1856-1935)
Some recent advances in the diagnosis and treatment of the abscess of the antrum of Highmore. [Richmond, 1890.] 15p. DNLM **90-0752**

BRYAN, Joseph Hammond (1856-1935)
Acute edema of the larynx, with the report of a case resulting from pyemia. [Philadelphia: Lea Bros. & Co., 1892.] 19p. DNLM **90-0753**

BRYAN, Joseph Hammond (1856-1935)
A case of suppurating ethmoiditis. [New York: D. Appleton & Co., 1893.] 7p. DNLM **90-0754**

BRYAN, Joseph Hammond (1856-1935)
The surgical treatment of chronic suppurating otitis media. Chicago: American Medical Association Press, 1895. 8p. DNLM **90-0755**

BRYAN, Joseph Hammond (1856-1935)
A further contribution to the study of suppurative disease of the accessory sinuses, with report of cases. New York, 1895. 19p. DNLM **90-0756**

BRYANT, Joseph Decatur (1845-1914)
Fracture of the patella treated by continuous extension; patients not confined to bed. [Philadelphia, 1893.] 13p. DNLM **90-0757**

BRYANT, Joseph Decatur (1845-1914)
The relation between the gross anatomy of the appendix and appendicitis. [Philadelphia, 1894.] 10p. DNLM **90-0758**

BRYANT, Joseph Decatur (1845-1914)
The Wesley M. Carpenter lecture. New York, 1895. 31p. DNLM **90-0759**

BRYANT, Joseph Decatur (1845-1914)
Operative surgery. . . . [3rd ed.] New York: D. Appleton & Co., 1899-1901. 2 v. col. and fold. plates. DLC; NNNAM; OCIM; PPC **90-0760**

BRYCE, Clarence A[rchibald] (*b.* 1849)
The physician's companion: a pocket reference book for physicians and students. . . . Richmond, Va.: The Southern Clinic, 1890. 160p. DLC **90-0761**

BRYSON, Louise Fiske
The present epidemic of influenza. [New York: D. Appleton & Co., 1890.] 20p. DNLM **90-0762**

BUCHANAN, Charles Milton (1868-1920)
The successful treatment of typhoid fever. A reply to Dr. Page [Charles E.]. St Louis, 1893. 8p. DNLM **90-0763**

BUCHANAN, Charles Milton (1868-1920)
Antisepsis and antiseptics, with an introduction by Augustus C. Bernays. Newark, N.J.: Terhune Co., 1895. 352p. 6 plates. DNLM; NNNAM; NjR **90-0764**

BUCHANAN, John
An encyclopedia of the practice of medicine, based on bacteriology. . . . 1st ed. New York: R. R. Russell, 1890. 1453p. DLC; NNNAM **90-0765**

BUCHANAN, Joseph Rodes (1814-1899)
Therapeutic sarcognomy. The application of sarcognomy, the science of the soul, brain and body, to the therapeutic philosophy and treatment of bodily and mental diseases by means of electricity, nervaura, medicine and haemospasia, with a review of authors on animal magnetism and massage and presentation of new instruments for electro-therapeutics. . . . Boston: J. G. Cupples Co., 1891. 671p. DLC; MBM **90-0766**

BUCK, Albert H[enry] (1842-1922)
A revised description of the anatomy of the elephant's ear. New Bedford: Mercury Publishing Co., 1890. 15p. DNLM **90-0767**

BUCK, Albert H[enry] (1842-1922)
The strongly counter-irritant effects of the usual mastoid operation. [New Bedford, 1893.] 14p. DNLM **90-0768**

BUCK. Albert H[enry] (1842-1922)
A manual of diseases of the ear. . . . 2nd rev. ed. New York: William Wood & Co., 1895. 457p. DLC; DNLM; NNNAM; PU **90-0769**

BUCK, Albert H[enry] (1842-1922)
A vest-pocket medical dictionary; embracing those terms and abbreviations which are commonly found in the medical literature of the day, but excluding the names of drugs and of many special anatomical terms. . . . New York: William Wood & Co., 1896. 529p. DLC; DNLM; NNNAM; PPC **90-0770**

BUCK, Albert H[enry] (1842-1922)
A treatise on diseases of the ear; together with a brief sketch of the anatomy and physiology of this organ. . . . 3rd rev. ed. New York: William Wood & Co., 1898. 592p. DLC; NNNAM; OCIM; PU **90-0771**

BUCK, Albert H[enry] (1842-1922)
First principles of otology; a text-book for medical students. . . . New York: William Wood & Co., 1899. 212p. DLC; MH-M; NNNAM; PPC **90-0772**

BUCK, J[irah] D[ewey] (1839-1916)
Address delivered at the forty-third annual session of the American Institute of Homoeopathy, at Waukesha, Wis., on the progress of homoeopathy. [Cincinnati, 1890.] 16p. DNLM **90-0773**

BUCKINGHAM, E[dward] M[arshall]
The medical treatment of diphtheria. Boston: Damrell & Upham, 1895. 16p. DNLM **90-0774**

BUCKLEY, J[ames] M[onroe] (1836-1920)
Faith-healing, Christian science, and kindred phenomena. New York: De Vinne Press, 1892. 308p. DNLM; MB; MH; NN **90-0775**

BUFFUM, Joseph Howard (*b.* 1849)
Manual of the essentials of diseases of the eye and ear. . . . Chicago: Gross & Delbridge Co., 1896. 315p. col. plates. DLC; IU-M; OCIM **90-0776**

BULKLEY, L[ucius] D[uncan] (1845-1928)
On the dangers arising from syphilis in the practice of dentistry. [New York, 1890.] 16p. DNLM **90-0777**

BULKLEY, L[ucius] D[uncan] (1845-1928)
Psorospermosis follicularis cutis. [Philadelphia, 1890.] 12p. DNLM **90-0778**

BULKLEY, L[ucius] D[uncan] (1845-1928)
On the treatment of eczema in elderly people. [New York, 1890.] 18p. DNLM **90-0779**

BULKLEY, L[ucius] D[uncan] (1845-1928)
On the treatment of eczema in elderly people. Philadelphia: W. J. Dornan, 1890. 16p. DNLM **90-0780**

BULKLEY, L[ucius] D[uncan] (1845-1928)
Clinical study of analysis of 1,000 cases of psoriasis. Baltimore, 1891. 16p. DNLM **90-0781**

BULKLEY, L[ucius] D[uncan] (1845-1928)
On the relation of eczema to disturbances of the nervous system. Philadelphia, 1891. 35p. DNLM **90-0782**

BULKLEY, L[ucius] D[uncan] (1845-1928)
Demilt Dispensary. Department of diseases of the skin. [Classification of diseases of the skin. Prepared for the use of classes in dermatology.] [New York, 1892?] 2 l. DNLM **90-0783**

BULKLEY, L[ucius] D[uncan] (1845-1928)
Acne und alopecia. . . . Detroit, Mich.: G. S. Davis, 1892. 85p. DLC; DNLM; OCIM **90-0784**

BULKLEY, L[ucius] D[uncan] (1845-1928)
Clinical notes on chancre of the tonsil, with analysis of fifteen cases. Philadelphia, 1893. 10p. DNLM **90-0785**

BULKLEY, L[ucius] D[uncan] (1845-1928)
The internal treatment of lupus erythematosus with phosphorus. Philadelphia, 1893. 6p. DNLM **90-0786**

BULKLEY, L[ucius] D[uncan] (1845-1928)
Syphilis in the innocent (syphilis insontium) clinically and historically considered, with a plan for the legal control of the disease. . . . The essay to which the College of Physicians of Philadelphia, in 1891, awarded the Alvarenga prize, for the best memoir of any medical subject. . . . New York: Bailey & Fairchild, [1894]. 398p. DLC; DNLM; NNNAM **90-0787**

BULKLEY, L[ucius] D[uncan] (1845-1928)
Clinical notes on psoriasis, with especial reference to its prognosis and treatment. Albany, 1895. 14p. DNLM **90-0788**

BULKLEY, L[ucius] D[uncan] (1845-1928)
Sleep in its relations to diseases of the skin. [New York, 1895.] 16p. DNLM **90-0789**

BULKLEY, L[ucius] D[uncan] (1845-1928)
Notes on some of the newer remedies used in diseases of the skin. Chicago, 1896. 11p. DNLM **90-0790**

BULKLEY, L[ucius] D[uncan] (1845-1928)
Manual of diseases of the skin, with an analysis of twenty thousand consecutive cases and a formulary. . . . 4th ed., rev. and enl. New York and London: G. P. Putnam's Sons, 1898. 362p. DLC; MBM; NNNAM; PPC **90-0791**

BULL, Charles Stedman (1844-1911)
Papillitis, or inflammation of the intra-ocular end of the optic nerve; its aetiology and connection with intracranial disease. [New York, 1891.] 16p. DNLM **90-0792**

BULL, Charles Stedman (1844-1911)
Gouty retinitis, chorio-retinitis, and neuro-retinitis. Hartford, 1893. 23p. DNLM **90-0793**

BULL, Charles Stedman (1844-1911)
Tumors of the orbit and neighboring cavities. New York, 1893. 40p. DNLM **90-0794**

BULL, Charles Stedman (1844-1911)
Recent experiences in the treatment of detached retina, with a detailed report of thirty-eight cases. Hartford, Conn., 1894. 35p. DNLM **90-0795**

BULL, Charles Stedman (1844-1911)
Preliminary report on six hundred and twelve cases of convergent squint, with the final results of operation. [Hartford, Conn., 1895.] 40p. DNLM **90-0796**

BULL, Charles Stedman (1844-1911)
Purulent inflammation of the eyeball and orbital issue and paralysis of the ocular muscles as possible complications or sequelae of influenza. Kansas City, 1895. 6p. DNLM **90-0797**

BULL, Charles Stedman (1844-1911)
Some unusual cases of orbital tumors emphasizing the necessity of careful differential diagnosis. New York, 1895. 18p. DNLM **90-0798**

BULL, Charles Stedman (1844-1911)
The course and prognosis of orbital tumors as influenced by surgical operations for their removal. Hartford, Conn., 1896. 30p. DNLM **90-0799**

BULL, William T[illinghast] (1849-1909)
Notes on cases of hernia which have relapsed after various operations for radical cure. [New York, 1891.] 9p. DNLM **90-0800**

BULL, William T[illinghast] (1849-1909)
On three cases of pylorectomy with gastro-enterostomy. New York: Trow's Co., 1891. 16p. DNLM **90-0801**

BULL, William T[illinghast] (1849-1909) and William B. COLEY
Observations on the mechanical and operative treatment of hernia at the Hospital for Ruptured and Crippled of New York. Philadelphia, 1893. 15p. 3 plates. DNLM **90-0802**

BULL, William T[illinghast] (1849-1909)
Further observations on chronic relapsing appendicitis; eighteen cases, with one death; list of four hundred and fifty operations. New York, 1894. 19p. DNLM **90-0803**

BULLARD, W[illiam] E.
Puerperal infection in New York City. Who is responsible? Can it be prevented? New York, 1894. 6p. DNLM **90-0804**

BULLARD, W[illiam] L.
Should not oculists be more careful in prescribing colored glasses? Chattanooga: Lane, Kuster & Chauncey, [1892]. 2 l. DNLM **90-0805**

BULLARD, William N[orton] (*b.* 1853)
Diffuse cortical sclerosis of the brain in children. [New York, 1890.] 11p. DNLM **90-0806**

BULLARD, William N[orton] (*b.* 1853)
The significance of paroxysmal running in childhood. Boston: Damrell & Upham, 1890. 18p. DNLM **90-0807**

BULLARD, William N[orton] (*b.* 1853)
Provision for the cure of adult pauper epileptics in Massachusetts. Boston: Damrell & Upham, 1891. 10p. DNLM **90-0808**

BULLARD, William N[orton] (*b.* 1853) and Edward H. BRADFORD
Cerebellar tumor; operation; haemorrhage from defect of occipital bone; death; general remarks. Boston: Damrell & Upham, 1891. 20p. DNLM **90-0809**

BULLARD, William N[orton] (*b.* 1853)
Consideration of some of the indications for operation in head injuries. Boston: Damrell & Upham, 1895. 9p. DNLM **90-0810**

BUNN, Walter S.
What to do until the doctor comes. A manual of instructions as to the proper method of managing cases of poisoning, sudden illness, accidents, etc. . . . Lawrence, Kansas: Journal Co., printers and binders, 1897. 120p. plates. DLC **90-0811**

BURCHARD, Henry H.
Compend of dental pathology and therapeutics. . . . Philadelphia: The S. S. White Dental Mfg. Co., 1896. 138p. DLC; MdU-D; PPC **90-0812**

BURCHARD, Henry H.
A text-book of dental pathology and therapeutics, including pharmacology. . . . Philadelphia and New York: Lea Bros. & Co., 1898. 587p. col. plates. DLC; NNNAM; PPC; PU **90-0813**

BURET, Frédéric
Syphilis in ancient and pre-historic times. Transl. from the French, with notes, by A. H. Ohmann-Dumesnil. Philadelphia & London: F. A. Davis, 1891. 226p. DNLM; ICU; MBM; PPC [Forms v. 1 of Syphilis today and among the ancients.] **90-0814**

BURET, Frédéric
Syphilis in the middle ages and in modern times. Transl. from the French, with notes, by A. H. Ohmann-Dumesnil. Philadelphia: F. A. Davis & Co., 1895. 289p. 1 p. l. DLC; DNLM; NNNAM; PPC [Forms v. 1 and 2 of: Syphilis today and among the ancients.] **90-0815**

BURGGRAEVE, Adolphe (1806-1902)
The diseases of women and their dosimetric treatment. . . . Transl. from the French. New York: W. J. Morrison, 1890. 77p. DLC; NNNAM **90-0816**

BURGGRAEVE, Adolphe (1806-1902)
The diseases of children and their dosimetric treatment. . . . Transl. from the French. New York: W. J. Morrison, 1890. 62p. DLC; NNNAM **90-0817**

BURGGRAEVE, Adolphe (1806-1902)
Phthisis and its dosimetric treatment. . . . Transl. from the French. New York: W. J. Morrison, 1891. 55p. DLC; NNNAM **90-0818**

BURGGRAEVE, Adolphe (1806-1902)
The essentials of dosimetric pharmacy and pharmacodynamia. . . . Transl. from the French. New York: W. J. Morrison, 1891. 45p. DLC; NNNAM; OCLloyd **90-0819**

BURGGRAEVE, Adolphe (1806-1902)
Fever and its dosimetric treatment. . . . Transl. from the French. New York: W. J. Morrison, 1891. 74p. DLC; NNNAM **90-0820**

BURGGRAEVE, Adolphe (1806-1902)
Manual of diathetic maladies and their dosimetric treatment. . . . Transl. from the French. N[ew] Y[ork]: W. J. Morrison, 1892. 39p. DLC; NNNAM **90-0821**

BURGHARDT, Joseph
Therapeutics of diphtheria. Transl. by Charles Raettig. New York: J. H. Vail & Co., 1891. 11p. DNLM; NNNAM **90-0822**

BURNET, R[obert] W[illiam] (1851-1931)
Foods and dietaries: a manual of clinical dietetics. Philadelphia: P. Blakiston, Son & Co., 1891. 196p. DNLM; NNNAM; PPC; PPJ **90-0823**

BURNETT, Charles H[enry], ed. (1842-1902)
System of diseases of the ear, nose, and throat. . . . Philadelphia, [etc.]: J. B. Lippincott Co., 1893. 2 v. col. plates. DLC; MBM; NNNAM; PPC **90-0824**

BURNETT, Charles H[enry] (1842-1902)
Partial myringectomy and removal of the incus and stapes for the relief of the lesions of chronic catarrhal otitis media. [Philadelphia, 1893.] 11p. DNLM **90-0825**

BURNETT, Charles H[enry] (1842-1902)
The surgical treatment of chronic tympanic vertigo, often miscalled Ménière's disease. [Philadelphia, 1893.] 8p. DNLM **90-0826**

BURNETT, Charles H[enry] (1842-1902)
Three cases of chronic tinnitus aurium and tympanic vertigo relieved by removal of the incus. [Philadelphia, 1894.] 8p. DNLM **90-0827**

BURNETT, D[aniel] L.
The management of pregnancy. New York, 1894. 5p. DNLM **90-0828**

BURNETT, E[dwin] C.
Report of a case of early obstruction of the ejaculatory ducts. New York: D. Appleton & Co., 1895. 4p. DNLM **90-0829**

BURNETT, James Compton (1840-1901)
The greater diseases of the liver: jaundice, gall-stones, enlargements, tumours, and cancer: and their treatment . . . Philadelphia: Hahnemann Publishing House, 1891. 186p. DLC; PPC; PPHa **90-0830**

BURNETT, James Compton (1840-1901)
The new cure of consumption by its own virus. Illustrated by numerous cases. . . . 2nd ed., rev. and enl. . . . Philadelphia: Boericke & Tafel, 1892 [1891]. 187p. DLC; NNNAM; PPC; PPHa **90-0831**

BURNETT, James Compton (1840-1901)
Ringworm: its constitutional nature and cure. . . . Philadelphia: Boericke & Tafel, [1892]. 126p. DLC; PPHa **90-0832**

BURNETT, James Compton (1840-1901)
Gout and its cure. . . . Philadelphia: Boericke & Tafel, 1895. 172p. DLC; PPC; PPHa **90-0833**

BURNETT, James Compton (1840-1901)
The diseases of the liver: jaundice, gall-stones, enlargements, tumours, and cancer: and their treatment. . . . 2nd rev. and enl. ed. . . . Philadelphia: Boericke & Tafel, 1895. 244p. DLC; NNNAM; PPC; PPHa **90-0834**

BURNETT, James Compton (1840-1901)
Delicate, backward, puny, and stunted children: their developmental defects, and physical, mental and moral peculiarities considered as ailments amenable to treatment by medicines. . . . Philadelphia: Boericke & Tafel, 1896. 164p. DLC; DNLM; PPC; PPHa **90-0835**

BURNETT, James Compton (1840-1901)
Organ diseases of women, notably enlargements and displacements of the uterus, and sterility, considered as curable by medicine. . . . Philadelphia: Boericke & Tafel, 1897. 156p. DLC; PPC; PPHa **90-0836**

BURNETT, James Compton (1840-1901)
Diseases of the skin; their constitutional nature and cure. . . . 3rd ed., rev. and enl. Philadelphia: Boericke & Tafel, 1898. 264p. DLC; PPC; PPHa **90-0837**

BURNETT, James Compton (1840-1901)
The change of life in women, and the ills and ailings incident thereto. . . . Philadelphia: Boericke & Tafel, 1898. 185p. DLC; NNNAM; PPHa **90-0838**

BURNETT, S. Grover
Points on the treatment of epilepsy. St. Joseph, 1890. 4 l. DNLM **90-0839**

BURNETT, S. Grover
The diagnosis of incipient melancholia. [New York, 1891.] 12p. 1 plate. DNLM **90-0840**

BURNETT, Swan M[oses] (1847-1906)
Reciprocal responsibilities. An address. Washington, 1890. 15p. DNLM **90-0841**

BURNETT, Swan M[oses] (1847-1906)
Some exceptional features in cataract extraction. Richmond, 1890 [1889]. 8p. DNLM **90-0842**

BURNETT, Swan M[oses] (1847-1906)
The physician as a man and a citizen. Chicago, 1891. 24p. DNLM **90-0843**

BURNETT, Swan M[oses] (1847-1906)
Recent views on the pathology of trachoma. [Nashville, 1891.] 5p. DNLM **90-0844**

BURNETT, Swan M[oses] (1847-1906)
On the reform in numbering prisms. [Philadelphia, 1891.] 7p. DNLM **90-0845**

BURNETT, Swan M[oses] (1847-1906)
The construction and use of the ophthalmometer; an explanation and a correction. [St. Louis, 1892.] 7p. DNLM **90-0846**

BURNETT, Swan M[oses] (1847-1906)
The general form of the human cornea and its relations to the refraction of the eye and visual acuteness. [Hartford, 1892.] 6p. DNLM **90-0847**

BURNETT, Swan M[oses] (1847-1906)
Recurrent iritis. [Kansas City, 1892.] 3p. DNLM **90-0848**

BURNETT, Swan M[oses] (1847-1906)
Some incidental phenomena of the shadow test. Philadelphia, 1892. 6p. DNLM **90-0849**

BURNETT, Swan M[oses] (1847-1906)
Ophthalmometry in America. St. Louis, 1893. 2p. DNLM **90-0850**

BURNETT, Swan M[oses] (1847-1906)
Tumor of the intervaginal space of the optic-nerve sheath. [n. p.], 1894. 9p. DNLM **90-0851**

BURNETT, Swan M[oses] (1847-1906)
The influence of country and race in the etiology of trachoma. New York, 1896. 8p. DNLM **90-0852**

BURNETT, Swan M[oses] (1847-1906)
The racial and geographic distribution of trachoma in the United States of America. [St. Louis, 1896.] 16p. DNLM **90-0853**

BURR, Albert H. (*b.* 1850)
Gonorrhea in the puerperium. Chicago, 1896. 8p. DNLM **90-0854**

BURR, Albert H. (*b.* 1850)
Gonorrhoea, its ravages and its prophylaxis. Chicago, [1896]. 19p. DNLM **90-0855**

BURR, Albert H. (*b.* 1850)
Infantile scorbutus. Chicago, 1896. 8 l. DNLM **90-0856**

BURR, Charles W[alts] (*b.* 1861)
Periodic paralysis, with the report of a case. [Philadelphia, 1893.] 4p. DNLM **90-0857**

BURR, Charles W[alts] (*b.* 1861)
The spinal cord in Pott's disease. Philadelphia, 1893. 8p. DNLM **90-0858**

BURR, Charles W[alts] (*b.* 1861)
Idiopathic muscular atrophy. Philadelphia: Lea Bros. & Co., 1894. 8p. DNLM **90-0859**

BURR, Charles W[alts] (*b.* 1861)
A contribution to the pathology of Friedreich's ataxia. Philadelphia, 1894. 7p. DNLM **90-0860**

BURR, Charles W[alts] (*b.* 1861)
Hysterical syncope, hemianesthesia, rapid respiration. [Philadelphia, 1895.] 5p. DNLM **90-0861**

BURR, C[olonel] Bell (1856-1931)
A primer of psychology and mental disease. Detroit, Mich.: G. S. Davis, 1894. 104p. DNLM; MH-M; NNNAM **90-0862**

BURR, C[olonel] Bell (1856-1931)
A primer of psychology and mental disease, for use in training-schools for attendants and nurses in medical classes. . . . 2nd ed., thoroughly rev. Philadelphia, New York, [etc.]: The F. A. Davis Co., 1898. 116p. DLC; NNNAM; PPC; PU **90-0863**

BURRAGE, Walter L[incoln] (1860-1935)
Treatment of chronic endometritis by curetting and gauze drainage, with a synopsis of twenty-seven cases. Boston: Damrell & Upham, 1893. 19p. 1 table. DNLM **90-0864**

BURRAGE, Walter L[incoln] (1860-1935)
A case of primary tuberculosis of the female bladder diagnosed and treated by Howard Kelly's new method of direct inspection with large endoscopes. Boston: Damrell & Upham, 1894. 13p. DNLM **90-0865**

BURRAGE, Walter L[incoln] (1860-1935)
Three years' experience with the electrical treatment of fibroid tumors of the uterus. New York: William Wood & Co., 1894. 24p. DNLM **90-0866**

BURRAGE, Walter L[incoln] (1860-1935)
Cases of retrodeviation of the pregnant uterus, including a case of pregnancy in an incarcerated cornu and a case complicated by an ovarian tumor. With remarks. Boston: Damrell & Upham, 1895. 11p. DNLM **90-0867**

BURRAGE, Walter L[incoln] (1860-1935)
Notes on the repair of rupture of the perineum through the sphincter ani. Boston: Damrell & Upham, 1895. 15p. DNLM **90-0868**

BURRAGE, Walter L[incoln] (1860-1935)
Congenital absence of uterus and vagina. Plastic operation for artificial vagina, taking flaps from nymphae and perineum. Philadelphia, 1897. 12p. DNLM **90-0869**

BURRELL, Herbert L[eslie] (1856-1910)
Abscesses in Pott's disease. Philadelphia, 1891. 11p. DNLM **90-0870**

BURRELL, Herbert L[eslie] (1856-1910) and Edwin W. DWIGHT
The treatment of compound fractures by modern methods. [Boston], 1892. 16p. 1 table. DNLM **90-0871**

BURRELL, Herbert L[eslie] (1856-1910)
A contribution to the anatomy of congenital equino-varus. Philadelphia, 1893. 2p. 1 plate. DNLM **90-0872**

BURROUGHS, James A.
Management and treatment of tuberculosis in the Asheville climate, with report of cases. Wilmington, 1896. 19p. DNLM **90-0873**

BURSTEIN, Maurice J.
Ideality of medical science. The evil events of the profession, and an available device for its reformation. New York, 1892. 14p. DNLM **90-0874**

BURSTEIN, Maurice J.
A review of ideality of medical science. A detailed plan of reformation of the practice and study of medicine. [New York, 1892.] 40p. DNLM; NNNAM **90-0875**

BURT, Stephen Smith (*b.* 1850)
Pulmonary consumption in the light of modern research. New York: Pusey & Troxell, 1890. 14p. DNLM **90-0876**

BURT, Stephen Smith (*b.* 1850)
Bacteriology and preventive medicine. New York: Pusey & Troxell, 1891. 10p. DNLM **90-0877**

BURT, Stephen Smith (*b.* 1850)
Bacteriology and preventive medicine. New York: Stettiner, Lambert & Co., [1891]. 7p. DNLM **90-0878**

BURT, Stephen Smith (*b.* 1850)
The ethics of experimentation upon living animals. New York, 1891. 2 l. DNLM **90-0879**

BURT, Stephen Smith (*b.* 1850)
The prevention of intemperance. New York, 1892. 2 l. DNLM **90-0880**

BURT, William H. (1836-1897)
Tuberculosis, or pulmonary consumption: its prophylaxis and cure by suralimentation of liquid food. . . . Chicago: W. T. Keener, 1890. 234p. DLC **90-0881**

BURT, William H. (1836-1897)
Characteristic materia medica memorizer. . . . Chicago: Halsey Bros. Co., 1895 [1894]. 391p. DLC **90-0882**

BURWELL, George
Obesity and its cure; a practical and common sense treatise on corpulency or excess of fat. Boston, 1892. 40p. DNLM; MBM **90-0883**

BUSEY, Samuel Clagett (1828-1901)
The Medical Society of the District of Columbia in 1894, with some important recommendations. Annual address of the president, . . . December 19, 1894. Pub. by order of the Society. Washington, D.C.: Gibson Bros., 1894. 22p. DLC; DNLM **90-0884**

BUSEY, Samuel Clagett (1828-1901)
Address of welcome to the Association of Military Surgeons, delivered at Washington, May 1, 1894. Washington, D.C.: Gibson Bros., 1894. 9p. DNLM **90-0885**

BUSEY, Samuel Clagett (1828-1901)
Addresses by the president at the celebration of the 75th anniversary of the Medical Society, D.C.; and at the banquet, February 16, 1894. Washington: Gibson Bros., 1894. 11p. DNLM **90-0886**

BUSEY, Samuel Clagett (1828-1901)
Compulsory reports of zymotic diseases: milk legislation; medical practice law; and society publication of its transactions. Annual address of the president of the Medical Society, District of Columbia, Dec. 18, 1895. Washington: Gibson Bros., 1895. 55p. DNLM **90-0887**

BUSEY, Samuel Clagett (1828-1901)
Address of welcome to the Southern Surgical and Gynecological Society, delivered at Washington, November 12, 1895. Washington: Gibson Bros., 1895. 8p. DNLM
90-0888

BUSEY, Samuel Clagett (1828-1901)
Personal reminiscences and recollections of forty-six years' membership in the Medical Society of the District of Columbia and residence in this city, with biographical sketches of many of the deceased members. . . . Washington, D.C.: [Philadelphia, Dornan, printer], 1895. 373p. DLC; DNLM; PPC
90-0889

BUSEY, Samuel Clagett (1828-1901)
The year 1896: An epoch in the history of the Medical Society of the District of Columbia. Annual address by the president, December 16, 1896. Washington, D.C.: Gibson Bros., 1896. 16p. DNLM **90-0890**

BUSEY, Samuel Clagett (1828-1901)
A souvenir with an autobiographical sketch of early life and selected miscellaneous addresses and communications. . . . City of Washington, D.C. [Philadelphia: Dornan, printer], 1896. 382p. DLC; DNLM; PPC **90-0891**

BUSEY, Samuel Clagett (1828-1901)
The organization, high esprit de corps, high standard of education and scientific attainments of the Army Medical Department. Address at the closing exercises of the Army Medical School, March 12, 1897, Washington, D.C. Washington, D.C.: Gibson Bros., 1897. 22p. DNLM **90-0892**

BUSEY, Samuel Clagett (1828-1901)
The duties of physicians to the profession and their relation to the medical charities of the District of Columbia. Annual address of the president, delivered . . . December 15, 1897. . . . [Washington]: Pub. by order of the Society, [1897]. 13p. DLC **90-0893**

BUSEY, Samuel Clagett (1828-1901)
Annual address of the president of the Medical Society of the District of Columbia, delivered 1894-95-96-97-98. . . . Washington, D.C.: [Philadelphia: Dornan, printer], 1899. 178p. fold. plate, 3 fold. maps. DLC; PPC **90-0894**

BUSHNELL, George E[nsign] (1853-1924)
Subpleural pulmonary abscess; with report of cases. Philadelphia, 1896. 18p. DNLM **90-0895**

BUSHONG, Charles H.
Modern gynecology; a treatise on diseases of women. . . . New York: E. B. Treat, 1893. 380p. DLC; NNNAM
90-0896

BUSHONG, Charles H.
Modern gynecology; a treatise on diseases of women, comprising the results of the latest investigations and treatment in the branch of medical science. . . . 2nd ed. enl. New York: E. B. Treat & Co., 1898. 404p. DLC; NNNAM
90-0897

BUTLER, F. W. P.
Vesico-vaginal fistula. [Charleston, S.C., 1890.] 2p. DNLM
90-0898

BUTLER, George Frank (1857-1921)
A text-book of materia medica, therapeutics, and pharmacology. Philadelphia: W. B. Saunders, 1896. 858p. DLC; DNLM; NNNAM; PPC **90-0899**

BUTLER, George Frank (1857-1921)
A text-book of materia medica, therapeutics, and pharmacology. . . . 2nd ed., revised. . . . Philadelphia: W. B. Saunders, 1898. 860p. 2 plates. DLC; NNNAM; OCLloyd; PPC
90-0900

BUTLER, Glentworth R[eeve] (1855-1926)
The methods and value of supervised exercise in the prophylaxis of pulmonary phthisis. New York: D. Appleton & Co., 1894. 16p. 4 plates. DNLM **90-0901**

BUTLER, Glentworth R[eeve] (1855-1926)
Membranous enteritis; its pathological character and treatment. [New York: D. Appleton & Co., 1895.] 23p. DNLM; NNNAM **90-0902**

BUTTS, H. Hoyle (*d.* 1906)
The removal of adenoid growths from the vault of the pharynx. [Philadelphia: Lea Bros. & Co., 1892.] 12p. DNLM
90-0903

BUTTS, H. Hoyle (*d.* 1906)
A new instrument for controlling tonsillar hemorrhage. New York: Trow's Co., 1893. 8p. 1 table. DNLM
90-0904

BUXTON, Dudley Wilmot (1855-1931)
Anaesthetics, their uses and administration. 2nd ed. Philadelphia: P. Blakiston, Son & Co., 1892. 222p. DNLM; NNNAM; PPC; PU **90-0905**

BUXTON, G. Edward (*b.* 1849)
Champagne and strychnin in chest troubles of the aged. Chicago, 1894. 7p. DNLM **90-0906**

BUXTON, G. Edward (*b.* 1849)
How invalids should come to southern California. National City, Cal., 1894. 8p. DNLM **90-0907**

BYERS, J. Wellington
The Metschnikovian theory of vital resistance. [Philadelphia: W. B. Saunders, 1892.] 15p. DNLM **90-0908**

BYFORD, H[enry] T[urman] (*b.* 1853)
Another twelve months of peritoneal surgery; fifty-seven cases. [Chicago, 1890.] 7p. DNLM **90-0909**

BYFORD, H[enry] T[urman] (*b.* 1853)
The cure of cystocele by inguinal suspension of the bladder; colpo-cystorrhaphy. [New York, 1890.] 3p. DNLM
90-0910

BYFORD, H[enry] T[urman] (*b.* 1853)
A new method of treating the stump in abdominal hysterectomy. Philadelphia: W. J. Dornan, 1890. 7p. DNLM
90-0911

BYFORD, H[enry] T[urman] (*b.* 1853)
Three peritoneal sections performed upon the same patient within nine months: vaginal section, ventral section, and inguinal section. [Chicago, 1890.] 4p. DNLM
90-0912

BYFORD, H[enry] T[urman] (*b.* 1853)
Abdominal hysterectomy for intraligamentous fibroid tumor; enucleation; vaginal fixation of the stump. [Philadelphia, 1891.] 8p. DNLM **90-0913**

BYFORD, H[enry] T[urman] (*b.* 1853)
Cases of extra-uterine pregnancy; abdominal section; remarks upon treatment. [New York, 1891.] 7p. DNLM **90-0914**

BYFORD, H[enry] T[urman] (*b.* 1853)
The technique of vaginal fixation of the stump in abdominal hysterectomy. Philadelphia: W. J. Dornan, 1891. 8p. DNLM **90-0915**

BYFORD, H[enry] T[urman] (*b.* 1853)
Unusual cases of abdominal section. Chicago: R. R. McCabe & Co., [1892]. 8p. DNLM **90-0916**

BYFORD, H[enry] T[urman] (*b.* 1853)
Manual of gynecology. Philadelphia: P. Blakiston, Son & Co., 1895. 488p. DLC; DNLM; NNNAM; PPC **90-0917**

BYFORD, H[enry] T[urman] (*b.* 1853)
Drainage of the stump and connective tissues in abdominal hysterectomy for fibroids and inflammatory disease. Philadelphia, 1896. 4p. DNLM **90-0918**

BYFORD, H[enry] T[urman] (*b.* 1853)
Drainage in peritoneal surgery. New York, [1896]. 4p. DNLM **90-0919**

BYFORD, H[enry] T[urman] (*b.* 1853)
Vaginal section for the cure of retroversion of the uterus. New York, 1896. 6p. DNLM **90-0920**

BYFORD, H[enry] T[urman] (*b.* 1853)
Anterior suspension of the uterus and shortening of the round ligaments by vaginal section. New York, 1896. 5p. DNLM **90-0921**

BYFORD, H[enry] T[urman] (*b.* 1853)
Extirpation of the rectum per vaginam, with utilization of the vagina to replace the lost rectal tissue. Philadelphia, 1896. 3p. DNLM **90-0922**

BYFORD, Henry T[urman] (*b.* 1853)
The microbic origin of fibroid and other benign tumors. Chicago, [1896]. 4p. DNLM **90-0923**

BYFORD, H[enry] T[urman] (*b.* 1853)
Manual of gynecology. . . . 2nd ed., containing three hundred and forty-one illustrations. . . . Philadelphia: P. Blakiston, Son & Co., 1897. 596p. DLC; NNNAM; PPC; PPJ **90-0924**

BYRNE, John (1825-1902)
An inquiry into the relative merits of vaginal hysterectomy and high amputation or partial extirpation by galvano-cautery in cancer of the cervix uteri. [Brooklyn, 1892.] 35p. 3 plates. DNLM; NNNAM **90-0925**

BYRNE, John (1825-1902)
The palliative treatment of utero-vaginal prolapse. New York, 1894. 8p. DNLM **90-0926**

BYRNE, John (1825-1902)
Vaginal hysterectomy by galvano-cautery. Remarks on the scope and limitations of the operation. New York: William Wood & Co., 1895. 12p. DNLM **90-0927**

CABOT, Arthur Tracy (1852-1912)
A case of cystitis, with the formation of a thick epidermal sheet in the bladder-pachydermia vesicae. Philadelphia, 1891. 8p. DNLM **90-0928**

CABOT, Arthur Tracy (1852-1912)
Papers upon abdominal surgery. I. Cases of laparotomy for tubercular peritonitis. II. Two cases of laparotomy for penetrating wounds of the abdomen. III. Notes on complications met with in cases of strangulated hernia. IV. Two cases of abscess of the liver implicating the pleural cavity; operation with recovery. V. A case of relapsing appendicitis, [etc.]. VI. Fifty-two cases of laparotomy undertaken for the removal of tumors. VII. Large papillomatous cyst with ascites; laparotomy, [etc.]. Boston: D. Clapp & Son, 1891. 59p. DNLM; MMB **90-0929**

CABOT, Arthur Tracy (1852-1912)
Cases of operation in spina bifida and encephalocele. Philadelphia, 1892. 3p. DNLM **90-0930**

CABOT, Arthur Tracy (1852-1912)
Papers upon genito-urinary surgery. I. Notes on the non-operative treatment of enlarged prostate. II. A contribution to the treatment of rupture of the bladder. III. A successful case of ureterolithotomy for an impacted calculus. IV. Observations upon the anatomy and surgery of the ureter. V. Pachydemia vesicae. VI. A case of calculous pyelitis; suppression of urine for seven days; operation; recovery. Boston: D. Clapp & Son, 1893. 59p. DNLM; MBM **90-0931**

CABOT, Arthur Tracy (1852-1912)
Remarks on the treatment of enlarged prostate. Boston: D. Clapp & Son, 1895. 22p. DNLM; MBM **90-0932**

CABOT, Arthur Tracy (1852-1912)
The question of castration for enlarged prostate. Philadelphia, 1896. 45p. DNLM; MBM **90-0933**

CABOT, Arthur Tracy (1852-1912)
Papers upon genito-urinary surgery. XIV. Five cases of rupture of the urethra treated by external urethrotomy and suture. XV. A case of cyst of the kidney, apparently cured by a single aspiration. XVI. A case of cancer of the urethra. XVII. A case of scirrhous cancer of the bladder . . . and a case of cystitis with ulceration. . . . XVIII. A case of sacculated bladder, with autopsy. Boston: D. Clapp & Son, 1896. 26p. DNLM; MBM **90-0934**

CABOT, Richard C[larke] (1868-1939)
The diagnostic and prognostic importance of leucocytosis. Boston: Damrell & Upham, 1894. 24p. DNLM **90-0935**

CABOT, Richard C[larke] (1868-1939)
The clinical uses of the preparations from the thyroid gland, pituitary body, suprarenal capsules, and bone marrow. Philadelphia, 1896. 11p. DNLM **90-0936**

CABOT, Richard C[larke] (1868-1939)
The myelocyte of Ehrlich. Boston: Damrell & Upham, 1896. 20p. DNLM **90-0937**

CABOT, Richard C[larke] (1868-1939)
A guide to the clinical examination of the blood for diagnostic purposes. New York: William Wood & Co., 1897. 405p. 4 plates. DLC; DNLM; NNNAM; PU **90-0938**

CABOT, Richard C[larke] (1868-1939)
A guide to the clinical examination of the blood for diagnostic purposes. . . . 2nd ed. New York: William Wood & Co., 1897. 439p. plates, diags. DLC; NNNAM; OCIM; PPC **90-0939**

CABOT, Richard C[larke] (1868-1939)
A guide to the clinical examination of the blood for diagnostic purposes. . . . With colored plates and engravings. 3rd rev. ed. New York: William Wood & Co., 1898. 440p. DLC; IU-M; NNNAM; PPJ **90-0940**

CABOT, Richard C[larke] (1868-1939)
The serum diagnosis of disease. . . . New York: William Wood & Co., 1899. 154p. plates, diags. DLC; NNNAM **90-0941**

CAILLÉ, Augustus (1854-1935)
Clinical notes for nurses, for use in the babies' wards of the Post-Graduate Hospital, by Augustus Caillé . . . and Robert Abbe. . . . [New York? 1895.] 24p. DLC; NNNAM **90-0942**

CAIRD, Francis M[itchell] (1853-1926)
Surgical handbook. . . . By F. M. Caird and Charles W. Cathcart. 5th ed. Philadelphia: P. Blakiston, Son & Co., 1890 [1889]. 262p. DNLM; MBM; PPC; PU **90-0943**

CALDWELL, John D.
A family hand book of specific treatment of disease. . . . McGregor, Ia.: J. F. Widman, printer and binder, 1894. 116p. DLC **90-0944**

CALDWELL, John J[abez] (*b.* 1836)
The erectile tissues; their physiology, pathology, and treatment. [Charlotte, N.C., 1893.] 8p. DNLM **90-0945**

CALDWELL, John L.
Liquor sedans, saw palmetto, damiana, pichi, and stylosanthes elatior; their uses in nervous diseases; their medico-legal relation; epilogue. [Richmond, 1894.] 10p. DNLM **90-0946**

CALDWELL, W[illiam] C.
The modes of action of emetics. New York, 1894. 7p. DNLM **90-0947**

CALE, George W.
Clinical report of six surgical cases. [St. Louis, 1892.] 8p. DNLM **90-0948**

CALL, Emma L[ouisa]
. . . Synopsis of lectures in anatomy and physiology. Arranged for the Boston Normal School of Gymnastics, by . . . . Boston: Press of G. H. Ellis, 1892. 53p. DLC; MB **90-0949**

CALLAN, Peter A.
Migraine and functional headaches from eye-strain. Chicago, 1891. 8p. DNLM **90-0950**

CALLAN, Peter A.
Four cases of orbital traumatism resulting in immediate monocular blindness through fracture into foramen opticum. In one of these cases the blow was over the left orbit, causing blindness of the right eye. Chicago, 1892. 7p. DNLM **90-0951**

CAMDEN (N.J.) DISTRICT MEDICAL SOCIETY
Report of the celebration of the fiftieth anniversary of the . . . held in Camden, N.J., February 11, 1896. Newark, N.J.: L. J. Hardham, 1896. 76p. 2 plates. DNLM; NjR **90-0952**

CAMMANN, D[onald] M[ühlenburg]
The physical diagnosis of the diseases of the heart and lungs and thoracic aneurism. . . . New York, [etc.]: G. P. Putnam's Sons, 1891. 188p. DLC; DNLM; NNNAM **90-0953**

CAMPBELL, G. Gordon (*b.* 1863)
Ether anaesthesia; clinical notes on three hundred cases. Philadelphia, 1894. 29p. DNLM **90-0954**

CAMPBELL, Henry Fraser (1824-1891)
Vesico-vaginal fistula with some aberrant cases, illustrating the causes of leakage after successful closure of the fistula; vesical calculi in connection with fistula; uretero-vaginal fistula. Philadelphia: W. J. Dornan, 1891. 29p. DNLM; PPC; PU **90-0955**

CAMPBELL, J[ames] B.
Three cases of pneumonia followed by mania. [Philadelphia, 1894.] 5p. DNLM **90-0956**

CAMPBELL, William A.
Outlines of anatomy for students. A guide to dissection based on Morris's text-book of anatomy. Philadelphia: P. Blakiston, Son & Co., 1895. 124p. DLC; DNLM; NNNAM; PPC **90-0957**

CANFIELD, Herman
The Azores as a health resort. [Providence, R.I.: Snow & Farnham, 1892.] 18p. 1 plate. DNLM **90-0958**

CANFIELD, Herman
Only nervousness. [New York: D. Appleton & Co., 1896.] 16p. DNLM **90-0959**

CANFIELD, William B[uckingham] (1857-1899)
The early detection of pulmonary consumption. Baltimore: Jour. Pub. Co., 1890. 11p. DNLM **90-0960**

CANFIELD, William B[uckingham] (1857-1899)
Practical notes on urinary analysis. [With additions.] Detroit, Mich.: G. S. Davis, 1891. 93p. 1 table, 1 plate. DNLM; OCIM **90-0961**

CANFIELD, William B[uckingham] (1857-1899)
The hygiene of the sick room. A book for nurses and others, being a brief consideration of asepsis, antisepsis, disinfection, bacteriology, immunity, heating and ventilation, and kindred subjects, for the use of nurses and other intelligent women. Philadelphia: P. Blakiston, Son & Co., 1892. 247p. DNLM; MdU-D; PPC; PU **90-0962**

CANNADY, Charles G[raham]
Subinvolution of uterus, and its treatment by electricity. [New York, 1893.] 4p. DNLM **90-0963**

CANNADY, Charles G[raham]
Chronic endometritis; its aetiology, modern methods in diagnosis, and treatment. [Richmond, 1893.] 12p. DNLM
90-0964

CANNADY, Charles G[raham]
The relation of tight lacing to uterine development and abdominal and pelvic disease. Toledo, 1894. 9p. DNLM
90-0965

CANTRELL, J. Abbott (*b.* 1863)
A case of painful subcutaneous neuroma (neuro-fibroma). Chicago, 1890. 7p. DNLM **90-0966**

CANTRELL, J. Abbott (*b.* 1863)
Unusual mode of transmission in a case of dermatitis venenata. [Philadelphia, 1891.] 1 galley sheet. DNLM
90-0967

CANTRELL, J. Abbott (*b.* 1863)
A case of eczema with urticaria as a complication. [Danbury, 1892.] 2 l. DNLM **90-0968**

CANTRELL, J. Abbott (*b.* 1863)
Notes on tinea circinata, tinea sycosis, and tinea tonsurans. [Philadelphia, 1892.] 6p. DNLM **90-0969**

CANTRELL, J. Abbott (*b.* 1863)
Remarks on and treatment of patients in the skin clinic of the Jefferson Medical College Hospital. Detroit: G. S. Davis, 1892. 9p. DNLM **90-0970**

CANTRELL, J. Abbott (*b.* 1863)
Acne, comedo, and acne rosacea. Philadelphia, 1893. 3p. DNLM **90-0971**

CANTRELL, J. Abbott (*b.* 1863)
Irritation from the local use of iodoform. [Philadelphia, 1893.] 2p. DNLM **90-0972**

CANTRELL, J. Abbott (*b.* 1863)
Scabies; its symptoms, diagnosis, and treatment. Detroit: G. S. Davis, 1893. 8p. DNLM **90-0973**

CANTRELL, J. Abbott (*b.* 1863)
Alumnol in dermatology. [New York, 1894.] 2p. DNLM
90-0974

CANTRELL, J. Abbott (*b.* 1863)
An unusual case of syphilis. Philadelphia: Lea Bros. & Co., 1894. 5p. DNLM **90-0975**

CANTRELL, J. Abbott (*b.* 1863)
Abnormalities in the color of the human hair, with a report of cases. Philadelphia, 1895. 21p. DNLM
90-0976

CANTRELL, J. Abbott (*b.* 1863)
A case of late syphilis showing unusual lesions of the skin. [Philadelphia, 1895.] 4p. DNLM **90-0977**

CANTRELL, J. Abbott (*b.* 1863)
Eczema of the scalp. Philadelphia, 1895. 7p. DNLM
90-0978

CANTRELL, J. Abbott (*b.* 1863)
Tinea circinata presenting two rings. New York: D. Appleton & Co., 1895. 2p. DNLM **90-0979**

CAPEN, John L.
The phrenological character . . . in a combination chart. . . . Philadelphia, Pa., 1894. 28p. DLC **90-0980**

CAPEN, John L.
Phrenological papers. . . . [Philadelphia?], 1896. 16p. DLC
90-0981

CAPP, William M.
The daughter: her health, education, and wedlock; homely suggestions for mothers and daughters. Philadelphia: F. A. Davis, 1893 [*c.* 1881]. 144p. ICU; MB; NN **90-0982**

CAREY, George W[ashington] (1845-1924)
The biochemic system of medicine, comprising the theory, pathological action, therapeutical application, materia medica, and repertory of Schuessler's twelve tissue remedies. St. Louis: F. A. Luyties, 1894. 444p. DLC **90-0983**

CAREY, George W[ashington] (1845-1924)
The biochemic system of medicine, comprising the theory, pathological action, therapeutical application, materia medica, and repertory of Scheussler's twelve tissue remedies. 3rd ed. St. Louis: F. A. Luyties, 1896. 444p. DNLM; OCIM
90-0984

CARHART, William Merle d'Aubigné (1863-1937)
The refraction of the eyes of one thousand school children, with particular reference to astigmatism, as shown by the Javal ophthalmometer. New York, 1897. 13p. DNLM
90-0985

CARHART, William Merle d'Aubigné (1863-1937)
The importance of the exact correction of refractive errors in school children. New York, 1897. 9p. DNLM
90-0986

CARLETON, Bukk G. (1856-1914)
A manual of genito-urinary and venereal diseases, by Bukk G. Carleton . . . with venereal diseases of the eye by Charles Deady . . . and vesical calculus and external urethrotomy, by Wm. Francis Honan. . . . New York: Boericke, Runyon & Ernesty, 1895. 315p. DLC; NNNAM; PPC; PPHa
90-0987

CARLETON, Bukk G. (1856-1914)
Medical and surgical diseases of the kidneys and ureters. . . . New York: Boericke, Runyon & Ernesty, 1898 [1897]. 253p. plates. DLC; DNLM; NNNAM **90-0988**

CARLETON, Bukk G. (1856-1914)
A practical treatise on the sexual disorders of men. . . . New York: Boericke, Runyon & Ernesty, 1898. 169p. DLC; NNNAM **90-0989**

CARMALT, William H. (1836-1929)
A brief consideration of the cases of appendicitis occurring in the practice of. [Bridgeport, 1894.] 13p. DNLM
90-0990

CARMALT, William H. (1836-1929)
Five gunshot wounds of the intestine and mesentery; laparotomy; sutures; recovery. New Haven, 1895. 2 l. DNLM
90-0991

CARMALT, William H. (1836-1929)
Report of a case of appendicitis presenting some peculiar and instructive features. New Haven, 1896. 2 l. DNLM
90-0992

CARMICHAEL, James
Disease in children. A manual for students and practitioners. New York: D. Appleton & Co., 1892. 591p. DNLM; NNNAM; PPC; PU **90-0993**

CARPENTER, John T., Jr.
Two cases of hyaline formations in the otpic nerve. [Philadelphia, 1893.] 5p. 1 plate. DNLM **90-0994**

CARPENTER, William B[enjamin] (1813-1885)
The microscope and its revelations. . . . Enlg., and rev. by W. H. Dalinger, 7th ed. Philadelphia: P. Blakiston, Son & Co., 1891. 1099p. plates. MBH; OCl; PPC; PU **90-0995**

CARR, Walter Lester (*b.* 1859)
Some manifestations of rachitis not always associated with severe bone changes. [Philadelphia, 1890.] 14p. DNLM **90-0996**

CARR, Walter Lester (*b.* 1859)
Laryngismus stridulus. New York, 1891. 8p. DNLM **90-0997**

CARR, Walter Lester (*b.* 1859)
A case of scorbutus in an infant. [New York, 1892.] 4p. DNLM **90-0998**

CARR, Walter Lester (*b.* 1859)
Sarcoma of the skin of the back in a baby. [New York, 1893.] 2p. DNLM **90-0999**

CARRIER, Albert E. (1841-1908)
Bald heads. [Detroit, 1891.] 9p. DNLM **90-1000**

CARRIER, Albert E. (1841-1908)
Pigmentation of the whole surface of the body, occurring suddenly during the treatment of a case of psoriasis; warty growths upon the palms and soles, following the internal use of arsenic. [Philadelphia, 1894.] 8p. DNLM **90-1001**

CARROLL, Alfred Ludlow (1833-1893)
Address on state medicine. Chicago, 1890. 20p. DNLM **90-1002**

CARROLL, Alfred Ludlow (1833-1893)
Remarks introductory to a discussion on acute diffuse peritonitis. **90-1003**

CARSON, J. C. and Alois F. HRDLICKA
An interesting case of pseudo-hermaphroditismus masculinus completus. Albany, 1897. 8p. 1 plate. DNLM **90-1004**

CARSON, N[orman] B.
Abscess of the brain. New York, 1895. 9p. DNLM **90-1005**

CARSTENS, J[ohn] H[enry] (1848-1920)
Three cases of hysterectomy following coeliotomy for pus-tubes. New York, 1895. 5p. DNLM **90-1006**

CARSTENS, J[ohn] H[enry] (1848-1920)
Some remarks upon a year's work in appendicitis. New York, 1896. 8p. DNLM **90-1007**

CARTER, Charles L.
A treatise on general pathology and its relation to practical medicine. 2nd ed., rev. St. Louis: Woodward & Tiernan Print. Co., 1891. 157p. DLC; DNLM **90-1008**

CARTER, J[ames] M[adison] (1843-1919)
The cause and treatment of pneumonia. [Chicago], 1890. 1p. DNLM **90-1009**

CARTER, J[ames] M[adison] (1843-1919)
Catarrhal diseases of the respiratory passages. Chicago: E. H. Colegrove & Co., 1895. 135p. DNLM; IU-M; OCIM **90-1010**

CARTER, William A.
A study of heat-production and heat-dissipation in the normal and febrile states. [New York, 1890.] 7p. DNLM **90-1011**

CARTER, William S.
Notes on the lectures of Prof. John Guitéras on general and special pathology, delivered before the second and third year students of the University of Pennsylvania; and on the lectures of Dr. Joseph McFarland on bacteriology, delivered before the third year class. Arranged by Dr. William S. Carter and Dr. David Riesman. . . . [Philadelphia: Avil Printing Co., 1895.] 246, 56p. DLC; PPC; PU **90-1012**

CARTLEDGE, A[biah] M[organ] (1858-1908)
The present status of drainage in surgery. [Philadelphia, 1893.] 11p. DNLM **90-1013**

CARTLEDGE, A[biah] M[organ] (1858-1908)
Hysterectomy in acute puerperal sepsis, with report of cases. [New York, 1896.] 9p. DNLM **90-1014**

A **CASE** of alleged criminal abortion; the consequences of a hasty assumption. New York, 1893. 10p. DNLM **90-1015**

A **CASE** of chronic Bright's disease (parenchymatous), with recovery; including the sworn statement of the patient. [New Orleans, 1893, *vel subseq.*] 32p. DNLM; LNT-M **90-1016**

A **CASE** of middle meningeal hemorrhage. Operation; recovery. An analysis of forty-eight cases of uncomplicated intra-cranial hemorrhage, by Charles L. Scudder, M.D., and Fred. B. Lund, M.D. II. Middle meningeal hemorrhage, by G. L. Walton, M.D. III. Localized hemorrhage beneath pia mater over upper third of Rolandic area, due to fall on the head; localized convulsions without loss of consciousness; later, slight mental confusion with paralysis of the affected limbs, followed by prolonged coma and death. By James J. Putnam, M.D. Philadelphia, 1895. 28p. DNLM; PPC **90-1017**

CASPARI, Charles (1850-1917)
A treatise on pharmacy for students and pharmacists. . . . With 288 illustrations. Philadelphia: Lea Bros. & Co., 1895. 679p. DLC; NNNAM; OCLloyd; PPC **90-1018**

CASSELBERRY, W[illiam] E[vans] (1858-1916)
Arthritis deformans of the larynx. [New York: D. Appleton & Co., 1893.] 7p. DNLM **90-1019**

CASSELBERRY, W[illiam] E[vans] (1858-1916)
Nasal polypus; its association with ethmoiditis and its treatment by resection of the middle turbinated body. New York, 1894, 19p. DNLM **90-1020**

CASSELBERRY, W[illiam] E[vans] (1858-1916)
Electrolysis by a current controller for the reduction of spurs of the nasal septum. New York, 1895. 13p. DNLM
90-1021

CASSELBERRY, W[illiam] E[vans] (1858-1916)
Intubation in the adult. With special reference to acute stenosis of the larynx. New York, 1896. 13p. DNLM
90-1022

CATHELL, Daniel Webster (1839-1925)
Book on the physician himself and things that concern his reputation and success. 9th ed., rev. and enl. Philadelphia: F. A. Davis Co., 1890. 298p. LNT-M; NNNAM; PPC; PPJ
90-1023

CATHELL, Daniel Webster (1839-1925)
Book on the physician himself and things that concern his reputation and success. 10th ed., carefully rev. and greatly enlarged. Philadelphia: F. A. Davis Co., 1892. 343p. DNLM; PPC; PPHa; PU **90-1024**

CATHELL, Daniel Webster (1839-1925)
A small but useful combination of medicines for vest pocket and office use. Baltimore, 1896. 4p. DNLM
90-1025

CATHELL, William T. (*b.* 1864)
Stammering. [Baltimore, 1890.] 3p. DNLM
90-1026

CATHELL, William T. (*b.* 1864)
The treatment of the nasal catarrhs. [Baltimore, 1891.] 8p. DNLM **90-1027**

CATHELL, William T. (*b.* 1864)
Catarrhal headache. [Baltimore, 1891.] 7p. DNLM
90-1028

CATHELL, William T. (*b.* 1864)
A study of two cases of paroxysmal sneezing, with the treatment. Baltimore: Friedenwald Co., [1893, *vel subseq.*]. 12p. DNLM **90-1029**

CATHELL, William T. (*b.* 1864)
Troches. [Baltimore, 1894.] 11p. DNLM
90-1030

CATHELL, William T. (*b.* 1864)
Over-fatness; a reliable and harmless way to diminish and cure it. Baltimore, 1897. 16p. DNLM
90-1031

CATLIN, A[rnold] W.
Oxygen as a distinct remedy for disease and a life-saving agent in extreme cases. New York: M. J. Rooney, 1892. 16p. DNLM
90-1032

CATTELL, Henry W[are] (1862-1936)
Notes on the demonstrations in morbid anatomy, including autopsies. Part I. [1892.] 24p. 1 plate. DNLM
90-1033

CATTELL, Henry W[are] (1862-1936)
Some who have suffered for pathology's sake. [Philadelphia, 1893.] 4p. DNLM **90-1034**

CATTELL, Henry W[are] (1862-1936)
Perforation of Meckel's diverticulum in a case of typhoid fever. [Philadelphia, 1893.] 2p. DNLM **90-1035**

CATTELL, Henry W[are] (1862-1936)
Some special points on the performance of autopsies on the new-born. [Philadelphia, 1893.] 6p. DNLM
90-1036

CATTELL, Henry W[are] (1862-1936)
Some practical post-mortem points. [Philadelphia, 1893.] 5p. DNLM **90-1037**

CATTELL, Henry W[are] (1862-1936)
Notes on the demonstrations in morbid anatomy (including autopsies), delivered in the Medical Department of the University of Pennsylvania before the third year class. . . . Philadelphia: International Medical Magazine Co., 1894. 172p. plates. DLC; PU **90-1038**

CAUTHORN, F[ranklin]
Successful removal of a large tumor of the mesentery, with resection of 43 inches of intestine; end-to-end anastomosis with Murphy button. Philadelphia, 1895. 5p. DNLM
90-1039

[CELSIUS, Robert C.]
Myopia for nearsightedness; its cause and chronic cure. Philadelphia, 1898. 8p. DLC **90-1040**

CERNA, David (*b.* 1857)
A study of the physiological action of kava-kava. Detroit: G. S. Davis, 1891. 28p. DNLM **90-1041**

CERNA, David (*b.* 1857)
Notes on the newer remedies, their therapeutic applications and modes of administration. . . . Philadelphia: W. B. Saunders, 1892. 177p. DLC; DNLM; NNNAM; PPC
90-1042

CERNA, David (*b.* 1857) and William S. CARTER
A study of the comparative actions of antipyrine, phenacetine and phenocoll on the circulation and heat phenomena. [Philadelphia, 1892.] 19p. DNLM **90-1043**

CERNA, David (*b.* 1857)
Typhus fever as met with in Mexico, with special reference to its treatment. St. Louis, 1893. 16p. DNLM
90-1044

CERNA, David (*b.* 1857)
The actions and uses of pental. [New York, 1893.] 36p. DNLM **90-1045**

CERNA, David (*b.* 1857)
The therapeutic uses of sparteine. New York, 1894. 24p. DNLM **90-1046**

CERNA, David (*b.* 1857)
Some thoughts on higher medical education and medical ethics. [New York, 1894.] 27p. DNLM
90-1047

CERNA, David (*b.* 1857)
The physiological actions of alcohol. Abstract of a paper presented to the section on therapeutics of the First Pan-American Medical Congress, held at Washington, D.C., September 5, 6, 7 and 8, 1893. Detroit, Mich.: G. S. Davis, 1894. 67p. DNLM; OCIM **90-1048**

CERNA, David (*b.* **1857)**
A contribution to the study of the physiological actions of sparteine. [New York, 1894.] 15p. DNLM
90-1049

CERNA, David (*b.* **1857)**
Notes on the newer remedies, their therapeutic applications and mode of administration. . . . 2nd ed. Philadelphia: W. B. Saunders, 1895. 253p. CtY-M; MBM; NNNAM; PPC
90-1050

CHADWICK, French Ensor (1844-1919)
Temperament, disease, and health. New York, London: G. P. Putnam's Sons, 1892. 85p. DNLM; NNNAM
90-1051

CHADWICK, James Read (1844-1905)
A case of nephro-lithotomy, in which no stone was found. Philadelphia: W. J. Dornan, 1890. 20p. 1 chart. DNLM; PPC
90-1052

CHAILLÉ, Stanford Emerson (1830-1911)
The practice of medicine as a money-making occupation. An address to the graduates at the annual commencement of the Medical Department, Tulane University, on April 14, 1897. New Orleans, 1897. 10p. DNLM; LNT-M
90-1053

CHAMBERLIN, Frank T.
Recurrence in a case of abscess of the epiglottis. [Richmond, 1893.] 4p. DNLM **90-1054**

CHAMBERLIN, Frank T.
Hypertrophy of the lingual tonsil. Richmond, 1894. 4p. DNLM **90-1055**

CHAMBERLIN, Frank T.
Notes on a case of round-celled sarcoma, treated by erysipelas and prodigiosus toxines, after excision. Richmond, 1895. 4p. DNLM **90-1056**

CHAMBERS, P. F.
Abortion as a cause of disease of the pelvic organs. New York, 1894. 5p. DNLM **90-1057**

CHANCELLOR, Charles Williams (1831-1915)
Observations on cholera and quarantine. A national quarantine implies national seclusion. [Baltimore, J. Murphy & Co., 1893.] 15p. DNLM **90-1058**

CHANCELLOR, Charles Williams (1831-1915)
Special consular report. Inoculation for diphtheria and croup. [Report on the treatment of diphtheria and croup by means of hypodermic injections of diphtheritic serum.] Oct. 14, 1894. [Washington, 1894.] 6p. DNLM **90-1059**

CHANNING, Walter (1849-1921)
Some remarks on the address delivered to the American Medico-Psychological Association, by S. Weir Mitchell, M.D., May 16, 1894. [Utica, N.Y., 1894?] 11p. DNLM
90-1060

CHANNING, Walter (1849-1921)
The importance of frequent observations of temperature in the diagnosis of chronic tuberculosis. (With illustrative charts.) [Boston, 1895.] 4p. DNLM **90-1061**

CHANNING, Walter (1849-1921)
[Report of] a case of tumor of the thalmus, with remarks on the mental symptoms. [New York: Raff & Co., 1896.] 8p. 2 plates. DNLM **90-1062**

CHANNING, Walter (1849-1921)
The relation of the medical profession to school education. [Cambridge: Harvard Printing Co., 1897.] 8p. DNLM
90-1063

CHANNING, Walter (1849-1921)
Characteristics of insanity; a lecture delivered to the students of Tufts College Medical School. . . . Boston: Damrell & Upham, 1897. 24p. DLC; MBM **90-1064**

CHAPIN, Charles V[alue] (1856-1941)
The purification of public water supplies. An address delivered before the Rhode Island Medical Society, June 1, 1893. [Providence, 1893.] 22p. DNLM **90-1065**

CHAPIN, Henry D[wight] (1857-1942)
The auriculo-ventricular (presystolic) sound. Some considerations on cardiac disease in early life. New York: Trow, 1890. 12p. DNLM **90-1066**

CHAPIN, Henry D[wight] (1857-1942)
Diphtheria. [New York, 1890.] 20p. DLC; DNLM
90-1067

CHAPIN, Henry D[wight] (1857-1942)
Studies in infant feeding. [Also:] A food for infants, with experiments, chemical and physiological. By Arnold Eiloart. [New York: D. Appleton & Co., 1890. 20p. DNLM
90-1068

CHAPIN, Henry D[wight] (1857-1942)
Paludism in children in New York. New York, 1894. 9p. DNLM **90-1069**

CHAPIN, John Bassett (1829-1918)
A compendium of insanity. . . . Philadelphia: W. B. Saunders, 1898. 234p. plates. DLC; PPC; PU
90-1070

CHAPMAN, A[ndrew] L.
The pathological signification of immunity. [Kansas City: Hudson Kimberly Publ. Co., 1893.] 11p. DNLM
90-1071

CHAPMAN, Henry Cadwalader (1845-1909)
Memoir of Joseph Leidy, M.D., LL.D. Philadelphia, 1891. 49p. port. DNLM; PPC; PU **90-1072**

CHAPMAN, Henry Cadwalader (1845-1909)
A manual of medical jurisprudence and toxicology. . . . With thirty-six illustrations, some of which are in colors. Philadelphia: W. B. Saunders, 1892. 237p. DLC; NNNAM; PPC; PU
90-1073

CHAPMAN, Henry Cadwalader (1845-1909)
A manual of medical jurisprudence and toxicology. . . . 2nd ed., rev. With 55 illustrations and 3 plates in colors. Philadelphia: W. B. Saunders, 1896. 254p. DLC: IU-M; PPC; PPJ
90-1074

CHAPMAN, Henry Cadwalader (1845-1909)
Treatise on human physiology. For the use of students and practitioners of medicine. . . . 2nd ed. Illustrated with 595 engravings. Philadelphia: Lea Bros. & Co., 1899. 924p. diags. DLC; NNNAM; PPC; PU **90-1075**

CHAPMAN, J. B.
Biochemistry: a domestic treatise on the application of Schuessler's twelve tissue remedies. St. Louis, Mo.: F. A. Luyties, [1897]. 307p. DNLM; OCIM; PPHa **90-1076**

CHAPMAN, W. Carroll (1841?-1910)
Resorcin as an antipyretic. Read before the Kentucky State Medical Society, May, 1891. [Louisville, 1891.] 12p. DNLM **90-1077**

CHAPMAN, W. Carroll (1841?-1910)
Diphtheria primarily a local, secondarily a constitutional disease. [Philadelphia, 1894.] 7p. DNLM **90-1078**

CHAPPELL, Walter F[ranklin]
Neurasthenia and neuralgia from traumatism of the nasal passages. [New York, 1890.] 13p. DNLM **90-1079**

CHAPPELL, Walter F[ranklin]
Results of the examination of the throat and nose of two thousand children to determine the frequency of certain abnormal conditions. 2nd ed. New York: N. Y. Inst. Deaf and Dumb, 1892. 11p. DNLM **90-1080**

CHAPPELL, Walter F[ranklin]
Treatment of oesophageal stricture by permanent tubage. [New York, 1892.] 11p. DNLM **90-1081**

CHAPPELL, Walter F[ranklin]
Hints on coughs, their causes and treatment. New York, 1892. 15p. DNLM **90-1082**

CHAPPELL, Walter F[ranklin]
Consumption at health resorts. [New York, 1892.] 8p. DNLM **90-1083**

CHAPPELL, Walter F[ranklin]
Two cases of congenital hypertrophy of the tongue. A case of tuberculosis of the thyroid gland. New York, 1894. 2 l. 2 plates. DNLM **90-1084**

CHAPPELL, Walter F[ranklin]
Short notes of unusual cases. [St. Louis], 1894. 8p. DNLM **90-1085**

CHAPPELL, Walter F[ranklin]
Vexed questions in the bacteriology of diphtheria. [New York, 1894.] 1 l. DNLM **90-1086**

CHAPPELL, Walter F[ranklin]
Cases of vaso-motor rhinitis from malarial poison. New York, 1894. 4p. DNLM **90-1087**

CHAPPELL, Walter F[ranklin]
The treatment of laryngeal tuberculosis by the application and submucous injection of creosote. Description of an automatic faryngeal syringe for making submucous injections. New York: D. Appleton & Co., 1895. 22p. DNLM **90-1088**

CHAPPELL, Walter F[ranklin]
Report of three cases of xerostomia or dry mouth. New York, 1896. 7p. DNLM **90-1089**

CHAPPELL, Walter F[ranklin]
Observations on the creosote treatment of tuberculosis of the upper air passages. New York, 1896. 7p. DNLM **90-1090**

CHAPPELL, Walter F[ranklin]
A new semifluid product, oleo-stearate of zinc. New York: D. Appleton & Co., 1896. 3p. DNLM **90-1091**

CHAREST, Remi
Painless parturition. A guide for women, how to avoid the pains and dangers of parturition. With a chapter on the laws of anti-natal influences. . . . [St. Cloud, Minn.: Gans & Fahnlender, 1891.] 48p. DLC **90-1092**

CHARLES, T[homas] William Cranstoun (1849-1894)
The elements of physiological and pathological chemistry. Philadelphia: Lea Bros. & Co., 1890 [1884]. 463p. plate. DNLM; ICU; PPC; PPJ **90-1093**

CHARTERIS, M[atthew] (1840-1897)
The student's guide to the practice of medicine. 6th ed. Philadelphia: P. Blakiston, Son & Co., 1891. 680p. 7 plates. CtY-M; DNLM; MBM; PPC **90-1094**

CHASE, Ira Carleton
A laboratory manual of medical chemistry; containing a systematic course of experiments in laboratory manipulation and chemical action, the non-metallic elements and the medicinal metals, quantitative processes applied to sanitary water analysis, medicinal organic compounds, proteids, digestion, blood, milk, urinalysis and toxicology. Fort Worth, Tex.: W. W. Underhill, 1897. 207p. DNLM **90-1095**

CHASE, Theodore L.
List of graduates of Hahnemann Medical College of Philadelphia, from 1849 to 1891. Arranged alphabetically, with year of graduation. Philadelphia, [1892?] 8p. PPHa **90-1096**

CHASE, Walter B[enaiah]
Remarks on the use of the uterine curette. [New York, 1890.] 11p. DNLM **90-1097**

CHASE, Walter B[enaiah]
The prevention of puerperal septicaemia. New York: Stuyvesant, 1893. 8p. DNLM **90-1098**

CHAVASSE, Pye Henry (1810-1879)
What every woman should know, containing facts of vital importance to every wife, mother and maiden. Adapted from the writings of Pye Henry Chavasse . . . Together with an introduction by Sarah Hackett Stevenson. . . . Chicago and Philadelphia: H. J. Smith & Co., 1892. 606p. plates. DLC; NNNAM; PU [In pocket: "Plates illustrating the female reproductive organs." Chicago: H. J. Smith & Co., 1892. [33]p. Second English edition published 1843, under title: Advice to wives on the management of themselves, during the periods of pregnancy, labour and suckling.] **90-1099**

CHAVASSE, Pye Henry (1810-1879)
Advice to a wife, and advice and counsel to a mother. Philadelphia: J. B. Lippincott Co., 1894. 309p. DNLM; NNNAM; PPC **90-1100**

CHAVASSE, Pye Henry (1810-1879)
Counsel to a mother; being a continuation and the completion of "Advice to a mother." Philadelphia: J. B. Lippincott Co., 1894. 169p. DNLM; NNNAM; PU **90-1101**

CHAVASSE, Pye Henry (1810-1879)
Chavasse's advice to a mother on the management of her children, and on the treatment on the moment of some of their more pressing illnesses and accidents. . . . New ed. Philadelphia: J. B. Lippincott Co., 1894. 408p. DNLM; IU-M; PPC; PU **90-1102**

CHAVASSE, Pye Henry (1810-1879)
Chavasse's Advice to a mother on the management of her children, and on the treatment on the moment of some of their more pressing illnesses and accidents, by George Carpenter. . . . Adapted for American readers by an American physician. . . . 15th ed. New York: G. Routledge & Sons, 1898. 435p. DLC: NNNAM [First English ed. published 1839 under title: Advice to mothers on the management of their offspring.] **90-1103**

CHAVASSE, Pye Henry (1810-1879)
Chavasse's Advice to a wife on the management of her own health and on the treatment of some of the complaints incidental to pregnancy, labor, and suckling; rev. by Fancourt Barnes. . . . 14th ed. New York: G. Routledge & Sons, 1898. 368p. DLC; NNNAM; PPC; PU **90-1104**

CHEATHAM, W[illiam]
Acute mania following the enucleation of an eye. [New York, 1890.] 1 l. DNLM **90-1105**

CHEATHAM, W[illiam]
Pyoktanin in diseases of the eye, ear, and throat. [Cincinnati], 1890. 7p. DNLM **90-1106**

CHEATHAM, W[illiam]
Uric acid diathesis in affections of the eye, ear, throat, and nose. Louisville: J. P. Morton & Co., 1890. 8p. DNLM **90-1107**

CHEATHAM, W[illiam]
The use of powdered jequirity in certain affections of the eye. [Chicago, 1890.] 4p. DNLM **90-1108**

CHEATHAM, W[illiam]
Trachoma and its treatment; powdered jequirity. [Nashville, 1891.] 4p. DNLM **90-1109**

CHEATHAM, W[illiam]
Tumors of the naso-pharynx, pharynx, larynx, and oesophagus. New York: D. Appleton & Co., 1891. 21p. DNLM **90-1110**

CHEATHAM, W[illiam]
The effect of diseases of the ear upon the general condition. Philadelphia: Penfield Bros., 1892. 10p. DNLM **90-1111**

CHEATHAM, W[illiam]
Leptothrix mycosis of the tonsil, pharynx, and base of the tongue. Louisville, 1893. 4p. DNLM **90-1112**

CHEATHAM, W[illiam]
Paralysis of laryngeal muscles, with cases. Louisville, 1893. 4p. DNLM **90-1113**

CHEATHAM, W[illiam]
A case of cysticercus of the vitreous. Kansas City, 1894. 3p. DNLM **90-1114**

CHEATHAM, W[illiam]
Eye symptoms in nephritis, as seen with the ophthalmoscope. Louisville, 1896. 2p. DNLM **90-1115**

CHEATHAM, W[illiam]
Hay fever; the best treatment for stay-at-homes. Louisville, 1896. 4p. DNLM **90-1116**

CHEATHAM, W[illiam]
Ophthalmia neonatorum. New York, 1896. 3p. DNLM **90-1117**

CHEATHAM, W[illiam]
Is there ever a serous iritis without an involvement of the ciliary body, or choroid, or both? Chicago, 1897. 2p. DNLM **90-1118**

CHEATHAM, W[illiam]
The present status of the serum treatment of diphtheria. Louisville, 1897. 6p. DNLM **90-1119**

CHEESMAN, Timothy Matlack (1853-1919)
A consideration of artesian well and surface waters from the standpoint of bacteriology and public health. [New York], 1893. 14p. DNLM **90-1120**

CHEEVER, David Williams (1831-1915)
Lectures on surgery. . . . Boston: Damrell & Upham, 1894. 591p. DLC; DNLM; MBM; NNNAM **90-1121**

CHEEVER, David Williams (1831-1915)
Lectures on surgery, and other papers. . . . 2nd ed.—rev. Boston: Damrell & Upham, 1898. 787p. DLC; MBM **90-1122**

CHENEY, Frederick E[dward] (1862-1924)
Errors of refraction and insufficiencies of the ocular muscles as causes of chorea, with cases. Boston: Damrell & Upham, 1890. 28p. DNLM **90-1123**

CHENEY, Frederick E[dward] (1862-1924)
Hysterical mydriasis, paralysis of the accommodation, and blindness, following the use of the hydrobromate of homatropine. Boston: Damrell & Upham, 1890. 12p. DNLM **90-1124**

CHENEY, Frederick E[dward] (1862-1924)
Purulent ophthalmia neonatorum as a cause of blindness. Boston: Damrell & Upham, 1892. 6p. DNLM **90-1125**

CHENEY, Frederick E[dward] (1862-1924)
Ocular headaches. Boston: Damrell & Upham, 1892. 7p. DNLM **90-1126**

CHENOWETH, James S.
Etiology of appendicitis; why is it more common in the Anglo-Saxon race? Louisville: J. P. Morton & Co., 1897. 42p. DNLM **90-1127**

CHETWOOD, Charles Howard (*b.* 1866)
. . . Genito-urinary and venereal diseases. A manual for students and practitioners. . . . Philadelphia: Lea Bros. & Co., [1892]. 178p. DLC; NNNAM; PPC; PU **90-1128**

CHEYNE, W[illiam] Watson (1852-1932)
The treatment of wounds, ulcers, and abscesses. Philadelphia: Lea Bros. & Co., 1895. 197p. CtY-M; DNLM; NNNAM; PPC **90-1129**

CHEYNE, W[illiam] Watson (1852-1932)
Tuberculous disease of bones and joints, its pathology, symptoms, and treatment. Philadelphia: J. B Lippincott Co., 1895. 374p. DNLM; NNNAM; PPC; PU **90-1130**

CHEYNE, W[illiam] Watson (1852-1932) and F. F. BURGHARD
A manual of surgical treatment. Philadelphia and New York: Lea Bros. & Co., 1899-1903. 7 v. NNNAM; OCIM; PPC; PU **90-1131**

CHILDREN'S HOSPITAL. BOSTON
Medical and surgical report of the . . . , 1869-1894. Edited by T. M. Rotch and Herbert L. Burrell. Boston, 1895. 367p. 1 plate. DNLM; MBM **90-1132**

CHISHOLM, Julian John (1830-1905)
Persistent headaches, and how to cure them. Baltimore: Guggenheimer, Weil & Co., 1890. 12p. DNLM **90-1133**

CHITTENDEN, R[ussell] H[enry] (1856-1943)
The importance of physiological chemistry as a part of medical education. [New York, 1893.] 15p. DNLM **90-1134**

CHITTENDEN, R[ussell] H[enry] (1856-1943)
On digestive proteolysis, being the Cartwright lectures for 1894. New Haven, Conn.: Tuttle, Morehouse & Taylor, 1896. 137p. CtY-M; DNLM; MH-M **90-1135**

CHITTENDEN, R[ussell] H[enry] (1856-1943)
1. A study of some infant foods in comparison with mothers' milk. 2. The deficiency of fat in dry milk foods for infants. 3. The content of fat in dry-milk foods for infants. New York, 1896. 28p. DNLM; NNNAM **90-1136**

CHRISTIAN, H[ilary] M.
The treatment of gonorrhoea by irrigation of the urethra. Detroit: G. S. Davis, 1894. 7p. DNLM **90-1137**

CHRISTIAN, H[ilary] M.
Posterior urethritis, acute and chronic. Philadelphia, 1894. 5p. DNLM **90-1138**

CHRISTINE, G[eorge] Maxwell (*d.* 1922)
The medical profession vs. criminal abortion (with comments on the legal phase of the question, by J. E. Scattergood). [Philadelphia, 1890.] 12p. DNLM **90-1139**

CHRISTINE, G[eorge] Maxwell (*d.* 1922)
The sequels of typhoid fever; with notes on a case by Horace F. Ivins. [Philadelphia, 1890.] 10p. DNLM **90-1140**

CHRISTINE, G[eorge] Maxwell (*d.* 1922)
Prostitution; no license, but prohibition. Philadelphia, 1896. 10p. DNLM **90-1141**

CHRISTINE, G[eorge] Maxwell (*d.* 1922)
Permanganate of potassium in the treatment of leg and other ulcers. New York, 1897. 10p. DNLM **90-1142**

CHRISTISON, John Sanderson (1856-1908)
. . . Drink and disease. . . . [Dell Rapids, S.D.: M. G. Christison], 1890. 23p. DLC **90-1143**

CHRISTOPHER, Walter Shield (1859-1905)
Summer complaint and infant feeding. . . . Chicago: Blakely & Rogers, printers, 1892. 92p. DLC **90-1144**

CHURCH, Archibald (*b.* 1861)
The nervous features and sequences of la grippe. [Chicago, 1891.] 11p. DNLM **90-1145**

CHURCH, Archibald (*b.* 1861)
Athetosis, with clinical cases. [Milwaukee, 1892.] 13p. DNLM **90-1146**

CHURCH, Archibald (*b.* 1861)
The vertigo of arterio-sclerosis. Philadelphia, 1892. 6p. DNLM **90-1147**

CHURCH, Archibald (*b.* 1861) and D. W. EISENDRATH
A contribution to spinal-cord surgery. [Philadelphia: Lea Bros. & Co., 1892.] 18p. DNLM **90-1148**

CHURCH, Archibald (*b.* 1861) and William HESSERT
Acromegaly, with the clinical report of a case. New York: Trow, 1893. 14p. DNLM **90-1149**

CHURCH, Archibald (*b.* 1861)
The hemiplegic state and its treatment. Chicago, 1897. 7p. DNLM **90-1150**

CHURCH, Archibald (*b.* 1861)
Nervous and mental diseases, by Archibald Church . . . and Frederick Peterson. . . . With 305 illustrations. Philadelphia: W. B. Saunders, 1899. 843p. DLC; NNNAM; OCIM; PPC **90-1151**

CLAIBORNE, John Herbert (1861-1922)
The functional examination of the eye. . . . Philadelphia: The Edwards & Docker Co., 1895. 96p. diags. DLC; DNLM; NNNAM; PPC **90-1152**

CLARK, Alexander (*b.* 1851)
The feet; how to take care of them. . . . [Philadelphia, 1896.] 36p. DLC; PPC **90-1153**

CLARK, Alexander (*b.* 1851)
Diseases of the human foot. Philadelphia, (1897). 62p. PPC **90-1154**

CLARK, Edward
Diagnosis and treatment of abscesses of the ano-rectal region. [Buffalo, 1892.] 8p. DNLM **90-1155**

CLARK, Elizabeth M.
The value of ichthyol in gynaecology. New York, 1895. 6p. DNLM **90-1156**

CLARK, Horace
Sarcoma of the nose; epithelioma of the larynx in a woman. Philadelphia, 1894. 6p. DNLM **90-1157**

CLARK, J[oseph] Payson
Papilloma of the larynx in adults. Boston: Damrell & Upham, 1893. 9p. DNLM **90-1158**

CLARK, J[oseph] Payson
Tubercular tumors of the larynx. Philadelphia, 1895. 11p. DNLM **90-1159**

CLARK, L. D. Pierce
Some observations on an epidemic of typhus fever. New York, 1894. 27p. DNLM **90-1160**

CLARK, L. D. Pierce
The Flechsig method in the treatment of insane epileptics. New York, 1895. 24p. DNLM **90-1161**

CLARK, L. D. Pierce
Mental automatism in epilepsy a psychological study. Boston: Damrell & Upham, 1897. 12p. DNLM **90-1162**

CLARK, L. D. Pierce
A study upon the disordered consciousness of epilepsy. New York, 1897. 14p. DNLM **90-1163**

CLARK, S. B.
Post-mortem demonstration of a case of pyemia, following a latent otitis media. Philadelphia, 1895. 3p. DNLM **90-1164**

CLARK, Talliaferro (*b.* 1867)
Acute anterior poliomyelitis. New York, 1896. 9p. DNLM **90-1165**

CLARKE, Augustus P[eck] (1833-1912)
Post-partem hemorrhage; its etiology and management. [Philadelphia, 1892.] 10p. DNLM **90-1166**

CLARKE, Augustus P[eck] (1833-1912)
The advantages of version in a certain class of obstetric cases. New York: William Wood & Co., 1892. 11p. DNLM **90-1167**

CLARKE, Augustus P[eck] (1833-1912)
Origin and development of modern gynecology. Chicago, 1892. 15p. DNLM **90-1168**

CLARKE, Augustus P[eck] (1833-1912)
The methods of drainage now prevailing in some of our Eastern seaboard municipalities, tending to the production and dissemination of disease. Chicago, 1896. 8p. DNLM **90-1169**

CLARKE, Augustus P[eck] (1833-1912)
Notes on my trip to attend the second Pan-American Medical Congress in Mexico City, Nov. 16-19, 1896. Chicago, 1897. 16p. DNLM **90-1170**

CLARKE, John Henry (1852-1931)
The prescriber: a dictionary of the new therapeutics. . . . American ed.: rev. and enl. . . . from the 4th English ed. Philadelphia: Boericke & Tafel, 1898. 258p. DLC; OCLloyd; PPC; PPHa **90-1171**

CLARKE, John H[enry] (1852-1931)
Catarrh, colds and grippe, including prevention and cure, with chapters on nasal polypus, hay fever and influenza. . . . American ed., rev. by the author from the 4th English ed. Philadelphia: Boericke & Tafel, 1899. 122p. DLC; PPC; PPHa **90-1172**

CLARKSON, Arthur
A text-book of histology, descriptive and practical, for the use of students. Philadelphia: W. B. Saunders, 1896. 554p. 88 plates. DNLM; MBM; NNNAM; PPC **90-1173**

CLEAVELAND, Charles H[arley] (1820-1863)
Pronouncing medical lexicon. . . . 33rd ed. Philadelphia: P. Blakiston, Son & Co., 1890. 302p. NNNAM; PPC; PPJ; PU [Original ed., Cincinnati: Longley Bros., 1855, 302p.] **90-1174**

CLEAVES, Margaret A[bigail] (1848-1917)
Electric light as a diagnostic and therapeutic agent. New York, 1894. 12p. DNLM **90-1175**

CLELAND, John (1835-1925) and John Yule MACKAY
Human anatomy, general and descriptive, for the use of students. New York: Macmillan Co., 1896. 833p. DLC; DNLM; ICU; MB **90-1176**

CLEVELAND, Clement (*b.* 1843)
Perineorrhaphy, a plea for immediate repair, with the description of a new method of suturing. New York: Trow's Co., 1891. 11p. DNLM **90-1177**

CLEVELAND, Clement (*b.* 1843)
An operating table for general and gynaecological surgery, adapted to give the Trendelenburg posture. New York: M. J. Rooney, 1892. 6p. DNLM **90-1178**

CLEVELAND, Clement (*b.* 1843)
The treatment of pelvic abscess by vaginal puncture and drainage. New York, 1894. 9p. DNLM **90-1179**

CLEVENGER, S[hobal] Vail (1843-1920)
Sleep, sleeplessness, and hypnotics. Chicago, 1894. 36p. DNLM **90-1180**

CLEVENGER, S[hobal] Vail (1843-1920)
Pain and its therapeusis. Chicago, 1897. 20p. DNLM **90-1181**

CLEVENGER, S[hobal] Vail (1843-1920)
Medical jurisprudence of insanity; or, Forensic psychiatry. . . . With an exhaustive presentation of the judicial decisions upon the subject. By F. H. Bowlby. . . . Rochester, N.Y.: The Lawyers' Co-operative Publishing Co., 1898. 2 v. DLC **90-1182**

CLOSE, Charles William (1859-1915)
. . . Phrenopathy; or rational mind cure. . . . Bangor, Me.: C. W. Close, 1894. 44p. DLC **90-1183**

CLOSE, Charles W[illiam] (1859-1915)
. . . Phrenopathy; or, Rational mind cure. . . . Bangor, Me.: C. W. Close, 1898. 48p. DLC **90-1184**

CLOUSTON, Thomas S[mith] (1840-1915)
Clinical lectures on mental diseases. . . . 4th ed. Philadelphia: Lea Bros. & Co., 1897. 736p. 15 col. plates. DLC; OCIM; NNNAM; PU **90-1185**

CLOUSTON, Thomas S[mith] (1840-1915)
Clinical lectures on mental diseases. . . . 5th ed. Philadelphia: Lea Bros. & Co., 1898. 727p. plates. IU-M; PPC; PPJ; PU **90-1186**

CLUNESS, W[illiam] R[obert] (*b.* **1845)**
An address delivered at the opening of the twenty-first annual meeting of the Medical Society of the State of California, April, 1891. Sacramento, 1891. 11p. 2 tables. DNLM
90-1187

COAKLEY, Cornelius Godfrey (1862-1934)
A manual of diseases of the nose and throat. . . . Illustrated with 92 engravings and 2 colored plates. New York and Philadelphia: Lea Bros. & Co., 1899. 536p. DLC; MBM; NNNAM; PPC **90-1188**

COBB, Frederic C.
Empyema of the antrum of Highmore. Boston: Damrell & Upham, 1896. 19p. DNLM **90-1189**

COBBE, William Rosser
Doctor Judas: A portrayal of the opium habit. Chicago: S. C. Griggs & Co., 1895. 324p. ICU **90-1190**

COBLENTZ, Virgil (1862-1932)
Handbook of pharmacy, embracing the theory and practice of pharmacy and the art of dispensing. . . . With three hundred and ninety-five illustrations. Philadelphia: P. Blakiston, Son & Co., 1894. 480p. diags. DLC; NNNAM; OCLloyd; PPC
90-1191

COBLENTZ, Virgil (1862-1932)
Handbook of pharmacy, embracing the theory and practice of pharmacy and the art of dispensing. . . . 2nd ed., rev. and enl., with four hundred and thirty-seven illustrations; Philadelphia: P. Blakiston, Son & Co., 1895. 572p. diags. DLC; OCLloyd; PPC; PU **90-1192**

COBLENTZ, Virgil (1862-1932)
The newer remedies. A reference manual for physicians, pharmacists and students. . . . New York: D. O. Haynes & Co., 1895. 64p. DLC; NNNAM **90-1193**

COBLENTZ, Virgil (1862-1932)
The newer remedies. A reference manual for physicians, pharmacists and students. . . . 2nd ed. rev. and enl. New York: D. O. Haynes & Co., 1896. 82p. DLC; NNNAM; PPC
90-1194

COBLENTZ, Virgil (1862-1932)
The newer remedies. . . . A reference book for physicians, pharmacists and students. 3rd ed., rev. and very much enl. Philadelphia: P. Blakiston's Son & Co., 1899. 147p. DLC; OCLloyd; PU **90-1195**

CODMAN, John T[homas]
Retrospect and prospect. Address delivered before the American Academy of Dental Science, at their twenty-second annual meeting, held in Boston, Nov. 13, 1889. Boston: Fort Hill Embossing & Print. Co., 1890. 10p. DNLM
90-1196

COE, Arthur H.
A remarkable case of suppurative otitis, with hemiplegia. Portland, Oregon, 1894. 6p. DNLM
90-1197

COE, Henry C[larke] (1856-1940)
Malignant disease of the corporeal endometrium. New York: Trow's, 1890. 24p. DNLM **90-1198**

COE, Henry C[larke] (1856-1940)
A second case of laparotomy for intestinal obstruction following vaginal hysterectomy. [New York, 1890.] 5p. DNLM
90-1199

COE, Henry C[larke] (1856-1940)
A unique case of vesico-utero-vaginal fistula. [Philadelphia, 1890.] 3p. DNLM **90-1200**

COE, Henry C[larke] (1856-1940)
The limits of vaginal hysterectomy for cancer of the uterus. New York, 1890. 13p. DNLM **90-1201**

COE, Henry C[larke] (1856-1940)
Concealed accidental hemorrhage during labor. New York: William Wood & Co., 1891. 8p. DNLM
90-1202

COE, Henry C[larke] (1856-1940)
The malarial element in oöphoralgia. [Philadelphia, 1891.] 3p. DNLM **90-1203**

COE, Henry C[larke] (1856-1940)
The care of the bladder before and after labor. New York: William Wood & Co., 1891. 11p. DNLM
90-1204

COE, Henry C[larke] (1856-1940)
Elevation of temperature of obscure origin during the puerperium. New York: William Wood & Co., 1891. 14p. DNLM
90-1205

COE, Henry C[larke] (1856-1940)
Adenoma uteri. [Philadelphia, 1891.] 8p. DNLM
90-1206

COE, Henry C[larke] (1856-1940)
Renal disease due to intra-pelvic obstruction of the ureter. [Philadelphia, 1891.] 7p. DNLM **90-1207**

COE, Henry C[larke] (1856-1940)
Accidental hemorrhage during the first state of labor at full term. Philadelphia: W. J. Dornan, 1891. 18p. DNLM
90-1208

COE, Henry C[larke] (1856-1940)
The elective Caesarean section; the most favorable time for operation. New York: William Wood & Co., 1892. 12p. DNLM
90-1209

COE, Henry C[larke] (1856-1940)
A contribution to the study of abdominal pregnancy. [Philadelphia, 1892.] 11p. DNLM **90-1210**

COE, Henry C[larke] (1856-1940)
The pathology of carcinoma; introducing a discussion on carcinoma before the Medical Society of the State of New York, February 3, 1893. [Philadelphia, 1893.] 9p. DNLM
90-1211

COE, Henry C[larke] (1856-1940)
Cancer of the cervix uteri complicating pregnancy. New York: William Wood & Co., 1893. 10p. DNLM **90-1212**

COE, Henry C[larke] (1856-1940)
Internal migration of the ovum; with report of a case of repeated ectopic gestation possibly supporting the theory. New York: William Wood & Co., 1893. 14p. DNLM
90-1213

COE, Henry C[larke] (1856-1940)
Acute localized vs. diffuse peritonitis in women from a clinical standpoint. New York: J. D. Emmet & A. H. Buckmaster, 1895. 8p. DNLM **90-1214**

COHEN, Jacob [da Silva] Solis (1838-1927)
A very irregular foreign body in the alimentary tract safely voided under the "potato" treatment. [Philadelphia, 1891.] 1 l. DNLM **90-1215**

COHEN, Jacob [da Silva] Solis (1838-1927)
The symptoms and pathological changes in the upper air passages in influenza. [New York: D. Appleton & Co., 1892.] 8p. DNLM **90-1216**

COHEN, Jacob [da Silva] Solis (1838-1927)
Multiple papillomata in a child; tracheotomy at four years of age; retention of canula thirteen years; evulsion of multiple laryngeal and pharyngeal neoplasms; closure of the tracheal fistule by a cutaneous flap; recurrent or repullulant growth at the anterior commissure of the glottis. [Philadelphia, 1893.] 3p. DNLM **90-1217**

COHEN, Jacob [da Silva] Solis (1838-1927)
Guaiacol externally in tuberculosis. Philadelphia, 1894. 3p. DNLM **90-1218**

COHEN, S[olomon] Solis (1857-1948)
Clinical notes in respiratory therapeutics. Philadelphia, 1890. 8p. DNLM **90-1219**

COHEN, S[olomon] Solis (1857-1948)
Two cases illustrating the therapeutic uses of the nitrites. Philadelphia, 1890. 7p. DNLM **90-1220**

COHEN, S[olomon] Solis (1857-1948)
Some of the therapeutic relations of the nervous system. Detroit: G. S. Davis, 1891. 19p. DNLM **90-1221**

COHEN, S[olomon] Solis (1857-1948) and Augustus A. ESHNER
Essentials of diagnosis, arranged in the form of questions and answers prepared especially for students of medicine. Philadelphia: W. B. Saunders, 1892. 382p. DNLM **90-1222**

COHEN, S[olomon] Solis (1857-1948)
Shall physicians become sales-agents for patent medicines? Philadelphia, 1892. 8p. DNLM **90-1223**

COHEN, S[olomon] Solis (1857-1948)
A case of akromegaly. [Philadelphia: Lea Bros. & Co., 1892.] 7p. DNLM **90-1224**

COHEN, S[olomon] Solis (1857-1948)
A case of uremia in an alcoholic patient with visceral complications, successfully treated by venesection, diaphoresis, and nitro-glycerin. [Reported by W. E. Bruner.] [Philadelphia, 1893.] 5p. DNLM **90-1225**

COHEN, S[olomon] Solis (1857-1948)
Some of the throat conditions observed in gouty subjects. [Philadelphia, 1893.] 12p. DNLM **90-1226**

COHEN, S[olomon] Solis (1857-1948)
An esophageal stethoscope; with remarks on intra-thoracic auscultation. [Philadelphia, 1893.] 4p. DNLM **90-1227**

COHEN, S[olomon] Solis (1857-1948)
Vasomotor ataxia; a contribution to the subject of idiosyncrasies. [Philadelphia, 1894.] 18p. DNLM **90-1228**

COHEN, S[olomon] Solis (1857-1948)
Pulmonary tuberculosis. Philadelphia: Lea Bros. & Co., 1894. 18p. DNLM **90-1229**

COHEN, S[olomon] Solis (1857-1948)
Glycosuria in connection with appendicitis; diabetes mellitus. New York: D. Appleton & Co., 1894. 17p. DNLM **90-1230**

COHEN, S[olomon] Solis (1857-1948)
Guaïacol, topically as a prophylactic against diphtheria. Philadelphia, 1895. 3p. DNLM **90-1231**

COHEN, S[olomon] Solis (1857-1948)
A simplified resistance valve for the pneumatic treatment of pulmonary affections. Philadelphia, 1895. 2p. DNLM **90-1232**

COHEN, S[olomon] Solis (1857-1948)
Some thoughts concerning disease and recovery in their relation to therapeutics. Annual address delivered before the Medical and Chirurgical Faculty of Maryland, at the 98th annual session, Baltimore, Md., April 30, 1896. [Baltimore, 1896.] 29p. DNLM **90-1233**

COLE, Carter S. (*b.* 1862)
A new method of reducing anterior dislocations of the humerus. [New York, 1891.] 8p. DNLM **90-1234**

COLEMAN, N[athaniel] R[unnels]
An appeal to the medical profession from the decision of the trustees of Columbia Medical College. [Columbus, Ohio, 1892.] 12p. DNLM **90-1235**

COLEMAN, Thomas D[avies]
The treatment of pulmonary phthisis. [Atlanta, 1891.] 24p. DNLM **90-1236**

COLEMAN, Warren (*b.* 1869)
A syllabus of materia medica, comp. . . . New York: William Wood & Co., 1899 [1898]. 169p. DLC; NNNAM; OCLloyd **90-1237**

COLEMAN, William Ludlow (1833-1904)
A history of yellow fever; indisputable facts pertaining to its origin and cause . . . with an addendum on its twin sister dengue, containing a parallel table of the most prominent symptoms of each disease. . . . [Chicago: The Clinic Publishing Co., 1898.] 141p. DLC; IU-M; OCIM **90-1238**

COLEY, William B[radley] (1862-1936)
A clinical report of operative surgery in the service of Dr. William T. Bull, at the New York Hospital, during October and November, 1889, and from February to June, 1890. New York: D. Appleton & Co., 1891. 109p. DNLM **90-1239**

COLEY, William B[radley] (1862-1936)
Contribution to the knowledge of sarcoma. [St. Louis, 1891.] 22p. DNLM **90-1240**

COLEY, William B[radley] (1862-1936)
Hydrocele in the female (with a report of fourteen cases). Philadelphia, 1892. 18p. DNLM **90-1241**

COLEY, William B[radley] (1862-1936)
The treatment of malignant tumors by repeated inoculations of erysipelas, with a report of ten original cases. [Philadelphia, 1893.] 25p. DNLM **90-1242**

COLEY, William B[radley] (1862-1936)
The operative treatment of hernia in children, with a report of fifty-one cases. New York: Trow's Directory, 1893. 8p. 1 table. DNLM **90-1243**

COLEY, William B[radley] (1862-1936)
A preliminary note on the treatment of inoperable sarcoma by the toxic products of erysipelas. Meriden, Conn., 1893. 8p. DNLM **90-1244**

COLEY, William B[radley] (1862-1936)
The treatment of inoperable malignant tumors with toxines of erysipelas and bacillus prodigiosus. [Philadelphia, 1894.] 30p. DNLM **90-1245**

COLEY, William B[radley] (1862-1936)
The treatment of inoperable malignant tumors with toxines of erysipelas and bacillus prodigiosus. Philadelphia: Lea Bros. & Co., 1894. 16p. DNLM **90-1246**

COLEY, William B[radley] (1862-1936)
The treatment of inoperable malignant tumors with the toxins of erysipelas and bacillus prodigiosus. New York: Trow's, 1895. 24p. DNLM **90-1247**

COLEY, William B[radley] (1862-1936)
The operative treatment of hernia in children, with a report of one hundred and thirty-three cases. Philadelphia, 1895. 13p. DNLM **90-1248**

COLEY, William B[radley] (1862-1936)
The operative treatment of hernia, with a report of two hundred cases. Philadelphia, 1895. 52p. DNLM **90-1249**

COLEY, William B[radley] (1862-1936)
The disadvantages of non-absorbable sutures in operations for the radical cure of hernia. New York, 1896. 8p. DNLM **90-1250**

COLEY, William B[radley] (1862-1936)
Therapeutic value of the mixed toxins of the streptococcus of erysipelas and bacillus prodigiosus in the treatment of inoperable malignant tumors, with a report of one hundred and sixty cases. Philadelphia, 1896. 32p. DNLM **90-1251**

COLEY, William B[radley] (1862-1936)
The radical cure of hernia, with a report of three hundred and sixty cases. Philadelphia, 1897. 36p. DNLM **90-1252**

COLGAN, James F[rancis] E[dward]
Gastric ulcer in a child two and half years old. [Philadelphia: Lea Bros. & Co., 1892.] 3p. DNLM **90-1253**

COLGAN, James F[rancis] E[dward]
Report of a case of right-angled deformity of knee resulting from tubercular arthritis. Detroit: G. S. Davis, 1892. 3p. DNLM **90-1254**

COLGROVE, W. E.
Some practical points on the diagnosis and treatment of pelvic haematocele, with report of a case. New York, 1895. 3p. DNLM **90-1255**

COLLEGE OF MEDICINE OF THE NATIONAL NORMAL UNIVERSITY OF LEBANON, OHIO
Announcement for 1891-1892. [Lebanon, 1891.] 12p. DNLM **90-1256**

COLLEGE OF PHARMACY OF THE CITY OF NEW YORK
Catalogue of the library of the . . . 1891. New York, 1891. 86p. DNLM **90-1257**

COLLEGE OF PHYSICIANS AND SURGEONS. BOSTON
Quarterly announcements of the . . . v. 15-17, spring session of 1895 to autumn session of 1897. Boston, 1895-1897. DNLM **90-1258**

COLLEGE OF PHYSICIANS AND SURGEONS OF CHICAGO
Non-resident course. Directions for students. [Chicago, 1891.] 6p. DNLM **90-1259**

COLLEGE OF PHYSICIANS AND SURGEONS OF CHICAGO
The laboratories of the . . . [Chicago, 1892.] 8p. DNLM **90-1260**

COLLEGE OF PHYSICIANS AND SURGEONS OF CHICAGO
[Time card for the session of 1892-1893.] [Chicago, 1892.] 5 l. DNLM **90-1261**

COLLEGE OF PHYSICIANS AND SURGEONS IN THE CITY OF NEW YORK. MEDICAL DEPARTMENT OF COLUMBIA UNIVERSITY
Annual catalogues of the officers and students, and announcements for the sessions of 1828-1829 (22.); 1837-1838 (31.); 1839-1840 (33.); 1842-1843 to 1884-1885 (36.-78.); 1886-1887 to 1889-1890 (80.-83.). New York, 1829-1890. DNLM; NNC [From 1842-1843 to 1865-1866, read: Annual catalogue. From 1866-1867 to 1889-1890, read: Annual catalogue and announcement. On July 1, 1891, the College of Physicians and Surgeons became, by authority of the legislature, an integral part of Columbia University.] **90-1262**

COLLEGE OF PHYSICIANS AND SURGEONS IN THE CITY OF NEW YORK. MEDICAL DEPARTMENT OF COLUMBIA UNIVERSITY
Annual announcements and circulars for the sessions of 1836-1837 (30.); 1837-1838 (31.); 1842-1843 (36.); 1845-1846 to 1861-1862 (39.-55.); 1866-1867 (60.); 1891-1892 to 1897-1898 (85.-81.). New York, 1836-1897. DNLM; NNC [The annual announcements for the years 1861-1862 to 1890-1891 are in the annual catalogues for the preceding years. From 1891-1892 to 1893-1894, read: Circulars of information.] **90-1263**

COLLEGE OF PHYSICIANS AND SURGEONS (MEDICAL DEPARTMENT OF KANSAS CITY UNIVERSITY) OF KANSAS CITY, KANSAS
Annual announcements for the sessions of 1894-1895 to 1896-1897 (1.-3.). Kansas City, Mo., 1894-1896. DNLM **90-1264**

COLLEGE OF PHYSICIANS AND SURGEONS. RICHMOND, VA.
Announcement for the session of 1893-1894 (1.). [Richmond, 1893.] 23p. DNLM [Organized and chartered in May, 1893.] **90-1265**

COLLEGE OF PHYSICIANS AND SURGEONS. RICHMOND, VA.
Summer school of medicine. [Circular for 1894.] Richmond, 1894. 2 l. DNLM [A supplementary clinical and didactic course.] **90-1266**

COLLIE, Alexander
A practical treatise on fevers, their history, etiology, diagnosis, prognosis, and treatment. Philadelphia: P. Blakiston, Son & Co., 1890. 288p. DLC; OCIM; PPC: PU **90-1267**

COLLINGS, Howard Paxton
Report of a case of reinfection of syphilis. New York, 1896. 2p. DNLM **90-1268**

COLLINGS, Howard Paxton
An unusual case of appendicitis. Hot Springs, 1897. 3p. DNLM **90-1269**

COLLINGS, S[amuel] P[osey]
Chronic seminal vesiculitis, with hemorrhage. [Cincinnati, 1895.] 5p. DNLM **90-1270**

COLLINS, George Lewis (1820-1889)
State control of medical practice. An address delivered at the annual meeting of the Rhode Island Medical Society, June 9, 1889. [Providence, 1890.] 20p. DNLM **90-1271**

COLLINS, Howard Dennis (*b.* 1868)
. . . Physiology. A manual for students and practitioners. By Howard D. Collins . . . and Wm. H. Rockwell, Jr. . . . Illustrated with one hundred and fifty-three engravings. Philadelphia and New York: Lea Bros. & Co., [1899]. 323p. DLC; NNNAM; PPC; PPJ **90-1272**

COLLINS, James (1831-1895)
Memoir of Elisha Bacon Shapleigh, M.D., of Philadelphia. (Died December 10, 1892.) Read before the Northern Medical Association, April 28, 1893. [Philadelphia: Avil Co., 1893.] 10p. DNLM; PPC **90-1273**

COLLINS, Joseph (1866-1950)
Fracture of the base of the skull with the escape of the cerebro-spinal fluid, followed by facial paralysis and recovery. [New York, 1892.] 7p. DNLM **90-1274**

COLLINS, Joseph (1866-1950)
Chloralamid; the treatment of insomnia. [New York, 1892.] 8p. DNLM **90-1275**

COLLINS, Joseph (1866-1950)
A contribution to the study of chronic myelitis, based on a record of twenty cases. [New York], 1892. 6p. DNLM **90-1276**

COLLINS, Joseph (1866-1950)
Acromegaly. [New York: Raff & Co., 1893.] 35p. DNLM **90-1277**

COLLINS, Joseph (1866-1950)
Haematomyelia and acute myelitis. New York: Trow, 1893. 22p. DNLM **90-1278**

COLLINS, Joseph (1866-1950)
A consideration of the paraesthesic neurosis. Boston: Damrell & Upham, 1893. 16p. DNLM **90-1279**

COLLINS, Joseph (1866-1950)
An analysis of one hundred and twenty-five cases of chorea. [Meriden, Conn., 1893.] 3 l. DNLM **90-1280**

COLLINS, Joseph (1866-1950)
A contribution to the arrangement and functions of the cells of the cervical spinal cord. To which is appended a note on central changes secondary to long-continued disuse of an extremity. [New York: D. Appleton & Co., 1894.] 46p. DNLM **90-1281**

COLLINS, Joseph (1866-1950)
On some affections of the nervous system occurring in the early and late stages of acquired syphilis. New York, 1895. 33p. DNLM **90-1282**

COLLINS, Joseph (1866-1950)
The genesis and dissolution of the faculty of speech, a clinical and psychological study of aphasia. New York: The Macmillan Co., 1898. 432p. DNLM; NNNAM **90-1283**

COLLINS, Samuel B.
Theriaki: a treatise on the habitual use of narcotic poison. La Porte, Indiana: The Author, [1887]. 64p. OCIM; InHi **90-1284**

COMEGYS, Cornelius George (1816-1896)
A healthy brain is necessary to a free will. Chicago: Office American Medical Association, 1892. 19p. DNLM **90-1285**

CONKLIN, William Judkins (1844-1916)
President's address. A page of medical history: Molière and the doctors. Toledo, 1891. 32p. DNLM **90-1286**

CONKLIN, William Judkins (1844-1916)
Splenectomy; with the report of a successful case. [Toledo, 1894.] 11p. DNLM **90-1287**

CONN, Granville Priest (1832-1916)
Prevention and cure of disease. Manchester, N.H.: J. B. Clarke, 1891. 17p. DNLM **90-1288**

CONNABLE & HARPER
Manufacturers of electrical and illuminating apparatus, cautery appliances, and electro-surgical instruments. Xenia, Ohio, 1891. 12p. DNLM **90-1289**

CONNECTICUT MEDICAL SOCIETY
Centennial index of the proceedings of the Connecticut Medical Society, 1792-1891. A complete catalogue of the members of the society. Hartford, Conn.: Case, Lockwood & Brainard Co., 1893. 165p. CtY-M; DNLM; MH **90-1290**

CONNECTICUT State medical directory. Containing a carefully prepared list of physicians, dentists, and druggists, together with colleges, hospitals, medical associations, and societies throughout the State. Danbury, Conn.: Danbury Med. Print. Co., 1893. 109p. CtY-M; DNLM **90-1291**

CONNOR, Leartus (1843-1911)
Tobacco amblyopia. Chicago, 1890. 29p. DNLM **90-1292**

CONNOR, Leartus (1843-1911)
Other methods of promoting the development of the sections. Chicago, 1891. 15p. DNLM **90-1293**

CONNOR, Leartus (1843-1911)
Three cases of enucleation of the eye; with remarks. Detroit, 1891. 7p. DNLM **90-1294**

CONNOR, Leartus (1843-1911)
Astigmatism as a factor in the causation of myopia. Detroit, 1895. 14p. DNLM **90-1295**

CONNOR, Leartus (1843-1911)
The technique of tenotomy of the ocular muscles. Chicago: American Medical Association Press, 1895. 8p. DNLM **90-1296**

CONNOR, Leartus (1843-1911)
Strabismus as a symptom; its causes and its practical management. Chicago, 1895. 11p. DNLM **90-1297**

CONNOR, Leartus (1843-1911)
Remarks on the causes of glaucoma. Chicago, 1896. 11p. DNLM **90-1298**

CONNOR, Leartus (1843-1911)
Remarks on the management of glaucoma. Chicago, 1896. 16p. DNLM **90-1299**

COOK, Frederick A[lbert] (1865-1940)
Medical observations among the Esquimaux. [New York, 1894.] 4p. DNLM **90-1300**

COOK, William Henry (1832-1899)
Man: his generative system and his marital relations. . . . Cincinnati: W. H. Cook, 1890. 160p. DLC; OC **90-1301**

COOK, William Henry (1832-1899)
A handbook of family medicine and hygiene. . . . Cincinnati: G. P. Houston, 1890. 750p. DLC; OC **90-1302**

COOK, William Henry (1832-1899)
A compend of the new materia medica together with additional description of some old remedies. . . . Chicago: W. H. Cook, [1896]. 157p. DLC; OCLloyd **90-1303**

COOKE, Joseph B. (*b.* 1868)
Preputial adhesions in children; with cases. Philadelphia, 1893. 8p. DNLM **90-1304**

COOKE, Joseph B. (*b.* 1868)
The use of chloroform as an anesthetic; with a case. [Philadelphia, 1893.] 8p. DNLM **90-1305**

COOLIDGE, A., Jr.
Deformities of the septal cartilage. Boston: Damrell & Upham, 1894. 9p. DNLM **90-1306**

COOMES, M[artin] F. (*b.* 1847)
Reports on nasal surgery, with illustrated cases. Louisville: J. P. Morton & Co., 1893. 8p. 1 plate. DNLM **90-1307**

COOMES, M[artin] F. (*b.* 1847)
Report of a case of gastrostomy, read before the Kentucky State Medical Society, 1896. Louisville, 1896. 7p. DNLM **90-1308**

COOMES, M[artin] F. (*b.* 1847)
Congenital ptosis; the operation devised by Panas for relief modified. Louisville, 1896. 2p. DNLM **90-1309**

COOP, W. A. H.
A curious anomaly of the female genitalia, with striking resemblance to some of the external male elements, converted by plastic surgery into a woman of normal appearance. New York, 1895. 4p. DNLM **90-1310**

COOPER, Alfred (1838-1908) and F. Swinford EDWARDS
Diseases of the rectum and anus. 2nd ed. Philadelphia: P. Blakiston, Son & Co., 1892. 324p. 11 plates. DNLM; MH-M; NNNAM; PPC **90-1311**

COOPER, Alfred (1838-1908)
Syphilis. . . . 2nd ed., enl. and illustrated by twenty full page plates, twelve of which are coloured. Ed. by Edward Cotterell. Philadelphia: P. Blakiston, Son & Co., 1896. 480p. DNLM; PPC; PPHa; PPJ **90-1312**

COPELAND, John Charles
The woman's medical guide, a medical treatise . . . for women. . . . Memphis: The Great South Press, 1897. 95p. DLC **90-1313**

COPLIN, William M[ichael] L[ate] (1864-1928) and David BEVAN
Acute infectious epiphysitis. Philadelphia, 1892. 29p. DNLM **90-1314**

COPLIN, William M[ichael] L[ate] (1864-1928), David BEVAN, and HENRY SOMMER, Jr.
The effects of heat as manifested in workmen in sugar refineries. [Philadelphia, 1892.] 18p. DNLM **90-1315**

COPLIN, William M[ichael] L[ate] (1864-1928)
A manual of practical hygiene. . . . By W. M. L. Coplin . . . and D. Bevan. . . . With an introduction by H. A. Hare. . . . Philadelphia: P. Blakiston, Son & Co., 1893. 456p. diags. DLC; DNLM; PPC; PU **90-1316**

COPLIN, William M[ichael] L[ate] (1864-1928) and Otho D. SEHAUL
Extensive fracture of the skull from an unusual cause. Philadelphia, 1893. 12p. DNLM **90-1317**

COPLIN, William M[ichael] L[ate] (1864-1928)
Lectures on pathology; delivered to the students at Jefferson Medical College, Philadelphia. Philadelphia: P. Blakiston, Son & Co., 1894, 612p. plate. DLC; PPJ **90-1318**

COPLIN, William M[ichael] L[ate] (1864-1928)
The element of malignancy in tumors. Philadelphia, 1894. 7p. DNLM **90-1319**

COPLIN, William M[ichael] L[ate] (1864-1928)
Manual of pathology, including bacteriology, the technic of postmortems, and methods of pathologic research . . . being a 2nd ed. of the author's "Lectures on pathology," rewritten and enl.; with two hundred and sixty-eight illustrations. . . . Philadelphia: P. Blakiston, Son & Co., 1897. 638p. DLC; DNLM; NNNAM; PPC **90-1320**

COPPENS, Charles (1835-1920)
Moral principles and medical practice, the basis of medical jurisprudence. . . . New York, Cincinnati, [etc.]: Benziger Bros., 1897. 222p. DLC; DNLM; ICU; MB
90-1321

CORDELL, Eugene F[auntleroy] (1843-1913)
Historical sketch of the University of Maryland School of Medicine (1807-1890), with an introductory chapter, notices of the schools of law, arts, and sciences, and theology, and the department of dentistry, and a general catalogue of medical alumni. Baltimore: I. Friedenwald, 1891. 218p. 1 plate, 19 port. DLC; DNLM; MdU-D **90-1322**

CORLETT, William Thomas (*b.* 1854)
Cold as an etiological factor in diseases of the skin, with a report of cases. . . . [New York, 1894.] 12p. col. plate. DLC
90-1323

CORNING, J[ames] Leonard (1853-1923)
A treatise on headache and neuralgia, including spinal irritation and a disquisition on normal and morbid sleep. . . . With an appendix. Eye strain, a cause of headache, by David Wedster [!]. . . . 3rd ed. New York: E. B. Treat; [etc., etc.], 1894. 275p. DLC; NNNAM **90-1324**

CORNING, J[ames] Leonard (1853-1923)
Pain in its neuro-pathological, diagnostic, medico-legal and neuro-therapeutic relations. . . . Philadelphia: J. B. Lippincott Co., 1894. 328p. DLC; DNLM; PPC; PU
90-1325

CORNING, J[ames] Leonard (1853-1923)
Experimental researches regarding the state of the mind in vertigo; vertigo as an aid to hypnotism and narcosis. New York, 1895. 13p. DNLM **90-1326**

COROMILAS, George
Action of quinine upon the internal genital organs during pregnancy and menstruation. New York, 1895. 5p. DNLM
90-1327

CORSON, Hiram (1804-1896)
A brief history of proceedings in the Medical Society of Pennsylvania, in the years 1859, 1860, 1866-1868, 1870, 1871, to procure the recognition of women physicians by the medical profession of the State; to which is added an account of the measures adopted by the society at its annual meetings, in, 1877-1879 to procure a law to authorize trustees of hospitals for the insane-poor, under the control of the State, to appoint women physicians to have entire medical control of the insane of their sex. 2nd ed. Norristown, Pa.: Herald Printing, 1894. 53p. DNLM; PPC **90-1328**

CORSON, Hiram (1804-1896)
Measles. Norristown, Pa., 1894. 19p. DNLM
90-1329

CORSON, Hiram (1804-1896)
Hydrophobia. Philadelphia, [1894]. 20p. DNLM
90-1330

CORWIN, Arthur Mills (*b.* 1864)
Outline of physical diagnosis of the thorax. . . . Chicago: The W. T. Keener Co., 1893. 111p. DLC
90-1331

CORWIN, Arthur Mills (*b.* 1864)
Essentials of physical diagnosis of the thorax. . . . 2nd ed., rev. and enl. Philadelphia: W. B. Saunders, 1896. 199p. DLC; DNLM; PPC; PU **90-1332**

CORWIN, Arthur Mills (*b.* 1864)
Essentials of physical diagnosis of the thorax. . . . 3rd ed., rev. and enl. Philadelphia: W. B. Saunders, 1899. 220p. DLC; NNNAM; PPC **90-1333**

COTTELL, H[enry] A.
The medical millenium. The doctorate address of the Medical Department of the University of Louisville, session of 1894-1895. Louisville: J. P. Morton & Co., 1895. 11p. DNLM
90-1334

COTTING, B[enjamin] E[ddy] (1812-1898)
Points noticeable in the [influenza] epidemic of 1889-1890. [Boston, 1890.] 2 l. DNLM; MBM **90-1335**

COTTING, B[enjamin] E[ddy] (1812-1898)
Questions to be answered by the family physician. [Boston, 1890.] 2 l. DNLM **90-1336**

COTTING, B[enjamin] E[ddy] (1812-1898)
Infleshed toe-nail; its radical relief. Boston: D. Clapp & Son, 1893. 15p. DNLM **90-1337**

COUES, Elliott (1842-1899)
"A woman in the case." An address, delivered at the annual commencement of the National Medical College, in the Congregational Church at Washington, March 16, 1887. . . . 2nd ed., with an introduction by Elizabeth Cavazza [*pseud.*]. Boston: The Occult Publishing Co., 1890. 54p. DLC
90-1338

COVEY, A[lfred] Dale (*b.* 1869)
The obtundine system of painless dentistry. . . . Lansing, Mich.: The Obtundine Dental Association, 1895. 42p. DLC
90-1339

COWL, Walter Y.
The factors of the respiratory rhythm, and the regulation of respiration. [New York, 1890.] 18p. DNLM
90-1340

COWL, Walter Y.
Is the cause of respiration the venosity of the blood and tissue fluid in the respiratory center of the medulla oblongata? [New York, 1891.] 23p. DNLM **90-1341**

COWLES, Edward (1837-1919)
Neurasthenia and its mental symptoms. The Shattuck lecture, 1891. Read before the Massachusetts Medical Society, June 9, 1891. Boston: D. Clapp & Son, 1891. 104p. DNLM; MBB
90-1342

COWLES, Edward (1837-1919)
Progress in the care and treatment of the insane during the half-century. Chicago: Rand, McNally & Co., 1894. 13p. DNLM **90-1343**

COWLES, Edward (1837-1919)
The advancement of psychiatry in America. Chicago: Rand, McNally & Co., 1896. 25p. DNLM
90-1344

COWPERTHWAITE, Allen C[orson] (*b.* 1848)
A text-book of materia medica and therapeutics. Characteristic, analytical, and comparative. 5th ed. Chicago: Gross & Delbridge, 1890. 772p. IU-M; OCLloyd; OCIM
90-1345

COWPERTHWAITE, Allen C[orson] (*b.* 1848)
A text-book of materia medica and therapeutics. Characteristic, analytical, and comparative. 6th ed. Entirely rewritten and revised, with clinical index. Chicago: Gross & Delbridge, 1891. 834p. DLC; OCLloyd; OCIM **90-1346**

COX, Charles N.
Some of the effects of chronic nasal obstruction. Brooklyn, 1896. 11p. DNLM **90-1347**

COX, George W. (1841?-1901)
Streptococcic infection and Marmorek's serum. Chicago, 1897. 17p. DNLM **90-1348**

CRAGIN, Edwin Bradford (1859-1918)
. . . Essentials of gynaecology. Arranged in the form of questions and answers, prepared especially for students of medicine. . . . With 58 illustrations. Philadelphia: W. B. Saunders; [etc., etc.], 1890. 192p. DLC; NNNAM; PPC; PU
90-1349

CRAGIN, Edwin Bradford (1859-1918)
. . . Essentials of gynaecology. Arranged in the form of questions and answers, prepared especially for students of medicine. . . . 2nd ed. Philadelphia: W. B. Saunders, 1891. 192p. DNLM; NNNAM; PPC; PPJ **90-1350**

CRAGIN, Edwin Bradford (1859-1918)
. . . Essentials of gynaecology. Arranged in the form of questions and answers, prepared especially for students of medicine. . . . 3rd ed. Philadelphia: W. B. Saunders, 1893. 192p. MBM; NNNAM; PPC; PU **90-1351**

CRAGIN, Edwin B[radford] (1859-1918)
Cases of haemato-salpinx and haematoma resembling ectopic gestation. New York, 1893. 6p. DNLM
90-1352

CRAGIN, Edwin B[radford] (1859-1918)
Operative experience with ectopic gestation. New York: William Wood & Co., 1893. 13p. DNLM
90-1353

CRAGIN, Edwin B[radford] (1859-1918)
. . . Essentials of gynaecology. Arranged in the form of questions and answers, prepared especially for students of medicine. . . . 4th ed. Philadelphia: W. B. Saunders, 1897. 200p. DLC; DNLM; NNNAM; PU **90-1354**

CRAIG, Charles Franklin (*b.* 1872)
Umbilical hemorrhage; etiology, pathology, and treatment. Report of a case. Philadelphia, 1894. 5p. DNLM
90-1355

CRAIG, Charles Franklin (*b.* 1872)
The parasitic origin of carcinoma. Bridgeport, 1896. 8p. 2 plates. DNLM **90-1356**

CRAIG, Charles Franklin (*b.* 1872)
Some remarks upon the uric acid diathesis, and its treatment. Danbury, Conn., 1897. 15p. DNLM
90-1357

CRAIG, Charles Franklin (*b.* 1872)
Notes on the pathology and bacteriology of appendicitis. Danbury, 1897. 11p. DNLM **90-1358**

CRAIG, Joseph D.
Epidemic intestinal diseases in Albany vicinity. Albany, N.Y.: Taylor & Roberts, 1891. 24p. DNLM
90-1359

CRANCH, Edward
First impressions of a medical examiner. Philadelphia, 1895. 3p. DNLM **90-1360**

CRANDALL, Floyd Milford (1858-1919)
A clinical study of one hundred and forty-two cases of heart disease in children. [Philadelphia, 1891.] 13p. DNLM
90-1361

CRANDALL, Floyd Milford (1858-1919)
Management of the new-born infant. New York, 1892. 21p. DNLM **90-1362**

CRANDALL, Floyd Milford (1858-1919)
The relation of rheumatism and chorea. New York, 1893. 7p. DNLM **90-1363**

CRANDALL, Floyd Milford (1858-1919)
Malarial fever in a new-born infant. New York, 1893. 7p. DNLM **90-1364**

CRANDALL, Floyd Milford (1858-1919)
Types of gastro-intestinal disease prevalent in New York. [New York: D. Appleton & Co., 1893.] 10p. DNLM
90-1365

CRANDALL, George
Care and treatment of the sick, in acute diseases. . . . Walton, N.Y., 1895. 200p. DLC **90-1366**

CRAVENS, Junius E. (*b.* 1844)
A treatise on pyorrhoea alveolaris (Riggs' disease); a system for its prompt positive and permanent cure. Indianapolis, Ind.: W. M. Herriott, 1894. 48p. DLC; DNLM
90-1367

CRAWFORD, Millard H.
Stricture of the male urethra. Chicago, 1894. 12p. DNLM
90-1368

CREIGHTON, Charles (1847-1927)
Jenner and vaccination. A strange chapter of medical history. . . . Providence: Snow & Farnham, 1892. 360p. RPB
90-1369

CRILE, George Washington (1864-1943)
An experimental research into surgical shock; an essay awarded the Cartwright prize for 1897. . . . Philadelphia: J. B. Lippincott Co., [1899]. 160p. DLC; DNLM; PPC; PU
90-1370

CRILE, George Washington (1864-1943)
Experimental research into the surgery of the respiratory system; an essay awarded the Nicholas Senn prize by the American Medical Association for 1898. . . . Philadelphia: J. B. Lippincott Co., [1899]. 113p. DLC; PPC
90-1371

CROCKER, Henry Radcliffe (1845-1909)
Diseases of the skin; their descriptions, pathology, diagnosis and treatment. . . . 2nd ed. Philadelphia: P. Blakiston, Son & Co., 1893. 987p. DNLM; NNNAM; PPC; PPJ
90-1372

CROCKETT ARSENIC-LITHIA SPRINGS COMPANY
(Crockett Warm Springs). Springs situated in Montgomery County, Va., seven miles from Norfolk and Western Railroad, at Shawsville. Roanoke, Va., 1893. 30p. DNLM
90-1373

CROCKETT, E[ugene] A[nthony]
A case of operation upon the lateral sinus, with remarks upon eight unoperated cases. New Bedford, Mass., 1894. 4p. 4 charts. DNLM **90-1374**

CROCKETT, E[ugene] A[nthony]
An acute syphilitic affection of the ear. Boston: Damrell & Upham, 1897. 7p. DNLM **90-1375**

CROOK, James K[ing] (*b.* 1859)
The diagnostic significance of the venous and arterial murmurs in the neck, based on examinations of fifteen hundred persons. Philadelphia, 1893. 7p. DNLM **90-1376**

CROOK, James K[ing] (*b.* 1859)
A clinical lecture on exophthalmic goitre (Graves's or Basedow's disease). New York, 1894. 6p. DNLM
90-1377

CROOK, James K[ing] (*b.* 1859)
The mineral waters of the United States and their therapeutic uses. With an account of the various mineral spring localities, their advantages as health resorts, means of access, etc., to which is added an appendix on potable waters. . . . New York and Philadelphia: Lea Bros. & Co., 1899. 588p. DLC; NNNAM; PPC; PU **90-1378**

CROOKSHANK, Edgar M[arch] (1858-1928)
Manual of bacteriology. . . . 3rd ed. New York: J. H. Vail & Co., 1891. 460p. 32 plates. CtY-M; DNLM; NNNAM; PPC
90-1379

CROOKSHANK, Edgar M[arch] (1858-1928)
A text-book of bacteriology. . . . 4th ed. Philadelphia: W. B. Saunders, 1897. 715p. 22 plates. DLC; DNLM; NNNAM; PPC
90-1380

CROTHERS, Thomas Davison (1842-1918)
Alcoholic heredity in diseases of children. [Hartford, 1890.] 8p. DNLM **90-1381**

CROTHERS, Thomas Davison (1842-1918)
Cerebral trance, or loss of consciousness and memory in inebriety. Hartford, 1890. 16p. DNLM
90-1382

CROTHERS, Thomas Davison (1842-1918)
Drift of American medical journalism. Detroit, 1890. 8p. DNLM **90-1383**

CROTHERS, Thomas Davison (1842-1918)
Some new medico-legal questions relating to inebriety. St. Louis, 1890. 13p. DNLM **90-1384**

CROTHERS, Thomas Davison (1842-1918)
The relation of life insurance to inebriety. Chicago, 1891. 12p. DNLM **90-1385**

CROTHERS, Thomas Davison (1842-1918)
Are inebriates curable? Danbury, 1892. 26p. DNLM
90-1386

CROTHERS, Thomas Davison (1842-1918)
The law of periodicity in inebriety. [St. Louis, 1892.] 11p. DNLM **90-1387**

CROTHERS, Thomas Davison (1842-1918)
The sanitary side of the drink problem. Chicago, 1892. 11p. DNLM **90-1388**

CROTHERS, Thomas Davison (1842-1918)
Some new studies of the opium disease. [Hartford, 1892.] 12p. DNLM **90-1389**

CROTHERS, Thomas Davison (1842-1918)
The drink problem. New York: D. Appleton & Co., 1893. 25p. DNLM **90-1390**

CROTHERS, Thomas Davison (1842-1918)
Sketch of the late Dr. Thomas Lee Wright, of Bellefontaine, Ohio. Hartford, Conn.: The Case, Lockwood & Brainard Comp., 1894. 9p. port. DNLM **90-1391**

CROTHERS, Thomas Davison (1842-1918)
Inebriety and imbecility. A medico-legal study. Hartford, Conn.: The Case, Lockwood & Brainard Comp., 1895. 12p. DNLM **90-1392**

CROTHERS, Thomas Davison (1842-1918)
Medical instruction in inebriety in medical colleges. Hartford, Conn.: The Case, Lockwood & Brainard Comp., 1895. 7p. DNLM **90-1393**

CROTHERS, Thomas Davison (1842-1918)
Inebriety and inebriate hospitals in America. [1896.] 7p. DNLM **90-1394**

CROWLEY, D. D.
A rapid method of locating intestinal wounds by the use of hydrogen gas and an antiseptic fluid. Sacramento, Cal., 1892. 11p. DNLM **90-1395**

CRUTCHER, Howard (*b.* 1865)
A practical treatise on appendicitis, prepared especially for the use of students and general practitioners. . . . Chicago: Hahnemann Publishing Co., 1897. 134p. DLC; ICJ
90-1396

CUFF, Herbert E[dmund] (*b.* 1864)
A course of lectures on medicine to nurses. Philadelphia: P. Blakiston, Son & Co., 1896. 232p. DNLM; NNNAM; PPC; PU **90-1397**

CULBRETH, David Marvel Reynolds (1856-1943)
A manual of materia medica and pharmacology . . . together with important allied species and useful synthetics. . . . Philadelphia & New York: Lea Bros. & Co., 1896. 818p. DLC; OCLloyd; PU **90-1398**

CULLEN, T[homas] S. (*b.* 1868)
Abscess (?) in the urethro-vaginal septum. [Baltimore, 1894.] 7p. 2 l., 1 plate. DNLM **90-1399**

CULLEN, T[homas] S. (*b.* 1868)
Angio-sarcoma of the ovary. Baltimore, 1894. 6p. 1 plate. DNLM **90-1400**

CULLEN, T[homas] S. (*b.* 1868)
Papillo-cystoma of the ovary. [Baltimore, 1894.] 4p. 2 plates. DNLM **90-1401**

CULLEN, T[homas] S. (*b.* 1868)
Hydrosalpinx, its surgical and pathological aspects, with a report of twenty-seven cases. Baltimore, [1895]. 60p. 9 plates. DNLM **90-1402**

CULLEN, T[homas] S. (*b.* 1868)
A rapid method of making permanent specimens from frozen sections by the use of formalin. Baltimore, 1895. 3p. DNLM **90-1403**

CULLEN, T[homas] S. (*b.* 1868)
Tumor developed from aberrant adrenal in the kidney. Baltimore, 1895. 6p. 1 plate. DNLM **90-1404**

CULLEN, T[homas] S. (*b.* 1868)
Adeno-myoma of the round ligament. Baltimore, 1896. 16p. 1 plate. DNLM **90-1405**

CULLEN, T[homas] S. (*b.* 1868)
Multilocular adeno-papillo-cystoma of the ovary; with sarcomatous nodules on the inner surface of one of the cysts. New York: William Wood & Co., 1896. 3p. 1 plate. DNLM **90-1406**

CULLEN, T[homas] S. (*b.* 1868)
Silkworm gut as a subcutaneous suture in closure of abdominal incisions. New York, 1897. 4p. DNLM **90-1407**

CULLINGWORTH, Charles J[ames] (1841-1908)
A manual of nursing, medical and surgical. 3rd rev. ed. Philadelphia: P. Blakiston, Son & Co., 1890. 190p. DLC; ICJ; PPC; PU **90-1408**

CULVER, Everett M.
Manual of venereal diseases . . . being an epitome of the most approved treatment. By E. M. Culver and J. R. Hayden. Philadelphia: Lea Bros. & Co., 1891. 294p. DLC; GU; LNT-M; PPC **90-1409**

CUMSTON, Charles Greene (1868-1927)
Multiple deviations of both legs in a rhachitic child; osteotomy of five bones performed in one séance; recovery. Philadelphia, 1894. 7p. DNLM **90-1410**

CUMSTON, Charles Greene (1868-1927)
Benign tumors of the breast. Boston, 1895. 8p. DNLM **90-1411**

CUMSTON, Charles Greene (1868-1927)
Metritis as a cause of miscarriage. Boston: Damrell & Upham, 1895. 48p. DNLM **90-1412**

CUMSTON, Charles Greene (1868-1927)
Neuralgia and uterine affections. Boston, 1895. 6p. DNLM **90-1413**

CUMSTON, Charles Greene (1868-1927)
Notes on the symptoms and diagnosis of tuberculosis of the bladder. Detroit, 1895. 5p. DNLM **90-1414**

CUMSTON, Charles Greene (1868-1927)
Parietal fibro-myomata of the uterus, and Prof. Vulliet's operation for their extraction. Boston, 1895. 36p. DNLM **90-1415**

CUMSTON, Charles Greene (1868-1927)
Pathology and treatment of osteomalacia, with report of a case cured by bilateral oöphorectomy. Boston, 1895. 8p. DNLM **90-1416**

CUMSTON, Charles Greene (1868-1927)
The treatment of gonorrhoeal affections in the female by permanganate of potassium. Boston, 1895. 8p. DNLM **90-1417**

CUMSTON, Charles Greene (1868-1927)
The treatment of inoperable uterine cancers. Boston, 1895. 7p. DNLM **90-1418**

CUMSTON, Charles Greene (1868-1927)
Tumors of the vagina considered from an obstetrical point of view. Boston, 1895. 10p. DNLM **90-1419**

CUMSTON, Charles Greene (1868-1927)
Amputation of the foot, with a dorsal flap. Philadelphia, 1896. 7p. DNLM **90-1420**

CUMSTON, Charles Greene (1868-1927)
Dosage of hemoglobin in gynaecological cases. Bartholinitis. Posterior vaginal coeliotomy. Medical treatment of dysmenorrhoea. Surgical treatment of prolapsus uteri. Boston, 1896. 4p. DNLM **90-1421**

CUMSTON, Charles Greene (1868-1927)
On Dr. Chaput's new anastomosis buttons for gastro-intestinal surgery. Louisville, 1896. 11p. DNLM **90-1422**

CUMSTON, Charles Greene (1868-1927)
Haemorrhagic metritis. Boston, 1896. 8p. DNLM **90-1423**

CUMSTON, Charles Greene (1868-1927)
Lumbar nephrectomy in anuria, due to uterine cancer. Boston, 1896. 8p. DNLM **90-1424**

CUMSTON, Charles Greene (1868-1927)
On primary malignant tumors of the clitoris. Boston, 1896. 12p. DNLM **90-1425**

CUMSTON, Charles Greene (1868-1927)
The urinary troubles produced by prolapsus of genital organs. Boston, 1896. 8p. DNLM **90-1426**

CUMSTON, Charles Greene (1868-1927)
Hydrocele muliebris, with the report of a case. Boston, 1897. 12p. **90-1427**

CUMSTON, Charles Greene (1868-1927)
Tertiary syphilitic epididymitis. Philadelphia, 1897. 9p. DNLM **90-1428**

CUMSTON, Charles Greene (1868-1927)
Tubercular cystitis in children. [Danbury, 1898.] 16p. DNLM **90-1429**

CUMSTON, Charles Greene (1868-1927)
Septic infection of ovarian cystoma. [New York, 1898.] 18p. DNLM **90-1430**

CUMSTON, Charles Greene (1868-1927)
Varicose veins and their treatment by Trendelenburg's operation. [Philadelphia, 1898.] 14p. DNLM
90-1431

CUMSTON, Charles Greene (1868-1927)
Pyonephrosis complicating gonorrhea. [Philadelphia, 1899.] 12p. DNLM **90-1432**

CUMSTON, Charles Greene (1868-1927)
Some points on the technique of cerebral operations. [Providence, 1899.] 4p. DNLM **90-1433**

CUMSTON, Charles Greene (1868-1927)
General considerations on the pathology of the serious forms of chronic osteomyelitis and their complications. [Philadelphia, 1899.] 36p. DNLM **90-1434**

CUMSTON, Charles Greene (1868-1927)
The gonorrheal puerperium. [New York, 1899.] 29p. DNLM
90-1435

CUMSTON, Charles Greene (1868-1927)
Premature separation of the placenta. [Boston, 1899.] 10p. DNLM **90-1436**

CURRAN, Martin W.
Information for nurses in home and hospital. Chicago: C. H. Kerr & Co., 1893. 333p. DNLM **90-1437**

CURRAN, Martin W.
Sickness and accidents; modern methods of treatment; information for nurses in home and hospital. Chicago: C. H. Kerr & Co., 1894. 333p. DNLM **90-1438**

CURRIER, Andrew F[ay] (*b.* 1851)
Importance of oedema of the vaginal portion of the cervix uteri, as a symptom of chronic disease. Philadelphia: W. J. Dornan, 1890. 9p. DNLM **90-1439**

CURRIER, Andrew F[ay] (*b.* 1851)
A new operation for prolapsus of the anterior vaginal wall. [Philadelphia, 1890.] 6p. DNLM **90-1440**

CURRIER, Andrew F[ay] (*b.* 1851)
Present status and tendency of gynaecological therapeutics. Danbury, 1890. 31p. DNLM **90-1441**

CURRIER, Andrew F[ay] (*b.* 1851)
What are the rational limitations of intra-uterine therapeutics? [New York, 1890.] 16p. DNLM **90-1442**

CURRIER, Andrew F[ay] (*b.* 1851)
Under what conditions can electricity be of positive service to the gynaecologist? Danbury, Conn., 1891. 20p. DNLM
90-1443

CURRIER, Andrew F[ay] (*b.* 1851)
The unrestricted evil of prostitution. New York, 1891. 19p. DNLM **90-1444**

CURRIER, Andrew F[ay] (*b.* 1851)
Amputation of the vaginal portion of the cervix uteri in cases of suspected carcinoma. [New York, 1892.] 11p. DNLM
90-1445

CURRIER, Andrew F[ay] (*b.* 1851)
The causes and treatment of sinuses resulting from abdominal section. [Philadelphia, 1892.] 6p. DNLM **90-1446**

CURRIER, Andrew F[ay] (*b.* 1851)
Certain forms of septicaemia resulting from abortion. [Philadelphia, 1893.] 6p. DNLM **90-1447**

CURRIER, Andrew F[ay] (*b.* 1851)
Constipation, especially in its relations to the diseases peculiar to women. New York, 1893. 16p. DNLM
90-1448

CURRIER, Andrew F[ay] (*b.* 1851)
Septicaemia and its treatment with oxygen. New York: William Wood & Co., 1893. 11p. DNLM **90-1449**

CURRIER, Andrew F[ay] (*b.* 1851)
Introduction to the debate on menstruation before the Medical Society of the State of New York, at Albany, February 6, 1894, with remarks concerning normal menstruation. New York, 1894. 11p. DNLM **90-1450**

CURRIER, Andrew F[ay] (*b.* 1851)
Puerperal septicaemia. Abdominal section followed by recovery. Abscess in right broad ligament. New York, 1895. 3p. DNLM **90-1451**

CURRIER, Andrew F[ay] (*b.* 1851)
The position or posture of the patient during parturition, with special reference to the merits of the Walcher position. Philadelphia, 1896. 16p. DNLM **90-1452**

CURRIER, Andrew F[ay] (*b.* 1851)
Supplementary report of a case of puerperal septicaemia of prolonged duration and with manifold complications. New York, 1896. 5p. 1 chart. DNLM **90-1453**

CURRIER, Andrew F[ay] (*b.* 1851)
Ventral hernia resulting after abdominal section and its treatment. Boston, 1897. 12p. DNLM **90-1454**

CURRIER, Andrew F[ay] (*b.* 1851)
The menopause; a consideration of the phenomena which occur to women at the close of the child-bearing period. . . . New York: D. Appleton & Co., 1897. 300p. DLC; DNLM; NNNAM **90-1455**

CURRIER, Charles G[ilman]
Self-purification of flowing water, and the influence of polluted water in the causation of disease. (A biological study.) [Philadelphia, 1890.] 19p. DNLM **90-1456**

CURRIER, Charles G[ilman]
The art of preserving health: outlines of practical hygiene adapted to American conditions. New York: E. B. Treat, 1893. 468p. DLC; DNLM; NNNAM **90-1457**

CURRIER, Charles G[ilman]
Outlines of practical hygiene. . . . 3rd ed., rev. and enl. New York: E. B. Treat & Co., 1898. 482p. DLC; NNNAM
90-1458

CURTIN, Roland G[ideon] (1839-1913)
Is herpes zoster a cause of pleurisy and peritonitis? New York, 1890. 6p. DNLM **90-1459**

CURTIN, Roland G[ideon] (1839-1913) and EDWARD W. WATSON
Papers on the epidemic of influenza from 1889 to 1892: 1. Relation between influenza and catarrhal fever. 2. The epidemic as seen in Philadelphia from 1889 to 1891. 3. The treatment of influenza and its sequelae. 4. The heart as influenced by the epidemic; with other notes. 5. Notes on the outbreak of influenza and its treatment during the fall and early winter of 1891. Philadelphia, 1892. 10, 18, 8, 6, 5p. DNLM **90-1460**

CURTIN, Roland G[ideon] (1839-1913)
Brief suggestions as to the prevention, recognition, and treatment of cholera. [Philadelphia, 1892.] 12p. DNLM **90-1461**

CURTIN, Roland G[ideon] (1839-1913)
Clinical teaching and clinical teachers in the Philadelphia Hospital. [Philadelphia, 1893.] 8p. DNLM; PU **90-1462**

CURTIN, Roland G[ideon] (1839-1913)
Hemorrhagic typhoid fever; treatment and a review of the tabulation of seventeen cases. Clinical lecture delivered at the Philadelphia Hospital, February 17, 1891. [Philadelphia, 1893.] 7p. DNLM **90-1463**

CURTIN, Roland G[ideon] (1839-1913) and Edward W. WATSON
The action of influenza poison on the heart, and a study of influenzal agina pectoris. Read before the American Climatological Association, Richfield Springs, New York, June 24, 1892. [Philadelphia: J. B Lippincott Co., 1893.] 8p. DNLM **90-1464**

CURTIN, Roland G[ideon] (1839-1913) and Edward W. WATSON
A brief study of some ancient epidemics, and their relations to influenza; with notes on the epidemic of 1893-1894, and recent methods of treatment. [Philadelphia, 1894.] 8p. DNLM; PU **90-1465**

CURTIS, B[enjamin] Farquhar (1857-1924)
The treatment of arterio-venous aneurism, with two cases treated by extirpation. [Philadelphia, 1891.] 17p. DNLM **90-1466**

CURTIS, Edward (1838-1912)
Manual of general medical technology including prescription-writing. . . . 3rd ed., confirmed to the U.S. Pharmacopoeia of 1890. New York: William Wood & Co., 1895. 235p. DLC; NNNAM; OCLloyd **90-1467**

CURTIS, G[eorge] Lenox (*b.* 1854)
Where dentistry looks over into oral surgery. [Philadelphia, 1892.] 7p. DNLM **90-1468**

CURTIS, G[eorge] Lenox (*b.* 1854)
Remarkable sequence of operation for necrosis at base of skull; a new method of resecting the third branch of the fifth nerve. Chicago: American Medical Assoc., 1893. 8p. DNLM **90-1469**

CURTIS, H[enry] Holbrook (1856-1920)
Voice building and tone placing, showing a new method of relieving injured vocal cords by tone exercises. New York: D. Appleton & Co., 1896. 215p. 1 plate. DNLM; NNNAM **90-1470**

CUSHING, Clinton (1840-1904)
Nine months' work in abdominal surgery. [San Francisco, 1890.] 7p. 1 table. DNLM **90-1471**

CUSHING, Clinton (1840-1904)
A review of forty-eight cases of abdominal surgery. [Philadelphia, 1891.] 12p. 1 table. DNLM **90-1472**

CUSHING, Clinton (1840-1904)
Abdominal section for diagnostic purposes. San Francisco, Cal.: W. A. Woodward & Co., [1892]. 7p. DNLM **90-1473**

CUSHING, Clinton (1840-1904)
Gynecology at the Lane Hospital, San Francisco. San Francisco: Woodward & Co., 1896. 8p. DNLM **90-1474**

CUSHING, E[rnest] W[atson] (1847-1916)
A case of extra-uterine pregnancy; operation at the ninth month; recovery. Boston, 1891. 2 l. 2 p. DNLM **90-1475**

CUSHING, E[rnest] W[atson] (1847-1916)
Vaginal hysterectomy for cancer, with reports of twenty-one cases (with nineteen recoveries). Philadelphia, 1891. 6p. 2 plates. DNLM **90-1476**

CUSHING, E[rnest] W[atson] (1847-1916)
The operative treatment of backward displacements of the uterus. Philadelphia, 1893. 27p. DNLM **90-1477**

CUSHING, E[rnest] W[atson] (1847-1916)
Irregular menstruation. New York, 1894. 4p. DNLM **90-1478**

CUSHING, H[enry] E.
A case of complete inversion of the uterus following labor. [Philadelphia: Lea Bros. & Co., 1892.] 3p. DNLM **90-1479**

CUSHNY, Arthur R[obertson] (1866-1926)
On the action of piperidine and some of its compounds. New York, 1896. 12p. DNLM **90-1480**

CUSHNY, Arthur R[obertson] (1866-1926)
A text-book of pharmacology and therapeutics; or, The action of drugs in health and disease. . . . Illustrated with forty-seven engravings. Philadelphia and New York: Lea Bros. & Co., 1899. 730p. DLC; NNNAM; OCLloyd; PPC **90-1481**

CUSTIS, Marvin A[shdowne] (*b.* 1866)
The practice of medicine, a condensed manual for the busy practitioner. . . . Philadelphia: Boericke & Tafel, 1896. 367p. DLC; PPC; PPHa **90-1482**

CUTLER, Condict W[alker] (1859-1930)
The use of iodine, carbolic acid, and chloral in dermatology. [New York, 1892.] 12p. DNLM **90-1483**

CUTLER, Condict W[alker] (1859-1930)
Practical lectures in dermatology; comprising a course of fifteen lectures delivered at the University of Vermont Medical Department during the session of 1892 and 1893. . . . New York: G. P. Putnam's Sons, 1894. 233p. DLC; DNLM; NNNAM **90-1484**

CUTLER, Condict W[alker] (1859-1930)
Suggestions by a general practitioner for the symptomatic treatment of skin diseases. New York, 1897. 19p. DNLM
90-1485

CUTLER, Condict W[alker] (1859-1930)
The treatment of typhoid fever. New York, 1897. 12p. DNLM
90-1486

CUTLER, Elbridge G[erry] (*b.* 1846)
Some cases of dilated stomach. Boston: Damrell & Upham, 1891. 15p. DNLM **90-1487**

CUTTER, Ephraim (1832-1917)
Some contributions to laryngology. I. Thyrotomy modified, 1866. II. Fibroid enlargement of arytenoid cartilages. III. A new name for the ventricular bands. Chicago, 1890. 8p. DNLM
90-1488

CUTTER, Ephraim (1832-1917) and John Ashburton CUTTER
Feeding in the wasting diseases. [New York, 1890.] 20p. DNLM **90-1489**

CUTTER, Ephraim (1832-1917)
Trophopathy in the fatty and fibroid degenerations: a joint paper by Ephraim Cutter . . . and John Ashburton Cutter. . . . Read by the junior writer before the Section of practice of medicine, materia medica and physiology of the American Medical Association, at its fortieth annual meeting, 1889. . . . New York: The Ariston, 1890. 8p. DLC
90-1490

CUTTER, Ephraim (1832-1917)
Food in motherhood. . . . New York: The Author, 1890. 144p. DLC; NNNAM **90-1491**

CUTTER, Ephraim (1832-1917)
The galvano cautery, its use in removal of piles and growths. Philadelphia, 1891. 7p. DNLM **90-1492**

CUTTER, Ephraim (1832-1917) and John Ashburton CUTTER
Diet in tumor and cancer. New York, 1891. 23p. DNLM
90-1493

CUTTER, Ephraim (1832-1917)
The esoteric beauty and utility of the microscope. With index and bibliography. New York, 1892. 43p. DNLM; NNNAM
90-1494

CUTTER, Ephraim (1832-1917)
Partial syllabic lists of the clinical morphologies of the blood, sputum, feces, skin, urine, vomitus, foods, (including potable waters, ice and the air), the clothing, uterine and vaginal discharges, and soils. . . . 2nd ed. New York: Pub. by the Author, 1892. 92p. DLC; NNNAM **90-1495**

CUTTER, Ephraim (1832-1917)
. . . The fatty and fibroid degenerations; Bright's disease, apoplexy, fatty heart, puerperal convulsions, cataract, locomotor ataxia, alcoholism; [by] Ephraim Cutter . . . [and] John A. Cutter. . . . New York, 1892. 21p. DLC; DNLM
90-1496

CUTTER, Ephraim (1832-1917)
The best waters to drink. New York, 1896. 12p. DNLM
90-1497

CUTTER, Ephraim (1832-1917)
The American blood test for cattle tuberculosis. [New York], 1896. 4 l. DNLM **90-1498**

CUTTER, Ephraim (1832-1917)
What makes the cures? [New York, 1897.] 8p. DNLM
90-1499

CUTTER, Ephraim (1832-1917)
The pre-asthmatic state. [New York, 1897.] 7p. DNLM
90-1500

CUTTER, Ephraim (1832-1917)
Fatty degeneration and its masquerades. New York, 1897. 21p. DNLM **90-1501**

CUTTER, Ephraim (1832-1917)
Systematic treatment of eyes; with description of a new mode of examination. New York, [1897]. 8p. DNLM
90-1502

CUTTER, Ephraim (1832-1917)
[Medical reprints.] The pre-apoplectic state, [etc.]. New York, 1897. 18p. DNLM **90-1503**

CUTTER, Ephraim (1832-1917)
Fatty ills and their masquerades, by Ephraim Cutter . . . and John Ashburton Cutter. . . . New York: Equitable Building, 1898. 194p. DLC; DNLM; NNNAM **90-1504**

CUTTER, John Ashburton (1867-1944)
Doctors' offices in business buildings. New York, 1896. 2p. DNLM **90-1505**

DABNEY, Charles W., Jr. (1855-1945)
Vivisection in the District of Columbia. [Washington, 1896.] 8p. DNLM **90-1506**

DABNEY, Samuel G.
Clinical reports in laryngology. [Philadelphia, 1893.] 4p. DNLM **90-1507**

DABNEY, T. S.
Sixteen years' experience in the treatment of syphilis by the hypodermic injection of bi-chloride of mercury. New Orleans, 1897. 11p. DNLM **90-1508**

DABNEY, T. S.
The treatment of yellow fever. [New Orleans], 1897. 12p. DNLM **90-1509**

DABNEY, T. S.
Diseases of tropical climates, their prevention, diagnosis, and treatment. New York, 1898. 18p. DNLM
90-1510

DABNEY, William Cecil (1849-1894)
The physiological action and therapeutic uses of the water of the Greenbrier White Sulphur Springs, W.Va. New York, 1890. 8p. DNLM **90-1511**

DABNEY, William Cecil (1849-1894)
An outbreak of typhoid fever presenting unusual features. [Philadelphia: Lea Bros. & Co., 1893.] 8p. DNLM
90-1512

DABNEY, William Cecil (1849-1894)
The aims and methods of medical education. [Philadelphia, 1893.] 10p. DNLM **90-1513**

DA COSTA, Jacob Mendes (1833-1900)
Medical diagnosis, with special reference to practical medicine. A guide to the knowledge and discrimination of diseases. . . . Illustrated with engravings on wood. 7th ed., rev. Philadelphia, [etc.] : J. B. Lippincott Co., 1890. 995p. diags. DLC; NNNAM; OCIM; PPC **90-1514**

DA COSTA, Jacob Mendes (1833-1900)
Professional aspirations. Valedictory address to the graduating class of Jefferson Medical College of Philadelphia. Philadelphia: J. B. Lippincott Co., 1891. 23p. DNLM **90-1515**

DA COSTA, Jacob Mendes (1833-1900)
Malarial paralysis. [Philadelphia, 1891.] 11p. DNLM **90-1516**

DA COSTA, Jacob Mendes (1833-1900)
The pulmonary complications of influenza. Philadelphia, [1892]. 22p. DNLM **90-1517**

DA COSTA, Jacob Mendes (1833-1900)
Address before the Harvard Medical Alumni Association. Boston: G. H. Ellis, 1893. 14p. DNLM **90-1518**

DA COSTA, Jacob Mendes (1833-1900)
The albuminuria and the Bright's disease of uric acid and of oxaluria. [Philadelphia, 1893.] 15p. DNLM **90-1519**

DA COSTA, Jacob Mendes (1833-1900)
Cardiac asthenia, or heat-exhaustion. [Philadelphia: Lea Bros. & Co., 1894.] 11p. DNLM **90-1520**

DA COSTA, Jacob Mendes (1833-1900)
Medical diagnosis, with special reference to practical medicine. A guide to the knowledge and discrimination of diseases. . . . Illustrated with engravings on wood. 8th ed., rev. Philadelphia, [etc.] : J. B. Lippincott Co., 1895. 1104p. diags. DLC; IU-M; NNNAM; PU **90-1521**

DA COSTA, Jacob Mendes (1833-1900)
Address delivered at the opening of the Garrett Memorial Building, Pennsylvania Hospital, on April 23, 1897. [Philadelphia: Times Print. House, 1897.] 12p. DNLM **90-1522**

DA COSTA, Jacob Mendes (1833-1900)
Tendencies in medicine. The president's address, delivered before the Association of American Physicians, Washington, D.C., May 4, 1897. 12p. DNLM **90-1523**

DA COSTA, Jacob Mendes (1833-1900)
The scholar in medicine. An address delivered before the Harvard Medical Alumni Association, June 29, 1897. Boston: G. H. Ellis, 1897. 14p. DNLM **90-1524**

DA COSTA, Jacob Mendes (1833-1900)
On the significance of jaundice in typhoid fever, and on the hepatic complications without jaundice. Philadelphia, 1898. 31p. DNLM **90-1525**

DA COSTA, John C[halmers] (1834-1910)
Absence of the vagina, with hematometra from retained menses. Philadelphia, 1894. 4p. DNLM **90-1526**

DA COSTA, John C[halmers] (1834-1910)
A case of pyaemia in a young infant. New York: William Wood & Co., 1897. 5p. DNLM **90-1527**

DA COSTA, John C[halmers] (1834-1910)
Clinical notes with specimens: I. Celiotomy during pregnancy. II. A large polyp with inversion of the uterus in a woman of advanced years. III. Removal of a large dermoid cyst nine weeks after labor. New York: William Wood & Co., 1897. 4p. DNLM **90-1528**

DA COSTA, John C[halmers] (1834-1910)
Two cases of fibroma of the broad ligament. New York: William Wood & Co., 1898. 4p. DNLM **90-1529**

DA COSTA, John Chalmers (1863-1933)
. . . A manual of modern surgery, general and operative. . . . With 188 illustrations in the text and 13 full page plates in colors and tints aggregating 276 separate figures. Philadelphia: W. B. Saunders, 1894. 809p. DLC; MH-M; NNNAM; PPC **90-1530**

DA COSTA, John Chalmers (1863-1933)
A manual of modern surgery, general and operative, by . . . . [2nd ed.]. Philadelphia: W. B. Saunders, 1898. 911p. plates. DLC; IEN-M; NNNAM; PPJ **90-1531**

DA COSTA, J[ohn] C., Jr. (1871-1920)
The serum diagnosis of enteric fever by the dried-blood method. New York: D. Appleton & Co., 1897. 30p. DNLM **90-1532**

DA COSTA, J[ohn] C., Jr. (1871-1920)
Blood staining. Philadelphia, [1897]. 3 l. DNLM **90-1533**

DAGGETT, B[yron] H.
Irrigation of the urethra and bladder by posture and continuous current. [Buffalo, 1893.] 7p. DNLM **90-1534**

DAGGETT, Charles H.
Daggett's book of medical reference comp. from lecture notes taken at the Massachusetts College of Pharmacy, sessions of 1886, '87, '88, '89, with additions taken from the authorities named on page 5. [Lynn, Mass., 1891.] 775p. DLC **90-1535**

DAGGETT, Charles H.
Daggett's school of pharmacy lecture course. A short and concise series of practical lessions in pharmacy. . . . 2nd ed., rev. and enl. Providence: Printed by J. F. Greene Co., 1899. 220p. DLC **90-1536**

DAILY, John Wesley
The home practice of medicine, for the use of families and everybody who can read the English language. . . . Boston: The Daily Publishing Co., 1898. 357p. DLC **90-1537**

DAILY, John Wesley
The home practice of medicine. . . . . Boston: The Daily Publishing Co., 1899. 436p. col. plates. DLC **90-1538**

DAKE, Jabez P[hilander] (1827-1894)
Civil government and the healers of the sick. An address delivered before the World's Congress of Homoeopathic Physicians, at Atlantic City, N.J., June 18, 1891. Philadelphia: The Hahnemann Monthly, 1891. 19p. PPC; PPHa
90-1539

DALAND, Judson
A volumetric study of the red and white corpuscles of human blood in health and disease, by aid of the haematokrit. [Philadelphia, 1891.] 18p. DNLM **90-1540**

DALAND, Judson
A clinical description of dysentery as it occurs in Nicaragua. Detroit: G. S. Davis, 1892. 7p. DNLM
90-1541

DALAND, Judson
A report on the origin and progress of the American Berlin Medical Society. [Philadelphia, 1892.] 2p. DNLM
90-1542

DALAND, Judson
A clinical study of eleven cases of Asiatic cholera treated by hypodermoclysis and enteroclysis. Philadelphia, 1893. 18p. DNLM **90-1543**

DALAND, Judson
Hysterical seizures relieved by hypnotic suggestions. [Philadelphia, 1893.] 8p. DNLM **90-1544**

DALAND, Judson
A new method of separating the white from the red blood corpuscles by means of the haematokrit. Philadelphia, 1893. 11p. 1 table. DNLM **90-1545**

DALAND, Judson
The treatment of cholera by hypodermoclysis and enteroclysis. Philadelphia, 1893. 8p. DNLM
90-1546

DALAND, Judson
In memoriam. John M. Keating. Philadelphia, 1894. 15p. port. DNLM **90-1547**

DALAND, Judson and W. Duffield ROBINSON
A clinical study of three cases of spontaneous haemophilia in brothers. [Philadelphia], 1895. 6p. DNLM
90-1548

DALAND, Judson
The treatment of malaria. Clinical lecture delivered at the Philadelphia Hospital. Philadelphia, [1896]. 15p. DLC; DNLM
90-1549

DALAND, Judson
Notes on examination of urine; based upon Prof. James Tyson's Handbook for practical examination of urine. 6th ed. [Philadelphia, 1896.] 1 l. DNLM
90-1550

DALBY, William B[artlett] (1840-1918)
Lectures on diseases and injuries of the ear . . . delivered at St. George's Hospital. 4th ed. Philadelphia: P. Blakiston, Son & Co., 1893. 279p. col. plates. DLC; MH-M; NNNAM; PU [1st ed., Philadelphia: Lindsay & Blakiston, 1873. 228p.]
90-1551

DALLAS, Alexander
The treatment of inguinal hernia. [Philadelphia, 1891.] 6p. DNLM **90-1552**

DALLAS, Alexander
New instrument for the cure of hernia. [Philadelphia: Lea Bros. & Co., 1892.] 3p. DNLM **90-1553**

DALLAS, Alexander
Hernia in infancy, and its correct treatment. New York: E. P. Coby & Co., 1892. 16p. DNLM
90-1554

DALLAS, Alexander
The treatment of inguinal hernia. [New York]. 1893. 16p. DNLM **90-1555**

DALLEY, Lawrence J.
Refractive and ophthalmic catechism, for the use of general practitioners, opticians, and students. Gloversville, N.Y.: Collins Pub. Co., 1898. 218p. DLC
90-1556

DALTON, H[enry] C.
A case of gastrostomy. [St. Louis, 1890.] 2 l. DNLM
90-1557

DALTON, H[enry] C.
Rupture of liver and kidney; excessive haemorrhage; laparotomy; recovery. [St. Louis, 1890.] 4p. DNLM
90-1558

DALTON, H[enry] C.
Cases of penetrating stab wounds of the abdomen; laparotomy; results. [Chicago, 1890.] 8p. DNLM
90-1559

DALTON, H[enry] C.
Three laparotomies on one patient; recovery. [St. Louis, 1890.] 6p. DNLM **90-1560**

DALTON, H[enry] C.
Some recent surgical cases. [St. Louis, 1890.] 6p. DNLM
90-1561

[DALTON, John Call] (1825-1889)
John Call Dalton, M.D., U.S.V. [Cambridge, Mass.]: Priv. print. [by H. O. Houghton & Co.], 1892. 195p. port. DLC; MB; MH **90-1562**

DALY, W[illiam] H[udson] (1842-1901)
A plea for early operation in diseases of the antrum of Highmore. [New York, 1894.] 8p. DNLM
90-1563

DALY, W[illiam] H[udson] (1842-1901)
A further discussion on malaria a waterborne disease. Chicago, 1895. 15p. DNLM **90-1564**

DANA, Charles L[oomis] (1852-1935)
A study of the anaesthesias of hysteria. [Philadelphia, 1890.] 12p. DNLM **90-1565**

DANA, Charles L[oomis] (1852-1935)
Text-book of nervous diseases, being a compendium for the use of students and practitioners of medicine by . . . . New York: William Wood & Co., 1892. 524p. DLC; DNLM; NNNAM; PPC **90-1566**

DANA, Charles L[oomis] (1852-1935)
Shaking palsy: a clinical and pathological study, with the reports of two autopsies. New York, 1893. 30p. 1 plate. DNLM **90-1567**

DANA, Charles L[oomis] (1852-1935)
Text-book of nervous diseases, being a compendium for the use of students and practitioners of medicine. . . . 2nd ed. . . . New York: William Wood & Co., 1893. 549p. DLC; NNNAM; OCIM; PU **90-1568**

DANA, Charles L[oomis] (1852-1935)
On the microbic origin of chorea. Report of a case with autopsy. [Philadelphia, 1894.] 8p. DNLM **90-1569**

DANA, Charles L[oomis] (1852-1935)
Text-book of nervous diseases, being a compendium for the use of students and practitioners of medicine. . . . 3rd ed. . . . New York: William Wood & Co., 1894. 549p. CtY-M; DLC; NNNAM; PPC **90-1570**

DANA, Charles L[oomis] (1852-1935)
On the new use of some older sciences, being a discourse on degeneration and its stigmata. New York: Trow Directory, Printing & Bookbinding Co., 1894. 19p. NN **90-1571**

DANA, Charles L[oomis] (1852-1935) and J. R. CONWAY
A case of successful operation for brain tumor. New York, 1895. 9p. DNLM **90-1572**

DANA, Charles L[oomis] (1852-1935)
Text-book of nervous diseases, being a compendium for the use of students and practitioners of medicine. . . . 4th ed., rev. and enl. New York: William Wood & Co., 1897. 628p. col. plates. DLC; DNLM; NNNAM; PPC **90-1573**

DANA, Charles L[oomis] (1852-1935)
Psychro-aesthesia (cold sensations) and psychro-algia (cold pains). New York, 1898. 11p. DNLM **90-1574**

DANDRIDGE, N[athaniel] P[endleton] (1846-1910)
Hospitals; their work and their obligations. Cincinnati: R. Blake & Co., 1893. 23p. DNLM **90-1575**

DANDRIDGE, N[athaniel] P[endleton] (1846-1910)
Report of two cases of amputation at the hip-joint, in which hemorrhage was controlled by transfixion pins and elastic compression. [Philadelphia, 1894.] 10p. DNLM **90-1576**

DANE, John
An apparatus for the correction of talipes equino varus. [Boston, 1891.] 3p. DNLM **90-1577**

DANE, John
A study of flat-foot; with special attention to the development of the arch of the foot. Boston: Damrell & Upham, 1892. 41p. DNLM; MBM **90-1578**

DANE, John
A study of the blood in cases of tuberculosis of the bones and joints. Boston: Damrell & Upham, 1896. 34p. 1 table. DNLM; MBM **90-1579**

DANE, John
Some effects upon the leg of pronation of the foot. [Philadelphia, 1897.] 13p. DNLM **90-1580**

DANFORTH, I[saac] N[ewton] (1835-1911)
Tube casts and their diagnostic value. Philadelphia, 1892. 12p. DNLM **90-1581**

DARLINGTON, Thomas (1858-1945)
The effect of the products of high explosives, dynamite and nitroglycerine on the human system. New York: Trow, 1890. 8p. NNNAM [The deleterious effects of nitroglycerine on tunnel workers, and the use of ammonia to counteract poisonous effects on nitrites in the blood.] **90-1582**

DARTMOUTH MEDICAL COLLEGE
Centennial exercises, Tuesday, June 29, 1897. [Historical address by Phineas S. Conner.] [1897.] 124p. MBM **90-1583**

DAVENPORT, Charles Benedict (1866-1944)
Experimental morphology. Part I: Effect of chemical and physical agents upon protoplasm. New York: Macmillan Co., 1897. 280p. DNLM; NN; NNNAM; PU **90-1584**

DAVENPORT, Francis H[enry] (*b.* 1851)
A case of incontinence of the urine, due to malposition of the ureter. Philadelphia: W. J. Dornan, 1890. 8p. DNLM **90-1585**

DAVENPORT, Francis H[enry] (*b.* 1851)
Diseases of women: a manual of non-surgical gynecology, designed especially for the use of students and general practitioners. . . . 2nd ed., rev. and enl. . . . Philadelphia: Lea Bros. & Co., 1892. 323p. DLC; DNLM; NNNAM; PPC **90-1586**

DAVENPORT, Francis H[enry] (*b.* 1851)
Diseases of women: a manual of gynecology designed especially for the use of students and general practitioners. . . . 3rd ed., rev. and enl. Philadelphia and New York: Lea Bros. & Co., 1898. 391p. DLC; DNLM; NNNAM; PU **90-1587**

DAVENPORT, George
Puerperal convulsions. [New York, 1895.] 8p. DNLM **90-1588**

DAVENPORT, Isaac B.
Articulation of the teeth. New York & Philadelphia, 1893. 8p. DNLM **90-1589**

DAVIES, Arthur Mercer (*b.* 1853)
A handbook of hygiene. Philadelphia: J. B. Lippincott & Co., 1895. 590p. DNLM; OCIM; PPC; PU **90-1590**

DAVIS, A[chilles] E[dward] (1866-1941)
Javal's ophthalmometer and atropine in determining errors of refraction. With an incidental notice of eye-strain and graduated tenotomies. [New York, 1892.] 30p. 1 table. DNLM **90-1591**

DAVIS, A[chilles] E[dward] (1866-1941)
Ophthalmometry in the United States and its championship. New York, 1893. 10p. DNLM **90-1592**

DAVIS, A[chilles] E[dward] (1866-1941)
The technics of the trial case; or subjective optometry. New York, 1896. 13p. DNLM **90-1593**

DAVIS, Andrew P. (*b.* 1835)
Osteopathy illustrated. A drugless system of healing. . . . Cincinnati: O. F. L. Rowe, 1899. 854p. plates. DLC **90-1594**

DAVIS, Byron B. (*b.* 1859)
A contribution to the surgery of gastroptosis and enteroptosis. Lincoln, Neb., 1897. 8p. DNLM **90-1595**

DAVIS, Byron B. (*b.* 1859)
Preparation of the patient for operation. Lincoln, Neb., 1898. 8p. DNLM **90-1596**

DAVIS, C[harles] G[ilbert] (1848-1928)
Vaginal hysterectomy; a review of sixty-six consecutive cases. Chicago, 1897. 8p. DNLM **90-1597**

DAVIS, C[harles] G[ilbert] (1848-1928)
Health and happiness. An address delivered at the commencement of the National Temperance Training School. [Chicago, 1897.] 10p. DNLM **90-1598**

DAVIS, C[harles] G[ilbert] (1848-1928)
The National Temperance Hospital. [Chicago, 1897.] 4p. DNLM **90-1599**

DAVIS, Edward P[arker] (*b.* 1856) and Thomas G. ASHTON
The value of the graduated bath and pack in the treatment of catarrhal pneumonia in children. Philadelphia, 1890. 22p. 3 tables. DNLM **90-1600**

DAVIS, Edward P[arker] (*b.* 1856)
A manual of practical obstetrics. Philadelphia: P. Blakiston, Son & Co., 1891. 298p. 10 plates. DLC; DNLM; NNNAM; PPC **90-1601**

DAVIS, Edward P[arker] (*b.* 1856)
Surgical treatment of labor delayed by rigidity of the os uteri. [Philadelphia, 1892.] 8p. DNLM **90-1602**

DAVIS, Edward P[arker] (*b.* 1856)
Scientific obstetrics in private practice. Philadelphia, 1893. 10p. DNLM **90-1603**

DAVIS, Edward P[arker] (*b.* 1856)
Mother and child. Pt. I. Mother. By Edward P. Davis. . . . Pt. II. Child. By John M. Keating. . . . Philadelphia, [etc.]: J. B. Lippincott Co., 1893. 472p. DLC; DNLM; NNNAM; PPC **90-1604**

DAVIS, Edward P[arker] (*b.* 1856)
A manual of practical obstetrics. 2nd ed. Philadelphia: P. Blakiston, Son & Co., 1894. 351p. 16 plates. DLC: DNLM; NNNAM; PU **90-1605**

DAVIS, Edward P[arker] (*b.* 1856)
Caesarean section and symphysiotomy for the relative indications, with a report of cases. [Philadelphia: Lea Bros. & Co., 1894.] 12p. DNLM **90-1606**

DAVIS, Edward P[arker] (*b.* 1856)
Fatal nausea and vomiting of pregnancy, with report of cases. [Philadelphia, 1894.] 13p. DNLM **90-1607**

DAVIS, Edward P[arker] (*b.* 1856)
The management of face-presentation. New York, 1894. 5p. DNLM **90-1608**

DAVIS, Edward P[arker] (*b.* 1856)
The prophylaxis and treatment of eclampsia. Detroit: G. S. Davis, 1895. 12p. DNLM **90-1609**

DAVIS, Edward P[arker] (*b.* 1856)
Celiotomy for painful abdominal growth of obscure nature—sacroma of the ovary with cystic degeneration. New York: William Wood & Co., 1895. 5p. DNLM **90-1610**

DAVIS, Edward P[arker] (*b.* 1856)
Puerperal sapraemia. [New York, 1895.] 5p. DNLM **90-1611**

DAVIS, Edward P[arker] (*b.* 1856)
Fatal post-partum hemorrhage. [Philadelphia, 1896.] 2p. DNLM **90-1612**

DAVIS, Edward P[arker] (*b.* 1856)
Post-mortem Caesarean section, with delivery of a living child. New York, 1896. 5p. DNLM **90-1613**

DAVIS, Edward P[arker] (*b.* 1856)
A treatise on obstetrics for students and practitioners. . . . Philadelphia and New York: Lea Bros. & Co., 1896. 553p. col. plates. DLC; DNLM; NNNAM; PPC **90-1614**

DAVIS, Gwilym G[eorge] (1857-1918)
The principles and practice of bandaging. Detroit: G. S. Davis, 1891. 61p. 23 plates. DLC; DNLM; NNNAM; PPC **90-1615**

DAVIS, Gwilym G[eorge] (1857-1918)
Operations for the correction of inveterate pes varus. [Philadelphia, 1894.] 10p. DNLM **90-1616**

DAVIS, Gwilym G[eorge] (1857-1918)
Rupture of the long head of the biceps brachii muscle associated with rheumatoid arthritis. Philadelphia, 1895. 8p. DNLM **90-1617**

DAVIS, Gwilym G[eorge] (1857-1918)
The effects of small-calibre bullets as used in military arms. Philadelphia, 1897. 15p. DNLM **90-1618**

DAVIS, J[ames] Aubrey (1865-1902)
Essentials of materia medica and prescription writing. So arranged as to conform with the classification adopted in the last ed. of Prof. H. C. Wood's "Therapeutics," making it of special value to students of those institutions, which the above work used as a textbook. . . . Philadelphia: P. Blakiston, Son & Co., 1892. 334p. DLC; OCLloyd; PPC; PU **90-1619**

DAVIS, John D[aniel] S[inkler] (*b.* 1859)
Epicystic surgical fistula for the relief of vesical catarrh. Chicago, 1890. 16p. DNLM **90-1620**

DAVIS, John D[aniel] S[inkler] (*b.* 1859)
An experimental study of intestinal anastomosis. Philadelphia, 1890. 41p. DNLM **90-1621**

DAVIS, Nathan Smith (1817-1904)
Report on the meteorological conditions and their relations to the epidemic influenza, and some other diseases in Chicago during the six months ending March 31, 1890. . . . Read in the Section of State Medicine of the American Medical Association, May 20, 1890. . . . Chicago: Printed at the Office of the Association, 1890. 16p. DLC **90-1622**

DAVIS, Nathan Smith (1817-1904)
Brief comments on the pathology of pneumonia and the principles that should guide in its treatment. . . . Read before the Chicago Medical Society, February 10th, 1892. . . . Chicago: Press of R. R. McCabe & Co., [1892]. 8p. DLC **90-1623**

DAVIS, Nathan Smith (1817-1904)
The history, present status, and future progress of practical medicine. . . . A lecture of the Post-Graduate Medical School and Hospital, of Chicago, Sept. 1st, 1893. Chicago, Ill., [1893]. 12p. DLC **90-1624**

DAVIS, Nathan Smith (1817-1904)
The importance of the study of medical jurisprudence by students of law, and the extent to which it should be taught in schools or colleges for the education of such students. Detroit, 1895. 9p. DLC; DNLM **90-1625**

DAVIS, Nathan Smith (1817-1904)
Address on the character of Dr. Edward Jenner, and the history of his discovery of the protective value of vaccination. Chicago, 1896. 15p. DLC; DNLM **90-1626**

DAVIS, Nathan Smith (1817-1904)
A brief history of the origin of the American Medical Association. Chicago, 1897. 11p. DNLM **90-1627**

DAVIS, Nathan Smith (1817-1904)
What are the characteristics of a true cardiac tonic? And what are the physiologic differences between a tonic and a stimulant? Chicago, 1898. 7p. DNLM **90-1628**

DAVIS, Nathan Smith (1817-1904)
The New York State Medical Society and ethics. [1899.] 5p. DNLM **90-1629**

DAVIS, N[athan] S[mith], Jr. (1858-1920)
Diseases of the lungs, heart, and kidneys. Philadelphia & London: F. A. Davis Co., 1892. 359p. DLC: DNLM; NNNAM; PPC **90-1630**

DAVIS, N[athan] S[mith], Jr. (1858-1920)
Remarks on the treatment of diabetes. Chicago, 1893. 12p. DNLM **90-1631**

DAVIS, N[athan] S[mith], Jr. (1858-1920)
Voluntary respiratory exercise in the treatment of phthisis. [Chicago, 1893.] 7p. DNLM **90-1632**

DAVIS, N[athan] S[mith], Jr. (1858-1920)
Animal extracts. [Chicago, 1894.] 12p. DNLM **90-1633**

DAVIS, N[athan] S[mith], Jr. (1858-1920)
Consumption: how to prevent it, and how to live with it. Its nature, its caues, its prevention, and the mode of life, climate, exercise, food, clothing necessary for its cure. Philadelphia: The F. A. Davis Company; London: F. J. Redman, 1894. 143p. DLC; DNLM; NNNAM; PU **90-1634**

DAVIS, N[athan] S[mith], Jr. (1858-1920)
Some statistics of diabetes mellitus. [Chicago, 1894.] 16p. DNLM **90-1635**

DAVIS, N[athan] S[mith], Jr. (1858-1920)
Pulmonary hypertrophic osteo-arthropathy. Chicago, 1895. 11p. DNLM **90-1636**

DAVIS, N[athan] S[mith], Jr. (1858-1920)
How to teach medicine. St. Louis, 1896. 6p. DNLM **90-1637**

DAVIS, N[athan] S[mith], Jr. (1858-1920)
Treatment of consumption. Detroit, 1896. 6p. DNLM **90-1638**

DAVIS, N[athan] S[mith], Jr. (1858-1920)
Trichomonas vaginalis. Chicago, 1896. 5p. DNLM **90-1639**

DAVIS, N[athan] S[mith], Jr. (1858-1920)
The cardio-vascular and renal relations and manifestations of gout. Chicago, 1897. 4p. DNLM **90-1640**

DAVIS, N[athan] S[mith], Jr. (1858-1920)
Cheyne-Stokes respiration phenomena. Chicago, 1897. 11p. DNLM **90-1641**

DAVIS, N[athan] S[mith], Jr. (1858-1920)
Diabetic gangrene. Chicago, 1898. 8p. DNLM **90-1642**

DAVIS, Wesley (1841?-1906)
The antiseptic treatment of typhoid fever. New York, 1896. 16p. DNLM **90-1643**

DAVIS, Wesley (1841?-1906)
Typhoid fever treated by the Woodbridge method. Chicago, 1896. 3p. DNLM **90-1644**

DAVIS, W[illiam] E[lias] B[rownlee] (1863-1903)
The treatment of local and general peritonitis. [Montgomery], 1890. 13p. DNLM **90-1645**

DAVIS, W[illiam] E[lias] B[rownlee] (1863-1903)
Operative procedures in acute general suppurative peritonitis. [New York, 1891.] 13p. DNLM **90-1646**

DAVIS, W[illiam] E[lias] B[rownlee] (1863-1903)
Annual lectures delivered before the Alumni Association of the College of Physicians and Surgeons of Baltimore. April 11 and 12, 1892. Baltimore: Friedenwald Co., 1892. 32p. DNLM; MdU-D **90-1647**

DAVISSON, J[ohn] H.
Restriction of tuberculosis. Chicago, 1894. 11p. DNLM **90-1648**

DAVISSON, J[ohn] H.
Sanitation of dwellings, public buildings, and thoroughfares. Sacramento: A. J. Johnston, 1894. 7p. DNLM **90-1649**

DAWBARN, Robert H[ugh] M[ackay] (1860-1915)
Water as a local anaesthetic. Its discovery American and not German. [New York, 1891.] 2 l. DNLM **90-1650**

DAWBARN, Robert H[ugh] M[ackay] (1860-1915)
A vegetable plate, also a new technique in intestinal anastomosis. [New York: Pusey & Troxell, 1891.] 20p. DNLM
90-1651

DAWBARN, Robert H[ugh] M[ackay] (1860-1915)
Arterial saline infusion. A report of three additional cases by the new technique, also of a case of infant diarrhoea treated by saline infusion. New York, 1892. 12p. DNLM
90-1652

DAWBARN, Robert H[ugh] M[ackay] (1860-1915)
Considerations upon medical haemorrhage surgically treated, with a successful case, by a new technique, of saline infusion for severe haemorrhage. [New York, 1892.] 20p. DNLM
90-1653

DAWBARN, Robert H[ugh] M[ackay] (1860-1915)
A new method of checking bleeding after tonsillotomy. New York, 1892. 4p. DNLM **90-1654**

DAWBARN, Robert H[ugh] M[ackay] (1860-1915)
Vegetable plates in bowel and stomach surgery; a discussion of the proper technique. Philadelphia, 1893. 16p. DNLM
90-1655

DAWBARN, Robert H[ugh] M[ackay] (1860-1915)
An aid to materia medica. . . . 3rd ed., rev. and enl. by Woolsey Hopkins, M.D. New York, [etc.]: G. P. Putnam's Sons, 1894. 133p. DLC; NNNAM; OCLloyd; PPC
90-1656

DAWBARN, Robert H[ugh] M[ackay] (1860-1915)
A curious case of appendicitis; with a discussion of certain points in operative technique. [New York, 1895.] 15p. DNLM **90-1657**

DAWBARN, Robert H[ugh] M[ackay] (1860-1915)
General considerations upon major anesthesia; threatened death during major anesthesia; a brief digression upon check. Danbury, Conn.: Danbury Med. Pr. Co., 1897. 47p. DNLM
90-1658

DAWBARN, Robert H[ugh] M[ackay] (1860-1915)
Three practical points in the management of fractures at the elbow-joint. Danbury, Conn.: Danbury Med. Print. Co., 1897. 8p. DNLM **90-1659**

DAWBARN, Robert H[ugh] M[ackay] (1860-1915)
Shock. . . . [New York, 1899.] 14p. DLC
90-1660

DEALE, Henry B. and Samuel S. ADAMS
Neurasthenia in young women. New York: William Wood & Co., 1894. 6p. DNLM **90-1661**

DEALE, Henry B.
Movable kidney. New York: William Wood & Co., 1896. 4p. DNLM **90-1662**

DEALE, Henry B.
The climatic treatment of pulmonary tuberculosis. Philadelphia, 1898. 12p. DNLM **90-1663**

DEAN, G. Edgar
The etiology and early management of glaucoma. Nashville, Tenn.: A. R. Gray & Son, 1894. 10p. DNLM
90-1664

DEAVER, John Blair (1855-1931)
The operative treatment of strictures of the male urethra. Detroit: G. S. Davis, 1890. 20p. DNLM
90-1665

DEAVER, John Blair (1855-1931)
The operative trestment of strictures of the male urethra. [With additions.] [Philadelphia, 1890.] 16p. 1 plate. DNLM
90-1666

DEAVER, John Blair (1855-1931)
The value of the Leiter incandescent-lamp urethroscope in the diagnosis and treatment of chronic urethral discharges. [Philadelphia, 1890.] 12p. DNLM **90-1667**

DEAVER, John Blair (1855-1931)
Examination of the bladder with the electric-light cystoscope. [Philadelphia, 1891.] 10p. DNLM **90-1668**

DEAVER, John Blair (1855-1931)
Lumbar versus iliac colotomy. [Philadelphia, 1891.] 7p. DNLM **90-1669**

DEAVER, John Blair (1855-1931)
The operative treatment of head injuries. [St. Louis, 1891.] 9p. DNLM **90-1670**

DEAVER, John Blair (1855-1931)
The operative treatment of some diseases and injuries of the nerves. [Philadelphia, 1891.] 21p. DNLM
90-1671

DEAVER, John Blair (1855-1931)
Thyroidectomy. [Detroit, 1891.] 10p. DNLM
90-1672

DEAVER, John Blair (1855-1931)
Inflammation in the right iliac fossa, associated with lesion of the cecum, the vermiform appendix, and adjacent tissues. Philadelphia, 1892. 18p. DNLM **90-1673**

DEAVER, John Blair (1855-1931)
Stone in the bladder. Abscess of the liver. [Philadelphia, 1892.] 6p. DNLM **90-1674**

DEAVER, John Blair (1855-1931)
Appendicitis in children. [New York, 1893.] 16p. DNLM
90-1675

DEAVER, John Blair (1855-1931)
Remarks upon the treatment of stricture of the sigmoid flexure and of the first portion of the rectum. [Philadelphia], 1893. 7p. DNLM **90-1676**

DEAVER, John Blair (1855-1931)
Treatment of appendicitis. [Philadelphia, 1893.] 10p. DNLM
90-1677

DEAVER, John Blair (1855-1931)
Treatment of appendicitis. [Philadelphia, 1893.] 8p. DNLM
90-1678

DEAVER, John Blair (1855-1931)
Acute appendicitis. With remarks, in opening discussion, by by J. M. Da Costa. Chronic appendicitis, by J. M. Da Costa. Chronic appendicitis, by John B. Deaver. Philadelphia, 1894. 50p. 1 table. DNLM **90-1679**

DEAVER, John Blair (1855-1931)
Further observations upon the etiology, diagnosis, and treatment of acute and chronic appendicitis. With the report of sixty-one chronic cases operated upon, with one death. [Philadelphia, 1894.] 24p. DNLM **90-1680**

DEAVER, John Blair (1855-1931)
Further observations upon the etiology, diagnosis, and treatment of acute and chronic appendicitis. With the report of sixty-one chronic cases operated upon, with one death. Philadelphia: Lea Bros. & Co., 1894. 15p. DNLM **90-1681**

DEAVER, John Blair (1855-1931)
Symptoms and treatment of tumors of the bladder. Chicago, 1894. 4p. DNLM **90-1682**

DEAVER, John Blair (1855-1931)
Appendicitis. Philadelphia: E. W. Eckel, 1895. 11p. DNLM **90-1683**

DEAVER, John Blair (1855-1931)
Appendicitis. [Richmond, 1895.] 8p. DNLM **90-1684**

DEAVER, John Blair (1855-1931)
The indications and nature of treatment in severe abdominal injuries and intra-abdominal hemorrhages unaccompanied by external evidence of violence. [Philadelphia], 1895. 10p. DNLM **90-1685**

DEAVER, John Blair (1855-1931)
Radical treatment of hernia, with 100 tabulated cases. Philadelphia, 1895. 15p. DNLM **90-1686**

DEAVER, John Blair (1855-1931)
Radical treatment of hernia, with 100 tabulated cases. Philadelphia, 1895. 6p. DNLM **90-1687**

DEAVER, John Blair (1855-1931)
Some salient points in the diagnosis, pathology, and treatment of appendicitis. Philadelphia, 1895. 17p. DNLM **90-1688**

DEAVER, John Blair (1855-1931)
A treatise on appendicitis. . . . containing 32 full-page plates and other illustrations. Philadelphia: P. Blakiston, Son & Co., 1896. 168p. DLC; DNLM; NNNAM; PPC **90-1689**

DEAVER, John Blair (1855-1931)
Surgical anatomy; a treatise on human anatomy in its application to the practice of medicine and surgery. . . . Philadelphia: P. Blakiston's Son & Co., 1899-1903. 3 v. plates. DLC; MBM; NNNAM; PPC **90-1690**

DE HART, John N.
The therapeutic value of oxygen and nitrous monoxide in the treatment of pneumonia, bronchitis, anemia, and chronic diseases. Baltimore, 1895. 6p. DNLM **90-1691**

DELAFIELD, Francis (1841-1915)
A handbook of pathological anatomy and histology with an introductory section on post-mortem examinations and the methods of preserving and examining diseased tissues, by Francis Delafield . . . and T. Mitchell Pruden. . . . 4th ed., illustrated by 300 wood engravings printed in black and colors. New York: William Wood & Co., 1892. 715p. col. illus. DLC; NNNAM; PPC; PPJ **90-1692**

DELAFIELD, Francis (1841-1915)
A handbook of pathological anatomy and histology, with an introductory section on post-mortem examinations and the methods of preserving and examining diseased tissues, by Francis Delafield . . . and T. Mitchell Prudden. . . . 5th ed. . . . New York: William Wood & Co., 1896. 846p. col. plate. DLC; DNLM; NNNAM; PPC **90-1693**

DELAVAN, D[avid] Bryson (1850-1942)
On the early diagnosis of malignant disease of the larynx. New York: D. Appleton & Co., 1890. 8p. DNLM **90-1694**

DELAVAN, D[avid] Bryson (1850-1942)
The withholding of reports of operations for the relief of cancer of the throat. New York: D. Appleton & Co., 1893. 9p. DNLM **90-1695**

DELAVAN, D[avid] Bryson (1850-1942)
The president's address, delivered before the American Laryngological Association, at its sixteenth annual congress. New York: D. Appleton & Co., 1894. 15p. DNLM **90-1696**

DELAVAN, D[avid] Bryson (1850-1942)
The prognosis in nasal operations performed during epidemics of la grippe and of allied conditions. New York, 1895. 4p. DNLM **90-1697**

DELAVAN, D[avid] Bryson (1850-1942)
Recent advances in the surgical treatment of malignant disease of the larynx. New York: D. Appleton & Co., 1896. 14p. DNLM **90-1698**

DELAVAN, D[avid] Bryson (1850-1942)
Tertiary ulceration simulating sarcoma of the tonsil. [New York]: D. Appleton & Co., [1897]. 5p. DNLM **90-1699**

DEMILT DISPENSARY. NEW YORK CITY
Department of Diseases of the Skin. Classification of diseases of the skin. [Prepared for the use of classes in dermatology, by L. Duncan Bulkley.] [New York, 1892?] 2 l. DNLM; NNNAM **90-1700**

DENCH, Edward Bradford (1864-1936)
Chronic purulent otitis media as a cause of persistent facial neuralgia. [New York, 1891.] 4p. DNLM **90-1701**

DENCH, Edward Bradford (1864-1936)
Removal of the membrana tympani, malleus and incus, for the relief of impaired hearing, due to chronic non-suppurative otitis media; report of a successful case. [New York, 1893.] 8p. DNLM **90-1702**

DENCH, Edward Bradford (1864-1936)
Operative measures for the relief of chronic suppurative and non-suppurative inflammation of the tympanum; the indications for the employment of such measures, and the results obtained. [New York, 1893.] 69p. DNLM **90-1703**

DENCH, Edward Bradford (1864-1936)
Diseases of the ear. A text-book. . . . New York: D. Appleton & Co., 1894. 645p. col. plates. DLC; DNLM; NNNAM; PPC **90-1704**

DENCH, Edward Bradford (1864-1936)
Affections of the sound-perceiving apparatus. [New York, 1894.] 86p. DNLM **90-1705**

DENCH, Edward Bradford (1864-1936)
Middle ear operations as a means of improving the organ of hearing. [New Bedford, 1894.] 21p. DNLM **90-1706**

DENCH, Edward Bradford (1864-1936)
What shall a general practitioner do for an acute otitis? [New York: Bailey & Fairchild, 1895.] 8p. DNLM **90-1707**

DENCH, Edward Bradford (1864-1936)
The treatment of acute inflammation of the middle ear and mastoid. [New York, 1895.] 21p. DNLM **90-1708**

DENCH, Edward Bradford (1864-1936)
Mastoid and intracranial complications of middle-ear suppuration. New York: William Wood & Co., 1896. 12p. DNLM **90-1709**

DENCH, Edward Bradford (1864-1936)
The differential diagnosis between diseases of the sound conducting and sound perceiving apparatus. New Bedford, Mass., 1897. 8p. DNLM **90-1710**

DENCH, Edward Bradford (1864-1936)
The technique of the mastoid operation. New York, 1898. 19p. DNLM **90-1711**

DENCH, Edward Bradford (1864-1936)
The surgical treatment of acute inflammations of the middle ear. Chicago, 1898. 7p. DNLM **90-1712**

DENCH, Edward Bradford (1864-1936)
The aural complications of influenza. Concord, N.H.: Rumford Press, 1898. 13p. DNLM **90-1713**

DENISON, Charles (1845-1909)
Abnormal intrathoracic air-pressures, and their treatment. New York, [1890]. 41p. DNLM **90-1714**

DENISON, Charles (1845-1909)
Tuberculin. The value and limitation of its use in consumption. Denver: Med. Times Publ. Co., 1892. 23p. DNLM **90-1715**

DENISON, Charles (1845-1909)
Tuberculin and the living cell. An inquiry as to how the one aids the other in the fight against tuberculosis. [Philadelphia, 1892.] 24p. DNLM **90-1716**

DENISON, Charles (1845-1909)
The Denison spirometer and manometer. Chicago, 1892. 2 l. DNLM **90-1717**

DENISON, Charles (1845-1909)
The mutual interest of the medical profession and insurance companies in the prolongation of life. Chicago, 1893. 4p. 2 l. DNLM **90-1718**

DENISON, Charles (1845-1909)
Exercise for pulmonary invalids. Read before the Congress of Medico-Climatology of World's Fair Congress Auxiliary, June 1, 1893, and printed in response to a resolution of the same. Denver, Col.: Chain & Hardy, 1893. 26p. DNLM **90-1719**

DENISON, Charles (1845-1909)
The air-pressure inhaler and exhaler. New York, 1894. 11p. DNLM **90-1720**

DENISON, Charles (1845-1909)
The diagnosis of tuberculosis by tuberculin injections. [New York, 1894.] 10p. 1 table. DNLM **90-1721**

DENISON, Charles (1845-1909)
Exercise and food for pulmonary invalids. . . . Denver: The Chain & Hardy Co., 1895. 71p. DLC **90-1722**

DENISON, Charles (1845-1909)
Favorable results of Koch's tuberculin treatment in tubercular affections that are not pulmonary. New York, 1895. 11p. DNLM **90-1723**

DENISON, Charles (1845-1909)
Degenerative heredity; or, some degenerative influences of modern civilization upon health. [New York: D. Appleton & Co., 1895.] 23p. DNLM **90-1724**

DENISON, Charles (1845-1909)
The microscopical proof of a curative process in tuberculosis; or, the reaction to tuberculin evidenced by blood changes hitherto unrecognized; and my latest improved binaural stethoscope. Denver, 1896. 14p. DNLM **90-1725**

DENISON, Charles (1845-1909)
New uses of the in- and exhaler. New York, 1897. 1 l. DNLM **90-1726**

DENISON, Charles (1845-1909)
The advantage of physical education as a prevention of disease. [Easton, Pa., 1898.] 10p. DNLM **90-1727**

DENISON, Charles (1845-1909)
The antitoxin treatment of tuberculosis of the direct (tuberculin preparations) versus the indirect (animal serum) method of immunization against tuberculosis. Chicago, 1898. 15p. DNLM **90-1728**

DENISON, Charles (1845-1909)
Modern treatment of tuberculosis. Chicago, 1898. 12p. DNLM **90-1729**

DENISON, Charles (1845-1909)
Chest examination chart. Designed for the purpose of studying lives impaired by chronic pulmonary diseases, with a view to the adaptation of climate to their special needs, for the use of life insurance companies and inquiring invalids. [Denver, 1899.] 1 l. 15 x 22 inches. DNLM **90-1730**

DENISON, Charles (1845-1909)
The chest diagnosis chart, and aid to climate selection. [1899.] 2 l. DNLM **90-1731**

DENISON, Charles (1845-1909)
. . . Air pressure limitations to intraboracic surgery. Also the illustrated use of new traction plasters for arresting pulmonary hemorrhages and for other purposes. . . . [New York, 1899.] 19p. DLC **90-1732**

DENISON, Charles (1845-1909)
. . . The tuberculosis crusade and its problems. . . . [Asheville], N.C., 1899.] 9p. DLC **90-1733**

DENNIS, Frederick S[hepard] (1850-1934)
The achievements of American surgery. New York, 1892. 47p. DNLM; NNNAM **90-1734**

DENNIS, Frederick S[hepard] (1850-1934)
Notes on surgery. [New York, 1893.] 74p. DNLM; NNNAM **90-1735**

DENNIS, Frederick S[hepard] (1850-1934)
Table showing nervous manifestations following traumatisms of the spine. [n. p., 1894.] 1 sheet. DNLM **90-1736**

DENNIS, Frederick S[hepard], ed. (1850-1934)
System of surgery. Edited by Frederick S. Dennis. . . . Assisted by John S. Billings. Philadelphia: Lea Bros. & Co., 1895-1896. 4 v. plates. DLC; DNLM; NNNAM; PPC **90-1737**

DENTAL register of the United States, comprising list of dentists, arranged by States, giving post-office address, with population and location, date and college of graduation, the various dental societies, dental colleges, a synopsis of the laws of registration, and other laws relating to the profession in each State. Dental journals with names of editors, frequency of publication, and subscription rates, and an index to the dentists in the United States, arranged alphabetically. 2nd ed. Detroit, Baltimore, & Chicago: R. L. Polk & Co., 1896-1897. 757p. DNLM; NNNAM; OCIM **90-1738**

DENTAL register of the United States, comprising list of dentists, arranged by States, giving post-office address, with population and location, date and college of graduation, the various dental societies, dental colleges, a synopsis of the laws of registration, and other laws relating to the profession in each State. Dental journals, with names of editors, frequency of publication, and subscription rates, and an index to the dentists in the United States, arranged alphabetically. 3rd ed. Detroit, Baltimore, & Chicago: R. L. Polk & Co., 1898-1899. 975p. DNLM; NNNAM; PPC **90-1739**

DERCUM, Clara T.
A case of hyperemesis gravidarum terminating in recovery after an induced abortion of twins. [Philadelphia, 1893.] 7p. DNLM **90-1740**

DERCUM, Francis X[avier] (1856-1931)
On the significance of optic neuritis, blindness, deafness, and the knee-jerk in cerebellar diseases. [New York, 1893.] 10p. DNLM **90-1741**

DERCUM, Francis X[avier] (1856-1931)
On the prognosis of "railway spine." [St. Louis, 1893.] 12p. DNLM **90-1742**

DERCUM, Francis X[avier] (1856-1931)
The treatment of neurasthenia, with special reference to the rest-cure. Detroit, Mich.: G. S. Davis, 1893. 21p. DNLM **90-1743**

DERCUM, Francis X[avier] (1856-1931)
A case of hemiplegia associated with atrophy of the muscles of the paralyzed side, and also with a partial motor aphasia, the patient having a good memory for substantives, but an absolute loss of all other parts of speech. [Philadelphia, 1893.] 4p. 1 plate. DNLM **90-1744**

DERCUM, Francis X[avier] (1856-1931)
A case of sporadic cretinism. [Philadelphia, 1893.] 2p. 1 plate. DNLM **90-1745**

DERCUM, Francis X[avier] (1856-1931)
A case of syringomyelia. New York, 1894. 6p. DNLM **90-1746**

DERCUM, Francis X[avier] (1856-1931) and W. W. KEEN
Two cases of ingravescent cerebral hemorrhage treated by ligation of the common carotid artery. New York, 1894. 3p. DNLM **90-1747**

DERCUM, Francis X[avier] (1856-1931)
The therapeutics of infectious processes in the nervous system. [Philadelphia, 1894.] 15p. DNLM **90-1748**

DERCUM, Francis X[avier] (1856-1931)
Address in mental disorders. Philadelphia, 1895. 11p. DNLM **90-1749**

DERCUM, Francis X[avier] (1856-1931)
A text-book on nervous diseases, by American authors. . . . Philadelphia: Lea Bros. & Co., 1895. 1056p. plates. DLC; DNLM; NNNAM; PPC **90-1750**

DESPRÉS, Armand (1834-1896)
A treatise on fractures. . . . Transl. by E. P. Hurd. . . . Detroit, Mich.: G. S. Davis, 1890. 112p. DLC **90-1751**

DESSAR, Leonard A.
Home treatment for catarrhs and colds; a handy guide for the prevention, care, and treatment of catarrhal troubles, cold in the head, sore throat, hay fever, hoarseness, ear affections, etc. Adapted for use in the household, or for vocalists, clergymen, lawyers, actors, lecturers, etc. New York: London: Bailliere, Tindall & Cox, 1894. 118p. DLC; DNLM; NNNAM [Also: New York: Home Series Publishing Co., 1894. 118p.] **90-1752**

DESSAU, S. Henry
The treatment of croupous pneumonia in children. [Philadelphia, 1891.] 9p. DNLM **90-1753**

DESSAU, S. Henry
Observations on rational therapeutics. New York: Trow's Co., 1891. 12p. DNLM **90-1754**

DETROIT DENTAL MFG. CO.
Illustrated catalogues, Nos. 6, 7, 8. Dental supplies. Detroit, 1893. 15, 16, 16p. NNNAM **90-1755**

DEW, J[ames] Harvie (*b.* 1843)
Establishing a new method of artificial respiration in asphyxia neonatorum. Corroborated by Geo. T. Harrison, Von Beverhout Thompson, [*et al.*]. New York: Stettiner, Lambert & Co., 1893. 16p. DNLM **90-1756**

DEWEES, William Bushy (1854-1912)
Malarial affections. [Philadelphia, 1890.] 11p. 2 diags. DNLM **90-1757**

DEWEY, Richard (1845-1933)
Old and new ideas with regard to the work and organization of institutions for the insane. Chicago: R. R. McCabe & Co., 1892. 11p. DNLM **90-1758**

DEWEY, Richard (1845-1933)
Presidential address. Our association and our associates. Some relations affecting medical officers of hospitals for the insane. Utica, 1896. 22p. DNLM **90-1759**

DEWEY, Willis Alonzo (1858-1938)
Essentials of homoeopathic materia medica: being a quiz compend. . . . Philadelphia: Boericke & Tafel, 1894. 269p. DLC; PPHa **90-1760**

DEWEY, Willis Alonzo (1858-1938)
Essentials of homoeopathic materia medica: being a quiz compend. . . . 2nd ed. Philadelphia: Boericke & Tafel, 1894. 269p. PPHa **90-1761**

DEWEY, Willis Alonzo (1858-1938)
Essentials of homoeopathic therapeutics; being a quiz compend upon the application of homoeopathic remedies to diseased states. . . . Philadelphia: Boericke & Tafel, 1895. 266p. DLC; DNLM; PPHa **90-1762**

DEWEY, Willis Alonzo (1858-1938)
Essentials of homoeopathic therapeutics; being a quiz compend of the application of homoeopathic remedies to diseased states. A companion to the Essentials of homoeopathic materia medica. Arranged and comp. especially for the use of students of medicine. . . . 2nd ed., rev. and enl. Philadelphia: Boericke & Tafel, 1898. 285p. DLC; OCLloyd; PPHa **90-1763**

DEWEY, Willis Alonzo (1858-1938)
Essential of homoeopathic materia medica: being a quiz compend. . . . 3rd ed. Philadelphia: Boericke & Tafel, 1899. 376p. DNLM **90-1764**

DEXTER, B. F.
Suggestions concerning the care of the insane. New York, [1890?]. 2 l. DNLM **90-1765**

DEXTER, Franklin (*b.* 1857)
The anatomy of the peritonaeum. New York: D. Appleton & Co., 1892. 86p. 35 plates. DLC; DNLM; NNNAM **90-1766**

DEYNARD, A. Britton
Rest in bed as a resource in the treatment of chronic non-suppurative catarrh of the middle ear. [New York, 1892.] 2 l. DNLM **90-1767**

DEYNARD, A. Britton
The value of Javal's ophthalmometer for the correction of astigmatism where marked amblyopia is present. New York, 1892. 4p. DNLM **90-1768**

DEYNARD, A. Britton
Cystic goitre; with cases in practice. [Philadelphia, 1893.] 4p. DNLM **90-1769**

DEYNARD, A. Britton
Granular lids; with cases in practice. [New York, 1895.] 2 l. DNLM **90-1770**

DICKINSON, Robert L[atou] (1861-1950)
The sheet-sling in forceps deliveries. New York, 1890. 1 l. DNLM **90-1771**

DICKINSON, Robert L[atou] (1861-1950)
The direction of the incision in episiotomy. [Philadelphia, 1892.] 4p. 4 plates. DNLM **90-1772**

DICKINSON, Robert L[atou] (1861-1950)
Details of a practical course of manikin instruction in obstetrics. [New York, 1892.] 14p. DNLM **90-1773**

DICKINSON, Robert L[atou] (1861-1950)
Does laceration through the sphincter ani ever occur in the median line? Seventeen cases of lateral injury. New York, 1895. 26p. DNLM **90-1774**

DILLER, Theodore (*b.* 1863)
Circular insanity; a contribution to the study of the affection; report of a case. [St. Louis, 1890.] 9p. DNLM **90-1775**

DILLER, Theodore (*b.* 1863)
Hypnotism in a religious meeting. [Philadelphia, 1890.] 11p. DNLM **90-1776**

DILLER, Theodore (*b.* 1863)
A case of paranoia, illustrating the feature of imperative conceptions. [St. Louis, 1890.] 7p. DNLM **90-1777**

DILLER, Theodore (*b.* 1863)
Fallacies in conclusions as to the efficacy of therapeutic measures for the relief of epilepsy. [Philadelphia, 1890.] 5p. DNLM **90-1778**

DILLER, Theodore (*b.* 1863)
Chorea in the adult as seen among the insane. [Philadelphia, 1890.] 21p. DNLM **90-1779**

DILLER, Theodore (*b.* 1863)
A plea for special state provision for epileptics. [Philadelphia, 1892.] 8p. DNLM **90-1780**

DILLER, Theodore (*b.* 1863)
The non-operative treatment of brain tumors. Philadelphia, 1894. 7p. DNLM **90-1781**

DILLER, Theodore (*b.* 1863)
A case of male hysteria characterized by recurrent attacks of motor aphasia and lethargy; apparent cure by hypnotism and suggestion. Philadelphia, 1894. 5p. DNLM **90-1782**

DILLER, Theodore (*b.* 1863)
Brain-syphilis; a report of seven cases. Philadelphia, 1895. 25p. DNLM **90-1783**

DIRECTORY of homoeopathic physicians in New York and vicinity, 1898; edited by G. A. Shepard. New York: J. A. Robinson, [1898]. [unp.] DLC; NNNAM **90-1784**

DIX, Archibald L.
A case of lupus successfully treated by an iodine compound. Philadelphia, 1897. 6p. 2 plates. DNLM **90-1785**

DIXON, Archibald
Recent advances in surgery. Report of the committee to the Kentucky State Medical Society. Danbury, 1890. 40p. DNLM **90-1786**

DIXON, Archibald
Gastrostomy for impermeable stricture of the cardiac end of the oesophagus; recovery; subseqeunt dilatation and retrograde dilatation of stricture. Danbury, Conn., 1891. 14p. DNLM
90-1787

DIXON, Samuel Gibson (1851-1918)
Establishing tolerance for tubercle bacillus. Philadelphia, 1890. 3p. DNLM **90-1788**

DIXON, Samuel Gibson (1851-1918)
Care in the use of tubercle bacillus as a remedy in tuberculosis. Philadelphia, 1891. 4p. DNLM **90-1789**

DIXON, Samuel Gibson (1851-1918)
Koch's method of treating tuberculosis. A lecture. Philadelphia, 1891. 10p. DNLM **90-1790**

DIXON, Samuel Gibson (1851-1918)
Annual address before the State Board of Health of Pennsylvania. Read May 15, 1891, at the Sanitary Convention at Altoona. [n. p., 1891.] 14p. DNLM
90-1791

DIXON, Samuel Gibson (1851-1918)
Apparatus for collecting water for bacteriological examination. Philadelphia: Am. Medical Press Co., 1891. 3p. DNLM
90-1792

DIXON, Samuel Gibson (1851-1918)
The bile salts, urea, etc., as therapeutic agents. [Philadelphia, 1893.] 4p. DNLM **90-1793**

DIXON, Samuel Gibson (1851-1918)
Involution form of the tubercle bacillus and the effect of subcutaneous injections of organic substances on inflammations. Philadelphia, 1893. 4p. DNLM **90-1794**

DIXON, Samuel Gibson (1851-1918)
Annual address before the State Board of Health of Pennsylvania. Harrisburg, Pa.: E. K. Meyers, 1893. 15p. DNLM
90-1795

DIXON, Samuel Gibson (1851-1918)
Address on hygiene; delivered at the meeting of the State Medical Society, Williamsport, Pa. [Philadelphia, 1893.] 16p. DNLM **90-1796**

DIXON, Samuel Gibson (1851-1918)
Possible relationship between the tubercular diathesis and nitrogenous metabolism. Detroit, Mich.: G. S. Davis, 1894. 10p. DNLM **90-1797**

DIXON, W. A. (*d.* 1899)
The morbid proclivities and retrogressive tendencies in the offspring of mulattoes. Philadelphia, 1892. 7p. DNLM
90-1798

DOCK, George (*b.* 1860)
Further studies in malarial disease. The parasites and the forms of disease as found in Texas. Philadelphia, 1891. 35p. DNLM
90-1799

DOCK, George (*b.* 1860)
Notes on the appendix vermiformis; anatomical and clinical. [Detroit, 1892.] 11p. DNLM **90-1800**

DOCK, George (*b.* 1860)
Chloroma and its relation to leukaemia. [Philadelphia, 1893.] 34p. 1 plate. DNLM **90-1801**

DOCK, George (*b.* 1860)
Gonorrhea of the rectum. [Philadelphia, 1893.] 5p. DNLM
90-1802

DOCK, George (*b.* 1860)
Flagellate protozoa in the freshly passed urine of a man. Philadelphia, 1894. 3p. DNLM **90-1803**

DOCK, George (*b.* 1860)
Goiter in Michigan. Philadelphia, 1895. 10p. DNLM
90-1804

DOCK, George (*b.* 1860)
Primary carcinoma of the gall-bladder. Philadelphia, 1895. 6p. DNLM **90-1805**

DOCK, George (*b.* 1860)
Staphylococcus-aureus infection with endocarditis simulating malarial intermittent fever (double quotidian). New York: D. Appleton & Co., 1897. 14p. 1 chart. DNLM
90-1806

DOCK, Lavinia L. (1858-1956)
Text-book of materia medica for nurses. . . . New York, [etc.] : G. P. Putnam's Sons, 1890. 201p. DLC; NNNAM; PPC; PU
90-1807

DOCK. Lavinia L. (1858-1956)
Text-book of materia medica for nurses. . . . 2nd ed., rev. and enl. New York: G. P. Putnam's Sons, 1897. 205p. NNNAM; OCIM; PPC **90-1808**

DOCK, Lavinia L. (1858-1956)
Text-book of materia medica for nurses. . . . 3rd ed., rev. and enl. 11th thousand. New York, London: G. P. Putnam's Sons, 1897. 240p. DLC; NNNAM; OCIM; PPC
90-1809

DODGE, William T.
Six cases of appendicitis. Philadelphia, 1894. 9p. DNLM
90-1810

DODGE, W[illiam] T.
The treatment of suppuration of the knee-joint, with illustrative cases. Philadelphia, 1897. 9p. DNLM; NN
90-1811

DOMVILLE, Edward J[ames] (1849-1925)
A manual for hospital nurses and others engaged in attending on the sick. 7th ed. Philadelphia: P. Blakiston, Son & Co., 1891. 104p. DNLM; NNNAM; PPC; PPJ
90-1812

DONDERS, F. C. (1818-1889)
An essay on the nature and the consequences of anomalies of refraction. Revised and edited by Charles A. Oliver. Philadelphia: P. Blakiston, Son & Co., 1899. 81p. CtY-M; NNNAM; PPC **90-1813**

DONNALLY, Williams
An opportunity for a great national dental museum and library. [Philadelphia, 1896.] 12p. DNLM
90-1814

DONNELLAN, P[atrick] S.
A case of electric shock of one thousand volts; insensibility of patient to pain; recovery. Philadelphia, 1894. 3p. DNLM
90-1815

DONNELLAN, P[atrick] S.
Exopthalmos (Graves' disease) without thyroid enlargement. Philadelphia, 1895. 4p. DNLM **90-1816**

DORLAND, W[illiam] A[lexander] N[ewman] (1864-1956)
The differential diagnosis of nasal ulcerations. Philadelphia, 1891. 3p. DNLM **90-1817**

DORLAND, W[illiam] A[lexander] N[ewman] (1864-1956) and F. Perceval GERSON
The treatment of chorea by large doses of quinine. Philadelphia, 1893. 9p. DNLM **90-1818**

DORLAND, W[illiam] A[lexander] N[ewman] (1864-1956)
Congenital absence of the uterus. Philadelphia, 1895. 2p. DNLM **90-1819**

DORLAND, W[illiam] A[lexander] N[ewman] (1864-1956)
Tetanus neonatorum. Philadelphia, 1895. 2p. DNLM
90-1820

DORLAND, W[illiam] A[lexander] N[ewman] (1864-1956)
A new classification of the possible terminations of extra-uterine gestation. New York, 1895. 11p. DNLM
90-1821

DORLAND, W[illiam] A[lexander] N[ewman] (1864-1956)
A manual of obstetrics.... Philadelphia: W. B. Saunders, 1896. 760p. plates. DLC; DNLM; NNNAM; PPC **90-1822**

DORLAND, W[illiam] A[lexander] N[ewman] (1864-1956)
A case of Ritter's disease. Philadelphia, 1896. 2p. DNLM
90-1823

DORLAND, W[illiam] A[lexander] N[ewman] (1864-1956)
Cystic disease of the chorion; with a tabulation of one hundred cases. Philadelphia, 1896. 27p. DNLM
90-1824

DORLAND, W[illiam] A[lexander] N[ewman] (1864-1956)
The incipient uterine carcinoma. Philadelphia, 1896. 4p. DNLM **90-1825**

DORLAND, W[illiam] A[lexander] N[ewman] (1864-1956)
A classification of puerperal sepsis. Philadelphia, 1896. 3p. DNLM **90-1826**

DORLAND, W[illiam] A[lexander] N[ewman] (1864-1956)
Gestational complications and dystocia subsequent to anterior fixation of the uterus. Philadelphia, 1896. 28p. DNLM
90-1827

DORLAND, W[illiam] A[lexander] N[ewman] (1864-1956)
A diprosopic monstrosity; a rare case of teratism. Philadelphia, 1896. 2p. 1 plate. DNLM **90-1828**

DORLAND, W[illiam] A[lexander] N[ewman] (1864-1956)
The statistics of malignant deciduoma. Philadelphia, 1897. 19p. DNLM **90-1829**

DORLAND, W[illiam] A[lexander] N[ewman], ed. (1864-1956)
Persistence of the umbilical cord. Philadelphia, 1897. 2p. DNLM **90-1830**

DORLAND, W[illiam] A[lexander] N[ewman], ed. (1864-1956)
American pocket medical dictionary. . . . Containing the pronunciation and definition of over 26,000 of the terms used in medicine and the kindred sciences, along with over 60 extensive tables. Philadelphia: W. B. Saunders, 1898. 518p. DLC; NNNAM; PPC; PU **90-1831**

DOTY, Alvah Hunt (*b.* 1854)
A manual of instruction in the principles of prompt aid to the injured; including a chapter on hygiene and the drill regulations for the hospital corps, U.S.A., designed for military and civil use. . . . 2nd ed., rev. and enl. New York, [etc.]: D. Appleton & Co., 1894. 304p. col. frontis. DLC; NNNAM
90-1832

DOTY, Alvah Hunt (*b.* 1854)
A manual of instruction in the principles of prompt aid to the injured; including a chapter on hygiene and the drill regulations for the hosptial corps, U.S.A., designed for military and civil use. . . . 3rd ed., rev. and enl. New York, London: D. Appleton & Co., 1898. 302p. col. frontis. and plate. DLC; NNNAM
90-1833

DOUBLEDAY, Edwin T., and J. Darwin NAGEL
Practice of medicine. A manual for students and practitioners. Series edited by Bern. B. Gallaudet. Philadelphia: Lea Bros. & Co., [1892]. 221p. DNLM; NNNAM; PPC; PU
90-1834

DOUGHTY, Francis E. (*b.* 1847)
A practical working handbook in the diagnosis and treatment of diseases of the genito-urinary system, and syphilis; being the rev. and enl. notes, with additions, by George Parker Holden, M.D., of clinical lectures delivered in Flower Hospital amphitheater, by F. E. Doughty. . . . Philadelphia: Boericke & Tafel, 1897. 461p. fold. frontis. DLC; NNNAM; PPHa
90-1835

DOUGLAS, James
History of a case of hydrophobia. New York, 1898. 10p. DNLM; NNNAM **90-1836**

DOUGLAS, Orlando B[enajah] (*b.* 1836)
Inaugural address of the president of the Medical Society of the County of New York, Nov. 24, 1890. New York: Stettiner, Lambert & Co., 1890. 10p. DNLM
90-1837

DOUGLAS, Orlando B[enajah] (*b.* 1836)
Is the cure of chronic nasal catarrh as difficult as has been supposed? [New York, 1890.] 11p. DNLM
90-1838

DOUGLAS, Orlando B[enajah] (*b.* 1836)
The upper air passages and their diseases. [New York, 1891.] 12p. DNLM **90-1839**

DOUGLAS, Orlando B[enajah] (*b.* 1836)
Modern methods of treating diseases of the nose and throat. New York, 1895. 10p. DNLM **90-1840**

DOUGLAS, Richard (1860-1908)
Acute peritonitis. New York, 1895. 11p. DNLM
90-1841

DOUGLASS, D[arwin] De Forrest
The Douglass patent artificial limbs. Springfield, Mass., 1896. 100p. DNLM; MBM; MWA **90-1842**

DOWD, Charles N[orth] (*b.* 1858)
The condition of the blood in chlorosis; notes on the course and secondary symptoms of chlorosis. [Philadelphia, 1890.] 19p. DNLM **90-1843**

DOWD, Charles N[orth] (*b.* 1858)
Some considerations on different types of exudative inflammation; a study based on bacterial examinations from one hundred and thirty-five surgical cases. New York: Trow, 1894. 15p. DNLM **90-1844**

DOWLING, Francis
Myopia in the schools of Cincinnati. [Chicago, 1891.] 4p. DNLM **90-1845**

DOWLING, Francis
The prevention of myopia. Chicago, 1891. 16p. DNLM **90-1846**

DOWN, John L[angdon] H[aydon] (1828-1896)
Mental affections of childhood and youth, and other papers. New York: William Wood & Co., 1891. 154p. DLC; IEN-M; LNT-M; NNNAM [Printed out of Wood's Medical & Surgical Monographs, vol. 10, No. 2 (1891), pp. 307-459] **90-1846A**

DRAKE, Olin M[ilton] (*b.* 1847)
Repertory of foot-sweat. [Philadelphia], 1894. 5p. DNLM **90-1847**

DRAPER, Andrew S[loan] (1848-1913)
The responsibilities of the medical profession. An address to the graduating class at the commencement of the Albany Medical College, March 16, 1887. Albany, N.Y.: W. Parsons & Co., 1892. 18p. DNLM **90-1848**

DRAPER, F[rank] W[inthrop] (1843-1909)
The medical profession and the commonwealth. Boston: D. Clapp & Son, 1892. 76p. DNLM; MBM; NNNAM **90-1849**

DRAPER, John C[hristopher] (1835-1885)
A text-book on anatomy, physiology, and hygiene. . . . 6th ed., rev. New York: Harper & Bros., [1894]. 260p. DLC: ICU; MH; NN **90-1850**

DRUITT, Robert (1814-1883)
The principles and practice of modern surgery. A new American, from the 12th London edition, ed. by Stanley Boyd. Philadelphia: Lea Bros. & Co., 1890 [1887]. 985p. DNLM; ICJ; PPC; PU **90-1851**

DUANE, Alexander (1858-1926)
The modern treatment of strabismus. [Richmond, 1890.] 10p. DNLM **90-1852**

DUANE, Alexander (1858-1926)
The students' dictionary of medicine and the allied sciences, comprising the pronunciation, derivation, and full explanation of medical terms, together with much collateral descriptive matter, numerous tables. . . . Philadelphia: Lea Bros. & Co., 1893. 650p. DNLM; MBM; NNNAM; PPC **90-1853**

DUANE, Alexander (1858-1926)
The treatment of heterophoria; an answer to Dr. Gould. St. Louis, 1894. 7p. DNLM **90-1854**

DUANE, Alexander (1858-1926)
The students' dictionary of medicine and the allied sciences, comprising the pronunciation, derivation, and full explanation of medical terms, together with much collateral descriptive matter, numerous tables. . . . With appendix. New York & Philadelphia: Lea Bros. & Co., 1896. 679p. DNLM; IU-M; NNNAM; PU **90-1855**

DUANE, Alexander (1858-1926)
A new classification of the motor anomalies of the eye based upon physiological principles, together with their symptoms, diagnosis, and treatment; the prize essay of the Alumni Association of the College of Physicians and Surgeons, New York, for 1896. New York: J. H. Vail & Co., 1897. 100p. 1 diag. DNLM; NNC **90-1856**

DUANE, Alexander (1858-1926)
When and why shall we operate in insufficiencies of the ocular muscles? New York, 1898, 37p. DNLM; NNNAM **90-1857**

DUDLEY, A[ugustus] Palmer (1853-1905)
The Caesarean operation, with the report of a case. New York: William Wood & Co., 1890. 10p. DNLM **90-1858**

DUDLEY, A[ugustus] Palmer (1853-1905)
Umbilical hernia in the female, with a report of five cases. [Philadelphia: Dornan, 1892.] 20p. DNLM **90-1859**

DUDLEY, E[millius] Clark (1850-1928)
A new operation for procidentia uteri. [New York, 1894.] 11p. DNLM **90-1860**

DUDLEY, E[millius] Clark (1850-1928)
Diseases of women; a treatise on the principles and practice of gynecology. Philadelphia & New York: Lea Bros. & Co., 1898. 637p. 2 col. plates. DLC; DNLM; NNNAM; PPC **90-1861**

DUDLEY, E[millius] Clark (1850-1928)
Diseases of women: a treatise on the principle and practice of gynecology. For students and practitioners. . . . 2nd ed., rev. and enl. With 453 illustrations of which 47 are in colors and 8 full-page plates in colors and monochrome. Philadelphia and New York: Lea Bros. & Co., [1899], 717p. DLC; NNNAM; PPC; PU **90-1862**

DUEL, Arthur B[aldwin] (1870-1936)
A preliminary note on a new method of dilating strictures of the Eustachian tube by means of the galvanic current. New York, 1897. 4p. DNLM **90-1863**

DUFF, John Milton (1846-1904)
The routine practice of administering ergot after the third stage of labor. Detroit: G. S. Davis, 1892. 5p. DNLM **90-1864**

DUFFIELD, George
Syphilis by conception. Philadelphia, 1894. 12p. DNLM **90-1865**

DUFFIELD, George
Prophylaxis of diphtheria. Detroit, 1895. 19p. DNLM **90-1866**

DUFFIELD, George
The treatment of typhoid fever. Detroit, 1896. 12p. DNLM
90-1867

DUFOUR, Clarence R.
The relation of general disease to the formation of cataract. Chicago, 1896. 12p. DNLM **90-1868**

DUFOUR, Clarence R.
Tumor of the brain involving the ocular nerves. Chicago: American Medical Assoc. Press, 1896. 3p. DNLM
90-1869

DUHRING, Louis Adolphus (1845-1913)
On the relation of impetigo herpetiformis (Hebra and Kaposi) to dermatitis herpetiformis (Duhring). [Philadelphia, 1890.] 7p. DNLM **90-1870**

DUHRING, Louis Adolphus (1845-1913)
A case of typical dermatitis herpetiformis. [Philadelphia, 1890.] 3p. DNLM **90-1871**

DUHRING, Louis Adolphus (1845-1913)
A case of lepra maculosa et tuberosa. [Philadelphia, 1890.] 6p. DNLM **90-1872**

DUHRING, Louis Adolphus (1845-1913)
A case of universal erythema multiforme. [New York, 1891.] 2 l. DNLM **90-1873**

DUHRING, Louis Adolphus (1845-1913)
Case of dermatitis vesiculosa neurotraumatica of forearm. Read before the College of Physicians, Philadelphia, Dec. 2, 1891. [Philadelphia, 1892.] 5p. DNLM **90-1874**

DUHRING, Louis Adolphus (1845-1913)
Experience in the treatment of chronic ringworm in an institution. [Philadelphia, 1892.] 8p. DNLM
90-1875

DUHRING, Louis Adolphus (1845-1913)
Notes of a visit to the leper hospital at San Remo, Italy. [Philadelphia, 1892.] 4p. DNLM **90-1876**

DUHRING, Louis Adolphus (1845-1913)
Morphoea with maculae atrophicae. [Philadelphia, 1892.] 3p. DNLM **90-1877**

DUHRING, Louis Adolphus (1845-1913)
Valedictory address to the graduating class in medicine, dentistry, and veterinary medicine of the University of Pennsylvania. Delivered June 7, 1894. Philadelphia: J. B. Lippincott Co., 1894. 12p. DNLM **90-1878**

DUHRING, Louis Adolphus (1845-1913)
The scope of dermatology. Chicago: Office American Medical Association, 1894. 11p. DNLM **90-1879**

DUHRING, Louis Adolphus (1845-1913)
Compound tincture of coal-tar. [Philadelphia: Lea Bros. & Co., 1894.] 7p. DNLM **90-1880**

DUHRING, Louis Adolphus (1845-1913) and Milton B. HARTZELL
A case of papulo-ulcerative, follicular, hypho-mycetic disease of the skin; an undescribed disease. [Philadelphia, 1895.] 4p. DNLM **90-1881**

DUHRING, Louis Adolphus (1845-1913)
Cutaneous medicine; a systematic treatise on the diseases of the skin. . . . Philadelphia: J. B. Lippincott Co., 1895-1898. 2 v. plates. CtY-M; DLC; DNLM; NNNAM
90-1882

DÜHRSSEN, [Jacob] Alfred (1862-1933)
A manual of gynaecological practice for students and practitioners. Transl. and edited from the 4th German ed. by John W. Taylor and Frederick Edge. Philadelphia: P. Blakiston, Son & Co., 1895. 241p. DNLM; NNNAM; PPC; PPJ
90-1883

DUJARDIN-BEAUMETZ, Georges Octave (1833-1895)
New medications. . . . Transl. by E. P. Hurd. . . . 2nd ed. Rev. and cor., with additions and illustrations. Detroit, Mich.: G. S. Davis, 1890. 2 v. DLC; NNNAM; OCIM
90-1884

DUKE, E. T.
Urinary analysis as a means of diagnosis. Baltimore, 1895. 8p. DNLM **90-1885**

DUKE, Henry Hunt
A substitute for iodoform. Louisville, 1897. 2 l. DNLM
90-1886

DUKEMAN, William H.
A neglected case of chronic pleurisy. San Francisco: W. A. Woodward & Co., 1892. 4p. DNLM
90-1887

DUKEMAN, William H.
The cure of stricture simplified. [Sacramento, 1892.] 3p. DNLM **90-1888**

DUKEMAN, William H.
Creosote carbonate in the treatment of pulmonary tuberculosis. Philadelphia, 1895. 15p. DNLM
90-1889

DULLES, Charles Winslow (1850-1921)
Curability of consumption. [Philadelphia, 1891.] 7p. DNLM
90-1890

DULLES, Charles Winslow (1850-1921)
Report of a case of akromegaly; with brief comments on this disorder. [Philadelphia, 1892.] 7p. DNLM
90-1891

DULLES, Charles Winslow (1850-1921)
Accidents and emergencies. A manual of the treatment of surgical and medical emergencies in the absence of a physician. . . . 4th ed., thoroughly rev. and enl., with new illustrations. Philadelphia: P. Blakiston, Son & Co., 1892. 154p. col. frontis. DLC; DNLM; NNNAM; PPC **90-1892**

DULLES, Charles Winslow (1850-1921)
A splint for fractures and luxations at the elbow-joint. Philadelphia, 1893. 4p. DNLM **90-1893**

DULLES, Charles Winslow (1850-1921)
Report on hydrophobia. Philadelphia, 1894. 9p. DNLM
90-1894

DULLES, Charles Winslow (1850-1921)
Treatment of typhoid fever. Philadelphia: Lea Bros. & Co., 1894. 12p. DNLM **90-1895**

DULLES, Charles Winslow (1850-1921)
Accidents and emergencies; a manual of the treatment of surgical and medical emergencies in the absence of a physician. . . . 5th ed., thoroughly rev. and enl., with new illustrations. Philadelphia: P. Blakiston, Son & Co., 1897. 166p. col. frontis. CtY-M; DLC; DNLM; MBM **90-1896**

DUNDAS, Thomas A.
A case of successful Sänger Caesarean operation. New York, 1894. 4p. DNLM **90-1897**

DUNDORE, Claude A.
Three cases of laminectomy. Philadelphia, 1894. 4p. DNLM **90-1898**

DUNDORE, Claude A.
The use of nosophen and antinosine in surgery. Philadelphia, 1897. 4 l. DNLM **90-1899**

DUNDORE, Claude A.
Nosophen and antinosine in the treatment of genito-urinary and venereal diseases, with report of cases. [New York, 1898.] 15p. DNLM **90-1900**

DUNGLISON, Richard James (1834-1901)
A new school physiology and hygiene, with special reference to the action of alcohol and narcotics. . . . Chicago, New York: The Werner Co., [1894]. 336p. DLC; NNNAM **90-1901**

DUNGLISON, Richard James (1834-1901)
An elementary physiology, with special reference to hygiene, alcohol and narcotics. . . . Chicago, New York: The Werner Co., [1894]. 208p. DLC; IU-M; NNNAM **90-1902**

DUNGLISON, Robley (1798-1869)
A dictionary of medical science; containing a full explanation of the various subjects and terms of anatomy, physiology, medical chemistry, pharmacy, pharmacology, therapeutics, medicine, hygiene, dietetics, pathology, bacteriology, surgery, ophthalmology, otology, laryngology, dermatology, gynecology, obstetrics, pediatrics, medical jurisprudence, dentistry, etc. 21st ed., thoroughly revised and greatly enlarged, with the pronunciation, accentuation, and derivation of the terms, by Richard J. Dunglison. Philadelphia: Lea Bros. & Co., 1893. 1181p. DLC; DNLM; NNNAM; PPC **90-1903**

DUNGLISON, Robley (1798-1869)
A dictionary of medical science. . . . 21st ed., with appendix, thoroughly rev. and greatly enl., with the pronunciation, accentuation, and derivation of the terms, by Richard J. Dunglison. . . . Philadelphia: Lea Bros. & Co., 1895. 1206p. DLC; IU-M; NNNAM; PU **90-1904**

DUNHAM, Edward K[ellogg] (1860-1922)
Histology; normal and morbid. New York & Philadelphia: Lea Bros. & Co., 1898. 448p. DNLM; NNNAM; PPC; PU **90-1905**

DUNHAM, Theodore
Surgical notes from the babies' wards, Post-Graduate Hospital, New York City. Report 1. [New York, 1894.] 8p. 2 plates. DNLM **90-1906**

[DUNHAM, William Russell] (*b.* 1833)
. . . Medical reform. Why do people drink alcoholic liquors? Medical doctrines responsible! By an American citizen. . . . Boston: [Press of H. G. Collins], 1890. 64p. DLC; MB **90-1907**

DUNHAM, W[illiam] R[ussell] (*b.* 1833)
Higher medical culture. Medical science based on the four vital properties and laws of organic force. . . . Cambridge, [Mass.]: Printed for the Author, 1892. 215p. DLC; MBM **90-1908**

DUNHAM, W[illiam] R[ussell] (*b.* 1833)
How does the cause of disease produce disease? A new interpretation of operative principles. Chicago, 1898. 16p. DNLM **90-1909**

DUNLAP, H[arley] M.
Treatment of disease of the respiratory organs by direct application to the parts affected. [Detroit], 1892. 12p. DNLM **90-1910**

DUNMIRE, G[eorge] B[enson] (*b.* 1837)
The deadly spur (Secale cornutum) in labor. [Philadelphia, 1890.] 7p. DNLM **90-1911**

DUNMIRE, G[eorge] B[enson] (*b.* 1837)
Some observations on treating cases of diphtheria. Chicago, 1893. 12p. DNLM **90-1912**

DUNN, B[erkley] Sherwood
Vaginal hysterectomy by the clamp method. New York, 1896. 11p. DNLM **90-1913**

DUNN, B[erkley] Sherwood
Some conservative operations upon the ovary. Los Angeles, 1896. 4p. DNLM **90-1914**

DUNN, B[erkley] Sherwood
Asepsis and antisepsis. Boston, 1898. 14p. DNLM **90-1915**

DUNN, John
Congenital chorea; two cases. [Richmond, 1893.] 11p. DNLM **90-1916**

DUNN, Thomas D[ewitt] (1854-1898)
Ligation of the common carotid artery in a child of three and one-half years, for hemorrhage following peritonsillar abscess; recovery. Philadelphia, 1891. 4p. DNLM **90-1917**

DUNN, Thomas D[ewitt] (1854-1898)
Peliosis rheumatica in a bleeder. [Philadelphia, 1893.] 2p. DNLM **90-1918**

DUNN, Thomas D[ewitt] (1854-1898)
A case of leukaemia, with rare lymphoid growths of orbits and parotid glands. [Philadelphia, 1894.] 7p. DNLM **90-1919**

DUNN, Thomas D[ewitt] (1854-1898)
Auto-infection. New York, 1895. 7p. DNLM **90-1920**

DUNNELL, W. B.
[Plan of the Third Hospital for Insane, Fergus Falls, Minnesota.] [Minneapolis, 1891?] Broadside, 10 by 13 inches. DNLM **90-1921**

DUNNING, L[ehman] H.
Chronic peritonitis. New York: D. Appleton & Co., 1891. 15p. DNLM **90-1922**

DUNNING, L[ehman] H.
Ruptured interstitial pregnancy. New York, 1895. 5p. DNLM **90-1923**

DUTTON, George (*b.* 1830)
Medical notes prepared expressly for his students. [1890?] 81p. DNLM; NNNAM **90-1924**

DUTTON, George (*b.* 1830)
The Vermont Medical College and its fight for life. Statement of facts by its founder. Montpelier: Argus & Patriot, pr., 1890. 24p. MB **90-1925**

DUTTON, George (*b.* 1830)
Ontology, or the science of being. A monograph, being an exposition of the mental cure; with a short chapter on hygiene. [Boston, 1890?] 20p. DNLM **90-1926**

DUTTON, George (*b.* 1830)
Consumption and rheumatism. A scientific statement in plain language of their origin, treatment, and cure. Boston: Cynosure Publishing Co., 1891. 59p. port. DLC; DNLM; MB **90-1927**

DUTTON, George (*b.* 1830)
Anatomy, scientific and popular. 2nd ed., with an appendix containing a complete alphabetical list of muscles, briefly and plainly described. Boston: Cynosure Publishing Co., 1892. 443, 25p. 4 plates. DLC; DNLM; MBM **90-1928**

DUTTON, George (*b.* 1830)
Medical notes, prepared expressly for his students. . . . [2nd enl. ed.] [Fall River, Mass., 1892.] 81p. DLC **90-1929**

DUTTON, George (*b.* 1830)
Key to the science of medicine; or, Medical terms alphabetically arranged with brief and plain definitions. . . . Boston: The Cynosure Publishing Co., 1894. 122p. DLC: MBM **90-1930**

DUTTON, George (*b.* 1830)
Etiopathy; or, Way of life, being an exposition of ontology, physiology, and therapeutics. A religious science and a scientific religion. . . . Boston: Cynosure Publishing Co., 1899. 517, 121p. frontis. plate. DLC; MBM **90-1931**

DWIGHT, Henry E[dwin]
Higher preliminary medical education. The influence of the German universities upon our profession. An address delivered before the American Academy of Medicine, December 4, 1890. [New York, 1890.] 12p. DNLM **90-1932**

DWIGHT, Henry E[dwin]
Higher preliminary medical education. The influence of the German universities upon our profession. An address delivered before the American Academy of Medicine, December 4, 1890. Philadelphia: G. F. Lasher, 1891. 16p. DNLM **90-1933**

DWIGHT, Thomas, Jr. (1843-1911)
The closure of the cranial sutures as a sign of age. Boston: Damrell & Upham, 1890. 12p. DNLM **90-1934**

DWIGHT, Thomas Jr. (1843-1911)
The scope and the teaching of human anatomy. Boston: Damrell & Upham, 1890. 13p. DNLM **90-1935**

DWIGHT, Thomas Jr. (1843-1911)
Fossa Praenasalis. [Philadelphia: Lea Bros. & Co., 1892.] 8p. DNLM **90-1936**

DWIGHT, Thomas Jr. (1843-1911)
Fusion of hands. Boston, 1892. 14p. 1 plate. DNLM **90-1937**

DWIGHT, Thomas, Jr. (1843-1911)
The Shattuck lecture. The range and significance of variation in the human skeleton. Boston: D. Clapp & Son, 1894. 29p. DNLM; MBM **90-1938**

DWIGHT, Thomas, Jr. (1843-1911)
Methods of estimating the height from parts of the skeleton. New York: Trow, 1894. 16p. DNLM **90-1939**

DWIGHT, Thomas, Jr. (1843-1911)
A case of anus vulvalis, with remarks on congenital communication of the vulva and rectum. Philadelphia, 1895. 4p. DNLM **90-1940**

DYAR, Harrison G[ray] (1866-1929)
A machine for tubing bacterial media. New York: D. Appleton & Co., 1895. 2p. DNLM **90-1941**

DYER, Isadore (1865-1920)
The treatment of acne. New Albany, Ind., 1894. 4p. DNLM **90-1942**

DYER, Isadore (1865-1920)
The use and abuse of arsenic in the treatment of skin diseases. Philadelphia: Lea Bros. & Co., 1894. 13p. DNLM **90-1943**

DYER, Isadore (1865-1920)
Report on the leprosy question in Louisiana. New Orleans, [1894]. 6p. DNLM **90-1944**

DYER, Isadore (1865-1920)
Leprosy. Galveston, 1894. 7p. DNLM **90-1945**

DYER, Isadore (1865-1920)
One year in a Southern skin clinic. New Orleans, 1894. 7p. DNLM **90-1946**

DYER, Isadore (1865-1920)
A case of hematidrosis combined with chromidrosis. Philadelphia, 1895. 3p. DNLM **90-1947**

DYER, Isadore (1865-1920)
Naevus. New Orleans, 1895. 7p. 1 plate. DNLM **90-1948**

DYER, Isadore (1865-1920)
On the differential diagnosis of varicella and variola, with the report of a case in point. New Orleans, 1896. 6p. DNLM **90-1949**

DYER, Isadore (1865-1920)
The eruptions of vaccination and re-vaccination. New Orleans, 1896. 6p. DNLM **90-1950**

DYER, Isadore (1865-1920)
A preliminary report on the use of anti-venene in the treatment of leprosy. New Orleans: L. Graham & Son, 1897. 24p. DNLM **90-1951**

DYER, Isadore (1865-1920)
Endemic leprosy in Louisiana, with a logical argument for the contagiousness of this disease. Philadelphia, 1898. 14p. DNLM **90-1952**

EAGLETON, S. Potts
A résumé of the history and practical application of hydrogen peroxide in surgical affections. Philadelphia, 1891. 2 l. DNLM **90-1953**

EAMES, George F[ranklin]
Relation of adenoid vegetations to irregularities of the teeth and associate parts. Chicago, 1898. 12p. DNLM **90-1954**

EAMES, George F[ranklin]
The practice of dental medicine. Philadelphia: S. S. White Mfg. Co., 1899. 240p. MdU-D; PPC; PU **90-1955**

[EARLE, Pliny] (1809-1892)
Memoirs of Pliny Earle, M.D., with extracts from his diary and letters (1830-1892) and selections from his professional writings (1839-1891). Edited, with a general introduction, by F. B. Sanborn, of Concord. Boston: Damrell & Upham, 1898. 409p. MBM; MWA; NNNAM **90-1956**

EASTMAN, Joseph (1842-1902)
Work in abdominal and pelvic surgery. [Indianapolis], 1890. 32p. DNLM **90-1957**

EASTMAN, Joseph (1842-1902)
Abdominal surgery and its evolution and involution. Chicago, 1893. 15p. DNLM **90-1958**

EASTMAN, Joseph (1842-1902)
A few points of interest to the family physician. Chicago, 1893. 12p. DNLM **90-1959**

EASTMAN, Joseph (1842-1902)
Vaginal extirpation of the uterus; forty consecutive cases. New York: Trow's Co., 1893. 16p. DNLM **90-1960**

EASTMAN, Joseph (1842-1902)
Chairman's address [on the present status of suprapubic hysterectomy]. Chicago: Office American Medical Association, 1894. 16p. DNLM **90-1961**

EASTMAN, Joseph (1842-1902)
Supra-pubic hysterectomy by enucleation of tumor and uterus, including cervix. Lansing, 1894. 12p. DNLM **90-1962**

EASTMAN, Joseph (1842-1902)
Report of a case of hysterectomy where the morphology of the tumor made total extirpation of the cervix the only possible procedure. New York, 1895. 4p. DNLM **90-1963**

EASTMAN, Joseph (1842-1902)
Diagnosis in abdominal disorders. [Denver, 1898.] 11p. DNLM **90-1964**

EASTMAN, Joseph (1842-1902)
The question of pelvic support. [New York, 1898.] 7p. DNLM **90-1965**

EASTMAN, J[oseph] S. (*b.* 1842)
Cure of masturbation in a woman by neurectomy. Philadelphia, 1893. 3p. DNLM **90-1966**

EASTMAN, J[oseph] S. (*b.* 1842)
Office gynecology. [Indianapolis, 1898.] 12p. DNLM **90-1967**

EASTMAN, Thomas B.
A case of fracture of the tyroid cartilage; recovery without tracheotomy. Chicago: American Medical Assoc. Press, 1895. 4p. DNLM **90-1968**

EBERT, Albert Ethelbert (1840-1906)
The standard formulary, a collection of over four thousand formulas for pharmaceutical preparations. . . . By Albert E. Ebert . . . and A. Emil Hiss. . . . Chicago: G. P. Engelhard & Co., 1896. 500p. DLC: OCLloyd **90-1969**

ECCLES, A. Symons (1855-1900)
The practice of massage, its physiological effects and therapeutic uses. 2nd ed. New York: William Wood & Co., 1898. 374p. DNLM; NNNAM; PU **90-1970**

ECCLES, Robert Gibson (1848-1934)
A report on new remedies, read before the New York State Pharmaceutical Association. Comp. by R. G. Eccles . . . and Prof. W. A. Viall. . . . Elmira, N.Y.: Advertiser Association, Printers, 1890. 24p. DLC **90-1971**

ECKLEY, William Thomas, ed.
Practical anatomy; including a special section on the fundamental principles of anatomy. Edited by W. T. Eckley . . . and Mrs. Corinne Buford Eckley. . . . With 347 illustrations, many of which are in colors. Philadelphia: P. Blakiston's Son & Co., 1899. 485p. col. illus. DLC; NNNAM; PPC; PU **90-1972**

EDEBOHLS, George M[ichael] (1853-1908)
Exploratory puncture of the female pelvic organs; a diagnostic study. New York: Trow, 1890. 32p. DNLM; NNNAM **90-1973**

EDEBOHLS, George M[ichael] (1853-1908)
A modified Alexander-Adams operation. [New York, 1890.] 14p. DNLM **90-1974**

EDEBOHLS, George M[ichael] (1853-1908)
A new method of suture in perineorrhaphy. New York: William Wood & Co., 1890. 10p. DNLM **90-1975**

EDEBOHLS, George M[ichael] (1853-1908)
A combined laparotomy and gynecological operating-table. [New York, 1891.] 11p. DNLM **90-1976**

EDEBOHLS, George M[ichael] (1853-1908)
Tubal and peritoneal tuberculosis, with special reference to diagnosis. Philadelphia: W. J. Dornan, 1891. 23p. DNLM **90-1977**

EDEBOHLS, George M[ichael] (1853-1908)
Ventral hernia; a plea for extraperitoneal operation, with case. New York: William Wood & Co., 1891. 13p. DNLM **90-1978**

EDEBOHLS, George M[ichael] (1853-1908)
Combined gynecological operations. [Philadelphia, 1892.] 18p. DNLM **90-1979**

EDEBOHLS, George M[ichael] (1853-1908)
Total extirpation of the uterus. Cases illustrating various indications for and different methods of performing the operation. Remarks upon removal of the uterus in diseases of the appendages. [New York, 1892.] 24p. DNLM **90-1980**

EDEBOHLS, George M[ichael] (1853-1908)
A menstrual dermato-neurosis. A vaginal irrigating speculum and leg-holder. New York, 1893. 6p. DNLM **90-1981**

EDEBOHLS, George M[ichael] (1853-1908)
Movable kidney; with a report of twelve cases treated by nephrorrhaphy. Philadelphia, 1893. 32p. 1 plate. DNLM **90-1982**

EDEBOHLS, George M[ichael] (1853-1908)
The operative treatment of complete prolapsus uteri et vaginae. [New York, 1893.] 7p. DNLM **90-1983**

EDEBOHLS, George M[ichael] (1853-1908)
The prevention of hernia after incision of the abdominal walls. New York, 1893. 6p. DNLM **90-1984**

EDEBOHLS, George M[ichael] (1853-1908)
The techique of total extirpation of the fibromatous uterus. [New York, 1893.] 7p. DNLM **90-1985**

EDEBOHLS, George M[ichael] (1853-1908)
Diagnostic palpation of the appendix vermiformis. Cases of appendicitis. New York, [1894]. 22p. DNLM **90-1986**

EDEBOHLS, George M[ichael] (1853-1908)
Pregnancy after ventral fixation; a report of four cases. New York, [1894]. 8p. DNLM **90-1987**

EDEBOHLS, George M[ichael] (1853-1908)
Report of five cases of acute appendicitis. [New York, 1894.] 7p. DNLM **90-1988**

EDEBOHLS, George M[ichael] (1853-1908)
Three cases of uterus bicornis septus; with report of operations performed upon them. New York, 1894. 8p. DNLM **90-1989**

EDEBOHLS, George M[ichael] (1853-1908)
Inversion of the vermiform appendix. Philadelphia, 1895. 8p. DNLM **90-1990**

EDEBOHLS, George M[ichael] (1853-1908)
Notes on movable kidney and nephrorrhaphy. [New York, 1895.] 8p. DNLM **90-1991**

EDEBOHLS, Geoge M[ichael] (1853-1908)
The technique of vaginal hysterectomy. [Philadelphia, 1895.] 8p. DNLM **90-1992**

EDEBOHLS, George M[ichael] (1853-1908)
Diagnositc palpation of the female pelvic organs. [New York, 1895.] 13p. DNLM **90-1993**

EDEBOHLS, George M[ichael] (1853-1908)
The indications for ventral fixation of the uterus. Philadelphia, 1896. 8p. DNLM **90-1994**

EDEBOHLS, George M[ichael] (1853-1908)
Shortening the round ligaments; indications, technics, and results. New York, 1896. 59p. DNLM **90-1995**

EDEBOHLS, George M[ichael] (1853-1908)
Shortening the round ligaments; indications, technics, and results. New York, 1896. 68p. DNLM **90-1996**

EDEBOHLS, George M[ichael] (1853-1908)
What is the best method of making and of closing the coeliotomy incision? New York, 1896. 13p. DNLM **90-1997**

EDEBOHLS, George M[ichael] (1853-1908)
The inguinal operation for femoral hernia. [New York, 1897.] 12p. DNLM **90-1998**

EDEBOHLS, George M[ichael] (1853-1908)
The other kidney in contemplated nephrectomy. [Philadelphia, 1898.] 8p. DNLM **90-1999**

EDEBOHLS, George M[ichael] (1853-1908)
. . . The hernia guarantee and the minimum of confinement after operations for appendicitis with and without pus. . . . [New York, 1899?] 7p. DLC **90-2000**

EDEBOHLS, George M[ichael] (1853-1908)
. . . Chronic appendicitis the chief symptom and most important complication of movable right kidney. . . . [New York: Press of C. C. Shelley & Son, 1899.] 14p. DLC **90-2001**

EDEBOHLS, George M[ichael] (1853-1908)
. . . Chronic nephritis affecting a movable kidney as an indication for nephropexy. . . . [New York?] 1899.] 8p. DLC **90-2002**

EDEBOHLS, George M[ichael] (1853-1908)
. . . The relations of movable kidney and appendicitis to each other and to the practice of modern gynaecology. . . . New York: The Publishers' Printing Co., 1899. 16p. DLC **90-2003**

EDES, Robert T[haxter] (1838-1923)
Tumor of the brain (thalamus and internal capsule). [New York, 1890.] 12p. DNLM **90-2004**

EDES, Robert T[haxter] (1838-1923)
Ovariotomy for nervous disease. Boston: Damrell & Upham, 1894. 11p. DNLM **90-2005**

EDES, Robert T[haxter] (1838-1923)
The Shattuck lecture, 1895: The New England invalid. Boston: D. Clapp & Son, 1895. 57p. DLC; DNLM **90-2006**

EDES, Robert T[haxter] (1838-1923)
Points in the diagnosis and treatment of some common neuroses. Chicago, 1896. 19p. DNLM **90-2007**

EDES, Robert T[haxter] (1838-1923)
Relation of neurasthenic symptoms to the general nutrition. Boston: Damrell & Upham, 1897. 24p. DNLM
90-2008

EDES, Robert T[haxter] (1838-1923)
The treatment of insomnia. Chicago, 1898. 16p. DNLM
90-2009

EDGAR, J. Clifton (*b.* 1859)
The manikin in the teaching of practical obstetrics. [New York, 1890.] 31p. DNLM **90-2010**

EDGAR, J. Clifton (*b.* 1859)
Intra-uterine injections of glycerine. A simple, safe, and efficient means for the induction of labor, and the stimulating of uterine contractions. New York, 1892. 11p. DNLM
90-2011

EDGAR, J. Clifton (*b.* 1859)
Conversion of a vertex into a shoulder presentation by a Champetier balloon dilator; direct podalic version with recovery for both mother and child. [New York, 1893.] 4p. DNLM
90-2012

EDGAR, J. Clifton (*b.* 1859)
The mechanism and diagnosis of vertex presentation. New York, 1893. 21p. DNLM **90-2013**

EDINGER, Ludwig (1855-1918)
Twelve lectures on the structure of the central nervous system. . . . 2nd rev. ed. With 133 illustrations. Transl. by Willis Hall Vittum. . . . Ed. by C. Eugene Riggs. Philadelphia and London: F. A. Davis, 1890. 230p. DLC; DNLM; PPC; PU
90-2014

EDINGER, Ludwig (1855-1918)
The anatomy of the central nervous system of man and of vertebrates in general. . . . Transl. from the 5th German ed. by Winfield S. Hall . . . assisted by Philo Leon Holland . . . and Edward P. Carlton. . . . Illustrated with 258 engravings. Philadelphia, New York, [etc.]: The F. A. Davis Co., 1899. 446p. DLC; NNNAM; PPC **90-2015**

EDIS, Arthur W[ellesley] (1840-1893)
Sterility in women, including its causation and treatment. Philadelphia: P. Blakiston, Son & Co., 1890. 112p. DNLM; NNNAM; PPC **90-2016**

EDSON, Cyrus (1857-1903)
La grippe and its treatment, for general readers. New York: D. Appleton & Co., 1891. 46p. DNLM; NNNAM
90-2017

EDSON, Cyrus (1857-1903)
The therapeutics of glycozone, composition and characteristics. Philadelphia, 1893. 1 l. DNLM
90-2018

EDSON, Cyrus (1857-1903)
Aseptolin. A formulated treatment for tuberculosis, septicaemia, malaria, and la grippe, with reports of cases. 2nd ed. New York, [1896]. 79p. DNLM; NNNAM
90-2019

EDWARDS, Arthur R[obin] (*b.* 1867)
The Chicago Medical Recorder prize essay for 1895. Chylous and adipose ascites; a clinical, historical, and experimental study. Chicago, 1895. 16p. DNLM [also: Detroit, 1895. 22p.]
90-2020

EDWARDS, Arthur R[obin] (*b.* 1867)
Cirrhosis of the liver. Clinical and pathological differential diagnosis, with case. Chicago, 1895. 15p. DNLM
90-2021

EDWARDS, Joseph F. (1853-1897)
Edwards' catechism of hygiene for use in schools. Philadelphia, 1893. 109p. DNLM; MB; MH; NN
90-2022

EDWARDS, Joseph F. (1853-1897)
Edwards' hygiene, with anatomy and physiology, being an amplification of Edwards' Catechism of hygiene. . . . Intended for school and general reading. New York: Catholic School Book Co., [1894]. 435p., col. frontis., plates. DLC; NNNAM
90-2023

EDWARDS, W[illiam] A[loysius] (*b.* 1860)
Subcutaneous rheumatic nodules. [Philadelphia, 1890.] 3p. DNLM **90-2024**

EDWARDS, W[illiam] A[loysius] (*b.* 1860)
The climate of southern California in relation to disease. [Philadelphia, 1891.] 14p. DNLM **90-2025**

EDWARDS, W[illiam] A[loysius] (*b.* 1860) and James Sears WATERMAN
Hepatic abscess; report of a case, with remarks upon the amoeba coli. San Francisco, 1892. 12p. DNLM
90-2026

EDWARDS, W[illiam] A[loysius] (*b.* 1860)
Acute enlargement of the thyroid gland; angio-neurotic oedema. Philadelphia, 1892. 2 l. DNLM
90-2027

EDWARDS, W[illiam] A[loysius] (*b.* 1860)
Acute retroversion of the virgin uterus; report of cases, with remarks upon the difficulty in their replacement. [Philadelphia, 1892.] 6p. DNLM **90-2028**

EDWARDS, W[illiam] A[loysius] (*b.* 1860)
The new lake in the desert; its apparent and unexpected effect upon the climate of San Diego and San Bernardino counties, California. [Philadelphia: W. B. Saunders, 1892.] 5p. DNLM
90-2029

EDWARDS, W[illiam] A[loysius] (*b.* 1860)
A remarkable respiration record in infantile pneumonia. [New York, 1892.] 2 l. DNLM **90-2030**

EDWARDS, W[illiam] A[loysius] (*b.* 1860)
A case of mediastino-pericarditis in a child; secondary empyema; operation; death. [Philadelphia, 1893.] 6p. DNLM
90-2031

EDWARDS, W[illiam] A[loysius] (*b.* 1860)
Acetanilid as an antiseptic surgical dressing. Los Angeles, 1895. 1 l. DNLM **90-2032**

EDWARDS, W[illiam] A[loysius] (*b.* 1860)
A practical low-priced device to secure the Trendelenburg posture. Philadelphia, 1895. 1 l. 1 plate.
90-2033

EDWARDS, W[illiam] A[loysius] (*b.* 1860)
Trachoma of the female genital tract; hydrocele of the labium majus. Los Angeles, 1895. 4p. DNLM **90-2034**

EDWARDS, W[illiam] A[loysius] (*b.* 1860) and William M. GRAY
Cirrhosis of the liver in childhood; with microscopic report. New York, 1895. 11p. DNLM **90-2035**

EDWARDS, W[illiam] A[loysius] (*b.* 1860) and Beatrice HARRADEN
Two health-seekers in southern California. Philadelphia: J. B. Lippincott Co., 1897. 144p. DNLM
90-2036

EGBERT, Seneca (*b.* 1863)
Report of an epidemic of typhoid fever in North Carolina, and its investigation. [Philadelphia, 1892.] 9p. DNLM
90-2037

EGBERT, Seneca (*b.* 1863)
The bicycle in its relation to the physician. [Philadelphia, 1892.] 11p. DNLM **90-2038**

EGBERT, Seneca (*b.* 1863)
Hygiene and tuberculosis. Philadelphia, 1895. 15p. DNLM **90-2039**

EGBERT, Seneca (*b.* 1863)
A manual of hygiene and sanitation. . . . Illustrated with sixty-three engravings. Philadelphia and New York: Lea Bros. & Co., 1898. 368p. DLC; DNLM; NNNAM; PPC
90-2040

EINHORN, Max (1862-1953)
A new method of obtaining small quantities of stomach contents for diagnostic purposes. New York: Trow, 1890. 8p. DNLM **90-2041**

EINHORN, Max (1862-1953)
Rumination in man. New York: Trow, 1890. 20p. DNLM **90-2042**

EINHORN, Max (1862-1953)
A new method for direct electrization of the stomach. New York: Trow's Co., 1891. 11p. DNLM
90-2043

EINHORN, Max (1862-1953)
On gastrodiaphany. [New York, 1892.] 14p. DNLM
90-2044

EINHORN, Max (1862-1953)
Therapeutic results of direct electrization of the stomach. New York: Trow Co., 1892. 41p. DNLM
90-2045

EINHORN, Max (1862-1953)
Ueber Achylia gastrica. New York: Cherouny Co., 1892. 15p. DNLM **90-2046**

EINHORN, Max (1862-1953)
Dietetics in diseases of the stomach. New York: Trow Co., 1893. 19p. DNLM **90-2047**

EINHORN, Max (1862-1953)
Enteroptosis, or Glénard's disease. New York: Stettiner, Lambert & Co., 1893. 8p. DNLM **90-2048**

EINHORN, Max (1862-1953)
Further experiences with direct electrization of the stomach. [New York: D. Appleton & Co., 1893.] 15p. 1 table. DNLM **90-2049**

EINHORN, Max (1862-1953)
Clinical observations on erosions of the stomach and their treatment. New York: Trow, 1894. 22p. DNLM
90-2050

EINHORN, Max (1862-1953)
The gastrograph: a new means of determining the mechanical action of the stomach. [New York: D. Appleton & Co., 1894.] 9p. DNLM **90-2051**

EINHORN, Max (1862-1953)
On functional disorders of the stomach accompanied with hypersecretion. 1. Hyperchlorhydria. 2. Gastro-succorrhoea continua periodica. 3. Gastro-succorrhoea continua chronica. New York: Trow Co., 1895. 24p. DNLM
90-2052

EINHORN, Max (1862-1953)
Diseases of the stomach; a text-book for practitioners and students. . . . New York: William Wood & Co., 1896. 478p. DLC; DNLM; NNNAM; PPC **90-2053**

EINHORN, Max (1862-1953)
The dimethylamidoazobenzol, or Toepfer's test for free hydrochloric acid. [New York: D. Appleton & Co.], 1896. 5p. DNLM **90-2054**

EINHORN, Max (1862-1953)
Enteroptosis. New York, 1896. 8p. DNLM
90-2055

EINHORN, Max (1862-1953)
Experiments upon the effects of direct electrization of the stomach. [New York: D. Appleton & Co.], 1896. 13p. DNLM **90-2056**

EINHORN, Max (1862-1953)
The state of the gastric mucosa in secretory disorders of the stomach. New York: Publishers' Print. Co., 1896. 11p. DNLM **90-2057**

EINHORN, Max (1862-1953)
The treatment of habitual constipation. New York, 1896. 7p. DNLM **90-2058**

EINHORN, Max (1862-1953)
The inspection of the oesophagus and the cardia. [New York, 1897.] 8p. DNLM **90-2059**

EINHORN, Max (1862-1953)
Diseases of the stomach; a text-book for practitioners and students. . . . 2nd rev. ed. New York: William Wood & Co., 1898. 486p. DLC; DNLM; NNNAM; PPC
90-2060

EINHORN, Max (1862-1953)
The early recognition and management of malignant disease of the digestive system. . . . [New York, 1899.] 8p. DLC
90-2061

EINHORN, Max (1862-1953)
Membranous enteritis and its treatment. . . . New York: The Publishers' Printing Co., 1899. 15p. DLC
90-2062

EINHORN, Max (1862-1953)
. . . Floating liver and its clinical significance. . . . New York: The Publishers' Printing Co., 1899. 23p. DLC
90-2063

EISENBERG, James (*b.* 1861)
Bacteriological diagnosis; tabular aids for use in practical work. Transl. and augmented, with the permission of the author, from the 2nd German ed., by Norval H. Pierce. Philadelphia & London: F. A. Davis Co., 1892. 184p. DNLM; NNNAM; OCIM; PPC **90-2064**

ELIOT, Charles W[illiam] (1834-1926)
Medical education of the future. [New York, 1896.] 28p. DNLM; MH **90-2065**

ELIOT, Ellsworth (*b.* 1827)
Remarks at the meeting of the board of managers of the New York Society for the Relief of Widows and Orphans of Medical Men, December 21, 1892. New York, 1893. 6p. DNLM
90-2066

ELIOT, Gustavus (1857-1932)
The use and abuse of pepsin. Bridgeport: Gould & Stiles, 1890. 6p. DNLM **90-2067**

ELIOT, Gustavus (1857-1932)
Cerebral arterial thrombosis. New York, 1895. 6p. DNLM
90-2068

ELIOT, Gustavus (1857-1932)
Chronic paroxysmal headache, commonly called migraine, hemicrania, or sick headache. [New York, 1897.] 13p. DNLM
90-2069

ELIOT, Llewellyn (*b.* 1853)
Is a child viable at six and a half months? [Richmond, 1891.] 11p. DNLM **90-2070**

ELIOT, Llewellyn (*b.* 1853)
Catheterization of the Fallopian tubes. New York: William Wood & Co., 1894. 4p. DNLM **90-2071**

ELIOT, Llewellyn (*b.* 1853)
The complications of the puerperal state. New York: William Wood & Co., 1894. 5p. DNLM **90-2072**

ELIOT, Llewellyn (*b.* 1853)
The treatment of fractures of the shaft of the femur. Detroit, Mich.: G. S. Davis, 1894. 8p. DNLM
90-2073

ELIOT, Llewellyn (*b.* 1853)
The use of vaccine-serum in the treatment of variola. Philadelphia, 1895. 14p. DNLM **90-2074**

ELIOT, Llewellyn (*b.* 1853)
Can the dispensary abuse be corrected? [Richmond, 1897.] 7p. DNLM **90-2075**

ELIOT, Llewellyn (*b.* 1853)
The suture-clamp operation for hemorrhoids. Detroit, Mich.: G. S. Davis, 1897. 4p. DNLM **90-2076**

ELIOT, Llewellyn (*b.* 1853)
A case of hysterical dysphagia. [Detroit: W. M. Warren, 1898.] 6p. DNLM **90-2077**

ELIOT, Llewellyn (*b.* 1853)
Presidential address, decennial anniversary of the Medical and Surgical Society of the District of Columbia, Oct. 31, 1898. Richmond, 1898. 6p. DNLM **90-2078**

ELIOT, Llewellyn (*b.* 1853)
Supra-public cystomy for hemorrhage into the bladder. Richmond, 1898. 4p. DNLM **90-2079**

ELLETT, E[dward] C[oleman] (*b.* 1869)
A case of rupture of the choroid coat. Nashville, 1897. 3p. DNLM **90-2080**

ELLETT, E[dward] C[oleman] (*b.* 1869)
A clinical report on the use of argonin in gonorrhoeal ophthalmia. Memphis, 1897. 2 l. DNLM
90-2081

ELLETT, E[dward] C[oleman] (*b.* 1869)
Hemorrhagic glaucoma. Report of a case, with micro-photographs. St. Louis, 1897. 15p. DNLM
90-2082

ELLETT, E[dward] C[oleman] (*b.* 1869)
Acute inflammation of the middle ear. Columbus, O.: Columbus Med. Publ. Co., 1898. 4p. DNLM
90-2083

ELLETT, E[dward] C[oleman] (*b.* 1869)
A case of tenonitis. Nashville, Tenn., 1898. 2p. 1 plate. DNLM
90-2084

ELLETT, E[dward] C[oleman] (*b.* 1869)
The determining cause of the site of ulcers on the nasal septum. St. Louis, 1898. 2 l. DNLM
90-2085

ELLINGWOOD, Finley (1852-1920)
A systematic treatise on materia medica and therapeutics with reference to the most direct action of drugs. . . . With a condensed consideration of pharmacy and pharmacognosy. By Prof. John Uri Lloyd. . . . Chicago: Chicago Medical Press Co., [1898]. 706p. DLC; OCLloyd; PU **90-2086**

ELLIOT, George T.
Bassorin paste; a new base for dermatological preparations. New York: D. Appleton & Co., [1891]. 8p. DNLM
90-2087

ELLIOT, George T.
Some cases of the dermatitis herpetiformis of Duhring, with remarks on their aetiology. [New York, 1892.] 25p. DNLM
90-2088

ELLIOT, George T.
Alopecia praematura; its most frequent cause eczema seborrhoicum. [New York, 1893.] 20p. DNLM
90-2089

ELLIOT, George T.
A case of idiopathic atrophy of the skin. New York, 1895. 3p. DNLM **90-2090**

ELLIOT, George T.
Three cases of dermatitis herpetiformis due to pregnancy (herpes gestationis). Philadelphia, 1895. 8p. DNLM **90-2091**

ELLIOT, George T.
Two cases of epidermolysis bullosa. New York, 1895. 9p. DNLM **90-2092**

ELLIOT, George T. and William H. MERRILL
A further study of alopecia praematura or praesenilis, and its most frequent cause, eczema seborrhoicum; and a preliminary bacteriological report on eczema seborrhoicum; for the first time successful production of the disease by inoculation of pure cultures of certain diplococci. New York, 1895. 20p. DNLM **90-2093**

ELLIOT, J[ohn] W[heelock] (1852-1925)
Papers on appendicitis. I. Appendicitis: a year's experience in private practice. II. Appendicitis: summary of cases. III. Excision of the vermiform appendix between the attacks in a case of chronic appendicitis. Boston: S. J. Parkhill & Co., 1892. 27p. DNLM; MBM **90-2094**

ELLIOT, J[ohn] W[heelock] (1852-1925)
Tubercular salpingitis, with cases treated by operation. New York: William Wood & Co., 1892. 8p. 1 plate. DNLM **90-2095**

ELLIOT, J[ohn] W[heelock] (1852-1925)
Intracranial hemorrhage; two cases trephined. Philadelphia, 1893. 8p. 2 plates. DNLM **90-2096**

ELLIOT, J[ohn] W[heelock] (1852-1925)
Strangulation of Meckel's diverticulum caused by volvulus of the ileum. Boston, 1894. 5p. DNLM **90-2097**

ELLIOT, J[ohn] W[heelock] (1852-1925)
Immediate suture of the gall-ducts and the gall-bladder after extraction of stones, with cases. Philadelphia, 1895. 13p. DNLM **90-2098**

ELLIOT, J[ohn] W[heelock] (1852-1925)
The operative relief of gangrene of intestine due to occlusion of the mesenteric vessels. [Philadelphia, 1895.] 15p. DNLM **90-2099**

ELLIOT, J[ohn] W[heelock] (1852-1925)
Successful laparotomy and Kraske operation on an infant two days old for imperforate rectum. Philadelphia, 1896. 2p. DNLM **90-2100**

ELLIOT, J[ohn] W[heelock] (1852-1925)
Nephro-ureterectomy; retroperitoneal extirpation of a kidney with its ureter. Boston: Damrell & Upham, 1897. 6p. 1 chart. **90-2101**

ELLIOT, J[ohn] W[heelock] (1852-1925)
Surgical treatment of tumor of the liver, with the report of a case. Philadelphia, 1897. 13p. DNLM **90-2102**

ELLIOT, Sydney Barrington (*b.* 1869)
Aedoecology. A treatise on generative life. Including pre-natal influence, prevention of conception, and hygiene of generative life. . . . New York: St. Clair Publishing Company, [1892]. 260p. DLC; NNNAM **90-2103**

ELLIOTT's hand-book of medical, hygienic, pharmaceutical and dental journals of the United States and Canada. . . . New York: A. R. Elliott, 1895. 144p. DLC; NNNAM **90-2104**

ELLIOTT, Arthur R. (*b.* 1869)
The importance of careful examination of the urine before surgical operations. Chicago, 1895. 14p. DNLM **90-2105**

ELLIOTT, Arthur R. (*b.* 1869)
A new method for the detection and estimation of sugar in the urine. New York, 1895. 5p. DNLM **90-2106**

ELLIOTT, Arthur R. (*b.* 1869)
Albumin testing. New York, 1896. 8p. DNLM **90-2107**

ELLIOTT, Arthur R. (*b.* 1869)
Urinary antiseptics in cystitis. Chicago, 1897. 7p. DNLM **90-2108**

ELLIOTT, Charles Sinclaire
Lectures on nervous and mental diseases. . . . New York: A. L. Chatterton & Co., 1897. 912p. col. plates. fold. table. DLC; NNNAM **90-2109**

ELLIS, John (1815-1896)
Personal experiences of a physician, with an appeal to the medical and clerical professions; and an appendix, a review of "Christ and the temperance question," in the Christian union. . . . Philadelphia: Hahnemann Publishing House, 1892. 134p. DLC; DNLM; PPC **90-2110**

ELLISON, Andrew (1846-1902)
Lectures on medical jurisprudence . . . to the graduating class, spring term, 1899. Of the American School of Osteopathy, Kirksville, Missouri. Reported by J. A. Quintal. Kirksville: Journal Printing Co., 1899. 52p. DLC **90-2111**

ELLWANGER, George Herman (1848-1906)
Meditations on gout; with a consideration of its cure through the use of wine. With a frontispeace & decoration by George Wharton Edwards. New York: Dodd, Mead & Co., [*c* 1897]. 208p. NNNAM **90-2112**

ELSNER, H[enry] L[eopold] (1857-1916)
On the practical value of the newer methods of examination in the diseases of the stomach, with a consideration of the indications given for diet and treatment by such examinations, being part of a discussion of the newer methods of diagnosis and treatment of stomach and intestinal diseases. New York: D. Appleton & Co., 1893. 54p. DNLM; NNNAM **90-2113**

ELSNER, H[enry] L[eopold] (1857-1916) and Hiram B. HAWLEY
On the clinical value of the centrifuge. [New York: D. Appleton & Co., 1894.] 16p. DNLM **90-2114**

ELSNER, H[enry] Leopold] (1857-1916)
The pathological factors of neurasthenia. New York, 1897. 7p. DNLM **90-2115**

ELWELL, John J. (1820-1900)
A medico-legal treatise on malpractice, medical evidence, and insanity, comprising the elements of medical jurisprudence. . . . 4th ed., rev. and enl. New York: Baker, Voorhies & Co., 1890 [1881]. 600p. ICJ; PPJ [1st ed., 1860; new ed., 1866; 3rd ed., 1871] **90-2116**

ELY, Albert H.
Acute inflammatory affections of the mammae, with special reference to treatment during lactation. [New York, 1892.] 14p. DNLM **90-2117**

ELY, John S[lade] (1860-1906)
A study of metastatic carcinoma of the stomach; report of a case of primary carcinoma of the testicle; secondary involvement of the vena cava inferior; metastases in the lungs, stomach, and falx cerebri. [Philadelphia, 1890.] 11p. DNLM **90-2118**

ELY, John S[lade] (1860-1906)
The dominant influence in the medical progress of the nineteenth century. [New York: D. Appleton & Co., 1895.] 11p. DNLM **90-2119**

ELY, John S[lade] (1860-1906)
Bacterial and allied tests as applied to the chemical diagnosis of typhoid fever. [New York], 1897. 16p. DNLM **90-2120**

THE EMERGENCY manual, for the treatment of simple diseases, accidents. . . . Auburn, N.Y.: R. Schicht, [1894]. 19p. DLC **90-2121**

EMERSON, Edward Waldo (1844-1930)
A history of the gift of painless surgery. Boston & New York: Houghton, Mifflin & Co., 1896. 9p. DNLM; MBM **90-2122**

EMERSON, Herbert C. (1865-1922)
Bacteriological diagnosis of diphtheria. [Concord], 1895. 5p. DNLM **90-2123**

EMMET, Thomas Addis (1828-1919)
Reminiscences of the founders of the Woman's Hospital Association. New York, 1893. 16p. 8 port., 1 plate. DNLM; NNNAM **90-2124**

EMMET, Thomas Addis (1828-1919)
The use of traction and morcellation in the removal of fibroids versus hysterectomy. New York, 1895. 20p. DNLM; NNNAM **90-2125**

EMMET, Thomas Addis (1828-1919)
A memoir of John Patten Emmet, M.D., formerly professor of chemistry and materia medica in the University of Virginia, with a brief outline of the Emmet family history. . . . New York: priv. print. [Bradstreet Press], 1898. 66p. 38 plates. DLC; DNLM; NNNAM **90-2126**

ENGEL, Hugo
A valuable discovery, the cure of impotence. Lansdale, Pa., 1895. 2 l. DNLM **90-2127**

ENGELMANN, George J[ulius] (1847-1903)
Menstruation and the removal of both ovaries. Philadelphia: W. J. Dornan, 1890. 20p. DNLM **90-2128**

ENGELMANN, George J[ulius] (1847-1903)
Thinness of the uterine wall during gestation simulating extra-uterine foetation. Philadelphia: W. J. Dornan, 1891. 15p. DNLM **90-2129**

ENGELMANN, George J[ulius] (1847-1903)
Annual address of the president. The health of the American girl as imperilled by the social conditions of the day. Philadelphia: W. J. Dornan, 1891. 29p. DNLM **90-2130**

ENGELMANN, George J[ulius] (1847-1903)
Medical education and legislation: from the valedictory address to the class of '92, Missouri Medical College. [St. Louis, 1892.] 8p. DNLM **90-2131**

ENGELMANN, George J[ulius] (1847-1903)
Recent investigations in faradic electricity. Variation and control of the current by rapidity of interruption and variation of coils, and the single wire high-tension current. Philadelphia, 1893. 12p. DNLM **90-2132**

ENGELMANN, George J[ulius] (1847-1903)
Vaginal hysterectomy and hysterectomy by morcellement; the vaginal route in pelvic operations in place of laparotomy or the abdominal method. [Philadelphia, 1894.] 16p. DNLM **90-2133**

ENGELMANN, George J[ulius] (1847-1903)
The interrupted high-voltage primary or mixed current. [Philadelphia, 1894.] 11p. DNLM **90-2134**

THE ERA dose book and reference tables for the prescription counter. Detroit, [1892]. 12p. DNLM **90-2135**

THE ERA dose book and reference tables for the prescription counter. 2nd ed. Detroit, 1893. 38p. DNLM **90-2136**

THE ERA dose book, compiled and arranged especially for use in writing and dispensing prescriptions, comprising a list, with doses of all remedies official in the pharmacopoeias of the United States, Great Britain, and Germany, and also those of the national formulary (revised edition), to which have been added many standard preparations, [etc.]. Compiled by the Pharmaceutical Era. 3rd ed. New York: D. O. Haynes & Co., [1898]. 45p. DNLM; NNNAM; OCLloyd **90-2137**

THE ERA druggists' directory. 5th ed. New York: Haynes, 1897. 256p. DNLM; OCLloyd **90-2138**

THE ERA formulary. Five thousand formulas for druggists. A collection of original and prize formulas to which has been added a selection of formulas from standard authorities in the English, French, and German, for application to pharmacy, in the household and the industries, making a complete and valuable reference work for all branches of the pharmacist's vocation. 1st ed. New York: D. O. Haynes & Co., [1893]. 462p. DNLM; OCLloyd **90-2139**

THE ERA key to U.S. P[harmacopoeia], 1893. Detroit, 1893. 75p. DNLM; OCLloyd **90-2140**

ERDMANN, John F. (*b.* **1864**)
Wound-infection with the bacillus aerogenes capsulatus. With discussion, by Edward K. Dunham, and bacteriologic report, by Harlow Brooks. New York, 1897. 22p. DNLM [also: New York, 1897. 17p.] **90-2141**

ERDMANN, John F. (*b.* **1864**)
Traumatic paralysis of the upper extremities. New York: Publ. Print. Co., 1897. 7p. DNLM **90-2142**

ERDMANN, John F. (*b.* **1864**)
Intestinal obstruction due to intussusception and volvulus. New York, 1898. 21p. DNLM **90-2143**

ERDMANN, John F. (*b.* **1864**)
Report of a case of intussusception due to a Merkel's diverticulum; also reports of three additional cases of diverticula. New York, 1898. 5p. DNLM **90-2144**

ESHNER, Augustus A[dolph] (*b.* **1862**)
Arterio-capillary fibrosis. [Philadelphia, 1891.] 4p. DNLM **90-2145**

ESHNER, Augustus A[dolph] (*b.* **1862**)
The diagnosis of cerebral haemorrhage. [Philadelphia, 1891.] 14p. DNLM **90-2146**

ESHNER, Augustus A[dolph] (*b.* **1862**)
Large aneurism of the thoracic aorta. [Philadelphia: Lea Bros. & Co., 1892.] 4p. DNLM **90-2147**

ESHNER, Augustus A[dolph] (*b.* **1862**)
A long toilet-pin accidently swallowed, and passed by the bowel after four days. [Philadelphia: Lea Bros. & Co., 1892.] Galley sheet. DNLM **90-2148**

ESHNER, Augustus A[dolph] (*b.* **1862**)
Achillodynia. [Philadelphia, 1893.] 4p. DNLM **90-2149**

ESHNER, Augustus A[dolph] (*b.* **1862**)
Congenital absence of the gall-bladder. Philadelphia, 1894. 7p. **90-2150**

ESHNER, Augustus A[dolph] (*b.* **1862**)
Influenza followed by pleuritis and endocarditis. [Philadelphia, 1894.] 3p. DNLM **90-2151**

ESHNER, Augustus A[dolph] (*b.* **1862**)
Fevers: including general considerations, typhoid fever, typhus fever, influenza, malarial fever, yellow fever, variola, relapsing fever, Weil's disease, thermic fever, dengue, miliary fever, mountain fever, etc. By James C. Wilson, M.D.; Solomon Solis-Cohen, M.D.; C. Meigs Wilson, M.D.; Augustus A. Eshner, M.D.; W. Reynolds Wilson, M.D. Comp. from the Annual of the universal medical sciences, from 1888 to 1894, inclusive, by Augustus A. Eshner, M.D. With copious commentaries and additions. Embellished by wood-engravings and lithographs. Philadelphia: F. A. Davis Co.; London: F. J. Rebman, 1895. 585p. col. plate. DLC; ICJ; PPC; PU **90-2152**

ESHNER, Augustus A[dolph] (*b.* **1862**)
A case of akromegaly. Philadelphia, 1895. 2 galley sheets. DNLM **90-2153**

ESHNER, Augustus A[dolph] (*b.* **1862**)
A case of renal calculus. Philadelphia, 1895. 2p. DNLM **90-2154**

ESHNER, Augustus A[dolph] (*b.* **1862**)
Congenital malformation of the heart. Philadelphia, 1895. 12p. DNLM **90-2155**

ESHNER, Augustus A[dolph] (*b.* **1862**)
Diminutive liver from an infant. [Philadelphia, 1895.] 3p. DNLM **90-2156**

ESHNER, Augustus A[dolph] (*b.* **1862**)
Further note on a case of renal calculus. Philadelphia, 1895. Galley sheet. DNLM **90-2157**

ESHNER, Augustus A[dolph] (*b.* **1862**)
A case of cerebro-spinal syphilis. Philadelphia, 1896. 3p. DNLM **90-2158**

ESHNER, Augustus A[dolph] (*b.* **1862**)
A case of mitral obstruction. Philadelphia, 1896. 1 l. DNLM **90-2159**

ESHNER, Augustus A[dolph] (*b.* **1862**)
Some considerations on the treatment of typhoid fever. Philadelphia, 1896. 10p. DNLM **90-2160**

ESHNER, Augustus A[dolph] (*b.* **1862**)
Typhoid fever with fatal relapse. Philadelphia, 1896. 2p. DNLM **90-2161**

ESHNER, Augustus A[dolph] (*b.* **1862**)
A case of congenital tremor. Detroit: G. S. Davis, 1897. 8p. DNLM **90-2162**

ESHNER, Augustus A[dolph] (*b.* **1862**)
A case of hyoscine intoxication. Detroit, Mich.: W. M. Warren, 1897. 4p. DNLM **90-2163**

ESHNER, Augustus A[dolph] (*b.* **1862**)
A case of obscure diagnosis, exhibiting hysteric stigmata. Detroit: W. M. Warren, 1897. 5p. DNLM **90-2164**

ESHNER, Augustus A[dolph] (*b.* **1862**)
A case of profound anemia, probably of gastro-intestinal origin. Philadelphia, 1897. 1 l. DNLM **90-2165**

ESHNER, Augustus A[dolph] (*b.* **1862**)
A case of uremia with high temperature. Philadelphia, 1897. 2p. DNLM **90-2166**

ESHNER, Augustus A[dolph] (*b.* **1862**)
Four cases of cerebral hemorrhage. Philadelphia, 1897. 5p. DNLM **90-2167**

ESHNER, Augustus A[dolph] (*b.* **1862**)
Hereditary laterial sclerosis. Philadelphia, 1897. 9p. DNLM **90-2168**

ESHNER, Augustus A[dolph] (*b.* **1862**)
Hysteria in early life. New York, 1897. 12p. DNLM **90-2169**

ESHNER, Augustus A[dolph] (*b.* **1862**)
Lateral sclerosis as a sequence of spinal meningitis. Philadelphia, 1897. 1p. DNLM **90-2170**

ESHNER, Augustus A[dolph] (*b.* **1862)**
Traumatic hysteria. Detroit, 1897. 6p. DNLM
90-2171

ESHNER, Augustus A[dolph] (*b.* **1862)**
Two cases of epilepsy. Philadelphia, 1897. 3p. DNLM
90-2172

ESHNER, Augustus A[dolph] (*b.* **1862)**
A case of adiposis dolorosa. Philadelphia, 1898. 10p. DNLM
90-2173

ESHNER, Augustus A[dolph] (*b.* **1862)**
A case of probable miliary tuberculosis. Philadelphia, 1898. 3p. DNLM **90-2174**

ESHNER, Augustus A[dolph] (*b.* **1862)**
A case of progressive muscular dystrophy. Baltimore, 1898. 4p. DNLM **90-2175**

ESHNER, Augustus A[dolph] (*b.* **1862)**
A case of renal calculus of more than ordinary interest. Philadelphia, 1898. 4p. DNLM **90-2176**

ESHNER, Augustus A[dolph] (*b.* **1862)**
A contribution to the statistics of exophthalmic goitre. Philadelphia, 1898. 2p. DNLM **90-2177**

ESHNER, Augustus A[dolph] (*b.* **1862)**
A contribution to the study of the muscular dystrophies. Philadelphia, 1898. 19p. DNLM **90-2178**

ESHNER, Augustus A[dolph] (*b.* **1862)**
Dilatation of the heart; atheroma of the aorta; pulmonary infarction. Philadelphia, 1898. 2p. DNLM
90-2179

ESHNER, Augustus A[dolph] (*b.* **1862)**
Enlarged cirrhotic liver. Philadelphia, 1898. 1 l. DNLM
90-2180

ESHNER, Augustus A[dolph] (*b.* **1862)**
Further communication upon a case of meningitis. Philadelphia, 1898. 2p. DNLM **90-2181**

ESHNER, Augustus A[dolph] (*b.* **1862)**
Orchitis, or epididymitis, as a complication or sequel of typhoid fever. Philadelphia, 1898. 17p. 1 table. DNLM
90-2182

ESHNER, Augustus A[dolph] (*b.* **1862)**
Typhoid fever with relapse; serum-reaction wanting in the primary attack. Philadelphia, 1898. 4p. DNLM
90-2183

ESHNER, Augustus A[dolph] (*b.* **1862)**
Erysipelas. Memphis, 1899. 4p. 10 charts. DNLM
90-2184

ESHNER, Augustus A[dolph] (*b.* **1862)**
Hemorrhage into pons Varolii. Chicago, 1899. 8p. DNLM
90-2185

ESHNER, Augustus A[dolph] (*b.* **1862)**
Pulmonary tuberculosis with intercurrent typhoid fever complicated by pneumonia; triple infection. Philadelphia, 1899. 5p. DNLM **90-2186**

ESHNER, Augustus A[dolph] (*b.* **1862)**
Some reflections upon cellular physiology and pathology. Chicago: American Medical Association Press, 1899. 7p. DNLM **90-2187**

ESHNER, Augustus A[dolph] (*b.* **1862)**
Two cases of protracted erysipelas. Detroit: W. W. Warren, 1899. 4p. DNLM **90-2188**

ESHNER, Augustus A[dolph] (*b.* **1862)**
Two cases of triple infection. Philadelphia, 1899. 3p. DNLM
90-2189

ESKRIDGE, Jeremiah Thomas (1848-1902)
Acute myelitis preceded by acute optic neuritis. New York: M. J. Rooney & Co., [1890]. 7p. DNLM
90-2190

ESKRIDGE, Jeremiah Thomas (1848-1902)
The medical expert. [Philadelphia, 1890.] 8p. DNLM
90-2191

ESKRIDGE, Jeremiah Thomas (1848-1902)
Nervous and mental diseases observed in Colorado. [New York, 1890.] 22p. DNLM **90-2192**

ESKRIDGE, Jeremiah Thomas (1848-1902)
Some points in the diagnosis of certain simulated mental and nervous diseases. [New York, 1890.] 16p. DNLM
90-2193

ESKRIDGE, Jeremiah Thomas (1848-1902)
A case of fracture of the twelfth dorsal vertebra, followed by injury to the spinal and sympathetic nerve-supply of the bowel in the region of the ileo-cecal valve. Intestinal hemorrhage and death on the seventh day. [Philadelphia, 1891.] 7p. DNLM
90-2194

ESKRIDGE, Jeremiah Thomas (1848-1902)
Chorea in relation to climate, especially the climate of Colorado. [Philadelphia, 1891.] 12p. DNLM
90-2195

ESKRIDGE, Jeremiah Thomas (1848-1902)
Hypnotism. New York, 1891. 36p. DNLM
90-2196

ESKRIDGE, Jeremiah Thomas (1848-1902)
Poliomyelitis with perineuritis. A clinical lecture. [New York, 1891.] 11p. DNLM **90-2197**

ESKRIDGE, Jeremiah Thomas (1848-1902)
Poliomyelitis with perineuritis. A clinical lecture. [New York, 1891.] 14p. DNLM **90-2198**

ESKRIDGE, Jeremiah Thomas (1848-1902)
Expert witnesses. [Denver, 1892.] 10p. DNLM
90-2199

ESKRIDGE, Jeremiah Thomas (1848-1902)
Myelitis in a case of incipient posterior spinal sclerosis. [Philadelphia, 1892.] 6p. DNLM **90-2200**

ESKRIDGE, Jeremiah Thomas (1848-1902)
Nervo-vascular disturbances in unacclimated persons in Colorado. [Philadelphia, 1892.] 11p. DNLM
90-2201

ESKRIDGE, Jeremiah Thomas (1848-1902)
Retroanterograde amnesia. With report of two cases. [St. Louis, 1892.] 37p. DNLM **90-2202**

ESKRIDGE, Jeremiah Thomas (1848-1902)
Some points in the diagnosis and nature of certain functional and organic nervous diseases. [St. Louis, 1892.] 16p. DNLM **90-2203**

ESKRIDGE, Jeremiah Thomas (1848-1902)
Subacute recurrent multiple neuritis. [New York, 1892.] 7p. DNLM **90-2204**

ESKRIDGE, Jeremiah Thomas (1848-1902)
Tumor of the brain. [Denver, 1892.] 9p. DNLM **90-2205**

ESKRIDGE, Jeremiah Thomas (1848-1902)
Chronic meningo-myelitis. Denver, 1893. 8p. DNLM **90-2206**

ESKRIDGE, Jeremiah Thomas (1848-1902)
Idiopathic muscular atrophy. New York, 1893. 11p. DNLM **90-2207**

ESKRIDGE, Jeremiah Thomas (1848-1902)
Polio-myelitis. [Austin, 1893.] 11p. DNLM **90-2208**

ESKRIDGE, Jeremiah Thomas (1848-1902)
(I) Polio-myelitis; (II) chorea, and (III) arthritis affecting the right sacro-iliac joint and the intervertebral substance in the lumbo-sacral region of the spine (probably rheumatic). [Richmond, 1893.] 12p. DNLM **90-2209**

ESKRIDGE, Jeremiah Thomas (1848-1902)
Report of cases of moral imbecility, of the opium habit, and of feigning, in which forgery is the offence committed. Philadelphia, 1893. 20p. DNLM **90-2210**

ESKRIDGE, Jeremiah Thomas (1848-1902)
Sarcoma of the pia and brain, simulating brain tumor; mono-spasm and mono-paresis; operation; death on the third day. Chicago, 1893. 12p. DNLM **90-2211**

ESKRIDGE, Jeremiah Thomas (1848-1902)
Some points in the diagnosis and treatment of intra-cerebral hemorrhage and in the treatment of chorea. [Philadelphia, 1893.] 19p. DNLM **90-2212**

ESKRIDGE, Jeremiah Thomas (1848-1902)
Tumor of the cerebellum. [Philadelphia, 1893.] 6p. DNLM **90-2213**

ESKRIDGE, Jeremiah Thomas (1848-1902)
Traumatic myelitis. A clinical lecture. Philadelphia, 1893. 14p. DNLM **90-2214**

ESKRIDGE, Jeremiah Thomas (1848-1902)
Bilateral cerebral thrombosis due to syphilitic arteritis, with incontinence of the vesical and anal sphincters. [Philadelphia, 1894.] 15p. DNLM **90-2215**

ESKRIDGE, Jeremiah Thomas (1848-1902)
Caries of the spine followed by compression of the cord. New York, 1894. 28p. DNLM **90-2216**

ESKRIDGE, Jeremiah Thomas (1848-1902)
Multiple neuritis, with the development of unilateral facial paralysis late in the course of the disease. Philadelphia, 1894. 11p. DNLM **90-2217**

ESKRIDGE, Jeremiah Thomas (1848-1902)
Tumor of the brain simulating a vascular lesion; to which is added an account of the autopsy, with remarks. [Philadelphia, 1894.] 14p. DNLM **90-2218**

ESKRIDGE, Jeremiah Thomas (1848-1902)
Trephining in three cases of epilepsy: two of the Jacksonian variety; one due to old meningeal hemorrhage; improvement. [Philadelphia, 1894.] 17p. DNLM **90-2219**

ESKRIDGE, Jeremiah Thomas (1848-1902)
Left hemiplegia followed by loss of the deep and superficial reflexes, considerable muscular atrophy, marked anaesthesia in the discal portions of the limbs, loss of faradaic irritability and reaction of degeneration of the muscles on the paralyzed side. With remarks by Frederick Peterson. [New York, 1895.] 10p. DNLM **90-2220**

ESKRIDGE, Jeremiah Thomas (1848-1902)
Report of cases of brain lesions; abscesses, meningitis, and sinus thrombosis, resulting from disease of the middle ear. Detroit, 1895. 7p. DNLM **90-2221**

ESKRIDGE, Jeremiah Thomas (1848-1902)
Syphilis and alcoholism of the brain, spinal cord, and probably of the nerves of the legs, followed by hysterical contractures of the flexors of the knees and a pronounced variability of certain reflexes. Philadelphia, 1895. 14p. DNLM **90-2222**

ESKRIDGE, Jeremiah Thomas (1848-1902) and F. F. McNAUGHT
Traumatic cyst of the brain from an injury received twenty-five years before; epilepsy; operation; recovery. New York, 1895. 6p. DNLM **90-2223**

ESKRIDGE, Jeremiah Thomas (1848-1902) and Clayton PARKHILL
Two abscesses of the brain caused by septic emboli resulting from an old gunshot wound of the right lung inflicted thirty-two years before; evacuation of one abscess; improvement; death from exhaustion, caused by primary abscess and old lung trouble. New York, 1895. 19p. DNLM **90-2224**

ESKRIDGE, Jeremiah Thomas (1848-1902) and Edmund J. A. ROGERS
Neuralgia of the right trigeminal nerve of eight years' duration. Philadelphia, 1895. 6p. DNLM **90-2225**

ESKRIDGE, Jeremiah Thomas (1848-1902)
Three cases of chronic abscess of the brain. Philadelphia, 1895. 19p. DNLM **90-2226**

ESKRIDGE, Jeremiah Thomas (1848-1902)
Tumor of the cerebellum with bulimia and recurrent apoplectiform seizures. Boston: Damrell & Upham, 1895. 16p. DNLM **90-2227**

ESKRIDGE, Jeremiah Thomas (1848-1902)
Tumor and large cyst of the cerebellum, with symptoms extending over several years. New York, 1895. 11p. DNLM **90-2228**

ESKRIDGE, Jeremiah Thomas (1848-1902)
Diagnosis of chronic abscess of the brain. Philadelphia, 1896. 31p. DNLM **90-2229**

ESKRIDGE, Jeremiah Thomas (1848-1902)
A series of articles on speech-defects as localizing symptoms, from a study of six cases of aphasia. Philadelphia, 1896. DNLM [Contents: Traumatic hemorrhage in the centrum ovale beneath the left angular gyrus. 21p.; Mind and word deafness after depressed fracture of the skull with subcortical hemorrhage; operation; complete recovery.13p.; Glioma of the left centrum ovale, monoplegia, hemiplegia, word-blindness, alexia, agraphia, partial apraxia, and color-blindness; operation; improvement. 18p.; Cyst of the brain in the foot of the left second frontal convolution; motor agraphia (?) from inability to spell; evacuation of the cyst; improvement; traumatic meningeal hemorrhage two months later; second operation; recovery. 26p.; Orolingual paralysis and slight motor disturbance in writing, of thrombotic origin; operation; recovery. 15p.; Motor and sensory aphasia of seven years' duration, due to probable thrombosis followed by angioma; operation; relief of pain; slight improvement in speech. 9p.; Speech defect as localizing symptoms, from a study of six cases of aphasia. 12p.] **90-2230**

ESKRIDGE, Jeremiah Thomas (1848-1902)
Glioma of the brain of twenty-seven months' duration, beginning in the middle of the left Rolandic region, with Jacksonian epilepsy; infiltration of the entire frontal lobe; dementia; aphasia; late operation; death from suppurative meningitis. Denver, 1896. 11p. DNLM **90-2231**

ESKRIDGE, Jeremiah Thomas (1848-1902)
Poliomyelitis occurring in an epidemic form, followed twelve years later by progressive muscular atrophy and lateral sclerosis. Denver, 1896. 8p. DNLM **90-2232**

ESKRIDGE, Jeremiah Thomas (1848-1902)
Temporary abulic agraphia probably due to partial obstruction of the superior longitudinal sinus. Denver, 1896. 8p. DNLM **90-2233**

ESKRIDGE, Jeremiah Thomas (1848-1902)
Difficulties in determining the causes of coma. Denver: Calhoun & Holmes, 1897. 19p. DNLM **90-2234**

ESKRIDGE, Jeremiah Thomas (1848-1902)
Hypnotism in general medicine. A few suggestions from personal experience. Lincoln, Neb., 1897. 6p. DNLM **90-2235**

ESKRIDGE, Jeremiah Thomas (1848-1902)
The professional and technical schools, especially those of medicine, in their relation to the college course. Denver, 1897. 15p. DNLM **90-2236**

ESKRIDGE, Jeremiah Thomas (1848-1902)
Report of a case of intradural spinal tumor extending through the foramen magnum, compressing the extreme upper portion of the cord and almost completely destroying it at the third cervical segment. Philadelphia, 1897. 17p. DNLM **90-2237**

ESKRIDGE, Jeremiah Thomas (1848-1902)
Mutual relations of the railway surgeon and the neurologist. Chicago, 1898. 8p. DNLM **90-2238**

ESKRIDGE, Jeremiah Thomas (1848-1902)
Some of the therapeutic properties of the thyreoid gland. Denver, 1898. 16p. DNLM **90-2239**

ESKRIDGE, Jeremiah Thomas (1848-1902)
Symptoms and diagnosis of caries of the spine. Philadelphia, 1898. 22p. DNLM **90-2240**

ESKRIDGE, Jeremiah Thomas (1848-1902) and Leonard FREEMAN
Intradural spinal tumor opposite the body of the fourth dorsal vertebra; complete paralysis of the parts below the lesion; operation; recovery, with ability to walk without assistance within three months. Philadelphia, 1898. 24p. DNLM **90-2241**

ESKRIDGE, Jeremiah Thomas (1848-1902) and Edmund J. A. RODGERS
Tumor of the spine; compression-myelitis; operation; death on the ninth day. Philadelphia, 1898. 8p. DNLM **90-2242**

ESPEY, John R.
Typhoid fever after double amputation; recovery. Philadelphia, 1895. 4p. DNLM **90-2243**

ESSIG, Charles James (1841-1901)
Dental metallurgy: a manual for the use of dental students.... 3rd ed., rev. Philadelphia: The S. S. White Dental Mfg. Co., 1893. 283p. DLC; MdU-D; PPC **90-2244**

ESSIG, Charles James, ed. (1841-1901)
The American textbook of prosthetic dentistry. In contributions by eminent American authorities. Philadelphia: Lea Bros. & Co., 1897. 760p. DLC; MdU-D; NNNAM; PU **90-2245**

ESTES, W[illiam] L[awrence] (*b.* 1855)
Seven amputations at the hip-joint. [Easton, Pa., 1893.] 10p. DNLM **90-2246**

ESTES, W[illiam] L[awrence] (*b.* 1855)
A contribution to the study of modern amputation. [New York: Trow, 1894.] 24p. DNLM **90-2247**

ESTES, W[illiam] L[awrence] (*b.* 1855)
Gold-foil in the shape of a conical cup introduced into a lacerated cavity of the cerebrum for the purpose of permanently stopping the outflow of cerebral tissue and closing a hole in the membranes. [Philadelphia, 1894.] 4p. DNLM **90-2248**

ESTES, W[illiam] L[awrence] (*b.* 1855)
Multiple synchronous amputations. New York, 1896. 12p. DNLM **90-2249**

ESTES, W[illiam] L[awrence] (*b.* 1855)
The use of gold-foil in fractures of the cranium and resulting hernia cerebri. Chicago, 1896. 8p. DNLM **90-2250**

ESTES, W[illiam] L[awrence] (*b.* 1855)
The address in surgery; State Medical Society of Pennsylvania, 1898. Detroit, Mich.: W. M. Warren, 1898. 14p. DNLM **90-2251**

ESTES, W[illiam] L[awrence] (*b.* 1855)
Surgical shock. Memphis, 1898. 10p. DNLM
90-2252

EVANS, B[ritton] D. (1858-1920)
Periodic insantiy, in which the exciting cause appears to be the menstrual function; report of a typical case. Philadelphia, 1893. 7p. DNLM **90-2253**

EVANS, E. C.
Acute articular rheumatism. Philadelphia, 1891. 2 l. DNLM
90-2254

EVANS, George (1844-1942)
Pulpless teeth and their treatment. [Philadelphia, 1893.] 10p. DNLM **90-2255**

EVANS, George (1844-1942)
A practical treatise on artificial crown- and bridge-work. . . . 3rd ed., rev. and enl. With 631 illustrations. Philadelphia: The S. S. White Dental Mfg. Co., 1893. 346p. DLC; NNNAM; PPC; PU **90-2256**

EVANS, George (1844-1942)
A practical treatise on artificial crown- and bridge-work. . . . 4th ed., rev. With 631 illustrations. Philadelphia: The S. S. White Dental Mfg. Co., 1893. 346p. DLC; MdU-D; PPC; PU
90-2257

EVANS, George (1844-1942)
A practical treatise on artificial crown- and bridge-work. . . . [5th ed.] Philadelphia: S. S. White Dental Mfg. Co., 1896. 337p. DNLM; MdU-D; NNNAM; PPC
90-2258

EVANS, George A[lfred] (1850-1925)
Mensuration in the physical diagnosis of pulmonary phthisis. [Brooklyn, 1893.] 32p. DNLM **90-2259**

EVANS, T[homas] C[rain] (*b.* 1860)
Report on otological progress. [St. Louis, 1893.] 7p. DNLM
90-2260

EVANS, T[homas] C[rain] (*b.* 1860)
Chancre of the tonsil; report of a case. New York: D. Appleton & Co., 1895. 3p. DNLM **90-2261**

EVANS, T[homas] C[rain] (*b.* 1860)
A new operation for congenital ptosis, with report of two cases. New York: D. Appleton & Co., 1895. 9p. DNLM
90-2262

EWALD, Carl Anton (1845-1915)
The diseases of the stomach. . . . Authorized transl. from the 2nd German ed. with special additions by the author; by Morris Manges. . . . New York: D. Appleton & Co., 1892. 497p. DLC; DNLM; NNNAM; PPC **90-2263**

EWALD, Carl Anton (1845-1915)
The diseases of the stomach. . . . Transl. and ed., with numerous additions, from the 3rd German ed. by Morris Manges. . . . 2nd rev. ed. New York: D. Appleton & Co., 1897. 602p. DLC; NNNAM; PPC; PU **90-2264**

EWART, William (1848-1929)
Cardiac outlines for clinical clerks and practitioners and first principles in the physical examination of the heart for the beginner. New York: G. P. Putnam's Sons, 1892. 165p. 7 plates. DLC **90-2265**

EWART, William (1848-1929)
Heart studies, chiefly clinical. I. The pulsations; a study in tactile sphygmology. New York: William Wood & Co., 1895. 486p. 3 plates. CtY-M; DNLM; NNNAM; PPC
90-2266

EWART, William (1848-1929)
Gout and goutiness, and their treatment. New York: William Wood & Co., 1896. 589p. DNLM; IU-M; NNNAM; PPC
90-2267

EWING, James (1866-1943)
A study of the leucocytosis of lobar pneumonia. New York: D. Appleton & Co., 1893. 17p. DNLM
90-2268

EWING, James (1866-1943)
Toxic hypoleucocytosis. New York: D. Appleton & Co., 1895. 19p. DNLM **90-2269**

EWING, James (1866-1943)
The leucocytosis of diphtheria under the influence of serum therapy. New York: D. Appleton & Co., 1895. 42p. 1 plate. DNLM; NNNAM **90-2270**

EWING, James (1866-1943)
The lymphatic constitution, and its relation to some forms of sudden death. New York: D. Appleton & Co., 1897. 21p. DNLM; NNNAM **90-2271**

EWING, James (1866-1943)
Studies on ganglion cells; a preliminary communication. New York, 1898. 16p. DNLM **90-2272**

EWING, James (1866-1943)
Preliminary report on the results of blood examinations at Camp Wikoff, August and September, 1898. New York, 1899. 23p. DNLM; NNNAM **90-2273**

EWING, James (1866-1943)
Studies on ganglion cells. Utica: State Hosp. Press, 1899. 181p. 6 plates. DNLM **90-2274**

EXMOUTH, Charles Ernest Pellew (*b.* 1863)
Manual of practical medical and physiological chemistry. . . . New York: D. Appleton & Co., 1892. 314p. col. plates. DLC; NNNAM **90-2275**

EXMOUTH, Charles Ernest Pellew (*b.* 1863)
Lessons in toxicology for laboratory use. . . . New York, 1895. 37p. DLC; NNNAM **90-2276**

EYER, Alvin
Injury to the thoracic duct, with an unique and inevitable death by inanition. New York: Troy Directory, 1891. 11p. DNLM; NNNAM **90-2277**

FAIRCHILD, Maria A[ugusta] (*b.* 1834)
Woman and health. A mother's hygienic hand book. . . . Quincy, Ill.: The Author; Peoria, Ill.: Printed by J. W. Franks & Sons, 1890. 384p. DLC **90-2278**

FAIRFIELD COUNTY MEDICAL ASSOCIATION
Centennial celebration. [Danbury, Conn., 1892.] 104p. DNLM
90-2279

FARLOW, J[ohn] W[oodford] (1853-1937)
Use of resorcine in whooping-cough. Boston: Damrell & Upham, 1890. 7p. DNLM **90-2280**

FARLOW, J[ohn] W[oodford] (1853-1937)
Hypertrophy in the post-nasal space, especially after childhood. Boston: Damrell & Upham, 1894. 8p. DNLM
90-2281

FARLOW, J[ohn] W[oodford] (1853-1937)
A case of subglottic fibroma; removal by tracheotomy and curetting. New York, 1897. 7p. DNLM **90-2282**

FARLOW, J[ohn] W[oodford] (1853-1937)
A case of disease of the antrum and the frontal and ethmoidal sinuses. New York, 1898. 4p. DNLM; NNNAM
90-2283

FARNHAM, Edwin
Season and deaths from certain diseases in Cambridge, 1880-89, inclusive. [Boston, 1892.] 1 sheet, 1 table. DNLM
90-2284

FARNHAM, Edwin
A table of mortalities. Cambridge. Mortality per 1,000 living in five-year periods. [Boston, 1892.] 1 galley sheet. DNLM
90-2285

FARNHAM, Edwin
Some conditions affecting the health of students. [Boston], 1893. 11p. DNLM **90-2286**

FARNUM, Edward J[ames] (*b.* 1860)
Deformities. A text-book on orthopedic surgery. Chicago: Med. Press Co., 1898. 544p. DNLM; IU-M; OCIM
90-2287

FARRAR, J[oseph] D.
Intestinal antisepsis in enteric fever by means of subiodide of bismuth and salol. [Baltimore, 1893.] 1 l. DNLM
90-2288

FARRINGTON, Ernest Albert (1847-1885)
A clinical materia medica. . . . 2nd ed. Philadelphia: Hahnemann Publishing House, 1890. 770p. OCLloyd; PPC; PPHa **90-2289**

FARRINGTON, Ernest Albert (1847-1885)
A clinical material medica. . . . 3rd ed. rev. Philadelphia: Boericke & Tafel, 1897. 770p. OCLloyd; PPHa
90-2290

FAULKNER, Richard B[iddle] (*b.* 1853)
Free hydrochloric acid; is its absence from the stomach a sign of cancer? Chicago, 1895. 8p. DNLM **90-2291**

FAULKNER, Thomas
The cottage physician. Best known methods of treatment in all diseases, accidents and emergencies of the home, prepared by the ablest physicians in the leading schools of medicine: allopathy, homoeopathy, etc., etc. By Thomas Faulkner . . . [and] J. H. Carmichael. . . . Assisted by other able physicians and surgeons of America and Europe. . . . Nearly 200 illustrations. Springfield, Mass., Cincinnati, [etc.]: King, Richardson & Co.; Omaha: Clark Publishing Co., 1892. 642p. DLC
90-2292

FAXON, Annie E.
A brief record of the physicians of Quincy, Massachusetts, from the earliest times, comp. and pub. by Annie E. Faxon, for the benefit of the hospital fund, June 17, 1890. [Boston: Press of Rockwell and Churchill], 1890. 31p. DLC; MBM
90-2293

FEICK BROTHERS
. . . Illustrated catalogue and price list of surgical instruments, artificial limbs, deformity apparatus, ... Pittsburgh, 1895. 104p. NNNAM **90-2294**

FELTER, Harvey Wickes (1865-1927) and J. U. LLOYD
King's American dispensatory. . . . Entirely rewritten and enlarged. [18th ed., 3rd rev.]. Cincinnati: Ohio Valley Co., 1898-1900. 2 v. DLC; OCLloyd **90-2295**

FENGER, Christian (1840-1902)
A case of elephantiasis of the scrotum; with remarks on its operative treatment. [Philadelphia, 1891.] 9p. DNLM
90-2296

FENGER, Christian (1840-1902)
Demonstration of specimens from operations on the kidney, with the presentation of patients. Chicago, 1893. 16p. DNLM
90-2297

FENGER, Christian (1840-1902)
Hyperplastic salpingitis and its operative treatment by drainage. New York: Trow, 1893. 23p. DNLM
90-2298

FENGER, Christian (1840-1902)
Remarks on appendicitis, with reports of cases. New York: William Wood & Co., 1893. 39p. DNLM
90-2299

FENGER, Christian (1840-1902)
Benignant tumors of the ileum. Chicago, 1894. 11p. DNLM
90-2300

FENGER, Christian (1840-1902)
Operation for the relief of valve-formation and stricture of the ureter in hydro- or pyonephrosis. Chicago, 1894. 28p. DNLM **90-2301**

FENGER, Christian (1840-1902)
Surgery of the ureter. Philadelphia, 1894. 40p. DNLM
90-2302

FENGER, Christian (1840-1902)
Basal hernias of the brain. Philadelphia, 1895. 16p. DNLM
90-2303

FENGER, Christian (1840-1902)
Cases of hernia of the bladder met with during operations for inguinal and femoral hernia. Philadelphia, 1895. 18p. DNLM
90-2304

FENGER, Christian (1840-1902)
Conservative operative treatment of sacculated kidneys; cystonephrosis. Philadelphia, 1896. 51p. DNLM
90-2305

FENGER, Christian (1840-1902)
Stones in the common duct and their surgical treatment; with remarks on the ball-valve action of floating choledochus-stones. Philadelphia, 1896. 51p. DNLM
90-2306

FENNER, B[yron] (*b.* 1844)
Fenner's complete formulary, containing original and selected working formulas for all preparations generally used or required in the practice of pharmacy and the business of the chemist, [etc.]. 10th ed. Westfield, N.Y., 1894. 1509p. DNLM; OCLloyd **90-2307**

FENNER, B[yron] (*b.* **1844)**
Fenner's hand-book of the United States Pharmacopoeia; seventh revision, 1890-93; a key to all official preparations; comparing the preparations of the present pharmacopoeia with those formerly official and converting the metric weight and measure directed in the pharmacopoeia into proportionate commercial weight and measure; with medicinal uses and doses of new preparations, convenient tables, etc., compiled and arranged by . . . . Westfield, N.Y.: B. Fenner, 1894. 221p. DNLM; OCLloyd **90-2308**

FENNER, B[yron] (*b.* **1844)**
Fenner's proprietary medicine, formulary, containing a complete line of formulas for patent or proprietary medicines similar to those most popular on the market, [ect.]. Westfield, N.Y., 1897. 68 l. fol. DNLM; OCLloyd
90-2309

FENWICK, Kenneth Neander (1852-1896)
Abdominal hysteropexy. New York, 1894. 3p. DNLM
90-2310

FENWICK, Samuel (1821-1902)
Medical diagnosis. 7th ed., revised and enlarged. Philadelphia: P. Blakiston, Son & Co., 1891. 352p. DNLM; NNNAM; PPC; PU **90-2311**

FENWICK, Samuel (1821-1902)
The student's guide to medical diagnosis. [8th ed.] By Samuel Fenwick and W. Soltan Fenwick. Philadelphia: P. Blakiston, Son & Co., 1897. 468p. CtY-M; DNLM; IU-M; PPC
90-2312

FERGUSON, John (1854-1939)
The treatment of internal hemorrhages. [New York, 1890.] 5p. DNLM **90-2313**

FERGUSON, John (1854-1939)
Epilepsia procursiva. [New York: D. Appleton & Co., 1891.] 10p. DNLM **90-2314**

FERGUSON, John (1854-1939)
Atheto-choreic movements. [New York, 1892.] 6p. DNLM
90-2315

FERNALD, Walter E[lmore] (1859-1924)
The history of the treatment of the feeble-minded. Boston: G. H. Ellis, 1893. 21p. DNLM **90-2316**

FERNANDEZ [de IBARRA], Augustin M.
Notes and remarks on the birth of a double foetus, somewhat resembling the Siamese twins. [Philadelphia, 1890.] 9p. DNLM
90-2317

FETTEROLF, George
Two thousand questions on practical anatomy; prepared for students of medicine and dentistry. . . . Philadelphia: F. W. S. Langmaid, 1899. 212p. DLC; PPC; PU
90-2318

FICK, Adolf Eugen (1829-1901)
Diseases of the eye and ophthalmoscopy. A handbook for physicians and students. Authorized transl. by Albert B. Hale. With a glossary. Philadelphia: P. Blakiston, Son & Co., 1896. 488p. DNLM; MBM; NNNAM; PPC **90-2319**

FILLEBROWN, Thomas (1836-1908)
Hypnotism as applied to dentistry. Chicago, 1892. 14p. DNLM
90-2320

FILLEBROWN, Thomas (1836-1908)
A new apparatus for continuing anesthesia while operating on or in the mouth. Philadelphia, 1895. 4p. DNLM
90-2321

FILLEBROWN, Thomas (1836-1908)
A study of the relation of the frontal sinus to the antrum. New York & Philadelphia, 1897. 6p. DNLM
90-2322

FILLEBROWN, Thomas (1836-1908)
Report of operations on hare-lip and cleft palate. Boston, 1898. 26p. DNLM **90-2323**

FINGER, Ernst (1856-1939)
Gonorrhoea: being the translation of Blenorrhoea of the sexual organs and its complications. . . . 3rd rev. and enl. ed. . . . New York: William Wood & Co., 1894. 324p. col. plates. DLC; NNNAM **90-2324**

FINKELPEARL, Harry
A syllabus of materia medica and pharmacognosy. With especial reference to the methods of prescribing, compounding and administering medicinal substances. . . . Pittsburgh, Pa.: Press of W. T. Nicholson, 1895. 338p. DLC; OCLloyd
90-2325

FIREBAUGH, Ellen M.
The physician's wife and the things that pertain to her life. . . . Philadelphia: The F. A. Davis Co.; [etc., etc.], 1894. 186p. DLC; ICU; MB; NN **90-2326**

FIRST annual nurse register. A book of reference for families and physicians. New York: J. H. Vail & Co., 1891. 33p. DNLM; NNNAM **90-2327**

FISCH, C[arl]
On the systematology of the bacteria. St. Louis, 1896. 14p. DNLM **90-2328**

FISCH, C[arl]
Infantile dysauxesis. St. Louis, 1897. 23p. DNLM
90-2329

FISCH, C[arl]
The antitoxic and bactericidal properties of the serum of horses treated with Koch's new tuberculin. Chicago, 1897. 24p. DNLM [*also*: Chicago: J. Hoban, 1897. 31p.]
90-2330

FISCH, C[arl]
Can tuberculosis be diagnosed from the blood? St. Louis, 1897. 16p. DNLM **90-2331**

FISCH, C[arl]
Experimental researches about mixed infection in chronic pulmonary tuberculosis. St. Louis, 1898. 20p. DNLM
90-2332

FISCH, C[arl]
Some experiments on the assimilation of diphtheria antitoxine. New York, 1898. 13p. DNLM
90-2333

FISCHER, Louis (*b.* **1864)**
The treatment of pertussis by bromoform. New York, 1890. 9p. DNLM **90-2334**

FISCHER, Louis (*b.* 1864)
An early method of diagnosis in diphtheria; with demonstrations. New York, 1891. 11p. DNLM **90-2335**

FISCHER, Louis (*b.* 1864)
An early method of diagnosis in diphtheria; with demonstrations. Frühzeitige Diagnose der Diphtherie, mit Demonstrationen. New York, 1891. 9p. DNLM **90-2336**

FISCHER, Louis (*b.* 1864)
The treatment of summer complaint, or gastro-enteritis catarrhalis acute, in children. New York, 1892. 5p. DNLM **90-2337**

FISCHER, Louis (*b.* 1864)
Antitoxine, its value in diphtheria; clinical experience in Berlin and New York. New York, 1894. 8p. DNLM **90-2338**

FISCHER, Louis (*b.* 1864)
Did stomatitis diphtheritica in an infant cause mastitis diphtheritica while nursing by infection? New York, 1894. 3p. DNLM **90-2339**

FISCHER, Louis (*b.* 1864)
Some practical points in infant feeding. New York, 1894. 3p. DNLM **90-2340**

FISCHER, Louis (*b.* 1864)
The modern treatment of diphtheria. New York, 1894. 8p. DNLM **90-2341**

FISCHER, Louis (*b.* 1864)
Antitoxine in diphtheria in Berlin, New York, and in the Municipal Hospital of Philadelphia. Philadelphia: Lea Bros. & Co., 1895. 14p. DNLM **90-2342**

FISCHER, Louis (*b.* 1864)
Behandlung der Lungentuberkulose bei Kindern. New York, 1895. 1 l. DNLM **90-2343**

FISCHER, Louis (*b.* 1864)
Clinical experience with antitoxin in private and hospital practice in the treatment of diphtheria (all forms). Chicago, 1895. 8p. DNLM **90-2344**

FISCHER, Louis (*b.* 1864)
A plea for the more extensive use of antitoxine in diphtheria; résumé of one year's experience; indications and contraindications for its use, with some practical points in the application of the same. New York: D. Appleton & Co., 1895. 31p. DNLM **90-2345**

FISCHER, Louis (*b.* 1864)
The treatment of pulmonary tuberculosis. New York, 1895. 12p. DNLM **90-2346**

FISCHER, Louis (*b.* 1864)
The treatment of summer complaint, or gastro-enteritis catarrhalis acuta, including cholera infantum in children. New York, 1895. 18p. DNLM **90-2347**

FISCHER, Louis (*b.* 1864)
The treatment of diphtheria: an inquiry into modern methods employed at Berlin in the summer of 1896. New York, 1896. 24p. DNLM **90-2348**

FISCHER, Louis (*b.* 1864)
The treatment of hyperpyrexia (high fever) in children; with some illustrative cases. New York, 1896. 24p. DNLM **90-2349**

FISCHER, Louis (*b.* 1864)
Some practical points on infant feeding and infant feces. Chicago, 1897. 15p. DNLM **90-2350**

FISCHER, Louis (*b.* 1864) and Herman POOLE
The clinical value and chemical results of using Professor Gaertner's mother milk in children. New York: Publ. Print. Co., 1897. 23p. DNLM **90-2351**

FISCHER, Louis (*b.* 1864)
Clinical experience with anti-streptococcus serum. New York, 1898. 12p. DNLM **90-2352**

FISCHER, Louis (*b.* 1864)
Infantile tuberculosis. Chicago, 1898. 8p. DNLM **90-2353**

FISCHER, Louis (*b.* 1864)
Dry antitoxine. A clinical study of its value in diphtheria. New York, 1899. 15p. DNLM **90-2354**

FISCHER, Louis (*b.* 1864)
Treatment of summer diarrhea in infants. Detroit, 1899. 10p. DNLM **90-2355**

FISH, Hamilton
The importance of blood examinations in reference to general anaesthetization and operative procedures. Philadelphia, 1899. 12p. DNLM **90-2356**

FISH, Hamilton
Asepsis in country and private practice; a new sterilizer. Denver, 1899. 7p. DNLM **90-2357**

FISHER, Charles Edmund (1853-1932)
A hand-book on the diseases of children and their homoeopathic treatment. . . . Chicago: Medical Century Co., 1895. 905p. plates. DLC; IU-M; OCIM **90-2358**

FISHER, Charles Edmund (1853-1932)
A homoeopathic text-book of surgery, ed. by Charles E. Fisher . . . and T. L. Macdonald. . . . Chicago: Medical Century Co.; New York, [etc.]: Boericke & Tafel, 1896. 1661p. col. plates. DLC; DNLM; NNNAM; PPC **90-2359**

FISHER, C[hester] Irving (*b.* 1847)
Hospital equipment. Albany, N.Y., 1898. 23p. DNLM **90-2360**

FISHER, John M.
Clinical observations on ventrofixation of the uterus. New York, 1896. 6p. DNLM **90-2361**

FISK, A[rthur] L[yman]
Photograph and skiagraph of a gouty hand. Philadelphia, 1897. 2 l. 2 plates. DNLM **90-2362**

FISK, Samuel A[ugustus], Jr.
Variations in typhoid fever, with illustrative charts. Boston: Damrell & Upham, 1893. 15p. 15 charts. DNLM **90-2363**

FISK, Samuel A[ugustus], Jr.
Abortive and afebrile typhoid fever. [Philadelphia: Lea Bros. & Co., 1894.] 12p. DNLM **90-2364**

FISK, Samuel A[ugustus], Jr.
Digestion vs. drugs in the treatment of pulmonary tuberculosis. [Philadelphia], 1897. 4p. DNLM **90-2365**

FITCH, Charles W[ellington] (1852-1934)
Diseases of women. Their causes, prevention and cure. . . . [Bridgeport, Conn.: City Steam Printing Co., 1890.] 48p. DLC **90-2366**

FITCH, Samuel Sheldon
Six lectures on the uses of the lungs, causes, prevention, and cure of pulmonary consumption, asthma, and diseases of the heart. . . . New York: Carlisle, 1897. 324p. NNNAM **90-2367**

FITE, C[ampbell] C.
Institutions for consumptives. A review of the newer and more successful method of treating this disease, together with a description of institutions especially adapted to this work. [New York, 1891.] 16p. DNLM **90-2368**

FITE, C[ampbell] C.
Anti-diphtheritic and anti-streptococcic serums. Their nature, method of production, and application for the relief of disease. Baltimore, 1896. 8p. DNLM **90-2369**

FITE, C[ampbell] C.
Diastase in therapeutics. [1897.] 18p. DNLM **90-2370**

FITE, C[ampbell] C.
A plea for a uniform diastase test. Chicago, 1897. 8p. DNLM **90-2371**

FITE, C[ampbell] C.
Solution of the proprietary medicine question. Philadelphia, 1898. 8p. DNLM **90-2372**

FITZ, George Wells (*b.* 1860)
Problems of physical education. Cambridge, 1893. 6p. DNLM **90-2373**

FITZ, George Wells (*b.* 1860)
A leg-apparatus for spastic and paralytic cases. [Philadelphia, 1895.] 3p. DNLM **90-2374**

FITZ, George Wells (*b.* 1860)
A study of types of respiratory movements. New York, 1896. 16p. 1 plate. DNLM **90-2375**

FITZ, George Wells (*b.* 1860)
Bed posture as an etiological factor in spinal curvature. [Philadelphia, 1898.] 3p. DNLM **90-2376**

FITZ, George Wells (*b.* 1860)
The hygiene of instruction in elementary schools. Cambridge, Mass.: Caustic & Claflin, 1898. 7p. DNLM **90-2377**

FITZ, George Wells (*b.* 1860)
Play as a factor in development. Boston, Mass.: J. P. Shults, 1898. 7p. DNLM **90-2378**

FITZ, Reginald H[eber] (1843-1913)
Intestinal perforation in typhoid fever; its prognosis and treatment. [Philadelphia, 1891.] 15p. DNLM **90-2379**

FITZ, Reginald H[eber] (1843-1913)
Annual address. Intra-peritoneal haemorrhage. Baltimore, 1893. 13p. DNLM [*also*: Baltimore, 1893. 9p.] **90-2380**

FITZ, Reginald H[eber] (1843-1913)
The legislative control of medical practice. Boston: D. Clapp & Son, 1894. 86p. DNLM; MBM; NNNAM **90-2381**

FITZ, Reginald H[eber] (1843-1913)
The rise and fall of the licensed physician in Massachusetts, 1781-1860. [Philadelphia, 1894.] 18p. DNLM **90-2382**

FITZ, Reginald H[eber] (1843-1913)
The significance of albumosuria in medical practice; suggested by a fatal case of albumosuric myxoedema treated with thyroid extract. Philadelphia, 1898. 13p. DNLM **90-2383**

FITZ, Reginald H[eber] (1843-1913) and Elliott P. JOSLIN
Diabetes mellitus at the Massachusetts General Hospital from 1824 to 1898. A study of the medical records. Chicago, 1898. 20p. DNLM **90-2384**

FITZPATRICK, Charles B[orromeo]
Notes on the preparation of diphtheria antitoxine. New York: D. Appleton & Co., 1895. 32p. 1 chart. DNLM; NNNAM **90-2385**

FITZPATRICK, Charles B[orromeo]
A preliminary note on the investigation and preparation of the antitoxine of the bubonic plague at the New York Quarantine Laboratory, Staten Island. New York: D. Appleton & Co., 1897. 7p. DNLM **90-2386**

FITZPATRICK, Thomas V.
Tonsillotomy and its after-treatment. [Cincinnati, 1891.] 12p. DNLM **90-2387**

FLAGG, J[osiah] F[oster] (1828-1903)
Plastics and plastic fillings; as pertaining to the filling of all cavities of decay in teeth below medium in structure, and to difficult and inaccessible cavities in teeth of all grades of structure. 3rd ed., revised. Philadelphia: P. Blakiston, Son & Co., 1890. 215p. DLC; DNLM; MdU-D; PPC **90-2388**

FLAGG, J[osiah] F[oster] (1828-1903)
Plastics and plastic fillings, as pertaining to the filling of all cavities of decay in teeth. . . . 4th ed., revised. 215p. 14 plates. DNLM; PPC; PU **90-2389**

FLAGG, J[osiah] F[oster] (1828-1903)
Preparation of pulp-cavity and canals. Philadelphia, 1896. 4p. DNLM **90-2390**

FLETCHER, Robert (1823-1912)
Anatomy and art. The annual address read before the Philosophical Society of Washington, December 12, 1894. Washington: Judd & Detweiler, 1895. 24p. DNLM **90-2391**

FLETCHER, Robert (1823-1912)
Medical lore in the older English dramatists and poets (exclusive of Shakespeare). Read before the Historical Club of the Johns Hopkins Hospital, May 13, 1895. Baltimore: Friedenwald Co., 1895. 35p. DNLM; PPC
90-2392

FLETCHER, Robert (1823-1912)
The witches' pharmacopoeia. Read before the Historical Club of the Johns Hopkins Hospital, April 13, 1896. Baltimore, 1896. 30p. DNLM **90-2393**

FLETCHER, Robert (1823-1912)
Scopelism. An essay read before the Anthropological Society of Washington, April 20, 1897. Washington: Judd & Detweiler, 1897. 15p. DNLM **90-2394**

FLETCHER, Robert (1823-1912)
A tragedy of the great plague of Milan in 1630. Baltimore: Friedenwald Co., 1898. 16p. 2 plates. DNLM
90-2395

FLETCHER, William B[aldwin] (1837-1907)
Purulent absorption considered as a cause of insanity. Indianapolis, 1892. 4p. DNLM **90-2396**

FLETCHER, William B[aldwin] (1837-1907)
Stray papers on cerebral subjects. [Indianapolis]: Cottman, 1892. 91p. DNLM **90-2397**

FLEXNER, Simon (1863-1946)
The diagnostic value of diphtheritic bacillus. [Louisville, 1891.] 22p. DNLM **90-2398**

FLEXNER, Simon (1863-1946)
A peculiar glioma (neuroepithelioma?) of the retina. [Baltimore, 1891.] 8 l. DNLM **90-2399**

FLEXNER, Simon (1863-1946)
Amobae in an abscess of the jaw. [Baltimore, 1892.] 4 l. DNLM **90-2400**

FLEXNER, Simon (1863-1946)
A case of primary carcinoma of the pancreas with multiple carcinosis. The organisms of cancer. [Baltimore, 1892.] 8 l. DNLM **90-2401**

FLEXNER, Simon (1863-1946)
Peritonitis caused by the Proteus vulgaris. [Baltimore, 1893.] 5 l. DNLM **90-2402**

FLEXNER, Simon (1863-1946)
Tuberculosis of the oesophagus. (Larvae of diptera in the uclers.) [Baltimore, 1893.] 7 l. DNLM **90-2403**

FLEXNER, Simon (1863-1946)
The pathologic changes caused by certain so-called toxalbumins. An experimental study. [Philadelphia: Lea Bros. & Co., 1894.] 27p. DNLM **90-2404**

FLEXNER, Simon (1863-1946) and Lewellys F[ranklin] BARKER
A contribution to our knowledge of epidemic cerebro-spinal meningitis. [Philadelphia: Lea Bros. & Co., 1894.] 34p. DNLM
90-2405

FLEXNER, Simon (1863-1946)
Bacillus pyogenes filiformis (nov. spec.). Baltimore, 1895. 7p. DNLM **90-2406**

FLEXNER, Simon (1863-1946)
The bacteriology and pathology of diphtheria. Baltimore, 1895. 15p. DNLM **90-2407**

FLEXNER, Simon (1863-1946) and Herbert D. PEASE
Primary diphtheria of the lips and gums. Baltimore, 1895. 10p. DNLM **90-2408**

FLEXNER, Simon (1863-1946)
A statistical and experimental study of terminal infections. New York, 1896. 18p. DNLM **90-2409**

FLEXNER, Simon (1863-1946)
A study of the bacillus (leptothrix?) pyogenes filiformis (nov. spec.) and of its pathogenic action. New York, 1896. 70p. 2 plates. DNLM **90-2410**

FLICK, Lawrence F[rancis] (1856-1938)
Special hospitals for the treatment of tuberculosis. Philadelphia, 1890. 37p. DNLM **90-2411**

FLICK, Lawrence F[rancis] (1856-1938)
The prevention of tuberculosis; a century's experience in Italy under the influence of the preventive laws of the kingdom of Naples, enacted in 1782. New York, [1891]. 14p. DNLM
90-2412

FLICK, Lawrence F[rancis] (1856-1938)
Some new points in the treatment of tuberculosis. [Philadelphia, 1891.] 6p. DNLM **90-2413**

FLICK, Lawrence F[rancis] (1856-1938)
Practical measures for the prevention of tuberculosis. [Philadelphia, 1893.] 20p. DNLM **90-2414**

FLICK, Lawrence F[rancis] (1856-1938)
The early recognition of tuberculosis. [Philadelphia, 1894.] 8p. DNLM **90-2415**

FLICK, Lawrence F[rancis] (1856-1938)
Prophylaxis in the treatment of tuberculosis. [Philadelphia, 1894.] 5p. DNLM **90-2416**

FLICK, Lawrence F[rancis] (1856-1938)
The control of tuberculosis. Harrisburgh: C. M. Busch, 1897. 7p. DNLM **90-2417**

FLICK, Lawrence F[rancis] (1856-1938)
Immunity as against heredity in tuberculosis. Asheville, N.C., 1899. 11p. DNLM **90-2418**

FLINT, Austin (1812-1886)
A manual of auscultation and percussion; embracing the physical diagnosis of diseases of the lungs and heart, and of thoracic aneurism. . . . 5th ed., thoroughly rev. By J. C. Wilson. . . . Philadelphia: Lea Bros. & Co., 1890. 268p. DLC; NNNAM; PPC; PU **90-2419**

FLINT, Austin (1812-1886)
A treatise on the principles and practice of medicine; designed for the use of practitioners and students of medicine. . . . 7th ed., thoroughly rev. by Frederick P. Henry. . . . Philadelphia: Lea Bros. & Co., 1894. 1143p. DLC; NNNAM; PPC; PPJ
90-2420

FLINT, Austin, Jr. (1836-1915)
Remarks on fermentative dyspepsia. New York: J. Wyeth & Bro., [1893]. 7p. DNLM **90-2421**

FLINT, Austin, Jr. (1836-1915)
The coming role of the medical profession in the scientific treatment of crime and criminals. New York, 1895. 32p. DNLM **90-2422**

FLINT, Austin, Jr. (1836-1915)
Stercorin and cholesteraemia. New York, 1897. 15p. DNLM **90-2423**

FLINT'S encyclopedia of medicine and surgery, by various writers; arranged upon a new system, which embodies the methods of treatment employed by eminent practitioners of medicine, compiled under the direction of the publishers. . . . 2nd rev. ed. New York: J. B. Flint & Co., 1898. 1558p. DLC; NNNAM **90-2424**

FLOWER, Sydney B[lanchard] (*b.* 1867)
A study in hypnotism. Chicago: Psychic Publ. Co., 1896. 226p. DNLM; ICU **90-2425**

FLOWER, Sydney B[lanchard] (*b.* 1867)
Hypnotism up to date. Chicago: C. H. Kerr & Co., 1896. 161p. DNLM; ICU **90-2426**

FLOWER, Sydney B[lanchard] (*b.* 1867)
A study in hypnotism. Chicago: C. H. Kerr & Co., 1897. 194p. DNLM; ICU **90-2427**

FOLSOM, Charles F[ollen] (1842-1907)
Henry Ingersoll Bowditch. [Boston, 1892.] 9p. DNLM **90-2428**

THE FOO & WING HERB COMPANY, LOS ANGELES
. . . The science of oriental medicine. A concise discussion of its principles and methods. . . . Comp. by the Foo and Wing Herb Company . . . Los Angeles, Cal.: G. Rice & Sons, 1897. 238p. DLC **90-2429**

THE FOO & WING HERB COMPANY, LOS ANGELES
. . . The practice of oriental medicine . . . with special reference to herb treatment. . . . Los Angeles, Cal.: The Foo & Wing Herb Co., [1898]. 126p. DLC **90-2430**

FOOTE, Charles J.
A bacteriologic study of oysters, with special reference to them as a source of typhoid infection. Philadelphia, 1895. 13p. DNLM **90-2431**

FOOTE, Edward Bliss (1829-1906)
Plain home talk about the human system—the habits of men and women—the causes and prevention of disease—our sexual relations and social natures. Embracing Medical common sense applied to causes, prevention, and cure of chronic diseases. . . . Rev. in 1896 by Drs. E. B. Foote, Sr. and Jr. . . . New York: Murray Hill Publishing Co., [etc., etc.], 1896. 959p. col. plates. DLC; NNNAM **90-2432**

FOOTE, Edward Bond (1854-1912)
Everybody's health primer; or, What the doctor says about ordinary habits of living favorable to maintaining good health and essential to regaining it. . . . New York: Murray Hill Publishing Co., 1891. 14p. DLC **90-2433**

FOOTE, Edward Bond (1854-1912)
. . . Food. "What's best to eat," together with Everybody's health primer, or What the doctor says about ordinary habits of living favorable to maintaining health and essential to regaining it. . . . New York: Murray Hill Publishing Co., 1891. 47, 13p. DLC **90-2434**

FOOTE, E[dward] B[ond] (1854-1912)
Auto-toxaemia, self-poisoned blood. Explaining the origin, relation and treatment of a variety of common ailments and chronic diseases. . . . New York: Murray Hill Publishing Co., 1893. 149p. DLC; NNNAM **90-2435**

FOOTE, E[dward] M[ilton] (*b.* 1866)
Operative surgery in the service of William T. Bull, M.D., at the New York Hospital, from July 1, 1890, to Jan. 1, 1895. New York, 1895. 128p. DNLM; NNNAM **90-2436**

FOOTE, E[dward] M[ilton] (*b.* 1866)
Ingrowing nail; a comparison of methods of operation. Philadelphia, 1899. 11p. DNLM **90-2437**

FORBES, W[illiam] S[mith] (1832-1905)
The removal of stone in the bladder. Philadelphia, 1894. 10p. DNLM **90-2438**

FORD, Campbell
An interrupted stitch by a continuous method. San Francisco, 1896. 3p. DNLM **90-2439**

FORD, Willis E.
The methods of administering galvanism in gynecology. [Philadelphia, 1892.] 8p. DNLM **90-2440**

FORD, Willis E.
The ultimate results of trachelorrhaphy. New York, 1895. 4p. DNLM **90-2441**

FORD, W. F.
Illustrated catalogue of orthopaedical apparatus and surgical instruments. New York, [*c.* 1891]. 182p. NNNAM **90-2442**

FORD, W. F.
Illustrated catalogue of orthopaedical apparatus. . . . New York, [*c.* 1897]. 57p. NNNAM **90-2443**

FORDYCE, John Addison (1858-1925)
Microscopic examination in Dr. Bronson's case of acne varioliformis of the extremities. New York: D. Appleton & Co., [1891]. 3 l. 2 plates. DNLM **90-2444**

FORDYCE, John Addison (1858-1925)
Multiple pigmented sarcoma of the skin (Kaposi). New York: D. Appleton & Co., [1891]. 7p. 1 plate. DNLM **90-2445**

FORDYCE, John Addison (1858-1925)
Peripheral neuritis of syphilitic origin. New York: D. Appleton & Co., [1891]. 4 l. DNLM **90-2446**

FORDYCE, John Addison (1858-1925)
Multiple benign cystic epithelioma of the skin. New York: D. Appleton & Co., [1892]. 15p. 1 plate. DNLM **90-2447**

FORDYCE, John Addison (1858-1925)
A contribution to the pathology of acne varioliformis Hebrae. New York: D. Appleton & Co., 1894. 10p. DNLM **90-2448**

FORDYCE, John Addison (1858-1925)
Adeno-carcinoma of the skin originating in the coil glands. New York: D. Appleton & Co., [1895]. 10p. 2 plates. DNLM **90-2449**

FORDYCE, John Addison (1858-1925)
Note on drug eruptions. New York: D. Appleton & Co., 1895. 4p. DNLM **90-2450**

FORDYCE, John Addison (1858-1925)
Angiokeratoma of the scrotum. Raynaud's disease of the ears. Lupus erythematosus disseminatus, disappearing during pregnancy. New York: D. Appleton & Co., 1896. 9p. 2 plates. DNLM **90-2451**

FORDYCE, John Addison (1858-1925)
A peculiar affection of the mucus membrane of the lips and oral cavity. New York, 1896. 7p. 3 plates. DNLM **90-2452**

FORDYCE, John Addison (1858-1925)
Hypertrophic lichen planus. New York, 1897. 8p. 5 plates. **90-2453**

FORDYCE, John Addison (1858-1925)
On the occurrence of nephritis in early syphilis; with the report of a case terminating fatally. New York, 1897. 7p. 2 plates. **90-2454**

FORDYCE, John Addison (1858-1925)
Report of a severe case of dermatitis herpetiformis, presenting many of the features of impetigo herpetiformis. New York, 1897. 12p. 4 plates. **90-2455**

FOREST, William E.
The new method in certain chronic diseases. . . . New York: M. L. Holbrook & Co., [1890]. 128p. DLC; NNNAM **90-2456**

FOREST, W[illiam] E.
A new method of artificial respiration in asphyxia of the new-born, with cases. New York: Trow's Co., 1892. 23p. DNLM; NNNAM **90-2457**

FOREST, William E.
From weakness to strength; a popular exposition of massage. . . . New York: Massage Appliance Co., [1894]. 48p. DLC; NNNAM **90-2458**

FOREST, W[illiam] E.
From weakness to strength. New York: [The Health Culture Co.], 1895. 72p. DNLM; NNNAM **90-2459**

FORMAD, H[enry] F. (1847-1892)
Pathological indications and suggestions as to the embryonal derivation of tissues. Part 1. Blastodermic layers with special reference to classification of tumors. Philadelphia, 1890. 8p. DNLM **90-2460**

FOSHAY, P. Max
The fertility of hybrids. [Philadelphia: Lea Bros. & Co., 1892.] 4p. DNLM **90-2461**

FOSHAY, P. Max
Changes in the urine subsequent to nephrectomy; two cases. [Philadelphia: J. B Lippincott & Co., 1893.] 4p. DNLM **90-2462**

FOSHAY, P. Max
Lithemia. Cleveland, O.: Buel & Hubbell, [1893]. 12p. DNLM **90-2463**

FOSHAY, P. Max
Some notes upon urinalysis. Philadelphia, 1893. 9p. DNLM **90-2464**

FOSTER, Burnside (1861-1917)
Rational medicine and charlatanry. St. Paul, 1894. 38p. DNLM **90-2465**

FOSTER, Burnside (1861-1917)
The bubo plague in China, with a brief account of the great plague of London. Chicago: American Medical Assoc. Press, 1894. 7p. DNLM **90-2466**

FOSTER, Burnside (1861-1917)
The history of the discovery of anaesthesia. [*Also*:] Fifty years of surgery under anaesthesia, by Theodore F. De Witt. [St. Paul, 1896.] 25p. DNLM **90-2467**

FOSTER, Charles C[hauncey]
A case of caries of the ankle treated conservatively. Philadelphia: W. J. Dornan, 1890. 4p. DNLM **90-2468**

FOSTER, Frank P[ierce] (1841-1911)
An illustrated encyclopedic medical dictionary. New York: D. Appleton & Co., 1890-1894. 4 v. DNLM; NNNAM; PPC; PU **90-2469**

FOSTER, Frank P[ierce], ed. (1841-1911)
Reference-book of practical therapeutics, by various authors; . . . New York: D. Appleton & Co., 1896-97. 2 v. DLC: MBM; NNNAM; PPC **90-2470**

FOSTER, Hal
Adenoid growths in the vault of the pharynx and their relation to diseases of the middle ear. Kansas City, 1895. 6p. DNLM **90-2471**

FOSTER, Michael (1836-1907)
A text-book of physiology. . . . 4th American, from the 5th English ed. . . . Philadelphia: Lea Bros. & Co., 1891. 1072p. DLC; DNLM; NNNAM; PPC **90-2472**

FOSTER, Michael (1836-1907)
Physiology for beginners. By M. Foster . . . and Lewis E. Shore. . . . New York and London: Macmillan & Co., 1894. 241p. DLC; ICU; MH; NN **90-2473**

FOSTER, Michael (1836-1907)
A text-book of physiology. . . . 6th American ed. . . . Philadelphia: Lea Bros. & Co., 1895. 929p. DLC; DNLM; NNNAM; PU **90-2474**

FOSTER, Michael (1836-1907)
A text book of physiology . . . rev. and abridged from the author's text book of physiology in five volumes; with an appendix on the chemical basis of the animal body, by A. Sheridan Lea. New York: The Macmillan Co.; [etc., etc.], 1896. 1351p. diags. DLC; MH-M; NNNAM; PPC **90-2475**

FOSTER, William D[avis] (*b.* 1841)
Operations on the intestines; cholecysto-enterostomy; gall-bladder and intestinal anatomosis; Murphy's button. Kansas City, [1893]. 7p. DNLM **90-2476**

FOSTER, William D[avis] (*b.* 1841)
Clinical contribution to the surgery of the appendix vermiformis; right inguinal hernia; operation; recovery. Kansas City: Hudson-Kimberly Publ. Co., [1894]. 3p. DNLM
90-2477

FOSTER, William L[awrence] (1823-1897)
Medical expert testimony. [Concord, N.H.], 1897. 29p. DNLM
90-2478

FOSTER, William S.
The mutual relations of the profession and the state, being the president's address. Philadelphia, 1896. 8p. DNLM
90-2479

FOTHERGILL, J[ohn] Milner (1841-1888)
A brief treatise on therapeutics. Edited for the U.S. Pharmacopoeia, by W. H. Rouse, with the addition of chapters on Diet for the sick, by Mrs. Emma Drant. Detroit, [1897]. 140p. DNLM; NNNAM; OCLloyd **90-2480**

FOWLER, George R[yerson] (1848-1906)
A treatise on appendicits. Philadelphia: J. B. Lippincott Co., 1894. 190p. 1 plate. DLC; DNLM; NNNAM; PPC
90-2481

FOWLER, George R[yerson] (1846-1906)
Two cases of rapidly progressive gangrene in which cultures of the bacillus pyocyaneus were found. New York: D. Appleton & Co., 1894. 12p. DNLM
90-2482

FOWLER, George R[yerson] (1848-1906)
A new method for the radical cure of inguinal hernia: intraperitoneal transplacement of the spermatic cord and typical obliteration of the internal ring and inguinal canal. Philadelphia, 1897. 21p. DNLM **90-2483**

FOLWER, George R[yerson] (1848-1906)
The radical cure of femoral hernia. [Brooklyn, 1897.] 13p. DNLM **90-2484**

FOWLER, J[ames] Kingston, ed. (1852-1934)
A dictionary of practical medicine, by various writers. Philadelphia: P. Blakiston, Son & Co., 1890. 942p. CtY-M; DNLM; NNNAM; PPC **90-2485**

FOWLER, Orson Squire (1809-1887)
The self-instructor in phrenology and physiology; with over one hundred new illustrations, including a chart for the use of practical phrenologists. By O. S. and L. N Fowler. Rev. by Nelson Sizer. . . . New York: Fowler & Wells Co., 1890 [1889]. 192p. DLC; NNNAM **90-2486**

FOWLER, Russel S[tory] (*b.* 1874)
The radical cure of hallux valgus. New York, 1899. 4p. DNLM
90-2487

FOWLER, S. Mills
Homoeopathy. A few thoughts for the intelligent. Gainsville: Yates Print. 23p. OCIM **90-2488**

FOX, George Henry (1846-1937)
Skin diseases of children. . . . With twelve photogravure and chromographic plates, and sixty illustrations in the text. New York: William Wood & Co., 1897. 166p. plates. DLC; DNLM; NNNAM **90-2489**

FOX, John J. (1853-1931)
The lungs: basic principles for their healing and development. New York: C. T. Hurlburt & Co., 1893. 217p. DNLM; NNNAM **90-2490**

FOX, L. Webster (1853-1931)
A history of spectacles. [Philadelphia, 1890.] 7p. DNLM
90-2491

FOX, L. Webster (1853-1931)
Resection of the optic nerve. [Philadelphia, 1891.] 9p. DNLM
90-2492

FOX, L. Webster (1853-1931)
Resection of the optic nerve. (Second paper.) Philadelphia: Bruder & Kelly, [1891]. 7p. DNLM **90-2493**

FOX, L. Webster (1853-1931)
A new astigmatic test chart. Nashville, Tenn., 1892. 1 l. DNLM
90-2494

FOX, L. Webster (1853-1931)
The surgical treatment of granular lids. Nashville, Tenn.: A. R. Gray & Son, 1892. 6p. DNLM **90-2495**

FOX, L. Webster (1853-1931)
Evisceration of the eyeball. Philadelphia: A. Van Horn, 1894. 2 l. 1 plate. DNLM **90-2496**

FOX, L. Webster (1853-1931)
History of the drop-bottle. Nashville, Tenn.: A. R. Gray & Son, 1894. 7p. DNLM **90-2497**

FOX, L. Webster (1853-1931)
Hygiene of the eye. New York, 1894. 20p. DNLM
90-2498

FOX, L. Webster (1853-1931)
Immediate capsulotomy following the removal of cataract. [Philadelphia, 1894.] 10p. DNLM **90-2499**

FOX, L. Webster (1853-1931)
An introductory address to the students of the Medico-Chirurgical College. Philadelphia, 1894. 4p. DNLM
90-2500

FOX, L. Webster (1853-1931)
Ophthalmia neonatorum; contraction of eyelids; glaucoma; grattage for granular lids. [Philadelphia, 1894.] 13p. DNLM
90-2501

FOX, L. Webster (1853-1931)
Retinitis albuminurica. [Philadelphia, 1894.] 15p. DNLM
90-2502

FOX, L. Webster (1853-1931)
Burns of the cornea; electric light explosion causing temporary blindness; traumatic injuries to eyes; hypopyon. Philadelphia, 1895. 4p. DNLM **90-2503**

FOX, L. Webster (1853-1931)
Evisceration of the eyeball. Philadelphia, 1895. 10p. DNLM
90-2504

FOX, L. Webster (1853-1931)
Lachrymal abscess; iridotomy; spontaneous expulsion of cataract; capsulotomy and wound of the cornea. Philadelphia, 1895. 4p. DNLM **90-2505**

FOX, L. Webster (1853-1931)
Ulcers of the cornea. Providence, 1895. 2 l. DNLM
90-2506

FOX, L. Webster (1853-1931)
Evisceration of the eyeball; Mule's operation; insertion of artificial vitreous (glass ball). Third paper. Philadelphia, [1896]. 8p. 8 plates. DNLM **90-2507**

FOX, L. Webster (1853-1931)
Implantation of a glass ball in the orbit after enucleation of an eye. Philadelphia, [1896]. 6p. 1 plate. DNLM
90-2508

FOX, L. Webster (1853-1931)
Intra-ocular growths. Philadelphia, 1896. 10p. DNLM
90-2509

FOX, L. Webster (1853-1931)
Operations performed in the eye department of the Medico-Chirurgical Hospital. Nashville, [1896]. 16p. DNLM
90-2510

FOX, L. Webster (1853-1931)
Retinitis and choroiditis. Philadelphia, 1896. 8p. DNLM
90-2511

FOX, L. Webster (1853-1931)
Sarcoma of the choroid, glioma of the retina, and new formed blood vessels in the vitreous. Nashville, [1896]. 8p. DNLM
90-2512

FOX, L. Webster (1853-1931)
Tattooing of the cornea. New York, 1896. 8p. DNLM
90-2513

FOX, L. Webster (1853-1931)
Valedictory address to the graduating class of the Medico-Chirurgical College of Philadelphia. Philadelphia, 1896. 4p. DNLM **90-2514**

FOX, L. Webster (1853-1931)
New ophthalmic operating table. Philadelphia: E. A. Yarnall & Co., 1897. 1 l. DNLM **90-2515**

FOX, L. Webster (1853-1931)
Ophthalmia neonatorum. [1897.] 3p. DNLM
90-2516

FOX, L. Webster (1853-1931)
Ophthalmia neonatorum. Philadelphia, 1897. 8p. DNLM
90-2517

FOX, L. Webster (1853-1931)
Ulcers of the cornea; implantation of a glass ball for the better support of an artificial eye. Philadelphia, 1897. 5p. DNLM **90-2518**

FOX, L. Webster (1853-1931)
Cataract operations; Mule's operation illustrated by skiagraphs; capsulotomy; operation for pterygium. Philadelphia, [1898]. 8p. 3 plates. DNLM **90-2519**

FOX, L. Webster (1853-1931)
Implantation of a glass ball for the support of an artificial eye and Mule's operation for the substitution of enucleation of an eyeball. Chicago, 1898. 8p. DNLM
90-2520

FOX, RULTZ & CO.
Catalog of bottles, corks, druggists' sundries, flint glassware, colognes, ovals, prescription bottles. . . . New York & Boston, [*c.* 1890]. 24p. MBM **90-2521**

FOX, Sidney Allan (1856-1890)
Naso-pharyngeal carcinoma. Report of a case, with a consideration of the treatment of this disease. [New York, 1890.] 7p. DNLM **90-2522**

FRANCIS, Richard P.
Tumor of the corpus callosum, with autopsy. With pathological memoranda, by M. Allen Starr and Ira Van Gieson. Philadelphia, 1895. 10p. DNLM **90-2523**

FRANCIS, Richard P.
Report of a case of removal of the appendix; coeliotomy for secondary pelvic abscess, followed by faecal fistula; intestinal resection (with the use of the Murphy button) in the same patient. New York, 1898. 7p. DNLM **90-2524**

FRANKLIN, George H.
. . . History of a case of incipient phthisis treated by hypodermic injections of silver nitrate over the vagi. . . . [Philadelphia? 1899.] 3p. DLC; DNLM **90-2525**

FRANKLIN, M[elvin] M.
Mania and catarrhal pneumonia following labor. Philadelphia, 1894. 4p. DNLM **90-2526**

FREEBORN, George C[ornell] (1850-1911)
A résumé of the uses of formalin. New York, 1896. 16p. DNLM **90-2527**

FREEMAN, Leonard (*b.* 1860)
Surgical diseases of the kidneys; cases illustrating some points in diagnosis and treatment. New York, 1899. 13p. DNLM
90-2528

FREEMAN, Rowland Godfrey (*b.* 1859)
On the sterilization of milk at low temperature, with description of a new and simple apparatus applying the principle of Pasteurization. [New York, 1892.] 8p. DNLM
90-2529

FREEMAN, Rowland Godfrey (*b.* 1859)
Sterilization of milk at 75°C. (Pasteurization) and its efficiency in destroying pathogenic organisms. New York: Trow, 1893. 11p. DNLM **90-2530**

FREEMAN, Rowland Godfrey (*b.* 1859)
Low temperature Pasteurization of milk at about 68°C. (155°F.). [New York, 1896.] 12p. DNLM
90-2531

FREEMAN, Rowland Godfrey (*b.* 1859)
Milk as an agency in the conveyance of disease. New York, 1896. 34p. DNLM **90-2532**

FREEMAN, Rowland Godfrey (*b.* 1859)
Dangers of the domestic use, other than drinking, of contaminated water. [New York, 1897.] 6p. DNLM
90-2533

FREER, James A. (*d.* 1905)
Some surgical causes of rheumatism. [New York, 1894.] 7p. DNLM **90-2534**

FREIBERG, Albert H[enry] (*b.* **1869)**
The treatment of club-foot. [Philadelphia: Lea Bros. & Co., 1892.] 17p. DNLM **90-2535**

FRENCH, George Hazen (1841-1935)
A manual of dissection and histology, for the use of classes in physiology in high schools, normal schools, and academies. . . . Philadelphia: J. B. Lippincott & Co., [1898]. 140p. plates. DLC; DNLM; NN **90-2536**

FRENCH, James M[agoffin] (1858-1907)
The dietetic treatment of typhoid fever. Cincinnati, [1890]. 15p. DNLM **90-2537**

FRENCH, James M[agoffin] (1858-1907)
The colitis of infants. Chicago, 1891. 10 l. DNLM **90-2538**

FRENCH, James M[agoffin] (1858-1907)
The treatment of alcoholism. Philadelphia, 1896-7. 7 l. DNLM **90-2539**

FRENCH, Thomas R[ushmore] (1849-1920)
Lymphoid growths in the vault of the pharynx. New York, 1893. 32p. DNLM **90-2540**

FRENCH, Thomas R[ushmore] (1849-1920)
The action of the glottis in singing. New York: D. Appleton & Co., 1891. 11p. DNLM **90-2541**

FRENCH, Thomas R[ushmore] (1849-1920)
Observations on some of the results of cutting operations on the nasal saeptum. New York: D. Appleton & Co., 1894. 15p. DNLM **90-2542**

FRENCH, Thomas R[ushmore] (1849-1920)
The relation of chronic diseases of the nose and throat to disorders of digestion. New York, 1896. 12p. DNLM **90-2543**

FRENCH, Thomas R[ushmore] (1849-1920)
Laryngeal and postnasal photography with the aid of the arc light. New York, 1897. 9p. DNLM **90-2544**

FRENCH, Thomas R[ushmore] (1849-1920)
The president's address delivered before the American Laryngological Association at its twentieth annual congress. New York: D. Appleton & Co., 1898. 22p. DNLM; NNNAM **90-2545**

FRENCH, William B.
The malarial organism, with report of cases. New York, 1896. 8p. 1 plate. DNLM **90-2546**

FRENCH, William B.
A contribution to the study and classification of malarial fevers in the District of Columbia. New York, 1897. 16p. DNLM **90-2547**

FREUDENTHAL, W[olff] (1858-1929)
Ueber da Ulcus septi nasi perforans. [New York, 1891.] 6p. DNLM **90-2548**

FREUDENTHAL, W[olff] (1858-1929)
Bermerkungen zu dem Artikel des Herrn Gleitzmann: "Ein neues und einfaches Verfahren zur Beseitigung der unangenchmen Folgezustände nach Gebrauch der Galvanocaustik bei Hypertrophien der Nase." [New York, 1892.] 3p. DNLM **90-2549**

FREUDENTHAL, W[olff] (1858-1929)
Poisoning by creosote. New York: S. & D. A. Huebsch, 1892. 8p. DNLM **90-2550**

FREUDENTHAL, W[olff] (1858-1929)
Asepsis or antisepsis in nasal surgery? [New York, 1893.] 14p. DNLM **90-2551**

FREUDENTHAL, W[olff] (1858-1929)
Is laryngitis sicca and Stoerk's blenorrhoea of the larynx one and the same disease? Kansas City, 1894. 9p. DNLM **90-2552**

FREUDENTHAL, W[olff] (1858-1929)
Severe haemorrhages from the nose. New York, 1894. 12p. DNLM **90-2553**

FREUDENTHAL, W[olff] (1858-1929)
The proposed city hospital for consumptives. New York, 1897. 6p. DNLM **90-2554**

FREUDENTHAL, W[olff] (1858-1929)
Contributions to the aetiology of pulmonary tuberculosis. St. Louis: D. A. Huebsch & Co., 1897. 36p. DNLM **90-2555**

FREUDENTHAL, W[olff] (1858-1929)
The climatic influence of our Southwestern States on diseases of the respiratory tract. New York, 1898. 27p. DNLM; NNNAM **90-2556**

FREUDENTHAL, W[olff] (1858-1929)
A modification of Laborde's method for resuscitation in deep asphyxia. New York, 1898. 3p. DNLM **90-2557**

FREUDENTHAL, W[olff] (1858-1929)
A case of chronic urticaria of the larynx. New York, 1898. 4p. DNLM **90-2558**

FREUND, H[enry] H.
Primary laryngeal diphtheria successfully treated with divided doses of Behring's antitoxin No. 1. [Philadelphia, 1895.] 3p. DNLM **90-2559**

FREYER, Peter J[ohnson] (1852-1921)
The modern treatment of stone in the bladder by litholapaxy. A description of the operation and instruments, with cases illustrative of the difficulties and complications met with. 2nd ed. New York: William Wood & Co., 1896. 120p. DNLM; NNNAM **90-2560**

FRIEDENWALD, A[aron] (1836-1902)
Jewish physicians and the contributions of the Jews to the science of medicine. Philadelphia, 1897. 61p. DNLM; PPC **90-2561**

FRIEDENWALD, Harry (1864-1950)
Recent investigations in strabismus. [New York, 1890.] 8p. DNLM **90-2562**

FRIEDENWALD, Harry (1864-1950)
Opening of the mastoid process. Read at the annual meeting of the Medical and Chirurgical Faculty of Maryland, April 29, 1892. [Baltimore, 1892.] 12p. DNLM **90-2563**

FRIEDENWALD, Harry (1864-1950)
The causation of inflammation. A review. [New York, 1893.] 15p. DNLM **90-2564**

FRIEDENWALD, Harry (1864-1950)
Cholesteatoma of the ear. Philadelphia, 1893. 21p. DNLM
90-2565

FRIEDENWALD, Harry (1864-1950)
Cranial deformity and optic-nerve atrophy. Philadelphia, 1893. 7p. DNLM **90-2566**

FRIEDENWALD, Harry (1864-1950) and Albert C. CRAWFORD
Calomel conjunctivitis. [St. Louis, 1893.] 8p. DNLM
90-2567

FRIEDENWALD, Harry (1864-1950)
Ante-partum ophthalmia neonatorum (intra-uterine opthalmia). [Philadelphia: Lea Bros. & Co., 1895.] 9p. DNLM
90-2568

FRIEDENWALD, Harry (1864-1950)
Necrosis of the labyrinth; report of a case; opening of the mastoid process; Küster's operation; finally, spontaneous elimination of a portion of the labyrinth. New York: D. Appleton & Co., 1895. 5p. DNLM
90-2569

FRIEDENWALD, Harry (1864-1950)
On movements of the eyelids associated with movements of the jaws and with lateral movements of the eyeballs. Baltimore, 1896. 9p. DNLM **90-2570**

FRIEDENWALD, Harry (1864-1950)
The early history of ophthalmology and otology in Baltimore (1800-50). Baltimore, 1897. 20p. DNLM
90-2571

FRIEDENWALD, Harry (1864-1950)
Joseph Friederich Piringer; his methods and investigations. Baltimore, 1897. 13p. DNLM **90-2572**

FRIEDENWALD, Julius (1866-1941)
Atony of the stomach. [Philadelphia, 1893.] 16p. DNLM
90-2573

FRIEDENWALD, Julius (1866-1941)
The diazo reaction of Ehrlich. New York: D. Appleton & Co., 1893. 13p. DNLM **90-2574**

FRIEDENWALD, Julius (1866-1941)
Electric illumination of the stomach. [Baltimore, 1894.] 4p. DNLM **90-2575**

FRIEDENWALD, Julius (1866-1941)
The use of the resorcin test for the detection and quantitative estimation of the free hydrochloric acid of the gastric juice. New York, 1894. 7p. DNLM **90-2576**

FRIEDENWALD, Julius (1866-1941)
The quantitative estimation of the rennet-zymogen; its diagnostic value in certin diseases of the stomach. Philadelphia, 1895. 12p. DNLM **90-2577**

FRIEND, Samuel H.
Routine cleanliness, isolation, and watchfulness of schools and children. Philadelphia, 1896. 6p. DNLM
90-2578

FRIEND, Samuel H.
The etiology and classification of tumors. Chicago, 1897. 20p. DNLM **90-2579**

FRIEND, Samuel H.
The thyroid-gland treatment of cretinism, with report of a case. Philadelphia, 1897. 15p. DNLM
90-2580

FRONCZAK, Francis Eustace (*b.* 1874)
Plica polonica. [University of Buffalo.] St. Louis, 1897-8. 39p. 1 plate. DNLM **90-2581**

FRONCZAK, Francis Eustace (*b.* 1874)
A case of post-mortem Caesarean section. Buffalo, 1898. 3p. DNLM **90-2582**

FRONCZAK, Francis Eustace (*b.* 1874)
Compound dislocations. Buffalo, 1899. 4p. DNLM
90-2583

FRONCZAK, Francis Eustace (*b.* 1874)
The pathogenesis of cholelithiasis in the light of latest investigations. Buffalo, 1899. 10p. DNLM
90-2584

FROTHINGHAM, George E[dward] (1836-1900)
Remarks on the need of more efficient protection of the eye after cataract extraction, and an improved apparatus for the purpose. Chicago: Office American Medical Assoc., 1891. 16p. DNLM **90-2585**

FROTHINGHAM, Langdon (1866-1935)
Laboratory guide for the bacteriologist. Philadelphia: W. B. Saunders, 1895. 61p., interleaved. 2 plates. DNLM; PPC; PU
90-2586

FRUITNIGHT, J[ohn] Henry (1851-1900)
Hyperemesis gravidarum as an indication for the induction of premature labor. New York: William Wood & Co., 1890. 10p. DNLM **90-2587**

FRUITNIGHT, J[ohn] Henry (1851-1900)
Puerperal phlegmasia alba dolens. [New York, 1891.] 5p. DNLM **90-2588**

FRUITNIGHT, J[ohn] Henry (1851-1900)
Perityphlitis in the young. [New York, 1891.] 13p. DNLM
90-2589

FRY, Henry D[avidson] (1853-1919)
Report of a successful Caesarean section. Philadelphia, 1890. 4p. DNLM **90-2590**

FRY, Henry D[avidson] (1853-1919)
A report of two cases. I. Symphysiotomy. II. Elective Caesarean section. New York, 1895. 8p. DNLM
90-2591

FRY, Henry D[avidson] (1853-1919)
The universal application of the principles of asepsis to private obstetric practice. New York, 1895. 14p. DNLM
90-2592

FRY, Henry D[avidson] (1853-1919)
On the indications for examinations of the uterus and the treatment of certain conditions immediately following childbirth. New York: William Wood & Co., 1896. 12p. DNLM
90-2593

FUCHS, Ernst (1851-1930)
Text-book of ophthalmology. . . . Authorized translation from the 2nd enl. and improved German ed. by A. Duane. . . . New York: D. Appleton & Co., 1892. 788p. DLC; NNNAM; OCIM; PPC **90-2594**

FUCHS, Ernst (1851-1930)
Text-book of ophthalmology. . . . authorized translation, revised from the seventh enlarged and improved German edition by A. Duane. . . . With two hundred and seventy-seven illustrations. 2nd American ed. New York: D. Appleton & Co., 1899. 800p. DLC; IU-M; NNNAM; PU **90-2595**

FULLER, Eugene (1858-1930)
Disorders of the male sexual organs. . . . Philadelphia: Lea Bros. & Co., 1895. 241p. plates. DLC; DNLM; NNNAM; PPC **90-2596**

FULLER, Eugene (1858-1930)
A case of cancer of the urethra. New York, 1895. 3p. DNLM **90-2597**

FULLER, Eugene (1858-1930)
Six successful and successive cases of prostatectomy. New York, 1895. 11p. DNLM **90-2598**

FULLER, Eugene (1858-1930)
Interesting points connected with a nephrectomy secondary to a nephrotomy. New York, 1896. 4p. DNLM **90-2599**

FULLER, Eugene (1858-1930)
Operative interference in aggravated instances of seminal vesiculitis. New York, 1896. 10p. DNLM **90-2600**

FULLER & FULLER
Prices current—chemicals, oils, proprietary medicines, sundries, furniture, glassware, moulds, signs, scales, counters, presses and trusses. Chicago, 1894. 915p. IU-M; OCIM **90-2601**

FULLER & FULLER
Prices current—chemicals, oils, proprietary medicines, sundries, furniture, glassware, moulds, signs, scales, counters, presses and trusses. Chicago, 1899. 1052p. OCIM **90-2602**

FULLER, GEORGE R., CO.
Artificial limbs. Rochester, N.Y.: The Company, 1897. 79p. NNNAM **90-2603**

FULLERTON, Anna Martha
A handbook of obstetrical nursing, for nurses, students and mothers. . . . Philadelphia: P. Blakiston, Son & Co., 1890. 214p. DLC; DNLM; NNNAM; PPC **90-2604**

FULLERTON, Anna Martha
The science of nursing, A plea. [Boston, 1890.] 10p. DNLM **90-2605**

FULLERTON, Anna Martha
The science of nursing. Buffalo, N.Y., 1890. 26p. DNLM **90-2606**

FULLERTON, Anna Martha
Surgery versus electricity in the management of salpingitis and allied conditions. [Philadelphia, 1890.] 12p. DNLM **90-2607**

FULLERTON, Anna Martha
A handbook of obstetrical nursing, for nurses, students and mothers. Comprising the course of instruction in obstetrical nursing given to the pupils of the training school for nurses connected with the Woman's Hospital of Philadelphia. . . . 2nd ed.—rev. Philadelphia: P. Blakiston, Son & Co., 1891. 222p. DLC; DNLM; NNNAM; PU **90-2608**

FULLERTON, Anna Martha
Nursing in abdominal surgery and diseases of women. A series of lectures delivered to the pupils of the training school for nurses connected with the Woman's Hospital of Philadelphia, comprising their regular course of instruction on such topics. . . . Philadelphia: P. Blakiston, Son & Co., 1891. 284p. DLC; DNLM; NNNAM; PPC **90-2609**

FULLERTON, Anna Martha
Women in medicine. Her duties and responsibilities. An address to the graduates of the Woman's Medical College of Pennsylvania, May 3, 1893. [Philadelphia, 1893.] 16p. PPC **90-2610**

FULLERTON, Anna Martha
A handbook of obstetrical nursing for nurses, students, and mothers. Comprising the course of instruction in obstetrical nursing given to the pupils of the training school for nurses connected with the Woman's Hospital of Philadelphia. . . . 3rd rev. ed. . . . Philadelphia: P. Blakiston, Son & Co., 1893. 264p. DLC; MBM; PPC; PU **90-2611**

FULLERTON, Anna Martha
Nursing in abdominal surgery and diseases of women. A series of lectures delivered to the pupils of the training school for nurses connected with the Woman's Hospital of Philadelphia, comprising their regular course of instruction on such topics. . . . 2nd ed., rev. and enl. . . . Philadelphia: P. Blakiston, Son & Co., 1893. 300p. DLC; DNLM; NNNAM; PPC **90-2612**

FULLERTON, Anna Martha
A handbook of obstetric nursing for nurses, students, and mothers. . . . 4th rev. ed. . . . Philadelphia: P. Blakiston, Son & Co., 1895. 254p. DLC; DNLM; NNNAM; PPC **90-2613**

FULLERTON, Anna Martha
A contribution to the clinical study of uterine fibroids. New York, 1895. 10p. DNLM **90-2614**

FULLERTON, Anna Martha
Chronic inversion of the uterus. New York, 1896. 4p. DNLM **90-2615**

FULLERTON, Anna M[artha]
A handbook of obstetric nursing for nurses, students, and mothers. Comprising the course of instruction in obstetric nursing given to the pupils of the training school for nurses connected with the Woman's Hospital of Philadelphia. 5th rev. ed. Philadelphia: P. Blakiston's Son & Co., 1899. 262p. DLC; DNLM; NNNAM; PPC **90-2616**

FULLERTON, Anna Martha
Surgical nursing; a compilation of the lectures upon abdominal surgery, gynaecology, and general surgical conditions and procedures, delivered to the classes in the training school for nurses connected with the Woman's Hospital of Philadelphia. . . . 3rd ed., rev. and enl., with 69 illustrations. Philadelphia: P. Blakiston's Son & Co., 1899. 294p. DLC; DNLM; NNNAM; PPC **90-2617**

FULLERTON, Erskine B[oles] (1842-1909)
Quinine in cholera. Columbus, Ohio: Nitschke Bros., 1893. 32p. DNLM **90-2618**

FULLERTON, W[illiam] S.
Modern abuses in our materia medica. A paper read before the St. Louis County Medical Society, accepted by the editors of the Northwestern Lancet for publication, by request of the society, and suppressed by the publisher of that journal. With an appendix containing some interesting correspondence. Duluth: [Christie & Collier], 1895. 8p. DNLM **90-2619**

FURNESS, Horace Howard (1833-1912)
University of Pennsylvania. Commencement, June 7, 1894. Address. Also a short address at the unveiling of the model of a statue of Provost Pepper. Philadelphia, 1894. 15p. DNLM; PPC **90-2620**

FURNISS, H[enry] W.
Diagnosis by blood examiantion. [Indianapolis, 1897.] 16p. DNLM **90-2621**

FÜTTERER, Gustav
The liver as an organ of elimination of corpuscular elements. Detroit: G. S. Davis, 1895. 4p. DNLM **90-2622**

FÜTTERER, Gustav
Primary carcinoma of the gall-bladder. Detroit, 1897. 20p. DNLM **90-2623**

FÜTTERER, Gustav
The elimination of bacteria from the general circulation by the liver and through the bile passages. A claim for priority in stating the presence of the bacillus typhi abdominalis in the gall-bladder. Detroit, 1898. 10p. DNLM **90-2624**

FÜTTERER, Gustav
How soon do bacteria which enter the portal vein become disseminated throughout the system, and when does their elimination commence? [Detroit]: W. M. Warren, 1898. 5p. DNLM **90-2625**

FÜTTERER, Gustav
Contributions to the histology, physiology, and pathology of the liver, bile passages, and bile. [Detroit]: W. M. Warren, 1898. 10p. 2 plates. DNLM **90-2626**

GAGE, Homer (1861-1938)
Movable kidney. Chicago, 1895. 12p. DNLM **90-2627**

GAGE, Homer (1861-1938)
Extra-uterine pregnancy. New York, 1896. 16p. DNLM **90-2628**

GAGE, Homer (1861-1938)
Treatment of cold abscesses. Boston, 1896. 7p. DNLM **90-2629**

GAGE, Simon Henry (1851-1944)
The microscope and histology, for the use of laboratory students in the anatomical department of Cornell University. . . . 3rd ed., entirely rewritten. Pt. I. The microscope and microscopical methods. Illustrated. Ithaca, N.Y.: [Printed by Andrus & Church, 1891.] 90p. diags. DLC **90-2630**

GAGE, Simon Henry (1851-1944)
The microscope and histology. . . . Pt. I. The microscope and microscopical methods. . . . 4th ed., rev. and enl. Philadelphia: J. W. Queen & Co., 1892. 90p. diags. DLC; PPC **90-2631**

GAGE, Simon Henry (1851-1944)
The microscope and microscopical methods. . . . 5th ed., rewritten, greatly enl. and illustrated by 103 figures in the text. Ithaca, N.Y.: Comstock Publishing Co., 1894. 156p. diags. DLC **90-2632**

GAGE, Simon Henry (1851-1944)
The microscope and microscopical methods. . . . 6th ed., rewritten, greatly enl., and illustrated by 165 figures in the text. Ithaca, N.Y.: Comstock Publishing Co., 1896. 237p. diags. DLC **90-2633**

GAGE, Simon Henry (1851-1944)
The microscope; an introduction to microscopic methods and to histology. . . . 7th ed. rev. Ithaca, N.Y.: Comstock Publishing Co., 1899. 237p. plates. DLC **90-2634**

GALLAUDET, Bern Budd (1860-1934)
. . . Surgery. A manual for students and practitioners. By Bern B. Gallaudet . . . and Charles N. Dixon-Jones. . . . Philadelphia: Lea Bros. & Co., [1893]. 301p. DLC; NNNAM; PPC; PU **90-2635**

GALLAVARDIN, M.
The homoeopathic treatment of alcoholism. By Dr. Gallavardin, of Lyons, France. Transl. by Irenaeus D. Foulon. Philadelphia: Hahnemann Publishing House, 1890. 136p. PPHa **90-2636**

GALLOUPE, Charles W[illiam]
A consideration of erysipelas occurring during the puerperium. [Boston, 1893.] 14p. DNLM **90-2637**

GALLOWAY, D[avid] H. (*b.* 1859)
Experience of an American physician in Mexico; operating for suppurative lymphangitis under difficulty; taking his own medicine; strychnia poisoning. Chicago, 1896. 11p. DNLM **90-2638**

GALLOWAY, D[avid] H. (*b.* 1859)
How anesthetization is taught in some places and how it is neglected in others. The relation of the anesthetizer to the surgeon. Chicago, 1897. 7p. DNLM **90-2639**

GALLOWAY, D[avid] H. (*b.* 1859)
The administration of anesthetics. Chicago, 1898. 15p. DNLM **90-2640**

GALLOWAY, D[avid] H. (*b.* 1859)
Death half an hour after chloroform-anesthesia in a case of aneurysm of the innominate artery and aorta. Philadelphia, 1898. 5p. DNLM **90-2641**

GALLOWAY, D[avid] H. (*b.* 1859)
. . . The anesthetizer as a specialist. . . . [Philadelphia, 1899.] 10p. DLC; DNLM **90-2642**

GALLOWAY, M. James
Electro-therapeutics, its marvellous cures. [Philadelphia], 1891. 16p. DNLM **90-2643**

GANT, Frederick J[ames] (1825-1905)
The student's surgery, a multum in parvo. Philadelphia: Lea Bros. & Co., 1890. 817p. DNLM; OCIM; PPC; PU
90-2644

GANT, Samuel Goodwin (1869-1944)
Diagnosis and treatment of diseases of the rectum, anus, and contiguous textures. . . . With two chapters on "cancer" and "colotomy," by Herbert William Allingham. . . . Philadelphia: The F. A. Davis Co., 1890. 399p. col. plates. DLC: DNLM; PPC; PU **90-2645**

GARCEAU, Edgar (1865-1913)
Vaginal hysterectomy, as done in France. New York, 1895. 42p. DNLM **90-2646**

GARCEAU, Edgar (1865-1913)
Vaginal hysterectomy for pelvic suppuration. Chicago, 1895. 12p. DNLM **90-2647**

GARCEAU, Edgar (1865-1913)
The influence of the catheter in causing vesical irritability. New York: William Wood & Co., 1896. 5p. DNLM
90-2648

GARCEAU, Edgar (1865-1913)
Some affections of the female bladder. Boston: Damrell & Upham, 1896. 11p. DNLM **90-2649**

GARCEAU, Edgar (1865-1913)
Some cases of cystitis in women. Boston: Damrell & Upham, 1897. 26p. DNLM; MBM **90-2650**

GARDENIER, A[delbert]
The standard physiology: with notes on anatomy and hygiene; aid to the injured; disinfectants, etc. Also containing explanatory index to the "standard" manikin. . . . New York and Chicago: E. L. Kellogg & Co., 1890. 94p. DLC; IU-M; OCIM
90-2651

GARDNER, Miriam
How far is retroversion of the uterus responsible for some of the functional neuroses? New York, 1899. 6p. DNLM
90-2652

GARDNER, R[obert] W[inslow] (1835-1911)
Syrup of hydriodic acid and its uses. [Danbury, 1893.] 1 l. DNLM **90-2653**

GARDNER, R[obert] W[inslow] (1835-1911)
Syrup of hydriodic acid; the facts. Danbury, Conn., 1893. 15p. DNLM **90-2654**

GARDNER, R[obert] W[inslow] (1835-1911)
Interstitial oxidation and nerve feeding. Nutrition of bone and nerve tissue by single, specially indicated phosphites. Delicate and weakly children. 11th ed. Danbury, Conn., 1894. 17p. DNLM **90-2655**

GARDNER, R[obert] W[inslow] (1835-1911)
Gardner's syrup of hydriodic acid as an internal antiseptic. Especially valuable in diseases of the genito-urinary tract. As a discutient in cataract. Therapeutic notes. 11th ed. Danbury, Conn., 1894. 14p. DNLM **90-2656**

GARDNER, R[obert] W[inslow], ed. (1835-1911)
Gardner's syrup of hydriodic acid. Therapeutical indications with clinical data. 12th ed. New York, 1895. 78p. DLC; NNNAM **90-2657**

GARDNER, William S[isson] (*b.* 1861)
Obstetric records. [New York: D. Appleton & Co., 1891.] 4p. DNLM **90-2658**

GARRETSON, James E[dmund] (1828-1895)
A system of oral surgery; being a treatise on the diseases and surgery of the mouth, jaws, and associate parts. 6th ed., thoroughly revised, with additions. Philadelphia: J. B. Lippincott Co., 1895. 1084p. DNLM; MdU-D; NNNAM; PPC
90-2659

GARRIGUES, Henry Jacques (1831-1913)
Ear presentation. [Philadelphia, 1890.] 3p. DNLM
90-2660

GARRIGUES, Henry Jacques (1831-1913)
The immediate closure of laceration of the cervix. New York: William Wood & Co., 1891. 4p. DNLM
90-2661

GARRIGUES, Henry Jacques (1831-1913)
So-called laceration of the perineum. [Philadelphia, 1891.] 20p. DNLM **90-2662**

GARRIGUES, Henry Jacques (1831-1913)
Intra-uterine packing forceps. New York: William Wood & Co., 1892. 2p. DNLM **90-2663**

GARRIGUES, Henry Jacques (1831-1913)
Reprehensible, debatable, and necessary antiseptic midwifery. [Philadelphia: Lea Bros. & Co., 1892.] 11p. DNLM
90-2664

GARRIGUES, Henry Jacques (1831-1913)
Stomatitis due to irritation of epithelial pearls in the mouths of newborn children. [Philadelphia: Lea Bros. & Co., 1892.] 7p. DNLM **90-2665**

GARRIGUES, Henry Jacques (1831-1913)
Symphysiotomy. New York: William Wood & Co., 1893. 9p. DNLM **90-2666**

GARRIGUES, Henry Jacques (1831-1913)
Symphysiotomy; with the report of a successful case. [Philadelphia, 1893.] 30p. DNLM **90-2667**

GARRIGUES, Henry Jacques (1831-1913)
A text-book of the diseases of women. . . . Containing three hundred and ten engravings and colored plates. Philadelphia: W. B. Saunders, 1894. 390p. col. plates. DLC; DNLM; NNNAM; PPC **90-2668**

GARRIGUES, Henry Jacques (1831-1913)
Colpoperineorrhaphy. Philadelphia, 1896. 13p. Philadelphia, 1896. 13p. DNLM **90-2669**

GARRIGUES, Henry Jacques (1831-1913)
Protection for the future wife and children. New York, 1896. 7p. DNLM **90-2670**

GARRIGUES, Henry Jacques (1831-1913)
A text-book of the diseases of women. . . . Containing three hundred and thirty-five engravings and colored plates. 2nd ed., thoroughly rev. Philadelphia: W. B. Saunders, 1897. 728p. col. plates. DLC; NNNAM; OCIM; PU
90-2671

GARRIGUES, Henry Jacques (1831-1913)
Anaesthesia-paralysis. Philadelphia, 1897. 9p. DNLM
90-2672

GARRIGUES, Henry Jacques (1831-1913)
Secondary operations. Boston, 1897. 7p. DNLM
90-2673

GARRIGUES, Henry Jacques (1831-1913)
The treatment of abortion. Philadelphia, 1897. 12p. DNLM
90-2674

GARRIGUES, Henry Jacques (1831-1913)
Electricity in gynecology. Philadelphia, 1898. 6p. DNLM
90-2675

GARRIGUES, Henry Jacques (1831-1913)
Fashions in gynecology. New Haven, 1898. 7p. DNLM
90-2676

GARROD, Alfred B[aring] (1819-1907)
Cullings from the Treatise on gout and rheumatic gout. St. Louis, Mo., 1892. 16p. DNLM **90-2677**

GARROD, Archibald E[dward] (1857-1936)
A treatise on rheumatism and rheumatoid arthritis. Philadelphia: P. Blakiston, Son & Co., 1890. 342p. 6 charts. DNLM; NNNAM; PPC; PPJ **90-2678**

GATCHELL, Charles (1851-1910)
Pocket medical dictionary. For the use of students of medicine, containing ten thousand words, including all the essential terms used in medicine and the allied sciences. Chicago: Era Publishing Co., 1891. 303p. IU-M; OCIM; PPHa
90-2679

GATCHELL, Charles (1851-1910)
Prevention and general treatment of pulmonary tuberculosis. Philadelphia, 1899. 17p. DNLM **90-2680**

GATCHELL, Charles (1851-1910)
Pocket-book of medical practice, including diseases of the kidneys, skin, nerves, eye, ear, nose, and throat, and obstetrics, gynecology, surgery, by special authors. Chicago, 1899. 384p. DNLM; IU-M; OCIM **90-2681**

GATTINGER, Augustin (1825-1903)
The medicinal plants of Tennessee exhibiting their commercial value, with an analytical key, descriptions in aid of their recognition, and notes relating to their distribution, time and mode of collection, and preparation for the drug market. Arranged and published under the direction of T. F. P. Allison. . . . Nashville, Tenn.: F. M. Paul, printer, 1894. 128p. DLC; OCLloyd **90-2682**

GAY, George W[ashington] (1842-1931)
Tracheotomy and intubation at one Boston City Hospital. Boston: Damrell & Upham, 1893. 7p. DNLM
90-2683

GAY, George W[ashington] (1842-1931)
Appendicitis. Boston: Damrell & Upham, 1895. 14p. DNLM
90-2684

GAY, George W[ashington] (1842-1931)
Circumstances under which chloroform is preferable to ether as an anesthetic. Boston: Damrell & Upham, 1895. 14p. DNLM
90-2685

GAY, George W[ashington] (1842-1931)
A case of ligature of the innominate artery for aneurism. Boston: Damrell & Upham, 1897. 18p. DNLM
90-2686

GAY, George W[ashington] (1842-1931)
When to call a surgeon in acute abdominal affections. Concord, N.H.: Evans, 1897. 17p. MB; MH
90-2687

GAY, George W[ashington] (1842-1931)
When to call a surgeon in appendicitis. Boston: Damrell & Upham, 1897. 18p. MB **90-2688**

GAYLE, Virginius W.
Typhoid fever. St. Louis, 1890. 7p. DNLM
90-2689

GEAR, Frank J.
Illustrated catalogue of invalid and sick room supplies, also surgical and electric apparatus and physicians' supplies. Boston, [*c.* 1890]. 44p. MBM **90-2690**

GEMMELL, G[eorge] H[arrison]
Chemical notes and equations, inorganic and organic. New York: William Wood & Co., 1896. 244p. DNLM; MB; MH; NN
90-2691

GENEVA OPTICAL COMPANY. CHICAGO
Wholesale priced and illustrated catalogue of optical goods, 1891-1892. [Chicago: Rogerson & Stockton, 1891.] 136p. DNLM **90-2692**

GENTRY, William D. (*b.* 1836)
The concordance repertory of the more characteristic symptoms of the materia medica. New York: A. L. Chatterton & Co., 1890. 6 v. OCLloyd; PPHa **90-2693**

GENTRY, William D. (*b.* 1836)
The rubrical and regional text-book of the homoeopathic materia medica. Section on the urine and urinary organs. Philadelphia: Hahnemann Publishing House, 1890. 240p. OCIM; OCLloyd; PPHa **90-2694**

GEORGEN, W. T.
Illustrated price list of modern ophthalmological apparatus for physicians and hospitals. New York, 1897. 16p. NNNAM
90-2695

GERRISH, Frederic H[enry] (1845-1920)
The medical dictionary. The introductory address before the medical department of Bowdoin College, at the opening of its 71st annual course of lectures in Brunswick, 8th February, 1891. Portland: Mitchell & Bickford, 1891. 42p. DNLM
90-2696

GERRISH, Frederic H[enry] (1845-1920)
The remedial uses of hypnotism. An essay. Portland, Maine: W. M. Marks, 1892. 24p. DNLM **90-2697**

GERRISH, Frederic H[enry] (1845-1920)
Suprapubic cystostomy; its frequent utility, and an appliance for preventing the chief annoyance attending a permanent opening in the bladder. Portland: W. M. Marks, 1892. 11p. DNLM **90-2698**

GERRISH, Frederic H[enry] (1845-1920) and E[dward] A. BALLOCH
Uniformity in the division of the abdominal regions. Boston: Damrell & Upham, 1893. 16p. DNLM
90-2699

GERRISH, Frederic H[enry] (1845-1920)
The best order of topics in a two-years' course of anatomy in a medical school. Portland, Me.: W. M. Marks, 1895. 15p. DNLM
90-2700

GERRISH, Frederick H[enry], ed. (1845-1920)
Prescription writing. Designed for the use of medical students who have never studied Latin. . . . 8th and rev. ed. Portland, Me.: Loring, Short & Harmon; Philadelphia: J. B. Lippincott & Co., 1895. 57p. DLC; PPC; PU **90-2701**

GERRISH, Frederick H[enry], ed. (1845-1920)
A text-book of anatomy by American authors. . . . Illustrated with 950 engravings in black and colors. Philadelphia and New York: Lea Bros. & Co., 1899. 917p. col. illus. DLC; DNLM; NNNAM; PPC **90-2702**

GERSTER, Arpad G[eyza] (1848-1923)
Essay upon the classification of the various forms of appendicitis and perityphlitic abscess, with practical conclusions. [New York, 1890.] 28p. DNLM; NNNAM
90-2703

GERSTER, Arpad G[eyza] (1848-1923)
The rules of aseptic and antiseptic surgery. A practical treatise for the use of students and the general practitioner. 3rd ed. New York: D. Appleton & Co., 1891. 365p. 3 plates. CtY-M; DNLM; NNNAM; PPC **90-2704**

GIBB, Joseph S.
Zinc stearate in the treatment of atrophic rhinitis. Philadelphia: Lea Bros. & Co., 1894. 12p. DNLM
90-2705

GIBBES, Heneage (*d.* 1912)
Miescher's or Rainey's corpuscles in actinomycosis. [St. Louis: J. H. Chambers & Co., 1890.] 6p. DNLM
90-2706

GIBBES, Heneage (*d.* 1912)
Some observations on the origin of ovarian cysts. Boston: Damrell & Upham, 1890. 7p. DNLM
90-2707

GIBBES, Heneage (*d.* 1912) and E. L. SHURLY
An investigation into the etiology of phthisis. I. On the histology of the tubercle, by Heneage Gibbes. [Philadelphia: Lea Bros. & Co., 1890.] 11p. DNLM
90-2708

GIBBES, Heneage (*d.* 1912) and E. L. SHURLY
An investigation into the etiology of phthisis. II. On the clinical history of phthisis pulmonalis, by E. L. Shurly. III. The tubercle bacillus by Heneage Gibbes. [Philadelphia, 1890.] 15p. DNLM **90-2709**

GIBBES, Heneage (*d.* 1912) and E. L. SHURLY
An investigation into the etiology of phthisis. IV. On the etiology and local treatment of phthisis pulmonalis, by E. L. Shurly. [Philadelphia, 1890.] 9p. DNLM
90-2710

GIBBES, Heneage (*d.* 1912) and E. L. SHURLY
An investigation into the etiology of phthisis. V. Tubercular peritonitis, by H. Gibbes. VI. Conclusions drawn from the first part of the investigation. [Philadelphia, 1890.] 14p. DNLM **90-2711**

GIBBES, Heneage (*d.* 1912) and E. L. SHURLY
On the value of the inhalation of chlorine gas and the use of iodine and chloride of gold and sodium hypodermically in the treatment of pulmonary consumption. With an abstract of the clinical history of twenty-seven cases. Detroit: G. S. Davis, 1891. 80p. DNLM; OCIM **90-2712**

GIBBES, Heneage (*d.* 1912)
On the etiology and pathology of tuberculosis. Philadelphia: W. J. Dornan, 1891. 8p. DNLM **90-2713**

GIBBES, Heneage (*d.* 1912)
Practical pathology and morbid histology. Philadelphia: Lea Bros. & Co., 1891. 320p. 1 plate. DNLM; NNNAM; PPC
90-2714

GIBBES, Heneage (*d.* 1912)
On the parasitic nature of cancer. Philadelphia, 1893. 7p. DNLM **90-2715**

GIBBONS, P[eter] J.
A method for resuscitation from electric shock. New York: D. Appleton & Co., 1895. 6p. DNLM
90-2716

GIBIER'S double antitoxin for malignant diphtheria. Tuberculosis, tetanus, and streptococcus antitoxins. The G. F. Harvey Company, manufacturing chemists. Saratoga Springs, N.Y., [1897]. 28 l. DNLM **90-2717**

GIBIER, Paul (1851-1900)
Three communications. 1. A new theory about temperaments. 2. Peroxide of hydrogen; ozone, their antiseptic properties. 3. On hydrophobia. Should Pasteur's method of inoculation against the risk of hydrophobia be practiced at a late period after an injury by a mad dog? New York, 1890. 8p. DNLM
90-2718

GIBNEY, V[irgil] P[endleton] (1847-1927)
Sprained ankle; a treatment that involves no loss of time, requires no crutches, and is not attended with any ultimate impairment of function. [New York: D. Appleton & Co., 1895.] 17p. DNLM **90-2719**

GIBSON, Charles L[angdon]
Local anaesthesia by ethyl chloride. [New York, 1893.] 8p. DNLM **90-2720**

GIBSON, Charles L[angdon]
Operative procedures in advanced age, based on a study of sixty-five cases aged 70 or more. Philadelphia, 1893. 8p. DNLM **90-2721**

GIBSON, Charles L[angdon]
Mortality and treatment of acute intussusception; with table of two hundred and thirty-nine cases. New York: Publishers' Print Co., 1897. 15p. DNLM **90-2722**

GIBSON, Charles L[angdon]
Empyema of the frontal sinuses and intracranial infection. Philadelphia, 1899. 8p. DNLM **90-2723**

GIBSON, George A[lexander] (1854-1913) and William RUSSELL
Physical diagnosis: a guide to methods of clinical investigation. New York: D. Appleton & Co., 1891. 376p. 1 plate. DNLM; NNNAM; PPC **90-2724**

GIBSON, Kasson C.
Treatment of fractures of the maxillae. Philadelphia, 1890. 21p. DNLM **90-2725**

GIBSON, Maris (*b.* 1841)
The axis traction forceps. Wilkesbarre, 1895. 8p. DNLM **90-2726**

GILCHRIST, James Grant (1842-1906)
The elements of surgical pathology with therapeutic hints. . . . Minneapolis: Minneapolis Pharmacy Co., 1895. 343p. DLC **90-2727**

GILLETTE, Arthur J.
Orthopedic surgery as a specialty. Diseases of the hip joint. [n. p., 1892.] 12p. DNLM **90-2728**

GILLETTE, Arthur J.
Pott's disease with special reference to treatment in the upper dorsal and cervical region. St. Paul, 1892. 11p. DNLM **90-2729**

GILLETTE, Arthur J.
Mechanical and surgical treatment of fractures of the neck of the femur. St. Paul, 1898. 20p. DNLM **90-2730**

GILLIAM, D[avid] Todd (1844-1923)
Abdominal tumors, and conditions simulating the same, with anomalous features. [New York: D. Appleton & Co., 1891.] 13p. DNLM **90-2731**

GILLIAM, D[avid] Todd (1844-1923)
Some recent cases of operation for uterine fibroids. [New York, 1891.] 6p. DNLM **90-2732**

GILLIAM, D[avid] Todd (1844-1923)
The operative treatment of ventral hernia resulting from abdominal section. Philadelphia, 1892. 7p. DNLM **90-2733**

GILLIAM, D[avid] Todd (1844-1923)
Report of abdominal operations. [New York, 1892.] 9p. DNLM **90-2734**

GILLIAM, D[avid] Todd (1844-1923)
The vaginal route for operations on the pelvic viscera. New York, 1895. 5p. DNLM **90-2735**

GILLIAM, D[avid] Todd (1844-1923)
A year's work in operative gynecology and abdominal surgery. Columbus, Ohio: Cott & Evans, 1896. 24p. DNLM **90-2736**

GIVENS, Amos J. (*b.* 1864)
Facts and figures concerning homoeopathy. Stamford, Conn., 1895. 6p. DNLM **90-2737**

GIVENS, Amos J. (*b.* 1864)
Climacteric insanity. [New York, 1898.] 6p. DNLM **90-2738**

GLASGOW, William Carr (1845-1907)
A septic and unusual form of lung disease, existing in the Mississippi Valley during the years 1886-90. [Philadelphia: Lea Bros. & Co., 1890.] 13p. DNLM **90-2739**

GLASGOW, William Carr (1845-1907)
A new and distinguishing sign of latent aneurysm of the aorta. New York: D. Appleton & Co., 1894. 8p. DNLM **90-2740**

GLASGOW, William Carr (1845-1907)
The physical signs of cellular oedema of the lung, considered in their relation to the pathological changes. Philadelphia, 1895. 5p. DNLM **90-2741**

GLASS, James H.
Report of fifty appendectomies. New York, 1896. 2 l. DNLM **90-2742**

GLASS, James H.
Immobilisation in the treatment of fractures at the elbow-joint. New York, 1897. 9p. DNLM **90-2743**

GLASS, James H.
Double intestinal anastomosis with Murphy buttons, with report of a successful case. New York, 1897. 6p. DNLM **90-2744**

GLASS, James H.
An experiment in transplantation of the entire human ovary. [Philadelphia, 1899.] 6p. DNLM **90-2745**

GLASS, James H.
Vaginal colpotomy in the treatment of pelvic disease. New York, 1899. 14p. DNLM **90-2746**

GLAZEBROOK, Larkin W. (1876-1943)
Stab-wound of the heart. Philadelphia, 1895. 2p. DNLM **90-2747**

GLEASON, E. B[aldwin] (1854-1934)
Polypoid disease of the nasal chambers. [Detroit, 1891.] 16p. DNLM **90-2748**

GLEASON, E. B[aldwin] (1854-1934)
Exostoses of the nasal septum, and their treatment by operative procedures. [Philadelphia, 1893.] 9p. DNLM **90-2749**

GLEASON, E. B[aldwin] (1854-1934)
Antipyrine as a local application in inflammation of the mucous membrane of the upper respiratory tract. New York: Schulze-Berge & Koechl, 1893. 16p. DNLM **90-2750**

GLEASON, E. B[aldwin] (1854-1934)
Necrosis of the palate process of the superior maxilliary bones; removal of a sequestrum representing much of the bony floor of both nasal chambers and a part of the septum; recovery without any deformity. [Philadelphia, 1893.] 12p. DNLM **90-2751**

GLEASON, E. B[aldwin] (1854-1934)
Essentials of the diseases of the ear. Arranged in the form of questions and answers, prepared especially for students of medicine and post-graduate students. Philadelphia: W. B. Saunders, 1894. 147p. 1 table. DLC; DNLM; ICJ; PPC **90-2752**

GLEASON, E. B[aldwin] (1854-1934)
Essentials of the diseases of the ear. Arranged in the form of questions and answers. Prepared especially for students of medicine and post-graduate students. 2nd ed., rev. and enl. Philadelphia: W. B. Saunders, [*c.* 1897]. 206p. IU-M; PPC; PU **90-2753**

GLEASON, Rachel B[rooks] (1820-1905)
Talks to my patients; hints on getting well and keeping well. New ed., enlarged with the addition of nineteen "letters to ladies" on health, education, society, etc. New York & London: M. L. Holbrook & Co.; L. N. Fowler & Co., 1895. 403p. DNLM; NNNAM **90-2754**

GLEITSMANN, [Joseph] William (1841-1914)
A case of primary tuberculosis of the pharynx terminating in cure. [New York, 1890.] 6p. DNLM **90-2755**

GLEITSMANN, [Joseph] William (1841-1914)
Asheville, N.C., and its advantages as a climatic resort for pulmonary disease. [New York, 1893.] 8p. DNLM **90-2756**

GLEITSMANN, [Joseph] William (1841-1914)
The importance of an early diagnosis of malignant tumors of the throat. [New York: D. Appleton & Co., 1894.] 8p. DNLM **90-2757**

GLEITSMANN, [Joseph] William (1841-1914)
Surgical treatment of laryngeal tuberculosis. New York, 1895. 29p. DNLM **90-2758**

GLEITSMANN, [Joseph] William (1841-1914)
A case of unusual laryngeal growth. New York, 1896. 6p. 1 plate. DNLM **90-2759**

GODFREY, E[dmund] L. B.
Pelvic cellulitis. [Philadelphia, 1891.] 2 l. DNLM **90-2760**

GODFREY, E[dmund] L. B.
The American physician in literature. [Philadelphia, 1892.] 12p. DNLM **90-2761**

GOELET, Augustin H. (1854-1910)
The conservative treatment of inflammatory diseases of the uterine appendages and sequelae by electricity. Boston: Rockwell & Churchill Press, 1890. 4 l. DNLM **90-2762**

GOELET, Augustin H. (1854-1910)
The rational treatment of uterine displacements, based upon a consideration of the pathological conditions present. New York: William Wood & Co., 1891. 18p. DNLM **90-2763**

GOELET, Augustin H. (1854-1910)
The electro-therapeutics of gynaecology. . . . Detroit, Mich.: G. S. Davis, 1892. 3 v. DLC; DNLM; NNNAM; OCIM **90-2764**

GOELET, Augustin H. (1854-1910)
Lecture upon metallic interstitial electrolysis. Philadelphia, [1893]. 12p. DNLM **90-2765**

GOELET, Augustin H. (1854-1910)
An operation for the radical cure of fistula in ano, by an improved method. New York, 1894. 8p. DNLM **90-2766**

GOELET, Augustin H. (1854-1910)
The treatment of uterine fibroids. New York, 1894. 11p. DNLM **90-2767**

GOELET, Augustin H. (1854-1910)
Electricity in gynecology. New York, 1895. 8p. DNLM **90-2768**

GOELET, Augustin H. (1854-1910)
The physiological effect and general therapeutic application of periodic induced currents in gynecology. New York, 1895. 13p. DNLM **90-2769**

GOELET, Augustin H. (1854-1910)
The treatment of metritis and endometritis. New York, 1895. 8p. DNLM **90-2770**

GOELET, Augustin H. (1854-1910)
A case of suspensio-uteri for adherent retroflexion of the uterus; a warning against vaginal operations for such conditions. New York, 1896. 4p. DNLM **90-2771**

GOELET, Augustin H. (1854-1910)
The indications for ventral suspension of the uterus. New York, 1896. 5p. DNLM **90-2772**

GOELET, Augustin H. (1854-1910)
The surgical treatment of uterine displacements. New York, 1896. 7p. DNLM **90-2773**

GOELET, Augustin H. (1854-1910)
Preparation of the patient for abdominal operations. Charlotte, N.C., 1898. 7p. DNLM **90-2774**

[GOLDMAN, S[ydney] Ormond]
Questions on physiology. Specially arranged for the students of College of Physicians and Surgeons, New York City. . . . New York: Press of Stettiner, Lambert & Co., 1894. 24p. DLC **90-2775**

GOLDMAN, S[ydney] Ormond
Questions on materia medica, therapeutics, etc. . . . New York: Press of Stettiner Bros., 1896. 32p. DLC **90-2776**

GOLDMAN, S[ydney] Ormond
A criticism of Dr. Kemp's article on the effects of different anaesthetics on the kidneys. New York, 1899. 6p. DNLM **90-2777**

GOLDMAN, S[ydney] Ormond
Anaesthesia; nitrous oxide; ether; chloroform. New York, 1899. 26p. DNLM; NNNAM **90-2778**

GOLDSMITH, Carrie
Massage for nurses. . . . Cincinnati: R. Clarke & Co., 1892. 59p. DLC; DNLM **90-2779**

GOLDSPOHN, Albert (*b.* 1851)
Errors and modern methods in minor gynecology. Chicago, 1895. 30p. DNLM **90-2780**

GOLDSPOHN, Albert (*b.* 1851)
The proper indications for repair of pathologic lacerations of the cervix uteri, and the proper operations to meet them. Chicago, 1896. 15p. DNLM **90-2781**

GOLDSPOHN, Albert (*b.* **1851**)
Tubo-ovarian cysts, with interesting cases. New York: William Wood & Co., 1896. 10p. DNLM
90-2782

GOLDSTEIN, M[ax] A[aron] (1870-1941)
The hospitals of Europe. St. Louis, 1894. 4p. DNLM
90-2783

GOLDSTEIN, M[ax] A[aron] (1870-1941)
Exfoliation of the cochlea, vestibule and semicircular canals. Kansas City, 1895. 12p. DNLM **90-2784**

GOLDSTEIN, M[ax] A[aron] (1870-1941)
Comparative value of the sense of hearing to the sense of sight. St. Louis, 1896. 4p. DNLM **90-2785**

GOLDSTEIN, M[ax] A[aron] (1870-1941)
Advanced method in teaching the deaf. St. Louis, 1897. 11p. DNLM **90-2786**

GOLDSTEIN, M[ax] A[aron] (1870-1941)
The Texas screw-worm and its invasion of the nasal cavities. St. Louis, 1897. 8p. DNLM **90-2787**

GOLDSTEIN, M[ax] A[aron] (1870-1941)
Bilateral syphilitic ulceration of the auricle. St. Louis, 1898. 6p. DNLM **90-2788**

GOLDSTEIN, M[ax] A[aron] (1870-1941)
The modern therapy of suppurative otitis media. St. Louis, 1898. 6p. DNLM **90-2789**

GOLDSTEIN, M[ax] A[aron] (1870-1941)
Nasal hemorrhage and the haemophilic diathesis. Memphis, 1898. 4p. DNLM **90-2790**

GOLDSTEIN, M[ax] A[aron] (1870-1941)
Modern therapy of the tympanic cavity. New York, 1899. 13p. DNLM **90-2791**

GOLDSTEIN, M[ax] A[aron] (1870-1941)
Otitis media; diagnosis and treatment. St. Louis, 1899. 7p. DNLM **90-2792**

GOLDSTEIN, S[amuel]
Creosote in tuberculosis. New York, 1899. 2 l. DNLM
90-2793

GOLDTHWAIT, Joel E[rnest] (*b.* **1866**)
The forcible straightening of angular defomities of the knee by means of special mechanical appliances. Boston: Damrell & Upham, 1892. 12p. 2 plates. DNLM
90-2794

GOLDTHWAIT, Joel E[rnest] (*b.* **1866**)
Forcible correction of angular deformities of the knee, with a report of cases. Boston, 1893. 8p. DNLM
90-2795

GOLDTHWAIT, Joel E[rnest] (*b.* **1866**)
Joint lesions due to disease of the spinal cord, with a report of two cases. [Philadelphia, 1893.] 10p. DNLM
90-2796

GOLDTHWAIT, Joel E[rnest] (*b.* **1866**)
The treatment of hallux valgus. Boston, 1893. 8p. DNLM
90-2797

GOLDTHWAIT, Joel E[rnest] (*b.* **1866**)
The anterior transverse arch of the foot. Its obliteration as a cause of metatarsalgia. Boston: Damrell & Upham, 1894. 6p. DNLM **90-2798**

GOLDTHWAIT, Joel E[rnest] (*b.* **1866**)
A case of acute osteo-arthritis involving the whole cervical region of the spine, in a woman nearly sixty years of age, with recovery. Boston, 1895. 4p. DNLM
90-2799

GOLDTHWAIT, Joel E[rnest] (*b.* **1866**)
Tendon transplantation in the treatment of paralytic deformities. Boston: Damrell & Upham, 1896. 16p. DNLM
90-2800

GOLDTHWAIT, Joel E[rnest] (*b.* **1866**)
The treatment of disabled joints resulting from the so-called rheumatoid diseases. Boston: Damrell & Upham, 1897. 16p. DNLM **90-2801**

GOLDTHWAIT, Joel E[rnest] (*b.* **1866**) **and C[harles] F. PAINTER**
Subtrochanteric osteotomy for the correction of deformities resulting from hip disease; report of cases. [Philadelphia, 1898.] 12p. DNLM **90-2802**

GOLDTHWAIT, Joel E[rnest] (*b.* **1866**)
The immediate correction of the deformities resulting from Pott's disease. [Philadelphia, 1898.] 20p. DNLM
90-2803

GOLDTHWAIT, Joel E[rnest] (*b.* **1866**)
A case of spinal caries followed by late suppuration, with discharge of the abscess through the bronchus. Boston, 1898. 3p. DNLM **90-2804**

GOLDTHWAIT, Joel E[rnest] (*b.* **1866**)
Permanent dislocation of the patella. The report of a case of twenty years' duration successfully treated by transplantation of the patella tendons, with the tubercle of the tibia. [Philadelphia, 1899.] 7p. DNLM **90-2805**

GOLDTHWAIT, Joel E[rnest] (*b.* **1866**)
Pott's paraplegia as affected by the correction of the spinal deformity; a report of cases. [Philadelphia], 1899. 8p. DNLM
90-2806

GOLDTHWAIT, Joel E[rnest] (*b.* **1866**)
Osteo-arthritis of the spine; spondylitis deformans. [Philadelphia], 1899. 21p. DNLM **90-2807**

GOLER, G[eorge] W[ashington] (*b.* **1864**)
Diphtheria; how is it propagated? Buffalo, 1894. 7p. DNLM
90-2808

GOODALE, Joseph L[incoln] (*b.* **1868**)
The preparation of diphtheria antitoxine. Boston, 1895. 13p. DNLM **90-2809**

GOODALE, Joseph L[incoln] (*b.* **1868**)
An experimental study of the respiratory functions of the nose. Boston: Damrell & Upham, 1896. 28p. DNLM
90-2810

GOODALE, Joseph L[incoln] (*b.* **1868**)
On the identity of the conditions commonly known as wandering rash of the tongue and Moeller's superficial glossitis. Philadelphia, 1896. 16p. DNLM **90-2811**

GOODALE, Joseph L[incoln] (*b.* 1868)
An etiologic study of atrophic disease of the upper air passages, based upon an examintion of two hundred cases. Chicago, 1898. 8p. DNLM **90-2812**

GOODALE, Joseph L[incoln] (*b.* 1868)
On the treatment of certain forms of cervical lymphadenitis by the introduction of medicinal substances into the crypts of the faucial tonsils. Boston, 1898. 7p. DNLM **90-2813**

GOODALE, Joseph L[incoln] (*b.* 1868)
The utilization of the normal tonsillar absorption in the treatment of tuberculosis of the angular lymphatic glands. Boston, 1898. 2p. DNLM **90-2814**

GOODALE, Joseph L[incoln] (*b.* 1868) and H[enry] F. HEWES
A case of isolated urticaria of the tongue associated with achlorhydria. Boston, 1898. 3p. DNLM **90-2815**

GOODALE, Joseph L[incoln] (*b.* 1868)
Acute suppurative processes in the faucial tonsils. New York, 1899. 12p. DNLM **90-2816**

GOODALE, Joseph L[incoln] (*b.* 1868)
A contribution to the pathological histology of acute tonsillitis. Boston, 1899. 8p. 3 plates. DNLM **90-2817**

GOODALE, Joseph L[incoln] (*b.* 1868)
A new method for the operative correction of exaggerated Roman nose. Boston, 1899. 4p. DNLM **90-2818**

GOODALL, E[dward] W[ilberforce] (*b.* 1861) and J[ohn] W[ychenford] WASHBOURN
A manual of infectious diseases. Philadelphia: P. Blakiston, Son & Co., [1896]. 368p. DNLM; NNNAM; PPC **90-2819**

GOODELL, William (1829-1894)
Lessons in gynecology. 3rd ed. Philadelphia & London: F. A. Davis, 1890. 579p. CtY-M; DNLM; PPC; PU **90-2820**

GOODELL, William (1829-1894)
What I have learned to unlearn in gynecology [Philadelphia, 1890.] 16p. DNLM **90-2821**

GOODELL, William (1829-1894)
Early diagnosis essential for the cure of uterine cancer. [Philadelphia, 1892.] 8p. DNLM **90-2822**

GOODELL, William (1829-1894)
The effect of castration on woman, and other problems in gynecology. [Philadelphia, 1893.] 15p. DNLM **90-2823**

GOODHART, James F[rederic] (1845-1916)
On common neuroses, or the neurotic element in disease and its rational treatment. Three lectures delivered before the Harveian Society of London, November, December, 1891. Philadelphia: P. Blakiston, Son & Co., 1892. 128p. DNLM; NNNAM; PPC **90-2824**

GOODHUE, E[dward] S[olon] (*b.* 1861)
Operation for the correction of deformity of the wrist caused by shortening of the radius after fracture. New York: Trow, 1894. 8p. DNLM **90-2825**

GOODNO, William C[olby]
The practice of medicine, with sections on diseases of the nervous system, by Clarence Bartlett. v. 1. Specific infectious diseases and diseases of the nervous system. Philadelphia: Hahnemann Press, 1894. 961p. DNLM; NNNAM; PPC; PPHa [Vol. II, 1895] **90-2826**

GOODWILLIE, D[avid] H[enderson] (*b.* 1834)
Nasal intubation. [New York, 1890.] 10p. DNLM **90-2827**

GOODWILLIE, D[avid] H[enderson] (*b.* 1834)
Fractures of the maxillary bones. [1891.] 3p. DNLM **90-2828**

GOODWIN, Charles H.
Treatment of diseases of the heart and lungs, with over three hundred and fifty formulae and prescriptions. . . . 4th ed., rev. New York: J. B. Flint & Co., 1897. 196p. DLC; NNNAM **90-2829**

GOODWIN, Charles H.
Treatment of diseases of infancy and childhood, with over four hundred formulae and prescriptions, as exemplified in the services of Drs. A. Jacobi, J. Lewis Smith . . . etc., etc., and in the hospitals of New York City. . . . 2nd ed., rev. New York: J. B. Flint & Co., 1897. 284p. DLC; NNNAM **90-2830**

GORDINIER, H[ermon] C. (*b.* 1864)
The gross and minute anatomy of the central nervous system. Philadelphia: P. Blakiston's Son & Co., 1890. 9p. DNLM; PPC; PU **90-2831**

GORDINIER, H[ermon] C. (*b.* 1864)
Injury to the cauda equina, probably due to intra-meningeal hemorrhage, with recovery. [Philadelphia, 1894.] 6p. DNLM **90-2832**

GORDINIER, H[ermon] C. (*b.* 1864)
Two cases of akromegaly. Philadelphia, 1895. 13p. DNLM **90-2833**

GORDON, Bernard (*b.* 1863)
The dangers of delaying intubation. New York: Stettiner, Lambert & Co., 1891. 4p. DNLM; NNNAM **90-2834**

GORDON, Henry Laing
Sir James Young Simpson and chloroform (1811-1870) by. . . . New York: Longmans, Green & Co., 1897. 233p. DLC; ICU; NN **90-2835**

GORDON, Joseph C[laybaugh] (1842-1903)
Notes and observations upon the education of the deaf; with a revised index to education of deaf children. Washington, D.C., 1892. 90p. DNLM **90-2836**

GORDON, Joseph C[laybaugh] (1842-1903)
Progress in the amelioration of certain forms of deafness and impaired hearing. Rochester, 1894. 25p. DNLM **90-2837**

GORDON, Joseph C[laybaugh] (1842-1903)
Address before the auricular section of the fourteenth Convention of American Instructors of the Deaf. [Flint, Mich., 1895.] 7p. DNLM **90-2838**

GORDON, Joseph C[laybaugh] (1842-1903)
Address upon the occasion of the opening of the first meeting of the oral section of the Convention of American Instructors of the Deaf, July 4, 1895. [Flint, Mich.], 1895. 11p. DNLM **90-2839**

GORDON, Joseph C[laybaugh] (1842-1903)
The difference between the two systems of teaching deaf-mute children the English language. Washington: Sanders, 1898. 4p. DNLM **90-2840**

GORDON, S[eth] C[hase] (*b.* 1830)
Peritonitis in the female; its causes, effects, and treatment both proplylactic and immediate. [New York, 1890.] 13p. DNLM **90-2841**

GORDON, S[eth] C[hase] (*b.* 1830)
Common sense in medicine. Boston: Damrell & Upham, 1891. 23p. DNLM **90-2842**

GORDON, S[eth] C[hase] (*b.* 1830)
Hysterectomy without pedicle. [New York, 1892.] 4p. DNLM **90-2843**

GORDON, S[eth] C[hase] (*b.* 1830)
Dangers and complications of uterine fibroids. New York: William Wood & Co., 1893. 5p. DNLM **90-2844**

GORDON, S[eth] C[hase] (*b.* 1830)
Recurrent appendicitis; six operations with six recoveries; treatment for acute attack in five cases. Boston: Damrell & Upham, 1893. 7p. DNLM **90-2845**

GORDON, S[eth] C[hase] (*b.* 1830)
Salines in appendicitis. Boston, 1893. 5p. DNLM **90-2846**

GORDON, S[eth] C[hase] (*b.* 1830)
Further experience and observations in hysterectomy for fibroids. New York, 1895. 6p. DNLM **90-2847**

GORDON, S[eth] C[hase] (*b.* 1830)
I. Two pregnancies following removal of both ovaries and tubes. II. Two peculiar cases of extra-uterine pregnancy. III. Effect of hysterectomy upon the vagina. New York, 1896. 5p. DNLM **90-2848**

GORGAS, Ferdinand James Samuel (1835-1914)
Dental medicine; a manual of dental materia medica and therapeutics. 4th ed. Rev. and enl. Philadelphia: P. Blakiston, Son & Co., 1891. 524p. DLC; DNLM; NNNAM; PPC **90-2849**

GORGAS, Ferdinand J[ames] S[amuel] (1835-1914)
A series of questions and answers for dental students, consisting of three parts: Part I. Pertaining to the freshman course. Part II. Pertaining to the junior course. Part III. Pertaining to the senior course. Baltimore: Snowden & Cowman, 1892. 3 v. DLC; DNLM; MdU-D; PPC **90-2850**

GORGAS, Ferdinand James Samuel (1835-1914)
Dental medicine; a manual of dental materia medica and therapeutics. . . . 5th ed. Rev. and enl. Philadelphia: P. Blakiston, Son & Co., 1895. 580p. DLC; DNLM; MdU-D; PPC **90-2851**

GORGAS, Ferdinand James Samuel (1835-1914)
Dental medicine: a manual of dental materia medica and therapeutics. . . . 6th ed. Rev. and enl. Philadelphia: P. Blakiston, Son & Co., 1898. 592p. DLC; DNLM; NNNAM; PU **90-2852**

GOTTHEIL, William S[amuel] (1859-1920)
Barber's itch. [Philadelphia, 1892.] 12p. DNLM **90-2853**

GOTTHEIL, William S[amuel] (1859-1920)
Two cases of labial chancre in cigar-makers. [Philadelphia]: Lea Bros. & Co., [1893]. 8p. DNLM **90-2854**

GOTTHEIL, William S[amuel] (1859-1920)
A manual of general histology. New York: Sabiston, Murray & Co., 1894. 148p. DNLM; NNNAM **90-2855**

GOTTHEIL, William S[amuel] (1859-1920)
Pseudo-chancre. New York, 1895. 12p. DNLM **90-2856**

GOTTHEIL, William S[amuel] (1859-1920)
Illustrated skin diseases; an atlas and textbook with special reference to diagnosis and the most approved methods of treatment. New York: E. B. Treat & Co., 1897. 424p. 45 plates. DNLM; NNNAM; PPC **90-2857**

GOTTHEIL, William S[amuel] (1859-1920)
A house epidemic of syphilis. New York, 1898. 7p. DNLM **90-2858**

GOTTHEIL, William S[amuel] (1859-1920)
The treatment of skin cancers. . . . New York: International Journal of Surgery Co., [1898]. 67p. plates. DLC; DNLM; NNNAM **90-2859**

GOTTHEIL, William S[amuel] (1859-1920)
Gummatous periostitis and osteitis, with record of a case of perforation of the cranial vault. New York, 1899. 10p. DNLM **90-2860**

GOULD, A[lfred] Pearce (1852-1922)
Elements of surgical diagnosis. . . . Philadelphia: Lea Bros. & Co., 1890. [1884]. 589p. DNLM; OCIM; PPC; PU **90-2861**

GOULD, George M[ilbry] (1848-1922)
A new medical dictionary; including all the words and phrases used in medicine, with their proper pronunciation and definitions. Based on recent medical literature. . . . Philadelphia: P. Blakiston, Son & Co., 1890. 519p. DLC; DNLM; NNNAM; PPC **90-2862**

GOULD, George M[ilbry] (1848-1922)
The abuse of a great charity. [Philadelphia, 1890.] 19p. DNLM **90-2863**

GOULD, George M[ilbry] (1848-1922)
Clinical illustrations of reflex ocular neuroses. [Philadelphia: Lea Bros. & Co., 1890.] 7p. DNLM **90-2864**

GOULD, George M[ilbry] (1848-1922)
The relation of eye strain to general medicine. [Philadelphia, 1890.] 21p. DNLM **90-2865**

GOULD, George M[ilbry] (1848-1922)
The statistics and lessons of fifteen hundred cases of refraction. Chicago, 1891. 15p. DNLM **90-2866**

GOULD, George M[ilbry] (1848-1922)
Amblyopiatrics. [Philadelphia, 1892.] 15p. DNLM **90-2867**

GOULD, George M[ilbry] (1848-1922)
The antiseptic dropper. [Philadelphia, 1892.] 2p. DNLM **90-2868**

GOULD, George M[ilbry] (1848-1922)
The etiology, diagnosis, and treatment of the prevalent epidemic of quackery. [Philadelphia, 1892.] 24p. DNLM **90-2869**

GOULD, George M[ilbry] (1848-1922)
Everybody's medical duty; an address to the Unitarian Club of Philadelphia, February 11, 1892. Philadelphia: W. A. Church, 1892. 22p. DNLM **90-2870**

GOULD, George M[ilbry] (1848-1922)
The function of the lachrymal puncta. Philadelphia, 1892. 3p. DNLM **90-2871**

GOULD, George M[ilbry] (1848-1922)
A method of infection, treatment, and prophylaxis of purulent ophthalmia. Philadelphia, 1892. 5p. DNLM **90-2872**

GOULD, George M[ilbry] (1848-1922)
A pocket medical dictionary, giving the pronunciation and definition of about 11,000 of the principal words used in medicine and the collateral sciences, including very complete tables of the arteries, msucles, nerves, [etc.]. Philadelphia: P. Blakiston, Son & Co., 1892. 317p. DNLM; PPC; PPJ; PU **90-2873**

GOULD, George M[ilbry] (1848-1922)
The practical adjustment of spectacles. [St. Louis, 1892.] 7p. DNLM **90-2874**

GOULD, George M[ilbry] (1848-1922)
A simple method of treating many cases of lachrymal obstruction. [New York, 1892.] 6p. DNLM **90-2875**

GOULD, George M[ilbry] (1848-1922)
An additional word as to the treatment of exophoria. [Philadelphia, 1893.] 5p. DNLM **90-2876**

GOULD, George M[ilbry] (1848-1922)
A case of homatropine susceptibility. [Philadelphia, 1893.] 1 l. DNLM **90-2877**

GOULD, George M[ilbry] (1848-1922)
The duty of the community to medical science. [Easton, Pa., 1893.] 12p. DNLM **90-2878**

GOULD, George M[ilbry] (1848-1922)
Homeochronous hereditary optic-nerve atrophy, extending through six generations. [St. Louis, 1893.] 5p. DNLM **90-2879**

GOULD, George M[ilbry] (1848-1922)
The meaning and the method of life; a search for religion in biology. New York & London: G. P. Putnam's Sons, 1893. 1 p. l. 297p. DNLM **90-2880**

GOULD, George M[ilbry] (1848-1922)
"The medical press." [Detroit, 1893.] 12p. DNLM **90-2881**

GOULD, George M[ilbry] (1848-1922)
The pernicious influence of albinism upon the eye. St. Louis, 1893. 10p. DNLM **90-2882**

GOULD, George M[ilbry] (1848-1922)
The spelling of some medical words. [Philadelphia, 1893.] 8p. DNLM **90-2883**

GOULD, George M[ilbry] (1848-1922)
A temporary change in the axis of astigmatism. [Philadelphia, 1893.] 1 l. DNLM **90-2884**

GOULD, George M[ilbry] (1848-1922)
An illustrated dictionary of medicine, biology and allied sciences. . . . Philadelphia: P. Blakiston, Son & Co., 1894. 1633p. DLC; DNLM; NNNAM; PPC **90-2885**

GOULD, George M[ilbry] (1848-1922)
Charity organization and medicine. [Philadelphia: Lea Bros. & Co., 1894.] 18p. DNLM **90-2886**

GOULD, George M[ilbry] (1848-1922)
A collective investigation as to the infuence of albinism upon the eye. [Circular.] [Philadelphia, 1894.] 2 l. DNLM **90-2887**

GOULD, George M[ilbry] (1848-1922) and E. M. HEWISH
A case of glaucoma simplex. Philadelphia, 1894. 5p. DNLM **90-2888**

GOULD, George M[ilbry] (1848-1922)
An illustrated dictionary of medicine, biology and allied sciences. . . . rev. ed. Philadelphia: P. Blakiston, Son & Co., 1895. 1633p. NNNAM; PU **90-2889**

GOULD, George M[ilbry] (1848-1922)
Hospitalism. Philadelphia, 1895. 32p. DNLM **90-2890**

GOULD, George M[ilbry] (1848-1922)
A study of muscae, with suggestions as to the physiology of intraocular nutrition, the etiology of cataract, glaucoma, etc. Philadelphia, 1895. 28p. DNLM; PPC **90-2891**

GOULD, George M[ilbry] (1848-1922)
An illustrated dictionary of medicine, biology and allied sciences. . . . 3rd rev. Philadelphia: P. Blakiston, Son & Co., 1896. 1633p. NNNAM; PPC; PU **90-2892**

GOULD, George M[ilbry] (1848-1922)
The student's medical dictionary, including all the words and phrases generally used in medicine, with their proper pronunciation and definitions, based on recent medical literature; with elaborate tables of the bacilli, micrococci, leucomains, ptomains, etc., of the arteries, ganglia, muscles, and nerves; of weights and measures, analyses of the mineral springs of the United States, etc. 10th ed., rewritten and enlarged. Philadelphia: P. Blakiston, Son & Co., 1896. 701p. DNLM; NNNAM; PPC; PU **90-2893**

GOULD, George M[ilbry] (1848-1922)
Borderland studies; miscellaneous addresses and essays pertaining to medicine and the medical profession, and their relations to general sciences and thought. . . . Philadelphia: P. Blakiston, Son & Co., 1896-1908. 2 v. DLC; DNLM; PPC; PU
90-2894

GOULD, George Milbry], ed. (1848-1922)
An American year-book of medicine and surgery, being a yearly digest of scientific progress and authoritative opinion in all branches of medicine and surgery, drawn from the journals, monographs, and text-books of the leading American and foreign authors and investigators; collected and arranged with critical editorial comments by J. M. Baldy, C. H. Burnett [*et al.*]. Philadelphia: W. B. Saunders, 1896. 1183p. 33 plates. DNLM; NNNAM; PPC; PU **90-2895**

GOULD, George M[ilbry] (1848-1922)
Law of refraction-change following increase or decrease of body weight. Philadelphia, 1897. 5p. DNLM
90-2896

GOULD, George M[ilbry] (1848-1922)
Retinitis pigmentosa without the characteristic pigmentation; a report of two cases. St. Louis, 1898. 16p. DNLM
90-2897

GOULD, George M[ilbry] (1848-1922)
Anomalies and curiosities of medicine; being an encyclopedic collection of rare and extraordinary cases, and of the most striking instances of abnormality in all branches of medicine and surgery, derived from an exhaustive research of medical literature from its origin to the present day, abstracted, classified, annotated, and indexed, by George M. Gould . . . and Walter L. Pyle. . . . With 295 illustrations in the text, and 12 half-tone and colored plates. Philadelphia: W. B. Saunders, 1897. 968p. DLC; DNLM; NNNAM; PPC
90-2898

GOULD, George M[ilbry] (1848-1922)
. . . A compend of the diseases of the eye and refraction including treatment and surgery, by George M. Gould . . . and Walter L. Pyle. . . . Philadelphia: P. Blakiston, Son & Co., 1897. 258p. col. frontis., diags. DLC; NNNAM; PPC; PU
90-2899

GOULD, George M[ilbry] (1848-1922)
A pocket medical dictionary, giving the pronunciation and definition of the principal words used in medicine and collateral sciences. . . . A new ed., entirely rewritten and enl. . . . Philadelphia: P. Blakiston's Son & Co., 1898. 580p. DLC; NNNAM; PPC; PU **90-2900**

GOULD, George M[ilbry] (1848-1922)
An illustrated dictionary of medicine, biology and allied sciences. . . . 4th ed. Philadelphia: P. Blakiston, Son & Co., 1898. 1633p. DNLM; NNNAM; PPC; PU
90-2901

GOULD, George M[ilbry] (1848-1922)
The biologic basis of ethics and religion. Philadelphia: E. Stern & Co., 1898. 30p. DNLM **90-2902**

GOULD, George M[ilbry] (1848-1922)
A case of mathematically perfect eyes. St. Louis, 1898. 6p. DNLM **90-2903**

GOULD, George M[ilbry] (1848-1922)
Some relations of author, publisher, editor, and profession. [Easton, Pa., 1899.] 11p. DNLM **90-2904**

GOULD, George M[ilbry] (1848-1922)
A pocket medical dictionary giving the pronunciation and definition of the principal words used in medicine and the collateral sciences. . . . 3rd ed. . . . rewritten and enlarged. . . . Philadelphia: P. Blakiston's Son & Co., 1899. 781p. DLC; IU-M; IEN-M; PPC **90-2905**

GOULD, George M[ilbry] (1848-1922)
. . . A compend of the diseases of the eye and refraction, including treatment and surgery, by George M. Gould . . . and Walter L. Pyle. . . . 2nd ed., rev. and enl. . . . Philadelphia: P. Blakiston's Son & Co., 1899. 295p. col. frontis. DLC; NNNAM; PPC; PPJ **90-2906**

GOULEY, John William Severin (1832-1920)
Retention of urine from prostatic obstruction in elderly men; its nature, diagnosis, and management. . . . [New York? 1890.] 18p. DLC; DNLM; NNNAM **90-2907**

GOULEY, John W[illiam] S[everin] (1832-1920)
A plea for the early extirpation of tumours. . . . New York: D. Appleton & Co., 1891. 53p. DLC; DNLM; NNNAM
90-2908

GOULEY, John William Severin (1832-1920)
Diseases of the urinary apparatus; phlegmasic affections. . . . New York: D. Appleton & Co., 1892. 342p. DLC; DNLM; NNNAM; PPC **90-2909**

GOULEY, John William Severin (1832-1920)
. . . Notes on American catheters and bougies. . . . [New York, 1893.] 11p. DLC **90-2910**

GOULEY, John W[illiam] S[everin] (1832-1920)
. . . Typhlenteritis versus appendicitis. . . . [New York]: D. Appleton & Co., 1894. 7p. DLC
90-2911

GOULEY, John William Severin (1832-1920)
Memoir of the late Alfred Ludlow Carroll, M.D. . . . Concord, N.H.: Printed by Republican Press Assoication, 1894. 23p. DLC **90-2912**

GOULEY, John William Severin (1832-1920)
The prognosis of malignant tumors as modified by their early detection and prompt ablation. . . . Read before the New York State Medical Association, October 16, 1895. Concord, N.H.: Printed by the Repub. Press Association, 1895. 23p. DLC
90-2913

GOULEY, John William Severin (1832-1920)
Retention of urine during urethritis and from urethral stricture. . . . Read before the New York State Medical Association, October 17, 1895. Concord, N.H.: Printed by the Republican Press Association, 1896. 13p. DLC
90-2914

GOULEY, John William Severin (1832-1920)
Prostate enlargement: remarks introductory to a discussion on it nature, diagnosis, and treatment. . . . Concord, N.H.: Printed by the Republican Press Association, 1896. 34p. DLC
90-2915

GOULEY, John William Severin (1832-1920)
Notes on intestinal obstruction from impaction of faeces, enteroliths, and foreign bodies. . . . [Concord? N.H., 1898.] 13p. DLC **90-2916**

GOULEY, John William Severin (1832-1920)
Urethral stricture; a few thoughts on its genesis and management. . . . [New York? 1898.] 3p. DLC **90-2917**

GOULEY, John William Severin (1832-1920)
Notes on urethral catheterism, catheters, and bougies. . . . [New York, 1899.] 36p. DLC; DNLM; NNNAM **90-2918**

GOWERS, William R[ichard] (1845-1915)
Neuralgia; its aetiology, diagnosis, and treatment. New York: William Wood & Co., 1890. 56p. CtY-M; IU-M [Separately printed out of Wood's Medical and Surgical Monographs, vol. 5 (1890), No. 1, pp. 1-56.] **90-2919**

GOWERS, William R[ichard] (1845-1915)
A manual and atlas of medical ophthalmoscopy. . . . 3rd ed., rev. throughout . . . ed. with the assistance of Marcus Gunn. Philadelphia: P. Blakiston, Son & Co., 1890. 330p. DNLM; ICU; PPC; PPJ **90-2920**

GOWERS, William R[ichard] (1845-1915)
Syphilis and the nervous system; being a revised reprint of the Lettsomian lectures for 1890, delivered before the Medical Society of London. Philadelphia: P. Blakiston, Son & Co., 1892. 131p. CtY-M; DLC; NNNAM; PPC **90-2921**

GOWERS, William R[ichard] (1845-1915)
A manual of diseases of the nervous system. 2nd ed., rev. and enl. Philadelphia: P. Blakiston, Son & Co., 1892-3. 2 v. DNLM; NNNAM; OCIM; PPC **90-2922**

GOWERS, William R[ichard] (1845-1915)
The dynamics of life; an address delivered before the Medical Society of Manchester, October 3, 1894. Philadelphia: P. Blakiston, Son & Co., 1894. 70p. DNLM; ICU; NNNAM; PPC **90-2923**

GOWERS, William R[ichard] (1845-1915)
Clinical lectures on diseases of the nervous system, delivered at the National Hospital for the Paralysed and Epileptic, London. Philadelphia: P. Blakiston, Son & Co., 1895. 279p. DLC; NNNAM; PPC; PU **90-2924**

GOWERS, William R[ichard] (1845-1915)
A manual of diseases of the nervous system. . . . 3rd ed., revised and enlarged; edited by Sir W. R. Gowers and James Taylor. Philadelphia: P. Blakiston, Son & Co., 1898-1899. 2 v. DNLM; OCIM; [v. 1, 3rd ed.; v. 2, 2nd ed.] **90-2925**

GRADY, Richard
Dental infirmary patients; use and abuse of dental charity. Chicago, 1891. 20p. DNLM **90-2926**

GRAHAM, Douglas (1848-1928)
Recent developments in massage; historical, physiological, medical, and surgical. New York: J. H. Vail & Co., [1890]. 18p. DNLM; NNNAM **90-2927**

GRAHAM, Douglas (1848-1928)
A treatise on massage, theoretical and practical; its history, mode of application and effects, indications and contra-indications, with results in over fifteen hundred cases. 2nd ed., revised and enlarged. New York: J. H. Vail & Co., 1890. 342p. DNLM; NNNAM; PPC **90-2928**

GRAHAM, Douglas (1848-1928)
Recent developments in message, historical, physiological, medical and surgical. . . . 2nd ed. . . . Detroit, Mich.: G. S. Davis, 1893. 128p. DLC; DNLM; NNNAM; OCIM **90-2929**

GRAHAM, Douglas (1848-1928)
Massage, movements, and bandaging in the treatment of displaced semilunar cartilages. Boston: Damrell & Upham, 1896. 12p. DNLM **90-2930**

GRAHAM, Edwin E. (*b.* 1864)
A case of neurotic oedema. [Philadelphia, 1894.] 1 l. DNLM **90-2931**

GRAHAM, Herbert
Cod-liver oil emulsion. [Philadelphia, 1890.] 1 galley-sheet. DNLM **90-2932**

GRAHAM, James
The medical treatment of appendicitis, and its limitations. Detroit: G. S. Davis, 1892. 9p. DNLM **90-2933**

GRAHAM, James E[lliot] (1847-1899)
Hydroa aestivale. New York, 1896. 6p. DNLM **90-2934**

GRAHAM, John
A plea for the continuation of outdoor sports in middle and advanced life. [Philadelphia: Lea Bros. & Co., 1892.] 4p. DNLM **90-2935**

GRAHAM, John
Some precautions against the spread of contagious diseases, especially in children. [Philadelphia, 1892.] 4p. DNLM **90-2936**

GRAHAM, J[ohn] T.
Address to the profession and the public, delivered at the 24th annual session of the Medical Society of Virginia, at Charlottesville, Tuesday, October 3, 1893. [Richmond, 1893.] 15p. DNLM **90-2937**

GRAHAM, N[eil] F. (*b.* 1840)
Simple fracture of the shaft of the femur, and its treatment with the long splint. Philadelphia, 1892. 13p. DNLM **90-2938**

GRAHAM, N[eil] F. (*b.* 1840)
Further considerations on the influence of old age in surgery. [Philadelphia: Lea Bros. & Co., 1895.] 9p. DNLM **90-2939**

GRANDIN, Egbert Henry (*b.* 1855)
Practical treatise on electricity in gynaecology, by Egbert H. Grandin . . . and Josephus H. Gunning. . . . New York: William Wood & Co., 1891. 171p. DLC; NNNAM **90-2940**

GRANDIN, Egbert Henry (*b.* 1855)
A clinical contribution to the subject of symphysiotomy. Philadelphia, 1893. 5p. DNLM **90-2941**

GRANDIN, Egbert Henry (*b.* 1855)
A clinical study of puerperal peritonitis. New York, 1893. 12p. DNLM **90-2942**

GRANDIN, Egbert Henry (*b.* 1855)
The relative value of certain obstetrical operations (embryotomy, Caesarean section, symphysiotomy). New York: William Wood & Co., 1893. 4p. DNLM
90-2943

GRANDIN, Egbert Henry (*b.* 1855)
Obstetric surgery. By Egbert H. Grandin . . . and George W. Jarman. . . . Philadelphia: The F. A. Davis Co.; [etc., etc.], 1894. 207p. plates. DLC; NNNAM; PPC
90-2944

GRANDIN, Egbert Henry (*b.* 1855)
Pregnancy, labor, and the puerperal state. By Egbert H. Grandin . . . and George W. Jarman. . . . Philadelphia: The F. A. Davis Co., [etc., etc.], 1895. 261p. col. plates. DLC; NNNAM; PPC **90-2945**

GRANDIN, Egbert Henry (*b.* 1855) and George W. JARMAN
Practical obstetrics. Philadelphia: F. A. Davis Co.; London: F. J. Rebman, 1895. 2 v. in 1. 15 plates. DNLM; NNNAM; PU
90-2946

GRANDIN, Egbert Henry (*b.* 1855)
Late infection in the puerperal state, being a plea for the routine manual examination of the interior of the uterus after the completion of the third stage of labor. Philadelphia, 1895. 5p. DNLM **90-2947**

GRANDIN, Egbert Henry (*b.* 1855)
Diseases of the intra-uterine life on the part of the mother. [Philadelphia, 1896.] 6p. DNLM
90-2948

GRANDIN, Egbert Henry (*b.* 1855)
A text-book of practical obstetrics, by Egbert H. Grandin . . . with the collaboration of George W. Jarman. . . . 2nd ed., rev. and enl. Illustrated with sixty-four full-page photographic plates and eighty-six illustrations in the text. Philadelphia, New York, [etc.]: The F. A. Davis Co., 1898. 461p. plates. DLC; NNNAM; PPC; PU **90-2949**

GRANT, H. Horace (*b.* 1853)
Suggestions as to the technique of intestinal anastomosis. [Louisville, 1892.] 5p. DNLM **90-2950**

GRANT, H. Horace (*b.* 1853)
Management of damaged intestine in strangulated hernia. [New York, 1893.] 8p. DNLM **90-2951**

GRANT, Thomas P[age]
A case of scirrus treated by internal medication. [Louisville, 1893.] 3p. DNLM **90-2952**

GRANVILLE, Joseph Mortimer (1833-1900)
Youth, its care and culture. An outline of principles for parents and guardians. New York: M. L. Holbrook, [1897]. 167p. DNLM; NNNAM **90-2953**

GRAVES, Schuyler C[olfax] (1858-1941)
A case of abdominal nephrectomy; with practical lessons thereon. [Philadelphia: Lea Bros. & Co., 1892.] 8p. DNLM
90-2954

GRAVES, Schuyler C[olfax] (1858-1941)
A case of lumbar nephrectomy for pyonephrosis. [Philadelphia: Lea Bros. & Co., 1892.] 5p. DNLM
90-2955

GRAVES, Schuyler C[olfax] (1858-1941)
Certain pelvic abscesses with a new apparatus for their successful drainage and cure. [Philadelphia: Lea Bros. & Co., 1895.] 6p. DNLM **90-2956**

GRAVES, Schuyler C[olfax] (1858-1941)
A rare dermoid. [Philadelphia: Lea Bros. & Co., 1895.] 3p. DNLM **90-2957**

GRAVES, Schuyler C[olfax] (1858-1941)
A new method of pedicle-ligation in abdominal surgery. [Philadelphia: Lea Bros. & Co., 1895.] 7p. DNLM
90-2958

GRAVES, William W[ashington] (1865-1949)
A preliminary report on a method of overcoming high resistance in Crookes' tubes; a possible step toward maximum radiance. St. Louis: Am. X-Ray Publ. Co., 1898. 15p. DNLM
90-2959

GRAY, Harry C.
A condensed compendium of pharmaceutical knowledge. A quiz book by H. C. Gray and C. H. Bryan. 6th ed. Chicago: Gray & Bryan, 1890. 114p. OCLloyd
90-2960

GRAY, Harry C.
Gray's prescriptionist. A treatise on the art of reading and compounding physicians' prescriptions, with tables of weights and measures, antidotes, abbreviations, etc. . . . Chicago, Ill.: Gray & Bryan, 1891. 87p. DLC; DNLM; OCLloyd
90-2961

GRAY, Harry C.
A condensed compendium of pharmaceutical knowledge. A quiz book by H. C. Gray and C. H. Bryan. 7th ed. Chicago: Gray & Bryan, 1891. 119p. IU-M; OCIM; OCLloyd
90-2962

GRAY, H[arry] C.
A condensed compendium of pharmaceutical knowledge; a quiz book by H. C. Gray, Ph.G., and C. H. Bryan, M.D. 8th ed. . . . Chicago, Ill.: Gray & Bryan, 1892. 130p. DLC; OCIM; OCLloyd **90-2963**

GRAY, Harry C.
A condensed compendium of pharmaceutical knowledge. A quiz book by H. C. Gray and C. H. Bryan. 9th ed. Chicago: Gray & Bryan, 1892. 154p. OCIM; OCLloyd
90-2964

GRAY, Harry C.
A condensed compendium of pharmaceutical knowledge. A quiz book. . . . 10th ed. . . . Chicago, Ill.: Gray & Bryan, 1893. 181p. DLC; OCIM **90-2965**

GRAY, Harry C.
A condensed compendium of pharmaceutical knowledge. A quiz book. . . . 11th ed. Revised to conform with the U.S. Pharmacopoeia of 1890. . . . Chicago, Ill.: Gray & Bryan, 1894. 206p. DLC; OCIM; OCLloyd
90-2966

GRAY, Harry C.
A condensed compendium of pharmaceutical knowledge. A quiz book. . . . 12th ed. Revised to conform with the U.S. Pharmacopoeia of 1890. . . . Chicago, Ill.: Gray & Bryan, 1895. 214p. DLC; OCIM; OCLloyd
90-2967

GRAY, Harry C.
A condensed compendium of pharmaceutical knowledge. A quiz book. . . . 12th ed. Revised to conform with the U.S. Pharmacopoeia of 1890. . . . Chicago, Ill.: Gray & Co., 1896. 215p. DLC; IU-M; OCLloyd **90-2968**

GRAY, Harry C.
Gray's prescriptionist. Revised. A treatise on the art of reading and compounding physicians' prescriptions, with tables of weights and measures, antidotes, abbreviations, etc., by H. C. Gray. . . . Revised by Geo. D. Oglesby. . . . Chicago, Ill.: Gray & Co., 1896. 212p. DLC; NNNAM; OCLloyd
90-2969

GRAY, Henry (1827-1861)
Anatomy, descriptive and surgical. . . . The drawings by H. V. Carter. . . . With additional drawings in later editions. A new American from the 13th English ed. Ed. by T. Pickering Pick. . . . Philadelphia: Lea Bros. & Co., 1893. 1129p. DLC; NNNAM; PPC; PPJ **90-2970**

GRAY, Henry (1827-1861)
Anatomy, descriptive and surgical. . . . New ed., thoroughly rev. by American authorities, from the 13th English ed. Ed. by T. Pickering Pick. . . . With 772 illustrations. . . . Philadelphia and New York: Lea Bros. & Co., 1897. 1249p. illus. (part. col.). DLC; NNNAM; OCIM; PPC **90-2971**

GRAY, John F. S.
Notes on the mineral waters of St. Clair Springs, Michigan; their efficacy in the treatment of diseases of a strumous origin; catarrhal affections, sub-acute and chronic maladies; rheumatism, gout, etc.; disorders of the nervous system and diseases of women. [Detroit: O. S. Gulley, Borman & Co., 1890.] 23p. 1 plate frontisp. DNLM **90-2972**

GRAY, John R. (*b.* 1859)
A guide to the study of pharmacognosy; or, The essentials of materia medica of the vegetable and animal kingdoms, for the use of junior and senior students in the Buffalo College of Pharmacy. . . . Buffalo: P. Paul Book Co., printers, 1894. 229p. DLC **90-2973**

GRAY, London C[arter] (1850-1900)
Can we diagnosticate hyperaemia or anaemia of the brain and cord? [New York, 1890.] 12p. DNLM
90-2974

GRAY, London C[arter] (1850-1900)
A treatise on nervous and mental diseases, for students and practitioners of medicine. . . . Philadelphia: Lea Bros. & Co., 1893. 687p. DLC; DNLM; NNNAM; PPC
90-2975

GRAY, London C[arter] (1850-1900)
Cases that should be operated upon by craniectomy. [Philadelphia, 1893.] 7p. DNLM **90-2976**

GRAY, London C[arter] (1850-1900)
Suggestions for a new method of taking expert testimony. New York, 1893. 11p. DNLM **90-2977**

GRAY, London C[arter] (1850-1900)
Persistent albuminuria and glycosuria, with frequent hyaline casts, in functional nervous diseases. [Philadelphia: Lea Bros. & Co., 1894.] 24p. DNLM **90-2978**

GRAY, London C[arter] (1850-1900)
A treatise on nervous and mental diseases, for students and practitioners of medicine. 2nd ed. Philadelphia: Lea Bros. & Co., 1895. 733p. 3 plates. DNLM; NNNAM; PPC; PU
90-2979

THE GRAY Mineral Springs and Hotel, Riverside, Cambridgeboro, Pa. A handbook of the early history of the spring, containing a discussion of its therapeutic properties, together with evidences of its marvelous healing power. Meadville, Pa., 1891. 20 l. oblong. DNLM **90-2980**

GRAYSON, Charles P[revost] (1859-1939)
General respiratory tuberculosis, pulmonary, laryngeal, nasal. Philadelphia, 1892. 7p. DNLM **90-2981**

GRAYSON, Charles P[revost] (1859-1939)
The galvano-cautery in nasal surgery; its injudicious application. [Philadelphia, 1893.] 5p. DNLM
90-2982

GRAYSON, Charles P[revost] (1859-1939)
An instance of spontaneous healing of an ulcerative tuberculous laryngitis. [Philadelphia, 1893.] 4p. DNLM
90-2983

GRAYSON, Charles P[revost] (1859-1939)
Carcinoma of the larynx, with consecutive epithelioma of the lip. [Philadelphia, 1894.] 7p. DNLM
90-2984

GREEN, Charles M[ontraville] (1850-1928)
Address on the duties and conduct of nurses in private nursing, delivered at the Boston City Hospital Training School for Nurses, June 7, 1889. Boston: Rockwell & Churchill, 1891. 20p. DNLM **90-2985**

GREEN, Charles M[ontraville] (1850-1928) and George HAVEN
A report of six months' work in the out-patient department for diseases of women, at the Boston City Hospital. Boston: Damrell & Upham, 1891. 16p. DNLM
90-2986

GREEN, Charles M[ontraville] (1850-1928)
The care of women in pregnancy. Boston: Damrell & Upham, 1892. 16p. DNLM **90-2987**

GREEN, Charles M[ontraville] (1850-1928)
The early physicians of Medford. Boston: Rockwell & Churchill, 1898. 20p. DNLM **90-2988**

GREEN, G[eorge] W.
Report of one thousand consecutive anaesthesias, observed in the service of Dr. A. J. Ochsner, at Augustana Hospital. Chicago, 1895. 8p. DNLM **90-2989**

GREEN, James S[proat] (1829-1892)
A view of modern surgery, from the standpoint of a general practitioner. Newark: L. F. Hardham, 1891. 22p. DNLM
90-2990

GREEN, John (1835-1913)
Dr. Henry Willard Williams. New York, 1896. 18p. port. DNLM **90-2991**

GREEN, J[ohn] Orne (1841-1922)
The treatment of inflammations of the mastoid; with an analysis of eighty operations. [Philadelphia, 1890.] 12p. DNLM **90-2992**

GREEN, J[ohn] Orne (1841-1922)
Personal experience in tympano-mastoid exenteration. New Bedford, 1899. 8p. DNLM **90-2993**

GREEN, Samuel Abbott (1830-1918)
An account of the physicians and dentists of Groton, Massachusetts: including three who, born there, have practiced their profession elsewhere. With an appendix. . . . Groton, 1890. 90p. DLC; DNLM; MBM **90-2994**

GREEN, Thomas Henry (1841-1923)
An introduction to pathology and morbid anatomy. . . . 7th American from the 8th English ed., rev. and enl. by H. Montague Murray. Philadelphia: Lea Bros. & Co., 1895. 598p. col. plate. DLC; DNLM; NNNAM; PPC
90-2995

GREEN, Thomas Henry (1841-1923)
An introduction to pathology and morbid anatomy. . . . Rev. and enl. by Montague Murray. . . . New (8th) American ed. Thoroughly rev. from the 8th English ed. By Walton Martin. . . . Illustrated with two hundred and sixteen engravings. . . . Philadelphia and New York: Lea Bros. & Co., 1898. 528p. DLC; DNLM; NNNAM; PPC **90-2996**

GREEN, W[illiam] O.
Report on rectal diseases. Louisville: J. P. Morton & Co., 1893. 7p. DNLM **90-2997**

GREENBAUM, Max (*b.* 1868)
Dentistry from a scientific standpoint. Philadelphia, 1893. 8p. DNLM **90-2998**

GREENE, Charles Lyman (*b.* 1862)
"Relation of druggist and physician." With "From the druggist's point of view." Lathrop Musseter, and an editorial from Journal of American Medical Association, Dec. 17, 1892. [Chicago, 1892.] 18p. DNLM
90-2999

GREENE, Charles Lyman (*b.* 1862)
The symptoms and diagnosis of chronic Bright's disease. St. Paul, 1893. 16p. DNLM **90-3000**

GREENE, Charles Lyman (*b.* 1862)
The diagnostic value of Ehrlich's diazo reaction. Chicago, 1894. 11p. DNLM **90-3001**

GREENE, Charles Lyman (*b.* 1862)
A suggestion bearing upon the treatment by a new method of persistent vomiting. Philadelphia, 1895. 6p. DNLM
90-3002

GREENE, Charles Lyman (*b.* 1862)
The treatment of chronic heart disease by the Schott method. St. Paul, 1895. 18p. DNLM **90-3003**

GREENE, Charles Lyman (*b.* 1862)
Recent aids in the differential diagnosis of typhoid fever (describing the author's modification of Ehrlich's test, with a preliminary report upon the serum test of Widal). New York, 1896. 10p. DNLM **90-3004**

GREENE, Charles Lyman (*b.* 1862)
The serum test of Widal and the possibility of its application without microscopic examination, with a report of cases and demonstration of method. New York, 1896. 8p. DNLM
90-3005

GREENE, Charles Lyman (*b.* 1862)
A case of Landry's paralysis; autopsy; pathologic report; life prolonged by artificial means for forty-one days after the establishment of respiratory paralysis; with pathologic reports by L. B. Wilson and J. L. Rothrock. Philadelphia, 1898. 13p. DNLM **90-3006**

GREENE, Charles Lyman (*b.* 1862)
The treatment of heart disease by saline baths and resisted movements; Schott method. Chicago: Am. Medical Assoc. Press, 1898. 11p. DNLM **90-3007**

GREENE, J[ames] B.
Report of two cases of uterine fibroid and one of stricture of the rectum. Treated by electrolysis and surgically. Also presentation of specimen of dermoid cyst. [Chicago, 1890.] 15p. DNLM **90-3008**

GREENE, J. M.
Whose are the falsehoods? An inquiry into the matter of how much pain is inflicted upon animals in physiological experiments; containing, on the one hand, the claims of vivisectors to the public; on the other hand, descriptions (written by the vivisectors themselves for the physiological journals) of some of their recent experiments upon animals. Boston, 1899. 8p. DNLM **90-3009**

GREENE, James S[umner]
The obscure origin and indeterminate course of acute infection, as illustrated by a case of malignant endocarditis. Boston: Damrell & Upham, 1894. 12p. DNLM
90-3010

GREENE, James S[umner]
The physician and his surrounding. Boston: Damrell & Upham, 1898. 20p. DNLM; MH-M **90-3011**

GREENE, Reuben (*b.* 1817)
Thoughts for the people; illustrating man's real relation, physically, politically, socially, and religiously, to the universe of God; with practical suggestions upon the origin and prevention of sickness, suffering, and premature death; the result of fifty-six years of professional experience and observation. Boston: Lee & Shepard, 1896. 272p. port. DNLM; MB; MH; NN **90-3012**

GREENLEAF, Charles Ravenscroft (1838-1911)
A digest of current orders and decisions, with extracts from Army regulations relating to the Medical Corps of the U.S. Army. Compiled under direction of the Surgeon-General. Washington: Government Printing Office, 1890. 125p. DNLM
90-3013

GREENLEAF, Charles Ravenscroft (1838-1911)
World's Columbian Exposition, Chicago, 1892-3. War Department exhibit. Medical Department, United States Army. No. 7. The personal identity of the soldier. Chicago, 1893. 10p. DNLM **90-3014**

GREENLEAF, Robert W[illard] (1856?-1901)
A medical clinic at the Boston Dispensary. Boston: Damrell & Upham, 1896. 19p. DNLM **90-3015**

GREENLEAF, Robert W[illard] (1856?-1901)
On the value of prompt cooperation with the municipal authorities for the prevention of the spread of diphtheria. Boston, 1897. 6p. DNLM **90-3016**

GREENLEAF, Robert W[illard] (1856?-1901)
A case of aconite poisoning. Boston, 1897. 8p. DNLM **90-3017**

GREENLEAF, Robert W[illard] (1856?-1901)
An historical report of the Boston Dispensary for one hundred and one years. 1796-1897. Boston: C. A. W. Spencer, 1898. 64p. DNLM **90-3018**

GREENOUGH, Robert B[attey] (1871-1937) and Elliott P. JOSLIN
Gastric ulcer at the Massachusetts General Hospital, 1888-98. Philadelphia, 1899. 16p. DNLM **90-3019**

GREENWOOD, Allen (*b.* 1866)
Ocular headaches. Waltham, Mass., 1898. 8p. DNLM **90-3020**

GREENWOOD, Allen (*b.* 1866)
Ophthalmia neonatorum. Nashville, Tenn., 1898. 2p. DNLM **90-3021**

GREENWOOD, T[homas] M.
Obstetrics as practiced in the mountains of north Georgia. New York, 1895. 8p. DNLM **90-3022**

GREER, J[oseph] H. (*b.* 1851)
A physician in the house for family and individual consultation; containing valuable articles on life and its preservation, the actions of the body in health and disease, the rules of hygiene and proper living, characteristics of foods, etc. Also a complete cyclopaedia of diseases and their treatment by non-poisonous remedies; with descriptions of medicinal agents and numerous formulas and special articles written in plain language. Chicago, [1897]. 800p. port. DNLM; OCIM **90-3023**

GRIEVES, Clarence J.
A case of progressive dentinal resorption. Philadelphia, 1899. 10p. DNLM **90-3024**

GRIFFIN, E[dwin] Harrison (*b.* 1860)
The treatment for the radical cure of polypi of the nose. New York: L. P. Kuhl, 1890. 10p. DNLM **90-3025**

GRIFFIN, E[dwin] Harrison (*b.* 1860)
Chancre of the mouth, with statistics and a report of twelve cases, three occurring in children in one family, and the local treatment for syphilitic manifestations of the throat. New York: L. P. Kuhl, 1892. 16p. DNLM **90-3026**

GRIFFIN, E[dwin] Harrison (*b.* 1860)
Abscess of the antrum of Highmore, with cases and their treatment. [New York: Trow, 1894.] 8p. DNLM **90-3027**

GRIFFIN, E[dwin] Harrison (*b.* 1860)
The occlusion of the post-nasal space by syphilitic adhesion. [New York: D. Appleton & Co., 1894.] 7p. DNLM **90-3028**

GRIFFIN, E[dwin] Harrison (*b.* 1860)
Chancres found in unusual localities. New York, 1896. 21p. DNLM **90-3029**

GRIFFIN, E[dwin] Harrison (*b.* 1860)
Deformities of the nasal septum. New York, 1897. 12p. DNLM **90-3030**

GRIFFIN, E[dwin] Harrison (*b.* 1860)
Polypus of the uvula. New York, 1899. 4p. DNLM **90-3031**

GRIFFITH, A[lexander] Hill
Diseases of the chorioid and vitreous. Philadelphia, 1898. 59p. 3 plates. DNLM **90-3032**

GRIFFITH, J[ohn] P. Crozer (1856-1941)
An additional note on the employment of antipyrine in pertussis. [Philadelphia, 1890.] 5p. DNLM **90-3033**

GRIFFITH, J[ohn] P. Crozer (1856-1941)
Climatic treatment of phthisis. [Philadelphia, 1891.] 15p. DNLM **90-3034**

GRIFFITH, J[ohn] P. Crozer (1856-1941) and Charles W. BURR
The pathology of pernicious anemia. [Philadelphia, 1891.] 18p. DNLM **90-3035**

GRIFFITH, J[ohn] P. Crozer (1856-1941)
Incontinence of urine in children. [Philadelphia, 1892.] 7p. DNLM **90-3036**

GRIFFITH, J[ohn] P. Crozer (1856-1941)
The care of the baby. A manual for mothers and nurses, containing practical directions for the management of infancy and childhood in health and disease. Philadelphia: W. B. Saunders, 1895. 392p. DLC; DNLM; NNNAM; PU **90-3037**

GRIFFITH, J[ohn] P. Crozer (1856-1941)
Forms of paralysis in children. [Philadelphia, 1895.] 15p. DNLM **90-3038**

GRIFFITH, J[ohn] P. Crozer (1856-1941)
Tetany in America, with a report of five cases. Philadelphia, 1895. 19p. DNLM **90-3039**

GRIFFITH, J[ohn] P. Crozer (1856-1941)
A case of varicella gangrenosa, diphtheria, and rubeola occurring at the same time. Philadelphia, 1896. 3p. DNLM **90-3040**

GRIFFITH, J[ohn] P. Crozer (1856-1941)
The care of the baby; a manual for mothers and nurses. . . . 2nd ed., revised. Philadelphia: W. B. Saunders, 1898. 404p. DLC; DNLM; NNNAM; PPC **90-3041**

GRIFFITH, J[ohn] P. Crozer (1856-1941)
The weight in the first two years of life with a description of a new chart weight. New York, 1899. 14p. 1 chart. DNLM
90-3042

GRIFFITH-DAVIS, J[osephine]
Notes on methyl-violet; its uses in malignant diseases. New York, 1896. 12p. DNLM **90-3043**

GRIFFITHS, A[rthur] B[ower] (*b.* 1859)
A report on certain experiments undertaken to ascertain the disinfecting and germicidal power of "Sanitas" preparations and appliances. New York, [1894]. 15p. DNLM
90-3044

GRIFFITHS, T[homas] M[ichael]
Non-secret formulas: a collection of over four thousand formulas and one thousand prize prescriptions for the use of physicians and druggists, to which has been added a selection of articles from standard authorities on photography, tablet triturates, compressed tablets, elixirs, proprietaries, and original formulas for toilet articles, perfumery and articles of household use, making a valuable book of reference on subjects appertaining to the business of an up-to-date pharmacist. 1st ed. St. Louis: Buxton & Skinner, 1897. 513p. DNLM; OCLloyd **90-3045**

GRINDON, Joseph (*b.* 1858)
The cutaneous phenomena of typhoid fever. St. Louis, 1893. 4p. DNLM **90-3046**

GRINDON, Joseph (*b.* 1858)
Recurrent zoster. New York, 1895. 18p. DNLM
90-3047

GROFF, George G. (1851-1910)
. . . What to do in home treatment of accidents and emergencies; what to do till the doctor comes. . . . New York: The Rural Publishing Co., 1892. 31p. DLC; NNNAM
90-3048

[GROSS, Samuel David] (1805-1884)
Autobiography of Samuel D. Gross with sketches of his contemporaries. Edited by his sons. . . . Preceded by a memoir of Dr. Gross by the late Austin Flint. Philadelphia: W. B. Saunders Co., 1893. 2 v. NNNAM; PPC; PPJ; PU
90-3049

[GROSS, Samuel David] (1805-1884)
Addresses at the unveiling of the bronze statue of the late Prof. Samuel D. Gross, M.D., erected by the American Surgical Association and the Jefferson Medical College, Washington, D.C., May 5, 1897. Philadelphia, 1897. 36p. PPJ
90-3050

GROSS, Samuel Weissell (1837-1889)
A practical treatise on impotence, sterility and all disorders of the male sexual organs. . . . 4th ed., rev. by F. R. Sturgis. Philadelphia: Lea Bros. & Co., 1890. 173p. DLC; NNNAM; PPC; PPJ **90-3051**

GUERNSEY, Joseph Colburn (*b.* 1849)
Urinalysis including blanks for recording the analysis and microscopic examination of the urine. . . . Philadelphia: J. B. Lippincott & Co., 1895. 512p. [inc. 502 forms]. DLC; NNNAM; PPC; PU **90-3052**

GUERNSEY, William Jefferson
The homoeopathic therapeutics of hemorrhoids. . . . 2nd ed. Philadelphia: Boericke & Tafel, 1892. 142p. DLC; PPC; PPHa
90-3053

GUILFORD, S[imeon] Hayden (1841-1919)
Orthodontia, or malposition of the human teeth; its prevention and remedy. 2nd ed. Philadelphia: Spangler & Davis, 1893. 228p. DNLM; MdU-D; PPC; PU [1st ed., 1889, 186p.]
90-3054

GUILFORD, S[imeon] Hayden (1841-1919)
An address to graduates of the Philadelphia Dental College at the twenty-first commencement, Academy of Music, Philadelphia, Feb. 19, 1894. Philadelphia, 1894. 8p. DNLM
90-3055

GUITERAS, Ramon B[enjamin] (1859-1917)
The present treatment of urethritis in New York. Philadelphia, 1895. 11p. DNLM **90-3056**

GUITERAS, Ramon B[enjamin] (1859-1917)
Report of a case of enuresis treated by injections of nitrate of silver. New York, 1895. 5p. DNLM
90-3057

GUITERAS, Ramon B[enjamin] (1859-1917)
The general treatment of syphilis in private practice. New York, 1896. 16p. DNLM **90-3058**

GUNN, John C. (1800-1863)
. . . Gunn and Jordan's newest revised physician: being the first New domestic physician, or, Home book of health; by John C. Gunn . . . [and] Johnson H. Jordan. . . . Cincinnati: Philadelphia, [etc.]: J. E. Moore & Co., 1893 [1892]. 1190p. plates. DLC **90-3059**

[GUNN, Robert Alexander] (*b.* 1844)
Confidential medical talks to women . . . diseases of women, general hygiene. . . . New York, Akron, O., [etc.]: The Werner Co., 1890. 378p. plates. DLC **90-3060**

GUNNING, Josephus Henry
Vaginismus: its causes and treatment. New York, 1895. 7p. DNLM **90-3061**

GÜNSBURG, Mark
The diagnosis and treatment of cystitis. New York, 1898. 21p. DNLM **90-3062**

GÜNSBURG, Mark
The technique of the Bottini operation. New York, 1899. 28p. DNLM **90-3063**

GUTTMAN, Oskar
Gymnastics of the voice for song and speech. A method for the cure of stuttering and stammering. 3rd ed. New York: Edgar S. Werner, 1893. 250p. NNNAM
90-3064

GUTTMANN, J.
Obstruction of the nose, and its influence upon the human organism. New York, 1898. 9p. DNLM
90-3065

GUTTMANN, J.
The use of holocaine as a local anaesthetic on the eye, ear, nose, and throat operations. New York, 1899. 11p. DNLM
90-3066

GWYER, Fred Walker
A guide to the study of surgical diagnosis during bedside instruction. For the use of senior students. [New York, 1894.] 7p. DNLM **90-3067**

GYNAECOLOGICAL AND OBSTETRICAL SOCIETY OF BALTIMORE
Extra-uterine pregnancy. The history of—by Dr. G. W. Miltenberger. Laparotomy for—with a report of a successful case, by Dr. T. A. Ashby. Review and discussion—by Dr. H. A. Kelly. General discussion. Papers read before the Obstetrical and Gynaecological Society of Baltimore City. January 14th and February 11th, 1890. Published by order of the Society. Baltimore: Press of Griffin, Curley & Co., 1890. 52p. DLC; MdU-D **90-3068**

HAAB, Otto (1850-1931)
Atlas of the external diseases of the eye, including a brief treatise on the pathology and treatment. . . . Authorized transl. from the German; edited by G. E. de Schweinitz. . . . With 76 colored plates and 6 engravings. Philadelphia: W. B. Saunders, 1899. 288p. DLC; NNNAM; PPC; PU **90-3069**

HACKENBERG, George P.
Medical consultation book, a pharmacological and clinical book of reference, containing the therapeutics of a full list of the officinal and non-officinal articles of the materia medica. . . . Austin, Tex.: E. Von Boeckmann, printer, 1893. 776p. frontis. port. DLC: OCLloyd **90-3070**

HACKER, Victor R. von (1852-1933)
Introduction to the antiseptic treatment of wounds, according to the method in use at Professor Billroth's clinic, Vienna. . . . Philadelphia: P. Blakiston, Son & Co., 1892. 66p. PPJ; PU **90-3071**

HADRA, B[erthold] E[rnest] (1842-1903)
Some reflections on morning sickness. Philadelphia: Medical Press Co., 1890. 7p. DNLM **90-3072**

HADRA, B[erthold] E[rnest] (1842-1903)
Wiring of the vertebrae as a means of immobilization in fracture and Pott's disease. Philadelphia, 1891. 8p. DNLM **90-3073**

HADRA, B[erthold] E[rnest] (1842-1903)
Omental tumours. [Philadelphia, 1891.] 10p. DNLM **90-3074**

HAHNEMANN HOMOEOPATHIC UNIVERSITY, WASHINGTON, D.C.
Annual announcement for the session of 1894-1895 (1.). [Washington, 1894.] 15p. DNLM **90-3075**

HAHNEMANN, Samuel Christian Friedrich (1755-1843)
Organon of medicine. Transl. from the 5th ed., with an appendix from R. E. Dudgeon. Chicago: Med. Advance Co., 1895. 178p. DNLM; OCIM; PPHa **90-3076**

HAHNEMANN, Samuel Christian Friedrich (1755-1843)
Organon of medicine. Transl. from the 5th ed., with an appendix from R. E. Dudgeon. Chicago: Hahnemann Publ. Co., 1896. 178p. DNLM; IU-M; OCIM; PPHa **90-3077**

HAHNEMANN, Samuel Christian Friedrich (1755-1843)
Hahnemann's defence of the Organon of rational medicine and of his previous homoeopathic works against the attacks of Professor Hecker. An explanatory commentary on the homoeopathic system. Translated by R. E. Dudgeon. . . . Philadelphia: Boericke & Tafel, 1896. 130p. frontis. port. DLC; DNLM; PPC; PPHa **90-3078**

HAHNEMANN, Samuel Christian Friedrich (1755-1843)
The chronic diseases, their peculiar nature and their homoeopathic cure. . . . Transl. from the 2nd enl. German ed. of 1835, by Prof. Louis H. Tafel. With annotations by Richard Hughes, M.D. Ed. by Pemberton Dudley, M.D. Philadelphia: Boericke & Tafel, 1896. 1600p. DLC: PPC; PPHa **90-3079**

HAIG, A[lexander] (1853-1924)
Some notes on the treatment of morbus cordis by iodides and other drugs which lower the blood-pressure. Detroit, Mich.: G. S. Davis, 1895. 12p. DNLM **90-3080**

HAIG, A[lexander] (1853-1924)
Uric acid as a factor in the causation of disease. A contribution to the pathology of high arterial tension, headache, epilepsy, mental depression, gout, rheumatism, diabetes, Bright's disease, and other disorders. 3rd ed. Philadelphia: P. Blakiston, Son & Co., 1896. 600p. DNLM; NNNAM; PPC; PU **90-3081**

HAIG, A[lexander] (1853-1924)
Uric acid as a factor in the causation of disease. A contribution to the pathology of high arterial tension, headache, epilepsy, mental depression, gout, rheumatism, diabetes, Bright's disease, and other disorders. 4th ed. Philadelphia: P. Blakiston, Son & Co., 1898. 698p. DNLM; PPC; PU **90-3082**

HAIG-BROWN, Florence A.
Hints on elementary physiology. Philadelphia: P. Blakiston, Son & Co., 1897. 121p. DNLM; PU **90-3083**

HALE, Edwin Moses (1829-1899)
On the toxic, pathogenetic, and therapeutic qualities of the cactaceae. New York: M. J. Rooney & Co., [1890]. 11p. DNLM **90-3084**

HALE, Edwin Moses (1829-1899)
The probable homoeopathic uses of unproven drugs. Are we justified in using them? Philadelphia, 1891. 7p. DNLM **90-3085**

HALE, Edwin Moses (1829-1899)
Hyoscyamine and hyoscine in nervous and mental disorders. Philadelphia, 1892. 4p. DNLM **90-3086**

HALE, Edwin Moses (1829-1899)
Primary and secondary symptoms and their relation to dose. Philadelphia, 1894. 11p. DNLM **90-3087**

HALE, Edwin Moses (1829-1899)
The geography of heart disease. Philadelphia, 1894. 6p. DNLM **90-3088**

HALE, Edwin Moses (1829-1899)
The practice of medicine. . . . Chicago: Gross & Delbridge, 1894. 1033p. frontis. port. DLC; OCIM **90-3089**

HALE, F. E[dwin]
Treatment of the uric acid diathesis. St. Louis, 1898. 7p. DNLM **90-3090**

HALE, F. E[dwin]
Anaemia. [*Also*:] How I quickly cured a cold in the head, by William H. Murray. [n. p., 1899.] 2 l. DNLM **90-3091**

HALE-WHITE, William (1857-1949)
Materia medica, pharmacy, pharmacology and therapeutics. . . . ed. by Reynold W. Wilcox. . . . Philadelphia: P. Blakiston, Son & Co., 1892. 607p. DLC; NNNAM; OCLloyd; PPC **90-3092**

HALE-WHITE, William (1857-1949)
Materia medica, pharmacy, pharmacology and therapeutics. . . . ed. by Reynold W. Wilcox. . . . 2nd American ed., thoroughly rev. Philadelphia: P. Blakiston, Son & Co., 1894. 661p. DLC; NNNAM; OCLloyd; PU **90-3093**

HALE-WHITE, William (1857-1949)
Materia medica, pharmacy, pharmacology and therapeutics. . . . ed. by Reynold W. Wilcox. . . . 3rd American ed., thoroughly revised. Philadelphia: P. Blakiston, Son & Co., 1895. 687p. DLC; IU-M; OCLloyd; PPC **90-3094**

HALE-WHITE, William (1857-1949)
Materia medica, pharmacy, pharmacology, and therapeutics; edited by R. W. Wilcox. 4th American ed., thoroughly revised. Philadelphia: P. Blakiston's Son & Co., 1898. 704p. DLC; IEN-M; PPC; PU **90-3095**

HALL, A[lbert] L.
The home treatment of hay fever. Buffalo, 1895. 4p. DNLM **90-3096**

HALL, Arthur J.
Treatment of puerperal eclampsia. Baltimore, 1898. 4p. DNLM **90-3097**

HALL, F[rancis] de Havilland (1847-1929)
Diseases of the nose and throat. . . . Philadelphia: P. Blakiston, Son & Co., 1895. 524p. DLC; DNLM; PPC; PPJ **90-3098**

HALL, H[arry] Newbery
A compend of general pathology and morbid anatomy. Philadelphia: P. Blakiston, Son & Co., 1894. 204p. 4 plates. DNLM; PPC; PPJ **90-3099**

HALL, Harry O[rville] (1846-1924)
Some rules which should be observed by editors and publishers of medical journals. Philadelphia, 1899. 6p. DNLM **90-3100**

HALL, Herbert J[ames] (1870-1923)
Notes on surgical gauzes. Boston, 1897. 10p. DNLM **90-3101**

HALL, Josiah N[ewhall] (*b.* 1859)
An undescribed heart-murmur. Philadelphia: Lea Bros. & Co., 1891. 3p. DNLM **90-3102**

HALL, Josiah N[ewhall] (*b.* 1859)
Certain points in the medico-legal investigation of gunshot wounds. Examination of weapon, body, and surroundings. New York, 1895. 10p. DNLM **90-3103**

HALL, Josiah N[ewhall] (*b.* 1859)
Report of three cases of phthisis pulmonalis following scald of the chest. New York, 1896. 2 l. DNLM **90-3104**

HALL, Josiah N[ewhall] (*b.* 1859)
A study of cicatrices with reference to right- and left-handedness and ambidexterity. Boston, 1896. 4p. DNLM **90-3105**

HALL, Josiah N[ewhall] (*b.* 1859)
The value of the pulmonic second sound. Chicago, 1896. 4p. DNLM **90-3106**

HALL, Josiah N[ewhall] (*b.* 1859)
A case of double pulmonic murmur, with a diastolic thrill. [Denver, 1897.] 2 l. DNLM **90-3107**

HALL, Josiah N[ewhall] (*b.* 1859)
A case of pulsating pleurisy. Philadelphia, 1897. 4p. DNLM **90-3108**

HALL, Josiah N[ewhall] (*b.* 1859)
Detection of foetal heart-murmur in gravida, with report of a case. [New York, 1897.] 4p. DNLM **90-3109**

HALL, Josiah N[ewhall] (*b.* 1859)
Interrupted respiration; a study of certain physical signs of disease of the chest. Chicago, 1897. 7p. DNLM **90-3110**

HALL, Josiah N[ewhall] (*b.* 1859) and H. L. TAYLOR
A case of partial dislocation of the occipito-atloidean articulation. [Denver, 1897.] 1 l. DNLM **90-3111**

HALL, Josiah N[ewhall] (*b.* 1859)
Phthisis originating in Colorado. Denver, Colo., 1897. 1 l. DNLM **90-3112**

HALL, Josiah N[ewhall] (*b.* 1859)
The physical signs of acute bronchitis. St. Louis, 1897. 4p. DNLM **90-3113**

HALL, Josiah N[ewhall] (*b.* 1859)
Acute pneumonia. Denver, [1898]. 4 l. DNLM **90-3114**

HALL, Josiah N[ewhall] (*b.* 1859)
Aortic stenosis with mitral regurgitation. A clinical lecture. [Denver, 1898.] 4p. DNLM **90-3115**

HALL, Josiah N[ewhall] (*b.* 1859)
A case of ruptured aortic aneurism; suit for accident insurance. New York, 1898. 8p. DNLM **90-3116**

HALL, Josiah N[ewhall] (*b.* 1859)
The causes of the inconstancy of mitral regurgitant murmurs. Chicago: Am. Med. Assoc. Press, 1898. 4p. DNLM **90-3117**

HALL, Josiah N[ewhall] (*b.* 1859)
Displacement of the heart in lung disease. [St. Louis, 1898.] 7p. DNLM **90-3118**

HALL, Josiah N[ewhall] (*b.* 1859)
Hepatic cirrhosis. Denver, [1898]. 2 l. DNLM **90-3119**

HALL, Josiah N[ewhall] (*b.* 1859)
Suggestions as to the use of digitalis. Philadelphia, [1898]. 8p. DNLM **90-3120**

HALL, Josiah N[ewhall] (*b.* 1859)
Thoracic aneurism. St. Louis, Mo., 1898. 6p. DNLM **90-3121**

HALL, Josiah N[ewhall] (*b.* 1859)
Bronchial obstruction by suppurating bronchial glands. Philadelphia, 1899. 5p. DNLM **90-3122**

HALL, Josiah N[ewhall] (*b.* 1859)
The climate of the plains. St. Louis, 1899. 4p. DNLM **90-3123**

HALL, Josiah N[ewhall] (*b.* 1859)
Three cases of leukemia. Boston, 1899. 8p. DNLM **90-3124**

HALL, Josiah N[ewhall] (*b.* 1859)
The valvular diseases of the left heart. Philadelphia, [1899]. 10p. DNLM **90-3125**

HALL, Winfield Scott (*b.* 1861)
A laboratory guide in physiology. Chapters I and II. On circulation and respiration. . . . Chicago: The W. T. Keener Co., 1896. 58p. diags. DLC **90-3126**

HALL, Winfield Scott (*b.* 1861)
A laboratory guide in physiology. . . . With appendices on organization and equipment. . . . Chicago: The W. T. Keener Co., 1897. 359p. col. plates, diags. DLC; OCIM **90-3127**

HALL, Winfield Scott (*b.* 1861)
A textbook of physiology. . . . Illustrated with 343 engravings and six colored plates. Philadelphia and New York: Lea Bros. & Co., 1899. 671p. col. plates. DLC; NNNAM; PPC; PU **90-3128**

HALLOCK, Frank K. (*b.* 1860)
Report of four cases of thyroid feeding. New Haven, 1896. 23p. DNLM **90-3129**

HALLOCK, Frank K. (*b.* 1860)
Thyroid feeding, with report of four cases. Hartford, 1896. 23p. DNLM **90-3130**

HALLOCK, Frank K. (*b.* 1860)
Equilibration and its relation to vertigo. Chicago, 1898. 14p. DNLM **90-3131**

HALLOCK, J. Henry
Results in the treatment of phthisis and late methods in diagnosis. Chicago, 1898. 6p. DNLM **90-3132**

HALLOCK, J. Henry
Tuberculosis in the Adirondacks. New York, 1898. 2 l. DNLM **90-3133**

HALPHIDE, Alvan C.
Mind and body; hypnotism and suggestion applied in therapeutics and education. Chicago: A. C. Halphide, [1899]. 231p. 5 plates, port. DNLM; ICU **90-3134**

HALSEY BROS CO., CHICAGO
Halsey Bros.' manual of homoeopathic medicine for popular use. [New and enl. ed.] Chicago: Halsey Bros. Co., 1896. 152p. DLC **90-3135**

HALSEY BROS. CO., CHICAGO
Halsey's homoeopathic label book for the use of physicians and pharmacists, containing a complete list of the preparations of the pharmacopoeia of the American Institute of Homoeopathy. . . . Chicago: Halsey Bros. Co., 1898. 42 l. DLC: OCLloyd **90-3136**

HALSTEAD, A. E[dward] (*b.* 1868)
Floating bodies in joints. Philadelphia, 1895. 16p. DNLM **90-3137**

HALSTEAD, A. E[dward] (*b.* 1868)
Metatarsalgia, with a report of three cases of what is termed Morton's painful affection of the feet. Detroit, 1896. 8p. DNLM **90-3138**

HALSTEAD, A. E[dward] (*b.* 1868)
Removal of Gasserian ganglion for the relief of trifacial neuralgia, with report of a case. Chicago, 1897. 16p. DNLM **90-3139**

HALSTEAD, A. E[dward] (*b.* 1868)
The treatment of acute abscess and gangrene of the lung. Detroit, 1898. 6p. DNLM **90-3140**

HALSTEAD, A. E[dward] (*b.* 1868) and E. R. LE COUNT
Tuberculosis of the mammary gland. Philadelphia, 1898. 23p. DNLM **90-3141**

HALSTEAD, A. E[dward] (*b.* 1868)
Movable kidney. Detroit, 1899. 16p. DNLM **90-3142**

HALSTEAD, A. E[dward] (*b.* 1868)
Three cases of perineal resection of the rectum for carcinoma. Chicago, 1899. 3 l. DNLM **90-3143**

HALSTED, T[homas] H.
Intubation in diphtheria before and since the use of antitoxine. New York: D. Appleton & Co., 1897. 11p. DNLM **90-3144**

HALSTED, William S[tewart] (1852-1922)
. . . The radical cure of inguinal hernia in the male. . . . [1893]. 15p. plates. NNC **90-3145**

HALSTED, William S[tewart] (1852-1922)
The radical cure of inguinal hernia in the male. [Baltimore, 1893.] 11 l. 3 plates. DNLM **90-3146**

HALSTED, William S[tewart] (1852-1922)
The results of operations for the cure of cancer of the breast performed at the Johns Hopkins Hospital from June, 1889 to Jan., 1894. Baltimore: Johns Hopkins Press, 1894. 53p. plates. DLC [The Johns Hopkins Hospital Reports, v. 4, No. 6] **90-3147**

HALSTED, William S[tewart] (1852-1922)
The operative treatment of hernia. Philadelphia, 1895. 5p. DNLM **90-3148**

HALSTED, William S[tewart] (1852-1922)
A clinical and histological study of certain adeno-carcinomata of the breast and a brief consideration of the supraclavicular operation and of the results of operations for cancer of the breast from 1889 to 1898 at the Johns Hopkins Hospital. Philadelphia, 1898. 19p. 5 plates. DNLM
90-3149

HAMILTON, Allan McLane (1848-1919)
A system of legal medicine, by Allan McLane Hamilton and Lawrence Godkin . . . with the collaboration of Prof. James F. Babcock, Lewis Balch [and others]. . . . New York: E. B. Treat, 1894. 2 v. col. plates, diags. DLC; NNNAM; PPC; PU
90-3150

HAMILTON, Allan McLane (1848-1919)
The connection of intestinal autotoxis with certain common forms of insanity. New York, 1896. 36p. DNLM; NNNAM
90-3151

HAMILTON, Allan McLane (1848-1919) and W. S. BROWN
A case of mild stuporous insanity in which it was possible to induce illusions, hallucinations, and automatic acts by suggestion. New York, 1896. 7p. DNLM **90-3152**

HAMILTON, Charles S.
Report of operations upon hernias. Philadelphia, 1892. 9p. DNLM **90-3153**

HAMILTON, Charles S.
Report of ten cases of supravaginal hysterectomy for fibroids of the uterus. [New York, 1894.] 2p. 1 l. DNLM
90-3154

HAMILTON, E[rnest] E.
The quarterly dioptry cylinder, some testimony for. St. Louis, Mo., 1895. 8p. DNLM **90-3155**

HAMILTON, Frank Hastings (1813-1886)
A practical treatise on fractures and dislocations. . . . 8th ed., revised and edited by Stephen Smith. . . . Illustrated with five hundred and seven wood-cuts. Philadelphia: Lea Bros. & Co., 1891. 849p. DLC; DNLM; NNNAM; PPC
90-3156

HAMILTON, Hugh (*b.* 1847)
Is the early recognition of cholera asiatica possible? [Philadelphia, 1892.] 2p. DNLM **90-3157**

HAMILTON, Hugh (*b.* 1847)
The application of graphics to the fetal heart sounds. New York: William Wood & Co., 1893. 4p. DNLM
90-3158

HAMILTON, Hugh (*b.* 1847)
Remarks upon the occasion of the presentation by Eli Houser Coover of portrait and paintings to the Harrisburg Academy of Medicine, April 28, 1899. [Harrisburg: Scheffer, 1899.] 7p. DNLM **90-3159**

HAMILTON, Hugh (*b.* 1847)
Medical tuberculosis. [1899.] 4 l. DNLM
90-3160

HAMILTON, John B. (1847-1898)
Lectures on tumors from a clinical standpoint. Detroit, Mich.: G. S. Davis, 1891. 138p. 2 plates. DNLM
90-3161

HAMILTON, John B. (1847-1898)
Address in surgery. The general principles of the surgery of the human brain and its envelopes. Chicago, 1892. 32p. DNLM
90-3162

HAMILTON, John B. (1847-1898)
Diverticulum of gall-bladder; herniotomy; bow-legs; osteotomy and osteoclasis compared. Selected cases from clinics at Rush Medical College, Chicago. Philadelphia, 1892. 2p. DNLM
90-3163

HAMILTON, John B. (1847-1898)
The establishment of a national quarantine station near New York Harbor. Chicago, 1892. 11p. DNLM
90-3164

HAMILTON, John B. (1847-1898)
The United States quarantine laws and their scope. Chicago, 1892. 16p. DNLM **90-3165**

HAMILTON, John B. (1847-1898)
Address of the executive president section on general surgery. Memorandum of a case of hydatids of the kidney, with some remarks. Summary of the surgery of the tendons. Chicago, 1893. 12p. DNLM **90-3166**

HAMILTON, John B. (1847-1898)
Biological department of Rush Medical College. Chicago, 1893. 6p. DNLM **90-3167**

HAMILTON, John B. (1847-1898)
Tumors of the bladder. Chicago, 1893. 16p. 1 table. DNLM
90-3168

HAMILTON, John B. (1847-1898)
The international scientific language. Chicago, 1895. 8p. DNLM **90-3169**

HAMILTON, John B. (1847-1898)
Surgical memoranda. I. Abdomino-inguinal supporter. II. Treatment of open factures. III. Case of cerebral clot, with blindness; recovery; IV. Case of hypertrophy of mammary glands. V. Normal situation of gall-bladder. Chicago, 1895. 19p. DNLM **90-3170**

HAMILTON, John B. (1847-1898)
Lectures on tumors from a clinical standpoint. Lectures on tumors. 3rd ed. Philadelphia: P. Blakiston's Son & Co., 1898. 143p. 1 plate. DNLM; ICJ; ICU **90-3171**

HAMILTON, W[illiam] D.
Five cases of removal of the jaw for tumor. Chicago, 1890. 8p. DNLM **90-3172**

HAMILTON, W[illiam] D.
A report of seven operations upon the kidney. [New York, 1890.] 11p. DNLM **90-3173**

HAMILTON, W[illiam] D.
Two recent cases of tubal pregnancy; abdominal section. [New York, 1890.] 7p. DNLM **90-3174**

HAMILTON, W[illiam] D.
Stormy convalescence after removal of intra-abdominal tumors. New York: Trow, 1891. 8p. DNLM
90-3175

HAMILTON, W. F[awcett] (*b.* 1865)
A case of congenital deficiency of both clavicles. Philadelphia, 1899. 4p. DNLM **90-3176**

HAMLINE UNIVERSITY
Catalogues for the years 1895-1896 to 1899-1900. Hamline, 1896-1900. DNLM [Contains the announcements of the Minneapolis College of Physicians and Surgeons for the years 1896-1897 to 1900-1901 (14.-18.). **90-3177**

HAMMARSTEN, Olof (1841-1932)
A textbook of physiological chemistry. Authorized trans. from the 2nd Swedish ed. and from the author's rev. German ed. by John A. Mandel. New York: John Wiley, 1893. 511p. ICU; MB; MH; NN **90-3178**

HAMMARSTEN, Olof (1841-1932)
A text-book of physiological chemistry. . . . Authorized transl. from the author's enlarged and revised third German edition, by John A. Mandel. . . . 2nd ed. 1st thousand. New York: J. Wiley & Sons; [etc., etc.], 1898. 705p. plate. DLC; MB; MH; NN **90-3179**

HAMMOND, Frederick Porter
Genital neuralgia and genito-reflex pains. Philadelphia, 1899. 14p. DNLM **90-3180**

HAMMOND, Graeme M[onroe]
Antipyrine for the relief of headaches. [New York, 1892.] 4p. DNLM **90-3181**

HAMMOND, Graeme M[onroe]
The bicycle in the treatment of nervous diseases. [New York, 1892.] 11p. DNLM **90-3182**

HAMMOND, L[evi] J.
Treatment of suppuration of the middle ear. [Philadelphia, 1890.] 4p. DNLM **90-3183**

HAMMOND, L[evi] J.
Stricture of the auditory canal; the result of a low-grade middle-ear suppuration. [Philadelphia, 1891.] 2p. DNLM **90-3184**

HAMMOND, L[evi] J.
Perforations of Shrapnell's membrane and their treatment. A report of twenty-five cases. [Philadelphia, 1892.] 3p. DNLM **90-3185**

HAMMOND, L[evi] J.
Three cases of attic suppuration in which operation was followed by facial paralysis [Bell's palsey]. Philadelphia, 1894. 5p. DNLM **90-3186**

HAMMOND, L[evi] J.
A case of appendicitis in a man seventy-two years of age, in which the pus had found its way through the abdominal wall, and was evacuated; recovery. Philadelphia, 1895. 2p. DNLM **90-3187**

HAMMOND, L[evi] J.
Report of four cases of pelvic abscess following labor. New York, 1896. 4p. DNLM **90-3188**

HAMMOND, Philip (1871-1937)
A case of necrosis of the mastoid with septicemia and gangrene of the lung; operation; recovery. Boston, 1898. 6p. DNLM **90-3189**

HAMMOND, William Alexander (1828-1900)
A treatise on the diseases of the nervous system . . . with the collaboration of Graeme M.Hammond. . . . 9th ed., with corrections and additions. New York: D. Appleton & Co., 1891. 932p. 3 plates. DLC; DNLM; NNNAM; PPC **90-3190**

HAMMOND, William Alexander (1828-1900)
Cardine; the extract of the heart. Its preparation and physiological and therapeutical effects. New York, 1893. 11p. DNLM **90-3191**

HAMMOND, William Alexander (1828-1900)
On certain organic extracts; their preparation and physiological and therapeutical effects. [New York, 1893.] 12p. DNLM **90-3192**

HAMMOND, William Alexander (1828-1900)
A further contribution to the subject of "animal extracts." New York, 1893. 7p. DNLM **90-3193**

HAMMOND, William Alexander (1828-1900)
Cerebral hyperaemia the result of mental strain or emotional disturbance the so-called nervous prostration or neurasthenia. . . . 2nd ed. enl. and improved. Washington: Brentano's, 1895. 118p. DLC **90-3194**

HAMMOND, William Alexander (1828-1900)
The American soldier and venereal diseases, a refutation of some of the statements of Edward Atkinson. New York, 1899. 22p. DNLM **90-3195**

HAMMOND, [W.] Isabel Adams (1859-1910)
Nursing; its principles and practice. For hospitals and private use. Philadelphia: W. B. Saunders, 1893. 484p. 6 plates. DNLM; NNNAM; PPC; PPJ **90-3196**

HANAWAY, H. D.
Illustrated catalogue of dental furniture, instruments and materials. New York, 1897. 594p. NNNAM **90-3197**

HANCHETT, Henry G[ranger] (1853-1918)
The elements of modern domestic medicine. .. . Carefully rev. by A. H. Laidlaw. . . . 2nd ed. Philadelphia: The Hahnemann Publishing House, 1891. 377p. DLC; PPHa **90-3198**

HANCHETT, Henry G[ranger] (1853-1918)
Sexual health; a companion to "Modern domestic medicine." . . . Carefully rev. by A. H. Laidlaw. . . . 3rd ed. Philadelphia: The Hahnemann Publishing House, 1891. 86p. DLC; PPHa **90-3199**

HANCOCK, Joseph L[ane] (1864-1922)
A case of quinin idiosyncrasy. [Philadelphia, 1894.] 1 l. DNLM **90-3200**

HANCOCK, Joseph L[ane] (1864-1922)
Vicarious menstruation from the breast. Philadelphia, 1895. 2p. DNLM **90-3201**

HANKS, H[orace] T[racy] (1837-1900)
The diagnosis and treatment of intestinal obstructions, and the management of greatly distended intestines during laparotomy. New York: William Wood & Co., 1891. 13p. DNLM **90-3202**

HANKS, H[orace] T[racy] (1837-1900)
The importance of understanding the function of the levator and muscle in the treatment of injuries of the floor of the vagina. Philadelphia: W. J. Dornan, 1891. 8p. DNLM
90-3203

HANKS, H[orace] T[racy] (1837-1900)
Rules to be followed in the effort to prevent mural abscesses, abdominal sinuses, and ventral hernia after laparotomy. Philadelphia: W. J. Dornan, 1891. 9p. DNLM
90-3204

HANKS, H[orace] T[racy] (1837-1900)
Secondary hemorrhage after ovariotomy, etc. Can we prevent it? Philadelphia: W. J. Dornan, 1891. 4p. DNLM
90-3205

HANKS, H[orace] T[racy] (1837-1900)
Counter-drainage after coeliotomy. [New York], 1893. 12p. DNLM **90-3206**

HANKS, H[orace] T[racy] (1837-1900)
The prevention and management of pelvic inflammation of puerperal women. [New York, 1893.] 36p. DNLM
90-3207

HANKS, H[orace] T[racy] (1837-1900)
A study of the pathological conditions of the pelvis which ought to be attacked from the vagina. New York, 1896. 12p. DNLM **90-3208**

HANKS, H[orace] T[racy] (1837-1900)
Retro-displacements of the uterus and its appendages; the cause, prevention, and cure. New York, 1897. 12p. DNLM
90-3209

HANKS, H[orace] T[racy] (1837-1900)
Intravenous injection of normal saline solution. New York, 1898. 12p. DNLM **90-3210**

HANSELL, Howard Forde (*b.* 1855)
A manual of clinical ophthalmology, by Howard F. Hansell . . . and James H. Bell. . . . Philadelphia: P. Blakiston, Son & Co., 1892. 231p. plates, diags. DLC; NNNAM; PPC; PU
90-3211

HANSELL, Howard Forde (*b.* 1855)
A practical handbook on the muscular anomalies of the eye; by Howard F. Hansell . . . and Wendell Reber. . . . Philadelphia: P. Blakiston's Son & Co., 1899. 182p. DLC; PPC; PPJ
90-3212

HARDAWAY, William Augustus (1850-1923)
Manual of skin diseases, with special reference to diagnosis and treatment. . . . St. Louis: T. F. Lange, 1890. 434p. DLC
90-3213

HARDAWAY, William Augustus (1850-1923)
Manual of skin diseases, with special reference to diagnosis and treatment; for the use of students and general practitioners. Philadelphia: Lea Bros. & Co., 1891. 467p. 1 plate. DNLM; NNNAM; PPC; PU **90-3214**

HARDAWAY, William A[ugustus] (1850-1923)
A clinical manual of skin diseases. With special reference to diagnosis and treatment. For the use of students and general practitioners. . . . 2nd ed., rev. and enl. . . . Philadelphia and New York: Lea Bros. & Co., 1898. 557p. plates. DLC; DNLM; MBM; PPC **90-3215**

HARDIE, T. Melville
Two cases of nasal hydrorrhoea. With a report of the eye symptoms by Casey A. Wood. [New York, 1890.] 12p. DNLM
90-3216

HARDY, Neal
Hip-joint amputation for recurrent lympho-sarcoma, preliminary laparotomy and direct compression of the aorta; recovery. [Philadelphia, 1891.] 3p. DNLM **90-3217**

HARE, Hobart Amory (1862-1931)
. . . Epilepsy: its pathology and treatment. Being an essay to which was awarded a prize of four thousand francs by the Académie royale de médécine [!] de Belgique, December 31, 1889. . . . Philadelphia and London: F. A. Davis, 1890. 228p. DLC; DNLM; NNNAM; PPC **90-3218**

HARE, Hobart Amory (1862-1931)
A text-book of practical therapeutics, with especial reference to the application of remedial measures to disease and their employment upon a rational basis. . . . Philadelphia: Lea Bros. & Co., 1890. 632p. DLC; DNLM; NNNAM; PPC
90-3219

HARE, Hobart Amory (1862-1931) and Arthur J. PATEK
Rare complications of typhoid fever. [Philadelphia, 1891.] 14p. DNLM **90-3220**

HARE, Hobart Amory (1862-1931)
. . . Fever: its pathology and treatment by antipyretics. Being an essay which was awarded the Boylston prize of Harvard University, July, 1890. . . . Philadelphia and London: F. A. Davis, 1891. 166p. diags. DLC; DNLM; NNNAM; PPC
90-3221

HARE, Hobart Amory (1862-1931)
A system of practical therapeutics. Ed. by Hobart Amory Hare. . . . Assisted by Walter Chrystie. . . . Philadelphia: Lea Bros. & Co., 1891-1897. 4 v. plates. DLC; NNNAM; OCIM; PPC
90-3222

HARE, Hobart Amory (1862-1931)
. . . Essentials of physiology arranged in the form of questions and answers, prepared especially for students of medicine. . . . 3rd ed., thoroughly rev. and enl. . . . Philadelphia: W. B. Saunders, 1891. 193p. plates. DLC; DNLM; NNNAM; PPC
90-3223

HARE, Hobart Amory (1862-1931)
A text-book of practical therapeutics, with especial reference to the application of remedial measures to diseases and their employment upon a rational basis. . . . 2nd ed., enl. and thoroughly rev. Philadelphia: Lea Bros. & Co., 1891. 658p. DLC; DNLM; NNNAM; PU **90-3224**

HARE, Hobart Amory (1862-1931)
A text-book of practical therapeutics, with especial reference to the application of remedial measures to disease and their employment upon a rational basis. . . . 3rd ed., enl. and thoroughly rev. Philadelphia: Lea Bros. & Co., 1892. 696p. DLC; DNLM; MBM; PPC **90-3225**

HARE, Hobart Amory (1862-1931) and E. Q[uin] THORNTON
A study of the influence of chloroform upon the respiration and circulation. Detroit, Mich.: G. S. Davis, 1893. 19p. 153 diag. on 21p. DNLM; OCIM **90-3226**

HARE, Hobart Amory (1862-1931)
A text-book of practical therapeutics, with especial reference to the application of remedial measures to disease and their employment upon a rational basis. . . . 4th ed., enl. and thoroughly rev. Philadelphia: Lea Bros. & Co., 1894. 740p. DLC; DNLM; NNNAM; PPC **90-3227**

HARE, Hobart Amory (1862-1931)
A text-book of practical therapeutics, with especial reference to the application of remedial measures to disease and their employment upon a rational basis. . . . 5th ed., enl. and thoroughly rev. Philadelphia: Lea Bros. & Co., 1895. 740p. DLC; DNLM; MH-M; PPC **90-3228**

HARE, Hobart Amory (1862-1931)
Practical diagnosis: the use of symptoms in the diagnosis of disease. . . . Illustrated with 191 engravings and 13 colored plates. Philadelphia and New York: Lea Bros. & Co., 1896. 573p. col. plates. DLC; DNLM; NNNAM; PU **90-3229**

HARE, Hobart Amory (1862-1931)
Practical diagnosis: the use of symptoms in the diagnosis of disease. 2nd ed., rev. and enl. . . . Illustrated with 201 engravings and 13 colored plates. Philadelphia and New York: Lea Bros. & Co., 1897. 605p. col. plates. DLC; DNLM; NNNAM; PU **90-3230**

HARE, Hobart Amory (1862-1931)
. . . Essentials of physiology, arranged in the form of questions and answers, prepared especially for students of medicine. . . . 4th ed., thoroughly rev. and enl. [by J. H. Raymond]. Philadelphia: W. R Saunders, 1897. 192p. plates. DNC; DNLM; PPC; PU **90-3231**

HARE, Hobart Amory (1862-1931)
The influence of digitalis on the heart muscle when the drug is administered for a long period of time, with a microscopical study and report by W. M. L. Coplin. Detroit, 1897. 12p. DNLM **90-3232**

HARE, Hobart Amory (1862-1931)
The rapidity of absorption and elmination of some commonly employed drugs as a guide to their administration. Detroit: W. M. Warren, 1897. 9p. DNLM **90-3233**

HARE, Hobart Amory (1862-1931)
A text-book of practical therapeutics, with especial reference to the application of remedial measures to disease and their employment upon a rational basis. . . . 6th ed., enl., thoroughly rev. and largely re-written. Philadelphia and New York: Lea Bros. & Co., 1897. 758p. DLC; DNLM; NNNAM; PPC **90-3234**

HARE, Hobart Amory (1862-1931) and Charles Adams HOLDER
The real value of the Brand bath in typhoid fever. Detroit: W. M. Warren, 1898. 14p. DNLM **90-3235**

HARE, Hobart Amory (1862-1931)
A text-book of practical therapeutics, with especial reference to the application of remedial measures to disease and their employment upon a rational basis. . . . 7th ed., enl., thoroughly rev. and largely re-written. Philadelphia and New York: Lea Bros. & Co., 1898. 776p. chart. DLC; DNLM; NNNAM; PPC **90-3236**

HARE, Hobart Amory (1862-1931)
Practical diagnosis: the use of symptoms in the diagnosis of disease. 3rd ed., rev. and enl. . . . Illustrated with 204 engravings and 13 colored plates. Philadelphia and New York: Lea Bros. & Co., 1898. 624p. plates. DLC; DNLM; NNNAM; PPC **90-3237**

HARE, Hobart Amory (1862-1931)
Practical diagnosis: the use of symptoms in the diagnosis of disease. 4th ed., rev. and enl. . . . Illustrated with 205 engravings and 14 colored plates. Philadelphia and New York: Lea Bros. & Co., 1899. 631p. plates. DLC; NNNAM; OCIM; PU **90-3238**

HARE, Hobart Amory (1862-1931)
The medical complication, accidents and sequelae of typhoid or enteric fever. . . . With a special chapter on the mental disturbances following typhoid fever. By F. X. Dercum. . . . Philadelphia and New York: Lea Bros. & Co., 1899. 286p. plates. DLC; DNLM; NNNAM; PPC **90-3239**

HARLAN, George C[uvier] (1835-1909)
The pupil reflex in absolute blindness. Philadelphia, 1896. 5p. DNLM **90-3240**

HARLAN, George C[uvier] (1835-1909)
Operations performed upon the eyelids. Philadelphia, 1898. 44p. DNLM **90-3241**

HARLAN, George C[uvier] (1835-1909)
Diseases of the eyelids. Philadelphia, 1898. 26p. DNLM **90-3242**

HARRIGAN, C[ornelius] P.
A plea for modern Caesarean section. New York, 1895. 5p. DNLM **90-3243**

HARRINGTON, A[rthur] H[udson] (*b.* 1856)
The legislative provisions for insane criminals in Massachusetts. Boston, 1895. 15p. DNLM **90-3244**

HARRINGTON, Charles (1856-1908)
Lectures on materia medica and therapeutics. Cambridge: The Cooperative Press, 1897. 242p. MBM **90-3245**

HARRINGTON, Charles (1856-1908)
A simple method for the sterilization of catgut. Philadelphia, 1898. 6p. DNLM **90-3246**

HARRINGTON, Charles (1856-1908)
The possibilities and limitations of formaldehyde as a disinfectant. Philadelphia, 1898. 14p. DNLM **90-3247**

HARRINGTON, F[rancis] B[ishop] (1854-1914)
On the feasibility of intraperitoneal cystotomy, with the report of a case. Philadelphia, 1893. 5p. DNLM **90-3248**

HARRINGTON, F[rancis] M.
Should medical registration laws cover the science of ophthalmology? New York, 1896. 7p. DNLM **90-3249**

HARRINGTON, Thomas F[rancis] (1866-1919)
Philosophy of sickness. Boston, 1899. 12p. DNLM **90-3250**

HARRIS, Chapin Aaron (1806-1860)
A dictionary of dental science. . . . 5th ed. Carefully rev. and enl. by Ferdinand J. S. Gorgas. . . . Philadelphia: P. Blakiston, Son & Co., 1891. 639p. DLC; DNLM; MdU-D; PPC **90-3251**

HARRIS, Chapin Aaron (1806-1860)
The principles and practice of dentistry including anatomy, physiology, pathology, therapeutics, dental surgery and mechanisms. . . . 13th ed. Rev. and ed. by Ferdinand J. S. Gorgas. . . . With twelve hundred and fifty illustrations. Philadelphia: P. Blakiston, Son & Co., 1896. 1180p. DLC; DNLM; NNNAM; PPC **90-3252**

HARRIS, Chapin Aaron (1806-1860)
A dictionary of dental science. . . . 6th ed., carefully rev. and enl. by Ferdinand J. S. Gorgas. . . . Philadelphia: P. Blakiston's Son & Co., 1898. 662p. DLC; NNNAM; PPC; PU **90-3253**

HARRIS, H[enry] F[auntleroy] (*b.* 1867)
Three cases of amebic dysentery. [Philadelphia: Lea Bros. & Co., 1892.] 7p. DNLM **90-3254**

HARRIS, H[enry] F[auntleroy] (*b.* 1867)
Some observations on a method of multiplication of the amoeba dysenteriae (amoeba coli). Philadelphia: Lea Bros. & Co., 1894. 6p. DNLM **90-3255**

HARRIS, H[enry] F[auntleroy] (*b.* 1867)
A case of diabetes mellitus quickly following mumps. On the pathological alterations of the salivary glands, closely resembling those found in the pancreas, in a case of diabetes mellitus. Boston, 1899. 17p. DNLM **90-3256**

HARRIS, M[alcolm] LaSalle (1862-1936)
A case of undescended ovary and tube, with sactosalpinx purulenta profluens. New York, 1896. 4p. DNLM **90-3257**

HARRIS, M[alcolm] LaSalle (1862-1936)
A new and simple method of obtaining the urine separately from the two kidneys in either sex. Chicago, 1898. 12p. DNLM **90-3258**

HARRIS, Philander A. (*b.* 1852)
A successful case of Caesarean section. New York, 1894. 3p. DNLM **90-3259**

HARRIS, Philander A. (*b.* 1852)
A method of performing rapid manual dilatation of the os uteri, and its advantages in the treatment of placenta previa. New York, 1894. 12p. DNLM **90-3260**

HARRIS, Philander A. (*b.* 1852)
Pelvimeters and the practice of pelvimetry as a means of discovering irregularities of the pelvis which are likely to embarrass parturition. Cambridge, Mass., 1895. 23p. DNLM **90-3261**

HARRIS, Robert P[atterson] (1822-1899)
Coeliotomy; this and not laparotomy is the proper Greek synonym of abdominal section, laparotomy being an incision of the flank only. Philadelphia: W. J. Dornan, 1890. 16p. DNLM **90-3262**

HARRIS, Robert P[atterson] (1822-1899)
Abdominal and uterine tolerance in pregnant women; as shown by the low rate of mortality under severe lacerated and other wounds, the result of direct violence. Philadelphia: W. J. Dornan, 1892. 20p. DNLM **90-3263**

HARRIS, Robert P[atterson] (1822-1899)
The remarkable results of antiseptic symphysiotomy. New York: William Wood & Co., 1892. 18p. DNLM **90-3264**

HARRIS, Robert P[atterson] (1822-1899)
The remarkable results of antiseptic symphysiotomy. [Philadelphia, 1892.] 20p. DNLM **90-3265**

HARRIS, Robert P[atterson] (1822-1899)
The symphysiotomies of the United States and of Canada. New York, 1895. 31p. DNLM **90-3266**

HARRIS, Robert P[atterson] (1822-1899)
Congenital absence of the penis, the urethra making its exit into or below the rectum, and emptying the bladder by, or exterior to, the anus. [Philadelphia, 1898.] 19p. DNLM **90-3267**

HARRIS, Vincent Dormer and Edwin Clifford BEALE
The treatment of pulmonary consumption: a practical manual. Philadelphia: P. Blakiston, Son & Co., 1895. 483p. CtY-M; DNLM; MdU-D; NNNAM **90-3268**

HARRISON, George Byrd (1844-1898)
A case of opium-poisoning treated with potassium permanganate. Philadelphia, 1895. 3p. DNLM **90-3269**

HARRISON, George T[ucker] (1835-1925)
Parametritis (or pelvic cellulitis); its pathological importance and clinical significance. New York, 1895. 8p. DNLM **90-3270**

HARRISON, George T[ucker] (1835-1925)
Indications of treatment in the case of uterine myomata. New York, 1896. 4p. DNLM **90-3271**

HARSHBERGER, John W. (1869-1929)
The botanists of Philadelphia and New York. Philadelphia: Press of T. C. Davis & Son, 1899. 457p. DLC; DNLM; PP; PPC **90-3272**

HART, Ernest [Abraham] (1835-1898)
The profession, the public, and the code. An address delivered by invitation before the third general meeting of the Pan-American Medical Congress, Washington, Sept. 7, 1893. 1893. 1 broadside. elephantine fol. DNLM **90-3273**

HART, James I.
Minute structure of dentine. Philadelphia, 1891. 13p. DNLM **90-3274**

HARTFORD MEDICAL SOCIETY
Fiftieth anniversary of the Hartford Medical Society. Founded September 15, 1846. Proceedings at the celebration, October 26, 1896, at Hartford, Connecticut. Hartford, 1897. 124p. CtY-M; DNLM **90-3275**

HARTFORD MEDICAL SOCIETY
Proceedings of the dedication of the Hunt Memorial Building by . . . February 1, 1898. Hartford: Plimpton Print. Co., 1898. 48p. 6 phot. CtY-M; DNLM **90-3276**

HARTIGAN, James W.
. . . Anatomy, physiology, and hygiene, with the effects of alcohol and narcotics on the human body. . . . Philadelphia: J. E. Potter & Co., [1890]. 419p. col. illus. DLC; DNLM; PPC **90-3277**

HARTMAN, Samuel B[rubaker] (*b.* 1830)
Diseases of the eye. Columbus, [1892]. 48p. DNLM **90-3278**

HARTMAN, Samuel B[rubaker] (*b.* 1830)
Paralysis and deformities. Columbus, [1894?]. 68p. DNLM; OCIM **90-3279**

HARTMAN, Samuel B[rubaker] (*b.* 1830)
The narcotic habit; as treated at the Surgical Hotel. Columbus, [1894?]. 13p. DNLM **90-3280**

HARTMAN, Samuel B[rubaker] (*b.* 1830)
Private counselor. For men only. Stricture of the urethra. Columbus, 1896. 16p. DNLM **90-3281**

HARTMAN, Samuel B[rubaker] (*b.* 1830)
A lecture on stammering. Columbus, [1895?]. 16p. DNLM **90-3282**

HARTMAN, Samuel B[rubaker] (*b.* 1830) and David R. SUMMY
A short treatise on pelvic surgery. Columbus, 1899. 34p. 6 plates. DNLM; OCIM **90-3283**

HARTMAN SANITARIUM, COLUMBUS
Department of the ear, Surgical Hotel. Columbus, [1895]. 63p. DNLM **90-3284**

HARTMAN SANITARIUM, COLUMBUS
Department of club feet, Surgical Hotel. Columbus, [1895]. 32p. DNLM **90-3285**

HARTMAN SANITARIUM, COLUMBUS
Department of spinal curvature, Surgical Hotel. Columbus, [1895]. 47p. DNLM **90-3286**

HARTMAN SANITARIUM, COLUMBUS
Department of joint diseases, Surgical Hotel. Columbus, [1895]. 47p. DNLM **90-3287**

HARTMAN SANITARIUM, COLUMBUS
Department of massage, Surgical Hotel. Columbus, [1895]. 68p. DNLM **90-3288**

HARTMAN SANITARIUM, COLUMBUS
Department of gynaecology, Surgical Hotel. Columbus, [1895]. 98p. DNLM **90-3289**

HARTMAN SANITARIUM, COLUMBUS
Department of cancer and skin diseases. Surgical Hotel. Columbus, 1896. 37p. DNLM **90-3290**

HARTMAN SANITARIUM, COLUMBUS
A visit to the . . . . By a physician and grateful patient. Souvenir No. 4. Columbus: Terry Eng. Co., 1899. 76p. DNLM; OC **90-3291**

HARTMAN, W. Louis
Gall-stones and abscess of liver. Philadelphia, 1899. 11p. DNLM **90-3292**

HARTMANN, Franz (1796-1853)
Occult science in medicine. New York, 1893. 100p. DNLM; NN **90-3293**

HARTMANN, Henri Albert Charles Antoine (1860-1952)
Bromide of ethyl, its qualities, its effects, its excellence as a general anaesthetic. Its history, its properties, its advantages, and mode of use . . . by Henry Hartmann and Henri Bourbon. Transl. from the French by G. Bouchard. Worcester, Mass.: Goessman, Gile & Co., 1899. 73p. DLC **90-3294**

HARTRIDGE, Gustavus (1849-1923)
The refraction of the eye. A manual for students. 4th ed. Philadelphia: P. Blakiston, Son & Co., 1890. 249p. 1 plate. DNLM; NNNAM; PPC; PPJ **90-3295**

HARTRIDGE, Gustavus (1849-1923)
The refraction of the eye. A manual for students. 5th ed. Philadelphia: P. Blakiston, Son & Co., 1890. 240p. NNNAM; PPC **90-3296**

HARTRIDGE, Gustavus (1849-1923)
The ophthalmoscope. A manual for students. Philadelphia: P. Blakiston, Son & Co., 1891. 128p. DLC; DNLM; PPC; PU **90-2397**

HARTRIDGE, Gustavus (1849-1923)
The refraction of the eye. A manual for students. 6th ed. Philadelphia: P. Blakiston, Son & Co., 1892. 251p. IU-M; NNNAM; PPJ **90-3298**

HARTRIDGE, Gustavus (1849-1923)
The refraction of the eye. A manual for students. 7th ed. Philadelphia: P. Blakiston, Son & Co., 1894. 259p. MBM; NNNAM; OCIM; PPC **90-3299**

HARTRIDGE, Gustavus (1849-1923)
The ophthalmoscope. A manual for students. 2nd ed. Philadelphia: P. Blakiston, Son & Co., 1895. 128p. DNLM; MdU-D; PPC: PU **90-3300**

HARTRIDGE, Gustavus (1849-1923)
The refraction of the eye, a manual for students. 8th ed. With additions by Dr. H. M. Martin, Dr. H. Culbertson, Dr. F. C. Hotz, [and] Dr. Chas. J. Oliver. Chicago: W. P. Dunn Co., 1895. 259, 35p. DLC; NNNAM; OCIM **90-3301**

HARTRIDGE, Gustavus (1849-1923)
The refraction of the eye. A manual for students. 8th ed. Philadelphia: P. Blakiston, Son & Co., 1896. 263p. 1 plate. DNLM; MBM; PPC; PU **90-3302**

HARTRIDGE, Gustavus (1849-1923)
The ophthalmoscope. A manual for students. 3rd ed. Philadelphia: P. Blakiston, Son & Co., 1897. 159p. 4 plates. DNLM; NNNAM; OCIM; PPC **90-3303**

HARTSHORNE, Henry (1823-1897)
The practical household physician. A cyclopedia of family medicine, surgery, nursing and hygiene. . . . New and rev. ed. Philadelphia, Pa.; Chicago, Ill. [etc.]: J. C. Winston & Co., 1891. 971p. col. plates. DLC; OCIM; PPC **90-3304**

HARTSHORNE, Henry (1823-1897)
Cholera and its migrations. [Philadelphia, 1892.] 12p. DNLM
90-3305

HARVARD UNIVERSITY. DENTAL SCHOOL (BOSTON)
Report of a meeting in behalf of a new building for the Dental Department of Harvard University. Held in Horticultural Hall, Boston, Nov. 30, 1893. Boton: W. H. Chandler, 1893. 20p. DNLM; MH-M **90-3306**

HARVEY MEDICAL COLLEGE, CHICAGO
Annual announcements for the sessions of 1895-1896 to 1899-1900 (5.-9.). Chicago, 1895-1899. DNLM
90-3307

HARVEY MEDICAL COLLEGE, CHICAGO
Mid-summer announcement of the session of 1896-1897. Chicago, 1896. 14 l. DNLM **90-3308**

HARVEY, N. Darrell
The dangers in removing foreign bodies from the cornea. Boston, 1895. 5p. DNLM **90-3309**

HARVIE, John B.
Fifty operations on the uterine cervix for lacerations. [New York, 1894.] 19p. DNLM **90-3310**

HARWOOD, Charles H.
The conservative phase of hypnotism in therapeutics. Boston, [1890]. 6p. DNLM **90-3311**

HASBROUCK, Edwin M.
The treatment of abscess by the Otis method, with a report of thirty-two cases. New York, 1896. 9p. DNLM
90-3312

HASBROUCK, Edwin M.
A case of hypertrophic pulmonary osteo-arthropathy. [New York, 1898.] 12p. 2 plates. DNLM
90-3313

HASKELL, Loomis P.
The student's manual and handbook for the dental laboratory. 2nd ed. . . . To which is appended Dr. E. H. Angle's system of appliances for correcting irregularities. Philadelphia: The Wilmington Dental Mfg. Co., 1890. 97p. DLC; MdU-D; PPC
90-3314

HASTINGS, Charles J. C. O.
Septicaemia in the puerperium. [New York, 1897.] 32p. DNLM **90-3315**

HASTINGS, Robert W.
Human food laws. Chicago, 1898. 8p. DNLM
90-3316

HASTINGS, Robert W.
Noise as a factor in the causation of disease. Chicago, 1898. 7p. DNLM **90-3317**

HASTINGS, Robert W.
Notes on vaccine rashes. [Boston, 1898.] 6p. DNLM
90-3318

HASTINGS, Robert W.
The digestion of amylaceous food. Boston, 1899. 8p. DNLM
90-3319

HATFIELD, Marcus P[atten] (1849-1909)
A compend of diseases of children. Especially adpated for the use of medical students. Philadelphia: P. Blakiston, Son & Co., 1890. 185p. 1 plate. DNLM; PPC; PPJ
90-3320

HAVEN, George (1861-1903)
The diagnosis of extra-uterine pregnancy. [Boston, 1893.] 6p. DNLM **90-3321**

HAVEN, George (1861-1903)
Caesarean section, with the report of a case. Boston: Damrell & Upham, 1895. 8p. DNLM **90-3322**

HAWKES, J[ohn] Marshall (1848?-1895)
Injury to the spine: invention and application of paper jacket. [Philadelphia: Lea Bros. & Co., 1892.] 9p. DNLM
90-3323

HAWKINS, J. A.
A case of diphtheria in which the membrane persisted for a long time, with nephritis as a sequence. [Philadelphia, 1892.] 5p. DNLM **90-3324**

HAWKINS, Thomas H.
State boards of medical examiners vs. medical colleges. Denver, 1895. 11p. DNLM **90-3325**

HAWKINS, Thomas H.
An improved method for the removal of intraligamentous cyst. [Denver, 1897.] 2 l. DNLM **90-3326**

HAWKINS, Thomas H.
Sterilized gauze in pelvic surgery. St. Louis, 1897. 8p. DNLM
90-3327

HAWKINS, Thomas H.
The advantages of vagino-abdominal section. [New York, 1897.] 5p. DNLM **90-3328**

HAWKINS, Thomas H.
Appendicitis or salpingitis with complications, and a report of some unusual cases. New York, 1899. 16p. DNLM
90-3329

HAWLEY, D[only] C[urtis] (*b.* 1855)
The radical cure of hydrocele. Chicago, 1895. 4p. DNLM
90-3330

HAWLEY, D[only] C[urtis] (*b.* 1855)
Thoughts on general and cardiac therapy. Chicago, 1896. 12p. DNLM **90-3331**

HAWLEY, R. Newton
The medical lore of Shakespeare. Detroit, 1892. 48p. DNLM
90-3332

HAY, C[harles] M.
Three types of cerebral syphilis producing mental disease. [Philadelphia, 1890.] 16p. DNLM **90-3333**

HAY, C[harles] M.
Hereditary chorea, with a contribution of eight additional cases of the disease. [Philadelphia, 1890.] 10p. DNLM
90-3334

HAY, C[harles] M.
Head injuries as a cause of insanity. [Philadelphia, 1891.] 12p. DNLM **90-3335**

HAYD, Herman E. (*b.* 1858)
Treatment of endometritis. New York, 1894. 4p. DNLM **90-3336**

HAYD, Herman E. (*b.* 1858)
Large hydronephrotic cyst simulating ovarian tumor; abdomianl nephrectomy; recovery. New York, 1895. 4p. DNLM **90-3337**

HAYD, Herman E. (*b.* 1858)
Intraperitoneal treatment of uterine displacements. New York, 1895. 6p. DNLM **90-3338**

HAYDEN, James Raynor (*b.* 1863)
A manual of veneral diseases. . . . New York and Philadelphia: Lea Bros. & Co., 1896. 267p. DLC; NNNAM; PPC **90-3339**

HAYDEN, James Raynor (*b.* 1863)
A manual of venereal diseases. . . . With fifty-four illustrations. [2nd ed.] New York and Philadelphia: Lea Bros. & Co., 1898. 304p. DLC; NNNAM; PPC; PU **90-3340**

HAYDEN'S VIBURNUM COMPOUND
Theory, practice, and demonstration. The thought and expression of many medical men in relation to the peculiar merits of Hayden's Viburnum Compound and the uric solvent. With much other interesting matter for physicians only. Bedford Springs, Mass., 1891. 126 l. DNLM **90-3341**

HAYDEN, W[illiam] R.
Anaesthesia by etherization, and the viburnum compound of Dr. Hayden. [Boston, 1891.] 30p. 4 plates. DNLM **90-3342**

HAYDEN, W[illiam] R.
History of anaesthesia or painless surgery. New York: J. MacDonald, 1896. 51p. 4 plates, port. DNLM; NNNAM **90-3343**

HAYEM, Georges (1841-1935)
Physical and natural therapeutics: the remedial uses of atmospheric pressure, climate, heat and cold, hydrotherapeutic measures, mineral waters, and electricity. . . . Ed. by Hobart Amory Hare. . . . Philadelphia: Lea Bros. & Co., 1895. 426p. DLC; DNLM; MBM; PPC **90-3344**

[HAYES, Albert Hamilton]
The diagnostician; or, Know thyself manual. By a humanitarian. [Former chief consulting physician to Peabody Medical Institute.] Boston: Peabody Medical Institute, 1898. 92p. col. plates. DLC; MBM **90-3345**

HAYES, J. R.
How to live longer and why we do not live longer. Philadelphia: J. B. Lippincott Co., 1897. 180p. DNLM; MH; NNNAM; PU **90-3346**

HAYES, Plymmon S[anford] (1850-1894)
Electricity and the methods of its employment in removing superfluous hair and other facial blemishes. Chicago: McIntosh Battery & Optical, 1894. 128p. OCIM **90-3347**

HAYNES, Celia M.
Elementary principles of electrotherapeutics for the use of physicians and students. With 135 illustrations. . . . Rev. ed. With an appendix, including recent discoveries in electrotherapeutics and diagnosis, profusely illustrated. Chicago: McIntosh Battery & Optical Co., 1890. 511p. DLC; OCIM **90-3348**

HAYNES, Celia M.
Elementary principles of electrotherapeutics for the use of physicians and students. With 145 illustrations. . . . Rev. ed. Chicago: The W. T. Kenner Co., 1896. 507p. DLC; OCIM **90-3349**

HAYNES, Francis L. (1850-1898)
Two cases in which the uterus was perforated by a curette, both recovering. New York, 1890. 1 l. DNLM **90-3350**

HAYNES, Francis L. (1850-1898)
Are ligature-fistulae after celiotomies avoidable? [Philadelphia: Lea Bros. & Co., 1894.] 3p. DNLM **90-3351**

HAYNES, Francis L. (1850-1898)
A uterine irrigating tube. Philadelphia, 1894. 1 l. DNLM **90-3352**

HAYNES, Irving S[amuel] (*b.* 1861)
Vicious union following Pott's fracture; operative treatment. Presentation of a case. [New York, 1892.] 8p. DNLM **90-3353**

HAYNES, Irving S[amuel] (*b.* 1861)
A clinical paper on some cases, with various interesting features. [New York, 1893.] 11p. DNLM **90-3354**

HAYNES, Irving S[amuel] (*b.* 1861)
Diphtheria; a new method of treatment. Ozone in the treatment of diphtheria, with reports of seven cases. [Chicago, 1893.] 12p. DNLM **90-3355**

HAYNES, Irving S[amuel] (*b.* 1861)
A practical guide for beginners to the dissection of the human body. New York: E. B. Treat, 1893. 123p. DLC; DNLM; NNNAM **90-3356**

HAYNES, Irving S[amuel] (*b.* 1861)
The diagnosis and treatment of tubal pregnancy. New York, 1894. 14p. DNLM **90-3357**

HAYNES, Irving S[amuel] (*b.* 1861)
A manual of anatomy. Philadelphia: W. B. Saunders, 1896. 680p. DLC; DNLM; NNNAM; PPC **90-3358**

HAYNES, Irving S[amuel] (*b.* 1861)
Appendicitis in children; a clinical paper. [New York, 1898.] 17p. DNLM **90-3359**

HAYNES, Irving S[amuel] (*b.* 1861)
The treatment of fractures of the patella by the purse-string suture. New York, 1898. 18p. DNLM **90-3360**

HAYNES, John R[andolph] (*b.* 1853)
Abdominal surgery. (1) Nephrorraphy. (2) Oophorectomy and hysterorraphy, etc. [*Also*:] Neuritis of the tibial nerves, requiring amputation of leg. History by Francis L. Haynes. [Los Angeles, 1890.] 7p. DNLM **90-3361**

HAYNES, John R[andolph] (*b.* 1853)
Gynecological memoranda. [Los Angeles, 1891.] 2 l. DNLM
90-3362

HAYNES, W[illiam] H[enry] (1856?-1902)
Obstetrical paralysis of infants. Brooklyn, 1897. 7p. DNLM
90-3363

HAYNES, W[illiam] H[enry] (1856?-1902)
Recurrent ptosis; report of a case, with anaesthesia of supra-orbital branch of the fifth cranial nerve. New York, 1897. 6p. DNLM **90-3364**

HAYNES, W[illiam] H[enry] (1856?-1902)
Complications affecting the nervous system in the treatment of typhoid fever. Brooklyn, 1898. 4p. DNLM
90-3365

HAYES, D. W[ilson]
Cystic degeneration of enlarged submaxillary glands. Philadelphia, 1893. 3p. DNLM **90-3366**

HAYT, Charles W[alker] (*d.* 1901)
Obstetrics. A manual for students and practitioners. Philadelphia: Lea Bros. & Co., [1892]. 190p. DLC; DNLM; PPC; PU
90-3367

HAZARD, Alexander
Pocket medical formulary, arranged therapeutically. . . . rev. and enl. by Abraham S. Gerhard. . . . With an appendix. . . . 3rd ed. Philadelphia: University of Pennsylvania Press, 1891. 334p. DLC; PU **90-3368**

HAZZARD, Charles
Lectures on principles of osteopathy. . . . Kirksville, Mo.: Advocate Book & Job Print, 1898. 209p. DLC
90-3369

HAZZARD, Charles
Principles of osteopathy. 2nd ed., rev. and enl. . . . Kirksville: Journal Printing Co., 1898. 2 pt. in 1 v. DLC
90-3370

HAZZARD, Charles
Principles of osteopathy. 3rd ed., thoroughly rev. . . . [Detroit: C. Hazzard, 1899.] 319p. DLC
90-3371

HEATH, Christopher (1835-1905)
Practical anatomy: a manual of dissections. Ed. by William Anderson. 8th ed. Philadelphia: P. Blakiston, Son & Co., 1893. 744p. DNLM; NNNAN; PPC; PU **90-3372**

HEATH, Christopher (1835-1905)
A manual of minor surgery. . . . 10th ed. Philadelphia: P. Blakiston, Son & Co., 1894. 389p. CtY-M; DNLM; NNNAM; PU **90-3373**

HEFFRON, John L[orenzo] (1851-1924)
Some effects of influenza on the heart. Philadelphia, 1895. 12p. DNLM **90-3374**

HEIMAN, Henry (*b.* 1865)
A clinical and bacteriological study of the gonococcus-Neisser as found in the male urethra and in the vulvo-vaginal tract of children; a paper based on experiments conducted in the Bacterial Laboratory, College of Physicians and Surgeons, Columbia College, New York. New York: Bloch & Conklin, 1895. 41p. DNLM; NNC **90-3375**

HEIMAN, Henry (*b.* 1865)
A further study of the biology of the gonococcus (Neisser), with contributions to the technique; a paper based on the morphological and biological examination of exudates in cases of chronic urethritis. New York, 1896. 24p. DNLM
90-3376

HEIMAN, Henry (*b.* 1865)
Further studies (third series) on the gonococcus (Neisser). New York, 1897. 8p. DNLM **90-3377**

HEIMAN, Henry (*b.* 1865)
An epitome of current methods of blood examination, with demonstrations. [New York, 1898.] 18p. DNLM
90-3378

HEISLER, John Clement (*b.* 1862)
A text-book of embryology for students of medicine. . . . With 190 illustrations, 26 of them in colors. Philadelphia: W. B. Saunders, 1899. 405p. col. plates. DLC; MBM; NNNAM; PPC
90-3379

HEITZMANN, C[arl] (1836-1896) and Frank ABBOTT
Senile atrophy of the upper jaw. Philadelphia, 1892. 11p. DNLM **90-3380**

HEITZMANN, Louis (*b.* 1864)
Urinary analysis and diagnosis by microscopical and chemical examination. . . . With one hundred and eight original illustrations. New York: William Wood & Co., 1899. 253p. DLC; NNNAM **90-3381**

HEKTOEN, Ludvig (1863-1951)
Carcinoma of oesophagus; secondary implantation; carcinoma in stomach; ulceration, death from hemorrhage. Rupture of portal vein from a fall; death. Loose bodies in the peritoneal cavity. Thoracic aneurism; varicose dilatation of subcutaneous thoracic and abdominal veins; rupture; death. Chicago: J. M. W. Jones, 1890. 18p. DNLM **90-3382**

HEKTOEN, Ludvig (1863-1951)
The pathological anatomy of acute arsenical poisoning. [Chicago, 1891.] 8p. DNLM **90-3383**

HEKTOEN, Ludvig (1863-1951)
Two interesting medico legal cases. [Chicago, 1891.] 9p. DNLM **90-3384**

HEKTOEN, Ludvig (1863-1951)
A contribution to the study of cystic kidney. Chicago: M. H. Kauffmann, [1892]. 15p. DNLM **90-3385**

HEKTOEN, Ludvig (1863-1951)
Embolism of the left coronary artery; sudden death. [Philadelphia, 1892.] 6p. DNLM **90-3386**

HEKTOEN, Ludvig (1863-1951)
Rupture of the aortic valves, with demonstration of specimen. Aneurisms of right auricular appendix. [Chicago, 1892.] 7p. DNLM **90-3387**

HEKTOEN, Ludvig (1863-1951)
Acute ulcerative endocarditis; a brief résumé of the pathology of eight cases. Chicago, 1893. 16p. DNLM
90-3388

HEKTOEN, Ludvig (1863-1951)
A case of amebic dysentery. [Chicago, 1893.] 7p. DNLM
90-3389

HEKTOEN, Ludvig (1863-1951)
Sarcoma of the pons, and glio-sarcoma of the cerebellum. Chicago, 1893. 11p. DNLM **90-3390**

HEKTOEN, Ludvig (1863-1951)
A specimen of four healed, ascending ileal invaginations, symmetrical and equidistant. [Philadelphia: J. B. Lippincott Co., 1893.] 9p. DNLM **90-3391**

HEKTOEN, Ludvig (1863-1951)
Three specimens of tumors of the heart; metastatic carcinomatous nodule in the myocardium, implantation-sarcoma of the right ventricle; primary round-celled sarcoma of the epicardium. [Philadelphia: Lea Bros. & Co., 1893.] 11p. DNLM **90-3392**

HEKTOEN, Ludvig (1863-1951)
Vitelline-duct remains at the navel. New York: William Wood & Co., 1893. 13p. DNLM **90-3393**

HEKTOEN, Ludvig (1863-1951)
The technique of post-mortem examination. . . . Chicago: The W. T. Keener Co., 1894 [1893]. 172p. plates. DLC; DNLM; NNNAM; OCIM **90-3394**

HEKTOEN, Ludvig (1863-1951)
The vascular changes of tuberculous meningitis, especially the tuberculous endarteritis. New York, 1896. 52p. DNLM **90-3395**

HELBRING, E.
Modern materia medica for pharmacists, medical men and students. New York: Lehn and Fink, 1892. 202p. NNNAM; OCLloyd **90-3396**

HELFERICH, Heinrich (1851-1945)
Atlas of traumatic fractures and luxations. . . . New York: William Wood & Co., 1896. 142p. NNNAM; OCIM; PPC; PU **90-3397**

HELLER, Edwin A.
Essentials of materia medica, pharmacy and prescription writing arranged in conformity with the classification in the last ed. of Prof. H. C. Wood's "Therapeutics" and following the course of pharmacy as taught in the University of Pennsylvania. . . . Philadelphia: P. Blakiston, Son & Co., 1897. 389p. DLC; DNLM; OCLloyd; PU **90-3398**

HELMUTH, William Tod (1833-1902)
Homoeopathy; its present relations to the people and to the old school. Address delivered in the Hospital Theatre at the inaugural exercises of the institution, January 7, 1890. New York: M. J. Rooney & Co., 1890. 18p. NNNAM **90-3399**

HELMUTH, William Tod (1833-1902)
A contribution to the study of renal surgery; nephrotomy for pyo-nephrosis; nephrolithotomy and nephrectomy for renal calculi. New York: M. J. Rooney, 1892. 11p. DNLM **90-3400**

HELMUTH, William Tod (1833-1902)
A glance at Japanese medicine, ancient and modern. New York, 1893. 22p. DNLM; NNNAM **90-3401**

HEMMETER, John C. (1863-1931)
An apparatus for washing out the stomach and sigmoid with a continuous current, with return stomach or rectal tube. New York, 1895. 8p. DNLM **90-3402**

HEMMETER, John C. (1863-1931)
Gastric lavage with a continuous current. An improved recurrent stomach tube, with history and technics of the subject. New York, 1895. 21p. DNLM **90-3403**

HEMMETER, John C. (1863-1931)
Diseases of the stomach; their special pathology, diagnosis and treatment. . . . Philadelphia: P. Blakiston & Co., 1897. 788p. col. plates. DLC; NNNAM; PPC; PU **90-3404**

HEMMETER, John C. (1863-1931)
Experimental basis of the dietetic and medicinal treatment of hyperacidity and gastritis. Chicago, 1897. 20p. DNLM **90-3405**

HEMMETER, John C. (1863-1931) and Delano AMES
A case of phlegmonous gastritis following ulcus carcinomatosum of the pylorus; dilatation, perforation, and peritonitis. A clinical history of fourteen months with chemical, bacteriological, and histopathological study. New York: Publ. Print. Co., 1897. 20p. DNLM **90-3406**

HENCKEL, George
Prescriptions and how to use them. An anatomical and physiological treatise on the human body. . . . Anatomy and physiology. . . . [with] diseases and their treatment, by Orville Juan Perkins. Chicago, Ill.: Henckel & Perkins, [1891]. 3 v. DLC **90-3407**

HENCKEL, George
The practical physician and home apothecary . . . with medical contributions by eminent physicians. Rev. by C. M. Spalding, M.D. Chicago, Ill.: Smucker & Co., 1891. 307p. plates. DLC; OCIM **90-3408**

HENCKEL, George
Prescriptions and how to use them. An anatomical and physiological treatise on the human body with a practical description of its diseases. . . . Anatomy and physiology by . . . . Diseases and their treatment by Orrville [!] Juan Perkins. . . . Chicago: Henckel & Co., [1892]. 3 v. DLC **90-3409**

HENDERSON, Frank Laramore (*b.* 1865)
Notes on the eye, for the use of students. . . . St. Louis, Mo.: Shultz Publishing Co., 1897. 103p. col. plate. DLC **90-3410**

HENKELS, AUCTIONEERS. PHILADELPHIA
Valuable medical and miscellaneous books . . . including the library of the late Dr. C. S. Boker. . . . Catalogue compiled by S. V. Henkels. Philadelphia: T. Birch's Sons [1895]. 40p. NN **90-3411**

HENROTIN, Fernand (1847-1906)
Conservative surgical treatment of para- and peri-uterine septic diseases. New York, 1895. 14p. DNLM **90-3412**

HENROTIN, Fernand (1847-1906)
The cure of septic pelvic diseases in women. New York, 1896. 18p. DNLM **90-3413**

HENROTIN, Fernand (1847-1906)
Vaginal section for extra-uterine pregnancy. New York, 1896. 9p. DNLM **90-3414**

HENROTIN, Fernand (1847-1906) and Maximilian HERZOG
Very early rupture in an ectopic gestation in a tubal diverticulum. New York, 1899. 9p. DNLM **90-3415**

HENROTIN, Fernand (1847-1906) and Maximilian HERZOG
Carcinoma developed in primarily non-malignant kyst-adenoma of the ovary. Chicago, 1899. 7p. DNLM **90-3416**

HENROTIN, Fernand (1847-1906) and Maximilian HERZOG
Myoma ovarii; endothelioma ovarii; calcified corpus luteum. New York: William Wood & Co., 1899. 12p. DNLM **90-3417**

HENRY, Clifford Elmore (*b.* 1873)
A manual of osteopathic therapeutics. . . . Minneapolis: The Author, 1898. 63p. DLC; DNLM **90-3418**

HENRY, Clifford E[lmore] (*b.* 1873)
A manual of osteopathic treatment of diseases of the eye. . . . [Minneapolis] : Pub. by the Author, 1899. 51p. DLC **90-3419**

HENRY, Frederick P[orteous] (1844-1919)
Digitalis in valvular disease of the heart. [Philadelphia, 1890.] 11p. DNLM **90-3420**

HENRY, Frederick P[orteous] (1844-1919)
Gastric ulcer: a clinical lecture delivered at the Woman's Hospital of Philadelphia. [New York: D. Appleton & Co., 1892.] 8p. DNLM **90-3421**

HENRY, Frederick P[orteous] (1844-1919)
Remarks on the pathology of the blood. [Philadelphia, 1893.] 11p. DNLM **90-3422**

HENRY, Frederick P[orteous] (1844-1919)
Clinical report of two cases of Raynaud's disease. Philadelphia, 1894. 11p. DNLM **90-3423**

HENRY, Frederick P[orteous] (1844-1919)
Remarks on chlorosis and its treatment. [Philadelphia], 1895. 8p. DNLM **90-3424**

HENRY, Frederick P[orteous] (1844-1919)
Report of a case of indigenous parasitic chyluria with filaria nocturna in the blood. Philadelphia, 1896. 20p. DNLM **90-3425**

HENRY, Frederick P[orteous] (1844-1919)
Treatment of rheumatism with the salicyl compounds. An historical note. Philadelphia, 1896. 3p. DNLM **90-3426**

HENRY, Frederick P[orteous] (1844-1919)
Standard history of the medical profession of Philadelphia. Chicago: Goodspeed Bros., 1897. 544p. ICU; NNNAM; PPC; PU **90-3427**

HENRY, Frederick P[orteous] (1844-1919)
Women in medicine. Philadelphia, 1897. 13p. DNLM **90-3428**

HENRY, Frederick P[orteous] (1844-1919)
A case of mitral stenosis, with fever (non-malarial) of relapsing type. Philadelphia, 1899. 4p. DNLM **90-3429**

HENRY, Frederick P[orteous] (1844-1919)
Extensive defect in the septum atriorum cordis, and malposition of the kidneys without symptoms or signs of heart disease. Philadelphia, 1899. 4p. 1 plate. DNLM **90-3430**

HENRY, John Norman (*b.* 1874)
A case of pure psychical epilepsy. New York, 1899. 7p. DNLM **90-3431**

HENRY, J. T.
A case of extra-uterine pregnancy. New York, 1896. 2p. DNLM **90-3432**

HENRY, M[orris] H[enry] (1835-1895)
Medical library of. . . . [New York, 1893.] 49p. DNLM; NNNAM **90-3433**

HENRY PHARMACAL COMPANY. LOUISVILLE
General and practical considerations of the pathology and therapy of gout and rheumatism. Louisville, Ky.: Henry Pharmacal Co., 1897. 16p. DNLM **90-3434**

HENRY, W[alter] O.
Indications for laparotomy. New York, 1895. 6p. DNLM **90-3435**

HENSHAW, George B.
The X-Ray with the new Holtz machine; some of its applications in medicine and surgery. Boston, 1897. 14p. skiagraphs. MBM **90-3436**

HERB, Ferdinand (*b.* 1866)
Female diseases, their prevention and cure. A popular scientific treatise of all diseases peculiar to women, with full directions for self-treatment. . . . Superior, Wisc.: Herb-Mussgang Publishing Co., 1896. 286p. DLC **90-3437**

HERDMAN, William James (1848-1896)
A laboratory manual of electrotherapeutics, by William James Herdman . . . and Frank W. Nagler. . . . Ann Arbor, Mich.: G. Wahr, [1898]. 163p. DLC **90-3438**

HERING, Constantin (1800-1880)
Condensed materia medica . . . rev., enl. and improved by E. A. Farrington. . . . 4th ed. Philadelphia: Boericke & Tafel, 1894. 968p. DLC; NNNAM; PPC; PPHa **90-3439**

HERING, Constantin (1800-1880)
A repertory of Hering's guiding symptoms of our materia medica, by Calvin B. Knerr, M.D. Philadelphia: F. A. Davis Co., for the estate of C. Hering, 1896. 1232p. DLC: PPC; PPHa; PU **90-3440**

HERMAN, G[eorge] Ernest (1849-1914)
First lines of midwifery; a guide to attendance on natural labor for medical students and midwives. Philadelphia: Lea Bros. & Co., [1891]. 191p. DNLM; NNNAM; OCIM; PPC **90-3441**

HERMAN, G[eorge] Ernest (1849-1914)
Difficult labor; a guide to its management for students and practitioners. New York: William Wood & Co., 1894. 443p. DNLM; MBM; PPC; PU **90-3442**

HERMAN, G[eorge] Ernest (1849-1914)
Diseases of women; a clinical guide to their diagnosis and treatment. New York: William Wood & Co., 1898. 886p. DNLM; OCIM; PPC; PU **90-3443**

HERMANN, Ludimar (1838-1914)
Experimental pharmacology. . . . Transl. by Robert Meade Smith. Philadelphia: Lea Bros. & Co., 1890 [1883]. 199p. DLC; IEN-M; MBM; PU **90-3444**

HEROLD, Justin (1861-1942)
Congenital induration or tumor of the sterno-mastoid. [Philadelphia, 1893.] 4p. DNLM **90-3445**

HEROLD, Justin (1861-1942)
A manual of legal medicine. For the use of practitioners and students of medicine and law. Philadelphia: J. B. Lippincott Co., 1898. 678p. CtY-M; DNLM; MBM; NNNAM **90-3446**

HEROLD, Justin (1861-1942)
Signs and tests of death. New Orleans, 1899. 50p. DNLM **90-3447**

HERRICK, A[lfred] B[irch]
A rare anomaly of the arch of the aorta, with an additional muscle in the neck. Baltimore, 1897. 5p. DNLM **90-3448**

HERRICK, C[larence] L[uther] (1858-1904)
Report upon the pathology of a case of general paralysis. [Granville, O., 1893.] 24p. 5 col. plates. DNLM **90-3449**

HERRICK, Clinton B. (*b.* 1859)
Rupture of the urethra in the male. [Philadelphia: Lea Bros. & Co., 1893.] 11p. DNLM **90-3450**

HERRICK, Clinton B. (*b.* 1859)
Railway surgery. A handbook of the management of injuries. New York: William Wood & Co., 1899. 265p. 1 plate. DNLM; NNNAM **90-3451**

HERRICK, James B[ryan] (1861-1954)
Diuretin. Chicago, 1893. 16p. DNLM **90-3452**

HERRICK, James B[ryan] (1861-1954)
Observations based on an experience with nearly one thousand cases of typhoid fever. Chicago, 1893. 16p. DNLM **90-3453**

HERRICK, James B[ryan] (1861-1954)
Report of seven cases of rupture of the urinary bladder, with observations on diagnosis. Philadelphia, 1893. 15p. DNLM **90-3454**

HERRICK, James B[ryan] (1861-1954)
A handbook of medical diagnosis for students. Philadelphia: Lea Bros. & Co., 1895. 432p. 2 plates. DNLM; NNNAM; PPC; PU **90-3455**

HERRICK, James B[ryan] (1861-1954)
On the importance of physical signs other than murmur in the diagnosis of valvular diseases of the heart. Detroit: G. S. Davis, 1896. 6p. DNLM **90-3456**

HERRICK, James B[ryan] (1861-1954)
Nervous shock and diseases of the nervous system as a cause of pernicious anemia. Chicago, 1896. 12p. DNLM **90-3457**

HERRICK, James B[ryan] (1861-1954)
Polymyositis acuta, with report of a case presumably of syphilitic origin (myositis syphilitica). Philadelphia, 1896. 17p. DNLM **90-3458**

HERRICK, James B[ryan] (1861-1954)
Report of a case of typhoid fever complicated by extrauterine pregnancy. New York, 1896. 3p. DNLM **90-3459**

HERRICK, James B[ryan] (1861-1954)
Thyroid therapy. Detroit: G. S. Davis, 1896. 7p. DNLM **90-3460**

HERRICK, S[tephen] S[olon] (1833-1906)
The plague four hundred years ago and now. [San Francisco, 1894.] 12p. DNLM **90-3461**

HERRICK, S[tephen] S[olon] (1833-1906)
The sanitary control of tuberculosis. San Francisco. A. J. Johnston, 1894. 8p. DNLM **90-3462**

HERROLD, Maude McKinley
Woman and disease. A collection of facts for women. By approved authorities. . . . Kansas City, Mo.: Published by the Author, 1896. 324p. plates. DLC; DNLM; OCIM **90-3463**

HERSHEY, E[dgar] P.
The prophylaxis of scarlet fever. Philadelphia, 1893. 4p. DNLM **90-3464**

HERSHEY, E[dgar] P.
The treatment of phthisis. New York, 1893. 12p. DNLM **90-3465**

HERSHEY, E[dgar] P.
The treatment of chronic enteritis. Denver, 1898. 4 l. DNLM **90-3466**

HERSMAN, C. C.
The relation between uterine disturbances and some of the insanities. Toledo, 1893. 8p. DNLM **90-3467**

HERTER, Christian A[rchibald] (1865-1910)
Clinical and pathological observations on cases of injury of the cervical spinal cord. [New York, 1891.] 21p. DNLM; NNNAM **90-3468**

HERTER, Christian A[rchibald] (1865-1910)
The diagnosis of diseases of the nervous system; a manual for students and practitioners. . . . New York, London: G. P. Putnam's Sons, 1892. 628p. DLC; DNLM; NNNAM; PPC **90-3469**

HERTER, Christian A[rchibald] (1865-1910) and E. E. SMITH
Observations on the excretion of uric acid in health and disease. [New York: D. Appleton & Co., 1892.] 38p. DNLM; NNNAM **90-3470**

HERTER, Christian A[rchibald] (1865-1910) and E. E. SMITH
Researches upon the aetiology of idiopathic epilepsy. A preliminary communication. [New York: D. Appleton & Co., 1892.] 48p. DNLM; NNNAM **90-3471**

HERTER, Christian A[rchibald] (1865-1910)
Some practical points regarding the excessive excretion of uric acid. New York, 1893. 21p. DNLM **90-3472**

HERTER, Christian A[rchibald] (1865-1910)
An experimental study of the toxic properties of indol. New York, 1898. 26p. 1 table. DNLM **90-3473**

HERZOG, Maximilian (1858-1918)
Cough of nasal origin, with report of a case. Philadelphia, 1893. 8p. DNLM **90-3474**

HERZOG, Maximilian (1858-1918)
Study of an early placenta in situ obtained from the living. New York, 1898. 20p. DNLM **90-3475**

HERZOG, Maximilian (1858-1918)
Superfetation in the human race. Chicago, [1898]. 22p. DNLM **90-3476**

HERZOG, Maximilian (1858-1918)
A case of lymphangioma cysticum. Chicago, 1899. 5p. DNLM **90-3477**

HERZOG, Maximilian (1858-1918)
A case of oestrus hominis. New York, 1899. 3p. DNLM **90-3478**

HERZOG, Maximilian (1858-1918)
A case of Paget's disease (malignant papillary dermatitis). Detroit, 1899. 9p. DNLM **90-3479**

HERZOG, Maximilian (1858-1918)
Lymphosarcoma of the mesentery. Chicago, 1899. 11p. DNLM **90-3480**

HERZOG, Maximilian (1858-1918)
Remarks on the histopathology of syphilis. Chicago, 1899. 4p. DNLM **90-3481**

HESSLER, Robert (*b.* 1867)
Norway itch (scabies Norvegia, H.). Report of a case. Philadelphia, 1893. 4p. DNLM **90-3482**

HESSLER, Robert (*b.* 1867)
Thyroid medication. A clinical report of a case. Indianapolis, 1896. 5p. DNLM **90-3483**

HESSLER, Robert (*b.* 1867)
Epilepsy and erysipelas. Chicago, 1898. 8p. DNLM **90-3484**

HESSLER, Robert (*b.* 1867)
Notes on thyroid medication from experience in the Northern Indiana Hospital for the Insane. Indianapolis, 1898. 3p. DNLM **90-3485**

HEWES, Henry F[ox] (*b.* 1867)
The chemical analysis of the gastric contents. I. Method of analysis for use in clinical work. II. Record of the analyses of the gastric contents of fifty healthy individuals. Boston: Damrell & Upham, 1897. 43p. DNLM; MBM **90-3486**

HEWES, Henry F[ox] (*b.* 1867)
On the classification of the leucocytes for clinical work. Boston, 1898. 9p. DNLM **90-3487**

HEWES, Henry F[ox] (*b.* 1867)
The examination of stained specimens of blood in its application to clinical work. Boston: Damrell & Upham, 1899. 28p. DNLM **90-3488**

HEWITT, Frederic W[illiam] (1857-1916)
The administration of nitrous oxide and oxygen for dental operations. Philadelphia, 1897. 108p. DNLM; MdU-D; PPC **90-3489**

HEWITT, G[eorge] A.
Glyco-thymoline (Kress) in nasal catarrh. Philadelphia, 1896. 1 l. DNLM **90-3490**

HEWLETT, Richard T[anner] (1856-1913)
A manual of bacteriology, clinical and applied; with an appendix on bacterial remedies, etc. Philadelphia: P. Blakiston, Son & Co., 1898. 439p. DNLM; NNNAM; PPC; PU **90-3491**

HEYDENFELDT, S[olomon], Jr.
The unison of the conscious forces. To the medical profession. Electro-magnetism; an outline of the secret of the Buddhists; subjectiveness, theosophy, spiritualism, eavesdropping, espionage; the doctrine of secrets, secret or cystic punishment. San Francisco: W. M. Hinton & Co., 1890. 15p. DNLM **90-3492**

HEYDENFELDT, S[olomon], Jr.
The unison of the conscious forces (continued). To the medical profession. Electromagnetism. The condition of being incysted; describing unfamiliar localities; telepsychological action; thought transference; mind reading; muscle reading, atmospheric telegraphing, etc.; phonomania; visualizing; transmission by sight; dreams. San Francisco: W. M. Hinton & Co., 1890. 12p. DNLM **90-3493**

HEYDENFELDT, S[olomon], Jr.
The unison of the conscious force. To the medical profession. Electro-magnetizing and hypnotism. Outline of the secret of the Buddhists. The doctrine of secrets. The augmentation of sound. [New York: J. J. Little & Co.], 1891. 105p. DNLM **90-3494**

HEYSINGER, Isaac W[inter] (1842-1917)
The scientific basis of medicine. Philadelphia: Boericke & Tafel, 1897. 122p. DNLM; PPHa **90-3495**

HIBBARD, Eugenie (*d.* 1946)
Diet for the sick, contributed by Miss E. Hibbard . . . and Mrs. Emma Drant. . . . To which have been added complete diet tables for various diseases and conditions. . . . Detroit, Mich.: The Illustrated Medical Journal Co., 1893. 81p. DLC **90-3496**

HIBBARD, Eugenie (*d.* 1946) and Emma DRANT
Diet for the sick. To which have been added diet tables for various diseases and conditions, as given by the highest authorities. 2nd ed. Detroit, [1897]. 103p. DNLM **90-3497**

HIBBS, Russell A[ubra] (*b.* 1869)
The treatment of abscess in connection with tuberculous joint disease. New York, 1897. 13p. DNLM **90-3498**

HIBBS, Russell A[ubra] (*b.* 1869)
The relation of suppuration to shortening of the limbs in tuberculous diseases of the hip joint; a study of 106 cases. New York, 1898. 9p. 1 table. DNLM
90-3499

HIBBS, Russell A[ubra] (*b.* 1869)
A study of shortening of the tibia and femur in fifty cases of tuberculous disease of the hip joint. New York, 1899. 12p. DNLM **90-3500**

HILDRETH, John L[ewis] (*b.* 1838)
The nurse's work from the point of view of a general practitioner. New York, 1895. 7p. DNLM
90-3501

HILDRETH, John L[ewis] (*b.* 1838)
The public care of the insane in Massachusetts. Cambridge, 1897. 43p. DNLM **90-3502**

HILL, Hibbert Winslow (*b.* 1871)
On the regulation requiring two consecutive negative cultures for the release of diphtheria cases. Boston, 1898. 7p. DNLM
90-3503

HILL, Hibbert Winslow (*b.* 1871)
A method of preparing test objects for disinfection experiments. Columbus, O., 1899. 4p. DNLM
90-3504

HILL, Hibbert Winslow (*b.* 1871)
A modification of the fermentation tube for bacteriological work. Boston, 1899. 2p. 1 plate. DNLM
90-3505

HILL, Hibbert Winslow (*b.* 1871)
Branching forms of bacillus diphtheriae. Boston, 1899. 7p. 1 plate. DNLM **90-3506**

HILL, Richard S.
Apioline in amenorrhoea and dysmenorrhoea. Richmond, 1891. 8p. DNLM **90-3507**

HILLMANTEL, Joseph L. (1863?-1899)
A case of distoma hematobium. Chicago: McClure Print. Co., 1893. 4p. DNLM **90-3508**

HILLSMAN, Blanton L. (1872-1935)
Notes on principles of surgery . . . from lectures by Stuart McGuire. Richmond, Va.: James E. Goode Printing Co., 1897. 224p. PPC; PU; ViRA **90-3509**

HINGSTON, William H[ales] (1829-1907)
Stone in the bladder; choice of operation. Philadelphia, 1894. 5p. DNLM **90-3510**

HINKEL, Frank Whitehill
A review of the relations between the state and the medical profession in New York, [Buffalo, 1894.] 11p. DNLM
90-3511

HINKEL, Frank Whitehill
Report of a death following immediately an operation for nasopharyngeal adenoids under chloroform, with remarks on chloroform anaesthesia in this operation. New York, 1898. 12p. DNLM **90-3512**

HINRICHSEN, Otto (*b.* 1870)
Statistics as to the frequency of simple acute mania with respect to its periodical forms. St. Louis, 1899. 17p. DNLM
90-3513

HINSDALE, Guy (*b.* 1858)
Acromegaly. [Boylston prize essay, 1898.] Detroit: W. M. Warren, 1898. 88p. DNLM **90-3514**

HINSDALE, Guy (*b.* 1858) and Howard S. ANDERS
A visit to the Loomis Sanitarium for Consumptives. Philadelphia, 1899. 6p. DNLM **90-3515**

HIRSCH, José L.
A report of four cases of epidemic cerebro-spinal meningitis, with special reference to the value of lumbar puncture as a means of diagnosis. New York, 1899. 13p. DNLM
90-3516

HIRSCH, William
Transitory disturbances of consciousness in their medico-legal aspects. New York, 1897. 24p. DNLM
90-3517

HIRSCH, William
A study of delirium. New York, 1899. 22p. DNLM
90-3518

HIRSCHFELDER, J. O.
A pocket manual of percussion and auscultation for physicians and students. Transl. from the 2nd German ed. by . . . . San Francisco: A. L. Bancroft & Co., 1890 [1873, *vel subseq.*] 52p. DLC **90-3519**

HIRST, Barton Cooke (1861-1935)
Human monstrosities. By Barton Cooke Hirst . . . and George A. Piersol. . . . Philadelphia: Lea Bros. & Co., 1891-1893. 4 v. plates. DLC: DNLM; PPC; PU **90-3520**

HIRST, Barton Cooke (1861-1935)
Large vaginal enterocele complicating pregnancy and obstructing labor. Philadelphia, 1891. 5p. DNLM
90-3521

HIRST, Barton Cooke (1861-1935)
The ultimate results of a pubeotomy; a ruptured uterus; injury to the lumbo-sacral plexus in labor; multiple abscesses in the abdominal cavity. [Philadelphia: Lea Bros. & Co., 1892.] 6p. DNLM **90-3522**

HIRST, Barton Cooke (1861-1935)
Symphysiotomy, with the report of an operation. [Philadelphia: Lea Bros. & Co., 1892.] 8p. DNLM
90-3523

HIRST, Barton Cooke (1861-1935)
Long-continued hemorrhage in the latter half of pregnancy, due to detachment of a normally situated placenta, and accompanied by septic intoxication; with a report of two cases. Philadelphia, 1893. 4p. DNLM **90-3524**

HIRST, Barton Cooke (1861-1935)
The lowest limit of pelvic contraction admitting of symphysiotomy. [Philadelphia: Lea Bros. & Co., 1893.] 2p. DNLM
90-3525

HIRST, Barton Cooke (1861-1935)
Symphysiotomy. [Philadelphia: Lea Bros. & Co., 1893.] 10p. DNLM **90-3526**

HIRST, Barton Cooke (1861-1935)
Suppurative metritis; ulcerative endometritis and metritis; double pyosalpinx and an ovarian abscess; embolic pneumonia following labor; hysterectomy; recovery. Philadelphia, 1894. 4p. DNLM **90-3527**

HIRST, Barton Cooke (1861-1935)
Obstetric memoranda. Philadelphia, 1894. 4p. DNLM **90-3528**

HIRST, Barton Cooke (1861-1935)
The influence of the habitual inclination of the pelvis in the erect posture upon the shape and size of the pelvic canal. Philadelphia, 1894. 3p. DNLM **90-3529**

HIRST, Barton Cooke (1861-1935)
Two Caesarean sections and three symphysiotomies. A year's work in the surgical treatment of insuperably obstructed labor. Philadelphia, 1894. 4p. 4 plates. DNLM **90-3530**

HIRST, Barton Cooke (1861-1935)
Dermoid cysts and pregnancy. New York, 1895. 1 l. DNLM **90-3531**

HIRST, Barton Cooke (1861-1935)
Clinical notes. New York, 1895. 10p. DNLM **90-3532**

HIRST, Barton Cooke (1861-1935)
A specimen of defective development of the abdominal wall and eventration, cyllosoma. Presented to the Wistar Museum, by Dr. I. Leopold. [Philadelphia, 1895.] 1 l. 2 plates. DNLM **90-3533**

HIRST, Barton Cooke (1861-1935)
Clinical notes. I. Large myoma of the ovarian ligament. II. Coincident ovarian and parovarian cysts. III. Report of a Caesarean section and of two symphysiotomies. New York, 1895. 8p. DNLM **90-3534**

HIRST, Barton Cooke (1861-1935)
A remarkable case of acquired atresia of the vagina. New York: William Wood & Co., 1895. 2p. DNLM **90-3535**

HIRST, Barton Cooke (1861-1935)
Colpocleisis. New York: William Wood & Co., 1896. 2p. DNLM **90-3536**

HIRST, Barton Cooke (1861-1935)
Clinical notes. New York, 1897. 5p. DNLM **90-3537**

HIRST, Barton Cooke (1861-1935)
A text-book of obstetrics. . . . With 653 illustrations. Philadelphia: W. B. Saunders, 1898. 846p. col. plates. DLC; DNLM; NNNAM; PU **90-3538**

HIRST, Barton Cooke (1861-1935)
The history of pain and the menstrual history of extrauterine pregnancy. New York, 1898. 7p. DNLM **90-3539**

HIRST, Barton Cooke (1861-1935)
The comparative value of celiohysterotomy and celiohysterectomy in cases requiring a Caesarean section. New York, 1898. 8p. DNLM **90-3540**

HIRT, Ludwig (1844-1907)
The diseases of the nervous system. A text-book for physicians and students. Transl. with permission of the author by August Hoch. Assisted by Frank R. Smith. With an introduction by William Osler. New York: D. Appleton & Co., 1899. 715p. NNNAM; OCIM; PPC; PU **90-3541**

HODENPYL, Eugene (1863-1910)
Actinomycosis of the lung, being the Joseph Mather Smith prize essay for 1890. New York, 1890. 12p. 4 plates. DNLM **90-3542**

HODENPYL, Eugene (1863-1910)
The anatomy and physiology of the faucial tonsils with reference to the absorption of infectious material. Philadelphia, 1891. 18p. DNLM **90-3543**

HODENPYL, Eugene (1863-1910)
On the aetiology of appendicitis. New York: D. Appleton & Co., 1893. 28p. DNLM **90-3544**

HODENPYL, Eugene (1863-1910)
On the occurrence of typhoid fever without characteristic lesions of the small intestine. Read at the meeting of the British Medical Association held at Montreal, September, 1897. New York: Knickerbocker Press, 1897. 8p. DNLM **90-3545**

HODENPYL, Eugene (1863-1910)
A case of apparent absence of the spleen, with general compensatory lymphatic hyperplasia. New York, 1898. 8p. DNLM **90-3546**

HODENPYL, Eugene (1863-1910)
A modification of Cullen's method of preparing fresh sections for microscopic work. New York, 1898. 2 l. DNLM **90-3547**

HODGDON, Alexander L.
Heredity; its relationship to mental disorders. [New York, 1893.] 7p. DNLM **90-3548**

HODGDON, Alexander L.
Some reasons for the performance of circumcision on all male infants. [New York, 1893.] 7p. DNLM **90-3549**

HODGDON, Alexander L.
Rheumatic conjunctivitis. [Baltimore, 1894.] 1 l. DNLM **90-3550**

HODGDON, Alexander L.
Alcoholic insanity and excess, with a reference to the opium habit. Baltimore, 1897. 10p. DNLM **90-3551**

HODGDON, Alexander L.
Circumcision, with a description of a pair of circumcision forceps. Baltimore, 1897. 8p. DNLM **90-3552**

HODGDON, Alexander L.
Post-febrile insanity. Baltimore, 1897. 6p. DNLM **90-3553**

HODGDON, Alexander L.
Preputial reflex epileptiform convulsions, with report of a case. St. Louis, 1897. 3p. DNLM **90-3554**

HODGDON, Alexander L.
A glance at psychiatry and neurology. Baltimore, 1898. 12p. DNLM **90-3555**

HODGDON, Alexander L.
The technique of radiography. Baltimore, 1899. 1 l. DNLM **90-3556**

HODGE, C[lifton] F[remont] (*b.* 1859)
The vivisection question. [New York, 1896.] 26p. DNLM **90-3557**

HODGE, C[lifton] F[remont] (*b.* 1859)
Experiments on the physiology of alcohol, made under the auspices of the Committee of Fifty. New York, 1897. 26p. DNLM **90-3558**

HODGEN, Joseph Dupuy
Practical dental metallurgy; a text and reference book for students and practitioners of dentistry. . . . San Francisco: The Hicks-Judd Co., 1896. 314p. DLC **90-3559**

HODGEN, Joseph Dupuy
Practical dental metallurgy. A text- and reference-book for students and practitioners of dentistry. . . . 2nd ed., completely rev., rearranged, and enl. San Francisco: The Hicks-Judd Co., 1897. 349p. DLC **90-3560**

HODGES, Fred Jenner
Some unusual fractures of the leg. [*Also*:] An aid to the diagnosis of surgical affections of the urinary bladder. [New York, 1891.] 11p. DNLM **90-3561**

HODGES, Fred Jenner
Reparative surgery of the peripheral nerves. [Philadelphia: Lea Bros. & Co., 1892.] 22p. DNLM **90-3562**

HODGES, Richard Manning (1827-1896)
A narrative of events connected with the introduction of sulphuric ether into surgical use. Boston: Little, Brown & Co., 1891. 159p. DLC; DNLM; MBM; MH **90-3563**

HODSON, Jane, ed.
How to become a trained nurse: a manual of information in detail. With a complete list of the various training schools for nurses in the United States and Canada. . . . New York: W. Abbatt, 1898. 265p. plates. DLC; DNLM; NNNAM **90-3564**

HOFF, John Van Rensselaer (1848-1920)
Outlines of sanitary organization of some of the great armies of the world. Detroit, 1895. 60p. DNLM **90-3565**

HOFF, John Van Rensselaer (1848-1920)
What is the most practicable plan of sanitary organization for the active service in the United States Army? Detroit, 1896. 12p. DNLM **90-3566**

HOFFA, Albert J. (1859-1907)
Scheme of the antiseptic method of wound treatment. . . . Transl. from the German, with additions, by special permission of the author, by Aug. Schachner. Louisville, Ky.: Bradley & Gilbert Co., 1890. 1 fold. sheet. DLC **90-3567**

HOFFMAN, Charles P.
A practical guide in electro-therapeutics, and special treatments given with the Hoffman-Van Houten electro-therapeutic cabinet bath, by Chas. P. Hoffman, M.D., and W. B. Van Houten. . . . New York: [The Mershon Co. Press, Rahway, N.J.], 1891. 64p. DLC; NNNAM **90-3568**

HOFFMAN, Charles S.
Gonorrhea of the vesiculae seminales. [Philadelphia, 1892.] 4p. DNLM **90-3569**

HOFFMANN, Philip
Original methods for detecting and measuring abduction and adduction of the thigh. St. Louis, 1897. 16p. DNLM **90-3570**

HOFMANN, E. Von (1837-1897)
Atlas of legal medicine. Authorized transl. from the German. Edited by Frederick Peterson, assisted by Aloysius O. J. Kelly. Philadelphia: W. B. Saunders, 1898. NNNAM; PPC; PPJ; PU [193 photographic figures and 56 chromolithographic plates with accompanying descriptive text]. **90-3571**

HOGAN, Louise E. (1855-1929)
How to feed children; a manual for mothers, nurses, and physicians. . . . Philadelphia: J. B. Lippincott Co., 1896. 236p. plates. DLC; MBM; NNNAM; PPC **90-3572**

HOGAN, Louise E. (1855-1929)
How to feed children; a manual for mothers, nurses, and physicians. . . . 2nd ed. Philadelphia: J. B. Lippincott Co., 1898. 236p. MB; PPC; PP **90-3573**

HOGAN, Louise E. (1855-1929)
How to feed children; a manual for mothers, nurses, and physicians. . . . 3rd ed. Philadelphia: J. B. Lippincott Co., 1899. 236p. plates. DLC; NNNAM; OCIM; PPC **90-3574**

HOGE, M. D., Jr.
Outlines of histology. Richmond: J. W. Ferguson & Sons, 1897. 82p. DNLM **90-3575**

HOISHOLT, A[ndrew] W[illiam] (*b.* 1858)
Some statistical observations on the etiology and symptomatology of dementia paralytica. Sacramento, Cal., 1897. 16p. DNLM **90-3576**

HOISHOLT, A[ndrew] W[illiam] (*b.* 1858)
Two cases of spontaneous rupture of the heart, with demonstrations of specimens. Sacramento, 1899. 4 l. DNLM **90-3577**

HOISHOLT, A[ndrew] W[illiam] (*b.* 1858)
A case of large solitary tubercles of the heart. San Francisco, [1899]. 6p. 1 plate. DNLM **90-3578**

HOLBROOK, M[artin] L[uther] (1831-1902)
The hygienic treatment of consumption. In three parts. Pt. I. Nature and causes of the disease. Pt. II. Prevention and treatment in its earlier stages. Pt. III. Treatment in more advanced stages. New York: M. L. Holbrook & Co., [1891]. 219p. DNLM; NNNAM **90-3579**

HOLBROOK, M[artin] L[uther] (1831-1902)
Liver complaint, nervous dyspepsia, and headache: their causes, prevention, and cure. 3rd ed. New York: M. L. Holbrook & Co., 1894. 141p. DNLM; NNNAM **90-3580**

HOLBROOK, M[artin] L[uther] (1831-1902)
Physical, intellectual, and moral advantages of chastity. New York & London: M. L. Holbrook & Co., & L. N. Fowler & Co., [1894]. 120p. DNLM; NNNAM
90-3581

HOLBROOK, M[artin] L[uther] (1831-1902)
Stirpiculture; or, the improvement of offspring through wiser generation. New York: M. L. Holbrook & Co., 1897. 192p. DNLM; NNNAM **90-3582**

HOLCOMBE, William Henry (1825-1893)
On the treatment, diet, and nursing of yellow fever. (For popular use.). . . . New York, Philadelphia, [etc.]: Boericke & Tafel, [189-?]. 19p. DLC; NNNAM
90-3583

HOLCOMBE, William Henry (1825-1893)
The truth about homoeopathy; a posthumous manuscript; also a sketch of the life of Dr. Holcombe. Philadelphia: Boericke & Tafel, 1894. 43p. DLC; DNLM; PPHa
90-3584

HOLDEN, Frederick C.
Note on the value of maceration in ether and ether solution of corrosive sublimate for the sterilization of catgut. [New York, 1894.] 6p. DNLM **90-3585**

HOLDEN, Luther (1815-1905)
Holden's Manual of the dissection of the human body; ed. by John Langton. . . . 6th ed. Rev. by A. Hewson. . . . Philadelphia: P. Blakiston, Son & Co., 1894 [1893]. 803p. 311 illustrations. DLC; DNLM; NNNAM; PPC
90-3586

HOLDEN, Ward A[ndrews] (*b.* 1866)
An outline of the embryology of the eye, with illustrations from original pen-drawings by the author. The Cartwright prize essay for 1893. New York & London: G. P. Putnam's Sons, 1893. 69p. 12 plates. DNLM; NNNAM
90-3587

HOLLAND, James William (1849-1922)
The urine, the common poisons, and the milk. Memoranda, chemical and microscopical, for laboratory use. . . . 4th ed., rev. and enl. Philadelphia: P. Blakiston, Son & Co., 1891. 94p. DLC; PPC; PU **90-3588**

HOLLAND, James William (1849-1922)
The urine and clinical chemistry of the gastric contents, the common poisons, and the milk. . . . Illustrated. 5th ed., rev. and enl. Philadelphia: P. Blakiston, Son & Co., 1895. 115p. DLC; PPC; PU **90-3589**

HOLLAND, James William (1849-1922)
The urine and clinical chemistry of the gastric contents, the common poisons, and milk. . . . 6th ed., rev. and enl. Philadelphia: P. Blakiston's Son & Co., 1899. 124p. DLC; PPC; PPJ; PU **90-3590**

HOLLAND, Mary A.
Our army nurses. Interesting sketches, addresses, and photographs of nearly one hundred of the noble women who served in hospitals and on battlefields during our civil war. . . . Boston, Mass.: B. Wilkins & Co., 1895. 548p. DLC; MB; MH; NN
90-3591

HOLLICK, Frederick (*b.* 1818)
The matron's manual of midwifery and the diseases of woman during pregnancy and in child bed. . . . New and improved ed. . . . New York: Excelsior Publishing House, [1890]. 448p. col. plates. DLC; NNNAM **90-3592**

HOLLOPETER, William Clarence (1855-1927)
Hay-fever and its successful treatment. . . . Philadelphia: P. Blakiston's Son & Co., 1898. 137p. DLC; PPC
90-3593

HOLLOPETER, William Clarence (1855-1927)
Hay-fever and its successful treatment. . . . 2nd ed., rev. and enl. Philadelphia: P. Blakiston's Son & Co., 1899. 151p. DLC; PPC **90-3594**

HOLMES, A. Mansfield
A case of dislocation of the fourth cervical vertebra without fracture. [Philadelphia, 1893.] 15p. DNLM
90-3595

HOLMES, A. Mansfield
The diagnosis of tuberculosis from the morphology of the blood: an original research, with report of cases. New York, 1896. 16p. DNLM **90-3596**

HOLMES, A. Mansfield
A study of the blood in tuberculosis. Chicago, 1897. 20p. DNLM **90-3597**

HOLMES, A. Mansfield
The technique of blood study and experiments in the physiological chemistry of leucocytes. A study in cell tissues and their significance in tuberculosis. Denver: Smith-Brooks Pr. Co., 1897. 16p. DNLM **90-3598**

HOLMES, A. Mansfield
A clinical study of tuberculous cases treated with the new antiphthisis serum T. R. (formula of Fish). Chicago, 1898. 19p. DNLM **90-3599**

HOLMES, Bayard Taylor (1852-1924)
The treatment of empyema. [Chicago, 1890.] 33p. DNLM
90-3600

HOLMES, Bayard Taylor (1852-1924)
Discussion of Dr. Vaughan's paper: [The kind and amount of laboratory work which should be required in our medical schools]. Chicago, 1892. 23p. DNLM
90-3601

HOLMES, Bayard Taylor (1852-1924)
The outlook for medicine. [New York, 1892.] 2 l. DNLM
90-3602

HOLMES, Bayard Taylor (1852-1924)
The forthcoming report of the Bureau of Education on professional education in the United States. Chicago, 1893. 19p. DNLM **90-3603**

HOLMES, Bayard Taylor (1852-1924)
Is it desirable and practicable in medical schools to teach methods of investigation in medical literature? [Philadelphia: Lea Bros. & Co., 1893.] 7p. DLC; DNLM
90-3604

HOLMES, Bayard Taylor (1852-1924)
The sources of the defective, dependent, and delinquent classes. [Easton, Pa., 1894.] 11p. DNLM **90-3605**

HOLMES, Bayard Taylor (1852-1924)
The medical library for the medical school or the small community. Easton, Pa., 1895. 55p. DLC; DNLM
90-3606

HOLMES, Bayard Taylor (1852-1924)
The seminar method in teaching surgery. Read before the American Academy of Medicine, Atlanta, May 4, 1896. . . . Chicago: American Medical Association Press, 1896. 4p. DLC **90-3607**

HOLMES, Bayard Taylor (1852-1924)
Surgery of the kidneys; being a study of a series of cases in which methods of diagnosis and treatment are illustrated. Chicago, 1899. 68p. 1 diag. DNLM
90-3608

HOLMES, Christian R[asmus] (1851-1920)
Extirpation of the lacrymal sac and gland. New York, 1899. 30p. DNLM; NNNAM **90-3609**

HOLMES, Edmund W[ales]
Outlines of anatomy; a guide to the methodical study of the human body in the dissecting room. Philadelphia: Avil Co., 1897. 183p. DNLM **90-3610**

HOLMES, Edmund W[ales]
The lateral route for the removal of cervical growths. Philadelphia, [1899]. 4p. DNLM **90-3611**

HOLMES, Oliver Wendell (1809-1894)
Lines on the presentation of his portrait to the Philadelphia College of Physicians, Saturday, April 30, 1892. [n. p., 1892.] 2 l. DNLM **90-3612**

HOLMES, Timothy (1825-1907)
Sir Benjamin Collins Brodie. . . . New York: Longmans, Green & Co., 1898. 255p. DLC; MB; MH; NN
90-3613

HOLSTEN, George D. (1857-1896)
Eruptions from iodide of potassium, with report of a case of dermatitis tuberosa from the iodide. [New York, 1892.] 19p. DNLM **90-3614**

HOLSTEN, George D. (1857-1896)
Acne. [Philadelphia: Lea Bros. & Co., 1893.] 14p. DNLM
90-3615

HOLSTEN, George D. (1857-1896)
Report of a case of dermatitis medicamentosa from iodoform, potassium iodide, and aristol. [Philadelphia, 1893.] 5p. DNLM
90-3616

[HOLT, Alfred F.] (1838-1890)
Catalogue of the medical library of the late Dr. . . . 1891. 8p. DNLM **90-3617**

HOLT, E[rastus] E[ugene] (*b.* 1849)
Otitis media suppurativa. Portland: S. Berry, 1890 [1878]. 15p. DNLM **90-3618**

HOLT, E[rastus] E[ugene] (*b.* 1849)
Orbital cellulitis. [Hartford, 1892.] 12p. DNLM
90-3619

HOLT, E[rastus] E[ugene] (*b.* 1849)
Removal of steel from the vitreous by the electro-magnet. [Hartford], 1893. 3p. DNLM **90-3620**

HOLT, Joseph (1839-1922)
An epitomized review of the principles and practice of maritime sanitation. New Orleans: L. Graham & Son, 1892. 93p. 1 plate. DNLM; LNT-M **90-3621**

HOLT, Joseph (1839-1922)
Pestilential foreign invasion, as a question of States' rights and the Constitution. The failure of the maritime States demands a common defense. An address delivered before the Tri-State Medical Society of Georgia, Alabama, and Tennessee, at Chattanooga, Oct. 26, 1892. New Orleans: L. Graham & Son, 1892. 35p. DNLM; LNT-M **90-3622**

HOLT, Joseph (1839-1922)
Quarantine control: State or National? the question. A speech delivered before the Chamber of Commerce and Industry of Louisiana, New Orleans, Jan. 11, 1893, and respectfully submitted to the honorable the Senate and House of Representatives of the United States in Congress assembled. New Orleans: L. Graham & Son, 1893. 21p. DNLM; LNT-M
90-3623

HOLT, Joseph (1839-1922)
The Charity Hospital and the alumni. Inaugural address. New Orleans: L. Graham & Son, 1895. 23p. 1 plate. DNLM; LNT-M
90-3624

HOLT, L[uther] Emmett (1855-1924)
A case of spina bifida with suppurative spinal meningitis and ependymitis, due to bacteria entering the wall of the sac. New York, 1890. 9p. 1 plate. DNLM
90-3625

HOLT, L[uther] Emmett (1855-1924)
The feeding of older infants and young children. [New York, 1890.] 19p. DNLM **90-3626**

HOLT, L[uther] Emmett (1855-1924)
Observations upon the capacity of the stomach in infancy. Philadelphia, 1890. 8p. DNLM **90-3627**

[HOLT, L[uther] Emmett] (1855-1924)
. . . Diet for young children. [New York: Babyhood Publishing Co., 1890.] 19p. DLC; NNNAM [Nursery health tracts, No. 2]
90-3628

HOLT, L[uther] Emmett (1855-1924)
The temperature in acute primary pneumonia of children. The diagnosis of acute broncho-pneumonia from bronchitis. [Philadelphia, 1891.] 22p. DNLM **90-3629**

HOLT, L[uther] Emmett (1855-1924)
The clinical examination of breast milk. New York: M. J. Rooney, 1893. 12p. DNLM **90-3630**

HOLT, L[uther] Emmett (1855-1924)
Three cases of acute pyelitis in infancy. [New York, 1894.] 16p. DNLM **90-3631**

HOLT, Luther] Emmett (1855-1924)
The care and feeding of children: a catechism for the use of mothers and children's nurses. . . . New York: D. Appleton & Co., 1894. 66p. DLC; NNNAM; PPC; PU
90-3632

HOLT, L[uther] Emmett (1855-1924) and C. A. HERTER
Rapid gliosis of the spinal cord, with a report of a case. Philadelphia, 1895. 15p. DNLM
90-3633

HOLT, L[uther] Emmett (1855-1924)
Artificial feeding. Extracts from: Diseases of infancy and childhood. New York: D. Appleton & Co., 1897. 8p. DNLM
90-3634

HOLT, L[uther] Emmett] (1855-1924)
The diseases of infancy and childhood, for the use of students and practitioners of medicine . . . with two hundred and four illustrations, including seven coloured plates. New York: D. Appleton & Co., 1897. 1117p. DLC; NNNAM; PPC; PU
90-3635

HOLT, L[uther] Emmett (1855-1924)
A report of five cases of abscess of the brain in infants, together with a summary of twenty-seven collected cases in infants and very young children. New York: E. B. Treat & Co., [1898]. 37p. DNLM **90-3636**

HOMAN, George (*b.* 1849)
Public health and the land question. [St. Louis, 1890.] 10p. DNLM **90-3637**

HOMAN, George (*b.* 1849)
The extension of the use of live steam to municipal and household disinfection. Concord: Republican Press Assoc., 1893. 6p. DNLM **90-3638**

HOMAN, George (*b.* 1849)
The fundamental conditions of public health in civilization. Concord, N.H.: Republican Press Assoc., 1893. 8p. DNLM
90-3639

HOMAN, George (*b.* 1849)
A contribution to the study of water-borne cholera. New York, 1895. 16p. DNLM **90-3640**

HOMAN, George (*b.* 1849)
The sanitary redemption of Havana: the need and the means. St. Louis, Mo., 1898. 16p. DNLM
90-3641

HOMANS, John (1836-1903)
A case of successful removal of a retroperitoneal fatty tumor. In the course of the operation a vein, supposed to be the left common iliac, torn and tied. [Philadelphia, 1891.] 4p. DNLM
90-3642

HOMANS, John (1836-1903)
The treatment of fibroid tumors of the uterus after the method of Dr. Apostoli. Boston, 1891. 38p. DNLM
90-3643

HOMANS, John (1836-1903) and George L. WALTON
A case of successful trephining for subdural haemorrhage produced by contre-coup. Boston: Damrell & Upham, 1891. 32p. DNLM **90-3644**

HOMANS, John (1836-1903)
An extraordinary case of twisting of the uterus as the pedicle of a large fibroid tumor of many years' existence. New York: William Wood & Co., 1892. 5p. DNLM
90-3645

HOMANS, John (1836-1903)
Fibroid tumors of the uterus. [Philadelphia, 1892.] 13p. DNLM **90-3646**

HOMANS, John (1836-1903)
Cases of extra-uterine pregnancy. [Boston, 1893.] 5p. DNLM
90-3647

HOMANS, John (1836-1903) and George HODGES
Addresses delivered at the annual meeting of the New England Cremation Society, January 15, 1895. Boston, Mass., 1895. 10p. DNLM **90-3648**

HOMANS, John (1836-1903)
The surgical treatment of fibroid tumors of the uterus. Boston, 1895. 12p. DNLM **90-3649**

HOMANS, John (1836-1903)
Recurrent gall-stones. Angioma of spleen. Excision of coecum. [n. p., 1897.] 8p. 3 plates. DNLM
90-3650

HOMANS, John (1836-1903)
Note book for cases of ovarian and other abdominal tumours. Adapted from the note books of Sir Spencer Wells and the Samaritan Hospital, London. Boston: Cupples, Upham & Co., [1897]. 23p. DNLM **90-3651**

[HOME MEDICINE COMPANY]
The home doctor. Compiled from the writings and practical experience of over one hundred famous physicians. . . . Mound City, Kan.: Republic Steam Printing House, 1895. 300p. DLC
90-3652

HOMOEOPATHIC HOSPITAL COLLEGE, CLEVELAND
Annual announcements for the sessions of 1854-1855 (5.); 1856-1857 (7.); 1858-1859 (9.); 1863-1864 (14.); 1864-1865 (15.); 1874-1875 (25.); 1876-1877 to 1893-1894 (27.-44.). Cleveland, 1852-1893. DNLM **90-3653**

HOMOEOPATHIC MEDICAL COLLEGE OF THE UNIVERSITY OF MICHIGAN, ANN ARBOR
Bulletin. Midwinter, 1897. 34p. Ann Arbor: Inland Press, 1897. 34p. DNLM **90-3654**

HOOD, Calvin Todd
A manual of electrotherapeutics. . . . Chicago: Gross & Delbridge Co., 1895. 181p. DLC; DNLM; OCIM
90-3655

HOOPER, Franklin Henry (1850-1892)
A case of tumor of the larynx, showing amyloid degeneration. New York: Trow, 1891. 8p. DNLM
90-3656

HOOPER, Franklin Henry (1850-1892)
Multiple papilloma of the larynx in young children, and its treatment. Philadelphia, 1891. 11p. DNLM
90-3657

HOOVER, Charles Franklin (1865-1927)
A clinical study of the pulse. Cleveland, 1897. 12p. DNLM
90-3658

HOOVER, Charles Franklin (1865-1927)
The diaphragm phenomenon, or Litten sign. Cleveland, 1897. 6p. DNLM **90-3659**

HOOVER, Charles Franklin (1865-1927)
Cardio-pulmonary murmurs. New York, 1898. 23p. DNLM
90-3660

HOPKINS, F[rederick] E.
The recurrence of lymphoid hypertrophy in the nasopharynx. [New York: D. Appleton & Co., 1895.] 16p. DNLM
90-3661

HOPKINS, F[rederick] E.
A case of adeno-carinoma of the nose. [New York, 1897.] 8p. DNLM **90-3662**

HOPKINS, F[rederick] E.
Recurrence of the tonsil after excision. New York, 1899. 12p. DNLM **90-3663**

HOPKINS, F[rederick] E.
A case of hysterical larynx. New York, 1899. 3p. DNLM
90-3664

HOPKINS, S[amuel] D.
A case of hysteria simulating organic disease of the brain. [St. Louis, 1897.] 8p. DNLM **90-3665**

HOPKINS, S[amuel] D.
Nervous disorders simulating peritonitis. [Denver, 1897.] 4p. DNLM **90-3666**

HOPKINS, S[amuel] D.
Respiratory paralysis from haemorrhage around the medulla. [Denver, 1897.] 4p. DNLM **90-3667**

HOPKINS, S[amuel] D.
Extradural spinal meningeal haemorrhage, with report of a case. New York, 1899. 5p. DNLM **90-3668**

HOPKINS, William Barton (*d.* 1904) and Charles E. PENROSE
On the organization and absorption of sterilized dead bone dowels. Chicago, 1890. 8p. DNLM **90-3669**

HOPKINS, William Barton (*d.* 1904)
Report of a case of detachment of the ligament of the patella; treatment by suture; recovery. [Philadelphia], 1893. 7p. DNLM **90-3670**

HOPKINS, William Barton (*d.* 1904)
A preliminary note on a new method of correcting inveterate talipes varus by the artificial production of Pott's fracture deformity. Philadelphia, 1895. 4p. DNLM
90-3671

HOPKINS, William Barton (*d.* 1904)
The roller bandage. With a chapter on surgical dressing. 4th ed. Philadelphia: J. B. Lippincott & Co., 1897. 130p. DNLM; PPC; PPJ **90-3672**

HORLBECK, Henry Buckingham (1839-1901)
American Public Health Association. October 26-29, 1897. Quarter centennial, Philadelphia. Address of Doctor Henry B. Horlbeck, President. [Concord? N.H.: The Rumford Press? 1897.] 26p. DLC **90-3673**

HORSLEY, J. Shelton (1870-1946)
Some remarks on amputation at the hip-joint, with report of a case by Wyeth's method. New York, 1895. 11p. DNLM
90-3674

HORSLEY, J. Shelton (1870-1946)
A new method of intestinal anastomosis. Some remarks on amputation at the hip-joint, with report of a case by Wyeth's method. Cocaine in surgery. Danbury, Conn., 1898. 24p. DNLM **90-3675**

HORSLEY, J. Shelton (1870-1946)
Reports of operations for the radical cure of three unusual cases of inguinal hernia. New York, 1899. 3p. DNLM
90-3676

HORSLEY, Victor [Alexander Hayden] (1857-1916)
The structure and functions of the brain and spinal cord. Being the Fullerian lectures for 1891. Philadelphia: P. Blakiston, Son & Co., 1892. 223p. DNLM; NNNAM; PPC
90-3677

HORWITZ, Orville (1859-1913)
. . . A compend of surgery. For students and physicians. Including minor surgery and a compelte section on bandaging. . . . 4th ed., rev. and enl., one hundred and thirty-six illustrations and eigty-four formulae. Philadelphia: P. Blakiston, Son & Co., 1890. 272p. DLC; DNLM; PPC; PPJ
90-3678

HORWITZ, Orville (1859-1913)
Reunion of a portion of an amputated finger. [Philadelphia, 1892.] 2p. DNLM **90-3679**

HORWITZ, Orville (1859-1913)
Spinal anaemia, due to syphilis. Detroit: G. S. Davis, 1892. 25p. DNLM **90-3680**

HORWITZ, Orville (1858-1913)
. . . A compend of surgery, for students and physicians. Including minor surgery and a complete section on bandaging. . . . 5th ed., rev. and enl. One hundred and sixty-seven illustrations and ninety-eight formulae. Philadelphia: P. Blakiston, Son & Co., 1893. 324p. DLC; NNNAM; PPC; PU
90-3681

HORWITZ, Orville (1859-1913)
A clinical investigation to determine the value of corrosive sublimate and the gray oil administered hypodermically in the treatment of syphilis. Detroit: G. S. Davis, 1894. 10p. DNLM
90-3682

HORWITZ, Orivlle (1859-1913)
Organic stricture of the urethra. Methods of treatment recommended, with indications for their employment. [Philadelphia, 1894.] 18p. DNLM **90-3683**

HORWITZ, Orville (1859-1913)
Complete extirpation of the penis for epithelial carcinoma. New York, 1896. 4p. DNLM **90-3684**

HORWITZ, Orville (1859-1913)
Hydrocele; its radical cure. New York, 1896. 8p. DNLM
80-3685

HORWITZ, Orville (1859-1913)
Ulcer of the rectum; stricture of the rectum due to syphilis. Philadelphia, 1898. 4p. DNLM **90-3686**

HOSPITAL formulary of the Department of Public Charities of the City of New York. 5th ed. New York, 1898. 95p. NNNAM; OCLloyd **90-3687**

THE HOT SPRINGS of Arkansas. An historical and legendary account of the famous health and pleasure resort. St. Louis, 1893. 33p. DNLM **90-3688**

HOTCHKISS, L[ucius] W.
Report of a case in which laparotomy was performed for intestinal perforation occurring in the course of typhoid fever. New York, 1896. 4p. DNLM
90-3689

HOTCHKISS, L[ucius] W.
Report of two successful cases of prostatectomy. New York, 1897. 9p. DNLM **90-3690**

HOUGHTON, E. Mark (*b.* 1867) and A. L. MUIRHEAD
A contribution to the study of strychnin-tetanus. Philadelphia, 1895. 8p. DNLM **90-3691**

HOUGHTON, E. Mark (*b.* 1867)
How can we increase the therapeutic reliability of medicinal agents? Chicago, 1897. 8p. DNLM
90-3692

HOUGHTON, E. Mark (*b.* 1867)
Ergot aseptic, a paper read before the Michigan State Medical Society, Detroit, May 6, 1898. Detroit, 1898. 4p. DNLM
90-3693

HOUGHTON, E. Mark (*b.* 1867)
The pharmacologic assay of the heart tonics. Chicago, 1898. 8p. DNLM **90-3694**

HOUGHTON, E. Mark (*b.* 1867)
An indispensable part of drug valuation; physiological assay necessary to pharmaceutical research; where the chemical test is futile the animal test affords the only safeguard; the bases of the newer pharmacy. Detroit, 1899. 8p. DNLM
90-3695

HOUGHTON, E. Mark (*b.* 1867) and T[homas] B. ALDRICH
Choloretone; a new hypnotic and anesthetic. Detroit: Parke, Davis & Co., 1899. 8p. DNLM **90-3696**

HOUSTON, Edwin J[ames] (1847-1914)
. . . Electricity in electro-therapeutics, by Edwin J. Houston, Ph.D., and A. E. Kennelly, Sc.D. New York: The W. J. Johnston Co., 1896. 402p. diags. DLC; NNNAM
90-3697

HOUSTON, Edwin J[ames] (1847-1914)
. . . Electricity in electro-therapeutics, by Edwin J. Houston . . . and A. E. Kennelly. . . . 2nd ed. New York: The W. J. Johnston Co., 1898. 452p. diags. DLC; NNNAM
90-3698

HOVELL, T[homas] Mark (1853-1925)
A treatise on the diseases of the ear . . . together with the treatment of the affections of the nose and pharynx which conduce to aural disease. Philadelphia: P. Blakiston, Son & Co., 1894. 720p. DNLM; ICJ; PPC; PPJ
90-3699

HOW, W. Storer
Cystic evacuation and irrigation. Philadelphia, 1894. 4p. DNLM **90-3700**

HOW, W. Storer
New bite-taking means and methods. Philadelphia, 1894. 11p. DNLM **90-3701**

HOWARD, E. M[elville] (*b.* 1848)
Causes of uterine displacements. Philadelpia, 1891. 6p. DNLM
90-3702

HOWARD, E. M[elville] (*b.* 1848), J. G. STREETS, and Wallace McGEORGE
Uterine displacements. Causes of uterine displacements, Dr. Howard. Mechanical treatment, Dr. Streets. Therapeutical treatment, Dr. McGeorge. Read before the New Jersey State Homoeopathic Medical Society, Atlantic City, N.J., September 10, 1890. Printed by the courtesy of E. A. Yarnall & Co., 1020 Walnut Street, Philadelphia, Pa., 1891. 28p. PPC; PPHa
90-3703

HOWARD, E. M[elville] (*b.* 1848)
List of vegetable substances used in medicine. Camden: Senseman, [1892]. 58p. DNLM **90-3704**

HOWARD, William Lee (1860-1918)
Hypnotism versus morphinism. [Baltimore, 1891.] 12p. DNLM **90-3705**

HOWARD, William Lee (1860-1918)
Hypnotism as a therapeutic agent. Baltimore: Am. Job Office, 1893. 36p. DNLM **90-3706**

HOWARD, William Lee (1860-1918)
Hypnotism: its uses and its medico-legal relations. Baltimore: Friedenwald Co., 1895. 24p. DNLM
90-3707

HOWARD, William Lee (1860-1918)
The practical uses of suggestive therapeutics. Chicago, 1896. 11p. DNLM **90-3708**

HOWARD, William Lee (1860-1918)
Alcoholic maniacal epilepsy. Transitory disturbance of consciousness mediating criminal acts. Baltimore, 1897. 4p. DNLM
90-3709

HOWARD, William Lee (1860-1918)
Psychical hermaphroditism. A few notes on sexual perversion, with two clinical cases of sexual inversion. St. Louis, 1897. 8p. DNLM **90-3710**

HOWARD, William Lee (1860-1918)
The pathologic impulse to drink; alcohol as a secondary factor in dipsomania. [Detroit, 1898.] 12p. DNLM
90-3711

HOWARD, William Lee (1860-1918)
Physiologic rhythms; the practical value of their recognition in treatment of functional neuroses. Chicago, 1899. 7p. DNLM
90-3712

HOWARD, William T[ravis], Jr. (1821-1907)
The ameba coli; its importance in diagnosis and prognosis, with the report of two cases. [Philadelphia: Lea Bros. & Co., 1892.] 17p. DNLM **90-3713**

HOWARD, William T[ravis], Jr. (1821-1907)
A case of congenital malformation of the heart; atresia of the pulmonary artery, with persistence of the foetal circulation. [Philadelphia, 1892.] 8p. DNLM **90-3714**

HOWARD, William T[ravis], Jr. (1821-1907)
The part played by leucocytes in inflammation in the light of recent bacteriological investigations. [Baltimore, 1892.] 8p. DNLM **90-3715**

HOWARD, William T[ravis], Jr. (1821-1907)
A case of acute ulcerative endocarditis due to the bacillus diphtheriae. Philadelphia, 1894. 13p. DNLM
90-3716

HOWARD, William T[ravis], Jr. (1821-1907)
The results of the treatment of forty cases of diphtheria with the antitoxin. Philadelphia, 1895. 14p. DNLM
90-3717

HOWARD, William T[ravis], Jr. (1821-1907)
The influence of cow's milk in the spread of diphtheria, with an account of a milk epidemic of diphtheria. Philadelphia, 1897. 14p. DNLM **90-3718**

HOWARD, William T[ravis], Jr. (1821-1907)
Acute fibrino-purulent cerebro-spinal meningitis, ependymitis, abscesses of the cerebrum, gas-cysts of the cerebrum, cerebro-spinal exudation, and of the liver, due to the bacillus aerogenes capsulatus. Baltimore, 1899. 10p. DNLM
90-3719

HOWE, Alexander C.
Report of a case of abscess on the interior surface of the epiglottis. New York, 1899. 3p. DNLM
90-3720

HOWE, Andrew Jackson (1825-1892)
Operative gynaecology. . . . Cincinnati: R. Clarke & Co., 1890. 336p. DLC; OCIM **90-3721**

HOWE, E. & CO.
Illustrated catalogue of trusses, supporters, braces, etc. Peterboro, N.H., 1890. 34p. DNLM
90-3722

HOWE, H[erbert] H.
A treatise on local anaesthesia. . . . Weston, Vt., 1894. 136p. DLC **90-3723**

HOWE, Lucien (1848-1928)
Legislation in the United States for the prevention of blindness. Chicago, 1893. 8p. DNLM **90-3724**

HOWE, Lucien (1848-1928)
The relation of the general health to ocular headaches. Chicago, 1896. 8p. DNLM **90-3725**

HOWE, Lucien (1848-1928)
On a compound microscope for viewing the eye. New York, 1899. 7p. DNLM **90-3726**

HOWE, William F. (*d.* 1899)
The electro-therapeutic guide. 3rd ed. [Indianapolis, Ind., 1897.] 49p. DNLM [1st ed., 1895. *Vel subseq.*]
90-3727

HOY, Albert Harris
Eating and drinking, the alkalinity of the blood, the test of food and drink in health and disease. Chicago: A. C. McClurg & Co., 1896. 304p. ICU; MB; MH; NN
90-3728

HOYNE, Temple S[toughton] (1841-1899)
Venereal and urinary diseases. . . . 2nd ed., rev. and enl. Chicago, Detroit and Buffalo: Halsey Bros., 1894. 133p. DLC; NNNAM **90-3729**

HOYT, E[ugene] F. (*b.* 1846)
Observations and experiences involving rectal diseases. [New York], 1890. 16p. DNLM; NNNAM
90-3730

HOYT, E[ugene] F. (*b.* 1846)
Office treatment of hemorrhoids and of fistula in ano. Chicago, 1899. 16p. DNLM **90-3731**

HOYT, E[ugene] F. (*b.* 1846)
Internal hemorrhoids. New York: Gilbert & Beittner, [1899]. 13p. DNLM **90-3732**

HRDLICKA, Alois F. (1869-1943)
The medico-legal aspect of the case of Maria Barbella. [Utica, 1897.] 87p. 19 plates. DNLM **90-3733**

HRDLICKA, Alois F. (1869-1943)
Pathological Institute of the New York State Hospitals. Department of Anthropology. Outline of its scope and exposition of the preliminary work. Utica, N.Y., 1897. 18p. DNLM
90-3734

HRDLICKA, Alois F. (1869-1943)
Study of the normal tibia. Washington, 1898. 6p. DNLM
90-3735

HRDLICKA, Alois F. (1869-1943)
Esquimo brain. New York, 1899. 7p. 7 plates. DNLM
90-3736

HRDLICKA, Alois F. (1869-1943)
Dimensions of the normal pituitary fossa or sella turcica in the white and the negro races; an anatomical study of fifty-seven normal skulls of white and sixty normal skulls of colored individuals. Utica, 1899. 20p. 1 plate, 2 diags. DNLM
90-3737

HUBBARD, Le Roy W.
Some points in the early diagnosis of vertebral tuberculosis. [Philadelphia: Lea Bros. & Co., 1892.] 12p. DNLM
90-3738

HUBBARD, Le Roy W.
Report of the treatment of a case of fracture of the femur during delivery. [Philadelphia, 1893.] 6p. DNLM
90-3739

HUBBARD, Le Roy W.
Cases of Pott's disease of the spine, presenting some unusual nervous symptoms. [Philadelphia: Lea Bros. & Co., 1895.] 8p. DNLM **90-3740**

HUBBARD, S[tephen] G[rosvenor] (1816-1905)
Biographical sketch of the life and writings of the late Professor Henry Bronson, M.D. [New Haven: Tuttle, Morehose & Tayler, 1895.] 117p. port. CtY-M; DNLM
90-3741

HUBBARD, Thomas
Epithelioma of the soft palate removed by injections of liquor potassae. New York, 1896. 4p. DNLM
90-3742

HUBBARD, Thomas
Some remarks on the principles of treatment of simple acute laryngitis and bronchitis. New York, 1896. 7p. DNLM
90-3743

HUBBARD, Thomas
Report of cases of peritonsillar abscess associated with diphtheria. New York, 1899. 4p. DNLM
90-3744

HUBBELL, Alvin A[llace] (1846-1911)
Extraction of steel from the interior of the eye with the electro-magnet. [New York, 1892.] 14p. DNLM
90-3745

HUBBELL, Alvin A[llace] (1846-1911)
Extraction of steel from the interior of the eye with the electro-magnet. [Buffalo, 1893.] 13p. DNLM
90-3746

HUBBELL, Alvin A[llace] (1846-1911)
Hysterical or functional blindness. New York, 1897. 7p. DNLM **90-3747**

HUBER, G[otthelf] Carl (1865-1934)
Nerve suturing and nerve implantation. Grand Rapids, Mich., 1896. 27p. DNLM **90-3748**

HUBER, G[otthelf] Carl (1865-1934)
Observations of the innervation of the sublingual and sub-maxillary glands. New York, 1896. 15p. 1 l. DNLM
90-3749

HUBER, G[otthelf] Carl (1865-1934)
The methylen-blue method for staining nerve tissues. Rochester, [1898]. 2 l. DNLM **90-3750**

HUBER, G[otthelf] Carl (1865-1934)
Notes on microscopical technique. Rochester, [1898]. 7 l. DNLM **90-3751**

HUBER, G[otthelf] Carl (1865-1934)
Sensory nerve-endings in striated muscle. Grand Rapids, 1898. 10p. DNLM **90-3752**

HUBER, G[otthelf] Carl (1865-1934)
The use of formalin in the silver nitrate method of staining endothelial cells. Rochester, [1898]. 1 l. DNLM
90-3753

HUDSON, Thompson Jay (1834-1903)
Hypnotism, a universal anaesthetic in surgery. New York, 1894. 16p. DNLM **90-3754**

HUDSON, Thompson Jay (1834-1903)
Hypnotism in its relations to criminal jurisprudence. [New York, 1895.] 14p. DNLM **90-3755**

HUDSON, Thompson Jay (1834-1903)
The law of psychic phenomena, a working hypothesis for the systematic study of hypnotism, spiritism, mental therapeutics, etc. 8th ed. Chicago: A. C. McClurg & Co., 1895. 409p. DNLM; ICJ; OCIM **90-3756**

HUDSON, Thompson Jay (1834-1903)
A scientific demonstration of the future life. Chicago: A. C. McClurg, 1895. 326p. DNLM; ICJ; OCIM
90-3757

HUEPPE, Ferdinand Adolph Theophil (1852-1938)
The principles of bacteriology . . . authorized transl. from the German by Dr. E. O. Jordan. . . . Chicago: The Open Court Publishing Co.; London: K. Paul, Trench, Trübner & Co., 1899. 467p. col. plates. DLC; IU-M; OCIM **90-3758**

HUGHES, C[harles] H[amilton] (1839-1916)
The psychopathic sequences of hereditary entailment. [St. Louis, 1890.] 13p. DNLM **90-3759**

HUGHES, C[harles] H[amilton] (1839-1916)
Notes on the virile reflex. [St. Louis, 1891.] 3p. DNLM
90-3760

HUGHES, C[harles] H[amilton] (1839-1916)
Psychical or physical. An inquiry into the mind and matter problem. [St. Louis, 1891.] 19p. DNLM
90-3761

HUGHES, C[harles] H[amilton] (1839-1916)
Report on neurology and psychiatry. [St. Louis, 1891.] 28p. DNLM **90-3762**

HUGHES, C[harles] H[amilton] (1839-1916)
Address of the president of the section on neurology and psychiatry of the first Pan-American Medical Congress. [St. Louis, 1893.] 35p. DNLM **90-3763**

HUGHES, C[harles] H[amilton] (1839-1916)
Address of the president at the banquet in honor of the first Pan-American Medical Congress, given by the American Medical Editors' Association, at the Arlington, Washington, U.S.A., Sept. 4, 1893. [St. Louis, 1893.] 6p. DNLM
90-3764

HUGHES, C[harles] H[amilton] (1839-1916)
Erotopathia; morbid erotism. [St. Louis, 1893.] 48p. DNLM
90-3765

HUGHES, C[harles] H[amilton] (1839-1916)
Neuratrophia, neurasthenia, and neuriatria. [St. Louis, 1894.] 11p. DNLM **90-3766**

HUGHES, C[harles] H[amilton] (1839-1916)
The successful management of inebriety without secrecy in therapeutics. [St. Louis, 1894.] 11p. DNLM
90-3767

HUGHES, C[harles] H[amilton] (1839-1916)
A neurologist's farewell. Valedictory to the graduating class, Barnes Medical College. St. Louis, 1896. 7p. DNLM
90-3768

HUGHES, C[harles] H[amilton] (1839-1916)
The sensory nerves system in diagnosis. The reflexes. A contribution for college students. St. Louis, 1896. 7p. DNLM
90-3769

HUGHES, C[harles] H[amilton] (1839-1916)
Cyclone neuroses. St. Louis, 1897. 5p. DNLM
90-3770

HUGHES, C[harles] H[amilton] (1839-1916)
Imperative conceptions. St. Louis, 1897. 5p. DNLM
90-3771

HUGHES, C[harles] H[amilton] (1839-1916)
Neurological progress in America. St. Louis, 1897. 30p. DNLM
90-3772

HUGHES, C[harles] H[amilton] (1839-1916)
Medical service and medical fees. The business side of the practice of medicine. St. Louis, 1898. 9p. DNLM
90-3773

HUGHES, C[harles] H[amilton] (1839-1916)
Progress in neurology. St. Louis, 1898. 11p. DNLM
90-3774

HUGHES, C[harles] H[amilton] (1839-1916)
The sanitary salvage of our soldiers in Cuba. St. Louis, 1898. 19p. DNLM **90-3775**

HUGHES, C[harles] H[amilton] (1839-1916)
Suicide. [Kansas City, 1898.] 8p. DNLM
90-3776

HUGHES, C[harles] H[amilton] (1839-1916)
Nutrition in general functional neurotrophia. [Louisville, 1898.] 4p. DNLM **90-3777**

HUGHES, Daniel E. (1851-1902)
A compend of the practice of medicine. . . . 5th physicians' ed. Thoroughly rev. and enl. Including a very complete section on skin diseases and a new section on mental diseases. Philadelphia: P. Blakiston, Son & Co., 1894. 568p. DLC; DNLM; PPC; PU **90-3778**

HUGHES, Daniel E. (1851-1902)
A compend of the practice of medicine. . . . 6th physicians' ed. Thoroughly revised and enlarged. Including a section on mental disease and a very complete section on skin diseases. Philadelphia: P. Blakiston's Son & Co., 1899. 625p. DLC; DNLM; NNNAM; PPC **90-3779**

HUGHES, Daniel E. (1851-1902)
. . . A compend of the practice of medicine. . . . 6th ed., rev. and enl. . . . Philadelphia: P. Blakiston's Son & Co., 1899. 2 v. DLC; NNNAM; PPC; PU **90-3780**

HUGHES, Richard
The drug-proving of the future. Philadelphia. Philadelphia, 1891. 10p. DNLM **90-3781**

HUMANE restraint appliances, consisting of the Lynch patent lock buckles, and the most humane and approved forms of restraints for the insane and delirious. In use in the U.S. Army and Navy and all important hospitals, asylums, police stations, etc. Madison, Wis., 1892. 8 l. DNLM
90-3782

HUMPHREYS, Frederick (1816-1900)
Mentor do Dr. Humphreys, ou Conselheiro de familia, para uso da medicina especifica. . . . Ed. corr. e augm. New York: Humphreys' Homeo. Medicine Company, 1890. 462p. DLC; NNNAM **90-3783**

HUMPHRY, Laurence (1856-1920)
A manual of nursing, medical and surgical. Philadelphia: P. Blakiston, Son & Co., 1890. [*vel subseq.*] 242p. DNLM; MdU-D; PPC; PU **90-3784**

HUMPHRY, Laurence (1856-1920)
A manual of nursing, medical and surgical. [4th ed.] Philadelphia: P. Blakiston, Son & Co., 1891. 243p. PPC; PU
90-3785

HUMPHRY, Laurence (1856-1920)
A manual of nursing, medical and surgical. 13th ed. Philadelphia: P. Blakiston, Son & Co., 1895. 250p. DNLM; NNNAM; PPC; PPJ **90-3786**

HUN, Henry (1854-1924)
The pathology of acute ascending (Landry's) paralysis. New York: D. Appleton & Co., 1891. 20p. DNLM
90-3787

HUN, Henry (1854-1924)
Two cases of traumatic hysteria. [Philadelphia, 1891.] 8p. DNLM **90-3788**

HUN, Henry (1854-1924)
Two cases of traumatic hysteria. [Philadelphia, 1891.] 12p. DNLM **90-3789**

HUN, Henry (1854-1924)
The objects and functions of a county medical society. Albany, 1892. 6p. DNLM **90-3790**

HUN, Henry (1854-1924)
Disease and immunity. Albany: C. F. Williams, 1893. 11p. DNLM **90-3791**

HUN, Henry (1854-1924)
The uses and abuses of animal extracts as medicines. [New York, 1894.] 16p. DNLM **90-3792**

HUN, Henry (1854-1924)
The nervous symptoms associated with Bright's disease. The unity of Bright's disease. Albany, 1895. 23p. DNLM
90-3793

HUN, Henry (1854-1924)
A sketch of the gradual perfecting of the methods of medical education in the Albany Medical College. Albany, 1896. 16p. DNLM **90-3794**

HUN, Henry (1854-1924)
The value of the antitoxin treatment in diphtheria. Albany, 1896. 15p. DNLM **90-3795**

HUN, Henry (1854-1924)
Analgesia, thermic anaesthesia, and ataxia, resulting from the foci of softening in the medulla oblongata and cerebellum, due to occlusion of the left inferior posterior cerebellum artery. A study of the coure of the sensory and co-ordinate tracts in the medulla oblongata. New York: D. Appleton & Co., 1897. 49p. 1 plate. DNLM **90-3796**

HUN, Henry (1854-1924)
A case of congenital stenosis of the pulmonary orifice and of the conus arteriosus. Albany, 1897. 10p. DNLM
90-3797

HUN, Henry (1854-1924)
A study of a hospital plan. Albany, 1897. 16, 2p. 9 plans. DNLM **90-3798**

HUNT, Joseph H[ill] (1849-1911)
John Baptist Morgagni, the father of pathological anatomy. Brooklyn, 1896. 7p. port. DNLM **90-3799**

HUNT, Joseph H[ill] (1849-1911)
Who discovered anaesthesia? St. Louis, 1897. 21p. DNLM **90-3800**

HUNT, R. Finley
Dentistry a distinct and independent profession; a position based upon undeniable historical and current facts, and not upon theories supported by arguments. [Washington, 1895.] 4p. DNLM **90-3801**

HUNT, William (1825-1896)
An address upon the late Joseph Leidy, his university career. [*Also*:] In memoriam, Dr. Joseph Leidy. . . . Personal history. Philadelphia: Collin's Printing House, 1892. 60p. 1 phot. DNLM; PPC; PPJ **90-3802**

HUNTER, John J[ames]
Renal calculus. New York, [1898]. 2 l. DNLM **90-3803**

HUNTER, J[oseph] W.
On asthma, its causation and treatment; with reports of cases. Alkalithia, as a positive cure. [Dallas, Tex., 1895.] 8p. DNLM **90-3804**

HUNTER, J[oseph] W.
Asthma; etiology and treatment. [Houston, 1898.] 12p. DNLM **90-3805**

HUNTINGTON, D[avid] L[ow] (1834-1899)
The Army Medical Museum and Library. (Read before the union meeting of the Maryland State and the Washington City Dental Societies, May 8, 1896.) [Washington, 1896.] 8p. DNLM **90-3806**

HURD, Edward Payson (1838-1899)
A treatise on neuralgia. . . . Detroit, Mich.: G. S. Davis, 1890. 153p. DLC; OCIM **90-3807**

HURD, Edward Payson (1838-1899)
Sleep, insomnia, and hypnotics. . . . Detroit, Mich.: G. S. Davis, 1891. 112p. DLC **90-3808**

HURD, Henry M[ills] (1843-1927)
Post-febrile insanity. [Baltimore], 1892. 6p. DNLM **90-3809**

HURD, Henry M[ills] (1843-1927)
Some mental disorders of childhood and youth. Baltimore: Friedenwald Co., 1895. 16p. DNLM **90-3810**

HURD, Henry M[ills] (1843-1927)
Laboratories and hospital work. Easton, Pa., 1896. 13p. DNLM **90-3811**

HUTCHINSON, Procter S[elby] (1863-1894)
A manual of diseases of the nose and throat, including the nose, naso-pharynx, pharynx, and larynx. Philadelphia: P. Blakiston, Son & Co., 1891. 127p. 2 plates. CtY-M; DNLM; NNNAM; PPC **90-3812**

HUTCHISON, Joseph Chrisman (1827-1887)
The laws of health: physiology, hygiene, stimulants, narcotics. For educational institutions and general readers. Illus. New York: Effingham Maynard, 1891. 223p. NNNAM **90-3813**

HUTCHISON, Robert (1871-1960) and Harry RAINY
Clinical methods, a guide to the practical study of medicine. Philadelphia: Lea Bros. & Co., 1897]. 552p. 7 plates. [*vel subseq.*] DNLM; NNNAM; PPC; PU **90-3814**

HYDE, Belcher
New drugs and pharmaceutical specialties, embracing new and important remedies, giving, where practicable, their composition, chemical formulae, solubility, physiological action, dosage, etc., together with indications for their therapeutic administration . . . under the direction and supervision of Belcher Hyde. . . . 1st ed. New York: Hyde & Co., 1893. 140p. DLC; NNNAM **90-3815**

HYDE, James Nevins (1840-1910)
Note relative to pemphigus vegetans. New York: D. Appleton & Co., 1891. 7 l. DNLM **90-3816**

HYDE, James Nevins (1840-1910)
A practical treatise on diseases of the skin, for the use of students and practitioners. 3rd ed., thoroughly rev. and enl. . . . Philadelphia: Lea Bros. & Co., 1893. 802p. col. plates. DLC; NNNAM; PPC; PU **90-3817**

HYDE, James Nevins (1840-1910)
A manual of syphilis and the venereal diseases, by James Nevins Hyde . . . and Frank H. Montgomery. . . . Philadelphia: W. B. Saunders, 1895. 618p. col. plates. DLC; DNLM; NNNAM; PPC **90-3818**

HYDE, James Nevins (1840-1910)
A new method in the local treatment of acne. New York, 1896. 3p. DNLM **90-3819**

HYDE, James Nevins (1840-1910) and Nicholas SENN
A contribution to the study of mycetoma of the foot as it occurs in America. New York, 1896. 15p. 1 plate. DNLM **90-3820**

HYDE, James Nevins (1840-1910)
A practical treatise on diseases of the skin, for the use of students and practitioners. 4th and rev. ed., by James Nevins Hyde . . . and Frank H. Montgomery. . . . Philadelphia and New York: Lea Bros. & Co., 1897. 808p. col. plates. DLC; DNLM; NNNAM; PPC **90-3821**

HYDE, Joel W[ilson] (*b.* 1839)
On the necessity of amputation of the cervix uteri in a certain class of cases of laceration. New York, 1893. 9p. DNLM **90-3822**

HYSLOP, Theophilus B[ulkeley] (1863-1933)
Mental physiology, especially in its relations to mental disorders. Philadelphia: P. Blakiston's Sons & Co., 1895. 552p. DNLM; MH; NIC **90-3823**

IMPEY, Samuel P[atton]
A handbook on leprosy. . . . Philadelphia: P. Blakiston, Son & Co., 1896. 116p. DLC; DNLM; PPC; PU **90-3824**

INGALS, Ephraim Fletcher (1848-1918)
The effects of dry atmosphere on chronic inflammation of the larynx and nares. Chicago, 1890. 8p. DNLM **90-3825**

INGALS, Ephraim Fletcher (1848-1918)
Supplemental report on cartilaginous tumors of the larynx and warty growths in the nose. Unilateral paralysis of the lateral crico-arytaenoid muscle. [New York, 1890.] 8p. DNLM **90-3826**

INGALS, Ephraim Fletcher (1848-1918)
The treatment of cystic goitre by electrolysis. Chicago, 1890. 7p. DNLM **90-3827**

INGALS, Ephraim Fletcher (1848-1918)
Hypertrophy of the pharyngeal tonsil. [Philadelphia, 1891.] 11p. DNLM **90-3828**

INGALS, Ephraim Fletcher (1848-1918) and John Edwin RHODES
The Shurley-Gibbes treatment of tuberculosis. Chicago: R. R. McCabe & Co., [1891]. 12p. DNLM **90-3829**

INGALS, Ephraim Fletcher (1848-1918)
Diseases of the chest, throat and nasal cavities. . . . 2nd ed., rev. and enl. . . . New York: William Wood & Co., 1892. 675p. DLC; NNNAM **90-3830**

INGALS, Ephraim Fletcher (1848-1918)
Cauterization of the nares, and accidents that may follow. [Chicago, 1894.] 11p. DNLM **90-3831**

INGALS, Ephraim Fletcher (1848-1918)
Hypertrophy of the pharyngeal or Luschka's tonsil. Chicago: American Med. Assoc. Press, 1894. 15p. DNLM **90-3832**

INGALS, Ephraim Fletcher (1848-1918)
Diseases of the chest, throat, and nasal cavities. . . . 3rd ed., rev. . . . New York: William Wood & Co., 1894. 686p. col. plate. DLC; NNNAM; OCIM **90-3833**

INGALS, Ephraim Fletcher (1848-1918)
The necessities of a modern medical college. Easton, Pa., [1894]. 12p. DNLM **90-3834**

INGALS, Ephraim Fletcher (1848-1918)
Orrhotherapy in diphtheria. Chicago, 1896. 11p. DNLM **90-3835**

INGALS, Ephraim Fletcher (1848-1918)
The antiseptic treatment and the limitation of climatic treatment of pulmonary tuberculosis. Chicago, 1897. 19p. DNLM **90-3836**

INGALS, Ephraim Fletcher (1848-1918)
Diseases of the chest, throat and nasal cavities. . . . Rev. 3rd ed., with appendix containing many important additions. Two hundred and forty illustrations. New York: William Wood & Co., 1898. 704p. col. plate. DLC; NNNAM; PPC; PU **90-3837**

INGLIS, David (*b.* 1850)
Some successful results in the treatment of epilepsy. [Detroit, 1893.] 7p. DNLM **90-3838**

IRWELL, Lawrence
Racial deterioration; the relation between phthisis and insanity. Brooklyn, N.Y., 1897. 29p. DNLM **90-3839**

IRWIN, B[ernard] J. D[owling] (1830-1917)
[Protest against the appointment of Edward P. Vollum as medical purveyor, U.S.A. Sent to the military committee of the U.S. Senate, Sept. 19, 1890.] San Francisco, 1890. 7p. DNLM **90-3840**

IRWIN, B[ernard] J. D[owling] (1830-1917)
Notes on the introduction of tent field hospitals in war. [St. Louis, 1894.] 28p. DNLM **90-3841**

IRWIN, J[ohn] A[rthur] (1853-1912)
Hydrotherapy at Saratoga. A treatise on natural mineral waters. New York: Cassell Publ. Co., [1892]. 270p. 1 plate. DNLM; NNNAM **90-3842**

IRWIN, J[ohn] A[rthur] (1853-1912)
The literature of sea-sickness. New York: Trow, 1893. 8p. DNLM **90-3843**

IRWIN, John L[inn] (1859-1912)
The Nu Sigma Nu Fraternity; its mission in the medical profession. Chicago, 1895. 16p. DNLM **90-3844**

IRWIN, J[oseph] W.
Evidence of arsenical poisoning in the Snook-Herr wedding guests. [New York, 1891.] 30p. DNLM **90-3845**

IRWIN, J[oseph] W.
Puerperal tetanus. New York, 1892. 5p. DNLM **90-3846**

ISAAC KNAPP DENTAL COTERIE, FORT WAYNE, INDIANA
An illustrated manual of popular dental instructions by the.... Fort Wayne: Aldine Printing House, 1894. 63p. DNLM **90-3847**

IVINS, Horace F[remont] (1856-1899)
Diseases of the nose and throat. A text book for students and practitioners. Philadelphia: F. A. Davis, 1893. 507p. 1 plate. DNLM; NNNAM; PPC; PU **90-3848**

JACK, Edwin E[verett] (*b.* 1863)
A case of recurrent paralysis of the oculo-motor nerve. Boston, 1893. 6p. DNLM **90-3849**

JACK, Edwin E[verett] (*b.* 1863)
Intraocular hemorrhage during or shortly after cataract extraction. Boston: Rockwell & Churchill, 1896. 14p. DNLM **90-3850**

JACK, Frederick L[afayette]
Adenoid growths in the naso-pharynx; results of their removal in seventy cases of middle-ear disease. Boston: Damrell & Upham, 1890. 7p. DNLM **90-3851**

JACK, Frederick L[afayette]
Operative treatment for the relief of chronic suppurative affections of the middle ear; report of three cases. Boston, 1892. 8p. DNLM **90-3852**

JACK, Frederick L[afayette]
Remarkable improvement in hearing by removal of the stapes. [New Bedford], 1892. 21p. 1 plate. DNLM **90-3853**

JACK, Frederick L[afayette]
Remarkable improvement in hearing by removal of the stapes. [Boston, 1892.] 24p. 1 plate. DNLM **90-3854**

JACK, Frederick L[afayette]
Further notes on removal of the stapes. Boston, 1897. 7p. DNLM **90-3855**

JACK, Frederick L[afayette]
A case of septic thrombosis of the lateral sinus. Nine cases of mastoid operation with complications. A case of osteoma of auditory canal. [New Bedford], 1894. 15p. DNLM
90-3856

JACK, Frederick L[afayette]
Some of the indications for opening the membrana tympani. Boston, 1897. 6p. DNLM **90-3857**

JACKSON, A[braham] Reeves (1827-1892)
On the choice of methods in the treatment of uteride cancer. [Philadelphia, 1890.] 12p. DNLM
90-3858

JACKSON, A[braham] Reeves (1827-1892)
Injuries of the bladder during laparotomy; including a report of sixty-seven cases. Chicago, 1890. 24p. DNLM
90-3859

JACKSON, Chevalier (1865-1958)
A satisfactory tongue depressor. [New York, 1892.] 4p. DNLM **90-3860**

JACKSON, Chevalier (1865-1958)
An aural masseur. Chicago, 1895. 4p. DNLM
90-3861

JACKSON, Chevalier (1865-1958)
The aural masseur in the Manhattan Eye and Ear Hospital. Chicago, 1895. 7p. DNLM **90-3862**

JACKSON, Edward (1856-1942)
. . . Essentials of refraction and the diseases of the eye. By Edward Jackson. . . . Essentials of diseases of the nose and throat. . . . By E. Baldwin Gleason. . . . Philadelphia: W. B. Saunders; [etc., etc.], 1890. 276p. diags. DLC; DNLM; PPC; PU **90-3863**

JACKSON, Edward (1856-1942)
The absolute static refraction of the eye. [Hartford, 1890.] 7p. DNLM **90-3864**

JACKSON, Edward (1856-1942)
Indirect massage of the lens for the artificial ripening of cataract. [New York: D. Appleton & Co., 1893.] 9p. DNLM
90-3865

JACKSON, Edward (1856-1942)
. . . Essentials of refraction and the diseases of the eye. By Edward Jackson. . . . Essentials of diseases of the nose and throat. By E. B. Gleason. . . . 2nd ed., rev. . . . Philadelphia: W. B. Saunders, 1894. 290p. diags. DLC; NNNAM; PPC; PPJ
90-3866

JACKSON, Edward (1856-1942)
Skiascopy and its practical application to the study of refraction. . . . With twenty-six illustrations. Philadelphia: The Edwards & Docker Co., 1895. 112p. diags. DLC; DNLM; PPC; PU **90-3867**

JACKSON, Edward (1856-1942)
Skiascopy and its practical application to the study of refraction. . . . 2nd ed. With twenty-seven illustrations. Philadelphia: The Edwards & Docker Co., 1896. 108p. diags. DLC; OCIM; PPC; PPJ **90-3868**

JACKSON, Edward (1856-1942)
Skiascopy and its practical application to the study of refraction. . . . 3rd ed. Philadelphia: Edwards & Docker Co., 1898. 108p. PU **90-3869**

JACKSON, Frank W[atson]
Some difficulties in the diagnosis of cardiac diseases. New York, 1894. 18p. DNLM **90-3870**

JACKSON, George Thomas (1852-1916)
Seborrhoea. [New York, 1890.] 11p. DNLM
90-3871

JACKSON, George Thomas (1852-1916)
Transitorische Erblindung bei Keuchhusten. [New York, 1891.] 8p. DNLM **90-3872**

JACKSON, George Thomas (1852-1916)
A dermatological bibliography. . . . Presented to the American Dermatological Association in 1889, and issued as part of its Transactions for 1890. New York: Press of Stettiner, Lambert & Co., 1891. 91p. DLC; DNLM; NNNAM
90-3873

JACKSON, George Thomas (1852-1916)
The ready reference handbook of diseases of the skin. . . . With fifty illustrations. Philadelphia: Lea Bros. & Co., 1892. 553p. col. frontis. DLC; DNLM; PPC; PU
90-3874

JACKSON, George Thomas (1852-1916)
A practical treatise on the diseases of the hair and scalp, by. . . . New, rev., and enl. ed. New York: E. B. Treat, 1894. 414p. DLC; DNLM; NNNAM **90-3875**

JACKSON, George Thomas (1852-1916)
Naevus lipomatoides; a report of a case. [New York, 1895.] 2p. DNLM **90-3876**

JACKSON, George Thomas (1852-1916)
Two cases of bromide eruption. New York: D. Appleton & Co., 1895. 4p. DNLM **90-3877**

JACKSON, George Thomas (1852-1916)
A case of Paget's disease of the nipple. New York: D. Appleton & Co., 1896. 11p. DNLM **90-3878**

JACKSON, George Thomas (1852-1916)
The ready-reference handbook of diseases of the skin. . . . With sixty-nine illustrations. 2nd ed., rev. and enl. New York and Philadelphia: Lea Bros. & Co., 1896. 594p. col. frontis. DLC; DNLM; NNNAM; PPC **90-3879**

JACKSON, George Thomas (1852-1916)
Chronic urticaria; with special reference to its aetiology and treatment. New York, [1897]. 8p. DNLM
90-3880

JACKSON, George Thomas (1852-1916)
Electrolysis in the treatment of diseases of the skin. New York: Publishers' Pr. Co., 1898. 16p. DNLM
90-3881

JACKSON, George Thomas (1852-1916)
The ready-reference handbook of diseases of the skin. . . . 3rd ed., rev. and enl. New York and Philadelphia: Lea Bros. & Co., 1899. 647p. col. frontis. DLC; DNLM; NNNAM; PU
90-3882

JACKSON, Shirls
A simple prismometer. Chicago, 1896. 4p. DNLM
90-3883

JACKSON, V[ictor] H[ugo] (*b.* 1850)
Correcting irregularities of the teeth. Philadelphia, 1890. 10p. DNLM **90-3884**

JACKSON, V[ictor] H[ugo] (*b.* 1850)
Methods of regulating teeth. Philadelphia, 1891. 15p. DNLM
90-3885

JACOBI, A[braham] (1830-1919)
Address delivered at the laying of the corner stone of the New York Academy of Medicine, October 2, 1889. [New York, 1890.] 8p. DNLM **90-3886**

JACOBI, A[braham] (1830-1919)
The Americans and the Tenth International Congress. New York: Trow, 1890. 12p. DNLM **90-3887**

JACOBI, A[braham] (1830-1919)
Enteralgia and chronic peritonitis. [Richmond, 1890.] 12p. DNLM **90-3888**

JACOBI, A[braham] (1830-1919)
The intestinal diseases of infancy and childhood. Physiology, hygiene, pathology and therapeutics. . . . 2nd ed. Detroit, Mich.: G. S. Davis, 1890. 2 v. DLC; OCIM; PPC
90-3889

JACOBI, A[braham] (1830-1919)
Inoculations with Professor Koch's tuberculin. New York: Trow, 1891. 44p. DNLM **90-3890**

JACOBI, A[braham] (1830-1919)
Infant diet; a lecture. . . . Delivered May 8, 1873. Revised, enlarged, and adapted to popular use by Mary Putnam Jacobi, M.D. New York: G. P. Putnam's Sons, 1891. 119p. DLC; NNNAM **90-3891**

JACOBI, A[braham] (1830-1919)
Non nocere. New York, 1894. 36p. DNLM
90-3892

JACOBI, A[braham] (1830-1919)
The production of diseases by sewer air. [New York: D. Appleton & Co., 1894.] 36p. DNLM
90-3893

JACOBI, A[braham] (1830-1919)
Rachitic deformities; etiology, clinical history, and lesions. A discussion at the meeting of the American Orthopedic Association, at Washington, D.C., May 30, 1894; stenographic report. [New York, 1894.] 7p. DNLM
90-3894

JACOBI, A[braham] (1830-1919)
Stomatitis neurotica chronica. [Philadelphia, 1894.] 9p. DNLM **90-3895**

JACOBI, A[braham] (1830-1919)
Hyperthermy in a man up to 148°F. (64.4°C.). Philadelphia, 1895. 31p. DNLM **90-3896**

JACOBI, A[braham] (1830-1919)
Dr. S. Tynberg's pygopagus. New York, [1895]. 9p. DNLM
90-3897

JACOBI, A[braham] (1830-1919)
Therapeutics of infancy and childhood. . . . Philadelphia: J. B. Lippincott Co., 1896. 518p. DLC; DNLM; NNNAM; PPC **90-3898**

JACOBI, A[braham] (1830-1919)
Infant feeding; a review. New York, 1896. 10p. DNLM
90-3899

JACOBI, A[braham] (1830-1919)
Dr. John Cooper's case of ischiopagus. New York, 1896. 3p. DNLM **90-3900**

JACOBI, A[braham] (1830-1919)
The muscles of rhachitical infants. New York, [1896]. 5p. DNLM **90-3901**

JACOBI, A[braham] (1830-1919)
Nephritis of the newly born. New York, 1896. 26p. DNLM
90-3902

JACOBI, A[braham] (1830-1919)
Nervous symptoms in rhachitis. New York, 1896. 6p. DNLM
90-3903

JACOBI, A[braham] (1830-1919)
The president's address delivered before the Association of American Physicians at its eleventh annual meeting, Washington, D.C., April 30, 1896. Philadelphia: Lea Bros. & Co., 1896. 12p. DNLM **90-3904**

JACOBI, A[braham] (1830-1919)
Hereditary syphilis. [Philadelphia: Dornan, 1897.] 20p. DNLM
90-3905

JACOBI, A[braham] (1830-1919)
Jacksonian epilepsy; adenoma of liver; acute ascites with tubercle bacilli. Philadelphia, 1897. 13p. DNLM
90-3906

JACOBI, A[braham] (1830-1919)
The semi-centennial of the New York Academy of Medicine; oration delivered by . . . . New York: Publishers' Pr. Co., 1897. 24p. DNLM **90-3907**

JACOBI, A[braham] (1830-1919)
Dermoid cyst over the centre of the large fontanelle. New York: E. B. Treat & Co., 1898. 3p. DNLM
90-3908

JACOBI, A[braham] (1830-1919)
Ergot in chronic malaria. Philadelphia, 1898. 21p. DNLM
90-3909

JACOBI, A[braham] (1830-1919)
Therapeutics of infancy and childhood. . . . 2nd ed. Philadelphia: J. B. Lippincott Co., 1898. 629p. DLC; DNLM; NNNAM; PU **90-3910**

JACOBI, A[braham] (1830-1919)
Three cases of amaurotic family idiocy. New York: E. B. Treat & Co., [1898]. 13p. DNLM **90-3911**

JACOBI, A[braham] (1830-1919)
Some preventives. Philadelphia, 1898. 43p. DNLM
90-3912

JACOBI, A[braham] (1830-1919) and James EWING
Septic perforation of the right-internal carotid artery; autopsy five months after death. Philadelphia, 1898. 8p. DNLM
90-3913

JACOBI, A[braham] (1830-1919)
European medicine about 1799. [Baltimore, 1899.] 17p. DNLM **90-3914**

JACOBI, A[braham] (1830-1919)
Typhoid fever in the young. New York, [1899]. 27p. DNLM; NNNAM **90-3915**

JACOBI, A[braham] (1830-1919)
Functional cardiac murmurs. [Philadelphia, 1899.] 14p. DNLM **90-3916**

JACOBI, A[braham] (1830-1919)
The disinfection of the alimentary canal. [Philadelphia: Dornan, 1899.] 19p. DNLM **90-3917**

JACOBSON, Henry
Gonorrhoea of the rectum. [New York, 1894.] 4p. DNLM
90-3918

JACOBSON, Nathan (1857-1913)
Some recent cases of appendicitis. [Philadelphia, 1893.] 16p. DNLM **90-3919**

JACOBSON, Nathan (1857-1913)
The treatment of Colles' fracture. New York, 1895. 8p. DNLM
90-3920

JACOBSON, Nathan (1857-1913)
Surgical tuberculosis. [Philadelphia: Lea Bros. & Co., 1895.] 16p. DNLM **90-3921**

JACOBSON, W[alter] H. A. (1847-1924)
Diseases of the male organs of generation. . . . Philadelphia: P. Blakiston, Son & Co., 1893. 766p. DLC; DNLM; PPC; PU
90-3922

JACOBY, George W. (1856-1940)
State care versus county care of the insane. Being the annual address delivered before the New York Neurological Society. May 7, 1889. New York, 1890. 11p. NN
90-3922A

JACOBY, George W. (1856-1940)
Subacute progressive polymyositis. . . . New York: M. J. Rooney, 1890. 28p. NCC; NN **90-3922B**

JACOBY, George W. (1856-1940)
Peripheral paralyses due to carbonic oxide poisoning. Read before the New York Neurological Society, June 4, 1889. New York, 1890. 10p. NN **90-3922C**

JACOBY, George W. (1856-1940)
The significance of the epiblastic origin of the central nervous system. Presidential address delivered at the annual meeting of the New York Neurological Society. May 1st, 1888. New York: L. Weiss, 1890. 15p. NN **90-3922D**

JACOBY, George W. (1856-1940)
Transitorische Erblindung bei Keuchhusten. Vorgetragen in der Deutschen Medicinischen Gesellschaft von New York, am 2. Februar 1891. New York, 1891. 8p. NN
90-3922E

JACOBY, George W. (1856-1940)
Thomsen's disease (Myotonia congenita). New York: William Wood & Co., 1891. 23p. NN **90-3922F**

JACOBY, George W. (1856-1940)
Einiges über den modernen Hypnotismus; Vortrag gehalten im Deutschen Gesellig-Wissenschaftlichen Verein von New York am 26. Februar 1891. New York: Druck der Cherouny Print. and Pub. Co., 1891. 48p. DLC; MB; NN
90-3922G

JACOBY, George W. (1856-1940)
Lumbar puncture of the subarachnoid space. Read before the New York Neurological Society, November 5, 1895. New York: D. Appleton & Co., 1896. 40p. NN
90-3922H

JACOBY, George W. (1856-1940)
On myotonia. Read before the American Neurological Association, May 27th, 1898. [New York: Raff & Co.], 1898. 21p. NN **90-3922I**

JAEGER, Gustav (1833-1917)
Selections from essays on health-culture and the sanitary woolen system. Transl. from the German. 2nd ed. New York: Dr. Jaeger's Sanitary Woolen System Co., 1891. 216p. DLC; NNNAM **90-3923**

JAKOB, Christfried (*b.* 1866)
Atlas of methods of clinical investigation, with an epitome of clinical diagnosis and of special pathology and treatment of internal diseases. . . . Authorized transl. from the German. Ed. by Augustus A. Eshner. . . . With 182 colored illustrations upon 68 plates, and 64 illustrations in the text. Philadelphia: W. B. Saunders, 1898. 15, [80]-259p.
90-3924

JAMESON, Henry
The science of medicine and its relation to people. Indianapolis, 1899. 38p. DNLM **90-3925**

JAMIESON, W[illiam] Allan (1839-1916)
Diseases of the skin. A manual for practitioners and students. 3rd ed., revised and enlarged. Philadelphia: Lea Bros. & Co., 1892. 644p. 8 plates. DNLM; MBM; NNNAM; PPC
90-3926

JAROS, L.
Jaros hygienic wear. The therapeutic and prophylactic application. [4th ed.] New York, [1890]. 79p. port. DNLM
90-3927

JAWORSKI, Walery (*b.* 1849)
The action, therapeutic value and use of the Carlsbad sprudel salt (powder form), and its relation to the Carlsbad thermal water. . . . With a dietary, by the translator, A. L. A. Toboldt. . . . Philadelphia: P. Blakiston, Son & Co., 1891. 100p. tables. DLC; PPC; PU **90-3928**

JAY, F[rank] W[ebster] (*b.* 1868)
Chromicized catgut as a means of direct fixation in the treatment of fractures and osteotomies, with a report of a case. Chicago, 1894. 20p. DNLM **90-3929**

JAY, F[rank] W[ebster] (*b.* 1868)
Cysts of the maxilla connected with the teeth, with report of a case. Philadelphia, 1895. 10p. DNLM
90-3930

JEFFERIS, Benjamin Grant (*b.* 1851)
The household guide; or, Domestic cyclopedia. A practical family physician. Home remedies and home treatment of all diseases. An instructor on nursing, housekeeping and home adornments. By Prof. B. G. Jefferis . . . and J. L. Nichols, A.M. Also a complete cook book, by Mrs. J. L. Nichols. 19th ed. Atlanta, Ga., Toronto, Ont., [etc.] : J. L. Nichols & Co., 1897. 539p. DLC **90-3931**

JEFFERSON MEDICAL COLLEGE, PHILADELPHIA
List of graduates for the years 1853; 1876-1894. Philadelphia, 1853-1894. DNLM; PPJ **90-3932**

JEFFERSON MEDICAL COLLEGE, PHILADELPHIA
. . . The new buildings of the Jefferson Medical College, 1899, to be completed for the 75th session, 1899-1900. [Philadelphia, 1899.] 18, [2] p. (incl. plans). DLC; DNLM; PPJ **90-3933**

JEFFRIES, John Amory (1859-1892)
Sulphonal in chorea. [Philadelphia, 1890.] 8p. DNLM **90-3934**

JEFFRIES, John Amory (1859-1892)
Two cases of syringomyelia. New York: J. Rooney & Co., [1890]. 17p. DNLM **90-3935**

JEFFRIES, John Amory (1859-1892)
A contribution to the study of the summer diarrhoeas of infancy. [Philadelphia, 1890.] 62p. DNLM; PPC **90-3936**

JEFFRIES, John Amory (1859-1892)
Eye paralyses. Boston: Damrell & Upham, 1892. 32p. DNLM; MBM **90-3937**

JELKS, James T[homas] (1849-1902)
Two cases of carcinoma of the uterus. [Little Rock, 1890.] 3p. DNLM **90-3938**

JELKS, James T[homas] (1849-1902)
Comparative value of mercury and the iodides in treatment of syphilis. Chicago: Office Am. Medical Assoc., 1890. 8p. DNLM **90-3939**

JELKS, James T[homas] (1849-1902)
Two cases of tubercular osteomyelitis of tibia. Hot Springs, Ark., 1891. 7p. DNLM **90-3940**

JELKS, James T[homas] (1849-1902)
Some effects of blennorrhoea in women. [Toledo, 1892.] 6p. DNLM **90-3941**

JELKS, James T[homas] (1849-1902)
Report of a case of gunshot wound of liver, stomach; laparotomy; recovery. Chicago, 1892. 4p. DNLM **90-3942**

JELKS, James T[homas] (1849-1902)
Blennorrhoea. [Atlanta, 1892.] 3p. DNLM **90-3943**

JELKS, James T[homas] (1849-1902)
The prevention of venereal disease. Annual address. [Little Rock, 1893.] 12p. DNLM **90-3944**

JELKS, James T[homas] (1849-1902)
The antiquity of syphilis, and Moses as a health officer. Chicago, 1893. 16p. DNLM **90-3945**

JELKS, James T[homas] (1849-1902)
The pathfinders. Chicago, 1896. 15p. DNLM **90-3946**

JELKS, John L.
The relationship between the genito-urinary tract and rectum; in operations of the female, which should receive priority? Memphis, 1898. 6p. DNLM **90-3947**

JELLETT, Henry (*b.* 1872)
A short practice of midwifery, embodying the treatment adopted in the Rotunda Hospital, Dublin. With a preface by W. J. Smyly. Philadelphia: P. Blakiston, Son & Co., 1897. 323p. DNLM; NNNAM; PPC; PU **90-3948**

JENKS, Edward W[atrous] (1833-1903)
The resemblance of some forms of benign disease to malignant. Philadelphia: W. J. Dornan, 1890. 13p. DNLM **90-3949**

JENKS, Edward W[atrous] (1833-1903)
The therapeutic aspect of some ovarian disorders. Philadelphia: W. J. Dornan, 1891. 13p. DNLM **90-3950**

JENKS, Edward W[atrous] (1833-1903)
Colpo-perineorrhaphy. Chicago, 1892. 16p. DNLM **90-3951**

JENKS, Edward W[atrous] (1833-1903)
The limits and requirements of gynecology. New York: Trow, 1893. 15p. DNLM **90-3952**

JENKS, Edward W[atrous] (1833-1903)
Perineo-vaginal restoration. New York: William Wood & Co., 1893. 10p. DNLM **90-3953**

JENNELLE, J[ohn] J.
Treatment of root canals. An essay read before the Southern Illinois Dental Society at Chester, Oct. 22, 1890. Cairo, Ill., 1890. 31p. DNLM **90-3954**

JENNER, William (1815-1898)
Lectures and essays on fevers and diphtheria, 1849-1879. New York: Macmillan & Co., 1893. 581p. DNLM; NNNAM **90-3955**

JENNINGS, Charles G[oodwin] (1857-1936)
A year's experience in the treatment of laryngeal diphtheria with antitoxin and intubation. Detroit, 1898. 5p. DNLM **90-3956**

JENNINGS, John Ellis
Color-vision and color-blindness. A practical manual for railroad surgeons. . . . Philadelphia: The F. A. Davis Co., 1896. 115p. col. frontis. DNLM; PPC; PU **90-3957**

JENNINGS, William Ellery
A case of colocynth poisoning. New York, 1899. 3p. DNLM **90-3958**

JERMAIN, PFLUEGER & KUEHMSTED CO.
Wholesale price list of drugs and pharmaceuticals. Milwaukee, 1896. 1408p. IU-M; OCIM **90-3959**

JEWETT, Charles (1839-1910)
Lecture notes in obstetrics, for the use of students in the Long Island College Hospital. . . . Brooklyn, N.Y.: E. A. Day, 1890. 162p. DLC; NNNAM **90-3960**

JEWETT, Charles (1839-1910)
Manual of childbed nursing. . . . New York: E. R. Pelton, 1891. 40p. DLC; NNNAM; PPC **90-3961**

JEWETT, Charles (1839-1910)
The application of the electric-light current in electro-therapeusis. [Brooklyn, 1892.] 14p. DNLM **90-3962**

JEWETT, Charles (1839-1910)
To what extent is the diagnosis of pregnancy possible in the early months? New York: M. J. Rooney, [1892]. 8p. DNLM **90-3963**

JEWETT, Charles (1839-1910)
Two successful cases of the conservative Caesarean section. [Philadelphia, 1892.] 9p. DNLM; PPC [*also*: New York: M. J. Rooney, 1892. 10p.] **90-3964**

JEWETT, Charles (1839-1910)
A case of symphysiotomy. Brooklyn, 1892. 2p. DNLM **90-3965**

JEWETT, Charles (1839-1910)
Outlines of obstetrics. A synopsis of lectures delivered at the Long Island College Hospital. . . . Ed. by H. F. Jewett. New York: Fairchild & Co., 1892. 177p. DLC; NNNAM; NNU-M **90-3966**

JEWETT, Charles (1839-1910)
Manual of childbed nursing. . . . 3rd ed. New York: Bailey & Fairchild Co., 1893. 40p. NNNAM **90-3967**

JEWETT, Charles (1839-1910)
Outlines of obstetrics, a syllabus of lectures delivered at the Long Island College Hospital. . . . Ed. by Harold F. Jewett, M.D. Philadelphia: W. B. Saunders, 1894. 264p. DLC; NNNAM; PPC; PU **90-3968**

JEWETT, Charles (1839-1910)
Manual of childbed nursing. 4th ed. New York: Bailey & Fairchild Co., 1895. 60p. DNLM; NNNAM **90-3969**

JEWETT, Charles (1839-1910)
A case of symphyseotomy. New York, 1895. 2p. DNLM **90-3970**

JEWETT, Charles (1839-1910)
Three recent symphyseotomies. New York, 1896. 5p. DNLM **90-3971**

JEWETT, Charles (1839-1910)
The question of puerperal self-infection. New York, 1896. 13p. DNLM **90-3972**

JEWETT, Charles (1839-1910)
Essentials of obstetrics. By Charles Jewett . . . assisted by Harold F. Jewett. . . . New York and Philadelphia: Lea Bros. & Co., 1897. 358p. col. plates. DLC; DNLM; NNNAM; PPC **90-3973**

JEWETT, Charles (1839-1910)
Syllabus of gynecology. . . . [Brooklyn: Eagle Press, 1899.] 3 v. DLC; NNNAM; NNU-M **90-3974**

JEWETT, Charles, ed. (1839-1910)
The practice of obstetrics; by American authors. . . . Illustrated with 441 engravings, 34 of which are in colors, and 22 colored plates. New York and Philadelphia: Lea Bros. & Co., 1899. 768p. DLC; DNLM; NNNAM; PPC **90-3975**

JOHNSON, G[eorge] W. (1861-1906)
A report of a case of anomalous thoracic aneurysm. Chicago, 1898. 8p. DNLM **90-3976**

JOHNSON, G[eorge] W. (1861-1906)
A report of the treatment of pulmonary tuberculosis by the inhalation of antiseptic vapors. Chicago, 1898. 8p. DNLM **90-3977**

JOHNSON, H. H[erbert]
Dental education. [Macon, 1895.] 6p. DNLM **90-3978**

JOHNSON, H[enry] L. E. (1858-1916)
A case of accidental hemorrhage from the gravid uterus. New York: William Wood & Co., 1890. 9p. DNLM **90-3979**

JOHNSON, H[enry] L. E. (1858-1916)
A case of placenta praevia marginalis with favorable termination without obstetric interference. Baltimore, 1890. 3p. DNLM **90-3980**

JOHNSON, H[enry] L. E. (1858-1916)
President's address, the completion of the second year of the active life of the Clinico-Pathological Society. Washington, 1890. 1 l. DNLM **90-3981**

JOHNSON, H[enry] L. E. (1858-1916)
A case of double ovariotomy. New York, 1895. 2p. DNLM **90-3982**

JOHNSON, H[enry] L. E. (1858-1916)
A contribution to the study of atresia of the uterine canal after the menopause; with a report of three cases. Chicago, 1895. 19p. DNLM **90-3983**

JOHNSON, H[enry] L. E. (1858-1916)
Appendicitis; with report of an interesting case. Chicago: Am. Medical Assoc. Press, 1897. 12p. DNLM **90-3984**

JOHNSON, H[enry] L. E. (1858-1916)
A case of pyosalpinx in a young girl, with specimens and remarks on special technique. Chicago: Am. Medical Assoc. Press, 1897. 4p. DNLM **90-3985**

JOHNSON, I. S., & CO., BOSTON
Treatment for diseases caused by or accompanied with inflammation. . . . Comp. and pub. by. . . . Boston, Mass.: I. S. Johnson & Co., 1894. 60p. DLC; MBM **90-3986**

JOHNSON, J[ames] C. (*fl.* 1895)
Aetiology and pathology of albuminuria of pregnancy, including puerperal eclampsia. New York, 1895. 4p. DNLM **90-3987**

JOHNSON, John G.
How shall a mother feed her baby if she is unable to nurse it or after she weans it? [n. p., 1894.] 8p. DNLM **90-3988**

JOHNSON, John Taber (1845-1921)
A record of eighty miscellaneous abdominal operations. New York: William Wood & Co., 1890. 18p. DNLM **90-3989**

JOHNSON, John Taber (1845-1921)
Report of a case of tetanus following ovariotomy. [Boston, 1890.] [1889] 3 l. DNLM **90-3990**

JOHNSON, John Taber (1845-1921)
Abortion and its effects. Baltimore, 1890. 27p. DNLM **90-3991**

JOHNSON, John Taber (1845-1921)
Brief observations based on an experience of eighty-seven abdominal sections. Philadelphia: W. J. Dornan, 1890. 10p. DNLM **90-3992**

JOHNSON, John Taber (1845-1921)
A record of eighty miscellaneous abdominal operations. Seventh annual address of the president, delivered before the Washington Obstetrical and Gynecological Society, October 4th, 1889. New York: William Wood & Co., 1890. 18p. DNLM **90-3993**

JOHNSON, John Taber (1845-1921)
Remarks on a series of one hundred laparotomies. Richmond, 1894. 8p. 2 tables. DNLM **90-3994**

JOHNSON, John Taber (1845-1921)
The growth of fibroid tumors of the uterus after the menopause. [Philadelphia, 1892.] 6p. DNLM **90-3995**

JOHNSON, John Taber (1845-1921)
A report of six cases of ovarian tumors with twisted pedicles. [New York, 1892.] 5p. DNLM **90-3996**

JOHNSON, John Taber (1845-1921)
Ovariotomy in old women. [Philadelphia, 1893.] 6p. DNLM **90-3997**

JOHNSON, John Taber (1845-1921)
Ectopic pregnancy in the later months. [Philadelphia, 1894.] 6p. DNLM **90-3998**

JOHNSON, John Taber (1845-1921)
Brief report of all the abdominal operations done in my private sanitarium up to July 1st 1895. New York, 1895. 5p. DNLM **90-3999**

JOHNSON, John Taber (1845-1921)
Hydro-pyonephrosis, with a case. [Philadelphia, 1895.] 4p. DNLM **90-4000**

JOHNSON, John Taber (1845-1921)
Battey's operation. Richmond, 1896. 11p. DNLM **90-4001**

JOHNSON, John Taber (1845-1921)
Chairman's address. Delivered in the section on obstetrics and diseases of women. Chicago, 1896. 15p. DNLM **90-4002**

JOHNSON, John Taber (1845-1921)
Seventeen cases of hysterectomy by the "Baer method." New York, 1896. 8p. DNLM **90-4003**

JOHNSON, John Taber (1845-1921)
Ninety cases of hysterectomy, with remarks on method and technique. Richmond, 1897. 15p. DNLM **90-4004**

JOHNSON, John Taber (1845-1921)
Pus in the pelvis. New York, 1898. 12p. DNLM **90-4005**

JOHNSON, John Taber (1845-1921)
Vaginal vs. abdominal operations, principally for pus in the pelvis. New York, 1898. 18p. DNLM **90-4006**

JOHNSON, John Taber (1845-1921)
The conservative treatment of the diseased ovary. New York, 1899. 6p. DNLM **90-4007**

JOHNSON, John Taber (1845-1921)
The president's address. Philadelphia, 1899. 16p. DNLM **90-4008**

JOHNSON, John Taber (1845-1921)
The president's address before the Southern Surgical and Gynecological Association, New Orleans, December, 1899. Philadelphia, 1899. 13p. DNLM **90-4009**

JOHNSON, John W[aldo]
Private lying-in hospital. [Circular announcing opening. Jan. 7, 1891.] [Boston, 1891.] 1 sheet. DNLM **90-4010**

JOHNSON & JOHNSON
Modern methods of antiseptic wound treatment. Compiled from notes and suggestions from the following surgeons: D. Hayes Agnew . . . A. C. Bernays . . . [and others]. New York: Johnson & Johnson, [1891]. 48p. plates. DLC; NNNAM **90-4011**

[JOHNSON, Laurence] (1845-1893)
Catalogue of the library of . . . . An interesting collection of books in general literature, with special collections on botany, medicine, and the literature of the rebellion. [New York, 1893.] 52p. DNLM **90-4012**

JOHNSON, Robert W.
The surgical care of workmen. [Philadelphia, 1892.] 16p. DNLM **90-4013**

JOHNSON, Robert W.
Healing under a moist blood-clot in accidental wounds. [Philadelphia, 1893.] 9p. DNLM **90-4014**

JOHNSON, Walter B[uckley]
Intubation of the larynx; with a report of eighteen cases. Newark: L. J. Hardham, 1891. 40p. DNLM **90-4015**

JOHNSON, Walter B[uckley]
Necrosis of the maxillae; with a report of three cases. Chicago, 1891. 16p. DNLM **90-4016**

JOHNSON, Walter B[uckley]
Abnormal living entozoa in the human ear. Nashville: A. R. Gray & Son, 1892. 7p. DNLM **90-4017**

JOHNSON, Walter B[uckley]
An original device for correcting deformities of the nose resulting from traumatism; with a report of two cases. New York: Trow's Co., 1892. 8p. DNLM
90-4018

JOHNSON, Walter B[uckley]
Peroxide of hydrogen, and its use in ear diseases. Chicago, 1892. 7p. DNLM **90-4019**

JOHNSON, Walter B[uckley]
Amblyopia from suppression of the visual image. Nashville, Tenn.: A. R. Gray & Son, 1893. 12p. DNLM
90-4020

JOHNSON, Walter B[uckley]
Intubation and tracheotomy in diphtheritic croup; with report of cases. Chicago, 1893. 19p. DNLM
90-4021

JOHNSON, Walter B[uckley]
Present status of legislation for the prevention of blindness. Newark, N.J., 1893. 13p. DNLM **90-4022**

JOHNSON, Walter B[uckley]
Quiescent foreign bodies within the eyeball; with report of cases. Chicago, 1893. 8p. DNLM **90-4023**

JOHNSON, Walter B[uckley]
Suppression of the visual image; also a permanent magnet for use in removing foreign bodies in the cornea. [Hartford, 1893.] 9p. DNLM **90-4024**

JOHNSON, Walter B[uckley]
Amblyopia from suppression of the visual image. St. Louis, 1894. 6p. DNLM **90-4025**

JOHNSON, Walter B[uckley]
A case of sarcoma of the palate successfully treated with the toxines of erysipelas. New York: Trow, 1894. 8p. DNLM
90-4026

JOHNSON, Walter B[uckley]
Foreign bodies in the orbital cavity. [Hartford, 1894.] 14p. DNLM **90-4027**

JOHNSON, Walter B[uckley]
Tonsillitis. Kansas City, 1894. 2p. DNLM
90-4028

JOHNSON, Walter B[uckley]
Removal of the superior maxillary bone for sarcoma, involving the cerebral and orbital cavities and the antrum of Highmore. St. Louis, 1895. 7p. DNLM **90-4029**

JOHNSON, Walter B[uckley]
Transplantation of skin in plastic operations of the eyelid. St. Louis, 1895. 8p. DNLM **90-4030**

JOHNSON, Walter B[uckley]
Description of a portable electro-magnet, an original device, to be used in connection with any incandescent electric-light current, for the removal of pieces of steel from the interior of the eyeball. New York, 1899. 4p. DNLM
90-4031

JOHNSON, Walter B[uckley]
Report of a case of optic neuritis. [New Bedford, 1899.] 7p. DNLM **90-4032**

JOHNSON, William N.
A case of depressed fracture of the skull in a child, with an enormous clot; operation; recovery. [Philadelphia: Lea Bros. & Co., 1893.] 3p. DNLM **90-4033**

JOHNSTON, Collins H.
Some points relative to the use of forceps, and antiseptics in obstetrical practice. The Walscher position. [New York, 1895.] 8p. DNLM **90-4034**

JOHNSTON, George Ben (1853-1916)
A successful case of nephrectomy. Richmond: J. W. Fergusson & Son, 1890. 8p. DLC; DNLM **90-4035**

JOHNSTON, George Ben (1853-1916)
Diagnosis and treatment of cholelithiasis. Richmond, 1895. 8p. DLC; DNLM **90-4036**

JOHNSTON, George Ben (1853-1916)
Imperforation of the rectum. [Huntington, W. Va., 1895.] 8p. DLC; DNLM **90-4037**

JOHNSTON, George Ben (1853-1916)
Movable kidney. [Philadelphia], 1895. 12p. DLC; DNLM
90-4038

JOHNSTON, George Ben (1853-1916)
Comparative frequency of stone in the bladder in the white and negro races. [Philadelphia, 1896.] 5p. DLC; DNLM
90-4039

JOHNSTON, George Ben (1853-1916)
Acquired umbilical hernia in adults. Richmond, 1897. 6p. DLC; DNLM **90-4040**

JOHNSTON, George Ben (1853-1916)
The prevalence of specialism, and who shall be specialists. Richmond, 1897. 7p. DLC; DNLM
90-4041

JOHNSTON, George Ben (1853-1916)
Splitting the capsule for the relief of nephralgia. Philadelphia, 1897. 11p. DLC; DNLM **90-4042**

JOHNSTON, George Ben (1853-1916)
Symptoms and treatment of hepatic abscess; with report of seventeen cases. Philadelphia, 1897. 24p. DLC; DNLM
90-4043

JOHNSTON, George Ben (1853-1916)
Symptoms and treatment of hepatic abscess; with report of seventeen cases. New York, 1897. 8p. DLC; DNLM
90-4044

JOHNSTON, George Ben (1853-1916)
Value to the public of state medical societies. Richmond, 1897. 9p. DLC; DNLM **90-4045**

JOHNSTON, George Ben (1853-1916)
Progress of renal surgery. Richmond, 1898. 18p. DLC; DNLM
90-4046

JOHNSTON, George Ben (1853-1916)
Some abdominal cases. Richmond: J. L. Hill Printing Co., 1898. 7p. 2 plates. DLC; DNLM **90-4047**

JOHNSTON, George Ben (1853-1916)
Gastrostomy for traumatic stricture of esophagus; report of case. Richmond, 1899. 6p. DLC; DNLM **90-4048**

JOHNSTON, James
The ambulance service in the war. New York, 1899. 19p. DNLM **90-4049**

JOHNSTON, James C[hew]
Xanthoma diabeticorum (so-called); its place among the dermatoses. New York: D. Appleton & Co., 1895. 9p. DNLM **90-4050**

JOHNSTON, J. Milton
Eye studies. A series of lessons on vision and visual tests. Chicago: J. M. Johnston, 1892. 228p. DNLM; IU-M; OCIM **90-4051**

JOHNSTON, W[illiam] W[aring] (1843-1902)
On the frequency of chronc diarrhea in women; its causes and treatment. New York: William Wood & Co., 1891. 12p. DNLM **90-4052**

JOHNSTON, W[illiam] W[aring] (1843-1902)
On the climatic treatment of chronic diarrhoea. [Philadelphia: W. B. Saunders, 1892.] 9p. DNLM **90-4053**

JOHNSTON, W[illiam] W[aring] (1843-1902)
On the nature and treatment of forms of disease characterized by indigestion, the presence of bile, urates, and uric acid in the urine, and by nervous symptoms. [Philadelphia: Lea Bros. & Co., 1892.] 27p. DNLM **90-4054**

JOHNSTON, W[illiam] W[aring] (1843-1902)
The treatment of acute dysentery by antiseptic rectal and colon irrigation. [Philadelphia: Lea Bros. & Co., 1892.] 10p. DNLM **90-4055**

JOHNSTON, W[illiam] W[aring] (1843-1902)
On whooping cough; its great fatality and the necessity for isolation and rest in its treatment. New York, 1895. 23p. DNLM **90-4056**

JOHNSTON, W[illiam] W[aring] (1843-1902)
The influence of school life upon the health of children. Washington, 1897. 12p. DNLM **90-4057**

JOHNSTON, W[illiam] W[aring] (1843-1902)
Errors in death returns from malarial and typho-malarial fevers; typhoid fever the prevailing continued fever of Washington. Washington, 1898. 6p. DNLM **90-4058**

JOHNSTON, W[illiam] W[aring] (1843-1902)
The continued fever of epidemic influenza. Philadelphia, 1899. 6p. DNLM **90-4059**

JOHNSTON, W[illiam] W[aring] (1843-1902)
The differential diagnosis of some diseases characterized by fever of intermittent type with more or less fixed intervals. [Philadelphia], 1899. 22p. DNLM **90-4060**

JOHNSTON, W[illiam] W[aring] (1843-1902)
John Hughes Bennett; his services to medicine. Baltimore, 1899. 10. DNLM **90-4061**

JOHNSTON, Wyatt [Galt] (1863-1902)
A new method for the culture of diphtheria-bacilli in hard-boiled eggs. Philadelphia,1892. 3p. DNLM **90-4062**

JOHNSTON, Wyatt [Galt] (1863-1902) and E. W. HAMMOND
A note upon serum diagnosis by means of dried-blood samples in (experimental) cholera. New York: D. Appleton & Co., 1896. 3p. DNLM **90-4063**

JOHNSTON, Wyatt [Galt] (1863-1902)
The use of the autoclave for sterilizing nutrient gelatin. New York, 1896. 2p. DNLM **90-4064**

JOHNSTON, Wyatt [Galt] (1863-1902)
On the application of the serum diagnosis of typhoid fever to the requirements of public health laboratories. New York: D. Appleton & Co., 1896. 11p. DNLM **90-4065**

JOHNSTON, Wyatt [Galt] (1863-1902)
An experiment with the serum reaction as a test for typhoid infection in water, etc. New York: D. Appleton & Co., 1897. 5p. DNLM **90-4066**

JOHNSTON, Wyatt [Galt] (1863-1902)
On the iodine test for semen. Boston, 1897. 6p. DNLM **90-4067**

JOHNSTON, Wyatt [Galt] (1863-1902)
Notes on the progress of legal medicine; the medico-legal study of injuries. Philadelphia, 1898. 7p. DNLM **90-4068**

JOHNSTONE, Alexander
Botany. A concise manual for students of medicine and science. New York: D. Appleton & Co., 1891. 260p. DNLM; NNNAM **90-4069**

JOHNSTONE, A[rthur] W[eir] (1835-1905)
Menopause; natural and artificial. New York, 1894. 6p. DNLM **90-4070**

JOHNSTONE, A[rthur] Weir] (1835-1905)
The relation of menstruation to other reproductive functions. New York: William Wood & Co., 1895. 15p. DNLM **90-4071**

JOHNSTONE, A[rthur] W[eir] (1835-1905)
The function and pathology of the reticular tissue. New York, 1896. 23p. DNLM **90-4072**

JONES, Allen A.
Gastric anacidity. New York, 1893. 9p. DNLM **90-4073**

JONES, Allen A.
The role of lactic acid in gastric digestion. [Philadelphia, 1893.] 5p. DNLM **90-4074**

JONES, Allen A.
The treatment of lactic-acid excess in the stomach. [Philadelphia, 1894.] 8p. DNLM **90-4075**

JONES, Allen A.
Painful gastric neuroses; their nature, symptomatology, etiology, diagnosis, and treatment. [Philadelphia: Lea Bros. & Co., 1894.] 16p. DNLM **90-4076**

JONES, Allen A.
Gastric conditions in renal disease. [New York: D. Appleton & Co., 1895.] 7p. DNLM **90-4077**

JONES, Charles E[dmond] (1849-1899)
Annual address of the president of the New York State Homoeopathic Society, delivered at Albany, N.Y., 1896. 41p. DNLM **90-4078**

JONES, H[enry] Lewis (1857-1915)
Medical electricity. A practical handbook for students and practitioners of medicine. 2nd ed. . . . P. Blakiston, Son & Co., 1895. 474p. DLC; MH-M; PPC; PU **90-4079**

JONES, Henry Macnaughton (1844-1918)
Practical manual of diseases of women and uterine therapeutics. For students and practitioners. 7th ed. New York: William Wood & Co., 1897. 909p. 28 plates. DNLM; MBM; OCIM; PPC **90-4080**

JONES, Isaac J.
Some observations, mainly clinical, upon the uric acid diathesis. Memphis, 1899. 2 l. DNLM **90-4081**

JONES, J[ohn] Harris (*b.* 1851)
Some stray thoughts in and out of medicine. Wilkes-Barre, 1899. 7p. DNLM **90-4082**

JONES, Louis H.
Crawford W. Long and his discovery. Atlanta: Franklin Pr. & Pub. Co., 1899. 14p. DNLM **90-4083**

JONES, Mary A[manda] Dixon (1828-1908)
Suppurating endothelioma; myofibroma in a condition of necrobiosis; remarks on the treatment of the pedicle, etc. New York: Trow, 1890. 32p. DNLM **90-4084**

JONES, Mary A[manda] Dixon (1828-1908)
Another hitherto undescribed disease of the ovaries; anomalous menstrual bodies. [New York, 1890.] 34p. DNLM **90-4085**

JONES, Mary A[manda] Dixon (1828-1908)
Sterility in woman. Causes, treatment, and illustrative cases. [New York, 1891.] 31p. DNLM **90-4086**

JONES, Mary A[manda] Dixon (1828-1908)
Microscopical studies in pelvic peritonitis. New York: Trow's Co., 1892. 31p. DNLM **90-4087**

JONES, Mary A[manda] Dixon (1828-1908)
Diagnosis and some of the clinical aspects of gyroma and endothelioma of the ovary. Buffalo, 1892. 19p. DNLM **90-4088**

JONES, Mary A[manda] Dixon (1828-1908)
Oophorectomy in diseases of the nervous system. [Philadelphia, 1893.] 12p. DNLM **90-4089**

JONES, Mary A[manda] Dixon (1828-1908)
Colpo-hysterectomy for malignant disease. Some considerations in regard to the operation, technique, etc. With a report of my first five cases. [New Yorik, 1893.] 56p. DNLM **90-4090**

JONES, Mary A[manda] Dixon (1828-1908)
Carcinoma of the floor of the pelvis. New York: Trow's Co., 1893. 22p. DNLM **90-4091**

JONES, Mary A[manda] Dixon (1828-1908)
Criminal abortion; its evils and sad consequences. New York, 1894. 32p. DNLM; NNNAM **90-4092**

JONES, Mary A[manda] Dixon (1828-1908)
Personal experiences in laparotomy. New York: Publishers' Pr. Co., 1897. 11p. DNLM **90-4093**

JONES, Samuel J. (1836-1901)
American Academy of Medicine. [Philadelphia]. The president's address. Chicago, 1891. 12p. DNLM; PPC **90-4094**

JONES, Stacy (1828-1905)
The bee-line repertory. . . . Philadelphia: Boericke & Tafel, 1894. 210p. DLC; PPC; PPHa **90-4095**

JONES, Stacy (1828-1905)
Bee-line therapia and repertory. . . . 2nd ed. Philadelphia: Boericke & Tafel, 1899. 333p. DLC; PPC; PPHa **90-4096**

JONES, William S.
Prolapse of the laryngeal ventricle. [Philadelphia, 1895.] 3p. DNLM **90-4097**

JONES, William S. and W. W. KEEN
Two unusual cases of surgery of the trachea. Philadelphia, 1899. 11p. DNLM **90-4098**

JORDAN, Edwin O[akes] (1866-1936)
The inheritance of certain bacterial diseases. Chicago: McCluer Pr. Co., 1898. 4p. DNLM **90-4099**

JORDAN, Edwin O[akes] (1866-1936)
The production of fluorescent pigment by bacteria. Chicago: Univ. of Chicago Press, 1899. 36p. DNLM **90-4100**

JORDAN, John W[oolf] (1840-1921)
The military hospitals at Bethlehem and Lititz during the Revolution. Philadelphia, 1896. 23p. DNLM; PPC **90-4101**

JORDAN, John W[oof] (1840-1921)
Continental hospital returns, 1777-80. Philadelphia, 1899. 32p. DNLM; PPC **90-4102**

JUDD, L. D.
Remarks based upon a further experience with calomel in diphtheria. New York, 1899. 5p. DNLM **90-4103**

JUDD, J. R[ichard]
Always strong and happy; a complete system of treatment for the general care of the body, with full directions for the development of the muscular system. Adapted to persons of sedentary habits, and those wishing a higher system of physical development. 3rd ed. New York, 1895. 201p. DNLM; NNNAM **90-4104**

JUDGE & DOLPH PHARMACEUTICAL CO.
Cut price list of drugs, hot water bottles, perfumes and sundries. St. Louis, 1895. 48p. OCIM **90-4105**

JUDKINS, William (*b.* 1847)
Odd methods of syphilitic inoculation. New York, 1893. 2p. DNLM **90-4106**

JUDSON, A[doniram] B[rown] (1837-1916)
A criticism of Willett's operation for talipes calcaneus. [New York, 1890.] 12p. DNLM **90-4107**

JUDSON, A[doniram] B[rown] (1837-1916)
The pendant limb in the treatment of joint diseases of the lower extremity. [Philadelphia, 1890.] 3p. DNLM **90-4108**

JUDSON, A[doniram] B[rown] (1837-1916)
I., The prevention of the short-leg hip disease. II. The after treatment of hip disease. Philadelphia: W. J. Dornan, 1890. 16p. DNLM **90-4109**

JUDSON, A[doniram] B[rown] (1837-1916)
The rotary element in lateral curvature of the spine. New York: Trow, 1890. 12p. DNLM **90-4110**

JUDSON, A[doniram] B[rown] (1837-1916)
Malignant disease of the vertebrae simulating Pott's disease. [New York, 1891.] 4p. DNLM **90-4111**

JUDSON, A[doniram] B[rown] (1837-1916)
Orthopaedic surgery as a specialty. The president's address, delivered before the American Orthopaedic Association at Washington, D.C., September 22, 1891. New York, 1891. 4p. DNLM **90-4112**

JUDSON, A[doniram] B[rown] (1837-1916)
Practical points in the treatment of club-foot. New York, 1892. 7p. DNLM **90-4113**

JUDSON, A[doniram] B[rown] (1837-1916)
The weight of the body in its relation to the pathology and treatment of club-foot. Boston: Damrell & Upham, 1892. 15p. DNLM **90-4114**

JUDSON, A[doniram] B[rown] (1837-1916)
A contribution to the treatment of white swelling of the knee. Chicago, 1893. 7p. DNLM **90-4115**

JUDSON, A[doniram] B[rown] (1837-1916)
Historical notes on the question of the value of traction in the treatment of hip disease. [New York: D. Appleton & Co., 1893.] 40p. DNLM **90-4116**

JUDSON, A[doniram] B[rown] (1837-1916)
The importance of early attention to the disability caused by infantile paralysis. Philadelphia, 1893. 12p. DNLM **90-4117**

JUDSON, A[doniram] B[rown] (1837-1916)
Practical points in the treatment of hip disease. New York, 1893. 15p. DNLM **90-4118**

JUDSON, A[doniram] B[rown] (1837-1916)
Early symptoms and diagnosis of tubercular joint-diseases. Chicago, 1894. 7p. DNLM **90-4119**

JUDSON, A[doniram] B[rown] (1837-1916)
Mechanical vs. operative surgery. New York, 1895. 3p. DNLM **90-4120**

JUDSON, A[doniram] B[rown] (1837-1916)
A method of preventing shortening after hip-disease. New York, 1895. 11p. DNLM **90-4121**

JUDSON, A[doniram] B[rown] (1837-1916)
Important trifles in the treatment of congenital club-foot. New York, 1896. 4p. DNLM **90-4122**

JUDSON, A[doniram] B[rown] (1837-1916)
Mensuration of the deformity of hip-disease. Chicago, 1896. 8p. DNLM **90-4123**

JUDSON, A[doniram] B[rown] (1837-1916)
Practical inferences from clinical observations in lateral curvature of the spine. New York, 1896. 6p. DNLM **90-4124**

JUDSON, A[doniram] B[rown] (1837-1916)
A study of the sitting posture and a proposed apparatus for patients shortened by Pott's disease. [Philadelphia, 1898.] 3p. DNLM **90-4125**

JUDSON, A[doniram] B[rown] (1837-1916)
Charles Fayette Taylor, M.D. New York, 1899. 1 l. port. DNLM **90-4126**

JUDSON, A[doniram] B[rown] (1837-1916)
A further view of the management of the deformity of hip disease. [Philadelphia, 1899.] 8p. DNLM **90-4127**

JUDSON, A[doniram] B[rown] (1837-1916)
The pathology and treatment of white swelling of the knee. New York, 1899. 9p. DNLM **90-4128**

JUDSON, A[doniram] B[rown] (1837-1916)
Subcutaneous tenotomy; biographical notes. [Philadelphia, 1899.] 5p. DNLM **90-4129**

JUDSON, Charles F[rancis]
Strangulated hernia; operation; recovery. New York: Bailey & Fairchild, 1894. 2p. DNLM **90-4130**

JULER, Henry E[dward] (1866-1921)
A handbook of ophthalmic science and practice. . . . 2nd ed. Philadelphia: Lea Bros. & Co., 1893. 549p. 17 plates. DNLM; MB; PPC; PU **90-4131**

KAHLER, Charles Otto (*b.* 1847)
How to treat your own feet; a treatise on the human foot. . . . New York: P. Kahler & Son, 1893. 78p. plates. DLC; NNNAM **90-4132**

KAHN, Adolph [J.]
Imperforate hymen with retention of menstrual fluid. [Philadelphia, 1893.] 2p. DNLM **90-4133**

KAHN, Cornelia
An incarcerated retroflexed pregnant uterus, with great distension of bladder; successful reposition; recovery. Philadelphia: Binder & Kelly, [1891]. 14p. DNLM **90-4134**

KAINS, Maurice G[renville] (1868-1946)
Ginseng. Its cultivation, harvesting, marketing, and market value; with a short account of its history and botany. New York: Judd, 1899. 53p. NNNAM **90-4135**

KALES, John Davis
The effects of ethyl alcohol of the affinity of haemoglobin for oxygen. [Chicago, 1894.] 6p. DNLM **90-4136**

KALES, John Davis
Rapid method of demonstrating tubercle bacilli in sputa. Chicago, 1894. 4p. DNLM **90-4137**

KALES, John Davis
Inflammation and microbes; a lecture. Chicago: Am. Medical Assoc. Press, 1895. 7p. DNLM **90-4138**

KALISH, Richard
The arrest and partial resorption of immature cataract with restoration of reading-power. New York: M. J. Rooney & Co., 1890. 11p. DNLM **90-4139**

KALISH, Richard
The absorption of immature cataract by manipulation conjoined with instillation. New York: M. J. Rooney, 1891. 16p. DNLM **90-4140**

KALISH, Richard
Ophthalmic suggestions for the general practitioner. [New York, 1894.] 13p. DNLM **90-4141**

KANSAS CITY book of the eighth annual meeting of the Association of Military Surgeons of the United States, June 1st to 3rd, 1898. Kansas City, Mo.: Hudson-Kimberly Publ. Co., 1898. 70p. DNLM **90-4142**

KANSAS CITY TRAINING SCHOOL FOR NURSES
Annual announcements for the sessions of 1894-5 to 1898-9 (1.-5.); 1901-2 (8.); 1902-3 (9.). Kansas City, 1894-1902. DNLM [Organized April 26, 1894.] **90-4143**

KANSAS CITY TRAINING SCHOOL FOR NURSES
Announcement. [With a list of questions to be answered by the applicant.] [Kansas City, 1895.] 2 l. DNLM **90-4144**

KANSAS CITY TRAINING SCHOOL FOR NURSES
Annual commencements. 3., 1897; 4., 1898. 6., 1900. 8., 1902. Kansas City, 1897-1902. DNLM **90-4145**

KANSAS MEDICAL COLLEGE, TOPEKA
Annual announcements for the sessions of 1890-91 to 1894-95 (1.-5.); 1897-98 to 1900-1901 (8.-11.); 1902-03 (13.). Topeka, 1890-1902. DNLM **90-4146**

KAPOSI, Moritz (1837-1902)
Pathology and treatment of diseases of the skin. . . . Translation of the last German edition, under the supervision of James C. Johnston. New York: William Wood & Co., 1895. 684p. col. plates. CtY-M; DLC; ICJ; PPJ **90-4147**

KAY, Thomas W[iles] (*b.* 1858)
A study of sterility; its causes and treatment. Chicago: Office Am. Medical Assoc., 1891. 56p. DNLM **90-4148**

KAYSAN, H. A.
Aseptic hospital furniture. [Catalogue.] Brooklyn, [1894.] 20p. DNLM; NNNAM **90-4149**

KAYSAN, H. A.
[Aseptic hospital furniture.] Special price list, No. 3. Brooklyn, [1895]. 16p. DNLM; NNNAM **90-4150**

KAYSAN, H. A.
[Aseptic hospital furniture.] Illustrated catalogue. Brooklyn: P. J. Collison & Co., [1896]. 52p. DNLM; NNNAM **90-4151**

KEATING, John M[arie] (1852-1893)
Diseases of the heart and circulation in infancy and childhood. With an appendix entitled "Clinical studies on the pulse in childhood," by J. M. Keating and William A. Edwards. Philadelphia: F. A. Davis, Publisher, 1890 [1889]. 225p. DLC; ICU; NNNAM; PPC **90-4152**

KEATING, John M[arie] (1852-1893)
Record of medical examinations. Designed by. . . . Philadelphia: F. A. Davis, Publishing, 1890 [1889]. [7 x 3¾ inches in two sizes, No. 1, covering 100 examinations; No. 2, covering 200 examinations] NNNAM; PPC **90-4153**

KEATING, John M[arie] (1852-1893)
How to examine for life insurance. Philadelphia: P. Blakiston, Son & Co., 1890. 211p. 2 plates. DNLM; PPC **90-4154**

KEATING, John M[arie] (1852-1893)
How to examine for life insurance. 2nd ed. Philadelphia: W. B. Saunders, 1891. 211p. DNLM; PPC **90-4155**

KEATING, John M[arie] (1852-1893)
Scarlet fever, and how to nurse it. [New York, 1890.] 11p. DLC; DNLM **90-4156**

KEATING, John M[arie] (1852-1893)
How to examine for life insurance. . . . Philadelphia: [Press of W. F. Fell & Co.], 1890. 211p. DLC; PPC **90-4157**

KEATING, John M[arie] (1852-1893)
Saunders' pocket medical lexicon. Being a dictionary of words and terms used in medicine and surgery. . . . By John M. Keating . . . and Henry Hamilton. . . . Philadelphia: W. B. Saunders, 1890. 280p. DLC; DNLM; PPC; PPL **90-4158**

KEATING, John M[arie], ed. (1852-1893)
Cyclopaedia of the diseases of children, medical and surgical. The articles written especially for the work by American, British, and Canadian authors. . . . Philadelphia: J. B. Lippincott Co., 1890-91. 4 v. DNLM; NNNAM; PPC; PU **90-4159**

KEATING, John M[arie] (1852-1893)
A new pronouncing dictionary of medicine. Being a voluminous and exhaustive hand-book of medical and scientific terminology. . . . By John M. Keating . . . and Henry Hamilton . . . With the collaboration of J. Chalmers Da Costa, M.D., and Frederick A. Packard. . . . Philadelphia: W. B. Saunders, 1892. 818p. DLC; DNLM; NNNAM; PPC **90-4160**

KEATING, John M[arie], ed. (1852-1893)
Clinical gynaecology, medical and surgical, by eminent American teachers; ed. by John M. Keating . . . and Henry C. Coe. . . . Philadelphia: J. B. Lippincott Co., 1895 [1894]. 904p. plates. DLC; DNLM; NNNAM; PPC **90-4161**

KEEFE, Daniel E.
Chloroform and ether, a criticism of Leonard Hill's address, with some remarks on syncope under anaesthetics. Boston: Damrell & Upham, 1897. 12p. DNLM
90-4162

KEEFE, Daniel E.
Sex in generation. The consideration of some factors exerting an influence in its determination. Danbury, Conn., 1898. 7p. DNLM **90-4163**

KEELEY, Leslie E. (1832?-1900)
A popular treatise on drunkenness and the opium habit, and their successful treatment with the double chloride of gold; the only cure. [Dwight, Ill., 1890.] 31p. DNLM
90-4164

KEELEY, Leslie E. (1832?-1900)
Drunkenness and heredity; and the inebriety of childhood. [Chicago, 1893.] 16p. DNLM **90-4165**

KEELEY, Leslie E. (1832?-1900)
The non-heredity of inebriety. Chicago: S. C. Griggs & Co., 1896. 359p. DNLM; OCIM **90-4166**

KEELEY, Leslie E. (1832?-1900)
Inebriety is a disease. [Boston, 1896.] 31p. DNLM
90-4167

KEELEY, Leslie E. (1832?-1900)
Inebriety is a disease. 2nd ed. Lexington, Mass., [1897]. 31p. DNLM **90-4168**

KEELEY, Leslie E. (1832?-1900)
Opium: its use, abuse, and cure; or from bondage to freedom. Chicago: Banner of Gold Co., 1897. 132p. ICU
90-4169

KEEN, William W[illiams] (1837-1932)
Craniectomy for microcephalus; the later history of a case of excision of the hard-centre for epilepsy. [Philadelphia, 1890.] 10p. DNLM **90-4170**

KEEN, William W[illiams] (1837-1932)
Intra-cranial lesions. Concord, N.H.: Republican Press Assoc., 1890. 27p. DNLM **90-4171**

KEEN, William W[illiams] (1837-1932)
Nephrorrhaphy. [St. Louis, 1890.] 35p. DNLM
90-4172

KEEN, William W[illiams] (1837-1932)
The new era in medicine and its demands upon the profession and the college. Philadelphia, 1890. 28p. DNLM
90-4173

KEEN, William W[illiams] (1837-1932)
Two suggestions in surgical technique. I. A new method of compressing the subclavian artery. II. A new method of ascertaining whether the bladder is or is not ruptured. Philadelphia: W. J. Dornan, 1890. 6p. DNLM **90-4174**

KEEN, William W[illiams] (1837-1932)
Five cases of suprapubic cystotomy; three for stone, one for tumor in the bladder, and one for exploration with catheterism of the ureters; one death. [Philadelphia, 1891.] 23p. DNLM
90-4175

KEEN, William W[illiams] (1837-1932)
Four congenital tumors of the head and spine, all submitted to operation. I. Meningocele. II. Cervical spina bifida. III. Sacral spina bifida. IV. A tumor of the post-anal gut, in connection with a dermoid cyst. [Philadelphia, 1891.] 14p. DNLM **90-4176**

KEEN, William W[illiams] (1837-1932)
Four operations for appendicitis; three recoveries, one death from a very small concealed abscess. [Philadelphia, 1891.] 6p. DNLM **90-4177**

KEEN, William W[illiams] (1837-1932)
A further communication on a new method of compressing the subclavian artery, with the report of two cases. Philadelphia, 1891. 3p. DNLM **90-4178**

KEEN, William W[illiams] (1837-1932)
The indications for early laparotomy in appendicitis. Philadelphia: W. J. Dornan, 1891. 8p. DNLM
90-4179

KEEN, William W[illiams] (1837-1932)
The indications for early laparotomy in appendicitis. [St. Louis, 1891.] 9p. DNLM **90-4180**

KEEN, William W[illiams] (1837-1932)
Linear craniotomy (miscalled craniectomy) for microcephalus. Philadelphia: Lea Bros. & Co., 1891. 7p. DNLM
90-4181

KEEN, William W[illiams] (1837-1932)
A new method of tenotomy, by which the tendons are lengthened to a definite extent, instead of the present haphazard method. [Philadelphia, 1891.] 5p. DNLM
90-4182

KEEN, William W[illiams] (1837-1932)
A new operation or spasmodic wry-neck. Namely, division or exsection of the nerves supplying the posterior rotator muscles of the head. [St. Louis, 1891.] 4p. DNLM
90-4183

KEEN, William W[illiams] (1837-1932)
The organization of an operation. [Philadelphia, 1891.] 12p. DNLM **90-4184**

KEEN, William W[illiams] (1837-1932)
An American text-book of surgery, for practitioners and students. By Charles H. Burnett, M.D., Phineas S. Conner, M.D. [and others] . . . . Ed. by William W. Keen . . . and J. William White. . . . Philadelphia: W. B. Saunders, 1892. 1209p. plates. DLC; DNLM; NNNAM; PPC **90-4185**

KEEN, William W[illiams] (1837-1932)
Amputation at the hip-joint by Wyeth's method, the patient being 5 months pregnant. [Philadelphia: Lea Bros. & Co., 1892.] 13p. DNLM **90-4186**

KEEN, William W[illiams] (1837-1932)
Arterio-venous aneurism of the common carotid artery and internal jugular veins; double ligature of both vessels; recovery. [Philadelphia, 1892.] 5p. DNLM
90-4187

KEEN, William W[illiams] (1837-1932) and David D. STEWART
Nephrotomy for calculus pyelitis. Nephrectomy rightly decided against because of the small percentage of urea; an apparently almost destroyed and useless kidney found to secrete over four and half times as much urine as the other kidney; death. Detroit: G. S. Davis, 1892. 10p. DNLM **90-4188**

KEEN, William W[illiams] (1837-1932)
Resection of the liver. [Boston, 1892.] 5p. 1 plate, 1 table. DNLM **90-4189**

KEEN, William W[illiams] (1837-1932)
Two cases of hernia, both treated by laparotomy. I. A properitoneal hernia. II. A femoral Littré's hernia. [Philadelphia, 1892.] 3p. DNLM **90-4190**

KEEN, William W[illiams] (1837-1932)
Umbilical hernia; operation; cure; Ligation of femoral artery for popliteal aneurism; cure. Fecal fistula caused by appendicitis; operation; cure. [Philadelphia: Lea Bros. & Co., 1892.] 13p. DNLM **90-4191**

KEEN, William W[illiams] (1837-1932)
Case of cancer of the hepatic flexure of the colon producing intestinal obstruction; temporary relief by an artificial anus; later re-establishment of the continuity of the bowel by ileocolostomy by means of Murphy's button. Philadelphia, 1893. 15p. DNLM **90-4192**

KEEN, William W[illiams] (1837-1932)
A case of suprapubic cystotomy in which the bladder was distended with air instead of water, and four hundred and ninety-five calculi removed. [Atlanta: Franklin Print. & Publ. Co., 1893.] 5p. DNLM **90-4193**

KEEN, William W[illiams] (1837-1932)
Laparotomy for apparent intestinal paralysis which caused arrest of the intestinal contents, and was equivalent to intestinal obstruction. Kansas City, 1893. 6p. DNLM **90-4194**

KEEN, William W[illiams] (1837-1932)
Medicine as a career for educated men. The commencement address at Lafayette College, June 13, 1893. Easton, Pa., [1893]. 19p. DNLM **90-4195**

KEEN, William W[illiams] (1837-1932)
Medicine as a career for educated men. The commencement address at Lafayette College, June 13, 1893. [Philadelphia], 1893. 9p. DNLM **90-4196**

KEEN, William W[illiams] (1837-1932)
The real rewards of medicine. Philadelphia, 1893. 4p. DNLM **90-4197**

KEEN, William W[illiams] (1837-1932)
An ovarian tumor weighing 111 pounds removed from a child of fifteen, whose weight was 68 pounds. [Philadelphia, 1893.] 3p. DNLM **90-4198**

KEEN, William W[illiams] (1837-1932)
Amputation of the entire upper extremity (including the scapula and clavicle) and of the arm at the shoulder-joint. With especial reference to methods of controlling hemorrhage. With report of one case of the former amputation and four of the latter. Philadelphia, 1894. 26p. DNLM **90-4199**

KEEN, William W[illiams] (1837-1932) and John K. MITCHELL
Removal of the Gasserian ganglion as the last of fourteen operations in thirteen years for tic douloureux. Philadelphia, 1894. 14p. DNLM **90-4200**

KEEN, William W[illiams] (1837-1932)
Amputation of the female breast. Cleveland, 1894. 16p. DNLM **90-4201**

KEEN, William W[illiams] (1837-1932)
Enormous oval hemorrhoid encircling the anus, Whitehead's operation; entire cure. Detroit, Mich., 1894. 4p. 2 plates. DNLM **90-4202**

KEEN, William W[illiams] (1837-1932)
Four cases of brain tumor, in three of which operation was done; two operative recoveries; ultimate death in all. [Philadelphia, 1894.] 28p. DNLM **90-4203**

KEEN, William W[illiams] (1837-1932)
Ligation of the common and external carotid arteries and the jugular vein, for arterio-venous aneurism of the internal carotid and jugular; with division of the optic nerve on the opposite side, the result of a gunshot wound. Philadelphia, 1894. 3p. DNLM **90-4204**

KEEN, William W[illiams] (1837-1932)
Operation wounds of the thoracic duct in the neck; with a résumé of the two prior recorded cases and two additional cases. [Philadelphia, 1894.] 10p. DNLM **90-4205**

KEEN, William W[illiams] (1837-1932)
Amputation of the entire upper extremity (including the clavicle and scapula) for sarcoma following fracture of the clavicle. Extensive thoracoplasty by Schede's method. [Philadelphia], 1895. 9p. 2 plates. DNLM **90-4206**

KEEN, William W[illiams], ed. (1837-1932)
An American text-book of surgery, for practitioners and students. By Charles H. Burnett, M.D., Phineas S. Conner, M.D. [and others] . . . . Ed. by William W. Keen . . . and J. William White. . . . 2nd ed., carefully rev. Philadelphia: W. B. Saunders, 1895. 1248p. plates. DLC; DNLM; NNNAM; PPC **90-4207**

KEEN, Williams W[illiams] (1837-1932)
Gangrene as a complication and sequel of the continued fevers, especially of typhoid. Shattuck lecture for 1896. Boston: Damrell & Upham, 1896. 33p. DNLM **90-4208**

KEEN, William W[illiams] (1837-1932)
Remarks on operations on the Gasserian ganglion, with a report of five additional cases. Philadelphia, 1896. 16p. DNLM **90-4209**

KEEN, William W[illiams] (1837-1932)
The surgical treatment of intra-cranial tumors. Philadelphia, 1896. 8p. DNLM **90-4210**

KEEN, William W[illiams] (1837-1932)
Three cases of plastic nasal surgery; for saddle-shaped nose, removal of entire nose, and arcned Roman nose. Detroit: G. S. Davis, 1896. 14p. DNLM **90-4211**

KEEN, William W[illiams] (1837-1932)
The treatment of traumatic lesions of the kidney; with tables of 155 cases. Philadelphia, 1896. 44p. DNLM
90-4212

KEEN, William W[illiams] (1837-1932)
Address in surgery. Chicago, 1897. 29p. DNLM
90-4213

KEEN, William W[illiams] (1837-1932)
Address on the unveiling of the bronze statue of the late Prof. Samuel David Gross, in Washington, D.C. Philadelphia, 1897. 8p. port. DNLM **90-4214**

KEEN, William W[illiams] (1837-1932)
The advantages of the Trendelenburg posture during all operations involving directly or indirectly, the cavities of the mouth, nose, and the trachea; with a report of two cases of epithelioma and sarcoma of the tonsil. Philadelphia, 1897. 7p. DNLM
90-4215

KEEN, William W[illiams] (1837-1932)
Clinical lecture on an obscure tumor of the abdomen; amputation of the breast for Paget's disease followed by cancer; tuberculosis of the tonsil and soft palate, by a method which avoided splitting of the cheek or dividing the jaw. Philadelphia, 1897. 6p. DNLM **90-4216**

KEEN, William W[illiams] (1837-1932)
Removal of and angioma of the liver by elastic constriction external to the abdominal cavity; with a table of 59 cases of operation for hepatic tumors. Pittsburgh, Pa., 1897. 12p. DNLM **90-4217**

KEEN, William W[illiams] (1837-1932)
Resection of the sternum for tumors; with a report of two cases and a table of seventeen previously reported cases. Philadelphia, 1897. 10p. DNLM
90-4218

KEEN, William W[illiams] (1837-1932)
Treatment of cancer of the rectum, with a report of twenty-five cases. Detroit, Mich.: G. S. Davis, 1897. 73p. DNLM
90-4219

KEEN, William W[illiams] (1837-1932)
Tuberculosis or carcinoma (?) of the stomach; exploratory coeliotomy; subsequent apparently complete cure. Philadelphia, 1897. 8p. DNLM **90-4220**

KEEN, William W[illiams] (1837-1932)
The advantages of a permanent abdominal anus and of total closure of the sacral end of the rectum, in operations for cancer of the rectum. Chicago, 1898. 11p. DNLM
90-4221

KEEN, William W[illiams] (1837-1932)
A case of appendicitis in which the appendix became permanently soldered to the bladder, like a third ureter, producing a urinary fecal fistula. Philadelphia, 1898. 9p. DNLM
90-4222

KEEN, William W[illiams] (1837-1932)
Remarks on resection of the Gasserian ganglion; with a pathological report on seven ganglia removed by Professor Keen. Philadelphia, 1898. 30p. DNLM **90-4223**

KEEN, William W[illiams] (1837-1932)
The surgical complications and sequels of typhoid fever, by. . . . Based upon tables of 1700 cases compiled by the author and by Thompson S. Westcott . . . with a chapter on the ocular complications of typhoid fever by George E. De Schweinitz. . . . And as an appendix, The Toner lecture, no. V. Philadelphia: W. B. Saunders, 1898. 386p. tables. DLC; DNLM; PPC; PU **90-4224**

KEEN, William W[illiams] (1837-1932)
The debt of the public to the medical profession. . . . [Philadelphia, 1899.] 24p. DLC; DNLM; PPJ **90-4225**

KEEN, William W[illiams], ed. (1837-1932)
An American text-book of surgery, for practitioners and students. By Phineas S. Conner, M.D., Frederic S. Dennis, M.D., William W. Keen, M.D., Charles B. Nancrede, M.D., Roswell Park, M.D., Lewis S. Pilcher, M.D., Nicholas Senn, M.D., Francis J. Shepherd, M.D., Lewis A. Stimson, M.D., J. Collins Warren, M.D., and J. William White, M.D. Ed. by William W. Keen . . . and J. William White. . . . 3rd ed., thoroughly rev. Philadelphia: W. B. Saunders, 1899. 1228p. plates. DLC; MH-M; NNNAM; PPC **90-4226**

KEEN, William W[illiams] (1837-1932)
Report of a case of resection of the liver for the removal of a neoplasm; with a table of seventy-six cases of resection of the liver for hepatic tumors. Philadelphia, 1899. 17p. DNLM
90-4227

KEITH, B. & CO.
Revised and enlarged manual of the active principles of indigenous and foreign medicinal plants, as prepared at the laboratory of. . . . Jersey City: Jersey City Print. Co., 1890. 72p. DNLM **90-4228**

KEITH, Skene (1858-1919)
Text book of abdominal surgery; a clinical manual for practitioners and students. By Skene Keith . . . assisted by George E. Keith. . . . With illustrations. Philadelphia: J. B. Lippincott Co., 1894. 508p. DLC; NNNAM; PPC; PU
90-4229

KEITH, Skene (1858-1919)
The management of the intestine after abdominal section. New York, 1894. 7p. DNLM
90-4230

KELLER, A. H.
Perpetual clinical index to materia medica, chemistry, and pharmacy charts. Philadelphia: F. A. Davis, Publisher, 1890 [1889]. 135p. DLC; MBM; PPC; PU
90-4231

KELLEY, S[amuel] W[alter] (1855-1929)
Clinic for diseases of children. Hurlbut Dispensary, Western Reserve University, 1891. [Cleveland, 1891.] 11p. DNLM
90-4232

KELLEY, S[amuel] W[alter] (1855-1929)
Present views on intubation of the larynx. Cleveland, O.: Buell & Hubbell, [1893]. 8p. DNLM
90-4233

KELLEY, S[amuel] W[alter] (1855-1929)
The profession of medicine as sketched from the outside and from the inside. Cleveland, O.: Buell & Hubbell, [1893]. 24p. DNLM **90-4234**

KELLEY, S[amuel] W[alter] (1855-1929)
Pediatrics; past, present, and prospective. Cleveland, 1896. 18p. DNLM **90-4235**

KELLEY, S[amuel] W[alter] (1855-1929)
About children; six lectures given to the nurses in the training school of the Cleveland General Hospital in February, 1896. Cleveland, 1897. 179p. DNLM; OCIM **90-4236**

KELLOGG, George M.
The physiology of decussation of nerves; a one-sided body means a one-sided brain. Chicago, 1896. 20p. DNLM **90-4237**

KELLOGG, George M.
The physiology of right- and left-handed. Chicago, 1898. 8p. DNLM **90-4238**

KELLOGG, John H[arvey] (1852-1943)
The influence of dress in producing the physical decadence of American women. [Detroit, 1891.] 39p. 5 plates. DNLM **90-4239**

KELLOGG, John H[arvey] (1852-1943)
A renal calculus of unusual size; nephrectomy; recovery. Battle Creek, 1892. 8p. DNLM **90-4240**

KELLOGG, John H[arvey] (1852-1943)
Sanitarium methods. Battle Creek, 1893. 12p. DNLM **90-4241**

KELLOGG, John Harvey (1852-1943)
Methods of precision in the investigation of disorders of digestion. Battle Creek, 1893. 74p. DNLM **90-4242**

KELLOGG, John Harvey (1852-1943)
The non-surgical treatment of ovarian diseases. Battle Creek, [1893]. 28p. 6 plates. DNLM **90-4243**

KELLOGG, John Harvey (1852-1943)
A new dynamometer for use in anthropometry. Battle Creek, 1894. 11p. 1 chart. DNLM **90-4244**

KELLOGG, John Harvey (1852-1943)
The relation of static disturbances of the abdominal viscera to displacements of the pelvic organs. Battle Creek, 1894. 43p. 2 tables. DNLM **90-4245**

KELLOGG, John Harvey (1852-1943)
The art of massage; its physiological effects and therapeutic application. Battle Creek: Mod. Med. Publ. Co., 1895. 282p. 43 plates, 1 table, 4 charts. DNLM **90-4246**

KELLOGG, John Harvey (1852-1943)
What is the matter with the American stomach? Battle Creek, [1895]. 34p. 1 table. DNLM **90-4247**

KELLOGG, John Harvey (1852-1943)
The cure of incurables. Battle Creek, 1896. 43p. DNLM **90-4248**

KELLOGG, John Harvey (1852-1943)
An exact method for determining the capacity of the stomach and the amount of residual contents. Battle Creek, 1896. 11p. DNLM **90-4249**

KELLOGG, John H[arvey] (1852-1943)
Physical chart. Classified and arranged according to heights from 64 to 72 inches. Battle Creek, 1896. 2 l. DNLM **90-4250**

KELLOGG, John H[arvey] (1852-1943)
The stomach; its disorders, and how to cure them. . . . 1st ed. Battle Creek, Mich., Chicago, [etc.]: Modern Medicine Pub. Co., 1896. 368p. col. frontis. DLC; DNLM; NNNAM; OCIM **90-4251**

KELLOGG, John H[arvey] (1852-1943)
The value of strength tests in the prescription of exercise. Battle Creek, 1896. 25p. 2 charts, 1 table. DNLM **90-4252**

KELLOGG, John H[arvey] (1852-1943)
A certain and successful method of shortening the round ligaments. [Grand Rapids, 1897.] 28p. DNLM **90-4253**

KELLOGG, John H[arvey] (1852-1943)
Special sanitariums for the treatment of disorders of the stomach. Battle Creek, Mich., 1897. 16p. DNLM **90-4254**

KELLOGG, John H[arvey] (1852-1943)
Outline views of the human figure. Chicago, London & Battle Creek, 1898. 20 plates. eleph. fol. DNLM **90-4255**

KELLOGG, Theodore H[arvey] (1841-1931)
Frequent disorders of pneumogastric functions, in insanity. Geneva, N.Y.: W. F. Humphrey, 1894. 12p. DNLM **90-4256**

KELLOGG, Theodore H[arvey] (1841-1931)
The pulse in insanity; original study of cases. Geneva, N.Y.: [W. F. Humphrey], 1895. 13p. DNLM **90-4257**

KELLOGG, Theodore H[arvey] (1841-1931)
A text-book on mental diseases, for the use of students and practitioners of medicine. . . . New York: William Wood & Co., 1897. 776p. diags. DLC; DNLM; NNNAM **90-4258**

KELLY, A[loysius] O[liver] J[oseph] (1870-1911)
The advantages presented by London to the American medical student. Philadelphia, 1893. 4p. DNLM **90-4259**

KELLY, A[loysius] O[liver] J[oseph] (1870-1911)
The opportunities offered by Prague, Heidelberg, and Dublin to the American medical student. Philadelphia, 1893. 4p. DNLM **90-4260**

KELLY, A[loysius] O[liver] J[oseph] (1870-1911)
Athetosis. Philadelphia, 1895. 4p. DNLM **90-4261**

KELLY, A[loysius] O[liver] J[oseph] (1870-1911)
Two cases of carcinoma of the pancreas. Philadelphia, 1895. 6p. DNLM **90-4262**

KELLY, A[loysius] O[liver] J[oseph] (1870-1911)
Venous phenomena. New York, 1896. 35p. DNLM **90-4263**

KELLY, Howard Atwood (1858-1943)
Cephalhaematoma. A case of sub-pericranial blood-tumor in the newborn child. Philadelphia, 1890. 6p. DNLM
90-4264

KELLY, Howard Atwood (1858-1943)
Cephalhaematoma verum externum. Philadelphia: W. J. Dornan, 1890. 79p. DNLM **90-4265**

KELLY, Howard Atwood (1858-1943)
On hysterorrhaphy. [Baltimore, 1890.] 4 l. DNLM
90-4266

KELLY, Howard Atwood (1858-1943)
Supra-vaginal hysterectomy. Hysteromyomectomy with suspension of the stump in the lower angle of the abdominal incision. [Philadelphia, 1890.] 9p. DNLM
90-4267

KELLY, Howard Atwood (1858-1943)
Antisepsis and asepsis before and after major gynecological operations. [Philadelphia, 1891.] 12p. DNLM
90-4268

KELLY, Howard Atwood (1858-1943)
Cancer of the cervix uteri in the negress, with pyo-physometra. Philadelphia, W. J. Dornan, 1891. 7p. DNLM
90-4269

KELLY, Howard Atwood (1858-1943)
A death caused by a uterine dilator, wih some remarks as to the proper method of using the dilator. New York: William Wood & Co., 1891. 7p. DNLM **90-4270**

KELLY, Howard Atwood (1858-1943)
Hand disinfection. New York: William Wood & Co., 1891. 8p. DNLM **90-4271**

KELLY, Howard Atwood (1858-1943)
The ideal dressing for the abdominal wound. New York: William Wood & Co., 1891. 5p. DNLM
90-4272

KELLY, Howard Atwood (1858-1943)
The palpation of normal ovaries. New York, 1891. 16p. DNLM
90-4273

KELLY, Howard Atwood (1858-1943)
The steps of the Caesarean section; the do's and don'ts. New York: William Wood & Co., 1891. 14p. DNLM
90-4274

KELLY, Howard Atwood (1858-1943)
The treatment of large myomatous tumors of the uterus. Myomotomy and hysteromyomectomy. Baltimore, 1891. 7p. DNLM **90-4275**

KELLY, Howard Atwood (1858-1943)
Address at the third annual commencement of the Training School for Nurses of the Wilkes-Barre City Hospital, July 1, 1892. Wilkes-Barre, Pa.: E. B. Yordz, 1892. 18p. DNLM
90-4276

KELLY, Howard Atwood (1858-1943)
Clinical report of cystectomy for polycystic ovarian tumor. [Philadelphia, 1892.] 6p. DNLM
90-4277

KELLY, Howard Atwood (1858-1943)
Gynaecological technique. A brief summary of the principles involved as well as the technique of the gynaecological operations performed in the Johns Hopkins Hospital. The significance of the operation and its technical surroundings to gynaecological practice. New York: M. J. Rooney, 1892. 8p. 14 plates. DNLM **90-4278**

KELLY, Howard Atwood (1858-1943)
A letter to my assistant on the methods of securing asepsis in the preparation of instruments, ligatures, and dressings in my private office. New York: William Wood & Co., 1892. 8p. DNLM **90-4279**

KELLY, Howard Atwood (1858-1943)
The ministry of nursing. An address delivered to the second class of nurses graduating at the Johns Hopkins Hospital, June 3, 1892. [Baltimore, 1892.] 14p. DNLM
90-4280

KELLY, Howard Atwood (1858-1943)
Abstract of a paper on urinalysis in gynaecology. New York, 1893. 3p. DNLM **90-4281**

KELLY, Howard Atwood (1858-1943)
The early treatment of carcinoma uteri. [New York: D. Appleton & Co., 1893.] 2p. DNLM
90-4282

KELLY, Howard Atwood (1858-1943)
The ethical side of the operation of oöphorectomy. New York, 1893. 2p. DNLM **90-4283**

KELLY, Howard Atwood (1858-1943)
The examination under anaesthesia; its uses and its limitations. [New York, 1893.] 7p. DNLM
90-4284

KELLY, Howard Atwood (1858-1943)
My recent ureteral work; catherterization of the ureters. [Philadelphia, 1893.] 16p. 6 plates. DNLM
90-4285

KELLY, Howard Atwood (1858-1943)
A preliminary report on the morphology of ovarian and myomatous tumors. New York, 1893. 22p. 1 plate. DNLM
90-4286

KELLY, Howard Atwood (1858-1943)
The advantage of atmospheric distention of the rectum, with dislodgment of the small intestines, in the bimanual examination of the uterus, ovaries, and tubes. New York: William Wood & Co., 1894. 3p. DNLM **90-4287**

KELLY, Howard Atwood (1858-1943)
The cystoscope. New York: William Wood & Co., 1894. 6p. DNLM **90-4288**

KELLY, Howard Atwood (1858-1943)
The diagnosis of pelvic inflammatory diseases. Philadelphia: Univ. Penn. Press, 1894. 5p. DNLM
90-4289

KELLY, Howard Atwood (1858-1943)
The direct examination of the female bladder with elevated pelvis; the catheterization of the ureters under direct inspection, with and without elevation of the pelvis. New York: William Wood & Co., 1894. 19p. DNLM
90-4290

KELLY, Howard Atwood (1858-1943)
Dysmenorrhoea. [New York, 1894.] 4p. DNLM
90-4291

KELLY, Howard Atwood (1858-1943)
Electric illumination of the field in abdominal surgery. New York: William Wood & Co., 1894. 6p. DNLM
90-4292

KELLY, Howard Atwood (1858-1943)
Results in hystero-myomectomy. The direct examination of the female bladder and catheterization of the ureters under direct inspection. [1894, *vel subseq.*] 8p. DNLM
90-4293

KELLY, Howard Atwood (1858-1943)
Resuscitation, from impending death due to concealed hemorrhage, by the infusion of a litre of normal salt solution centrally into the radial artery. New York: William Wood & Co., 1894. 8p. DNLM **90-4294**

KELLY, Howard Atwood (1858-1943)
A study of intra-abdominal pressure, with practical deductions. Cleveland, 1894. 8p. DNLM **90-4295**

KELLY, Howard Atwood (1858-1943)
Uretero-ureteral anastomosis; uretero-preterostomy. [Philadelphia, 1894.] 8p. DNLM **90-4296**

KELLY, Howard Atwood (1858-1943)
Diagnosis of renal calculus in women. Philadelphia, 1895. 12p. DNLM **90-4297**

KELLY, Howard Atwood (1858-1943)
A new method of examination and treatment of diseases of the rectum and sigmoid flexure. Philadelphia, 1895. 12p. DNLM **90-4298**

KELLY, Howard Atwood (1858-1943)
Suspension of the uterus. Chicago, 1895. 11p. DNLM
90-4299

KELLY, Howard Atwood (1858-1943)
Conservatism in ovariotomy. Chicago: Amer. Medical. Assoc. Press, 1896. 11p. DNLM **90-4300**

KELLY, Howard Atwood (1858-1943)
Delivery by traction on the scalp of the child. New York: William Wood & Co., 1896. 2p. DNLM
90-4301

KELLY, Howard Atwood (1858-1943)
Five case of ovariotomy in women over seventy years of age. New York: William Wood & Co., 1896. 6p. DNLM
90-4302

KELLY, Howard Atwood (1858-1943)
Personal purity. [Washington], 1896. 16p. DNLM
90-4303

KELLY, Howard Atwood (1858-1943)
Some recent important advances in the diagnosis and treatment of urinary diseases in women. Pittsburgh, 1896. 8p. DNLM **90-4304**

KELLY, Howard Atwood (1858-1943)
State regulation of the social evil. Washington: Purity Publ. Co., 1896. 15p. DNLM **90-4305**

KELLY, Howard Atwood (1858-1943)
The treatment of backward displacements of the uterus. Philadelphia, 1896. 20p. DNLM **90-4306**

KELLY, Howard Atwood (1858-1943)
The treatment of extra-uterine pregnancy, ruptured in the early months, by vaginal puncture and drainage. New York, 1896. 23p. DNLM **90-4307**

KELLY, Howard Atwood (1858-1943)
The conservative treatment of myomatous uteri. Chicago, 1897. 4p. DNLM **90-4308**

KELLY, Howard Atwood (1858-1943)
The sources and diagnosis of pyuria. Philadelphia, 1897. 19p. DNLM **90-4309**

KELLY, Howard Atwood (1858-1943)
The catheterization of the ureters in the male through an open cystoscope with the bladder distended with air by posture. Baltimore, 1898. 2p. DNLM **90-4310**

KELLY, Howard Atwood (1858-1943)
Cystoscopy and catheterization of the ureters in the male. Philadelphia, 1898. 12p. DNLM **90-4311**

KELLY, Howard Atwood (1858-1943)
The hand basin in use in surgical operating rooms. New York: William Wood & Co., 1898. 6p. DNLM
90-4312

KELLY, Howard Atwood (1858-1943)
A preliminary report upon the examination of the bladder and the catheterization of ureters in men. Philadelphia, 1898. 3p. DNLM **90-4313**

KELLY, Howard Atwood (1858-1943)
Operative gynecology. . . . With twenty-four plates and over five hundred and fifty original illustrations. New York: D. Appleton & Co., 1898. 2 v. plates. DLC; DNLM; NNNAM; PPC **90-4314**

KELLY, Howard Atwood (1858-1943) and W. G. MacCALLUM
Pneumaturia. Chicago, 1898. 23p. DNLM
90-4315

KELLY, Howard Atwood (1858-1943)
The preservation of the hymen. New York: William Wood & Co., 1898. 8p. DNLM **90-4316**

KELLY, Howard Atwood (1858-1943)
A curette for cervical cancer. New York, 1899. 2p. DNLM
90-4317

KELLY, Howard Atwood (1858-1943)
The dissection and liberation of the sphincter and muscle followed by its direct suture in cases of complete tearing of the perineum, with a splinting suture passing between the outer and inner margins of the muscle. Baltimore, 1899. 19p. 4 plates. DNLM **90-4318**

KELLY, Howard Atwood (1858-1943)
The exploration of the abdomen as an adjunct to every celiotomy. New York, 1899. 6p. DNLM **90-4319**

KELLY, Howard Atwood (1858-1943)
A new handle and grip for scissors for plastic and other delicate work. New York, 1899. 2p. DNLM **90-4320**

KELLY, Howard Atwood (1858-1943)
The recognition of the poisonous serpents of North America. Baltimore, 1899. 11p. 6 plates. **90-4321**

KELLY, Howard Atwood (1858-1943)
The reflux of air into the ureters through the air-distended bladder in the knee-breast posture. New York, 1899. 2p. DNLM **90-4322**

KELLY, Howard Atwood (1858-1943)
Some new instruments to facilitate the operation of myomectomy. New York, 1899. 4p. DNLM **90-4323**

KELLY, Howard Atwood (1858-1943)
Operative gynecology. . . . [2nd ed.] New York: D. Appleton & Co., 1899-1900. 2 v. plates. DNLM; NNNAM; PPC; PU **90-4324**

KELSEY, Charles B[oyd] (1850-1917)
Stricture of the rectum; intestinal obstruction; inguinal colotomy. [Philadelphia, 1890.] 13p. DNLM **90-4325**

KELSEY, Charles B[oyd] (1850-1917)
Stricture of the rectum; a study of ninety-six cases. [New York, 1890.] 46p. DNLM **90-4326**

KELSEY, Charles B[oyd] (1850-1917)
The diagnosis and treatment of haemorrhoids, with general rules as to the examination of rectal diseases. . . . Detroit, Mich.: G. S. Davis, 1890. 78p. DLC; OCIM **90-4327**

KELSEY, Charles B[oyd] (1850-1917)
Diseases of the rectum and anus; their pathology, diagnosis, and treatment. . . . 3rd ed., rewritten and enlarged. . . . New York: William Wood & Co., 1890. 483p. col. plates. DLC; DNLM; NNNAM; PPC **90-4328**

KELSEY, Charles B[oyd] (1850-1917)
Stricture of the rectum; a study of ninety-six cases. [2nd ed.] [New York, 1891.] 48p. DNLM **90-4329**

KELSEY, Charles B[oyd] (1850-1917)
The choice between extirpation and colotomy in cancer of the rectum. New York, 1892. 8p. DNLM **90-4330**

KELSEY, Charles B[oyd] (1850-1917)
The indications for colotomy. Detroit: G. S. Davis, 1892. 6p. DNLM **90-4331**

KELSEY, Charles B[oyd] (1850-1917)
The second year's work in diseases of the rectum at the New York Post-Graduate Hospital. [New York, 1892.] 7p. DNLM **90-4332**

KELSEY, Charles B[oyd] (1850-1917)
Diseases of the rectum and anus; their pathology, diagnosis, and treatment. . . . 4th ed., rev. and enl. New York: William Wood & Co., 1893. 490p. col. plates. DLC; DNLM; NNNAM **90-4333**

KELSEY, Charles B[oyd] (1850-1917)
Abscess around the rectum. Detroit: G. S. Davis, 1893. 8p. DNLM **90-4334**

KELSEY, Charles B[oyd] (1850-1917)
Colotomy. A clinical lecture. Detroit: G. S. Davis, 1893. 8p. DNLM **90-4335**

KELSEY, Charles B[oyd] (1850-1917)
Four years' work in diseases of the rectum at the Post-Graduate Hospital Clinic. [New York, 1893.] 8p. DNLM **90-4336**

KELSEY, Charles B[oyd] (1850-1917)
How to operate for hemorrhoids. A clinical lecture. Detroit: G. S. Davis, 1893. 16p. DNLM **90-4337**

KELSEY, Charles B[oyd] (1850-1917)
The third year's work at the clinic for diseases of the rectum in the New York Post-Graduate Hospital. [New York, 1893.] 7p. DNLM **90-4338**

KELSEY, Charles B[oyd] (1850-1917)
Five years' work in diseases of the rectum at the New York Post-Graduate Hospital. [New York: D. Appleton & Co., 1894.] 10p. DNLM **90-4339**

KELSEY, Charles B[oyd] (1850-1917)
Surgery of the rectum and pelvis. . . . With two hundred and eighty-one illustrations and half-tone plates. New York: R. Kettles & Co., 1897. 573p. DLC; DNLM; NNNAM **90-4340**

KELSEY, Charles B[oyd] (1850-1917)
The office treatment of hemorrhoids, fistula, etc., without operation; together with remarks on the relation of diseases of the rectum to other diseases in both sexes, but especially in women, and the abuse of the operation of colostomy. New York: E. R. Pelton, 1898. 68p. DNLM **90-4341**

KEMP, Robert C[oleman] (*b.* 1865)
Indications for the use of the double-current rectal irrigator; position of the patient, temperature of the fluid, solutions employed, etc. New York, 1897. 24p. DNLM **90-4342**

KEMP, Robert C[oleman] (*b.* 1865)
Further experimental researches on the effects of different anaesthetics on the kidneys. New York, 1899. 38p. 1 plate, 8 diags. DNLM **90-4343**

KEMPER, W[illiam] H[arrison] (1839-1927)
One thousand cases of labor, and their lessons. [Philadelphia, 1891.] 27p. DNLM **90-4344**

KEMPTER, J. Elmond
Ethyl bromide as an anesthetic in minor surgery. Baltimore, 1899. 3p. DNLM **90-4345**

KENISTON, J[ames] M[ortimer] (*b.* 1848)
Analgesia in insanity. [Utica, N.Y., 1890.] 10p. DNLM **90-4346**

KENISTON, J[ames] M[ortimer] (*b.* 1848)
Report of two interesting cases. Word-blindness; localized muscular spasms illustrating cerebral localization. New York, 1895. 13p. DNLM **90-4347**

KENNEDY, Catherine M. and Charles F. J. KENNEDY
Cystic degeneration of the chorionic villi. [Philadelphia, 1894.] 4p. DNLM **90-4348**

KENNEDY, James
Resection of both ulnar bones, with an experiment in bone-grafting. Philadelphia, 1892. 6p. DNLM
90-4349

KENNEDY, James C.
Why we should operate early in appendicitis. New York, 1896. 8p. DNLM **90-4350**

KENNEDY, James C.
Hydatidiform mole. New York, 1898. 4p. DNLM
90-4351

KENNEDY, James S.
Irregular gout. New York, 1898. 2p. DNLM
90-4352

KENNEDY, Samuel (*d.* 1900)
Gunshot wound of the chest; report of a case; recovery. New York, 1897. 8p. DNLM **90-4353**

KENNER, Robert C. (*b.* 1859)
Contributions of physicians to English and American literature. Detroit: G. S. Davis, 1892. 93p. DNLM; NNNAM; OCIM
90-4354

KENNER, Robert C. (*b.* 1859)
The treatment of typhoid fever; with clinical reports. New Albany, Ind., 1898. 6p. DNLM **90-4355**

KENSINGTON HOSPITAL FOR WOMEN. PHILADELPHIA
Facts concerning the . . . of interest to the public. Philadelphia: Craig, Finley & Co., [1890]. 7p. DNLM
90-4356

KENSINGTON HOSPITAL FOR WOMEN. PHILADELPHIA
Special report of the. . . . From its organization in 1883 until 1896. By Charles P. Noble, surgeon in chief. [Philadelphia: R. E. Lynch, 1896.] 22p. DNLM; PPC
90-4357

KENT, James Tyler (1849-1916)
Repertory of the homoeopathic materia medica. . . . Lancaster, Pa.: Examiner Printing House, 1897-[-99]. 1349p. DLC; OCLloyd; PPHa **90-4358**

KENTUCKY UNIVERSITY. MEDICAL DEPARTMENT, LOUISVILLE
Annual announcements for the sessions of 1899-1901 (1.-3.); 1903 (5.). Louisville, 1898-1902. DNLM
90-4359

KENWOOD, H[enry] R[ichard] (*b.* 1862)
Public health; laboratory work. Including methods employed in bacteriological research, with special reference to the examination of air, water, and food, contributed by Rubert Boyce. Philadelphia: P. Blakiston, Son & Co., 1893. 491p. 3 plates. DNLM; NNNAM; PPC; PU **90-4360**

KEOKUK MEDICAL COLLEGE, IOWA
Annual announcements for the sessions of 1890-91 to 1893-94 (1.-4.); 1895-96 to 1898-99 (6.-9.). Keokuk, 1890-98. DNLM [Organized 1890. In 1899 the College of Physicians and Surgeons, Keokuk, united with this school under the following title: Keokuk Medical College, College of Physicians and Surgeons, Keokuk.] **90-4361**

KEOKUK MEDICAL COLLEGE, COLLEGE OF PHYSICIANS AND SURGEONS, KEOKUK
Annual announcements for the sessions of 1899-1900 (59.); 1902-03 (62.). Keokuk, 1899-1902. DNLM [The title of this school is formed by the union of two medical schools located at Keokuk, viz.: The Keokuk Medical College, established in 1899, and the College of Physicians and Surgeons, established in 1849, under the title: College of Physicians and Surgeons of the Upper Mississippi, at Davenport. The numbering of the announcements dates from 1849, including the eight summer sessions held in 1863-65 and 1873-77, which makes the session of 1899-1900 the fifty-ninth. The announcement for 1902-03 contains a list of the alumni of the College of Physicians and Surgeons from its organization in 1849, and the alumni of the united school from 1900 to 1902.] **90-4362**

KERLEY, Charles G[ilmore] (*b.* 1863)
Clinical history of a "Walker-Gordon baby." New York, 1895. 4p. DNLM **90-4363**

KERLEY, Charles G[ilmore] (*b.* 1863)
Acute gastro-intestinal infection in infants. New York, 1898. 13p. DNLM **90-4364**

KERLIN, Isaac N[ewton] (1834-1893)
The moral imbecile. [Boston, 1890.] 13p. DNLM
90-4365

KERR, James
A case of intra-peritoneal rupture of the bladder; recovery after laparotomy. [Philadelphia, 1893.] 7p. DNLM
90-4366

KERR, James
Report of some of the surgical work at the new Emergency Hospital during the past year. [Washington, D.C., 1893.] 16p. DNLM **90-4367**

KERR, James
A case of rupture of the lung, unassociated with fractures of the ribs, with early subsequent recovery. Reported by W. L. Pyle. [Philadelphia, 1894.] 3p. DNLM
90-4368

KERR, Norman (1834-1899)
Inebriety or narcomania. Its etiology, pathology. Treatment and jurisprudence. New York: H. K. Lewis, 1894. 646p. NN; NNNAM **90-4369**

KERSHAW, J. Martine
Long continued congestion of the brain is the forerunner of paralysis. Auxiliary measures in the treatment of congestion of the brain. St. Louis, 1890. 3p. DNLM
90-4370

KERSHNER, Edward
Yellow fever prophylaxis in infected ports. [New York, 1894.] 16p. DNLM **90-4371**

KEYES, Edward Lawrence (1843-1924)
Some fallacies concerning syphilis. . . . Detroit, Mich.: G. S. Davis, 1890. 71p. DLC; OCIM **90-4372**

KEYES, Edward Lawrence (1843-1924)
The tonic treatment of syphilis. . . . Rev. ed. New York: D. Appleton & Co., 1896. 78p. DLC; NNNAM
90-4373

KEYES, Thomas Bassett
Hypnotic anesthesia. New York, 1896. 2p. DNLM
90-4374

KEYES, Thomas Bassett
Hypnotic suggestion as a cure for asthma. Philadelphia, 1896. 2 l. DNLM **90-4375**

KEYES, Thomas Bassett
The treatment of dipsomania, morphiomania, and onanism by hypnotism. New York, 1896. 2 l. DNLM
90-4376

KEYES, Thomas Bassett
Osteopathic treatment in the hypnotic state; or, Suggestion-massage: the cure for incurables. . . . Chicago, [1899]. 46p. plates. DLC **90-4377**

KILMER, Fred B[arnett] (*b.* 1851)
Modern surgical dressings. Philadelphia, 1897. 16p. DNLM
90-4378

KILNER, Walter B.
A compendium of modern pharmacy and druggists' formulary. 6th ed. Springfield, 1890-95. 2 v. DNLM; OCLloyd
90-4379

KIMBER, Diana Clifford
Text-book of anatomy and physiology for nurses. . . . New York and London: Macmillan & Co., 1894. 268p. DLC; NNNAM **90-4380**

KIMBERLEY, William T.
A new system of medicine for domestic practice. . . . [Guthrie, Okl.: Representative Print], 1896. 31p. DLC
90-4381

KIME, R[ufus] R. (*b.* 1857)
The drainage-tube in puerperal infection. New York, 1895. 3p. DNLM **90-4382**

KIME, R[ufus] R. (*b.* 1857)
The present status of puerperal infection. Boston, 1897. 15p. DNLM **90-4383**

KIME, R[ufus] R. (*b.* 1857)
Some practical thoughts on the development of the human race and obstetric nursing. Atlantic: Franklin Print. & Publ. Co., [1898]. 21p. DNLM **90-4384**

KING, Albert Freeman Africanus (1841-1914)
The nervous autonomy of the human body in health and disease. Philadelphia, 1891. 7p. DNLM
90-4385

KING, Albert Freeman Africanus (1841-1914)
Hysteria. New York: William Wood & Co., 1891. 22p. DNLM
90-4386

KING, Albert Freeman Africanus (1841-1914)
A manual of obstetrics. . . . 5th ed. Philadelphia: Lea Bros. & Co., 1892. 450p. DLC; DNLM; PPC; PU
90-4387

KING, Albert Freeman Africanus (1841-1914)
A manual of obstetrics. . . . 6th ed. Philadelphia: Lea Bros. & Co., 1895. 533p. DNLM; NNNAM; PPC; PPJ
90-4388

KING, Albert Freeman Africanus (1841-1914)
A manual of obstetrics. . . . 7th ed., with two hundred and twenty-three illustrations. Philadelphia and New York: Lea Bros. & Co., 1898. 574p. DLC; DNLM; MBM; PPC
90-4389

KING, E[lbridge] H.
An unusual accident after celiotomy. [Philadelphia, Lea Bros. & Co., 1894.] 2p. DNLM **90-4390**

KING, Emil
The antiseptic treatment of typhoid fever with the chlorin-quinin solution. [Philadelphia, 1895.] 10p. DNLM
90-4391

KING, Ferdinand
Flushing the colon. New York, 1894. 7p. DNLM
90-4392

KING, George W.
The physician's responsibility in the treatment of fractures. [New York, 1892.] 7p. DNLM **90-4393**

KING, Herbert Maxon
Suppurative disease of the necessary sinuses of the nose. [New York, 1894.] 12p. DNLM **90-4394**

KING, Herbert Maxon
A case of renal phthisis complicating pulmonary tuberculosis. New York, 1896. 10p. DNLM **90-4395**

KING, John (1813-1893)
The American family physician; or, domestic guide to health. Prepared expressly for the use of families, in language adapted to the understanding of the people. Arranged in two divisions. Indianapolis: R. Douglas, 1892. 2 v. in 1. [792p., 14 plates, 348p.] DNLM; OCLloyd **90-4396**

KING, John (1813-1893)
King's eclectic obstetrics. Rewritten, rev. and enl. by Robert C. Wintermute. . . . 9th ed. Cincinnati: The Ohio Valley Co., 1892. 747p. DLC; DNLM; OCIM **90-4397**

KING, John (1813-1893) and John H. LLOYD
The American dispensatory . . . rev. and enl. with supplement. [17th ed.] Cincinnati: The Ohio Valley Co., 1895. 1439p. OCLloyd **90-4398**

KING, John Henry (*b.* 1843)
Dr. King's medical prescriptions carefully compiled and formulated. Containing the favorite formulas of the most eminent medical authorities, collected from their published writings. . . . Atlanta, Ga.: J. P. Harrison & Co., 1890. 346p. DLC
90-4399

KING, John H[enry] (*b.* 1843)
Man, an organic community; being an exposition of the law that the human personality in all its phases in evolution, both coordinate and discoordinate, is the multiple of many sub-personalities. New York: G. P. Putnam's Sons, 1893. 2 v. DNLM; NNNAM **90-4400**

KING, John H[enry] (*b.* 1843)
Dr. King's medical prescriptions, containing the favorite formulas of the most eminent medical authorities, collected from their published writings. 2nd ed. New York: Bailey & Fairchild, 1896. 346p. DNLM; NNNAM
90-4401

KING, R. B.
How to examine absorbent cotton. [Chicago, 1898.] 1 galley sheet. DNLM **90-4402**

KING, Willis P[ercival] (1839-1909)
Stories of a country doctor. Philadelphia: Hummel & Parmele, 1891. 397p. DNLM; PU **90-4403**

KING, Willis P[ercival] (1839-1909)
Intracranial aneurism of the carotid; recovery. [Kansas City, 1891.] 14p. DNLM **90-4404**

KINGMAN, R[ufus] A[nderson]
Report of a second case of double ovariotomy during pregnancy, with hydatiform mole. Boston: [Damrell & Upham], 1899. 6p. DNLM **90-4405**

KING'S American Dispensatory. By Harvey Wickes Felter and John Uri Lloyd. Entirely rewritten and enlarged. 18th ed., third revision. Cincinnati: Ohio Valley Co., 1898. v. 1 [904p.] DNLM; OCLloyd **90-4406**

[KINGSBURY, Charles A.]
The valuable library of the late . . . , to be sold by Thos. Birch's Sons. Philadelphia, 1891. 24p. DNLM
90-4407

KINGSLEY, Adriel S.
A bold arraignment of the medical profession, for the practice of false theories, false pretenses, fraudulent claims for a false science, and for their determined purpose to oppose the cold bath in all fevers. . . . With the papers attached of Drs. Simon Baruch and G. C. Smythe, read before their respective medical societies, on the treatment of typhoid fever with cold water. . . . Indianapolis, Ind.: Indianapolis Printing Co., 1890. 361p. port. DLC **90-4408**

KINGSLEY, Norman W[illiam] (1829-1913)
Adenoid growths, mouth-breathing, and thumb-sucking in their relation to deformities of the jaws and irregular teeth. Philadelphia: S. S. White Dental Mfg. Co., 1892. 31p. port. DNLM; PPC **90-4409**

KINGSLEY, Norman W[illiam] (1829-1913)
Cleft palate. Philadelphia, 1894. 15p. DNLM
90-4410

KINLOCH, R[obert] A[lexander] (1826-1891)
Drainage of wounds, with special reference to drainage after urethrotomy. [Charleston, 1891.] 11p. DNLM
90-4411

KINNEAR, B[everley] O.
Neurasthenia or neurosthenia, which? and an efficient treatment. New York, 1898. 8p. DNLM
90-4412

KINNEAR, B[everley] O.
Pneumonia, treated by heat over the spine and by the inhalation of pure oxygen. New York, 1898. 8p. DNLM
90-4413

KINNEY, C. Spencer
Melancholia and its treatment. Utica, 1897. 40p. DNLM **90-4414**

KIPP, Charles J[ohn] (1835-1911)
A case of acute purulent inflammation of the middle ear with double optic neuritis, but without tenderness or swelling of, or spontaneous pain in, the mastoid process, in which the opening of the mastoid cells was followed by a rapid subsidence of the optic neuritis and cure of the ear disease. [New Bedford, 1892.] 5p. DNLM **90-4415**

KIPP, Charles J[ohn] (1835-1911)
A case of bilateral recurrent inflammation of Ténon's capsule in connection with profound mercurial poisoning. [Hartford, 1892.] 4p. DNLM **90-4416**

KIPPAX, John Robert (*b.* 1849)
A hand-book of diseases of the skin, and their homoeopathic treatment. . . . 4th ed.; rev. and enl. Chicago: Gross & Delbridge, 1890. 294p. diags. DLC; DNLM; OCIM
90-4417

KIPPAX, John Robert (*b.* 1849)
A hand-book of diseases of the skin, and their homoeopathic treatment. . . . 5th ed., revised and enlarged. Chicago: Gross & Delbridge, 1893. 294p. DNLM; OCIM
90-4418

KIRBY, Ellwood R.
Manual of genito-urinary diseases. Philadelphia: F. W. S. Langmaid, 1899. 143p. 60 plates. CtY-M; DNLM; PPC; PPJ **90-4419**

KIRCHHOFF, Friedrich A[ugust] T[heodor] (1853-1922)
Handbook of insanity for practitioners and students. New York: William Wood & Co., 1893. 362p. 11 plates. DNLM; MBM; NNNAM; PPC **90-4420**

KIRK, Edward C[ameron] (1856-1933)
The manual-training idea as a factor in dental education. [Philadelphia, 1890.] 26p. DNLM **90-4421**

KIRK, Edward C[ameron] (1856-1933)
On coagulants in the treatment of the pulp-chamber and canals. Philadelphia, 1894. 10p. DNLM
90-4422

KIRK, Edward C[ameron], ed. (1856-1933)
The American text-book of operative dentistry. In contributions by eminent authorities. . . . Philadelphia and New York: Lea Bros. & Co., 1897. 702p. DLC; NNNAM; PPC; PU
90-4423

KIRK, Eleanor (1831-1908)
The prevention and cure of old age. Brooklyn: E. Kirk, [1899]. 156p. DNLM; NN **90-4424**

KIRKENDALL, John S.
Epilepsy and eye strain. New York, 1897. 4p. DNLM
90-4425

KIRKES, William Senhouse (1823-1864)
Manual of physiology. . . . 13th ed. Philadelphia: P. Blakiston, Son & Co., 1892. 884p. 3 plates. DNLM; MBM; NNNAM; PPC **90-4426**

KIRKES, William Senhouse (1823-1864)
Manual of physiology. . . . By W. D. Halliburton, 14th ed. Philadelphia: P. Blakiston, Son & Co., 1896. 851p. 2 plates. CtY-M; DNLM; IEN-M; NNNAM
90-4427

KIRKES, William Senhouse (1823-1864)
Kirkes' handbook of physiology. Handbook of physiology by W. M. Baker and V. D. Harris. American revision of chapters on the nervous system by C. L. Dana. New York: William Wood & Co., 1896. 847p. DLC; DNLM; NNNAM; PU **90-4428**

KIRKES, William Senhouse (1823-1864)
Manual of physiology. . . . By W. D. Halliburton. 15th ed. Philadelphia: P. Blakiston, Son & Co., 1899. 872p. 3 plates. DNLM; NNNAM; PPC; PPJ **90-4429**

KIRKES, William Senhouse (1823-1864)
Handbook of physiology, by W. Morrant Baker . . . and Vincent Dormer Harris. . . . 15th American ed., rev. by Warren Coleman . . . and Charles L. Dana. . . . With upwards of five hundred illustrations including many in colors. New York: William Wood & Co., 1899. 840p. col. frontis. DLC; DNLM; NNNAM; PPC **90-4430**

KIRSTEIN, Alfred (*b.* 1863)
Autoscopy of the larynx and trachea (direct examination without mirror). Authorized transl. (altered, enlarged, and revised by the author) by Max Thorner. Philadelphia: F. A. Davis & Co., 1897. 68p. DNLM; PPC **90-4431**

KIRWIN, G[eorge] H[enry] (1856-1895)
Modern surgery of the pelvic floor in women. New York, 1895. 18p. DNLM **90-4432**

KITCHEL, Edwin M. (*d.* 1897)
Notes on the fixation of nerve fibres by formalin. New York: D. Appleton & Co., 1895. 3p. DNLM **90-4433**

KLEBS, E[dwin] Th. A. (1834-1913)
The treatment of tuberculosis with tuberculocidin. A preliminary communication. [New York: G. Wirsing, 1892.] 24p. DNLM **90-4434**

KLEBS, E[dwin] Th. A. (1834-1913)
Anatomic researches on yellow fever. Chicago, 1898. 12p. DNLM **90-4435**

KLEEN, Emil [A. G.] (1847-1923)
Handbook of massage. Authorized translation from the Swedish, by Edward Mussey Hartwell, Philadelphia: P. Blakiston, Son & Co., 1892. 316p. DNLM; PPC **90-4436**

KLEEN, Emil [A. G.] (1847-1923)
Carlsbad. A medico-practical guide. New York & London, 1893. 101p. DNLM; NNNAM **90-4437**

KLEIN, Carl H. von
Intubation of the larynx. Cleveland, O.: Buel, Mather & Hubell, 1891. 7p. DNLM **90-4438**

KLEIN, [Edward] Emanuel (1844-1925)
Elements of histology. Revised and enlarged ed., by E. Klein and J. S. Edkins. Philadelphia & New York: Lea Bros. & Co., [1898]. 500p. DNLM; IU-M; NNNAM; PPC **90-4439**

KLEMPERER, Georg (1865-1946)
The elements of clinical diagnosis. . . . 1st American from the 7th (last) German ed., with sixty-one illustrations. Authorized transl. by Nathan E. Brill . . . and Samuel M. Brickner. . . . New York: The Macmillan Co.; London: Macmillan & Co., Ltd., 1893. 292p. diags. DLC; NNNAM **90-4440**

KLINGENSMITH, I[srael] P[utnam] (1850?-1904)
The care of the injured by the Pennsylvania Railroad. Blairesville, Pa., 1892. 6p. DNLM **90-4441**

KLINGENSMITH, I[srael] P[utnam] (1850?-1904)
Strangulated hernia; the importance of its early recognition, and advantages of prompt operative interference. Blairsville, Pa., 1894. 5p. DNLM **90-4442**

KLOPHEL, C. G. Buchanan
Urinary, urethral, catheter or urine fever; with the report of a case. Detroit: G. S. Davis, 1890. 28p. DNLM **90-4443**

KLOTZ, Hermann G[ustav] (*b.* 1844)
Notes on pilocarpine in dermatology. [New York, 1890.] 8p. DNLM **90-4444**

KLOTZ, Hermann G[ustav] (*b.* 1844)
A case of pemphigus foliaceus ending fatally within eight months. [Philadelphia, 1891.] 8p. DNLM **90-4445**

KLOTZ, Hermann G[ustav] (*b.* 1844)
On the occurrence of tertiary lesions of syphilis as the result of direct local infection, with general remarks on syphilis as an infectious disease. [New York, 1893.] 16p. DNLM **90-4446**

KLOTZ, Hermann G[ustav] (*b.* 1844)
Endoscopic studies on vegetations, polyps, angeioma, membranes, and diphtheritic urethritis, suppuration from the ejaculatory ducts, cyst of the colliculus seminalis, etc. [New York: D. Appleton & Co., 1895.] 24p. DNLM **90-4447**

KNAPP, J[akob] H[ermann] (1832-1911)
Operations usually performed in eye-surgery. Philadelphia, 1898. 163p. 1 plate. DNLM; NNNAM; PPC **90-4448**

KNAPP, Miland A[ustin] (*b.* 1868)
Teeth regulation, with finely made original devices ready for immediate operative application without soldering. . . . Philadelphia, Pa.: The S. S. White Dental Manufacturing Co., 1899. 53p. DLC; MdU-D **90-4449**

KNAPP, Philip Coombs (1858-1920)
Accidents from the electric current; a contribution to the study of the action of currents of high potential upon the human organism. Boston: Damrell & Upham, 1890. 43p. DNLM **90-4450**

KNAPP, Philip Coombs (1858-1920)
The insanity of doubt. [Worcester, 1890.] 23p. DNLM **90-4451**

KNAPP, Philip Coombs (1858-1920)
Astasia-abasia. With the report of a case of paroxysmal trepidant abasia associated with paralysis agitans. [New York, 1891.] 31p. DNLM **90-4452**

KNAPP, Philip Coombs (1858-1920)
A contribution from brain surgery to the study of the localization of the sensory centres in the cerebral cortex. Boston: Damrell & Upham, 1891. 12p. DNLM **90-4453**

KNAPP, Philip Coombs (1858-1920)
The pathology, diagnosis, and treatment of intra-cranial growths. Fiske fund prize essay. Boston: Rockwell & Churchill, 1891. 165p. DNLM **90-4454**

KNAPP, Philip Coombs (1858-1920)
A case of tumor of the cerebellum, in which trephining was done for the relief of increased intra-cranial pressure. [New York, 1892.] 10p. DNLM **90-4455**

KNAPP, Philip Coombs (1858-1920)
The nervous and mental sequelae of influenza. [Boston, 1892.] 17p. DNLM **90-4456**

KNAPP, Philip Coombs (1858-1920)
Sudden death from affections of the nervous system. Boston: Damrell & Upham, 1892. 8p. DNLM **90-4457**

KNAPP, Philip Coombs (1858-1920)
Traumatic nervous affections. An attempt of their classification based on a study of ninety cases. Philadelphia, 1892. 15p. DNLM **90-4458**

KNAPP, Philip Coombs (1858-1920) and Abner POST
Two cases of trephining for traumatic epilepsy. Boston: Damrell & Upham, 1892. 20p. DNLM **90-4459**

KNAPP, Philip Coombs (1858-1920)
Simulation in traumatic nervous diseases. Boston: Damrell & Upham, 1893. 14p. DNLM **90-4460**

KNAPP, Philip Coombs (1858-1920)
Recurrent oculo-motor paralysis. Report of a case with recurrent anaesthesia in the distribution of the fifth nerve. Boston: Damrell & Upham, 1894. 19p. DNLM **90-4461**

KNAPP, Philip Coombs (1858-1920)
Spinal concussion. Traumatic spinal sclerosis. Boston: Damrell & Upham, 1894. 18p. DNLM **90-4462**

KNAPP, Philip Coombs (1858-1920)
The alleged reflex causes of nervous diseases. Philadelphia, 1895. 9p. DNLM **90-4463**

KNAPP, Philip Coombs (1858-1920)
President's address delivered at the twenty-first annual meeting of the American Neurological Association, Boston, June 5, 1895. Boston: Damrell & Upham, 1895. 8p. DNLM **90-4464**

KNAPP, Philip Coombs (1858-1920)
The treatment of chorea, with especial reference to the use of quinine. Boston: Damrell & Upham, 1895. 8p. DNLM **90-4465**

KNAPP, Philip Coombs (1858-1920)
The nature of neurasthenia, and its relation to morbid fears and imperative ideas. Boston: Damrell & Upham, 1896. 12p. DNLM **90-4466**

KNAPP, Philip Coombs (1858-1920)
Anesthesia in diseases of the spinal cord. New York, 1897. 20p. DNLM **90-4467**

KNAPP, Philip Coombs (1858-1920)
Three cases of general paralysis preceded by optic atrophy. Boston: Damrell & Upham, 1899. 22p. DNLM **90-4468**

KNAPP, Philip Coombs (1858-1920)
The treatment of cerebral tumors. Boston: Damrell & Upham, 1899. 13p. DNLM **90-4469**

KNEIPP, E. H. Sebastian (1821-1897)
The Kneipp cure; an absolute verbal and literal translation of Meine Wasserkur (My Water Cure). New York: Kneipp Cure Publication Co., [1897?]. 451p. DNLM; NNNAM **90-4470**

KNIES, Max (1851-1917)
Relations of diseases of the eye to general diseases. . . . forming a supplementary volume to every manual and text-book of practical medicine and ophthalmology; ed. by Henry D. Noyes. . . . New York: William Wood & Co., 1895. 467p. DLC; DNLM; NNNAM **90-4471**

KNIGHT, Arthur L.
Brain tumor. Report of a case of psammoma of the right frontal lobe. Cincinnati, 1898. 4p. DNLM **90-4472**

KNIGHT, Charles Huntoon (1849-1913)
Cyst of the middle turbinated bone. [New York, 1892.] 8p. 1 plate. DNLM **90-4473**

KNIGHT, Charles Huntoon (1849-1913)
Intubation for stenosis of the larynx in a boy twelve years old; retention of tube for ten weeks. tracheotomy; death from general tuberculosis. New York, 1892. 6p. DNLM **90-4474**

KNIGHT, Charles Huntoon (1849-1913)
A case of cyst of the epiglottis. New York, 1894. 6p. DNLM **90-4475**

KNIGHT, Charles Huntoon (1849-1913)
A case of torticollis following removal of adenoids of the rhinopharynx, with remarks on nasal reflexes. St. Louis, 1894. 7p. DNLM **90-4476**

KNIGHT, Charles Huntoon (1849-1913)
Three cases of laryngeal neoplasm. [New York: D. Appleton & Co., 1894.] 8p. DNLM **90-4477**

KNIGHT, Charles Huntoon (1849-1913)
Cyst of the maxillary sinus. New York, 1896. 7p. DNLM **90-4478**

KNIGHT, Charles Huntoon (1849-1913)
The sequelae of syphilis and their treatment; nasal sequelae. New York, 1896. 14p. DNLM **90-4479**

KNIGHT, Charles Huntoon (1849-1913)
Exostosis of the septum as a cause of chronic naso-pharyngitis. St. Louis, 1897. 4p. DNLM **90-4480**

KNIGTH, Charles Huntoon (1849-1913)
The president's address, delivered before the American Laryngological Association at its nineteenth annual congress. New York, 1897. 11p. DNLM **90-4481**

KNIGHT, Charles Huntoon (1849-1913)
Three case of obscure laryngeal disease; tuberculosis, syphilis, epithelioma. Philadelphia, 1897. 6p. DNLM **90-4482**

KNIGHT, Frederick Irving (1841-1909)
On the return of cured tubercular patients from high altitudes. New York, 1890. 7p. DNLM **90-4483**

KNIGHT, Frederick Irving (1841-1909)
Henry Ingersoll Bowditch, M.D. The memorial meeting of the section for clinical medicine, pathology, and hygiene of the Massachusetts Medical Society. Boston, 1892. 40p. DNLM **90-4484**

KNIGHT, Frederick Irving (1841-1909)
Remarks on sending patients away from home. Boston: Damrell & Upham, 1893. 6p. DNLM **90-4485**

KNIGHT, Frederick Irving (1841-1909)
Shall anything be done by legal authority to prevent the spread of tuberculosis? Philadelphia, 1894. 5p. DNLM **90-4486**

KNIGHT, Frederick Irving (1841-1909)
Singers' nodes. [New York: D. Appleton & Co., 1894.] 6p. DNLM **90-4487**

KNIGHT, Frederick Irving (1841-1909)
Intermittent dysphonia spastica. New York, 1896. 3p. DNLM **90-4488**

KNIGHT, Frederick Irving (1841-1909)
The treatment of bronchial asthma. Boston: Damrell & Upham, 1897. 10p. DNLM **90-4489**

KNIGHT, Frederick Irving (1841-1909)
Common errors of general practitioners in dealing with cases of pulmonary tuberculosis. [Philadelphia], 1898. 4p. DNLM **90-4490**

KNOPF, S[iegmund] A[dolphus] (1857-1940)
Are sanatoriums for consumptives a danger to the neighborhood? New York, 1896. 7p. DNLM **90-4491**

KNOPF, S[iegmund] A[dolphus] (1857-1940)
Should we treat pulmonary tuberculosis as a contagious or as a communicable disease? Los Angeles, 1896. 4p. DNLM **90-4492**

KNOPF, S[iegmund] A[dolphus] (1857-1940)
The hygienic, educational, and symptomatic treatment of pulmonary tuberculosis. With a plea for sanatoriums for the poor. New York, 1897. 16p. DNLM **90-4493**

KNOPF, S[iegmund] A[dolphus] (1857-1940)
The present status of preventative means against the spread of tuberculosis in the various states of the Union critically reviewed. New York, 1897. 16p. DNLM **90-4494**

KNOPF, S[iegmund] A[dolphus] (1857-1940)
The urgent need of sanatoria for the consumptive poor of our large cities. New York, 1897. 11p. DNLM **90-4495**

KNOPF, S[iegmund] A[dolphus] (1857-1940)
State and municipal care of consumptives. New York, 1898. 15p. DNLM **90-4496**

KNOPF, S[iegmund] A[dolphus] (1857-1940)
Early recognition of pulmonary tuberculosis. Chicago, 1899. 20p. DNLM **90-4497**

KNOPF, S[iegmund] A[dolphus] (1857-1940)
Pulmonary tuberculosis; its modern prophylaxis and the treatment in special institutions and at home; Alvarenga prize essay of the College of Physicians of Philadelphia for the year 1898; rev. and enl. by . . . with descriptions and illustrations of the most important sanatoria of Europe, the United States, and Canada. Philadelphia: P. Blakiston's Son & Co., 1899. 343p. plates. DLC; DNLM; NNNAM; PPC **90-4498**

KNOTT, J[ames] J[errold] (*b.* 1839)
Phosphorus. The cause of yellow fever; its prevention and cure. Atlanta: S. W. Postell, [1893]. 27p. DNLM **90-4499**

KNOTT, J[ames] Proctor (1830-1911)
Kentucky School of Medicine; doctorate address, 1890. Louisville: Courier-Journal Job Print. Co., 1890. 8p. DNLM **90-4500**

KOBER, George Martin (1850-1931)
The etiology and prevention of tuberculosis. [Sacramento, 1890.] 8p. DNLM **90-4501**

KOBER, George Martin (1850-1931)
The etiology and prevention of infectious diseases. [Richmond, 1892.] 18p. DNLM **90-4502**

KOBER, George Martin (1850-1931)
The etiology, distribution, and prevention of land and ship cholera. [Sacramento, 1893.] 6p. DNLM **90-4503**

KOBER, George Martin (1850-1931)
A plea for the prevention of tuberculosis. Sacramento: A. J. Johnston, 1894. 12p. DNLM **90-4504**

KOBER, George Martin (1850-1931)
A study of the soil in relation to health and disease. Richmond, 1894. 29p. DNLM **90-4505**

KOBER, George Martin (1850-1931)
A study of water in relation to health and disease. Sacramento: A. J. Johnston, 1894. 37p. DNLM **90-4506**

KOBER, George Martin (1850-1931)
Impure milk in relation to infantile mortality. Chicago, 1895. 15p. DNLM **90-4507**

KOBER, George Martin (1850-1931)
A plea for vaccination. Richmond, 1895. 16p. DNLM **90-4508**

KOBER, George Martin (1850-1931)
A review of Max Bartels's work. "Die Medicin der Naturvölker, ethnologische Beiträge zur Urgeschichte der Medicin," Leipzig, 1893. With a condensation of the subject matter on primitive minor and major surgery. Richmond, 1895. 12p. DNLM **90-4509**

KOBER, George Martin (1850-1931)
A study of milk in relation to health and disease. Sacramento: A. J. Johnston, 1896. 51p. DNLM **90-4510**

KOBER, George Martin (1850-1931)
The place of military medicine and surgery in the medical college curriculum. Columbus, O., 1897. 8p. DNLM
90-4511

KOBER, George Martin (1850-1931)
Predisposition and immunity. New York, 1897. 7p. DNLM
90-4512

KOBER, George Martin (1850-1931)
Prevention of puerperal fever. Richmond, 1897. 16p. DNLM
90-4513

KOBER, George Martin (1850-1931)
The progress and achievements of hygiene. New York, 1897. 12p. DNLM **90-4514**

KOBER, George Martin (1850-1931)
Higher medical education and a plea for better training of the volunteer medical officer. Richmond, 1898. 5p. DNLM
90-4515

KOBER, George Martin (1850-1931)
Complimentary dinner to Joseph J. Kinyoun . . . by members of the medical profession, Washington, D.C., Saturday, May 20, 1899. Address delivered by . . . . Georgetown, 1899. 12p. DNLM **90-4516**

KOBER, George Martin (1850-1931)
Sarcoma of the testicle. Conclusions based upon one hundred and fourteen cases. Philadelphia, 1899. 18p. DNLM
90-4517

KOCHER, Emil Theodor (1841-1917)
Operative surgery. New York: William Wood & Co., 1894. 279p. NNNAM; OCIM; PPC; PU **90-4518**

KOLIPINSKI, Louis
Case of suicidal poisoning with hydrocyanic acid. Baltimore, 1898. 1 l. DNLM **90-4519**

KOLIPINSKI, Louis
Typhoid fever in a man of sixty-eight. Baltimore, 1898. 1 l. DNLM **90-4520**

KOLIPINSKI, Louis
Cases illustrating the contagiousness of inherited syphilis. Baltimore, 1899. 2p. DNLM **90-4521**

KOLIPINSKI, Louis
On the free use of drinking water in acute hemorrhage. Baltimore, 1899. 2p. DNLM **90-4522**

KOLIPINSKI, Louis
Note on the treatment of typhoid fever, and special indications for the use of copper arsenite in this disease. Baltimore, 1899. 3p. DNLM **90-4523**

KOLIPINSKI, Louis
The treatment of croupous pneumonia with hot-water bags. Baltimore, 1899. 4p. DNLM **90-4524**

KOLIPINSKI, Louis
The treatment of epidemic cerebro-spinal meningitis with arsenite of copper. Baltimore, 1899. 5p. DNLM
90-4525

KOLLE, Frederick Strange (1871-1929)
The X-rays. Their production and application. . . . New York: J. S. Ogilvie Publishing Co., [1898]. 191p. plates. DLC; DNLM; NNNAM **90-4526**

KOPLIK, Henry (1858-1927)
Arthritis complicating vulvo-vaginal inflammation in children. [New York, 1890.] 9p. DNLM **90-4527**

KOPLIK, Henry (1858-1927)
The etiology of empyema in children. [Philadelphia, 1890.] 11p. 4 plates. DNLM **90-4528**

KOPLIK, Henry (1858-1927)
The etiology of empyema in children; an experimental and clinical study. [Philadelphia, 1891.] 24p. DNLM
90-4529

KOPLIK, Henry (1858-1927)
The sterilization of milk and the status of our knowledge upon the subject. [Philadelphia, 1891.] 17p. DNLM
90-4530

KOPLIK, Henry (1858-1927)
Acute alcoholic intoxication in infants and the abuse of alcohol in the gastrointestingal disorders of infancy. [Philadelphia, 1893.] 8p. DNLM **90-4531**

KOPLIK, Henry (1858-1927)
Malarial fever in infants and children from a study of the plasmodium malariae. New York: D. Appleton & Co., 1893. 17p. DNLM **90-4532**

KOPLIK, Henry (1858-1927)
Urogenital blenorrhoea in children. Vulvo-vaginitis in girls; urethritis in boys. A clinical and bacteriological study. [n. p., 1893.] 25p. DNLM **90-4533**

KOPLIK, Henry (1858-1927)
Acute lacunar diphtheria of the tonsils, with studies on the relation of the real to the pseudo bacillus diphtheriae. New York, 1894. 20p. DNLM **90-4534**

KOPLIK, Henry (1858-1927)
The rapid bacteriological and clinical diagnosis of diphtheria. New York, 1896. 12p. DNLM **90-4535**

KOPLIK, Henry (1858-1927)
Sporadic cretinism, and its distinction from forms of idiocy and other diseases. New York, 1897. 29p. DNLM
90-4536

KRAFFT-EBING, Richard von (1840-1902)
Psychopathia sexualis, with special reference to contrary sexual instinct: a medico-legal study. . . . Authorized translation of the 7th enlarged and rev. German ed. by Charles G. Chaddock. Philadelphia and London: F. A. Davis Co., 1892. 436p. DLC; DNLM; NNNAM; PU **90-4537**

KRAFFT-EBING, Richard von (1840-1902)
An experimental study in the domain of hypnotism. Transl. from the German by Charles G. Chaddock. New York & London: G. P. Putnam's Sons, 1896. 129p. DNLM; ICU; MH; NN **90-4538**

KRAFFT-EBING, Richard von (1840-1902)
Hemicrania and its relations to epilepsy and hysteria. (Transl. by W. Alfred McCorn.) St. Louis, 1899. 25p. DNLM
90-4539

KRAFFT-EBING, Richard von (1840-1902)
Relations between neuralgia and transitory psychoses. Transl. by W. Alfred McCorn. St. Louis, 1899. 31p. DNLM
90-4540

KREIDER, George N[oble] (*b.* 1856)
A case of movable or floating liver. Philadelphia, 1893. 3p. DNLM **90-4541**

KREIDER, George N[oble] (*b.* 1856)
Surgical cleanliness; an address. New York, 1896. 11p. DNLM
90-4542

KREIDER, George N[oble] (*b.* 1856)
Cases in hospital practice: Ligation of the gastro-epiploica artery; disturbances of the thyroid gland complicating fibroid tumors of the uterus. Chicago, 1899. 7p. DNLM
90-4543

KREISSEL, F[ilip] (*b.* 1859)
Bottini's operation for senile enlargement of the prostate. Chicago, 1898. 1 l. 1 plate. DNLM
90-4544

KREUTZMANN, H[enry] (*b.* 1855)
Albuminuria during pregnancy, without convulsions of the mother, but with eclampsia of the new-born infant. New York, [1898]. 5p. DNLM **90-4545**

KREUTZMANN, H[enry] (*b.* 1855)
Cystic degeneration of the chorion villi with coincident cystic tumour of both ovaries. New York: William Wood & Co., 1898. 8p. DNLM **90-4546**

KREUTZMANN, H[enry] (*b.* 1855)
Diabetes mellitus and carcinoma uteri; hysterectomy; recovery. New York, 1898. 4p. DNLM **90-4547**

KREUTZMANN, H[enry] (*b.* 1855)
Torsion of the pedicle of an ovarian tumor with acute symptoms. San Francisco, 1898. 4p. DNLM
90-4548

KRIEGER, Georg E. (*b.* 1859)
Blood serum therapy and antitoxins. . . . Chicago: E. H. Colegrove & Co., 1895. 69p. plates. DLC
90-4549

KRUG, Florian
Atreasiae of the genital tract. [Philadelphia: W. J. Dornan, 1891.] 10p. DNLM **90-4550**

KRUG, Florian
My personal experience with vaginal hysterectomy. New York: William Wood & Co., 1891. 13p. DNLM
90-4551

KRUG, Florian
Transperitoneal hysterorrhaphy; a new method of ventral fixation of the uterus without opening the peritoneal cavity. [New York, 1891.] 12p. DNLM **90-4552**

KRUG, Florian
Trendelenburg's posture in gynecology. [Philadelphia, 1892.] 8p. 1 plate. DNLM **90-4553**

KRUG, Florian
Double pyosalpinx; ovarian abscess; curettement during acute stage of purulent inflammation; subsequent laparotomy; recovery. New York: M. J. Rooney, [1892]. 7p. DNLM
90-4554

KRUG, Florian
Total extirpation versus leaving a stump in operation for uterine fibro-myomata. [New York, 1892.] 11p. DNLM
90-4555

KRUG, Florian
Trendelenburg's posture in gynaecology, demonstration of a convenient apparatus for obtaining the same. Philadelphia, 1892. 5p. DNLM **90-4556**

KRUG, Florian
Hysterectomy in ectopic gestation with disease of the other appendages. New York, 1894. 7p. DNLM
90-4557

KRUSEN, Wilmer
Two cases of parotiditis following coeliotomy. New York, 1896. 3p. DNLM **90-4558**

KRUSEN, Wilmer
Treatment of uterine prolapse, with illustrative cases. New York, 1897. 10p. DNLM **90-4559**

KRUSEN, Wilmer
Sequelae of abdominal operations. New York, 1898. 7p. DNLM **90-4560**

KRUSEN, Wilmer
A case of thyroidectomy. Detroit: W. M. Warren, 1898. 3p. DNLM **90-4561**

KRUSEN, Wilmer
Difficult points in gynecologic diagnosis. Philadelphia, 1899. 11p. DNLM **90-4562**

KRUSEN, Wilmer
The causation of uterine retrodisplacements. New York, 1899. 3p. DNLM **90-4563**

KUFLEWSKI, W[ladyslaw] A.
Fracture of femur and its treatment. Chicago, 1898. 2 l. DNLM **90-4564**

KUH, Edwin [J.] (1858-1940)
A common etiology in the inflammatory diseases of the respiratory tract. [Philadelphia: Lea Bros. & Co., 1893.] 3p. DNLM **90-4565**

KUH, Edwin [J.] (1858-1940)
A topical treatment of bronchitis. Chicago, 1893. 5p. DNLM
90-4566

KUH, Edwin [J.] (1858-1940)
Sectarianism in medicine; distinctive features of existing medical sects. Chicago: Office Am. Medical Assoc., 1894. 8p. DNLM **90-4567**

KUH, Edwin [J.] (1858-1940)
Some additional experiences with Behring's diphtheria-antitoxin, and some remarks on the use of Loeffler's toluol-solution. [Philadelphia, 1895.] 6p. DNLM
90-4568

KUH, Edwin [J.] (1858-1940)
Primary cancer of the nasopharynx cured by injections of alcohol. New York, 1897. 8p. DNLM
90-4569

KUH, Edwin [J.] (1858-1940)
A second contribution to the treatment of cancer by injections of alcohol. Philadelphia, 1898. 13p. DNLM
90-4570

KUH, Sidney (*b.* 1866)
The pathology of locomotor ataxia. [Philadelphia: Lea Bros. & Co., 1894.] 9p. DNLM **90-4571**

KUH, Sidney (*b.* 1866)
Syphilis of the central nervous system. St. Louis, 1897. 28p. DNLM **90-4572**

KUH, Sidney (*b.* 1866)
The medico-legal aspects of hypnotism. Philadelphia, 1898. 11p. DNLM **90-4573**

KUHNE, Louis
The new science of healing; or, the doctrine of the oneness of all diseases forming the basis of a uniform method of cure, without medicines and without operations: an instructor and adviser for the healthy and the sick. Transl. from the third greatly augmented German edition by Th. Baker, Leipzig; published by Louis Kuhne; New York: International News Co., [1892]. 458p. NNNAM **90-4574**

KYLE, David Braden (1863-1916)
The effect of fluids on the strength of catgut. Detroit: G. S. Davis, 1892. 3p. DNLM **90-4575**

KYLE, David Braden (1863-1916)
The pathology and treatment of tetanus; including a series of investigations in regard to the micro-organism of the disease and the influence of disinfectant substances on the same. A study from the pathological laboratory of the Jefferson Medical College. Detroit: G. S. Davis, 1892. 49p. 1 plate, 1 table. DNLM **90-4576**

KYLE, David Braden (1863-1916)
The treatment of hay-fever by means of cocaine phenate. Philadelphia, 1892. 4p. DNLM **90-4577**

KYLE, David Braden (1863-1916)
Phenate or carbolate of cocaine as a local anaesthetic. Detroit: G. S. Davis, 1893. 6p. DNLM **90-4578**

KYLE, David Braden (1863-1916)
Resterilized sponges, with bacteriological investigation. Detroit: G. S. Davis, 1893. 3p. DNLM
90-4579

KYLE, David Braden (1863-1916)
The etiology, pathology, and treatment of ozena. Philadelphia, 1894. 7p. DNLM **90-4580**

KYLE, David Braden (1863-1916)
Illumination and examination of the anterior and posterior nasal cavities. [Philadelphia: Lea Bros. & Co., 1894.] 3p. DNLM **90-4581**

KYLE, David Braden (1863-1916)
Bacteriological study of four cases of diphtheria treated with artitoxine by Louis Fischer at the Municipal Hospital, Philadelphia. Philadelphia, 1895. 9p. 1 plate. DNLM
90-4582

KYLE, David Braden (1863-1916)
Fibrino-plastic exudates; with reports of two cases of laminated fibrino-plastic rhinitis, including laboratory investigation. New York, 1895. 12p. DNLM **90-4583**

KYLE, David Braden (1863-1916)
A study of the mode of action of ichthyol in inflammatory conditions. Detroit: G. S. Davis, 1895. 5p. DNLM
90-4584

KYLE, David Braden (1863-1916)
A text-book of diseases of the nose and throat. . . . With 175 illustrations, 23 of them in colors. Philadelphia: W. B. Saunders, 1899. 646p. col. plates. DLC; MBM; NNNAM; PPC
90-4585

KYLE, John J[ohnson] (1869-1920)
An oculist's experience in the army. St. Louis, 1899. 4 l. DNLM **90-4586**

KYLE, John J[ohnson] (1869-1920)
Typhoid fever. Louisville, 1899. 4 l. DNLM
90-4587

LADD, George Trumbull (1842-1921)
Outlines of physiological psychology; a text-book of mental science for academies and colleges. New York: C. Scribner's Sons, 1891. 505p. DNLM; ICU; MB; NN
90-4588

LADD, George Trumbull (1842-1921)
Psychology, descriptive and explanatory: A treatise on the phenomena, laws, and development of human mental life. New York: C. Scribner's Sons, 1894. 676p. ICU; MH; NN
90-4589

LA GARDE, Louis Anatole (1849-1920)
The difference between certain wounds inflicted by the projectiles of large and small calibre hand-weapons. Philadelphia, 1894. 10p. DNLM **90-4590**

LA GARDE, Louis Anatole (1849-1920)
The medical department in time of war. [Boston, 1896.] 8p. DNLM **90-4591**

LAGORIO, Aleksander E[ugenievich] (*b.* 1852)
Chicago Pasteur Institute, for the preventive treatment of hydrophobia. [Statement of the number of patients treated to date, April 12, 1892.] [Chicago, 1892.] 1 sheet. DNLM
90-4592

LAIDLAW, Alexander H[amilton] (1828-1908) and Frederick LAIDLAW
Mustard in therapeutics. Chicago, 1893. 8p. DNLM
90-4593

LAIDLAW, George Frederick (*b.* 1871)
The diagnosis of substances passed from the bowels. New York, 1895. 4p. DNLM **90-4594**

LAIDLAW, George Frederick (*b.* 1871)
Six cases of hemorrhage. New York, 1896. 8p. DNLM
90-4595

LAIDLEY, L[eonidas] H. (1844-1881)
Suppurative appendicitis. Chicago, 1893. 8p. DNLM
90-4596

LAJOIE, M. T.
Dyspepsia and how to cure it. Description of the digestive organs and of the different kinds of food. . . . By. . . . 6th ed. Nashua, N.H.: Telegraphic Publishing Co., 1895. 124, 14p. DLC **90-4597**

LAKE, Richard (*b.* 1861)
A contribution to the pathology of laryngeal phthisis. Philadelphia, 1895. 12p. DNLM **90-4598**

LAMB, Daniel Smith (1843-1929)
The hygiene of school studies. Chicago, 1891. 8p. DNLM
90-4599

LAMB, Daniel Smith (1843-1929)
Osteomalacia. Chicago, 1892. 8p. DNLM
90-4600

LAMB, Daniel Smith (1843-1929)
The deadly microbe and its destruction. Washington, 1893. 28p. DNLM **90-4601**

LAMB, Daniel Smith (1843-1929)
The Meckel diverticulum. Philadelphia, 1893. 8p. DNLM
90-4602

LAMB, Daniel Smith (1843-1929)
The female external genital organs; a criticism on current anatomical description. New York, 1894. 7p. DNLM
90-4603

LAMB, Daniel Smith (1843-1929)
Polyorchism. Tubercle in trochanteric fossa. Philadelphia, 1895. 15p. DNLM **90-4604**

LAMB, Daniel Smith (1843-1929)
Precolumbian syphilis. [Washington, 1897.] 6p. DNLM
90-4605

LAMBERT, Alexander (*b.* 1861)
A study of tetanus, and its treatment. New York, 1897. 29p. DNLM; NNNAM **90-4606**

LAMBERT, Alexander (*b.* 1861)
Sunstroke as it occurred in New York City during 1896. [New York, 1897.] 32p. 1 plate. DNLM; NNNAM
90-4607

LAMBERT, W[alter] E[yre]
Retinoscopy as a means of estimating astigmatism. [New York, 1892.] 6p. DNLM **90-4608**

LAND, [Charles Henry] (1847-1922)
Land system of dental practice. . . . [Detroit, Mich., 1893.] 25p. DLC **90-4609**

LANDESMANN, Ernst
Therapy of the clinics of the Royal and Imperial Hospital of Vienna, Austria. Transl. and revised from the last two compilations of . . . by John H. Metzerott. Chicago: Fergus Print. Co., 1897. 765p. DNLM; ICRM **90-4610**

LANDIS, Henry Gardner (1848-1886)
. . . A compend of obstetrics. Especially adapted to the use of medical students and physicians. . . . 4th ed. . . . Philadelphia: P. Blakiston, Son & Co., 1891. 118p. DLC; PPC; PU
90-4611

LANDIS, Henry Gardner (1848-1886)
. . . A compend of obstetrics. Especially adapted to the use of medical students and physicians. . . . Rev. and ed. by William H. Wells. . . . 5th ed. . . . Philadelphia: P. Blakiston, Son & Co., 1893. 174p. col. plates. DLC; NNNAM; PPC
90-4612

LANDIS, Henry Gardner (1848-1886)
. . . A compend of obstetrics. Especially adapted to the use of medical students and physicians. . . . Revised and edited by William H. Wells. . . . 6th ed. . . . Philadelphia: P. Blakiston's Son & Co., 1893. 188p. col. plates. DLC; NNNAM; PPC; PU
90-4613

LANDIS, Henry Gardner (1848-1886)
How to use the forceps. With an introductory account of the female pelvis and of the mechanism of delivery. . . . Rev. and enl. by Charles H. Bushong. . . . New York: E. B. Treat, 1894. 203p. DLC; NNNAM **90-4614**

LANDOIS, Leonard (1837-1902)
Text-book of human physiology, including histology and microscopical anatomy, with special reference to the practice of medicine. 4th American ed. transl. from the 7th German ed., with additions by William Stirling. Philadelphia: P. Blakiston, Son & Co., 1892. 1156p. DLC; ICRM; MBM; PPC
90-4615

LANDOIS, Leonard (1837-1902)
A text-book of human physiology. . . . 5th American, translated from the last German ed., with additions by Wm. Stirling. Philadelphia: P. Blakiston, Son & Co., 1894. 1156p. CtY-M; DLC; PPC; PU **90-4616**

LANE, Edward B[inney]
Hallucinations in the insane. Boston: Damrell & Upham, 1891. 14p. DNLM **90-4617**

LANE, Edward B[inney]
The so-called motor area of the cortex. Utica, 1891. 11p. DNLM **90-4618**

LANE, Edward B[inney]
Observations upon hebephrenia. Chicago: Rand, McNally & Co., 1895. 9p. DNLM **90-4619**

LANE HOSPITAL, SAN FRANCISCO
Annual report of the . . . , including dispensary clinics of Cooper Medical College as out-patient department. 1, 1895. San Francisco: William A. Woodward & Co., 1895. 46p. DNLM **90-4620**

LANE, L[evi] C[ooper] (1830-1902) and Edward R. TAYLOR
Addresses delivered on the occasion of the commencement exercises of Cooper Medical College, Nov. 13, 1890. San Francisco: Goodwin & Taylor, [1890]. 45p. DNLM
90-4621

LANE, L[evi] C[ooper] (1830-1902)
Rudolph Virchow. An address. Sacramento, [1893]. 12p. DNLM **90-4622**

LANE, L[evi] C[ooper] (1830-1902)
An address delivered at the opening of Lane Hospital, January 2, 1895. Sacramento, 1895. 11p. DNLM
90-4623

LANE, L[evi] C[ooper] (1830-1902)
The surgery of the head and neck. . . . [San Francisco]: Pub. by the Author, [1896]. 1180p. DLC
90-4624

LANE, L[evi] C[ooper] (1830-1902)
The surgery of the head and neck. 2nd ed. Philadelphia: P. Blakiston, Son & Co., 1898. 1180p. DNLM; PPC; PU
90-4625

LANE, W[illiam] Arbuthnot (1856-1943)
Antrectomy as a treatment for chronic purulent otitis media. New York, 1892. 7p. DNLM **90-4626**

LANGDON, F[rank] W[arren] (1851-1933)
Tenotomy to increase the mobility and power of the musician's ring-finger. Cincinnati, 1890. 3p. DNLM
90-4627

LANGDON, F[rank] W[arren] (1851-1933)
Tenotomy to increase the mobility and power of the musician's ring-finger. Cincinnati: Spencer & Craig, 1893. 8p. 1 l., 1 plate. DNLM **90-4628**

LANGDON, F[rank] W[arren] (1851-1933)
Applied anatomy of the brain. Cincinnati: Spencer & Craig, 1893. 14p. DNLM **90-4629**

LANGDON, F[rank] W[arren] (1851-1933)
Epilepsy and other convulsive diseases; a study in neurodynamics and pathogenesis. Philadelphia, 1896. 16p. DNLM
90-4630

LANGDON, F[rank] W[arren] (1851-1933)
Focal cord lesions. I. Lumbar poliomyelitis anterior subacuta unilateralis in a man of forty-four. II. Traumatic cervicodorsal poliomyelitis without vertebral fracture. New York, 1897. 15p. DNLM **90-4631**

LANGDON, F[rank] W[arren] (1851-1933)
Locomotor ataxia; its newer pathology and treatment. Cincinnati, 1897. 7p. DNLM **90-4632**

LANGDON, F[rank] W[arren] (1851-1933)
Treatment of insanity. Cincinnati, 1898. 7p. DNLM
90-4633

LANGDON, F[rank] W[arren] (1851-1933)
Facial paralysis, congenital, unilateral, and of unique distribution. New York, 1899. 10p. DNLM **90-4634**

LANGDON, F[rank] W[arren] (1851-1933)
Paranomia visual and myotactic; nonrecollection aphasia for names of objects seen and felt. Philadelphia, 1899. 12p. DNLM
90-4635

LANGDON, F[rank] W[arren] (1851-1933) and Albert H. FREIBERG
Pachymeningitis spinalis externa; recovery complete. Chicago, 1899. 15p. DNLM **90-4636**

LANPHEAR, Emory (*b.* 1859)
The new treatment of peritonitis. [Kansas City, 1890.] 8p. DNLM **90-4637**

LANPHEAR, Emory (*b.* 1859)
Amputation at the hip-joint. How should it be performed? [Philadelphia, 1891.] 4p. DNLM **90-4638**

LANPHEAR, Emory (*b.* 1859)
Treatment of penetrating wounds of the abdomen. [Kansas City, 1891.] 8p. DNLM **90-4639**

LANPHEAR, Emory (*b.* 1859)
Chloralamid in surgery. [New York, 1891.] 1 l. DNLM
90-4640

LANPHEAR, Emory (*b.* 1859)
Gastrotomy in carcinoma of the cardiac orifice. [Philadelphia, 1892.] 3p. DNLM **90-4641**

LANPHEAR, Emory (*b.* 1859)
Report of an operation for removal of the Gasserian ganglion. [Kansas City, 1892.] 4p. DNLM **90-4642**

LANPHEAR, Emory (*b.* 1859)
When shall we trephine in fractures of the skull? [Kansas City, 1892.] 8p. DNLM **90-4643**

LANPHEAR, Emory (*b.* 1859)
Treatment of post-operative conditions. . . . [New York: M. J. Breitenbach Co., 1898.] 8p. DNLM
90-4644

LAPLACE, Ernest (*b.* 1861)
Causes of failure in the treatment of appendicitis. [Philadelphia, 1892.] 8p. DNLM **90-4645**

LAPLACE, Ernest (*b.* 1861)
Penetrating wound of the base of the brain through the left orbit; hemiplegia; removal of clots from the base of the brain; recovery. [Philadelphia, 1892.] 4p. DNLM
90-4646

LAPLACE, Ernest (*b.* 1861)
A new forceps for intestinal anastomosis. Philadelphia, 1899. 9p. 11 plates on 6 l. DNLM **90-4647**

LARTIGAN, August Jerome
The Bacillus pyocyaneus as a pathogenic factor in human pathology, with the report of three cases. Philadelphia, 1898. 17p. DNLM **90-4648**

LARTIGAN, August Jerome
Xerostomia, or dry-mouth; report of a case. New York: Lea Bros. & Co., 1898. 7p. DNLM **90-4649**

LARTIGAN, August Jerome
A contribution to the study of the micrococcus tetragenus in acute angina. Philadelphia, 1899. 8p. DNLM
90-4650

LATIMER, Thomas S[argent] (1839-1906)
A brief summary of the clinical history and treatment of two thousand and twelve cases of alcoholism, of which eighty-seven were maniacal. [Philadelphia, 1892.] 12p. DNLM
90-4651

LAUGHLIN, William Ross
Anatomy in a nutshell, or questions and answers with explanatory notes. . . . Kirksville, Mo.: Democrat Print, 1899. 152p. DLC **90-4652**

LAURA MEMORIAL WOMAN'S MEDICAL COLLEGE, CINCINNATI
Annual announcements for the sessions of 1892-93 (3.); 1898-99 (9.); 1900-01 to 1902-03 (11.-13). Cincinnati, 1892-1902. DNLM [Organized in 1890 under the title of Presbyterian Hospital and Woman's Medical College, Cincinnati. In 1895 the Woman's Medical College of Cincinnati merged with it.] **90-4653**

LAUTENBACH, Louis J. (*b.* 1860)
A few thoughts about ophthalmometry, as to what the Javal instrument will do, and what it will not do. Nashville, Tenn.: A. R. Gray & Son, 1893. 7p. DNLM **90-4654**

LAUTENBACH, Louis J. (*b.* 1860)
Phlyctenular conjunctivitis, with special reference to the pathology and prophylaxis of the disease. Providence: E. A. Johnson & Co., 1893. 8p. DNLM **90-4655**

LAUTENBACH, Louis J. (*b.* 1860)
The value of the ophthalmometer in the determination of the axis and the amount of astigmatism. [New York, 1893.] 4p. DNLM **90-4656**

LAUTENBACH, Louis J. (*b.* 1860)
A new tongue-depressor and an ear-screw for the removal of foreign bodies. [Philadelphia, 1894.] 6p. DNLM **90-4657**

LAUTENBACH, Louis J. (*b.* 1860)
The nose as a frequently unrecognized cause of disease. Philadelphia, [1894]. 4p. DNLM **90-4658**

LAUTENBACH, Louis J. (*b.* 1860)
Some observations on corneal astigmatism and conditions that change corneal curvature. Philadelphia, 1894. 4p. DNLM **90-4659**

LAUTENBACH, Louis J. (*b.* 1860)
The treatment of the various forms of conjunctivitis as practiced at the German Hospital; to which is added a report of the new patients in the eye, ear, and throat departments of the German Hospital from their inception. Philadelphia: J. B. Smith, 1894. 12p. DNLM **90-4660**

LAUTENBACH, Louis J. (*b.* 1860)
Non-suppurative cases of diseases of the ear; massage vs. removal of the sound-conducting apparatus in such cases. Philadelphia, 1895. 8p. DNLM **90-4661**

LAUTENBACH, Louis J. (*b.* 1860)
Gonorrheal conjunctivitis; its treatment. Chicago, 1896. 7p. DNLM **90-4662**

LAUTENBACH, Louis J. (*b.* 1860)
Oto-massage in suppuration of the ear; its value for the relief of deafness and in the treatment of the suppuration. Chicago, 1896. 8p. DNLM **90-4663**

LAUTENBACH, Louis J. (*b.* 1860)
Phono- and pneumo-massage in suppurative disease of the ear. Philadelphia, 1896. 8p. DNLM **90-4664**

LAUTENBACH, Louis J. (*b.* 1860)
The treatment of epidemic conjunctivitis or pink eye. Nashville, [1896]. 8p. DNLM **90-4665**

LAUTENBACH, Louis J. (*b.* 1860)
The influence of nasal disease in modifying the quantity and axis of corneal astigmatism. Nashville, 1897. 4p. DNLM **90-4666**

LAUTENBACH, Louis J. (*b.* 1860)
Prompt attention to earaches in infancy and early childhood. Chicago, 1898. 8p. DNLM **90-4667**

LAUTENBACH, Louis J. (*b.* 1860)
Rupture of the drum head not necessarily incurable. Pittsburgh, Pa., 1898. 16p. DNLM **90-4668**

LAUTENBACH, Louis J. (*b.* 1860)
Some results in cases of tobacco amblyopia. Chicago, 1898. 8p. DNLM **90-4669**

LAUTENBACH, Louis J. (*b.* 1860)
The attitude of the family physician to his patients in respect to opticians. Pittsburgh, 1899. 8p. DNLM **90-4670**

LAUTENBACH, Louis J. (*b.* 1860)
Some further results in treating ears by massage method. Philadelphia, 1899. 8p. DNLM **90-4671**

LAUTENBACH, Louis J. (*b.* 1860)
Suppurative disease of the ear. The presence of polypi and granulations therein not an unfavorable indication. Chicago, 1899. 8p. DNLM **90-4672**

LAUTENBACH, Louis J. (*b.* 1860)
Tretment of nasopharyngeal adenoids. [Chicago, 1899.] 8p. DNLM **90-4673**

LAW, Hartland
The Viavi gynecological plates, designed to educate mothers and daughters concerning diseases of the uterine organs. Constructed under the supervision of Hartland Law and Herbert E. Law. . . . San Francisco, Cal.: The "Viavi" Co., [1891]. 24p. col. plates. CtY-M; DLC **90-4674**

LAW, Hartland
The Viavi manager's guide by Hartland Law, M.D. [and] Herbert E. Law, F.C.S. San Francisco, Cal.: The Viavi Co., 1897. 186p. DLC **90-4675**

LAW, Hartland
Viavi hygiene for women, men, and children. By Hartland Law, M.D., Herbert E. Law, F.C.S. San Francisco, Calif.: The Viavi Co., 1899. 610p. DLC [*vel subseq.*] **90-4676**

LAWLESS, E[dmond] J[ames]
The bearer's companion. First aid to the injured, and management of the sick; an ambulance handbook and elementary manual of nursing for volunteer bearers and others. Philadelphia: J. B. Lippincott Co., 1894. 253p. DNLM; PU **90-4677**

LAZARUS-BARLOW, Walter S[ydney] (1865-1950)
A manual of general pathology for students and practitioners. Philadelphia: P. Blakiston, Son & Co., 1898. 795p. DNLM; NNNAM; PPC; PU **90-4678**

LEA BROS. & CO. PHILADELPHIA
Classified catalogue of medical and surgical publications. Philadelphia, 1890. 31p. DNLM; PPC
90-4679

LEAMAN, H[enry] (*b.* 1839)
Gonorrhoeal labor. New York, 1896. 4p. DNLM
90-4680

LEAMING, J[ames] R[osebrugh] (1820-1892)
Contributions to the study of the heart and lungs. New York: E. B. Treat; London: H. K. Lewis, 1890. 300p. DNLM; NNNAM **90-4681**

LEAVITT, Sheldon (1848-1933)
The science and art of obstetrics. . . . 2nd ed. rewritten and enl. Chicago: Gross & Delbridge, 1892. 769p. DLC; PPHa
90-4682

LEAVITT, Sheldon (1848-1933)
The use of obstetric forceps. Chicago: Era Publishing Co., 1897. 112p. ICU **90-4683**

LEDERLE, Ernst J[oseph] (*b.* 1865)
Formaldehyde, with special reference to its chemistry in disinfection. New York, 1897. 12p. DNLM
90-4684

LEDERMAN, M[oses] D. (*b.* 1868)
Sarcoma of the nasal cavity; ligation of both external carotids; decided beneficial effect. New York, 1895. 8p. DNLM
90-4685

LEDERMAN, M[oses] D. (*b.* 1868)
Diffuse external otitis following the careless use of carbolic acid. New York, 1895. 5p. DNLM **90-4686**

LEDERMAN, M[oses] D. (*b.* 1868)
Foreign bodies in the ear and nose. [St. Louis], 1895. 5p. DNLM **90-4687**

LEDERMAN, M[oses] D. (*b.* 1868)
Cerebral disease following middle-ear suppuration. Chicago, 1896. 12p. DNLM **90-4688**

LEDERMAN, M[oses] D. (*b.* 1868)
. . . Angina Ludovici complicating acute suppurative otitis; recovery. . . . New York: The Publishers' Printing Co., 1898. 4p. DLC **90-4689**

LEDERMAN, M[oses] D. (*b.* 1868)
An unusual case of sinus thrombosis and epidural abscess complicated by malaria—operation—recovery. . . . New York: Publishers' Printing Co., 1899. 8p. DLC
90-4690

LEE, Arthur Bolles (1849-1927)
The microtomist's vade-mecum. A handbook of the methods of microscopic anatomy. 3rd ed. Philadelphia: P. Blakiston, Son & Co., 1893. 509p. DNLM; PPC; PU
90-4691

LEE, Arthur Bolles (1849-1927)
The microtomist's vade-mecum. A handbook of the methods of microscopic anatomy. 4th ed. Philadelphia: P. Blakiston, Son & Co., 1896. 536p. CtY-M; DNLM; NNNAM; PPC
90-4692

LEE, Benjamin (1833-1913)
A brief memoir of Henry Hollingsworth Smith. [Philadelphia, 1890.] 9p. DNLM **90-4693**

LEE, Benjamin (1833-1913)
An analysis of the statistics of forty-one thousand five hundred cases of epidemic influenza. Chicago, 1891. 12p. DNLM
90-4694

LEE, Benjamin (1833-1913)
Extract from remarks made before the State Sanitary Convention at Pittsburgh, May 30, 1889. [On boards of health.] Harrisburg: E. K. Meyers, 1891. 6p. DNLM
90-4695

LEE, Benjamin (1833-1913)
The nervous and muscular elements in the caustion of idiopathic lateral curvature. [Philadelphia, 1891.] 4p. DNLM
90-4696

LEE, Benjamin (1833-1913)
Sacro-iliac disease. [Philadelphia, 1891.] 7p. DNLM
90-4697

LEE, Benjamin (1833-1913)
The ability of the State to prevent an epidemic of cholera. Philadelphia, 1892. 10p. DNLM **90-4698**

LEE, Benjamin (1833-1913)
Responsibility of the National and State governments for the protection of the purity of the water supplies. Chicago, 1892. 20p. DNLM **90-4699**

LEE, ELLWOOD J., CO.
. . . Annual retail catalogue, . . . metallic splints, trusses, electric batteries, orthopaedic supplies. . . . Conshohocken, Pa., 1891. 88p. PU **90-4700**

LEE, ELLWOOD J., CO.
Wholesale catalogue of specialties. Conshohocken, Pa., 1892. 72p. NNNAM **90-4701**

LEE, ELLWOOD J., CO.
Illustrated catalogue of medical and surgical plasters. Conshohocken, Pa., 1897. 94p. NNNAM
90-4702

LEFFINGWELL, Albert [Tracy] (1845-1916)
A dangerous ideal. [Providence, R.I., 1895?] 7p. DNLM
90-4703

LEFFINGWELL, Albert [Tracy] (1845-1916)
Does science need secrecy? A reply to Prof. Porter and others of Harvard Medical School. With statement concerning vivisection, by Prof. W. T. Porter. Providence, R.I., 1896. 25p. DNLM **90-4704**

LEFFMANN, Henry (1847-1930)
. . . A compend of chemistry, inorganic and organic; including urinary analysis. . . . 3rd ed. rev. Philadelphia: P. Blakiston, Son & Co., 1890. 193p. DLC; DNLM; PPC; PU
90-4705

LEFFMANN, Henry (1847-1930) and William BEAM
Progressive exercises in practical chemistry. Philadelphia: P. Blakiston, Son & Co., 1890. 104p. DNLM; PPC
90-4706

LEFFMANN, Henry (1847-1930) and William BEAM
A modification of the Reichert distillation process for butter. [Philadelphia, 1891.] 4p. DNLM **90-4707**

LEFFMANN, Henry (1847-1930) and William BEAM
Analytic notes on commercial codliver-oil emulsions. [Philadelphia, 1892.] 4p. DNLM **90-4708**

LEFFMANN, Henry (1847-1930) and William BEAM
Analysis of milk and milk products. Philadelphia: P. Blakiston, Son & Co., 1893. 92p. DNLM; PU **90-4709**

LEFFMANN, Henry (1847-1930)
Analytic notes on liquid malt extracts. Philadelphia, 1893. 4p. DNLM **90-4710**

LEFFMANN, Henry (1847-1930)
Analytic notes on some commercial disinfectants. Philadelphia, 1893. 5p. DNLM **90-4711**

LEFFMANN, Henry (1847-1930)
The water supply of Philadelphia. [Philadelphia, 1893.] 16p. DNLM **90-4712**

LEFFMANN, Henry (1847-1930)
The commercial forms of hydrogen dioxid. Philadelphia, 1894. 2 l. DNLM **90-4713**

LEFFMANN, Henry (1847-1930)
Food colors and food preservatives. New York, [1894]. 11p. DNLM **90-4714**

LEFFMANN, Henry (1847-1930)
Examination of water for sanitary and technic purposes. 3rd ed. Philadelphia: P. Blakiston, Son & Co., 1895. 154p. DNLM **90-4715**

LEFFMANN, Henry (1847-1930)
The filtration of public water supplies. [Philadelphia], 1895. 8p. DNLM **90-4716**

LEFFMANN, Henry (1847-1930)
Milk inspection and milk-standards. [Philadelphia: Lea Bros. & Co., 1895.] 9p. DNLM **90-4717**

LEFFMANN, Henry (1847-1930)
Note on hydrogen dioxide as furnished to practicing dentists. [New York & Philadelphia, 1895.] 3p. DNLM **90-4718**

LEFFMANN, Henry (1847-1930) and William BEAM
Analysis of milk and milk products. 2nd ed., revised and enlarged, with illustrations. Philadelphia: P. Blakiston, Son & Co., 1896. 120p. DNLM; PPC **90-4719**

LEFFMANN, Henry (1847-1930)
Handbook of structural formulae for use of students, containing 180 structural and stereochemic formulae. Philadelphia: P. Blakiston, Son & Co., 1897. 57p. DNLM **90-4720**

LEFFMANN, Henry (1847-1930)
Examination of water for sanitary and technic purposes. 4th ed., revised and enlarged. Philadelphia: P. Blakiston's Son & Co., 1899. 145p. DNLM **90-4721**

LEFFMANN, Henry (1847-1930)
Digestive ferments, with especial reference to the effects of food preservatives. Philadelphia, 1899. 12p. DNLM **90-4722**

LEGG, J[ohn] Wickham (1843-1921)
Practical guide to the examination of urine. . . . 7th ed., enl. Edited and rev. by H. Lewis Jones. Philadelphia: P. Blakiston, Son & Co., 1893. 139p. DNLM; PPC; PU **90-4723**

LE HARDY, J[ulius] C[aesar] (*b.* 1831)
Yellow fever, the American plague; thorough drainage and municipal cleanliness the only means of insuring its extinction. [New York, 1894.] 12p. DNLM **90-4724**

LEHLBACH, Charles F. J. (1835-1896)
Diet and therapy of typhoid fever. Philadelphia: Binder & Kelly, [1891]. 20p. DNLM **90-4725**

LEHLBACH, Charles F. J. (1835-1896)
The true pathology of sudden death in acute pneumonia, and the best means of averting it. [Philadelphia, 1892.] 19p. DNLM **90-4726**

LEHMANN, Karl Bernhard (1858-1940) and Rudolf NEUMANN
Atlas and essentials of bacteriology. New York: William Wood & Co., 1897. 204p. 63 plates. DNLM; NNNAM; OCIM; PPC **90-4727**

LEIDY, Joseph, Jr. (*b.* 1866)
Fracture of the body of the scapula through muscular violence. [Philadelphia, 1891.] 2p. DNLM **90-4728**

LEISHMAN, William (1834-1894)
A system of midwifery, including the diseases of pregnancy and the puerperal state. . . . 4th American ed. . . . Philadelphia: Lea Bros. & Co., 1890 [1888]. 2 v. (paged continuously) DNLM; LNT-M; NNNAM; PU **90-4729**

[LEONARD, Charles Henri] (1850-1925)
Over one thousand prescriptions or favorite formulae of various authors. . . . Detroit, Mich.: Illustrated Medical Journal Co., 1892. 132p. DLC; OCIM **90-4730**

LEONARD, Charles Henri (1850-1925)
A case of infantile scurvy caused by prolonged use of sterilized food. Providence, 1893. 4p. DNLM **90-4731**

LEONARD, C[harles] Henri (1850-1925)
The pocket anatomist (founded upon Gray). 19th ed., containing dissection hints and visceral anatomy. Detroit, [1897]. 297p. DNLM **90-4732**

LEONARD, C[harles] Henri (1850-1925)
The hair; its growth, care, diseases, and treatment. Detroit & London, [1897]. 316p. DNLM; OCIM **90-4733**

LEONARD, C[harles] Henri (1850-1925)
A manual of bandaging. Adapted for self-instruction. 6th ed. Detroit, [1897]. 159p. DNLM; OCIM **90-4734**

LEONARD, Charles Lester (1861-1913)
A demonstration of the endogenous formation of the malarial parasite. Philadelphia, 1895. 4p. 3 plates. DNLM **90-4735**

LEONARD, Charles Lester (1861-1913)
A new method of studying cell motion. Philadelphia, 1895. 4p. DNLM **90-4736**

LEONARD SCHOOLS OF MEDICINE AND PHARMACY, SHAW UNIVERSITY, RALEIGH, N.C.
Annual announcements and catalogues for the sessions of 1896-97 to 1898-99 (16.-18.); 1900-1901 to 1903-04 (20.-23.). Raleigh, 1896-1903. DNLM [List of students and graduates for the sessions of 1896-97 to 1898-99; 1900-1901 to 1903-04 in announcements for subsequent years.] **90-4737**

LEONARD, William E[dwin] (1855-1935)
Homoeopathic medical education. Philadelphia, 1891. 5p. DNLM **90-4738**

LEONARD, William E[dwin] (1855-1935)
Inaugural address: What constitutes a homoeopathic physician? Opening of fourth annual course of lectures, College of Homoeopathic Medicine and Surgery, University of Minnesota, October 6, 1891. [Minneapolis, 1891.] 9p. DNLM **90-4739**

LESZYNSKY, William M.
A contribution to the clinial study of spontaneous degenerative neuritis of the brachial plexus. [New York, 1890.] 25p. DNLM **90-4740**

LESZYNSKY, William M.
The use of atropine in the treatment of localized muscular spasm. [New York, 1891.] 6p. DNLM **90-4741**

LESZYNSKY, William M.
The management and care of patients with hemiplegia, resulting from cerebral haemorrhage. [New York, 1892.] 10p. DNLM **90-4742**

LESZYNSKY, William M.
A case of sporadic myxoedematous cretinism. [New York, 1894.] 2 l. DNLM **90-4743**

LESZYNSKY, William M.
Electricity in diagnosis and prognosis of affections of the peripheral nerves. [New York, 1894.] 12p. DNLM **90-4744**

LESZYNSKY, William M.
The knee-jerk in diagnosis. New York, 1895. 11p. DNLM **90-4745**

LESZYNSKY, William M.
Bilateral neuritis of the brachial plexus following acute croupous pneumonia. New York, 1896. 5p. DNLM **90-4746**

LESZYNSKY, William M.
Congenital absence of outward movement of both eyes. New York, 1897. 13p. DNLM **90-4747**

LESZYNSKY, William M.
Unilateral loss of the pupillary light reflex (reflex iridoplegia); its pathology and clinical significance. [New York, 1898.] 29p. 1 table. DNLM **90-4748**

LEVIS, M[inford]
944 examination questions on anatomy with their correct answers. . . . By M. Levis and W. Henry Price. . . . Philadelphia: University of Pennsylvania Press, 1892. 109p. DLC; PPC; PU **90-4749**

LEVY, Robert (*b.* 1864)
Treatment of laryngeal phthisis. Philadelphia: Avil Print. Co., [1891]. 19p. DNLM **90-4750**

LEVY, Robert (*b.* 1864)
Two cases of laryngeal neoplasms. Chicago, 1893. 8p. DNLM **90-4751**

LEVY, Robert (*b.* 1864)
Inoperable sarcoma of the nose. New York, 1894. 5p. DNLM **90-4752**

LEVY, Robert (*b.* 1864)
The treatment of laryngeal tuberculosis, with a report of cases. New York: D. Appleton & Co., 1895. 16p. 1 table. DNLM **90-4753**

LEVY, Robert (*b.* 1864)
Direct autoscopy; Kirstein. With demonstration. [Denver], 1896. 2 l. DNLM **90-4754**

LEVY, Robert (*b.* 1864)
Exaggerated arytenoid movement; anchylosis of the crico-arytenoid articulation. [St. Louis, 1896.] 3p. DNLM **90-4755**

LEVY, Robert (*b.* 1864)
Fatal hemorrhage from the nose and pharynx from unusual cause; with exhibition of specimen. St. Louis, 1896. 4p. DNLM **90-4756**

LEVY, Robert (*b.* 1864)
Pharyngeal tuberculosis. Denver, 1896. 7p. DNLM **90-4757**

LEVY, Robert (*b.* 1864)
Medical education. [Denver], 1897. 12p. DNLM **90-4758**

LEVY, Robert (*b.* 1864)
Prognosis of laryngeal tuberculosis. Chicago, 1899. 7p. DNLM **90-4759**

LEVY, Robert (*b.* 1864)
Sinus-thrombosis; cure without opening the sinus. St. Louis, 1899. 4p. DNLM **90-4760**

LEWERS, Arthur [Hamilton Nicholson]
A practical text-book of the diseases of women. 2nd ed. Philadelphia: P. Blakiston, Son & Co., 1890. 444p. DNLM; PPC; PU **90-4761**

LEWERS, Arthur [Hamilton Nicholson]
A practical text-book of the diseases of women. 3rd ed., rev. Philadelphia: P. Blakiston, Son & Co., 1892. 444p. NNNAM; PPC; PU **90-4762**

LEWERS, Arthur [Hamilton Nicholson]
A practical text-book of the diseases of women. 4th ed. Philadelphia: P. Blakiston, Son & Co., 1896. 439p. PPC; PPJ **90-4763**

LEWERS, Arthur [Hamilton Nicholson]
A practical text-book of the diseases of women. 5th ed. Philadelphia: P. Blakiston, Son & Co., 1897. 526p. 4 plates. DNLM; NNNAM; PPC; PU **90-4764**

LEWI, Emily
Rhythmic head-movements associated with nystagmus occurring in infants and young children. [Philadelphia: Lea Bros. & Co., 1894.] 14p. DNLM **90-4765**

LEWIS, Bertha
Case of supra spinous dislocation of the right shoulder, presumably occurring at birth. [Philadelphia, 1895.] 4p. DNLM **90-4766**

LEWIS, Bransford (*b.* 1862)
A consideration of sexual neurasthenia. [St. Louis, 1890.] 16p. DNLM **90-4767**

LEWIS, Bransford (*b.* 1862)
A materialistic view of sexual impotence. [Philadelphia: Lea Bros. & Co., 1892.] 10p. DNLM **90-4768**

LEWIS, Bransford (*b.* 1862)
The role of the posterior urethra in chronic urethritis. [New York, 1893.] 7p. DNLM **90-4769**

LEWIS, Bransford (*b.* 1862)
Why chronic urethritis is ordinarily difficult of cure, and an efficacious method of curing it. [Keokuk, 1894.] 7p. DNLM **90-4770**

LEWIS, Bransford (*b.* 1862)
The infiltration method of local anesthesia in genito-urinary surgery. [St. Louis, 1896.] 2 l. DNLM **90-4771**

LEWIS, Bransford (*b.* 1862)
Conservative yet effectual treatment of hypertrophied prostate by electro-incision done through the urethra; presentation of specimens of hypertrophied prostate; demonstration of Bottini-Freudenberg electro-incisor. St. Louis, 1899. 15p. DNLM **90-4772**

LEWIS, Daniel (1846-1919)
The anniversary address before the Medical Society of the State of New York. Philadelphia: W. J. Dornan, 1890. 14p. DNLM **90-4773**

LEWIS, Daniel (1846-1919)
Cancer and its treatment. Detroit, Mich.: G. S. Davis, 1892. 127p. 2 plates. DNLM; OCIM **90-4774**

LEWIS, Daniel (1846-1919)
The caustic treatment of cancer. New York: Trow, 1892. 11p. DNLM **90-4775**

LEWIS, Daniel (1846-1919)
Memoir of Laurence Johnson. [New York, 1893.] 7p. DNLM **90-4776**

LEWIS, Daniel (1846-1919)
The use and place of caustics in the treatment of cancer. [New York, 1893.] 6p. DNLM **90-4777**

LEWIS, F[rancis] Park (1855-1940)
Consideration of the legal status of midwifery in the state of New York. [New York, 1891.] 5p. DNLM **90-4778**

LEWIS, F[rancis] Park (1855-1940)
A new spectacle lens; a compound achromatic periscope. New York, 1896. 4p. DNLM **90-4779**

LEWIS, F[rancis] Park (1855-1940)
Artificial light in its effect on the eyes. New York, 1897. 21p. DNLM **90-4780**

LEWIS, George Andrew (1870-1915)
The origin and treatment of stammering. 5th ed., enlarged and revised. Detroit, 1899. 200p. DNLM **90-4781**

LEWIS, G[eorge] Griffin (*b.* 1865)
A few interesting eye cases. St. Louis, 1897. 3p. DNLM **90-4782**

LEWIS, G[eorge] Griffin (*b.* 1865)
A new instrument for testing the external ocular muscles. [St. Louis], 1897. 2p. DNLM **90-4783**

LEWIS, G[eorge] Griffin (*b.* 1865)
A peculiar case of sarcoma of the choroid. [St. Louis], 1897. 2p. DNLM **90-4784**

LEWIS, G[eorge] Griffin (*b.* 1865)
Some statistics on blindness and deafness, with a comparison of the inconveniences of each. New York: D. Appleton & Co., 1897. 9p. DNLM **90-4785**

LEWIS, G[eorge] Griffin (*b.* 1865)
Otology; its relation to general medicine. New York, 1899. 13p. DNLM **90-4786**

LEWIS, G[eorge] Griffin (*b.* 1865)
The relation of ophthalmology to general medicine. New York, 1899. 12p. DNLM **90-4787**

LEWIS, H[arry] Edwin (*b.* 1875)
The philosophy of sex. Burlington, Vt., 1896. 51p. DNLM **90-4788**

LEWIS, H[arry] Edwin (*b.* 1875)
Irregular menstruation in young women due to anaemic conditions. New York: M. J. Breitenbach Co., [1897]. 7p. DNLM **90-4789**

LEWIS, Henry F[oster] (1864-1929)
Iniencephalus. New York, 1897. 43p. DNLM **90-4790**

LEWIS, Henry F[oster] (1864-1929)
Aberrant tendinous cords of the heart. Philadelphia, 1898. 12p. DNLM **90-4791**

LEWIS, Henry F[oster] (1864-1929)
Uraemia in the process of child-bearing. New York: William Wood & Co., 1898. 32p. DNLM **90-4792**

LEWIS, Henry F[oster] (1864-1929)
Maternal impressions. New York, 1899. 8p. DNLM **90-4793**

LEWIS PHONO-METRIC INSTITUTE AND SCHOOL FOR STAMMERERS, DETROIT
Announcement of the principal. Detroit: The Phono-Meter, [1899?]. 6 l. (illustr.). DNLM **90-4794**

LEWIS, Robert
A remarkable angeioneurosis of the tongue, due to the application of chromic acid to granulations of the upper and posterior portions of the tympanic membrane. A contribution to the physiology of the chorda tympani nerve. New York, 1897. 9p. DNLM **90-4795**

LEWIS SCHOOL FOR STAMMERERS, DETROIT
Circular. Detroit: Richmond & Backus, [1899?]. 13 l. (illustr.). DNLM **90-4796**

LEWIS, W[illiam] Bevan (1847-1929)
A text-book of mental diseases; with special reference to the pathological aspects of insanity. Philadelphia: P. Blakiston, Son & Co., 1890. 552p. 18 plates, 3 charts. DNLM; NNNAM; PPC; PU **90-4797**

LEWIS, W[illiam] Bevan (1847-1929)
Mental diseases. A text-book having special reference to pathoIgoical aspects of insanity. 2nd ed. Philadelphia: P. Blakiston, Son & Co., 1893. 297p. NNNAM; PPC; PU **90-4798**

LEWIS, W[illiam] Bevan (1847-1929)
A text-book of mental diseases; with special reference to the pathological aspects of insanity. 2nd ed., thoroughly revised, enlarged, and in part re-written. Philadelphia: P. Blakiston's Son & Co., 1899. 609p. DNLM; MBM; PPC; PU **90-4799**

LEWIS, W[illiam] M.
Injuries to the head. [Philadelphia, 1892.] 5p. DNLM **90-4800**

LIEBERTHAL, David
Case of vitiligo presenting unusual features. [St. Louis], 1897. 2 l. DNLM **90-4801**

LIEBERTHAL, David
A case of leprosy. Chicago, 1898. 1 l. 1 plate. DNLM **90-4802**

LIEBERTHAL, David
Prevention of venereal diseases. Chicago, 1899. 7p. DNLM **90-4803**

LILIENTHAL, Howard (1861-1946)
A case of traumatic meningocele; operation, followed by perfect recovery. [Philadelphia, 1895.] 2p. DNLM **90-4804**

LILIENTHAL, Howard (1861-1946)
Unintentional neglect in the treatment of surgical diseases. New York, 1895. 9p. DNLM **90-4805**

LILIENTHAL, Howard (1861-1946)
Surgical hints for the surgeon and general practitioner. New York, 1897. 29p. DNLM **90-4806**

LILIENTHAL, Howard (1861-1946)
Clinical observations on acute sepsis. New York: D. Appleton & Co., 1898. 12p. DNLM **90-4807**

LILIENTHAL, Samuel (1815-1891)
Homoeopathic therapeutics. 3rd, rewritten and enl. ed. . . . Philadelphia: Hahnemann Publishing House, 1890. 1154p. DLC; PPHa **90-4808**

LILLARD, John F. B.
The medical muse, grave and gay. A collection of rhymes up to date, by the doctor, for the doctor, and against the doctor. New York: L. E. Booth, 1895. 141p. DNLM; NN **90-4809**

LILLIE, James
Homeopathy vindicated, in a letter to J. V. C. Smith, containing a reply to his review of Drs. C. and L.'s "Epitome of homeopathic practice," with the acceptance of J. V. C. Smith's and C. A. Lee's challenges and the consequences. New York, 1895. 8p. DNLM **90-4810**

LILLY, ELI & CO.
Illustrated catalogue of formaldehyde disinfectors, deodorizers, sterilizers, chemicals. Indianapolis, 1898. 32p. NNNAM **90-4811**

LILLY's hand book of pharmacy and therapeutics. 5th revision, 13th ed. Indianapolis: E. Lilly & Co., 1898. 336p. DNLM; OCLloyd **90-4812**

LINCOLN MEDICAL COLLEGE OF COTNER UNIVERSITY, LINCOLN, NEB.
Annual announcements for the sessions of 1890-91 to 1892-93 (1.-3.); 1897-98 (8.); 1903-04 (14.). Lincoln, 1890-1903. DNLM [Organized in 1890 as the Medical Department of Nebraska Christian University. In 1891 became the Medical Department of Cotner University.] **90-4813**

LINCOLN, R[ufus] P[ratt] (1841-1900)
The use of pyoctanin, an antiseptic in diseases of the upper air-passages. [New York, 1891.] 6p. DNLM **90-4814**

LINCOLN, R[ufus] P[ratt] (1841-1900)
Recurrence at a new site of a laryngeal growth (papilloma) in a new site already under the title "Evulsion of a laryngeal tumor which returned twenty-two years after its removal by laryngotomy"; with an analysis of thirty-four cases. New York: D. Appleton & Co., 1893. 10p. 1 table. DNLM **90-4815**

LINCOLN, William
Abscess of the nasal septum; with a report of two cases. Cleveland, 1896. 6p. DNLM **90-4816**

LINK, W[illiam] H.
Object lessons in gynaecology. III. [Philadelphia, 1892.] 4p. DNLM **90-4817**

LINK, W[illiam] H.
Object lessons in gynaecology. IV. [Philadelphia, 1893.] 3p. DNLM **90-4818**

LINN, S[amuel] H.
Specialties in medicine and surgery. New York, 1893. 4p. DNLM **90-4819**

LIPPINCOTT, E[ldridge]
Angina Ludovici. New York, 1891. 6p. DNLM **90-4820**

LIPPINCOTT, E[ldridge]
Our public institutions as sources of impairment of vision. [Philadelphia, 1892.] 19p. DNLM **90-4821**

LIPPINCOTT, J[ames] A[udrey] (*b.* 1847)
Intra-ocular syringing in cataract extraction, with a report of fifty-three operations. Philadelphia: W. J. Dornan, 1890. 19p. DNLM **90-4822**

LIPPINCOTT, J[ames] A[udrey] (*b.* 1847)
New tests for binocular vision. [New York, 1890.] 7p. DNLM **90-4823**

LIPPINCOTT'S medical dictionary, a complete vocabulary of the terms used in medicine and the allied sciences, with their pronunciation, etymology, and signification, including much collateral information of a descriptive and encyclopaedic character; prepared on the basis of Thomas's complete medical dictionary, by Ryland W. Greene, with the editorial collaboration of John Ashhurst, George A. Piersol, Joseph P. Remington. Philadelphia & London: J. B. Lippincott Co., 1897. 1154p. DNLM; NNNAM; PPC; PU **90-4824**

LITTLEJOHN, James B.
Notes on histology. . . . Kirksville, Mo.: Weekly Advocate Print, 1899. 53p. DLC **90-4825**

LITTLEJOHN, James B.
Outlines of pathology. . . . Kirksville, Mo.: Weekly Advocate Print, 1899. 124p. DLC **90-4826**

LITTLEJOHN, J[ohn] M[artin] (*b.* 1867)
Lecture notes on physiology, delivered before the January and April classes of the American School of Osteopathy. . . . Kirskville, Mo.: Advocate Book and Job Print, 1898. 277p. DLC **90-4827**

LITTLEJOHN, J[ohn] M[artin] (*b.* 1867)
Physiology, exhaustive and practical. A series of practical lectures delivered . . . in the American School of Osteopathy at Kirksville, Missouri. Especially adapted for students of osteopathy. Kirksville: Journal Printing Co., 1898. 285p. DLC **90-4828**

LITTLEJOHN, John Martin (*b.* 1867)
Lectures on psycho-physiology. Kirksville, Mo.: American School of Osteopathy, 1899. 12p. DLC **90-4829**

LIVINGSTON, Louis J.
Medical and dental red book. A register of all the physicians, surgeons, dentists, druggists, nurses, etc., of Cleveland and vicinity, together with a digest of the state laws, and the city laws pertaining to these professions and other miscellaneous matter. . . . Cleveland: The Helman-Taylor Co., 1899. 372p. DLC; OCIM **90-4830**

LLOYD, James Hendrie (*b.* 1853)
A case of tumor of the mid-brain and left optic thalamus. Philadelphia, 1892. 6p. DNLM **90-4831**

LLOYD, James Hendrie (*b.* 1853)
Forms of pseudo-tabes due to lead, alcohol, diphtheria, etc. Philadelphia, 1892. 6p. DNLM **90-4832**

LLOYD, James Hendrie (*b.* 1853)
Report of a case of syringomyelia, with exhibition of sections of the spinal cord. [Philadelphia, 1893.] 13p. 3 plates. DNLM **90-4833**

LLOYD, James Hendrie (*b.* 1853) and David RIESMAN
Infectious endocarditis, with septicaemia, complicated with multiple neuritis. [Philadelphia, 1895.] 11p. DNLM **90-4834**

LLOYD, John U[ri] (1849-1936)
Elixirs and flavoring extracts: their history, formulae, and methods of preparation. [3rd rev. ed.] New York: William Wood & Co., 1892. 191p. NNNAM; OCLloyd **90-4835**

LOBB, Henry W.
A treatise on the errors of youth and diseases of the sexes. . . . Philadelphia, Pa., 1894. 191p. DLC; PPC **90-4836**

LOCKE, F[rank] S[piller]
On the action of ether on contracture and of positive kathodic polarization of vertebrate voluntary muscle. New York, 1896. 26p. 4 plates. **90-4837**

LOCKE, Frederick John (1829-1903)
Notes from lectures of F. J. Locke, M.D., Professor of materia medica and therapeutics, Eclectic Medical Institute, Cincinnati, Ohio. By students of class 1895. Cincinnati, [1894]. 170p. DLC; OCLloyd **90-4838**

LOCKE, Frederick J[ohn] (1829-1903)
Syllabus of eclectic materia medica and therapeutics, compiled from notes taken from the lectures of . . . . Edited with pharmacological additions by Harvey W. Felter, with notes on specific medicines, by John Uri Lloyd. Cincinnati: J. M. Scudder's Sons, 1895. 461p. DNLM; OCLloyd **90-4839**

LOCKETT, W[illiam] R.
The use of gloves in surgery; with a report on an investigation as to the efficacy of cotton gloves. Philadelphia, 1899. 7p. DNLM **90-4840**

LOCKHART, F[rederick] A[lbert] L[awton]
Artificial dilatation of the non-pregnant uterine canal. New York, 1896. 7p. DNLM **90-4841**

LOCKHART, F[rederick] A[lbert] L[awton]
Second laparotomy. New York, 1896. 2p. DNLM **90-4842**

LOCKHART, F[rederick] A[lbert] L[awton]
The operative treatment of uterine fibroids. New York, 1899 11p. DNLM **90-4843**

LOCKWOOD, Charles E.
A study of alcohol, tobacco, coffee, and tea as causative factors in the production of nervous disorders. New York: D. Appleton & Co., 1898. 36p. DNLM; NNNAM **90-4844**

LOCKWOOD, George Roe
Purpura haemorrhagica. New York: Trow, 1891. 16p. DNLM **90-4845**

LOCKWOOD, George Roe
A manual of the practice of medicine. . . . Philadelphia: W. B. Saunders, 1896. 935p. col. plates. DLC; DNLM; PPC; PU **90-4846**

LOMBARD, Warren P[limpton] (1855-1939)
The effect of fatigue on voluntary muscular contractions. [Worcester, 1890.] 19p. 2 plates.
90-4847

LONG, Charles
A case of acromegaly. [Easton, Pa., 1891.] 8p. 1 plate. DNLM
90-4848

LONG, Eli Herr (*b.* 1860)
Tables for doctor and druggist. . . . 2nd ed., rev. and enl. . . . Detroit, G. S. Davis, 1894. 149p. DLC; DNLM; OCLloyd
90-4849

LONG, J[ohn] H[arper] (1856-1918)
Laboratory manual of elementary chemical physiology and urine analysis. Chicago: E. H. Colegrove & Co., 1894. 366p. DNLM; ICU **90-4850**

LONG, J[ohn] W[esley] (1859-1926)
An ideal uterine dilator and a new haemostatic forceps. [Asheville, N.C., 1890.] 1 l. DNLM **90-4851**

LONG, J[ohn] W[esley] (1859-1926)
What kind of instruments are demanded by modern surgery? [Philadelphia, 1890.] 8p. DNLM **90-4852**

LONG, J[ohn] W[esley] (1859-1926)
Two cases illustrating the use of the curette after labor and abortion. [Richmond, 1891.] 4p. DNLM
90-4853

LONG, J[ohn] W[esley] (1859-1926)
Character the true test of the physician. Baltimore, 1892. 14p. DNLM **90-4854**

LONG, J[ohn] W[esley] (1859-1926)
The indications for operation in appendicitis. St. Louis, 1894. 16p. DNLM **90-4855**

LONG, J[ohn] W[esley] (1859-1926)
The value of Hegar's sign of pregnancy. [Buffalo, 1894.] 2 l. DNLM **90-4856**

LONG, J[ohn] W[esley] (1859-1926)
Surgery on the wing; three successful abdominal sections. Wilmington, 1895. 4p. DNLM **90-4857**

LONG, J[ohn] W[esley] (1859-1926)
Syllabus of gynecology, based on American text-book of gynecology. Philadelphia: W. B. Saunders, [1895]. 133p., interleaved. DNLM **90-4858**

LONG, J[ohn] W[esley] (1859-1926)
The technique of abdominal and pelvic surgery. [New York], 1895. 9p. DNLM **90-4859**

LONG, J[ohn] W[esley] (1859-1926)
The value of plastic work in operations involving the peritonaeum. [New York, 1895.] 6p. DNLM
90-4860

LONG, J[ohn] W[esley] (1859-1926)
Vaginal incision and drainage. New York, 1896. 7p. DNLM
90-4861

LONG ISLAND COLLEGE HOSPITAL. BROOKLYN, N.Y.
History of the Long Island College Hospital and its graduates, together with the Hoagland Laboratory and the Polhemus Memorial Clinic. By Joseph Howard Raymond. Brooklyn: Association of the Alumni, 1899. 433p. NNNAM
90-4862

LONGLEY, Elias (1822-1899)
Pocket medical dictionary. . . . new ed. Philadelphia: P. Blakiston, Son & Co., 1890. 303p. NNC; NNNAM; PPC; PU [Original ed., 1879] **90-4863**

LOOKER, J. K. M.
A lecture on the circulation of the blood by electromagnetism or polarity, with a textbook lesson annexed. . . . Bonaparte, Ia., 1896. 25p. DLC **90-4864**

LOOMIS, Alfred L[ebbeus] (1831-1895)
Valedictory address. Philadelphia, 1893. 12p. DNLM
90-4865

LOOMIS, Alfred Lebbeus (1831-1895)
Lessons in physical diagnosis. . . . rev. by Alexander Lambert. . . . 10th ed. New York: William Wood & Co., 1893. 278p. DNLM; NNNAM **90-4866**

LOOMIS, Alfred Lebbeus (1831-1895)
A text-book of practical medicine, designed for the use of students and practitioners of medicine. . . . 3rd ed., revised and enlarged. New York: William Wood & Co., 1895. 1134p. DNLM; NNNAM; PPC **90-4867**

LOOMIS, Alfred Lebbeus (1831-1895)
A text-book of practical medicine, designed for the use of students and practitioners of medicine. . . . Rev. and enl. . . . [11th ed.] New York: William Wood & Co., 1895. 1134p. plates. DLC; NNNAM **90-4868**

LOOMIS, Alfred Lebbeus, ed. (1831-1895)
A system of practical medicine, by American authors. Ed. by Alfred L. Loomis . . . and William Gilman Thompson. . . . New York and Philadelphia: Lea Bros. & Co., 1897-98. 4 v. col. plates. DLC; NNNAM; PPC; PU **90-4869**

LOOMIS, Alfred Lebbeus (1831-1895)
Lessons in physical diagnosis . . . rev. by Alexander Lambert. . . . 11th ed., rev. and enl. New York: William Wood & Co., 1899. 341p. DLC; DNLM; NNNAM
90-4870

LOOMIS, Henry Patterson (1859-1907)
A study of the processes which result in the arrest or cure of phthisis. New York: Trow, 1892. 27p. DNLM
90-4871

LOOMIS, Henry Patterson (1859-1907)
A new preparation of iron in the treatment of anaemia, with effect shown by increase in number of red corpuscles and amount of haemoglobin. [New York: M. J. Breitenbach Co., 1893.] 8p. DNLM **90-4872**

LOOMIS, Henry Patterson (1859-1907)
The successful treatment of anaemia, with effect shown by increase of red corpuscles and haemoglobin. [New York], 1893. 8p. DNLM **90-4873**

LOOMIS SANITARIUM FOR CONSUMPTIVES, LIBERTY, N.Y.
Annual reports of the officers to the society. And Branch Hospital and Dispensary for Incurables. New York City. 2., 1897-98; 3., 1898-99. New York: The De Vinne Press, 1898-1899. 35p. 12p., 37p. DNLM [Incorporated in 1895, and opened in the summer of 1896.] **90-4874**

LORING, Edward G[reely] (1837-1888)
Text-book of ophthalmoscopy. Part I. The normal eye, determination of refraction, diseases of the media, physiological optics, and theory of the ophthalmoscope. New York: D. Appleton & Co., 1893. 274p. CtY-M; NNNAM; PPC; PPJ **90-4875**

LOUISVILLE CITY HOSPITAL TRAINING SCHOOL FOR NURSES
Circulars for 1897; 1900. Louisville, 1897-1900. 12p.; 11p. DNLM **90-4876**

LOUISVILLE CITY HOSPITAL TRAINING SCHOOL FOR NURSES
Circular of information. [Louisville, 1898.] 2 l. DNLM **90-4877**

LOUISVILLE CITY HOSPITAL TRAINING SCHOOL FOR NURSES
Questions to be answered by candidate. [Louisville, 1898.] 1 sheet. DNLM **90-4878**

LOUISVILLE CITY HOSPITAL TRAINING SCHOOL FOR NURSES
Rules for the admission of pupils. [Louisville, 1898.] 1 sheet. DNLM **90-4879**

LOUISVILLE NATIONAL MEDICAL COLLEGE
Annual announcements for the sessions of 1894-95 (7.); 1896-97 (9.); 1898-99 (11.); 1899-1900 (12.); 1902-03 (15.); 1903-04 (16.). Louisville, 1894-1903. DNLM [List of students and graduates for the sessions of 1893-94; 1895-96; 1897-98; 1898-99; 1901-02; 1902-03, in Announcements for subsequent years. List of graduates from 1889 to 1903 in Announcement for 1903-04.] DNLM **90-4880**

LOVE, I[saac] N[ewton] (1848-1903)
Painful menstruation in virgins. [St. Louis, 1890.] 10 l. DNLM **90-4881**

LOVE, I[saac] N[ewton] (1848-1903)
Practical points in the management of some of the diseases of children. Detroit, Mich.: G. S. Davis, 1891. 141p. DNLM **90-4882**

LOVE, I[saac] N[ewton] (1848-1903)
"Children's rights." Valedictory address delivered to the graduating class of the Marion-Sims College of Medicine, St. Louis, 1893. Louisville: Renz & Henry, [1893]. 48p. DNLM **90-4883**

LOVELAND, Bradford C[hurchill] (*b.* 1862)
Food versus medicine as a blood-maker. New York, 1896. 7p. DNLM **90-4884**

LOVELAND, Bradford C[hurchill] (*b.* 1862)
Hysteria. Buffalo, 1897. 6p. DNLM **90-4885**

LOVELAND, Bradford C[hurchill] (*b.* 1862)
A contribution to the study of melancholia, with a table showing the results of an examination of the blood in fifty-seven cases. New York: D. Appleton & Co., 1898. 10p. 1 table. DNLM **90-4886**

LOVELAND, Bradford C[hurchill] (*b.* 1862)
A few interesting psycho-neuroses. New York: D. Appleton & Co., 1899. 5p. DNLM **90-4887**

LOVETT, Robert W[illiamson] (1859-1924)
High temperature in chronic joint disease. [Boston, 1890.] 6p. DNLM **90-4888**

LOVETT, Robert W[illiamson] (1859-1924)
Lateral deviation of the spine as a diagnostic symptom in Pott's disease. Boston: Damrell & Upham, 1890. 9p. DNLM **90-4889**

LOVETT, Robert W[illiamson] (1859-1924)
The diagnosis of Pott's disease. Philadelphia, 1891. 8p. DNLM **90-4890**

LOVETT, Robert W[illiamson] (1859-1924)
The etiology, pathology, and treatment of diseases of the hip joint. Boston: G. H. Ellis, 1891. 220p. DNLM **90-4891**

LOVETT, Robert W[illiamson] (1859-1924)
The place of fixation in the traction treatment of hip disease. [New York: D. Appleton & Co., 1891.] 11p. DNLM **90-4892**

LOVETT, Robert W[illiamson] (1859-1924) and John L. MORSE
A transient or ephemeral form of hip-disease; with a report of cases. Boston: Damrell & Upham, 1892. 6p. DNLM **90-4893**

LOVETT, Robert W[illiamson] (1859-1924)
A clinical classification of hip-disease. Boston: Damrell & Upham, 1892. 11p. DNLM **90-4894**

LOVETT, Robert W[illiamson] (1859-1924)
Intubation versus tracheotomy. Being a study of 858 cases operated on at the Boston City Hospital. [Philadelphia, 1892.] 12p. DNLM **90-4895**

LOVETT, Robert W[illiamson] (1859-1924)
The surgical aspect of the paralysis of new-born children. Boston: Damrell & Upham, 1892. 12p. DNLM **90-4896**

LOVETT, Robert W[illiamson] (1859-1924)
The mechanics and treatment of the broken-down foot. New York, 1896. 16p. DNLM **90-4897**

LOVETT, Robert W[illiamson] (1859-1924) and John DANE
The affections of the arch of the foot commonly classified as flat-foot. New York, 1896. 18p. DNLM **90-4898**

LOVETT, Robert W[illiamson] (1859-1924)
Bursitis of the deep pretibial bursa, with a report of cases. Boston: Rockwell & Churchill, 1897. 8p. DNLM **90-4899**

LOVETT, Robert W[illiamson] (1859-1924)
Late excision of the hip. Boston: Damrell & Upham, 1897. 14p. DNLM **90-4900**

LOVETT, Robert W[illiamson] (1859-1924)
The prevention of flat-foot and similar affections. Boston: Damrell & Upham, 1897. 12p. DNLM **90-4901**

LOVETT, Robert W[illiamson] (1859-1924)
Spondylolisthesis, with description of a case. [Philadelphia], 1897. 16p. DNLM **90-4902**

LUDLAM, R[euben] (1831-1899)
An address on homoeopathy and the public health. [Chicago, 1893.] 8p. DNLM **90-4903**

LUFF, Arthur P[earson] (1855-1938)
Manual of chemistry, inorganic and organic . . . for the use of students of medicine. Philadelphia: Lea Bros. & Co., [1892]. 522p. ICJ; NN; PPJ; PU **90-4904**

LUFF, Arthur P[earson] (1855-1938)
Gout, its pathology and treatment. Founded on the Goulstonian lectures on the chemistry and pathology of gout delivered . . . before the Royal College of Physicians of London in 1897. . . . New York: William Wood & Co., 1899. 248p. CtY-M; NNNAM; OCIM; PPC **90-4905**

LUNDY, Charles J. (1846-1892)
Hypodermic medication in diseases of the eye. . . . Detroit: J. F. Eby & Co., printers, 1890. 16p. DLC **90-4906**

LUSK, Graham (1866-1932)
Influence of the carbohydrates on proteid catabolism, with special reference to diabetes. An abstract. New York: [D. Appleton & Co., 1891.] 7p. DNLM **90-4907**

LUSK, Graham (1866-1932)
Formation of glycogen after taking different varieties of sugar. An abstract. [New York: D. Appleton & Co., 1892.] 10p. DNLM **90-4908**

LUSK, William T[hompson] (1838-1907)
The science and art of midwifery. New edition with numerous illustrations. New York: D. Appleton & Co., 1890. 763p. NNC; NNNAM; PPC **90-4909**

LUSK, William T[hompson] (1838-1907)
The science and art of midwifery. . . . New [4th] ed., rev. and enl. . . . New York: D. Appleton & Co., 1892. 761p. col. plates. DLC; DNLM; NNNAM **90-4910**

LUSK, William T[hompson] (1838-1907)
The illustrious Boerhaave. New York: D. Appleton & Co., 1895. 12p. port. DNLM; NNNAM **90-4911**

LUSK, William T[hompson] (1838-1907)
The science and art of midwifery. . . . New ed., rev. and enl. . . . New York: D. Appleton & Co., 1896. 797p. col. plates. DLC; NNNAM; OCIM; PU **90-4912**

LUSK, Z[era] J.
Mistral stenosis in pregnancy, with cases. Philadelphia, 1893. 12p. DNLM **90-4913**

LUYTIES HOMOEOPATHIC PHARMACY CO.
Price list and reference book for druggists. St. Louis, 1896. 164p. OCIM **90-4914**

LYDSTON, G[eorge] Frank (1858-1923)
Addresses and essays. [Chicago: F. Klein & Co., 1890.] 86p. DNLM **90-4915**

LYDSTON, G[eorge] Frank (1858-1923)
The local treatment of syphilitic phenomena. [Chicago, 1890.] 7p. DNLM **90-4916**

LYDSTON, G[eorge] Frank (1858-1923)
Addresses and essays. 2nd ed. Louisville: Renz & Henry, [1892]. 289p. DNLM **90-4917**

LYDSTON, G[eorge] Frank (1858-1923)
Varicocele and its treatment. Chicago: W. T. Keener, 1892. 126p. DNLM; OCIM **90-4918**

LYDSTON, G[eorge] Frank (1858-1923)
Gonorrhoea and urethritis. . . . Detroit, Mich.: G. S. Davis, 1892. 216p. DLC; DNLM; OCIM **90-4919**

LYDSTON, G[eorge] Frank (1858-1923)
The etiology of prostatic hypertrophy. Philadelphia: R. C. Penfield, 1893. 11p. DNLM **90-4920**

LYDSTON, G[eorge] Frank (1858-1923)
Homoeopathy and its congeners. Louisville: Renz & Henry, [1893]. 27p. DNLM **90-4921**

LYDSTON, G[eorge] Frank (1858-1923)
Stricture of the urethra. . . . Chicago: The W. T. Keener Co., 1893. 334p. plates. DLC; DNLM; OCIM **90-4922**

LYDSTON, G[eorge] Frank (1858-1923)
Over the hookah; the tales of a talkative doctor. Chicago: F. Klein, 1896. 618p. DNLM; ICU **90-4923**

LYDSTON, G[eorge] Frank (1858-1923)
The surgical diseases of the genito-urinary tract, venereal and sexual diseases; a text-book for students and practitioners. . . . Illustrated iwth 235 engravings. Philadelphia, New York, [etc.]: The F. A. Davis Co., 1899. 1011p. DLC; DNLM; NNNAM; PPC **90-4924**

LYDSTON, James A.
A petrified eye. [Philadelphia, 1893.] 7p. DNLM **90-4925**

LYMAN, C[harles] B[aldwin]
Simplicity in the treatment of fractures. [New York: D. Appleton & Co., 1894.] 12p. DNLM **90-4926**

LYMAN, C[harles] B[aldwin]
The hand in railway surgery. Chicago, 1895. 8p. DNLM **90-4927**

LYMAN, C[harles] B[aldwin]
Intestinal approximation, with report of a case of gastro-enterostomy and one of end-to-end approximation. [Philadelphia: Lea Bros. & Co., 1895.] 8p. DNLM **90-4928**

LYMAN, C[harles] B[aldwin]
Omphalorrhagia; umbilical hemorrhage. [Denver, 1895.] 6p. DNLM **90-4929**

LYMAN, G[eorge] H[inckley] (1819-1890)
Some aspects of the medical service in the armies of the United States during the war of the Rebellion. Boston: S. J. Parkhill & Co., 1891. 40p. DNLM; MBM **90-4930**

LYMAN, Henry Munson (1835-1904)
The practical home physician. . . . Written by Henry M. Lyman . . . Christian Fenger . . . H. Webster Jones . . . W. T. Belfield. . . . Rev. and enl. ed. . . . Chicago: Star Publishing Co., 1891. 1157p. col. plates. DLC; ICU; OCIM **90-4931**

LYMAN, Henry Munson (1835-1904)
A text-book of the principles and practice of medicine, for the use of medical students and practitioners. . . . Philadelphia: Lea Bros. & Co., 1892. 923p. DLC; DNLM; PPC; PU **90-4932**

LYMAN, Henry M[unson] (1835-1904)
The book of health, a reliable family physician giving in detail the cause, symptoms, treatment and history of all diseases of the human body. . . . Rev. ed., 1898. Providence, R.I.: W. P. Mason, [1898]. 1157p. DLC **90-4933**

LYNDS, James G.
Hernia of the placenta through the muscular coat of the uterus during labor. Philadelphia, 1893. 2p. DNLM **90-4934**

LYON, Irving Phillips
Combined typhoid and malarial infection. Report of a case, and review of the literature, with special reference to the so-called typho-malarial fever. Philadelphia, 1899. 17p. DNLM **90-4935**

LYON, Irving Phillips
Types of normal and morbid blood. [Philadelphia], 1899. 1 l. 1 plate. DNLM **90-4936**

LYONS, Albert Brown (1841-1926)
Hand book of practical assaying of drugs and galenicals. . . . Detroit: Nelson, Baker & Co., 1899. 237p. DLC; OCLloyd **90-4937**

MABBOTT, J. Milton
Three warnings of interest to obstetricians. New York, 1896. 6p. DNLM **90-4938**

MABON, William
Trional and tetronal. Clinical observations on their action as hypnotics and sedatives for the insane. Utica, N.Y., 1893. 13p. DNLM **90-4939**

MACALESTER, Richard K.
The hydriatic treatment of pneumonia. Denver, 1899. 8p. DNLM **90-4940**

MACALESTER, Richard K.
Some clinical observations on the action of the thermal waters of Glenwood Springs in gout and lithemia. Detroit, 1899. 23p. DNLM **90-4941**

MACALISTER, Alexander (1844-1919)
A textbook of human anatomy: systematic and typographical. . . . Philadelphia: P. Blakiston, Son & Co., 1890 [1889]. 775p. ICJ; PPC; PPHa **90-4942**

McBRIDE, J[ames] H.
Epileptic insanity. [Milwaukee, 1893.] 20p. DNLM **90-4943**

MACBRIDE, Nathaniel L.
Diseases of the eye. . . . New York: Boericke, Runyon & Ernesty, 1897. 310p. col. frontis. DLC; NNNAM **90-4944**

McBRIDE, Peter (1854-1946)
Diseases of the throat, nose, and ear. A clinical manual for students and practitioners. Philadelphia: P. Blakiston [and others], 1892. 640p. CtY-M; DNLM; IU-M; PPC **90-4945**

McBURNEY, Charles (1845-1913) and M. Allen STARR
A contribution to cerebral surgery. Diagnosis, localization, and operation for removal of three tumors of the brain; with some comments upon the surgical treatment of brain tumors. Philadelphia, 1893. 27p. DNLM; PPC **90-4946**

McCAHEY, Peter
The atmospheric tractor. A new instrument and some new theories in obstetrics. [Philadelphia: J. T. O'Callaghan, 1890.] 8p. DNLM **90-4947**

McCAHEY, Peter
Parturition rendered safe and comparatively painless. The atmospheric tractor and the uterine safety tube. Philadelphia: J. T. O'Callaghan, 1891. 14p. DNLM **90-4948**

McCALLUM, H[ugh]
Chloroform inhalation. [Philadelphia: Lea Bros. & Co., 1892.] 20p. DNLM **90-4949**

McCALLUM, H[ugh]
Four cases of appendicitis presenting some points of interest. Philadelphia, 1892. 5p. DNLM **90-4950**

McCALLUM, H[ugh]
The physiologic and therapeutic action of iron, with a discussion of its newer pharmaceutic compounds. [Philadelphia, 1895.] 6p. DNLM **90-4951**

MacCALLUM, John Bruce (1876-1906)
On the histogenesis of the striated muscle fibre, and the growth of the human sartorius muscle. Baltimore, 1898. 20p. DNLM **90-4952**

McCASKEY, G[eorge] W[ashington] (1853-1935)
Disinfection during and after the acute infectious diseases. St. Louis, 1890. 14p. DNLM **90-4953**

McCASKEY, G[eorge] W[ashington] (1853-1935)
Bio-chemistry in its relation to nervous diseases. New York, 1895. 6 l. DNLM **90-4954**

McCASKEY, G[eorge] W[ashington] (1853-1935)
Case of brain traumatism with focal symptoms, trephining and death. Peoria, 1896. 3 l. DNLM **90-4955**

McCASKEY, G[eorge] W[ashington] (1853-1935)
The diagnosis and treatment of cerebral meningeal haemorrhage. New York, 1896. 10p. DNLM **90-4956**

McCASKEY, G[eorge] W[ashington] (1853-1935)
Clinical examination of the blood. Fort Wayne, 1897. 2 l. DNLM **90-4957**

McCASKEY, G[eorge] W[ashington] (1853-1935)
The diagnosis of stomach disease. Fort Wayne, 1897. 13p. DNLM **90-4958**

McCASKEY, G[eorge] W[ashington] (1853-1935)
Physical therapeutics; electricity; hydro-therapeutics; massage; Schott treatment of heart disease. Fort Wayne, 1897. 9p. DNLM **90-4959**

McCASKEY, G[eorge] W[ashington] (1853-1935)
The neurasthenic symptoms of gastro-intestinal disease. New York, 1898. 11p. DNLM **90-4960**

McCASKEY, G[eorge] W[ashington] (1853-1935)
The toxemic factor in diabetes mellitus; a clinical study. [Detroit, 1899.] 11p. DNLM **90-4961**

McCASKEY, G[eorge] W[ashington] (1853-1935)
The toxic origin of certain neuroses and psychoses. [New York, 1899.] 2 l. DNLM **90-4962**

McCASSY, J[ohn] H.
Deformities of the nasal septum. New York, 1896. 7p. DNLM **90-4963**

McCASSY, J[ohn] H.
Footwear in relation to catarrh. New York, 1896. 8p. DNLM **90-4964**

McCASSY, J[ohn] H.
Nasal affections as a cause of headaches. Cincinnati, 1896. 3p. DNLM **90-4965**

McCASSY, J[ohn] H.
A trial frame. New York, 1897. 3p. DNLM **90-4966**

McCASSY, J[ohn] H.
Odor as a symptom of disease. Detroit, Mich.: W. M. Warren, 1898. 2p. DNLM **90-4967**

McCAW, James Francis
Adenoid vegetations of the pharynx. New York, 1898. 9p. DNLM **90-4968**

McCAW, James Francis
Mastoiditis; the importance of early surgical treatment. New York, 1899. 6p. DNLM **90-4969**

McCLELLAN, George (1849-1913)
Regional anatomy in its relation to medicine and surgery. Philadelphia: J. B. Lippincott Co., 1891-1892. 2 v. col. plates. MBM; NNNAM; PPC; PPJ [97 photographic plates hand-colored by the author] **90-4970**

McCLELLAN, George (1849-1913)
Regional anatomy in its relation to medicine and surgery. . . . Illustrated from photographs taken by the author of his own dissections, expressly designed and prepared for this work, and colored by him after nature. . . . In two volumes. Philadelphia: J. B. Lippincott Co., 1892-1893 [i.e., v. 1, 1893]. 2 v. 97 col. plates. NcD; NIC [Plates accompanied by leaf with descriptive letterpress.] **90-4971**

McCLELLAN, George (1849-1913)
Regional anatomy in its relation to medicine and surgery. . . . Philadelphia: Published by the Author, 1894. 2 v. 97 col. plates. DNLM; NN; PPC; PU ["2nd ed."] **90-4972**

McCLELLAN, George (1849-1913)
Regional anatomy in its relation to medicine and surgery. 3rd ed. Philadelphia: The Author, 1896. 2 v. illustrated. DNLM; ICJ; PPHa; PPJ **90-4973**

McCLELLAN, George (1849-1913)
Regional anatomy in its relation to medicine and surgery. 4th ed. Philadelphia: The Author, 1898. 2 v. PPL; PPJ **90-4974**

McCLELLAND, J[ames] H[enderson]
Jubilee address delivered before the American Institute of Homoeopathy upon the occasion of the fiftieth anniversary. Denver, 1891. 48p. DNLM **90-4975**

McCLINTOCK, Charles T[homas] (1860-1921)
Corrosive sublimate as a germicide. [Philadelphia, 1892.] 32p. DNLM **90-4976**

McCLINTOCK, Charles T[homas] (1860-1921)
A new, practical disinfecting material. Detroit: Parke, Davis & Co., 1897. 10p. DNLM **90-4977**

MacCLURE, Theodore R. (*b.* 1869)
The State Board of Health and a quarter century of public-health work in Michigan. Lansing, Mich.: R. Smith Print. Co., [1898]. 48p. DNLM **90-4978**

MacCLURE, Theodore R. (*b.* 1869)
The State Board of Health and a quarter century of public-health work in Michigan, 1873-98. Lansing: R. Smith Print. Co., 1898. 48p. 1 plate. DNLM **90-4979**

McCOLLOM, John H[ildreth]
Antitoxin in the treatment of diphtheria. [Boston, 1896.] 16p. DNLM **90-4980**

McCOLLOM, John H[ildreth]
The treatment of diphtheria at the South Department of the Boston City Hospital. Boston: Rockwell & Churchill, 1897. 30p. DNLM; MBM **90-4981**

McCOLLOM, J. M.
A clinical study of eight hundred cases of diphtheria at the South Department of the Boston City Hospital. Boston, 1898. 32p. 1 plate, 3 charts. DNLM; MBM **90-4982**

McCOLLOM, William (*b.* 1831)
Phthisis pulmonalis. Chicago, 1891. 16p. DNLM **90-4983**

McCOLLOM, William (*b.* 1831)
Criminal abortion. Chicago, 1896. 7p. DNLM **90-4984**

McCONKEY, E.
Cyclopedia of medicine; or, The household friend; containing valuable prescriptions and formulae. . . . Chicago, Ill.: [Fergus Printing Co.], 1892. 61p. DLC; OCIM **90-4985**

McCONNELL, Carl Philip
Notes on osteopathic therapeutics, prepared . . . . Kirksville, Mo.: Journal Printing Co., 1898. 237p. DLC
90-4986

McCONNELL, Carl Philip
The practice of osteopathy; designed for the use of practitioners and students of osteopathy. . . . [Chicago: W. B. Conkey Co.], 1899. 766p. DLC; OCIM
90-4987

McCOOK, Henry C[hristopher] (1837-1911)
Address delivered on the occasion of the opening of the new lecture hall of the Academy of Natural Sciences, Philadelphia, Feb. 22, 1892. 4p. [Philadelphia, 1892.] 4p. DNLM
90-4988

McCORMICK, Charles N. (*b.* 1858)
Practical optics for beginners. . . . Chicago: A. L. Swift & Co., printers, 1895. 101p. diags. DLC **90-4989**

McCORMICK, Charles N. (*b.* 1858)
Optical truths. Illustrated. . . . Chicago: McCormick Optical College, [1898]. 152p. col. plates. DLC; DNLM; OCIM
90-4990

McCORMICK, H[orace] G.
The effect of the local application of guaiacol in the reduction of the temperature in typhoid fever. [Philadelphia, 1895.] 13p. DNLM **90-4991**

McCOSH, A[ndrew] J[ames] (1858-1908)
The surgical treatment of movable kidney, with report of four nephrorraphies. [New York, 1890.] 20p. 1 table. DNLM
90-4992

McCOSH, A[ndrew] J[ames] (1858-1908)
Excision of cancer of the rectum. [New York: D. Appleton & Co., 1892.] 27p. DNLM **90-4993**

McCOSH, A[ndrew] J[ames] (1858-1908)
Results of vaginal hysterectomy. [Philadelphia, 1893.] 19p. DNLM **90-4994**

McCOSH, A[ndrew] J[ames] (1858-1908)
A case of congenital umbilical hernia. New York: D. Appleton & Co., 1897. 3p. DNLM **90-4995**

McCOURT, P[eter] J.
Medical terminology, its etymology and errors. New York, 1895. 21p. DNLM **90-4996**

McCUEN, A. G.
Synopsis of a lecture on evolution of the diet. Or, Man's developmental history and dentition. . . . Lindsborg, Kan., [1898]. 31p. DLC **90-4997**

McCURDY, Stewart Le Roy (1859-1931)
Hip-joint disease, with cases. [Cleveland, 1890.] 8p. DNLM
90-4998

McCURDY, Stewart Le Roy (1859-1931)
The mechanical treatment of synovitis. [Pittsburgh], 1890. 15p. DNLM **90-4999**

McCURDY, Stewart Le Roy (1859-1931)
The treatment of compound fracture. [Columbus, 1891.] 7p. DNLM **90-5000**

McCURDY, Stewart Le Roy (1859-1931)
A modification of Wyeth's method of bloodless amputation at the hip-joint. [New York: D. Appleton & Co., 1892.] 6p. DNLM **90-5001**

McCURDY, Stewart Le Roy (1859-1931)
New York letters on orthopedic surgery. The scope of orthopedic surgery. Tubercular abscesses and their treatment. Columbus, O.: A. C. Berlin & Co., [1892]. 34p. DNLM
90-5002

McCURDY, Stewart Le Roy (1859-1931)
A few things that may add to the convenience of railroad surgeons; with which is printed an article on bloodless amputation at the hip-joint at one sitting and with one needle. Chicago, [1893, *vel subseq.*]. 10p. DNLM
90-5003

McCURDY, Stewart Le Roy (1859-1931)
A retaining splint for excisions of the hip-joint, with a case. Pittsburgh, [1893]. 4p. DNLM **90-5004**

McCURDY, Stewart Le Roy (1859-1931)
Old and neglected deformities following infantile spinal paralysis. Columbus, 1894. 8p. DNLM **90-5005**

McCURDY, Stewart Le Roy (1859-1931)
The use of traction in the treatment of joint diseases. Pittsburgh: Murdoch, Kerr & Co., 1894. 7p. DNLM
90-5006

McCURDY, Stewart Le Roy (1859-1931)
Manual of orthopedic surgery. Pittsburgh, Pa.: Nicholson Press, 1898. 339p. DLC; NNNAM; PPC
90-5007

McDILL, John R[ich] (*b.* 1860)
A report on the present status of the treatment and prognosis of accessible surgical tuberculosis. Chicago, 1895. 22p. DNLM
90-5008

McDILL, John R[ich] (*b.* 1860)
Continuation of a report on the present status of the treatment and prognosis of accessible surgical tuberculosis. Chicago, 1897. 39p. DNLM **90-5009**

McDILL, John R[ich] (*b.* 1860) and C. H. VAN ALSTINE
Localized infectious diseases following slight injuries as the proximate cause, and their medico-legal relations. Chicago, 1898. 24p. DNLM **90-5010**

McDILL, John R[ich] (*b.* 1860)
Hospitals, their construction, organization and management. Chicago, 1899. 32p. DNLM **90-5011**

MACDONALD, J[ohn] W[illiam] (*b.* 1844)
A clinical text-book of surgical diagnosis and treatment for practitioners and students of surgery and medicine. Philadelphia: W. B. Saunders, 1898. 798p. DNLM; NNNAM; PPC; PU
90-5012

MACDONALD, T[homas] L.
Laughing gas as an anaesthetic in general surgery. [Baltimore, 1893.] 8p. DNLM **90-5013**

MACDONALD, T[homas] L.
Nitrous oxide anaesthesia. A further contribution to the subject of nitrous oxide in general surgery. Chicago: Med. Century Co., [1894]. 7p. DNLM **90-5014**

MACDONALD, T[homas] L.
Am I an orificialist? Boston, [1896]. 6p. DNLM **90-5015**

McDONALD, William O.
Paralysis of the muscles of the abdominal wall due to injury to nerve trunks during operation. [New York, 1898, *vel subseq.*] 20p. DNLM **90-5016**

McDONALD, William O.
Rupture of the plantaris. Chicago, 1898. 11p. DNLM **90-5017**

McDONALD, William O.
Pelvic neuritis, or inflammation of the pudic nerve in women. New York, 1899. 6p. DNLM **90-5018**

MACDONALD, Willis Goss (*b.* 1863)
A case of congenital umbilical hernia; abdominal section six hours after delivery; recovery. New York: William Wood & Co., 1890. 9p. DNLM **90-5019**

MACDONALD, Willis Goss (*b.* 1863)
The present status of ectopic pregnancy; a surgical disease. Chicago: Am. Medical Assoc. Press, 1896. 15p. DNLM **90-5020**

McFARLAND, Joseph (1868-1945)
The nervous form of mercurial poisoning. [Philadelphia, 1892.] 12p. DNLM **90-5021**

McFARLAND, Joseph (1868-1945)
A text-book upon the pathogenic *Bacteria*. . . . With 113 illustrations. Philadelphia: W. B. Saunders, 1896. 359p. col. frontis. DLC; PPC; PPJ **90-5022**

McFARLAND, Joseph (1868-1945)
A text-book upon the pathogenic *Bacteria*. . . . 2nd ed. Philadelphia: W. B. Saunders, 1898. 497p. PU **90-5023**

McFARLAND, Joseph (1868-1945)
Antituberculin. Philadelphia, 1897. 7p. DNLM **90-5024**

McFARLAND, Joseph (1868-1945)
A simple method of securing a measured quantity of blood for making the quantitative typhoid reaction. New York, 1897. 7p. DNLM **90-5025**

MACFARLANE, Andrew (*d.* 1906)
The duty of the state to the insane. [New York: D. Appleton & Co., 1893.] 13p. DNLM **90-5026**

MACFARLANE, Andrew (*d.* 1906)
A clinical manual. A guide to the practical examination of the excretions, secretions, and the blood, for the use of physicians and students. New York & London: G. P. Putnam's Sons, 1894. 139p. 4 plates. DNLM; NNNAM **90-5027**

MACFARLANE, A. W.
Insomnia and its therapeutics. New York: William Wood & Co., 1891. 298p. NNNAM **90-5028**

McGAHAN, Charles
The sanitorium treatment of pulmonary phthisis. Richmond, 1897. 14p. DNLM **90-5029**

McGANNON, M[atthew] C.
Extraperitoneal shortening of the round ligaments. (The Alexander-Adams operation.) New York, 1896. 8p. DNLM **90-5030**

McGEE, Anita Newcomb (1864-1940)
Standard for army nurses. New York, 1899. 4p. DNLM **90-5031**

McGEE, J[ohn] B[ernard] (*b.* 1853)
Urotropin in cystitis. Cleveland, O., 1899. 3p. DNLM **90-5032**

McGILLICUDDY, Timothy J. (1857-1899)
Notes on some interesting cases at the New York Mothers' Home Maternity Hospital. Chicago, 1892. 11p. DNLM **90-5033**

McGILLICUDDY, Timothy J. (1857-1899)
Enormous ovarian tumor, two hundred and two pounds in weight. [New York, 1895.] 2p. DNLM **90-5034**

McGILLICUDDY, Timothy J. (1857-1899)
Functional disorders of the nervous system in women. New York: William Wood & Co., 1896. 367p. 2 plates, 10 charts. DNLM; NNNAM **90-5035**

McGILLICUDDY, Timothy J. (1857-1899)
Some obstetric accessories. New York, 1896. 5p. DNLM **90-5036**

McGINNIS, E[dward] L. H. (*b.* 1862)
A case of extra-uterine pregnancy. [New York, 1894.] 3p. DNLM **90-5037**

McGINNIS, E[dward] L. H. (*b.* 1862)
Menorrhagia and metrorrhagia as caused by conditions other than fibroids. New York, 1895. 2p. DNLM **90-5038**

McGRATH, John J.
Report of a case of tuberculosis of the bladder, with some observations. New York, 1899. 9p. DNLM **90-5039**

McGRAW, Theodore A[ndrews] (1839-1921)
Resection of the intestine for chronic obstruction. Detroit, 1890. 14p. DNLM **90-5040**

McGRAW, Theodore A[ndrews] (1839-1921)
Upon the use of the elastic ligature in the surgery of the intestines. Chicago, 1891. 32p. DNLM **90-5041**

McGRAW, Theodore A[ndrews] (1839-1921)
Intestinal obstruction by immense gallstone. Detroit, [1894]. 4p. DNLM **90-5042**

McGRAW, Theodore A[ndrews] (1839-1921)
The treatment of obstruction of the common gall-duct. [Philadelphia], 1895. 14p. DNLM **90-5043**

McGUIRE, Hunter Holmes (1835-1900)
Address of the president before the Southern Surgical and Gynecological Association, at the meeting held in Nashville, Tenn., Nov. 13, 1889. Philadelphia: W. J. Dornan, 1890. 14p. DNLM **90-5044**

McGUIRE, Hunter Holmes (1835-1900)
A report of twenty-one cases of supra-pubic cystotomy. Philadelphia, 1890. 12p. DNLM **90-5045**

McGUIRE, Hunter Holmes (1835-1900)
Case of tuberculosis cured by cancrum oris. Richmond, 1897. 1 l. DNLM **90-5046**

McGUIRE, J[ames] Clark
Lupus vulgaris, in its relation to tuberculosis. New York: D. Appleton & Co., [1891]. 4 l. DNLM **90-5047**

McGUIRE, J[ames] Clark
The care of the skin. Richmond, 1894. 32p. DNLM **90-5048**

McGUIRE, J[ames] Clark
Electrolysis in the treatment of diseases of the skin. Richmond, 1896. 10p. DNLM **90-5049**

McGUIRE, J[ames] Clark
Freaks, as pertaining to diseases of the skin. Richmond, 1896. 12p. DNLM **90-5050**

McINTIRE, Charles (*b.* 1847)
State requirements for the practice of medicine. A guide to the qualifications and methods of procedure to enter upon the practice of medicine in the United States. Easton, Pa., 1897. 85p. DNLM **90-5051**

McINTIRE, Charles (*b.* 1847)
State requirements for the practice of medicine. A guide to the qualifications and methods of procedure to enter upon the practice of medicine in the United States. 1898 supplement. Pt. II. Indicating changes in the laws and procedures during 1897. Easton, Pa., 1898. 26p. DNLM **90-5052**

McINTIRE, Charles (*b.* 1847)
State requirements for the practice of medicine. A guide to the qualifications and methods of procedure to enter upon the practice of medicine in the United States. 1899 supplement. Pt. III. Indicating changes in the laws and procedures during 1898. Easton, Pa., 1899. 18p. DNLM **90-5053**

McINTOSH BATTERY AND OPTICAL CO.
Electro-therapeutical catalogue. 18th ed. Chicago, 1897. 288p. DNLM **90-5054**

MacINTOSH, J. S.
Funeral address and memorial discourse in memory of D. Hayes Agnew, M.D., LL.D., delivered in the Second Presbyterian Church, March 25 [and] April 3, 1892. [Philadelphia, 1892.] 8p. PPC **90-5055**

McINTOSH, W. Page
Laparotomy and removal of cystic tumor (cysto-adenoma) of peritoneum. Formation of artificial anus; subsequent laparotomy and resection of colon; closure of artificial anus; recovery. Philadelphia, 1893. 6p. DNLM **90-5056**

McINTYRE, John H[oge] (*b.* 1833)
A report of ten selected case of laparotomy. [Chicago, 1891.] 12p. 1 plate. DNLM **90-5057**

MACK, Charles S[amuel]
Kali chloricum. A lecture. [Philadelphia, 1891.] 10p. DNLM **90-5058**

MACK, Charles S[amuel]
Empiricism; rational practice; practice under guidance of law. A lecture to medical students. [New York, 1892.] 12p. DNLM **90-5059**

MACK, Charles S[amuel]
Some considerations bearing upon practice with dynamic antagonists in cases of drug-poisoning. [New York, 1894.] 6p. DNLM **90-5060**

MACK, Charles S[amuel]
Principles of medicine, designed for use as a text-book in medical colleges, and for consideration by practitioners generally. Chicago: W. T. Keener Co., 1897. 133p. DNLM; IU-M; OCIM **90-5061**

McKAY, W. J. Stewart (*b.* 1866)
Lawson Tait's perineal operations and an essay on curettage of the uterus. New York: William Wood & Co., 1897. 69p. DNLM; NNNAM **90-5062**

McKEE, Edward S.
Abortion. New York: William Wood & Co., 1891. 9p. DNLM **90-5063**

McKEE, Edward S.
Habitual abortion. New York: William Wood & Co., 1892. 7p. DNLM **90-5064**

McKENDRICK, John G[ray] (1841-1926)
Hermann Ludwig Ferdinand von Helmholtz. . . . Masters of medicine. New York: Longmans, Green & Co., 1899. 299p. ICU; NN **90-5065**

MACKENZIE, John N[oland] (*b.* 1853)
A contribution to the pathological anatomy of ethmoid disease. New York, 1897. 11p. 1 plate. DNLM **90-5066**

MACKENZIE, John N[oland] (*b.* 1853)
The physiological and pathological relations between the nose and the sexual apparatus of man. Baltimore, 1898. 23p. DNLM **90-5067**

MACKENZIE, Morell, ed. (1837-1892)
The pharmacopoeia of the London Hospital for Diseases of the Throat. 5th ed., rev. and imp. by F. G. Harvey. Philadelphia: P. Blakiston, Son & Co., 1894. 112p. DNLM; OCLloyd; PPC; PU **90-5068**

McKERNON, James F.
Report of a case of severe hemorrhage following paracentesis of the drum membrane. St. Louis, Mo., 1898. 4p. DNLM **90-5069**

MACKIE, William (*b.* 1855)
Clinical observations on the healing of aseptic bone cavities by Senn's method of implantation of antiseptic decalcified bone. [Philadelphia, 1890.] 28p. DNLM **90-5070**

MACKIE, William (*b.* **1855)**
Renal neoplasms, with report of two cases of nephrectomy. [Philadelphia, 1893.] 22p. DNLM **90-5071**

McKONE, James J.
Ventral hernia; rupture of the coverings; escape of intestines and their exposure for eighteen hours; recovery. Philadelphia, 1891. 3p. DNLM **90-5072**

McLAIN, John S.
Narcotics and narcosis in children. New York: M. J. Rooney, 1893. 13p. DNLM **90-5073**

McLAREN, A[rchibald] (1858-1924)
Vaginal hysterectomy. St. Paul, 1893. 12p. DNLM **90-5074**

McLAREN, A[rchibald] (1858-1924)
Ovariotomy; report of thirty-nine cases. St. Paul, 1894. 15p. DNLM **90-5075**

McLAREN, A[rchibald] (1858-1924)
The best method of the sterilization of catgut. New York, 1895. 3p. DNLM **90-5076**

McLAREN, A[rchibald] (1858-1924)
Catgut for ligation of the pedicle. New York, 1895. 17p. DNLM **90-5077**

McLAREN, A[rchibald] (1858-1924)
Some considerations on the subject of hysterectomy; with the report of fifty consecutive cases. St. Paul, [1897]. 4 l. DNLM **90-5078**

McLAREN, A[rchibald] (1858-1924)
Rupture of the urinary bladder; with reprot of a case of extra-peritoneal rupture complicated with fracture of the pelvis. Chicago, 1898. 8p. DNLM **90-5079**

McLAREN, A[rchibald] (1858-1924)
Cases suitable for vaginal section. St. Paul, 1899. 12p. DNLM **90-5080**

McLAREN, A[rchibald] (1858-1924)
Ectopic pregnancy; with report of fourteen cases. St. Paul, Minn., 1899. 12p. DNLM **90-5081**

McLAREN, A[rchibald] (1858-1924)
Hernia, Minneapolis, [1899]. 14p. DNLM **90-5082**

McLAREN, A[rchibald] (1858-1924)
Interstitial pregnancy; with report of a case operated upon thirteen months after conception. New York, 1899. 8p. DNLM **90-5083**

McLAUGHLIN, J[ames] W[harton] (1840-1909)
An explanation of the phenomena of immunity and contagion, based upon the action of physical and biological laws. [Austin, 1890.] 36p. DNLM **90-5084**

McLAUGHLIN, J[ames] W[harton] (1840-1909)
The fermentation theory of infection and immunity. [Austin, 1890.] 32p. DNLM **90-5085**

McLAUGHLIN, J[ames] W[harton] (1840-1909)
Fermentation, infection, and immunity; a new theory of these processes, which unifies their primary causation and places the explanation of their phenomena in chemistry, biology, and the dynamics of molecular physics. Austin, Texas: E. Von Boeckmann, 1892. 240p. DNLM **90-5086**

McLAUGHLIN, J[ames] W[harton] (1840-1909)
The kinetic and therapeutic energy of drugs. A theoretic explanation of the causes of drug energy, and the rationale of its action on the living tissue elements of the body. Galveston, 1895. 23p. DNLM **90-5087**

McLAUGHLIN, J[ames] W[harton] (1840-1909)
An outline of the physical theory of fermentation, immunity, and infection, and its bearing on the rationale of serum therapy. Galveston, 1895. 14p. DNLM **90-5088**

McLAUGHLIN, J[ames] W[harton] (1840-1909)
The bacteriology of dengue. Austin, [1896]. 4p. 1 plate. DNLM **90-5089**

McLAUGHLIN, Thomas N.
Drug eruptions. Chicago, 1890. 2 l. DNLM **90-5090**

McLAUGHLIN, Thomas N.
Realgar-arsenic di-sulphide in the treatment of skin diseases. Richmond, 1890. 4p. DNLM **90-5091**

McLAURY, William M[uir] (*d.* **1896)**
Hallucinations and delusions. [St. Louis, 1894.] 26p. 4 l. DNLM **90-5092**

McLAUTHLIN, H[erbert] W[eston]
Report of a case of Addison's disease. Philadelphia, 1895. 9p. DNLM **90-5093**

MACLEAN, Donald (1839-1903)
Personal reminiscences of Syme. Detroit: W. M. Warren, 1898. 14p. DNLM **90-5094**

McLEAN HOSPITAL TRAINING SCHOOL FOR NURSES. WAVERLY
Application for admission (With questions to be answered by the candidate.) [Boston, 189-.] 2 l. DNLM **90-5095**

McLEAN HOSPITAL TRAINING SCHOOL FOR NURSES. WAVERLY
List of questions to be answered by those recommending a candidate for admission as a pupil. Confidential. For males. [Boston, 189-.] 2 l. DNLM **90-5096**

McLEAN HOSPITAL TRAINING SCHOOL FOR NURSES. WAVERLY
List of questions to be answered by those recommending a candidate for admission as a pupil. Confidential. For females. [Boston, 189-.] 2 l. DNLM **90-5097**

McLEAN HOSPITAL TRAINING SCHOOL FOR NURSES. WAVERLY
Organization, terms of admission, course of instruction, and other information. [Boston, 189-.] 4 l. DNLM **90-5098**

McLEAN HOSPITAL TRAINING SCHOOL FOR NURSES. WAVERLY
Annual reports of the medical superintendent to the trustees of the Massachusetts General Hospital. 7.-14., 1889-96; 16.-18., 1898-1900. Boston, 1890-1901. DNLM
90-5099

McLEISH, J[ohn] and Charles WEBER
Cancer and tumors scientifically treated and cured. The knife discarded. Cincinnati, O.: Spenger & Craig, [1890]. 48p. 1 plate. DNLM; OC **90-5100**

McMANUS, Charles
One of the present needs of the profession. A history. Philadelphia, 1898. 8p. DNLM **90-5101**

McMANUS, James
Notes on the history of anaesthesia. The Wells memorial celebration at Hartford, 1894. Early record of dentists in Connecticut. Hartford: Clark & Smith, 1896. 116p. CtY-M; DNLM; MH-M **90-5102**

McMANUS, James
A professional review, 1864-98. Hartford, Conn.: Clark & Smith, 1898. 45p. 27 blank l. DNLM; MBM
90-5103

McMICHAEL, Arkell Roger
A compendium of materia medica, therapeutics and repertory of the digestive system. . . . Philadelphia: Boericke & Tafel, 1892. 359p. DLC; DNLM; OCLloyd; PPHa
90-5104

MacMONAGLE, Beverly (1855-1912)
Ectopic pregnancy, with cases. Sacramento, 1896. 8p. DNLM
90-5105

MacMONAGLE, Beverly (1855-1912)
The management of surgical injuries to the ureters. Philadelphia, 1899. 10p. DNLM **90-5106**

McMURTRY, Lewis S[amuel] (1850-1924)
Twenty consecutive cases of abdominal section. Philadelphia: W. J. Dornan, 1890. 15p. DNLM
90-5107

McMURTRY, Lewis S[amuel] (1850-1924)
A manual on nursing in pelvic surgery. Louisville: J. P. Morton & Co., 1894. 92p. 1 plate. DNLM
90-5108

McMURTRY, Lewis S[amuel] (1850-1924)
The evolution and perfection of the aseptic surgical technique. Louisville: J. P. Morton & Co., 1897. 16p. DNLM
90-5109

McMURTRY, Lewis S[amuel] (1850-1924)
The operation itself in appendicitis. Philadelphia, 1897. 15p. DNLM **90-5110**

MACNAMARA, N[ottridge] C[harles] (1832-1918)
Diseases and refraction of the eye by N. C. Macnamara and Gustavus Hartridge. 5th ed. Philadelphia: P. Blakiston, Son & Co., 1891. 604p. DNLM; MBM; NNNAM; PPC
90-5111

McNAUGHTON, George and William MADDREN
Treatment of true croup by intubation of the larynx. Statistics of the different methods of treating true croup, compiled by Geo. McNaughton and Wm. Maddren. Treatment of true croup by the sublimation of calomel (Corbin or Brooklyn method), by Wm. Madden. New York: M. J. Rooney & Co., [1892]. 26p., 5p. DNLM **90-5112**

MacNEILL, J. E[dward]
Dosimetry in Colorado. New York: W. J. Morrison, 1890. 12p. DNLM **90-5113**

McNEILL, R[oger]
The prevention of epidemics and the construction and management of isolation hospitals. Philadelphia: P. Blakiston, Son & Co., 1895. 247p. 27 plates. DNLM; NNNAM; PPC; PU
90-5114

McNUTT, W[illiam] F[letcher] (*b.* 1839)
Five cases of vaginal hysterectomy for malignant diseases of the uterus; all recovered. [San Francisco, 1890.] 8p. DNLM
90-5115

McNUTT, W[illiam] F[letcher] (*b.* 1839)
Elixir chloroform compositus. San Francisco, [1891]. 1 l. DNLM **90-5116**

McNUTT, W[illiam] F[letcher] (*b.* 1839)
Diseases of the kidneys and bladder: a text-book for students of medicine. . . . Philadelphia: J. B. Lippincott Co., 1893. 242p. DLC; PPC; PU **90-5117**

McNUTT, W[illiam] F[letcher] (*b.* 1839)
Cremation as the only sanitary method of disposing of the dead. Sacramento: A. J. Johnston, 1894. 8p. DNLM
90-5118

McNUTT, W[illiam] F[letcher] (*b.* 1839)
Vaginal hysterectomy for cancer; 23 cases. San Francisco, 1894. 7p. DNLM **90-5119**

McPHEDRAN, A[lexander]
Pernicious anaemia, with a report of five cases. [Philadelphia, 1890.] 12p. DNLM **90-5120**

McPHEDRAN, A[lexander]
Pulmonary and other internal hemorrhage. Philadelphia, 1898. 6p. DNLM **90-5121**

MACREADY, Jonathan F. C. H.
A treatise on ruptures. . . . Philadelphia: P. Blakiston, Son & Co., 1893. 442p. CtY-M; DNLM; ICJ; NNNAM
90-5122

MADDEN, Frank S.
Tumor of the cortex. [New York, 1893.] 4p. DNLM
90-5123

MADDEN, John
Shall we drink wine? A physician's study of the alcohol question. Milwaukee: Owen & Weihbrecht Co., 1899. 220p. 6 plates. DNLM **90-5124**

MADDEN, Thomas More (1838-1902)
Clinical gynaecology: being a handbook of diseases peculiar to women. . . . Philadelphia: J. B. Lippincott Co., 1893. 562p. DLC; NNNAM; PPC; PU **90-5125**

MAGRUDER, E[dward] M.
A guide to physical diagnosis. . . . [Charlottesville, Va.: Charlottesville Printing Co.], 1897. 177p. DLC; DNLM
90-5126

MAGRUDER, G[eorge] L[loyd] (1848-1914) and C. W. STILES
An extreme case of leucoderma in a Negro, with a comparison of similar conditions in various animals. New York: Trow, 1894. 16p. DNLM **90-5127**

MAISCH, John Michael (1831-1903)
A manual of organic materia medica. Being a guide to materia medica of the vegetable and animal kingdoms for the use of students, druggists, pharmacists and physicians. . . . 4th ed. With two hundred and fifty-nine illustrations. Philadelphia: Lea Bros. & Co., 1890. 539p. DLC; DNLM; OCLloyd
90-5128

MAISCH, John Michael (1831-1903)
A manual of organic materia medica. Being a guide to materia medica of the vegetable and animal kingdoms, for the use of students, druggists, pharmacists, and physicians. . . . 5th ed. . . . Philadelphia: Lea Bros. & Co., 1892. 556p. DLC; DNLM; OCLloyd; PU **90-5129**

MAISCH, John Michael (1831-1903)
A manual of organic materia medica. Being a guide to materia medica of the vegetable and animal kingdoms, for the use of students, druggists, pharmacists, and physicians. . . . 6th ed. Rev. by Henry C. C. Maisch. . . . Philadelphia: Lea Bros. & Co., 1895. 526p. DLC; DNLM; NNNAM; OCLloyd
90-5130

MAISCH, John Michael (1831-1903)
A manual of organic materia medica; being a guide to materia medica of the vegetable and animal kingdoms, for the use of students, druggists, pharmacists, and physicians. . . . 7th ed. Rev. by Henry C. C. Maisch. . . . Philadelphia and New York: Lea Bros. & Co., 1899. 523p. DLC; DNLM; NNNAM; PPC
90-5131

MAJOR, George W.
Notes on an interesting case of aneurysm. [New York, 1890.] 5p. DNLM **90-5132**

MAKUEN, G[eorge] Hudson (*b.* 1855)
The breathing movements in relation to voice production. [Boston, 1890.] 11p. DNLM **90-5133**

MAKUEN, G[eorge] Hudson (*b.* 1855)
A modification of Gottstein's curette. Philadelphia, 1893. 3p. DNLM **90-5134**

MAKUEN, G[eorge] Hudson (*b.* 1855)
Exhibition of a case of stammering, with demonstration of the methods employed in treatment. New York, 1899. 7p. DNLM
90-5135

MAKUEN, G[eorge] Hudson (*b.* 1855)
Falsetto voice in the male. Report of five cases. Chicago, 1899. 7p. DNLM **90-5136**

MAKUEN, G[eorge] Hudson (*b.* 1855)
Report of a case in which defective speech results in some interesting derangements of cerebral functions. Philadelphia, 1899. 6p. DNLM **90-5137**

MALCOLM, John Gilmore (*b.* 1830) and Oscar Burnham MOSS
A regional and comparative materia medica. Chicago: Malcolm & Moss, 1895. 919p. DNLM; OCIM; OCLloyd
90-5138

MALL, Franklin P[aine] (1862-1917)
Early human embryos and the mode of their presentation. [Baltimore, 1893.] 17p. DNLM; MdBJ-W
90-5139

MALL, Franklin P[aine] (1862-1917)
The anatomical course and laboratory of the Johns Hopkins University. Baltimore, 1896. 31p. 13 plates. DNLM; MdBJ-W
90-5140

MALL, Franklin P[aine] (1862-1917)
Development of the internal mammary and deep epigastric arteries in man. Baltimore, 1898. 10p. DNLM; MdBJ-W
90-5141

MALL, Franklin P[aine] (1862-1917)
The lobule of the spleen. Baltimore, 1898. 6p. DNLM; MdBJ-W
90-5142

MALL, Franklin P[aine] (1862-1917)
The value of embryological specimens. Baltimore, 1898. 5p. DNLM; MdBJ-W **90-5143**

MALL, Franklin P[aine] (1862-1917)
Liberty in medical education Philadelphia, 1899. 15p. DNLM; MdBJ-W **90-5144**

MALLETT, E. Pierre
The use of parotid gland extract in the treatment of ovarian disease. New York, 1899. 15p. DNLM
90-5145

MALLORY, F[rank] B[urr] (1862-1941)
Sacrococcygeal dimples, sinuses, and cysts. Philadelphia, 1892. 15p. DNLM **90-5146**

MALLORY, F[rank] B[urr] (1862-1941)
A case of actinomycosis. Boston: Rockwell & Churchill, 1895. 13p. 1 plate. DNLM **90-5147**

MALLORY, Frank] B[urr] (1862-1941) and James Homer WRIGHT
Pathological technique. A practical manual for the pathological laboratory. Philadelphia: W. B. Saunders, 1897. 397p. DNLM; NNNAM; PPC; PU **90-5148**

MALONEY, J[ames] A. (*b.* 1846)
Sound as a therapeutic agent in deafness and tinnitus aurium. [Philadelphia: Lea Bros. & Co., 1892.] 3p. DNLM
90-5149

MALONEY, J[ames] A. (*b.* 1846)
Sound waves in the treatment of deafness and tinnitus aurium. [Washington, 1892.] 12p. DNLM **90-5150**

MANDEL, John A[lfred] (*b.* 1865)
Handbook for the bio-chemical laboratory, including methods of preparation and numerous tests, arranged alphabetically. New York: J. Wiley & Sons, 1896. 101p. DNLM; NNNAM; OCIM; PPC **90-5151**

MANGES, Morris
Cylindroids or so-called mucous casts in the urine. [New York, 1893.] 19p. DNLM **90-5152**

MANGES, Morris and Howard LILIENTHAL
A stenosing carcinoma of the transverse colon; excision; Murphy-button anastomosis (end to end). New York: D. Appleton & Co., 1894. 6p. DNLM **90-5153**

MANGES, Morris
The phonendoscope. New York: D. Appleton & Co., 1897. 11p. DNLM **90-5154**

MANGES, Morris
The treatment of coughs with heroin. New York, 1898. 80p. DNLM **90-5155**

MANLEY, Thomas H[enry] (1851-1905)
Cocaine analgesia; its extended application in general surgery when hypodermically employed. [Boston, 1890.] 12p. DNLM **90-5156**

MANLEY, Thomas H[enry] (1851-1905)
The early operation for hare-lip; with the report of a case, illustrations, etc. [Detroit, 1890.] 8p. DNLM **90-5157**

MANLEY, Thomas H[enry] (1851-1905)
Radical operation for hernia. Abstract of a clinical lecture delivered at the Harlem Hospital, New York. [Philadelphia, 1890.] 4p. DNLM **90-5158**

MANLEY, Thomas H[enry] (1851-1905)
Some of the uses of the temporary-transfixion ligature. Concord, N.H., 1890. 20p. DNLM **90-5159**

MANLEY, Thomas H[enry] (1851-1905)
Two cases of fractured skull; recovery in one, death from chloroform in the other. [Philadelphia, 1890.] 14p. DNLM **90-5160**

MANLEY, Thomas H[enry] (1851-1905)
Fractures at the elbow joint. [New York: D. Appleton & Co., 1891.] 30p. DNLM **90-5161**

MANLEY, Thomas H[enry] (1851-1905)
The report of a case of a large interstitial fibroid of the uterus removed by abdominal section, with some observations in relation to the most rational methods of dealing with neoplastic formations which originate in the muscular fibre of the uterus. [Brooklyn, 1891.] 7p. DNLM **90-5162**

MANLEY, Thomas H[enry] (1851-1905)
Resection as a substitute for primary amputation. Danbury, 1891. 19p. DNLM **90-5163**

MANLEY, Thomas H[enry] (1851-1905)
Cocaine analgesia in the treatment of hemorrhoids, of ulcers, fistulae, and fissures in the ano-rectal region. St. Louis, 1892. 8p. DNLM **90-5164**

MANLEY, Thomas H[enry] (1851-1905)
Extensive railroad injury; amputation; fistula in ano; peritonitis. [Philadelphia, 1892.] 3p. DNLM **90-5165**

MANLEY, Thomas H[enry] (1851-1905)
Something more on the pathology and treatment of hemorrhoids, fissures, fistulas, and ulcers in the ano-rectal region, with a few notes on prolapsus ani and neoplasm. St. Louis, 1892. 7p. DNLM **90-5166**

MANLEY, Thomas H[enry] (1851-1905)
The therapeutical value of the mercurial salts in general surgery. Philadelphia: Med. Press Co., 1892. 20p. DNLM **90-5167**

MANLEY, Thomas H[enry] (1851-1905)
Fibro-myoma of the uterus and broad ligament of forty-five years' duration. [Toledo, 1893.] 8p. 1 plate. DNLM **90-5168**

MANLEY, Thomas H[enry] (1851-1905)
Hernia; its palliative and radical treatment in adults, children, and infants. Philadelphia: Med. Press Co., 1893. 231p. DNLM **90-5169**

MANLEY, Thomas H[enry] (1851-1905)
Notes on cases of homoeo-osteoplasty in the shattering disorganization of compound fracture of the leg, thigh, and hand. New York, 1893. 11p. DNLM **90-5170**

MANLEY, Thomas H[enry] (1851-1905)
The pathology, symptomatology and treatment of hemorrhoids, simple and complicated. [St. Louis, 1893.] 12p. DNLM **90-5171**

MANLEY, Thomas H[enry] (1851-1905)
Surgical therapy of rectal cancer. [New York, 1893.] 22p. DNLM **90-5172**

MANLEY, Thomas H[enry] (1851-1905)
Contusion of the abdomen, with rupture of the thoracic duct. [Philadelphia: Lea Bros. & Co., 1894.] 5p. DNLM **90-5173**

MANLEY, Thomas H[enry] (1851-1905)
Surgical treatment of tumors of the neck. St. Louis, 1894. 4p. DNLM **90-5174**

MANLEY, Thomas H[enry] (1851-1905)
Various fractures, simple and compound; a clinical report of fifteen cases. New York, 1894. 27p. DNLM **90-5175**

MANLEY, Thomas H[enry] (1851-1905)
Deformities following fractures of the shafts of bones, with observations on treatment. New York, 1895. 6p. DNLM **90-5176**

MANLEY, Thomas H[enry] (1851-1905)
The element of causation in abdominal contusions. [New York, 1895.] 10p. DNLM **90-5177**

MANLEY, Thomas H[enry] (1851-1905)
The element of elimination and assimilation in pus formation. New York, 1895. 3p. DNLM **90-5178**

MANLEY, Thomas H[enry] (1851-1905)
The limitation of surgical operations as a means of relief or cure in epilepsy. New York, 1895. 13p. DNLM **90-5179**

MANLEY, Thomas H[enry] (1851-1905)
On the treatment of fractured shafts of bone in children; simple, complicated, and compound. Chicago, 1896. 16p. DNLM **90-5180**

MANLEY, Thomas H[enry] (1851-1905)
Contribution to traumatic abdominal surgery. Philadelphia, 1897. 16p. DNLM **90-5181**

MANLEY, Thomas H[enry] (1851-1905)
Renal suppuration, catarrhal, specific, and traumatic, and the value of micro-uranalysis of the urinary sediment as an aid to definite diagnosis of it. Chicago: American Med. Association Press, 1897. 37p. DNLM **90-5182**

MANN, Edward C[ox] (1850-1908)
A treatise on the medical jurisprudence of insanity. Albany, N.Y.: M. Bender, 1893. 420p. DNLM; NNNAM **90-5183**

MANN, John
Puerperal septicaemia in the practice of the country physician. New York, 1895. 6p. DNLM **90-5184**

MANN, J[ohn] Dixon (1840-1912)
Forensic medicine and toxicology. . . . Philadelphia: P. Blakiston, Son & Co., 1893. 639p. DNLM; ICJ; PPC; PPJ **90-5185**

MANN, M[atthew] D[arbyshire] (1845-1921)
Inflammation of the ureters in women. [Philadelphia, 1894.] 22p. DNLM **90-5186**

MANN, M[atthew] D[arbyshire] (1845-1921)
Perforation of the uterus after abortion with prolapse of intestine, with a report of three cases, operation in two. New York: William Wood & Co., 1895. 4p. DNLM **90-5187**

MANN, M[atthew] D[arbyshire] (1845-1921)
The president's address. The relations of lithaemia to diseases of the pelvic organs in women. [Philadelphia], 1895. 17p. DNLM **90-5188**

MANN, M[atthew] D[arbyshire] (1845-1921)
Two cases of ectopic gestation. Retention of the fetus for eight and thirteen years, respectively; operation; cure. Buffalo, 1895. 7p. DNLM **90-5189**

MANN, M[atthew] D[arbyshire] (1845-1921)
The choice of operation in ectopic gestation. New York, 1896. 5p. DNLM **90-5190**

MANN, M[atthew] D[arbyshire] (1845-1921)
The sloughing of uterine fibroids after abortion and labor. New York, 1896. 8p. DNLM **90-5191**

MANN, M[atthew] D[arbyshire] (1845-1921)
Intra-abdominal shortening of the round ligaments for posterior displacements of the uterus. [Philadelphia], 1897. 8p. DNLM **90-5192**

MANN, M[atthew] D[arbyshire] (1845-1921)
The surgical treatment of irreducible retroflexion of the pregnant uterus. New York, 1898. 3p. DNLM **90-5193**

MANNING, Frederick A[rnold] (1859-1896)
Physiology. A manual for students and practitioners. Philadelphia: Lea Bros. & Co., [1892]. 213p. DNLM; PPC; PPJ; PU **90-5194**

MANSELL-MOULLIN, Charles William (1851-1940)
Sprains; their consequences and treatment. New York: William Wood & Co., 1891. 221p. DNLM **90-5195**

MANSON, Otis F[rederick] (1822-1888)
Catalogue of the medical library of the late. . . . Richmond: Whittet & Sheperson, 1890 [1889]. 31p. DNLM **90-5196**

MANSON, Patrick (1844-1922)
Tropical diseases; a manual of the diseases of warm climates. New York: William Wood & Co., 1898. 607p. 2 plates. DNLM; NNNAM **90-5197**

MANTON, W[alter] P[orter] (1858-1925)
Sudden emptying of the bladder as a cause of cystorrhagia. [Detroit, 1890.] 7p. DNLM **90-5198**

MANTON, W[alter] P[orter] (1858-1925)
Abortion; its immediate and remote effects with reference to treatment. [Detroit, 1892.] 8p. DNLM **90-5199**

MANTON, W[alter] P[orter] (1858-1925)
Can adhesion of the intestines to the abdominal wall following laparotomy give rise to obstruction? Toledo, [1892]. 3p. DNLM **90-5200**

MANTON, W[alter] P[orter] (1858-1925)
On a certain cause of sterility and its cure. New York: William Wood & Co., 1892. 9p. DNLM **90-5201**

MANTON, W[alter] P[orter] (1858-1925)
On the management of the third stage of labor and its relation to postpartum haemorrhage. Toledo, [1892]. 4p. DNLM **90-5202**

MANTON, W[alter] P[orter] (1858-1925)
Syllabus of lectures on human embryology; an introduction to the study of obstetrics and gynaecology. For medical students and practitioners. With a glossary of embryological terms. Philadelphia: F. A. Davis & Co.; London, 1894. 125p. 1 plate, interleaved. DLC; DNLM; PPC **90-5203**

MANTON, W[alter] P[orter] (1858-1925)
Syllabus of lectures on human embryology; an introduction to the study of obstetrics and gynaecology. For medical students and practitioners. With a glossary of embryological terms. . . . 2nd ed. Philadelphia: The F. A. Davis Co.; [etc., etc.], 1895. 125p. DLC; NN; PPC; PU **90-5204**

MANTON, W[alter] P[orter] (1858-1925)
So-called puerperal eclampsia in its relation to insanity. New York: William Wood & Co., 1895. 3p. DNLM **90-5205**

MANTON, W[alter] P[orter] (1858-1925)
The relation of visceral disorders to the delusions of the insane. New York, 1896. 6p. DNLM **90-5206**

MARCHAND, Charles
The therapeutical applications of hydrozone and glycozone. . . . Treatment of diseases caused by germs, bacteria, microbes. New York, 1890. 32p. DNLM; NNNAM **90-5207**

MARCHAND, Charles
The therapeutical applications of peroxide of hydrogen (medicinal) and glycozone. Treatment of diseases caused by germs, bacteria, microbes. Revised ed. New York: J. J. Little & Co., 1890. 56p. DLC; DNLM **90-5208**

MARCHAND, Charles
The therapeutical applications of peroxide of hydrogen (medicinal) and glycozone. Treatment of diseases caused by germs, bacteria, microbes. 2nd ed. New York, 1891. 72p. DNLM **90-5209**

MARCHAND, Charles
The therapeutical applications of peroxide of hydrogen (medicinal) and glycozone. Treatment of diseases caused by germs, bacteria, microbes. 4th ed. New York, 1892. 80p. DNLM **90-5210**

MARCHAND, Charles
The therapeutical applications of peroxide of hydrogen (medicinal) and glycozone. Treatment of diseases caused by germs, bacteria, microbes. 5th ed. New York, 1893. 95p. DNLM **90-5211**

MARCHAND, Charles
The therapeutical applications of peroxide of hydrogen (medicinal) and glycozone. Treatment of diseases caused by germs, bacteria, microbes. 8th ed. New York, 1894. 168p. DNLM **90-5212**

MARCHAND, Charles
The therapeutical applications of peroxide of hydrogen (medicinal) and glycozone. Treatment of diseases caused by germs, bacteria, microbes. 9th ed. New York, 1895. 188p. 2 l. DNLM **90-5213**

MARCHAND, Charles
The therapeutical applications of peroxide of hydrogen (medicinal) and glycozone. Treatment of diseases caused by germs, bacteria, microbes. 11th ed. New York, 1896. 215p. DNLM **90-5214**

MARCHAND, Charles
The therapeutical applications of peroxide of hydrogen (medicinal) and glycozone. Treatment of diseases caused by germs, bacteria, microbes. 13th ed. New York, 1898. 257p. DNLM **90-5215**

MARCHAND, Charles
The therapeutical applications of peroxide of hydrogen (medicinal) and glycozone. Treatment of diseases caused by germs, bacteria, microbes. 14th ed. New York, 1899. 278p. DNLM **90-5216**

MARCHAND, Charles
The rational treatment of gastric and intestinal disorders. [New York, 1897.] 28p. DNLM **90-5217**

MARCHAND, Charles
The rational treatment of acute and chronic diseases of the genito-urinary tract. [New York, 1898.] 27p. DNLM **90-5218**

MARCHAND, Charles
Rational treatment and prevention of hay fever. Poisonous drugs do more harm than good. [New York, 1898.] 24p. DNLM **90-5219**

MARCY, Henry O[rlando] (1837-1924)
Surgical relief for biliary obstruction. Chicago: Office Amer. Med. Assoc., 1890. 28p. DNLM **90-5220**

MARCY, Henry O[rlando] (1837-1924)
The surgical treatment of non-pedunculated abdominal tumors. Chicago: Office Amer. Med. Assoc., 1890. 15p. DNLM **90-5221**

MARCY, Henry O[rlando] (1837-1924)
In what class of wounds shall we use drainage? Philadelphia: W. J. Dornan, 1890. 8p. DNLM **90-5222**

MARCY, Henry O[rlando] (1837-1924)
I. Femoral and ventral hernia in women. II. The kangaroo suture. Philadelphia: W. J. Dornan, 1891. 27p. DNLM **90-5223**

MARCY, Henry O[rlando] (1837-1924)
Kangaroo tendons. Philadelphia, 1891. 4p. DNLM **90-5224**

MARCY, Henry O[rlando] (1837-1924)
The scientific rationale of modern wound treatment. Chicago, 1891. 24p. DNLM **90-5225**

MARCY, Henry O[rlando] (1837-1924)
The anatomy and surgical treatment of hernia. New York: D. Appleton & Co., 1892. 521p. 66 plates, 11 outline plates. DLC; DNLM; NNNAM **90-5226**

MARCY, Henry O[rlando] (1837-1924)
The president's address; evolution of medicine. Chicago, 1892. 30p. DNLM **90-5227**

MARCY, Henry O[rlando] (1837-1924)
The reconstruction of the pelvic structures in woman; the advantages of the buried tendon suture. New York: William Wood & Co., 1892. 26p. DNLM **90-5228**

MARCY, Henry O[rlando] (1837-1924)
The reconstruction of the pelvic structures in woman; the advantages of the buried tendon suture. Philadelphia, 1893. 22p. 2 plates. DNLM **90-5229**

MARCY, Henry O[rlando] (1837-1924)
Analysis of one hundred and thirty-three cases of hernia operated upon for the purpose of radical cure. Chicago, 1893. 16p. DNLM **90-5230**

MARCY, Henry O[rlando] (1837-1924)
The cure of inguinal hernia in the male. [Philadelphia, 1893.] 9p. DNLM **90-5231**

MARCY, Henry O[rlando] (1837-1924)
The surgical treatment of inguinal hernia. Concord, N.H.: Republican Press Assoc., 1894. 21p. DNLM **90-5232**

MARCY, Henry O[rlando] (1837-1924)
Personal service as the especial exponent of a great profession. Boston: Damrell & Upham, 1895. 20p. DNLM **90-5233**

MARCY, Henry O[rlando] (1837-1924)
Sanitation in street pavement. Chicago, 1895. 14p. DNLM **90-5234**

MARCY, Henry O[rlando] (1837-1924)
The surgical technique of aseptic wounds. Chicago, 1895. 16p. DNLM **90-5235**

MARCY, Henry O[rlando] (1837-1924)
The surgical treatment of hemorrhoids by excision and closure with the buried animal suture. New York: William Wood & Co., 1895. 16p. DNLM **90-5236**

MARCY, Henry O[rlando] (1837-1924)
The surgical treatment of spina bifida. Philadelphia, 1895. 16p. 1 plate. DNLM **90-5237**

MARCY, Henry O[rlando] (1837-1924)
Intestinal obstruction after laparotomy. Chicago, 1896. 19p. DNLM **90-5238**

MARCY, Henry O[rlando] (1837-1924)
The technics of the buried tendon suture. New York: D. Appleton & Co., 1896. 13p. DNLM **90-5239**

MARCY, Henry O[rlando] (1837-1924)
The cure of hernia. Boston: Damrell & Upham, 1897. 10p. DNLM **90-5240**

MARCY, Henry O[rlando] (1837-1924)
The cure of inguinal hernia in the male. Norwalk: Laning Print. Co., 1897. 16p. DNLM **90-5241**

MARCY, Henry O[rlando] (1837-1924)
The cure of vesico-vaginal fistula by the free dissection of the bladder from its vaginal attachments and closure with the buried continuous tendon suture. Chicago, 1897. 8p. DNLM **90-5242**

MARCY, Henry O[rlando] (1837-1924)
The aseptic animal suture; its place in surgery. Chicago, 1898. 20p. DNLM **90-5243**

MARCY, Henry O[rlando] (1837-1924)
The milk-supply of cities; can it be improved? Chicago, 1898. 27p. DNLM **90-5244**

MARCY, Henry O[rlando] (1837-1924)
The surgical treatment of uterine myomsis. Chicago: Amer. Med. Assoc. Press, 1898. 24p. DNLM **90-5245**

MARCY, Henry O[rlando] (1837-1924)
The reconstruction of the pelvic structures incident to lesions of perineum. Chicago, 1899. 15p. DNLM **90-5246**

MARCY, W[illiam] H.
Caesarean section. New York, 1898. 4p. DNLM **90-5247**

MARION-SIMS-BEAUMONT MEDICAL COLLEGE OF MEDICINE, ST. LOUIS, MO.
Annual announcements for the sessions of 1890-91 to 1896-97 (1.-7.); 1898-99 (9.); 1903-04 (14.); 1904-05 (15.). St. Louis, 1890-1904. DNLM [Organized in 1890. List of students and graduates for the years 1890-91 to 1895-96; 1897-98; 1902-03; 1903-04, in announcements for subsequent years. On May 1, 1901, title was adopted by the consolidation of the Marion-Sims College of Medicine with the Beaumont Hospital Medical College.] **90-5248**

MARION-SIMS DENTAL COLLEGE, ST. LOUIS
Annual announcements for the sessions of 1894-95 to 1897-98 (1.-4.); 1904-05 (11.). St. Louis, 1894-1904. DNLM [List of students and graduates for the years 1893-94 to 1896-97; 1903-04, in announcements for subsequent years.] **90-5249**

MARKS, A. A.
Patent artificial limbs with india-rubber hands and feet. New York, 1891. 106p. DNLM; NNNAM **90-5250**

[MARKS, George Edwin] (1853-1932)
A treatise on Marks' patent artificial limbs with rubber hands and feet. New York: A. A. Marks, 1894. 445p. DLC; NNNAM **90-5251**

MARKS, George E[dwin] (1853-1932)
Amputations prothetically considered. New York, 1894. 16p. DNLM **90-5252**

[MARKS, George E[dwin]] (1853-1932)
A treatise on artificial limbs. . . . [Special ed.] New York: A. A. Marks, 1896. 544p. DLC; NNNAM **90-5253**

[MARKS, George E[dwin]] (1853-1932)
A treatise on artificial limbs with rubber hands and feet. . . . New York: A. A. Marks, 1899. 530p. DLC; NNNAM **90-5254**

MARKS, Heine
Rest in gunshot wounds of the chest. [St. Louis] , 1894. 32p. DNLM **90-5255**

MARLOW, F[rank] W[illiam] (*b.* 1858)
Some remarks on heterophoria and its treatment. New York, 1893. 19p. DNLM **90-5256**

MARLOW, F[rank] W[illiam] (*b.* 1858)
A case of retinitis pigmentosa, with extreme contraction of the visual fields and without night blindness. New York: D. Appleton & Co., 1894. 3p. DNLM **90-5257**

MARLOW, F[rank] W[illiam] (*b.* 1858)
The errors of refraction in a series of two thousand eyes, and some of the symptoms related thereto. New York, 1895. 16p. DNLM **90-5258**

MARLOW, F[rank] W[illiam] (*b.* 1858)
Spontaneous absorption of senile cataract, with restoration of vision. Dislocation of nucleus and capsule into the anterior chamber. New York, 1899. 3p. DNLM **90-5259**

MARSH, E[lias] J. (*b.* 1835)
Insured lives as affected by gout. New York, 1895. 18p. DNLM **90-5260**

MARSH, E[lias] J. (*b.* 1835)
Reports on asthma and on biliary and renal colic and calculus. New York, 1895. 12p. DNLM **90-5261**

MARSH, E[lias] J. (*b.* 1835)
Syphilis as affecting life-insurance risks. New York, 1895. 13p. DNLM **90-5262**

MARSH, E[lias] J. (*b.* 1835)
Value of family history and personal condition in estimating a liability to consumption. New York, 1895. 23p. DNLM
90-5263

MARSH, E[lias] J. (*b.* 1835)
Mortality from casualties. New York, 1896. 36p. DNLM
90-5264

MARSH, E[lias] J. (*b.* 1835)
Report on the mortality resulting from suicides. New York, 1896. 16p. DNLM **90-5265**

MARSHALL, Arthur Milnes (1852-1893)
Vertebrate embryology; a text-book for students and practitioners. . . . New York: G. P. Putnam's Sons; London: Smith, Elder & Co., 1893. 640p. DLC; NNNAM
90-5266

MARSHALL, Clara (1848-1931)
The Woman's Medical College of Pennsylvania. An historical outline. . . . Philadelphia: P. Blakiston, Son & Co., 1897. 142p. DLC; PPC; PPJ; PU **90-5267**

MARSHALL, John (1818-1891)
Physiological diagrams . . . designed for demonstration before the class. Philadelphia: P. Blakiston, Son & Co., 1894. DLC [Eleven life-size diagrams (each 7 feet by 3 feet, 7 inches): No. 1, the Skeleton and Ligaments; No. 2, the Muscles and Joints, with animal mechanics; No. 3, the Viscera in Position; No. 4, the Heart and Principal Blood-Vessels; No. 5, the Lymphatics or Absorbents; No. 6, the Digestive Organs; No. 7, the Brain and Nerves; Nos. 8 and 9, the Organs of the Senses; Nos. 10 and 11, the Microscopic Structure of the Textures and Organs.] **90-5268**

MARSHALL, John (1855-1925)
Notes on the chemical lectures in the medical department of the University of Pennsylvania for first year students. Published by authority of Prof. Theo. G. Wormley. . . . Philadelphia: Press of W. F. Fell & Co., 1890 [1889]. 166p. DLC; PPPH **90-5269**

MARSHALL, John (1855-1925)
Notes on the chemical lectures in the medical department of the University of Pennsylvania for first year students. Published by authority of Prof. Theo. G. Wormley. . . . 2nd ed., rev. Philadelphia: Press of W. F. Fell & Co., 1890. 165p. DLC **90-5270**

MARSHALL, John (1855-1925)
Notes on the chemical lectures in the medical department of the University of Pennsylvania for first year students. Published by authority of Prof. Theo. G. Wormley. . . . 3rd ed., rev. Philadelphia: Avil Printing Co., 1894. 165p. PU
90-5271

MARSHALL, John Sayre (1846-1922)
Electricity as a therapeutic agent in the treatment of hyperemia and congestion of the pulp and peridental membrane. Philadelphia, 1891. 5p. DNLM **90-5272**

MARSHALL, John Sayre (1846-1922)
A manual of the injuries and surgical diseases of the face, mouth and jaws. . . . Philadelphia: The S. S. White Dental Mfg. Co., 1897. 716p. DLC; DNLM; PPC
90-5273

MARTIN, August Eduard (1847-1933)
Pathology and therapeutics of the diseases of women. . . . Transl. from the 2nd rev. and enl. ed. . . . with notes and appendix, by Dr. Ernest W. Cushing. 2nd American ed. Boston: E. W. Cushing [Press of Rockwell and Churchill], 1890. 681p. plates. DLC; MBM; NNNAM; PPC **90-5274**

MARTIN, Edward (1859-1938)
. . . Essentials of surgery, together with a full description of the handkerchief and roller bandage. Arranged in the form of questions and answers, prepared especially for students of medicine. . . . 2nd ed. With ninety illustrations. Philadelphia: W. B. Saunders, 1890. 314p. DLC; PPC; PU
90-5275

MARTIN, Edward (1859-1938)
. . . Essentials of minor surgery and bandaging, with an appendix on venereal diseases. Arranged in the form of questions and answers. . . . Philadelphia: W. B. Saunders, 1890. 166p. DLC; DNLM; PPC; PU **90-5276**

MARTIN, Edward (1859-1938)
. . . Essentials of minor surgery and bandaging, with an appendix on venereal diseases. Arranged in the form of questions and answers. . . . 4th ed., revised and enlarged by an appendix, containing full directions and prescriptions for the preparation of the various materials used in antiseptic surgery; also several hundred receipts covering the medical treatment of surgical affections. Philadelphia: W. B. Saunders, 1891. 334p. DNLM; PPC **90-5277**

MARTIN, Edward (1859-1938) and H. A. HARE
The surgical treatment of wounds and obstruction of the intestines. Philadelphia: W. B. Saunders, 1891. 169p. DNLM; PPC [Fiske Fund Prize Essay for 1890] **90-5278**

MARTIN, Edward (1859-1938)
Impotence and sexual weakness in the male and female. . . . Detroit, Mich.: G. S. Davis, 1893. 102p. DLC; DNLM; OCIM [2nd ed., 1895] **90-5279**

MARTIN, Edward (1859-1938)
. . . Essentials of minor surgery and bandaging, with an appendix on venereal diseases. Arranged in the form of questions and answers. . . . 2nd ed., rev. and enl. 78 illustrations. Philadelphia: W. B. Saunders, 1893. 166p. DLC; PPC; PU
90-5280

MARTIN Edward (1859-1938)
Epithelioma of the penis. [New York, 1895.] 7p. DNLM
90-5281

MARTIN, Edward (1859-1938)
. . . Essentials of minor surgery and bandaging, with an appendix on venereal diseases. Arranged in the form of questions and answers. . . . 6th ed. Philadelphia: W. B. Saunders, 1897. 338p. DNLM; PPC; PU **90-5282**

MARTIN, Francis C[offin]
The propagation, preservation, and use of vaccine virus. New York, 1896. 12p. DNLM **90-5283**

MARTIN, Franklin H[enry] (1857-1935)
Electricity in diseases of women and obstetrics. Chicago: W. T. Keener Co., 1893. 278p. DNLM; IU-M
90-5284

MARTIN, Franklin H[enry] (1857-1935)
Alexander's operation without buried sutures. New York, 1896. 2p. DNLM **90-5285**

MARTIN, H[enry] Newell (1848-1896)
Recent discoveries in the physiology of ganglion cells. Baltimore, 1891. 6p. DNLM **90-5286**

MARTIN, H[enry] Newell (1848-1896)
Vaso-motor nerves of the heart. Baltimore, 1891. 4p. DNLM **90-5287**

MARTIN, H[enry] Newell (1848-1896)
The human body; an elementary text-book of anatomy, physiology, and hygiene. New York: H. Holt & Co., 1892. 399p. DNLM; NN **90-5288**

MARTIN, H[enry] Newell (1848-1896)
Physiological papers. Baltimore: Johns Hopkins Press, 1895. 264p. 15 plates. DNLM; MdBJ-W **90-5289**

MARTIN, S[olomon] C[laiborne] (1837-1906)
Chronic cutaneous ulcers, and treatment. St. Louis, 1898. 1 l. DNLM **90-5290**

MARTIN, S[olomon] C[laiborne] (1837-1906)
Scrofuloderma and its treatment. St. Louis, 1898. 2 l. DNLM **90-5291**

MARTIN, Thomas Charles (1864-1926)
A new stitch securing the rectal mucous membrane to the skin at the anus after removal of a cylindrical part of its lower third. Chicago, 1895. 4p. 2 plates. DNLM **90-5292**

MARTIN, Thomas Charles (1864-1926)
New evidence that the rectal valve is an anatomical fact. Louisville: J. P. Morton & Co., 1896. 25p. DNLM **90-5293**

MARTIN, Thomas Charles (1864-1926)
Procto colonoscopy and its possibilities, by a new method. Louisville: J. P. Morton & Co., 1896. 23p. 7 plates. DNLM **90-5294**

MARTIN, Thomas Charles (1864-1926)
Difficult defecation in infants. Chicago, 1898. 28p. DNLM **90-5295**

MARTIN, Thomas Charles (1864-1926)
A pictorial demonstration of a new method for ballooning the rectum and for the removal of foreign bodies from the anus and rectum without anesthesia. Philadelphia, 1899. 6p. DNLM **90-5296**

MARX, S[imon] (*b.* 1864)
Care and treatment of the nipple in the gravid and puerperal states. New York: Trow, 1893. 17p. DNLM **90-5297**

MARX, S[imon] (*b.* 1864)
Contribution to the study of face presentations. New York, 1894. 8p. DNLM **90-5298**

MARX, S[imon] (*b.* 1864)
Placenta praevia; its rational treatment. New York, 1895. 8p. DNLM **90-5299**

MARYLAND MEDICAL COLLEGE OF BALTIMORE
Annual announcements for the sessions of 1898-99 to 1904-05 (1.-7.). Baltimore, 1898-1904. DNLM [Organized in July, 1898. List of students and graduates for the years 1898-99 to 1904-04 in: Announcements for subsequent years.] **90-5300**

MARYOTT, E[rastus] Edgar (1845-1904)
The new medical world. A book for reference and consultation, containing a thorough description of disease, with the latest and best methods for its treatment. . . . Springfield, Mass.: The Hampden Publishing Co., 1897. 1898 [*vel subseq.*] 583p. plates. DLC; DNLM; MBM **90-5301**

MASLAND, H[arvey] C.
Ovarian cyst with internal hemorrhage; operation; recovery. [Philadelphia, 1893.] 3p. DNLM **90-5302**

MASLAND, H[arvey] C.
A case of exstrophy of the bladder. [Philadelphia: Lea Bros. & Co., 1894.] 6p. DNLM **90-5303**

MASON, A[mos] L[awrence] (1842-1914)
Notes on typhoid from 676 cases admitted to the Boston City Hospital in 1890 and 1891. Boston: Damrell & Upham, 1892. 28p. DNLM; MBM **90-5304**

MASON, A[mos] L[awrence] (1842-1914)
Subphrenic abscess, with special reference to those cases which simulate pyo-pneumothorax. [Philadelphia, 1893.] 32p. DNLM **90-5305**

MASON, Lewis D[uncan] (*b.* 1843)
An address delivered at a meeting of the American Association for the Study and Cure of Inebriety, held at Burlington, N.J., to celebrate the seventy-first birthday of Joseph Parish, president and founder of the association. Hartford: Case, Lockwood & Brainard Co., 1890. 11p. DNLM **90-5306**

MASON, Lewis D[uncan] (*b.* 1843)
A study of the social statistics of 4,663 cases of alcoholic inebriety. [Hartford, 1890.] 8p. DNLM **90-5307**

MASON, Lewis D[uncan] (*b.* 1843)
An address on the twentieth anniversary of the American Association for the Study and Cure of Inebriety, delivered before the association at a meeting held in the New York Academy of Medicine, Dec. 10, 1890. Hartford: Case, Lockwood & Brainard Co., 1891. 14p. DNLM **90-5308**

MASON, Lewis D[uncan] (*b.* 1843)
The absence of reasonable motive in the so-called "criminal acts" of the confirmed inebriate. [Hartford, 1892.] 14p. DNLM **90-5309**

MASON, Lewis D[uncan] (*b.* 1843)
The aetiology and therapeutics of alcoholic inebriety. [n. p., 1893.] 7p. DNLM; NN **90-5310**

MASON, Lewis D[uncan] (*b.* 1843)
Differential diagnosis of alcoholic coma from other forms of coma, with especial reference to the care of persons found by the police on the streets in a comatose or semi-comatose condition. Hartford, 1894. 26p. DNLM **90-5311**

MASON, Lewis D[uncan] (*b.* **1843)**
The pauper inebriate; his legal status, care, and control. Hartford, 1899. 21p. NN **90-5312**

MASON, R[ufus] D[odd] (1859-1911)
The importance of rectal examinations in life insurance. St. Louis, 1897. 4p. DNLM **90-5313**

MASON, R[ufus] D[odd] (1859-1911)
Quinine in malaria. Charlotte, N.C., 1898. 3p. DNLM **90-5314**

MASSACHUSETTS MEDICAL SOCIETY
. . . A catalogue of its officers, fellows and licentiates, 1781-1893. Boston: The Society, 1894. 204p. DLC; MBM; MH **90-5315**

MASSEY, G[eorge] Betton (1856-1927)
. . . Electricity in the diseases of women, with special reference to the application of strong currents. . . . 2nd ed. Rev. and enl. Philadelphia and London: F. A. Davis, 1890. 240p. DLC; DNLM; PPC; PU **90-5316**

MASSEY, G[eorge] Betton (1856-1927)
The electrical treatment of fibroid tumors, with an analysis of forty-six cases. [Philadelphia, 1891.] 11p. DNLM **90-5317**

MASSEY, G[eorge] Betton (1856-1927)
Modern electrical methods as a substitute for surgery in certain pelvic affections. Richmond, 1892. 8p. DNLM **90-5318**

MASSEY, G[eorge] Betton (1856-1927)
Notes of some fibroid tumors treated by electricity. Philadelphia, 1892. 8p. DNLM **90-5319**

MASSEY, G[eorge] Betton (1856-1927)
A case illustrating the treatment of painful prolapsed ovaries in young girls. [Philadelphia, 1893.] 3p. DNLM **90-5320**

MASSEY, G[eorge] Betton (1856-1927)
Prevalent errors in the treatment of the diseases of women. Detroit: G. S. Davis, 1893. 9p. DNLM **90-5321**

MASSEY, G[eorge] Betton (1856-1927)
Recent progress in electro-gynecology. Chicago: American Med. Assoc., 1893. 8p. DNLM **90-5322**

MASSEY, G[eorge] Betton (1856-1927)
Certain erroneous principles and methods in gynaecology. Philadelphia, 1894. 6p. DNLM **90-5323**

MASSEY, G[eorge] Betton (1856-1927)
The electrical treatment of fibroid tumors. Chicago, 1894. 8p. DNLM **90-5324**

MASSEY, G[eorge] Betton (1856-1927)
Electricity in the treatment of chronic prostatitis and other conditions underlying impotence in men. Philadelphia, 1894. 5p. DNLM **90-5325**

MASSEY, G[eorge] Betton (1856-1927)
A large oedematous myoma treated by abdominal electropuncture. New York, 1895. 2p. DNLM **90-5326**

MASSEY, G[eorge] Betton (1856-1927)
Local electrolysis and zinc-amalgam cataphoresis in malignant and non-malignant tumors. [Philadelphia: Lea Bros. & Co., 1895.] 9p. DNLM **90-5327**

MASSEY, G[eorge] Betton (1856-1927)
Menorrhagia and its rational treatment. New York, 1896. 3p. DNLM **90-5328**

MASSEY, G[eorge] Betton (1856-1927)
The new cataphoric treatment of cancer. New York, 1898. 6p. DNLM **90-5329**

MASSEY, G[eorge] Betton (1856-1927)
Conservative gynecology and electro-therapeutics; a practical treatise on the diseases of women and their treatment by electricity. . . . 3rd ed., rev., rewritten, and greatly enl. Illustrated with twelve (12) original full-page chromo-lithographic plates and twelve (12) full-page half-tone plates of photographs taken from nature and numerous engravings in the text. Philadelphia, New York [etc.]: The F. A. Davis Co., 1898. 394p. plates. DLC; DNLM; NNNAM; PPC **90-5330**

MASTERS, J[ames] M.
Charge to the graduating class, Tennessee Medical College. Delivered at the third annual commencement, Knoxville, Tenn., March 17, 1892. Knoxville: S. B. Newman & Co., 1892. 12p. DLC **90-5331**

MASTERS, J[ames] M.
The duty of the present to future generations from a reproductive point of view. [Richmond, 1893.] 6p. DNLM **90-5332**

MASTIN, Claudius H[enry] (1826-1898)
Address of the president. "The past, the present, and future of our association." Philadelphia: W. J. Dornan, 1891. 15p. DNLM **90-5333**

MASTIN, Claudius H[enry] (1826-1898)
Two interesting surgical cases. Philadelphia, 1895. 6p. DNLM **90-5334**

MASTIN, Claudius H[enry] (1826-1898)
President's address before the tenth annual meeting of the American Association of Genito-Urinary Surgeons. New York: D. Appleton & Co., 1896. 6p. DNLM **90-5335**

MATAS, Rudolph (1860-1957)
The present status of the operations of intestinal anastomosis and enterorrhaphy, and the comparative merits of the various "aids" that have been recently suggested in the performance of these operations. New Orleans, 1890. 35p. DNLM **90-5336**

MATAS, Rudolph (1860-1957)
A clinical report on intravenous saline infusion in the wards of the New Orleans Charity Hospital from June, 1888, to June, 1891. New Orleans: L. Graham & Son, [1891]. 44p. DNLM **90-5337**

MATAS, Rudolph (1860-1957)
Large cavernous angioma involving the integument of an entire auricle, successfully treated by dissection, free resection of diseased tissue, and ligation of the afferent trunks in situ by a special method. Philadelphia, 1892. 17p. DNLM **90-5338**

MATAS, Rudolph (1860-1957)
Notes on some congenital anomalies connected with the branchial apparatus. [Philadelphia: Lea Bros. & Co., 1893.] 91p. DNLM **90-5339**

MATAS, Rudolph (1860-1957)
Traumatisms and traumatic aneurisms of the vertebral artery, and their surgical treatment; with the report of a cured case. Philadelphia, 1893.] 40p. DNLM **90-5340**

MATAS, Rudolph (1860-1957)
Remarks on the continued fevers of Louisiana. [Philadelphia, 1894.] 5p. DNLM **90-5341**

MATAS, Rudolph (1860-1957)
Fracture of the zygomatic arch. A simple method of reduction and fixation, with remarks on the prevalence, symptomatology, and treatment of this fracture. New Orleans, 1896. 19p. DNLM **90-5342**

MATAS, Rudolph (1860-1957)
The surgical peculiarities of the American Negro. A statistical inquiry based upon the records of the Charity Hospital of New Orleans, La., decenium 1884-94. Philadelphia, 1896. 130p. DNLM **90-5343**

MATAS, Rudolph (1860-1957)
The surgical treatment of ano-rectal imperforation in the light of modern operative procedures. [Philadelphia, 1897.] 101p. DNLM **90-5344**

MATAS, Rudolph (1860-1957)
Multiple (triple) stricture of probable tubercular origin within thirteen inches (33 cm.) of the jetjunum. Resection and circular enterorrhaphy by Maunsell's method, followed by complete recovery; with remarks on multiple intestinal strictures. Philadelphia, 1898. 22p. DNLM **90-5345**

MATAS, Rudolph (1860-1957)
The surgery of the chest, and some of the problems related to the treatment of its penetrating traumatisms and their immediate complications. New Orleans: L. Graham & Son, [1898]. 70p. DNLM **90-5346**

MATAS, Rudolph (1860-1957)
Remarks on the operative treatment of cancer of the breast, with a synopsis of 27 cases operated on. Philadelphia, 1898. 18p. DNLM **90-5347**

MATAS, Rudolph (1860-1957)
Extrauterine (tubal) pregnancy with rupture of sac; repeated hemorrhage; laparotomy; convalescence complicated by secondary abscess of the liver; transpleural hepatotomy; recovery. Chicago, 1899. 11p. DNLM **90-5348**

MATAS, Rudolph (1860-1957)
Exstrophy of the bladder. Operative treatment, with special reference to Maydi's operation. Chicago, 1899. 11p. DNLM **90-5349**

MATHEWS, Joseph McDowell (*b.* 1847)
The address on surgery. Chicago, 1891. 32p. DNLM **90-5350**

MATHEWS, Joseph McDowell (*b.* 1847)
A treatise on diseases of the rectum, anus, and sigmoid flexure. . . . New York: D. Appleton & Co., 1892. 537p. col. plates. DLC; DNLM; NNNAM **90-5351**

MATHEWS, Joseph McDowell (*b.* 1847)
Our diagnostic resources in rectal and allied diseases. Chicago, 1893. 24p. DNLM **90-5352**

MATHEWS, Joseph McDowell (*b.* 1847)
A treatise on diseases of the rectum, anus, and sigmoid flexure. . . . 2nd ed., rev. New York: D. Appleton & Co., 1896. 545p. col. plates. DLC; DNLM; NNNAM **90-5353**

MATTHEWS, Samuel Alexander (*b.* 1866)
Syllabus of lectures on pharmacology and therapeutics in the University of Michigan. . . . Ann Arbor, Mich.: G. Wahr, [1896]. 114p. DLC; DNLM **90-5354**

MATTISON, J[ansen] B[eemer] (*b.* 1845)
The treatment of the morphine disease. Detroit: G. S. Davis, 1890. 24p. DNLM **90-5355**

MATTISON, J[ansen] B[eemer] (*b.* 1845)
Triple narcotic addiction; Opium, alcohol, cocaine. Philadelphia, 1890. 4p. DNLM **90-5356**

MATTISON, J[ansen] B[eemer] (*b.* 1845)
Chloralism. New York, 1891. 8p. DNLM **90-5357**

MATTISON, J[ansen] B[eemer] (*b.* 1845)
Cocaine poisoning. [Philadelphia, 1891.] 21p. DNLM **90-5358**

MATTISON, J[ansen] B[eemer] (*b.* 1845)
Hypnal, the new nervine. Brooklyn, 1891. 3 l. DNLM **90-5359**

MATTISON, J[ansen] B[eemer] (*b.* 1845)
New and improved galvanic and faradic batteries, with new and original electrodes, in the treatment of narcotic habitués. [St. Louis, 1891.] 2 l. DNLM **90-5360**

MATTISON, J[ansen] B[eemer] (*b.* 1845)
Papers by . . . . [List of works.] [1891.] 2 l. DNLM **90-5361**

MATTISON, J[ansen] B[eemer] (*b.* 1845)
The prevention of morphinism. A therapeutic revolution; codeine and narceine, vice morphine. [New York, 1891.] 7p. DNLM **90-5362**

MATTISON, J[ansen] B[eemer] (*b.* 1845)
Cocaine inebriety. [New York, 1893.] 24p. DNLM **90-5363**

MATTISON, J[ansen] B[eemer] (*b.* 1845)
The etiology of narcotic inebriety. [St. Louis, 1893.] 4p. DNLM **90-5364**

MATTISON, J[ansen] B[eemer] (*b.* 1845)
The Mattison method in morphinism. [Philadelphia, 1893.] 6 l. DNLM **90-5365**

MATTISON, J[ansen] B[eemer] (*b.* 1845)
The modern and humane treatment of the morphine disease. New York, 1893. 8p. DNLM **90-5366**

MATTISON, J[ansen] B[eemer] (*b.* **1845**)
Trional, the new hypnotic. Its use in narcotic habitués. [Philadelphia, 1893.] 2 l. DNLM **90-5367**

MATTISON, J[ansen] B[eemer] (*b.* **1845**)
Twenty-seven years' addiction to opium; recovery; relapse. Danbury, Conn., 1893. 4p. DNLM **90-5368**

MATTISON, J[ansen] B[eemer] (*b.* **1845**)
Morphinism in medical men. Chicago, 1894. 7p. DNLM **90-5369**

MATTISON, J[ansen] B[eemer] (*b.* **1845**)
The post-active treatment of narcotic habitués. Chicago, 1895. 7p. DNLM **90-5370**

MATTISON, J[ansen] B[eemer] (*b.* **1845**)
The diagnosis of the morphin disease. [New York, 1896.] 4p. DNLM **90-5371**

MATTISON, J[ansen] B[eemer] (*b.* **1845**)
Morphinism: Morphinism in the young; a tale of the poppy and its moral; morphinism in the old, cases at three score and ten, recovery; morphinism in women. [Providence, 1896.] 10, 10, 8, 13p. DNLM **90-5372**

MATTISON, J[ansen] B[eemer] (*b.* **1845**)
Narcotic inebriety in America. [1898.] 2p. MB **90-5373**

THE MATTISON Prize. Opium addiction as related to renal disease. [Brooklyn, 1890.] 1 sheet. DNLM **90-5374**

MAUDSLEY, Henry (1835-1918)
Responsibility in mental disease. New York: D. Appleton & Co., 1896. 313p. CtY-M; NNNAM; PPC **90-5375**

[MAXEN, R. A.]
The home doctor, a complete manual of family medicine. . . . New York City: Home Treatment Co., [1895]. 272p. DLC; NNNAM **90-5376**

MAXWELL, Theodore, ed.
Terminologia medica polyglotta . . . a concise international dictionary of medical terms. . . . Philadelphia: P. Blakiston, Son & Co., 1890. 459p. DNLM; NNNAM; PPC; PPL **90-5377**

MAY, Charles Henry (1861-1943)
May's Diseases of women, being a concise and systematic exposition of the theory and practice of gynecology. For the use of students and practitioners. 2nd ed., rev. by Leonard S. Rau. . . . Philadelphia: Lea Bros. & Co., 1890. 373p. DLC; NNNAM; PPC; PU **90-5378**

MAY, Charles H[enry] (1861-1943)
The early eye-symptoms in chronic alcoholism. [Minneapolis, 1892.] 6p. DNLM **90-5379**

MAY, Charles H[enry] (1861-1943)
The prevention and treatment of ophthalmia neonatorum, and the necessity for more efficient legislation to prevent blindness from this cause. [New York, 1895.] 16p. DNLM **90-5380**

MAY, Charles H[enry] (1861-1943)
Mixed forms of trachoma and spring catarrh. St. Louis, 1896. 8p. DNLM **90-5381**

MAY, Charles H[enry] (1861-1943)
The treatment of contusions of the lids ("black eye"). New York, 1897. 7p. DNLM **90-5382**

MAY, Charles H[enry] (1861-1943)
Acute inflammation of the middle ear complicating scarlet fever and measles. New York, 1899. 10p. DNLM **90-5833**

MAY, Charles H[enry] (1861-1943)
Restoration of the conjunctival cul-de-sac in a case of total symblepharon by means of Thiersch skin grafts. New York, 1899. 9p. DNLM **90-5384**

MAYER, Emil (1854-1931)
Catarrh of the upper air passages. New York, 1892. 8p. DNLM **90-5385**

MAYER, Emil (1854-1931)
Congenital stricture of the oesophagus, with report of a case. Philadelphia, 1893. 5p. DNLM **90-5386**

MAYER, Emil (1854-1931)
Deviation of the cartilaginous nasal septum; its cure. New York, 1895. 8p. DNLM **90-5387**

MAYER, Emil (1854-1931)
The nasal mucous membrane. A plea for the greater care of it in intranasal operations. New York, 1896. 7p. DNLM **90-5388**

MAYER, Emil (1854-1931)
The Asch operation for deviations of the cartilaginous nasal septum, with a report of two hundred operations. New York, 1898. 16p. DNLM **90-5389**

MAYER, Emil (1854-1931)
Primary lupus of the larynx. New York, 1898. 15p. DNLM **90-5390**

MAYER, Emil (1854-1931)
Tuberculosis of the upper air-passages. New York, 1898. 10p. DNLM **90-5391**

MAYER, Emil (1854-1931)
On the use of Schleich's mixtures for anaesthesia in operations on the nose and throat. New York, 1898. 12p. DNLM **90-5392**

MAYER, Emil (1854-1931)
Adenoid vegetations. How and when shall we operate for them? Chicago, 1899. 7p. DNLM **90-5393**

MAYER, Emil (1854-1931)
Section on laryngology and otology. Chicago, 1899. 7p. DNLM **90-5394**

MAYER, Emil (1854-1931)
The tonsils as portals of infections. Chicago, 1899. 11p. DNLM **90-5395**

MAYER, Emil (1854-1931)
Clinical memoranda from the throat department. New York, 1899. 5p. DNLM **90-5396**

MAYLARD, A[lfred] Ernest
A treatise on the surgery of the alimentary canal, comprising the oesophagus, the stomach, the small and large intestines, and the rectum. Philadelphia: P. Blakiston's Son & Co., 1896. 724p. 27 plates. DNLM; NNNAM; PCC; PU
90-5397

MAYO, William J. (1861-1939)
Observations upon the diagnosis and surgical treatment of certain diseases of the stomach, based upon personal experience. New York, 1898. 11p. DNLM **90-5398**

MAYO, William J. (1861-1939)
Localized tuberculosis of the intestine, with a report of seven operated cases. New York, 1899. 20p. DNLM
90-5399

MAYS, Thomas Jefferson (1846-1918)
Pulmonary consumption, a nervous disease: considered as such from a practical, a clinical, and a therapeutic standpoint. . . . Detroit, Mich.: G. S. Davis, 1891. 185p. DLC; OCIM
90-5400

MAYS, Thomas Jefferson (1846-1918)
. . . The hypodermic injection of silver nitrate over the course of the vagi in the treatment of pulmonary consumption. A preliminary report. . . . [Philadelphia? 1899.] 6p. fold. tab. DLC **90-5401**

MEADOWCROFT, William H. (1853-1937)
The A B C of the X rays. New York, [1896]. 189p. 7 plates. DNLM; NNNAM **90-5402**

MEARS, J. Ewing (1838-1919)
Practical surgery. . . . 2nd ed., rev. and enl. Philadelphia: F. A. Davis, Publisher, 1890 [1889]. 794p. DLC; NNNAM; PPC; PPJ
90-5403

MEARS, J. Ewing (1838-1919)
Cleft of the hard and soft palates. [Philadelphia, 1893.] 8p. DNLM **90-5404**

MEARS, J. Ewing (1838-1919)
Naso- or retro-pharyngeal growths. [Philadelphia, 1893.] 6p. 1 plate. DNLM **90-5405**

MEARS, J. Ewing (1838-1919)
Address of the president, American Surgical Association, 1894. [Philadelphia, 1894.] 9p. DNLM
90-5406

MEARS, J. Ewing (1838-1919)
Ligature of the spermatic cord in the treatment of hypertrophy of the prostate gland. [Philadelphia, 1894.] 5p. DNLM
90-5407

MEARS, J. Ewing (1838-1919)
Ligature of the spermatic cord for conditions other than hypertrophy of the prostate gland. Philadelphia, 1895. 4p. DNLM **90-5408**

MEARS, J. Ewing (1838-1919)
The operative treatment in occlusion of the jaws. Chicago, 1897. 15p. DNLM **90-5409**

THE MEDICAL colleges and the hospital fee. [Nashville, 1892.] 7p. DNLM **90-5410**

MEDICAL and Dental Red Book. A register of all the physicians, surgeons, dentists, druggists, nurses, etc., of Cleveland and vicinity, together with a digest of the State laws and the city laws pertaining to these professions and other miscellaneous matter. Compiled by Louis J. Livingston. Cleveland: Helman-Taylor Co., 1899. 372p. DNLM; OCIM **90-5411**

MEDICAL directory for New England, 1892. Physicians', dentists', and druggists' directory of the New England States. Chicago: Gonesir, 1892. 381p. DNLM **90-5412**

MEDICAL INVESTIGATION CLUB OF BALTIMORE
A pathogenetic materia medica, based upon Drs. Hughes' and Dake's cyclopaedia of drug pathogenesy. By the Medical Investigation Club of Baltimore, Md. . . . Philadelphia: Boericke & Tafel, 1895. 347p. DLC; OCLloyd; PPHa
90-5413

MEDICAL SOCIETY OF THE DISTRICT OF COLUMBIA
Report on typhoid fever in the District of Columbia, submitted by the Medical Society of the District of Columbia to the Committee on the District of Columbia of the U.S. House of Representatives, June 14, 1894. . . . Washington: Government Printing Office, 1894. 18p. fold. maps. DLC
90-5414

MEDICAL and surgical directory of the homoeopathic physicians of the United States and Canada. Issued annually. 1., 1897. New York: A. L. Chatterton & Co., 1897. 29p. 33 l. DLC; NNNAM **90-5415**

MEDICAL and surgical register of the United States, comprising list of physicians and surgeons, arranged by localities, giving post-office address, with population, the school practiced, date and college of graduation; all the existing and extinct medical colleges in the United States and Canada. 2nd ed. Detroit: R. L. Polk & Co., 1890. 1708p. DNLM; NNNAM
90-5416

MEDICAL and surgical register of the United States, comprising a list of physicians and surgeons, arranged by localities, giving post-office address, with population, the school practiced, date and college of graduation; all the existing and extinct medical colleges in the United States and Canada. 3rd ed., revised. Detroit: R. L. Polk & Co., 1893. 1492p. DNLM; NNNAM **90-5417**

MEDICAL and surgical register of the United States, comprising a list of physicians and surgeons, arranged by localities, giving post-office address, with population, the school practiced, date and college of graduation; all the existing and extinct medical colleges in the United States and Canada. 4th ed. Detroit & Chicago: R. L. Polk & Co., 1896. 2351p. DNLM; NNNAM **90-5418**

MEDICAL and surgical register of the United States, comprising a list of physicians and surgeons, arranged by localities, giving post-office address, with population, the school practiced, date and college of graduation; all the existing and extinct medical colleges in the United States and Canada. Medical and surgical register of the United States and Canada. 5th ed. Detroit & Chicago: R. L. Polk & Co., 1898. 2502p. DNLM; NNNAM **90-5419**

MEDICO-CHIRURGICAL COLLEGE, KANSAS CITY, MO.
Annual announcements for the sessions of 1899-1900 (3.); 1902-03 (6.); 1903-04 (7.). Kansas City, 1899-1903. DNLM [List of graduates, 1898-1903, in: Announcement for 1903-04.] **90-5420**

MEDICO-CHIRURGICAL COLLEGE OF PHILADELPHIA. DEPARTMENT OF DENTISTRY
Annual announcements for the sessions of 1897-98 to 1903-04 (1.-7.). Philadelphia, 1897-1903. DNLM [List of graduates, 1989-1903, in: Announcement for 1903-04.] **90-5421**

MEDICO-CHIRURGICAL HOSPITAL OF PHILADELPHIA
Annual reports of the board of trustees and officers to the contributors. 12., 1896; 16., 1900; 18., 1902; 19., 1903. Philadelphia, 1897-1904. DNLM [Incorporated Oct. 21, 1882.] **90-5422**

MEDICO-CHIRURGICAL HOSPITAL OF PHILADELPHIA
Annual reports of the board of trustees and officers to the contributors. An illustrated description of the clinical ampitheatre of the . . . . [Philadelphia: C. A. Dixon], 1897. 35p. DNLM; PPC **90-5423**

MEDICO-LEGAL CONGRESS, NEW YORK
Bulletin of the Medico-Legal Congress held . . . in the city of New York, September 4th, 5th and 6th, 1895. New York: Pub. under the auspices of the Medico-Legal Society by the Medico-Legal Journal, 1898. 481p. plates. DLC; DNLM **90-5424**

MEIGS, Arthur V[incent] (1850-1912) and Harvey SHOEMAKER
Further experiments in weighing before and after feeding as a means of determining the amount of food taken. [Philadelphia, 1890.] 3p. DNLM **90-5425**

MEIGS, Arthur V[incent] (1850-1912)
The microscopical anatomy of the human heart, showing the existence of capillaries within the muscular fibres. [Philadelphia], 1891. 14p. DNLM **90-5426**

MEIGS, Arthur V[incent] (1850-1912)
Cystic degeneration of the muscular fibres of the heart, a form of disease hitherto undescribed. [Philadelphia, 1892.] 8p. 1 plate. DNLM **90-5427**

MEIGS, Arthur V[incent] (1850-1912) and G. E. de SCHWEINITZ
Round-celled sarcoma of the anterior mediastinum; extensive metastasis, including the brain, both choroid coats, oculomotor and optic nerves, and external ocular muscles. [Philadelpia, 1894.] 13p. DNLM **90-5428**

MEIGS, Arthur V[incent] (1850-1912)
Feeding in early infancy. . . . Philadelphia: W. B. Saunders, 1896. 15p. DLC **90-5429**

MEIGS, Arthur V[incent] (1850-1912)
The origin of disease, especially of disease resulting from intrinsic as opposed to extrinsic causes. With chapters on diagnosis, prognosis, and treatment. . . . With one hundred and thirty-seven original illustrations. Philadelphia [etc.]: J. B. Lippincott Co., 1897. 229p. 61 plates. DLC; DNLM; NNNAM; PPC **90-5430**

MELLIN'S FOOD COMPANY, BOSTON
Anweisung fur mütter bei der pflege und ernährung der kinder. . . . Mellin's nahrungsmittel für kinder und unvaliden; seine beschreibung und analyse. Boston, Mass.: Doliber-Goodale Co., 1895. 78p. DLC; MBM **90-5431**

MELTZER, Samuel J[ames] (1851-1920)
Some remarks on my hypothesis of the self-regulation of respiration, and Dr. Cowl's discussion of it. [New York, 1890.] 11p. DNLM **90-5432**

MELTZER, Samuel J[ames] (1851-1920)
Theories of respiration. [New York: D. Appleton & Co., 1891.] 6p. DNLM **90-5433**

MELTZER, Samuel J[ames] (1851-1920)
Eine Atropin-Intoxication nach epidermatischem Gebrauch einer Belladonna-Salbe. [New York, 1892.] 4p. DNLM **90-5434**

MELTZER, Samuel J[ames] (1851-1920)
Eine Haarnadel in einer männlichen Harnröhre. [New York, 1892.] 4p. DNLM **90-5435**

MELTZER, Samuel J[ames] (1851-1920)
On the self-regulation of the beat of the heart. New York, 1893. 17p. DNLM **90-5436**

MELTZER, Samuel J[ames] (1851-1920)
On subphrenic abscess. New York, 1893. 16p. DNLM **90-5437**

MELTZER, Samuel J[ames] (1851-1920)
Recent experimental contributions to the physiology of deglutition. New York, 1894. 22p. DNLM **90-5438**

MELTZER, Samuel J[ames] (1851-1920)
On the thyreoid therapy; its history and its use in internal medicine. New York, 1895. 19p. DNLM **90-5439**

MELTZER, Samuel J[ames] (1851-1920)
On absorption of strychnine and hydrocyanic acid from the mucous membrane of the stomach. An experimental study on rabbits. New York, 1896. 8p. DNLM **90-5440**

MELTZER, Samuel J[ames] (1851-1920)
On congenital hypertrophic stenosis of the pylorus in infants. New York, 1898. 24p. DNLM **90-5441**

MELTZER, Samuel J[ames] (1851-1920)
Otitis media and earache in lobar pneumonia of children. Philadelphia, 1899. 16p. DNLM **90-5442**

MEMMINGER, Allard (*b.* 1854)
The practical examination of urine, with special reference to diagnosis. Philadelphia: P. Blakiston, Son & Co., 1892. 77p. CtY-M; DLC; DNLM **90-5443**

MEMMINGER, Allard (*b.* 1854)
The practical examination of urine, with special reference to diagnosis. 2nd ed., enl. and rev. Philadelphia: P. Blakiston, Son & Co., 1899. 124p. DLC; PPC; PPJ **90-5444**

MERCK & CO.
Merck's Market Report. Prices of drugs and chemicals. . . . New York, 1892. 52p. NNNAM **90-5445**

. . . **MERCK'S** 1896 index. An encyclopedia for the physician and the pharmacist. . . . [2nd ed.] New York: Merck & Co., [1895]. 268p. DLC; NNNAM **90-5446**

MERIWETHER, Frank T.
A large meningocele. New York, 1894. 3p. DNLM **90-5447**

MERIWETHER, Frank T.
Climate in the treatment of phthisis. Charlotte, 1896. 3p. DNLM **90-5448**

MERIWETHER, Frank T.
Puerperal sepsis. Charlotte, 1896. 4p. DNLM **90-5449**

MERIWETHER, Frank T.
A report of some interesting surgical cases seen during the past year. Charlotte, 1897. 8p. DNLM **90-5450**

MERIWETHER, Frank T.
The treatment of chronic endometritis. Charlotte, N.C., 1897. 7p. DNLM **90-5451**

MERIWETHER, Frank T.
The surgical treatment of appendicitis. Charlotte, N.C., 1898. 11p. DNLM **90-5452**

MERIWETHER, Frank T.
A study of 61 cases of appendicitis, 30 of whom were operated upon. Boston, 1899. 11p. DNLM **90-5453**

MERRELL, A. F. & CO.
Catalogue of pharmacy goods, drugs, glassware, implements, . . . Philadelphia, 1894. 32p. PPC; PU **90-5454**

MESSINGER, W. C.
. . . Illustrated catalogue of dental furniture, ...instruments and materials. Hartford, 1897. 594p. DNLM **90-5455**

METHOD of examining the bladder and catheterizing the ureters in women. Claim to its discovery by Prof. Pawlik, Prague. With a reply by Howard A. Kelly. New York: William Wood & Co., 1896. 8p. DNLM; NNNAM **90-5456**

METTLER, Lee Harrison (*b.* 1863)
A plea for the medical expert. Chicago: Office Amer. Med. Assoc., 1892. 15p. DNLM **90-5457**

METTLER, Lee Harrison (*b.* 1863)
The sensory-motor functions of the brain. New York: Trow's Co., 1892. 32p. DNLM **90-5458**

METTLER, Lee Harrison (*b.* 1863)
Some remarks on pneumonia and the cause of heart failure, with report of a case. [New York: D. Appleton & Co., 1892.] 16p. DNLM **90-5459**

METTLER, Lee Harrison (*b.* 1863)
Hemiparaplegia; with report of a case completely recovered after one year's duration. Chicago: Amer. Med. Assoc., 1893. 12p. DNLM **90-5460**

METTLER, Lee Harrison (*b.* 1863)
Spontaneous gangrene following typhoid fever. New York, 1895. 9p. DNLM **90-5461**

METTLER, Lee Harrison (*b.* 1863)
The neuroses of gout. St. Louis, Mo., 1897. 12p. DNLM **90-5462**

MEYER, Bernard
Illustrated catalogue of druggists' pill and powder boxes, standard drugs, . . . New York, 1894. 32p. NNNAM **90-5463**

MEYER, Willy (*b.* 1858)
The operative treatment of erysipelas. New York: Trow, 1890. 11p. DNLM **90-5464**

MEYER, Willy (*b.* 1858)
Operative treatment of flat-foot by supra-malleolar osteotomy. [New York, 1890.] 20p. DNLM **90-5465**

MEYER, Willy (*b.* 1858)
Review of Nitze's textbook on cystoscopy. [St. Louis, 1890.] 8p. DNLM **90-5466**

MEYER, Willy (*b.* 1858)
Trendelenburg's new operating table, designed for operations in the posture bearing his name. New York: Trow's Print. & Bookbind. Co., 1890. 8p. DNLM **90-5467**

MEYER, Willy (*b.* 1858)
Notes on the effect of the aniline dyes, especially the blue pyoktanin, in the treatment of inoperable malignant growths. New York: Trow's Co., 1891. 23p. DNLM **90-5468**

MEYER, Willy (*b.* 1858)
External oesophagotomy in the operative treatment of cicatricial stricture of the oesophagus. With a proposition for improving the method of performing internal oesophagotomy. New York, 1892. 24p. 1 plate. DNLM **90-5469**

MEYER, Willy (*b.* 1858)
Nephrotomy for the relief of sudden total suppression of urine occurring some time after nephrectomy. [With the report of a successful case.] Philadelphia, 1892. 16p. DNLM **90-5470**

MEYER, Willy (*b.* 1858)
The progress of cystoscopy in the last three years. [New York, 1892.] 57p. DNLM **90-5471**

MEYER, Willy (*b.* 1858)
Roser's sound and Trendelenburg's catheter-sound. [New York: D. Appleton & Co., 1892.] 3p. DNLM **90-5472**

MEYER, Willy (*b.* 1858)
The results obtained from the use of aniline products in the treatment of carcinoma. Philadelphia, 1893. 24p. DNLM **90-5473**

MEYER, Willy (*b.* **1858)**
An improved method of the radical operation for carcinoma of the breast. New York, 1894. 16p. DNLM
90-5474

MEYER, Willy (*b.* **1858)**
A portable sterilizer for private operations. New York, 1894. 11p. DNLM **90-5475**

MEYER, Willy (*b.* **1858)**
Practical and efficient sterilization of materials for private operations. The finished portable sterilizer. New York, 1894. 12p. DNLM **90-5476**

MEYER, Willy (*b.* **1858)**
Recent methods of gastrostomy for stricture of the oesophagus. Philadelphia, 1894. 27p. DNLM
90-5477

MEYER, Willy (*b.* **1858)**
Simultaneous ligation of both internal iliac arteries for hypertrophy of the prostate gland (Bier's method). Philadelphia, 1894. 8p. DNLM **90-5478**

MEYER, Willy (*b.* **1858)**
A case of gastrostomy performed according to Kader's method. New York, 1896. 14p. DNLM **90-5479**

MEYER, Willy (*b.* **1858)**
Catheterism of the ureters in the male and in the female with the help of Casper's ureter cystoscope. New York, 1896. 15p. DNLM **90-5480**

MEYER, Willy (*b.* **1858)**
The early diagnosis of tuberculosis of the kidney. Philadelphia: Lea Bros. & Co., 1896. 9p. DNLM
90-5481

MEYER, Willy (*b.* **1858)**
Further experience in the effect of the simultaneous ligation of both internal iliac arteries for hypertrophy of the prostate gland. Philadelphia, 1896. 12p. DNLM
90-5482

MEYER, Willy (*b.* **1858)**
Incision of retro-pharyngeal abscess according to antiseptic principles: from the neck. New York, 1896. 12p. DNLM
90-5483

MEYER, Willy (*b.* **1858)**
When shall we operate for appendicitis? New York, 1896. 24p. DNLM **90-5484**

MEYER, Willy (*b.* **1858)**
The place of the Murphy button in gastro-enterostomy. St. Louis, 1897. 35p. 1 plate. DNLM **90-5485**

MEYER, Willy (*b.* **1858)**
Personal experience with Bottini's operation in the radical treatment of hypertrophy of the prostate. New York, 1899. 56p. DNLM **90-5486**

MEYROWITZ, E. B.
Illustrated catalogue of surgical instruments, ophthalmological apparatus, and eye, ear, nose and throat instruments. . . . [Pts. 2, 3]. New York, 1895. 153p. NNNAM
90-5487

MEYROWITZ, E. B.
Illustrated catalogue of surgical instruments, ophthalmological apparatus, and eye, ear, nose and throat instruments. . . . [Pts. 2, 3]. 4th ed. New York, 1898. 281p. NNNAM
90-5488

MICHEL, Middleton (1822-1894)
Trephining for the cure of epilepsy. Montgomery, Ala.: Brown Co., 1892. 10p. DNLM **90-5489**

MICHEL, Middleton (1822-1894)
Two cervical muscle anomalies in the Negro. New York, 1892. 8p. DNLM **90-5490**

MICHIGAN. UNIVERSITY OF MICHIGAN, ANN ARBOR. HOMOEOPATHIC MEDICAL COLLEGE
Bulletin. Midwinter, 1897. Ann Arbor: Inland Press, 1897. 34p. DNLM **90-5491**

MICHIGAN. UNIVERSITY OF MICHIGAN, ANN ARBOR. HOMOEOPATHIC MEDICAL COLLEGE
Phials. Published annually by the junior class of the Homoeopathic Department of the University of Michigan. Nos. 1, 2, v. 1. Ann Arbor, 1899-1900. 42 l.; 44 l., (illustr.) DNLM
90-5492

MILBURY, Frank S[tephen] (1858-1900)
Methods of diagnosticating diseases of the antrum of Highmore, and their treatment. New York, 1896. 10p. DNLM
90-5493

MILES, Albert B[aldwin] (1852-1894)
Memorial address on Warren Stone. New Orleans, 1895. 20p. DNLM **90-5494**

MILES, George W.
Tetany, with illustrative case. Philadelphia, 1896. 7p. DNLM
90-5495

MILLIANO, G.
The equable scrotal compressor, or resolvent suspensory, for the relief and cure of varicocele and vascular swellings of the testicles and scrotum. [New York, 1892.] 2 l. DNLM
90-5496

MILLARD, Henry B. (1832-1893)
On albumina minima, transient and dietetic, and the so-called physiological albuminuria, and their relations to health and to life assurance. New York: D. Appleton & Co., 1891. 21p. DNLM **90-5497**

MILLARD, Henry B. (1832-1893)
A treatise on Bright's disease of the kidneys; its pathology, diagnosis, and treatment, with chapters on the anatomy of the kidney, albuminuria and the urinary secretion. . . . 3rd ed. Rev. and enl. New York: William Wood & Co., 1892. 322p. DLC; NNNAM **90-5498**

MILLER, Adam (1810-1901)
A new system of muscular flexion and hygienic treatment. For health and long life. . . . Chicago, 1890. 16p. DLC
90-5499

MILLER, B. Curtis
Six successful operations for biliary calculi. Philadelphia, 1890. 6p. DNLM **90-5500**

MILLER, D. J. Milton
A fatal case of purpura haemorrhagica. [Philadelphia, 1891.] 6p. DNLM **90-5501**

MILLER, D. J. Milton
Primary carcinoma of the head of the pancreas, with hour-glass contraction of the stomach, simulating, during life, pyloric stenosis. New York, 1895. 8p. DNLM **90-5502**

MILLER, D. J. Milton
Remarks on the use of the farinacea in the diet of later infancy. New York, 1898. 6p. DNLM **90-5503**

MILLER, D. J. Milton
Acute articular rheumatism in infants under one year, with the report of a case. New York, 1899. 11p. DNLM **90-5504**

MILLER, D. J. Milton
Bilateral swelling of the submaxillary (salivary) glands in typhoid fever, without enlargement of the parotids. Philadelphia, 1899. 2p. 1 plate. DNLM **90-5505**

MILLER, D. J. Milton
Report of a case of perforation in typhoid fever, closed by an adherent tag of omentum, followed by a relapse, second perforation, and death. Boston, 1899. 8p. DNLM **90-5506**

MILLER, Frank E. (1859-1932), James P. McEVOY and John E. WEEKS
Diseases of the eye, ear, throat, and nose. A manual for students and practitioners. Philadelphia: Lea Bros. & Co., [1892]. 228p. 2 plates. DNLM; NNNAM; PPC; PU **90-5507**

MILLER, G. Brown
The bacteriology of the cavity of the corpus uteri of the non-pregnant woman. A report of 68 cases. Baltimore, 1899. 17p. DNLM **90-5508**

MILLER, George B.
The use of thermol in typhoid fever. Philadelphia, 1899. 12p. DNLM **90-5509**

MILLER, George R.
Infantile scorbutus. New York, 1895. 11p. DNLM **90-5510**

MILLER, John Alexander
Home treatment for diseases of women and some favorite prescriptions. . . . [San Francisco]: Published for the Author, [1891]. 309p. plates. DLC **90-5511**

MILLER, John S.
Nephrorrhaphy for floating kidney. Philadelphia: W. J. Dornan, 1891. 8p. DNLM **90-5512**

MILLER, John S.
An improved shot compressor. [New York, 1892.] 6p. DNLM **90-5513**

MILLER, John S.
The modern treatment of fracture of the patella. [Philadelphia, 1893.] 6p. DNLM **90-5514**

MILLER, John S.
The application of heat in anticipation of surgical shock as a prophylactic measure. Philadelphia: A. Van Horn, 1896. 2 l. DNLM **90-5515**

MILLER, John S.
Hemothorax from stab-wound of an intercostal artery; operation; recovery. [Philadelphia, 1896.] 4p. DNLM **90-5516**

MILLER, John S.
A contribution to the study of anastomosis of the hollow viscera; a modified Murphy button. [Philadelphia, 1897.] 7p. DNLM **90-5517**

MILLER, Lewis H.
Pemphigus chronicus vulgaris of the mouth and epiglottis. New York, 1897. 8p. 1 plate. DNLM **90-5518**

MILLER, Maurice Norton (1838-1888)
Students' histology; a course of normal histology for students and practitioners of medicine. . . . Rev. by Herbert U. Williams. . . . 3rd rev. ed. . . . New York: William Wood & Co., 1898. 250p. DLC; DNLM; NNNAM **90-5519**

MILLER, W[illoughby] D[ayton] (1853-1907)
The micro-organisms of the human mouth. The local and general diseases which are caused by them. Philadelphia: The S. S. White Dental Mfg. Co., 1890. 364p. 3 plates. DNLM; MdU-D **90-5520**

MILLER, W[illoughby] D[ayton] (1853-1907)
The decomposition of the contents of the dentinal tubules as a disturbing factor in the treatment of pulpless teeth. Philadelphia, 1890. 8p. DNLM **90-5521**

MILLER, W[illoughby] D[ayton] (1853-1907)
Experiments on the comparative value of various antiseptics in the treatment of diseased teeth. Philadelphia, 1890. 16p. DNLM **90-5522**

MILLER, W[illoughby] D[ayton] (1853-1907)
Decay of a replanted tooth. Philadelphia, 1891. 4p. DNLM **90-5523**

MILLER, W[illoughby] D[ayton] (1853-1907)
The disinfection of dental and surgical instruments. Philadelphia, 1891. 13p. DNLM **90-5524**

MILLER, W[illoughby] D[ayton] (1853-1907)
The human mouth as a focus of infection. Philadelphia, 1891. 47p. 5 plates. DNLM **90-5525**

MILLER, W[illoughby] D[ayton] (1853-1907)
Concerning combined fillings. Philadelphia, 1892. 10p. DNLM **90-5526**

MILLER, W[illoughby] D[ayton] (1853-1907)
Asepsis and antisepsis in practice. Philadelphia, 1893. 4p. DNLM **90-5527**

MILLER, W[illoughby] D[ayton] (1853-1907)
The iodoform question. Philadelphia, 1893. 6p. DNLM **90-5528**

MILLER, W[illoughby] D[ayton] (1853-1907)
The iodoform question; or, the value of iodoform in the treatment of diseased conditions of the teeth. Philadelphia, 1893. 10p. DNLM 90-5529

MILLER, W[illoughby] D[ayton] (1853-1907)
Experiments relative to the form in which arsenious acid may be best applied for devitalizing the pulps of teeth. Philadelphia, 1894. 7p. DNLM 90-5530

MILLER, W[illoughby] D[ayton] (1853-1907)
An introduction to the study of the bacterio-pathology of the dental pulp. Philadelphia, 1894. 24p. DNLM 90-5531

MILLIKEN, S[amuel] E.
Lateral curvature of the spine and its association with hernia. New York: D. C. Gardner, 1892. 2 l. DNLM 90-5532

MILLIKEN, S[amuel] E.
The radical cure of inguinal hernia; Bassini's method illustrated, with remarks on recurrent and ventral hernia. New York: Trow's Co., 1892. 12p. DNLM 90-5533

MILLIKEN, S[amuel] E.
Herniotomy; osteotomy. New York: E. P. Coby & Co., 1895. 6p. DNLM 90-5534

MILLIKEN, S[amuel] E.
Tendon grafting. A new operation for deformities following infantile paralysis, with report of a successful case. New York, 1895. 8p. DNLM 90-5535

MILLIKIN, Dan (1845-1896)
A study in credulity. Toledo, 1896. 23p. DNLM 90-5536

MILLIKIN, Dan (1845-1896)
Paracelsus and his tribe. An address introductory to the lectures at the Miami Medical College. [Hamilton, O.: Brown & Whitaker, [1896].] 16p. DNLM 90-5537

MILLS, Brooker
Umbilical hemorrhage, with report of two cases. Philadelphia, 1899. 5p. DNLM 90-5538

MILLS, Charles K[arsner] (1845-1931) and Charles J. HOBAN
Remarks on two cases simulating hydrophobia and occurring after dog-bites. [New York, 1890.] 2p. DNLM 90-5539

MILLS, Charles K[arsner] (1845-1931)
Lesions of the cauda equina. Haemorrhage into the cauda equina. Fracture of the spine with haemorrhage into the cauda equina. Fracture of the spine with haemorrhage into the lumbo-sacral spinal cord and cauda equina. A clinical lecture. [Philadelphia, 1890.] 15p. DNLM 90-5540

MILLS, Charles K[arsner] (1845-1931)
Notes on some cases of chorea and tremor. [New York, 1890.] 12p. DNLM 90-5541

MILLS, Charles K[arsner] (1845-1931)
Spasmodic torticollis; different forms of spasm affecting the muscles of the neck. [Philadelphia, 1890.] 7p. DNLM 90-5542

MILLS, Charles K[arsner] (1845-1931)
Unilateral ophthalmoplegia, probably dependent upon thrombosis of the cavernous sinus, with associated basic meningitis. [Philadelphia, 1890.] 9p. DNLM 90-5543

MILLS, Charles K[arsner] (1845-1931)
Aphasia and other affections of speech in some of their medico-legal relations, studied largely from the standpoint of localization. [Milwaukee, 1891.] 81p. DNLM 90-5544

MILLS, Charles K[arsner] (1845-1931) and W. W. KEEN
Jacksonian epilepsy; trephining; removal of small tumor and excision of cortex. [Philadelphia, 1891.] 13p. DNLM 90-5545

MILLS, Charles K[arsner] (1845-1931)
Myotonia and athetoid spasm. Clinical lecture delivered at the Philadelphia Hospital. [Philadelphia, 1891.] 20p. 2 plates. DNLM 90-5546

MILLS, Charles K[arsner] (1845-1931)
Subcortical hemorrhagic cyst beneath the arm and leg areas. [New York, 1891.] 4p. DNLM 90-5547

MILLS, Charles K[arsner] (1845-1931)
Multiple neuritis and some of its complications. Clinical lecture delivered at the Philadelphia Hospital. [Philadelphia, 1892.] 18p. DNLM 90-5548

MILLS, Charles K[arsner] (1845-1931)
The nervous and mental phenomena and sequelae of influenza. [Philadelphia, 1892.] 17p. DNLM 90-5549

MILLS, Charles K[arsner] (1845-1931)
Neuritis and myelitis and the forms of paralysis and pseudo-paralysis following labor. Philadelphia, 1893. 28p. DNLM 90-5550

MILLS, Charles K[arsner] (1845-1931)
Some phases of syphilis of the brain. Philadelphia: Lea Bros. & Co., 1895. 21p. DNLM 90-5551

MILLS, Charles K[arsner] (1845-1931) and William G. SPILLER
A case of cerebral abscess situated at the posterior part of the external capsule. New York: Raff & Co., 1896. 7p. DNLM 90-5552

MILLS, Charles K[arsner] (1845-1931) and G. E. de SCHWEINITZ
The association of hemianopsia with certain symptom-groups, chiefly with reference to the diagnosis of the site of the lesion. Philadelphia, 1896. 15p. DNLM 90-5553

MILLS, Charles K[arsner] (1845-1931) and Mary A. SHIVELY
Preliminary report, clinical and pathological, of a case of progressive dementia. Baltimore, 1897. 4p. 7 plates. DNLM 90-5554

MILLS, Charles K[arsner] (1845-1931)
Suggestions regarding a laboratory of neurology and psychology at the University of Pennsylvania. Philadelphia, 1898. 4p. DNLM 90-5555

MILLS, Charles K[arsner] (1845-1931)
The nervous system and its diseases. A practical treatise on neurology for the use of physicians and students. . . . Diseases of the brain and cranial nerves, with a general introduction on the study and treatment of nervous diseases. . . . Philadelphia, [etc.]: J. B. Lippincott Co., 1898. 1056p. DLC; DNLM; NNNAM; PPC **90-5556**

MILLS, Charles K[arsner] (1845-1931)
Some points of special interest in the study of the deep reflexes of the lower extremities. New York, 1899. 30p. 3 plates. DNLM **90-5557**

MILLS, Charles K[arsner] (1845-1931)
Syphilitic insanities and pseudo-insanities, with especial reference to their prognosis and treatment. Philadelphia, 1899. 11p. DNLM **90-5558**

MILLS, T[homas] Wesley (1845-1915)
The blood and blood-vessels in health and disease. [New York, 1890.] 10p. DNLM **90-5559**

MILLSPAUGH, Charles F[rederick] (1854-1923)
Medicinal plants: an illustrated and descriptive guide to plants indigenous to and naturalized in the United States which are used in medicine. . . . Philadelphia: John C. Horston & Co., 1892. 2 v. 180 col. plates. CtY-M; DLC; MB; MB-H **90-5560**

MILROY, W[illiam] F.
An undescribed variety of hereditary oedema. [New York, 1892.] 12p. DNLM **90-5561**

MILWAUKEE MEDICAL COLLEGE. DENTAL DEPARTMENT
Annual announcements for the sessions of 1894-95 to 1898-99 (1.-5.). Milwaukee, 1894-1898. DNLM [Prior to 1898-99 called Milwaukee Medical College and School of Dentistry. List of students and graduates for the years 1894-95 to 1897-98, in: Announcements for subsequent years.] DNLM **90-5562**

MILWAUKEE MEDICAL COLLEGE. MEDICAL DEPARTMENT
Annual announcements for the sessions 1894-95 to 1898-99 (1.-5.); 1901-02 (8.); 1902-03 (9.); 1904-05 (11.). Milwaukee, 1894-1904. DNLM [Organized in 1894 under the title Milwaukee Medical College and School of Dentistry. In 1898 the School of Dentistry became distinct from the medical department, and the above title was adopted. List of graduates from 1895 to 1904 in: Announcement for 1904-05.] **90-5563**

MINNESOTA. STATE BOARD OF MEDICAL EXAMINERS
Official register of physicians, 1883-90, containing the names, residences, and college of graduation of all physicians and surgeons duly licensed to practice in the State ot Minnesota. St. Paul: Lancet Print, 1890. 94p. DNLM **90-5564**

MINNESOTA. THIRD HOSPITAL FOR THE INSANE, FERGUS FALLS
[Plan of the hospital. By W. B. Dunnell, architect.] [Minneapolis, 1891?] broadside, 10 by 13 inches. DNLM **90-5565**

MINNESOTA. UNIVERSITY OF MINNESOTA. COLLEGE OF MEDICINE AND SURGERY, MINNEAPOLIS
Annual announcements for the sessions of 1891-92 to 1901-02 (4.-14.); 1903-04 (16.). Minneapolis, 1891-1903. DNLM [List of students and graduates for the years 1890-91 to 1900-1901; 1902-03, in announcements for subsequent years.] **90-5566**

MINNESOTA. UNIVERSITY OF MINNESOTA. COLLEGE OF PHARMACY, MINNEAPOLIS
Annual announcements for the session of 1892-93 to 1904-05 (1.-13.). Minneapolis, 1892-1904. 41p. DNLM **90-5567**

MINOR, Charles L.
Hygiene versus drugs in the treatment of pulmonary tuberculosis. New York, 1899. 27p. DNLM **90-5568**

MINOR, James L.
Aural complications in mumps; with report of eight cases. New York, 1897. 7p. DNLM **90-5569**

MINOR, James L.
Learning to see at forty; first with one eye, and later with both. New York, 1898. 8p. DNLM **90-5570**

MINOT, C[harles] S[edgwick] (1852-1914)
On certain phenomena of growing old. Salem, Mass., 1891. 21p. DNLM **90-5571**

MINOT, C[harles] S[edgwick] (1852-1914)
Human embryology. New York: William Wood & Co., 1892. 815p. DNLM; NNNAM **90-5572**

MINOT, C[harles] S[edgwick] (1852-1914)
Structural plan of the human brain. [New York: D. Appleton & Co., 1893.] 12p. DNLM **90-5573**

MINOT, C[harles] S[edgwick] (1852-1914)
The work of the naturalist in the world. New York, 1895. 13p. DNLM **90-5574**

MINOT, C[harles] S[edwick] (1852-1914)
Human embryology. New York: The Macmillan Co., 1897. 815p. DNLM; NNNAM **90-5575**

MITCHELL, Clifford (1854-1939)
A clinical study of diseases of the kidneys. . . . Chicago: W. T. Keener, 1890. 431p. DLC; DNLM; PPC; PPJ **90-5576**

MITCHELL, Clifford (1854-1939)
. . . Dental chemistry and metallurgy. Being the 2nd ed. of The dentist's manual of special chemistry, rev. [and] rewritten. . . . Chicago: W. T. Keener, 1890. 411p. DLC; DNLM; OCIM **90-5577**

MITCHELL, Clifford (1854-1939)
The biologist as a practitioner. [Philadelphia, 1891.] 3p. MB **90-5578**

MITCHELL, Clifford (1854-1939)
Blood in the urine. Diagnosis and treatment. Philadelphia, 1893. 13p. PPC **90-5579**

MITCHELL, Clifford (1854-1939)
The treatment of "nerve waste," as indicated by the urine. Philadelphia, 1894. 6p. DNLM **90-5580**

MITCHELL, Clifford (1854-1939)
The action of certain therapeutic agents in the urine. Chicago, 1895. 4p. ICJ **90-5581**

MITCHELL, Clifford (1854-1939)
Manual of urinary analysis, containing a systematic course in didactic and laboratory instruction for students, together with reference tables and clinical data for practitioners. Chicago: Era Pub. Co., 1897. 327p. 1 plate. DNLM; OCIM; PPHa **90-5582**

MITCHELL, Clifford (1854-1939)
Dental chemistry and metallurgy. . . . 4th ed. Chicago: Chicago Medical Book Co., 1898. 586p. DNLM; OCIM **90-5583**

MITCHELL, Clifford (1854-1939)
Renal therapeutics; including also a study of the etiology, pathology, diagnosis and medical treatment of diseases of the urinary tract. . . . Philadelphia: Boericke & Tafel, 1898. 365p. col. plate. DLC; PPHa **90-5584**

MITCHELL, Giles S. (1852-1904) and James G. HYNDMAN
A study of the Snook-Herr poisoning case. [Philadelphia, 1891.] 23p. DNLM **90-5585**

MITCHELL, Hubbard Winslow (*d.* 1913)
The evolution of life, or causes of change in animal forms. A study in biology. New York & London: G. P. Putnam's Sons, 1891. 460p. DNLM; ICU; NN **90-5586**

MITCHELL, John Kearsley, Jr. (1859-1917)
Preliminary note on the effect of massage on the blood-count. [Philadelphia, 1893.] 4p. DNLM **90-5587**

MITCHELL, John Kearsley, Jr. (1859-1917)
The effect of massage on the number and haemoglobine value of the red blood-cells. Philadelphia, 1894. 14p. DNLM **90-5588**

MITCHELL, John Kearsley, Jr. (1859-1917) and G. E. de SCHWEINITZ
A further study of hysterical cases, and their fields of vision. New York, [1894]. 49p. DNLM **90-5589**

MITCHELL, John Kearsley, Jr. (1859-1917)
Remote consequences of injuries of nerves, and their treatment. An examination of the present condition of wounds received 1863-65, with additional illustrative cases. Philadelphia: Lea Bros. & Co., 1895. 245p. DLC; DNLM; NNNAM; PPC **90-5590**

MITCHELL, John Kearsley, Jr. (1859-1917) and J. H. Wallace RHEIN
Case of primary combined column disease. Chicago: Amer. Med. Assoc. Press, 1898. 16p. DNLM **90-5591**

MITCHELL, John Kearsley, Jr. (1859-1917) and J. H. Wallace RHEIN
A case of transverse myelitis with an unusual form of descending degeneration in the posterior columns. Chicago: Amer. Med. Assoc. Press, 1898. 15p. DNLM **90-5592**

MITCHELL, John Kearsley, Jr. (1859-1917)
Seborrhoea nigricans, an unusual hysterical disorder. Philadelphia, 1898. 11p. DNLM **90-5593**

MITCHELL, John Kearsley, Jr. (1859-1917)
A study of a case of family periodic paralysis. Philadelphia, 1899. 18p. DNLM **90-5594**

MITCHELL, Louis J. and John A. WESENER
Two fatal cases of sausage poisoning. Detroit: G. S. Davis, 1895. 3p. DNLM **90-5595**

MITCHELL, Louis J. and E. R. LE COUNT
Report of a necropsy in a case of acromegaly, with a critical review of the recorded pathologic anatomy. New York, 1899. 42p. DNLM **90-5596**

MITCHELL, S[ilas] Weir (1829-1914)
Suspension in locomotor ataxia. With summary of twenty-three cases from the clinical service of Dr. Mitchell, reported by Guy Hinsdale from the tables of the resident, Caspar W. Sharples. Philadelphia, 1890. 5p. DNLM **90-5597**

MITCHELL, S[ilas] Weir (1829-1914)
Address on opening of the Institute of Hygiene of the University of Pennsylvania. Philadelphia: Univ. Penn. Press, 1892. 16p. DNLM **90-5598**

MITCHELL, S[ilas] Weir (1829-1914)
A talk about nurses and nursing, delivered before the nurses of the Philadelphia Orthopaedic Hospital and Infirmary for Nervous Diseases. April 4, 1892. Philadelphia, [1892]. 15p. DNLM **90-5599**

MITCHELL, S[ilas] Weir (1829-1914)
Verses read on the presentation by . . . to the Philadelphia College of Physicians of Sarah W. Whitman's portrait of Oliver Wendell Holmes, associate fellow. April 30, 1892. [Philadelphia: Univ. Penn. Press, 1892. 6 l. DNLM **90-5600**

MITCHELL, S[ilas] Weir (1829-1914)
The early history of instrumental precision in medicine. New Haven: Tuttle, Morehouse & Tuttle, 1892. 42p. CtY-M; DNLM **90-5601**

MITCHELL, S[ilas] Weir (1829-1914)
Two lectures on the conduct of the medical life, addressed to the students of the University of Pennsylvania and the Jefferson Medical College. Philadelphia: Univ. Penn. Press, 1893. 51p. DNLM **90-5602**

MITCHELL, S[ilas] Weir (1829-1914)
A catalogue of the scientific and literary work of . . . . [Philadelphia, 1894.] 40p. DNLM; PPC; PU **90-5603**

MITCHELL, S[ilas] Weir (1829-1914)
Clinical lessons on nervous diseases. . . . Philadelphia and New York: Lea Bros. & Co., 1897. 305p. col. plates. DLC; DNLM; NNNAM; PPC **90-5604**

MITCHELL, S[ilas] Weir (1829-1914)
Fat and blood: an essay on the treatment of certain forms of neurasthenia and hysteria. . . . 7th ed. Philadelphia, [etc.]: J. B. Lippincott & Co., 1898. 177p. DLC; NNNAM; PPC; PU **90-5605**

MIX, Charles L[ouis] (1869-1935)
Origin of the red blood-corpuscles. Boston: Damrell & Upham, 1892. 27p. DNLM **90-5606**

MIXTER, S[amuel] J[ason] (1855-1926)
Resection of second and third divisions of fifth nerve at the foramina rotundum and ovale. Boston, 1891. 7p. DNLM **90-5607**

MOHR, Charles (1844-1907)
The medicinal plants of Alabama. Systematic list of the medicinal plants occurring within the limits of the State, with notes on their distribution and proper time of collecting the parts used. Mobile, [1890]. 17p. DNLM **90-5608**

MOHR, Charles (1844-1907)
Beliefs concerning materia medica. [Also: Homoeopathic treatment of goitre.] [Philadelphia, 1890.] 8p. DNLM **90-5609**

MOHR, Charles (1844-1907)
Homoeopathy as related to paedology. Philadelphia, 1899. 7p. DNLM **90-5610**

MOHR, Charles (1844-1907)
Valedictory to the class of 1899 of the Hahnemann Medical College and Hospital of Philadelphia. Philadelphia, 1899. 12p. DNLM **90-5611**

MOHR, Charles (1844-1907)
Treatment of intermittent fever. [Philadelphia, [1899].] 2p. DNLM **90-5612**

MONELL, S[amuel] H[oward] (1857-1918)
A brief synopsis of the therapeutics of static electricity. New York: D. Appleton & Co., 1894. 5p. DNLM **90-5613**

MONELL, S[amuel] H[oward] (1857-1918)
Practical chapters on static electricity, collected and reprinted from various medical journals, etc. New York: [Van Houten & Ten Broeck, 1895.] 40p. 1 plate. DNLM **90-5614**

MONELL, S[amuel] H[oward] (1857-1918)
Manual of static electricity in X-ray and therapeutic uses, . . . 2nd ed., with appendix. New York: W. B. Harison, 1897. 636p. plates. DLC; DNLM; NNNAM **90-5615**

MONELL, S[amuel] H[oward] (1857-1918)
The treatment of disease by electric currents. A handbook of plain instructions, for the general practitioner. . . . New York: W. B. Harison, 1897. 1100p. plates. DLC; DNLM; NNNAM **90-5616**

MONKS, George H[oward] (*b.* 1853)
A cae of appendicitis in the scrotum; removal of pus by aspiration; excision of the appendix during a remission; recovery. Boston: Damrell & Upham, 1890. 4p. DNLM **90-5617**

MONKS, George H[oward] (*b.* 1853)
Fragments of glass removed from the popliteal space, where they had lodged for over three years. [Boston, 1891.] 4p. DNLM **90-5618**

MONKS, George H[oward] (*b.* 1853)
Operations for correcting the deformity due to prominent ears. Boston: Damrell & Upham, 1891. 10p. DNLM **90-5619**

MONKS, George H[oward] (*b.* 1853)
The remains of a broken lead pencil (surrounded by phosphatic deposits), and the metal tip of the pencil removed from the bladder by perineal section. [Boston, 1891.] 4p. DNLM **90-5620**

MONKS, George H[oward] (*b.* 1853)
A method for applying pressure to the seat of a fracture, for the purpose of bringing the bony fragments into accurate apposition and retaining them there until consolidation has taken place. Boston: Damrell & Upham, 1893. 5p. DNLM **90-5621**

MONKS, George H[oward] (*b.* 1853)
Unilateral laryngectomy; a case of excision of the right half of the larynx for carcinoma; recovery; no recurrence at the end of the year. Philadelphia: Univ. Penn. Press, 1893. 8p. 1 plate. DNLM **90-5622**

MONKS, George H[oward] (*b.* 1853)
A case of stab wound of the abdomen, with wounds of the intestine; protrusion of the intestine through the wound; operation; recovery. Boston, 1895. 3p. DNLM **90-5623**

MONKS, George H[oward] (*b.* 1853)
Fracture of the humerus from an unusual cause. Boston: Rockwell & Churchill, 1895. 5p. DNLM **90-5624**

MONKS, George H[oward] (*b.* 1853)
Unilateral laryngectomy for cancer; no recurrence after three years. Philadelphia, 1895. 2p. 1 plate. DNLM **90-5625**

MONKS, George H[oward] (*b.* 1853)
Another case of fracture of the humerus from an unusual cause. Boston, 1896. 4p. 1 plate. DNLM **90-5626**

MONKS, George H[oward] (*b.* 1853)
A case of fracture of the upper end of the humerus just below the tuberosities, with dislocation of the head of the bone into the axilla. Boston, 1896. 4p. DNLM **90-5627**

MONKS, George H[oward] (*b.* 1853)
A plastic operation on the nose, by Tagliacozzi's method. Boston, 1896. 7p. DNLM **90-5628**

MONKS, George H[oward] (*b.* 1853)
Resection of the head of the humerus for old irreducible dislocation. Boston, 1896. 3p. DNLM **90-5629**

MONKS, George H[oward] (*b.* 1853)
Correction, by operation, of some nasal deformities and disfigurements. 1898. 14p., 3 p. DNLM **90-5630**

MONKS, George H[oward] (*b.* 1853)
The restoration of a lower eyelid by a new method. Boston, 1898. 6p. DNLM **90-5631**

MONTEIRO, Aristides (1829-1911)
War reminiscences by the surgeon of Mosby's Command. 2nd ed. Richmond, Va., 1890. 236p. ViRA
90-5632

MONTEZUMA UNIVERSITY MEDICAL COLLEGE, BESSEMER, ALABAMA
Announcement for the session of 1898-99 (3.). Bessemer: Judson Ptg. House, 1898. 22p. DNLM
90-5633

MONTGOMERY, Douglass W[illiam] (1859-1941) and H. M. SHERMAN
Tuberculosis of cervical lymphatic glands; with an illustrative case. [Sacramento, 1890.] 4p. DNLM
90-5634

MONTGOMERY, Douglass W[illiam] (1859-1941)
Bleeding cavernous angioma with commencing epithelioma of the upper lip. [San Francisco, 1890.] 2p. DNLM
90-5635

MONTGOMERY, Douglass W[illiam] (1859-1941)
Enlargement of sub-cutaneous lymphatic glands in tertiary syphilis. [San Francisco, 1891.] 4p. DNLM
90-5636

MONTGOMERY, Douglass W[illiam] (1859-1941)
Pemphigus neurotico-traumaticus. Sacramento, 1891. 4p. DNLM **90-5637**

MONTGOMERY, Douglass W[illiam] (1859-1941)
Primary carcinoma of the liver. [Sacramento, 1891.] 4p. DNLM **90-5638**

MONTGOMERY, Douglass W[illiam] (1859-1941)
Address delivered before the San Francisco County Medical Society on retiring from the presidency, Nov. 8, 1892. [San Francisco, 1892.] 4p. DNLM **90-5639**

MONTGOMERY, Douglass W[illiam] (1859-1941)
An American leper. [San Francisco, 1892.] 4p. DNLM
90-5640

MONTGOMERY, Douglass W[illiam] (1859-1941)
Case of a small and large papular syphilide associated with miliary gummata of the iris. [San Francisco, 1892.] 2p. DNLM
90-5641

MONTGOMERY, Douglass W[illiam] (1859-1941)
Parasitelike bodies in cancer. [San Francisco: W. A. Woodward & Co., 1892.] 7p. DNLM **90-5642**

MONTGOMERY, Douglass W[illiam] (1859-1941)
A case of extirpation of the uterus per vaginam for epithelioma of the cervix, complicated by sarcoma of the body. [Sacramento, 1893.] 2p. DNLM **90-5643**

MONTGOMERY, Douglass W[illiam] (1859-1941)
Some cases of leucoplasia. [San Francisco: W. A. Woodward & Co., 1893.] 8p. DNLM **90-5644**

MONTGOMERY, Douglass W[illiam] (1859-1941)
An ulcus elevation of the face. [Philadelphia, 1893.] 5p. DNLM **90-5645**

MONTGOMERY, Douglass W[illiam] (1859-1941)
Unilateral hypertrophy of the face. [Philadelphia, 1893.] 13p. DNLM **90-5646**

MONTGOMERY, Douglass W[illiam] (1859-1941)
Atheroma. [Philadelphia, 1894.] 5p. DNLM
90-5647

MONTGOMERY, Douglass W[illiam] (1859-1941)
An erythema of lepra containing giant cell-like structures, simulating somewhat the giant-cells found in tuberculosis. [Philadelphia: Lea Bros. & Co., 1894.] 6p. DNLM
90-5648

MONTGOMERY, Douglass W[illiam] (1859-1941)
Diarrhea from potassium iodid. [Philadelphia, 1894.] 3p. DNLM **90-5649**

MONTGOMERY, Douglass W[illiam] (1859-1941)
Leprosy in San Francisco. Chicago, 1894. 8p. DNLM
90-5650

MONTGOMERY, Douglass W[illiam] (1859-1941)
Report of a case of epithelioma of the skin of the face, with unusual course of infection of lymph-nodes. Philadelphia: Univ. Penn. Press, 1898. 6p. DNLM
90-5651

MONTGOMERY, Douglass W[illiam] (1859-1941)
A maculo-anesthetic lepride of the palm. New York, 1899. 55p. DNLM **90-5652**

MONTGOMERY, Edmund B.
Typhoid fever in very young children; with a report of three cases with unusual complications. New York, 1899. 13p. DNLM **90-5653**

MONTGOMERY, Edward Emmet (1849-1927)
Vaginal hysterectomy. Philadelphia: W. J. Dornan, 1890 [1889]. DNLM **90-5654**

MONTGOMERY, Edward Emmet (1849-1927)
A report of six cases of vaginal hysterectomy. Philadelphia: W. J. Dornan, 1890. 8p. DNLM **90-5655**

MONTGOMERY, Edward Emmet (1849-1927)
The application of sacral resection to gynecological work. Philadelphia: W. J. Dornan, 1891. 17p. 2 plates. DNLM
90-5656

MONTGOMERY, Edward Emmett (1849-1927)
Conditions following parturition requiring abdominal section. [Philadelphia, 1891.] 9p. DNLM **90-5657**

MONTGOMERY, Edward Emmett (1849-1927)
Bromide of ethyl. Detroit: G. S. Davis, 1892. 4p. DNLM
90-5658

MONTGOMERY, Edward Emmett (1849-1927)
Some mooted points in obstetrics and gynecology. President's address. Chicago, 1892. 12p. DNLM
90-5659

MONTGOMERY, John
Medical Society of Franklin County; its history, and sketches of early practitioners of the county. Published by Medical Society of Franklin County, Pa. Chambersburg, Pa.: J. R. Kerr & Bro., 1892. 62p. DNLM; PPC **90-5660**

MONTGOMERY, J[ohn] C.
Some methods in the treatment of nasal troubles. Charlotte, N.C., 1897. 2 l. DNLM **90-5661**

MOOR, William
The treatment of opium-poisoning by potassium permanganate. Philadelphia, 1895. 5p. DNLM **90-5662**

MOORE, H[enry] B. (*d.* 1900)
The early recognition and the climatic treatment of pulmonary tuberculosis. Philadelphia: Lea Bros. & Co., 1895. 8p. DNLM **90-5663**

MOORE, James E[dward] (1852-1918)
Orthopedic surgery, by . . . . With 177 illustrations. Philadelphia: W. B. Saunders, 1898. 354p. DLC; DNLM; NNNAM; PPC **90-5664**

MOORE, John William (1845-1937)
Text-book of the eruptive and continued fevers. New York: William Wood & Co., 1892. 535p. 2 plates, 17 diags. DNLM; NNNAM **90-5665**

MOORE, Veranus Alva (1859-1931)
Laboratory directions for beginners in bacteriology. Ithaca, N.Y.: Andrus & Church, 1898. 89p. DNLM **90-5666**

MOORE, Veranus Alva (1859-1931)
The nature and prevention of infectious entero-hepatitis. Ithaca, N.Y., 1898. 2 l. DNLM **90-5667**

MOORE, Veranus Alva (1859-1931)
The natural in disease. [Buffalo], 1899. 20p. DNLM **90-5668**

MOORE, William Oliver (*b.* 1852)
The after-treatment of cataract-extraction. [Philadelphia: Lea Bros. & Co., 1893.] 15p. DNLM **90-5669**

MOORE, William Oliver (*b.* 1852)
Rheumatic and gouty affections of the eye. New York, 1893. 28p. DNLM **90-5670**

MORGAN, A[lonzo] R[ichardson] (*b.* 1830)
Repertory of the urinary organs and prostate gland, including condylomata. Philadelphia: Boericke & Tafel, 1899. 318p. DNLM; PPC; PPHa **90-5671**

MORGAN, Edwin L[ee] (*b.* 1855)
Case of idiosyncrasy from ipecac. [Richmond, 1892.] 3 l. DNLM **90-5672**

MORGAN, Edwin L[ee] (*b.* 1855)
Circumcision; short review of the origin and history of this custom. Richmond, 1895. 14p. DNLM **90-5673**

MORGAN, Edwin L[ee] (*b.* 1855)
Case of obstruction of the bowel from carcinoma. [Richmond, 1897.] 10p. DNLM **90-5674**

MORGAN, James D[udley] (1862-1919)
Need of care in the diagnosis of the spitting of blood, and remarks on typhoid fever. [Richmond, 1894.] 11p. DNLM **90-5675**

MORGAN, James D[udley] (1862-1919)
The consideration of urea in the urine. Richmond, 1896. 8p. DNLM **90-5676**

MORGAN, James D[udley] (1862-1919)
Angina pectoris. Chicago, 1899. 11p. DNLM **90-5677**

MORGAN, James E[thelbert] (1822-1889)
Tuberculosis of fascia. Chicago, 1899. 12p. DNLM **90-5678**

MORGAN, John C[oleman] (1831-1899)
The study of homoeopathy, a distinct and commanding department of medicine. Philadelphia: Sherman & Co., 1893. 58p. DNLM; PPC **90-5679**

MORIARTA, Douglas C.
Diphtheria and anti-toxine. [New York, 1898.] 10p. DNLM **90-5680**

MORIARTY, Patrick W[illiam]
Congenital cleft palate and its treatment. New York, 1892. 7p. DNLM **90-5681**

MORRILL, F[erdinand] Gordon
The immunizating effects of antitoxin. Boston: Damrell & Upham, 1895. 14p. DNLM; MB; NN **90-5682**

MORRILL, F[erdinand] Gordon
The treatment of typhoid fever in children. New York: E. B. Treat, [1897]. 4p. DNLM **90-5683**

MORRILL, F[erdinand] Gordon
For what period of time can immunity from diphtheria be conferred by a single injection of antitoxin? The dosage. Boston: Damrell & Upham, 1898. 11p. DNLM; MB; NN **90-5684**

MORRIS, Henry (1844-1926)
. . . Essentials of practice of medicine. Arranged in the form of questions and answers. . . . With a very complete appendix, on the examination of urine, by Lawrence Wolff. . . . Philadelphia: W. B. Saunders, 1890. 368, 66p. col. frontis. . . . DLC; PPC; PU **90-5685**

MORRIS, Henry (1844-1926)
Surgical diseases of the kidney. . . . Philadelphia: Lea Bros. & Co., 1890 [1884]. 554p. col. plates. MBM; NNNAM; OCIM; PPC [Each plate accompanied by leaf with descriptive letter-press] **90-5686**

MORRIS, Henry (1844-1926)
. . . A compend of gynaecology. . . . Philadelphia: P. Blakiston, Son & Co., 1891 [1890]. 178p. DLC; DNLM; PPC **90-5687**

MORRIS, Henry (1844-1926)
. . . Essentials of practice of medicine. . . . With a very complete appendix, on the examination of urine, by Lawrence Wolff. . . . 2nd ed., enlarged by some three hundred essential formulae, selected from the writings of the most eminent authorities of the medical profesion. Collected and arranged by William M. Powell. . . . Philadelphia: W. B. Saunders, 1891. 368, 66p. col. frontis. DLC; DNLM; PPC **90-5688**

MORRIS, Henry (1844-1926)
Essentials of materia medica, therapeutics, and prescription writing, arranged in the form of questions and answers; prepared especially for students of medicine. 2nd ed. Philadelphia: W. B. Saunders, 1891. 250p. DNLM; PPC **90-5689**

MORRIS, Henry (1844-1926)
Essentials of materia medica, therapeutics, and prescription writing, arranged in the form of questions and answers; prepared especially for students of medicine. 3rd ed. Philadelphia: W. B. Saunders, 1893. 250p. CtY-M
90-5690

MORRIS, Henry, ed. (1844-1926)
Human anatomy; a complete systematic treatise by various authors, including a special section on surgical and topographical anatomy. . . . Philadelphia: P. Blakiston, Son & Co., 1893. 1286p. DLC; DNLM; NNNAM; PPC
90-5691

MORRIS, Henry (1844-1926)
Essentials of materia medica, therapeutics, and prescription writing, arranged in the form of questions and answers; prepared especially for students of medicine. 4th ed. Philadelphia: W. B. Saunders, 1894. 250p. CtY-M; PPC
90-5692

MORRIS, Henry (1844-1926)
. . . Essentials of practice of medicine. Arranged in the form of questions and answers. . . . With a very complete appendix, on the examination of urine, by Lawrence Wolff. . . . 3rd ed., rev. and enlarged by some three hundred essential formulae, selected from the writings of the most eminent authorities of the medical profession. Collected and arranged by William M. Powell. . . . Philadelphia: W. B. Saunders, 1894. 374, 66p. col. frontis. DLC **90-5693**

MORRIS, Henry (1844-1926)
Human anatomy; a complete systematic treatise by various authors, including a special section on surgical and topographical anatomy. Philadelphia: P. Blakiston, Son & Co., 1895. 1310p. PPJ **90-5694**

MORRIS, Henry (1844-1926)
Injuries and diseases of the genital and urinary organs. New York: William Wood & Co., 1895. 478p. DNLM; NNNAM; PPJ **90-5695**

MORRIS, Henry (1844-1926)
On the origin and progress of renal surgery, with special reference to stone in the kidney and ureter and to the surgical treatment of calculous anuria. Being the Hunterian lectures for 1898. Together with a critical examination of subparietal injuries of the ureter. Philadelphia: P. Blakiston, Son & Co., 1898. 288p. DNLM; PPC; PPPH; PU
90-5696

MORRIS, Henry (1844-1926)
. . . Essentials of materia medica, therapeutics, and prescription writing, arranged in the form of questions and answers; prepared especially for students of medicine. . . . 5th ed., rev. and enl. Philadelphia: W. B. Saunders, 1898. 288p. DLC; DNLM; PPC; PU **90-5697**

MORRIS, Henry, ed. (1844-1926)
Human anatomy; a complete systematic treatise by various authors, including a special section on surgical and topographical anatomy. . . . [2nd ed.] Illustrated by seven hundred and ninety woodcuts, the greater part of which are original and made expressly for this work by special artists, over 200 printed in colors. Philadelphia: P. Blakiston's Son & Co., 1898. 1274p. DLC; DNLM; NNNAM; PPC
90-5698

MORRIS, J[ames] Cheston (1831-1923)
On vital molecular vibrations. Detroit, 1891. 7p. DNLM
90-5699

MORRIS, J[ames] Cheston (1831-1923)
[Abstr.] [On vital molecular vibrations.] [Philadelphia, 1891.] 1 l. DNLM **90-5700**

MORRIS, Lewis R.
The therapeutic action of hot sulpho-saline waters, with some personal observations at Glenwood Hot Springs. New York, 1895. 16p. DNLM **90-5701**

MORRIS, Malcolm [Alexander] (1849-1924)
Diseases of the skin; an outline of the principles and practice of dermatology. Philadelphia: Lea Bros. & Co., 1894. 556p. 8 plates. DNLM; NNNAM; OCIM; PPC
90-5702

MORRIS, Malcolm [Alexander] (1849-1924)
Diseases of the skin; an outline of the principles and practice of dermatology. New and revised ed. Philadelphia: Lea Bros. & Co., [1898]. 589p. 10 plates. DNLM; IU-M; PPC; PU
90-5703

MORRIS, Robert T[uttle] (1857-1945)
The necessary peroxide of hydrogen. [Also:] Peroxide of hydrogen and ozone. Their antiseptic properties, by Paul Gibier. [1890.] 2 l. DNLM **90-5704**

MORRIS, Robert T[uttle] (1857-1945)
How we treat wounds today; a treatise on the subject of antiseptic surgery which can be understood by beginners. 4th ed. New York: G. P. Putnam's Sons, 1890. 165p. NNNAM; PPC; PU **90-5705**

MORRIS, Robert T[uttle] (1857-1945)
A fourth series of one hundred consecutive operations, showing the results of antiseptic methods of work. New York: Kettiner, Lambert & Co., 1892. 21p. DNLM
90-5706

MORRIS, Robert T[uttle] (1857-1945)
Another method for palpation of the kidney. [Philadelphia, 1892.] 3p. DNLM **90-5707**

MORRIS, Robert T[uttle] (1857-1945)
Is evolution trying to do away with the clitoris? New York: William Wood & Co., 1892. 12p. DNLM
90-5708

MORRIS, Robert T[uttle] (1857-1945)
The prevention of secondary peritoneal adhesions by means of an aristol film. [Philadelphia, 1892.] 3p. DNLM
90-5709

MORRIS, Robert T[uttle] (1857-1945)
Appendicitis. Danbury, 1893. 30p. DNLM
90-5710

MORRIS, Robert T[uttle] (1857-1945)
Appendicitis. Clinical lecture at the New York Post-Graduate Medical School, Feb. 11, 1893. [New York, 1893.] 16p. DNLM **90-5711**

MORRIS, Robert T[uttle] (1857-1945)
Infectious appendicitis. [Washington, 1895.] 18p. DNLM
90-5712

MORRIS, Robert T[uttle] (1857-1945)
Lectures on appendicitis and notes on other subjects. . . . With illustrations by Henry Macdonald, M.D. New York [etc.]: G. P. Putnam's Sons, 1895. 163p. DLC; DNLM; NNNAM **90-5713**

MORRIS, Robert T[uttle] (1857-1945)
Correspondence between a layman and a surgeon on the subject of appendicitis. New York, 1898. 16p. DNLM **90-5714**

MORRIS, Robert T[uttle] (1857-1945)
Best method in the treatment of appendicitis. Chicago, 1899. 16p. DNLM **90-5715**

MORRISON, William Alexander
The value of the stomach-tube in feeding after intubation, based upon 28 cases; also its use in post-diphtheritic paralysis. Boston: Damrell & Upham, 1895. 7p. 1 tab. DNLM **90-5716**

MORRISON, William H.
Linear craniotomy for defective mental development. New York: Trow, 1891. 7p. DNLM **90-5717**

MORRISON, William H.
Severe puerperal eclampsia. The immediate induction of labor; recovery. [Philadelphia, 1891.] 4p. DNLM **90-5718**

MORRISON, William H.
Report of a case of large intra-cranial tumor (weight, five ounces) compressing the left frontal lobe. [Philadelphia, 1892.] 12p. DNLM **90-5719**

MORRISON, William H.
Three cases of cranial surgery. I. Linear craniotomy for defective mental development; report of a case thirteen months after operation; decided mental improvement. II. Exploratory trephining for epilepsy; negative results. III. Trephining for abscess of the brain; evacuation of one ounce of pus; recovery. [Philadelphia, 1892.] 11p. DNLM **90-5720**

MORRISON, William H.
Extra-uterine pregnancy simulated by a small tumor of the ovary; operation; recovery. Philadelphia, 1894. 4p. DNLM **90-5721**

MORROW, Prince A[lbert] (1846-1913)
Note on a new method of skin grafting. [New York, 1891.] 10p. DNLM **90-5722**

MORROW, Prince A[lbert] (1846-1913)
The removal of necrotic and carious bone with hydrochloric acid and pepsin. New York, 1892. 1 l. DNLM **90-5723**

MORROW, Prince A[lbert] (1846-1913)
Some differential points in the diagnosis of syphilis and tuberculosis, with illustrative cases. [New York, 1892.] 12p. DNLM **90-5724**

MORROW, Prince A[lbert] (1846-1913)
A system of genito-urinary diseases, syphilology and dermatology, by various authors. . . . New York: D. Appleton & Co., 1893-1894. 3 v. col. plates. DLC; DNLM; NNNAM; PPC **90-5725**

MORROW, Prince A[lbert] (1846-1913)
Venereal memoranda. A manual for the student and practitioner. New York: William Wood & Co., 1894. 332p. DNLM; NNNAM **90-5726**

MORROW, Prince A[lbert] (1846-1913)
Report of a case of urticaria pigmentosa of over twenty years' duration. New York: D. Appleton & Co., 1895. 10p. DNLM **90-5727**

MORROW, Prince A[lbert] (1846-1913)
A case of symmetrical morphoea attended with the formation of bullae and extensive ulceration. New York, 1896. 9p. DNLM **90-5728**

MORROW, Prince A[lbert] (1846-1913)
Notes on syphilis. Syphiloma of the nose of unusual form and evolution. The diagnostic value of syphilitic cicatrices. Extra-genital chancres, prognostic significance of. Professional syphilis. New York, 1896. 16p. DNLM **90-5729**

MORROW, Prince A[lbert] (1846-1913)
A report of two cases of linear naevus, with remarks on its nature and nomenclature. New York, 1898. 12p. 2 plates. DNLM **90-5730**

MORSE, Frank L.
Diphtheria. Boston, 1897. 23p. DNLM **90-5731**

MORSE, John Lovett (1865-1940)
A bacteriological study of four hundred cases of inflammation of the throat, occurring in diphtheria and scarlet fever, with especial reference to pathogenesis. Boston: Rockwell & Churchill, 1894. 28p. DNLM **90-5732**

MORSE, John Lovett (1865-1940)
Leukemia in infants. Boston, 1894. 8p. DNLM **90-5733**

MORSE, John Lovett (1865-1940)
A clinical and experimental study of the leucocytosis of diphtheria. Boston: Rockwell & Churchill, 1895. 23p. 1 plate. DNLM **90-5734**

MORSE, John Lovett (1865-1940)
The home modification of milk. Boston, 1896. 8p. DNLM **90-5735**

MORSE, John Lovett (1865-1940)
A study of the changes produced in the kidneys by the toxins of the Staphylococcus pyogenes aureus. New York, 1896. 10p. 2 plates. DNLM **90-5736**

MORSE, John Lovett (1865-1940)
Typhoid fever in childhood, with an analysis of two hundred and eighty-four cases. Boston: Damrell & Upham, 1896. 26p. DNLM **90-5737**

MORSE, John Lovett (1865-1940)
The non-operative treatment of phimosis in infancy. Boston, 1897. 6p. DNLM **90-5738**

MORSE, John Lovett (1865-1940)
Precocious maturity. [New York, 1897.] 10p. DNLM **90-5739**

MORSE, John Lovett (1865-1940)
A study of the blood in rickets. Boston, 1897. 23p. DNLM
90-5740

MORSE, John Lovett (1865-1940)
Acute leucaemia in childhood. New York: E. B. Treat & Co., [1898]. 5p. DNLM **90-5741**

MORSE, John Lovett (1865-1940)
A consideration of the Professor Gaetner-mother-milk. [Boston, 1898.] 5p. DNLM **90-5742**

MORSE, John Lovett (1865-1940)
The principle and limitations of the home modification of milk. Boston, 1898. 7p. DNLM **90-5743**

MORSE, John Lovett (1865-1940)
Remarks on the classification of the anaemias of infancy, with a report of a severe case. [New York, 1898.] 11p. DNLM
90-5744

MORSE, John Lovett (1865-1940)
A study of thirty-seven fatal cases of cirrhosis of the liver. Boston: Municipal Printing Office, 1898. 11p. DNLM
90-5745

MORSE, John Lovett (1865-1940)
Tetany in infancy, with a report of six cases. Chicago, 1898. 16p. DNLM **90-5746**

MORSE, John Lovett (1865-1940)
A case of erysipelas migrans. Boston, 1899. 6p. DNLM
90-5747

MORSE, John Lovett (1865-1940)
The renal complications of the acute enteric diseases of infancy. New York, 1899. 18p. DNLM
90-5748

MORSE, John Lovett (1865-1940)
The treatment of the acute diarrheas of childhood. Boston, 1899. 13p. DNLM **90-5749**

MORSE, John T[orrey], Jr. (1840-1937)
Life and letters of Oliver Wendell Holmes. Boston and New York: Houghton, Mifflin & Co., 1896. 2 v. DNLM; MB; MH; NN **90-5750**

MORTON, A[ndrews] Stanford (1847-1925)
On refraction of the eye. Its diagnosis and correction of its errors. With a chapter on keratoscopy, and test types. 4th ed., rev. and enl. Philadelphia: P. Blakiston, Son & Co., 1891. 71p. DLC; NNNAM; PU **90-5751**

MORTON, A[ndrews] Stanford (1847-1925)
On refraction of the eye. Its diagnosis and correction of its errors. With a chapter on keratoscopy, and test types. 5th ed., rev. and enl. Philadelphia: P. Blakiston, Son & Co., 1894. 72p. DNLM; NcD **90-5752**

MORTON, A[ndrews] Stanford (1847-1925)
On refraction of the eye. Its diagnosis and correction of its errors. With a chapter on keratoscopy, and test types. 6th ed., rev. and enl. Philadelphia: P. Blakiston, Son & Co., 1897. 74p. DLC; PPC; PU **90-5753**

MORTON, Bowditch (1857-1909)
Handbook of first aid to the injured: prepared at the request of the Society for Instruction in First Aid to the Injured. Revised under the authority of the Society by George A. Richards, and Henry A. Griffin. 1st revised ed. New York: The Society, 1896. 106p. MB; PPC **90-5754**

MORTON, Henry H[oldich] (*b.* 1861)
Treatment of syphilis. [Brooklyn, 1893.] 8p. DNLM
90-5755

MORTON, Henry H[oldich] (*b.* 1861)
Raynaud's disease, with report of three cases. New York, 1894. 8p. DNLM **90-5756**

MORTON, Henry H[oldich] (*b.* 1861)
Bottini's operation for enlarged prostate, with report of five cases. New York, 1898. 15p. DNLM
90-5757

MORTON, Howard McI.
The insertion of an artificial globe into Tenon's capsule, with preservation of the function of the ocular muscles; an operation for certain cases in which Mule's method is inadvisable or impracticable. New York, 1897. 6p. DNLM
90-5758

MORTON, Thomas George (1835-1903)
Inflammation of the vermiform appendix; its results, diagnosis, and treatment, together with the reports of seven cases of excision of the vermiform appendix for perforative appendicitis; with exhibition of five of the patients. Philadelphia: J. B. Lippincott Co., 1890. 44p. DNLM; PPC
90-5759

MORTON, Thomas George (1835-1903)
Progress in surgery in 1891. Philadelphia, 1892. 56p. DNLM; PPC **90-5760**

MORTON, Thomas George (1835-1903)
Some medico-legal experiences in railway cases. Chicago, 1893. 8p. DNLM **90-5761**

MORTON, Thomas George (1835-1903) and William HUNT
Cystic growth within the internal condyle of the femur. [Philadelphia, 1893.] 8p. DNLM **90-5762**

MORTON, Thomas George (1835-1903)
The history of the Pennsylvania Hospital, 1751-1895, by Thomas G. Morton . . . assisted by Frank Woodbury. . . . Publication authorized by the contributors at their annual meeting May, 1893, and directed by the Board of Managers. Philadelphia: Times Printing House, 1895. 575p. plates. DLC; DNLM; PPC; PU **90-5763**

MORTON, Thomas George (1835-1903)
Memoir of William Hunt. Philadelphia, 1897. 20p. DNLM
90-5764

MORTON, Thomas S. K.
Abdominal section for traumatism, with tables of two hundred and thirty-four cases. Chicago, 1890. 16p. DNLM
90-5765

MORTON, Thomas S. K.
The operative treatment of appendicitis. [Philadelphia, 1891.] 9p. DNLM **90-5766**

MORTON, Thomas S. K.
Radical treatment of hydrocele. [Philadelphia, 1892.] 8p. DNLM **90-5767**

MORTON, Thomas S. K.
The treatment of leg ulcers. [Philadelphia, 1892.] 7p. DNLM **90-5768**

MORTON, Thomas S. K.
Metatarsalgia (Morton's painful affection of the foot), with an account of six cases cured by operation. Philadelphia, 1893. 18p. DNLM **90-5769**

MORTON, Thomas S. K.
Metatarsalgia (Morton's painful affection of the foot), with an account of six cases cured by operation. Its causes, symptoms, and treatment, with illustrative cases and bibliography. 2nd ed. Philadelphia, 1895. 35p. DNLM **90-5770**

MORTON, Thomas S. K.
Tumors of the peripheral nerves; with the report of a case of sarcoma of the sciatic. [Philadelphia, 1893.] 7p. DNLM **90-5771**

MORTON, Thomas S. K.
Acetanilid as an antiseptic; with observations upon its use in one thousand surgical cases. [Philadelphia, 1894.] 6p. DNLM **90-5772**

MORTON, Thomas S. K.
Conditions justifying removal of the testicle in radical operations for inguinal hernia, with a report of three successful cases. [Philadelphia, 1894.] 11p. DNLM **90-5773**

MORTON, Thomas S. K.
Fibrous bodies in the tunica vaginalis testis; with a report of three cases. [Philadelphia, 1894.] 5p. DNLM **90-5774**

MORTON, Thomas S. K.
Kocher's method of reducing sub-coracoid dislocations of the shoulder; with cases of fracture incident to the procedure in old displacements. [Philadelphia, 1894.] 2 l. DNLM **90-5775**

MORTON, Thomas S. K.
A new method for reduction of fractures of the lower end of the radius. [Philadelphia, 1894.] 3p. DNLM **90-5776**

MORTON, Thomas S. K.
Treatment of traumatic shock. [Philadelphia, 1894.] 8p. DNLM **90-5777**

MORTON, Thomas S. K.
Two cases of congenital hypertrophy of the fingers. [Philadelphia: Lea Bros. & Co., 1894.] 6p. DNLM **90-5778**

MORTON, Thomas S. K.
A case of abdominal section for multiple gunshot wounds of the intestine, complicated by tuberculous peritonitis. Philadelphia, 1895. 6p. DNLM **90-5779**

MORTON, Thomas S. K.
Fracture of thyroid and cricoid cartilages and hyoid bone; asphyxia; tracheotomy; death. Philadelphia, 1895. 3p. DNLM **90-5780**

MORTON, Thomas S. K.
A successful case of castration for prostatic hemorrhage and hypertrophy. Philadelphia, 1895. 1 l. DNLM **90-5781**

MORTON, Thomas S. K.
A case of removal of the major portion of the lower jaw for sarcoma. Philadelphia, 1896. 2p. DNLM **90-5782**

MORTON, Thomas S. K.
Extracts from the proceedings of the section on general surgery of the College of Physicians of Philadelphia. Meeting of May 8, 1896. Philadelphia, 1896. 6p. DNLM **90-5783**

MORTON, Thomas S. K.
Modern gastrostomy. Philadelphia, 1896. 15p. DNLM **90-5784**

MORTON, Thomas S. K.
Intra-venous saline infusion for hemorrhage; with report of a case of rupture, extra-uterine pregnancy, and a case of stab-wound of the thorax apparently saved by its employment. Detroit: G. S. Davis, 1896. 14p. DNLM **90-5785**

MORTON, Thomas S. K.
Extracts from the proceedings of the Philadelphia County Medical Society meeting of February 10, 1897. Presentation of cases. [Philadelphia, 1897.] 4p. DNLM **90-5786**

MORTON, Thomas S. K.
Fractured ribs in the aged. [Philadelphia,1897.] 2p. DNLM **90-5787**

MORTON, Thomas S. K.
Removal of certain benign breast tumors by Thomas' trap-door incision and hidden cicatrix method. [Philadelphia, 1898.] 3p. DNLM **90-5788**

MORTON, Thomas S. K.
Trans-peritoneal ligation of the iliac arteries; with report of seven new cases and statistics of twenty-nine operations. Chicago, 1898. 8p. 1 tab. DNLM **90-5789**

MORTON, William J[ames] (1846-1920)
The Franklinic interrupted current, or my new system of therapeutic administration of static electricity. New York: Trow's, 1891. 8p. DNLM **90-5790**

MORTON, William J[ames] (1846-1920)
Upon a possible electric polarity of metabolism, and its relations to electro-therapeutics and electro-physiology. A suggested basis and guide for medical treatment by electric energy. New York, 1892. 32p. DNLM **90-5791**

MORTON, William J[ames] (1846-1920)
Ozone and its uses in medicine. New York, 1894. 58p. DNLM **90-5792**

MORTON, William J[ames] (1846-1920)
Electric medicamental diffusion. Metallic electrolysis, cataphoresis, soluble metallic electrodes, with illustrative cases of tinnitus aurium, trachoma, nasal and post-nasal catarrh, urethritis, tonsillitis, vascular tumor, dermoid cyst, naevi, sycosis, etc. Chicago, 1895. 27p. DNLM **90-5793**

MORTON, William J[ames] (1846-1920)
Memoranda relating to the "discovery of anaesthesia." [New York, 1895.] 4 galley sheets. DNLM
90-5794

MORTON, William J[ames] (1846-1920) and Edwin W. HAMMER
The X-ray, or photography of the invisible, and its value in surgery. New York, 1896. 196p. 32 plates. DNLM
90-5795

MORTON, William J[ames] (1846-1920)
"Cataphoresis"; or, Electric medicamental diffusion as applied in medicine, surgery and dentistry. . . . New York: American Technical Book Co., 1898. 267p. col. frontis. DLC; DNLM
90-5796

MORTON, William J[ames] (1846-1920)
Cases of sciatic and brachial neuritis and neuralgia; treatment and cure by electro-static currents. Cases compiled from records by W. B. Snow. New York, 1899. 24p. DNLM
90-5797

MORTON, William J[ames] (1846-1920)
Electrostatic currents and the cure of locomotor ataxia, rheumatoid arthritis, neuritis, migraine, incontinence of urine, sexual impotence, and uterine fibroids. New York, 1899. 16p. DNLM
90-5798

LUCRETIA MOTT Dispensary, Infirmary and Hospital. A brief general review of its work. [New York, 1894.] 12p. NNNAM
90-5799

MOULLIN, C[harles] W[illiam] Mansell (1851-1940)
Sprains; their consequence and treatment. New York: William Wood & Co., 1891. 221p. DLC; DNLM; NIC
90-5800

MOULLIN, C[harles] W[illiam] Mansell (1851-1940)
Surgery; a practical treatise, with special reference to treatment; by . . . , assisted by various writers on special subjects. Philadelphia: P. Blakiston, Son & Co., 1891. 1180p. CtY-M; DNLM; PPC; PU
90-5801

MOULLIN, C[harles] W[illiam] Mansell (1851-1940)
Surgery; a practical treatise, with special reference to treatment; by . . . , assisted by various writers on special subjects. 2nd American ed., revised and edited by John B. Hamilton. Philadelphia: P. Blakiston, Son & Co., 1893. 1238p. 3 plates. DNLM; ICJ; NNNAM; PU
90-5802

MOULLIN, C[harles] W[illiam] Mansell (1851-1940)
Enlargement of the prostate: its treatment and radical cure. Philadelphia: P. Blakiston, Son & Co., 1894. 176p. ICJ; PPC; PPJ
90-5803

MOULLIN, C[harles] W[illiam] Mansell (1851-1940)
Surgery; a practical treatise, with special reference to treatment; by . . . , assisted by various writers on special subjects. 3rd American ed. Philadelphia: P. Blakiston, Son & Co., 1895. 1250p. 1 plate. DNLM; NNNAM; OCIM; PPC
90-5804

MOULLIN, C[harles] W[illiam] Mansell (1851-1940)
Inflammation of the bladder, and urinary fever. Philadelphia: P. Blakiston, Son & Co., 1898. 156p. DNLM; PPC; PU
90-5805

MOULLIN, C[harles] W[illiam] Mansell (1851-1940)
Enlargement of the prostate: its treatment and radical cure. 2nd ed. Philadelphia: P. Blakiston, Son & Co., 1899. 211p. ICJ; PPPH
90-5806

MOYER, Harold N[icholas] (1858-1923)
Catarrhal gastritis. [Philadelphia, 1892.] 9p. DNLM
90-5807

MRACEK, Franz (1848-1908)
Atlas of syphilis and the venereal diseases, including a brief treatise on the pathology and treatment . . . authorized translation from the German; edited by L. Bolton Bangs. . . . With 71 colored plates. Philadelphia: W. B. Saunders & Co., 1898. 1p., 7-16p., 73 l., 122p. DNLM; NNNAM; PPC; PU
90-5808

MRACEK, Franz (1848-1908)
Atlas of diseases of the skin, including an epitome of pathology and treatment . . . authorized translation from the German; ed. by Henry W. Stelwagon. . . . With 63 colored plates. . . . Philadelphia: W. B. Saunders & Co., 1899. 199p. 65 l. DNLM; NNNAM; OCIM; PPJ
90-5809

MUDD, Henry H[odgen] (1844-1899)
The Hodgen suspension-splint. [Philadelphia], 1890. 16p. DNLM
90-5810

MUDD, Henry H[odgen] (1844-1899)
Echinococcus multilocularis of the brain. Philadelphia, 1892. 10p. 1 plate. DNLM
90-5811

MULFORD, H. K. CO.
Catalogue of pharmaceutical and biological products. Philadelphia, 1899. 216p. PPC; PU
90-5812

MULHALL, Joseph C. (1851-1900)
The general health and the upper air-passages. New York, 1898. 11p. DNLM
90-5813

MUMFORD, J[ames] G[regory] (1863-1914)
Salol; its antiseptic use in diseases of the genito-urinary system. A report of nine consecutive cases. Boston, 1890. 4p. DNLM
90-5814

MUMFORD, J[ames] G[regory] (1863-1914)
Fractures of the skull. Conclusions drawn from three hundred cases. Boston, 1893. 13p. DNLM
90-5815

MUMFORD, J[ames] G[regory] (1863-1914)
Compound fractures. A study of three hundred cases. Boston, 1894. 16p. DNLM
90-5816

MUMFORD, J[ames] G[regory] (1863-1914)
Sir Astley Cooper, Bart. An estimate of his character and career. Boston, 1898. 22p. DNLM
90-5817

MUNCASTER, Magruder (1859-1901)
The importance of pleasant medication. New York, 1894. 8p. DNLM
90-5818

MUNDÉ, Paul F[ortunatus] (1846-1902)
The present treatment of uterine displacements. New York, 1895. 14p. DNLM
90-5819

MUNDÉ, Paul F[ortunatus] (1846-1902)
A report of the gynecological service of Mount Sinai Hospital, New York, for the twelve years from Jan. 1, 1883, to Dec. 31, 1894. New York: William Wood & Co., 1895. 116p. DNLM; NNNAM **90-5820**

MUNDÉ, Paul F[ortunatus] (1846-1902)
Torsion of the pedicle of an ovarian tumor. New York: D. Appleton & Co., 1899. 16p. DNLM **90-5821**

MUNDORFF, George Theodore
The value of electrolysis in the treatment of urethritis chronica glandularis. New York: Publ. Print. Co., 1898. 15p. DNLM **90-5822**

MUNN, H[oward] E.
Pathology of cancer. Toledo: Samsey & Fister, 1894. 7p. DNLM **90-5823**

MUNN, William P[hipps] (1865-1903)
Diphtheria; a clinical study. [Philadelphia, 1893.] 42p. DNLM **90-5824**

MUNN, William P[hipps] (1865-1903)
Legislative restriction of the practice of medicine. Pittsburgh, 1893. 8p. DNLM **90-5825**

MUNN, William P[hipps] (1865-1903)
The operative treatment of inflammatory phimosis and the use of the sharp curet and strong bichlorid solution for chancroids. [Philadelphia, 1894.] 4p. DNLM **90-5826**

MUNN, William P[hipps] (1865-1903)
Phimosis and the conditions that it complicates in the adult. [Philadelphia: Lea Bros. & Co., 1894.] 8p. DNLM **90-5827**

MUNRO, John C[ummings] (1858-1910)
Some indications for external urethrotomy. Boston, 1893. 8p. DNLM **90-5828**

MUNRO, John C[ummings] (1858-1910)
Inguinal colotomy for malignant adenoma of rectum. With autopsy. Boston: Damrell & Upham, 1893. 7p. DNLM **90-5829**

MUNRO, Walter Lee (*b.* 1857)
The physician upon the witness stand. New York, 1897. 30p. DNLM **90-5830**

MUNSON, Edward L[yman] (*b.* 1868)
Emergency diet for the sick in the military services. Washington: Government Printing Office, 1899. 45p. DNLM **90-5831**

MUNYON'S HOMOEOPATHIC REMEDIES
Guide to health and treatise on the use of Munyon's homoeopathic home remedies. Published by Munyon's Homoeopathic Home Remedy Co., 1324 Walnut St., Philadelphia, Pa., 1891. 48p. PPC; PPHa **90-5832**

MURDOCH, Frank H[all]
Stomach digestion. Pittsburgh: Murdoch, Kerr & Co., 1896. 7p. DNLM **90-5833**

MURDOCH, Frank H[all]
The diagnosis and treatment of chronic gastric catarrh. New York, 1897. 7p. DNLM **90-5834**

MURDOCH, Frank H[all]
The use and abuse of the stomach tube. New York, 1897. 5p. DNLM **90-5835**

MURDOCH, Frank H[all]
Nervous dyspepsia, with report of cases. New York, 1898. 10p. DNLM **90-5836**

MURDOCH, J[ames] B[issett] (1830-1896)
A contribution to the study of amputation at the hip-joint. [Philadelphia, 1893.] 15p. DNLM **90-5837**

MURPHY, Charles W.
Abortion; accompanied with unusual reflex motor disturbance of the arm. [St. Louis, 1892.] 2 l. DNLM **90-5838**

MURPHY, Charles W.
The coal tar derivatives; their use and abuse. Philadelphia, 1892. 1 l. DNLM **90-5839**

MURPHY, Charles W.
The sequelae of la grippe. [St. Louis,1892.] 2 l. DNLM **90-5840**

MURPHY, J[ohn] B[enjamin] (1857-1916)
Cholecysto-intestinal, gastro-intestinal, entero-intestinal anastomosis and approximation without sutures. (Original search.) New York, 1892. 47p. DNLM **90-5841**

MURPHY, J[ohn] B[enjamin] (1857-1916)
Appendicitis; with original report and analysis of one hundred and forty-one histories and laparotomies for that disease under personal observation. Chicago, 1894. 56p. 1 tab. DNLM **90-5842**

MURPHY, J[ohn] B[enjamin] (1857-1916)
Intestinal approximation; pathological histology of reunion and statistical analysis. New York: Trow Co., 1894. 24p. DNLM **90-5843**

MURPHY, J[ohn] B[enjamin] (1857-1916)
Operative surgery of the gall tracts, with original report of twenty successful cholecyst-enterostomies by means of the anastomosis button. [Chicago, 1894.] 51p. DNLM **90-5844**

MURPHY, J[ohn] B[enjamin] (1857-1916)
Appendicitis; further consideration of this subject, with tabulated report of cases not previously published. [Philadelphia: Lea Bros. & Co., 1895.] 21p. DNLM **90-5845**

MURPHY, J[ohn] B[enjamin] (1857-1916)
Surgical clinic and demonstration. Chicago, 1894. 24p. DNLM **90-5846**

MURPHY, J[ohn] B[enjamin] (1857-1916)
Traumatism of the urinary tract. Chicago, 1895. 47p. DNLM **90-5847**

MURPHY, J[ohn] B[enjamin] (1857-1916)
Fibromyoma complicating pregnancy; fibroma of vaginal wall. Chicago, 1896. 12p. DNLM **90-5848**

MURPHY, J[ohn] B[enjamin] (1857-1916)
Ileus. Chicago, 1896. 36p. DNLM **90-5849**

MURPHY, J[ohn] B[enjamin] (1857-1916)
Surgery of the Gasserian ganglion, with demonstration and report of two cases. Lincoln, 1896. 12p. DNLM
90-5850

MURPHY, J[ohn] B[enjamin] (1857-1916)
Resection of arteries and veins injured in continuity; end-to-end suture; experimental and clinical research. New York, 1897. 31p. DNLM **90-5851**

MURPHY, J[ohn] B[enjamin] (1857-1916)
Surgery of the lung. Chicago, 1898. 144p. 12 plates. DNLM
90-5852

MURPHY, J[ohn] B[enjamin] (1857-1916)
Surgery of the lung. Chicago, 1898. 64p. 12 plates. DNLM
90-5853

MURRAY, George R[edmayne] (*b.* 1865)
Organotherapy. No. 5. The Goulstonian lectures on the pathology of the thyroid gland. Chicago: Armour & Co., [1899]. 37p. DNLM **90-5854**

MURRAY, J[ohn] A.
Ligation of the dorsal vein of the penis for functional impotence, with a report of five cases. Chicago, 1897. 8p. DNLM **90-5855**

MURRELL, William (1853-1912)
Chronic bronchitis and its treatment. . . . A clinical study. Philadelphia: P. Blakiston, Son & Co., 1890. 176p. CtY-M; DNLM; PPC; PU **90-5856**

MURRELL, William (1853-1912)
Nitro-glycerine as a remedy for angina pectoris. . . . Detroit: G. S. Davis, 1890 [1882, *vel subseq.*] 78p. DNLM; ICJ; OCIM; PPC **90-5857**

MURRELL, William (1853-1912)
Massotherapeutics, or massage as a mode of treatment. 5th ed. Philadelphia: P. Blakiston, Son & Co., 1890. 264p. DNLM; NNNAM; PPC **90-5858**

MURRELL, William (1853-1912)
What to do in cases of poisoning. 7th ed., enl. and rev. Philadelphia: P. Blakiston, Son & Co., 1893. 276p. DNLM
90-5859

MURRELL, William (1853-1912)
Clinical lectures on the prevention of consumption. Delivered at the Westminster Hospital. New York: William Wood & Co., 1895. 103p. DNLM; ICJ; NNNAM
90-5860

MURRELL, William (1853-1912)
A manual of pharmacology and therapeutics. . . . Rev. by Frederick A. Castle. . . . New York: William Wood & Co., 1896. 516p. DLC; NNNAM; PPHa; PU
90-5861

MUSKETT, Philip Edward
Prescribing and treatment in the diseases of infants and children. Philadelphia: P. Blakiston, Son & Co., 1891. 293p. DNLM; MBM; NNNAM; PU **90-5862**

MUSSER, John H[err] (1856-1912)
Some clinical remarks on dysentery. [Philadelphia, 1890.] 9p. DNLM **90-5863**

MUSSER, John H[err] (1856-1912)
Tuberculous ulcer of the stomach. [Philadelphia, 1890.] 8p. DNLM **90-5864**

MUSSER, John H[err] (1856-1912)
On the gastric disorders of pulmonary tuberculosis. [Philadelphia: Univ. Penn. Press, 1891.] 7p. DNLM
90-5865

MUSSER, John H[err] (1856-1912)
Grave forms of purpura haemorrhagica. [Philadelphia, 1801.] 12p. DNLM **90-5866**

MUSSER, John H[err] (1856-1912)
Note on pernicious anaemia and chlorosis in the Negro. [Philadelphia, 1891.] 2p. DNLM **90-5867**

MUSSER, John H[err] (1856-1912)
Whooping-cough: its management; its climatic treatment. [Philadelphia: W. B. Saunders, 1891.] 4p. DNLM
90-5868

MUSSER, John H[err] (1856-1912)
The address in medicine. The limitations and the powers of therapeutics. [Philadelphia, 1892.] 11p. DNLM
90-5869

MUSSER, John H[err] (1856-1912)
The address in medicine. The limitations and the powers of therapeutics. [Philadelphia: Univ. Penn. Press, 1892.] 8p. DNLM **90-5870**

MUSSER, John H[err] (1856-1912)
Universal melanotic sarcomata. Philadelphia, 1892. 6p. DNLM
90-5871

MUSSER, John H[err] (1856-1912)
Notes on the summer diseases of the gastro-intestinal tract in children. Detroit: G. S. Davis, 1892. 16p. DNLM
90-5872

MUSSER, John H[err] (1856-1912)
Notes on the treatment of dysmenorrhoea. Detroit: G. S. Davis, 1892. 13p. DNLM **90-5873**

MUSSER, John H[err] (1856-1912)
The uses of fever heat; the occasional dangers of antipyretics in typhoid fever. Philadelphia, 1892. 12p. DNLM
90-5874

MUSSER, John H[err] (1856-1912)
The uses of fever heat; the occasional dangers of antipyretics in typhoid fever. [Philadelphia: Lea Bros. & Co., 1892.] 8p. DNLM **90-5875**

MUSSER, John H[err] (1856-1912) and De Forest WILLARD
A case of abscess of the liver following amoebic dysentery. [Philadelphia, 1893.] 6p. DNLM **90-5876**

MUSSER, John H[err] (1856-1912)
The mild character and diminished prevalence of syphilis, and the infrequency of visceral syphilis. Philadelphia, 1894. 6p. DNLM **90-5877**

MUSSER, John H[err] (1856-1912)
The mild character and diminished prevalence of syphilis, and the infrequency of visceral syphilis. Philadelphia, 1894. 8p. DNLM **90-5878**

MUSSER, John H[err] (1856-1912)
Notes on tuberculous pleurisy. Philadelphia, 1894. 5p. DNLM
90-5879

MUSSER, John H[err] (1856-1912)
A practical treatise on medical diagnosis for students and physicians. . . . Illustrated with 162 woodcuts and 2 colored plates. Philadelphia: Lea Bros. & Co., 1894. 881p. col. plates. DLC; DNLM; PPC; PU **90-5880**

MUSSER, John H[err] (1856-1912)
A case of aspiration broncho-pneumonia in an infant. New York, 1895. 2p. DNLM **90-5881**

MUSSER, John H[err] (1856-1912)
A case of secondary carcinoma of the bones. Multiple fracture; associated duodenal ulcer; polyuria. Philadelphia, 1895. 9p. DNLM **90-5882**

MUSSER, John H[err] (1856-1912)
Subdiaphragmatic abscess due to abscess of the pancreas, with remarks on effusions in the lesser peritoneal cavity. Philadelphia, 1895. 5p. DNLM **90-5883**

MUSSER, John H[err] (1856-1912)
A case of secondary carcinoma of the bones; multiple fractures; associated duodenal ulcer; polyuria. Philadelphia: University of Pennsylvania Press, 1895. 8p. DNLM
90-5884

MUSSER, John H[err] (1856-1912)
A protracted case of typhoid fever; some features of treatment. Philadelphia, 1895. 5p. DNLM **90-5885**

MUSSER, John H[err] (1856-1912) and Thomas S. K. MORTON
Case of carcinoma of descending colon; excision and anastomosis; recovery. Philadelphia, 1896. 5p. 1 plate. DNLM
90-5886

MUSSER, John H[err] (1856-1912)
A practical treatise on medical diagnosis for students and physicians. . . . 2nd ed., rev. and enl. Illustrated with 177 woodcuts and 11 colored plates. Philadelphia and New York: Lea Bros. & Co., 1896. 938p. col. plates. DLC; DNLM; NNNAM; PPC **90-5887**

MUSSER, John H[err] (1856-1912) and J. Dutton STEELE
A case of aneurism of the abdominal aorta with thrombosis of the right renal artery. [Philadelphia], 1896. 4p. DNLM
90-5888

MUSSER, John H[err] (1856-1912) and Joseph SAILER
A case of leucaemia. [Philadelphia], 1896. 7p. DNLM
90-5889

MUSSER, John H[err] (1856-1912) and John M. SWAN
A clinical study of Widal's serum diagnosis of typhoid fever. Chicago, Amer. Med. Assoc., 1897. 7p. DNLM
90-5890

MUSSER, John H[err] (1856-1912)
Angina pectoris; its relation to dilatation of the heart. Philadelphia, 1897. 10p. DNLM **90-5891**

MUSSER, John H[err] (1856-1912)
Angina pectoris; its relation to dilatation of the heart. [Philadelphia], 1897. 9p. DNLM **90-5892**

MUSSER, John H[err] (1856-1912) and J. Dutton STEELE
Symposium on the pathology of the diseases of the cardiovascular system. The myocardium. Philadelphia, [1898]. 7p. DNLM **90-5893**

MUSSER, John H[err] (1856-1912) and Joseph SAILER
A case of Malta fever. Philadelphia, 1898. 7p. DNLM
90-5894

MUSSER, John H[err] (1856-1912)
The diagnostic importance of fever in late syphilis. Philadelphia: Avil Print. Co., 1898. 11p. DNLM **90-5895**

MUSSER, John H[err] (1856-1912)
The essential of the art of medicine. Chicago: Amer. Med. Assoc. Press, 1898. 28p. DNLM **90-5896**

MUSSER, John H[err] (1856-1912)
The essential of the art of medicine. Philadelphia, 1898. 27p. DNLM **90-5897**

MUSSER, John H[err] (1856-1912)
Renal calculus. Philadelphia, 1898. 14p. DNLM
90-5898

MUSSER, John H[err] (1856-1912)
Amyloid disease of the liver, with an abnormally enlarged left lobe. Pittsburgh, 1899. 6p. DNLM **90-5899**

MUSSER, John H[err] (1856-1912)
Cancer of the common bile-duct. Philadelphia, 1899. 4p. DNLM **90-5900**

MUSSER, John H[err] (1856-1912) and Joseph SAILER
Hemorrhagic diathesis in typhoid fever. Philadelphia, 1899. 2 l. DNLM **90-5901**

MUSSER, John H[err] (1856-1912)
A practical treatise on medical diagnosis for students and physicians. . . . 3rd ed., rev. and enl. . . . Philadelphia and New York: Lea Bros. & Co., [1899]. 1082p. col. plates. DLC; DNLM; NNNAM; PU **90-5902**

MYERS, Randolph M.
Cramps as affecting stokers. Richmond, Va., 1897. 3p. DNLM
90-5903

MYERS, T[alleyrand] D.
Some of the pecularities of the climate of California, and their relation to the treatment of consumption of the lungs. Philadelphia: W. F. Fell & Co., 1891. 14p. DNLM
90-5904

MYERS, T[alleyrand] D.
A study of the modern pathology and the treatment of chronic granulation of the eyelids. Philadelphia: W. F. Fell & Co., 1891. 12p. DNLM **90-5905**

MYERS, T. Halsted
The prognosis of pressure-paralysis. [Philadelphia, 1890.] 4p. DNLM **90-5906**

MYERS, William H.
The limitation of craniotomy. New York, 1895. 8p. DNLM
90-5907

MYNTER, Herman (1845-1903)
Appendicitis and its surgical treatment, with a report of seventy-five operated cases. . . . Philadelphia [etc.]: J. B. Lippincott Co., 1897. 303p. DLC; DNLM; NNNAM; PPC
90-5908

NAGLE, John Thomas (1842-1919)
The acting assistant surgeon of the United States Army in the war of the rebellion. . . . New York: Trow's Printing & Bookbinding Co., 1890. 16p. DLC; NNNAM
90-5909

NAGLE, John Thomas (1842-1919)
The status of acting assistant surgeons of the United States Army, who served in the late civil war, being a reply to the ruling of the War Department. . . . New York: M. B. Brown, printer, 1893. 90p. DLC; NNNAM **90-5910**

NANCREDE, Charles B[eylard] Guerard de (1847-1921)
. . . Essentials of anatomy and manual of practical dissection. . . . 3rd ed., rev. and enl. [8th thousand] Based upon the last ed. of Gray's Anatomy. . . . Philadelphia: W. B. Saunders; [etc., etc.], 1890. 388p. 30 col. plates. DLC; DNLM; NNNAM; PPC **90-5911**

NANCREDE, Charles B[eylard] Guerard de (1847-1921)
. . . Essentials of anatomy and manual of practical dissection, together with the anatomy of the viscera. . . . 4th ed. rev. and enl. by an appendix containing hints on dissection, by J. Chalmers Da Costa, M.D., based upon the last edition of Gray's Anatomy. 30 handsome full-page lithographic plates, in color, and 188 fine woodcuts. Philadelpha: W. B. Saunders, 1891. 388p. DLC; DNLM; PPC; PU **90-5912**

NANCREDE, Charles B[eylard] Guerard de (1847-1921)
Annual address of the orator of the section of surgery. The modern anti-bacillary treatment of tubercular joint disease. [Detroit, 1892.] 12p. DNLM **90-5913**

NANCREDE, Charles B[eylard] Guerard de (1847-1921)
Surgical cases illustrating some facts of clinical interest. [Lansing, 1893.] 10p. DNLM **90-5914**

NANCREDE, Charles B[eylard] Guerard de (1847-1921)
Surgical treatment of cervical, thoracic, and abdominal aneurism. [Philadelphia, 1893.] 10p. DNLM
90-5915

NANCREDE, Charles B[eylard] Guerard de (1847-1921)
Essentials of anatomy, including the anatomy of the viscera; arranged in the form of questions and answers prepared especially for students of medicine. . . . 5th ed. Philadelphia: W. B. Saunders, 1895. 388p. 30 col. plates. DNLM; OCIM; PPC; PPJ **90-5916**

NANCREDE, Charles B[eylard] Guerard de (1847-1921)
. . . Essentials of anatomy, including the anatomy of the viscera; arranged in the form of questions and answers prepared especially for students of medicine. . . . 6th ed., thoroughly revised by Fred J. Brockway. Philadelpha: W. B. Saunders, 1899. 419p. DLC; DNLM; PPC; PU
90-5917

NANCREDE, Charles B[eylard] Guerard de (1847-1921)
Lectures upon the principles of surgery; delivered at the University of Michigan. . . . With an appendix containing a resume of the principal views held concerning inflammation, by Wm. A. Spitzley. . . . Philadelphia: W. B. Saunders, 1899. 398p. DLC; DNLM; PPC; PU **90-5918**

NAPHEYS, George Henry (1842-1876)
Napheys' Modern therapeutics, medical and surgical, including the diseases of women and children, a compendium of recent formulae and therapeutical directions from the practice of eminent contemporary physicians, American and foreign. 9th ed., rev. and enl. . . . By Allen J. Smith . . . and J. Aubrey Davis. . . . Philadelphia: P. Blakiston, Son & Co., 1892-1893. 2 v. DLC; DNLM; PPC; PPJ **90-5919**

NAPHEYS, George Henry (1842-1876)
Transmission of life. Counsels on the nature and hygiene of the masculine function. . . . Philadelphia: D. McKay, 1898. 362p. DLC; PPC **90-5920**

NASH, Eugene Beauharnais (*b.* 1838)
Leaders in homoeopathic therapeutics. . . . Philadelphia: Boericke & Tafel, 1899. 381p. DLC; PPC; PPHa
90-5921

NASH, Francis Smith
Reminiscences, medical and hygienic, of the Arctic. Richmond, 1897. 12p. DNLM **90-5922**

NASH, Henry S. (1832-1901)
Loosening teeth, or chronic alveolitis. . . . Its causes, clinical history and treatment. . . . New York: B. F. Welles, 1897. [vol. 1, 299p.] DLC; DNLM; NNNAM
90-5923

NATIONAL COLLEGE OF ELECTRO-THERAPEUTICS, INDIANAPOLIS
Announcement for 1897. Indianapolis, [1896]. 32p. DNLM
90-5924

NATIONAL DENTAL ASSOCIATION
Transactions of the . . . , including minutes of the convention, resulting in the formation of the National Dental Association, and the first meeting, held at Old Point Comfort, Va., August 5 and 6, 1897. Proceedings of the second annual session, held at Omaha, Neb., commencing August 30, 1898. Proceedings of the first annual session of the Southern Dental Association, branch of the National Dental Association, held at St. Augustine, Fla., commencing February 22, 1898. Philadelphia: S. S. White Dent. Mfg. Co., 1899. 406p. DNLM; MdU-D; PPC
90-5925

NATIONAL DENTAL ASSOCIATION
Report of the committee on history. [n. p., 1899.] 22p. DNLM **90-5926**

THE NATIONAL formulary of unofficial preparations. Revised ed. By authority of the American Pharmaceutical Association. [n. p.], 1896. 195p. DNLM; OCLloyd; PPC; PU
90-5927

NATIONAL HOMOEOPATHIC MEDICAL COLLEGE, WASHINGTON, D.C.
Annual announcement for the session of 1895-96 (3.). Washington: Beresford, 1895. 26p. DNLM
90-5928

NATIONAL INSTITUTE OF PHARMACY. CHICAGO
Semi-annual announcement for 1891-92 (2.). Chicago: G. P. Engelhard & Co., 1891. 16p. DNLM [A system of home study. Lectures semi-monthly by mail.]
90-5929

NATIONAL MEDICAL UNIVERSITY, CHICAGO
Annual announcements for the sessions of 1891-92 (1.); 1897-98 (7.); 1901-02 to1903-04 (11.-13.). Chicago, 1891-1903. DNLM [Organized in 1891 as the National Homeopathic Medical College. The word "Homeopathic" dropped from the title in 1895. List of graduates from 1892 to 1903, in announcement for 1903-04.] **90-5930**

NAULTEUS, F[rancis]
Medical compendium on all acute and chronic, all female and children, eye, ear, nose and throat diseases. . . . Hastings, Neb.: E. Watkins, 1899. 321p. DLC **90-5931**

[NEILL, John] (1819-1880)
Valuable medical library of the late John Neill. [Philadelphia, 1890.] 19p. DNLM **90-5932**

NEISWANGER, Charles S[herwood] (*b.* 1849)
Electro-therapeutical practice. A ready reference guide for physicians in the use of electricity. . . . Chicago: E. H. Colegrove & Co., 1895. 80p. DLC; OCIM; PPC; PPHa [*vel subseq.*] **90-5933**

NEISWANGER, Charles S[herwood] (*b.* 1849)
Electro-therapeutical practice. A ready reference guide for physicians in the use of electricity. 5th ed. Rev., rewritten, and greatly enl. Chicago: E. H. Colegrove & Co., 1898. 134p. DLC; OCIM **90-5934**

NELSON, A[biel] W.
Topical treatment of diphtheria and chemical solution of the membrane. Sulphate of iron and salicylic acid. Chicago: Office Amer. Medical Assoc., 1890. 7p. DNLM **90-5935**

NELSON, Daniel T[hurber] (*b.* 1839)
Dermoid cyst, complicated by a twisted pedicle and consequent peritonitis. Oöphorectomy during pregnancy for hystero-epilepsy. Philadelphia, 1890. 8p. DNLM **90-5936**

NETTLESHIP, Edward (1845-1913)
Diseases of the eye. . . . 4th American from the 5th English ed. With a chapter on examination for color-perception. By William Thomson. . . . Philadelphia: Lea Bros. & Co., 1890. 508p. 2 plates. DLC; DNLM; OCIM; PPC **90-5937**

NETTLESHIP, Edward (1845-1913)
Diseases of the eye. . . . Rev. and ed. by W. T. Holmes Spicer. . . . 5th American from the 6th English ed. With a supplement on color-blindness by William Thomson. . . . Philadelphia and New York: Lea Bros. & Co., 1897. 528p. col. plates. DLC; DNLM; NNNAM; PPC **90-5938**

NEVIUS, Laird W.
The discovery of modern anaesthesia: By whom was it made? A brief statement of facts. New York: George W. Nevius, Cooper Institute, 1894. 111p. NNNAM **90-5939**

NEW YORK ACADEMY OF MEDICINE
List of resident fellows. Jan. 1, 1892. [New York, 1892.] 20p. DNLM; NNNAM **90-5940**

NEW YORK [CITY]. DEPARTMENT OF PUBLIC CHARITIES
Hospital formulary of . , boroughs of Manhattan and the Bronx, 5th ed., revised. New York: Printing Bureau, 1898. 95p. DNLM; OCLloyd **90-5941**

NEW YORK COLLEGE OF DENTISTRY. NEW YORK CITY
Catalogue of graduates [from 1867 to] 1894. [New York, 1894.] 19p. DNLM; NNNAM **90-5942**

NEW YORK DENTAL COLLEGE. NEW YORK CITY
Annual announcements for the sessions of 1894-95 to 1897-98 (2.-5.). New York, 1894-1897. DNLM; NNNAM [Chartered June 8, 1892. An institution in the University of the State of New York. Co-educational.] **90-5943**

NEW YORK MEDICAL BOOK COMPANY
Catalogue No. 1. Choice and valuable sets of medical journals, publications of the Government and learned societies. Medical books and pamphlets. Appendix: New American Medical Publications, [1898]. 40p. NNNAM **90-5944**

NEWCOMB, James E[dward] (1857-1912)
Syphilis of the lingual tonsil. [Philadelphia, 1892.] 9p. DNLM **90-5945**

NEWCOMB, James E[dward] (1857-1912)
Ludwig's angina. New York: D. Appleton & Co., 1895. 12p. DNLM **90-5946**

NEWCOMB, James E[dward] (1857-1912)
Guaicol as a local anaesthetic in minor operations on the nose and throat. New York, 1897. 9p. DNLM **90-5947**

NEWCOMB, James E[dward] (1857-1912)
Adeno-carcinoma of the nose; report of a case. New York, 1899. 8p. DNLM **90-5948**

NEWELL, H. L.
Care of patients during gestation and confinement. [New York, 1895.] 7p. DNLM **90-5949**

NEWELL, Otis K[imball]
Apparatus for the preparation of bone specimens, and for the arterial and other injections. Boston: Damrell & Upham, 1890. 8p. DNLM **90-5950**

NEWELL, Otis K[imball]
The improvement of evacuators for litholapaxy and the later developments of the operation. [New York, 1891.] 8p. DNLM **90-5951**

NEWELL, Otis K[imball]
The treatment of urethral stricture and a new divulsor for rapid dilatation. New York: Trow's Co., 1891. 8p. DNLM **90-5952**

NEWELL, Otis K[imball]
The intermittent rapid dilatation of urethral stricture. New York: Trow, 1894. 11p. DNLM **90-5953**

NEWMAN, Robert (*d.* 1903)
Electrolysis in the treatment of stricture of the rectum. Chicago, 1890. 19p. DNLM **90-5954**

NEWMAN, Robert (*d.* 1903)
Electricity in carcinoma. Philadelphia, 1891. 29p. DNLM **90-5955**

NEWMAN, Robert (*d.* 1903)
Cremation and its importance in cholera. New York, 1893. 9p. DNLM **90-5956**

NEWMAN, Robert (*d.* 1903)
Cremation and its importance in cholera. Danbury, Conn., 1893. 81p. DNLM **90-5957**

NEWMAN, Robert (*d.* 1903)
The present status of electrolysis in the treatment of urethral strictures. With statistics of one hundred cases (third series). Chicago, 1893. 11p. DNLM **90-5958**

NEWMAN, Robert (*d.* 1903)
Electricity in the treatment of exophthalmic goitre. Chicago, 1895. 12p. DNLM **90-5959**

NEWMAN, Robert (*d.* 1903)
Hydro-galvanism of the urethra. [n. p., 1895.] 8p. DNLM **90-5960**

NEWMAN, Robert (*d.* 1903)
Supplementary report on the success of electrolysis in the treatment of urethral strictures. Chicago, 1895. 7p. DNLM **90-5961**

NEWMAN, Robert (*d.* 1903)
The want of college instruction in electro-therapeutics. Chicago, 1896. 8p. DNLM **90-5962**

NEWMAN, Robert (*d.* 1903)
Electric treatment in gout and the uric-acid diathesis. New York, 1897. 16p. DNLM **90-5963**

NEWMAN, Robert (*d.* 1903)
Results of (chemical) electrolysis versus divulsion or cutting in the treatment of urethral strictures. New York: Publishers' Print. Co., 1897. 12p. DNLM **90-5964**

NEWMARK, Leo
A case of Brown-Séquard's paralysis. [Philadelphia: Lea Bros. & Co., 1892.] 8p. DNLM **90-5965**

NEWMARK, Leo
Syringomyelia. [Philadelphia, 1893.] 16p. DNLM **90-5966**

NEWMARK, Leo
Lead palsy in children. Philadelphia, 1895. 8p. DNLM **90-5967**

NEWMARK, Leo
Trophic lesions of the jaws in tabes dorsalis. [Philadelphia: Lea Bros. & Co., 1895.] 13p. DNLM **90-5968**

NEWTON, Alonzo Eliot (1822-1889)
Pre-natal culture. Suggestions to parents relative to systematic methods of moulding the tendencies of offspring before birth. . . . Introduction by Alice B. Stockham. Chicago: A. B. Stockham & Co., 1893. [*vel subseq.*] 73p. DLC [Originally: Washington: Moral Education Society, 1879. 67p. CtY-M; DNLM] **90-5969**

NICHOLS, J[ohn] Benjamin (*b.* 1867)
The eclectic medical system. Philadelphia, 1895. 7p. DNLM **90-5970**

NICHOLS, J[ohn] Benjamin (*b.* 1867)
Physio-medicalism. [Philadelphia: Lea Bros. & Co., 1895.] 8p. DNLM **90-5971**

NICHOLS, J[ohn] Benjamin (*b.* 1867)
The Thomsonian and botanic medical systems. [Philadelphia: Lea Bros. & Co., 1895.] 11p. DNLM **90-5972**

NICHOLS, J[ohn] Benjamin (*b.* 1867)
Notes on the reactions and tests of bile pigments in urine and other organic fluids. New York, 1896. 7p. DNLM **90-5973**

NICHOLS, J[ohn] Benjamin (*b.* 1867)
Permanent separation of the amnion and chorion in the mature after birth, forming double fetal sacs. New York, 1899. 3p. DNLM **90-5974**

NICHOLS, J[ohn] Benjamin (*b.* 1867)
The histology of Dupuytren's contraction of the palmar fascia; report of microscopic examination in two additional cases. New York, 1899. 6p. DNLM **90-5975**

NICHOLS, J[ohn] Benjamin (*b.* 1867)
Notes on the histology of the amnion. Rochester, [1899]. 2 l. DNLM **90-5976**

NICHOLS, J[ohn] Benjamin (*b.* 1867) and Frank Palmer VALE
Histology and pathology. A manual for students and practitioners. Series edited by Bern B. Gallaudet. Philadelphia & New York: Lea Bros. & Co., 1899. 458p. DNLM; NNNAM; PPC; PU **90-5977**

NIEDERKORN, Joseph Stephen (*b.* 1861)
The physician's and student's ready guide to specific medication. . . . Bradford, O.: The Little Printing Co., 1892. 115p. DLC **90-5978**

NILES, H[arry] D[orr] (1856-1909)
Surgical conception of peritonitis. Lincoln, Neb., 1898. 16p. DNLM **90-5979**

NOBLE, Charles P[ercy] (1863-1935)
Primary perineorraphy. [Detroit, 1890.] 12p. DNLM **90-5980**

NOBLE, Charles P[ercy] (1863-1935)
Report of a case of abdominal section. Boston, 1890. 8p. DNLM **90-5981**

NOBLE, Charles P[ercy] (1863-1935)
Abdominal surgery at the Kensington Hospital for Women. [Philadelphia, 1891.] 16p. DNLM **90-5982**

NOBLE, Charles P[ercy] (1863-1935)
The dangers of leaving the products of inflammation in the female pelvis. Philadelphia, 1891. 44p. DNLM **90-5983**

NOBLE, Charles P[ercy] (1863-1935)
Minor uterine surgery. Philadelphia, 1891. 16p. DNLM **90-5984**

NOBLE, Charles P[ercy] (1863-1935)
The peroxide of hydrogen; its uses in abdominal surgery. [Philadelphia, 1891.] 4p. DNLM **90-5985**

NOBLE, Charles P[ercy] (1863-1935)
Pyosalpinx in relation to sterility in women. Philadelphia, 1891. 12p. DNLM **90-5986**

NOBLE, Charles P[ercy] (1863-1935)
Salpingitis considered in its relation to pregnancy and the puerperal state. [Philadelphia, 1891.] 13p. DNLM
90-5987

NOBLE, Charles P[ercy] (1863-1935)
Unique case of Caesarean section. New York: William Wood & Co., 1891. 6p. DNLM **90-5988**

NOBLE, Charles P[ercy] (1863-1935)
A year's work in abdominal surgery at the Kensington Hospital for Women. Philadelphia: Univ. Penn. Press, 1891. 48p. DNLM
90-5989

NOBLE, Charles P[ercy] (1863-1935)
Case of true pelvic abscess. Philadelphia: Univ. Penn. Press, 1892. 5p. DNLM **90-5990**

NOBLE, Charles P[ercy] (1863-1935)
Certain aspects of gonorrhoea in women. [Philadelphia, 1892.] 15p. DNLM **90-5991**

NOBLE, Charles P[ercy] (1863-1935)
Early diagnosis and operation in cancer of the uterus. Toledo, O., 1892. 4p. DNLM **90-5992**

NOBLE, Charles P[ercy] (1863-1935)
Endometritis considered clinically. [Philadelphia, 1892.] 13p. DNLM **90-5993**

NOBLE, Charles P[ercy] (1863-1935)
Points in office practice in the treatment of the diseases of women. [Philadelphia, 1892.] 9p. DNLM
90-5994

NOBLE, Charles P[ercy] (1863-1935)
A year's work in minor surgical gynecology at the Kensington Hospital for Women. [Philadelphia, 1892.] 9p. DNLM
90-5995

NOBLE, Charles P[ercy] (1863-1935)
The Caesarean section and its substitutes. New York: William Wood & Co., 1893. 10p. DNLM **90-5996**

NOBLE, Charles P[ercy] (1863-1935)
The causation of the diseases of women. [Philadelphia, 1893.] 8p. DNLM **90-5997**

NOBLE, Charles P[ercy] (1863-1935)
The causation of the diseases of women. [Chicago, 1893.] 16p. DNLM **90-5998**

NOBLE, Charles P[ercy] (1863-1935)
Certain problems in abdominal surgery, based on one hundred coeliotomies done at the Kensington Hospital for Women. [Philadelphia, 1893.] 24p. DNLM **90-5999**

NOBLE, Charles P[ercy] (1863-1935)
Report of a successful elective Caesarean section. Philadelphia: Univ. Penn. Press, 1893. 3p. DNLM **90-6000**

NOBLE, Charles P[ercy] (1863-1935)
Report of two years' work in abdominal surgery at the Kensington Hospital for Women, Philadelphia. [Philadelphia, 1893.] 18p. DNLM **90-6001**

NOBLE, Charles P[ercy] (1863-1935)
The relations of urinary conditions to gynaecological surgery. [New York, 1893.] 12p. DNLM **90-6002**

NOBLE, Charles P[ercy] (1863-1935)
Report of a year's work in minor gynecological surgery in the Kensington Hospital for Women, Philadelphia. [Philadelphia, 1893.] 8p. DNLM **90-6003**

NOBLE, Charles P[ercy] (1863-1935)
Symphysiotomy versus its substitutes; with the report of a case of symphysiotomy. Philadelphia, 1893. 19p. DNLM
90-6004

NOBLE, Charles P[ercy] (1863-1935)
Vaginal hysterectomy for cancer, with a report of four cases. Philadelphia: Univ. Penn. Press, 1893. 4p. DNLM
90-6005

NOBLE, Charles P[ercy] (1863-1935)
Acute puerperal cellulitis and true pelvic abscess. [New York, 1894.] 10p. DNLM **90-6006**

NOBLE, Charles P[ercy] (1863-1935)
The diagnosis of pregnancy during the first three months. Philadelphia, 1894. 4p. DNLM **90-6007**

NOBLE, Charles P[ercy] (1863-1935)
A new method of examining the kidney, especially for stone. [Philadelphia, 1894.] 3p. DNLM **90-6008**

NOBLE, Charles P[ercy] (1863-1935)
A new uterine curetting forceps. [Philadelphia, 1894.] 1 l. DNLM **90-6009**

NOBLE, Charles P[ercy] (1863-1935)
The perfect needle-holder. [Philadelphia, 1894.] 2p. DNLM
90-6010

NOBLE, Charles P[ercy] (1863-1935)
Procidentia uteri. [Philadelphia, 1894.] 8p. DNLM
90-6011

NOBLE, Charles P[ercy] (1863-1935)
Profuse menstruation. [Philadelphia, 1894.] 7p. DNLM
90-6012

NOBLE, Charles P[ercy] (1863-1935)
Remarks on the treatment of inevitable abortion. Philadelphia, 1894. 2 l. DNLM **90-6013**

NOBLE, Charles P[ercy] (1863-1935)
Surgical shock. Philadelphia: Univ. of Penn. Press, 1894. 6p. DNLM **90-6014**

NOBLE, Charles P[ercy] (1863-1935)
Symphyseotomy versus the induction of premature labor. [Philadelphia, 1894.] 10p. DNLM **90-6015**

NOBLE, Charles P[ercy] (1863-1935)
Uterine fibroids. Philadelphia, 1894. 8p. DNLM
90-6016

NOBLE, Charles P[ercy] (1863-1935) and Joseph P. TUNIS
A case of dermoid tumor of both ovaries complicated by a deposit of bone upon each side of the true pelvis, having no connection with the tumors. Philadelphia, 1895. 6p. DNLM
90-6017

NOBLE, Charles P[ercy] (1863-1935)
Appendicitis of mild type. [New York, 1895.] 4p. DNLM
90-6018

NOBLE, Charles P[ercy] (1863-1935)
Coeliotomy for puerperal septicaemia and peritonitis. New York, 1895. 8p. DNLM **90-6019**

NOBLE, Charles P[ercy] (1863-1935)
A consideration of some of the newer problems in abdominal and pelvic surgery in women. New York: William Wood & Co., 1895. 20p. DNLM **90-6020**

NOBLE, Charles P[ercy] (1863-1935)
Movable kidney. New York, [1895]. 7p. DNLM **90-6021**

NOBLE, Charles P[ercy] (1863-1935)
Puerperal pelvic cellulitis and puerperal peritonitis. [New York, 1895.] 8p. DNLM **90-6022**

NOBLE, Charles P[ercy] (1863-1935)
The relation of certain urinary conditions to gynecological surgery. [Washington, 1895.] 10p. DNLM **90-6023**

NOBLE, Charles P[ercy] (1863-1935)
Remarks on ectopic pregnancy. [New York, 1895.] 4p. DNLM **90-6024**

NOBLE, Charles P[ercy] (1863-1935)
Technique of emptying the uterus in inevitable abortion. Philadelphia, 1895. 2 l. DNLM **90-6025**

NOBLE, Charles P[ercy] (1863-1935)
A clinical report on the course of pregnancy and labor as influenced by suspensio uteri. New York: J. D. Emmet, 1896. 8p. DNLM **90-6026**

NOBLE, Charles P[ercy] (1863-1935)
A consideration of certain doubtful points in the management of abortion. Detroit, 1896. 11p. DNLM **90-6027**

NOBEL, Charles P[ercy] (1863-1935)
Drainage versus radical operation in the treatment of large pelvic abscesses. Chicago, 1896. 7p. DNLM **90-6028**

NOBLE, Charles P[ercy] (1863-1935)
A new operation for certain cases of procidentia uteri. New York, 1896. 3p. DNLM **90-6029**

NOBLE, Charles P[ercy] (1863-1935)
Remarks on the use of the buried permanent suture in abdominal surgery. New York: J. D. Emmet, 1896. 6p. DNLM **90-6030**

NOBLE, Charles P[ercy] (1863-1935)
Suspensio uteri with reference to its influence upon pregnancy and labor. New York: William Wood & Co., 1896. 19p. DNLM **90-6031**

NOBLE, Charles P[ercy] (1863-1935)
Suspensio uteri, or ventrofixation of the uterus; its influence upon pregnancy and labor. New York, 1896. 1 l. DNLM **90-6032**

NOBLE, Charles P[ercy] (1863-1935)
A contribution to the technique of operations for the cure of laceration of the pelvic floor in women. New York: J. D. Emmet, 1897. 10p. DNLM **90-6033**

NOBLE, Charles P[ercy] (1863-1935)
The development and the present status of hysterectomy for fibro-myomata. Boston, 1897. 40p. 1 plate. DNLM **90-6034**

NOBLE, Charles P[ercy] (1863-1935)
Ectropion of the cervix in nulliparae resembling laceration of the cervix. New York: J. D. Emmet, 1897. 6p. DNLM **90-6035**

NOBLE, Charles P[ercy] (1863-1935)
A new method of suturing the abdominal wall in celiotomy. New York: William Wood & Co., 1897. 4p. 1 plate. DNLM **90-6036**

NOBLE, Charles P[ercy] (1863-1935)
Some further observations concerning movable kidney. New York, 1897. 10p. DNLM **90-6037**

NOBLE, Charles P[ercy] (1863-1935)
Vaginal incision and drainage of suppurating haematoceles due to ectopic gestation. New York: J. D. Emmet, 1897. 3p. DNLM **90-6038**

NOBLE, Charles P[ercy] (1863-1935)
Abdominal section on a patient suffering from exophthalmic goitre. New York, 1898. 2p. DNLM **90-6039**

NOBLE, Charles P[ercy] (1863-1935)
Closure of vesico-vaginal fistuale following vaginal hysterectomy and other operative procedures by the vaginal route. New York, 1898. 4p. DNLM **90-6040**

NOBLE, Charles P[ercy] (1863-1935)
The conservative treatment of fibroid tumors by myomectomy. [Pittsburgh, 1898.] 11p. DNLM **90-6041**

NOBLE, Charles P[ercy] (1863-1935)
The conservative treatment of pelvic suppuration of puerperal origin. Philadelphia, 1898. 13p. DNLM **90-6042**

NOBLE, Charles P[ercy] (1863-1935)
Shall absorbable or nonabsorbable ligatures and sutures be employed in hysterectomy and salpingo-oophorectomy? New York, 1898. 13p. DNLM **90-6043**

NOBLE, Charles P[ercy] (1863-1935) and W. Wayne BABCOCK
A new method of diagnosis of tuberculosis of the kidney. New York, 1899. 5p. DNLM **90-6044**

NOBLE, Charles P[ercy] (1863-1935)
Alexander's operation. New York, 1899. 6p. DNLM **90-6045**

NOBLE, Charles P[ercy] (1863-1935)
The history of the early operations for fibroid tumors. New York: William Wood & Co., 1899. 32p. DNLM **90-6046**

NOBLE, Charles P[ercy] (1863-1935)
Operations during pregnancy. New York, 1899. 7p. DNLM **90-6047**

NOBLE, Charles P[ercy] (1863-1935)
Progress in gynecology; an address. Baltimore, 1899. 5p. DNLM **90-6048**

NOBLE, Charles P[ercy] (1863-1935)
Remarks on nephrectomy, with a plea for the more certain and earlier diagnosis of conditions requiring it. Pittsburgh, 1899. 24p. DNLM **90-6049**

NOBLE, Charles P[ercy] (1863-1935)
True conservatism in gynecology. Pittsburgh, 1899. 24p. DNLM **90-6050**

NOBLE, George Henry (1860-1932)
A case of carcinoma of the parturient uterus removed three days after confinement; recovery. [New York, 1895.] 4p. DNLM **90-6051**

NOBLE, George Henry (1860-1932)
A remarkable case of ruptured ectopic pregnancy; late operation; recovery. New York, 1895. 3p. DNLM **90-6052**

NOBLE, George Henry (1860-1932)
One hundred and sixty-six cases of cancer of the pregnant uterus occurring since 1886. Atlanta, 1896. 29p. DNLM **90-6053**

NOBLE, George Henry (1860-1932)
A remarkable case of ventral hernia, cured by a flap operation. New York, 1896. 7p. DNLM **90-6054**

NOBLE, George Henry (1860-1932)
Four cases of abscess of the uterus treated by incision, curretement, sterilization with carbolic acid, and drainage. [1897.] 12p. DNLM **90-6055**

NOBLE, George Henry (1860-1932)
Ureteral anastomosis. New York, 1899. 16p. DNLM **90-6056**

NOBLE, William H.
Report of an operation for the removal of the stomach for carcinoma. New York, 1898. 7p. DNLM **90-6057**

NORRIS, Charles (*b.* 1867)
A report on six cases in which the Bacillus aërogenes capsulatus was isolated. Philadelphia, 1899. 28p. DNLM **90-0658**

NORRIS, Henry S.
The internal administration of ozone in the treatment of phthisis. Report of cases. [New York], 1892. 16p. DNLM **90-6059**

NORRIS, Richard Cooper (*b.* 1863)
Syllabus of the obstetrical lectures in the Medical Department of the University of Pennsylvania. Philadelphia: W. B. Saunders; [etc., etc.], 1890. 154p. DLC; NNNAM; PPC; PU **90-6060**

NORRIS, Richard C[ooper] (*b.* 1863)
Syllabus of the obstetrical lectures in the Medical Department of the University of Pennsylvania. 2nd ed. Philadelphia: W. B. Saunders, 1891. 198p., interleaved. DLC; DNLM; PPC **90-6061**

NORRIS, Richard C[ooper] (*b.* 1863)
The Preston Retreat. [New York], 1895. 3p. DNLM **90-6062**

NORRIS, Richard C[ooper] (*b.* 1863)
Puerperal infection of the urinary tract and of the rectum. [New York, 1895.] 7p. DNLM **90-6063**

NORRIS, Richard C[ooper], ed. (*b.* 1863)
An American text-book of obstetrics. For practitioners and students by James C. Cameron, M.D., Edward P. Davis, M.D., Robert L. Dickinson, M.D. . . . Richard C. Norris, M.D., editor, Robert L. Dickinson, M.D., art editor. Philadelphia: W. B. Saunders, 1895. 1009p., col. plates. DLC; DNLM; NNNAM; PPC **90-6064**

NORRIS, Richard C[ooper] (*b.* 1863)
A report of two years' work at the Preston Retreat. New York, 1896. 38p. DNLM **90-6065**

NORRIS, William Fisher (1839-1901)
Foreign bodies in the orbit. Hartford, 1890. 5p. 1 plate. DNLM **90-6066**

NORRIS, William Fisher (1839-1901)
Two cases of brain tumor with interesting eye symptoms. [Hartford, 1890.] 10p. 1 plate. DNLM **90-6067**

NORRIS, William Fisher (1839-1901) and Charles A. OLIVER
A text-book of ophthalmology. Philadelphia: Lea Bros. & Co., 1893. 641p. 5 plates. DLC; DNLM; NNNAM; PPC **90-6068**

NORRIS, William Fisher (1839-1901) and James WALLACH
A contribution to the anatomy of the human retina, with a special consideration of the terminal loops of the rods and cones. Philadelphia: Univ. Penn. Press, 1894. 6p. DNLM **90-6069**

NORRIS, William Fisher (1839-1901)
The terminal loops of the cones and rods of the human retina. [Hartford, 1895.] 8p. 5 plates. DNLM **90-6070**

NORRIS, William Fisher, ed. (1839-1901)
System of diseases of the eye. By American, British, Dutch, French, German, and Spanish authors. Ed. by William F. Norris . . . and Charles A. Oliver. . . . Philadelphia and London: J. B. Lippincott Co., 1897-1900. 4 v. col. plates. DLC; DNLM; NNNAM; PPC **90-6071**

NORSTRÖM, G[ustaf Mauritz] (*b.* 1840)
Cephalalgy and massage. New York, 1896. 68p. DNLM; NNNAM **90-6072**

NORTHROP, H[erbert] L.
The technique of wound treatment. Philadelphia, 1893. 8p. DNLM **90-6073**

NORTHROP, H[erbert] L.
The intracirculatory injecton of saline solution. Philadelphia, 1894. 7p. DNLM **90-6074**

NORTHROP, H[erbert] L.
Reasons for the administration of oxygen with chloroform when the latter is used as an anaesthetic. Philadelphia, 1895. 8p. DNLM **90-6075**

NORTHRUP, William P[erry]
Sclerema neonatorum; report of a case. [New York, 1890.] 6p. DNLM **90-6076**

NORTHRUP, William P[erry]
Tuberculosis in children. Primary infection in bronchial lymph nodes, with exhibition of illustrative specimens. New York: D. Appleton & Co., 1891. 10p. 1 plate. DNLM **90-6077**

NORTHRUP, William P[erry]
Scorbutus in infants; American cases. New York: M. J. Rooney, 1892. 18p. DNLM **90-6078**

NORTHRUP, William P[erry] and Floyd M. CRANDALL
Scorbutus in infants. New York, 1894. 14p. 1 tab. DNLM **90-6079**

NORTHRUP, William P[erry]
Infantile scorbutus. New York, 1895. 3p. DNLM **90-6080**

NORTHRUP, William P[erry]
Typhoid fever in children under two years. Is it frequent? Jersey City, 1895. 3p. DNLM **90-6081**

NORTHRUP, William P[erry]
Typhoid fever in young children, being a report of cases occurring at Stamford, Conn., during the epidemic of 1895. [New York, 1896.] 9p. DNLM **90-6082**

NORTHRUP, William P[erry]
The tuberculin test for the presence of tuberculosis. New York, 1898. 25p. DNLM **90-6083**

NORTHRUP, William P[erry]
Intussusception in an infant nine months old; high rectal injection; recovery. New York, 1899. 2 l. DNLM **90-6084**

NORTHRUP, William P[erry] and C. A. HERTER
Carcinoma of the pancreas; exploratory operation; study of the fat absorption. Philadelphia, 1899. 8p. DNLM **90-6085**

NORTON, A[rthur] B[righam] (1856-1919)
Acute glaucoma. Boston: O. Clapp & Son, 1890. 12p. DNLM **90-6086**

NORTON, A[rthur] B[righam] (1856-1919)
Can headaches and asthenopia, resulting from hyperopia, be relieved without glasses? New York: A. L. Chatterton & Co., 1890. 11p. DNLM **90-6087**

NORTON, Rupert (1867-1914)
Augeioneurotic oedema. New York: D. Appleton & Co., 1897. 18p. DNLM **90-6088**

NORTON, Rupert (1867-1914)
How does malaria enter the human body? Albany, 1897. 11p. DNLM **90-6089**

NORTON, Rubert (1867-1914)
Is malaria a water-borne disease? Baltimore, 1897. 22p. DNLM **90-6090**

NORTON, Rupert (1867-1914)
Malaria as a causative factor in other diseases. Philadelphia, 1898. 23p. DNLM **90-6091**

NORTON, Rupert (1867-1914)
The thymus gland and its relation to sudden death in children. Philadelphia, 1898. 14p. DNLM **90-6092**

NORWOOD, W[esley] C.
The therapeutical powers and properties of veratrum viride. 6th ed. New York, [1899]. 16p. DNLM; NNNAM **90-6093**

NOTES on the therapeutic uses of europhen. New York: W. H. Schieffelin & Co., 1894. 16p. DNLM; NNNAM **90-6094**

NOTES on the therapeutic uses of the new iodine compound aristol. New York: W. H. Schieffelin & Co., 1890. 24p. DNLM; NNNAM **90-6095**

NOTTER, J[ames] Lane (1843-1923)
The theory and practice of hygiene . . . by J. L. Notter and R. H. Firth. Philadelphia: P. Blakiston's Son & Co., 1896. 1034p. DNLM; ICJ; PPC; PU **90-6096**

NOTTINGHAM, D. M.
Address delivered before the Twenty-first Annual Meeting of the Homoeopathic Medical Society of the State of Michigan, May 20, 1890. By the President. Lansing, Mich.: S. A. Ray & Co., 1890. 11p. OCIM **90-6097**

NOVY, Frederick G[eorge] (*b.* 1864)
Directions for laboratory work in bacteriology, for the use of the medical class in the University of Michigan. Ann Arbor: G. Wahr, [1894]. 209p. 1 plate. DNLM **90-6098**

NOVY, Frederick G[eorge] (*b.* 1864)
The etiology of diphtheria. [Philadelphia], 1895. 23p. DNLM **90-6099**

NOVY, Frederick G[eorge] (*b.* 1864)
The causation of diphtheria. Lansing, 1896. 14p. DNLM **90-6100**

NOVY, Frederick G[eorge] (*b.* 1864)
The immunizing power of nucleohiston and of histon. New York, 1896. 24p. DNLM **90-6101**

NOVY, Frederick G[eorge] (*b.* 1864)
Toxins and antitoxins. Lansing, 1896. 8p. DNLM **90-6102**

NOVY, Frederick G[eorge] (*b.* 1864)
Laboratory work in bacteriology. 2nd ed., revised and enlarged. Ann Arbor: G. Wahr, 1899. Front., 563p. DNLM **90-6103**

NOYES BROTHERS & CUTLER
Illustrated catalogue of drugs and pharmaceuticals, surgical and dental instruments, galvanic batteries, artificial limbs, microscopes and sundries. St. Paul, 1890. 476p. OCIM **90-6104**

NOYES, Henry Drury (1832-1900)
The therapeutic effect of prisms in ophthalmic practice; a study of one hundred cases in which they were prescribed. [Hartford, 1896.] 41p. DNLM **90-6105**

NOYES, Henry Drury (1832-1900)
A text-book on diseases of the eye. New York: William Wood & Co., 1890. 733p. 12 plates. DLC; DNLM; NNNAM
90-6106

NOYES, Henry Drury (1832-1900)
Hemianopsia. New York: Trow, 1891. 23p. DNLM
90-6107

NOYES, Henry Drury (1832-1900)
Clinical contributions. [New York, 1894.] 11p. DNLM
90-6108

NOYES, Henry Drury (1832-1900)
A text-book on diseases of the eye. 2nd ed. New York: William Wood & Co., 1894. 816p. 10 plates, 5 charts. DNLM; NNNAM
90-6109

NOYES, William (1874-1915)
On certain peculiarities of the knee-jerk in sleep in a case of terminal dementia. [Baltimore, 1892.] 19p. 1 plate. DNLM
90-6110

NOYES, William B.
Enteric fever in infancy. Chicago, 1895. 22p. DNLM
90-6111

NUNN, R[ichard] J. (1831-1900)
The proabable cause of the epidemic of typhoid fever in Savannah, Ga., in 1892. How to avoid it and other filth diseases in the future. Savannah, 1893. 10p. DNLM
90-6112

OBERSTEINER, Heinrich (1847-1922)
The anatomy of the central nervous organs in health and disease. . . . Transl. with annotations and additions by Alex Hill. Philadelphia: P. Blakiston, Son & Co., 1890. 432p. ICJ; MBM; PPC; PU **90-6113**

OCHSNER, A[lbert] John (1858-1925)
Practical ideas on antiseptic and aseptic methods in the treatment of wounds, with a report of forty-seven consecutive operations for non-suppurative conditions in the Augustana Hospital during the past year. Chicago: R. R. McCabe & Co., 1892. 18p. DNLM **90-6114**

OCHSNER, A[lbert] John (1858-1925)
Demonstration of actinomyces. [Chicago, 1893.] 3p. DNLM
90-6115

OCHSNER, A[lbert] John (1858-1925)
Three cases of acute intestinal obstruction treated by abdominal section. I. Intussusception. II. Volvulus of sigmoid. III. Strangulation of Meckel's diverticulum. Chicago, 1893. 12p. DNLM **90-6116**

OCHSNER, A[lbert] John (1858-1925)
Demonstration of pathological specimens. Chicago, 1894. 5p. DNLM **90-6117**

OCHSNER, A[lbert] John (1858-1925)
The surgical treatment of cleft palate. Chicago, 1894. 2 l. DNLM **90-6118**

OCHSNER, A[lbert] John (1858-1925)
The treatment of erysipelas with strong alcohol. Kansas City, 1894. 4p. DNLM **90-6119**

OCHSNER, A[lbert] John (1858-1925)
Report of cases of resection of the cecum. Chicago, 1895. 6p. DNLM **90-6120**

OCHSNER, A[lbert] John (1858-1925)
Umbilical and ventral hernia. Chicago, 1896. 8p. DNLM
90-6121

OCHSNER, A[lbert] John (1858-1925)
Multiple symmetrical lipomata. Detroit: G. S. Davis, 1897. 6p. DNLM **90-6122**

OCHSNER, A[lbert] John (1858-1925)
The treatment of hernia in old men. New York, 1897. 10p. DNLM **90-6123**

OCHSNER, A[lbert] John (1858-1925)
Appendicitis. Chicago, 1899. 16p. 1 tab. DNLM
90-6124

OCHSNER, A[lbert] John (1858-1925)
Report of surgical clinic. Kansas City, [1899]. 4 l. DNLM
90-6125

O'CONNOR, Joseph T.
American homoeopathic pharmacopoeia. . . . 4th ed. New York: Boericke & Tafel, 1890. 521p. OCLloyd
90-6126

O'CONNOR, Joseph T.
Nervous diseases with homoeopathic treatment. New York: Boericke, Runyon & Ernesty, 1898. 416p. CtY-M; DLC; ICJ; PPHa **90-6127**

O'CONOR, John
Traumatic haemarthrosis of knee joint. [1896.] 10p. DNLM
90-6128

OGDEN, J[ay] Bergen (*b.* 1868)
Tuberculosis of the urinary tract; an important element in diagnosis. [Philadelphia], 1898. 6p. DNLM
90-6129

OHIO COLLEGE OF DENTAL SURGERY. DENTAL DEPARTMENT OF THE UNIVERSITY OF CINCINNATI
[Sixteen photographs of the building and working rooms.] Cincinnati, [1898]. DNLM **90-6130**

THE OHIO Medical University imbroglio. personal malice, jealousy, ambition vs. the demands for higher standards. Cincinnati: Curts & Jennings, [1899]. 43p. DNLM; OC
90-6131

OHIO MEDICAL UNIVERSITY, COLUMBUS
Annual announcements of the department of medicine, dentistry, and pharmacy for the sessions of 1892-93 to 1904-05 (1.-13.). Columbus, 1892-1904. DNLM [Directory of alumni from 1893 to 1903 in announcement for 1904-05.]
90-6132

[OHIO] physicians', dentists', and druggists' directory. Cincinnati: G. Gonser, 1890. 304p. DLC; ICJ [Includes list of physicians and surgeons, dentists and druggists alphabetically arranged; physicians's school and year of graduation; all medical, dental and pharmaceutical colleges with their officers, faculty, etc.; medical, dental and pharmaceutical societies, hospitals, asylums, etc.] **90-6133**

OHLEMANN, [Friedrich Wilhelm] M[ax]
Ocular therapeutics for physicians and students. . . . Transl. and ed. by Charles A. Oliver. Philadelphia: P. Blakiston's Son & Co., 1899. 274p. DLC; DNLM; NNNAM; PPC
90-6134

OHLMACHER, A[lbert] P. (1861-1916)
A brief résumé of the carcinoma organism question. [Chicago, 1892.] 8p. DNLM **90-6135**

OHLMACHER, A[lbert] P. (1861-1916)
Laboratory instruction in elementary comparative anatomy and embryology with large classes of medical students. New York: D. Appleton & Co., 1894. 26p. DNLM
90-6136

OHLMACHER, A[lbert] P. (1861-1916)
A detailed report of some experiments in the production of the diphtheria-antitoxin. [Philadelphia: Lea Bros. & Co., 1895.] 19p. DNLM **90-6137**

OHLMACHER, A[lbert] P. (1861-1916)
The importance of a knowledge of the diphtheria culture test. Cleveland, 1895. 8p. DNLM **90-6138**

OHLMACHER, A[lbert] P. (1861-1916)
Some notes on the use of formalin as a mordant in anilin-staining. [Philadelphia, 1895.] 5p. DNLM
90-6139

OHLMACHER, A[lbert] P. (1861-1916)
Some suggestions in bacteriological technique. [New York, 1895.] 6p. DNLM **90-6140**

OHLMACHER, A[lbert] P. (1861-1916)
On the importance of technical instruction in the medical college laboratories. New York, 1896. 10p. DNLM
90-6141

OHLMACHER, A[lbert] P. (1861-1916)
The bacterium vulgare in a case of cerebellar abscess and leptomeningitis following middle-ear disease. Cincinnati, 1897. 7p. DNLM **90-6142**

OHLMACHER, A[lbert] P. (1861-1916)
Clinical and pathologic features of two cases of typhoid meningitis. Cleveland, 1897. 12p. DNLM
90-6143

OHLMACHER, A[lbert] P. (1861-1916)
Technical note. I. A modified fixing fuid for general histological and neuro-histological purposes. II. A staining combination of gentian violet and picro-acid fuchsin. New York, 1897. 8p. DNLM **90-6144**

OHMANN-DUMESNIL, A[mant] H[enry] (*b.* 1857)
Alopecia areata due to traumatism. St. Louis, 1890. 5p. DNLM
90-6145

OHMANN-DUMESNIL, A[mant] H[enry] (*b.* 1857)
A case of rhinophyma; operation. [St. Louis, 1890.] 7p. DNLM **90-6146**

OHMANN-DUMESNIL, A[mant] H[enry] (*b.* 1857)
A case of ringworm of the scalp, complicated by pustular eczema; cure. [Cincinnati, 1890.] 4p. DNLM
90-6147

OHMANN-DUMESNIL, A[mant] H[enry] (*b.* 1857)
A peculiar case of Addison's disease. Atlanta, Ga.: Franklin, 1890. 5p. DNLM **90-6148**

OHMANN-DUMESNIL, A[mant] H[enry] (*b.* 1857)
Scarlatiniform erythema in typhoid fever. [New York, 1890.] 8p. DNLM **90-6149**

OHMANN-DUMESNIL, A[mant] H[enry] (*b.* 1857)
The treatment of sycosis. [St. Louis, 1890.] 6p. DNLM
90-6150

OHMANN-DUMESNIL, A[mant] H[enry] (*b.* 1857)
An unusual case of atrophy of the skin. [St. Louis, 1890.] 5p. DNLM **90-6151**

OHMANN-DUMESNIL, A[mant] H[enry] (*b.* 1857)
A case of striae et maculae atrophicae following typhoid fever. [St. Louis, 1891.] 6p. DNLM **90-6152**

OHMANN-DUMESNIL, A[mant] H[enry] (*b.* 1857)
A case of intra-urethral chancroid. [St. Louis, 1891.] 4p. DNLM **90-6153**

OHMANN-DUMESNIL, A[mant] H[enry] (*b.* 1857)
Disseminate parasitic peri-folliculitis. [New Orleans, 1891.] 7p. DNLM **90-6154**

OHMANN-DUMESNIL, A[mant] H[enry] (*b.* 1857)
A treatment for pruritis ani. [St. Louis, 1891.] 4p. DNLM
90-6155

OHMANN-DUMESNIL, A[mant] H[enry] (*b.* 1857)
Rheumatism and gout as factors in the causation of eczema and the management of those conditions. [St. Louis, 1891.] 7p. DNLM **90-6156**

OHMANN-DUMESNIL, A[mant] H[enry] (*b.* 1857)
Some points in the diagnosis of diseases of the skin. Cincinnati, 1891. 7p. DNLM **90-6157**

OHMANN-DUMESNIL, A[mant] H[enry] (*b.* 1857)
Elastic skin. [Philadelphia, 1892.] 3p. DNLM
90-6158

OHMANN-DUMESNIL, A[mant] H[enry] (*b.* 1857)
Double chancre à distance. [St. Louis, 1892.] 12p. DNLM
90-6159

OHMANN-DUMESNIL, A[mant] H[enry] (*b.* 1857)
Some successful methods of treating alopecia and alopecia areata. [New Orleans, 1892.] 11p. DNLM
90-6160

OHMANN-DUMESNIL, A[mant] H[enry] (*b.* 1857)
The commoner animal parasites of the skin. [St. Louis] 1893. 23p. 4 plates. DNLM; MB; NN
90-6161

OHMANN-DUMESNIL, A[mant] H[enry] (*b.* 1857)
Tattooing and its successful removal. Danburgy, Conn., 1893. 14p. DNLM **90-6162**

OHMANN-DUMESNIL, A[mant] H[enry] (*b.* 1857)
Rhinophyma: a case in which operation a good result; a new pathological condition found. Philadelphia, 1894. 8p. DNLM
90-6163

OHMANN-DUMESNIL, A[mant] H[enry] (*b.* 1857)
Handbook of dermatology, for the use of students. . . . 2nd ed., rev. and enl. . . . St. Louis: Quarterly Atlas Co., 1894. 276p. plates. DLC; OCIM **90-6164**

OHMANN-DUMESNIL, A[mant] H[enry] (*b.* 1857)
A case of pemphigus. Atlanta, 1895. 4p. DNLM **90-6165**

OHMANN-DUMESNIL, A[mant] H[enry] (*b.* 1857)
Vitiligo: its cause and treatment. St. Louis, 1896. 7p. DNLM **90-6166**

OHMANN-DUMESNIL, A[mant] H[enry] (*b.* 1857)
Cornu cutaneum and cornu unguale. St. Louis, 1896. 9p. DNLM **90-6167**

OHMANN-DUMESNIL, A[mant] H[enry] (*b.* 1857)
Condylomata lata. Keokuk [Iowa], 1896. 6p. DNLM **90-6168**

OHMANN-DUMESNIL, A[mant] H[enry] (*b.* 1857)
The pustulo-crustaceous syphilide of the end of the nose. St. Louis, 1896. 20p. DNLM **90-6169**

OHMANN-DUMESNIL, A[mant] H[enry] (*b.* 1857)
A rapid and successful treatment of herpes zoster. St. Louis, 1896. 8p. DNLM **90-6170**

OHMANN-DUMESNIL, A[mant] H[enry] (*b.* 1857)
Syphilitic ulcers of the pharynx. St. Louis, 1896. 6p. DNLM **90-6171**

OHMANN-DUMESNIL, A[mant] H[enry] (*b.* 1857)
Rupia. St. Louis, 1896. 7p. DNLM **90-6172**

OHMANN-DUMESNIL, A[mant] H[enry] (*b.* 1857)
Syphilitic perforations of the bones. St. Louis, 1896. 8p. DNLM **90-6173**

OHMANN-DUMESNIL, A[mant] H[enry] (*b.* 1857)
The chancre and its treatment. St. Louis, 1896. 8p. DNLM **90-6174**

OHMANN-DUMESNIL, A[mant] H[enry] (*b.* 1857)
Favus. St. Louis, 1896. 8p. DNLM **90-6175**

OHMANN-DUMESNIL, A[mant] H[enry] (*b.* 1857)
Zona. St. Louis, 1897. 7p. DNLM **90-6176**

OHMANN-DUMESNIL, A[mant] H[enry] (*b.* 1857)
Elephantiasis. St. Louis, 1897. 6p. DNLM **90-6177**

OHMANN-DUMESNIL, A[mant] H[enry] (*b.* 1857)
The pustulo-crustaceous syphilide. St. Louis, 1897. 8p. DNLM **90-6178**

OHMANN-DUMESNIL, A[mant] H[enry] (*b.* 1857)
The varioliform syphilide. St. Louis, 1897. 8p. DNLM **90-6179**

OHMANN-DUMESNIL, A[mant] H[enry] (*b.* 1857)
Syphilitic pigmentation. St. Louis, 1897. 7p. DNLM **90-6180**

OHMANN-DUMESNIL, A[mant] H[enry] (*b.* 1857)
The squamous syphilide. St. Louis, 1897. 8p. DNLM **90-6181**

OHMANN-DUMESNIL, A[mant] H[enry] (*b.* 1857)
Ulcero-crustaceous syphilide. [1897.] 8p. DNLM **90-6182**

OHMANN-DUMESNIL, A[mant] H[enry] (*b.* 1857)
A rapid treatment of chancroid and ulcerative syphilitic lesions. St. Louis, 1898. 16p. DNLM **90-6183**

OHMANN-DUMESNIL, A[mant] H[enry] (*b.* 1857)
Erythematous lupus of the hand. [Chicago, 1898.] 9p. DNLM **90-6184**

OHMANN-DUMESNIL, A[mant] H[enry] (*b.* 1857)
A rapid and successful treatment of chronic ulcers of the leg. St. Louis, 1899. 16p. DNLM **90-6185**

OLDBERG, Oscar (1846-1913)
1,500 prescriptions of all kinds, right and wrong. Chicago: Apothecaries' Co., 1892. 244p. DNLM; OCLloyd **90-6186**

OLDBERG, Oscar (1846-1913)
A course of home study for pharmacists; first lessions in the study of pharmacy. 2nd ed. Chicago: Chicago Med. Book Co., 1898. 571p. 2 plates. DNLM **90-6187**

OLESON, Charles Wilmot (*d.* 1906)
Secret nostrums and systems of medicne: a book of formulas comp. . . . Chicago: Oleson & Co., 1890. 206p. DLC **90-6188**

OLESON, Charles Wilmot (*d.* 1906)
Secret nostrums and systems of medicine: a book of formulas comp. . . . 2nd ed. Chicago: Oleson & Co., 1890. 206p. DLC **90-6189**

OLESON, Charles Wilmot (*d.* 1906)
Secret nostrums and systems of medicine: a book of formulas. . . . 3rd ed., rev. and enl. Chicago: Oleson & Co., 1891. 240p. DLC **90-6190**

OLESON, Charles Wilmot (*d.* 1906)
Secret nostrums and systems of medicine: a book of formulas. . . . 4th ed. Chicago: Oleson & Co., 1892. 240p. DLC; DNLM **90-6191**

OLESON, Charles Wilmot (*d.* 1906)
Secret nostrums and systems of medicine, a book of formulas. . . . 5th ed., rev. and enl. Chicago: Oleson & Co., 1894. 241p. DLC **90-6192**

OLESON, Charles Wilmot (*d.* 1906)
Secret nostrums and systems of medicine, a book of formulas. . . . 6th ed., rev. and enl. Chicago: Oleson & Co., 1896. 255p. DLC **90-6193**

OLESON, Charles Wilmot (*d.* 1906)
Secret nostrums and systems of medicine; a book of formulas. 7th ed. Chicago: Oleson & Co., 1897. 255p. DNLM **90-6194**

OLIVER, Charles A[ugustus] (1853-1911)
An analysis of the motor symptoms and conditions of the ocular apparatus, as observed in imbecility, epilepsy, and the second stage of general paralysis of the insane. [Philadelphia, 1890.] 5p. DNLM **90-6195**

OLIVER, Charles A[ugustus] (1853-1911)
An analysis of the ocular symptoms found in the third stage of paralysis of the insane. Hartford: Case, Lockwood & Brainard Co., 1890. 7p. DNLM **90-6196**

OLIVER, Charles A[ugustus] (1853-1911)
A case of intracranial neoplasm with localizing eye symptoms; position of tumor verified at autopsy. Hartford: Case, Lockwood & Brainard Co., 1890. 7p. 1 plate. DNLM **90-6197**

OLIVER, Charles A[ugustus] (1853-1911)
Analysis of the sensory changes and conditions of the ocular appartus as found in imbecility, epilepsy, and general paralysis of the insane. Chicago, 1891. 12p. DNLM **90-6198**

OLIVER, Charles A[ugustus] (1853-1911)
A clinical study of the ocular symptoms found in the so-called Mongolian type of idiocy. [Philadelphia, 1891.] 6p. DNLM **90-6199**

OLIVER, Charles A[ugustus] (1853-1911)
A clinical study of the ocular symptoms found in the so-called Mongolian type of idiocy. [Hartford, 1891.] 10p. DNLM **90-6200**

OLIVER, Charles A[ugustus] (1853-1911)
History of a case of sarcoma of the genu of the corpus callosum, presenting symptoms of profound hysteria; with autopsy. [Philadelphia, 1891.] 6p. DNLM **90-6201**

OLIVER, Charles A[ugustus] (1853-1911)
Cases of symmetrically placed opacities of the corneae, occurring in mother and son. [Hartford, 1892.] 5p. DNLM **90-6202**

OLIVER, Charles A[ugustus] (1853-1911)
Clinical history of a case of successful extraction of a piece of steel from an iris and lens by an iridectomy, with subsequent absorption of the lens and recovery of normal vision. Chicago, 1892. 3p. DNLM **90-6203**

OLIVER, Charles A[ugustus] (1853-1911)
Clinical history of a case of successful extraction of a piece of steel from an iris and lens by an iridectomy, with subsequent absorption of the lens and recovery of normal vision. [Philadelphia, 1892.] 3p. DNLM **90-6204**

OLIVER, Charles A[ugustus] (1853-1911)
The clinical value of repeated careful correction of manifest refractive error in plastic iritis. [Hartford, 1892.] 12p. DNLM **90-6205**

OLIVER, Charles A[ugustus] (1853-1911)
History of a case of gunpowder injuries to both corneae, irides, and lenses, with subsequent restoration of vision to almost full acuity. [Philadelphia, 1892.] 4p. DNLM **90-6206**

OLIVER, Charles A[ugustus] (1853-1911)
The significance of ocular symptoms in intra-cranial disease. [Philadelphia, 1892.] 8p. DNLM **90-6207**

OLIVER, Charles A[ugustus] (1853-1911)
Clinical history of a case of spindle-celled sarcoma of the choroid, with a study of the microscopic condition of the growth. [Hartford, 1893.] 9p. 1 plate. DNLM **90-6208**

OLIVER, Charles A[ugustus] (1853-1911)
Clinical history of a case of spindle-celled sarcoma of the choroid, with a study of the microscopic condition of the growth. [Philadelphia, 1893.] 6p. DNLM **90-6209**

OLIVER, Charles A[ugustus] (1853-1911)
The clinical value of repeated careful correction of manifest refractive error in plastic iritis. Philadelphia, [1893]. 8p. DNLM **90-6210**

OLIVER, Charles A[ugustus] (1853-1911)
Obituary notice of Joseph Zentmayer. [Philadelphia, 1893.] 7p. port. DNLM **90-6211**

OLIVER, Charles A[ugustus] (1853-1911)
The relation of the patellar tendon-reflex to some of the ocular reflexes found in general paralysis of the insane. [Philadelphia, 1893.] 4p. DNLM **90-6212**

OLIVER, Charles A[ugustus] (1853-1911)
The relation of the patellar tendon-reflex to some of the ocular reflexes found in general paralysis of the insane. [Hartford, 1893.] 4p. DNLM **90-6213**

OLIVER, Charles A[ugustus] (1853-1911)
A series of wools for the ready detection of "color blindness." [Hartford, 1893.] 6p. DNLM **90-6214**

OLIVER, Charles A[ugustus] (1853-1911)
A series of wools for the ready detection of "color blindness." [and package of wool]. New York, [1893]. 2 l. DNLM **90-6215**

OLIVER, Charles A[ugustus] (1853-1911)
Description of an artificial eye intended for the study of ophthalmoscopy and the objective determination of ametropia. [Hartford, 1894.] 4p. DNLM **90-6216**

OLIVER, Charles A[ugustus] (1853-1911)
Description of a new trial-frame. [St. Louis, 1894.] 3p. DNLM **90-6217**

OLIVER, Charles A[ugustus] (1853-1911)
History of a case of indurated (Hunterian) chancre of the eyelid. Philadelphia: A. Van Horn, 1894. 2 l. DNLM **90-6218**

OLIVER, Charles A[ugustus] (1853-1911)
The relation of ophthalmoscopic findings to diseases of the cerebral cortex, as illustrated by a series of observations upon nearly two hundred cases of epilepsy and general paralysis of the insane. [Philadelphia, 1894.] 4p. DNLM **90-6219**

OLIVER, Charles A[ugustus] (1853-1911)
A short note upon so-called "hereditary optic-nerve atrophy," as a contribution to the question of transmission of structural peculiarity. Philadelphia, 1894. 3p. DNLM
90-6220

OLIVER, Charles A[ugustus] (1853-1911)
Some additional studies upon the clinical value of repeated careful correction of manifest refractive error in plastic iritis. [Philadelphia, 1894.] 3p. DNLM **90-6221**

OLIVER, Charles A[ugustus] (1853-1911)
Preliminary note upon a few of the changes found in the fields of vision while the eyes are placed at right angles to their ordinary position. [Philadelphia, 1895.] 2p. DNLM
90-6222

OLIVER, Charles A[ugustus] (1853-1911)
A clinical study of three hundred and fifty-four cases of foreign bodies situated on and in the cornea. Philadelphia, 1895. 2 l. DNLM **90-6223**

OLIVER, Charles A[ugustus] (1853-1911)
Description of a case showing the late ophthalmoscopic appearances of supposed emoblism of the central retinal artery. [Philadephia, 1895.] 2p. 1 plate. DNLM
90-6224

OLIVER, Charles A[ugustus] (1853-1911)
A description of some of the most important ophthalmic methods employed for the recognition of peripheral and central nerve disease. Philadelphia, 1895. 47p. DNLM
90-6225

OLIVER, Charles A[ugustus] (1853-1911)
A series of clinical cases. Philadelphia, 1895. 12p. 1 plate. DNLM **90-6226**

OLIVER, Charles A[ugustus] (1853-1911)
The action of hydrobromate of scopolamine upon the iris and ciliary muscle. Philadelphia, 1896. 3p. DNLM
90-6227

OLIVER, Charles A[ugustus] (1853-1911)
Brief report of a case of traumatic pterygium, with a comparative study of the refractive condition of the eye before and after operation. St. Louis, 1896. 2p. DNLM
90-6228

OLIVER, Charles A[ugustus] (1853-1911)
A brief résumé of a comparative study of the ophthalmoscopic conditions seen in interstitial nephritis as found in dispensary service and in general hospital practice. Philadelphia, 1896. 2p. DNLM **90-6229**

OLIVER, Charles A[ugustus] (1853-1911)
A brief study of the ophthalmic conditions in a case of cerebellar tumor; autopsy. Philadelphia, 1896. 4p. DNLM
90-6230

OLIVER, Charles A[ugustus] (1853-1911)
A clinical study of a case of double chorio-retinitis in the macular regions following a flash of lightning and a flash from burning lycopodium. Philadelphia, 1896. 12p. 7 plates. DNLM **90-6231**

OLIVER, Charles A[ugustus] (1853-1911)
Description of a successful operation for blepharoplasty, embracing the outer halves of both the upper and the lower lids by a single split flap taken from the forehead for epithelioma. Philadelphia, 1896. 6p. DNLM
90-6232

OLIVER, Charles A[ugustus] (1853-1911)
History of a case, in which five years previously a piece of steel was successfully removed from the vitreous chamber by means of an electro-magnet. St. Louis, 1896. 4p. DNLM
90-6233

OLIVER, Charles A[ugustus] (1853-1911)
An ophthalmoscopic study of a case of hemorrhagic neuro-retinitis. Philadelphia, 1896. 3p. 1 plate. DNLM
90-6234

OLIVER, Charles A[ugustus] (1853-1911)
Some of the inefficiencies of the methods ordinarily employed by railway surgeons for the detection of subnormal color-perception (color-blindness). St. Louis, 1896. 8p. DNLM
90-6235

OLIVER, Charles A[ugustus] (1853-1911)
The therapeutic value of hydrobromate of scopolamine in plastic iritis. Philadelphia, 1896. 4p. DNLM
90-6236

OLIVER, Charles A[ugustus] (1853-1911)
A case of reparation from extensive injury involving the inner angle of the eyelids. Nashville, 1897. 2p. DNLM
90-6237

OLIVER, Charles A[ugustus] (1853-1911)
Clinical history of a case of subconjunctival dislocation of the crystalline lens. Nashville, 1897. 3p. DNLM
90-6238

OLIVER, Charles A[ugustus] (1853-1911)
Clinical history of an operation for cicatricial ectropium with advancement of the levator palpebrae. St. Louis, 1897. 3p. DNLM **90-6239**

OLIVER, Charles A[ugustus] (1853-1911)
Clinical history of a series of operative procedures for the cure of cicatricial ectropium from antral disease. Philadelphia, 1897. 2p. DNLM **90-6240**

OLIVER, Charles A[ugustus] (1853-1911)
Clinical notes of a case of injury producing as the most prominent symptom luxation of the eyeball into the orbit (so-called traumatic enophthalmos). Nashville, 1897. 1 l. DNLM **90-6241**

OLIVER, Charles A[ugustus] (1853-1911)
A clinical study of the ophthalmic symptoms seen in a case of fracture of the anterior base of the skull. Philadelphia, 1897. 7p. DNLM **90-6242**

OLIVER, Charles A[ugustus] (1853-1911)
The ocular expressions of gout. Philadelphia, 1897. 3p. DNLM
90-6243

OLIVER, Charles A[ugustus] (1853-1911)
Ophthalmoscopic representation of a case of traumatic rupture of the inferior temporal vein of the right retina. St. Louis, 1897. 3p. 1 plate. DNLM **90-6244**

OLIVER, Charles A[ugustus] (1853-1911)
A perfected series of test-type. Philadelphia, 1897. 1 l. DNLM **90-6245**

OLIVER, Charles A[ugustus] (1853-1911)
Resection and advancement of the levator palpebrae muscle in traumatic ptosis. Philadelphia, 1897. 3p. DNLM **90-6246**

OLIVER, Charles A[ugustus] (1853-1911)
Removal of a piece of steel from the vitreous chamber, the position of the foreign body being determined by the presence of a scotoma in the field of vision. Chicago, 1897. 3p. DNLM **90-6247**

O'MALLEY, Austin
Diphtheria and the serum therapy. New York, 1894. 13p. DNLM **90-6248**

ONE aspect of the subject of medical examination as set forth in the work of the North Carolina board of medical examiners. [Washington, N.C., 1894.] 34p. DNLM **90-6249**

O'NEILL, James B.
Symphyseotomy. A paper read before the Maine Medical Association, June 14, 1894. 12p. Portland: S. Berry, 1894. 12p. DNLM **90-6250**

O'NEILL, John W.
On the use of gauze in place of tongue forceps during the administration of anaesthetics, and a new mouth gag. Chicago: Amer. Medical Assoc., 1894. 4p. DNLM **90-6251**

OPINIONS concerning vivisection and dissection in schools. Chicago, 1895. 12p. DNLM **90-6252**

OPINIONS of the press on a bill to establish a Bureau of Public Health within the Department of the Interior of the United States. Prepared by the national quarantine committee of the New York Academy of Medicine. New York: J. J. O:Brien & Son, 1894. 7p. 2 sheets. DNLM; NNNAM **90-6253**

OPPENHEIMER, Seymour (*b.* 1871)
The advocation of a new method of operation for marked diffuse cartilaginous deflection of the nasal septum. St. Louis, 1895. 4p. DNLM **90-6254**

OPPENHEIMER, Seymour (*b.* 1871)
Tuberculosis of the tonsil. Philadelphia, 1898. 9p. DNLM **90-6255**

OPPENHEIMER, Seymour (*b.* 1871)
The effect of atmospheric changes on the hearing in chronic catarrhal otitis media. New York: D. Appleton & Co., 1899. 11p. DNLM **90-6256**

OPPENHEIMER, Seymour (*b.* 1871)
The effect of certain occupations on the pharynx. New York: Publishers' Print. Co., 1899. 12p. DNLM **90-6257**

ORME, Henry S[ayre] (*b.* 1837)
Leprosy; its extent and control, origin and geographical distribution. [n. p. 1890?] 38p. DNLM **90-6258**

ORMEROD, Joseph A[nderne] (1848-1925)
Diseases of the nervous system. . . . Philadelphia: P. Blakiston, Son & Co., 1892. 343p. plates. DLC; PPC; PPHa; PU **90-6259**

OSBORNE, O[liver] T[homas] (*b.* 1862)
Diphtheria, follicular tonsilitis, and membranous sore throat and their relations to each other, with cases. Bridgeport, Conn.: Gould & Stiles, 1890. 26p. DNLM **90-6260**

OSBORNE, O[liver] T[homas] (*b.* 1862)
A case of acromegaly. Philadelphia, 1892. 8p. DNLM **90-6261**

OSBORNE, O[liver] T[homas] (*b.* 1862)
A case of Morton's metatarsalgia; neuritis; exsection of joint; cure. [New York], 1895. 4p. DNLM **90-6262**

OSBORNE, O[liver] T[homas] (*b.* 1862)
A case of acromegaly; autopsy; skeleton. Philadelphia, 1897. 16p. 8 plates. DNLM **90-6263**

OSBORNE, O[liver] T[homas] (*b.* 1862)
A case of acromegaly; autopsy; skeleton. Part II. Pathology and etiology. New Haven, 1897. 15p. 1 plate. DNLM **90-6264**

OSBORNE, O[liver] T[homas] (*b.* 1862)
Drugs versus cardiac insufficiency. New Haven, 1898. 9p. DNLM **90-6265**

OSBORNE, O[liver] T[homas] (*b.* 1862)
A case of acromegaly. New Haven, 1899. 1 l. DNLM **90-6266**

OSBORNE, O[liver] T[homas] (*b.* 1862)
The clinical significance of fever. Philadelphia, 1899. 12p. DNLM **90-6267**

OSBORNE, O[liver] T[homas] (*b.* 1862)
Medical shock or heart failure. New Haven, 1899. 8p. DNLM **90-6268**

OSBORNE, O[liver] T[homas] (*b.* 1862)
The progress of medicine. New Haven, 1899. 9p. DNLM **90-6269**

OSBURN, William
Manual of histology and bacteriology; including a concise statement of the important facts of microscopic technique and urinalysis, and a laboratory course of seventy practical exercises, with provision for notes and drawings. . . . Nashville, Tenn.: Marshall & Bruce Co., 1899. 188p. DLC **90-6270**

OSGOOD, Hamilton (*b.* 1839)
The therapeutic value of suggestion during the hypnotic state; with an historical sketch of hypnotism and a report of thirty-five cases. Boston: Damrell & Upham, 1890. 46p. DNLM; MBM **90-6271**

OSGOOD, Hamilton (*b.* 1839)
The winter and its dangers. . . . Philadelphia: P. Blakiston, Son & Co., 1890. 160p. DLC; DNLM; PP; PPC [American Health Primers; original printing, 1879, *vel subseq.*] **90-6272**

OSLER, William (1849-1919)
On fever of hepatic origin, particularly the intermittent pyrexia associated with gallstones. Baltimore, 1890. 29p. DNLM
90-6273

OSLER, William (1849-1919)
Cases of post-febrile insanity. Baltimore, 1890. 5p. DNLM
90-6274

OSLER, William (1849-1919)
Rare forms of cardiac thrombi. Baltimore, 1890. 6p. DNLM
90-6275

OSLER, William (1849-1919)
Note on endocarditis in phthisis. Baltimore, 1890. 3p. DNLM
90-6276

OSLER, William (1849-1919)
Tubercular peritonitis; general considerations, tubercular abdominal tumors; curability. Baltimore, 1890. 47p. DNLM
90-6277

OSLER, William (1849-1919)
Acute nephritis in typhoid fever. Baltimore, 1890. 10p. DNLM
90-6278

OSLER, William (1849-1919)
On the amoeba coli in dysentery and in dysenteric liver abscess. Baltimore, 1890. 5p. DNLM
90-6279

OSLER, William (1849-1919)
On the form of convulsive tic associated iwth coprolalia, etc. Philadelphia, 1890. 8p. DNLM **90-6280**

OSLER, William (1849-1919)
A case of sensory apliasia, word-blindness with heimanopsia. Philadelphia, 1891. 6p. DNLM **90-6281**

OSLER, William (1849-1919)
Rudolf Virchow; the man and the student. Boston, 1891. 9p. DNLM **90-6282**

OSLER, William (1849-1919)
Doctor and nurse; remarks to the first class of graduates from the Training School for Nurses, at the Johns Hopkins Hospital. Baltimore: J. Murphy & Co., 1891. 11p. DNLM
90-6283

OSLER, William (1849-1919)
Remarks on specialism. Boston: Damrell & Upham, 1892. 9p. DNLM **90-6284**

OSLER, William (1849-1919)
The healing of tuberculosis. Philadelphia, 1892. 5p. DML
90-6285

OSLER, William (1849-1919)
On the association of congenital wry-neck, with marked facial symmetry. New York: M. J. Rooney, 1892. 5p. DNLM
90-6286

OSLER, William (1849-1919)
The principles and practice of medicine. New York: D. Appleton & Co., 1892. 1079p. 19 charts and 5 woodcut figures. DLC; DNLM; NNC; PPC [FIRST EDITION, *first issue*, has misprint "Georgias" on page VI and the publishers' catalogue at end dated November, 1891. Of the first printing 3000 copies were sold in a month; through triennial revisions, the book became a standard text for students and practitioners over a period of thirty years, not only in English, but also in German, Spanish, French, and Chinese translations. For Dr. Osler's own account of the preparation of this book see *Bibliotheca Osleriana*, No. 3544.] **90-6287**

OSLER, William (1849-1919)
The cold-bath treatment of typhoid fever. Philadelphia, 1892. 8p. DNLM **90-6288**

OSLER, William (1849-1919)
Tuberculous pericarditis. [Philadelphia, 1893.] 18p. DNLM
90-6289

OSLER, William (1849-1919)
On dilatation of the colon in young children. New York: M. J. Rooney, 1893. 8p. DNLM **90-6290**

OSLER, William (1849-1919)
Physic and physicians as depicted in Plato. Boston: Damrell & Upham, 1893. 20p. DNLM **90-6291**

OSLER, William (1849-1919)
Case of arterio-venous aneurism of the axillary artery and vein of fourteen years' duration. Philadelphia, 1893. 4p. DNLM
90-6292

OSLER, William (1849-1919)
The chronic intermittent fever of endocarditis. Baltimore, 1893. 12p. DNLM **90-6293**

OSLER, William (1849-1919)
Remarks on the varieties of chronic chorea, and a report upon two families of the hereditary form, with one autopsy. [New York, 1893.] 15p. DNLM **90-6294**

OSLER, William (1849-1919)
Note on a remarkable house epidemic of typhoid fever. Philadelphia, 1893. 3p. DNLM **90-6295**

OSLER, William (1849-1919)
Shattuck lecture, 1893. Tuberculous pleurisy. Boston: D. Clapp & Son, 1893. 66p. DNLM **90-6296**

OSLER, William (1849-1919)
On sporadic cretinism in America. Philadelphia, 1893. 16p. DNLM **90-6297**

OSLER, William (1849-1919)
Notes on tuberculosis in children. New York, 1893. 8p. DNLM
90-6298

OSLER, William (1849-1919)
Teacher and student. An address delivered on the occasion of the opening of the new building of the College of Medicine and Surgery of the University of Minnesota, Minneapolis, October 4th, 1894. Baltimore: J. Murphy & Co., 1894. 22p. DNLM **90-6299**

OSLER, William (1849-1919)
On chorea and choreiform affections. Philadelphia: P. Blakiston, Son & Co., 1894. 125p. DNLM **90-6300**

OSLER, William (1849-1919)
Parotitis in pneumonia. Case of pericarditis treated by incision and drainage. Philadelphia, 1894. 5p. DNLM
90-6301

OSLER, William (1849-1919)
I. General analysis and summary of two hundred and twenty-nine cases of typhoid fever. II. The treatment of typhoid fever. III. A study of the fatal cases. IV. Special symptoms, complications, and sequelae. Baltimore, 1894. 72p. 3 charts. DNLM
90-6302

OSLER, William (1849-1919)
Lectures on the diagnosis of abdominal tumors, delivered to the post-graduate class, Johns Hopkins University, 1893. New York: D. Appleton & Co., 1894. 192p. DNLM
90-6303

OSLER, William (1849-1919)
The army surgeon. An address delivered at the closing exercises of the Army Medical School, Washington, D.C., Feb. 28, 1894. [Philadelphia: Lea Bros. & Co., 1894.] 12p. DNLM
90-6304

OSLER, William (1849-1919)
The leaven of science. An address delivered at the opening of the Wistar Institute of Anatomy and Biology of the University of Pennsylvania, May 21, 1894. Philadelphia, 1894. 16p. DNLM **90-6305**

OSLER, William (1849-1919)
Oliver Wendell Holmes. Baltimore, 1894. 10p. DNLM
90-6306

OSLER, William (1849-1919)
Introductory remarks to course of clinical demonstrations on typhoid fever. Baltimore, 1894. 4p. DNLM
90-6307

OSLER, William (1849-1919)
Cancer of the stomach with very rapid course. Philadelphia, 1895. 5p. DNLM **90-6308**

OSLER, William (1849-1919)
Case of sporadic cretinism (infantile myxoedema) treated successfully with thyroid extract. New York, 1895. 4p. DNLM
90-6309

OSLER, William (1849-1919)
Typhoid fever in country districts. Baltimore, 1895. 3p. DNLM
90-6310

OSLER, William (1849-1919)
The practical value of Laveran's discoveries. New York, 1895. 10p. DNLM **90-6311**

OSLER, William (1849-1919)
On the visceral complications of erythema exudativum multiforme. Philadelphia, 1895. 18p. DNLM
90-6312

OSLER, William (1849-1919)
The principles and practice of medicine, designed for the use of practitioners and students of medicine. . . . 2nd ed. New York: D. Appleton & Co., 1895. 1143p. col. illus., diags. DNLM; NNNAM; PU **90-6313**

OSLER, William (1849-1919)
John Keats, the apothecary poet. Baltimore: Friedenwald Co., 1896. 18p. DNLM **90-6314**

OSLER, William (1849-1919)
Thomas Dover (of Dover's powder), physician and buccaneer. Baltimore: Friedenwald Co., 1896. 18p. DNLM
90-6315

OSLER, William (1849-1919)
An Alabama student. Baltimore: Friedenwald Co., 1896. 19p. DNLM **90-6316**

OSLER, William (1849-1919)
On six cases of Addison's disease, with the report of a case greatly benefited by the use of the supra-renal extract. Philadelphia, 1896. 8p. DNLM **90-6317**

OSLER, William (1849-1919)
Addison's disease. Philadelphia, 1896. 4p. DNLM
90-6318

OSLER, William (1849-1919)
On the association of enormous heart hypertrophy, chronic proliferative peritonitis, and recurring ascites, with adherent pericardium. New York, 1896. 8p. DNLM
90-6319

OSLER, William (1849-1919)
Hemiplegia in typhoid fever. New York, 1896. 12p. DNLM
90-6320

OSLER, William (1849-1919)
The cerebral complications of Raynaud's disease. Philadelphia, 1896. 8p. DNLM **90-6321**

OSLER, William (1849-1919)
On the classification of the tics or habit movement. [New York, 1897. 5]. DNLM **90-6322**

OSLER, William (1849-1919)
On certain features in the prognosis of pneumonia. [Philadelphia, 1897.] 9p. DNLM **90-6323**

OSLER, William (1849-1919)
The diagnosis of malarial fever. [New York, 1897.] 13p. DNLM **90-6324**

OSLER, William (1849-1919)
The functions of a state faculty. [Baltimore, 1897.] 9p. DNLM **90-6325**

OSLER, William (1849-1919)
Nurse and patient. An address. [Baltimore, 1897.] 17p. DNLM **90-6326**

OSLER, William (1849-1919)
Influence of Louis on American medicine. [Baltimore, 1897.] 18p. DNLM **90-6327**

OSLER, William (1849-1919)
Internal medicine as a vocation. [New York, 1897.] 14p. DNLM **90-6328**

OSLER, William (1849-1919)
Pneumonia. [Washington, 1897.] 10p. DNLM
90-6329

OSLER, William (1849-1919)
Occasional notes on American medical classics. [Philadelphia, 1897.] 4p. DNLM **90-6330**

OSLER, William (1849-1919)
Lectures on angina pectoris and allied states. New York: D. Appleton & Co., 1897. 160p. DLC; NcD; PPC; PPHa **90-6331**

OSLER, William (1849-1919)
On chronic symmetrical enlargement of the salivary and lachrymal glands. [Philadelphia, 1898.] 4p. DNLM **90-6332**

OSLER, William (1849-1919)
On some of the intestinal features of typhoid fever. [Philadelphia, 1898.] 9p. DNLM **90-6333**

OSLER, William (1849-1919)
The principles and practice of medicine, designed for the use of practitioners and students of medicine. . . . 3rd ed. New York: D. Appleton & Co., 1898. 1181p. illus. DLC; DNLM; NNNAM; PPC **90-6334**

OSLER, William (1849-1919)
Leprosy in the United States, with the report of a case. [Baltimore, 1898.] 7p. DNLM **90-6335**

OSLER, William (1849-1919)
On diffuse scleroderma; with special reference to diagnosis and to the use of the thyroid-gland extract. [New York, 1898.] 26p. 1 plate. DNLM **90-6336**

OSLER, William (1849-1919)
Cerebro-spinal fever. [Baltimore, 1898.] 7p. DNLM **90-6337**

OSLER, William (1849-1919)
The arthritis of cerebro-spinal fever. [Boston, 1898.] 14p. DNLM **90-6338**

OSLER, William (1849-1919)
On the study of pneumonia. [St. Paul, 1899.] 6p. DNLM **90-6339**

OSLER, William (1849-1919)
The problem of typhoid fever in the United States. Baltimore, 1899. 13p. DNLM **90-6340**

OSLER, William (1849-1919)
An acute myxoedematous condition, with tachycardia, glycosuria, melaena, mania, and death. [New York, 1899.] 7p. DNLM **90-6341**

OSLER, William (1849-1919)
The clinical features of sporadic trichinosis. [Philadelphia, 1899.] 15p. DNLM **90-6342**

OSLER, William (1849-1919)
In memoriam William Pepper. [Philadelphia, 1899.] 16p. DNLM **90-6343**

OSLER, William (1849-1919)
The diagnosis of typhoid fever. [New York, 1899.] 12p. DNLM **90-6344**

OSTROM, Homer I[rwin] (*b.* 1852)
Vaginal hystero-oophorectomy for other than malignant diseases of the uterus and adnexa. Abdominal hysterectomy. [New York, 1894.] 32p. DNLM **90-6345**

OSTROM, Kurre W[ilhelm] (*b.* 1856)
Massage and the original Swedish movements; their application to various diseases of the body. Philadelphia: P. Blakiston, Son & Co., 1890. 97p. DLC: DNLM; PPC **90-6346**

OSTROM, Kurre W[ilhelm] (*b.* 1856)
Massage and the original Swedish movements; their application to various diseases of the body. Lectures before the training schools for nurses connected with the hospital of the University of Pennsylvania, [etc.]. 2nd ed. Philadelphia: P. Blakiston, Son & Co., 1891. 139p. DLC; DNLM **90-6347**

OSTROM, Kurre W[ilhelm] (*b.* 1856)
Massage and the original Swedish movements; their application to various diseases of the body. 3rd ed. Philadelphia: P. Blakiston, Son & Co., 1895. 149p. DNLM **90-6348**

OSTROM, Kurre W[ilhelm] (*b.* 1856)
Massage and the original Swedish movements; their application to various diseases of the body. 4th ed., revised and enlarged. Philadelphia: P. Blakiston's Son & Co., 1899. 168p. DLC; DNLM **90-6349**

OTIS, Edward O[sgood] (1848-1933)
Gymnastic exercise as a prophylactic and curative remedy in chest diseases. [Philadelphia, 1891.] 12p. DNLM **90-6350**

OTIS, Edward O[sgood] (1848-1933)
A case of broken neck. Boston: Damrell & Upham, 1892. 6p. DNLM **90-6351**

OTIS, Edward O[sgood] (1848-1933)
Pulmonary tuberculosis, with special reference to its prophylaxis, hygienic and climatic treatment. Concord, N.H.: Republican Press. Assoc., 1893. 28p. DNLM **90-6352**

OTIS, Edward O[sgood] (1848-1933)
Pulmonary tuberculosis, with special reference to its prophylaxis, hygienic and climatic treatment. Boston: Damrell & Upham, 1893. 29p. DNLM **90-6353**

OTIS, Edward O[sgood] (1848-1933)
Climatic therapeutics in the treatment of pulmonary tuberculosis. Boston: Damrell & Upham, 1894. 16p. DNLM **90-6354**

OTIS, Edward O[sgood] (1848-1933)
Measurements of the chest and lung capacity. Philadelphia, 1895. 3p. DNLM **90-6355**

OTIS, Edward O[sgood] (1848-1933)
Methods of chest examination, supplementary to auscultation and percussion. Boston: Damrell & Upham, 1895. 13p. DNLM **90-6356**

OTIS, Edward O[sgood] (1848-1933)
The treatment of advanced (hopeless) cases of phthisis. Boston: Damrell & Upham, 1895. 12p. DNLM **90-6357**

OTIS, Edward O[sgood] (1848-1933)
The sanatorium or closed treatment of phthisis. New York, 1896. 21p. DNLM **90-6358**

OTIS, Edward O[sgood] (1848-1933)
The value of respiratory gymnastics in maintaining the integrity of the lungs, and as an aid in the treatment of diseases of these organs. Boston: Damrell & Upham, 1896. 12p. DNLM **90-6359**

OTIS, Edward O[sgood] (1848-1933)
Are especial hospitals or homes for consumptives a source of danger to their neighborhood? Boston, 1897. 8p. DNLM **90-6360**

OTIS, Edward O[sgood] (1848-1933)
Auenbrugger and Laennec, the discoverers of percussion and auscultation. Boston: Damrell & Upham, 1898. 29p. DLC; DNLM **90-6361**

OTIS, Edward O[sgood] (1848-1933)
The causes and conditions of pulmonary tuberculosis, and how to avoid them. Philadelphia, 1898. 28p. DNLM **90-6362**

OTIS, Edward O[sgood] (1848-1933)
Hospitals and sanatoria for consumption abroad. Boston, 1898. 28p. 2 plates. DNLM **90-6363**

OTIS, Edward O[sgood] (1848-1933)
Some modern methods of the treatment of phthisis, and its symptoms. [Boston, 1898.] 28p. DNLM **90-6364**

OTIS, Edward O[sgood] (1848-1933)
The tuberculin test in cervical adenitis. New York, 1898. 9p. DNLM **90-6365**

OTIS, Edward O[sgood] (1848-1933)
Some notes upon the tuberculin test. [Philadelphia], 1899. 10p. DNLM **90-6366**

OTIS, Edward O[sgood] (1848-1933)
The struggle against tuberculosis. Boston: Damrell & Upham, 1899. 15p. DNLM **90-6367**

OTIS, Walter J[oseph]
Clinical features and treatment of external piles. Boston: Damrell & Upham, 1895. 10p. DNLM **90-6368**

OTIS, Walter J[oseph]
External piles and their relation to the external hemorrhoidal veins. [Philadelphia, 1895.] 11p. DNLM **90-6369**

OTT, I[saac] (1847-1916)
An improved calorimeter. [New York, 1890.] 4p. DNLM **90-6370**

OTT, I[saac] (1847-1916)
The function of the tuber cinerum. [New York, 1891.] 2p. DNLM **90-6371**

OTT-Isaac] (1847-1916)
The modern antipyretics; their action in health and disease. Easton, Pa.: E. D. Vogel, 1891. 52p. 3 charts. DNLM **90-6372**

OTT, I[saac] (1847-1916)
Vaso-tonic centres in the thalami. [New York, 1891.] 6p. DNLM **90-6373**

OTT, I[saac] (1847-1916)
The modern antipyretics; their action in health and disease. 2nd ed. Easton, Pa.: E. D. Vogel, 1892. 124p. 1 plate. DNLM **90-6374**

OTT, I[saac] (1847-1916)
Phenocoll hydrochlorate. [New York, 1892.] 6p. DNLM **90-6375**

OTT, I[saac] (1847-1916)
The seat of absinthic epilepsy. [New York, 1892.] 3p. DNLM **90-6376**

OTT, I[saac] (1847-1916)
How does atropin elevate the temperature of the body? [New York, 1893.] 6p. DNLM **90-6377**

OTT, I[saac] (1847-1916)
The relation of the nervous system to heat production. [New York, 1893.] 8p. DNLM **90-6378**

OTT, I[saac] (1847-1916)
A vesical detrusor centre in the cerebral peduncles. [Philadelphia, 1894.] 3p. DNLM **90-6379**

OTT, I[saac] (1847-1916)
The thermogenic centre in the tuber cinereum. [Philadelphia, 1895.] 7p. DNLM **90-6380**

OTT, I[saac] (1847-1916)
Dr. Brown-Séquard. An introductory address to the students of the Medico-Chirurgical College of Philadelphia, Oct. 1, 1896. Philadelphia, 1896. 7p. DNLM **90-6381**

OTT, I[saac] (1847-1916)
Glucinum; its physiological action. Philadelphia, 1898. 7p. DNLM **90-6382**

OTT, I[saac] (1847-1916)
How does beta-tetrahydronaphylamin elevate the temperature of the body? Philadelphia, 1898. 2p. DNLM **90-6383**

OTT, I[saac] (1847-1916)
Plassiflora incarnata: its physiological action. [Philadelphia, 1898.] 7p. DNLM **90-6384**

OTT, I[saac] (1847-1916)
The peristaltic action of the intestine. Action of certain agents upon it. New function of the spleen. Philadelphia, 1898. 7p. DNLM **90-6385**

OTT, I[saac] (1847-1916)
Heroin. Philadelphia, 1899. 11p. DNLM **90-6386**

OVERALL, G[eorge] W[hitfield]
Practical electricity in medicine and surgery. Memphis, 1890. 128p. DNLM; OCIM **90-6387**

OVERHOLSER, M. P.
The ultimate physiological units of the organism. New York, 1896. 22p. DNLM **90-6388**

OVERLACH, Martin
Migranin, an approved remedy in the severest cases of migraine. [New York, 1893.] 7p. DNLM **90-6389**

OWENS, John E. (*b.* 1838)
Address in surgery. [Chicago, 1891.] 16p. DNLM **90-6390**

OWENS, John E. (*b.* 1838)
Sketch of the medical bureau, World's Columbian Exposition. Chicago, 1895. 24p. DNLM **90-6391**

PACKARD, Francis R[andolph] (1870-1950)
Scarlatiniform eruptions following operation or traumatism. [New York, 1897.] 18p. DLC; NNNAM **90-6392**

PACKARD, Francis R[andolph] (1870-1950)
A healthy regiment, and the reason it was so. By . . . , assistant surgeon Second Pennsylvania Volunteer Infantry. . . . Charlotte, N.C., 1898. 9p. DLC **90-6393**

PACKARD, Francis R[andolph] (1870-1950)
The care of the sick and wounded in the revolution; by . . . . [Charlotte? N.C., 1899.] 23p. DLC **90-6394**

PACKARD, Francis R[andolph] (1870-1950)
Early methods of medical education in North America. Read before the H. C. Wood Medical Society of the University of Pennsylvania, Jan. 12, 1899. . . . Chicago: American Medical Association Press, 1899. 28p. DLC **90-6395**

PACKARD, Frederick A. (1862-1902)
The signs and symptoms of aortic aneurism. Philadelphia, 1897. 9p. DNLM **90-6396**

PACKARD, Horace (*b.* 1855)
A review of abdominal surgery, with a report of one hundred and twelve cases. Boston: C. A. White & Co., 1890. 31p. DNLM; MBM **90-6397**

PACKARD, Horace (*b.* 1855)
Annual report of surgical operations performed by . . . , for the year 1891; with a report of a third series of abdominal operations, comprising sixty-seven cases. Montpelier, Vt., 1892. 61, 2p. DNLM; MBM **90-6398**

PACKARD, Horace (*b.* 1855)
Annual report of surgical operations for the year 1892; with a report of a fourth series of abdominal operations, comprising twenty-five cases. Boston: A Mudge & Son, 1893. 48p. DNLM; MBM **90-6399**

PACKARD, Horace (*b.* 1855)
A colostomy, a Kraske operation, and a circular enterorrhaphy, all on the same patient. New York, 1899. 3p. DNLM; MBM **90-6400**

PACKARD, Horace (*b.* 1855)
Osteomyelitis. Philadelphia, 1899. 20p. DNLM; MBM **90-6401**

PACKARD, John H[ooker] (1832-1907)
Traumatic separation of the lower epiphysis of the femur. [Philadelphia, 1890.] 10p. DNLM **90-6402**

PACKARD, John H[ooker] (1832-1907)
On surgical shock. Philadelphia: W. J. Dornan, 1892. 16p. DNLM **90-6403**

PACKARD, John H[ooker] (1832-1907)
On the anatomy of oblique inguinal hernia, with special reference to the operation for its radical cure, and a description of modified procedure for this purpose. Philadelphia, 1895. 7p. DNLM **90-6404**

PACKARD, John H[ooker] (1832-1907)
On a modification of the "invagination" method of operating for the radical cure of hernia. [Philadelphia, 1895.] 4p. DNLM **90-6405**

PAGE, Charles E[dward] (*b.* 1840)
Pneumonia and typhoid fever; a study. 2nd ed., revised. Boston: A. Mudge & Son, 1891. 28p. DNLM **90-6406**

PAGE, Charles E[dward] (*b.* 1840)
Pneumonia and typhoid fever; a study. 4th ed., revised. Boston: Damrell & Upham, 1891. 30p. DNLM **90-6407**

PAGE, Charles E[dward] (*b.* 1840)
Typhoid fever; a study. Boston: A Mudge & Son, 1891. 28p. DNLM **90-6408**

PAGE, Charles E[dward] (*b.* 1840)
Some checks to the introduction of the cold-bath treatment. [New York, 1893.] 4p. DNLM **90-6409**

PAGE, Charles E[dward] (*b.* 1840)
Hygienic vs. drug treatment for typhoid fever. New York: Troy Directory Pr. Co., 1894. 12p. DNLM **90-6410**

PAGE, Charles E[dward] (*b.* 1840)
Measles and phenacetin; which killed the patient, the disease or the treatment? Philadelphia, 1894. 5p. DNLM **90-6411**

PAGE, Charles E[dward] (*b.* 1840)
Should therapeutic fasting be termed starving? Its employment in typhoid fever and other diseases. New York: Trow Directory Pr. Co., 1894. 12p. DNLM **90-6412**

PAGE, Henry
Pneumonia with persistent hyperpyrexia, followed by tetany; another case of tetany. Philadelphia, 1895. 6p. DNLM **90-6413**

PAGE, Herbert W[illiam] (1845-1926)
Railroad injuries, special reference to those of the back and nervous system, in their medico-legal and clinical aspects. Philadelphia: P. Blakiston, Son & Co., 1891. 148p. ICJ; MBM; PPC; PU **90-6414**

PAGE, R[ichard] C[hanning] M[oore] (1841-1898)
A handbook of physical diagnosis of diseases of the organs of respiration and heart, and of aortic aneurism. 2nd ed. New York: J. H. Vail & Co., 1890. 291p. NNNAM **90-6415**

PAGE, R[ichard] C[hanning] M[oore] (1841-1898)
A handbook of physical diagnosis of diseases of the organs of respiration and heart, and of aortic aneurism. 3rd ed. New York: J. H. Vail & Co., 1891. 291p. NNNAM
90-6416

PAGE, R[ichard] C[hanning] M[oore] (1841-1898)
A handbook of physical diagnosis of diseases of the organs of respiration and heart, and of aortic aneurism. 4th ed. New York: J. H. Vail & Co., 1891. 291p. NNNAM
90-6417

PAGE, R[ichard] C[hanning] M[oore] (1841-1898)
A handbook of physical diagnosis of diseases of the organs of respiration and heart, and of aortic aneurism. 5th ed. New York: J. H. Vail & Co., 1891. 291p. NNNAM
90-6418

PAGE, R[ichard] C[hanning] M[oore] (1841-1898)
A text-book of the practice of medicine for the use of students and practitioners. New York: William Wood & Co., 1892. 600p. DNLM; NNNAM **90-6419**

PAGE, R[ichard] C[hanning] M[oore] (1841-1898)
Functional dyspepsia, so-called. [New York, 1893.] 8p. DNLM **90-6420**

PAGE, R[ichard] C[hanning] M[oore] (1841-1898)
A handbook of physical diagnosis of diseases of the organs of respiration and heart, and of aortic aneurism. 6th ed. New York: J. H. Vail & Co., 1893. 291p. NNNAM
90-6421

PAGE, R[ichard] C[hanning] M[oore] (1841-1898)
A handbook of physical diagnosis of diseases of the organs of respiration and heart, and of aortic aneurism. 7th ed. New York: J. H. Vail & Co., 1894. 291p. NNNAM
90-6422

PAGE, R[ichard] C[hanning M[oore] (1841-1898)
A handbook of physical diagnosis of diseases of the organs of respiration and heart, and of aortic aneurism. 8th ed. New York: J. H. Vail & Co., 1895. 345p. 7 plates. DNLM; NNNAM
90-6423

PAGE, R[ichard] C[hanning] M[oore] (1841-1898)
A handbook of physical diagnosis of diseases of the organs of respiration and heart, and of aortic aneurism. 9th ed. New York: J. H. Vail & Co., 1895. 345p. NNNAM
90-6424

PAGE, R[ichard] C[hanning] M[oore] (1841-1898)
A handbook of physical diagnosis of diseases of the organs of respiration and heart, and of aortic aneurism. 10th ed. New York: J. H. Vail & Co., 1896. 345p. 8 plates. DNLM: NNNAM
90-6425

PAGET, Stephen (1855-1926)
Ambroise Paré and his times, 1510-1590. New York & London: G. P. Putnam's Sons, 1897. 309p. DNLM; ICU; MH; NN **90-6426**

PAGET, Stephen (1855-1926)
John Hunter, man of science and surgeon. . . . Masters of Medicine Series. New York: Longmans, Green, 1898. 272p. ICU; NIC; MH; NN **90-6427**

PAGE, Stephen (1855-1926)
Essays for students. New York: William Wood & Co., 1899. 177p. DNLM; NNNAM **90-6428**

PAINE, N[athanial] Emmons (*b.* 1853)
Homoeopathy and the insane. Boston: C. A. White & Co., 1892. 14p. DNLM **90-6429**

PALMER, Benjamin W[ood] (*d.* 1895)
Favorite prescriptions of distinguished practitioners, and notes on treatment; compiled from the pulished writings or unpublished records of Drs. Fordyce Barker, Roberts Bartholow. . . . New York: E. B. Treat & Co., 1892. 256p. DNLM; NNNAM [*vel subseq.*] **90-6430**

PALMER, Charles Follen
Inebriety: its source, prevention and cure. New York: Fleming H. Revell Co., 1898. 114p. NIC; NN
90-6431

PALMER, E[dward] R[ush] (1842-1895)
Cases of successful operation for bulbo-membranous close stricture by internal urethrotomy. [New York, 1890.] 4p. DNLM **90-6432**

PALMER, E[dward] R[ush] (1842-1895)
A contribution to the physiology of sexual impotence. New York, 1892. 12p. DNLM **90-6433**

PALMER, Sarah Ellen
The method of Dr. Apostoli. [Portland, 1891.] 7p. DNLM
90-6434

PALMER, Sarah Ellen
Report of four cases of hysterectomy for fibroids. Boston: Damrell & Upham, 1898. 20p. DNLM
90-6435

PALMER, Sarah Ellen
Caesarian section in a generally contracted pelvis, with a true conjugate of seven centimetres minus. Boston: Heintzemann Press, 1899. 2 sheets. DNLM **90-6436**

PALMER, S[tuart] B[ailey] (1822-1903)
Abstract of present office practise. Philadelphia, 1897. 8p. DNLM **90-6437**

PAN-AMERICAN MEDICAL CONGRESS
Preliminary announcement of the first Pan-American Medical Congress, to be held at Washington, D.C., U.S.A., Sept. 5-8, A.D. 1893. [Executive edition.] [1893.] 100p. DNLM
90-6438

PAN-AMERICAN MEDICAL CONGRESS
Hand-book of the first . . . , Washington, D.C., U.S.A., Sept. 5-8, 1893. Philadelphia: Anvil Printing Co.,[1893]. 239p. DNLM; PPC **90-6439**

PAN-AMERICAN MEDICAL CONGRESS
Transactions of the first . . . , held in the city of Washington, D.C., U.S.A., Sept. 5-8, A.D. 1893. Washington: Government Printing Office, 1895. 2 v. [paged consecutively]. DNLM
90-6440

PAN-AMERICAN MEDICAL CONGRESS
Report of committee of the first Pan-American Medical Congress on department of public health for the United States. 55th Cong., 1st sess. S. Doc. No. 38. April 14, 1897. Presented by Mr. Gallinger. [Washington, 1897.] 4p. DNLM
90-6441

PANCOAST, John Ross
Approaching maternity. . . . 10th ed. Philadelphia: The Pancoast Co., 1897. 37p. DLC **90-6442**

PANCOAST, Seth (1823-1889)
. . . The ladies' new medical guide; an instructor, counsellor and friend . . . To which is added much valuable hygienic instruction. . . . By C. C. Vanderbeck. . . . Philadelphia: J. E. Potter & Co., [1890] . 682p. plates. DLC: PPC
90-6443

PARK, J. Walter
A case of acute purulent inflammation of middle ear with two attacks of double optic neuritis, no mastoid complication, frequent delirium, two operations, and recovery. [St. Louis, 1895.] 7p. DNLM **90-6444**

PARK, J. Walter
The medico-legal aspect of eye and ear cases. Chicago, 1896. 7p. DNLM **90-6445**

PARK, J. Walter
Ocular symptoms in cerebral disturbances; with a report of ten cases, and a translation of Dr. Magnus's "Anleitung zur Diagnostic der centralen Störungen des optischen Apparetes." Boston, 1897. 20p. DNLM **90-6446**

PARK, Roswell (1852-1914)
Clinical contributions to the subject of brain surgery. [Philadelphia: Lea Bros. & Co., 1892.] 20p. DNLM
90-6447

PARK, Roswell (1852-1914)
The Mütter lectures on surgical pathology. St. Louis: J. H. Chambers & Co., 1892. 293p. DNLM; NNNAM
90-6448

PARK, Roswell (1852-1914)
The parasitic theory of the aetiology of carcinoma. [New York, 1893.] 16p. DNLM **90-6449**

PARK, Roswell (1852-1914)
The forms of peritonitis, their relation to appendicitis and the aetiology of each. [Detroit, 1894.] 31p. DNLM
90-6450

PARK, Roswell (1852-1914)
On the value of antipyrin to the surgeon. New York: V. Koechel & Co., 1894. 4p. DNLM **90-6451**

PARK, Roswell (1852-1914)
On calcification of the tunica vaginalis as a complication of old hydrocele, orchidomeningitis calcificans. New York: D. Appleton & Co., 1895. 8p. DNLM
90-6452

PARK, Roswell, ed. (1852-1914)
A treatise on surgery by American authors. For students and practitioners of surgery and medicine, edited by Roswell Park. Philadelphia & New York: Lea Bros. & Co., 1896. 2 v. col. plates. DLC; DNLM; NNNAM; PPC
90-6453

PARK, Roswell (1852-1914)
An epitome of the history of medicine. . . . Based upon a course of lectures delivered in the University of Buffalo. Illustrated with portraits and other engravings. Philadelphia, New York [etc.]: The F. A. Davis Co., 1897. 348p. DLC; DNLM; NNNAM; PPC **90-6454**

PARK, Roswell, ed. (1852-1914)
A treatise on surgery; by American authors. For students and practitioners of surgery and medicine. . . . Condensed ed., with revisions. With 625 engravings and 37 full-page plates in colors and monochrome. New York and Philadelphia: Lea Bros. & Co., 1899. 1262p. DLC; NNNAM; PPC; PU
90-6455

PARK, Roswell (1852-1914)
An epitome of the history of medicine. . . . Based upon a course of lectures delivered in the University of Buffalo. 2nd ed. Illustrated with portraits and other engravings. Philadelphia, New York, [etc.]: The F. A. Davis Co., 1899. 370p. DLC; NNNAM; OCIM; PU **90-6456**

PARK, William Hallock (1863-1939)
Diphtheria and allied pseudo-membranous inflammations. A clinical and bacteriological study. New York: Trow, 1892. 48p. 1 plate. DNLM; NNNAM **90-6457**

PARK, William Hallock (1863-1939)
Diphtheria and allied pseudo-membranous inflammations. A clinical and bacteriological study. Second paper. New York, 1893. 23p. DNLM; NNNAM **90-6458**

PARK, William Hallock (1863-1939) and A. W. WILLIAMS
The production of diphtheria toxin. New York, 1896. 22p. DNLM **90-6459**

PARK, William Hallock (1863-1939)
Bacteriology in medicine and surgery. A practical manual for physicians, health officers, and students. By Wm. Hallock Park . . . assisted by A. R. Guerard. . . . New York and Philadelphia: Lea Bros. & Co., [1899] . 693p. 11 col. plates. DLC; DNLM; NNNAM; PPC **90-6460**

PARKE, DAVIS & CO.
A souvenir of the visit of the American Medical Association to Detroit. Detroit, 1892. 59 l. DNLM **90-6461**

PARKE, DAVIS & CO.
Complete catalogue of the products of the laboratories. Revised Feb. 25, 1893. Detroit, 1893. 200p. 14 plates. DNLM; OCIM **90-6462**

PARKE, DAVIS & CO.
Pepsin cordial. Detroit & New York, [1893] . 7 l. DNLM
90-6463

PARKE, DAVIS & CO.
Complete price list of laboratory products. Detroit, 1893. 200p. DNLM **90-6464**

PARKE, DAVIS & CO.
Descriptive catalogue of laboratory products, compressed tablets and tablet triturates. Detroit, 1894. 48p. DLC
90-6465

PARKE, W[illiam] E. (*b.* 1867)
Some complications and sequelae of gynecological operations. New York, 1896. 9p. DNLM **90-6466**

PARKER, Edward F[rost] (*b.* 1867)
Vomiting induced by an elongated uvula; operation; relief. [Philadelphia, 1892.] 3p. DNLM **90-6467**

PARKER, Edward F[rost] (*b.* 1867)
Interesting manifestations of syphilis in the eye and throat; ulcers of the epiglottis, strabismus, and paralysis of ocular muscles. [Philadelphia, 1893.] 6p. DNLM **90-6468**

PARKER, Edward F[rost] (*b.* 1867)
A history of surgery in South Carolina. Being the essay to which the prize offered by Joseph Price, of Philadelphia, was awarded by the South Carolina Medical Association, April, 1893. [Wilmington, 1893.] 20p. DNLM **90-6469**

PARKER, Edward F[rost] (*b.* 1867)
Spurs of the nasal septum and their influence on the respiratory tract. New York: D. Appleton & Co., 1897. 7p. DNLM **90-6470**

PARKER, H[enry] J.
A Rip Van Winkle in the practice of medicine; the efficacy of venesection, cold water, starvation, and some other of the older means of cure in certain diseases. Clayton, Ill., 1899. 132p. DNLM **90-6471**

PARKER, Le Roy (1844-1926) and Robert WORTHINGTON
The law of public health and safety, and the powers and duties of boards of health. Albany, N.Y.: M. Bender, 1892. 471p. DNLM; NN **90-6472**

PARKER, William E.
Bullet-wounds of the abdomen. New Orleans, 1896. 24p. DNLM **90-6473**

PARKER, W[illiam] Thornton (1849-1925)
The regimental Red Cross corps. A manual for medical officers of the U.S. militia. Salem, 1890. 24p. DNLM **90-6474**

PARKER, W[illiam] Thornton (1849-1925)
Boroglyceride in the treatment of diseases of women. [New York], 1891. 8p. DNLM **90-6475**

PARKER, W[illiam] Thornton (1849-1925)
A clothing-case for the Army and Navy and a device for transporting the wounded. Philadelphia, 1894. 4p. 1 plate. DNLM **90-6476**

PARKER, W[illiam] Thornton (1849-1925)
Concerning immunity and the use of normal non-immunized serums. Philadelphia, 1899. 4 l. DNLM **90-6477**

PARKER, William W. (1824-1899)
The rise and decline of homoeopathy. [Richmond, 1890?] 12p. DLC **90-6478**

PARKER, William W. (1824-1899)
The ancient and modern physicians, St. Luke and Jenner. [Richmond, 1891.] 18p. DNLM **90-6479**

PARKER, William W. (1824-1899)
Was Hahnemann insane? Read in the section on neurology and medical jurisprudence at the 46th annual meeting of the American Medical Association at Baltimore, Md., May 7-10, 1895. Chicago: American Medical Association Press, 1896. 8p. DLC **90-6480**

PARKES, Charles T[heodore] (1842-1891)
Uterine myoma, renal calculus, and surgical operations upon the kidney. Chicago: Office Amer. Medical Assoc., 1891. 42p. DNLM **90-6481**

PARKES, Charles T[heodore] (1842-1891)
Clinical lectures on abdominal surgery and other subjects. . . . Ed. by Dr. A. J. Ochsner. Chicago: The W. T. Keener Co., 1896. 477p. DLC; DNLM; OCIM **90-6482**

PARKES, Louis C[oltman]
Hygiene and public health . . . 2nd ed. Philadelphia: P. Blakiston, Son & Co., 1890. 485p. PCC; PU **90-6483**

PARKES, Louis C[oltman]
Hygiene and public health. . . . 3rd ed. Philadelphia: P. Blakiston, Son & Co., 1892. 523p. DNLM; PPC; PU **90-6484**

PARKES, Louis C[oltman]
Hygiene and public health. . . . 4th ed. Philadephia: P. Blakiston, Son & Co., 1895. 531p. DNLM; PPC **90-6485**

PARKES, Louis C[oltman]
The elements of health; an introduction to the study of hygiene. Philadelphia: P. Blakiston, Son & Co., 1895. 246p. DNLM; NNNAM; PPC; PU **90-6486**

PARKES, Louis C[oltman]
Hygiene and public health. . . . 5th ed. Philadelphia: P. Blakiston, Son & Co., 1897. 551p. DNLM; PPC; PU **90-6487**

PARKHILL, Clayton (1860-1902)
A new apparatus for the treatment of fracture of the inferior maxilla. Chicago, 1894. 7p. DNLM **90-6488**

PARKHILL, Clayton (1860-1902)
A case of ileocolostomy by the Murphy method. Excision of the cecum; total exclusion of a portion of the ileum (enteroapokleisis). Philadelphia, 1895. 6p. DNLM **90-6489**

PARKHILL, Clayton (1860-1902)
A new method of closing a laryngeal fistula. Philadelphia, 1895. 2p. 1 plate. DNLM **90-6490**

PARKHILL, Clayton (1860-1892)
Two cases of fracture of the skull. Denver, 1897. 5p. DNLM **90-6491**

PARKHILL, Clayton (1860-1902)
A new apparatus for the fixation of bones after resection and in fractures with a tendency to displacement, with report of cases. [Philadelphia], 1897. 6p. DNLM **90-6492**

PARKHILL, Clayton (1860-1902)
Further observations regarding the use of the bone-clamp in ununited fractures, fractures with mal-union, and recent fractures with a tendency to displacement. Philadelphia, 1898. 18p. DNLM **90-6493**

PARRISH, William H.
Coeliotomy after labor. [Philadelphia, 1892.] 9p. DNLM **90-6494**

PARRISH, William H.
Minute on the death of William Goodell. [New York, 1895.] 1 l. DNLM **90-6495**

PARRISH, William H.
Reopening of the abdomen during the few days following coeliotomy. New York, 1895. 3p. DNLM **90-6496**

PARSONS, Frank S.
Acute rheumatism in children. Chicago, 1890. 12p. DNLM **90-6497**

PARSONS, Frank S.
A contribution to the subject of acute pleurisy; its pathology, etiology, symptomatology, and treatment. [Philadelphia, 1893.] 29p. DNLM; PPC **90-6498**

PARSONS, Frank S.
A practical theory and treatment of pulmonary tuberculosis. Philadelphia, [1895]. 77p. DNLM; PPC; PU **90-6499**

PARSONS, Ralph L[yman] (1828-1914)
Points, facts, opinions, and experiences in favor of the reception of voluntary patients for care and treatment in hospitals for the insane and more especially for care and treatment in private hospitals for the insane. [New York, 1891.] 12p. DNLM **90-6500**

PARSONS, Ralph L[yman] (1828-1914)
A contribution to the study of syphilis of the nervous system. [New York, 1894.] 4p. DNLM **90-6501**

PARSONS, Ralph L[yman] (1828-1914)
Report of a case of acromegaly. [New York, 1894.] 7p. DNLM **90-6502**

PARSONS, Ralph L[yman] (1828-1914)
On the mode of procedure under the new lunacy law of the State of New York, with suggstions of methods under which its provisions can most easily be carried into effect, and also of improvements in the law itself. New York, 1896. 16p. DNLM **90-6503**

PARSONS, Ralph L[yman] (1828-1914)
Objections to and criticisms on the majority report of the committee of the Medico-Legal Society on the existing law for the commitment of the insane. New York, [1896]. 16p. 1 l. DNLM **90-6504**

PARSONS, Ralph L[yman] (1828-1914)
Practical points regarding the senile insanities, with special reference to prophylaxis and management. New York, 1896. 14p. DNLM **90-6505**

PARSONS, Ralph Wait
Some reasons why more original investigation and more literary work is not done by the physicians in large public hospitals for the insane, with a suggestion of certain remedial measures. [New York, 1895.] 8p. DNLM **90-6506**

PARSONS, Stoyell C.
Dr. S. C. Parsons' family physician, contains 200 practical receipts. . . . Savannah, [Ga.]: The Morning News Print, 1890. 197p. DLC **90-6507**

PARSONS, Stoyell C.
The family physician, written in plain language, for practical home use, containing over 200 practical receipts. . . . Savannah, Ga., [1891]. 363p. DLC **90-6508**

PARVIN, Theophilus (1829-1898)
The science and art of obstetrics. . . . 2nd ed. rev. and enl. . . . Philadelphia: Lea Bros. & Co., 1890. 704p. col. plates. DLC; NNNAM; PPC; PU **90-6509**

PARVIN, Theophilus (1829-1898) and F. von WINCKEL
I. The president's address. II. The necessity of the union of obstetrics and gynecology as branches of medical instruction. [Philadelphia, 1893.] 35p. DNLM **90-6510**

PARVIN, Theophilus (1829-1898)
Congratulatory address, delivered at the seventy-fifth anniversary of the Medical Society of the District of Columbia at Rifles' Armory Hall, Washington, D.C., February 16, 1894. Washington, 1894. 6p. DNLM **90-6511**

PARVIN, Theophilus (1829-1898)
Hygiene of the sexual functions. A lecture delivered in the regular course at Jefferson Medical College of Philadelphia. Philadelphia: W. F. Fell & Co., 1894. 16p. DNLM **90-6512**

PARVIN, Theophilus (1829-1898)
In memoriam William Goodell. New York: William Wood & Co., 1894. 11p. DNLM **90-6513**

PARVIN, Theophilus (1829-1898)
The science and art of obstetrics. . . . 3rd ed., carefully rev. . . . Philadelphia: Lea Bros. & Co., 1895. 685p. col. plates. DLC; NNNAM; PPC; PU **90-6514**

PARVIN, Theophilus (1829-1898)
The science and art of obstetrics. 4th ed. Philadelphia: Lea Bros. & Co., 1895. 685p. 2 plates. DNLM; OCIM; PPC; PU **90-6515**

PARVIN, Theophilus (1829-1898)
A physician on vivisection. Extracts from the annual address before the American Academy of Medicine, Washington, May 4, 1891. . . . Cambridge, [Mass.]: J. Wilson & Son, 1895. 16p. DLC; DNLM **90-6516**

PARVIN, Theophilus (1829-1898)
Schleich's local anaesthesia in surgery. [Philadelphia], 1896. 8p. DNLM **90-6517**

PARVIN, Theophilus (1829-1898)
Alumni oration, 1897: The sciences and modern languages in the college curriculum. An address delivered in the auditorium of Pardee Hall, before the alumni, trustees, and faculty, at the sixty-second commencement of Lafayette College, June 22, 1897. Easton, Pa.: Chem. Publ. Co., 1897. 18p. DNLM **90-6518**

PATON, Stewart (1865-1942)
The early diagnosis of dementia paralytica. New York: D. Appleton & Co., 1898. 11p. DNLM **90-6519**

PATRICK, Hugh T[albot] (1860-1939)
Vibratory medicine. Chicago, 1894. 4p. DNLM **90-6520**

PATRICK, Hugh T[albot] (1860-1939)
The Bryson symptom in exophthalmic goitre, with a report of forty cases. [New York: D. Appleton & Co., 1895.] 8p. DNLM **90-6521**

PATRICK, Hugh T[albot] (1860-1939)
The combination of hysteria and organic disease. Detroit: G. S. Davis, 1895. 7p. DNLM **90-6522**

PATRICK, Hugh T[albot] (1860-1939)
Hypnotism at Nancy. [Chicago, 1895.] 10p. DNLM **90-6523**

PATRICK, Hugh T[albot] (1860-1939)
The diagnosis of hysteria. New York, 1896. 48p. DNLM **90-6524**

PATRICK, Hugh T[albot] (1860-1939)
Hysteria blindness and pseudomeningitis, with report of a case treated by hypnotism. Chicago, 1896. 12p. DNLM **90-6525**

PATRICK, Hugh T[albot] (1860-1939)
Anaesthesia of the trunk in locomotor ataxia. New York, 1897. 20p. DNLM **90-6526**

PATRICK, Hugh T[albot] (1860-1939)
A case of syringomyelia with trunk anesthesia. [New York], 1897. 7p. DNLM **90-6527**

PATRICK, Hugh T[albot] (1860-1939)
Remarks on spinal irritation. [Detroit], 1897. 8p. DNLM **90-6528**

PATRICK, Hugh T[albot] (1860-1939)
Neurology in relation to general medicine. [Chicago, 1898.] 4p. DNLM **90-6529**

PATRICK, Hugh T[albot] (1860-1939)
The points of distinction between cerebral syphilis and general paralysis of the insane; two lectures delivered to the medical staff of the Illinois Eastern Hospital for the Insane. New York: D. Appleton & Co., 1898. 64p. DNLM **90-6530**

PATTON, Joseph McIntyre (*b.* 1860)
Some clinical notes on the so-called alkaloids of cod liver oil. Detroit: F. Stearns & Co., 1895. 8p. DNLM **90-6531**

PATTON, Joseph McIntyre (*b.* 1860)
Clinical lectures on the diseases of the heart, lungs, and pleura, designed for the use of practitioners and advanced students of medicine. Chicago: The Clinical Review Publishing Co., 1899. 395p. DNLM; ICJ; IU-M **90-6532**

PAYNTER, J. C[ollins]
Practical treatise on the mouth and its constituents. . . . Philadelphia: [Spangler & Davis, prs.], 1896. 88p. DLC; PPC **90-6533**

PEABODY, Philip G[lendower] (*b.* 1857)
The cruel vivisector, Pasteur, of Paris. [Summer of 1893.] Statement of an eyewitness. Aurora, Ill.: J. Siegmund, [1893?] 7p. DNLM **90-6534**

PEABODY, Philip G[lendower] (*b.* 1857)
Vivisectional cruelties of today. [Summer of 1893] as reported by an eye-witness; address delivered at London, June 14, 1893, with an introduction by Col. Robt. G. Ingersoll. Aurora, Ill.: J. Siegmund, [1893?] 24p. DNLM **90-6535**

PEARCE, Richard Mills, Jr. (1874-1930)
The bacteriology of lobar and lobular pneumonia; various infections due to the diplococcus lanceolatus. Boston: Damrell & Upham, 1897. 15p. DNLM **90-6536**

PEARCE, Richard Mills, Jr. (1874-1930)
The bacteriology of the accessory sinuses of the nose in diphtheria and scarlet fever. Boston, 1899. 9p. DNLM **90-6537**

PEARCE, Richard Mills, Jr. (1874-1930)
Scarlet fever; its bacteriology and gross and minute anatomy. Boston: Municipal Print. Office, 1899. 44p. 2 plates. DNLM **90-6538**

PEASE, Charls G[iffin] (*b.* 1854)
Hints and suggestions as aids in the care and preservation of the teeth and the relation of the dental organs to our health. . . . New York: Boericke, Runyon & Ernesty, 1895. 46p. DLC **90-6539**

PEASE, Edward Allen
A new method of introducing a plate for restoring a depressed nose. Remarks on nephrorraphy; with report of a case of wandering kidney anchored in position through abdominal incision. Boston: Damrell & Upham, 1896. 7p. 3 plates. DNLM **90-6540**

PECKHAM, Adelaide Ward
Study of a case of erysipelas genitalium due to the use of infected ointment. Philadelphia, 1893. 10p. DNLM **90-6541**

PEIRCE, C[yrus] N[ewlin] (1829-1908)
The gouty origin of pyorrhea alveolaris. Philadelphia, 1894. 6p. DNLM **90-6542**

PELLEW, Charles Ernest (*b.* 1863)
Manual of practical medical and physiological chemistry. New York: D. Appleton & Co., 1892. 314p. 8 plates. DNLM; OCIM; PPC; PU **90-6543**

PENNELL, William W[esley] (*b.* 1853)
The genesis of croupous pneumonia. [Philadelphia, 1892.] 9p. DNLM **90-6544**

PENNELL, William W[esley] (*b.* 1853)
Valvular disease of the heart and chronic rheumatism. Philadelphia: Lea Bros. & Co., 1894. 7p. DNLM **90-6545**

PENNINGTON, J. Rawson (1858-1927)
Recent observations in colotomy, with cases in London. Chicago, 1893. 8p. DNLM **90-6546**

PENNINGTON, J. Rawson (1858-1927)
Hygiene of the anus and contiguous parts. Chicago, 1895. 8p. DNLM **90-6547**

PENNINGTON, J. Rawson (1858-1927)
Diseases of the rectum as a cause of auto-infection, with report of cases. Chicago, 1897. 8p. DNLM **90-6548**

PENROSE, Charles Bingham (1862-1925)
Drainage in abdominal surgery. Chicago: Office Amer. Med. Assoc., 1890. 15p. DNLM **90-6549**

PENROSE, Charles Bingham (1862-1925)
The treatment of certain forms of gangrene of the intestine. [Philadelphia: Lea Bros. & Co., 1890.] 11p. DNLM **90-6550**

PENROSE, Charles Bingham (1862-1925)
The treatment of haemorrhoids by excision. [Philadelphia: Lea Bros. & Co., 1890.] 7p. DNLM **90-6551**

PENROSE, Charles Bingham (1862-1925)
Acute peritonitis from gonorrhoea. [Philadelphia: Lea Bros. & Co., 1890.] 5p. DNLM **90-6552**

PENROSE, Charles Bingham (1862-1925) and H. D. BEYEA
Tuberculosis of the Fallopian tubes. (Preliminary paper.) [Philadelphia, 1894.] 20p. DNLM **90-6553**

PENROSE, Charles Bingham (1862-1925)
A case of abdominal hysterectomy in which the ureter was resected and implanted into the bladder. [Philadelphia, 1894.] 3p. DNLM **90-6554**

PENROSE, Charles Bingham (1862-1925)
Hysterectomy for other conditions than fibroid and malignant tumors. Philadelphia, 1894. 12p. DNLM **90-6555**

PENROSE, Charles Bingham (1862-1925)
The work of the gynecological clinic of the hospital of the University of Pennsylvania, 1893-94. [Philadelphia, 1894.] 5p. DNLM **90-6556**

PENROSE, Charles Bingham (1862-1925)
Bacteriology in pelvic surgery. [New York], 1895. 13p. 1 plate. DNLM **90-6557**

PENROSE, Charles Bingham (1862-1925)
Syllabus of the lectures on gynecology, delivered in the medical department of the University of Pennsylvania. Arranged by W. A. N. Dorland. Philadelphia: W. F. Fell & Co., 1896. 149p. DNLM; PU **90-6558**

PENROSE, Charles Bingham (1862-1925)
A textbook of diseases of women. . . . Philadelphia: W. B. Saunders & Co., 1897. 529p. CtY-M; IU-M; NNNAM; PPC **90-6559**

PENROSE, Charles Bingham (1862-1925)
A textbook of diseases of women. . . . 2nd ed. Philadelphia: W. B. Saunders & Co., 1897. 529p. NNNAM; OCIM; PPC; PU **90-6560**

PENROSE, George H. (*b.* 1861)
The treatment of pulmonary tuberculosis by creosote. New York: Trow's Co., 1892. 8p. DNLM **90-6561**

PEPPER, William (1843-1898)
Benjamin Rush. . . . An address delivered before the American Medical Association at its annual meeting in Newport, R.I., June, 1889. . . . Chicago: Printed at the Office of the Association, 1890. 24p. DLC; DNLM **90-6562**

PEPPER, William (1843-1898) and J. P. Crozer GRIFFITH
Varicose aneurisms of the aorta and superior vena cava. [Philadelphia, 1890.] 31p. DNLM **90-6563**

PEPPER, William (1843-1898)
Hepatic fever. The Middleton-Goldsmith lecture for 1890, delivered before the New York Pathological Society, Jan. 15, 1890. [Philadelphia: Lea Bros. & Co., 1890.] 30p. DNLM **90-6564**

PEPPER, William (1843-1898)
The university in modern life; an address delivered before the College Association of the Middle States and Maryland, at its annual meeting at the University of Pennsylvania, November, 1889. Remarks made at the banquet of the alumni of Columbia College, New York, February 3, 1890, in response to the toast: The ideal university. [Philadelphia, 1890.] 20p. DNLM **90-6565**

PEPPER, William (1843-1898)
The address of the president of the Association of American Physicians. [Philadelphia, 1891.] 4p. DNLM **90-6566**

PEPPER, William (1843-1898)
The relation of undergraduate to post-graduate curricula. An address read before the National Educational Association, at Saratoga, July 12th, 1892. . . . Philadelphia: Allen, Lane & Scott's Printing House, 1892. 24p. DLC; DNLM **90-6567**

PEPPER, William (1843-1898)
An epitome of the theory and practice of medicine. Being an outline of lectures delivered at the University of Pennsylvania. . . . Arranged and classified in convenient form for the use of students at the university, from notes taken by the author, James Hawley Burtenshaw. . . . Philadelphia: Press of W. F. Fell & Co., 1892. 391p. DLC; PPC; PU **90-6568**

PEPPER, William (1843-1898)
An address before the first Pan-American Medical Congress, September 6, 1893, in the city of Washington, D.C. Philadelphia: Allen, Lane & Scott, 1893. 34p. DNLM **90-6569**

PEPPER, William (1843-1898)
Higher medical education, the true interest of the public and of the profession; inaugural address at the opening of the four-year course of medical study in the University of Pennsylvania, October 2, 1893. . . . [Philadelphia, 1893.] 16p. DLC; PU **90-6570**

PEPPER, William, ed. (1843-1898)
A text-book of the theory and practice of medicine. By American teachers. . . . Philadelphia: W. B. Saunders, 1893-94. 2 v. col. plates. DLC; DNLM; NNNAM; PPC **90-6571**

PEPPER, William (1843-1898)
Higher medical education, the true interest of the public and of the profession. Two addresses delivered before the Medical Department of the University of Pennsylvania on October 1, 1877, and October 2, 1893. . . . Philadelphia: J. B. Lippincott Co., 1894. 100p. DLC; DNLM; PPC; PU **90-6572**

PEPPER, William (1843-1898)
Daniel Drake; or then and now. The address in medicine delivered before the Mississippi Valley Medical Association, Detroit, Mich., Sept. 4, 1895. Chicago, 1895. 29p. DNLM
90-6573

PEPPER, William (1843-1898) and Alfred STENGEL
Diagnosis of dilatation of the stomach. Philadelphia, 1897. 32p. DNLM **90-6574**

PEPPER, William (1843-1898) and Alfred STENGEL
Abrupt onset in typhoid fever. Philadelphia, 1898. 10p. DNLM
90-6575

PERKINS, Jay
The treatment of pulmonary tuberculosis. [Providence], 1896. 18p. DNLM **90-6576**

PERKINS, Jay
Air embolism; with report of cases, clinical and experimental. Boston: Damrell & Upham, 1897. 20p. DNLM
90-6577

PERKINS, John W.
A case of impacted gallstone with abscess formation; cholecystotomy; recovery. Kansas City, 1891. 8p. DNLM
90-6578

PERKINS, John W.
A hot operating table and its advantages. New York, 1895. 5p. DNLM **90-6579**

PERKINS, John W.
The mechanism and diagnosis of traumatic cerebral lesions. Chicago: Amer. Medical Assoc. Press, 1896. 22p. DNLM
90-6580

PERRY, Alfred W.
Causes, prevention, and treatment of camp diarrhoea. San Francisco, 1898. 4p. DNLM **90-6581**

PERRY, C[harles] H[umphrey] (*b.* 1844)
Astigmatism, according to and contrary to the rule. [Nashville, 1895.] 7p. DNLM **90-6582**

PERRY, Middleton L.
Some studies of the blood in thyroid feeding in insanity. New York, 1896. 18p. DNLM **90-6583**

PERRY, Safford G.
Professional fees. Philadelphia, 1896. 12p. DNLM
90-6584

PERSHING, Edward Hamilton
The treatment of compound fractures. [Philadelphia: Lea Bros. & Co., 1895.] 18p. DNLM **90-6585**

PERSHING, Howell T. (*b.* 1858)
Auditory aphasia. Chicago, 1897. 15p. DNLM
90-6586

PETER, Robert (1805-1894)
Restorative and tonic medicine. Toledo, 1897. 2 l. DNLM
90-6587

PETERS, Hermann (1847-1920)
Pictorial history of ancient pharmacy, with sketches of early medical practice. Transl. from the German and rev. with numerous additions by William Netter. Chicago: G. P. Engelhard & Co., 1899. 184p. DLC; DNLM; PPC; PPHa
90-6588

PETERSON, Frederick (1859-1938)
A case of locomotor ataxia associated with nuclear cranial nerve palsies and with muscular atrophies. New York: M. J. Rooney & Co., [1890]. 8p. DNLM
90-6589

PETERSON, Frederick (1859-1938)
A clinical study of forty-seven cases of paralysis agitans. [New York, 1890.] 18p. DNLM **90-6590**

PETERSON, Frederick (1859-1938)
Homonymous hemiopic hallucinations. [New York, 1890.] 3p. DNLM **90-6591**

PETERSON, Frederick (1859-1938)
Paranoia in two sisters. [St. Louis, 1890.] 12p. DNLM
90-6592

PETERSON, Frederick (1859-1938)
A farther study of anodal diffusion as a therapeutic agent. New York: Trow's, 1891. 11p. DNLM
90-6593

PETERSON, Frederick (1859-1938)
A second note upon homonymous hemiopic hallucinations. [New York]: D. Appleton & Co., 1891. 7p. DNLM
90-6594

PETERSON, Frederick (1859-1938) and A. E. KENNELLY
Some physiological experiments with magnets at the Edison Laboratory. [New York, 1892.] 13p. DNLM
90-6595

PETERSON, Frederick (1859-1938)
Outline of a plan for an epileptic colony. [New York, 1892.] 4p. DNLM **90-6596**

PETERSON, Frederick (1859-1938)
Progress in the care and colonization of epileptics. [New York: Raff & Co., 1892.] 11p. DNLM **90-6597**

PETERSON, Frederick (1859-1938)
Some practical points in the diagnosis of spinal-cord lesions. New York: Trow's Co., 1892. 12p. DNLM
90-6598

PETERSON, Frederick (1859-1938)
The treatment of epilepsy. [Buffalo, 1892.] 6p. DNLM
90-6599

PETERSON, Frederick (1859-1938)
Three cases of acute mania from inhaling carbon bisulphide. Boston: Damrell & Upham, 1892. 7p. DNLM
90-6600

PETERSON, Frederick (1859-1938)
Wintering in Egypt. New York: Trow Co., 1892. 16p. DNLM
90-6601

PETERSON, Frederick (1859-1938)
Hydrotherapy in the treatment of nervous and mental diseases. [Philadelphia, 1893.] 9p. DNLM **90-6602**

PETERSON, Frederick (1859-1938)
Tetra-ethyl-ammonium. A solvent for uric acid discovered at the Edison Laboratory. [New York, 1893.] 9p. DNLM
90-6603

PETERSON, Frederick (1859-1938)
The treatment of alcoholic inebriety. [Chicago, 1893.] 12p. DNLM **90-6604**

PETERSON, Frederick (1859-1938) and Charles H. LANGDON
A study of the temperature in twenty-five cases of general paralysis of the insane. [New York, 1893.] 23p. DNLM
90-6605

PETERSON, Frederick (1859-1938)
The treatment of the insane outside of asylums. [Philadelphia, 1893.] 15p. DNLM **90-6606**

PETERSON, Frederick (1859-1938)
Notes upon some kymographic tracings of tremor. New York, 1894. 71p. DNLM **90-6607**

PETERSON, Frederick (1859-1938)
Deformities of the hard palate in degenerates. New York & Philadelphia, 1895. 16p. DNLM **90-6608**

PETERSON, Frederick (1859-1938)
Hydrocephalic idiocy. New York: D. Appleton & Co., 1896. 19p. DNLM **90-6609**

PETERSON, Frederick (1859-1938) and Pearce BAILEY
Results of thyreoid treatment in sporadic cretinism. New York, 1896. 12p. DNLM **90-6610**

PETERSON, Frederick (1859-1938)
The psychology of the idiot. Utica, 1896. 25p. DNLM
90-6611

PETERSON, Frederick (1858-1938)
The stigmata of degeneration. Utica, N.Y., 1896. 19p. 10 plates. DNLM **90-6612**

PETERSON, Frederick (1859-1938)
Beneficial effects of the withdrawal of bromides in the treatment of epilepsy. New York: D. Appleton & Co., 1897. 9p. DNLM **90-6613**

PETERSON, Frederick (1859-1938)
Katatonia (Katatonie of Kahlbaum; katatonische Verrücktheit of Schüle). [Baltimore, 1897.] 22p. DNLM
90-6614

PETERSON, Frederick (1859-1938)
A case of amaurotic family idiocy, with autopsy. [New York, 1898.] 11p. DNLM **90-6615**

PETERSON, Frederick (1859-1938)
Colonies for epileptics. Philadelphia, 1898. 12p. DNLM
90-6616

PETERSON, Frederick (1859-1938)
New paths in psychiatry. Philadelphia, 1898. 6p. DNLM
90-6617

PETERSON, Frederick (1859-1938)
Vibratory therapeutics. Philadelphia, 1898. 7p. DNLM
90-6618

PETERSON, Reuben (1862-1942)
A review of twenty-five consecutive cases of abdominal section. Toledo, 1892. 16p. DNLM **90-6619**

PETERSON, Reuben (1862-1942)
A review of twenty-five consecutive cases of abdominal section. [Detroit, 1892.] 15p. 1 table. DNLM
90-6620

PETERSON, Reuben (1862-1942)
A case of appendicitis occurring on the seventh day following labor; rupture into the bowel; recovery. [Philadelphia, 1893.] 8p. DNLM **90-6621**

PETERSON, Reuben (1862-1942)
A case of rupture of an ovarian cyst. New York: William Wood & Co., 1893. 3p. DNLM **90-6622**

PETERSON, Reuben (1862-1942)
The treatment of pus in the pelvis by vaginal incision. Detroit & Ann Arbor, 1893. 3p. DNLM **90-6623**

PETERSON, Reuben (1862-1942)
Tubal and peritoneal tuberculosis. New York: William Wood & Co., 1893. 15p. DNLM **90-6624**

PETERSON, Reuben (1862-1942)
Pelvic abscess and its treatment. Detroit & Ann Arbor, [1894]. 6p. DNLM **90-6625**

PETERSON, Reuben (1862-1942)
A surgical kit containing all the essentials for aseptic operations at private residences. New York, 1894. 6p. DNLM
90-6626

PETERSON, Reuben (1862-1942)
Abdominal nephrectomy, with case. [Detroit, 1895.] 8p. DNLM **90-6627**

PETERSON, Reuben (1862-1942)
Abdominal nephrectomy, with case. Grand Rapids, Mich.: Seymour & Muir, 1895. 6p. DNLM
90-6628

PETERSON, Reuben (1862-1942)
Hysterectomy for puerperal infection. Chicago, 1895. 12p. DNLM **90-6629**

PETERSON, Reuben (1862-1942)
The influence of pregnancy upon dental caries. Philadelphia, 1895. 6p. DNLM **90-6630**

PETERSON, Reuben (1862-1942)
The need of more medical reference libraries, and the way in which they can be established. New York, 1895. 14p. DNLM
90-6631

PETERSON, Reuben (1862-1942)
Suspension of the retrodisplaced uterus by the utero-ovarian ligaments, with a report of seventeen cases. New York: William Wood & Co., 1895. 17p. DNLM **90-6632**

PETERSON, Reuben (1862-1942)
Hysterectomy as an accompaniment to bilateral removal of the appendages. New York, 1896. 8p. DNLM
90-6633

PETERSON, Reuben (1862-1942)
The prevention of pelvic disease. Chicago, 1896. 12p. DNLM **90-6634**

PETERSON, Reuben (1862-1942)
Treatment of pelvic suppuration by abdominal section without hysterectomy. New York, 1896. 6p. DNLM **90-6635**

PETERSON, Reuben (1862-1942)
A case of beginning tuberculosis of the mesenteric lymph glands revealed by an exploratory coeliotomy. New York, 1897. 2p. DNLM **90-6636**

PETERSON, Reuben (1862-1942)
Tuberculosis of the mesenteric lymph-glands, and its treatment by abdominal section. Philadelphia, 1897. 19p. DNLM **90-6637**

PETERSON, Reuben (1862-1942)
The need of more medical reference libraries, and the way in which they can be established. Easton, Pa., 1897. 9p. DNLM **90-6638**

PETERSON, Reuben (1862-1942)
A clinical and pathological study of five recent cases of hysterectomy for fibromata. New York, 1898. 11p. DNLM **90-6639**

PETERSON, Reuben (1862-1942)
The etiology of non-malignant rectal stricture in women. Philadelphia, 1899. 12p. 3 plates. DNLM **90-6640**

PETERSON, Reuben (1862-1942)
Peripheral nerve transplantation, with the report of a case in which the sciatics of a dog were transplanted successfully between the severed ends of the median and ulnar nerves of a man. Philadelphia, 1899. 29p. DNLM **90-6641**

PETERSON, Reuben (1862-1942)
Right inguinal hernia of the vermiform appendix. Chicago, 1899. 4p. DNLM **90-6642**

PETTYJOHN, E[lmore] S[loan] (*b.* 1855)
Rheumatism; its pathology and modern treatment. St. Louis, 1895. 6p. DNLM **90-6643**

PETTYJOHN, E[lmore] S[loan] (*b.* 1855)
Constipation; some of its effects and its non-medical treatment. Chicago, 1896. 8p. DNLM **90-6644**

PETTYJOHN, E[lmore] S[loan] (*b.* 1855)
Erb's primary muscular atrophy. Chicago, 1896. 11p. DNLM **90-6645**

PETTYJOHN, E[lmore] S[loan] (*b.* 1855)
Internal cerebral meningitis chronica; notes on diagnosis and treatment. Chicago, 1898. 8p. DNLM **90-6646**

PETTYJOHN, E[lmore] S[loan] (*b.* 1855)
Sleeplessness; its cause and treatment. Detroit & Ann Arbor, 1898. 4p. DNLM **90-6647**

PEYER, Alexander
On affections of the stomach in diseases of the male genital organs. New York: William Wood & Co., 1890. 35p. NNNAM; NN [Printed out of Wood's medical and surgical monographs, vol. 8, no. 2, pp. 473-508 (1890)] **90-6648**

PEYER, Alexander
An atlas of clinical microscopy. . . . Transl. by Alfred C. Girard. 1st American from the manuscript of the 2nd German ed., with additions. Ninety plates with one hundred and five illustrations. New York: D. Appleton & Co., 1890 [1885]. 194p. DLC; NcD; PPL; PU **90-6649**

PEYSER, Mark W[allace]
Manual of the physics of physiology. Prepared for students of medicine. Richmond: H. T. Ezekiel, [1899]. 119p. DLC **90-6650**

PHARMACEUTICAL ERA
The era formulary. 5000 formulas for druggists. A collection of original and prize formulas, to which has been added a selection of formulas from standard authorities in the English, French and German. . . . 1st ed. . . . Comp. and ed. by the Pharmaceutical Era. New York: D. O. Haynes & Co., [1893]. 462p. DLC; NNNAM; OCLloyd **90-6651**

THE PHARMACOPOEIA of the United States of America. 7th decennial revision (1890). By authority of the National Convention for Revising the Pharmacopoeia, held at Washington, A.D., 1890. Philadelphia: J. B. Lippincott Co., 1893. 602p. DLC; DNLM; PPC; PU **90-6652**

THE PHARMACOPOEIA of the United States of America. Seventh decennial revision (1890). Published by the committee of revision and publication (1890-1900). Part I. Comprising abstracts of papers up to July 1, 1896. New York, 1897. 183p. DNLM; NNNAM **90-6653**

PHELPS, A[bel] M[ix] (1851-1902)
The question of what produces and what prevents ankylosis of joints. New York, 1890. 12p. DNLM **90-6654**

PHELPS, A[bel] M[ix] (1851-1902)
Congenital dislocation of the hip. [Philadelphia, 1891.] 11p. DNLM **90-6655**

PHELPS, A[bel] M[ix] (1851-1902)
The present status of the open incision method for talipes varo-equinus. Danbury, Conn., 1891. 13p. DNLM **90-6656**

PHELPS, A[bel] M[ix] (1851-1902)
Transplantation of tissue from lower animals to man, and a report of the case of bone-transplantation at Charity Hospital, Blackwell's Island, N.Y. New York: Trow, 1891. 22p. DNLM **90-6657**

PHELPS, A[bel] M[ix] (1851-1902)
The wood corset. With improvements, for the treatment of lateral curvature and Pott's disease of the spine. Danbury, Conn., 1892. 8p. DNLM **90-6658**

PHELPS, A[bel] M[ix] (1851-1902)
A clinical lecture on hip-joint disease and club-foot. [New York], 1893. 8p. DNLM **90-6659**

PHELPS, A[bel] M[ix] (1851-1902)
An address delivered before the American Orthopedic Association, Washington, D.C., in May, 1894. [Philadelphia, 1894.] 12p. DNLM **90-6660**

PHELPS, A[bel] M[ix] (1851-1902)
Etiology of the deformities occurring in knee-joint disease. [Philadelphia, 1894.] 8p. DNLM **90-6661**

PHELPS, A[bel] M[ix] (1851-1902)
A new operation for hernia. New York: D. Appleton & Co., 1894. 18p. DNLM **90-6662**

PHELPS, A[bel] M[ix] (1851-1902)
What shall we do for hip-joint disease? Philadelphia, 1894. 5p. DNLM **90-6663**

PHELPS, A[bel] M[ix] (1851-1902)
Modern orthopedic surgery. A reply to Dr. Shaffer. New York, 1895. 21p. DNLM **90-6664**

PHELPS, A[bel] M[ix] (1851-1902)
Modern orthopedic surgery, what it is and what it should be, as the members of the American Orthopedic Association by a vast majority proclaim. An answer to an attack made upon me personally and upon orthopedic surgeons. Danbury, Conn., 1895. 35p. DNLM **90-6665**

PHELPS, A[bel] M[ix] (1851-1902)
The plaster of Paris; wood, aluminum, and other spinal supports. New York, 1895. 12p. DNLM **90-6666**

PHELPS, A[bel] M[ix] (1851-1902)
Purulent tuberculosis and rheumatic hip-joint disease. Peoria, 1898. 16p. DNLM **90-6667**

PHELPS, Charles (1834-1913)
The treatment of simple fracture of the patella by wiring. New York, 1890. 58p. 1 tab. DNLM; NNNAM **90-6668**

PHELPS, Charles (1834-1913)
A clinico-pathological study of injuries of the head, with special reference to lesions of the brain substance. [New York, 1893.] 98p. DNLM; NNNAM **90-6669**

PHELPS, Charles (1834-1913)
The treatment of certain forms of fracture. [New York, 1893.] 27p. DNLM; NNNAM **90-6670**

PHELPS, Charles (1834-1913)
A case of intra-abdominal sarcoma. New York, 1894. 3p. DNLM; NNNAM **90-6671**

PHELPS, Charles (1834-1913)
Two cases of malignant disease; an osteosarcoma involving an interior cranial fossa, and an epithelioma of the larynx. New York, 1894. 9p. DNLM; NNNAM **90-6672**

PHELPS, Charles (1834-1913)
The differential diagnosis of traumatic intracranial lesions. [New York, 1895.] 150p. DNLM; NNNAM **90-6673**

PHELPS, Charles (1834-1913)
The medical profession at the close of the nineteenth century. An address. New York: D. Appleton & Co., 1897. 38p. DNLM; NNNAM **90-6674**

PHELPS, Charles (1834-1913)
Traumatic injuries of the brain and its membranes, with a special study of pistol-shot wounds of the head in their medico-legal and surgical relations. New York: D. Appleton & Co., 1897. 582p. DNLM; NNNAM **90-6675**

PHELPS, Charles (1834-1913)
The history of a case of cerebral abscess of unusual origin. New York, 1898. 16p. 1 plate. DNLM; NNNAM **90-6676**

PHELPS, Charles (1834-1913)
The results of open operation in the treatment of recent fracture of the patella. New York: D. Appleton & Co., 1898. 21p. DNLM; NNNAM **90-6677**

PHELPS, Charles (1834-1913)
The Sheldon murder trial. A review of the medical evidence relating to pistol-shot wounds of the head. New York, 1899. 51p. DNLM; NNNAM **90-6678**

PHELPS, R[obert] M.
A consideration of knee-jerk symptom. [St. Paul, 1892.] 6 l. DNLM **90-6679**

PHELPS, R[obert] M.
A new consideration of hereditary chores. [New York, 1892.] 12p. DNLM **90-6680**

PHELPS, R[obert] M.
Are there degrees of insanity? St. Paul, 1894. 10p. DNLM **90-6681**

PHELPS, R[obert] M.
Inebriety as a disease analytically studied. Philadelphia, 1894. 8p. DNLM **90-6682**

PHILADELPHIA COLLEGE OF PHARMACY
Annual announcements for the sessions of 1890-91 to 1899-1900 (70.-79.); 1901-02 to 1907-08 (81.-87.). Philadelphia, 1890-1907. DNLM **90-6683**

PHILADELPHIA COLLEGE OF PHARMACY
Condensed history, with the original and revised constitution; by-laws of the College and Board of Trustees, with resolutions pertaining thereunto; roll of members, officers, and standing committees. [Philadelphia], 1891. 65p. PPC; PU **90-6684**

PHILADELPHIA COUNTY MEDICAL SOCIETY
Annual meeting in the interest of the Mutual Aid Association; De Forest Willard, president of the County Society, in the chair. Philadelphia, 1893. 11p. DNLM **90-6685**

PHILADELPHIA COUNTY MEDICAL SOCIETY
[Circular against advertisements of secret nostrums in medical journals.] [Philadelphia, 1895.] 7p. DNLM **90-6686**

PHILADELPHIA COUNTY MEDICAL SOCIETY
Semi-centennial anniversary, January 16, 1899. [Philadelphia, 1899?] 95p. DNLM **90-6687**

PHILADELPHIA DISPENSARY FOR SKIN DISEASES
Medical reports, covering a period of ten years and nine months (February, 1880 to November, 1890) by Henry W. Stelwagon. [Philadelphia, 1893.] 23p. DNLM; PHi; PPHa **90-6688**

PHILADELPHIA POLYCLINIC AND COLLEGE FOR GRADUATES IN MEDICINE
Annual reports of the board of trustees and officers to the corporation. 7.-16., 1889-98. Including the Polyclinic Hospital, the College Department, the Training School for Nurses, and the Ladies' Aid Society. Philadelphia, 1890-99. DNLM
90-6689

PHILADELPHIA POLYCLINIC AND COLLEGE FOR GRADUATES IN MEDICINE
Annual announcements for the sessions of 1891-92 to 1893-94 (9.-11.); 1896-97 (14.); 1897-98 (15.); 1899-1900 (17.); 1902-03 (20.); 1903-04 (21.). Philadelphia, 1891-1903. DNLM
90-6690

PHILADELPHIA POLYCLINIC AND COLLEGE FOR GRADUATES IN MEDICINE
A week in ophthalmology at the Philadelphia Polyclinic, Dec. 15 to 22, 1892. [Philadelphia, 1893.] 4 l. DNLM
90-6691

PHILADELPHIA POLYCLINIC AND COLLEGE FOR GRADUATES IN MEDICINE
Department of practical instruction in massage. [Philadelphia, 1893.] 1 sheet. DNLM **90-6692**

PHILADELPHIA POLYCLINIC AND COLLEGE FOR GRADUATES IN MEDICINE
The polyclinic laboratories. Department of photo-therapy and radiography. Announcement. [Philadelphia, 1893.] 1 sheet. DNLM **90-6693**

PHILLIPS, George Marquet (*b.* 1862)
A handbook of genito-urinary surgery and venereal diseases. . . . [St. Louis: Shallcross-McCallum Co., printers, 1898.] 313p. DLC **90-6694**

PHILLIPS, R[ichard] J[ones] (*b.* 1861)
Spectacles and eyeglasses. Their forms, mounting, and proper adjustment. Philadelphia: P. Blakiston, Son & Co., 1892. 97p. DLC; DNLM; PPC; PU **90-6695**

PHILLIPS, R[ichard] J[ones] (*b.* 1861)
Spectacles and eyeglasses. Their forms, mounting, and proper adjustment. 2nd ed. Philadelphia: P. Blakiston, Son & Co., 1895. 105p. DLC; DNLM; PPC **90-6696**

PHILLIPS, S. Latimer
Rupture of the membrana tympani by the injection of warm water into the auditory canal for the removal of impacted cerumen. [Atlanta, 1891.] 2 l. DNLM
90-6697

PHILLIPS, S. Latimer
A peculiar form of iritis characterized by a gelatinous mass in anterior chamber at times resembling a cataractous lens. Atlanta, 1896. 4p. DNLM **90-6698**

PHILLIPS, Wendell C. (*b.* 1857)
Translumination of the antrum of Highmore, nasal cavities, frontal sinuses, and larynx, with remarks on the treatment of empyema of the antrum. Philadelphia, 1891. 6p. DNLM
90-6699

PHILLIPS, Wendell C. (*b.* 1857)
A case of so-called laryngeal vertigo or laryngeal epilepsy. [Philadelphia, 1892.] 6p. DNLM
90-6700

PHILLIPS, Wendell C. (*b.* 1857)
Some observations upon the sequelae of adenoid or lymphoid tissue in the naso- and oro-pharynx. Philadelphia, 1899. 8p. DNLM **90-6701**

PHYSICIANS', dentists', and druggists' directory of Maryland, District of Columbia, and Virginia. Comprising list of physicians and surgeons, dentists, and druggists, arranged alphabetically by post-offices. Baltimore: G. Gonsier & Co., 1892. 232p. DNLM; MdU-D **90-6702**

PHYSICIANS', dentists', and druggists' directory of New York and Connecticut. Comprising list of physicians and surgeons, dentists, and druggists, arranged alphabetically by post-office, with population and location. The physician's school practice is indicated by the appellations: (R) Regular, (H) Homoeopathic, and (E) Eclectic, together with his college and year of graduation. Chicago: G. Gonsier & Co., 1895. 398p. DNLM; IU-M; OCIM **90-6703**

PHYSICIANS' interpreter in four languages, English, French, German, and Italian. . . . Specially arranged for diagnosis. . . . Philadelphia: F. A. Davis, Publisher, 1890 [1889]. 206p. DLC; MB; NN; PPC **90-6704**

PICK, T[homas] Pickering (1841-1919)
Fractures and dislocations. . . . Philadelphia: Lea Bros. & Co., 1890 [1885]. 530p. 93 engravs. CtY-M; ICJ; OCIM; PPC
90-6705

PICKEL, J. W.
A case of complete inversion and prolapsus of the uterus. New York, 1894. 2p. DNLM **90-6706**

PIERCE, Norval H[arvey] (1863-1946)
Syphilis of the nose; with reports of cases. New York, 1895. 22p. DNLM **90-6707**

PIERCE, Norval H[arvey] (1863-1946)
Chronic suppurative otitis media. New York, 1898. 12p. DNLM **90-6708**

PIERCE, Ray Vaughn (*b.* 1840)
The people's common sense medical adviser in plain English; or, Medicine simplified. . . . 30th ed. 710th thousand. . . . Buffalo, N.Y.: World's Dispensary Printing Office & Bindery, 1895. 1008p. col. plates. DLC **90-6709**

PIERSOL, G[eorge] A[rthur] (1856-1924)
Development of pigment within the epidermis. [Philadelphia, 1890.] 9p. 1 plate. DNLM **90-6710**

PIERSOL, G[eorge] A[rthur] (1856-1924)
The advancement of American medicine. Philadelphia: G. H. Buchanan & Co., 1890. 25p. DNLM; PPC
90-6711

PIERSOL, G[eorge] A[rthur] (1856-1924)
Text-book of normal histology, including an account of the development of the tissues and of the organs. Philadelphia: J. B. Lippincott Co., 1893. 439p. DNLM; NNNAM; PPC; PU
90-6712

PIERSOL, G[eorge] A[rthur] (1856-1924)
Text-book of normal histology, including an account of the development of the tissues and of the organs. 2nd ed. Philadelphia: J. B. Lippincott Co., 1894. 439p. DNLM; IU-M; PPC; PU
90-6713

PIERSOL, G[eorge] A[rthur] (1856-1924)
Text-book of normal histology, including an account of the development of the tissues and of the organs. 3rd ed. Philadelphia: J. B. Lippincott, 1895. 439p. DNLM; NNNAM; PPC; PU
90-6714

PIERSOL, G[eorge] A[rthur] (1856-1924)
Text-book of normal histology, including an account of the development of the tissues and of the organs. 4th ed. Philadelphia: J. B. Lippincott Co., 1896. 439p. NNNAM; PPC; PU
90-6715

PIERSOL, G[eorge] A[rthur] (1856-1924)
Text-book of normal histology, including an account of the development of the tissues and of the organs. 5th ed. Philadelphia: J. B. Lippincott Co., 1898. 439p. CtY-M; MBM; PPC; PU
90-6716

PIERSOL, G[eorge] A[rthur] (1856-1924)
Text-book of normal histology, including an account of the development of the tissues and of the organs. 6th ed. Philadelphia: J. B. Lippincott Co., 1899. 439p. ICU; IEN-M; PPC; PU
90-6717

PIERSOL, G[eorge] A[rthur] (1856-1924)
Text-book of normal histology, including an account of the development of the tissues and of the organs. 7th ed. Philadelphia: J. B. Lippincott Co., 1899. 439p. NNNAM; PPJ; PPC; PU
90-6718

PIFFARD, Henry Granger (1842-1910)
The modern treatment of eczema. . . . Detroit, Mich.: G. S. Davis, 1890. 54p. DLC **90-6719**

PIFFARD, Henry Granger (1842-1910)
A practical treatise on diseases of the skin, by Henry G. Piffard . . . assisted by Robert M. Fuller. . . . New York, [etc.]: D. Appleton & Co., 1891. 157p. 50 plates. DLC; DNLM; NNNAM **90-6720**

PIFFARD, Henry Granger (1842-1910)
Further improvements in the adaptation of the Edison current to general office use. [New York: D. Appleton & Co., 1891.] 16p. DNLM **90-6721**

PIFFARD, Henry Granger (1842-1910)
Feeding fat into milk. New York, 1896. 8p. DNLM
90-6722

PILCHER, James Evelyn (1857-1911)
First aid in illness and injury; comprised in a series of chapters on the human machine, its structure, its implements of repair, and the accidents and emergencies to which it is liable. . . . New York: C. Scribner's Sons, 1892. 304p. DLC; DNLM; NNNAM **90-6723**

PILCHER, James Evelyn (1857-1911)
First aid in illness and injury; comprised in a series of chapters on the human machine, its structure, its implements of repair, and the accidents and emergencies to which it is liable. . . . Revised ed. New York: C. Scribner's Sons, 1894. 322p. 1 plate. DNLM; NNNAM **90-6724**

PILCHER, James Evelyn (1857-1911)
Chauliac and Mondeville; a surgical retrospect. Philadelphia, 1895. 19p. DNLM **90-6725**

PILCHER, James Evelyn (1857-1911)
Notes on the present status of military medicine and surgery. [Columbus, 1896.] 6p. DNLM **90-6726**

PILCHER, James Evelyn (1857-1911)
Felix Würtz and Pierre Franco; a glimpse of sixteenth century surgery. Philadelphia, 1896. 30p. DNLM; PPC
90-6727

PILCHER, James Evelyn (1857-1911)
First aid in illness and injury; comprised in a series of chapters on the human machine, its structure, its implements of repair, and the accidents and emergencies to which it is liable. . . . 3rd ed. New York: C. Scribner's Son, 1897. 322p. NNNAM
90-6728

PILCHER, James Evelyn (1857-1911)
First aid in illness and injury; comprised in a series of chapters on the human machine, its structure, its implements of repair, and the accidents and emergencies to which it is liable. . . . 4th ed. New York: C. Scribner's Sons, 1897. 322p. 2 plates. DNLM; NNNAM **90-6729**

PILCHER, James Evelyn (1857-1911)
First aid in illness and injury; comprised in a series of chapters on the human machine, its structure, its implements of repair, and the accidents and emergencies to which it is liable. . . . 5th ed. New York: C. Scribner's Sons, 1898. 322p. NNNAM
90-6730

PILCHER, James Evelyn (1857-1911)
First aid in illness and injury; comprised in a series of chapters on the human machine, its structure, its implements of repair, and the accidents and emergencies to which it is liable. . . . 6th ed., rev. with 175 illustrations. New York: C. Scribner's Sons, 1899. 322p. DLC; NNNAM **90-6731**

PILCHER, Lewis Stephen (1845-1934)
Castration for prostatic hypertrophy. [n. p., 1893, *vel subseq.*] 2 galley sheets. DNLM **90-6732**

PILCHER, Lewis Stephen (1845-1934)
The treatment of wounds: its principles and practice, general and special . . . with one hundred and forty-two wood engravings. . . . New York: William Wood & Co., 1899. 453p. DLC; DNLM; NNNAM **90-6733**

PINTO, Viviato J.
A case of adipocere of a foetus. New York, 1894. 2p. DNLM
90-6734

PINTO, Viviato J.
The puerperium. [New York], 1895. 2p. DNLM
90-6735

PINTO, Viviato J.
Midwifery in Goa. New York, 1896. 5p. DNLM
90-6736

PITTSBURGH DENTAL COLLEGE. DENTAL DEPARTMENT OF THE WESTERN UNIVERSITY OF PENNSYLVANIA
Catalogues and circulars of information for the sessions of 1897-98 (2.); 1899-1900 to 1903-04 (4.-8.); 1905-06 (10.); 1906-07 (11.). Pittsburgh, 1897-1906 DNLM [List of graduates from 1897 to 1905 in announcement for 1906-07.]
90-6737

PLATT, Charles (*b.* 1869)
Laboratory notes in qualitative analysis and medical chemistry. . . . Philadelphia: J. J. McVey, 1895. 109p. DLC; PU
90-6738

PLATT, Isaac Hull
A case of rheumatic fever without joint symptoms. Philadelphia, 1893. 5p. DNLM **90-6739**

PLATT, S[mith] H.
The secrets of health, or how not to be sick and how to get well from sickness. New York: O. Judd Co., 1895. 576p. DNLM; NNNAM **90-6740**

PLATT, Walter B.
Baron von Langenbeck, surgeon-general of the German army, professor of surgery in the University of Berlin. Baltimore, 1894. 6p. DNLM **90-6741**

PLATT, Walter B.
Some account of Baron Larrey, surgeon to the armies of France under Napoleon First. Baltimore, 1894. 6p. DNLM
90-6742

PLATT, Walter B.
Medicine as a profession. Boston: Damrell & Upham, 1899. 12p. DNLM **90-6743**

PLATT, Walter B.
A report of thirty-five cases of hip-joint disease treated at the Robert Garrett Hospital for Children, Baltimore. [Philadelphia], 1899. 11p. DNLM **90-6744**

PLAYFAIR SCHOOL OF MIDWIFERY, CHICAGO
Annual announcements for the sessions of 1898; 1899. Chicago: Rogers & Hall Co., 1898-99. 16p.; 20p. DNLM
90-6745

PLAYFAIR, William Smoult (1836-1903)
A treatise on the science and practice of midwifery. . . . 6th American from the 8th English ed. With notes and additions by Robert P. Harris. . . . Philadelphia: Lea Bros. & Co., 1893. 697p. plates. DLC; NNNAM; PPC; PU **90-6746**

PLAYFAIR, William Smoult (1836-1903)
A treatise on the science and practice of midwifery. . . . 7th American from the 9th English ed., with 7 plates and 207 illustrations. Philadelphia and New York: Lea Bros. & Co., 1898. 687p. col. plates. DLC; OCIM; PPC; PU
90-6747

PLUMMER, Edward M[ark]
Intubation, with an analysis of fifty cases. Portland: S. Berry, 1896. 24p. DNLM **90-6748**

PLUMMER, Edward M[ark]
Intubation, with an analysis of fifty cases. Boston, 1897. 16p. DNLM **90-6749**

PLUMMER, Edward M[ark]
Athletics and games of the ancient Greeks. Cambridge, Mass., 1898. 61p. DNLM **90-6750**

PLUMMER, S[amuel] C. (1821?-1900)
Punctured wounds of the feet. A report of two hundred and three cases treated at the Medical Bureau, World's Columbian Exposition, during the "construction period," June 1st, 1891, to May 1st, 1893. Chicago, 1893. 8p. DNLM
90-6751

POLAK, John O[sborn] (1870-1931)
Report of two cases of puerperal fever. [Philadelphia: Lea Bros. & Co., 1892.] 6p. DNLM **90-6752**

POLAK, John O[sborn] (1870-1931)
A case of vomiting of pregnancy, resulting in the induction of abortion. [Philadelphia, 1893.] 4p. DNLM
90-6753

POLAK, John O[sborn] (1870-1931)
Treatment of eclampsia. New York, 1895. 7p. DNLM
90-6754

POLAK, John O[sborn] (1870-1931)
A contribution to the study of occipito-posterior position of the vertex. [Philadelphia: Lea Bros. & Co., 1895.] 6p. DNLM
90-6755

POLITZER, Adam (1835-1920)
The membrana tympani in health and disease. . . . Clinical contributions to the diagnosis and treatment of diseases of the ear, with Supplement. . . . Transl. by A. Mathewson . . . and H. G. Newton. New York: William Wood & Co., 1890 [1869.] 183p. col. plates. DLC; KU; NNNAM; PPC
90-6756

POLITZER, Adam (1835-1920)
A text-book on the diseases of the ear and adjacent organs. . . . 2nd American from the 3rd German ed. Transl. by Oscar Dodd, and ed. by William Dalby. Philadelphia: Lea Bros. & Co., 1894. 748p. 330 engrvs. CtY-M; DNLM; ICJ; PPC [1st ed., Philadelphia: H. C. Lea's Son & Co., 1883, 800p.]
90-6757

POLK, R. L. & CO.
Medical and surgical register of the United States. [2nd ed.] Detroit, Philadelphia & Chicago, 1890. 1707p. DNLM; NNNAM **90-6758**

POLK, R. L. & CO.
Medical and surgical register of the United States. 3rd ed., revised. Detroit, Philadelphia & Chicago, 1893. 1889p. DNLM; NNNAM **90-6759**

POLK, R. L. & CO.
Medical and surgical register of the United States. 4th ed. Detroit & Chicago: R. L. Polk & Co., 1896. 2351p. DNLM; NNNAM **90-6760**

POLK, R. L. & CO.
Dental register of the United States. 2nd ed. Detroit, Baltimore & Chicago, 1896. 808p. DNLM; NNNAM **90-6761**

POLK, R. L. & CO.
Medical and surgical register of the United States and Canada. 5th ed. Detroit & Chicago, 1898. 2502p. DNLM; NNNAM
90-6762

POLK, R. L. & CO.
Dental register of the United States. 3rd ed. Detroit, Baltimore & Chicago, 1898. 976p. DNLM; NNNAM **90-6763**

POLK, William M[ecklenburg] (1844-1918)
Drainage with gauze-packing as applied to the uterus in chronic endometritis and chronic metritis, not only when these conditions exist independently of salpingitis or other forms of perimetritis, but also where they are associated with such disorders; 40 cases. New York, 1892. 10p. DNLM; NNNAM
90-6764

POLK, William M[ecklenburg] (1844-1918)
The relation of hysterectomy to conservative operations upon the appendages. New York, 1894. 12p. DNLM
90-6765

POLK, William M[ecklenburg] (1844-1918)
Remarks upon hysterectomy, with description of specimens. New York, 1894. 2p. DNLM **90-6766**

POLK, William M[ecklenburg] (1844-1918)
Surgical treatment of suppurative disease of the appendages. New York, 1896. 10p. DNLM **90-6767**

POLLAK, Simon (*b.* 1814)
Report of a case of ophthalmia albuminurica. With a report of the histological examination of the eye by Adolf Alt. [St. Louis, 1893.] 10p. DNLM **90-6768**

POLLITZER, S[igmund] (1859-1937)
Remarks on the histology of xeroderma pigmentosum. [New York, 1892.] 6p. DNLM **90-6769**

POLLITZER, S[igmund] (1859-1937)
Prickly heat, lichen tropicus, miliaria papulosa, rubra, etc. [New York, 1893.] 7p. DNLM **90-6770**

POLLITZER, S[igmund] (1859-1937)
The nature of the xanthomata. New York, 1899. 26p. DNLM
90-6771

POMEROY, Oren Day (1834-1902)
On some points in the pathogenesis of aural vertigo. [New York: D. Appleton & Co., 1891.] 13p. DNLM
90-6772

POMEROY, Oren Day (1834-1902)
A report of fifty cases of extraction of cataract without iridectomy. [New York, 1892.] 10p. DNLM
90-6773

POMEROY, Oren Day (1834-1902)
On operations for divergent strabismus, illustrated by twenty-five cases. [New York, 1893.] 11p. DNLM
90-6774

POMEROY, Ralph H.
A case of symphyseotomy. New York, 1896. 5p. DNLM
90-6775

POOLE, William H[enry] (1820-1896)
Rhinolith, or nasal calculus. Report of a case and exhibition of pathological specimen. [New York, 1898.] 5p. DNLM
90-6776

POOLEY, Thomas Rickett (1841-1926)
Removal of a large exostosis of the orbit with preservation of the eye. [Also:] Operation for ectropion of the lower lid by the sliding-flap method. Hartford: Lockwood & Brainard Co., 1890. 12p.; 6p. DNLM **90-6777**

POORE, Charles T[albot] (1846-1911)
Contributions from the surgical service of St. Mary's Hospital for Children. [New York, 1892.] 75p. DNLM; NNNAM
90-6778

POPE, Benjamin Franklin (1843-1902) and D. S. LAMB
Mycetoma, the fungus foot of India. New York: D. Appleton & Co., 1896. 8p. DNLM
90-6779

POPE, Curran (*b.* 1866)
Insomnia. [New York, 1893.] 15p. DNLM
90-6780

POPE, Curran (*b.* 1866)
Therapeutics of degenerative diseases of the spinal cord. New York: Stettiner, Lambert & Co., 1893. 7p. DNLM
90-6781

PORCHER, F[rancis] Peyre (1825-1895)
Address before the Association of the Survivors of the Confederate Surgeons, of South Carolina, at the annual meeting held at Columbia, S.C., November, 1889. Charleston: Walker [*et al.*], 1890. 14p. DNLM **90-6782**

PORCHER, F[rancis] Peyre (1825-1895)
A pathological condition of the lungs hitherto undescribed in this country, but which is not infrequent. Chicago, 1891. 7p. DNLM **90-6783**

PORCHER, W. Peyre
The prevention of colds, and their sequelae by surgical methods. Read before South Carolina Medical Association, June 9, 1891. [Charleston, 1891.] 7p. DNLM
90-6784

PORCHER, W. Peyre
A case of complete glottic spasm in an adult, followed by unconsciousness and prolonged drowsiness. [New York, 1893.] 4p. DNLM **90-6785**

PORTEOUS, J. Lindsay
Posture in parturition. [New York, 1892.] 5p. DNLM
90-6786

PORTEOUS, J. Lindsay
Eclampsia gravidarum et parturientium. Philadelphia, 1893. 5p. DNLM **90-6787**

PORTEOUS, J. Lindsay
Myxedema; its history, etiology, pathology, and treatment. With particulars of a case successfully treated. [New York, 1893.] 8p. DNLM **90-6788**

PORTER, Charles B[urnham] (1840-1909)
Recurring appendicitis: Is excision of the appendix during a remission a justifiable operation? If so, when and how? Boston: Damrell & Upham, 1891. 18p. DLC
90-6789

PORTER, Charles B[urnham] (1840-1909)
A case of diffuse fibroma, with a tendency to intra-canalicular growth of both breasts; operation on each with an interval of three weeks; recovery. Philadelphia, 1891. 7p. DLC
90-6790

PORTER, Joshua H[enry] (*d.* 1880)
The surgeon's pocket book: an essay on the best treatment of wounded in war; for which a prize was awarded by Her Majesty the Queen of Prussia and Empress of Germany. Specially adapted for the public medical services. 3rd [2nd] ed. Philadelphia: P. Blakiston, Son & Co., 1893. 257p. DLC; PPHa
90-6791

PORTER, Miles H.
Surgical diseases of the gall-bladder and gall-ducts; with a report of five cases. [Philadelphia, 1892.] 8p. DNLM
90-6792

PORTER, Miles F.
Some moot points in the treatment of appendicitis. [Philadelphia: Lea Bros. & Co.], 1895. 7p. DNLM
90-6793

PORTER, Miles F.
Coeliotomy in general suppurative peritonitis, with report of a case. New York, 1895. 3p. DNLM
90-6794

PORTER, William (1852-1921)
The early diagnosis of aneurism of the arch. New York: D. Appleton & Co., 1899. 7p. DNLM **90-6795**

PORTER, W. Evelyn
Malignant diseases of the uterus, with especial reference to operative treatment. [New York, 1892.] 20p. DNLM
90-6796

PORTER, W[illiam] G[ibbs] (1846-1906)
The progress of modern surgery in twenty-five years. Philadelphia, 1891. 23p. DNLM; PPC **90-6797**

PORTER, William Henry (*b.* 1853)
The formation and the clinical significance of albumin and casts in the urine. Philadelphia, 1898. 27p. DNLM; PPC
90-6798

PORTER, William Townsend (1862-1949)
Further researches on the closure of the coronary arteries. New York: D. Appleton & Co., 1896. 24p. DNLM
90-6799

PORTER, William Townsend (1862-1949)
A new method for the study of the intracardiac pressure curve. New York, 1896. 8p. DNLM **90-6800**

PORTER, William Townsend (1862-1949)
I. On the cause of the heart beat. II. The recovery of the heart from fibrillary contractions. III. Note on the relation between the beat of the ventricle and the flow of blood through the coronary arteries. Boston, 1897. 7p. DNLM
90-6801

PORTER, William Townsend (1862-1949)
The teaching of physiology in medical schools. Boston: Damrell & Upham, 1898. 20p. DNLM
90-6802

PORTER, William Townsend (1862-1949)
The teaching of physiology in medical schools. [Boston, 1899.] 16p. DNLM **90-6803**

POSSE, Nils (1862-1895)
The therapeutic application of medical gymnastics. A paper read before the . . . Massachusetts Medical Society (Suffolk), March 13, 1889. . . . Boston: T. R. Marvin & Son, printers, 1891. 30p. DLC; MBM **90-6804**

POSSE, Nils (1862-1895)
The special kinesiology of educational gymnastics. With 276 illustrations and an analytic chart. Boston: Lothrop, Lee & Shepard [1894]. 380p. MB; MH **90-6805**

POST, Sarah E.
Massage, a primer for nurses. . . . New York: The Nightingale Publishing Co., 1890. 47p. DLC; NNNAM
90-6806

POTTER, H. N.
Tubercular meningitis; with report of a peculiar case. Boston, 1897. 8p. DNLM **90-6807**

POTTER, Samuel Otway L[ewis] (1846-1914)
Handbook of materia medica, pharmacy, and therapeutics, including the physiological action of drugs, the special therapeutics of disease, official and extemporaneous pharmacy, and minute directions for prescription writing. . . . 2nd ed., rev. and enl. Philadelphia: P. Blakiston, Son & Co., 1890. 766p. DLC; PPC; PU **90-6808**

POTTER, Samuel Otway L[ewis] (1846-1914)
. . . A compend of human anatomy, including the anatomy of the viscera. . . . 5th ed., rev. and enl. With 117 wood engravings; also an appendix containing numerous tables and sixteen lithographic plates of the nerves and arteries. Philadelphia: P. Blakiston, Son & Co., 1890. 315p. DLC; NNNAM; PPC; PU
90-6809

POTTER, Samuel Otway L[ewis] (1846-1914)
Handbook of materia medica, pharmacy, and therapeutics, including the physiological action of drugs, the special therapeutics of disease, official and practical pharmacy, and minute directions for prescription writing. . . . 3rd ed., rev. Philadelphia: P. Blakiston, Son & Co., 1891. 767p. DLC; OCLloyd; PU
90-6810

POTTER, Samuel Otway L[ewis] (1846-1914)
Handbook of materia medica, pharmacy, and therapeutics, including the physiological action of drugs, the special therapeutics of disease, official and practical pharmacy, and minute directions for prescription writing. . . . 4th ed., rev. Philadelphia: P. Blakiston, Son & Co., 1893. 781p. DLC; NNNAM; PPC; PPJ **90-6811**

POTTER, Samuel Otway L[ewis] (1846-1914)
Handbook of materia medica, pharmacy, and therapeutics, including the physiological action of drugs, the special therapeutics of disease, official and practical pharmacy, and minute directions for prescription writing. . . . 5th ed., rev. and enl. Philadelphia: P. Blakiston, Son & Co., 1894. 805p. DLC; IEN-M; PPC; PU **90-6812**

POTTER, Samuel Otway L[ewis] (1846-1914)
. . . A compend of materia medica, therapeutics and prescription writing, with especial reference to the physiological actions of drugs. Based on the seventh revision of the U.S. Pharmacopoeia, 1890, including also many unofficial remedies. . . . 6th ed., rewritten and enl. Philadelphia: Blakiston, Son & Co., 1894. 255p. DLC; NNNAM; PPC; PPJ
90-6813

POTTER, Samuel Otway L[ewis] (1846-1914)
Handbook of materia medica, pharmacy, and therapeutics, including the physiological action of drugs, the special therapeutics of disease, official and practical pharmacy, and minute directions for prescription writing. . . . 6th ed., fully rev. and greatly enl. Philadelphia: P. Blakiston, Son & Co., 1897. 900p. DLC; NNNAM; PPC; PU **90-6814**

POTTER, Samuel Otway L[ewis] (1846-1914)
Handbook of materia medica, pharmacy, and therapeutics, including the physiological action of drugs, the special therapeutics of disease, official and practical pharmacy, and minute directions for prescription writing. . . . 7th ed. Rev. and enl. Philadelphia: P. Blakiston's Son & Co., 1899. 929p. DLC; IU-M; PPC; PU **90-6815**

POTTER, Samuel Otway L[ewis] (1846-1914)
A compend of human anatomy, including the anatomy of the viscera. 6th ed. Philadelphia: P. Blakiston's Son & Co., 1890. 289p. 15 plates. DNLM; PPC; PU **90-6816**

POTTER, Theodore (1861-1915)
Essays on bacteriology and its relation to the progress of medicine. Indianapolis: Indiana M. J. Publ. Co., 1898. 161p. DNLM **90-6817**

POTTER, William Warren (1838-1911)
What is the present medico-legal status of the abdominal surgeon? New York: William Wood & Co., 1890. 12p. DNLM **90-6818**

POTTER, William Warren (1838-1911)
How should girls be educated? A public health problem for mothers, educators, and physicians. Philadelphia: W. J. Dornan, 1891. 17p. DNLM **90-6819**

POTTER, William Warren (1838-1911)
Pelvic inflammation in women; a pathological study. Toledo, O., 1891. 10p. DNLM **90-6820**

POTTER, William Warren (1838-1911)
Asepsis and antisepsis as applied in the lying-in chamber. [Philadelphia, 1892.] 9p. DNLM **90-6821**

POTTER, William Warren (1838-1911)
Specialism in medicine, particularly as related to surgery and gynecology. [Philadelphia, 1892.] 14p. DNLM **90-6822**

POTTER, William Warren (1838-1911)
Posture in relation to obstetrics and gynecology. Philadelphia: W. J. Dornan, 1893. 31p. 5 plates. DNLM **90-6823**

POTTS, Charles S[ower] (1864-1930)
A case of acute delirium, with autopsy and bacteriologic examination of cerebro-spinal fluid. Philadelphia, 1894. 4p. DNLM **90-6824**

POWELL, Charles H.
Diabetes mellitus. St. Louis, 1898. 4p. DNLM **90-6825**

POWELL, Richard Douglas (1842-1925)
On diseases of the lungs and pleurae, including consumption. 4th ed. Philadelphia: P. Blakiston, Son & Co., 1893. 600p. 4 plates. CtY-M; DNLM; NNNAM; PPC **90-6826**

POWELL, William M[cCauley] (*b.* 1862)
. . . Essentials of the diseases of children, arranged in the form of questions and answers, prepared especially for students of medicine. . . . Philadelphia: W. B. Saunders, 1890. 222p. DLC; DNLM; PPC; PU **90-6827**

POWELL, William M[cCauley] (*b.* 1862)
Saunders' pocket medical formulary. With an appendix containing posological table; formulae and doses for hypodermic medication; poisons and their antidotes; diameters of the female pelvis and foetal head; diet list for various diseases; obstetrical table; materials and drugs used in antiseptic surgery, etc. Philadelphia: W. B. Saunders, 1891. 261p. DLC; DNLM; PPC; PU **90-6828**

POWELL, William M[cCauley] (*b.* 1862)
Saunders' pocket medical formulary. With an appendix containing posological table; formulae and doses for hypodermic medication; poisons and their antidotes; diameters of the female pelvis and foetal head; diet list for various diseases; obstetrical table; materials and drugs used in antiseptic surgery, etc. 2nd ed. Philadelphia: W. B. Saunders, 1892. 285p. CtY-M; NNNAM; PPC; PU [3rd ed., 1894. 285p.; 4th ed., 1896, 285p.] **90-6829**

POWELL, William M[cCauley] (*b.* 1862)
Saunders' pocket medical formulary. With an appendix containing posological table; formulae and doses for hypodermic medication; poisons and their antidotes; diameters of the female pelvis and foetal head; diet list for various diseases; obstetrical table; materials and drugs used in antiseptic surgery, etc. 5th ed. Philadelphia: W. B. Saunders, 1899. 290p. DLC; DNLM; PU **90-6830**

POWELSON, A. Palen
Counterfeit science. Philadelphia, 1897. 4p. DNLM **90-6831**

POWER, D'Arcy (1855-1941)
Ununited fracture in children. Philadelphia, 1892. 7p. DNLM **90-6832**

POWER, D'Arcy (1855-1941)
The surgical diseases of children and their treatment by modern methods. Philadelphia: P. Blakiston, Son & Co., 1895. 548p. DNLM; NNNAM; PPC; PU **90-6833**

POWER, Henry (1829-1911)
Elements of human physiology. . . . 2nd ed. Philadelphia: Lea Bros. & Co., 1890. 396p. 4 engravs. DNLM; NN; PPC; PPHa **90-6834**

POWERS, Charles A.
On conical stump after amputation in children, with especial reference to its physiological causes and prognosis. New York: Trow, 1890. 20p. DNLM **90-6835**

POWERS, Charles A.
On dermatol, a proposed substitute for iodoform; its use in surgical practice. [New York, 1891.] 8p. DNLM **90-6836**

POWERS, Charles A.
A brief note on some cases recently admitted to the surgical service at the New York Cancer Hospital. [New York, 1894.] 2 l. DNLM **90-6837**

POWERS, Charles A.
Further observations on the physiological occurrence of conical stump after amputation in children. New York: Trow, 1894. 12p. DNLM **90-6838**

POWERS, Charles A.
The relative age-occurrence of Colles' fracture; a table of nine hundred and eighty-eight cases. [Philadelphia: Lea Bros. & Co., 1895.] 6p. DNLM **90-6839**

POWERS, Charles A. and George R. WHITE
Excision of the larynx; six cases hitherto unreported, together with the analysis of three hundred additional cases gathered from literature. New York, 1895. 24p. DNLM; NNNAM **90-6840**

POWERS, Charles A.
The question of position in the treatment of fractures of the lower end of the humerus. The testimony of 650 cases under the care of Hartley [*et al.*]. New York, 1896. 10p. DNLM
90-6841

POWERS, Charles A.
Early diagnosis and mistaken diagnosis in cases of tumor of the breast. New York, 1897. 7p. DNLM
90-6842

POWERS, Charles A.
A further case of primary tuberculosis of the breast. Philadelphia, 1897. 2p. DNLM **90-6843**

POWERS, Charles A.
A preliminary comparison of methods and results in operative surgery at the sea-level (New York) and in places of high altitude (Denver). Philadelphia, 1897. 10p. DNLM
90-6844

POWERS, Charles A.
Methods and results in four hundred and fifty cases of fractures of the forearm bones. Denver, Col., 1897. 23p. DNLM
90-6845

POWERS, Charles A.
Branchial carcinoma. Philadelphia, 1898. 6p. DNLM
90-6846

POWERS, Charles A.
External esophagotomy for impacted foreign body. Two recent cases, with recovery in each. Boston: Damrell & Upham, 1898. 11p. DNLM **90-6847**

POWERS, Charles A.
The question of operative interference in recent, simple fractures of the patella. Philadelphia, 1898. 43p. DNLM
90-6848

POWERS, Charles A.
Methods and results in one hundred and seventy-five cases of simple fracture of the femur. Denver, Col., 1899. 8p. DNLM
90-6849

POWERS, Charles A.
Wound of the urinary tract during an operation for acute appendicitis; spontaneous closure of urinary fistula; recovery. Philadelphia, 1899. 3p. DNLM **90-6850**

POZZI, Samuel Jean (1846-1918)
Treatise on gynecology, medical and surgical. . . . Transl. from the French ed. under the supervision of, and with additions by, Brooks H. Wells. . . . New York: William Wood & Co., 1891-92. 2 v. col. plates. DLC; DNLM; NNNAM; PPC
90-6851

POZZI, Samuel Jean (1846-1918)
A system of gynaecology with 359 illus. based upon a translation from the French of S. Pozzi. Revised by C. M. Beebe. New York: J. B. Flint & Co., 1894. 604p. NNNAM
90-6852

POZZI, Samuel Jean (1846-1918)
A treatise on gynaecology, medical and surgical. . . . 2nd American ed., transl. from the 3rd French ed. under the supervision of Brooks H. Wells. . . . New York: William Wood & Co., 1897. 936p. DLC; DNLM; NNNAM
90-6853

PRACTICAL anatomy, including a special section of the fundamental principles of anatomy. Edited by W. T. Eckley and Mrs. Corinne Buford Eckley. Philadelphia: P. Blakiston's Son & Co., 1899. 485p. DNLM; PPC; PU **90-6854**

A PRACTICAL treatise on thialion, with complete bibliography. Danbury, Conn.: The Vass Chemical Co., 1898. 45p. DNLM
90-6855

A PRACTICAL treatise on thialion, with complete bibliography. 2nd ed. Danbury, Conn.: The Vass Chemical Co., 1898. 73p. DNLM **90-6856**

PRAEGER, Emil Arnold (1855-1898)
Is so-called conservatism in gynaecology conducive to the best results to the patient? New York, 1895. 9p. DNLM
90-6857

PRATT, E[dwin] Hartley (1849-1930)
Orificial surgery, and its application to the treatment of chronic diseases. . . . Chicago: Halsey Bros., 1890. 164p. DLC; ICJ; PPC; PPHa **90-6858**

PRATT, E[dwin] Hartley (1849-1930)
Practical hints in orificial surgery. 1st series. Chicago: C. N. Trivess, [1892]. 39p. DNLM **90-6859**

PRATT, E[dwin] Hartley (1849-1930)
Continuation of the report on hysterectomies. Nine more cases of hysterectomy performed by the new method. [Chicago, 1893.] 16p. DNLM **90-6860**

PRATT, E[dwin] Hartley (1849-1930)
Hysterectomy by a new method, which is simple, safe, bloodless, and entirely obviates the necessity of either clamp, cautery, or ligature; a major operation converted into a minor one by a simple process of easy dissection. [Chicago, 1893.] 12p. DNLM **90-6861**

PRATT, E[dwin] Hartley (1849-1930)
Uterine pathology. [Chicago, 1894.] 15p. DNLM
90-6862

PRATT, E[dwin] Hartley (1849-1930)
A needed reform in abdominal surgery. Chicago, 1894. 9p. DNLM **90-6863**

PRATT, Isaac Hull
Obstacles to a national quarantine. Philadelphia, 1893. 2p. DNLM **90-6864**

PRATT, Joseph Hersey (1872-1956)
Secondary infection of the skin and subcutaneous tissues by the bacillus typhosus. Boston, 1899. 4p. DNLM
90-6865

PRENDERGAST, James F.
A simple remedy for enuresis. New York: D. Appleton & Co., 1896. 7p. DNLM **90-6866**

PRENTICE, Chalmers
The eye in its relation to health. . . . Chicago: A. C. McClurg & Co., 1895. 214p. DLC **90-6867**

PRENTICE, Chalmers
Repression treatment and differential test for visual nerve strain. New York: D. Appleton & Co., 1898. 17p. DNLM
90-6868

PRENTISS, D[aniel] W[ebster] (1843-1899)
Purpura hemorrhagica rheumatica (peliosis rheumatica; morbus maculosus Werholfii). [Philadelphia, 1890.] 4p. DNLM
90-6869

PRENTISS, D[aniel] W[ebster] (1843-1899)
Report of three cases of remarkably slow pulse; to which is appended brief abstracts of ninety-three cases of slow pulse found recorded in medical journals in the Library of the Surgeon-General's Office, Washington, D.C. Detroit: G. S. Davis, 1890. 26p. DNLM **90-6870**

PRENTISS, D[aniel] W[ebster] (1843-1899)
A case of slow pulse; with the report of the autopsy, by Robert T. Edes. Detroit: G. S. Davis, 1891. 5p. DNLM
90-6871

PRENTISS, D[aniel] W[ebster] (1843-1899)
The Medical Society of the District of Columbia. Washington: Rothrock, [1891]. 20p. DNLM **90-6872**

PRENTISS, D[aniel] W[ebster] (1843-1899)
Three cases of cerebral apoplexy, one case of progressive coma, and one case of rheumatic meningitis following the grip. [Philadelphia: Lea Bros. & Co., 1891.] 8p. DNLM
90-6873

PRESTISS, D[aniel] W[ebster] (1843-1899)
Address to the graduating class at the annual commencement of the Medical Department of the Columbian University, District of Columbia, March 17, 1892. Washington, 1892. 15p. DNLM **90-6874**

PRESTISS, D[aniel] W[ebster] (1843-1899)
Address delivered at the opening of the Medical Department of the Columbian University, District of Columbia, October 1, 1892. With a sketch of life and work of Edward T. Fristoe. Washington, 1892. 16p. DNLM **90-6875**

PRENTISS, D[aniel] W[ebster] (1843-1899)
Report of cases of poisoning from exalgine, cannabis indica, arsenic, and camphor. Detroit: G. S. Davis, 1892. 9p. DNLM
90-6876

PRENTISS, D[aniel] W[ebster] (1843-1899)
Pilocarpine; its physiological action and therapeutic uses, with exhibition of specimens showing change in the color of the hair. Detroit: G. S. Davis, 1893. 41p. DNLM
90-6877

PRENTISS, D[aniel] W[ebster] (1843-1899)
Sarcoma of the right lung diagnosticated during life by use of the microscope; secondary to sarcoma of the testicle which had been removed four years previously. [Philadelphia, 1893.] 5p. DNLM **90-6878**

PRENTISS, D[aniel] W[ebster] (1843-1899) and Francis P. MORGAN
Anhalonium Lewinii (mescal buttons). A study of the drug, with especial reference to its physiological action upon man, with report of experiments. Detroit: Geo. S. Davis, 1895. 24p. DNLM **90-6879**

PRENTISS, D[aniel] W[ebster] (1843-1899) and Francis P. MORGAN
Mescal buttons, Anhalonium Lewinii; Henning's Lophophora Williamsii Lewinii; Coulter. New York, 1896. 31p. DNLM
90-6880

PRENTISS, D[aniel] W[ebster] (1843-1899) and Francis P. MORGAN
Therapeutic uses of the mescal buttons (Anahalonium Lewinii). The mescal plant and ceremony by James Mooney. Detroit, 1896. 24p. DNLM **90-6881**

PRENTISS, D[aniel] W[ebster] (1843-1899)
Report of two cases of erythromelalgia (red neuralgia Mitchell). [Washington], 1897. 13p. DNLM
90-6882

PRENTISS, D[aniel] W[ebster] (1843-1899)
Five cases of mushroom poisoning, three of which proved fatal; treatment of the poisoning. Philadelphia, 1898. 16p. DNLM **90-6883**

PRENTISS, D[aniel] W[ebster] (1843-1899)
A case of syphilitic fever, with a discussion of the diagnosis of fevers. Philadelphia, 1899. 13p. DNLM
90-6884

PRESBYTERIAN HOSPITAL. NEW YORK CITY
Outline of the work of the . . . . [New York: W. C. Martin], 1894. 19p. DNLM; NNC **90-6885**

PRESCOTT, W[illiam] H[erbert] and Joel E. GOLDTHWAIT
Report of three hundred and ninety-two cases of intubation and one hundred and thirty-nine cases of tracheotomy done at the Boston City Hospital. Boston: Damrell & Upham, 1892. 9p. DNLM **90-6886**

THE PRESENT status of diphtheria antitoxic serum. Philadelphia & Chicago: H. K. Mulford Co., [1897]. 40p. DNLM; PPC
90-6887

THE PRESENT status of diphtheria antitoxic serum. 3rd ed. Philadelphia & Chicago: H. K. Mulford Co., [1897]. 40p. DNLM; PPC **90-6888**

PRESTON, George J. (1858-1908)
The differential diagnosis and treatment of multiple neuritis. [Baltimore, 1891.] 7p. DNLM **90-6889**

PRESTON, George J. (1858-1908)
The effect of arterio-sclerosis upon the central nervous system. Report on the ophthalmoscopic examination of Dr. Preston's cases, by Harry Friedenwald. Chicago, 1891. 20p. DNLM
90-6890

PRESTON, George J. (1858-1908)
A case of probable meningeal haemorrhage with symptoms resembling general paresis. [Baltimore, 1893.] 3p. DNLM
90-6891

PRESTON, George J. (1858-1908)
Importance of arterio-sclerosis in the etiology of posterior spinal sclerosis. [Philadelphia, 1893.] 5p. DNLM
90-6892

PRESTON, George J. (1858-1908)
Traumatic lesions of the spinal cord. [Philadelphia, 1893.] 15p. DNLM **90-6893**

PRESTON, George J. (1858-1908)
Cerebral oedema. [New York, 1894.] 12p. DNLM
90-6894

PRESTON, George J. (1858-1908)
Detention wards for cases of suspected insanity. [Baltimore, 1894.] 3p. DNLM **90-6895**

PRESTON, George J. (1858-1908)
Clinical notes on the diagnosis and treatment of apoplexy. [Baltimore, 1894.] 4p. DNLM **90-6896**

PRESTON, George J. (1858-1908)
Hysterical pyrexia. [Baltimore, 1894.] 4p. DNLM **90-6897**

PRESTON, George J. (1858-1908)
Tetany; with the report of a typical case. [New York], 1895. 6p. DNLM **90-6898**

PRESTON, George J. (1858-1908)
Hysteria and certain allied conditions; their nature and treatment, with special reference to the application of the rest cure, massage, electrotherapy, hypnotism, etc. Philadelphia: P. Blakiston, Son & Co., 1897. 298p. DNLM; PPC; PU **90-6899**

PRICE, Eldridge C. (*b.* 1854)
The significance of a reconstructed materia medica. New York: H. B. Elkins, 1890. 15p. NNNAM **90-6900**

PRICE, Joseph (1853-1911)
Ectopic pregnancy and puerperal peritonitis. Philadelphia, 1890. 14p. 4 plates. DNLM **90-6901**

PRICE, Joseph (1853-1911)
Analysis of fifteen months' abdominal work in the Gynaecean Hospital, Philadelphia. Richmond, 1890. 11p. DNLM **90-6902**

PRICE, Joseph (1853-1911)
Certain causes of major pelvic troubles traceable to minor gynecology. [Philadelphia, 1890.] 12p. DNLM **90-6903**

PRICE, Joseph (1853-1911)
Cleanliness in maternities. [Philadelphia, 1890.] 8p. DNLM **90-6904**

PRICE, Joseph (1853-1911)
Early operations in purulent peritonitis. Philadelphia, 1890. 8p. DNLM **90-6905**

PRICE, Joseph (1853-1911)
Ectopic pregnancy and puerperal peritonitis. [Philadelphia, 1890.] 14p. 4 plates. DNLM **90-6906**

PRICE, Joseph (1853-1911)
The motive and method of pelvic surgery. [Philadelphia, 1890.] 9p. DNLM **90-6907**

PRICE, Joseph (1853-1911)
The present status of abdominal surgery. [Richmond], 1890. 8p. DNLM **90-6908**

PRICE, Joseph (1853-1911)
A retrospect of abdominal surgery. [Philadelphia, 1890.] 11p. DNLM **90-6909**

PRICE, Joseph (1853-1911)
An educational need. Philadelphia, 1892. 7p. DNLM **90-6910**

PRICE, Joseph (1853-1911)
Intestinal lesions in abdominal and pelvic surgery. [Philadelphia, 1892.] 9p. DNLM **90-6911**

PRICE, Joseph (1853-1911)
Motive, preparation, and results in abdominal and pelvic surgery. Philadelphia, 1892. 8p. DNLM **90-6912**

PRICE, Joseph (1853-1911)
Disputed points in hysterectomy. [Philadelphia, 1893.] 4 galley sheets. DNLM **90-6913**

PRICE, Joseph (1853-1911)
Sexual function and insanity. Philadelphia: R. C. Penfield, 1893. 8p. DNLM **90-6914**

PRICE, Joseph (1853-1911)
Discussion of methods in pelvic surgery. New York, 1894. 6p. DNLM **90-6915**

PRICE, Joseph (1853-1911)
How to do abdominal section without fuss, feathers, and foolishness, with immunity from sepsis. New York, 1895. 6p. DNLM **90-6916**

PRICE, Joseph (1853-1911)
Opium in gynaecology. [New York, 1895.] 3p. DNLM **90-6917**

PRICE, Joseph (1853-1911)
"Physician, heal thyself." [New York], 1895. 5p. DNLM **90-6918**

PRICE, Joseph (1853-1911)
The Preston Retreat controversy. Richard C. Norris versus The Preston Retreat. New York, 1895. 11p. DNLM **90-6919**

PRICE, Joseph (1853-1911)
The surgical management of suppurative forms of tubal and ovarian disease. New York, 1895. 5p. DNLM **90-6920**

PRICE, Joseph (1853-1911)
Presentation of post-operative sequelae and how they favor mortality. New York, 1896. 2p. DNLM **90-6921**

PRICE, Joseph (1853-1911)
Report of a mixed group of abdominal sections, with a discussion of methods. [Philadelphia, 1897.] 3 galley sheets. DNLM **90-6922**

PRICE, Joseph (1853-1911)
Pus in the pelvis, and how to deal with it. [Philadelphia, 1899.] 12p. DNLM **90-6923**

PRICE list of surgical instruments and physicians' supplies. Manufactured and imported by Richard Kny & Co. New York, [1894]. 128p. DNLM; NNNAM **90-6924**

PRICE, Mordecai (1844-1904)
Extra-uterine pregnancy. Philadelphia, 1893. 8p. DNLM **90-6925**

PRICE, Mordecai (1844-1904)
Hysterectomy for puerperal infection. New York, 1895. 3p. DNLM **90-6926**

PRICE, W[illiam] Henry and S. Potts EAGLETON
The nervo-vascular system, arranged by . . . in three sheets. Examined and approved by John B. Deaver. Revised ed. Philadelphia: F. A. Davis, [1890]. fol. DNLM; PPC; PU
90-6927

PRICE, W[illiam] Henry
Essentials of physical diagnosis for medical students. . . . Philadelphia, 1893. 81p. DLC; PPC
90-6928

PRINCE, J. A.
Obstruction of the bowel from Meckel's diverticulum. A cholecystotomy. [Philadelphia, 1893.] 7p. DNLM
90-6929

PRINCE, L[awrence] H. (*b.* 1858)
The fire protection of hospitals for the insane. Chicago: C. H. Blakely & Co., 1891. 122p. DNLM
90-6930

PRINCE, L[awrence] H. (*b.* 1858)
Observations in five hundred consecutive anaesthesias in the service of A. J. Ochsner, at the Augustana Hospital. Chicago, 1895. 14p. DNLM **90-6931**

PRINCE, Morton (1854-1929)
Idiopathic internal hydrocephalus (serous meningitis) in the adult. With reports of three cases (two with autopsies). New York, 1897. 20p. DNLM **90-6932**

PRINCE, Morton (1854-1929)
The educational treatment of neurasthenia and certain hysterical states. [Boston], 1898. 22p. DNLM
90-6933

PRINCE, Morton (1854-1929)
Sexual perversion or vice? A pathological and therapeutic inquiry. New York, 1898. 20p. DNLM
90-6934

PRITCHARD, Urban (*b.* 1845)
Handbook of diseases of the ear for the use of students and practitioners. 2nd ed. Philadelphia: P. Blakiston, Son & Co., 1891. 238p. 1 plate. DNLM; PPC; PU
90-6935

PRITCHARD, Urban (*b.* 1845)
On systematic procedure in operations for the relief of intercranial disease secondary to ear suppuration. New York, 1894. 34p. DNLM; NNNAM **90-6936**

PRITCHARD, Urban (*b.* 1845)
Handbook of diseases of the ear for the use of students and practitioners. 3rd ed. Philadelphia: P. Blakiston, Son & Co., 1896. 238p. 1 plate. DNLM; NNNAM
90-6937

PRITCHARD, William Broaddus (*d.* 1915)
A case of traumatic neuritis illustrating the medico-legal value of electricity in diagnosis. [New York, 1890.] 5p. DNLM
90-6938

PRITCHARD, William Broaddus (*d.* 1915)
Melancholia; its diagnosis and treatment at home. A clinical lecture delivered at the New York Polyclinic. [Philadelphia, 1891.] 10p. DNLM **90-6939**

PRITCHARD, William Broaddus (*d.* 1915)
The importance of early diagnosis in locomotor ataxia, as affected by the newer pathology. New York, 1899. 15p. DNLM **90-6940**

PROCTOR, Bernard Simpson (1827-1903)
Lectures on practical pharmacy. Philadelphia: P. Blakiston, Son & Co., 1892. 539p. 32 plates. DNLM; MBM; PPC; PU
90-6941

PROUT, Thomas P.
A case of acute delirium, with some considerations on its pathologic aspect. Philadelphia, 1894. 6p. DNLM
90-6942

PROUT, Thomas P.
Some minor studies in nerve-cell degeneration, as presented by a case of localized cerebral atrophy. New York, 1895. 6p. 1 plate. DNLM **90-6943**

A PROVISIONAL hand-book of haematherapy, or auxiliary blood supply in medicine and surgery. Compiled and reprinted from numerous medical journals and correspondents, including the entire records up to date of Sound View Hospital, Stamford, Conn. New York: Borinine Co., [1898]. 240p. DNLM; NNNAM
90-6944

A PROVISIONAL hand-book of haematherapy, or auxiliary blood supply in medicine and surgery. Compiled and reprinted from numerous medical journals and correspondents, including the entire records up to date of Sound View Hospital, Stamford, Conn. New York, [1898]. 256p. DNLM; NNNAM
90-6945

PRUDDEN, T[heophil] Mitchell (1849-1924)
Bacterial studies on the influenza and its complicating pneumonia. New York: Trow, 1890. 7p. DNLM
90-6946

PRUDDEN, T[heophil] Mitchell (1849-1924)
Dust and its dangers. New York & London: G. P. Putnam's Sons, 1890. 111p. 4 plates. DNLM; NNNAM
90-6947

PRUDDEN, T[heophil] Mitchell (1849-1924)
Drinking-water and ice supplies and their relations to health and disease. New York & London: G. P. Putnam, 1891. 148p. DNLM; NNNAM **90-6948**

PRUDDEN, T[heophil] Mitchell (1849-1924)
Studies on the etiology of diphtheria. Second series. New York: Trow's, 1891. 19p. 2 plates. DNLM
90-6949

PRUDDEN, T[heophil] Mitchell (1849-1924)
A study of experimental pneumonitis in the rabbit induced by the intratracheal injection of dead tubercle bacilli. New York: D. Appleton & Co., 1891. 18p. DNLM
90-6950

PRUDDEN, T[heophil] Mitchell (1849-1924)
The element of contagion in tuberculosis. New York: D. Appleton & Co., 1892. 9p. DNLM **90-6951**

PRUDDEN, T[heophil] Mitchell (1849-1924)
On the poisonous products of the tubercle bacillus. New York: D. Appleton & Co., 1892. 11p. DNLM
90-6952

PRUDDEN, T[heophil] Mitchell (1849-1924)
A study on the aetiology of exudative pleuritis. New York: D. Appleton & Co., 1893. 13p. DNLM
90-6953

PRUDDEN, T[heophil] Mitchell (1849-1924)
A case of pyaemia following the incision of an urethral stricture; with a note of certain biological peculiarities in the Staphylococcus pyogenes aureus. [New York: D. Appleton & Co., 1894.] 2p. DNLM **90-6954**

PRUDDEN, T[heophil] Mitchell (1849-1924)
Concurrent infections and the formation of cavities in acute pulmonary tuberculosis; an experimental study. [New York: D. Appleton & Co., 1894.] 30p. 2 plates. DNLM
90-6955

PRUDDEN, T[heophil] Mitchell (1849-1924)
New outlooks in the science and art of medicine. New York, 1896. 16p. DNLM **90-6956**

PRYOR, W[illiam] R[ice] (1858-1904)
Septic endometritis with peritonitis and their treatment by means of the curette, and its antiseptic dressings. New York: William Wood & Co., 1892. 21p. DNLM
90-6957

PRYOR, W[illiam] R[ice] (1858-1904)
Mr. Lawson Tait and the germ theory of disease. [New York: D. Appleton & Co., 1894.] 11p. DNLM
90-6958

PRYOR, W[illiam] R[ice] (1858-1904)
The cure of ventral hernia by connective-tissue granulation. New York, 1894. 4p. DNLM **90-6959**

PRYOR, W[illiam] R[ice] (1858-1904)
A new and rapid method of dealing with intra-ligamentous fibromyomata. Philadelphia, 1894. 5p. DNLM
90-6960

PRYOR, W[illiam] R[ice] (1858-1904)
Latent gonorrhoea in women. [New York, 1895.] 7p. DNLM
90-6961

PRYOR, W[illiam] R[ice] (1858-1904)
A new method of treating adherent retroposed uteri. New York, 1895. 8p. DNLM **90-6962**

PRYOR, W[illiam] R[ice] (1858-1904)
The treatment of gonorrhoea in women. New York, 1895. 6p. DNLM **90-6963**

PRYOR, W[illiam] R[ice] (1858-1904)
The anatomy of the endometrium and the technique of its removal by curettage. New York, 1896. 6p. DNLM
90-6964

PRYOR, W[illiam] R[ice] (1858-1904)
A method of examining the pelvic contents which renders exploratory laparotomy unnecessary in inflammatory conditions of the adnexa uteri and in certain other diseased states of the pelvic viscera. New York, 1896. 16p. 1 plate. DNLM
90-6965

PRYOR, W[illiam] R[ice] (1858-1904)
The treatment of pelvic inflammations through the vagina. Philadelphia: W. B. Saunders, 1899. 248p. 18 plates. DNLM; PPC; PU **90-6966**

PULFORD, Alfred (*b.* 1863)
Repertory of the symptoms of rheumatism, sciata, et cetera. . . . Tiffin, O.: B. B. Krammes, [1898]. 211p. DLC
90-6967

PUNTON, John (*b.* 1853)
The social and medical aspects of insanity. [Kansas City, Mo., 1891.] 8p. DNLM **90-6968**

PUNTON, John (*b.* 1853)
"The neuropathic constitution, education, and marriage as factors in the causation and propagation of nervous diseases." [St. Joseph, 1893.] 14p. DNLM **90-6969**

PUNTON, John (*b.* 1853)
The modern crank and mental responsibility. Keokuk, 1894. 9p. DNLM **90-6970**

PUNTON, John (*b.* 1853)
Review of recent advances in our knowledge of the anatomy and physiology of the nervous system. Kansas City, 1894. 8p. DNLM **90-6971**

PUNTON, John (*b.* 1853)
The treatment and prophylaxis of insanity. St. Louis, 1894. 16p. DNLM **90-6972**

PUNTON, John (*b.* 1853)
The civic duties and responsibilities of the physician to his community, State, and nation. St. Louis, 1897. 10p. DNLM
90-6973

PUNTON, John (*b.* 1853)
The relation of the science of medicine to public school education. Kansas City, Mo.: Gate City Print. Co., [1897]. 8p. DNLM **90-6974**

PUNTON, John (*b.* 1853)
The diagnosis and treatment of neurasthenia. [n. p.], 1899. 8p. DNLM **90-6975**

PUNTON, John (*b.* 1853)
The pathogenesis of functional nervous diseases and their prophylactic indication. New York, 1899. 8p. DNLM
90-6976

PURDY, Charles W[esley] (1846-1901)
Diabetes; its causes, symptoms, and treatment. Philadelphia & London: F. A. Davis, 1890. 184p. DLC; DNLM; PPC
90-6977

PURDY, Charles W[esley] (1846-1901)
The influences of climate in the United States over Bright's disease. [New York, 1890.] 14p. DNLM
90-6978

PURDY, Charles W[esley] (1846-1901)
Examination of the urine for life-insurance. A lecture delivered at the opening of the new building of the Chicago Post-Graduate Medical School. [New York, 1891.] 25p. DNLM; NNNAM **90-6979**

PURDY, Charles W[esley] (1846-1901)
Quantitative testing for sugar in the urine. [Chicago, 1891, *vel subseq.*] 2 l. DNLM; NNNAM
90-6980

PURDY, Charles W[esley] (1846-1901)
Practical uranalysis and urinary diagnosis. A manual for the use of physicians, surgeons and students. Philadelphia: F. A. Davis Co., 1894. 357p. 1 plate. DLC; DNLM; PU
90-6981

PURDY, Charles W[esley] (1846-1901)
Practical uranalysis and urinary diagnosis. A manual for the use of physicians, surgeons, and students. . . . 2nd ed. . . . Philadelphia: The F. A. Davis Co.; London: F. J. Rebman, 1895. 357p. col. plates. DLC; NNNAM; PPC; PU
90-6982

PURDY, Charles W[esley] (1846-1901)
Practical uranalysis and urinary diagnosis. A manual for the use of physicians, surgeons, and students. . . . 3rd ed. Philadelphia: The F. A. Davis Co., 1896. 383p. 6 plates. DLC; DNLM; PPC
90-6983

PURDY, Charles W[esley] (1846-1901)
Utility and recent developments in centrifugal methods. New York, 1896. 16p. DNLM **90-6984**

PURDY, Charles W[esley] (1846-1901)
Practical uranalysis and urinary diagnosis. A manual for the use of physicians, surgeons, and students. . . . 4th ed. Philadelphia, New York & Chicago: F. A. Davis Co., 1898. 365p. 7 plates. DLC; DNLM; NNNAM; PPC **90-6985**

PURDY, Charles W[esley] (1846-1901)
Principles of the dietetic treatment of diabetes mellitus. Chicago, 1898. 16p. DNLM **90-6986**

PURDY, Charle W[esley] (1846-1901)
Quantitative determination of albumin in the urine. New York, 1899. 10p. DNLM **90-6987**

PURRINGTON, William Archer (1852-1926)
A review of recent legal decisions affecting physicians, dentists, druggists and the public health, together with a brief for the prosecution of unlicensed practitioners of medicine, dentistry, or pharmacy, with a paper upon manslaughter, Christian science and the law and other matter. . . . New York: E. B. Treat & Co., 1899 [1907]. 105p. DLC; NNNAM
90-6988

PUTNAM, James J[ackson] (1846-1919)
Cases of cerebral tumor, with autopsy. Boston: Damrell & Upham, 1890. 16p. DNLM **90-6989**

PUTNAM, James J[ackson] (1846-1919)
A form of polyneuritis, probably analogous to, or identical with, beri-beri, occurring in seafaring men in northern latitudes. New York: M. J. Rooney & Co., 1890. 11p. DNLM
90-6990

PUTNAM, James J[ackson] (1846-1919)
The frequency with which arsenic is found in the urine; with notes on some new cases of poisoning from wallpaper and fabrics. Boston: Damrell & Upham, 1890. 8p. DNLM
90-6991

PUTNAM, James J[ackson] (1846-1919)
Intra-cranial lesions. A discussion of the question, What are the present means of localizing intra-cranial lesions? Concord, N.Y., 1890. 17p. DNLM **90-6992**

PUTNAM, James J[ackson] (1846-1919)
The character of the evidence as to the injuriousness of arsenic as a domestic poison. Boston: Damrell & Upham, 1891. 12p. DNLM **90-6993**

PUTNAM, James J[ackson] (1846-1919)
A group of cases of scleroses of the spinal cord, associated with diffuse collateral degeneration; occurring in enfeebled persons past middle life, and especially in women. Studied with particular reference to etiology. [New York, 1891.] 42p. DNLM **90-6994**

PUTNAM, James J[ackson] (1846-1919)
Personal observations on the pathology and treatment of neuralgias of the fifth pair. Boston: Damrell & Upham, 1891. 23p. DNLM **90-6995**

PUTNAM, James J[ackson] (1846-1919)
On the relation of epilepsy to injury of the head. Boston: Damrell & Upham, 1892. 16p. DNLM
90-6996

PUTNAM, James J[ackson] (1846-1919)
Case of myxoedema and acromegalia treated with sheep's thyroids; recent observations respecting the pathology of the cachexias following disease of the thyroid; clinical relationships of Graves's disease and acromegalia. [Philadelphia], 1893. 32p. DNLM **90-6997**

PUTNAM, James J[ackson] (1846-1919)
Cases of myxoedema and acromegalia treated with sheep's thyroids; recent observations respecting the pathology of the cachexias following disease of the thyroid; clinical relationships of Graves's disease and acromegalia. Philadelphia, 1893. 24p. DNLM **90-6998**

PUTNAM, James J[ackson] (1846-1919)
On certain peculiarities in the reactions of the musculo-spiral nerve to electrical currents, and their practical significance. Boston, 1893. 5p. DNLM **90-6999**

PUTNAM, James J[ackson] (1846-1919)
The treatment of Graves's disease by thyroidectomy. New York, 1893. 23p. DNLM **90-7000**

PUTNAM, James J[ackson] (1846-1919)
Notes on two additional cases of thyroidectomy for Graves's disease. New York, 1894. 8p. DNLM **90-7001**

PUTNAM, James J[ackson] (1846-1919)
Relation of infectious processes to diseases of the nervous system; pathology and etiology. Philadelphia, 1895. 24p. DNLM **90-7002**

PUTNAM, James J[ackson] (1846-1919)
Remarks on the psychical treatment of neurasthenia. Boston: [Damrell & Upham], 1895. 24p. DNLM
90-7003

PUTNAM, James J[ackson] (1846-1919)
Hyperostosis cranii, with the reports of four new cases; a fifth case contributed by Morton Prince; and photographs of a specimen in the Army Medical Museum. Philadelphia, 1896. 21p. DNLM **90-7004**

PUTNAM, James J[ackson] (1846-1919)
On the etiology and pathogenesis of the post-traumatic psychoses and neuroses. New York, 1898. 31p. DNLM
90-7005

PUTNAM, James J[ackson] (1846-1919)
The relation between trigeminal neuralgias and migraine. [n. p., 1898, *vel subseq.*] 6p. DNLM
90-7006

PUTNAM, James J[ackson] (1846-1919)
Remarks on the desirability of a more careful study and extended use of hydrotherapeutics. Boston: Damrell & Upham, 1899. 13p. DNLM **90-7007**

PUTNAM, James J[ackson] (1846-1919)
The Shattuck lecture. Not the disease only, but also the man. [Boston, 1899.] 33p. DNLM; MB; MH
90-7008

PUTNAM, James J[ackson] (1846-1919) and Maurice H. RICHARDSON
A case of cerebral sarcoma of great extent; extirpation; marked amelioration of symptoms; recurrence and death at the end of six months. Remarks on the advantages of palliative operations in cerebral tumors. Boston: Damrell & Upham, 1899. 16p. DNLM **90-7009**

PUTNAM, James J[ackson] (1846-1919) and J. Collins WARREN
The surgical treatment of tumors within the spinal canal. Philadelphia, 1899. 16p. DNLM **90-7010**

PYE, Walter (1853-1932)
Pye's surgical handicraft. . . . 1st American from 3rd London ed., rev. and ed. by T. H. R. Crowle. [Vol. I] New York: E. B. Treat, 1892. 276p. MBM; NNNAM; PU
90-7011

PYE, Walter (1853-1932)
Elementary bandaging and surgical dressing, with directions concerning the immediate treatment of cases of emergency; for the use of dressers and nurses. Revised and in part rewritten by G. Bellingham Smith. 7th ed. Philadelphia: W. B. Saunders, 1897. 218p. DNLM; NNNAM; PPC; PU [Earlier editions appeared as Pye's Surgical handicraft. . . .]
90-7012

PYE-SMITH, Philip Henry (1839-1914)
An introduction to the study of diseases of the skin. Philadelphia: Lea Bros. & Co., 1893. 408p. DNLM; NNNAM; OCIM; PPC **90-7013**

PYLE, J[ohn] S.
Emptying the uterine cavity by artificial dilation; a new bag for its accomplishment. New York, 1893. 4p. DNLM
90-7014

PYLE, J[ohn] S.
A plea for the appropriation of criminals condemned to capital punishment to the experimental physiologist. [Keokuk, 1893.] 8p. DNLM **90-7015**

PYLE, J[ohn] S.
A new surgical table. New York: D. Appleton & Co., 1899. 10p. DNLM **90-7016**

PYLE, J[ohn] S.
Pneumonectomy, the future treatment of incipient pulmonary tuberculosis. New York, 1899. 6p. DNLM
90-7017

[PYLE, Walter L[ytle]] (1871-1921)
3000 questions on medical subjects, arranged for self-examination. With the proper reference to standard works in which the correct replies will be found. Philadelphia: P. Blakiston, Son & Co., 1891. 144p. DLC; PPC
90-7018

PYLE, Walter L[ytle] (1871-1921)
Four cases of opium poisoning in which potassium permanganate was administered. Philadelphia, 1894. 5p. DNLM
90-7019

PYLE, Walter L[ytle] (1871-1921)
Ainhum. [Philadelphia: Lea Bros. & Co., 1895.] 12p. DNLM **90-7020**

PYLE, Walter L[ytle] (1871-1921)
The treatment of syphilis with intravenous injection of mercuric chlorid. [Philadelphia: Lea Bros. & Co., 1895.] 11p. DNLM **90-7021**

PYLE, Walter L[ytle] (1871-1921)
The therapeusis of the saints. Philadelphia, 1896. 12p. DNLM **90-7022**

PYLE, Walter L[ytle] (1871-1921)
Unilateral albuminuric retinitis; with report of a case. Philadelphia, 1898. 9p. DNLM **90-7023**

PYLE, Walter L[ytle] (1871-1921)
The diagnosis of iritis. New York: E. B. Treat & Co., 1899. 2 l. DNLM **90-7024**

PYLE, Walter L[ytle] (1871-1921)
Functional disturbances of the ocular muscles. New York: E. B. Treat & Co., 1899. 2 l. DNLM
90-7025

PYLE, Walter L[ytle] (1871-1921)
Hydrophthalmos; a bibliographic, clinical, and pathologic study. Philadelphia, 1899. 28p. DNLM
90-7026

PYLE, Walter L[ytle] (1871-1921)
Hydrophthalmos; a bibliographic, clinical, and pathologic study. St. Louis, 1899. 30p. 1 plate. DNLM
90-7027

PYLE, Walter L[ytle] (1871-1921)
A new model of a small ophthalmoscope. Philadelphia, 1899. 4p. DNLM **90-7028**

[PYLE, Walter L[ytle]] (1871-1921)
3,000 questions on medical subjects, arranged for self-examination. With the proper reference to standard works in which the correct replies will be found. 2nd ed., enl. Philadelphia: P. Blakiston's Son & Co., 1899. 189p. DLC; NNNAM; PPC **90-7029**

PYNCHON, Edwin (1853-1914)
Removal of tonsillar hypertrophy by electro-cautery dissection. Chicago: Office Amer. Med. Assoc., 1890. 12p. DNLM **90-7030**

PYNCHON, Edwin (1853-1914)
The post-partum douche (showing new instrument). Chicago: R. R. Donnelley & Sons, 1891. 1p. DNLM
90-7031

PYNCHON, Edwin (1853-1914)
The post-partum douche (showing new instrument). Anniston, Ala., 1891. 8p. DNLM **90-7032**

PYNCHON, Edwin (1853-1914)
How can diseases of the nose and throat affect the teeth? Chicago: Regan, 1892. 16p. DNLM **90-7033**

PYNCHON, Edwin (1853-1914)
Anterior soft hypertrophies of the nasal septum. St. Louis, 1896. 4p. DNLM **90-7034**

PYNCHON, Edwin (1853-1914)
Colono-enteric irrigation in the treatment of intestinal obstruction. Chicago, 1896. 8p. DNLM **90-7035**

PYNCHON, Edwin (1853-1914)
Solutions Dobell. Kansas City, Mo., 1896. 7p. DNLM **90-7036**

PYNCHON, Edwin (1853-1914)
The absolute and permanent cure of tonsillitis. Chicago, 1897. 4 l. DNLM **90-7037**

PYNCHON, Edwin (1853-1914)
The evolution of the Buttles inhaler. St. Louis, 1897. 7p. DNLM **90-7038**

PYNCHON, Edwin (1853-1914)
Hydrastis in the treatment of catarrhal dyspepsia. Chicago, 1897. 3p. DNLM **90-7039**

PYNCHON, Edwin (1853-1914)
Impaired ventilation and drainage of the nose the most common causes of nasal catarrh. Chicago, 1897. 8p. DNLM **90-7040**

PYNCHON, Edwin (1853-1914)
Instruments used in tonsillotomy by electro-cautery dissection. St. Louis, 1897. 4p. DNLM **90-7041**

PYNCHON, Edwin (1853-1914)
Intussusception treated by colono-enteric irrigation. Louisville, 1897. 8p. DNLM **90-7042**

PYNCHON, Edwin (1853-1914)
Nasal bougies and drainage-tubes. [New York, 1897.] 4p. DNLM **90-7043**

PYNCHON, Edwin (1853-1914)
A new nebulizing device. St. Louis, 1897. 4p. DNLM **90-7044**

PYNCHON, Edwin (1853-1914)
Either a pocket inhaler or a middle-ear inflater. New York, 1898. 4p. DNLM **90-7045**

PYNCHON, Edwin (1853-1914)
Improved rhinological furniture. St. Louis, 1898. 4p. DNLM **90-7046**

PYNCHON, Edwin (1853-1914)
The submerged tonsil. Chicago: McClure Pr. Co., [1898]. 11p. DNLM **90-7047**

PYNCHON, Edwin (1853-1914)
The technique of tympanic inflation. St. Louis, 1898. 8p. DNLM **90-7048**

PYNCHON, Edwin (1853-1914)
A new nasal septometer. St. Louis, 1899. 1 l. DNLM **90-7049**

PYNCHON, Edwin (1853-1914)
The offending middle turbinal. [St. Louis, 1899.] 8p. DNLM **90-7050**

PYNCHON, Edwin (1853-1914)
The bête noir of the vocalist. Chicago, 1899. 24p. DNLM **90-7051**

QUACKENBOS, John Duncan (1848-1926)
Causes and recent treatment of neurasthenia. New York, [1897]. 19p. DNLM **90-7052**

QUAIN, Richard, ed. (1816-1898)
A dictionary of medicine including general pathology, general therapeutics, hygiene, and the diseases peculiar to women and children by various authors. New York: D. Appleton & Co., 1890. 1816p. CtY-M; NNNAM; OCIM; PU **90-7053**

QUAIN, Richard, ed. (1816-1898)
A dictionary of medicine, including general pathology, general therapeutics, hygiene . . . by various writers . . . assisted by Frederick Thomas Roberts . . . and J. Mitchell Bruce . . . with an American appendix by Samuel Treat Armstrong. . . . New ed., rev. throughout and enl. New York: D. Appleton & Co., 1894. 2 v. plates. DLC; NNNAM; PPC; PU **90-7054**

QUEEN, JAMES W., & CO. PHILADELPHIA
Priced and illustrated catalogue of microscopes and accessories, magnifying glasses, stereoscopes, graphoscopes, etc. Philadelphia, 1890. 107p. DNLM; PPC **90-7055**

QUEEN, JAMES W., & CO. PHILADELPHIA
A pocket catalogue of microscopes, magnifiers, microscopical accessories, mounting materials, etc. Philadelphia, 1892. 20p. DNLM; PU **90-7056**

QUIMBY, Charles E.
The penumatic cabinet in the treatment of pulmonary phthisis. [Philadelphia], 1893. 16p. DNLM **90-7057**

QUIMBY, Charles E.
Pneumotherapy in pulmonary hemorrhage. New York: D. Appleton & Co., 1896. 12p. DNLM **90-7058**

QUINLAN, Francis J.
Nasal obstruction as a factor of tinnitus aurium. [New York, 1895.] 8p. DNLM **90-7059**

RABAGLIATI, Andrea C[arlo] F[rancesco] (*b.* 1843)
On some symptoms which simulate disease of the pelvic organs in women, and their treatment by allopiesto-myo-kinetics (massage) and by auto-piesto-myo-kinetics (self-movements of muscles under pressure). New York: William Wood & Co., 1895. 77p. 11 plates. DNLM; NNNAM **90-7060**

RABAGLIATI, Andrea C[arlo] F[rancesco] (*b.* 1843)
Air, food, and exercise; an essay on the predisposing causes of disease. New York: William Wood & Co., 1898. 220p. DNLM; NNNAM **90-7061**

RACHFORD, Benjamin Knox (1857-1929)
Anaemia of tuberculosis. New York: M. J. Rooney, 1892. 24p. DNLM; NNNAM **90-7062**

RACHFORD, Benjamin Knox (1857-1929)
Fat digestion. Philadelphia, 1892. 9p. DNLM **90-7063**

RACHFORD, Benjamin Kox (1857-1929)
Purpura hemorrhagica. [Philadelphia, 1892.] 8p. DNLM **90-7064**

RACHFORD, Benjamin Knox (1857-1929)
The etiology of chorea. [n. p., 1893.] 14p. DNLM **90-7065**

RACHFORD, Benjamin Knox (1857-1929)
Tuberculous neuroses of childhood. New York, 1893. 17p. DNLM **90-7066**

RACHFORD, Benjamin Knox (1857-1929)
Paraxanthin as a factor in the etiology of certain obscure nervous conditions. [Philadelphia: Lea Bros. & Co., 1894.] 17p. DNLM **90-7067**

RACHFORD, Benjamin Knox (1857-1929)
Uric-acid leukomains as factors in the etiology of migraine and kindred nervous diseases. [Philadelphia: Lea Bros. & Co., 1894.] 13p. DNLM **90-7068**

RACHFORD, Benjamin Knox (1857-1929)
Comparative anatomy of the bile and pancreatic ducts in mammals, studied from the physiologic standpoint of fat digestion. Detroit: Geo. S. Davis, 1895. 11p. DNLM **90-7069**

RACHFORD, Benjamin Knox (1857-1929)
Leucomain poisoning. New York, 1895. 21p. DNLM **90-7070**

RACHFORD, Benjamin Knox (1857-1929)
Treatment of leukomain poisoning. Philadelphia: Lea Bros. & Co., 1895. 11p. DNLM **90-7071**

RACHFORD, Benjamin Knox (1857-1929)
Some physiological factors of the neuroses of childhood. . . . Cincinnati: The R. Clarke Co., 1895. 112p. DLC **90-7072**

RACHFORD, Benjamin Knox (1857-1929)
A case of superficial gangrene. New York, 1896. 8p. DNLM **90-7073**

RACHFORD, Benjamin Knox (1857-1929)
Leukomain poisoning. New York, 1896. 18p. DNLM **90-7074**

RADCLIFFE, Samuel J. (1828-1903)
The relation of tonsillitis to rheumatism. Chicago, 1890. 8p. DNLM **90-7075**

RADCLIFFE, Samuel J. (1828-1903)
Ichthyol as a remedy for facial erysipelas. Detroit, Mich.: G. S. Davis, 1892. 7p. DNLM **90-7076**

RADCLIFFE, Samuel J. (1828-1903)
Foreign bodies in the nasal cavities. [St. Louis, 1893.] 6p. DNLM **90-7077**

RADCLIFFE, Samuel J. (1828-1903)
Cold water as a hygienic measure in health and disease. [n. p., 1893.] 4p. DNLM **90-7078**

RAINEAR, A. Rusling
The electro-therapeutics of rheumatism. [Philadelphia], 1897. 2 l. DNLM **90-7079**

RAKE, Beaven (1858-1894)
The value of surgery in leprosy. St. Louis, 1893. 24p. DNLM **90-7080**

RAMBAUD, George Gibier (*b.* 1875)
The treatment of tetanus by means of intracerebral injections of antitoxine; with a résumé of reports of cases, and a few remarks on the technique of the injection. New York, 1898. 14p. DNLM **90-7081**

RAMDOHR, C. A. von
Results from the administration of iron in a readily assimilated form after gynaecological operations. New York, 1897. 2 l. DNLM **90-7082**

RAMSAY, William (1852-1916)
A system of inorganic chemistry. Philadelphia: P. Blakiston, Son & Co., 1891. 700p. ICU; MB; MH; NN **90-7083**

RAND, H[enry] W[alter] (1851-1895)
Observations on the treatment of urethral stricture, and a modification of Otis's urethrotome. [New York: D. Appleton & Co., 1891.] 11p. DNLM **90-7084**

RAND, H[enry] W[alter] (1851-1895)
External perineal urethrotomy. [Brooklyn], 1894. 5p. DNLM **90-7085**

RAND, J[ohn] P[rentice] (1857-1923)
The significance of germs in pulmonary disease. New York, 1895. 9p. DNLM **90-7086**

RAND, J[ohn] P[rentice] (1857-1923)
Obligations of the physician. Annual oration delivered before the Massachusetts Homoeopathic Medical Society, October 13, 1897. Boston: O. Clapp, 1897. 12p. DNLM **90-7087**

RANDALL, Burton Alexander (1858-1932)
Can hypermetropia be healthfully outgrown? Hartford, Conn., 1890. 12p. DNLM **90-7088**

RANDALL, Burton Alexander (1858-1932)
The perforation in Shrapnell's membrane. New Bedford: Mercury Publ. Co., 1890. 15p. 1 plate. DNLM **90-7089**

RANDALL, Burton Alexander (1858-1932)
The corrosion method in the study of the anatomy of the ear. [Philadelphia, 1890.] 7p. 1 plate. DNLM **90-7090**

RANDALL, Burton Alexander (1858-1932)
Suppuration of the tympanic attic and perforation in Shrapnell's membrane. New York, 1890. 20p. DNLM **90-7091**

RANDALL, Burton Alexander (1858-1932)
The corrosion method in the study of the anatomy of the ear. [Philadelphia, 1891.] 4p. DNLM **90-7092**

RANDALL, Burton Alexander (1858-1932)
Mastoid abscess breaking into the digastric fossa. Detroit, 1892. 10p. DNLM **90-7093**

RANDOLPH, Robert L[ee] (1860-1919)
A series of fifty consecutive operations for cataract. [Baltimore, 1892.] 6 l. DNLM **90-7094**

RANDOLPH, Robert L[ee] (1860-1919)
A case of panophthalmitis caused by the bacillus coli communis. [Philadelphia, 1893.] 4p. DNLM **90-7095**

RANDOLPH, Robert L[ee] (1860-1919)
Sympathetic ophthalmia. Philadelphia, 1898. 55p. 1 plate. DNLM **90-7096**

RANKIN, Egbert Guernsey
A digest of external therapeutics; with numerous formulae arranged for reference. . . . New York: Boericke & Runyon Co., 1899. 647p. DLC; NNNAM; PPHa; PU **90-7097**

RANKIN, Francis H[untington] (1845-1896)
Hygiene of childhood: suggestions for the care of children after the period of infancy to the completion of puberty. . . . New York: D. Appleton & Co., 1890. 140p. DLC; NNNAM **90-7098**

RANNEY, Ambrose L[oomis] (1848-1905)
Lectures on nervous diseases from the stand-point of cerebral and spinal localization, and the later methods employed in the diagnosis and treatment of these affections. Philadelphia: F. A. Davis, 1890. 778p. CtY-M; NNNAM; PPC; PU **90-7099**

RANNEY, Ambrose L[oomis] (1848-1905)
Sleeplessness; facts relating to its causes and cure. New York: D. Appleton & Co., 1891. 22p. DNLM; NNNAM **90-7100**

RANNEY, Ambrose L[oomis] (1848-1905)
Some prevalent errors relating to "eyestrain" as a cause of nervous derangements. With illustrative cases. [New York, 1892.] 51p. 1 tab. DNLM; NNNAM **90-7101**

RANNEY, Ambrose L[oomis] (1848-1905)
The eye treatment of epileptics. A critical review of certain factors that may lead to convulsive seizures, and the treatment of epilepsy without drugs. [New York: D. Appleton & Co.], 1894. 73p. 1 tab. DNLM; NNNAM **90-7102**

RANNEY, Ambrose L[oomis] (1848-1905)
Eye-strain as a cause of epilepsy, and the results of eye treatment. (A reply to Frederick Peterson.) New York, 1897. 50p. 1 tab. DNLM; NNNAM **90-7103**

RANNEY, Ambrose L[oomis] (1848-1905)
Eye-strain in health and disease. With special reference to the amelioration or cure of chronic nervous derangements without the aid of drugs. . . . Philadelphia, New York, [etc.]: The F. A. Davis Co., 1897. 321p. diags. DLC; DNLM; NNNAM; PPC **90-7104**

RANNEY, George E[mery] (1839-1915)
President's annual address. Death a universal law. [Lansing, 1892.] 21p. DNLM **90-7105**

RANSOHOFF, Joseph (1853-1921)
Rupture of middle meningeal artery without fracture; ligation of common carotid artery. Philadelphia: W. J. Dornan, 1890. 15p. DNLM **90-7106**

RANSOHOFF, Joseph (1853-1921)
Tuberculous disease of the tarsus. Philadelphia, 1890. 10p. 1 tab. DNLM **90-7107**

RANSOHOFF, Joseph (1853-1921)
Linear craniotomy for microcephalus. [Philadelphia, 1891.] 6p. DNLM **90-7108**

RANSOHOFF, Joseph (1853-1921)
The treatment of gangrenous hernia. [Philadelphia, 1892.] 16p. 2 plates. DNLM **90-7109**

RANSOHOFF, Joseph (1853-1921)
Trephining for abscess of the brain. [Cincinnati, 1892.] 8p. DNLM **90-7110**

RANSOHOFF, Joseph (1853-1921)
The extirpation of aneurisms. [Philadelphia, 1894.] 7p. DNLM **90-7111**

RANSOHOFF, Joseph (1853-1921)
Thyroid abscess; thyroidectomy; recovery. [Philadelphia, 1894.] 8p. DNLM **90-7112**

RANSOHOFF, Joseph (1853-1921)
Treatment of strangulated hernia. Chicago: Amer. Med. Assoc. Press, 1894. 24p. DNLM **90-7113**

RANSOHOFF, Joseph (1853-1921)
Concerning stone in the kidney and its operative treatment, with report of cases. Chicago, 1895. 24p. DNLM **90-7114**

RANSOHOFF, Joseph (1853-1921)
Considerations on the diagnosis and operative treatment of gall-stones. Cincinnati, 1898. 10p. DNLM **90-7115**

RANSOHOFF, Joseph (1853-1921)
Decortication of the tongue in the treatment of lingual psoriasis. Philadelphia, 1899. 7p. DNLM **90-7116**

RANSOHOFF, Joseph (1853-1921)
Gall-stones; consideration of their etiology, diagnosis, and operative treatment. Chicago, 1899. 24p. DNLM **90-7117**

RANSOHOFF, Joseph (1853-1921)
Nephrectomy vs. nephrotomy. Philadelphia, 1899. 34p. DNLM **90-7118**

RANSOHOFF, Joseph (1853-1921)
Nephrectomy vs. nephrotomy. Philadelphia, 1899. 33p. DNLM **90-7119**

RANSOM, Charles C[ook] (*b.* 1860)
Removal of large fragment of glass from larynx after lodgment for twenty-one months. New York, 1891. 4p. DNLM **90-7120**

RANSOM, Charles C[ook] (*b.* 1860)
Diseases of the skin. A manual for students and practitioners. Series editd by Bern B. Gallaudet. Philadelphia: Lea Bros. & Co., [1893]. 201p. DNLM; NNNAM; PPC; PU **90-7121**

RANSOM, Charles C[ook] (*b.* 1860)
An unusual case of naevus unius lateris. New York, 1896. 6p. DNLM **90-7122**

RANSOM, Charles C[ook] (*b.* 1860)
The treatment of gout. New York: W. R. Jenkins, 1897. 16p. DNLM **90-7123**

RAU, Leonard S.
A comparative study of the different methods of treating posterior displacements of the uterus, both mechanical and operative. [New York, 1894.] 7p. DNLM **90-7124**

RAUCH, John H[enry] (1828-1894)
Medical educatio , medical colleges, and the regulation of the practice of the medicine in the United States and Canada, 1765-1891. (Illinois State Board of Health.) Springfield, Ill.: H. W. Rokker, 1891. 222p. IU-M; NNNAM; OCIM; PU **90-7125**

RAUE, Charles Godlove (1820-1896)
Special pathology and diagnostics, with therapeutic hints. . . . 4th ed., rev. and augm. Philadelphia: Boericke & Tafel, 1896. 1039p. DLC; PPC; PPHa **90-7126**

RAUE, Charles Sigmund (*b.* 1873)
Diseases of children. . . . Philadelphia: Boericke & Tafel, 1899. 473p. DLC; ICJ; PPC; PPHa **90-7127**

RAVENEL, Mazÿck Porcher (1861-1946)
Trichorexis nodosa; a preliminary note. [Philadelphia, 1892.] 1 galley sheet. DNLM **90-7128**

RAVENEL, Mazÿck Porcher (1861-1946)
A contribution to the study of the etiology of membranous rhinitis. Philadelphia: Lea Bros. & Co., 1895. 27p. DNLM; PPC **90-7129**

RAVOGLI, Augustus (*b.* 1851)
The influence of the nervous system on certain disturbances of the skin. [Philadelphia, 1892.] 13p. DNLM **90-7130**

RAVOGLI, Augustus (*b.* 1851)
Psorospermosis cutis. Chicago, 1894. 12p. DNLM **90-7131**

RAVOGLI, Augustus (*b.* 1851)
Chairman's address. Chicago, 1898. 12p. DNLM **90-7132**

RAVOGLI, Augustus (*b.* 1851)
Nature and treatment of cutaneous cancer. Chicago, 1899. 30p. **90-7133**

RAVOGLI, Augustus (*b.* 1851)
The treatment of gonorrhea in the female. New York, 1899. 14p. DNLM **90-7134**

RAY, J. Morrison (*b.* 1861)
Observations upon eye diseases and blindness in the colored race. New York, 1896. 9p. DNLM **90-7135**

RAY, Richard
Uric acid and its elimination; with clinical reports of seven cases. [Kansas City, 1890.] 8p. DNLM **90-7136**

RAY, Richard
Anemic conditions due to imperfect nutrition. [1890.] 8p. DNLM **90-7137**

RAYMOND, Joseph Howard (1845-1915)
Preparation of the city of Brooklyn for the anticipated epidemic of cholera in 1884 and 1885. New York: M. J. Rooney, [1892]. 7p. DNLM **90-7138**

RAYMOND, Joseph Howard (1845-1915)
Sulphur fumigation in cholera. [New York, 1892.] 11p. DNLM **90-7139**

RAYMOND, Joseph Howard (1845-1915)
A manual of human physiology, prepared with special reference to students of medicine. Philadelphia: W. B. Saunders, 1894. 382p. 4 plates. DLC; DNLM; PPC; PU **90-7140**

REBER, [James] Wendell (1867-1916)
Six instances of color-blind women occurring in two generations of one family. [Philadelphia, 1895.] 6p. DNLM **90-7141**

REDLINGTON & CO.
Prices current of druggists' proprietary articles and sundries. San Francisco, 1891. 345p. OCLloyd **90-7142**

REED, Boardman (1842-1917)
The climatic treatment of gastro-intestinal disease in children. [Philadelphia, 1890.] 8p. DNLM **90-7143**

REED, Boardman (1842-1917)
Note on the contagiousness of la grippe. Philadelphia, 1891. 3p. DNLM **90-7144**

REED, Boardman (1842-1917)
The teachings of experience and of rational therapeutics as to the treatment of pneumonia. Detroit, Mich.: G. S. Davis, 1892. 40p. DNLM **90-7145**

REED, Boardman (1842-1917)
The diagnosis and treatment of the early stages of chronic Bright's disease. New York: Trow, 1893. 8p. DNLM **90-7146**

REED, Boardman (1842-1917)
The classes of invalids most benefited at Atlantic City. Detroit, Mich.: G. S. Davis, 1894. 5p. DNLM **90-7147**

REED, Boardman (1842-1917)
The ratio that alimentation should bear to oxygenation in disease of the lungs. [Philadelphia, 1894.] 18p. DNLM **90-7148**

REED, Boardman (1842-1917)
A new pleximeter. [Philadelphia], 1895. 1 sheet. DNLM **90-7149**

REED, Boardman (1842-1917)
The diagnosis of changes in the size, position, and motility of the stomach in cases where intragastric instruments cannot be used. Philadelphia, 1896. 15p. DNLM **90-7150**

REED, Boardman (1842-1917)
The frequent dependence of insomnia, mental depression, and other neurasthenic symptoms upon disease of the gastro-intestinal tract. Chicago, 1896. 12p. DNLM
90-7151

REED, Boardman (1842-1917)
Diet in the chronic catarrhs of the gastro-intestinal tract. Chicago, 1898. 11p. DNLM **90-7152**

REED, Boardman (1842-1917)
Important indications and contra-indications for massage of the abdomen, with report of cases showing its effect upon the secretion of the gastric juice. [Philadelphia], 1898. 7p. DNLM
90-7153

REED, Boardman (1842-1917)
A plea for the more frequent resort to analysis of the stomach-contents for diagnostic purposes. [Philadelphia], 1898. 5p. DNLM **90-7154**

REED & CARNRICK
An abstract of the symptoms, with the latest dietetic and medicinal treatment of various diseased conditions. The food products. Digestion and assimilation. New York: Reed & Carnrick, 1891. 79p. 1 tab. DNLM; NNNAM
90-7155

REED, Charles A[lfred] L[ee] (1856-1928)
The genital factor in certain cases of neurasthenia in women. [New York, 1898.] 8p. DNLM **90-7156**

REED, Charles B. (*b.* 1866) and Frederick B. NOYES
A quiz manual of histology, general and dental. Chicago: W. T. Keener Co., 1897. 203p. DNLM; OCIM
90-7157

REED, Charles B. (*b.* 1866) and Frederick B. NOYES
A quiz manual of histology, general and dental. 2nd ed. Chicago: Chicago Medical Book Co., 1898. 203p. DLC
90-7158

REED, R. Harvey (1851-1907)
A case of haematoma of the ovary following chronic catarrhal salpingitis; with operation and recovery. Cincinnati, 1890. 8p. DNLM **90-7159**

REED, R. Harvey (1851-1907)
The surgical treatment of chronic catarrhal appendicitis. [Toledo, 1891.] 9p. DNLM **90-7160**

REED, R. Harvey (1851-1907)
A contribution to the study of some of the diseases peculiar to the right iliac fossa, with reference to their relief by surgical interference. Toledo, 1892. 19p. DNLM
90-7161

REED, R. Harvey (1851-1907)
Experimental research on the implantation of the ureters into the rectum. [Philadelphia, 1892.] 18p. 4 plates. DNLM
90-7162

REED, R. Harvey (1851-1907)
A unique case of traumatic neurosis. [Philadelphia, 1893.] 6p. DNLM **90-7163**

REED, R. Harvey (1851-1907)
The diagnosis and treatment of floating kidney. [Columbus, O., 1894.] 8p. DNLM **90-7164**

REED, R. Harvey (1851-1907)
A new method for anchoring the kidney. Chicago: Amer. Med. Assoc. Press, 1894. 8p. DNLM **90-7165**

REED, R. Harvey (1851-1907)
Post-operative insanity. Chicago, 1898. 12p. DNLM
90-7166

REED, R. Harvey (1851-1907)
The X-ray from a medico-legal standpoint. Chicago, 1898. 11p. DNLM **90-7167**

REED, R. Harvey (1851-1907)
The higher the order of railway surgery, the greater the protection to the employe, the passenger, and the company. Chicago, 1899. 11p. DNLM **90-7168**

REED, R. Harvey (1851-1907)
Some of the rare forms of hernia and their radical treatment. Chicago, 1899. 12p. DNLM **90-7169**

REED, Walter (1851-1902)
An investigation into the so-called lymphoid nodules of the liver in abdominal typhus. Philadelphia, 1895. 17p. DNLM
90-7170

REED, Walter (1851-1902) and James CARROLL
Bacillus icteroides and bacillus cholerae suis. A preliminary note. New York, 1899. 6p. DNLM **90-7171**

REED, Walter (1851-1902) and James CARROLL
The specific cause of yellow fever. A reply to Dr. G. Sanarelli. New York, 1899. 9p. DNLM **90-7172**

REED, Walter (1851-1902)
The germicidal value of trikresol. Washington, 1899. 8p. DNLM **90-7173**

REESE, John James (1818-1892)
The post-mortem imbibition of poisons in its medico-legal bearings. [Philadelphia, 1890.] 16p. DNLM
90-7174

REESE, John James (1818-1892)
Text-book of medical jurisprudence and toxicology. 3rd ed., revised and enlarged. Philadelphia: P. Blakiston, Son & Co., 1891. 666p. DLC; DNLM; PPC **90-7175**

REESE, John James (1818-1892)
Text-book of medical jurisprudence and toxicology. 4th ed., revised by Henry Leffmann. Philadelphia: P. Blakiston, Son & Co., 1894. 624p. DLC; DNLM; NNNAM; PU
90-7176

REESE, John James (1818-1892)
Text-book of medical jurisprudence and toxicology. 5th ed., revised by Henry Leffmann. Philadelphia: P. Blakiston, Son & Co., 1898. 645p. DLC: DNLM; PPC; PPJ
90-7177

REEVE, J[ohn] Charles (1826-1920)
Chloroform and the Hyderabad commission. [Philadelphia, 1890.] 21p. DNLM **90-7178**

REEVE, J[ohn] Charles (1826-1920)
The A. C. E. mixture. Cleveland, O.: Lowing & Prescott, [1891]. 14p. DNLM **90-7179**

REEVE, J[ohn] Charles (1826-1920)
Some surgery of the liver and gall-bladder. [New York, 1892.] 14p. DNLM **90-7180**

REEVE, J[ohn] Charles (1826-1920)
In memoriam. Alexander Dunlap. A.M., M.D. [New York, 1894.] 10p. port. DNLM **90-7181**

REEVE, J[ohn] Charles (1826-1920)
The entrance of woman into medicine. Cleveland, O., 1895. 18p. DNLM **90-7182**

REEVES, James Edmund (1829-1896)
Some points in the natural history of enteric or typhoid fever. Philadelphia: W. J. Dornan, 1890. 26p. DNLM; PPC **90-7183**

REEVES, James Edmund (1829-1896)
A hand-book of microscopy for students and general practitioners, including chapters on bacteriology, neoplasms, and urinary examinations; with a glossary. Philadelphia: P. Blakiston, Son & Co., 1894. 237p. DLC; DNLM; PPC; PU **90-7184**

RÉGIS, Emmanuel (1855-1918)
A practical manual of mental medicine . . . with a preface by M. Benjamin Ball. . . . A work crowned by the Faculty of Medicine of Paris Chateauvillard Prize, 1886. 2nd ed. thoroughly rev. and largely re-written. Authorized translation by H. M. Bannister. . . . Utica, N.Y.: Press of American Journal of Insanity, 1894. 692p. CtY-M; IU-M; OCIM; PPC **90-7185**

RÉGIS, Emmanuel (1855-1918)
A practical manual of mental medicine. With a preface by Benjamin Ball. 2nd ed., thoroughly and largely re-written. Authorized translation by H. M. Bannister, with an introduction by the author. Philadelphia: P. Blakiston, Son & Co., 1895. 692p. DNLM; ICJ; MB; MH **90-7186**

REHFUSS, William F.
A treatise on dental jurisprudence, for dentists and lawyers. Philadelphia: The Wilmington Dental Mfg. Co., 1892. 468p. DLC **90-7187**

REICHERT, Edward T[yson] (*b.* 1865)
The action of alcohol on animal heat functions. Detroit: G. S. Davis, 1890. 15p. DNLM **90-7188**

REICHERT, Edward T[yson] (*b.* 1865)
Heat phenomena in normal animals. Part I. Calorimetry. [Philadelphia, 1890.] 12p. DNLM **90-7189**

REICHERT, Edward T[yson] (*b.* 1865)
Heat phenomena in normal animals. Part II. Heat production in relation to body weight. [Philadelphia, 1890.] 10p. DNLM **90-7190**

REICHERT, Edward T[yson] (*b.* 1865)
Heat phenomena in normal animals. Part III. Normal variations in heat production. [Philadelphia, 1890.] 14p. DNLM **90-7191**

REICHERT, Edward T[yson] (*b.* 1865)
The knee-jerk after section of the spinal cord. [New York, 1890.] 4p. DNLM **90-7192**

REINGER, GEBBERT & SCHALL
Electro-medical instruments, an illustrated catalogue of apparatus. 5th ed. Chicago, 1893. 101p. NNNAM **90-7193**

REINHOLD, August F.
Nature vs. drugs. A challenge to the drugging fraternity. New York: A. F. Reinhold, 1898. 546p. NN; NNNAM **90-7194**

REMINGTON, Joseph Price (1847-1918)
The practice of pharmacy. A treatise on the modes of making and dispensing official, unofficial, and extemporaneous preparations, with descriptions of their properties, uses, and doses. Intended as a hand-book for pharmacists and physicians and a text-book for students. 3rd ed. Enl. and thoroughly rev. . . . With over six hundred illustrations. Philadelphia, [etc.]: J. B. Lippincott Co., [1894]. 1497p. diags. DLC; DNLM; NNNAM; PPC **90-7195**

REMONDINO, P[eter] C[harles] (1846-1926)
Longevity and climate. Relations of climatic conditions to longevity, history, and religion. Relations of climate to national and personal habits. The climate of California and its effects in relation to longevity. San Francisco: Woodward & Co., 1890. 44p. DNLM; NN **90-7196**

REMONDINO, P[eter] C[harles] (1846-1926)
The social evil. Some observations on its causes, orign, and progress in history. How far is woman chargeable with its existence? [Los Angeles, 1890.] 16p. DNLM **90-7197**

REMONDINO, P[eter] C[harles] (1846-1926)
History of circumcision from the earliest times to the present. Moral and physical reasons for its performance, with a history of eunuchism, hermaphrodism, etc., and of different operations practiced upon the prepuce. Philadelphia & London: F. A. Davis, 1891. 346p. 1 plate. DNLM; NNNAM; PPC; PU **90-7198**

REMONDINO, P[eter] C[harles] (1846-1926)
An interesting and instructive case of uraemia, combining coma and mania, with marked local toxaemic manifestations. [New York, 1891.] 8p. DNLM **90-7199**

REMONDINO, P[eter] C[harles] (1846-1926)
Ventilation and impure air as prophylactic or causative of disease. Concord, N.H., 1891. 25p. DNLM **90-7200**

REMONDINO, P[eter] C[harles] (1846-1926)
. . . History of circumcision from the earliest times to the present. Moral and physical reasons for its performance. . . . Philadelphia and London: F. A. Davis, 1891. 346p. CtY-M; DLC; ICJ; NIC **90-7201**

REMONDINO, P[eter] C[harles] (1846-1926)
The Mediterranean shores of America. Southern California: climate, physical and meteorological conditions. Philadelphia & London: F. A. Davis Co., 1892. 160p. 2 maps. DNLM; PPC **90-7202**

REMONDINO, P[eter] C[harles] (1846-1926)
The mild climatic treatment of invalids with pulmonary consumpton in Southern California. Detroit, Mich.: G. S. Davis, 1893. 126p. 2 charts, 1 plate. DNLM; OCIM **90-7203**

REMONDINO, P[eter] C[harles] (1846-1926)
The evolution of relic worship. a page from the history of medicine. Detroit, 1895. 11p. DNLM
90-7204

REMONDINO, P[eter] C[harles] (1846-1926)
Pancreatic cysts. Los Angeles, 1895. 7p. DNLM
90-7205

REMONDINO, P[eter] C[harles] (1846-1926)
History of the evolutionary processes that led to the discovery of the circulation of the blood by William Harvey. Philadelphia, 1899. 27p. DNLM; PPC **90-7206**

REMONDINO, P[eter] C[harles] (1846-1926)
A study in retrospective therapeutics. The evolutionary processes through which have traveled transfusion, infusion, subcutaneous injection, enteroclysis, peritoneoclysis, and cystoclysis in the treatment of Asiatic cholera, from 1830 to 1895. Philadelphia, 1899. 57p. DNLM; PPC
90-7207

REMSEN, Ira (1846-1927)
The principles of theoretical chemistry, with special reference to the constitution of chemical compounds. 4th ed. Philadelphia: Lea Bros. & Co., 1892. 322p. DNLM; NNNAM; PPC; PPJ **90-7208**

REMSEN, Ira (1846-1927)
The principles of theoretical chemistry, with special reference to the constitution of chemical compounds. 5th ed. Philadelphia & New York: Lea Bros. & Co., 1897. 326p. DNLM; MdBJ-W; PPC: PU **90-7209**

REYBURN, Robert (1833-1909)
Curiosities of homoeopathic pharmacy. Chicago, 1890. 7p. DNLM **90-7210**

REYBURN, Robert (1833-1909)
The life-history of micro-organisms, with its relation to the theory of evolution. (Read before the Washington Microscopical Society.) [n. p., 1890.] 4p. DNLM
90-7211

REYBURN, Robert (1833-1909)
Type of disease among the freed people of the United States. Consolidated reports of sick and wounded freed people and white refugees under treatment from 1865 to June 30, 1872, by medical officers on duty in Bureau of Refugees, Freedmen and Abandoned Lands. Washington: Gibson, 1891. 15p. 8 tab. DNLM **90-7212**

REYBURN, Robert (1833-1909)
Aseptic surgery in the hospitals of Paris in 1892. [Philadelphia, 1892.] 7p. DNLM **90-7213**

REYBURN, Robert (1833-1909)
Diphtheria treated by the early local use of germicides. [Philadelphia, 1893.] 8p. DNLM **90-7214**

REYBURN, Robert (1833-1909)
Laws of growth of the cell applied to human anatomy. [Baltimore, 1893.] 4p. DNLM **90-7215**

REYBURN, Robert (1833-1909)
Type of disease among the freed people (mixed Negro races) of the United States. [Philadelphia, 1893.] 14p. DNLM
90-7216

REYBURN, Robert (1833-1909)
Clinical history of the case of President James Abram Garfield. Chicago, 1894. 108p. 1 chart. DNLM **90-7217**

REYBURN, Robert (1833-1909)
The operation of vaginal hysterectomy by enucleation due to Langenbeck. [Philadelphia, 1894.] 3p. DNLM
90-7218

REYBURN, Robert (1833-1909)
Vaginal hysterectomy for carcinoma of the uterus performed by enucleation without hemorrhage. [Philadelphia, 1894.] 5p. DNLM **90-7219**

REYBURN, Robert (1833-1909)
Life history of bacillus tuberculosis in its relations to the treatment by tuberculin. Chicago, 1898. 12p. DNLM
90-7220

REYBURN, Robert (1833-1909)
Treatment of purulent tubercular peritonitis by incision, with illustrative case. Chicago, 1898. 7p. DNLM **90-7221**

REYNDERS, JOHN & CO. NEW YORK
Illustrated catalogue and price-list of surgical instruments, orthopaedical apparatus, trusses, etc. 6th ed. New York, [1890, *vel subseq.*] 398p. DNLM; NNNAM
90-7222

REYNDERS, JOHN & CO. NEW YORK
Illustrated compendium and price-list of instrumentalities for surgery, therapeutics and biology . . . manufactured and imported by John Reynders & Co. . . . 7th ed. [New York], 1895. 617p. DLC; NNNAM **90-7223**

REYNOLDS, Dudley S[harpe] (1842-1915)
Granular lids. Chicago, 1896. 12p. DNLM
90-7224

REYNOLDS, Edward (*b.* 1860)
Modern methods in teaching clincial obstetrics. Read at the annual meeting of the Massachusetts Medical Society, June 12, 1889. [n. p., 1890?] 21p. NN **90-7225**

REYNOLDS, Edward (*b.* 1860)
On the frequency of contracted pelvis among American women, as deduced from 2,227 cases of labor. [Philadelphia, 1890.] 11p. DNLM **90-7226**

REYNOLDS, Edward (*b.* 1860)
The relations of the anatomy of the perineum to the mechanics of its laceration. Philadelphia: W. J. Dornan, 1891. 11p. 8 plates. DNLM **90-7227**

REYNOLDS, Edward (*b.* 1860)
The essentials of success in repair of the pelvic floor in primary and secondary operations. Boston: Damrell & Upham, 1892. 11p. DNLM **90-7228**

REYNOLDS, Edward (*b.* 1860)
The value of electricity in minor gynecology. Boston: Damrell & Upham, 1892. 17p. DNLM **90-7229**

REYNOLDS, Edward (*b.* 1860)
Practical midwifery; a handbook of treatment. . . . New York: William Wood & Co., 1892. 421p. DLC; DNLM; NNNAM; PPC **90-7230**

REYNOLDS, Edward (*b.* 1860)
Extra-uterine pregnancy. [Boston, 1893.] 15p. DNLM
90-7231

REYNOLDS, Edward (*b.* 1860)
A case of concealed accidental haemorrhage during the first stage of labor, with recovery of mother under conservative treatment. Boston, 1894. 3p. DNLM **90-7232**

REYNOLDS, Edward (*b.* 1860)
The treatment of face presentation. New York: William Wood & Co., 1894. 11p. DNLM **90-7233**

REYNOLDS, Edward (*b.* 1860)
A case of accidental concealed hemorrhage. Boston, 1894. 5p. DNLM **90-7234**

REYNOLDS, Edward (*b.* 1860)
Practical midwifery; a handbook of treatment. . . . [2nd ed.] New York: William Wood & Co., 1894. 421p. NNNAM; NNU-M; PPC; PPJ **90-7235**

REYNOLDS, Edward (*b.* 1860)
The results obtained by examination of the air-distended bladder in females, with remarks upon the technique and a summarized report of cases. Boston: Damrell & Upham, 1896. 15p. DNLM **90-7236**

REYNOLDS, Edward (*b.* 1860)
Tuberculosis of the bladder; its appearance and treatment through the Kelly cystoscope; with a report of cases. New York, 1896. 20p. DNLM **90-7237**

REYNOLDS, Edward (*b.* 1860)
A case of sacculated bladder. Boston, 1896. 7p. DNLM
90-7238

REYNOLDS, Edward (*b.* 1860)
Some aspects of ureteritis in women. Philadelphia, 1896. 11p. DNLM **90-7239**

REYNOLDS, Edward (*b.* 1860)
Practical midwifery; a handbook of treatment. . . . 3rd rev. ed. . . . New York: William Wood & Co., 1896. 427p. DLC; DNLM; ICJ; PPC **90-7240**

REYNOLDS, Edward (*b.* 1860)
The diagnosis of the condition of each kidney by inoculation of the separated sediments into guinea-pigs in suspected renal tuberculosis. Baltimore, 1898. 12p. 1 plate. DNLM
90-7241

REYNOLDS, Edward (*b.* 1860)
A new growth of the bladder. [Savannah, 1898.] 2 l. DNLM
90-7242

REYNOLDS, Edward (*b.* 1860)
Nephrectomy for renal tuberculosis, with report of a case. St. Paul, Minn., 1899. 7p. DNLM **90-7243**

REYNOLDS, Henry J.
On the identity of so-called specific and non-specific urethritis. [Philadelphia, 1891.] 6p. DNLM
90-7244

REYNOLDS, John P.
The limiting of childbearing among the married; the president's annual address. Philadelphia: W. J. Dornan, 1890. 24p. DNLM [Am. Gynaec. Soc.] **90-7245**

RHEIN, M[eyer] L.
Amputation of roots as a radical cure in chronic alveolar abscess: in pyorrhoea alveolaris complicated by alveolar abscess. Chicago: H. D. Justi, [1890]. 10p. DNLM
90-7246

RHEIN, M[eyer] L.
The value of intense cold in dentistry, and its production by the chloride of methyl spray. [Philadelphia, 1890.] 5p. DNLM
90-7247

RHEIN, M[eyer] L.
Ideal bridge-work. [Philadelphia, 1894.] 14p. DNLM
90-7248

RHEIN, M[eyer] L.
Dental Society of the State of New York. Report of the committee on practice. Philadelphia, 1895. 8p. DNLM
90-7249

RHEIN, M[eyer] L.
An etiological classification of pyorrhea alveolaris. Philadelphia, 1895. 3p. DNLM **90-7250**

RHEIN, M[eyer] L.
Alveolar abscess; preventive and curative treatment. [Philadelphia, 1896.] 7p. DNLM **90-7251**

RHEIN, M[eyer] L.
The oral expressions of malnutrition. [Philadelphia, 1896.] 12p. DNLM **90-7252**

RHOADS, Thomas Leidy (*b.* 1870)
The necessity for investigation and observation by the general practitioner. Chicago, 1897. 11p. DNLM
90-7253

RHOADS, Thomas Leidy (*b.* 1870)
The technique of Professor Keen's surgical clinic in the Jefferson Medical College Hospital. Detroit: G. S. Davis, 1897. 46p. DNLM **90-7254**

RHOADS, Thomas Leidy (*b.* 1870)
The post-operative treatment of surgical cases. Detroit: W. M. Warren, 1898. 73p. DNLM **90-7255**

RHOADS, Thomas Leidy (*b.* 1870)
Treatment of acromio-clavicular dislocation. Philadelphia, 1898. 6p. DNLM **90-7256**

RHODE ISLAND HOSPITAL TRAINING SCHOOL FOR NURSES, PROVIDENCE
Directions for infant diet, from birth to first year. [Providence, 1893?] 2 l. DNLM **90-7257**

RHODES, John Edwin (1851-1925)
Pocket dose book, compiled by . . . . Chicago, Ill.: Sharp & Smith, 1893. 98 l. DNLM **90-7258**

RHODES, John Edwin (1851-1925)
Atrophic rhinitis. Chicago: Amer. Med. Assoc. Press, 1897. 19p. DNLM **90-7259**

RHODES, John Edwin (1851-1925)
Spasm of the tensors of the vocal cords. New York, 1899. 12p. DNLM **90-7260**

RIBOT, Théodule A[rmand] (1839-1916)
The diseases of personality. Authorized transl. Chicago: The Open Court Publishing Co., 1891. 151p. DNLM; ICU; NN; NNC **90-7261**

RIBOT, Théodule A[rmand] (1839-1916)
Diseases of memory: an essay in the positive psychology. Transl. from the French by William Huntington Smith. New York: D. Appleton & Co., 1893. 209p. DLC: ICJ; MBM; PU **90-7262**

RIBOT, Théodule A[rmand] (1839-1916)
The diseases of personality. . . . Authorized translation. 2nd rev. ed. Chicago: The Open Court Publishing Co., 1895. 163p. DLC; IU-M; NcD; PU **90-7263**

RIBOT, Théodule A[rmand] (1839-1916)
The diseases of personality. 3rd rev. ed. Chicago: The Open Court Publishing Co., 1898. 163p. DLC; IEN-M; MBM; PPC **90-7264**

RICE, Charles (1841-1901)
The study of pharmacy. Introduction. New York, 1895. 16p. DNLM **90-7265**

RICE, Clarence C.
Atrophic catarrh. A new method of treatment. The use of ozone in atrophic catarrh. New York, [1893]. 12p. DNLM **90-7266**

RICE, Clarence C.
In what conditions of the nose, pharynx, and larynx the galvano-cautery should and should not be employed. [New York, 1898.] 11p. DNLM **90-7267**

RICHARDS, George Lyman (*b.* 1863)
Paramonochlorophenol; its use in the local treatment of laryngeal tuberculosis. Chicago, 1896. 8p. DNLM **90-7268**

RICHARDS, George Lyman (*b.* 1863)
Bleeding polyp of the septum (telangiectoma); report of a case. St. Louis, 1898. 4p. DNLM **90-7269**

RICHARDS, George Lyman (*b.* 1863)
Consumption; cases that should go to Colorado and cases that should stay at home. Fall River, Mass., 1898. 16p. DNLM **90-7270**

RICHARDS, George Lyman (*b.* 1863)
Perichondritis of the larynx; with a report of two cases, and the description of a new tracheotomy-tube. Philadelphia, 1898. 12p. DNLM **90-7271**

RICHARDS, George Lyman (*b.* 1863)
The minor surgery of the nose and throat. New York, 1899. 11p. DNLM **90-7272**

RICHARDS, Huntington
Mastoid sclerosis as illustrated by a very typical and a fatal case. New Bedford, 1890. 16p. DNLM **90-7273**

RICHARDSON, Alonzo Blair (1853-1903)
Alcoholism; a consideration of the symptomatology with reference to the pathological anatomy. [Cincinnati, 1890.] 8p. DNLM **90-7274**

RICHARDSON, Alonzo Blair (1853-1903)
The therapeutic value of hypnotism. [Cincinnati, 1891.] 7p. DNLM **90-7275**

RICHARDSON, Benjamin Ward (1828-1896)
Diseases of modern life. New York: D. Appleton & Co., 1895. 520p. ICU; MB; MH; NN **90-7276**

RICHARDSON, Charles H.
Rubber gloves in aseptic abdominal surgery, with a new method of sterilization and bacteriological provings. New York, 1899. 7p. DNLM **90-7277**

RICHARDSON, Charles Williamson (1861-1929)
The importance of surgical means applied to the naso-pharynx in the relief of naso-pharyngeal and middle-ear catarrh. Chicago, 1890. 12p. DNLM **90-7278**

RICHARDSON, Charles Williamson (1861-1929)
A pharyngeal aneurism. [Chicago, 1890.] 4p. DNLM **90-7279**

RICHARDSON, Charles Williamson (1861-1929)
Nasal cystomata; report of two cases. Chicago, 1891. 11p. DNLM **90-7280**

RICHARDSON, Charles Williamson (1861-1929)
Spastic contraction of tensor tympani muscle. Chicago, 1892. 7p. DNLM **90-7281**

RICHARDSON, Charles Williamson (1861-1929)
Foreign bodies in bronchus. New York: M. J. Rooney, 1893. 5p. DNLM **90-7282**

RICHARDSON, Charles Williamson (1861-1929)
A case of myxo-sarcoma. St. Louis, 1894. 4p. DNLM **90-7283**

RICHARDSON, Charles Williamson (1861-1929)
Report of a case of double pediculated myxo-fibroma. St. Louis, 1895. 4p. DNLM **90-7284**

RICHARDSON, Charles Williamson (1861-1929)
A case of hemorrhage from external auditory canal. St. Louis: J. H. Parker, 1896. 4p. DNLM **90-7285**

RICHARDSON, Charles Williamson (1861-1929)
A case of laryngectomy, with specimen. St. Louis, 1897. 4p. DNLM **90-7286**

RICHARDSON, Charles Williamson (1861-1929)
The after treatment of restored deflected nasal septum. St. Louis, 1898. 4p. DNLM **90-7287**

RICHARDSON, Charles Williamson (1861-1929)
A case of chronic abscess of the tongue. Chicago, 1898. 3p. DNLM **90-7288**

RICHARDSON, Charles Williamson (1861-1929)
Septic thrombosis of the sigmoid sinus. [New Bedford], 1899. 6p. DNLM **90-7289**

RICHARDSON, David Dorrington (1832-1906)
Nervous and mental diseases, their primary causes, their effects, their course and cure. Chicago: Richardson & Co., 1898. 21p. DNLM **90-7290**

RICHARDSON, Joseph (1824-1890)
A practical treatise on mechanical dentistry. . . . 6th ed. Rev. and ed. by George W. Warren. . . . Philadelphia: P. Blakiston, Son & Co., 1893. 662p. DLC; DNLM; MdU-D; PPC
90-7291

RICHARDSON, Joseph (1824-1890)
A practical treatise on mechanical dentistry. . . . 7th ed., rev., enl. and ed by George W. Warren. . . . Philadelphia: P. Blakiston, Son & Co., 1897. 677p. DLC; DNLM; PPC; PU
90-7292

RICHARDSON, J. Julius
Aural reflex phenomena. New York, 1894. 6p. DNLM
90-7293

RICHARDSON, Mark Wyman (*b.* 1867)
A case of cholecystitis due to the typhoid bacillus. Boston, 1897. 6p. DNLM **90-7294**

RICHARDSON, Mark Wyman (*b.* 1867)
On the bacteriological examination of the stools in typhoid fever, and its value in diagnosis. Boston: Damrell & Upham, 1897. 16p. DNLM **90-7295**

RICHARDSON, Mark Wyman (*b.* 1867)
Recent bacteriological studies in typhoid fever. Boston, 1898. 8p. DNLM **90-7296**

RICHARDSON, Mark Wyman (*b.* 1867)
Recent progress in the bacteriology of typhoid fever. Read at the Massachusetts Medical Society, June 7, 1898. Boston, 1898. 13p. DNLM **90-7297**

RICHARDSON, Maurice Howe (1851-1912)
I. Gall-bladder surgery; (a) one case of impacted gall-stones; perforation; death without operation; (b) four exploratory operations on the gall-bladder; (c) six cholecystotomies for gallstones. II. Large echinococcus cyst of the liver successfully obliterated by laparotomy and drainage. Boston: Damrell & Upham, 1892. 31p. DNLM **90-7298**

RICHARDSON, Maurice Howe (1851-1912)
Remarks on the surgical treatment of appendicitis. Boston: Damrell & Upham, 1892. 22p. DNLM
90-7299

RICHARDSON, Maurice Howe (1851-1912)
Acute abdominal symptoms demanding immediate operative interference. Boston: Damrell & Upham, 1893. 14p. 1 tab. DNLM **90-7300**

RICHARDSON, Maurice Howe (1851-1912)
Case of chronic intestinal obstruction. Boston: Damrell & Upham, 1893. 24p. DNLM **90-7301**

RICHARDSON, Maurice Howe (1851-1912)
A contribution to the surgery of the gall-bladder. Philadelphia, 1893. 23p. DNLM **90-7302**

RICHARDSON, Maurice Howe (1851-1912)
Four successful nephrectomies. Boston: Damrell & Upham, 1893. 16p. DNLM **90-7303**

RICHARDSON, Maurice Howe (1851-1912)
Hysterectomy for cancer of the cervix by combined abdominal and vaginal dissection. Boston: Damrell & Upham, 1893. 10p. DNLM **90-7304**

RICHARDSON, Maurice Howe (1851-1912)
Ten days' experience with inflammations of the vermiform appendix. Boston: Damrell & Upham, 1893. 16p. DNLM
90-7305

RICHARDSON, Maurice Howe (1851-1912) and George L. WALTON
Contribution to the study of cerebral surgery based on an operation for the removal of a tumor. Philadelphia, 1893. 9p. DNLM **90-7306**

RICHARDSON, Maurice Howe (1851-1912) and George L. WALTON
Removal of the Gasserian ganglion for facial neuralgia; a successful case. Boston: Damrell & Upham, 1894. 14p. DNLM
90-7307

RICHARDSON, Maurice Howe (1851-1912)
Extra-uterine pregnancy and pelvic haemorrhage; cases and remarks. Philadelphia, 1894. 26p. DNLM
90-7308

RICHARDSON, Maurice Howe (1851-1912)
Remarks upon appendicitis based upon a personal experience of 181 cases. Revised and corrected from the American Journal of the Medical Sciences, January, 1894. With 213 tabulated cases. [Philadelphia, 1894.] 44p. DNLM
90-7309

RICHARDSON, Maurice Howe (1851-1912) and George L. WALTON
The operative treatment of spasmodic torticollis, with cases. [Philadelphia: Lea Bros. & Co., 1895.] 15p. DNLM
90-7310

RICHARDSON, Maurice Howe (1851-1912)
A case of pancreatic cyst treated by drainage; recovery. Boston, 1895. 4p. DNLM **90-7311**

RICHARDSON, Maurice Howe (1851-1912)
Two cases of dermoid cyst of the ovary involving the larger intestine; removal of cysts, resection of intestine and end to end suture; recovery. Boston: Damrell & Upham, 1895. 10p. DNLM **90-7312**

RICHARDSON, Maurice Howe (1851-1912)
Three cases of lateral anastomosis by means of the Murphy button. Boston: Damrell & Upham, 1896. 10p. DNLM
90-7313

RICHARDSON, Maurice Howe (1851-1912)
Two cases of intraperitoneal suprapubic cystotomy for stone. Philadelphia, 1896. 8p. 1 plate. DNLM **90-7314**

RICHARDSON, Maurice Howe (1851-1912) and George L. WALTON
Further observations on the treatment of spasmodic torticollis. Philadelphia, 1896. 14p. DNLM **90-7315**

RICHARDSON, Maurice Howe (1851-1912)
Two cases of perforating gunshot wound of the kidney. Philadelphia, 1896. 9p. DNLM **90-7316**

RICHARDSON, Maurice Howe (1851-1912)
A case of chronic intestinal obstruction from incomplete volvulus of the sigmoid flexure. Philadelphia, 1897. 5p. DNLM **90-7317**

RICHARDSON, Maurice Howe (1851-1912)
A successful case of ureteroplasty for intermittent hydronephrosis. Philadelphia, 1897. 5p. DNLM
90-7318

RICHARDSON, Maurice Howe (1851-1912) and G. W. W. BREWSTER
Appendicitis; remarks based upon a personal experience of 757 cases, including 151 consecutive cases successfully operated upon in the interval. Boston: Damrell & Upham, 1898. 23p. DNLM; MBM **90-7319**

RICHARDSON, Maurice Howe (1851-1912)
Acute inflammation of the gall-bladder. Philadelphia, 1898. 21p. DNLM **90-7320**

RICHARDSON, Maurice Howe (1851-1912)
A successful gastrectomy for cancer of the stomach. Boston: Damrell & Upham, 1898. 19p. DNLM
90-7321

RICHARDSON, Maurice Howe (1851-1912)
A successful pylorectomy, with removal of a portion of the pancreas, for cancer of the pylorus. Boston: [Damrell & Upham], 1898. 5p. DNLM **90-7322**

RICHARDSON, Maurice Howe (1851-1912)
Acute abdominal symptoms demanding immediate surgical intervention. Oration before the Maine Medical Association, June 8, 1899. Portland: S. Berry, 1899. 33p. DNLM
90-7323

RICHARDSON, Maurice Howe (1851-1912)
The complete history of a case of total extirpation of the stomach, with remarks upon the surgical treatment of gastric cancer. Boston: Damrell & Upham, 1899. 20p. DNLM
90-7324

RICHARDSON, William Lambert (1842-1932)
Report on midwifery and gynaecology; pregnancy. [1890.] 13p. DNLM **90-7325**

RICHARDSON, William Lambert (1842-1932)
Report on obstetrics and diseases of women; obstetrics. [1891.] 14p. DNLM **90-7326**

RICHARDSON, William Lambert (1842-1932) and George Lincoln WALTON
Case of temporo-sphenoidal tumor, presenting symptoms suggestive of abscess. Boston: Damrell & Upham, 1897. 11p. DNLM **90-7327**

RICHEY, Stephen Olin
The prime etiological factor of glaucoma is constitutional. [Philadelphia, 1892.] 11p. DNLM **90-7328**

RICHEY, Stephen Olin
The disease process, glaucoma. [Philadelphia, 1893.] 6p. DNLM **90-7329**

RICHEY, Stephen Olin
The halo symptom in glaucoma. Washington, 1894. 3p. DNLM
90-7330

RICHEY, Stephin Olin
Chronic interstitial ophthalmitis (chronic simple glaucoma). [Kansas City, Mo.], 1895. 20p. DNLM
90-7331

RICHEY, Stephen Olin
The fads and fashions of surgery. St. Louis, 1896. 15p. DNLM
90-7332

RICHEY, Stephen Olin
The management of glaucoma: chronc simple glaucoma (chronic interstitial ophthalmitis). St. Louis, 1896. 8p. DNLM
90-7333

RICHEY, Stephen Olin
Gout and rheumatism as factors in the etiology of glaucoma. [St. Louis], 1897. 12p. DNLM **90-7334**

RICHEY, Stephen Olin
Taxis in increased intra-ocular tension. Chicago, 1897. 4p. DNLM **90-7335**

RICHEY, Stephen Olin
The nature of acute and chronic glaucoma; their common origin. Philadelphia, 1899. 4p. DNLM
90-7336

RICKETTS, Benjamin M[errill] (*b.* 1858)
Atypic herpes zoster gangrenosa, with report of two cases. Chicago, 1890. 8p. DNLM **90-7337**

RICKETTS, Benjamin M[errill] (*b.* 1858)
External surgery of the nose. Chicago, 1890. 11p. DNLM
90-7338

RICKETTS, Benjamin M[errill] (*b.* 1858)
The use and abuse of soap and water. [New York, 1890.] 7p. DNLM **90-7339**

RICKETTS, Benjamin M[errill] (*b.* 1858)
Osteo-penthesis. Chicago, 1891. 11p. DNLM
90-7340

RICKETTS, Benjamin M[errill] (*b.* 1858)
The radical opertion for hernia, with the report of two unique cases. [Cincinnati, 1891.] 4p. DNLM
90-7341

RICKETTS, Benjamin M[errill] (*b.* 1858)
The surgery of cleft palate. Read before the Mississippi Valley Dental Society, held at Cincinnati, March, 1891. Toledo, O.: Andrews, Myers & Busse, 1891. 7p. DNLM
90-7342

RICKETTS, Benjamin M[errill] (*b.* 1858)
The surgical treatment of epilepsy, with the report of a case and presentation of the patient. [Cincinnati, 1891.] 3p. DNLM
90-7343

RICKETTS, Benjamin M[errill] (*b.* 1858)
Eczema infantile. Cincinnati, 1892. 7p. DNLM
90-7344

RICKETTS, Benjamin M[errill] (*b.* 1858)
One hundred and fifty circumcisions, and the lessons they teach. [Cincinnati, 1892.] 8p. DNLM
90-7345

RICKETTS, Benjamin M[errill] (*b.* 1858)
Report of a case of talipes equino varus. Chicago, 1892. 12p. DNLM **90-7346**

RICKETTS, Benjamin M[errill] (*b.* **1858)**
Report of twelve cases of herniotomy. Cincinnati, 1892. 7p. DNLM **90-7347**

RICKETTS, Benjamin M[errill] (*b.* **1858)**
Circular-saw injury. [Philadelphia, 1893.] 2p. DNLM **90-7348**

RICKETTS, Benjamin M[errill] (*b.* **1858)**
The early removal of tubercular foci of the bone. [New York], 1893. 8p. DNLM **90-7349**

RICKETTS, Benjamin M[errill] (*b.* **1858)**
Excision of the hip-joint in tubercular disease. Cincinnati, O., 1893. 3p. DNLM **90-7350**

RICKETTS, Benjamin M[errill] (*b.* **1858)**
Lupus; its extirpation. With report of cases. New York, 1893. 8p. DNLM **90-7351**

RICKETTS, Benjamin M[errill] (*b.* **1858)**
Primary syphilis and gonorrhea in children. Chicago, 1893. 4p. DNLM **90-7352**

RICKETTS, Benjamin M[errill] (*b.* **1858)**
Report of a case of carcinoma of ileum; intestinal obstruction relieved by anastomosis with a Murphy button. [Cincinnati, O., 1893.] 3p. 1 fig. DNLM **90-7353**

RICKETTS, Benjamin M[errill] (*b.* **1858)**
Varicocele, with a report of nineteen radical operations, and the different ways in which they were done. [New York, 1893.] 4p. DNLM **90-7354**

RICKETTS, Benjamin M[errill] (*b.* **1858)**
Castration for hypertrophied prostate. [Philadelphia, 1894.] 8p. DNLM **90-7355**

RICKETTS, Benjamin M[errill] (*b.* **1858)**
Circumcision. The last fifty of a series of two hundred circumcisions. Cincinnati: D. Appleton & Co., 1894. 5p. DNLM **90-7356**

RICKETTS, Benjamin M[errill] (*b.* **1858)**
Colotomy and the Kraske operation. Cincinnati, 1894. 3p. DNLM **90-7357**

RICKETTS, Benjamin M[errill] (*b.* **1858)**
Direct fixation in fractures. Philadelphia, 1894. 4p. DNLM **90-7358**

RICKETTS, Benjamin M[errill] (*b.* **1858)**
Dislocation and double fracture of the upper third of the humerus. Chicago, 1894. 7p. DNLM **90-7359**

RICKETTS, Benjamin M[errill] (*b.* **1858)**
Fifty cases of rectal surgery. Louisville: J. P. Morton & Co., 1894. 5p. DNLM **90-7360**

RICKETTS, Benjamin M[errill] (*b.* **1858)**
Obliteration of congenital pigmentations. Chicago: Office of the Association, 1894. 7p. DNLM **90-7361**

RICKETTS, Benjamin M[errill] (*b.* **1858)**
Removal of the head of the femur from the lesser sciatic notch. [Philadelphia, 1894.] 8p. DNLM **90-7362**

RICKETTS, Benjamin M[errill] (*b.* **1858)**
The removal, by trephine, of fluid as the result of acute cerebral meningitis, with report of a case. [Philadelphia, 1894.] 8p. DNLM **90-7363**

RICKETTS, Benjamin M[errill] (*b.* **1858)**
Brain surgery for epilepsy. Cincinnati, 1894. 7p. DNLM **90-7364**

RICKETTS, Benjamin M[errill] (*b.* **1858)**
Flat-foot; its correction and comparative study, with foot of the orang, chimpanzee, gorilla, and baboon (illustrated by photographs). Lupus treated by galvanism (illustrated by photographs). Double club feet and hands; treatment (illustrated by photographs). Chicago, 1895. 36p. DNLM **90-7365**

RICKETTS, Benjamin M[errill] (*b.* **1858)**
Modern surgery of serous cavities. Chicago, [1895]. 31p. DNLM **90-7366**

RICKETTS, Benjamin M[errill] (*b.* **1858)**
Neuralgia of the fifth nerve; treatment. Cincinnati, 1895. 2p. DNLM **90-7367**

RICKETTS, Benjamin M[errill] (*b.* **1858)**
Removal of the head of the femur from the lesser sciatic notch. St. Louis, 1895. 7p. DNLM **90-7368**

RICKETTS, Benjamin M[errill] (*b.* **1858)**
Rupture of left lateral ventricle. Detroit, 1895. 2p. DNLM **90-7369**

RICKETTS, Benjamin M[errill] (*b.* **1858)**
I. Typhoid ulcer; perforation (?); operation; death. II. Cerebral cyst; operation; recovery. Cincinnati, 1895. 4p. DNLM **90-7370**

RICKETTS, Benjamin M[errill] (*b.* **1858)**
Surgical mélange. Cincinnati, [1896?]. 7p. DNLM **90-7371**

RICKETTS, Benjamin M[errill] (*b.* **1858)**
Abdominal incision for ascites. Cincinnati, 1897. 3p. DNLM **90-7372**

RICKETTS, Benjamin M[errill] (*b.* **1858)**
Appendicitis; report of four cases. Cincinnati, 1897. 3p. DNLM **90-7373**

RICKETTS, Benjamin M[errill] (*b.* **1858)**
Craniectomies; with report of four cases. Cincinnati, 1897. 3p. DNLM **90-7374**

RICKETTS, Benjamin M[errill] (*b.* **1858)**
Ligation of the common carotid artery for trifacial neuralgia, with experiments and observations upon dogs. Chicago, 1897. 7p. DNLM **90-7375**

RICKETTS, Benjamin M[errill] (*b.* **1858)**
Aneurysm of the aortic arch; ligation of right subclavian and common carotid arteries. Chicago, 1898. 8p. DNLM **90-7376**

RICKETTS, Benjamin M[errill] (*b.* **1858)**
Deaths (ten), surgical and causes. [Also:] Prostate hypertrophy; emasculation, nine cases. Cincinnati, 1898. 6p. DNLM **90-7377**

RICKETTS, Benjamin M[errill] (*b.* **1858)**
Serpents and their venom; copperhead, coral, and rattlesnake. Cincinnati, 1898. 6p. DNLM **90-7378**

RICKETTS, Benjamin M[errill] (*b.* **1858)**
Cranial injuries of childhood, and their treatment. Richmond, 1899. 8p. DNLM **90-7379**

RICKETTS, Benjamin M[errill] (*b.* **1858)**
Femoral artery and vein; their destruction without loss of leg. Chicago, 1899. 7p. DNLM **90-7380**

RICKETTS, Benjamin M[errill] (*b.* **1858)**
Ovarian pregnancy; report of a case at full term. St. Louis, 1899. 4 l. DNLM **90-7381**

RICKETTS, Benjamin M[errill] (*b.* **1858)**
Rectal carcinoma with subsequent colotomy. Philadelphia, 1899. 2p. DNLM **90-7382**

RICKETTS, Edwin
Cholecystotomy. [Pittsburgh, 1890.] 10p. DNLM
90-7383

RICKETTS, Edwin
Cholecystotomy. Read before the Southern Surgical and Gynecological Association. [Philadelphia], 1892. 8p. DNLM **90-7384**

RICKETTS. Edwin
Chloroform in labor. Richmond, 1895. 7p. DNLM
90-7385

RICKETTS, Edwin
Operation for appendicitis; report of a case. [Cincinnati, 1892.] 4p. DNLM **90-7386**

RICKETTS, Edwin
Early diagnosis of cancer of the uterus. A paper read before the Cincinnati Obstetrical Society, June 14, 1894. [Cincinnati], 1894. 8p. DNLM **90-7387**

RICKETTS, Joseph V.
Vascular tumors of the anterior nares, with the report of a case. A paper read before the Academy of Medicine, Nov. 10, 1890. [Cincinnati, 1891.] 7p. DNLM
90-7388

RIDENBAUGH, Mary Young
The biography of Ephraim McDowell, M.D., "the father of ovariotomy." By his granddaughter. . . . Together with valuable scientific treatises and articles relating to ovariotomy and eulogistic letters from eminent members of the medical profession in Europe and America. New York: C. L. Webster & Co., 1890. 558p. plates. DLC; DNLM; NN
90-7389

RIDLON, John (1852-1936)
A report of sixty-two cases of hip disease. [New York, 1890.] 6p. DNLM **90-7390**

RIDLON, John (1852-1936)
The non-operative treatment of delayed union in fractures of the leg. New York: Trow's, 1891. 12p. DNLM
90-7391

RIDLON, John (1852-1936)
Supracotyloid dislocation. [New York, 1891.] 6p. DNLM **90-7392**

RIDLON, John (1852-1936)
Syphilitic spondylitis in children. [Philadelphia, 1891.] 8p. DNLM **90-7393**

RIDLON, John (1852-1936)
. . . Spondylitis. By John Ridlon . . . and Robert Jones. . . . Reprinted from "The Journal of the American Medical Association," December 10, 1892. Chicago: Pub. at the Office of the Association, 1892. 24p. MB
90-7394

RIDLON, John (1852-1936)
. . . Hip disease. By John Ridlon . . . and Robert Jones. . . . Reprinted from "The Journal of the American Medical Association," February 18 and March 4, 1893. Chicago: The Association, 1893. 66p. DLC **90-7395**

RIDLON, John (1852-1936)
Chronic joint disease: (some preliminary papers). By John Ridlon . . . and Robert Jones. . . . Chicago: C. J. Burroughs, printer, 1894. 179p. plates. DLC **90-7396**

RIDLON, John (1852-1936)
Lectures on orthopedic surgery, by John Ridlon . . . and Robert Jones. . . . Philadelphia: E. Stern & Co., Inc., 1899. 358p. DLC; ICJ; NcD; PPC **90-7397**

RIEDER, Hermann (1858-1932)
Atlas of urinary sediments with special reference to their clinical significance. Transl. by F. Moore. Edited and annotated by A. S. Delephine. Philadelphia: J. B. Lippincott, 1899. 111p. MBM; NNNAM; PPC; PU **90-7398**

RIES, Emil (*b.* **1865)**
The anatomy of the endometrium. New York, 1896. 4p. DNLM **90-7399**

RIES, Emil (*b.* **1865)**
Complicated laparotomies. Chicago, 1896. 12p. DNLM
90-7400

RIES, Emil (*b.* **1865)**
How to improve the prognosis of carcinoma uteri. [Chicago, 1896.] 13p. DNLM **90-7401**

RIES, Emil (*b.* **1865)**
Ichthyosis uteri. New York, 1896. 10p. DNLM
90-7402

RIES, Emil (*b.* **1865)**
On membranes discharged from the uterus. Chicago, 1896. 16p. DNLM **90-7403**

RIES, Emil (*b.* **1865)**
On vaginal celiotomy, with report of cases. Chicago, 1897. 10p. DNLM **90-7404**

RIES, Emil (*b.* **1865)**
Plastic operations on the tubes. Boston, 1898. 4p. DNLM **90-7405**

RIGGS, C[harles] Eugene (1853-1930?)
A résumé of lectures upon the structure and physiology of the central nervous system, with a localization of its lesions, including Dr. Starr's review of Flechsig's plan of the human brain. [1890, *vel subseq.*] 78p. DNLM
90-7406

RIGGS, C[harles] Eugene (1853-1930?)
The value of voltaic alternatives in optic nerve atrophy. St. Paul, 1893. 9p. DNLM **90-7407**

RIGGS, C[harles] Eugene (1853-1930?)
The spinal cord in a case of pernicious anaemia. Philadelphia, 1896. 4p. 2 plates. DNLM **90-7408**

RIGGS, C[harles] Eugene (1853-1930?)
A quiz upon lectures on static, galvanic, and faradic electricity, electro-physiology, electro-diagnosis, and electro-therapy. St. Paul: H. L. Collins Co., [1896]. 47p. DNLM **90-7409**

RILEY, Henry A[lsop]
Who can be medical experts? [Philadelphia, 1891.] 10p. DNLM **90-7410**

RILEY, J. B.
Antikamnia and the atmospheric tractor in obstetrics. St. Joseph, Mo., 1891. 3p. DNLM **90-7411**

RING, Charles Augustus (1854-1907)
Our insane patients and their hospital relations. Buffalo, 1894-95. 7p. DNLM **90-7412**

RINGER, Sydney (1835-1910)
A handbook of therapeutics. By Sydney Ringer . . . and Harrington Sainsbury. . . . 13th ed. New York: William Wood & Co., 1897. 746p. DLC; NNNAM **90-7413**

RISHMILLER, John H.
A series of interesting cases in the service of Horace Tracy Hanks at the Woman's Hospital. [New York, 1894.] 24p. DNLM **90-7414**

RISHMILLER, John H.
The employment of gauze in the uterine cavity. New York: J. D. Emmet, 1896. 5p. DNLM **90-7415**

RISHMILLER, John H.
The limitation of hysterectomy for carcinoma of the uterus. [New York, 1898.] 4p. DNLM **90-7416**

RISLEY, S[amuel] D[oty] (1845-1920)
A new apparatus for detecting and measuring the anomalies of ocular muscles. Philadelphia: Binder & Kelly, [1891]. 8p. DNLM **90-7417**

RISLEY, S[amuel] D[oty] (1845-1920)
The mydriatics in ophthalmology. [Philadelphia, 1893.] 9p. DNLM **90-7418**

RITTER DENTAL MFG. CO.
Catalogue of new Columbia dental chairs, electric dental engines and appliances. New York & Rochester, 1898. 16p. NNNAM **90-7419**

RIVERS, E[dmund] C.
Cataract extraction. [New York, 1893.] 9p. DNLM **90-7420**

RIVES, William C[abell] (1858-1938)
The baths of Nauheim in the treatment of diseases of the heart, and the therapeutic methods of the Doctors Schott. New York, 1896. 30p. DNLM; NNNAM **90-7421**

ROBB, Hunter (1863-1940) and Albert A. GHRISKEY
Coeliotomy for myoma of the uterus, hystero-myomectomy, infection by bacterium coli commune. [Baltimore, 1891.] 2 l. DNLM **90-7422**

ROBB, Hunter (1863-1940) and Albert A. GHRISKEY
Infection through the drainage tube, the result of the bacteriological examination of drainage-tube fluids in sixteen consecutive cases of coeliotomy. [Baltimore, 1891.] 4 l. DNLM **90-7423**

ROBB, Hunter (1863-1940)
Improved gynecological instruments. New York: William Wood & Co., 1891. 15p. DNLM **90-7424**

ROBB, Hunter (1863-1940)
Mme. Lachapelle, midwife. [Baltimore, 1891.] 3 l. DNLM **90-7425**

ROBB, Hunter (1863-1940)
Ruptured right tubal pregnancy, associated with perforation of the vermiform appendix. Confirmatory diagnosis by aspiration; colon bacillus in the aspirated fluid; operation; death. With remarks by W. H. Welch. [Baltimore, 1891.] 8 l. DNLM **90-7426**

ROBB, Hunter (1863-1940) and Albert A. GHRISKEY
The bacteria in wounds and skin-stitches. Baltimore, 1892. 4 l. DNLM **90-7427**

ROBB, Hunter (1863-1940)
A case of associated streptococcus infection of the vermiform appendix and Fallopian tube. [Baltimore, 1892.] 4 l. DNLM **90-7428**

ROBB, Hunter (1863-1940)
Conclusions regarding the use of drainage tubes and ligatures, and the possibilities of skin disinfection based upon bacteriological investigations. New York: William Wood & Co., 1892. 15p. DNLM **90-7429**

ROBB, Hunter (1863-1940)
Hysterectomy, with a report of four cases. [Baltimore, 1892.] 6 l. DNLM **90-7430**

ROBB, Hunter (1863-1940)
Rupture of the sac of an extra-uterine pregnancy through the fimbriated extremity without tearing the Fallopian tube; operation; recovery. New York: M. J. Rooney, [1892]. 5p. DNLM **90-7431**

ROBB, Hunter (1863-1940)
The use of morphine and other strong sedatives in gynecological practice. [Baltimore, 1892.] 4p. DNLM **90-7432**

ROBB, Hunter (1863-1940)
Hysteromyomectomy for large myomata of the uterus. Baltimore, 1893. 4p. DNLM **90-7433**

ROBB, Hunter (1863-1940)
Importance to the surgeon of a bacteriological training. Baltimore, 1893. 7p. DNLM **90-7434**

ROBB, Hunter (1863-1940)
Maintenance of an aseptic technique in gynecological operations outside of hospitals. Baltimore, 1893. 10p. DNLM **90-7435**

ROBB, Hunter (1863-1940)
Remarks on the writings of Louyse Bourgeois. Baltimore, 1893. 10 l. DNLM **90-7436**

ROBB, Hunter (1863-1940)
Abstract of two articles treating of progress in midwifery. Baltimore, 1894. 6p. DNLM **90-7437**

ROBB, Hunter (1863-1940)
Asepsis in minor procedures. Baltimore, 1894. 4p. DNLM **90-7438**

ROBB, Hunter (1863-1940)
A case of double vagina, with operation. Baltimore, 1894. 3p. DNLM **90-7439**

ROBB, Hunter (1863-1940)
The limitations of the use of the pessary. Baltimore, 1894. 5p. DNLM **90-7440**

ROBB, Hunter (1863-1940)
Madame Boivin. Baltimore, 1894. 10p. DNLM **90-7441**

ROBB, Hunter (1863-1940)
A new spigot attachment to facilitate asepsis. Philadelphia, 1894. 3p. DNLM **90-7442**

ROBB, Hunter (1863-1940)
Notes on gynaecological technique. New York, 1894. 4p. DNLM **90-7443**

ROBB, Hunter (1863-1940)
An operating table. Baltimore, 1894. 2p. 1 plate. DNLM **90-7444**

ROBB, Hunter (1863-1940)
Practical application of the principles of sterilization. New York: William Wood & Co., 1894. 10p. DNLM **90-7445**

ROBB, Hunter (1863-1940)
Some impressions of gynecology in Europe. Cleveland, 1894. 10p. DNLM **90-7446**

ROBB, Hunter (1863-1940)
The surgery of the ureters and kidneys. [Cleveland, 1894.] 7p. DNLM **90-7447**

ROBB, Hunter (1863-1940)
The works of Justine Siegemundin, the midwife. Baltimore, 1894. 28p. DNLM **90-7448**

ROBB, Hunter (1863-1940)
Aseptic surgical technique; with especial reference to gynaecological operations, together with notes on the technique employed in certain supplementary procedures. . . . Philadelphia: J. B. Lippincott Co., 1894. 264p. col. plates. DLC; DNLM; PPC; PU **90-7449**

ROBB, Hunter (1863-1940)
Case of double pyosalpinx. Cleveland, 1895. 6p. DNLM **90-7450**

ROBB, Hunter (1863-1940)
A case of hydrosalpinx. Removal of the right tube and ovary without rupture of the sac. Cleveland, 1895. 6p. DNLM **90-7451**

ROBB, Hunter (1863-1940)
The early recognition of carcinoma of the cervix. New York, 1895. 6p. DNLM **90-7452**

ROBB, Hunter (1863-1940)
The influences of operative procedures in peritoneal tuberculosis. Cleveland, 1895. 8p. DNLM **90-7453**

ROBB, Hunter (1863-1940)
Pruritus of the genitals. [Cleveland, 1895.] 6p. DNLM **90-7454**

ROBB, Hunter (1863-1940)
Some impressions of gynecology in Europe. Cleveland, 1895. 10p. DNLM **90-7455**

ROBB, Hunter (1863-1940)
A successful case of Porro-Caesarian section (modified). Cleveland, 1895. 6p. DNLM **90-7456**

ROBB, Hunter (1863-1940)
Thoroughness in medical education. Cleveland, 1895. 7p. DNLM **90-7457**

ROBB, Hunter (1863-1940)
The writings of Mauriceau. Baltimore, 1895. 19p. 1 plate. DNLM **90-7458**

ROBB, Hunter (1863-1940)
The surgery of the ureters and kidneys. Cleveland, 1895-96. 7p. DNLM **90-7459**

ROBB, Hunter (1863-1940)
A case of double salpingo-oöphorectomy, excessive loss of blood from separated adhesions necessitating a second operation within three hours; infusion with sterile normal salt solution during second operation; recovery. New York: William Wood & Co., 1896. 7p. DNLM **90-7460**

ROBB, Hunter (1863-1940)
A brief description of the New Lakeside Hospital. Cleveland, 1896. 8p. DNLM **90-7461**

ROBB, Hunter (1863-1940)
A case of multiple myomata of the uterus; ulcerated varicose veins of left leg; hysteromyomectomy; recovery. Cleveland, 1896. 2 l. DNLM **90-7462**

ROBB, Hunter (1863-1940)
The causes and mechanism of retroflexion and retroversion of the uterus. Cleveland, 1896. 9p. DNLM **90-7463**

ROBB, Hunter (1863-1940)
Formalin catgut. Cleveland, 1896. 3p. DNLM **90-7464**

ROBB, Hunter (1863-1940)
Tears of the rectum in abdominal operations for pyosalpinx and their treatment. [Abstr.] Cleveland, 1896. 4p. DNLM **90-7465**

ROBB, Hunter (1863-1940) and Albert A. GHRISKEY
The bacillus proteus Zenkeri in an ovarian abscess. Baltimore, 1897. 8p. DNLM **90-7466**

ROBB, Hunter (1863-1940)
The bacteria occurring in the female genital canal and their relations to endometritis. [Abstr.] Cleveland, 1897. 10p. DNLM **90-7467**

ROBB, Hunter (1863-1940)
Case of papilloma of the ovary. Cleveland, 1897. 5p. 1 plate. DNLM **90-7468**

ROBB, Hunter (1863-1940)
The conservative treatment of the myomatous uterus. New York: William Wood & Co., 1897. 6p. DNLM **90-7469**

ROBB, Hunter (1863-1940)
The importance of a systematic microscopical examination of uterine scrapings and of excised pieces as an aid to diagnosis; based upon the analysis of one hundred cases. Philadelphia, 1897. 20p. DNLM **90-7470**

ROBB, Hunter (1863-1940)
The intra-uterine application of chlorid of zinc. [Abstr.] Cleveland, 1897. 4p. DNLM **90-7471**

ROBB, Hunter (1863-1940)
Resection and ignipuncture of the ovaries. [Abstr.] Cleveland, 1897. 6p. DNLM **90-7472**

ROBB, Hunter (1863-1940)
Secondary abdominal pregnancy attaining to maturity after traumatic rupture of the uterus in the fourth month; laparotomy; recovery. [Abstr.] Cleveland, 1897. 4p. DNLM **90-7473**

ROBB, Hunter (1863-1940)
The treatment of retrodisplacements of the uterus. [St. Louis, 1897.] 4 l. DNLM **90-7474**

ROBB, Hunter (1863-1940)
A case of endothelioma lymphangiomatodes of the cervix uteri. Philadelphia, 1898. 8p. DNLM **90-7475**

ROBB, Hunter (1863-1940)
Infection after abdominal operations, and its treatment. Cleveland, 1898. 10p. DNLM **90-7476**

ROBB, Hunter (1863-1940)
The influence of extirpation of the ovaries upon structural changes in the uterus. [Abstr.] Cleveland, 1898. 9p. DNLM **90-7477**

ROBB, Hunter (1863-1940)
Irrigation with salt solution and other fluids in surgical practice. New York: William Wood & Co., 1898. 5p. DNLM **90-7478**

ROBB, Hunter (1863-1940)
Notes on the care of the newborn infant. Cleveland, 1898. 4p. DNLM **90-7479**

ROBB, Hunter (1863-1940)
The opening of the new Lakeside Hospital. Cleveland, 1898. 4p. DNLM **90-7480**

ROBB, Hunter (1863-1940)
Suture materials and methods in coeliotomy. Cleveland, 1898. 6p. DNLM **90-7481**

ROBB, Hunter (1863-1940)
The treatment of retrodisplacements of the uterus. Philadelphia, 1898. 10p. DNLM **90-7482**

ROBB, Hunter (1863-1940)
Abdominal section under cocaine anaesthesia for retroverted adherent uterus in a case with marked cardiac symptoms and goitre. Cleveland, 1899. 3p. DNLM **90-7483**

ROBB, Hunter (1863-1940)
A case of complete prolapse of the uterus; hysterectomy; sudden death on the seventeenth day after operation, proved by necropsy to be due to a congenital cyst of the brain. Cleveland, 1899. 4p. DNLM **90-7484**

ROBB, Hunter (1863-1940)
A case of gall-stones in the cystic duct in which the diagnosis was obscured by symptoms due to pelvic disturbances. [Cleveland, 1899.] 2p. DNLM **90-7485**

ROBB, Hunter (1863-1940)
A case of submucous myoma. Cleveland, 1899. 4p. DNLM **90-7486**

ROBB, Hunter (1863-1940)
Ninety-three consecutive abdominal sections witout a death, with clinical and pathological reports. Philadelphia, 1899. 12p. DNLM **90-7487**

ROBBINS, Henry Alfred (1839-1911)
Non-venereal syphilis; a clinical lecture. Philadelphia, 1892. 10p. DNLM **90-7488**

ROBBINS, Henry Alfred (1839-1911)
Third act of the drama of syphilis; a clinical lecture. Richmond, 1892. 8p. DNLM **90-7489**

ROBBINS, Henry Alfred (1839-1911)
Organic syphilis; a lecture. Washington: Gibson Bros., 1893. 10p. DNLM **90-7490**

ROBBINS, Henry Alfred (1839-1911)
Unmerited syphilis, and the third act of the drama of syphilis. Richmond, 1894. 24p. DNLM **90-7491**

ROBBINS, Henry Alfred (1839-1911)
Cerebral syphilis. Richmond, 1895. 16p. DNLM **90-7492**

ROBBINS, Henry Alfred (1839-1911)
Lues venerea. [Richmond, 1895.] 16p. DNLM **90-7493**

ROBBINS, Henry Alfred (1839-1911)
Syphilis of the vital organs; cerebral syphilis. Richmond, 1895. 36p. DNLM **90-7494**

ROBBINS, Henry Alfred (1839-1911)
Lues venerea and the third act of the drama of syphilis. Washington: Gibson Bros., 1896. 24p. DNLM **90-7495**

ROBBINS, Henry Alfred (1839-1911)
Syphilis of the innocent. Baltimore, 1896. 4p. DNLM **90-7496**

ROBBINS, Henry Alfred (1839-1911)
Cerebral syphilis. Baltimore, 1897. 8p. DNLM
90-7497

ROBBINS, Henry Alfred (1839-1911)
Cerebral syphilis; inunction treatment. Baltimore, 1897. 5p. DNLM **90-7498**

ROBBINS, Henry Alfred (1839-1911)
Non-venereal syphilis. New York, 1897. 4p. DNLM
90-7499

ROBBINS, Henry Alfred (1839-1911)
Syphilis. Baltimore, 1897. 7p. DNLM
90-7500

ROBBINS, Henry Alfred (1839-1911)
Syphilis of the abdominal organs. [Baltimore], 1897. 6p. DNLM **90-7501**

ROBBINS, Henry Alfred (1839-1911)
Syphilis of the eye, ear and throat. Baltimore, 1897. 6p. DNLM **90-7502**

ROBBINS, Henry Alfred (1839-1911)
Syphilis of the nose and buccal cavity. Baltimore, 1897. 6p. DNLM **90-7503**

ROBBINS, Henry Alfred (1839-1911)
Syphilis of the thoracic organs. [Baltimore], 1897. 7p. DNLM
90-7504

ROBBINS, Henry Alfred (1839-1911)
The toxine of syphilis. [Baltimore], 1897. 5p. DNLM
90-7505

ROBBINS, Henry Alfred (1839-1911)
The treatment of syphilis. Baltimore, 1897. 4p. DNLM
90-7506

ROBBINS, Henry Alfred (1839-1911)
Dangers of the barber shop. [Baltimore], 1898. 4p. DNLM
90-7507

ROBBINS, Henry Alfred (1839-1911)
Hereditary syphilis. Baltimore, 1898. 4p. DNLM
90-7508

ROBBINS, Henry Alfred (1839-1911)
Lues venerea. Washington, [1898]. 5 l. DNLM
90-7509

ROBBINS, Henry Alfred (1839-1911)
A case of polymorphism. Baltimore, 1899. 3p. 2 plates. DNLM
90-7510

ROBBINS, Henry Alfred (1839-1911)
Gonococcus Neisser. Baltimore, 1899. 7p. DNLM
90-7511

ROBBINS, Henry Alfred (1839-1911)
The mercurial vapor bath. Baltimore, 1899. 2p. DNLM
90-7512

ROBE, R[obert] C.
A plea for national medical legislation. Denver. [1899]. 8p. DNLM **90-7513**

ROBERTS, A[lgernon] Sydney (1855-1896)
Contributions to orthopedic surgery; with a brief biographical sketch by James K. Young. Philadelphia: W. J. Dornan, 1898. 298p. DNLM; NNNAM; PPC; PU **90-7514**

ROBERTS, Deering J. (1840-1925)
Anaemia and its treament. Nashville, 1898. 7p. DNLM
90-7515

ROBERTS, Frederick T[homas] (1838-1919)
The theory and practice of medicine. . . . 9th ed. Philadelphia: P. Blakiston, Son & Co., 1894. 1168p. DNLM; ICJ; PPC; PPJ
90-7516

ROBERTS, John B[ingham] (1852-1924)
A manual of modern surgery; an exposition of the accepted doctrines and approved operative procedures of the present time. For the use of students and practitioners. Philadelphia: Lea Bros. & Co., 1890. 800p. DNLM; MBM; PPC; PPJ
90-7517

ROBERTS, John B[ingham] (1852-1924)
A retrospect or short history of the Philadelphia Polyclinic. Extracted from the reports of the proceedings at the laying of the cornerstone of the new building, on November 4, 1889. Philadelphia, 1890. 4p. DNLM **90-7518**

ROBERTS, John B[ingham] (1852-1924)
Need of a state board of medical examiners. [Philadelphia, 1890.] 14p. DNLM **90-7519**

ROBERTS, John B[ingham] (1852-1924)
The relation of bacteria to practical surgery. Philadelphia: W. J. Dornan, 1890. 16p. DNLM **90-7520**

ROBERTS, John B[ingham] (1852-1924)
Clinical contributions to brain surgery. [Philadelphia, 1891.] 16p. DNLM **90-7521**

ROBERTS, John B[ingham] (1852-1924)
The compend of anatomy. For use in the dissecting room, and in preparing for examinations. . . . Philadelphia: C. C. Roberts & Co., 1892. 191p. DLC; PPC; PU
90-7522

ROBERTS, John B[ingham] (1852-1924)
The after-treatment in operative surgery. [Philadelphia, 1892.] 6p. DNLM **90-7523**

ROBERTS, John B[ingham] (1852-1924)
The cosmetic surgery of the nose. Chicago, 1892. 7p. DNLM
90-7524

ROBERTS, John B[ingham] (1852-1924)
Intra-cranial neurectomy of the second and third divisions of the fifth nerve immediately in front of the Gasserian ganglion. Philadelphia, 1892. 3p. DNLM **90-7525**

ROBERTS, John B[ingham] (1852-1924)
Treatment of fractures of the lower end of the humerus and of the base of the radius. [Philadelphia, 1892.] 41p. DNLM
90-7526

ROBERTS, John B[ingham] (1852-1924)
Tumor of the liver in which removal was attempted. Philadelphia, 1892. 4p. DNLM **90-7527**

ROBERTS, John B[ingham] (1852-1924)
The cure of complete prolapse of the rectum by posterior proctectomy. [Philadelphia, 1893.] 6p. DNLM **90-7528**

ROBERTS, John B[ingham] (1852-1924)
Points of similarity between us and homoeopathic physicians. [Philadelphia, 1893.] 12p. DNLM **90-7529**

ROBERTS, John B[ingham] (1852-1924)
Simplicity in the treatment of fractures. [Philadelphia, 1893.] 9p. DNLM **90-7530**

ROBERTS, John B[ingham] (1852-1924)
A case of primary tuberculosis of the laminae and spinous processes of the vertebral column. Philadelphia, 1894. 6p. DNLM **90-7531**

ROBERTS, John B[ingham] (1852-1924)
Recent experience with tumors of the liver. [Philadelphia: Lea Bros. & Co., 1894.] 12p. DNLM **90-7532**

ROBERTS, John B[ingham] (1852-1924)
Some defects in anatomical teaching in the medical schools of the United States. New York: D. Appleton & Co., 1894. 13p. DNLM **90-7533**

ROBERTS, John B[ingham] (1852-1924)
Modern medicine and homoeopathy; two addresses. Philadelphia: Edwards & Docker Co., 1895. 69p. DNLM **90-7534**

ROBERTS, John B[ingham] (1852-1924)
Cases of artificial anus and fecal fistule treated by intraperitoneal operation. Philadelphia, 1896. 5p. DNLM **90-7535**

ROBERTS, John B[ingham] (1852-1924)
A clinical, pathological, and experimental study of fracture of the lower end of the radius, with displacement of the carpal fragment toward the flexor or anterior surface of the wrist. . . . Philadelphia: P. Blakiston, Son & Co., 1897. 76p. plate. DLC; DNLM; PPC **90-7536**

ROBERTS, John B[ingham] (1852-1924)
Exploratory incision in the treatment of closed fractures and dislocations. Philadelphia, 1897. 11p. DNLM **90-7537**

ROBERTS, John B[ingham] (1852-1924)
The surgical treatment of suppurative pericarditis. [Philadelphia], 1897. 23p. 1 plate. DNLM **90-7538**

ROBERTS, John B[ingham] (1852-1924)
Cases illustrating the beneficial effect of plastic operations upon the face for the cure of cicatricial and congenital deformities. Philadelphia, 1898. 2p. DNLM **90-7539**

ROBERTS, John B[ingham] (1852-1924)
Intestinal anastomosis for fecal fistula in the lumbar region. Philadelphia, 1898. 3p. DNLM **90-7540**

ROBERTS, John B[ingham] (1852-1924)
An outline of the proper organization of the surgical teaching in a medical school. Philadelphia, 1898. 2p. DNLM **90-7541**

ROBERTS, John B[ingham] (1852-1924)
Recent advances in the treatment of fractures of the extremities. Pittsburgh, 1898. 5p. DNLM **90-7542**

ROBERTS, John B[ingham] (1852-1924)
The surgical treatment of common deformities of the face. Detroit: W. W. Warren, 1898. 5p. DNLM **90-7543**

ROBERTS, John B[ingham] (1852-1924)
A manual of modern surgery; an exposition of the accepted doctrines and approved operative procedures of the present time. For the use of students and practitioners. 2nd ed. Philadelphia & New York: Lea Bros. & Co., [1899]. 842p. 8 plates. NNNAM; PPC; PU **90-7544**

ROBERTS, John B[ingham] (1852-1924)
Notes on the modern treatment of fractures. New York: D. Appleton & Co., 1899. 162p. DNLM **90-7545**

ROBERTS, John B[ingham] (1852-1924)
The success of operative treatment in facial disfigurement. [Philadelphia, 1899.] 8p. DNLM **90-7546**

[ROBERTS, Milton Josiah] (1850-1893)
Schedule of lectures on mechanical and operative orthopedic surgery. [New York, 1890.] 10p. DNLM **90-7547**

[ROBERTS, Milton Josiah] (1850-1893)
Catalogue of the library of the late Dr. Milton Josiah Roberts, including a portion of the library of the late Mrs. Martha J. Lamb. New York, 1893. [unpag.] DNLM; NNNAM **90-7548**

ROBERTS, William (1830-1899)
Collected contributions on digestion and diet. Philadelphia: Lea Bros. & Co., 1891. 261p. DNLM; PPC **90-7549**

ROBERTSON, John W[ooster] (*b.* 1856)
The Keeley treatment of alcoholism. San Francisco, 1893. 7p. DNLM **90-7550**

ROBERTSON, John W[ooster] (*b.* 1856)
Cerebral localization; what is known, what surmised, and what is its surgical value? Chicago, 1894. 16p. DNLM **90-7551**

ROBERTSON, John W[ooster] (*b.* 1856)
Brain surgery and operations, based on cerebral localization. New York, 1896. 12p. DNLM **90-7552**

ROBINS, Charles R. (*b.* 1868)
Stone in the kidney. [Richmond, 1897.] 15p. DNLM **90-7553**

ROBINSON, A[ndrew] R[ose] (1845-1924)
Some considerations on the treatment of cutaneous malignant epithelioma (cancers). New York. E. P. Coby & Co., 1892. 40p. DNLM; NNNAM **90-7554**

ROBINSON, A[ndrew] R[ose] (1845-1924)
Hydrocystoma. New York: D. Appleton & Co., [1893]. 11p. 1 plate. DNLM; NNNAM **90-7555**

ROBINSON, Beverley (1844-1924)
Notes on general versus local treatment of catarrhal inflammations of the upper air-tract. [Philadelphia, 1891.] 16p. DNLM
90-7556

ROBINSON, Beverley (1844-1924)
On the use of creosote in the treatment of pulmonary phthisis. New York: Trow, 1892. 16p. DNLM
90-7557

ROBINSON, Beverley (1844-1924)
A contribution to the treatment of organic diseases of the heart. [Philadelphia: Lea Bros. & Co., 1894.] 23p. DNLM
90-7558

ROBINSON, Beverley (1844-1924)
The treatment of certain symptoms of croupous pneumonia, particularly in adults. Philadelphia, 1894. 18p. DNLM
90-7559

ROBINSON, Beverley (1844-1924)
Suggestions as to prophylaxis, contagion, and treatment of pneumonia. New York, 1898. 13p. DNLM
90-7560

ROBINSON, Beverley (1844-1924)
The nasal douche; what it accomplishes and what it does not. [New York, 1899.] 2 l. DNLM **90-7561**

ROBINSON, David H[amilton]
The Latin grammar of pharmacy and medicine. With an introduction by L. E. Sayre. Philadelphia: P. Blakiston, Son & Co., 1890. 271p. CtY-M; DNLM; PPC; PU
90-7562

ROBINSON, David H[amilton]
The Latin grammar of pharmacy and medicine. With an introduction by L. E. Sayre. 2nd ed. Philadelphia: P. Blakiston, Son & Co., 1893. 277p. NcD; PPC; PPJ; PU
90-7563

ROBINSON, David H[amilton]
The Latin grammar of pharmacy and medicine. With an introduction by L. E. Sayre. 3rd ed., rev. with elaborate vocabularies. Philadelphia: P. Blakiston, Son & Co., 1896. 277p. OCIM; PPJ; PU **90-7564**

ROBINSON, D. W.
Dakota for health-seekers. A climatic sketch. A part of the program (with additions) of the tenth annual meeting of the American Climatological Association, Philadelphia, Pa., May 25, 26, 27, 1893. Pierre, 1893. 20p. DNLM
90-7565

ROBINSON, Fred Byron (1854-1910)
Accidents, anomalies, and unrecognized matters in abdominal surgery. No. 1. [Chicago, 1891.] 11p. DNLM
90-7566

ROBINSON, Fred Byron (1854-1910)
Circular enterorrhaphy by a new method. [Philadelphia, 1891.] 15p. DNLM **90-7567**

ROBINSON, Fred Byron (1854-1910)
Automatic menstrual ganglia. A new theory of menstruation. [New York, 1891.] 16p. DNLM **90-7568**

ROBINSON, Fred Byron (1854-1910)
Practical intestinal surgery. Detroit, Mich.: G. S. Davis, 1891. 2 v. 1 plate. DNLM; OCIM **90-7569**

ROBINSON, Fred Byron (1854-1910)
Tait's perineal flap operation. Chicago, 1893. 8p. DNLM
90-7570

ROBINSON, Fred Byron (1854-1910)
Critique of macroscopic examination of specimens removed in thirty-two consecutive laparotomies [with one death]. Chicago, 1894. 32p. DNLM **90-7571**

ROBINSON, Fred Byron (1854-1910)
Landmarks in gynaecology. Detroit, Mich.: G. S. Davis, 1894. 2 v. DNLM; NNNAM **90-7572**

ROBINSON, Fred Byron (1854-1910)
Peritoneal adhesions after laparotomy. New York, 1895. 6p. DNLM **90-7573**

ROBINSON, Fred Byron (1854-1910)
The peritonaeum. [New York, 1895.] 7p. DNLM
90-7574

ROBINSON, Fred Byron (1854-1910)
The peritoneum. Part I. Histology and physiology. Bibliography. Chicago: The W. T. Keener Co., 1897. 406, 103p. DNLM
90-7575

ROBINSON, Fred Byron (1854-1910)
Colpoperineorrhaphy and the structures involved; the vagina and perineum and how to mend them. Chicago, 1899. 134p. DNLM; OCIM **90-7576**

ROBINSON, Fred Byron (1854-1910)
The abdominal, brain and automatic visceral ganglia. Chicago: Clinic Pub. Co., 1899. 261p. DNLM; OCIM
90-7577

ROBINSON, Fred Byron (1854-1910)
The peritoneum. Part I: Histology and physiology. With 247 illustrations. Chicago: Medical Book Co., 1899. 528p. DLC; ICJ; ICRM; NNNAM **90-7578**

ROBINSON, W[illiam] F[rancis]
Electro-therapeutics of neurasthenia. Detroit, Mich.: G. S. Davis, 1893. 72p. DNLM; OCIM **90-7579**

ROBINSON, William J[osephus] (1867-1936)
The therapeutics of methylene blue, with special reference to its employment in urethritis. [New York], 1895. 5p. DNLM
90-7580

ROBINSON, William J[osephus] (1867-1936)
The remarkable action of ichthyol-glycerin on a severe, apparently hopeless, case of lymphangeio-phlebitis. New York: D. Appleton & Co., 1896. 4p. DNLM
90-7581

ROBINSON, William J[osephus] (1867-1936)
Painless operations without ether, or chloroform, or the method of infiltration anaesthesia, etc. New York, 1897. 8p. DNLM **90-7582**

ROBISON, John A.
Chicago's need of special hospitals for consumptives. Chicago: J. H. White & Co., 1894. 3p. DNLM
90-7583

ROBSON, A[rthur] W[illiam] Mayo (1853-1933)
Diseases of the gall-bladder and bile-ducts. New York: William Wood & Co., 1897. 150p. CtY-M; DNLM; NNNAM; PU **90-7584**

ROCKWELL, A[lphonso] D[avid] (1840-1908)
The nervous origin of jaundice. [Philadelphia, 1893.] 7p. DNLM **90-7585**

ROCKWELL, A[lphonso] D[avid] (1840-1908)
Some causes and characteristics of neurasthenia. [New York, 1893.] 8p. DNLM **90-7586**

ROCKWELL, A[lphonso] D[avid] (1840-1908)
The medical and surgical uses of electricity. . . . Illustrated with two hundred engravings. New ed. New York: William Wood & Co., 1896. 612p. plate. DLC; DNLM; NNNAM **90-7587**

ROCKWELL T[homas] H.
The early recognition of kidney disease, especially in its reference to life insurance. New York, 1899. 8p. DNLM **90-7588**

ROCKWOOD, Elbert William (*b.* 1860)
A laboratory manual of physiological chemistry. . . . Philadelphia, New York, [etc.]: The F. A. Davis Co., 1899. 204p. plates. DLC; DNLM; NNNAM; PPC **90-7589**

ROE, John Orlando (1848-1915)
Stricture of the oesophagus from interstitial thickening of its walls, a fibroid hypertrophy. New York: D. Appleton & Co., 1891. 10p. 1 plate. DNLM **90-7590**

ROE, John Orlando (1848-1915)
The aseptic method as applied to intranasal surgery. New York, 1891. 10p. DNLM **90-7591**

ROE, John Orlando (1848-1915)
Aetiology of deviations, spurs, and ridges of the nasal saeptum. New York: D. Appleton & Co., 1896. 18p. DNLM **90-7592**

ROE, John Orlando (1848-1915)
The correction of nasal deformities by subcutaneous operations. New York, 1899. 31p. DNLM **90-7593**

ROGERS, Edmund J[ames] A[rmstrong] (*b.* 1852)
Neuroma. (With report of a case.) [Philadelphia, 1892.] 12p. DNLM **90-7594**

ROGERS, Edmund J[ames] A[rmstrong] (*b.* 1852)
Conservatism in accidental surgery. Read before the Colorado State Medical Society, 1893. [Denver, 1893.] 9p. DNLM **90-7595**

ROGERS, Edmund J[ames] A[rmstrong] (*b.* 1852)
Fracture of the skull; trephining; retro-anterograde amnesia; recovery; death one month subsequently from other causes; autopsy. Philadelphia: Lea Bros. & Co., 1894. 14p. DNLM **90-7596**

ROGERS, Edmund J[ames] A[rmstrong] (*b.* 1852)
Successful operation for intestinal obstruction in an infant sixty-four hours old. Denver: Calhoun & Holmes, 1897. 7p. DNLM **90-7597**

ROGERS, Henry Raymond (1822-1901)
Cholera; its nature and its cure. Chicago, 1893. 7p. DNLM **90-7598**

ROGERS, James Goodwin (1841-1908)
First aid for the insane. Read, on invitation, before the Marion County Medical Society at the Central Hospital for Insane, Indianapolis, April 10, 1898. Indianapolis, [1898]. 26p. DNLM **90-7599**

ROGERS, Joseph Goodwin (1841-1908)
The state and its insane. Read before the State Conference of Charities and Corrections, Nov. 17, 1898, Indianapolis. Indianapolis, [1898]. 14p. DNLM **90-7600**

ROGERS, Loyal Dexter (*b.* 1856)
Rogers' homoeopathic guide, a popular treatise containing a brief description of all diseases, with practical hints for their prevention and cure. Designed for the guidance of intelligent laymen; also, for the ready reference of students and practitioners, by L. D. Rogers . . . and Ida Wright Rogers. . . . Chicago: People's Health Journal Co., 1893. 351p. DLC **90-7601**

ROGERS, Oscar H. (*b.* 1857)
A graphic standard table of heights and weights. New York, 1899. 8p. 1 tab. DNLM **90-7602**

ROGERS, Shep. A.
Address to the graduating class of Memphis Hospital Medical College. [Memphis, 1892.] 8p. DNLM **90-7603**

ROGERS, W[illiam] B[oddie] (*b.* 1856)
Appendicitis; report of fifteen cases. Memphis, [1893]. 8p. DNLM **90-7604**

ROGERS, W[illiam] B[oddie] (*b.* 1856)
External perineal urethrotomy. A review of nine cases. Philadelphia, 1894. 16p. DNLM **90-7605**

ROGERS, W[illiam] B[oddie] (*b.* 1856)
Laryngo-tracheotomy for foreign body. A clinical lecture presenting two cases. Operations successful. Memphis, 1895. 6p. DNLM **90-7606**

ROGERS, W[illiam] B[oddie] (*b.* 1856)
Multilocular cystic tumor of inferior maxilla. Memphis, 1897. 7p. DNLM **90-7607**

ROHÉ, George H. (1851-1899) and William J. TODD
One hundred consecutive cases of labor at the Maryland Maternité, with a description of the methods practiced in that institution. Baltimore, 1890. 22p. DNLM **90-7608**

ROHÉ, George H. (1851-1899)
Text-book of hygiene; a comprehensive treatise on the principles and practice of preventive medicine from an American stand-point. . . . 2nd ed., thoroughly rev. and largely rewritten, with many illustrations and valuable tables. Philadelphia and London: F. A. Davis, 1890. 421p. diags. DLC; DNLM; MH; PPC **90-7609**

ROHÉ, George H. (1851-1899)
The influence of parturient lesions of the uterus and vagina in the causation of puerperal insanity. Chicago, 1892. 8p. DNLM **90-7610**

ROHÉ, George Henry (1851-1899)
. . . A practical manual of diseases of the skin, By George H. Rohé . . . assisted by J. Williams Lord. . . . Philadelphia and London: The F. A. Davis Co., 1892. 303p. DLC; DNLM; PPC; PU **90-7611**

ROHÉ, George Henry (1851-1899)
Further observations on the relation of pelvic disease and psychical disturbances in women. [Philadelphia, 1893.] 7p. DNLM **90-7612**

ROHÉ, George Henry (1851-1899)
Lactational insanity. Chicago, 1893. 8p. DNLM **90-7613**

ROHÉ, George Henry (1851-1899)
Intestinal obstruction following operations in which the peritoneal cavity is opened. Philadelphia, 1894. 12p. DNLM **90-7614**

ROHÉ, George Henry (1851-1899)
Text-book of hygiene. . . . 3rd ed., thoroughly rev. and largely rewritten. . . . Philadelphia: The F. A. Davis Co., [etc., etc.], 1894. 553p. diags. DLC; NNNAM; PPC; PU **90-7615**

ROHÉ, George Henry (1851-1899)
Clinical observations upon the relation of somatic diseases to mental derangement. Baltimore, 1895. 11p. DNLM **90-7616**

ROHÉ, George Henry (1851-1899)
Total extirpation of uterus and adnexa per vaginam in inflammatory diseases of the pelvis. Richmond, 1895. 14p. DNLM **90-7617**

ROHMER, J[oseph] (1856-1921)
Resection of the optic nerve. [Transl. from the French.] Nashville, Tenn.: A. R. Gray & Son, 1893. 10p. DNLM **90-7618**

ROLLINS, William (1852-1929)
Notes on X-light. Boston: the Author, 1894. 400p. 152 plates. MBM; MWA **90-7619**

ROOSA, Daniel Bennett St. John (1838-1908)
The determination of the necessity for wearing glasses. . . . Detroit, Mich.: G. S. Davis, 1890. 73p. DLC **90-7620**

ROOSA, Daniel Bennett St. John (1838-1908)
The relation of errors of refraction and insufficiency of the ocular muscles to functional diseases of the nervous system. New York: Trow, 1890. 24p. DNLM; NNNAM **90-7621**

ROOSA, Daniel Bennett St. John (1838-1908)
A pocket medical lexicon, being a dictionary of the words, terms, and symbols of medical science, collated from the best authorities, with the addition of new words not before introduced into a lexicon. 4th revised and enlarged ed. New York: William Wood & Co., [1890]. 323p. DNLM; NNNAM; PPC; PPJ **90-7622**

ROOSA, Daniel Bennett St. John (1838-1908)
Ophthalmic and otic memoranda. By D. B. St. John Roosa . . . and Edward T. Ely. . . . 4th rev. ed. New York: William Wood & Co., 1891. 339p. DLC; DNLM; NNNAM; NNU-M **90-7623**

ROOSA, Daniel Bennett St. John (1838-1908)
A practical treatise on the diseases of the ear, including a sketch of aural anatomy and physiology. . . . 7th rev. ed. New York: William Wood & Co., 1891. 741p. col. plates. DLC; NNNAM; OCIM; PPC **90-7624**

ROOSA, Daniel Bennett St. John (1838-1908)
The causes of asthenopia. [Albany, 1891.] 5p. DNLM **90-7625**

ROOSA, Daniel Bennett St. John (1838-1908)
Constitutional conditions combined with ametropia the cause of asthenopia. [New York, 1891.] 13p. DNLM **90-7626**

ROOSA, Daniel Bennett St. John (1838-1908)
A clinical manual of diseases of the eye, including a sketch of its anatomy. New York: William Wood & Co., 1894. 621p. 2 plates. DNLM; NNNAM; PPC; PU **90-7627**

ROOSA, Daniel Bennett St. John (1838-1908)
Defective eyesight; the principles of its relief by glasses. . . . New York: The Macmillan Co.; [etc., etc.], 1899. 193p. fold. plate. DLC; DNLM; NNNAM; PPC **90-7628**

ROOSEVELT HOSPITAL TRAINING SCHOOL FOR NURSES, NEW YORK CITY
Circular of information. [New York, 1896.] 7p. DNLM; NNNAM **90-7629**

ROOSEVELT, J[ames] West (1858-1896)
The frequency of the localization of phthisis pulmonalis in the upper lobes. [New York: D. Appleton & Co., 1891.] 20p. DNLM; NNNAM **90-7630**

ROOSEVELT, J[ames] West (1858-1896)
A study. The anatomy of the lungs as shown by corrosion, considered in relation to pulmonary phthisis. New York: [D. Appleton & Co., 1891.] 22p. DNLM; NNNAM **90-7631**

ROOSEVELT, J[ames] West (1858-1896)
Acquired immunity from certain infectious diseases a result of heredity and natural selection. [New York: D. Appleton & Co., 1893.] 7p. DNLM; NNNAM **90-7632**

ROOSEVELT, J[ames] West, ed. (1858-1896)
In sickness and in health; a manual of domestic medicine and surgery, hygiene, dietetics, and nursing. . . . By George Waldo Crary, M.D., Frederic S. Lee, Ph.D., Josiah Royce, Ph.D. [and others] and J. West Roosevelt, M.D., editor. New York: D. Appleton & Co., 1896. 991p. col. plates. DLC; NNNAM **90-7633**

ROSE, A[chilles] (1839-1916)
What is the significance of the splashing sound of the stomach? New York, 1895. 5p. 1 tab. DNLM **90-7634**

ROSE WILLIAM (1847-1910) and Albert CARLESS
A manual of surgery for students and practitioners. New York: William Wood & Co., 1898. 1162p. DNLM; NNNAM **90-7635**

ROSE, William (1847-1910) and Albert CARLESS
A manual of surgery for students and practitioners. 2nd ed. New York: William Wood & Co., 1899. 1190p. DNLM; NNNAM **90-7636**

ROSENHEIMER, M[eyer]
Peanuts in the vermiform appendix; operation; complete removal of the appendix; recovery. [Philadelphia, 1892.] 3p. DNLM **90-7637**

ROSENHEIMER, M[eyer]
Dermoid cyst of the ovary simulating appendicitis. Philadelphia, 1894. 3p. DNLM **90-7638**

ROSENSTIRN, Julius (*b.* 1850)
Treatment of stricture of the male urethra. Chicago, 1894. 8p. DNLM **90-7639**

[ROSENTHAL, Charles A.]
The blood, its rotary motion and centrifugal force. [San Francisco, 1892.] 32p. DNLM **90-7640**

ROSENTHAL, Edwin
A report of a series of cases of laryngeal diphtheria treated with the antitoxin, and without intubation. Philadelphia, 1895. 7p. DNLM **90-7641**

ROSENTHAL, Edwin
The treatment of diphtheria with diphtheria antitoxin. Read before the Philadelphia County Medical Society, Sept. 11, 1895. Philadelphia, 1895. 43p. DNLM **90-7642**

ROSENTHAL, Edwin
Reduced period of intubation by the serum treatment of laryngeal diphtheria. Philadelphia, 1896. 8p. DNLM **90-7643**

ROSENTHAL, Edwin
The influence of antitoxine in the treatment of laryngeal diphtheria with and without intubation. Baltimore, 1898. 2p. 1 tab. DNLM **90-7644**

ROSENTHAL, Edwin
Injuries to the new born in cross, complex, and breech presentation. Baltimore, 1898. 5p. DNLM **90-7645**

ROSENTHAL, Edwin
Subnormal temperature in typhoid fever. Philadelphia, 1898. 5p. DNLM **90-7646**

ROSENWASSER, Marcus (1846-1910)
What are the indications for abdominal section in intra-pelvic hemorrhage? Philadelphia, 1893. 19p. DNLM **90-7647**

ROSENWASSER, Marcus (1846-1910)
Clinical fragments. Cleveland, 1894. 44p. DNLM **90-7648**

ROSENWASSER, Marcus (1846-1910)
Exceptional location of the blood clot in a case of ruptured ectopic pregnancy. New York, 1895. 3p. DNLM **90-7649**

ROSENWASSER, Marcus (1846-1910)
A plea against the meddlesome treatment of acute gonorrhea in women. Cleveland, 1896. 6p. DNLM **90-7650**

ROSENWASSER, Marcus (1846-1910)
A practical consideration of gonorrhea in women. Cleveland, 1896. 6p. DNLM **90-7651**

ROSSENWASSER, Marcus (1846-1910)
A case of intraperitoneal gestation at term; operation after death of fetus; recovery. New York, 1897. 8p. DNLM **90-7652**

ROSENWASSER, Marcus (1846-1910)
The ideal medical society. Cleveland, 1897. 7p. DNLM **90-7653**

ROSENWASSER, Marcus (1846-1910)
The treatment of circumscribed pelvic hemorrhage. Chicago, 1897. 7p. 1 tab. DNLM **90-7654**

ROSENWASSER, Marcus (1846-1910)
The treatment of circumscribed pelvic hemorrhage. New York, 1897. 6p. 1 tab. DNLM **90-7655**

ROSEWATER, Charles
Electrolysis in gynaecology. [Omaha, 1891.] 18p. DNLM **90-7656**

ROSS, James F[rederick] W[illiam] (1856-1911)
How should we proceed when abdominal tumors are complicated by pregnancy? Philadelphia: W. J. Dornan, 1891. 27p. DNLM **90-7657**

ROSS, James F[rederick] W[illiam] (1856-1911)
An inquiry into our present knowledge of the progress of myomatous tumors: 1. After the use of electricity. 2. After removal of the ovaries and tubes. 3. After the old treatment by ergot, rest, etc. New York: D. Appleton & Co., 1891. 18p. DNLM **90-7658**

ROSS, James F[rederick] W[illiam] (1856-1911)
Abdominal section for purulent peritonitis resulting from ectopic gestation. Toledo, O., 1892. 7p. DNLM **90-7659**

ROSS, James F[rederick] W[illiam] (1856-1911)
Cases requiring abdominal operations. New York: William Wood & Co., 1892. 21p. DNLM **90-7660**

ROSS, John W.
Three amputations of the thigh; two in the upper third, one at the middle. Philadelphia, 1894. 9p. DNLM **90-7661**

ROSSE, Irving C[ollins] (1847-1901)
Clinical evidence of borderland insanity. Washington: Gedney & Roberts, 1891. 16p. DLC; DNLM **90-7662**

ROSSE, Irving C[ollins] (1847-1901)
The neuroses from a demographic point of view. [New York, 1891.] 14p. DNLM **90-7663**

ROSSE, Irving C[ollins] (1847-1901)
Triple personality. [New York], 1892. 6p. DNLM **90-7664**

ROSSE, Irving C[ollins] (1847-1901)
Brief mention of a few cases of nervous and mental malady in which a medico-legal question was involved. [Richmond, 1894.] 14p. DNLM **90-7665**

ROSSE, Irving C[ollins] (1847-1901)
The conservative value of the play impulse. Boston: Damrell & Upham, 1895. 15p. DNLM **90-7666**

ROSSE, Irving C[ollins] (1847-1901)
The importance of early diagnosis in some forms of nervous disease. Charlotte, N.C., 1895. 7p. DNLM
90-7667

ROSSE, Irving C[ollins] (1847-1901)
Words not usually found in medical dictionaries. Richmond, 1895. 8p. DNLM **90-7668**

ROSSE, Irving C[ollins] (1847-1901)
Brief mention of neurological cases successfully treated. [Richmond, 1898.] 8p. DNLM **90-7669**

ROTCH, Thomas Morgan (1849-1914)
Notes on infant feeding. New York, 1890 [1889]. 22p. DNLM
90-7670

ROTCH, Thomas Morgan (1849-1914)
The management of human breast-milk in cases of difficult infantile digestion. New York, 1890. 13p. DNLM
90-7671

ROTCH, Thomas Morgan (1849-1914)
The president's address before the American Pediatric Society, on iconoclasm and original thought in the study of pediatrics. Philadelphia, 1891. 6p. DNLM **90-7672**

ROTCH, Thomas Morgan (1849-1914)
A case of double movable kidney. Boston: Damrell & Upham, 1892. 10p. DNLM **90-7673**

ROTCH, Thomas Morgan (1849-1914)
The value of milk laboratories for the advancement of our knowledge of artificial feeding. New York, 1893. 12p. DNLM
90-7674

ROTCH, Thomas Morgan (1849-1914) and L. E. HOLT
The nomenclature of diseases of the gastro-enteric tract. The report of the committee of the American Pediatric Society, May, 1894. [New York, 1894.] 4p. 1 tab. DNLM
90-7675

ROTCH, Thomas Morgan (1849-1914)
The substitute feeding of infants. Philadelphia, 1896. 16p. DNLM **90-7676**

ROTCH, Thomas Morgan (1849-1914)
Pediatrics: the hygienic and medical treatment of children. . . . Philadelphia: J. B. Lippincott Co., 1896. 1124p. col. plates. DLC; DNLM; NNNAM; PPC **90-7677**

ROTCH, Thomas Morgan (1849-1914)
Pediatrics: the hygienic and medical treatment of children. . . . 2nd ed. Philadelphia: J. B. Lippincott Co., 1897. 1132p. col. plates. MBM; NNNAM; PPC; PU
90-7678

ROTCH, Thomas Morgan (1849-1914)
The differential diagnosis of the acute exanthemata, with especial reference to scarlet fever. Boston: Damrell & Upham, 1897. 31p. DNLM **90-7679**

ROTCH, Thomas Morgan (1849-1914)
The use of modified milk in health and disease. New York, 1897. 18p. DNLM **90-7680**

ROTCH, Thomas Morgan (1849-1914)
Perforation of the stomach in an infant seven weeks old. Philadelphia, 1899. 4p. DNLM **90-7681**

ROWE, George H[oward] M[alcolm] (1841-1916)
Public health; better legislation and enforcement. Boston, 1890. 21p. DNLM **90-7682**

ROWE, George H[oward] M[alcolm] (1841-1916)
A plea for trained nurses for almshouse hospitals. Boston: G. H. Ellis, 1895. 11p. DNLM **90-7683**

ROWLEY, W. S.
Preliminary report on Stafford mineral spring, near Vossburg, Mississippi. New Orleans, [1896]. 39p. DNLM
90-7684

von RUCK, Karl (1849-1922)
The detrimental effects of over-exertion in pulmonary phthisis. Detroit: G. S. Davis, 1890. 18p. DNLM
90-7685

von RUCK, Karl (1849-1922)
Phthisical patients at climatic resorts. Philadelphia, 1890. 11p. DNLM **90-7686**

von RUCK, Karl (1849-1922)
Prognosis in pulmonary tuberculosis, based upon an analysis of five hundred and fifteen cases. [Philadelphia, 1890.] 26p. DNLM **90-7687**

von RUCK, Karl (1849-1922)
The prophylaxis of tuberculosis. Detroit: G. S. Davis, 1890. 26p. DNLM **90-7688**

von RUCK, Karl (1849-1922)
Some observations upon the gastro-intestinal disorders and the diet in pulmonary phthisis. Detroit: G. S. Davis, 1890. 18p. DNLM **90-7689**

von RUCK, Karl (1849-1922)
The terminations of croupous pneumonia. Wilmington, 1890. 10p. DNLM **90-7690**

von RUCK, Karl (1849-1922)
The cure of pulmonary tuberculosis upon the principles of nutrition. [New York, 1891.] 24p. DNLM
90-7691

von RUCK, Karl (1849-1922)
Professor Koch's method, and the results of its application in twenty-five cases of pulmonary and laryngeal tuberculosis. Detroit, Mich.: G. S. Davis, 1891. 40p. DNLM
90-7692

von RUCK, Karl (1849-1922)
The choice of climatic resorts for tubercular patients. [New York, 1892.] 10p. DNLM **90-7693**

von RUCK, Karl (1849-1922)
The climatic treatment of phthisis, with a description of the climate of Asheville, N.C. Asheville, N.C., 1893. 16p. DNLM
90-7694

von RUCK, Karl (1849-1922)
A contribution to the treatment of pulmonary tuberculosis with Professor Koch's tuberculin. Detroit, 1893. 16p. DNLM
90-7695

von RUCK, Karl (1849-1922)
Results in ninety cases of pulmonary tuberculosis. Treated at the Winyah Sanitarium at Asheville, N.C., from May 1, 1891, to May 1, 1892, with a comparison of results obtained with and without the use of tuberculin. [Philadelphia, 1893.] 8p. DNLM **90-7696**

von RUCK, Karl (1849-1922)
The climate of western North Carolina; with a consideration of the relative value of high and medium levels in the treatment of pulmonary tuberculosis. New York, 1893. 3p. DNLM **90-7697**

von RUCK, Karl (1849-1922)
Rest as a therapeutic agent in chronic pulmonary tuberculosis. New York, 1893. 1 l. DNLM **90-7698**

von RUCK, Karl (1849-1922)
The therapeutic uses of the pneumatic cabinet. [St. Paul], 1894. 7p. DNLM **90-7699**

von RUCK, Karl (1849-1922)
The use of pepto-mangan for anaemia in pulmonary tuberculosis. [New York, 1894.] 3 l. DNLM **90-7700**

von RUCK, Karl (1849-1922)
The etiological treatment of pulmonary tuberculosis. Detroit, 1895. 21p. DNLM **90-7701**

von RUCK, Karl (1849-1922)
The present status of pulmonary tuberculosis. [Asheville, N.C., 1895.] 24p. DNLM **90-7702**

von RUCK, Karl (1849-1922)
The present status of pulmonary tuberculosis. Cincinnati, 1895. 16p. DNLM **90-7703**

von RUCK, Karl (1849-1922)
What is tuberculin? [New York: D. Appleton & Co., 1895.] 15p. DNLM **90-7704**

von RUCK, Karl (1849-1922)
Report of 182 cases of pulmonary tuberculosis treated in the Winyah Sanitarium, Asheville, N.C., with tuberculocidin and anti-phthisin, Klebs. Detroit, 1896. 7p. DNLM **90-7705**

von RUCK, Karl (1849-1922)
The clinical value of the culture products of the bacillus of tuberculosis. Detroit, 1897. 10p. DNLM **90-7706**

von RUCK, Karl (1849-1922)
Pulmonary tuberculosis. [New York, 1897.] 29p. DNLM **90-7707**

von RUCK, Karl (1849-1922)
Clinical report from the Winyah Sanitarium. Seventy-eight cases of pulmonary tuberculosis treated and discharged in 1898. Asheville, N.C., 1899. 21p. DNLM **90-7708**

RUDDIMAN, Edsel A[lexander] (*b.* **1864**)
Incompatibilities in prescriptions. 1st ed. 1st thousand. New York: J. Wiley & Sons, 1897. 264p. DLC; DNLM; NNNAM **90-7709**

RUGH, J. Torrance
A case of concurrent sarcoma and hip-joint disease. Philadelphia, 1895. 5p. DNLM **90-7710**

RUMBOLD, Thomas F[razier] (1830-1901)
The functions of the tensor tympani and stapedius muscles and incidentally the mechanism of the tinnitus aurium. St. Louis, 1897. 16p. DNLM **90-7711**

RUMBOLD, Thomas F[razier] (1830-1901)
The hygiene of the voice. . . . St. Louis, Mo.: Witt Pub. Co., 1898. 144p. DLC **90-7712**

RUNNELS, Moses T[hurston] (1830-1902)
Health and study. The science of physical life and mental development. Delivered before the 14th annual session of the Missouri Institute of Homoeopathy. Kansas City, Mo., 1890. 27p. DNLM **90-7713**

RUPP, Adolph (1856-1907)
On syphilis of the external ear. New York: D. Appleton & Co., 1891. 5 l. DNLM; NNNAM **90-7714**

RUPP, Adolph (1856-1907)
Aphthae and diphtheria, their association and differentiation. New York, 1894. 13p. DNLM; NNNAM **90-7715**

RUPP, Adolph (1856-1907)
Fish bones in the throat, and what they suggest concerning deglutition. New York, 1894. 16p. DNLM; NNNAM **90-7716**

RUPP, Adolph (1856-1907)
Perforations of the nasal septum; etiology, clinical significance, and treatment. New York: Trow, 1894. 24p. DNLM; NNNAM **90-7717**

RUPP, Adolph (1856-1907)
Concerning the aims and methods of hospital alumni societies. New York, 1895. 7p. DNLM; NNNAM **90-7718**

RUPP, Adolph (1856-1907)
Concerning bedsores; their aetiology, pathology, and treatment. New York, 1895. 15p. DNLM **90-7719**

RUPP, Adolph (1856-1907)
Remarks on antitoxin, diphtheria, the practitioner, and history. A practical view of antitoxin and diphtheria in private practice. Antitoxin, diphtheria, and statistics. New York, 1899. 48p. DNLM; NNNAM **90-7720**

RUPTURE relieved by Rorick air-cushion truss. Washington, [1893]. 32p. DNLM [also: Washington, (1893), 40p., *vel subseq.*] **90-7721**

RUSCHENBERGER, William Samuel Waithman (1807-1895)
A sketch of the life of Casper Wister. Philadelphia: W. J. Dornan, 1891. 34p. port. DNLM; PPC **90-7722**

RUSCHENBERGER, William Samuel Waithman (1807-1895)
A sketch of the life of Dr. Gouverneur Emerson. Philadelphia: MacCalla & Co., 1891. 26p. port. DNLM; PPC **90-7723**

RUSH, Benjamin (1745-1813)
Old family letters relating to yellow fever. Series B. Philadelphia: J. B. Lippincott Co., 1892. 108p. CtY-M; DNLM; PPC; PU **90-7724**

RUSH MEDICAL COLLEGE, CHICAGO. MEDICAL DEPARTMENT OF LAKE FOREST UNIVERSITY
Triennial catalogue. Containing the names of the trustees, presidents, instructors, and alumni from 1843 [to date of issue]. Chicago: Rogers & Wells, 1895. 42p. DNLM; ICRM **90-7725**

RUSHBY, Henry H[urd] (1855-1940)
The botanical names of the U.S. Pharmacopoeia. [Detroit, 1892.] 20p. DNLM **90-7726**

RUSHBY, Henry H[urd] (1855-1940)
Vegetable medicines of the ipecac class. [New York, 1893.] 15p. DNLM **90-7727**

RUSHBY, Henry H[urd] (1855-1940)
Comparative action of the green and brown strophanthus seeds. Philadelphia, 1899. 7p. DNLM **90-7728**

RUSSELL, Francis A[lbert] R[olls] (1849-1914)
The atmosphere in relation to human life and health. Washington: Smithsonian Inst., 1896. 148p. DNLM **90-7729**

RUSSELL, Gurdon Wadsworth (1815-1909)
. . . Early medicine and early medical men in Connecticut. Read at the centennial meeting of the Connecticut Medical Society, at New Haven, May 25, 1892. . . . [Hartford], 1892. 158p. CtY-M; DLC **90-7730**

RUSSELL, John F[rancis] (*b.* 1855)
The composition of the Russell emulsion of mixed fats, and a consideration of the importance of fat as a constituent of diet in acute febrile conditions. New York, 1898. 7p. DNLM **90-7731**

RUSSELL, John F[rancis] (*b.* 1855)
On the use of the Russell emulsion (emuls. sevi et olei comp.) in diseases other than phthisis pulmonalis, and methods of administration. New York, 1898. 8p. DNLM **90-7732**

RUSSELL, W[illiam] W.
Hemorrhagic infarction of the Fallopian tube. New York: William Wood & Co., 1894. 8p. DNLM **90-7733**

RUSSELL, W[illiam] W.
The clinical course of forty-seven cases of carcinoma of the uterus subsequent to hysterectomy. Baltimore, 1895. 8p. DNLM **90-7734**

RUSSELL, W[illiam] W.
The operative significance of metastases and post-operative recurrences in carcinoma of the uterus. New York, 1896. 14p. 3 plates. DNLM **90-7735**

RYAN, Charles Edward (1850-1925)
With an ambulance during the Franco-German War; personal experiences and adventures with both armies, 1870-1871. New York: Charles Scribner's Sons, 1896. 368p. NN; NNC; PPL; RPB **90-7736**

RYDER, John Adam (1852-1895)
The synthetic museum of comparative anatomy as the basis for a comprehensive system of research. Philadelphia, 1893. 15p. DNLM; PPC **90-7737**

SACHS, Bernard (1858-1944)
Progressive facial hemiatrophy with some unusual symptoms. New York: Trow, 1890. 8p. DNLM **90-7738**

SACHS, Bernard (1858-1944) and F. PETERSON
A study of cerebral palsies of early life, based upon an analysis of one hundred and forty cases. New York: M. J. Rooney & Co., [1890]. 38p. DNLM; NNNAM **90-7739**

SACHS, Bernard (1858-1944)
Contributions to the pathology of infantile cerebral palsies. [New York, 1891.] 24p. 3 plates. **90-7740**

SACHS, Bernard (1858-1944) and S. T. ARMSTRONG
Morvan's disease. [New York, 1892.] 13p. DNLM **90-7741**

SACHS, Bernard (1858-1944)
What can we expect from the surgical treatment of epilepsy? [New York, 1892.] 18p. DNLM **90-7742**

SACHS, Bernard (1858-1944)
A treatise on the nervous diseases of children for physicians and students. . . . New York: William Wood & Co., 1895. 666p. col. plates. DLC; DNLM; NNNAM; PU **90-7743**

SACHS, Bernard (1858-1944)
A family form of idiocy, generaly fatal, and associated with early blindness (amaurotic family idiocy). Being part of a presidential address delivered before the New York Neurological Society, May 5, 1896. New York, 1896. 22p. DNLM **90-7744**

SACHS, Bernard (1858-1944)
The early recognition of general paresis (progressive dementia). [1898.] 29p. DNLM **90-7745**

SADTLER, Samuel Philip (1847-1923) and Henry TRIMBLE
A text-book of chemistry, intended for the use of pharmaceutical and medical students. Philadelphia: J. B. Lippincott Co., 1895. 950p. DNLM; NN; NNNAM; PU **90-7746**

SADTLER, Samuel Philip (1847-1923) and Henry TRIMBLE
A text-book of chemistry, intended for the use of pharmaceutical and medical students. 2nd revised and enlarged ed. Philadelphia: J. B. Lippincott Co., [1898?]. [2 v.] v. 1: General Chemistry. 842p. DNLM; NNNAM; PPC; PU **90-7747**

SAINT LOUIS COLLEGE OF PHARMACY
Annual prospectuses for the sessions of 1890-91 to 1895-96 (25.-30.); 1897-98 (32.); 1898-99 (33.); 1900-01 (35.). St. Louis, 1890-1900. DNLM [List of graduates from 1867-1900, in announcement for 1900-1901.] **90-7748**

SAINT LOUIS MEDICAL COLLEGE
Annual announcements and catalogues for the sessions of 1842-43 (1.); 1890-91 to 1898-99 (49.-57.). St. Louis, 1842-98. DNLM [Became the medical department of Washington University April 14, 1891. In 1899 the faculty of this school united with the faculty of the Missouri Medical College, forming the Medical Department of Washington University.] **90-7749**

SAINT LOUIS POST-GRADUATE SCHOOL OF MEDICINE, POLYCLINIC AND HOSPITAL
Annual announcements and catalogues for the sessions of 1892 (10.); 1893 (11.). St. Louis: Commercial Ptg. Co., 1892-93. 16p. DNLM **90-7750**

SAINT LOUIS SCHOOL OF SUGGESTIVE THERAPEUTICS AND MEDICAL ELECTRICITY
Annual announcements for the years 1897 to 1898-99 (1.-3.); 1901 (6.). [St. Louis, Mo., and Los Angeles, Cal., 1897-1901.] DNLM [Session of 1897-99, held at St. Louis, Mo.; 1901, at Los Angeles, Cal.] **90-7751**

SAJOUS, Charles E[ucharisté] de Médicis (1852-1929)
Lectures on the diseases of the nose and throat delivered during the spring session of Jefferson Medical College. 2nd ed. Philadelphia: F. A. Davis, 1890. 439p. 8 plates. CtY-M; NNNAM; PPC; PU **90-7752**

SAJOUS, Charles E[ucharisté] de Médicis, ed. (1852-1929)
Annual and analytical cyclopaedia of practical medicine; by Charles E. de M. Sajous, M.D., and one hundred associate editors, assisted by corresponding editors, collaborators, and correspondents. . . . Philadelphia, New York, [etc.] : The F. A. Davis Co., 1898-1901. 6 v. col. plates. DLC; NNNAM; PPC; PPJ **90-7753**

SANBORN, Franklin B[enjamin], ed. (1831-1917)
Memoirs of Pliny Earle, M.D., with extracts from his diary and letters (1830-1892) and selections from his professional writings (1839-1891). Edited, with a general introduction. . . . Boston: Damrell & Upham, 1898. 409p. MB; MH; MH-M; MSaE **90-7754**

SANSON, A[rthur] Ernest (1839-1907)
The diagnosis of diseases of the heart and thoracic aorta, and the pathology which serves for the recognition of morbid states of the organs of circulation. Philadelphia: P. Blakiston, Son & Co., 1892. 567p. 13 charts. DNLM; OCIM; PPC; PU **90-7755**

SANTEE, Harris E[llett] (1864-1936)
A syllabus of lectures on the brain and spinal cord. . . . [Chicago: Rogers & Hall Co., 1898.] 117p. DLC **90-7756**

SARGENT INVALID FURNITURE CO.
Illustrated catalogue of invalid supplies. Boston, 1897. 48p. MBM **90-7757**

SATTERLEE, Francis Le Roy (1847-1917)
Rheumatism and gout. . . . Detroit, Mich.: G. S. Davis, 1890. 83p. DLC; OCIM **90-7758**

SATTERTHWAITE, Thomas E[dward] (*b.* 1843)
Corpulence and the fatty heart. New York, 1899. 12p. DNLM **90-7759**

SATTERTHWAITE, Thomas E[dward] (*b.* 1843)
Displacement of the heart in lateral curvature. New York, 1899. 22p. DNLM **90-7760**

SATTERTHWAITE, Thomas E[dward] (*b.* 1843)
Pericardial diseases illustrated clinically. Philadelphia, 1899. 12p. DNLM **90-7761**

SAUNDBY, Robert (*b.* 1849)
Lectures on diabetes; including the Bradshaw lecture, delivered before the Royal College of Physicians on August 18, 1890. New York: E. B. Treat, 1891. 232p. DNLM; NNNAM; PPC; PU **90-7762**

SAUNDBY, Robert (*b.* 1849)
Lectures on renal and urinary diseases. 2nd ed. Philadelphia: W. B. Saunders & Co., 1897. 434p. 4 plates. DNLM; MBM; NNNAM; OCIM **90-7763**

SAUNDERS' complete catalogue. Medical and surgical books. Philadelphia: W. B. Saunders & Co., [1894?] 80p. DNLM; PPC **90-7764**

SAUNDERS, Robert R.
A case of gunshot injury involving both eyes, studied nine years after the accident. St. Louis, 1895. 3p. DNLM **90-7765**

SAVAGE, George H[enry] (1842-1921)
Insanity and allied neuroses, practical and clinical. 2nd and enl. ed. Philadelphia: Lea Bros. & Co., 1890. 551p. DLC; NNC; NNNAM; PU [1st ed., Philadelphia: H. C. Lea's Son & Co., 1884. 531p.] **90-7766**

SAVAGE, Giles Christopher (1854-1930)
The harmonious symmetrical action of the oblique muscles in all cases of oblique astigmatism. Nashville, 1891. 15p. DNLM **90-7767**

SAVAGE, Giles Christopher (1854-1930)
Heterophoria; a safe line drawn between operative and non-operative cases. Nashville: A. R. Gray & Son, 1892. 14p. DNLM **90-7768**

SAVAGE, Giles Christopher (1854-1930)
Insufficiencies of the oblique muscles and how to correct them. Nashville: A. R. Gray & Son, 1892. 8p. DNLM **90-7769**

SAVAGE, Giles Christopher (1854-1930)
New truths in ophthalmology, as developed by G. C. Savage. . . . Thirty-two illustrations. Nashville, Tenn.: Pub. by the Author, 1893. 152p. DLC; DNLM; OCIM; PU [2nd ed., 1893. 152p. DLC; NcD] **90-7770**

SAVAGE, Giles Christopher (1854-1930)
New truths in ophthalmology, as developed by G. C. Savage. . . . Nashville, Tenn.: Pub. by the Author, 1896. 270p. DLC; MH; NcD; PU **90-7771**

SAVIDGE, Eugene Coleman (*b.* 1863)
The post-partum management of uterine displacements. New York, 1899. 9p. DNLM **90-7772**

SAVITT, Thomas Dixon (1856-1910)
Clinical lectures on neurasthenia. New York: William Wood & Co., 1899. 144p. DNLM; NNNAM **90-7773**

SAYRE, Lewis A[lbert] (1820-1900)
Results in cases of hip-joint diseases treated by the portable traction splint, without immobilization, except during the inflammatory stage of the disease. [New York, 1892.] 17p. 6 plates. DNLM; NNNAM **90-7774**

SAYRE, Lewis A[lbert] (1820-1900)
A practical manual of the treatment of club-foot. 4th ed. New York: D. Appleton & Co., 1894. 143p. DNLM; NNNAM; NNU-M **90-7775**

SAYRE, Lewis A[lbert] (1820-1900)
The history of the treatment of spondylitis and scoliosis by partial suspension and retention by means of plaster-of-Paris bandages. [Also] The plaster of Paris, wood, aluminum, and other spinal supports by A. M. Phelps. New York, 1895. 58p. DNLM; NNNAM **90-7776**

SAYRE, Lucius Elmer (1847-1925)
. . . Essentials of practice of pharmacy. Arranged in the form of questions and answers. . . . Philadelphia: W. B. Saunders, 1890. 179p. DLC; DNLM; NNNAM; PPC **90-7777**

SAYRE, Lucius Elmer (1847-1925)
. . . Essentials of practice of pharmacy. Arranged in the form of questions and answers. . . . (2nd ed., rev.) . . . Philadelphia: W. B. Saunders, 1894. 200p. DLC; NNNAM; PPC; PU **90-7778**

SAYRE, Lucius Elmer (1847-1925)
A manual of organic materia medica and pharmacognosy; an introduction to the study of the vegetable kingdom and the vegetable and animal drugs. . . . With 543 illustrations, the majority of which are from original drawings. Philadelphia: P. Blakiston, Son & Co., 1895 [1894]. 555p. DLC; DNLM; NNNAM; PPC **90-7779**

SAYRE, Lucius Elmer (1847-1925)
A manual of organic materia medica and pharmacognosy; an introduction to the study of the vegetable kingdom and the vegetable and animal drugs. . . . 2nd ed., rev., with histology and microtechnique by William C. Stevens. . . . With 374 illustrations. Philadelphia: P. Blakiston's Sons & Co., 1899. 684p. DLC; DNLM; OCLloyd; PU **90-7780**

SAYRE, Reginald H[all] (1859-1929)
Spondylitis of second cervical vertebra, with report of cases and instruments for treatment. [Philadelphia, 1892.] 8p. DNLM **90-7781**

SAYRE, Reginald H[all] (1859-1929)
The necessity of thorough examination in suspected Pott's disease. Danbury, Conn., 1893. 16p. DNLM **90-7782**

SAYRE, Reginald H[all] (1859-1929)
The treatment of neglected cases of rotary lateral curvature of the spine. New York: D. Appleton & Co., 1893. 10p. 3 plates on 2 l. DNLM **90-7783**

SAYRE, Reginald H[all] (1859-1929)
Posture in the diagnosis of disease. New York, 1897. 54p. DNLM **90-7784**

SCHACHNER, August (1865-1941)
Studies upon injuries of the kidney, nephrolithotomy, and nephrorraphy. [Philadelphia, 1891.] 70p. DNLM; PPC **90-7785**

SCHACHNER, August (1865-1941)
Three illustrative cases of abdominal section. New York: William Wood & Co., 1894. 10p. DNLM **90-7786**

SCHACHNER, August (1865-1941)
The Murphy button; with a report of an unsuccessful cholecystduodenostomy. New York, 1895. 11p. DNLM **90-7787**

SCHACHNER, August (1865-1941)
Suggestions for a portable instrument-bag; operating overalls; a bandage for supra-pubic dressings; a blanket for protection of patients during operations; a table for the Trendelenburg posture; the sterilization of sponges; an antiseptic soap paste. Philadelphia, 1895. 17p. DNLM **90-7788**

SCHACHNER, August (1865-1941)
An improved surgical bed. Philadelphia, 1896. 3p. 4 plates. DNLM **90-7789**

SCHACHNER, August (1865-1941)
Transfusion infusion and autotransfusion; their comparative merits and indications. Louisville, 1896. 7p. DNLM **90-7790**

SCHAEFER, Frederick C. (1849-1904)
Vertebral surgery, with reports of three cases, and a new method of operating in the dorsal region. [Chicago, 1891.] 10p. DNLM **90-7791**

SCHAEFER, Frederick C. (1849-1904)
Traumatic synovitis of knee-joint with hemorrhage into joint cavity; four ounces of blood encapsuled sixteen months. [Chicago, 1892.] 4 l. DNLM **90-7792**

SCHAEFER, Frederick (1849-1904)
Brain surgery, with report of nine cases. Chicago, 1893. 23p. DNLM **90-7793**

SCHAEFER, Frederick C. (1849-1904)
Brain surgery; injury received five years ago, followed three years later by convulsions and paralysis; blood clot found under the dura mater and removed; patient improving. [Chicago, 1893.] 8p. DNLM **90-7794**

SCHAEFER, Frederick (1849-1904)
Perityphlitis; report of three cases of perforating "caecitis" and "pericaecitis." Chicago, 1893. 16p. DNLM **90-7795**

SCHAEFER, Frederick C. (1849-1904)
Skin grafting upon the cranium. [Chicago, 1893.] 11p. DNLM **90-7796**

SCHAEFER, Frederick C. (1849-1904)
Laminectomy for paraplegia from Pott's disease; tenotomy of contractured hamstring tendons of both legs; amputation at the hip-joint; appendicitis; stone in the bladder; supra-pubic lithotomy. [Philadelphia, 1894.] 6p. DNLM **90-7797**

SCHAEFER, Theodore William
The therapeutic uses of the salts of cesium and rubidum. Philadelphia, 1894. 3p. DNLM **90-7798**

SCHAEFER, Theodore William
The commercialization of medicine, or the physician as tradesman; a sociological study. Boston: Damrell & Upham, 1894. 7p. DNLM **90-7799**

SCHAEFER, Theodore William
The sociological status of medical practice. [New York, 1894.] 16p. DNLM **90-7800**

SCHAEFER, Theodore William
The poisonous sting of the "electric light-bug," or Belostoma, as it is called by entomologists. Kansas City, Mo., 1895. 2 l. DNLM **90-7801**

SCHAEFER, Theodore William
Examination of the urine as a means of diagnosis. Kansas City, Mo., 1897. 8p. DNLM **90-7802**

SCHAEFFER, Oskar (*b.* 1863)
Anatomical atlas of obstetric diagnosis and treatment. . . . With 145 illustrations. New York: William Wood & Co., 1896. 234p. col. plates. CtY-M; DNLM; ICJ; PPC [On cover; Wood's medical hand atlases.] **90-7803**

SCHAEFFER, Oskar (*b.* 1863)
Atlas and essentials of gynecology. New York: William Wood & Co., 1897. 288p. illus., col. plates. DNLM; IU-M; PPC; PPHa [Wood's medical hand atlases.] **90-7804**

SCHÄFER, Edward Albert (1850-1935)
The essentials of histology and descriptive and practical for the use of students. 3rd ed. Philadelphia: Lea Bros. & Co., 1892. 301p. DNLM; OCIM; PPC; PU **90-7805**

SCHÄFER, Edward Albert (1850-1935)
The essentials of histology descriptive and practical for the use of students. 4th ed. Philadelphia: Lea Bros. & Co., 1895. 340p. DLC; MBM; PPC; PU **90-7806**

SCHÄFER, Edward Albert (1850-1935)
A course of practical histology. 2nd ed. Philadelphia: Lea Bros. & Co., 1897. 298p. DNLM; NNNAM; OCIM; PPC **90-7807**

SCHÄFER, Edward Albert (1850-1935)
The essentials of histology descriptive and practical for the use of students. New (5th) ed., revised and enlarged. Philadelphia & New York: Lea Bros. & Co., 1898. 359p. DNLM; NNNAM; PPC; PPJ **90-7808**

SCHAMBERG, Jay Frank (1870-1934)
Xanthoma diabeticorum, with report of a case. New York, 1895. 7p. DNLM **90-7809**

SCHAMBERG, Jay Frank (1870-1934)
Impetigo contagiosa annulata et serpiginosa. New York, 1896. New York, 1896. 5p. DNLM **90-7810**

SCHAMBERG, Jay Frank (1870-1934)
. . . A compend of diseases of the skin. . . . Philadelphia: P. Blakiston's Son & Co., 1898. 307p. DLC; NNNAM; PPC; PU **90-7811**

SCHAMBERG, Jay Frank (1870-1934)
A clinical study of the lymphatic glands in one hundred cases of scarlet fever. Boston, 1899. 6p. DNLM **90-7812**

SCHAPPS, John C.
Orthopedics for the poor. Brooklyn, 1892. 8p. DNLM **90-7813**

SCHAPPS, John C.
I. A combination of steel and plaster of Paris for fixation of ankle and tarsus. II. Deformity following excision of the knee joint. New York: M. J. Rooney, [1892]. 7p. DNLM **90-7814**

SCHAPPS, John C.
Recumbency in the treatment of Pott's disease. [New York, 1893.] 22p. DNLM **90-7815**

SCHAPPS, John C.
A garment for rectum patients. New York, 1895. 3p. DNLM **90-7816**

SCHAPPS, John C.
The mechanical treatment of Pott's disease of the spine in the subacute or convalescent stage. New York, 1895. 11p. DNLM **90-7817**

SCHAPPS, John C.
An elastic tourniquet. New York, 1895. 2p. DNLM **90-7818**

SCHAPPS, John C.
Some apparatus for the treatment of Pott's disease. New York: D. Appleton & Co., 1896. 24p. DNLM; NNNAM **90-7819**

SCHAPRINGER, Alois
Ueber Vaccine-Blepharitis. [New York, 1890.] 4p. DNLM **90-7820**

SCHAPRINGER, Alois
Enophthalmus traumaticus mit dem Ausgange in Genesung. [New York, 1890.] 7p. DNLM **90-7821**

SCHAPRINGER, Alois
The proximate cause of the transient form of myopia associated with iritis. With remarks on other forms of symptomatic ametrophia. [New York, 1893.] 10p. DNLM **90-7822**

SCHARMAN, Gustav
Catalogue of dental specialties. New York, [c. 1898]. 16 l. NNNAM **90-7823**

SCHEPPEGRELL, William (*b.* 1860)
Hypertrophy of the lingual tonsil, with report of fifteen cases. [Philadelphia: Lea Bros. & Co., 1892.] 7p. DNLM **90-7824**

SCHEPPEGRELL, William (*b.* 1860)
Deformities of the nasal septum and their influence in diseases of the ear and throat. New Orleans: L. Graham & Son, [1893]. 15p. 3 plates. DNLM **90-7825**

SCHEPPEGRELL, William (*b.* 1860)
Non-malignant tumors of the larynx. [New Orleans, 1893.] 15p. 9 plates. DNLM **90-7826**

SCHEPPEGRELL, William (*b.* 1860)
The influence of diseases of the nose and naso-pharynx on other parts of the body. New Orleans: L. Graham & Son, 1894. 14p. 2 plates. DNLM **90-7827**

SCHEPPEGRELL, William (*b.* 1860)
Congenital occlusion of the posterior nares. Kansas City, 1894. 5p. DNLM **90-7828**

SCHEPPEGRELL, William (*b.* 1860)
A new and simple method by which cautery-irons may be electrically heated almost instantaneously. Philadelphia, 1895. 4p. DNLM **90-7829**

SCHEPPEGRELL, William (*b.* 1860)
Papillomata of the soft palate. New York, 1896. 4p. DNLM
90-7830

SCHEPPEGRELL, William (*b.* 1860)
Keloid tumors of the external ear. New York: D. Appleton & Co., 1896. 9p. DNLM **90-7831**

SCHEPPEGRELL, William (*b.* 1860)
The progress of laryngology. [St. Louis, 1897.] 3p. DNLM
90-7832

SCHEPPEGRELL, William (*b.* 1860)
Transillumination in diseases of the nose, throat and ear. [St. Louis, 1897.] 22p. DNLM **90-7833**

SCHEPPEGRELL, William (*b.* 1860)
The treatment of laryngeal tuberculosis with cupric interstitial cataphoresis, with report of cases; the advantages of direct laryngoscopy in this method. New York, 1897. 12p. DNLM
90-7834

SCHEPPEGRELL, William (*b.* 1860)
The abuse and dangers of cocain. New York, 1898. 19p. DNLM **90-7835**

SCHEPPEGRELL, William (*b.* 1860)
Bronchitis, with special reference to abnormal nasal respiration as an aetiological factor. New York, 1898. 9p. DNLM
90-7836

SCHEPPEGRELL, William (*b.* 1860)
Case of recurrent headache, each attack being relieved by the discharge through right nostril of a fluid from the cranial cavity. Chicago: Amer. Med. Assoc. Press, 1898. 8p. DNLM
90-7837

SCHEPPEGRELL, William (*b.* 1860)
Electricity in the diagnosis and treatment of disease of the nose, throat and ear, with 161 illustrations. . . . New York, London: G. P. Putnam's Sons, 1898. 403p. DLC; DNLM; NNNAM **90-7838**

SCHEPPEGRELL, William (*b.* 1860)
Perichondritis and necrosis of the arytenoid cartilage. (Transl. from the Rev. internat. de rhinol., otol. et laryngol., Par., 1898, July.) St. Louis, 1898. 6p. DNLM **90-7839**

SCHEPPEGRELL, William (*b.* 1860)
The progress of rhino-laryngology. St. Louis, 1899. 14p. DNLM **90-7840**

SCHEPPEGRELL, William (*b.* 1860)
The Schleich method of general anesthesia, with special reference to nose, throat and ear practice. . . . [Memphis, 1899.] 6p. DLC; DNLM **90-7841**

SCHIMMELBUSCH, Curt (1860-1895)
A guide to the aspetic treatment of wounds. . . . Preface by E. Von Bergmann. Transl. from the 2nd German ed. by Frank J. Thornbury. New York: G. P. Putnam's Sons, 1895. 233p. DLC; ICJ; NNNAM; PU **90-7842**

SCHIMPF, Henry W[illiam] (*b.* 1868)
A text-book of volumetric analysis with special reference to the volumetric processes of the Pharmacopoeia of the United States. Designed for the use of pharmacists and pharmaceutical students. New York: J. Wiley & Sons, 1894. 400p. DNLM; NNNAM; OCIM; OCLloyd **90-7843**

SCHIMPF, Henry W[illiam] (*b.* 1868)
A text-book of volumetric analysis with special reference to the volumetric processes of the Pharmacopoeia of the United States. Designed for the use of pharmacists and pharmaceutical students. 2nd ed. New York: J. Wiley & Sons, 1895. 400p. NNNAM; PPC; PU **90-7844**

SCHIMPF, Henry W[illiam] (*b.* 1868)
A text-book of volumetric analysis with special reference to the volumetric process of the Pharmacopoeia of the United States. Designed for the use of pharmacists and pharmaceutical students. 3rd ed. New York: J. Wiley & Sons, 1898. 522p. DNLM; NNNAM; OCLloyd **90-7845**

SCHLEIF, William (*b.* 1868)
The administration of drugs. A guide for the pharmaceutical laboratory. . . . Philadelphia: Press of Avil Printing Co., 1898. 105p. DLC; PU **90-7846**

SCHLEIF, William (*b.* 1868)
Materia medica, therapeutics, medical pharmacy, prescription writing, and medical Latin. A manual for students and practitioners. . . . Philadelphia and New York: Lea Bros. & Co., [1899]. 354p. DLC; NNNAM; PPC; PU
90-7847

SCHOFIELD, Alfred T[aylor] (1846-1929)
Elementary physiology for students. Philadelphia: Lea Bros. & Co., 1893. 380p. CtY-M; NNNAM; PPC; PU
90-7848

SCHOOLFIELD, Charles B.
Cholelithiasis. New York: J. D. Emmet, 1896. 4p. DNLM
90-7849

SCHREIBER, August (1853-1924)
General orthopedics, including surgical operations. New York: William Wood & Co., 1891. 348p. CtY-M; IU-M; NNNAM; PU [Printed out of Wood's Medical and Surgical Monographs, vol. 2., No. 3, pp. (569)-912 (1889)] **90-7850**

von SCHRENCK-NOTZING, Albert (1862-1929)
Therapeutic suggestion in psychopathia sexualis (pathological manifestations of the sexual sense), with especial reference to contrary sexual instinct. Authorized transl. from the German by Charles Gilbert Chaddock. Philadelphia: F. A. Davis; London: F. J. Rebmar, 1895. 320p. DNLM; ICU; MH; NNNAM **90-7851**

SCHUESSLER, Wilhelm Heinrich (1821-1898)
An abridged therapy. Manual for the biochemical treatment of disease. . . . 25th ed., in part rewritten. Transl. by Prof. Louis H. Tafel. Philadelphia: Boericke & Tafel, 1898. 179p. DLC; NNNAM; PPC; PPHa **90-7852**

SCHULTZE, Bernhard S[igmund] (1827-1919)
The pathology and treatment of displacements of the uterus. Transl. from the German by Jameson J. Macan and ed. by Arthur V. Macan. New York: D. Appleton & Co., 1890 [1888-1889]. 378p. DNLM; ICJ; OCIM; PPC
90-7853

de SCHWEINITZ, Emil Alexander (1866-1904)
The production of immunity in guinea-pigs from hog-cholera by the use of blood-serum from immunified animals. [Philadelphia: Lea Bros. & Co., 1892.] 7p. DNLM
90-7854

de SCHWEINITZ, Emil Alexander (1866-1904)
The enzymes or soluble ferments of the hog-cholera germ. [Philadelphia: Lea Bros. & Co., 1892.] 4p. DNLM
90-7855

de SCHWEINITZ, Emil Alexander (1866-1904)
Culture media for biochemic investigations. [New York, 1893.] 1 l. DNLM **90-7856**

de SCHWEINITZ, Emil Alexander (1866-1904)
The attenuated bacillus tuberculosis; its use in producing immunity to tuberculosis in guinea-pigs. New York, 1894. 13p. DNLM **90-7857**

de SCHWEINITZ, Emil Alexander (1866-1904)
The production of immunity to hog-cholera by means of the blood serum of immune animals. Antitoxic serums for hog-cholera and swine plague. New York: D. Appleton & Co., 1896. 8p. DNLM **90-7858**

de SCHWEINITZ, Emil Alexander (1866-1904)
The war with the microbes. New York, 1897. 20p. DNLM
90-7859

de SCHWEINITZ, Emil Alexander (1866-1904)
Some products of the tuberculosis bacillus and the treatment of experimental tuberculosis with antitoxic serum. Philadelphia, 1897. 15p. DNLM **90-7860**

de SCHWEINITZ, Emil Alexander (1866-1904) and Marion DORSET
Some products of the tuberculosis bacillus and the treatment of experimental tuberculosis with antitoxic serum. New York, 1897. 18p. DNLM; NNNAM **90-7861**

de SCHWEINITZ, Emil Alexander (1866-1904)
Laboratory guide. Methods for the examination of urine for the students of the Columbian Medical School, Washington, D.C. Washington, D.C.: N. T. Elliott, 1898. 37p. DNLM; PPC; PU **90-7862**

de SCHWEINITZ, G[eorg] E[dmund] (1858-1938)
Erysipelas of the eyelids spreading extensively to face and scalp; orbital cellulitis; recovery without impairment of vision. [Philadelphia, 1890.] 6p. DNLM **90-7863**

de SCHWEINITZ, G[eorg] E[dmund] (1858-1938)
The ocular complications of malaria. [Philadelphia, 1890.] 21p. DNLM **90-7864**

de SCHWEINITZ, G[eorg] E[dmund] (1858-1938)
A series of cases presenting minor lesions of the macula lutea. Chicago, 1890. 16p. DNLM **90-7865**

de SCHWEINITZ, G[eorg] E[dmund] (1858-1938)
Some experiments to determine the lesion in quinine-blindness. A preliminary note. [Philadelphia, 1890.] 9p. DNLM
90-7866

de SCHWEINITZ, G[eorg] E[mund] (1858-1938)
Symblepharon as a sequel of purulent ophthalmia. [Philadelphia, 1890.] 2p. DNLM **90-7867**

de SCHWEINITZ, G[eorg] E[dmund] (1858-1938)
Additional experiments to determine the lesion of quinine blindness. With photo-micrographic studies by William M. Gray. [Hartford, 1891.] 7p. 3 plates. DNLM
90-7868

de SCHWEINITZ, G[eorg] E[dmund] (1858-1938)
A case of homonymous hemiopic hallucinations, with lesion of the right tract. [New York, 1891.] 3p. DNLM
90-7869

de SCHWEINITZ, G[eorg] E[dmund] (1858-1938)
A case of persistent hemorrhage from the conjunctiva of a new-born infant, following the instillation of a solution of nitrate of silver. [New York, 1891.] 3p. DNLM
90-7870

de SCHWEINITZ, G[eorg] E[dmund] (1858-1938)
Coloboma of the iris, polycoria, and primary glaucoma. [Hartford, 1891.] 6p. 1 plate. DNLM
90-7871

de SCHWEINITZ, G[eorg] E[dmund] (1858-1938)
The indications for some of the applications commonly used in the treatment of chronic granular lids. [Philadelphia, 1891.] 11p. DNLM **90-7872**

de SCHWEINITZ, G[eorg] E[dmund] (1858-1938)
Neuroma of the right upper eyelid and adjacent temporal region. [Hartford, 1891.] 10p. 2 plates. DNLM
90-7873

de SCHWEINITZ, G[eorg] E[dmund] (1858-1938)
A note on fluorescin-coloring and the actual cautery in corneal ulcers. [Philadelphia, 1891.] 4p. DNLM **90-7874**

de SCHWEINITZ, G[eorg] E[dmund] (1858-1938)
One hundred cases of hypermetropic astigmatism contrary to the rule, and the associated symptoms. Chicago, 1891. 56p. DNLM **90-7875**

de SCHWEINITZ, G[eorg] E[dmund] (1858-1938)
Perimetric observations on the influence of eserine and iridectomy in chronic glaucoma. Chicago, 1891. 24p. DNLM
90-7876

de SCHWEINITZ, G[eorg] E[dmund] (1858-1938)
Pyoktanin in dacryocystitis. [Philadelphia, 1891.] 2p. DNLM
90-7877

de SCHWEINITZ, G[eorg] E[dmund] (1858-1938)
The treatment of corneal ulcers by the actual cautery. Philadelphia: W. J. Dornan, 1891. 8p. DNLM
90-7878

de SCHWEINITZ, G[eorg] E[dmund] (1858-1938)
Diseases of the eye. A hand-book of ophthalmic practice, for students and practitioners. . . . Philadelphia: W. B. Saunders, 1892. 641p. col. plates. DLC; ICRM; NNNAM; PPC
90-7879

de SCHWEINITZ, G[eorg] E[dmund] (1858-1938)
Embolism of the central artery of the retina, with the report of three cases. Chicago, 1892. 16p. DNLM
90-7880

de SCHWEINITZ, G[eorg] E[dmund] (1858-1938)
Hyaline bodies (Drusen) in the nervehead. (Photo-micrographs by William M. Gray.) [Hartford, 1892.] 12p. 2 plates. DNLM
90-7881

de SCHWEINITZ, G[eorg] E[dmund] (1858-1938)
A note on asthenopia and intra-nasal disease. [Philadelphia, 1892.] 6p. DNLM **90-7882**

de SCHWEINITZ, G[eorg] E[dmund] (1858-1938)
A note on the treatment of vitreous opacities with the fluid extract of jaborandi. Detroit: G. S. Davis, 1892. 9p. DNLM **90-7883**

de SCHWEINITZ, G[eorg] E[dmund] (1858-1938)
Ophthalmia neonatorum; its treatment and prophylaxis. [Philadelphia, 1892.] 6p. DNLM **90-7884**

de SCHWEINITZ, G[eorg] E[dmund] (1858-1938)
Post-diphtheritic paralysis of the external recti; with a case. [Kansas City, 1892.] 6p. DNLM **90-7885**

de SCHWEINITZ, G[eorg] E[dmund] (1858-1938)
Some cases of obstructive disease of the lachrymal passages and the associated intra-nasal lesions. [Philadelphia, 1892.] 8p. DNLM **90-7886**

de SCHWEINITZ, G[eorg] E[dmund] (1858-1938)
Some notes on the corneal astigmatism in two hundred eyes measured with the ophthalmometer of Javal, in comparison with the total subjective astigmatism after complete mydriasis. Detroit: G. S. Davis, 1892. 10p. DNLM **90-7887**

de SCHWEINITZ, G[eorg] E[dmund] (1858-1938)
Ophthalmic memoranda. [St. Louis: J. P. Parker, 1893.] 7p. DNLM **90-7888**

de SCHWEINITZ, G[eorg] E[dmund] (1858-1938)
Subconjunctival injections of corrosive sublimate. Detroit: G. S. Davis, 1893. 9p. DNLM **90-7889**

de SCHWEINITZ, G[eorg] E[dmund] (1858-1938)
Sympathetic irritation and sympathetic serous iritis. Detroit: G. S. Davis, 1893. 14p. DNLM **90-7890**

de SCHWEINITZ, G[eorg] E[dmund] (1858-1938) and Emil Alexander de SCHWEINITZ
Some results of a bacteriological examination of the pipettes and collyria taken from a treatment case used in ophthalmic practice, with the effects of inoculations; a preliminary communication. [Philadelphia, 1893.] 12p. DNLM **90-7891**

de SCHWEINITZ, G[eorg] E[dmund] (1858-1938) and Emil Alexander de SCHWEINITZ
A further communication on the results of a bacteriological examination of the pipettes and collyria taken from a treatment case used in ophthalmic practice, with the effects of inoculations. 1894. 4p. DNLM **90-7892**

de SCHWEINITZ, G[eorg] E[dmund] (1858-1938)
Diseases of the eye. A hand-book of ophthalmic practice, for students and practitioners. . . . 2nd ed., thoroughly rev. Philadelphia: W. B. Saunders, 1896. 679p. col. plates. DLC; IEN-M; MBM; PPC **90-7893**

de SCHWEINITZ, G[eorg] E[dmund] (1858-1938)
The toxic amblyopias: their classification, history, symptoms, pathology, and treatment. Being an essay to which was awarded the Alvarenga prize of the College of Physicians of Philadelphia, October, 1894. . . . With forty-six illustrations and nine plates. Philadelphia: Lea Bros. & Co., 1896. 238p. plates. DLC; DNLM; PPC; PU **90-7894**

de SCHWEINITZ, G[eorg] E[dmund] (1858-1938)
Diseases of the eye. A hand-book of ophthalmic practice, for students and practitioners. . . . With 255 illustrations and two chromo-lithographic plates. 3rd ed., thoroughly revised. Philadelphia: W. B. Saunders, 1899. 696p. DLC; DNLM; NNNAM; PPC **90-7895**

de SCHWEINITZ, G[eorg] E[dmund] (1858-1938)
An American text-book of diseases of the eye, ear, nose and throat; ed. by G. E. De Schweinitz . . . and B. Alex. Randall. . . . Illustrated with 766 engravings, 59 of them in colors. Philadelphia: W. B. Saunders, 1899. 1251p. DLC; MBM; NNNAM; PPC **90-7896**

SCHWYZER, A.
Removal of the whole transverse colon and partial resection of the pancreas and large curvature of the stomach for carcinoma, with lateral suture of the superior and inferior mesenteric veins. St. Paul, Minn., 1899. 12p. 3 plates. DNLM **90-7897**

SCHWYZER, Fritz
Blood diagnosis, and some of the most important advances in the study of blood. New York, 1896. 23p. DNLM **90-7898**

SCHWYZER, Fritz
A case of congenital hypertrophy and stenosis of the pylorus. New York, 1896. 9p. DNLM **90-7899**

SCOTT, Alfred J.
A new treatment for pneumonia. Milwaukee, Wis., 1899. 2 l. DNLM **90-7900**

SCOTT, James Foster (*b.* 1863)
Hydrothiomina, or the phenomenon of sulphuretted-hydrogen gas in urine; four cases; a review of the literature. [New York: D. Appleton & Co., 1893.] 21p. DNLM; NNNAM **90-7901**

SCOTT, James Foster (*b.* 1863)
Pathology and treatment of periuterine pelvic inflammations. New York: William Wood & Co., 1894. 9p. DNLM **90-7902**

SCOTT, James Foster (*b.* 1863)
Bacteriology and treatment of puerperal tetanus. New York: William Wood & Co., 1895. 8p. DNLM **90-7903**

SCOTT, James Foster (*b.* 1863)
Criminal abortion. New York: William Wood & Co., 1896. 18p. DNLM **90-7904**

SCOTT, James Foster (*b.* 1863)
The sexual instinct, its use and dangers as affecting heredity and morals. New York: E. B. Treat & Co., 1899. 436p. DNLM; NNNAM **90-7905**

SCOTT, J[oseph] B.
Asthma and anemia relieved by removal of nasal polypi. [Philadelphia, 1895.] 3p. DNLM **90-7906**

SCOTT, Matthew Thompson (1855-1894)
Laparotomy for gunshot wound of intestine. Four perforations by large bullet; various complications; complete recovery. New York: Trow, 1890. 8p. DNLM **90-7907**

SCOTT, Matthew Thompson (1855-1894)
A case of compound comminuted fracture of the patella into the knee joint. [New York, 1890.] 1 galley sheet. DNLM **90-7908**

SCOTT, Matthew Thompson (1855-1894)
Suppurative perityphlitis; report of case; rupture into bladder and rectum; operation; recovery. New York: Trow, 1892. 11p. DNLM **90-7909**

SCOTT, N. Stone (*b.* 1863)
Rectal stricture of puerperal origin, relieved by laparotomy. [New York, 1893.] 7p. DNLM **90-7910**

SCOTT, N. Stone (*b.* 1863)
Non-malignant stenosis of the pylorus and duodenum. Cleveland, 1897. 14p. DNLM **90-7911**

SCOTT, N. Stone (*b.* 1863)
Why does the surgeon fail to find the appendix? Cleveland, 1899. 8p. DNLM **90-7912**

SCOVIL, Elisabeth Robinson (*b.* 1849)
The care of children. Revised ed. Philadelphia: H. Altemus, 1895. 360p. port. DNLM; PPC; PU **90-7913**

SCOVIL, Elisabeth Robinson (*b.* 1849)
Preparation for motherhood. Philadelphia: H. Altemus, [1896]. 316p. port. DNLM; NN; PU **90-7914**

SCOVILLE, Wilbur Lincoln (1865-1942)
The art of compounding. A textbook for students and a reference book for pharmacists at the prescription counter. Philadelphia: P. Blakiston, Son & Co., 1895. 264p. DNLM; OCLloyd; PPC; PU **90-7915**

SCUDDER, Charles Locke (1860-1949)
Congenital dislocation of the shoulder-joint; a report of two cases. [Philadelphia, 1890.] 10p. 1 plate. DNLM **90-7916**

SCUDDER, Charles Locke (1860-1949)
A report of eighteen cases of chronic disease of the ankle and tarsus, with observations upon the operative treatment. Boston, 1890. 23p. 1 tab. DNLM **90-7917**

SCUDDER, Charles Locke (1860-1949)
Diphtheria; tracheotomy, persistent and increasing dyspnoea; systematic curetting of the trachea; recovery. Boston, 1893. 3p. DNLM **90-7918**

SCUDDER, Charles Locke (1860-1949)
A study of four hundred and four cases of divulsion of urethral stricture. The results in twenty-eight cases. New York, 1893. 16p. DNLM **90-7919**

SCUDDER, Charles Locke (1860-1949)
White swelling of the knee; report of results after excision of the knee in thirteen cases done at the Massachusetts General Hospital by different operators. Boston: Damrell & Upham, 1894. 14p. DNLM **90-7920**

SCUDDER, Charles Locke (1860-1949) and Fred P. LUND
I. A case of middle meningeal hemorrhage; operation; recovery; an analysis of forty-eight cases of uncomplicated intra-cranial hemorrhage. II. Middle meningeal hemorrhage, by G. L. Walton. III. Localized hemorrhage beneath pia mater over upper third of Rolandic area, due to fall on the head; localized convulsions without loss of consciousness; later, slight mental confusion with paralysis of the affected limbs, followed by prlonged coma and death, by James J. Putnam. Philadelphia & New York, 1895. 28p. DNLM **90-7921**

SCUDDER, Charles Locke (1860-1949)
Compound depressed fracture of the skull; absence of unconsciousness; paralysis of one-half the body; operation; recovery. [Philadelphia, 1896.] 2p. DNLM **90-7922**

SCUDDER, Charles Locke (1860-1949)
Nephrectomy for cystic adenoma in a pregnant woman; recovery. [Philadelphia, 1896.] 6p. DNLM **90-7923**

SCUDDER, Charles Locke (1860-1949)
The treatment of caries of the ankle joint. Boston, 1896. 4p. DNLM **90-7924**

SCUDDER, Charles Locke (1860-1949)
The ambulatory treatment of fractures. Boston, 1898. 10p. DNLM **90-7925**

SCUDDER, Charles Locke (1860-1949)
A case of tuberculosis of the breast, with analysis of all cases of tuberculosis of the breast recorded in medical literature. Philadelphia, 1898. 10p. DNLM **90-7926**

SCUDDER, Charles Locke (1860-1949)
Major amputations at the Massachusetts General Hospital. A study of the mortality from 1822 to 1896. Boston, 1898. 8p. DNLM **90-7927**

SCUDDER, Charles Locke (1860-1949)
Middle meningel hemorrhage in a woman sixty-nine years old; operation; recovery. New York, 1898. 7p. DNLM **90-7928**

SCUDDER, Charles Locke (1860-1949)
Acute hemorrhagic gangrenous pancreatitis; operation after the second and twenty-eighth day; death. [Boston, 1899.] 3p. DNLM **90-7929**

SCUDDER, Charles Locke (1860-1949)
Emergency cases at the Massachusetts General Hospital. Boston, 1899. 6p. DNLM **90-7930**

SCUDDER, John K[ing] (*b.* 1865)
Numerical strength of the different schools of medicine in the United States. [Cincinnati, Ohio, 1894.] 2p. DNLM **90-7931**

SCUDDER, John Milton (1829-1894)
On the reproductive organs and the venereal. 3rd ed. Cincinnati: J. M. Scudder, 1890. 393p. 6 plates. DNLM; OCIM **90-7932**

SCUDDER, John Milton (1829-1894)
Specific diagnosis; a study of diseases with special reference to the administration of remedies. 9th ed. [Cincinnati]: J. M. Scudder, 1891. 387p. DNLM; OCIM **90-7933**

SCUDDER, John Milton (1829-1894)
The American eclectic. Materia medica and therapeutics. 11th ed. Cincinnati: J. M. Scudder, 1891. 748p. DNLM; OCLloyd
90-7933A

SCUDDER, John Milton (1829-1894)
The eclectic practice of medicine. . . . 13th ed. 3rd revision. Cincinnati: J. M. Scudder, 1891. 813p. DLC; NNNAM; OCLloyd **90-7934**

SCUDDER, John Milton (1829-1894)
A practical treatise on the diseases of women. Illustrated by colored plates and numerous wood engravings. . . . With a paper on the diseases of the breasts. By Robert S. Newton. . . . 15th ed., thoroughly rev. Cincinnati: J. M. Scudder, 1891. 533p. col. plates. DLC: DNLM; OCIM
90-7935

SCUDDER, John Milton (1829-1894)
Specific medication and specific medicines. Fourth revision, with an appendix containing the articles published on the subject since the first edition, and a report of cases illustrating specific medication. 14th ed. Cincinnati: J. M. Scudder & Sons, 1893. 432p. DNLM; OCLloyd **90-7936**

SCUDDER, John Milton (1829-1894)
. . . On the use of medicated inhalations in the treatment of diseases of the respiratory organs. . . . With an Appendix on diseases of the nose and throat, by Wm. Byrd Scudder. . . . 4th ed. Cincinnati, O.: J. M. Scudder & Sons, 1895. 159p. DLC; DNLM; OCIM **90-7937**

SEAMAN, Gilbert E[dmund] (*b.* 1869)
Importance of surgical treatment in chronic purulent otitis media. Madison, Wis.: Tracy, Gibbs & Co., 1894. 11p. DNLM
90-7938

SEAMAN, Gilbert E[dmund] (*b.* 1869)
Rheumatic affections of the throat and nose. Milwaukee, 1897. 13p. DNLM **90-7939**

SEAMAN, Louis Livingston (1851-1932)
The U.S. army ration and its adaptability for use in tropical climates. A paper read before the New York Academy of Medicine at its stated meeting, February 2, 1899. New York: Hayes & Wright, 1899. 23p. DNLM; NNNAM
90-7940

SEARS, George G. (*b.* 1859)
The treatment of pregnancy complicated by heart disease. Boston: Damrell & Upham, 1894. 12p. DNLM
90-7941

SEARS, George G. (*b.* 1859)
Cases of pregnancy complicated by heart disease. Boston: Damrell & Upham, 1895. 10p. DNLM
90-7942

SEARS, George G. (*b.* 1859)
Acute pericarditis; a study of one hundred cases. Boston: Damrell & Upham, 1897. 11p. DNLM
90-7943

SEARS, George G. (*b.* 1859)
Endocarditis from gonorrhoea. Boston: Municipal Pr. Office, 1898. 11p. DNLM **90-7944**

SEARS, George G. (*b.* 1859)
A case of hemorrhagic pericarditis due to the pneumococcus; aspiration; recovery. Boston, 1898. 5p. DNLM
90-7945

SEDGWICK, William Thompson (1855-1921)
Investigation of recent epidemics of typhoid fever in Massachusetts. Boston, 1892. 78p. 7 maps, 6 plates. DNLM; MBM
90-7946

SEDGWICK, William Thompson (1855-1921) and Allen HAZEN
Typhoid fever in Chicago. New York, 1892. 21p. DNLM
90-7947

SEDGWICK, William Thompson (1855-1921)
On methods used and results obtained in making germicidal efficiency tests of a disinfectant for use in railway sanitation. Boston: T. Todd, 1893. 23p. DNLM; MBM
90-7948

SEDGWICK, William Thompson (1855-1921)
Quarantine vs. sanitation. Boston: Damrell & Upham, 1893. 5p. DNLM **90-7949**

SEGUIN, Edward Constant (1843-1898)
Lectures on some points in the treatment and management of neuroses, delivered before the Medical Society of the University of Toronto, March 11 and 12, 1890. . . . New York: D. Appleton & Co., 1890. 100p. DLC: DNLM; NNNAM
90-7950

SEGUIN, Edward Constant (1843-1898)
Lectures on some points in the treatment and management of neuroses. New York: D. Appleton & Co., 1890. 100p. DNLM; NNNAM **90-7951**

SEGUIN, Edward Constant (1843-1898)
Early diagnosis of some serious diseases of the nervous system; its importance and feasibility. Boston: Damrell & Upham, 1891. 37p. DNLM; MBM **90-7952**

SEGUIN, Edward Constant (1843-1898)
Eye-strain and its relations to "cerebral hyperaemia," etc. [New York, 1892.] 9p. DNLM **90-7953**

SEIBERT, August (1854-1926)
A submembranous local treatment of pharyngeal diphtheria. [New York, 1890.] 17p. DNLM; NNNAM
90-7954

SEIBERT, August (1854-1926)
A reform in artificial infant feeding, with an improved and inexpensive sterilizer and nursing bottles. [New York: W. S. Gottsberger & Co., 1890.] 11p. DNLM
90-7955

SEIBERT, August (1854-1926)
The prevention and treatment of gastro-enteritis in children. New York, 1898. 14p. DNLM **90-7956**

SEIBERT, William H.
Antitoxin and diphtheria. Chicago, 1897. 12p. DNLM
90-7957

SEIFERT, Otto (1853-1933)
Manual of clinical diagnosis, by Dr. Otto Seifert . . . and Dr. Friedrich Müller. . . . Transl. from the 5th German ed., enl. and rev. . . . by William Buckingham Canfield. . . . 2nd English ed. rev. and enl., with fifty illustrations and one colored plate. New York, [etc.]: G. P. Putnam's Sons, 1890. 185p. DLC; DNLM; NNNAM; PU **90-7958**

SEILER, Carl (1849-1905)
Handbook of the diagnosis and treatment of diseases of the throat, nose and naso-pharynx. . . . 4th ed., thoroughly rev. and greatly enl. Illustrated with two lithographic plates containing ten figures, and one hundred and seven wood engravings. Philadelphia: Lea Bros. & Co., 1893. DLC; DNLM; NNNAM; PPC **90-7959**

SEILER, Carl (1849-1905)
The prophylaxis of nasal catarrh. New York: D. Appleton & Co., 1896. 6p. DNLM **90-7960**

SELECTED reports on orthoform from American physicians. New York: V. Koechl & Co., 1899. 10p. DNLM **90-7961**

SEMON, Felix (1849-1921)
On the alleged special liability of benign laryngeal growths to undergo degeneration after intralaryngeal operations. New York: D. Appleton & Co., 1894. 4p. DNLM **90-7962**

SEMON, Felix (1849-1921)
On the alleged special liability of benign laryngeal growths to undergo malignant degeneration after intralaryngeal operations, with an appendix by David Newman. New York: D. Appleton & Co., 1894. 16p. DNLM **90-7963**

SEMPLE, C[harles] E[dward] Armand (1845-1895)
Essentials of pathology and morbid anatomy. Philadelphia: W. B. Saunders, 1890. 160p. DNLM; PPC; PU **90-7964**

SENN, Emanuel John (*b.* 1869)
Olive oil as a remedy in the treatment of gastric ulcer. Chicago, 1894. 7p. DNLM **90-7965**

SENN, Emanuel John (*b.* 1869)
Tenorrhaphy, by means of the suture à distance of catgut, with a report of a case. Chicago, 1894. 11p. DNLM **90-7966**

SENN, Emanuel John (*b.* 1869)
Gastrostomy by a circular valve method. Chicago, 1896. 11p. DNLM **90-7967**

SENN, Emanuel John (*b.* 1869)
Inflammation of joints in gonorrhoeal patients. New York, 1897. 20p. DNLM **90-7968**

SENN, Emanuel John (*b.* 1869)
Amputation of the breast by means of the anterior ancillary incision. Chicago: Am. Medical Assoc., 1899. 4p. DNLM **90-7969**

SENN, Emmanuel John (*b.* 1869)
Traumatic rupture of the urethra. Philadelphia, 1899. 12p. DNLM **90-7970**

SENN, Nicholas (1844-1908)
Principles of surgery. . . . Illustrated with 109 wood engravings. Philadelphia and London: F. A. Davis, 1890. 611p. DLC; DNLM; PPC; PU **90-7971**

SENN, Nicholas (1844-1908)
Diagnosis and operative treatment of gunshot wounds of the stomach and intestines. Chicago, 1890. 83p. DNLM **90-7972**

SENN, Nicholas (1844-1908)
Two cases of resection of the caecum for carcinoma, with remarks on intestinal anastomosis in the iliocaecal region. Chicago, 1890. 45p. DNLM **90-7973**

SENN, N[icholas] (1844-1908)
Away with Koch's lymph! Chicago: R. R. McCabe & Co., [1891]. 38p. DNLM **90-7974**

SENN, N[icholas] (1844-1908)
The chair of surgery in Rush Medical College. Chicago, 1891. 8p. DNLM **90-7975**

SENN, N[icholas] (1844-1908)
Intra-peritoneal myo-fibroma of the rectum, weighing twelve pounds, successfully removed by laparotomy. [St. Louis, 1891.] 8p. DNLM **90-7976**

SENN, N[icholas] (1844-1908)
Surgical bacteriology. 2nd ed. Philadelphia: Lea Bros. & Co., 1891. 271p. 13 plates. DLC; DNLM; PPC; PU **90-7977**

SENN, N[icholas] (1844-1908)
The surgical treatment of pyloric stenosis, with a report of fifteen operations for this condition. New York: Trow's Co., 1891. 56p. DNLM; NNNAM **90-7978**

SENN, N[icholas] (1844-1908)
An experimental inquiry concerning elastic construction as a haemostatic measure. [Philadelphia, 1892.] 8p. DNLM **90-7979**

SENN, N[icholas] (1844-1908)
Gastrostomy. [Chicago, 1892.] 15p. DNLM **90-7980**

SENN, N[icholas] (1844-1908)
Clinical lecture delivered at the second annual meeting of the Association of Military Surgeons of the United States. St. Louis: Nixon-Jones, 1892. 24p. DNLM **90-7981**

SENN, N[icholas] (1844-1908)
The mission of the Association of the Military Surgeons of the National Guard of the United States. Chicago, 1892. 19p. DNLM **90-7982**

SENN, N[icholas] (1844-1908)
The treatment of tuberculosis of bones and joints by parenchymatous and intra-articular injections. [Philadelphia, 1892.] 39p. DNLM **90-7983**

SENN, N[icholas] (1844-1908)
Tuberculosis of bones and joints. Philadelphia & London: F. A. Davis Co., 1892. 504p. 7 plates. DLC; DNLM; PPC; PU **90-7984**

SENN, N[icholas] (1844-1908)
Bloodless amputation at the hip-joint by a new method. Chicago, 1893. 12 l. DNLM **90-7985**

SENN, N[icholas] (1844-1908)
Enterorrhaphy; its history, technique and present status. President's address delivered at the meeting of the Association of Military Surgeons of the National Guard of the United States, Chicago, August 8, 1893. Chicago, 1893. 23p. roy. DNLM **90-7986**

SENN, N[icholas] (1844-1908)
Intestinal surgery. Chicago: W. T. Keener Co., 1893. 269p. DNLM **90-7987**

SENN, N[icholas] (1844-1908)
Laparo-hysterotomy; its indications and technique. Philadelphia, 1893. 13p. DNLM **90-7988**

SENN, N[icholas] (1844-1908)
A new method of direct fixation of the fragments in compound and ununited fractures. [Philadelphia, 1893.] 27p. DNLM **90-7989**

SENN, N[icholas] (1844-1908)
Some further remarks on elastic constriction as a haemostatic measure, with a letter from Professor von Esmarch. New York, 1893. 8p. DNLM **90-7990**

SENN, N[icholas] (1844-1908)
Supra-pubic cystotomy in two stages. [Philadelphia, 1893.] 10p. DNLM **90-7991**

SENN, N[icholas] (1844-1908)
Surgical clinic. Chicago, [1893]. 24p. DNLM **90-7992**

SENN, N[icholas] (1844-1908)
Abdominal surgery on the battle-field. St. Louis, 1894. 15p. DNLM **90-7993**

SENN, N[icholas] (1844-1908)
Appendicitis obliterans. Chicago, 1894. 11p. DNLM **90-7994**

SENN, N[icholas] (1844-1908)
The etiology, pathology and treatment of intestinal fistula and artificial anus. New York: William Wood & Co., 1894. 27p. DNLM; NNNAM **90-7995**

SENN, N[icholas] (1844-1908)
Operative treatment of myofibroma uteri. Chicago: McClure Print. Co., [1894]. 19p. DNLM **90-7996**

SENN, N[icholas] (1844-1908)
Syllabus of lectures on the practice of surgery, arranged in conformity with the American text-book of surgery. Philadelphia: W. B. Saunders, 1894 [1893]. 221p. DLC; DNLM **90-7997**

SENN, N[icholas] (1844-1908)
Conservative surgery on the battlefield and first aid to the wounded. Chicago, 1895. 42p. DNLM **90-7998**

SENN, N[icholas] (1844-1908)
The early history of vaginal hysterectomy. Chicago, 1895. 23p. DNLM **90-7999**

SENN, N[icholas] (1844-1908)
The pathology and surgical treatment of tumors. Philadelphia: W. B. Saunders, 1895. 700p. 13 plates. DLC; DNLM; PPC; PU **90-8000**

SENN, N[icholas] (1844-1908)
Pompeian surgery and surgical instruments. Philadelphia, 1895. 8p. DNLM **90-8001**

SENN, N[icholas] (1844-1908)
Principles of surgery. 2nd ed., thoroughly revised. Philadelphia: F. A. Davis Co., 1895. 656p. DLC; DNLM; PPC; PU **90-8002**

SENN, N[icholas] (1844-1908)
The treatment of malignant tumors by the toxins of the streptococcus of erysipelas. Chicago, 1895. 8p. DNLM **90-8003**

SENN, N[icholas] (1844-1908)
The indications and modes of drainage after abdominal and vaginal section. New York, 1896. 5p. DNLM **90-8004**

SENN, N[icholas] (1844-1908)
Lumbar nephropexy without suturing. Chicago, 1897. 8p. DNLM **90-8005**

SENN, N[icholas] (1844-1908)
Military surgery in Greece and Turkey. Chicago, 1897. 16p. DNLM **90-8006**

SENN, N[icholas] (1844-1908)
A new method of nerve resection for amputation-neuroma. [New Haven], 1897. 2 l. DNLM **90-8007**

SENN, N[icholas] (1844-1908)
The presidential address: The American Medical Association; its past, present, and future. Chicago: Amer. Med. Assoc. Press, 1897. 15p. DNLM **90-8008**

SENN, N[icholas] (1844-1908)
Treatment of chronic empyema of the antrum of Highmore by temporary osteo-plastic resection of the anterior antral wall. [San Francisco], 1897. 4p. DNLM **90-8009**

SENN, N[icholas] (1844-1908)
Tuberculosis of the genito-urinary organs, male and female. Philadelphia: W. B. Saunders, 1897. 317p. 6 plates. DLC; DNLM; PPC; PU **90-8010**

SENN, N[icholas] (1844-1908)
On the frequency of varicocele and the limitations of operative treatment for this affection. Philadelphia, 1898. 5p. DNLM **90-8011**

SENN, N[icholas] (1844-1908)
I. Intestinal tuberculosis; etiology, pathology, and diagnosis. II. Surgical treatment. Chicago, 1898. 19p. DNLM **90-8012**

SENN, N[icholas] (1844-1908)
The invasion of Porto Rico, from a medical standpoint. New York: Lea Bros. & Co., 1898. 13p. DNLM **90-8013**

SENN, N[icholas] (1844-1908)
The modern treatment of gunshot wounds in military practice. Chicago: Amer. Med. Assoc. Press, 1898. 12p. DNLM
90-8014

SENN, N[icholas] (1844-1908)
The modern treatment of gunshot wounds in military practice. Washington, 1898. 19p. DNLM **90-8015**

SENN, N[icholas] (1844-1908)
A new incision for arthrectomy resection and for reduction of irreducible dislocation of the shoulder-joint. Philadelpia, 1898. 10p. DNLM **90-8016**

SENN, N[icholas] (1844-1908)
Restitution of skin by plastic operation in cases of extensive traumatic surface defects of the scrotum and penis. Philadelphia, 1898. 6p. DNLM **90-8017**

SENN, N[icholas] (1844-1908)
Excision of high rectal carcinoma without sacral resection. Philadelphia, 1899. 10p. DNLM **90-8018**

SENN, N[icholas] (1844-1908)
On the frequency of cryptorchism and its results. [New Orleans, 1899.] 1 sheet. DNLM **90-8019**

SENN, N[icholas] (1844-1908)
War correspondence (Hispano-Amercan war). Chicago, 1899. 278p. 1 plate, 1 tab., 1 plan. DNLM; ICU; NN
90-8020

SEUFERT, Edward Constant (*b.* 1873)
The treatment of forty-three cases of typhoid fever, with no deaths, and with complications in but one case. New York, 1899. 3 l. DNLM **90-8021**

SEWALL, Henry (1855-1936)
Infectious disease in cities; with especial reference to Denver. [Philadelphia, 1892.] 23p. DNLM **90-8022**

SEWALL, Henry (1855-1936)
The value of stethoscopic percussion in medical diagnosis. [Philadelphia, 1893.] 11p. DNLM **90-8023**

SEWALL, Henry (1855-1936)
On the causes of edema. [Denver, 1893.] 8p. DNLM
90-8024

SEWALL, Henry (1855-1936)
Remittent fever in Colorado, illustrated by a case. Denver, 1896. 4p. DNLM **90-8025**

SEWALL, Henry (1855-1936)
A strange case of blood infection. Denver, 1896. 4p. DNLM
90-8026

SEWALL, Henry (1855-1936)
How may the dissemination of tuberculosis in Colorado be prevented? Denver, 1897. 4p. DNLM
90-8027

SEWALL, Henry (1855-1936)
On the use of stethoscopic pressure in physical examination of the heart. New York, 1897. 15p. DNLM
90-8028

SEWALL, Henry (1855-1936)
The clinical significance of reduplication of the heart sounds. Philadelphia, 1898. 30p. DNLM **90-8029**

SEWALL, Henry (1855-1936)
A case of persistent foramen ovale with auscultatory signs. Denver, 1899. 2 l. DNLM **90-8030**

SEWALL, Henry (1855-1936)
On the clinical relations of the papillary muscles of the heart. Philadelphia, 1899. 38p. DNLM **90-8031**

SEWARD, W. M.
A case of intubation of the larynx of unusual interest. New York: D. Appleton & Co., 1894. 5p. DNLM
90-8032

SEWILL, Henry [also: Sewell, Henry]
Dental surgery, including special anatomy and pathology. A manual for students and practitioners. 3rd ed. Philadelphia: P. Blakiston, Son & Co., 1890. 400p. DNLM; KU; NNC; PU [2nd ed. appeared as Handbook of dental anatomy and surgery. . . . Philadelphia: P. Blakiston, Son & Co., 1882. 203p.; 1st ed. published as The Students' guide to dental anatomy and surgery. . . . Philadelphia: P. Blakiston, Son & Co., 1881. 203p.] **90-8033**

SEXTON, Samuel (1833-1896)
The classification and treatment of over two thousand consecutive cases of ear diseases at Dr. Sexton's aural clinic, New York Eye and Ear Infirmary. By Samuel Sexton . . . and W. A. Bartlett . . . and Robert Barclay. . . . Detroit, Mich.: G. S. Davis, 1890. 91p. DLC; NNNAM **90-8034**

SEXTON, Samuel (1833-1896)
Deafness and discharge from the ear; the modern treatment for the radical cure of deafness, otorrhoea . . . By Samuel Sexton . . . assisted by Alexander Duane, M.D. New York: J. H. Vail & Co., 1891. 89p. DLC; NNNAM **90-8035**

SEYMOUR, William W[otkyns] (1853-1904)
Personal experiences with gallstones and the operation for their relief. Philadelphia: W. J. Dornan, 1890. 12p. DNLM
90-8036

SEYMOUR, William W[otkyns] (1853-1904)
A report of a case of total laryngectomy for carcinoma. Philadelphia, 1897. 4p. 1 plate. DNLM
90-8037

SHAFFER, Newton M[elman] (1846-1928)
What is orthopedic surgery? Read before the orthopaedic section of the Tenth International Medical Congress, Berlin, August 5, 1890. New York: G. P. Putnam's Sons, 1890. 18p. DNLM; NNNAM **90-8038**

SHAFFER, Newton M[elman] (1846-1928)
On the definition and scope of orthopaedic surgery. Remarks on Dr. Gibney's paper. [New York: D. Appleton & Co., 1891.] 9p. DNLM **90-8039**

SHAFFER, Newton M[elman] (1846-1928)
The relation of orthopaedic surgery to general surgery. Boston: Damrell & Upham, 1891. 7p. DNLM **90-8040**

SHAFFER, Newton M[elman] (1846-1928)
On the benign course of abscess in Pott's disease under efficient mechanical treatment. [New York, 1892.] 6p. DNLM
90-8041

SHAFFER, Newton M[elman] (1846-1928)
The present needs and future demands of orthopaedic surgery. A portion of an address delivered before the trustees of the New York Orthopaedic Dispensary and Hospital upon the occasion of their twenty-ninth annual meeting, held November 16, 1896. New York: D. Appleton & Co., 1896. 8p. DNLM; NNNAM **90-8042**

SHAFFER, Newton M[elman] (1846-1928)
Flat-foot; its causes and treatment. New York: D. Appleton & Co., 1897. 18p. DNLM; NNNAM **90-8043**

SHAFFER, Newton M[elman] (1846-1928)
On mechanical treatment of united fracture of the neck of the femur with traction apparatus producing abduction of the thigh, and direct lateral pressure over the trochanter major. New York, 1897. 12p. DNLM; NNNAM **90-8044**

SHAFFER, Newton M[elman] (1846-1928)
Brief essays on orthopaedic surgery, including a consideration of its relation to general surgery, its future demands, and its operative as well as its mechancial aspects, with remarks on specialism. New York: D. Appleton & Co., 1898. 81p. DLC; DNLM; NNNAM **90-8045**

SHAFFER, Newtom M[elman] (1846-1928)
On the care of crippled and deformed children. New York, 1898. 14p. DNLM; NNNAM **90-8046**

SHAKESPEARE, Edward O[ram] (1846-1900)
Report on cholera in Europe and India. 49th Cong., 2nd sess. Senate. Mis. Doc. No. 92. Washington: Government Printing Office, 1890. 945p. 16 plates, 5 maps. 2 charts, 2 plans, 21 diags. DNLM; PPC **90-8047**

SHAKESPEARE, Edward O[ram] (1846-1900)
The national government should have supreme control of quarantine at all frontiers. [Philadelphia, 1892.] 21p. DNLM **90-8048**

SHAKESPEARE, Edward O[ram] (1846-1900)
Preventive measures for the individual during times of actual threatened prevalence of cholera. [Philadelphia, 1892.] 21p. DNLM **90-8049**

SHALLER, John M. (1856-1931)
A therapeutic guide to alkaloid dosimetric medication. . . . Chicago: W. C. Abbott, 1895. 212p. DLC; DNLM **90-8050**

SHALLER, John M. (1856-1931)
A therapeutic guide to alkaloidal, dosimetric medication. 2nd ed. Chicago: Alkaloidal Clinic Pub. Co., 1897. 216p. DNLM; OCIM **90-8051**

SHANDS, Aurelius Rives (*b.* 1860)
Treatment of clubfoot by Wolff's method. Richmond, 1894. 8p. DNLM **90-8052**

SHANDS, Aurelius Rives (*b.* 1860)
Compression myelitis from Pott's disease. Richmond, 1895. 11p. DNLM **90-8053**

SHANDS, Aurelius Rives (*b.* 1860)
Severe pain and spasm of inflammatory rheumatism of the ankle relieved by immobilization of the joint. New York, 1895. 6p. DNLM **90-8054**

SHANDS, Aurelius Rives (*b.* 1860)
Gant's femoral osteotomy for the correction of hip deformity in adults. With a report of cases. Richmond, 1896. 6p. DNLM **90-8055**

SHANDS, Aurelius Rives (*b.* 1860)
Case of harelip complicated with intermaxillary fissure. Richmond, 1897. 5p. DNLM **90-8056**

SHANDS, Aurelius Rives (*b.* 1860)
Treatment of flexion deformities of the knee-joint. Richmond, 1897. 12p. DNLM **90-8057**

SHANDS, Aurelius Rives (*b.* 1860)
Cases illustrating the value of the X-ray in the treatment of fractures of long bones with displacement. Richmond, 1898. 6p. 8 plates. DNLM **90-8058**

SHANDS, Aurelius Rives (*b.* 1860)
Prognosis and treatment of lateral spinal curvature. Richmond, 1898. 14p. DNLM **90-8059**

SHANDS, Aurelius Rives (*b.* 1860)
Excision of the shoulder-joint. [New Orleans], 1899. 4p. 1 plate. DNLM **90-8060**

SHANDS, Aurelius Rives (*b.* 1860)
Treatment of club-foot, with report of six cases. Richmond, 1899. 15p. DNLM **90-8061**

SHARPE, Norvelle Wallace
Peculiarities and treatment of electric injuries. Philadelphia, 1898. 8p. DNLM **90-8062**

SHARPE, Norvelle Wallace
Municipal medical inspection of schools. Philadelphia, 1899. 24p. 1 diag., 1 tab. DNLM **90-8063**

SHARPLES, Caspar W[istar]
Cerebral palsy of childhood following diphtheria. Philadelphia: Lea Bros. & Co., 1894. 7p. DNLM **90-8064**

SHARPLESS, W. T.
Three cases from private practice. [Philadelphia, 1892.] 4p. DNLM **90-8065**

SHASTID, Thomas Hall (1866-1947)
A new myringotome. New York, 1895. 1 l. DNLM **90-8066**

SHASTID, Thomas Hall (1866-1947)
A new operation for chronic catarrhal and chronic suppurative deafness. New York, 1895. 8p. DNLM **90-8067**

SHASTID, Thomas Hall (1866-1947)
Some observations made during the treatment of chronic catarrhal deafness. Chicago, 1896. 4p. DNLM **90-8068**

SHASTID, Thomas Hall (1866-1947)
Eucane in atrophic rhinitis. New York, 1897. 4p. DNLM **90-8069**

SHATTINGER, Charles
A plea for the treatment of typhoid fever by cold baths. St. Louis, 1899. 7p. DNLM **90-8070**

SHATTOCK, Samuel G. (1853-1924)
An atlas of the bacteria pathogenic in man with descriptions of their morphology and modes of microscopic examintion, with an introductory chapter on bacteriology, its practical value to the general practitioner by W. Wayne Babcock. New York: E. B. Treat & Co., 1899. 82p. 16 plates. DNLM; NNNAM
90-8071

SHATTUCK, Frederick Cheever (1847-1929)
The relation of pneumonia to influenza in Boston. [New York, 1890.] 12p. DNLM; MBM **90-8072**

SHATTUCK, Frederick Cheever (1847-1929)
Auscultation and percussion. Detroit: G. S. Davis, 1890. 121p. 7 plates. DNLM; NNNAM; OCIM; PU
90-8073

SHATTUCK, Frederick Cheever (1847-1929)
Methods of teaching clinical medicine. Chicago, 1893. 11p. DNLM **90-8074**

SHATTUCK, Frederick Cheever (1847-1929)
Some remarks on arsenical poisoning, with special reference to domestic sources. [Philadelphia, 1893.] 12p. DNLM
90-8075

SHATTUCK, Frederick Cheever (1847-1929)
The treatment of pneumonia. [Boston, 1893.] 12p. DNLM
90-8076

SHATTUCK, Frederick Cheever (1847-1929)
Four cases of myxoedema treated by thyroid extract. Boston: Damrell & Upham, 1894. 15p. DNLM
90-8077

SHATTUCK, Frederick Cheever (1847-1929)
The frequency of renal albuminuria as shown by albumen and casts apart from Bright's disease, fever, or obvious cause of renal irritation. Boston: Damrell & Upham, 1894. 8p. DNLM
90-8078

SHATTUCK, Frederick Cheever (1847-1929)
Diet in typhoid fever. Chicago, 1897. 8p. DNLM
90-8079

SHATTUCK, Frederick Cheever (1847-1929)
Pericarditis; some points in its diagnosis and treatment, with discussion. Philadelphia, 1897. 20p. DNLM
90-8080

SHATTUCK, Frederick Cheever (1847-1929)
Specialism, the laboratory, and practical medicine. Boston, 1897. 15p. DNLM **90-8081**

SHATTUCK, Frederick Cheever (1847-1929), C. B. PORTER and James H. WRIGHT
Atonic dilatation of stomach; gastrorraphy. Philadelphia, 1897. 10p. DNLM **90-8082**

SHATTUCK, Frederick Cheever (1847-1929)
Some remarks on hospital abuse. President's address. [Philadelphia, 1898.] 7p. DNLM **90-8083**

SHATTUCK, George Brune (1844-1923)
Influenza in Massachusetts. Boston, 1890. 61p. DNLM; MBM
90-8084

SHATTUCK, George Brune (1844-1923)
Pneumonia in Boston during the recent epidemic of influenza. Boston: Damrell & Upham, 1892. 16p. DNLM; MBM
90-8085

SHATTUCK, Lemuel (1793-1859)
Bills of mortality 1810-1849, city of Boston. With an essay of the vital statistics of Boston from 1810 to 1841. Boston, 1893. 87p. DNLM; MBM; MH; MHi **90-8086**

SHAW, Arthur J.
A few clinical and anatomical points relating to the ear. St. Louis, 1898. 3p. DNLM **90-8087**

SHAW, Arthur J.
Histological methods in ophthalmology. St. Louis, 1898. 4p. DNLM **90-8088**

SHAW, Arthur J.
Spontaneous hemorrhage into the orbit. Nashville, 1898. 1 l. DNLM **90-8089**

SHAW, Arthur J.
A few anatomical and clinical points in the ear of the new-born infant. Boston, 1899. 16p. DNLM **90-8090**

SHAW, John C[argyll] (1845-1900)
. . . Essentials of nervous diseases and insanity: their symptoms and treatment. A manual for students and practitioners. . . . Philadelphia: W. B. Saunders, 1892. 194p. DLC; NNNAM; PPC; PU **90-8091**

SHAW, John C[argyll] (1845-1900)
. . . Essentials of nervous diseases and insanity: their symptoms and treatment. A manual for students and practitioners. . . . 2nd ed., rev. Philadelphia: W. B. Saunders, 1894. 194p. DLC; IU-M; PPC; PPJ **90-8092**

SHAW, John C[argyll] (1845-1900)
. . . Essentials of nervous diseases and insanity: their symptoms and treatment. A manual for students and practitioners. . . . 3rd ed., rev. . . . Philadelphia: W. B. Saunders, 1898. 204p. DLC; MBM; NBM; PPC **90-8093**

SHAWS, Rosalind Gillette
Notes for visiting nurses. . . . With an appendix . . . by Mrs. Helen C. Jenks. Philadelphia: P. Blakiston, Son & Co., 1893. 144p. DLC; PPC; PU **90-8094**

SHEFFIELD, Herman B[ernard] (*b.* 1871)
Intermittent fever in children, with special reference to its origin in New York. New York, 1897. 14p. DNLM
90-8095

SHEFFIELD, Herman B[ernard] (*b.* 1871)
A simple method of preparing nutrient agar-agar. New York: D. Appleton & Co., 1897. 4p. DNLM
90-8096

SHEFFIELD, Herman B[ernard] (*b.* 1871)
A contribution to the study of hysteria in childhood as it occurs in the United States of America. New York, 1898. 21p. 1 tab. DNLM **90-8097**

SHEFFIELD, Herman B[ernard] (*b.* 1871)
An easy and effective method of treatment of tinea tonsurans. New York, 1898. 6p. DNLM **90-8098**

SHEFFIELD, Herman B[ernard] (*b.* **1871)**
Diphtheria. Remarks on clinical diagnosis and treatment. New York, 1899. 8p. DNLM **90-8099**

SHEILD, A[rthur] Marmaduke (1858-1922)
Surgical anatomy for students. New York: D. Appleton & Co., 1891. 226p. DLC; DNLM; NNNAM; PU **90-8100**

SHEPARD, Charles Henry (1825-1910)
Rheumatism and its treatment by Turkish baths. Brooklyn, N.Y., 1892. 32p. DNLM [*Vel subseq.*] **90-8101**

SHEPARD, Charles Henry (1825-1910)
Rheumatism and its treatment by Turkish baths. 5th ed. Brooklyn, N.Y, 1898. 32p. DNLM **90-8102**

SHEPARD, Charles Henry (1825-1910)
Alcohol in the grippe. Chicago, 1895. 8p. DNLM **90-8103**

SHEPARD, Charles Henry (1825-1910)
The bath in modern medicine. Chicago, 1895. 11p. DNLM **90-8104**

SHEPARD, Charles Henry (1825-1910)
Chairman's address, delivered in the Section on State Medicine at the forty-seventh annual meeting of the Amrican Medical Association at Atlanta, Ga., May 5-8, 1896. Chicago, 1896. 15p. DNLM **90-8105**

SHEPARD, Charles Henry (1825-1910)
Public Turkish baths needed. Chicago, 1896. 7p. DNLM **90-8106**

SHEPARD, Charles Henry (1825-1910)
Teaching temperance in public schools. Chicago, 1896. 4p. DNLM **90-8107**

SHEPARD, Charles Henry (1825-1910)
Alcohol versus animal poison. Chicago, 1897. 7p. DNLM **90-8108**

SHEPARD, Charles Henry (1825-1910)
Hydrophobia. Chicago, 1897. 15p. DLC; DNLM **90-8109**

SHEPARD, Charles Henry (1825-1910)
The first inebriate asylum and its founder. [Hartford], 1898. 23p. DNLM **90-8110**

SHEPARD, L[uther] D[immick]
Annual address before the Massachusetts Dental Society, July 7, 1892. Cambridge, Mass.: Harvard Pr. Co., 1892. 26p. DNLM; MH-M **90-8111**

SHEPARD'S SANITARIUM, COLUMBUS
[Circular of the proprietor, Wm. Shepard. Two separate departments, nervous and chronic diseases, and mental diseases.] Columbus: Nitschke Bros., [1896?]. 16p. DLC; DNLM **90-8112**

SHEPHERD, Francis J[ohn] (1851-1924)
A case of cholecystenterostomy performed with Murphy's button; death from hemorrhage on fourth day. Philadelphia, 1865. 4p. DNLM **90-8113**

SHEPHERD, Francis J[ohn] (1851-1924)
A remarkable case of purpuric eruption ending in gangrene, apparently caused by salium salicylate. New York, 1896. 6p. DNLM **90-8114**

SHEPHERD, Francis J[ohn] (1851-1924)
Some causes of feigned eruptions. New York, 1897. 8p. DNLM **90-8115**

SHEPHERD, Francis J[ohn] (1851-1924)
Some remarks on the symptoms of bronchocele and the results of operative treatment. Philadelphia, 1899. 7p. 2 plates. DNLM **90-8116**

SHEPPARD, J. E.
Removal of the ossicles. [St. Louis, 1893.] 10p. DNLM **90-8117**

SHEPPARD, J. E.
Three cases of hysterical mastoiditis. New York, 1896. 5p. DNLM **90-8118**

SHERMAN, Frank M.
Operation for perforated gastric ulcer; perforation not found; drainage; recovery. Boston, 1899. 5p. 1 chart. DNLM **90-8119**

SHERMAN, Harry Mitchell (*b.* **1854)**
Erosion of the knee in children, with conservation of the epiphyseal cartilages. [Philadelphia], 1897. 7p. 4 plates. DNLM **90-8120**

SHERMAN, Harry Mitchell (*b.* **1854)**
Scorbutus in infants; some California cases. [San Francisco], 1897. 8p. DNLM **90-8121**

SHERMAN, Harry Mitchell (*b.* **1854)**
A preliminary report on the treatment of congenital dislocation of the hip by operative and manipulative methods. San Francisco, 1898. 8p. DNLM **90-8122**

SHERMAN, Harry Mitchell (*b.* **1854)**
Traumatic dislocation of the hip in children, old and recent. Philadelphia, 1898. 7p. DNLM **90-8123**

SHERMAN, Harry Mitchell (*b.* **1854) and Harold BRUNN**
A case of forcible reduction of the deformity of vertebral tuberculosis; death after three months, and the autopsy report. San Francisco, 1898. 10p. DNLM **90-8124**

SHERWELL, Samuel (1841-1927)
Cases of favus contagion from the lower animals. New York: Holt Bros., 1892. 5p. DNLM **90-8125**

SHERWELL, Samuel (1841-1927)
Multiple sarcomata. History of a case showing modification and amelioration of symptoms under large doses of arsenic. [Philadelphia, 1892.] 7p. DNLM **90-8126**

SHERWELL, Samuel (1841-1927)
Ichthyosis congenita (so-called harlequin foetus); history of a case still living. New York, 1894. 5p. DNLM **90-8127**

SHERWOOD-DUNN, B[erkeley] (*b.* **1857)**
Conservation of the ovaries. Boston, 1898. 31p. DNLM **90-8128**

SHERWOOD-DUNN, B[erkeley] (*b.* **1857)**
The relation of diseases of the female generative organs to nervous and mental affections. [Also:] The graver nerve disturbances due to organic changes in the genital organs. By William H. Humiston. Philadelphia, 1898. 41p. DNLM; PPC
90-8129

SHIELDS, Charles M. (1856-1897)
Conservatism in nasal surgery. Richmond, 1890. 8p. DNLM
90-8130

SHIELDS, N. T., and L. N. SHIELDS
A system of crown- and bridge-work. Philadelphia, 1893. 14p. DNLM **90-8131**

SHIELDS, T. E.
The effect of colours, irritant vapours, and mental work upon the blood flow. New York, 1896. 42p. 7 plates. DNLM; NNNAM **90-8132**

SHLENKER, Milton A.
Clinical observations of a new antipyretic kryofine. New York: C. Bischoff & Co., 1898. 4p. DNLM
90-8133

SHOBER, John B.
Anomalous positions of the colon. With report of a case discovered by exploratory operation. Philadelphia, 1898. 18p. DNLM **90-8134**

SHOBER, John B.
Mammary gland therapy in gynecology. Philadelphia, 1899. 11p. 1 chart. DNLM **90-8135**

SHOEMAKER, George E[rety]
Drainage in abdominal surgery. [Philadelphia, 1890.] 8p. DNLM **90-8136**

SHOEMAKER, George E[rety]
Malignant degeneration in dermoid cysts. Philadelphia: W. J. Dornan, 1890. 8p. DNLM **90-8137**

SHOEMAKER, George E[rety]
Three cases of extrauterine pregnancy; ligation of ureter. [Philadelphia, 1892.] 8p. 1 plate. DNLM
90-8138

SHOEMAKER, George E[rety]
Suppurative pylephlebitis and hepatic abscess secondary to appendicitis; with a report of two cases. [Philadelphia, 1893.] 12p. DNLM **90-8139**

SHOEMAKER, George E[rety]
A case of congenital deficiency of the lower extremities. [Philadelphia, 1893.] 4p. 1 plate. DNLM
90-8140

SHOEMAKER, George E[rety]
Dermoid cyst; broad ligament cyst; vicious union of cervix with vagina. Philadelphia, 1894. 1 l. DNLM
90-8141

SHOEMAKER, George E[rety]
Celiotomy under unusual conditions, with a report of ten cases. Philadelphia: Lea Bros. & Co., 1894. 15p. DNLM
90-8142

SHOEMAKER, George E[rety]
A patient cured five and half years after coeliotomy for tubercular peritonitis. Philadelphia, 1894. 3p. DNLM
90-8143

SHOEMAKER, George E[rety]
Case of hysterectomy by ligation for fibroma. New York, 1895. 4p. DNLM **90-8144**

SHOEMAKER, George E[rety]
The relations of nervous disorders in women to pelvic disease. Philadelphia, 1897. 4p. DNLM **90-8145**

SHOEMAKER, George E[rety]
Forty-one consecutive peritoneal operations, with one death; including twelve hysterectomies. Philadelphia, 1897. 17p. DNLM **90-8146**

SHOEMAKER, George E[rety]
Papillary cancer of the body of the uterus; absence of cardinal symptoms. New York: William Wood & Co., 1897. 3p. DNLM
90-8147

SHOEMAKER, George E[rety]
Remarks on the relation of the uterus to descent of the pelvic floor, and genital prolapse. Chicago: Amer. Med. Assoc., 1897. 4p. DNLM **90-8148**

SHOEMAKER, George E[rety]
Clinical report. Ovarian cyst of unusual shape and history. New York, 1898. 7p. DNLM **90-8149**

SHOEMAKER, George E[rety]
(a.) Extrauterine pregnancy; temporary arrest of hemorrhage by placental tissue; operation; recovery. (b.) Interstitial fibroma; hysterectomy; recovery. (c.) Intraligamentary fibroma; hysterectomy; recovery. New York: William Wood & Co., 1898. 7p. DNLM **90-8150**

SHOEMAKER, George E[rety]
A study of results in one hundred abdominal operations. Philadelphia, 1898. 12p. DNLM **90-8151**

SHOEMAKER, George E[rety]
The importance of chronic irritability of the colon with mucous stools as a symptom of appendicitis. Philadelphia, 1898. 8p. DNLM **90-8152**

SHOEMAKER, John Vietch (1852-1910)
Heredity, health, and personal beauty. Philadelphia & London: F. A. Davis, 1890. 422p. DNLM; NNNAM; PPC; PU
90-8153

SHOEMAKER, John Vietch (1852-1910)
Ointments and oleates, especially in diseases of the skin. 2nd ed. Philadelphia & London: F. A. Davis, 1890. 298p. DNLM; PPC; PPJ; PU **90-8154**

SHOEMAKER, John Vietch (1852-1910)
Valedictory address to the graduating class of the Medico-Chirurgical College. Advice to young men beginning the practice of medicine. [1890.] 4p. DNLM; PPC
90-8155

SHOEMAKER, John Veitch (1852-1910)
A practical treatise on diseases of the skin. . . . 2nd ed., rev. and enl. with chromogravure plates and other illustrations. New York: D. Appleton & Co., 1892. 878p. plates. DLC; NNNAM; OCIM; PPC **90-8156**

SHOEMAKER, John Vietch (1852-1910)
A practical treatise on materia medica and therapeutics, with especial reference to the clinical application of drugs. . . . 2nd ed., thoroughly rev. . . . Philadelphia and London: The F. A. Davis Co., 1893. 2 v. DLC; OCLloyd; PPC; PU
90-8157

SHOEMAKER, John Vietch (1852-1910)
The clinical application of ingluvin. Philadelphia, 1893. 24p. DNLM **90-8158**

SHOEMAKER, John Vietch (1852-1910)
A clinical review of the value of kumysgen. Philadelphia, 1893. 5p. DNLM **90-8159**

SHOEMAKER, John Vietch (1852-1910)
Ointment bases. [Philadelphia, 1893.] 12p. DNLM
90-8160

SHOEMAKER, John Vietch (1852-1910)
Electricity as a cosmetic. Philadelphia: Lea Bros. & Co., 1894. 11p. DNLM **90-8161**

SHOEMAKER, John Vietch (1852-1910)
An interesting case of leprosy. Philadelphia, 1895. 16p. DNLM **90-8162**

SHOEMAKER, John Vietch (1852-1910)
Paget's disease. New York, 1895. 7p. DNLM
90-8163

SHOEMAKER, John Vietch (1852-1910)
A practical treatise on materia medica and therapeutics, with especial reference to the clinical application of drugs. . . . 3rd ed., thoroughly rev. Philadelphia: The F. A. Davis Co., [etc., etc.], 1895. 1108p. DLC; OCLloyd; PPC: PU
90-8164

SHOEMAKER, John Vietch (1852-1910)
A practical treatise on materia medica and therapeutics, with especial reference to the clinical application of drugs. . . . 4th ed., revised. Philadelphia: The F. A. Davis Co., 1896. 1108p. DLC; PPC; PPJ; PU **90-8165**

SHOEMAKER, John Vietch (1852-1910)
A practical treatise on diseases of the skin. . . . 3rd ed., rev. and enl. . . . New York: D. Appleton & Co., 1897. 894p. plates. DLC; NNNAM; PPC; PPJ **90-8166**

SHOEMAKER, John Vietch (1852-1910)
Acute gonorrhoea. Philadelphia, 1897. 7p. DNLM
90-8167

SHOEMAKER, John Vietch (1852-1910)
Progress and problems of medicine today. New York, 1897. 16p. DNLM **90-8168**

SHOEMAKER, John Vietch (1852-1910)
Clinical lectures; a series of lectures to members of the American Medical Association. Chicago, 1898. 42p. DNLM **90-8169**

SHOEMAKER, John Vietch (1852-1910)
Mycosis fungoides; with reference to a case. Chicago, 1898. 8p. DNLM **90-8170**

SHOEMAKER, John Vietch (1852-1910)
Questions in the treatment of congenital dislocations of the hip. Chicago: Amer. Med. Assoc. Press, 1898. 12p. DNLM **90-8171**

SHOEMAKER, John Vietch (1852-1910)
Judicial methods; medico-legal testimony; the Zelner case. Philadelphia, 1899. 8p. DNLM **90-8172**

SHOEMAKER, John Vietch (1852-1910)
The medical expert's duty and where he most frequently fails in it, with illustrations from the Zelner case. Philadelphia, 1899. 15p. DNLM **90-8173**

SHURLY, Burt Russell (*b.* 1871)
Measles complicated by laryngeal diphtheria; intubation; recovery. New York, 1897. 2p. DNLM
90-8174

SHURLY, Ernest L[orenzo] (1845-1913)
Tuberculosis and phthisis. [Detroit, 1890.] 3p. DNLM
90-8175

SHURLY, Ernest L[orenzo] (1845-1913)
The address in medicine. Chicago: Office Amer. Med. Assoc., 1891. 24p. DNLM **90-8176**

SHURLY, Ernest L[orenzo] (1845-1913)
The treatment of phthisis. A lecture. Chicago: Office Amer. Med. Assoc., 1891. 12p. DNLM **90-8177**

SHURLY, Ernest L[orenzo] (1845-1913)
The treatment of tuberculosis as related to therapeutics. [New York, 1891.] 9p. DNLM **90-8178**

SHURLY, Ernest L[orenzo] (1845-1913)
A study of the sputum in pulmonary consumption. [Philadelphia: W. B. Saunders, 1892.] 11p. DNLM
90-8179

SHURLY, Ernest L[orenzo] (1845-1913)
Remarks on the nature and treatment of tuberculosis. [Detroit, 1892.] 10p. DNLM **90-8180**

SHURLY, Ernest L[orenzo] (1845-1913)
Artificial opening of pulmonary cavities, insertion of rubber tube and injection of chlorine gas. Chicago, 1893. 12p. DNLM **90-8181**

SHURLY, Ernest L[orenzo] (1845-1913)
Discussion on the prevention and communicability of phthisis pulmonalis. Detroit, 1894. 8p. DNLM
90-8182

SHURLY, Ernest L[orenzo] (1845-1913)
Remarks on some of the features of the grippe and influenza. Detroit, [1895]. 7p. DNLM **90-8183**

SHURLY, Ernest L[orenzo] (1845-1913)
Questions concerning the etiology and prevention of pulmonary consumption. Detroit, [1896]. 3p. DNLM
90-8184

SHURLY, Ernest L[orenzo] (1845-1913)
Present status and prospects of the art of medicine. Detroit, [1897]. 4p. DNLM **90-8185**

SHURLY, Ernest L[orenzo] (1845-1913)
The contagiousness of pulmonary consumption. Detroit & Ann Arbor, 1899. 5p. DNLM **90-8186**

SIDIS, Boris (1867-1923)
The psychology of suggestion; a research into the subconscious nature of man and society; with an introduction by Prof. William James. New York: D. Appleton & Co., 1898. 386p. DNLM; ICU; MH; NN **90-8187**

SIEGFRIED, Charles A. (1850-1900)
The recent inventions of new optical glass. Philadelphia, [1892]. 10p. DNLM **90-8188**

SIEGFRIED, Charles (1850-1900)
Some observations on the etiology and treament of diphtheria. New York: Trow Directory, 1892. 16p. DNLM; NNNAM **90-8189**

SIEGFRIED, Charles A. (1850-1900)
The work of the medical department on board United States naval vessels; together with a description of a new United States Navy portable operating table and a new portable dressing and instrument table. Columbus, O.: Berlin Pr. Co., 1897. 29p. DNLM: OCIM **90-8190**

SIMMONS, C. W.
The etiology and pathology of delirium. Philadelphia, 1898. 3p. DNLM **90-8191**

SIMMONS, C. W.
The caustic action of arsenic in treating carcinomatous growths accessible from the surface of the body. Philadelphia, 1899. 4p. DNLM **90-8192**

SIMMONS, George H.
Analgesia in labor. New York, 1895. 8p. DNLM **90-8193**

SIMMONS, T. W. (1836-1905)
The preventive treatment of tetanus. [Philadelphia, 1892.] 6p. DNLM **90-8194**

SIMON, Charles E[dmund] (1866-1927)
Acute angioneurotic oedema. Baltimore, 1891. 12p. DNLM **90-8195**

SIMON, Charles E[dmund] (1866-1927)
A manual of clinical diagnosis by means of microscopic and chemical methods, for students, hosptial physicians, and practitioners. . . . With 132 illustrations on wood and 10 colored plates. Philadelphia and New York: Lea Bros. & Co., 1896. 504p. DLC; DNLM; NNNAM; PPC **90-8196**

SIMON, Charles E[dmund] (1866-1927)
A manual of clinical diagnosis by means of microscopic and chemical methods, for students, hospital physicians, and practitioners. . . . 2nd ed., rev. and enl. With 133 illustrations on wood and 14 colored plates. Philadelphia and New York: Lea Bros. & Co., 1897. 563p. DLC; DNLM; NNNAM; PPC **90-8197**

SIMON, William (1844-1916)
Manual of chemistry. A guide to lectures and laboratory work for beginners in chemistry. A text-book specially adapted for students of pharmacy and medicine. . . . 3rd ed., thoroughly rev. With forty-four illustrations and seven colored plates representing fifty-six chemical reactions. Philadelphia: Lea Bros. & Co., 1891. 479p. DLC; NNNAM; PPC; PU **90-8198**

SIMON, William (1844-1916)
Manual of chemistry. A guide to lectures and laboratory work for beginners in chemistry. A text-book specially adapted for students of medicine and pharmacy. . . . 4th ed., thoroughly rev. With forty-four illustrations and seven colored plates, representing fifty-six chemical reactions. Philadelphia: Lea Bros. & Co., 1893. 493p. DLC; MBM; NNNAM; PPC **90-8199**

SIMON, William (1844-1916)
Manual of chemistry. A guide to lectures and laboratory work for beginners in chemistry. A text-book specially adapted for students of medicine, pharmacy, and dentistry. . . . 5th ed., thoroughly rev. With forty-four illustrations and eight colored plates, representing sixty-four chemical reactions. Philadelphia: Lea Bros. & Co., 1895. 502p. DLC; IU-M; LNT-M; PPC **90-8200**

SIMON, William (1844-1916)
Manual of chemistry. A guide to lectures and laboratory work for beginners in chemistry. A text-book specially adapted for students of medicine, pharmacy, and dentistry. . . . 6th ed., thoroughly revised. With forty-six illustrations and eight colored plates. . . . Philadelphia and New York: Lea Bros. & Co., 1898. 536p. DLC; ICRM; NNNAM; PPC **90-8201**

SIMPSON, Frank F. (*b.* 1868)
Post-operative acute toxic hyperemia and inflammation of the kidneys. New York, 1899. 14p. DNLM **90-8202**

SIMPSON, William
Woman: her health and destiny; a popular treatise. [Detroit, Mich.: Dr. Simpson Co., 1893.] 80p. DLC; ICJ **90-8203**

SIMPSON, William Kelly (1855-1914)
A consideration of some of the more important principles of intra-nasal surgery. New York, 1895. 9p. DNLM **90-8204**

SIMPSON, William Kelly (1855-1914)
Specialism in medicine. New York, 1895. 7p. DNLM **90-8205**

SIMPSON, William Kelly (1855-1914)
The sequelae of syphilis of the larynx and their treatment. New York, 1896. 10p. DNLM **90-8206**

SIMPSON, William Kelly (1855-1914)
Intubation in diphtheria. New York, 1898. 16p. DNLM **90-8207**

SIMPSON, William Kelly (1855-1914)
The use of the Bernays asceptic sponge in the nose and naso-pharynx, with special reference to its use as a pressure hemostatic. New York, 1898. 6p. DNLM **90-8208**

SINKLER, Wharton (1845-1910)
Recent observations in the etiology and treatment of migraine. [Philadelphia, 1890.] 24p. DNLM **90-8209**

SINKLER, Wharton (1845-1910) and C. W. BURR
A case of acute spinal paralysis; death on the twelfth day; autopsy showing transverse cervical myelitis. With a report of the microscopical examination. Philadelphia, 1891. 17p. DNLM **90-8210**

SINKLER, Wharton (1845-1910)
A case of brain tumor situated in the motor region; autopsy. Philadelphia, 1892. 3p. DNLM **90-8211**

SINKLER, Wharton (1845-1910)
On hereditary chorea, with a report of three additional cases and details of an autopsy. New York, 1892. 21p. DNLM **90-8212**

SINKLER, Wharton (1845-1910)
The remote results of removal of the tubes and ovaries. Philadelphia, [1892]. 13p. DNLM **90-8213**

SINKLER, Wharton (1845-1910)
A case of tumor of the optic thalamus. Philadelphia, 1893. 7p. 2 plates. DNLM **90-8214**

SINKLER, Wharton (1845-1910)
Insanity in early childhood. Philadelphia, 1893. 8p. DNLM **90-8215**

SINKLER, Wharton (1845-1910)
Long remissions in epilepsy and their bearing on prognosis. New York, 1893. 7p. DNLM **90-8216**

SINKLER, Wharton (1845-1910)
Pathology and treatment of paralysis from Pott's disease. [Philadelphia, 1893.] 22p. DNLM **90-8217**

SINKLER, Wharton (1845-1910)
A case of lesion of the thalamus. Death from intestinal hemorrhage. New York, 1894. 8p. DNLM **90-8218**

SINKLER, Wharton (1845-1910)
On lead-palsy in children; with a report of three cases. Philadelphia, 1894. 14p. DNLM **90-8219**

SINKLER, Wharton (1845-1910)
Sporadic cretinism, and its treatment by thyroid extract. Philadelphia, 1894. 9p. 1 plate. DNLM **90-8220**

SINKLER, Wharton (1845-1910)
The treatment of acro-paresthesia (numbness of the extremities). Philadelphia, 1894. 8p. DNLM **90-8221**

SINKLER, Wharton (1845-1910) and Augustus A. ESHNER
Three cases of essential anaemia in one family, father and two daughters. Philadelphia, 1896. 7p. DNLM **90-8222**

SINKLER, Wharton (1845-1910)
Case of Erb's paralysis, upper-arm type, in a child of seven years. [1896.] 2p. PU **90-8223**

SINKLER, Wharton (1845-1910)
A case of trophoneurosis of the hands (acrotrophoneurosis), with spontaneous amputation of the fingers. New York, 1897. 12p. DNLM **90-8224**

SINKLER, Wharton (1845-1910)
A case of sporadic cretinism. Philadelphia, 1898. 6p. DNLM **90-8225**

SINKLER, Wharton (1845-1910)
Rumination in man. Chicago, 1898. 12p. DNLM **90-8226**

SINKLER, Wharton (1845-1910)
Asthenic bulbar paralysis. New York, 1899. 8p. DNLM **90-8227**

SINNETT, Alfred Percy (1840-1921)
The rationale of mesmerism. Boston & New York: Houghton, Mifflin & Co., 1892. 232p. DNLM; MB; MH; NN **90-8228**

SKENE, Alexander J[ohnston] C[halmers] (1837-1900)
Intraligamentous ovarian cystomata. New York: Trow, 1890. 12p. DNLM; NNNAM **90-8229**

SKENE, Alexander J[ohnston] C[halmers] (1837-1900)
Notes on the galvano-cautery in the treatment of urethral and vesical diseases. New York, 1892. 8p. DNLM **90-8230**

SKENE, Alexander J[ohnston] C[halmers] (1837-1900)
Treatment before and after laparotomy. Philadelphia, 1892. 8p. DNLM **90-8231**

SKENE, Alexander J[ohnston] C[halmers] (1837-1900)
Pathology and treatment of injuries of the pelvic floor. New York: Stuyvesant Press, 1893. 15p. DNLM **90-8232**

SKENE, Alexander J[ohnston] C[halmers] (1837-1900)
Treatise on the diseases of women for the use of students and practitioners. 2nd ed., revised and enlarged. New York: D. Appleton & Co., 1893. 968p. 4 col. plates. DLC; DNLM; NNNAM; PPC **90-8233**

SKENE, Alexander J[ohnston] C[halmers] (1837-1900)
Senile endometritis. New York, 1894. 11p. DNLM **90-8234**

SKENE, Alexander J[ohnston] C[halmers] (1837-1900)
Medical gynecology. A treatise on the diseases of women from the standpoint of the physician. New York: D. Appleton & Co., 1895. 529p. DLC; DNLM; NNNAM; PPC **90-8235**

SKENE, Alexander J[ohnston] C[halmers] (1837-1900)
Electro-cautery as a haemostatic. New York: D. Appleton & Co., 1897. 16p. DNLM; NNNAM **90-8236**

SKENE, Alexander J[ohnston] C[halmers] (1837-1900)
The haemostatic forceps in exsecting the appendix. New York, 1898. 9p. DNLM **90-8237**

SKENE, Alexander J[ohnston] C[halmers] (1837-1900)
Treatise on the diseases of women for the use of students and practitioners. 3rd ed., revised and enlarged. New York: D. Appleton & Co., 1898. 991p. 4 plates. DLC; DNLM; NNNAM; PU **90-8238**

SKENE, Alexander J[ohnston] C[halmers] (1837-1900)
Electro-haemostasis in operative surgery. New York: D. Appleton & Co., 1899. 173p. DLC; DNLM; NNNAM
90-8239

SKINNER, Clarence Edward (*b.* 1868)
Medical examination for life insurance in the field. [New York, 1898.] 30p. DNLM; NNNAM **90-8240**

SKINNER, Clarence Edward (*b.* 1868)
Dry heat of high degree as a therapeutic agent. New York, 1899. 54p. DNLM; NNNAM **90-8241**

SKINNER, Cornelius (*b.* 1866)
Report of some cases in practice. [Louisville, 1892.] 15p. DNLM **90-8242**

SKINNER, David Nevens (1841-1892)
The care of the eyes in health and disease. . . . Boston: J. G. Cupples Co., 1891. 116p. DLC; DNLM; MBM
90-8243

SKINNER, Winslow Warner (1856-1900)
Recent studies in naupathia, or seasickness; symptomatology, diagnosis, pathogenesis, and treatment by a new and efficacious method. New York: D. Appleton & Co., 1894. 48p. DNLM; NNNAM **90-8244**

SLAGLE, Charles D. (*b.* 1871)
The exact treatment of malarial fevers. Detroit: W. W. Warren, 1897. 12p. DNLM **90-8245**

SLIFER, Henry F. (*b.* 1852)
Artificial feeding of infants. Philadelphia, [1896]. 6p. DNLM
90-8246

SLIFER, Henry F. (*b.* 1852)
Angioneurotic edema. Philadelphia, 1899. 8p. DNLM
90-8247

SLOCUM, Harris A. (*b.* 1857)
A case of extreme puerperal anemia and nephritis; delivery at term with forceps applied, under chloroform, above the superior strait; recovery of mother and child. Philadelphia, 1892. 4p. DNLM **90-8248**

SLOCUM, Harris A. (*b.* 1857)
A problem in abdominal surgery: Why is the uterus retained after the ovaries are removed? Philadelphia, 1893. 10p. DNLM
90-8249

SMALL, Alvan E[dmond] (1811-1866)
The decline of manhood. Its causes, the best means of preventing their effects and bringing about a restoration to health. 4th ed. Chicago: Gross and Delbridge, 1890. 99p. PPHa [1st ed., Chicago: Clindinning & Co., 1873, 59p.; 2nd ed., Chicago, 1881, 112p.; 3rd ed., Chicago: Duncan, 1885, 112p.]
90-8250

SMALL, J. W.
The therapeutic action of tonica water, with the history of twenty-six cases where it has been used. Chicago, 1891. 16p. DNLM **90-8251**

SMALL, J. W.
The treatment of the first stage of acute lobar pneumonia. Chicago, 1891. 8p. DNLM **90-8252**

SMART, Charles (1841-1905)
The connection of the Army Medical Department with the development of meteorology in the United States. Chicago, 1893. 10p. DNLM **90-8253**

SMART, Charles (1841-1905)
How to keep well. The Chicago Record's hygienic manual. For United States soldiers in the field. [Chicago, 1898.] 31p. DNLM **90-8254**

SMART, Charles (1841-1905)
Handbook for the Hospital Corps of the U.S. Army and state military forces. . . . Approved by the Surgeon-General of the Army. New York: William Wood & Co., 1898. 350p. DLC; NNNAM; NBM; PU **90-8255**

SMITH, Andrew H[eermance] (1837-1910)
Some considerations in regard to acute obstructive diseases of the lungs. New York, 1890. 12p. DNLM
90-8256

SMITH, Andrew H[eermance] (1837-1910)
Pneumonia. Clinical lecture delivered at the New York Post-Graduate School. [Philadelphia, 1892.] 8p. DNLM
90-8257

SMITH, Andrew H[eermance] (1837-1910)
The reaction of ether with urine. [Philadelphia, 1893.] 6p. DNLM **90-8258**

SMITH, Andrew H[eermance] (1837-1910)
Alimentation in pulmonary disease. Philadelphia, 1894. 5p. DNLM **90-8259**

SMITH, Andrew H[eermance] (1837-1910)
The clinical divisions of pneumonia. [New York, 1894, *vel subseq.*] 15p. DNLM **90-8260**

SMITH, Andrew H[eermance] (1837-1910)
The use of the differential stethoscope in the study of cardiac murmurs. Philadelphia, 1895. 3p. DNLM
90-8261

SMITH, Andrew H[eermance] (1837-1910)
Some points on the physical examination of the chest. New York: Pusey & Troxell, 1896. 12p. DNLM
90-8262

SMITH, Andrew H[eermance] (1837-1910)
Prognosis in pneumonia. [Philadelphia], 1896. 7p. DNLM
90-8263

SMITH, Andrew H[eermance] (1837-1910)
Can we diagnosticate obliteration of the receptaculum chyli? New York, 1899. 8p. DNLM **90-8264**

SMITH, Andrew H[eermance] (1837-1910)
The treatment of pneumonia as based upon recent views as to its pathology. Philadelphia, 1899. 25p. DNLM; NNNAM
90-8265

SMITH, Andrew H[eermance] (1837-1910)
Lobar pneumonia. New York, [1899]. 139p. DNLM; NNNAM
90-8266

SMITH, A[rthur] Lapthorn (*b.* 1855)
A new and improved method of performing Alexander's operation. Philadelphia: Lea Bros. & Co., 1896. 6p. DNLM
90-8267

SMITH, A[rthur] Lapthorn (*b.* 1855)
Rapid decrease in the size of a fibroid tumor of the uterus following its treatment by electricity. New York, 1897. 4p. DNLM **90-8268**

SMITH, A[rthur] Lapthorn (*b.* 1855)
Five cases of pyosalpingitis. New York: William Wood & Co., 1894. 9p. DNLM **90-8269**

SMITH, A[rthur] Lapthorn (*b.* 1855)
What has sewer gas got to do with bad results in obstetrics and gynaecology? Boston, 1895. 8p. DNLM **90-8270**

SMITH, A[rthur] Lapthorn (*b.* 1855)
Ventrofixation and Alexander's operation compared. New York: William Wood & Co., 1895. 7p. DNLM **90-8271**

SMITH, A[rthur] Lapthorn (*b.* 1855)
Recto-vaginal fistulae and fistulae about the anus in women. Louisville, 1895. 6p. DNLM **90-8272**

SMITH, Charles Emory (1842-1908)
Alumni oration delivered before the Alumni Association of the Medico-Chirurgical College of Philadelphia. Philadelphia, 1894. 12p. DNLM; PPC **90-8273**

SMITH, Charles D[ennison] (*b.* 1855)
Cases of Chickamauga typhoid treated at the Maine General Hospital. Portland: S. Berry, 1899. 16p. DNLM **90-8274**

SMITH, Charles N[orth] (1860-1921)
Electricity in gynecology: the galvanic apparatus. [Toledo, 1890.] 6p. DNLM **90-8275**

SMITH, Charles N[orth] (1860-1921)
The treatment of ectopic gestation by abdominal section. New York, 1896. 6p. DNLM **90-8276**

SMITH, Charles N[orth] (1860-1921)
Tubal abortion. New York, 1896. 5p. DNLM **90-8277**

SMITH, D[avid] D.
The dental pulp; its office and eccentricities. [Philadelphia], 1895. 6p. DNLM **90-8278**

SMITH, D[avid] T[homas] (*b.* 1840)
Obstetric problems; being an inquiry into the nature of the forces determining head presentation, internal rotation, and also the development of the amnion. Louisville: J. P. Morton & Co., 1892. 60p. DNLM; KyLoJM **90-8279**

SMITH, Edgar F[ahs] (1854-1928)
Electro-chemical analysis. Philadelphia: P. Blakiston, Son & Co., 1890. 116p. DLC; DNLM; PU **90-8280**

SMITH, Edgar F[ahs] (1854-1928)
Electro-chemical analysis. 2nd ed. Philadelphia: P. Blakiston, Son & Co., 1894. 143p. CtY-M; DLC; ICJ; PPC **90-8281**

SMITH, Eugene
Cataract; how shall we deal with the capsule? New cystitome forceps. Chicago, 1891. 4p. DNLM **90-8282**

SMITH, Eustace (1835-1914)
On the wasting diseases of infants and children. 6th ed. Philadelphia: P. Blakiston's Son & Co., 1899. 377p. DNLM; MBM; PPC; PU **90-8283**

SMITH, E. Franklin
Text-book of anatomy, physiology, and hygiene. New York: W. R. Jenkins, [1898]. 198p. DNLM; NNNAM **90-8284**

SMITH, Frank Trester (*b.* 1854)
Gonorrhoeal ophthalmia; report of a case treated with argonin. Chicago, 1897. 1 sheet. DNLM **90-8285**

SMITH, Frederick A. A.
Keep your mouth shut. A popular treatise on mouth breathing; its causes, effects, and treatment. To which is added an appendix on ophthalmia in new-born children, by Dr. Smith and Swan M. Burnett. Boston: Roberts Bros., 1893. 73p. DNLM; MBM **90-8286**

SMITH, Frederick K[insman] (*b.* 1859)
Presentations of the parietal bone. Cleveland, 1894. 6p. DNLM **90-8287**

SMITH, Frederick K[insman] (*b.* 1859)
An operation for phimosis. [Cleveland], 1897. 8p. DNLM **90-8288**

SMITH, Frederick K[insman] (*b.* 1859)
The development of the test card. Cleveland, 1896. 12p. 1 chart. DNLM **90-8289**

SMITH, Gouverneur Mather (1832?-1898)
An international congress of microbes at Berlin. [New York, 1891.] 3p. DNLM **90-8290**

SMITH, Henry H[ollingsworth] (1815-1890)
A case of accidental hemorrhage in the first stage of labor at full term. Philadelphia, 1893. 3p. DNLM **90-8291**

SMITH, Herbert E[ugene] (*b.* 1857)
Report on the cause of the recent outbreak of typhoid fever in Waterbury, made to the Connecticut State Board of Health. [New Haven, 1890.] 10p. DNLM **90-8292**

SMITH, H[erbert] L. (*b.* 1863)
Position in the treatment of elbow-joint fracture. An experimental study. Boston: Damrell & Upham, 1894. 28p. DNLM; MBM **90-8293**

SMITH, J[ames] Greig (1834-1897)
Abdominal surgery. 4th ed. Philadelphia: P. Blakiston, Son & Co., 1891. 806p. CtY-M; DNLM; PPC; PU **90-8294**

SMITH, J[ames] Greig (1834-1897)
Abdominal surgery. 5th ed. Philadelphia: P. Blakiston, Son & Co., 1896. 2 v. PPC; PPJ; PU **90-8295**

SMITH, J[ames] Greig (1834-1897)
Abdominal surgery. 6th ed. Philadelphia: P. Blakiston, Son & Co., 1897. 2 v. [continuous pagination] DNLM; IU-M; NNNAM **90-8296**

SMITH, J[ames] Greig (1834-1897)
Was Robert Houston, of Glasgow, the first ovariotomist? Baltimore, 1897. 16p. DNLM; MdU-D **90-8297**

SMITH, J[ob] Lewis (1827-1897)
A treatise on the diseases of infancy and childhood. . . . 7th ed., thoroughly rev. . . . Philadelphia: Lea Bros. & Co., 1890. 900p. DLC; NNNAM; PPC; PPJ **90-8298**

SMITH, J[ob] Lewis (1827-1897), [*et al.*]
Summer complaints of infants and children. [St. Louis, 1891.] 16 l. DNLM; NNNAM **90-8299**

SMITH, J[ob] Lewis (1827-1897)
A treatise on the medical and surgical diseases of infancy and childhood. . . . 8th ed., thoroughly rev. and greatly enl. . . . New York and Philadelphia: Lea Bros. & Co., 1896. 987p. plates. DLC; DNLM; NNNAM; PPC **90-8300**

SMITH, J[oseph] Heber (1842-1898)
The desirability of disposing of infected bodies by cremation. Boston, 1896. 8p. DNLM **90-8301**

SMITH, Joseph R[owe] (1831-1911)
Statistical reports, Medical Department, U.S. Army. [Review of the plan proposed by Surgeon J. S. Billings, Nov. 8, 1890.] [Los Angeles, 1890.] 20p. DNLM **90-8302**

SMITH, Q[uintius] Cincinnatus (*b.* 1842)
The treatment of chronic tubercular pulmonary consumption, and the importance of the recognition of its curability, and early diagnosis, and prompt diligent treatment by home hygiene and drugs. [Austin, Texas, 1890.] 22p. DNLM **90-8303**

SMITH, S[eth] MacCuen (*b.* 1863)
Employment of pilocarpine muriate in labyrinthine disease, with report of case. [Philadelphia, 1891.] 8p. DNLM **90-8304**

SMITH, S[eth] MacCuen (*b.* 1863)
The class of cases in which we may expect good results from excision of the membrana tympani and ossicles. Detroit: G. S. Davis, 1893. 10p. DNLM **90-8305**

SMITH, S[eth] MacCuen (*b.* 1863)
The necessity for early recognition and treatment of suppurative diseases of the tympanum, and their relation to cerebral complications. Philadelphia, 1893. 8p. DNLM **90-8306**

SMITH, S[eth] MacCuen (*b.* 1863)
The radical cure of aural polypi. St. Louis, 1893. 4p. DNLM **90-8307**

SMITH, S[eth] MacCuen (*b.* 1863)
Incipient inflammation of the ear in early life, and their sequelae. New York, 1894. 12p. DNLM **90-8308**

SMITH, S[eth] MacCuen (*b.* 1863)
Fununculosis of the external auditory canal. [Philadelphia: Lea Bros. & Co., 1895.] 9p. DNLM **90-8309**

SMITH, Thomas C[roggon] (1842-1913)
The use of ergot in the second stage of labor. New York: William Wood & Co., 1892. 13p. DNLM **90-8310**

SMITH, Thomas C[roggon] (1842-1913)
Case of excessive secretion of milk. New York, 1894. 6p. DNLM **90-8311**

SMITH, Thomas C[roggon] (1842-1913)
A case of hypertrophic elongation of the infravaginal portion of the cervix uteri complicating pregnancy and obstructing labor. New York: William Wood & Co., 1896. 7p. DNLM **90-8312**

SMITH, Vannie E. (*b.* 1869)
Cerebral hyperemia. [St. Louis], 1897. 8p. DNLM **90-8313**

SMITH, William F.
I. Case of corneal transplantation from the rabbit's to the human eye. II. A singular case of injury. New York, 1890. 6p. DNLM **90-8314**

SMITH, W. Harvey
Scopolamine; its value in ophthalmic practice. New York, 1894. 9p. DNLM **90-8315**

SMYTHE, Gonzalvo C[ordova] (1836-1897)
Influence of heredity in producing disease and degeneracy. The remedy. Insanity, inebriety, crime, and pauperism considered as physical diseases. Acquired physical conditions transmitted to offspring. An unprejudiced discussion of the alcohol question. All sin reduced to a physical basis. Indianapolis: W. B. Burford, 1891. 24p. DNLM **90-8316**

SNADER, Edward R.
Stoop and round shoulders; their relation to chest expansion and phthisis pulmonalis. [Philadelphia], 1890. 11p. DNLM **90-8317**

SNADER, Edward R.
Some practical observations concerning examinations of the heart. [Philadelphia], 1891. 18p. DNLM **90-8318**

SNADER, Edward R.
On the impossibility of diagnosing phthisis pulmonalis in the earlier stages with certainty, without the evidence afforded by physical signs. Philadelphia, 1893. 10p. DNLM **90-8319**

SNADER, Edward R.
On the coexistence of phthisis pulmonalis and valvular disease of the heart. An arraignment of Flint's plea of incompatibility. [Philadelphia, 1893.] 7p. DNLM **90-8320**

SNIVELY, I[saac] Newton (1862-1909)
A case of congenital deformity of the upper and lower extremities and of the spinal column. Philadelphia, 1894. 6p. DNLM **90-8321**

SNIVELY, I[saac] Newton (1862-1909)
Personal observations and experience with diphtheria antitoxic serum. Chicago, 1897. 12p. DNLM **90-8322**

SNOW, Sargent F.
Hemicrania and other neuralgic affections of the head relieved by intra-nasal surgery. New York, 1894. 6p. DNLM **90-8323**

SNOW, Sargent F.
Headaches from nasal causes. New York, 1897. 11p. DNLM **90-8324**

SNOW, Sargent F.
Modern possibilities in chronic catarrhal deafness. St. Louis, Mo., 1898. 8p. DNLM **90-8325**

SNOW, Sargent F.
Nasal and aural complications in epidemic influenza. Chicago, 1899. 7p. DNLM **90-8326**

SNYDER, Walter Hamilton
The color sense and color blindness . . . ; with practical test for color-blindness. Toledo, 1896. 3p. DNLM **90-8327**

SNYDER, Walter Hamilton
Traumatic symblepharo-pterygium. St. Louis, 1899. 2p. 1 plate. DNLM **90-8328**

SOLLY, S[amuel] Edwin (1845-1906)
The personal equation in the treatment of phthisis. Philadelphia, 1891. 15p. DNLM **90-8329**

SOLLY, S[amuel] Edwin (1845-1906)
Neglect of the early diagnosis and treatment of pulmonary tuberculosis. [Philadelphia, 1893.] 14p. DNLM **90-8330**

SOLLY, S[amuel] Edwin (1845-1906)
The relation of chronic nasal and laryngeal diseases to pulmonary tuberculosis. Chicago, 1894. 8p. DNLM **90-8331**

SOLLY, S[amuel] Edwin (1845-1906)
Principles of medical climatology. Chicago: Amer. Medical Assoc. Press, 1895. 8p. DNLM **90-8332**

SOLLY, S[amuel] Edwin (1845-1906)
The comparative merits of resorts in New Mexico, Colorado, and Arizona. Detroit: W. M. Warren, 1897. 18p. DNLM **90-8333**

SOLLY, S[amuel] Edwin (1845-1906)
A handbook of medical climatology, embodying its principles and therapeutic application, with scientific data of the chief health resorts of the world. Philadelphia & New York: Lea Bros. & Co., 1897. 470p. DNLM; NNNAM; PPC; PU **90-8334**

SOLOMON, Leon L. (*b.* 1872)
Analysis of gastric contents, with special reference to hydrochloric acid and the ferments of the stomach. Louisville, 1896. 8p. DNLM **90-8335**

SOLOMON, Leon L. (*b.* 1872)
The study of medicine in Europe. Benefits which the American derives therefrom. Charlotte, N.C., 1897. 15p. DNLM **90-8336**

SOME apparatus to facilitate the work of the histological and embryological laboratory. Rochester, N.Y., 1898. 4 l. DNLM **90-8337**

SOMERS, Lewis S[ummerl] (*b.* 1871)
Nasal syphilis with extensive lesions. Philadelphia, 1896. 3p. DNLM **90-8338**

SOMERS, Lewis S[ummerl] (*b.* 1871)
The use of menthol in pharyngitis. St. Louis, 1896. 5p. DNLM **90-8339**

SOMERS, Lewis S[ummerl] (*b.* 1871)
The use of nitrate of silver in the pharynx. Philadelphia, 1896. 11p. DNLM **90-8340**

SOMERS, Lewis S[ummerl] (*b.* 1871)
Acetanilide as an antiseptic in chronic suppurative otitis. New York, 1896. 8p. DNLM **90-8341**

SOMERS, Lewis S[ummerl] (*b.* 1871)
Aural herpes. New York, 1896. 8p. DNLM **90-8342**

SOMERS, Lewis S[ummerl] (*b.* 1871)
Membranous rhinitis. Philadelphia, 1896. 5p. DNLM **90-8343**

SOMERS, Lewis S[ummerl] (*b.* 1871)
Tuberculosis of the tonsils, pharynx and larynx. Philadelphia, 1897. 14p. DNLM **90-8344**

SOMERS, Lewis S[ummerl] (*b.* 1871)
A study of lingual tonsil. St. Louis, 1897. 11p. DNLM **90-8345**

SOMERS, Lewis S[ummerl] (*b.* 1871)
Traumatic performance of the membrana tympani. Philadelphia, 1897. 1p. DNLM **90-8346**

SOMERS, Lewis S[ummerl] (*b.* 1871)
Adductor vocal paralysis. Philadelphia, 1897. 6p. DNLM **90-8347**

SOMERS, Lewis S[ummerl] (*b.* 1871)
Atrophic rhinitis. St. Louis, 1897. 7p. DNLM **90-8348**

SOMERS, Lewis S[ummerl] (*b.* 1871)
Eucaine hydrochlorate as a local anesthetic in hypertrophic rhinitis. Detroit: G. S. Davis, 1897. 3p. DNLM **90-8349**

SOMERS, Lewis S[ummerl] (*b.* 1871)
Hereditary deafness. Detroit, 1897. 7p. DNLM **90-8350**

SOMERS, Lewis S[ummerl] (*b.* 1871)
The influence of diseases of the nares and pharynx on aural affections; a study of six hundred cases of middle-ear disease. Philadelphia, 1897. 5p. DNLM **90-8351**

SOMERS, Lewis S[ummerl] (*b.* 1871)
Pharyngitis herpetica associated with menstruation. [Philadelphia], 1898. 5p. DNLM **90-8352**

SOMERS, Lewis S[ummerl] (*b.* 1871)
The treatment of chronic naso-pharyngitis. Memphis, 1898. 7p. DNLM **90-8353**

SOMERS, Lewis S[ummerl] (*b.* 1871)
Entotical sound perceptions. Detroit: W. M. Warren, 1898. 8p. DNLM **90-8354**

SOMERS, Lewis S[ummerl] (*b.* 1871)
The effect of hypertrophy of the inferior turbinal on the nasal septum. Philadelphia, 1898. 4p. DNLM **90-8335**

SOMERS, Lewis S[ummerl] (*b.* 1871)
The differential diagnosis of pharyngeal syphilitic lesions and diphtheria. Philadelphia, 1899. 7p. DNLM **90-8356**

SOMERS, Lewis S[ummerl] (*b.* 1871)
The influence of turbinal hyptertrophy upon the pharynx. Philadelphia, 1899. 4p. DNLM **90-8357**

SOMERS, Lewis S[ummerl] (*b.* 1871)
Late consecutive oro-pharyngeal syphilis. Philadelphia, 1899. 2 l. DNLM **90-8358**

SONDERN, Frederic E[wald] (1867-1947)
The value of the centrifugal apparatus for diagnostic purposes. [New York, 1893.] 7p. DNLM **90-8359**

SONDERN, Frederic E[wald] (1867-1947)
Remarks on the technique of analysis of small quantities of urine as obtained by the ureter-catheter. New York, 1897. 5p. DNLM **90-8360**

SORENSON, [James] S.
Practical removal of hairs, moles, etc., by electrolysis. [Philadelphia, 1893.] 13p. DNLM **90-8361**

SOTHORON, Elmer (*b.* 1868)
Things we should remember in the application of the forceps. Richmond, 1895. 8p. DNLM **90-8362**

SOTHORON, Elmer (*b.* 1868)
Hour-glass contraction of the uterus. Richmond, 1898. 7p. DNLM **90-8363**

SOUCHON, Edmond (1841-1924)
A new apparatus for administering anaesthetics, in face and mouth operations. [Chicago, 1894.] 4p. DNLM **90-8364**

SOUCHON, Edmond (1841-1924)
A plea for a methodically written textbook on anatomy. Philadelphia, 1894. 12p. DNLM **90-8365**

SOUCHON, Edmond (1841-1924)
Reminiscences of J. Marion Sims in Paris. New York: Trow, 1894. 15p. DNLM **90-8366**

SOUCHON, Edmond (1841-1924)
On the drilling of capillary holes through the skull, for the purpose of exploring the brain with a needle and syringe. (Read at a meeting of the Louisiana State Medical Society.) New Orleans: L. Graham & Son, [1895]. 8p. DNLM **90-8367**

SOUCHON, Edmond (1841-1924)
Operative treatment of aneurisms of the third portion of the subclavian artery. [With two additional cases.] Philadelphia, 1895. 80p. 1 l., 1 plate. DNLM **90-8368**

SOUCHON, Edmond (1841-1924)
Simultaneous double aneurism of the femorals on the same side of the femorals and popliteal at the same time, also cases of simultaneous triple and quadruple aneurism on the same lower side. [Philadelphia], 1895. 31p. DNLM **90-8369**

SOUCHON, Edmond (1841-1924)
Uninterrupted anesthesia in operations upon the face and mouth. Philadelphia, 1895. 11p. DNLM **90-8370**

SOUCHON, Edmond (1841-1924)
The methodic description of a surgical disease. Chicago: Amer. Med. Assoc. Press, 1896. 31p. DNLM **90-8371**

SOUCHON, Edmond (1841-1924)
The methodic description of a surgical diseases and the methodic report of a surgical case. New Orleans: Southern Stationery Co., 1896. 20p. DNLM **90-8372**

SOUCHON, Edmond (1841-1924)
Peculiarities of the surgical diseases and injuries of the neck. Philadelphia, 1896. 87p. DNLM **90-8373**

SOUCHON, Edmond (1841-1924)
Places rendered famous by Marion Sims, in Montgomery, Ala. Notes on a trip to the meeting of the American Surgical Association in New York, May, 1895. New Orleans, 1896. 18p. DNLM **90-8374**

SOUCHON, Edmond (1841-1924)
Reminiscences of T. G. Richardson. New Orleans, 1896. 11p. 1 plate, port. DNLM **90-8375**

SOUCHON, Edmond (1841-1924)
Peculiarities of the surgical diseases and injuries of the neck. Chicago, 1897. 93p. DNLM **90-8376**

SOUCHON, Edmond (1841-1924)
Operative diagnosis of tumors. Philadelphia, [1897]. 11p. DNLM **90-8377**

SOUCHON, Edmond (1841-1924)
Operative treatment of irreducible dislocations of the shoulder-joint, recent or old, simple or complicated. [Philadelphia], 1897. 138p. DNLM **90-8378**

SOUCHON, Edmond (1841-1924)
Instructions to laymen who may have to manage yellow fever cases in default of a physician; also recommendations to physicians inexperienced in the treatment of yellow fever with regard to the use of medicines. New Orleans: L. Graham & Son, 1898. 14p. DNLM **90-8379**

SOUDER, C. Fletcher
The injection treatment for the relief and cure of hernia. Philadelphia, 1896. 4p. DNLM **90-8380**

SOUDER, C. Fletcher
Acute insanity; its management and treatment. Read before the Homoeopathic Medical Society of the County of Philadelphia. [Philadelphia, 1896.] 2 l. DNLM **90-8381**

SOUTER, William Norwood (1861-1935)
Handbook of optics for students of ophthalmology. . . . New York: The Macmillan Co.; London: Macmillan & Co., 1899. 209p. diags. DLC; ICJ; MB; PU **90-8382**

THE SOUTH-WEST and New Mexico for phthisis, weak lungs, asthma, bronchitis, etc. Chicago: Vandercook & Co., [1891]. 46p. 1 l. DNLM **90-8383**

SOUTHWESTERN HOMOEOPATHIC MEDICAL COLLEGE, LOUISVILLE, KY.
Annual announcements for the sessions of 1896-97 (4.); 1900-1901 (8.); 1908-09 (16.). Louisville, 1896-1908. DNLM **90-8384**

SOUTHWICK, George R[inaldo] (1859-1930)
A practical manual of gynaecology. 2nd ed. Boston: O. Clapp & Son, 1890. 532p. DLC; MBM; NNNAM; PPHa **90-8385**

SOUTHWICK, George R[inaldo] (1859-1930)
A domestic handbook of the diseases of women and of midwifery, with supplementary chapters. Boston: Hygienic Pub. Co., 1892. 350p. DLC; DNLM **90-8386**

SOUTHWICK, George R[inaldo] (1859-1930)
Suggestions for mothers. . . . Cambridge, [Mass.] : Cambridge Cooperative Press, [1896]. 32p. DLC
90-8387

SOUTHWORTH, Thomas S. (*b.* 1861)
The technique and diagnostic value of Ehrlich's method of staining the white blood-corpuscles. [New York, 1893.] 18p. DNLM **90-8388**

SOUTHWORTH, Thomas S. (*b.* 1861)
Acute pneumonia in childhood. New York: D. Appleton & Co., 1894. 20p. DNLM; NNNAM **90-8389**

SPALDING, James A[lfred] (*b.* 1846)
Glaucoma and mastoid inflammation as sequelae of epidemic of influenza [la grippe]. [Portland, 1899.] 8p. DNLM
90-8390

SPEAR, Edmund D[oe] (*b.* 1852)
The function of the semicircular canals. Philadelphia, 1892. 3p. DNLM **90-8391**

SPEAR, Edmund D[oe] (*b.* 1852)
Nomenclatura morborum auris et nomenclatura morborum nasi et naso-pharyngis. Boston, 1892. 10p. DNLM
90-8392

SPEAR, Edmund D[oe] (*b.* 1852)
The relation of the thyroid gland to certain diseases of the ear with a theory of its function. Boston: Rockwell & Churchill, 1896. 16p. DNLM **90-8393**

SPEAR, Edmund D[oe] (*b.* 1852)
Earache in children; its relation to adenoid disease. Boston, [1897]. 4p. DNLM **90-8394**

SPEAR, Edmund D[oe] (*b.* 1852)
The relation of the thyroid gland to certain diseases of the ear, with a theory of its functions. Boston, 1897. 15p. DNLM
90-8395

SPECIAL articles on yellow fever. The etiology and pathology, by R. Matas. The symptomatology and diagnosis, by F. W. Parham. The treatment, by T. S. Dabney. New Orleans: L. Graham & Son, 1897. 50p. DNLM; LNT-M
90-8396

SPECIAL bulletin from the "University Medical Magazine" on the clinical results of Koch's treatment of tuberculosis, and on the method to be pursued in investigating the value of the remedy in the University Hospital. [Philadelphia, 1891.] 10p. DNLM **90-8397**

SPENCE, Arnot (1863-1907)
The results of expectant treatment in three hundred and twenty-three cases of typhoid fever. New York: Trow's Co., 1892. 11p. DNLM **90-8398**

SPENCE, Arnot (1863-1907)
The treatment of pneumonia in St. Francis Hospital, with results in two hundred and twenty-eight cases. New York: Trow's Co., 1893. 16p. DNLM **90-8399**

SPENCER, George W[icks] (*b.* 1870)
Wounds of the hand. New York, 1897. 18p. DNLM
90-8400

SPENCER, H[oratio] N[elson] (*b.* 1842)
Clinical observations on the effects of quinine in acute inflammation of the ear. St. Louis, 1892. 7p. DNLM
90-8401

SPENCER, Walter G[eorge] (1858-1940)
Outlines of practical surgery. New York: William Wood & Co., 1899. 694p. DNLM; NNNAM **90-8402**

SPENZER, John George (*b.* 1864)
The principles of pharmacology, wiht practical exercises. . . . Adapted for self-study. Author's ed. Cleveland, O., 1899. 375p. DLC; OCIM **90-8403**

SPERRY, Lyman B[eecher] (1841-1923)
Brief treatise on narcotics; their sources, nature, physiological effects, medicinal uses, etc. Northfield, Minn., 1890. 75p. DLC **90-8404**

SPERRY, Lyman B[eecher] (1841-1923)
Confidential talks with young men. . . . Chicago, New York: F. H. Revell Co., 1892. 179p. DLC; NN [*vel subseq.*]
90-8405

SPERRY, Lyman B[eecher] (1841-1923)
Confidential talks with young women. . . . Chicago, New York: F. H. Revell Co., [1893]. 137p. DLC [*vel subseq.*]
90-8406

SPIERS, Henry H.
Tuberculosis or consumption. [1st] ed. [Ravenna, Ohio, 1898.] 66p. DNLM **90-8407**

SPILLER, William G[ibson] (1863-1940)
A contribution to the study of spinal syphilis. New York, 1897. 21p. DNLM; NNNAM **90-8408**

SPILLER, William G[ibson] (1863-1940)
On amyloid, colloid, hyaloid, and granular bodies in the central nervous system. [New York, 1898.] 1p. DNLM
90-8409

SPITZKA, Edward Charles (1852-1914)
The legal disabilities of natural children justified biologically and historically. St. Louis, 1899. 26p. DNLM
90-8410

SPIVAK, Charles David (1861-1927)
Menstruation, a brief summary of the theories of the ancients, with special reference to the views held by the Talmudists. Philadelphia, 1891. 12p. DNLM **90-8411**

SPIVAK, Charles David (1861-1927)
Varicella complicated by gangrene of the scrotum. Philadelphia, 1895. 4p. DNLM **90-8412**

SPIVAK, Charles David (1861-1927)
A case of imperforate anus. New York, 1896. 4p. DNLM
90-8413

SPIVAK, Charles David (1861-1927)
Delivery at term after ten previous consecutive abortions. New York, 1896. 4p. DNLM **90-8414**

SPIVAK, Charles David (1861-1927)
Gastrodiaphany, or electrical trans-illumination of the stomach, with demonstrations. Denver, 1896. 4p. DNLM
90-8415

SPIVAK, Charles David (1861-1927)
Hyperacidity and hypersecretion of the gastric juices. Denver, 1896. 4p. DNLM **90-8416**

SPIVAK, Charles David (1861-1927)
Kephir. New York, 1896. 18p. DNLM
90-8417

SPIVAK, Charles David (1861-1927)
Nasal affections as factors in chronic gastritis. Philadelphia, 1896. 1 l. DNLM **90-8418**

SPIVAK, Charles David (1861-1927)
Chelidonium majus in the treatment of cancer. Detroit, 1897. 9p. DNLM **90-8419**

SPIVAK, Charles David (1861-1927)
How every town may secure a medical library. Philadelphia, 1897. 5p. DNLM **90-8420**

SPIVAK, Charles David (1861-1927)
The union catalogue of medical books, and some of the private medical libraries in the city of Denver. Denver, 1897. 4p. DNLM **90-8421**

SPIVAK, Charles David (1861-1927)
Rest; a neglected factor in the treatment of gastro-intestinal disorder. Chicago, 1898. 15p. DNLM
90-8422

SPIVAK, Charles David (1861-1927)
The ancient and modern instruments used in the diagnosis and treatment of diseases of the oesophagus and stomach. New York, 1898. 15p. DNLM **90-8423**

SPIVAK, Charles David (1861-1927)
The medical libraries of the United States. Philadelphia, 1898. 14p. 3 charts. DNLM **90-8424**

SPIVAK, Charles David (1861-1927)
Union catalogue and statistics of medical libraries. [Denver, 1898.] 8p. DNLM **90-8425**

SPIVAK, Charles David (1861-1927)
Medical treatment of intestinal obstruction. Chicago, 1899. 8p. DNLM **90-8426**

SPOTSWOOD, Dillon J.
Yellow fever and the abuses of quarantine in the South during the epidemic of 1897. New York: Lea Bros. & Co., 1898. 12p. DNLM **90-8427**

SPRAGUE, W[illiam] B. (1836-1891)
Electricity vs. the knife in the treatment of pelvic disease. [Detroit, 1890.] 26p. DNLM **90-8428**

SPRATLING, Edgar J.
The nodes of Ranvier. New York, [1898]. 6p. DNLM
90-8429

SPRATLING, William P[hilip] (1863-1915)
Moral insanity. [New York, 1890.] 7p. DNLM
90-8430

SPRATLING, William P[hilip] (1863-1915)
The treatment of the acutely insane in general hospitals. New York: Trow, 1890. 8p. DNLM
90-8431

SPRATLING, William P[hilip] (1863-1915)
The formation of a national association or society for the study of epilepsy and the care and treatment of epileptics. Opinions and suggestions bearing on its formation and purposes. Sonyea, N.Y., [1898]. 16p. DNLM
90-8432

SPRINGSTEEN, Wallace S.
Illustrated gynecological study of the diseases of women. . . . Cleveland, O.: The Springsteen Medicine Co., [1894]. 53p. col. illus. DLC; OCIM **90-8433**

SQUIBB, Edward R[obinson] (1819-1900)
Semi-annual price list of standard pharmaceutical preparations and pharmacopoeial reagents. No. 81. [Brooklyn, N.Y., 1899.] DNLM; NNNAM **90-8434**

STALL, Sylvanus (1847-1915)
What a young husband ought to know. Philadelphia, [1897]. 300p. DNLM; PU **90-8435**

STALL, Sylvanus (1847-1915)
What a young boy ought to know. Philadelphia, [1897]. 190p. DNLM; PU **90-8436**

STALL, Sylvanus (1847-1915)
What a young man ought to know. Philadelphia, [1897]. 281p. DNLM; PU **90-8437**

STALL, Sylvanus (1847-1915)
What a young husband ought to know. Philadelphia & London, [1899]. 300p. DNLM; PU **90-8438**

STAMM, M[artin] (1847-1918)
A case of intestinal anastomosis with cartilage plates, for traumatic stricture of the ileum; recovery. [Philadelphia: Lea Bros. & Co., 1891.] 8p. DNLM **90-8439**

STAMM, M[artin] (1847-1918)
Report of a case of a large abdominal echinococcus cyst; with remarks. [Philadelphia, 1893.] 15p. DNLM
90-8440

STAPLES, Franklin (1833-1904)
Concerning the present condition of state medicine in the United States. Chicago, 1897. 8p. DNLM
90-8441

STAPLES, Franklin (1833-1904)
State medicine to the present time. Chicago, 1897. 8p. DNLM
90-8442

STAPLES, Franklin (1833-1904)
Bacteriology in the progress of medicine; a few notes from current history. New York: D. Appleton & Co., 1898. 16p. DNLM **90-8443**

STAPLES, Franklin (1833-1904)
Enteric fever; its infection, pathology and present treatment. Chicago, 1899. 12p. DNLM **90-8444**

STAPLES, Franklin (1833-1904)
The advance of medical education in the United States. St. Paul, [1899], 15p. DNLM **90-8445**

STARLING, Ernest H[enry] (1866-1927)
Elements of human physiology. Philadelphia: P. Blakiston, Son & Co., 1892. 437p. DNLM; PU **90-8446**

STARR, Louis (1849-1925)
Diseases of the digestive organs in infancy and childhood, with chapters on the investigation of disease; the diet and general management of children, and massage in paediatrics. . . . 2nd ed. . . . Philadelphia: P. Blakiston, Son & Co, 1891. 396p. plates. DLC; DNLM; PPC; PU **90-8447**

STARR, Louis (1849-1925)
Hygiene of the nursery. . . . Including the general regimen and feeding of infants and children, and the domestic management of the ordinary emergencies of early life. 3rd ed. Philadelphia: P. Blakiston, Son & Co., 1891. 293p. DNLM; NNNAM; PPC; PU **90-8448**

STARR, Louis (1849-1925)
Hygiene of the nursery. Including the general regimen and feeding of infants and children; massage, and the domestic management of the ordinary emergies of early life. . . . 4th ed. With twenty-five illustrations. Philadelphia: P. Blakiston, Son & Co., 1894. 293p. DLC; DNLM; IU-M; PPC **90-8449**

STARR, Louis, ed. (1849-1925)
An American text-book of the diseases of children, including special chapters on essential surgical subjects; diseases of the eye, ear, nose, and throat; diseases of the skin; and on the diet, hygiene, and general management of children, by American teachers. Edited by Louis Starr, assisted by Thompson S. Westcott. Philadelphia: W. B. Saunders, 1894. 1190p. 28 plates. DLC; DNLM; NNNAM; PPC **90-8450**

STARR, Louis (1849-1925)
Hygiene of the nursery. Including the general regimen and feeding of infants and children; massage, and the domestic management of the ordinary emergencies of early life. . . . 5th ed. With twenty-five illustrations. Philadelphia: P. Blakiston, Son & Co., 1896. 293p. DLC; MB: PPC; PU **90-8451**

STARR, Louis (1849-1925)
Diets for infants and children in health and in disease. Philadelphia: W. B. Saunders, 1896. 234 l. DNLM; PPC; PU **90-8452**

STARR, Louis, ed. (1849-1925)
An American test-book of the diseases of children. . . . By American teachers. Ed. by Louis Starr . . . assisted by Thompson S. Westcott. . . . 2nd ed., rev. Philadelphia: W. B. Saunders, 1898. 1244p. col. plates. DLC; ICRM; PPC; PPJ **90-8453**

STARR, Moses Allen (1854-1932)
Familiar forms of nervous disease . . . with illustrations, diagrams, and charts. New York: William Wood & Co., 1890. 339p. diags. DLC; DNLM; NNNAM; PPC **90-8454**

STARR, Moses Allen (1854-1932)
Familiar forms of nervous disease . . . with illustrations, diagrams, and charts. 2nd ed. . . . New York: William Wood & Co., 1891. 339p. DNLM; MdBJ-W; NNNAM **90-8455**

STARR, Moses Allen (1854-1932)
Lectures upon diseases of the mind, delivered at the College of Physicians and Surgeons, New York. Printed for the use of the students. New York: Trow, 1891. 52, 11p. NNC [Bound with Francis Delafield. Lectures on practical medicine and pathology. New York, 1891.] **90-8456**

STARR, Moses Allen (1854-1932)
The cerebral atrophies of childhood. With special reference to the operation of craniotomy for imbecility, epilepsy, and paralysis. New York, 1892. 24p. DNLM; NNNAM **90-8457**

STARR, Moses Allen (1854-1932)
Brain surgery. . . . New York: William Wood & Co., 1893. 295p. DLC; DNLM; NNNAM; PU **90-8458**

STARR, Moses Allen (1854-1932)
Megalo-cephaly, or leontiasis ossea. Philadelphia: Lea Bros. & Co., 1894. 7p. DNLM **90-8459**

STARR, Moses Allen (1854-1932)
Myxedema and its differential diagnosis from chronic nephritis. Philadelphia: Lea Bros. & Co., 1894. 13p. DNLM **90-8460**

STARR, Moses Allen (1854-1932)
A contribution to the localization of the muscular sense. Philadelphia, 1894. 3p. DNLM **90-8461**

STARR, Moses Allen (1854-1932)
Atlas of nerve cells, by M. Allen Starr . . . With the cooperation of Oliver S. Strong . . . and Edward Leaming. . . . With fifty-three plates and thirteen diagrams. New York, London: Pub. for the Columbia University Press by Macmillan & Co., 1896. 78p. DLC; DNLM; NNC; NNNAM **90-8462**

STARR, Moses Allen (1854-1932)
Lectures upon diseases of the mind, delivered at the College of Physicians and Surgeons, New York. . . . New York, 1897. 48p. CtY-M; NNC [Interleaved with blank pages for notes. Bound with is Synopsis of lectures upon diseases of the nervous system. . . . New York, c. 1898] **90-8463**

STARR, Moses Allen (1854-1932)
Synopsis of lectures upon diseases of the nervous system, delivered at the College of Physicians and Surgeons, Medical Department of Columbia University, New York. New York: Doughtery, c. 1898. 81p. CtY-M; NNC **90-8464**

STARR, William Martin
In defense of medical botany. 3rd ed. . . . Washington, [1891]. 102p. DLC; DNLM **90-8465**

STARR, William Martin
Medical botany or specific remedies from nature's own cures. Defending botanic practice of medicine. To U.S. Congress. . . . Washington, D.C.: [Beckert & McCurdy, prs.], 1895. 100p. DLC **90-8466**

STAVELY, Albert L[ivingston] (*b.* 1863)
A case of congenital deformity. Baltimore, 1891. 2 l. DNLM **90-8467**

STAVELY, Albert L[ivingston] (*b.* 1863)
Myomectomy during pregnancy. New York, 1891. 12p. DNLM
90-8468

STEARNS, Henry Putnam (1828-1905)
Lectures on mental diseases, designed especially for medical students and general practitioners. Philadelphia: P. Blakiston, Son & Co., 1893. 636p. 1 plate. DLC; DNLM; NNNAM; PPC
90-8469

STEAVENSON, W[illiam] E[dward] (1850-1891) and H[enry] Lewis JONES
Medical electricity; a practical handbook for students and practitioners. 2nd ed. Philadelphia: P. Blakiston, Son & Co., [1895]. 474p. DNLM; NNNAM; PPC; PU
90-8470

STEDMAN, C[harles] Ellery (1831-1909)
The profession as viewed by the public. Boston, 1895. 20p. DNLM; MBM **90-8471**

STEDMAN, Henry R[ust] (1849-1926)
The selection of cases of insanity for different methods of private care. [Philadelphia, 1891.] 11p. DNLM
90-8472

STEDMAN, Henry R[ust] (1849-1926)
The management of convalescence and the after-care of the insane. Chicago, 1894. 18p. DNLM **80-8473**

STEDMAN, Henry R[ust] (1849-1926)
The prognosis and duration of attacks of mental disease. Boston: Damrell & Upham, 1897. 12p. DNLM
90-8474

STEDMAN, Joseph (1835-1898)
Vomiting of obscure origin in young children. Boston: Damrell & Upham, 1890. 8p. DNLM; MBM
90-8475

STEDMAN, Joseph (1835-1898)
Cerebral tumors; with clinical cases. Boston: Damrell & Upham, 1891. 19p. DNLM; MBM **90-8476**

STEDMAN, Joseph (1835-1898)
Some general observations on rectal diseases. Boston: Damrell & Upham, 1896. 19p. DNLM; MBM **90-8477**

STEDMAN, Thomas Lathrop, ed. (1853-1938)
Twentieth century practice; an international encyclopedia of modern medical science by leading authorities of Europe and America. . . . New York: William Wood & Co., 1895-1903. 21 v. plates, charts, diags. DLC; DNLM; NNNAM; PU
90-8478

STEELE, [Aaron] John (1835-1917)
Plaster-of-Paris in orthopedics. [Philadelphia, 1893.] 15p. DNLM **90-8479**

STEELE, [Aaron] John (1835-1917)
The osteopathic fad. Columbia, Mo.: E. W. Stephens, 1895. 15p. DNLM **90-8480**

STEELE, D[aniel] A[tkinson] K[ing] (1852-1931)
Report of a case of cerebral tumor, diagnosed by focal symptoms, with operation, successful removal of tumor and exhibition of specimen. Chicago, 1894. 8p. DNLM
90-8481

STEIN, Alexander W. (1841-1897)
Valedictory lecture, class of 1890, New York College of Dentistry. [New York, 1890.] 12p. DNLM; NNNAM
90-8482

STELWAGON, Henry Weightman (1853-1919)
. . . Essentials of diseases of the skin, including the syphilodermata. Arranged in the form of questions and answers. . . . Philadelphia: W. B. Saunders; [etc., etc.], 1890. 270p. DLC; DNLM; NNNAM; PPC **90-8483**

STELWAGON, Henry Weightman (1853-1919)
Dermatitis herpetiformis; a report of three cases. [n. p., 1890.] 7p. DNLM **90-8484**

STELWAGON, Henry Weightman (1853-1919)
Notes on the hospital treatment of psoriasis. Philadelphia, 1892. 4p. DNLM **90-8485**

STELWAGON, Henry Weightman (1853-1919)
On the increasing prevalence of scabies. Philadelphia, 1893. 11p. DNLM **90-8486**

STELWAGON, Henry Weightman (1853-1919)
Medical report of the Philadelphia Dispensary for Skin Diseases, covering a period of ten years and nine months (February, 1880, to November, 1891). [Philadelphia, 1893.] 32p. DNLM; PPC **90-8487**

STELWAGON, Henry Weightman (1853-1919)
. . . Essentials of diseases of the skin, including the syphilodermata. Arranged in the form of questions and answers. . . . 3rd ed., rev. and enl. . . . Philadelphia: W. B. Saunders, 1894. 270p. plates. DLC; NNNAM; PPC; PPJ
90-8488

STELWAGON, Henry Weightman (1853-1919)
The question of contagiousness or molluscum contagiosum. [New York, 1895.] 13p. DNLM **90-8489**

STELWAGON, Henry Weightman (1853-1919)
. . . Essentials of diseases of the skin, including the syphilodermata, arranged in the form of questions and answers, prepared especially for students of medicine. . . . 4th ed., thoroughly rev. . . . Philadelphia: W. B. Saunders, 1899. 276p. plates. DLC; DNLM; PPC; PU **90-8490**

STEMEN, C[hristian] B[erry] (1836-1915)
Railway surgery. A practical work on the special department of railway surgery; for railway surgeons, and practitioners in the general practice of surgery. St. Louis: J. H. Chambers & Co., [1890]. 315p. DNLM; IU-M; OCIM; PPC
90-8491

STENGEL, Alfred (1868-1939)
Nature, diagnosis, and treatment of pernicious anaemia. Detroit: G. S. Davis, 1894. 28p. DNLM
90-8492

STENGEL, Alfred (1868-1939)
Fever in the course of Bright's disease and in uraemia. Philadelphia, 1895. 15p. DNLM **90-8493**

STENGEL, Alfred (1868-1939)
Arsenical neuritis; with the report of a case occurring in a lad of five years. New York: E. B. Treat, 1897. 6p. DNLM
90-8494

STENGEL, Alfred (1868-1939)
The blood in the diseases of the cardio-vascular system. Philadelphia, [1897]. 6p. DNLM **90-8495**

STENGEL, Alfred (1868-1939)
Gonorrheal endocarditis. Philadelphia, 1897. 23p. 2 plates. DNLM **90-8496**

STENGEL, Alfred (1868-1939)
A text-book of pathology. . . . With 372 illustrations. . . . Philadelphia: W. B. Saunders, 1898. 848p. col. plates. DLC; DNLM; NNNAM; PPC **90-8497**

STENGEL, Alfred (1868-1939)
The medical treatment of movable kidney. Philadelpia, 1899. 7p. DNLM **90-8498**

STENGEL, Alfred (1868-1939) and Henry D. BEYEA
Gastroptosis; report of a case in which a new operation was undertaken and the patient greatly improved. Philadelphia, 1899. 12p. DNLM **90-8499**

STENGEL, Alfred (1868-1939)
A text-book of pathology. . . . 2nd ed. Philadelphia: W. B. Saunders 1899. 848p. col. plates. DLC; MdBJ-W; PPC; PPJ **90-8500**

STEPHENSON, Frank H[alleck] (*b.* 1856)
Melancholia, with reports of cases. New York, 1895. 10p. DNLM **90-8501**

STEPHENSON, Frank H[alleck] (*b.* 1856)
Neuritis. New York, 1895. 6p. DNLM **90-8502**

STERN, Heinrich (1868-1918)
An, as yet, undefined fact in pharmacology. St. Louis: L. A. Turnbull, 1894. 7p. DNLM **90-8503**

STERN, Heinrich (1868-1918)
A rational diabetic flour. Philadelphia, 1895. 10p. DNLM **90-8504**

STERN, Heinrich (1868-1918)
A case of crossed hemiplegia. Most prominent phenomenon, paralysis of the pharynx; syphilitic basis. New York, 1897. 3p. DNLM **90-8505**

STERN, Heinrich (1868-1918)
Urinalysis, a guide for the busy practitioner. New York: E. R. Pelton, 1897. 61p. DLC; DNLM; NNNAM **90-8506**

STERNBERG, George Miller (1838-1915)
. . . Report on the etiology and prevention of yellow fever. . . . Pub. by order of the Secretary of the Treasury, in accordance with an act of Congress approved March 3, 1887. Washington: Government Printing Office, 1890. 271p. col. plates. DLC; DNLM **90-8507**

STERNBERG, George Miller (1838-1915)
A manual of bacteriology. . . . Illustrated by heliotype and chromolithographic plates and two hundred and sixty-eight engravings. New York: William Wood & Co., 1892. 836p. DLC; DNLM; MdU-D; NNNAM **90-8508**

STERNBERG, George M[iller] (1838-1915)
Protective inoculations in infectious diseases. Concord, N.H., 1893. 21p. DNLM **90-8509**

STERNBERG, George M[iller] (1838-1915)
Address to members of Pan-American Medical Congress. Chicago, 1893. 19p. DNLM **90-8510**

STERNBERG, George M[iller] (1838-1915)
How can we prevent cholera? [New York, 1893.] 8p. DNLM **90-8511**

STERNBERG, George M[iller] (1838-1915)
Immunity, protective inoculations in infectious diseases, and serum-therapy. . . . New York: William Wood & Co., 1895. 325p. DLC; DNLM; NNC; PPC **90-8512**

STERNBERG, George M[iller] (1838-1915)
A text-book of bacteriology. New York: William Wood & Co., 1896. 693p. 9 plates. NNNAM; PPC; PU **90-8513**

STERNBERG, George M[iller] (1838-1915)
Scientific researches relating to the specific infectious agent of small-pox and the production of artificial immunity from this disease. Chicago, 1896. 30p. DNLM **90-8514**

STERNBERG, George M[iller] (1838-1915)
The address of the president, delivered at the forty-ninth annual meeting of the American Medical Association, held at Denver, Colo., June 7-10, 1898. Chicago, 1898. 24p. DNLM **90-8515**

STERNBERG, George M[iller] (1838-1915)
Sanitary lessons of the war. Chicago: American Medical Assoc. Press, 1899. 24p. DNLM **90-8516**

STEVENS, A[rthur] A[lbert] (1865-1944)
A manual of the practice of medicine, prepared especially for students. Philadelphia: W. B. Saunders, 1893. 501p. DNLM; NNNAM; PPC; PU **90-8517**

STEVENS, A[rthur] A[lbert] (1865-1944)
A manual of the practice of medicine, prepared especially for students. . . . 2nd ed., rev. Philadelphia: W. B. Saunders, 1893 [1892]. 501p. DLC; NNNAM; PPC; PU **90-8518**

STEVENS, A[rthur] A[lbert] (1865-1944)
A manual of the practice of medicine, prepared especially for students. . . . 3rd ed., rev. . . . Philadelphia: W. B. Saunders, 1894. 501p. DLC; MBM; PPC; PPJ **90-8519**

STEVENS, A[rthur] A[lbert] (1865-1944)
A manual of therapeutics. Philadelphia: W. B. Saunders, 1894. 435p. DNLM; NNC; PPC; PU **90-8520**

STEVENS, A[rthur] A[lbert] (1865-1944)
A manual of therapeutics. 2nd ed. Philadelphia: W. B. Saunders, 1896. 445p. MdU-D; NNNAM; PPC; PU **90-8521**

STEVENS, A[rthur] A[lbert] (1865-1944)
A manual of the practice of medicine, prepared especially for students. . . . 4th ed., rev. and enl. Philadelphia: W. B. Saunders, 1896. 511p. DLC; NBM; NNNAM; PPC **90-8522**

STEVENS, A[rthur] A[lbert] (1865-1944)
A manual of the practice of medicine, prepared especially for students. 5th ed. Philadelphia: W. B. Saunders, 1898. 519p. DNLM; NNC; OCIM; PPC **90-8523**

STEVENS, A. Jay (*b.* **1866)**
. . . The star quizzer on pharmacy, chemsitry and materia medica. . . . By A. Jay Stevens . . . and Chas. W. Mallory. . . . Ada, O.: Stevens & Mallory, [1896]. 160p. DLC
90-8524

STEVENS, Edward S[ommerville] (*b.* **1857)**
Fractured clavicle; a new dressing. Philadelphia, 1892. 6p. DNLM **90-8525**

STEVENS, Edward S[ommerville] (*b.* **1857)**
The obscure cases of gall-bladder disease. New York, 1898. 8p. DNLM **90-8526**

STEVENS, George T[homas] (1832-1921)
L'influence de l'état des muscles moteurs de l'oeil sur l'expression du visage. New York, 1892. 20p. 3 plates. DNLM
90-8527

STEVENS, George T[homas] (1832-1921)
The relation of the function of accommodation to that of convergence. [New York: D. Appleton & Co., 1895.] 7p. DNLM **90-8528**

STEVENS, George T[homas] (1832-1921)
Historical notes of strabismus and other anomalies of the eye muscles. St. Louis, 1899. 24p. DNLM
90-8529

STEVENS, J[ames] H[erbert] (*b.* **1871)**
Report of five cases of wounds by the Mauser bullet. Boston, 1898. 6p. DNLM **90-8530**

STEVENSON, Thomas (1838-1908) and Shirley F. MURPHY, eds.
A treatise on hygiene and public health. Philadelphia, 1892-94. 3 v. DNLM; PPC; PU **90-8531**

STEVENSON, W[illiam] F[lack] (1844-1922)
Wounds in war, the mechanism of their production and their treatment. New York: William Wood & Co., 1898. 437p. DNLM; NNNAM **90-8532**

STEWART, A[lonzo] H. (*b.* **1867)**
A new cover-slip forceps. Philadelphia, 1895. 2p. DNLM
90-8533

STEWART, Colin C[ampbell] (*b.* **1873)**
Influence of acute alcohol poisoning on nerve cells. New York, 1896. 7p. 1 plate. DNLM **90-8534**

STEWART, David Denison (1859-1905)
On the utility of suspension in diseases of the spinal cord. Illustrated by a case. [Philadelphia, 1891.] 7p. DNLM
90-8535

STEWART, David Denison (1859-1905)
. . . Essentials of medical electricity. By D. D. Stewart . . . and E. S. Lawrance. . . . Philadelphia: W. B. Saunders, 1892 [1891]. 158p. DLC; DNLM; PPC; PU
90-8536

STEWART, David Denison (1859-1905)
Hydronaphthol in the prophylaxis and treatment of cholera; report of laboratory experiments. Philadelphia, 1892. 7p. DNLM **90-8537**

STEWART, David Denison (1859-1905)
Treatment of sacculated aortic aneurism by electrolysis through introduced wire. Report of a case. Philadelphia, 1892. 17p. DNLM **90-8538**

STEWART, David Denison (1859-1905)
A consideration of some modern therapeutic agents in the treatment of diseases of the stomach. Detroit, 1893. 28p. DNLM **90-8539**

STEWART, David Denison (1859-1905)
Treatment of typhoid fever. . . . Detroit, Mich.: G. S. Davis, 1893. 104p. DLC; OCIM **90-8540**

STEWART, David Denison (1859-1905)
The identity of the proprietary, so-called "hydro-naphthol" and impure beta-naphthol. With a special report of an analysis of hydro-naphthol, by Chas. P. Beckwith. [Philadelphia, 1893.] 10p. DNLM **90-8541**

STEWART, David Denison (1859-1905)
The measured effects of certain therapeutic agents, among which are lavage, HCl, and intragastric electricity, upon the secretory and motor functions of the stomach in cases of chronic catarrh (glandular gastritis). Detroit: G. S. Davis, 1893. 25p. DNLM **90-8542**

STEWART, David Denison (1859-1905)
Piperazin in the treatment of stone in the kidney; report of cases. Detroit: G. S. Davis, 1893. 9p. DNLM
90-8543

STEWART, David Denison (1859-1905)
The prevention and treatment of cholera by the naphthols, and bacteriological report by George M. Sternberg. Philadelphia, 1893. 6p. DNLM **90-8544**

STEWART, David Denison (1859-1905)
A résumé of some modern methods of diagnosis of diseases of the stomach. Philadelphia, 1893. 25p. DNLM
90-8545

STEWART, David Denison (1859-1905)
Further remarks on the occurrence of a form of non-albuminous nephritis other than typical fibroid kidney. Philadelphia: Lea & Bros., 1894. 27p. DNLM **90-8546**

STEWART, David Denison (1859-1905)
The reactions of nucleo-albumin (erroneously styled mucin) with the commonly employed urinary albumin tests; the difficulty of distinguishing these reactions from those of serum-albumin, globulin, etc. Philadelphia: Lea Bros. & Co., 1894. 29p. DNLM **90-8547**

STEWART, David Denison (1859-1905)
A serious fallacy attending the employment of certain delicate tests for the detection of serum-albumin in the urine, especially in the trichloracetic acid test. Philadelphia, 1894. 19p. DNLM
90-8548

STEWART, David Denison (1859-1905)
A new diagnostic sign for the early recognition of carcinoma of the stomach. [Philadelphia: Lea Bros. & Co., 1895.] 16p. DNLM **90-8549**

STEWART, David Denison (1859-1905)
A further account of the treament of aneurysm by the conjoint use of galvanism through introduced coil wire; report of cases. Philadelphia, 1898. 27p. DNLM **90-8550**

STEWART, F[rancis] Edward (1853-1941)
Haemoglobin compound or bullock's blood in therapeutics. Detroit & New York: Parke, Davis & Co., 1890. 25p. DNLM **90-8551**

STEWART, F[rancis] Edward (1853-1941)
Haemoglobin compound or bullock's blood in therapeutics. New York & Detroit: Parke, Davis & Co., [1890?]. 27p. DNLM **90-8552**

STEWART, F[rancis] Edward (1853-1941)
Is pharmacy a profession or a trade? [Wilmington, 1890?] 12p. DNLM **90-8553**

STEWART, F[rancis] Edward (1853-1941)
A compend of pharmacy. . . . Based upon Prof. Joseph P. Remington's "Textbook of Pharmacy." 3rd rev. ed. . . . Philadelphia: P. Blakiston, Son & Co., 1890. 171p. DNLM; NNNAM; PPC; PPJ **90-8554**

STEWART, F[rancis] Edward (1853-1941)
A compend of pharmacy. . . . Based upon Prof. Joseph P. Remington's "Textbook of Pharmacy." 4th rev. ed. . . . Philadelphia: P. Blakiston, Son & Co., 1894. 181p. DNLM; MBM; PPC; PU **90-8555**

STEWART, F[rancis] Edward (1853-1941)
A compend of pharmacy. . . . Based upon Prof. Joseph P. Remington's "Textbook of Pharmacy." 5th rev. ed. . . . Philadelphia: P. Blakiston, Son & Co., 1895. 187p. DNLM; IU-M; PPC; PU **90-8556**

STEWART, F[rancis] Edward (1853-1941)
Some recent discoveries in regard to the mode of action and chemistry of cod liver oil. Chicago, 1896. 16p. DNLM **90-8557**

STEWART, G[eorge] N[eil] (1860-1930)
A manual of physiology. With practical exercises. For students and practitioners. Philadelphia: W. B. Saunders & Co., 1897. 796p. CtY-M; NNNAM; IU-M; PU **90-8558**

STEWART, G[eoge] N[eil] (1860-1930)
A manual of physiology. With practical exercises. For students and practitioners. 2nd rev. ed. Philadelphia: W. B. Saunders & Co., 1898. 848p. CU-M; ICRM; NNNAM; PPC **90-8559**

STEWART, G[eorge] N[eil] (1860-1930)
A manual of physiology. With practical exercises. For students and practitioners. 3rd rev. ed. Philadelphia: W. B. Saunders & Co., 1898. 848p. MBM; MdBJ-W; NNC; PU **90-8560**

STEWART, George Taylor
Alimentation of the sick. New York, 1895. 6p. DNLM **90-8561**

STEWART, James (1846-1906)
The symptomatology of tumors involving the hypophysis cerebri. Philadelphia, 1899. 13p. DNLM **90-8562**

STEWART, John Pope (*b.* 1864)
Evolution from a scientific standpoint. Read before the Tri-State Medical Association at its annual meeting, October, 1891, in the city of Chattanooga. Birmingham, Ala.: R. E. Jones, 1891. 14p. DNLM **90-8563**

STEWART, R[obert] W. (*b.* 1853)
Direct and oblique inguinal hernia on the same side. [Philadelphia, 1893.] 3p. DNLM **90-8564**

STEWART, R[obert] W. (*b.* 1853)
A report of four surgical cases. 1. Excision of the superior maxillary nerve. 2. Intracranial neurectomy of the fifth nerve. 3. Cholecystectomy. 4. Esophagotomy. Philadelphia, 1895. 12p. DNLM; PPC **90-8565**

STEWART, R[obert] W. (*b.* 1853)
The diseases of the male urethra. New York: William Wood & Co., 1896. 221p. DNLM; NNNAM; ScU **90-8566**

STEWART, R[obert] W. (*b.* 1853)
Toxicity of urine of last month of pregnancy. New York, 1897. 10p. DNLM **90-8567**

STEWART, R[obert] W. (*b.* 1853)
Occipito-dextro-posterior position of the fetal head. New York, 1897. 8p. DNLM **90-8568**

STEWART, R[obert] W. (*b.* 1853)
Puerperal eclampsia. Report of a case, with the treatment of same patient during a subsequent pregnancy. New York, 1899. 14p. DNLM; NNNAM **90-8569**

STEWART, William Blair (*b.* 1867)
Hepatic abscess, with the report of a clinical case. [Philadelphia, 1892.] 8p. DNLM **90-8570**

STEWART, William Blair (*b.* 1867)
Albuminate of iron. [New York, 1893.] 12p. DNLM **90-8571**

STEWART, William Blair (*b.* 1867)
A synopsis of the practice of medicine. New York: E. B. Treat, 1894. 433p. DLC; DNLM; NNNAM **90-8572**

STEWART, William Blair (*b.* 1867)
Arsenite of copper as an antispasmodic. New York, 1894. 8p. DNLM **90-8573**

STEWART, William Blair (*b.* 1867)
Functional constipation. Danbury, Conn., 1894. 7 l. DNLM **90-8574**

STEWART, William Blair (*b.* 1867)
Spindle-cell sarcoma and epithelioma; a report of cases. New York, 1894. 8p. DNLM **90-8575**

STEWART, William Blair (*b.* 1867)
The treatmnet of symptomatic anaemia. Philadelphia, 1895. 11p. DNLM **90-8576**

STIEREN, Edward (*b.* 1873)
Oedematous changes in the epithelium of the cornea in a case of uveitis following gonorrhoeal ophthalmia. [Baltimore, 1898.] 6p. 1 plate. DNLM **90-8577**

STILES, Charles Wardell (1867-1941)
Address to medical graduates. Delivered before the graduating class of the Medical Department of Georgetown University, Washington, D.C., 1896. Philadelphia, 1896. 8p. DNLM **90-8578**

STILL, Andrew Taylor (1828-1917)
Autobiography of Andrew T. Still, with a history of the discovery and development of the science of osteopathy, together with an account of the founding of the American School of Osteopathy. . . . Kirksville, Mo.: The Author, 1897. 460p. plates, ports. DLC; OCIM **90-8579**

STILL, Andrew Taylor (1828-1917)
Philosophy of osteopathy. . . . Kirksville, Mo.: A. T. Still, 1899. 268p. DLC **90-8580**

STILLÉ, Alfred (1813-1900)
The national dispensatory. Containing the natural history, chemistry, pharmacy, actions, and uses of medicines. Including those recognized in the pharmacopoeias of the United States, Great Britain, and Germany, with numerous references to the French codex. By Alfred Stillé . . . John M. Maisch . . . Charles Caspari . . . and Henry C. C. Maisch. . . . 5th ed., enl. and rev. in accordance with the 7th decennial revision of the United States pharmacopoeia. With three hundred and twenty illustrations. Philadelphia: Lea Bros. & Co., 1894. 1903p. DLC; NNNAM; OCLloyd; PPC **90-8581**

STILLÉ, Alfred (1813-1900)
The national dispensatory. Containing the natural history, chemistry, pharmacy, actions, and uses of medicines. Including those recognized in the pharmacopoeias of the United States, Great Britain, and Germany, with numerous references to the French codex. By Alfred Stillé . . . John M. Maisch . . . Charles Caspari, Jr. . . . and Henry C. C. Maisch. 5th ed., enl. and rev. in accordance with the 7th decennial revision of the United States Pharmacopoeia, to which is added the National formula (New ed.) Philadelphia and New York: Lea Bros. & Co., 1896. 1790, 115, 1791-1903p. DLC; IU-M; MBM; OCLloyd **90-8582**

STILLMAN, Charles F[rederick] (1853-1892)
A practical résumé of modern methods employed in the treatment of chronic articular ostitis of the hip. Detroit: G. S. Davis, 1891. 118p. DNLM; OCIM **90-8583**

STIMSON, J. Coplin (*d.* 1906)
Appendicitis; a report of 54 consecutive operative cases; when to operate; points in technique. New York, 1896. 11p. DNLM **90-8584**

STIMSON, J. Coplin (*d.* 1906)
The operative treatment of inguinal hernia, with a review of ninety-seven cases; preferable method of operation. New York, 1896. 2 l. DNLM **90-8585**

STIMSON, J. Coplin (*d.* 1906)
The radical cure of femoral hernia; preferable operation; the surgical anatomy of the transversalis fascia at the internal inguinal and femoral rings. New York, 1896. 4 l. DNLM **90-8586**

STIMSON, J. Coplin (*d.* 1906)
Another method of fixation of a kidney. New York, 1897. 3 l. DNLM **90-8587**

STIMSON, J. Coplin (*d.* 1906)
Ectopic gestation; a report of operative cases; when to operate; points of technique. Detroit, 1897. 4 l. DNLM **90-8588**

STIMSON, J. Coplin (*d.* 1906)
Conservative operations upon the uterine appendages, with illustrative cases. Sacramento, 1897. 3p. DNLM **90-8589**

STIMSON, J. Coplin (*d.* 1906)
Ovarian cyst removed by enucleation without ligature, clamp or cautery. Vaginal hystero-salpyngo-oophorectomy by a modification of Pratt's method by unucleation for puerperal metritis, intramural abscess, etc. San Francisco, 1897. 8p. DNLM **90-8590**

STIMSON, J. Coplin (*d.* 1906)
Multiple calculi and hyperdistension of the gall bladder; calculous obstruction of the cystic duct; cholecystotomy. Los Angeles, 1897. 1 sheet. DNLM **90-8591**

STIMSON, J. Coplin (*d.* 1906)
The radical cure of inguinal hernia; some points in technique; concise review of the several methods of operation. San Francisco, 1897. 10 l. DNLM **90-8592**

STIMSON, Lewis A[tterbury] (1844-1917)
A contribution to the study of appendicitis. [New York, 1890.] 28p. DNLM **90-8593**

STIMSON, Lewis A[tterbury] (1844-1917)
On the treatment of some old unreduced dislocations of the elbow. [New York: D. Appleton & Co., 1891.] 11p. DNLM **90-8594**

STIMSON, Lewis A[tterbury] (1844-1917)
The treatment of fracture of the humerus involving the elbow-joint. [Philadelphia, 1891.] 19p. DNLM **90-8595**

STIMSON, Lewis A[tterbury] (1844-1917)
Pott's fracture at the ankle. [New York, 1892.] 13p. 3 plates. DNLM; NNNAM **90-8596**

STIMSON, Lewis A[tterbury] (1844-1917)
Pasteur's life and work in relation to the advancement of medical science. New York: Stettiner, Lambert & Co., 1893. 28p. DNLM; NNNAM **90-8597**

STIMSON, Lewis A[tterbury] (1844-1917)
A manual of operative surgery. By Lewis A. Stimson . . . and John Rogers, Jr. . . . 3rd ed. With three hundred and thirty-four illustrations. Philadelphia: Lea Bros. & Co., 1895. 398p. DLC; DNLM; NNNAM; PPC **90-8598**

STIMSON, Lewis A[tterbury] (1844-1917)
A practical treatise on fractures and dislocations. . . . With 326 illustrations and 20 plates in monotint. New York and Philadelphia: Lea Bros. & Co., 1899. 822p. col. plates. DLC; DNLM; NNNAM; PPC [also, 2 v. ed.] **90-8599**

STIMSON, Lewis A[tterbury] (1844-1917)
A practical treatise on fractures and dislocations. . . . With 326 illustrations and 20 plates in monotint. [2nd ed.] New York and Philadelphia: Lea Bros. & Co., 1899. 822p. col. plates. NNNAM; PPC; PPJ; PU **90-8600**

STIRLING, Alexander W.
Glaucoma; its symptoms, varieties, pathology and treatment. St. Louis: J. H. Parker, 1898. 177p. DNLM; OCIM **90-8601**

STIRLING, Alexander W.
Sarcoma of the orbit. Nashville, 1898. 4p. 1 plate. DNLM **90-8602**

STIRLING, Alexander W.
Albuminuria and its relation to diseases of the eye. Nashville, 1899. 7p. DNLM **90-8603**

STIRLING, William (1851-1932)
Outlines of practical histology; a manual for students. . . . Philadelphia: P. Blakiston, Son & Co., 1890. 339p. CtY-M; DNLM; PPC; PU **90-8604**

STIRLING, William (1851-1932)
Outlines of practical histology. Being a manual for the physiological laboratory, including chemical and experimental physiology with reference to practical medicine. 2nd ed. Philadelphia: P. Blakiston, Son & Co., 1893. 419p. CtY-M; DNLM; NNC; PU **90-8605**

STIRLING, William (1851-1932)
Outlines of practical histology. Being a manual for the physiological laboratory, including chemical and experimental physiology with reference to practical medicine. 3rd ed. Philadelphia: P. Blakiston, Son & Co., 1895. 402p. DNLM; KyLoJM; PPC; PPJ **90-8606**

STOCKTON, Charles G. (1853-1931)
Simplified directions for examining the stomach. [Philadelphia, 1892.] 10p. DNLM **90-8607**

STOCKTON, Charles G. (1853-1931)
Misconceptions and misnomers revealed by modern gastric research. [Philadelphia, 1892.] 20p. DNLM **90-8608**

STOCKTON, Charles G. (1853-1931)
The etiology of gastric ulcer. [Philadelphia, 1893.] 13p. DNLM **90-8609**

STOCKTON, Charles G. (1853-1931)
The nature and management of functional gastric disorders. Philadelphia: Lea Bros. & Co., 1894. 10p. DNLM **90-8610**

STOCKWELL, G. Archie
A study of the organic extracts cerebrine and cerebrin. Philadelphia: Lea Bros. & Co., 1893. 7p. 1 tab. DNLM **90-8611**

STOCKWELL, G. Archie
Cholera, its Protean aspects and its management. Detroit, Mich.: G. S. Davis, 1893. 2 v. [paged consecutively]. 306p. DLC; DNLM **90-8612**

STÖHR, Philipp (1849-1911)
Text-book of histology, including the microscopical technique. . . . 6th ed. Transl. by Emma L. Bilstein. . . . Ed., with additions, by Dr. Alfred Schaper. With 268 illustrations. Philadelphia: P. Blakiston, Son & Co., 1896. 344p. DLC; DNLM; PPC; PU **90-8613**

STÖHR, Philipp (1849-1911)
Text-book of histology, including the microscopic technic. . . . 2nd American from 7th German ed. Transl. by Dr. Emma L. Bilstein. . . . Ed., with additions, by Alfred Schaper . . . with 292 illustrations. Philadelphia: P. Blakiston's Son & Co., 1898. 424p. DLC; DNLM; NNNAM; PPJ **90-8614**

STOKES, William (1839-1900)
William Stokes, his life and work (1804-1878); by his son William Stokes. . . . New York: Longmans, Green & Co., 1898. 355p. port. DLC; DNLM; ICU; NN **90-8615**

STONE, Arthur K[ingsbury] (*b.* 1861)
Clinical value of the bacillus of tuberculosis. Boston, 1890. 6p. DNLM **90-8616**

STONE, Arthur K[ingsbury] (*b.* 1861)
Why the sputa of tuberculous patients should be destroyed. An observation on the viability of the bacilli of tuberculosis. Philadelphia: Lea Bros. & Co., 1891. 5p. DNLM **90-8617**

STONE, Arthur K[ingsbury] (*b.* 1861)
Bacteriological and clinical investigations into the new antiseptic, dermatol. [Boston, 1892.] 16p. DNLM **90-8618**

STONE, Arthur K[ingsbury] (*b.* 1861)
The hygienic argument for cremation considered from a bacteriological standpoint. Boston: Damrell & Upham, 1893. 22p. DNLM; MB **90-8619**

STONE, Arthur K[ingsbury] (*b.* 1861)
A study of anemia cases with the aid of the hemometer and blood counter. Reported by Anna G. Richardson, Elliot P. Joslin, and Francis P. Denny. Boston, 1894. 9p. DNLM **90-8620**

STONE, Arthur K[ingsbury] (*b.* 1861)
Transverse septa of the vagina. Boston, 1895. 12p. DNLM **90-8621**

STONE, Arthur K[ingsbury] (*b.* 1861)
Gummata of the pelvis, with report of cases. St. Paul, 1899. 8p. DNLM **90-8622**

STONE, Charles Granville (*b.* 1846)
Venesection. Detroit, 1894. 15p. DNLM **90-8623**

STONE, I[saac] S[cott] (*b.* 1851)
The importance of a correct clinical history in operative gynecological cases. [New York, 1890.] 2p. DNLM **90-8624**

STONE, I[saac] S[cott] (*b.* 1851)
Posterior displacements of the uterus; remarks upon pathology and treatment. Philadelphia, 1890. 8p. DNLM **90-8625**

STONE, I[saac] S[cott] (*b.* 1851)
Psychical results of gynecological operations. Chicago, 1890. 11p. DNLM **90-8626**

STONE, I[saac] S[cott] (*b.* 1851)
The diagnosis of pelvic disease; or, when to operate. [Richmond, 1890.] 8p. DNLM **90-8627**

STONE, I[saac] S[cott] (*b.* 1851)
Can the gynecologist aid the alienist in institutions for the insane? Chicago, 1891. 16p. DNLM **90-8628**

STONE, I[saac] S[cott] (*b.* 1851)
The pedicle in hysterectomy. How formed; its subsequent behavior; its final condition. New York: William Wood & Co., 1891. 9p. 1 col. plate. DNLM **90-8629**

STONE, I[saac] S[cott] (*b.* 1851)
A case of obscure abdominal hemorrhage. [Philadelphia], 1892. 2p. DNLM **90-8630**

STONE, I[saac] S[cott] (*b.* 1851)
My operative experience in "pus cases." Chicago, 1892. 12p. DNLM **90-8631**

STONE, I[saac] S[cott] (*b.* 1851)
Note on drainage after laparotomy. New York: William Wood & Co., 1893. 2p. DNLM **90-8632**

STONE, I[saac] S[cott] (*b.* 1851)
One hundred operations for severe structural disease of the abdominal and pelvic organs of women. New York, 1893. 10p. 1 tab. DNLM **90-8633**

STONE, I[saac] S[cott] (*b.* 1851)
Pelvic abscess. Laparotomy for twenty cases. [St. Louis, 1893.] 8p. 1 tab. DNLM **90-8634**

STONE, I[saac] S[cott] (*b.* 1851)
The significance of pyrexia in surgical cases; with special reference to the temperature curve before and after laparotomy. [Toledo, O., 1893.] 7p. DNLM **90-8635**

STONE, I[saac] S[cott] (*b.* 1851)
A case of hydronephrosis; nephrectomy; recovery. Philadelphia, 1894. 2p. DNLM **90-8636**

STONE, I[saac] S[cott] (*b.* 1851)
How to remove pus tubes without rupture. Chicago, 1896. 4p. DNLM **90-8637**

STONE, I[saac] S[cott] (*b.* 1851)
Nephroptosis; movable kidney. New York, 1896. 13p. DNLM **90-8638**

STONE, I[saac] S[cott] (*b.* 1851)
Synoptical report of one hundred consecutive abdominal operations. Richmond, 1896. 4p. DNLM **90-8639**

STONE, I[saac] S[cott] (*b.* 1851)
Cholelithotomy; report of seven cases. New York: Lea Bros. & Co., 1897. 8p. DNLM **90-8640**

STONE, I[saac] S[cott] (*b.* 1851)
The surgical technique of operations for pus in the pelvis. New York: William Wood & Co., 1897. 11p. DNLM **90-8641**

STONE, I[saac] S[cott] (*b.* 1851)
Twenty-five consecutive successful supra-vaginal hysterectomies for fibroid tumors. New York, 1897. 4p. DNLM **90-8642**

STONE, I[saac] S[cott] (*b.* 1851)
Emmet's operation for lacerated perineum and relaxed vaginal outlet. New York: William Wood & Co., 1898. 5p. DNLM **90-8643**

STONE, I[saac] S[cott] (*b.* 1851)
One hundred abdominal sections. Richmond, 1898. 4p. DNLM **90-8644**

STONE, I[saac] S[cott] (*b.* 1851)
The rarity of ovarian cysts in Negresses. Philadelphia, 1899. 6p. DNLM **90-8645**

STONE, I[saac] S[cott] (*b.* 1851)
Surgical diseases of the liver. Richmond, 1899. 4 l. DNLM **90-8646**

STONE, I[saac] S[cott] (*b.* 1851)
Tumors of the kidneys. Report of four cases of nephrectomy. Richmond, 1899. 4p. DNLM **90-8647**

STONE, J[ames] S. (*b.* 1868)
Deformities of the chest in rickets. Philadelphia, 1898. 10p. DNLM **90-8648**

STONE, Richard French, ed. (1844-1913)
Biography of eminent American physicians and surgeons, illustrated with fine photo-engraved portraits. . . . Indianapolis: Carlon & Hollenbeck, 1894. 729p. ports. DLC; OCIM; NNNAM **90-8649**

STONE, Richard French (1844-1913)
Biography of eminent Americn physicians and surgeons. 2nd ed., representing all schools of medicine. Indianapolis: C. E. Hollenbeck, 1898. 857p. DNLM; MH-M; NNC; PPC **90-8650**

STONE, William Stephen (*b.* 1867)
Malignant adenoma of the uterus. New York: D. Appleton & Co., 1895. 15p. DNLM **90-8651**

STONEY, Emily M[arjory] A[rmstrong]
Some practical points in nursing for nurses in private practice. . . . Boston: Printed by J. Cashman & Co., 1895. 166p. DLC; MBM **90-8652**

STONEY, Emily M[arjory] A[rmstrong]
Practical points in nursing for nurses in private practice. . . . Philadelphia: W. B. Saunders, 1896. 456p. col. plates. DLC; NNNAM; PPC; PU **90-8653**

STONEY, Emily M[arjory] A[rmstrong]
Practical points in nursing, for nurses in private practice; with an appendix. . . . 2nd ed., thoroughly rev. Illustrated with 73 engravings in the text and a colored and half-tone plates. Philadelphia: W. B. Saunders, 1897. 456p. DLC; IEN-M; LNT-M; PPC **90-8654**

STONEY, Emily M[arjory] A[rmstrong]
Practical materia medica for nurses, with an appendix containing poisons and their antidotes . . . mineral waters; weights and measures; dose-list; and a glossary. . . . Philadelphia: W. B. Saunders, 1899. 306p. DLC; NNNAM; OCLloyd; PU **90-8655**

STORER, Horatio R[obinson] (1830-1922)
Volunteer sanitary organizatins as an aid to official boards of health. Chicago, 1890. 23p. DNLM **90-8656**

STORER, Horatio R[obinson] (1830-1922)
The medallic medical history of the United States. [Providence], 1891. 4p. DNLM **90-8657**

STORER, Horatio R[obinson] (1830-1922)
1796-1896: The memorials of Edward Jenner. Address delivered at the centennial, celebration, held at Atlanta, Ga., May, 1896. Chicago, 1896. 19p. DNLM **90-8658**

STORER, Horatio R[obinson] (1830-1922)
Criminal abortion; its prevalence, its prevention, and its relation to the medical examiner; based on the summary of the vital statistics of the New England States for the year 1892 by the six secretaries of the New England State boards of health. Providence, 1897. 34p. DNLM **90-8659**

STORER, Malcolm (*b.* 1862)
Ichthyol in gynecology. Boston, [1894]. 12p. DNLM; MBM **90-8660**

STORER, Malcolm (*b.* 1862)
A study of axis rotation, with especial reference to the torsion of ovarian tumors. Boston: Damrell & Upham, 1896. 14p. DNLM; MBM **90-8661**

STORER, Malcolm (*b.* 1862)
The traumatic rupture of ovarian cysts, with report of a case. Boston: Damrell & Upham, 1896. 13p. DNLM; MBM **90-8662**

STORER, Malcolm (*b.* 1862)
Fibroma of the vulva. Boston, 1898. 5p. DNLM; MBM **90-8663**

STORER, Malcolm (*b.* 1862)
On vulvo-vaginitis in children. Boston: Damrell & Upham, 1898. 12p. DNLM; MBM **90-8664**

STORER, Malcolm (*b.* 1862)
On retrodisplacements of the pregnant uterus. Boston: Damrell & Upham, 1899. 15p. DNLM; MBM **90-8665**

STOUT, Emanuel J. (*b.* 1878)
Six cases of labial chancre. New York: D. Appleton & Co., 1896. 6p. DNLM **90-8666**

STOUT, F. J.
Leukopathia unguium. Philadelphia: Lea Bros. & Co., 1894. 6p. DNLM **90-8667**

STOUTENBURGH, John A. (*b.* 1870)
Report of treatment of secondary anemias, with cases. New York, 1897. 4 sheets. DNLM **90-8668**

STOVER, Charles (*b.* 1854)
Mental inhibition, or self-control; and its relation to legal responsibility. Amsterdam, N.Y., 1895. 11p. DNLM **90-8669**

STOVER, George Henry (1871-1915)
A case of angina Ludovici. Philadelphia, 1894. 2p. DNLM **90-8670**

STOVER, George Henry (1871-1915)
Two cases of cutaneous vaso-motor neurosis, with speculations thereupon. Denver, 1896. 4p. DNLM **90-8671**

STOWELL, Sidney S.
Local exercise and dietetic influence upon the teeth. Philadelphia, 1895. 5p. DNLM **90-8672**

STRAHAN, Samuel A[lexander] K[enry] (*d.* 1902)
Marriage and disease. A study of heredity and the more important family degenerations. New York: D. Appleton & Co., 1892. 326p. DNLM; ICU; MH; NN **90-8673**

STRAIGHT, Howard S.
Syphilis and "apex-catarrh." Philadelphia: Lea Bros. & Co., 1894. 8p. DNLM **90-8674**

STRAIGHT, Howard S.
Unresolved amygdalitis. New York, 1896. 9p. DNLM **90-8675**

STRAIGHT, Howard S.
Headaches and upper air-passages. Cleveland, 1898. 7p. DNLM **90-8676**

STRAIGHT, Howard S.
Facts not generally appreciated concerning adenoid growths. Cleveland, 1899. 6p. DNLM **90-8677**

STREETER, John Williams (1841-1905)
The ideal physician. To the class of '92, Chicago Homoeopathic College. . . . [Chicago? 1892.] 32p. DLC **90-8678**

STRICKLER, David A. (*b.* 1869)
President's address before the Minnesota State Homoeopathic Institute, at their 26th annual session, held at Duluth, Minn., May 17th and 18th, 1892. The work of Homoeopathy. Minneapolis, Minn., 1892. 16p. DNLM **90-8679**

STRONG, Charles Pratt (1855-1893)
Cases illustrative of some of the more unusual forms of bladder disease among women. [Boston, 1890.] 11p. DNLM **90-8680**

STRONG, Charles Pratt (1855-1893)
Congenital malformation of the genital tract; persistence of the sinus uro-genitalis as a common opening with the urethra; bicornate uterus. Philadelphia: W. J. Dornan, 1891. 7p. DNLM **90-8681**

STRONG, Charles Pratt (1855-1893)
Cases of laparotomy presenting features of unusual interest. Boston: Damrell & Upham, 1892. 9p. DNLM **90-8682**

STRONG, Charles Pratt (1855-1893)
Ectopic gestation. [Boston, 1892.] 3p. DNLM **90-8683**

STRONG, Charles Pratt (1855-1893)
Hyperaesthesia of the vaginal orifice a cause of reflex pelvic pain. Boston: Damrell & Upham, 1892. 5p. DNLM **90-8684**

STRONG, Charles Pratt (1855-1893)
The relief of salpingitis by dilatation and drainage of the uterus. Boston: Damrell & Upham, 1892. 8p. DNLM **90-8685**

STRONG, Charles Pratt (1855-1893)
Total extirpation of the uterus; improved method of treating the stump. Boston: Damrell & Upham, 1892. 7p. DNLM **90-8686**

STRONG, Charles Pratt (1855-1893)
The influence of morbid conditions of the uterine adnexa upon reflex phenomena. Boston: Damrell & Upham, 1893. 5p. DNLM **90-8687**

STRONG, Charles Pratt (1855-1893)
The pelvic conditions found at a coeliotomy four years subsequent to an ectopic gestation. [Boston, 1893.] 3p. DNLM **90-8688**

STRONG, Lawrence Watson (*b.* 1870)
A study of the encapsulated bacilli. Boston, 1899. 12p. DNLM **90-8689**

STRONG, Walter (*b.* 1870)
The operative treatment of wandering spleen. Philadelphia, 1898. 5p. DNLM **90-8690**

STROUD, Bert Brenette
On the anatomy of the anus. Philadelphia, 1896. 15p. DNLM **90-8691**

STRÜMPELL, Adolf von (1853-1925)
Short guide for the clinical examination of patients, comp. for the practical students of the clinic. . . . Transl. . . . from the 3rd German ed. by Jos. L. Abt. Ann Arbor, Mich.: G. Wahr, [1892]. 39p. DLC; DNLM; ICJ; PU **90-8692**

STRÜMPELL, Adolf von (1853-1925)
A text-book of medicine, for students and practitioners. . . . 2nd American ed., transl. by permission from the 2nd and 3rd, and thoroughly rev. from the 6th German ed., by Herman F. Vickery . . . and Philip Coombs Knapp. . . . With editorial notes by Frederick C. Shattuck. . . . New York: D. Appleton & Co., 1893. 1043p. diags. DLC; IU-M; NNNAM; NcD **90-8693**

STUART, James (*b.* 1865)
The local treatment of abscesses and phlegmonous conditions. New York, 1897. 11p. DNLM **90-8694**

STUBBERT, J[ames] Edward (*b.* 1859)
The pernicious malarial fever of the Tropics. New York: Lea Bros. & Co., 1898. 6p. DNLM **90-8695**

STUBBERT, J[ames] Edward (*b.* 1859)
Sanitarium treatment of pulmonary tuberculosis. New York, 1898. 19p. DNLM **90-8696**

STUBBERT, J[ames] Edward (*b.* 1859)
Semi-annual report of the Loomis Sanatorium for Consumptives, at Liberty, Sullivan County, New York. [Includes:] Report of consulting laryngologist, by Walter F. Chappell. Philadelphia, 1898. 12p. DNLM **90-8697**

STUBBERT, J[ames] Edward (*b.* 1859)
Some statistics upon sero-therapy in tuberculosis. Philadelphia, 1898. 17p. DNLM **90-8698**

STUBBERT, J[ames] Edward (*b.* 1859)
Yellow-fever; its diagnosis and treatment. New York, 1898. 10p. DNLM **90-8699**

STUBBERT, J[ames] Edward (*b.* 1859)
Annual report of the Loomis Sanatorium for Consumptives. Philadelphia, 1899. 7p. DNLM **90-8700**

STUBBERT, J[ames] Edward (*b.* 1859)
Some auxiliaries to climatic treatment of phthisis. New York, 1899. 23p. DNLM **90-8701**

STUCKY, Thomas Hunt (*b.* 1860)
Some remarks concerning mercauro (mercuric bromide of gold and arsenic) with especial reference to its use in the treatment of neurotic conditions of specific origin. Danbury, Conn.: Danbury M. Pr. Co., 1894. 16p. DNLM **90-8702**

STUCKY, Thomas Hunt (*b.* 1860)
The gold combinations as alteratives. New York, 1895. 15p. 2 plates. DNLM **90-8703**

STUDIES in diphtheria. A contribution to the pathology of experimental diphtheria, by A. C. Abbott and A. A. Ghriskey. Diphtheria with bronchopneumonia, by Simon Flexner. Acute ulcerative endocarditis due to the bacillus diphtheriae, by W. T. Howard, Jr. Remarks by W. H. Welch. Baltimore, 1893. 7 l. 1 plate. DNLM; MdU-D **90-8704**

STURGIS, Frederic R[ussell] (1844-1919)
The student's manual of venereal disease. . . . 6th ed. . . . New York: G. P. Putnam's Sons, 1891. 196p. DLC; NNNAM; NNU-M; PU **90-8705**

STURGIS, Frederic R[ussell] (1844-1919)
On the physical causes of sexual debility in the male, as distinguished from the psychical causes. New York, 1894. 10p. DNLM **90-8706**

STURGIS, Frederic R[ussell] (1844-1919)
Are complete castrates capable of procreation? New York: Lea Bros. & Co., 1898. 15p. DNLM **90-8707**

STURGIS, Frederic R[ussell] (1844-1919)
Prostatorrhea simplex and urethrorrhea ex libidine. New York, 1898. 17p. DNLM **90-8708**

STURGIS, Frederic R[ussell] (1844-1919)
Cystoid disease of the testicle; teratoma testis? New York: I. H. Blanchard, 1899. 17 l. 3 plates. DNLM **90-8709**

STURGIS, Russell, Jr. (1856-1899)
The use of hypnotism to the first-degree, as a means of modifying or of completely eliminating a fixed idea. Boston: S. J. Parkhill & Co., 1894. 27p. DNLM **90-8710**

STURGIS, Russell, Jr. (1856-1899)
Results of further experience in the use of the suggestion under slight hypnosis. Boston: S. J. Parkhill & Co., 1899. 24p. DNLM **90-8711**

SUITER, A. Walter (*b.* 1850)
The inaugural address before the Medical Society of the State of New York. Philadelphia: W. J. Dornan, 1892. 16p. DNLM **90-8712**

SUKER, George F. (*b.* 1869)
Thiosinamine; a clinical contribution to its study. [Nashville], 1898. 7p. DNLM **90-8713**

SUKER, George F. (*b.* 1869)
Excision of the superior cervical sympathetic ganglion for glaucoma, with a report of a case. Nashville, 1899. 4p. DNLM **90-8714**

SULLIVAN, J[ohn] D. (*b.* 1841)
Clinical observations on appendicitis, with report of cases illustrating different forms of the disease. [New York: D. Appleton & Co., 1893.] 15p. DNLM **90-8715**

SUMMA, Hugo (*b.* 1859)
On xerostomia. [St. Louis, 1890.] 8p. DNLM **90-8716**

SUMMA, Hugo (*b.* 1859)
The influence of medicine on human culture. [St. Louis, 1891.] 8p. DNLM **90-8717**

SUMMA, Hugo (*b.* 1859)
The value of Gude's pepto-mangan in the treatment of anaemia. [New York: D. Appleton & Co., 1895.] 5p. DNLM **90-8718**

SUMMERS, John Edward (*b.* 1858)
The treatment of appendicitis, with illustrative cases. [Omaha, 1891.] 20p. NN **90-8719**

SUMMERS, John Edward (*b.* 1858)
Recent experience in abdominal surgery; sixteen consecutive cases. [Omaha, 1891.] 15p. DNLM **90-8720**

SUMMERS, John Edward (*b.* 1858)
The indications for amputation in chronic disease of the larger bones and joints; with a report of seventeen recent cases, including three successful amputations at the hip-joint. [Omaha, 1893.] 11p. DNLM **90-8721**

SUMMERS, John Edward (*b.* 1858)
[Clinical lectures.] [Omaha, 1894.] 10p. 1 plate. DNLM **90-8722**

SUMMERS, John Edward (*b.* 1858)
Surgery of the bile-ducts. St. Louis, [1897]. 8p. DNLM **90-8723**

SUMMERS, John Edward (*b.* 1858)
Stricture of the esophagus as a complication and sequel of typhoid fever. Report of a case cured by Abbe's operation. Philadelphia, 1899. 4p. DNLM **90-8724**

SUMMERS, John Edward (*b.* 1858)
The modern treatment of wounds. Omaha, 1899. 149p. 9 plates. CtY-M; ICJ; PPC **90-8725**

SUMMERS, John Edward (*b.* 1858)
Empyema of the gall-bladder. Lincoln, Neb., 1899. 9p. DNLM **90-8726**

SUMMERS, John Edward (*b.* 1858)
Nephro-ureterectomy for traumatic haemato-hydro-nephro-ureterosis. New York, 1899. 7p. DNLM **90-8727**

SUMMERS, John Edward (*b.* 1858)
Rubber gloves or gauntlets. Their use by physicians and surgeons. Chicago, 1899. 4p. DNLM **90-8728**

SURGERY two hundred years ago; illustrated from original copper plates. New York: T. Neely, [1895]. 23 l. 12 plates. DNLM; NNNAM **90-8729**

SUTER, William Norwood
Handbook of optics for students of ophthalmology. New York & London: The Macmillan Co., 1890. 209p. DNLM; GU; NNNAM; PU **90-8730**

SUTTON, Francis (1831-1917)
A systematic handbook of volumetric analysis. . . . 6th ed. Philadelphia: P. Blakiston's Son & Co., 1890. 554p. NNC; PPL; PU **90-8731**

SUTTON, Francis (1831-1917)
A systematic handbook of volumetric analysis. . . . 7th ed. Philadelphia: P. Blakiston's Son & Co., 1896. 587p. DNLM; MB; PPF; PU **90-8732**

SUTTON, Henry Gawen (1836-1891)
Lectures on pathology delivered at the London Hospital, edited by Maurice Eden Paul, and revised by Samuel Wilks. Philadelphia: P. Blakiston [and others], 1891. 503p. CtY-M; DNLM; PPC; PU **90-8733**

SUTTON, R[hoades] Stansbury (1841-1906)
Address before the Pittsburgh Obstetrical and Gynecological Society, Jan. 9, 1890. [Some remarks upon one hundred completed abdominal sections.] Pittsburgh: Murdoch, Kerr & Co., 1890. 7p. DNLM **90-8734**

SUTTON, R[hoades] Stansbury (1841-1906)
Simplicity an element of success in surgery. St. Louis, 1892. 4p. DNLM **90-8735**

SUTTON, R[hoades] Stansbury (1841-1906)
Last one hundred abdominal sections for removal of ovarian tumors and diseased uterine appendages. [Pittsburgh, 1894.] 7p. DNLM **90-8736**

SWAIN, Henry L[aurence] (*b.* 1846)
Adenoid tissue in the naso-pharynx and pharynx; preliminary report. [New York, 1890.] 12p. DNLM **90-8737**

SWAIN, Henry L[aurence] (*b.* 1846)
Some remarks on acute disease of the lingual tonsil. New York: D. Appleton & Co., 1896. 16p. DNLM; NNNAM **90-8738**

SWAIN, Henry L[aurence] (*b.* 1846)
The local use of the aqueous extract of the suprarenal glands of the sheep in the nose and throat. New York: D. Appleton & Co., 1898. 10p. DNLM; NNNAM **90-8739**

SWAIN, Henry L[aurence] (*b.* 1846)
Nasal and other polypi. New York, 1898. 18p. DNLM; NNNAM **90-8740**

SWAIN, Henry L[aurence] (*b.* 1846)
The relation of pathological conditions of the ethmoid region of the nose to asthma. The pathology. New York: Appleton & Co., 1899. 11p. DNLM; NNNAM **90-8741**

SWAIN, William Paul (1834-1916)
Surgical emergencies, together with the emergencies attendant on parturition and the treatment of poisoning. A manual for the use of general practitioners. 5th ed. Philadelphia: P. Blakiston, Son & Co., 1896. 254p. CU-M; DNLM; PPC; PU **90-8742**

SWAN, John M[umford] (*b.* 1870)
Anomalies occurring in the anatomical room of the University of Pennsylvania during the session of 1897-1898. [Philadelphia, 1898.] 8p. PPC; PU **90-8743**

SWAN, John M[umford] (*b.* 1870)
A manual of human anatomy, arranged for second year students. Philadelphia: F. W. S. Langmaid, 1898. 277p. DNLM; PU **90-8744**

SWAN, William E[dward] (*d.* 1906)
Report of two cases of large suppurating ovarian cysts. New York, 1898. 9p. DNLM **90-8745**

SWAN, William E[dward] (*d.* 1906)
A plea for the more frequent digital exploration of the uterine cavity, and the histological study of uterine scrapings as an aid to the diagnosis of the diseases of the uterus. New York, 1899. 18p. DNLM; NNNAM **90-8746**

SWANZY, Henry R[osborough] (1843-1913)
A handbook of the diseases of the eye and their treatment. 3rd ed. Philadelphia: P. Blakiston, Son & Co., 1890. 508p. 1 plate, 1 card explanatory of Holmgren's test. CtY-M; DNLM; NNNAM; PPC **90-8747**

SWANZY, Henry R[osborough] (1843-1913)
A handbook of the diseases of the eye and their treatment. . . . 4th ed. . . . Philadelphia: P. Blakiston, Son & Co., 1892. 518p. col. plates. DLC; DNLM; PPC; PU **90-8748**

SWANZY, Henry R[osborough] (1843-1913)
A handbook of the diseases of the eye and their treatment. 1 test card. 5th ed. Edited under supervision of the author, by Louis Werner. Philadelphia: P. Blakiston, Son & Co., 1896. 582p. 1 plate. DNLM; MBM; NNNAM; PU **90-8749**

SWANZY, Henry R[osborough] (1843-1913)
A handbook of the diseases of the eye and their treatment. . . . 6th ed., with illustrations. Philadelphia: P. Blakiston, Son & Co., 1897. 629p. fold. plate. DLC; NNNAM; PPC; PPJ **90-8750**

SWEEMER, William (*b.* 1853)
The contagion, mortality and prevention of whooping cough. Madison, Wis.: Tracy, Gibbs & Co., 1895. 6p. DNLM **90-8751**

SWEENEY, Arthur (*b.* 1858) and Charles F. DENNY
Rabies. St. Paul, 1896. 18p. DNLM **90-8752**

SWEENEY, Arthur (*b.* 1858)
Rabies; with report of cases. Minneapolis, 1897. 23p. DNLM **90-8753**

SWINBURNE, George Knowles (*b.* 1858)
The use of argonin in the acute stages of gonorrhoea; a preliminary report. New York, 1896. 13p. DNLM **90-8754**

SYMONDS, Brandreth
Tests for sugar in urine. New York, 1890. 7p. DNLM **90-8755**

SYMONDS, Brandreth
Manual of chemistry for medical students. . . . Philadelphia: P. Blakiston, Son & Co., 1890 [1889]. 154p. DLC; DNLM; PPC; PPF **90-8756**

SYMONDS, Brandreth
Manual of chemistry for medical students. . . . 2nd ed. Philadelphia: P. Blakiston, Son & Co., 1891. 154p. NN; NNNAM; PPC; PU **90-8757**

SYMPOSIUM of homoeopathic prescribing. [Chicago: Medical Advance Co., 1896.] 16p. DNLM **90-8758**

SYMPSON, E[dward] Mansel (1860-1921)
Typhlitis in the young, with notes of three cases. Read before the Lincoln Medical Society. October 29, 1890. [Philadelphia, 1891.] 10p. DNLM **90-8759**

SYMS, Parker (*b.* 1860)
The arthropathies of locomotor ataxia. [New York: D. Appleton & Co., 1895.] 12p. DNLM **90-8760**

SYMS, Parker (*b.* 1860)
Actinomycosis. Philadelphia, 1897. 17p. DNLM **90-8761**

SYMS, Parker (*b.* 1860)
Appendicitis; when to operate and how to operate. New York: D. Appleton & Co., 1897. 16p. DNLM **90-8762**

SYMS, Parker (*b.* 1860)
Bunion; its aetiology, anatomy, and operative treatment. New York, 1897. 8p. DNLM **90-8763**

SYMS, Parker (*b.* 1860)
The operative treatment of haemorrhoids. New York, 1898. 6p. DNLM **90-8764**

SYMS, Parker (*b.* 1860)
The surgery of tuberculosis of the peritoneum. New York, 1898. 8p. DNLM **90-8765**

SYMS, Parker (*b.* 1860)
Prostatectomy. Philadelphia, 1899. 7p. DNLM **90-8766**

TAFT, Charles H.
The progress of science and its influence in modern civilization. Address delivered before the American Academy of Dental Science, at its twenty-third annual meeting, Boston, Nov. 12, 1890. Boston: Rockwell & Churchill, 1891. 16p. DNLM; MBM **90-8767**

TALAMON, Charles (*b.* 1850)
Appendicitis and perityphlitis. . . . Transl. by E. P. Hurd, M.D. Detroit, Mich.: G. S. Davis, 1893. 210p. DLC; OCIM **90-8768**

TALBOT, Eugene S[olomon] (1847-1924)
Irregularities of the teeth and their treatment. . . . 2nd ed., rev. and enl. With two hundred and thirty-four illustrations. . . . Philadelphia: P. Blakiston, Son & Co., 1890. 261p. DLC; MdU-D; PPC; PU **90-8769**

TALBOT, Eugene S[olomon] (1847-1924)
Mouth-breathing not the cause of contracted jaws and high vaults. [Philadelphia, 1891.] 29p. DNLM; PPC **90-8770**

TALBOT, Eugene S[olomon] (1847-1924)
The differentiation of anterior protrusions of the upper maxilla and teeth. Philadelphia, 1891. 8p. DNLM
90-8771

TALBOT, Eugene S[olomon] (1847-1924)
Chart of typical forms of constitutional irregularities of the teeth. Philadelphia: The Wilmington Dent. Manuf. Co., 1891. 16 plates. fol. DNLM; MdU-D **90-8772**

TALBOT, Eugene S[olomon] (1847-1924)
The etiology of osseous deformities of the head, face, jaws, and teeth. 3rd ed. Chicago: W. T. Keener Co., 1894. 487p. 42 plates. DLC; DNLM; IU-M; OCIM
90-8773

TALBOT, Eugene S[olomon] (1847-1924)
Interstitial gingivitis, or so-called pyorrhoea alveolaris . . . with seventy-three illustrations. Philadelphia: The S. S. White Dental Manufacturing Co., 1899. 192p. plates. DLC; PU
90-8774

TALMEY, B[ernard] S[imon] (1862-1926)
Contributions to the study of the aetiology of varicocele. New York: D. Appleton & Co., 1894. 10p. DNLM
90-8775

TALMEY, B[ernard] S[imon] (1862-1926)
Contribution to the study of the simultaneous development of two different exanthematic diseases. New York: D. Appleton & Co., 1894. 7p. DNLM **90-8776**

TALMEY, B[ernard] S[imon] (1862-1926)
Note on a case of gallstone. New York, 1897. 10p. DNLM
90-8777

TANNER, Thomas Hawkes (1824-1871)
Memoranda on poisons. . . . 7th American from the last London ed. Rev. by John J. Reese. . . . Philadelphia: P. Blakiston, Son & Co., 1892. 177p. DLC; DNLM; NNNAM; PPC
90-8778

TAYLOR, Alfred Swaine (1806-1880)
A manual of medical jurisprudence. . . . Rev. and ed. by Thomas Stevenson. . . . 11th American, ed. with citations and additions from the 12th English ed. By Clark Bell. . . . Philadelphia: Lea Bros. & Co., 1892. 790p. DLC; DNLM; IU-M; PPC **90-8779**

TAYLOR, Alfred Swaine (1806-1880)
A manual of medical jurisprudence. . . . Rev. and ed. by Thomas Stevenson. . . . 12th American, ed with citations and additions from the 12th English ed. By Clark Bell. . . . New York and Philadelphia: Lea Bros. & Co., 1897. 832p. plates. DLC; NNNAM; PPC; PU **90-8780**

TAYLOR, Charles Fayette (1827-1899)
Climate and health. New York: D. Appleton & Co., 1895. 14p. DNLM **90-8781**

TAYLOR, Charles Fayette (1827-1899)
The spinal assistant. Autobiographical reminiscences. Philadelphia, 1899. 13p. DNLM **90-8782**

TAYLOR, Edward H[enry] (*d.* 1922)
The operative treatment of cancer of the rectum. Philadelphia, 1897. 45p. DNLM; PPC **90-8783**

TAYLOR, Edward Wyllys (1866-1932)
The mental element in the treatment of disease. Prize essay of Boylston Medical Society of Harvard University. Boston: D. Clapp & Son. 1891. 31p. DNLM; MBM **90-8784**

TAYLOR, Edward Wyllys (1866-1932)
Two cases of tumor of the brain, with autopsy. Boston: Damrell & Upham, 1896. 14p. DNLM **90-8785**

TAYLOR, Edward Wyllys (1866-1932)
Immediate effects upon the spinal cord of fractures or dislocations of the vertebrae. Boston, 1898. 3p. DNLM
90-8786

TAYLOR, Edward Wyllys (1866-1932)
Tumors of the frontal lobes; with special reference to a case with predominant symptoms of a neurasthenic type. Boston, 1898. 30p. DNLM **90-8787**

TAYLOR, Edward Wyllys (1866-1932)
Types of habit neuro-psychoses. Boston, 1898. 12p. DNLM
90-8788

TAYLOR, Edward Wyllys (1866-1932)
The hospital for chronic diseases. Boston, 1899. 11p. DNLM
90-8789

TAYLOR, Edward Wyllys (1866-1932)
Syphilitic and the parasyphilitic affections: two cases. Boston, 1899. 12p. DNLM **90-8790**

TAYLOR, Frederick (1847-1920)
A manual of the practice of medicine. Philadelphia: P. Blakiston's Son & Co., 1890. [*vel subseq.*] 895p. DNLM; PPC; PPJ; PU **90-8791**

TAYLOR, George H[erbert] (1821-1896)
Illustrated catalogue and price list of remedial apparatus. [New York], 1890. 31p. DNLM; NNNAM **90-8792**

TAYLOR, George H[erbert] (1821-1896)
Mechanical aids in the treatment of chronic forms of disease. New York: G. W. Rogers, 1893. 109p. DNLM; NNNAM
90-8793

TAYLOR, Henry Ling (1857-1923)
The rational treatment of hip-joint disease. Philadelphia: Med. Press Co., 1890. 8p. DNLM **90-8794**

TAYLOR, Henry Ling (1857-1923)
A ready method for counter-extension at the knee. Boston: Damrell & Upham, 1890. 6p. DNLM **90-8795**

TAYLOR, Henry Ling (1857-1923)
The treatment of pes equino-varus by continuous leverage. New York: Trow, 1890. 14p. DNLM **90-8796**

TAYLOR, Henry Ling (1857-1923)
The treatment of lateral curvature of the spine. [New York, 1890.] 12p. DNLM **90-8797**

TAYLOR, Henry Ling (1857-1923)
Adjusted locomotion in the treatment of the recovering stage of hip-joint disease. [New York, 1891.] 13p. DNLM; NNNAM
90-8798

TAYLOR, Henry Ling (1857-1923)
Two cases of peculiar type of primary crural asymmetry. Philadelphia, 1891. 7p. DNLM **90-8799**

TAYLOR, Henry Ling (1857-1923)
The value of mechanical treatment in old and neglected cases of Potts' disease. [Philadelphia, 1891.] 11p. DNLM
90-8800

TAYLOR, Henry Ling (1857-1923)
American childhood from a medical standpoint. New York, 1892. 16p. DNLM **90-8801**

TAYLOR, Henry Ling (1857-1923)
The treatment of club-foot by continuous leverage. [New York, 1892.] 7p. DNLM **90-8802**

TAYLOR, Henry Ling (1857-1923)
Improved long traction hip-splint with proper method of applying adhesive plaster. Augusta, Ga.: Mutal Print. Co., 1893. 4p. DNLM **90-8803**

TAYLOR, Henry Ling (1857-1923)
The mechanical treatment of osteitis of the knee. New York: D. Appleton & Co., 1893. 12p. DNLM **90-8804**

TAYLOR, Henry Ling (1857-1923)
Orthopedic papers. New York, 1893. 1 l. DNLM
90-8805

TAYLOR, Henry Ling (1857-1923)
Osteitis deformans (Paget), with report of two cases. New York: Trow, 1893. 15p. DNLM **90-8806**

TAYLOR, Henry Ling (1857-1923)
Remarks on the management of suppuration, complicating tuberculous disease of the bones and joints. New York, 1893. 11p. DNLM **90-8807**

TAYLOR, Henry Ling (1857-1923)
Infantile scorbutus. [New York, 1894.] 12p. DNLM
90-8808

TAYLOR, Henry Ling (1857-1923)
Infantile scorbutus and its relations to orthopaedic practice. New York, 1894. 8p. DNLM **90-8809**

TAYLOR, Henry Ling (1857-1923)
Congenital luxation of the knee. Philadelphia, 1895. 6p. DNLM **90-8810**

TAYLOR, Henry Ling (1857-1923)
Ingrown toe-nail mechanically treated. New York, 1896. 7p. DNLM **90-8811**

TAYLOR, Henry Ling (1857-1923)
A bivalve plastic splint for Potts' disease. New York, 1898. 7p. DNLM **90-8812**

TAYLOR, Henry Ling (1857-1923)
Exercise and vigor. New York, 1898. 6p. DNLM
90-8813

TAYLOR, Henry Ling (1857-1923)
Growth in spondylitics. New York, 1898. 5p. 1 diag. DNLM
90-8814

TAYLOR, Henry Ling (1857-1923)
The work of Charles Fayette Taylor in the field of therapeutic exercises. Boston, 1899. 13p. DNLM
90-8815

TAYLOR, Henry Ling (1857-1923)
Notes on orthopedic cases. New York, [1899-1900]. 27p. DNLM **90-8816**

TAYLOR, H[enry] Longstreet (*b.* 1857)
The results of the Shurly-Gibbes treatment of tuberculosis at Asheville, N.C. Detroit: G. S. Davis, 1891. 11p. DNLM
90-8817

TAYLOR, H[enry] Longstreet (*b.* 1857)
The situation and climate of Asheville, N.C. A paper read before the Academy of Medicine of Cincinnati, Oct. 15, 1891. [n. p., 1891.] 4p. DNLM **90-8818**

TAYLOR, H[enry] Longstreet (*b.* 1857)
The necessity of special institutions for the consumptive poor. The first step toward the complete eradication of tuberculosis. St. Paul, 1893. 13p. DNLM **90-8819**

TAYLOR, Hugh M[cGuire] (*b.* 1856)
Post-operative intestinal obstruction. Richmond, 1895. 14p. DNLM **90-8820**

TAYLOR, Hugh M[cGuire] (*b.* 1856)
Abdominal contusions with visceral lesion. [Richmond], 1896. 10p. DNLM **90-8821**

TAYLOR, Hugh M[cGuire] (*b.* 1856)
Diagnosis of bullet wounds of the abdomen. Richmond, 1898. 14p. DNLM **90-8822**

TAYLOR, Hugh M[cGuire] (*b.* 1856)
Delay as a factor in unsuccessful surgery. Savannah, 1899. 10p. DNLM **90-8823**

TAYLOR, Hugh M[cGuire] (*b.* 1856)
Perforating ulcer of duodenum; operation; recovery. Richmond, 1899. 10p. DNLM **90-8824**

TAYLOR, Hugh M[cGuire] (*b.* 1856)
Typhoid perforation; operation; recovery. Richmond, 1899. 13p. DNLM **90-8825**

TAYLOR, James H.
How shall we rear our babies? [New York, 1895.] 6p. DNLM
90-8826

TAYLOR, John Jay (*b.* 1853)
The physician as a business man; or, How to obtain the best financial results in the practice of medicine. . . . Philadelphia: The Medical World, 1891. 144p. DLC; DNLM; PPC; PU
90-8827

TAYLOR, John Madison (*b.* 1855)
The treatment of exophthalmic goiter. [Philadelphia: Lea Bros. & Co., 1893.] 23p. DNLM; PPC **90-8828**

TAYLOR, John Madison (*b.* 1855)
The insane disorders of childhood. [New York, 1893.] 16p. DNLM **90-8829**

TAYLOR, John Madison (*b.* 1855)
An epidemic of poliomyelitis. Philadelphia, 1898. 5p. DNLM
90-8830

TAYLOR, John Madison (*b.* 1855) and William H. WELLS
Manual of the diseases of children. Philadelphia: P. Blakiston's Son & Co., 1898. 743p. DNLM; NNNAM; PPC; PU
90-8831

TAYLOR, John Madison (*b.* 1855)
Hypnotic suggestion as a practical aid to medicine. Philadelphia, 1899. 7p. DNLM **90-8832**

TAYLOR, Lewis H. (*b.* 1850)
Cases and treatment of mastoid disease. [Easton, Pa., 1891.] 11p. DNLM **90-8833**

TAYLOR, Lewis H. (*b.* 1850)
Cases and treatment of mastoid disease. [Wilkesbarre, 1891.] 11p. DNLM **90-8834**

TAYLOR, Lewis H. (*b.* 1850)
The medical specialist. [Easton, Pa., 1891.] 11p. DNLM **90-8835**

TAYLOR, Lewis H. (*b.* 1850)
Typhoid fever and impure milk. [Philadelphia, 1892.] 11p. DNLM **90-8836**

TAYLOR, Lewis H. (*b.* 1850)
Double consciousness. Wilkesbarre, 1897. 14p. DNLM **90-8837**

TAYLOR, Robert W[illiam] (1842-1908)
Chronic inflammation, infiltration and ulceration of the external genitals of women, with a cosideration of the question of esthiomène, or lupus, of these parts. New York: D. Appleton & Co., 1890. 19p. 1 plate. DNLM **90-8838**

TAYLOR, Robert W[illiam] (1842-1908)
A contribution to the study of multiple neuritis of syphilitic origin. New York: D. Appleton & Co., 1890. 8p. 1 plate. DNLM **90-8839**

TAYLOR, Robert W[illiam] (1842-1908)
Some unusual modes of infection with syphilis. [New York, 1890.] 16p. DNLM **90-8840**

TAYLOR, Robert W[illiam] (1842-1908) and Ira VAN GIESON
Observations on prurigo, clinical and pathological. New York: D. Appleton & Co., 1891. 20p. 7 plates. DNLM; NNNAM **90-8841**

TAYLOR, Robert W[illiam] (1842-1908)
The pigmentary syphilide. New York: D. Appleton & Co., 1893. 6p. 3 plates. DNLM **90-8842**

TAYLOR, Robert W[illiam] (1842-1908)
The pathology and treatment of venereal diseases. Philadelphia: Lea Bros. & Co., 1895. 1002p. 7 plates. DNLM; MBM; PPC; PU **90-8843**

TAYLOR, Robert W[illiam] (1842-1908)
A practical treatise on sexual disorders of the male and female. . . . New York and Philadelphia: Lea Bros. & Co., 1897. 451p. col. plates. DLC; DNLM; NNNAM; PPC **90-8844**

TAYLOR, Seymour (*b.* 1851)
Index of medicine. A manual for the use of senior students and others. Philadelphia: Lea Bros. & Co., 1894. 794p. DNLM; NNNAM; OCIM; PPC **90-8845**

TAYLOR UNIVERSITY, FORT WAYNE, INDIANA
Catalogue for the session of 1889-1890. With prospectus for 1890-91 (including the medical department). Fort Wayne: Archer, House & Co., 1890. 29p. DNLM **90-8846**

TAYLOR, William J. (*b.* 1861)
Some anatomical and surgical relations of the parts involved in the operation of intra-cranial neurectomy of the fifth pair of nerves and removal of the Gasserion ganglion. Philadelphia, 1894. 6p. DNLM **90-8847**

TAYLOR, William W[ood] (*b.* 1854)
Brief review of my last year's work in abdominal surgery and vaginal hysterectomy. Memphis, 1898. 6p. DNLM **90-8848**

TENNESSEE MEDICAL COLLEGE, KNOXVILLE
Annual announcements for the sessions of 1890-91 to 1897-98 (2.-9.); 1899-1900 (11.); 1903-04 to 1908-09 (15.-21.). Knoxville, 1890-1903. DNLM **90-8849**

TENNESSEE MEDICAL COLLEGE, KNOXVILLE
Dental Department. Annual announcement for the session of 1894-95. Knoxville, 1894. 15p. DNLM **90-8850**

THACHER, John S[eymour] (*b.* 1856)
The diagnosis of pancreatic disease. [New York, 1892.] 13p. DNLM. NNNAM **90-8851**

THAYER, Alfred I.
A prescription of exercise for health and grace; a manual of movements for healthful and harmonious development. . . . Newark, [N.J.]: Advertiser Printing House, 1892. 46p. DLC; NN **90-8852**

THAYER, C[armi] C[asander] (1840-1916)
Extra-uterine haemorrhage in parturition. New York, 1896. 7p. DNLM **90-8853**

THAYER, O[rson] V[alentine]
Concentrated rays of the sun (solar cautery) as a remedial agent. [San Francisco: W. R. Woodward & Co., 1893.] 8p. DNLM **90-8854**

THAYER, William Henry (1822-1897)
Observations on rheumatism, especially as involving the tonsils. [New York, 1890.] 11p. DNLM **90-8855**

THAYER, William Henry (1822-1897)
Errors in ventilation. No. 2. [New York, 1892.] 4p. DNLM **90-8856**

THAYER, William Henry (1822-1897)
Veratrum viride in puerperal convulsions. Boston, 1897. 4p. DNLM **90-8857**

THAYER, William Sidney (1864-1932)
A case of super-secretion of the gastric juice. Baltimore, 1892. 6 l. DNLM **90-8858**

THAYER, William Sidney (1864-1932)
Remarks on the clinical value of Ehrlich's methods of examination of the blood. Boston, 1893. 31p. DNLM **90-8859**

THAYER, William Sidney (1864-1932)
Note on the increase in the number of the leucocytes in the blood after cold baths. [Baltimore, 1893.] 3 l. 1 tab. DNLM
90-8860

THAYER, William Sidney (1864-1932)
Note on a case of cicatricial stenosis of the pylorus following a peptic ulcer. [Baltimore, 1893.] 4p. DNLM
90-8861

THAYER, William Sidney (1864-1932)
Note on the value of guiacol applied externally as an antipyretic. [Philadelphia, 1894.] 12p. DNLM
90-8862

THAYER, William Sidney (1864-1932)
Types of malarial fever observed in Baltimore, and their relations to the season of the year. [Baltimore, 1895.] 7 l. DNLM
90-8863

THAYER, William Sidney (1864-1932)
Acute pancreatitis; parapancreatic abscess; disseminated fat-necrosis. Philadelphia, 1895. 10p. DNLM
90-8864

THAYER, William Sidney (1864-1932) and John HEWETSON
The malarial fevers of Baltimore. Baltimore, 1895. 218p. 2 plates, 5 diags. DNLM; MdU-D **90-8865**

THAYER, William Sidney (1864-1932)
Hypertrophic pulmonary osteoarthropathy and acromegaly. A clinical lecture with the histories and photographs of four cases. New York, 1896. 24p. 8 plates. DNLM
90-8866

THAYER, William Sidney (1864-1932) and George BLUMER
Ulcerative endocarditis due to the gonoccocus; gonorrhoeal septicaemia. Baltimore, 1896. 19p. DNLM
90-8867

THAYER, William Sidney (1864-1932)
Lectures on the malarial fevers. New York: D. Appleton & Co., 1897. 326p. 9 plates. DNLM **90-8868**

THAYER, William Sidney (1864-1932)
Post-diphtheritic paralysis. [Baltimore, 1897.] 5p. DNLM
90-8869

THAYER, William Sidney (1864-1932)
An address on malarial fever, delivered before the Cleveland Medical Society. Cleveland, 1897. 15p. DNLM
90-8870

THAYER, William Sidney (1864-1932)
On the parasites of malarial fevers. [New Haven, 1898.] 16p. DNLM **90-8871**

THAYER, William Sidney (1864-1932)
A third case of trichinosis with remarkable increase in the eosinophilic cells. Philadelphia, 1898. 5p. DNLM
90-8872

THAYER, William Sidney (1864-1932)
On nephritis of malarial origin. Philadelphia, 1898. 37p. DNLM
90-8873

THAYER, William Sidney (1864-1932)
Hypertrophic pulmonary osteo-arthropathy and akromegaly. Philadelphia, 1898. 16p. 1 plate. DNLM **90-8874**

THAYER, William Sidney (1864-1932)
Recent investigations concerning the haematozoa of malaria. [Richmond, 1899.] 11p. DNLM **90-8875**

THAYER, William Sidney (1864-1932)
Remarks on Cushing's paper on laparotomy for intestinal perforation in typhoid fever. [Baltimore, 1899.] 1 l. DNLM
90-8876

THAYER, William Sidney (1864-1932)
Alfredo Antunes Kanthack. [Baltimore, 1899.] 5p. DNLM
90-8877

THAYER, William Sidney (1864-1932)
Malaria. [Baltimore, 1899.] 7p. DNLM
90-8878

THAYER, William Sidney (1864-1932)
Recent investigations upon malaria. [Baltimore, 1899.] 4p. DNLM **90-8879**

THEISEN, Clement F[rank] (*b.* 1871)
A new powder for acute coryza. Albany, 1897. 2 l. DNLM
90-8880

THEISEN, Clement F[rank] (*b.* 1871)
Nasal obstruction. With particular reference to deviations of the nasal septum and hypertrophic rhinitis, and a report of three hundred and fifty operations. Albany, 1897. 16p. DNLM
90-8881

THEOBALD, Samuel (1846-1930)
Some partially successful attempts to promote the healing of old perforations of the tympanal membrane. [Hartford, Conn.], 1891. 9p. DNLM **90-8882**

THEOBALD, Samuel (1846-1930)
Subnormal accommodative power in young persons a not infrequent cause of asthenopia. [Hartford, Conn.], 1891. 9p. DNLM **90-8883**

THEOBALD, Samuel (1846-1930)
Marked impairment of central vision following prolonged use of the affected eye. [Hartford, Conn.], 1897. 5p. DNLM
90-8884

THEOBALD, Samuel (1846-1930)
Two cases of vernal catarrh in which the roller forceps was employed with good effect. [Hartford, Conn., 1897.] 3p. DNLM **90-8885**

THEOBALD, Samuel (1846-1930)
Diseases of the lacrymal apparatus. Philadelphia, 1898. 39p. 3 plates. DNLM **90-8886**

THEOBALD, Samuel (1846-1930)
Remarks upon the treatment of otomycosis by the insufflation of boracic acid and oxide of zinc. Washington, 1898. 4p. DNLM **90-8887**

THEOBALD, Samuel (1846-1930)
The treatment of entropion of the lower lid with caustic potash. St. Louis, 1898. 3p. DNLM **90-8888**

THEOBALD, Samuel (1846-1930)
A case of atrophy of the optic nerves following hemorrhage from the stomach, with a consideration of the causes of post-hemorrhagic blindness. Baltimore, 1899, 8p. 1 diag. DNLM
90-8889

THEOBALD, Samuel (1846-1930)
Report of one hundred consecutive cases of cataract extraction. New York, 1899. 23p. DNLM **90-8890**

THOMAS, A[mos] R[ussell] (1826-1895)
Evolution of the earth and man. A lecture before the Hahnemannian Institute to the students of the Hahnemannian Medical College of Philadelphia, February 2, 1892. Philadelphia, 1892. 30p. DNLM; PPHa **90-8891**

THOMAS, A[mos] R[ussell] (1826-1895)
History of anatomy. Introductory address delivered at the opening of the 45th session of the Hahnemann Medical College of Philadelphia, October 3, 1893. Philadelphia: D. J. Gallagher & Co., [1893]. 25p. DNLM; PPHa **90-8892**

THOMAS, A[mos] R[ussell] (1826-1895)
In memoriam James Kitchen, Philadelphia. Philadelphia, 1894. 8p. port. DNLM; PPHa **90-8893**

THOMAS, Charles Hermon (*b.* 1839)
The construction and adaptation of spectacle-frames. Philadelphia: W. J. Dornan, [1891]. 10p. DNLM **90-8894**

THOMAS, Charles Hermon (*b.* 1839)
An operation for the radical cure of the stricture of the lachrymal duct, with description of a stricturotome. [Philadelphia, 1892.] 7p. DNLM **90-8895**

THOMAS, Charles Hermon (*b.* 1839)
Lachrymal obstruction and its treatment. Detroit, Mich.: G. S. Davis, 1893. 10p. DNLM **90-8896**

THOMAS, Charles Hermon (*b.* 1839)
Three cases of strabismus and anomalous diplopia; an original and acquired fixation-spot in the same eve. [Hartford], 1894. 6p. DNLM **90-8897**

THOMAS, C[harles] P[reston] (*b.* 1864)
Anti-streptococcus serum. Chicago, 1897. 4p. DNLM **90-8898**

THOMAS, Eb. W. (*b.* 1858)
Rotators of the femur and their other functions. Philadelphia, 1899. 40p. DNLM; PPC **90-8899**

THOMAS, Henry M. (*b.* 1861) and Simon FLEXNER
Alveolar sarcoma of the cerebellum. Baltimore, 1896. 14p. DNLM **90-8900**

THOMAS, Henry M. (*b.* 1861) and William W. KEEN
A successful case of removal of a large brain-tumor from the left frontal region; opening and packing of the lateral ventrical and iodoform-gauze. Philadelphia, 1896. 20p. DNLM; PPC **90-8901**

THOMAS, Jerome B[eers] (*b.* 1867)
A book of detachable diet lists for albuminuria, anaemia and debility, constipation, diabetes, diarrhoea, dyspepsia, fevers, gout or uric acid diathesis, obesity, tuberculosis, and a sickroom dietary. Philadelphia: W. B. Saunders, 1895, unp. DNLM; PPC [Contains 160 detachable diet lists; and 40 detachable sheets for sickroom dietary] **90-8902**

THOMAS, John D. (*b.* 1868)
Wisdom teeth. Philadelphia: S. Loag, 1890 [1886]. 12p. DNLM; PPC **90-8903**

THOMAS, John D. (*b.* 1868)
Nitrous oxide gas viewed from a practical standpoint. [Philadelphia, 1891.] 20p. DNLM; PPC **90-8904**

THOMAS, John D. (*b.* 1868)
The anesthetic zone in nitrous-oxid anesthesia. [Philadelphia, 1893.] 5p. DNLM **90-8905**

THOMAS, John D. (*b.* 1868)
Extracting teeth, and conditions warranting such procedure. Philadelphia, 1893. 10p. DNLM **90-8906**

THOMAS, John D. (*b.* 1868)
Cold baths; their use and abuse. Chicago, 1896. 19p. DNLM **90-8907**

THOMAS, John Jenks (*b.* 1861)
Two cases of tumor of the spinal cord. New York, 1895. 20p. DNLM **90-8908**

THOMAS, John Jenks (*b.* 1861)
Diphtheritic hemiplegia. Philadelphia, 1896. 20p. DNLM **90-8909**

THOMAS, John Jenks (*b.* 1861)
Nephritis in infantile scurvy. Boston: Damrell & Upham, 1896. 15p. DNLM **90-8910**

THOMAS, John Jenks (*b.* 1861)
Two cases of acute ascending paralysis, with autopsy. Philadelphia, 1898. 28p. DNLM **90-8911**

THOMAS, John Jenks (*b.* 1861)
Acute degeneration of the nervous system in diphtheria. Boston: Damrell & Upham, 1898. 37p. DNLM; MBM **90-8912**

THOMAS, John Jenks (*b.* 1861)
A case of bone formation in the human brain, due to the presence of coccidia oviformia. [Abstr.] Boston, 1899. 3p. DNLM **90-8913**

THOMAS, John Jenks (*b.* 1861)
Two cases of injury in the cord resulting from fracture of the spine. Boston, 1899. 25p. DNLM **90-8914**

THOMAS, Joseph (1811-1891)
Lippincott's medical dictionary: a complete vocabulary of the terms used in medicine and the allied sciences; with their pronunciation, etymology, and significance . . . prepared on the basis of Thomas's Complete Medical Dictionary by Ryland W. Greene, with the editorial collaboration of John Ashhurst, Jr. . . . George A. Piersol . . . Joseph P. Remington. . . . Philadelphia, London: J. B. Lippincott Co., 1897. 1154p. DLC; NNNAM; PPC; PU **90-8915**

THOMAS, J[oseph] D.
How long is syphilis contagious? Chicago, 1894. 4p. DNLM **90-8916**

THOMAS, J[oseph] D.
The management of filiform structure of the urethra, with some observations on structure. New York, 1896. 7p. DNLM **90-8917**

THOMAS, T[heodore] Gaillard (1832-1903)
Cornelius Rea Agnew. A memorial address. New York, [1890]. 31p. NN; NNNAM **90-8918**

THOMAS, T[heodore] Gaillard (1832-1903)
Annual report of the New York Medical and Surgical Society. [1890.] 24p. DNLM **90-8919**

THOMAS, T[heodore] Gaillard (1832-1903)
A practical chart of auscultation and percussion, for the use of students. New York: J. A. Gray, [1890]. 1 l. Broadside fol. DNLM **90-8920**

THOMAS, T[heodore] Gaillard (1832-1903)
Abortion and its treatment, from the stand-point of practical experience; a special course of lectures delivered at the College of Physicians and Surgeons, New York, session of 1889-90. From notes by P. Brynberg Porter, revised by the author. New York: D. Appleton & Co., 1890. 112p. DNLM; NNNAM **90-8921**

THOMAS, T[heodore] Gaillard (1832-1903)
An address delivered before the New York Orthopaedic Dispensary and Hospital, on the occasion of its twenty-fifth anniversary, December 10, 1891. [New York, 1891.] 8p. DNLM **90-8922**

THOMAS, T[heodore] Gaillard (1832-1903)
A practical treatise on the diseases of women. . . . 6th ed., enl. and thoroughly rev. by Paul F. Mundé . . . containing three hundred and forty-seven engravings on wood. Philadelphia: Lea Bros. & Co., 1891. 826p. DLC; MBM; NNNAM; PPC **90-8923**

THOMAS, T[heodore] Gaillard (1832-1903)
The possibilities of medicine. An address. New York: J. J. O'Brien & Son, 1891. 16p. DNLM; NNNAM **90-8924**

THOMAS, T[heodore] Gaillard (1832-1903)
A successful case of Caesarean section. New York: Trow's Co., 1892. 8p. DNLM **90-8925**

THOMPSON, Alton Howard (1849-1914)
Facial expression, and its psychology. [n. p., 1890.] 7p. DNLM **90-8926**

THOMPSON, Alton Howard (1849-1914)
A manual of comparative dental anatomy for dental students; prepared by request of the National Association of Dental Faculties and adopted as a text-book for colleges August 27, 1898. Philadelphia: S. S. White Dental Mfg. Co., 1899. 176p. DNLM; MdU-D; PPC **90-8927**

THOMPSON, C[harles] O. (*b.* 1862)
Horsehair in minor surgery. Boston: W. S. Best & Co., 1893. 9p. DNLM **90-8928**

THOMPSON, Edward P[ruden]
Roentgen rays and phenomena of the anode and cathode. Principles, applications and theories. . . . Concluding chapter by Prof. William A. Anthony. . . . New York: D. Van Nostrand, [1896]. 190p. NNNAM; NNC; PPJ; PU **90-8929**

THOMPSON, Henry (1820-1904)
The preventive treatment of calculous disease, and the use of solvent remedies. [3rd ed.] Philadelphia: P. Blakiston, Son & Co., 1890 [1889]. 87p. DNLM; IU-M; PPC [1st American ed., Philadelphia: Lindsay & Blakiston, 1873. 72p.] **90-8930**

THOMPSON, Henry (1820-1904)
Diet in relation to age and activity. [Also:] Hygiene of the aged, by L. H. Watson. Philadelphia: L. S. Filbert, [1890?] 53p. DNLM; PPC **90-8931**

THOMPSON, John H[arry] (*b.* 1828)
The diseases and injuries of the conjunctiva, especially the so-called granulated lids. 1st ed. Kansas City, Mo.: H. Kimberly, 1897. 216p. DNLM; KU **90-8932**

[THOMPSON, Mary Harris] (1829-1895)
In Memoriam: Mary Harris Thompson. Chicago: Chicago Hospital for Women and Children, 1896. 59p. ICU; IU-M; [Dr. Thompson founded the Chicago Hospital for Women and Children in 1865.] **90-8933**

THOMPSON, W[illiam] Gilman (1856-1927)
Three cases of tumor of the frontal lobe. [Philadelphia, 1890.] 11p. DNLM **90-8934**

THOMPSON, W[illiam] Gilman (1856-1927)
Successful brain grafting. [New York, 1890.] 8p. DNLM **90-8935**

THOMPSON, W[illiam] Gilman (1856-1927)
Somnal; a new hypnotic. Danbury, Conn.: Danbury Med. Print. Co., 1891. 14p. DNLM **90-8936**

THOMPSON, W[illiam] Gilman (1856-1927)
A study of Addison's disease and of the adrenals. Philadelphia, 1893. 20p. DNLM; PPC **90-8937**

THOMPSON, W[illiam] Gilman (1856-1927)
Notes on the observation of malarial organisms in connection with enteric fever. Philadelphia, 1894. 6p. DNLM **90-8938**

THOMPSON, W[illiam] Gilman (1856-1927)
Practical dietetics, with special reference to diet in disease. . . . New York: D. Appleton & Co., 1895. 802p. col. plates. DLC; DNLM; NNNAM; OCIM **90-8939**

THOMSON, A[rchibald] G.
A case of accidental sponge-grafting of the conjunctiva of eighteen months' duration; with some suggestions upon sponge-grafting in eye-surgery. Philadelphia, 1895. 6p. DNLM **90-8940**

THOMSON, H[erbert] Campbell (1870-1940)
An introduction to diseases of the nervous system. New York: William Wood & Co., 1899. 123p. DNLM; NNNAM **90-8941**

THOMSON, John (1856-1926)
Guide to the clinical examination and treatment of sick children. Philadelphia & New York: Lea Bros. & Co., 1898. 336p. 12 plates. DNLM; NNNAM; OCIM; PPC **90-8942**

THOMSON, J[ohn] Arthur (*b.* 1861)
The science of life, an outline of the history of biology and its recent advances. Chicago & New York: H. S. Stone & Co., 1899. 246p. DNLM; ICU; MB; NN **90-8943**

THOMSON, Samuel (1769-1843)
New guide to health; or, Botanic family physician, containing a complete system of practice on a plan entirely new; with a description of the vegetables made use of, and directions for preparing and administering them to cure disease. . . . A reprint from 3rd ed. . . . Boston: Printed for the Author, by J. Howe, 1831; Indianapolis, Ind.: A. I. Berninger, 1894. 154p. port. DLC: OCLloyd **90-8944**

THOMSON, William (1833-1907)
A new wool-test for the detection of color-blindness. [Philadelphia, 1894.] 11p. DNLM **90-8945**

THOMSON, William (1833-1907)
Cases illustrative of different forms of color-blindness. Case I. Congenital color-blindness. Case II. Tobacco color-blindness. Case III. Traumatic color-blindness. Chicago, 1896. 12p. DNLM **90-8946**

THOMSON, William H[anna] (1833-1918)
Notes on materia medica and therapeutics taken from lectures delivered by . . . . Edited by W. M. H. Mc Enroe. 4th ed. New York: Stettiner, Lambert & Co., 1890. 303p. DNLM; NNNAM; OCLloyd **90-8947**

THOMSON, William H[anna] (1833-1918)
Notes on materia medica and therapeutics, taken from lectures delivered by . . . . Edited by William H. McEnroe. . . . 5th ed., completely rev. and enl. New York: Trow Directory, Printing & Bookbinding Co., 1894. 376p. DLC; DNLM; NNNAM **90-8948**

THOMSON, William H[anna] (1833-1918)
Original lecture on the significance of cough with reference to treatment. Danbury, Conn., 1894. 16p. DNLM **90-8949**

THOMSON, W[illiam] H[anna] (1833-1918)
Modern experimental medicine. New York: D. Appleton & Co., 1894. 32p. DNLM **90-8950**

THOMSON, W[illiam] H[anna] (1833-1918)
Further notes on the pathology and treatment of Graves's disease. New York, 1896. 32p. DNLM **90-8951**

THOMSON, W[illiam] H[anna] (1833-1918) and James EWING
A case of acute leukaemia. New York, 1898. 6p. DNLM **90-8952**

THOMSON, W[illiam] H[anna] (1833-1918) and Robert Coleman KEMP
Experimental researches on the effects of different anesthetics on the kidneys. New York, 1898. 20p. DNLM **90-8953**

THOMSON, W[illiam] H[anna] (1833-1918)
Inaugural address. New York, 1899. 15p. DNLM **90-8954**

THORBURN, William (1861-1923)
A contribution to the study of surgery of the spinal cord. Philadelphia: P. Blakiston, Son & Co., 1890 [1889]. 230p. ICJ; MBM; NNNAM; PU **90-8955**

THORINGTON, James (*b.* 1858)
An axonometer. Philadelphia, 1894. 3p. DNLM **90-8956**

THORINGTON, James (*b.* 1858)
Retinoscopy (or shadow test) in the determination of refraction at one meter distance, with the plane mirror. . . . Twenty-four illustrations. Philadelphia: P. Blakiston, Son & Co., 1897. 66p. DLC; PPC; PU **90-8957**

THORINGTON, James (*b.* 1858)
Retinoscopy (or shadow test) in the determination of refraction at one meter distance, with the plane mirror. . . . 2nd ed., rev. & enl. Thirty-eight illustrations, twelve of which are colored. Philadelphia: P. Blakiston, Son & Co., 1898. 72p. DLC; PPC; PPJ **90-8958**

THORINGTON, James (*b.* 1858)
Retinoscopy (or shadow test) in the determination of refraction at one meter of distance, with the plane mirror. . . . 3rd ed., rev. and enl., forty-three illustrations, twleve of which are colored. Philadelphia: P. Blakiston's Son & Co., 1899. 86p. DLC; PPC; PU **90-8959**

THORNBURY, Frank J.
Advances in aseptic surgery. Chicago, 1892. 19p. DNLM **90-8960**

THORNBURY, Frank J.
The demands for sterilization. New York: D. Appleton & Co., 1892. 14p. DNLM **90-8961**

THORNBURY, Frank J.
Inert tubercle bacilli; other more dangerous organisms in the sputum and lungs. [Buffalo, 1892.] 1 l. DNLM **90-8962**

THORNBURY, Frank J.
A new combination sterilizer for asepticizing simultaneously water, instruments, and dressings. New York: D. Appleton & Co., 1892. 4p. DNLM **90-8963**

THORNBURY, Frank J.
Tricuspid insufficiency. Buffalo, 1893. 3p. DNLM **90-8964**

THORNBURY, Frank J.
I. Demands for sterilization. II. A new combination sterilizer for asepticizing simultaneously water, instruments, and dressings. [New York, 1893.] 18p. DNLM **90-8965**

THORNBURY, Frank J.
The specific cure of diphtheria by antitoxin. [New York, 1894.] 22p. DNLM **90-8966**

THORNBURY, Frank J.
The pathology of trichinosis. Original observations. Philadelphia, 1897. 16p. DNLM **90-8967**

THORNDIKE, Augustus (*b.* 1863)
Spastic hemiplegia treated by open tenotomy or myotomy in the forearm and hand. [Philadelphia, 1892.] 7p. DNLM **90-8968**

THORNDIKE, Augustus (*b.* 1863)
A modification of the long traction splint for hip disease, designed to provide a light apparatus for little children. Boston, 1893. 3p. DNLM **90-8969**

THORNDIKE, Augustus (*b.* 1863)
Treatment of club-foot. Boston, 1896. 7p. DNLM **90-8970**

THORNDIKE, Augustus (*b.* 1863)
Joint-disease in infancy. [Philadelphia], 1896. 8p. DNLM
90-8971

THORNDIKE, Augustus (*b.* 1863)
Four cases of rupture of spina bifida sac, three during childbirth. [Boston, 1898.] 16p. DNLM **90-8972**

THORNDIKE, Augustus (*b.* 1863)
Congenital absence of the patella, or its tardy development. Summary of fifty-one cases, old and new. [Philadelphia], 1898. 13p. DNLM **90-8973**

THORNDIKE, Augustus (*b.* 1863)
Voluntary lateral dislocaiton of the knees in infants with lax ligaments; two cases. [Philadelphia], 1898. 3p. DNLM
90-8974

THORNDIKE, Paul (*b.* 1863)
Remarks on the disturbances that may follow instrumentation upon the male urethra and bladder. Philadelphia, 1891. 16p. DNLM **90-8975**

THORNDIKE, Paul (*b.* 1863)
A case of nephro-lithotomy, with remarks on the operation. Boston: Damrell & Upham, 1892. 8p. DNLM
90-8976

THORNDIKE, Paul (*b.* 1863)
Long-continued bladder drainage. Boston: Damrell & Upham, 1893. 7p. DNLM **90-8977**

THORNDIKE, Paul (*b.* 1863)
Remarks on pre-vesical inflammation. [New York, 1893.] 8p. DNLM **90-8978**

THORNDIKE, Paul (*b.* 1863)
Notes on phosphaturia. Boston: Damrell & Upham, 1894. 11p. DNLM **90-8979**

THORNDIKE, Paul (*b.* 1863)
A case of cystin calculus in the male bladder. [Also:] Remarks on cystinuria; examination of the urine and calculus. By J. Bergen Ogden. Boston: Damrell & Upham, 1898. 12p. DNLM
90-8980

THORNDIKE, Paul (*b.* 1863)
A few remarks on the diagnosis and treatment of rupture of the bladder. New York, 1899. 8p. DNLM
90-8981

THORNE, William Bezly (*d.* 1917)
The Schott methods of the treatment of chronic diseases of the heart, with an account of the Nauheim baths, and of the therapeutic exercises. [2nd ed.] Philadelphia: P. Blakiston's Son & Co., 1896. 83p. CtY-M; IU-M; MH; PPC
90-8982

THORNE, William Bezly (*d.* 1917)
The Schott methods of the treatment of chronic diseases of the heart, with an account of the Nauheim baths, and of the therapeutic exercises. [3rd ed.] Philadelphia: P. Blakiston's Son & Co., 1899. 132p. 15 plates. DNLM; PPC
90-8983

THORNER, Max (1859-1899)
Report of a case of partial laryngectomy for carcinoma of the larynx. Chicago, 1890. 7p. DNLM **90-8984**

THORNER, Max (1859-1899)
The object of medical societies. President's address, delivered before the Cincinnati Medical Society, Nov. 11, 1890. [Cincinnati, 1891.] 11p. DNLM **90-8985**

THORNER, Max (1859-1899)
Benign tumors of the larynx; with report of cases. [Cincinnati, 1892.] 8p. DNLM **90-8986**

THORNER, Max (1859-1899)
Intubation in an adult followed by a fatal oedema of the larynx after extraction of the tube. [St. Louis, 1893.] 1 l. DNLM **90-8987**

THORNER, Max (1859-1899)
The management of foreign bodies in the air-passages. New York, 1893. 7p. DNLM **90-8988**

THORNER, Max (1859-1899)
Pathological conditions following piercing of the lobules of the ear. Chicago: Office Amer. Med. Assoc., 1894. 7p. DNLM
90-8989

THORNER, Max (1859-1899)
Multiple papillomata of the larynx. Cincinnati, 1894. 3p. DNLM **90-8990**

THORNER, Max (1859-1899)
A new mastoid retractor. New York: Trow, 1895. 4p. DNLM
90-8991

THORNER, Max (1859-1899)
Syphilis of the nose. Cincinnati, 1896. 7p. DNLM
90-8992

THORNER, Max (1859-1899)
Serious complications of suppuration of the middle ear. [Cincinnati, 1896.] 6p. DNLM **90-8993**

THORNER, Max (1859-1899)
Uncommon accidents following operations in the nose and throat. Chicago, 1896. 4p. DNLM **90-8994**

THORNER, Max (1859-1899)
Autoscopy of the larynx and of the trachea. Chicago: Amer. Med. Assoc. Press, 1896. 8p. DNLM **90-8995**

THORNER, Max (1859-1899)
Primary syphilis of the tonsil; report of a case. St. Louis, 1897. 4p. DNLM **90-8996**

THORNER, Max (1859-1899)
Practical experience with autoscopy. Examination of the air-passages without mirror. St. Louis, 1897. 4p. DNLM
90-8997

THORNER, Max (1859-1899)
Intubation with improved instruments. Cincinnati, 1898. 3p. DNLM **90-8998**

THORNTON, E[dward] Q[uin] (*b.* 1866)
Clinical study of syrup of hydriodic acid. [Philadelphia, 1892?] 7p. DNLM **90-8999**

THORNTON, E[dward] Q[uin] (*b.* 1866)
. . . Dose-book and manual of prescription-writing, with a list of the official drugs and preparations, and also many of the newer remedies now frequently used, with their doses. . . . Philadelphia: W. B. Saunders, 1895. 334p. plates. DLC; DNLM; NNNAM; PPC **90-9000**

THORNTON, E[dward] Q[uin] (*b.* 1866)
The Medical news pocket formulary for 1899. . . . Philadelphia and New York: Lea Bros. & Co., 1899. 272p. DLC; NNNAM; PPC; PU **90-9001**

THORNTON, G[ustavus] B. (*b.* 1835)
Diphtheria; pseudo-membranous croup. [Memphis, 1895.] 8p. DNLM **90-9002**

THORNTON, John Knowdey (1845-1904)
The surgery of the kidneys. . . . Being the Harveian lectures, 1889. Philadelphia: P. Blakiston, Son & Co., 1890. 102p. DLC; NNNAM; PPC; PU **90-9003**

THORNTON, William (*b.* 1846)
The cause and cure of malignancy; an important announcement to the medical profession. [Boston, 1894.] 26p. DNLM **90-9004**

THOROUGH room disinfection by means of Schering's formalin lamp and Schering's formalin disinfector. New York, 1898. 47p. DNLM; NNNAM **90-9005**

THREE thousand questions on medical subjects arranged for self-examination; with the proper references to standard works in which the correct replies will be found. 2nd ed. Philadelphia: P. Blakiston's Son & Co., 1899. 189p. DNLM; NNNAM; OCIM; PPC **90-9006**

THRESH, John C[lough] (1850-1932)
Water and water supplies. Philadelphia: W. B. Saunders, 1896. 438p. DNLM; NNNAM; PU **90-9007**

TIERS, M. C.
A compend of anatomy and physiology. Illustrated by the New model anatomical manikin including a key, a glossary of medical terms, and incidental notes on pathology. Ed. and comp. from standard works. . . . New York: Fowler & Wells Co., 1891. 271p. DLC; NNNAM **90-9008**

TIFFANY, Flavel B[enjamin] (1846-1918)
Optometry. [St. Louis, 1893.] 24p. DNLM **90-9009**

TIFFANY, Flavel B[enjamin] (1846-1918)
Anomalies of refraction and of the muscles of the eye. Kansas City, Mo.: Hudson-Kimberly Pub. Co., 1894. 307p. PPC **90-9010**

TIFFANY, Flavel B[enjamin] (1846-1918)
Anomalies of refraction and of the muscles of the eye. Author's 2nd ed. Kansas City, Mo.: Hudson-Kimberly Pub. Co., 1896. 307p. 12 plates. DNLM; KU; OCIM **90-9011**

TIFFANY, Flavel B[enjamin] (1846-1918)
Sojourn among the oculists of Europe. Kansas City, Mo.: Hudson-Kimberly Pub. Co., 1896. 125p. DNLM; KU; NNC; PPC **90-9012**

TIFFANY, Flavel B[enjamin] (1846-1918)
Anomalies of refraction and of the muscles of the eye. Author's 3rd ed. Kansas City, Mo.: Hudson-Kimberly Pub. Co., 1898. 307p. PPC; PU **90-9013**

TIFFANY, Louis McLane (1844-1916)
The expediency of operating at one sitting upon the bladder and kidney, with report of a case in which the double operation was done. [Philadelphia, 1890.] 4p. DNLM **90-9014**

TIFFANY, Louis McLane (1844-1916)
Removal of a small solid tumor from the liver. [Philadelphia, 1892.] 4p. DNLM **90-9015**

TIFFANY, Louis McLane (1844-1916)
Osteo-sarcoma of the femur. [Philadelphia, 1892.] 4p. 1 plate. DNLM **90-9016**

TIFFANY, Louis McLane (1844-1916)
Report of additional cases of intracranial neurectomy. Philadelphia, 1895. 9p. DNLM **90-9017**

TILDEN, John Henry (1851-1940)
Cursed before birth. A few straight tips regarding our social conditions. . . . Denver, Col.: The Author, [1895] [*vel subseq.*]. 314p. DLC; DNLM; NNC **90-9018**

TILLMANNS, R[obert] Hermann (1844-1927)
The principles of surgery and surgical pathology; general rules governing operations and the application of dressings. . . . Transl. from the 3rd German ed. by John Rogers . . . and Benjamin Tilton. . . . Ed. by Lewis A. Stimson. . . . New York: D. Appleton & Co., 1894. 800p. col. illus. DLC; NNNAM; PPJ; PU **90-9019**

TILLMANNS, R[obert] Hermann (1844-1927)
A text-book of surgery . . . transl. from the . . . German ed. by John Rogers . . . and Benjamin T. Tilton . . . edited by Lewis A. Stimson. . . . New York: D. Appleton & Co., 1897-98. 3 v. DLC; MH-M; NNNAM; OCIM **90-9020**

TILLMANNS, R[obert] Hermann (1844-1927)
A text-book of surgery . . . transl. from the 7th German ed. by Benjamin T. Tilton and John Rogers. Ed. by Lewis A. Stimson. New York: D. Appleton & Co., 1897-1901. 3 v. NNNAM; PPC; PPJ; PU **90-9021**

TODD, Frank C. (*b.* 1869)
The implantation of an artificial vitreous as a substitute for enucleation of the eyeball. New York, 1898. 10p. DNLM **90-9022**

TODD, J[ames] S[cott] (*b.* 1847)
Dysentery (so called), entero-colitis. Atlanta, 1890 [1888]. 4p. DNLM **90-9023**

TOEPLITZ, Max
Clinical contribution to the study of aural syphilis. [New York, 1893.] 5p. DNLM **90-9024**

TOEPLITZ, Max
Mycosis pharyngis leptothricia. New York, 1898. 16p. DNLM **90-9025**

TOLEDO MEDICAL COLLEGE
Annual announcements for the sessions of 1892-93 to 1897-98 (12.-17.); 1900-1901 to 1902-03 (20.-22.); 1904-05 (24.); 1906-07 to 1907-08 (26.-27.). Toledo & Attica, 1892-1907. DNLM **90-9026**

TOMES, Charles S[issmore] (1846-1928)
A manual of dental anatomy, human and comparative. 3rd ed. Philadelphia: P. Blakiston, Son & Co., 1890. 492p. 1 plate. DNLM; NNNAM; PPC; PU **90-9027**

TOMES, Charles S[issmore] (1846-1928)
A manual of dental anatomy, human and comparative. 4th ed. Philadelphia: P. Blakiston, Son & Co., [1895?]. 540p. DLC; MdU-D; PU **90-9028**

TOMES, Charles S[issmore] (1846-1928)
A manual of dental anatomy, human and comparative. 5th ed. Philadelphia: P. Blakiston, Son & Co., 1898. 596p. 1 plate. DNLM; IU-M; MdU-D; PPC **90-9029**

TOMES, John (1815 1895)
A system of dental surgery. 4th ed. Philadelphia: P. Blakiston, Son & Co., 1897. 717p. DNLM; MdU-D; PPC: PU **90-9030**

TOMLINSON, H[arry] Ashton (1855-1913)
Hysterical mania? A clinical study based upon six cases under treatment at the same time in the Friends' Asylum. New York, 1891. 13p. DNLM **90-9031**

TOMLINSON, H[arry] Ashton (1855-1913)
A study of the sensory and sensory-motor disturbances associated with insanity, from a biological and physiological standpoint. New York, 1892. 14p. DNLM **90-9032**

TOMLINSON, H[arry] Ashton (1855-1913)
The genesis of hallucination, illusion and delusion. New York, 1894. 12p. DNLM **90-9033**

TOMLINSON, H[arry] Ashton (1855-1913)
A consideration of the subject of training schools, with a record of the development of the training school in this hospital [St. Peter State Hospital, St. Peter, Minn.]. [St. Peter, Minn., 1898.] 12p. DNLM **90-9034**

TOMLINSON, H[arry] Ashton (1855-1913)
Some of the problems of professional life and their relation to success in practice. St. Paul, 1899. 10p. DNLM **90-9035**

TOMPKINS, Christopher (1847-1918)
Notes on obstetrics and diseases of the puerperal state; collected and arranged by Charles R. Robins. Richmond: J. L. Hill Printing Co., 1896. 288p. DNLM; ViRA **90-9036**

TOMS, S[amuel] W[illiam] S[pencer] (*b.* 1861)
Tetanus complicating vaccinia. Philadelphia: Lea Bros. & Co., 1894. 11p. DNLM **90-9037**

TOMS, S[amuel] W[illiam] S[pencer] (*b.* 1861)
Nervous hemorrhages. A contribution to their study. Philadelphia, 1899. 9p. DNLM **90-9038**

TOOKER, Robert Newton (1841-1902)
The diseases of children and their homoeopathic treatment. A text-book for students, colleges, and practitioners. . . . Chicago: Gross & Delbridge, 1895. 813p. DLC; IU-M; OCIM; PPC **90-9039**

TOOKER, Robert N[ewton] (1841-1902)
All about the baby and preparations for its advent, together with the homoeopathic treatment of its ordinary ailments. A book for mothers. Chicago & New York: Rand, McNally & Co., [1896]. 331p. col. plate. DLC; DNLM; IU-M; OCIM **90-9040**

TOUATRE, Just [Charles] (1838-1901)
Yellow fever. Clinical notes. . . . Transl. from the French by Charles Chassaignac. . . . New Orleans: New Orleans Medical and Surgical Journal, 1898. 206p. DLC; LNT-M **90-9041**

TOUSEY, Sinclair (*b.* 1864)
Thiosinamine; a treatment for inoperable tumors and cicatricial contractions. New York, 1896. 13p. DNLM **90-9042**

TOUSEY, Sinclair (*b.* 1864)
Thiosinamine; a further study of its use in the treatment of keloid, "inoperable tumors" and cicatricial conditions, including deafness. New York, 1897. 12p. DNLM **90-9043**

TOUSEY, Sinclair (*b.* 1864)
Empyema; incision and drainage successful in two cases of very long standing, with perforation of the lung and the thoracic wall. New York, 1899. 5p. DNLM **90-9044**

TOWLES, William Beverly (1847-1893)
Notes on anatomy. 2 pts. Charlottesville, Va.: Anderson Bros., 1893. 640p. DNLM; NNNAM; PPC **90-9045**

TOWNES, W. C.
Chattanooga as a health resort. [Chicago, 1890.] 12p. DNLM **90-9046**

TOWNSEND, Charles W[endell] (*b.* 1859)
Notes on the infectious nature of acute lobar pneumonia. Boston: Damrell & Upham, 1890. 8p. DNLM **90-9047**

TOWNSEND, Charles W[endell] (*b.* 1859)
Summer diarrhoea in infants: being an analysis of the cases treated at the Sea-Shore Home during the summers of 1887, 1888, 1889. [Philadelphia, 1890.] 9p. DNLM **90-9048**

TOWNSEND, Charles W[endell] (*b.* 1859)
An epidemic of measles; with remarks on Rötheln. [Philadelphia, 1890.] 12p. DNLM **90-9049**

TOWNSEND, Charles W[endell] (*b.* 1859)
Haemorrhages in the new-born. Boston: Damrell & Upham, 1891. 11p. DNLM **90-9050**

TOWNSEND, Charles W[endell] (*b.* 1859)
The treatment of incontinence of urine in children. Boston: Damrell & Upham, 1892. 10p. DNLM **90-9051**

TOWNSEND, Charles W[endell] (*b.* **1859)**
Malaria in Boston and vincinity. Boston: Damrell & Upham, 1893. 8p. DNLM **90-9052**

TOWNSEND, Charles W[endell] (*b.* **1859)**
Placenta praevia at the Boston Lying-in Hospital. Boston: Damrell & Upham, 1893. 8p. DNLM **90-9053**

TOWNSEND, Charles W[endell] (*b.* **1859)**
Primary nasal diphtheria. Boston: Damrell & Upham, 1894. 11p. DNLM **90-9054**

TOWNSEND, Charles W[endell] (*b.* **1859)**
Chlorosis, with especial reference to its treatment by intestinal antiseptics. Boston, 1896. 7p. DNLM **90-9055**

TOWNSEND, Charles W[endell] (*b.* **1859)**
Remarks on the treatment of placenta previa, with especial reference to the use of the intra-uterine tampon after delivery. Boston, 1896. 4p. DNLM **90-9056**

TOWNSEND, Charles W[endell] (*b.* **1859)**
Scurvy in infants; a report of twelve cases. Boston, 1896. 8p. DNLM **90-9057**

TOWNSEND, Charles W[endell] (*b.* **1859)**
Congenital heart disease; a study of thirty cases. New York, 1899. 6p. DNLM **90-9058**

TOWNSEND, Charles W[endell] (*b.* **1859)**
Remarks on infant feeding, with special reference to the home modifications of milk. Read before the Boston Society for Medical Improvement. Boston: Damrell & Upham, 1899. 8p. DNLM **90-9059**

TOWNSEND, George H. (*d.* **1869)**
The relation of food to health and premature death. With collaboration of F. J. Levy, H. G. Nicks, and G. C. Crandall. St. Louis: Witt Pub. Co., 1898. 427p. 3 plates. DNLM; OCIM **90-9060**

TOWNSEND, Wisner R[obinson] (*b.* **1857)**
The diagnosis of chronic joint diseases. New York: D. Appleton & Co., 1895. 13p. DNLM **90-9061**

TOWNSEND, Wisner R[obinson] (*b.* **1857)**
The prevention of deformity after excision of the knee in children. New York, 1899. 14p. DNLM **90-9062**

TRACY, Edward A[loysius] (*b.* **1863)**
A new material for surgical splints and jackets, with a method for applying it. Chicago, 1893. 7p. DNLM **90-9063**

TRACY, Edward A[loysius] (*b.* **1863)**
A brief splint-technology for surgeons. [Philadelphia, 1894.] 12p. DNLM **90-9064**

TRACY, Edward A[loysius] (*b.* **1863)**
List of surgical splints exhibited at the Columbian Exposition, Chicago, 1893. Boston, 1894. 4 l. DNLM **90-9065**

TRACY, Edward A[loysius] (*b.* **1863)**
The new surgical splinting. A further report of cases exemplifying it. Boston: Damrell, 1895. 5p. MB **90-9066**

TRACY, Edward A[loysius] (*b.* **1863)**
The control of the spine by a new method. Boston, 1896. 5p. 1 plate. DNLM **90-9067**

TRACY, Edward A[loysius] (*b.* **1863)**
Treatment of Colles' fracture. Chicago, 1897. 4p. DNLM **90-9068**

TRACY, Edward A[loysius] (*b.* **1863)**
The passing of plaster. Chicago, 1897. 7p. DNLM **90-9069**

TRACY, Edward A[loysius] (*b.* **1863)**
The fallacies of X-ray pictures. Chicago, 1897. 7p. DNLM **90-9070**

TRACY, Edward A[loysius] (*b.* **1863)**
Modern treatment of fractures. Chicago, 1899. 4p. DNLM **90-9071**

TRACY, Edward A[loysius] (*b.* **1863)**
A safe and quick method of joint and bone fixation. Boston, 1899. 12p. DNLM **90-9072**

TRACY, Evert E. (*b.* **1870)**
Ligation of the dorsal vein of the penis for impotency. Chicago, 1897. 3 l. DNLM **90-9073**

TRACY, Roger S[herman] (1841-1926)
Hand-book of sanitary information for householders, containing facts and suggestions about ventilation, drainage, care of contagious diseases, disinfection, food, and water. With appendices on disinfectants and plumbers' materials. New York: D. Appleton & Co., 1895. 114p. DNLM; NNNAM **90-9074**

TRALL, Russell Thacher (1812-1877)
Sexual physiology and hygiene. . . . Rev. and greatly enl. New York: M. L. Holbrook Co.; [etc., etc.], 1895. 399p. DLC; NNNAM **90-9075**

TRANSACTIONS of the Antiseptic Club. Reported by Albert Abrams, a member of the San Francisco medical profession. New York: E. B. Treat, 1895. 206p. 16 plates. DNLM; NNNAM **90-9076**

TRAU, Adam
Typhoid fever complicated by twin abortion; recovery. [Reported by Arthur J. Patek.] Philadelphia, 1894. 1 l. DNLM **90-9077**

TRAWICK, A[ndrew] M.
Hippocratic oath. Memphis, 1899. 1 l. DNLM **90-9078**

A TREATISE on the Greenbrier White Sulphur Springs and its waters. Richmond: A. Hoenx Co., 1893. 34p. 1 plan. DNLM **90-9079**

TREATMENT of choleraic diarrhoea. St. Louis, Mo.: Lambert Pharmacal Co., 1893. 32p. DNLM **90-9080**

TREATMENT of uric acid manifestations with tartarlithine, and tartarlithine and sulphur. New York, [1896]. 32p. DNLM; NNNAM **90-9081**

TREVES, Frederick (1853-1923) and Hugo LANG
A German-English dictionary of medical terms. Philadelphia: P. Blakiston, Son & Co., 1890. 402p. DNLM; NNNAM; PPC; PU **90-9082**

TREVES, Frederick (1853-1923)
A manual of operative surgery. Philadelphia: Lea Bros. & Co., 1892. 2 v. CtY-M; DNLM; OCIM; PPC **90-9083**

TREVES, Frederick (1853-1923)
The student's handbook of surgical operations. (Abridged from the author's "Manual of operative surgery.") Philadelphia: Lea Bros. & Co., 1892. 495p. DNLM; IU-M; NNNAM; PPC **90-9084**

TREVES, Frederick, ed. (1853-1923)
A system of surgery, by Charles B. Ball, Arthur E. Barker [et al.]. Edited by Frederick Treves. Philadelphia: Lea Bros. & Co., 1895-96. 2 v. DNLM; NNNAM; OCIM; PPC **90-9085**

TREVES, Frederick (1853-1923)
Intestinal obstruction; its varieties with their pathology, diagnosis, and treatment. New and revised ed. New York: William Wood & Co., 1899. 565p. CtY-M; DNLM; NNNAM; OCIM **90-9086**

TROUESSART, Edouard Louis (1842-1927)
Microbes, ferments, and moulds. New York: D. Appleton & Co., 1890. 314p. ICU; MH; NIC; NN **90-9087**

TRUAX, Charles, Green & Co.
Illustrated price list of physicians' supplies, surgical instruments and drugs. 6th ed. Chicago, 1893. 1568p. NNNAM **90-9088**

TRUDEAU, E[dward] L[ivingston] (1848-1915)
The tuberculin test in incipient and suspected pulmonary tuberculosis. Philadelphia, 1897. 13p. DNLM; PPC **90-9089**

TRUDEAU, E[dward] L[ivingston] (1848-1915)
Sanitaria for the treatment of incipient tuberculosis. New York, 1897. 14p. DNLM; PPC **90-9090**

TRUDEAU, E[dward] L[ivingston] (1848-1915) and E. R. BALDWIN
A résumé of experimental studies on the preparation and effects of antitoxic serum in tuberculosis. From the Saranac Laboratory for the Study of Tuberculosis, Saranac Lake, N.Y. [Philadelphia, 1898.] 13p. DNLM; PPC **90-9091**

TRUDEAU, E[dward] L[ivingston] (1848-1915) and E. R. BALDWIN
Experimental studies on the preparation and effects of antitoxin for tuberculosis. Philadelphia, 1899. 36p. DNLM; PPC **90-9092**

TRUMAN, Henry S.
Household hand-book of medicine. . . . Chicago: Spaulding & Co., 1898. 156p. DLC **90-9093**

TUCKER, Ernest Fanning (*b.* 1861)
The mechanism of lacerations of the pelvic floor. [New York, 1894.] 5p. DNLM **90-9094**

TUCKER, Ernest Fanning (*b.* 1861)
Two cases of acute intestinal obstruction; operation; death. [New York, 1894.] 8p. DNLM **90-9095**

TUCKER, Ernest Fanning (*b.* 1861)
The treatment of prolapsus uteri. Portland, Oreg., 1894. 6p. DNLM **90-9096**

TUCKER, Ernest Fanning (*b.* 1861)
Retro-displacements of the uterus, their treatment by a new method. Portland, Oreg., [1895]. 5p. DNLM **90-9097**

TUCKER, Ernest Fanning (*b.* 1861)
The use of the curette in gynecology. Portland, Oreg., 1899. 8p. DNLM **90-9098**

TUCKER, Ervin Alden (1862-1902)
Some unusual cases of obstetrics. New York, 1896. 11p. DNLM **90-9099**

TUCKER, Genevieve
Mother, baby, and nursery. A manual for mothers. Boston: Roberts Bros., 1896. 161p. 12 plates. DNLM; MBM **90-9100**

TUCKER, James L.
A remarkable case of laryngeal oedema. Chicago: R. R. McCabe & Co., 1892. 5p. DNLM **90-9101**

TUCKER, Willis Gaylor (1849-1922)
Some educational problems. The introductory address to the eleventh lecture course at the Albany College of Pharmacy, delivered October 5, 1891. Albany, 1891. 16p. DNLM **90-9102**

TUCKER, Willis Gaylord (1849-1922)
The purification of water by chemical treatment. Albany, N.Y.: G. H. Reynolds, [1892]. 13p. DNLM **90-9103**

TUCKER, Willis Gaylord (1849-1922)
Report as director State Board of Health Laboratory, on analysis of drugs, foods, water, etc. Albany, 1894. 125p. DNLM **90-9104**

TUCKER, Willis Gaylord (1849-1922)
Pharmacy a science. The introductory address to the fourteenth lecture course at the Albany College of Pharmacy, delivered October 1, 1894. Albany: C. F. Williams, 1894. 21p. DNLM **90-9105**

TUCKER, Willis Gaylord (1849-1922)
State control in medicine. Albany: C. F. Williams, [1895]. 20p. DNLM **90-9106**

TUCKER, Willis Gaylord (1849-1922)
The adulteration of drugs. Albany: C. F. Williams, 1895. 30p. DNLM **90-9107**

TUCKER, Willis Gaylord (1849-1922)
Note on diastatic preparations. Albany, 1898. 3p. DNLM **90-9108**

TUFTS COLLEGE MEDICAL SCHOOL, BOSTON
Annual announcements for the years 1893-94 to 1896-97; 1898-99; 1899-1900; 1901-02 & 1902-03. Boston, 1893-1902. DNLM **90-9109**

TUFTS COLLEGE MEDICAL SCHOOL, BOSTON
Catalogues for the years 1893-94 to 1895-96; 1897-98; 1898-99; 1900-01 to 1901-02. Boston, 1893-1901. DNLM
90-9110

TUHOLSKE, H[erman] (*b.* 1848)
Gastro-enterestomy and pylorectomy. Philadelphia, 1890. 11p. DNLM **90-9111**

TUHOLSKE, H[erman] (*b.* 1848)
Pyloric obstruction. Philadelphia, 1893. 14p. DNLM
90-9112

TUKE, D[aniel] Hack (1827-1895)
The influence of the mind upon the body in health and disease. 2nd ed. Philadelphia: Lea Bros. & Co., 1890 [1884]. 482p. col. plates. DLC; ICJ; PPJ; PU **90-9113**

TUKE, D[aniel] Hack, ed. (1827-1895)
Dictionary of psychological medicine giving the definition, etymology, and synonyms of the terms used in medical psychology. . . . Philadelphia: P. Blakiston, Son & Co., 1892. 2 v. [paged continuously]. DNLM; IU-M; NcD; OC [Bibliography compiled by A. R. Urquhart, II, 1382-1405]
90-9114

TULANE UNIVERSITY OF LOUISIANA, NEW ORLEANS. MEDICAL DEPARTMENT
Annual report of the dean of the medical department to the president of the University, for the years 1889-90 to 1894-95; 1898-99 to 1900-01. New Orleans, 1890-1901. DNLM; LNT-M
90-9115

TULANE UNIVERSITY OF LOUISIANA, NEW ORLEANS. MEDICAL DEPARTMENT
The Tulane Medical School, 1892 (Richardson Memorial). Floor plans designed by Prof. Edmond Souchon, M.D. [New Orleans, 1892.] 9 plans. 1 phot. DNLM; LNT-M
90-9116

TULANE UNIVERSITY OF LOUISIANA, NEW ORLEANS. MEDICAL DEPARTMENT
Catalogues for the sessions of 1898-99-1908-09. New Orleans, 1899-1909. DNLM; LNT-M **90-9117**

TULEY, Henry Enos (1870-1923)
Clinical aspects of pneumonia in children. Philadelphia, 1893. 3p. DNLM **90-9118**

TULEY, Henry Enos (1870-1923)
The differentiation of acute bronchopneumonia and bronchitis in children. Louisville, 1893. 3p. DNLM
90-9119

TULEY, Henry Enos (1870-1923)
Stomach-washing in infants. Philadelphia, 1893. 9p. DNLM
90-9120

TUNIS, Joseph P[rice] (*b.* 1866)
Rib fracture from muscular action, with forty collected cases. [Philadelphia, 1890.] 9p. DNLM **90-9121**

TUNIS, Joseph P[rice] (*b.* 1866)
Traumatic tetanus in a child; recovery. [Philadelphia, 1892.] 4p. 1 plate. DNLM **90-9122**

TURCK, Fenton Benedict (1857-1932)
Diseases of the mouth, nose, and throat as aetiological factors in chronic glandular gastritis, with bacteriological studies of the pharyngeal vault. New York: D. Appleton & Co., 1895. 16p. DNLM **90-9123**

TURCK, Fenton Benedict (1857-1932)
A clinical lecture on the treatment of chronic glandular gastritis, first stage, at the Cook County Hospital, Chicago. Detroit, Mich.: G. S. Davis, 1895. 10p. DNLM
90-9124

TURCK, Fenton Benedict (1857-1932)
The treatment of the second and third stages of chronic glandular gastritis. Detroit, Mich.: G. S. Davis, 1895. 11p. DNLM **90-9125**

TURCK, Fenton Benedict (1857-1932)
Demonstration of new methods of diagnosis and treatment of diseases of the stomach and intestines. New York, 1895. 14p. DNLM **90-9216**

TURCK, Fenton Benedict (1857-1932)
The early diagnosis of carcinoma of the stomach, with the bacteriology of the stomach contents. Chicago, 1895. 8p. 1 plate. DNLM **90-9127**

TURCK, Fenton Benedict (1857-1932)
Modern method of treatment of diseases of the intestines. New York, 1897. 27p. DNLM **90-9128**

TURCK, Fenton Benedict (1857-1932)
Experimental and clinical observations on erosions of the stomach. Fort Wayne, 1897. 9p. DNLM
90-9129

TURCK, Fenton Benedict (1857-1932)
Experiments and technique of a new hydrotherapeutic method. Louisville, 1898. 4p. DNLM
90-9130

TURCK, Fenton Benedict (1857-1932)
Treatment of the abdominal viscera through the colon. Chicago, 1899. 16p. 1 plate. DNLM **90-9131**

TURCK, Raymond Custer
Surgical anatomy of hernia; observations thereon, with results of fifty dissections. Chicago: Amer. Med. Assoc. Press, 1899. 23p. DNLM **90-9132**

TURNBULL, Laurence (1821-1900)
Artificial anaesthesia. A manual of anaesthetic agents and their employment in the treatment of disease. . . . 3rd ed. Rev. and enl. . . . Philadelphia: P. Blakiston, Son & Co., 1890. 531p. fold. tab. DLC; DNLM; NNNAM; PPC
90-9133

TURNBULL, Laurence (1821-1900)
Deaths from chloroform and ether since the Hyderabad commission. With conclusions. Chicago, 1891. 24p. 1 tab. DNLM
90-9134

TURNBULL, Laurence (1821-1900)
Aural massage by condensation and rarefaction of the air in the external meatus and middle ear; its value in the treatment of various diseases of the ear. [Philadelphia, 1894.] 16p. DNLM; PPC **90-9135**

TURNBULL, Laurence (1821-1900)
Artificial anaesthesia. A manual of anaesthetic agents and their employment in the treatment of disease. . . . 4th ed. Rev. and enl. Philadelphia: P. Blakiston, Son & Co., 1896. 550p. fold. tab. DLC; DNLM; PPC; PU **90-9136**

TURNER, Dawson [Fryers Duckworth] (1857-1928)
A manual of practical medical electricity. 2nd ed. New York: William Wood & Co., 1898. 335p. 19 plates. DNLM; NNNAM [1st ed., London: Baillière, Tindall & Cox, 1893] **90-9137**

TURNER, James Edward (1822-1889)
The history of the first inebriate asylum in the world by its founder, an account of his indictment, also a sketch of the Woman's National Hospital by its projector. New York, 1898. 503p. 1 plate. DNLM; NNNAM **90-9138**

TUSSEY, A. Edgar
Principles or guides for a better selection or classification of consumptives amenable to high altitude treatment and to the selection of patients who may be more successfully treated in the environment to which they were accustomed previous to their illness. Philadelphia: P. Blakiston, Son & Co., 1896. 141p. DNLM; PPC; PPJ **90-9139**

TUTTLE, Albert H[enry] (*b.* 1861)
Animal ligatures and sutures, their variety, preparation and uses. Chicago, 1892. 12p. DNLM **90-9140**

TUTTLE, Albert H[enry] (*b.* 1861)
The surgical anatomy and surgery of the ear. Detroit, Mich.: G. S. Davis, 1892. 96p. 22 plates. DLC; DNLM; OCIM **90-9141**

TUTTLE, Albert H[enry] (*b.* 1861)
A study of the radical cure of hernia by Marcy's method. Chicago, 1893. 8p. DNLM **90-9142**

TUTTLE, Albert H[enry] (*b.* 1861)
Total extirpation of the uterus by a new method. Boston: Damrell & Upham, 1894. 11p. DNLM **90-9143**

TUTTLE, Albert H[enry] (*b.* 1861)
Two cases of disease of the Fallopian tubes, with complications, and notes on diagnosis. Boston, 1895. 7p. 2 plates. DNLM **90-9144**

TUTTLE, Albert H[enry] (*b.* 1861)
Total hysterectomy by a new vagino-abdominal method. Boston, 1895. 11p. 4 plates. DNLM **90-9145**

TUTTLE, George M[arvine] (*b.* 1866)
Diseases of children. A manual for students and practitioners. Series edited by Bern B. Gallaudet. Philadelphia & New York: Lea Bros. & Co., 1899. 386p. plates. DLC; DNLM; NNNAM; PPC **90-9146**

TUTTLE, George T. (*b.* 1850)
Kidney disease and insanity. Utica, N.Y., 1895. 12p. DNLM **90-9147**

TUTTLE, J[ames] B.
Homoeopathy vs. allopathy, in the Michigan State Prison. Jackson, Mich., 1896. 2 l. DNLM **90-9148**

TUTTLE, James P. (1857-1913)
The treatment of anorectal fistula. New York, 1893. 25p. DNLM **90-9149**

TUTTLE, James P. (1857-1913)
The rectum and urethra as related in disease. [New York, 1894.] 14p. DNLM **90-9150**

TUTTLE, James P. (1857-1913)
Extreme local dilatation in the treatment of urethral stricture and its allied conditions. [New York: D. Appleton & Co., 1895.] 6p. 1 tab. DNLM **90-9151**

TUTTLE, James P. (1857-1913)
Syphilitic ulceration of the rectum. Chicago: Amer. Med. Assoc. Press, 1896. 11p. DNLM **90-9152**

TUTTLE, James P. (1857-1913)
Cancer of the rectum. Chicago, 1897. 30p. DNLM **90-9153**

TUTTLE, James P. (1857-1913)
Local examination and treatment of diseases of the upper rectum and sigmoid flexure. [New York, 1898.] 19p. 1 plate. DNLM **90-9154**

TWOMBLY, Edward L[ambert] (*b.* 1859)
A case of anencephalia. Boston, 1896. 8p. plates. DNLM **90-9155**

TWOMBLY, Edward L[ambert] (*b.* 1859)
Vaginal myomectomy. Boston: Damrell & Upham, 1897. 15p. DNLM **90-9156**

TYNDALE, J[ulius] Hilgard (*b.* 1843)
A plea for physical diagnosis. Boston, 1890. 6p. DNLM **90-9157**

TYNDALE, J[ulius] Hilgard (*b.* 1843)
Pulmonary phthisis treated by inoculation with animal virus. [New York, 1890.] 5p. DNLM **90-9158**

TYRRELL, Charles A[lfred] (1846-1918)
The royal road to health or the secret of health without medicine. New York, 1899. 204p. DNLM; NN **90-9159**

TYSON, James (1841-1919)
A guide to the practical examination of urine. For the use of physicians and students. 7th ed. Rev. and cor. Philadelphia: P. Blakiston, Son & Co., 1890. 255p. DNLM; IUM; NNNAM; PPC **90-9160**

TYSON, James (1841-1919)
Some considerations preliminary to the study of medicine. Being the introductory address to the 124th annual session of the medical department of the University of Pennsylvania. Philadelphia: Univ. of Pennsylvania Press, 1890. 16p. DNLM; PU **90-9161**

TYSON, James (1841-1919)
The Bright's disease of pregnancy, with especial reference to its management. New York: Trow, 1891. 8p. DNLM; NNNAM **90-9162**

TYSON, James (1841-1919)
Manual of physical diagnosis, for the use of students and physicians. . . . Philadelphia: P. Blakiston, Son & Co., 1891. 136p. DLC; DNLM; PPC; PU **90-9163**

TYSON, James (1841-1919)
Valedictory address to the graduating classes in medicine and dentistry of the University of Pennsylvania. Philadelphia: W. F. Fell & Co., [1891]. 14p. DNLM; PU
90-9164

TYSON, James (1841-1919)
A guide to the practical examination of urine. For the use of physicians and students. 8th ed. Rev. and cor. Philadelphia: P. Blakiston, Son & Co., 1893. 272p. DNLM; MBM; PPC; PU
90-9165

TYSON, James (1841-1919)
Manual of physical diagnosis for the use of student and physicians. . . . 2nd ed., rev. and enl. Philadelphia: P. Blakiston, Son & Co., 1893. 241p. DLC; NNNAM; PPC; PU
90-9166

TYSON, James (1841-1919)
A clinical lecture on chlorosis. Philadelphia: Univ. Pennsylvania Press, 1893. 7p. DNLM **90-9167**

TYSON, James (1841-1919)
Heart disease or kidney disease? [Philadelphia, 1893.] 15p. DNLM **90-9168**

TYSON, James (1841-1919)
Treatment of chronic valvular disease of the heart. Detroit: G. S. Davis, 1893. 12p. DNLM **90-9169**

TYSON, James (1841-1919)
The relation between renal disease and disease of the circulatory system. [Philadelphia, 1893.] 11p. DNLM
90-9170

TYSON, James (1841-1919)
The primary or essential anaemias. [Philadelphia, 1893.] 2p. 1 plate. DNLM **90-9171**

TYSON, James (1841-1919)
A guide to the practical examination of urine. For the use of physicians and students. 9th ed. Rev. and cor. Philadelphia: P. Blakiston, Son & Co., 1895. 272p. DNLM; GU; ICRM; PPC
90-9172

TYSON, James (1841-1919)
A case of mycotic endocarditis. [Philadelphia: Lea Bros. & Co., 1895.] 15p. DNLM **90-9173**

TYSON, James (1841-1919)
The practice of medicine; a textbook for practitioners and students with special reference to diagnosis and treatment. . . . Philadelphia: P. Blakiston, Son & Co., 1896. 1184p. col. plates. DLC: DNLM; IU-M; PPC **90-9174**

TYSON, James (1841-1919)
Diagnosis in ascites. Chicago, 1897. 4p. DNLM
90-9175

TYSON, James (1841-1919)
Haematuria. Philadelphia, 1897. 7p. DNLM
90-9176

TYSON, James (1841-1919)
Report of a (i) case of hypertrophic or biliary cirrhosis, with comments on its etiology; also a (ii) case of persistent crepitant râle. [Richmond], 1897. 11p. DNLM
90-9177

TYSON, James (1841-1919)
Manual of physical diagnosis, for the use of students and physicians. . . . 3rd ed., rev. and enl. . . . Philadelphia: P. Blakiston, Son & Co., 1898. 278p. DLC; NNNAM; OCIM; PPC **90-9178**

TYSON, James (1841-1919)
The treatment of obstinate dropsies. Detroit, Mich.: W. M. Warren, 1898. 32p. DNLM **90-9179**

TYSON, James (1841-1919)
Is the uric-acid diathesis an important factor in pathology? Philadelphia, 1898. 12p. DNLM **90-9180**

TYSON, James (1841-1919)
Treatment of diabetes mellitus. Charlotte, N.C., 1898. 9p. DNLM **90-9181**

TYSON, James (1841-1919)
The use of iron and opium in Bright's disease. Chicago, 1898. 7p. DNLM **90-9182**

TYSON, James (1841-1919)
The selection of food for the sick. Philadelphia, 1898. 4p. DNLM **90-9183**

TYSON, James (1841-1919)
The general practitioner. Philadelphia, 1898. 16p. DNLM
90-9184

TYSON, James (1841-1919)
Address of the retiring president of the Philadelphia County Medical Society. Philadelphia, 1898. 3p. DNLM
90-9185

ULZER, F[erdinand] & A. FRAENKEL
Introduction to chemical-technical analysis. (Authorized translation.) With appendix by the translator, Hermann Fleck. Philadelphia: P. Blakiston's Son & Co., 1898. 188p. DNLM; NNNAM; PPC; PU **90-9186**

UNION UNIVERSITY. DEPARTMENT OF PHARMACY. ALBANY COLLEGE OF PHARMACY
Catalogues and announcements for the sessions of 1892-93 to 1912-13. Albany, 1892-1912. DNLM
90-9187

UNION UNIVERSITY. MEDICAL DEPARTMENT. ALBANY MEDICAL COLLEGE
Annual catalogues and announcements for the sessions of 1894-95 to 1913-14. Albany, 1894-1913. DNLM
90-9188

U.S. SURGEON-GENERAL'S OFFICE. LIBRARY
Alphabetical list of abbreviations of titles of medical periodicals employed in the Index-Catalogue of the library of the Surgeon-General's office, United States Army, from volume I to volume XVI inclusive. Washington: Government Printing Office, 1895. 282p. DLC; DNLM **90-9189**

U.S. SURGEON-GENERAL'S OFFICE. LIBRARY
Index-Catalogue of the library of the Surgeon-General's office, United States Army. Authors and subjects. . . . 2nd series. . . . Washington: Government Printing Office, 1896-1916. 21 v. CU-M; DNLM; MBM; OCIM **90-9190**

UNNA, Paul G[erson] (1850-1929)
Ichthyol and resorcin as representatives of the group of reducing remedies. Philadelphia: J. B. Lippincott Co., 1890. 64p. DNLM; PPC **90-9191**

UNNA, Paul G[erson] (1850-1929)
Inflammation and chemotaxis. Transl. by C. Bernard Wolff. [St. Louis, 1893.] 12p. DNLM **90-9192**

UPHAM, Henry L[auriston]
Pleasure and pain. Read at the annual meeting of Harvard Odontological Society, Boston. [Boston], 1891. 6p. DNLM **90-9193**

UPHAM, J[abez] Baxter (1820?-1902)
Some observations on the nature, treatment, and prevention of malarial fever. New York, 1896. 31p. DNLM; NNNAM **90-9194**

UPSHUR, John N[ottingham] (1848-1924)
A new cervical dilator. New York, 1895. 2p. DNLM **90-9195**

UPSON, Henry S[wift] (*b.* 1859)
On certain forms of tremor. Philadelphia, 1891. 12p. DNLM **90-9196**

UPSON, Henry S[wift] (*b.* 1859)
Report on progress in neurology. Cleveland: Bull & Hubbell, 1893. 7p. DNLM **90-9197**

UPSON, Henry S[wift] (*b.* 1859)
The spleen as a bactericide. Philadelphia, 1895. 4p. DNLM **90-9198**

UPSON, Henry S[wift] (*b.* 1859)
Intestinal indigestion in its clinical aspects. New York: D. Appleton & Co., 1897. 10p. DNLM **90-9199**

THE USE and abuse of dental charity. [New York, 1891.] 2 l. DNLM **90-9200**

[VACCINATION]
Terrible results of vaccination. By eminent authors. Providence: Snow and Farnham, printers, 1892. 8 pts. DNLM; RPB [Contents: Wilkinson, James John Garth. Small pox and vaccination. Providence, Snow & Farnham, 1892. 44p.; —— Compulsory vaccination, its wickedness to the poor. 1892. 48p.; Testimonies concerning vaccination and its enforcement: by scientists, statisticians, philosophers, publicists, and vaccine physicians. 1892. vi, [7]-38p.; The case against compulsory vaccination. [N.d.] 201-14p.; Tebb, William. The results of vaccination, and the inequity and injustice of its enforcement. 1892. vi, [7]-37p., [2] p. advts.; Wilkinson. Pasetur and Jenner, an example and a warning. [N.d.] 8p.; St. Pancras Anti-Compulsory Vaccination Society. [N.d.] 16p.; Taylor, Peter Alfred. Speeches of Mr. P. A. Taylor and Mr. C. H. Hopwood on vaccination. 1892. 44p.] **90-9201**

VALDIRI, Alcides
What is disease and how it can be cured? Essay. Philadelphia: G. S. Harris & Sons, 1894. 12p. DNLM; PPC **90-9202**

VALENTINE, Ferdinand C[arl] (1851-1910)
When may gonorrheal patients marry? New York: G. A. Sykes, 1895. 6p. DNLM **90-9203**

VALENTINE, Ferdinand C[arl] (1851-1910)
Urethroscopy in chronic urethritis. The largest catheter always. New York: G. A. Sykes, 1895. 8p. DNLM **90-9204**

VALENTINE, Ferdinand C[arl] (1851-1910)
The protection of the innocent from gonorrhea. St. Louis, 1896. 4p. DNLM **90-9205**

VALENTINE, Ferdinand C[arl] (1851-1910)
The rapid cure of gonorrhoea. New York, 1896. 8p. DNLM **90-9206**

VALENTINE, Ferdinand C[arl] (1851-1910)
A contribution to the study of the symptoms of chronic urethritis. Chicago, 1898. 19p. DNLM **90-9207**

VALENTINE, Ferdinand C[arl] (1851-1910)
Advice to gonorrheal patients. Philadelphia, 1899. 18p. DNLM **90-9208**

VALENTINE'S MEAT JUICE CO.
Medical reports on Valentine's meat-juice as a nutrient in phthisis, pneumonia, and allied diseases. [Richmond, Va., 1893.] 23p. DNLM **90-9209**

VALK, Francis (1845-1919)
Lectures on the errors of refraction and their correction with glasses, delivered at the New York Post-Graduate Medical School, with illustrative cases from practice, both private and clinical 3rd ed. New York: G. P. Putnam, 1892. 257p. illus., diags. DLC; NNC; NNNAM; PU [2nd ed. (1890, 241p.) is a reprint of 1st ed. (1889) with no change] **90-9210**

VALK, Francis (1845-1919)
Cataract extraction with the iris retractor. [New York: D. Appleton & Co., 1893.] 12p. DNLM **90-9211**

VALK, Francis (1845-1919)
Strabismus, or crossed eyes. How shall we treat them? [New York: D. Appleton & Co., 1894.] 12p. DNLM **90-9212**

VALK, Francis (1845-1919)
Lectures on the errors of refraction and their correction with glasses, delivered at the New York Post-Graduate Medical School, with illustrative cases from practice, both private and clinical. 4th ed. New York: G. P. Putnam, 1895. 257p. plates (part. col.). DNLM; NcD; PPC: PU **90-9213**

VALK, Francis (1845-1919)
An operation for shortening the ocular muscles in asthenopia, etc. New York, 1896. 10p. DNLM **90-9214**

VALK, Francis (1845-1919)
The curvature of a cornea in reference to the refractive condition of the dioptric apparatus in the two principal meridians. [Chicago, 1897.] 14p. DNLM **90-9215**

VAN ARSDALE, William Waldo (1856?-1899)
Nitrogen monoxide and oxygen for anaesthesia in minor surgical operations. With a report of fifty cases. [Philadelphia, 1891.] 20p. DNLM **90-9216**

VAN ARSDALE, William Waldo (1856?-1899)
Sprains; a report of twelve hundred and thirty-one recent cases treated by massage at the Good Samaritan and Eastern Dispensaries, reported by A. Ernest Gallant. Philadelphia, 1895. 17p. DNLM; PPC **90-9217**

VAN BRAUN, William W.
Inordinate paroxysmal palpitation of the heart and its treatment. Philadelphia, 1890. 6p. DNLM **90-9218**

VAN BRAUN, William W.
The treatment of endocardial complications in the diseases of children. Philadelphia, 1890. 6p. DNLM **90-9219**

VAN BRAUN, William W.
Causticum in laryngeal affections. Philadelphia, 1891. 3p. DNLM **90-9220**

VAN BRAUN, William W.
Where shall we send our consumptives? Philadelphia, 1891. 10p. DNLM **90-9221**

VAN BRAUN, William W.
Some points bearing upon the prognosis and treatment of valvular heart diseases. Philadelphia, 1892. 7p. DNLM **90-9222**

VANDERBECK, C[ornelius] C. (*b.* 1852)
Narcotic inebriety. Paper No. 1. Opium. [San Francisco, 1894?] 16p. DNLM **90-9223**

VANDERBILT UNIVERSITY, NASHVILLE. DEPARTMENT OF DENTISTRY
Annual announcements for the sessions of 1892-93 to 1905-06. Nashville, 1893-1906. DNLM **90-9224**

VANDERBILT UNIVERSITY, NASHVILLE. DEPARTMENT OF DENTISTRY
Requirements for admission. Nashville, 1899. 1 l. DNLM **90-9225**

VANDERBILT UNIVERSITY, NASHVILLE. MEDICAL DEPARTMENT
Annual announcements for the sessions of 1895-96 (23.); 1900-01 to 1903-04 (28.-31.); 1905-06 (33.). Nashville, 1896-1906. DNLM **90-9226**

VANDERPOEL, Waldron B.
Albuminuria without manifest organic renal lesion. New York: Trow Directory, 1893. 30p. DNLM; NNNAM **90-9227**

VANDER VEER, Albert (1841-1929)
The medico-legal aspect of abdominal section. "She thought it was her change of life." Chicago, 1890. 19p. DNLM **90-9228**

VANDER VEER, Albert (1841-1929)
Comparison between perineal and supra-pubic cystotomy, with report of cases. Albany, N.Y.: Burdick & Taylor, [1890]. 15p. DNLM **90-9229**

VANDER VEER, Albert (1841-1929)
Appendicitis: the relation of the physician and the surgeon in the care of cases. [Philadelphia, 1891.] 4p. DNLM **90-9230**

VANDER VEER, Albert (1841-1929)
The relation of the board of health to the public. . . . An address delivered before the Albany Institute, May, 1891. Albany: Taylor & Roberts, 1891. 15p. N **90-9231**

VANDER VEER, Albert (1841-1929)
Report of cases of molecystotomy, with special reference to the treatment of calculus lodging in the common duct. [Philadelphia, 1891.] 8p. DNLM **90-9232**

VANDER VEER, Albert (1841-1929)
Report on a case of haematophilia, or a family of bleeders. [Philadelphia, 1891.] 4p. DNLM **90-9233**

VANDER VEER, Albert (1841-1929)
Tubercular peritonitis. [Richmond, 1891.] 8p. DNLM **90-9234**

VANDER VEER, Albert (1841-1929)
Retro-peritoneal tumors; their anatomical relations, pathology, diagnosis, and treatment. With a report of cases. [Philadelphia, 1892.] 13p. DNLM **90-9235**

VANDER VEER, Albert (1841-1929)
Hystero-epilepsy, with report of cases. [Philadelphia, 1892.] 8p. DNLM **90-9236**

VANDER VEER, Albert (1841-1929)
Some considerations in reference to uterine hemorrhage, puerperal and non-puerperal. Toledo, O., 1892. 18p. DNLM **90-9237**

VANDER VEER, Albert (1841-1929)
The use of the curette in uterine surgery. Albany: C. F. Williams, 1892. 17p. DNLM **90-9238**

VANDER VEER, Albert (1841-1929)
Report of one hundred and forty-five operations done for the removal of ovarian tumors and pathological conditions associated with the ovaries and uterine appendages only. Albany, 1895. 52p. DNLM; NNNAM **90-9239**

VANDER VEER, Albert (1841-1929)
Tuberculosis of the female genital organs, including tuberculosis of the kidney. [Detroit, 1896.] 24p. DNLM **90-9240**

VANDER VEER, Albert (1841-1929)
Report of seven cases of abdominal surgery in which the Murphy button was applied. Louisville, Ky., 1896. 12p. DNLM **90-9241**

VANDER VEER, Albert (1841-1929)
Presentation of two pathological specimens. Boston, 1897. 7p. DNLM **90-9242**

VANDER VEER, Albert (1841-1929)
A description of hospital buildings on the pavilion plan. Albany, 1898. 15p. 3 plans, 1 plate. DNLM **90-9243**

VANDER VEER, Albert (1841-1929)
Foreign bodies in the oesophagus, with report of cases. Chicago, 1899. 12p. DNLM **90-9244**

VANDER VEER, Albert (1841-1929)
Some unusual cases of appendicitis with complications. New York, 1899. 19p. DNLM **90-9245**

VAN DE WARKER, [Edward] Ely (1841-1910)
Stricture of the urethra in women. New York: Trow's Printing & Bookbinding Co., 1890. 16p. DNLM
90-9246

VAN DE WARKER, [Edward] Ely (1841-1910)
Temporary compression of the stump in laparo-hysterectomy. A new method. Toledo, O., [1891]. 8p. DNLM
90-9247

VAN DE WARKER, [Edward] Ely (1841-1910)
The treatment of chronic pelvic pain. [Toledo, 1893.] 7p. DNLM **90-9248**

VAN DE WARKER, [Edward] Ely (1841-1910)
Rare complications in two cases of hysterectomy. New York: J. D. Emmet, 1896. 6p. DNLM **90-9249**

VAN DE WARKER, [Edward] Ely (1841-1910)
Intravenous transfusion of saline solution with a new apparatus. New York, 1896. 12p. DNLM
90-9250

VAN DE WARKER, [Edward] Ely (1841-1910)
Psoas abscess in women. Buffalo, 1898. 5p. DNLM
90-9251

VAN DE WARKER, [Edward] Ely (1841-1910)
The relations of pelvic cellulitis to recent pelvic surgery. New York, 1899. 36p. DNLM **90-9252**

VAN DE WARKER, [Edward] Ely (1841-1910)
Formalin; its good and bad qualities. New York, 1899. 4p. DNLM **90-9253**

VAN DE WARKER, [Edward] Ely (1841-1910)
The diagnosis of tuberculosis of the peritoneum. New York, 1890. 24p. DNLM **90-9254**

VAN FLEET, Frank (*b.* 1860)
Ophthalmic reprints. New York: Van Fleet, 1892. 40p. DNLM; NNNAM **90-9255**

VAN FLEET, Frank (*b.* 1860)
The purpose and necessity of medical laws, with a brief history of the so-called optometry bill. Albany, 1897. 18p. 1 tab. DNLM **90-9256**

VAN GIESON, Ira T[hompson] (1866-1913)
A contribution to the pathology of the laryngeal and other crises in tabes dorsalis. New York: M. J. Rooney & Co., [1890]. 14p. DNLM; NNNAM **90-9257**

VAN GIESON, Ira T[hompson] (1866-1913)
Alternate paralysis due to multiple areas of softening in the pons Varolii. [New York, 1891.] 3p. DNLM
90-9258

VAN GIESON, Ira T[hompson] (1866-1913)
A report of the gross and microscopical examinations in six cases of death by strong electrical currents. New York: D. Appleton & Co., 1892. 19p. 1 plate. DNLM; NNNAM
90-9259

VAN GIESON, Ira T[hompson] (1866-1913)
A case of traumatic myelitis in the lower dorsal region with a central column of necrosis extending above the lesion throughout the whole dorsal and cervical regions. [New York, 1892.] 4p. 1 plate. DNLM **90-9260**

VAN GIESON, Ira T[hompson] (1866-1913)
A study of the artefacts of the nervous system, the topographical alterations of the gray and white matters of the spinal cord caused by autopsy bruises, and a consideration of heterotopia of the spinal cord. New York: D. Appleton & Co., 1892. 119p. 9 plates. CtY-M; DNLM; NNNAM; PPC
90-9261

VAN GIESON, Ira T[hompson] (1866-1913)
A contribution to the pathology of traumatic epilepsy, comprising the report of the microscopical examination in two cases operated upon by trephining. New York, 1893. 32p. DNLM; NNNAM **90-9262**

VAN GIESON, Ira T[hompson] (1866-1913)
Discussion of the papers on auto-intoxication of the nervous system. Boston, 1897. 5p. DNLM **90-9263**

VAN GIESON, Ira T[hompson] (1866-1913)
Haemato-myelopore, a new spinal cord disease. [New York, 1897.] 3p. DNLM **90-9264**

VAN GIESON, Ira T[hompson] (1866-1913)
Remarks on the scope and organization of the Pathological Institute of the New York State Hospitals. Utica, [1897]. 20p. DNLM **90-9265**

VAN GIESON, Ira T[hompson] (1866-1913)
A brief résumé of some of the relations of the scientific investigations of the insane to public medicine as presented in the first report of the Pathological Institute of the New York State Hospitals. New York, 1897. 7p. DNLM **90-9266**

VAN GIESON, Ira T[hompson] (1866-1913) and Boris SIDIS
Epilepsy and expert testimony. [Utica, 1897.] 24p. DNLM
90-9267

VAN HARLINGEN, Arthur (1845-1936)
Handbook of the diagnosis and treatment of skin diseases. . . . 3rd ed., enl. and rev. . . . Philadelphia: P. Blakiston, Son & Co., 1895. 577p. col. plats. DLC; DNLM; NNNAM; PPC
90-9268

VAN HOOK, Weller (*b.* 1862)
The prostatectomies. Celiotomy for tuberculous salpingitis. Philadelphia, 1893. 7p. DNLM **90-9269**

VAN HOOK, Weller (*b.* 1862)
The surgery of the ureters; a clinical, literary and experimental research. Chicago, 1893. 16p. DNLM
90-9270

VAN HOOK, Weller (*b.* 1862)
Experimental reunion of the transversely divided vas deferens. Philadelphia, 1894. 5p. DNLM **90-9271**

VAN HOOK, Weller (*b.* 1862)
The advantages and technique of capillary abdominal drainage. New York, 1896. 6p. DNLM **90-9272**

VAN HOOK, Weller (*b.* 1862)
Strangulated inguinal hernia of a cystic appendix vermiformis. New York, 1896. 13p. DNLM **90-9273**

VAN HOUTEN & TEN BROECK
The Morton-Wimshurst-Holtz influence machine for x-ray purposes. . . . New York, 1898. 15p. NNNAM
90-9274

VAN LENNEP, G[ustav] A.
Dislocation forward of the head of the ulna at the wrist-joint; fracture of the styloid process of the ulna. Philadelphia, 1897. 4p. 2 plates. DNLM **90-9275**

VAN LENNEP, William B. (1853-1919)
Cases of abdominal surgery. [Philadelphia, 1890.] 11p. DNLM **90-9276**

VAN LENNEP, William B. (1853-1919)
Suprapubic drainage of the bladder. Philadelphia, 1890. 7p. DNLM **90-9277**

VAN LENNEP, William B. (1853-1919)
A new surgical bag. [Philadelphia, 1891.] 10p. DNLM **90-9278**

VAN LENNEP, William B. (1853-1919)
Inflammations of the right iliac fossa and their surgical treatment. [Philadelphia, 1891.] 22p. DNLM **90-9279**

VAN LENNEP, William B. (1853-1919)
Notes on intestinal surgery. Philadelphia, 1891. 6p. DNLM **90-9280**

VAN LENNEP, William B. (1853-1919)
Cases of cranial fracture, with remarks and presentation of cases. Philadelphia, 1892. 11p. DNLM **90-9281**

VAN LENNEP, William B. (1853-1919)
A modification in the technique of operations for the repair of complete perineal lacerations. Philadelphia, 1892. 2p. DNLM **90-9282**

VAN LENNEP, William B. (1853-1919)
Cases of cranial fracture, with remarks and presentation of cases. [Philadelphia, 1892.] 11p. DNLM **90-9283**

VAN LENNEP, William B. (1853-1919)
A modification in the technique of operations for the repair of complete perineal lacerations. Philadelphia, 1892. 2p. DNLM **90-9284**

VAN LENNEP, William B. (1853-1919)
The rectal mucous membrane as a means of preventing infection in operations about the anus. [n. p., 1892.] 4p. DNLM **90-9285**

VAN LENNEP, William B. (1853-1919)
A contribution to plastic surgery. Philadelphia, 1893. 12p. 4 plates. DNLM **90-9286**

VAN LENNEP, William B. (1853-1919)
Closure of wounds in large veins. Philadelphia, 1893. 6p. DNLM **90-9287**

VAN LENNEP, William B. (1853-1919)
Appendicitis. Philadelphia, 1893. 12p. DNLM **90-9288**

VAN LENNEP, William B. (1853-1919)
Inaugural address on surgery. Philadelphia, 1893. 12p. DNLM **90-9289**

VAN LENNEP, William B. (1853-1919)
A contribution to plastic surgery. Philadelphia, 1893. 12p. 4 plates. DNLM **90-9290**

VAN LENNEP, William B. (1853-1919)
Closure of wounds in large veins. Philadelphia, 1893. 6p. DNLM **90-9291**

VAN LENNEP, William B. (1853-1919)
Early operations in head injuries. Chicago: Med. Century Co., [1894]. 15p. DNLM **90-9292**

VAN LENNEP, William B. (1853-1919)
Appendicitis, with especial reference to its diagnosis and the indications for operation. Philadelphia: Sherman & Co., [1895]. 22p. DNLM **90-9293**

VAN LENNEP, William B. (1853-1919)
History of surgery; introductory lecture to the forty-eighth session of the Hahnemann Medical College. [Philadelphia, 1895.] 12p. DNLM **90-9294**

VAN LENNEP, William B. (1853-1919)
Clinical lecture. Intracapsular fracture of the right femoral neck. Philadelphia, 1896. 8p. DNLM **90-9295**

VAN LENNEP, William B. (1853-1919)
Clinical lecture. Fracture of the skull. Necrosis of the skull. Microcephalus. Philadelpia, 1897. 9p. DNLM **90-9296**

VAN LENNEP, William B. (1853-1919)
A few thoughts concerning fractures. Philadelphia, 1897. 16p. 10 plates. DNLM **90-9297**

VAN LENNEP, William B. (1853-1919)
Clinical lecture. Hernia. Subcoracoid luxation of right humerus. Philadelphia, 1897. 8p. DNLM **90-9298**

VAN LENNEP, William B. (1853-1919)
Clinical lecture. Exostosis of the tibia. Secondary sarcoma of the skull. Philadelphia, 1897. 10p. DNLM **90-9299**

VAN LENNEP, William B. (1853-1919)
Some unusual cases of appendicitis. New York, 1897. 4p. DNLM **90-9300**

VAN LENNEP, William B. (1853-1919)
Appendicitis. Philadelphia, 1897. 33p. DNLM **90-9301**

VAN LENNEP, William B. (1853-1919)
An unusual case of abdominal hemorrhage. New York, 1898. 5p. DNLM **90-9302**

VAN LENNEP, William B. (1853-1919)
Three cases of bladder tumor. Philadelphia, 1898. 10p. DNLM **90-9303**

VAN LENNEP, William B. (1853-1919)
A plea for early operation in mammary tumors. Philadelphia, 1898. 12p. DNLM **90-9304**

VAN LENNEP, William B. (1853-1919)
A few desultory remarks on femoral hernia. Chicago, 1898. 19p. DNLM **90-9305**

VAN LENNEP, William B. (1853-1919)
Amputation at the hip joint. Chicago, 1898. 12p. DNLM **90-9306**

VAN LENNEP, William B. (1853-1919)
The present status of the surgery of the kidney and ureter. Philadelphia, 1899. 16p. DNLM **90-9307**

VAN NÜYS, Thomas C[harlton]
Chemical analysis of healthy and diseased urine, qualitative and quantitative. Philadelphia: P. Blakiston, Son & Co., 1890 [1888]. 187p. DLC; DNLM; ICJ; PPC **90-9308**

VANSANT, E[ugene] Larue (*b.* 1859)
A case of syphilitic cicatricial adhesion of the tongue to the palate and pharyngeal walls, with notes of operation. [Philadelphia: Lea Bros. & Co., 1894.] 7p. DNLM **90-9309**

VANSANT, E[ugene] Larue (*b.* 1859)
Removal of a needle from the larynx. Philadelphia, 1894. 4p. DNLM **90-9310**

VANSANT, E[ugene] Larue (*b.* 1859)
A new and successful treatment of certain forms of headache. Philadelphia, 1898. 10p. DNLM **90-9311**

VAN SCHAICK, George Gray (*b.* 1861)
Insomnia in surgery, and its treatment. [New York: D. Appleton & Co., 1895.] 7p. DNLM **90-9312**

VAN VALZAH, William W[ard] (*b.* 1849)
The modern management of dyspepsia and chronic gastritis. [New York, 1891.] 20p. DNLM **90-9313**

VAN VALZAH, William W[ard] (*b.* 1849)
The chronic disorders of the digestive tube. New York: J. H. Vail & Co., 1892. 151p. DLC; DNLM; NNNAM **90-9314**

VAN VALZAH, William W[ard] (*b.* 1849)
On the nature and preventive treatment of seasickness. [New York, 1892.] 18p. DNLM; NNNAM **90-9315**

VAN VALZAH, William W[ard] (*b.* 1849)
The diseases of the stomach, by William W. Van Valzah . . . and J. Douglas Nisbet. . . . Philadelphia: W B. Saunders, 1898. 674p. DLC; NNNAM; PPC; PU **90-9316**

VAUGHAN, B[ernard] E.
A new method of treating acute urethritis. [New York: D. Appleton & Co., 1892.] 35p. 1 tab. DNLM; NNNAM **90-9317**

VAUGHAN, George Tully (1859-1948)
Hepatic abscess. Philadelphia, 1894. 6p. DNLM **90-9318**

VAUGHAN, George Tully (1859-1948)
A new operation for the radical cure of inguinal hernia. Chicago, 1896. 3p. DNLM **90-9319**

VAUGHAN, George Tully (1859-1948)
Gunshot wound of the abdomen; ten intestinal perforations and twelve perforations of the mesentery; operation; recovery. [New York], 1898. 4p. DNLM **90-9320**

VAUGHAN, George Tully (1859-1948)
Excision of the right clavicle for osteosarcoma. Philadelphia, 1898. 3p. DNLM **90-9321**

VAUGHAN, Paul Turner
Material infection as a factor in causing eye disease. New York, 1899. 6p. DNLM **90-9322**

VAUGHAN, Victor C[larence] (1851-1929) and Frederick G. NOVY
Ptomaines, leucomaines, and bacterial proteids; or the chemical factors in the causation of disease. 2nd ed. Philadelphia: Lea Bros. & Co., 1891. 391p. 1 tab. DNLM; OCIM; PPC **90-9323**

VAUGHAN, Victor C[larence] (1851-1929)
The infection of food. Detroit, 1892. 15p. DNLM **90-9324**

VAUGHAN, Victor C[larence] (1851-1929) and Charles T. McCLINTOCK
The nature of the germicidal constituent of blood-serum. [Philadelphia, 1893.] 22p. DNLM; PPC **90-9325**

VAUGHAN, Victor C[larence] (1851-1929) Frederick G. NOVY, and Charles T. McCLINTOCK
The germicidal properties of nucleins. A preliminary contribution from the laboratory of hygiene of Michigan University. [Philadelphia, 1893.] 6p. DNLM **90-9326**

VAUGHAN, Victor C[larence] (1851-1929)
The treatment of tuberculosis with yeast-nuclein. [Philadelphia: Lea Bros. & Co., 1894.] 32p. DNLM **90-9327**

VAUGHAN, Victor C[larence] (1851-1929)
[Circular letter to prominent men of both schools, soliciting an opinion on the expediency of abolishing the Homoeopathic School, as a department, owing to the reduced number of students attending, and that a professor of homoeopathic materia medica and therapeutics, as the only distinctive feature of the system, be appointed in the medical department. Feb. 11, 1895.] [Ann Arbor, 1895.] 1 sheet. DNLM **90-9328**

VAUGHAN, Victor, C[larence] (1851-1929) and George D. PERKINS
Food-infection with toxicogenic germs. New York, 1895. 14p. DNLM **90-9329**

VAUGHAN, Victor C[larence] (1851-1929) and George D. PERKINS
A poison-producing bacillus found in ice-cream and cheese. Philadelphia, 1896. 17p. DNLM **90-9330**

VAUGHAN, Victor C[larence] (1851-1929)
William Beaumont and his work. Detroit, 1896. 13p. DNLM **90-9331**

VAUGHAN, Victor C[larence] (1851-1929) and Frederick G. NOVY
Ptomains, leucomains, toxins and antitoxins; or the chemical factors in the causation of disease. 3rd ed. Philadelphia & New York: Lea Bros. & Co., 1896. 604p. 1 tab. CtY-M; DNLM; PPC; PPJ **90-9332**

VAUGHAN, Victor C[larence] (1851-1929)
The physiological action and therapeutic uses of yeast nucleinic acid, with special reference to its employment in tuberculosis. New York, 1897. 105p. DNLM **90-9333**

VAUGHAN, Victor C[larence] (1851-1929)
The physiologic chemistry of uric acid. Philadelphia, 1898. 18p. DNLM **90-9334**

VAUGHAN, Victor C[larence] (1851-1929)
Some remarks on typhoid fever among our soldiers during the late war with Spain. New York, 1899. 15p. DNLM **90-9335**

VEASEY, Clarence A[rchibald] (*b.* 1869)
Ophthalmia neonatorum. [Philadelphia, 1892.] 24p. DNLM **90-9336**

VEASEY, Clarence A[rchibald] (*b.* 1869)
The use of subconjunctival injections of mercuric bichloride in various ocular affections, with a report of fifteen cases so treated. Detroit: G. S. Davis, 1894. 12p. DNLM **90-9337**

VEASEY, Clarence A[rchibald] (*b.* 1869)
The importance of active treatment of the naso-pharynx, in the treatment of obstructive disease of the lachrymal passages. [Nashville, Tenn., 1895.] 6p. DNLM **90-9338**

VEASEY, Clarence A[rchibald] (*b.* 1869)
The treatment of simple ulcers of the cornea. Philadelphia, 1895. 4p. DNLM **90-9339**

VEASEY, Clarence A[rchibald] (*b.* 1869)
A case of albuminuric retinitis. [Philadelphia, 1895.] 2p. DNLM **90-9340**

VEASEY, Clarence A[rchibald] (*b.* 1869)
Ophthalmia neonatorum. [Philadelphia: Lea Bros. & Co., 1893.] 12p. DNLM **90-9341**

VEASEY, Clarence A[rchibald] (*b.* 1869)
Concerning sub-conjunctival injections of sodium chloride versus mercuric chloride in various ocular diseases, with cases. St. Louis, 1896. 7p. DNLM **90-9342**

VEASEY, Clarence A[rchibald] (*b.* 1869)
Ophthalmic operations as practiced on animals' eyes. Philadelphia: The Edwards & Docker Co., 1896. 99p. DNLM **90-9343**

VEASEY, Clarence A[rchibald] (*b.* 1869)
A case of duboisin poisoning. Philadelphia, 1896. 2p. DNLM **90-9344**

VEASEY, Clarence A[rchibald] (*b.* 1869)
Episcleritis and its treatment. Detroit, 1896. 9p. DNLM **90-9345**

VEASEY, Clarence A[rchibald] (*b.* 1869)
A new eye model for use in ophthalmoscopy and skiascopy. St. Louis, 1896. 4p. DNLM **90-9346**

VEASEY, Clarence A[rchibald] (*b.* 1869)
A knife protector. Chicago, 1896. 1 l. DNLM **90-9347**

VEASEY, Clarence A[rchibald] (*b.* 1869)
The treatment of complicated ulcers of the cornea. Detroit: G. S. Davis, 1897. 12p. DNLM **90-9348**

VEASEY, Clarence A[rchibald] (*b.* 1869)
Cases of paralysis of some of the ocular muscles. Philadelphia, 1897. 5p. DNLM **90-9349**

VEASEY, Clarence A[rchibald] (*b.* 1869)
Binasal hemianopsis, with the report of an additional case. Nashville, 1897. 8p. DNLM **90-9350**

VEASEY, Clarence A[rchibald] (*b.* 1869)
Primary sarcoma of the iris. A statistical study, with the report of an additional case, in which the growth was successfully removed by iridectomy. St. Louis, 1897. 23p. DNLM **90-9351**

VEASEY, Clarence A[rchibald] (*b.* 1869)
The importance of the early recognition and treatment of acute inflammatory glaucoma. Detroit: W. M. Warren, 1898. 6p. DNLM **90-9352**

VEASEY, Clarence A[rchibald] (*b.* 1869)
The employment of solutions of toluidin-blue as collyria, and as a stain for corneal abrasions and ulcers. Philadelphia, 1898. 4p. DNLM **90-9353**

VEASEY, Clarence A[rchibald] (*b.* 1869)
A case of hypopyon kerato-iritis occurring in a patient during an attack of typhoid fever. [Nashville, 1898.] 2p. DNLM **90-9354**

VEASEY, Clarence A[rchibald] (*b.* 1869)
Central amblyopia in a dye-worker probably produced by inhalation of the aniline dyes. [St. Louis, 1898.] 4p. DNLM **90-9355**

VEASEY, Clarence A[rchibald] (*b.* 1869)
A case of bilateral syphilitic ulceration of the palpebral conjunctiva. [Philadelphia, 1898.] 1 l. 1 plate. DNLM **90-9356**

VEASEY, Clarence A[rchibald] (*b.* 1869)
A note on the employment of solutions of toluidin-blue in external inflammatory diseases of the eye. Detroit: W. M. Warren, 1899. 4p. DNLM **90-9357**

VEASEY, Clarence A[rchibald] (*b.* 1869)
A case of primary nonpigmented sarcoma of the left upper lid. Philadelphia, 1899. 4p. DNLM **90-9358**

VEASEY, Clarence A[rchibald] (*b.* 1869)
A clinical study of double choked discs in a case of quiet otitic thrombosis of the sigmoid sinus, without pyaemia. Nashville, 1899. 10p. DNLM **90-9359**

VEASEY, Clarence A[rchibald] (*b.* 1869)
Concerning the bacteriology of acute catarrhal conjunctivitis. New York, 1899. 7p. DNLM **90-9360**

VECKI, Victor G. (1857-1938)
The pathology and treatment of sexual impotence. . . . From the author's 2nd German ed., rev. and rewritten. Philadelphia: W. B. Saunders, 1899. 291p. DLC; DNLM; PPC; PU
90-9361

VEEDER, Major Albert (1848-1915)
Three unusual cases of abscess. Philadelphia, 1894. 2p. DNLM; NN **90-9362**

VEEDER, Major Albert (1848-1915)
A dressing for fractures of the lower extremity. Philadelphia, 1895. 2 l. DNLM; NN **90-9363**

VEEDER, Major Albert (1848-1915)
Neuritis complicating dislocations of the shoulder and elbow. New York, 1896. 6p. DNLM; NN **90-9364**

VERDI, Tullio S[uzzara] (1829-1902)
Special diagnosis and homoeopathic treatment of disease for popular use, including such functional disturbances as are peculiar to girls and to maternity. Philadelphia: Boericke & Tafel, 1893. 579p. DNLM; NNNAM; PPC; PPHa
90-9365

VERHOEFF, Frederick Herman (*b.* 1874)
Two new astigmatic charts. Chicago, 1899. 3p. DNLM
90-9366

VERHOEFF, Frederick Herman (*b.* 1874)
A description of the reflecting phorometer and a discussion of the possibilities concerning torsion of the eyes. New York, 1899. 15p. 4 plates. DNLM **90-9367**

VETTER, J. C. & CO.
Illustrated catalogue of the Vetter galvanic and faradic batteries and standard electro-medical apparatus. New York, 1893. 56p. NNNAM **90-9368**

VICTOR ELECTRIC CO.
Illustrated catalogue of high grade electrical, dental and surgical specialties. 3rd ed. Chicago, 1898. 48p. NNNAM
90-9369

VIERORDT, Oswald (1856-1906)
A clinical text-book of medical diagnosis for physicians and students, based on the most recent methods of examination. Authorized transl. from the 2nd German ed., with additions by Francis H. Stuart. Philadelphia: W. B. Saunders 1891. 700p. CU-M; DNLM; IU-M; NNNAM
90-9370

VIERORDT, Oswald (1856-1906)
A clinical text-book of medical diagnosis for physicians and students, based on the most recent methods of examination. Authorized transl., with additions, by Francis H. Stuart. 3rd ed. Philadelphia: W. B. Saunders, 1896. 700p. DNLM; NNNAM; PPC; PPJ **90-9371**

VIERORDT, Oswald (1856-1906)
A clinical text-book of medical diagnosis for physicians and students, based on the most recent methods of examination. Authorized transl., with additions, by Francis H. Stuart. 4th American ed. from the 5th German revised and enlarged. Philadelphia: W. B. Saunders, 1898. 603p. DNLM; LNT-M; MBM; NNNAM **90-9372**

VIETOR, Agnes C.
The diagnosis of some common injuries in the shoulder region. Boston: Damrell & Upham, 1897. 25p. DNLM; MBM
90-9373

VIETOR, Agnes C.
A case of septicemia (gonotoxemia?) treated with the streptococcus antitoxin; recovery. Boston: Damrell & Upham, 1898. 10p. DNLM; MBM **90-9374**

VIETOR, Agnes C.
The abuse of medical charity; the passing of the charity hospital and dispensary. Boston: Damrell & Upham, 1899. 22p. DNLM; MBM **90-9375**

VIETOR, Agnes C.
The making of a woman surgeon. Boston, [1899]. 11p. DNLM; MBM **90-9376**

VILAS, Charles H[arrison] (*b.* 1846)
Diseases of the eye and ear. . . . Chicago: For sale by Boericke & Tafel, [1890]. 117p. DLC; DNLM; PPHa
90-9377

VINEBERG, Hiram N. (*b.* 1857)
Practical points in the diagnosis and treatment of malaria in children. [Philadelphia, 1890.] 24p. DNLM; PPC
90-9378

VINEBERG, Hiram N. (*b.* 1857)
A plea for a just estimate of the value of electro-therapeutics in gynaecology. [New York, 1893.] 11p. DNLM
90-9379

VINEBERG, Hiram N. (*b.* 1857)
Two years' experience with pelvic massage in gynecological cases, with report of cases. New York: William Wood & Co., 1893. 37p. DNLM; NNNAM **90-9380**

VINEBERG, Hiram N. (*b.* 1857)
Anterior vagino-fixation of the uterus for backward displacements; a new operation. [New York, 1894.] 8p. DNLM
90-9381

VINEBERG, Hiram N. (*b.* 1857)
Congenital annular stenosis of the vagina; an improved method of operating. New York: Trow, 1894. 11p. DNLM
90-9382

VINEBERG, Hiram N. (*b.* 1857)
The technique and indications of vagino-fixation (Mackenrodt's operation). [New York: D. Appleton & Co., 1894.] 16p. DNLM **90-9383**

VINEBERG, Hiram N. (*b.* 1857)
Tubal mode pregnancy, with some remarks on the differential diagnosis of ectopic gestation. New York, 1895. 12p. DNLM
90-9384

VINEBERG, Hiram N. (*b.* 1857)
Vaginal coeliotomy, with remarks on the new field it opens up for the treatment of backward displacements of the uterus with diseased annexa by vagino-fixation. New York: Stettiner, Lambert & Co., 1895. 9p. DNLM **90-9385**

VINEBERG, Hiram N. (*b.* 1857)
Notes on three interesting cases presented before the New York Obstetrical Society. New York, 1895. 4p. DNLM
90-9386

VINEBERG, Hiram N. (*b.* 1857)
The surgical treatment of backward displacements of the uterus with special reference to vaginal fixation. New York: Stettiner, Lambert & Co., 1896. 15p. DNLM
90-9387

VINEBERG, Hiram N. (*b.* 1857)
Indications for vaginal fixation, with especial reference to the behavior of pregnancy and labor after the operation. Philadelphia, 1896. 9p. DNLM **90-9388**

VINEBERG, Hiram N. (*b.* 1857)
Acute catarrhal salpingitis; its resemblance to appendicitis; differential diagnosis; treatment. New York, 1896. 18p. DNLM **90-9389**

VINEBERG, Hiram N. (*b.* 1857)
Conservative surgery upon the uterus and its annexa through the vaginal route. New York, 1896. 15p. DNLM
90-9390

VINEBERG, Hiram N. (*b.* 1857)
A contribution to the study of lactation-atrophy of the uterus. Philadelphia, 1896. 14p. DNLM **90-9391**

VINEBERG, Hiram N. (*b.* 1857)
A new method of performing vaginal fixation. New York, 1896. 4p. DNLM **90-9392**

VINEBERG, Hiram N. (*b.* 1857)
Hysterectomy for acute puerperal septic metritis. New York, 1898. 18p. DNLM **90-9393**

VINEBERG, Hiram N. (*b.* 1857)
Castration for rudimentary uterus, absence of vagina, menstrual molimina. New York: William Wood & Co., 1898. 12p. DNLM **90-9394**

VINEBERG, Hiram N. (*b.* 1857)
The diagnosis and treatment of the more common bladder affections in women by means of Kelly's method. New York, 1899. 16p. DNLM **90-9395**

VIRCHOW, Rudolf (1821-1902)
Cellular pathology as based upon physiological and pathological histology. . . . Transl. from the 2nd edition of the original by Frank Chance. With notes and numerous emendations, principally from manuscript notes of the author. . . . 7th American ed. New York: De Witt Publishing House [1890?]. 554p. IU-M; NNNAM; NNU-M; OC
90-9396

VISCHER, Carl V.
The supra-pubic removal of an enormous vesical calculus, together with the pathology of stone in the bladder. Philadelphia, 1893. 7p. 1 plate. DNLM **90-9397**

VOSWINKEL, Bertha M.
Surgical nursing, a manual for nurses. Philadelphia: P. Blakiston, Son & Co., 1895. 168p. DLC; DNLM; PPC; PU
90-9398

VOSWINKEL, Bertha M.
Surgical nursing, a manual for nurses. 2nd ed., rev. and enl. Philadelphia: P. Blakiston's Son & Co., 1899. 206p. DLC; DNLM; PPC; PU **90-9399**

VOUGHT, Walter (1862-1893)
A chapter on cholera for lay readers. History, symptoms, prevention, and treatment of the disease. Philadelphia & London: The F. A. Davis Co., 1893. 107p. 2 plates. CU-M; DNLM; MBM; PPC **90-9400**

WACHENHEIM, Frederick L. (*b.* 1870)
The administration of atropine in epilepsy. New York, 1899. 6p. DNLM **90-9401**

WADE, John Alexander (1859-1908)
Nasal catarrh; its treatment. Danbury, Conn., 1898. 2 l. DNLM
90-9402

WADE, John Alexander (1859-1908)
Gravel. Toledo, O., 1898. 2p. DNLM
90-9403

WADSWORTH, William S[cott] (*b.* 1868)
The pathology of color perception. [Philadelphia, 1898.] 7p. MH **90-9404**

WADSWORTH, William S[cott] (*b.* 1868)
A case of symmetric deformity of both hands, probably congenital. [Philadelphia, 1899.] 4p. MH
90-9405

WAGGAMAN, Samuel
A lexicon for the use of druggists and students in pharmacy. . . . Washington, D.C.: W. H. Morrison, 1890. 104p. DLC
90-9406

WAGGAMAN, Samuel
A compendium of botanic materia medica for the use of students in medicine and pharmacy. . . . Washington, D.C.: W. H. Morrison, 1891 [1890]. 325p. DLC **90-9407**

WAGGAMAN, Samuel
A compendium of botanic materia medica for use of students in medicine and pharmacy. With a glossary. . . . Rev. and cor. ed. Washington, D.C. W. H. Lowdermilk & Co, 1895. 504p. DLC **90-9408**

WAGNER, Clinton (1837-1914)
Papillomatous growths of the palatal arches and uvula. New York, 1893. 3p. DNLM **90-9409**

WAGNER, Henry Lewis (*b.* 1859)
Seropurulent maxillary sinusitis in chronic lead poisoning. New York, 1896. 4p. DNLM **90-9410**

WAGNER, Henry Lewis (*b.* 1859)
Natural immunity of the mucous membranes of the respiratory tract. New York, 1898. 4p. DNLM
90-9411

WAGNER, Henry Lewis (*b.* 1859)
Early diagnosis in whooping-cough. New York, 1898. 3p. DNLM **90-9412**

WAGNER, William C.
A few remarks upon Wagner's infant food. (For the medical profession.) Brooklyn, N.Y., [1890]. 26p. DNLM
90-9413

WAGONER, George W[ashington] (1856-1919)
How the physicians of Johnston were relieved after the flood. Philadelphia, W. J. Dornan, 1890. 11p. DNLM
90-9414

WAINWRIGHT, John W[illiam] (*b.* 1850)
Recent therapeutic application of the valerianates of creosote and guaiacol. Chicago, 1898. 12p. DNLM
90-9415

WAITE & BARTLETT MFG. CO.
Illustrated price list of electro-medical and electro-surgical instruments. New York, 1890. 48p. NNNAM
90-9416

WAITE & BARTLETT MFG. CO.
Illustrated price list of electro-medical and electro-surgical instruments. New York, 1890. 8p. DNLM
90-9417

WAITE & BARTLETT MFG. CO.
Illustrated price list of electro-medical and electro-surgical instruments. New York, [1892?]. 48p. NNNAM
90-9418

WAITE & BARTLETT MFG. CO.
Illustrated price list of electro-medical and electro-surgical instruments. New York, 1893. 47p. NNNAM
90-9419

WAKEFIELD, W. Francis B. (*b.* 1866)
The treatment of retrodisplacements of the uterus. Oakland, Cal.: Jordan, 1897. 8p. DNLM **90-9420**

WAKEFIELD, W. Francis B. (*b.* 1866)
The radical vaginal operation for bilateral disease of the ovaries and tubes. [Sacramento, 1898.] 7p. DNLM
90-9421

WALKER, D[avid] Ernest (*b.* 1850)
The early recognition of uterine cancer, with some remarks on its treatment. New York: D. Appleton & Co., 1896. 8p. DNLM **90-9422**

WALKER, Edwin (*b.* 1853)
Some remarks on one phase of puerperal sepsis. [St. Louis, 1891.] 3p. DNLM **90-9423**

WALKER, Gertrude A[nnie] (*b.* 1863)
Students' aid in ophthalmology. Philadelphia: P. Blakiston, Son & Co., 1895. 183p. col. plate. DLC; DNLM; PPC; PPJ
90-9424

WALKER, Gulielmus M.
I. Lectures on rectal and gastro-intestinal surgery, with demonstrations. II. A modification of Kraske's method of excision of the rectum. III. A tunneled fistulatome. IV. Gastro-enterostomy within two minutes without suture, ligature, or forceps, with a modification of the Murphy's button. Louisville: J. P. Morton & Co., 1894. 19p. DNLM; KyLoJM
90-9425

WALKER, H[enry] O. (1843-1912)
Brain surgery, with report of eleven cases. [Philadelphia, 1890.] 26p. DNLM; PPC **90-9426**

WALKER, H[enry] O. (1843-1912)
Report of seven cases of double castration for relief of enlarged prostate gland. [New York: D. Appleton & Co., 1895.] 6p. DNLM **90-9427**

WALKER, H[enry] O. (1843-1912)
Surgical clinic at St. Mary's Hospital, September 23, 1896. Detroit, 1896. 20p. 2 photos. DNLM **90-9428**

WALKER, H[enry] O. (1843-1912)
The surgery of the gall-bladder and its ducts. Detroit, 1898. 6p. DNLM **90-9429**

WALKER, H[enry] O. (1843-1912)
The radical cure of inguinal hernia by Fowler's method, with reports of cases. Detroit, [1898]. 16p. DNLM
90-9430

WALKER, H[enry] O. (1843-1912)
Some remarks and reports upon specimens in abdominal surgery. Detroit & Ann Arbor, 1898. 10p. DNLM
90-9431

WALKER, H[enry] O. (1843-1912)
Appendicitis. Detroit, 1899. 10p. 11 plates on 2 l. DNLM
90-9432

WALKER, John B. (*b.* 1860)
Hernia and its mechanical treatment. New York, 1894. 11p. DNLM **90-9433**

WALKER, M[ahlon] M[urphy] (1845-1896)
Fifty consecutive cases of typhoid fever. [Philadelphia, 1891.] 18p. DNLM **90-9434**

WALKER, Maurice A.
A case of pseudo-hermaphroditism. New York: D. Appleton & Co., 1894. 6p. DNLM; NNNAM **90-9435**

WALKER, Norman (1862-1942)
An introduction to dermatology. New York: William Wood & Co., 1899. 247p. 30 plates. CtY-M; DNLM; MBM; NNNAM
90-9436

WALKER, S. T.
The modicum of hearing of deaf mutes; how to use it and how to improve it. St. Louis, 1896. 7p. DNLM
90-9437

WALKER, S. T.
Clinical examination of deaf mutes. Cincinnati, 1896. 9p. DNLM **90-9438**

WALKER, W[illiam] A.
Vegetable dyspepsia. Detroit: G. S. Davis, 1896. 4p. DNLM
90-9439

WALKER, W[illiam] A.
Faulty metabolism; nutrition and growth. [New York, 1898.] 4p. DNLM **90-9440**

WALKER, W[illiam] E.
Prothetic dentistry; the glenoid fossa; the movements of the mandible; the cusps of the teeth. Philadelphia, 1896. 10p. DNLM **90-9441**

WALKER, W[illiam] E.
Movements of the mandibular condyles and dental articulation. Philadelphia, 1896. 10p. DNLM **90-9442**

WALL, Otto Augustus (1846-1922)
The prescription, therapeutically, pharmaceutically, grammatically and historically considered. . . . 2nd and rev. ed. St. Louis, Mo.: A. Gast Bank Note & Litho. Co., 1890. 206p. col. plate. DLC **90-9443**

WALL, Otto Augustus (1846-1922)
Notes on pharmacognosy. Junior work. . . . St. Louis, Mo.: A. Gast Bank Note & Litho. Co., 1897. 180p. DLC
90-9444

WALL, Otto Augustus (1846-1922)
The prescription, therapeutically, pharmaceutically, grammatically and historically considered. . . . 3rd and rev. ed. St. Louis, Mo.: A. Gast Bank Note & Litho. Co., 1898. 211p. col. plate. DLC **90-9445**

WALLACE, James
The physical and physiological basis of color. Philadelphia, 1894. 7p. 1 plate. DNLM **90-9446**

WALLIAN, Samuel S[pencer] (1836-1907)
A study of aerotherapeutics. [New York: D. Appleton & Co., 1891.] 11p. DNLM **90-9447**

WALLIAN, Samuel S[pencer] (1836-1907)
Hydrogen dioxide. [New York, 1892.] 23p. DNLM
90-9448

WALLIAN, Samuel S[pencer] (1836-1907)
A national system of sanatoria; a plea and a prophecy. [Philadelphia, 1892.] 12p. DNLM **90-9449**

WALLIAN, Samuel S[pencer] (1836-1907)
The influence of climate on the breathing-habit, with a comparison of American climatic resorts. [Philadelphia, 1893.] 23p. DNLM **90-9450**

WALLIAN, Samuel S[pencer] (1836-1907)
Where to send invalids and semi-invalids for the winter. New York, 1896. 11p. DNLM **90-9451**

WALSH, David
Excretory irritation, and the action of certain internal remedies on the skin. New York: William Wood & Co., 1898. 68p. DNLM; NNNAM; ICJ; PPC **90-9452**

WALSH, David
Premature burial; fact or fiction? New York: William Wood & Co., 1898. 49p. DNLM; NNNAM **90-9453**

WALSH, David
. . . The Röntgen rays in medical work. With an introductory section upon electrical apparatus and methods, by J. E. Greenhill. New York: William Wood & Co., 1898. 144p. 28 plates. DNLM; NNNAM; PPC; PU
90-9454

WALSH, David
. . . The Röntgen rays in medical work. With an introductory section upon electrical apparatus and methods, by J. E. Greenhill. 2nd ed. New York: William Wood & Co., 1899. 257p. NcD **90-9455**

WALSH, J. Francis
The anatomy and functions of the muscles of the hand and of the extensor tendons of the thumb. Essay awarded by "Boylston" prize for 1897, department of anatomy and physiology, by the Boylston medical committee, Boston, Mass. Philadelphia: C. H. Walsh, 1897. 51p. DNLM; MBM; PPC **90-9456**

WALSH, James Joseph (1865-1942)
Some features of the year's work in orthopedic surgery. Philadelphia, 1896. 12p. DNLM **90-9457**

WALSH, James Joseph (1865-1942)
Some notes on an epidemic of chicken-pox in the orthopedic ward of the Hospital of the University of Pennsylvania; service of De Forest Willard. Detroit: G. S. Davis, 1896. 8p. DNLM
90-9458

WALSH, John E.
Celiotomy for abscess of the pancreas; with the report of a case. [Philadelphia, 1893.] 5p. DNLM
90-9459

WALSH, John E.
A case of ruptured ectopic gestation; celiotomy; recovery. [Philadelphia, 1893.] 6p. DNLM **90-9460**

WALSH, John E. (*b.* 1865)
Diphtheria. Richmond, 1898. 17p. DNLM
90-9461

WALSHAM, William J[ohnson] (1847-1903)
Surgery; its theory and practice. . . . 3rd ed. Philadelphia: P. Blakiston, Son & Co., 1891. 748p. CtY-M; DNLM; PPC; PU **90-9462**

WALSHAM, William J[ohnson] (1847-1903)
Surgery: its theory and practice. . . . 4th ed. Philadelphia: P. Blakiston, Son & Co., 1893. 748p. DLC; PPC; PPJ; PU
90-9463

WALSHAM, William J[ohnson] (1847-1903) and William Kent HUGHES
The deformities of the human foot, with their treatment. New York: William Wood & Co., 1895. 550p. DNLM; NNNAM; PPC; PPJ **90-9464**

WALSHAM, William J[ohnson] (1847-1903)
Surgery, its theory and practice. . . . 5th ed., rev. and enlarged. . . . Philadelphia: P. Blakiston, Son & Co., 1896. 815p. NNNAM; OCIM; PPC; PU **90-9465**

WALSHAM, William J[ohnson] (1847-1903)
Nasal obstruction; the diagnosis of the various conditions causing it and their treatment. New York: William Wood & Co., 1898. 256p. DLC; DNLM; NNNAM; PU
90-9466

WALSHAM, William J[ohnson] (1847-1903)
Surgery: its theory and practice. . . . 6th ed. Philadelphia: P. Blakiston, Son & Co., 1899. 846p. DNLM: IUM; NNNAM; PPC **90-9467**

WALTER, Robert (*b.* 1841)
Outlines of a common-sense system of treatment without drugs, based on recent important discoveries, adapted to every phase of health and disease; to the sick that they may get well; to the well that they may keep well. Reading, Pa.: B. F. Owen, 1890. 69p. DNLM **90-9468**

WALTER, Will (*b.* 1866)
General considerations on the treatment and management of ophthalmia neonatorum. New York: D. Appleton & Co., 1897. 11p. DNLM **90-9469**

WALTER, Will (*b.* 1866)
On asthenopia as a fatigue neurosis and its analogy to the professional neuroses. Chicago, 1897. 7p. DNLM
90-9470

WALTON, Alice
The cult of Asklepios. [Boston: Published for the University by Ginn & Co., 1894.] 136p. DLC; MH
90-9471

WALTON, George L[incoln] (1854-1941)
Contribution to the study of the traumatic neuropsy choses. [New York, 1890.] 18p. DNLM **90-9472**

WALTON, George L[incoln] (1854-1941)
Dislocation of cervical vertebrae without fatal results. Boston: Damrell & Upham, 1890. 11p. DNLM
90-9473

WALTON, George L[incoln] (1854-1941)
Fatal case of lead-poisoning in which ataxia was the principal symptom (pseudo-tabes). Boston: Damrell & Upham, 1890. 6p. DNLM **90-9474**

WALTON, George L[incoln] (1854-1941) and Cyrus Faulkner CARTER
The etiology of epilepsy; with special reference to the connection between the epilepsy and infantile convulsions. Boston: Damrell & Upham, 1891. 12p. DNLM
90-9475

WALTON, George L[incoln] (1854-1941)
A case of metastatic abscess of the brain; operation; death. Boston: Damrell & Upham, 1892. 11p. DNLM
90-9476

WALTON, George L[incoln] (1854-1941) and Frederick E. CHENEY
The improtance of correcting ocular defects in functional nervous disorders. Boston: Damrell & Upham, 1892. 19p. DNLM **90-9477**

WALTON, George L[incoln] (1854-1941) and Frederick E. CHENEY
The importance of correcting ocular defects in functional nervous disorders. Boston, 1892. 19p. DNLM
90-9478

WALTON, George L[incoln] (1854-1941)
A new method of reducing dislocation of the cervical vertebrae. New York: Raff & Co., 1893. 3p. DNLM
90-9479

WALTON, George L[incoln] (1854-1941)
Reduction of cervical dislocation; a successful case. Boston: Damrell & Upham, 1893. 23p. DNLM
90-9480

WALTON, George L[incoln] (1854-1941)
The etiology of obstetrical paralysis. Boston, 1896. 8p. DNLM **90-9481**

WALTON, George L[incoln] (1854-1941)
Multiple neuritis the essential element in Landry's paralysis; an illustrative case. Boston, 1896. 15p. DNLM
90-9482

WALTON, George L[incoln] (1854-1941) and William A. BROOKS, Jr.
Observation on brain surgery suggested by a case of multiple cerebral hemorrhage. Boston: Damrell & Upham, 1897. 16p. DNLM **90-9483**

WALTON, George L[incoln] (1854-1941)
The nature and treatment of spasmodic torticollis. Philadelphia, 1898. 6p. DNLM **90-9484**

WALTON, George L[incoln] (1854-1941) and Frederick E. CHENEY
Tumor of the pituitary body. Boston: Damrell & Upham, 1899. 15p. DNLM **90-9485**

WALTON, J[ames] T.
The comparative mortality of the white and colored races in te South. Charlotte, N.C., 1897. 10p. DNLM
90-9486

WARBASSE, James Peter (*b.* 1866)
Are the parasitic theories of etiology of carcinoma tenable? [Brooklyn, 1894.] 10p. DNLM **90-9487**

WARBASSE, James Peter (*b.* 1866)
The treatment of fractures of the lower extremity. Clinical report of four hundred and fifty cases treated in the Methodist Episcopal Hospital in the city of Brooklyn. Philadelphia, 1898. 25p. DNLM **90-9488**

WARBASSE, James Peter (*b.* 1866)
Original studies in the bacteriology of chronic endometritis. Philadelphia, 1898. 5p. DNLM **90-9489**

WARBASSE, James Peter (*b.* 1866)
Plastic operation for saddle-nose. Brooklyn, N.Y., 1898. 3p. DNLM **90-9490**

WARD, Charles H.
Nasal characteristics, human and comparative. [n. p.], 1895. 20p. DNLM **90-9491**

WARD, Charles H.
The evolution of the patient. Philadelphia, 1899. 12p. DNLM
90-9492

WARD, George Gray, Jr. (*b.* 1868)
Atresia vaginae complicating labor. With report of a case. New York, 1899. 11p. DNLM **90-9493**

WARD, Henry A[ugustus] (1834-1906)
Catalogue of human skeletons, human and comparative anatomical models, botanical models, busts and masks. 6th ed. Rochester, N.Y., [1893]. 79p. DNLM
90-9494

WARD, Henry B[ascom] (*b.* 1876)
The Asiatic lung-distome in the United States. [Philadelphia: Lea Bros. & Co., 1895.] 10p. DNLM
90-9495

WARD, James W[illiam] (*b.* 1861)
A contribution to the surgical study of ectopia vesicae. . . . [San Francisco: J. Winterburn Co.], 1899. 16p. DLC
90-9496

WARD, Jessie M.
Notes on massage, including elementary anatomy and physiology. Philadelphia: P. Blakiston, Son & Co., 1898. 97p. 1 plate. DNLM; PPC; PPJ **90-9497**

WARD, M[arshall] R.
Septic thrombo-phlebitis as a complication of peritonsillar abscess. New York, 1899. 12p. DNLM
90-9498

WARD, Milo B[uell] (1848-1901)
Should exploratory incisions be resorted to as a means of diagnosis in obscure diseases of the abdominal cavity? [New York, 1895.] 5p. DNLM **90-9499**

WARD, Samuel B[aldwin] (*b.* 1842)
Carcinomatous papilloma of bladder. Occlusion of orifices of ureters. Death by uraemic coma. New York: G. P. Putnam's Sons, [1892]. 17p. DNLM; NNNAM **90-9500**

WARD, Samuel B[aldwin] (*b.* 1842)
Climatic treatment of pulmonary phthisis. [Philadelphia, 1891.] 4p. DNLM **90-9501**

WARD, Whitfield
Diseases of the nasal organs and naso-pharynx. New York & London: G. P. Putnam's Sons, 1891. 165p. DLC; DNLM; NNNAM; PPC **90-9502**

WARE, Martin Wiener (*b.* 1869)
Local anesthesia with special reference to the infiltration method. Philadelphia, 1898. 12p. DNLM **90-9503**

WARING, Edward John (1819-1891)
A manual of practical therapeutics, considered with reference to articles of the materia medica. . . . Ed. by Dudley W. Buxton. 4th ed. rev. Philadelphia: P. Blakiston, Son & Co., 1890. 666p. NNNAM; OCLloyd; PPC; PU **90-9504**

WARK, David
Prevention and cure of consumptions. New York: Fowler & Wells Co., 1891. 56p. illus. NN [Human Nature Library, No. 3, 1891.] **90-9505**

WARK, David
The practical home doctor for women and children, to which is added a valuable appendix, containing a list of medicinal herbs and their value, with chapters explaining poisons and their antidotes, how to resuscitate the drowned, how to proceed in cases of accidents and emergencies, the skin and its care, the teeth and their care, etc. New York: Gay Bros., 1892. [*c.* 1882.] 554p. CtY-M; DNLM **90-9506**

WARNER, A[mos] G[riswold] (1861-1900)
Syllabus of a course of ten lectures on pauperism [at the University of Wisconsin]. Madison: Tracy, Gibbs & Co., 1892. 32p. DNLM **90-9507**

WARNER, Levi Farr (1822-1889)
Materia medica and therapeutics. A manual for students and practitioners. Philadelphia: Lea Bros. & Co., 1892. 223p. CtY-M; DNLM; PPC; PU **90-9508**

WARNER, WILLIAM R., & CO. (PHILADELPHIA & N.Y.C.)
Wm. R. Warner's therapeutic handy reference book for physicians. Philadelphia: W. R. Warner & Co., 1890 [*c.* 1889.] 119p. tables. IU-M; NcU; NNC; PPC [*vel subseq., e.g.,* 8th ed., 1896, 119p.] **90-9509**

WARNER, WILLIAM R., & CO. (PHILADELPHIA & N.Y.C.)
Warner's pocket medical dictionary of to-day, comprising pronunciation and definition of ten thousand essential words and terms used in medicine and associated sciences. Philadelphia: W. R. Warner & Co., 1897. 338p. DNLM; NNNAM; PPC; PPJ **90-9510**

WARNER, WILLIAM R., & CO. (PHILADELPHIA & N.Y.C.)
To the medical profession. Liquid pancreopepsine. Philadelphia: W. R. Warner & Co., [1898]. 38p. DNLM; PPC **90-9511**

WARNER, WILLIAM R., & CO. (PHILADELPHIA & N.Y.C.)
Pocket medical dictionary of today, comprising pronunciation and definition of 10,000 essential words and terms used in medicine and associated sciences. . . . [2nd ed. rev.] Philadelphia, 1898. 374p. DNLM; NN; PPC; PU **90-9512**

WARREN, George W[ashington] (*b.* 1863)
A compend of dental pathology and dental medicine, containing the most noteworthy points upon the subjects of interest to the dental student. Philadelphia: P. Blakiston, Son & Co., 1890. 109p. DLC; DNLM; PPC; PPJ **90-9513**

WARREN, George W[ashington] (*b.* 1863)
. . . A compend of dental pathology and dental medicine. . . . 2nd ed. Philadelphia: P. Blakiston, Son & Co., 1893. 163p. DLC; DNLM; NNNAM; PU **90-9514**

WARREN, George W[ashington] (*b.* 1863)
Crown- and bridge-work as a means of regulation combined with restoration. Philadelphia, 1893. 8p. DNLM **90-9515**

WARREN, George W[ashington] (*b.* 1863)
A compend of dental prosthesis and metallurgy . . . with one hundred and twenty-nine illustrations. Philadelphia: P. Blakiston, Son & Co., 1894. 265p. DLC; DNLM; PPC; PPJ **90-9516**

WARREN, George W[ashington] (*b.* 1863)
. . . A compend of dental pathology and dental medicine. . . . 3rd ed. . . . Philadelphia: P. Blakiston, Son & Co., 1898. 176p. DLC; NNNAM; OCIM; PPC **90-9517**

WARREN, Ira (1806-1864)
New Warren's household physician, enlarged and revised, being a brief description . . . of all the diseases of men, women and children, with the latest and most approved methods of treatment. Allopathic department by Ira Warren . . . rev. by William Thorndike. . . . Homoeopathic department by A. E. Small . . . rev. by J. Heber Smith. . . . Boston: A. I. Bradley & Co., 1898. 984p. col. plates. DLC; MBM **90-9518**

WARREN, John Collins (1842-1927)
A case of fracture of the temporal bone, with remarks on trephining for fracture of the base of the skull. [Philadelphia, 1890.] 11p. DNLM **90-9519**

WARREN, John Collins (1842-1927)
A case of enlarged accessory thyroid gland at the base of the tongue. Philadelphia, 1892. 6p. DNLM **90-9520**

WARREN, John Collins (1842-1927)
Laparotomy for extra-uterine pregnancy; removal of macerated foetus of eight months. [Boston, 1892.] 4p. DNLM
90-9521

WARREN, John Collins (1842-1927)
The operative treatment of goitre. Boston: Damrell & Upham, 1892. 17p. DNLM **90-9522**

WARREN, John Collins (1842-1927)
Two cases of congenital umbilical hernia into the cord; operation; recovery. Philadelphia, 1893. 7p. 2 plates. DNLM
90-9523

WARREN, John Collins (1842-1927)
A case of laminectomy for depressed fracture of the spine. [Philadelphia, 1893.] 3p. 1 plate. DNLM
90-9524

WARREN, John Collins (1842-1927)
Hypertrophies and degenerations of cicatrices and cicatricial tissue. [Philadelphia, 1893.] 30p. 1 plate. DNLM
90-9525

WARREN, John Collins (1842-1927)
I. Laparotomy for extra-uterine pregnancy; removal of macerated foetus of eight months. II. Solid tumor of ovary. Boston: Damrell & Upham, 1893. 7p. DNLM
90-9526

WARREN, John Collins (1842-1927)
Medical education in the United States. Chicago, 1893. 24p. DNLM **90-9527**

WARREN, John Collins (1842-1927)
Two cases of congenital umbilical hernia into the cord; operation; recovery. [New York, 1893.] 9p. DNLM
90-9528

WARREN, John Collins (1842-1927)
Cases of abdominal surgery at the Massachusetts General Hospital, during the winter of 1892-93. Reported by Charles L. Scudder. Boston: Damrell & Upham, 1894. 28p. DNLM
90-9529

WARREN, John Collins (1842-1927)
Tumors of the breast. Boston: Damrell & Upham, 1894. 16p. DNLM **90-9530**

WARREN, John Collins (1842-1927)
Clinical experience in abdominal surgery at the Massachusetts General Hospital. Boston: Damrell & Upham, 1895. 51p. DNLM **90-9531**

WARREN, John Collins (1842-1927)
Surgical pathology and therapeutics. . . . Philadelphia: W. B. Saunders, 1895. 832p. col. plates. DLC; DNLM; NNNAM; PPC
90-9532

WARREN, John Collins (1842-1927)
Cervical ribs and other cases. Boston: Damrell & Upham, 1896. 32p. DNLM **90-9533**

WARREN, John Collins (1842-1927)
Tumors of the breast. Boston: Damrell & Upham, 1897. 45p. 1 tab. DNLM **90-9534**

WARREN, John Collins (1842-1927)
The influence of anaesthesia on the surgery of the nineteenth century. Address of the president. Philadelphia, 1897. 25p. DNLM **90-9535**

WARREN, John Collins (1842-1927)
The surgery of gastric ulcer, with the report of a case of gastrolysis. Boston: Damrell & Upham, 1898. 16p. DNLM
90-9536

WARREN, John Collins (1842-1927)
The question of the curability of cancer of the breast. Boston, 1898. 13p. DNLM **90-9537**

WARREN, Stanley P[erkins] (*b.* 1846)
The principles and application of axis-traction forceps, with special reference to the instrument devised by Tarnier. Portland, Me.: Brown, Thurston Co., [1892]. 16p. DNLM
90-9538

WARREN, Stanley P[erkins] (*b.* 1846)
Plans for delivery of occipito-posterior positions. New York: William Wood & Co., 1896. 12p. DNLM
90-9539

WARREN, Stanley P[erkins] (*b.* 1846)
Dystocia due to accidental hemorrhage. New York: William Wood & Co., 1899. 12p. DNLM **90-9540**

WARTHIN, Aldred Scott (1866-1931)
Additional notes on the diazo-reaction. [Philadelphia, 1893.] 12p. DNLM **90-9541**

WARTHIN, Aldred Scott (1866-1931)
Some physiologic effects of music in hypnotized subjects. [Philadelphia: Lea Bros. & Co., 1894.] 13p. DNLM
90-9542

WARTHIN, Aldred Scott (1866-1931)
Accentuation of the pulmonary second sound an important sign in the diagnosis of pericarditis. Philadelphia, 1895. 15p. DNLM **90-9543**

WARTHIN, Aldred Scott (1866-1931)
Report of a case of ectopic gestation associated with tuberculosis of the tubes, placenta, and fetus. New York, 1896, 16p. DNLM **90-9544**

WARTHIN, Aldred Scott (1866-1931)
The diagnosis of primary sarcoma of the pleura from the cells found in the pleuritic exudate. Philadelphia, 1897. 16p. DNLM
90-9545

WARTHIN, Aldred Scott (1866-1931)
Some experimenal investigations as to the effects of the administration of yeast nuclein upon the leucocytes. New York, 1897. 43p. DNLM **90-9546**

WARTHIN, Aldred Scott (1866-1931)
The minute pathology of acute hemorrhagic pancreatitis associated with multiple fat-necrosis. Philadelphia, 1898. 19p. DNLM **90-9547**

WARTHIN, Aldred Scott (1866-1931)
Multiple primary carcinoma; report of two cases. Chicago, 1899. 20p. DNLM **90-9548**

WARTHIN, Aldred Scott (1866-1931)
The statistics of fifty autopsies on tuberculous subjects. Philadelphia, 1899. 9p. DNLM **90-9549**

WARTHIN, Aldred Scott (1866-1931)
The pathology of the Pacinian corpuscle. Philadelphia, 1899. 20p. DNLM **90-9550**

WARTHIN, Aldred Scott (1866-1931)
The coexistence of carcinoma and tuberculosis of the mammary gland. Philadelphia, 1899. 11p. DNLM **90-9551**

WARTHIN, Aldred Scott (1866-1931)
Unusual localization of tuberculosis. Philadelphia, 1899. 7p. DNLM **90-9552**

WARTHIN, Aldred Scott (1866-1931)
A primary polymorphous-cell sarcoma of the nose, with universal metastasis and formation of a free sarcomatous mass in the right ventricular cavity. New York, 1899. 18p. DNLM **90-9553**

WASDIN, Eugene (1869-1911)
The value of the autopsic findings in cases that have died of suspected yellow fever. Washington: Government Printing Office, 1898. 11p. DNLM **90-9554**

WASHBURN, George H[amlin]
The sedative action of electricity. Boston, 1890. 9p. DNLM **90-9555**

WASHINGTON DENTAL COLLEGE AND HOSPITAL OF ORAL SURGERY, WASHINGTON, D.C.
General announcement for the session of 1898-99. Washington, 1898. DNLM **90-9556**

WATERMAN, Jerome Hilton
Observations on the local use of hydrochloric acid in bone necrosis of tuberculous origin; with report of cases. New York: D. Appleton & Co., 1896. 7p. DNLM **90-9557**

WATERS, Bertram H[oward] (*b.* 1867)
A report on salophen. [New York: D. Appleton & Co., 1895.] 10p. DNLM **90-9558**

WATHEN, William H[udson] (1846-1913)
Treatment of ectopic pregnancy, with report of a case. [New York, 1890.] 4p. DNLM **90-9559**

WATHEN, William H[udson] (1846-1913)
Abdominal and pelvic surgery. [n. p., 1891.] 8p. DNLM **90-9560**

WATHEN, William H[udson] (1846-1913)
Complications during and after the operation in a few recent cases of abdominal and pelvic surgery. [New York, 1892.] 8p. DNLM **90-9561**

WATHEN, William H[udson] (1846-1913)
Report on abdominal and pelvic surgery, including thirty-two successful cases. of laparotomy. Chicago, 1892. 9p. DNLM **90-9562**

WATHEN, William H[udson] (1846-1913)
Results of aseptic celiotomy. [New York: William Wood & Co., 1893. 9p. DNLM **90-9563**

WATHEN, William H[udson] (1846-1913)
Umbilical and ventral hernia. New York: William Wood & Co., 1893. 6p. DNLM **90-9564**

WATHEN, William H[udson] (1846-1913)
Intraligamentous and retroperitoneal tumors of the uterus and its adnexa. Philadelphia, 1894. 14p. DNLM **90-9565**

WATHEN, William H[udson] (1846-1913)
Treatment of intraligamentous and retroperitoneal uterine myomata. New York, 1896. 4p. DNLM **90-9566**

WATHEN, William H[udson] (1846-1913)
Treatment of uterine myomata and diseases of the uterine annexa per vaginam. [New York, 1897.] 6p. DNLM **90-9567**

WATHEN, William H[udson] (1846-1913)
Vaginal hysterectomy for uterine myomata and diseases of the adnexa. Philadelphia, 1897. 12p. DNLM **90-9568**

WATHEN, William H[udson] (1846-1913)
Operation for uterine myoma by the vagino-abdominal method; iodoform poisoning. [New York, 1898.] 4p. DNLM **90-9569**

WATHEN, William H[udson] (1846-1913)
Abdominal and pelvic surgery. Extracts from clinical lectures and society transactions. Louisville, Ky.: J. P. Morton & Co., 1898. 24p. DNLM **90-9570**

WATHEN, William H[udson] (1846-1913)
Curettage of the uterus. [Philadelphia, 1898.] 6p. DNLM **90-9571**

WATHEN, William H[udson] (1846-1913)
Congenital imperforate anus with fecal impaction extending above the umbilicus. [Louisville, 1898.] 1 l. DNLM **90-9572**

WATKINS, Lyman (1854-1912)
An eclectic compendium of the practice of medicine. Cincinnati: J. M. Scudder's Sons, 1895. 457p. DLC; DNLM; OC; OCIM **90-9573**

WATKINS, T[homas] J[ames] (1863-1925)
Vaginal section and drainage for pelvic abscess, with report of cases. New York, 1895. 8p. DNLM **90-9574**

WATKINS, T[homas] J[ames] (1863-1925)
Technic of abdominal salpingo-oöphorectomy without pedicle. New York, 1896. 19p. DNLM **90-9575**

WATKINS, T[homas] J[ames] (1863-1925)
Drainage in abdominal section for pelvic disease. New York, 1896. 6p. DNLM **90-9576**

WATKINS, T[homas] J[ames] (1863-1925)
Treatment of endometritis. New York, 1897. 7p. DNLM **90-9577**

WATKINS, T[homas] J[ames] (1863-1925)
Tampons and pessaries in the treatment of displacement of the uterus. New York, 1899. 4p. DNLM **90-9578**

WATKINS, T[homas] J[ames] (1863-1925)
Gynecologic diseases. Some points in the diagnosis of the more common ones. Chicago, 1899. 11p. DNLM
90-9579

WATKINS, T[homas] J[ames] (1863-1925)
1. Gonorrhea in women. [Also:] 2. Gonorrhea in children, by I. A. Abt. 3. Pathology of gonorrhea and treatment of some surgical complications, by D. N. Eisendrath. 4. Why is gonorrhea still a much dreaded disease? By F. Kreissl. [Chicago, 1899.] 30p. DNLM; OCIM **90-9580**

WATKINS, William J.
A compend of human physiology, arranged in the form of questions and answers. Louisville, Ky.: W. J. Watkins, 1891. 243p. DNLM; KyLoJM **90-9581**

WATSON, Arthur W.
The operation for deviation of the nasal septum. New York: D. Appleton & Co., 1896. 6p. DNLM
90-9582

WATSON, Beriah André (1836-1892)
Concussion of the spinal cord, brain, etc. Chicago, 1890. 2p. 1 plate. DNLM **90-9583**

WATSON, Beriah André (1836-1892)
An experimental study of lesions arising from severe concussions. Philadelphia: P. Blakiston, Son & Co., 1890. 76p. DNLM; PPC; PU **90-9584**

WATSON Beriah André (1836-1892)
A historical sketch of surgery, ancient, mediaeval, and modern. [New York, 1890.] 47p. DNLM; NNNAM
90-9585

WATSON, Beriah André (1836-1892)
The diagnosis of traumatic lesions in the cerebro-spinal axis and the detection of malingering referred to this centre. [Philadelphia, 1891.] 22p. DNLM **90-9586**

WATSON, Beriah André (1836-1892)
The relation of concussion of the brain and spinal cord to inflammatory and other morbid conditions of these organs. Chicago, 1891. 23p. DNLM **90-9587**

WATSON, Beriah André (1836-1892)
Expert examinations and testimony in railway cases. [Philadelphia, 1892.] 16p. DNLM **90-9588**

WATSON, D[ouglas] Chalmers (1870-1946)
Practical hand-book of the diseases of the eye. New York: Macmillan Co., 1897. 236p. DNLM; IU-M; NNNAM; NNU-M
90-9589

WATSON, Edward W[illard] (1843-1925) and Roland G. CURTIN
The treatment of influenza and its sequelae. Philadelphia, 1892. 8p. DNLM **90-9590**

WATSON, Edward W[illard] (1843-1925)
Some observations on influenzal neuritis. Philadelphia, 1894. 8p. DNLM **90-9591**

WATSON, Francis Sedgwick (1853-1942)
Diagnosis and surgical treatment of embolism and thrombosis of the mesenteric blood-vessels; with reports of cases. Boston: Damrell & Upham, 1894. 22p. DNLM
90-9592

WATSON, Francis Sedgwick (1853-1942)
The clinical features of primary tuberculosis of the genito-urinary organs. Boston: Damrell & Upham, 1895. 14p. DNLM
90-9593

WATSON, Francis Sedgwick (1853-1942)
Hour-glass stomach due to cicatrization of gastric ulcer. Operation by anastomosis between the cardiac and pyloric portions by a new method. Recovery, with restoration of health. Boston: Damrell & Upham, 1896. 8p. DNLM
90-9594

WATSON, Irving A[llison] (1849-1918)
Tuberculosis; its prevalence, communicability, and prevention. Concord, N.H.: E. N. Pearson, 1894. 23p. DNLM
90-9595

WATSON, Irving A[llison], ed. (1849-1918)
Physicians and surgeons of America. (Illustrated). A collection of biographical sketches of the regular medical profession. . . . Concord, N.H.: Republic Press Association, 1896. 843p. DLC; DNLM; MBM; NNNAM **90-9596**

WATSON, W. H.
The student's course in pharmacy, a series of lectures for the use of drug clerks and home students in pharmacy. . . . Nashville, Tenn.: F. M. Paul, 1890. 312p. DLC
90-9597

WAUGH, William F[rancis] (1849-1918)
Practice of medicine. Lectures delivered at the Medico-Chirurgical College [October 1888-February 1889]. . . . [Philadelphia, 1890.] 128p. PPC [MS. unfinished]
90-9598

WAUGH, William F[rancis] (1849-1918) and Ferdinand LASCAR
Laryngeal cough succeeding la grippe. The diastasic and nutritive qualities of malt preparations. [n. p., 1892.] 5p. DNLM
90-9599

WAUGH, W[illiam] F[rancis] (1849-1918)
Outline of treatment with dosimetric granules: from the standpoint of the general practitioner. . . . Philadelphia: The Medical World, 1892. 103p. DLC; OCLloyd; PPC
90-9600

WAUGH, William F[rancis] (1849-1918)
Manual of treatment by active principles, concentrations, and new remedies. . . . Philadelphia: The Medical Press Co., Limited, 1893. 251p. DLC; ICJ; PPC; PPHa
90-9601

WAUGH, William F[rancis] (1849-1918)
The treatment of the sick; a system of applied therapeutics. . . . Chicago: The Alkaloidal Clinic Co., 1897. 527p. DNLM; MH **90-9602**

WAUGH, William F[rancis] (1849-1918)
The treatment of the sick. A system of applied therapeutics. 2nd ed. Chicago: Clinic Publishing Co., 1899. 547p. DLC; ICRM; IEN-M **90-9603**

WAXHAM, F[rank] E[ndoras] (1852-1911)
Report of three hundred cases of intubation of the larynx. [Chicago, 1890.] 8p. DNLM **90-9604**

WAXHAM, F[rank] E[ndoras] (1852-1911)
The treatment of diphtheria. Chicago, 1893. 7p. DNLM
90-9605

WEAVER, B[enjamin] F[ranklin] (*b.* 1839)
Disease chart; or, The silent doctor, revealing diseases by means of illustrated symptoms. . . . Bucyrus, O.: Pub. by the Author, 1893. 32p. DLC **90-9606**

WEAVER, B[enjamin] F[ranklin] (*b.* 1839)
Dr. Weaver's new illustrated family atlas of human diseases. . . . Bucyrus, O.: Pub. by the Author, 1896. 32p. DLC **90-9607**

WEAVER, W[illiam] H.
The primary lesion of tuberculosis; how located. New York, 1899. 6p. DNLM **90-9608**

WEBBER, Samuel G[ilbert] (1838-1926)
Cases of hysteria treated by hypnotism. [New York, 1890.] 12p. DNLM **90-9609**

WEBBER, Samuel G[ilbert] (1838-1926)
Lead paralysis. Boston: Damrell & Upham, 1891. 14p. DNLM **90-9610**

WEBBER, Samuel G[ilbert] (1838-1926)
The condition of the blood in certain mental states. Boston: Damrell & Upham, 1892. 8p. DNLM **90-9611**

WEBBER, Samuel G[ilbert] (1838-1926)
A case of neuralgia. Boston, 1893. 6p. DNLM **90-9612**

WEBBER, Samuel G[ilbert] (1838-1926)
Report of one hundred and sixty cases of epilepsy. Boston: Damrell & Upham, 1893. 24p. DNLM **90-9613**

WEBER, Frederick Parkes (*b.* 1863)
Muscular cramp, in relation with the phenomena of angina pectoris and "intermittent claudication of the extremities." Philadelphia, 1894. 8p. DNLM **90-9614**

WEBER, Frederick Parkes (*b.* 1863)
On the pathology of arterio-sclerosis. [Philadelphia, 1894.] 6p. DNLM **90-9615**

WEBER, Frederick Parkes (*b.* 1863)
Syphilis and lardaceous disease. [Philadelphia, 1895.] 6p. DNLM **90-9616**

WEBER, Frederick Parkes (*b.* 1863)
Syphilis and the etiology of atheroma. Philadelphia, 1896. 7p. DNLM **90-9617**

WEBSTER, David (*b.* 1842)
Foreign bodies in the eye. New York, 1890. 11p. DNLM **90-9618**

WEBSTER, David (*b.* 1842)
The introductory lecture at the opening of the ninety-fifth annual lecture course of Dartmouth Medical College, Hanover, N.H., July 15, 1891. [New York: D. Appleton & Co., 1891.] 11p. DNLM **90-9619**

WEBSTER, David (*b.* 1842)
A case of sarcoma of the ciliary body and chorioid. Clinical history and operation. Pathological examination and remarks by H. Davison Schwarzschild. New York, 1894. 5p. DNLM **90-9620**

WEBSTER, David (*b.* 1842)
Two cases of destruction of vision by foreign bodies; restoration of sight in one out of four eyes operation. New York: D. Appleton & Co., 1894. 3p. DNLM **90-9621**

WEBSTER, David (*b.* 1842) and H. Davison SCHWARZSCHILD
A case of ciliary wound followed by sympathetic irritation. Clinical history and enucleation; pathological report. [New York: D. Appleton & Co., 1895.] 4p. DNLM **90-9622**

WEBSTER, George Washington (*b.* 1857)
. . . Lectures on physical diagnosis. [Chicago, 1895-1897.] 140 l. ICJ **90-9623**

WEBSTER, Herbert Tracy (*b.* 1836)
The principles of medicine as applied to dynamical therapeutics. . . . Designed as an introduction to the study of eclectic medicine. Oakland, Cal.: Pub. by the Author, 1891. 168p. DLC; DNLM **90-9624**

WEBSTER, Herbert Tracy (*b.* 1836)
Dynamical therapeutics; a work devoted to the theory and practice of specific medication, with special reference to the newer remedies, with a clinical index, adapting it to the needs of the busy practitioner, by Herbert T. Webster . . . assisted by J. U. Lloyd . . . and Kent O. Foltz. . . . Oakland, Cal.: Pub. and for sale by the Author, [1893]. 173, 680p. DLC; ICJ **90-9625**

WEBSTER, Herbert Tracy (*b.* 1836)
Dynamical therapeutics; a work devoted to the theory and practice of specific medication, with special reference to the newer remedies, with a clinical index, adapting it to the needs of the busy practitioner, by Herbert T. Webster . . . with notes on practical pharmacy by Prof. J. U. Lloyd and therapeutics of the eye and ear by Prof. Kent O. Foltz, M.D. 2nd ed., rev. and enl. . . . San Francisco, Cal.: Webster Medical Publishing Co., [1898]. 184, 758p. DLC; DNLM **90-9626**

WEBSTER, Herbert Tracy (*b.* 1836)
New eclectic medical practice; designed for students and practitioners. . . . Oakland, Cal.: Webster Medical Publishing Co., [1899-1902]. 2 v. DLC **90-9627**

WEBSTER, J[ohn] Clarence (*b.* 1863)
Ectopic pregnancy. Its etiology, classification, embryology, diagnosis, and treatment. New York: Macmillan & Co., 1895. 240p. 22 plates. DNLM; NNNAM **90-9628**

WEDDERBURN, Alexander J.
A compilation of the pharmacy and drug laws of the several States and Territories. Washington: Government Printing Office, 1894. 152p. DNLM **90-9629**

WEEKS, Clara S[haw]
A text-book of nursing; for the use of training schools, families, and private students. New York: D. Appleton & Co., 1892. 391p. 2 plates, 1 tab. DNLM; NNNAM **90-9630**

WEEKS, Clara S[haw]
A text-book of nursing, for the use of training schools, families, and private students. . . . 2nd ed., rev. and enl. New York: D. Appleton & Co., 1892. 391p. col. plate, fold. diag. DLC; NNNAM **90-9631**

WEEKS, John E[lmer] (1853-1949)
"La grippe" as a cause of retro-bulbar-neuritis and other nerve lesions. [New York: D. Appleton & Co., 1891.] 18p. DNLM **90-9632**

WEEKS & POTTER
Revised catalogue of foreign and domestic drugs. Boston: Cashman, Keating & Co., 1890. 468, 128p. DNLM; MBM **90-9633**

WEEKS & POTTER
Revised catalogue. . . . [Druggists' sundries.] Boston, 1890. 131p. DNLM; MBM **90-9634**

WEEKS & POTTER
Illustrated catalogue. . . . [Druggists' sundries.] Boston, 1890. 468, 131p. DNLM **90-9635**

WEEKS, Stephen H. (1835-1909)
Gangrene of the foot due to uterine myoma. Portland, Me.: W. M. Marks, 1898. 15p. DNLM **90-9636**

WEIGEL, Louis A. (1854?-1906)
Apparatus for recording the curve of rotation in scoliosis. New York, 1893. 2 l. DNLM **90-9637**

WEILAND, Carl (*b.* 1860)
A critical study of the main defects of Javal's ophthalmometer. [Philadelphia, 1892.] 10p. DNLM **90-9638**

WEILAND, Carl (*b.* 1860)
A new eye-model (anaklasimeter) for determining the refraction by ophthalmoscopy and retinoscopy. [Philadelphia, 1893.] 6p. DNLM **90-9639**

WEILAND, Carl (*b.* 1860)
A simple and efficient test for binocular reading. Philadelphia, 1894. 3p. DNLM **90-9640**

WELCH, George T[heodore] (*b.* 1845)
Therapeutical superstition. Newark: L. J. Hardham, 1893. 29p. DNLM **90-9641**

WELCH, William H[enry] (1850-1934)
Report of [his] remarks and exhibition of specimens of animal parasites at the meeting of the Johns Hopkins Hospital Medical Society, on March 17, 1890. Report of [his] remarks on Diplococcus pneumoniae at the meeting of the Johns Hopkins Hospital Medical Society, on Feb. 17, 1890. [Baltimore, 1890.] 4 l. DNLM **90-9642**

WELCH, William H[enry] (1850-1934) and Alexander C. ABBOTT
The etiology of diphtheria. Baltimore, 1891. 10 l. DNLM **90-9643**

WELCH, William H[enry] (1850-1934)
Rudolph Virchow, pathologist. Boston: Damrell & Upham, 1891. 19p. DNLM **90-9644**

WELCH, William H[enry] (1850-1934)
Cirrhosis anthracotica. [Baltimore, 1891.] 3 l. DNLM **90-9645**

WELCH, William H[enry] (1850-1934)
Annual address. The causation of diphtheria. [Baltimore, 1891.] 27p. DNLM **90-9646**

WELCH, William H[enry] (1850-1934)
Some considerations concerning antiseptic surgery. [Baltimore, 1891.] 13p. DNLM **90-9647**

WELCH, William H[enry] (1850-1934) and Simon FLEXNER
The histological changes in experimental diphtheria. Preliminary communication. [Baltimore, 1891.] 4 l. DNLM **90-9648**

WELCH, William H[enry] (1850-1934)
Conditions underlying the infection of wounds; including a discussion of disinfection with reference to treatment of wounds, of the relation of bacteria to suppuration, of the resistance of tissues to the multiplication of bacteria, and of the effects of antiseptic agents on wounds. [New Haven, 1892.] 12p. DNLM **90-9649**

WELCH, William H[enry] (1850-1934)
Sanitation in relation to the poor. An address delivered before the Charity Organization Society of Baltimore, November 14, 1892. [Baltimore, 1892.] 14p. DNLM **90-9650**

WELCH, William H[enry] (1850-1934)
President's address. The etiology of acute lobar pneumonia, considered from a bacteriological point of view. [Baltimore, 1892.] 29p. DNLM **90-9651**

WELCH, William H[enry] (1850-1934) and George H. F. NUTTALL
A gas-producing bacillus (Bacillus aerogenes capsulatus, nov. spec.) capable of rapid development in the blood-vessels after death. [Baltimore, 1892.] 15 l. DNLM **90-9652**

WELCH, William H[enry] (1850-1934) and Simon FLEXNER
The histological lesions produced by the toxalbumen of diphtheria. [Baltimore, 1892.] 2 l. DNLM **90-9653**

WELCH, William H[enry] (1850-1934)
Asiatic cholera in its relation to sanitary reform. [Washington, D.C., 1893.] 7p. DNLM **90-9654**

WELCH, William H[enry] (1850-1934)
The Johns Hopkins Medical School. An address delivered at the graduating exercises of the Johns Hopkins University, June 13, 1893. [Baltimore], 1893. 6p. DNLM **90-9655**

WELCH, William H[enry] (1850-1934)
Higher medical education and the need of its endowment. Philadelphia, 1894. 24p. DNLM **90-9656**

WELCH, William H[enry] (1850-1934)
Bacteriological investigations of diphtheria in the United States. A report in behalf of the American committee on diphtheria to the eighth International Congress of Hygiene and Demography, held in Budapest, September 1 to 9, 1894. Philadelphia, 1894. 35p. DNLM **90-9657**

WELCH, William H[enry] (1850-1934) and A. W. CLEMENT
Remarks on hog cholera and swine plague. [Philadelphia, 1894.] 37p. DNLM **90-9658**

WELCH, William H[enry] (1850-1934)
The treatment of diphtheria by antitoxin. [Philadelphia, 1895.] 64p. DNLM **90-9659**

WELCH, William H[enry] (1850-1934)
The treatment of diphtheria by antitoxin. Baltimore, 1895. 62p. 2 charts. DNLM **90-9660**

WELCH, William H[enry] (1850-1934)
The evolution of modern scientific laboratories. Baltimore, 1896. 16p. DNLM **90-9661**

WELCH, William H[enry] (1850-1934)
The influence of anesthesia upon medical science. Boston: Damrell & Upham, 1896. 10p. DNLM **90-9662**

WELCH, William H[enry] (1850-1934)
Principles underlying the serum diagnosis of typhoid fever and the methods of its application. Chicago, 1897. 32p. DNLM **90-9663**

WELCH, William H[enry] (1850-1934) and William S. THAYER
Malaria. New York & Philadelphia, 1897. 154p. DNLM **90-9664**

WELCH, William H[enry] (1850-1934)
Adaptation in pathological processes. Philadelphia, 1897. 24p. DNLM **90-9665**

WELCH, William H[enry] (1850-1934)
Remarks at the presentation of the candidates for the degree of doctor of medicine at the commencement of the Johns Hopkins University, June 14, 1898. Baltimore, 1898. 8p. DNLM **90-9666**

WELCH, William M[iller] (*b.* 1837)
A statistical record of five thousand cases of small-pox. New York, 1894. 20p. DNLM **90-9667**

WELLES, Charles Stuart
Practical dietetics and outline of medicine. . . . New York, [etc.] : F. V. Doane, 1893. 79p. DLC; NNNAM **90-9668**

WELLS, David Washburn (*b.* 1862)
Keratometry and astigmatism. New York, 1899. 6p. DNLM **90-9669**

WELLS, David Washburn (*b.* 1862)
Squint. Boston, 1899. 8p. DNLM **90-9670**

WELLS, Edward F[ranklin] (*b.* 1853)
Pneumonia fever; its mortality, with a consideration of some of the elements of prognosis. Chicago, 1892. 23p. DNLM **90-9671**

WELLS, Edward F[ranklin] (*b.* 1853)
Hospitals for the insane; their scope and design. Chicago: Amer. Med. Assoc. Press, 1895. 32p. DNLM **90-9672**

WELLS, Frank
The address of the president of the Michigan State Board of Health. Lansing, 1895. 4p. DNLM **90-9673**

WELLS, Frank
Suggestions on public health work in Michigan. Presidential address to the Michigan State Board of Health, Lansing, April 9, 1897. Lansing, 1897. 8p. DNLM **90-9674**

WELLS, Samuel R[oberts] (1820-1875)
New physiognomy, or signs of character. New York: Fowler & Wells, 1896. 768p. DLC; NN [Originally, 1867, *vel subseq.*] **90-9675**

WELLS, Walter A[ugustine] (*b.* 1870)
Negative histological examination of the blood as a factor in differential diagnosis. Philadelphia, 1896. 13p. DNLM **90-9676**

WELLS, Walter A[ugustine] (*b.* 1870)
Some nervous and mental manifestations occurring in connection with nasal disease. Philadelphia, 1898. 15p. DNLM **90-9677**

WELLS, Walter A[ugustine] (*b.* 1870)
The pathogenesis of the nasal reflex neuroses. Philadelphia, 1898. 12p. DNLM **90-9678**

WELLS, Walter A[ugustine] (*b.* 1870)
The significance of uric acid in the nasal reflex neuroses. New York, 1898. 12p. DNLM **90-9679**

WELLS, Walter A[ugustine] (*b.* 1870)
On the relationship of the nose to diseases of the skin. New York, 1898. 10p. DNLM **90-9680**

WELLS, Walter A[ugustine] (*b.* 1870)
The breath of life. New York, 1898. 11p. DNLM **90-9681**

WELLS, Walter A[ugustine] (*b.* 1870)
The value of thiol in nose and throat practice. Philadelphia, 1899. 2 l. DNLM **90-9682**

WELLS, Walter S[cott] (*d.* 1897)
Uterine osmosis. [Philadelphia, 1892.] 12p. DNLM **90-9683**

WELLS, William Hughes (1859-1919)
A compend of gynecology. Philadelphia: P. Blakiston, Son & Co., 1896. 262p. CtY-M; DNLM; PPC; PU **90-9684**

WELLS, William Hughes (1859-1919)
. . . A compend of gynecology. . . . Philadelphia: P. Blakiston's Son & Co., 1899. 279p. DLC; NNNAM; PPC; PU **90-9685**

WELT, Sara
A contribution on the occurrence of mental disturbances following acute diseases in childhood. [New York, 1893.] 10p. DNLM **90-9686**

WENDE, Ernest (1853-1910)
The death-dealing long-tube nursing bottle. Chicago, 1899. 7p. DNLM **90-9687**

WENDE, Grover William (*b.* 1866)
An interesting case of tinea favosa epidermidis. New York, 1896. 8p. DNLM **90-9688**

WENDE, Grover William (*b.* 1866)
A case of rhinoscleroma originating in the United States. New York, 1896. 4p. DNLM **90-9689**

WENDE, Grover William (*b.* 1866)
Porokeratosis, with report of a case. [New York, 1898.] 9p. DNLM **90-9690**

WENDT, Edmund Charles (1857-1903)
Case of large-round-celled sarcoma of the testicle in a unilateral cyptorchis; extirpation; cure. [New York, 1891.] 9p. DNLM **90-9691**

WENDT, Edmund Charles (1857-1903)
The new Rome, and the question of Roman fever. New York: Trow Co., 1892. 24p. DNLM **90-9692**

WENNER, Ralph Jay (1870-1900)
Lumbar puncture of the subarachnoid space, with report of cases. Cleveland, 1896. 7p. DNLM **90-9693**

WENNER, Ralph Jay (1870-1900)
Acute empyema of the frontal sinus, with report of cases. Cleveland, 1898. 7p. DNLM **90-9694**

WENTWORTH, A[rthur] H[oward] (*b.* 1864)
Two cases of infection of the lungs proceeding from the pleura. [Philadelphia], 1895. 11p. DNLM **90-9695**

WENTWORTH, A[rthur] H[oward] (*b.* 1864)
Two cases of malignant growth in the kidney. [Philadelphia], 1896. 21p. DNLM **90-9696**

WENTWORTH, A[rthur] H[oward] (*b.* 1864)
Observations on meningitis in infants and children. Boston: Damrell & Upham, 1898. 43p. 4 charts. DNLM **90-9697**

WENTWORTH, A[rthur] H[oward] (*b.* 1864)
Epidemic cerebro-spinal meningitis. Boston, 1898. 27p. DNLM **90-9698**

WENTWORTH, A[rthur] H[oward (*b.* 1864)
A case of meningitis due to the typhoid bacillus. Boston, 1899. 8p. DNLM **90-9699**

WENZEL, Henry P.
Placenta previa, its causes, diagnosis, and treatment; with three cases, all mother and two children saved. [New York, 1890.] 15p. DNLM **90-9700**

WENZEL, Henry P.
Caesarean section performed at term successfully, both mother and child remaining alive and in good health. [Philadelphia, 1891.] 14p. DNLM **90-9701**

WERDER, X[avier] O. (1857-1919)
Etiology of pelvic diseases in women, and their prophylaxis. Pittsburgh: Murdoch, Kerr & Co., 1893. 8p. DNLM **90-9702**

WERDER, X[avier] O. (1857-1919)
Pregnancy following a partial suprapubic hysterectomy, complicated by hemorrhage through the abdominal cicatrix. Philadelphia, 1893. 5p. DNLM **90-9703**

WERDER, X[avier] O. (1857-1919)
The present status of the treatment of uterine fibroids. Philadelphia, 1893. 8p. DNLM **90-9704**

WERDER, X[avier] O. (1857-1919)
Two interesting cases of intestinal resection with end-to-end anastomosis by means of the Murphy button, with recovery. Pittsburgh: Murdoch, Kerr & Co., 1897. 5p. DNLM **90-9705**

WERDER, X[avier] O. (1857-1919)
Tonic and spasmodic intestinal contractions, with report of cases. Boston, 1897. 12p. DNLM **90-9706**

WERDER, X[avier] O. (1857-1919)
Appendicitis complicating ovarian cyst and simulating torsion of the pedicle, with three cases. Chicago, 1898. 4p. DNLM **90-9707**

WERDER, X[avier] O. (1857-1919)
A new operation for the radical treatment of cancer of the cervix, consisting of the removal of the uterus and vagina en masse by the supra-pubic method; with report of a case. New York, 1898. 4p. DNLM **90-9708**

WESCOTT, Casius D. (*b.* 1861)
Report of a case of sudden death from coronary obstruction, with specimen. [Chicago, 1892.] 7p. DNLM **90-9709**

WESCOTT, Cassius D. (*b.* 1861)
Injuries to the eye and its appendages. [Chicago, 1893.] 8p. DNLM **90-9710**

WESCOTT, Cassius D. (*b.* 1861)
On the necessity of repeated examination in the correction of errors of refraction. Nashville, 1898. 4p. DNLM **90-9711**

WESCOTT, Cassius D. (*b.* 1861)
An additional case of double congenital microphthalmos. Chicago, 1898. 8p. DNLM **90-9712**

WESCOTT, Cassius D. (*b.* 1861)
What should the general practitioner know about the eye? Chicago, 1898. 8p. DNLM **90-9713**

WESCOTT, Cassius D. (*b.* 1861)
Traumatism of the eyeball involving the crystalline lens. Chicago, 1899. 15p. DNLM **90-9714**

WEST, James N[ephew] (*b.* 1866)
A successful secondary laparotomy for haemorrhage following abdominal hysterectomy. New York, 1896. 4p. DNLM **90-9715**

WEST SIDE GERMAN DISPENSARY OF THE CITY OF NEW YORK
Annual report of the board of trustees and officers to the subscribers for the year 1892-93. New York: G. Lauter, 1894. 37p. DNLM; NNNAM [German and English text.] **90-9716**

WESTCOTT, Thompson S[eiser] (*b.* 1862)
A case of influenza with persistent respiratory failure in an infant of four weeks. New York: E. B. Treat & Co., 1897. 7p. DNLM **90-9717**

WESTERN RESERVE UNIVERSITY, CLEVELAND, OHIO
Annual catalogues of the officers and students [including the Medical Department, at Cleveland] for the years 1894-95; 1909-10. Cleveland, 1895-1910. DNLM **90-9718**

WESTERN RESERVE UNIVERSITY, COLLEGE OF DENTISTRY, CLEVELAND, OHIO
Annual announcements for the sessions of 1895-96 to 1903-04. Cleveland, 1896-1904. DNLM **90-9719**

WESTERN RESERVE UNIVERSITY, MEDICAL DEPARTMENT, CLEVELAND, OHIO
Annual announcements for the sessions of 1893-94 to 1912-13. Cleveland, 1894-1913. DNLM **90-9720**

WESTLAND, Albert (1853-1915)
The wife and mother. A handbook for mothers. . . . Philadelphia: P. Blakiston, Son & Co., 1896. 282p. DNLM; NNNAM; PPC; PPJ **90-9721**

WETHERED, Frank J[oseph] (1860-1928)
Medical microscopy. A guide to the use of the microscope in medical practice. Philadelphia: P. Blakiston, Son & Co., 1892. 406p. DNLM; OCIM; PPC; PU **90-9722**

WETHERILL, Horace G. (1856-1941)
The insane and the asylums. Trenton, N.J.: MacCrellish & Quigley, 1892. 26p. DNLM **90-9723**

WETHERILL, Horace G. (1856-1941)
Health resorts of the West and Southwest. [Philadelphia, 1893.] 10p. DNLM **90-9724**

WETHERILL, Horace G. (1856-1941)
Some noteworthy hysterectomies. A retrospective view. New York, 1896. 10p. DNLM **90-9725**

WEYL, Theodor (1851-1913)
The coal-tar colors, with especial reference to their injurious qualities and the restriction of their use. A sanitary and medico-legal investigation, with a preface by Professor Sell. Transl. with permission of the author by Henry Leffmann. Philadelphia: P. Blakiston, Son & Co., 1892. 154p. DNLM; PPC; PPJ **90-9726**

WEYSSE, Arthur Wisswald (*b.* 1867)
An epitome of human histology; for the use of students in connection with lectures and laboratory work. . . . New York, [etc.]: Longmans, Green & Co., 1898. 90p. DLC; NNNAM **90-9727**

WHARTON, Henry Redwood (1853-1925)
Minor surgery and bandaging, including the treatment of fractures and dislocations. . . . With four hundred and three illustrations. Philadelphia: Lea Bros. & Co., 1891. 497p. DLC; DNLM; NNNAM; PPC **90-9728**

WHARTON, Henry Redwood (1853-1925)
Minor surgery and bandaging, including the treatment of fractures and dislocations. . . . 2nd ed., thoroughly rev. and enl., with four hundred and sixteen illustrations. Philadelphia: Lea Bros. & Co., 1893. 529p. DLC; IEN-M; MBM; PPC **90-9729**

WHARTON, Henry Redwood (1853-1925)
Minor surgery and bandaging, including the treatment of fractures and dislocations. . . . 3rd ed., thoroughly rev. and enl., with 475 illustrations. Philadelphia, and New York: Lea Bros. & Co., 1896. 597p. DLC; DNLM; MH-M; NNNAM **90-9730**

WHARTON, Henry Redwood (1853-1925)
The practice of surgery; a treatise on surgery for the use of practitioners and students, by Henry R. Wharton . . . and B. Farquhar Curtis. . . . Philadelphia: J. B. Lippincott Co., 1898. 1240p. col. plates. CtY-M; DLC; DNLM; PPC; PU **90-9731**

WHARTON, Henry Redwood (1853-1925)
Minor surgery and bandaging; including the treatment of fractures and dislocations, the ligation of arteries, amputations, excisions and resections, intestinal anastomosis, operations upon nerves and tendons, tracheotomy, intubation of the larynx, etc. . . . 4th ed., thoroughly rev. and enl., with 502 illustrations. Philadelphia and New York: Lea Bros. & Co., 1899. 594p. DLC; LNT-M; PPC; PU **90-9732**

WHARTON, Henry Redwood (1853-1925)
The practice of surgery; a treatise on surgery for the use of practitioners and students, by Henry R. Wharton . . . and B. Farquhar Curtis. . . . Rev. ed. Philadelphia, London: J. B. Lippincott Co., [1899]. 1244p. col. plates. DLC; NNNAM; PPC; PU **90-9733**

WHEELER, Alexander (*d.* 1903)
Handbook of medicine and therapeutics. New York: William Wood & Co., 1894. 512p. MBM; NNNAM; PPC; PU **90-9734**

WHEELER, C[harles] Gilbert (1836-1912)
Medical chemistry, including outlines of organic and physiological chemistry. Based in part on Riche's "Manuel de Chimie." 5th ed. Chicago: S. J. Wheeler, 1890. 424p. DNLM; ICU; ICRM; NNC **90-9735**

WHEELER, John Brooks (*b.* 1853)
Appendicitis. Danbury, 1893. 30p. DNLM **90-9736**

WHEELER, John Brooks (*b.* 1853)
The necessity of prompt operative treatment in appendicitis. New York: D. Appleton & Co., 1894. 7p. DNLM **90-9737**

WHEELER, John Brooks (*b.* 1853)
Surgery in its relations to the female pelvic organs. Boston, 1899. 6p. DNLM **90-9738**

WHEELER, Leonard A. (*b.* 1845)
The treatment of uterine fibroids, with report of cases. Boston: Damrell & Upham, 1895. 13p. DNLM **90-9739**

WHELPLEY, H[enry] M[ilton] (1861-1926)
Synopsis of a course in microscopy for pharmacists. [Philadelphia, 1890.] 6p. DNLM **90-9740**

WHELPLEY, H[enry] M[ilton] (1861-1926)
Chemical lecture notes. Taken from Prof. C. O. Curtman's lectures at the St. Louis College of Pharmacy. . . . 3rd ed. With over one hundred illustrations. St. Louis, Mo.: The Author, 1890. 211p. diags. DLC **90-9741**

WHELPLEY, H[enry] M[ilton] (1861-1926)
Trichina spiralis. St. Louis: Nixon-Jones Printing Co., [1891]. 6p. DNLM **90-9742**

WHELPLEY, H[enry] M[ilton] (1861-1926)
Chemical lecture notes. Taken from Prof. C. O. Curtman's lectures at the St. Louis College of Pharmacy. . . . 4th ed. with over one hundred illustrations. St. Louis, Mo.: The Author, 1892. 211p. diags. DLC **90-9743**

WHELPLEY, H[enry] M[ilton] (1861-1926)
Therapeutic terms for pharmacists and physicians. St. Louis, Mo., 1894. 67p. DLC; DNLM **90-9744**

WHELPLEY, H[enry] M[ilton] (1861-1926)
Board of pharmacy examinations. Also: The government of students in colleges of pharmacy. [St. Louis, 1894.] 1 l. DNLM **90-9745**

WHELPLEY, H[enry] M[ilton] (1861-1926)
A consideration of the pharmacist of today. [St. Louis, 1895.] 2 l. DNLM **90-9746**

WHELPLEY, H[enry] M[ilton] (1861-1926)
A metric system report; statistics based upon 233,000 prescriptions. [St. Louis, 1897.] 1 l. DNLM **90-9747**

WHELPLEY, H[enry] M[ilton] (1861-1926)
Report on the use of the metric system in 545,000 prescriptions. [St. Louis, 1899.] 1 l. DNLM **90-9748**

WHIPPLE, Farrington H[asham]
A guide to the clinical examination of the urine. . . . Boston: Damrell & Upham, 1891. 206p. tables. DLC; DNLM; MBM **90-9749**

WHIPPLE, George Chandler (1866-1924)
The microscopy of drinking water. 1st ed. New York: J. Wiley & Sons; London: Chapman & Hall, 1899. 300p. 19 plates. DNLM; NNNAM **90-9750**

WHIPPLE, Leander Edmund (*d.* 1916)
Absent treatment in metaphysical healing. . . . [New York]: American Bank Note Co., 1891. 16p. DLC **90-9751**

WHIPPLE, Leander Edmund (*d.* 1916)
The philosophy of mental healing. A practical exposition of natural restorative power. New York: Metaphysical Pub. Co., 1893. 234p. DLC; DNLM; MB; NN [*vel subseq.*] **90-9752**

WHITACRE, Horace J. (*b.* 1869)
A laboratory text-book of pathology for the use of students and practitioners of medicine. Philadelphia: P. Blakiston, Son & Co., 1897. 172p. DNLM; PPC **90-9753**

WHITALL, TATUM & CO.
Illustrated catalogue, with supplement. [Druggists' supplies.] Philadelphia & New York, 1890. 198, 32p. PPC **90-9754**

WHITALL, TATUM & CO.
Illustrated catalogue. [Druggists' supplies.] Philadelphia & New York, 1891. 200p. PPC; PU **90-9755**

WHITALL, TATUM & CO.
Illustrated catalogue. [Druggists' supplies]. Philadelphia & New York, 1893. 206p. PU **90-9756**

WHITALL, TATUM & CO.
Illustrated catalogue. [Druggists' supplies.] Philadelphia & New York, 1894. 206p. PU **90-9757**

WHITALL, TATUM & CO.
Illustrated catalogue. [Druggists' supplies.] Philadelphia & New York, 1895. 206p. PU **90-9758**

WHITALL, TATUM & CO.
Illustrated catalogue. [Druggists' supplies.] Philadelphia & New York, 1896. 206p. PPC; PU **90-9759**

WHITALL, TATUM & CO.
Illustrated catalogue. [Druggists' supplies.] Philadelphia & New York, 1897. 206p. PPC; PU **90-9760**

WHITALL, TATUM & CO.
Illustrated catalogue. [Druggists' supplies]. Philadelphia & New York, 1898. 206p. PPC **90-9761**

WHITALL, TATUM & CO.
Illustrated catalogue. [Druggists' supplies]. Philadelphia & New York, 1899. 202p. PPC **90-9762**

WHITE, Charles J[ames] (*b.* 1868)
The study of dermatology in Europe. Boston: Damrell & Upham, 1895. 29p. DNLM **90-9763**

WHITE, Charles J[ames] (*b.* 1868)
Dystrophia unguium et pilorum hereditaria. New York, 1896. 8p. DNLM **90-9764**

WHITE, Charles J[ames] (*b.* 1868)
Ringworm as it exists in Boston. New York, 1899. 17p. 3 plates. DNLM **90-9765**

WHITE, David Kirk (*b.* 1865)
A case of dermatitis of exfoliativa neonatorum. [New York]: D. Appleton & Co., 1895. 2p. DNLM **90-9766**

WHITE, FIRM, DENTAL MANUFACTURERS, PHILADELPHIA
. . . Catálogo condensado con ilustraciones. Dientes, instrumentos, máquinas. . . . [Marzo, 1892] Philadelphia: The S. S. White Dental Mfg. Co., [1892]. 316p. DLC **90-9767**

WHITE, FIRM, DENTAL MANUFACTURERS, PHILADELPHIA
. . . Catálogo condensado con ilustraciones. Dientes, instrumentos, máquinas. . . . [Philadelphia: The S. S. White Dental Mfg. Co.], 1895. 359p. DLC **90-9768**

WHITE, Franklin W[arren] (*b.* 1869)
The diagnostic value of tuberculin. Boston: Damrell & Upham, 1898. 11p. DNLM **90-9769**

WHITE, Franklin W[arren] (*b.* 1869)
A case of sporadic cretinism. Boston, 1899. 7p. DNLM **90-9770**

WHITE, Franklin W[arren] (*b.* 1869)
Experiments upon the germicidal properties of bloody serum. Boston: Damrell & Upham, 1899. 24p. DNLM **90-9771**

WHITE, Franklin W[arren] (*b.* 1869)
A case of tetany. [Boston, 1899.] 6p. DNLM **90-9772**

WHITE, Franklin W[arren] (*b.* 1869)
Blood cultures in septicemia, pneumonia, meningitis, and chronic disease. Boston, 1899. 8p. DNLM **90-9773**

WHITE, James C[larke] (1833-1916)
Keratosis follicularis (psorospermose folliculaire végétante). A second case. [New York, 1890.] 8p. DNLM **90-9774**

WHITE, James C[larke] (1833-1916)
The relations of the Massachusetts Medical Society to medical education. A plea for professional independence. The annual discourse delivered in Boston before the Massachusetts Medical Society, June 11, 1890. Boston: D. Clapp & Son, 1890. 47p. DNLM **90-9775**

WHITE, James C[larke] (1833-1916)
Clinical aspects and etiological relations of cutaneous tuberculosis. Boston: Damrell & Upham, 1891. 30p. DNLM **90-9776**

WHITE, James C[larke] (1833-1916)
Some dangers of infection incidental to professional life. Boston: Damrell & Upham, 1892. 13p. DNLM **90-9777**

WHITE, James C[larke] (1833-1916)
The contagiousness and control of leprosy. Boston: Damrell & Upham, 1894. 12p. DNLM; MBM **90-9778**

WHITE, James C[larke] (1833-1916)
Cases of pityriasis rubra pilaris (Besnier); érythème indure des scrofuleux; lymphangioma circumscriptum; multiple benign cystic epithelioma; angioma speriginosum (Crocker). New York, 1894. 30p. DNLM **90-9779**

WHITE, James C[larke] (1833-1916)
The prevalence of germ dermatoses. Boston: Damrell & Upham, 1896. 11p. DNLM **90-9780**

WHITE, James C[larke] (1833-1916)
Prurigo. New York, 1897. 11p. DNLM **90-9781**

WHITE, James C[larke] (1833-1916)
Notes on dermatitis venenata. Boston: Damrell & Upham, 1897. 9p. DNLM **90-9782**

WHITE, James C[larke] (1833-1916)
The president's address before the American Dermatological Association at the twenty-first annual meeting, at Washington, May 4, 1897. New York, 1897. 9p. DNLM **90-9783**

WHITE, James C[larke] (1833-1916)
Lupus erythematosus; its amenability to treatment. New York, 1898. 9p. DNLM **90-9784**

WHITE, James C[larke] (1833-1916)
Hydroa vacciniforme. New York, 1898. 9p. DNLM **90-9785**

WHITE, James C[larke] (1833-1916) and Charles J. WHITE
A case of lymphangioma of labia majora vulvae. New York, 1898. 6p. DNLM **90-9786**

WHITE, James William (1826-1891)
Los dientes: naturales y artificiales. . . . Philadelphia: The S. S. White Dental Mfg. Co., 1898. 32p. DLC **90-9787**

WHITE, J[ames] William (1850-1916)
Electrical execution. [Philadelphia: Lea Bros. & Co., 1890.] 15p. DNLM **90-9788**

WHITE, J[ames] William (1850-1916)
A method of applying antisepsis in the treatment of recent anterior urethritis. [Philadelphia: Lea Bros. & Co., 1890.] 15p. DNLM **90-9789**

WHITE, J[ames] William (1850-1916)
The modern treatment of vesical calculus in male children. [Philadelphia: Lea Bros. & Co., 1890.] 12p. DNLM **90-9790**

WHITE, J[ames] William (1850-1916)
On the removal of enormous vesical calculi by the suprapubic route, with report of a recent successful case. [St. Louis, 1890.] 16p. DNLM **90-9791**

WHITE, J[ames] William (1850-1916)
Two cases of prostatectomy. [Philadelphia, 1890.] 12p. DNLM **90-9792**

WHITE, J[ames] William (1850-1916)
Valedictory address to graduating class of the medical department of the University of Pennsylvania, May, 1890. [Philadelphia, 1890.] 11p. DNLM **90-9793**

WHITE, J[ames] William (1850-1916)
Glandular tumors of the neck. Detroit: G. S. Davis, 1890. 11p. DNLM **90-9794**

WHITE, J[ames] William (1850-1916)
Memorandum of a rare complication of litholapaxy. [Philadelphia, 1891.] 3p. DNLM **90-9795**

WHITE, J[ames] William (1850-1916)
Notes on six cases of perineal section; with some remarks on the technique of the operation. [Philadelphia, 1891.] 8p. DNLM **90-9796**

WHITE, J[ames] William (1850-1916)
The supposed curative effect of operations per se. [St. Louis, 1891.] 76p. DNLM **90-9797**

WHITE, J[ames] William (1850-1916)
The treatment of stricture of the male urethra. [Philadelphia, 1891.] 22p. DNLM **90-9798**

WHITE, J[ames] William (1850-1916)
The present position of antiseptic surgery. St. Louis, 1891. 30p. DNLM **90-9799**

WHITE, J[ames] William (1850-1916)
The surgery of the spine. Detroit, 1891. 98p. 1 plate. DNLM **90-9800**

WHITE, J[ames] William (1850-1916)
Memoir of D. Hayes Agnew, M.D., LL.D. Philadelphia, 1893. 30p. 3 plates. DNLM **90-9801**

WHITE, J[ames] William (1850-1916) and Alfred C. WOOD
Surgical methods and results in cases of tubercular disease, aneurism, ununited fractures, head injuries, neoplasms, vesical calculi, and diseases of the bones and joints. [Philadelphia: Lea Bros. & Co., 1893.] 46p. DNLM **90-9802**

WHITE, J[ames] William (1850-1916)
An address on appendicitis. Detroit, Mich.: G. S. Davis, 1894. 55p. DNLM **90-9803**

WHITE, J[ames] William (1850-1916) and Alfred C. WOOD
The treatment of empyema, with seclected cases. Detroit, Mich.: G. S. Davis, 1894. 19p. DNLM
90-9804

WHITE, J[ames] William (1850-1916)
Castration for the cure of hypertrophied prostate. Philadelphia, 1894. 7p. DNLM 90-9805

WHITE, J[ames] William (1850-1916)
In re White's operation for hypertrophied prostate. Philadelphia, 1895. 7p. DNLM 90-9806

WHITE, J[ames] William (1850-1916)
As to castration for hypertrophied prostate; a protest against a protest. [Philadelphia, 1895.] 4p. DNLM
90-9807

WHITE, J[ames] William (1850-1916)
The results of double castration in hypertrophy of the prostate with a consideration of allied methods and a table of cases. Philadelphia: Univ. Penn. Press, 1895. 80p. DNLM
90-9808

WHITE, J[ames] William (1850-1916)
A foreign body in the esophagus detected and located by the Röntgen rays. Philadelphia, 1896. 6p. DNLM
90-9809

WHITE, J[ames] William (1850-1916)
Genito-urinary surgery and venereal diseases. By J. William White . . . and Edward Martin. . . . Philadelphia, [etc.] : J. B. Lippincott Co., 1897. 1061p. col. plates. DLC; DNLM; NNNAM; PPC 90-9810

WHITE, J[ames] William (1850-1916)
Genito-urinary surgery and venereal diseases. By J. William White . . . and Edward Martin. . . . 2nd ed. Philadelphia: J. B. Lippincott Co., 1898. 1061p. col. plates. PPC; PPJ
90-9811

WHITE, J[ames] William (1850-1916)
Genito-urinary surgery and venereal diseases. By J. William White . . . and Edward Martin. . . . 3rd ed. Philadelphia: J. B. Lippincott Co., 1898. 1061p. col. plates. NNNAM; PPC; PPJ; PU 90-9812

WHITE, John Blake (*b.* 1850)
A case of stricture followed by rupture of the urethra and extravasation of urine. External urethrotomy; recovery. [New York, 1890.] 4p. DNLM 90-9813

WHITE, John Blake (*b.* 1850)
Value of the subcutaneous administration of gold and manganese in the treatment of tuberculosis. New York, 1891. 24p. DNLM 90-9814

WHITE, John Blake (*b.* 1850)
An antiseptic syringe for hypodermic injection. New York, 1891. 1 l. DNLM 90-9815

WHITE, John Blake (*b.* 1850)
Observations on the syphilitic cachexia. [New York, 1892.] 5p. DNLM 90-9816

WHITE, John Blake (*b.* 1850)
Pneumotomy twice n the same patient for the relief tuberculous abscess and gangrene of the lungs; recovery. [Philadelphia, 1893.] 12p. DNLM 90-9817

WHITE, John Blake (*b.* 1850)
The tubercular diathesis controlled by gold and manganese in combination. New York, 1894. 12p. DNLM
90-9818

WHITE, Joseph A.
Mistaken impressions about nasal catarrh and its treatment. Richmond, Va., 1891. 6p. DNLM 90-9819

WHITE, Leon Edward (*b.* 1867)
Classification and prognosis of cases of long-standing deafness. Baltimore, 1899. 8p. DNLM 90-9820

WHITE, William A[lanson] (1870-1937)
The physical basis of insanity and the insane diathesis. Utica, N.Y., 1894. 8p. DNLM 90-9821

WHITE, William Hale (1857-1949)
Materia medica, pharmacy, pharmacology, and therapeutics. Edited by Reynold W. Wilcox. Philadelphia: P. Blakiston, Son & Co., 1892. 607p. CtY-M; DNLM; MH-M; PPC
90-9822

WHITE, William Hale (1857-1949)
Materia medica, pharmacy, pharmacology, and therapeutics. 2nd ed. Edited by Reynold W. Wilcox. Philadelphia: P. Blakiston, Son & Co., 1894. 661p. DLC; PPC; PPJ
90-9823

WHITE, William Hale (1857-1949)
Materia medica, pharmacy, pharmacology, and therapeutics. 3rd ed. Edited by Reynold W. Wilcox. Philadelphia: P. Blakiston, Son & Co., 1895. 687p. DLC; DNLM; PPC; PU
90-9824

WHITE, William Hale (1857-1949)
Materia medica, pharmacy, pharmacology, and therapeutics. 4th American ed. Edited by Reynold W. Wilcox. Philadelphia: P. Blakiston, Son & Co., 1898. 704p. DNLM; NNNAM; OCLloyd; PPC 90-9825

WHITEHEAD, William Riddick (1831-1902)
The autobiography of a Western surgeon. Denver, Col.: W. F. Robinson & Co., 1890. 32p. port. DNLM
90-9826

WHITEHOUSE, Henry H[oward] (*b.* 1864)
A case of ringworm of the scalp simulating alopecia areata. New York, 1892. 4p. DNLM 90-9827

WHITEHOUSE, Henry H[oward] (*b.* 1864)
A case of impetigo herpetiformis (Hebra) in the male. New York, 1898. 10p. DNLM 90-9828

WHITING, A[lbert] D[raper] (*b.* 1869)
Aids to aseptic technique. Philadelphia: J. B. Lippincott Co., 1898. 157p. DLC; DNLM; PPC; PU
90-9829

WHITLA, William (1851-1933)
A dictionary of treatment; or, Therapeutic index, including medical and surgical therapeutics. . . . Rev. and adapted to the pharmacopoeia of the United States. Philadelphia: Lea Bros. & Co., 1892. 921p. DLC; NNNAM; PPC; PU
90-9830

WHITMAN, Charles Otis (1842-1910)
Some of the functions and features of a biological station. New York, 1898. 16p. DNLM 90-9831

WHITMAN, Royal (1857-1946)
The rational treatment of flat-foot. [New York, 1890.] 7p. DNLM **90-9832**

WHITMAN, Royal (1857-1946)
The treatment of persistent abduction of the foot, commonly known as chronic sprain of the ankle. [New York, 1890.] 7p. DNLM **90-9833**

WHITMAN, Royal (1857-1946)
The prevention of unnecessary deformity in Pott's disease. [Philadelphia, 1891.] 3p. DNLM **90-9834**

WHITMAN, Royal (1857-1946)
Observations on torticollis, with particular reference to the significance of the so-called hematoma of the sterno-mastoid muscle. Philadelphia, 1891. 17p. DNLM **90-9835**

WHITMAN, Royal (1857-1946)
A consideration of some of the affections of tendon-sheaths and bursae, and their relations to injuries and diseases of the joints. New York, 1892. 12p. DNLM **90-9836**

WHITMAN, Royal (1857-1946)
Observations on tuberculous knee-joint disease in childhood. New York, 1892. 11p. DNLM **90-9837**

WHITMAN, Royal (1857-1946)
Observations on the ultimate deformities of Pott's disease: their modification and prevention, with special reference to the middle region of the spine. [Philadelphia, 1892.] 14p. DNLM **90-9838**

WHITMAN, Royal (1857-1946)
Observations on the ultimate deformities of Pott's disease: their modification and prevention, with special reference to the middle region of the spine. [Philadelphia, 1892.] 9p. DNLM **90-9839**

WHITMAN, Royal (1857-1946)
The radical cure of confirmed flat-foot. [New York, 1892.] 18p. DNLM **90-9840**

WHITMAN, Royal (1857-1946)
Additional notes on forcible over-correction in the treatment of rigid flat-foot. Philadelphia, 1893. 9p. DNLM **90-9841**

WHITMAN, Royal (1857-1946)
The elements of the differential diagnosis of Pott's disease in childhood. New York, 1893. 16p. DNLM **90-9842**

WHITMAN, Royal (1857-1946)
Observations on Pott's disease, with reference to the principles of treatment and their application. [New York, 1893.] 15p. DNLM **90-9843**

WHITMAN, Royal (1857-1946)
Observations on fracture of the neck of the femur in childhood, with especial reference to treatment and differential diagnosis from separation of the epiphysis. New York: Trow, 1893. 16p. DNLM **90-9844**

WHITMAN, Royal (1857-1946)
Observations on bending of the neck of the femur in adolescence, with particular reference to the diagnosis and significance of the affection. New York: D. Appleton & Co., 1894. 18p. 1 plate. DNLM **90-9845**

WHITMAN, Royal (1857-1946)
A study of the weak foot, with reference to its causes, its diagnosis, and its cure; with an analysis of a thousand cases of so-called flat-foot. New York: D. Appleton & Co., 1895. 42p. DNLM **90-9846**

WHITMAN, Royal (1857-1946)
A definition of the scope of orthopaedic surgery, as indicated by its origin, by its development, and by the work of the American Orthopaedic Association. New York, 1896. 11p. DNLM **90-9847**

WHITMAN, Royal (1857-1946)
Further observations on coxa vara, with particular reference to its aetiology and treatment. New York, 1899. 30p. DNLM **90-9848**

WHITMAN, Walt (1819-1892)
The wound dresser, a series of letters written from the hospitals in Washington during the war of the rebellion. Edited by Richard Maurice Bucke. Boston: Small, Maynard & Co., 1898. 201p. MB; MH; NN; PU **90-9849**

WHITMORE, Benjamin T.
Professor Behring's patent on diphtheria antitoxins. [New York, 1898.] 5p. DNLM **90-9850**

WHITNEY, Charles Melville (*b.* 1862)
Intubation of the larynx in private practice; results in seventy-eight cases. Boston: Damrell & Upham, 1893. 19p. DNLM **90-9851**

WHITNEY, H[erbert] B. (*b.* 1856)
Diagnosis of pleuritic effusion. New York, 1894. 10p. DNLM **90-9852**

WHITNEY, H[erbert] B. (*b.* 1856)
The normal praecordia in childhood. New York, 1894. 6p. DNLM **90-9853**

WHITNEY, H[erbert] B. (*b.* 1856)
Two cases of abscess of the liver, with remarks on diagnosis. [Denver, 1895.] 11p. DNLM **90-9854**

WHITNEY, H[erbert] B. (*b.* 1856)
Cyclic vomiting; a brief review of this affection as illustrated by a typical case. New York: E. B. Treat & Co., [1898]. 7p. DNLM **90-9855**

WHITNEY, H[erbert] B. (*b.* 1856)
An unusual form of bronchiectasis. [Boston, 1898.] 11p. DNLM **90-9856**

WHITNEY, H[erbert] B. (*b.* 1856)
Acute pulmonary edema successfully treated by venesection. [New York, 1898.] 6p. DNLM **90-9857**

WHITNEY, H[erbert] B. (*b.* 1856)
Some practical considerations concerning pneumothorax, based on a brief report of cases. Philadelphia, 1899. 14p. DNLM **90-9858**

WHITNEY, William Fiske (1850-1921)
Extra-uterine pregnancy. [Boston, 1893.] 4p. DNLM
90-9859

WHITNEY, William Fiske (1850-1921)
Address to the students of Harvard Veterinary School. New York, 1896. 7p. DNLM **90-9860**

WHITTAKER'S anatomical model. A pictorial representation of the human frame and its organs. With descriptive text by Dr. Schmidt. English edition by William S. Furneaux. New York: T. Whittaker, [1896?]. 16p. superimposed plates. DNLM; NNNAM **90-9861**

WHITTAKER, James T. (*d.* 1900)
Valedictory address, delivered to the students of the graduating class of the seventy-first annual session of the Medical College of Ohio. [1891?] 8p. DNLM **90-9862**

WHITTAKER, James T. (*d.* 1900)
The theory and practice of medicine, prepared for students and practitioners. New York: William Wood & Co., 1893. 821p. 1 col. plate. DLC; DNLM; NNNAM; PPC
90-9863

WHITTAKER, James T. (*d.* 1900)
Annual oration, Medical College of Ohio Alumni Association. [Cincinnati, 1893.] 20p. DNLM **90-9864**

WHITTAKER, James T. (*d.* 1900)
Predisposition to phthisis. Baltimore, 1894. 24p. DNLM
90-9865

WHITTAKER, James T. (*d.* 1900)
Pneumonia; how regarded in 1895. Cincinnati, 1895. 24p. DNLM **90-9866**

WHITTAKER, James T. (*d.* 1900)
Medicine and surgery of the Queen City. Chicago, 1896. 32p. DNLM **90-9867**

WHITTAKER, James T. (*d.* 1900)
Arterio-sclerosis. Pittsburgh, 1899. 12p. DNLM
90-9868

WIENER, Alexander C.
The extension corset and its indications. Chicago, 1896. 23p. DNLM **90-9869**

WIENER, Alexander C.
Treatment of fractures of the lower extremities in ambulando. Chicago, 1896. 16p. DNLM **90-9870**

WIENER, Alfred (*b.* 1865)
A case of subacute unilateral bulbar palsy, with autopsy. New York: D. Appleton & Co., 1894. 19p. DNLM
90-9871

WIENER, Joseph (1828-1904)
The present status of gynaecology abroad. New York: D. Appleton & Co., 1897. 93p. DNLM; NNNAM
90-9872

WIESNER, Oscar E. A.
New illustrated catalogue of white porcelite enameled steel aseptic hospital furniture, opeating room equipment. . . . Brooklyn, [*c.* 1893]. 38p. NNNAM
90-9873

WIGGIN, Frederick Holme (1853-1910)
Intestinal obstructions; diagnosis and treatment. New York: Trow Directory Pr. Bk. Co., 1892. 28p. DNLM
90-9874

WIGGIN, Frederick Holme (1853-1910)
A case of contusion and rupture of the ileum with peritonitis, without external wound, successfully treated by coeliotomy and primary interectomy, followed by circular enterorrhaphy (Maunsell's method). New York, 1894. 18p. DNLM
90-9875

WIGGIN, Frederick Holme (1853-1910)
Coeliotomy for bilateral pyosalpinx, followed four days later by appendicitis. Operation; recovery. A case of bilateral ovarian fibrosarcoma. New York, 1894. 6p. DNLM
90-9876

WIGGIN, Frederick Holme (1853-1910)
A case of chronic peritonitis, with intestinal and abdominal fistulae, enterorrhaphy; recovery. New York: Trow Directory Co., 1894. 7p. DNLM **90-9877**

WIGGIN, Frederick Holme (1853-1910)
Intestinal anastomosis. With report of a case. New York, 1894. 18p. 1 table. DNLM **90-9878**

WIGGIN, Frederick Holme (1853-1910)
Intestinal anastomosis. New York, 1894. 1 l. DNLM
90-9879

WIGGIN, Frederick Holme (1853-1910)
A case of contusion and rupture of the ileum with peritonitis, without external wound, successfully treated by coeliotomy and primary enterectomy, followed by circular enterorrhaphy (Maunsell's method); exhibition of patient and specimen. New York: D. Appleton & Co., 1894. 16p. DNLM
90-9880

WIGGIN, Frederick Holme (1853-1910)
Intestinal anastomosis; with the report of a case. New York, 1894. 18p. 1 table. DNLM **90-9881**

WIGGIN, Frederick Holme (1853-1910)
Perforation in enteric fever; its surgical treatment. [Bridgeport, 1895.] 6p. DNLM **90-9882**

WIGGIN, Frederick Holme (1853-1910)
Treatment of uterine retrodisplacements by vaginofixation, with reports of cases. [Danbury, Conn., 1895.] 4 l. DNLM
90-9883

WIGGIN, Frederick Holme (1853-1910)
Cystic tumors of the vaginal vault, with reports of two cases. [New York: D. Appleton & Co., 1895.] 7p. DNLM
90-9884

WIGGIN, Frederick Holme (1853-1910)
The technics of Maunsell's method of intestinal anastomosis, with a résumé of the cases of operation to date. [New York: D. Appleton & Co., 1895.] 22p. DNLM
90-9885

WIGGIN, Frederick Holme (1853-1910)
The necessity of complete extirpation of tumors and the importance of rapid cicatrization of the wound. Read at the twelfth annual meeting of the New York State Medical Association, October 16th, 1895, as a part of the discussion on surgery. New York, 1895. 7p. DNLM **90-9886**

WIGGIN, Frederick Holme (1853-1910)
Notes on the treatment of faecal fistulae. New York, 1896. 14p. DNLM **90-9887**

WIGGIN, Frederick Holme (1853-1910)
Infantile intussusception, a study of one hundred and three cases treated by intestinal distention or laparotomy, and a report of two cases. New York, 1896. 42p. DNLM **90-9888**

WIGGIN, Frederick Holme (1853-1910)
Report of five cases of uterine retrodisplacement treated by vaginal fixation (Mackenrodt). New York, 1896. 10p. DNLM **90-9889**

WIGGIN, Frederick Holme (1853-1910)
Hysterectomy, with special reference to the vaginal route; a report of eight cases. New York, 1896. 16p. DNLM **90-9890**

WIGGIN, Frederick Holme (1853-1910)
The abuse of medical charity. Philadelphia: Lea Bros. & Co., 1897. 22p. DNLM **90-9891**

WIGGIN, Frederick Holme (1853-1910)
The country doctor. New York, 1897. 9p. DNLM **90-9892**

WIGGIN, Frederick Holme (1853-1910)
Notes on the operative treatment of complete vaginal and uterine prolapse; with reports of two cases. Philadelphia, 1897. 7p. DNLM **90-9893**

WIGGIN, Frederick Holme (1853-1910) and John A. FORDYCE
Report of a case of malignant papillary dermatitis, with especial reference to its pathology. New York, 1897. 14p. DNLM **90-9894**

WIGGIN, Frederick Holme (1853-1910)
The management of patients before and after laparotomy. New York, 1898. 16p. DNLM **90-9895**

WIGGIN, Twing Brooks (*b.* 1865)
Outlines of physiology. . . . Chicago: Henson Bros., 1894. 63p. DLC **90-9896**

WIGGIN, Twing Brooks (*b.* 1865)
Outlines of physiology. . . . Chicago: [Henson Bros.], 1897. 155p. DLC **90-9897**

WIGHT, Jervis [Sherman] (1834-1901)
Some measurements of skulls and heads, showing that development, growth and education increase the volume of the anterior parts of the cerebrum—indicated by the masto-frontal angle. . . . New York, [1890]. 32p. NN [Originally, 1878. *vel subseq.*] **90-9898**

WIGHT, Jervis [Sherman] (1834-1901)
A memorial of O. W. Wight, sanitarian, lawyer, and author. Cambridge: Riverside Press, 1890. 266p. port. DLC; DNLM; MB; PU **90-9899**

WIGHT, Jervis [Sherman] (1834-1901)
Address to the graduates of the training school for nurses at the Long Island College Hospital, on Thursday evening, June 4th, 1891. Brooklyn: Press of Eagle Book Printing Dept., 1891. 24p. DLC; KU **90-9900**

WIGHT, Jervis [Sherman] (1834-1901)
Suggestions to the medical witness. . . . Cambridge: Printed at the Riverside Press, 1891. 228p. DNLM; DLC; ICJ; NN **90-9901**

WIGHT, Jervis [Sherman] (1834-1901)
The weight and size of the body and its organs. . . . For the use of medical students. Brooklyn: Tremplett & Co., printers, 1891. 26p. DLC; NN [Originally, 1881. *vel subseq.*] **90-9902**

WIGHT, Jervis [Sherman] (1834-1901)
Report of eighty operations performed before the medical class of the College Hospital during the regular session of 1891-92. [Brooklyn, 1892.] 22p. DNLM; NNNAM **90-9903**

WIGHT, Jervis [Sherman] (1834-1901)
Report of one hundred and nine operations, performed at the Long Island College Hospital during the regular session of 1892-93. New York: M. J. Rooney, [1893]. 35p. DNLM; MB; NNNAM **90-9904**

WILBUR, Cressy L[ivingston] (1865-1928)
A provisional arrangement of causes of death. [Concord, N.H., 1895.] 10p. DNLM **90-9905**

WILBUR, Cressy L[ivingston] (1865-1928)
How the establishment of a permanent census bureau will improve the vital statistics of the United States. Chicago, 1897. 8p. DNLM **90-9906**

WILCOX, Reynold W[ebb] (1856-1931)
Hydrastis, viburnum, and piscidia in the diseases of the female organs of generation. [New York, 1890.] 7p. DNLM; NNNAM **90-9907**

WILCOX, Reynold W[ebb] (1856-1931)
Anaemia: its treatment by a new preparation of iron. New York, 1892. 24p. DNLM; NNNAM **90-9908**

WILCOX, Reynold W[ebb] (1856-1931)
Syrup of hydriodic acid and its uses. A reply thereto by R. W. Gardner, New York, and subsequent correspondence. [New York, 1893.] 24p. DNLM; NNNAM **90-9909**

WILCOX, Reynold W[ebb] (1856-1931)
An improved stethoscope. [New York, 1894.] 1 l. DNLM **90-9910**

WILCOX, Reynold W[ebb] (1856-1931)
A new method of administering creosote. New York, 1894. 8p. DNLM **90-9911**

WILCOX, Reynold W[ebb] (1856-1931)
Cod-liver oil: What is it? [New York, 1894.] 4p. DNLM **90-9912**

WILCOX, Reynold W[ebb] (1856-1931)
The therapeutics of kola. Detroit, Mich.: Parke, Davis & Co., [1895]. 6p. DNLM **90-9913**

WILCOX, Reynold W[ebb] (1856-1931)
The treatment of pulmonary tuberculosis by hypodermic injections of nuclein. Detroit: G. S. Davis, 1895. 5p. DNLM **90-9914**

WILCOX, Reynold W[ebb] (1856-1931)
The use of vaso-constrictors in cardiac disease. [New York, 1895.] 12p. DNLM **90-9915**

WILCOX, Reynold W[ebb] (1856-1931)
The indigestion of starchy foods. New York: Parke, Davis & Co., 1896. 18p. DNLM **90-9916**

WILCOX, Reynold W[ebb] (1856-1931)
The newer preparations of bismuth. [New York, 1897.] 2 l. DNLM **90-9917**

WILCOX, Reynold W[ebb] (1856-1931)
A phase of the treatment of goutiness. [New York], 1897. 15p. DNLM **90-9918**

WILCOX, Reynold W[ebb] (1856-1931)
Strophanthus; a clinical study. Philadelphia, 1897. 16p. DNLM **90-9919**

WILCOX, Reynold W[ebb] (1856-1931)
Strophanthus; a clinical study. Chicago, 1897. 19p. DNLM **90-9920**

WILCOX, Reynold W[ebb] (1856-1931)
Diet for consumptives. Philadelphia, 1898. 10p. DNLM **90-9921**

WILCOX, Reynold W[ebb] (1856-1931)
An old remedy for diabetes mellitus. [St. Louis, 1898.] 5 l. DNLM **90-9922**

WILCOX, Reynold W[ebb] (1856-1931)
The treatment of typhoid fever by chlorin. New York, 1899. 12p. DNLM **90-9923**

WILCOX, Reynold W[ebb] (1856-1931)
The modern use of synthetics. [St. Louis, 1899.] 12p. DNLM **90-9924**

WILDER, Burt Green (1841-1925)
The morphological importance of the membranous or other thin portions of the parieties on the encephalic cavities. Cincinnati, 1891. 1 l. DNLM **90-9925**

WILDER, Burt Green (1841-1925)
Exhibition of a suicide's brain, with two pistol-ball wounds; remarks on its fissured anomalies. New York, 1894. 4p. DNLM **90-9926**

WILDER, Burt Green (1841-1925)
The cerebral fissures of two philosophers, Chauncey Wright and James Edward Oliver. [Granville, O.], 1895. 1 sheet. DNLM **90-9927**

WILDER, Burt Green (1841-1925)
What is the morphologic status of the olfactory portion of the brain? New York, 1898. 6p. DNLM **90-9928**

WILDER, William Hamlin (*b.* 1860)
Operation for ptosis. St. Louis, 1898. 5p. DNLM **90-9929**

WILE, William C[onrad] (1847-1913)
The Soden water and pastiles in the treatment of some of the chronic diseases of the air passages. Danbury, Conn., 1890. 32p. DNLM **90-9930**

WILE, William C[onrad] (1847-1913)
The ideal place for those suffering from pulmonary troubles. [Southern Pines, N.C.]. Danbury, 1891. 28p. DNLM **90-9931**

WILE, William C[onrad] (1847-1913)
Three cases of lead poisoning and their treatment. [New York], 1898. 6p. DNLM **90-9932**

WILKINS, George
The treatment of typhoid fever by cold baths. [Philadelphia, 1892.] 8p. DNLM **90-9933**

WILKINSON, A[lonzo] D. (*b.* 1857)
Phlegmasia dolens. New York: J. D. Emmet, 1896. 9p. DNLM **90-9934**

WILKINSON, George
The voice, a musical instrument, as by disease affected. Some papers on applied acoustics (medical). [1. Acoustic color in medical aspect. 2. Pitch and timbre. 3. The voice, as a musical instrument, by disease affected.] [Omaha, 1892.] 36p; 12p; 24p. DNLM **90-9935**

WILLIAMETTE UNIVERSITY, SALEM. MEDICAL DEPARTMENT
List of graduates from 1867-93. Announcement for 1893-94. [1893.] DNLM **90-9936**

WILLARD, DE FOREST (1846-1910)
Erasion (arthrectomy) in diseases of the joints. Philadelphia: Univ. of Penn. Press, 1890. 10p. DNLM **90-9937**

WILLARD, DE FOREST (1846-1910)
The operative treatment of hip disease. [n. p., 1890.] 30p. DNLM **90-9938**

WILLARD, DE FOREST (1846-1910)
I. Operative treatment of hip-disease. II. Rest and fixation in joint-disease. Philadelphia: W. J. Dornan, 1890. 30p. DNLM **90-9939**

WILLARD, DE FOREST (1846-1910) and Lewis H. ADLER
Artificial anaesthesia and anaesthetics. Detroit, Mich.: G. S. Davis, 1891. 144p. DNLM **90-9940**

WILLARD, DE FOREST (1846-1910)
Intra-thoracic surgery; bronchotomy through the chest-wall for foreign bodies impacted in the bronchi. [Philadelphia: Lea Bros. & Co., 1891.] 14p. DNLM **90-9941**

WILLARD, DE FOREST (1846-1910)
Operative treatment of the deformities resulting from infantile spinal and cerebral spastic paralysis. [Philadelphia, 1891.] 19p. DNLM **90-9942**

WILLARD, DE FOREST (1846-1910)
Operative treatment of spinal caries. [Philadelphia, 1891.] 10p. DNLM **90-9943**

WILLARD, DE FOREST (1846-1910)
Surgical and mechanical treatment of the deformities following infantile spinal paralysis. [Philadelphia, 1891.] 8p. DNLM **90-9944**

WILLARD, DE FOREST (1846-1910)
Two cases of removal of laminae for spinal fracture. [Philadelphia, 1891.] 10p. DNLM **90-9945**

WILLARD, DE FOREST (1846-1910)
Gluck's ivory joints for replacing excised articulations. Philadelphia, 1891. 3p. DNLM **90-9946**

WILLARD, DE FOREST (1846-1910)
Report of a case of a dissecting aneurism of the aorta; rupture and death. Philadelphia, 1891. 2p. DNLM **90-9947**

WILLARD, DE FOREST (1846-1910)
Experiments in pneumonectomy and pneumonotomy. [Philadelphia, 1891.] 10p. DNLM **90-9948**

WILLARD, DE FOREST (1846-1910)
Ligation of the internal jugular vein for profuse hemorrhage caused by a sloughing adenitis, which followed malignant scarlet fever. Philadelphia, 1891. 2p. DNLM **90-9949**

WILLARD, DE FOREST (1846-1910) and James Hendrie LLOYD
A case of porencephalon in which trephining was done for the relief of local symptoms: death from scarlet fever. Philadelphia, 1892. 7p. DNLM **99-9950**

WILLARD, DE FOREST (1846-1910)
Comparison of operative methods in the treatment of club-foot. [Philadelphia], 1892. 7p. DNLM **90-9951**

WILLARD, DE FOREST (1846-1910)
D. Hayes Agnew. Biographical sketch. Philadelphia, 1892. 16p. port. DNLM **90-9952**

WILLARD, DE FOREST (1846-1910)
D. Hayes Agnew. A short sketch of his life and services. [Philadelphia, 1892.] 8p. DNLM **90-9953**

WILLARD, DE FOREST (1846-1910)
D. Hayes Agnew, M.D., LL.D.: A biographical sketch by his pupil, friend and assistant. . . . Read before the Philadelphia County Medical Society, April 13, 1892. [Philadelphia, 1892.] 16p. port. PPC; PPHa; PU **90-9954**

WILLARD, DE FOREST (1846-1910)
Experiments in pneumonotomy and pneumonectomy; suturing of lung. [Philadelphia, 1892.] 8p. DNLM **90-9955**

WILLARD, DE FOREST (1846-1910)
Operative treatment of knee-joint disease. Philadelphia, 1893. 8p. DNLM **90-9956**

WILLARD, DE FOREST (1846-1910)
The early management of club-foot. Detroit, Mich.: G. S. Davis, 1893. 15p. DNLM **90-9957**

WILLARD, DE FOREST (1846-1910)
Nerve-suturing – neurorrhaphy, nerve-grafting. Philadelphia, 1894. 17p. DNLM **90-9958**

WILLARD, DE FOREST (1846-1910) and Guy HINSDALE
Antero-lateral sclerosis; posterior sclerosis; pathology and treatment of locomotor ataxia by suspension and by apparatus. Philadelphia, 1894. 17p. DNLM **90-9959**

WILLARD, DE FOREST (1846-1910) and Guy HINSDALE
Anterior poliomyelitis. Philadelphia, 1894. 8p. DNLM **90-9960**

WILLARD, DE FOREST (1846-1910)
Correction of rachitic deformities and of the deformities following infantile and spastic paralyses. Philadelphia, 1894. 2 l. DNLM **90-9961**

WILLARD, DE FOREST (1846-1910)
Operative treatment of paralytic deformities. [Philadelphia], 1894. 8p. DNLM **90-9962**

WILLARD, DE FOREST (1846-1910)
Annual address by the president of the Philadelphia County Medical Society. Philadelphia, 1894. 4p. DNLM **90-9963**

WILLARD, DE FOREST (1846-1910)
Rachitic deformities. Operative treatment. [Philadelphia], 1894. 5p. DNLM **90-9964**

WILLARD, DE FOREST (1846-1910)
Rachitic deformities. Operative treatment. New York, 1894. 5p. DNLM **90-9965**

WILLARD, DE FOREST (1846-1910) and James J. JOHNSTON
Cephalic tetanus; general tetanus associated with hemifacial paralysis; recovery. Philadelphia, 1895. 12p. 1 plate. DNLM **90-9966**

WILLARD, DE FOREST (1846-1910)
Treatment of paralytic deformities. [Philadelphia, 1895.] 5p. DNLM **90-9967**

WILLARD, DE FOREST (1846-1910)
Erasion, excision and amputation in joint disease. Chicago, 1895. 15p. DNLM **90-9968**

WILLARD, DE FOREST (1846-1910)
Laminectomy in spinal caries paraplegia. New York, 1896. 7p. DNLM **90-9969**

WILLARD, DE FOREST (1846-1910)
Surgical and mechanical relief of so-called hopeless paralytic cripples. Philadelphia, 1896. 6p. DNLM **90-9970**

WILLARD, DE FOREST (1846-1910)
Tuberculosis of the superficial lymphatic glands. Philadelphia, 1896. 13p. DNLM **90-9971**

WILLARD, DE FOREST (1846-1910)
Röntgen-ray skiagraphs; tubercular knees; club-foot; glass in finger; deformed hand; knock-knees, etc. Philadelphia, 1896. 4p. 7 plates. DNLM **90-9972**

WILLARD, DE FOREST (1846-1910)
Congenital anterior displacement of the hip. Philadelphia, 1896. 4p. DNLM **90-9973**

WILLARD, DE FOREST (1846-1910)
Roentgen ray skiagraphy. Chicago, 1897. 7p. DNLM
90-9974

WILLARD, DE FOREST (1846-1910) and Wm. G. SPILLER
Concussion of the spinal cord (railway-spine). New York: D. Appleton & Co., 1897. 11p. DNLM
90-9975

WILLARD, DE rOREST (1846-1910)
Errors of diagnosis in orthopedic practice. Philadelphia, 1898. 7p. DNLM **90-9976**

WILLARD, DE FOREST (1846-1910)
Children's orthopedic ward; Agnew Memorial Pavilion, University Hospital, special equipment. [Philadelphia], 1898. 4p. 2 plates. DNLM **90-9977**

WILLARD, DE FOREST (1846-1910)
Osteotomy. Chicago, 1899. 16p. DNLM
90-9978

WILLARD, DE FOREST (1846-1910) and Samuel M. WILSON
Ovarian multiocular cystic tumor, existing for thirty-five years without destroying life, the woman dying from influenzal bronchitis at the age of seventy-four years; repeated tappings. Philadelphia, 1899. 6p. DNLM **90-9979**

WILLARD NERVINE HOME, BURLINGTON, VERMONT
[Circular of the proprietor, Dr. A. J. Willard.] [Burlington, 1890.] 2 l. DNLM [*Also*: Burlington, 1894, 6 l.]
90-9980

WILLETTS, Joseph E. (*b.* 1860)
Horny epithelium or summer granulations; its relation to *conjunctivitis* trachomatosa; impracticability of treatment by expression. [Philadelphia, 1893.] 8p. DNLM
90-9981

WILLETTS, Joseph E. (*b.* 1860)
The halo, or rainbow symptom in glaucoma. [St. Louis, 1895.] 5p. DNLM **90-9982**

WILLETTS, Joseph E. (*b.* 1860)
A preliminary report of a perimeter based on a new principle. St. Louis, 1896. 7p. DNLM **90-9983**

WILLETTS, Joseph E. (*b.* 1860)
Address in ophthalmology. Personal observations in antiseptics and anaesthetics in ocular operations; perimetry; and corneal corpuscular activity. [Pittsburgh]: Murdoch-Kerr, [1897]. 22p. DNLM **90-9984**

WILLIAM, Charles B[aeder] (*b.* 1865)
A study of aneurism of the pulmonary artery; with the report of a case. Philadelphia: W. J. Dornan, 1890. 10p. DNLM
90-9985

WILLIAM, Charles B[aeder] (*b.* 1865)
Euthanasia. [Philadelphia, 1894.] 4p. DNLM
90-9986

WILLIAMS, Charles B[aeder] (*b.* 1865)
Influenza and its treatment. [Philadelphia, 1894.] 3p. DNLM
90-9987

WILLIAMS, Charles B[aeder] (*b.* 1865)
A surgical clinic in the early days of the Pennsylvania Hospital, Philadelphia. [Philadelphia: Univ. Penn. Press, 1895.] 5p. DNLM **90-9988**

WILLIAMS, Daniel H.
The treatment of the retroverted uterus, with special reference to the value of massage and the author's application of the uterine respiratory movement. Philadelphia, 1893. 9p. DNLM
90-9989

WILLIAMS, Daniel H.
Stab wound of the heart and pericardium; suture of the pericardium; recovery; patient alive three years afterward. New York: Publishers' Print. Co., 1897. 8p. DNLM
90-9990

WILLIAMS, Dawson (*b.* 1854)
Medical diseases of infancy and childhood. Philadelphia & New York: Lea Bros. & Co., [1898]. 634p. 18 plates. DNLM; NNNAM; PPC; PPJ **90-9991**

WILLIAMS, E. H.
Low-power objectives in microscopic diagnosis. [Philadelphia, 1893.] 2p. DNLM **90-9992**

WILLIAMS, Francis H. (1852-1936)
Early, local treatment of diphtheria. [Boston, 1892.] 13p. DNLM **90-9993**

WILLIAMS, Francis H. (1852-1936)
Some suggestions about nourishment in acute disease. [Boston], 1893. 8p. DNLM **90-9994**

WILLIAMS, Francis H. (1852-1936)
The intermittent administration of quinine in malaria with the temperature as a guide. [Boston, 1893.] 12p. DNLM
90-9995

WILLIAMS, Francis H. (1852-1936)
Diphtheria and other membranous affections of the throat. [Philadelphia, 1893.] 21p. DNLM **90-9996**

WILLIAMS, Francis H. (1852-1936)
Observations on the diagnosis of diphtheria; and a study of its local treatment. Boston: Rockwell & Churchill, 1895. 33p. DNLM **90-9997**

WILLIAMS, Francis H. (1852-1936)
A more comfortable way of using cold in fevers. Philadelphia, 1895. 6p. **90-9998**

WILLIAMS, Francis H. (1852-1936)
A method for more fully determining the outline of the heart by means of the fluoroscope, together with other uses of this instrument in medicine. Boston: Damrell & Upham, 1896. 6p. 1 plate. DNLM **90-9999**

WILLIAMS, Francis H. (1852-1936)
Notes on X-rays in medicine. Philadelphia, 1896. 6p. 2 plates.
90-10,000

WILLIAMS, Francis H. (1852-1936)
A study of the adaptation of the X-rays to medical practice. Boston, 1897. 59p. DNLM
90-10,001

WILLIAMS, Francis H. (1852-1936)
The Röntgen rays in thoracic disease. [Philadelphia], 1897. 23p. DNLM **90-10,002**

WILLIAMS, Francis H. (1852-1936)
An outline of some of the medical uses of the Röntgen light. [Philadelphia], 1898. 24p. 16 plates. **90-10,003**

WILLIAMS, Francis H. (1852-1936)
The importance of knowing the size of the heart; inaccuracy of percussion in determining it as shown by X-ray examinations. [Boston], 1899. 15p. 4 plates. DNLM **90-10,004**

WILLIAMS, Francis H. (1852-1936)
Röntgen-ray examinations in incipient pulmonary tuberculosis. [Philadelphia], 1899. 16p. DNLM **90-10,005**

WILLIAMS, Hadley
Normal and surgical anatomy of the vermiform appendix. Philadelphia, 1895. 22p. DNLM; PPC **90-10,006**

WILLIAMS, Harold
Hypnotism. Boston: Damrell & Upham, 1891. 8p. DNLM **90-10,007**

WILLIAMS, Harold and Horace D. ARNOLD
The effects of violent and prolonged muscular exercise upon the heart. Philadelphia, 1899. 20p. DNLM; PPC **90-10,008**

WILLIAMS, Herbert F. (*b.* 1850)
A vaporizer, sublimer, and air-sterilizer. [New York, 1890.] 6p. DNLM **90-10,009**

WILLIAMS, Herbert U[pham] (*b.* 1866)
A manual of bacteriology. . . . With seventy-eight illustrations. Philadelphia: P. Blakiston, Son & Co., 1898. 263p. DLC; DNLM; NNNAM; PPC **90-10,010**

WILLIAMS, Herbert U[pham] (*b.* 1866)
Experimental production of fat necrosis; fat necrosis about the pancreas of the hog. Boston, 1897. 4p. 1 plate. DNLM **90-10,011**

WILLIAMS, J[ames] Leon (1852-1932)
A contribution to the study of pathology of enamel. New York, 1897. 82p. DNLM; NNNAM **90-10,012**

WILLIAMS, J[ohn] Whitridge (1866-1931)
Contributions to the normal and pathological histology of the Fallopian tubes. [Philadelphia, 1891.] 12p. DNLM **90-10,013**

WILLIAMS, J[ohn] Whitridge (1866-1931)
Contributions to the histogenesis of the papillary cystomata of the ovary. [Baltimore, 1891.] 13 l. 1 plate. DNLM **90-10,014**

WILLIAMS, J[ohn] Whitridge (1866-1931)
Pelvimetry for the general practitioner. [Philadelphia, 1891.] 13p. DNLM **90-10,015**

WILLIAMS, J[ohn] Whitridge (1866-1931)
The premature induction of labor in contracted pelves. [Baltimore, 1891.] 7p. DNLM **90-10,016**

WILLIAMS, J[ohn] Whitridge (1866-1931)
Diphtheria. Read before the Richmond Academy of Medicine and Surgery, Feb. 16, 1892. Richmond, Va.: J. L. Hill, [1892]. 10p. DNLM **90-10,017**

WILLIAMS, J[ohn] Whitridge (1866-1931)
Puerperal infection considered from a bacteriological point of view, with special reference to the question of auto-infection. Philadelphia, 1893. 14p. DNLM **90-10,018**

WILLIAMS, J[ohn] Whitridge (1866-1931)
Calcified tumors of the ovary. New York: William Wood & Co., 1893. 18p. DNLM **90-10,019**

WILLIAMS, J[ohn] Whitridge (1866-1931)
The frequency of contracted pelves in the first thousand women delivered in the obstetrical department of the Johns Hopkins Hospital. New York, [1894]. 13p. 4 tab. DNLM **90-10,020**

WILLIAMS, J[ohn] Whitridge (1866-1931)
Contribution to the histology and histogenesis of sarcoma of the uterus. New York: William Wood & Co., 1894. 44p. DNLM **90-10,021**

WILLIAMS, J[ohn] Whitridge (1866-1931)
Deciduoma malignum. Baltimore: Johns Hopkins Press, 1895. 44p. DNLM **90-10,022**

WILLIAMS, J[ohn] Whitridge (1866-1931)
Diphtheria of the vulva. [Baltimore], 1897. 6p. DNLM **90-10,023**

WILLIAMS, J[ohn] Whitridge (1866-1931)
Teaching obstetrics. [Easton, Pa., 1898.] 12p. DNLM **90-10,024**

WILLIAMS, J[ohn] Whitridge (1866-1931)
The bacteria of the vagina and their practical significance; based upon the bacteriological examination of the vaginal secretion of ninety-two pregnant women. New York: William Wood & Co., 1898. 35p. DNLM **90-10,025**

WILLIAMS, J[ohn] Whitridge (1866-1931)
The cause of the conflicting statements concerning the bacterial contents of the vaginal secretion of the pregnant woman. New York: William Wood & Co., 1898. 10p. DNLM **90-10,026**

WILLIAMS, J[ohn] Whitridge (1866-1931)
Forty cases of fever in the puerperium, with bacteriological examination of the uterine contents. New York: William Wood & Co., 1898. 9p. DNLM **90-10,027**

WILLIAMS, J[ohn] Whitridge (1866-1931)
A case of spondylolisthesis, with description of the pelvis. Philadelphia, 1899. 31p. 6 plates. DNLM **90-10,028**

WILLIAMS, J. W. Hume
On unsoundness of mind, in its legal and medical considerations. New York: William Wood & Co., 1892. 179p. DNLM; NNNAM **90-10,029**

WILLIAMS, Seward W[hiting] (*b.* 1861)
Should pharmacy and chemistry speak the same language? With special reference ot the nomenclature of alkaloidal salts. New York, 1897. 29p. DNLM **90-10,030**

WILLIAMS, Talcott (1849-1928)
Oriental medicine. [Philadelphia, 1890.] 3p. DNLM **90-10,031**

WILLIAMS, W[illiam] Roger
A monograph on diseases of the breast, their pathology and treatment with special reference to cancer. New York: William Wood & Co., 1895. 572p. DNLM; NNNAM **90-10,032**

WILLIAMSON, A[llan] N.
Epilepsy; a brief account of the disease, and a description of the most successful mode of treatment. New London, Conn.: Day, 1892. 12p. DNLM **90-10,033**

WILLIAMSON, A[llan] N.
Observations on the treatment of epilepsy. New London, Conn., 1895. 15p. DNLM **90-10,034**

[WILLIS, L. M.]
Catalogue of the library of the late Dr. L. M. Willis. For sale by C. L. Libbie & Co., Boston, 1893. 86p. DNLM; MBM **90-10,035**

WILLS, William Lemoyne (*b.* 1853)
Experimental study in thoracic surgery. Report of committee on surgery. [San Francisco, 1892.] 12p. DNLM **90-10,036**

WILLS, William Lemoyne (*b.* 1853)
The radical cure of hernia. Los Angeles, 1897. 8p. 1 tab. DNLM **90-10,037**

WILMARTH, A[lfred] W.
Report on the examination of one hundred brains of feeble-minded children. [St. Louis, 1890.] 16p. DNLM **90-10,038**

WILMARTH, A[lfred] W.
The medical organization of general institutions for the feeble-minded. [Philadelphia, 1892.] 10p. DNLM **90-10,039**

WILMINGTON DENTAL MFG. CO.
Catalogue of dental materials and supplies. Philadelphia, 1890. 376p. PU **90-10,040**

WILSON, Edmund Beecher (*b.* 1856)
The cell in development and inheritance. New York: The Macmillan Co., 1896. 371p. DNLM; NNNAM **90-10,041**

WILSON, Erasmus (1809-1884)
The anatomist's vade mecum; a system of human anatomy. 11th ed. Edited by Henry Edward Clark. Philadelphia: P. Blakiston, Son & Co., 1892. 840p. 26 col. plates. CU-M; DNLM; PPC; ViRA **90-10,042**

WILSON, Ezra H[erbert] (1858-1905) and R. B. F. RANDOLPH
Incubator for the maintenance of constant low tempeature. Brooklyn, 1899. 7p. DNLM **90-10,043**

WILSON, George (1811-1897)
A handbook of hygiene and sanitary science. 7th ed. Philadelphia: P. Blakiston, Son & Co., 1892. 751p. DNLM; PPC; PU **90-10,044**

WILSON, George R.
Clinical studies in vice and in insanity. New York: The Macmillan Co., 1899. 234p. DNLM; ICU; MB; NN **90-10,045**

WILSON, Harry Augustus (1853-1919)
The aseptic closure of long-standing sinuses having their origin in tubercular joints. [Philadelphia, 1891.] 9p. DNLM **90-10,046**

WILSON, Harry Augustus (1853-1919)
Illustrative cases of congenital club-foot. [Philadelphia, 1891.] 21p. 4 plates. DNLM **90-10,047**

WILSON, Harry Augustus (1853-1919)
Report of a case of spina bifida, with partial motor and sensory paralysis of both extremities, complete paralysis of the sphincters of the bladder and rectum, double equinovarus, and purulent bursitis. [Philadelphia, 1891.] 6p. DNLM **90-10,048**

WILSON, Harry Augustus (1853-1919)
Scope of orthopedics; the forms of club-foot; tenotomy. The etiology of club-foot; the treatment of club-foot; the plaster-of-Paris bandage. Philadelphia: Binder & Kelly, 1891. 26p. DNLM **90-10,049**

WILSON, Harry Augustus (1853-1919)
Clinical lecture. Deformity of hip and knee following acute osteitis; lumbar abscess resembling incipient hip-joint disease. [Detroit, 1892.] 8p. DNLM **90-10,050**

WILSON, Harry Augustus (1853-1919)
Clinical lecture. 1. Subcutaneous osteotomy of femur. 2. Incipient hip-joint disease. New York: M. J. Rooney, 1892. 7p. DNLM **90-10,051**

WILSON, Harry Augustus (1853-1919)
Clinical lecture: tenotomy by open incision for talipes equinus; torticollis from rheumatoidal arthritis; subcutaneous tenotomy of sterno-cleido-mastoid for torticollis. [Detroit, 1892.] 12p. DNLM **90-10,052**

WILSON, Harry Augustus (1853-1919)
A demonstration of some of the causes of rotary lateral curvature of the spine. Chicago: Office Amer. Med. Assoc., 1892. 11p. DNLM **90-10,053**

WILSON, Harry Augustus (1853-1919)
Early symptoms of hip disease and aetiology of hip disease. Treatment of abscess in hip disease. [New York, 1892.] 8p. DNLM **90-10,054**

WILSON, Harry Augustus (1853-1919)
Mechanical support in fracture and dislocation of the sixth cervical vertebra. [Philadelphia, 1892.] 11p. DNLM **90-10,055**

WILSON, Harry Augustus (1853-1919)
The necessity for early correction in congenital club-foot. [New York & Philadelphia, 1892.] 10p. DNLM **90-10,056**

WILSON, Harry Augustus (1853-1919)
Tenotomy by open and subcutaneous incision, tubercular synovitis and osteitis of shoulder. Detroit. G. S. Davis, 1892. 8p. DNLM **90-10,057**

WILSON, Harry Augustus (1853-1919)
Tubercular ostitis of tarsus; rheumatoidal arthritis of tarsus. [Detroit, 1892.] 11p. DNLM **90-10,058**

WILSON, Harry Augustus (1853-1919)
At what age should the first treatment of congenital club-foot be instituted? [Philadelphia, 1892.] 12p. DNLM **90-10,059**

WILSON, Harry Augustus (1853-1919)
Bone operations for the correction of club-foot, based upon an analysis of 434 operations by 108 operators. [Philadelpia, 1893.] 36p. DNLM **90-10,060**

WILSON, Harry Augustus (1853-1919)
A clinical lecture on the prevention of idiopathic rotary lateral curvatures of the spine. [Philadelphia, 1893.] 10p. 3 plates. DNLM **90-10,061**

WILSON, Harry Augustus (1853-1919)
Fixation after excision of the knee. Philadelphia, 1893. 10p. DNLM **90-10,062**

WILSON, Harry Augustus (1853-1919)
Free incision of abscess of ostitis of hip; and closure without drainage. [Philadelphia, 1893.] 6p. DNLM **90-10,063**

WILSON, Harry Augustus (1853-1919)
Suturing the tendo Achillis in the correction of deformities of the feet. [Philadelphia, 1893.] 6p. 2 plates. DNLM **90-10,064**

WILSON, Harry Augustus (1853-1919)
Can physicians honorably accept commissions from orthopedic instrument makers? Philadelphia, 1894. 14p. DNLM **90-10,065**

WILSON, Harry Augustus (1853-1919)
Excision of tubercular knee joint. A case of incipient hip-joint disease. [Kansas City, 1894?] 8p. DNLM **90-10,066**

WILSON, Harry Augustus (1853-1919)
Rotary lateral curvature of the spine, and its treatment by remedial gymnastics. [Philadelphia, 1894.] 5p. 1 plate. DNLM **90-10,067**

WILSON, Harry Augustus (1853-1919)
1. Can physicians honorably accept commissions from orthopedic instrument makers? 2. Commissions to physicians upon the scale of orthopedic apparatus from the manufacturer's standpoint. Philadelphia, 1895. 32p. DNLM; PPC **90-10,068**

WILSON, Harry Augustus (1853-1919)
The pathology of hip-joint disease, with illustrative cases. [Philadelphia, 1895?] 14p. DNLM **90-10,069**

WILSON, H. M., Jr.
A contribution to the study of atrophic rhinitis. [New York, 1892.] 7p. DNLM **90-10,070**

WILSON, H[enry] P[arke] C[ustis] (1827-1898)
The indiscriminate use of opiates in the pelvic diseases of women. Philadelphia: W. J. Dornan, 1891. 8p. DNLM **90-10,071**

WILSON, H[enry] P[arke] C[ustis] (1827-1898)
Retro-displacements of the uterus. Richmond: J. W. Ferguson & Son, 1891. 12p. DNLM **90-10,072**

WILSON, I[srael] P.
Pathological conditions of the ethmoid bone resulting from dental lesion. Read before the Iowa State Dental Society, May 7, 1890. [n. p., 1890.] 8p. DNLM **90-10,073**

WILSON, I[srael] P.
Abscess of the antrum, with cases and treatment. [n. p., 1891.] 8p. DNLM **90-10,074**

WILSON, I[srael] P.
Heredity. A paper read before the Iowa State Dental Society, at its thirtieth annual session, held at Des Moines, May, 1892. [Des Moines], 1892. 11p. DNLM **90-10,075**

WILSON, J[ames] C[ornelius] (1847-1934)
The treatment of enteric fever, with special reference to the method of Brand. [Philadelphia, 1890.] 20p. DNLM **90-10,076**

WILSON, J[ames] C[ornelius] (1847-1934)
. . . Fever-nursing: designed for the use of professional and other nurses, and especially as a text-book for nurses in training. . . . 2nd ed. Philadelphia: J. B. Lippincott Co., 1891. 210p. PPC; PU **90-10,077**

WILSON, J[ames] C[ornelius] (1847-1934)
The complete medical pocket-formulary and physician's vade-mecum; containing upwards of 2500 prescriptions. . . . Collated for the use of practitioners. . . . Philadelphia: J. B. Lippincott Co., 1892. 261p. DLC; NNNAM; PPC; PU **90-10,078**

WILSON, J[ames] C[ornelius] (1847-1934), E. O. SHAKESPEARE & R. A. CLEEMAN
An address, from a special committee of the College of Physicians of Philadelphia, to the medical societies of the United States: concerning the dangers to which the country is exposed by the ineffectual methods of quarantine at its ports, and in regard to the necessity of national control of maritime quarantine. [Philadelphia, 1892?] 20p. DNLM; PPC **90-10,079**

WILSON, J[ames] C[ornelius] (1847-1934)
A further report in regard to the treatment of enteric or typhoid fever, by means of systematic cold bathing, in the German Hospital, Philadelphia. [Philadelphia, 1892.] 12p. DNLM **90-10,080**

WILSON, J[ames] C[ornelius] (1847-1934)
Report of a fifth series of cases of enteric or typhoid fever treated by systematic cold bathing in the German Hospital, Philadelphia. [Philadelphia, 1893.] 11p. DNLM **90-10,081**

WILSON, J[ames] C[ornelius] (1847-1934)
Wilson's pocket visiting list. Sixty patients each week. Perpetual. Arranged for the use of practitioners. Philadelphia: J. B. Lippincott Co., [1894]. 328p. DNLM; PPC
90-10,082

WILSON, J[ames] C[ornelius] (1847-1934), ed.
An American text-book of applied therapeutics. . . . Ed. by J. C. Wilson . . . assisted by Augustus A. Eshner. . . . Philadelphia: W. B. Saunders, 1896. 1326p. plates. DLC; NNNAM; PPC; PU **90-10,083**

WILSON, J[ames] C[ornelius] (1847-1934)
Modern medical education. Easton, Pa., 1897. 3 galley sheets. DNLM **90-10,084**

WILSON, J[ames] C[ornelius] (1847-1934)
The complete medical pocket-formulary and physician's vade-mecum: containing upwards of 2,500 prescriptions. . . . Collated for the use of practitioners. . . . Rev. by Henry Tucker, M.D. Philadelphia: J. B. Lippincott Co., [1899]. 267p. DLC; NNNAM; PPC; PPJ **90-10,085**

WILSON, J[ames] C[ornelius] (1847-1934)
. . . Fever-nursing: designed for the use of professional and other nurses, and especially as a text-book for nurses in training. . . . 3rd ed., rev. and enl. Philadelphia and London: J. B. Lippincott Co., [1899]. 241p. DLC; DNLM; NNNAM; PPC **90-10,086**

WILSON, John T. (1846-1910)
Plastic operations in carcinoma of the breast. New York, 1895. 5p. DNLM **90-10,087**

WILSON, John T. (1846-1910)
Mental complications following surgical operation. New York, 1897. 9p. DNLM **90-10,088**

WILSON, L. N.
Latent gout of the menopause. Danbury, Conn., 1898. 2p. DNLM **90-10,089**

WILSON, Norton L[uther] (*b.* 1861)
Purulent discharges from the middle ear. New York, 1896. 10p. DNLM **90-10,090**

WILSON, Norton L[uther] (*b.* 1861)
Chronic diseases of the tonsils. New York, 1896. 8p. DNLM
90-10,091

WILSON, Norton L[uther] (*b.* 1861)
Uric acid as a factor in the production of hay fever. New York: D. Appleton & Co., 1896. 12p. DNLM
90-10,092

WILSON, W[illiam] Reynolds (*b.* 1863)
A case of congenital cystic elephantiasis. New York: William Wood & Co., 1891. 7p. DNLM **90-10,093**

WILSON, W[illiam] Reynolds (*b.* 1863)
A report of two cases of symptomatic dermatitis in the puerperal state. Philadelphia, 1891. 12p. DNLM
90-10,094

WILSON, W[illiam] Reynolds (*b.* 1863)
The use of morphia in eclampsia, with a report of two cases. Philadelphia, 1892. 7p. DNLM **90-10,095**

WILSON, W[illiam] Reynolds (*b.* 1863)
Uterine thrombosis following post-partum haemorrhage and its relation to puerperal infection. Philadelphia: Univ. Penn. Press, 1893. 7p. DNLM **90-10,096**

WILSON, W[illiam] Reynolds (*b.* 1863)
The morbid changes in the puerperal endometrium due to local infection, and their relation to general symptoms. New York, 1895. 5p. DNLM **90-10,097**

WILSON, W[illiam] Reynolds (*b.* 1863)
Recent surgical advances and their relation to conservative obstetrics. Read before the section on obstetrics, Pan-American Medical Congress. [n. p., 1895.] 9p. DNLM
90-10,098

WILSON-PREVOST, Charles A.
Hyperkerato-mycosis of the pharynx. Danbury, Conn.: Danbury Medical Printing Co., 1898. 61p. DNLM
90-10,099

WILSON-PREVOST, Charles A.
Treatment of atonic fatigue and strain of the vocal organs by local applications of cold water and massage of the larynx. New York: G. L. Goodman & Co., [1899]. 10p. DNLM
90-10,100

WILTROUT, Irving D.
Somnal; a hypnotic. [St. Paul, 1890?] 1 l. DNLM
90-10,101

WILTROUT, Irving D.
Melancholia. [St. Paul, 1890.] 12p. DNLM
90-10,102

WIMMER, Sebastian J.
Tables and notes on human osteology. . . . With a preface by Prof. William F. Waugh. . . . Philadelphia: The Medical Publishing Co., 1894. 239p. DLC; PPC **90-10,103**

WIMMER, Sebastian J.
The physician's vade mecum. Being a hand-book of medical and surgical reference, with other useful information and tables. . . . With additions by Frank S. Parsons. . . . Philadelphia: The Medical Publishing Co., 1894. 483p. DLC; PPC
90-10,104

WINANS, William Wallace
Sophomore and junior notes from lectures on materia medica, delivered in Hahnemann Medical College, Philadelphia, Pa., session of 1896-97. . . . Rochester, N.Y.: Burnett Printing Co., 1897. 190p. DLC **90-10,105**

WINANS, William W[allace]
Quiz-compend on surgery; with the collaboration, on special and regional surgery of R. M. Haehl; with a section on venereal diseases by J. L. Thorpe. Philadelphia: The Morris Press, 1898. 338p. DLC; PPC **90-10,106**

WINANS, William W[allace]
Examination questions in anatomy, delivered in Hahnemann Medical College, Philadelphia, Pa., with answers. Corrected and approved by H. L. Northrop. . . . Comp. by W. W. Winans, '99. [Philadelphia, 1898.] 60p. DLC; PPC; PU
90-10,107

WINCKEL, Franz Karl Ludwig Wilh. von (1837-1911)
A text-book of obstetrics, including the pathology and therapeutics of the puerperal state; designed for practitioners and students of medicine. Transl. from the first German ed. with permission of the author under the supervision of J. Clifton Edgar. Philadelphia: P. Blakiston, Son & Co., 1890. 927p. DNLM; NNNAM; PPC; PU **90-10,108**

WINCKEL, Franz Karl Ludwig Wilh. von (1837-1911), ed.
Cyclopaedia of obstetrics and gynecology. New York: William Wood & Co., 1890 [1887- .] 12 v. col. plates. MH-M; NNNAM; PPC; PU **90-10,109**

WINCKEL, Franz Karl Ludw. Wilh. von (1837-1911)
Diseases of women . . . including the diseases of the bladder and urethra. Transl. by special authority of the author and publisher, under the supervison of, and with an introduction by Theophilus Parvin. 3rd ed., rev. and enl. Philadelphia: P. Blakiston, Son & Co., 1891. 766p. DLC: ICJ; NIC; PPJ **90-10,110**

WINFIELD, James Macfarlane (*b.* 1859)
The treatment of acne in both sexes by relief of genital irritation; a generalization of Sherwell's method. New York: D. Appleton & Co., 1891. 7p. DNLM **90-10,111**

WINFIELD, James Macfarlane (*b.* 1859)
Blood examinations regarding the malarial origin of zoster. New York: D. Appleton & Co., 1895. 10p. DNLM **90-10,112**

WINGATE, Uranus O[wen] B[rackett] (1849-1911)
Address delivered before the first graduating class of the Wisconsin Training School for Nurses, September 4th, 1890. Milwaukee: Corbit & Skidmore Co., 1890. 11p. DNLM **90-10,113**

WINGATE, Uranus O[wen] B[rackett] (1849-1911)
The etiology, prevalence and treatment of hysteria. Madison, Wis.: Tracy, Gibbs & Co., 1898. 8p. DNLM **90-10,114**

WINGATE, Uranus O[wen] B[rackett] (1849-1911)
Tumors of the brain, with reference to disturbances of vision. St. Louis, 1899. 19p. DNLM **90-10,115**

WINSLOW, Lyttleton Stewart Forbes (1844-1913)
Mad humanity; its forms, apparent and obscure. New York: M. F. Mansfield & Co., [1898]. 451p. 13 plates. DNLM; NNNAM **90-10,116**

WINTER, John Thomas (1842-1902)
Jaundice during pregnancy. New York: William Wood & Co., 1890. 9p. DNLM **90-10,117**

WINTERS, Joseph E[dell] (*d.* 1922)
Remarks on the use of antitoxine in diphtheria. New York, 1896. 11p. DNLM **90-10,118**

WIRT, William Edgar
A theoretical and practical demonstration of the action and tension of the tendo Achillis in supporting the body on tiptoe. New York, 1890. 7p. DNLM **90-10,119**

WIRT, William Edgar
Radical cure of hernia. Discussion of F. C. Larimore's paper. [Toledo], 1891. 2 l. DNLM **90-10,120**

WIRT, William Edgar
Case of double club-foot, double club-hand and multiple deformities. Philadelphia, 1891. 2 l. DNLM **90-10,121**

WIRT, William Edgar
Pott's disease. Cleveland, O., 1891. 5p. DNLM **90-10,122**

WIRT, William Edgar
Congenital dislocation of the hip, illustrated by three cases. Cleveland, 1891. 8p. DNLM **90-10,123**

WIRT, William Edgar
The treatment of certain forms of club-foot. Cincinnati, 1892. 7p. DNLM **90-10,124**

WIRT, William Edgar
Hip-disease; operative treatment in old and neglected cases—sixteen cases reported. Columbus, 1892. 13p. DNLM **90-10,125**

WIRT, William Edgar
Conservative treatment of joint diseases. Philadelphia, 1893. 8p. DNLM **90-10,126**

WIRT, William Edgar
Rickets, and the treatment of its resulting deformities. [Chicago, 1893.] 4 l. DNLM **90-10,127**

WIRT, William Edgar
Treatment of initial cases of club-foot. [Cincinnati], 1893. 5p. DNLM **90-10,128**

WIRT, William Edgar
Phelps' method for the cure of club-foot in adults. [New York], 1894. 7p. DNLM **90-10,129**

WIRT, William Edgar
Hernia in children. Phildelphia, 1894. 8p. DNLM **90-10,130**

WIRT, William Edgar
Treatment of old cases of hip disease. Philadelphia, 1894. 6p. DNLM **90-10,131**

WIRT, William Edgar
Inaugural address, Cleveland Medical Society. Cleveland, 1895. 7p. DNLM **90-10,132**

WIRT, William Edgar
Treatment of tubercular disease of the knee-joint. Columbus, 1895. 8p. DNLM **90-10,133**

WIRT, William Edgar
Clinical reports. Cleveland, 1896. 13p. DNLM **90-10,134**

WIRT, William Edgar
An original method of using dry heat of high temperature in the treatment of chronic joint affections. Cleveland, 1896. 6p. DNLM **90-10,135**

WIRT, William Edgar
Cleveland Medical Society. Address of the retiring president, at the annual banquet. Cleveland, 1896. 7p. DNLM **90-10,136**

WIRT, William Edgar
The use of dry heat of high temperature in the treatment of chronic joint affections, with report of cases. [Norwalk, 1897.] 10p. DNLM **90-10,137**

WIRT, William Edgar
Lateral curvature of the spine and other affections benefited by systematic gymnastic exercise. Cleveland, 1897. 8p. DNLM **90-10,138**

WIRT, William Edgar
The treatment of scoliosis, spinal irritation, chorea, infantile and other paralysis, and the poorly developed, by gymnastic exercise, massage, electricity, etc. St. Louis, 1898. 28p. DNLM **90-10,139**

WIRT, William Edgar
Surgical treatment of Pott's disease. Cleveland, 1899, 10p. DNLM **90-10,140**

WIRT, William Edgar
Rectification of club-foot in adults, with the presentation of a case. [Cleveland, 1899.] 8p. DNLM **90-10,141**

WISE, Peter M. (1851-1907)
Medical work in wards of hospitals for the insane. Chicago: Rand, McNally & Co., 1895. 11p. DNLM **90-10,142**

WISE, Peter M. (1851-1907)
A text-book for training schools for nurses, including physiology and hygiene and the principles and practice of nursing, with an introduction by Edward Cowles. New York: G. Putnam's Sons, 1896. 2 v. DNLM; NNNAM **90-10,143**

WISE, Peter M. (1851-1907)
The construction of hospitals. [Albany], 1898. 8p. DNLM **90-10,144**

WISE, Peter M. (1851-1907)
The past, present and prospective treatment of insanity in the State of New York. With an appendix containing a directory of the State hospital system and licensed institutions for the insane in the State of New York. Utica: State Hosp. Print, 1898. 16p. DNLM **90-10,145**

WISHARD, William N.
Perineal operations on the prostate, with a brief report of a new method of removing the lateral lobes. New York: D. Appleton & Co., [1892]. 4p. DNLM **90-10,146**

WISHARD, William N.
The palliative and operative treatment of the enlarged prostate. Read before the Indiana State Medical Society, June 12, 1892. Indianapolis, 1892. 8p. DNLM **90-10,147**

WISHART, Charles A.
A form of total third nerve paralysis, typical of a unilateral nuclear lesion; with a case. [New York, 1897.] 6p. DNLM **90-10,148**

WITHINGTON, Charles Francis (1852-1917)
Cases of multiple sarcoma. Boston: Rockwell & Churchill, 1897. 24p. DNLM **90-10,149**

WITHINGTON, Charles Francis (1852-1917)
Pulmonary abscess and gangrene. Boston: Damrell & Upham, 1898. 18p. DNLM **90-10,150**

WITTHAUS, R[udolph] A[ugust] (1846-1915)
Essentials of chemistry and toxicology, for the use of students in medicine. . . . 11th ed. New York: William Wood & Co., 1890. 299p. DLC; NNNAM; PPC; PU **90-10,151**

WITTHAUS, R[udolph] A[ugust] (1846-1915)
The medical student's manual of chemistry. . . . 3rd ed. New York: William Wood & Co., 1890. 528p. DLC; DNLM; NNNAM; PPC **90-10,152**

WITTHAUS, R[udolph] A[ugust] (1846-1915)
The medical student's manual of chemistry. . . . 4th ed. New York: William Wood & Co., 1893. 543p. DLC; NNNAM; OCIM; PU **90-10,153**

WITTHAUS, R[udolph] A[ugust] (1846-1915)
A laboratory guide in urinalysis and toxicology. . . . 3rd ed. New York: William Wood & Co., 1893. 96 l. col. front. DLC; NNNAM; OCIM; PPC **90-10,154**

WITTHAUS, R[udolph] A[ugust] (1846-1915)
Essentials of chemistry and toxicology, for the use of students in medicine. . . . 12th ed. New York: William Wood & Co., 1894. 314p. DLC; NNNAM; OCIM; PPC **90-10,155**

WITTHAUS, R[udolph] A[ugust] (1846-1915)
Medical jurisprudence, forensic medicine and toxicology, by R. A. Witthaus . . . and Tracy C. Becker. . . . With the collaboration of August Becker, Esq., Chas. A. Boston, Esq. [a. o.] . . . New York: William Wood & Co., 1894-96. 4 v. col. plates. DLC; DNLM; MBM; NNNAM **90-10,156**

WITTHAUS, R[udolph] A[ugust] (1846-1915)
A laboratory guide in urinalysis and toxicology. . . . 4th ed. New York: William Wood & Co., 1898. 111 l. col. front. DLC; DNLM; NNNAM **90-10,157**

WOCHER, MAX & SON
Illustrated catalogue and price list of surgical instruments, orthopaedic apparatus, trusses, elastic hosiery, electrical batteries, microscopes, hospital & laboratory supplies. . . . 2nd ed. Cincinnati, (1896). 533p. DNLM **90-10,158**

WÖHLER, Friedrich (1800-1882)
Wöhler's outlines of organic chemistry . . . by Rudolph Fittig. Transl. from the 8th German ed., by Ira Remsen. Philadelphia: Lea Bros. & Co., 1890 [1873]. 550p. CtY-M; DLC; PPC; PU **90-10,159**

WOLDERT, Albert (*b.* 1867)
The use of quinin in malarial hemoglobinuria. New York, 1898. 13p. DNLM **90-10,160**

WOLDERT, Albert (*b.* 1867)
Naphthalin in typhoid fever; a remedy in preventing intestinal putrefaction and tympanites. Chicago, 1899. 12p. DNLM **90-10,161**

WOLFE, Samuel (*b.* 1851)
Treatment of insomnia. [New York, 1894.] 6p. DNLM **90-10,162**

WOLFE, Samuel (*b.* 1851)
Polio-encephalitis superior acuta. New York: Alliance Press, 1894. 8p. DNLM **90-10,163**

WOLFE, Samuel (*b.* 1851)
Auto-intoxication. Philadelphia, 1897. 5p. DNLM **90-10,164**

WOLFE, Samuel (*b.* 1851)
Remedial measures proposed for Pennsylvania. [New York], 1898. 11p. DNLM **90-10,165**

WOLFE, Samuel (*b.* 1851)
The bearing of the neurotrophic function on cutaneous conditions. Philadelphia, 1899. 10p. DNLM **90-10,166**

WOLFENSTEIN, Julius
Cocaine in the treatment of acute inflammations of the ear. [New York, 1892.] 5p. DNLM **90-10,167**

WOLFENSTEIN, Julius
Paresthesia of the pharynx and larynx as a premonitory symptom of tuberculosis of the lungs. [Philadelphia, 1893.] 11p. DNLM **90-10,168**

WOLFENSTEIN, Julius
A case of acute empyema of the antrum of Highmore of nasal origin. [New York, 1893.] 8p. DNLM **90-10,169**

WOLFF, Lawrence (1845?-1901)
The examination of urine, chemical and microscopical, for clinical purposes. Arranged in the form of questions and answers. . . . Philadelphia: W. B. Saunders; [etc., etc.], 1890. 66p. col. front. DLC; DNLM; PPC; PU **90-10,170**

WOLFF, Lawrence (1845?-1901)
. . . Essentials of medical chemistry, organic and inorganic. . . . 3rd and rev. ed., with an appendix. Philadelphia: W. B. Saunders, 1891. 218p. DLC; DNLM; NNNAM; PPC **90-10,171**

WOLFF, Lawrence (1845?-1901)
Naphthalin in typhoid fever; based on its employment in one hundred consecutive cases. [Philadelphia, 1891.] 13p. DNLM **90-10,172**

WOLFF, Lawrence (1845?-1901)
Gastrectasis. Detroit, Mich.: G. S. Davis, 1891. 18p. DNLM **90-10,173**

WOLFF, Lawrence (1845?-1901)
. . . Essentials of medical chemistry, organic and inorganic. . . . 4th and rev. ed., with an appendix. Philadelphia: W. B. Saunders, 1893. 218p. DLC; NNNAM; PPC; PU **90-10,174**

WOLFF, Lawrence (1845?-1901)
The dyspepsia of hyperacidity. [Philadelphia, 1893.] 13p. DNLM **90-10,175**

WOLFF, Lawrence (1845?-1901)
Ulcer of the stomach. [Philadelphia, 1893.] 13p. DNLM **90-10,176**

WOLFF, Lawrence (1845?-1901)
Two cases of rupture of the esophagus. Philadelphia, 1894. 8p. DNLM **90-10,177**

WOLFF, Lawrence (1845?-1901)
Two cases of typhoid fever in the same person. Reported by Alfred Hand and Arthur J. Patek. [Philadelphia, 1894.] 2p. DNLM **90-10,178**

WOLFF, Lawrence (1845?-1901)
. . . Essentials of medical chemistry, organic and inorganic. . . . prepared especially for students of medicine. . . . 5th ed., thoroughly rev. by Smith Ely Jelliffe. . . . Philadelphia: W. B. Saunders, 1899. 222p. DLC; MBM; PPC; PPJ **90-10,179**

WOLFSTEIN, David I. (*b.* 1862)
The histological basis of the neuron theory. Cincinnati, 1897. 15p. 20 plates. DNLM **90-10,180**

WOLFSTEIN, David I. (*b.* 1862)
The neuron theory as related to brain and nerve diseases, in the light of the most recent investigations. Providence: Snow & Farnham, 1899. 176p. DNLM **90-10,181**

WOMAN'S MEDICAL COLLEGE OF BALTIMORE
Annual announcements and catalogues for the sessions of 1896 to 1907-08. Baltimore, 1896-1908. DNLM **90-10,182**

WOMAN'S MEDICAL COLLEGE OF CINCINNATI
Annual announcements for the sessions of 1892-93; 1894-95. Cincinnati, 1893-95. DNLM [Merged into Laura Memorial College, 1895.] **90-10,183**

WOMAN'S MEDICAL COLLEGE OF KANSAS CITY, MISSOURI
Annual announcements for the sessions 1895-96, 1898-99 to 1900-1901; 1902-03. Kansas City, Mo., 1895-1903. DNLM **90-10,184**

WOMAN'S MEDICAL COLLEGE OF THE NEW YORK INFIRMARY, NEW YORK CITY
Annual announcements and catalogues for the years 1892-93 to 1898-99. New York, 1893-99. DNLM [Merged into Cornell University Medical College, 1899.] **90-10,185**

WOMAN'S MEDICAL COLLEGE OF THE NEW YORK INFIRMARY, NEW YORK CITY
A brief history of . . . . New York, 1897. 11p. DNLM; NIC **90-10,186**

WOMAN'S MEDICAL COLLEGE AND WOMAN'S HOSPITAL, ST. LOUIS
Annual announcement and catalogue for the session 1895-96. St. Louis, 1895. 24p. DNLM **90-10,187**

WOMAN'S MEDICAL SCHOOL OF NORTHWESTERN UNIVERSITY, CHICAGO
Annual announcement for the session of 1891-92, with catalogue of student for 1890-91. Chicago, 1891. 24p. DNLM **90-10,188**

WOMAN'S MEDICAL SCHOOL OF NORTHWESTERN UNIVERSITY, CHICAGO
Circulars of information for the years 1892 to 1901. Chicago, 1892-1901. DNLM **90-10,189**

WOMAN'S MEDICAL SCHOOL OF NORTHWESTERN UNIVERSITY, CHICAGO
The institution and its founders. Class histories. 1870-96. Chicago, 1896. 162p. 5 port. DNLM; ICU
90-10,190

WOOD, Albert (*b.* 1833)
Appendicitis as it affects life insurance risks. New York, 1896. 23p. DNLM; NNNAM **90-10,191**

WOOD, Casey A[lbert] (1856-1942)
Lessons in the diagnosis and treatment of eye diseases. Detroit, Mich.: G. S. Davis, 1891. 154p. DLC; DNLM; OCIM
90-10,192

WOOD, Casey A[lbert] (1856-1942)
Solid mixtures of homatropine and cocaine as substitute for atropine and duboisine in determining refractive errors. [St. Louis, 1891. 7p. DNLM **90-10,193**

WOOD, Csaey A[lbert] (1856-1942)
Solid mixtures of homatropine and cocaine as a substitute for atropine and duboisine in determining refractive errors. [Also] the use of compressed and other discs in ophthalmic practice. Philadelphia, 1891. 6 l. DNLM **90-10,194**

WOOD, Casey A[lbert] (1856-1942)
The effect of kindergarten work on the eyesight of the children. New York: D. Appleton & Co., 1897. 10p. DNLM
90-10,195

WOOD, Edward Addison
Gold in therapy. New York: E. M. Johnson & Co., 1893. 13p. DNLM **90-10,196**

WOOD, Edward Stickney (1846-1905)
Renal albuminuria not due to organic disease of the kidneys. Boston: Damrell & Upham, 1892. 14p. DNLM; MBM
90-10,197

WOOD, George B[acon] (1797-1879)
The elimination of ether and its relation to the kidney. Philadelphia, 1894. 9p. DNLM **90-10,198**

WOOD, Georbe B[acon] (1797-1879)
The dispensatory of the United States of America. By George B. Wood . . . and Franklin Bache. . . . 17th ed. Thoroughly rev. and largely rewritten. . . . By H. C. Wood . . . Joseph P. Remington . . . and Samuel P. Sadtler. . . . Philadelphia: J. B. Lippincott Co., 1894. 1930p. DLC; NNNAM; OCLloyd; PPC
90-10,199

WOOD, George Bacon (1797-1879)
The dispensatory of the United States of America. By Dr. Geo. B. Wood and Dr. Franklin Bache, 18th ed. Thoroughly rev. and largely rewritten . . . by H. C. Wood . . . Joseph P. Remington . . . and Samuel P. Sadtler. . . . Philadelphia: J. B. Lippincott Co., [1899]. 1999p. DLC; MBM; OCIM; PU
90-10,200

WOOD, Horatio C. (1841-1920)
Therapeutics: its principles and practice; a work on medical agencies, drugs and poisons, with especial reference to the relations between physiology and clinical medicine. 7th ed. of "A treatise on therapeutics." Philadelphia: J. B. Lippincott Co., 1890. 908p. CtY-M; DNLM; OCLloyd; PPC
90-10,201

WOOD, Horatio C. (1841-1920) and David CERNA
A research to determine the action of nitrous oxide, nitrogen, oxygen, and carbonic acid upon the circulation, with especial reference to nitrous oxide anaesthesia. Detroit, Mich.: G. S. Davis, 1890. 43p. DNLM; OCIM **90-10,202**

WOOD, Horatio C. (1841-1920) and H. A. HARE
The cause of death from chloroform. [Philadelphia, 1890.] 26p. DNLM; PPC **90-10,203**

WOOD, Horatio C. (1841-1920)
Therapeutics: its principles and practice. . . . 8th ed. . . . Philadelphia: J. B. Lippincott Co., 1890. 937p. DLC; ICJ; NcD; PPJ **90-10,204**

WOOD, Horatio C. (1841-1920) and David CERNA
Physiological study of chloralamid. The new hypnotic. [New York, 1891.] 11p. DNLM **90-10,205**

WOOD, Horatio C. (1841-1920)
Cardiac nerve storms. Essential tachycardia. Philadelphia, 1891. 10p. DNLM **90-10,206**

WOOD, Horatio C. (1841-1920)
The relation of neuropathic insanity to crime. [Philadelphia, 1892.] 10p. DNLM **90-10,207**

WOOD, Horatio C. (1841-1920)
Brain work and overwork. . . . Philadelphia: P. Blakiston, Son & Co., 1893. 126p. DLC; PPC; PPF; PPL [American Health Primers, first printing, 1880] **90-10,208**

WOOD, Horatio C. (1841-1920)
The choreic movement. [New York: Raff & Co., 1893.] 13p. DNLM; NNNAM **90-10,209**

WOOD, Horatio C. (1841-1920)
An investigation into the action of convulsants. [1893?] 12p. DNLM **90-10,210**

WOOD, Horatio C. (1841-1920)
Original memoirs and clinical lectures. [Philadelphia, 1893?] 4p. DNLM **90-10,211**

WOOD, Horatio C. (1841-1920)
On potassium permanganate as an antidote to vegetable poisons. Philadelphia, 1894. 6p. DNLM
90-10,212

WOOD, Horatio C. (1841-1920)
Therapeutics: its principles and practice. . . . The 9th ed. of A treatise on therapeutics, thoroughly revised. Philadelphia, [etc.]: J. B. Lippincott Co., 1894. 1007p. DLC; NNNAM; OCIM; PU **90-10,213**

WOOD, Horatio C. (1841-1920)
Strontium salicylate. Philadelphia, 1895. 5p. DNLM
90-10,214

WOOD, Horatio C. (1841-1920) and J. William WHITE
Subcortical glioma of the cerebrum affecting principally the arm centre; removal; recurrence of the growth; second operation; recovery. Reported by Alfred C. Wood. Philadelphia, 1895. 8p. DNLM **90-10,215**

WOOD, Horatio C. (1841-1920)
An expiscation of acute delirium. Philadelphia, 1895. 19p. DNLM **90-10,216**

WOOD, Horatio C. (1841-1920)
The practice of medicine. By Horatio C. Wood . . . and Reginald H. Fitz. . . . Philadelphia: J. B. Lippincott Co; [etc., etc.], 1897. 1088p. charts. CtY-M; DLC; DNLM; PPC
90-10,217

WOOD, Horatio C. (1841-1920)
Therapeutics: its principles and practice. . . . The 10th ed. of A treatise on therapeutics, thoroughly revised. Philadelphia, [etc.]: J. B. Lippincott Co., 1897. 1033p. DLC; MBM; NNNAM; PPC **90-10,218**

WOOD, Horatio C. (1841-1920)
Memoir of Harrison Allen. [Philadelphia], 1898. 15p. DNLM
90-10,219

WOOD, Horatio C. (1841-1920)
Judicial methods; medico-legal testimony; the Zelner case. Philadelphia, 1899. 22p. DNLM; PPC
90-10,220

WOOD, Horatio C. (1841-1920)
Nostrums. Chicago, 1899. 12p. DNLM
90-10,221

WOOD, Horatio C. (1841-1920)
The proposed law governing expert testimony. Philadelphia, 1899. 6p. DNLM **90-10,222**

WOOD, Horatio C. (1841-1920) and Horatio C. WOOD, Jr.
Should the United States Pharmacopoeia recognize veratrum album and veratrum viride as one drug? Philadelphia, 1899. 7p. DNLM **90-10,223**

WOOD, Horatio C. (1841-1920) and John P. ARNOLD
Strontium; a study in physiological therapeutics. Philadelphia, 1899. 18p. DNLM **90-10,224**

WOOD, Horatio C[harles], Jr. (*b.* 1874)
A study of the effect of minute doses of ether and chloroform. Philadelphia, 1898. 7p. DNLM **90-10,225**

WOOD, Horatio C[harles], Jr. (*b.* 1874)
The origin of the "Traube" waves. Boston, 1899. 3p. DNLM
90-10,226

WOOD, Horatio C[harles], Jr. (*b.* 1874)
Benzine in anesthetic mixtures. Philadelphia, 1899. 6p. DNLM
90-10,227

WOOD, James C[raven] (*b.* 1858)
Epilepsy as a hystero-neurosis. Chicago: The Era Publishing Co., 1891. 20p. ICU; IU-M; PPHa **90-10,228**

WOOD, James C[raven] (*b.* 1858)
Three cases of acute intestinal obstruction. . . . Philadelphia, 1891. 8p. PPHa **90-10,229**

WOOD, James C[raven] (*b.* 1858)
Three cases of acute intestinal obstruction. . . . Philadelphia, 1891. 7p. DLC **90-10,230**

WOOD, James C[raven] (*b.* 1858)
Epoche in medicine. . . . Boston: C. A. White & Co., 1892. 18p. MH **90-10,231**

WOOD, James C[raven] (*b.* 1858)
A textbook of gynecology. . . . Philadelphia: Boericke & Tafel, 1894. 858p. CtY-M; DLC; ICJ; PPHa **90-10,232**

WOOD, James C[raven] (*b.* 1858)
Reflex epilepsy from pelvic lesions. [n. p., 1895, *vel subseq.*] 8p. DNLM **90-10,233**

WOOD, James C[raven] (*b.* 1858)
A plea for the removal of all lesions of the lower orifices of the body at one sitting. New York, 1895. 17p. DNLM
90-10,234

WOOD, James C[raven] (*b.* 1858)
The present state of antisepsis in the homoeopathic school. Cleveland, 1898. 10p. DNLM **90-10,235**

WOOD, James C[raven] (*b.* 1858)
A textbook of gynecology. . . . 2nd ed., rev. and enl. Philadelphia: Boericke & Tafel, 1898. 964p. col. plates. ICJ; PPHa
90-10,236

WOOD, James C[raven] (*b.* 1858)
Exophthalmic goitre as a hystero-neurosis. New York, 1899. 7p. DNLM **90-10,237**

WOOD, James C[raven] (*b.* 1858)
The relations of homoeopathy to allied systems of therapeutics. Philadelphia, 1899. 12p. DNLM
90-10,238

WOOD, James C[raven] (*b.* 1858)
Obstruction of the bowel due to abnormal contents. [1899.] 7p. DNLM **90-10,239**

WOOD, Wallace (*d.* 1916)
A new method in brain study; fissura calcarina; cerebral eidola; prothymia; intention; the anthemion. New York, 1899. 48p. DNLM **90-10,240**

WOOD, William B.
The after-treatment of obstetric cases. [New York, 1890.] 7p. DNLM **90-10,241**

WOOD-ALLEN, Mary (1841-1908) and Sylvanus STALL
What a young woman ought to know. Philadelphia: Vir Pub. Co., [1898]. 264p. DNLM; ICU; MH; NN
90-10,242

WOODARD, Robert Lee (*b.* 1874)
Aseptic surgery in the country. New York: D Appleton & Co., 1899. 4p. DNLM **90-10,243**

WOODBRIDGE, John Eliot (1846?-1901)
Can typhoid fever be aborted? Second paper. Chicago, 1894. 12p. DNLM **90-10,244**

WOODBRIDGE, John Eliot (1846?-1901)
Can typhoid fever be aborted? Third paper, with the records of the reported cases continued to date of recovery; also of three other members of the family who were attacked after the reading of this paper. Chicago, 1894. 20p. DNLM
90-10,245

WOODBRIDGE, John Eliot (1846?-1901)
Can typhoid fever be aborted? Fourth paper, with clinical data. Toledo, 1894. 9p. DNLM **90-10,246**

WOODBRIDGE, John Eliot (1846?-1901)
Can typhoid fever be aborted? Fifth paper. Chicago, 1894. 8p. DNLM **90-10,247**

WOODBRIDGE, John Eliot (1846?-1901)
Can typhoid fever be aborted? Eighth paper, Toledo, 1895. 23p. DNLM **90-10,248**

WOODBRIDGE, John Eliot (1846?-1901)
Further reports on the abortion of typhoid fever. Chicago, 1895. 16p. DNLM **90-10,249**

WOODBRIDGE, John Eliot (1846?-1901)
Reports on typhoid fever. Chicago, 1895. 44p. DNLM **90-10,250**

WOODBRIDGE, John Eliot (1846?-1901)
Typhoid fever and its abortive treatment. . . . Cleveland: L. Leavengood & Co., 1896. 368p. col. plates. DLC; DNLM; OCIM **90-10,251**

WOODBRIDGE, John Eliot (1846?-1901)
Typhoid fever. . . . A report from the Transactions of the fifty-second annual meeting of the Ohio State Medical Society held at Cleveland, O. Norwalk, O.: The Laning Printing Co., 1897. 50p. DNLM **90-10,252**

WOODBURY, Frank (1848-1927)
On the employment of the cataphoric action of the galvanic current for the removal of syphilitic new growths. A contribution to the medical treatment of tumors. [Philadelphia, 1890.] 6p. DNLM **90-10,253**

WOODBURY, Frank (1848-1927)
On the use of nitrogenized food in fever and wasting diseases, especially in the form of peptonized beef powder. (Mosquera's beef meal). Detroit, 1890. 8p. DNLM **90-10,254**

WOODBURY, Frank (1848-1927)
A note on two new creosote compounds, creosote valerianate and guaiacol valerianate. New York: D. Appleton & Co., 1897. 12p. DNLM **90-10,255**

WOODBURY, John H. (*b.* 1832)
What dermatology has to do with beauty. How to remove all imperfections of the skin. New York, [1894]. 151p. DNLM; NNNAM **90-10,256**

WOODHEAD, G[erman] Sims (1855-1921)
Practical pathology. . . . Philadelphia: J. B. Lippincott & Co., 1892. 652p. CtY-M; NNNAM; PPC; PU **90-10,257**

WOODHULL, Alfred A[lexander] (1837-1921)
The enlisted soldier. (Prize essay.) Washington: Government Printing Office, 1890. 44p. DNLM **90-10,258**

WOODHULL, Alfred A[lexander] (1837-1921)
Notes on military hygiene, for officers of the line: a syllabus of lectures at the U.S. Infantry and Cavalry School. New York: J. Wiley & Sons, 1890. 150p., interleaved. DNLM; NNNAM **90-10,259**

WOODHULL, Alfred A[lexander] (1837-1921)
The place of the Medical Department in the Army. Governor's Island, N.Y.H., 1890. 22p. DNLM **90-10,260**

WOODHULL, Alfred A[lexander] (1837-1921)
Observations upon the medical department of the British army, made in 1891. Abridged from an official report. St. Louis: Buxton & Skinner Stationery Co., 1894. 160p. DNLM; IU-M **90-10,261**

WOODHULL, Alfred [Alexander] (1837-1921)
[Report of the Medical Department of the Colorado for the fiscal year 1896.] Denver, 1896. 23p. DNLM **90-10,262**

WOODHULL, Alfred A[lexander] (1837-1921)
The better type of medical officer. Columbus, O.: Berlin Print. Co., 1897. 7p. DNLM **90-10,263**

WOODHULL, Alfred [Alexander] (1837-1921)
Notes on military hygiene, for officers of the line. A syllabus of lectures formerly delivered at the U.S. Infantry and Cavalry School. . . . New ed., rev. and augm. 1st thousand. New York: J. Wiley & Sons; London: Chapman & Hall, 1898. 181p. DLC; NNNAM **90-10,264**

WOODMAN, W[illiam] Bathhurst (1836-1877)
Forensic medicine and toxicology. A comprehensive work on medical jurisprudence. By W. B. Woodman and Charles M. Tidy. . . . Philadelphia: P. Blakiston, Son & Co., 1890. 1083p. [Originally, Philadelphia: Lindsay & Blakiston, 1877, 1083p. *vel subseq.*] **90-10,265**

WOODRUFF, Charles E[dward] (1860-1915)
The causes of the explosive effects of the modern small-caliber bullets. New York, 1898. 29p. DNLM **90-10,266**

WOODS, Hiram (1857-1931)
Diphtheritic conjunctivitis; report of two cases, with the bacteriologic study of the false membrane. [Philadelphia, 1892.] 15p. DNLM **90-10,267**

WOODWARD, Alfred W. (1839-1902)
The systemic functions and their reciprocal influence in disease. Being preliminary to a study of pharmaco-dynamics. . . [Chicago: C. E. Crandall, printer], 1893. 46p. DLC **90-10,268**

WOODWARD, Julius H[ayden] (*b.* 1858)
Chronic nasal catarrh in Vermont. [New York, 1890.] 6p. DNLM **90-10,269**

WOODWARD, Julius H[ayden] (*b.* 1858)
Eye-strain and functional nervous diseases. Burlington, 1890. 25p. DNLM **90-10,270**

WOODWARD, Julius H[ayden] (*b.* 1858)
Glaucoma; its nature and treatment. Nashville: A. R. Gray & Son, 1892. 8p. DNLM **90-10,271**

WOODWARD, Julius H[ayden] (*b.* 1858)
The ophthalmometer of Javal and Schlötz, and the diagnosis of astigmatism. [New York, 1892.] 6pl 1 tab. **90-10,272**

WOODWARD, Julius H[ayden] (*b.* 1858)
Some observations of general interest regarding the course and management of cataract. New York: G. L. Goodman & Co., 1898. 17p. DNLM; NNNAM **90-10,273**

WOODWARD, Julius H[ayden] (*b.* 1858)
A case of cerebellar abscess; autopsy. New York, 1898. 5p. DNLM **90-10,274**

WOODWARD, Julius H[ayden] (*b.* 1858)
A case of pulsating exophthalmus; rupture of the left carotid into the cavernous sinus; cured. New York: D. Appleton & Co., 1898. 4p. DNLM **90-10,275**

WOODWARD, Julius H[ayden] (*b.* 1858)
Epiphora, or the watery eye; its complications, etiology, and management. New York: Publishers' Print Co., 1899. 12p. DNLM; NNNAM **90-10,276**

WOODY, Samuel E[lisha] (*b.* 1854)
Essentials of medical chemistry and urinalysis. 3rd ed. Philadelphia: P. Blakiston, Son & Co., 1890. 157p. CtY-M; DNLM; NNNAM; PU **90-10,277**

WOOLSEY, Abby Howland (1828-1893)
Hand-book for hospitals. 3rd ed. New York & London: G. P. Putnam's Sons, 1895. 267p. DNLM; NNNAM **90-10,278**

WOOLSEY, E[lliott] H. (*b.* 1844)
Colles's fracture. Illustrated by photographs of splints used in treatment, and by photographs of cases. Oakland: San Francisco & New York, 1892. 45p. 12 plates. DNLM **90-10,279**

WOOLSEY, George (*b.* 1861)
Some considerations on prostatectomy. [New York, 1895.] 16p. DNLM **90-10,280**

WOOLSEY, George (*b.* 1861)
A clinical lecture on a case operated upon for the radical cure of inguinal hernia and for urethro-rectal fistula. New York: D. Appleton & Co., 1896. 10p. DNLM **90-10,281**

WOOLSEY, George (*b.* 1861)
Massage in the treatment of fractures. New York, 1897. 20p. DNLM **90-10,282**

WOOLSEY, George (*b.* 1861)
Some considerations on abdominal incisions. Philadelphia, 1898. 13p. DNLM **90-10,283**

WOOLSEY, George (*b.* 1861)
Report of three cases of multiple pistol-shot wounds of the intestine. New York, 1899. 14p. DNLM **90-10,284**

WORCESTER, Alfred (1855-1951)
Monthly nursing. 2nd ed. New York: D. Appleton & Co., 1890. 250p. 1 plate. DNLM; NNNAM **90-10,285**

WORCESTER, Alfred (1855-1951)
The treatment of occipito-posterior positions. Chicago: Office Amer. Med. Assoc., 1891. 8p. DNLM **90-10,286**

WORCESTER, Alfred (1855-1951)
The treatment of appendicitis. [Philadelphia: Univ. Penn. Press, 1892.] 6p. DNLM **90-10,287**

WORCESTER, Alfred (1855-1951)
Training schools for nurses in small cities. Boston: G. H. Ellis, [1893]. 68p. 1 plate, 1 plan. DNLM; ICJ; MB **90-10,288**

WORCESTER, Alfred (1855-1951)
A case of Caesarean section. Boston: Damrell & Upham, 1893. 6p. DNLM **90-10,289**

WORCESTER, Alfred (1855-1951)
Cases of extra-uterine pregnancy. [Boston, 1893.] 15p. DNLM **90-10,290**

WORCESTER, Alfred (1855-1951)
The treatment of puerperal septic peritonitis; report of cases. [Boston, 1893.] 8p. DNLM **90-10,291**

WORCESTER, Alfred (1855-1951)
Small hospitals. Establishment and maintenance, and suggestions for hospital architecture; with plans for a small hospital, by William Atkinson. New York: J. Wiley & Sons, 1894. 114p. 1 plate. DLC; DNLM; NIC; NNNAM **90-10,292**

WORCESTER, Alfred (1855-1951)
The physician's extra-professional duties. The annual discourse delivered before the Massachusetts Medical Society, June 12, 1895. . . . Boston: D. Clapp & Son, printers, 1895. 27p. NN **90-10,293**

WORCESTER, William Leonard (1845-1901)
Is puerperal insanity a distinct clinical form? Utica, N.Y., 1890. 7p. DNLM **90-10,294**

WORCESTER, William Leonard (1845-1901)
Cases of multiple neuritis. Utica, N.Y., 1893. 6p. DNLM **90-10,295**

WORCESTER, William Leonard (1845-1901)
Sclerosis of the cornu ammonis in epilepsy. [n. p.], 1896. 32p. DNLM **90-10,296**

WORCESTER, William Leonard (1845-1901)
The psychology of insane delusions. Baltimore, 1897. 7p. DNLM **90-10,297**

WORCESTER, William Leonard (1845-1901)
The relations of renal disease to mental derangement. New York, 1899. 9p. DNLM **90-10,298**

WORMLEY, Theodore G[eorge] (1826-1897)
Recovery of absorbed morphine from the urine, the blood, and the tissues. [Philadelphia, 1890.] 11p. DNLM **90-10,299**

WORMLEY, Theodore G[eorge] (1826-1897)
Notes on some of the chemical properties of the mydriatic alkaloids. Philadelphia, 1894. 4p. DNLM **90-10,300**

WORMLEY, Theodore G[eorge] (1826-1897)
On some of the tests for quinine. Philadelphia, 1894. 13p. DNLM **90-10,301**

WORSTER, Willard Parker
The treatment and cure of chancre with peroxide of hydrogen. New York, 1894. 4p. DNLM **90-10,302**

WOSSIDLO, Hans [R.] (1854-1918)
Practical urethroscopy. New York: Trow, 1895. 30p. DNLM **90-10,303**

WRIGHT, Charles D'A. (*b.* 1863)
A hand book of the refraction of the eye, its anomalies and their correction. Ann Arbor, Mich.: Sheehan & Co., [1896]. 128p. DNLM **90-10,304**

WRIGHT, Edward W[illiam] (*b.* 1860)
(1) Eserine. (2) The relation of eye symptoms to urinary excretion, a clinical study. (3) Readers' cramp. [Brooklyn, 1897.] 16p. DNLM **90-10,305**

WRIGHT, James Homer (1869-1928)
Studies in the pathology of diphtheria. [Boston, 1894.] 12p. 1 tab. DNLM **90-10,306**

WRIGHT, James Homer (1869-1928)
On the cultivation of the gonococcus from cases of gonorrhoea, ophthalmia purulenta, and pyosalpinx. Philadelphia, 1895. 11p. DNLM **90-10,307**

WRIGHT, James Homer (1869-1928)
The histological lesions of acute glanders in man and of experimenal glanders in the guinea-pig. New York, 1896. 18p. 2 plates. DNLM **90-10,308**

WRIGHT, James Homer (1869-1928) and W[illiam] Royal STOKES
A report on the bacteriological investigations of autopsies. Boston, 1895. 40p. DNLM **90-10,309**

WRIGHT, John S[hepard] (*b.* 1870)
A guide to the organic drugs of the United States Pharmacopoeia 1890. Containing, in addition to the brief accounts of organic drugs, a conspectus of the natural orders of plants mentioned, and glossaries of the botanical and medical terms used. Comp. and arr. by John S. Wright. Indianapolis: Botanical Department of E. Lilly & Co., 1895. 118p. DLC; DNLM; ICU; NIC **90-10,310**

WRIGHT, John S[hepard] (*b.* 1870)
A guide to the organic drugs of the United States Pharmacopoeia 1890. Indianapolis: Lilly & Co., 1896. 162p. MB; OCLloyd **90-10,311**

WRIGHT, John S[hepard] (*b.* 1870)
A guide to the organic drugs of the United States Pharmacopoeia, 1890, rev. with app. Indianapolis: E. Lilly & Co., 1899. 179p. DNLM; OCLloyd **90-10,312**

WRIGHT, John W[estley] (1842-1935)
A text-book of ophthalmology. Columbus: J. L. Trauger, 1896. 405p. PPJ **90-10,313**

WRIGHT, Jonathan (1860-1928)
Salol in acute tonsillitis and pharyngitis. [Philadelphia, 1890.] 8p. DNLM **90-10,314**

WRIGHT, Jonathan (1860-1928)
Lymphoid hypertrophy in the pharyngeal vault. Chicago: Amer. Med. Assoc., 1890. 16p. DNLM **90-10,315**

WRIGHT, Jonathan (1860-1928)
Nasal papillomata. [New York: D. Appleton & Co., 1891.] 14p. DNLM **90-10,316**

WRIGHT, Jonathan (1860-1928)
Subglottic neoplasms. [Chicago, 1891.] 16p. DNLM **90-10,317**

WRIGHT, Jonathan (1860-1928)
A case of primary lupus of the pharynx. [Philadelphia, 1892.] 10p. DNLM **90-10,318**

WRIGHT, Jonathan (1860-1928)
Papillary hypertrophy of the nasal mucous membrane compared with a true papilloma. New York: D. Appleton & Co., 1894. 7p. DNLM **90-10,319**

WRIGHT, Jonathan (1860-1928)
A consideration of the vascular mechanism of the nasal mucous membrane and its relations to certain pathological processes. Philadelphia, 1895. 7p. DNLM **90-10,320**

WRIGHT, Jonathan (1860-1928)
A cyst of the nasopharynx and a cyst of the oropharynx. New York, 1895. 6p. DNLM **90-10,321**

WRIGHT, Jonathan (1860-1928)
A few remarks on some cases of mycosis of the nose and throat. [New York: D. Appleton & Co., 1895.] 5p. 1 plate. **90-10,322**

WRIGHT, Jonathan (1860-1928)
Tuberculosis of the upper air-passages; aetiology. [New York: D. Appleton & Co., 1895.] 14p. DNLM **90-10,323**

WRIGHT, Jonathan (1860-1928)
Tuberculous infection of the lymphoid tissue in the pharynx, with some remarks on laryngeal infection. New York, 1896. 9p. 1 plate. DNLM **90-10,324**

WRIGHT, Jonathan (1860-1928)
Papillary oedematous nasal polypi and their relation to adenomata. [New York, 1897.] 16p. DNLM **90-10,325**

WRIGHT, Jonathan (1860-1928)
The nose and throat in medical history. St. Louis: L. S. Matthews. [1898, *vel subseq.*] 244. DNLM; ICU; NNC **90-10,326**

WRIGHT, Thomas Lee (1825-1893)
Some principles involved in the nature and treatment of inebriety. St. Louis, 1892. 7p. DNLM **90-10,327**

WYETH, John Allan (1845-1922)
A text-book on surgery, general, operative, and mechanical. . . . 2nd ed., rev. and enl. New York: D. Appleton & Co., 1890. 887p. col. illus. DLC; DNLM; NNNAM; PU **90-10,328**

WYETH, John Allan (1845-1922)
Bloodless amputation at the hip-joint; a report of forty-two cases by the author's method. New York, 1894. 19p. DNLM; NNNAM **90-10,329**

WYETH, John Allan (1845-1922)
A text-book on surgery, general, operative, and mechanical. . . . 3rd ed., rev. and enl. New York: D. Appleton & Co., 1898. 997p. col. illus. DLC; DNLM; NNNAM; OCIM **90-10,330**

WYETH, JOHN & BRO.
Therapeutic notes; sevetol. Philadelphia, [1890?] 6p. DNLM **90-10,331**

WYETH, JOHN & BRO.
Price list of the most elegant pharmaceutical preparations. Philadelphia, 1891. 90p. DNLM; PPC **90-10,332**

WYLIE, Robert Hawthorne (*b.* 1863)
Fourteen hysterectomies. New York, 1894. 11p. DNLM
90-10,333

WYMAN, Hal C. (1852-1908)
A failure in brain surgery. [Philadelphia, 1890.] 6p. DNLM
90-10,334

WYMAN, Hal C. (1852-1908)
Diseases of the bladder and prostate. Detroit, Mich.: G. S. Davis, 1891. 132p. DNLM; OCIM
90-10,335

WYMAN, Hal C. (1852-1908)
Septicaemia treated by foods, drainage, and rest. Chicago: Cameron, Amberg & Co., 1891. 16p. DNLM
90-10,336

WYMAN, Hal C. (1852-1908)
Some cases of brain surgery. [Detroit, 1898.] 11p. DNLM
90-10,337

WYMAN, Morrill (1812-1903)
Cottage hospitals. Boston: Damrell & Upham, 1895. 24p. DNLM
90-10,338

WYMAN, Walter (1848-1911)
National control of leprosy. Philadelphia, 1894. 7p. DNLM
90-10,339

WYNTER, W[alter] Essex (1860-1928) and Frank J. WETHERED
A manual of clinical and practical pathology. Philadelphia: P. Blakiston, Son & Co., 1890. 310p. DNLM; NNNAM; PPC; PU
90-10,340

YALE UNIVERSITY. MEDICAL DEPARTMENT, NEW HAVEN
Annual announcements and circulars, for the seasons of 1839-40 to 1841-42 (27.-29.); 1852-53 (40.); 1853 (41.); 1866-67 to 1877-78 (54.-65.); 1879-80 (67.); 1882-83 (70.); 1887-88 to 1893-94 (75.-81). New Haven, 1839-94. CtY-M; DNLM
90-10,341

YANDELL, David W[endell] (1826-1898)
Pioneer surgery in Kentucky; a sketch. Louisville: J. P. Morton & Co., 1890. 33p. DLC; ICJ; OC
90-10,342

YANDELL, David W[endell] (1826-1898)
Temperament: an address. Louisville: J. P. Morton & Co., 1892. 21p. DLC; OC; OCIM
90-10,343

YARNALL, E. A. & CO.
Illustrated catalogue of medical supplies. Philadelphia, 1892. 344p. NNNAM; PPC
90-10,344

YARNALL, E. A. & CO.
Illustrated catalogue of surgical and medical apparatus and supplies. 2nd ed. Philadelphia, 1894. 384p. DNLM
90-10,345

THE YEARBOOK of treatment for 1890. A critical review for practitioners of medicine and surgery. Philadelphia: Lea Bros. & Co., 1890-. 324p. NNNAM; OCIM; PPC; PPJ [English work imported by Lea and published under the Lea imprint.]
90-10,346

YEO, Gerald Francis (1845-1909)
A manual of physiology. . . . 6th American from the 3rd rev. English ed. . . . Philadelphia: P. Blakiston, Son & Co., 1893. 759p. col. front. DLC; DNLM; PPC; PU
90-10,347

YEO, I[saac] Burney (1835-1914)
Food in health and disease. . . . Philadelphia: Lea Bros. & Co., 1892. 569p. CtY-M; PPC; PPJ; PU
90-10,348

YEO, I[saac] Burney (1835-1914)
A manual of medical treatment or clinical therapeutics. Philadelphia: Lea Bros. & Co., 1893. 2 v. DNLM; NNNAM; PPC; PU
90-10,349

YEO, I[saac] Burney (1835-1914)
A manual of medical treatment or clinical therapeutics. Rev. ed. Philadelphia: Lea Bros. & Co., 1895. 2 v. PPC; PPJ
90-10,350

YEO, I[saac] Burney (1835-1914)
Food in health and disease. . . . New and rev. ed. Philadelphia: Lea Bros. & Co., [1896]. 592p. CtY-M; MH; PPC; PU
90-10,351

YINGLING, William A. (*b.* 1851)
The accoucheur's emergency manual. . . . Philadelphia: Boericke & Tafel, 1895. 323p. DLC; PPC; PPHa
90-10,352

YOUNG, Adelbert A.
Amoebic catarrh of the intestinal tract. Buffalo, 1896. 5p. DNLM
90-10,353

YOUNG, Albion G. (*b.* 1843)
Notes on disinfectants and disinfection. Augusta: Kennebec Journal Print, 1898. 218p. DNLM
90-10,354

YOUNG, Hugh H[ampton] (1870-1945)
Long, the discoverer of anaesthesia. A presentation of his original documents. [Baltimore, 1897.] 22p. DNLM
90-10,355

YOUNG, Hugh H[ampton] (1870-1945)
On the presence of nerves in tumors and of other structures in them as revealed by a modification of Ehrlich's method of "vital staining" with methylene blue. New York, 1897. 12p. DNLM
90-10,356

YOUNG, James Kelly (1862-1923)
A practical treatise on orthopedic surgery. . . . Philadelphia: Lea Bros. & Co., 1894. 446p. DLC; DNLM; NNNAM; PPC
90-10,357

YOUNGMAN, Maurice D.
The classes of cases of pulmonary disease in which the climate of Atlantic City, N.J., is beneficial. Philadelphia, 1897. 7p. DNLM
90-10,358

ZAHORSKY, John (*b.* 1871)
A critical study of infant feeding based on recent analyses of human milk. New York & London, 1898. 13p. DNLM
90-10,359

ZAHORSKY, John (*b.* 1871)
A study of migraine. St. Louis, 1898. 16p. DNLM
90-10,360

ZAHORSKY, John (*b.* 1871)
A case of diverticulum oesophagi. St. Louis, 1899. 3 l. DNLM
90-10,361

ZAHORSKY, John (*b.* 1871)
A contribution to the study of meteolologic states etiologically related to influenza epidemics. St. Louis, 1899. 10p. DNLM
90-10,362

ZAHORSKY, John (*b.* 1871)
General infection by the diplococcus intracellularis in an infant. Charlotte, N.C., 1899. 4p. DNLM
90-10,363

ZERVAS, Josef
A manual on the treatment of diseases by electricity. . . . New York: F. G. Otto, 1890. [1888] 48p. DLC
90-10,363A

ZIEGLER, Ernst (1849-1905)
General pathology; or, The science of the causes, nature and course of the pathological disturbances which occur in the living subject. . . . Transl. from the 8th rev. German ed. by Dr. Leonard Woolsey Bacon, Jr. . . . Drs. B. Meade Bolton and Henry W. Cattell . . . [and others]. Editor: Dr. Albert H. Buck. . . . New York: William Wood & Co., 1895. 588p. col. plates. DLC; DNLM; NNNAM; PU
90-10,364

ZIEGLER, Ernst (1849-1905)
A text-book of special pathological anatomy. . . . Transl. and ed. from the 8th German ed. by Donald MacAlister . . . and Henry W. Cattell. . . . Sections I-XV. New York: The Macmillan Co.; London: Macmillan & Co., Ltd., 1896-97. 2 v. col. plates. DLC; DNLM; MBM; NNNAM
90-10,365

ZIEGLER, Ernst (1849-1905)
General pathology, or the science of the causes, nature, and course of the pathological disturbances which occur in the living subject. Transl. from the 9th revised German ed. by Theodore Dunham, Edward M. Foote [et al.]. Editor: Albert H. Buck. New York: William Wood & Co., 1899. 578p. DNLM; NNNAM **90-10,366**

ZIEGLER, S[amuel] Lewis (1861-1926)
A convenient prism scale. [St. Louis, 1893.] 11p. DNLM; MB
90-10,367

ZIEGLER, S[amuel] Lewis (1861-1926)
The treatment of corneal ulcer by the general practitioner. [New York: D. Appleton & Co., 1893.] 9p. DNLM; MB
90-10,368

ZIEGLER, S[amuel] Lewis (1861-1926)
A note on the use of Dr. Zeng's refractometer. [Chicago, 1897.] 12p. MB; PPHa **90-10,369**

ZIMMERMANN, Charles (*b.* 1856)
The eye-symptoms of brain disease. Madison: Tracy, Gibbs & Co., 1891. 12p. DNLM **90-10,370**

ZIMMERMANN, Charles (*b.* 1856)
The relation of the ocular nerves to the brain. Madison: Tracy, Gibbs & Co., 1892. 8p. DNLM **90-10,371**

ZIMMERMANN, Charles (*b.* 1856)
The medicinal treatment of granular conjunctivitis. [Philadelphia, 1894.] 3p. DNLM **90-10,372**

ZIMMERMANN, Charles (*b.* 1856)
Traumatic paresis of left inferior rectus combined with traumatic insufficiency of left external rectus. Kansas City, 1894. 2p. DNLM **90-10,373**

ZIMMERMANN, Charles (*b.* 1856)
Etiology and pathology of sympathetic ophthalmia. Philadelphia, 1895. 7p. DNLM **90-10,374**

ZIMMERMANN, Charles (*b.* 1856)
Prevention of ophthalmia neonatorum. [Detroit]: G. S. Davis, [1896]. 3p. DNLM **90-10,375**

ZIMMERMANN, Charles (*b.* 1856)
Tuberculous parenchymatous keratitis. [Detroit]: W. H. Warren, [1897]. 7p. DNLM **90-10,376**

ZIMMERMANN, Charles (*b.* 1856)
Hemorrhage following tonsillotomy. New York, 1898. 6p. DNLM **90-10,377**

ZINKE, [Ernst] G[ustav] (*b.* 1846)
Symphyseotomy vs. embryotomy upon the living fetus, accompanied by a tabulated record of 389 symphyseotomies performed from 1777 to 1894. Cincinnati, O.: Earhart & Richardson, [1895]. 65p. DNLM; OC
90-10,378

IX. AMERICAN MEDICAL IMPRINTS, 1900-1910

It may seem a work of supererogation to study anew a subject which has already been so ably discussed by Allis, Roberts, Stimson, Lane, Cotton, Chutro, Mouchet, Destot, Vignard, Barlatier, and other surgeons of experience; and this, indeed, was my own opinion until recently. But evidences which constantly recur, both in literature and in practical work, demonstrating the actual ignorance of otherwise well-informed surgeons anent the anatomy and surgery of the elbow region, have convinced me that a further study of this subject is really of importance. To limit the scope of this essay, it has seemed best to confine it to a discussion of recent fractures involving the lower end of the humerus.

The older surgeons gained their experience of these injuries in the period before the use of the X-rays made possible the control and correction of a diagnosis; and many of the younger surgeons, taught by them, are growing up with the idea that after any such fracture a stiff elbow is to be anticipated; and that to prevent its development the most important thing is to encourage early motion—even to insist upon it to the extent of attempting to secure it by repeated and forcible manipulations.

Astley Paston Cooper Ashhurst,
An Anatomical and Surgical Study of Fractures of the Lower End of the Humerus
(1910)
[The Samuel D. Gross Prize Essay of the Philadelphia Academy of Surgery]

ABBOTT, Alexander C[rever] (1860-1935)
The hygiene of transmissible diseases: their causation, modes of dissemination, and methods of prevention. 2nd ed. Philadelphia: W. B. Saunders & Co., 1901. 350p. CtY-M; MBM; NNNAM; PPC **00-0001**

ABBOTT, Alexander C[rever] (1860-1935)
The principles of bacteriology: a practical manual. . . . 6th ed. Philadelphia: Lea Bros. & Co., 1902. 641p. MBM; NNNAM; PPC; PPJ **00-0002**

ABBOTT, Alexander C[rever] (1860-1935)
The principles of bacteriology: a practical manual. . . . 7th ed. Philadelphia: Lea Bros. & Co., 1905. 689p. NNNAM; OCIM; PPC; PU **00-0003**

ABBOTT, Alexander C[rever] (1860-1935)
The principles of bacteriology: a practical manual. . . . 8th ed. Philadelphia: Lea & Febiger, 1909. 631p. CU-M; ICRM; NNNAM; PPC **00-0004**

ABBOTT, Maude E[lizabeth] S[eymour] (1869-1940)
Congenital cardiac disease [Philadelphia: Lea & Febiger, 1908.] 104p. DLC; ICJ; MBM; PU [Reprinted out of Osler & McCrea, Modern Medicine (7 v., 1907-1910)] DLC; ICJ; MH-M; PPC **00-0005**

ABBOTT, Wallace C[alvin] (1857-1921)
Alkaloidal digest, a brief therapeutics of some of the principal alkaloidal medicaments with suggestions for clinical application, embodying various articles on important special agents and certain great phases of alkaloidal therapy that have been developed in my personal practice. Chicago: Clinic Pub. Co., 1904. 248p. OCLloyd; PPC; PU **00-0006**

ABBOTT, Wallace C[alvin] (1857-1921)
Abbott's *Alkaloidal* digest; a brief description of the therapeutics of some of the principal alkaloidal medicaments and other success-makers, with suggestions for their clinical application. Chicago: Clinic Pub. Co., 1905. 248p. ICJ; OCLloyd; PU **00-0007**

ABBOTT, Wallace C[alvin] (1857-1921)
Abbott's alkaloidal digest. A brief description of the therapeutics of some of the principal alkaloidal medicaments and other success-makers in active-principal lines with suggestions for their clinical application. Chicago: Clinic Pub. Co., 1907. 258p. MH; OCLloyd **00-0008**

ABBOTT, Wallace C[alvin] (1857-1921)
An appeal for a square deal; to the medical profession of America. Dr. Abbott's reply to his critics. [An answer to attacks made in the Journal of the American Medical Association.] Chicago, 1908. 48p. MH; NN **00-0009**

ABBOTT, Wallace C[alvin] (1857-1921)
A digest of positive therapeutics. Chicago: The Clinic Publishing Co., [1908?]. 258p. CtY-M; OCLloyd **00-0010**

ABDERHALDEN, Emil (1877-1950)
Textbook of physiological chemistry in thirty lectures. . . . Transl. by William T. Hall. New York: J. Wiley & Sons, 1908. 722p. NNNAM; PU **00-0011**

ABEL, Karl (*b.* 1863)
Gynecological pathology: a manual of microscopic technique and diagnosis in gynecological practice. . . . Transl. and edited by Samuel Wyllis Bandler. . . . New York: William Wood & Co., 1901. 237p. IEN-M; NNNAM; PPC; PU **00-0012**

ABRAMS, Albert (1863-1924)
Diseases of the heart: their diagnosis and treatment. . . . Chicago: G. P. Engelhard & Co., 1900. 170p. ICJ; IU-M; NNNAM; OCIM **00-0013**

ABRAMS, Albert (1863-1924)
Scattered leaves from a physician's diary. St. Louis: Fortnightly Press, 1900. 59p. ICJ; IU-M; NN; OCIM **00-0014**

ABRAMS, Albert (1863-1924)
The blues (splanchnic neurasthenia); causes and cure. New York: E. B. Treat & Co., 1904. 240p. NNNAM **00-0015**

ABRAMS, Albert (1863-1924)
The blues (splanchnic neurasthenia); causes and cure. 2nd ed. New York: E. B. Treat & Co., 1905. 254p. ICJ; NN; NNNAM; PU **00-0016**

ABRAMS, Albert (1863-1924)
Man and his poisons: a practical exposition of the causes, symptoms and treatment of self-poisoning. New York: E. B. Treat & Co., 1906. 268p. IU-M; NNNAM; PPC; PU **00-0017**

ABRAMS, Albert (1863-1924)
The blues (splanchnic neurasthenia); causes and cure. 3rd ed. New York: E. B. Treat & Co., 1908. 287p. ICJ; NNNAM; PPC; PU **00-0018**

ABRAMS, Albert (1863-1924)
Diagnostic therapeutics; a guide for practitioners in diagnosis by aid of drugs and methods other than drug-giving. . . . New York: Rebman Co., 1910. 1039p. CtY-M; NNNAM; PPC; PU **00-0019**

ABRAMS, Albert (1863-1924)
Spondylotherapy: spinal concussion and the application of other methods to the spine in the treatment of disease. San Francisco: The Philopolis Press, 1910. 400p. CU-M; ICJ; NNNAM; PU **00-0020**

ACADEMY OF MEDICINE OF CINCINNATI
The Academy of Medicine of Cincinnati; its history, constitution, and by-laws, with a brief historical sketch of the medical organizations that preceded it. Rev. by A. G. Drury, [Cincinnati], 1910. 42p. ICJ; OC; OCHP **00-0021**

ACHORN, John W[arren] (*b.* 1857)
Some physical disorders having mental origins. Boston: Emmanuel Church, 1908. 32p. DLC; ICJ [Also: New York: Moffat, Yard & Co., 1908, 32p. DNLM] **00-0022**

ACHORN, John W[arren] (*b.* 1857)
Nature's help to happiness; or ground treatment. New York: Moffat, Yard & Co., 1909. 45p. NN **00-0023**

ADAIR, Bethenia Angelina [Owens] (1840-1926)
Dr. Owens-Adair; some of her life experiences. [Portland, Ore.]: Mann & Beach, printers, [1906?]. 4p. MBM
00-0024

ADAIR, Bethenia Angelina [Owens] (1840-1926)
Human sterilization [by] Dr. B. Owens Adair, author of the famous "Human Sterilization" Bill of Oregon. [Warrenton, Oregon, 1910?] 60p. DLC; ICU
00-0025

ADAMI, J[ohn] George (1862-1926)
Inflammation. An article by J. G. Adami. . . . New York: The Macmillan Co., 1907. [4, 54]-139p. ICJ [Reprinted from Prof. Clifford Allbutt's New system of medicine, for private circulation.] **00-0026**

ADAMI, J[ohn] George (1862-1926)
Inflammation. An introduction to the study of pathology. Being the reprint (revised and enlarged) of an article in Professor Allbutt's "System of medicine." New York: The Macmillan Co., 1907. 240p. CtY-M; DLC; ICJ; OCIM
00-0027

ADAMI, J[ohn] George (1862-1926)
Charles White: surgeon and obstetrician. New York: Eagle Press, 1907. 18p. NN **00-0028**

ADAMI, J[ohn] George (1862-1926)
Sir John Harington. [Baltimore], 1908. 31p. NN
00-0029

ADAMI, J[ohn] George (1862-1926)
The principles of pathology. . . . Philadelphia: Lea & Febiger, 1908-1909. 2 v. CtY-M; NNNAM; PPC; PU
00-0030

ADAMI, J[ohn] George (1862-1926)
The principles of pathology. 2nd ed., rev. and enl. Philadelphia: Lea & Febiger, 1910-1911. 2 v. ICRM; NNNAM; PPC; PU **00-0031**

ADAMS, Ernest O.
Diseases of the digestive system. [Cleveland]: The Cleveland Homoeopathic Publishing Co., 1910. 349p. ICJ; OCIM
00-0032

ADAMS, James F[orster] A[lleyne] (1844-1914)
The segregation of consumptives. . . . Delivered at the annual meeting of the Massachusetts Medical Society, June 12, 1907. [Boston, 1907.] 10p. DLC; DNLM; MB
00-0033

ADAMS, Samuel H[opkins] (1871-1958)
The great American fraud; a series of articles on the patent medicine evil, reprinted from Collier's Weekly [Oct. 7, 1905-Feb. 17, 1906]. Also, the patent medicine conspiracy against the freedom of the press. [Chicago?]: P. F. Collier, [1906]. 95p. DLC; ICJ; KU; NN **00-0034**

ADAMS, Samuel H[opkins] (1871-1958)
The great American fraud; articles on the nostrum evil and quacks. . . . [New York, 1906.] 146p. DLC; MB; NcD
00-0035

ADAMS, Samuel H[opkins] (1871-1958)
The great American fraud: articles on the nostrum evil and quacks. . . . [4th ed.] Chicago: American Medical Association, 1907. 166p. DNLM; ICJ; NcU; OCIM **00-0036**

ADAMS, Samuel S[hugert] (1853-1928)
The diploma of the nurse, and what she owes to it. Washington: R. O. Polkinhorn, 1901. 6p. DNLM; KU [1891. *vel subseq.*] **00-0037**

ADAMS, Samuel S[hugert] (1853-1928)
The evolution of pediatric literature in the United States. [New York, 1900.] 29p. DLC; DNLM [1897. *vel subseq.*]
00-0038

AIKENS, Charlotte A[lbina] (*b.* 1868)
Hospital training-school methods and the head nurse. Philadelphia: W. B. Saunders Co., 1907. 267p. ICJ; NNNAM; PPC; PU
00-0039

AIKENS, Charlotte A[lbina] (*b.* 1868)
Primary studies for nurses; a textbook for first year pupil nurses, containing courses of studies. . . . Philadelphia: W. B. Saunders Co., 1909. 428p. ICJ; PPC; PPJ; PU
00-0040

AIKENS, Charlotte A[lbina] (*b.* 1868)
Clinical studies for nurses; a textbook for second and third year pupil nurses and a handbook for all who are engaged in caring for the sick. Philadelphia: W. B. Saunders Co., 1909. 510p. ICJ; NNNAM; PPC; PU **00-0041**

AIKENS, Charlotte A[lbina] (*b.* 1868)
Hospital housekeeping. . . . 2nd ed. Detroit: D. T. Sutton, 1910. 162p. ICJ; IU-M; OCIM; PU **00-0042**

ALBERT, Eduard (1841-1900)
The diagnosis of surgical diseases. Authorized transl. from the 8th enl. and rev. ed. by Robert T. Frank. New York: D. Appleton & Co., 1902. 419p. NNNAM; OCIM; PPC; PU
00-0043

ALBRECHT, Johann
Primer of eye diseases and their treatment; from the German of the 5th rev. ed.... Transl. and notes by Otto G. Haussmann. Philadelphia: Ware Bros. Co., Printers, 1909. 78p. PPC
00-0044

ALBRIGHT, Jacob D.
The general practitioner as a specialist. A treatise devoted to the consideration of medical specialties. 2nd ed., rev., enl. Pottsville (Pa.): Pottsville Republican Print., 1901. 299p. DLC; PPC **00-0045**

ALBRIGHT, Jacob D.
The general practitioner as a specialist. A treatise devoted to the consideration of medical specialties. 3rd ed., rev., enl. and illustrated. Philadelphia: the Author, 1904. 367p. DLC; PPC
00-0046

ALBRIGHT, Jacob D.
A practical treatise on rectal diseases, their diagnosis and treatment by ambulant methods. Philadelphia: the Author, 1909. 455p. DLC; PPC; PU **00-0047**

ALGER, Ellice Murdoch (1870-1945)
Refraction and motility of the eye, with chapters on color blindness and the field of vision, designed for students and practitioners . . . with one hundred and twenty-two illustrations. Philadelphia: F. A. Davis Co., 1910. 380p. DLC; NNNAM; PPC; PU **00-0048**

ALLCHIN, William H[enry] (1846-1912)
A manual of medicine. New York: The Macmillan Co., 1900-1902. 4 v. DNLM; MBM; NNNAM; PPC
00-0049

ALLEN, Charles Warrenne (1854-1906)
The practitioner's manual; a condensed system of general medical diagnosis and treatment. . . . 2nd ed., rev. and enl. . . . New York: William Wood & Co., 1902. 889p. tables. DLC; ICJ; NNNAM; PPC **00-0050**

ALLEN, Charles Warrenne (1854-1906)
Radiotherapy and phototherapy, including radium and high-frequency currents, their medical and surgical applications in diagnosis and treatment. For students and practitioners. By Charles Warrenne Allen . . . with the co-operation of Milton Franklin . . . and Samuel Stern . . . illustrated with 131 engravings and 27 plates in colors and monochrome. New York and Philadelphia: Lea Bros. & Co., 1904. 618p. plates. DLC; NNNAM; PPC; PU **00-0051**

ALLEN, Henry C. (1836-1909)
The therapeutics of fevers: continued, bilious, intermittent, malarial, remittent, pernicious, typhoid, typhus, septic, yellow, zymotic, etc. . . . Philadelphia: Boericke & Tafel, 1902. 541p. DLC; PPC; PPHa; PU **00-0052**

ALLEN, Henry C. (1836-1909)
The materia medica of the nosodes with provings of the X-ray. . . . Philadelphia: Boericke & Tafel, 1910. 583p. DLC: ICJ; PPC; PU **00-0053**

ALLEN, J[ames] Henry (*b.* 1854)
Diseases and therapeutics of the skin. . . . Philadelphia: Boericke & Tafel, 1902. 353p. DLC; ICJ; PPC; PPHa
00-0054

ALLEN, Richard William (1876-1921)
Vaccine therapy, its theory and practice. . . . 3rd ed. Philadelphia: P. Blakiston's Sons & Co.; [London: H. K. Lewis], 1910. 277p. DLC; NNNAM; PPC; PU **00-0055**

ALLINGHAM, William (1829-1908)
The diagnosis and treatment of diseases of the rectum; being a practical treatise on fistula, piles, fissure and painful ulcer. 7th ed. New York: William Wood & Co., 1901. 471p. ICJ; NNNAM; PPHa; PU [6th ed. (1896), 485p. ICJ; PPC]
00-0056

ALLISON, W. D. & CO.
Illustrated catalogue of the Allison line of physicians' appliances, operating tables, chairs, cabinets. . . . Indianapolis, 1900. 42p. ICJ; OCIM **00-0057**

AMBLER, Henry L[ovejoy]
Facts, fads and fancies about teeth. Cleveland: Helman-Taylor, 1900. 310p. ICJ; OCIM **00-0058**

AMBLER, Henry L[ovejoy]
Around the world dentistry. Cleveland, O.: The Judson Printing Co., 1910. 63p. DLC; DNLM; PU
00-0059

AMERICAN ACADEMY OF MEDICINE
Prevention of infant mortality; being the papers and discussions of a conference held at New Haven, Conn., November 11, 12, 1909, under the auspices of the American Academy of Medicine. . . . [Easton, Pa., 1909?] 347p. diags. CtY-M; DLC
00-0060

THE AMERICAN homoeopathic pharmacopoeia. 7th ed. Enlarged by the addition of a supplement containing the more important remedies added to the homoeopathic materia medica since the publication of the 3rd rev. and enl. ed. Philadelphia: Boericke & Tafel, 1904. 538p. DLC; OCLloyd; PPC; PU
00-0061

THE AMERICAN homoeopathic pharmacopoeia. 8th ed. Enl. by the addition of a supplement containing the more important remedies added to the homoeopathic materia medica since the publication of the 3rd rev. and enl. ed. Philadelphia: Boericke & Tafel, 1906. 549p. DLC; OCLloyd; PPC; PU
00-0062

AMERICAN INSTITUTE OF HOMOEOPATHY. COMMITTEE ON PHARMACOPOEIA
The homoeopathic pharmacopoeia of the United States. Published under the direction of the Committee on Pharmacopoeia of the American Institute of Homoeopathy. 2nd ed. Boston: O. Clapp & Son, 1901. 674p. DLC; MBM; OCLloyd; PU **00-0063**

AMERICAN MEDICAL ASSOCIATION
The propaganda for reform in proprietary medicines. 6th ed. Chicago: American Medical Association, [1905-06?]. 292p. ICM; IU-M; NNNAM; PPC **00-0064**

AMES, Azel (1845-1908)
Compulsory vaccination essential; the example of Porto Rico. New York, 1902. 8p. MH **00-0065**

AMES, Azel (1845-1908)
A medical reserve corps for the United States Army; . . . Carlisle, Pa.: Cornman Printing Co., 1905. 22p. DLC; NN
00-0066

ANDERS, Howard S[chultz] (*b.* 1866)
Physical diagnosis, with case examples of the inductive method, . . . with eighty-eight illustrations in the text and thirty-two plates. New York and London: D. Appleton & Co., 1907. 456p. plates. DLC; NNNAM; PPC; PPJ
00-0067

ANDERS, James M[eschter] (1854-1936)
A textbook of the practice of medicine. 4th ed. Philadelphia: W. B. Saunders & Co., 1900. 1292p. NNNAM; NNU-M; NcD; PPC **00-0068**

ANDERS, James M[eschter] (1854-1936)
A textbook of the practice of medicine. 5th ed. Philadelphia: W. B. Saunders, 1901. 1297p. GU; ICRM; PPC; PU
00-0069

ANDERS, James M[eschter] (1854-1936)
A textbook of the practice of medicine. 6th ed. Philadelphia: W. B. Saunders & Co., 1903. 1295p. IEN-M; IU-M; MH-M; PPC **00-0070**

ANDERS, James M[eschter] (1854-1936)
A textbook of the practice of medicine. 7th ed. Philadelphia: W. B. Saunders & Co., 1905. 1297p. KU; MBM; NNC; PU
00-0071

ANDERS, James M[eschter] (1854-1936)
A textbook of the practice of medicine. 8th ed. Philadelphia: W. B. Saunders & Co., 1907. 1317p. MdBJ-W; NcU; OC; PPC
00-0072

ANDERS, James M[eschter] (1854-1936)
A textbook of the practice of medicine. 9th ed. Philadelphia: W. B. Saunders & Co., 1909. 1326p. CU-M; NjR; NNNAM; PPC **00-0073**

ANDERS, James M[eschter] (1854-1936)
A textbook of the practice of medicine. 10th ed. Philadelphia: W. B. Saunders & Co., 1910 [1911]. 1326p. DLC; DNLM; MH-M; PU **00-0074**

ANDERS, James M[eschter] (1854-1936)
A textbook of medical diagnosis. By James M. Anders and L. Napoleon Boston. Philadelphia: W. B. Saunders & Co., 1910 [1911]. 1175p. col. plates. DLC; DNLM; NcD; PU **00-0075**

ANDERSON, John F. (1873-1958)
. . . I. The presence of tubercle bacilli in the circulating blood in clinical and experimental tuberculosis, by John F. Anderson. II. The viability of the tubercle bacillus, by M. J. Rosenau. Washington: Government Printing Office, 1909. 42p. DLC **00-0076**

ANDERSON, John F. (1873-1958)
. . . Studies upon anaphylaxis, with special reference to the antibodies concerned, by John F. Anderson and W. H. Frost. Washington: Government Printing Office, 1910. 56p. DLC **00-0077**

[ANESTHESIA]
Chloroform anesthesia. . . . [Philadelphia, 1905.] 47p. DLC; ICJ [Contributors include Lauder Brunton, Victor Horsley, F. W. Hewitt and others] **00-0078**

[ANESTHESIA]
Preliminary report of the Anesthesia Commission of the American Medical Association. [Chicago: American Medical Association, 1908.] unp. DLC; ICJ **00-0079**

ANGLE, Edward Hartley (1855-1930)
Treatment of malocclusion of the teeth and fractures of the maxillae. Angle's system. 6th ed., greatly enl. and entirely rewritten, with two hundred and ninety-nine illustrations. . . . Philadelphia: The S. S. White Dental Manufacturing Co., 1900. 315p. DLC; MdU-D; NNNAM; PPC **00-0080**

ANGLE, Edward Hartley (1855-1930)
Treatment of malocclusion of the teeth. Angle's system. 7th ed., greatly enl. and entirely rewritten, with six hundred and forty-one illustrations. . . . Philadelphia: The S. S. White Dental Manufacturing Co., 1907. 626p. DLC; NNC; PPC; PU **00-0081**

ANSHUTZ, Edward Pollock, ed. (1846-1918)
New, old, and forgotten remedies. Papers by many writers. Collected, arranged and ed. Philadelphia: Boericke & Tafel, 1900 386p. DLC; KU; PPC; PU **00-0082**

ANSHUTZ, Edward Pollock (1846-1918)
A guide to the twelve tissue remedies of biochemistry, the cell-salts, biochemic or Schuessler remedies. . . . Philadelphia: Boericke & Tafel, 1909. 91p. DLC; ICJ; PPC; PPHa **00-0083**

[ANTISEPSIS]
Modern methods of antiseptic treatment. New York: Johnson & Johnson, [*c.* 1900]. 48p. DLC; NN ["A compilation of recent notes and suggestions from eminent surgeons" on antiseptic wound treatment] **00-0084**

ARNDT, Hugo Emil Rudolph (*b.* 1848)
The Hahnemannian oration . . . at the jubilee meeting of California State Homoeopathic Medical Society . . . May 13, 1896. [no imprint.] 15p. PPHa [1900. *vel subseq.*] **00-0085**

ARNDT, Hugo Emil Rudolph (*b.* 1848)
A practice of medicine. . . . Philadelphia: Boericke & Tafel, 1900 [1899]. 1331p. DLC; ICJ; PPC; PPHa **00-0086**

ARNDT, Hugo Emil Rudolph (*b.* 1848)
First lessons in the symptomatology of leading homoeopathic remedies. . . . Philadelphia: Boericke & Tafel, 1904. 271p. DLC; DNLM; PPC; PPHa **00-0087**

ARNOLD, H. D.
Medical diet charts. . . . Philadelphia: W. B. Saunders. Co., [1901]. unp. *vel subseq.* DLC **00-0088**

ARNY, Henry V[inecome] (*b.* 1868)
A home study course in pharmacy. . . . Cleveland, 1902. 175 l. DLC; DNLM [Originally issued in 176 separate sheets, most of them printed on one side only] **00-0089**

ARNY, Henry V[inecome] (*b.* 1868)
Principles of pharmacy . . . with 246 original illustrations. Philadelphia and London: W. B. Saunders Co., 1909. 1175p. DLC; OCLloyd; PPC; PU **00-0090**

ASHBURN, Percy Moreau (1872-1940)
The elements of military hygiene, especially arranged for officers and men of the line. . . . Boston and New York: Houghton Mifflin Co., 1909. 314p. DLC; ICJ; NNNAM; PU **00-0091**

ASHBY, Henry (1846-1908)
The diseases of children, medical and surgical, by Henry Ashby . . . and G. A. Wright. . . . 4th ed., edited for American students by William Perry Northrop. . . . New York: Longmans, Green & Co., [etc., etc.], 1900. 894p. plates. DLC; GU; NNNAM; PPC **00-0092**

ASHHURST, Astley Paston Cooper (1876-1932)
An anatomical and surgical study of fractures of the lower end of the humerus. . . . The Samuel D. Gross prize essay of the Philadelphia Academy of Surgery, 1910. Philadelphia and New York: Lea & Febiger, 1910. 163p. DLC; NNNAM; PPC; PU **00-0093**

ASHTON, William Easterly (1859-1933)
. . . Essentials of obstetrics; arranged in the form of questions and answers, prepared especially for students of medicine. . . . 5th ed., rev. and enl. Seventy-five illustrations. Philadelphia: W. B. Saunders & Co., 1900. 256p. DLC; NNNAM; PPC; PU **00-0094**

ASHTON, William Easterly (1859-1933)
. . . Essentials of obstetrics arranged in the form of questions and answers, prepared especially for students of medicine. . . . 6th ed., rev. Seventy-five illustrations. Philadelphia and London: W. B. Saunders & Co., 1905. 256p. DLC; IU-M; MBM; PU **00-0095**

ASHTON, William Easterly (1859-1933)
A text-book on the practice of gynecology, for practitioners and students . . . with ten hundred and forty-six new line drawings illustrating the text, by John V. Alteneder. Philadelphia and London: W. B. Saunders & Co., 1905. 1079p. DLC; NNNAM; PPC; PU **00-0096**

ASHTON, William Easterly (1859-1933)
A text-book on the practice of gynecology, for practitioners and students . . . with ten hundred and forty-six new line drawings illustrating the text, by John V. Alteneder. 2nd ed. Philadelphia and London: W. B. Saunders & Co., 1906. 1079p. DLC; MH-M; NNNAM; PPC **00-0097**

ASHTON, William Easterly (1859-1933)
A text-book on the practice of gynecology, for practitioners and students . . . with ten hundred and fifty-seven new line drawings illustrating the text by John V. Alteneder. 3rd ed., rev. and enl. Philadelphia and London: W. B. Saunders & Co., 1906. 1097p. DLC; NNNAM; NjR; PPC **00-0098**

ASHTON, William Easterly (1859-1933)
A text-book on the practice of gynecology, for practitioners and students . . . with ten hundred and fifty-eight new line drawings illustrating the text by John V. Alteneder. 4th ed., rev. and enl. Philadelphia and London: W. B. Saunders & Co., 1909. 1099p. DLC; OCIM; PPC; PPJ **00-0099**

ASSOCIATION OF MILITARY SURGEONS OF THE UNITED STATES
Proceedings of the ninth annual meeting of the . . . held at New York City, May 31, June 1, and 2, 1900. Chicago: R. Donnelley Co., 1901. 514p. ICJ; IU-M; NNNAM **00-0100**

ATKINS, Albert J. (*b.* 1868)
Electrical physiology; or, Electro-chemic energy vs. oxygenation of the human blood. A lecture delivered before the National Eclectic Medical Association at Indianapolis, Ind., June 11, 1903. . . . San Francisco, 1903. 16p. DLC **00-0101**

ATTFIELD, John (1835-1911)
Chemistry: general medical, and pharmaceutical, including the chemistry of the U.S. pharmacopoeia. A manual on the science of chemistry, and its applications in medicine and pharmacy. . . . Ed. by Leonard Dobbin. . . . 19th ed. Philadelphia and New York: Lea Bros. & Co., 1906. 756p. fold. tables. DLC; NNNAM; PPC; PU **00-0102**

ATWATER, Wilbur Olin (*b.* 1844) and Francis Gano BENEDICT
A respiration calorimeter with appliances for the direct determination of oxygen. Washington: Carnegie Institution, 1905. 193p. 16 plates. DNLM; PP; PU **00-0103**

AUGUSTIN, George
History of yellow fever. . . . New Orleans: Pub. for the Author by Searcy & Pfaff, 1909. 14p. charts. DLC; LNT-M **00-0104**

AUGUSTIN, George
History of yellow fever. With contributions by 13 other authors. New Orleans: The Author, 1909. 1194p. LNT-M **00-0105**

AUSTIN, George Lowell (1849-1893)
A doctor's talk with maiden, wife, and mother. . . . With recommendatory letters from Mrs. Mary A. Livermore and Miss Frances E. Willard. . . . Boston: Lothrop, Lee & Shepard Co., [1907]. 240p. DLC; MB; MH; NN **00-0106**

AUTENRIETH, Wilhelm (1863-1926)
The detection of poisons and strong drugs including the quantitative estimation of medicinal principles in certain crude materials. Transl. by W. H. Warren from the 3rd German ed. Philadelphia: P. Blakiston's Son & Co., 1905. 272p. CtY-M; NNNAM; PPC; PU **00-0107**

AXENFELD, [Karl] Theodor (1867-1930)
The bacteriology of the eye. . . . Transl. by Angus Macnab. . . . With 87 illustrations, some of which are coloured, and 3 coloured plates. New York: William Wood & Co., 1908. 402p. 3 col. pates. DLC; ICJ; NNNAM; PU **00-0108**

AYERS, Edward A[ugustus] (1855-1917)
Physical diagnosis in obstetrics. A guide in ante-partum, partum, and postpartum examinations for the use of physicians and undergraduates. . . . New York: E. B. Treat & Co., 1901. 283p. DLC; ICJ; NNNAM; PU **00-0109**

BAAR, Gustav (*b.* 1872)
The modern view of syphilis and its treatment. . . . New York and London: D. Appleton & Co., 1910. 285p. DLC: ICJ; NNNAM; PU **00-0110**

BABCOCK, Robert H[all] (*b.* 1851)
Diseases of the heart and arterial system, designed to be a practical presentation of the subject for the use of students and practitioners of medicine . . . with three coloured plates and one hundred and thirty-nine illustrations. New York and London: D. Appleton & Co., 1903. 853p. DLC; GU; NNNAM; PPC **00-0111**

BABCOCK, Robert H[all] (*b.* 1851)
Diseases of the heart and arterial system, designed to be a practical presentation of the subject for the use of students and practitioners of medicine . . . with three coloured plates and one hundred and thirty-nine illustrations. 2nd ed., rev. New York and London: D. Appleton & Co., 1905. 853p. DLC; KU; NNNAM; PU **00-0112**

BABCOCK, Robert H[all] (*b.* 1851)
Diseases of the lungs; designed to be a practical presentation of the subject for the use of students and practitioners of medicine . . . with twelve colored plates and one hundred and four text illustrations. 1st ed. New York and London: D. Appleton & Co., 1907. 809p. DLC; ICJ; NNNAM; PPC **00-0113**

BABCOCK, Robert H[all] (*b.* 1851)
Diseases of the heart and arterial system, designed to be a practical presentation of the subject for the use of students and practitioners of medicine . . . with three coloured plates and one hundred and thirty-nine illustrations. 3rd ed. rev. New York and London: D. Appleton & Co., 1909. 856p. DLC; ICJ; NNNAM; PU **00-0114**

BACON, Francis (1831-1912)
Address of Dr. Francis Bacon at the dedication of the Gaylord Farm Sanitorium, October 29, 1904. [1904.] 9p. CtY-M **00-0115**

BACON, Gorham (*b.* 1855)
A manual of otology. . . . With an introductory chapter by Clarence John Blake. 2nd ed., rev. and enl. New York and Philadelphia: Lea Bros. & Co., 1900. 422p. plates. DLC; NNNAM; PPC; PU **00-0116**

BACON, Gorham (*b.* 1855)
A manual of otology. . . . With an introductory chapter. By Clarence John Blake. . . . 3rd ed., rev. and enl. . . . New York and Philadelphia: Lea Bros. & Co., [1902]. 445p. plates. DLC; IU-M; NNNAM; PPC **00-0117**

BACON, Gorham (*b.* 1855)
A manual of otology. . . . With an introductory chapter by Clarence John Blake. . . . 4th ed., rev. and enl. With 134 illustrations and 11 plates. New York and Philadelphia: Lea Bros. & Co., 1906. 485p. DLC; IEN-M; MBM; PPJ **00-0118**

BACON, Gorham (*b.* 1855)
A manual of otology. . . . With an introductory chapter. By Clarence John Blake. . . . 5th ed., rev. and enl. With 147 illustrations and 12 plates. New York and Philadelphia: Lea & Febiger, 1909. 508p. DLC; MdBM; PPC; PU **00-0119**

BAILEY, Benjamin F[ranklin], ed. (*b.* 1860)
The present status of pediatrics . . . , ed. by B. F. Bailey and Allison Clokey. Lincoln [Nebraska]: State Journal Co., 1900 [*c.* 1896]. 304p. DLC; ICJ; NcD; PPHa **00-0120**

BAILEY, Benjamin F[ranklin] (*b.* 1860)
Homoeopathy in the public service. Lincoln [Nebraska, 1901.] 10p. DNLM; PPHa **00-0121**

BAILEY, Frederick Randolph (1871-1923)
A text-book of histology. . . . New York: William Wood & Co., 1904. 481p. CtY-M; DLC; NNNAM; PU **00-0122**

BAILEY, Frederick Randolph (1871-1923)
A text-book of histology. . . . 2nd and rev. ed. . . . New York: William Wood & Co., 1906. 497p. diags. CU-M; DLC; NNNAM; PPC **00-0123**

BAILEY, Frederick Randolph (1871-1923)
Text-book of embryology, by Frederick Randolph Bailey . . . and Adam Marion Miller . . . with five hundred and fifteen illustrations. New York: William Wood & Co., 1909. 672p. CtY-M; DLC; NNNAM; PPC **00-0124**

BAILEY, Frederick Randolph (1871-1923)
A text-book of histology . . . 3rd rev. ed. . . . New York: William Wood & Co., 1910. 589p. DLC; ICJ; NNNAM; PPC **00-0125**

BAILEY, Pearce (1865-1922)
Diseases of the nervous system resulting from accident and injury. . . . New York and London: D. Appleton & Co., 1906. 627p. CU-M; DLC; NNNAM; PU **00-0126**

BAILEY, Pearce (1865-1922)
Diseases of the nervous system resulting from accident and injury, . . . 2nd ed. New York and London: D. Appleton & Co., 1908. 627p. DLC: ICJ; NNNAM; PU **00-0127**

BALDWIN, James Fairchild (1850-1936)
Class-book of operative gynecology. . . . Illustrated by 147 cuts. Columbus, O.: Columbus Medical Publishing Co., 1900 [*c.* 1898]. 256p. DNLM; ICJ; OCIM; PPC **00-0128**

BALDWIN, James Fairchild (1850-1936)
Formation of an artificial vagina by intestinal transplantation. . . . New York: William Wood & Co., 1907. 5p. NNNAM **00-0129**

BALDWIN, L[auris] Blake (*b.* 1870)
Syphilis in dentistry, by L. Blake Baldwin . . . and Ezra Read Larned. . . . Chicago: F. H. Colegrove, 1903. 120p. col. plates. DLC; ICJ; OCIM **00-0130**

BALL, Charles B[ent] (1851-1916)
The rectum and anus, their diseases and treatment. 2nd ed. Philadelphia: Lea Bros. & Co., 1900. [*c.* 1895]. 439p. DNLM; MBM; NNNAM; PPC [1st ed., Philadelphia: H. C. Lea, 1887. 410p.] **00-0131**

BALL, James Moores (*b.* 1862)
Modern ophthalmology; a practical treatise on the anatomy, physiology, and disease of the eye. . . . with 417 illustrations in the text and numerous figures on colored plates. Philadelphia: F. A. Davis Co., 1904. 820p. DLC; NNNAM; PPC; PPJ **00-0132**

BALL, James Moores (*b.* 1862)
Modern ophthalmology; a practical treatise on anatomy, physiology, and diseases of the eye. . . . 2nd ed., with 417 illustrations in the text and numerous figures on 21 colored plates. Philadelphia: F. A. Davis Co., 1908. 820p. DLC; IU-M; MBM; PU **00-0133**

BALL, Michael Valentine (*b.* 1868)
. . . Essentials of bacteriology; being a concise and systematic introduction to the study of micro-organisms, by . . . . 5th ed., thoroughly rev. by Karl M. Vogel. . . . With ninety-six illustrations, some in colors, and six plates. Philadelphia, [etc.]: W. B. Saunders & Co., 1904. 243p. DLC; MH-M; NNNAM; PPC **00-0134**

BALL, Michael Valentine (*b.* 1868)
. . . Essentials of bacteriology; being a concise and systematic introduction to the study of bacteria and allied microörganisms. . . . 6th ed., thoroughly rev. With 135 illustrations, some in colors. Philadelphia and London: W. B. Saunders & Co., 1908. 290p. DLC; IEN-M; NNNAM; PPC **00-0135**

BALLENGER, Edgar Garrison (1877-1945)
Genito-urinary diseases and syphilis . . . with 86 illustrations. Atlanta, Ga.: E. W. Allen & Co., 1908. 276p. DLC **00-0136**

BALLENGER, William Lincoln (1861-1915)
. . . Eye, ear, nose, and throat. A manual for students and practitioners. By William Lincoln Ballenger . . . and A. G. Wippern. . . . Illustrated with one hundred and fifty engravings and six colored plates. Philadelphia and New York: Lea Bros. & Co., [1900]. 511p. DLC; ICRM; NNNAM; PPC **00-0137**

[BALTIMORE GENERAL DISPENSARY]
One hundred years of history of the Baltimore General Dispensary [1801-1901]. Baltimore: A Hoen & Co., [1901]. 27p. DLC; MdBM; MdU-D **00-0138**

BANDLER, Samuel W[yllis] (1869-1932)
Uterine and tubal gestation; a study of the embedding and development of the human ovum, the early growth of the embryo, and the development of the syncytium and placental gland. . . . New York: William Wood & Co., 1903. 159p. CtY-M; DNLM; ICJ; PPC **00-0139**

BANDLER, Samuel W[yllis] (1869-1932)
Associated nervous conditions in gynecology, with especial reference to the climacterium and allied states. [New York: William Wood & Co., 1906.] 54p. NN **00-0140**

BANDLER, Samuel W[yllis] (1869-1932)
Medical gynecology . . . with original illustrations. Philadelphia and London: W. B. Saunders & Co., 1908. 676p. plates. DLC; ICJ; NNNAM; PPC **00-0141**

BANDLER, Samuel W[yllis] (1869-1932)
Medical gynecology . . . 2nd rev. ed., with original illustrations. Philadelphia and London: W. B. Saunders & Co., [1909]. 698p. plates. DLC; MBM; NNC; PU **00-0142**

BANDLER, Samuel W[yllis] (1869-1932)
How to enter the peritoneal cavity by the anterior vaginal route. New York, 1909. 29p. NN **00-0143**

BANDLER, Samuel W[yllis] (1869-1932)
Vaginal celiotomy . . . with 148 original illustrations. Philadelphia and London: W. B. Saunders & Co., 1910 [*c.* 1911]. 450p. plates. DLC; ICJ; PPC; PU **00-0144**

BARDELEBEN, Karl H[einrich] von (1849-1919) and H. HAECKEL
Atlas of applied human anatomy. . . . New York: Rebman Co., 1906. 166p. 204 col. plates. DNLM; ICJ; OCIM; PPC **00-0145**

BARKER, Anthony
Physical culture simplified. A safe and rapid way to health and strength. Published by the Author. New York, [1902]. 111p. NN; PU **00-0146**

BARKER, George F[rederick], ed. (1835-1910)
Röntgen rays; memoirs by Röntgen, Stokes, and J. J. Thomson, transl. and ed. by . . . . New York and London: Harper & Bros., 1900 [*c.* 1899]. 75p. DLC; ICJ; MBM; PU **00-0147**

BARKER, Lewellys F[ranklin] (1867-1943)
Medicine and the universities. [1902.] 5p. ICJ; ICU; MH; NN **00-0148**

BARKER, Lewellys F[ranklin] (1867-1943)
. . . A description of the brains and spinal cords of two brothers dead of hereditary ataxia; cases XVIII and XX of the series in the family described by Dr. Sanger Brown. With a clinical introduction by Dr. Sanger Brown . . . Chicago: The University of Chicago Press, 1903. 50p. plates. DLC; ICJ; ICU **00-0149**

BARKER, Lewellys F[ranklin] (1867-1943)
Anatomical terminology, with special reference to the "BNA" . . . with vocabularies in Latin and English and illustrations. Philadelphia: P. Blakiston's Son & Co., 1907. 103p. CtY-M; DLC; PPC; PU **00-0150**

BARNHILL, John Flach (*b.* 1865)
Principles and practice of modern otology, by John F. Barnhill . . . and Ernest de Wolfe Wales . . . with 305 original illustrations, many in colors. Philadelphia and London: W. B. Saunders & Co., 1907. 575p. DLC; NNNAM; PPC; PU **00-0151**

BARNUM, Henry Weston (*b.* 1859)
Lessons in vibratory therapeutics; the practical application of mechanical vibration in the treatment of disease. . . . Poughkeepsie, N.Y.: Press of The A. V. Haight Co., [1904]. 26p. plates. DLC; DNLM **00-0152**

BARNUM, Henry Weston (*b.* 1859)
Lessons in vibratory therapeutics. (2nd ed.) The practical application of mechanical vibration in the treatment of disease. . . . Poughkeepsie, N.Y.: The Author, [1905]. 129p. DLC; NN **00-0153**

BARNUM, Henry Weston (*b.* 1859)
Lessons in vibratory therapeutics. 3rd ed. The practical application of mechanical vibration in the treatment of disease. . . . Poughkeepsie, N.Y.: The Author, [1907]. 152p. DLC; DNLM **00-0154**

BARR, Martin W. (1860-1938)
Mental defectives, their history, treatment and training. Philadelphia: P. Blakiston's Son & Co., 1904. 386p. ICJ; NN; PPC; PU **00-0155**

BARRET, Frederic Allen
Barret's medical hand book; what to do before the doctor comes. A book of practical information, giving full and simple instructions in case of sickness or accident. . . . St. Louis, Mo.: Barret Chemical Co., 1902. 66p. DLC; ICJ **00-0156**

BARRETT, A[shley] William
Dental surgery for general practitioners and students of medicine and dentistry. . . . 4th ed. Philadelphia: P. Blakiston, Son & Co., 1905. 159p. DNLM; MdU-D; PPC; PU **00-0157**

BARRETT, William C[ary] (1834-1903)
Oral pathology and practice. A text-book for the use of students in dental colleges and a hand-book for dental practitioners. . . . 2nd ed., rev., enl. and illustrated. Philadelphia: The S. S. White Dental Mfg. Co., 1901. 319p. DLC; MdU-D; PPC; PU **00-0158**

BARTHOLOMEW, Elmer J[efferson]
Lesions other than mechanical. Chicago, [*c.* 1907.] 17p. DNLM **00-0159**

BARTHOLOMEW, Elmer J[efferson]
The two causes of disease. Chicago, [*c.* 1907.] 163p. illus. DNLM **00-0160**

BARTHOLOMEW, Elmer J[efferson]
Man, woman, know thyself! An illustrated treatise on practical psychology for both the medical profession and the laity. . . . Chicago, Ill.: [Press of Grant's Printery, 1908.] 221p. plates. DLC; ICJ **00-0161**

BARTHOLOW, Roberts (1831-1904)
A practical treatise on materia medica and therapeutics. . . . 11th ed., rev. and enl. New York and London: D. Appleton & Co., 1903. 866p. DLC; NNNAM; OCLloyd; PU **00-0162**

BARTHOLOW, Roberts (1831-1904)
A practical treatise on materia medica and therapeutics. . . . With new articles and additions by Paul Bartholow. . . . 12th ed., rev. and enl. New York and London: D. Appleton & Co., 1906. 890p. DLC; IU-M; NNNAM; OCLloyd
00-0163

BARTLETT, Clarence (1858-1935)
A text-book of clinical medicine. Principles of diagnosis. . . . With 245 illustrations, including six colored plates. Philadelphia: Boericke & Tafel, 1903. 976p. DLC; NNNAM; PPC; PPHa **00-0164**

BARTLETT, Clarence (1858-1935)
A text-book of clinical medicine. Treatment. . . . Philadelphia: Boericke & Tafel, 1908. 1223p. DLC; NNNAM; PPC; PU
00-0165

BARTLEY, Elias Hudson (1849-1937)
Manual of physiological and clinical chemistry. . . . 2nd ed., rev. and enl.; with 47 illustrations. Philadelphia: P. Blakiston's Son & Co., 1904. 188p. DLC; IU-M; PPC; PU
00-0166

BARTON, Clara (1821-1912)
The story of my childhood. . . . New York: The Baker & Taylor Co., 1907. 125p. ICU; MB; NIC; NN
00-0167

BARTON, Wilfred Mason (1871-1930)
A thesaurus of medical words and phrases, by Wilfred M. Barton . . . and Walter A. Wells. . . . Philadelphia, [etc.]: W. B. Saunders & Co., 1903. 534p. DLC; MBM; NNNAM; PPC
00-0168

BARUCH, Simon (1840-1921)
The principles and practice of hydrotherapy; a guide to the application of water in disease, for students and practitioners of medicine. . . . 2nd ed., rev. and enl. . . . New York: William Wood & Co., 1903. 496p. DLC; MBM; NNNAM; PU
00-0169

BARUCH, Simon (1840-1921)
The principles and practice of hydrotherapy; a guide to the application of water in disease, for students and practitioners of medicine. . . . 3rd ed., rev. and enl., with numerous illustrations. New York: William Wood & Co., 1908. 544p. DLC; MBM; NNNAM; PPC **00-0170**

BASE, Daniel (*b.* 1869)
Elements of vegetable histology, for the use of students of pharmacy, preparatory to the study of pharmacognosy, with 62 illustrations. . . . 2nd ed., rev. and enl. Baltimore, Md.: The Author, 1905. 112p. DLC; MdU-D
00-0171

BASHORE, Harvey B[rown] (1864-1934)
Outlines of rural hygiene for physicians, students, and sanitarians. With an appendix on the normal distribution of chlorine, by Herbert E. Smith. Philadelphia: F. A. Davis Co., 1900 [*c.* 1897]. 84p. CtY-M; DNLM; ICJ; PPC
00-0172

BASHORE, Harvey B[rown] (1864-1934)
Our rural water supplies. A word for the thoughtful. . . . New York: William Wood & Co., 1904? 3p. NN
00-0173

BASHORE, Harvey B[rown] (1864-1934)
The sanitation of a country house. . . . With sixteen illustrations. 1st ed. 1st thousand. New York: J. Wiley & Sons; [etc., etc.], 1905. 103p. DLC; ICJ; MB; PP
00-0174

BASHORE, Harvey B[rown] (1864-1934)
Outlines of practical sanitation, for students, physicians and sanitarians . . . with forty-two illustrations. 1st ed. 1st thousand. New York: J. Wiley & Sons; [etc., etc.], 1906. 208p. DLC; ICJ; MB; NN **00-0175**

BASHORE, Harvey B[rown] (1864-1934)
The sanitation of recreation camps and parks. New York: John Wiley & Sons, 1908. 109p. DLC; ICJ; NcD; NN
00-0176

BASSLER, Anthony (*b.* 1874)
Diseases of the stomach and upper alimentary tract, by . . . copiously illustrated with numerous half-tones and line text-engravings and 56 full-page half-tone plates (with nearly 100 figures) plain and in colors, from original photographs and drawings. Philadelphia: F. A. Davis Co., 1910. 836p. DLC; ICJ; NNNAM; PPC **00-0177**

BAUM, William L[ouis], ed. (1867-1932)
. . . Skin and venereal diseases; miscellaneous topics. Ed. by W. L. Baum, M. D., Harold N. Moyer, M.D. . . . Chicago: The Year Book Publishers, 1908. 248p. plats. DLC; ICJ; NNNAM; OCIM **00-0178**

BAUM, William L[ouis], ed. (1867-1932)
. . . Skin and venereal diseases; miscellaneous topics. Ed. by W. L. Baum, M.D., Harold N. Moyer, M.D. . . . Chicago: The Year Book Publishers, [1909]. 240p. plates. DLC; ICJ; NNNAM; OCIM **00-0179**

BAUSCH & LOMB OPTICAL CO.
Microtomes and accessories. 18th ed. [Rochester], 1908. 22p. DLC; MB; NN; NNNAM **00-0180**

BAUSCH & LOMB OPTICAL CO.
Bacterial apparatus. Rochester, N.Y., 1909. 55p. DLC; MH; NNNAM; PU **00-0181**

BEAL, James Hartley (*b.* 1861)
Notes on equation writing and chemical and pharmaceutical arithmetic. 3rd ed., rev. and enl. . . . Columbus, O.: The Midland Publishing Co., [1904]. 139p. DLC; OC
00-0182

BEAL, James Hartley (*b.* 1861)
Prescription practice and general dispensing, an elementary treatise for students of pharmacy. . . . [Columbus?]: The Author, 1908. 217p. DLC **00-0183**

BEAL, James Hartley (*b.* 1861)
Elementary principles of the theory and practice of pharmacy. [Columbus]: J. H. Beal, 1910. unp. DLC
00-0184

BEARD, Charles H[eady] (1855-1906)
Ophthalmic surgery; a treatise on surgical operations pertaining to the eye and its appendages, with chapters on para-operative technic and management of instruments. . . . With 9 plates, showing 100 instruments and 300 other illustrations. Philadelphia: P. Blakiston's Son & Co., 1910. 674p. DLC; PPC; PU; ScCM **00-0185**

BEARD, George Miller (1839-1883)
A practical treatise on nervous exhaustion (neurasthenia), its symptoms, nature, sequences, treatment. . . . Ed., with notes and additions, by A. D. Rockwell. . . . 4th ed., enl. New York: E. B. Treat & Co., 1901. 274p. DLC; ICJ; NNNAM; PPC
00-0186

BEARD, George Miller (1839-1883)
A practical treatise on nervous exhaustion (neurasthenia), its symptoms, nature, sequences, treatment. . . . Ed., with notes and additions, by A. D. Rockwell. . . . 5th ed.—enl. New York: E. B. Treat & Co., 1905. 288p. DLC; MBM; NNNAM; PU
00-0187

BEARD, George Miller (1839-1883)
Sexual neurasthenia (nervous exhaustion), its hygiene, causes, symptoms and treatment, with a chapter on diet for the nervous. . . . Ed., with notes and additions, by A. D. Rockwell. . . . 6th ed.—with formulas. New York: E. B. Treat & Co., 1905. 316p. DLC; GU; NNNAM; PPC
00-0188

BEARD, Sidney Hartnell (*b.* 1862)
A comprehensive guide-book to natural, hygienic and humane diet. . . . New York: T. Y. Crowell & Co., [1902]. 169p. DLC; NNNAM; PPL **00-0189**

BEARD, Sidney Hartnell (*b.* 1862)
A comprehensive guide-book to natural, hygienic and humane diet. . . . [2nd ed.] New York: T. Y. Crowell & Co., [1902]. 169p. DLC; ICJ; MB; NN **00-0190**

BECK, Amanda Kathryn
A reference hand-book for nurses. . . . Philadelphia and London: W. B. Saunders & Co., 1905. 177p. DLC; NcU; PPC; PU **00-0191**

BECK, Amanda Kathryn
A reference hand-book for nurses. . . . 2nd ed., rev. Philadelphia and London: W. B. Saunders & Co., 1908. 199p. DLC; ICJ; PPC; PU **00-0192**

BECK, Carl (1856-1911)
Is appendicitis a surgical disease? New York, 1900 [*c.* 1898]. 72p. NN **00-0193**

BECK, Carl (1856-1911)
Fractures . . . with an appendix on the practical use of the Röntgen rays. . . . Philadelphia: W. B. Saunders & Co., 1900. 355p. DLC; NNNAM; PPC; PU **00-0194**

BECK, Carl (1856-1911)
A case of double penis, combined with exstrophy of the bladder and showing four ureteral orifices. [New York], 1901. 4p. NN; NNNAM **00-0195**

BECK, Carl (1856-1911)
. . . Some new points in regard to Raynaud's disease. . . . [1901]. 3p. NNC; NNNAM **00-0196**

BECK, Carl (1856-1911)
Practical applications of Roentgen rays. [Scranton, 1903.] 108p. plates. MB **00-0197**

BECK, Carl (1856-1911)
. . . The utilization of the lower lip in rhinoplasty, a new procedure. . . . [1904.] 5p. NNC **00-0198**

BECK, Carl (1856-1911)
Röntgen ray diagnosis and therapy . . . with 322 illustrations in the text. New York and London: D. Appleton & Co., 1904. 460p. DLC; ICJ; NNNAM; PPC **00-0199**

BECK, Carl (1856-1911)
Heidelberg und studententhum. Philadelphia: German American Press, [1904]. 24p. DNLM; MH
00-0200

BECK, Carl (1856-1911)
The medicolegal aspect of accidents caused by the Röntgen rays. New York: William Wood & Co., 1904. 6p. MH
00-0201

BECK, Carl (1856-1911)
Recent advances in Roentgen ray diagnosis, with especial reference to the use of the diaphragm and osteoscope in venal skiagraphy. New York: Rebman, [1905]. 8p. 4 plates. MH
00-0202

BECK, Carl (1856-1911)
Principles of surgical pathology, for the use of the student. . . . Chicago: W. T. Keener & Co., 1905. 134p. DLC; OCIM
00-0203

BECK, Carl (1856-1911)
. . . Further observations on extensive separation of the periosteum in displaced bone fragments. . . . [1906.] 1p. plate. NNC **00-0204**

BECK, Carl (1856-1911)
. . . On extensive separation of the periosteum in displaced bone fragments. . . . [1906.] 3p. NNC
00-0205

BECK, Carl (1856-1911)
Surgical diseases of the chest . . . with 16 colored and 162 other illustrations. Philadelphia: P. Blakiston's Son & Co., 1907. 371p. DLC; NNNAM; PPC; PU
00-0206

BECK, Carl (1856-1911)
The Roentgen method in the surgery of the chest. [Chicago, 1907?] 14p. NN **00-0207**

BECK, Carl (1856-1911)
. . . The significance of the various enlargements of the thyreoid gland with special reference to Basedow's disease. . . . [*c.* 1910.] 33p. NNC **00-0208**

BECKWITH, David H[errick] (1825-1909)
The Erie Street Medical College sixty years ago. . . . Annual address delivered before the Cleveland Medical Library Association, December, 1908. [Cleveland: The Cleveland Medical Library Association, 1908.] 10p. OCIM
00-0209

BECKWITH, David H[errick] (1825-1909)
History of the Western College of Homoeopathic Medicine from 1850 to 1860. [Cleveland, 1908.] 72p. OCIM
00-0210

BEEBE, Silas Palmer (*b.* 1876)
Outlines of physiological chemistry, by S. P. Beebe and B. H. Buxton. . . . New York: The Macmillan Co.; London: Macmillan & Co., Ltd., 1904. 195p. DLC; ICJ; NN; PPC
00-0211

BEEBE, Silas Palmer (*b.* 1876)
The effect of alcohol and alcoholic fluids upon the excretion of uric acid in man. [1904.] n.p. 24p. MH
00-0212

BELL, Victor Charles (*b.* 1867)
. . . Our teeth, and how to take care of them. . . . New York: Young America Publishing Co., [1900]. 70p. DLC; NNNAM
00-0213

BELL, Victor Charles (*b.* 1867)
Our teeth; how to take care of them . . . with an introduction by O. H. Lang . . . 2nd ed. New York: Young America Publishing Co., [1901]. 77p. DLC; NNNAM
00-0214

BELL, Victor Charles (*b.* 1867)
Our teeth; how to take care of them . . . with an introduction by O. H. Lang . . . 3rd ed. New York: Young America Publishing Co., 1901. 76p. CtY-M; PU
00-0215

BELL, Victor Charles (*b.* 1867)
Popular essays upon the care of the teeth and mouth . . . 5th ed. New York: V. C. Bell, 1902. 112p. NNNAM
00-0216

BELL, Victor Charles (*b.* 1867)
Popular essays upon the care of the teeth and mouth . . . 6th ed. New York: V. C. Bell, 1903. 112p. NNNAM
00-0217

BELL, Victor Charles (*b.* 1867)
Our teeth; how to take care of them . . . 4th ed., carefully rev. . . . New York: V. C. Bell, 1907. 79p. DLC; NNNAM
00-0218

BELL, Victor Charles (*b.* 1867)
Popular essays upon the care of the teeth and mouth . . . 7th ed., carefully rev. New York: V. C. Bell, 1907. 112p. DLC; NNNAM
00-0219

[BELSHAW, William]
Smallpox, its external treatment and prevention. . . . Snohomish, Wash.: Press of W. Maw, 1904. 13p. DLC; DNLM
00-0220

BENEDICT, Arthur L[incoln] (1865-1950)
Golden rules of dietetics. . . . St. Louis: The C. V. Mosby Medical Book & Pub. Co., [1906]. 350p. DLC; ICJ; OCIM
00-0221

BENEDICT, Francis Gano (1870-1957)
The influence of inanition on metabolism. Washington: Carnegie Institution, 1907. 542p. DLC; DNLM
00-0222

BENNETT, Homer Clark (*b.* 1865)
The electro-therapeutic guide; or, A thousand questions asked and answered . . . 8th ed., rev. and condensed. . . . Lima, O.: Literary Department of the National College of Electro-Therapeutics, [1907]. 319p. DLC; ICJ; NcD
00-0223

BENNETT, William Henry (1852-1931)
Injuries and diseases of the knee-joint, considered from the clinical aspect. New York: William Wood & Co., 1909. 236p. 14 plates. MBM; NNNAM; OCIM; PU
00-0224

BENNIE, P[eter] Bruce
Rational and effective treatment of hip-disease . . . founded on experience of numerous cases in hospital practice during 28 years. Compiled by Alex. B. Bennie. New York: William Wood & Co., 1907. 108p. 9 plates. DNLM; NNNAM; PPC; PU
00-0225

BERGEY, David H[endricks] (1860-1937)
Handbook of practical hygiene. Easton, Pa.: The Chemical Publishing Co., 1900 [1899]. 164p. DLC; PLF; PPF; PU
00-0226

BERGEY, David H[endricks] (1860-1937)
The principles of hygiene: a practical manual for students, physicians, and health officers. Philadelphia: W. B. Saunders & Co., 1901. 495p. DLC; NN; OC; PPC
00-0227

BERGEY, David H[endricks] (1860-1937)
The source and nature of bacteria in milk. [Harrisburg]; W. S. Ray, State Printer, 1904. 40p. DLC
00-0228

BERGEY, David H[endricks] (1860-1937)
The principles of hygiene: a practical manual for students, physicians, and health officers. 2nd ed., thoroughly rev. and enl. Philadelphia: W. B. Saunders & Co., 1904. 536p. DLC; ICRM; PPC
00-0229

BERGEY, David H[endricks] (1860-1937)
The principles of hygiene: a practical manual for students, physicians, and health officers. 3rd ed., rev. and enl. Philadelphia: W. B. Saunders & Co., 1909. 555p. DLC; NIC; NN; PU
00-0230

BERGMANN, Ernst von (1836-1907)
A system of practical surgery. By E. von Bergmann, Paul von Bruns, and J. von Mikulicz. Transl. and ed. by William T. Bull and Walton Martin. New York & Philadelphia: Lea Bros. & Co., 1904. 5 v. DNLM; NNNAM; PPC; PU
00-0231

BERNAYS, Augustus Charles (1854-1907)
Golden rules of surgery: aphorisms, observations, and reflections on the science and art of surgery. . . . St. Louis: C. V. Mosby, 1906. 203p. NNNAM; OCIM; PPC; PU
00-0232

BERNHEIM, Hippolyte (1840-1919)
Suggestive therapeutics, a treatise on the nature and uses of hypnotism. . . . Transl. from the 2nd and rev. French ed., by Christian A. Herter. . . . Twelfth impression. New York, [etc.]: G. P. Putnam's Sons, 1900. 420p. CtY-M; DLC; ICJ; NNNAM
00-0233

BERRY, Richard J[ames] A[rthur] (*b.* 1867)
Outlines of applied anatomy, with special reference to surface landmarks. Philadelphia: J. B. Lippincott, 1906. 244p. CtY-M; RPM [Simultaneously published: Edinburgh: W. Green, 1906]
00-0234

BERTELING, L. A.
Instructions for L. A. Berteling's compound optometer for correcting errors of refraction. San Francisco: G. Spaulding & Co., 1900. 18p. CtY-M; CU-M; PPHa [Originally, 1885, *vel subseq.*]
00-0235

BICKHAM, Warren S[tone] (*b.* 1861)
A textbook of operative surgery, covering the surgical anatomy and operative technic involved in the operations of general surgery, written for students and practitioners . . . with 559 illustrations. Philadelphia: W. B. Saunders & Co., 1903. 984p. DLC; MBM; NNNAM; PU **00-0236**

BICKHAM, Warren S[tone] (*b.* 1861)
A textbook of operative surgery, covering the surgical anatomy and operative technic involved in the operations of general surgery, written for students and practitioners. . . . 2nd ed., with 559 illustrations. Philadelphia: W. B. Saunders & Co., 1904. 984p. DLC; IEN-M; PPC; PPJ **00-0237**

BICKHAM, Warren S[tone] (*b.* 1861)
A textbook of operative surgery, covering the surgical anatomy and operative technic involved in the operations of general surgery, written for students and practitioners. . . . 3rd ed., greatly enl., containing 854 illustrations. Philadelphia: W. B. Saunders & Co., 1908. 1206p. DLC; MH-M; NNNAM; PPC **00-0238**

BIDDLE, JAMES G. CO. (PHILADELPHIA)
. . . "Roentgen" induction coils and other X-ray apparatus. [Catalogue 480, 1903] Philadelphia: J. G. Biddle, [1903]. 32p. DLC; PPC **00-0239**

BIDDLE, JAMES G. CO. (PHILADELPHIA)
. . . "Roentgen" induction coils and other X-ray apparatus. James G. Biddle, general sales agent . . . Philadelphia, [1904]. 52p. DLC **900-0240**

BIER, August Karl Gustav (1861-1945)
Hyperemia as a therapeutic agent. . . . Authorized translation ed. by Dr. Gustavus M. Blech . . . with eleven illustrations. Chicago: A. Robertson & Co., 1905. 239p. DLC; ICJ; IU-M; OCIM **00-0241**

[BIER, August Karl Gustav] (1861-1945)
Bier's hyperemic treatment in surgery, medicine, and the specialties . . . by Willy Meyer and Victor Schmieden. Philadelphia: W. B. Saunders & Co., 1908. 209p. CtY-M; NNNAM; PPC; PU **00-0242**

[BIER, August Karl Gustav] (1861-1945)
Bier's hyperemic treatment in surgery, medicine, and the specialties . . . by Willy Meyer and Victor Schmieden. 2nd ed. Philadelphia: W. B. Saunders & Co., 1909. 280p. DLC; PPC; PPJ; PU **00-0243**

[BIGELOW, Henry Jacob] (1818-1890)
A memoir of . . . . Boston: Little, Brown & Co., 1900. 297p. MB; MH; NN **00-0244**

BIGELOW, Henry Jacob (1818-1890)
I. The mechanism of dislocations and fracture of the hip. II. Litholapaxy: or, Rapid lithotrity with evacuation. . . . Boston: Little, Brown & Co., 1900. 366p. DLC; MBM; PPC; PU **00-0245**

BIGELOW, Henry Jacob (1818-1890)
Orthopedic surgery and other medical papers. . . . Boston: Little, Brown & Co., 1900. 371p. plates. DLC; MBM; NNNAM; PU **00-0246**

BIGELOW, Henry Jacob (1818-1890)
Surgical anaesthesia; addresses and other papers. . . . Boston: Little, Brown & Co., 1900. 378p. DLC; MH-M; NNNAM; PPC **00-0247**

BIGELOW, Horatio Ripley, ed.
An international system of electrotherapeutics, for students, general practitioners, and specialists, by numerous associated authors. . . . 2nd ed., thoroughly rev. and brought up to the present date, with several entirely new departments embodying the most recent developments of the science, ed. by C. Betton Massey. . . . Thoroughly illustrated. Philadelphia: F. A. Davis Co., 1901. 1160p. plates. DLC; NNNAM; OCIM; PPC **00-0248**

BIGSBY, Myron Houghton (*b.* 1872)
Osteopathic diagnosis and technique, with chapters on osteopathic landmarks. . . . Vineland, N.J.: Commercial Printing House, 1907. 262p. plates. DLC **00-0249**

BILLINGS, Frank (1854-1932)
. . . General medicine, ed. by Frank Billings . . . with the collaboration of S. C. Stanton. . . . Chicago: The Year Book Publishers, 1901. 270p. plates. DLC; ICJ; PPC; PU **00-0250**

BILLINGS, Frank, ed. (1854-1932)
. . . General medicine; ed. by Frank Billings . . . and J. H. Salisbury. . . . Chicago: The Year Book Publishers, 1902. 358p. DLC; ICJ; NNNAM; PU **00-0251**

BILLINGS, Frank, ed. (1854-1932)
. . . Diseases of the digestive system . . . an authorized translation from "Die deutsche klinik" under the general editorial supervision of Julius L. Salinger, M.D.; with forty-five illustrations in the text. New York: D. Appleton & Co., 1906. 824p. col. plates. CtY-M; DLC; ICJ; NNNAM **00-0252**

BILLINGS, Frank, ed. (1854-1932)
. . . General medicine, ed. by Frank Billings . . . and J. H. Salisbury. . . . Chicago: The Year Book Publishers, 1906. 369p. plates. DLC; ICJ; NNNAM; PU **00-0253**

BILLINGS, Frank, ed. (1854-1932)
. . . General medicine, ed. by Frank Billings . . . and J. H. Salisbury. . . . Chicago: The Year Book Publishers, 1907. 359p. plates. DLC; GU; ICJ; PPC **00-0254**

BILLINGS, Frank, ed. (1854-1932)
. . . General medicine, ed. by Frank Billings . . . and J. H. Salisbury. . . . Chicago: The Year Book Publishers, 1908. 408p. plates. DLC; ICU; MBM; PU **00-0255**

BILLINGS, Frank, ed. (1854-1932)
. . . General medicine, ed. by Frank Billings . . . and J. H. Salisbury. . . . Chicago: The Year Book Publishers, [1909]. 358p. plates. CtY-M; DLC; ICJ; PU **00-0256**

BILLINGS, Frank, ed. (1854-1932)
. . . Diseases of the digestive system . . . an authorized translation from "Die deutsche klinik" under the general editorial supervision of Julius L. Salinger, M.D., with forty-five illustrations in the text. [2nd ed.] New York and London: D. Appleton & Co., 1909. 824p. col. plates. DLC; IU-M; NNNAM; PPC **00-0257**

BILLINGS, Frank, ed. (1854-1932)
. . . General medicine, ed. by Frank Billings . . . and J. H. Salisbury. . . . Chicago: The Year Book Publishers, [1910]. 352p. plates. DLC; ICJ; PPC; PU **00-0258**

BILLINGS, Frank, ed. (1854-1932)
. . . General medicine, ed. by Frank Billings . . . and J. H. Salisbury. . . . Chicago: The Year Book Publishers, [1910]. 406p. DLC; ICJ; NNC; PU **00-0259**

BILLINGS, John S[edgwick] (1869-1928)
The leucocytes in malarial fever. [Baltimore], 1900 [1894]. 10p. NN **00-0260**

BILLINGS, John S[edgwick] (1869-1928)
The leucocytes in croupous pneumonia. [Baltimore], 1900 [1894]. 22p. NN **00-0261**

BILLINGS, John S[edgwick] (1869-1928)
Therapeutic use of extract of bone marrow. [Baltimore], 1900 [1894]. 6p. 3 diags. NN **00-0262**

BILLINGS, John S[edgwick] (1869-1928)
A case of infantile malarial fever, with grave anemia. New York: Lea Bros. & Co., 1900 [1897]. 5p. NN **00-0263**

BILLINGS, John S[edgwick] (1869-1928)
The clinic for the communicable pulmonary diseases. [Dept. of Health, City of New York, 1906.] 46p. NNNAM **00-0264**

BILLINGS, John S[haw] (1838-1913)
Some library problems of tomorrow. . . . President's address to the American Library Association, June 17, 1902. [New York, 1902.] 10p. DLC; NN **00-0265**

BILLINGS, John S[haw] (1838-1913)
The military medical officer at the opening of the twentieth century: address to the graduating class of the Army Medical School at Washington, April 14, 1903. . . . Carlisle, Pa.: Assoc. of Military Surgeons, 1903. 11p. NN **00-0266**

BILLINGS, John S[haw] (1838-1913)
The relation of milk to typhoid fever in New York City. [New York, 1905.] 10p. NN **00-0267**

BINET, Alfred (1857-1911)
The psychic life of micro-organisms. A study in experimental psychology. Chicago: Open Court Pub., 1903. 120p. ICU; MB; NN **00-0268**

BINNIE, John Fairbairn (1865-1936)
Manual of operative surgery . . . with 559 illustrations, a number of which are printed in colors. Philadelphia: P. Blakiston's Son & Co., [1905] [1904]. 644p. DLC; ICJ; NNNAM; PPC **00-0269**

BINNIE, John Fairbairn (1865-1936)
Manual of operative surgery. . . . 2nd ed., rev. and enl., with 567 illustrations, a number of which are printed in colors. Philadelphia: P. Blakiston's Son & Co., 1905. 655p. DLC; IU-M; PPC; PU **00-0270**

BINNIE, John Fairbairn (1865-1936)
Manual of operative surgery. . . . 3rd ed., rev. and enl., with 678 illustrations, a number of which are printed in colors. Philadelphia: P. Blakiston's Son & Co., 1907. 743p. DLC; NNNAN; OCIM; PU **00-0271**

BINNIE, John Fairbairn (1865-1936)
Manual of operative surgery. . . . v. 1 . . . 4th ed., rev. and enl. . . . Philadelphia: P. Blakiston's Son & Co., 1909. 1150p. col. plates. DLC; NNNAM; PPC; PPJ **00-0272**

BISHOP, Edward S[tanmore] (1848-1912)
Uterine fibromyomata; their pathology, diagnosis, and treatment. . . . With 49 illustrations. Philadelphia: P. Blakiston's Son & Co., 1901. 323p. plates. DLC; ICJ; PPC; PPJ **00-0273**

BISHOP, Edward S[tanmore] (1848-1912)
Uterine fibromyomata; their pathology, diagnosis, and treatment. New York: A. R. Elliott, 1904. 323p. illus. ICJ; NN; PU **00-0274**

BISHOP, Hudson D. (*b.* 1866)
The obstetric duties of mother and nurse; a monograph on the management of pregnancy, the aseptic and antiseptic technique of labor, the care of mother and child after labor and the principles and methods of infant feeding. . . . 2nd ed., rev. and enl. Cleveland: Press of J. H. Lamb, 1904. 96p. DLC; DNLM; PPC; PPHa **00-0275**

BISHOP, Hudson D. (*b.* 1866)
Motherhood; a manual on the management of pregnancy . . . and the principles and methods of infant feeding up to the third year of the child's life. Prepared especially for mothers, nurses and students of medicine. . . . Cleveland: Rose Publishing Co., 1910. 244p. DLC; PPHa **00-0276**

BISHOP, Irving Prescott (1849-1913)
Methods and outlines for teaching physiology. . . . Buffalo, N.Y.: The Author, 1903. 66p. DLC; DNLM **00-0277**

BISHOP, Irving Prescott (1849-1913)
Methods and outlines for teaching physiology. . . . Rev. and enl. Buffalo, N.Y.: The Author, 1910. 78p. DLC **00-0278**

BISHOP, Louis Faugeres (1864-1931)
Blood pressure as affecting heart, brain, kidneys, and general circulation; a practical consideration of theory and treatment. . . . New York: E. B. Treat & Co., 1904. 112p. DLC; NNNAM; PPC **00-0279**

BISHOP, Louis Faugeres (1864-1931)
Heart disease and blood pressure; a practical consideration of theory and treatment. . . . 2nd ed. New York: E. B. Treat & Co., 1907. 120p. DLC; ICJ; NNNAM; PU **00-0280**

BISHOP, Louis Faugeres (1864-1931)
Heart disease, blood-pressure, and the Nauheim-Schott treatment. . . . 3rd ed. New York: E. B. Treat & Co., 1909. 284p. CtY-M; DLC; NNNAM; PPC **00-0281**

BISHOP, Seth Scott (1852-1923)
Diseases of the nose, throat, and ear, and their accessory cavities. . . . 3rd ed. Thoroughly rev. and enl. Illustrated with ninety-four colored lithographs and two hundred and thirty additional illustrations. Philadelphia: F. A. Davis Co., 1904. 564p. DLC; NNNAM; OCIM; PPC **00-0282**

BISHOP, Seth Scott (1852-1923)
The ear and its diseases; a text-book for students and physicians. . . . Illustrated with twenty-seven colored lithographs and two hundred additional illustrations. Philadelphia: F. A. Davis Co., 1906. 439p. DLC; IU-M; PPC; PU
00-0283

BISHOP, Seth Scott (1852-1923)
Diseases of the nose, throat, and ear, and their accessory cavities. . . . 4th rev. ed. Illustrated with ninety-four colored lithographs and two hundred and thirty additional illustrations. Philadelphia: F. A. Davis Co., 1908. 564p. DLC; NNNAM; OCIM; PU **00-0284**

BISSELL, J. Dougal (*b.* 1864)
Sterility and its surgical treatment. New York: William Wood & Co., 1906. 11p. ScU **00-0285**

BISSELL, J. Dougal (*b.* 1864)
Intra-abdominal route for the removal of calculi from the pelvic portion of the female ureter. New York: William Wood & Co., 1908. 13p. ScU **00-0286**

BLACK, Carl E[llsworth] (*b.* 1862)
The card system in medical practice. . . . [St. Louis, 1903.] 23p. ICJ **00-0287**

BLACK, Carl E[llsworth] (*b.* 1862)
System in medical practice. n. p., [1903]. 17p. NN
00-0288

BLACK, Carl E[llsworth] (*b.* 1862)
Injuries to the spinal column. A review of the comparative results of the operative and non-operative treatment of 551 cases. Jacksonville, 1905. 15p. DNLM
00-0289

BLACK, Carl E[llsworth] (*b.* 1862)
Classification of medicine. [1908.] 18 l. ICJ
00-0290

BLACK, Greene V[ardiman] (1836-1915)
Descriptive anatomy of the human teeth. 5th ed. Philadelphia: S. S. White Dental Mfg. Co., 1902. 169p. MdU-D; PPC; PU **00-0291**

BLACK, Greene V[ardiman] (1836-1915)
The technical procedures in filling teeth. . . . Chicago: The Blakely Printing Co., 1903. 196p. DLC; ICJ
00-0292

BLACK, Greene V[ardiman] (1836-1915)
A work on operative dentistry. . . . Chicago: Medico Dental Publishing Co. 2 v. plates. DLC; ICJ
00-0293

BLACK, John Janvier (1837-1909)
Forty years in the medical profession, 1858-1898. . . . Philadelphia: J. B. Lippincott Co., 1900. 498p. DLC; NN; PPC; PU
00-0294

BLACK, John Janvier (1837-1909)
Eating to live, with some advice to the gouty, the rheumatic, and the diabetic; a book for everybody. . . . Philadelphia and London: J. B. Lippincott Co., 1906. 412p. DLC; PP; PPC; PPL **00-0295**

BLACKBURN, Isaac W[right] (1851-1911)
Intracranial tumors among the insane. A study of 29 intracranial tumors found in 1,642 autopsies in cases of mental disease. Washington: Government Printing Office, 1903. 94p. CtY-M; DLC; DNLM; PU **00-0296**

BLACKBURN, Isaac W[right] (1851-1911)
Illustrations of the gross morbid anatomy of the brain in the insane. A selection of 75 plates showing the pathological conditions found in post-mortem examinations of the brain in mental diseases. Washington: Government Printing Office, 1908. CtY-M; DLC; DNLM; PU [Quarto. 75 photographic plates with explanation on facing page.]
00-0297

BLACKWOOD, Alexander Leslie (1862-1924)
Diseases of the heart. . . . Chicago and St. Paul: Halsey Bros. Co., 1901. 261p. DLC; ICJ **00-0298**

BLACKWOOD, Alexander Leslie (1862-1924)
Diseases of the heart. . . . Chicago and St. Paul: Halsey Bros. Co., 1901. 261p. DLC; ICJ [2nd ed.] **00-0299**

BLACKWOOD, Alexander Leslie (1862-1924)
Diseases of the lungs. . . . Chicago and St. Paul: Halsey Bros. Co., 1902. 338p. DLC; ICJ **00-0300**

BLACKWOOD, A[lexander] L[eslie] (1862-1924)
A manual of materia medica, therapeutics and pharmacology, with clinical index. . . . Philadelphia: Boericke & Tafel, 1906. 592p. DLC; OCLloyd; PPC; PPHa **00-0301**

BLACKWOOD, Alexander Leslie (1862-1924)
Diseases of the liver, pancreas, and ductless glands, ... Philadelphia: Boericke & Tafel, 1907. 200p. DLC; PPC
00-0302

BLACKWOOD, Alexander Leslie (1862-1924)
The food tract, its ailments and diseases of the peritoneum. . . . Philadelphia: Boericke & Tafel, 1909. 359p. DLC; PPC
00-0303

BLACKWOOD, Alexander Leslie (1862-1924)
Contagious, constitutional and blood diseases. . . . Philadelphia: Boericke & Tafel, 1910. 367p. DLC; PPC; PPHa
00-0304

BLAIR, Thomas S[tewart] (*b.* 1867)
A practitioner's handbook of materia medica and therapeutics, based upon established physiological actions and the indications in small doses. To which is added some pharmaceutical data and the most important therapeutic developments of sectarian medicine as explained along rational lines. . . . Philadelphia, Pa.: The Medical Council, [1907]. 253p. CU-M; DLC; ICJ; PPC **00-0305**

BLAIR, Vilray Papin (1871-1955)
Essentials of oral surgery, by Vilray Papin Blair . . . and Robert Henry Ivy . . . with the collaboration of James Barrett Brown. . . . 2nd ed. St. Louis: The C. V. Mosby Co., 1906. 606p. DLC; MdU-D **00-0306**

BLAIR, Vilray Papin (1871-1955)
Laboratory guide for the modeling of the human bones in clay. St. Louis: Cooperative Association of the Medical Dept. of Washington University, 1906. 69p. NNU-M; PPC
00-0307

BLAIR, Vilray Papin (1871-1955)
Underdeveloped lower jaw, with limited excursion. [1909.] 6p. 13 photo. illus. NN **00-0308**

BLAISDELL, Frank (*b.* 1852)
One hundred years of New Hampshire surgery. A brief sketch of the life and work of New Hampshire surgeons from 1800 to 1900. Read before the New Hampshire Surgical Club at Plymouth, N.H., September 18, 1907. Goffstown, N.H., [1907]. 40p. NN **00-0309**

BLAISDELL, Frank (*b.* 1852)
One hundred years of New Hampshire surgery. A brief sketch of the life and work of New Hampshire surgeons from 1800 to 1900, read before the New Hampshire Surgical Club at Plymouth, N.H., September 18, 1907. . . . [Manchester, N.H.: Printed by the J. B. Clarke Co., 1907.] 40p. DLC; ICJ **00-0310**

BLAKE, Clarence John (1843-1919)
Operative otology; surgical pathology and treatment of diseases of the ear, by Clarence John Blake . . . and Henry Ottridge Reik. . . . New York and London: D. Appleton & Co., 1906. 359p. plates. DLC; ICJ; NNNAM; PPC **00-0311**

BLAKE, Wyatt Heffin
The need of a separate prison for consumptive convicts. . . . Read before the Medical Association of the State of Alabama, April, 1900. Birmingham, Ala.: Leslie Printing Co., [1900]. 6p. DLC **00-0312**

BLAND-SUTTON, John (1855-1936)
Surgical diseases of the ovaries and fallopian tubes. Including abdominal pregnancy. Philadelphia: Lea Bros. & Co., 1900 [*c.* 1891]. 513p. CtY-M; DNLM; ICJ; IU-M **00-0313**

BLAND-SUTTON, John (1855-1936)
Tumours, innocent and malignant; their clinical characters and appropriate treatment. 3rd ed. Chicago: W. T. Keener & Co., [1903]. 556p. ICJ; KU; OC; PPJ **00-0314**

BLAND-SUTTON, John (1855-1936)
Tumours, innocent and malignant; their clinical characters and appropriate treatment. 4th ed. Chicago: W. T. Keener & Co., 1907. 675p. ICJ; PPC; PPJ; PU **00-0315**

BLAND-SUTTON, John (1855-1936)
Gall-stones and diseases of the bile-ducts. New York: William Wood & Co., 1907. 233p. 1 plate. CtY-M; DNLM; NNNAM; PPC **00-0316**

BLECH, Gustavus M[aximillian] (*b.* 1870)
The practitioner's guide to the diagnosis and treatment of diseases of women. Chicago: M. Robertson & Co., 1903. 112p. ICJ; IU-M; OCIM **00-0317**

BLECH, Gustavus M[aximillian] (*b.* 1870)
Practical suggestions in borderland surgery for the use of students and practitioners. . . . Philadelphia: Professional Publishing Co., 1910. 219p. DLC; PPC; PU **00-0318**

BLOODGOOD, Joseph C[olt] (1867-1935)
Operations on 459 cases of hernia in the Johns Hopkins Hospital from June, 1889 to January 1, 1899. The special consideration of 268 cases operated on by the Halsted Method, and the transplantation of the rectus muscle in certain cases of inguinal hernia. . . . Baltimore: Johns Hopkins Press, 1900 [1899]. 340p. 17 plates. DLC; MdBJ-W **00-0319**

BLOODGOOD, Joseph C[olt] (1867-1935)
Pamphlets prepared for the teaching of surgical, clinical and pathological diagnosis. [1903.] 2 v. DLC; DNLM; MdBJ-W **00-0320**

BLUE, Rupert (*b.* 1867)
. . . The conduct of a plague campaign. . . . [Chicago: American Medical Association, 1908.] 8p. DLC; ICJ **00-0321**

BLUE, Rupert (*b.* 1867)
. . . The underlying principles of anti-plague measures. . . . [San Francisco, 1908?] 10p. DLC **00-0322**

BLUE, Rupert (*b.* 1867)
Anti-plague measures in San Francisco, California, U.S.A. . . . Cambridge: The University Press, [1909]. 8p. DLC **00-0323**

BOAS, Ismar [Isidor] (1858-1938)
Diseases of the intestines. . . . Authorized transl. from the 1st German ed., with special additions by Seymour Basch. . . . With forty-seven illustrations. New York: D. Appleton & Co., 1901. 562p. DLC: ICJ; NNNAM; PU **00-0324**

BOAS, Ismar [Isidor] (1858-1938)
Diseases of the intestines. . . . 2nd rev. and enl. American ed., transl. by permission from the German ed., with special notations and additions, by Seymour Basch . . . with forty-eight illustrations. New York and London: D. Appleton & Co., 1904. 600p. CtY-M; DLC; NNNAM; PU **00-0325**

BOAS, Ismar [Isidor] (1858-1938)
Diseases of the stomach . . . the sole authorized English-American ed. from the latest German ed., by Albert Bernheim. . . . Illustrated with five full-page plates and sixty-five engravings in the text. Philadelphia: F. A. Davis Co., 1907. 730p. DLC; NNNAM; PPC; PPJ **00-0326**

BOCKENHEIMER, Philipp (*b.* 1875)
Atlas of typical operations in surgery, by Dr. Ph. Bockenheimer and Dr. Fritz Frohse; sixty illustrations from water colours by Franze Frohse . . . adapted English version by J. Howell Evans. . . . New York: Rebman Co.; [etc., etc.], 1906. 250p. DLC; MBM; NNNAM; PPC **00-0327**

BOCKENHEIMER, Philipp (*b.* 1875)
Atlas of clinical surgery, with special reference to diagnosis and treatment for practitioners and students. . . . English adaptation by C. F. Marshall. . . . With 150 colored figures from models by F. Kolbow in the Pathoplastic Institute of Berlin. New York: Rebman Co., [1908]. 3 v. CtY-M; DLC; NNNAM; PPC **00-0328**

BOERICKE, Felix Aerial (*b.* 1857)
The elements of homoeopathic theory, materia medica, practice and pharmacy. Comp. and arranged from homoeopathic text-books. By Dr. F. A. Boericke and E. P. Anshutz. Philadelphia: Boericke & Tafel, 1905. 196p. CtY-M; DLC; PPC; PPHa **00-0329**

BOERICKE, Felix Aerial (*b.* 1857)
The elements of homoeopathic theory, materia medica, practice and pharmacy. Comp. and arranged from homoeopathic text-books. By Dr. F. A. Boericke and E. P. Anshutz. Philadelphia: Boericke & Tafel, 1907. 218p. DNLM; PPC; PPHa **00-0330**

BOERICKE, William (1849-1929)
Pocket manual of homoeopathic materia medica . . . 1st ed. . . . San Francisco: Boericke & Runyon Co., 1901. 572p. CtY-M; MBM; OCLloyd; PPHa **00-0331**

BOERICKE, William (1849-1929)
Pocket manual of homoeopathic materia medica comprising the characteristic and cardinal symptoms of all remedies. Second ed. revised and enlarged. San Francisco: Homoeopathic Publishing, 1903. 682p. CU-M; OCLloyd; PPHa **00-0332**

BOERICKE, William (1849-1929)
The management and care of children, including homoeopathic treatment. San Francisco: Homoeopathic Pub. Co., 1903. 199p. ICJ; NN **00-0333**

BOERICKE, William (1849-1929)
Pocket manual of homoeopathic materia medica, comprising the characteristic and guiding symptoms of all remedies . . . 3rd ed., rev. and enl., with the addition of a repertory by Oscar E. Boericke. . . . New York: Boericke & Runyon, 1906. 1049p. CtY-M; DLC; NNNAM; PU **00-0334**

BOERICKE & TAFEL (NEW YORK AND PHILADELPHIA)
The physiological treatment of disease, and guide to health and long life. . . . Philadelphia, New York, etc.: Boericke & Tafel, 1908. 40p. NN; PPHa **00-0335**

BÖHM, Alexander A.
A text-book of histology, including microscopic technic, by A. A. Böhm, M.D., and M. von Davidoff, M.D. . . . ed., with extensive additions to both text and illustrations by G. Carl Huber . . . authorized transl. from the 2nd rev. German ed. by Herbert H. Cushing. . . . With 351 illustrations. Philadelphia, [etc.]: W. B. Saunders & Co., 1900. 501p. DLC; NNNAM; PPC; PU **00-0336**

BÖHM, Alexander A.
A text-book of histology, including microscopic technic, by A. A. Böhm, M.D., and M. von Davidoff, M.D. . . . . Ed., with extensive additions to both text and illustrations, by G. Carl Huber . . . 2nd ed., thoroughly rev. and enl. with 377 illustrations. Philadelphia, London, [etc.]: W. B. Saunders & Co., 1904. 528p. DLC; NNNAM; OCIM; PU **00-0337**

BOLLER, William George
Vigorous manhood. A manual of drugless self-treatment for sexual diseases of men, together with self-treatment by natural means for indigestion, dyspepsia, constipation and piles. Rev., enl. and rewritten from the author's previous work. Men's pocket physician. . . . New York City: [Home Treatment Publishing Co.], 1903. 80p. DLC; NNC; NNNAM **00-0338**

BONNEY, Sherman Grant (*b.* 1864)
Pulmonary tuberculosis and its complications, with special reference to diagnosis and treatment, for general practitioners and students. . . . With 189 original illustrations, including 20 in colors, and 60 X-ray photographs. Philadelphia: W. B. Saunders & Co., 1908. 778p. 15 col. plates. DLC; NNNAM; PPC; PU **00-0339**

BONNEY, Sherman Grant (*b.* 1864)
Pulmonary tuberculosis and its complications, with special reference to diagnosis and treatment for general practitioners and students. . . . 2nd ed., thoroughly rev., with 243 original illustrations, including 31 in colors and 73 X-ray photographs. Philadelphia and London: W. B. Saunders & Co., 1910. 955p. DLC; OCIM; PPC; PPJ **00-0340**

BÖNNINGHAUSEN, Clemens Maria Franz von (1785-1864)
A systematic, alphabetic repertory of homoeopathic remedies. . . . Transl. from the 2nd German ed., by C. M. Boger. . . . Philadelphia: Boericke & Tafel, 1900-. DLC; ICJ; PPC; PU **00-0341**

BOOTH, Emmons Rutledge (1851-1934)
History of osteopathy, and twentieth-century medical practice. . . . Cincinnati: Press of Jennings and Graham, [1905]. 428p. plates. DLC; ICJ; MB; MH **00-0342**

BOOTH, Emmons Rutledge (1851-1934)
History of osteopathy and twentieth-century medical practice. 2nd ed., partially rev. Cincinnati: Press of Jennings and Graham, 1905. 428p. illus., ports. ICJ; KU; OC **00-0343**

BORDEN, W[illiam] C[line] (1858-1934)
The use of the Rontgen ray by the medical department of the United States Army in the war with Spain. (1898) Prepared under the direction of Surgeon-General George M. Sternberg. Washington: Government Printing Office, 1900. 98p. DLC; DNLM; PU **00-0344**

BORDEN, W[illiam] C[line] (1858-1934)
The education of the medical officer of the army. . . . Carlisle, Pa.: The Association of Military Surgeons, 1902. 8p. DLC; DNLM **00-0345**

BORDEN, W[illiam] C[line] (1858-1934)
Military surgery. [Washington: Government Printing Office, 1905.] 68p. illus. DLC; DNLM [Enno Sander – Prize Essay, Association of Military Surgeons of the United States, 1900.] **00-0346**

BORDLEY, James
Trachoma in the American Negro race. [Philadelphia, 1907.] 8p. PU **00-0347**

BOSANQUET, W[illiam] Cecil (1866-1941)
Serums, vaccines and toxines in treatment and diagnosis. . . . Chicago: W. T. Keener & Co., 1905. 344p. ICJ; NNNAM; PU **00-0348**

BOSANQUET, W[illiam] Cecil (1866-1941)
Nature of diabetes mellitus. [1905.] 7p. DNLM **00-0349**

BOSANQUET, W[illiam] Cecil (1866-1941)
Spirochaetes: a review of recent work, with some original observations. Philadelphia: W. B. Saunders & Co., 1910 [*c.* 1911]. 152p. CLM; ICRM; NNNAM; PU **00-0350**

[BOSTON CITY HOSPITAL]
A history of the Boston City Hospital from its foundation until 1904. Authorized by the trustees and edited by a committee of the hospital staff: David W. Cheever, George Gay, A. Lawrence Mason, J. Bapst Blake. . . . Boston: Municipal Printing Office, 1906. 422p. ICJ; MB; MBM; NN **00-0351**

BOSTON. CONSUMPTIVES' HOSPITAL
Tuberculosis; nature of the disease, danger and sources of contagion, how to prevent, how to cure, and advice to the well and the sick, together with the mayor's order to the heads of city departments in regard to consumption among city employees. Prepared under the supervision of the trustees of the Boston Consumptives' Hospital. . . . [Boston, 1906.] 12p. DLC; MBM **00-0352**

BOSTON, Leonard N[apoleon] (*b.* **1871)**
A text-book of clinical diagnosis by laboratory methods; for the use of students, practitioners, and laboratory workers. . . . with 320 illustrations, many of them in colors. Philadelphia: W. B. Saunders & Co., 1904. 549p. DLC; MBM; NNNAM; PPC **00-0353**

BOSTON, Leonard N[apoleon] (*b.* **1871)**
A text-book of clinical diagnosis by laboratory methods for the use of students, practitioners, and laboratory workers. . . . 2nd ed., rev. and enl., with 330 illustrations. Philadelphia and London: W. B. Saunders & Co., 1905. 563p. DLC; NNNAM; PPC; PU **00-0354**

BOSTON, Leonard N[apoleon] (*b.* **1871)**
History of the stomach-tube devised by Philip S. Physick, M.D. of Philadelphia. Manufactured 1803. [Philadelphia, 1905?] 4p. PPC **00-0355**

BOUCHARD, Charles (1837-1915)
Lectures on auto-intoxication in disease, or self-poisoning of the individual. 2nd ed., rev. Transl. with preface and new chapters added by Thomas Oliver. Philadelphia: F. A. Davis Co., 1906. 342p. DLC; ICJ; MBM; NN **00-0356**

BOVÉE, John Wesley, ed. (1861-1927)
. . . The practice of gynecology, in original contributions by American authors . . . illustrated with 382 engravings and 60 full-page plates. Philadelphia and New York: Lea Bros. & Co., 1906. 836p. DLC; DNLM; NNNAM; PPC **00-0357**

[BOWDITCH, Henry Ingersoll] (1808-1892)
Life and correspondence of Henry Ingersoll Bowditch. By his son Vincent Y. Bowditch. Boston: Houghton Mifflin Co., 1902. 2 v. MB; MBM; MWA; NN **00-0358**

BOWDITCH, Henry P[ickering] (1840-1911)
The medical school of the future. [Boston, 1900.] 45p. MH **00-0359**

BOYCE, Rupert W. (*b.* **1864)**
Yellow fever and its prevention. A manual for medical practitioners and students. New York: E. P. Dutton, 1910. 380p. 61 plates, maps, charts. CtY-M; DLC; NNNAM; PU [Simultaneously published in England: London: J. Murray (*c.* 1911), 380p.] **00-0360**

BRADFORD, Edward Hickling (1848-1926)
Case teaching in orthopedic surgery, by Edward H. Bradford . . . and John D. Adams. Boston: F. H. Thomas Co., 1905. 34p. MBM; MH **00-0361**

BRADFORD, Edward Hickling (1848-1926)
Treatise on orthopedic surgery, by Edward H. Bradford . . . and Robert W. Lovett. . . . 3rd ed., illustrated by five hundred and ninety-two engravings. New York: William Wood & Co., 1905. 669p. CtY-M; DLC; NNNAM; PPC **00-0362**

BRADFORD, Thomas Lindsley (1847-1918)
Index to homoeopathic provings. . . . Philadelphia: Boericke & Tafel, 1901. 305p. DLC; ICJ; PPHa **00-0363**

BRAINERD, Henry Clark (*b.* **1845)**
The old family doctor. . . . Cleveland: The A. H. Clark Co., 1905. 117p. DLC; MB; NcD; OCIM **00-0364**

BRAISTED, William C[larence] (1864-1941)
Report on the Japanese naval medical and sanitary features of the Russo-Japanese War to the Surgeon-General, U.S. Navy. Washington: Government Printing Office, 1906. 82p. plates. DLC; DNLM; MH; NN **00-0365**

BREWER, George Emerson (1861-1939)
A text-book of surgery. For students and practitioners. . . . Illustrated with 280 engravings in the text and 7 plates in colors and monochrome. New York and Philadelphia: Lea Bros. & Co., 1903. 706p. DLC; NNNAM; PPC; PU **00-0366**

BREWER, George Emerson (1861-1939)
A text-book of surgery. For students and practitioners. . . . Illustrated with 415 engravings in the text and 14 plates in colors and monochrome. 2nd ed., thoroughly rev. and much enl. New York and Philadelphia: Lea & Febiger, 1909. 915p. DLC; NNNAM; OCIM; PPC **00-0367**

BREWER, Isaac W[illiams] (*b.* **1867)**
. . . Notes on the vital statistics of the Philippine census of 1903. . . . [Philadelphia, 1906.] 9p. DLC **00-0368**

BREWER, Isaac W[illiams] (*b.* **1867)**
Altitude and pneumonia. . . . [Los Angeles, 1906.] 4p. DLC **00-0369**

BREWER, Isaac W[illiams] (*b.* **1867)**
. . . Tuberculosis among the Indians of Arizona and New Mexico. . . . [New York, 1906.] 8p. DLC **00-0370**

BREWER, Isaac W[illiams] (*b.* **1867)**
The winter climate of Tucson, Pima County, Arizona. [Boston, 1906.] 6p. DLC **00-0371**

BREWER, Isaac W[illiams] (*b.* **1867)**
The mortality from lobar pneumonia in high altitudes. A summary of the statistics at three military hospitals in Arizona and New Mexico. . . . New York: William Wood & Co., [1906]. 4p. DLC **00-0372**

BREWER, Isaac W[illiams] (*b.* **1867)**
Observations on the treatment of tuberculosis in Arizona. . . . New York: William Wood & Co., [1907]. 12p. DLC; NNNAM **00-0373**

BREWER, Isaac W[illiams] (*b.* **1867)**
An American school of tropical medicine. Shall there be one? Where shall it be located? What shall be its organization? . . . [New Orleans, 1907.] 7p. DLC **00-0374**

BREWER, Isaac W[illiams] (*b.* **1867)**
Personal hygiene in tropical and semi-tropical countries; a popular manual, written for the use of foreigners residing in the Philippines, Cuba, and other portions of the tropics. . . . Philadelphia: F. A. Davis Co., [1908]. 130p. DLC; ICJ; PPC; PU **00-0375**

BREWER, Isaac W[illiams] (b. 1867)
Rural hygiene; a hand-book of sanitation designed for the use of students in the agricultural schools and colleges, and for the residents of the rural districts of the United States. . . . Philadelphia and London: J. B. Lippincott Co., 1909. 226p. illus., plates. DLC: ICJ; MB; NN **00-0376**

BRICKNER, Walter M[ax] (1875-1930)
The surgical assistant, a manual for students, practitioners, hospital internes and nurses. . . . with 123 original illustrations. New York: International Journal of Surgery Co., [1905]. 363p. DLC; DNLM; NNNAM; ICJ **00-0377**

BRICKNER, Walter M[ax] (1875-1930)
Surgical suggestions; practical brevities in diagnosis and treatment, by Walter M. Brickner . . . and Eli Moschcowitz. . . . New York: Surgical Publishing Co., 1906. 58p. DLC; DNLM; NNNAM; PU **00-0378**

BRICKNER, Walter M[ax] (1875-1930)
500 surgical suggestions; practical brevities in diagnosis and treatment, by Walter M. Brickner . . . and Eli Moschcowitz. . . . 2nd series. New York: Surgery Publishing Co., 1907. 108p. DLC; ICJ; NNNAM; PPC **00-0379**

BRICKNER, Walter M[ax] (1875-1930)
The surgical assistant; a manual for students, practitioners, hospital internes and nurses. 2nd ed. New York: Internat. Jour. of Sur. Co., 1907. 363p. CtY-M; NNNAM; PPC; PPJ **00-0380**

BRICKNER, Walter M[ax] (1875-1930)
700 surgical suggestions; practical brevities in diagnosis and treatment, by Walter M. Brickner . . . Eli Moschcowitz . . . and Harold M. Hays. . . . 3rd series. New York: Surgery Publishing Co., 1909. 150p. CtY-M; DLC; NNNAM; PPJ **00-0381**

BRINKERHOFF, William Carey (*b.* 1861)
Diseases of the rectum: their consequences and non-surgical treatment. . . . Chicago: Orban Publishing Co., 1907. 207p. plates. DLC; ICJ; IU-M; PPC **00-0382**

BROADBENT, William H[enry] (1835-1907)
Heart disease: with special reference to prognosis and treatment. By William H. Broadbent . . . and John F. H. Broadbent. . . . 3rd ed. New York: William Wood & Co., 1900. 420p. plates. DLC; OCIM; PPC; PPH **00-0383**

BROADBENT, William H[enry] (1835-1907)
Heart disease: with special reference to prognosis and treatment. By William H. Broadbent . . . and John F. H. Broadbent. . . . 4th ed. New York: William Wood & Co., 1906. 479p. plates. CtY-M; DLC; NcD; PU **00-0384**

BROOMELL, Isaac Norman (*b.* 1858)
Anatomy and histology of the mouth and teeth, by . . . . 2nd ed., rev. and enl., with 337 illustrations. Philadelphia: P. Blakiston's Son & Co., 1902. 500p. DLC; MdU-D; PPC; PU **00-0385**

BROOMELL Isaac Norman, ed. (*b.* 1858)
Practical dentistry, by practical dentists. . . . Philadelphia: The L. D. Caulk Co., 1908. 461p. DLC; GU; PPC; PU **00-0386**

BROOMELL, Isaac Norman (*b.* 1858)
Anatomy and histology of the mouth and teeth, by I. Norman Broomell . . . and Philipp Fischelis. . . . 3rd ed., rev. with 357 illustrations. Philadelphia: P. Blakiston's Son & Co., 1909. 454p. CtY-M; DLC; PPC; PU **00-0387**

BROUARDEL, Paul C[amille] H[ippolyte] (1837-1906)
Death and sudden death. Transl. by F. Lucas Benham. 2nd ed. New York: William Wood & Co., 1902. 336p. DLC; MH-M; NNNAM; PU [1st ed., transl. by F. Lucas Benham, New York: William Wood & Co., 1897. 270p. NNNAM] **00-0388**

BROWER, Daniel Roberts (1839-1909)
A practical manual of insanity for the medical student and general practitioner by Daniel R. Brower . . . and Henry M. Bannister. . . . Philadelphia and London: W. B. Saunders & Co., 1902. 428p. plates. DLC; NNNAM; OCIM; PPC **00-0389**

BROWN, Christian Henry (1857-1933)
The optician's manual. . . . A treatise on the science and practice of optics. . . . Philadelphia: The Keystone, 1902. 2 v. col. plates. DLC; ICJ; PPC; PPJ **00-0390**

BROWN, Christian Henry (1857-1933)
Clinics in optometry; a compilation of eye clinics covering fully all errors of refraction and anomalies of muscles, with methods of examination, tests and corrections, as used in actual practice. A text-book of the practice of optometry. . . . Philadelphia: The Keystone Publishing Co., 1907. 254p. DLC; NN; PPC; PU **00-0391**

BROWN, Jacob Rhodes
Brown's system of treating and preventing contagious sexual diseases. . . . [Joplin? Mo., 1904?] 79p. DLC **00-0392**

BROWN, John James Graham (1853-1925)
Medical diagnosis; a manual of clinical methods for practitioners and students. Fifth edition, greatly enlarged and revised to date, by J. J. Graham Brown . . . and W. T. Ritchie. . . . With 200 illustrations and 8 full-page plates. New York: Imperial Publishing Co., 1907. 508p. CtY-M; ICJ; NNNAM; OCIM **00-0393**

BROWN, John Price (1844-1938)
Diseases of the nose and throat. . . . Illustrated with 159 engravings, including 6 full-page color-plates and 9 color-cuts in the text, many of them original. Philadelphia, New York, [etc.]: The F. A. Davis Co., 1900. 471p. DLC; ICJ; OCIM; PPC **00-0394**

BROWN, Samuel Horton (1878-1940)
Eczema; a consideration of its course, diagnosis, and treatment, embracing many points of practical importance, and containing 146 prescriptions, illustrating dosage in local application. . . . Philadelphia: P. Blakiston's Son & Co., 1906. 105p. CtY-M; DLC; PPC; PU **00-0395**

[BROWNING, Walter C.] (*b.* 1856)
Oxygen; its discovery, history & uses. [Philadelphia, 1900.] 56p. DLC [Originally 1888. *vel subseq.*] **00-0396**

BROWNING, Walter C. (*b.* 1856)
The rectum: its diseases and complications. . . . [Philadelphia? 1903.] 54p. DLC; PPC **00-0397**

BRUBAKER, Albert Philson (1852-1943)
. . . A compend of human physiology, especially adapted for the use of medical students. . . . 10th ed., rev. and enl. . . . Philadelphia: P. Blakiston's Son & Co., 1900. 270p. CtY-M; DLC; PPC; PU **00-0398**

BRUBAKER, Albert Philson (1852-1943)
. . . A compend of human physiology; especially adapted for the use of medical students. . . . 11th ed., rev. and enl., with illustrations and a table of physiologic constants. Philadelphia: P. Blakiston's Son & Co., 1902. 270p. CU-M; DLC; PPC; PU **00-0399**

BRUBAKER, Albert Philson (1852-1943)
A text-book of human physiology. . . . With colored plates and 354 illustrations. Philadelphia: P. Blakiston's Son & Co., 1904. 699p. CtY-M; DLC; PPC; PU **00-0400**

BRUBAKER, Albert Philson (1852-1943)
. . . A compend of human physiology; especially adapted for the use of medical students. . . . 12th ed.—rev. and enl. . . . Philadelphia: P. Blakiston's Son & Co., 1905. 286p. DLC; NN; PPC; PU **00-0401**

BRUBAKER, Albert Philson (1852-1943)
A text-book of human physiology. Including a section on physiologic apparatus. . . . 2nd ed. Philadelphia: P. Blakiston's Son & Co., 1906. 708p. CtY-M; NN; PPC; PU **00-0402**

BRUBAKER, Albert Philson (1852-1943)
A text-book of human physiology. Including a section on physiologic apparatus. . . . 3rd ed. Rev. and enl. With colored plates and 383 illustrations. Philadelphia: P. Blakiston's Son & Co., 1908. 752p. DLC; NNNAM; PPC; PU **00-0403**

BRUCE, John Mitchell (1846-1929)
Materia medica and therapeutics. An introduction to the rational treatment of diseases. . . . [New edition.] Philadelphia: Lea Bros. & Co., [1900]. 582p. ICJ; NNNAM; PPJ; PU [Pref., 1893] **00-0404**

BRUCE, John Mitchell (1846-1929)
Materia medica and therapeutics. . . . Rev. ed. Philadelphia: Lea Bros. & Co., 19-. 609p. CtY-M; NN; PPC; PPJ **00-0405**

BRUCE, John Mitchell (1846-1929)
Materia medica and therapeutics. An introduction to the rational treatment of diseases. . . . New and enlarged edition, revised throughout, and containing the Indian and colonial addendum to the British pharmacopoeia. . . . Chicago: W. T. Keener & Co., 1905. 632p. ICJ; OCLloyd; PPJ; PU **00-0406**

BRUCE, John Mitchell (1846-1929)
Materia medica and therapeutics. . . . New and enl. ed. rev. throughout, and containing the Indian and colonial addendum to the British pharmacopoeia. 49th thousand. 1st American ed. with the formulae adapted to the U.S. pharmacopoeia, by Oscar Oldberg. New York, [1905]. CtY-M; NNC; NjR; PU **00-0407**

BRUCK, Alfred (*b.* 1865)
Diseases of the nose, mouth, pharynx and larynx. Transl. by F. W. Forbes Ross. New York: Rebman Co., [1910]. 615p. DLC; ICJ; PPC **00-0408**

BRÜHL, Gustav (*b.* 1871)
Atlas and epitome of otology . . . with the collaboration of Prof. Dr. A. Politzer . . . authorized transl. from the German; ed. by S. MacCuen Smith . . . with 244 colored figures on 39 lithographic plates, and 99 text illustrations. Philadelphia and London: W. B. Saunders & Co., 1902. 292p. DLC; ICJ; OCIM; PPC **00-0409**

BRUNDAGE, Albert H[arrison] (*b.* 1862)
A manual of toxicology; a concise presentation of the principal facts relating to poisons, with detailed directions for the treatment of poisoning. Also a table of doses of the principal and many new remedies. . . . Brooklyn, N.Y.: [The H. Harrison Co.], 1901. 354p. DLC; NN; NNNAM **00-0410**

BRUNDAGE, Albert H[arrison] (*b.* 1862)
A manual of toxicology; a concise presentation of the principal facts relating to poisons, with detailed directions for the treatment of poisoning. Also a table of doses of the principal and many new remedies. . . . 2nd ed., rev. and enl. New York: The Henry Harrison Co.; [etc., etc.], 1902. 375p. DLC; NN; NNNAM; PU **00-0411**

BRUNDAGE, Albert H[arrison] (*b.* 1862)
A manual of toxicology. . . . 3rd ed., rev. and enl. New York: The H. Harrison Co.; London: Baillière, Tindall & Cox, 1903. 401p. DLC; DNLM; ICJ; NNNAM **00-0412**

BRUNDAGE, Albert H[arrison] (*b.* 1862)
Practical points in physiology; a collection and arrangement of some of the most important physiological facts. With which are presented certain associated anatomical features. . . . 2nd ed., rev. and improved. New York: The H. Harrison Co., 1904. 73p. DLC; ICJ; NNNAM; PPC **00-0413**

BRUNDAGE, Albert H[arrison] (*b.* 1862)
A manual of toxicology. . . . 4th ed., rev. and profusely illustrated. New York: The H. Harrison Co.; London: Baillière, Tindall & Cox, 1904. 401p. col. plates. DLC; DNLM; NN; NNNAM **00-0414**

BRUNDAGE, Albert H[arrison] (*b.* 1862)
A manual of toxicology; a concise presentation of the principal facts relating to poisons, with detailed directions for the treatment of poisoning. Also a table of doses of the principal and many new remedies. . . . 5th ed., rev. and profusely illustrated. New York: The H. Harrison Co.; [etc., etc.], 1907. 401p. col. plates. DLC; DNLM; NNNAM; PU **00-0415**

BRUNDAGE, Albert H[arrison] (*b.* 1862)
A manual of toxicology; a concise presentation of the principal facts relating to poisons, with detailed directions for the treatment of poisoning. Also a table of doses of the principal and many new remedies. . . . 6th ed., rev. and profusely illustrated. New York: The H. Harrison Co.; [etc., etc.], 1908. 401p. col. plates. DLC; DNLM; NNNAM; OCIM **00-0416**

BRUNDAGE, Albert H[arrison] (*b.* 1862)
A manual of toxicology; a concise presentation of the principal facts relating to poisons, with detailed directions for the treatment of poisoning. Also a table of doses of the principal and many new remedies. . . . 7th ed., rev. . . . New York: The H. Harrison Co.; [etc., etc.], 1909. 428p. col. plates. DLC; DNLM; ICJ; NNNAM **00-0417**

BRUNTON, T[homas] Lauder (1844-1916)
Lectures on the action of medicines; being the course of lectures on pharmacology and therapeutics delivered at St. Bartholomew's Hospital during the summer session of 1896. . . . New York, London: The Macmillan Co., 1903. 673p. DLC; NN; NNNAM; PU **00-0418**

BRUNTON, T[homas] Lauder (1844-1916)
Therapeutics of the circulation. Eight lectures delivered in the Spring of 1905 in the physiological laboratory of the University of London. . . . Philadelphia: P. Blakiston's Son & Co., 1908. 280p. DLC; ICJ; MWiW; PU **00-0419**

BRUSH, Edmund C[one] (1852-1930)
The pioneer physicians of the Muskingum Valley. . . . Zanesville? O.: Zanesville Times Recorder Print, 1900 [1890.] 10p. DNLM **00-0420**

BRUSH, Edmund C[one] (1852-1930)
Report of twenty cases of fractures of the skull. Zanesville, O., 1900. 15p. DNLM **00-0421**

BRUSH, Edmund C[one] (1852-1930)
The place and work of the medical profession. Zanesville, O., 1900. [*c.* 1899]. 12p. DNLM **00-0422**

BRUSH, Edward F.
Tuberculosis and tuberculin. . . . [New York: Wynkoop Hallenbeck Crawford Co., 1900.] 13p. NNC **00-0423**

BRUSH, E[dward] F.
Aphithae and herpes contracted by children drinking milk from cows suffering from foot and mouth disease. . . . Chicago: Press of Amer. Medical Assoc., 1903. 11p. DLC **00-0424**

BRUSH, Edward F.
How to produce milk for infant feeding. Read at the fifty-fifth annual session of the American Medical Association. Chicago: Amer. Med. Assoc., 1904. 7p. NN **00-0425**

BRUSH, Edward F.
Kumyss, in the intestinal disorders of infants and young children. Mt. Vernon, N.Y.: Chronicle Print, 1904. [1879. *vel subseq.*] 17p. DNLM **00-0426**

BRUSH, Edward F.
Milk delusions. . . . Mt. Vernon, N.Y., [1906?] 15p. DNLM **00-0427**

BRYANT, Joseph Decatur (1845-1914)
Operative surgery. . . . 4th ed., printed from new plates, entirely rev. and rewritten. . . . New York and London: D. Appleton & Co., 1905. 2 v. col. plates. DLC; NNNAM; PPC; PU **00-0428**

BRYANT, Joseph Decatur, ed. (1845-1914)
American practice of surgery; a complete system of the science and art of surgery, by representative surgeons of the United States and Canada. Editors: Joseph D. Bryant, M.D., Albert H. Buck, M.D. . . . New York: William Wood & Co., 1906-11. 8 v. col. plates. DLC: ICJ; NNNAM; PU [Includes a 65p. Introduction on "The Evolution of American Surgery" with portrait inserts by Stephen Smith] **00-0429**

BUCHANAN, Robert Andrew (*b.* 1877)
Mother's family physician; a method of treating diseases according to symptoms, and a guide to the use of H. H. H. family remedies. . . . Lima, O.: The J. U. Heiniger Remedy Co., [1908]. 64p. DLC; ICJ **00-0430**

BUCK, Albert H[enry], ed. (1842-1922)
A reference handbook of the medical sciences, embracing the entire range of scientific and practical medicine and allied science, by various writers. A new ed., completely revised and rewritten. New York: William Wood & Co., 1900-1908. 8 v., and Supp. (v. 9). CtY-M; DLC; NNNAM; PU **00-0431**

BUCK, Albert H[enry], ed. (1842-1922)
First principles of otology; a text-book for medical students. . . . 2nd ed. New York: William Wood & Co., 1903. 216p. DLC; NNNAM; PPC; PPJ **00-0432**

BUCKLEY, John Peter (*b.* 1873)
Modern dental materia medica, pharmacology and therapeutics . . . forty-six illustrations. Philadelphia: P. Blakiston's Son & Co., 1909. 383p. DLC; ICJ; MdU-D; PPC **00-0433**

BUCKLEY, John Peter (*b.* 1873)
Modern dental materia medica, pharmacology and therapeutics, including the practical application of drugs and remedies in the treatment of disease . . . 2nd ed., forty-six illustrations. Philadelphia: P. Blakiston's Son & Co., 1910. 383p. CtY-M; DLC; PPC; PU **00-0434**

BUCKMASTER, George A.
The morphology of normal and pathological blood. . . . Philadelphia: P. Blakiston's Son & Co., 1906. 244p. col. plates. DLC; ICJ; PPC; PPJ **00-0435**

BUDGETT, Sidney Payne (*b.* 1862)
. . . Essentials of physiology, prepared especially for students of medicine . . . arranged with questions following each chapter. . . . Philadelphia and London: W. B. Saunders & Co., 1901. 233p. DLC; PPC; PU; ScU **00-0436**

BUDGETT, Sidney Payne (*b.* 1862)
. . . Essentials of physiology, prepared especially for students of medicine . . . 2nd ed., thoroughly rev. by Haven Emerson. . . . Arranged with questions following each chapter. . . . Philadelphia and London: W. B. Saunders & Co., 1905. 240p. DLC; PPC; PPJ; PU **00-0437**

BUDGETT, Sidney Payne (*b.* 1862)
. . . Essentials of physiology, prepared especially for students of medicine . . . 3rd ed., thoroughly rev. by Haven Emerson. . . . Arranged with questions following each chapter. . . . Philadelphia and London: W. B. Saunders & Co., 1909. 250p. DLC; NNNAM; PPC; PU **00-0438**

BUFFUM, Joseph Howard (*b.* 1849)
Manual of the essentials of diseases of the eye and ear. [2nd ed.] . . . . Chicago: Halsey Bros. Co., 1901. 315p. col. plates. DLC; ICJ; OCIM **00-0439**

BULKLEY, Lucius Duncan (1845-1928)
. . . Eczema, with an analysis of eight thousand cases of the disease. . . . 3rd ed. of Eczema and its management, entirely rewritten. New York & London: G. P. Putnam's Sons, 1901. 368p. CU-M; DLC; NNNAM; PPC **00-0440**

BULKLEY, Lucius Duncan (1845-1928)
The influence of the menstrual function on certain diseases of the skin. . . . New York: Rebman Co.; [etc., etc.], 1906. 108p. CtY-M; DLC; NNNAM; PPC **00-0441**

BULKLEY, Lucius Duncan (1845-1928)
On the relations of diseases of the skin to internal disorders, with observations on diet, hygiene and general therapeutics. . . . New York: Rebman Co.; [etc., etc.], 1906. 175p. DLC; MBM; NNNAM; PPC **00-0442**

BULKLEY, Lucius Duncan (1845-1928)
Principles and application of local treatment in diseases of the skin. . . . New York: Rebman Co., [1907]. 130p. CtY-M; DLC; NNNAM; PU **00-0443**

BUNGE, Gustav von (1844-1920)
Text-book of physiological and pathological chemistry. . . . 2nd English ed.; transl. from the 4th German ed. by Forence A. Starling and ed. by Ernest H. Starling. . . . Philadelphia: P. Blakiston's Son & Co., 1902. 470p. CtY-M; DLC; PPC; PU **00-0444**

BUNGE, Gustav von (1844-1920)
Text-book of organic chemistry for medical students ... transl. with additions by R. H. Aders Plimmer. . . . London, New York, Bombay, and Calcutta: Longmans, Green & Co., 1907. 260p. DLC; MH-M; NNNAM; PU **00-0445**

BURCHARD, Henry H.
A text-book of dental pathology and therapeutics, for students and practitioners . . . rev. by Otto E. Inglis. . . . 2nd ed., illustrated with 545 engravings and a colored plate. Philadelphia and New York: Lea Bros. & Co., 1904. 639p. DLC; ICJ; NNNAM; PPC **00-0446**

BURCHARD, Henry H.
A text-book of dental pathology and therapeutics, for students and practitioners, based upon the original of Henry H. Burchard . . . rewritten by Otto E. Inglis . . . 3rd ed., thoroughly rev., illustrated with 567 engravings and a colored plate. Philadelphia and New York: Lea & Febiger, 1908. 717p. DLC; ICJ; PPC; PU **00-0447**

BURDICK, Gordon Granger
X-ray and high frequency in medicine. . . . [Chicago?]: Physical Therapy Library Publishing Co., [1909]. 313p. DLC; ICJ **00-0448**

BURGESS, William Harvey (*b.* 1842)
Chronic disease; the natural method of diagnosis and successful treatment. . . . (Avondale) Chattanooga, Tenn., [1907]. 320p. DLC; DNLM; ICJ **00-0449**

BURKHOLDER, Jacob F. (*b.* 1861)
The anatomy of the brain; a manual for students and practitioners of medicine. The brain of the sheep (ovis aries) being selected for description and illustration because of its availability and its practical identity with the human brain for laboratory use. . . . With an introduction by Prof. Henry H. Donaldson. . . . With thirty-six full page plates (five of them colored) from original drawings by the author. Chicago: G. P. Engelhard & Co., 1904. 174p. DLC: ICJ; NcD; PPC **00-0450**

BURKHOLDER, Jaocb F. (*b.* 1861)
. . . Ear, nose, throat. Chicago, Ill.: Manhattan School of Preventive Medicine and Home Hygiene, [1910]. 24p. DLC [Extension lecture] **00-0451**

BURNETT, Charles Henry (1842-1902)
A text-book on diseases of the ear, nose and throat, by Charles H. Burnett, M.D., E. Fletcher Ingals, M.D., James E. Newcomb, M.D. . . . Philadelphia and London: J. B. Lippincott Co., 1901. 716p. col. plates. DLC; NNNAM; PPC; PPJ **00-0452**

BURNETT, J[ames] Compton (1840-1901)
The new cure for consumption by its own virus. Illustrated by numerous cases. . . . 4th ed. . . . Philadelphia: Boericke & Tafel, 1900. 323p. DLC: ICJ; PPC; PPHa **00-0453**

BURNETT, J[ames] Compton (1840-1901)
Enlarged tonsils cured by medicines. . . . Philadelphia: Boericke & Tafel, 1901. 100p. DLC; PPC; PPHa **00-0454**

BURNETT, J[ames] Compton (1840-1901)
Curability of tumours by medicine. . . . 2nd ed., rev. Philadelphia: Boericke & Tafel, 1901. 345p. DLC; NNNAM; PPC; PPHa **00-0455**

BURNETT, Swan M[oses] (1847-1906)
An exposition of the principles of refraction in the human eye, based on the laws of conjugate foci. With 17 original illustrations. . . . [St. Louis?], 1903. 30p. DLC **00-0456**

BURNETT, Swan M[oses] (1847-1906)
The principles of refraction in the human eye, based on the laws of conjugate foci. . . . Illustrated with 25 original diagrams, by Chas. F. Prentice, M.E. Philadelphia: The Keystone, 1904. 67p. DLC; PPC **00-0457**

BURR, Colonel Bell (1856-1931)
A primer of psychology and mental disease, for use in training-schools for attendants and nurses and in medical classes, and as a ready reference for the practitioner. . . . 3rd ed., thoroughly rev. Philadelphia: F. A. Davis Co., 1906. 183p. DLC; ICJ; PPC; PPJ **00-0458**

BURRAGE, Walter Lincoln (1860-1935)
Gynecological diagnosis . . . with two hundred and seven text illustations. New York: D. Appleton & Co., 1910. 656p. DLC; NNNAM; PPC; PU **00-0459**

BURT, Stephen Smith (*b.* 1850)
Recollections and reflections of a quarter of a century. New York: Press of Pusey & Troxell, 1900 [1899]. 12p. DLC **00-0460**

BURT, Stephen Smith (*b.* 1850)
Exploration of the chest in health and disease. . . . New York: D. Appleton & Co., 1901. 306p. plates. ICJ; NNNAM; PPC; PU **00-0461**

BURT, Stephen Smith (*b.* 1850)
Bacteriology and preventive medicine. New York: Press of Pusey & Co., 1906. 104p. NNNAM **00-0462**

BUSCH, Frederick Carl (1873-1914)
Laboratory manual of physiology. . . . New York: William Wood & Co., 1905. 206p. DLC; MBM; NNNAM; PPC **00-0463**

BUSEY, Samuel Clagett (1828-1901)
The code of American medical ethics; annual address of the president of the Medical Society of the District of Columbia before the Washington Academy of Sciences, delivered December 29, 1899. . . . Washington, D.C., 1900. 16p. DLC
00-0464

BUTLER, George Frank (1857-1921)
A text-book of materia medica, therapeutics, and pharmacology. . . . 4th ed., thoroughly rev. . . . Philadelphia: W. B. Saunders & Co., 1902. 896p. DLC; OCLloyd; PPC; PU
00-0465

BUTLER, George F[rank], ed. (1857-1921)
. . . Materia medica and therapeutics; preventive medicine; climatology; forensic medicine; ed. by George F. Butler . . . Henry B. Favill . . . Norman Bridge . . . Harold N. Moyer. . . . Chicago: The Year Book Publishers, 1902. 270p. DLC: ICJ; OCLloyd **00-0466**

BUTLER, George Frank (1857-1921)
A text-book of materia medica, therapeutics and pharmacology. . . . 5th ed., thoroughly rev. and rewritten and adapted to the eighth revision (1905) of the U.S. pharmacopoeia by Smith Ely Jelliffe. . . . Philadelphia: W. B. Saunders & Co., 1906. 604p. DLC; NNNAM; PPC; PU
00-0467

BUTLER, George Frank, ed. (1857-1921)
. . . Materia medica and therapeutics; Preventive medicine; Climatology. Ed. by George F. Butler . . . Henry B. Favill . . . Norman Bridge. . . . Chicago: The Year Book Publishers, 1908. 360p. DLC; ICJ; OCIM **00-0468**

BUTLER, George Frank (1857-1921)
A text-book of materia medica, pharamcology and therapeutics. . . . 6th ed., thoroughly rev. and enl. and adapted to the eighth revision (1905) of the U.S. pharmacopoeia. Philadelphia: W. B. Saunders & Co., 1908. 706p. DLC; MBM; PPC; PPJ **00-0469**

BUTLER, George Frank (1857-1921)
The exploits of a physician detective. . . . Chicago: Clinic Publishing Co., 1908. 322p. DLC: IU-M; OCIM; NN
00-0470

BUTLER, Glentworth Reeve (1855-1926)
The diagnostics of internal medicine; a clinical treatise upon the recognized principles of medical diagnosis, prepared for the use of students and practitioners of medicine . . . with five coloured plates and two hundred and forty-six illustrations and charts in the text. New York: D. Appleton & Co., 1901. 1050p. DLC; NNNAM; OCIM; PPC **00-0471**

BUTLER, Glentworth Reeve (1855-1926)
The diagnostics of internal medicine; a clinical treatise upon the recognized principles of medical diagnosis, prepared for the use of students and practitioners of medicine. . . . With five coloured plates and two hundred and eighty-eight illustrations and charts in the text. 2nd rev. ed. New York: D. Appleton & Co., 1905. 1168p. DLC; MBM; NNNAM; PU
00-0472

BUTLER, Glentworth Reeve (1855-1926)
The diagnostics of internal medicine; a clinical treatise upon the recognized principles of medical diagnosis, prepared for the use of students and practitioners of medicine . . . with five coloured plates and two hundred and seventy-two illustrations and charts in the text. 3rd rev. ed. New York: D. Appleton & Co., 1909. 1193p. DLC; IU-M; NNNAM; PPC
00-0473

BUTLER, William Morris
Mental diseases and their homoeopathic treatment, for the student and practitioner of medicine. . . . New York: Boericke & Runyon, 1910. 504p. plates. ICJ; NNNAM; PPHa; PU
00-0474

BUTTNER, Jacques Louis (*b.* 1876)
A fleshless diet; vegetarianism as a rational dietary. . . . New York: F. A. Stokes Co., [1910]. 287p. DLC: ICJ; MB; NN
00-0475

BYFORD, Henry Turman (*b.* 1853)
Manual of gynecology. . . . 3rd rev. ed., containing three hundred and sixty-three illustrations, many of which are original. Philadelphia: P. Blakiston's Son & Co., 1902. 598p. DLC; NNNAM; OCIM; PPC **00-0476**

BYRAM, John Quincy (*b.* 1871)
Principles and practice of filling teeth with procelain; with 132 illustrations. . . . New York: Consolidated Dental Manufacturing Co.; [etc., etc., 1908]. 120p. DLC; ICJ; NNNAM; PU
00-0477

CABOT, A[rthur] T[racy] (1852-1912)
Papers upon genito-urinary surgery. . . . Boston: D. Clapp & Son, 1907. 48p. plates. fold. tab. ICJ; PU
00-0478

CABOT, Richard C[larke] (1868-1939)
Physical diagnosis of diseases of the chest. . . . With one hundred and forty-two illustrations. New York: William Wood & Co., 1900. 310p. DLC; NNNAM; PPC; PU
00-0479

CABOT, Richard C[larke] (1868-1939)
A guide to the clinical examination of the blood for diagnostic purposes. . . . With colored plates and engravings. 4th rev. ed. New York: William Wood & Co., 1901. 494p. DLC; NcD; NNNAM; PPC **00-0480**

CABOT, Richard C[larke] (1868-1939)
Physical diagnosis of diseases of the chest. . . . 2nd rev. ed., with one hundred and forty-seven illustrations. New York: William Wood & Co., 1903. 319p. DLC; NNNAM; OCIM; PPC
00-0481

CABOT, Richard C[larke] (1868-1939)
A guide to the clinical examination of the blood for diagnostic purposes. . . . With colored plates and engravings. 5th rev. ed. New York: William Wood & Co., 1904. 549p. CtY-M; DLC; NNNAM; PPC **00-0482**

CABOT, Richard C[larke] (1868-1939)
Physical diagnosis. . . . 3rd ed., rev. and enl. With five plates, and two hundred and forty figures in the text. New York: William Wood & Co., 1905. 577p. CtY-M; DLC; NNNAM; PU
00-0483

CABOT, Richard C[larke] (1868-1939)
Case teaching in medicine; a series of graduated exercises in the differential diagnosis, prognosis and treatment of actual cases of disease. . . . Boston: D. C. Heath & Co., 1906. 214p. DLC; MBM; NNNAM; PU **00-0484**

CABOT, Richard C[larke] (1868-1939)
Social service and the art of healing. . . . New York: Moffat, Yard & Co., 1909. 192p. DLC; NN; NNNAM; NNU-M **00-0485**

CABOT, Richard C[larke] (1868-1939)
. . . Diseases of metabolism and of the blood, animal parasites, toxicology. . . . An authorized translation from "Die deutsche klinik" under the general editorial supervision of Julius L. Salinger, M.D. With one colored plate and fifty-eight illustrations in the text. New York and London: D. Appleton & Co., 1909. 649p. DLC; NNNAM; OCIM; PU **00-0486**

CABOT, Richard C[larke] (1868-1939)
Physical diagnosis. . . . 4th ed., rev. and enl., with five plates, and two hundred and forty figures in the text. New York: William Wood & Co., 1909. 579p. DLC; MBM; NNNAM; PU **00-0487**

CABOT, Richard C[larke] (1868-1939)
Differential diagnosis. . . . Presented through an analysis of 385 cases. Philadelphia: W. B. Saunders & Co., 1910 [1911]. 753p. DNLM; ICJ; MBM; PPC **00-0488**

CADWALLADER, Rawlins (*b.* 1866)
Hand-book of obstetrics. . . . with 104 illustrations in the text. Philadelphia: F. A. Davis Co., 1908. 370p. DLC; NNNAM; PPC; PU **00-0489**

CAILLÉ, Augustus (1854-1935)
Differential diagnosis and treatment of disease; a text-book for practitioners and advanced students . . . with two hundred and twenty-eight illustrations in the text. New York and London: D. Appleton & Co., 1906. 867p. DLC; ICJ; NNNAM; PU **00-0490**

[CALIFORNIA]
Paso Robles Hot Springs. . . . [Frank W. Sawyer, M.D., Director.] Paso Robles, [*c.* 1905]. 64p. ICJ **00-0491**

CALMETTE, Leon C[harles] A[lbert] (1863-1933)
Venomous animals and anti-venomous serum-therapeutics. Transl. by Ernest E. Austen. New York: William Wood & Co., 1908. 403p. MBM; NNNAM; PPC; PU **00-0492**

CAMAC, Charles N. B. (1868-1940)
Epoch-making contributions to medicine, surgery and the allied sciences. Being reprints of those communications which first conveyed epoch-making observations to the scientific world together with biographical sketches of the observers. Philadelphia: W. B. Saunders & Co., 1909. 435p. ICU; MB; NIC; NN **00-0493**

CAMPBELL, Harry (1860?-1938)
On treatment. New York: William Wood & Co., 1907. 421p. DLC; NNNAM; PPC; PU **00-0494**

CAMPBELL, William A.
Dissection outline and index for students; a systematic outline for the dissection of the human body and an arranged index adapted for use with Morris's Anatomy. . . . 2nd ed., rev. Philadelphia: P. Blakiston's Son & Co., 1901. 160p. DLC; NNNAM; PPC; PU **00-0495**

CAMPBELL, William B.
Hand-book of modern treatment and medical formulary; a condensed and comprehensive manual of practical formulae and general remedial measures. . . . Philadelphia: F. A. Davis Co., 1908. 483p. CtY-M; DLC; ICJ; PPC **00-0496**

CAMPBELL, William B.
Hand-book of modern treatment and medical formulary; a condensed and comprehensive manual of practical formulae and general remedial measures compiled. . . . 2nd rev. ed. Philadelphia: F. A. Davis Co., 1910. 483p. CtY-M; DLC; PPC; PPJ **00-0497**

CAMPBELL, William F[rancis] (*b.* 1865)
A text-book of surgical anatomy . . . with 319 original illustrations. Philadelphia and London: W. B. Saunders & Co., 1908. 675p. DLC; ICJ; PPC; PU **00-0498**

CAMPBELL, William F[rancis] (*b.* 1865)
A text-book of surgical anatomy . . . with 319 original illustrations. 2nd ed. Philadelphia: W. B. Saunders & Co., 1910 [1911]. 675p. DLC; OCIM; PPC; PU **00-0499**

CAMPBELL, William F[rancis] (*b.* 1865)
The surgical anatomy of the Gasserian ganglion, with special reference to the deep injection of the nerve roots for trifacial neuralgia. [New York, 1910.] 15p. NN **00-0500**

CANDLER, George Henry (*b.* 1867)
The every-day diseases of children and their rational treatment. . . . Chicago, Ill.: The Clinic Publishing Co., 1907. 386p. DLC; IU-M; OCIM; PU **00-0501**

CAREY, George Washington (1845-1924)
Course of instruction in the biochemic disease. . . . Boston, Mass., [1904?]. 44p. DLC; MBM **00-0502**

CARLETON, Bukk G. (1856-1914)
Uropoietic diseases. . . . 2nd ed., rev. and enl. Illustrated with 33 photomicrographs and 6 lucotype figures. New York: Boericke & Runyon Co., 1900. 384p. DLC; ICJ; NNNAM; PPHa **00-0503**

CARLETON, Bukk G. (1856-1914)
A treatise on urological and venereal diseases. . . . With one hundred and seventy-one illustrations. Philadelphia: Boericke & Tafel, 1905. 795. CU-M; DLC; PPC; PPHa **00-0504**

CARPENTER, William Benjamin (1813-1885)
Principles of mental physiology, with their applications to the training and discipline of the mind, and the study of its morbid conditions. . . . New York: D. Appleton & Co., 1900. 737p. DLC; NNNAM; PU; ScCM **00-0505**

CARPENTER, William Benjamin (1813-1885)
The microscope and its revelations. . . . 8th ed. in which the first seven and the twenty-third chapters have been entirely rewritten, and the text throughout reconstructed, enlarged, and revised by the Rev. W. H. Dallinger. . . . With XXII plates and nearly nine hundred wood engravings. Philadelphia: P. Blakiston's Sons & Co., 1901. 1181p. CtY-M; DLC; NNNAM; PPC **00-0506**

CARR, Walter L[eslie], ed. (*b.* 1859)
The practice of pediatrics in original contributions by American and English authors. . . . Philadelphia & New York: Lea Bros. & Co., 1906. 1014p. 32 plates. DLC; NNNAM; PPC; PU **00-0507**

CARREL, Alexis (1873-1944)
The transplantation of organs. [1905.] 2p. NN **00-0508**

CARREL, Alexis (1873-1944)
Results of the transplantation of blood vessels, organs, and limbs. [1908.] 5p. ICJ **00-0509**

CARREL, Alexis (1873-1944)
Further studies on transplantation of vessels and organs. [Chicago, 1908.] 22p. ICJ; NN **00-0510**

CARREL, Alexis (1873-1944)
Results of the transplantation of blood vessels, organs, and limbs. New York, 1909. 31p. 8 plates. DNLM; NNNAM **00-0511**

CARROLL, James (1854-1907)
The treatment of yellow fever. . . . [Washington, 1902.] 24p. NcD **00-0512**

CARROLL, James (1854-1907)
The transmission of yellow fever. Chicago: Amer. Med. Assoc., 1903. 15p. NN **00-0513**

CARROLL, James (1854-1907)
The aetiology of yellow fever: an addendum. [1903.] 11p. DLC; DNLM **00-0514**

CARROLL, James (1854-1907)
Remarks on the history, cause, and mode of transmission of yellow fever and the occurrence of similar types of fatal fevers in places where yellow fever is not known to have existed. . . . Pennsylvania: The Association of Military Surgeons, 1903. 36p. DLC; KU **00-0515**

CARROLL, James (1854-1907)
. . . Yellow fever; a popular lecture. Austin: The University of Texas, 1905. 32p. DLC; MB; NN; PU ["Delivered at Galveston, Texas, April 12, 1905, under the auspices of the University of Texas."] **00-0516**

CARROLL, James (1854-1907)
Lessons to be learned from the present outbreak of yellow fever in Louisiana. . . . [Boston, 1905.] 6p. NcD **00-0517**

CARTER, Arthur Brewster
The prevention and cure of obesity. . . . Boston: Rockwell and Churchill Press, 1901. 15p. DLC **00-0518**

CARVER, Willard (1866-1943)
Carver's chiropractic analysis as applied to anatomy, physiology, chiropractic principles, symptomatology and diagnosis. . . . Oklahoma City, Okla.: Printed by Warden-Ebright Printing Co., [1909]. 486p. DLC; ICJ **00-0519**

CASE, Calvin Suverill (*b.* 1847)
A practical treatise on the technics and principles of dental orthopedia, including drawings and working details of appliances and apparatus for all forms of irregularities of the teeth. . . . Chicago: The C. S. Case Co., 1908. 406p. DLC; OCIM **00-0520**

CASPARI, Charles (1850-1917)
A treatise on pharmacy for students and pharmacists. . . . 2nd ed., rev. and enl. . . . Philadelphia and New York: Lea Bros. & Co., 1901. 776p. DLC; NNNAM; PPC; PU **00-0521**

CASPARI, Charles (1850-1917)
A treatise on pharmacy for students and pharmacists. . . . 3rd ed., enl. and thoroughly rev. Illustrated with 301 engravings. Philadelphia and New York: Lea Bros. & Co., 1906. 834p. DLC; IEN-M; PPC; PU **00-0522**

CASPARI, Charles (1850-1917)
A treatise on pharmacy for students and pharmacists. . . . 4th ed., enl. and rev. Illustrated with 350 engravings. Philadelphia and New York: Lea & Febiger, 1910. 913p. DLC; OCLloyd; PPC; PPJ **00-0523**

CASPER, Leopold (*b.* 1859)
Functional diagnosis of kidney disease with especial reference to renal surgery; clinical experimental investigations by Dr. Leopold Casper . . . and Dr. Paul Friedrich Richter . . . transl. by Dr. Robert C. Bryan . . . and Dr. Henry L. Sanford. . . . Philadelphia: P. Blakiston's Son & Co., 1903. 233p. DLC: ICJ; PPC; PU **00-0524**

CASPER, Leopold (*b.* 1859)
A text-book of genito-urinary diseases, including functional sexual disorders in man . . . transl. and ed. with additions by Charles W. Bonney. . . . With 213 illustrations and 23 full page plates, of which 7 are in colors. Philadelphia: P. Blakiston's Son & Co., 1906. 618p. DLC; ICJ; NNNAM; PPC **00-0525**

CASPER, Leopold (*b.* 1859)
A text-book of genito-urinary diseases, including functional sexual disorders in man . . . transl. and ed. with additions by Charles W. Bonney. . . . 2nd ed., rev. and enl., with 230 illustrations and 24 full-page plates, of which 8 are in colors. Philadelphia: P. Blakiston's Son & Co., 1909. 645p. CtY-M; DLC; ICJ; PPC **00-0526**

CATHELL, Daniel Webster (1839-1925)
Book on the physician himself and things that concern his reputation and success. . . . The twentieth century ed., being the eleventh ed. rev. and enl. by the author and his son William T. Cathell. . . . Philadelphia: F. A. Davis Co., 1902. 411p. DLC; ICJ; PPC; PU **00-0527**

CATTELL, Henry Ware (1862-1936)
Post-mortem pathology; a manual of post-mortem examinations and the interpretations to be drawn thereform; a practical treatise for students and practitioners . . . with 162 illustrations. . . . Philadelphia and London: J. B. Lippincott Co., 1903. 372p. plates. DLC; NNNAM; NNC; PPC **00-0528**

CATTELL, Henry Ware (1862-1936)
Post-mortem pathology; a manual of post-mortem examinations and the interpretations to be drawn therefrom; a practical treatise for students and practitioners. . . . 2nd, rev. and enl. ed. . . . Philadelphia and London: J. B. Lippincott Co., 1905. 551p. plates. DLC; NcD; PPC; PU **00-0529**

CATTELL, Henry Ware (1862-1936)
Post-mortem pathology; a manual of the technic of post-mortem examinations and the interpretations to be drawn therefrom; a practical treatise for students and practitioners. . . . 3rd ed. . . . Philadelphia and London: J. B. Lippincott Co., 1906. 547p. plates. CtY-M; DLC; NNNAM; PPC **00-0530**

CATTELL, Henry Ware (1862-1936)
"606"; Ehrlich's new preparation, arsenobenzol ("606"), in the treatment of syphilis. . . . True syphilitic iritis (iritis papulosa) treated with an injection of Ehrlich's "606," by G. E. De Schweinitz . . . and E. A. Sumway. . . . [Philadelphia: J. B. Lippincott Co., 1910.] 9p. plates. DLC **00-0531**

CATTELL, Henry Ware (1862-1936)
Lippincott's new medical dictionary, a vocabulary of the terms used in medicine and the allied sciences, with their pronunciation, etymology, and signification, including much collateral information of a descriptive and encyclopaedic character . . . freely illustrated with figures in the text. Philadelphia & London: J. B. Lippincott Co., [1910]. 1100p. DLC; NNNAM; PPC; PU **00-0532**

CHADDOCK, Charles Gilbert (*b.* 1861)
Outlines of psychiatry: introductory lessons designed for the use of students of medicine . . . St. Louis: Commercial Printing Co., 1904. 228p. DLC; DNLM; ICJ; PPC **00-0533**

CHADWICK, James Read (1844-1905)
"Medical libraries." Annual oration delivered before the Maine Medical Association, June 5, 1902. . . . Portland: S. Berry, printer, 1902. 7p. DLC **00-0534**

CHAPIN, Henry Dwight (1857-1942)
The theory and practice of infant feeding, with notes on development. . . . New York: William Wood & Co., 1902. 326p. CtY-M; DLC; NNNAM; PPC **00-0535**

CHAPIN, Henry Dwight (1857-1942)
The theory and practice of infant feeding, with notes on development. . . . 2nd ed., rev. New York: William Wood & Co., 1904. 342p. DLC; NNNAM; PPC; PU **00-0536**

CHAPIN, Henry Dwight (1857-1942)
The theory and practice of infant feeding, with notes on development. . . . 3rd ed., rev. . . . New York: William Wood & Co., 1909. 350p. DLC; ICJ; NNNAM; PU **00-0537**

CHAPIN, Henry Dwight (1857-1942)
Diseases of infants and children, by Henry Dwight Chapin . . . and Godfrey Roger Pisek . . . with 179 illustrations and eleven colored plates. New York: William Wood & Co., 1909. 609p. DLC; NNNAM; OCIM; PPC **00-0538**

[CHAPIN, John Bassett] (1829-1918)
Addresses at the dinner given to John B. Chapin, in celebration of the completion of half a century in hospitals for the insane. Philadelphia, [1904]. 67p. DLC; NN; PPC **00-0539**

CHAPMAN, Henry Cadwalader (1845-1909)
A manual of medical jurisprudence, insanity and toxicology. . . . 3rd ed., thoroughly rev., with 64 illustrations, and 4 plates in colors. Philadelphia, London, [etc.]: W. B. Saunders & Co., 1903. 329p. DLC; NNNAM; PPC; PU **00-0540**

CHAPMAN, Rose W[ood] Allen] (1875-1923)
. . . Helps for mothers of boys. . . . Cooperstown, N.Y.: Crist, Scott & Parshall, 1907. 10p. DLC [American motherhood leaflets: No. 6] **00-0541**

CHAPMAN, Rose W[ood] Allen] (1875-1923)
Dr. Mary Wood-Allen; a life sketch. Chicago: Ruby I. Gilbert, 1908. 96p. ICU [Dr. Wood-Allen received her M.D. from the University of Michigan in 1875, and was editor of American Motherhood.] **00-0542**

CHARTIER, M[elite E[lysée]
Monograph of a stimulant, sedative, antispasmodic expectorant. New York, [1900, *vel subseq.*] 8p. DNLM **00-0543**

CHASE, Alvin Wood (1817-1885)
Dr. Chase's recipes; or, Information for everybody. An invaluable collection of over one thousand practical recipes. . . . Illustrated ed., rev. and enl. in 1900. . . . Chicago: Thompson & Thomas, [1900]. 669p. DLC; ICJ **00-0544**

CHASE, Robert Howland (1845-1921)
General paresis, practical and clinical. . . . Philadelphia: P. Blakiston's Son & Co., 1902. 291p. plates. CtY-M; DLC; NNNAM; PPJ **00-0545**

CHAVASSE, Pye Henry (1810-1879)
Advice to a married woman on the management of her own health and on the treatment of some of the complaints incidental to pregnancy, labor and suckling, by . . . . Philadelphia: Continental Co., 1904. 280p. DLC; NN; PPC; PP **00-0546**

CHEEVER, David Williams (1831-1915)
The new surgery. The Shattuck Lecture delivered at the annual meeting of the Massachusetts Medical Society, June 8, 1897. [Boston, 1900.] 17p. MB **00-0547**

CHEEVER, David Williams (1831-1915)
Privileged medical communications. Read at the annual meeting of the Massachusetts Medical Society, June 10, 1903. [Boston?], 1903. 6p. NN **00-0548**

CHEEVER, David Williams (1831-1915)
Medicine and religion: a lecture delivered at the Old South Church in Boston, April 2, 1905. Boston: D. Clapp & Son, 1905. 11p. DNLM; MB; MH **00-0549**

CHEEVER, David Williams (1831-1915)
A history of the Boston City Hospital from its foundation until 1904, authorized by the trustees and edited by a committee of the hospital staff: David W. Cheever, M.D., George W. Gay, M.D., A. Lawrence Mason, M.D., J. Bapst Blake, M.D. Boston: Municipal Printing Office, 1906. 422p. MB; MH **00-0550**

CHEW, Samuel Claggett (1837-1915)
Addresses on several occasions. Baltimore: Deutsch Co., 1906. 137p. MdBJ-W; MdU-D; NNNAM **00-0551**

CHILD, Charles Gardner (*b.* 1873)
. . . Diseases of women; a manual for students and practitioners. . . . Illustrated with 101 engravings. Philadelphia and New York: Lea & Febiger, [1909]. 219p. DLC; NNNAM; PPC; PU **00-0552**

CHITTENDEN, Russell Henry, ed. (1856-1943)
Studies in physiological chemistry; being reprints of the more important studies issued from the laboratory of physiological chemistry, Sheffield Scientific School of Yale University during the years 1897-1900. . . . New York: Scribner's Sons; [etc., etc.], 1901. 424p. CtY-M; DLC; NNNAM; OCIM **00-0553**

CHITTENDEN, Russell Henry (1856-1943)
Physiological economy in nutrition, with special reference to the minimal proteid requirement of the healthy man; an experimental study. . . . New York: F. A. Stokes Co., 1904. 478p. DLC; MH; NNNAM; PU **00-0554**

CHITTENDEN, Russell Henry (1856-1943)
Some problems of intermediary metabolism. [The Shattuck Lectures, 1905] Boston, 1905. 43p. DNLM; MBM; MH; NN **00-0555**

CHITTENDEN, Russell Henry (1856-1943)
The nutrition of man. . . . New York: F. A. Stokes Co., [1907]. 321p. DLC; NcD; NN; PPL **00-0556**

CHRISTISON, John Sanderson (1856-1908)
Epilepsy, responsibility and the Czolgosz case; was the assassin sane or insane? . . . [Chicago, 1902?] 15p. DLC **00-0557**

CHURCH, Archibald (*b.* 1861)
Nervous and mental diseases, by Archibald Church . . . and Frederick Peterson. . . . With 305 illustrations. 2nd ed. Philadelphia: W. B. Saunders, 1900. 843p. diags. DLC; NNNAM; PPC; PPJ **00-0558**

CHURCH, Archibald (*b.* 1861)
Nervous and mental diseases, by Archibald Church . . . and Frederick Peterson. . . . Wth 322 illustrations. 3rd ed., thoroughly rev. Philadelphia and London: W. B. Saunders & Co., 1901. 869p. plates. DLC; IU-M; PPC; PU **00-0559**

CHURCH, Archibald (*b.* 1861)
Nervous and mental diseases, by Archibald Church . . . and Frederick Peterson. . . . With 338 illustrations. 4th ed., thoroughly rev. Philadelphia, [etc.]: W. B. Saunders & Co., 1903. 922p. DLC; IEN-M; NNNAM; PPC **00-0560**

CHURCH, Archibald (*b.* 1861)
Nervous and mental diseases, by Archibald Church . . . and Frederick Peterson. . . . with 341 illustrations. 5th ed., thoroughly rev. Philadelphia and London: W. B. Saunders & Co., 1905. 937p. plates. DLC; IU-M; PPC; PU **00-0561**

CHURCH, Archibald (*b.* 1861)
Nervous and mental diseases, by Archibald Church . . . and Frederick Peterson . . . with 341 illustrations. 6th ed., thoroughly rev. Philadelphia and London: W. B. Saunders & Co., 1908. 945p. CtY-M; DLC; NNNAM; PPC **00-0562**

CHURCH, Archibald, ed. (*b.* 1861)
. . . Diseases of the nervous system . . . an authorized translation from "Die deutsche klinik" under the general editorial supervision of Julius L. Salinger, M.D. With one hundred and ninety-five illustrations in the text and five colored plates. New York and London: D. Appleton & Co., 1908. 1205p. DLC; NNNAM; PPC; PU **00-0563**

CLAIBORNE, John Herbert, ed. (1861-1922)
Cataract extraction; being a series of papers with discussion and comments read before the Ophthalmological Section of the New York Academy of Medicine, 1907-1908. . . . New York: William Wood & Co., 1908. 169p. CtY-M; DLC; MBM; NNNAM **00-0564**

CLARK, Alexander (*b.* 1851)
The feet and hands. How to take care of them. . . . Philadelphia, Pa.: The National Printing Co., 1901. 41p. DLC; PU **00-0565**

CLARK, Charles H[erbert] (*b.* 1854)
Practical methods in microscopy. . . . 3rd ed. Boston: D. C. Heath & Co., 1900. 261p. ICJ; NN; PU **00-0566**

CLARK, Charles H[erbert] (*b.* 1854)
Practical methods in microscopy. 4th ed. Boston: D. C. Heath & Co., 1907. 261p. ICJ; MH; NN; PU [1st ed., 1894; 2nd ed., rev. and enl., 1896] **00-0567**

CLARK, George Hardy (*b.* 1860)
. . . The ABC manual of materia medica and therapeutics. . . . Philadelphia: Boericke & Tafel, 1901. 197p. DNLM; PPC **00-0568**

CLARK, George Hardy (*b.* 1860)
The ABC manual of materia medica and therapeutics. . . . 2nd ed., enl. Philadelphia: Boericke & Tafel, 1905. 301p. DLC; DNLM; ICJ; PPC **00-0569**

CLARK, Marion E[dward]
Diseases of women: a manual of gynecology designed for the use of osteopathic students and practitioners. 2nd ed., rev. Kirksville, Mo.: Journal Printing Co., 1904. 539p. DNLM; ICJ; PU **00-0570**

CLARK, Marion E[dward]
Applied anatomy. Designed for the use of osteopathic students and practitioners as an aid in the anatomical explanation of disease from an osteopathic viewpoint. Kirksville, Mo.: Journal Printing Co., 1906. 687p. DNLM; PU **00-0571**

CLARK, Marion E[dward]
2000 questions and answers on osteopathy applied anatomy, obstetrics and gynecology, taken from lectures and quizzes given by Dr. M. E. Clark. . . . Falls City: Press of Tribune [1906]. 162p. DLC; PU **00-0572**

CLARKE, John Henry (1852-1931)
Indigestion; its causes and cure. American ed. Rev. and enl. by the author. From the 5th English ed. Philadelphia: Boericke & Tafel, 1900. 147p. DLC; ICJ; NNNAM; PPC
00-0573

CLARKE, John H[enry] (1852-1931)
A dictionary of domestic medicine. Giving a description of diseases, directions for their general management and homoeopathic treatment, with a special section on diseases of infants. . . . American ed., rev. and enl. by the author. Philadelphia: Boericke & Tafel, 1901. 363p. DLC; NNNAM; PPC; PU
00-0574

CLEAVES, Margaret A[bigail] (1848-1917)
Light energy: its physics, physiological action and therapeutic applications. New York: Rebman Co., [1904]. 827p. DLC; DNLM; ICJ; PPC **00-0575**

CLEAVES, Margaret A[bigail] (1848-1917)
The autobiography of a neurasthene as told by one of them and recorded by Margaret A. Cleaves. Boston: R. G. Badger, 1910. 246p. DLC; GU; NIC; PPC **00-0576**

[CLEMENS, Samuel Langhorne, 1835-1910]
Christian science, with notes containing corrections to date, by Mark Twain [pseud.]. Hartford, Conn.: American Pub. Co., 1907. 362p. plates, port. MB; NN **00-0577**

[CLEMENS, Samuel Langhorne, 1835-1910]
Christian science, with notes containing corrections to date, by Mark Twain [pseud.] . . . . New York and London: Harper & Bros., [1907]. 263p. DLC; MB; MH; NcD
00-0578

CLEVENGER, Shobal Vail (1843-1920)
Therapuetics, materia medica and the practice of medicine. . . . Atlantic City, N.J.: Evolution Publishing Co., 1905. 307p. DLC; PPC **00-0579**

CLOSE, Charles William (1859-1915)
. . . Phrenopathy, or Rational mind cure. . . . 3rd ed., Bangor, Me.: C. W. Close, 1900. 54p. DLC **00-0580**

CLOSE, Charles William (1859-1915)
. . . Phrenopathy, or Rational mind cure. . . . 4th ed. Bangor, Me.: C. W. Close, 1906. 64p. DLC **00-0581**

CLOUSTON, Thomas Smith (1840-1915)
The hygiene of mind. 4th ed. New York: E. P. Dutton, 1907. 284p. ICU; MA; NIC; NNNAM **00-0582**

CLYMER, R[euben] Swinburne (*b.* 1878)
Vaccination brought home to you. . . . Terre Haute, Ind.: Press of G. H. Hebb, 1904. 92p. DLC; DNLM
00-0583

CLYMER, R[euben] Swinburne (*b.* 1878)
The Thomsonian system of medicine, with complete rules for the treatment of disease. Also a short materia medica. . . . Allentown, Pa.: The Philosophical Publishing Co., [1906]. 196p. DLC **00-0584**

CLYMER, R[euben] Swinburne (*b.* 1878)
The international system of direct medication, giving the causes and symptoms of different diseases and their treatment by ozone, direct medication, the diet, internal bath and the nature cure. . . . Allentown, Pa.: R. S. Clymer, [1907]. 2 v. DLC **00-0585**

CLYMER, R[euben] Swinburne (*b.* 1878)
The international system of magnetic (alchemic) therapeutics. . . . Allentown, Pa.: R. S. Clymer, [1909]. 152p. DLC
00-0586

COAKLEY, Cornelius Godfrey (1862-1934)
A manual of diseases of the nose and throat. . . . 2nd ed., rev. and enl. Illustrated with 103 engravings and 4 colored plates. New York and Philadelphia: Lea Bros. & Co., 1901. 566p. DLC; NNNAM; OCIM; PPC **00-0587**

COAKLEY, Cornelius Godfrey (1862-1934)
A manual of diseases of the nose and throat. . . . 3rd ed., rev. and enl. Illustrated with 118 engravings and five colored plates. New York and Philadelphia: Lea Bros. & Co., 1905. 594p. DLC; IU-M; NNNAM; PPC **00-0588**

COAKLEY, Cornelius Godfrey (1862-1934)
A manual of diseases of the nose and throat. . . . 4th ed., rev. and enl. Illustrated with 126 engravings and 7 colored plates. New York and Philadelphia: Lea Bros. & Co., 1908. 604p. DLC; GU; NNNAM; PPC **00-0589**

COBB, Elizabeth Emma
The medical adviser is a reliable guide for the management of diseases, giving the causes of diseases, the symptoms of the various diseases, the prevention and treatment of all diseases of both sexes of all ages. . . . Decatur, Ill.: Hostetler Printing House, 1903. 880p. DLC **00-0590**

COBLENTZ, Virgil (1862-1932)
A manual of volumetric analysis; treating on the subjects of indicators, test-papers, alkalimetry, acidimetry, analysis by oxidation and reduction, iodometry, assay processes for drugs with the tirimetric estimation of alkaloids, estimation of phenol, sugar, tables of atomic and molecular weights. . . . Philadelphia: P. Blakiston's Son & Co., 1901. 181p. DLC; OCLloyd; PPC; PU **00-0591**

COBLENTZ, Virgil (1862-1932)
The newer remedies, including their synonyms, sources, tests, solubilities, incompatibles, medicinal properties and doses as far as known, together with such proprietaries as have similar titles; a reference manual for physicians, pharmacists and students. . . . 4th ed., rev. and enl. Boston: The Apothecary Publishing Co., 1908. 133p. DLC; MBM; PPC
00-0592

COBLENTZ, Virgil (1862-1932)
A manual of volumetric analysis, treating on the subjects of indicators, test-papers, alkalimetry, including assay of drugs by titration, acidimetry, analysis of oxidation and reduction, iodometry, determinations by precipitation, and by color comparison. . . . 2nd ed., rev., completely reconstructed and enl., by Anton Vorisek . . . with 87 illustrations. Philadelphia: P. Blakiston's Son & Co., 1909. 234p. DLC; NNNAM; PPC; PU
00-0593

COHEN, S[olomon] Solis (1857-1948)
Essentials of diagnosis. . . . 2nd ed. By S. Solis Cohen and A. A. Eshner. Philadelphia: W. B. Saunders & Co., 1900. 382p. DLC; NNNAM; PPC; PU **00-0594**

COHEN, S[olomon] Solis (1857-1948)
Progress in therapeutics. Address of the retiring president of the Philadelphia County Medical Society, delivered March 14, 1900. Detroit: W. M. Warren, 1900. 20p. PPHa; PU
00-0595

COHEN, S[olomon] Solis (1857-1948)
The true role of drugs in the management of tuberculosis. [Chicago? 1901.] 10p. DLC **00-0596**

COHEN, S[olomon] Solis, ed. (1857-1948)
A system of physiologic therapeutics. . . . Philadelphia: P. Blakiston's Sons & Co., 1901-02. 11 v. DLC; NNNAM; PPC; PU [Contents. — v. 1-2. Electrotherapy [by] George W. Jacoby. — v. 3. Climatology, health resorts-mineral springs [by] Frederick P. Weber. — v. 5. Prophylaxis-personal hygiene-civic hygiene-care of the sick [by] Joseph McFarland. — v. 6. Dictotherapy and food in health [by] Nathan S. Davis. — v. 7. Mechanotherapy and physical education [by] John K. Mitchell. — v. 8. Rest, mental therapeutics, suggestion [by] Francis X. Dercum. — Hydrotherapy, thermotherapy and phototherapy [by] William Winternitz. — v. 10. Pneumotherapy including aerotherapy and inhalation methods and therapy [by] Paul Louis A. Tissier. — v. 11. Serum therapy . . . [by] Joseph McFarland. **00-0597**

COHEN, S[olomon] Solis (1857-1948)
The proper scope of scientific (so called expert) testimony in trials involving pharmacological questions. [1905.] 6p. DLC **00-0598**

COHEN, S[olomon] Solis (1857-1948)
Hypodermic use of quinine and urea hydro-chloride in the diagnosis and treatment of acute and chronic malarial infections. [Philadelphia], 1908. 12p. DLC **00-0599**

COHN, Lassar (1858-1922)
The praxis of urinary analysis. A guide to the chemical analysis of urine. With directions for preparing artificial pathological urines for practicing various tests and an appendix on the analysis of stomach contents. . . . Authorized transl. from the author's enl. and rev. 2nd ed. by H. W. F. Lorenz . . . 1st thousand. New York: J. Wiley & Sons; [etc., etc.], 1903. 58p. CtY-M; DLC; NNNAM; PU **00-0600**

COHNHEIM, Paul (*b.* 1867)
Diseases of the digestive canal (oesophagus, stomach, intestines) . . . from the 2nd German ed., edited and transl. by Dudley Fulton. . . . Philadelphia and London: J. B. Lippincott Co., [1909]. 373p. DLC; NNNAM; PPC; PU **00-0601**

COLEMAN, Warren (*b.* 1869)
A syllabus of materia medica . . . 2nd ed. New York: William Wood & Co., 1905. 189p. CU-M; DLC; NNNAM; PP **00-0602**

COLEMAN, Warren (*b.* 1869)
A syllabus of materia medica . . . 3rd ed., revised to conform to the eighth decennial revision of the U.S. pharmacopoeia. New York: William Wood & Co., 1906. 186p. DLC; ICJ; NNNAM; PPC **00-0603**

COLLINS, Edward T[reacher] (*b.* 1862) and M. S. MAYOU
Pathology and bacteriology of the eye. Edited by Walter L. Pyle. Philadelphia: P. Blakiston's Son & Co., 1910 [1911]. 558p. NNNAM; OCIM; PPC; PU **00-0604**

COLLINS, Joseph (1866-1950)
The treatment of diseases of the nervous system; a manual for practitioners. . . . Illustrated by twenty-three engravings. New York: William Wood & Co., 1900. 602p. CtY-M; DLC; NNNAM; PU **00-0605**

COLLINS, Joseph (1866-1950)
Letters to a neurologist, to which are appended brief replies purporting to set forth concisely the nature of the ailments therein described, with remarks on their appropriate treatment. . . . New York: William Wood & Co., 1908. 143p. DLC; MBM; NNNAM; PPC **00-0606**

COLLINS, Joseph (1866-1950)
Mind and malady: The general practitioner and the functional nervous diseases. . . . Chicago: American Medical Association, 1909. 16p. DLC **00-0607**

COMBE, Adolphe (1859-1916)
Intestinal auto-intoxication . . . together with an appendix on the lactic ferments with particular reference to their application in intestinal therapeutics, by Albert Fournier. . . . Only authorized English adaptation by William Gaynor States . . . with eighteen figures in the text, four of which are colored. New York: Rebman Co., [1908]. 461p. DLC; ICJ; NNNAM; PPJ **00-0608**

CONGER, Horace O.
Obstetrics and womanly beauty. A treatise on the physical life of woman, embracing full information on all important matters for both mothers and maidens . . . by Horace O. Conger, M.D., and Caroline P. Crane, M.D. Chicago: American Publishing House, [1900]. 541p. DLC; DNLM; ICJ **00-0609**

CONKLIN, William J[udkins] (1844-1916)
Medical libraries. Chicago: American Medical Association, [*c.* 1909]. 7p. ICU **00-0610**

CONSOLIDATED DENTAL MANUFACTURING CO.
Illustrated and descriptive catalogue and price list of dental supplies. . . . [1908.] 485p. NNNAM **00-0611**

COOK, William H.
Woman's hand-book of health; a guide for the wife, mother and nurse. With addenda of favorite prescriptions. Charleroi, Pa., 1902. 408p. DLC; NN **00-0612**

COOKE, Joseph Brown (*b.* 1868)
A manual of obstetrical technique as applied to private practice; with a chapter on abortion, premature labor, and curettage. . . . Philadelphia: J. B. Lippincott Co., 1900. 169p. DLC; MBM; PPC; PU **00-0613**

COOKE, Joseph Brown (*b.* 1868)
A manual of obstetrical technique as applied to private practice; with a chapter on abortion; premature labor, and curettage. . . . 2nd ed. Philadelphia: J. B. Lippincott Co., 1901. 169p. DLC; PPJ; PU **00-0614**

COOKE, Joseph Brown (*b.* 1868)
A manual of obstetrical technique as applied to private practice; with a chapter on abortion, premature labor, and curettage. . . . 3rd ed. Philadelphia: J. B. Lippincott Co., 1902. 169p. DLC; NNNAM; PPHa **00-0615**

COOKE, Joseph Brown (*b.* 1868)
A manual of obstetrical technique as applied to private practice; with a chapter on abortion, premature labor, and curettage. . . . 4th ed., rev. and enl. Philadelphia: J. B. Lippincott Co., 1902. 200p. DLC; NN; PPC; PU **00-0616**

COOKE, Joseph Brown (*b.* 1868)
A nurse's handbook of obstetrics, for use in training-schools. . . . Philadelphia: J. B. Lippincott Co., 1903. 391p. plates. CtY-M; DLC; PPC; PU **00-0617**

COOKE, Joseph Brown (*b.* 1868)
A nurse's handbook of obstetrics, for use in training-schools . . . 2nd ed., rev. Philadelphia: J. B. Lippincott Co., 1905. 403p. plates. DLC; MBM; PPC; PU **00-0618**

COOKE, Joseph Brown (*b.* 1868)
A manual of obstetrical technique as applied to private practice, with a chapter on abortion, premature labor, and curettage . . . 5th ed. Philadelphia: J. B. Lippincott Co., 1906. 209p. DLC; NNNAM; PPC; PU **00-0619**

COOKE, Joseph Brown (*b.* 1868)
A nurse's handbook of obstetrics, for use in training-schools. . . . 3rd ed., rev. Philadelphia: J. B. Lippincott Co., [1907]. 408p. plates. DLC; GU; NNNAM; PU **00-0620**

COOKE, Joseph Brown (*b.* 1868)
A manual of obstetrical technique as applied to private practice, with a chapter on abortion, premature labor, and curettage . . . .6th ed., enl. and fully rev. Philadelphia: J. B. Lippincott Co., 1908. 258p. col. plates. DLC; MBM; PPC; PU **00-0621**

COOKE, Joseph Brown (*b.* 1868)
A nurse's handbook of obstetrics, for use in training schools . . . 4th ed., rev. Philadelphia: J. B. Lippincott Co., [1909]. 403p. plates. CU-M; DLC; PPC; PPJ **00-0622**

[COOPER, John G.]
Biographical sketch of the late James G. Cooper, M.D. of Hayward, Alameda Co., California. [Santa Clara? Calif.], 1902. 31p. plates. DLC **00-0623**

COOPER, William Colby (*b.* 1835)
Preventive medicine, including a disquisition on therapeutic philosophy. . . . Cleveland, O.: The Author, 1905. 147p. DLC; DNLM; ICJ; OCIM **00-0624**

COPLIN, William M[ichael] L[ate] (1864-1928)
Manual of pathology, including bacteriology, the technic of postmortems, and methods of pathologic research. . . . 3rd ed., rev. and enl., with three hundred and thirty illustrations and seven colored plates. . . . Philadelphia: P. Blakiston's Son & Co., 1900. 846p. CtY-M; DLC; PPC; PU **00-0625**

COPLIN, William M[ichael] L[ate] (1864-1928)
Manual of pathology, including bacteriology, the technic of postmortems, and methods of pathologic research. . . . 4th ed., rewritten and enl. With four hundred and ninety-five illustrations, many of which are original, and ten colored plates. Philadelphia: P. Blakiston's Son & Co., 1905. 994p. DLC; NN; PPC; PPJ **00-0626**

COPLIN, William M[ichael] L[ate] (1864-1928)
Manual of pathology, including bacteriology, the technic of postmortems, and methods of pathologic research. . . . 4th ed., rewritten and enl., reprinted with corrections, with four hundred and ninety-five illustrations and twenty-three plates, ten of which are in colors. Philadelphia: P. Blakiston's Son & Co., 1910. 994p. DLC; NNNAM; PPC; PU **00-0627**

CORDELL, Eugene Fauntleroy (1843-1913)
Charles Frederick Wiesenthal, medicinae practicus, the father of the medical profession of Baltimore. . . . [Baltimore: The Johns Hopkins Press, 1900.] 13p. DLC; MdBJ-W **00-0628**

CORDELL, Eugene Fauntleroy (1843-1913)
The medical annals of Maryland, 1799-1899; prepared for the centennial of the Medical and Chirurgical Faculty. . . . Baltimore: Press of Williams & Wilkins Co., 1903. 889p. plates. DLC; MdBM; MdBJ-W; MdU-D **00-0629**

CORLETT, William Thomas (1854-1948)
A treatise on the acute, infectious exanthemata; including variola, rubeola, scarlatina, rubella, varicella, and vaccinia, with especial reference to diagnosis and treatment. . . . Illustrated by twelve colored plates, twenty-eight half-tone plates from life, and two engravings. Philadelphia: F. A. Davis Co., 1901. 392p. DLC; KU; MBM; PPC **00-0630**

CORNARO, Luigi (1467-1566)
The art of living long; a new and improved English version of the treatise by the celebrated Venetian centenarian Louis Cornaro, with essays by Joseph Addison, Lord Bacon, and Sir William Temple. . . . Milwaukee: W. F. Butler, 1905. 214p. 4 ports. DLC; OCIM; PP; PPL **00-0631**

CORNELIUS, Elias (1758-1823)
Journal of Dr. Elias Cornelius, a revolutionary surgeon. Graphic description of his sufferings while a prisoner in Provost Jail, New York, 1777 and 1778, with biographical sketch. Washington, D.C.: C. M. Tompkins and C. T. Sherman, 1903. 27p. DLC **00-0632**

CORSON, Eugene R[ollin] (*b.* 1855)
A case of Colles' fracture treated prone on a flat splint, with chief regard to ruptured ligaments. [New York, 1900 [1898].] 8p. NN **00-0633**

CORSON, Eugene R[ollin] (*b.* 1855)
The centennial anniversary of the Georgia Medical Society. Savannah, 1905. 7p. DNLM; GU **00-0634**

CORSON, Eugene R[ollin] (*b.* 1855)
Sir Charles Bell, the man and his work. [Baltimore, 1910.] 31p. MB; GU **00-0635**

COSGROVE, John J[oseph] (*b.* 1869)
History of sanitation. Pittsburgh: Standard Sanitation Co., 1909. 124p. DLC; MB; NN; PPC **00-0636**

COTTON, Alfred Cleveland (1847-1916)
Lessons on the anatomy, physiology and hygiene of infancy and childhood for junior students. Consisting of extracts from lectures given at Rush Medical College. . . . Chicago: Doctor's Magazine Publishing Co., 1900. 174p. plates. DLC; ICJ; ICRM **00-0637**

COTTON, Alfred Cleveland (1847-1916)
. . . The medical diseases of infancy and childhood, with points on the anatomy, physiology, and hygiene peculiar to the developing period. . . . Philadelphia and London: J. B. Lippincott Co., 1906. 670p. plates. DLC; NNNAM; PPC; PU **00-0638**

COTTON, Frederic Jay (1869-1938)
Causes of disability after fractures of the lower leg and ankles. [Boston, 1907.] 12p. MB **00-0639**

COTTON, Frederic Jay (1869-1938)
Dislocations and joint-fractures . . . with 1201 illustrations, 830 from drawings by the author. Philadelphia and London: W. B. Saunders & Co., 1910. 654p. DLC; ICJ; NNNAM; OCIM; PPC **00-0640**

COUNCILMAN, William Thomas (1854-1933), F. B. MALLORY, and J. H. WRIGHT
Epidemic cerebro-spinal meningitis and its relation to other forms of meningitis. Sears Path. Lab. and Lab. of the Boston City Hospital and the Massachusetts Gen. Hospital. [1901?] 178p. DLC; MBM **00-0641**

COUNCILMAN, William Thomas (1854-1933)
Pathology; a syllabus, by W. T. Councilman, M.D., and F. B. Mallory, M.D. . . . Boston: Printed by J. L. Fairbanks & Co., 1902. 174p. DLC; MBM **00-0642**

COVEY, Alfred Dale (*b.* 1869)
The secrets of specialists. . . . 1st ed. Detroit, Mich.: Physicians Supply Co., [1903]. 304p. DLC; ICJ **00-0643**

COVEY, Alfred Dale (*b.* 1869)
The secrets of specialists. . . . 2nd ed. Detroit, Mich.: Physicians Supply Co., [1905]. 330p. DLC **00-0644**

COWPERTHWAITE, Allen Corson (*b.* 1848)
A text-book of the practice of medicine . . . including a section on Diseases of the nervous system, by N. B. Delamater. . . . Chicago: Halsey Bros. Co., 1901. 1039p. DLC; ICJ; NN **00-0645**

COWPERTHWAITE, A[llen] C[orson] (*b.* 1848)
A text-book on materia medica and therapeutics. Characteristic, analytical, and comparative. . . . 9th ed. With an appendix including the new remedies. Chicago: J. B. Delbridge & Son, 1905. 860p. DLC; ICJ; IU-M; OCLloyd **00-0646**

COWPERTHWAITE, Allen Corson (*b.* 1848)
A text-book of materia medica and therapeutics, characteristic, analytical and comparative. . . . 10th ed., with an appendix, enl., including new remedies. Philadelphia: Boericke & Tafel, 1909. 864p. DLC; MBM; OCIM; PPC **00-0647**

COX, Joseph A[bram] (*b.* 1858)
Practical paragraphs for patients and physicians. Wheeling, W. Va.: Mitchell Printing House, 1902. 126p. DLC **00-0648**

COX, Marvin Earl
Elementary instructions in vital magnetic therapeutics, Fargo, N.D.: World's College of Therapeutics, [1901]. 39p. DLC **00-0649**

COX, Marvin Earl
Child life. A scientific and practical treatise on the study of life and the care, education and development of children from conception to maturity. . . . Fargo, N.D.: The World's College of Therapeutics, 1902. 174p. DLC **00-0650**

COX, Marvin Earl
. . . Complete and special mail course of the world's system of therapeutics; comprising several complete courses. . . . Personal magnetism and magnetic healing. . . . [2nd ed., rev., enl. and illustrated] [Fargo? N.D., 1902.] 275p. DLC [First edition was private and not copyrighted.] **00-0651**

CRAGIN, Edwin B[radford] (1859-1918)
. . . Essentials of gynecology, arranged in the form of questions and answers prepared especially for students of medicine. . . . 5th ed., thoroughly rev. by F. S. Mathews. . . . Philadelphia and London: W. B. Saunders & Co., 1901. 207p. DLC; MH-M; NN; PPC **00-0652**

CRAGIN, Edwin B[radford] (1859-1918)
. . . Essentials of gynecology, arranged in the form of questions and answers, prepared especially for students of medicine. . . . 6th ed., thoroughly rev., by Frank S. Mathews. . . . With 57 illustrations. Philadelphia and London: W. B. Saunders & Co., 1905. 215p. DLC; GU; PPC; PU **00-0653**

CRAGIN, Edwin B[radford] (1859-1918)
. . . Essentials of gynecology, arranged in the form of questions and answers, prepared especially for students of medicine. . . . 7th ed., thoroughly rev. by Frank S. Mathews . . . with 59 illustrations. Philadelphia and London: W. B. Saunders & Co., 1909. 232p. DLC; MBM; NNNAM; PPC **00-0654**

CRAIG, Arthur Still
Atlas of sectional anatomy for student and practitioner, . . . ; a uniform series of life-size, tri-color sections of the body and two one-half size outline skeletal drawings, with explanation. [Maryville? Mo., 1907.] 93p. 2 fold. col. plates. DLC **00-0655**

CRAIG, Charles Franklin (*b.* 1872)
The estivo autumnal (remittent) malarial fevers. . . . Illustrated by two colored plates and twenty-one clinical charts. New York: William Wood & Co., 1901. 221p. CtY-M; DLC; ICJ; NNNAM **00-0656**

CRAIG, Charles Franklin (*b.* 1872)
The malarial fevers, haemoglobinuric fever and the blood protozoa of man . . . illustrated by four colored plates, twenty-five clinical charts, and twenty-eight photomicrographs and drawings. New York: William Wood & Co., 1909. 477p. CtY-M; DLC; NNNAM; PU **00-0657**

CRAIG, Charles Franklin (*b.* 1872)
Importance to the army of diseases transmitted by mosquitoes and methods for their prevention. . . . Washington: The Association of Military Surgeons, 1910. 17p. DLC **00-0658**

CRAIG, Joseph D.
A consideration of some tendencies in modern medical education. Address before the Association of the Alumni of the Albany Medical College, May 3, 1904. [Albany? 1904?] 12p. NN **00-0659**

CRAIG, Maurice (1866-1935)
Psychological medicine. A manual on mental diseases for practitioners and students. Philadelphia: P. Blakiston, Son & Co., 1905. 449p. NNNAM; OCIM; PPC; PU **00-0660**

CRANDALL, Floyd M[ilford] (1858-1918)
How to keep well: an explanation of modern methods of preventing disease. . . . New York: Doubleday, Page & Co., 1903. 511p. DLC; NN; NNNAM; PU **00-0661**

CRANDON, Le Roi G[oddard] (*b.* 1873)
Surgical after-treatment. A manual of the conduct of surgical convalescence. Philadelphia: W. B. Saunders & Co., 1910. 803p. DLC; DNLM; PPC; PPJ **00-0662**

CRILE, George W[ashington] (1864-1943)
Experimental research into the surgery of the respiratory system. An essay awarded the Nicholas Senn Prize by the American Medical Association for 1898. 2nd ed. Philadelphia: J. B. Lippincott Co., 1900. 114p. DLC; PP; PPC; PU **00-0663**

CRILE, George W[ashington] (1864-1943)
An experimental and clinical research into certain problems relating to surgical operations; an essay awarded the Alvarenga Prize for 1901 by the College of Physicians of Philadelphia. . . . Philadelphia: J. B. Lippincott Co., 1901. 200p. DLC; PPC; PPJ; PU **00-0664**

CRILE, George W[ashington] (1864-1943)
Blood-pressure in surgery; an experimental and clinical research; the Cartwright Prize Essay for 1903. . . . Philadelphia and London: J. B. Lippincott Co., 1903. 442p. diags. DLC; DNLM; NNNAM; PPC **00-0665**

CRILE, George W[ashington] (1864-1943)
Hemorrhage and transfusion; an experimental and clinical research. . . . New York and London: D. Appleton & Co., 1909. 560p. tables, charts. DLC; NNC; NNNAM; PPC **00-0666**

CRILE George W[ashington] (1864-1943)
Phylogenetic association in relation to certain medical problems. . . . Ether day address, 1910. [Boston: Barta Press, 1910.] 41p. DLC; MBM **00-0667**

CROCKETT, M[ontgomery] Adams
. . . Gynecology. A manual for students and practitioners. . . . Philadelphia and New York: Lea Bros. & Co., [1900]. 368p. DLC; NNNAM; OCIM; PPC **00-0668**

CROFTAN, Alfred Careño (*b.* 1871)
Clinical urinology. . . . New York: William Wood & Co., 1904. 298p. CtY-M; dlc; NNNAM; PU **00-0669**

CROFTAN, Alfred Careño (*b.* 1871)
Clinical therapeutics; a handbook on the special treatment of internal diseases. . . . Chicago: Cleveland Press, 1906. 626p. DLC; NNNAM; OCIM; PU **00-0670**

CROFTAN, Alfred Careño (*b.* 1871)
Clinical urinology; a treatise on the urinary aspect of disease. . . . Chicago: Cleveland Press, 1907. 298p. DLC; ICJ; OCIM; PPC **00-0671**

CROFTAN, Alfred Careño (*b.* 1871)
Clinical therapeutics; a handbook on the special treatment of internal disease. . . . 2nd ed., rev. . . . Chicago: Cleveland Press, 1907. 626p. DLC; ICJ; NN; PPC **00-0672**

CROFTAN, Alfred Careño (*b.* 1871)
Clinical therapeutics; a handbook on the special treatment of internal disease. . . . 3rd ed., rev. . . . Chicago: Cleveland Press, 1910. 626p. DLC; ICJ; OCIM; PU **00-0673**

CROOK, Herbert Evelyn
High frequency currents: their production, physical properties, physiological effects, and therapeutical uses. New York: William Wood & Co., 1906. 206p. DLC; ICJ; NNNAM; PU **00-0674**

CROSSEN, Harry Sturgeon (*b.* 1869)
The diagnosis and treatment of diseases of women . . . with seven hundred illustrations. St. Louis: C. V. Mosby Medical Book & Pub. Co., 1907. 799p. DLC; ICJ; NNNAM; PU **00-0675**

CROSSEN, Harry Sturgeon (*b.* 1869)
Diagnosis and treatment of diseases of women. . . . 2nd ed., rev. and enl., with seven hundred and forty-four engravings. St. Louis: C. V. Mosby Co., 1910. 1025p. DLC; ICJ; OCIM; PPC **00-0676**

CROTHERS, Thomas Davison (1842-1918)
Morphinism and narcomaniacs from other drugs; their etiology, treatment, and medicolegal relations. . . . Philadelphia and London: W. B. Saunders & Co., 1902. 351p. DLC; MBM; NNNAM; PPC **00-0677**

CROTHERS, Thomas Davison (1842-1918)
The drug habits and their treatment; a clinical summary of some of the general facts recorded in practice. . . . Chicago: G. P. Engelhard & Co., 1902. 94p. DLC; OCIM **00-0678**

CRYER, Matthew H[enry] (*b.* 1840)
Studies of the internal anatomy of the face. Philadelphia: S. S. White Dental Mfg. Co., 1901. 176p. CtY-M; DLC; KU; PPC **00-0679**

CULBRETH, David Marvel Reynolds (1856-1943)
A manual of materia medica and pharmacology. Comprising all organic and inorganic drugs which are and have been official in the United States pharmacopoeia, together with important allied species and useful synthetics. . . . 2nd ed., enl. and thoroughly rev. With four hundred and sixty-four illustrations. Philadelphia and New York: Lea Bros. & Co., 1900. 885p. DLC; NN; OCLloyd; PPC **00-0680**

CULBRETH, David Marvel Reynolds (1856-1943)
A manual of materia medica and pharmacology. Comprising all organic and inorganic drugs which are or have been official in the United States pharmacopoeia, together with important allied species and useful synthetics, especially designed for students of pharmacy and medicine, as well as for druggists, pharmacists, and physicians. . . . 3rd ed., enl. and thoroughly rev. With four hundred and seventy-three illustrations. Philadelphia and New York: Lea Bros. & Co., 1903. 916p. DLC; NNNAM; PPC; PU **00-0681**

CULBRETH, David Marvel Reynolds (1856-1943)
A compend of materia medica . . . of the University of Baltimore. Baltimore: Fleet-McGinley Co., 1905. 96p. MdBJ-W; MdU-D; PU **00-0682**

CULBRETH, David Marvel Reynolds (1856-1943)
A manual of materia medica and pharmacology. Comprising all organic and inorganic drugs which are or have been official in the United States pharmacopoeia, together with important allied species and useful synthetics, especially designed for students of pharmacy and medicine, as well as for druggists, pharmacists, and physicians. . . . 4th ed., enl. and thoroughly rev. With four hundred and eighty-seven illustrations. Philadelphia and New York: Lea Bros. & Co., 1906. 976p. DLC; KU; PPC; PU **00-0683**

CULBRETH, David Marvel Reynolds (1856-1943)
A manual of materia medica and pharmacology. Comprising all organic and inorganic drugs which are or have been official in the United States pharmacopoeia, together with important allied species and useful synthetics. . . . 5th ed., enl. and thoroughly rev. With four hundred and eighty-seven illustrations. Philadelphia and New York: Lea & Febiger, 1910. 986p. DLC; OCLloyd; PPC; PU **00-0684**

CULLEN, Thomas Stephen (1868-1953)
Cancer of the uterus; its pathology, symptomatology, diagnosis, and treatment; also the pathology of diseases of the endometrium . . . with eleven lithographic plates and over three hundred coloured and black illustrations in the text; by Max Brödel and Hermann Becker. New York: D. Appleton & Co., 1900. 693p. DLC; NNNAM; PPC; PU
00-0685

CULLEN, Thomas Stephen (1868-1953)
Surgery of the liver: a series of liver cases in which it was necessary to remove a segment of the liver or to suture torn areas. [1907.] 12p. 11 illus. DLC; DNLM
00-0686

CULLEN, Thomas S[tephen] (1868-1953)
Adenomyoma of the uterus . . . illustrated by Herman Becker and August Horn. Philadelphia and London: W. B. Saunders Co., 1908. 270p. DLC; PPC; PU; PPJ
00-0687

CULLER, Joseph Albertus (1858-1937)
. . . The second book of anatomy, physiology and hygiene of the human body. . . . Philadelphia and London: J. B. Lippincott Co., 1904. 275p. DLC; NN; PPC; PU
00-0688

CULLER, Joseph Albertus (1858-1937)
. . . The third book of anatomy, physiology and hygiene of the human body. . . . Philadelphia and London: J. B. Lippincott Co., 1904. 364p. DLC; MB; NN; PU
00-0689

CULLER, Joseph Albertus (1858-1937)
. . . The second book of anatomy, physiology and hygiene of the human body. . . . Philadelphia and London: J. B. Lippincott Co., [1909]. 315p. DLC; MH; NN; PPC
00-0690

CULVER, Everett M.
A manual of venereal diseases. Being an epitome of the most approved treatment. By Everett M. Culver . . . and James R. Hayden. . . . Philadelphia: Lea Bros. & Co., 1900 [*c.* 1891]. 294p. DLC; GU; NNNAM; PPC **00-0691**

CUMSTON, Charles Greene (1868-1927)
Pregnancy complicated by suppuration of fibroids. [Detroit, 1900.] 4p. MB **00-0692**

CUMSTON, Charles Greene (1868-1927)
Injuries of the nerves due to fracture. [New York, 1900.] 7p. MB **00-0693**

CUMSTON, Charles Greene (1868-1927)
General remarks on the pathology and treatment of stricture of the urethra. [New York, 1900.] 27p. MB
00-0694

CUMSTON, Charles Greene (1868-1927)
General remarks on the pathology and symptomatology of acute pelvic suppurative processes in the female and their treatment by posterior colpotomy. Boston, 1900. 22p. MB
00-0695

CUMSTON, Charles Greene (1868-1927)
Prolapsus of the rectum in children. [Philadelphia, 1900.] 16p. MB **00-0696**

CUMSTON, Charles Greene (1868-1927)
Neoplasms of the thyroid gland. [Boston, 1900.] 11p. MB
00-0697

CUMSTON, Charles Greene (1868-1927)
The indications for operation in malignant neoplasms of the stomach. Boston: Damrell & Upham, 1901. 12p. MB
00-0698

CUMSTON, Charles Greene (1868-1927)
Lesions of the bladder during abdominal and vaginal hysterectomy. Boston: Damrell & Upham, 1901. 19p. MB
00-0699

CUMSTON, Charles Greene (1868-1927)
The pathology and treatment of bilocular stomach. With a report of two cases. [Philadelphia, 1901.] 30p. MB
00-0700

CUMSTON, Charles Greene (1868-1927)
A brief resume of the life and work of Ambroise Paré. With biographical notes on men of his time. Boston: Damrell & Upham, 1901. 44p. port. MB; MH
00-0701

CUMSTON, Charles Greene (1868-1927)
Fibroids and pregnancy. [New York, 1901.] 11p. MB
00-0702

CUMSTON, Charles Greene (1868-1927)
The surgical aspects of carcinoma uteri complicating pregnancy, labor, and the puerperium. [New York, 1902.] 26p. MB **00-0703**

CUMSTON, Charles Greene (1868-1927)
Intestinal invagination in infants and children with the report of a case successfully treated by laparotomy. Boston: Damrell & Upham, 1902. 16p. MB **00-0704**

CUMSTON, Charles Greene (1868-1927)
Notes on the life and writings of Geronimo Cardano. Boston: Damrell & Upham, 1902. 17p. MB; MH
00-0705

CUMSTON, Charles Greene (1868-1927)
The symptomatology, diagnosis, and treatment of carcinoma of the caecum, with a report of two cases. [Philadelphia, 1902.] 58p. illus. plates. MB **00-0706**

CUMSTON, Charles Greene (1868-1927)
. . . Henry de Mondeville, the man and his writings, with translation of several chapters of his works. . . . [Buffalo], 1903. 50p. ICU **00-0707**

CUMSTON, Charles Greene (1868-1927)
Chloride of ethyl as a general anesthetic. Boston: Old Corner Book Store, 1903. 16p. NcD **00-0708**

CUMSTON, Charles Greene (1868-1927)
The question of "justifiable homicide." Boston, 1907. 55p. MH-M **00-0709**

CUMSTON, Charles Greene (1868-1927)
A biography of Michel Servetus, the discoverer of pulmonary circulation. Boston: D. C. Heath & Co., 1907. 34p. DNLM **00-0710**

CUMSTON, Charles Greene (1868-1927)
The medical history of Edgar Allan Poe. . . . Boston, [1909]. 18p. RPB **00-0711**

CUMSTON, Charles Greene (1868-1927)
Benjamin Franklin from the medical viewpoint. [New York]: A. R. Elliott Publishing Co., 1909. 32p. MB **00-0712**

CUMSTON, Charles Greene (1868-1927)
Remarks on the history of forensic medicine from the Renaissance to the XIX century. New York: William Wood & Co., [1910?]. 15p. DNLM **00-0713**

CUNNINGHAM, Daniel John (1850-1909)
Manual of practical anatomy. . . . 3rd ed. . . . Philadelphia: J. B. Lippincott Co., 1903. 2 v. plates. DLC; NNNAM; OCIM; PU **00-0714**

CUNNINGHAM, Daniel John (1850-1909)
Imperial stereoscopic anatomy of the head and neck, by Professor D. J. Cunningham . . . David Waterston . . . and Professor M. H. Cryer . . . adapted to the use of the specialist on diseases of the brain and nervous system, the head surgeon, the ear, nose and throat specialist, the dentist, etc., etc. . . . New York City: Imperial Publishing Co., [1909]. DLC; PPC [102 cards in 3 cases. illus., mounted photos. The photographs consist of 100 stereograms, each mounted on card with descriptive text; the remaining two cards have titles to sections I-II. Accompanied by prospectus with table of contents.] **00-0715**

CUNNINGHAM, Daniel John, ed. (1850-1909)
Textbook of anatomy. . . . 3rd ed. New York: William Wood & Co., 1909. 1427p. DNLM; NNNAM; OCIM; PPC **00-0716**

CUNNINGHAM, R[ichard] H[oope] (*b.* 1865)
The preparation of aseptic catgut by means of formalin. 1900. [New York, 1895.] 2p. NN **00-0717**

CUNNINGHAM, R[ichard] H[oope] (*b.* 1865)
Aseptic formalin catgut. 1900. [New York, 1898.] 4p. NN **00-0718**

CURSCHMANN, Heinrich (*b.* 1846)
. . . Typhoid fever and typhus fever . . . ed., with additions by William Osler. . . . Authorized transl. from the German, under the editorial supervision of Alfred Stengel. . . . Philadelphia: W. B. Saunders & Co., 1901. 646p. col. plates. DLC; NNNAM; PPC; PU [Nothnagel's encyclopedia of practical medicine. (American ed.)] **00-0719**

CURTIN, Roland Gideon (1839-1913)
A study of ancient and modern secret medical fraternities. [Philadelphia, 1907.] 24p. DLC; DNLM; ICJ; PU **00-0720**

CURTIS, Edward (1838-1912)
Nature and health; a popular treatise on the hygiene of the person and the home. . . . New York: H. Holt & Co., 1906. 313p. NN **00-0721**

CURTIS, W[alter] G[ilman]
. . . Reminiscences, by Dr. W. C. Curtis, 1848-1900. For thirty years state quarantine surgeon for the port of Wilmington. . . . Southport, N.C.: Herald Job Office, [1905]. 64p. DLC; MB; NcD; NN **00-0722**

CUSHING, Harvey W[illiams] (1869-1939)
Acute diffuse gonococcus peritonitis. [Baltimore, 1900.] 6p. MdBJ-W **00-0723**

CUSHING, Harvey W[illiams] (1869-1939)
Thrombosis of carotid artery. [Baltimore, 1900.] 1 l. MdBJ-W **00-0724**

CUSHING, Harvey W[illiams] (1869-1939)
A comparative study of some members of a pathogenic group of bacilli of the hog cholera . . . type. [Baltimore, 1900.] 16p. MdBJ-W **00-0725**

CUSHING, Harvey W[illiams] (1869-1939)
Experimental and surgical notes upon the bacteriology of the upper portion of the alimentary canal, with observations on the establishment there of amicrobic state as a preliminary to operative procedures on the stomach and small intestine. [Baltimore, 1900.] 49p. MdBJ-W **00-0726**

CUSHING, Harvey W[illiams] (1869-1939)
Observations upon the origin of gall-bladder infections and upon the experimental formation of gall-stones. [Baltimore, 1900.] 4p. MdBJ-W **00-0727**

CUSHING, Harvey W[illiams] (1869-1939)
Concerning a definite regulatory mechanism of the vasomotor centre which controls blood pressure during cerebral compression. [Baltimore, 1901.] 4p. MdBJ-W **00-0728**

CUSHING, Harvey W[illiams] (1869-1939)
On routine determinations of arterial tension in operating room and clinic. [Baltimore, 1903.] 6p. MdBJ-W **00-0729**

CUSHING, Harvey W[illiams] (1869-1939)
The sensory distribution of the fifth cranial nerve. [Baltimore, 1904.] 30p. MdBJ-W **00-0730**

CUSHING, Harvey W[illiams] (1869-1939)
Perineal zoster. [Baltimore, 1904.] 1 l. MdBJ-W **00-0731**

CUSHING, Harvey W[illiams] (1869-1939)
Comparative surgery. Second series of reports. [Baltimore, 1906.] 71p. MdBJ-W **00-0732**

CUSHING, Harvey W[illiams] (1869-1939)
Dr. Garth: The kit-kat poet. [Baltimore, 1906.] 17p. MdBJ-W **00-0733**

CUSHING, Harvey W[illiams] (1869-1939)
Instruction in operative medicine. With the description of a course given in the Hunterian Laboratory of Experimental Medicine. [Baltimore, 1906.] 29p. MdBJ-W; MH **00-0734**

CUSHING, Harvey W[illiams] (1869-1939)
Technical methods of performing certain cranial operations. [Baltimore, 1908.] 20p. photo. ills. MdBJ-W
00-0735

CUSHING, Harvey W[illiams] (1869-1939)
The hypophysis cerebri clinical aspects of hyperpituitarism and of hypopituitarism. [Baltimore, 1909.] 6p. MdBJ-W
00-0736

CUSHING, Harvey W[illiams] (1869-1939)
Observations on experimentally induced choked disc. [Baltimore, 1909.] 7p. MdBJ-W **00-0737**

CUSHING, Harvey W[illiams] (1869-1939)
Is the pituitary gland essential to the maintenance of life? [Baltimore, 1909.] 2p. MdBJ-W **00-0738**

CUSHING, Harvey W[illiams] (1869-1939)
The functions of the pituitary body. Philadelphia, 1910. 12p. MdBJ-W **00-0739**

CUSHING, Harvey W[illiams] (1869-1939)
The special field of neurological surgery: five years later. [Baltimore, 1910.] 16p. MdBJ-W **00-0740**

CUSHING, Harvey W[illiams] (1869-1939), S. J. CROWE, and John HOMANS
Experimental hypophysectomy. [Baltimore, 1910.] 42p. MdBJ-W **00-0741**

CUSHNY, Arthur Robertson (1866-1926)
A textbook of pharmacology and therapeutics; or, The action of drugs in health and disease. . . . 2nd ed., rev. and enl. Illustrated with forty-seven engravings. Philadelphia and New York: Lea Bros. & Co., 1901. 782p. DLC; NNNAM; PPC; PU
00-0742

CUSHNY Arthur Robertson (1866-1926)
A textbook of pharmacology and therapeutics; or, The action of drugs in health and disease. . . . 3rd ed., rev. and enl.; illustrated with fifty-two engravings. Philadelphia and New York: Lea Bros. & Co., [1903]. 756p. DLC; NNNAM; OCIM; PU **00-0743**

CUSHNY, Arthur Robertson (1866-1926)
A textbook of pharmacology and therapeutics; or, The action of drugs in health and disease. . . . 4th ed., thoroughly rev. Illustrated with fifty-two engravings. Philadelphia and New York: Lea Bros. & Co., 1906. 752p. DLC; IU-M; NNNAM; PPC **00-0744**

CUSHNY, Arthur Robertson (1866-1926)
A textbook of pharmacology and therapeutics; or, The action of drugs in health and disease. . . . 5th ed., thoroughly rev., illustrated with sixty-one engravings. Philadelphia and New York: Lea & Febiger, 1910. 744p. DLC; IEN-M; PPC; PU
00-0745

CUTLER, Manasseh (1742-1823)
. . . An account of some of the vegetable productions, naturally growing in this part of America, botanically arranged by the Rev. Manasseh Cutler. . . . Cincinnati, O.: J. U. & C. G. Lloyd, 1903. 3-8; 396-493p. DLC; DNLM; ICJ; OCLloyd [Originally published in 1785] **00-0746**

CUTTEN, George B[arton] (*b.* 1874)
The psychology of alcoholism. New York: Scribner's Sons, 1907. 382p. MH; NN **00-0747**

CUTTER, Ephraim (1832-1917)
Food; its relation in health and disease, by Ephraim Cutter . . . and John Ashburton Cutter. . . . New York: The Gazette Publishing Co., 1907. 334p. DLC; ICJ; NN; NNNAM
00-0748

DA COSTA, Jacob Mendes (1833-1900)
Medical diagnosis, with special reference to practical medicine; a guide to the knowledge and discrimination of diseases . . . 9th ed., rev. Philadelphia and London: J. B. Lippincott Co., 1900. 966p. col. plates. DLC; NNNAM; OCIM; PPC
00-0749

DA COSTA, John Chalmers (1863-1933)
Modern surgery, general and operative . . . with 493 illustrations. 3rd ed., rev. and enl. Philadelphia and London: W. B. Saunders & Co., 1900. 1117p. col. plates. DLC; IU-M; NNNAM; PPC **00-0750**

DA COSTA, John Chalmers (1863-1933)
Modern surgery, general and operative. . . . 4th ed., rewritten and enl., with 707 illustrations, some of them in colors. Philadelphia, New York, London: W. B. Saunders & Co., 1903. 1099p. DLC; ICRM; MBM; PU **00-0751**

DA COSTA, John Chalmers (1863-1933)
Dickens's doctors; a paper read before the Philobiblon Club, May 28, 1903. Philadelphia: Philobiblon Club, 1905. 52p. MH; NN; PP; PU **00-0752**

DA COSTA, John C[halmers] (1863-1933)
Baron Larrey: a sketch. [Baltimore, 1906.] 19p; NN; PPC
00-0753

DA COSTA, John C[halmers] (1863-1933)
Modern surgery, general and operative . . . 5th ed., thoroughly rev. and enl., with 872 illustrations, some of them in colors. Philadelphia and London: W. B. Saunders & Co., 1907. 1283p. DLC; KyLoJM; NNNAM; PPC **00-0754**

DA COSTA, John C[halmers] (1863-1933)
Modern surgery, general and operative . . . 6th ed., thoroughly rev. and enl., with 966 illustrations, some of them in colors. Philadelphia and London: W. B. Saunders & Co., 1910. 1502p. DLC; MdU-D; NNNAM; PPC **00-0755**

DA COSTA, John C[halmers] (1871-1920)
Clinical hematology; a practical guide to the examination of the blood with reference to diagnosis. . . . Containing eight full-page colored plates, three charts, and forty-eight other illustrations. Philadelphia: P. Blakiston's Son & Co., 1901. 474p. DLC; ICJ; PPC; PU **00-0756**

DA COSTA, John C[halmers] (1871-1920)
Clinical hematology; a practical guide to the examination of the blood with reference to diagnosis . . . 2nd ed., rev. and enl., containing nine full-page colored plates, three charts, and sixty-four other illustrations. Philadelphia: P. Blakiston's Son & Co., 1905. 591p. DLC; NNNAM; OCIM; PU
00-0757

DA COSTA, John C[halmers] (1871-1920)
Opsonic index in diabetes mellitus. Philadelphia, 1907. 14p. PPJ **00-0758**

DA COSTA, John C[halmers] (1871-1920)
The Old Blockley Hospital; its characters and characteristics. . . . Chicago: American Medical Association, 1908. 6p. PU
00-0759

DA COSTA, John C[halmers] (1871-1920)
Principles and practice of physical diagnosis . . . with 212 original illustrations. Philadelphia and London: W. B. Saunders & Co., 1908. 548p. DLC; NNNAM; PPC; PU
00-0760

DA COSTA, John C[halmers] (1871-1920)
Principles and practice of physical diagnosis . . . with 212 original illustrations. 2nd ed. Philadelphia: W. B. Saunders & Co., 1910 [1911]. 557p. DLC; DNLM; NcD; PPC
00-0761

DAGGETT, Charles H.
Theory of pharmaceutical chemistry. . . . Philadelphia and New York: Lea & Febiger, 1910. 540p. DLC; ICJ; NN; PU
00-0762

DALAND, Judson
Observations upon leprosy occurring in Japan, Iceland and Norway. . . . [Philadelphia, 1903.] 8p. DLC
00-0763

DANA, Charles Loomis (1852-1935)
Text-book of nervous diseases; being a compendium for the use of students and practitioners of medicine . . . 5th ed. . . . New York: William Wood & Co., 1901. 633p. plates. DLC; MBM; NNNAM; PU **00-0764**

DANA, Charles Loomis (1852-1935)
Inebriety. A study of its causes, duration . . . and management. . . . New York: Wynkoop Hallenbeck Crawford Co., [1901]. 11p. NN **00-0765**

DANA, Charles Loomis (1852-1935)
Text-book of nervous diseases and psychiatry, for the use of students and practitioners of medicine . . . 6th rev. and enl. ed. Illustrated by two hundred and forty-four engravings and three plates in black and colors. New York: William Wood & Co., 1904. 690p. plates. DLC; NNNAM; PPC; ScCM
00-0766

DANA, Charles Loomis (1852-1935)
Text-book of nervous diseases and psychiatry, for the use of students and practitioners of medicine . . . 7th ed. Illustrated by two hundred and sixty-one engravings and three plates in black and colors. New York: William Wood & Co., 1908. 782p. plates. DLC; MBM; NNNAM; PPC **00-0767**

DARIER, Armand (*b.* 1854)
Ophthalmic therapeutics according to the most recent discoveries. . . . Transl. by Sidney Stephenson. Edited by Walter L. Pyle. Philadelphia: P. Blakiston's Son & Co., 1910. 440p. DLC; NNNAM; PPC; PPJ **00-0768**

DARLING, Samuel T[aylor] (1872-1925)
The relapsing fever of Panama. [1908.] 36p. charts, tables. DLC; MH **00-0769**

DARLING, Samuel T[aylor] (1872-1925)
Histoplasmosis: a fatal infectious disease resembling Kala-azar found among natives of tropical America. [1908.] 16p. DLC
00-0770

DARLING, Samuel T[aylor] (1872-1925)
Studies in relation to malaria. Washington: Government Printing Office, 1910. 38p. DLC; ICJ; NN; PU [At head of title: Isthmian Canal Commission]
00-0771

DAVENPORT, Francis Henry (*b.* 1851)
Diseases of women: a manual of gynecology, designed especially for the use of students and general practitioners. . . . 4th ed., rev. and enl. . . . With 154 illustrations. Philadelphia and New York: Lea Bros. & Co., 1902. 405p. DLC; NNNAM; PPC; PU
00-0772

DAVIES, Porter
The doctor's leisure hour; facts and fancies of interest to the doctor and his patient; Charles Wells Moulton, general editor; arranged by Porter Davies, M.D. Akron, O.: Chicago, [etc.]: The Saalfield Publishing Co., 1904. 352p. DLC; ICJ; IU-M; NN
00-0773

DAVIES, Porter
Doctors of the old schools; being curiosities of medicine and ancient practice, arranged by Porter Davies, M.D. Akron, O.; Chicago, [etc.]: The Saalfield Publishing Co., 1905. 251p. plates. DLC; DNLM; ICJ; OCIM **00-0774**

DAVIS, A[chilles] Edward (1866-1941)
The refraction of the eye; including a complete treatise on ophthalmometry; a clinical text-book for students and practitioners . . . with one hundred and nineteen engravings, ninety-seven of which are original. New York, London: The Macmillan Co., 1900. 431p. CtY-M; DLC; NNNAM; PU
00-0775

DAVIS, A[chilles] Edward (1866-1941)
Congenital absence of the iris (aniridia) in each eye. Report of a case. [New York, 1900?] 4p. CtY-M
00-0776

DAVIS, A[chilles] Edward (1866-1941)
Report of recovery of a case of hemorrhagic albuminuric retinitis. Remarks as to etiology and pathology. [New York, 1900?] 6p. CtY-M **00-0777**

DAVIS, A[chilles] Edward (1866-1941)
Eye, ear, nose, and throat nursing, by A. Edward Davis . . . and Beaman Douglass. . . . With 32 illustrations. Philadelphia: F. A. Davis Co., 1905. 318p. DLC; ICJ; NNC; PPC
00-0778

DAVIS, Andrew P. (*b.* 1835)
Neurology, embracing neuro-ophthalmology, the new science for the successful treatment of all functional human ills. Neuropathy, chiropractic, magnetism, suggestive therapeutics, phrenology and palmistry, as related to neuropathy. . . . Cincinnati: F. L. Rowe, 1905. 242p. DLC; ICJ; OCIM
00-0779

DAVIS, Andrew P. (*b.* 1835)
Neuropathy; the new science of drugless healing amply illustrated and explained, embracing ophthalmology, osteopathy, chiropractic science, suggestive therapeutics, magnetism, instructions on diet, deep breathing, bathing, etc. Advice to mothers—how to care for children—physical manipulations to cure chronic and acute disease. Many invaluable recipes for home use—instructions how to cure diseases without medicine, and some conditions where certain domestic remedies are useful. . . . Cincinnati, O.: F. L. Rowe, 1909. 715p. DLC; ICJ; OC **00-0780**

DAVIS, Charles H[enry] S[tanley] (1840-1917)
The self-cure of consumption without medicine, with a chapter on the prevention of consumption and other diseases. . . . New York: E. B. Treat & Co., 1904. 176p. DLC; ICJ; NNNAM; PU
00-0781

DAVIS, Charles H[enry] S[tanley] (1840-1917)
The voice as a musical instrument; with medical hints as to its proper training and culture. . . . Boston: O. Ditson Co.; New York: C. H. Ditson & Co.; [etc., etc.], 1907. 41p. illus., plates. DLC; ICJ; PP [First published in 1879]
00-0782

DAVIS, Charles H[enry] S[tanley] (1840-1917)
Consumption, its prevention and cure without medicine; with chapters on sanitation and prevention of other diseases. . . . 2nd ed., enl. New York: E. B. Treat & Co., 1908. 218p. CtY-M; DLC; NNNAM; PPC **00-0783**

DAVIS, David John (1875-1954)
. . . The bacteriology of whooping-cough. . . . Chicago, 1906. 36p. DLC **00-0784**

DAVIS, Edward Parker (*b.* 1856)
Obstetric and gynecologic nursing. . . . Philadelphia: W. B. Saunders & Co., 1901. 402p. col. plates. DLC; ICJ; NNNAM; PPC **00-0785**

DAVIS, Edward Parker (*b.* 1856)
Mother and child . . . Philadelphia: J. B. Lippincott Co., 1902. 264p. plates. DLC; NN; PPC; PU **00-0786**

DAVIS, Edward Parker (*b.* 1856)
A treatise on obstetrics, for students and practitioners. . . . 2nd ed., illustrated with 274 engravings and 39 plates in colors and monochrome. Philadelphia and New York: Lea Bros. & Co., 1904. 809p. DLC; NNNAM; PPC; PU
00-0787

DAVIS, Edward Parker (*b.* 1856)
Obstetric and gynecologic nursing. . . . 2nd ed.,rev. Philadelphia, London, [etc.]: W. B. Saunders & Co., 1904. 402p. plates. CU-M; DLC; NNC; PPC **00-0788**

DAVIS, Edward Parker (*b.* 1856)
Mother and child. . . . 2nd ed. Philadelphia: J. B. Lippincott Co., 1905. 270p. DLC; NNC; PPC; PU
00-0789

DAVIS, Edward Parker (*b.* 1856)
Obstetric and gynecologic nursing . . . 3rd ed., thoroughly rev. Philadelphia and London: W. B. Saunders & Co., 1908. 436p. plates. DLC; NNNAM; PPC; PU **00-0790**

DAVIS, Gwilym George (1857-1918)
The principles and practice of bandaging . . . illustrated from original drawings by the author. Philadelphia: P. Blakiston's Son & Co., 1902. 146p. DLC; NNNAM; PPC; PU
00-0791

DAVIS, Gwilym George (1857-1918)
Applied anatomy; the construction of the human body considered in relation to its functions, diseases, and injuries . . . with six hundred and thirty illustrations, mostly from original dissections and many in color, by Erwin F. Faber. Philadelphia: J. B. Lippincott Co., [1910]. 630p. DLC; NNNAM; OCIM; PPC **00-0792**

DAVIS, John S[taige] (1866-1933)
A syllabus of lectures on general pathology. . . . Charlottesville, Va.: G. W. Olivier, [1900]. 178p. DLC; ICJ
00-0793

DAVIS, John S[taige] (1866-1933)
The transplantation of free flaps of fascia. An experimental study. . . . [1910.] 25p. DLC **00-0794**

DAVIS, Nathan Smith (1871-1904)
History of medicine, with code of medical ethics. . . . Chicago: Cleveland Press, [1903]. 209p. DLC; IU-M; OCIM; PPC
00-0795

DAVIS, Nathan Smith, Jr. (1858-1920)
History of experimental investigations concerning the influence of alcohol and alcoholic drinks on the functions and structures of the living animal body, by American investigators. [Chicago, 1900.] 20p. DLC; ICJ [Prepared for the tenth annual meeting of the American Medical Temperance Association in Atlantic City, June 5-8, 1900.] **00-0796**

DAVIS, Nathan Smith, Jr. (1858-1920)
. . . Dietotherapy and food in health. . . . Philadelphia: P. Blakiston's Son & Co., 1901. 372p. DLC; NN; PPC; PU
00-0797

DAVIS, Nathan Smith, Jr. (1858-1920)
The treatment of pneumonia. [Chicago? 1902.] 11p. DNLM
00-0798

DAVIS, Nathan Smith, Jr. (1858-1920)
Consumption; how to prevent it and how to live with it. Its nature, its causes, its prevention, and the mode of life, climate, exercise, food, clothing necessary for its cure. . . . [1st ed.] Philadelphia: F. A. Davis Co., 1902. 143p. CtY-M; NNNAM; PPC; PU **00-0799**

DAVIS, Nathan Smith, Jr. (1858-1920)
Consumption; how to prevent it and how to live with it. Its nature, its causes, its prevention, and the mode of life, climate, exercise, food, clothing necessary for its cure. . . . 2nd ed., thoroughly rev. Philadelphia: F. A. Davis Co., 1908. 172p. DLC; NNNAM; PPC; PU **00-0800**

DAVIS, Nathan Smith, Jr. (1858-1920)
Dietotherapy and food in health. Edited by Solomon Solis Cohen. Philadelphia: P. Blakiston's Son & Co., [1909]. 372p. CtY-M; DLC; ICJ; PU **00-0801**

DAVIS, Thomas D[avis] (*b.* 1846)
Pioneer physicians of western Pennsylvania. Philadelphia, 1901. 8p. DNLM **00-0802**

DAWBARN, Robert Hugh Mackey (1860-1915)
The treatment of certain malignant growths by excision of the external carotids. . . . Philadelphia: F. A. Davis Co., 1903. 192p. CtY-M; DLC; PPC; PU **00-0803**

DAWBARN, Robert Hugh Mackey (1860-1915)
An aid to materia medica . . . 4th ed., rev. and enl., by Eden V. Delphey, M.D. New York: The Macmillan Co., 1908. 338p. DLC; OCLloyd; NNNAM; PU **00-0804**

DAYTON, Hughes (*b.* 1873)
. . . Practice of medicine. A manual for students and practitioners. . . . New York and Philadelphia: Lea Bros. & Co., [1905]. 324p. DLC;ICJ; NNNAM; PPC
00-0805

DEADERICK, William H[eiskell] (*b.* 1876)
A practical study of malaria. Philadelphia: W. B. Saunders & Co., 1909. 402p. col. plates. DLC; DNLM; PPJ; PU
00-0806

DEARBORN, Henry M. (1846-1904)
Diseases of the skin. Their symptomatology, etiology and diagnosis with special reference to principles of treatment including full indications for drug remedies. New York: Boericke & Runyon, 1903. 834p. DLC; ICJ; NNNAM; PPHa
00-0807

DEARBORN, Henry M. (1846-1904)
Diseases of the skin, with special reference to principles of treatment for the use of advanced students and general practitioners. . . . 3rd ed., rev., enl. and ed. by Frederick M. Dearborn . . . with one hundred and thirty-five illustrations, including ninety-eight full page engravings. New York: Boericke & Runyon, 1906. 655p. DLC; MBM; NNNAM; PU
00-0808

DEASON, J[ohn]
Practical bacteriology. . . . Kirksville, Mo.: Journal Printing Co., 1910. 50p. forms. DLC **00-0809**

DEAVER, John Blair (1855-1931)
A treatise on appendicitis. . . . 2nd ed., thoroughly rev. and considerably enl. . . . Philadelphia: P. Blakiston's Son & Co., 1900. 300p. col. plates. DLC; NNNAM; PPC; PU
00-0810

DEAVER, John Blair (1855-1931)
Surgical anatomy. A treatise on human anatomy in its application to the practice of medicine and surgery. . . . Philadelphia: P. Blakiston's Son & Co., 1901-1903. 3 v. NNNAM: OCIM; PPC; PU **00-0811**

DEAVER, John Blair (1855-1931)
Surgical anatomy of the head and neck . . . illustrated by 177 plates nearly all drawn from original dissections. Neck; mouth; pharynx; larynx; nose; orbit; eyeball; organ of hearing; brain; back of neck; cranium; scalp; face. Philadelphia: P. Blakiston's Son & Co., 1904. 770p. DLC; MBM; NNNAM; PPC
00-0812

DEAVER, John Blair (1855-1931)
Appendicitis; its history, anatomy, aetiology, pathology, symptomatology, diagnosis, prognosis, treatment, technique of operation, complications and sequels. . . . 3rd ed., thoroughly rev. and enl. Containing sixty-four full-page plates, eight of which are coloured. Philadelphia: P. Blakiston's Son & Co., 1905. 492p. DLC; NNNAM; OCIM; PPC
00-0813

DEAVER, John Blair (1855-1931)
Enlargement of the prostate; its history, anatomy, aetiology, pathology, clinical causes, symptoms, diagnosis, prognosis, treatment, technique of operations, and after-treatment, by John B. Deaver . . . assisted by Astley Paston Cooper Ashhurst . . . illustrated with 108 full-page plates and a coloured frontispiece. Philadelphia: P. Blakiston's Son & Co., 1905. 266p. DLC; MBM; NNNAM; PPC **00-0814**

DEAVER, John Blair (1855-1931)
Surgery of the upper abdomen . .. by John B. Deaver . . . and Astley Paston Cooper Ashhurst. . . . Philadelphia: P. Blakiston's Son & Co., 1909-13. 2 v. col. plates. DLC; NNNAM; PPC; PU
00-0815

DEBIERRE, Charles M[arie] (*b.* 1853)
Malformations of the genital organs of women. Transl. by J. Henry Simes. Philadelphia: P. Blakiston's Son & Co., 1905. 182p. 85 woodcuts. DLC; ICJ; MBM; PU
00-0816

DE CAMP, E. J. (*d.* 1910)
Nature's law of health and disease and the ladies' toilet; a concise up-to-date family medical work and ladies' companion. . . . Rochester, N.Y.: G. W. Winkelman, [1910]. 177p. plates. DLC; NNC **00-0817**

DE FORD, William H. (*b.* 1858)
Lectures on general anaesthetics in dentistry, advocating painless dental operations by use of nitrous oxid, nitrous oxid and oxygen, chloroform analgesia, ethyl chloride and somnoform. St. Louis: J. Nolde, [1908]. 297p. DLC; KyLoJM; MdU-D; NNC **00-0818**

DE GARMO, William Burton (*b.* 1849)
Abdominal hernia, its diagnosis and treatment. . . . Philadelphia and London: J. B. Lippincott Co., [1907]. 458p. DLC; NNNAM; PPC; PU **00-0819**

DELAFIELD, Francis (1841-1915)
A handbook of pathological anatomy and histology, with an introductory section on post-mortem examintions and the methods of preserving and examining diseased tissues, by Francis Delafield . . . and T. Mitchell Prudden. . . . 6th ed. . . . New York: William Wood & Co., 1901. 819p. col. plates. DLC; NNNAM; OCIM; PU **00-0820**

DELAFIELD, Francis (1841-1915)
Lectures on the practice of medicine, with cases and charts. . . . New York: J. T. Dougherty, [1903]. 2 v. DLC; ICJ; NNNAM; PPC **00-0821**

DELAFIELD, Francis (1841-1915)
A handbook of pathological anatomy and histology, with an introductory section on post-mortem examinations and the methods of preserving and examining diseased tissues, by Francis Delafield . . . and T. Mitchell Prudden. . . . 7th ed., with 13 full page plates and 545 illustrations in the text in black and colors. New York: William Wood & Co., 1904. 885p. col. plates. DLC; MBM; NNNAM; PPC
00-0822

DELAFIELD, Francis (1841-1915)
A text-book of pathology, with an introductory section on post-mortem examinations and the methods of preserving and examining diseased tissues, by Francis Delafield . . . and T. Mitchell Prudden. . . . 8th ed., with thirteen full-page plates and six hundred and fifty illustrations in the text, in black and colors. New York: William Wood & Co., 1907. 1067p. col. plates. DLC; NNNAM; PPC; ScCM **00-0823**

DE LEE, Joseph B[olivar] (1869-1942)
Notes on obstetrics, for the junior and senior classes. Northwestern University Medical School. Chicago: Press of Kenfield Publishing Co., 1904. 475p. DLC; ICJ; NNNAM
00-0824

DE LEE, Joseph B[olivar] (1869-1942)
Obstetrics for nurses. . . . Philadelphia, London, [etc.]: W. B. Saunders & Co., 1904. 460p. plates. DLC; NNNAM; PPC; PU
00-0825

DE LEE, Joseph B[olivar] (1869-1942)
. . . Obstetrics . . . with the collaboration of D. Roehler, M.D., and Herbert M. Stowe, M.D. . . . Chicago: The Year Book Publishers, 1906. 256p. plates. DLC: ICJ
00-0826

DE LEE, Joseph B[olivar] (1869-1942)
Obstetrics for nurses. . . . 2nd ed., thoroughly rev. and enl. Philadelphia and London: W. B. Saunders & Co., 1906. 510p. plates. DLC; IU-M; PPC; PU **00-0827**

DE LEE, Joseph B[olivar], ed. (1869-1942)
. . . Obstetrics . . . with the collaboration of Henry D. Roehler, M.D. and Herbert M. Stowe, M.D. . . . Chicago: The Year Book Publishers, 1907. 243p. plates. DLC: ICJ **00-0828**

DE LEE, Joseph B[olivar] (1869-1942)
Obstetrics for nurses. . . . 3rd ed., thoroughly rev. and enl. Philadelphia and London: W. B. Saunders & Co., 1908. 512p. plates. DLC; LNT-M; NNNAM; PPC **00-0829**

DENCH, Edward Bradford (1864-1934)
Ossiculectomy. New York, 1903. 23p. NN **00-0830**

DENCH, Edward Bradford (1864-1934)
Diseases of the ear; a text-book for practitioners and students of medicine . . . with fifteen plates and one hundred and fifty-eight illustrations in the text. 3rd ed., rev. and enl. New York and London: D. Appleton & Co., 1903. 718p. DLC; NNNAM; PPC; PU **00-0831**

DENCH, Edward Bradford (1864-1934)
Diseases of the ear; a text-book for practitioners and students of medicine . . . with nineteen plates and one hundred and fifty-eight illustrations in the text. 4th ed., rev. and enl. New York and London: D. Appleton & Co., 1909. 718p. DLC; MBM; NNNAM; PPC **00-0832**

DENISON, Charles (1845-1909)
The tuberculin test, and the need of a more complete diagnosis of tuberculosis. . . . [Chicago, 1900.] 8p. DLC **00-0833**

DENISON, Charles (1845-1909)
Educational and legislative control of tuberculosis, degenerative results of deficient ventilation. . . . [Chicago, 1900?] 15p. DLC **00-0834**

DENISON, Charles (1845-1909)
. . . Degenerative results of defective heredity. . . . [Denver?], 1900. 16p. DLC **00-0835**

DENISON, Charles (1845-1909)
Devitalized air toxaemia, a prime cause of tuberculosis. . . . [New York, 1901.] 24p. DLC; NNNAM **00-0836**

DENISON, Charles (1845-1909)
. . . Ten years' experience with the tuberculins. . . . [Asheville, N.C., 1901.] 8p. DLC **00-0837**

DENNIS, Frederic S[hepard] (1850-1934)
The history and development of surgery during the past century. [New York, 1905.] 86p. DNLM; NN [Text of an address before the International Congress of Arts and Sciences (St. Louis), September 1904] **00-0838**

DENTAL MEDICINE CO. (PHILADELPHIA)
Catalogue of dental pharmaceutical preparations, specialties and instruments. Philadelphia, [1900]. 19p. ICJ; NNNAM **00-0839**

DERCUM, Francis Xavier (1856-1931)
. . . Rest, mental therapeutics, suggestion. . . . Philadelphia: P. Blakiston's Son & Co., 1903. 332p. DLC; NN; PPC; PU **00-0840**

DETROIT PHARMACAL COMPANY
Catalogue of physicians' supplies, including drugs and chemicals . . . manufactured, imported and sold by Detroit Pharmacal Company. . . . Detroit, Mich.: Aldine Printing Works, 1900 [*c.* 1894.] 635p. DLC; ICJ; OCIM; NN **00-0841**

DEWEY, Edward H[ooker] (1837?-1904)
Chronic alcoholism: its radical cure without money, without price. [Meadville, Pa.] For the Author, 1900 [*c.* 1899]. 75p. DLC **00-0842**

DEWEY, Edward H[ooker] (1837?-1904)
The no-breakfast plan and the fasting cure. Meadville, Pa.: The Author, 1900. 207p. DLC **00-0843**

DEWEY, Edward H[ooker] (1837?-1904)
The true science of living. The new gospel of health, practical and physiological. Story of an evolution of natural law in the cure of disease, for physicians and laymen. How the sick get well; how the well get sick. Alcoholics freshly considered. Norwich, Conn.: Henry Bill Publishing Co., 1900. 323p. [*c.* 1895. *vel subseq.*] DLC **00-0844**

DEWEY, Willis Alonzo (1858-1938)
Practical homoeopathic therapeutics. . . . Philadelphia: Boericke & Tafel, 1901. 379p. DLC; ICJ; PPC; PPHa **00-0845**

DEWEY, Willis Alonzo (1858-1938)
Essentials of homoeopathic materia medica and homoeopathic pharmacy; being a quiz compend upon the principles of homoeopathy, homoeopathic pharmacy, and homoeopathic materia medica, arranged and compiled especially for the use of students of medicine. . . . 4th rev. ed. Philadelphia: Boericke & Tafel, 1908. 372p. DLC; NN; PPC; PPHa **00-0846**

DE WITT, Charles Howard (*b.* 1873)
A laboratory guide to histology. . . . Valparaiso, Ind.: C. H. De Witt, 1904. 88p. DLC **00-0847**

DE WITT, Charles Howard (*b.* 1873)
A laboratory guide and outlines in histology. Rev. ed. . . . Valparaiso, Ind.: C. H. De Witt, 1908. 174p. DLC: ICJ **00-0848**

DIBBLE, Frederick L.
Vagaries of sanitary science. . . . Philadelphia: J. B. Lippincott Co., 1900 [*c.* 1893]. 462p. DLC; ICJ; MH; NN **00-0849**

DIEFFENBACH, William Hermann (*b.* 1865)
Hydrotherapy; a brief summary of the practical value of water in disease, for students and practicians of medicine. . . . New York: Rebman Co., [1909]. 267p. plates. DLC; ICJ; NN; NNNAM **00-0850**

DIENST, George Elias (*b.* 1858)
What to do for the stomach; a careful arrangement of the most important symptoms in diseased conditions of the stomach and the remedy indicated in the cure of these symptoms. . . . Philadelphia: Boericke & Tafel, 1907. 202p. DLC; NN; PPC; PPHa **00-0851**

DIEUDONNÉ, Adolf (1864-1944)
Bacterial food poisoning: a concise exposition of the etiology, bacteriology, pathology, symptomatology, prophylaxis, and treatment of so-called ptomaine poisoning . . . transl. and ed., with additions, by Dr. Charles Frederick Bolduan. . . . Authorized translation. New York: E. B. Treat & Co., 1909. 128p. DLC; ICJ; NNNAM; PU **00-0852**

DITMAN, Norman Edward
Opsonins and vaccines in medicine and surgery [by] Norman Edward Ditman . . . in collaboration with Nathaniel B. Potter, M.D., and Ernest B. Bradley. . . . [Chicago: American Medical Association Press, 1908?] 35p. diags. DLC; ICJ; NN; PU **00-0853**

DOCK, George (*b.* 1860)
Sarcoma of the stomach. Read by title at the meeting of the Association of Americn Physicians, Washington, D.C., May 3, 1900. [n. p., 1900?] 8p. MH-M **00-0854**

DOCK, George (*b.* 1860)
Cancer of the stomach in early life, and the value of cells in effusions in the diagnosis of cancer of the serous membranes. Read before the Association of American Physicians at the meeting in Washington, May 4-6, 1897. [Philadelphia, 1900.] 14p. DNLM **00-0855**

DOCK, George (*b.* 1860)
A case of fatal epistaxis, from endothelioma of the nose, with a study of the blood. [Washington? 1900.] 12p. DLC **00-0856**

DOCK, George (*b.* 1860)
Outlines for the case taking, as used in the medical clinic of the University of Michigan. . . . Ann Arbor, Mich.: G. Wahr, [1902]. 31p. DLC; DNLM **00-0857**

DOCK, George (*b.* 1860)
A new case of chloroma with leucemia, with a study of cases reported since 1893. By George Dock and Alfred Scott Warthin. [1904.] 84p. DLC **00-0858**

DOCK, George (*b.* 1860)
The medical library of the University of Michigan. . . . Brooklyn, 1905. 9p. DLC **00-0859**

DOCK, George (*b.* 1860)
Medical considerations of gastric surgery. Read before the Yale Medical Alumni Association, New Haven, March 29, 1905. New Haven, Conn., 1905. 24p. CtY-M **00-0860**

DOCK, George (*b.* 1860)
Medical classics in medical meeting. [1906.] 7p. DLC **00-0861**

DOCK, George, ed. (*b.* 1860)
. . . Diseases of the heart, by Prof. Th. v. Jürgensen . . . Prof. L. v. Schrötter . . . Prof. L. Krehl. . . . Ed., with additions, by George Dock . . . authorized translation from the German, under the editorial supervision of Alfred Stengel. . . . Philadelphia and London: W. B. Saunders & Co., 1908. 848p. plates. DLC; NNNAM; PPC; PU [American ed., Nothnagel's encyclopedia of practical medicine] **00-0862**

DOCK, George (*b.* 1860)
Hookworm disease: etiology, pathology, diagnosis, prognosis, prophylaxis, and treatment, by George Dock . . . and Charles C. Bass . . . illustrated with forty-nine special engravings and colored plate. St. Louis: C. V. Mosby Co., 1910. 250p. DLC; DNLM; ICJ; PU **00-0863**

DOCK, L[avinia] L. (1858-1956)
Short papers on nursing subjects. . . . New York: M. L. Longeway, 1900. 57p. DLC; NNC; NNNAM; PU **00-0864**

DOCK, L[avinia] L. (1858-1956)
Text-book of materia medica for nurses. . . . 4th ed., rev. and enl. New York: G. P. Putnam's Sons, 1905. 330p. DLC; NNNAM; OCLloyd; PU **00-0865**

DOCK, L[avinia] L. (1858-1956)
Hygiene and mortality; a manual for nurses and others, giving an outline of the medical, social, and legal aspects of the venereal diseases. . . . New York: G. P. Putnam's Sons, 1910. 200p. DLC; ICJ; NNNAM; PU **00-0866**

THE DOCTOR says; a book of advice for the household, with practical hints for the preservation of health and the prevention of disease. Philadelphia: G. W. Jacobs & Co., [1909]. 342p. DLC; NN; PPC **00-0867**

DOLLEY, Sara R. A[damson] (1829-1909)
Address . . . at the second annual meeting of the Woman's Medical Society of New York State, held in Rochester, N.Y., March 11, 1908. [Rochester, N.Y.: Democrat & Chronicle Press, 1908.] 16p. DLC **00-0868**

DOMVILLE, Edward J[ames] (*b.* 1849)
Manual for nurses and others engaged in attending to the sick. . . . 8th ed., rev. With recipes for sickroom cookery. Philadelphia: P. Blakiston's Son & Co., 1904. 152p. DLC; ICJ; NN; PU **00-0869**

DOMVILLE, Edward J[ames] (*b.* 1849)
Manual for nurses and others engaged in attending to the sick. . . . 9th ed., rev. with recipes for sickroom cookery. Philadelphia: P. Blakiston's Son & Co., 1907. 152p. DLC; DNLM; NN; PU **00-0870**

DONAHOE, Margaret Frances
A manual of nursing. . . . New York: D. Appleton & Co., 1910. 489p. DLC; NNC; NNNAM; PPC **00-0871**

DORLAND, W[illiam] A[lexander] N[ewman] (1864-1956)
The American illustrated medical dictionary; a new and complete dictionary of the terms used in medicine, surgery, dentistry, pharmacy, chemistry, and the kindred branches, with their pronunciation, derivation, and definition. . . . With numerous illustrations and 24 colored plates. . . . Philadelphia and London: W. B. Saunders & Co., 1900. 770p. plates. DLC; MBM; NNNAM; PPC **00-0872**

DORLAND, W[illiam] A[lexander] N[ewman] (1864-1956)
Modern obstetrics; general and operative . . . with 201 illustrations. 2nd ed., rev. and enl. Philadelphia and London: W. B. Saunders & Co., 1901. 797p. plates. DLC; NNNAM; PPC;; PU **00-0873**

DORLAND, W[illiam] A[lexander] N[ewman] (1864-1956)
The American illustrated medical dictionary; a new and complete dictionary of the terms used in medicine, surgery, dentistry, pharmacy, chemistry, and the kindred branches, with their pronunciation, derivation, and definition. . . . 2nd ed., rev. Philadelphia and London: W. B. Saunders & Co., 1901. 770p. plates. CU-M; DLC; IU-M; PPC
00-0874

DORLAND, W[illiam] A[lexander] N[ewman] (1864-1956)
American pocket medical dictionary. . . . 4th ed., rev. and enl. Philadelphia and London: W. B. Saunders & Co., 1903. 566p. DLC; NNNAM; PPC; PU **00-0875**

DORLAND, W[illiam] A[lexander] N[ewman] (1864-1956)
The American illustrated medical dictionary; a new and complete dictionary of the terms used in medicine, surgery, dentistry, pharmacy, chemistry, and the kindred branches, with their pronunciation, derivation, and definition, including much collateral information on an encyclopedic character. . . . 3rd ed., rev. and enl. Philadelphia: London, [etc.]: W. B. Saunders & Co., 1903. 798p. DLC; IEN-M; LNT-M; PPC
00-0876

DORLAND, W[illiam] A[lexander] N[ewman], ed. (1864-1956)
American pocket medical dictionary . . . containing the pronunciation and definition of all the principal terms used in medicine and the kindred sciences, along with over 60 extensive tables. 5th ed., rev. and enl. Philadelphia and London: W. B. Saunders & Co., 1906. 578p. DLC; MBM; OCIM; PPC
00-0877

DORLAND, W[illiam] A[lexander] N[ewman] (1864-1956)
The American illustrated medical dictionary; a new and complete dictionary of the terms used in medicine, surgery, dentistry, pharmacy, chemistry, and the kindred branches, with their pronunciation, derivation, and definition, including much collateral information of an encyclopedic character. . . . 4th ed., rev. and enl. Philadelphia and London: W. B. Saunders & Co., 1906. 836p. plates. DLC; ICRM; NNNAM; PPC
00-0878

DORLAND, W[illiam] A[lexander] N[ewman], ed. (1864-1956)
American pocket medical dictionary . . . containing the pronunciation and definition of all the principal terms used in medicine and the kindred sciences, along with over 60 extensive tables. 6th ed., rev. and enl. Philadelphia and London: W. B. Saunders & Co., 1909. 598p. DLC; NNNAM; PPC; PU
00-0879

DORLAND, W[illiam] A[lexander] N[ewman] (1864-1956)
The American illustrated medical dictionary; a new and complete dictionary of the terms used in medicine, surgery, dentistry, pharmacy, chemistry, nursing, and kindred branches, with the pronunciation, derivation, and definition, including much collateral information of an encyclopedic character. . . . 5th ed., rev. and enl. Philadelphia and London: W. B. Saunders & Co., 1909. 876p. plates. CtY-M; DLC; NNNAM; OCIM; PPC
00-0880

DOTY, Alvah Hunt (*b.* 1854)
A manual of instruction in the principles of prompt aid to the injured; including a chapter on hygiene and the drill regulations for the hospital corps, U.S.A., designed for military and civil use. . . . 4th ed., rev. and enl. New York, [etc.] : D. Appleton & Co., 1902. 302p. plates. CtY-M; DLC; NNNAM; PU
00-0881

DOUGLAS, Charles (*b.* 1843)
A treatise on feeding and nursing the baby, for mothers and nurses. . . . Detroit, Mich.: Baby Book Co., 1901. 611p. col. plates. DLC; ICJ; OC **00-0882**

DOUGLAS, Charles (*b.* 1843)
Feeding rules for healthy infants. . . . Containing educational and record charts showing practical percentage feeding without laboratory assistance. Detroit, Mich.: Baby Book Co., 1906. 279p. DLC; ICJ; OCIM **00-0883**

DOUGLAS, James (1800-1886)
Journals and reminiscences of James Douglas, M.D., ed. by his son. New York: Priv. Printed, 1910. 245p. DLC; ICJ; NN; PPC **00-0884**

DOUGLAS, Richard (1860-1908)
Surgical diseases of the abdomen, with special reference to diagnosis. . . . Illustrated by 20 full page plates. Philadelphia: P. Blakiston's Son & Co., 1903. 883p. CtY-M; DLC; PPC; PU
00-0885

DOUGLAS, Richard (1860-1908)
Surgical diseases of the abdomen, with special reference to diagnosis. . . . illustrated by 20 full page plates. 2nd ed., rev. and enl., edited by Richard A. Barr. . . . Philadelphia: P. Blakiston's Son & Co., 1909. 897p. DLC; NNNAM; PPC; PU
00-0886

DOWD, J[ames] Henry
A practical treatise on simple and chronic specific urethritis. . . . Buffalo, N.Y.: A. W. Landsittel, 1901. 135p. col. plate. DLC; DNLM **00-0887**

DRAPER, Frank W[inthrop] (1843-1909)
A text-book of legal medicine. . . . Philadelphia, London, [etc.]: W. B. Saunders & Co., 1905. 573p. plates. DLC; NNNAM; PPC; PU **00-0888**

DRESSER, Horatio W[illis] (*b.* 1866)
Health and the inner life: an analytical and historical study of spiritual healing theories with an account of the life and technique of P. P. Quimby. New York: G. P. Putnam's Sons, 1906. 255p. DLC; ICJ; MH; NN **00-0889**

DRESSER, Horatio W[illis] (*b.* 1866)
A physician to the soul. New York: G. P. Putnam's Sons, 1908. 171p. DLC; MH; NN; PP **00-0890**

DREWRY, William Francis (1860-1934)
Commitment of the insane in the southern states. . . . [1900?] 8p. DLC **00-0891**

DREWRY, William Francis (1860-1934)
Evolution of psychiatry, or, Progress in the care and treatment of the insane. Raleigh, N.C.: Edwards & Broughton, [1904]. 48p. DNLM; NcD **00-0892**

DREWRY, William Francis (1860-1934)
Evolution of psychiatry, or, Progress in the care and treatment of the insane. [Richmond? Va., 1905?] 34p. DLC
00-0893

DREWRY, William Francis (1860-1934)
Historical sketch of the Central State Hospital and the care of the colored insane of Virginia, 1870-1905. . . . Richmond: E. Waddey Co., printers, [1905]. 18p. plates. DLC
00-0894

DREWRY, William Francis (1860-1934)
Correlation of the physician and the layman. Address of the president. . . . [Richmond, Va.: Williams Printing Co., 1908?] 31p. DLC; DNLM; NN **00-0895**

DREWRY, William Francis (1860-1934)
Care and condition of the insane in Virginia. . . . (Read at the 35th National Conference of Charities and Correction, Richmond, Va., May, 1908.] [1908.] 8p. DLC **00-0896**

DREYFUS, W[olfram] E., ed. (*b.* 1864)
The Hospital Formulary of the Department of Public Charities and the Department of Bellevue and Allied Hospitals of the City of New York. 6th rev. ed. New York, 1903. 160p. OCLloyd; NNNAM; NNU-M; PU **00-0897**

THE DRUGGISTS CIRCULAR
The modern materia medica. The source, chemical and physical properties, therapeutic action, dosage, antidotes and incompatibles of all additions to the newer materia medica that are likely to be called for on prescriptions. New York: The Druggists Circular, 1906. 306p. DLC; ICJ; NNNAM; OCLloyd **00-0898**

DUANE, Alexander (1858-1926)
A dictionary of medicine and the allied sciences. Comprising the pronunciation, derivation, and full explanation of medical, pharmaceutical, dental, and veterinary terms. . . . 3rd ed., enl. and thoroughly rev. With eight full page colored plates. Philadelphia and New York: Lea Bros. & Co., 1900. 646p. DLC; NNNAM; PPC; PU **00-0899**

DUANE, Alexander (1858-1926)
Listing's law. What does it mean and what is its practical value in diagnosis? [New York: The Knickerbocker Press, 1900?] 8p. DLC **00-0900**

DUANE, Alexander (1858-1926)
The nomenclature of ocular movements. [Chicago, 1900?] 4p. DLC **00-0901**

DUANE, Alexander (1858-1926)
Angio-neurotic oedema of the conjunctiva. [Chicago, 1900?] 1 l. DLC **00-0902**

DUANE, Alexander (1858-1926)
A dictionary of medicine and the allied sciences. . . . 4th ed., rev. with appendix. . . . Philadelphia and New York: Lea Bros. & Co., [1902]. 678p. col. plates. DLC; NNNAM; OCIM; PPC **00-0903**

DUBOIS, Paul (1848-1918)
The psychic treatment of nervous disorders. (The psychoneuroses and their moral treatment) . . . transl. and ed. by Smith Ely Jelliffe . . . and William A. White. . . . New York and London: Funk & Wagnalls Co., 1905. 466p. DLC; ICJ; NNNAM; PU **00-0904**

DUBOIS, Paul (1848-1918)
The influence of the mind on the body; translated from the 5th French ed. by L. B. Gallatin. New York: Funk & Wagnalls, 1908. 63p. MB; MH; NN; PU **00-0905**

DUBOIS, Paul (1848-1918)
The psychic treatment of nervous disorders (the pyschoneuroses and their moral treatment) . . . transl. and ed. by Smith Ely Jelliffe . . . and William A. White. . . . 6th ed., rev. New York and London: Funk & Wagnalls Co., 1909. 466p. DLC; ICJ; NNNAM; PU **00-0906**

DUBOIS, Paul (1848-1918)
Nervous states, their nature and causes. . . . Authorized translation by Edward G. Richards. New York: Funk & Wagnalls Co., 1910. 385p. CtY-M; DLC; NNNAM; PU **00-0907**

DUBOIS, Paul (1848-1918)
Self-control and how to secure it (L'éducation de soi-même); translated by Harry Hutcheson Boyd. New York: Funk & Wagnalls Co., 1910. 337p. DLC; OCIM; NN; PU **00-0908**

DUBOIS, Paul (1848-1918)
Reason and sentiment; an address delivered in the aula of the University of Berne, March 3, 1910 . . . authorized translation by Edward G. Richards. New York and London: Funk & Wagnalls Co., [1910]. 82p. DLC; ICJ; MB; PPC **00-0909**

DUDLEY, Emilius Clark (1850-1928)
The principles and practice of gynecology. For students and practitioners. . . . 3rd ed., rev. and enl. With 474 illustrations, of which 60 are in colors and 22 full-page plates in colors and monochrome. Philadelphia and New York: Lea Bros. & Co., 1902. 761p. DLC; NNNAM; PPC; PU **00-0910**

DUDLEY, Emilius Clark, ed. (1850-1928)
. . . Gynecology; ed. by Emilius C. Dudley . . . with the collaboration of William Healy. . . . Chicago: The Year Book Publishers, 1902. 212p. DLC; ICJ **00-0911**

DUDLEY, Emilius Clark (1850-1928)
The principles and practice of gynecology. For students and practitioners. . . . 4th ed., rev. With 419 illustrations in colors and monochrome, of which 18 are full-page plates. Philadelphia and New York: Lea Bros. & Co., 1904. 771p. DLC; NNNAM; OCIM; PPC **00-0912**

DUDLEY, Emilius C[lark], ed. (1850-1928)
. . . Gynecology, ed. by Emilius C. Dudley . . . and C. von Bachellé. . . . Chicago: The Year Book Publishers, [1905]. 224p. DLC; ICJ **00-0913**

DUDLEY, Emilius Clark, ed. (1850-1928)
. . . Gynecology, ed. by Emilius C. Dudley . . . and C. von Bachellé. . . . Chicago: The Year Book Publishers, 1908. 236p. DLC; ICJ **00-0914**

DUDLEY, Emilius Clark (1850-1928)
The principles and practice of gynecology. For students and practitioners. . . . 5th ed., rev. and enl. With 431 illustrations and 20 full-page plates in colors and monochrome. Philadelphia and New York: Lea & Febiger, 1908. 806p. DLC; MBM; NNNAM; PPC **00-0915**

DUDLEY, Emilius Clark, ed. (1850-1928)
. . . Gynecology, ed. by Emilius C. Dudley . . . and C. von Bachellé. . . . Chicago: The Year Book Publishers, 1909. 225p. DLC; ICJ **00-0916**

DUGAN, William James (*b.* 1869)
Manual of electro-therapeutics . . . with ninety-one illustrations. Philadelphia: F. A. Davis Co., 1910. 242p. plates. DLC; ICJ; NNNAM; PPC **00-0917**

DULLES, Charles Winslow (1850-1921)
Accidents and emergencies; a manual of the treatment of surgical and medical emergencies in the absence of a physician. . . . 6th ed., thoroughly rev. and enl., with new illustrations. Philadelphia: P. Blakiston's Son & Co., 1904. 209p. DLC; NN; PPC; PU **00-0918**

DULLES, Charles Winslow (1850-1921)
Accidents and emergencies; a manual of the treatment of surgical and medical emergencies in the absence of a physician. . . . 7th ed., thoroughly rev. and enl., with 44 illustrations. Philadelphia: P. Blakiston's Son & Co., 1909. 205p. DLC; MBM; NNNAM; PPC **00-0919**

DUNCAN, Thomas C[ation]
Children, acid, and alkaline. . . . The law of diet selection, contraria. The therapeutic law, similia. . . . Philadelphia: Boericke & Tafel, 1900. 148p. DLC; MH-M; PPC; PPHa **00-0920**

DUNGLISON, Richard James (1834-1901)
A new school physiology and hygiene, with special reference to the action of alcohol and narcotics. . . . New York, Cincinnati, [etc.]: American Book Co., [1908]. 336p. DLC; ICU; MB; NNNAM **00-0921**

DUNGLISON, Robley (1798-1869)
A dictionary of medical science. . . . 22nd ed., with appendix, thoroughly rev. and greatly enl., and with the pronunciation, accentuation, and derivation of the terms, by Richard Dunglison. . . . Philadelphia and New York: Lea Bros. & Co., 1900. 1376p. DLC; NNNAM; PPC; PU **00-0922**

DUNHAM, William Russell (*b.* 1833)
Biologic science. Vital force the only power and active principle that can operate the living human organism. Thought exercise for the nineteenth century. A criticism in the teachings of Prof. Rudolph Virchow of the University of Berlin, and Prof. Jacques Loeb of the University of Chicago. . . . Keene, N.H.: The Author, 1902. 50p. DLC; MH **00-0923**

DUNHAM, William Russell (*b.* 1833)
. . . Fundamental principles that persuade to a new education of medical science. . . . [Cambridge, U.S.A.]: The Author, 1907. 37p. DLC; MBM; MH **00-0924**

DÜRCK, Hermann (*b.* 1869)
Atlas and epitome of special pathologic histology. . . . Authorized transl. from the German; ed. by Ludvig Hektoen. . . . Circulatory organs; respiratory organs; gastro-intestinal tract. Philadelphia: W. B. Saunders & Co., 1900. 158p. 62 col. plates. DLC; DNLM; NNC; PPC **00-0925**

DÜRCK, Hermann (*b.* 1869)
Atlas and epitome of special pathologic histology. . . . Liver; urinary organs; sexual organs; nervous system; skin; muscles; bones. Edited, with additions, by Ludvig Hektoen. Philadelphia: W. B. Saunders & Co., 1901. 192p. 123 col. figs. on 60 plates. DLC; DNLM; PPJ; PU **00-0926**

DÜRCK, Hermann (*b.* 1869)
Atlas and epitome of general pathologic histology. . . . Edited, with additions, by Ludvig Hektoen. Philadelphia: W. B. Saunders & Co., 1904. 371p. 176 col. figs. on 80 lithographic plates. DLC; DNLM; PPC; PU **00-0927**

DUVAL, Mathias Marie (1844-1907)
Duval's artistic anatomy. Completely rev. . . . by A. Melville Paterson. New York: Funk & Wagnalls Co., 1905. 348p. DLC; NN; NNNAM; PPC **00-0928**

DWIGHT, Edwin Welles (*b.* 1863)
. . . Medical jurisprudence. A manual for students and practitioners. . . . Philadelphia and New York: Lea Bros. & Co., [1903]. 249p. DLC; ICJ; NNNAM; PPC **00-0929**

DWIGHT, Edwin Welles (*b.* 1863)
. . . Toxicology. A manual for students and practitioners. . . . Philadelphia and New York: Lea Bros. & Co., [1904]. 298p. DLC; NNNAM; PPC; PU **00-0930**

DWIGHT, Thomas (1843-1911)
A clinical atlas. Variations of the bones of the hands and feet. Philadelphia: J. B. Lippincott Co., 1907. 25p. 35 plates. DLC; ICJ; NNNAM; PU [The verso of each plate contains letterpress description of plate opposite.] **00-0931**

EALES, Irving James
Healthology (health study) in three parts. Part I. Practical dietetics. How, when and what to eat. Part II. History of the evolution of the fasting cure, healthopathy. Part III. History of the author's thirty-one days without food. . . . Healthopathy (the fasting cure, health treatment). . . . . London, Eng.: L. N. Fowler & Co.; [Belleville, Ill.: The Author], 1907. 211p. DLC **00-0932**

EARLE, Pliny (1809-1892)
The curability of insanity: a series of studies. Philadelphia: J. B Lippincott Co., 1900 [*c.* 1887]. 232p. DLC; MBM; NNNAM; PPC **00-0933**

EASTMAN, Crystal
Work-accidents and the law. . . . New York: Charities Publication Committee, 1910. 345p. ICU; MB; NIC; NN **00-0934**

EBERHART, Noble M[urray] (*b.* 1870)
Practical x-ray therapy. . . . Chicago: G. P. Engelhard & Co., 1907. 344p. ICJ; IU-M; MH; NN **00-0935**

EBERHART, Noble M[urray] (*b.* 1870)
A brief guide to vibratory technique. Chicago: G. P. Engelhard & Co., 1908. 124p. CtY-M; DNLM **00-0936**

EBERHART, Noble M[urray] (*b.* 1870)
Practical x-ray therapy. . . . 2nd ed., rev. and enl. Chicago: New Medicine Pulbishing Co., 1909. 256p. DLC; DNLM; ICJ **00-0937**

EBERHART, Noble M[urray] (*b.* 1870)
A brief guide to vibratory technique. 2nd ed., rev. and enl. Chicago: New Medicine Publishing Co., 1910. 160p. DLC; ICJ; PPC **00-0938**

EBERT, Albert Ethelbert (1840-1906)
The standard formulary; a collection of nearly five thousand formulas for pharmaceutical preparations, family remedies, toilet articles, veterinary remedies, soda fountain requisites, and miscellaneous preparations especially adapted to the requirements of retail druggists. 17th ed., rev. By Albert E. Ebert . . . and A. Emil Hiss. Chicago: G. P. Engelhard & Co., 1906. 500p. DLC; ICJ; OCLloyd; PU **00-0939**

ECCLES, William McAdam
Hernia, its etiology, symptoms and treatment. New York: William Wood & Co., 1900. 231p. DLC; ICJ; NN; PU
00-0940

ECCLES, William McAdam
The imperfectly descended testis; its anatomy, physiology and pathology. New York: William Wood & Co., 1903. 140p. DNLM; ICJ; IU-M; NNNAM **00-0941**

ECKELS, Howard S[amuel] (*b.* 1865)
The practical embalmer; a practical and comprehensive treatise on embalming, together with a complete description of the anatomy of the human body, designed to accompany Eckels' Anatomical aid, prepared by Howard S. Eckels. . . . Philadelphia, Pa.: H. S. Eckels & Co., Inc., [1903]. 196p. DLC; DNLM; ICJ; PU **00-0942**

ECKELS, Howard S[amuel] (*b.* 1865)
Sanitary science; a reference and text-book for the communicable diseases, disinfection and chemistry for the undertaker. . . . Philadelphia: G. F. Lasher, printer, 1904. 393p. plates. DLC; ICJ; PPF; PPL **00-0943**

ECKELS, Howard S[amuel] (*b.* 1865)
Derma surgery, with a complete catalogue of embalmers' supplies. Lawrenceburg, Ind.: Ohio Valley Casket Co., [*c.* 1904]. 317p. illus. ICJ; OCIM **00-0944**

ECKELS, Howard S[amuel], ed. (*b.* 1865)
The Eckels-Genung method and practical embalmer; a practical and comprehensive treatise on embalming, together with a complete description of the anatomy and circulation of the human body. Ed. by Howard S. Eckels . . . and Charles A. Genung. . . . Philadelphia, Pa.: H. S. Eckels & Co., Inc., [1906]. 248p. DLC; ICJ; PPL; PU **00-0945**

ECKLEY, William Thomas
Comments on anatomical nomenclature, by William T. Eckley . . . and Corinne B. Eckley. . . . Chicago: E. H. Colegrove, 1902. 129p. DLC **00-0946**

ECKLEY, William Thomas
Regional anatomy of the head and neck, for students and practitioners of dentistry, by William T. Eckley . . . and Corinne Buford Eckley. . . . With twenty plates in black and colors and thirty-six illustrations in the text. Philadelphia and New York: Lea Bros. & Co., [1902]. 240p. DLC; NNNAM; PPC **00-0947**

ECKLEY, William Thomas
A manual of dissection and practical anatomy. Founded on Gray and Gerrish. By William T. Eckley . . . and Corinne B. Eckley. . . . Illustrated with 220 engravings, 116 of which are colored. Philadelphia and New York: Lea Bros. & Co., 1903 [1902]. 408p. DLC; NNNAM; PPC; PU
00-0948

EDEBOHLS, George M[ichale] (1853-1908)
The cure of chronic Bright's disease by operation. . . . New York: William Wood & Co., 1901. 32p. DLC; NNNAM
00-0949

EDEBOHLS, George M[ichael] (1853-1908)
Renal decapsulation for chronic Bright's disease. . . . [New York?] 1903.] 29p. DLC; NNNAM
00-0950

EDEBOHLS, George M[ichael] (1853-1908)
The surgical treatment of Bright's disease. . . . New York: F. F. Lisiecki, 1904. 327p. 2 plates. DLC; NN; NNNAM **00-0951**

EDGAR, James Clifton (*b.* 1859)
The practice of obstetrics, designed for the use of students and practitioners of medicine . . . with 1221 illustrations, many of which are printed in colors. Philadelphia: P. Blakiston's Son & Co., 1903. 1111p. DLC; NNNAM; OCIM; PPC
00-0952

EDGAR, James Clifton (*b.* 1859)
The practice of obstetrics, designed for the use of students and practitioners of medicine. . . . 2nd ed., rev. With 1264 illustrations, including five colored plates and 38 figures printed in colors. Philadelphia: P. Blakiston's Son & Co., 1904. 1153p. DLC; MBM; NNNAM; PU **00-0953**

EDGAR, James Clifton (*b.* 1859)
The practice of obstetrics, designed for the use of students and practitioners of medicine. . . . 3rd ed., rev. With 1279 illustrations, including five colored plates and 38 figures printed in colors. Philadelphia: P. Blakiston's Son & Co., 1907. 1071p. DLC; IU-M; PPC; ScCM **00-0954**

EDMUNDS, Charles Wallis (1873-1941)
Laboratory guide in experimental pharmacology; directions for the course given in the University of Michigan, by Charles W. Edmunds . . . and Arthur R. Cushny. . . . Ann Arbor, Mich.: G. Wahr, [1905]. 246p. DLC; ICJ
00-0955

EDMUNDS, Charles Wallis (1873-1941)
. . . The physiological standardization of digitalis, by Charles Wallis Edmunds and Worth Hale. . . . Washington: Government Printing Office, 1909. 61p. DLC; DNLM
00-0956

EDWARDS, Arthur R[obin] (*b.* 1867)
Notes on therapeutics. . . . Chicago: A. W. Skelsey, [1901]. 82p. DLC; ICJ **00-0957**

EDWARDS, Arthur R[obin] (*b.* 1867)
A treatise on the principles and practice of medicine . . . illustrated with 101 engravings and 19 plates. Philadelphia and New York: Lea Bros. & Co., 1907. 1328p. DLC; NNNAM; PPC; PU **00-0958**

EDWARDS, Arthur R[obin] (*b.* 1867)
A treatise on the principles and practice of medicine . . . 2nd and thoroughly rev. ed., illustrated with 100 engravings and 21 plates. New York and Philadelphia: Lea & Febiger, 1909. 1257p. DLC; MBM; NNNAM; PPC
00-0959

EDWARDS, William A[loysius], ed. (*b.* 1860)
Diseases of children, medical and surgical, the articles written especially for the work by American, British, and Canadian authors. . . . A supplement to Keating's Cyclopaedia of the diseases of children. . . . Philadelphia and London: J. B. Lippincott Co., [1901]. 1368p. col. plates. DLC; NNNAM; PPC; PU **00-0960**

EGBERT, Seneca (*b.* 1863)
A manual of hygiene and sanitation. . . . 2nd ed., enl. and thoroughly rev. . . . Philadelphia and New York: Lea Bros. & Co., 1900. 435p. DLC: MBM; NNNAM; PPC
00-0961

EGBERT, Seneca (*b.* 1863)
A manual of hygiene and sanitation. . . . 3rd ed., enl. and thoroughly rev. Illustrated with 86 engravings. Philadelphia and New York: Lea Bros. & Co., [1903]. 473p. DLC; NNNAM; PPC; PU **00-0962**

EGBERT, Seneca (*b.* 1863)
A manual of hygiene and sanitation. . . . 4th ed., enl. and thoroughly rev. Illustrated with 93 engravings. Philadelphia and New York: Lea Bros. & Co., 1907. 498p. DLC; IU-M; NNNAM; PPC **00-0963**

EGBERT, Seneca (*b.* 1863)
A manual of hygiene and sanitation. . . . 5th ed., enl. and thoroughly rev. Illustrated with 97 engravings. Philadelphia and New York: Lea & Febiger, 1910. 508p. DLC; IEN-M; NNNAM; PPC **00-0964**

EICHBERG, Louis Robert (*b.* 1879)
. . . Catarrh, its cause, treatment and cure. . . . New York: Laymen's Medical Publishing Co., [1900]. 76p. DLC: NN; NNNAM **00-0965**

EICHHORST, Hermann Ludwig (1849-1921)
A text-book of the practice of medicine . . . authorized transl. from the German, edited by Augustus A. Eshner. . . . Philadelphia and London: W. B. Saunders & Co., 1901. 2 v. DLC; MBM; NNNAM; PPC **00-0966**

EINHORN, Max (1862-1953)
Diseases of the intestines; a text-book for practitioners and students of medicine. . . . New York: William Wood & Co., 1900. 391p. DLC; ICJ; NNNAM; PPC **00-0967**

EINHORN, Max (1862-1953)
A new case of syphilitic tumor of the stomach. . . . [Philadelphia? 1902?] 3p. DLC **00-0968**

EINHORN, Max (1862-1953)
Remarks on achylia gastrica and pernicious anaemia. . . . New York: William Wood & Co., [1903]. 18p. DLC; NNNAM **00-0969**

EINHORN, Max (1862-1953)
Cardioptosis and its association with floating liver. . . . New York: William Wood & Co., [1903]. 14p. DLC; NNNAM **00-0970**

EINHORN, Max (1862-1953)
Diseases of the stomach; a text-book for practitioners and students . . . 3rd rev. ed. New York: William Wood & Co., 1903. 534p. DLC; NNNAM; OCIM; PPC **00-0971**

EINHORN, Max (1862-1953)
The treatment of gastric and duodenal haemorrhages. . . . [New York, 1903.] 10p. DLC **00-0972**

EINHORN, Max (1862-1953)
Diseases of the intestines; a text-book for practitioners and students of medicine . . . 2nd, rev. ed. New York: William Wood & Co., 1904. 397p. DLC; MBM; NNNAM; PPC **00-0973**

EINHORN, Max (1862-1953)
Practical problems of diet and nutrition. . . . New York: William Wood & Co., 1905. 64p. DLC; NN; NNNAM **00-0974**

EINHORN, Max (1862-1953)
Diseases of the stomach; a text-book for practitioners and students . . . 4th rev. ed. New York: William Wood & Co., 1906. 559p. DLC; NNNAM; OCIM; PU **00-0975**

EISENDRATH, Daniel N[athan] (*b.* 1867)
A text-book of clinical anatomy for students and practitioners. . . . Philadelphia, New York, [etc.]: W. B. Saunders & Co., 1903. 515p. col. plates. DLC; NNNAM; PPC; PU **00-0976**

EISENDRATH, Daniel N[athan] (*b.* 1867)
A text-book of clinical anatomy, for students and practitioners. . . . 2nd ed., thoroughly rev. Philadelphia and London: W. B. Saunders & Co., 1907. 535p. CtY-M; DLC; NNNAM; PPC **00-0977**

EISENDRATH, Daniel N[athan] (*b.* 1867)
Surgical diagnosis . . . with four hundred and eighty-two original illustrations, fifteen of them in colors. Philadelphia and London: W. B. Saunders & Co., 1907. 776p. DLC; NNNAM; PPC; PPJ **00-0978**

EISENDRATH, Daniel N[athan] (*b.* 1867)
Surgical diagnosis . . . 2nd ed., thoroughly rev. and enl., with 574 original illustrations, 25 of them in colors. Philadelphia and London: W. B. Saunders & Co., 1909. 885p. DLC; IU-M; NNNAM; PPC **00-0979**

ELIOT, Charles W[illiam] (1834-1926)
The fruits of medical research with the aid of anesthesia and asepticism. [Boston: Barta Co., 1910.] 15p. MH **00-0980**

ELLINGWOOD, Finley (1852-1920)
A systematic treatise on materia medica and therapeutics with reference to the most direct action of drugs. . . . With a condensed consideration of pharmacy and pharmacognosy by Prof. John Uri Lloyd. . . . 5th ed. Chicago: Chicago Medical Times Publishing Co., 1905. 811p. DLC; OCLloyd **00-0981**

ELLINGWOOD, Finley (1852-1920)
A manual for the eclectic treatment of disease, designed for the many students and practitioners who are now diligently searching for knowledge of the most direct action of drugs, as applied to specific conditions of disease. . . . Chicago: Chicago Medical Times Publising Co., 1906-07. 2 v. DLC; OCLloyd; NNNAM **00-0982**

ELLIOTT, Charles Sinclaire
Electro-therapeutics and X-rays. . . . Philadelphia, Pa.: Boericke & Tafel, 1900. 349p. DLC; PPC **00-0983**

ELLIS, George V[iner] (1812-1900)
Demonstrations of anatomy being a guide to the knowledge of the human body by dissection. [12th ed.] New York: William Wood & Co., 1906. 851p. DLC; IJC; PPC **00-0984**

ELLIS, Havelock (1859-1939)
. . . The evolution of modesty; the phenomena of sexual periodicity; auto-erotism. . . . Philadelphia, New York, [etc.]: The F. A. Davis Co., 1900. 275p. DLC; MB: NIC; NN **00-0985**

ELLIS, Havelock (1859-1939)
. . . Sexual inversion. . . . Philadelphia: F. A. Davis Co., 1901. 272p. DLC; MH; NN; PU **00-0986**

ELLIS, Havelock (1859-1939)
. . . Analysis of the sexual impulse; love and pain; the sexual impulse in women. . . . Philadelphia: F. A. Davis Co., 1903. 266p. DLC; MB: NIC; NN **00-0987**

ELLIS, Havelock (1859-1939)
. . . Sexual selection in man: I. Touch. II. Smell. III. Hearing. IV. Vision. . . . Philadelphia: F. A. Davis Co., 1905. 270p. DLC; ICU; MH; NN **00-0988**

ELLIS, Havelock (1859-1939)
. . . Erotic symbolism; the mechanism of detumescence; the psychic state of pregnancy. . . . Philadelphia: F. A. Davis Co., 1906. 285p. DLC; ICJ; ICU; NN **00-0989**

ELLIS, Havelock (1859-1939)
. . . The evolution of modesty, the phenomena of sexual periodicity, auto-erotism . . . 3rd ed., rev. and enl. Philadelphia: F. A. Davis Co., 1910. 352p. DLC; MH; NNC; NN **00-0990**

ELLIS, Havelock (1859-1939)
. . . Sex in relation to society. . . . Philadelphia: F. A. Davis Co., 1910. 656p. DLC; ICU; MH; NN **00-0991**

EMERSON, Charles Phillips (1872-1928)
Clinical diagnosis; a text-book of clinical microscopy and clinical chemistry for medical students, laboratory workers, and practitioners of medicine. . . . Philadelphia and London: J. B. Lippincott Co., [1906]. 641p. plates. DLC; NNNAM; PPC; PU **00-0992**

EMERSON, Charles Phillips (1872-1928)
Clinical diagnosis; a text-book of clinical microscopy and clinical chemistry for medical students, laboratory workers, and practitioners of medicine. . . . 2nd ed. Philadelphia and London: J. B. Lippincott Co., 1908. 686p. plates. DLC; MBM; NNNAM; PPC **00-0993**

EMERSON, Charles Phillips (1872-1928)
Essentials of medicine; a text-book of medicine, for students beginning a medical course, for nurses, and for all others interested in the care of the sick . . . illustrated by the author. Philadelphia and London: J. B. Lippincott Co., [1908]. 383p. DLC; ICJ; PPC; PU **00-0994**

EMERSON, Robert Leonard (*b.* 1872)
Legal medicine and toxicology. . . . New York and London: D. Appleton & Co., 1909. 593p. col. plates. DLC; ICJ; NNNAM; PU **00-0995**

EMERY, Walter d'Este (1870-1923)
Handbook of bacteriological diagnosis for practitioners, including instructions for the clinical examination of the blood. . . . Philadelphia: P. Blakiston's Son & Co., 1902. 215p. col. plates. DLC; DNLM; PPC; PU **00-0996**

EMERY, Walter d'Este (1870-1923)
Immunity and specific therapy. With illustrations. New York: P. B. Hoeber, 1909. 448p. 71 illus. incl. diags. ICJ; NN; PPJ **00-0997**

[EMMETT, Thoams Addis] (1828-1919)
The birthday dinner to Thomas Addis Emmet given by his professional friends at Delmonico's, New York, May 29, 1905. With an autobiographical narrative. New York: Bradstreet Press, 1905. 176p. DLC; NN [16 photolithographs on Japan paper, mostly of individual participants] **00-0997A**

ESHNER, Augustus A[dolph] (*b.* 1862)
A possible second attack of acute anterior poliomyelitis in the same patient. [Read before the American Neurological Assoication, May 4, 1910.] New York: William Wood & Co., [1910]. 12p. NN **00-0998**

ESHNER, Augustus A[dolph] (*b.* 1862)
The treatment of aneurysm of the aorta by the introduction of wire and the passage of a galvanic current. [Philadelphia, 1910.] 10p. NN **00-0999**

ESMARCH, Friedrich von (1823-1908)
Surgical technic; a text-book on operative surgery, by Fr. von Esmarch . . . and E. Kowalzig . . . transl. by Professor Ludwig H. Grau . . . and William N. Sullivan . . . edited by Nicholas Senn. . . . With fourteen hundred and ninety-seven Illustrations and fifteen colored plates. New York: The Macmillan Co.; London: Macmillan & Co., 1901. 866p. DLC; NNNAM; OCIM **00-1000**

ESSIG, Charles James, ed. (1841-1901)
The American text-book of prosthetic dentistry. In contributions by eminent authorities. . . . 2nd ed., rev. and enl. Illustrated with 1089 engravings. Philadelphia and New York: Lea Bros. & Co., 1900 817p. DLC; MBM; NNNAM; PPC **00-1001**

ESSIG, Charles James (1841-1901)
Dental metallurgy: a manual for the use of dental students and practitioners. . . . Revised by Augustus Koenig . . . 4th ed., rev. and enl. . . . Philadelphia and New York: Lea Bros. & Co., 1904. 286p. DLC; MdU-D; PPC; PU **00-1002**

ESSIG, Charles James (1841-1901)
Dental metallurgy: a manual for the use of dental students and practitioners. By Charles J. Essig . . . and Augustus Koenig . . . 5th ed., rev. and enl. Illustrated with 76 engravings. Philadelphia and New York: Lea Bros. & Co., 1904. 318p. DLC; MdU-D; NNNAM; PPC **00-1003**

ESSIG, Charles James (1841-1901)
Dental metallurgy: a manual for the use of dental students and practitioners. By Charles J. Essig . . . and Augustus Koenig . . . 6th ed., rev. and enl. Illustrated with 77 engravings. Philadelphia and New York: Lea & Febiger, 1909. 355p. DLC; MBM; NNNAM; PU **00-1004**

ESTES, William Lawrence (*b.* 1855)
The treatment of fractures. . . . New York: International Journal of Surgery Co., [1900]. 216p. DLC; ICJ; NNNAM; PPC **00-1005**

EVANS, David James (*b.* 1868)
. . . Obstetrics. A manual for students and practitioners. . . . illustrated with one hundred and forty-nine engravings. Philadelphia and New York: Lea Bros. & Co., [1900]. 430p. DLC; NNNAM; PPC; PU **00-1006**

EVANS, David James (*b.* 1868)
Obstetrics. A manual for students and practitioners . . . 2nd ed., rev. and enl. Illustrated with one hundred and seventy-two engravings. Philadelphia and New York: Lea & Febiger, 1909. 440p. DLC; NNNAM; OCIM; PPC
00-1007

EVANS, George (1844-1942)
A practical treatise on artificial crown- and bridge-work and procelain dental art. . . . 6th ed., rev. With 651 illustrations. Philadelphia: The S. S. White Dental Mfg. Co., 1900. 367p. DLC; MdU-D; PPC **00-1008**

EVANS, George (1844-1942)
A practical treatise on artificial crown-, bridge-, and porcelain work . . . 7th ed., rev. and enl. With 754 illustrations. Philadelphia: The S. S. White Dental Mfg. Co., 1905. 448p. DLC; PPC; PU **00-1009**

EWING, Arthur Eugene (1855-1929)
An operation for atrophic entropion, especially of the lower lid. . . . [Boston? 1900?] 4p. plate. DLC
00-1010

EWING, James (1866-1943)
Clinical pathology of the blood; a treatise on the general principles and special applications of hematology. . . . Illustrated with thirty engravings, and fourteen colored plates drawn by the author. Philadelphia and New York: Lea Bros. & Co., 1901. 432p. DLC; MBM; PPC; PU
00-1011

EWING, James (1866-1943)
Clinical pathology of the blood; a treatise on the general principles and special applications of hematology. . . . 2nd ed., rev. and enl. Illustrated with forty-three engravings, and eighteen colored plates drawn by the author. New York and Philadelphia: Lea Bros. & Co., 1903. 495p. DLC; IU-M; NNNAM; PPC **00-1012**

EYRE, John William Henry (1869-1944)
The elements of bacteriological technique; a laboratory guide for the medical, dental, and technical student. . . . With 170 illustrations. Philadelphia: W. B. Saunders & Co., 1902. 371p. DLC; MdU-D; NNNAM; PPC **00-1013**

FAHNSTOCK, Joseph C.
A manual of homoeopathic materia medica. . . . Piqua, O.: The Author, 1901. 264p. DLC; ICJ; PPHa
00-1014

FANTUS, Bernard (1874-1940)
A laboratory manual and syllabus of lectures on pharmacognosy, pharmacy and prescription writing. . . . Chicago, Ill., 1902. 516p. DLC; ICJ; PPC **00-1015**

FANTUS, Bernard (1874-1940)
Essentials of prescription-writing. . . . Chicago: Chicago Medical Book Co., 1906. 136p. DLC; ICJ; PPJ
00-1016

FANTUS, Bernard (1874-1940)
A text book on prescription-writing and pharmacy, with practice in prescription writing, laboratory exercises in pharmacy and a reference list of the official drugs, especially designed for medical students. . . . 2nd ed., thoroughly rev. and adapted to the eighth (1905) edition of the United States pharmacopoeia. Chicago: Chicago Medical Book Co., 1906. 404p. DLC; DNLM; ICJ; PPC **00-1017**

FARMACOPOEA de los Estados Unidos de América. Octava revision decenal. Autorizada por la Convención de la farmacopea de los Estados Unidos, reunida en Washington el año 1900 A.D. Rev. por el comité de revisión y publicada por la junta directiva. Oficial desde septiembre 1 de 1905 incluyente adiciones y correcciones hasta 1 de junio 1907. Nueva York: American Druggist Publishing Co., [1909]. 715p. DLC; ICJ OCLloyd **00-1018**

FARRINGTON, Ernest Albert (1847-1885)
A clinical materia medica; being a course of lectures delivered at the Hahnemann Medical College, of Philadelphia. . . . Reported phonographically by Clarence Bartlett, M.D., with a memorial sketch of the author, by Aug. Korndoerfer, M.D. 4th ed., rev. and enl. by Harvey Farrington, M.D. Philadelphia: Boericke & Tafel, 1908. 826p. DLC; ICJ; PPC; PPHa
00-1019

FARRINGTON, Ernest Albert (*b.* 1880)
The relation of the physical body to mental subnormality. [n. p., 1908.] 8p. DLC **00-1020**

FARRINGTON, Ernest Albert (*b.* 1880)
The role of systematic motor and sensory training in certain mental diseases of children. . . . [New York, 1909?] 8p. DLC
00-1021

FAUGHT, Francis Ashley (*b.* 1881)
Essentials of laboratory diagnosis, designed for students and practitioners . . . containing an indican scale in colors, six full-page plates and numerous engravings in the text. Philadelphia: F. A. Davis Co., 1909. 309p. plates. DLC; NNNAM; OCIM; PPC **00-1022**

FAUGHT, Francis Ashley (*b.* 1881)
The sphygmomanometer and its practical application, prepared for studens and practitioners of medicine. . . . Philadelphia: G. P. Pilling & Son Co., 1909. 60p. IU-M
00-1023

FAUGHT, Francis Ashley (*b.* 1881)
Essentials of laboratory diagnosis designed for students and practitioners . . . containing an indican scale in colors; eight full-page plates and numerous engravings in the text. 2nd rev. ed. Philadelphia: F. A. Davis Co., 1910. 336p. plates. DLC; MBM; NNNAM; PPC **00-1024**

FAUGHT, L[uther] Ashley (*b.* 1857)
Some studies of dental education in the United States . . . read before the Central Dental Association of Northern New Jersey, Nov. 15, 1897. 1900 [1897]. 11p. DLC
00-1025

FAULKNER, Richard B[iddle] (*b.* 1853)
Tonsil research. New York: William Wood & Co., 1910. 14p. DLC; NN **00-1026**

FAY, Edward A[llen] (1843-1923)
Marriages of the deaf in America. An inquiry concerning the results of marriages of the deaf. Washington, D.C.: Gibson Bros., Printers, 1900 [*c.* 1898]. 527p. DLC; ICJ; MH; NN
00-1027

FEIDLER, Francis J[ohn] (*b.* 1851)
The household osteopath, written for sick people. New York: Broadway Publishing Co., [1906]. 211p. DLC; NN
00-1028

FEIDLER, Francis J[ohn] (*b.* 1851)
Osteopathic first aids to the sick; written for the sick people. New York: Broadway Publishing Co., [1906]. 211p. DLC; NN **00-1029**

FELTER, Henry Wickes (1865-1927)
History of the Eclectic Medical Institute, Cincinnati, Ohio, 1845-1902; including the Worthington Medical College (1830-1842), the Reformed Medical School of Cincinnati (1842-1845), and the Eclectic College of Medicine (1856-1859), with biographical sketches of members of the various faculties and list of graduates arranged alphabetically and by classes. . . . Cincinnati, Ohio: [Published for the Alumni Association of the Eclectic Medical Institute], 1902. 203p. DLC; ICJ; OCLloyd **00-1030**

FELTER, Henry Wickes (1865-1927) and J. U. LLOYD
King's American dispensatory. . . . Entirely rewritten and enl. 19th ed., 3rd rev. Cincinnati: Ohio Valley Co., 1905. 2 v. OCLloyd **00-1031**

FELTER, Henry Wickes (1865-1927) and J. U. LLOYD
King's American dispensatory. . . . Entirely rewritten and enl. 19th ed., 4th rev. Cincinnati: Ohio Valley Co., 1909. 2 v. OCLloyd **00-1032**

FENWICK, William Soltau
Dyspepsia, its varieties and treatment. . . . Philadelphia and London: W. B. Saunders & Co., 1910. 485p. plates. DLC; NNNAM; PPC; PU **00-1033**

FERGUSON, J. Bruce
. . . Diseases of the nose and throat. . . . Philadelphia and New York: Lea Bros. & Co., [1906]. 343p. DLC; NNNAM; PPC; PPJ **00-1034**

FERGUSON, Jeremiah S[weetser] (*b.* 1871)
Normal histology and microscopical anatomy. New York: D. Appleton & Co., 1905. 738p. DLC; MBM; NNNAM; OCIM **00-1035**

FERRIER, David (1843-1928)
The localization of brain diseases, being the Gulstonian lectures of the Royal College of Physicians for 1878. . . . New York: G. P. Putnam's Sons, 1900 [*c.* 1879]. 148p. KU; NNNAM; PPC; PU **00-1036**

FERRIER, David (1843-1928)
On tabes dorsalis; the Lumleian lectures delivered before the Royal College of Physicians, London, March, 1906. New York: William Wood & Co., 1906. 122p. DNLM; ICJ; IU-M; NN **00-1037**

FILATOV, Nil Fedorovich (1847-1902)
Semeiology and diagnosis of diseases of children, together with a therapeutic index. . . . Transl. from the Russian by G. B. Hassin . . . with extensive additions, by Frank B. Earle. . . . Chicago: Cleveland Press, 1904. 2 v. 87 textual illus. DLC; IU-M; OCIM; PU **00-1038**

FINCH, Edwin Ward (*b.* 1831)
The frontier, army and professional life of Edwin W. Finch, M.D., with suggestive thoughts from his own personal experiences in the treatment of pneumonia, etc. [New York: Press of Simmons, Manning & Dawson, 1909.] 119p. DLC; ICJ; NcD; NN **00-1039**

FINCH, PAUL V. & CO.
Cut rate catalog — drugs, herbs, patent medicines, chemicals, pharmaceuticals. . . . Grand Rapids, [*c.* 1900]. 80p. OCIM **00-1040**

FINDLEY, Palmer (*b.* 1868)
The diagnosis of diseases of women. A treatise for students and practitioners. . . . Illustrated with 210 engravings in the text and 45 plates in colors and monochrome. Philadelphia and New York: Lea Bros. & Co., 1903. 494p. plates. DLC; ICJ; OCIM; PPC **00-1041**

FINDLEY, Palmer (*b.* 1868)
The diagnosis of diseases of women. A treatise for students and practitioners. . . . 2nd ed., rev. and enl. Illustrated with 222 engravings in the text and 59 plates in colors and monochrome. Philadelphia and New York: Lea Bros. & Co., 1905. 588p. plates. DLC; IU-M; ICJ; PPC **00-1042**

FINDLEY, Palmer (*b.* 1868)
Gonorrhoea in women. . . . St. Louis, Mo.: C. V. Mosby Medical Book & Pub. Co., 1908. 112p. DLC; ICJ; IU-M; PPC **00-1043**

FIREBAUGH, Ellen M.
The physician's wife and the things that pertain to her life. Philadelphia: F. A. Davis Co., 1906. 186p. DLC; ICU; MB; NN **00-1044**

FISCHER, Louis (*b.* 1864)
Infant-feeding in its relation to health and disease. . . . Philadelphia, Chicago: F. A. Davis Co., 1901. 359p. plates. DLC; NNNAM; PPC; PU **00-1045**

FISCHER, Louis (*b.* 1864)
Infant-feeding in its relation to health and disease. . . . 2nd ed. Philadelphia: F. A. Davis Co., 1901. 343p. plates. DLC; MBM; PPC; PU **00-1046**

FISCHER, Louis (*b.* 1864)
The health-care of the baby; a handbook for mothers and nurses. . . . New York and London: Funk & Wagnalls Co., 1906. 144p. DLC; MBM; NNNAM; PPC **00-1047**

FISCHER, Louis (*b.* 1864)
Infant-feeding in its relation to health and disease . . . containing 54 illustrations, with 24 charts and tables, mostly original. 3rd ed. Philadelphia: F. A. Davis Co., 1906. 367p. plates. DLC; NNNAM; PPC; PU **00-1048**

FISCHER, Louis (*b.* 1864)
Diseases of infancy and childhood, their dietetic, hygienic, and medical treatment; a text-book designed for practitioners and students in medicine. . . . With three hundred and three illustrations, several in colors, and twenty-seven full-page half-tone and color plates. Philadelphia: F. A. Davis Co., 1907. 979p. DLC; NNNAM; OCIM; PPC **00-1049**

FISCHER, Louis (*b.* 1864)
Diseases of infancy and childhood, their dietetic, hygienic, and medical treatment; a text-book designed for practitioners and students in medicine. . . . 2nd ed., with three hundred and three illustrations, several in colors, and twenty-seven full-page half-tone and color plates. Philadelphia: F. A. Davis Co., 1908. 979p. DLC; MBM; NNNAM; PPC **00-1050**

FISCHER, Louis (*b.* 1864)
Diseases of infancy and childhood, their dietetic, hygienic, and medical treatment; a text-book designed for practitioners and students in medicine. . . . 3rd ed. With three hundred and three illustrations, several in colors, and twenty-nine full-page half-tone and color plates. Philadelphia: F. A. Davis Co., 1910. 980p. DLC; NNNAM; PPC; PU
00-1051

FISCHER, Martin Henry (1879-1962)
The physiology of alimentation . . . 1st ed. 1st thousand. New York: J. Wiley & Sons; [etc., etc.], 1907. 348p. plates. DLC; MH-M; NNNAM; PU **00-1052**

FISCHER, Martin Henry (1879-1962)
Oedema; a study of the physiology and the pathology of water absorption by the living organism. . . . The 1909 Nathan Lewis Hatfield prize essay of the College of Physicians of Philadelphia. Republished with the consent of the Board of Trustees from the transactions of the College. New York: J. Wiley & Sons; [etc., etc.], 1910. 209p. plates. CtY-M; DLC; NNNAM; PPC **00-1053**

FISHER, Charles Perry (*b.* 1857)
An account of the library of the College of Physicians of Philadelphia, [1788-1906]. . . . [Philadelphia, 1907.] 12p. DLC; ICJ; PPC **00-1054**

FISHER, George B[atchelder] (*b.* 1859)
Murdering God is the science of obtaining health, with a blending of foods, drinks, brain, lung and stomach gymnastics, massaging and percussion . . . [1st ed]. [Denver], 1904. 79p. plates. DLC **00-1055**

FISHER, George B[atchelder] (*b.* 1859)
Murdering God is the science of obtaining health, with a blending of food, drinks, brain, lung and stomach gymnastics, massaging and percussion. . . . [Denver? Col.], 1904-06. 202p. plates. DLC **00-1056**

FISHER, Irving (1867-1947)
The modern crusade against consumption. New York, 1903. 8p. DNLM; NN **00-1057**

FISHER, Irving (1867-1947)
The modern crusade against tuberculosis. Chicago: Illinois State Association for the Prevention of Tuberculosis, 1908. 15p. DNLM; ICJ **00-1058**

FISHER, Irving (1867-1947)
The modern crusade against tuberculosis. 2nd ed. New Haven: National Health Month, 1909. 24p. DNLM; NN
00-1059

FITZ, Reginald H[eber], ed. (1843-1913)
Diseases of the pancreas, suprarenals, and liver. . . . . By L. Oser . . . E. Neusser . . . H. Quincke . . . G. Hopper-Seyler . . . edited with additions by Reginald H. Fitz and Frederick A. Packard. Philadelphia: W. B. Saunders & Co., 1903. 918p. DLC; MB; NcD; PPJ [American ed., Nothnagel's encyclopedia of practical medicine] **00-1060**

FITZ, Reginald H[eber] (1843-1913)
The pancreas and pancreatic diseases. The symptomatology and diagnosis of diseases of the pancreas. New Haven, 1903. 18p. MB **00-1061**

FITZ, Reginald H[eber] (1843-1913)
Intrapleural lipoma: acute pericarditis; pericardial exploration. [Boston, 1906.] 11p. MB **00-1062**

FITZ, Reginald H[eber] (1843-1913)
The borderline of medicine and surgery. New Haven, 1907. 30p. MH; NN **00-1063**

[FITZ, Reginald H[eber] (1843-1913)
Medical papers dedicated to Reginald Heber Fitz. . . . Boston, 1908. 556p. MB; MBM; NNNAM; PU
00-1064

FLAGG, J[osiah] Foster (1828-1903)
Amalgams. Philadelphia, 1900. 4p. DNLM
00-1065

FLAVELL, G. W. & BROS.
Manufacturers of elastic stockings, abdominal supporters, trusses, etc. Philadelphia [1901?] 34p. NN; PPC
00-1066

FLEXNER, Abraham (1866-1859)
Medical education in the United States and Canada; a report to the Carnegie Foundation for the Advancement of Teaching . . . with an introduction by Henry S. Pritchett, president of the Foundation. . . . New York City, [1910]. 346p. maps, tables. DLC; NNNAM; OCIM; PU
00-1067

FLEXNER, Abraham (1866-1959)
The plethora of doctors. Boston, 1910. 6p. DNLM
00-1068

FLEXNER, Abraham (1866-1959)
Report on the Johns Hopkins Medical School. [Baltimore, 1910.] 25p. MdBJ-W [On the clinical full-time system; a "confidential" excerpt from the Report]
00-1069

FLEXNER, Simon (1863-1946)
Perforation of the inferior vena cava in amoebic abscesses of the liver. n. p., 1900. [1897.] 6p. NN
00-1070

FLEXNER, Simon (1863-1946)
Infection and intoxication. Boston: Ginn & Co., 1900? 10p. NN **00-1071**

FLEXNER, Simon (1863-1946)
On the prevalent diseases in the Philippines. A report to the committee of the Johns Hopkins Medical School. [Baltimore, 1900.] 12p. DNLM **00-1072**

FLEXNER, Simon (1863-1946)
The pancreas and pancreatic diseases. The pathology of pancreatitis, diabetes and fat necrosis. [New Haven, 1903.] 17p. MB **00-1073**

FLEXNER, Simon (1863-1946)
On the occurrence of spirochaeta pallida. Schaudinn, in syphilis. New York: Rockefeller Institute, 1905. 4p. NN
00-1074

FLEXNER, Simon (1863-1946)
An aspect of modern pathology. . . . [Baltimore, 1903.] 21p. DLC **00-1075**

FLEXNER, Simon (1863-1946) and Hidayo NOGUCHI
On the plurality of cytolysins in snake venom. [1903.] 32p. DLC **00-1076**

FLEXNER, Simon, ed. (1863-1946)
Bacteriological and clinical studies of the diarrheal diseases of infancy with reference to the Bacillus dysenteriae (Shiga) from the Rockefeller Institute for Medical Research, ed. by Simon Flexner and L. Emmett Holt. [New York], 1904. 202p. DNLM; ICJ; NIC; NN **00-1077**

FLEXNER, Simon (1863-1946) and J. W. JOBLING
Serum treatment of epidemic cerebrospinal meningitis. [Lancaster, Pa., 1908.] 64p. NN **00-1078**

FLEXNER, Simon (1863-1946)
Studies upon a transplantable rat tumor . . . by Simon Flexner and J. W. Jobling. New York: Rockefeller Institute, 1901. 51p. OCIM; NN **00-1079**

FLICK, Lawrence F[rancis] (1856-1938)
. . . Consumption a curable and preventable disease; what a layman should know about it. . . . Philadelphia: D. McKay, 1903. 295p. DLC; ICJ; PPC; PP [*vel subseq.* A 6th ed. appeared in 1908] **00-1080**

FLINT, Austin (1836-1915)
Collected essays and articles on physiology and medicine [1855-1902]. . . . New York: D. Appleton & Co., 1903. 2 v. plates. DLC; MH-M; NNNAM; PU **00-1081**

FLINT, Austin (1836-1915)
Handbook of physiology, for students and practitioners of medicine . . . with two hundred and forty-seven illustrations in the text—including four in colors—and an atlas of sixteen color-plates, including forty-eight original figures taken from actual stained microscopical preparations. New York, London: The Macmillan Co., 1905. 877p. DLC; NNNAM; OCIM; PU **00-1082**

FLINT, Austin (1836-1915)
Notes and citations on the homicidal insanities and feigned insanity. . . . New York: Priv. print, 1907. 90p. DLC; ICJ; NNNAM; PU **00-1083**

FOLSOM, Charles F[ollen] (1842-1907)
Studies of criminal responsibility and limited responsibility. [New York?]: Privately Printed, 1909. 153p. DLC; NN; NNNAM **00-1084**

FOLTZ, Kent Oscanyan (*b.* 1857)
. . . Diseases of the eye, a hand-book of ophthalmic practice for students and practitioners, in which particular attention is given the treatment of diseases of the eye by eclectic medication. . . . With 193 illustrations and 4 plates in color, and chromo-lithographic frontispiece. . . . Cincinnati: The Scudder Bros. Co., 1900. 566p. DLC; ICJ; OC; OCIM **00-1085**

FOLTZ, Kent Oscanyan (*b.* 1857)
Diseases of the nose, throat and ear. For students and practitioners, in which particular attention is given the treatment of diseases by eclectic medication. . . . Cincinnati: The Scudder Bros. Co., 1906. 643p. DLC; ICJ; OC; OCIM **00-1086**

THE FOO & WING HERB CO., LOS ANGELES
. . . The science of oriental medicine, its principles and methods comprising biographical sketches of its leading practitioners, its treatment of various prevalent diseases, useful information on matters of diet, exercise, and hygiene; a guide to health, compiled by the Foo & Wing Herb Co. . . . [Los Angeles: Times-Mirror Printing and Binding House, 1902.] 296p. DLC **00-1087**

FOOTE, Edward Bliss (1829-1906)
Dr. Foote's new plain home talk on love, marriage, and parentage. A fair and earnest discussion of human, social, and marital relations. . . . Rev. and enl. by the author. . . . Embracing also Tocology for mothers. By A. Westland. . . . New York: Murray Hill Publishing Co., 1901. 1248p. col. plates. DLC; NN; NNNAM **00-1088**

FOOTE, Edward B[liss] (1829-1906)
Dr. Foote's new book on health and disease, with recipes, including sexology. . . . Rev. and enl. by the author. . . . New York: Murray Hill Pub. Co., 1901. 806p. col. plates. DLC; NN; NNNAM **00-1089**

FOOTE, Edward Bliss (1829-1906)
Dr. Foote's home cyclopedia of popular medical, social, and sexual science, embracing his New book on health and disease . . . also embracing Plain home talk on love, marriage and parentage. . . . Twentieth century rev. and enl. ed. . . . New York: Murray Hill Pub. Co.; London: L. N. Fowler & Co., 1901. 1248p. col. plates. DLC; NN; NNNAM **00-1090**

FOOTE, Edward Milton (*b.* 1866)
A text-book of minor surgery . . . illustrated by four hundred and seven engravings from original drawings and photographs. New York and London: D. Appleton & Co., 1908 [1907]. 752p. DLC; NN; NNNAM **00-1091**

FOOTE, Edward Milton (*b.* 1866)
A text-book of minor surgery . . . 2nd ed., illustrated by four hundred and seven engravings from original drawings and photographs. New York and London: D. Appleton & Co., 1909. 752p. DLC; NN; NNNAM; PU **00-1092**

FOOTE, James Stephen (1851-1925)
A constructive method in histology, based upon the tube plan of structure of the animal body, with case of models for demonstration. . . . Naugatuck, Conn.: F. L. Bradbury, 1907. 152p. atlas [4p.]. DLC; MH-M **00-1093**

FOOTE, John Ambrose (1874-1931)
The essentials of materia medica and therapeutics. . . . Philadelphia and London: J. B. Lippincott Co., 1910. 194p. DLC; NN; PPC; PU **00-1094**

FORCHHEIMER, Frederick (1853-1913)
The prophylaxis and treatment of internal diseases, designed for the use of practitioners and of advanced students of medicine. . . . New York and London: D. Appleton & Co., 1906. 652p. DLC; NNNAM; PPC; PU **00-1095**

FORCHHEIMER, Frederick (1853-1913)
The prophylaxis and treatment of internal diseases, designed for the use of practitioners and of advanced students of medicine . . . 2nd ed. New York and London: D. Appleton & Co. 1910. 712p. DLC; MBM; NNNAM; PPC **00-1096**

FORD, Francis Chipman
Handbook of regional anatomy. . . . Chicago: F. C. Ford, 1910. 193p. DLC; ICJ; NN **00-1097**

FOREL, Auguste Henri (1848-1931)
Hygiene of nerves and mind in health and disease . . . authorised transl. from the second German edition by Hubert Austin Aikins. . . . New York: G. P. Putnam's Sons, 1907. 343p. DLC; ICJ; NNNAM; PU **00-1098**

FOREL, Auguste Henri (1848-1931)
Hypnotism; or, Suggestion and psychotherapy; a study of the psychological, psycho-physiological and therapeutic aspects of hypnotism . . . transl. from the 5th German ed. by H. W. Armit . . . American ed., rev. and cor. New York: Rebman Co., [1907]. 323p. DLC; MB; NNNAM; PU **00-1099**

FOREL, Auguste Henri (1848-1931)
The sexual question; a scientific, psychological, hygienic and sociological study for the cultured classes. . . . English adaptation by C. F. Marshall. . . . 1st to 2nd thousand. New York: Rebman Co., [1908]. 536p. col. plates. DLC; IU-M; NNNAM; PU **00-1100**

FOREST, William E.
Massotherapy; or, The use of massage rollers in functional disorders. New York: Health-Culture Co., [1900]. 88p. NN **00-1101**

FOREST, William E.
The new method in health culture; a guide to home treatment of the sick . . . 16th ed., edited, enl. and illustrated by Albert Turner. . . . New York: The Health-Culture Co., 1902. 328p. plates. DLC; DNLM; NN; NNNAM **00-1102**

FORSTER, Edward J[acob] (1846-1896)
A sketch of the medical profession, from the professional and industrial history of Suffolk County. Boston: Boston History Co., 1900 [1894]. 111p. DNLM; MB; MH; NN **00-1103**

FOSTER, Frank Pierce, ed. (1841-1911)
Appleton's medical dictionary; an illustrated dictionary of medicine and allied subjects in which are given the derivation, accentuation, and definition of terms used throughout the entire field of medical science. . . . New York and London: D. Appleton & Co., 1904. 1991p. plates. DLC; MBM; NNNAM; PPC **00-1104**

FOSTER, M[ichael] (1836-1907)
Nociones de fisiologia. . . . Nueva ed., castellana por el doctor A. Soler. . . . Nueva York: D. Appleton y Cia., 1900. 156p. DLC; MH-M; NNNAM; PU **00-1105**

FOURNIER, Alfred (1832-1914)
The treatment and prophylaxis of syphilis. . . . English transl. of the 2nd ed. rev. and enl. by C. F. Marshall . . . American ed., rev. and cor., with an appendix by George M. MacKee. . . . New York: Rebman Co., [1907]. 601p. DLC; ICJ; MBM; NNNAM **00-1106**

FOWLER, George Ryerson (1848-1906)
A treatise on appendicitis. . . . 2nd ed., rev. and enl. Philadelphia and London: J. B. Lippincott Co., 1900 235p. col. plates. DLC; NNNAM; PPC **00-1107**

FOWLER, George R[yerson] (1848-1906)
A treatise on surgery . . . containing 888 text-illustrations and four colored plates, all original. Philadelphia and London: W. B. Saunders & Co., 1906. 2 v. DLC; MBM; NNNAM; PPC **00-1108**

FOWLER, Russell S[tory] (*b.* 1874)
The operating room and the patient. . . . Philadelphia: W. B. Saunders & Co., 1906. 172p. DLC; NNNAM; PPC; PU **00-1109**

FOWLER, Russell S[tory] (*b.* 1874)
The operating room and the patient. . . . 2nd ed., rev. and enl. Philadelphia: W. B. Saunders & Co., 1907. 284p. DLC; NNNAM; PPC; PU **00-1110**

FOX, George Henry (1846-1937)
. . . Photographic atlas of the diseases of the skin; a series of eighty plates, comprising more than one hundred illustrations, with descriptive text, and a treatise on cutaneous therapeutics. . . . [Physician's ed.] Philadelphia and London: J. B. Lippincott Co., 1904. 224p. col. plates. DLC; NNNAM; PPC; PPJ **00-1111**

FOX, George Henry (1846-1937)
. . . Photographic atlas of the diseases of the skin . . . a series of ninety-six plates, comprising nearly two hundred illustrations, with descriptive text, and a treatise on cutaneous therapeutics. . . . [Physicians' ed.] Philadelphia and London: J. B. Lippincott Co., [1908]. 4 v. DLC; MBM; NNNAM; PPC **00-1112**

FOX, Lawrence Webster (1853-1931)
Diseases of the eye . . . with five coloured plates and two hundred and ninety-six illustrations in the text. New York and London: D. Appleton & Co., 1904. 584p. DLC; NNNAM; OCIM; PU **00-1113**

FOX, Lawrence Webster (1853-1931)
Massage, an occupation for the blind. Chicago: Press of the American Medical Association, 1906. 8p. DLC; NN **00-1114**

FOX, Lawrence Webster (1853-1931)
A practical treatise on ophthalmology. . . . With six coloured plates and three hundred illustrations in text. New York and London: D. Appleton & Co., 1910. 807p. DLC; MBM; NNNAM; PPC **00-1115**

FRENCH, James Magoffin (1858-1907)
A test-book on the practice of medicine, designed for the use of students . . . illustrated by ten full-page plates and fifty wood engravings. New York: William Wood & Co., 1903. 780p. DLC; MH-M; NNNAM; PU **00-1116**

FRENCH, James Magoffin (1858-1907)
A text-book on the practice of medicine, for students and practitioners. . . . 2nd rev. ed. Illustrated by eleven full-page plates and fifty wood-engravings. New York: William Wood & Co., 1905. 780p. DLC; MBM; NNNAM; PPC **00-1117**

FRENCH, James Magoffin (1858-1907)
A text-book of the practice of medicine, for students and practitioners. . . . 3rd rev. ed., illustrated by one hundred and ten engravings in the text and twenty-five full-page plates in tints and colors. New York: William Wood & Co., 1907. 1253p. DLC; MBM; NNNAM; PPC **00-1118**

FRENCH, James Magoffin (1858-1907)
A text-book of the practice of medicine for students and practitioners . . . rev. by Charles Spencer Williamson. . . . 4th rev. ed., illustrated by 133 engravings in the text and 28 full-page plates in tints and colors. New York: William Wood & Co., 1910. 1301p. DLC; NNNAM; OCIM; PU
00-1119

FRENKEL, Heinrich S. (1860-1931)
The treatment of tabetic ataxia by means of systematic exercise. . . . Transl. by L. Freyberger. Philadelphia: P. Blakiston's Son & Co., 1902. 185p. ICJ; NNNAM; PPC; PU
00-1120

FRERICHS, Friedrich T[heodor] von (1819-1885)
A clinical treatise on diseases of the liver. Transl. by Charles Murchison. New York: William Wood & Co., 1900 [1879]. 3 v. CtY-M; NcD; NN; PPJ [A reissue of the Sydenham Society's 1860-1861 London ed. The 1st German ed. was published in 1858] **00-1121**

FREUD, Sigmund (1856-1939)
Selected papers on hysteria and other psychoneuroses . . . authorized transl. by A. A. Brill. . . . New York: The Journal of Nervous and Mental Disease Publishing Co., 1909. 200p. DLC; ICJ; NNNAM; PU **00-1122**

FREUD, Sigmund (1856-1939)
Three contributions to the sexual theory. . . . Authorized transl. by A. A. Brill . . . with introduction by James J. Putnam, M.D. New York: The Journal of Nervous and Mental Disease Publishing Co., 1910. 91p. DLC; MH; NNNAM; PU
00-1123

FREUND, Leopold (1868-1944)
Elements of general radio-therapy for practitioners. Transl. by G. H. Lancashire. New York: Rebman Co., 1904. 538p. MH-M; NNNAM; PU [Bound with Clarence A. Wright, notes on instrumentation.] **00-1124**

FRIDENBERG, Percy H.
The ophthalmic patient: a manual of therapeutics and nursing in eye disease. New York: The Macmillan Co., 1900. 312p. DLC; ICJ; MH-M; NNNAM **00-1125**

[FRIEDENWALD, Aaron] (1836-1902)
Life, letters, and addresses of Aaron Friedenwald, M.D., by his son Harry Friedenwald, M.D. . . . Baltimore, Md.: The Lord Baltimore Press, 1906. 356p. plates. DLC; MdU-D; PPC; PU
00-1126

FRIEDENWALD, Julius (1866-1941)
Diet in health and disease, by Julius Friedenwald . . . and John Ruhräh. . . . Philadelphia, London, [etc.]: W. B. Saunders & Co., 1905 [1904]. 689p. DLC; MH-M; PPC; PU
00-1127

FRIEDENWALD, Julius (1866-1941)
Guide to clinical laboratory diagnosis, by Julius Friedenwald . . . Harvey G. Beck . . . and Hubert C. Knapp. . . . [2nd ed.] Baltimore: Williams & Wilkins Co., 1904. 140p. DLC; MdBJ-W; MdU-D; PU **00-1128**

FRIEDENWALD, Julius (1866-1941)
Dietetics for nurses, by Julius Friedenwald . . . and John Ruhräh. . . . Philadelphia and London: W. B. Saunders & Co., 1905. 363p. DLC; MBM; PPC; PU
00-1129

FRIEDENWALD, Julius (1866-1941)
Diet in health and disease, by Julius Friedenwald . . . and John Ruhräh. . . . 2nd ed., thoroughly rev. and enl. Philadelphia and London: W. B. Saunders & Co., 1906. 728p. DLC; MBM; NNNAM; PPC **00-1130**

FRIEDENWALD, Julius (1866-1941)
Diet in health and disease, by Julius Friedenwald . . . and John Ruhräh. . . . 3rd ed., thoroughly rev. and enl. Philadelphia and London: W. B. Saunders & Co., 1909. 765p. DLC; MBM; NNNAM; PPC **00-1131**

FRIEDENWALD, Julius (1866-1941)
Dietetics for nurses, by Julius Friedenwald . . . and John Ruhräh. . . . 2nd ed., rev. and enl. Philadelphia and London: W. B. Saunders & Co., 1909. 395p. DLC; NN; PPC; PU
00-1132

FRIEDRICH, Ernest Paul (1867-1925)
Rhinology, laryngology, and otology, and their significance in general medicine. . . . Authorized transl. from the German; ed. by H. Holbrook Curtis. . . . Philadelphia and London: W. B. Saunders & Co., 1900. 348p. DLC; NNNAM; PPC; PU
00-1133

FRITSCH, Heinrich (1844-1915)
The diseases of women. . . . Transl. by Isidor Furst. New York: William Wood & Co., 1900 [*c.* 1883]. 355p. DLC: ICJ; MBM; NNNAM [159 woodcuts] **00-1134**

FRONCZAK, Francis Eustace (*b.* 1874)
On the resuscitation of apparently dead newborn by Laborde's method. Buffalo, 1900 4p. DNLM **00-1135**

FROST, William Dodge (1867-1957)
A laboratory guide in elementary bacteriology. . . . Madison, Wis.: The Author, 1901. 205p. DLC: ICJ
00-1136

FROST, William Dodge (1867-1957)
A laboratory guide in elementary bacteriology. . . . 2nd rev. ed. Madison, Wis.: The Author, 1902. 355p. DLC
00-1137

FROST, William Dodge (1867-1957)
A laboratory guide in elementary bacteriology. . . . 3rd rev. ed. New York: The Macmillan Co.; London: Macmillan & Co., 1903. 395p. DLC: ICJ; NNNAM; PU
00-1138

FROST, William Dodge (1867-1957)
. . . Tuberculosis or consumption, with special reference to Wisconsin conditions. . . . Madison, Wis., 1909. 75p. DLC; NN; PP **00-1139**

FROST, William Dodge (1867-1957)
A text-book of general bacteriology, by William Dodge Frost . . . and Eugene Franklin McCampbell. . . . New York: The Macmillan Co., 1910. 340p. DLC: ICJ; NNNAM; PU
00-1140

FRÜHWALD, Ferdinand (1854-1908)
Diseases of children. A practical reference book for students and practitioners. Edited, with additions by Thompson S. Wescott. Philadelphia: W. B. Saunders & Co., 1905. 533p. DLC; ICRM; MBM; PU **00-1141**

FUCHS, Ernst (1851-1930)
Text-book of ophthalmology. . . . Authorized transl. from the 11th rev. and greatly enl. German ed., with numerous additions, by Alexander Duane. . . . With four hundred and forty-one illustrations. 3rd ed. Philadelphia and London: J. B. Lippincott Co., [1908]. 908p. col. plates. DLC; MBM; NNNAM; PPC **00-1142**

FULLER, Eugene (1858-1930)
Diseases of the genito-urinary system; a thorough treatise on urinary and sexual surgery. . . . New York: The Macmillan Co.; London: Macmillan & Co., 1900. 774p. DLC; DNLM; ICJ; PPC **00-1143**

FULLER, William (*b.* 1842)
36 vertical sections of the brain. Grand Rapids, Mich.: Press of Seymour & Muir Co., [1900?] 37 plates. DLC **00-1144**

FULLER, William (*b.* 1842)
Architecture of the brain. . . . Grand Rapids, Mich.: [Press of Seymour & Muir Printing Co.], 1900 [*c.* 1896]. 182p. plates. DLC **00-1145**

FULLER, William (*b.* 1842)
Illustrations of anatomy of the brain. [Grand Rapids, 1900?] 1p. 7 plates. DLC **00-1146**

FULLERTON, Anna M[artha]
A handbook of obstetric nursing for nurses, students and mothers. Comprising the course of instruction in obstetric nursing given to the pupils of the training school for nurses connected with the Woman's Hospital of Philadelphia. . . . 6th rev. ed. . . . Philadelphia: P. Blakiston's Son & Co., 1903. 270p. DLC; ICJ; PPC; PU **00-1147**

FULTON, Henry D.
Variation of type in diphtheria and scarlet fever. Philadelphia, 1900. 8p. DLC; DNLM **00-1148**

FULTON, Henry D.
Should we burn our dead? [Philadelphia, 1901.] 5p. MB **00-1149**

GAGE, Simon Henry (1851-1944)
The microscope; an introduction to microscopic methods and to histology. . . . 8th ed., rev., enl. and illustrated by over two hundred figures. Ithaca, N.Y.: Comstock Publishing Co., 1901. 299p. plates. DLC; ICJ; MH; NN **00-1150**

GAGE, Simon Henry (1851-1944)
The microscope; an introduction to microscopic methods and to histology. . . . 9th ed., rev., enl. and illustrated by over two hundred figures. Ithaca, N.Y.: Comstock Publishing Co., 1904. 299p. plates. DLC: ICJ; NIC; PPC **00-1151**

GAGE, Simon Henry (1851-1944)
The microscope; an introduction to microscopic methods and to histology. . . . 10th ed., rev. and illustrated by over two hundred figures. Ithaca, N.Y.: Comstock Publishing Co., 1908. 350p. plates. DLC; ICJ; MH; NIC **00-1152**

GALBRAITH, Anna M[ary] (*b.* 1859)
Are the dangers of the menopause natural or acquired? A physiological study. New York, 1900 [1899]. 24p. DNLM; NN **00-1153**

GALBRAITH, Anna M[ary] (*b.* 1859)
The four epochs of woman's life: a study in hygiene with an introductory note by John H. Musser. Philadelphia: W. B. Saunders & Co., 1901. 200p. MBM; NN; PPC; PU **00-1154**

GALBRAITH, Anna M[ary] (*b.* 1859)
The four epochs of woman's life: a study in hygiene with an introductory note by John H. Musser. 2nd ed. Philadelphia: W. B. Saunders & Co., 1903. 244p. DLC; DNLM; PPC; PU **00-1155**

GALVIN, George W[illiam] (1854-1928)
The doctor, the hospital, and the patient. Boston: Rockwell & Churchill Press, 1908 [*c.* 1898. *vel subseq.*] 15p. DNLM; MH-M; NN **00-1156**

GANT, Samuel G[oodwin] (1869-1944)
Diseases of the rectum and anus, designed for students and practitioners of medicine. . . . 2nd ed., rewritten and enl. With thirty-seven full-page plates, twenty of which are in colors, and two hundred and twelve smaller engravings and half-tones. Philadelphia: F. A. Davis Co., 1902. 687p. DLC; DNLM; NcD; PPC **00-1157**

GANT, Samuel G[oodwin] (1869-1944)
Diseases of the rectum and anus. Designed for students and practitioners of medicine. . . . Third ed., revised and enlarged. With thirty-seven full-page plates, twenty of which are in colors, and two hundred and twelve smaller engravings and half-tones. Philadelphia: F. A. Davis Co., 1905. 697p. DNLM; ICJ; PPHa; PPJ **00-1158**

GANT, Samuel G[oodwin] (1869-1944)
Constipation and intestinal obstruction (obstipation) . . . with 250 original illustrations. Philadelphia and London: W. B. Saunders & Co., 1909. 559p. DLC; DNLM; PPC; PPJ **00-1159**

GARCEAU, Edgar (1865-1913)
Renal, ureteral, perirenal and adrenal tumors, and actinomycosis and echinococcus of the kidney . . . with seventy-two illustrations in text. New York and London: D. Appleton & Co., 1909. 421p. DLC; MH-M; NNNAM; PU **00-1160**

GARDINER, Charles Fox (*b.* 1857)
The care of the consumptive; a consideration of the scientific use of natural therapeutic agencies in the prevention and cure of consumption; together with a chapter on Colorado as a resort for invalids. . . . New York and London: G. P. Putnam's Sons, 1900. 182p. DLC; DNLM; NNC; NNNAM **00-1161**

GARDNER, R[obert] W[inslow] (1835-1911)
Internal administration of iodine. Hydriodic acid. New York, 1900. 24p. DLC; DNLM; NN **00-1162**

GARDNER, Robert W[inslow] (1835-1911)
Chemically pure hypophosphites. Therapeutical indications with clinical data. New York, 1900. 147p. DLC: ICJ; PU [12th-16th eds., 1895-1899] **00-1163**

GARDNER, Robert W[inslow] (1835-1911)
Why hydriodic acid is superior to all other forms of iodine for internal use. New York, 1900. 16p. DNLM; NN **00-1164**

GARDNER, Robert W[inslow] (1835-1911)
Iodine and phosphorus. . . . Part I: Iodine for internal use. . . . Part II: Phosphorus and the hypophosphites. New York, 1902. 150p. DLC; ICJ; NN; PU **00-1165**

GARDNER, Robert W[inslow] (1835-1911)
Special therapeutic notes on syrup hydriodic acid. . . . [New York? 1902.] 18p. DLC **00-1166**

GARDNER, Robert W[inslow] (1835-1911)
Autobiography. Orange, N.J.: [Privately Printed], 1910. 101p. DLC; NN **00-1167**

GARRIGUES, Henry Jacques (1831-1913)
A text-book of the diseases of women. . . . 3rd ed., thoroughly rev. Philadelphia: W. B. Saunders & Co., 1900 756p. col. plates. DLC; DNLM; NNNAM; PPC **00-1168**

GARRIGUES, Henry Jacques (1831-1913)
A text-book of the science and art of obstetrics. . . . Philadelphia and London: J. B. Lippincott Co., 1902. 844p. col. plates. DLC; MBM; NNNAM; PPC **00-1169**

GARRIGUES, Henry Jacques (1831-1913)
Gynecology, medical and surgical; outlines for students and practitioners . . . with three hundred and forty-three illustrations. Philadelphia and London: J. B. Lippincott Co., 1905. 461p. DLC; NNNAM; PPC; PU **00-1170**

GARRIGUES, Henry Jacques (1831-1913)
A text-book of the science and art of obstetrics. . . . 2nd ed., thoroughly rev., with five hundred and twenty-five illustrations. Philadelphia and London: J. B. Lippincott Co., [1907]. 868p. col. plates. DLC; MBM; NNNAM; PPC **00-1171**

GATEWOOD, James Duncan (1857-1924)
Notes on naval hospitals, medical schools, and training school for nurses, with a sketch of hospital history. . . . Baltimore: Press of the Friedenwald Co., 1900 [*c.* 1893]. 2 v. DLC; ICJ; MH-M; PPC **00-1172**

GATEWOOD, James Duncan (1857-1924)
Naval hygiene. . . . Prepared by direction of the Bureau of Medicine and Surgery, and published by permission of the Navy Department. With eight colored plates and 105 other illustrations. Philadelphia: P. Blakiston's Son & Co., 1909. 779p. DLC; ICJ; PPC; PU **00-1173**

GATHMANN, Henry (*b.* 1864)
Medicine vs. quackery. 1. Glimpses into the world of medicine. 2. Glimpses into the world of quackery. 3. The evils of self-drugging. By H. Gathmann, M.D. [and] J. J. Seelman, M.D. Milwaukee: Western Pub. Co., 1901. 55p. DLC; DNLM; ICJ; NN **00-1174**

GAUCHER, Ernest (1855-1918)
Diseases of the skin. Including radiotherapy and radium therapy. Transl. and ed. by C. F. Marshall. New York: D. Appleton & Co., 1910. 460p. CtY-M; IU-M; PPC; PU **00-1175**

GAY, Frederick P[arker] (1844-1939)
Immunology: a medical science developed through animal experimentation. [Chicago, 1910.] 19p. DNLM; MB **00-1176**

GAY, George W[ashington] (1842-1931)
Abuse of medical charity. Boston: Old Corner Book Store, 1905. 68p. NN **00-1177**

GAY, George W[ashington] (1842-1931)
Reminiscences of the Boston City Hospital. Boston: Municipal Printing Office, 1906. 36p. MB **00-1178**

GAY, George W[ashington] (1842-1931)
When to call the physician. Boston: Health Education League, [1909]. 15p. NN **00-1179**

GAYLORD, Harvey R[ussell] (*b.* 1872)
The principles of pathological histology, by Harvey R. Gaylord . . . and Ludwig Aschoff. . . . With an introductory note by William H. Welch. . . . Illustrated with 81 engravings in the text and forty full-page plates. Philadelphia and New York: Lea Bros. & Co., [1901]. 359p. DLC; ICJ; PPC; PU **00-1180**

GAYLORD, Harvey R[ussell] (*b.* 1872)
The principles of pathology. . . . By Harvey Gaylord and Ludwig Aschoff. Introduction by William Welch. Philadelphia: Lea Bros. & Co., 1901. 2 v. plates. NNNAM; OCIM; PPC; PU **00-1181**

GEDDES, Patrick (1854-1932)
The evolution of sex. By Patrick Geddes and J. Arthur Thomson. Rev. ed. New York: C. Scribner's Sons, 1901. 342p. DLC; NIC; NN; PP **00-1182**

GEDDINGS, Henry Downes (1859-1913)
The prevention of the spread of scarlet fever. . . . [Prepared under the direction of the Surgeon-General] . . . . Washington: Government Printing Office, 1902. 8p. DLC; ICJ; NN **00-1183**

GEDDINGS, Henry Downes (1859-1913)
. . . Precis on the management of outbreaks of smallpox, diphtheria, and scarlet fever. . . . Washington: Government Printing Office, 1909. 18p. DLC; DNLM **00-1184**

GERRISH, Frederick Henry (1845-1920)
A text-book of anatomy by American authors. . . . 2nd ed., rev. and enl. Illustrated with 1003 engravings in black and colors. Philadelphia and New York: Lea Bros. & Co., 1902. 943p. DLC; DNLM; NNNAM; PPC **00-1185**

GETCHELL, Albert C[olby] (*b.* 1857)
The medical knowledge of Shakespeare. Boston: D. C. Heath, 1907. 40p. MB; MH **00-1186**

GETCHELL, Frank Horace, ed. (1836-1907)
An illustrated encyclopaedia of the science and practice of obstetrics. Illustrated with the celebrated Moreau's atlas of (84) folio plates, and one hundred and thirty-three woodcuts. . . . Philadelphia: Gebbie & Co., 1900 [*c.* 1884]. 276p. DLC; ICJ; NNC; PPC **00-1187**

GIBBONS, Edward Engler (*b.* 1871)
The eye, its refraction and diseases. . . . New York: The Macmillan Co.; London: Macmillan & Co., Ltd. 1904-05. 2 v. DLC; MBM; NNNAM; PU **00-1188**

GIBSON, George A[lexander], ed. (1854-1913)
Practice of medicine, by eminent medical specialists and authorities. Philadelphia: J. B. Lippincott Co., 1901. 2 v. DNLM; NNNAM; PPC; PU **00-1189**

GILBERT BROTHERS & CO.
Catalogue of drugs and chemicals, bottles, glassware and sundries. Baltimore, 1900. 228p. DLC; MdU-D; PPC **00-1190**

GILBERT, George Abner (*b.* 1859)
A text book on uric acid and its congeners, with special reference to its physical and chemical properties, its metabolism and accumulation in the organism, together with the disease processes arising therefrom and their aetiological therapy; for medical students and practitioners. . . . 1st ed. Danbury, Conn.: The Danbury Medical Printing Co., 1907. 310p. CtY-M; DLC; MH-M; PU **00-1191**

GILLIAM, David Tod (1844-1923)
A text-book on practical gynecology for practitioners and students. . . . Illustrated with 350 engravings, a colored frontispiece, and 7 full-page half-tone plates. Philadelphia: F. A. Davis Co., 1903. 634p. DLC; NNNAM; OCIM; PPC **00-1192**

GILLIAM, David Tod (1844-1923)
A text-book of practical gynecology, for practitioners and students. . . . 2nd ed. Philadelphia: F. A. Davis Co., 1907. 642p. plates. DLC; DNLM; PPC; PU **00-1193**

GILLIAM, David Tod (1844-1923)
A text-book of practical gynecology, for practitioners and students. . . . 3rd rev. ed. Illustrated with 350 engravings, a colored frontispiece, and 13 full-page and half-tone plates. Philadelphia: F. A. Davis Co., 1908. 642p. DLC; MBM; NNNAM; PPC **00-1194**

GILMAN, Daniel C[oit] (1831-1908)
The Sheffield Scientific School of Yale University: a semicentennial discourse. New Haven, 1900 [*c.* 1897]. 39p. MH; NN **00-1195**

GILSON, Charles L[lewellyn] (*b.* 1852)
The law of natural healing. The embodiment of a theory and practice which are combined into a system of developing the body, mind and spirit of man, through the agency of the forces within himself. Worcester, Mass.: The Hamilton Press, 1905. 154p. DLC; MH **00-1196**

GLEASON, E[dward] B[aldwin] (1854-1934)
. . . Essentials of diseases of the nose and throat, arranged in the form of questions and answers. . . . 3rd ed., rev. and enl. Philadelphia and London: W. B. Saunders & Co., 1901. 241p. DLC; NN; PPC; PPJ **00-1197**

GLEASON, E[dward] B[aldwin] (1854-1934)
. . . Essentials of the diseases of the ear. Arranged in the form of questions and answers. Prepared especially for students of medicine and post-graduate students. . . . 3rd ed., thoroughly rev. Philadelphia and London: W. B. Saunders & Co., 1902. 214p. DLC; PPC; PPJ; PU **00-1198**

GLEASON, E[dward] B[aldwin] (1854-1934)
. . . Essentials of diseases of the nose and throat, arranged in the form of questions and answers. . . . 4th ed., rev. and enl. 120 illustrations. Philadelphia and London: W. B. Saunders & Co., 1906. 259p. DLC; PPC; PPJ; PU **00-1199**

GLEASON, E[dward] B[aldwin] (1854-1934)
A manual of diseases of the nose, throat, and ear. . . . Philadelphia and London: W. B. Saunders & Co., 1907. 556p. col. plates. DLC; NNNAM; OCIM; PPC **00-1200**

GLEASON, E[dward] B[aldwin] (1854-1934)
A manual of diseases of the nose, throat, and ear. . . . 2nd ed., thoroughly rev. Philadelphia and London: W. B. Saunders & Co., 1910. 563p. DLC; ICJ; MBM; PPC **00-1201**

GLENISTER, John W.
Home physician and medical instructor. An invaluable collection of information that should be possessed by everybody. . . . [Jamaica Plain: The Brookside Print, 1905.] 200p. DLC; NN **00-1202**

GOAT LYMPH SANITARIUM ASSOCIATION
Goat lymph; a journal of special information concerning the goat-lymph treatment. . . . Gilbert White, M.D., medical director. 2nd ed. Chicago: Goat Lymph Sanitarium Association, 1903. 47p. DLC; ICJ **00-1203**

GODFREY, Edmund L. B.
History of the medical profession of Camden County, New Jersey, including a brief review of the charitable institutions within the County. Philadelphia: F. A. Davis, 1900 [*c.* 1896]. 303p. DLC; NcD; NjR; PP **00-1204**

GODFREY, Hollis (1874-1936)
Elementary chemistry. . . . New York, [etc.]: Longmans, Green, & Co., 1909. 456p. DLC; MB; NN; PU **00-1205**

GODFREY, Hollis (1874-1936)
The health of the city. Boston: Houghton Mifflin Co., 1910. 372p. DLC; MB; NN; PP **00-1206**

GODFREY, Hollis (1874-1936)
A laboratory manual to accompany Godfrey's elementary chemistry. . . . New York, [etc.]: Longmans, Green, & Co., 1910. 110p. DLC; MH; NN; PU **00-1207**

GOELET, Augustin H. (1854-1910)
The technique of surgical gynecology, devoted exclusively to a description of the technique of gynecological operations. . . . New York: International Journal of Surgery Co., [1900]. 340p. plates. DLC; NN; NNNAM; PU **00-1208**

GOELET, Augustin H. (1854-1910)
Therapeutic uses of electricity in gynecology. [Scranton, 1903.] 123p. plates. MB **00-1209**

GOEPP, R[udolph] Max (1866-1950)
State board questions and answers. . . . Philadelphia and London: W. B. Saunders & Co., 1908. 684p. DLC; MH-M; NNNAM; PPC **00-1210**

GOLDMAN, S[idney] Ormond
. . . Questions on anatomy, physiology, medicine and pathology, surgery, materia medica, therapeutics, etc., obstetrics and gynecology, clinical subjects, embracing paediatrics, ophthalmology, laryngology, and rhinology, dermatology, otology, venereal diseases. Specially arranged for the students of the College of Physicians and Surgeons, New York, [4th ed.] [New York?], 1901. 132p. DLC; NN; NNNAM **00-1211**

GOLDMAN, S[idney] Ormond
. . . Apparatus without automatic valves for the administration of different anaesthetics by various methods for medical, surgical, and dental purposes, with special reference to the gas-ether method of anaesthesia. . . . [New York: Press of Stettiner Bros.], 1903. 19p. DLC; NN; NNNAM
00-1212

GOLDSON, Malinda
Family medical book on morality, the diseases of women and children, and miscellaneous diseases. . . . Oakland, Cal.: Pacific Press Pub. Co., 1901. 886p. DLC
00-1213

GOLDSTEIN, M[ax] A[aron] (1870-1941)
One hundred years of medicine and surgery in Missouri: historical and biographical review of the careers of the physicians and surgeons of the State of Missouri, and sketches of some of its notable medical institutions. St. Louis: St. Louis Star, 1900. 364p. DLC; DNLM; ICJ; KU
00-1214

GOLDSTEIN, M[ax] A[aron] (1870-1941)
What not to do in ear, nose, and throat work. St. Louis, 1900. 8p. DNLM **00-1215**

GOLDSTEIN, M[ax] A[aron] (1870-1941)
The radical treatment of follicular tonsilitis. St. Louis, 1900. 4p. DNLM **00-1216**

GOLDSTEIN, M[ax] A[aron] (1870-1941)
The cosmetic and plastic surgery of the ear. [St. Louis, 1908.] 28p. NNC **00-1217**

GOLDTHWAIT, Joel Ernest (*b.* 1866)
Diseases of the bones and joints; clinical studies, by Joel E. Goldthwait, M.D., Charles F. Painter, M.D., Robert B. Osgood, M.D. . . . Boston: D. C. Heath & Co., 1909. 675p. CtY-M; DLC; MBM; NN **00-1218**

GOLEBIEWSKI, Eduard (1856-1901)
Atlas and epitome of diseases caused by accidents. . . . Edited with editorial notes and additions, by Pearce Bailey. Philadelphia: W. B. Saunders & Co., 1900. 549p. 40 col. plates. DLC; ICJ; NN; OCIM **00-1219**

GOODHUE, E[dward] S[olon] (*b.* 1861)
State care of leprosy. Philadelphia, 1900. 7p. DLC; DNLM
00-1220

GOODWIN, E. J.
A history of medicine in Missouri. St. Louis: W. L. Smith, 1905. 284p. DLC; ICJ **00-1221**

GORDINIER, Hermon C. (*b.* 1864)
The gross and minute anatomy of the central nervous system. Philadelphia: P. Blakiston's Son & Co., 1902 [*c.* 1899]. 589p. 48 plates. DLC; ICJ; MH-M; PPC **00-1222**

GORDON, Alfred (*b.* 1869)
The semeiotic value of the different symptoms in cancer of the stomach. New York, 1900 [*c.* 1898]. 8p. DNLM
00-1223

GORDON, Alfred (*b.* 1869)
Special provisions for management of certain forms of mental disorder. New York: William Wood & Co., 1906. 10p. PPC
00-1224

GORDON, Alfred (*b.* 1869)
Diseases of the nervous system, for the general practitioner and student . . . with one hundred and thirty-six illustrations. Philadelphia: P. Blakiston's Son & Co., 1908. 487p. DLC; ICJ; PPC; PU **00-1225**

GORDON, Alfred (*b.* 1869)
Mental responsibility in acute and chronic intoxication with alcohol and other drugs. [Philadelphia], 1909. 10p. PPC
00-1226

GORDON, Alfred (*b.* 1869)
Diseases of the optic nerve as an early or earliest symptom of multiple sclerosis. Philadelphia, 1909. 7p. PPC
00-1227

GORDON, Henry Laing
The modern mother, a guide to girlhood, motherhood, and infancy. . . . Fully illustrated by René Walker. New York: R. F. Fenno & Co., [1909]. 277p. DLC; NN; NNNAM
00-1228

GORGAS, Ferdinand J[ames] S[amuel] (1835-1914)
Questions and answers embracing the curriculum of the dental student, divided into three parts. . . . Philadelphia: P. Blakiston's Son & Co., 1901. 531p. DLC; NN; PPC; PU
00-1229

GORGAS, Ferdinand J[ames] S[amuel] (1835-1914)
Dental medicine; a manual of dental materia medica and therapeutics . . . 7th ed., rev. and enl. Philadelphia: P. Blakiston's Son & Co., 1901. 624p. DLC; MdU-D; NNNAM; PPC
00-1230

GORGAS, Ferdinand J[ames] S[amuel] (1835-1914)
Dental medicine; a manual of dental materia medica and therapeutics. . . . 8th ed. Rev. and enl. Philadelphia: P. Blakiston's Son & Co., 1909. 627p. DLC; IU-M; NNNAM; PPC
00-1231

GORGAS, William Crawford (1854-1920)
The work of the Sanitary Department of Havana; with special reference to the repression of yellow fever. . . . New York: William Wood & Co., 1901. 15p. DLC; ICJ; NN; NNNAM
00-1232

GORGAS, William Crawford (1854-1920)
Methods of quarantine against yellow fever adopted in Havana, Cuba, during the year 1901. . . . New York: William Wood & Co., [1903]. 11p. DLC; ICJ; NNNAM; PU
00-1233

GORGAS, William Crawford (1854-1920)
. . A few general directions with regard to destroying mosquitoes, particularly the yellow fever mosquito. . . . Washington: Government Printing Office, 1904. 14p. DLC; DNLM
00-1234

GORGAS, William Crawford (1854-1920)
Health conditions in the Canal Zone. . . . Chicago: Press of American Medical Association, [1905]. 6p. DLC
00-1235

GORHAM, Frederic P[oole] (1871-1933)
A laboratory course in bacteriology, for the use of medical, agricultural, and industrial students. . . . With 97 illustrations. Philadelphia and London: W. B. Saunders & Co., 1901. 192p. DLC; NNNAM; PPC; PU **00-1236**

GORTON, David A[llyn] (1832-1916)
Dyspepsia. A brief treatise on the nature, cause, and cure of the prevailing disease of America, upon hygienic principles. . . . Peekskill, N.Y..: Peekskill Hygeopathic Institute, 1900. 35p. DLC [First published, 1860. *vel subseq.*]
00-1237

GORTON, David A[llyn] (1832-1916)
Neurasthenia or nervous exhaustion. New York: G. P. Putnam's Sons, 1900. 23p. CtY-M; NN; PPC **00-1238**

GORTON, David A[llyn] (1832-1916)
The history of medicine, philosophical and critical, from its origins to the twentieth century. New York: G. P. Putnam's Sons, 1910. 2 v. ICU; MB; NIC; NN
00-1239

GOSLEE, Hart J[ohn] (1871-1930)
Principles and practice of crowning teeth; a practical, systematic and modern treatise upon the requirements and technique of artificial crown work, including some incidental reference to bridgework. With 459 illustrations. . . . New York: The Consolidated Dental Mfg. Co.; London: C. Ash & Sons, 1903. 292p. DLC: ICJ; OCIM; PU
00-1240

GOSLEE, Hart J[ohn] (1871-1930)
Principles and practice of crown and bridgework; a practical, systematic and modern treatise upon the requirements and technique of artificial crown and bridgework. With 917 illustrations, 2nd ed. . . . New York: The Consolidated Dental Mfg. Co.; [etc., etc.], 1907. 505p. DLC; MdU-D; NNNAM; PU
00-1241

GOSLEE, Hart J[ohn] (1871-1930)
Principles and practice of crown and bridgework; a practical, systematic and modern treatise upon the requirements and technique of artificial crown and bridgework. With 1141 illustrations. 3rd ed. . . . New York: The Consolidated Dental Mfg. Co.; [etc., etc.], 1910. 600p. DLC; ICJ; NN; NNNAM
00-1242

GOSS, Isham H[amilton] (1853-1921)
[Crawford Williamson] Long (1815-1878) and his discovery. [n. p., 1908] 8p. GU; NcD **00-1243**

GOSSE, Philip H[enry] (1810-1888)
Evenings at the microscope, or researches among the minute organs and forms of animal life. New York: P. F. Collier & Son, 1900. 468p. DLC; NN; NIC; PU
00-1244

GOSSELIN, Leon
Clinical lectures on surgery. Transl. from the French by Lewis A. Stimson. Philadelphia: Lea Bros. & Co., 1900 [*c.* 1878.] 350p. MBM; ICJ; NNNAM; PU **00-1245**

GOTTHEIL, William S[amuel] (1859-1920)
Syphilis: its diagnosis and treatment. . . . Chicago: G. P. Engelhard & Co., 1901. 216p. DLC; ICJ; OCIM; PU
00-1246

GOTTHEIL, William S[amuel] (1859-1920)
The treatment of skin cancers. [Second edition.] New York: International Journal of Surgery Co., 1901. 67p. ICJ; NN
00-1247

GOTTHEIL, William S[amuel] (1859-1920)
A manual of general histology. . . . 2nd ed., rev. New York: W. R. Jenkins, 1905. 152p. DLC: ICJ; NNNAM; PPC
00-1248

GOTTHEIL, William S[amuel] (1859-1920)
Illustrated skin diseases; an atlas and text-book, with special references to modern diagnosis and the most approved methods of treatment. . . . 2nd ed., rev. and enl. New York: E. B. Treat & Co., 1906. 446p. DLC; ICJ; NNNAM; PU
00-1249

GOTTHEIL, William S[amuel] (1859-1920)
The treatment of skin cancers. . . . 3rd ed., rev. and enl. New York: International Journal of Surgery Co., [1907]. 89p. plates. DLC; NN; NNNAM **00-1250**

GOTTSCHALK, Franklin B[enjamin] (*b.* 1867)
Practical electro-therapeutics. Chicago: T. Eisele, [1904]. 331p. DLC; DNLM; ICJ; NcD **00-1251**

GOULD, Alfred H[enry]
The technic of operations upon the intestines and stomach . . . with 190 illustrations, mostly original, several of them in colors. Philadelphia and London: W. B. Saunders & Co., 1906. 302p. DLC; NcD; PPC; PU **00-1252**

GOULD, A[lfred] Pearce (1852-1922)
Elements of surgical diagnosis. . . . 3rd ed., rev. and enl. Chicago: W. T. Keener & Co., 1904. 607p. ICU; IEN-M; IU-M; PU **00-1253**

GOULD, George M[ilbry] (1848-1922)
Suggestions to medical writers. . . . Philadelphia: The Philadelphia Medical Publishing Co., 1900. 185p. DLC; ICJ; PPJ; NN
00-1254

GOULD, George M[ilbry] (1848-1922)
A pocket medical dictionary; giving the pronunciation and definition of the principal words used in medicine and the collateral sciences . . . 4th ed., rev. and enl. 30,000 words. Philadelphia: P. Blakiston's Son & Co., 1900. 837p. DLC; DNLM; MBM; PPC **00-1255**

GOULD, George M[ilbry] (1848-1922)
An illustrated dictionary of medicine, biology and allied sciences . . . based upon recent scientific literature; 5th ed., with additions and corrections. Philadelphia: P. Blakiston's Son & Co., 1900. 1688p. DLC; NNNAM; OCIM; PPC
00-1256

GOULD, George M[ilbry] (1848-1922)
The student's medical dictionary; including all the words and phrases generally used in medicine, with their proper pronunciation and definitions; based on recent medical literature . . . 11th ed., enl. . . . Philadelphia: P. Blakiston's Son & Co., 1900. 840p. DLC; NNNAM; PPC; PU **00-1257**

GOULD, George M[ilbry] (1848-1922)
A cyclopedia of practical medicine and surgery: a concise reference book, alphabetically arranged, of medicine, surgery, obstetrics, materia medica, therapeutics, and the various specialties, with particular reference to diagnosis and treatment, comp. under the editorial supervision of George M. Gould, M.D. and Walter L. Pyle, M.D. . . . Philadelphia: P. Blakiston's Son & Co., 1900. 986p. DLC; MBM; NNNAM; PPC **00-1258**

GOULD, George M[ilbry] (1848-1922)
A pocket cyclopedia of medicine and surgery, based upon "A cyclopedia of practical medicine and surgery"; ed. by George M. Gould . . . and Walter L. Pyle. . . . Philadelphia: P. Blakiston's Son & Co., 1902 [1901]. 567p. DLC; MH-M; PPC; PPJ **00-1259**

GOULD, George M[ilbry] (1848-1922)
. . . A compend of the diseases of the eye and refraction, including treatment and surgery, by George M. Gould and Walter L. Pyle. . . . 2nd ed., rev. and enlarged. Philadelphia: P. Blakiston's Son & Co., 1903. 295p. MBM; NNNAM; PPC; ScCM **00-1260**

GOULD, George M[ilbry] (1848-1922)
A dictionary of new medical terms, including upwards of 38,000 words and many useful tables, being a supplement to "An illustrated dictionary of medicine, biology, and allied sciences." . . . Based upon recent scientific literature. Philadelphia: P. Blakiston's Son & Co., 1904. 571p. DLC; IU-M; NNNAM; PPC **00-1261**

GOULD, George M[ilbry] (1848-1922)
. . . A compend of the diseases of the eye and refraction, including treatment and surgery, by George M. Gould . . . and Walter L. Pyle. . . . 3rd ed., rev. and cor. One hundred and nine illustrations, several of which are in colors. Philadelphia: P. Blakiston's Son & Co., 1904. 295p. DLC; NNNAM; PPC; PU **00-1262**

GOULD, George M[ilbry] (1848-1922)
Jefferson Medical College of Philadelphia; benefactors, alumni, hospital, etc., its founders, officers, instructors, 1826-1904. A history. Chicago: Lewis Publising Co., 1904. 2 v. NNNAM; PPC; PPJ; PU **00-1263**

GOULD, George M[ilbry] (1848-1922)
The practitioner's medical dictionary; an illustrated dictionary of medicine and allied subjects, including all the words and phrases generally used in medicine, with their proper pronunciation, derivation, and definition based on recent medical literature. . . . Philadelphia: P. Blakiston's Son & Co., 1907. 1043p. DLC; IU-M; NNNAM; PPC
00-1264

GOULD, George M[ilbry] (1848-1922)
A pocket medical dictionary, giving the pronunciation and definition of the principal words used in medicine and the collateral sciences . . . 5th ed. 30,000 words pronounced and defined. Philadelphia: P. Blakiston's Son & Co., 1909. 863p. DLC; NNNAM; OCIM; PPC **00-1265**

GOULD, George M[ilbry] (1848-1922)
Fifty-seven varieties of medical and ophthalmic blunders. . . . Ithaca, N.Y.: Andrus & Church, 1909. 23p. DLC
00-1266

[GOULD, George Milbry] (1848-1922)
Bibliography of the contributions of George M. Gould, M.D., to ophthalmology, general medicine, literature, etc. Ithaca, N.Y.: Andrus & Church, 1909. 62p. DLC; DNLM; NIC; NNNAM **00-1267**

GOULD, George M[ilbry] (1848-1922)
An illustrated dictionary of medicine, biology and allied sciences . . . 6th ed., with additions and corrections and a supplement including upwards of 38,000 additional words based upon recent scientific literature. Philadelphia: P. Blakiston's Son & Co., 1910. 1633p. CtY-M; DLC; NNNAM; PPC **00-1268**

GOULD, George M[ilbry] (1848-1922)
The practitioner's medical dictionary; an illustrated dictionary of medicine and allied subjects, including all the words and phrases generally used in medicine, with their proper pronunciation, derivation, and definition, based on recent medical literature . . . 2nd ed., illustrated. Philadelphia: P. Blakiston's Son & Co., 1910. 1043p. DLC; MBM; NNNAM; PU
00-1269

[GOULEY, John William Severin] (1832-1920)
Conference on the moral philosophy of medicine, prepared by an American physician. . . . New York, [etc.]: Rebman Co., [1906]. 368p. DLC; ICJ; NNNAM; PU
00-1270

GOULEY, John William Severin (1832-1920)
Surgery of genito-urinary organs. . . . New York: Rebman Co., [1907]. 531p. DLC; MBM; NNNAM; PPC
00-1271

GOWERS, William R[ichard] (1845-1915)
A manual of diseases of the nervous system. . . . rev. and enl. Ed. by Sir W. R. Gowers and James Taylor. . . . Philadelphia: P. Blakiston's Son & Co., 1900. 2 v. CtY-M; DLC; NIC; PPPH [v. 1, 3rd ed.; v. 2, 2nd ed.] **00-1272**

GOWERS, William R[ichard] (1845-1915)
Epilepsy and other chronic convulsive diseases. . . . 2nd ed. Philadelphia: P. Blakiston's Son & Co., 1901. 320p. CtY-M; MB; NN; PPC **00-1273**

GOWERS, William R[ichard] (1845-1915)
. . . Subjective sensations of sight and sound, abiotrophy, and other lectures. . . . Philadelphia: P. Blakiston's Son & Co., 1904. 250p. DLC; KU; NcD; PPJ **00-1274**

GOWERS, William R[ichard] (1845-1915)
A manual and atlas of medical ophthalmoscopy. 4th ed. Ed. by the author and Marcus Gunn. Philadelphia: P. Blakiston's Son & Co., 1904. 318p. plates. IU-M; NcD; NIC; PPC
00-1275

GOWERS, William R[ichard] (1845-1915)
The border-land of epilepsy. Faints, vagal attacks, vertigo, migraine, sleep symptoms, and their treatment. . . . Philadelphia: P. Blakiston's Son & Co., 1907. 121p. CtY-M; DNLM; ICJ; NcU **00-1276**

GRADLE, Henry (1855-1911)
Diseases of the nose, pharynx, and ear. . . . Philadelphia and London: W. B. Saunders & Co., 1902. 547p. plates. DLC; MBM; PPC; PU **00-1277**

GRADY, Richard
Cooperation of the public schools in teaching "good teeth, good health." New York, 1900. 13p. DNLM
00-1278

GRAETZER, Eugen
Practical pediatrics; a manual of the medical and surgical diseases of infancy and childhood . . . authorized transl., with numerous additions and notes, by Herman B. Sheffield. . . . Philadelphia: F. A. Davis Co., 1905. 544p. DLC; NNNAM; PPC; PU **00-1279**

GRAFSTROM, Axel V.
A text-book of mechano-therapy (massage and medical gymnastics) prepared for the use of medical students, trained nurses, and medical gymnasts . . . 2nd ed., rev. and enl. Philadelphia, [etc.]: W. B. Saunders & Co., 1904. 200p. plates. CtY-M; DLC; DNLM; PU **00-1280**

GRAHAM, Douglas (1848-1928)
Manual therapeutics; a treatise on massage; its history, mode of application and effects, indications and contraindications . . . 3rd ed., rev., enl., and illustrated. Philadelphia and London: J. B. Lippincott Co., 1902. 462p. plates. DLC; NNNAM; PPC; PU **00-1281**

GRANDIN, Egbert Henry (*b.* 1855)
A text-book on practical obstetrics, by Egbert H. Grandin . . . with the collaboration of George W. Jarman . . . 3rd ed., rev. and enl. Illustrated with fifty-two full-page photographic plates and one hundred and five illustrations in the text. Philadelphia, New York, [etc.]: F. A. Davis Co., 1900. 511p. DLC; MBM; NNNAM; PPC **00-1282**

GRANDIN, Egbert Henry (*b.* 1855)
A text-book on practical obstetrics, by Egbert H. Grandin . . . with the collaboration of George W. Jarman . . . and Simon Mars . . . 4th ed., rev. and enl. Illustrated with forty-seven full-page photographic plates and one hundred and sixteen illustrations in the text. Philadelphia: F. A. Davis Co., 1909. 538p. DLC; IU-M; PPC; PU **00-1283**

GRANT, H[enry] Horace (*b.* 1853)
A text-book of surgical principles and surgical diseases of the face, mouth, and jaws, for dental students. . . . Philadelphia and London: W. B. Saunders & Co., 1902. 231p. DLC; MdU-D; PPC; PU **00-1284**

GRASSET, Joseph (1849-1918)
The diagnosis of diseases of the cord. Location of lesions. . . . Transl. by Jeanne C. Solis. . . . Ann Arbor, Mich.: G. Wahr, [1901]. 96p. DLC; ICJ **00-1285**

GRASSET, Joseph (1849-1918)
The semi-insane and the semi-responsible. . . . Authorized American ed., transl. by Smith Ely Jellife, New York and London: Funk & Wagnalls Co., 1907. 415p. fold. tab. diag. DLC; ICJ; NNNAM; PU **00-1286**

GRASSET, Joseph (1849-1918)
The marvels beyond science . . . being a record of progress made in the reduction of occult phenomena to a scientific basis. . . . With a preface by Emile Faguet. . . . Authorized English translation of the 2nd rev. and enl. French ed. by René Jacques Tubeuf. New York and London: Funk & Wagnalls Co., 1910. 387p. DLC; ICJ; MH; NN **00-1287**

GRAY, Harry C.
A condensed compendium of pharmaceutical knowledge; a quiz book . . . 14th ed., rev. to conform with the U.S. pharmacopoeia, eighth decennial revision. . . . Chicago, Ill.: M. M. Gray & Co., 1905. 254p. DLC; ICJ; OCLloyd **00-1288**

GRAY, Harry C.
Gray's prescriptionist; a treatise on the art of reading and compounding physician's prescriptions, with tables of weights and measures, antidotes, abbreviations, etc. . . . Revised by George D. Oglesby. . . . Chicago, Ill.: M. M. Gray & Co., 1906. 236p. DLC; OCIM; OCLloyd **00-1289**

GRAY, Henry (1825-1861)
Anatomy, descriptive and surgical. . . . Edited by T. Pickering Pick . . . and Robert Howden. . . . A revised American, from the 15th English edition, with 780 illustrations. . . . Philadelphia and New York: Lea Bros. & Co., 1901. 1249p. DLC; NNNAM; PPC; PPJ **00-1290**

GRAY, Henry (1825-1861)
Anatomy, descriptive and surgical. . . . Ed. by T. Pickering Pick . . . and Robert Howden . . . New American ed. Thoroughly rev. and re-edited with additions by John Chalmers Da Costa . . . Illustrated with 1132 elaborate engravings. Philadelphia and New York: Lea Bros. & Co., 1905. 1600p. DLC; IU-M; PPC; PU **00-1291**

GRAY, Henry (1825-1861)
Anatomy, descriptive and surgical . . . 17th ed., thoroughly rev. and re-edited with additions, by John Chalmers Da Costa . . . and Edward Anthony Spitzka . . . illustrated with 1149 engravings. Philadelphia and New York: Lea & Febiger, 1908. 1614p. CtY-M; DLC; NNNAM; PPC **00-1292**

GRAY, Henry (1825-1861)
Anatomy, descriptive and applied . . . 18th ed., thoroughly rev. and re-edited with additions, by Edward Anthony Spitzka . . . illustrated with 1298 engravings. Philadelphia and New York: Lea & Febiger, 1910. 1496p. CU-M; DLC; NNNAM; PPC **00-1293**

GRAYSON, Charles Prevost (1859-1939)
The diseases of the nose, throat, and ear. . . . Illustrated with 120 engravings and 8 plates in colors and monochrome. Philadelphia and New York: Lea Bros. & Co., 1902. 540p. DLC; MBM; NNNAM; PPC **00-1294**

GRAYSON, Charles Prevost (1859-1939)
The diseases of the nose, throat, and ear. . . . 2nd ed., rev. and enl. Illustrated with 152 engravings and 15 plates in colors and monochrome. Philadelphia and New York: Lea Bros. & Co., 1906. 532p. DLC; NNNAM; PPC; PU **00-1295**

GREEFF, Richard (1862-1938)
Atlas of external diseases of the eye for physicians and students . . . only authorized English transl. by P. W. Shedd . . . with 84 illustrations in color from wax models printed on 54 plates with explanatory text. The illustrations are from models in the Pathoplastic Institute in Berlin, art director: F. Kolbow. New York: Rebman Co., [1909]. 140p. + plates. DLC; ICJ; NNNAM; PPC **00-1296**

GREEN, Samuel Sweet (1837-1918) and John GREEN
Medical education in Boston and New York in 1827. An old letter read at the meeting of the American Antiquarian Society, October 21, 1902. [Worcester], [1902]. 6p. MBM **00-1297**

GREEN, Thomas Henry (1841-1923)
Pathology and morbid anatomy. . . . Rev. and enl. by H. Montague Murray . . . 9th American, rev. from the 9th English ed. by Walton Martin. . . . With 4 colored plates and 339 illustrations. Philadelphia and New York: Lea Bros. & Co., 1900. 585p. DLC; NNNAM; PPC; PU **00-1298**

GREEN, Thomas Henry (1841-1923)
Pathology and morbid anatomy. . . . 10th American revised from the 10th English ed. Rev. and enl. by W. Cecil Bosanquet. . . . With a colored plate and 348 illustrations in the text. Philadelphia and New York: Lea Bros. & Co., 1905. 610p. DLC; MBM; NNNAM; PPC **00-1299**

GREENE, Charles Lyman (*b.* 1862)
The medical examination for life insurance and its associated clinical methods, with chapters on the insurance of substandard lives and accident insurance. Philadelphia: P. Blakiston's Son & Co., 1900. 426p. DLC; DNLM; PPC; PU **00-1300**

GREENE, Charles Lyman (*b.* 1862)
Medical diagnosis; a manual for students and practitioners. . . . With 7 colored plates and 230 illustrations. Philadelphia: P. Blakiston's Son & Co., 1907. 683p. DLC; ICJ; MBM; PPC **00-1301**

GREENE, Charles Lyman (*b.* 1862)
Medical diagnosis; a manual for students and practitioners. . . . 2nd ed., rev., with 7 colored plates and 241 illustrations. Philadelphia: P. Blakiston's Son & Co., 1907. 691p. DLC; MBM; PPC; PU **00-1302**

GREENE, Charles Lyman (*b.* 1862)
Medical diagnosis, a manual for students and practitioners . . . 3rd ed., rev., with 7 colored plates and 248 illustrations. Philadelphia: P. Blakiston's Son & Co., 1910. CtY-M; DLC; NNNAM; PPC **00-1303**

[GREENE, Charles Wilson] (1866-1947)
Experimental pharmacology; a laboratory guide for the study of the physiological action of drugs. Laboratory of physiology and pharmacology. University of Missouri, Columbia, Missouri. [Columbus, Mo.: Press of E. W. Stephens, 1905.] 54p. DLC **00-1304**

GREENE, Charles Wilson (1866-1947)
Experimental pharmacology, a laboratory guide for the study of the physiological action of drugs . . . 3rd ed., rev., with 37 new illustrations. Philadelphia: P. Blakiston's Son & Co., 1909. 76p. DLC; PPC; OCLloyd **00-1305**

GREENE, Robert Holmes (*b.* 1861)
Diseases of the genito-urinary organs and the kidney, by Robert Holmes Greene . . . and Harlow Brooks . . . with 292 illustrations. Philadelphia and London: W. B. Saunders & Co., 1907. 536p. plates. DLC; NNNAM; PPC; PU **00-1306**

GREENE, Robert Holmes (*b.* 1861)
Diseases of the genito-urinary organs and the kidney, by Robert Holmes Greene . . . and Harlow Brooks . . . 2nd ed., rev. and enl., with 323 illustrations. Philadelphia and London: W. B. Saunders & Co., 1908. 605p. plates. DLC; ICRM; NNNAM; PPC **00-1307**

GRIEVES, Clarence J.
Cemented inlays or contact fillings, which? Toledo: Franklin, 1906. 9p. PU **00-1308**

GRIFFITH, Frederic R[ichardson]
A hand-book of surgery for students and practitioners . . . with 417 illustrations. Philadelphia, London, [etc.] : W. B. Saunders & Co., 1904. 579p. CtY-M; DLC; PPC; ScCM **00-1309**

GRIFFITH, John Price Crozer (1856-1941)
The care of the baby; a manual for mothers and nurses, containing practical directions for the management of infancy and childhood in health and in disease . . . 3rd ed., thoroughly rev. Philadelphia, New York [etc.] : W. B. Saunders & Co., 1903. 436p. plates. DLC; NNNAM; PPC; PU [4th ed., 1907, 455p.] **00-1310**

GRIFFITHS, T[homas] M[ichael]
Non-secret formulas. . . . 2nd ed. [St. Louis, Mo.: Printed by Interstate Printing Co., 1910.] 514p. DLC; ICJ; MB; NN **00-1311**

GRINDON, Joseph (*b.* 1858)
. . . Diseases of the skin. A manual for students and practitioners . . . illustrated with thirty-nine engravings. Philadelphia and New York: Lea Bros. & Co., [1902]. 377p. DLC; MH-M; NN; PPC **00-1312**

GROFF, John Eldred (*b.* 1854)
Handbook of materia medica, for trained nurses; including sections on therapeutics and toxicology and a glossary of terms with dose and use of each drug. . . . Philadelphia: P. Blakiston's Son & Co., 1900 [*c.* 1898]. 235p. DLC: DNLM; NN; PP **00-1313**

GROFF, John Eldred (*b.* 1854)
Materia medica for nurses. . . . 2nd ed., rev. and rewritten. Philadelphia: P. Blakiston's Son & Co., 1903. 160p. DLC; OCLloyd; PPC; PU **00-1314**

GROFF, John Eldred (*b.* 1854)
Materia medica for nurses. . . . 3rd ed. rev., with an appendix giving list of questions for self-examination, based upon 8th decennial revision of the U.S. pharmacopoeia. Philadelphia: P. Blakiston's Son & Co., 1905. 176p. DLC; PPC; PU **00-1315**

GROFF, John Eldred (*b.* 1854)
Materia medica for nurses; with an epitome of official drugs, preparations and chemicals, giving their medicinal uses and doses; and questions for self-examination. . . . 4th rev. ed., rearranged by Lucy C. Ayers. . . . Sections on therapeutics rewritten by Herman C. Pitts. . . . Philadelphia: P. Blakiston's Son & Co., 1908. 221p. DLC; ICJ; PPC; PU **00-1316**

GROFF, John Eldred (*b.* 1854)
Materia medica for nurses, with an epitome of offical drugs, preparations and chemicals, giving their medicinal uses and doses; and questions for self-examination . . . 5th rev. ed., with an appendix on solutions, rearranged by Lucy C. Ayers. . . . Sections on therapeutics rewritten by Herman C. Pitts. . . . Philadelphia: P. Blakiston's Son & Co., 1909. 223p. DLC; ICJ; PPC; PU **00-1317**

GROVES, Ernest W[illiam] H[ey] (1872-1944)
A synopsis of surgery. . . . 2nd ed. New York: William Wood & Co., 1910. 579p. NNNAM; NNU-M; NjR; OCIM **00-1318**

GRUNER, Oskar C[ameron] (*b.* 1877)
Studies in puncture fluids: a contribution to clinical pathology. Philadelphia: P. Blakiston's Son & Co., 1910. 289p. DLC; MBM; NNNAM; PPC **00-1319**

GUERINI, Vincenzo (*b.* 1859)
A history of dentistry from the most ancient times until the end of the eighteenth century. Philadelphia and New York: Lea & Febiger, 1909. 355p. 20 plates. DLC; DNLM; MdU-D; PPC **00-1320**

GUFFEY, Don Carlos
Notes on general and medical chemistry, based on Dr. Marshall's lectures, Marshall's notes, and various works on general and medical chemistry. . . . Unionville, Mo.: Conger & Martin, printers, 1902. 233p. DLC **00-1321**

GUILFORD, S[imeon] Hayden (1841-1919)
Orthodontia, or malposition of the human teeth, its prevention and remedy. 4th ed. Philadelphia: T. C. Davis, 1905. 220p. DLC; MdU-D; NNC; PU [3rd ed., 1898. 254p. CtY-M; DLC; DNLM; PU] **00-1322**

GUILFORD, William M.
Notes and medical history of Lebanon County; paper read before the Lebanon County Historical Society, April 24, 1908. . . . [Lebanon, Pa., 1908.] 15p. DLC **00-1323**

GULICK, Charlotte Emily (*b.* 1865)
Emergencies. . . . Boston: Ginn & Co., [1909]. 173p. DLC; MB; MH; NN [Half-title: The Gulick Hygiene Series by L. H. Gulick] **00-1324**

GULICK, Luther H[alsey] (1865-1918)
The bicycle as a therapeutic agent. Boston, 1904. 19p. MH; NN **00-1325**

GULICK, Luther H[alsey] (1865-1918)
Physical education by muscular exercise. . . . Philadelphia: P. Blakiston's Son & Co., 1904. 67p. DLC; MH; PP; NN **00-1326**

GULICK, Luther H[alsey] (1865-1918)
Muscle building; practical points for practical people. New York: American Sports Publishing Co., 1905. 43p. DLC; NN **00-1327**

GULICK, Luther H[alsey] (1865-1918)
Health of school children. Statement of the endeavors of the Board of Education to conserve the health of children under its care. . . . New York: William Wood & Co., [1906]. 28p. DLC; NN; NNNAM; PP **00-1328**

GULICK, Luther H[alsey] (1865-1918)
The argument for medical inspection of schools and significant facts about medical inspection. . . . New York: Dept. of Child Hygiene, Russell Sage Foundation, [1908]. 9p. DLC; NN **00-1329**

GULICK, Luther H[alsey] (1865-1918)
. . . Medical inspection of schools, by Luther Halsey Gulick . . . and Leonard P. Ayres. . . . New York: Charities Publication Committee, 1908. 276p. DLC; ICJ; MH; NN **00-1330**

GULICK, Luther H[alsey] (1865-1918)
Mind and work. . . . New York: Doubleday, Page & Co., 1908. 201p. DLC; MB; NN; PP **00-1331**

GULICK, Luther H[alsey] (1865-1918)
Tuberculosis and the public schools. [New York: New York Charities Publication Committee, 1908?] 8p. DLC; NN **00-1332**

GULICK, Luther H[alsey] (1865-1918)
Children of the century. . . . New York: Dept. of Child Hygiene, Russell Sage Foundation, [1909?]. 9p. DLC; NN **00-1333**

GULICK, Luther H[alsey] (1865-1918)
Exercise and rest. . . . New York: Dept. of Child Hygiene, Russell Sage Foundation, [1910]. 7p. DLC; NN **00-1334**

HAAB, Otto (1850-1931)
Atlas and epitome of ophthalmoscopy and ophthalmoscopic diagnosis. . . . Authorized transl. from the 3rd rev. and enl. German ed. Ed. by G. E. De Schweinitz. . . . With 152 colored lithographic illustrations. Philadelphia and London: W. B. Saunders & Co., 1901. 85p. 80 col. plates. DLC; NNNAM; PPC; PU **00-1335**

HAAB, Otto (1850-1931)
Atlas of the external diseases of the eye, including a brief treatise on the pathology and treatment. . . . Authorized transl. from the German. 2nd ed., rev., edited by G. E. De Schweinitz. . . . With 98 colored lithographic illustrations on 48 plates. Philadelphia, London, [etc.]: W. B. Saunders & Co., 1903. 232p. DLC; IU-M; NNNAM; PPC **00-1336**

HAAB, Otto (1850-1931)
Atlas and epitome of operative ophthalmology . . . authorized transl. from the German, with editorial notes and additions; ed. by G. E. De Schweinitz . . . with 300 colored lithographic plates and 154 textcuts. Philadelphia, New York, [etc.]: W. B. Saunders & Co., 1905. 377p. 30 col. plates. DLC; MBM; NNNAM; PPC **00-1337**

HAAB, Otto (1850-1931)
Atlas and epitome of ophthalmoscopy and ophthalmoscopic diagnosis . . . 2nd American ed. from the 5th rev. and enl. German ed. Edited by G. E. De Schweinitz . . . with 125 colored lithographic illustrations. Philadelphia and London: W. B. Saunders & Co., 1909. 94p. col. plates. DLC; NNNAM; OCIM; PPC **00-1338**

HAAB, Otto (1850-1931)
Atlas of the external diseases of the eye, including a brief treatise on the pathology and treatment. . . . Authorized transl. from the German. 3rd ed., rev., edited by G. E. De Schweinitz . . . with 101 colored lithographic illustrations on 46 plates. Philadelphia and London: W. B. Saunders & Co., 1909. 244p. 46 col. plates. DLC; LNT-M; NNNAM; PU **00-1339**

HADRA, Berthold Ernest (1842-1908)
The public and the doctor. By a regular physician. Dallas, Tex.: B. E. Hadra, [1902]. 149p. DLC **00-1340**

[HAHNEMANN, Samuel] (1755-1843)
Historic sketch of the monument erected in Washington City under the auspicies of the American Institute of Homoeopathy to the honor of Samuel Hahnemann and for the ornamentation of the national capitol. Dedicated June 21, 1900 in the presence of the President of the United States and with the active participation of public officials, civil and military. Washington, D.C., 1900. [unp.] DLC **00-1341**

HAHNEMANN, Samuel (1755-1843)
The chronic diseases, their peculiar nature and their homoeopathic cure. (Theoretical part only in this volume). . . . Transl. from the 2nd enl. German ed. of 1835, by Prof. Louis H. Tafel. Philadelphia: Boericke & Tafel, 1904. 269p. DLC; ICJ; PPC; PPHa **00-1342**

HAIG, A[lexander] (1853-1924)
Diet and food considered in relation to strength and power of endurance, training, and athletics. 2nd ed. Philadelphia: P. Blakiston's Son & Co., 1900. 102p. DLC; DNLM; ICJ; PPC **00-1343**

HAIG, A[lexander] (1853-1924)
Uric acid as a factor in the causation of disease. A contribution to the pathology of high arterial tension, headache, epilepsy, mental depression, gout, rheumatism, diabetes, Bright's disease, and other disorders. 5th ed. Philadelphia: P. Blakiston's Son & Co., 1900. 846p. ICJ; KU; NcD; PPC **00-1344**

HAIG, A[lexander] (1853-1924)
Uric acid as a factor in the causation of disease. A contribution to the pathology of high arterial tension, headache, epilepsy, mental depression, gout, rheumatism, diabetes, Bright's disease, and other disorders. 6th ed. Philadelphia: P. Blakiston's Son & Co., 1903. 947p. DNLM; ICJ; PPC; PU **00-1345**

HAIG, A[lexander] (1853-1924)
Uric acid: an epitome of the subject. 2nd ed. Philadelphia: P. Blakiston's Son & Co., 1906. 162p. CtY-M; DLC; PPC; PU **00-1346**

HALBERT, Homer V[almore] (*b.* 1858)
The practice of medicine. . . . Chicago: P. H. Mallen Co., 1905. 1110p. CtY-M; DLC; ICJ; OCIM **00-1347**

HALE-WHITE, William (1857-1949)
Materia medica, pharmacy, pharmacology and therapeutics. . . . ed. by Reynold W. Wilcox. . . . 5th American ed., thoroughly revised. Philadelphia: P. Blakiston's Son & Co., 1901. 744p. DLC; NNNAM; OCLloyd; PPC **00-1348**

HALE-WHITE, William (1857-1949)
Common affections of the liver. New York: William Wood & Co., 1908. 302p. DLC; ICJ; MBM; NN **00-1349**

HALL, G[ranville] Stanley (1844-1924)
Adolescence. Its psychology and its relations to physiology, anthropology, sociology, sex, crime, religion, and education. New York: D. Appleton & Co., 1904. 2 v. ICU; MH; NIC; NN **00-1350**

HALL, I[saac] Walker (*b.* 1868)
The purin bodies of food stuffs and the role of uric acid in health and disease. 2nd ed., rev. Philadelphia: P. Blakiston's Son & Co., 1904. 201p. 2 col. plates. DLC; ICJ; MBM; NNNAM **00-1351**

HALL, I[saac] Walker (*b.* 1868)
Methods of morbid histology and clinical pathology. Philadelphia: J. B. Lippincott Co., 1905. 290p. DLC; ICJ; NN; PU **00-1352**

HALL, Winfield Scott (*b.* 1861)
A manual of experimental physiology for students of medicine. . . . With 89 illustrations and a colored plate. Philadelphia and New York: Lea Bros. & Co., 1904. 245p. col. plate. CtY-M; DLC; ICJ; PPC **00-1353**

HALL, Winfield Scott (*b.* 1861)
A text-book of physiology, normal and pathological. For students and practitioners of medicine. . . . 2nd ed., rev. and enl. Illustrated with engravings and three colored plates. Philadelphia and New York: Lea Bros. & Co., 1905. 795p. DLC; NNNAM; PPC; PU **00-1354**

HALL, Winfield Scott (*b.* 1861)
Nutrition and dietetics; a manual for students of medicine, for trained nurses, and for dietitians in hospitals and other institutions. . . . New York and London: D. Appleton & Co., 1910. 315p. DLC; ICJ; NNNAM; PU **00-1355**

HALLIBURTON, William D[obinson] (1860-1931)
Ten lectures on biochemistry of muscle and nerve. . . . Philadelphia: P. Blakiston's Son & Co., 1904. 160p. plates. DLC; ICJ; NN; PPC **00-1356**

HALSTEAD, A. E[dward] (*b.* 1868)
Report of a case of recovery after ligation of the first portion of the right subclavian artery for aneurism of the third portion. Philadelphia, 1900. 4p. DLC **00-1357**

HALSTEAD, A. E[dward] (*b.* 1868)
Surgical cases. Chicago, 1900. 11p. DLC **00-1358**

HALSTEAD, A. E[dward] (*b.* 1868)
Carcinoma of the thyroid gland. Detroit, 1901. 9p. DLC **00-1359**

HALSTED, William S[tewart] (1852-1922)
Circular suture of the intestines; an experimental study. [1900?] 24p. [Originally, Amer. J. Med. Sci., 94 (1887): 436-461] **00-1360**

HALSTED, William S[tewart] (1852-1922)
Contributions to the surgery of the bile passages, especially of the common bile-duct. Baltimore, 1900. 40p. DNLM; MdBJ-W **00-1361**

HALSTED, William S[tewart] (1852-1922)
The cure of the more difficult as well as the simpler inguinal ruptures. . . . Baltimore: The Lord Baltimore Press, 1903. 18p. plates. NNC **00-1362**

HALSTED, William S[tewart] (1852-1922)
The training of the surgeon; the annual address in medicine delivered at Yale University, June 27, 1904 . . . [1904?] 25p. MH; NNC **00-1363**

HALSTED, William S[tewart] (1852-1922)
Hypoparathyreosis, status parathyreoprivus and transplantation of the parathyroid glands. [1907.] 15p. plate. DNLM; NNC **00-1364**

HALSTED, William S[tewart] (1852-1922)
The results of radical operations for the cure of carcinoma of the breast. [1907.] 19p. NNC **00-1365**

HALSTED, William S[tewart] (1852-1922)
Partial, progressive and complete occlusion of the aorta and other large arteries in the dog by means of the metal band. [1909.] 19p. 3 plates. MdBJ-W; NNNAM **00-1366**

HALSTED, William S[tewart] (1852-1922)
Auto- and isotransplantation, in dogs, of the parathyroid glandules. [1909.] 24p. NNC; NN; NNNAM
00-1367

HALSTED, William St[ewart] (1852-1922)
End-to-end suture of the intestine by a bulkhead method. Preliminary communication. [1910.] 6p. NNC
00-1368

HAMBLY, Charles R.
The practice builder. A treatise on the conduct and enlargement of a dental practice. . . . Bradford, [Pa.]: American Dental Publishing Co., 1902. 668p. CtY-M [1st ed., 1897, 668p., DLC; PU] **00-1369**

HAMILTON, Allan McLane (1848-1919)
A system of legal medicine, by Allan McLane Hamilton and Lawrence Godkin . . . and others. . . . Illustrated . . . 2nd ed. New York: E. B. Treat & Co., 1900. 2 v. plates. DLC; ICJ; NNNAM; PPC **00-1370**

HAMILTON, Allan McLane (1848-1919)
Railway and other accidents with relation to injury and disease of the nervous system; a book for court use. . . . With 15 plates, 2 superimposed charts and 36 illustrations. New York: William Wood & Co., 1904. 351p. DLC; MBM; NNNAM; PU
00-1371

HAMILTON, Hugh (*b.* 1847)
The address of the retiring president, January 30, 1903. Harrisburg, Pa., 1903. 8p. NN [Pennsylvania State Medical Society]. **00-1372**

HAMMARSTEN, Olof (1841-1932)
A text-book of physiological chemistry. . . . Authorized transl. from the author's enl. and rev. 4th German ed., by John A. Mandel. . . . 3rd ed. 1st thousand. New York: J. Wiley & Sons; [etc., etc.], 1900. 628p. CtY-M; DLC; ICU; NN
00-1373

HAMMARSTEN, Olof (1841-1932)
A text-book of physiological chemistry. . . . Authorized transl. from the author's enl. and rev. 5th German ed., by John A. Mandel. . . . 4th ed. 1st thousand. New York: J. Wiley & Sons; London: Chapman & Hall, 1904. 703p. DLC; ICJ; NN; PU
00-1374

HAMMARSTEN, Olof (1841-1932)
A text-book of physiological chemistry. . . . Authorized transl. from the author's enlarged and revised 6th German ed., by John A. Mandel. . . . 5th ed., 1st thousand. New York: J. Wiley & Sons, [etc., etc.], 1908. 845p. DLC; MA; MBM; NN
00-1375

HAMMER, William J[oseph] (*b.* 1858)
Radium, and other radio-active substances: polonium, actinium and thorium, with a consideration of phosphorescent and fluorescent substances, the properties and applications of selenium and the treatment of disease by ultra-violet light. New York: D. Van Nostrand Co., 1903. 72p. DLC; ICJ; NN; PU **00-1376**

HAMMOND, Phillip (1871-1937)
Diseases of the ear of interest to insurance examiners. [Boston], 1902. 6p. MH **00-1377**

HAMMOND, Phillip (1871-1937)
Some acute diseases of the ear; their diagnosis and treatment. [Boston, 1902.] 12p. MH **00-1378**

HAMMOND, Phillip (1871-1937)
The palliative treatment of acute mastoiditis and its limitations. Chicago, 1904. 6p. MH **00-1379**

HAMMOND, Phillip (1871-1937)
Some recent experiences with chronic suppurations of the ear. Chicago, 1904. 6p. MH **00-1380**

HAMMOND, Phillip (1871-1937)
Technic in the after care of the radical mastoid operation. Chicago, 1906. 6p. MH **00-1381**

HAMMOND, Phillip (1871-1937)
Headaches due to aural disease. Chicago: American Med. Ass'n., 1906. 4p. NN **00-1382**

A HANDBOOK on the prevention of tuberculosis, being the first annual report of the Committee on the Prevention of Tuberculosis. . . . New York: The Charity Organization Society, 1903. 388p. NN; NNNAM; NNU-M; PP **00-1383**

HANNEY, P. M.
How to gain health and long life. Chicago: The Hazel Pure Food Co., 1910. 178p. DLC; ICJ [1st ed., 1899, 114p.]
00-1384

HANSELL, Howard F[orde] (*b.* 1855)
Text-book of diseases of the eye, for student and practitioners of medicine, by Howard F. Hansell . . . and William M. Sweet . . . with chapters by Christian R. Holmes, M.D., Casey A. Wood . . . Wendell Reber, M.D. With 256 illustrations, including colored plates. Philadelphia: P. Blakiston's Son & Co., 1903. 532p. DLC; NNNAM; PPC; PU **00-1385**

HANSELL, Howard F[orde] (*b.* 1855)
Diseases of the eye. . . . A treatise on the principles and practice of ophthalmic medicine and surgery. By Howard F. Hansell and William M. Sweet. . . . Philadelphia: P. Blakiston's Son & Co., 1906. 515p. col. plates. CU-M; NNNAM; PPC; PU
00-1386

HANSELL, Howard F[orde] (*b.* 1855)
The ocular muscles. . . . A practical handbook of the muscular anomalies of the eye. Philadelphia: P. Blakiston's Son & Co., 1910. 223p. DLC; MBM; PPC; PU **00-1387**

HARDAWAY, William A[ugustus] (1850-1923)
Handbook of cutaneous therapeutics, including sections on the X-ray, high-frequency current and the minor surgery of the skin, for the use of general practitioners, by W. A. Hardaway . . . and Joseph Grindon. . . . Philadelphia and New York: Lea Bros. & Co., 1907. 606p. DLC; NNNAM; PPC; PU
00-1388

HARDESTY, Irving (*b.* 1866)
Neurological technique; some special histological methods employed for the study of the nervous system, together with a laboratory outline for the dissection of the central nervous system and the neurological nomenclature "[bna]" arranged in a classified list. . . . Chicago: The University of Chicago Press; [etc., etc.], 1902. 183p. DLC: ICJ; ICU; PPJ
00-1389

HARDESTY, Irving (*b.* **1866)**
A laboratory guide for histology; laboratory outlines for the study of histology and microscopic anatomy. . . . With a chapter on laboratory drawing by Adelebert Watts Lee. . . . With 30 illustrations 9 of which are in colors. Philadelphia: P. Blakiston's Son & Co., 1908. 193p. DLC; DNLM; IU-M; PPC **00-1390**

HARDESTY, Irving (*b.* **1866)**
A class model of the spinal cord. [1908.] 15p. PU **00-1391**

HARDING, Arthur R[obert] (*b.* **1871)**
Ginseng and other medicinal plants. A book of valuable information for growers as well as collectors of medicinal roots, barks, leaves . . . [rev. ed.]. Columbus: The Author, 1908. 367p. MH; NN; OCLloyd; PU [1st ed., 1908, 317p.] **00-1392**

HARE, Hobart Amory (1862-1931)
A text-book of practical therapeutics, with especial reference to the application of remedial measures to disease and their employment upon a rational basis. . .. 8th ed., enl., thoroughly rev. and largely re-written. Illustrated with 37 engravings and 3 colored plates. Philadelphia and New York: Lea Bros. & Co., 1900. 798p. DLC; NNNAM; PPC; PPJ **00-1393**

HARE, Hobart Amory, ed. (1862-1931)
A system of practical therapeutics. . . . 2nd ed., rev. and largely rewritten. . . . Philadelphia and New York: Lea Bros. & Co., 1901. 3 v. plates. DLC; NNNAM; PPC; PU **00-1394**

HARE, Hobart Amory (1862-1931)
Practical diagnosis: the use of symptoms and physical signs in the diagnosis of disease. 5th ed., rev. and enl. . . . Illustrated with 236 engravings and 25 plates. Philadelphia and New York: Lea Bros. & Co., 1902. 698p. DLC; MBM; NNNAM; PPC **00-1395**

HARE, Hobart Amory (1862-1931)
A text-book of practical therapeutics, with especial reference to the application of remedial measures to disease and their employment upon a rational basis. . . . 9th ed., enl., thoroughly rev. and largely re-written. Illustrated with 105 engravings and 4 colored plates. Philadelphia and New York: Lea Bros. & Co., 1902. 857p. DLC; IU-M; NNNAM; PPC **00-1396**

HARE, Hobart Amory (1862-1931)
A text-book of practical therapeutics, with especial reference to the application of remedial measures to disease and their employment upon a rational basis. . . . 10th ed., enl., thoroughly rev. and largely re-written. Illutrated with 113 engravings and 4 colored plates. Philadelphia and New York: Lea Bros. & Co., 1904. 908p. CtY-M; DLC; NNNAM; PPC **00-1397**

HARE, Hobart Amory (1862-1931)
A text-book of practical therapeutics, with especial reference to the application of remedial measures to disease and their employment upon a rational basis. . . . 11th ed., enl., thoroughly rev. and largely re-written. Illustrated with 113 engravings and 4 colored plates. Philadelphia and New York: Lea Bros. & Co., 1905. 910p. DLC; ICRM; NNNAM; PU **00-1398**

HARE, Hobart Amory (1862-1931)
A text-book of the practice of medicine. For students and practitioners. . . . Illustrated with 129 engravings and 10 plates in colors and monochrome. Philadelphia and New York: Lea Bros. & Co., 1905. 1119p. DLC; NNNAM; PPC; PU **00-1399**

HARE, Hobart Amory (1862-1931)
The national standard dispensatory. Containing the natural history, chemistry, pharmacy, actions, and uses of medicines. . . . In accordance with the eighth decennial revision of the United States pharmacopoeia, 1905. By Hobart Amory Hare . . . Charles Caspari, Jr. . . . Henry H. Rusby . . . Joseph F. Geisler . . . Edward Kremers . . . and Daniel Base. . . . Philadelphia and New York: Lea Bros. & Co., 1905. 1860p. DLC; NNNAM; OCLloyd; PPC ["This dispensatory is designed to succeed the National dispensatory of Stillé and Maisch."—Author's pref.] **00-1400**

HARE, Hobart Amory (1862-1931)
A text-book of practical therapeutics, with especial references to the application of remedial measures to disease and their employment on a rational basis. . . . 12th ed., enl., thoroughly rev. and largely re-written. Illustrated with 114 engravings and 4 colored plates. Philadelphia and New York: Lea Bros. & Co., 1907. 939p. DLC; MdBM; NNNAM; PU **00-1401**

HARE, Hobart Amory (1862-1931)
Practical diagnosis; the use of symptoms and physical signs in the diagnosis of disease . . . 6th ed., rev. and enl., illustrated with 203 engravings and 16 plates. Philadelphia and New York: Lea Bros. & Co., 1907. 616p. DLC; MBM; PPC; PU **00-1402**

HARE, Hobart Amory (1862-1931)
A text-book of the practice of medicine. For students and practitioners. . . . 2nd ed., rev. and enl. Illustrated with 131 engravings and 11 plates in colors and monochrome. Philadelphia and New York: Lea Bros. & Co., 1907. 1132p. DLC; NNNAM; PPC; PPJ **00-1403**

HARE, Hobart Amory (1862-1931)
The national standard dispensatory. Containing the natural history, chemistry, pharmacy, actions, and uses of medicines. . . . In accordance with the eight decennial revision of the United States pharmacopoeia, as amended to 1908. By Hobart Amory Hare . . . Charles Caspari, Jr. . . . Henry H. Rusby . . . Joseph F. Geisler . . . Edward Kremers . . . and Daniel Base . . . 2nd ed., thoroughly rev. and much enl. Philadelphia and New York: Lea & Febiger, 1909 [1908]. 2011p. DLC; NNNAM; OCLloyd; PU **00-1404**

HARE, Hobart Amory (1862-1931)
The medical complications, accidents and sequels of typhoid fever and the other exanthemata, by Hobart Amory Hare . . . and E. J. G. Beardsley . . . with a special chapter on the mental disturbances following typhoid fever, by F. X. Dercum . . . with 26 illustrations and 2 plates. 2nd ed. Philadelphia and New York: Lea & Febiger, [1909]. 406p. DLC; NNNAM; PPC; PU **00-1405**

HARE, Hobart Amory (1862-1931)
A text-book of practical therapeutics, with especial reference to the application of remedial measures to disease and their employment upon a rational basis. . . . 13th ed., enl., thoroughly rev., and largely re-written. Illustrated with 122 engravings and 4 colored plates. Philadelphia and New York: Lea & Febiger, 1909. 958p. CU-M; DLC; GU; PPC **00-1406**

HARE, Hobart Amory, ed. (1862-1931)
Modern treatment; the management of disease with medicinal and non-medicinal remedies, in contributions by American and foreign authorities . . . assisted by H. R. M. Landis. . . . Philadelphia and New York: Lea & Febiger, [1910-11]. 2 v. plates. DLC; MBM; NNNAM; PPC **00-1407**

HARLEY, George (1829-1896)
On sounding for gall-stones and the extrusion of gall-stones by digital manipulation. New York: William Wood & Co., [1900]. 26p. IU-M; NN [Printed out of Wood's Medical and Surgical Monographs, vol. 4, No. 3, pp. 851-877, 1889] **00-1408**

HARLEY, George (1829-1896)
The urine and its derangements. With the application of physiological chemistry to the diagnosis and treatment of constitutional as well as local diseases. Being a course of original lectures delivered at University College, London. Philadelphia: P. Blakiston's Son & Co., 1900. 334p. CtY-M; ICJ; NNC; PPJ [First American ed., Philadelphia: Lindsay & Blakiston, 1872] **00-1409**

HARLEY, George (1829-1896)
Diseases of the liver, with and without juandice, with the special application of physiological chemistry to their diagnosis and treatment. Philadelphia: P. Blakiston's Son & Co., 1900. 751p. DLC; ICJ; NN; PPC [1st American ed., 1883] **00-1410**

HARRINGTON, Charles (1856-1908)
A manual of practical hygiene, for students, physicians, and medical officers. . . . Illustrated with twelve plates and one hundred and five engravings. Philadelphia and New York: Lea Bros. & Co., 1901. 729p. DLC; DNLM; NNNAM; PPC **00-1411**

HARRINGTON, Charles (1856-1908)
A manual of practical hygiene for students, physicians, and medical officers. . . . 2nd ed., rev. and enl. Illustrated with twelve plates in colors and monochrome, and one hundred and thirteen engravings. Philadelphia and New York: Lea Bros. & Co., 1902. 760p. DLC; MBM; NNNAM; PPC **00-1412**

HARRINGTON, Charles (1856-1908)
A manual of practical hygiene for students, physicians, and medical officers. . . . 3rd ed., rev. and enl. Illustrated with twelve plates in colors and monochrome, and one hundred and eighteen engravings. Philadelphia and New York: Lea Bros. & Co., 1905. 793p. DLC; IU-M; NNNAM; PPC **00-1413**

HARRINGTON, Thomas Francis (1866-1919)
Dr. Samuel Fuller, of the Mayflower (1620), the pioneer physician. . . . [Baltimore: The Friedenwald Co., 1903.] 21p. DLC; MdU-D; PPC **00-1414**

HARRINGTON, Thomas Francis (1866-1919)
The Harvard Medical School; a history, narrative and documentary. 1782-1905. By Thomas Francis Harrington, M.D., class of 1888; ed. by James Gregory Mumford, M.D., class of 1888. . . . New York, Chicago: Lewis Publishing Co., 1905. 3 v. plates. DLC; MH; NN; PP **00-1415**

HARRIS, Malcolm LaSalle (1862-1936)
Tuberculosis of the kidney. Read by invitation before the Suffolk County Medical Society, Boston, Mass., March 17, 1909. Chicago: American Medical Association, 1909. 15p. NN **00-1416**

HARRIS, Malcolm LaSalle (1862-1936)
A new operation for prolapse of the uterus. Chicago: American Medical Association. 1910. 7p. NN **00-1417**

HARRISON, Eveleen
Home nursing; modern scientific methods for the care of the sick. New York and London: Macmillan & Co., 1900. 235p. DLC; DNLM; NNNAM; PPC **00-1418**

HART, D[avid] Berry (1851-1920)
Manual of gynecology, by D. Berry Hart and A. H. Barbour. 5th ed. New York: J. H. Vail, 1900 [*c.* 1897]. 743p. DLC; PPC; PPJ; PU [Vail also published the 4th ed. (1890), 722p.] **00-1419**

HART, D[avid] Berry (1851-1920)
Manual of gynecology, by D. Berry Hart and A. H. Barbour. 6th ed. New York: William Wood & Co., 1904. 736p. DNLM; ICJ; NN; PPC [1st-6th ed., New York: William Wood & Co., 1883-1904] **00-1420**

HART, D[avid] Berry (1851-1920)
Manual of gynecology, by D. Berry Hart . . . and A. H. Freeland Barbour . . . with 12 lithographs and 359 woodcuts. 6th ed. Chicago: W. T. Keener & Co., 1905. 736p. DLC: ICJ; PPC; PU **00-1421**

HART, D[avid] Berry (1851-1920)
Phases of evolution and heredity. New York: Rebman Co., 1910. 259p. CtY-M; DNLM; ICJ; PPC **00-1422**

HARTMAN, Samuel B[rubaker] (*b.* 1830)
The confidential physician, or the theory and practice of medicine simplified. Columbus, O.: Dr. S. B. Hartman & Co., 1900. 174p. DLC [1st ed., 1885; 107p.] **00-1423**

HARTRIDGE, Gustavus (1849-1923)
The refraction of the eye. A manual for students. 10th ed. Philadelphia: P. Blakiston's Son & Co., 1900. 269p. 1 plate. DNLM; NNNAM; PPC; PU **00-1424**

HARTRIDGE, Gustavus (1849-1923)
The ophthalmoscope. A manual for students. 4th ed. Philadelphia: P. Blakiston's Son & Co., 1901. 153p. NNNAM; OCIM; PPC; PU **00-1425**

HARTRIDGE, Gustavus (1849-1923)
The refraction of the eye. A manual for students. 11th ed. Philadelphia: P. Blakiston's Son & Co., 1902. 271p. NNNAM; PPC; PU; ScCM **00-1426**

HARTRIDGE, Gustavus (1849-1923)
The refraction of the eye. A manual for students. 12th ed. Philadelphia: P. Blakiston's Son & Co., 1903. 271p. IU-M; PPC; PPJ; ScMS **00-1427**

HARTRIDGE, Gustavus (1849-1923)
The refraction of the eye. A manual for students. 13th ed. Philadelphia: P. Blakiston's Son & Co., 1905. 271p. NNNAM; OCIM; PPC; PU **00-1428**

HARTRIDGE, Gustavus (1849-1923)
The refraction of the eye. A manual for students. 14th ed. Philadelphia: P. Blakiston's Son & Co., 1907. 273p. CtY-M; NNNAM; PPC; PU **00-1429**

HARTRIDGE, Gustavus (1849-1923)
The ophthalmoscope. A manual for students. 5th ed. Philadelphia: P. Blakiston's Son & Co., 1907. 153p. MBM; NNNAM; PPC; PPJ **00-1430**

HARVARD UNIVERSITY. MEDICAL SCHOOL
The Harvard Medical School, 1782-1906. [Boston? 1906] 212p. DLC; MB; MH; NN **00-1431**

HARVARD UNIVERSITY. MEDICAL SCHOOL
Dedication of the new buildings of the Harvard Medical School, September twenty-fifth and twenty-sixth, nineteen hundred and six. Boston: Pub. by the Faculty of Medicine, [1906]. 49p. DLC; MB; MH **00-1432**

HASKELL, Loomis P.
Haskell's manual of plate work; or, Hand-book for the dental laboratory. . . . Rev. ed. . . . Chicago, 1910. 63p. DLC: ICJ **00-1433**

HATCHER, Robert A[nthony] (1868-1944)
A text-book of materia medica, including laboratory exercises in the histologic and chemic examinations of drugs for pharmaceutic and medical schools and for home study, by Robert A. Hatcher . . . and Torald Sollmann. . . . Philadelphia, [etc.]: W. B. Saunders & Co., 1904. 411p. DLC; NNNAM; OCLloyd; PPC **00-1434**

HATCHER, Robert A[nthony] (1868-1944)
The pharmacopoeia and the physician; a series of articles which originally appeared in the Journal of the American Medical Association, discussing the chief substances in the United States pharmacopoeia, classifying them according to their uses and describing their methods of combination and how they may take the place of many proprietary preparations for which extravagant claims have been made. By Robert A. Hatcher . . . and Martin I. Wilbert. . . . Chicago: American Medical Association Press, 1907; 410p. DLC; ICU; NNNAM; OCLloyd **00-1435**

HATCHER, Robert A[nthony] (1868-1944)
The pharmacopoeia and the physician; a series of articles which originally appeared in the Journal of the American Medical Association, discussing the chief substances in the United States pharmacopoeia, classifying them according to their uses and describing their methods of combination and how they may take the place of many proprietary preparations for which extravagant claims have been made. By Robert. A. Hatcher . . . and Martin I. Wilbert. . . . 2nd ed., rev. and enl. Chicago: American Medical Association, 1908. 485p. MBM; IU-M; NNNAM; PPC **00-1436**

HAUBOLD, Herman A[rthur] (1867-1931)
Preparatory and after treatment in operative cases. New York: D. Appleton & Co., 1910. 650p. CtY-M; NNNAM; PPC; PU **00-1437**

HAVARD, Valery (1846-1927)
The most practicable organization for the medical department of the United States Army in active service. . . . Eno Sander Prize Essay. . . . Carlisle, Pa.: The Association of Military Surgeons, 1902. 110p. 1 diag., cut of medal. DLC; DNLM **00-1438**

HAVARD, Valery (1846-1927)
The venereal peril. Prepared by Lieutenant Colonel Valery Havard, deputy surgeon general, U.S. Army. Pub. by authority of the Secretary of War. Washington: Government Printing Office, 1903. 16p. DLC; DNLM **00-1439**

HAVARD, Valery (1846-1927)
Manual of military hygiene for the military services of the United States . . . Illustrated with seven plates and two hundred and twenty-eight engravings. New York: William Wood & Co., 1909. 481p. CtY-M; DLC: MBM; NNNAM **00-1440**

HAWES, Alfred T[aylor] (*b.* 1874)
Talks to first year nurses. . . . Boston: Whitcomb & Barrows, 1907. 191p. DLC; ICJ; MBM; NN **00-1441**

HAWES, Alfred T[aylor] (*b.* 1874)
Observations of symptoms . . . arranged for the use of nurses. Boston: Whitcomb & Barrows, 1908. 82p. DLC; ICJ; MBM **00-1442**

HAWES, Alfred T[aylor] (*b.* 1874)
Care of the patient; a book for nurses . . . with 6 illustrations. Philadelphia: P. Blakiston's Son & Co., 1910 [*c.* 1911]. 173p. DLC; ICJ; PPC; PPJ **00-1443**

HAWK, Philip Bovier (*b.* 1874)
The influence of hemorrhage upon metabolism. . . . Easton, Pa.: The Chemical Publishing Co., 1905. 73p. DLC; NN; PU **00-1444**

HAWK, Philip Bovier (*b.* 1874)
Practical physiological chemistry; a book designed for use in courses in practical physiological chemistry in schools of medicine and of science . . . with two full page plates of absorption spectra in colors, four additional full page color plates and one hundred and twenty-six figures of which twelve are in colors. Philadelphia: P. Blakiston's Son & Co., 1907. 416p. CtY-M; DLC; PPC; PU **00-1445**

HAWK, Philip Bovier (*b.* 1874)
Practical physiological chemistry; a book designed for use in courses in practical physiological chemistry in schools of medicine and of science . . . with two full page plates of absorption spectra in colors, four additional full page color plates and one hundred and twenty-six figures of which twelve are in colors. 2nd ed., rev. and enl. Philadelphia: P. Blakiston's Son & Co., 1909. 447p. DLC; DNLM; ICJ; PU **00-1446**

HAWK, Philip Bovier (*b.* 1874)
Practical physiological chemistry; a book designed for use in courses in practical physiological chemistry in schools of medicine and of science . . . 3rd ed., rev. and enl., with two full-page plates of absorption spectra in colors, four additional full-page color plates and one hundred and twenty-seven figures of which twelve are in colors. Philadelphia: P. Blakiston's Son & Co., 1910. 400p. CtY-M; DLC; DNLM; PPC **00-1447**

HAWKINS, Thomas H.
Intraligamentous growths. New York, 1900. 18p. DNLM **00-1448**

HAYDEN, James R[aynor] (*b.* 1863)
. . . Venereal diseases. A manual for students and practitioners. . . . 3rd and rev. ed. . . . Philadelphia and New York: Lea Bros. & Co., [1901]. 301p. DLC; NNNAM; PPC; PU **00-1449**

[HAYES, P. Harold]
Asthma and hay fever cured to stay cured. [Buffalo, N.Y.: The Courier Co., printers, 1900.] 100p. DLC
00-1450

HAYS, Harold Melvin (1880-1940)
Questions and answers in physiological chemistry, with common tests, formulae, equations and past examination papers, founded on the course in physiological chemistry, given at the College of Physicians and Surgeons, Columbia University, New York City. . . . New York: J. D. Abraham & Son, [1902]. 84p. DLC; ICJ; NNC; NNNAM **00-1451**

HAZEN, E[dward] H[amlin] (*b.* 1834)
New findings in ophthalmology and otology, with description of two new instruments, illustrated, . . . [Des Moines, Ia.: G. A. Miller Printing Co., 1903.] 87p. DLC; DNLM; ICJ; PPC **00-1452**

HAZZARD, Charles
The practice and applied therapeutics of osteopathy. . . . Kirksville, Mo.: American School of Osteopathy, 1900 [1901]. 266p. DLC; ICJ **00-1453**

HAZZARD, Charles
The practice and applied therapeutics of osteopathy. (2nd rev. ed.). . . . Kirksville, Mo.: Journal Printing Co., 1901. 444p. DLC; ICJ **00-1454**

HAZZARD, Charles
The practice and applied therapeutics of osteopathy. . . . (Third revised edition.) Kirksville: Journal Printing Co., 1905. 442p. DLC: ICJ **00-1455**

HEALD, George Henry (1861-1934)
Colds, their cause, prevention, and cure. . . . Washington, D.C.: Review and Herald Publishing Assn., 1905. 58p. DLC; PPC
00-1456

HEALD, George Henry (1861-1934)
Colds, their cause, prevention, and cure. . . . Washington, D.C.: Review and Herald Publishing Assn., 1907. 62p. DLC; PPC
00-1457

HEATH, Christopher (1835-1905)
A manual of minor surgery and bandaging for the use of house-surgeons, dressers and junior practitioners. 12th ed. rev. by Bilton Pollard. Philadelphia: P. Blakiston's Son & Co., 1901. 420p. ICJ; NNNAM; PPC; PU **00-1458**

HEATH, Christopher (1835-1905)
Practical anatomy: a manual of dissections. Ed. by J. Ernest Lane. . . . 9th ed. Philadelphia: P. Blakiston's Son & Co., 1902. 696p. DLC; NNNAM; PPC; ScCM **00-1459**

HECKER, Rudolf (*b.* 1868)
Atlas and epitome of diseases of children, by Dr. R. Hecker and Dr. J. Trumpp . . . authorized transl. from the German; ed. by Isaac A. Abt . . . with 48 colored plates and 147 black and white illustrations. Philadelphia and London: W. B. Saunders & Co., 1907. 453p. DLC; NNNAM; PPC; PU
00-1460

HEINEMANN, Paul G[ustav]
A laboratory guide in bacteriology, for the use of students, teachers, and practitioners. . . . Chicago: The University of Chicago Press, 1905. 143p. DLC; ICJ; ICU; NN
00-1461

HEISLER, John Clement (*b.* 1862)
A text-book of embryology for students of medicine. . . . 2nd ed., thoroughly rev. Philadelphia and London: W. B. Saunders & Co., 1901. 405p. col. plates. DLC; NNNAM; PPC; PU
00-1462

HEISLER, John Clement (*b.* 1862)
A text-book of embryology, for students of medicine. . . . with 212 illustrations, 32 of them in colors. 3rd ed., thoroughly rev. Philadelphia and London: W. B. Saunders & Co., 1907. 452p. col. plates. DLC; IU-M; NNNAM; PPC
00-1463

HEITZMANN, Louis (*b.* 1864)
Urinary analysis and diagnosis by microscopical and chemical examination . . . 2nd rev. and enl. ed., with one hundred and thirty-one illustrations, mostly original. New York: William Wood & Co., 1906. 319p. plates. DLC; DNLM; NNNAM; PPC
00-1464

HEKTOEN, Ludvig, ed. (1863-1951)
An American text-book of pathology, for the use of students and practitioners of medicine and surgery, ed. by Ludvig Hektoen . . . and David Riesman . . . with 448 illustrations, many of them in colors. Philadelphia and London: W. B. Saunders & Co., 1901. 1245p. col. plates. DLC; MBM; NNNAM; PPC **00-1465**

HELFERICH, Heinrich (1851-1945)
Atlas and epitome of traumatic fractures and dislocations . . . authorized transl. from the German; ed. by Joseph C. Bloodgood . . . 5th ed., rev. and enl. With 216 colored illustrations on 64 lithographic plates, and 190 figures in the text. Philadelphia and London: W. B. Saunders & Co., 1902. 353p. DLC; NNNAM; PPC; PU **00-1466**

HEMMETER, John C[onrad] (1863-1931)
Diseases of the stomach; their special pathology, diagnosis, and treatment. . . . 2nd enl. and rev. ed., with new chapters. . . . Philadelphia: P. Blakiston's Son & Co., 1900. 898p. 14 plates. DLC; DNLM; NNNAM; PPC **00-1467**

HEMMETER, John C[onrad] (1863-1931)
Diseases of the intestines; their special pathology, diagnosis and treatment. . . . Philadelphia: P. Blakiston's Son & Co., 1901-02. 2 v. plates. DLC; NNNAM; PPC; PU
00-1468

HEMMETER, John C[onrad] (1863-1931)
Diseases of the stomach; their special pathology, diagnosis, and treatment, with sections on anatomy, physiology, chemical and microscopical examination of stomach contents, dietetics, surgery of the stomach, etc. . . . With many original illustrations, a number of which are in colors, and a lithographic frontispiece. 3rd enl. and rev. ed. Philadelphia: P. Blakiston's Son & Co., 1902. 894p. col. plates. DLC; MBM; NNNAM; PPC
00-1469

HENDERSON, Frank Laramore (*b.* 1865)
Notes on the eye, for the use of undergraduate students. . . . 2nd ed. St. Louis, Mo.: Nixon-Jones Printing Co., 1900. 151p. col. front. DLC; ICJ **00-1470**

HENDERSON, Frank Laramore (*b.* 1865)
Lessons on the eye, for the use of undergraduate students. . . . 3rd ed. Philadelphia: P. Blakiston's Son & Co., 1903. 205p. col. front. CU-M; DLC; PPC; PU **00-1471**

HENDERSON, Frank Laramore (*b.* 1865)
Lessons on the eye for the use of undergraduate students. . . . 4th ed., rev. Philadelphia: P. Blakiston's Son & Co., 1910. 238p. DLC; ICJ; PPC; PPJ **00-1472**

HENKEL, Alice (1869-1916)
. . . Weeds used in medicine. . . . Washington: Government Printing Office, 1904. 47p. DLC: DNLM **00-1473**

HENKEL, Alice (1869-1916)
. . . Wild medicinal plants of the United States. . . . Washington: Government Printing Office, 1906. 76p. DLC; DNLM **00-1474**

HENKEL, Alice (1869-1916)
. . . American root drugs. . . . Washington: Government Printing Office, 1907. 80p. plates. DLC; DNLM **00-1475**

HENKEL, Alice (1869-1916)
. . . American medicinal barks. . . . Washington: Government Printing Office, 1909. 59p. DLC; DNLM; OCLloyd **00-1476**

HENRY, Frederick P[orteous] (1844-1919)
Clinical notes on cases of pernicious anaemia. Philadelphia, 1900. 14p. DNLM **00-1477**

HENRY, Frederick P[orteous], ed. (1844-1919)
The treatment of pneumonia by hypodermoclysis. Philadelphia, [1900]. 14p. DNLM **00-1478**

HENRY, Frederick P[orteous] (1844-1919)
Founders' week memorial volume, containing an account of the two hundred and twenty-fifth anniversary of the founding of the city of Philadelphia and histories of its principal scientific institutions, medical colleges, hospitals, etc. Ed. by Frederick P. Henry. . . . Pub. by the city of Philadelphia in commemoration of the two hundred and twenty-fifth anniversary of its founding. Philadelphia: F. A. Davis Co., 1909. [v. p.] DLC; NNNAM; PPC; PU **00-1479**

HENSEL, Otto
The urine and feces in diagnosis. By Otto Hensel and Richard Weil. In collaboration with Smith Ely Jelliffe. Philadelphia: Lea Bros. & Co., 1905. 334p. 10 col. plates. DLC; DNLM; ICJ; PPC **00-1480**

HERB, Ferdinand (*b.* 1866)
The care-feeding of the baby. A handbook for mothers, midwives and nurses. . . . Superior, Wis.: The R. & S. Publ. Co., [1907]. 267p. DLC; ICJ **00-1481**

HERB, Ferdinand (*b.* 1866)
Gonorrhea and sexual debility in men. . . . Superior, Wis.: The R. & S. Publ. Co., [1908]. 228p. DLC; ICJ **00-1482**

HERBERT, John Frederick
Anatomy and physiology of the eye, with hints for the preservation of the eye sight. . . . Philadelphia, Pa.: The Author, [1901]. 72p. DLC; DNLM; PPC **00-1483**

HERBERT, John Frederick
Anatomy and physiology of the eye, with hints for the preservation of the eyesight. . . . 2nd ed. Philadelphia, Pa. [1901]. 68p. DLC; PPC; PU **00-1484**

HERMAN, G[eorge] Ernest (1849-1914)
Diseases of women. A clinical guide to their diagnosis and treatment. Rev. ed. New York: William Wood & Co., 1903. 884p. DNLM; NNC; NNNAM; NNU-M **00-1485**

HERMAN, G[eorge] Ernest (1849-1914)
Diseases of women. A clinical guide to their diagnosis and treatment. [3rd ed.] New York: William Wood & Co., 1907. 900p. DNLM; ICJ; NN; PPC **00-1486**

HERMAN, G[eorge] Ernest (1849-1914)
Difficult labor; a guide to its management for students and practitioners. Enl. ed. New York: William Wood & Co., 1910. 547p. DNLM; ICJ; PPC; PPHa **00-1487**

HERRICK, James B[ryan], ed. (1861-1954)
Diseases of kidneys and spleen, and hemorrhagic diatheses. . . . By H. Senator . . . M. Litten . . . edited with additions by James B. Herrick. Philadelphia: W. B. Saunders & Co., 1905. 815p. DLC; NNNAM; PPC; PU [American ed., Nothnagel's encyclopedia of practical medicine] **00-1488**

HERROLD, Maude McKinley
Woman: diseases and remedies; a collection of facts for woman; by approved authorities the statements contained in this book are proved. . . . Kansas City, Mo.: The Woman's Publishing Co., 1902. 650p. DLC; ICJ **00-1489**

HERSEY, George D.
The medical library as a factor in medical progress. Providence, 1901. 11p. DNLM **00-1490**

HERTER, Christian A[rchibald] (1865-1910)
Lectures on chemical pathology in relation to practical medicine, delivered at the University and Bellevue Medical School, New York City. . . . Philadelphia: Lea Bros. & Co., 1902. 461p. DLC; NNNAM; NNU-M; PPC **00-1491**

HERTER, Christian A[rchibald] (1865-1910)
The influence of Pasteur on medical science; an address delivered before the Medical School of Johns Hopkins University. . . . New York: Dodd, Mead & Co., 1904. 77p. CtY-M; DLC; NNNAM; PU **00-1492**

HERTER, Christian A[rchibald] (1865-1910)
The common bacterial infections of the digestive tract and the intoxications arising from them. . . . New York: The Macmillan Co.; London: Macmillan & Co., 1907. 560p. DLC; MBM; NNNAM; PU **00-1493**

HERTER, Christian A[rchibald] (1865-1910)
Diagnosis of organic nervous diseases. . . . Rev. and enl. by L. Pierce Clark . . . with 109 illustrations. [2nd ed.] New York and London: G. P. Putnam's Sons, 1907. 690p. DLC; ICJ; NNNAM; PU **00-1494**

HERTER, Christian A[rchibald] (1865-1910)
On infantilism from chronic intestinal infection, characterized by the overgrowth and persistance of flora of the nursing period; a study of the clinical course, bacteriology, chemistry and therapeutics of arrested development in infancy. . . . New York: The Macmillan Co., 1908. 118p. DLC: ICJ; NN; NNNAM **00-1495**

HERTER, Christian A[rchibald] (1865-1910)
The action of sodium benzoate and benzoic acid on the human organism. . . . [New York? Privately printed], 1910. 18p. DLC; NNNAM **00-1496**

HERTER, Christian A[rchibald] (1865-1910)
Imagination and idealism in the medical sciences. . . . An address delivered to the College of Physicians and Surgeons, Columbia University, Sept. 23, 1909, at the opening of the Medical School. Chicago: American Medical Association, 1910. 40p. DLC; NNC **00-1497**

HERZOG, Maximilian Joseph (1858-1918)
A text-book on disease-producing microorganisms, especially intended for the use of veterinary students and practitioners . . . with 214 illustrations in black and 14 colored plates. Philadelphia and New York: Lea & Febiger, 1910. 644p. col. plates. DLC; ICJ; LNT-M; PPC **00-1498**

HILL, Charles (*b.* 1862)
A manual of normal histology and organography. . . . Philadelphia and London: W. B. Saunders & Co., 1906. 463p. col. plates. DLC; NNNAM; PPC; PU **00-1499**

HILL, Charles (*b.* 1862)
A manual of normal histology and organography . . . 2nd ed., thoroughly rev. Philadelphia and London: W. B. Saunders & Co., 1909. 468p. col. plates. DLC; MBM; PPC; PU **00-1500**

HILL, Edward Curtis (*b.* 1863)
A chart of diseases of the lungs, pleurae, bronchi. . . . Ansonia, Conn.: The McArthur Hypophosphite Co., 1901. 12p. DNLM; MH **00-1501**

HILL, Edward Curtis (*b.* 1863)
Temperature as a guide to diagnosis. . . . St. Louis, U.S.A.: Lambert Pharmacal Co., 1903. 39p. col. plate. DLC; NN **00-1502**

HILL, Edward Curtis (*b.* 1863)
A reference chart of diseases of nervous system and muscles. . . . [St. Louis: The Antikamnia Chemical Co., 1903.] 7 fold. numb 1., [i.e., 15p.] [Each leaf printed on both sides. Part of text on lining-papers] CtY-M; MB; NN; PPC **00-1503**

HILL, Edward Curtis (*b.* 1863)
A text-book of chemistry, for students of medicine, pharmacy, and dentistry . . . with seventy-eight illustrations, including nine full-page halftone and colored plates. Philadelphia: F. A. Davis Co., 1903. 523p. DLC; NNNAM; PPC; PU **00-1504**

HILL, Edward Curtis (*b.* 1863)
Pain and its indications; an analytical outline of diagnosis and treatment. . . . Chicago: G. P. Engelhard & Co., 1904. 328p. DLC; OCIM; PPC; PPJ **00-1505**

HILL, Leonard E[rskine], ed. (*b.* 1866)
Recent advances in physiology and bio-chemistry. New York: Longmans, Green & Co., 1906. 740p. DLC; ICJ; MB; NjR **00-1506**

HILL, Leonard E[rskine], ed. (*b.* 1866)
Further advances in physiology. . . . New York: Longmans, Green & Co., 1909. 440p. DLC; NIC; PPC; PU **00-1507**

HINSDALE, Guy (*b.* 1858)
Acromegaly; syringomyelia; crossed knee-jerk; anterior poliomyelitis. Philadelphia, 1900. 88, 74, 8p. plates. CtY-M; DLC; ICJ; PPC **00-1508**

HINSDALE, Guy (*b.* 1858)
Tuberculosis in Pennsylvania. Chicago, 1900. 14p. DLC; DNLM **00-1509**

HINSDALE, Guy (*b.* 1858)
Hydrotherapy . . . its application to special affections, the technic or processes employed, and the use of waters internally. Philadelphia: W. B. Saunders & Co., 1910. 466p. DLC; ICJ; NcD; PPC **00-1510**

HIPPOCRATES
The genuine works of Hippocrates. Transl. from the Greek with a preliminary discourse and annotations by Francis Adams. New York: William Wood & Co.,, 1900. 2 v. 8 plates. DLC; MH; NIC; NN [First appeared in Wood's Library of Standard Medical Authors in 1886. First published by the Sydenham Society, London, 1849] **00-1511**

HIRSCH, Charles Solomon (*b.* 1879)
. . . A compend of genito-urinary diseases and syphilis, including their surgery and treatment. . . . Philadelphia: P. Blakiston's Son & Co., 1906. 351p. DLC; ICJ; PPC; PU **00-1512**

HIRSCHFELDER, Arthur Douglass (*b.* 1879)
Diseases of the heart and aorta . . . with an introductory note by Lewellys F. Barker. . . . 329 illustrations by the author. Philadelphia & London: J. B. Lippincott Co., [1910]. 632p. col. plates. DLC; NNNAM; OCIM; PPC **00-1513**

HIRSCHMAN, Louis Jacob (*b.* 1878)
Hand-book of diseases of the rectum . . . with one hundred and forty-seven illustrations, mostly original, including two colored plates. St. Louis: C. V. Mosby Medical Book & Publishing Co., 1909. 374p. DLC; ICJ; OCIM; PPC **00-1514**

HIRSHBERG, Leonard K[eene] (*b.* 1877)
Practical bacteriology. . . . Baltimore: The Friedenwald Co., 1904. 204p. DLC; MdBM; MdU-D; PPC
00-1515

HIRSHBERG, Leonard K[eene] (*b.* 1877)
What you ought to know about your baby. . . . A text-book for mothers on the care and feeding of babies, with questions and answers. New York: The Butterick Publishing Co., 1910. 97p. DLC; NNNAM; PPC; PU **00-1516**

HIRST, Barton Cooke (1861-1935)
A text-book of obstetrics . . . 3rd ed., thoroughly rev. . . . Philadelphia and London: W. B. Saunders & Co., 1901. 873p. col. plates. DLC; IU-M; PPC; PU **00-1517**

HIRST, Barton Cooke (1861-1935)
A text-book of diseaees of women . . . with 655 illustrations, many of them in colors. Philadelphia, New York, [etc.] : W. B. Saunders & Co., 1903. 683p. col. plates. DLC; LNT-M; MBM; PPC **00-1518**

HIRST, Barton Cooke (1861-1935)
A text-book of obstetrics . . . 4th ed., rev. and enl., with 746 illustrations, 39 of them in colors. Philadelphia, [etc.] : W. B. Saunders & Co., 1903. 899p. DLC; KyLoJM; NNNAM; NcU
00-1519

HIRST, Barton Cooke (1861-1935)
A text-book of diseases of women . . . 2nd ed., rewritten and enl., with 701 illustrations, many of them in colors. Philadelphia and London: W. B. Saunders & Co., 1905. 741p. DLC; GU; NNNAM; PPC **00-1520**

HIRST, Barton Cooke (1861-1935)
A text-book of obstetrics . . . 5th ed., rev. and enl., with 767 illustrations, 40 of them in colors. Philadelphia and London: W. B. Saunders & Co., 1906. 915p. DLC; MBM; MdU-D; PPC
00-1521

HIRST, Barton Cooke (1861-1935)
A text-book of obstetrics . . . 6th ed., rev. and enl., with 847 illustrations, 43 of them in colors. Philadelphia and London: W. B. Saunders & Co., 1909. 992p. CU-M; DLC: IEN-M; PPC
00-1522

HIS, Wilhelm (1831-1904)
Anatomical terminology with special reference to the [B. N. A.], by Lewellys F. Barker. Philadelphia: P. Blakiston's Son & Co., 1907. 103p. CtY-M; DLC; NNNAM; PPC
00-1523

HISS, A. Emil
Thesaurus of proprietary preparations and pharmaceutical specialties, including "patent" medicines, proprietary pharmaceuticals, open-formula specialties, synthetic remedies. . . . Chicago: G. P. Engelhard & Co., 1900 [*c.* 1898]. 279p. DNLM; ICJ; NN; NNC **00-1524**

HISS, Philip Hanson (1868?-1913)
A text-book of bacteriology, a practical treatise for students and practitioners of medicine, by Philip Hanson Hiss, Jr. . . . and Hans Zinsser . . . with one hundred and fifty-six illustrations in the text, some of which are colored. New York and London: D. Appleton & Co., 1910. 745p. DLC; ICJ; NNNAM; PU **00-1525**

HOAG, Ernest B[ryant] (1868-1924)
Health studies; applied physiology and hygiene . . . with a prefatory note by David Starr Jordan. Boston: D. C. Heath & Co., 1909. 223p. DLC: ICU; MH; NN **00-1526**

HOAG, Ernest B[ryant] (1868-1924)
The health index of children . . . with a prefatory note by Frank F. Bunker. San Francisco: Whitaker & Ray-Wiggin Co., 1910. 188p. DLC; ICJ **00-1527**

HOBBS, Arthur G.
Adenoids, with a description of new instruments. [Atlanta, 1900?] 7p. DNLM **00-1528**

HOBBS, Arthur G.
An epitome of eye, ear, throat, and nose diseases. 2nd ed. Philadelphia: S. M. Miller, 1900. 200p. DLC; NN [1st ed., 1885, 202p; 2nd ed., 1886, 200p.]
00-1529

HODSON, Jane, ed.
How to become a trained nurse: a manual of information in detail. With a complete list of the various training schools for nurses in the United States and Canada. 2nd ed. . . . New York: W. Abbatt, 1905. 265p. plates. DLC; DNLM; MB; NNNAM
00-1530

HOFF, John Van Rensselaer (1848-1920)
The share of the white man's burden that has fallen to the medical departments of the public services in Puerto Rico. Philadelphia, 1900. 11p. DLC; DNLM
00-1531

HOFF, Nelville Soulé (1854-1926)
Lectures on dental materia medica and therapeutics. Delivered during the session 1899 and 1900 at the University of Michigan . . . reported by G. W. Clapp. . . . Ann Arbor, Mich.: Edwards Bros., 1900. 324p. DLC: DNLM; ICJ
00-1532

HOFF, Nelville Soulé (1854-1926)
Lectures on dental materia medica and therapeutics. Delivered during the session 1902 and 1903 at the University of Michigan. . . . Reported by G. W. Clapp. . . . Ann Arbor, Mich.: Edwards Bros., 1902. 1p. 312 numb. 1. [Mimeographed copy] DLC
00-1533

HOFFMAN, C. H.
Essentials of pathology, general and special. . . . Kirksville, Mo.: J. F. Janisch Supply House, [1905]. 149p. DLC; ICJ
00-1534

HOFFMANN, Philip
A treatment of acute serous synovitis permitting of joint functions. New York, 1900. 7p. DNLM
00-1535

HOFHEIMER, Justinian A.
Alcoholic gastritis. St. Louis, [1900]. 2 l. DNLM
00-1536

HOGAN, Louise E. (1855-1929)
Children's diet in home and school, with classified recipes and menus; a reference book for parents, nurses, teachers, women's clubs, and physicians. . . . Philadelphia: H. T. Coates & Co., 1902. 176p. DLC; NN; PPC; PU **00-1537**

HOGAN, Louise E. (1855-1929)
How to feed children; a manual for mothers, nurses, and physicians. . . . 8th ed., newly rev. Philadelphia: J. B. Lippincott Co., 1906. 239p. DLC: ICJ; PPC; PU
00-1538

HOGAN, Louise E. (1855-1929)
How to feed children; a manual for mothers, nurses, and physicians. . . . 9th ed., newly rev. Philadelphia: J. B. Lippincott Co., 1909. 249p. plates. DLC; NN; PPC; PU
00-1539

HOLDEN, Luther (1815-1905)
Landmarks, medical and surgical. 4th ed. Philadelphia: P. Blakiston's Son & Co., 1900. 79p. DNLM; NNNAM; PPC; PPJ
00-1540

HOLDEN, Luther (1815-1905)
Holden's anatomy; a manual of the dissection of the human body; ed. by John Langton. . . . 7th ed. rev. by A. Hewson. . . . Philadelphia: P. Blakiston's Son & Co., 1901. 2 v. DLC; DNLM; PPC; PU **00-1541**

HOLLAND, James William (1849-1922)
The urine and clinical chemistry of the gastric contents, the common poisons, and milk. . . . Forty-one illustrations. 7th ed., rev. and enl. Philadelphia: P. Blakiston's Son & Co., 1904. 172p. DLC; ICJ; PPC; PU **00-1542**

HOLLAND, James William (1849-1922)
A text-book of medical chemistry and toxicology. . . . Philadelphia and London: W. B. Saunders & Co., 1905. 592p. col. plates. DLC; NNNAM; PPC; PU **00-1543**

HOLLAND, James William (1849-1922)
A text-book of medical chemistry and toxicology . . . 2nd ed., rev. and enl. Philadelphia and London: W. B. Saunders & Co., 1908. 655p. col. plates. DLC; MBM; NNNAM; PPC
00-1544

HOLLAND, James William (1849-1922)
The urine and clinical chemistry of the gastric contents, the common poisons, and milk . . . forty-illustrations. 8th ed., rev. and enl. Philadelphia: P. Blakiston's Son & Co., 1908. 160p. DLC; DNLM; PPC; PU
00-1545

HOLLAND, James William (1849-1922)
The Jefferson Medical College of Philadelphia from 1825 to 1908. . . . [Philadelphia? 1909?] 27p. plates. DLC; PPJ
00-1546

HOLLANDER, Bernard (1864-1934)
The revival of phrenology. The mental functions of the brain; an investigation into their localisation and their manifestation in health and disease. . . . New York and London: G. P. Putnam's Sons, 1901. 507p. plates. DLC; MH; NNNAM; PU
00-1547

HOLLANDER, Bernard (1864-1934)
Hypnotism and suggestion in daily life, education, and medical practice. . . . New York: G. P. Putnam's Sons, 1910. 295p. DLC; ICJ; NNNAM; PPC **00-1548**

HOLLANDER, Bernard (1864-1934)
The mental symptoms of brain disease; an aid to the surgical treatment of insanity, due to injury, haemorrhage, tumours, and other circumscribed lesions of the brain, by Bernard Hollander. . . . With preface by Dr. Jul. Morel. . . . New York: Rebman Co., 1910. 237p. ICJ; NN; PPC; PPJ
00-1549

HOLLICK, Frederick (*b.* 1818)
The origin of life and process of reproduction in plants and animals, with the anatomy and physiology of the human generative system, male and female. . . . New ed. with additions. Philadelphia: D. McKay, [1902]. 932p. DLC; NN; PP; PU [44 plates (some in color); anatomical mannequin with fold-out parts in color of a pregnant woman; 200 textual engravings. The individual works making up this volume were all originally published in the period 1845-1850 and passed through hundreds of editions before this combined printing.]
00-1550

HOLLISTER, John Hamilcar (1824-1911)
Biographical sketches of some of the early physicians of Illinois. [Springfield, 1907.] 33p. DNLM; ICJ **00-1551**

HOLMAN, John Hamilton (*b.* 1869)
Laboratory methods of histology and bacteriology. . . . Nashville, Tenn.: National Baptist Publishing Board, 1908. 227p. DLC; ICJ **00-1552**

HOLMES, Bayard Taylor (1852-1924)
. . . The surgery of the head. . . . New York: D. Appleton & Co., 1903. 569p. plates. DLC; NNNAM; PPC; PPJ
00-1553

HOLMES, Bayard Taylor (1852-1924)
Echinoccus cyst of the liver, with report of a case with operation and recovery. Chicago, 1904. 14p. illus. DLC
00-1554

HOLMES, Bayard Taylor (1852-1924)
. . . The surgery of the abdomen, pt. 1— . . . . New York: D. Appleton & Co., 1904- . Plates. DLC; ICJ; NNNAM; PPC
00-1555

HOLMES, Bayard Taylor (1852-1924)
The friends of the insane, The soul of medical education, and other essays. . . . Cincinnati: The Lancet-Clinic Publishing Co., 1910-1911. 270p. DLC; DNLM; ICJ; MH-M
00-1556

HOLMES, Christian R[asmus] (1857-1920)
Hypertrophy of the turbinated bodies and their relations to inflammation of the middle ear. New York, 1900. 24p. DNLM
00-1557

HOLMES, Christian R[asmus] (1857-1920)
Laryngology and otology. Chicago, 1900. 14p. DNLM
00-1558

HOLT, E[rastus] Eugene (1849-1931)
Portland Medical Club, 1876-1902. History and statistics. Portland, Me., 1903. 13p. 1 plate. DNLM; MH
00-1559

HOLT, L[uther] Emmett (1855-1924)
The diseases of infancy and childhood, for the use of students and practitioners of medicine. . . . 2nd ed., rev. and enl. New York: D. Appleton & Co., 1902. 1161p. plates. DLC; NNNAM; PPC; PU **00-1560**

HOLT, L[uther] Emmett (1855-1924)
The care and feeding of children; a catechism for the use of mothers and children's nurses. . . . 3rd ed., rev. and enl. New York and London: D. Appleton & Co., 1903. 149p. DLC; NNNAM; PP; PU **00-1561**

HOLT, L[uther] Emmett (1855-1924)
The diseases of infancy and childhood, for the use of students and practitioners of medicine . . . with two hundred and forty-one illustrations, including eight coloured plates. 3rd ed., rev. and enl. New York and London: D. Appleton & Co., 1906. 1174p. DLC; IU-M; NNNAM; PPC **00-1562**

HOLT, L[uther] Emmett (1855-1924)
The diseases of infancy and childhood, for the use of students and practitioners of medicine . . . with two hundred and forty-one illustrations, including eight coloured plates. 4th ed., rev. and enl. New York and London: D. Appleton & Co., 1908 [1907]. 1171p. DLC; GU; NNNAM; PU
00-1563

HOLT, L[uther] Emmett (1855-1924)
The care and feeding of children; a catechism for the use of mothers and children's nurses. . . . 4th ed., rev. and enl. New York and London: D. Appleton & Co., 1907. 192p. CU-M; DLC; ICRM; PPC **00-1564**

HOLT, L[uther] Emmett (1855-1924)
Cuidado y alimentación de los niños desde recién nacidos hasta los diez años, cartilla en forma de catecismo para uso de las madres y amas de cria. . . . Chicago, New York, [etc.]: D. Appleton & Compañía, 1908. 203p. CU-M; DLC; ICJ; NNNAM **00-1565**

HOLT, L[uther] Emmett (1855-1924)
The care and feeding of children; a catechism for the use of mothers and children's nurses. . . . 5th ed., rev. and enl. New York and London: D. Appleton & Co., 1909. 195p. DLC; NNNAM; OCIM; PPC **00-1566**

HOLT, L[uther] Emmett (1855-1924)
The diseases of infancy and childhood, for the use of students and practitioners of medicine . . . with two hundred and thirty-nine illustrations including eight coloured plates. 5th ed., rev. and enl. New York and London: D. Appleton & Co., 1909. 1171p. CtY-M; DLC; NNNAM; PPC
00-1567

HOMAN, George (*b.* 1849)
Some medical and other gleanings from old-time chronicles and records. St. Louis, 1900. 12p. DNLM
00-1568

HOME and health; a household manual containing two thousand recipes and helpful suggestions on the building and care of the home in harmony with sanitary laws . . . and the home treatment of the more simple ailments and diseases . . . prepared and edited by a competent committee of home-makers and physicians. Mountain View, Cal., Portland, Ore., [etc.]: Pacific Press Publishing Co., 1907. 589p. DLC
00-1569

HOME REMEDY COMPANY. IOWA CITY, IA.
Health at home; a digest of modern medical science. Compiled from standard authorities. . . . [Iowa City, Ia.: Iowa Citizen Publishing Co.], 1900. 446p. DLC **00-1570**

HOOD, Calvin T[odd]
The heart and its diseases. Chicago. F. H. Mallen Co., 1904. 104p. ICRM; ICU **00-1571**

HOOD, Calvin T[odd]
The management of the ordinary heart cases. . . . [Chicago, 1904?] 8p. ICJ **00-1572**

HOOD, G. Durant
Dr. Hood's plain talks, about the human system, the habits of men and women, the causes and prevention of disease, our sexual relations, and social natures; embracing common sense medical adviser. Chicago: Hood Medical Book Co., [1901]. 1080p. DNLM [Also issued under title: The practical family physician] **00-1573**

HOOD, G. Durant
The practical family physician; a complete treatise on the human system . . . embracing common sense medical adviser. . . . Chicago: The Hood Medical Book Co., [1901]. 1072p. DLC [Also issued under title: Dr. Hood's plain talks about the human system. . . .] **00-1574**

HOOD, G. Durant
Dr. Hood's plain talks about the human system—the habits of men and women—the causes and prevention of disease—our sexual relations and the social natures—embracing common sense medical adviser. . . . Chicago: The Hood Medical Book Co., [1902]. 1060p. plates. DLC **00-1575**

HOOD, JOHN & CO. (BOSTON)
Dental catalogue of gold foil and other dental supplies. . . . Boston, [*c.* 1900]. 675p. MH-M
00-1576

HOOPER, Robert (1773-1835)
. . . Hooper's Physician's vade-mecum: a manual of the principles and practice of physic; with an outline of general pathology, therapeutics, and hygiene. 10th ed. Rev. by William Augustus Guy . . . and John Barley. . . . New York: William Wood & Co., 1900. 2 v. CtY-M; ICJ; NIC: PP [First appeared in Wood's Library of Standard Medical Authors, 1884]
00-1577

HOOPER, William F[ranklin] (*b.* 1866)
A practical treatise on typhoid and all other slow fevers broken in fourteen days. . . . Booneville, Ark.: The Booneville Incorporated Book Co., [1910]. 186p. DLC: ICJ **00-1578**

HOPKINS, T[homas] A[ndrews], ed.
Willcox's reference book and formulary. Designed for the use of physicians and students. . . . St. Louis: C. D. Willcox, 1900. 291p. DLC; DNLM; ICJ; PP **00-1579**

HOPKINS, T[homas] A[ndrews]
Willcox's emergency practice . . . a book designed for ready reference in case of accident and injury, written by twenty-five of the leading physicians and surgeons of St. Louis. St. Louis: The C. V. Mosby Medical Book and Pub. Co., [1906]. 300p. ICJ; OCIM; PU **00-1580**

HOPKINS, William Barton (1853-1904)
A clinical treatise on fractures. . . . Philadelphia: J. B. Lippincott & Co., 1900. 268p. DLC; DNLM; NNNAM; PPC
00-1581

HOPKINS, William Barton (1853-1904)
The roller bandage. . . . 5th ed., rev. Philadelphia: J. B. Lippincott Co., 1902. 162p. DLC; MBM; NNNAM; PPC
00-1582

HORT, Edward C[ollett] (1868-1922)
Rational immunization in the treatment of pulmonary tuberculosis and other diseases. New York: William Wood & Co., 1909. 75p. DLC; DNLM; NN **00-1583**

HORWITZ, Orville (1859-1913)
A brief account of a few surgical cases of unusual interest. Philadelphia, 1900. 13p. DNLM **00-1584**

HORWITZ, Orville (1859-1913)
Some points of interest in connection with chronic urethritis. Detroit: W. M. Warren, 1900. 12p. DNLM
00-1585

HORWITZ, Orville (1859-1913)
. . . Compend of surgery, for students and physicians; including minor surgery and a complete section on bandaging. . . . 6th ed., rev. and enl. One hundred and ninety-five illustrations and one hundred and four formulae. Philadelphia: P. Blakiston's Son & Co., 1907. 334p. DLC; NNNAM; PPC; PU
00-1586

THE HOUSEHOLD physician. A book of popular information on health and disease. Originated, comp. and ed. by eminent physicians and able medical writers. . . . Boston, Mass.: The Household Medical Company, [1905]. 195p. DLC; MBM
00-1587

THE HOUSEHOLD physician, a twentieth century medica; a practical description in plain language of all the diseases of men, women and children. . . . By a corps of eminent specialists, practising physicians and surgeons: Herbert E. Buffum . . . A. T. Lovering . . . Ira Warren . . . A. E. Small . . . William Thorndike . . . J. Heber Smith . . . Charles P. Lyman . . . Boston: Physicians' Publishing Co., 1905. 1434p. plates. DLC; MBM **00-1588**

THE HOUSEHOLD physician, a twentieth century medica; a practical description in plain lanugage pf all the diseases of men, women and children. . . . By a corps of eminent specialists, practising physicians and surgeons: Herbert E. Buffum . . . A. T. Lovering . . . Ira Warren . . . A. E. Small . . . William Thorndike . . . J. Heber Smith . . . Charles P. Lyman . . . New ed. Boston: Woodruff Publishing Co., Inc. [1909]. 1440p. plates. DLC; MBM **00-1589**

THE HOUSEHOLD physician, a twentieth century medica; a practical description in plain language of all the diseases of men, women and children. . . . By a corps of eminent specialists, practising physicians and surgeons: Herbert E. Buffum . . . A. T. Lovering . . . Ira Warren . . . A. E. Small . . . William Thorndike . . . J. Heber Smith . . . Charles P. Lyman . . . Fully illustrated with manikins, colored and half-tone plates. . . . New ed. Boston: Woodruff Publishing Co., Inc., [1910]. 1440p. col. plates. DLC **00-1590**

HOUSTON, Edwin James (1847-1914)
. . . Electricity in electro-therapeutics, by Edwin J. Houston, Ph.D. and A. E. Kennelly, C.D. 3rd ed., enl. New York: McGraw Publishing Co., 1906. 467p. CtY-M; DLC; NNNAM; PU **00-1591**

HOVELL, T[homas] Mark (1853-1925)
A treatise on the diseases of the ear, including the anatomy and physiology of the organ, together with a treatment of the affections of the nose and pharynx which conduce to aural disease. 2nd ed. Philadelphia: P. Blakiston's Son & Co., 1901. 808p. CtY-M; DNLM; NNNAM; PPC
00-1592

HOWARD, L[eland] O[ssian] (1857-1950)
Mosquitoes: how they live; how they carry disease; how they are classified; how they may be destroyed. New York: McClure, Phillips, 1901. 241p. ICU; MH; NIC; NN
00-1593

HOWARD, L[eland] O[ssian] (1857-1950)
Concerning the geographic distribution of the yellow fever mosquito. Washington: Government Printing Office, 1903. 7p. NN [U.S. Public Health & Marine Hospital Service]
00-1594

HOWARD, L[eland] O[ssian] (1857-1950)
. . . Concerning the geographic distribution of the yellow fever mosquito. . . . (Revised to September 10, 1905.) Washington: Government Printing Office, 1905. 9p. fold. chart. DLC; DNLM **00-1595**

HOWARD UNIVERSITY, WASHINGTON, D.C. SCHOOL OF MEDICINE
Howard University Medical Department, Washington, D.C. A historical, biographical and statistical souvenir, compiled and edited for and by authority of the medical faculty of Howard University by Daniel Smith Lamb. . . . Washington: Printed by R. Beresford, 1900. 301p. DLC; DNLM
00-1596

HOWE, Joseph W[illiam] (1843-1890)
Excessive venery, masturbation, and continence. The etiology, pathology, and treatment of the diseases resulting from venereal excesses, masturbation, and continence. New York: E. B. Treat Co., 1907. 299p. DLC; MBM; NN; PPC [1st ed., 1883]
00-1597

HOWE, Lucien (1848-1928)
The muscles of the eye. I: Anatomy and physiology, including instruments for testing and methods of measurement. II. Pathology and treatment. New York: G. P. Putnam's Sons, 1907-1908. 2 v. DLC: ICJ; MB; NNNAM
00-1598

HOWE, Maud (1854-1948) and Florence Howe HALL
Laura Bridgman. Dr. Howe's famous pupil and what he taught her. . . . Boston: Little, Brown & Co., 1903. 394p. MB; MH; NN [Dr. Samuel G. Howe of the Perkins Institute in Boston]
00-1599

HOWE, William F. (*d.* 1899)
The electro-therapeutic guide. By Wm. F. Howe and H. C. Bennett. 6th ed., rev. Lima, O.: National College of Electro-therapeutics, 1902. 178p. ICJ **00-1600**

HOWELL, William Henry, ed. (1860-1945)
An American text-book of physiology, by Henry P. Bowditch . . . John G. Curtis . . . Henry H. Donaldson . . . W. H. Howell . . . Frederic S. Lee . . . Warren P. Lombard . . . Graham Lusk . . . W. T. Porter . . . Edwart T. Reichart . . . Henry Sewall. Ed. by William H. Howell. . . . Philadelphia: W. B. Saunders & Co., 1900-01. 1052p. col. plates. DLC; NNNAM; PPC; PU
00-1601

HOWELL, William Henry, ed. (1860-1945)
An American text-book of physiology by Henry P. Bowditch . . . John G. Curtis . . . Henry H. Donaldson . . . W. H. Howell . . . Frederic S. Lee . . . Warren P. Lombard . . . Graham Lusk . . . W. T. Porter . . . Edwart T. Reichert . . . Henry Sewall. Ed. by William H. Howell . . . 2nd ed., rev. . . . Philadelphia: W. B. Saunders & Co., 1900-01. 2 v. col. plates. DLC; IU-M; MBM; PPC **00-1602**

HOWELL, William Henry (1860-1945)
A text-book of physiology, for medical students and physicians. . . . Philadelphia and London: W. B. Saunders & Co., 1905. 905p. col. plates. DLC; LNT-M; NNNAM; PU
00-1603

HOWELL, William Henry (1860-1945)
A text-book of physiology, for medical students and physicians. . . . 2nd ed., thoroughly rev. Philadelphia and London: W. B. Saunders & Co., 1907. 939p. col. plates. DLC; MdU-D; NNNAM; PPC **00-1604**

HOWELL, William Henry (1860-1945)
A text-book of physiology for medical students and physicians. . . . 3rd ed., thoroughly rev. Philadelphia and London: W. B. Saunders & Co., 1909. 998p. col. plates. CU-M; DLC; GU; PPC **00-1605**

HOXIE, George Howard (*b.* 1872)
Practice of medicine for nurses; a text-book for nurses and students of domestic science, and a hand-book for all those who care for the sick . . . with a chapter on the technic of nursing by Pearl L. Laptad. . . . Philadelphia and London: W. B. Saunders & Co., 1908. 284p. plates. DLC; KU; PPC; PU
00-1606

HOXIE, George Howard (*b.* 1872)
Symptomatic and regional therapeutics . . . with fifty-eight illustrations in text. New York and London: D. Appleton & Co., 1910. 499p. DLC; ICJ; NNNAM; PPC
00-1607

HRDLICKA, Alois F. (1869-1943)
Arrangement and preservation of large collections of human bones for purposes of investigation. Boston: Ginn & Co., 1900. 15p. DLC: DNLM; MH; NN **00-1608**

HRDLICKA, Alois F. (1869-1943)
Diseases of the Indians, more especially of the southwest United States and southern Mexico. . . . [n. p., 1905?] 21p. DLC; NN **00-1609**

HRDLICKA, Alois F. (1869-1943)
Skeletal remains suggesting or attributed to early man in North America. Washington: Government Printing Office, 1907. 113p. DLC;; ICJ; NIC; NN **00-1610**

HRDLICKA, Alois F. (1869-1943)
Physiological and medical observations among the Indians of southwestern United States and northern Mexico. Smithsonian Institution, Bureau of American Ethnology, Bulletin 34. Washington: Government Printing Office, 1908. 460p. DLC; DNLM; ICJ; NN **00-1611**

HRDLICKA, Alois F. (1869-1943)
. . . Tuberculosis among certain Indian tribes of the United States. . . . Washington: Government Printing Office, 1909. 48p. DLC; ICJ; NN; PU [Smithsonian Institution. Bureau of American Ethnology, Bulletin 42] **00-1612**

HUBBELL, Alvin A[llace] (*b.* 1846)
The development of ophthalmology in America, 1800 to 1870. . . . Chicago: American Medical Association, 1908. 197p. DLC; DNLM; ICJ [also: Chicago: W. T. Keener Co., 1908. 197p. DNLM; NcD] **00-1613**

HUBER, G[otthelf] Carl (1865-1934)
Laboratory work in histology. 3rd ed. Ann Arbor: G. Wahr, 1900. 204p. DLC; DNLM; ICJ; OCIM [1st ed., Directions for work in the histological laboratory for the use of medical classes in the University of Michigan, 1892, 119p; 2nd ed., 1895, 191p.] **00-1614**

HUBER, G[otthelf] Carl (1865-1934)
An historical sketch of the Department of Medicine and Surgery in the University of Michigan. [New York, 1901.] 12p. DLC; NN **00-1615**

HUBER, G[otthelf] Carl (1865-1934)
On the development and shape of uriniferous tubules of certain of the higher mammals. . . . With 24 figures. [Baltimore, 1905.] 98p. DLC **00-1616**

HUBER, John Bessner (*b.* 1864)
Consumption; its relation to man and his civilization; its prevention and cure. . . . Philadelphia and London: J. B. Lippincott Co., [1906]. 536p. col. plates. CtY-M; DLC; PPC; PU **00-1617**

HUDSON, Thomson J[ay] (1834-1903)
The law of mental medicine; the correlation of the facts of psychology and histology in their relation to mental therapeutics. Chicago: A. C. McClurg & Co., 1903. 281p. DLC; ICJ; ICU; NIC **00-1618**

HUDSON, Thomson J[ay] (1834-1903)
The law of psychic phenomena: a working hypothesis for the systematic study of hypnotism, spiritism, mental therapeutics. . . . Chicago: A. C. McClurg & Co., 1909 [*c.* 1894]. 409p. DLC; ICJ; ICU; NN **00-1619**

HUGHES, Daniel E. (1851-1902)
A compend of the practice of medicine . . . 7th rev. ed., edited, rev. and in parts rewritten by Samuel Horton Brown. . . . Philadelphia: P. Blakiston's Son & Co., 1904. 779p. plates. DLC; KU; PPC; PU **00-1620**

HUGHES, Daniel E. (1851-1902)
A compend of the practice of medicine . . . 8th rev. ed., edited, rev. and enl. by Samuel Horton Brown . . . including a section on mental diseases and a very complete section on skin diseases. . . . Philadelphia: P. Blakiston's Son & Co., 1905. 780p. plates. DLC; NNNAM; PPC; PPJ **00-1621**

HUGHES, Daniel E. (1851-1902)
A compend of the practice of medicine, including a section on mental diseases and diseases of the skin. . . . 9th rev. ed., edited, rev. and enl. by Samuel Horton Brown. . . . Philadelphia: P. Blakiston's Son & Co., 1905. 785p. plates. CtY-M; DLC; MBM; PPC **00-1622**

HULETT, Guy Dudley (*b.* 1874)
A text-book of the principles of osteopathy. . . . Kirksville, Mo.: Journal Printing Co., 1903. 366p. DLC **00-1623**

HULETT, Guy Dudley (*b.* 1874)
A text-book of the principles of osteopathy . . . 2nd ed. . . . Kirksville, Mo.: Monotyped by Journal Printing Co., 1904. 373p. DLC: ICJ **00-1624**

HULETT, Guy Dudley (*b.* 1874)
A text-book of the principles of osteopathy . . . 3rd ed. . . . Kirksville, Mo.: Journal Printing Co., [1905]. 372p. DLC; ICJ **00-1625**

HULETT, Guy Dudley (*b.* 1874)
A text-book of the principles of osteopathy . . . 4th ed. . . . Kirskville, Mo.: Journal Printing Co., [1906]. 372p. DLC; PU **00-1626**

HUMPHREYS, Frederick (1816-1900)
Manual of specific homoeopathy for the administration of medicine and cure of disease. New York: Humphreys, [1900]. 144p. DNLM; NNNAM **00-1627**

HUNT, Reid (1870-1948)
. . . Changes in the pharmacopoeia of the United States of America. Eighth decennial revision. (Official from September 1, 1905) By Reid Hunt and Murray Galt Motter. Washington: Government Printing Office, 1905. 122p. DLC; DNLM; OCLloyd; PU **00-1628**

HUNTINGTON, George Sumner (1861-1927)
The anatomy of the human peritoneum and abdominal cavity considered from the standpoint of development and comparative anatomy . . . illustrated with 300 full-page plates containing 582 figures, many in colors. Philadelphia and New York: Lea Bros. & Co., 1903. 292p. col. plates. DLC: IEN-M; NNNAM; PU **00-1629**

HURD, Henry M[ills] (1843-1927)
The duty and responsibility of the university in medical education. [1903.] 16p. ICJ; NN **00-1630**

HURD, Henry M[ills] (1843-1927)
Is nursing a profession? [1904.] 13p. NN **00-1631**

HURD, Henry M[ills] (1843-1927)
Florence Nightingale—a force in medicine . . . address . . . May 19, 1910. Baltimore, 1910. 13p. DLC **00-1632**

HUTCHINSON, Jonathan (1828-1913)
Illustrations of clinical surgery. . . . Illustrating surgical diseases, symptoms and accidents, also operative and other methods of treatment. . . . Philadelphia: P. Blakiston's Son & Co., 1900 [*c.* 1888]. 2 v. DLC; IU-M; NN; PU **00-1633**

HUTCHINSON, Jonathan (1828-1913)
The surgical treatment of facial neuralgia. New York: William Wood & Co., 1905. 151p. illus. DLC; DNLM; ICJ; NNNAM **00-1634**

HUTCHINSON, Jonathan (1828-1913)
Syphilis. . . . New and enlarged edition. With twelve coloured and twenty-four black-and-white plates. New York: Funk & Wagnalls Co., 1910. 583p. ICJ; NN; PPJ; PU **00-1635**

HUTCHINSON, Woods (1862-1930)
The economics of prostitution. [New York, 1900.] 28p. DLC; NN [Originally, 1895. *vel subseq.*] **00-1636**

HUTCHINSON, Woods (1862-1930)
Preventable diseases. . . . Boston and New York: Houghton Mifflin Co., 1909. 442p. DLC; MBM; NNNAM: PU **00-1637**

HUTCHINSON, Woods (1862-1930)
The conquest of consumption. . . . Boston and New York: Houghton Mifflin Co., 1910. 138p. plates. DLC; MBM; NNNAM; PPC **00-1638**

HUTCHISON, Robert (1871-1960)
Food and the principles of dietetics. New York: William Wood & Co., 1901. 548p. 3 plates. DLC; DNLM; NNNAM; PPC
00-1639

HUTCHISON, Robert (1871-1960)
Clinical methods: a guide to the practical study of medicine. By Robert Hutchison . . . and Harry Rainy . . . 5th ed. Chicago: W. T. Keener & Co., 1902. 612p. col. plates. DLC; PPC; PPL; PU **00-1640**

HUTCHISON, Robert (1871-1960)
Clinical methods: a guide to the practical study of medicine. By Robert Hutchison . . . and Harry Rainy . . . 6th ed. Chicago: W. T. Keener & Co., 1902. 612p. col. plates. DLC; PPC; PPL; PU **00-1641**

HUTCHISON, Robert (1871-1960)
Clinical methods: a guide to the practical study of medicine. By Robert Hutchison . . . and Harry Rainy . . . 7th ed. Chicago: W. T. Keener & Co., 1903. 612p. col. plates. DLC; PPC; PPL; PU **00-1642**

HUTCHISON, Robert (1871-1960)
Clinical methods: a guide to the practical study of medicine. By Robert Hutchison . . . and Harry Rainy . . . 8th ed. Chicago: W. T. Keener & Co., 1904. 612p. col. plates. DLC; PPC; PPL; PU **00-1643**

HUTCHISON, Robert (1871-1960)
Clinical methods: a guide to the practical study of medicine. By Robert Hutchison . . . and Harry Rainy . . . 9th ed. Chicago: W. T. Keener & Co., 1905. 634p. col. plates. DLC; PPC; PPL; PU **00-1644**

HUTCHISON, Robert (1871-1960)
Clinical methods: a guide to the practical study of medicine. By Robert Hutchison . . . and Harry Rainy . . . 10th ed., 19th thousand. Chicago: W. T. Keener & Co., 1906. 634p. col. plates. DLC; IEN-M; ICJ **00-1645**

HYDE, James Nevins (1840-1910)
A manual of syphilis and the venereal diseases, by James Nevins Hyde . . . and Frank Hugh Montgomery . . . 2nd ed., rev. and enl. With 58 illustrations in the text, and 19 full-page lithographic plates. Philadelphia: W. B. Saunders & Co., 1900. 594p. col. plates. DLC; DNLM; PPC; PU
00-1646

HYDE, James Nevins (1840-1910)
Touching the symptoms and diagnosis of the epidemic of modified small-pox; an open letter to the State Board of Health of Illinois. [Chicago], 1900. 24p. DNLM; ICJ
00-1647

HYDE, James Nevins (1840-1910)
A practical treatise on diseases of the skin; for the use of students and practitioners, by J. N. Hyde . . . and F. H. Montgomery . . . 5th rev. ed. Philadelphia and New York: Lea Bros. & Co., 1900. 863p. col. plates. CU-M; NNNAM; PPC; PU **00-1648**

HYDE, James Nevins (1840-1910)
A practical treatise on diseases of the skin; for the use of students and practitioners by J. N. Hyde . . . and F. H. Montgomery . . . 6th and rev. ed. . . . Philadelphia and New York: Lea Bros. & Co., 1901. 828p. col. plates. DLC; DNLM; NNNAM; PPC **00-1649**

HYDE, James Nevins (1840-1910)
A practical treatise on diseases of the skin, for the use of students and practitioners, by James Nevins Hyde . . . and Frank Hugh Montgomery . . . 7th and rev. ed., illustrated with 107 engravings and 34 plates in colors and monochrome. Philadelphia and New York: Lea Bros. & Co., 1904. 938p. DLC; IU-M; MBM; PPC **00-1650**

HYDE, James Nevins (1840-1910)
A practical treatise on diseases of the skin, for the use of students and practitioners . . . 8th and rev. ed., illustrated with 223 engravings and 58 plates in colors and monochrome. Philadelphia and New York: Lea & Febiger, 1909. 1126p. DLC; NNNAM; NjR; PPC **00-1651**

INGALS, Ephraim F[letcher] (1848-1918)
Diseases of the chest, throat and nasal cavities. . . . 4th ed. . . . New York: William Wood & Co., 1900. 765p. col. plates. DLC; DNLM; ICJ; NNNAM **00-1652**

INGLIS, William D. (*b.* 1874)
Obstetrics in abstract. . . . Pittsburgh, Pa.: Medical Abstract Publishing Co., [1908]. 171p. DLC. ICJ
00-1653

INGLIS, William D. (*b.* 1874)
Obstetrics in abstract. . . . Pittsburgh, Pa.: Medical Abstract Publishing Co., [1910]. 183p. DLC; ICJ
00-1654

INTERNATIONAL CONGRESS OF MILITARY SURGEONS. ST. LOUIS, 1904
Program of the International Congress of Military Surgeons. World's Fair, 1904. Association of Military Surgeons of the United States of America. Thirteenth annual meeting. Saint Louis, Missouri, October 10-15. [St. Louis? 1904.] 15p. DLC **00-1655**

INTERNATIONAL CONGRESS ON TUBERCULOSIS. 6th, WASHINGTON, 1908
Provisional program of the international Congress of Tuberculosis. Washington, D.C., U.S.A. September 21 to October 12, 1908. [Washington, 1908.] 69p. DLC
00-1656

INTERNATIONAL CONGRESS ON TUBERCULOSIS. 6th, WASHINGTON, D.C., 1908
Anuncio preliminar. L'annonce preliminaire. Vorläufige anzeige. Preliminary announcement of the International Congress on Tuberculosis. Washington, D.C., 1908. 153p. DLC
00-1657

INTERNATIONAL CONGRESS ON TUBERCULOSIS. 6th, WASHINGTON, 1908
Anuncio preliminar. L'annonce preliminaire. Vorläufige anzeige. Preliminary announcement of the International Congress on Tuberculosis. Washington, D.C., U.S.A. September 21 to October 12, 1908. 9th ed. July 1, 1908. [Washington, 1908.] 188p. DLC **00-1658**

INTERNATIONAL CONGRESS ON TUBERCULOSIS. 6th, WASHINGTON, 1908
Program of the International Congress on Tuberculosis. Washington, D.C., U.S.A. Section meetings September 28 to Oct. 3, 1908. [Baltimore, 1908.] 120p. DLC
00-1659

INTERNATIONAL CONGRESS ON TUBERCULOSIS. 6th, WASHINGTON, 1908
General catalogue of the European and American exhibits intended to illustrate the world's work in its struggle against tuberculosis. Collected and arranged in connection with the Sixth International Congress on Tuberculosis held in . . . Washington, D.C., U.S.A., Sept. 21 to Oct. 12, 1908. [Baltimore, 1908.] 298p. DLC; ICJ; MdU-D; MH **00-1660**

INTERNATIONAL CONGRESS ON TUBERCULOSIS. 6th, WASHINGTON, 1908
Special catalogue of the State of Rhode Island exhibit, supplementary to the general catalogue of the Sixth International Congress on Tuberculosis, held in the National Museum, Washington, D.C., U.S.A., Sept. 21 to Oct. 12, 1908. [Washington? 1908.] 13p. DLC **00-1661**

INTERNATIONAL CONGRESS ON TUBERCULOSIS. 6th, WASHINGTON, 1908
Transactions of the Sixth International Congress on Tuberculosis. Washington, September 28 to October 5, 1908. With an account and catalogue of the tuberculosis exhibition, Washington, September 21 to October 12, 1908. Philadelphia: W. F. Fell Co., 1908. 6 v in 8. plates. DLC; DNLM; ICJ; MH
00-1662

IOWA COLLEGE OF PHYSICIANS AND SURGEONS [MEDICAL DEPARTMENT OF DRAKE UNIVERSITY, DES MOINES]
Annual announcements for sessions of 1885-1886 (4.); 1886-1887 (5.); 1889-1890 (8.); 1891-1892 to 1893-1894 (10.-12.); 1895-1896 to 1897-1898 (14.-16.); 1901-1902 to 1902-1903 (20.-21.). Des Moines, [1885]-1902. DNLM [List of graduates from 1884 to 1891 in announcement for 1891-1892]
00-1663

IOWA. STATE UNIVERSITY OF IOWA. COLLEGE OF DENTISTRY
Annual announcements for the sessions of 1900-1901 to 1902-1903 (20.-22.). Iowa City, 1900-1902. DNLM
00-1664

IOWA. STATE UNIVERSITY OF IOWA. COLLEGE OF MEDICINE
Annual announcements for the sessions of 1886-1887 to 1897-1898 (17.-28.); 1900-1901 to 1902-1903 (31.-33.). Des Moines, Chicago, and Iowa City, 1886-1902. DNLM
00-1665

IOWA. STATE UNIVERSITY OF IOWA
University Hospital. Training School for Nurses. Rules for the admission of pupils. [Iowa City, 1900?] 2 l. DNLM
00-1666

IOWA. STATE UNIVERSITY OF IOWA
University Homoeopathic Hospital. Annual announcement of clinics, 1901-1902. Iowa City: University Press, 1901. 1 l. DNLM **00-1667**

IOWA. STATE UNIVERSITY OF IOWA
College of Pharmacy. Annual announcements for 1900-1901 (16.); 1902-1903 (18.). Iowa City: The University Press, 1900-1902. 18p., 14 plates, 2 plans. 32p., 14 plates, 2 plans. DNLM
00-1668

IOWA. STATE UNIVERSITY OF IOWA
University Hospital. Annual announcements of clinics, 1901-1902. Iowa City: University Press, 1901. 1 l. DNLM
00-1669

IRELAND, William W[otherspoon] (1832-1909)
The mental affections of children, idiocy, imbecility, and insanity. 2nd ed. Philadelphia: P. Blakiston's Son & Co., 1900. 450p. 15 plates. DNLM; IU-M; NNNAM; PPC
00-1670

IRISH, John C[arroll] (*b.* 1843)
Treatment of complete prolapse of the uterus. Boston: Damrell & Upham, 1900 [*c.* 1893]. 6p. DNLM
00-1671

IRISH, John C[arroll] (*b.* 1843)
Surgical treatment of uterine neoplasms. New York, 1900 [*c.* 1894]. 11p. NN **00-1672**

IRISH, John C[arroll] (*b.* 1843)
Laparotomy for pus in the abdominal cavity, and for peritonitis. [Boston, 1900?] 16p. DLC; DNLM; NN
00-1673

IRISH, John C[arroll] (*b.* 1843)
Treatment of uterine fibro-myomata by abdominal hysterectomy. Boston: Damrell & Upham, 1900. [1890]. 15p. NN
00-1674

IRISH, John C[arroll] (*b.* 1843)
Abdominal hysterectomy for cancer of the cervix. Boston: Damrell & Upham, 1900 [*c.* 1899]. 10p. MB
00-1675

IRISH, John C[arroll] (*b.* 1843)
Medical expert testimony. Boston: [Damrell & Upham], 1900 [*c.* 1899]. 6p. DNLM **00-1676**

IVY, Robert H[enry] (*b.* 1881)
Applied anatomy and oral surgery, for dental students. . . . Philadelphia and London: W. B. Saunders & Co., 1910 [*c.* 1911]. 280p. DLC; DNLM; PPC; PPJ
00-1677

JACK, Frederick L[afayette]
Successful operation upon a case of brain abscess following suppurative middle ear disease. Boston: Damrelll & Upham, 1901. 19p. MB **00-1678**

JACK, Frederick L[afayette]
Report of four cases showing the result of Killian's operation. [Chicago, 1906.] 8p. ICU **00-1679**

JACK, George N.
. . . Asthma of blood origin and not nerve or reflex. . . . [New York, 1902.] 23p. DLC; NNNAM **00-1680**

JACKSON, Chevalier (1865-1958)
Notes on turbinotomy. St. Louis, 1900. 3p. DNLM
00-1681

JACKSON, Chevalier (1865-1958)
An overlooked nasal factor in ear disease. Chicago, 1901. 4p. DNLM **00-1682**

JACKSON, Chevalier (1865-1958)
Primary carcinoma of the nasopharynx; a table of cases. Chicago, 1901. 16p. DNLM **00-1683**

JACKSON, Chevalier (1865-1958)
Deviation of the nasal septum. Why do our corrective operations often fail? St. Louis, 1902. 8p. DNLM
00-1684

JACKSON, Chevalier (1865-1958)
. . . Thyrotomy vs. laryngectomy: . . . [1905.] 8p. DLC
00-1685

JACKSON, Chevalier (1865-1958)
Fibroma of the nasopharynx. Tracheotomy, external carotid ligation, extirpation, cure. . . . Chicago: Press of the American Medical Association, 1906. 3p. DLC
00-1686

JACKSON, Chevalier (1865-1958)
Tracheo-bronchoscopy, esophagoscopy and gastroscopy. . . . With five colored plates and many illustrations. St. Louis, Mo.: The Laryngoscope Co., 1907. 199p. col. plates. DLC: ICJ; OCIM; PPC **00-1687**

JACKSON, Chevalier (1865-1958)
The bronchoscope as an aid in general diagnosis. [St. Louis, 1908.] 7p. col. plate. DLC; ICJ; NN
00-1688

JACKSON, Edward (1856-1942)
A manual of the diagnosis and treatment of the diseases of the eye. . . . With 178 illustrations and 2 colored plates. Philadelphia: W. B. Saunders & Co., 1900 [*c.* 1899]. 604p. col. plates. DLC, DNLM, NNNAM; PPC **00-1689**

JACKSON, Edward (1856-1942)
Microscope for the examination of the anterior segment of the eye. [Nashville, 1900 (1899).] 3p. MB
00-1690

JACKSON, Edward (1856-1942)
Symmetrical aberration of the eye, meridional astigmatism. [1900; originally, 1888. *vel subseq.*] 10p. PU
00-1691

JACKSON, Edward (1856-1942)
. . . Essentials of refraction and of diseases of the eye, with a consideration of ocular injuries and the ocular symptoms of general diseases . . . 3rd ed., rev. and enl. 82 illustrations. Philadelphia and London: W. B. Saunders & Co., 1901. 261p. DLC; DNLM; PPC; PU
00-1692

JACKSON, Edward, ed. (1856-1942)
The Ophthalmic year book . . . containing a digest of the literature of ophthalmology . . . edited by Edward Jackson [and others]. . . . Denver, Col.: Herrick Book and Stationery Co., 1904-[Irregular]. ICJ; PPC; NNNAM
00-1693

JACKSON, Edward (1856-1942)
The relations of ophthalmology to other departments of science. St. Louis, 1904. 11p. MB **00-1694**

JACKSON, Edward (1856-1942)
Skiascopy and its practical application to the study of refraction . . . 4th ed., rev. and enl. With twenty-eight illustrations. Denver, Col.: The Herrick Book and Stationery Co., 1905. 120p. DLC; ICJ **00-1695**

JACKSON, Edward (1856-1942)
. . . Essentials of refraction and of diseases of the eye, with a consideration of ocular injuries and the ocular symptoms of general diseases . . . 4th ed., rev. and enl., 82 illustrations. Philadelphia and London: W. B. Saunders & Co., 1906. 261p. DLC; NNNAM; PPC; PPJ **00-1696**

JACKSON, Edward (1856-1942)
A manual of the diagnosis and treatment of the diseases of the eye . . . 2nd ed., thoroughly rev. With 182 illustrations and 2 colored plates. Philadelphia and London: W. B. Saunders & Co., 1907. 615p. col. plates. CU-M; DLC; NNNAM; PPC
00-1697

JACKSON, George Thomas (1852-1916)
The ready reference handbook of diseases of the skin . . . 4th ed., thoroughly rev. New York and Philadelphia: Lea Bros. & Co., 1901. 642p. plates. CU-M; DLC; PPC; PU
00-1698

JACKSON, George Thomas (1852-1916)
The ready reference handbook of diseases of the skin. . . . With 91 illustrations and 3 plates. 5th ed., thoroughly rev. New York and Philadelphia: Lea Bros. & Co., [1905]. 676p. DLC; NNNAM; PPC; PU **00-1699**

JACKSON, George Thomas (1852-1916)
The ready reference handbook of diseases of the skin. . . . With 99 illustrations and 4 plates. 6th ed., thoroughly rev. New York and Philadelphia: Lea & Febiger, 1908. 737p. DLC; IU-M; NNNAM; PPC **00-1700**

JACKSON, Shirls
Photographing the eye-ground. Chicago, 1901. 3p. DLC; DNLM **00-1701**

JACKSON, Victor Hugo (*b.* 1850)
Orthodontia and orthopaedia of the face . . . with seven hundred and sixty original illustrations. Philadelphia and London: J. B. Lippincott Co., 1904. 517p. plates. DLC; MdU-D; NN; PPC **00-1702**

[JACOBI, Abraham] (1830-1919)
Proceedings and addresses at the complimentary dinner tendered to Dr. A. Jacobi on the occasion of the seventieth anniversary of his birthday. [New York, 1900.] [unp.] DNLM; NN; NNNAM **00-1703**

[JACOBI, Abraham] (1830-1919)
International contributions to medical literature. "Festschrift" in honor of Abraham Jacobi, M.D., LL.D. to commemorate the seventieth anniversary of his birth, May sixth, 1900. New York: The Knickerbocker Press, 1900. 496p. port., plates. DLC; DNLM; NNNAM; PP **00-1704**

JACOBI, Abraham (1830-1919)
Functional and organic heart murmurs in infancy and in childhood. New York, 1900. 13p. DLC; DNLM; NN
00-1705

JACOBI, Abraham (1830-1919)
German text-books half a century ago. History and reminiscences. New York, 1901. 22p. DLC; NN
00-1706

JACOBI, Abraham (1830-1919)
Notes on cow's milk and infant tuberculosis. New York, 1902. 9p. DNLM **00-1707**

JACOBI, Abraham (1830-1919)
History of American pediatrics before 1800. [1902.] 25p. DLC; NN; PP **00-1708**

JACOBI, Abraham (1830-1919)
Prolonged medication, with special reference to digitalis. New York, 1902. 9p. DNLM; NN **00-1709**

JACOBI, Abraham (1830-1919)
Therapeutics of infancy and childhood . . . 3rd ed. Philadelphia and London: J. B. Lippincott Co., 1903. 560p. DLC; NNNAM; PPC; PU **00-1710**

JACOBI, Abraham (1830-1919)
Tuberculosis and children. . . . [New York]: The Committee on the Prevention of Tuberculosis of the Charity Organization Society, 1903. 10p. DLC; NN; PPC **00-1711**

JACOBI, Abraham (1830-1919)
The modern doctor. . . . New York, 1905. 39p. DLC; NN **00-1712**

JACOBI, Abraham (1830-1919)
Exile and drugs in the treatment of tuberculosis. New York, 1905. 17p. DLC; NN **00-1713**

JACOBI, Abraham (1830-1919)
Portrait of Dr. Paul Fortunatus Mundé. Delivered before the Academy of Medicine, New York, at the presentation of Dr. Mundé's portrait. [New York]: A. R. Elliott Publ. Co., 1906. 2p. NN **00-1714**

JACOBI, Abraham (1830-1919)
The role of pure cow's milk in infant-feeding. Annual oration. [New York, 1906.] 20p. NN **00-1715**

JACOBI, Abraham (1830-1919)
Some of the benefits derived from medical libraries. [New York? 1906.] 19p. NN **00-1716**

JACOBI, Abraham (1830-1919)
The tonsil as a portal of microbic and toxic invasion. Presidential address at the eighteenth annual meeting of the American Pediatric Society, Atlantic City, N.J., May 30, 1906. New York: E. B. Treat & Co., 1906. 4 l. NN **00-1717**

JACOBI, Abraham (1830-1919)
. . . The physical cost of woman's work. . . . New York: The Charity Organization Society, 1907. 8p. DLC; NN **00-1718**

JACOBI, Abraham (1830-1919)
Gastric ulcer in the young. New York, 1909. 13p. DLC; NN **00-1719**

JACOBI, Abraham (1830-1919)
Dr. Jacobi's works. Collected essays, addresses, scientific papers and msicellaneous writings of A. Jacobi . . . ed. by William J. Robinson, M.D. New York: [The Critic and Guide Co.], 1909. 8 v. Half-title: Collectanea Jacobi. DLC; ICJ; NcD; PPJ [Contents—I-III. Contributions to pediatrics.—IV. Contributions to theraeputics.—V. Contributions to pathology—VI. Medical addresses—VII-VIII. Miscellaneous addresses and writings.] **00-1720**

JACOBI, Abraham (1830-1919)
Miscellaneous addresses and writings. . . . Edited by William J. Robinson. . . . New York: The Critic and Guide Co., 1909. 2 v. ICJ; NN **00-1721**

JACOBI, Abraham (1830-1919)
Medical addresses. . . . Edited by William J. Robinson. . . . New York: The Critic and Guide Co., 1909. 467p. ICJ; NN **00-1722**

JACOBI, Abraham (1830-1919)
Contributions to therapeutics. . . . Edited by William J. Robinson. . . . New York: The Critic and Guide Co., 1909. 454p. ICJ; NN **00-1723**

JACOBI, Abraham (1830-1919)
Contributions to pediatrics. . . . Edited by William J. Robinson. . . . New York: The Critic and Guide Co., 1909. 3 v. ICJ; NN **00-1724**

JACOBI, Abraham (1830-1919)
Contributions to pathology. . . . Edited by William J. Robinson. . . . New York: The Critic and Guide Co., 1909. 381p. ICJ; NN **00-1725**

JACOBI, Abraham, ed. (1830-1919)
. . . Diseases of children. . . . An authorized translation from "Die deutsche klinik" under the general editorial supervision of Julius L. Salinger, M.D. With thirty-four illustrations in the text. New York and London: D. Appleton & Co., 1910. 828p. CtY-M; DLC; MBM; NNNAM **00-1726**

JACOBI, Eduard (1862-1915)
Portfolio of dermochromes, by Professor Jacobi . . . English adaptation of text by J. J. Pringle . . . with 155 colored and 13 black and white illustrations on 91 plates. 2nd rev. and enl. ed. . . . New York: Rebman Co. [etc., etc.], 1904. 2 v. DLC; ICJ; MBM; NN [Supplement; containing 76 additional coloured illustrations. New York: Rebman Co. [etc., etc.], 1906] **00-1727**

JACOBI, Eduard (1862-1915)
Portfolio of dermochromes, by Professor Jacobi . . . English adaptation of text of the 1st and 2nd editions by J. J. Pringle . . . with 243 colored and 2 black and white illustrations on 132 plates. 3rd rev. and enl. ed. New York: Rebman Co., [1909]. 216p. DLC; ICJ; LNT-M; MH-M **00-1728**

JACOBI, Eduard (1862-1915)
Portfolio of dermochromes, by Professor Jacobi . . . English adaptation of text of the 1st and 2nd editions by J. J. Pringle . . . 4th ed., rev. and enl., with 246 colored and 2 black and white figures on 134 plates, with explanatory text. . . . New York: Rebman Co., [1910]. 3 v. CtY-M; DLC; ICJ; MBM **00-1729**

[JACOBI, Mary Putnam] (1842-1906)
In memory of Mary Putnam Jacobi. New York: [New York] Academy of Medicine. [1907?] 85p. DLC; NN; NNNAM **00-1730**

JACOBS, Philip P[eter] (1879-1940)
Ambulance service in Greater New York. State Charities Aid Association of New York, Publication No. 99. New York: State Charities Aid Association of New York, 1907. 36p. NN **00-1731**

JACOBS, Philip P[eter] (1879-1940)
The campaign against tuberculosis in the United States, including a directory of institutions dealing with tuberculosis in the United States and Canada. . . . New York: Charities Publication Committee, 1908. 67p. MH; NIC; NN; PU **00-1732**

JACOBSON, W[alter] H[amilton] A[cland] (1847-1924)
The operations of surgery, intended especially for the use of those recently appointed on a hospital staff and for those preparing for the higher examinations. By W. H. A. Jacobson and F. J. Steward. . . . 4th ed. With five hundred and fifty illustrations. Philadelphia: P. Blakiston's Son & Co., 1902. 2 v. DLC; DNLM; NNNAM; PPC **00-1733**

JACOBY, George W. (1856-1940)
. . . Electrotherapy. . . . Philadelphia: P. Blakiston's Son & Co., 1901. 2 v. DLC; PPC; PU **00-1734**

JACOBY, George W. (1856-1940)
The sign of the orbicularis in peripheral facial paralysis. Read at the meeting of the American Neurological Association, May 12, 13, and 14, 1903. [New York], 1903. 10p. NN **00-1735**

JACOBY, George W. (1856-1940)
Peripheral facial diplegia and palatal involvement. Read . . . at the meeting of the American Neurological Association, June 4 and 5, 1906. New York, [1907]. 13p. NN **00-1736**

JACOBY, George W. (1856-1940)
Sanatorium cure for the impecunious neurasthenic. New York, 1906. 6p. NN **00-1737**

JACOBY, George W. (1856-1940)
Intradural resection of the posterior roots of a number of spinal nerves for the relief of intractable pain. With a report of a case of resection of all the roots which go to make up the brachial plexus. Read at the meeting of the American Neurological Association held in Washington, D.C., May 7, 1907. New York: A. R. Elliott Pub. Co., 1907. 27p. NN **00-1738**

JACOBY, George W. (1856-1940)
Psychiatric expert evidence in criminal proceedings; its imperfection and remedy. Read before the New York Neurological Society . . . March 3, 1908. [New York: A. R. Elliott Pub. Co., 1908.] 23p. NN **00-1739**

JAKOB, Christfried (*b.* 1866)
An atlas of the normal and pathological nervous system. Together with a sketch of the anatomy, pathology, and therapy of the same. Introduction by A. von Strümpell. Transl. and ed. by Joseph Collins. New York: William Wood & Co., 1900 [*c.* 1896]. 232p. 78 plates. DLC; ICJ; MH-M; PPC **00-1740**

JAKOB, Christfried (*b.* 1866)
Atlas of the nervous system, including an epitome of the anatomy, pathology and treatment . . . with a preface by Prof. Dr. Ad. v. Strümpell. . . . Authorized transl. from the 2nd rev. German edition; ed. by Edward D. Fisher. . . . With 112 colored lithographic figures and 139 other illustrations, many of them in colors. Philadelphia and London: W. B. Saunders & Co., 1901. 218p. DLC; NNNAM; OCIM; PPC **00-1741**

JAMES, Walter B[elknap], ed. (1858-1927)
Tuberculosis and acute general miliary tuberculosis. . . . By G. Cornet . . . edited with additions by Walter B. James. Philadelphia: W. B. Saunders & Co., 1904. 806p. DLC; NNNAM; PPC; PU [American ed., Nothnagel's encyclopedia of practical medicine] **00-1742**

JAMISON, Alcinous B[urton] (*b.* 1851)
Intestinal ills; chronic constipation, indigestion, autogenetic poisons, diarrhea, piles, etc. Also auto-infection, auto-intoxication, anemia emaciation, etc., due to proctitis and colitis. New York: Knickerbocker Press, 1901. 244p. DLC; DNLM; NNNAM; PU **00-1743**

JAMISON, Alcinous B[urton] (*b.* 1851)
Intestinal irrigation; or, Why, how, and when to flush the colon, treated in connection with other matters of physiological interest and importance. . . . New York: The Author, 1903. 185p. DLC; NN; NNNAM; PU **00-1744**

JANEWAY, Theodore C[aldwell] (1872-1917)
The clinical study of blood-pressure. . . . New York: D. Appleton & Co., 1907. 300p. DLC; MBM; ICJ; PPC **00-1745**

JEFFERIS, Benjamin Grant (*b.* 1851)
Know thyself; or, The royal path to health and happiness; a concise treatise on the laws of perfect life—love, courtship and marriage, by Prof. B. G. Jefferis . . . and J. L. Nichols. Naperville, Ill., Atlanta, Ga., [etc.]: J. L. Nichols & Co., [1903]. 288p. DLC; GU **00-1746**

JEFFERSON MEDICAL COLLEGE, PHILADELPHIA
Post-graduate instruction. Summer course, 1907. Philadelphia, 1906. 8p. PHi; PPJ **00-1747**

JEFFERYS, W[illiam] Hamilton (1871-1945)
. . . Practical ideals in medical mission work. . . . New York: The Domestic and Foreign Missionary Society of the Protestant Episcopal Church, [1906]. 27p. DLC **00-1748**

JEFFERYS, W[illiam] Hamilton (1871-1945)
Hospital dialogue in Mandarin, New York [and Shanghai]: American Presbyterian Mission Press, 1909. 93, [12]p. DLC; NIC **00-1749**

JEFFERYS, W[illiam] Hamilton (1871-1945)
The diseases of China, including Formosa and Korea, by W. Hamilton Jefferys . . . and James L. Maxwell . . . with 5 colored plates, 11 noso-geographical plates, and 360 illustrations in the text. Philadelphia: P. Blakiston's Son & Co., 1910. 716p. DLC; ICJ; KU; PPC **00-1750**

JELKS, John L.
Some complications met with before and after operations for hemorrhoids; their causes, prevention, and treatment. Louisville, Ky., 1900. 8p. DLC; DNLM **00-1751**

JELKS, John L.
Three months' office experience in the treatment of chronic dysentery. Memphis, 1902. 12p. DLC; DNLM **00-1752**

JELLIFFE, Smith Ely (1866-1945)
An introduction to pharmacognosy. . . . Philadelphia, London, [etc.]: W. B. Saunders & Co., 1904. 265p. DLC; OCLloyd; PPC; PU **00-1753**

JENNINGS, I. H.
How to photograph microscopic objects. A manual for the practical microscopist. New York: E. & H. T. Anthony & Co. [*c.* 1900]. 32p. DLC; NN **00-1754**

JENNINGS, John Ellis
A manual of ophthalmoscopy, for students and general practitioners. . . . Philadelphia: P. Blakiston's Son & Co., 1902. 180p. DLC; DNLM; PPC; PU **00-1755**

JENNINGS, John Ellis
Color-vision and color-blindness. A practical manual for railroad surgeons. . . . 2nd ed., thoroughly rev. . . . Philadelphia: F. A. Davis Co., 1905. 132p. DLC; NNNAM; PPC; PU **00-1756**

JENNINGS, Oscar (1851-1914)
On the cure of the morphia habit without suffering (physiological demorphinisation), with a note on the physiological method of relieving the craving for drink. New York: William Wood & Co., 1901. 211p. DNLM; ICJ; NNNAM; PU **00-1757**

JEWETT, Charles (1839-1910)
Syllabus of gynecology. . . . [Brooklyn, 1900]. 132p. DLC; NN; NNNAM **00-1758**

JEWETT, Charles (1839-1910)
Essentials of obstetrics, by Charles Jewett . . . assisted by Harold F. Jewett, M.D. Illustrated by 80 woodcuts and 5 colored plates. [2nd ed.] New York and Philadelphia: Lea Bros. & Co., 1901. 386p. 5 plates. DNL; DNLM; NNNAM; PPC **00-1759**

JEWETT, Charles, ed. (1839-1910)
The practice of obstetrics; by American authors. . . . 2nd ed., rev. and enl. Illustrated with 445 engravings, 48 of which are in colors, and 36 colored plates. New York and Philadelphia: Lea Bros. & Co., [1901]. 786p. DLC; DNLM; NNNAM; PPC **00-1760**

JEWETT, Charles (1839-1910)
Manual of childbed nursing, with notes on infant feeding. . . . 5th ed., rev. and enl. New York: E. B. Treat & Co., 1902. 84p. DLC; DNLM; NNNAM; PU **00-1761**

JEWETT, Charles (1839-1910)
Essentials of obstetrics, by Charles Jewett . . . assisted by Harold F. Jewett, M.D. 3rd ed., rev. and enl. Illustrated by 80 illustrations and 5 colored plates. New York and Philadelphia: Lea Bros. & Co., 1907. 413p. DLC: IU-M; NNNAM; PPC **00-1762**

JEWETT, Charles, ed. (1839-1910)
The practice of obstetrics by American authors. . . . 3rd ed., rev. and enl. Illustrated with 484 engravings, 46 of which are in colors, and 36 colored plates. New York and Philadelphia: Lea Bros. & Co., 1907. 820p. DLC; GU; NNNAM; PPC **00-1763**

JEWETT, Charles (1839-1910)
Syllabus of gynecology. . . . Brooklyn, N.Y., 1907. 178p. DLC; NN; NNNAM **00-1764**

JEWETT, Charles (1839-1910)
Syllabus of gynecology. . . . Brooklyn, N.Y., 1909. 191p. DLC; NN; NNNAM **00-1765**

JOHNSON, Alexander B[ryan] (1860-1917)
Surgical diagnosis. . . . New York: D. Appleton & Co., 1909-1910. 3 v. col. plates. DLC; ICJ; NcD; PPHa **00-1766**

JOHNSON, Charles Nelson (1860-1938)
Principles and practice of filling teeth. . . . Philadelphia: The S. S. White Dental Manufacturing Co., 1900. 283p. DLC; MdU-D; PPC; PU **00-1767**

JOHNSON, Charles Nelson (1860-1938)
Principles and practice of filling teeth. . . . 2nd ed., rev. and enl. Philadelphia: The S. S. White Dental Mfg. Co., [etc., etc.], 1902. 299p. DLC; PPC; PU **00-1768**

JOHNSON, Charles Nelson (1860-1938)
Success in dental practice; a few suggestions relative to the most approved methods of conducting a practice. . . . Philadelphia and London: J. B. Lippincott Co., 1903. 159p. DLC; NNNAM; PPC; PU **00-1769**

JOHNSON, Charles Nelson (1860-1938)
Principles and practice of filling teeth. . . . 3rd ed., rev. and enl. Philadelphia: The S. S. White Dental Mfg. Co., [etc., etc.], 1906. 299p. DLC; MdU-D; PPC; PU **00-1770**

JOHNSON, Charles Nelson, ed. (1860-1938)
A text-book of operative dentistry, by various authors . . . with six hundred and eighteen illustrations. Philadelphia: P. Blakiston's Son & Co., 1908. 755p. DLC: MdU-D; PPC; PU **00-1771**

JOHNSON, Charles Nelson, ed. (1860-1938)
A text-book of operative dentistry, by various authors . . . 2nd ed., rev. and enl., with six hundred and forty-eight illustrations. Philadelphia: P. Blakiston's Son & Co., 1910. 769p. DLC; DNLM; MdU-D; PPC **00-1772**

JOHNSON, John Taber (1845-1921)
The complications of gonorrhoea in women and their prophylactic treatment. New York, 1901. 15p. DLC; DNLM **00-1773**

JOHNSON & LUND (PHILADELPHIA)
Illustrated catalogue and price list of dental materials. [Philadelphia, 1900.] 250p. ICJ; PP; PPF; PPL **00-1774**

JOHNSON, Wallace and Walter H. MERRILL
The x-rays in the treatment of carcinoma. Philadelphia, 1900. 12p. DLC; DNLM **00-1775**

JOHNSON, Walter B[uckley]
The prevention of blindness by the adoption of laws compelling hygienic precautions. Columbus, 1900. 7p. DLC; DNLM **00-1776**

JOHNSTON, George Ben (1853-1916)
Treatment of cancer of the cervix of the uterus complicated by pregnancy. New York, 1900. 5p. DLC; DNLM **00-1777**

JOHNSTON, James C[hew]
Atlas of venereal and skin diseases. 2nd ed., with additional new plates and half-tone illustrations; text entirely rewritten by James C. Johnston. . . . With the addition of chapters on acute and chronic gonorrhea, by George Knowles Swinburne. New York: William Wood & Co., 1900. 240p. 76 plates. DLC; DNLM; NNNAM; PPC **00-1778**

JOHNSTON, James C[hew]
A case of multiple angiosarcoma of the skin. New York, 1901. 3p. DNLM **00-1779**

JOHNSTON, James C[hew]
Sarcoma and the sarcoid growths of the skin. New York, 1901. 21p. 2 plates. DNLM **00-1780**

JOHNSTON, William B[ernard] (*b.* 1878)
A reconstruction of a glomerulus of the human kidney. Baltimore, 1900. 8p. DLC; DNLM **00-1781**

JOHNSTON, W[illiam] W[aring] (1843-1902)
Aneurism of ascending aorta of great size; treatment by gelatin injections and electrolysis, with effect of coagulating most of the contained blood. Philadelphia, 1901. 7p. DNLM **00-1782**

JOHNSTON, W[illiam] W[aring] (1843-1902)
On the evils arising from the failure to recognize the true nature of neurasthenia, and some causes of this failure. [Philadelphia, 1901.] 8p. DNLM **00-1783**

JOHNSTON, W[illiam] W[aring] (1843-1902)
Synopsis of methods employed in the examination of patients for the purpose of arriving at a diagnosis. For the use of the clinical class, University Hospital. Washington: B. S. Adams, [1901]. 6 l. DNLM **00-1784**

JOLLY, Rudolf (*b.* 1875)
Atlas of microscopic diagnosis in gynaecology, with preface and explanatory text by Dr. Rudolf Jolly. . . . Only authorized English translation by P. W. Shedd . . . with 52 lithographs in color and 2 textual figures. New York: Rebman Co., [1910]. 192p. DLC; DNLM; ICJ; PU **00-1785**

JONES, Edward Groves (1874-1921)
Outlines of physiology. . . . Philadelphia: P. Blakiston's Son & Co., 1901. 442p. DLC; DNLM; PPC; PU **00-1786**

JONES, Edward Groves (1874-1921)
Outlines of physiology, by Edward Groves Jones . . . and Robert Grier Stephens . . . 2nd ed., rev., 107 illustrations. Philadelphia: P. Blakiston's Son & Co., 1908 [1907]. 883p. DLC; PPC; PU **00-1787**

JONES, H[enry] Lewis (1857-1915)
Medical electricity. A practical handbook for students and practitioners of medicine. 4th ed. Philadelphia: P. Blakiston's Son & Co., 1904. 536p. DNLM; ICU; NN; PU **00-1788**

JONES, H[enry] Lewis (1857-1915)
Medical electricity. A practical handbook for students and practitioners of medicine. 5th ed. Philadelphia: P. Blakiston's Son & Co., 1906. 519p. DNLM; MBM; PPC; PU **00-1789**

JONES, Henry Macnaughton (1844-1918)
Practical manual of diseases of women and uterine therapeutics. For students and practitioners. 8th ed. New York: William Wood & Co., 1900. 974p. 28 plates. CtY-M; DNLM; NNNAM; PPC **00-1790**

JONES, Henry Macnaughton (1844-1918)
Points of practical interest in gynaecology. New York: William Wood & Co., 1901. 124p. 12 plates. CU-M; DNLM; NNNAM; PPC **00-1791**

JONES, Henry Macnaughton (1844-1918)
Points of practical interest in gynaecology. 2nd ed. New York: William Wood & Co., 1901. 157p. 18 plates. DNLM; MBM; OCIM; PPC **00-1792**

JONES, Henry Macnaughton (1844-1918)
Practical manual of diseases of women and uterine therapeutics. For students and practitioners. 9th ed. New York: William Wood & Co., 1905. 1044p. DNLM; PPHa **00-1793**

JORDAN, David S[tarr], ed. (1851-1931)
Leading American men of science. New York: Henry Holt & Co., 1910. 471p. Portraits. DLC; MH; NIC; NN **00-1794**

JORDAN, Edwin Oakes (1866-1936)
A text-book of general bacteriology. . . . Philadelphia and London: W. B. Saunders & Co., 1908. 557p. DLC; NNNAM; PPC; PU **00-1795**

JORDAN, Edwin Oakes (1866-1936)
A text-book of general bacteriology. . . . 2nd ed., thoroughly rev. Philadelphia and London: W. B. Saunders & Co., 1910. 594p. DLC; NNNAM; OCIM; PPC **00-1796**

JOUSSET, Pierre (1818-1910)
Practice of medicine, containing the homoeopathic treatment of diseases. . . . Transl. from the 3rd rev. and profusely enl. non-published French ed., with valuable additions and annotations, by John Arschagouni. . . . New York: A. L. Chatterton & Co., 1901. 1115p. DLC; NNNAM; PPC; PPHa **00-1797**

JOUSSET, Pierre (1818-1910)
The pathogenic microbes. . . . Authorized transl. of Horace P. Holmes, M.D. Philadelphia: Boericke & Tafel, 1903. 192p. DLC; ICJ; PPC; PPHa **00-1798**

JUDD, Aspinwall (*b.* 1868)
Practical points in the use of x-ray and high frequency currents. New York: Rebman Co., [1909]. 189p. 10 plates. DLC; ICJ; MH-M; NNNAM **00-1799**

JUDD, Charles
The life and work of Lister. [Baltimore, 1910.] 12p. NN; PU **00-1800**

JUDSON, A[doniram] B[rown] (1837-1916)
The question of spinal braces in lateral curvature. Philadelphia, 1901. 5p. DNLM **00-1801**

JUDSON, Charles Francis
The artificial feeding of infants, including a critical review of the recent literature of the subject, by Charles F. Judson . . . and J. Claxton Gittings. . . . Philadelphia: J. B. Lippincott Co., 1902. 368p. DLC; NNNAM; PPC; PU **00-1802**

JUETTNER, Otto (1865-1922)
Modern physio-therapy. A system of drugless therapeutic methods, including a chapter on X-ray diagnosis. . . . Cincinnati, O.: Harvey Publishing Co., [1906]. 513p. DLC; ICJ; OC; OCIM **00-1803**

JUETTNER, Otto (1865-1922)
1785-1909. Daniel Drake and his followers; historical and biographical sketches. . . . Cincinnati: Harvey Publishing Co., [1909]. 496p. ports. DLC; OC; OCHP; OCIM **00-1804**

JULER, Henry E[dward] (1866-1921)
A handbook of ophthalmic science and practice. 3rd ed. Philadelphia: Lea Bros. & Co., 1904. 733p. plates. DLC; IEN-M; NNNAM; PPC **00-1805**

JUNG, Carl Gustav (1875-1961)
The psychology of dementia praecox. . . . authorized transl. with an introduction by Frederick Peterson . . . and A. A. Brill. . . . New York: The Journal of Nervous and Mental Disease Publishing Co., 1909. 153p. DLC; ICU; MB; NN **00-1806**

JUNG, Franz August Richard (*b.* 1869)
The work of the digestive glands (Pawlow) and estimation of pepsin digestion by modern instruments of precision. . . . [Chicago, 1902.] 18p. DLC; ICJ **00-1807**

KAHLER, Charles O[tto] (*b.* 1847)
Our feet; a treatise on the human foot and its clothing . . . With 25 illustrations. . . . New York: P. Kahler's Sons, 1903. 89p. plates. DLC; NN; NNNAM **00-1808**

KAHLER, Charles O[tto] (*b.* 1847)
Our feet; a treatise on the human foot and its clothing . . . [2nd ed.] New York: P. Kahler, 1903. 89p. illus. DNLM; NN; PP; PPC **00-1809**

KAHLER, Charles O[tto] (*b.* 1847)
Surgical chiropody . . . with 48 illustrations picturing various ailments of the feet and showing the chiropodist how to operate. . . . [3rd ed.] New York: Priv. print. for Dr. P. Kahler's Sons [by the Winthrop Press], 1904. 223p. plates. DLC; NN; NNNAM **00-1810**

KAHN, Robert J[ohnstone] (*b.* 1860)
Man's mission on earth; a series of lectures on diseases of the genito-urinary organs as delivered at Dr. Kahn's museum of anatomy and medical science by Drs. Kahn and [Louis J.] Jordan. New York: I. Goldmann & Co., Printers, 1902. 123p. DLC; NN **00-1811**

KAHN, Robert J[ohnstone] (*b.* 1860)
Man's mission on earth; a short treatise on diseases of the genito-urinary organs and accompanying nervous diseases, with a chapter on syphilis. By R. J. Kahn and Louis J. Jordan. New York: Isaac Goldmann Co., Printers, 1909. 203p. DLC; NN **00-1812**

KASSABIAN, Mihran Krikor (1870-1910)
. . . Röntgen rays and electro-therapeutics, with chapters on radium and phototherapy. . . . Philadelphia and London: J. B. Lippincott Co., [1907]. 545p. col. plates. DLC; MBM; NNNAM; PPC **00-1813**

KASSABIAN, Mihran Krikor (1870-1910)
. . . Röntgen rays and electro-therapeutics, with chapters on radium and phototherapy . . . 2nd ed. Philadelphia and London: J. B. Lippincott Co., [1910]. 540p. col. plates. DLC; IU-M; NNNAM; PPC **00-1814**

KEAN, Jefferson Randolph (1860-1950)
The prevention of disease in the army and the best method of accomplishing that result; the Seaman prize essay. . . . Carlisle, Pa.: The Association of Military Surgeons, 1906. 36p. DLC; DNLM **00-1815**

KEAY, J[ohn] H[ay] (1849-1914)
The medical treatment of gallstones. Philadelphia: P. Blakiston's Son & Co., 1902. 126p. CtY-M; DLC; NNNAM; PPC **00-1816**

KEEN, William W[illiams] (1837-1932) and Randle C. ROSENBERGER
The surgical use of celluloid thread. Philadelphia, 1900. 5p. DNLM **00-1817**

KEEN, William W[illiams] (1837-1932)
A case of ligature of the abdominal aorta just below the diaphragm, the patient surviving for forty-eight days; with a proposed instrument for the treatment of aneurisms of the abdominal aorta by temporary compression. Philadelphia, 1900. 27p. DNLM **00-1818**

KEEN, William W[illiams] (1837-1932)
I. A bullet in the popliteal space. II. A case of dilated esophagus. Two cases showing the value of the x-rays and at the same time that in the first case they were misleading. Philadelphia, 1900. 14p. DNLM **00-1819**

KEEN, William W[illiams] (1837-1932)
The endowment of medical colleges. Philadelphia, 1900. 19p. DNLM **00-1820**

KEEN, William W[illiams] (1837-1932)
The ideal physician. Chicago, 1900. 7p. DNLM **00-1821**

KEEN, William W[illiams] (1837-1932)
Nephrectomy for a large aneurysm of the right renal artery; with a résumé of the twelve formerly reported cases of renal aneurysm. Philadelphia, 1900. 16p. 1 plate. DNLM **00-1822**

KEEN, William W[illiams] (1837-1932)
The president's address, delivered at the fifty-first annual meeting of the American Medical Association, held at Atlantic City, N.J., June 5-8, 1900. Chicago, 1900. 19p. DNLM **00-1823**

KEEN, William W[illiams] (1837-1932)
Surgical treatment of perforation of the bowel in typhoid fever; with a table of 158 cases. Chicago, 1900. 12p. 1 table. DNLM **00-1824**

KEEN, William W[illiams] (1837-1932) and W. G. SPILLER
A case of multiple neuro-fibromata of the ulnar nerve. Philadelphia, 1900. 14p. DNLM **00-1825**

KEEN, William W[illiams] (1837-1932) and W. G. SPILLER
Peripheral resection of the fifth nerve. Three cases with microscopic examination of the portions of nerves removed, and report on the later conditions of patients. Philadelphia, 1900. 12p. DNLM **00-1826**

KEEN, William W[illiams] (1837-1932)
The progress of surgery as influenced by vivisection. . . . [Philadelphia, 1901.] 26p. DLC; MH; NN; PPJ **00-1827**

KEEN, William W[illiams] (1837-1932)
Misstatements of antivivisectionists; correspondence with American Humane Association. . . . Philadelphia, [1901]. 20p. DLC; NN; PPJ **00-1828**

KEEN, William W[illiams] (1837-1932)
Misstatements of the antivivisectionists again. . . . Philadelphia, [1901]. 8p. DLC **00-1829**

KEEN, William W[illiams] (1837-1932)
An American text-book of surgery, for practitioners and students, by Phineas S. Conner, M.D., Frederic S. Dennis, M.D., William W. Keen, M.D., Charles B. Nancrede, M.D., Roswell Park, M.D., Lewis S. Pilcher, M.D., Nicholas Senn, M.D., Francis J. Shepherd, M.D., Lewis A. Stimson, M.D., J. Collins Warren, M.D. and J. William White, M.D.; edited by William W. Keen . . . and J. William White . . . 4th ed., thoroughly rev. and enl. Philadelphia, [etc.] : W. B. Saunders & Co., 1903. 1363p. col. plates. DLC; NNNAM; PPC; PPJ **00-1830**

KEEN, William W[illiams] (1837-1932)
Address and other papers. Philadelphia: W. B. Saunders & Co., 1905. 441p. plates. DLC; NNNAM; PPC; PPJ [Twenty-six papers, including: The early history of practical anatomy; The history of the Philadelphia School of Anatomy and its relation to medical teaching; Our recent debts to vivisection; Vivisection and brain surgery; Samuel D. Gross; Surgical reminiscences of the Civil War; and The ideal physician] **00-1831**

KEEN, William W[illiams] (1837-1932)
Some reminiscences of students days in the Jefferson. [Philadelphia], 1905. [unp.] PPJ **00-1832**

KEEN, William W[illiams], ed. (1837-1932)
Surgery, its principles and practice by various authors. . . . Philadelphia: W. B. Saunders & Co., 1906-1921. 8 v. DLC; NNNAM; PPC; PPJ [Vols. 4-5 edited by W. W. Keen and John Chalmers da Costa; *also*: Complete Index to Keen's Surgery, vols. I-VIII, Philadelphia: W. B. Saunders & Co., 1921. Consists of 6 original vs., 2 supplements, and index volume; includes Harvey Cushing's 260p. monograph on Surgery of the Head, and a 65p. History of Surgery by J. G. Mumford] **00-1833**

KEEN, William W[illiams] (1837-1932)
Samuel David Gross: the lesson of his life and labors; a eulogy pronounced at the eighty-fifth annual commencement of the Jefferson Medical College, June 6th, 1910. Philadelphia, 1910. 14p. PPJ **00-1834**

KEEN, William W[illiams] (1837-1932)
Modern antiseptic surgery and the role of experiment in its discovery and development [Philadelphia, 1910.] 19p. PPJ **00-1835**

KEEN, William W[illiams] (1837-1932)
What vivisection has done for humanity. [Philadelphia, 1910.] 15p. PPJ **00-1836**

KEIBEL, Franz K. J. (1861-1929) and Franklin P. MALL, eds.
Manual of human embryology. Philadelphia: J. B. Lippincott Co., 1910-1912. 2 v. CtY-M; IU-M; NNNAM; PPC **00-1837**

KEIRLE, Nathaniel G[arland] (1833-1919)
Studies in rabies: collected writings. Introduction by Wm. H. Welch, and a biographical sketch by Harry Friedenwald. Baltimore: Lord Baltimore Press, 1909. 386p. DLC; DNLM; ICJ; NN **00-1838**

KEITH, Skene (1858-1919)
Cancer; relief of pain and possible cure, by Skene Keith . . . and E. Keith. . . . New York: The Macmillan Co., 1908. 155p. DLC; ICJ; NNNAM; PU **00-1839**

KELLEY, Samuel W[alter] (1855-1929)
Surgical diseases of children. A modern treatise on pediatric surgery. New York: E. B. Treat & Co., 1909. 765p. DLC; DNLM; ICJ; PU **00-1840**

KELLOGG, John H[arvey] (1852-1943)
The home handbook of domestic hygiene and rational medicine. 55th thousand, revised and enlarged. Battle Creek, 1900. 1675p. 1 superposed plate, 34 plates. DLC; DNLM **00-1841**

KELLOGG, John H[arvey] (1852-1943)
Man the masterpiece, or plain truths plainly told about boyhood, youth, and manhood. Battle Creek, 1900. 604p. 20 plates. DLC; DNLM **00-1842**

KELLOGG, John H[arvey] (1852-1943)
Ladies' guide in health and disease. Girlhood, maidenhood, wifehood, motherhood. Battle Creek, 1901. 690p. 1 superposed plate, 37 plates. DLC; DNLM **00-1843**

KELLOGG, John H[arvey] (1852-1943)
Rational hydrotherapy; a manual of the physiological and therapeutic effects of hydriatic procedures, and the technique of their application in the treatment of disease. . . . With two hundred ninety-three illustrations, eighteen in colors. Philadelphia: The F. A. Davis Co., 1901. 1193p. DLC; DNLM; ICJ; PPC **00-1844**

KELLOGG, John H[arvey] (1852-1943)
Rational hydrotherapy, a manual of the physiological and therapeutic effects of hydriatic procedures, and the technique of their application in the treatment of disease . . . with two hundred ninety-three illustrations, eighteen in colors. 2nd ed. Philadelphia: F. A. Davis Co., 1902. 1193p. DLC; ICJ; NNNAM; PPC **00-1845**

KELLOGG, John H[arvey] (1852-1943)
Rational hydrotherapy; a manual of the physiological and therapeutic effects of hydriatic procedures, and the technique of their application in the treatment of disease . . . with two hundred ninety-three illustrations, nineteen in colors. 3rd rev. ed. Philadelphia: F. A. Davis Co., 1906. 1217p. DLC; NN; OCIM; PPC **00-1846**

KELLOGG, John H[arvey] (1852-1943)
The home book of modern medicine; a family guide in health and disease. . . . Battle Creek, Mich.: Modern Medicine Publishing Co., [1906]. 1676p. col. plates. DLC; ICJ; OCIM; PU **00-1847**

KELLOGG, John H[arvey] (1852-1943)
The Battle Creek sanitarium system; history, organization, methods. . . . Battle Creek, Mich.: Gage Printing Co., 1908. 210p. DLC; ICJ **00-1848**

KELLOGG, John H[arvey] (1852-1943)
The Battle Creek sanitarium diet list. . . . Battle Creek, Mich.: Modern Medicine Pub. Co., 1909. 71p. DLC; ICJ **00-1849**

KELLOGG, John H[arvey] (1852-1943)
Rational hydrotherapy; a manual of the physiological and therapeutic effects of hydriatic procedures, and the technique of their application in the treatment of disease . . . with two hundred ninety-three illustrations, nineteen in colors. 4th rev. ed. Philadelphia: F. A. Davis Co., 1910. 1247p. DLC; ICJ; NNNAM; PPC **00-1850**

KELLOGG, Theodore H[arvey] (1841-1931)
The histrionic element of mental disease. [New York, 1902.] 11p. MB; MH **00-1851**

KELLOGG, Theodore H[arvey] (1841-1931)
The relation of certain extreme emotional states to insanity. . . . [New York: A. R. Elliott Publishing Co., 1905.] 10p. DLC; NN; NNNAM **00-1852**

KELLY, Aloysius Oliver Joseph (1870-1911)
The practice of medicine; a guide to the nature, discrimination and management of disease. . . . Philadelphia and New York: Lea & Febiger, 1910. 945p. col. plates. DLC; NNNAM; OCIM; PPC **00-1853**

KELLY, Howard A[twood] (1858-1943)
The evolution of my technique in the treatment of fibroid uterine tumors. New York: William Wood & Co., 1900. 19p. 2 plates. DNLM **00-1854**

KELLY, Howard A[twood] (1858-1943)
An improved vesical speculum. New York, 1900. 6p. DNLM **00-1855**

KELLY, Howard A[twood] (1858-1943)
Methods of teaching gynecology. Philadelphia, 1900. 8p. DNLM **00-1856**

KELLY, Howard A[twood] (1858-1943)
A new method of making applciations to the vaginal vault and a new instrument to facilitate cleansing the vagina in leucorrhoea. New York, 1900. 3p. DNLM **00-1857**

KELLY, Howard A[twood] (1858-1943)
Normal prophylactic appendectomy. St. Louis, 1900. 3p. DNLM **00-1858**

KELLY, Howard A[twood] (1858-1943)
A note on a series of new vesical specula. Baltimore, 1900. 1 l. 1 plate. DNLM **00-1859**

KELLY, Howard A[twood] (1858-1943)
Notes on an improved method of removing the cancerous uterus by the vagina. Baltimore, 1900. 4p. DNLM **00-1860**

KELLY, Howard A[twood] (1858-1943)
What precautions shall we take to avoid leaving foreign bodies in the abdomen after operations? New York, 1900. 1p. DNLM **00-1861**

KELLY, Howard A[twood] (1858-1943)
A preliminary report on the surgical treatment of complicated fibroid tumors of the womb; with a description of two methods of operating. Baltimore, 1900. 6p. DNLM **00-1862**

KELLY, Howard A[twood] (1858-1943)
The present status of operations for cancerous uteri. Chicago, 1900. 16p. DNLM **00-1863**

KELLY, Howard A[twood] (1858-1943)
A rapid and simple operation for gallstones found by exploring the abdomen in the course of a lower abdominal operation. Philadlephia, 1900. 13p. DNLM **00-1864**

KELLY, Howard A[twood] (1858-1943)
Resection and anastomosis of the divided ureter. Baltimore, 1900. 11p. DNLM **00-1865**

KELLY, Howard A[twood] (1858-1943)
The removal of pelvic inflammatory masses by the abdomen after bisection of the uterus. New York: William Wood & Co., 1900. 22p. DNLM **00-1866**

KELLY, Howard A[twood] (1858-1943)
Ureteral calculus; its diagnosis by means of the wax-tipped bougie. Escape of the calculus per vias naturales after forcible dilatation of the ureteral orifice. Chicago, 1900. 10p. DNLM **00-1867**

KELLY, Howard A[twood] (1858-1943)
Exhibition of methods of medical instruction in the Johns Hopkins Medical School and Hospital. Philadelphia, 1901. 3p. DNLM **00-1868**

KELLY, Howard A[twood] (1858-1943)
A historical note upon Diptera as carriers of diseases; Paré, Déclat. Baltimore, 1901. 7p. DNLM **00-1869**

KELLY, Howard A[twood] (1858-1943)
How to deal with the vermiform appendix. Some forms of complicated appendicitis. Philadelphia, 1901. 6p. DNLM **00-1870**

KELLY, Howard A[twood] (1858-1943)
Jules Lemaire. The first to recognize the true nature of wound infection and inflammation and the first to use carbolic acid in medicine and surgery. Chicago, 1901. 16p. DNLM **00-1871**

KELLY, Howard A[twood] (1858-1943)
A new and better method of opening and of draining the bladder in women. New York, 1901. 3p. 2 plates. DNLM **00-1872**

KELLY, Howard A[twood] (1858-1943)
The removal of pelvic inflammatory masses by the abdomen after bisection of the uterus. Baltimore, 1901. 4p. 2 plates. DNLM **00-1873**

KELLY, Howard A[twood] (1858-1943)
Scratch-marks on the wax-tipped catheter as a means of determining the presence of stone in the kidney and in the ureter. New York, 1901. 13p. 2 plates. DNLM **00-1874**

KELLY, Howard A[twood] (1858-1943)
Some further notes on the extension of the principle of bisection in abdominal surgery. St. Paul, 1901. 7p. DNLM **00-1875**

KELLY, Howard A[twood] (1858-1943)
The vermiform appendix and its diseases, by Howard A. Kelly . . . and Elizabeth Hurdon. . . . With 399 original illustrations, some in colors, and 3 lithographic plates. Philadelphia and London: W. B. Saunders & Co., 1905. 827p. DLC; NNNAM; PPC; PU **00-1876**

KELLY, Howard A[twood] (1858-1943)
Some lessons from the life of Major Walter Reed. [Baltimore, 1906.] 7p. DLC; NN **00-1877**

KELLY, Howard A[twood] (1858-1943)
Walter Reed and yellow fever. . . . New York: McClure, Phillips & Co., 1906. 293p. ports. DLC; ICU; MB; NN **00-1878**

KELLY, Howard A[twood] (1858-1943)
Walter Reed and yellow fever. . . . New and rev. ed. Baltimore: Medical Standard Book Co., 1906. 310p. MdU-D; MdBJ-W; NNNAM; PU **00-1879**

KELLY, Howard A[twood] (1858-1943)
Operative gynecology . . . with eleven plates and seven hundred and three original illustrations for the most part by Max Brödel. . . . 2nd ed., rev. and enl. New York and London: D. Appleton & Co., 1906. 2 v. col. plates. DLC; IU-M; NNNAM; PPC **00-1880**

KELLY, Howard A[twood] (1858-1943)
Gynecology and abdominal surgery, ed. by Howard A. Kelly . . . and Charles P. Noble . . . illustrated by Hermann Becker, Max Brödel and others. . . . Philadelphia and London: W. B. Saunders & Co., 1907-08. 2 v. col. plates. DLC; MdU-D; NNNAM; PPC **00-1881**

KELLY, Howard A[twood] (1858-1943)
Medical gynecology . . . with one hundred and sixty-three illustrations, for the most part by Max Brödel and A. Horn. New York and London: D. Appleton & Co., 1908. 662p. DLC; NNNAM; PPC; ScCM **00-1882**

KELLY, Howard A[twood] (1858-1943)
Appendicitis, and other diseases of the vermiform appendix . . . with 215 original illustrations, some in colors, and three lithographic plates. [New ed.] Philadelphia and London: J. B. Lippincott Co., [1909]. 502p. DLC; MBM; NNC; PPC **00-1883**

KELLY, Howard A[twood] (1858-1943)
Myomata of the uterus, by Howard A. Kelly . . . and Thomas S. Cullen . . . illustrated by August Horn and Hermann Becker. Philadelphia and London: W. B. Saunders & Co., 1909. 723p. col. plates. DLC; NNNAM; PPC; PU **00-1884**

KELLY, Howard A[twood] (1858-1943)
Operative gynecology . . . with eleven plates and seven hundred and three original illustrations for the most part by Max Brödel. . . . 2nd ed., rev. and enl. New York and London: D. Appleton & Co., 1909 [1908]. 2 v. DLC; MBM; NNNAM; PPC **00-1885**

KELSEY, Charles B[oyd] (1850-1917)
Stricture of the rectum; a study of ninety-six cases. [New York, 1900.] 46p. DNLM; NNNAM [Reprinted from Wood's Medical and Surgical Monographs, vol. 7 (1890)] **00-1886**

KELSEY, Charles B[oyd] (1850-1917)
The office treatment of hemorrhoids, fistula, etc., without operation; together with remarks on the relation of diseases of the rectum to other diseases in both sexes, but especially in women, and the abuse of the operation of colostomy. New York: E. R. Pelton, 1900. 80p. ICJ; NNNAM; PPC; PU **00-1887**

KELSEY, Charles B[oyd] (1850-1917)
The surgery of the rectum . . . 6th ed., illustrated by two hunded and fifteen engravings. New York: William Wood & Co., 1902. 402p. DLC; DNLM; ICJ; NNNAM **00-1888**

KELSEY, Charles B[oyd] (1850-1917)
The office treatment of diseases of the rectum, with a description of some new methods. New York: William Wood & Co., [1905]. 16p. NN **00-1889**

KELYNACK, T[heophilus] N[ichols] (1866-1944)
Tuberculosis in infancy and childhood, its pathology, prevention. and treatment. By various writers. Edited by T. N. Kelynack. New York: William Wood & Co., 1908. 376p. DNLM; ICJ; NNNAM; PU **00-1890**

KEMP, Robert C[oleman] (*b.* 1865)
Enteroclysis, hypodermoclysis and infusion. . . . New York: James T. Dougherty, 1900. 349p. DLC; NN; NNNAM; PU **00-1891**

KEMP, Robert C[oleman] (*b.* 1865)
Diseases of the stomach and intestines. . . . Philadelphia: W. B. Saunders & Co., 1901. 766p. col. pates. DLC; NcD; PPJ; PU **00-1892**

KEMPER, [General] William Harrison (1839-1927)
The world's anatomists; concise biographies of anatomic masters, from 300 B.C. to the present time, whose names have adorned the literature of the medical profession. . . . Revised and enlarged from the original serial publication in the Medical Book News; with eleven illustrations nine of which are portraits. Philadelphia: P. Blakiston's Son & Co., 1905. 79p. DLC: ICJ; KU; PPC **00-1893**

KENT, James T[yler] (1849-1916)
Lectures on homoeopathic philosophy. Lancaster, Pa.: Examiner Printing House, 1900. 190p. DLC; DNLM **00-1894**

KENT, James T[yler] (1849-1916)
Lectures on homoeopathic materia medica. . . . Philadelphia: Boericke & Tafel, 1905. 965p. DLC; ICJ; PPC; PPHa **00-1895**

KENT, James T[yler] (1849-1916)
Repertory of the homoeopathic materia medica. . . . 2nd rev. ed. Lancaster, Pa.: Examiner Printing House, 1908. 1380p. DLC **00-1896**

KERLEY, Charles Gilmore (*b.* 1863)
Short talks with young mothers on the management of infants and young children. New York and London: G. P. Putnam's Sons, 1901. 262p. CtY-M; DLC; MB; OCIM **00-1897**

KERLEY, Charles Gilmore (*b.* 1863)
Treatment of the diseases of children. . . . Philadelphia and London: W. B. Saunders & Co., 1907. 597p. DLC; DNLM; PPC; PPJ **00-1898**

KERLEY, Charles Gilmore (*b.* 1863)
Personal observations in scarlet fever. Read in the Section on Diseases of Chidlren of the American Medical Association, at the 59th annual session, held at Chicago, June 1908. Chicago: Amer. Med. Association, 1908. 11p. NN **00-1899**

KERLEY, Charles Gilmore (*b.* 1863)
Public school education. New York: E. B. Treat & Co., [1908]. 11p. NN **00-1900**

KERLEY, Charles Gilmore (*b.* 1863)
Treatment of the diseases of children . . . 2nd ed., rev. Philadelphia and London: W. B. Saunders & Co., 1909. 629p. DLC; NcD; PPJ; PU **00-1901**

KERLEY, Charles Gilmore (*b.* 1863)
Short talks with young mothers on the management of infants and young children . . . 2nd ed., rev. and enl. New York and London: G. P. Putnam's Sons, 1909. 327p. DLC; ICJ; PPC **00-1902**

KERR, Abram T[ucker] (1873-1938)
On the preservation of anatomical material in America by means of cold storage. Baltimore, 1901. 17p. 1 plate. DLC; DNLM **00-1903**

KERR, LE GRAND (*b.* 1870)
Diagnostics of the diseases of children. . . . Philadelphia and London: W. B. Saunders & Co., 1907. 542p. DLC; ICJ; PPC; PU **00-1904**

KERR, LE GRAND (*b.* 1870)
The baby, its care and development, for the use of mothers. . . . Brooklyn, N.Y.: A. T. Huntington, 1908. 150p. DLC; DNLM; ICJ; PPJ **00-1905**

KERR, LE GRAND (*b.* 1870)
The care and training of children. . . . New York and London: Funk & Wagnalls Co., 1910. 233p. DLC; ICJ; NNNAM; PU **00-1906**

KEYES, Edward Lawrence (1843-1924)
Venereal diseases; their complications and sequelae, by Edward L. Keyes . . . and Charles H. Chetwood. . . . Illustrated by eight full-page plates in black and colors and one hundred and seven engravings. New York: William Wood & Co., 1900. 356p. DLC; DNLM; NcD; PPC **00-1907**

KEYES, Edward Lawrence (1843-1924)
The surgical diseases of the genito-urinary organs, by E. L. Keyes . . . and E. L. Keyes, Jr. . . . A revision of Van Buren and Keyes's text-book, with one hundred and seventy-four illustrations in the text and ten plates, eight of which are coloured. New York and London: D. Appleton & Co., 1903. 827p. DLC; ICJ; PPHa; PU **00-1908**

KEYES, Edward Lawrence (1843-1924)
The surgical diseases of the genito-urinary organs, by E. L. Keyes . . . and E. L. Keyes, Jr. . . . 2nd ed., rev., with one hundred and seventy-four illustrations in the text and ten plates, eight of which are coloured. New York and London: D. Appleton & Co., 1905. 827p. DLC; MBM; NcD; PPHa **00-1909**

KEYES, Edward Lawrence (1843-1924)
The fear of death. . . . New York: Privately printed [at the Scribner Press], 1910. [unp.] CtY-M; DNLM; NN **00-1910**

KEYES, Edward Loughborough (*b.* 1873)
Syphilis; a treatise for practitioners. . . . With sixty-nine illustrations in the text and nine plates, seven of which are colored. New York and London: D. Appleton & Co., 1908. 577p. DLC; ICJ; NjR; PPC **00-1911**

KEYES, Edward Loughborough (*b.* 1873)
Diseases of the genito-urinary organs considered from a medical and surgical standpoint, including a description of gonorrhea in the female and conditions peculiar to the female urinary organs . . . with one hundred and ninety-five illustrations in the text and seven plates, four of which are colored. New York and London: D. Appletôn & Co., 1910. 975p. DLC; ICJ; OCIM; PPC **00-1912**

KEYES, Thomas Bassett
The cure of consumption with subcutaneous injections of oils. [Chicago, 1907?] 96p. NN **00-1913**

KEYES, Thomas Bassett
The renewal of life; arguments for subcutaneous injections of oil in the cure and prevention of senility and disease; for the making of the acme of abundant health, stamina, vigor, vitality and constitution; for the cure of consumption and other diseases, particularly those of a chronic nature. . . . Chicago, Ill.: The Tubercle Press Bureau, 1909-10. 206p. DLC; DNLM; ICJ **00-1914**

KEYSOR, William W[inchester] (*b.* 1852)
A medico-legal manual. Omaha: Burkley, 1901. 316p. DLC; DNLM **00-1915**

KILMER, Theoron W[endell] (*b.* 1872)
The practical care of the baby . . . with sixty-eight illustrations. Philadelphia: F. A. Davis Co., 1903. 158p. DLC; GU; MdU-D; NcD **00-1916**

KILMER, Theoron W[endell] (*b.* 1872)
The physical examination of infants and young children. . . . Illustrated with 59 half-tone engravings. Philadelphia: F. A. Davis Co., 1906. 86p. DLC: ICJ; MBM; NNNAM **00-1917**

KIMBER, Diana Clifford
Text-book of anatomy and physiology for nurses. . . . New York, London: The Macmillan Co., 1902. 276p. DLC; MBM; NNNAM; PU **00-1918**

KIMBER, Diana Clifford
Text-book of anatomy and physiology for nurses. . . . 2nd ed. New York: The Macmillan Co., 1905. 276p. DLC: NNNAM; PPC; PU **00-1919**

KIMBER, Diana Clifford
Text-book of anatomy and physiology for nurses. . . . 3rd ed., rev. by Carolyn E. Gray. . . . New York: The Macmillan Co., 1909. 438p. DLC; ICJ; NNNAM; PU **00-1920**

KING, Albert F[reeman] A[fricanus] (1841-1914)
A manual of obstetrics, 8th ed., rev. and enl. Philadelphia and New York: Lea Bros. & Co., 1900. 612p. DLC; DNLM; NNNAM; PPC **00-1921**

KING, Albert F[reeman A[fricanus] (1841-1914)
A new factor in the etiology of malarial fever, indicating new methods of treatment. [Philadelphia, 1902.] 5p. DNLM **00-1922**

KING, Albert F[reeman] A[fricanus] (1841-1914)
A new factor in the etiology and treatment of intermittent fever; destruction of the parasite by ultra-violet rays of fluorescent light. Washington, 1902. 28p. DNLM **00-1923**

KING, Albert F[reeman] A[fricanus] (1841-1914)
A manual of obstetrics. . . . 9th ed., rev. and enl. With two hundred and seventy-five illustrations. Philadelphia and New York: Lea Bros. & Co., 1903. 622p. CtY-M; DLC; NNNAM; PPC **00-1924**

KING, Albert F[reeman] A[fricanus] (1841-1914)
A manual of obstetrics. . . . 10th ed., rev. and enl. With three hundred and one illustrations in text and three plates. Philadelphia and New York: Lea Bros. & Co., 1907. 688p. DLC; GU; NNNAM; PPC **00-1925**

KING, Albert F[reeman] A[fricanus] (1841-1914)
A manual of obstetrics. . . . 11th ed., rev. and enl. With three hundred and forty-one illustrations in text and three plates. Philadelphia and New York: Lea & Febiger, 1910. 713p. DLC; IU-M; NNNAM; PPC **00-1926**

KING, John B[lair] S[mith] (*b.* 1855)
Practical observations upon the chemistry of food and dietetics. . . . [Chicago]: The Blakely Printing Co., 1906. 140p. DLC; ICJ; PPHa **00-1927**

KING, John B[lair] S[mith] (*b.* 1855)
Practical observations upon the chemistry of food and dietetics. 2nd rev. and enl. ed. . . . Philadelphia: Boericke & Tafel, 1907. 147p. DLC; PPC **00-1928**

KING, JULIUS (OPTICAL CO.)
[Catalogue] New York: Berdan & Redcliffe, [1900]. 203p. DNLM **00-1929**

KING, JULIUS (OPTICAL CO.)
Directions for King's elite test lenses in the correction of defective vision. [Cleveland, O., 1900.] unp. 3 l. DLC [Originally, 1888, *vel subseq.*] **00-1930**

KING, JULIUS (OPTICAL CO.)
Synopsis of instructions in the use of King's elite test case . . . Julius King Optical Co., New York, Cleveland . . . [New York?], 1900. 32p. DLC [Originally, 1895, *vel subseq.*] **00-1931**

KING, William Harvey (*b.* 1861)
Treatise on spermatorrhea, impotence, and sterility. . . . New York: A. L. Chatterton & Co., 1900 [*c.* 1897]. 172p. NNNAM **00-1932**

KING, William Harvey (*b.* 1861)
Electricity in medicine and surgery, including the X-ray; with a section on electro-physiology, by W. Y. Cowl; and a section on the Bottini operation, by Albert Freudenberg. New York: Boericke & Runyon, 1901. 2 v. DNLM; ICJ; PPC; PU **00-1933**

KING, William Harvey (*b.* 1861)
Electricity in medicine and surgery, including the X-ray. . . . Second edition. With a section on electro-physiology by W. Y. Cowl . . . and a section on the Bottini operation by Albert Freudenberg. . . . New York: Boericke & Runyon, 1902. 2 v. in 1. diags., illus., plates. CtY-M; ICJ; NN; PPHa **00-1934**

KING, William Harvey (*b.* 1861)
Medical union number six. . . . New York: The Monograph Press, 1904. 58p. DLC; NN; PPC **00-1935**

KING, William Harvey, ed. (*b.* 1861)
History of homoeopathy and its institutions in America; their founders, benefactors, faculties, officers, hospitals, alumni, etc., with a record of achievement of its representatives in the world of medicine. . . . New York, Chicago: The Lewis Publishing Co., 1905. 4 v. DLC; ICJ; KU; NcU **00-1936**

KING, William Harvey (*b.* 1861)
Static, high frequency, radio, photo and radium therapy. New York: Boericke & Runyon, 1905. 291p. illus. CtY-M; ICJ **00-1937**

KING, William Harvey (*b.* 1861)
The treatment of chronic appendicitis with high frequency currents. New York: William Wood & Co., [1910]. 18p. NN **00-1938**

KINGMAN, R[ufus] A[nderson]
Two cases illustrating conservative operations for uterine fibroids. Boston: Damrell & Upham, 1900. 18p. DNLM **00-1939**

KINGMAN, R[ufus] A[nderson]
Anteflexion. Its importance and its operative treatment. Boston, 1901. 10p. DNLM **00-1940**

KINGSBURY, Jerome (*b.* 1871)
The neurotic element in infantile eczema. Philadelphia, 1901. 6p. DNLM **00-1941**

KINGSBURY, Jerome (*b.* 1871)
The conjunctival tuberculin reaction in certain diseases of the skin. New York: The Grafton Press, 1909. 8p. NN **00-1942**

KINGSLEY, Sherman C[olver] (*b.* 1866)
Open air crusaders: a report of the Elizabeth McCormick open air school, together with a general account of open air school work in Chicago and a chapter on school ventilation. . . . Chicago, Ill.: United Charities of Chicago, [1910]. 107p. DLC; ICJ; MB; NN **00-1943**

KINTZING, Pearce
The signs of internal disease. With a brief consideration of the principal symptoms thereof. Chicago: The Cleveland Press, 1906. 374p. DLC; ICJ; MH; NN **00-1944**

KINTZING, Pearce
Long life and how to attain it. New York: Funk & Wagnalls Co., 1908. 285p. DLC; NIC; NN **00-1945**

KIRBY, Ellwood R[obert]
Manual of surgery. Philadelphia: F. W. Langmaid, 1900. 372p. DNLM; ICJ; NNNAM; PU **00-1946**

KIRK, Edward Cameron, ed. (1856-1933)
The American text-book of operative dentistry. In contributions of eminent authorities. . . . 2nd ed. rev. and enl. Illustrated with 897 engravings. Philadelphia and New York: Lea Bros. & Co., 1900. 852p. DLC; MdU-D; NNNAM; PPC **00-1947**

KIRK, Edward Cameron, ed. (1856-1933)
The American text-book of operative dentistry. In contributions by eminent authorities. . . . 3rd ed., rev. and enl. Illustrated with 875 engravings. Philadelphia and New York: Lea Bros. & Co., 1905. 899p. DLC; MdU-D; PPC; PU **00-1948**

KIRKES, William Senhouse (1823-1864)
Kirkes' handbook of physiology. . . . By William D. Halliburton [16th ed.] Philadelphia: P. Blakiston's Son & Co., 1900. 872p. 3 plates. CtY-M; DNLM; PPC; PU
00-1949

KIRKES, William Senhouse (1823-1864)
Kirkes' handbook of physiology. Handbook of physiology by W. Morrant Baker . . . and Vincent Dormer Harris . . . 16th American ed. Revised by Warren Coleman . . . and Charles L. Dana . . . with upwards of five hundred illustrations including many in colors. New York: William Wood & Co., 1900. 840p. DLC; IU-M; NNNAM; PPC **00-1950**

KIRKES, William Senhouse (1823-1864)
Kirkes' handbook of physiology. . . . By William D. Halliburton. Philadelphia: P. Blakiston's Son & Co., 1901. 888p. DLC; NNNAM; PPC; PU **00-1951**

KIRKES, William Senhouse (1823-1864)
Kirkes' handbook of physiology. Handbook of physiology, rev. by William H. Rockwell, Jr., M.D. and Charles L. Dana . . . 4th American ed., with upwards of five hundred illustrations, including many in colors. New York: William Wood & Co., 1902. 854p. DLC; DNLM; NNNAM; PU
00-1952

KIRKES, William Senhouse (1823-1864)
Kirkes' handbook of physiology. . . . By William D. Halliburton. Philadelphia: P. Blakiston's Son & Co., 1904. 902p. CtY-M; NNNAM; PPC; PU **00-1953**

KIRKES, William Senhouse (1823-1864)
Kirkes' handbook of physiology. Handbook of physiology, revised by Frederick C. Busch . . . 5th American revision, with five hundred and thirty-five illustrations, including many in colors. New York: William Wood & Co., 1904. 862p. DLC; GU; NNNAM; PPC **00-1954**

KIRKES, William Senhouse (1823-1864)
Kirkes' handbook of physiology, revised and rewritten by Charles Wilson Greene . . . 6th American revision, with five hundred and seven illustrations, including many in colors. New York: William Wood & Co., 1907. 723p. DLC; MBM; NNNAM; PPC **00-1955**

KIRKES, William Senhouse (1823-1864)
Kirkes' handbook of physiology, revised and rewritten by Charles Wilson Greene . . . 7th American revision. With five hundred and seven illustrations, including many in colors. New York: William Wood & Co., 1910. 761p. DLC; LNT-M; NNNAM; ScCM **00-1956**

KISCH, Enoch Heinrich (1841-1918)
The sexual life of woman in its physiological, pathological and hygienic aspects. . . . Only authorized transl. into the English language from the German by M. Eden Paul, M.D. With 97 illustrations in the text. New York: Rebman Co., [1910]. 686p. DLC; DNLM; PPC; PU **00-1957**

KLEBS, Arnold C[arl], ed. (1870-1943)
Tuberculosis; a treatise by American authors on its etiology, pathology, frequency, semeiology, diagnosis, prognosis, prevention, and treatment. Edited by Arnold C. Klebs. New York and London: D. Appleton & Co., 1900. 939p. 3 plates. DLC; DNLM; NcD; PPC **00-1958**

KLEBS, E[dwin] Th. A. (1834-1913)
Studies on internal antisepsis. New York, 1900. 30p. DLC; DNLM; ICJ; NNNAM **00-1959**

KLEEN, Emil [A. G.] (1847-1923)
On diabetes mellitus and glycosuria. Philadelphia: P. Blakiston's Son & Co., 1900. 313p. CtY-M; DNLM; PPC; PU
00-1960

KLOTZ, Hermann G[ustav] (*b.* 1844)
Syphilitic lesions of the wheal type. New York, 1901. 5p. DLC; DNLM **00-1961**

KNAPP, Miland Austin (*b.* 1868)
Teeth regulation; with finely made original devices ready for immediate operative application without soldering. . . . 2nd ed., rev., and enl. Philadelphia, Pa.: The S. S. White Dental Manufacturing Co., 1900. 78p. DLC; MdU-D; PPC; PU
00-1962

KNAPP, Miland Austin (*b.* 1868)
Orthodontia practically treated; designed for the use of both practitioner and student. . . . 1st ed., with five hundred and sixty-four illustrations. Minneapolis, Minn.: Press of Harrison & Smith Co., 1904. 406p. plates. DLC; ICJ; NN; PU
00-1963

KNAPP, Miland Austin (*b.* 1868)
The Knapp system of teeth regulation for major protrusion; with instructions for the application and operation of the protrusion set "B." . . . [Minneapolis?], 1905. 24p. DLC; NN
00-1964

KNAPP, Philip Coombs (1858-1920)
The problem of Boston's insane. Boston: Damrell & Upham, 1900. 9p. DLC; DNLM **00-1965**

KNAPP, Philip Coombs (1858-1920)
The unity of the acute psychoses. Boston: Damrell & Upham, 1900. 18p. DLC; DNLM **00-1966**

KNAPP, Philip Coombs (1858-1920) and John Jenks THOMAS
Landry's paralysis. [New York, 1900.] 18p. DLC; DNLM
00-1967

KNIGHT, Charles Huntoon (1849-1913)
Diseases of the nose and throat. . . . 147 illustrations. Philadelphia: P. Blakiston's Son & Co., 1903. 423p. DLC; GU; NNNAM; PPC **00-1968**

KNIGHT, Charles Huntoon (1849-1913)
Diseases of the nose, throat and ear, by Charles Huntoon Knight . . . and W. Sohier Bryant . . . 2nd ed., rev., with 239 illustrations. Philadelphia: P. Blakiston's Son & Co., 1909. 631p. DLC: MdU-D; NNNAM; PPC
00-1969

KNOPF, S[iegmund] A[dolphus] (1857-1940)
Neglected clinical opportunities in American medical centers. New York, 1900. 13p. DNLM; NN **00-1970**

KNOPF, S[iegmund] A[dolphus] (1857-1940)
The tenement and tuberculosis; an address delivered before a conference held under the auspices of the tenement house committee of the Charity Organization Society, New York, Feb. 20, 1900. [New York, 1900.] 7p. DNLM; NN
00-1971

KNOPF, S[iegmund] A[dolphus] (1857-1940)
Tuberculosis as a disease of the masses and how to combat it. . . . New York: Fred P. Flori, 1901. 86p. *vel subseq.* DLC; DNLM; NN; NNNAM [Prize essay of the International Tuberculosis Congress, Berlin, 1899.] **00-1972**

KNOPF, S[iegmund] A[dolphus] (1857-1940)
Tuberculosis a preventable and curable disease; modern methods for the solution of the tuberculosis problem. . . . New York: Moffat, Yard & Co., 1909. 394p. col. plate. DLC; ICJ; NNNAM; PU **00-1973**

KNOPF, S[iegmund] A[dolphus] (1857-1940)
Tuberculosis a preventable and curable disease; modern methods for the solution of the tuberculosis problem. . . . 2nd ed. New York: Moffatt, Yard & Co., 1910. 394p. col. plate. DLC; MH; NNNAM; PU **00-1974**

THE KNY-SCHEERER CO. (NEW YORK CITY)
Illustrated . . . price list of surgical and orthopaedic apparatus and appliances, artificial limbs, trusses, supporters, crutches and invalid furniture. New York, 1900. 192p. DNLM; ICJ; NNNAM **00-1975**

THE KNY-SCHEERER CO. (NEW YORK CITY)
. . . Illustrated and descriptive catalogue of aseptic surgical supplies for the equipment of operating rooms, sterilizing rooms, hospital wards, physicians' offices, sanitaria and sick rooms. New York: The Kny-Scheerer Co., [1904]. 336p. DLC; NNNAM **00-1976**

KOBER, George M[artin] (1850-1931)
Filtration. The pollution of streams and the purification of public water supplies. Washington, 1900. 8p. DLC; DNLM **00-1977**

KOBER, George M[artin] (1850-1931)
Protest from the Civic Center of the District of Columbia against the passage of Senate Bill No. 34, providing for the further prevention of cruelty to animals. Washington, 1900. 9p. DLC; DNLM **00-1978**

KOBER, George M[artin] (1850-1931)
Shall alcohol be considered as a food? Richmond, 1900. 7p. DLC; DNLM **00-1979**

KOBER, George M[artin] (1850-1931)
Conclusions based upon three hundred and thirty outbreaks of infectious diseases spread through the milk supply. Philadelphia, 1901. 6p. DLC; DNLM **00-1980**

KOBER, George M[artin] (1850-1931)
The pollution of streams and the purification of public water supplies. Comparative efficiency of slow sand and mechanical filters. Chicago, 1901. 8p. 1 tab. DLC; DNLM **00-1981**

KOBER, George M[artin] (1850-1931)
The progress and tendency of hygiene and sanitary science in the nineteenth century. Chicago, 1901. 31p. DLC; DNLM **00-1982**

KOBER, George M[artin] (1850-1931)
Recent books on hygiene. New York, 1901. 6p. DLC; DNLM **00-1983**

KOBER, George M[artin] (1850-1931)
The causation of disease. Washington, 1902. 63p. DLC; DNLM **00-1984**

KOBER, George M[artin] (1850-1931)
Milk in relation to public health. The necessity for the enactment of Senate bill entitled "A bill to regulate the production and sale of milk and cream in and for the District of Columbia." Washington: Government Printing Office, 1902. 235p. 15 plates. DLC; DNLM **00-1985**

KOCH, Charles R[udloph] E[dward], ed.
History of dental surgery, contributions by various authors. . . . Chicago, Ill.: The National Art Publishing Co., 1909. 3 v. DLC; ICJ; PPC; PU **00-1986**

KOCH, Charles R[udolph] E[dward], ed.
History of dental surgery, contributions by various authors. . . . Ft. Wayne, Ind.: National Art Pub. Co., 1910 [*c.* 1909]. 3 v. CtY-M; DNLM; NcD **00-1987**

KOHBERGER, Henry Paul (*b.* 1879)
Physical diagnosis and laboratory diagnosis. . . . Pittsburgh, Pa.: Medical Abstract Publishing Co., [1908]. 64p. DLC; DNLM; NN **00-1988**

KOHBERGER, Henry Paul (*b.* 1879)
Medicine in abstract. Pittsburgh: Medical Abstract Pub. Co., [*c.* 1909]. 218p. DLC; DNLM; ICJ **00-1989**

KOLIPINSKI, Louis
Chronic enteritis and tuberculous enteritis treated with hypodermic injections of arsenic. New York, 1900. 15p. DLC; DNLM **00-1990**

KOLIPINSKI, Louis
Exstrophy of the bladder from ulcerative destruction of the scar of a suprapubic cystotomy. Baltimore, 1900. 2p. DLC; DNLM **00-1991**

KOLIPINSKI, Louis
The appearance of the soft palate a pathognomonic symptom of epidemic influenza. Philadelphia, 1901. 4p. DLC; DNLM **00-1992**

KOLIPINSKI, Louis
Artificial milks. New York, 1901. 9p. DLC; DNLM **00-1993**

KOLIPINSKI, Louis
Lager beer in acute vomiting. Philadelphia, 1901. 2p. DLC; DNLM **00-1994**

KOLIPINSKI, Louis
A study of sex production in man. New York, 1902. 13p. DLC; DNLM **00-1995**

KOLIPINSKI, Louis
Therapeutics of chromium sulphate. Green chronic sulphate. Philadelphia, 1902. 8p. DLC; DNLM **00-1996**

KOLLE, F[rederick] Strange (1871-1929)
The grown baby book. . . . Boston: R. G. Badger, 1903. 71p. incl. front. 5 plates. DLC; MH; NIC; NN **00-1997**

KOLLE, F[rederick] Strange (1871-1929)
Subcutaneous hydrocarbon protheses. New York: The Grafton Press, [1908]. 153p. plates. DLC; ICJ; PPC
00-1998

KOLLE, F[rederick] Strange (1871-1929)
Subcutaneous hydrocarbon protheses. [2nd ed.] New York: The Grafton Press, [1908]. 153p. NN **00-1999**

KOPLIK, Henry (1858-1927)
The diseases of infancy and childhood. Designed for the use of students and practitioners of medicine . . . with 169 engravings and 30 plates in color and monochrome. New York and Philadelphia: Lea Bros. & Co., 1902. 675p. DLC; MBM; NNNAM; PPC **00-2000**

KOPLIK, Henry (1858-1927)
The diseases of infancy and childhood. Designed for the use of students and practitioners of medicine . . . 2nd ed., thoroughly rev. and enl. Illustrated with 184 engravings and 33 plates in color and monochrome. New York and Philadelphia: Lea Bros. & Co., 1906. 885p. DLC; IU-M; PPC; PU
00-2001

KOPLIK, Henry (1858-1927)
The diseases of infancy and childhood. Designed for the use of students and practitioners of medicine. . . . 3rd ed., rev. and enl. Illustrated with 204 engravings and 30 plates in color and monochrome. New York and Philadelphia: Lea & Febiger, [1910]. 944p. DLC; IEN-M; NNNAM; PPC
00-2002

KRAEMER, Henry (1868-1924)
A course in botany and pharmacognosy . . . illustrated with plates from original drawings by the author. Philadelphia: [Press of E. Stearn & Co.], 1902. 384p. DLC; OCLloyd; PPC; PU **00-2003**

KRAEMER, Henry (1868-1924)
A text-book of botany and pharmacognosy, intended for the use of students of pharmacy, as a reference book for pharmacists, and as a handbook for food and drug analysts. . . . Illustrated with 331 plates comprising upward of 1500 figures. 2nd rev. and enl. ed. Philadelphia and London: J. B. Lippincott Co., [1907]. 840p. DLC; NNNAM; OCIM; PPC
00-2004

KRAEMER, Henry (1868-1924)
A text-book of botany and pharmacognosy; intended for the use of students of pharmacy, as a reference book for pharmacists, and as a hand-book for food and drug analysts . . . illustrated with over 300 plates comprising about 2000 figures. 3rd rev. and enl. ed. Philadelphia and London: J. B. Lippincott Co., [1908]. 850p. DLC; NNNAM; OCLloyd; PPC
00-2005

KRAEMER, Henry (1868-1924)
A text-book of botany and pharmacognosy, intended for the use of students of pharmacy, as a reference book for pharmacists, and as a handbook for food and drug analysts . . . illustrated with over 300 plates comprising about 2000 figures. 4th rev. and enl. ed. Philadelphia and London: J. B. Lippincott Co., [1910]. 888p. DLC; IU-M; OCLloyd; PU
00-2006

KRAEPELIN, Emil (1856-1926)
The duty of the state in the care of the insane. Transl. by Stewart Paton. [Utica, 1900.] 45p. DNLM; MH
00-2007

KRAEPELIN, Emil (1856-1926)
The duty of the state in the care of the insane. [New York], 1900. 46p. NNNAM **00-2008**

KRAEPELIN, Emil (1856-1926)
Clinical psychiatry. A textbook for students and physicians. Abstracted and adapted from the 6th German ed. by A. Ross Diefendorf. New York: The Macmillan Co., 1902. 490p. 11 plates. DNLM; MBM; OCIM; PPC
00-2009

KRAEPELIN, Emil (1856-1926)
Lectures on clinical psychiatry. Transl. from the 2nd German ed., rev. and ed. by Thomas Johnstone. New York: Rebman Co., 1906. 352p. DLC; ICU; NIC; NN
00-2010

KRAEPELIN, Emil (1856-1926)
Clinical psychiatry . . . abstracted and adapted from the 7th German edition by A. Ross Diefendorf. New ed., rev. and aug. The Macmillan Co., 1907. 562p. DLC; ICU; MH; NN
00-2011

KRAEPELIN, Emil (1856-1926)
The university man and the alcohol question, by Prof. Emil Kraepelin. . . . Westerville, O.: Amer. Issue Pub. Co., [1910?] 14p. MH; NN **00-2012**

KRAFFT-EBING, Richard von (1840-1902)
Psychopathia sexualis, with especial reference to antipathetic sexual instinct; a medico-forensic study. . . . Only authorized English transl. of the 10th German ed. Chicago: W. T. Keener & Co., 1900. 585p. DLC; ICU; MH; NN
00-2013

KRAFFT-EBING, Richard von (1840-1902)
Transitory mental disorder in hemicrania. (Transl. by W. Alfred McCorn.) St. Louis, 1900. 29p. DNLM
00-2014

KRAFFT-EBING, Richard von (1840-1902)
Pseudopastic paresis. (Simulation of spastic spinal paresis by hysteria.) St. Louis, 1902. 20p. DNLM
00-2015

KRAFFT-EBING, Richard von (1840-1902)
Simulation of tabes dorsalis. Transl. St. Louis, 1903. 21p. DNLM **00-2016**

KRAFFT-EBING, Richard von (1840-1902)
The suggestive treatment of hysteria gravis. Transl. St. Louis, 1903. 7p. DNLM **00-2017**

KRAFFT-EBING, Richard von (1840-1902)
Text-book of insanity, based on clinical observations for practitioners and students of medicine . . . authorized transl. from the last German ed. by Charles Gilbert Chaddock. . . . With an introduction by Frederick Peterson. . . . Philadelphia: F. A. Davis Co., 1905. 638p. DLC; NNNAM; PPC; PU
00-2018

KRAFFT-EBING, Richard von (1840-1902)
Psychopathia sexualis, with especial reference to the antipathic sexual instinct; a medico-forensic study. . . . Only authorized English adaptation of the 12th German ed. by F. J. Rebman. With author's portrait as frontispiece. New York, London: Rebman Co., [1906]. 617p. DLC; MB; NNNAM; OCIM
00-2019

KRAUSE, Fedor (1856-1937)
Surgery of the brain and spinal cord, based on personal experience . . . transl.by Prof. Herman A. Haubold. . . . New York: Rebman Co., [1909-12]. 3 v. plates. DLC; ICJ; MH-M; NNNAM **00-2020**

KREHL, Ludolf von (1861-1937)
The principles of clinical pathology; a text-book for students and physicians . . . authorized transl. from the 3rd German ed., by Albion Walter Hewlett . . . with an introduction by William Osler. . . . Philadelphia and London: J. B. Lippincott Co., 1905. 504p. DLC: NNNAM; PPC; PU **00-2021**

KREHL, Ludolf von (1861-1937)
The principles of clinical pathology; a text-book for students and physicians . . . authorized transl. from the fourth German edition, by Albion Walter Hewlett . . . with an introduction by William Osler . . . 2nd ed. Philadelphia and London: J. B. Lippincott & Co., 1907. 520p. DLC; NNNAM; OCIM; PPC **00-2022**

KREISSEL, Filipp (*b.* 1859)
Urogenital therapeutics, medical and surgical; a treatise on the practical treatment of diseases of the urinary and genital systems. . . . Chicago: Cleveland Press, 1908. 461p. plates. DLC; IU-M; OCIM **00-2023**

KUEPPER, Wilhelmine H.
Nature cure (formerly called water cure); or, Home treatment without medicine. . . . Philadelphia, Chicago, [etc.] : The J. C. Winston Co., 1905. 254p. plates. DLC; ICJ; PP; PU **00-2024**

KUH, Syndey (*b.* 1866)
Treatment of acromegaly with pituitary bodies. Chicago, 1902. 15p. DLC; DNLM **00-2025**

KULP, John S[tewart]
A Manila military hospital. Carlisle, Pa., 1901. 12p. DLC; DNLM **00-2026**

KULP, John S[tewart]
The relation of personnel to bed-capacity in military hospitals. Carlisle, Pa., 1902. 19p. DLC; DNLM **00-2027**

KULP, John S[tewart]
The sanitary service of the English army. Carlisle, Pa., 1902. 24p. DLC; DNLM **00-2028**

KYLE, David Braden (1863-1916)
A text-book of diseases of the nose and throat. . . . With 175 illustrations, 23 of them in colors. 2nd ed. Philadelphia: W. B. Saunders & Co., 1900. 646p. DLC; NNNAM; OCIM; PPC **00-2029**

KYLE, David Braden (1863-1916)
A text-book of diseases of the nose and throat . . . with 175 illustrations, 24 of them in colors. 3rd ed., rev. and enl. Philadelphia, London, [etc.] : W. B. Saunders & Co., 1904. 669p. DLC; NNNAM; PPC; PU **00-2030**

KYLE, David Braden (1863-1916)
A text-book of diseases of the nose and throat . . . with 219 illustrations, 26 of them in colors. 4th ed., thoroughly rev. and enl. Philadelphia and London: W. B. Saunders & Co., 1907. 797p. DLC; MBM; NNNAM; PPC **00-2031**

KYLE, John Johnson (1869-1920)
. . . Compend of diseases of the ear, nose and throat . . . 85 illustrations. Philadelpia: P. Blakiston's Son & Co., 1903. 280p. DLC; NN; PPC; PU **00-2032**

KYLE, John Johnson (1869-1920)
Manual of diseases of the ear, nose and throat. . . . With 160 illustrations. Philadelphia: P. Blakiston's Son & Co., 1906. 595p. DLC; ICJ; PPC; PU **00-2033**

KYLE, John Johnson (1869-1920)
Manual of diseases of the ear, nose and throat . . . 2nd ed., rev. and enl. With 169 illustrations. Philadelphia: P. Blakiston's Son & Co., 1907. 627p. CtY-M; DLC; GU; PPC **00-2034**

LA FLESCHE, Francis (1860-1932)
Who was the medicine man? Address by . . . [of the Omaha tribe]. . . . Reprinted, with an introduction from the 32nd annual report of the Fairmount Park Art Association, Philadelphia, 1904. Hampton, Va.: Hampton Institute Press, 1905. 13p. DLC; PPC **00-2035**

LA GARDE, Louis Anatole (1849-1920)
Gunshot injuries by the rifles of reduced calibre. Boston, 1900. 8p. DNLM **00-2036**

LA GARDE, Louis Anatole (1849-1920)
Gunshot injuries by the weapons of reduced calibre. [Baltimore, 1900.] 11p. DNLM **00-2037**

LA GARDE, Louis Anatole (1849-1920)
Remarks upon the gunshot wounds of the reduced-calibre rifles in the Santiago campaign. [Boston, 1900.] 8p. DNLM **00-2038**

LA GARDE, Louis Anatole (1849-1920)
Gunshot wounds of the chest and abdomen from a military standpoint. New York, 1902. 10p. DNLM **00-2039**

LA GARDE, Louis Anatole (1849-1920)
Gunshot wounds of the head and cranium. [Boston, 1902.] 6p. DNLM **00-2040**

LA GARDE, Louis Anatole (1849-1920)
Gunshot wounds of the hip joint by reduced caliber projectiles. New York, 1902. 2 l. DNLM **00-2041**

LA GARDE, Louis Anatole (1849-1920)
Gunshot wounds of the knee-joint by the projectile of reduced caliber. Boston, 1902. 8p. DNLM **00-2042**

LA GARDE, Louis Anatole (1849-1920)
Poisoned wounds by the implements of warfare. The Mütter lecture delivered at the College of Physicians of Philadelphia, Dec. 2, 1902. Chicago, 1903. 45p. DNLM **00-2043**

LAKE, Richard (*b.* 1861)
Laryngeal phthisis, or consumption of the throat. Philadelphia: P. Blakiston's Son & Co., 1901. 94p. 6 plates. DNLM; MBM; PPC; PU **00-2044**

LAMB, Daniel Smith (1943-1929) and Isabel Haslup LAMB
Rules of health. Hampton: Institute Press, 1900. 32p. DLC; DNLM **00-2045**

LAMB, Daniel Smith (1943-1929)
The daily medical inspection of schools. New York, 1901. 52p. DLC; DNLM **00-2046**

LAMB, Daniel Smith (1843-1929)
Spiculum of bone from shot fracture of skull which rested against the brain for forty-four years. New York, 1901. 3p. DLC; DNLM **00-2047**

LAMB, Daniel Smith (1843-1929)
Spiculum of bone from shot fracture of skull, which rested against the brain for forty-four years. New York, 1903. 3p. DLC; DNLM **00-2048**

LAMB, Daniel Smith, ed. (1843-1929)
History of the Medical Society of the District of Columbia, 1817-1909. Washington: The Society, 1909. 501p. 79 plates. DLC; ICJ; MdBM; NN **00-2049**

LAMBERT, Adrian Van Sinderen (*b.* 1872)
A terminology of disease, to facilitate the classification of histories in hospitals, adopted by the managers of the Vanderbilt Clinic of the College of Physicians and Surgeons of Columbia University, New York. Comp. by Adrian V. S. Lambert, M.D. and Walton Martin, M.D. . . . New York, 1910. 122p. DLC; NNC; NNNAM; PU **00-2050**

LANDIS, Henry Gardner (1848-1886)
A compend of obstetrics. Especially adapted to the use of medical students and physicians. . . . Rev. and ed. by W. H. Wells . . . 7th ed. . . . Philadelphia: P. Blakiston's Son & Co., 1901. 205p. plates. DLC; NN; PPC; PU
00-2051

LANDIS, Henry Gardner (1848-1886)
. . . A compend of obstetrics, especially adapted to the use of medical students and physicians. . . . Rev. and ed. by William H. Wells. . . . 8th ed. . . . Philadelphia: P. Blakiston's Son & Co., 1906. 227p. plates. DLC; NNNAM; PPC; PU
00-2052

LANDIS, Henry R[obert] M[urray] (1872-1937)
The history of the development of medical science in America. Philadelphia: Lea Bros. & Co., 1901. 24p. DLC; NN; PPC; PU
00-2053

LANDOIS, Leonard (1837-1902)
Text-book of human physiology, including histology and microscopical anatomy, with especial reference to the practice of medicine. . . . 10th rev. and enl. ed., edited by Albert P. Brubaker . . . transl. by Augustus A. Eshner. . . . With 394 illustrations. Philadelphia: P. Blakiston's Son & Co., 1904. 1027p. DLC; ICJ; PPC: PPJ **00-2054**

LANE, Henry E[dward]
Diagnosis from the eye, a new art of diagnosing with perfect certainty from the iris of the eye the normal and abnormal conditions of the organism in general and of the different organs in particular; a scientific essay for the public and medical profession. . . . Chicago, Ill.: Kosmos Publishing Co.; London: L. N. Fowler & Co., [1904]. 156p. DLC; ICJ
00-2055

LANG, Hugo
German-English medical dictionary. Rev., enl. and ed. by Bertram L. Abrahams. Philadelphia: P. Blakiston's Son & Co., 1907. 598p. CtY-M; NNNAM; PPC; PPJ
00-2056

LANGDON, F[rank] W[arren] (1851-1933)
The plantar reflex and Babinski's sign, their diagnostic value in spinal disease. Cincinnati, 1900. 6p. 1 plate,1 tab. DLC; DNLM **00-2057**

LANGDON, F[rank] W[arren] (1851-1933)
Some problems concerning nervous disease. Brooklyn, 1900. 15p. DLC; DNLM **00-2058**

LANGDON, F[rank] W[arren] (1851-1933)
Syringomyelia; a clinical lecture. [Cincinnati, 1900.] 8p. DLC; DNLM **00-2059**

LANGDON, F[rank] W[arren] (1851-1933)
"The most useful citizen." A study of human dynamics. Philadelphia, 1901. 8p. DLC; DNLM
00-2060

LANGDON, F[rank] W[arren] (1851-1933)
Syphilis of the nervous system, its general pathology, with remarks on treatment. Chicago, 1901. 16p. DLC; DNLM
00-2061

LANGDON, F[rank] W[arren] (1851-1933)
Paramyoclonus multiplex; a report of a new case, with further history of a case reported in 1896, wihch has since recovered. New York, 1902. 8p. DLC; DNLM
00-2062

LANGDON, F[rank] W[arren] (1851-1933)
Neurologic progress and prospects. Chicago, 1903. 19p. DLC; DNLM **00-2063**

LANGFELD, Millard (1872-1937)
Introduction to infectious and parasitic diseases, including their cause and manner of transmission. . . . With an introduction by Lewellys F. Barker . . . with thrity-three illustrations. Philadelphia: P. Blakiston's Son & Co., 1907. 260p. DLC; MBM; PPC; PU **00-2064**

LANPHEAR, Emory (*b.* 1859)
Surgical therapeutics. . . . Chicago: The Clinic Publishing Co., 1907. 396p. DLC; ICJ; IU-M; OCIM
00-2065

LARTIGAN, August Jerome
Typhoid infection of the uterus. New York, 1900. 12p. DNLM
00-2066

LARTIGAN, August Jerome
Primary sarcoma of the thyroid gland. Philadelphia, 1901. 10p. DNLM **00-2067**

LARTIGAN, August Jerome
A study of a case of gonorrhoeal ulcerative endocarditis, with cultivation of the gonococcus. Philadelphia, 1901. 8p. DNLM
00-2068

LARTIGAN, August Jerome
The bacillus coli communis in human infections. [Chicago, 1902.] 24p. DNLM **00-2069**

LATSON, William R[ichard] C[unningham] (*b.* 1866)
Practical dietetics; food value of meat. Flesh food not essential to mental or physical vigor. New York: Health-culture Co., [*c.* 1900]. 72p. DNLM; NN; PPC [Health Culture Library No. 19] **00-2070**

LATSON, William R[ichard] C[unningham] (*b.* **1866)**
Common disorders with rational methods of treatment, including diet, exercise, masso-therapy, baths, etc. . . . New York: Health-Culture Co., [1904]. 325p. DLC; NNNAM
00-2071

LATSON, William R[ichard] C[unningham] (*b.* **1866)**
The attainment of efficiency; rational methods of developing health and personal power. New York: Health-Culture Co., 1910. 93p. DNLM; PP **00-2072**

LATSON, William R[ichard] C[unningham] (*b.* **1866)**
The enlightened life and how to live it. . . . New York: The Health-Culture Co., [1910]. 356p. NN; PP ["This book is made up of reprints of certain editorials which have appeared from time to time in Health-Culture"]
00-2073

LAUGHLIN, William Ross
Anatomy in a nutshell; a treatise on human anatomy in its relation to osteopathy. . . . Illustrated by two hundred and ninety plates. [2nd ed.] Kirkeville: V. R. Laughlin, 1905. 616p. DLC; ICJ **00-2074**

DE LAURENCE, L. W.
Hypnotism, a complete system of method, application, and use; including all that is known in the art and practice of mesmerism and mental healing, prepared for the self-instruction of beginners as well as for the use of advanced students and practitioners. Chicago, 1900. 188p. 5 plates. DLC; DNLM; ICJ; OCIM **00-2075**

LAUTENBACH, Louis J. (*b.* **1860)**
A few thoughts indicating a causative connection between the uric-acid diathesis and astigmatism against the rule. Philadelphia, 1900. 8p. DNLM **00-2076**

LAUTENBACH, Louis J. (*b.* **1860)**
Increasing therapeutic value of cod-liver oil by the addition of free iodine and free phosphorous. Philadelphia, 1900. 8p. DNLM **00-2077**

LAVINDER, Claude Hervey (*b.* **1872)**
. . . Pellagra; a précis. . . . Prepared by direction of the Surgeon-General. Washington: Government Printing Office, 1908. 22p. DLC **00-2078**

LAVINDER, Claude Hervey (*b.* **1872)**
. . . Notes on the prognosis and treatment of pellagra. . . . Washington: Government Printing Office, 1909. 10p. DLC; ICJ; NcD; NN **00-2079**

THE LAW and the doctor. A compilation of the fundamental legal principles governing the relation of the physician to his patients and community at large. Vol. I. The physician's civil liability for malpractice. Yonkers, N.Y., 1903. 47p. DLC; DNLM **00-2080**

LAW, Hartland
Viavi hygiene for women, men and children, by Hartland Law . . . [and] Herbert E. Law. . . . San Francisco, Cal.; Cleveland, O.: The Viavi Co., 1903. 610p. DLC; ICJ [*vel subseq.*]
00-2081

[LAW, Hartland]
Viavi hygiene, explaining the natural principles upon which the Viavi system of treatment for men, women and children is based. (Rev. ed.). San Francisco, Cal.: The Viavi Co., 1908. 416p. DLC; ICJ **00-2082**

LAWRENCE, Charles (*b.* **1837)**
History of the Philadelphia almshouses and hospitals from the beginning of the eighteenth to the ending of the nineteenth centuries . . . showing the mode of distributing public relief through the management of the boards of overseers of the poor, guardians of the poor and the directors of the Department of Charities and Correction; with an appendix, containing a list of former visiting and resident physicians; illustrated from photographs. Comp. . . . by Charles Lawrence, superintendent from 1891 to 1900. [Philadelphia]: C. Lawrence, 1905. 398p. DLC; LNT-M; PP; PPC
00-2083

LAZARUS-BARLOW, Walter S[ydney] (1865-1950)
The elements of pathological anatomy and histology for students. Philadelphia: P. Blakiston's Son & Co., 1903. 705p. 7 plates. CtY-M; DNLM; NNNAM; PPC
00-2084

[LEA, Arthur Henry] (*b.* **1859)**
Henry Charles Lea. 1825-1909. Privately printed. Philadelphia, 1910. 24p. port. DLC; NN; PPC; PU
00-2085

LEALE, Charles Augustus (*b.* **1842)**
Lincoln's last hours. . . . [Address delivered before the commandery of the state of New York. Military order of the loyal legion of the United States, at the regular meeting, February, 1909, city of New York, in observance of the one hundredth anniversary of the birth of President Abraham Lincoln.] [New York? 1909.] 16p. DLC; NN **00-2086**

LEAVITT, Sheldon (1848-1933)
The science and art of obstetrics. . . . 3rd ed., rev. and enl. Chicago: Halsey Bros. Co., 1901. 797p. DLC; DNLM; ICJ; OCIM **00-2087**

LEAVITT, Sheldon (1848-1933)
Psycho-therapy in the practice of medicine and surgery. . . . Chicago: Garner-Taylor Press, 1903. 247p. DLC; DNLM; ICJ; OCIM **00-2088**

LEAVITT, Sheldon (1848-1933)
The absent treatment of disease, with particular reference to telepathy. . . . Chicago: Magnum Bonum Co., 1906. 112p. DLC; ICJ **00-2089**

LEAVITT, Sheldon (1848-1933)
Psycho-therapy in the practice of medicine and surgery. . . . 2nd ed. Chicago: Garner-Taylor Press, 1907. 247p. OCIM
00-2090

LEAVITT, Sheldon (1848-1933)
The essentials of the unity of life. . . . New York: Progressive Literature Co., 1907. 102p. DLC; ICJ; NN
00-2091

LEAVITT, Sheldon (1848-1933)
The psychic solution of the problem of cure. . . . Chicago: Magnum Bonum Co., [1908]. 182p. DLC; ICJ
00-2092

LEAVITT, Sheldon (1848-1933)
Auto-suggestion: the methods by which it is made effective, together with a list of affirmations for daily use. Chicago: Magnum Bonum Co., [1910]. 44p. ICJ; NN
00-2093

LEDERMAN, M[oses] D. (*b.* 1868)
A clinical report on the use of argyrol (silver vitelline) in diseases of the nose, throat, and ear. New York, 1902. 2 l. DNLM **00-2094**

LEE, Arthur B[olles] (1849-1927)
The microtomist's vade-mecum; a handbook of the methods of microscopic anatomy, . . . 5th rev. ed. Philadelphia: P. Blakiston's Son & Co., 1901. 526p. DLC; DNLM; PPC; PU **00-2095**

LEE, ELLWOOD J., CO.
. . . 17th annual illustrated catalogue. [Medical and surgical supplies] . . . . Conshohocken, Pa., 1900. 136p. ICJ; NNNAM **00-2096**

LEFFINGWELL, Albert (1845-1916)
Some mistakes of scientists. . . . [Providence?] : Printed for the American Human Association, 1900. 18p. DLC; PU **00-2097**

LEFFINGWELL, Albert (1845-1916)
Is science advanced by deceit? A question and a criticism. . . . [Providence] : The American Human Association, 1900. 32p. DLC; PU **00-2098**

LEFFINGWELL, Albert (1845-1916)
The lesson of reform; an address before the American Human Association, Pittsburgh, Pa., Ocotber 12, 1900. . . . [Pittsburgh] : The American Human Association, 1901. 32p. DLC; PU **00-2099**

LEFFINGWELL, Albert (1845-1916)
The vivisection question. New Haven: The Tuttle, Morehouse & Taylor Co., 1901. 267p. DLC; MH; NN **00-2100**

LEFFINGWELL, Albert (1845-1916)
The rise of the vivisection controversy; a chapter of history. New York: [American Human Association], 1903. 32p. DNLM; MH; NcD **00-2101**

LEFFINGWELL, Albert (1845-1916)
The vivisection question. 2nd ed. Chicago: The Vivisection Reform Society, 1907. 267p. DLC; ICJ; ICU; NN **00-2102**

LEFFINGWELL, Albert (1845-1916)
The vivisection problem; a controversy between Charles S. Myers . . . and Albert Leffingwell. . . . [Philadelphia?] : Printed for the Vivisection Reform Society, 1907. 10p. DLC **00-2103**

LEFFINGWELL, Albert (1845-1916)
American meat; its methods of production and influence on public health. . . . New York: T. E. Schulte [etc., etc.], 1910. 208p. ICJ; NN **00-2104**

LEFFINGWELL, Albert (1845-1916)
American meat and its influence upon the public health. . . . New York: T. E. Schulte [etc., etc.], 1910. 208p. DLC; NIC; PPC **00-2105**

LEFFMANN, Henry (1847-1930)
Under the yellow flag; an account of some experiences of Henry Leffmann as Port Physician of the Port of Philadelphia, to which have been added a few notes and comments on the history of the Port of Philadelphia. Philadelphia: W. Fell & Co., 1900 [*c.* 1896] . 35p. DLC; NN; PHi; PPC [Also: Philadelphia: the Author, 1896. 68p. CtY-M] **00-2106**

LEFFMANN, Henry (1847-1930) and William BEAM
Select methods in food analysis. Philadelphia: P. Blakiston's Son & Co., 1901. 383p. 4 plates. DNLM; NNNAM; PPC; PU **00-2107**

LEFFMANN, Henry (1847-1930)
Examination of water for sanitary and technic purposes. . . . 5th ed., rev. and enl. . . . Philadelphia: P. Blakiston's Son & Co., 1903. 140p. DLC; DNLM; MB; PU **00-2108**

LEFFMANN, Henry (1847-1930)
Analysis of milk and milk products . . . 3rd ed., rev. and enl. . . . Philadelphia: P. Blakiston's Son & Co., 1905. 78p. DLC; ICJ; PPC; PU **00-2109**

LEFFMANN, Henry (1847-1930)
. . . A compend of medical chemistry, inorganic and organic, including urinary analysis. . . . 5th ed.—rev. Philadelphia: P. Blakiston's Son & Co., 1905. 200p. DLC; NN; PPC; PU **00-2110**

[LEFFMANN, Henry] (1847-1930)
Outline autobiography of Henry Leffmann . . . of Philadelphia. With reference index of contributions to science and literature. . . . Philadelphia, 1905. 21p. DLC; PP; PPC; PPJ **00-2111**

LEFFMANN, Henry (1847-1930)
Examination of water for sanitary and technic purposes, by chemical and bacteriological methods. . . . 6th ed., rev. and enl., with illustrations. Philadelphia: P. Blakiston's Son & Co., 1909. 144p. DLC; DNLM; NN; PPC **00-2112**

LEHMANN, Karl Bernhard (1858-1940) and Rudolf NEUMANN
Atlas and epitome of bacteriology and textbook of special bacteriologic diagnosis. Authorized transl. from the 2nd enlarged and revised German ed. Edited by George H. Weaver. Philadelphia: W. B. Saunders & Co., 1901. Pt. 1: Atlas, 7p., 69 plates; Pt. 2: text, 511p., 1 table. DNLM; MBM; NNNAM; PU **00-2113**

LENHARTZ, Hermann (1854-1910)
Manual of clinical microscopy and chemistry, prepared for the use of students and practitioners of medicine, by . . . authorized transl. from the 4th and last German ed., with notes and additions by Henry T. Brooks . . . with 148 illustrations in the text and 9 colored plates. . . . Philadelphia: F. A. Davis Co., 1904. 412p. DLC; NNNAM; OCIM; PPC **00-2114**

LENTZ, CHARLES, & SONS (PHILADELPHIA)
Catalogue of microscopes and accessories, microtomes, bacteriological apparatus, laboratory supplies and instruments for clinical diagnosis. Philadelphia: Edward Stern & Co., 1900. 135p. DLC; ICJ; PP **00-2115**

LENTZ, CHARLES, & SONS (PHILADELPHIA)
Illustrated catalogue and price list of surgical instruments, orthopaedical apparatus, trusses, etc., 6th ed. Philadelphia: Charles Lentz & Sons, [1906?] 598p. DLC; PP [1st ed., 1884, 26p.] **00-2116**

LENTZ, CHARLES, & SONS (PHILADELPHIA)
. . . Illustrated catalogue and price list of surgical instruments, hospitals supplies, orthopedic apparatus, trusses, etc. 7th ed. Philadelphia: Charles Lentz & Sons, 1910. 610p. illus., plates (1 double), port. Plates printed on both sides. DLC; ICJ; PP **00-2117**

LEOPOLD, [Christian] Gerhard (1846-1911)
A very young ovum in situ. Authorized English transl. by W. H. Vogt. St. Louis: C. V. Mosby Co., 1907. 69p. 16 plates. DLC; ICJ **00-2118**

LEOPOLD, F. B.
Filtration of water in its relations to the health and prosperity of a municipality. [Pittsburgh: Pittsburgh Filter Mfg. Co., 1905.] 29p. DLC **00-2119**

LEROY, Louis (*b.* 1874)
Essentials of histology; arranged with questions following each chapter. . . . Philadelphia and London: W. B. Saunders & Co., 1900. 231p. DLC; NNNAM; PPC; PU **00-2120**

LEROY, Louis (*b.* 1874)
Smallpox. Its diagnosis, treatment, restriction, and prevention. With a few remarks on the present epidemic. Nashville, [1900. *vel subseq.*] 30p. 25 plates. DNLM **00-2121**

LEROY, Louis (*b.* 1874)
. . . Essentials of histology . . . arranged with questions following each chapter . . . 2nd ed., rev. and enl. Philadelphia and London: W. B. Saunders & Co., 1902. 263p. CtY-M; DLC; NN; PPC **00-2122**

LEROY, Louis (*b.* 1874)
. . . Essentials of histology . . . arranged with questions following each chapter. 106 illustrations. 3rd ed., rev. and enl. Philadelphia and London: W. B. Saunders & Co., 1905. 278p. DLC; NNNAM; PPC; PPJ **00-2123**

LEROY, Louis (*b.* 1874)
. . . Essentials of histology . . . arranged with questions following each chapter; 114 illustrations. 4th ed., rev. and enl. Philadelphia and London: W. B. Saunders & Col, 1909. 284p. CtY-M; DLC; PPC; PU **00-2124**

LEROY, Louis (*b.* 1874)
Pulmonary tuberculosis. . . . Issued by the Tennessee State Board of Health (2nd ed.) 1910. Nashville: Foster, Webb & Parkes, 1910. 93p. plates. DLC: ICJ **00-2125**

LESSER, Ladislaus L[eon] von (1846-1925)
Surgical emergencies . . . 12 lectures delivered at the University of Leipsic. . . . Transl. and rev. by Frederick A. Lyons. New York, [1901?] 215p. DLC; ICJ; MBM; PU [1st American ed., New York: Bermingham & Co., 1883, 215p. DLC] **00-2126**

LESTER, [William]
. . . Dr. Lester's encyclopedia and guide to health . . . assisted by other eminent physicians and practitioners. Chicago: Harper-Adams Co., [1902]. 446p. DLC; ICJ **00-2127**

LEUBE, Wilhelm Olivier von (1842-1922)
Medical diagnosis; special diagnosis of internal medicine, a handbook for physicians and students . . . authorized transl. from the 6th German edition, ed., with annotations, by Julius L. Salinger . . . with five colored plates and seventy-four illustrations in the text. New York and London: D. Appleton & Co., 1904. 1058p. DLC; ICJ; NcD; PPC **00-2128**

LEUF, Alexander H[ubert] P[rovidence] (*b.* 1867)
Practical first principles, simplifying the study of normal and abnormal structure and function, and aiding diagnosis, designed for the use of students and practitioners of medicine. . . . Philadelphia: The Medical Council, 1901. 105p. DLC; ICJ; PPC; PPHa **00-2129**

LEUF, Alexander H[ubert] P[rovidence] (*b.* 1867)
Gynecology, obstetrics, menopause. Part I. The general practitioner his own gynecologist. Part II. Common sense in obstetrics. Part III. The change of life in woman. . . . Philadelphia: The Medical Council, 1902. 326p. CtY-M; ICJ; NNC; PPJ **00-2130**

LEVERETT, John
. . . A few cases of diphtheria and what they taught me. . . . [Philadelphia? 1900] 6p. DLC **00-2131**

LEVY, Ernest C[oleman] (*b.* 1868)
Bacteriological report of mechanical filtration plant at Danville, Virginia. . . . Pittsburgh: Pittsburgh Filter Manufacturing Co., 1905. 6p. DLC **00-2132**

LEVY, Ernst (*b.* 1864)
Elements of clinical bacteriology for physicians and students, by Dr. Ernst Levy . . . and Dr. Felix Klemperer . . . 2nd enl. and rev. ed. Authorized transl. by Augustus A. Eshner. . . . Philadelphia: W. B. Saunders & Co., 1900. 441p. col. plate. DLC; NNNAM; PPC; PU **00-2133**

LEWERS, Arthur [Hamilton Nicholson]
Cancer of the uterus; a clinical monograph on its diagnosis and treatment. . . . Philadelphia: P. Blakiston's Son & Co., 1902. 328p. 3 plates. CU-M; DNLM; NNNAM; PPC **00-2134**

LEWIS, Bransford (*b.* 1862)
Report of a case of exstrophy of the bladder, with remarks upon the operative treatment of that condition. Philadelphia, 1900. 10p. DNLM **00-2135**

LEWIS, Bransford (*b.* 1862)
Preliminary report on argyrol in gonorrhoeic infections. New York, 1902. 2 l. DNLM **00-2136**

LEWIS, Bransford (*b.* 1862)
Surgery of the bladder. Philadelphia, 1908. 62p. DNLM **00-2137**

LEWIS, Bransford (*b.* 1862)
Originality and priority in modern cystoscopes: a reply to Dr. F. Tilden Brown. St. Louis, [1908?] 17p. NN **00-2138**

LEWIS, Bransford (*b.* 1862)
Practical cystoscopy: its scope and limitations. With a review of the prominent cystoscopes of the present day. [St. Louis, 1908?] 23p. NN **00-2139**

LEWIS, Charles A[lbert] (*b.* 1858)
The only osteopractic method of treating diseases at home. . . . Combining osteopathy, magnetic healing and massage. . . . Afton, Ia.: Star Enterprise Print, 1902. 324p. DLC; ICJ **00-2140**

LEWIS, Denslow (1856-1913)
The gynecologic consideration of the sexual act. . . . Chicago: The Henry O. Shepard Co., 1900. 49p. DLC; DNLM; ICJ **00-2141**

LEWIS, Denslow (1856-1913)
Obstetric clinic. . . . A series of clinical lectures on practical obstetrics delivered to students and practitioners in Cook County Hospital, Chicago. . . . Chicago: E. H. Colegrove, [1900]. 652p. col. plates. DLC; DNLM; ICJ; OCIM
00-2142

LEWIS, Eugene Richards
Importance of early treatment of convergent squint. Detroit, 1902. 11p. DNLM **00-2143**

LEWIS, Eugene Richards
The conservation of binocular single vision. St. Louis, 1903. 42p. DNLM **00-2144**

LEWIS, F[rancis] Park (1855-1940)
The necessity of frequent examinations of the eyes of children. [New York, 1901.] 13p. DNLM **00-2145**

LEWIS, F[rancis] Park (1855-1940)
Ocular incoordination and cerebral reflexes. New York, 1903. 12p. DNLM **00-2146**

LEWIS, F[rancis] Park (1855-1940)
Squint and its modern treatment. Buffalo, 1903. 5p. DNLM
00-2147

LEWIS, George A[ndrew] (1870-1915)
The origin and treatment of stammering. (6th ed., enl. and rev.). . . . [Detroit: Phonometer Press], 1900. 202p. DLC; ICJ [1st ed., Detroit: J. F. Eby & Co., 1896. 90p. DLC. *vel subseq.*]
00-2148

LEWIS, George A[ndrew] (1870-1915)
The practical treatment of stammering and stuttering, with suggestions for practice and helpful exercises . . . and a treatise on the cultivation of the voice, with a discussion of principles and suggestions for practice, by George B. Hynson. . . . Detroit: G. A. Lewis, 1902. 415p. DLC; ICJ
00-2149

LEWIS, George A[ndrew] (1870-1915)
Methods of attack, a text book for students of the Lewis Phono-metric Institute and School for Stammerers, intended especially for class use . . . by Geo. Andrew Lewis and Geo. B. Hynson. Rev. ed. Detroit: The Phonometer Press, 1902. 64p. DLC **00-2150**

LEWIS, George A[ndrew] (1870-1915)
The origin and treatment of stammering (7th ed., enl. and rev.). . . . [Detroit: Phometer Press], 1903. 202p. DLC
00-2151

LEWIS, George A[ndrew] (1870-1915)
Home care for stammerers, by George Andrew Lewis (an inveterate stammerer for more than twenty years). . . . A compilation of extended views and advice by forty writers and authorities on the subject of stammering and stuttering, with specific directions for home treatment and cure. . . . Detroit: G. A. Lewis, 1907. 415p. DLC; ICJ
00-2152

LEWIS, G[eorge] Griffin (*b.* 1865)
Hemorrhage of the retina. St. Louis, 1901. 5p. DNLM
00-2153

LEWIS, G[eorge] Griffin (*b.* 1865)
Tinnitus aurium. Philadelphia, 1902. 12p. DNLM
00-2154

LEWIS, G[eorge] Griffin (*b.* 1865)
Muscular anomalies of the eye. Syracuse, N.Y., [1902]. 9p. DNLM **00-2155**

LEWIS, H[arry] Edwin (*b.* 1875)
Pulmonary tuberculosis. A brief consideration of its etiology, symptomatology, diagnosis and treatment. St. Louis, 1901. 28p. DNLM **00-2156**

LEWIS, H[arry] Edwin (*b.* 1875)
The development of tuberculosis in the individual, with some remarks on the tubercle bacillus and certain allied forms of bacilli. Asheville, 1902. 12p. DNLM
00-2157

LEWIS, James J[ohn] (*b.* 1868)
Pocket optical dictionary, including pronunciation and definition of the principal words used in optometry and ophthalmology, together with a complete description of the light wave theory, anatomy of the eye, functions and nerve supply of the different parts. . . . 2nd ed., rev. and enl. . . . [Chicago?], 1907. 207p. DLC; ICJ; ICU; NN **00-2158**

LEWIS, James J[ohn] (*b.* 1868)
Pocket optical dictionary, including pronunciation and definition of the principal words used in optometry and ophthalmology, together with a complete description of the light wave theory, anatomy of the eye, functions and nerve supply of the different parts. . . . 3rd ed., rev. and enl. . . . [Chicago?], 1908. 232p. DLC; ICJ; MH; PPC **00-2159**

LEWIS, LE ROY
Anatomy and physiology for nurses. Philadelphia: W. B. Saunders & Co., 1905. 317p. DLC; NNC; PPJ; PU
00-2160

LEWIS, LE ROY
Anatomy and physiology for nurses. 2nd ed., rev. and enl. Philadelphia: W. B. Saunders & Co., 1910. 344p. DLC; DNLM; ICJ; PU **00-2161**

LEWIS, Warren H[armon] (1870-1964)
Observations on the pectoralis major muscle in man. Baltimore, 1901. 13p. DNLM **00-2162**

LEXER, Ehrich (1867-1937)
General surgery; a presentation of the scientific principles upon which the practice of modern surgery is based . . . American ed., edited by Arthur Dean Bevan . . . an authorized transl. of the 2nd German ed., by Dean Lewis . . . with four hundred and forty-nine illustrations in the text, partly in color, and two colored plates. New York and London: D. Appleton & Co., 1908. 1015p. DLC; NNNAM; OCIM; PPC
00-2163

LEXER, Ehrich (1867-1937)
General surgery; a presentation of the scientific principles upon which the practice of modern surgery is based . . . American ed., edited by Arthur Dean Bevan . . . and authorized transl. of the 2nd German ed. by Dean Lewis . . . with four hundred and forty-nine illustations in the text, partly in color, and two colored plates. New York and London: D. Appleton & Co., 1910. 1041p. DLC; ICJ; PPC; PPL **00-2164**

LIEBERTHAL, David
A case of epithelioma developed on the basis of a healed lupus vulgaris treated by X-rays. Chicago, 1901. 6p. DNLM; NN
00-2165

LIEBERTHAL, David
Remarks on primary and secondary syphilis, and a few remarks as to the application of mercury. St. Louis, 1901. 2 l. DNLM; NN **00-2166**

LIEBERTHAL, David
Lichen planus hypertrophicus. Chicago, 1902. 12p. DNLM; NN **00-2167**

LIEBERTHAL, David
Sarcomatosis cutis. Chicago, 1902. 14p. DNLM; NN **00-2168**

LIEBERTHAL, David
Acne rosacea. [Chicago, 1904.] 7p. DNLM; NN **00-2169**

LIEBIG, Gustav A.
Practical electricity in medicine and surgery. . . . By G. A. Liebig and George H Rohé. Philadelphia: F. A. Davis Co., 1900 [*c.* 1890]. 383p. DLC; MBM; NNNAM; PPC **00-2170**

LILIENTHAL, Howard (1861-1946)
Imperative surgery; for the general practitioner, the specialist, and the recent graduate. New York and London: Macmillan Co., 1900. 412p. DNLM; NNNAM **00-2171**

LILIENTHAL, Howard (1861-1946)
The closure of cutaneous wounds without suture. New York, 1901. 4p. DNLM **00-2172**

LILIENTHAL, Howard (1861-1946)
Treatment of biliary disease as determined at the operation. [New York: A. R. Elliott Publishing Co., 1908.] 7p. NN **00-2173**

LILLIE, C[harles] W. (1848-1922)
Use of fats in wasting diseases. New York: C. N. Crittenden Co., [1901]. 2 l. DNLM **00-2174**

LINCOLN, Harry Warren
General remarks on diseases of the stomach. New York, 1903. 4p. DNLM **00-2175**

LINN, S[amuel] H.
Hernia (rupture). Its etiology, strangulation, treatment, and radical cure by electro-cataphoric, chemical, hypodermic, and surgical methods. [Rochester, 1901.] 30p. 1 plate. DLC; DNLM; NN **00-2176**

LISCHER, Benno Edward (*b.* 1876)
Elements of orthodontia; a laboratory note book for students and beginners, comprising a series of exercises in orthodontia technology. . . . St. Louis: The C. V. Mosby Co., 1909. 96p. DLC; MdU-D; NNNAM; PPC **00-2177**

LITTLE, Seelye W[illiam] (*b.* 1867)
Nephritis; a manual of the disease commonly called nephritis or Bright's disease, and of allied disorders of the kidneys. . . . New York: The Grafton Press, 1907. 134p. DLC; NN; NNNAM; PP **00-2178**

LITTLEFIELD, James E[dwin]
The Littlefield system of eye and nerve measurements. . . . [Saco? Me., 1905.] 108p. col. plates. DLC **00-2179**

LITTLEFIELD, James E[dwin]
Optometry; the Littlefield system of eye and nerve measurements. . . . [Biddeford, Me.: Press of the Biddeford Journal, 1905.] 240p. col. plates. DLC ["Fifth edition of the Littlefield system of eye and nerve measurements."—Introductory.] **00-2180**

LLOYD, John U[ri] (1849-1936)
Do physicians and pharmacists live on the misfortunes of humanity? An essay. . . . [Boston, 1900.] 9p. DLC; OCLloyd **00-2181**

[LLOYD, John Uri] (1849-1936)
. . . Life and medical discoveries of Samuel Thomson, and a history of the Thomsonian materia medica, as shown in "The new guide to health," (1835), and the literature of that day. Including portraits of Samuel Thomson; fac-simile of Thomson's "patent" to the practice of medicine; the famous letters of Professor Benjamin Waterhouse, M.D.; the celebrated "Trial of Dr. Frost," and other features of a remarkable epoch in American medical history. Cincinnati, O.: J. U. & C. G. Lloyd, [1909]. 63-106, 137-140p. DLC: OCLloyd; NcD; NN **00-2182**

[LLOYD, John Uri] (1849-1936)
. . . The eclectic alkaloids, resins, resinoids, oleo-resins and concentrated principles. Including portraits and biographies of John King, William Stanley Merrell, Alexander Wilder, William Tully, Grover Coe, Robert Stafford Newton, Edward S. Wayne, Calvin Newton and John Coakley Lettsom. Cincinnati, O.: J. U. & C. G. Lloyd, [1910]. 54p. DLC; ICJ; OCLloyd; PU **00-2183**

LLOYD, John U[ri] (1849-1936)
. . . History of the vegetable drugs of the Pharmacopoeia of the United States . . . with portraits of Charles Rice . . . and Joseph P. Remington. . . . Cincinnati, O.: J. U. & C. G. Lloyd, [1910-1911]. 135p. DLC; NcD; OCLloyd; PU **00-2184**

LOCKE, Edwin A[llen] (*b.* 1874)
The clinical value of the iodine reaction in the leucocytes of the blood. . . . Boston, 1902. 22p. RPB **00-2185**

LOCKE, Edwin A[llen] (*b.* 1874)
Crusade against tuberculosis in Germany. Boston, 1907. 33p. RPB **00-2186**

LOCKE, Edwin A[llen] (*b.* 1874)
Treatment of non-tuberculous chronic arthiritis, [by] E. A. Locke and R. B. Osgood. Chicgo, 1907. 12p. RPB **00-2187**

LOCKE, Edwin A[llen] (*b.* 1874)
The municipal hospital for advanced consumptives in Boston by Edwin A. Locke . . . and Simon F. Cox. [Boston, 1908.] 21p. MBM **00-2188**

LOCKE Edwin A[llen] (*b.* 1874)
Tuberculosis in Massachusetts. Boston: Wright & Potter, 1908. 223p. MBM; MH [Prepared by the Massachusetts State Committee for the International Congress on Tuberculosis, Washington, D.C., September 21 to October 12, 1908.] **00-2189**

LOCKE, Edwin A[llen] (*b.* 1874)
The municipal anti-tuberculosis work in Boston. Boston, [1908?] 27p. MBM **00-2190**

LOCKE, Edwin A[llen] (*b.* **1874)**
The municipal anti-tuberculosis work in Boston. n. p., [1908]. 18p. NN **00-2191**

LOCKE, Edwin A[llen] (*b.* **1874)**
An economic study of 500 consumptives treated in the Boston consumptives' hospital, by Edwin A. Locke and Cleaveland Floyd. [Boston, 1909?] 9p. RPB **00-2192**

LOCKE, Edwin A[llen] (*b.* **1874)**
Boston's hospital school for tuberculous children [by] Edwin A. Locke . . . and Timothy J. Murphy. . . . [Boston? 1910.] 11p. DLC; MBM **00-2193**

LOCKE, Edwin A[llen] (*b.* **1874)**
Food values; practical tables for use in private practice and public institutions. . . . New York and London: D. Appleton & Co., 1910. 110p. DLC; ICJ; NN; PPJ **00-2194**

LOCKHART-MUMMERY, John Percy (1875-1957)
The after-treatment of operations. . . . New York: William Wood & Co., 1903. 221p. MBM; NNNAM; PPC; PPJ **00-2195**

LOCKWOOD, George Roe
A manual of the practice of medicine . . . 2nd ed., rev. . . . Philadelphia and London: W. B. Saunders & Co., 1901. 847p. plates. DLC; DNLM; NNNAM; PPC **00-2196**

LOCKWOOD, Robert M[inturn] (*b.* **1857)**
The principles of optometry; an illustrated text book with questions, for use in optical schools and for private students. . . . New York: F. Boger Pub. Co., [1903]. 144p. DLC; NN **00-2197**

LOCKWOOD, R[obert] M[inturn] (*b.* **1857)**
Subjectives tests for difficult cases, a practical treatise for optometrists. . . . New York: F. Boger Pub. Co., [1904]. 84p. DLC; NN; NNNAM; PPC **00-2198**

LOCKWOOD, R[obert] M[inturn] (*b.* **1857)**
The trial case and how to use it; a practical treatise for optometrists. . . . New York: F. Boger Pub. Co., [1904]. 69p. DLC; NN **00-2199**

LOCKWOOD, R[obert] M[inturn] (*b.* **1857)**
The trial case and how to use it; a practical treatise for optometrists. Illustrated 2nd ed. . . . New York: F. Boger Pub. Co., [1904]. 78p. DLC; NN **00-2200**

LOCKWOOD, R[obert] M[inturn] (*b.* **1857)**
The human eye. With two dissected sectional models in colors, containing fifteen separate plates, with a clear and detailed explanation of the various parts of the eye and their functions. Transl. and adapted from the German of Dr. Securio. . . . New York: F. Boger Pub. Co., [1905]. 16p. col. plates. DLC; NN; NNNAM; PP **00-2201**

LOCKWOOD, R[obert] M[inturn] (*b.* **1857)**
The trial case and how to use it. A practical treatise for optometrists. . . . 3rd ed., enl. and rev. New York: Optical Pub. Co., [1905?] 85p. DLC **00-2202**

LOCKWOOD, R[obert] M[inturn] (*b.* **1857)**
Frames and lenses, a practical treatise for optometrists. . . . New York: F. Boger Pub. Co., [1905]. 87p. DLC; ICJ; NN; PP **00-2203**

LOCKWOOD, Robert M[inturn] (*b.* **1857)**
Skiascopy without the use of drugs; a practical treatise for optometrists. New York: F. Boger Pub. Co., [1906]. 112p. DLC; ICJ **00-2204**

LOCKWOOD, Robert M[inturn] (*b.* **1857)**
The trial case and how to use it; a practical treatise for optometrists. 4th ed., enl. and rev. New York: Optical Pub. Co., [1906?]. 85p. MH **00-2205**

LOCKWOOD, Robert M[inturn] (*b.* **1857)**
Transpositions; a practical treatise for optometrists and opticians. . . . New York: F. Boger Pub. Co., [1907]. 32p. DLC; ICJ **00-2206**

LOCKWOOD, Robert M[inturn] (*b.* **1857)**
The human eye. . . . New York: Optical Pub. Co., [*c.* 1910]. 16p. DLC **00-2207**

LOEB, Jacques (1859-1924)
Comparative physiology of the brain and comparative psychology. . . . New York: G. P. Putnam's Sons, 1900. 300p. DLC; ICJ; MH; NN **00-2208**

LOEB, Jacques (1859-1924)
Studies in general physiology. Chicago: University of Chicago Press, 1905. 2 v. DLC; IEN-M; LNT-M; MH-M **00-2209**

LOEB, Jacques (1859-1924)
The dynamics of living matter. . . . New York: Columbia University Press, 1906. 233p. DLC; ICJ; NIC; PU **00-2210**

LOMBROSO, Cesare (1835-1909)
The female offender, by Prof. Caesar Lombroso and William Ferrero; with an introduction by W. Douglas Morrison. . . . New York: D. Appleton & Co., 1900. 313p. plates. tables. DLC; MH; NN; PP [1st Appleton ed., 1895?] **00-2211**

LOMBROSO, Cesare (1835-1909)
The man of genius. . . . New York: C. Scribner's Sons, 1908. 370p. fold. map, plates. DLC; MH; NN; PU [1st Scribner ed., 1891] **00-2212**

LOMBROSO, Cesare (1835-1909)
After death—what? Spiritistic phenomena and their interpretation. . . . Rendered into English by William Sloane Kennedy. . . . Illustrated by photographs, diagrams, etc. Boston: Small, Maynard & Co., [1909]. 364p. plates. DLC; MB; NN; PU **00-2213**

LONG, Eli Herr (*b.* **1860)**
Dental materia medica, therapeutics and prescription writing . . . illustrated with 6 engravings and 18 colored diagrams. Philadelphia and New York: Lea Bros. & Co., 1903. 321p. DLC; MdU-D; NNNAM; PPC **00-2214**

LONG, Eli Herr (*b.* 1860)
Dental materia medica, therapeutics and prescription writing . . . 2nd ed., thoroughly rev. and enl. Illustrated with seven engravings and eighteen colored diagrams. Philadelphia and New York: Lea Bros. & Co., 1905. 298p. DLC; MBM; NNNAM; PPC **00-2215**

LONG, Eli Herr (*b.* 1860)
Dental materia medica, therapeutics and prescription writing . . . 3rd ed., rev. and enl. Illustrated with six engravings and eighteen colored diagrams. Philadelphia and New York: Lea & Febiger, 1909. 311p. DLC; MBM; NNNAM; PPC **00-2216**

LONG, John Harper (1856-1918)
A text-book of urine analysis; for students and practitioners of medicine. . . . Easton, Pa.: The Chemical Publishing Co., 1900. 249p. DLC; DNLM; MBM; PPC **00-2217**

LONG, John Harper (1856-1918)
A text-book of physiological chemistry, for students of medicine. . . . Philadelphia: P. Blakiston's Son & Co., 1905. 424p. DLC; NNNAM; PPC; PU **00-2218**

LONG, John Harper (1856-1918)
A text-book of physiological chemistry for students of medicine . . . 2nd ed., rev., with 42 illustrations. Philadelphia: P. Blakiston's Son & Co., 1909. 396p. CtY-M; DLC; NNNAM; PPC **00-2219**

LONG, Joseph Ragland (1870-1932)
The prevention and cure of tuberculosis; a collection of articles of a popular character on the subject of tuberculosis, by S. A. Knopf, M.D., J. H. Huddleston, M.D. . . . and others. Comp. by Joseph R. Long. Denver: H. M. Brinker, 1905. 246p. DLC; ICJ **00-2220**

LONG, Margaret (*b.* 1873)
On the development of the unclei pontis during the second and third months of embryonic life. Baltimore, 1901. 8p. 3 plates. DNLM **00-2221**

LONG, S[eely] F.
Circumcision; a consideration of the subject, with new methods of treatment of the infant and adult. San Francisco, 1902. 9p. DNLM **00-2222**

LONG, Stephen M.
Tropical dysenteries. New York, 1901. 10p. DNLM **00-2223**

LONGCOPE, Warfield T[heobald] (*b.* 1877)
Hepatic infarctions. Philadelphia, 1901. 14p. DNLM **00-2224**

LOOMIS SANITARIUM FOR CONSUMPTIVES (LIBERTY, NEW YORK)
Statistics of the Loomis Sanatorium, at Liberty, N.Y. By J. Edward Stubbert, physician in charge. [New York, 1900.] 7p. DNLM; NN **00-2225**

LOOMIS SANITARIUM FOR CONSUMPTIVES (LIBERTY, NEW YORK)
Descriptive pamphlet of the Loomis Sanatorium. [n. p., 1903.] 4p. (illus.) DNLM; NN **00-2226**

LORAND, Arnold
Old age deferred, the causes of old age and its postponement by hygienic and therapeutic measrues. . . . Philadelphia: F. A. Davis Co., 1910. 458p. DLC; ICJ; MB; PPC **00-2227**

LOTHROP, Howard A[ugustus] (1864-1928)
The anatomy and surgery of the frontal sinus and anterior ethmoidal cells. Boston, 1900 [1909]. 134p. illus. (plates). PPJ **00-2228**

LOTHROP, Howard A[ugustus] (1864-1928) and Joseph H. PRATT
A report of two cases of filariasis; operation for lymphatic varices and chylous hydrocele, with removal of adult worms. Philadelphia, 1900. 29p. DNLM **00-2229**

LOTHROP, Howard A[ugustus] (1864-1928)
The anatomy of the inferior ethmoidal turbintate bone with particular reference to cell formation. [Philadelphia, 1903.] 6p. MH **00-2230**

LOTHROP, Howard A[ugustus] (1864-1928)
Neuralgia of the superior maxillary nerve. A peripheral operation to reach the dental branches. [Boston, 1903?] 6p. MH **00-2231**

LOTHROP, Howard A[ugustus] (1864-1928)
The results of treatment of cancer in and about the mouth at the Boston City Hospital. Boston, 1905. 10p. MBM **00-2232**

LOTHROP, Howard A[ugustus] (1864-1928)
Fractures of the superior maxillary bone caused by direct blows over the malar bone. A method for the treatment of such fractures. Boston, 1906. 8p. MBM **00-2233**

LOVELAND, Bradford C[hurchill] (*b.* 1862)
Rheumatic gout. New York, 1900. 13p. DNLM **00-2234**

LOVETT, Robert W[illiamson] (1859-1924)
The mechanics of lateral curvature as applied to the treatment of severe cases. (Second paper.) Boston, 1901. 6p. DNLM **00-2235**

LOVETT, Robert W[illiamson] (1859-1924)
The diagnosis of hip disease; an analysis of ninety-five cases. Boston: Damrell & Upham, 1902. 19p. DNLM **00-2236**

LOVETT, Robert W[illiamson] (1859-1924)
A frame for the application of plaster-of-Paris jackets in Pott's disease. Philadlephia, 1902. 5p. DNLM **00-2237**

LOVETT, Robert W[illiamson] (1859-1924)
Rotation in lateral curvature. New York, 1902. 7p. DNLM **00-2238**

LOVETT, Robert W[illiamson] (1859-1924)
Round shoulders and faulty attitude; a method of observation and record, with conclusions as to treatment. Boston: Damrell & Upham, 1902. 11p. DNLM **00-2239**

LOVETT, Robert W[illiamson] (1859-1924)
Lateral curvature of the spine and round shoulders, by . . . with 154 illustrations. Philadelphia: P. Blakiston's Son & Co., 1907. 188p. DLC; ICJ; PPC; PU **00-2240**

LUCAS, William P[almer] (1880-1960)
A review of recent experimental work on hemorrhagic conditions. . . . Boston: D. C. Heath & Co., 1909. 14p. DLC; MH **00-2241**

LUCAS, William P[almer] (1880-1960)
The diagnosis of infantile paralysis in the prodromal and early acute stage as found in the experimental study of acute poliomyelitis in monkeys, with report of findings in four human cases. . . . [Boston? 1910.] 12p. DLC; MBM **00-2242**

LUCAS, William P[almer] (1880-1960)
The diagnosis of infantile paralysis in the prodromal and early acute stage as found in the experimental study of acute poliomyelitis in monkeys, with report of findings in four human caes. Boston: W. M. Leonard, 1910. 7p. NN **00-2243**

LUCAS, William P[almer] (1880-1960)
Methods of serum diagnosis in bacillary dysentery (infectious diarrhea) in infants [by] W. P. Lucas . . . J. G. Fitzgerald . . . and E. H. Schorer. . . . [Chicago, 1910.] 16p. DLC **00-2244**

LUCKETT, William H[enry] (1872-1929)
Paraffin in surgery; a critical and clinical study, by William H. Luckett . . . and Frank I. Horn. . . . With thirty-eight illustrations. New York: Surgery Publishing Co., 1907. 118p. DLC; ICJ; NNNAM; PU **00-2245**

LUDY, Robert B[orneman] (1870?-1936)
Answers to questions prescribed by dental state boards. . . . Philadelphia: Conover Publishing House, 1902. 396p. DLC; NN; PP; PPC **00-2246**

LUDY, Robert B[orneman] (1870?-1936)
Answers to questions prescribed by medical state boards. . . . Philadelphia: J. J. McVey, 1903. 661p. DLC; NN; PPC; PU **00-2247**

LUDY, Robert B[orneman] (1870?-1936)
Answers to questions prescribed by medical state boards. . . . 2nd ed., rewritten and enl. Philadelphia: J. J. McVey, 1905. 713p. DLC; NN; PP; PPC **00-2248**

LUDY, Robert B[orneman] (1870?-1936)
Answers to questions prescribed by dental state boards. . . . 2nd ed., rewritten and enl. Philadelphia: J. J. McVey, 1905. 462p. DLC; PP; PPC; PU **00-2249**

LUDY, Robert B[orneman] (1870?-1936)
Answers to questions prescribed by dental state boards. . . . 3rd ed., rewritten and enl. Philadelphia: J. J. McVey, 1907. 490p. DLC; MH; NN; PPC **00-2250**

LUDY, Robert B[orneman] (1870?-1936)
Answers to questions prescribed by medical state boards. . . . 3rd ed., rewritten and enl. Philadelphia: J. J. McVey, 1907. 709p. DLC; NN; PPC; PU **00-2251**

LUDY, Robert B[orneman], ed. (1870?-1936)
Answers to questions prescribed by dental state boards. . . . 4th ed., rewritten and enl. Philadelphia: J. J. McVey, 1909. 500p. DLC; NN; PP; PPC **00-2252**

LUDY, Robert B[orneman], ed. (1870?-1936)
Answers to questions prescribed by medical state boards. . . . 4th ed., rewritten and enl. Philadelphia: J. J.McVey, 1910. 768p. DLC; NNNAM; PPC **00-2253**

LUFF, Arthur P[earson] (1855-1938)
Gout, its pathology and treatment. Founded on the Goulstonian lectures on the chemistry and pathology of gout delivered . . . . before the Royal College of Physicians of London in 1897. . . . [3rd ed.] New York: William Wood & Co., 1907. 290p. MBM; NNC; NNNAM; PPC **00-2254**

LUKE, Thomas D[avey]
Anesthesia in dental surgery. . . . With 28 illustrations. New York: Rebman Co., 1903. 78p. ICJ; NN; PP; PU **00-2255**

LUKE, Thomas D[avey]
Anesthesia in dental surgery. . . . 2nd ed. New York: Rebman Co., 1906. 227p. KU; MBM; NNNAM; PU **00-2256**

LUKE, Thomas D[avey]
Guide to anaesthetics, for the student and general practitioner. 3rd ed. Philadelphia: J. B. Lippincott, 1906. 136p. KU; NN; PPC; PPJ **00-2257**

LUKE, Thomas D[avey]
A manual of natural therapy. . . . With thirty plates and one hundred and twenty-five illustrations, many of which are original. New York: William Wood & Co., 1908. 303p. DNLM; ICJ; IU-M; PPC **00-2258**

LUSK, Graham (1866-1932)
The elements of the science of nutrition. . . . Philadelphia and London: W. B. Saunders & Co., 1906. 326p. DLC; NNNAM; PPC; PU **00-2259**

LUSK, Graham (1866-1932)
The elements of the science of nutrition . . . 2nd ed., rev. and enl. Philadelphia and London: W. B. Saunders & Co., 1909. 402p. DLC; NNNAM; PPC; PU **00-2260**

LUSK, Graham (1866-1932)
Metabolism in diabetes. [Philadelphia, 1910.] 28p. DLC; NN; PPC **00-2261**

LUYTIES' physicians price list and reference book of the materia medica. St. Louis: Luyties Pharmacy Co., [*c.* 1903.] 506p. OCIM; OCLloyd **00-2262**

LYDSTON, G[eorge] Frank (1856-1923)
Medicine as a business proposition. Chicago, 1900. 32p. DNLM **00-2263**

LDYSTON, G[eorge] Frank (1856-1923)
Panama and the Sierras; a doctor's wander days. Chicago: Riverton Press, 1900. 283p. 42 plates. DLC; ICJ; MH; NN **00-2264**

LYDSTON, G[eorge] Frank (1858-1923)
Exceptional cases of empyaema. 1900. 4p. DNLM **00-2265**

LYDSTON, G[eorge] Frank (1858-1923)
Modern sanitation. Some of its fallacies and relations to the zymotic diseases, with especial reference to the defects of our so-called "modern improvements." Chicago: M. Stern & Co., [1902]. 14p. DNLM **00-2266**

LYDSTON, G[eorge] Frank (1858-1923)
The practice of athletics as a conservator of health. [1904.] 1 l. DNLM **00-2267**

LYDSTON, G[eorge] Frank (1858-1923)
The diseases of society (the vice and crime problem). . . . Philadelphia and London: J. B. Lippincott Co., 1904. 626p. plates. DLC; ICJ; MH-M; PPC **00-2268**

LYDSTON, G[eorge] Frank (1858-1923)
The surgical diseases of the genito-urinary tract, venereal and sexual diseases; a text-book for students and practitioners. . . . Rev. ed. Illustrated with 233 engravings and 7 colored plates. Philadelphia: F. A. Davis Co., 1904. 1008p. DLC; NNNAM; OCIM; PPC **00-2269**

LYDSTON, G[eorge] Frank (1858-1923)
The diseases of society (the vice and crime problem). . . . [2nd ed.] Philadelphia and London: J. B. Lippincott Co., 1905. 626p. plates. DLC; NNNAM; PPC; PU **00-2270**

LYMAN, Henry Munson (1835-1904)
20th century family physician; a reliable family physician giving in detail the cause, symptoms, treatment and history of all diseases of the human body. . . . Written by Henry M. Lyman . . . Christian Fenger . . . H. Webster Jones . . . W. T. Belfield. . . . Chicago: Thompson & Thomas, [1900]. 1157p. col. plates. DLC; ICJ; ICRM **00-2271**

LYMAN, Henry Munson (1835-1904)
The practical home physician . . . giving the history, cause, means of prevention and symptoms of all diseases of men, women and children, and the most approved methods of treatment. . . . Written by Henry M. Lyman . . . Christian Fenger . . . H. Webster Jones . . . W. T. Belfield. . . . Rev. and enl. ed. . . . Chicago: Star Publishing Co., 1907. 1157p. col. plates. DLC; ICJ **00-2272**

LYNCH, Charles (*b.* 1868)
Medical department of the Japanese army. . . . Boston: Old Corner Book Store, 1906. 49p. DLC; MBM; MH **00-2273**

LYNCH, Charles (*b.* 1868)
What is the most effective organization of the American national Red Cross for war and what should be its relations with the medical departments of the army and navy? The Enno Sander prize essay. . . . Carlisle, Pa.: The Association of Military Surgeons, 1907. 32p. DLC; DNLM; PU **00-2274**

LYNCH, Charles (*b.* 1868)
American Red Cross abridged text-book on first aid. General ed. A manual of instruction. . . . Prepared for and endorsed by the American Red Cross. With 55 illustrations. Philadelphia: P. Blakiston's Son & Co., 1910. 183p. DLC; NNNAM; PPC; PU **00-2275**

LYON, Irving Phillips and Alfred B. WRIGHT
An inquiry into the existence of autochthonus malaria in Buffalo and its environs. Preliminary report on species of mosquitoes and blood examinations. [Buffalo, 1900.] 10p. DNLM **00-2276**

LYON, Irving Phillips
The inoculation of malaria by the mosquito; a review of the literature. New York, 1900. 23p. DNLM **00-2277**

LYON, Irving Phillips
Arterio-sclerosis and the kidney. Albany, 1903. 3p. DNLM **00-2278**

LYON, Irving Phillips
Blood examination in general practice. New York, 1903. 8p. DNLM **00-2279**

LYONS, Albert Brown (1841-1926)
Plant names, scientific and popular, including in the case of each plant the correct botanical name in accordance with the reformed nomenclature, together with botanical and popular synonyms. . . . Comp. from the most authentic sources. . . . Detroit: Nelson, Baker & Co., 1900. 489p. DLC; ICJ; MH; OCLloyd **00-2280**

[LYONS, Albert Brown] (1841-1926)
Urine testing up to date. A concise and comprehensive manual of urinary analysis, including many tests not given in the standard text books. Detroit: Nelson, Baker & Co., 1902. 23p. DLC; ICJ; ICRM **00-2281**

LYONS, Albert Brown (1841-1926)
Plant names, scientific and popular, including in the case of each plant the correct botanical name in accordance with the reformed nomenclature, together with botanical and popular synonyms. . . . Comp. from the most authentic sources. . . . 2nd ed., thoroughly rev. with much added matter. Detroit: Nelson, Baker & Co., 1907. 630p. DLC; ICJ; NN; OCLloyd **00-2282**

MABEE, Charles Ralph
The physician's business and financial adviser. . . . 4th ed. Cleveland, O.: Continental Publishing Co., 1900. 256p. DLC; DNLM; ICJ [Reprint of 1st ed. (1899); 2nd ed. (1899); 3rd ed. (1899) with no change] **00-2283**

MABEE, Charles Ralph
The physician's business and financial adviser. 5th ed. Cleveland: Continental Publishing Co., 1901. 269p. DLC; PPC; ICJ **00-2284**

MacADAM, Henry Graham
The benefits of medical school inspection. New York, 1900. 10p. DLC; DNLM **00-2285**

MACALESTER, Richard K.
Gouty affections of the kidneys. New York, 1901. 5p. DNLM **00-2286**

McBRIDE, J[ames] H.
The good nurse. Chicago, 1900. 12p. DNLM **00-2287**

McBRIDE, J[ames] H.
The treatment of the morphine habit. Can it be cured? New York, 1900. 14p. DNLM **00-2288**

McBRIDE, J[ames] H.
The mental symptoms of cerebral syphilis. Chicago, 1901. 15p. DNLM **00-2289**

MacCALLUM, John B[ruce] (1876-1906)
On the mechanism of the physiological action of the cathartics. Berkeley: The University Press, 1906. 91p. DLC; ICJ; MH; NN [Includes a 3p. preface-obituary by Jacques Loeb]
00-2290

McCARTHY, Daniel J[oseph] (*b.* 1874)
Contributions to the study of (a) Iron infiltration in the ganglion cells; (b) Forced movements due to cellular degeneration of the cerebellum following rattlesnake poisoning. 1900. 8p. PU **00-2291**

McCARTHY, Daniel J[oseph] (*b.* 1874)
Cerebral lesions in experimental lead intoxication. Philadelphia, 1902. 6p. DNLM **00-2292**

McCARTHY, Daniel J[oseph] (*b.* 1874) and A. P. FRANCINE
Focal facial epilepsy, followed by temporary unilateral paralysis of the face and tongue. Philadelphia, 1902. 6p. DNLM
00-2293

McCARTHY, Daniel J[oseph] (*b.* 1874) and Mazÿck P. RAVENEL
Melanoses of the cerebro-spinal meninges. Philadelphia, 1902. 2p. 1 plate. DNLM **00-2294**

McCARTHY, Daniel J[oseph] (*b.* 1874)
Fat crystals in the spinal cord. n. p., [1903]. 4p. PU
00-2295

McCARTHY, Daniel J[oseph] (*b.* 1874)
The changes in peripheral nerves produced by toxic substances applied to the skin; a medicolegal study. Philadelphia, 1903. 7p. DNLM; PU **00-2296**

McCARTHY, Daniel J[oseph] (*b.* 1874)
Formation of hemolymph glands from a dipose tissue in man. 1903. 4p. PU **00-2297**

McCARTHY, Daniel J[oseph] (*b.* 1874)
Cholesteatoma vasculosa of the chorid plexus of the lateral cerebral vertricle. n. p., 1906. 5p. PU
00-2298

MacCARTHY, Francis H[amilton] (*b.* 1871)
Hygiene for mother and child; a manual for mothers and nurses, including hygiene for the prospective mother and practical directions for the care and feeding of children. . . . New York and London: Harper & Bros., 1910. 295p. DLC; MB; MH; NNNAM **00-2299**

MacCARTHY, Francis H[amilton] (*b.* 1871)
Hygiene for mother and child; a manual for mothers and nurses, including hygiene for the prospective mother and practical directions for the care and feeding of children. . . . [2nd ed.] New York and London: Harper & Bros., 1910. 295p. DLC; DNLM; ICJ; MB **00-2300**

McCASKEY, G[eorge] W[ashington] (1853-1935)
Hysteric lethargy, with report of cases. [Chicago, 1900.] 7p. DNLM **00-2301**

McCASKEY, G[eorge] W[ashington] (1853-1935)
Neurasthenia; some points in its pathology and treatment. Chicago, 1900. 16p. DNLM **00-2302**

McCASKEY, G[eorge] W[ashington] (1853-1935)
A new method for the clinical determination of the position of the cardia. Philadelphia, 1900. 8p. DNLM
00-2303

McCASKEY, G[eorge] W[ashington] (1853-1935)
Report of a case of tumor of the cerebellum with drainage of fluid through the nose. New York, 1900. 14p. DNLM
00-2304

McCASKEY, G[eorge] W[ashington] (1853-1935)
Simple and ethereal sulphates. A simple and rapid method for their separate determination, thirty minutes. Fort Wayne, 1900. 8p. DNLM **00-2305**

McCASKEY, G[eorge] W[ashington] (1853-1935)
A case of combined gastric and aural vertigo, with a discussion of the pathology of such cases. Chicago, 1901. 11p. DNLM
00-2306

McCASKEY, G[eorge] W[ashington] (1853-1935)
The clinical laboratory as an aid to diagnosis. Fort Wayne, 1901. 4 l. DNLM **00-2307**

McCASKEY, G[eorge] W[ashington] (1853-1935)
Hysterical dissociation of temperature senses, with reversal of sensibility to cold. New York, 1901. 7p. DNLM
00-2308

McCASKEY, G[eorge] W[ahington] (1853-1935)
Physiology the basis of clinical medicine; a plea for scientific methods. Fort Wayne, 1901. 15p. DNLM
00-2309

McCASKEY, G[eorge] W[ashington] (1853-1935)
Alexia from cyst caused by bullet wound; operation; death. Chicago, 1902. 7p. DNLM **00-2310**

McCASKEY, G[eorge] W[ashington] (1853-1935)
Anemias secondary to gastro-intestinal disease, with report of two cases. Chicago, 1902. 7p. DNLM
00-2311

McCASKEY, G[eorge] W[ashington] (1853-1935)
A case of leucemia preceded by mucosanguinolent colitis and physiological leucocytosis. New York, 1902. 10p. DNLM
00-2312

McCASKEY, G[eorge] W[ashington] (1853-1935)
The clinical association of cancer and tuberculosis, with report of a case. Philadelphia, 1902. 8p. DNLM
00-2313

McCASKEY, G[eorge] W[ashington] (1853-1935)
Electrical reactions of the gastro-intestinal musculature, and their therapeutic value. New York: William Wood & Co., 1902. 20p. DNLM **00-2314**

McCASKEY, G[eorge] W[ashington] (1853-1935)
Chronic gastritis; a clinical study of six hundred cases. [New York, 1903.] 16p. DNLM **00-2315**

McCASKEY, G[eorge] W[ashington] (1853-1935)
Localization in brain disease with a view to surgical intervention. Fort Wayne, 1903. 2 l. DNLM
00-2316

McCASKEY, G[eorge] W[ashington] (1853-1935)
Tuberculosis of bronchial glands; tuberculin; chest pain. [Philadelphia, 1903.] 8p. DNLM **00-2317**

McCASKEY, G[eorge] W[ashington] (1853-1935)
Weakness and dilatation of the heart in chronic nutritional disease. [Chicago, 1903.] 13p. DNLM **00-2318**

McCASKEY, G[eorge] W[ashington] (1853-1935) and Miles F. PORTER
A case of brain abscess due to latent typhoid infection; operation; death from cardiac complication [and] brain tumor developing in a case of peripheral neuritis, the latter obscuring diagnosis; operative removal of tumor; recovery. [Chicago, 1903.] 15p. DNLM **00-2319**

McCASSY, J[ohn] H.
School life in relation to health. [New York, 1903.] 7p. DNLM; NN **00-2320**

[McCAW, Walter Drew] (1863-1939)
Walter Reed. A memoir. Washington, D.C.: The Walter Reed Memorial Association, 1904. 11p. DLC; DNLM; MB; NN **00-2321**

McCAW, Will
How to use a trial case of lenses for the proper adjustment of glasses to defective refractions. Geneva, N.Y.: W. F. Humphrey, printer, 1900 [*c.* 1898]. 97p. fold. plate. DLC **00-2322**

McCLELLAN, George (1849-1913)
Anatomy in its relation to art: an exposition of the bones and muscles of the human body with especial reference to their influence upon its actions and external form . . . illustrated by three hundred and thirty-eight original drawings and photographs made by the author and expressly prepared for this work. . . . Philadelphia: The Author, 1900. 142p. plates. DLC; DNLM; PPC; PU **00-2323**

McCLELLAN, George (1849-1913)
Anatomy in its relation to art. . . . Philadelphia: W. B. Saunders & Co., 1901. 142p. DLC; NN; PHi; PP **00-2324**

McCLELLAN, George (1849-1913)
Regional anatomy in its relation to medicine and surgery. . . . Illustrated from photographs taken by the author of his own dissections, expressly designed and prepared for this work, and colored by him after nature. . . . Philadelphia and London: W. B. Saunders & Co., 1901. 2 v. 97 col. plates. DLC; NNNAM; OCIM; PU ["4th ed."] **00-2325**

McCLINTOCK, John C[alhoun] (*b.* 1855)
An abstract of lectures on hernia. Topeka, 1902. 28p. DLC; DNLM **00-2326**

McCLINTOCK, John C[alhoun] (*b.* 1855)
A Kansas surgeon in Karlsbad. Topeka: Crane & Co., 1910. 122p. DLC; DNLM; ICJ; NN **00-2327**

McCOLLOM, John H[ildreth]
A plea for larger doses of antitoxin in the treatment of diphtheria. Boston, 1900. 15p. DLC; DNLM **00-2328**

McCOMBS, Robert S[helmerdine] (*b.* 1860)
Diseases of children for nurses; including infant feeding, therapeutic measures employed in childhood, treatment for emergencies, prophylaxis, hygiene, and nursing. . . . Philadelphia and London: W. B. Saunders & Co., 1907. 431p. col. plates. DLC; NNNAM; OCIM; PPC **00-2329**

McCONNELL, Carl Philip
The practice of osteopathy [by] Carl Philip McConnell . . . and Charles Clayton Teall . . . 2nd ed., completely rewritten and rev., containing much new and original material from authentic sources never before published. Kirksville, Mo.: Journal Printing Co., 1906. 780p. DLC: DNLM; ICJ; PP **00-2330**

McCONNELL, Carl Philip
The practice of osteopathy [by] Carl Philip McConnell . . . [and] Charles Clayton Teall . . . 3rd ed., completely rewritten and rev., containing much new and original matter from authentic sources never before published. Kirksville, Mo.: Journal Printing Co., 1906. 781p. DLC; DNLM; ICJ; PPC **00-2331**

McCONNELL, Guthrie (1875-1923)
A manual of pathology. . . . Philadelphia and London: W. B. Saunders & Co., 1906. 523p. DLC; PPC; PPJ; PU **00-2332**

McCORMICK, Arthur T.
Instrumental and operative obstetrics. Louisville, 1901. 15p. DNLM **00-2333**

McCORMICK, Charles N. (*b.* 1858)
Optical truths. 2nd ed. . . . Chicago: McCormick Neurological College, [1906]. 193p. col. plates. DLC: ICJ **00-2334**

McCORMICK, John H[enry], ed. (*b.* 1870)
Century book of health; the maintenance of health, prevention and cure of disease, motherhood, care, feeding and diseases of children, modern home nursing, accidents and emergencies, injurious habits; a complete practical guide based upon the latest medical practice, recent discoveries in science and U.S. pharmacopoeia revision of 1905. . . . Springfield, Mass., Chicago, [etc.]: The King-Richardson Co., [1906]. 872p. plates. DLC; ICJ; MBM; NNNAM **00-2335**

McCOSH, A[ndrew] J[ames] (1858-1908)
Myomectomy vs. hysterectomy. New York, 1902. 21p. 4 plates. DLC: DNLM; NN **00-2336**

MacCOY, Alexander
A clinical study of the use of antitoxine serum (Dunbar's) in hay fever during the season of 1903. A new and distinct advance in its management. New York, 1903. 8p. DLC; DNLM **00-2337**

McCOY, John
Consumption or pulmonary tuberculosis; how to stay its ravages, how to prevent it, how to cure it, how to eradicate it from civilization; in language that the masses can understand. . . Los Angeles, Cal.: B. R. Baumgardt & Co., 1900. 83p. DLC; DNLM **00-2338**

McCOY, John
A report of three cases of laryngeal growth removed by direct laryngolcopy. [St. Louis, 1908.] 4p. NN **00-2339**

McCOY, John
Symptoms of internal ear suppuration with report and presentation of two cases; operation; recovery. [St. Louis, 1910.] 2 l. NN **00-2340**

McCRAE, Thomas and James F. MITCHELL
Surgical features of typhoid fever. Philadelphia, 1902. 32p. DLC; DNLM; PU **00-2341**

McCRUDDEN, Francis H[enry] (*b.* 1879)
Uric acid: chemistry, physiology and pathology of uric acid and the physiologically important purin bodies. With a discussion on the metabolism of gout. Boston, 1906. 318p. DLC; ICJ; MH-M; NN **00-2342**

McCULLY, Charles H[arvey] (*b.* 1868)
Sanitation and disinfection: a concise treatise on disease prevention with special reference to the communicable diseases. Chicago: H. S. Fassett, 1906. 184p. DLC; ICJ; NN **00-2343**

[McCURDY, Richard A.]
Poisons—remedies; a manual for reference, issued by the Mutual Life Insurance of New York. . . . [New York: The Company, 1903.] 45p. DLC; ICJ; NIC; NN [*vel subseq.*] **00-2344**

McCURDY, Stewart Le Roy (1859-1931)
Oral surgery; a text-book on general medicine and surgery as applied to dentistry. Pittsburgh: The Calumet Publishing Co., 1901. 368p. DNLM; ICJ; PPC; PU **00-2345**

McCURDY, Stewart Le Roy (1859-1931)
The wiring of bone for recent and ununited fracture, with report of cases. New York, 1904. 17p. DNLM **00-2346**

McCURDY, Stewart Le Roy (1859-1931)
Anatomy in abstract. . . . Pittsburgh, Pa.: Medical Abstract Publishing Co., 1905. 215p. DLC; ICJ **00-2347**

McCURDY, Stewart Le Roy (1859-1931)
Surgical and medical emergencies in abstract. . . . Pittsburgh, Pa.: Medical Abstract Publishing Co., 1906. 153p. DLC: ICJ **00-2348**

McCURDY, Stewart Le Roy (1859-1931)
Arthrosteopedic surgery (extremities and skeleton). . . . Pittsburgh, Pa.: Medical Abstract Publishing Co., [1909]. 210p. DLC; DNLM; ICJ **00-2349**

McCURDY, W. D.
Eating to live or how I got sick and how I got well, by natural methods. Containing facts in regard to cooked and uncooked food. No breakfast plan. One meal a day. Breathing. Physical culture exercises, and the use of water as a curative agent. San Francisco: Whitaker & Ray Co., 1903. 122p. DNLM **00-2350**

MacDONALD, Robert (*b.* 1866)
Mind, religion and health, with an appreciation of the Emmanuel movement; how its principles can be applied in promoting health and in the enriching of our daily life, by. . . . New York and London: Funk & Wagnalls Co., 1908. 368p. DLC; ICJ; MB; NN **00-2351**

MacDONALD, Robert (*b.* 1866)
Mind, religion and health, with an appreciation of the Emmanuel movement; how its principles can be applied in promoting health and in the enriching of our daily life. 2nd ed.—rev. New York: Funk & Wagnalls Co., 1909. 368p. ICU; MB; MH; NN **00-2352**

MACDONALD, Willis G[oss] (*b.* 1863)
The relation of the clinical laboratory to modern surgery. New York, 1900. 11p. DNLM **00-2353**

MACDONALD, Willis G[oss] (*b.* 1863)
Medical education. New York, 1904. 21p. DNLM **00-2354**

MACEWEN, William (1848-1924)
Atlas of head sections. . . . New York: Macmillan Co., 1900 [*c.* 1893]. 4p. + 53 plates. MBM; ICJ; NNNAM; PU [53 engraved copper plates of frozen sections of the head, and 53 key plates with descriptive texts] **00-2355**

McFARLAND, Joseph (1868-1945)
A text-book upon the pathogenic *Bacteria*; for students of medicine and physicians. . . . With 142 illustrations. 3rd ed., rev. and enl. Philadelphia: W. B. Saunders & Co., 1900. 621p. plates. DLC; NNNAM; PPC; PU **00-2356**

McFARLAND, Joseph (1868-1945)
Mulford's diphtheria antitoxic serum. [Philadelphia, 1900?] 4p. DNLM **00-2357**

McFARLAND, Joseph (1868-1945)
A text-book upon the pathogenic bacteria, for students of medicine and physicians . . . with 153 illustrations, a number of them in colors. 4th ed., rewritten and enl. Philadelphia, London, [etc.]: W. B. Saunders & Co., 1903. 629p. DLC; MBM; NNNAM; PPC **00-2358**

McFARLAND, Joseph (1868-1945)
A text-book of pathology, for practitioners and students . . . with 350 illustrations, a number in colors. Philadelphia, London, [etc.]: W. B. Saunders & Co., 1904. 818p. DLC; NNNAM; PPC; PU **00-2359**

McFARLAND, Joseph (1868-1945)
. . . Serum therapy, by Joseph McFarland. . . . Organotherapy, by Oliver T. Osborne. . . . Radium, thorium, and radioactivity, by Samuel G. Tracy. . . . Counterirritation, external applications, bloodletting, by Frederick A. Packard. . . . An outline of the principles of therapeutics, by the editor; with addendum on X-ray therapy and an Index-digest of the complete system of eleven volumes [by R. M. Goepp and C. W. Bonney]. . . . Philadelphia: P. Blakiston's Son & Co., 1905. 388p. DLC: ICJ; PPC; PU [Vol. 11 of S. S. Cohen, ed., A system of physiologic therapeutics] **00-2360**

McFARLAND, Joseph (1868-1945)
A text-book upon the pathogenic bacteria, for students of medicine and physicians. . . . With 190 illustrations, a number of them in colors. 5th ed., thoroughly rev. Philadelphia and London: W. B. Saunders & Co., 1906. 647p. DLC: IU-M; MBM; PPC **00-2361**

McFARLAND, Joseph (1868-1945)
A text-book upon the pathogenic bacteria, for students of medicine and physicians . . . with 211 illustrations, a number of them in colors. 6th ed., thoroughly rev. Philadelphia and London: W. B. Saunders & Co., 1909. 709p. DLC; NNNAM; PPC; PU **00-2362**

McFARLAND, Joseph (1868-1945)
A text-book of pathology, for practitioners and students . . . 2nd ed., thoroughly rev., with 437 illustrations, a number in colors. Philadelphia and London: W. B. Saunders & Co., 1910. 856p. DLC; NNNAM; PPC; PU **00-2363**

McFARLAND, Joseph (1868-1945)
Biology, general and medical . . . with 160 illustrations. Philadelphia and London: W. B. Saunders & Co., 1910. 440p. plates. DLC; MBM; NIC; PPC **00-2364**

MACFARLANE, Catharine (*b.* 1877)
A reference hand-book of gynecology for nurses. . . . Philadelphia and London: W. B. Saunders & Co., 1908. 150p. plates. DLC; NNNAM; PPC; PU **00-2365**

McGAVREN, Charles William
"The physician's medicine case." A book of instructions to fathers and mothers of the household. Comprising two parts: Part I for adults, and Part II for children. . . . [Missouri Valley? Ia., 1901.] 77p. DLC **00-2366**

McGAVREN, C[harles] W[illiam]
"The physician's medicine case." A book of plain instructions for the care of the sick, to father and mothers of the household. . . . [2nd ed.] [Missouri Valley? Ia., 1902.] 92p. DLC **00-2367**

McGEE, Anita N[ewcomb] (1864-1940)
Women nurses in the American Army. Columbus: Berlin Print. Co., 1900. 7p. DNLM **00-2368**

McGEE, Anita N[ewcomb] (1864-1940)
The growth of the nursing profession in the United States. New York, 1900. 4 l. DNLM **00-2369**

McGEE, Anita N[ewcomb] (1864-1940)
The standard of trained nursing in America. New York, 1900. 4 l. DNLM **00-2370**

McGEE, Anita N[ewcomb] (1864-1940)
The nurse corps of the Army. Carlisle, 1902. 9p. DNLM **00-2371**

McGEE, Anita N[ewcomb] (1864-1940)
The Red Cross. New York, 1903. 4p. DNLM **00-2372**

McGLANNAN, Alexius (1872-1940)
. . . Physics and inorganic chemistry. A manual for students and practitioners. . . . illustrated with twenty engravings. Philadelphia and New York: Lea Bros. & Co., [1903]. 216p. CtY-M; DLC; PPC; PU **00-2373**

McGLANNAN, Alexius (1872-1940)
. . . Organic and physiologic chemistry: a manual for students and practitioners. . . . Illustrated with nine engravings. Philadelphia and New York: Lea Bros. & Co., [1903]. 246p. DLC; NNNAM; PPC; PU **00-2374**

McGLANNAN, Alexius (1872-1940)
The Whitehead operation for hemorrhoids. Richmond: Old Dominion Publishing Corporation, 1910. 6p. NN **00-2375**

MacGOWAN, Granville
The present state of the galvano-caustic operation of Bottini for ischuria. New York, 1900. 30p. DLC; DNLM **00-2376**

MacGOWAN, Granville
Report of ten cases of vesical tumor, with some remarks upon the cleansing of foul bladders and the technic of suprapubic cystotomy. New York, 1900. 27p. DNLM **00-2377**

MacGOWAN, Granville
The surgery of the prostate from the standpoint of personal experience. New York, 1903. 38p. DLC; DNLM **00-2378**

McGRATH, John J[oseph] (*b.* 1866)
Surgical anatomy and operative surgery for students and practitioners. Philadelphia: F. A. Davis Co., 1902. 559p. plates. CtY-M; DLC; DNLM; PPC **00-2379**

McGRATH, John J[oseph] (*b.* 1866)
Operative surgery, for students and practitioners . . . 2nd ed., thoroughly rev. With 265 illustrations, including many full-page plates in colors and half-tone. Philadelphia: F. A. Davis Co., 1906. 628p. DLC; MH-M; PPC; PU **00-2380**

McGRATH, John J[oseph] (*b.* 1866)
Operative surgery, for students and practitioners . . . 3rd rev. ed. With 276 illustrations, including many full-page plates in color and half-tone, Philadelphia: F. A. Davis Co., 1909. 653p. CtY-M; DLC; NNNAM; PPC **00-2381**

McGUIRE, Stuart (*b.* 1867)
Syllabus of lectures on principles of surgery. Richmond, Va.: Hunter & Co., [1900?] 46 l. DLC **00-2382**

McGUIRE, Stuart (*b.* 1867)
Lectures on principles of surgery. Baltimore: Southern Medical Publishing Co., 1908. 480p. DLC; MdU-D; MH-M; NN **00-2383**

MACH, Ernst (1838-1916)
Contributions to the analysis of the sensations. Transl. by Cora May Williams. Chicago: Open Court Publishing Co., 1901 [*c.* 1896]. DLC; ICJ; NIC; PU **00-2384**

McILVAINE, Charles (1840-1909)
Toadstools, mushrooms, *Fungi*, edible and poisonous. One thousand American *Fungi*; how to select and cook the edible; how to distinguish and avoid the poisonous; giving full botanic descriptions . . . by Charles McIlvaine . . . assisted by Robert K. Macadam. Toadstool poisons and their treatment, instructions to students, recipes for cooking, etc., etc. Indianapolis: The Bowen-Merrill Co., [1900]. 704p. col. plates. DLC; ICJ; MH; NN **00-2385**

McINTIRE, Charles (*b.* 1847)
Physic and its practisers in old Northampton, an historical sketch for the jubilee meeting of the Medical Society of Northampton County. Easton, Pa., 1900. 64p. DLC; DNLM; PU **00-2386**

McINTOSH, Herbert (1857-1917)
Practice handbook of medical electricity for students and practitioners . . . containing over two hundred illustrations. Boston, Mass.: The Therapeutic Publishing Co., 1909. 510p. DLC; ICJ; MBM; PPJ **00-2387**

McINTYRE, E. R.
Stepping stones to neurology. A manual for the student and general practitioner. Philadelphia: Boericke & Tafel, 1903. 205p. DLC; NNNAM; PPC; PU **00-2388**

McISAAC, Isabel
Primary nursing technique for first-year pupil nurses. New York: The Macmillan Co., 1907. 197p. DLC; DNLM; ICJ; PP
00-2389

McISAAC, Isabel
Hygiene for nurses. . . . New York: The Macmillan Co., 1908. 208p. DLC; ICJ; MB; NN **00-2390**

McISAAC, Isabel
Bacteriology for nurses. New York: The Macmillan Co., 1909. 179p. DLC; ICJ; MB; PPC **00-2391**

McISAAC, Isabel
The elements of hygiene for schools. New York: The Macmillan Co., 1909. 172p. DNLM; NN **00-2392**

MACK, Charles H.
A few practical hints on the teeth and how to take care of them. Salem, Ore.: Printed by Frank Conover, 1900 [*c.* 1898]. 16p. DLC **00-2393**

MACK, Charles S[amuel]
Are we to have a united medical profession? La Porte, Ind.: The Author, [*c.* 1904]. 44p. DLC; DNLM **00-2394**

McKAY, W[illiam] J[ohn] Stewart (1866-1948)
The history of ancient gynecology. New York: William Wood & Co., 1901. 302p. DNLM; MH-M; NNNAM; PU
00-2395

McKAY, W[illiam] J[ohn] Stewart (1866-1948)
Operations upon the uterus, perineum, and round ligaments. New York: William Wood & Co., 1909. 454p. 148 plates. CtY-M; ICJ; LNT-M; NNNAM **00-2396**

MACKENZIE, James (1853-1925)
Diseases of the heart. 2nd ed. New York: Oxford University Press (American Branch), 1910. 419p. DNLM; NcD; NIC [Oxford Medical Publications] **00-2397**

[MACKENZIE, John Kenneth] (1850-1888)
John Kenneth Mackenzie, medical missionary to China. [2nd ed.] By Mrs. [Mary Isabella] Bryson. New York and Chicago: F. H. Revell Co., [1900?] 404p. port. DLC; DNLM; NIC; NN
00-2398

McKENZIE, R. Tait (1867-1938)
Exercise in education and medicine. Philadelphia: W. B. Saunders & Co., 1909. 406p. DLC; ICJ; OCIM; PPC
00-2399

McKIM, W[illiam] Duncan (1855-1935)
Heredity and human progress. New York and London: G. P. Putnam's Sons, 1900. 283p. DNLM; ICU; KU; NN
00-2400

McLAREN, A[rchibald] (1858-1924)
The relationship between cholecystitis, jaundice, and gallstones. Philadelphia, 1900. 7p. DNLM
00-2401

McLAREN, A[rchibald] (1858-1924)
The relationship between dysmenorrhoea and appendicitis. New York, 1900. 6p. DNLM **00-2402**

McLAREN, A[rchibald] (1858-1924)
The surgical importance of jaundice. New York, 1900. 12p. DNLM **00-2403**

McLAREN, A[rchibald] (1858-1924)
A clinical study of the surgery of the kidney. St. Paul, 1901. 10p. DNLM **00-2404**

McLAREN, A[rchibald] (1858-1924)
Prostatectomy. St. Paul, 1901. 5p. DNLM
00-2405

McLAUGHLIN, Allen J[oseph] (*b.* 1872)
Inefficiency of ferrous sulphate as an antiseptic and germicide. Washington: Government Printing Office, 1903. 7p. DLC: DNLM **00-2406**

McLAUGHLIN, Allen J[oseph] (*b.* 1872)
. . . Cholera: its nature, detection, and prevention. . . . United States Public Health and Marine Hospital Service. Prepared by direction of the Surgeon-General. Washington: Government Printing Office, 1910. 20p. DLC; DNLM
00-2407

McLAUGHLIN, Candor (*b.* 1864)
An abridgement of practical medicine and allied sciences. Arranged in alphabetical order with definitions of principal medical terms. . . . [2nd ed. Rearranged, rev. and enl.] [Kansas City, Mo.: Grant Printing Co., 1909.] 677p. DLC: ICJ
00-2408

McMANUS, Charles
Edward Hudson; a biographical sketch. [Philadelphia, 1902.] 7p. port. DNLM **00-2409**

McMANUS, Charles
Biographical sketch of Royal William Varney. Philadelphia, 1902. 4p. port. DNLM **00-2410**

McMECHAN, F[rancis] H[oeffer] (1879-1939)
Anesthesia for prostatectomy. Boston, [1910]. 13p. MBM
00-2411

MacMILLAN, James A[lexander] (*b.* 1864)
Chronic constipation and allied conditions, pathology, etiology, diagnosis and treatment. . . . Kansas City, Mo.: The Burton Co., 1908. 257p. DLC; KyLoJM
00-2412

McMURRICH, J[ames] Playfair (1859-1939)
The development of the human body; a manual of human embryology. Philadelphia: P. Blakiston's Son & Co., 1902. 527p. CtY-M; DLC; DNLM; PPC **00-2413**

McMURRICH, J[ames] Playfair (1859-1939)
The development of the human body; a manual of human embryology . . . 2nd ed., rev. and enl. With two hundred and seventy-two illustrations. Philadelphia: P. Blakiston's Son & Co., 1904. 539p. DLC; ICJ; PPC; PU
00-2414

McMURRICH, J[ames] Playfair (1859-1939)
The development of the human body; a manual of human embryology . . . 3rd ed., rev. and enl. With two hundred and seventy-seven illustrations. Philadelphia: P. Blakiston's Son & Co., 1907. 528p. DLC; ICJ; NNNAM; PPC
00-2415

McMURTRIE, Henry (1793-1865)
A compendium of domestic medicine, and health adviser. . . . Chicago: Alhambra Book Co., [1900]. 256p. plates. DLC; DNLM **00-2416**

McMURTRIE, Henry (1793-1865)
Plain medical talks for women and nursery adviser.... Chicago: Alhambra Book Co., [1902]. 299p. DLC; DNLM
00-2417

McOSCAR, James R[iley] (*b.* 1864)
The all around specialist. . . . Techniques of specialists in most branches of medicine. Philadelphia: J. B. Lippincott Co., 1904. 342p. col. plates. CtY-M; MBM; NNNAM; PPC
00-2418

McOSCAR, James R[iley] (*b.* 1864)
The all around specialist. . . . Techniques of specialists in most branches of medicine. 2nd ed. Philadelphia: J. B. Lippincott Co., 1904. 342p. col. plates. PPC; PU
00-2419

McOSCAR, James R[iley] (*b.* 1864)
The all around specialist. . . . Techniques of specialists in most branches of medicine. 3rd ed. Philadelphia: J. B. Lippincott Co., 1905. 448p. col. plates. DLC; NNNAM; PPJ; PU
00-2420

MAGNUS, Hugo F[riedrich] (1842-1907)
Visual economies, with rules for estimation of the earning ability after injuries to the eyes. By H. Magnus . . . and H. V. Würdemann . . . for the use of the medical and legal professions, business corporations and insurance officials. Milwaukee, Wis.: C. Porth, 1902. 144p. 5 diags. (1 col.) DLC; DNLM; ICJ; PU **00-2421**

MAGNUS, Hugo F[riedrich] (1842-1907)
Superstition in medicine, by Prof. Dr. Hugo Magnus; authorized translation from the German, ed. by Dr. Julius L. Salinger. . . . New York and London: Funk & Wagnalls Co., 1905. 205p. CtY-M; DLC; KU; NcD **00-2422**

MAGRUDER, Edward M.
Guide to physical diagnosis. . . . Charlottesville, Va.: The Michie Co., printers, 1907. 238p. DLC; ICJ; NcD [1st ed., 1897. 177p.] **00-2423**

MAGRUDER, Ernest Pendleton (1875-1915)
Case of aortic regurgitation and floating liver.... [New York: A. R. Elliott Publishing Co., 1908.] 10p. DLC; NN
00-2424

MAGRUDER, Ernest Pendleton (1875-1915)
Uraemia, with terminal cerebral haemorrhage.... [New York: A. R. Elliott Publishing Co., 1910.] 13p. DLC; NN
00-2425

MAGRUDER, Ernest Pendleton (1875-1915)
. . . Fracture of the patella: the operation of choice. . . . Chicago: American Medical Association, 1910. 15p. DLC; NN
00-2426

MAGRUDER, Ernest Pendleton (1875-1915)
. . . Bone-grafting and osteoplasty; a case of the latter presented.... [Chicago], 1910. 3p. DLC; NN
00-2427

MAGRUDER, W[illiam] E[dward] (*b.* 1873)
Claims arising from results of personal injuries; the relation injury bears to disease and disease to injury; a treatise showing how personal injury may affect various diseases, and how certain diseases may add to claims for accidents by protracting recovery. Chicago: The Spectator Co., [1910]. 266p. DLC; ICJ; NN **00-2428**

MAHER, Stephen J[ohn] (1860-1939)
Some investigations of a bacterial treatment of tuberculosis. New York, 1904. 41p. DNLM; ICJ; MH-M; NNNAM
00-2429

MAKUEN, G[eorge] Hudson (*b.* 1855)
Defects of speech. Philadelphia, [1900]. 8p. DLC
00-2430

MAKUEN, G[eorge] Hudson (*b.* 1855)
How to prevent stammering. Philadelphia, 1906. 6p. PU
00-2431

MAKUEN, G[eorge] Hudson (*b.* 1855)
. . . The essentials of speech production.... Philadelphia: A. R. Elliott Publishing Co., 1908. 7p. DLC **00-2432**

MAKUEN, G[eorge] Hudson (*b.* 1855)
Stammering and its treatment. [Read by invitation before the Chicago Medical Society, April 6, 1910. Philadelphia, 1910.] 3p. NN **00-2433**

MAKUEN, G[eorge] Hudson (*b.* 1855)
The physiology and psychology of hearing with special reference to development of speech. [St. Louis, 1910.] 7p. NN
00-2434

MALL, Franklin P[aine] (1862-1917)
A contribution to the study of the pathology of early human embryos. Baltimore, 1900. 68p. 6 plates. DLC; DNLM
00-2435

MALL, Franklin P[aine] (1862-1917)
On the development of the human diaphragm. Baltimore, 1901. 38p. DLC; DNLM **00-2436**

MALL, Franklin P[aine] (1862-1917)
Note on the basement membranes of the tubules of the kidney. Baltimore, 1901. 5p. DLC; DNLM **00-2437**

MALL, Franklin P[aine] (1862-1917)
On the origin of the lymphatics in the liver. Baltimore, 1901. 8p. DLC; DNLM **00-2438**

MALL, Franklin P[aine] (1862-1917)
Notes on the collection of human embryos in the anatomical laboratory of Johns Hopkins University. Baltimore, 1903. 12p. DLC; DNLM **00-2439**

MALL, Franklin P[aine] (1862-1917)
Second contribution to the study of the pathology of early human embryos. [Ann Arbor, 1903.] 28p. DLC; DNLM
00-2440

MALLORY, Frank B[urr] (1862-1941)
Pathological technique; a practical manual for workers in pathological histology and bacteriology. . . . By Frank Burr Mallory . . . and James Homer Wright . . . 2nd ed. rev. and enl. . . . Philadelphia, London: W. B. Saunders & Co., 1901. 432p. col. plates. DLC; MBM; NNNAM; PPC **00-2441**

MALLORY, Frank B[urr] (1862-1941)
Pathological technique; a practical manual for workers in pathological histology and bacteriology including directions for the performance of autopsies and for clinical diagnosis by laboratory methods, by Frank Burr Mallory and James Homer Wright . . . 3rd ed., rev. and enl., with 156 illustrations. Philadelphia, [etc.]: W. B. Saunders & Co., 1904. 469p. plates. CU-M; DLC; NNNAM; PU **00-2442**

MALLORY, Frank B[urr] (1862-1941)
Pathological technique; a practical manual for workers in pathological histology and bacteriology including directions for the performance of autopsies and for clinical diagnosis by laboratory methods, by Frank Burr Mallory . . . and James Homer Wright . . . 4th ed., rev. and enl., with 152 illustrations. Philadelphia and London: W. B. Saunders & Co., 1908. 480p. plates. DLC; IU-M; NNNAM; PPC **00-2443**

MALTBIE, Birdsey L[ucius] (*b.* 1864)
Practical pharmacy for pharmacists and physicians; a text book for students in medicine and pharmacy. . . . Newark, N.J.: Physicians' Drug News Co., [1910]. 434p. CtY-M; DLC; DNLM; NjR **00-2444**

MANGES, Morris
The diet in typhoid fever. New York, 1900. 24p. DLC; DNLM **00-2445**

MANGES, Morris
A second report on the therapeutics of heroine. New York, 1900. 20p. DLC; DNLM **00-2446**

MANGES, Morris
Some general considerations on the treatment of typhoid fever. New York, 1904. 16p. DLC; DNLM **00-2447**

MANGES, Morris
Complications and sequelae of gastric ulcer. [New York, 1905.] 31p. MB **00-2448**

MANN, M[atthew] D[arbyshire] (1845-1921)
Experiences in intestinal surgery. New York, 1900. 19p. DNLM **00-2449**

MANN, M[atthew] D[arbyshire] (1845-1921)
A new operation for removal of cancer of the rectum. Chicago, 1901. 6p. DNLM **00-2450**

MANN, M[atthew] D[arbyshire] (1845-1921)
Removal of the female urinary bladder for malignant disease. [Philadelphia], 1901. 16p. DNLM **00-2451**

MANN, M[atthew] D[arbyshire] (1845-1921)
Removal of the female urinary bladder for malignant disease. Philadelphia, 1901. 13p. DNLM **00-2452**

MANN, M[atthew] D[arbyshire] (1845-1921)
In memoriam. Paul F. Mundé, M.D., LL.D. Died February 7, 1902. [New York, 1902.] 14p. port. DNLM **00-2453**

MANN, M[atthew] D[arbyshire] (1845-1921)
A manual of prescription writing, with a full explanation of the methods of correctly writing prescriptions, a table of doses expressed in both apothecaries' and metric system; rules for avoiding incompatibilities and for combining medicines. . . . Rev. by Edward Cox Mann . . . 6th ed., rev., enl., and cor. according to the U.S. pharmacopoeia of 1906. New York and London: G. P. Putnam's Sons, 1907. 232p. DLC: ICJ; MH-M; NNNAN **00-2454**

MANNABERG, Julius (*b.* 1860)
Malaria, influenza and dengue, by Dr. Julius Mannaberg . . . Dr. O. Leichtenstern . . . ed. with additions by Major Ronald Ross . . . J. W. W. Stephens . . . and Albert S. Grünbaum. Authorized transl. from the German, under the editorial supervision of Alfred Stengel. Philadelphia: W. B. Sanders & Co., 1905. 769p. 8 plates (incl. maps), diags. DLC; ICJ; MBM; NN [Nothnagel's encyclopedia of practical medicine. American ed.] **00-2455**

MANQUET, Alfred
Principles of therapeutics . . . transl. by M. Simbad Gabriel, M.D. New York and London: D. Appleton & Co., 1910. 298p. DLC; DNLM; ICJ; NNNAM **00-2456**

MANSON, Patrick (1844-1922)
Tropical diseases. A manual of the diseases of warm climates. . . . With 114 illustrations and two coloured plates. Revised and enlarged edition. New York: William Wood & Co., 1900. 684p. DNLM; ICJ; LNT-M; PU **00-2457**

MANSON, Patrick (1844-1922)
Tropical diseases; a manual of the diseases of warm climates. New and enlarged ed. New York: William Wood & Co., 1903. 756p. 2 plates. DNLM; LNT-M; NNNAM; PU **00-2458**

MANSON, Patrick (1844-1922)
Lectures on tropical diseases, being the Lane Lectures for 1905 delivered at Cooper Medical College; San Francisco, U.S.A., August 1905. Chicago: W. T. Keener & Co., 1905. 230p. illus. DNLM; ICJ; IU-M; KU **00-2459**

MANSON, Patrick (1844-1922)
Tropical diseases. A manual of the diseases of warm climates. . . . With illustrations and coloured plates. Fourth edition. New York: William Wood & Co., 1907. 876p. 7 plates. DNLM; ICJ; LNT-M; PPC **00-2460**

MANTON, Walter P[orter] (1858-1925)
. . . Obstetrics. A manual for students and practitioners . . . illustrated with eighty-two engravings. Philadelphia and New York: Lea Bros. & Co., [1903]. 265p. DLC:NNNAM; PPC; PU **00-2461**

MANTON, Walter P[orter] (1858-1925)
Syllabus of lectures on human embryology; an introduction to the study of obstetrics and gynaecology. For medical students and practitioners. With a glossary of embryological terms. . . . 3rd ed. Rev. and enl. Illustrated with numerous outline drawings. Philadelphia: F. A. Davis Co., 1906. 136p. col. front. DLC; MBM; PPC; PU **00-2462**

MARCHAND, Charles
Therapeutical applications of peroxide of hydrogen (medicinal) and glycozone. . . . 15th ed. New York, 1900. 292p. DLC; ICJ; MH-M; PU **00-2463**

MARCHAND, Charles
Hydrozone and glycozone in diseases caused by germs. New York, [1900]. 40p. DLC; DNLM **00-2464**

MARCHAND, Charles
Hydrozone and glycozone in diseases of the genito-urinary organs. [New York], 1902. 32p. DLC: DNLM **00-2465**

MARCHIAFAVA, Ettore (1847-1935)
Malaria and micro-organisms. By Ettore Marchiafava . . . Amico Bignami . . . Simon Flexner . . . Eugene L. Opie. . . . Specially reprinted from "Twentieth century practice," for the use of the United States Government. New York: William Wood & Co., 1900. 828p. 11 plates. DLC; DNLM; ICJ; NN **00-2466**

MARCY, Henry O[rlando] (1837-1924)
On the principles involved in the immediate hermetic sealing of aseptic wounds. Philadelphia, 1900. 10p. DNLM **00-2467**

MARCY, Henry O[rlando] (1837-1924)
The essential factors for the cure of hernia in the male. Chicago, 1900. 14p. DNLM **00-2468**

MARCY, Henry O[rlando] (1837-1924)
Gynecology; its contribution to general surgery. Chicago, 1901. 11p. DNLM **00-2469**

MARCY, Henry O[rlando] (1837-1924)
Obstructive diseases of the lower bowel. New York, 1901. 8p. DNLM **00-2470**

MARCY, Henry O[rlando] (1837-1924)
The restoration of the perineum. Chicago, 1903. 12p. DNLM **00-2471**

MARCY, Henry O[rlando] (1837-1924)
. . . A brief sketch of one of Baltimore's greatest men, Horatio Gates Jameson, M.D. His most valuable contribution to surgery: the occlusion of arteries by the buried animal ligature. . . . [Philadelphia, 1906.] 24p. DLC; DNLM; MdU-D; PPC **00-2472**

MARCY, Henry O[rlando] (1837-1924)
The early history of abdominal surgery in America. [Chicago, 1910.] 16p. DLC; ICJ **00-2473**

MARIANI, Angelo
Coca and its therapeutic application. New York: J. N. Jaros, 1901 [*c.* 1890]. 78p. double col. plate. DLC; NN **00-2474**

MARIE, A[rmand] (*b.* 1865)
Pellagra. Introductory notes by Prof. [C.] Lombroso. Transl. from the French by C. H. Lavinder and J. W. Babcock, with additions. . . . Columbia, S.C.: The State Co., 1910. 434p. DLC; LNT-M; ScCM; ScU **00-2475**

MARION-SIMS-BEAUMONT COLLEGE OF MEDICINE. ST. LOUIS, MO.
Bulletin for the session of 1904-05. St. Louis. The University, 1904. 23p. DNLM; ICJ **00-2476**

MARION-SIMS HOSPITAL, CHICAGO
Announcement. [Also, announcement of the Marion-Sims Training School for Nurses.] Chicago: Amer. Med. Assoc. Press, [1900?] 30p. DNLM; ICJ **00-2477**

MARION-SIMS HOSPITAL, CHICAGO
Report of medical, surgical, and obstetrical cases treated at the . . . from November, 1894. to November, 1900. [Chicago, 1900.] 2 l. DNLM; ICJ **00-2478**

MARK, Ernest G[utheric] (*b.* 1878)
The present status of spinal subarachnoid cocainization. New York, 1903. 17p. DLC; DNLM; NN **00-2479**

[MARKS, George Edwin] (1853-1932)
A treatise on artificial limbs with rubber hands and feet. . . . Eight hundred illustrations. New York City: A. A. Marks, 1901. 530p. DLC; NN; NNNAM **00-2480**

[MARKS, George Edwin] (1853-1932)
Manual of artificial limbs . . . an exhaustive exposition of prothesis. New York: A. A. Marks, 1905. 255p. DLC; ICJ; NNNAM; PU **00-2481**

[MARKS, George Edwin] (1853-1932)
Manual of artificial limbs . . . an exhaustive exposition of prothesis. New York: A. A. Marks, 1907. 430p. DLC; ICJ; NNNAM; PPL **00-2482**

[MARKS, George Edwin] (1853-1932)
Manual of artificial limbs . . . an exhaustive exposition of prothesis. New York: A. A. Marks, 1910. 414p. DLC; NN NNNAM **00-2483**

MARSH, E[ias] J. (*b.* 1835) and Granville M. WHITE
Report on the mortality records of the Mutual Life Insurance Company of New York, for fifty-six years from 1843 to 1898. New York, 1900. 245p. 6 diags. DNLM; NN; NNNAM **00-2484**

MARSH, Frederick H[oward] (1839-1915)
Diseases of the joints and spine. New ed., rev. by the author and C. Gordon Watson. Chicago: Chicago Medical Book Co., 1910. 632p. ICJ; IU-M; OCIM; PU **00-2485**

MARSHALL, John S[ayre] (1846-1922)
Principles and practice of operative dentistry. . . . Philadelphia and London: J. B. Lippincott Co., 1901. 635p. plates. DLC; MBM; MdU-D; PPC **00-2486**

MARSHALL, John S[ayre] (1846-1922)
A manual of the injuries and surgical diseases of the face, mouth, and jaws. . . . 2nd ed., rev. and enl. Philadelphia: The S. S. White Dental Mfg. Co., 1902. 715p. col. plates. DLC; DNLM; MdU-D; PPC **00-2487**

MARSHALL, John S[ayre] (1846-1922)
Principles and practice of operative dentistry. . . . 2nd ed. Philadelphia and London: J. B. Lippincott Co., [1905]. 651p. plates. DLC; MdU-D; PPC; PU **00-2488**

MARSHALL, John S[ayre] (1846-1922)
A manual of the injuries and surgical diseases of the face, mouth, and jaws. . . . 3rd ed., rev. and enl. Philadelphia: The S. S. White Dental Mfg. Co., 1909. 717p. col. plates. DLC; MdU-D; PPC; PU **00-2489**

MARSHALL, John S[ayre] (1846-1922)
Principles and practice of operative dentistry . . . 3rd ed. Philadelphia and London: J. B. Lippincott Co., [1909]. 654p. plates. DLC; MdU-D; NNNAM; PU **00-2490**

MARTIN, Edward (1859-1938)
Case of castration for the relief of obstructive symptoms cause of prostatic enlargement. 1900, [*c.* 1896]. 5p. PU **00-2491**

MARTIN, Edward (1859-1938)
. . . Essentials of surgery, together with a full description of the handkerchief and roller bandage. Arranged in the form of questions and answers; prepared especially for students of medicine. . . . 7th ed., rev. and enl., with appendix. . . . Philadelphia: W. B. Saunders & Co., 1900. 342p. DLC; DNLM; PPC; PU **00-2492**

MARTIN, Edward (1859-1938), [*et al.*]
The surgical treatment of sterility due to obstruction of the epididymis, together with a study of the morphology of human spermatozoa. Philadelphia, 1902. 14p. 2 plates. DNLM
00-2493

MARTIN, Edward (1859-1938)
Sterility from obstruction at the epididymis cured by operative means. New York, 1903. 4p. DNLM
00-2494

MARTIN, Edward (1859-1938)
Surgical diagnosis . . . illustrated with 445 engravings and 18 plates in colors and monochrome. Philadelphia and New York: Lea & Febiger, 1909. 772p. DLC; MBM; NNNAM; PU
00-2495

MARTIN, Franklin H[enry] (1857-1935)
A treatise on gynecology; being a guide-book for practitioners. . . . Chicago: Cleveland Press, 1903. 639p. plates. DLC; ICJ; IU-M; OCIM **00-2496**

MARTIN, Walton (*b.* 1869) and William H. ROCKWELL
Chemistry and physics, a manual for students and practitioners. Philadelphia and New York: Lea Bros. & Co., [1900]. 374p. CtY-M; DNLM; NNNAM; PU **00-2497**

MARYLAND. UNIVERSITY OF MARYLAND
The centennial celebration of the foundation of the University of Maryland (1807-1907). Memorial volume. Baltimore: Williams and Wilkins, 1908. 267p. DLC; MdU-D; PPC; PU [Includes memoriam to James Carroll of the U.S. Fever Commission; a history of the School of Dentistry; and an address by Samuel Chew on the medical school]
00-2498

MARYOTT, E[rastus] Edgar (1845-1904)
The new medical world. A book for reference and consultation, containing a thorough description of disease, with the latest and best methods for its treatment. . . . 5th ed., rev. . . . Springfield, Mass.: The Hampton Publishing Co., 1906. 593p. plates. DLC; MBM; MH **00-2499**

MASON, Charles [Field] (1864-1922)
A complete handbook for the hospital corps of the U.S. army and navy and state military forces. . . . New York: William Wood & Co., 1906. 545p. col. plates. DLC; ICJ; NNNAM; PU
00-2500

MASON, Charles [Field] (1864-1922)
A complete handbook for the hospital corps of the U.S. army and navy and state military forces. . . . Approved by the Surgeon-Generals of the army and navy. . . . [2nd ed.] New York: William Wood & Co., 1909. 573p. DLC; MB; MH-M; NNNAM **00-2501**

MASON, Enoch M.
Pellagra; its etiology, diagnosis, and treatment. . . . [Montgomery, Ala., 1910.] 4p. DLC **00-2502**

MASON, Lewis D[uncan] (*b.* 1843)
Inebriety a disease. Hartford, 1903. 12p. DLC; MH; NN
00-2503

MASON, Lewis D[uncan] (*b.* 1843)
Patent and proprietary medicines as the cause of the alcohol and opium habit or other forms of narcomania, with some suggestions as to how the evil may be remedied. Hartford, 1903. 12p. DLC; DNLM **00-2504**

MASON, Lewis D[uncan] (*b.* 1843)
The psychic treatment of inebriety and its relation to so-called cures. . . . Chicago: Press of American Medical Association, 1907. 10p. DLC; NN **00-2505**

MASON, Lewis D[uncan] (*b.* 1843)
Moderate drinking. Its dangers and possibilities. An address delivered before the World's Centennial Congress held at Saratoga Springs, New York, June 18, 1908. . . . New York: National Temperance Soc. and Publ. House, [1908]. 12p. MH; NN **00-2506**

MASON, Rufus D[odd] (1859-1911)
The office treatment of rectal diseases explained and simplified. Being an exposition of the treatment of all those diseases, both medical and surgical, of the rectum, anus and sig-moid flexure, the cure of which may be accomplished without surgical anesthesia. . . . Omaha: [F. B. Festner, printer], 1901]. 83p. DLC; DNLM; ICJ; MH-M [2nd ed., 1903, 83p.]
00-2507

MASON, Rufus D[odd] (1859-1911)
The office treatment of rectal diseases explained and simplified; being an exposition of the treatment of all those diseases, both medical and surgical, of the rectum, anus, and sigmoid flexure, the cure of which may be accomplished without surgical anaesthesia. . . . 3rd ed. Minneapolis, Minn.: The Burton Co., 1905. 222p. DLC; ICJ
00-2508

MASON, Rufus D[odd] (1859-1911)
The office treatment of rectal diseases explained and simplified; being an exposition of the treatment of all those diseases, both medical and surgical, of the rectum, anus, and sigmoid flexure, the cure of which may be accomplished without surgical anaesthesia. . . . 4th ed. . . . Kansas City, Mo.: The Burton Co., 1908. 354p. DLC; ICJ; KU
00-2509

MASSEY, G[eorge] Betton (1856-1927)
Cases of carcinoma and sarcoma recently treated by electric sterilization. Philadelphia, 1902. 10p. DLC; DNLM
00-2510

MASSEY, G[eorge] Betton (1856-1927)
The cataphoric treatment of cancer. [n. p.], 1902. 30p. DLC; DNLM **00-2511**

MASSEY, G[eorge] Betton (1856-1927)
Chronic inflammation of the uterine appendages; its treatment by mercuric cataphoresis. Chicago, 1902. 4p. DLC; DNLM
00-2512

MASSEY, G[eorge] Betton (1856-1927)
Report of a case of carcinoma of the breast treated by massive mercuric cataphoresis. New York, 1903. 8p. DLC; DNLM
00-2513

MASSEY, G[eorge] Betton (1856-1927)
Conservative gynecology and electro-therapeutics; a practical treatise on the diseases of women and their treatment by electricity . . . 4th ed., rev., rewritten, and greatly enl. Illustrated with twelve (12) original, full-page, chromo-lithographic plates and twelve (12) full-page half-tone plates of photographs taken from nature, and numerous engravings in the text. Philadelphia: F. A. Davis Co., 1905. 467p. DLC; NNNAM; PPC; PU **00-2514**

MASSEY, G[eorge] Betton (1856-1927)
Conservative gynecology and electro-therapeutics; a practical treatise on the diseases of women and their treatment by electritity . . . 5th rev. ed. Illustrated with twelve (12) original, full-page, chromo-lithographic plates and fifteen (15) full-page half-tone plates of the photographs taken from nature, and numerous engravings in the text. Philadelphia: F. A. Davis Co., 1906. 467p. DLC; MBM; PPC; PPJ
00-2515

MASSEY, G[eorge] Betton (1856-1927)
Conservative gynecology and electro-therapeutics; a practical treatise on the diseases of women and their treatment by electricity . . . 6th rev. ed. Illustrated with twelve (12) original, full-page, chromo-lithographic plates and fifteen (15) full-page half-tone plates of photographs taken from nature, and numerous engravings in the text. Philadelphia: F. A. Davis Co., 1909. 462p. DLC; ICJ; NN; PPC **00-2516**

MASSEY, G[eorge] Betton (1856-1927)
Ionic surgery in the treatment of cancer, with a chapter on ionization in surgical tuberculosis and hemorrhoids. . . . New York: The A. L. Chatterton Co., 1910. 243p. DLC; GU; ICJ; NNNAM **00-2517**

MATAS, Rudolph (1860-1957)
Intralaryngeal insufflation; for the relief of acute surgical pneumothorax. Its history and methods, with a description of the latest devices for this purpose. Chicago, 1900. 32p. DLC; LNT-M **00-2518**

MATAS, Rudolph (1860-1957)
Local and regional anesthesia with cocain and other analgesic drugs. The latest methods. Report of the chairman of the section of surgery of the Louisiana State Medical Society, contributed to the proceedings of the meeting held in New Orleans, April 19-21, 1900. [New Orleans, 1900.] 78p. 3 plates. DNLM; LNT-M **00-2519**

MATAS, Rudolph (1860-1957)
The treatment of abdominal aortic aneurism by a preliminary exploratory coeliotomy and peritoneal exclusion of the sac, followed at a later sitting by wiring and electrolysis. [Philadelphia, 1901.] 59p. DNLM; LNT-M **00-2520**

MATAS, Rudolph (1860-1957)
Massive infiltration anesthesia with weak analgesic solutions. (Modified Schleich Method). [n. p., 1901.] 6p. DLC; LNT-M
00-2521

MATAS, Rudolph (1860-1957)
Artificial respiration by direct intralaryngeal intubation with a modified O'Dwyer tube and a new graduated air-pump, in its applications to medical and surgical practice. [n. p., 1902.] 23p. DLC; LNT-M **00-2522**

MATAS, Rudolph (1860-1957)
Operation for the radical cure of aneurism based upon arteriorraphy. Philadelphia, 1903. 36p. DNLM; LNT-M
00-2523

MATAS, Rudolph (1860-1957)
Introductory remarks; some of the problems related to the surgery of the vasculary system. . . . The president's address before the American Surgical Association, Washington, D.C., May, 1910. [Washington]: American Surgical Assoc., 1910. 48p. NN **00-2524**

MATHER, Sedgwick
Anatomy and physiology of the nervous system. . . . Philadelphia: J. J. McVey, 1909. 154p. plates. DLC; NN; PPC; PU
00-2525

MATHEWS, Joseph McDowell (*b.* 1847)
How to succeed in the practice of medicine, by . . . . Louisville: J. P. Morton & Co., 1902. 215p. plates, port. DLC; DNLM; NNNAM; OCIM **00-2526**

MATHEWS, Joseph McDowell (*b.* 1847)
A treatise on diseases of the rectum, anus, and sigmoid flexure . . . with six chromo-lithographs and numerous illustrations. 3rd ed., rev. New York: D. Appleton & Co., 1903. 589p. DLC; ICJ; NNNAM; PPC **00-2527**

MATHEWS, Joseph McDowell (*b.* 1847)
How to succeed in the practice of medicine. . . . Philadelphia and London: W. B. Saunders & Co., 1905. 215p. port. DLC; NNNAM; PPC; PU **00-2528**

MATTISON, J[ansen] B[eemer] (*b.* 1845)
The Mattison method in morphinism. A modern and humane treatment of morphin disease. New York: E. B. Treat, 1902. 40p. CtY-M; DLC; MB; NNNAM **00-2529**

MAY, Charles H[enry] (1861-1943)
Manual of the diseases of the eye; for students and general practitioners. . . . New York: William Wood & Co., 1900. 406p. col. plates. DLC; DNLM; NNNAM; PPC
00-2530

MAY, Charles H[enry] (1861-1943)
Manual of the diseases of the eye, for students and general practitioners . . . 2nd ed., rev. New York: William Wood & Co., 1901. 408p. col. plates. DLC; DNLM; NNNAM; OCIM
00-2531

MAY, Charles H[enry] (1861-1943)
Manual of the diseases of the eye, for students and general practitioners . . . 3rd ed., revised. New York: William Wood & Co., 1903. 408p. col. plates. DNLM; NNNAM; OCIM; PPC
00-2532

MAY, Charles H[enry] (1861-1943)
Manual of the diseases of the eye, for students and general practitioners . . . 4th ed., rev. With 360 original illustrations including 21 plates, with 60 colored figures. New York: William Wood & Co., 1905. 391p. col. plates. DLC; MBM; NNNAM; PPC **00-2533**

MAY, Charles H[enry] (1861-1943)
Manual of the diseases of the eye, for students and general practitioners . . . 5th ed., rev. With 362 original illustrations including 22 plates, with 62 colored figures. New York: William Wood & Co., 1907. 391p. col. plates. DLC; LNT-M; NNNAM; PU **00-2534**

MAY, Charles H[enry] (1861-1943)
Manual of the diseases of the eye, for students and general practitioners . . . 6th ed., rev., with 362 original illustrations, including 22 plates, with 62 colored figures. New York: William Wood & Co., 1909. 391p. col. plates. DLC; IU-M; NNNAM; PPC **00-2535**

MAYER, Emil (1854-1931)
Laryngeal stenosis due to comminution of the thyroid cartilages. Chicago, 1900. 7p. DLC; DNLM
00-2536

MAYER, Emil (1854-1931)
Some points in the differential diagnosis of laryngeal diphtheria in children. New York, 1900. 5p. DLC; DNLM
00-2537

MAYER, Emil (1854-1931)
Clinical experience with adrenalin. Philadelphia, 1901. 7p. DLC; DNLM **00-2538**

MAYER, Emil (1854-1931)
Empyema of the antrum of Highmore in young infants. New York, 1901. 13p. DLC; DNLM **00-2539**

MAYER, Emil (1854-1931)
Adenoma of the nose, with incipient sarcomatous metamorphosis. Philadelphia, 1902. 4p. DLC; DNLM
00-2540

MAYER, Emil (1854-1931)
Affections of the mouth and throat, associated with the fusiform bacillus and spirillum of Vincent. Philadelphia, 1902. 7p. DLC; DNLM **00-2541**

MAYER, Emil (1854-1931)
The Asch operation for deviations of the cartilaginous nasal septum, with some conditions complicating its performance. Chicago, 1903. 6p. DLC; DNLM
00-2542

MAYER, Emil (1854-1931)
The cause and specific treatment of hay fever; a preliminary report on the uses of the toxines and antitoxines of Professor Dunbar. [New York, 1903.] 4p. DLC; DNLM
00-2543

MAYER, Emil (1854-1931)
Morris J. Asch. St. Louis, 1903. 8p. DLC; DNLM
00-2544

MAYER, Emil (1854-1931)
Perichondritis of the larynx, with report of a case. New York, 1903. 16p. DLC; DNLM **00-2545**

MAYER, Emil (1854-1931)
Neuroses of the larynx. St. Louis, 1904. 16p. DLC; DNLM
00-2546

MAYER, Emil (1854-1931)
Post-typhoid perichondritis of the larynx. [New York], 1904. 4p. DLC; DNLM **00-2547**

MAYLARD, A[lfred] Ernest
The student's handbook of the surgery of the alimentary canal, being an abridged and amended edtion of the author's treatise on the same subject. Philadelphia: P. Blakiston's Son & Co., 1900. 510p. 1 plate. DNLM; NNNAM; OCIM; PPC
00-2548

MAYLARD, A[lfred] Ernest
Abdominal pain, its causes and clinical significance. 2nd ed. (rev.) Philadelphia: P. Blakiston's Son & Co., 1906. 310p. ICJ; MBM; NNNAM; PPC **00-2549**

MAYLARD, A[lfred] Ernest
Abdominal tuberculosis. Philadelphia: P. Blakiston's Son & Co., 1908. 360p. CtY-M; ICJ; IU-M; PPC
00-2550

MAYO, C[harles] H[orace] (1865-1939)
Hypospadias. Chicago, 1901. 16p. DNLM; ICJ
00-2551

MAYO, William J[ames] (1861-1939)
Cholecystectomy, with especial reference to the removal of the mucous membrane of the gall-bladder as a substitute. Report of a case in which the gall-bladder was removed for malignant disease. Chicago, 1900. 4p. DNLM
00-2552

MAYO, William J[ames] (1861-1939)
Limitations of surgical work for the insane. New York, 1901. 8p. DNLM **00-2553**

MAYO, William J[ames] (1861-1939)
An operation for the radical cure of umbilical hernia. Philadelphia, 1901. 5p. 1 plate. DNLM **00-2554**

MAYO, William J[ames] (1861-1939)
Pre-existing heart disease in reference to surgical operations. Philadelphia, 1901. 6p. DNLM **00-2555**

MAYO, William J[ames] (1861-1939)
The medical and surgical aspects of the diseases of the gall bladder and bile ducts. A study of 534 operations upon the gall bladder and bile passages, with tabulated report of 547 operated cases. [New Haven, 1903.] 8p. MB
00-2556

MAYO, William J[ames] (1861-1939)
The causes of the occasional failure to cure gallstone disease. Chicago, 1904. 7p. DNLM **00-2557**

MAYO, William J[ames] (1861-1939)
Radical operations for the cure of cancer of the pyloric end of the stomach. Philadelphia, 1904. 12p. 4 plates. DNLM
00-2558

MAYO, William J[ames] (1861-1939)
Some observations on the surgery of the common duct of the liver. New York: William Wood & Co., 1904. 16p. DNLM
00-2559

MAYO, William J[ames] (1861-1939)
Cholecystotomy with removal of gallstones. [Troy, N.Y.: Southworth Co., 1910.] 19p. 11 stereos. DNLM
00-2560

MAYO, William J[ames] (1861-1939)
Gastrojejunostomy. [Troy, N.Y.: Southworth Co., 1910.] 30p. 19 stereos. DNLM **00-2561**

MAYS, Thomas J[efferson] (1846-1918)
. . . Notes on the silver-nitrate injections in the treatment of phthisis and Report of seven cases of pulmonary disease which were treated with silver-nitrate injections, with exhibition of cases. . . . [Philadelphia, 1900.] 14p. DLC; PPC
00-2562

MAYS, Thomas J[efferson] (1846-1918)
Pulmonary consumption, pneumonia, and allied diseases of the lungs, their etiology, pathology and treatment, with a chapter on physical diagnosis. . . . New York: E. B. Treat & Co., 1901. 539p. DLC; ICJ; MBM; NNNAM **00-2563**

MEARS, J[ames] Ewing (1838-1919)
The evolution of surgery. . . . Read before the meeting of the American Surgical Association, at St. Louis, June 16, 1904. Philadelphia: W. J. Dornan, printer, 1904. 15p. DLC; DNLM; PPC **00-2564**

MEARS, J[ames] Ewing (1838-1919)
Reminiscences of the early days of the American Surgical Association. . . . Read before the meeting of the American Surgical Association held in Richmond, Virginia, May 4, 1908. [Philadelphia? 1908.] 20p. DLC; PPC **00-2565**

MEARS, J[ames] Ewing (1838-1919)
The triumph of American medicine in the construction of the Panama Canal. Philadelphia: J. Dornan, 1910-1911. 25p. DLC; NN **00-2566**

MEDICAL directory, containing list of physicians, dentists, and druggists of Maryland and District of Columbia; also a list of trained nurses. Arranged alphabetically, and giving the school of medicine practiced by each physician, together with his college and year of graduation, 1900-1901. Compiled by Leverrier & Mitchell. Baltimore: Guggenheimer, Weil & Co., 1900. 250, 138p. 1 map. DNLM; ICJ; MdU-D; NN **00-2567**

MEDICAL RECORD
Post graduate guide; what to do after you graduate. How to secure salaried positions and appointments after you graduate. . . . New York: William Wood & Co., [1909]. 244p. DLC; NN; NNNAM; PU **00-2568**

MEDICAL SOCIETY OF THE COUNTY OF BROOME, BINGHAMTON, N.Y.
The proceedings of the centennial meeting of the Medical Society of the County of Broome, held October 24, 1906, with a list of members and officers of the Society from 1806 to 1906. [Binghamton?]: The Society, [1908?] 74p. DLC **00-2569**

MEDICAL SOCIETY OF THE COUNTY OF NEW YORK
Report of the Committee of seven on the prophylaxis of venereal disease in New York City. By the chairman. [Prince A. Morrow]. [New York, 1901.] 33p. DLC; NNNAM **00-2570**

MEDICAL SOCIETY OF THE DISTRICT OF COLUMBIA
. . . Rabies. Report of the Committee on Public Health. . . . Washington: Government Printing Office, 1900. 29p. DLC; DNLM **00-2571**

MEDICAL SOCIETY OF THE DISTRICT OF COLUMBIA
Medical educational standards. . . . Memorial of the Medical Society . . . protesting against the passage of the Bill (S. 5221, Calendar No. 2635) to regulate the practice of osteopathy. . . . [Washington: Government Printing Office, 1906.] 6p. DLC **00-2572**

MEDICAL SOCIETY OF THE DISTRICT OF COLUMBIA
History of the Medical Society of the District of Columbia, 1817-1909. Washington: The Society, 1909. 501p. plates, ports. DLC; MdBM; MdHi; PPC **00-2573**

MEDICO-CHIRURGICAL COLLEGE. PHILADELPHIA
The medico-collegian; a year book of the Medico-Chirurgical College, and a complete record of the medical class of 1906, with over 300 half-tone engravings and illustrations. The medical class of 1906. Philadelphia: Medico-Chirurgical college, [1906]. 433p. DLC; PP; PPC **00-2574**

MEIGS, Arthur V[incent] (1850-1912)
Analysis of human milk the basis of the artificial feeding of infants. New York: E. B. Treat & Co., 1902. 10 l. DNLM **00-2575**

MEIGS, Arthur V[incent] (1850-1912)
A study of the human blood-vessels in health and disease; a supplement to "The origin of disease." . . . With one hundred and three original illustrations. Philadelphia and London: J. B. Lippincott Co., [1907]. 136p. col. plates. DLC; NNNAM; PPC; PU **00-2576**

MELENDY, Mary R[ies] (*b.* 1842)
Cure of disease simplified. A modern vade-mecum for the household. [Chicago: Guiding Star Publishing House], 1901 [*c.* 1893]. 368p. DLC; ICJ **00-2577**

MELENDY, Mary R[ies] (*b.* 1842)
Perfect womanhood for maidens, wives, mothers. A book giving full information on all the mysterious and complex matters pertaining to women. Chicago: Monarch Book Co., 1903. 448p. plates. DLC; ICJ **00-2578**

MELENDY, Mary R[ies] (*b.* 1842)
Vivlore, the pathway to mental and physical perfection; the twentieth century book for every woman. [Chicago? 1904.] 648p. col. plates. DLC: ICJ **00-2579**

MELENDY, Mary R[ies] (*b.* 1842)
Perfect health and beauty for parents and children; a pure, searching and scholarly treatment of the life relation between the sexes. [Chicago? 1906.] 591p. DLC: ICJ **00-2580**

MELLER, Josef (*b.* 1874)
Ophthalmic surgery; a handbook of the surgical operations on the eyeball and its appendages as practiced at the clinic of Prof. Hofrat Fuchs. . . . the transl. reviewed by Walter L. Pyle . . . with 118 original illustrations. Philadelphia: P. Blakiston's Son & Co., 1908. 262p. DLC; NNNAM; PPC; PU **00-2581**

MELLIN'S FOOD COMPANY. BOSTON
The care and feeding of infants. Boston: Mellin's Food Co., 1900. 68p. DLC; MBM **00-2582**

MELLIN'S FOOD COMPANY. BOSTON
El cuidado y la alimentación de los niños. Boston, Mass.: Mellin's Food Co., 1901. 70p. plate. DLC; MB **00-2583**

MELLIN'S FOOD COMPANY. BOSTON
Les soins et alimentation des enfants. Boston, Mass.: Mellin's Food Co., 1901. 71p. plate. DLC; MB **00-2584**

MELLIN'S FOOD COMPANY. BOSTON
Diet after weaning; a manual for the care and feeding of children between the ages of one and two years. Boston, Mass.: Mellin's Food Co., 1905. 46p. DLC; MB **00-2585**

MELTZER, S[amuel] J[ames] (1851-1920)
Haemolysis. New York: Wynkoop, Hallenbeck, Crawford Co., 1901. 28p. DNLM **00-2586**

MELTZER, S[amuel] J[ames] (1851-1920)
Paratyphoid. New York, 1902. 15p. DNLM **00-2587**

MELTZER, S[amuel] J[ames] (1851-1920)
The role of inhibition in the normal and in some of the pathological phenomena of life. New York, 1902. 47p. DNLM; NNNAM **00-2588**

MELTZER, S[amuel] J[ames] (1851-1920)
On the contraction of the iliopsoas muscle as an aid in the diagnosis of the contents of the iliac fossa. New York, 1902. 10p. DNLM **00-2589**

MELTZER, S[amuel] J[ames] (1851-1920)
The influence of alcohol upon infection and its use in the treatment of acute infectious diseases. Philadelphia, 1902. 16p. DNLM **00-2590**

MEMMINGER, Allard (*b.* 1854)
The practical examination of urine, with special reference to diagnosis. 3rd ed., enl. and rev. Philadelphia: P. Blakiston's Son & Co., 1908. 116p. DLC; DNLM; PPC; PPJ **00-2591**

MENDEL, Emanuel (1839-1907)
Text-book of psychiatry: a psychological study of insanity for practitioners and students. . . . Authorized transl. edited and enlarged by William C. Krauss. . . . Philadelphia: F. A. Davis Co., 1907. 311p. DLC; ICU; NNNAM; PU **00-2592**

MERCK's 1901 manual of the materia medica. . . . New York: Merck & Co., 1900. 282p. NNNAM [Annual] **00-2593**

MERCK'S 1907 index (3rd ed.) An encyclopedia for the chemist, pharmacist and physician. . . . New York, St. Louis, Mo., [etc.] : Merck & Co., [1907] . 472p. DLC: ICJ; NNNAM; PU **00-2594**

MERCK'S report ready-reference, designed for use at the prescription counter and pharmaceutical laboratory. . . . New York: Merck & Co., 1900. 107p. DLC; NNNAM **00-2595**

MERTON, Holmes W[hittier] (*b.* 1860)
Descriptive mentality from the head, face and hand. Philadelphia: D. McKay, 1901. 224p. DLC; MH; NN [1st ed. pub. in 1893] **00-2596**

METCHNIKOFF, Elie (1845-1916)
The nature of man. Studies in optimistic philosophy. Transl. by P. Chalmers Mitchell. New York: G. P. Putnam's Sons, 1903. 309p. DLC; ICJ; NNNAM; PU [Gives view on intestinal auto-intoxication] **00-2597**

METCHNIKOFF, Elie (1845-1916)
Old age. [Washington, 1905.] 17p. DLC **00-2598**

METCHNIKOFF, Elie (1845-1916)
The new hygiene; three lectures on the prevention of infectious diseases. With a preface by E. Ray Lankester. New York: G. P. Putnam's Sons, 1906. 104p. DLC; NN [The Heinemann (London, 1906) ed., with the Putnam title page tipped in] **00-2599**

METCHNIKOFF, Elie (1845-1916)
Scientifically soured milk; its influence in arresting intestinal putrefaction and its action in the treatment of diseases caused by auto-intoxication. . . . New York: The Lacto-Bacilline Co. of New York, [1907] . 16p. DLC; NN **00-2600**

METCHNIKOFF, Elie (1845-1916)
The prolongation of life. Optimistic studies. The English transl. edited by P. Chalmers Mitchell. New York: G. P. Putnam's Sons, 1908. 343p. ICU; MH; NIC; NN **00-2601**

METCHNIKOFF, Elie (1845-1916)
The prolongation of life; optimistic studies . . . the English transl. edited by P. Chalmers Mitchell. . . . Popular ed., with an introduction by Charles S. Minot. New York and London: G. P. Putnam's Sons, 1910. 343p. DLC; MH; NIC; NN **00-2602**

METTLER, Lee H[arrison] (*b.* 1863)
Imperative conceptions: a study in differential diagnosis. . . . New York: William Wood & Co., 1903. 22p. DLC; DNLM; NN **00-2603**

METTLER, Lee H[arrison] (*b.* 1863)
A treatise on diseases of the nervous system. . . . Chicago: Cleveland Press, 1905. 989p. col. plates. DLC; DNLM; NNNAM; OCIM **00-2604**

MEYER, Willy (*b.* 1858)
The improvement of general anaesthesia on the basis of Schleich's principles. With special reference to anaesthol. [Chicago: American Medical Association, 1903.] 29p. NN **00-2605**

MEYER, Willy (*b.* 1858)
Carcinoma of the breast. Ten years' experience with my method of radical operation. [Chicago, 1905.] 16p. ICJ; NN **00-2606**

MEYER, Willy (*b.* 1858)
The improvement of general anesthesia on basis of the principle of adapting the boiling point of the anaesthetic to the temperature of the body (Schleich)—ten years' experience at the German Hospital. New York: William Wood & Co., 1908. 8p. NcD; NN **00-2607**

MEYER, Willy (*b.* 1858)
Esophagogastrostomy after intrathoracic resection of the esophagus. [Philadelphia, 1909.] 31p. NN **00-2608**

MEYER, Willy (*b.* 1858)
Some observations regarding thoracic surgery on human beings. [Read before the American Surgical Assoc. May 3, 1910.] [Philadelphia, 1910.] 25p. 4 plates. NN **00-2609**

MIAMI MEDICAL COLLEGE. CINCINNATI
Alumni catalogue. Including members of the faculty. 1852-1900. Compiled for the college by Archibald I. Carson. 2nd ed. Cincinnati, 1900. 134p. DNLM; OC **00-2610**

MIAMI MEDICAL COLLEGE. CINCINNATI
Addresses delivered at the forty-second annual commencement, May 1, 1903. By W. C. Cochran and Rev. David Philipson. Cincinnati: The McDonald Press, 1903. 14p. DNLM; OC **00-2611**

MICHIGAN. UNIVERSITY OF MICHIGAN, ANN ARBOR. DEPARTMENT OF MEDICINE AND SURGERY
Laying of the corner-stone of the new medical building. October 15, 1901. [Ann Arbor?], 1901. 64p. 2 plates. (in pagination). DNLM **00-2612**

MILBURY, Frank S[tephen] (1858-1900)
Suppurative ethmoiditis and its treatment. New York, 1900. 7p. DNLM **00-2613**

MILLER, Caspar W.
Specific gravity of the urine, and nitrogen elimination in pregnancy. Philadelphia, 1902. 3p. DNLM **00-2614**

MILLER, Charles C[onrad] (*b.* 1880)
Excision of the frenum preputii following laceration during a suspicious intercourse. New York, 1904. 6p. DNLM **00-2615**

MILLER, Charles C[onrad] (*b.* 1880)
The correction of featural imperfections. Chicago: The Author, [1907]. 134p. DLC **00-2616**

MILLER, Charles C[onrad] (*b.* 1880)
Cosmetic surgery. The correction of featural imperfections . . . 2nd ed., enlarged. [n. p.], 1908. 134p. CtY-M; ICJ; PPJ **00-2617**

MILLER, Charles C[onrad] (*b.* 1880)
The cure of rupture by paraffin injections. . . . Chicago: Oak Printing Co., 1908. 82p. DLC; ICJ; PU **00-2618**

MILLER, D. J. Milton
The prophylaxis of the summer diarrheas of infants. New York, 1900. 2 l. DNLM **00-2619**

MILLER, D. J. Milton
Three cases of head-nodding and head-rotation in rachitic infants. New York, 1900. 8p. DNLM **00-2620**

MILLER, D. J. Milton
A case of taenia saginata in a child of twenty-four months from the use of raw beef for the relief of chronic intestinal disturbance. New York, 1901. 3p. DNLM **00-2621**

MILLER, D. J. Milton
A case of acute hemorrhagic nephritis complicating influenza in an infant of thirteen months; with an analysis of 40 cases of influenzal nephritis. New York, 1902. 16p. DNLM **00-2622**

MILLER, D. J. Milton
A case of pneumococcic arthritis, accompanying acute croupous pneumonia. Philadelphia, 1902. 6p. DNLM **00-2623**

MILLER, D. J. Milton
Note of a case in which the time required by an inappropriate food to produce scorbutic symptoms was accurately noted. Philadelphia, 1902. 3p. DNLM **00-2624**

MILLER, D. J. Milton
A case of femoral thrombosis in acute croupous pneumonia. Philadelphia, 1903. 6p. DNLM **00-2625**

MILLER, D. J. Milton
The trained nurse. New York, 1903. 8p. DNLM **00-2626**

MILLER, D. J. Milton
Address to the members of the Philadelphia Pediatric Society at its eighth annual meeting, January 12, 1904. Philadelphia, 1904. 9p. DNLM **00-2627**

MILLER, D. J. Milton
The inaccuracy of the common spoon as a milk-sugar measure in the home modification of milk. New York, 1904. 3p. DNLM **00-2628**

MILLER, J. Preston
Primary sarcoma of the omentum. The clinical report of a case. Philadelphia, 1902. 14p. DNLM **00-2629**

MILLER, Oliver L.
Thermol in typhoid fever. Philadelphia, 1901. 8p. DNLM **00-2630**

MILLER PUBLISHING COMPANY. OMAHA, NEB.
Miller's prescriptions and formulas; containing 231 up-to-date prescriptions from the most reliable authorities of the medical profession, with full instructions as to preparation and use in the various diseases. Also 89 scientific pharmaceutical formulas. . . . Omaha, Neb.: Miller Publishing Co., [1906]. 106p. DLC **00-2631**

MILLER, R[obert] Gibson (1862-1919)
A synopsis of homoeopathic philosophy. Philadelphia, 1900. 21p. DNLM **00-2632**

MILLER, R[obert] Gibson (1862-1919)
Relationship of remedies. [1901.] 15p. DNLM **00-2633**

MILLS, Charles K[arsner] (1845-1931)
Publications of . . . , 1872-1900. [Philadelphia, 1900.] 16p. DNLM **00-2634**

MILLS, Charles K[arsner] (1845-1931), W. W. KEEN and W. G. SPILLER
Tumor of the superior parietal convolution accurately localized and removed by operation. New York, 1900. 21p. DNLM **00-2635**

MILLS, Charles K[arsner] (1845-1931)
Some neurological and medico-legal experiences and reflections. Denver, 1900. 14p. DNLM **00-2636**

MILLS, Charles K[arsner] (1845-1931)
A case of peripheral pseudo-tabes with exaggerated reflexes. Autopsy and microscopical examination showing degeneration of the peripheral nerves and no lesions of the spinal cord. New York, 1901. 6p. DNLM **00-2637**

MILLS, Charles K[arsner] (1845-1931)
The Czolgosz trial; a unique event. Philadelphia, 1901. 3p. DNLM **00-2638**

MILLS, Charles K[arsner] (1845-1931)
Political assassinations in some of their relations to psychiatry and legal medicine. Philadelphia, 1901. 16p. DNLM **00-2639**

MILLS, Charles K[arsner] (1845-1931)
The separate localization in the cortex and subcortex of the cerebrum of the representation of movements and of muscular and cutaneous sensibility. New York, 1901. 13p. DNLM **00-2640**

MILLS, Charles K[arsner] (1845-1931)
The surgery of brain tumors from the point of view of the neurologist; with notes on a recent case. Philadelphia, 1902. 20p. DNLM **00-2641**

MILLS, Charles K[arsner] (1845-1931) and William G. SPILLER
Case of external spinal pachymeningitis, implicating the entire ventral surface of the spinal dura. Philadelphia, 1902. 8p. 2 plates. **00-2642**

MILLS, Charles K[arsner] (1845-1931) and William G. SPILLER
A case of progressively developing hemiplegia, later becoming triplegia, resulting from primary degeneration of the pyramidal tracts. New York, 1903. 13p. DNLM **00-2643**

MILLS, Charles K[arsner] (1845-1931) and William G. SPILLER
Paralysis of all four limbs and of one side of the face with dislocation of sensation, developing in a few hours and resulting from meningo-encephalitis. [New York], 1903. 12p. DNLM **00-2644**

MILLS, Charles K[arsner] (1845-1931)
Neurology in Philadelphia from 1874-1904. New York, 1904. 15p. DNLM **00-2645**

MILLS, Charles K[arsner] (1845-1931)
The physiological areas and centres of the cerebral cortex of man, with new diagrammatic schemes. Philadelphia, 1904. 23p. DNLM **00-2646**

MILLS, Charles K[arsner] (1845-1931)
Subdivisions of the concrete concept area of the human cerebrum. New York, 1904. 28p. DNLM **00-2647**

MILLS, Charles K[arsner] (1845-1931)
Practical lessons in nursing. The nursing and care of the nervous and the insane. . . . New ed. Philadelphia, London: J. B. Lippincott Co., 1904. 132p. DLC; NN; PPC; PU **00-2648**

MILLS, Charles K[arsner] (1845-1931)
Treatment of aphasia by training. Chicago: Amer. Med. Assoc. Press, 1905. 22p. DNLM **00-2649**

MILLS, Charles K[arsner] (1845-1931)
Unilateral ascending paralysis and unilateral descending paralysis. Their clinical varieties and their pathologic causes. . . . Chicago: Press of the American Medical Association, 1906. 22p. DLC; ICJ **00-2650**

MILLS, Charles K[arsner] (1845-1931)
The Philadelphia Almshouse and the Philadelphia Hospital from 1854 to 1908. . . . [Philadelphia, 1909.] 52p. plates. DLC; PP; PPC; PU **00-2651**

MILLS, Charles K[arsner] (1845-1931)
Historical memoranda concerning the Philadelphia Hospital for the Insane. . . . An address at the semi-annual meeting of the Association of trustees and superintendents of the state and incorporated hospitals for the insane and feeble-minded of Pennsylvania, May 14, 1909, at the Philadelphia Hospital for the Insane. [Philadelphia, 1909.] 14p. DLC; PP; PPC; PU **00-2652**

MILWAUKEE COUNTY HOSPITAL TRAINING SCHOOL FOR NURSES, WANWATOSA
Annual announcements for the sessions of 1902-03 to 1904-05. Wanwatosa, 1902-04. DNLM [In association with Milwaukee County Hospital.] **00-2653**

MINNESOTA. STATE BOARD OF MEDICAL EXAMINERS
Official register of physicians, 1883-1903. [With lists of candidates licensed in April, June, and October, 1903; January, April, July, and October, 1904. January, April, 1905.] Minneapolis: Northwestern Lancet, 1903. 100p. DNLM; ICJ **00-2654**

MINOT, C[harles] S[edgwick] (1852-1914)
The embryological basis of pathology. Boston, 1901. 39p. DNLM **00-2655**

MINOT, C[harles] S[edgwick] (1852-1914)
A further study of the unit system of laboratory construction. New York, 1901. 7p. DNLM **00-2656**

MINOT, C[harles] S[edgwick] (1852-1914)
The problem of consciousness in biological aspects. [New York, 1902.] 26p. MB; NN **00-2657**

MINOT, C[harles] S[edgwick] (1852-1914)
The problem of consciousness in its biological aspects; address of the president of the American Association for the Advancement of Science, Pittsburgh, Pa., June 1, 1902. [Pittsburgh, 1902.] 26p. MH **00-2658**

MINOT, C[harles] S[edgwick] (1852-1914)
A laboratory text-book of embryology. Philadelphia: P. Blakiston's Son & Co., 1903. 380p. 2 plates. DNLM; PPC; PU **00-2659**

MINOT, C[harles] S[edgwick] (1852-1914)
The implantation of the human ovum in the uterus. [Philadelphia], 1904. 8p. DNLM **00-2660**

MINOT, C[harles] S[edgwick] (1852-1914)
The Harvard embryological collection. [1905.] 24p. MH **00-2661**

MINOT, C[harles] S[edgwick] (1852-1914)
The relations of embryology to medical progress. Oration delivered before the Maine State Medical Association, June 14, 1906. Boston, 1906. 20p. NN **00-2662**

MINOT, C[harles] S[edgwick] (1852-1914)
The problem of age, growth and death. Six lectures delivered at the Lowell Institute. Boston, [March, 1907.] 121p. DLC; MB; MH; MHi **00-2663**

MINOT, C[harles] S[edwick] (1852-1914)
The problem of age, growth and death: a study of Cytomorphosis. New York: G. P. Putnam's Sons, 1908. 280p. 73 textual illus. DLC; MH; NIC; NN **00-2664**

MINOT, C[harles] S[edgwick] (1852-1914)
Certain ideals of medical education. Chicago, 1909. 6p. MH; NN **00-2665**

MINOT, C[harles] S[edgwick] (1852-1914)
A laboratory text-book of embryology. . . . 2nd ed., rev., with 262 illustrations, chiefly original. Philadelphia: P. Blakiston's Son & Co., 1910. 402p. DLC; NcD; NjP; PU **00-2666**

MINOT, C[harles] S[edgwick] (1852-1914)
Henry Pickering Bowditch. [New York, 1910?] 6p. MB
00-2667

MISSOURI. UNIVERSITY OF MISSOURI. COLUMBIA
Graduates of the University of Missouri from its foundation to 1902, including the School of Mines, at Rolla, and the medical graduates, at St. Louis, Missouri. [Jefferson City, 1902.] 60p. DNLM **00-2668**

MITCHELL, C[harles] Ainsworth (*b.* 1867)
Flesh foods, with methods for their chemical microscopical, and bacteriological examination. A practical handbook for medical men, analysts, inspectors, and others. London: C. Griffin & Co.; Philadelphia: J. B. Lippincott, 1900. 336p. 1 plate. DNLM; NN; PPC; PU **00-2669**

MITCHELL, Clifford (1854-1939)
Manual of urinary analysis, containing a systematic course in didactic and laboratory instruction for students, together with reference tables and clinical data for practitioners, by . . . 3rd ed. . . . Philadelphia: Boericke & Tafel, 1902. 363p. DLC; ICJ; PPC; PPHa **00-2670**

MITCHELL, Clifford (1854-1939)
Diseases of the urinary organs, including diabetes mellitus and insipidus. . . . Philadelphia: Boericke & Tafel, 1903. 716p. DLC; ICJ; PPC; PU **00-2671**

MITCHELL, James F[arnandis]
The surgical treatment of tuberculous cervical adenitis. Baltimore, 1902. 18p. 5 plates. DLC; DNLM
00-2672

MITCHELL, John K[earsley] (1859-1917)
A case of myelitis exhibiting the results of coordination exercises. New York, 1902. 3p. DNLM
00-2673

MITCHELL, John K[earsley] (1859-1917)
Some points in the treatment of locomotor ataxia. Philadelphia, 1902. 4p. DNLM **00-2674**

MITCHELL, John K[earsley] (1859-1917)
Two unusual forms of clonus; toe-clonus and lateral ankle-clonus. New York, 1902. 4p. DNLM
00-2675

MITCHELL, John K[earsley] (1859-1917)
. . . Mechanotherapy and physical education, including massage and exercise, by John K. Mitchell . . . and Physical education by muscular exercise, by Luther Halsey Gulick . . . with special chapters on Orthopedic apparatus, by James K. Young . . . on Corrective manipulations in orthopedic surgery (including the 'Lorenz method'), by H. Augustus Wilson . . . and on Physical methods in ophthalmic therapeutics, by Walter L. Pyle. . . . With 229 illustrations. Philadelphia: P. Blakiston's Son & Co., 1904. 420p. DLC; ICJ; PPC; PU **00-2676**

MITCHELL, John K[earsley] (1859-1917)
Self help for nervous women; familiar talks on economy in nervous expenditure. . . . Philadelphia: J. B. Lippincott Co., [1909]. 201p. 1 plate. DLC; ICJ; PP; PPC
00-2677

MITCHELL, S[ilas] Weir (1829-1914)
A case of erythromelalgia, with microscopical examination of the tissue from an amputated toe. By S. Weir Mitchell . . . and William G. Spiller. . . . (From the William Pepper Laboratory of Clinical Medicine, University of Pennsylvania.) [Philadelphia and New York], 1900 [*c.* 1899]. 13p. CtY-M; DLC
00-2678

MITCHELL, S[ilas] Weir (1829-1914)
Dr. North and his friends. New York: The Century Co., 1900. 499p. MA; MB; MH; NN **00-2679**

MITCHELL, S[ilas] Weir (1829-1914)
The autobiography of a quack, and the case of George Dedlow. New York: The Century Co., 1900. 149p. 8 plates. DNLM; KU; MH; NN **00-2680**

MITCHELL, S[ilas] Weir (1829-1914)
Abraham Jacobi: medicus, magister, amicus. [1900.] 1 l. CtY-M **00-2681**

MITCHELL, S[ilas] Weir (1829-1914)
Doctor and patient. . . . 3rd ed. Philadelphia: J. B. Lippincott Co., 1901. 177p. CtY-M; NNNAM; OCIM; PPC
00-2682

MITCHELL, S[ilas] Weir (1829-1914)
Fat and blood: an essay on the treatment of certain forms of neurasthenia and hysteria. . . . 8th ed. Ed., with additions, by John K. Mitchell, M.D. Philadelphia, [etc.]: J. B. Lippincott Co., 1902. 236p. DLC; NNNAM; PPC; PU
00-2683

MITCHELL, S[ilas] Weir (1829-1914)
Nurses and their education. [1902.] 9p. DLC
00-2684

MITCHELL, S[ilas] Weir (1829-1914)
Historical notes of Dr. Benjamin Rush, 1777. Philadelphia, 1903. 22p. DLC; NN; PPL; PU **00-2685**

MITCHELL, S[ilas] Weir (1829-1914)
A case of uncomplicated hysteria in the male lasting thirty years, with postmortem examination. By S. Weir Mitchell . . . and William G. Spiller. . . . [Philadelphia], 1904. 13p. CtY-M; DLC; PPC; PU **00-2686**

MITCHELL, S[ilas] Weir (1829-1914)
Doctor and patient. . . . 4th ed. Philadelphia and London: J. B. Lippincott Co., 1904. 177p. DLC; MBM; NNNAM; PPC
00-2687

MITCHELL, S[ilas] Weir (1829-1914)
Books and the man. Read to the Charaka Club of New York, March 4, 1905. [n. p., 1905.] 11p. CtY-M; NcD; NN; RPB
00-2688

MITCHELL, S[ilas] Weir (1829-1914)
Address delivered at the commencement exercises, class '05, of the School of Nursing, the Presbyterian Hospital in the city of New York, Florence Nightingale Hall, May eleventh, nineteen hundred and five. [New York, 1905.] 11p. MH; NN
00-2689

MITCHELL, S[ilas] Weir (1829-1914)
Fat and blood, and how to make them. . . . Philadelphia and London: J. B. Lippincott Co., 1905. 236p. DLC; MBM; NNNAM; PU **00-2690**

MITCHELL, S[ilas] Weir (1829-1914)
Address of Dr. S. Weir Mitchell to the nurse-graduates of the Philadelphia Orthopaedic Hospital and Infirmary for Nervous Diseases, November 16, 1906. [n. p., 1906.] 17p. DLC; DNLM; NcD; NN **00-2691**

MITCHELL, S[ilas] Weir (1829-1914)
Toast: to the surviving members of the Pathological Society. Boston: Office of the Journal of Medical Research, [1907]. 3p. NN **00-2692**

MITCHELL, S[ilas] Weir (1829-1914)
The treatment by rest, seclusion, etc., in relation to psychotherapy. . . . Chicago: American Medical Association, 1908. 15p. DLC; PPL; PU **00-2693**

MITCHELL, S[ilas] Weir (1829-1914)
Address . . . to the graduating class of the New York Hospital Training School for Nurses, February 28th, 1908. [n. p.], 1908. 27p. DNLM; MH; NcD **00-2694**

MITCHELL, S[ilas] Weir (1829-1914)
Address to the American Neurological Association, by the president, S. Weir Mitchell. . . . [Chicago, 1909.] 16p. DLC **00-2695**

MITCHELL, S[ilas] Weir (1829-1914)
Address by S. Weir Mitchell. . . . Delivered on the opening of the new hall of the College of Physicians of Philadelphia, November 11th, 1909. [Philadelphia], 1909. 18p. DLC; DNLM; NcD; NN **00-2696**

MITCHELL, S[ilas] Weir (1829-1914)
Address delivered before the Medical and Chirurgical Society of Maryland, on the occasion of the dedication of its building. [n. p., 1909.] 7p. NN **00-2697**

MONELL, Samuel H[oward] (1857-1918)
Elements of correct technique. Clinics from the New York School of Special Electro-therapeutics. . . . New York: E. R. Pelton, 1900. 314p. DLC; MBM; NNNAM; PU **00-2698**

MONELL, Samuel H[oward] (1857-1918)
Rudiments of modern medical electricity. Arranged in the form of questions and answers prepared especially for students of medicine. . . . New York: E. R. Pelton, 1900. 165p. DLC; ICJ; NNNAM; PU **00-2699**

MONELL, Samuel H[oward] (1857-1918)
The treatment of disease by electric currents, a handbook of plain instructions for the general practitioner . . . 2nd ed. New York: E. R. Pelton, 1900. 1100p. plates. DLC; MBM; NNNAM; PPC **00-2700**

MONELL, Samuel H[oward] (1857-1918)
The treatment of disease by electric currents, a handbook of plain instructions for the general practitioner . . . 3rd ed. New York: E. R. Pelton, 1902. 1100p. CtY-M; NNNAM; PPC; PU **00-2701**

MONELL, Samuel H[oward] (1857-1918)
A system of instruction in X-ray methods and medical uses of light, hot-air, vibration and high-frequency currents . . . prepared especially for the post-graduate home-study of surgeons, general physicians, dentists, [etc.] . . . . New York: E. R. Pelton, [1902]. 656, 987-1010p. plates. DLC; NNNAM; PPC; PU **00-2702**

MONELL, Samuel H[oward] (1857-1918)
. . . Thirty chapters on static electricity, selected from the original Manual of static electricity in X-ray and therapeutic uses. . . . New York: E. R. Pelton, 1903. 366p. DLC; ICJ; NN; NNNAM **00-2703**

MONELL, Samuel H[oward] (1857-1918)
Electricity in health and disease; a treatise on authentic facts for general readers, in which is shown how electric currents are made to act as curative remedies, together with an account of the principal diseases which are benefited by them. Presenting also the solution of the problem of tuberculosis in the United States. . . . New York: McGraw Publishing Co., 1907. 321p. plates. DLC; MH-M; NNNAM; PU **00-2704**

MONELL, Samuel H[oward] (1857-1918)
High frequency electric currents in medicine and dentistry, their nature and actions and simplified uses in external treatments . . . finely illustrated with special instruction plates. New York: W. R. Jenkins Co., 1910. 465p. plates. DLC; MBM; NNNAM; PPC **00-2705**

MONKS, George H[oward] (*b.* 1853)
Intestinal localization; a study on the cadaver for the purpose of determining to what extent the various parts of the small intestine may be identified through an abdominal wound. Philadelphia, 1903. 19p. 6 plates, 1 tab. DNLM; PPC **00-2706**

MONKS, George H[oward] (*b.* 1853) and David D. SCANNELL
A case of acute pancreatitis, and necrosis of fat tissue laparotomy; drainage; death nine days after the operation; autopsy. Boston, 1903. 11p. DNLM; MH **00-2707**

MONTGOMERY, Douglass W[illiam] (1859-1941)
The cause of the streak in naevus linearis. [New York, 1901.] 10p. DNLM **00-2708**

MONTGOMERY, Douglass W[illiam] (1859-1941)
Instances of spontaneous cure in a leper family. New York, 1902. 19p. DNLM **00-2709**

MONTGOMERY, Douglass W[illiam] (1859-1941)
Leucloplasia in secondary syphilis. New York, 1903. 7p. DNLM **00-2710**

MONTGOMERY, Douglass W[illiam] (1859-1941)
Papilloma of the sole. [Chicago, 1903.] 7p. DNLM **00-2711**

MONTGOMERY, Edmund B.
The general practitioner and his relation to early surgical operations. New York, 1903. 12p. DNLM **00-2712**

MONTGOMERY, Edmund B.
Intestinal obstruction following appendiceal abscess; anastomosis with Murphy button; recovery. Chicago, 1904. 8p. DNLM **00-2713**

MONTGOMERY, Edmund B.
Report of a case of tetanus treated with anti-tetanic serum; recovery. Chicago: G. P. Englehard & Co., 1904. 4p. DNLM **00-2714**

MONTGOMERY, Edmund B.
Symphysiotomy in persistent mento-posterior (face) presentation. New York, 1904. 4p. DNLM
00-2715

MONTGOMERY, Edward E[mmet] (1849-1927)
Practical gynecology; a comprehensive text-book for students and physicians. . . . Philadelphia: P. Blakiston's Son & Co., 1900. 819p. DLC; DNLM; PPC; PU **00-2716**

MONTGOMERY, Edward E[mmet] (1849-1927)
Practical gynecology; a comprehensive text-book for students and physicians . . . 2nd rev. ed., with five hundred and thirty-nine illustrations, the greater number of which have been drawn and engraved specially for this work, for the most part from original sources. Philadelphia: P. Blakiston's Son & Co., 1903. 900p. DLC; DNLM; NNNAM; PPC
00-2717

MONTGOMERY, Edward E[mmet] (1849-1927)
The disturbances of menstruation, and their significance. New York, 1904. 11p. DLC; DNLM **00-2718**

MONTGOMERY, Edward E[mmet] (1849-1927)
Practical gynecology; a comprehensive text-book for students and physicians . . . 3rd rev. ed. With five hundred and seventy-four illustrations, the greater number of which have been drawn and engraved specially for this work, for the most part from original sources. Philadelphia: P. Blakiston's Son & Co., 1907. 970p. DLC; MBM; PPC; PU **00-2719**

MONTGOMERY, Frank H[ugh] (*b.* 1862)
A brief summary of the clinical, pathologic, and bacteriologic features of cutaneous blastomycosis (blastomycetic dermatitis of Gilchrist). From the observations of James Nevins Hyde and the writer; with illustrations from thirteen cases, three of them hitherto unpublished. Chicago, 1902. 16p. 8 plates on 4 l. DNLM; ICJ **00-2720**

MOODY, Charles S[tuart]
Backwoods surgery and medicine. New York: Outing Publishing Co., 1910. 100p. DLC; NN **00-2721**

MOORE, Albertus A[dair]
Placenta praevia centralis. Profuse haemorrhage; collapse; podalic version; manual extraction of placenta; recovery of mother. New York, 1904. 7p. DNLM
00-2722

MOORE, Alfred
Origin of the vermiform appendix. A preliminary report. New York, 1904. 5p. DNLM **00-2723**

MOORE, John T.
Nephritis in malaria. Philadelphia, 1901. 5p. DNLM
00-2724

MOORE, John T.
Malaria; marked cerebral and spinal symptoms; Kernig's sign present; double tertian. St. Louis, 1902. 8p. DNLM
00-2725

MOORE, John T.
An observation showing that the flagella of the malarial parasite are fertilizing elements. Baltimore, 1902. 3p. DNLM
00-2726

MOORE, John T.
Typhoid fever. Chicago: G. P. Englehard & Co., 1902. 155p. DNLM; ICJ; OCIM; PU **00-2727**

MOORE, John T. and W. S. ALLISON
A comparative study of the value of methylene blue and quinine in the treatment of malarial fever. New York, 1902. 10p. DNLM **00-2728**

MOORE, John W[illiam], ed. (1845-1937)
Smallpox (including vaccination), varicella, cholera asiatica, cholera nostras, erysipelas, erysipeloid, pertussis, and hay fever. . . . By H. Immermann . . . Th. von Jürgensen . . . C. Liebermeister . . . H. Lenhartz . . . G. Sticker . . . edited with additions by J. W. Moore. Philadelphia: W. B. Saunders & Co., 1902. 682p. col. plates. DLC; MH; NcD; PPHa [American ed., Nothnagel's encyclopedia of practical medicine]
00-2729

MOORE, Richard C[anning]
President's address. The sanatorium for treatment of pulmonary tuberculosis. St. Joseph, 1902. 8p. DNLM
00-2730

MOORE, Veranus A[lva] (1859-1931)
The preparation of tuberculin; its value as a diagnostic agent, and remarks on the human and bovine tubercle bacilli. Philadelphia, 1900. 22p. DNLM **00-2731**

MOORE, Veranus A[lva] (1859-1931)
An introduction to practical bacteriology for students and practitioners of comparative and of human medicine. 2nd ed. Boston: Ginn & Co., 1900. 143p. 1 plate. DNLM; MBM; MH; NNNAM **00-2732**

MOORE, Veranus A[lva] (1859-1931)
An introduction to practical bacteriology for students and practitioners of comparative and of human medicine. 3rd ed., enlarged and revised. Boston: Ginn & Co., 1905. 151p. 1 plate. DNLM; MBM; PPC; PU **00-2733**

MOOREHOUSE, George W[ilton]
Feeding in typhoid fever; with a report of cases. Boston, 1900. 20p. DNLM **00-2734**

MOOREHOUSE, George W[ilton]
Tuberculin reactions. Cleveland, 1900. 14p. DNLM
00-2735

MOOREHOUSE, George W[ilton]
A report of two cases of typhoid spine. Boston, 1902. 15p. DNLM **00-2736**

MORGAN, Francis P[atterson] (*b.* 1867)
Cerebral rheumatism. Philadelphia, 1900. 17p. DNLM
00-2737

MORGAN, Francis P[atterson] (*b.* 1867)
Glosso-labio-laryngeal paralysis, with report of a case. Philadelphia, 1900. 5p. DNLM **00-2738**

MORGAN, Francis P[atterson] (*b.* 1867)
Suggestions concerning the use of the metric system in prescription writing. Philadelphia, 1901. 8p. DNLM
00-2739

MORGAN, James D[udley] (1862-1919)
Symmetrical gangrene (Raynaud's) versus endarteritis obliterans. Chicago, 1902. 13p. DNLM **00-2740**

MORGAN, James D[udley] (1862-1919)
A study of gout. Chicago, 1904. 7p. DNLM
00-2741

MORGAN, John (1735-1789)
The journal of Dr. John Morgan of Philadelphia, from the city of Rome to the city of London, 1764, together with a fragment of a journal, written at Rome, 1764, and a biographical sketch [by Julia Morgan Harding]. Philadelphia: Printed for private circulation by J. P. Lippincott Co., 1907. 258p. plate, ports. DLC; NN; PPC; PU **00-2742**

MORRIS, Henry (1844-1926)
Surgical diseases of the kidney and ureter. Including injuries, malformations and misplacements . . . with two coloured plates, and upwards of two hundred engravings. New York: William Wood & Co., 1901. 2 v. DLC; ICJ; NNNAM; PPC
00-2743

MORRIS, Henry, ed. (1844-1926)
Human anatomy; a complete systematic treatise by various authors, including a special section on surgical and topographical anatomy; . . . 3rd ed., rev. and enl. Philadelphia: P. Blakiston's Son & Co., 1902. 1328p. DLC; DNLM; NNNAM; PPC **00-2744**

MORRIS, Henry (1844-1926)
Surgical diseases of the kidney and ureter including injuries, malformations and misplacements. . . . With two coloured plates and upwards of two hundred engravings. Chicago: W. T. Keener & Co., 1903. 2 v. ICJ; IEN-M; PPJ
00-2745

MORRIS, Henry (1844-1926)
. . . Essentials of materia medica, therapeutics and prescription writing, arranged in the form of questions and answers, prepared especially for students of medicine . . . 6th ed., thoroughly rev., by W. A. Bastedo. . . . Philadelphia, London, [etc.]: W. B. Saunders & Co., 1904. 294p. DLC; DNLM; PPC; PU **00-2746**

MORRIS, Henry (1844-1926)
. . . Essentials of materia medica, therapeutics and prescription writing, arranged in the form of questions and answers; prepared especially for students of medicine . . . 7th ed., thoroughly rev. and adapted to the eighth revision (1905) of the United States pharmacopoeia [!] by W. A. Bastedo. . . . Philadelphia and London: W. B. Saunders & Co., 1905. 300p. DLC; NNNAM; PPC; PPJ **00-2747**

MORRIS, Henry, ed. (1844-1926)
Morris's Human anatomy; a complete systematic treatise by English and American authors, ed. by Henry Morris . . . and J. Playfair McMurrich . . . ten hundred and twenty-five illustrations, three hundred and nineteen printed in colors. 4th ed., rev. and enl. . . . Philadelphia: P. Blakiston's Son & Co., 1902. 5 v. DLC; NNNAM; PPC; PU **00-2748**

MORRIS, Henry, ed. (1844-1926)
Morris's Human anatomy; a complete systematic treatise for English and American authors, edited by Henry Morris . . . and J. Playfair McMurrich . . . ten hundred and twenty-five illustrations, three hundred and nineteen printed in colors. 4th ed., rev. and enl. Philadelphia: P. Blakiston's Son & Co., 1907. 1530p. DLC; MBM; NNNAM; PPC **00-2749**

MORRIS, John Little
Pulmonary disease. An original article, with histories of cases. Chicago, 1904. 2 l. DNLM **00-2750**

MORRIS, Robert T[uttle] (1857-1945)
Diabetes in surgery. New York, 1901. 4p. DNLM
00-2751

MORRIS, Robert T[uttle] (1857-1945)
Normal involution of the appendix as a matter of surgical interest. New York, 1902. 5p. DNLM
00-2752

MORRIS, Robert T[uttle] (1857-1945)
Some of the avoidable causes of disaster in appendicitis work. Philadelphia, 1902. 3p. DNLM **00-2753**

MORRIS, Robert T[uttle] (1857-1945)
Dawn of the fourth era in surgery and other articles. Philadelphia: W. B. Saunders & Co., 1910. 145p. plates. DLC; ICJ; NN; PU **00-2754**

MORROW, Albert S[idney] (*b.* 1878)
The immediate care of the injured. Philadelphia: W. B. Saunders & Co., 1906. 340p. illus. (partly col.); DLC; ICJ; PPC; PU **00-2755**

MORROW, Albert S[idney] (*b.* 1878)
Diagnostic and therapeutic technic. . . . Philadelphia: W. B. Saunders & Co., 1910. 775p. DLC; NNNAM; PPC; PPJ
00-2756

MORROW, Joseph E.
A new method of holding in place the retained catheter. Indianapolis, 1902. 4p. DNLM **00-2757**

MORROW, Prince A[lbert] (1846-1913)
The prophylaxis and control of leprosy in this country. New York, 1900. 21p. DNLM **00-2758**

MORROW, Prince A[lbert] (1846-1913)
The prophylaxis of venereal diseases. Philadelphia, 1901. 20p. DNLM **00-2759**

MORROW, Prince A[lbert] (1846-1913)
Report of the committee of seven on the prophylaxis of venereal diseases in New York. New York, 1901. 33p. DNLM; NN; NNNAM **00-2760**

MORROW, Prince A[lbert] (1846-1913)
Social diseases and marriage, social prophylaxis. . . . New York and Philadelphia: Lea Bros. & Co., 1904. 390p. DLC; DNLM; NNNAM; PPC **00-2761**

MORSE, John L[ovett] (1865-1940)
An analysis of fifty-one cases of pneumothorax. Philadelphia, 1900. 7p. DNLM **00-2762**

MORSE, John L[ovett] (1865-1940)
Chronic enlargement of the spleen in infancy. Boston, 1900. 8p. DNLM **00-2763**

MORSE, John L[ovett] (1865-1940)
Fetal and infantile typhoid. Chicago: Amer. Med. Assoc. Press, 1900. 29p. DNLM **00-2764**

MORSE, John L[ovett] (1865-1940)
The frequency of rickets in infancy in Boston and vicinity. Chicago, 1900. 8p. DNLM **00-2765**

MORSE, John L[ovett] (1865-1940)
The leucocyte count in serous pleurisy. Philadelphia, 1900. 4p. DNLM **00-2766**

MORSE, John L[ovett] (1865-1940)
Rickets. Philadelphia, 1900. 14p. DNLM
00-2767

MORSE, John L[ovett] (1865-1940)
An analysis of thirty-two cases of congenital heart disease. New York, 1901. 7p. DNLM **00-2768**

MORSE, John L[ovett] (1865-1940)
A case of chronic arsenical poisoning in an infant of seven months. New York, 1901. 3p. DNLM
00-2769

MORSE, John L[ovett] (1865-1940)
A case of secondary anemia with splenic tumor. New York, 1901. 5p. DNLM **00-2770**

MORSE, John L[ovett] (1865-1940)
The diagnosis of typhoid fever in the laboratory. Chicago, 1901. 7p. DNLM **00-2771**

MORSE, John L[ovett] (1865-1940)
The feeding of infants. Philadelphia, 1901. 10p. DNLM
00-2772

MORSE, John L[ovett] (1865-1940)
Infantile atrophy. New York, 1901. 8p. DNLM
00-2773

MORSE, John L[ovett] (1865-1940)
Infantile scorbutus. Boston, 1901. 14p. DNLM
00-2774

MORSE, John L[ovett] (1865-1940)
A study of the plantar reflex in infancy. New York, 1901. 5p. DNLM **00-2775**

MORSE, John L[ovett] (1865-1940)
Three cases of epidemic cerebro-spinal meningitis in infants. Boston, 1901. 8p. DNLM **00-2776**

MORSE, John L[ovett] (1865-1940)
Value of the Widal reaction in infancy and childhood. New York, 1901. 7p. DNLM **00-2777**

MORSE, John L[ovett] (1865-1940)
A case of chondrodystrophy fetalis. New York, 1902. 7 l. 1 plate. DNLM **00-2778**

MORSE, John L[ovett] (1865-1940)
Cirrhosis of the liver in childhood. Boston: Damrell & Upham, 1902. 10p. DNLM **00-2779**

MORSE, John L[ovett] (1865-1940)
Notes on some diseases of the kidney and bladder in infancy. Philadelphia, 1902. 13p. DNLM **00-2780**

MORSE, John L[ovett] (1865-1940)
Fetal congenital and infantile typhoid. New York, 1903. 23p. DNLM **00-2781**

MORSE, John L[ovett] (1865-1940)
A note on the transmission of whooping-cough by indirect contagion. Boston, 1903. 4p. DNLM
00-2782

MORSE, John L[ovett] (1865-1940)
Otitis media in infancy. Chicago, 1903. 7p. DNLM
00-2783

MORRIS, John L[ovett] (1865-1940)
The relation of chronic enlargement of the spleen to anemia in infancy. Boston, 1903. 32p. 1 tab. DNLM
00-2784

MORSE, John L[ovett] (1865-1940)
A report of eight cases of pneumonia in infancy treated with antipneumococcic serum. New York, 1903. 7 l. DNLM
00-2785

MORSE, John L[ovett] (1865-1940)
Retropharyngeal abscess in infancy. Chicago, 1903. 7p. DNLM
00-2786

MORSE, John L[ovett] (1865-1940)
The treatment of the acute diarrheas of infancy. New York, 1903. 13p. DNLM **00-2787**

MORSE, John L[ovett] (1865-1940)
An analysis of one hundred and eighteen cases of lobar pneumonia in infancy. New York, 1904. 6 l. DNLM
00-2788

MORSE, John L[ovett] (1865-1940)
A case of traumatic hemopericardium. Boston, 1904. 7p. DNLM **00-2789**

MORSE, John L[ovett] (1865-1940)
The diagnosis of metapneumonic empyema in infancy and early childhood. Philadelphia, 1904. 6p. DNLM
00-2790

MORSE, John L[ovett] (1865-1940)
Hematuria as the earliest or only symptom of infantile scurvy. Chicago: American Medical Assoc., 1904. 8p. DNLM
00-2791

MORSE, John L[ovett] (1865-1940)
Milk laboratories. Detroit, 1904. 3p. DNLM
00-2792

MORSE, John L[ovett] (1865-1940)
Rheumatoid disease in children. Boston, 1904. 5p. DNLM
00-2793

MORSE, John L[ovett] (1865-1940)
A study of the caloric needs of premature infants. Philadelphia, 1904. 15p. DNLM **00-2794**

MORSE, John L[ovett] (1865-1940)
Tonsilitis a cause of acute nephritis. New York, 1904. 3 l. DNLM **00-2795**

MORSE, John L[ovett] (1865-1940)
The care and feeding of premature infants. New York: William Wood & Co., 1905. 10p. DNLM **00-2796**

MORSE, John L[ovett] (1865-1940)
Lobar pneumonia in infancy. Philadelphia, 1905. 7p. DNLM
00-2797

MORSE, John L[ovett] (1865-1940)
The treatment of acute nephritis in childhood. Philadelphia: J. B. Lippincott Co., 1905. 13p. DNLM
00-2798

MORSE, Nathan C[lark] (1856-1919)
Postoperative treatment; an epitome of the general management of postoperative care and treatment of surgical cases as practised by prominent American and European surgeons. Together with suggestions concerning the technique of certain operations with a view to securing better postoperative results. . . . Containing 5 plates and 155 other illustrations. Philadelphia: P. Blakiston's Son & Co., 1905. 468p. plates. DLC; MH-M; PPC; PU **00-2799**

MORSE, Nathan C[lark] (1856-1919)
Postoperative treatment; an epitome of the general management of postoperative care and treatment of surgical cases as practiced by prominent American and European surgeons. Together with suggestions concerning the technic of certain operations with a view to securing better postoperative results . . . 2nd ed., rev. and enl. Containing 5 plates and 175 other illustrations. Philadelphia: P. Blakiston's Son & Co., 1907. 490p. plates. DLC; NNNAM; PPC; PU
00-2800

MORTON A[ndrews] Stanford (1847-1925)
On refraction of the eye. Its diagnosis and correction of its errors. With a chapter on keratoscopy, and test types. 7th ed., rev. and enl. Philadelphia: P. Blakiston's Son & Co., 1906. 96p. DNLM; ICJ; PU **00-2801**

MORTON, Bowditch (1857-1909)
Handbook of first aid to the injured, prepared at the request of the Society for Instruction in First Aid to the Injured . . . revised under the authority of the Society, by Ellsworth Eliot . . . and Louis Faugères Bishop . . . 2nd rev. ed. New York: The Society, [1903]. 110p. CtY-M; MH; NN; NNNAM
00-2802

MORTON, Henry H[oldich] (*b.* 1861)
Genito-urinary diseases and syphilis . . . illustrated with half-tones and full-page color-plates. Philadelphia: F. A. Davis Co., 1902. 372p. col. plates. DLC; DNLM; NN; PPC
00-2803

MORTON, Henry H[oldich] (*b.* 1861)
Genito-urinary diseases and syphilis . . . illustrated with 158 half-tones and photo-engravings, and 7 full-page color-plates. 2nd ed., rev. and enl. Philadelphia: F. A. Davis Co., 1906. 500p. col. plates. DLC; NNNAM; PPC; PU
00-2804

MORTON, William J[ames] (1846-1920)
The use of electricity in chronic rheumatism. New York, 1900. 12p. DLC; DNLM **00-2805**

MORTON, William J[ames] (1846-1920)
Radiotheraphy for cancer and other diseases. New York: William Wood & Co., 1902. 19p. DLC; DNLM
00-2806

MORTON, William J[ames] (1846-1920)
Artificial fluorescence of living tissue in relation to disease. New York, 1904. 24p. DLC; DNLM
00-2807

MORTON, William J[ames] (1846-1920)
Memoranda relating to the discovery of surgical anesthesia, and William T. G. Morton's relation to this event. New York, 1905. 21p. 1 plate, port. New York, 1905. DLC; DNLM
00-2808

MORTON, William J[ames] (1846-1920)
Recent advances in electrotherapeutics. New York, 1905. 14p. DLC; DNLM **00-2809**

MOSSO, Angelo (1846-1910)
Fatigue. . . . Transl. by Margaret Drummond. New York: G. P. Putnam's Sons, 1904. 334p. DLC; ICJ; MH; NN
00-2810

MOTT, J. L., IRON WORKS. (NEW YORK)
Hospital fixtures. . . . New York: J. L. Mott Iron Works. [*c.* 1905.] 131p. DLC; ICJ; NNNAM [Operating theaters and rooms, sterilizing rooms, laboratories, morgues, autopsy tables, hydrotherapeutic apparatus, shampoo tables, slop sinks, etc.]
00-2811

MOTT, J. L., IRON WORKS. (NEW YORK)
Hospital appliances and fixtures. 2nd ed. . . . [New York: J. L. Mott Iron Works], 1905. 52p. DLC; ICJ; NNNAM; PU
00-2812

[MOTT, J. L., IRON WORKS. (NEW YORK)]
Hospital appliances and fixtures. . . . [New York: J. L. Mott Iron Works], 1905. 36p. DLC; MH; NNNAM; PU
00-2813

MOTTER, Murray G[alt] (1866-1926)
Medical education, with special reference to the subject of physiology. Chicago, 1905. 12p. DNLM; ICJ
00-2814

MOULLIN, C[harles] W[illiam] Mansell (1851-1940)
Enlargement of the prostate, its treatment and radical cure. 3rd ed. Philadelphia: P. Blakiston's Son & Co., 1904. 204p. 3 plates. DNLM; NNNAM; PPC; PU
00-2815

MOULTON, Charles W[ells], ed. (1859-1913)
The Doctor's red lamp: a book of short stories concerning the doctor's daily life. Akron: The Saalfield Publishing Co., 1904. 343p. 4 plates. DLC; MH; NIC; NN
00-2816

MOULTON, Charles W[ells], ed. (1859-1913)
The doctor's who's who. . . . New York, Akron, O., [etc.]: The Saalfield Publishing Co., 1906. 269p. DLC; MH; NN; PP
00-2817

MOULTON, Charles W[ells], ed. (1859-1913)
A biographical cyclopedia of medical history. Akron, O.: The Saalfield Publishing Co., 1906. 367p. NNNAM; OC; OCIM; PU
00-2818

MOURE, Jean G[abriel] É[mile] (1855-1941)
Elementary practical treatise on diseases of the pharynx and larynx. . . . Transl. and adapted by J. Malcolm Farquharson. . . . New York: Rebman Co., 1909. 403p. DNLM; ICJ; NNNAM; PU **00-2819**

MOURE, Jean G[abriel] É[mile] (1855-1941)
The abuse of the singing and speaking voice; causes, effects, and treatment, by E. J. Moure . . . [and] A. Bouyer, fils. . . . Transl. by Macleod Yearsley. . . . New York: Rebman Co., 1910. 130p. DNLM; ICJ; NN; PPC
00-2820

MOUNTOUX, Charles [George Reinhard] (*b.* 1859)
Health and disease. A popular exposition on the essentials of health, the causes of disease, the care of the sick and convalescent, with addenda. And also an appendix containing essays on the gradual physical degeneration of the human race, the causes of the increasing occurrence of childlessness, and the principles of sexual physiology. . . . Oakland, Cal.: The Author, 1905. 222p. DLC **00-2821**

MOYER, Harold N[icholas] (1858-1923)
The relation of the medical editor to original communications. Philadelphia, 1901. 5p. DNLM **00-2822**

MOYNIHAN, Berkeley [George Andrew] (1865-1936)
Diseases of the pancreas and their surgical treatment. By B. G. A. Moynihan and A. W. Robson. Philadelphia: W. B. Saunders & Co., 1903. 293p. DLC; ICJ; MBM; PPC **00-2823**

MOYNIHAN, Berkeley [George Andrew] (1865-1936)
Gall-stones and their surgical treatment. . . . Philadelphia, London: W. B. Saunders & Co., 1904. 386p. col. plates. DLC; NNNAM; PPC; PU **00-2824**

MOYNIHAN, Berkeley [George Andrew] (1865-1936)
Gall-stones and their surgical treatment. . . . 2nd ed., rev. and enl. Philadelphia and London: W. B. Saunders & Co., 1905. 458p. col. plates. DLC; DNLM; NNNAM; PU **00-2825**

MOYNIHAN, Berkeley [George Andrew] (1865-1936)
Abdominal operations. . . . Philadelphia and London: W. B. Saunders & Co., 1905. 694p. DLC; DNLM; NNNAM; PPC **00-2826**

MOYNIHAN, Berkeley [George Andrew] (1865-1936)
Abdominal operations . . . 2nd ed., thoroughly rev. Philadelphia and London: W. B. Saunders & Co., 1906. 815p. DLC; IU-M; NNNAM; PPC **00-2827**

MOYNIHAN, Berkeley [George Andrew] (1865-1936)
The pathology of the living, and other essays. . . . Philadelphia and London: W. B. Saunders & Co., 1910. 260p. CtY-M; DLC; PPC; PU **00-2828**

MOYNIHAN, Berkeley [George Andrew] (1865-1936)
Duodenal ulcer. . . . Philadelphia and London: W. B. Saunders & Co., 1910. 379p. DLC; NNNAM; PPC; PPJ **00-2829**

MRACEK, Franz (1848-1908)
Atlas and epitome of diseases of the skin . . . authorized translation from the German. 2nd ed., rev. and enl., ed. by Henry W. Stelwagon . . . with 77 colored plates by the artists, J. Fink and A. Schmitson. . . . Philadelphia: W. B. Saunders & Co., 1905. 273p. 113 plates. DNLM; NNNAM; PPC; PU **00-2830**

MUDD, Samuel A[lexander] (1833-1883)
The life of Dr. Samuel A. Mudd, containing his letters from Fort Jefferson, Dry Tortugas Island, where he was imprisoned for a period of 4 years for his alleged complicity in the assassination of Abraham Lincoln, with statements from Mrs. Samuel A. Mudd, Dr. Samuel A. Mudd, and Edward Spangler regarding the assassination and the argument of General Ewing on the question of the jurisdiction of the military commission, and on the law and facts of the case. Also: "Diary of John Wilkes Booth." Edited by his daughter, Nettie Mudd, with preface by Dr. Eldgridge Monroe of the Baltimore Bar. New York: The Neale Publishing Co., 1906. 326p. DLC; ICJ; MH; NN **00-2831**

MUENSTERBERG, Hugo (1863-1916)
Psychotherapy, New York: Moffat, Yard & Co., 1909. 401p. DLC; MH; NIC; NN **00-2832**

MUIR, Edwin S[tanton] (*b.* 1858)
Manual of materia medica and pharmacy, specially designed for the use of practitioners and medical, pharmaceutical, dental, and veterinary students . . . 3rd ed., rev. and enl. Philadelphia: F. A. Davis Co., 1904. 192p. DLC; PPC; PPHa; PU **00-2833**

MUIR, Robert (*b.* 1864) and James RITCHIE
Manual of bacteriology . . . by Robert Muir and James Ritchie. American edition (with additions) rev. and ed. from the 3rd English edition by Norman MacLeod Harris. . . . New York: The Macmillan Co., 1903. 565p. CtY-M; DNLM; NNNAM; PPC **00-2834**

MUIR, Robert (*b.* 1864) and James RITCHIE
Manual of bacteriology . . . by Robert Muir and James Ritchie. American edition (with additions) rev. and ed. from the 4th English edition by Norman MacLeod Harris. . . . New York: The Macmillan Co., 1907. 605p. CtY-M; DNLM; ICU; MH **00-2835**

MUIR, Robert (*b.* 1864) and James RITCHIE
Manual of bacteriology . . . by Robert Muir and James Ritchie. 5th ed. New York: The Macmillan Co., [1910]. 688p. DLC; MH; NN; PU **00-2836**

MUMFORD, J[ames] G[regory] (1863-1914)
On a certain lack of mechanical facility in surgeons. St. Paul, 1900. 4p. DNLM **00-2837**

MUMFORD, J[ames] G[regory] (1863-1914)
Is there a decadence of our ethical standard? St. Paul, Minn., 1901. 10p. DNLM **00-2838**

MUMFORD, J[ames] G[regory] (1863-1914)
The story of the Boston Society for Medical Improvement. Boston, 1901. 25p. DNLM **00-2839**

MUMFORD, James G[regory] (1863-1914)
A narrative of medicine in America. . . . Philadelphia and London: J. B. Lippincott Co., 1903. 508p. DLC; MH; NN; PPC **00-2840**

MUMFORD, James G[regory] (1863-1914)
Clinical talks on minor surgery. . . . Boston: The Old Corner Bookstore, [1903]. 115p. DLC; MBM; NNNAM; PPC **00-2841**

MUMFORD, James G[regory] (1863-1914)
Surgical aspects of digestive disorders, by James G. Mumford . . . in association with Arthur K. Stone. . . . New York: The Macmillan Co.; London: Macmillan & Co., 1905. 395p. DLC; MBM; NNNAM; PU **00-2842**

MUMFORD, James G[regory] (1863-1914)
Surgical aspects of digestive disorders, by James G. Mumford . . . in association with Arthur K. Stone. . . . 2nd ed. New York, London: The Macmillan Co., 1907. 395p. DLC; ICJ; NNNAM; PPC **00-2843**

MUMFORD, James G[regory] (1863-1914)
Surgical memoirs, and other essays. . . . New York: Moffat, Yard & Co., 1908. 358p. ports. DLC; ICJ; NNNAM; PU **00-2844**

MUMFORD, James G[regory] (1863-1914)
. . . Some end-results of surgery. . . . New York: Moffat, Yard & Co., 1908. 19p. DLC; MB; NNNAM; PU
00-2845

MUMFORD, James G[regory] (1863-1914)
The practice of surgery . . . with 682 illustrations. Philadelphia and London: W. B. Saunders & Co., 1910. 1015p. col. plate. DLC; MBM; NNNAM; PPC **00-2846**

MUMMERY, [John] P[ercy] Lockhart (*b.* 1875)
The after-treatment of operations. A manual for practitioners and house surgeons. New York: William Wood & Co., 1903. 221p. DNLM; NNNAM; PPC; PU **00-2847**

MUMMERY, [John] P[ercy] Lockhart (*b.* 1875)
The after-treatment of operations. A manual for practitioners and house surgeons. 2nd ed. New York: William Wood & Co., 1905. 240p. DNLM; MBM; PPC; PU
00-2848

MUMMERY, [John] P[ercy] Lockhart (*b.* 1875)
Diseases of the colon and their surgical treatment. . . . Illustrated by coloured and other plates, and numerous figures in the text, many of which are reproduced from the author's sketches. New York: William Wood & Co., 1910. 322p. DLC; ICJ; PPC; PU **00-2849**

MUNCASTER, S[tuart] B.
A new method of treatment for chronic intraocular diseases, such as atrophy of the optic nerve, choroidal troubles, etc. Chicago, 1902. 3p. DNLM **00-2850**

MUNDORF, George T[heodore]
Hereditary abnormity of the little finger. New York, 1904. 3p. DNLM **00-2851**

MUNDORF, George T[heodore]
The Kollmann five-glass test. New York, 1904. 7p. DNLM **00-2852**

MUNDY, William N[elson] (*b.* 1860)
. . . The eclectic practice in diseases of children for students and practitioners. . . . Cincinnati: The Scudder Bros. Co., 1902. 631p. DLC; NcD; OC; OCLloyd
00-2853

MUNDY, William N[elson] (*b.* 1860)
The eclectic practice in diseases of children, for students and practitioners . . . 2nd ed., rev., rewritten and enl. Cincinnati: The Scudder Bros. Co., 1908. 512p. DLC; ICJ; OCLloyd; OCIM **00-2854**

MUNRO, Henry S[umner] (*b.* 1869)
A handbook of suggestive therapeutics, applied hypnotism, psychic science. . . . St. Louis: C. V. Mosby Medical Book & Publishing Co., 1907. 353p. CtY-M; ICJ; IU-M; PPC
00-2855

MUNRO, Henry S[umner] (*b.* 1869)
A handbook of suggestive therapeutics, applied hypnotism, psychic science . . . 2nd ed. St. Louis: C. V. Mosby Medical Book & Publishing Co., 1908. 360p. DLC; ICJ; PPHa; PPJ **00-2856**

MUNRO, John C[ummings] (1858-1910)
Laminectomy. Chicago, 1900. 24p. 1900. DNLM
00-2857

MUNRO, John C[ummings] (1858-1910)
Surgical treatment of hemorrhagic pachymeningitis. Boston, 1902. 11p. DNLM **00-2858**

MUNRO, John C[ummings] (1858-1910)
The clinical diagnosis of typhoid perforation. Boston, 1903. 17p. DNLM **00-2859**

MUNRO, John C[ummings] (1858-1910)
Empyema from a surgical standpoint. [Philadelphia, 1903.] 6p. DNLM **00-2860**

MUNSON, Edward L[yman] (*b.* 1868)
The theory and practice of military hygiene. Illustrated by eight plates and nearly four hundred engravings. New York: William Wood & Co., 1901. 971p. plates. DLC; DNLM; NNNAM; PP **00-2861**

MUNSON, Edward L[yman] (*b.* 1868)
The civil sanitary function of the Army medical department in territory under military control. Washington: The Association of Military Surgeons, 1909. 34p. DLC; DNLM
00-2862

MUNSON, Edward L[yman] (*b.* 1868)
The principles of sanitary tactics. A handbook on the use of medical department detachments and organizations in campaign. [Menasha, Wis.: Press of Banta Publishing Co., 1910.] 306p. fold. maps. DLC; ICJ; MH; NIC
00-2863

MUNSON, Edward L[yman] (*b.* 1868)
A study in camp sanitation by Major Edward L. Munson and Captain LeRoy Eltinge. Fort Leavenworth, Kans.: Army Service Schools Press, 1910. 15p. maps, diags. DLC
00-2864

MUNSON, J. F.
A study of the stomach function in pulmonary tuberculosis. New York, 1905. 7p. DNLM **00-2865**

MURDOCH, Frank H[all]
The diagnosis of gastric ulcer, with report of cases. Philadelphia, 1900. 5p. DNLM **00-2866**

MURDOCH, Frank H[all]
Further remarks on orthoform in the diagnosis of gastric ulcer. New York, 1904. 5p. DNLM; MB
00-2867

MURDY, Robert L.
The obstetric guide; being a treatise on pregnancy and childbirth, prepared especially for the laity. . . . Aberdeen, S.D.: News Printing Co., 1907. 94p. DLC; ICJ
00-2868

MURPHY, Fred T.
Experiments with the McGraw elastic ligature. Boston: Old Corner Book Store, 1904. 5p. 2 plates. DNLM
00-2869

MURPHY, J[ohn] B[enjamin] (1857-1916)
Tuberculosis of the testicle, with special consideration of its conservative treatment. Chicago, 1900. 56p. DNLM
00-2870

MURPHY, J[ohn] B[enjamin] (1857-1916)
Fibroma of the mesentery. Philadelphia, 1901. 13p. DNLM **00-2871**

MURPHY, J[ohn] B[enjamin] (1857-1916)
Resection of the rectum per vaginam. Philadelphia, 1901. 19p. DNLM **00-2872**

MURPHY, J[ohn] B[enjamin] (1857-1916)
General surgery. . . . Chicago: The Year Book Publishers, [1901]. 551p. ICJ; OCIM [The . . . Year book of general surgery. Chicago: The Year Book Publishers, 1901-.] **00-2873**

MURPHY, J[ohn] B[enjamin] (1857-1916) and J. M. NEFF
Perforating ulcers of the duodenum. New York, 1902. 43p. DNLM **00-2874**

MURPHY, J[ohn] B[enjamin] (1857-1916)
General surgery. . . . Chicago: The Year Book Publishers, 1902. 553p. ICJ; OCIM **00-2875**

MURPHY, J[ohn] B[enjamin] (1857-1916)
The prostate. Chicago, 1902. 44p. DNLM **00-2876**

MURPHY, J[ohn] B[enjamin] (1857-1916)
The diagnosis of gall-stones. New York, 1903. 24p. 1 tab. **00-2877**

MURPHY, J[ohn] B[enjamin], ed. (1857-1916)
General surgery . . . November, 1903. Chicago: The Year Book Publishers, 1903. 556p. ICJ; NNNAM; OCIM **00-2878**

MURPHY, J[ohn] B[enjamin] (1857-1916)
Report of a case of typhoid perforation with peritoneal infection, and five other consecutive cases of general suppurative peritonitis; all recovered. Chicago, 1903. 13p. DNLM **00-2879**

MURPHY, J[ohn] B[enjamin] (1857-1916)
Tuberculosis of the female genitalia and peritoneum. [Chicago], 1903. 119p. DNLM **00-2880**

MURPHY, J[ohn] B[enjamin] (1857-1916)
Two thousand operations for appendicitis, with deductions from his personal experience. Philadelphia, 1904. 24p. DNLM **00-2881**

MURPHY, J[ohn] B[enjamin] (1857-1916)
Ankylosis. Arthroplasty—clinical and experimental. . . . [Chicago]: Press of the American Medical Association, [1905]. 77p. ICJ **00-2882**

MURPHY, J[ohn] B[enjamin] (1857-1916)
General surgery. . . . Chicago: The Year Book Publishers, [1906]. 583p. DLC; ICJ **00-2883**

MURPHY, J[ohn] B[enjamin], ed. (1857-1916)
General surgery. . . . Chicago: The Year Book Publishers, [1907]. 608p. ICJ; NNNAM; OCIM; PPC **00-2884**

MURPHY, J[ohn] B[enjamin], ed. (1857-1916)
General surgery. . . . Chicago: The Year Book Publishers, [1909]. 617p. ICJ; OCIM **00-2885**

MURRAY, Charles H[enry] (*b.* 1863)
Practice of osteopathy, its practical applications in the various diseases of the human body. Elgin, Ill.: [Brethren Publishing House], 1909. 338p. DLC; ICJ **00-2886**

MURRAY, Dwight H[enderson]
Rectocolonic lavage, with description of new and improved tubes. New York, 1904. 10p. DNLM **00-2887**

MURRAY, William (1839-1920)
Rough notes on remedies. [4th ed.] Philadelphia, P. Blakiston's Son & Co., 1901. 176p. PPJ **00-2888**

MUSSER, John H[err] (1856-1912)
A practical treatise on medical diagnosis for students and physicians. . . . 4th ed., rev. and enl. . . . Philadelphia and New York: Lea Bros. & Co., 1900. 1105p. col. plates. DLC; DNLM; NNNAM; PPC **00-2889**

MUSSER, John H[err] (1856-1912) and J. DUTTON STEELE
Some cases of dilatation of the stomach. Philadelphia, 1900. 16p. DNLM **00-2890**

MUSSER, John H[err] (1856-1912) and Joseph SAILER
Meralgia paresthetica. New York, 1900. 25p. DNLM **00-2891**

MUSSER, John H[err] (1856-1912)
Diagnosis of medical and surgical diseases of the liver and biliary passages. Philadelphia, 1900. 11p. DNLM **00-2892**

MUSSER, John H[err] (1856-1912)
The indications for the use of alcoholic stimulants in typhoid fever. Detroit: W. M. Warren, 1900. 5p. DNLM **00-2893**

MUSSER, John H[err] (1856-1912)
Subpectoral abscess. Philadelphia, 1900. 11p. DNLM **00-2894**

MUSSER, John H[err] (1856-1912)
On the use and abuse of lavage. Detroit: W. M. Warren, 1900. 5p. DNLM **00-2895**

MUSSER, John H[err] (1856-1912)
On the use of antitoxin in diphtheria, with special reference to small and frequently repeated doses. Philadelphia, 1900. 13p. DNLM **00-2896**

MUSSER, John H[err] (1856-1912), R. M. PEARCE and Norman GWYN
Two cases of streptothrical infection; demonstration of a streptothrix, or branched tubercle bacillus, in the sputum. Abscess of the brain due to a streptothrix. Philadelphia, 1901. 8p. 4 plates, 1 chart. DNLM **00-2897**

MUSSER, John H[err] (1856-1912) and Henry R. WHARTON
Perforating ulcer of the stomach; operation; recovery. Philadelphia, 1901. 5p. DNLM **00-2898**

MUSSER, John H[err] (1856-1912) and Aloysius O. J. KELLY
Hemoglobinuria complicating typhoid fever. Philadelphia, 1901. 6p. DNLM **00-2899**

MUSSER, John H[err] (1856-1912)
Notes on the fever of Hodgkin's disease; recurrent (Rückfall) fever; Ebstein's disease. Philadelphia, 1901. 18p. DNLM **00-2900**

MUSSER, John H[err] (1856-1912)
Notes on the fever of Hodgkin's disease; recurrent (Rückfall) fever; Ebstein's disease. Philadelphia, 1902. 15p. DNLM **00-2901**

MUSSER, John H[err] (1856-1912)
Notes on tropical dysentery. Chicago, 1901. 8p. 1 chart. DNLM **00-2902**

MUSSER, John H[err] (1856-1912)
On streptothrical infections. Philadelphia, 1901. 18p. DNLM **00-2903**

MUSSER, John H[err] (1856-1912)
Chronic myocarditis. 1. Morbid anatomy and physical signs. New York, 1902. 15p. DNLM **00-2904**

MUSSER, John H[err] (1856-1912)
Clinical expression of chronic myocarditis. New York, 1902. 27p. DNLM **00-2905**

MUSSER, John H[err], ed. (1856-1912)
Diseases of the bronchi, diseases of the pleura, and inflammation of the lungs. . . . By F. A. Hoffmann . . . O. Rosenbach . . . F. Aufrecht . . . edited with additions by John H. Musser. Philadelphia: W. B. Saunders & Co., 1902. 1029p. col. plates. DLC; NNNAM; PPC; PU [American ed., Nothnagel's encyclopedia of practical medicine] **00-2906**

MUSSER, John H[err] (1856-1912)
Primary cancer of the lung. Philadelphia, 1903. 19p. DNLM **00-2907**

MUSSER, John H[err] (1856-1912)
Abdominal pain. [Philadelphia], 1904. 11p. DNLM **00-2908**

MUSSER, John H[err] (1856-1912)
Motives in medicine. Philadelphia, 1904. 13p. DNLM **00-2909**

MUSSER, John H[err] (1856-1912)
Some aspects of medical education, president's address. Chicago: American Medical Assoc. Press, 1904. 23p. DNLM **00-2910**

MUSSER, John H[err] (1856-1912)
The treatment of pneumococci infection of the lung, or croupous pneumonia; a clinical lecture. Philadelphia: J. B. Lippincott Co., 1904. 14p. DNLM **00-2911**

MUSSER, John H[err] (1856-1912) and W. W. KEEN
Perforating gastric ulcer; posterior gastro-enterostomy; Fowler's position. Chicago: Amer. Medical Assoc., 1904. 4p. DNLM **00-2912**

MUSSER, John H[err] (1856-1912) and J. T. ULLOM
A case of status lymphaticus. Detroit: E. G. Swift, 1904. 23p. DNLM **00-2913**

MUSSER, John H[err] (1856-1912)
A practical treatise on medical diagnosis for students and physicians. . . . 5th ed., rev. and enl. Illustrated with 395 wood-cuts and 63 colored plates. Philadelphia and New York: Lea Bros. & Co., 1904. 1213p. col. plates. DLC; DNLM; NNNAM; PPC **00-2914**

MUSSER, John H[err], ed. (1856-1912)
A handbook of practical treatment. By 82 eminent specialists. Edited by John H. Musser and A. O. J. Kelly. Philadelphia: W. B. Saunders & Co., 1910-1917. 4 v. DLC; MH; NcD; PPC [Complete index to Vols. 1-4, W. B. Saunders & Co., 1917. 218p.] **00-2915**

MYNTER, Herman (1845-1903)
Appendicitis and its surgical treatment; with a report of one hundred and eighty-five operated cases. . . . 3rd rev. ed. Philadelphia, [etc.]: J. B. Lippincott Co., 1900. 231p. CtY-M; DLC; NNNAM; PPC **00-2916**

NAGEL, Joseph Darwin (*b.* 1867)
. . . Nervous and mental diseases. A Manual for students and practitioners. With an appendix on insomnia. . . . Illustrated with 46 engravings. Philadelphia and New York: Lea Bros. & Co., [1904]. 276p. DLC; DNLM; NNNAM; PPC **00-2917**

NAGLE, John Thomas (1842-1919)
An appeal to President Roosevelt for justice to a class of acting assistant surgeons of the United States Army, who served in the Civil War. . . . [New York: M. B. Brown Press, 1908.] 194p. DLC; ICJ; NNNAM; PPC **00-2918**

NAMMACK, Charles E.
The state care of consumptives. Philadelphia, 1900. 7p. DNLM **00-2919**

NAMMACK, Charles E.
Diagnosis and treatment of gastric ulcer. New York: A. R. Elliott, 1905. 13p. DNLM; NNNAM **00-2920**

NANCREDE, Charles Beylard [Guerard de] (1847-1921) and W. H. HUTCHINGS
Boiling as a method of sterilizing catheters. New York, 1903. 12p. DNLM **00-2921**

NANCREDE, Charles Beylard [Guerard de] (1847-1921)
. . . Essentials of anatomy, including the anatomy of the viscera arranged in the form of questions and answers, prepared especially for students of medicine. . . . 7th ed., thoroughly rev. Philadelphia, London, [etc.]: W. B. Saunders & Co., 1904. 419p. DLC; DNLM; NNNAM; PPC **00-2922**

NANCREDE, Charles Beylard [Guerard de] (1847-1921)
Lectures upon the principles of surgery, delivered at the University of Michigan . . . with an appendix containing a résumé of the principal views held concerning inflammation, by William A. Spitzley . . . 2nd ed., thoroughly rev. Philadelphia and London: W. B. Saunders & Co., 1905. 407p. DLC; DNLM; PPC; PU **00-2923**

NANCREDE, Charles Beylard [Guerard de] (1847-1921)
Influences and conditions which should be taken into account before one decides to operate. New York: William Wood & Co., 1908. 8p. DNLM **00-2924**

NANCREDE, Charles Beylard [Guerard de] (1847-1921)
Surgical diseases, certain abnormities, and wounds of the face. New York: William Wood & Co., 1908. 83p. DNLM **00-2925**

NASCHER, I[gnatz] L[eo] (*b.* 1863)
Geriatrics. [New York]: A. R. Elliott Publishing Co., 1909. 3p. NN **00-2926**

NASH, Eugene Beauharnais (*b.* 1838)
Leaders in typhoid fever. . . . Philadelphia: Boericke & Tafel, 1900. 135p. DLC; DNLM; PPC; PPHa **00-2927**

NASH, Eugene Beauharnais (*b.* 1838)
Leaders in homoeopathic therapeutics. 2nd ed. Philadelphia: Boericke & Tafel, 1901. 420p. DLC; ICJ; PPHa
00-2928

NASH, Eugene Beauharnais (*b.* 1838)
Regional leaders. . . . Philadelphia: Boericke & Tafel, 1901. 282p. DLC; PPHa **00-2929**

NASH, Eugene Beauharnais (*b.* 1838)
Leaders for the use of sulphur, with comparisons. . . . Philadelphia: Boericke & Tafel, 1907. 159p. DLC; ICJ; PPC; PPHa
00-2930

NASH, Eugene Beauharnais (*b.* 1838)
How to take the case and to find the similimum. . . . Philadelphia: Boericke & Tafel, 1907. 54p. DLC; PPC; PPHa
00-2931

NASH, Eugene Beauharnais (*b.* 1838)
Regional leaders . . . 2nd ed., rev. and enl. Philadelphia: Boericke & Tafel, 1908. 315p. DLC; PPHa **00-2932**

NASH, Eugene Beauharnais (*b.* 1838)
Leaders in respiratory organs. . . . Philadelphia: Boericke & Tafel, 1909. 188p. DLC; ICJ; PPC; PPHa **00-2933**

NASH, Eugene Beauharnais (*b.* 1838)
The testimony of the clinic. Philadelphia: Boericke & Tafel, 1910 [*c.* 1911]. 209p. DLC; DNLM; ICJ; PPHa
00-2934

NEAL, E. Virgil, ed.
Hypnotism and hypnotic suggestion: a scientific treatise on the uses and possibilities of hypnotism, suggestion and allied phenomena. By thirty authors. Ed. by E. Virgil Neal . . . and Charles S. Clark. Rochester, N.Y.: New York State Publishing Co., [1900]. 103p. DLC; NN [Issued by the American College of Sciences. *vel subseq.*] **00-2935**

NEESEN, Victor (*b.* 1872)
Six cases of chronic heart diseases successfully treated by the Schott method. New York, 1900. 13p. DNLM
00-2936

NEESEN, Victor (*b.* 1872)
Dr. Neesen's book on wheeling; hints and advice to men and women from the physician's standpoint. . . . New York: New Amsterdam Book Co., 1900 [*c.* 1899]. 106p. DLC; MB; NN; PPL **00-2937**

NEFF, M[ary] L[awson] (*b.* 1862)
A brief manual of prescription writing in Latin and English, for the use of physicians, pharmacists, and medical and pharmacal students. Philadelphia: F. A. Davis Co., 1901. 136p. DLC; DNLM; ICJ; PPC **00-2938**

NEFF, M[ary] L[awson] (*b.* 1862)
Mental hygiene. . . . [Detroti, Mich.]: Swift, 1904. 34p. ICJ; OCIM **00-2939**

NEFF, Wallace
The surgery of the Gasserian ganglion. Philadelphia, 1900. 15p. DLC; DNLM **00-2940**

NEFF, Wallace
Diagnosis and treatment of some of the ordinary fractures, with report of cases. Richmond, 1901. 18p. DLC; DNLM
00-2941

NEFF, Wallace
Ruptured traumatic aneurism of the femoral artery due to gunshot wound; with report of a case. Philadelphia, 1901. 7p. DLC; DNLM **00-2942**

NEFF, Wallace
Tuberculosis of the peritoneum. Richmond, 1901. 12p. DLC; DNLM **00-2943**

NEFF, Wallace
Multiple fistulae of the perineum, with report of a case. [Washington, 1903.] 7p. DLC **00-2944**

NEFF, Wallace
Furuncle and carbuncle. [Washington, 1903?] 4p. DLC
00-2945

NEISWANGER, Charles Sherwood (*b.* 1849)
Electro-therapeutical practice. A ready reference guide for physicians in the use of electricity. 7th ed. Revised, rewritten and greatly enlarged. . . . Chicago: E. H. Colgrove & Co., 1902. 202p. DLC; ICJ; NcD; PPJ **00-2946**

NEISWANGER, Charles Sherwood (*b.* 1849)
Electro-therapeutical practice; a ready reference guide for physicians in the use of electricity. 12th ed., rev., rewritten and greatly enl. . . . Chicago: Ritchie & Co., 1905. 276p. CtY-M; DLC; DNLM; ICJ **00-2947**

NEISWANGER, Charles Sherwood (*b.* 1849)
Electro-therapeutical practice; a ready reference guide for physicians in the use of electricity. 14th ed., rev., rewritten, and greatly enl. . . . Chicago: Ritchie & Co., 1907. 276p. DLC; ICJ; ICRM **00-2948**

NEISWANGER, Charles Sherwood (*b.* 1849)
Electro-therapeutical practice; a ready reference guide for physicians in the use of electricity. 15th ed., rev., rewritten and greatly enl. . . . Chicago: Ritchie & Co., 1908. 276p. DLC; ICJ **00-2949**

NEISWANGER, Charles Sherwood (*b.* 1849)
Electro-therapeutical practice; a ready reference guide for physicians in the use of electricity. 16th ed., rev. . . . Chicago: Ritchie & Co., 1909. 284p. DLC; ICJ
00-2950

NEISWANGER, Charles Sherwood (*b.* 1849)
Electro-therapeutical practice; a ready reference guide for physicians in the use of electricity. 17th ed., rev. . . . Chicago: Ritchie & Co., 1910. 285p. DLC; ICJ; PPHa
00-2951

NETTLESHIP, Edward (1845-1913)
Diseases of the eye. . . . Rev. and ed. by Wm. Campbell Posey . . . 6th American from the 6th English ed. With a supplement on examinations for color-blindness and acuity of vision and hearing, by William Thomson. . . . With 5 colored plates and 192 engravings. Philadelphia and New York: Lea Bros. & Co., 1900. 500p. plates. DLC; DNLM; NNNAM; PPC
00-2952

NEUSSER, Edmund von (1852-1912)
Clinical treatises on the symptomatology and diagnosis of disorders of respiration and circulation. . . . Authorized English translation by Andrew MacFarlane. . . . New York: E. B. Treat & Co., 1907-09. 3 v. CtY-M; DLC; PPJ; PU
00-2953

[NEW MEXICO]
New Mexico health resorts. [1900?] 87p. ICJ
00-2954

NEW YORK ACADEMY OF MEDICINE
Transactions of the . . . , 1896-1901. Semi-centennial celebration. New York, 1903. 471p. DNLM; NNNAM
00-2955

NEW YORK ACADEMY OF MEDICINE
List of current medical periodicals on file in the library. New York, 1904. 46p. DNLM; NNNAM **00-2956**

NEW YORK ACADEMY OF MEDICINE
List of current medical periodicals on file in the library. New York, 1904. 24p. (double col.) DNLM; NNNAM
00-2957

NEW YORK (CITY). DEPARTMENT OF PUBLIC CHARITIES
Bellevue Hospital formulary. City and county of New York. 5th revised ed. New York, 1901. 95p. DNLM; NNNAM; NNU-M **00-2958**

NEW YORK (CITY). DEPARTMENT OF PUBLIC CHARITIES
The hospital formulary of the department of public charities and the department of Bellevue and allied hospitals of the city of New York. 6th revised ed. W. E. Dreyfus, editor. New York, 1903. 160p. 2 plates. DNLM; NNNAM; NNU-M
00-2959

NEW YORK (CITY). DEPARTMENT OF PUBLIC CHARITIES
A nomenclature of diseases, and conditions and rules for the recording and filing of histories for Bellevue and allied hospitals. Adopted by the board of trustees. New York: M. B. Brown, 1903. 101p. DLC; DNLM; NNNAM: NNU-M
00-2960

NEWELL, Franklin S[pilman] (*b.* 1871)
The contraindications of the elective Caesarean section. Report of eight cases. Philadelphia, 1904. 18p. DNLM **00-2961**

NEWELL, Franklin S[pilman] (*b.* 1871)
The treatment of eclampsia. New York, 1905. 9p. DNLM
00-2962

NEWMAN, George (1870-1948)
Bacteriology and the public health. 3rd ed. Philadelphia: P. Blakiston's Son & Co., 1904. 497p. col. plates. DLC; MH; NN; PU [1st American ed., Bacteria, especially as they are related . . . to the public health. New York: G. P. Putnam's Sons, 1899. 348p.] **00-2963**

NICHOLS, C[harles] F[essenden]
Vaccination: a blunder in poisons. [Boston, 1902.] 65p. DNLM; MBM **00-2964**

NICHOLS, C[harles] F[essenden]
Vaccination: a blunder in poisons. [New York?], 1902. 65p. DLC; DNLM **00-2965**

NICHOLS, C[harles] F[essenden]
Vaccination; a blunder in poisons. [2nd ed.] [Boston: Rockwell and Churchill Press, 1903?] 69p. DLC
00-2966

NICHOLS, C[harles] F[essenden]
Homoeopathy and modern serum therapy, and homoeopathy's claim as a science in medicine. [Boston? 1905.] 7p. MB
00-2967

NICHOLS, C[harles] F[essenden]
The outrage vaccination. The arraignment of vaccination by eminent men, and by medical specialists. 3rd ed. Boston, 1908. 4p. DNLM [*vel subseq.*] **00-2968**

NICHOLS, Edward H[all] (1864-1922) and
Edward H. BRADFORD
The surgical anatomy of congenital dislocation of the hip-joint. Philadelphia, 1900. 22p. DNLM; PPC
00-2969

NICHOLS, Edward H[all] (1864-1922)
Diseases of the bones. [Philadelphia, 1907.] 58p. DNLM
00-2970

NICHOLS, Edward H[all] (1864-1922)
Surgical pathology; syllabus. Boston: Printed by J. L. Fairbanks, 1908. 43p. MH-M; N **00-2971**

NICHOLS, Edward H[all] (1864-1922)
Arthritis deformans [by] E. H. Nichols and F. L. Richardson. Boston, [1909]. 73p. 25 plates. MH-M
00-2972

NICHOLS, Henry J[ames] (1877-1927)
The relation between anthracosis and pulmonary tuberculosis. Philadelphia, 1905. 8p. DNLM **00-2973**

NICHOLS, Henry J[ames] (1877-1927)
Thrombosis of the receptaculum chyli and chylous ascites as a complication of cirrhosis of the liver. New York: Lea Bros. & Co., 1905. 16p. DNLM **00-2974**

NICHOLS, Henry J[ames] (1877-1927)
Tinea versicolor in an institution. Philadelphia, 1905. 9p. DNLM **00-2975**

NICHOLS, J[ohn] Benjamin (*b.* 1867)
A manual of clinical laboratory methods. New York: William Wood & Co., 1902. 303p. DNLM; ICJ; NNNAM; PU
00-2976

NICHOLS, J[ohn] Benjamin (*b.* 1867)
Acute leukemia. Philadelphia, 1903. 29p. DNLM
00-2977

NICHOLS, J[ohn] Benjamin (*b.* 1867)
The etiology of leukemia. Philadelphia, 1903. 22p. DNLM **00-2978**

NICHOLS, J[ohn] Benjamin (*b.* 1867)
The diet in typhoid fever. Philadelphia, 1905. 31p. DNLM
00-2979

NICHOLS, J[ohn] Benjamin (*b.* 1867)
. . . Diet in typhoid fever. . . . Providence: Snow & Farnham Co., printers, 1907. 92p. fold. chart. CtY-M; DLC; DNLM; ICJ **00-2980**

NICHOLS, J[ohn] Benjamin (*b.* 1867)
. . . The life of Thomas Sydenham, M.D., 1624-1689. . . . [Washington? D.C., 1909?] 12p. DLC
00-2981

NILES, George McCallum (*b.* 1864)
Pellegra, an American problem. . . . Philadelphia: W. B. Saunders & Co., 1910 [*c.* 1911]. 253p. DLC: ICJ; NcD; PU
00-2982

NILES, H[arry] D[orr] (1856-1909)
Surgical diseases of the sigmoid. New York: A. R. Elliott Co., 1904. 13p. DNLM **00-2983**

NOBLE, Charles P[ercy] (1863-1935)
Address in obstetrics. Pittsburgh, 1900. 29p. DNLM **00-2984**

NOBLE, Charles P[ercy] (1863-1935)
Nephrorrhaphy. [Chicago], 1900. 11p. DNLM **00-2985**

NOBLE, Charles P[ercy] (1863-1935)
Remarks on extra-uterine pregnancy. New York, 1900. 5p. DNLM **00-2986**

NOBLE, Charles P[ercy] (1863-1935)
Remarks on the influence of technique upon the results of closure of wounds of the abdominal wall. Boston, 1900. 16p. DNLM **00-2987**

NOBLE, Charles P[ercy] (1863-1935)
Report of a case of nephrectomy for pyonephrosis due to the impaction of a stone in the ureter, with remarks on the importance of the early diagnosis and treatment of renal calculi. New York, 1900. 4p. 1 plate DNLM **00-2988**

NOBLE, Charles P[ercy] (1863-1935)
Report of two cases of epithelioma of the vulva. New York, 1900. 3p. 1 plate. DNLM **00-2989**

NOBLE, Charles P[ercy] (1863-1935)
The complications and degenerations of fibroid tumors of the uterus as bearing upon the treatment of these growths. New York, 1901. 16p. DNLM **00-2990**

NOBLE, Charles P[ercy] (1863-1935)
General considerations of treatment of placenta previa. Detroit, 1901. 10p. DNLM **00-2991**

NOBLE, Charles P[ercy] (1863-1935)
The new formation of the female urethra, with report of a case. New York, 1901. 8p. DNLM **00-2992**

NOBLE, Charles P[ercy] (1863-1935)
The ultimate results of operation for cancer of the uterus. Philadelphia, 1901. 11p. DNLM **00-2993**

NOBLE, Charles P[ercy] (1863-1935)
Clinical report upon ureteral surgery. Philadelphia, 1902. 9p. DNLM **00-2994**

NOBLE, Charles P[ercy] (1863-1935)
The half-hitch suture; a new suture for use in anterior colporrhaphy. New York, 1902. 4p. DNLM **00-2995**

NOBLE, Charles P[ercy] (1863-1935)
Report of a case of epithelioma of the clitoris, with operation. New York, 1902. 4p. DNLM **00-2996**

NOBLE, Charles P[ercy] (1863-1935)
Two cases of deciduoma malignum. New York, 1902. 8p. DNLM **00-2997**

NOBLE, Charles P[ercy] (1863-1935)
The operative cure of procidentia uteri. Philadelphia, 1902. 5p. DNLM **00-2998**

NOBLE, Charles P] ercy] (1863-1935)
The treatment of suppuration in the uterine appendages. Philadelphia, 1902. 5p. DNLM **00-2999**

NOBLE, Charles P[ercy] (1863-1935)
The ultimate results of nephrorrhaphy. New York: E. B. Treat & Co., 1902. 2 l. DNLM **00-3000**

NOBLE, Charles P[ercy] (1863-1935) and W. Wayne BABCOCK
Report of three rare operations upon the urinary organs: 1. Hypernephroma of the kidney; nephrectomy. 2. Papillary carcinoma of the pelvis of the kidney; nephrectomy. 3. Stone in the left ureter; extraperitoneal operation; removal of the stone. [New York, 1902.] 11p. 2 plates. DNLM; NNNAM **00-3001**

NOBLE, Charles P[ercy] (1863-1935)
The use of the electric cautery clamp in the treatment of cancer of the uterus. New York, 1902. 6p. DNLM **00-3002**

NOBLE, Charles P[ercy] (1863-1935)
Exhibition of a specimen of abdominal pregnancy removed at the end of twenty-one months by coeliotomy. Philadelphia, 1903. 2p. DNLM **00-3003**

NOBLE, Charles P[ercy] (1863-1935)
Personal experience in operations upon diabetic patients. Philadelphia, 1903. 5p. DNLM **00-3004**

NOBLE, Charles P[ercy] (1863-1935)
Preliminary report of an operation for abdominal pregnancy of twenty-one months' duration. Philadelphia, 1903. 4p. DNLM **00-3005**

NOBLE, Charles P[ercy] (1863-1935)
The role of the cystoscope in the diagnosis and treatment of some diseases of the urinary tract. Pittsburgh, 1903. 10p. DNLM **00-3006**

NOBLE, Charles P[ercy] (1863-1935)
The significance of the temperature in the diagnosis of extra-uterine pregnancy during the period of collapse from hemorrhage. Philadelphia, 1903. 2p. DNLM **00-3007**

NOBLE, Charles P[ercy] (1863-1935)
A study of the degenerations and complications of fibroid tumors of the uterus from the standpoint of the treatment of these growths. New York, 1903. 14p. DNLM **00-3008**

NOBLE, Charles P[ercy] (1863-1935)
The Downes electrothermic clamps. Further experience in their use in the treatment of cancer of the uterus. Chicago, 1904. 6p. DNLM **00-3009**

NOBLE, Charles P[ercy] (1863-1935)
The nature of the indications for operation for fibroid tumors of the uterus. Philadelphia, 1904. 6p. DNLM **00-3010**

NOBLE, Charles P[ercy] (1863-1935)
Observations upon gastric, intestinal, and liver surgery in the German clinics. Philadelphia, 1904. 13p. DNLM **00-3011**

NOBLE, Charles P[ercy] (1863-1935)
Overlapping the aponeuroses in the closure of wounds of the abdominal wall. New York, 1904. 8p. DNLM
00-3012

NOBLE, Charles P[ercy] (1863-1935)
Report of a case of the invasion of a fibromyoma of the uterus by an adenocarcinoma, which by metaplasia had assumed the appearance of a squamous cell carinoma. New York, 1904. 5p. 1 plate. DNLM **00-3013**

NOBLE, Charles P[ercy] (1863-1935)
Some of the more unusual results of movable kidney. New York, 1904. 12p. DNLM **00-3014**

NOBLE, Charles P[ercy] (1863-1935)
The treatment of fibroid tumors of the uterus. Chicago, 1904. 8p. DNLM **00-3015**

NOBLE, Charles P[ercy] (1863-1935)
Cancer of the uterus. (Transactions of the New York State Medical Association, 1905.) New York, 1905. 8p. DNLM
00-3016

NOBLE, Charles P[ercy] (1863-1935)
Extrauterine pregnancy. [New York], 1905. 13p. DNLM
00-3017

NOBLE, Charles P[ercy] (1863-1935)
The treatment of retrodisplacements of the uterus. [Scranton], 1905. 16p. DNLM **00-3018**

NOBLE, George Henry (1860-1932)
I. Seventeen years of congenital nocturnal incontinence of urine cured by operation. II. Suspension of the uterus by intramural shortening of the round ligaments. III. An operation of cystocele. IV. Pregnancy in uterus bicornis. Philadelphia: W. J. Dornan, 1900. 53p. DNLM; PPC
00-3019

NOBLE, George Henry (1860-1932)
A flap operation for atresia of the vagina. Atlanta: Foote & Davies Co., 1900. 8p. DNLM **00-3020**

NOBLE, George Henry (1860-1932)
I. Seventeen years of congenital nocturnal incontinence of urine cured by operation. II. Suspension of the uterus by intramural shortening of the round ligaments. III. An operation for cystocele. IV. Pregnancy in uterus bicornis. Philadelphia: W. J. Dornan, printer, 1900. 55p. DNLM
00-3021

NOBLE, George Henry (1860-1932)
A new method of suturing the fascia and levator and muscle in perineorrhaphy; also an operation for complete laceration of the perineum designed for the purpose of eliminating danger of infections from the rectum. New York, 1903. 29p. DNLM; NNNAM **00-3022**

NOBLE, Richard B.
Rhythmic breathing plus olfactory nerve influence on respiration. Boston: R. B. Noble, 1908. 143p. MH; NN
00-3023

NOBLES, Newman T[homas] B[ritton] (*b.* 1874)
A text-book of minor surgery, including bandaging. Philadelphia: Boericke & Tafel, 1903. 325p. DNLM; ICJ; PPC; PPHa
00-3024

NOCARD, Edmond I[sadore] É[tienne] (1850-1903)
The animal tuberculoses and their relation to human tuberculosis. . . . Transl. by H. Scurfield. New York: W. R. Jenkins, 1901. 143p. diag. DLC; ICJ; MH-M; NN
00-3025

NOGUCHI, Hideyo (1876-1928)
The action of snake venom upon cold-blooded animals. . . . Washington: The Carnegie Institution, 1904. 16p. DLC [on *verso* of t. p.: Carnegie Institution of Washington, Publication, No. 12] **00-3026**

NOGUCHI, Hideyo (1876-1928)
Snake venoms, an investigation of venomous snakes with special reference to the phenomena of their venoms. Washington, D.C.: Carnegie Institution of Washington, 1909. 315p. 33 plates. DLC; DNLM; MH; NN [Plates 21-22 preceded by leaf with letterpress] **00-3027**

NOGUCHI, Hideyo (1876-1928)
Serum diagnosis of syphilis and the butyric acid test for syphilis . . . 14 illustrations. Philadelphia and London: J. B. Lippincott Co., [1910]. 173p. 3 plates. DLC; DNLM; PPC; PU **00-3028**

NOORDEN, Karl Harko von (1858-1944)
Clinical treatises on the pathology and therapy of disorders of metabolism and nutrition, by Prof. Dr. Carl von Noorden . . . pt. I-IX. . . . Authorized American edition. . . . New York: E. B. Treat & Co., 1903-1910. 9 v. DLC; ICJ; PPC; PPJ [Contents — I. Obesity, the indications for reduction cures — II. Nephritis — III. Membranous catarrh of the intestines (Colka mucosa) — IV. The acid autointoxication. — V. Concerning the effects of saline waters (Kissingen, Homburg) on metabolism. — VI. Drink restriction (thirst-cures) particularly in obesity. — VII. Diabetes mellitus, its pathological chemistry and treatment. Lectures delivered in the University and Bellevue Hospital Medical College, New York. Herter Lectureship Foundation. — VIII. Inanition and fattening cures. — IX. Technique of reduction cures and gout.]
00-3029

NOORDEN, Karl Harko von (1858-1944)
Metabolism and practical medicine. By Carl von Noorden . . . Anglo-American issue under the editorship of I. Walker Hall. . . . Chicago: W. T. Keener & Co., 1907. 3 v. CtY-M; ICJ; NcD; PPJ **00-3030**

NOORDEN, Karl Harko von (1858-1944)
New aspects of diabetes; pathology and treatment. . . . Lectures delivered at the New York Post-Graduate Medical School, New York. New York: E. B. Treat & Co., [1910?] 160p. diags. DLC; ICRM; NNU-M; PU **00-3031**

NORRIS, Charles C[amblos] (*b.* 1876)
Primary carcinoma of the vermiform appendix, and the report of a case. Philadelphia, 1903. 7p. DLC; DNLM
00-3032

NORRIS, George W[illiam] (*b.* 1875)
Some remarks on catalepsy, with notes on a case. Philadelphia, 1900. 8p. DNLM **00-3033**

NORRIS, George W[illiam] (*b.* 1875)
Croupous pneumonia. A clinical study of five hundred cases from the recent records of the Pennsylvania Hospital. Philadelphia, 1901. 7p. DNLM **00-3034**

NORRIS, George W[illiam] (*b.* 1875)
A contribution to the study of the human blood pressure in some pathological conditions. Philadelphia, 1903. 15p. DNLM
00-3035

NORRIS, George W[illiam] (*b.* 1875)
The diagnosis of incipient pulmonary tuberculosis. New York, 1904. 15p. DNLM **00-3036**

NORRIS, George W[illiam] (*b.* 1875)
The differential diagnosis between incipient pulmonary tuberculosis, healed cavities, and non-tuberculous fibrosis. New York, 1904. 6p. DNLM **00-3037**

NORRIS, George W[illiam] (*b.* 1875)
Tuberculosis and heart disease, based upon the study of 1,764 autopsies, 1,276 clinical histories, and a review of the literature. Philadelphia, 1904. 20p. DNLM; PPC **00-3038**

NORRIS, George W[illiam] (*b.* 1875)
Tuberculous pericarditis, based upon a study of 7,219 autopsies in Philadelphia hospitals. Philadelphia, 1904. 47p. DNLM; PPC **00-3039**

NORRIS, George W[illiam] (*b.* 1875)
Studies in cardiac pathology. Philadelphia: W. B. Saunders & Co., 1910. 235p. CtY-M; ICRM; NNNAM; PU
00-3040

NORRIS, Henry and J. M. ASHER
Urethral chancre. Philadelphia, 1902. 9p. DLC; DNLM
00-3041

NORRIS, Richard Cooper, ed. (*b.* 1863)
The American text-book of obstetrics for practitioners and students, by James C. Cameron, M.D., Edward P. Davis, M.D. . . . Richard C. Norris, M.D., editor, Robert L. Dickinson, M.D., art editor. With nearly 900 illustrations . . . 2nd ed., rev. Philadelphia, [etc.]: W. B. Saunders & Co., 1902. 2 v. col. plates. DLC; NNNAM; OCIM; PPC **00-3042**

NORRISS, H. C. R.
Toxins; their origin, their influence, their evidences, and their treatment by a new and rational process. With especial reference to cancers, tuberculosis, etc. [n. p., 1902.] 14p. port. DNLM; NNNAM **00-3043**

NORSTRÖM, G[ustaf Mauritz] (*b.* 1840)
The manual treatment of diseases of women. New York: G. E. Stechert, 1900. 230p. DNLM; ICJ; NNNAM; PU
00-3044

NORSTRÖM, G[ustaf Mauritz] (*b.* 1840)
Chronic headache, and its treatment by massage. New York: G. E. Stechert, 1903. 59p. DNLM; NNNAM
00-3045

NORSTRÖM, G[ustaf Mauritz] (*b.* 1840)
Diseases of the joints, and their treatment by massage. New York, 1904. 22p. DNLM; NNNAM **00-3046**

NORSTRÖM, G[ustaf Mauritz] (*b.* 1840)
A study of the affection writer's cramp. New York, 1904. 21 p. DNLM **00-3047**

NORSTRÖM, G[ustaf Mauritz] (*b.* 1840)
Chronic headache, and its treatment by massage. New York: A. R. Elliott Pub. Co., 1905. 43p. DNLM; NNNAM
00-3048

NORTHRUP, William P[erry], ed.
Diphtheria, measles, scarlet fever, and rötheln. . . . By William P. Northrup . . . Th. von Jurgensen . . . edited with additions by William P. Northrup. Philadelphia: W. B. Saunders & Co., 1902. 672p. col. plates. DLC; ICJ; NcD; PPHa [American ed., Nothnagel's encyclopedia of practical medicine]
00-3049

NORTHRUP, William P[erry]
Skin lesions associated with rapid growth of long bones, lineae albicantes (les vergetures de croissance, Jules Comby). New York, 1903. 8p. DNLM **00-3050**

NORTHRUP, William P[erry]
Joseph O'Dwyer. His methods of work on intubation; the measure of his success; the interest of both to young graduates. New York, 1904. 16p. DNLM **00-3051**

NORTHRUP, William P[erry]
Nervous exhaustion in infants. New York, 1905. 3 l. DNLM
00-3052

NORTHRUP, William P[erry]
The theory and practice of percentage feeding in infancy. Philadelphia, 1905. 10p. DNLM **00-3053**

NORTHRUP, William P[erry]
The strenuous life of school girls. New York, 1906. 11p. DNLM **00-3054**

NORTON, Alice [Peloubet] (*b.* 1860)
Food and dietetics. . . . Chicago: American School of Home Economics, 1907. 231p. tables, plates. DLC; ICJ; ICU
00-3055

NORTON, Alice [Peloubet] (*b.* 1860)
Food and dietetics. . . . [text book ed.]. Chicago: American School of Economics, 1910. 266p. tables, diags., plates. DLC; ICJ; ICU **00-3056**

NORTON, A[rthur] B[righam] (1856-1919)
Ophthalmic diseases and therapeutics. . . . With fifty-three illustrations and twelve chromolithographic figures. Philadelphia: Boericke & Tafel, 1901. 555p. col. plates. DLC; ICJ; NIC; PPC [1st printing, 1892] **00-3057**

NORTON, A[rthur] B[righam] (1856-1919)
Ophthalmic diseases and therapeutics. . . . 2nd ed., rev. and enl. Philadelphia: Boericke & Tafel, 1902. 647p. col. plates. DLC; MH-M; OC; PP [1st printing, 1898]
00-3058

NORTON, A[rthur] B[righam] (1856-1919)
Ophthalmic diseases and therapeutics. 3rd ed., rev. and enl. Philadelphia: Boericke & Tafel, 1902. 659p. CtY-M; ICJ; NNNAM; PPHa **00-3059**

NORTON, A[rthur] B[righam] (1856-1919)
Essentials of diseases of the eye. Philadelphia: Boericke & Tafel, 1904. 349p. DLC; MH-M; PPC; PPHa
00-3060

NORTON, George Mosse
Anaemia and chlorosis, and the rationale of chalybeate therapy in their treatment. New York: Eisner & Mendelson & Co., [1901?] 14p. DNLM; NNNAM **00-3061**

NORTON, John P[ease] (*b.* 1877)
The economic advisability of inaugurating a national department of health. . . . Chicago: Press of the American Medical Association, 1906. 15p. DLC; ICJ **00-3062**

NOTABLE physicians and surgeons of the present. [Medical World biographical sketches] New York: Berlin Publishing Co., 1910? unp. DNLM; IU-M; NIC **00-3063**

NOTES on physical diagnosis, for use in the College of Physicians and Surgeons, Columbia University, New York. New York: J. F. Dougherty, 1902. 72p. DNLM; NNC; NNNAM; NNU-M **00-3064**

NOTHNAGEL, Hermann (1841-1905)
. . . Diseases of the intestines and peritoneum . . . ed., with additions, by Humphrey [!] D. Rolleston. . . . Authorized translation from the German, under the editorial supervision of Alfred Stengel. . . . Philadelphia, New York, [etc.]: W. B. Saunders & Co., 1904. 1032p. 20 plates. DLC; DNLM; NNNAM; PPC [American ed., Nothnagel's encyclopedia of practical medicine] **00-3065**

NOTHNAGEL, Hermann (1841-1905)
. . . Diseases of the intestines and peritoneum . . . ed., with additions, by H. D. Rolleston . . . 2nd ed., thoroughly rev. Authorized translation from the German under the editorial supervision of Alfred Stengel. . . . Philadelphia and London: W. B. Saunders & Co., 1907. 1059p. plates. DLC; NNNAM; OCIM; PPC [American ed., Nothnagel's encyclopedia of practical medicine] **00-3066**

NOYES BROTHERS & CUTLER. (ST. PAUL, MINN.)
Illustrated catalogue of surgical and dental instruments. 4th ed. St. Paul, 1900. 1200p. ICJ; PU **00-3067**

NOYES BROTHERS & CUTLER. (ST. PAUL, MINN.)
General catalogue of . . . , importers and wholesale dealers in drugs, chemicals, patent medicines, pharmaceutical preparations, paints, oils, varnishes and window glass. . . . St. Paul, Minn., [1904-1909]. unp. ICJ [Library has vol. 27, 28, 32, 1904, 1905, 1909-1910. illus., col. plates.] **00-3068**

NOYES, Parker J[ewitt] (*b.* 1842)
Why Doctor Dobson became a quack and other stories. New York: Cochrane Publishing Co., 1910. 280p. DLC; MH; NN; NIC **00-3069**

NOYES, William B.
The criminal equivalent of insanity. New York: [Lea Bros. & Co.], 1902. 16p. NN **00-3070**

NUTT, John Joseph (*b.* 1870)
Health and hygiene for the household. . . . New York, London, [etc.]: The Abbey Press, [1901]. 69p. DLC; NN **00-3071**

NUTTALL, George H[enry] F[alkiner] (1862-1937)
. . . On the role of insects, arachnids and myriapods, as carriers in the spread of bacterial and parasitic diseases of man and animals. A critical and historical study. . . . Baltimore: The Johns Hopkins Press, 1900 [*c.* 1899]. 154p. plates. DLC; MH-M; MdBJ-W; MdU-D **00-3072**

NUTTALL, George H[enry] F[alkiner] (1862-1937)
Hygienic measures in relation to infectious diseases. . . . New York, [etc.]: G. P. Putnam's Sons, 1901. 112p. DLC; ICJ; NIC; NN [1st printing, 1893] **00-3073**

NUTTALL, George H[enry] F[alkiner] (1862-1937)
Blood immunity and blood relationship; a demonstration of certain blood relationships among animals by means of the precipitin test for blood, by George H. F. Nuttall . . . Including original researches by G. S. Graham-Smith . . . and T. S. P. Strangeways. . . . New York: G. P. Putnam's Sons, Inc. 1904. 444p. plates. DLC; MH; NIC; NNNAM **00-3074**

NUTTALL, George H[enry] F[alkiner] (1862-1937)
The bacteriology of diphtheria including sections on the history, epidemiology and pathology of the disease, the mortality caused by it, the toxins and antitoxins and the serum disease, by F. Loeffler . . . Arthur Newsholme . . . F. B. Mallory . . . G. S. Graham-Smith . . . George Dean . . . William H. Park . . . Charles F. Goldman. . . . Ed. by G. H. F. Nuttall . . . and G. S. Graham-Smith . . . New York: G. P. Putnam's Sons, Inc., 1908. 718p. 16 plates, 4 port, diags. DLC; ICJ; MH-M; NNNAM **00-3075**

NUTTING, M[ary] Adelaide (*b.* 1858)
. . . The education and professional position of nurses. . . . Washington: Government Printing Office, 1907. 60p. DLC **00-3076**

NUTTING, M[ary] Adelaide (*b.* 1858)
A history of nursing. The evolution of nursing systems from the earliest times to the foundation of the first English and American training schools for nurses by M. A. Nutting and Lavinia L. Dock. New York: G. P. Putnam's Sons, 1907-1912. 4 v. DLC; DNLM; MB; PU **00-3077**

NUTTING, Perley G[ilman] (*b.* 1873)
Outlines of applied optics. Philadelphia: P. Blakiston's Son & Co., 1910. 234p. DLC; PPC **00-3078**

O'BRIEN, H[enry] J[oseph], ed. (1862-1931)
Medical and surgical nursing; a treatise on modern nursing from the physician's and surgeon's standpoint for the guidance of graduate and student nurses, together with practical instruction in the art of cooking for the sick. . . . New York and London: G. P. Putnam's Sons, 1900. 287p. DLC; DNLM; MH-M; NNNAM **00-3079**

THE OBSTETRICAL SOCIETY OF BOSTON
Papers read at the meeting in commemoration of the fortieth anniversary of the foundation of the society. [Boston, 1901.] 85p. DNLM; MBM; MH; MHi **00-3080**

OCHSNER, A[lbert] J[ohn] (1858-1925)
The relation between gallstones and appendicitis. Philadelphia, 1900. 9p. 1 tab. DNLM **00-3081**

OCHSNER, A[lbert] J[ohn] (1858-1925)
Essentials in the construction of hospitals for large cities. Chicago, 1902. 16p. DNLM **00-3082**

OCHSNER, A[lbert] J[ohn] (1858-1925)
A handbook of appendicitis. Chicago: G. P. Engelhard & Co., 1902. 182p. DLC; DNLM; ICJ; OCIM **00-3083**

OCHSNER, A[lbert] J[ohn] (1858-1925)
Clinical observations on the surgery of the gall-bladder. Philadelphia: J. B. Lippincott Co., 1902. 25p. DNLM
00-3084

OCHSNER, A[lbert] J[ohn] (1858-1925)
The surgical treatment of tuberculous peritonitis. Philadelphia, 1902. 14p. DNLM **00-3085**

OCHSNER, A[lbert] J[ohn] (1858-1925)
Clinical surgery for the instruction of practitioners and students of surgery. . . . Chicago: Cleveland Press (The Clinical Review Publishing Co.), [1902]. 481p. plates. DLC; DNLM; IU-M; OCIM **00-3086**

OCHSNER, A[lbert] J[ohn] (1858-1925)
The construction of hospitals for the treatment of contagious diseases. [Chicago, 1904.] 16p. DNLM
00-3087

OCHSNER, A[lbert] J[ohn] (1858-1925)
Hospital construction in American cities and towns. Chicago, 1904. 26p. DNLM **00-3088**

OCHSNER, A[lbert] J[ohn] (1858-1925)
Minimum requirements for aseptic surgical operating in a hospital in which the personnel of the operating-room is permanent. Philadelphia, 1904. 12p. DNLM
00-3089

OCHSNER, A[lbert] J[ohn] (1858-1925)
A review of the histories of one thousand consecutive cases of appendicitis operated on at the Augustana Hospital during the thirty-three months from July 1, 1901, to April 1, 1904. 25p. DNLM **00-3090**

OCHSNER, A[lbert] J[ohn] (1858-1925)
Clinical surgery for the instruction of practitioners and students of surgery. . . . 2nd ed., rev. and enl. Chicago: Cleveland Press, 1904. 757p. plates. DLC; DNLM; ICJ; NcD
00-3091

OCHSNER, A[lbert] J[ohn] (1858-1925)
Hospitals for smaller cities and towns. . . . 1905. 18p. DNLM; ICJ **00-3092**

OCHSNER, A[lbert] J[ohn] (1858-1925)
A handbook of appendicitis. . . . [2nd ed.] Chicago: G. P. Engelhard & Co., 1906. 264p. ICJ; PPC
00-3093

OCHSNER, A[lbert] J[ohn] (1858-1925)
The organization, construction and management of hospitals, with numerous plans and details, by Albert J. Ochsner . . . and Meyer J. Sturm. . . . Chicago: Cleveland Press, 1907. 600p. plans, diags. DLC; ICJ; OCIM; PPC **00-3094**

OCHSNER, A[lbert] J[ohn] (1858-1925)
The organization, construction and management of hosptials, by Albert J. Ochsner and Meyer J. Sturm. 2nd ed., rev. and enl. Chicago: Cleveland Press, 1909. 654p. plans, diags. IU-M; NNC; PPC **00-3095**

OCHSNER, A[lbert] J[ohn] (1858-1925)
The surgery and pathology of the thyroid and parathyroid glands, by Albert J. Ochsner . . . and Ralph L. Thompson . . . with 57 illustrations in the text and 40 full-page plates, 4 of the plates being in colors. St. Louis: C. V. Mosby Co., 1910. 391p. DLC; ICJ; IU-M; OCIM **00-3096**

O'CONNOR, Joseph T.
American homoeopathic pharmacopoeia. . . . 8th ed. Philadelphia: Boericke & Tafel, 1906. 549p. OCLloyd; PPHa
00-3097

OERTEL, Horst (*b.* 1873)
On a case of leukaemia. . . . New Haven, Conn., [1900]. 6p. DNLM **00-3098**

OERTEL, Horst (*b.* 1873)
The anatomic histological processes of Bright's disease and their relation to the functional changes; lectures delivered in the Russell Sage Institute of Pathology, City Hospital, New York, during the winter of 1909. . . . Philadelphia and London: W. B. Saunders & Co., 1910. 227p. col. plates. DLC; ICJ; NNNAM; PPC **00-3099**

OERTEL, Horst (*b.* 1873)
On the determination of the cause of death and some cases of sudden death. [New York: A. R. Elliott Pub. Co., 1910.] 30p. illus. NN **00-3100**

OERTEL, Theodore Eugene (*b.* 1864)
Medical microscopy; designed for students in laboratory work and for practitioners . . . with 131 illustrations, some of which are colored. Philadelphia: P. Blakiston's Son & Co., 1902. 362p. DLC; ICJ; PPC; PU **00-3101**

OGDEN, J[ay] Bergen (*b.* 1868)
Clinical examination of the urine and urinary diagnosis, a clinical guide for the use of practitioners and students of medicine and surgery. Philadelphia: W. B. Saunders & Co., 1900. 416p. 11 plates. DNLM; ICJ; PPC; PU
00-3102

OGDEN, J[ay] Bergen (*b.* 1868)
Clinical examination of the urine and urinary diagnosis, a clinical guide for the use of practitioners and students of medicine and surgery. 2nd ed., thoroughly revised. Philadelphia: W. B. Saunders & Co., 1903. 418p. 11 plates. DNLM; MBM; PPC; PU **00-3103**

OGDEN, J[ay] Bergen (*b.* 1868)
The significance of oxaluria. New York, 1903. 8p. DNLM
00-3104

OGDEN, J[ay] Bergen (*b.* 1868)
Functional albuminuria, with a report of a case. Boston, 1904. 16p. DNLM **00-3105**

OGDEN, J[ay] Bergen (*b.* 1868)
A plea for uniformity of tests for albumin and sugar among medical examiners. New York, 1907. 12p. DNLM
00-3106

OGDEN, J[ay] Bergen (*b.* 1868)
Clinical examination of the urine and urinary diagnosis. . . . 3rd ed. Philadelphia: W. B. Saunders & Co., 1909. 427p. DLC; DNLM; PPJ; PU **00-3107**

OGILVY, Charles
The treatment of Pott's disease, and of rotary lateral curvature, by the plaster of Paris jacket and the aluminum corset. New York: A. R. Elliott, 1905. 30p. DNLM; NNNAM
00-3108

O'HANLON, Philip F.
Delayed results of a wound of the brain. New York, 1905. 4p. DLC; DNLM **00-3109**

O'HARA, M[ichael]
A method of performing anastomosis of hollow viscera by means of a new instrument. New York, 1900. 10p. DLC; DNLM **00-3110**

OHIO COLLEGE OF DENTAL SURGERY. DENTAL DEPARTMENT OF THE UNIVERSITY OF CINCINNATI
Annual announcements for the sessions of 1888-89 to 1906-07. (43.-61.). Cincinnati, 1888-1906. DNLM; OC **00-3111**

[OHIO] physicians' and dentists' directory of the State of Ohio. Comprising a list of physicians and surgeons and dentists. . . . Cincinnati: Gonsier, 1905. [101]-455p. ICJ; OC **00-3112**

OHMANN-DUMESNIL, Amant Henry (*b.* 1857)
Collier's methods exposed. Pipe dreams versus facts. St. Louis, [1906]. 8p. DNLM **00-3113**

OHMANN-DUMESNIL, Amant Henry (*b.* 1857)
Diseases of the skin . . . 3rd ed., thoroughly rev. and enl., 140 original illustrations. St. Louis: C. V. Mosby Medical Book & Pub. Co., 1908. 606p. DLC; ICJ; OCIM; PU **00-3114**

OLESON, Charles Wilmot (*d.* 1906)
Secret nostrums and systems of medicine, a book of formulas . . . 8th ed. Chicago: Oleson & Co., 1901 [*c.* 1896]. 255p. DLC; ICJ [Probably an unrevised reprint of the 6th ed., 1896.] **00-3115**

OLESON, Charles Wilmot (*d.* 1906)
Secret nostrums and systems of medicine, a book of formulas . . . [9th ed.] Chicago: Oleson & Co., 1902 [*c.* 1896]. 255p. ICJ **00-3116**

OLESON, Charles Wilmot (*d.* 1906)
Secret nostrums and systems of medicine, a book of formulas . . . 10th ed., rev. and enl. Chicago: Oleson & Co., 1902. 264p. DLC; ICRM; ICJ; PU **00-3117**

OLIVER, Charles A[ugustus] (1853-1911)
Color perception, normal and subnormal. [New York], 1901. 14p. DNLM **00-3118**

OLIVER, Charles A[ugustus] (1853-1911)
Memoir of William Fisher Norris. Philadelphia, 1901. 7p. port. DNLM **00-3119**

OLIVER, Charles A[ugustus] (1853-1911)
Report of a successful case of extensive blepharoplasty for the removal of an epithelioma. Philadelphia, 1901. 3p. DNLM **00-3120**

OLIVER, Charles A[ugustus] (1853-1911) and George B. WOOD
Orbital abscess associated with antral and ethmoidal disease. Philadelphia, 1902. 6p. DNLM **00-3121**

OLIVER, Charles A[ugustus] (1853-1911)
Blindness from congenital malformation of the skull. [Philadelphia, 1902.] 14p. 1 plate. DNLM **00-3122**

OLIVER, Charles A[ugustus] (1853-1911)
Clinical history of a case of blindness from congenital deformity of the occiput. Philadelphia, 1902. 7p. DNLM **00-3123**

OLIVER, Charles A[ugustus] (1853-1911)
An experimental study of the effects of change of color upon pigment bacteria. Philadelphia, 1902. 5p. DNLM **00-3124**

OLIVER, Charles A[ugustus] (1853-1911)
A histologic study of the crystalline lenses of a hanged criminal. [Philadelphia, 1902.] 6p. 1 plate. DNLM **00-3125**

OLIVER, Charles A[ugustus] (1853-1911)
A modification of the Abney pellet test for the ready detection of central scotomata. St. Louis, 1902. 3p. DNLM **00-3126**

OLIVER, Charles A[ugustus] (1853-1911)
A preliminary study of the ocular changes produced by the injection of pure cultures of the bacillus typhosus into the vitreous chambers of rabbits and guinea pigs. Philadelphia, 1902. 8p. DNLM **00-3127**

OLIVER, Charles A[ugustus] (1853-1911)
The teaching of ophthalmology in China. St. Louis, 1903. 8p. DNLM **00-3128**

OLIVER, Charles A[ugustus] (1853-1911)
Brief report upon the treatment of gonococcal conjunctivitis. [Philadelphia], 1904. 2 l. DNLM **00-3129**

OLIVER, Charles A[ugustus] (1853-1911)
A case illustrating the inadequacies of the present methods for the recognition of distant color signals, with a series of brief plans for remedying the same. [Philadelphia, 1904.] 8p. DNLM **00-3130**

OLIVER, Charles A[ugustus] (1853-1911)
Clinical and histologic study of the ophthalmic conditions in a case of cerebellar neoplasm occurring in a subject with renal disease. Philadelphia, 1904. 9p. DNLM **00-3131**

OLIVER, Charles A[ugustus] (1853-1911)
Regulation of color signals in marine and naval service. Philadelphia, 1904. 4p. DNLM **00-3132**

OLIVER, Charles A[ugustus] (1853-1911)
Right pulsating exophthalmos; ligation of both the right common carotid artery and the left internal carotid artery; accidental traumatism; cure. New York, 1904. 6p. DNLM **00-3133**

OLIVER, Charles A[ugustus] (1853-1911)
Sketch of the external appearances of uveitis from congenital syphilis. Philadelphia, 1904. 2p. DNLM **00-3134**

OLIVER, Charles A[ugustus] (1853-1911)
A brief note of the relative virulencies of differently tinted colonies of chromogenic bacteria. [Chicago], 1905. 4p. DNLM **00-3155**

OLIVER, Charles A[ugustus] (1853-1911)
A plea for governmental supervision of posts necessitating normal perception of color. [Philadelphia], 1905. 2p. DNLM **00-3136**

OLIVER, Charles A[ugustus] (1853-1911)
A study of simultaneous contrast color images. [Philadelphia], 1905. 3p. DNLM **00-3137**

OLIVER, Charles A[ugustus] (1853-1911)
The teaching of specialties in medicine. [Philadelphia], 1905. 1 l. DNLM **00-3138**

OLIVER, Charles A[ugustus] (1853-1911)
The requirements and the regulation of signalling by color. Abstract. [Philadelphia, Pa., 1909.] 10p. NN [Read before the Eleventh International Congress of Ophthalmology, in Naples, Italy, April 1909.] **00-3139**

OLIVER, George (1841-1915)
On bedside urine-testing; a clinical guide to the observation of urine in the course of work. New York: J. H. Vail & Co., 1901. 254p. plate, diags. DLC; ICJ; NNNAM [1st American from the 3rd English edition, 1885] **00-3140**

OLIVER, James (1836-1918)
Early intrauterine death, with undue delay in the occurrence of abortion thereafter (missed abortion). New York, 1904. 10p. DLC; DNLM **00-3141**

OLIVER, Thomas, ed. (1853-1942)
Dangerous trades: the historical, social, and legal aspects of industrial occupations as affecting health, by a number of experts; edited by Thomas Oliver. . . . New York: E. P. Dutton & Co., 1902. 891p. plates, tables, diags. DLC; NN; PPC; PPJ **00-3142**

OLIVER, Thomas (1853-1942)
Diseases of occupation. From the legislative, social and medical points of view. New York: E. P. Dutton & Co., 1908. 427p. DLC; MBM; NNNAM; PU [2nd ed., without change, 1909] **00-3143**

O'MALLEY, Austin (1858-1932)
Human terata. Philadelphia, 1903. 10p. DNLM **00-3144**

O'MALLEY, Austin (1858-1932)
Ethics of foeticide. Philadelphia, [1910]. 16p. PPC **00-3145**

O'MALLEY, Joseph
Diphtheria antitoxin in the infectious or bacterial broncho-pneumonia of childhood. Philadelphia, 1903. 8p. DNLM **00-3146**

O'MALLEY, Joseph and Austin O'MALLEY
Splenic anaemia, with haemoglobinaemia and decreasing splenomegaly. New York, 1905. 14p. DNLM **00-3147**

ONEAL, Oren
Eye and ear diseases cured at home. A treatise on diseases of the eye and ear and the Oneal dissolvent or natural method treatment. Chicago, Ill.: [Hollister, 1908?] 80p. DLC; ICJ **00-3148**

ONEAL, Oren
A treatise on diseases of the eye and the Oneal dissolvent treatment. Chicago, Ill.: [Hollister, 190?] 55p. ICJ **00-3149**

O'NEIL, Richard F[rothingham]
A case of stone in the bladder in a boy of fifteen. Boston, 1904. 5p. DNLM **00-3150**

O'NEIL, Richard F[rothingham]
Hematuria due to the Bilharzia hematobia, with the report of a case. Boston, 1904. 11p. 2 plates on 1 l. DNLM **00-3151**

OPHÜLS, W[ilhelm] (1871-1933) and Herbert C. MOFFITT
A new pathogenic mould (formerly described as a protozoon, Coccidiodes immitis pyogenes). Preliminary report. Philadelphia, 1900. 6p. DLC; DNLM **00-3152**

OPHÜLS, W[ilhelm] (1871-1933)
Infection of the rectum, with secondary infection of the liver, caused by the bacillus influenzae similis. Philadelphia, 1901. 10p. DLC; DNLM **00-3153**

OPIE, Eugene L[indsay] (1873-1962) and V. H. BASSETT
Typhoid infection without lesion of the intestine. A case of haemorrhagic typhoid fever with atypical intestinal lesions. Baltimore, 1901. 15p. DLC; DNLM **00-3154**

OPIE, Eugene L[indsay] (1873-1962)
The etiology of acute hemorrhagic pancreatitis. Baltimore, 1901. 20p. DLC; DNLM **00-3155**

OPIE, Eugene L[indsay] (1873-1962)
Filarial lymphatic varix. Philadelphia, 1901. 16p. DLC; DNLM **00-3156**

OPIE, Eugene L[indsay] (1873-1962)
The relation of cholethiasis to disease of the pancreas and to fat necrosis. Philadelphia, 1901. 16p. DLC; DNLM **00-3157**

OPIE, Eugene L[indsay] (1873-1962)
Disease of the pancreas; its cause and nature. Philadelphia & London: J. B. Lippincott Co., 1903. 359p. 11 plates. DLC; DNLM; PPC; PU **00-3158**

OPIE, Eugene L[indsay] (1873-1962)
An experimental study of the relation of cells with eosinophile granulation to infection with an animal parasite (trichina spiralis). Philadelphia, 1904. 17p. DLC; DNLM **00-3159**

OPIE, Eugene L[indsay] (1873-1962)
The occurrence of cells with eosinophile granulation and their relation to nutrition. Philadelphia, 1904. 22p. DLC; DNLM **00-3160**

OPIE, Eugene L[indsay] (1873-1962)
The relation of cells with eosinophile granulation to bacterial infection. Philadelphia, 1904. 28p. 1 plate. DLC; DNLM **00-3161**

OPIE, Eugene L[indsay] (1873-1962)
Zonal necrosis of the liver. Philadelphia, 1904. 20p. DLC; DNLM **90-3162**

OPIE, Eugene L[indsay] (1873-1962)
Disease of the pancreas, its cause and nature . . . 2nd ed., rewritten. . . . Philadelphia & London: J. B. Lippincott Co., 1910. 387p. plates. DLC; MBM; NNNAM; PPC **00-3163**

OPIE, Thomas (*b.* 1840)
Thirty-two unselected abdominal sections. [Philadelphia, 1901.] 33p. DLC; DNLM; PPC **00-3164**

OPPENHEIM, Hermann (1858-1919)
Diseases of the nervous system; a text-book for students and practitioners of medicine . . . authorized translation by Edward E. Mayer . . . 1st American from the 2nd rev. and enl. German ed., with two hundred and ninety-three illustrations. Philadelphia and London: J. B. Lippincott Co., 1900. 899p. DLC; IU-M; NNNAM; PPC **00-3165**

OPPENHEIM, Hermann (1858-1919)
Diseases of the nervous system; a text-book for students and practitioners of medicine . . . transl. and ed. by Edward E. Mayer . . . 2nd American ed., rev. and enl. With three hundred and forty-three illustrations. Philadelphia and London: J. B. Lippincott Co., 1904. 953p. plates. DLC; MBM; PPC; PU **00-3166**

OPPENHEIMER, Seymour (*b.* 1871)
On the use of suprarenal extract in diseases of the nose and throat. New York, 1900. 15p. DLC; DNLM **00-3167**

OPPENHEIMER, Seymour (*b.* 1871)
A general consideration on hyperplasia of the lingual tonsil. New York, 1902. 15p. DLC; DNLM **00-3168**

OPPENHEIMER, Seymour (*b.* 1871)
[Collected essays.] 106p. New York, 1903. 106p. DLC; MH; NN; NNNAM **00-3169**

OPPENHEIMER, Seymour (*b.* 1871)
The surgical treatment of chronic suppuration of the middle ear and mastoid . . . illustrated by forty-six half-tone plates containing sixty-four figures and twenty-seven key plates, all engraved from original drawings prepared from special dissections under the supervision of the author. Philadelphia: P. Blakiston's Son & Co., 1906. 425p. DLC; DNLM; PPC; PPJ **00-3170**

ORDRONAUX, John (1830-1908)
Address delivered to the medical graduates of the University of Vermont. Burlington: Free Press Association, 1901. 12p. DNLM; VtHi **00-3171**

ORDRONAUX, John (1830-1908)
Celebration of the semi-centennial anniversary of the founding of the Old Colony Historical Society of Massachusetts. Commemorative oration delivered at Taunton, Massachusetts, May 4, 1903. . . . Taunton, Mass.: The Old Colony Historical Society, 1903. 44p. DLC **00-3172**

O'REILLY, Brefney R[olph]
A manual of physical diagnosis . . . with 6 plates and 49 other illustrations. Philadelphia: P. Blakiston's Son & Co., 1910 [*c.* 1911]. 369p., illus. (partly col.), 3 plates. DLC; MH-M; NNNAM; PU **00-3173**

ORTNER, Norbert (1865-1935)
Treatment of internal diseases, for physicians and students . . . ed. by Nathaniel Bowditch Potter . . . transl. by Frederic H. Bartlett, M.D., from the 4th German ed. Philadelphia & London: J. B. Lippincott Co., [1908]. 658p. DLC: NNNAM; PPC; PU **00-3174**

OSBORNE, O[liver] T[homas] (*b.* 1862)
Introduction to materia medica and prescription writing. . . . [New York: Stettiner Bros.], 1900. 64p. DLC; MBM; NNNAM; OCLloyd **00-3175**

OSBORNE, O[liver] T[homas] (*b.* 1862)
Chronic endocarditis or valvular disease. New Haven, 1900. 9p. DNLM **00-3176**

OSBORNE, O[liver] T[homas] (*b.* 1862)
Graves' thyroid disease. New York, 1900. 22p. DNLM **00-3177**

OSBORNE, O[liver] T[homas] (*b.* 1862)
Therapeutic indications suggested by the condition of the blood. Chicago, 1901. 13p. DNLM **00-3178**

OSBORNE, O[liver] T[homas] (*b.* 1862)
A case of primary carcinoma of the lung. New Haven, 1902. 3p. DNLM **00-3179**

OSBORNE, O[liver] T[homas] (*b.* 1862)
A case of tumor of the cerebellum; autopsy, New York, 1902. 3p. DNLM **00-3180**

OSBORNE, O[liver] T[homas] (*b.* 1862)
A case of unusual cerebral hemorrhage. New York, 1902. 3p. DNLM **00-3181**

OSBORNE, O[liver] T[homas] (*b.* 1862)
The pathologic relations of the white blood corpuscles; a case of Hodgkin's disease of tuberculous origin; a case of lymphatic leukemia. Philadelphia, 1902. 17p. DNLM **00-3182**

OSBORNE, O[liver] T[homas] (*b.* 1862)
Therapeutic uses of the organic extracts. New York, 1902. 17p. DNLM **00-3183**

OSBORNE, O[liver] T[homas] (*b.* 1862)
The significance of variations in the internal secretions. New York, 1903. 14p. DNLM **00-3184**

OSBORNE, O[liver] T[homas] (*b.* 1862)
The aetiology and treatment of arteriosclerosis. New York, 1904. 13p. DNLM **00-3185**

OSBORNE, O[liver] T[homas] (*b.* 1862)
The management of pneumonia. New York: A. R. Elliott Co., 1905. 17p. DNLM **00-3186**

OSBORNE, O[liver] T[homas] (*b.* 1862)
The treatment of cerebrospinal meningitis. New York, 1906. 15p. DNLM **00-3187**

OSBORNE, O[liver] T[homas] (*b.* 1862)
Introduction to materia medica and pharmacology, including the elements of medical pharmacy, prescription writing, medical Latin, toxicology, and methods of local treatment. . . . Philadelphia and New York: Lea Bros. & Co., 1906. 167p. DLC; NNNAM; OCLloyd; PU **00-3188**

OSBORNE, O[liver] T[homas] (*b.* 1862)
Handbook of therapy . . . with a chapter on prescription writing by George W. Hall . . . 2nd ed. Chicago: The Journal of the American Medical Association, [1910]. 452p. CtY-M; DNLM; ICJ; PPC **00-3189**

OSGOOD, Charles (1808-1881)
The causes, treatment, and cure of fever and ague, and other diseases of bilious climates. Norwich, Conn., 1902. 15p. CtY-M; DNLM **00-3190**

OSGOOD, Robert B[ayley] (1873-1956)
Lesions of the tibial tubercle occurring during adolescence. Boston, 1903. 10p. 6 plates. DNLM; MBM **00-3191**

OSLER, William (1849-1919) and Thomas McCRAE
Cancer of the stomach. A clinical study. Philadelphia: P. Blakiston's Son & Co., 1900. 157p. DNLM; NNNAM; PPC; PU **00-3192**

OSLER, William (1849-1919)
On splenic anaemia. [Philadelphia, 1900.] 19p. DNLM **00-3193**

OSLER, William (1849-1919)
The home treatment of consumption. [Baltimore, 1900.] 4p. DNLM **00-3194**

OSLER, William (1849-1919)
A case of multiple gangrene in malarial fever. [Baltimore, 1900.] 4p. 2 plates. DNLM **00-3195**

OSLER, William (1849-1919)
Latent cancer of the stomach. [Philadelphia, 1900.] 9p. DNLM **00-3196**

OSLER, William (1849-1919)
Elisha Bartlett, A Rhode Island philosopher. An address delivered before the Rhode Island Medical Society, Dec. 7, 1899. With an appendix containing Dr. Bartlett's sketch of Hippocrates. Providence: Snow & Farnham, 1900. 43p. DNLM **00-3197**

OSLER, William (1849-1919)
On the study of tuberculosis. [Philadelphia, 1900.] 5p. DNLM **00-3198**

OSLER, William (1849-1919)
The principles and practice of medicine, designed for the use of practitioners and students of medicine . . . 4th ed. New York: D. Appleton & Co., 1901. 1182p. DLC: DNLM; NNNAM; PPC **00-3199**

OSLER, William (1849-1919)
On perforation and perforative peritonitis in typhoid fever. [Philadelphia, 1901.] 11p. DNLM **00-3200**

OSLER, William (1849-1919)
Books and men. [Boston, 1901.] 6p. DNLM **00-3201**

OSLER, William (1849-1919)
The progress of medicine in the nineteenth century. [New York, 1901.] 23 l. DNLM **00-3202**

OSLER, William (1849-1919)
The medical aspects of carcinoma of the breast; with a note on the spontaneous disappearance of secondary growth. [Philadelphia, 1901.] 19p. DNLM **00-3203**

OSLER, William (1849-1919)
On the advantages of a trace of albumin and a few tube casts in the urine of certain men above fifty years of age. [New York, 1901.] 5p. DNLM **00-3204**

OSLER, William (1849-1919)
Congenital absence of the abdominal muscles with distended and hypertrophied urinary bladder. [Baltimore, 1901.] 4 l. DNLM **00-3205**

OSLER, William (1849-1919)
On a family form of recurring epistaxis, associated with multiple telangiectases of the skin and mucous membranes. [Baltimore, 1901.] 6 l. DNLM **00-3206**

OSLER, William (1849-1919)
Alfred Stillé. Philadelphia, 1902. 18p. DNLM **00-3207**

OSLER, William (1849-1919)
A case of chronic purpuric erythema, eight years duration, with pigmentation of skin and enlargement of liver and spleen. New York: Grafton Press, [1902]. 5p. col. plate. NcD **00-3208**

OSLER, William (1849-1919)
The principles and practice of medicine, designed for the use of practitioners and students of medicine, . . . 5th ed. New York: D. Appleton & Co., 1902. 1182p. DLC; DNLM; IU-M; PU **00-3209**

OSLER, William (1849-1919)
On amebic abscess of the liver. New York, 1902. 15p. DNLM **00-3210**

OSLER, William (1849-1919)
Amebic dysentery. Detroit, 1902. 3p. DNLM **00-3211**

OSLER, William (1849-1919)
Chauvinism in medicine. An address before the Canadian Medical Association, Montreal, Sept. 17, 1902. Baltimore: Williams & Wilkins Co., 1902. 23p. DNLM **00-3212**

OSLER, William (1849-1919)
On the diagnosis of bilateral cystic kidney. Philadelphia, 1902. 6p. DNLM **00-3213**

OSLER, William (1849-1919)
On heredity in bilateral cystic kidney. Philadelphia, 1902. 2p. DNLM **00-3214**

OSLER, William (1849-1919)
Notes on aneurism. Chicago, 1902. 12p. DNLM **00-3215**

OSLER, William (1849-1919)
Some aspects of American medical bibliography. Baltimore, 1902. 16p. DNLM **00-3216**

OSLER, William (1849-1919)
William Beaumont, a pioneer American physiologist. An address before the St. Louis Medical Society, Oct. 4, 1902. [St. Louis], 1902. 29p. DNLM **00-3217**

OSLER, William (1849-1919)
Aneurism of the descending thoracic aorta. Philadelphia: J. B. Lippincott Co., 1903. 40p. 5 plates [4 plates on 2 l.] DNLM **00-3218**

OSLER, William (1849-1919)
On the educational value of the medical society. Boston, 1903. 16p. DNLM **00-3219**

OSLER, William (1849-1919)
The home in its relation to the tuberculosis problem. New York, 1903. 6p. DNLM **00-3220**

OSLER, William (1849-1919)
The master-word in medicine. Baltimore: J. Murphy Co., 1903. 33p. DNLM **00-3221**

OSLER, William (1849-1919)
On the need of a radical reform in our methods of teaching senior students. New York, 1903. 14p. DNLM **00-3222**

OSLER, William (1849-1919)
The principles and practice of medicine, designed for the use of practitioners and students of medicine . . . 5th ed. New York and London: D. Appleton & Co., 1903. 1182p. DLC; NNNAM; NNU-M; PU [Differs slightly from the 5th edition, published in 1902. cf. pp. 907-908.] **00-3223**

OSLER, William (1849-1919)
On obliteration of the superior vena cava. [Baltimore, 1903.] 14p. 3 plates. NcD **00-3224**

OSLER, William (1849-1919)
Aequanimitas, with other addresses to medical students, nurses, and practitioners of medicine. Philadelphia: P. Blakiston's Son & Co., 1904. 388p. DLC; DNLM; NNNAM; PPC **00-3225**

OLSER, William (1849-1919)
Science and immortality. Boston: Houghton, Mifflin & Co., 1904. 54p. DLC: DNLM; NNNAM; PPC **00-3226**

OSLER, William (1849-1919)
Counsels and ideals from the writings of . . . [Selected and edited by C. N. B. Camac.] Boston and New York: Houghton, Mifflin & Co., 1905. 277p. DLC; DNLM; NNNAM; PPC **00-3227**

OSLER, William (1849-1919)
The principles and practice of medicine, designed for the use of practitioners and students of medicine . . . 6th ed., thoroughly rev. from new plates. New York and London: D. Appleton & Co., 1905. 1143p. CtY-M; DLC; DNLM; PPC **00-3228**

[OSLER, William] (1849-1919)
Charaka Club. Folia of the Charaka Club to Dr. Osler. A record of things once said (and not regretted) by Dr. . . . and of things put before him at the dinner given in his honor. . . . New York, 1905. [unp.] PPC **00-3229**

OSLER, William (1849-1919)
Aequanimitas, with other addresses to medical students, nurses, and practitioners of medicine. [2nd ed.] Philadelphia: P. Blakiston's Son & Co., 1906. DLC; DNLM; NNNAM; PPC **00-3230**

OSLER, William, ed. (1849-1919)
Modern medicine, its theory and practice, in original contributions by American and foreign authors; ed. by William Osler . . . assisted by Thomas McCrae. . . . Philadelphia and New York: Lea Bros. & Co. [& Lea & Febiger], 1907-1910. 7 v. DLC; NNNAM; PPC; PU **00-3231**

OSLER, William (1849-1919)
An Alabama student, and other biographical essays. . . . New York: Oxford University Press, American Branch; [etc., etc.], 1908. 334p. plates. DLC; ICU; MA; NN **00-3232**

OSLER, William (1849-1919)
Vienna after thirty-four years. [Boston: Merrymount Press, 1908?] 18p. N **00-3233**

OSLER, William (1849-1919)
The principles and practice of medicine, designed for the use of practitioners and students of medicine . . . 7th ed., thoroughly rev. New York and London: D. Appleton & Co., 1909. 1143p. DLC: IU-M; MBM; NNNAM **00-3234**

OSLER, William (1849-1919)
Michael Servetus. [Baltimore, 1909.] 31p. plates. NN **00-3235**

OSLER, William (1849-1919)
In memoriam: Dr. John Hewetson, 1867-1910 [by W. O. and Lewellys F. Barker. Baltimore], 1910. 4p. NcD **00-3236**

OSTEOPATHIC ASSOCIATION OF THE DISTRICT OF COLUMBIA
. . . Answer of the Osteopathic Association of the District of Columbia to Senate Document No. 436, entitled "Medical Educational Standards." [Washington: Government Printing Office, 1906.] 16p. DLC **00-3237**

[OSTEOPATHY]
Home study course in osteopathy, massage, and manual therapeutics. [2nd ed.] Chicago, 1902. 130p. ICJ **00-3238**

OSTHEIMER, Maurice
A case of congenital rachitis. New York: E. B. Treat & Co., 1902. 1 sheet. DNLM **00-3239**

OSTHEIMER, Maurice
The death of Virchow. Philadelphia, 1902. 7p. port. DLC; DNLM; PU **00-3240**

OSTROM, Henry (*b.* 1862)
Rich in yesterdays; a message to the aged . . . ; illustrations by Wilbur Kurtz and Esther Chapman. Fairbury, Ill., Philadelphia, Pa.: The Praise Publishing Co., [1909]. 111p. frontis. (port.). DLC; PU **00-3241**

OSTROM, Homer I[rvin] (*b.* 1852)
The diseases of the uterine cervix. Philadelphia: Boericke & Tafel, 1904. 386p. DLC; DNLM; ICJ; PPC; PPHa **00-3242**

OSTROM, Homer I[rvin] (*b.* 1852)
Leucorrhoea and other varieties of gynaecological catarrh; a treatise on the catarrhal affections of the genital canal of women; their medical and surgical treatment. . . . Philadelphia, Pa.: Boericke & Tafel, 1910. 179p. DLC; ICJ; PPC; PPHa **00-3243**

OSTROM, Kurre W[ilhelm] (*b.* 1856)
Massage and the original Swedish movements; their application to various diseases of the body . . . 5th ed., rev. and enl., with one hundred and fifteen illustrations. Philadelphia: P. Blakiston's Son & Co., 1902. 181p. DLC: ICJ; PPC; PU **00-3244**

OSTROM, Kurre W[ilhelm] (*b.* 1856)
Massage and the original Swedish movements. . . . Lectures before the training school for nurses connected with the hospital of the University of Pennsylvania. 6th ed., revised and enlarged. Philadelphia: P. Blakiston's Son & Co., 1905. 184p. DLC; DNLM; PPC; PU **00-3245**

OSWALD, Felix L[eopold] (1845-1906)
Vaccination, a crime; with comments on other sanitary superstitions. New York: Physical Culture Pub. Co., 1901. 195p. DLC; PPC **00-3246**

OTIS, Edward O[sgood] (1848-1933)
The duty of state and municipality in the care of pulmonary tuberculosis among the poor. Albany, 1900. 13p. DLC; DNLM **00-3247**

OTIS, Edward O[sgood] (1848-1933)
Especial hospitals for consumption among the poor in our cities. Philadelphia, 1900. 9p. DLC; DNLM **00-3248**

OTIS, Edward O[sgood] (1848-1933)
Further notes upon the diagnostic test of tuberculin. New York, 1901. 6p. DLC; DNLM **00-3249**

OTIS, Edward O[sgood] (1848-1933)
Dispensaries for tuberculosis, wiht a description of the tuberculosis department of the Boston Dispensary. [Asheville, N.C.], 1903. 11p. DLC; DNLM **00-3250**

OTIS, Edward O[sgood] (1848-1933)
The significance of the tuberculosis crusade, and its future. Boston, 1904. 17p. DLC; DNLM **00-3251**

OTIS, Edward O[sgood] (1848-1933)
Chronic bronchitis in the adult as influenced by a change of climate. Boston, 1905. 8p. DLC; DNLM **00-3252**

OTIS, Edward O[sgood] (1848-1933)
The early diagnosis of pulmonary tuberculosis. St. Louis, 1905. 1 l. DLC; DNLM **00-3253**

OTIS, Edward O[sgood] (1848-1933)
The municipal control of tuberculosis. Boston, 1905. 11p. DLC; DNLM **00-3254**

OTIS, Edward O[sgood] (1848-1933)
Home treatment of tuberculosis either in favorable or unfavorable climates. [New York], 1906. 10p. DLC; DNLM **00-3255**

OTIS, Edward O[sgood] (1848-1933)
The methods and aims of the physician. Boston, 1906. 19p. DLC; DNLM **00-3256**

OTIS, Edward O[sgood] (1848-1933)
The great white plague, tuberculosis. . . . New York: T. Y. Crowell & Co., [1909]. 321p. DLC; NN **00-3257**

OTIS, Edward O[sgood] (1848-1933)
The medical achievements of Dr. [Oliver Wendell] Holmes. Boston, 1909. 22p. MH **00-3258**

OTIS, William K. (1870-1906)
Concerning the new electrocystoscope. New York, 1905. 12p. DLC; DNLM; MBM **00-3259**

OTT, Isaac (1847-1916)
Animal extracts; effects upon the circulation. Philadelphia, 1900. 8p. DNLM **00-3260**

OTT, I[saac] (1847-1916) and S. B. HARRIS
Iodothyrin and glycosuria. Philadelphia, 1903. 2p. DNLM **00-3261**

OTT, I[saac] (1847-1916) and S. B. HARRIS
The physiological action of adrenalin chloride. Detroit, 1903. 14p. DNLM **00-3262**

OTT, I[saac] (1847-1916)
Intestinal peristalsis in its nervous relations. Baltimore, 1904. 4p. DNLM **00-3263**

OTT, I[saac] (1847-1916) and Joseph F. ULMAN
Intestinal peristalsis. Action of different agents upon it. [n. p., 1904.] 9p. DNLM **00-3264**

OTT, Isaac (1847-1916)
A text-book of physiology . . . with 137 illustrations. Philadelphia: F. A. Davis Co., 1904. 563p. DLC; DNLM; NNNAM; PU **00-3265**

OTT, Isaac (1847-1916)
A text-book of physiology . . . 2nd ed., rev. and enl. Illustrated with 393 half-tone and other engravings, many in colors. Philadelphia: F. A. Davis Co., 1907. 813p. DLC; IU-M; NNNAM: PPC **00-3266**

OTT, Isaac (1847-1916)
A text-book of physiology . . . 3rd ed., rev. and enl., illustrated with 419 half-tone and other engravings, many in colors. Philadelphia: F. A. Davis Co., 1909. 891p. CU-M; DLC; IEN-M; PPC **00-3267**

OTT, Isaac (1847-1916)
Internal secretions from a physiological and therapeutical standpoint. . . . Easton, Pa.: E. D. Vogel, 1910. 133p. plates. DLC; ICJ; MH-M; PPC **00-3268**

OUTLINES of anatomy; a guide to the dissection of the human body; based on the text-book of anatomy by American authors. Ann Arbor, Mich.: G. Wahr, [1900]. 57p. DLC; ICJ **00-3269**

OVERALL, G[eorge] W[hitfield]
A non-surgical treatise on diseases of the prostate gland and adnexa. Chicago: Marsh & Grant Co., 1903. 207p. CtY-M; DLC; ICJ; PPC **00-3270**

OVERALL, G[eorge] W[hitfield]
A non-surgical treatise on diseases of the prostate gland and adnexa. [2nd ed.] Chicago: Rowe Publishing Co., 1906. 228p. DNLM; MB; NN **00-3271**

OVERALL, G[eorge] W[hitfield]
A non-surgical treatise on diseases of the prostate gland and adnexa. 3rd ed. [Chicago]: Rowe Publishing Co., 1906. 228p. CtY-M; DLC; ICJ; PU **00-3272**

OVERHOLSER, M. P.
On laboratory diagnosis. New York, 1904. 37p. DLC; DNLM; NNNAM **00-3273**

OVERMAN, David R.
Womanhood; or, The physical life of maiden, wife and mother, with illustrated treatise on the physiology of the female body. . . . St. Louis: The Thompson Publishing Co., [1910]. 478p. illus., plates. DLC **00-3274**

OVERTON, Frank (*b.* 1867)
Applied physiology, including the effects of alcohol and narcotics. . . . Advanced grade. New York, Cincinnati, [etc.]: American Book Company, 1901 [*c.* 1897]. 432p. DLC; MB; NN **00-3275**

OVERTON, Frank (*b.* 1867)
Applied physiology, including the effects of alcohol and narcotics. . . . Intermediate grade. New York, Cincinnati, [etc.]: American Book Company, 1901 [*c.* 1898]. 464p. DLC; ICJ **00-3276**

OVERTON, Frank (*b.* 1867)
. . . Elementary physiology. Baltimore: W. J. C. Dulany Co., [1904]. 188p. DLC **00-3277**

OVERTON, Frank (*b.* 1867)
Applied physiology, including the effects of alcohol and narcotics. . . . Advanced grade. New York, Cincinnati, [etc.]: American Book Company, [1908]. 448p. DLC; ICJ; NIC **00-3278**

OVERTON, Frank (*b.* 1867)
Applied physiology, including the effects of alcohol and narcotics. . . . Advanced grade. New York, Cincinnati, [etc.]: American Book Company, [1910]. 464p. DLC; MH; NN **00-3279**

OVINGTON, Irene H.
Helps for home nursing. . . . Chicago: C. H. Kerr & Co., 1900. 114p. DLC; ICJ; ICRM [*c.* 1891. *vel subseq.*] **00-3280**

OWEN, W[illiam] O[tway] (1854-1924)
Preventable disease in the Army of the United States; cause, effect, and remedy. Cincinnati, 1901. 14p. DLC; DNLM; NN **00-3281**

OWEN, W[illiam] O[tway] (1854-1924)
Preventable disease in the Army of the United States – Cause, effect and remedy. [New York? 1901.] 45p. NN **00-3282**

OWSLEY, J. R[obert]
Outlines of physiology, anatomy, and hygiene. . . . Dearborn, Mo.: J. R. Owsley, 1900. 60p. DLC **00-3283**

PACIFIC COAST REGULAR COLLEGE OF MEDICINE, SAN FRANCISCO
Annual announcement for the session of 1900 (1.). San Francisco: Mysell-Rollins Co., 1900. 15p. DNLM **00-3284**

PACKARD, A[lpheus] S[pring] (1839-1905)
Lamarck, the founder of evolution; his life and work, with translations of his writings on organic evolution, . . . New York, [etc.]: Longmans, Green, & Co., 1901. 451p. DLC; MB; NIC; NN **00-3285**

PACKARD, A[lpheus] S[pring] (1839-1905) and Robert G. LE CONTE
The medical and surgical aspects of gangrene of the lung. Philadelphia, 1902. 19p. DNLM **00-3286**

PACKARD, A[lpehus] S[pring] (1839-1905) and R. N. WILLSON
Antitubercle serum. Philadelphia, 1902. 4p. DNLM **00-3287**

PACKARD, Francis R[andolph] (1870-1950)
The history of medicine in the United States; a collection of facts and documents relating to the history of medical science in this country, from the earliest English colonization to the year 1800; with a supplemental chapter on the discovery of anaesthesia. . . . Philadelphia and London: J. B. Lippincott Co., 1901. 542p. 7 plates. DLC; DNLM; NNNAM; PPC **00-3288**

PACKARD, Francis R[andolph] (1870-1950)
Crawford Williamson Long (1815-1878), '39M, the pioneer in the use of ether as an anesthetic. Philadelphia, 1902. 6p. DNLM **00-3289**

PACKARD, Francis R[andolph] (1870-1950)
. . . Text-book of diseases of the nose, throat and ear, for the use of students and general practitioners. . . . Philadelphia & London: J. B. Lippincott Co., [1909]. 369p. plates. DLC; NNNAM; PPC; PU **00-3290**

PACKARD, Horace (*b.* 1855) and J. Emmons BRIGGS
The involution of the appendix; acute suppurative appendicitis as a sequel thereto; a report of a series of cases, with deductions. New York, [1902]. 27p. DNLM; MBM **00-3291**

PACKARD, Horace (*b.* 1855)
A safe, simple, and efficient method of prostatectomy, followed by perfect results. Boston, 1904. 16p. 2 plates on 1 l. DNLM; MBM **00-3292**

PADDOCK, Charles E[vart] (*b.* 1859)
Maternitas: a book concerning the care of the prospective mother and her child. Chicago: C. J. Head & Co., [1905]. 191p. DLC; ICJ; NN; PP **00-3293**

PAGE, Logan Waller
. . . How to prevent typhoid fever. By Logan Waller Page, John R. Mohler, and Erwin F. Smith. Washington: Government Printing Office, 1910. 8p. DLC **00-3294**

PAGET, Stephen (1855-1926)
Experiments on animals. With an introduction by Lord Lister. New York: William Wood & Co., 1900. 274p. 3 plates. DNLM; ICJ; NNNAM; PU **00-3295**

PAGET, Stephen (1855-1926)
Ambroise Paré and his times, 1510-1590. New York and London: G. P. Putnam's Sons, 1901 [*c.* 1897]. 309p. plates. DLC; ICJ; MH; NN **00-3296**

PAGET, Stephen (1855-1926)
Experiments on animals, by Stephen Paget, with an introduction by Lord Lister. New and rev. ed. New York: G. P. Putnam's Sons, [etc., etc.], 1903. 307p. DLC; MH; NIC; NN **00-3297**

PAGET, Stephen (1855-1926)
Confessio medici, by the writer of "The young people" . . . New York: The Macmillan Co., 1908. 232p. DLC; NIC; NN **00-3298**

PAGET, Stephen (1855-1926)
The faith and works of Christian science, by the writer of "Confessio medici" . . . New York: The Macmillan Co., 1909. 232p. DLC; ICJ; MB; NN **00-3299**

PAIGE, Harry W[orthington] (*b.* **1864)**
Diseases of the lungs, bronchi and pleura, by . . . . Philadelphia: Boericke & Tafel, 1904. 100p. DLC; MH-M; PPC; PPHa
00-3300

PAINE, Horace M[arshfield] (1827-1903)
History of the organization, purposes and progress, of the Homoeopathic Medical Society of the State of New York. The work accomplished by the society during fifty years—1850 to 1900. . . . An historical address, presented at the jubilee meeting of the society, held at Brooklyn, N.Y., October 3rd and 4th, 1900, by the only surviving representative of its charter membership. Atlanta, Ga.: Franklin Printing & Publishing Co., [1900?]. 29p. ports. DLC **00-3301**

PAINE, N[athaniel] Emmons (*b.* **1853)**
Bad Nauheim; some observations. West Newton, [1903]. 8p. DNLM **00-3302**

PAINE, N[athaniel] Emmons (*b.* **1853)**
Instruction in psychiatry in American medical colleges. Utica, [1903?]. 9p. MB **00-3303**

PAINTER, Charles F[airbank] (*b.* **1869)**
The operative treatment of intercostal neuralgia occurring in the deformities of the chest following Pott's disease and scoliosis. Philadelphia, 1901. 7p. DNLM
00-3304

PAINTER, Charles F[airbank] (*b.* **1869)**
The pathology of rheumatoid arthritis; a preliminary report. [Philadelphia, 1901.] 16p. DNLM; PPC
00-3305

PAINTER, Charles F[airbank] (*b.* **1869)**
I. Infantile paralysis, an epidemic of thirty-eight cases. II. The malignancy of joint tuberculosis, illustrated by a series of forty-seven cases. [Philadelphia, 1902.] 40p. DNLM; PPC
00-3306

PAINTER, Charles F[airbank] (*b.* **1869) and Robert B. OSGOOD**
Cases of rupture of the spinal ligaments. Boston: Damrell & Upham, 1902. 17p. DNLM; MBM **00-3307**

PAINTER, Charles F[airbank] (*b.* **1869) and William G. ERVING**
Lipoma arborescens. Boston: Old Cor. Book Store, 1903. 14p. 2 plates. DNLM; MBM **00-3308**

PALMER, Benjamin W[ood], ed. (*d.* **1895)**
Favorite prescriptions of distinguished practitioners, with notes on treatment; compiled from the published writings or unpublished records of Drs. Fordyce Barker, Roberts Bartholow . . . 7th ed. New York: E. B. Treat & Co., 1901. 248p. DLC; ICJ; NcD; PPJ **00-3309**

PALMER, Charles Follen
Inebriety; its source, prevention, and cure. . . . Philadelphia: The Union Press, [1900?] 109p. fold. diag. DLC; ICJ; NcU; NN **00-3310**

PALMER, Daniel David (1842-1913)
The science of chiropractic; its principles and adjustments, by Dr. D. D. Palmer . . . and B. J. Palmer . . . illustrated with 117 illustrations. Davenport, Ia.: The Palmer School of Chiropractic, 1906. 413p. plates. DLC; DNLM; ICJ
00-3311

PALMER, Daniel David (1842-1913)
Text-book of the science, art and philosophy of chiropractic for students and practitioners . . . founded on tone. Portland, Or.: Portland Printing House Co., 1910. 1007p. DLC; ICJ
00-3312

PALMER, Daniel David (1842-1913)
The chiropractor. . . . Los Angeles, Cal.: Press of Beacon Light Printing Co., [1910?] 115p. port. DLC; DNLM
00-3313

PALMER, Henry B[owman] (1862-1907)
Surgical asepsis, especially adapted to operations in the home of the patient . . . with ninety illustrations. Philadelphia: F. A. Davis Co., 1903. 231p. DLC; ICJ **00-3314**

PALMER, Margaret D.
Lessons on massage. New York: William Wood & Co., 1901. 234p. DNLM; NNNAM **00-3315**

PALMER, Margaret D.
Lessons on massage. 2nd ed. New York: William Wood & Co., 1904. 261p. 2 plates. DNLM; NNNAM
00-3316

PALMER, Margaret D.
Lessons on massage. . . . 3rd ed. New York: William Wood & Co., 1907. 261p. DNLM; ICJ; NNNAM
00-3317

PALMER, Owen Abraham (*b.* **1847)**
Physical perfection. . . . Warren, O.: F. W. Perry, [1900?] 212p. DLC; DNLM **00-3318**

PALMER, Owen Abraham (*b.* **1847)**
Diseases of the digestive organs, for students and practitioners of medicine. . . . Cleveland, O., 1907. 524p. plates. DLC; ICJ; OCIM **00-3319**

PAMMEL, Louis H[ermann] (*b.* **1862)**
A manual of poisonous plants, chiefly of eastern North America, with brief notes on economic and medicinal plants, and numerous illustrations. . . . Cedar Rapids, Ia.: The Torch Press, 1910. 150p. front., illus., plates. DLC; OCLloyd
00-3320

PAN AMERICAN SANITARY CONFERENCE. 1st, WASHINGTON, D.C., 1902
. . . Transactions of the first general International Sanitary Convention of the American Republics, held at . . . Washington, D.C., December 2, 3, and 4, 1902, under the auspices of the governing board of the International Union of the American Republics. Washington: Government Printing Office, 1903. 356p. DLC [English and Spanish] **00-3321**

PAN AMERICAN SANITARY CONFERENCE 2nd, WASHINGTON, D.C., 1905
. . . Sanitary convention. Message from the President of the United States, transmitting a sanitary convention signed ad referendum on October 14, 1905, by the delegates of the United States, Chile, Costa Rica, Cuba, the Dominican Republic, Ecuador, Guatemala, Mexico, Nicaragua, Peru, and Venezuela. [Washington: Government Printing Office, 1905] 18p. DLC **00-3322**

PAN AMERICAN SANITARY CONFERENCE. 2nd, WASHINGTON, D.C., 1905
Transactions of the second International Sanitary Convention of the American Republics, held at . . . Washington, D.C., October 9, 10, 12, 13, and 14, 1905, under the auspices of the governing board of the International Union of the American Republics. Washington: Government Printing Office, 1906. 400p. DLC [English and Spanish] **00-3323**

PAN AMERICAN SANITARY CONFERENCE. 2nd, WASHINGTON, D.C., 1905
. . . Second general International Sanitary Convention of the American Republics. Sanitary convention ad referendum. . . . Washington: Government Printing Office, 1907. 9p. DLC **00-3324**

PAN AMERICAN SANITARY CONFERENCE. 3rd, MEXICO, 1907
Transactions of the third International Sanitary Conference of the American Republics . . . Mexico, December 2-3-4-5-6-7, 1907. Pub. and distributed under the auspices of the International Bureau of the American Republics. Washington, D.C.: [Press of B. S. Adams], 1909. 251p. DLC **00-3325**

PAN AMERICAN SANITARY CONFERENCE. 4th, SAN JOSÉ, COSTA RICA, 1909-10
Transactions of the fourth International Sanitary Conference of the American Republics, held in San José, Costa Rica, December 25, 1909, to January 3, 1910. Published and distributed under the auspices of the Pan American Union, John Barrett, Director-General. . . . Washington, D.C., 1910. 200p. plates, ports. DLC [Plates printed on both sides.] **00-3326**

PARDO DE TAVERA, Trinidad [Hermenegildo] (1857-1925)
The medicinal plants of the Philippines. Transl. and rev. by Jerome B[eers] Thomas. Philadelphia: P. Blakiston's Son & Co., 1901. 269p. DLC; ICJ; OCLloyd; PU **00-3327**

PARK, Roswell (1852-1914)
Poisoning by animals and plants. Acute intoxications, including delirium tremens. New York, 1901. 7p. MB **00-3328**

PARK, Roswell (1852-1914)
Scurvy and rickets. New York, 1901. 3p. plate. MB **00-3329**

PARK, Roswell (1852-1914)
Shock and collapse. New York, 1901. 2p. MB **00-3330**

PARK, Roswell (1852-1914)
Surgical aspects and sequelae of other infections and diseases. New York, 1901. 5p. MB **00-3331**

PARK, Roswell (1852-1914)
Surgical diseases common to man and the domestic animals. New York, 1901. 26p. illus. col. plates. MB **00-3332**

PARK, Roswell (1852-1914)
Surgical diseases of the osseous system. New York, 1901. 32p. illus. plates. MB **00-3333**

PARK, Roswell (1852-1914)
The surgical fevers and septic infections. New York, 1901. 17p. MB **00-3334**

PARK, Roswell (1852-1914)
Ulcer and ulceration. New York, 1901. 10p. illus. plates. MB **00-3335**

PARK, Roswell, ed. (1852-1914)
A treatise on surgery, by American authors. For students and practitioners of surgery and medicine. . . . 3rd ed., enl. and thoroughly rev. . . . New York and Philadelphia: Lea Bros. & Co., [1901]. 1408p. 65 plates. DLC; DNLM; NNNAM; PPC **00-3336**

PARK, Roswell (1852-1914)
Surgical pathology of the blood. New York, 1901. 12p. illus. plate. MB **00-3337**

PARK, Roswell (1852-1914)
The pancreas and pancreatic diseases. The surgical consideration of cysts and other neoplasms of the pancreas. New Haven, 1903. 24p. MB **00-3338**

PARK, Roswell (1852-1914)
The principles and practice of modern surgery . . . with 722 engravings and 60 full-page plates in colors and monochrome. Philadelphia and New York: Lea Bros. & Co., 1907. 1074p. col. plates. DLC; NNNAM; OCIM; PPC **00-3339**

PARK, William Hallock (1863-1939)
I. A practical method for differentiating between variola and varicella by means of the inoculation of monkeys. II. Negative results of attempts to cause the active principles of vaccine and small-pox virus to pass through filters impervious to bacteria. Philadelphia, 1902. 5p. DNLM **00-3340**

PARK, William Hallock (1863-1939) and L. Emmett HOLT
Report upon the results, with different kinds of pure and impure milk, in infant feeding in tenement houses and institutions of New York City; a clinical and bacteriological study. New York, 1903. 29p. DNLM; NNNAM **00-3341**

PARK, William Hallock (1863-1939)
Pathogenic micro-organisms, including bacteria and protozoa. A practical manual for students, physicians, and health officers . . . assisted by Anna W. Williams. New York and Philadelphia: Lea Bros. & Co., 1905. 556p. 4 plates. DLC; DNLM; NNNAM; PU **00-3342**

PARK, William Hallock (1863-1939)
Pathogenic micro-organisms, including bacteria and *Protozoa*; a practical manual for students, physicians and health officers . . . assisted by Anna W. Williams . . . 2nd ed., enl. and thoroughly rev. With 165 engravings and 4 full-page plates. New York and Philadelphia: Lea Bros. & Co., 1905. 566p. 4 plates. DLC; MBM; NNNAM; PPC **00-3343**

PARK, William Hallock (1863-1939)
Some observations upon the agglutination of bacteria. Chicago, 1906. 9p. DNLM **00-3344**

PARK, William Hallock (1863-1939)
Pathogenic micro-organisms, including bacteria and *Protozoa*; a practical manual for students, physicians and health officers . . . assisted by Anna W. Williams . . . 3rd ed., enl. and thoroughly rev., with 176 engravings and 5 full-page plates. New York and Philadelphia: Lea & Febiger, 1908. 642p. 5 plates. DLC; IU-M; NNNAM; PU **00-3345**

PARK, William Hallock (1863-1939)
Pathogenic micro-organisms, including bacteria and protozoa; a practical manual for students, physicians and health officers, by . . . and Anna W. Williams . . . 4th ed., enl. and thoroughly rev., with 196 engravings and 8 full-page plates. New York and Philadelphia: Lea & Febiger, 1910. 670p. 8 plates. CU-M; DLC; NNNAM; PPC **00-3346**

PARKE, DAVIS & COMPANY
Sueros antidiftérico, antitetánico y antiestreptocócico. Detroit, Mich., Nueva York: Parke, Davis & Compaña, [1902]. 63p. DLC; ICJ **00-3347**

PARKE, DAVIS & COMPANY
Manual of therapeutics, referring especially to the products of the pharmaceutical and biological laboratories of . . . . Detroit, Mich., 1909. 643p. DLC; ICJ **00-3348**

PARKE, J[oseph] Richardson (*b.* 1854)
Human sexuality. A medico-literary treatise on the laws, anomalies, and relations of sex with especial reference to contrary sexual desire. Philadelphia: Professional Publishing Co., 1906. 476p. DLC; ICJ; PPC; PU **00-3349**

PARKE, J[oseph] Richardson (*b.* 1854)
[Human sexuality, a medico-literary treatise on the history and pathology of the sex instinct, for the use of physicians and jurists. . . .] [2nd ed.] [Philadelphia: Professional Publishing Co., *c.* 1907.] 476p. DLC; ICJ; PPC **00-3350**

PARKE, J[oseph] Richardson (*b.* 1854)
Human sexuality; a medico-literary treatise on the laws, anomalies, and relations of sex, with especial reference to contrary sexual desire. . . . 3rd ed. . . . Philadelphia: Professional Publishing Co., 1908. 476p. DLC **00-3351**

PARKE, J[oseph] Richardson (*b.* 1854)
Human sexuality, a medico-literary treatise on the history and pathology of the sex instinct, for the use of physicians and jurists. 4th rev. ed. . . . Philadelphia: Professional Publishing Co., 1909. 476p. DLC; DNLM; PPC **00-3352**

PARKER, Delos L.
The etiology of alopecia. New York: Wynkoop, Hallenbeck, Crawford Co., 1901. 25p. DNLM; NNNAM **00-3353**

PARKER, Harry C[aldwell] (*b.* 1877)
Refraction of the eye . . . with 106 illustrations. Philadelphia and London: W. B. Saunders & Co., 1908. 201p. diags. DLC; NNNAM; PPC; PU **00-3354**

PARKER, Harry C[aldwell] (*b.* 1877)
Hand-book of diseases of the eye; a text-book for students and practitioners . . . illustrated with 115 text engravings, a half-tone frontispiece and 5 full-page chromolithographic plates, with 26 figures. Philadelphia: F. A. Davis Co., 1910. 303p. col. plates. DLC; IU-M; NNNAM; PPC **00-3355**

PARKER MEMORIAL HOSPITAL, UNIVERSITY OF MISSOURI, COLUMBIA
Circular by the superintendent. [Columbia, 1902.] 4p. DNLM **00-3356**

PARKER, Nelson H.
Dr. Parker's Indian recipe book containing a complete system of practice upon an entirely new plan, with a description of the vegetables made use of, and directions for preparing and administering them to cure disease; to which is added a description of several cases of diseases attended by the author, with the mode of treatment and cure. . . . [Mancelona, Mich.: Mancelona Herald Stream Print, 1905.] 40p. DLC **00-3357**

PARKER, W[illiam] Thornton (1849-1925)
A medico-religious charity. The Guild of Mercy. Atlanta, 1900. 5p. DNLM **00-3358**

PARKER, W[illiam] Thornton (1849-1925)
A medico-religious society. Richmond, 1900. 6p. DLC; DNLM **00-3359**

PARKES, Louis Coltman
Hygiene and public health, by Louis Parkes . . . and Henry Kenwood. . . . Philadelphia: P. Blakiston's Son & Co., 1901. 732p. DNLM; ICJ; MBM; PPC [Cover title: Parkes' practical hygiene. Sixth edition. First edition under joint authorship.] **00-3360**

PARKES, Louis Coltman
Hygiene and public health, by Louis Parkes . . . and Henry Kenwood . . . [2nd ed.] Philadelphia: P. Blakiston's Son & Co., 1902. 763p. DLC; ICJ; PPC; PU **00-3361**

PARKYN, Herbert A[rthur]
Therapeutic suggestion; what is it? Chicago: Chicago School of Psychology, 1900. 8p. DNLM [1898. *vel subseq.*] **00-3362**

PARKYN, Herbert A[rthur]
Suggestive therapeutics and hypnotism; being a special mail course of thirty-eight lessons on the uses and abuses of suggestion. . . . Chicago: Suggestion Publishing Co., 1900. 334p. DLC [*vel subseq.*] **00-3363**

PARKYN, Herbert A[rthur]
Suggestive therapeutics and hypnotism; being a special mail course of forty-one lessons on the uses and abuses of suggestion . . . 3rd ed. Chicago, Ill.: Suggestion Publishing Co., 1900. 366p. DLC; DNLM **00-3364**

PARKYN, Herbert A[rthur]
Auto-suggestion; what it is and how to use it for health, happiness and success; a book for practical self-development. Chicago: Suggestion Publishing Co., 1905. 174p. DLC [*vel subseq.*] **00-3365**

PARKYN, Herbert A[rthur]
Auto-suggestion; what it is and how to use it for health, happiness and success, a book for practical self-development. . . . Chicago: Suggestion Publishing Co., 1905. 190p. NN **00-3366**

PARKYN, Herbert A[rthur]
Auto-suggestion; what it is and how to use it for health, happiness and success . . . 4th ed. [completing the 10th thousand] Chicago: Suggestion Publishing Co., 1906. 190p. DLC: ICJ **00-3367**

PARKYN, Herbert A[rthur]
Auto-suggestion; what it is and how to use it for health, happiness and success . . . 6th ed. [completing the 35th thousand] Chicago, Ill.: Suggestion Publishing Co., 1909. 190p. DLC; ICJ **00-3368**

PARSONS, J[ohn] Herbert (1868-1957)
Elementary ophthalmic optics, including ophthalmoscopy and retinoscopy. Philadelphia: P. Blakiston's Son & Co., 1902. 162p. DNLM; NNNAM; PPC; PU **00-3369**

PARSONS, J[ohn] Herbert (1868-1957)
The pathology of the eye. . . . New York: G. Putnam's Sons, 1904-1908. 4 v. DLC; ICJ; NcD; PU **00-3370**

PARSONS, J[ohn] H[erbert] (1868-1957)
Diseases of the eye. . . . Philadelphia: P. Blakiston's Son & Co., 1910. 684p. col. plates. DLC; MH-M; NN; PU **00-3371**

PARSONS, J[ohn] Inglis (*b.* 1857)
The arrest of growth in cancer by the interrupted voltaic current (electro-atrophy). New York: William Wood & Co., 1900. 16p. DNLM; IU-M [Originally in Wood's Medical and Surgical Monographs, vol. 5 (1890), No. 3, pp. 587-602] **00-3372**

PARSONS, J[ohn] Inglis (*b.* 1857)
The operative treatment of prolapse and retroversion of the uterus. New York: William Wood & Co., 1906. 90p. 6 plates. DNLM; ICJ; NNNAM; PU **00-3373**

PASCHKIS, Heinrich (1849-1923)
Cosmetics: a treatise for physicians. New York: William Wood & Co., 1900. 202p. DLC; ICJ; NN; PU [Reprinted out of Wood's Medical & Surgical Monographs, vol. 7, No. 2 (1890), pp. 217-472] **00-3374**

PATCHEN, G[eorge] H[enry] (*b.* 1845)
How should we breathe? A physiological study. New York: The Improved Movement Cure Institute, 1903. 56p. DLC; NN **00-3375**

PATCHEN, G[eorge] H[enry] (*b.* 1845)
The chiropractic idea: the new method of analyzing the symptoms and adjusting the physical cause of disease. New York: The Improveed Movement Cure Institute, 1908. 12p. DLC; NN **00-3376**

PATERSON, Herbert J[ohn] (1868-1940)
Gastric surgery. Being the Hunterian lectures, delivered before the Royal College of Surgeons of England, on Feb. 19, 21, and 23, 1906. New York: William Wood & Co., 1906. 181p. 2 plates. DNLM; ICJ; NNNAM; PU **00-3377**

PATERSON, Herbert J[ohn] (1868-1940)
The surgery of the stomach. A handbook of diagnosis and treatment, by Herbert J. Paterson. . . . With plates. New York: William Wood & Co., 1910 [*c.* 1911]. 312p. 32 plates. ICJ; IU-M; PPJ **00-3378**

PATON, Stewart (1865-1942)
The hospitals for the insane and the study of mental diseases. Philadelphia, 1900. 16p. DNLM; PPC **00-3379**

PATON, Stewart (1865-1942)
The histogenesis of the cellular elements of the cerebral cortex. [Baltimore, 1901.] 4p. DNLM **00-3380**

PATON, Stewart (1865-1942)
Acute paresis with report of a case . . . by S. Paton and G. K. Rusk. [n. p., 1903.] 6p. NN **00-3381**

PATON, Stewart (1865-1942)
Psychiatry. A text-book for students and physicians. Philadelphia: J. B. Lippincott Co., 1905. 618p. 20 plates. DNLM; NNNAM; OCIM; PPC **00-3382**

PATTEE, Alida Frances
Practical dietetics, with reference to diet in disease . . . as arranged for and used at Bellevue Hospital. [New York: Press of J. J. Little & Co., 1903.] 56p. DLC; DNLM; NNNAM; PU **00-3383**

PATTEE, Alida Frances
Practical dietetics, with reference to diet in disease . . . 2nd ed., rev. and enl. New York: The Author, [1904]. 340p. DLC; ICJ; MB; NNNAM **00-3384**

PATTEE, Alida Frances
Practical dietetics, with reference to diet in disease . . . 3rd ed. New York: A. F. Pattee, [1905]. 352p. DLC; MB: NNNAM; PPJ **00-3385**

PATTEE, Alida Frances
Practical dietetics, with reference to diet in disease . . . 4th ed. Mt. Vernon, N.Y.: A. F. Pattee, [1905]. 312p. NNNAM; NNU-M **00-3386**

PATTEE, Alida Frances
Practical dietetics, with reference to diet in disease . . . 5th ed. Mt. Vernon, N.Y.: A. F. Pattee, [1906]. 312p. NNNAM; NNU-M **00-3387**

PATTEE, Alida Frances
Practical dietetics, with reference to diet in disease . . . 6th ed., rev. and enl. Mt. Vernon, N.Y.: A. F. Pattee, 1910. 527p. DLC; ICJ; NNNAM; PU **00-3388**

PATTERSON, Francis Denison (*b.* 1875)
A statistical digest of epithelioma of the penis. Philadelphia, 1901. 19p. DNLM; NNNAM **00-3389**

PATTERSON, Francis Denison (*b.* 1875)
Spinal analgesia. The present position of the method, based on a review of the literature. 1904. 61p. DNLM; NNNAM **00-3390**

PATTERSON, Francis Denison (*b.* 1875)
Extra-genital chancre, infection from a barber. Detroit: E. G. Swift, 1905. 4p. DNLM **00-3391**

PATTERSON, Francis Denison (*b.* 1875)
Acute appendicitis the result of a foreign body. Philadelphia, 1906. 14p. DNLM **00-3392**

PATTON, Joseph McIntyre (*b.* 1860)
Clinical lectures on the diseases of the heart, lungs, and pleura, designed for the use of practitioners and advanced students of medicine . . . 2nd ed., rev. and enl. Chicago: The Clinical Review Publishing Co., 1900. 428p. DLC; ICJ; IU-M; OCIM **00-3393**

PATTON, Joseph McIntyre (*b.* 1860)
Anaesthesia and anaesthetics general and local, for practitioners and students of medicine and dentistry. . . . Chicago: Cleveland Press, 1903. 207p. DLC; DNLM; ICJ; OCIM
00-3394

PATTON, Joseph McIntyre (*b.* 1860)
Anaesthesia and anaesthetics, general and local, for practitioners and students of medicine and dentistry . . . 2nd ed., rev. and enl. . . . Chicago: Cleveland Press, 1906. 225p. DLC; ICJ **00-3395**

PATTON, Joseph McIntyre (*b.* 1860)
Anaesthesia and anaesthetics, general and local, for practitioners and students of medicine and dentistry. 3rd ed., rev. and enl. Chicago: Cleveland Press, 1910. 225p. illus. ICJ
00-3396

PAUL, George P[hillip] (*b.* 1879)
Nursing in the acute infectious fevers. Philadelphia: W. B. Saunders & Co., 1906. 200p. DLC; NN; PPC; PU
00-3397

PAUL, George P[hillip] (*b.* 1879)
A text-book of materia medica for nurses, including therapeutics and toxicology. . . . Philadelphia and London: W. B. Saunders & Co., 1907. 242p. DLC; OCLloyd; PPC; PU
00-3398

PAUL, George P[hillip] (*b.* 1879)
A text-book of materia medica for nurses, including therapeutics and toxicology . . . 2nd ed., thoroughly rev. Philadelphia: W. B. Saunders & Co., 1910 [*c.* 1911]. 282p. DLC; GU; ICJ; PU **00-3399**

PAUL, George P[hillip] (*b.* 1879)
Nursing in the acute infectious fevers. 2nd ed., thoroughly rev. Philadelphia: W. B. Saunders & Co., 1910 [*c.* 1911]. 246p. col. plates, diags. DLC; ICJ; MBM; NNNAM
00-3400

PAUL, W[alter] E[verard]
Notes from the neurological department of the Massachusetts General Hospital. Cases of myasthenia gravis pseudoparalytica. Boston, 1900. 7p. DNLM; MH **00-3401**

PAUL, W[alter] E[verard]
Notes from the neurological department of the Massachusetts General Hospital. Sudden (apoplectiform) bulbar paralysis; hemiplegia; astereognosis. Boston, 1901. 4p. DNLM; MH
00-3402

PAYNE, Joseph F[rank] (1840-1910)
Thomas Sydenham. New York: Longmans, Green & Co., 1900. 264p. ICJ; MB; MH; PP **00-3403**

PEABODY, Frederick W[illiam] (*b.* 1862)
A complete exposé of Eddyism, or Christian Science, and the plain truth in plain terms regarding Mary Baker G. Eddy, founder of Christian Science. An address at Tremont Temple, Boston, Aug. 1, 1901. [Boston, 1901.] 68p. port. DNLM; MB; MH; McD **00-3404**

PEABODY, Frederick W[illiam] (*b.* 1862)
Complete exposure of Eddyism or Christian Science. The plain truth in plain terms regarding Mary Baker G. Eddy. . . . 2nd ed., enl. [Boston, 1904.] 53p. DLC; ICJ; MB; NN
00-3405

PEABODY, Frederick W[illiam] (*b.* 1862)
Complete exposure of Eddyism or Christian Science. The plain truth in plain terms regarding Mary Baker G. Eddy. 3rd, enl. ed. [Boston, 1904.] 53p. MH [Inserted is "Extract from letter of 'Mark Twain' to F. W. Peabody," 1 sheet, printed for private circulation.] **00-3406**

PEABODY, Frederick W[illiam] (*b.* 1862)
The religio-medical masquerade; a complete exposure of Christian Science. . . . Boston, Mass.: The Hancock Press, [1910]. 97p. DLC; MH **00-3407**

PEABODY, James Edward (*b.* 1869)
Laboratory exercises in anatomy and physiology . . . 2nd ed., rev. New York: H. Holt & Co., 1902. 117p. Interleaved. DLC; MB; NN; NIC [1st ed., 1898. 79p.] **00-3408**

PEABODY, James Edward (*b.* 1869)
Studies in physiology, anatomy and hygiene. . . . [New ed.] New York: The Macmillan Co., 1907. 322p. DLC; MH; NIC; NN **00-3409**

PEARCE, F[rank] Savary (1867-1904)
Notes on the lectures on pathology of Prof. John Guiteras, delivered before the first year students, University of Pennsylvania. 2nd ed. Philadelphia, 1901? [*c.* 1895]. 55p. PPC
00-3410

PEARCE, F[rank] Savary (1867-1904)
A practical treatise on nervous diseases, for the medical student and general practitioner . . . ninety-one illustrations in the text, many in colours. New York and London: D. Appleton & Co., 1904. 401p. DLC; ICJ; NcD; PPJ **00-3411**

PEARCE, Richard Mills, Jr. (1874-1930)
An experimental study of nephrotoxins. Philadelphia, 1903. 54p. DNLM **00-3412**

PEARCE, Richard Mills, Jr. (1874-1930)
Concerning hemagglutinins of bacterial origin and their relation to hyaline thrombi and liver necroses. Albany, 1904. 10p. DNLM **00-3413**

PEARCE, Richard Mills, Jr. (1874-1930) and Charles K. WINNE, Jr.
Concerning hemagglutinins of bacterial origin and their relation to hyaline thrombi and liver necroses. Albany, 1904. 10p. DNLM **00-3414**

PEARCE, Richard Mills, Jr. (1874-1930)
Cancer of the pancreas and glycosuria. Albany, 1904. 8p. DNLM **00-3415**

PEARCE, Richard Mills, Jr. (1874-1930)
Cancer of the pancreas and glycosuria. An histological study of the changes in the islands of Langerhans. Philadelphia, 1904. 6p. DNLM **00-3416**

PEARCE, Richard Mills, Jr. (1874-1930)
Concerning the specificity of the somatogenic cytotoxins. Albany, 1904. 16p. DNLM **00-3417**

PEARCE, Richard Mills, Jr. (1874-1930)
Concerning the specificity of the somatogenic cytotoxins. Boston, 1904. 15p. DNLM **00-3418**

PEARCE, Richard Mills, Jr. (1874-1930)
Experimental pancreatitis considered in its relation to the acute forms of pancreatitis in man. Albany, 1904. 16p. DNLM
00-3419

PEARCE, Richard Mills, Jr. (1874-1930)
The experimental production of liver necroses by the intravenous injection of haemagglutinins. Albany, 1904. 10p. DNLM
00-3420

PEARCE, Richard Mills, Jr. (1874-1930)
The islands of Langerhans in congenital syphilitic pancreatitis. Albany, 1904. 7p. 1 plate. DNLM **00-3421**

PEARCE, Richard Mills, Jr. (1874-1930)
The pathology of diabetes. Albany, 1904. 12p. DNLM
00-3422

PEARCE, Richard Mills, Jr. (1874-1930)
The scientific method in medicine. Albany, 1905. 18p. DNLM
00-3423

PEARCE, Richard Mills, Jr. (1874-1930) and E. MacD. STANTON
Experimental arteriosclerosis. New York, 1906. 13p. 2 plates. DNLM **00-3424**

PEARCE, Richard Mills, Jr. (1874-1930)
Medical research in American universities; present facilities, needs, and opportunities. . . . [1910?] 24p. NNC
00-3425

PEARSON, Karl (1857-1936)
The grammar of science . . . with 25 figures in the text. New York: C. Scribner's Sons, 1901. 493p. illus., diags. (Half-title: The contemporary science series). DLC; MH; NIC; NN [first published 1892.] **00-3426**

PECKHAM, Fenner H.
Address of Dr. Fenner H. Peckham on the purification of the water supply of the city of Providence, before the Joint Special Committee of the City Council appointed to consider and report on the best method of filtration. [Providence] : Snow & Farnham, Printers, 1902. 11p. DLC **00-3427**

PEEBLES, James Martin (1822-1922)
Death defeated; or, The psychic secret of how to keep young . . . 4th ed. . . . Battle Creek, Mich.: Dr. Peebles' Institute of Health, 1908. 216p. DLC; ICJ **00-3428**

PELS-LEUSDEN, Friedrich (*b.* 1866)
Surgical operations; a hand-book for students and practitioners . . . only authorized English translation, by Faxton E. Gardner . . . with six hundred and sixty-eight illustrations. New York: Rebman Co., [1910?] 726p. DLC; ICJ; MBM; NNNAM
00-3429

PEMBERTON, Henry
The path of evolution through ancient thought and modern science. . . . Philadelphia: H. Altemus Co., [1902]. 374p. DLC; MH; NIC; NN **00-3430**

PENNINGTON, J[ohn] Rawson (1858-1927)
New points in the anatomy, histology, and pathology of the rectum and colon. Chicago, [1900?] 16p. DNLM
00-3431

PENNINGTON, J[ohn] Rawson (1858-1927)
Narrowing of the anus; stricture; hemorrhoids. A clinical lecture at the Chicago Policlinic. Chicago, [1901]. 13p. 1 plate. **00-3432**

PENNINGTON, J[ohn] Rawson (1858-1927)
A simple operation for the radical treatment of hemorrhoids. Chicago, 1901. 8p. DNLM **00-3433**

PENNINGTON, J[ohn] Rawson (1858-1927)
New and improved rectal instruments. Louisville, 1902. 5p. DNLM **00-3434**

PENNINGTON, J[ohn] Rawson (1858-1927)
Obstipation; hemorrhoids; fissure ani. Philadelphia, 1902. 7p. DNLM **00-3435**

PENNINGTON, J[ohn] Rawson (1858-1927)
X-ray tube-shields and specula for treating cancer of the rectum and other cavities. Philadelphia, 1902. 7p. DNLM
00-3436

PENNINGTON, J[ohn] Rawson (1858-1927)
New X-ray tube. Chicago, 1903. 2p. DNLM
00-3437

PENNINGTON, J[ohn] Rawson (1858-1927)
X-ray as applied to malignant growths in cavities. Chicago, 1903. 14p. DNLM **00-3438**

PENNINGTON, J[ohn] Rawson (1858-1927)
Roetngen rays in the treatment of pruritus ani. New York, 1904. 6p. DNLM **00-3439**

PENNINGTON, J[ohn] Rawson (1858-1927)
Address of the president of the American Proctologic Society. Philadelphia, 1905. 9p. DNLM **00-3440**

PENNINGTON, J[ohn] Rawson (1858-1927)
Normal salt solution and other local analgesics in the office treatment of anorectal diseases. Chicago, 1905. 8p. DNLM
00-3441

PENNINGTON, J[ohn] Rawson (1858-1927)
Regional analgesia in the surgical treatment of anorectal diseases. Philadelphia, 1905. 8p. DNLM
00-3442

PENNINGTON, J[ohn] Rawson (1858-1927)
Remarks on the etiology of fissure in the ano. New York, 1905. 11p. DNLM **00-3443**

PENROSE, Charles B[ingham] (1862-1925)
A textbook of diseases of women. 3rd ed. Philadelphia: W. B. Saunders & Co., 1900. 531p. DNLM; NNNAM; PPC; PPJ
00-3444

PENROSE, Charles B[ingham] (1862-1925)
A textbook of diseases of women. 4th ed. Philadelphia: W. B. Saunders & Co., 1901. 539p. CU-M; DNLM; NNNAM; PPC
00-3445

PENROSE, Charles B[ingham] (1862-1925)
A textbook of diseases of women. 5th ed. Philadelphia: W. B. Saunders & Co., 1904. 550p. DNLM; IU-M; LNT-M; PPC
00-3446

PENROSE, Charles B[ingham] (1862-1925)
A textbook of diseases of women. 6th ed. Philadelphia: W. B. Saunders & Co., 1908. 550p. KyLoJM; MBM; NNNAM; PU
00-3447

PEPPER, William, Jr. (1874-1947)
A study of congenital sarcoma of the liver and suprarenals. Philadelphia, 1901. 14p. DNLM **00-3448**

PEPPER, William, Jr. (1874-1947)
A manual of clinical laboratory methods for the use of the third and fourth year and post graduate medical students, by William Pepper and John A. Kolmer. Philadelphia: Dolbey, [1906?] 56p. DNLM; PPC; PPL; PU
00-3449

PEPPER, William, Jr. (1874-1947)
The medical side of Benjamin Franklin. . . . Philadelphia: W. J. Campbell, 1910 [*c.* 1911]. 122p. front., plates, ports., facsims. DLC; ICJ; MB; NcD **00-3450**

PERKINS, Jay (*b.* 1864)
A state sanatorium for tuberculosis in Rhode Island. What would it accomplish? Providence, 1901. 7p. DNLM
00-3451

PERKINS, Jay (*b.* 1864)
The community and tuberculosis. Providence, 1903. 8p. 2 charts. DNLM **00-3452**

PERKINS, Jay (*b.* 1864) and Pearl WILLIAMS
Report of the department of pulmonary tuberculosis (out-patient of the R. I. Hospital) for the year ending June 30, 1905. [New York, 1906.] 9p. DNLM
00-3453

PERKINS, Roger G[riswold] (*b.* 1874)
Report of two cases of angiosarcoma of the brain. Cleveland, 1901. 12p. DNLM **00-3454**

PERRY, Alfred W. and Albert ABRAMS
Nutrition in pulmonary tuberculosis. Asheville, N.C., 1902. 10p. DNLM **00-3455**

PERRY, Safford G.
Where are we at? Philadelphia, 1901. 30p. DNLM
00-3456

PERSHING, Howell T[erry] (*b.* 1858)
The diagnosis of nervous and mental diseases. Philadelphia: P. Blakiston's Son & Co., 1901. 223p. DNLM; NNNAM; PPC; PU **00-3457**

PERSHING, Howell T[erry] (*b.* 1858)
Mental therapeutics and the need of psychology in the medical curriculum. Chicago, 1902. 8p. DNLM; ICJ
00-3458

PETER, Robert (1805-1894)
. . . The history of the Medical Department of Transylvania University . . . prepared for publication by his daughter, Miss Johanna Peter. . . . Louisville, Ky.: J. P. Morton & Co., printers, 1905. 193p. ports. DLC; ICJ; KyLoJM [Filson Club Publications, No. 20] **00-3459**

[PETERS, Franklin Daniel] (*b.* 1873)
. . . How to read eyes, with instruction, how to cultivate pretty eyes. By Martini [*pseud.*] . . . . Allentown, Pa.: The Author, 1903. 38p. front. (port.) DLC **00-3460**

PETERS, Hermann (1847-1920)
Pictorial history of ancient pharmacy, with sketches of early medical practice. Transl. from the German and rev. with numerous additions by William Netter. 3rd ed. Chicago: G. P. Engelhard & Co., 1902. 210p. GU; OCIM; OCLloyd; PPC
00-3461

PETERS, H[oratio] G[ates]
Eighty-eight celebrated remedies, by celebrated physicians . . . a valuable book for every home. [Mt. Gilead? O., 1900.] 35p. DLC **00-3462**

PETERSON, Fred Julius (*b.* 1863)
Materia medica and clinical therapeutics. . . . Los Olivos, Cal.: F. J. Petersen, [1905]. 400p. CU-M; DLC; ICJ
00-3463

PETERSON, Edward W.
Acute intestinal obstruction. Brief mention of illustrative cases. New York, 1906. 10p. DNLM **00-3464**

PETERSON, Frederick (1859-1938)
The care of the insane. Address before the Neurological Section of the Medical and Chirurgical Faculty of Maryland, January, 1903. [Baltimore, Md., 1903.] 10p. NN
00-3465

PETERSON, Frederick (1859-1938) and Walter S. HAINES, eds.
A text-book of legal medicine and toxicology. . . . Philadelphia: W. B. Saunders & Co., 1903-04. 2 v. col. plates. DLC; NNNAM; PPC; PPJ **00-3466**

PETERSON, Reuben (1862-1942)
Anastomosis of the ureters with the intestine. An historical and experimental research. Chicago, 1900. 70p. 7 plates. DNLM **00-3467**

PETERSON, Reuben (1862-1942)
Appendicitis and pelvic disease. New York, 1902. 6p. DNLM
00-3468

PETERSON, Reuben (1862-1942)
Clinical notes on some recent abdominal cases. Philadelphia, 1902. 6p. DNLM **00-3469**

PETERSON, Reuben (1862-1942)
A consideration of ovarian fibromata, based on a study of two recent cases and eighty-two collected from the literature. New York, 1902. 24p. DNLM **00-3470**

PETERSON, Reuben (1862-1942)
Infected ovarian cysts. New York, 1902. 10p. DNLM
00-3471

PETERSON, Reuben (1862-1942)
The use and abuse of the uterine curette. Ann Arbor & Detroit, 1902. 8p. DNLM **00-3472**

PETERSON, Reuben (1862-1942)
The value of plaster casts for accurate case records and as aids in the teaching of the differential diagnosis of abdominal tumors; with demonstrations. Detroit, 1902. 2 l. DNLM
00-3473

PETERSON, Reuben, ed. (1862-1942)
. . . Obstetrics . . . 1902-1910. Chicago: The Year Book Publishers, 1902-1910. DLC; ICJ
00-3474

PETERSON, Reuben (1862-1942)
Pelvic inflammation from the standpoint of the general practitioner. Ann Arbor & Detroit, 1903. 7p. DNLM
00-3475

PETERSON, Reuben (1862-1942)
The surgical treatment of procidentia uteri. Ann Arbor & Detroit, 1903. 5p. DNLM **00-3476**

PETERSON, Reuben (1862-1942)
The relation of the appendix to pelvic disease, based upon a clinical and microscopic study in 200 cases. New York: William Wood & Co., 1904. 20p. DNLM **00-3477**

PETERSON, Reuben (1862-1942)
Ascites and pelvic disease. Detroit, 1905. 3 l. DNLM
00-3478

PETERSON, Reuben (1862-1942)
Edward Swift Dunster. A biographical sketch. Ann Arbor & Detroit, 1905. 12p. DNLM **00-3479**

PETERSON, Reuben (1862-1942)
The indications for operation in pelvic disease. Ann Arbor & Detroit, 1905. 8p. DNLM **00-3480**

PETERSON, Reuben (1862-1942)
Migratory uterine fibroids. New York: William Wood & Co., 1905. 15p. 2 plates. DNLM **00-3481**

PETERSON, Reuben (1862-1942)
Urinary incontinence. Chicago, 1906. 7p. ICJ
00-3482

PETERSON, Reuben, ed. (1862-1942)
. . . The practice of obstetrics in original contributions by American authors. . . . Illustrated with 523 engravings and 30 full-page plates. Philadelphia and New York: Lea Bros. & Co., 1907. 454p. CtY-M; DNLM; NNNAM; PPC
00-3483

PETIT, Julius C.
Woman; her physical condition, sufferings and maternal relations. A course of parlor lectures to ladies. . . . [St. Louis, Mo.]: The Author, 1901 [*c.* 1895]. 112p. illus., facsim. DLC
00-3484

[PETTIGREW, Richard R.]
Pettigrew's New England professional directory. . . . Containing a directory of physicians, and information regarding the hospitals, societies, dispensaries, and training schools of New England, and other information of interest to the medical profession. . . . Boston: The Garden Press, W. B. Libby, 1904. ICJ; MHi **00-3485**

PETTUS, W[illiam] J. (*b.* 1863)
Some observations on the movability of the apex of the heart. Richmond, 1904. 2p. DNLM **00-3486**

PFAUNDLER, Meinhard von, ed. (1872-1947)
The diseases of children; a work for the practising physician, ed. by Dr. M. Pfaundler . . . Dr. A. Schlossmann . . . English translation ed. by Henry L. K. Shaw . . . Linnaeus La Fétra. . . . With an introduction by L. Emmett Holt. . . . Philadelphia & London: J. B. Lippincott Co., [1908-14]. 7 v. col. plates, tables, diags. DLC; ICJ; NNNAM; PPC
00-3487

PFENDER, Charles Alexander (1878-1926)
A review of recent observations on treponema pallidum of syphilis. Philadelphia, 1906. 14p. DNLM
00-3488

PHARMACEUTICAL ERA
The Era dose book, comp. and arranged especially for use in writing and dispensing prescriptions. Comprising a list with doses, of all remedies official in the pharmacopoeias of the United States (eighth revision), Great Britain (1898) and Germany (vierte ausgabe), and also those of the National formulary (third edition), to which have been added many standard preparations. . . . Comp. by the Pharmaceutical Era. To which is added an appendix by Prof. A. B. Stevens, being a compilation of U.S.P. and N.F. preparations, and showing the percentages of alcohol and the quantities of narcotic drugs which must be declared on the labels of these compounds, as prescribed by the Food and Drugs Act of June 30, 1906. 5th ed., rev. and enl. New York: D. O. Haynes & Co., 1907. 80p. DLC; NNNAM; OCLloyd; PU **00-3489**

PHARMACEUTICAL ERA
Philadelphia section of the Era album; reprinted from the Pharmaceutical Era. New York: D. O. Haynes & Co., 1908. 109p. DLC; PP; PPC; PU **00-3490**

THE PHARMACEUTICAL syllabus. 1st ed., recommended by the National Committee representing the boards and schools of pharmacy of the United States for the first syllabus period August 1, 1910 to July 31, 1915. . . . [Albany, N.Y.]: The New York State Board of Pharmacy, 1910. 146p. col. plate. DLC **00-3491**

THE PHARMACOPOEIA of the United States of America. 8th decennial revision. By authority of the United States Pharmacopoeial Convention held at Washington, A.D., 1900. Rev. by the committee of revision and pub. by the Board of Trustees. Official from September 1st, 1905. Philadelphia: P. Blakiston's Son & Co., agents [etc., etc., 1905]. 692p. DLC; DNLM; PPC; PU [also: Changes in the Pharmacopoeia of the United States of America, 8th decennial rev., Washington, D.C., 122p.] **00-3492**

THE PHARMACOPOEIA of the United States of America. Physicians' manual of the Pharmacopoeia and the National Formulary; an epitome of all the articles contained in the U.S.P. VIII and the National Formulary, by C. S. N. Hallberg . . . and J. H. Salisbury. . . . Chicago: American Medical Association, 1907. 198p. DLC; OCLloyd; PPC; PU **00-3493**

THE PHARMACOPOEIA of the United States of America. Physicians' manual of the Pharmacopoeia and the National Formulary; an epitome of all the articles contained in the U.S.P. (eighth revision) and the National Formulary (third revision) by C. S. N. Hallberg . . . and J. H. Salisbury . . . 2nd ed. – rev. Chicago: American Medical Association, 1908. 198p. DLC; OCLloyd; PPC; PU **00-3494**

THE PHARMACOPOEIA of the United States of America. Physicians' manual of the Pharmacopoeia and the National Formulary; an epitome of all the articles contained in the U.S.P. (eighth revision) and the National Formulary (third edition). By C. S. N. Hallberg . . . and J. H. Salisbury . . . 3rd ed. – rev. Chicago: American Medical Association, 1909. 198p. DLC; NNNAM; OCLloyd; PPC **00-3495**

PHELPS, Charles (1834-1913)
Injuries of the brain and its membranes from external violence; with a special study of pistol-shot wounds of the head in their medico-legal and surgical relations . . . 2nd ed. with forty-nine illustrations. New York: D. Appleton & Co., 1900. 602p. DLC; DNLM; NNNAM; PPC **00-3496**

PHELPS, Charles (1834-1913)
An analytical and statistical review of one thousand cases of head injury. [Philadelphia, 1909.] 140p. ICJ **00-3497**

PHELPS, Edward Bunnell (1863-1915)
A statistical study of infant mortality. . . . [Boston? 1908?] 40p. DLC; MH **00-3498**

PHELPS, Edward Bunnell (1863-1915)
A statistical survey of infant mortality's urgent call for action. . . . [Baltimore? 1910?] 27p. DLC **00-3499**

PHELPS, R[obert] M.
A text-book on nursing in bodily and mental diseases. . . . Ed. and pub. by R. M. Phelps . . . and Sarah L. Phelps. . . . Rochester, Minn., 1902 [*c.* 1895]. 140p. DLC **00-3500**

PHILADELPHIA as a medical centre. With sketch of the early history of medical education in Philadelphia. Philadelphia, [1905]. 38p. DNLM; PP; PPC; PU **00-3501**

PHILLIPS, George Marquet (*b.* 1862)
Prostatic hypertrophy from every surgical standpoint, by George M. Phillips, M.D. and forty distinguished authorities; ed. and comp. by S. C. Martin, Jr., M.D. St. Louis: The Ajod Co., [1903]. 176p. DLC; ICJ; OCIM **00-3502**

PHILLIPS, Richard Jones (*b.* 1861)
Spectacles and eyeglasses, their forms, mounting and proper adjustment . . . 3rd ed., rev., with 52 illustrations. Philadelphia: P. Blakiston's Son & Co., 1902. 109p. DLC; DNLM; MBM; PPJ **00-3503**

PHILLIPS, Richard Jones (*b.* 1861)
Spectacles and eyeglasses, their forms, mounting, and proper adjustment . . . 4th ed., rev., with 56 illustrations. Philadelphia: P. Blakiston's Son & Co., 1908. 91p. CtY-M; DLC; DNLM; PPC **00-3504**

PHILLIPS, Wendell C[hristopher] (*b.* 1857)
Diseases of the ear, nose and throat, medical and surgical . . . illustrated with 545 half-tone and other text engravings, many of them original; including 31 full-page plates, some in colors. Philadelphia: F. A. Davis Co., 1910 [*c.* 1911]. 847p. DLC; GU; ICJ; NNNAM **00-3505**

PHIN, John (1830-1913)
Practical hints on the selection and use of the microscope, intended for beginners. 4th ed. New York: Industrial Publication Co., 1900. 231p. [1st ed., 1875. *vel subseq.*] **00-3506**

PHYSICIANS' defense company. An x-ray on the defense of malpractice suits. Fort Wayne, Ind., [1903]. 16p. DNLM **00-3507**

PHYSICIANS' manual of therapeutics; referring especially to the products of the pharmaceutical and biological laboratories of Parke, Davis & Co. Detroit, Mich., 1900. 526p. DLC; ICJ **00-3508**

PHYSICIAN'S PROTECTIVE LEAGUE OF CORTLAND COUNTY, CORTLAND, N.Y.
Constitution and by-laws of the Physician's League of Cortland County, New York. [Cortland, N.Y.], 1901. 30 l. DLC **00-3509**

PHYSICIANS' PUBLISHING COMPANY, (BOSTON)
A complete course of jiu-jitsu and physical culture. . . . Boston, Mass.: Physicians' Publishing Co., [1905]. 118p. DLC [Cover-title: The Japanese secret science jiu-jitsu, demonstrated by John J. O'Brien, the ex-supt. of police at Nagasaki, Japan, and instructor of Pres. Roosevelt.] **00-3510**

PHYSICIANS' register and reference handbook of Philadelphia, including Camden, Atlantic City, etc. Ed. of 1902. Ed. and comp. by G. E. Raymond. Moorestown, N.J.: The Lovell Printing Co., 1902 – Irreg. DLC **00-3511**

PHYSICIAN'S SUPPLY AND DRUG COMPANY
Illustrated catalogue. Chicago, 2nd ed. [*c.* 1906]. 576p. DLC; ICJ; OCIM **00-3512**

PHYSIOLOGICAL aspects of the liquor problem. Investigations made by and under the direction of W. O. Atwater, J. S. Billings, H. P. Bowditch, R. H. Chittenden, and W. H. Welch. Boston: Houghton Mifflin & Co., 1903. 2 v. DLC; MH; NIC; NN **00-3513**

PICK, Alois (1859-1945)
Clinical symptomatology, with special reference to life-threatening symptoms and their treatment, by Alois Pick . . . and Adolph Hecht . . . an authorized translation under the editorial supervision of Karl Konrad Koessler. . . . New York and London: D. Appleton & Co., 1910 [*c.* 1911]. 833p. DLC; ICJ; MH-M; PU **00-3514**

PICKETT, William C. (1868-1907)
Paresis; a clinical study of one hundred and forty-nine cases occurring at the Philadelphia Hospital. Philadelphia, 1902. 24p. DNLM; PPC **00-3515**

PICKETT, William [C.] (1868-1907)
Acute combined degeneration of the spinal cord with perinicious anemia. Detroit, 1902. 10p. 1 plate. DNLM **00-3516**

PIERCE, Nathaniel N.
Directions for cleansing the blood and curing all forms of disease that the human family is subject to, without the use of any medicine whatever. . . . Philmont, N.Y.: Printed at the Office of the Sentinel, [1901?] 32p. DLC [Preface, dated 1883] **00-3517**

PIERCE, Ray Vaughn (*b.* 1840)
The people's common sense medical adviser in plain English; or, Medicine simplified. . . . 72nd ed. . . . Buffalo, N.Y.: World's Dispensary Printing Office and Bindery, [1909]. 1006p. col. plates. DLC; NN **00-3518**

PIERCE, Ray Vaughn (*b.* **1840)**
The people's common sense medical adviser in plain English; or, Medicine simplified. . . . 77th ed., two million five hundred and ninety thousand. Carefully rev. by the author. . . . . Buffalo, N.Y.: World's Dispensary Printing Office and Bindery, [1909]. 1008p. col. plates. DLC; MB; NN
00-3519

PIERSOL, George Arthur, ed. (1856-1924)
Human anatomy, including structure and development and practical considerations, by Thomas Dwight . . . J. Playfair McMurrich . . . Carl A. Hamann . . . George A. Piersol . . . and J. William White . . . with seventeen hundred and thirty-four illustrations, of which fifteen hundred and twenty-two are original and largely from dissections by John C. Heisler. . . . Ed. by George A. Piersol. Philadelphia: J. B. Lippincott Co., [1907]. 2088p. DLC; NNNAM; PPC; PU
00-3520

PIERSOL, George Arthur, ed. (1856-1924)
Human anatomy, including structure and development and practical considerations, by Thomas Dwight . . . J. Playfair McMurrich . . . Carl A. Hamann . . . George A. Piersol . . . and J. William White . . . with seventeen hundred and thirty-four illustrations, of which fifteen hundred and twenty-two are original and largely from dissections by John C. Heisler . . . ed. by George A. Piersol. Philadelphia & London: J. B. Lippincott Co., [1908]. 2 v. [paged continuously] DLC; GU; NNNAM; PPC **00-3521**

PIERSOL, George Arthur, ed. (1856-1924)
Human anatomy, including structure and development and practical considerations, by Thomas Dwight . . . J. Playfair McMurrich . . . Carl A. Hamann . . . George A. Piersol . . . and J. William White . . . with seventeen hundred and thirty-four illustrations, of which fifteen hundred and twenty-two are original and largely from dissections by John C. Heisler . . . ed. by George A. Piersol. 3rd ed. Philadelphia & London: J. B. Lippincott Co., 1910 [*c.* 1911]. 2104p. DLC: ICJ; NN; PU **00-3522**

PIERSOL, G[eorge] A[rthur] (1856-1924)
Normal histology, with special reference to the structure of the human body . . . 438 illustrations, many of which are in colors. 8th ed. (rewritten). Philadelphia & London: J. B. Lippincott Co., [1910]. 418p. DLC; IU-M; OC; PU
00-3523

PIERSON, Edward L.
Acetone and diacetic acid as a cause of persistent recurrent vomiting of children. [New York: E. B. Treat, 1903.] 4 l. DNLM **00-3524**

PIFFARD, Henry G[ranger] (1842-1910)
Elementary studies in ortho-chromatic photography. . . . [New York? 1904?] 8p. DNLM . **00-3525**

PIFFARD, Henry G[ranger] (1842-1910)
A safety X-ray tube. New York, 1905. 8p. DNLM
00-3526

PIFFARD, Henry G[ranger] (1842-1910)
Aids to accuracy and efficiency in radiotherapy. New York, 1906. 12p. DNLM **00-3527**

PIFFARD, Henry G[ranger] (1842-1910)
The d'Arsonval and other high-frequency currents; what they are and what they will do. New York, 1906. 19p. DNLM
00-3528

PIFFARD, Henry G[ranger] (1842-1910)
Hand protection in Roentgen praxis. New York, 1906. 18p. DNLM **00-3529**

PIFFARD, Henry G[ranger] (1842-1910)
The milk problem. [New York, 1906.] 18p. DNLM
00-3530

PIFFARD, Henry G[ranger] (1842-1910)
Some new high-frequency devices. New York: A. R. Elliott Co., 1907. 11p. DNLM **00-3531**

PIFFARD, Henry G[ranger] (1842-1910)
A study of sour milks. New York, 1908. 6p. 2 plates. DNLM
00-3532

PIKE, Frank Henry
. . . Resuscitation of the respiratory and other bulbar nervous mechanisms, with special reference to the question of their automaticity. . . . Chicago, 1907. 31p. DLC; ICJ [Abstract, Ph.D. thesis, University of Chicago]
00-3533

PILCHER, James Evelyn (1857-1911)
First aid in illness and injury; comprised in a series of chapters on the human machine, its structure, its implements of repair, and the accidents and emergencies to which it is liable. . . . 7th ed. New York: C. Scribner's Sons, 1903. 322p. NNNAM
00-3534

PILCHER, James Evelyn (1857-1911)
First aid in illness and injury; comprised in a series of chapters on the human machine, its structure, its implements of repair, and the accidents and emergencies to which it is liable. . . . 8th ed. New York: C. Scribner's Sons, 1904. 322p. 1 plate. DNLM; NNNAM **00-3535**

PILCHER, James Evelyn (1857-1911)
First aid in illness and injury; comprised in a series of chapters on the human machine, its structure, its implements of repair, and the accidents and emergencies to which it is liable. . . . 9th ed., rev., with 208 illustrations. New York: C. Scribner's Sons, 1905. 356p. DLC; DNLM; NNNAM; PPC
00-3536

PILCHER, James Evelyn (1857-1911)
The surgeon generals of the army of the United States of America: a series of biographical sketches of the senior officers of the military medical service from the American Revolution to the Philippine pacification. . . . Carlisle, Pa.: The Association of Military Surgeons, 1905. 114p. ports. DLC; DNLM; NNNAM; PU **00-3537**

PILCHER, James Evelyn (1857-1911)
The training of the medical officer of the State forces to best qualify him for local service and for mobilization with national troops. Carlisle, Pa., 1907. 32p. DNLM
00-3538

PILCHER, Lewis S[tephen] (1845-1934)
Clinical studies of the surgical diseases of the female generative organs from observations made during ten years work in the Method Episcopal Hospital in Brooklyn. . . . Philadelphia: J. B. Lippincott Co., 1900 [*c.* 1898]. 96p. PPC **00-3539**

PILCHER, Lewis S[tephen] (1845-1934)
Jacobus Berengarius Carpensi and his commentaries on Mundinus. [Brooklyn, N.Y.? 1903.] 8p. 1 illus., facsim. NN
00-3540

PILCHER, Lewis S[tephen] (1845-1934)
Obstructive hypertrophy body. . . . By L. S. Pilcher and Paul M. Pilcher. Philadelphia: J. B. Lippincott, 1905. 40p. DLC; PU [Includes Pathology and etiology by P. M. Pilcher, and Methods and results of prostatectomy by L. S. Pilcher]
00-3541

PILCHER, Lewis S[tephen] (1845-1934)
The cure of carcinoma of the breast. Brooklyn, 1905. 10p. DNLM **00-3542**

PILCHER, Lewis S[tephen] (1845-1934)
Remarks made in presenting the Fowler memorial tablet in the library building of the Medical Society of the County of Kings, N.Y., May 27, 1906. Brooklyn, 1906. 9p. DNLM
00-3543

PILCHER, Lewis S[tephen] (1845-1934)
Some observations upon the removal of the prostate for the cure of prostatic dysuria. New York, 1906. 12p. DNLM
00-3544

PILCHER, Lewis S[tephen] (1845-1934) and St. Clair McKELWAY
Tribute to George Ryerson Fowler. With historical record, by William Schroeder. Brooklyn, 1906. 27p. DNLM
00-3545

PILCHER, Lewis S[tephen] (1845-1934)
The Mondino myth; a study of the conditions attending the revival in the thirteenth and fourteenth centuries of the practical study of human anatomy from the cadaver. . . . [Brooklyn, N.Y.: Eagle Press, 1907?] 24p. plates. DLC; NN
00-3546

PILCHER, Lewis S[tephen] (1845-1934)
The cure of cancer. . . . Philadelphia: J. B. Lippincott Co., 1909. 29p. PPC **00-3547**

PILCHER, Lewis S[tephen] (1845-1934)
Odium medicum and other addresses and studies in medical life and affairs. Philadelphia: J. B. Lippincott Co., 1910 [*c.* 1911]. 234p. DLC; DNLM; ICJ; NcD
00-3548

PILCHER, Lewis S[tephen] (1845-1934)
Epigastric incisions in dealing with cancer of the breast. Philadelphia: Press of J. B. Lippincott Co., 1910. 5p. NIC
00-3549

PILGRIM, Maurice F[lescher] (1858-1903)
Clinical history and progress of a case of pulmonary disease treated exclusively by mechanical vibratory stimulation. New York: A. L. Chatterton, 1903. 3p. DNLM
00-3550

PILGRIM, Maurice F[lescher] (1858-1903)
A consideration of the scientific application of mechanical vibratory stimulation in the treatment of disease. New York: Lea Bros. & Co., 1903. 10p. DNLM
00-3551

PILGRIM, Maurice F[lescher] (1858-1903)
Mechanical vibration: Its theory and application in the treatment of disease. Boston: Old Corner Book Store, 1903. 7p. illus. DNLM; NN **00-3552**

PILGRIM, Maurice F[lescher] (1858-1903)
Mechanical vibratory stimulation, its theory and application in the treatment of disease. New York: The Lawrence Press, [1903]. 152p. 8 col. plates. DLC; ICJ; NN; PP
00-3553

PILLING, GEORGE P., & SON (PHILADELPHIA)
. . . Illustrated dental catalogue of George P. Pilling & Son, manufacturers and exporters of surgical, dental and veterinary instruments [1901]. Philadelphia: G. P. Pilling & Son, 1901. [unp.] DLC **00-3554**

PILLING, GEORGE P., & SON (PHILADELPHIA)
. . . Pilling eye, ear, nose, throat and bronchoscopic instruments and equipment. Philadelphia, Pa., [1902?] [unp.] DLC ["Catalog of instruments and apparatus for surgeons and hospitals."] **00-3555**

PILSBURY, Lawrence B[ell] (*b.* 1874)
The degree to which substances agglutinating the dysentery bacilli are present in the blood of non-infected persons. New York, 1903. 13p. 1 table. DNLM; NNNAM
00-3556

PILSBURY, Lawrence B[ell] (*b.* 1874)
Rhinoplasty by the Indian method; report of a case. Lincoln, Neb., 1904. 3p. DNLM **00-3557**

[PILZ, D.]
Anatomical model of the eye, ear, nose and throat. New York: Thermo-Ware Co., [1901?] 8p. DLC [Fold-out color charts which lift up to show complete anatomical models]
00-3558

PINARD, Adolphe (1844-1934)
A treatise on abdominal palpation, as applied to obstetrics and version by external manipulation. . . . Transl. by L. E. Neale. . . . New York: J. H. Vail & Co., [1901?] 101p. DLC; MdU-D; MH-M; PU [1st printing, 1885. *vel subseq.*]
00-3559

PIPER, Edward W[ester]
The mariner's medical companion, symptoms, diseases, treatment, with plain and simple directions for the use of the medicines and appliances in Nelson's medicine chest. . . . New York: The Fraser Press, 1901. 65p. DLC; DNLM; NNNAM
00-3560

PITFIELD, Robert Lucas (*b.* 1870)
A new method of staining flagella. [Philadelphia, 1900?] 2p. DNLM **00-3561**

PITFIELD, Robert Lucas (*b.* 1870)
. . . A compend on bacteriology, including animal parasites . . . with 4 plates and 80 other illustrations. Philadelphia: P. Blakiston's Son & Co., 1907. 232p. DLC; ICJ; PPC; PU
00-3562

PITTSBURGH MEDICAL LIBRARY ASSOCIATION
Catalogue of the Pittsburgh Medical Library Association, which is located in rooms 10 and 17 of the Pittsburgh Free Dispensary Building. . . . Pittsburgh, Pa.: Pub. by order of the Library Committee, [1901]. 36p. DLC **00-3563**

PITZER, George C[alvin]
Therapeutic suggestion applied . . . 2nd ed. St. Louis, Mo.: [St. Louis School of Suggestive Therapeutics and Medical Electricity], 1901. 206p. front. port. DLC
00-3564

PLATT, Charles (*b.* 1869)
A manual of qualitative analysis and of clinical medical chemistry, for physicians and students. . . . 3rd ed., rev. and enl. Philadelphia: J. J. McVey, 1900. 179p. DLC; MB; PP; PU
00-3565

PLATT, Charles (*b.* 1869)
Practical notes in qualitative analysis and in clinical medical chemistry. . . . 2nd ed. rev. and enl. Philadelphia: J. J. McVey, 1901 [*c.* 1896]. DLC; ICJ; NN; PU **00-3566**

PLATT, Charles (*b.* 1869)
A manual of qualitative analysis and of clinical medical chemistry, for physicians and students. . . . 4th ed., rev. and enl. Philadelphia: J. J. McVey, 1902. 190p. DLC; PP; PPJ; PU
00-3567

PLATT, Charles (*b.* 1869)
A manual of qualitative analysis and of medical chemistry, for physicians and students. . . . 5th ed., rewritten and enl. Philadelphia: J. J. McVey, 1906. 243p. DLC; NN; PP; PU
00-3568

PLATT, Charles (*b.* 1869)
Practical medical chemistry, for physicians and students. By Charles Platt . . . and William A. Pearson . . . 6th ed., rewritten and enl. Philadelphia: J. J. McVey, 1910 [*c.* 1911]. 300p. DLC; MH; NIC; PU **00-3569**

PLATT, S[mith] H.
The secrets of health; or, How not to be sick and how to get well from sickness. Color plate ed. New York: O. Judd Co., 1900. 536p. DLC; NN **00-3570**

PLATT, S[mith] H.
Home treatment with the cell-salts. Southern Pines, N.C.: E. F. Barnes, 1901 [*c.* 1897]. 363p. front. (port.). DLC
00-3571

PODMORE, Frank (1856-1910)
Mesmerism and Christian Science, a short history of mental healing. . . . Philadelphia: G. W. Jacobs & Co., [1909]. 306p. DLC; MA; NN; PU **00-3572**

POISONS; remedies. A manual for reference issued by the Mutual Life Insurance Co., of New York. New York, 1903. 45p. DNLM; NNNAM **00-3573**

POLAK, John O[sborn] (1870-1931)
Observations on fibromyomatous tumors of the uterus. New York, 1906. 11p. DNLM **00-3574**

POLITZER, Adam (1835-1920)
Atlas and epitome of otology. Edited by S. MacCuen Smith. Philadelphia: W. B. Saunders & Co., 1902. 16p. 39 plates, 24 l. 292p. DNLM; ICRM; NNNAM; PPC
00-3575

POLITZER, Adam (1835-1920)
A text-book of the diseases of the ear. . . . Transl. . . . and edited by Milton J. Ballin and Clarence L. Heller . . . 4th ed., rev. and enl. Philadelphia: Lea Bros. & Co., 1903. 884p. CtY-M; DNLM; ICJ; PPC **00-3576**

POLITZER, Adam (1835-1920)
A text-book of the diseases of the ear for students and practitioners. Transl. at the personal request of the author, and edited by Milton J. Ballin and Clarence L. Heller. With 337 original illustrations. 6th ed., rev. and enl. Philadelphia: Lea & Febiger, 1909. 892p. DNLM; ICJ; MH-M; PU
00-3577

POLK, John Metcalfe (1875-1904)
Notes on physical diagnosis, by John Metcalfe Polk . . . ed. by C. N. B. Camac. . . . New York: Cornell University Medical College, 1905. 178p. DLC; ICJ; NIC; NNNAM
00-3578

POLK, R. L. & CO.
Dental register of the United States. 4th ed. Detroit, Baltimore & Chicago, 1900. 1006p. DNLM; ICJ
00-3579

POLK, R. L. & CO.
Polk's medical and surgical register of the United States and Canada. 6th ed. Detroit, Baltimore & Chicago: R. L. Polk & Co., 1900. 2748p. DNLM; PPC **00-3580**

POLK, R. L. & CO.
Polk's medical register and directory of the United States and Canada. 7th ed. Detroit, Baltimore & Chicago, 1902. 3008p. DNLM; NN **00-3581**

POLK, R. L. & CO.
Dental register and directory of the United States and Canada. 5th ed. Detroit, Baltimore & Chicago, 1902. 1150p. DNLM; ICJ **00-3582**

POLK, R. L. & CO.
Dental register and directory of the United States and Canada. 6th ed. Detroit, Baltimore & Chicago, 1904. 1286p. DNLM; ICJ **00-3583**

POLK, R. L. & CO.
Polk's medical register and directory of North America. 8th rev. ed. Detroit, Baltimore & Chicago, 1904. 3076p. DNLM; PPC **00-3584**

POLK, R. L. & CO.
Dental register and directory of the United States and Canada. 7th ed. Detroit, Baltimore & Chicago, 1906. 1400p. DNLM; ICJ **00-3585**

POLK, R. L. & CO.
Polk's medical register and directory of North America. 9th ed. Detroit, Baltimore & Chicago, 1906. 3166p. DNLM; ICJ; PP **00-3586**

POLLITZER, S[igmund] (1859-1937)
Serum therapy and serum diagnosis in syphilis. New York, 1907. 11p. DNLM **00-3587**

POOLEY, Thomas Rickett (1841-1926)
The operations for the artificial maturation of the immature senile cataract. New York, 1907. 4p. DNLM
00-3588

POORE, George V[ivian] (1843-1904)
A treatise on medical jurisprudence. Based on lectures delivered at University College, London. New York: Longmans, Green & Co., 1901. 533p. 18 plates, forms. ICJ; MH; NN; PU
00-3589

POPE, Amy Elizabeth (*b.* 1869)
Home care of the sick. . . . Chicago: American School of Home Economics, 1907. 190p. DLC; ICU; NN
00-3590

POPE, Amy Elizabeth (*b.* 1869)
Essentials of dietetics in health and disease; a textbook for nurses and a practical dietary guide for the household, by Amy Elizabeth Pope . . . and Mary L. Carpenter. . . . New York & London: G. P. Putnam's Sons, 1908. 249p. DLC; ICJ; MB; NN
00-3591

POPE, Amy Elizabeth (*b.* 1869)
A quiz book of nursing for teachers and students, by Amy Elizabeth Pope . . . and Thirza A. Pope . . . together with chapters on visiting nursing, by Margaret A. Bewley . . . hospital planning, construction, and equipment, by Bertrand E. Taylor, A.A.I.A., and hospital book-keeping and statistics, by Frederic B. Morlok. . . . New York and London: G. P. Putnam's Son, 1909. 469p. fold. plan, fold. forms. DLC; ICJ; NNNAM **00-3592**

POPE, Amy Elizabeth (*b.* 1869)
Home care of the sick. . . . [Text book ed.] Chicago: American School of Home Economics, 1910 [*c.* 1911]. 190p. DLC; ICRM; KU; NNNAM **00-3593**

POPE, Curran (*b.* 1866)
The treatment of anaemia. New York, 1907. 11p. DNLM
00-3594

POPE, Curran (*b.* 1866)
Practical hydrotherapy, a manual for students and practitioners. . . . Cincinnati: Cincinnati Medical Book Co., 1909. 646p. plates, plans, diags. CtY-M; DLC; ICJ
00-3595

PORTER, Eugene Hoffman (1856-1929)
The fight against preventable diseases: an address delivered at the fourth annual meeting of the Association of Life Insurance Presidents in Chicago, Ill., on December 10, 1910. . . . Albany: New York State Department of Health, Division of Publicity and Education, [1910?] 13p. DLC; NN
00-3596

PORTER, Eugene Hoffman (1856-1929)
. . . Unity in health work: an address delivered before the Conference of Mayors at Schenectady, June 24, 1910. . . . Albany: New York State Department of Health, Division of Publicity and Education, 1910. 11p. NN
00-3597

PORTER, Eugene Hoffman (1856-1929)
The purity of natural ice; an address. . . . New York, N.Y.: The Natural Ice Association of America, [1910?] 4p. DLC; NN
00-3598

PORTER, Eugene Hoffman (1856-1929)
Progress in medical education. An address. . . . Albany, N.Y., [1910?] 5p. DLC **00-3599**

PORTER, Miles F.
Cornual pregnancy; rupture in the fourth month; operation; recovery. New York: William Wood & Co., 1901. 6p. DNLM
00-3600

PORTER, Miles F.
Management of fibromyomata complicated by pregnancy. Boston, 1902. 8p. DNLM **00-3601**

PORTER, William H[enry] (*b.* 1853)
A practical treatise on renal diseases and urinary analysis. . . . New York: William Wood & Co., 1900. 349p. CtY-M; DLC; ICJ; PPC [1st printing, 1887] **00-3602**

PORTER, William H[enry] (*b.* 1853)
The physiological importance of the proximate principles and their practical utility in the foodstuffs and in the nutritive processes of the system. . . . [Philadelphia? 1900?] 19p. NN **00-3603**

PORTER, William H[enry] (*b.* 1853)
Intestinal indigestion and its consequences. Philadelphia, 1900. 29p. DLC; DNLM **00-3604**

PORTER, William H[enry] (*b.* 1853)
Physiological and artificial sleep, with remarks upon a new hypnotic, chloretone. New York, 1900. 8p. DLC; DNLM
00-3605

PORTER, William H[enry] (*b.* 1853)
A college course on tuberculosis. St. Louis, 1905. 2 l. DLC; DNLM **00-3606**

PORTER, William H[enry] (*b.* 1853)
Tuberculosis. The problem of the general practitioner. St. Louis, 1905. 9p. DLC; DNLM **00-3607**

PORTER, William H[enry] (*b.* 1853)
Hygiene and diet in the cure of the consumptive. New York, 1905. 16p. DLC; DNLM **00-3608**

PORTER, William H[enry] (*b.* 1853)
Clinical studies at Mount St. Rose. St. Louis, 1905. 12p. DLC; DNLM **00-3609**

PORTER, William H[enry] (*b.* 1853)
Some phenomena of tuberculosis infection. Chicago, 1906. 8p. DLC; DNLM **00-3610**

PORTER, William H[enry] (*b.* 1853)
Tuberculosis in the Mississippi Valley. St. Louis, 1906. 8p. DLC; DNLM **00-3611**

PORTER, William H[enry] (*b.* 1853)
The effects of uric acid on the genito-urinary tract. New York, 1906. 19p. 1 table. DLC; DNLM
00-3612

[PORTER, William Sydney] (1862-1910)
. . . Let me feel your pulse, by O. Henry [*pseud.*]; illustrations by W. W. Fawcett. New York: Doubleday, Page & Co., 1910. 38p. front., plates. DLC; MH; NIC; NN [At head of title: Adventures in neurasthenia.] **00-3613**

PORTER, William Townsend (1862-1949)
The relation of the depressor nerve to the vasomotor centre by W. T. Porter and H. G. Bayer. [1900.] 4p. DNLM
00-3614

PORTER, William Townsend (1862-1949)
Experiments concerning the prolonged inhibition said to follow injury of the spinal chord by W. T. Porter and W. Muhlberg. [1900.] 6p. DNLM **00-3615**

PORTER, William Townsend (1862-1949)
Introduction to physiology. Cambridge, Mass.: The University Press, 1900. 577p. PPJ; PU
00-3616

PORTER, William Townsend (1862-1949)
The teaching of physiology. Philadelphia, 1900. 16p. DNLM; MH **00-3617**

PORTER, William Townsend (1862-1949)
An introduction to physiology. Part IV. Physiological optics. Cambridge, Mass.: The University Press, 1901. 96p. DLC; DNLM; MH-M **00-3618**

PORTER, William Townsend (1862-1949)
The laboratory teaching of physiology. New York, 1901. 4p. DNLM; NN **00-3619**

PORTER, William Townsend (1862-1949)
An introduction to physiology. . . . Cambridge, Mass.: The University Press, 1901. 314p. DLC; ICJ; NN; PPJ **00-3620**

PORTER, William Townsend (1862-1949)
Experiments for students in the Harvard Medical School. Third series. . . . Cambridge, Mass.: The University Press, 1901. 93p. DLC; MH-M **00-3621**

PORTER, William Townsend (1862-1949)
Physiology at Harvard. . . . Cambridge, Mass.: The University Press, 1902. 66p. DLC; DNLM; MH-M; PPC **00-3622**

PORTER, William Townsend (1862-1949)
Physiology at Harvard. . . . 2nd ed. Cambridge, Mass.: The University Press, 1903. 101p. DNLM; ICJ; MH-M; PPC **00-3623**

PORTER, William Townsend (1862-1949)
Experiments for students in the Harvard Medical School. 3rd ed. Cambridge, Mass.: The University Press, 1903. 108p. MH-M; NIC **00-3624**

PORTER, William Townsend (1862-1949)
Physiology at Harvard. . . . 3rd ed. Cambridge, Mass.: The University Press, 1904. 117p. DLC; DNLM; ICJ; MH-M **00-3625**

PORTER, William Townsend (1862-1949)
Physiology at Harvard. . . . 4th ed. Cambridge, Mass.: The University Press, 1905. 117p. DLC; DNLM; MH-M **00-3626**

PORTER, William Townsend (1862-1949)
Physiology at Harvard. . . . 5th ed. Cambridge, Mass.: The University Press, 1906. 124p. DLC; MH-M **00-3627**

PORTER, William Townsend (1862-1949)
An introduction to physiology. . . . [2nd ed.] Cambridge, Mass.: The University Press, 1906. 587p. DLC; ICJ; MH-M; PPC **00-3628**

POSEY, William Campbell (1866-1934)
Papilloma of the caruncle, with a report of a case. Philadelphia, 1902. 8p. DNLM **00-3629**

POSEY, William Campbell (1866-1934) and
Edward A. SHUMWAY
Carcinoma of the eyelids, with secondary involvement of the eyeball; removal of the growth by extensive plastic operations; recurrence. Philadelphia, 1902. 3p. DNLM **00-3630**

POSEY, William Campbell, ed. (1866-1934)
A treatise on diseases of the eye. For students and practitioners. By various authors. Edited by William Campbell Posey. . . . Volume I. of a treatise on diseases of the eye, nose, throat, and ear. Edited by William Campbell Posey, M.D., and Jonathan Wright, M.D. Illustrated with 358 engravings and 19 plates in colors and monochrome. Philadelphia and New York: Lea Bros. & Co., [1902]. 685p. ICJ; NNC; PPC; PU **00-3631**

POSEY, William Campbell, ed. (1866-1934)
A treatise on diseases of the eye, nose, throat and ear. For students and practitioners. By various authors. Ed. by William Campbell Posey . . . and Jonathan Wright. . . . Illustrated with 650 engravings and 35 plates in colors and monochrome. Philadelphia and New York: Lea Bros. & Co., 1903. 1238p. 35 plates. DLC; DNLM; NNNAM; PPC **00-3632**

POSEY, William Campbell (1866-1934) and
H. Maxwell LANGDON
Some observations upon the non-operative treatment of squint; the Worth amblyoscope. New York, 1904. 32p. DNLM **00-3633**

POSEY, William Campbell (1866-1934)
Unusual success from iridotomy in eyes practically blind from iridocyclitis and complicated cataract. New York, 1906. 6p. DNLM **00-3634**

POSEY, William Campbell, ed. (1866-1934)
The eye and nervous system, their diagnostic relations, by various authors; ed. by William Campbell Posey . . . and William G. Spiller. . . . Philadelphia and London: J. B. Lippincott Co., [1906]. 988p. col. plates. DLC; NNNAM; PPC; PU **00-3635**

POSEY, William Campbell (1866-1934)
The accessory sinuses of the nose from an ophthalmological standpoint. New York: A. R. Elliott Co., 1907. 11p. DNLM **00-3636**

POST, Wilber E.
A classified nomenclature of diseases, designed for use as a diagnosis index in the central free dispensary. Rush Medical College. . . . [Chicago? 1909.] 137p. DLC; ICJ; ICRM **00-3637**

POTTENGER, Francis M[arion] (*b.* 1869)
A study of the diagnosis of incipient pulmonary tuberculosis based upon the pathology of the disease. Asheville, N.C., 1902. 16p. DNLM; MB **00-3638**

POTTENGER, Francis M[arion] (*b.* 1869)
The rhinologist; an important factor in the prevention of tuberculosis. St. Louis, 1902. 8p. DNLM; MB **00-3639**

POTTENGER, Francis M[arion] (*b.* 1869)
Culture products in the treatment of tuberculosis. Asheville, N.C., 1902. 22p. DNLM; MB **00-3640**

POTTENGER, Francis M[arion] (*b.* 1869)
Tuberculosis of childhood, with especial reference to infection. Los Angeles, 1902. 12p. DNLM; MB **00-3641**

POTTENGER, Francis M[arion] (*b.* 1869)
Some suggestions relative to the treatment of tuberculosis. New York, 1902. 11p. MB **00-3642**

POTTENGER, Francis M[arion] (*b.* **1869)**
When and how should the tuberculous patient be treated. New York, 1905. 14p. DNLM **00-3643**

POTTENGER, Francis M[arion] (*b.* **1869)**
The diagnosis and treatment of pulmonary tuberculosis. . . . New York: William Wood & Co., 1908. 377p. plates. DLC; DNLM; NNNAM; PU **00-3644**

POTTER, Samuel Otway Lewis (1846-1914)
A handbook of materia medica, pharmacy, and therapeutics, including the physiological action of drugs, the special therapeutics of disease, official and practical pharmacy, and minute directions for prescription writing . . . 8th ed., rev. and enl. Philadelphia: P. Blakiston's Son & Co., 1901. 950p. DLC; DNLM; NN; PU **00-3645**

POTTER, Samuel Otway Lewis (1846-1914)
A handbook of materia medica, pharmacy and therapeutics, including the physiological action of drugs, the special therapeutics of disease, official and practical pharmacy, and minute directions for prescription writing . . . 9th ed., rev. and enl. Philadelphia: P. Blakiston's Son & Co., 1902. 951p. DLC; NNNAM; PPC; PU **00-3646**

POTTER, Samuel Otway Lewis (1846-1914)
A compend of human anatomy . . . 7th ed., rev. and enl., with 138 wood engravings; also numerous tables and 16 plates of the arteries and nerves. Philadelphia: P. Blakiston's Son & Co., 1903. 372p. DLC; NNNAM; PPC; PU **00-3647**

POTTER, Samuel Otway Lewis (1846-1914)
. . . A compend of materia medica, therapeutics and prescription writing, with especial reference to the physiological action of drugs; based on the eighth revision of the U.S. pharmacopoeia including also many unofficial remedies . . . 7th ed. — Rev. and enl. Philadelphia: P. Blakiston's Son & Co., 1906. 292p. DLC; DNLM; NNNAM; PPC **00-3648**

POTTER, Samuel Otway Lewis (1846-1914)
Materia medica, pharmacy and therapeutics, including the physiological action of drugs, the special therapeutics of disease, official and practical pharmacy, minute directions for prescription writing and avoiding incompatibility, also the antidotal and antagonistic treatment of poisoning. . . . 10th ed., rev., and in greater part rewritten. Philadelphia: P. Blakiston's Son & Co., 1906. 914p. DLC; DNLM; OCLloyd; PU **00-3649**

POTTER, Samuel Otway Lewis (1846-1914)
Therapeutics, materia medica, and pharmacy, including the special therapeutics of diseases and symptoms, the physiological and therapeutical action of drugs, the modern materia medica, official and practical pharmacy, minute directions for prescription writing, also the antidotal and antagonistic treatment of poisoning . . . 11th ed., rev. and enl. Philadelphia: P. Blakiston's Son & Co., 1909. 937p. DLC; NNNAM; PPC; PU **00-3650**

POTTER, William (1852-1926)
Address introductory to the seventy-ninth session of the Jefferson Medical College. September 24, 1903. 16p. PPJ; PPC **00-3651**

POTTER, William (1852-1926)
Address introductory to the eightieth session of Jefferson Medical College. September 26th, 1904. [Philadelphia, 1904.] 24p. PPJ **00-3652**

POTTER, William (1852-1926)
Addresses at opening of new Jefferson Medical College, June 7-8, 1907 by William Potter, J. Chalmers Da Costa, and William H. Welch. Chicago, 1907. 36p. PPJ **00-3653**

POTTS, Barton H.
Foreign body in the maxillary antrum. [St. Louis, 1905.] 3p. DNLM **00-3654**

POTTS, Barton H.
Report of a case of septic meningo-encephalitis or cerebritis. New York, 1907. 5p. DNLM **00-3655**

POTTS, Charles S[ower] (1864-1930)
Clinical notes on the analgesic effect of Lactophenin. New York: C. F. Bochringer & Seehowe, [1900?]. 16p. NN **00-3656**

POTTS, Charles S[ower] (1864-1930)
Nervous and mental diseases; a manual for students and practitioners. Philadelphia & New York: Lea Bros. & Co., [1900]. 455p. DLC; DNLM; NNNAM; PU **00-3657**

POTTS, Charles S[ower] (1864-1930) and William G. SPILLER
A case of solitary tubercle of the pons; remarks on the pathway for sensations of taste from the anterior portion of the tongue; with pathological report and remarks on palsy of associated ocular movements. Philadelphia, 1903. 11p. DNLM **00-3658**

POTTS, Charles S[ower] (1864-1930) and William G. SPILLER
Pseudo-sclerosis, diffuse sclerosis, with the report of a case with necropsy. Chicago, 1905. 14p. DNLM **00-3659**

POTTS, Charles S[ower] (1864-1930)
A case of traumatic cervical hematomyelia and complete division of the cord, with probable dislocation of the fifth cervical vertebra; remarks on the location of the center for the biceps reflex. New York, 1905. 7p. DNLM **00-3660**

POTTS, Charles S[ower] (1864-1930)
Nervous and mental diseases, for students and practitioners . . . 2nd ed., rev. and enl.; illustrated with 133 engravings and 9 plates. Philadelphia and New York: Lea & Febiger, 1908. 570p. col. plates. DLC: NNNAM; OCIM; PPC **00-3661**

POTTS, Charles S[ower] (1864-1930)
Electricity; its medical and surgical applications, including radiotherapy and phototherapy, by Charles S. Potts . . . with a section on electrophysics, by Horace Clark Richards . . . and a section on X-rays, by Henry K. Pancoast . . . with 356 illustrations and 6 plates. Philadelphia and New York: Lea & Febiger, 1910 [*c.* 1911]. 509p. 7 plates. DLC; ICJ; PPJ; PPC **00-3662**

POWELL, Charles H.
Some clinical experience. Nashville, 1904. 8p. DNLM **00-3663**

POWELL, Lyman P[ierson] (*b.* 1866)
The Emmanuel Movement in a New England town: a systematic account of experiments and reflections designed to determine the proper relationship between the minister and the doctor in the light of modern needs. New York & London: G. P. Putnam's Sons, 1909. 194p. DLC; ICJ; NNNAM; PP
00-3664

POWELL, Seneca D. (1847-1907)
Carbolic acid in surgery. [Philadelphia, 1900.] 34p. DNLM; PPC **00-3665**

POWELL, Seneca D. (1847-1907)
A new dilator. [New York, 1901?] 1 l. DNLM
00-3666

POWELL, William M. (*b.* 1862)
Saunders' pocket medical formulary . . . 6th ed., thoroughly rev. Philadelphia: W. B. Saunders & Co., 1900. 298p. CU-M; DLC; PPC; PU **00-3667**

POWELL, William M. (*b.* 1862)
. . . Essentials of the diseases of children, arranged in the form of questions and answers prepared especially for students of medicine . . . 3rd ed., thoroughly rev. by Alfred Hand, Jr. . . . Philadelphia and London: W. B. Saunders & Co., 1901. 259p. DLC; DNLM; NNNAM; PU [2nd ed., 1895. 222p.; 1st ed., 1890. 222p.] **00-3668**

POWELL, William M. (*b.* 1862)
Saunders' pocket medical formulary. With an appendix. . . . 7th ed., thoroughly rev. and enl. Philadelphia and London: W. B. Saunders & Co., 1905. 301p. DLC; DNLM; GU; PPC
00-3669

POWELL, William M. (*b.* 1862)
Saunders' pocket medical formulary. . . . 8th ed., thoroughly rev., enl. and adapted to the eighth revision (1905) of the U.S. pharmacopoeia. Philadelphia and London: W. B. Saunders & Co., 1906. 299p. DLC; DNLM; NNNAM; PU
00-3670

POWELL, William M. (*b.* 1862)
Saunders' pocket medical formulary. . . . 9th ed., thoroughly rev., enl. and adapted to the eighth revision (1905) of the U.S. pharmacopoeia. Philadelphia and London: W. B. Saunders & Co., 1909. 308p. DLC; IU-M; NNNAM; PPC
00-3671

POWER, D'Arcy (1855-1941)
William Harvey. New York: Longmans, Green & Co., 1900 [*c.* 1898]. 282p. DLC; MH; NIC; NN
00-3672

POWERS & ANDERSON
Abridged catalogue and price list of surgical instruments, orthopaedic apparatus, trusses, elastic hosiery, electrical batteries, microscopes, hospital and laboratory supplies. Richmond, Va., 1900. 179p. DNLM; PPF
00-3673

POWERS, Charles A.
Conical stump after amputation in childhood. Philadelphia, 1900. 3p. DNLM **00-3674**

POWERS, Charles A.
Early diagnosis in carcinoma. Chicago, 1901. 15p. DNLM
00-3675

POWERS, Charles A.
Giant sacro-coccygeal tumors. An account of one which pursued an atrophic course. New York, 1901. 13p. DNLM
00-3676

POWERS, Charles A.
Permanent suprapubic drainage for advanced tuberculosis of the bladder; report of a case at end of five years. Philadelphia, 1902. 5p. DNLM **00-3677**

POWERS, Charles A.
The surgeon's heritage. Chairman's address. Chicago, 1904. 10p. DNLM **00-3678**

POWERS, Charles A.
On the present status of our knowledge of serotherapy in surgical affections. New York, 1906. 8p. DNLM
00-3679

POWERS, Samuel A.
Variola. A series of twenty-one heliotype plates illustrating the progressive stages of the eruption. Boston: S. A. Powers [1901?] 2p. 21 plates. DLC; MH-M **00-3680**

POZZI-ESCOT, [Marius] Emmanuel (*b.* 1880)
The toxins and venoms and their antibodies. Transl. by Alfred I. Cohn. New York: John Wiley & Sons, 1906. 101p. DLC; ICJ; NNNAM; PU **00-3681**

PRACTICAL lessons in nursing. Maternity, infancy, childhood. Hygiene of pregnancy; nursing and weaning of infants; the care of children in health and disease. Adapted especially to the use of mothers or those intrusted with the bringing up of infants and children, and training schools for nurses, as an aid to the teaching of the nursing of women and children. 3rd ed. Philadelphia: J. B. Lippincott Co., 1906. 221p. DNLM; PP; PPC **00-3682**

THE PRACTICAL medicine series, comprising ten volumes on the year's progress in medicine and surgery . . . 1901-. Chicago: The Year Book Publishers, 1901-1910. DLC; ICJ [Issued from 1901-1905 under title: The practical medicine series of year books, comprising the volumes on the year's progress in medicine and surgery. Ten volumes issued each year; each volume has special editors; the contents of earlier issues of Vol. VII-X differ somewhat from later issues. General editor: 1901-1909, G. P. Head. Contents: I. General medicine. — II. General surgery. — III. The eye, ear, nose and throat. — IV. Gynecology. — V. Obstetrics. — VI. General medicine. — VII. Pediatrics; orthopedic surgery. — VIII. Materia medica and therapeutics; preventive medicine; climatology. — IX. Skin and venereal diseases; miscellaneous topics. — X. Nervous and mental diseases.] **00-3683**

A PRACTICAL treatise on thialion . . . 13th ed. Danbury: The Vass Chemical Co., 1904. 259p. DNLM; MH
00-3684

A PRACTICAL treatise on uric acid toxemia in all its phases, including its treatment with thialion (a laxative salt of lithia) with a complete bibliography and index. 15th ed. Danbury: The Vass Chemical Co., 1906. 153p. DNLM; MH
00-3685

PRATT, E[dwin] Hartley (1849-1930)
The composite man as comprehended in fourteen anatomical impersonations. 2nd ed. Chicago, 1901. 150p. 14 plates. Chicago, 1901. DNLM; OCIM **00-3686**

PRATT, E[dwin] Hartley (1849-1930)
Sores and sinuses in the light of modern surgical thought. New York: The Bovinine Co., [1901]. 2 l. DNLM
00-3687

PRATT, E[dwin] Hartley (1849-1930)
The composite man as comprehended in fourteen anatomical impersonations. . . . Chicago, Ill., 1901. 153p. DLC; ICJ
00-3688

PRATT, E[dwin] Hartley (1849-1930)
The composite man as comprehended in fourteen anatomical impersonations . . . [3rd ed.] Chicago: New Age Publishing House, 1902. 233p. CtY-M; ICJ; NNC; PP
00-3689

PRATT, E[dwin] Hartley (1849-1930)
Proceedings of the fourth free clinic in orificial surgery and first free clinic in suggestive therapeutics. . . . Chicago, Illinois, September 22-26, 1908. Twenty-first annual session of the American Association of Orificial Surgeons, Chicago, Ill., September 23-24, 1908. Chicago, Ill.: Nanetta L. McCall, [1908]. 291p. 3 col. plates. ICJ **00-3690**

PRATT, E[dwin] Hartley (1849-1930)
A synthetic clinic including a three days' course in orificial surgery . . . September 27-October 2, 1909. Twenty-second annual session of the American Association of Orificial Surgeons, Chicago, Illinois, September 29-30, 1909. Chicago, Ill.: N. L. McCall, [1910]. 343p. DLC; ICJ
00-3691

PRATT, Joseph Hersey (1872-1956) and F. T. FULTON
Report of cases in which the bacillus aerogenes capsulatus was found. Boston: Damrell & Upham, 1900. 15p. DNLM
00-3692

PRATT, Joseph Hersey (1872-1956)
Typhoid cholecystitis, with observations upon gallstone formation. Philadelphia, 1901. 10p. DNLM
00-3693

PRATT, Joseph Hersey (1872-1956)
On the classification of the benign thyroid tumors. Boston, 1902. 9p. DNLM **00-3694**

PRATT, Joseph Hersey (1872-1956)
On parathyphoid fever and its complications. Boston, 1903. 20p. DNLM **00-3695**

PRATT, Joseph Hersey (1872-1956)
On the causes of cardiac insufficiency. Baltimore, 1904. 24p. DNLM **00-3696**

PRATT, Joseph Hersey (1872-1956)
Hydrotherapeutic prescriptions. Boston, 1904. 13p. DNLM
00-3697

PRATT, Joseph Hersey (1872-1956)
The present status of hydrotherapy and other forms of physical therapeutics. Boston, 1904. 14p. DNLM
00-3698

PRATT, Joseph Hersey (1872-1956)
Clinical report of the year's work at the medical baths. [n. p.], 1904. 5p. DNLM **00-3699**

PRATT, Joseph Hersey (1872-1956)
A critical study of the various methods employed for enumerating blood platelets. [Chicago, 1906.] 10p. DNLM
00-3700

PRATT, Joseph Hersey (1872-1956)
Recent advances in the bacteriology of typhoid fever. Boston, 1906. 29p. DNLM **00-3701**

PRATT, Joseph Hersey (1872-1956)
On the development of scientific hydrotherapy. Boston, 1906. 21p. DNLM **00-3702**

PRATT, Joseph Hersey (1872-1956)
The home sanatorium treatment of consumption. Boston, 1906. 19p. DNLM **00-3703**

PREBLE, Robert Bruce
Pneumonia and pneumonococcus infections. . . . Chicago: C. J. Head & Co., 1905. 211p. plates, diags. DLC; ICJ
00-3704

PREISWERK, Gustav (*b.* 1866)
Atlas and text-book of dentistry, including diseases of the mouth. . . . Authorized translation from the German. Ed. by George W. Warren. . . . With 103 colored figures on 44 plates and 152 text-illustrations. Philadelphia and London: W. B. Saunders & Co., 1906. 343p. col. plates. CtY-M; DLC; KU; PU
00-3705

PRENTICE, Charles F[rederick] (*b.* 1854)
The perfected prismometer, its practical advantage, construction, and various applications. Rochester: Bausch & Lomb Optical Co., 1900. [*c.* 1891, *vel subseq.*] 8p. NN
00-3706

PRENTICE, Charles F[rederick] (*b.* 1854)
On the practical execution of ophthalmic prescriptions involving prisms. . . . St. Louis, [1900?] 8p. NN
00-3707

PRENTICE, Charles F[rederick] (*b.* 1854)
Ophthalmic lenses. Dioptric formulae for combined cylindrical lenses. The prism-dioptry and other optical papers. Philadelphia: The Keystone, 1900. 192p. DNLM; ICJ; MdBJ-W; PPC
00-3708

PRENTICE, Charles F[rederick] (*b.* 1854)
Ophthalmic lenses, dioptric formulae for combined cylindrical lenses, the prism-dioptry, and other optical papers. With . . . diagrams. [2nd ed.] Philadelphia: The Keystone Publishing Co., 1907. 192p. NN; PU **00-3709**

PRENTICE, Charles F[rederick] (*b.* 1854)
The standardization of trial cases. . . . [New York? 1909?] 6p. NN **00-3710**

PRENTICE, Charles F[rederick] (*b.* 1854)
The prism-dioptry in elementary optics. A lecture delivered before the Optometrical Society of the City of New York, April 13, 1910. . . . New York, 1910. 5p. NN
00-3711

[PRENTISS, Daniel Webster] (1843-1899)
Memorial meeting of the Medical Society of the District of Columbia, held November 22, 1899, in honor of Daniel Webster Prentiss. Washington: The Society, [1900?] unp. DLC; DNLM **00-3712**

PRENTISS, D[aniel] W[ebster] (1843-1899)
A case of fever during the puerperium caused by a large lumbricoid worm in the intestine. New York: William Wood & Co., 1901. 4p. DNLM; NN **00-3713**

PRENTISS, D[aniel] W[ebster] (1843-1899)
The kidney of pregnancy, with the report of one case. New York, 1906. 7p. DNLM **00-3714**

PRESCOTT, Samuel C[ate] (*b.* 1872)
A note on methods of isolating colon bacilli. New York, 1902. 2p. DNLM **00-3715**

PRESCOTT, Samuel C[ate] (*b.* 1872)
On certain precautions required in making and interpreting the so-called colon test for potable waters. Detroit: W. M. Warren, 1903. 10p. DNLM **00-3716**

PRESCOTT, Samuel C[ate] (*b.* 1872) and Charles Edward Amory WINSLOW
Elements of water bacteriology, with special reference to sanitary water analysis. New York: J. Wiley & Sons, 1904. 162p. DNLM; ICJ; NNNAM; PU **00-3717**

PRESCOTT, Samuel C[ate] (*b.* 1872)
The occurrence of organisms of sanitary significance on grains. Boston, 1906. 9p. MB **00-3718**

PRESCOTT, Samuel C[ate] (*b.* 1872) and Charles Edward Amory WINSLOW
Elements of water bacteriology, with special reference to sanitary water analysis. 2nd ed., rewritten. New York: J. Wiley & Sons, 1908. 258p. CtY-M; DLC; ICJ; PP **00-3719**

THE PREVENTION of disease. Translated from the German. With an introduction by H. Timbrell Bulstrode. New York: Funk & Wagnalls Co., 1903. 2 v. DLC; NNNAM; NNU-M; PPC **00-3720**

PRICE, Eldridge C. (*b.* 1854)
A philosophy of therapeutics. The foundation of which rests upon the two postulates: first, that it is the human organism that is the active factor in healing of the sick and not drugs; and second, that there are two therapeutic laws. Baltimore: Nunn & Co., 1904. 336p. DLC; ICJ; MdU-D; PU **00-3721**

PRICE, Eldridge C. (*b.* 1854)
The ethical relations of the dominant schools of medicine . . . annual address of the president of the Maryland State Homoeopathic Medical Society . . . May 17, 1904. 8p. MdBM **00-3722**

PRICE, George B[acon] (*b.* 1860)
Gaining health in the West (Colorado, New Mexico, Arizona) being impressions of a layman, based on seven years' personal experience with "climate." . . . New York: B. W. Huebsch, 1907. 139p. DLC; ICJ; NN **00-3723**

PRICE, G[eorge] E.
Lesions of the neurofibrils in pathologic states, with report of neurofibrillar changes in a case of hydrophobia and one of pernicious anemia. [Philadelphia, 1906.] 8p. DNLM **00-3724**

PRICE, G[eorge] E.
An unusual symptom in chorea. Philadlephia, 1907. 3p. DNLM **00-3725**

PRICE, George M[oses] (1864-1942)
Handbook on sanitation. A manual of theoretical and practical sanitation. For students and physicians: for health, sanitary, tenement-house, plumbing, factory, food, and other inspectors; as well as for candidates for all municipal sanitary positions. . . . 1st ed. 1st thousand. New York: J. Wiley & Sons; [etc., etc.], 1901. 317p. DLC; ICJ; NIC; NN **00-3726**

PRICE, George M[oses] (1864-1942)
Handbook on sanitation. A manual of theoretical and practical sanitation. . . . 2nd ed., rev. and partly rewritten. New York: J. Wiley & Sons; [etc., etc.], 1905. 307p. plans. DLC; MH; NIC; PU **00-3727**

PRICE, George M[oses] (1864-1942)
Handbook on sanitation. A manual of theoretical and practical sanitation. For students and physicians; for health, sanitary, tenement-house, plumbing, factory, food, and other inspectors; as well as for candidates for all municipal sanitary positions. By George M. Price . . . 2nd ed., rev. and partly rewritten. . . . New York: J. Wiley & Sons, 1910 [*c.* 1911]. 305p. plans. DLC; MH; NIC; NN **00-3728**

PRICE, George M[oses] (1864-1942)
. . . Hygiene and public health. . . . Philadelphia and New York: Lea & Febiger, [1910]. 255p. DLC; MH; NNNAM; PPC **00-3729**

PRICE, James Russell
Universal health and longevity without the use of drugs. . . . By James Russell Price . . . and T. Julian. . . . Chicago: Universal Health Co., [1900?] 48p. DLC; ICJ [The prevention and cure of disease by the use of enemata.] **00-3730**

PRICE, Marshall Langton
Occurrence of the strongyloids intestinalis in the United States. Chicago, 1903. 31p. DNLM **00-3731**

PRICE-BROWN, J[ohn] (1844-1938)
Diseases of the nose and throat. Philadelphia, New York & Chicago: F. A. Davis Co., 1900. 471p. 6 plates. CtY-M; DNLM; IU-M; PPC **00-3732**

PRINCE, Morton (1854-1929)
A contribution to the study of hysteria and hypnosis. . . . New York, 1900 [*c.* 1898]. 19p. DLC **00-3733**

PRINCE, Morton (1854-1929)
The great toe (Babinski) phenomenon. A contribution to the study of the normal plantar reflex based on the observation of one hundred and fifty-six healthy individuals. Boston, 1901. 7p. DNLM **00-3734**

PRINCE, Morton (1854-1929)
Physiological dilatation and the mitral sphincter as factors in functional and organic disturbances of the heart. Philadelphia, 1901. 21p. DNLM **00-3735**

PRINCE, Morton (1854-1929)
Osteitis deformans and hyperostosis caranii; a contribution to their pathology, with a report of cases. Philadelphia, 1902. 18p. DNLM **00-3736**

PRINCE, Morton (1854-1929)
The course of the sensory fibers in the spinal cord and some points in spinal localization based on a case of section of the cord. New York, 1905. 20p. DNLM **00-3737**

PRINZ, Hermann (*b.* 1868)
Dental formulary; a practical guide for the preparation of chemical and technical compounds and accessories used in the office and laboratory by the dental practitioner, with an index to oral diseases and their treatment including the modern methods of local anesthesia. . . . St. Louis, Mo.: The Author, 1907. 308p. CU-M; DLC; ICJ; PU **00-3738**

PRINZ, Hermann (*b.* 1868)
Dental materia medica and therapeutics, with special reference to the rational application of remedial measures to dental diseases; a text book for students and practitioners. . . . St. Louis: The C. V. Mosby Medical Book & Publishing Co., 1909. 595p. DLC; ICJ; MB; PU **00-3739**

PRINZ, Hermann (*b.* 1868)
Dental materia medica and therapeutics, with special reference to the rational application of remedial measures to dental diseases; a text book for students and practitioners . . . 2nd rev. ed. St. Louis: C. V. Mosby Co., [1910]. 595p. DLC; ICJ; MH-M; NNNAM **00-3740**

PRITCHARD, Edward R[andolph]
Health hints and health talks. . . . Chicago: The Reilly & Britton Co., [1910]. 153p. DLC; ICJ **00-3741**

PROTHERO, James Harrison
Prosthetic dentistry. . . . Chicago, Ill., 1904. 358p. DLC; ICJ **00-3742**

PRUDDEN, T[heophil] Mitchell (1849-1924)
Tuberculosis and its prevention. New York, 1902. 24p. MB **00-3743**

PRUDDEN, T[heophil] Mitchell (1849-1924)
The story of the bacteria and their relations to health and disease . . . 2nd ed., rev. and enl. New York and London: G. P. Putnam's Sons, 1910. 232p. plates. DLC; NN; NNNAM; PU **00-3744**

PRUDDEN, T[heophil] Mitchell (1849-1924)
Dust and its dangers . . . 2nd ed., illustrated. New York and London: G. P. Putnam's Sons, 1910. 113p. illus., plates. DLC; ICJ; NN; PPC **00-3745**

PRYOR, John H.
Deep breathing as a therapeutic and preventive measure in certain diseases of the lungs. [n. p.], 1906. 11p. DNLM **00-3746**

PRYOR, John H.
Recurring pleural empyema. New York, 1907. 11p. DNLM **00-3747**

PRYOR, J[oseph] W[illiam] (*b.* 1856)
Development of the bones of the hand as shown by the X-ray method. Lexington, Ky., 1905. 5p. 19 plates. DNLM; KU; NNC **00-3748**

PRYOR, J[oseph] W[illiam] (*b.* 1856)
Ossification of the epiphyses of the hand. X-ray method. [20 photos in text.] Lexington, Ky., 1906. 33p. DNLM **00-3749**

PRYOR, J[oseph] W[illiam] (*b.* 1856)
The X-ray in the study of congenital malformations. . . . New York: William Wood & Co., [1906?] 12p. DLC **00-3750**

PRYOR, W[illiam] R[ice] (1858-1904)
Gynaecology. A text-book for students and a guide for practitioners. New York: D. Appleton & Co., 1903. 380p. DLC; DNLM; NcD; NNNAM **00-3751**

PRYOR, W[illiam] R[ice] (1858-1904)
Puerperal sepsis, and its treatment by iodine. New York, 1904. 21p. DNLM; NN **00-3752**

PSYCHOTHERAPEUTICS, a symposium by Morton Prince . . . Frederic H. Gerrish . . . James J. Putnam . . . E. W. Taylor . . . Boris Sidis . . . George A. Waterman . . . John E. Donley . . . Ernest Jones . . . Tom A. Williams. . . . Boston & Toronto: R. G. Badger, 1910. 204p. DLC; MH; NIC; NN **00-3753**

PUBLIC HEALTH DEFENSE LEAGUE
. . . Brief history—Resolution adopted at Public Health Conference, New York City, November 15, 1906; charter; list of societies appointing delegates to the conference; conference committee. [New York, 1906.] 13p. DLC **00-3754**

PUNTON, John (*b.* 1853)
The relative value of medical advertising. Kansas City, 1901. 5p. DNLM **00-3755**

PUNTON, John (*b.* 1853)
The criminal responsibility of the epileptic. New York: William Wood & Co., 1902. 11p. DNLM **00-3756**

PUNTON, John (*b.* 1853)
A gigantic medical fraud detected and exposed. Kansas City, 1903. 15p. DNLM **00-3757**

PUNTON, John (*b.* 1853)
The trend of modern psychiatry and its relation to general medicine. Chicago, 1904. 10p. DNLM **00-3758**

PUNTON, John (*b.* 1853)
The principles of diagnosis of medical malingering. New York, 1904. 20p. DNLM **00-3759**

PUNTON, John (*b.* 1853)
The borderland of insanity in its clinical aspects. [Kansas City], 1907. 30p. DNLM **00-3760**

PURDY, Charles W[esley] (1846-1901)
Practical urinalysis and urinary diagnosis. A manual for the use of physicians, surgeons, and students. 5th ed. Philadelphia, New York & Chicago: F. A. Davis Co., 1900. 392p. 7 plates. DLC; DNLM; NNNAM; PPC **00-3761**

PURDY, Charles W[esley] (1846-1901)
Practical urinalysis and urinary diagnosis. A manual for the use of physicians, surgeons, and students. 6th ed., thoroughly revised. Philadelphia: F. A. Davis Co., 1901. 392p. 7 plates. DLC; DNLM; PPC; PPJ **00-3762**

[PURPLE, Samuel Smith] (1822-1900)
Catalogue of the genealogical library of the late. . . . Boston, 1909. 252p. port. DNLM; MB; MH; NN **00-3763**

PUSEY, Brown (*b.* 1869)
A new ophthalmoscope, combined with which there is a plain mirror for retinoscopy; intended as a pocket instrument for ophthalmologists and practitioners. Chicago, 1901. 1 l. DNLM **00-3764**

PUSEY, Brown (*b.* 1869)
The genesis of glioma retinae in neuroglia. Baltimore, 1902. 14p. 1 plate. DNLM **00-3765**

PUSEY, Brown (*b.* 1869)
An old-time quack eye doctor, the Chevalier John Taylor. Chicago: Press of American Medical Association, 1903. 7p. MB **00-3766**

PUSEY, William A[llen] (1865-1940)
Lupus healed with Roentgen rays. Chicago, 1900. 7p. DNLM **00-3767**

PUSEY, William A[llen] (1865-1940)
Roentgen rays in the treatment of skin diseases and for the removal of hair. Chicago, 1900. 14p. DNLM **00-3768**

PUSEY, William A[llen] (1865-1940)
Roentgen rays in the treatment of diseases of the skin. A review of recent literature and a personal experience. Chicago, 1901. 23p. DNLM **00-3769**

PUSEY, William A[llen] (1865-1940) and Eugene Wilson CALDWELL
The practical application of the Röntgen rays in therapeutics and diagnosis. Philadelphia: W. B. Saunders & Co., 1903. 591p. 3 plates. DLC; DNLM; PPC; PU **00-3770**

PUSEY, William A[llen] (1865-1940) and Eugene Wilson CALDWELL
The practical application of the Röntgen rays in therapeutics and diagnosis. 2nd ed., thoroughly revised and enlarged. Philadelphia: W. B. Saunders & Co., 1904. DLC; DNLM; NNNAM; PPC **00-3771**

PUSEY, William A[llen] (1865-1940)
The principles and practice of dermatology. Designed for students and practitioners. New York & London: D. Appleton & Co., 1907. 1021p. DLC; DNLM; NNNAM; PU **00-3772**

PUSEY, William A[llen] (1865-1940)
The principles and practice of dermatology, designed for students and practitioners . . . with five plates, one in color, and three hundred and eighty-four text illustrations. 2nd ed. New York and London: D. Appleton & Co., 1910 [*c.* 1911]. 1021p. DLC; ICJ; PPC; PPJ **00-3773**

PUTNAM, James J[ackson] (1846-1918) and Franz PFAFF
Experimental research showing that uric acid secretion is not regularly diminished in the period preceding epileptic seizures. Philadelphia, 1900. 3p. DNLM **00-3774**

PUTNAM, James J[ackson] (1846-1918)
A case of family periodic paralysis. Philadelphia, 1900. 11p. DNLM **00-3775**

PUTNAM, James J[ackson] (1846-1918)
Vivisection in Harvard Medical School; a reply. Boston: Damrell & Upham, 1900. 28p. DNLM; MH-M **00-3776**

PUTNAM, James J[ackson] (1846-1918)
Theoretical and practical considerations on the treatment of Jacksonian epilepsy by operation, with the report of five cases. Philadelphia, 1901. 20p. DNLM **00-3777**

PUTNAM, James J[ackson] (1846-1918) and Edward R. WILLIAMS
On tumors involving the corpus callosum. [New York], 1901. 46p. DNLM **00-3778**

PUTNAM, James J[ackson] (1846-1918)
Studies in neurological diagnosis, by James J. Putnam, M.D., and George A. Waterman, M.D. Boston: G. H. Ellis Co., printers, 1902. 214p. plates. DLC; ICJ; MBM; MH **00-3779**

PUTNAM, James J[ackson] (1846-1918) and J. W. ELLIOTT
Three cases of tumor involving the spinal cord; treated by operation. New York, 1903. 12p. DNLM **00-3780**

PUTNAM, James J[ackson] (1846-1918)
The clinical associations and significance of the cardio-pulmonary murmur. Boston, 1903. 10p. DNLM **00-3781**

PUTNAM, James J[ackson] (1846-1918)
A consideration of mental therapeutics as employed by special students of the subject. Boston, 1904. 15p. DNLM **00-3782**

PUTNAM, James J[ackson] (1846-1918)
Abstract of a report on the medical baths. [Boston], 1904. 3p. DNLM **00-3783**

PUTNAM, James J[ackson] (1846-1918)
The value of the physiological principle in the study of neurology. Philadelphia, 1904. 18p. DNLM **00-3784**

PUTNAM, James J[ackson] (1846-1918) and George A. WATERMAN
Notes on some unusual forms of infectious disease of the central nervous system. New York, 1904. 11p. DNLM **00-3785**

PUTNAM, James J[ackson] (1846-1918)
A memoir of Dr. James Jackson; with sketches of his father, Hon. Jonathan Jackson, and his brothers, Robert, Henry, Charles, and Patrick Tracy Jackson; and some account of their ancestry. Boston: Houghton, Mifflin Co., 1905. 456p. DLC; MH; NN; PU **00-3786**

PUTNAM, James J[ackson] (1846-1918)
A memoir of James Jackson. With sketches of his father, Jonathan Jackson, and his brothers, Robert, Henry, Charles, and Patrick Tracy Jackson; and some account of their ancestry. Boston & New York: Houghton, Mifflin & Co., 1905. 456p. 16 port., 8 plates. DLC; DNLM; MBM; MH **00-3787**

PUTNAM, James J[ackson] (1846-1918)
The treatment of psychasthenia from the standpoint of the social consciousness. Philadelphia, 1908. 20p. DNLM; PPC **00-3788**

PUTNAM, James J[ackson] (1846-1918)
Memoir of Charles Follen Folsom. Cambridge: Wilson, 1908. 23p. port. ICJ; MB; MBM; NN **00-3789**

PUTNAM, James J[ackson] (1846-1918)
Personal impressions of Sigmund Freud and his work, with special reference to his recent lectures at Clark University. [Boston? 1910.] 26p. MH **00-3790**

PUTNAM, James W., William C. KRAUSS and Roswell PARK
Sarcoma of the third cervical segment; operation; removal; continued improvement. Philadelphia, 1903. 5p. DNLM
00-3791

PYLE, Walter Lytle, ed. (1871-1921)
A manual of personal hygiene. . . . Philadelphia: W. B. Saunders & Co., 1900. 344p. DLC; DNLM; NNNAM; PPC
00-3792

PYLE, Walter L[ytle] (1871-1921)
The spontaneous disappearance of senile cataract, with report of a case. Philadelphia, 1900. 15p. DNLM
00-3793

PYLE, Walter L[ytle] (1871-1921)
The treatment of blepharitis. New York: E. B. Treat & Co., 1900. 2 l. DNLM **00-3794**

PYLE, Walter L[ytle] (1871-1921)
Extensive laceration of the external ocular muscles; diplopia; spontaneous recovery. Chicago, 1901. 4p. DNLM
00-3795

PYLE, Walter L[ytle] (1871-1921)
The necessity of expert supervision of medical items printed in the daily newspapers. Easton, Pa., [1901]. 3p. DNLM
00-3796

PYLE, Walter L[ytle] (1871-1921)
Postpartum metastatic panophthalmitis, with a clinical and pathological study of a case. Philadelphia, 1901. 10p. DNLM
00-3797

PYLE, Walter L[ytle] (1871-1921)
The treatment of acute catarrhal conjunctivitis. New York: E. B. Treat & Co., 1901. 2 l. DNLM **00-3798**

PYLE, Walter L[ytle] (1871-1921)
The disappearance of opacities of the crystalline lens. Chicago, 1902. 12p. DNLM **00-3799**

PYLE, Walter L[ytle] (1871-1921)
The first treatment of penetrating wounds of the eyeball. Philadelphia, 1902. 2 l. DNLM **00-3800**

PYLE, Walter L[ytle] (1871-1921)
Ocular affections associated with glycosuria, with especial reference to central amblyopia. Philadelphia, 1902. 14p. DNLM **00-3801**

PYLE, Walter L[ytle] (1871-1921)
The significance of intraocular lesions associated with albuminuria. New York: E. B. Treat & Co., 1902. 1 l. DNLM
00-3802

PYLE, Walter L[ytle] (1871-1921)
Bilateral acute glaucoma following artifical mydriasis. Chicago, 1903. 3p. DNLM **00-3803**

PYLE, Walter L[ytle] (1871-1921)
An interesting case of pigmentary degeneration of the retina (retinitis pigmentosa). Philadelphia, 1903. 4p. DNLM
00-3804

PYLE, Walter L[ytle] (1871-1921)
The teaching of personal hygiene. Philadelphia, 1903. 8p. DNLM **00-3805**

PYLE, Walter L[ytle], ed. (1871-1921)
A manual of personal hygiene; proper living upon a physiologic basis, by American authors . . . 2nd ed., rev. and enl. Philadelphia, London, [etc.]: W. B. Saunders & Co., 1904. 441p. DLC; NNNAM; PPC; PPJ **00-3806**

PYLE, Walter L[ytle] (1871-1921)
Myopia associated with opacities of the cornea. Chicago: Amer. Medical Assoc. Press, 1907. 10p. DNLM
00-3807

PYLE, Walter L[ytle], ed. (1871-1921)
A manual of personal hygiene; proper living upon a physiologic basis, by American authors . . . 3rd ed., rev. and enl. Philadelphia and London: W. B. Saunders & Co., 1907. 451p. DLC; IU-M; NNNAM; PPC **00-3808**

PYLE, Walter L[ytle] (1871-1921)
Microphthalmus, with extensive colobomata and other congenital defects in both eyes. Chicago, 1908. 3p. DNLM
00-3809

PYLE, Walter L[ytle], ed. (1871-1921)
A manual of personal hygiene; proper living upon a physiologic basis, by American authors . . . 4th ed., rev. and enl. Philadelphia and London: W. B. Saunders & Co., 1910. 472p. DLC; MBM; NNNAM; PPC **00-3810**

PYNCHON, Edwin (1853-1914)
Nosophen and antinosine in the treatment of diseases of the nose, throat, and ear. Birmingham, Ala., 1900. 7p. DLC; DNLM **00-3811**

PYNCHON, Edwin (1853-1914)
Slight irregularities of the nasal septum. [St. Louis, 1900.] 4p. DLC; DNLM **00-3812**

PYNCHON, Edwin (1853-1914)
Some improved nose, throat, and ear instruments. St. Louis, 1900. 2 l. DLC; DNLM **00-3813**

PYNCHON, Edwin (1853-1914)
The attic of the nose. St. Louis, 1901. 8p. DLC; DNLM
00-3814

PYNCHON, Edwin (1853-1914)
The home treatment of nasal catarrh. Philadelphia, 1901. 21p. DLC; DNLM **00-3815**

PYNCHON, Edwin (1853-1914)
The rhinological corner. Chicago, 1901. 6p. DLC; DNLM
00-3816

PYNCHON, Edwin (1853-1914)
Pneumatic massage in aural practice. [St. Louis, 1902.] 8p. DLC; DNLM **00-3817**

PYNCHON, Edwin (1853-1914)
The degenerate tonsil. Chicago, 1903. 8p. DLC; DNLM
00-3818

PYNCHON, Edwin (1853-1914)
The principles of rhinologic practice. St. Louis, 1903. 16p. DLC; DNLM **00-3819**

QUACKENBOS, John D[uncan] (1848-1926)
Hypnotism in mental and moral culture. New York: Harper & Bros., 1900. 291p. CtY-M; DLC; MB; NN
00-3820

QUACKENBOS, John D[uncan] (1848-1926)
Standing forests in their relation to the public health. n. p., 1901. 14p. DLC **00-3821**

QUACKENBOS, John D[uncan] (1848-1926)
Hypnotic therapeutics in theory and practice with numerous illustrations of treatment by suggestion. New York: Harper & Bros., 1908. 336p. DLC; ICJ; MB; NNNAM **00-3822**

QUACKS and grafters, by Ex-osteopath; being an expose of the state of therapeutics at the present time, with some reasons why such grafters flourish, and suggestions to remedy the deplorable muddle. Cincinnati, O.: The Cincinnati Medical Book Co., 1908. 126p. DLC **00-3823**

QUAIN, Richard (1816-1898)
A dictionary of medicine, including general pathology, general therapeutics, hygiene, and the diseases of women and children, by various writers. Edited by H. Montague Murray, assisted by John Harold and W. Cecil Bosanquet. New York: D. Appleton & Co., 1903. 1892p. 21 plates. CU-M; DNLM; NNNAM; PPC **00-3824**

QUIMBY, Charles E.
The president's address before the society of alumni of Bellevue Hospital. New York, 1900. 19p. DNLM **00-3825**

QUIMBY, Charles E.
Pneumatic differentiation in the treatment of organic disease of the heart. Chicago, 1902. 24p. DNLM **00-3826**

QUIMBY, Charles E.
The relation of intestinal toxemia to arteriorenal disease. New York, 1902. 15p. DNLM **00-3827**

QUIMBY, William C.
Sterility in the male; its operative treatment when due to bilateral epididymitis. Boston, 1906. 7p. 1 plate. DNLM **00-3828**

QUINAN, Clarence
The relations of specific gravity and osmotic pressure to hemolysis. Boston, 1903. 10p. DNLM **00-3829**

QUINAN, Clarence
. . . On the quantitative separation of the globulins of hemolytic serum, with special reference to the carbon dioxide group. . . . Berkeley: The University Press, 1903. 5p. DNLM; ICJ; MB; NN **00-3830**

QUINLAN, Francis J.
Paraffin injections for nasal and other facial deformities, with exhibition of a new instrument. St. Louis, 1902. 7p. DNLM **00-3831**

QUINLAN, Francis J.
Benign tumors of the nasopharynx. St. Louis, 1902. 12p. DNLM **00-3832**

RABAGLIATI, Andrea C[arlo] F[rancesco] (*b.* 1843)
Aphorisms, definitions, reflections, and paradoxes, medical, surgical, and dietetic. New York: William Wood & Co., 1901. 291p. CtY-M; DNLM; ICJ; PPC **00-3833**

RABAGLIATI, Andrea C[arlo] F[rancesco] (*b.* 1843)
Air, food and exercises; an essay on the predisposing causes of disease. . . . 3rd ed., greatly enl. and almost entirely re-written. New York: William Wood & Co., 1904. 559p. DNLM; ICU; IU-M; PPC **00-3834**

RACHFORD, Benjamin Knox (1857-1929)
Studies in pancreatic digestion, made with pancreatic juice. Cincinnati, 1900. 99p. DNLM **00-3835**

RACHFORD, Benjamin Knox (1857-1929)
Study of a typhoid fever epidemic. Detroit, 1901. 13p. DNLM **00-3836**

RACHFORD, Benjamin Knox (1857-1929)
Acute influenzal nephritis in childhood. New York, 1902. 8p. DNLM **00-3837**

RACHFORD, Benjamin Knox (1857-1929) and W. H. CRANE
Comparative toxicity of ammonium compounds; a study in auto-intoxication. New York, 1902. 17p. DNLM **00-3838**

RACHFORD, Benjamin Knox (1857-1929)
Treatment of migraine. New York, 1903. 12p. DNLM **00-3839**

RACHFORD, Benjamin Knox (1857-1929)
Neurotic disorders of childhood, including a study of auto and intestinal intoxication, chronic anaemia, fever, eclampsia, epilepsy, migraine, chorea, hysteria, asthma, etc. . . . New York: E. B. Treat & Co., 1905. 440p. DLC: ICJ; NNNAM; PPC **00-3840**

RACHFORD, Benjamin Knox (1857-1929)
Gonococcus vaginitis in children. Cincinnati, 1906. 4p. DNLM **00-3841**

RACHFORD, Benjamin Knox (1857-1929)
Pseudomasturbation in infants. New York, 1907. 20p. DNLM **00-3842**

RACHFORD, Benjamin Knox (1857-1929)
Lithemia; its pathology, etiology, symptomatology, and treatment. [Cincinnati, 1907.] 48p. DNLM **00-3843**

RADASCH, Henry E[rdmann] (*b.* 1874)
Ectopia of the adrenal. Philadelphia, 1902. 12p. DNLM **00-3844**

RADASCH, Henry E[rdmann] (*b.* 1874)
An interesting tumor and its relations to heredity. Philadelphia, 1905. 8p. DNLM **00-3845**

RADASCH, Henry E[rdmann] (*b.* 1874)
. . . A compend of histology. . . . With ninety-eight illustrations. Philadelphia: P. Blakiston's Son & Co., 1905. 304p. illus. (partly col.) CtY-M; DLC; PPC; PPJ **00-3846**

RADASCH, Henry E[rdmann] (*b.* 1874)
Observations upon the form of the red blood corpuscle of man. [Philadelphia, 1906.] 7p. DNLM **00-3847**

RADASCH, Henry E[rdmann] (*b.* 1874)
An unusual anomaly of the palmaris longus muscle. [Philadelphia, 1906.] 4p. DNLM **00-3848**

RADASCH, Henry E[rdmann] (*b.* 1874)
. . . A compend of histology . . . 2nd ed., rev. and enl., with one hundred and seven illustrations. Philadelphia: P. Blakiston's Son & Co., 1909. 350p. illus. (part col.) CU-M; DLC; PPC; PPJ **00-3849**

RADUE, William Ferdinand (*b.* 1862)
A manual of treatment of the diseases of children. . . . Chicago: The Clinic Publishing Co., 1907. 165p. DLC; ICJ; OCIM; PPC **00-3850**

RAINEAR, A. Rusling
The treatment of the enlarged prostate gland by electricity. [Philadelphia, 1903?] 2 l. DNLM **00-3851**

RAINEAR, A. Rusling
The proper recognition of electro-therapeutics. New York, 1903. 9p. DNLM **00-3852**

RAINEAR, A. Rusling
Some results of Röntgen-ray treatment. Philadelphia, 1904. 2 l. DNLM **00-3853**

RAINEAR, A. Rusling
Electricity in the treatment of rheumatism. Philadelphia, 1907. 7p. DNLM **00-3854**

RAINEAR, A. Rusling
Electricity in the treatment of neuralgia of the arm. [Philadelphia, 1907?] 3p. DNLM **00-3855**

RAINFORTH, S[elden] Irwin (*b.* 1879)
The stereoscopic skin clinic. An atlas of diseases of the skin, consisting of colored stereoscopic illustrations and a text in the form of clinical lectures designed for the use of practitioners and students of medicine. New York: Medical Arts Publishing, 1910. DLC; NNNAM; ICJ [128 5" x 7" stereographic cards with dermochromes on one side, text explanation on reverse; in cloth covered box with stereoscope viewer. The stereoscopic pictures were made from photographs of patients at the Vanderbilt Clinic and the Presbyterian Hospital Dispensary where they were under the care of Dr. Augustus F. Buchler and Prof. George T. Jackson. Each card has text on the reverse.] **00-3856**

RALSTON COMPANY
. . . Ralston meals for every day in the year and how to prepare them. The luxury of eating for health without dieting. Washington, D.C.: Ralston Co., [1905]. 63p. DLC [*vel subseq.*] **00-3857**

RALSTON HEALTH CLUB
First book of the Ralston Health Club containing all the principles of Ralstonism and the natural laws of life and death. . . . Washington, D.C.: Ralston Co., 1907. 224p. DLC [*vel subseq.*] **00-3858**

RALSTON HEALTH CLUB
Universal system of the Ralston Health Club. [Washington?]: Ralston Health Club, 1909. 342p. DLC [*vel subseq.*] **00-3859**

RALSTON HEALTH CLUB
Personal book of the Ralston Health Club, introducing its "personal system" . . . Washington, D.C.: Ralston University Co.; Hopewell, N.J.: Ralston Co., [1910]. 158p. DLC [*vel subseq.*] **00-3860**

RAMBAUD, George G[ibier] (*b.* 1875)
The antirabic vaccinations at the New York Pasteur Institute during 1900 and 1901. New York, 1902. 23p. DNLM; NNNAM **00-3861**

RAMDOHR, C. A. von
Clinical observations on the use of cotarnine phthalate. New York, 1907. 4p. DNLM **00-3862**

RAMSAY, A[rthur] Maitland (*b.* 1859)
Atlas of external diseases of the eye. . . . New York: The Macmillan Co., 1900 [*c.* 1898]. 195p. illus., plate. CtY-M; DNLM; IU-M; NcD **00-3863**

RAMSAY, A[rthur] Maitland (*b.* 1859)
Eye injuries and their treatment. . . . New York: The Macmillan Co., 1907. 210p. plate (part col.) DNLM; ICJ; NcD; PPC **00-3864**

RAMSAY, A[rthur] Maitland (*b.* 1859)
Diathesis and ocular diseases. New York: William Wood & Co., 1909. 184p. DLC; ICJ; NNNAM; PPC [Later editions published under title: The eye in general medicine, the constitutional factor in the causation of disease] **00-3865**

RAMSEY, Westley Carle
Dr. W. C. Ramsey's famous prescription "Lilies of the valley" for the cure of diseases of women. . . . Constructed under the direction of . . . . [Cleveland, O., [1901]. 23p. col. plates. DLC **00-3866**

RANDOLPH, B[enjamin] M.
A case of spontaneous arrest of growth in an endothelioma, with subsequent inflammatory absorption. Philadelphia, 1905. 4p. DNLM **00-3867**

RANKLIN, Egbert Guernsey
A digest of external therapeutics, with numerous formulae arranged for reference . . . 2nd ed. New York: Boericke & Runyon, 1900. 722p. CtY-M; DLC; PPJ **00-3868**

RANKIN, Egbert Guernsey
A digest of external therapeutics, with numerous formulae arranged for reference . . . 3rd ed. New York: Boericke & Runyon, 1904. 754p. DLC; PPC; PPHa; PU **00-3869**

RANKIN, Egbert Guernsey
A text-book of diseases of the chest; pericardium, heart, aorta, bronchi, lungs, mediastinum and pleura . . . with 63 illustrations. Philadelphia: Boericke & Tafel, 1905. 744p. plates. DLC; ICJ; PPC; PPHa **00-3870**

RANNEY, Ambrose L[oomis] (1848-1905)
Anatomical plates, arranged as a companion volume for "The essentials of anatomy." (William Darling and A. L. Ranney) Comprising four hundred and thirty-nine designs on steel by Prof. J. N. Masse. Ed., with revisions, from the original translation of Prof. Granville Sharp Pattison. New York: G. P. Putnam's Sons, 1901 [*c.* 1881]. xvi columns, 124 plates. DLC; ICJ; PPHa; PU **00-3871**

RANNEY, Ambrose L[oomis] (1848-1905)
Epilepsy and its modern treatment. Danbury: Danbury Ped. Pr. Co., 1902. 32p. DNLM **00-3872**

RANNEY, Ambrose L[oomis] (1848-1905)
Is epilepsy an organic disease? New York, 1904. 4p. DNLM
00-3873

RANNEY, Ambrose L[oomis] (1848-1905)
Cases of epilepsy cured without drugs, with explanatory remarks concerning the modern treatment of this disease. New York, 1904. 30p. DNLM **00-3874**

RANSOHOFF, Joseph (1853-1921)
Cystadenoma of pancreas; extirpation. Philadelphia, 1901. 8p. DNLM **00-3875**

RANSOHOFF, Joseph (1853-1921)
Nephrolithiasis; its diagnosis and surgical treatment. Cincinnati, 1901. 6p. DNLM **00-3876**

RANSOHOFF, Joseph (1853-1921)
The prerectal curvilinear incision for prostatic abscess; with a report of three cases. Philadelphia, 1902. 10p. DNLM
00-3877

RANSOHOFF, Joseph (1853-1921)
Trephining for brain tumors; report of two successful cases, one of nine years. Chicago, 1902. 8p. DNLM
00-3878

RANSOHOFF, Joseph (1853-1921) and A. V. PHELPS
An unusual and fatal hemorrhage from trephining. Philadelphia, 1903. 6p. 2 plates. DNLM **00-3879**

RANSOHOFF, Joseph (1853-1921)
Unilateral disease of the kidney simulating stone. Chicago, 1903. 7p. DNLM **00-3880**

RANSOHOFF, Joseph (1853-1921)
Hepatectomy for tuberculoma of the liver. New York, 1904. 9p. DNLM **00-3881**

RANSOHOFF, Joseph (1853-1921)
Stone in the kidney; its diagnosis and operative treatment. New York, 1904. 15p. DNLM **00-3882**

RANSOHOFF, Joseph (1853-1921)
Pulsating exophthalmos; ligature of the common carotid, external carotid, and superior thyroid arteries. Chicago, 1906. 3p. 1 plate. DNLM **00-3883**

RANSOHOFF, Joseph (1853-1921)
Pistol-shot wounds of the brain. [Cincinnati, 1906.] 11p. DNLM **00-3884**

RANSOM, Charles C[ook] (*b.* 1860)
Spa treatment of gout. New York, 1902. 15p. DNLM
00-3885

RAUE, Charles S[igmund] (*b.* 1873)
Acute poliomyelitis or infantile spinal paralysis. [1900.] 6p. PPHa **00-3886**

RAUE, Charles S[igmund] (*b.* 1873)
Clinical importance of early differentiation of true and false diphtheria. [1900.] 6p. PPHa **00-3887**

RAUE, Charles S[igmund] (*b.* 1873)
Clinical importance of early differentiation of true and false diphtheria. [1900.] 4p. PPHa **00-3888**

RAUE, Charles S[igmund] (*b.* 1873)
Prescribing in diseases of children. [Detroit], 1900? 8p. DNLM; PPHa **00-3889**

RAUE, Charles S[igmund] (*b.* 1873)
The relationship of the distribution of the artereal and venous blood in the heart chambers to the development of endocarditis. Philadelphia, 1902? 6p. PPHa
00-3890

RAUE, Charles S[igmund] (*b.* 1873)
Diseases of children; a text-book for the use of students and practitioners of medicine . . . 2nd ed., rev., enl. and illustrated. Philadelphia: Boericke & Tafel, 1906. 776p. DLC; ICJ; PPC; PPHa **00-3891**

RAVENBYRNE, Ervie Mary (*b.* 1870)
Good health, with suggestive questions and notes. Chicago: Ainsworth & Co., 1910. 99p. DLC; ICJ
00-3892

RAVENBYRNE, Ervie Mary (*b.* 1870)
Good health and good manners, with suggestive questions and notes. Chicago: Ainsworth & Co., 1910. 127p. DLC; ICJ
00-3893

RAVENEL, Mazÿck Porcher (1861-1946)
An experiment in the transmission of syphilis to calves. [n. p., 1900.] 4p. DNLM **00-3894**

RAVENEL, Mazÿck Porcher (1861-1946)
. . . Rabies. . . . [Harrisburg]: W. S. Ray, State Printer of Pennsylvania, 1901. 28p. illus. PP; PPC **00-3895**

RAVENEL, Mazÿck Porcher (1861-1946) and Daniel J. McCARTHY
The rapid diagnosis of rabies. Philadelphia, 1901. 10p. DNLM **00-3896**

RAVENEL, Mazÿck Porcher (1861-1946)
The intercommunicability of human and bovine tuberculosis. Philadelphia, 1902. 61p. DNLM; NN
00-3897

RAVENEL, Mazÿck Porcher (1861-1946)
The intercommunicability of human and bovine tuberculosis. [Detroit]: W. M. Warren, 1902. 34p. 1 plate. NN
00-3898

RAVENEL, Mazÿck Porcher (1861-1946)
A case of tuberculosis of the skin following accidental inoculation with the bovine tubercle bacillus. Philadelphia, 1902. 2p. DNLM **00-3899**

RAVENEL, Mazÿck Porcher (1861-1946)
The etiology of tuberculosis. Philadelphia, 1907. 14p. DNLM
00-3900

RAVENEL, Mazÿck Porcher (1861-1946)
Disinfection and commercial disinfectants. Madison, [1909]. 19p. NN **00-3901**

RAVOGLI, Augustus (*b.* 1851)
The hygiene of the skin; or, The art of preventing skin diseases. . . . Cincinnati: Central Medical Publishing Co., [1900?] 299p. DLC; ICJ; OC; PPJ [1st printing, 1888]
00-3902

RAVOGLI, Augustus (*b.* 1851)
Case of fibroma molluscum. [Cincinnati], [1900.] 8p. DLC
00-3903

RAVOGLI, Augustus (*b.* 1851)
Tuberculin in dermatology. Cincinnati, O., [1900?] 8p. DLC
00-3904

RAVOGLI, Augustus (*b.* 1851)
Tuberculosis of the skin. Cincinnati, 1900. 8p. DLC; DNLM
00-3905

RAVOGLI, Augustus (*b.* 1851)
A few notes on syphilitic bubo. New York, 1902. 20p. DLC; DNLM **00-3906**

RAVOGLI, Augustus (*b.* 1851)
A case of progressive idiopathic atrophy of the skin. Chicago, 1903. 12p. DLC; DNLM **00-3907**

RAVOGLI, Augustus (*b.* 1851)
On the reflex eruptions of the skin from morbid alterations in the male urethra. New York, 1903. 14p. DLC; DNLM
00-3908

RAVOGLI, Augustus (*b.* 1851)
A false or cicatricial keloid. Chicago, 1904. 11p. DLC; DNLM
00-3909

RAVOGLI, Augustus (*b.* 1851)
A few considerations on the etiology and pathology of cutaneous cancer. Cincinnati, 1904. 10p. 1 plate. DLC; DNLM
00-3910

RAVOGLI, Augustus (*b.* 1851)
Lichen planus verrucosus. New York, 1904. 8p. DLC; DNLM
00-3911

RAVOGLI, Augustus (*b.* 1851)
Alterations in the posterior urethra as a factor in nuerasthenia. New York, 1905. 11p. DLC; DNLM **00-3912**

RAVOGLI, Augustus (*b.* 1851)
Irritation of the bladder. Cincinnati, 1906. 6p. DLC; DNLM
00-3913

RAVOGLI, Augustus (*b.* 1851)
Syphilis in relation to crime. Columbus, 1906. 7p. DLC; DNLM **00-3914**

RAVOGLI, Augustus (*b.* 1851)
Valedictory address, delivered to the graduating class of the Medical College of Ohio, 1905-06. Cincinnati, 1906. 4p. DLC; DNLM **00-3915**

RAVOGLI, Augustus (*b.* 1851)
Syphilis in its medical, medico-legal, and sociological aspects. New York: Grafton Press, [1907]. 518p. 15 plates. DNLM; ICJ; NNNAM; PPC **00-3916**

RAY, J[ames] Morrison (*b.* 1861)
Experiences with operations for secondary capsular membranes. [Nashville, 1900?] 7p. DNLM
00-3917

RAY, J[ames] Morrison (*b.* 1861)
The cosmetic and visual results in squint. Chicago, 1901. 8p. DNLM **00-3918**

RAY, J[ames] Morrison (*b.* 1861)
Some of the failures immediate and remote met with after cataract extraction. [Louisville, 1902?] 11p. CtY-M; MB
00-3919

RAY, J[ames] Morrison (*b.* 1861)
The blind of Kentucky: based on a study of one hundred and seventy-five pupils of the Kentucky Institution for the Education of the Blind [Louisville, 1902?] 6p. CtY-M
00-3920

RAY, W. W., [*et al.*]
What are pellagra and pellagrous insanity? Does such a disease exist in South Carolina, and what are its causes? An inquiry and preliminary report. Columbia, S.C., 1907. 20p. DNLM; ScCM **00-3921**

RAYMOND, Joseph H[oward] (1845-1915)
Human physiology, prepared with special reference to students of medicine . . . 2nd ed., entirely rewritten. 443 illustrations, some of them in colors, and 4 full-page lithographic plates. Philadelphia and London: W. B. Saunders & Co., 1901. 668p. col. plates. DLC; DNLM; NNNAM; PPC
00-3922

RAYMOND, Joseph H[oward] (1845-1915)
Human physiology, prepared with special reference to students of medicine . . . 3rd ed., thoroughly rev. 444 illustrations, some of them in colors, and 4 full-page lithographic plates. Philadelphia and London: W. B. Saunders & Co., 1905. 687p. col. plates. DLC; DNLM; PPC: PU **00-3923**

REBER, [James] Wendell (1867-1916)
A clinical and statistical study of convergent strabismus. New York: A. R. Elliott Pub. Co., 1904. 20p. DNLM; NNNAM
00-3924

REBER, [James] Wendell (1867-1916)
The present status of preliminary iridectomy as related to cataract extraction. New York, 1907. 29p. DNLM; NNNAM
00-3925

RECORD of a memorial meeting of the late Surgeon-General William A. Hammond, held at the New York Post-Graduate Medical School and Hospital, February 23, 1900. New York, 1900. 51p. port. DNLM; NNNAM **00-3926**

RED CROSS. THE AMERICAN NATIONAL RED CROSS
The American national Red Cross emergency chart; first aid to the injured. . . . New York: First Aid Department, American National Red Cross, [1903]. 30p. DLC; NN
00-3927

REDFIELD, Harold Hamilton
A compend of the active principles, with symptomatic indications for their therapeutic use. . . . Chicago, Ill.: The Clinic Publishing Co., 1910. 115p. DLC; ICJ **00-3928**

REDGROVE, H[erbert] Stanley (*b.* 1887)
Alchemy: ancient and modern. . . . Philadelphia: David McKay, [1910?] 141p. 16 plates. DLC; MH; NcD; PPC
00-3929

REED, Boardman (1842-1917)
Lectures to general practitioners on the diseases of the stomach and intestines, with an account of their relations to other diseases and of the most recent methods applicable to the diagnosis and treatment of them in general; also "The gastro-intestinal clinic," in which all such diseases are separately considered. . . . New York: E. B. Treat & Col., 1904. 1021p. DLC; DNLM; NNNAM; NNU-M **00-3930**

REED, Boardman (1842-1917)
Lectures to general practitioners on the diseases of the stomach and intestines, with an account of their relations to other diseases and of the most recent methods applicable to the diagnosis and treatment of them in general; also "The gastro-intestinal clinic," in which all such diseases are separately considered. . . . 2nd ed. New York: E. B. Treat & Co., 1907. 1021p. DLC; IU-M; NNNAM; PPC **00-3931**

REED, Boardman (1842-1917)
Lectures to general practitioners on the diseases of the stomach and intestines. With an account of their relations to other diseases and of the most recent methods applicable to the diagnosis and treatment of them in general; also "The gastro-intestinal clinic," in which all such diseases are separately considered. 3rd ed. New York: E. B. Treat & Co., 1910 [*c.* 1911]. 1037p. illus. ICJ; IU-M; PPC; PPJ **00-3932**

REED, Charles A[lfred] L[ee] (1856-1928)
A text-book of gynecology . . . illustrated by R. J. Hopkins. New York: D. Appleton & Co., 1901. 900p. DLC: DNLM; NNNAM; PU **00-3933**

REED, Charles A[lfred] L[ee] (1856-1928)
Rudolf Virchow; an appreciation, pronounced before the Medical Society of the State of New York, at Albany, January 28, 1903, by Charles A. L. Reed. . . . [Buffalo: A. T. Brown Press], 1903. 30p. port. DLC **00-3934**

REED, Charles A[lfred] L[ee] (1856-1928)
Christian Science, a sociological study. Cincinnati: McClelland, 1903. 32p. DLC **00-3935**

REED, Charles A[lfred] L[ee], ed. (1856-1928)
A text-book of gynecology . . . illustrated by R. J. Hopkins. 2nd ed., rev. New York and London: D. Appleton & Co., 1904. 900p. DLC; MBM; NNNAM; PPC **00-3936**

REED, Charles A[lfred] L[ee] (1856-1928)
The Panama Canal mismanagement; report to the government showing how the commission makes efficient sanitation impossible . . . Chicago: Press of the American Medical Association, 1905. 18p. DLC; ICJ **00-3937**

REED, Charles A[lfred] L[ee] (1856-1928)
An address on the smoke problem. . . . [Cincinnati, 1905?] 13p. DLC **00-3938**

REED, Charles A[lfred] L[ee] (1856-1928)
Medical legislators of two republics. Chicago: American Medical Assoc., 1907. 14p. DNLM **00-3939**

REED, R[obert] Harvey (1851-1907)
Pelvic injuries. Columbus, O., 1901. 7p. DNLM **00-3940**

REED, R[obert] Harvey (1851-1907)
A case resembling locomotor ataxia. Death, post-mortem, with exhibition of specimens. [n. p., 1901?] 7p. DNLM **00-3941**

REED, R[obert] Harvey (1851-1907)
Grave abdominal injuries without external evidences of traumatism. Boston, 1902. 7p. DNLM **00-3942**

REED, Thomas E. (*b.* 1844)
Cyclic law; its influence over man in both health and disease, determining the sex. . . . Middletown, O.: Editor Publishing Co., [1900?] 167p. fold. tab. DLC: PP; PPC; PPHa **00-3943**

REED, Thomas E. (*b.* 1844)
The sex cycle of the germ plasm; its relation to sex determination. New York, 1907. 40p. DNLM; NNNAM **00-3944**

REED, Thomas E. (*b.* 1844)
The sex cycle of the germ plasm; its relation to sex determination. [Middletown, O., 1907.] 40p. NN **00-3945**

REED, Thomas E. (*b.* 1844)
Sex, its origin and determination; a study of the metabolic cycle and its influence in the origin and determination of sex, the course of acute disease, parturition, etc. . . . New York: Rebman Co., [1910?] 313p. diags. DLC; ICJ; NN; PU **00-3946**

REED, Walter (1851-1902)
Notes on pathology, lectures of Maj. Walter Reed, U.S.A., professor of pathology and bacteriology, medical department, Columbia University and James Carroll, associate professor of bacteriology and pathology. [1900?] 171p. NcU **00-3947**

REED, Walter (1851-1902)
Yellow fever; an address before the Michigan Academy of Medicine. [1900?] 45p. DNLM [Typewritten] **00-3948**

REED, Walter (1851-1902)
A comparative study of the biological character and pathogenesis of bacillus X (Sternberg), bacillus icteroids (Sanarelli) and the hog-cholera bacillus (Salmon and Smith). By Walter Reed and James Carroll. [n. p.], 1900. 45p. plate. NcD **00-3949**

REED, Walter (1851-1902), Victor C. VAUGHAN, and Edward O. SHAKESPEARE
Abstract of report on the origin and spread of typhoid fever in U.S. military camps during the Spanish War of 1898. Washington: Government Printing Office, 1900. 239p. DLC; DNLM; ICJ; NN **00-3950**

REED, Walter (1851-1902), James CARROLL, Aristide AGRAMONTE, and Jesse W. LAZEAR
The etiology of yellow fever. A preliminary note. Philadelphia, 1900. 18p. 1 tab. DLC; DNLM **00-3951**

REED, Walter (1851-1902)
Experimental yellow fever. By Walter Reed, James Carroll, and A. Agramonte. [Philadelphia, 1901.] 26p. charts. DNLM; MB; NcD **00-3952**

REED, Walter (1851-1902)
A comparative study of the biological characters and pathogenesis of Bacillus X (Sternberg), Bacillus icteroides (Sanarelli), and the hog-cholera bacillus (Salmon and Smith), by Walter Reed and James Carroll. [New York, 1901?] 45p. plate, tables. DLC; NcD **00-3953**

REED, Walter (1851-1902)
. . . The etiology of yellow fever. – A preliminary note. By Walter Reed . . . James Carroll . . . A. Agramonte . . . and Jesse W. Lazear. . . . Columbus, O.: The Berlin Printing Co., 1901. 16p. tables, diags. DLC; NcD **00-3954**

REED, Walter (1851-1902), James CARROLL, and Aristide AGRAMONTE
Experimental yellow fever. [Philadelphia], 1901. 9p. DLC; DNLM [*also*: Philadelphia, 1901, 26p.] **00-3955**

REED, Walter (1851-1902), James CARROLL, and Aristide AGRAMONTE
The etiology of yellow fever. Chicago, 1901. 24p. DLC; DNLM; MB **00-3956**

REED, Walter (1851-1902)
The propagation of yellow fever based on recent researches. Annual address delivered before the Medical and Chirurgical Faculty of Maryland, at the 103rd annual session, Baltimore, Md., April 1901. [n. p.], 1901. 31p. NcD **00-3957**

REED, Walter (1851-1902)
The propagation of yellow fever; observations based on recent researches. New York: William Wood & Co., 1901. 35p. DNLM; ICJ; NNNAM; PPC **00-3958**

REED, Walter (1851-1902) and James CARROLL
The prevention of yellow fever. New York: William Wood & Co., 1901. 34p. DNLM; NNNAM **00-3959**

REED, Walter (1851-1902) and James CARROLL
The etiology of yellow fever. A supplemental note. Philadelphia, 1902. 16p. DNLM; PPC **00-3960**

REED, Walter (1851-1902)
Recent researches concerning the etiology, propagation, and prevention of yellow fever, by the United States Army Commission. By Walter Reed. . . . Cambridge: At the University Press, [1902?] 18p. tables, diags. DLC; MH **00-3961**

REED, Walter (1851-1902)
The etiology of yellow fever; an additional note [by] Walter Reed, Jas. Carroll and Aristide Agramonte. Chicago: American Medical Association, 1903. 19p. fold. plate. NcD **00-3962**

REED, Walter (1851-1902)
The prevention of yellow fever. By Walter Reed and James Carroll. New York: William Wood & Co., 1903. 33p. NcD **00-3963**

REED, Walter (1851-1902)
The etiology of yellow fever; a preliminary note, by Walter Reed, James Carroll, A. Agramonte [and] Jesse W. Lazear. Columbus, O.: Berlin Print. Co., 1903. 19p. NcD **00-3964**

REED, Walter (1851-1902), Victor C. VAUGHAN, and Edward O. SHAKESPEARE
Report on the origin and spread of typhoid fever in U.S. military camps during the Spanish War of 1898. Prepared in accordance with Act of Congress, under the direction of Surgeon-General Robert M. O'Reilly. Washington: Government Printing Office, 1904. 2 v. DLC; DNLM; NNNAM; PPC **00-3965**

WALTER REED MEMORIAL ASSOCIATION, WASHINGTON, D.C.
[Extracts from reports and papers in reference to Major Walter Reed, surgeon, U.S. Army.] [Washington, 1904.] 7p. DLC; DNLM **00-3966**

WALTER REED MEMORIAL ASSOCIATION, WASHINGTON, D.C.
Proposed commemoration of the services of Major Walter Reed, surgeon, U.S.A., respecting the origin and suppression of yellow fever. [Washington, 1904.] 1 l. DLC; DNLM **00-3967**

REEDER, Albert
Obesity and the cure. . . . [Boston], 1901 [*c.* 1891]. 16p. DLC; MH **00-3968**

REEDER, Albert
The treatment of disease by passive and active exercise; or, Massage and the Swedish movements. . . . [Boston], 1902 [*c.* 1891]. 19p. DLC; MH **00-3969**

REEDER, David H.
Home health club. Dr. David H. Reeder's practical hygienic lectures . . . (3rd series). Laport, Ind.: Home Health Club, 1900. 96p. DLC [1st ed., 1898] **00-3970**

REEDER, David H.
. . . Home Health club. [2nd ed.] . . . . Laporte, Ind.: The Home Health Club, 1907. 96p. DLC **00-3971**

REES, Charles M.
Tubercular ulceration of the cervix uteri. Charleston, S.C.: Walker, Evans & Cogswell Co., 1904. 4p. DNLM **00-3972**

REESE, John James (1818-1892)
Text-book of medical jurisprudence and toxicology . . . 6th ed., rev. by Henry Leffmann. . . . Philadelphia: P. Blakiston's Son & Co., 1902. 660p. DLC; DNLM; PPC; PU **00-3973**

REESE, John James (1818-1892)
Text-book of medical jurisprudence and toxicology . . . 7th ed., rev. by Henry Leffmann. . . . Philadelphia: P. Blakiston's Son & Co., 1906. 656p. DLC; DNLM; NNNAM; PPC **00-3974**

REESE, John James (1818-1892)
Text-book of medical jurisprudence and toxicology . . . 8th ed., rev. by D. J. McCarthy. . . . Philadelphia: P. Blakiston's Son & Co., 1910 [*c.* 1911]. 660p. DLC; DNLM; ICJ; PPC **00-3975**

REGISTER, Edward C[hauncey] (*b.* 1860)
A text-book on practical fever nursing. Philadelphia: W. B. Saunders & Co., 1907. 352p. plates, charts. DLC; DNLM; ICJ; PU **00-3976**

REID, Mary Eliza
Bacteriology in a nutshell; a primer for junior nurses; comp. and arranged by Mary E. Reid. . . . Cincinnati, O., 1904. 114p. DLC; ICJ; OCIM **00-3977**

REID, Mary Eliza
Bacteriology in a nutshell, a primer for junior nurses; comp. and arranged by Mary E. Reid. . . . Rev. and enl. 1907. . . . Cincinnati, O., 1904 [1907]. 160p. DLC; OC **00-3978**

REID, Mary Eliza
Bacteriology in a nutshell; a primer for nurses. Comp. and arranged by Mary E. Reid . . . 4th ed., rev. and enl. . . . Charleston-on-Kanawha, W. Va., 1907-1910. 206p. DLC; ICJ **00-3979**

REISSIG, Carl
The standard family physician; a practical international encyclopedia of medicine and hygiene especially prepared for the household, by Prof. Carl Reissig . . . and Smith Ely Jelliffe . . . with the assistance of many American and German specialists in the treatment of diseases and experts in medicine and surgery . . . , New York and London: Funk & Wagnalls Co., 1907. 2 v. col. plates. DLC; ICJ; NN; NNNAM **00-3980**

REISSIG, Carl
The standard family physician; a practical international encyclopedia of medicine and hygiene, especially prepared for the household. Appendix comp. and ed. by eminent physicians. This volume embraces home remedies, emergency treatment, health and beauty culture, etc. New York: Funk & Wagnalls, 1908, 100p. DNLM; PU **00-3981**

REISSIG, Carl
The standard family physician; a practical international encyclopedia of medicine and hygiene especially prepared for the household, by Prof. Carl Reissig . . . Smith Ely Jelliffe . . . Sr. William Broadbent, bart. . . . Sir James Crichton-Browne . . . with the assistance of many American, British, Canadian and German specialists in the treatment of diseases and experts in medicine and surgery. . . . New York and London: Funk & Wagnalls Co., 1909. 3 v. col. plates. DLC; NIC; NNNAM; PU **00-3982**

REMINGTON, Joseph P[rice] (1847-1918)
The practice of pharmacy; a treatise on the modes of making and dispensing official, unofficial, and extemporaneous preparations, with descriptions of medicinal substances, their properties, uses, and doses; intended as a hand-book for pharmacists and physicians and a text-book for students. 4th ed. . . . with over eight hundred illustrations. Phladelphia, [etc.]: J. B. Lippincott Co., [1905]. 1504p. DLC; NNNAM; OCLloyd; PPC **00-3983**

REMINGTON, Joseph P[rice] (1847-1918)
The practice of pharmacy; a treatise on the modes of making and dispensing official, unofficial, and extemporaneous preparations, with descriptions of medicinal substances, their properties, uses, and doses; intended as a hand-book for pharmacists and physicians and a text-book for students. 5th ed. . . . assisted by E. Fullerton Cook. . . . With over eight hundred illustrations. Philadelphia and London: J. B. Lippincott Co., [1907]. 1541p. DLC; NNNAM; PPC; PU **00-3984**

REMONDINO, Peter C[harles] (1846-1926)
The relations of state boards of medical examiners and medical practice acts to medical education, medical colleges, medical students and the profession. . . . San Diego, Cal.: Frye & Smith, 1908. 247p. CU-M; ICJ; IEN-M; NN **00-3985**

REMSEN, Charles M.
A case of syphilis of the peripheral nerves and lungs. Baltimore, 1903. 9p. 1 l. DNLM **00-3986**

RENNER, W[illiam] Scott (*b.* 1861)
Infection through upper air passages. Buffalo: Brown, 1900. 15p. DNLM; PPC [Paper read at the meeting of the Medical Club of Buffalo, Nov. 1899.] **00-3987**

RENNER, W[illiam] Scott (*b.* 1861)
The indications for the radical mastoid operation, with a description of its technique. Buffalo, 1902. 20p. DNLM **00-3988**

RENNER, W[illiam] Scott (*b.* 1861)
Tertiary syphilis of the nose and pharynx. New York, 1904. 57p. DNLM **00-3989**

RENNER, W[illiam] Scott (*b.* 1861)
Treatment of acute otitis media. Buffalo, 1905. 7p. DNLM **00-3990**

REPORT of the Tuberculosis Commission of the State of Maryland, 1902-1904. Baltimore: Sun Job Printing Office, 1904. 110p. DNLM; MdHi; MdU-D; PU **00-3991**

REUTERDAHL, Arvid
Electrolysis according to the energonic hypothesis. . . . Providence: The Franklin Press, 1904. 16p. plates. DLC; RPJCB **00-3992**

REYBURN, Robert (1833-1909)
Address by Dr. Robert Reyburn on the anniversary of the emancipation in the District of Columbia, April 16, 1901. [1901.] 7p. DNLM **00-3993**

REYBURN, Robert (1833-1909)
The case of President James A. Garfield; an abstract of the clinical history. Philadelphia, 1901. 13p. DNLM; NcD; NN **00-3994**

REYBURN, Robert (1833-1909)
Failure of the knife in the treatment of cancer. New York: William Wood & Co., 1901. 7p. DNLM **00-3995**

REYBURN, Robert (1833-1909)
Causes of cancer. New York, 1902. 7p. DNLM **00-3996**

REYBURN, Robert (1833-1909)
Assassination of President Garfield twenty-four years ago. Story of the tragedy told by the sole survivor of his attending physicians and surgeons. [Washington, D.C.: R. Beresford, printer, 1905.] 24p. NcD; NN **00-3997**

REYBURN, Robert (1833-1909)
Causes and cure of cancer, and some of the causes of failure in treating malignant growths by X-rays and electric currents. New York, 1906. 8p. DNLM **00-3998**

REYBURN, Robert (1833-1909)
Fifty years in the practice of medicine and surgery, 1856-1906. Autobiography. Washington, 1907. 39p. NN; PU
00-3999

REYNOLDS, Edward (*b.* 1860)
The conditions which govern success in the Sänger Caesarian section, from the standpoint of a personal experience of fifteen cases without mortality. New York, 1900. 12p. 1 tab. DNLM
00-4000

REYNOLDS, Edward (*b.* 1860) and L. V. FRIEDMAN
The scope of vaginal section in the treatment of pus in the pelvis, with a report of eighty-two abdominal sections without mortality; and eighteen vaginal sections with one death due to accidental causes. [Boston, 1901.] 15p. DNLM
00-4001

REYNOLDS, Edward (*b.* 1860)
A case of vesical implantation of the ureter by Dudley's forceps method after the failue of several plastics. Boston, 1901. 7p. DNLM **00-4002**

REYNOLDS, Edward (*b.* 1860)
The major obstetrical operations, from the standpoint of the general practitioner; with a tabular report of twenty-three consecutive successful cases. Chicago, 1901. 14p. DNLM
00-4003

REYNOLDS, Edward (*b.* 1860)
Circumstances which render the elective section justifiable in the interest of the child alone. Philadelphia, 1901. 4p. DNLM
00-4004

REYNOLDS, Edward (*b.* 1860)
Practical obstetrics. A text-book for practitioners and students. By Edward Reynolds . . . and Franklin S. Newell. . . . Illustrated with 252 engravings and 3 colored plates. Philadelphia and New York: Lea Bros. & Co., 1902. 553p. DLC; ICJ; PPC; PU **00-4005**

REYNOLDS, Edward (*b.* 1860)
Cases of extra-uterine pregnancy illustrating difficulties in the diagnosis of the condition. Boston, 1902. 10p. DNLM
00-4006

REYNOLDS, Edward (*b.* 1860)
The indications for myomectomy in young married women; with a report of four cases of strangulation of fibroids during puerperal involution. [Chicago], 1902. 11p. DNLM
00-4007

REYNOLDS, Edward (*b.* 1860)
The use of gynecology by the general practitioner. [Portland, 1902.] 19p. DNLM **00-4008**

REYNOLDS, Edward (*b.* 1860)
The principles underlying the repair of cystocele and an operation founded thereon. Philadelphia, 1902. 7p. DNLM
00-4009

REYNOLDS, Edward (*b.* 1860)
Conservative surgery of the ovaries. Chicago: Amer. Med. Assoc., 1906. 15p. DNLM **00-4010**

REYNOLDS, Edward (*b.* 1860) and Richard G. WADSWORTH
Retroperitoneal perirenal lipomata; a study of large retroperitoneal lipomata of perirenal origin; the technique of their removal, based on anatomical studies, with the report of a case. Philadelphia, 1906. 78p. DNLM
00-4011

REYNOLDS, Edward (*b.* 1860)
The menopause in fable and in fact. Detroit: E. G. Swift, 1906. 14p. DNLM **00-4012**

REYNOLDS, Edward (*b.* 1860)
The causes and treatment of sterility in women. Philadelphia, 1907. 12p. DNLM **00-4013**

REYNOLDS, Edward (*b.* 1860)
Constitutional ill-equipment of the patient as a factor in determining the performance of the primary Caesarean section. Chicago, 1907. 7p. DNLM **00-4014**

REYNOLDS, Edward (*b.* 1860)
Primary operations for obstetrical debility; the delivery of debilitated women by operative methods, intrapelvic or abdominal, before labor, in the absence of mechanical impediments and as a method of choice. Chicago, 1907. 13p. DNLM
00-4015

REYNOLDS, Edward (*b.* 1860)
The superiority of primary over secondary Caesarean sections, and the feasibility and advantages of a predetermination of the method of delivery. Philadelphia, 1907. 22p. 10 charts. DNLM
00-4016

REYNOLDS, Frederick P.
The most practicable organization for the Medical Department of the United States Army in active service. Carlisle, 1902. 51p. DNLM **00-4017**

REYNOLDS, Frederick P.
The training of medical officers of the state forces from a regular army standpoint. Carlisle, Pa., 1908. 10p. DNLM
00-4018

REYNOLDS, John Russell (1828-1896)
Essays and addresses. . . . New York: Macmillan & Co., 1901 [*c.* 1896]. 307p. front. (port.) DLC; ICU; NIC; NN ["A brief sketch of the life of Sir John Russell Reynolds": p. [vii]-xxi.]
00-4019

RHEA, Lawrence J[oseph] (*b.* 1877) and Arthur B. EMMONS
A series of ninety-one consecutive blood cultures. Boston, 1907. 15p. DNLM **00-4020**

RHEIN, John H. W[allace] (*b.* 1869)
Encephalitis and other nervous affections complicating scarlatina. Philadelphia, 1905. 13p. DNLM
00-4021

RHEIN, John H. W[allace] (*b.* 1869)
A pathological study of acute myelitis, with a report of two cases. Philadelphia, 1905. 25p. DNLM
00-4022

RHEIN, John H. W[allace] (*b.* 1869)
Four cases of hemiplegia (syphilitic encephalitis, cerebrospinal syphilis), with autopsy. Philadelphia, 1906. 15p. DNLM
00-4023

RHEIN, John H. W[allace] (*b.* **1869)**
A pathologic study of seven cases of paralysis without gross anatomic change in relation to the cause or causes of uremic hemiplegia. [Chicago], 1906. 15p. DNLM
00-4024

RHEIN, John H. W[allace] (*b.* **1869)**
The treatment of arthritis deformans. Detroit, 1907. 9p. DNLM **00-4025**

RHEIN, John H. W[allace] (*b.* **1869) and Charles S. POTTS**
Post-apoplectic tremor (symmetrical areas of softening in both lenticular nuclei and external capsules). Chicago, 1907. 12p. DNLM **00-4026**

RHOADS, Thomas Leidy (*b.* **1870)**
Diagnosis and treatment of abscess of the liver. [Philadelphia, 1903.] 28p. DLC; DNLM; PPC **00-4027**

RHODES, John Edwin (1851-1925)
Notes on recent progress in laryngology and rhinology. New York, 1904. 22p. DNLM; NNNAM
00-4028

RIBOT, Théodule A[rmand] (1839-1916)
The diseases of personality. . . . Authorized translation, 4th rev. ed. Chicago: The Open Court Publishing Co., 1906. 163p. DLC; ICJ; IU-M; PU **00-4029**

RIBOT, Théodule A[rmand] (1839-1916)
Diseases of the personality. . . . Transl. (with homoeotherapeutic annotations) by P. W. Shedd. . . . Philadelphia: Boericke & Tafel, 1909. 142p. CtY-M; DLC; ICJ; PPJ
00-4030

RICE, May Cushman (*b.* **1863)**
Electricity in gynecology, the practical uses of electricity in diseases of women. . . . Chicago: L. I. Laing & Co., 1909. 159p. DLC; ICJ; ICRM; PPC **00-4031**

RICHARDIÈRE, Henri Alphonse (*b.* **1857)**
Whooping-cough. . . . Transl. by Joseph Helfman. . . . Detroit, Mich.: G. S. Davis, 1901 [*c.* 1893]. 2 v. DLC: ICJ; ICRM; PU [Physicians' leisure library] **00-4032**

RICHARDS, Ellen Henrietta (1842-1911)
Air, water, and food from a sanitary standpoint. By Ellen H. Richards and Alpheus G. Woodman . . . 1st ed., 1st thousand. New York: J. Wiley & Sons, 1900. 226p. plates, tables, fold. map. DLC; DNLM; ICJ; MH **00-4033**

RICHARDS, Ellen Henrietta (1842-1911)
The cost of food: a study in dietaries. . . . 1st ed. 1st thousand. . . . New York: J. Wiley & Sons, 1901. 161p. DLC; ICJ; MB; Nh **00-4034**

RICHARDS, Ellen Henrietta (1842-1911)
The art of right living. . . . Boston: Whitcomb & Barrows, 1904. 50p. ICJ; MB; NN **00-4035**

RICHARDS, Ellen Henrietta (1842-1911)
Air, water, and food from a sanitary standpoint. By Ellen H. Richards and Alpheus G. Woodman. . . . 2nd ed., rev. and enl. 1st thousand. New York: J. Wiley & Sons, 1904. 262p. plates, fold. map. DLC; ICJ; PPL **00-4036**

RICHARDS, Ellen Henrietta (1842-1911)
The chemistry of cooking and cleaning; a manual for housekeepers [by] Ellen H. Richards [and] S. Marie Elliott. 3rd ed., rev. and enl. Boston: Whitcomb & Barrows, 1907. 186p. DLC; ICJ; NIC; PU **00-4037**

RICHARDS, Ellen Henrietta (1842-1911)
Sanitation in daily life. Boston: Whitcomb & Barrows, 1907. 82p. DLC; MB; MH; NN **00-4038**

RICHARDS, Ellen Henrietta (1842-1911)
The cost of cleanness. . . . 1st ed. 1st thousand. New York: J. Wiley & Sons, 1908. 109p. DLC; DNLM; MB; PPL
00-4039

RICHARDS, Ellen Henrietta (1842-1911)
The cost of food: a study in dietaries. 2nd ed. New York: J. Wiley & Sons, 1908. 167p. DNLM; MH; NN; PU
00-4040

RICHARDS, George L[yman] (*b.* **1863)**
A brief report of a case of cerebral abscess of otitic origin; operation; death. Boston, 1900. 4p. DNLM
00-4041

RICHARDS, George L[yman] (*b.* **1863)**
Syphilis of the upper air-tract. Some remarks on its diagnosis and treatment. Chicago, 1900. 10p. DNLM
00-4042

RICHARDS, George L[yman] (*b.* **1863)**
Is it the duty of the State to care for the tuberculous individual? The experience of Massachusetts. St. Paul, 1901. 6p. DNLM **00-4043**

RICHARDS, George L[yman] (*b.* **1863)**
Chronic suppurative otitis media; when should radical surgery be employed in its treatment, and of what should this consist? St. Louis, 1902. 16p. DNLM **00-4044**

RICHARDS, George L[yman] (*b.* **1863)**
Empyema of the frontal sinus; some observations on its treatment. Chicago, 1902. 18p. DNLM **00-4045**

RICHARDS, George L[yman] (*b.* **1863)**
Is the adenoid operation a justifiable surgical procedure; and, if so, shall it be done in accordance with the rules of general surgery? Chicago, 1903. 7p. DNLM **00-4046**

RICHARDS, George L[yman] (*b.* **1863)**
The use of gelato-glycerin bougies in the treatment of acute earache in young children. Chicago, 1903. 4p. DNLM
00-4047

RICHARDS, George L[yman] (*b.* **1863)**
Nose and throat work for the general practitioner. New York: International Journal of Surgery Co., 1903. 330p. 6 plates. DNLM; MH; NNNAM; PPC **00-4048**

RICHARDS, George L[yman] (*b.* **1863)**
The significance of pus in the nose, with special reference to the affections of the accessory sinuses and their proper treatment. Philadelphia, 1904. 29p. DNLM
00-4049

RICHARDS, George L[yman] (*b.* **1863)**
The non-operative treatment of chronic otitis media purulenta, with special reference to the use of pyoktanin. St. Louis, 1905. 8p. DNLM **00-4050**

RICHARDS, George L[yman] (*b.* 1863)
Personal experiences with empyemata of the frontal sinus. Philadelphia, 1905. 24p. DNLM **00-4051**

RICHARDS, George L[yman] (*b.* 1863)
The treatment of empyemata of the maxiliary sinus through the nose. Chicago, 1905. 8p. DNLM **00-4052**

RICHARDS, John D[avid]
Report of a case of infective sigmoid sinus thrombosis and jugular vein infection of otitic origin without apparent mastoid involvement in an adult; operation; recovery. New York, 1905. 6p. DNLM **00-4053**

RICHARDS, John D[avid]
On the operative treatment of infective sigmoid-sinus thrombosis. . . . [New York: The Knickerbocker Press, 1905.] 44p. DLC; DNLM ["Read in part before the Otological Section of the New York Academy of Medicine, April 13, 1905."] **00-4054**

RICHARDS, John D[avid]
A case illustrating the effect of long continued pressure upon the interior of the mastoid by a fluid of low infectivity. New York: A. R. Elliott Co., 1906. 3p. DNLM **00-4055**

RICHARDS, John D[avid]
Report of a case of cerebellar abscess. New York: A. R. Elliott Co., 1907. 6p. DNLM **00-4056**

RICHARDSON, Alonzo Blair (1853-1903)
The influence of military campaigns in tropical climates in the production of insanity. Richmond, 1900. 11p. DNLM **00-4057**

RICHARDSON, Benjamin W[ard] (1828-1896)
Disciples of Aesculapius. With a life of the author by his daughter, Mrs. George Martin. New York: E. P. Dutton, 1901. 2 v. DLC; MB; NIC; NN **00-4058**

RICHARDSON, Benjamin W[ard] (1828-1896)
Vita medica: chapters of medical life and work. . . . . New York, [etc.]: Longmans, Green & Co., 1901 [*c.* 1897]. 495p. DLC; MH; NIC; NN **00-4059**

RICHARDSON, Charles H.
Private-house operations. The preparation and after treatment of the patient; the preparation of the rooms, etc. New York: A. R. Elliott, 1905. 14p. DNLM **00-4060**

RICHARDSON, Charles Williamson (1861-1929)
Pathology of adenoid growths. St. Louis, 1900. 4p. DNLM **00-4061**

RICHARDSON, Charles Williamson (1861-1929)
Early treatment of mastoiditis. St. Louis, 1901. 4p. DNLM **00-4062**

RICHARDSON, Charles Williamson (1861-1929)
Three cases illustrating cerebral complications of otitis media suppurativa. Chicago, 1901. 15p. DNLM **00-4063**

RICHARDSON, Charles Williamson (1861-1929)
Keratosis of the pharynx. Philadelphia, 1902. 8p. DNLM **00-4064**

RICHARDSON, Charles Williamson (1861-1929)
Medical education. Philadelphia, 1902. 7p. DNLM **00-4065**

RICHARDSON, Charles Williamson (1861-1929)
Etiology of catarrh of the nasopharynx. New York: E. B. Treat & Co., 1903. 2 l. DNLM **00-4066**

RICHARDSON, Charles Williamson (1861-1929)
Etiology, pathology, and symptomatology of chronic suppurative otitis. St. Louis, 1903. 7p. DNLM **00-4067**

RICHARDSON, Charles Williamson (1861-1929)
Report of two cases of cerebral abscess with recovery. [New Bedford], 1903. 8p. 1 chart. DNLM **00-4068**

RICHARDSON, Charles Williamson (1861-1929)
Acute osteomyelitis of the temporal bone. [New Bedford], 1904. 7p. DNLM **00-4069**

RICHARDSON, Charles Williamson (1861-1929)
The collodium dressing for intra-nasal surgery. St. Louis, 1904. 4p. DNLM **00-4070**

RICHARDSON, Charles Williamson (1861-1929)
Osteo-myelitis of the temporal and adjacent bones of the skull as a sequel of otitis media suppurativa. New York, 1904. 7p. DNLM **00-4071**

RICHARDSON, Charles Williamson (1861-1929)
Gangrene of the tonsil. Philadelphia, 1905. 6p. DNLM **00-4072**

RICHARDSON, Charles Williamson (1861-1929)
The accessory sinuses of the nose from the rhinological standpoint. New York: A. R. Elliott Co., 1907. 7p. DNLM **00-4073**

RICHARDSON, Delmer D[alton] (*b.* 1868)
Special diseases . . . 11th ed., rev. and enl. Chicago, 1906. 134p. col. plates. DLC; ICJ **00-4074**

RICHARDSON, Delmer D[alton] (*b.* 1868)
A treatise on diseases of the rectum, prostate and associate organs. . . . Containing one hundred illustrations, seventy colored plates. 2nd ed., rev. Chicago: [The Campbell Co.], 1908. 111p. DLC; ICJ **00-4075**

RICHARDSON, Frank L.
Effect of severe hemorrhage on the number of blood plates in blood from the peripheral circulation of rabbits. Boston, [1904?] 5p. diag. DNLM **00-4076**

RICHARDSON, Frank L.
A clinical report of 75 cases of arthritis deformans (chronic, non-tubercular arthritis). Boston, 1905. 19p. 6 plates on 3 l. DNLM **00-4077**

RICHARDSON, Hubert
The clinical value of blood pressure. New York, 1903. 11p. DNLM **00-4078**

RICHARDSON, Hubert
On the clinical importance of the specific gravity and alkalinity of the blood. Detroit, 1904.15p. DNLM **00-4079**

RICHARDSON, Hubert
Sodium glycocholate in diseases of the liver. New York: A. R. Elliott Pub. Co., 1905. 11p. DNLM **00-4080**

RICHARDSON, Hubert
The thyroid and parathyroid glands. Philadelphia: P. Blakiston's Son & Co., 1905. 261p. DNLM; ICJ; PPC; PU **00-4081**

RICHARDSON, Hubert
The functions of the testicles. New York, 1906. 13p. DNLM **00-4082**

RICHARDSON, Hubert
Metabolism of water. Philadelphia, 1906. 11p. DNLM **00-4083**

RICHARDSON, Joseph Gibbons (1836-1886)
Medicology; or, Home encyclopedia of health; a complete family guide. . . . By Joseph G. Richardson . . . William H. Ford . . . C. C. Vanderbeck . . . managing editor, J. P. Wood, M.D., assisted by a large and able corps of medical practitioners, lecturers and teachers. . . . New York, Philadelphia, [etc.]: University Medical Society, 1901. 1421p. col. plates. DLC; PPC; CU-M [Published in 1885 under title: The modern family physician and hygienic guide.] **00-4084**

RICHARDSON, Joseph Gibbons (1836-1886)
Medicology, or Home encyclopedia of health; a complete family guide. . . . by Joseph G. Richardson . . . William H. Ford . . . C. C. Vanderbeck . . . managing editor, James P. Wood, M.D., assisted by a large and able corps of medical practitioners, lecturers and teachers. . . . New York, Philadelphia, [etc.]: University Medical Society, 1903. 1735p. plates. DLC; ICJ; MH; NNNAM **00-4085**

RICHARDSON, Joseph Gibbons (1836-1886)
Medicology; or, Home encylcopedia of health. A complete family guide. . . . by Joseph G. Richardson . . . William H. Ford . . . C. C. Vanderbeck . . . managing editor, James P. Wood, M.D., assisted by a large and able corps of medical practitioners, lecturers and teachers. . . . New York, Philadelphia, [etc.]: University Medical Society, 1908. 1432p. plates. DLC; MB; NNNAM; PPC **00-4086**

RICHARDSON, Joseph Gibbons (1836-1886)
Health and longevity / by Joseph G. Richardson, assisted by B. F. Scholl . . . [et al.] — New York: Home Health Society, 1910. 1382p. [63] leaves of plates, ill. (some col.), port. DLC; ICJ; NN; PU [Published in 1885 and 1889 under title: The modern family physician and hygiene guide.] **00-4087**

RICHARDSON, J. Julius
Button in the ear 27 years; deafness cured by its removal. Philadelphia, 1904. 1 l. DNLM **00-4088**

RICHARDSON, J. Julius
Endotracheal medication. Philadelphia, 1904. 6p. DNLM **00-4089**

RICHARDSON, J. Julius
Hypertrophy of the lingual tonsil. Philadelphia, 1904. 5p. DNLM **00-4090**

RICHARDSON, J. Julius
Electricity in otology. New York: A. R. Elliott, 1905. 8p. DNLM **00-4091**

RICHARDSON, Mark W[yman] (*b.* 1867)
On the cultivation of the typhoid bacillus from rose-spots. Philadelphia, 1900. 6p. DNLM **00-4092**

RICHARDSON, Mark W[yman] (*b.* 1867)
Diagnosis between appendicitis and typhoid fever. Read before the Providence Medical Association, March 4, 1901. Providence, 1901. 12p. DNLM **00-4093**

RICHARDSON, Mark W[yman] (*b.* 1867)
The treatment of typhoid fever with specific sera, filtrates, and residues (Vaughan). Boston, 1907. 19p. DNLM **00-4094**

RICHARDSON, Mark W[yman] (*b.* 1867)
Fact and speculation concerning the nature of typhoid fever. . . . Boston: D. C. Heath & Co., 1908. 12p. NN **00-4095**

RICHARDSON, Mark W[yman] (*b.* 1867)
The present status of serum and vaccine therapy. [Philadelphia], 1908. 15p. NN **00-4096**

RICHARDSON, Mark W[yman] (*b.* 1867)
Ophthalmia neonatorum: facts concerning the disease and its prevention as affecting the State of Massachusetts. [New York, 1910.] 7p. NN **00-4097**

RICHARDSON, Mark W[yman] (*b.* 1867)
The importance of animal experimentation in the development of our knowledge of dysentery, cholera and typhoid fever. [Chicago, 1910.] 7p. MB **00-4098**

RICHARDSON, Maurice H[owe] (1851-1912)
Remarks on the surgery of uterine fibroids with especial reference to the importance of early removal in the young. Boston, 1900. 12p. DLC; MB **00-4099**

RICHARDSON, Maurice H[owe] (1851-1912)
A case of acute tuberculosis of the mesenteric glands of the ileocaecal coil; removal; permanent recovery. Philadelphia, 1900. 6p. DNLM **00-4100**

RICHARDSON, Maurice H[owe] (1851-1912)
The importance of early operation in gall-stones. Chicago, 1900. 12p. DNLM **00-4101**

RICHARDSON, Maurice H[owe] (1851-1912)
On lesions of the pancreas simulating gall-stone impactions of the common duct. Philadelphia, 1900. 16p. DNLM **00-4102**

RICHARDSON, Maurice H[owe] (1851-1912)
Remarks upon obscure non-traumatic tumors of the lower abdomen suddenly appearing where none had previously been detected. Boston: Damrell & Upham, 1900. 24p. DNLM **00-4103**

RICHARDSON, Maurice H[owe] (1851-1912)
Remarks on the surgery of uterine fibroids with especial reference to the importance of early removal in the young. Boston: Damrell & Upham, 1900. 12p. DNLM **00-4104**

RICHARDSON, Maurice H[owe] (1851-1912)
On the surgical treatment of gall-stones; an address before the Chicago Medical Society at its annual meeting, June, 1900. Chicago, 1900. 32p. DNLM **00-4105**

RICHARDSON, Maurice H[owe] (1851-1912)
Two cases of oesophageal diverticulum, with remarks. Philadelphia, 1900. 22p. DNLM **00-4106**

RICHARDSON, Maurice H[owe] (1851-1912)
A case of idiopathic dilatation of the colon. Boston, 1901. 6p. DNLM **00-4107**

RICHARDSON, Maurice H[owe] (1851-1912)
A case of obliteration of the right ureter by a calcified fibroid; removal of fibroid and implantation of the ureter into the bladder; recovery. Boston, 1901. 4p. DNLM **00-4108**

RICHARDSON, Maurice H[owe] (1851-1912)
Conservatism in surgery. Detroit: W. M. Warren, 1901. 18p. DNLM **00-4109**

RICHARDSON, Maurice H[owe] (1851-1912)
Remarks on the diagnosis between acute appendicitis and some atypical cases of typhoid fever. Boston: Damrell & Upham, 1902. 28p. DNLM **00-4110**

RICHARDSON, Maurice H[owe] (1851-1912)
Indications for the extirpation of the gall-bladder. Philadelphia, 1903. 14p. DNLM **00-4111**

RICHARDSON, Maurice H[owe] (1851-1912)
On certain unavoidable calamities following surgical operation. Boston, 1904. 19p. DNLM **00-4112**

RICHARDSON, Maurice H[owe] (1851-1912)
Diseases of the bile passages, including the liver, gall-bladder and pancreas. 1906. 30p. DNLM **00-4113**

RICHARDSON, Maurice H[owe] (1851-1912)
The importance to the surgeon of the study of anatomical appearances in the living. St. Louis, 1906. 30p. DNLM **00-4114**

RICHARDSON, Maurice H[owe] (1851-1912)
On the responsibilities of the general practitioner. St. Louis, 1906. 49p. DNLM **00-4115**

RICHARDSON, Maurice H[owe] (1851-1912)
A consideration of contra-indications in surgery. [St. Paul], 1907. 7p. DLC **00-4116**

RICHARDSON, Maurice H[owe] (1851-1912)
Diseases of the bile passages, including the liver, gallbladder, and pancreas. [Boston, 1907.] 34p. DNLM; MB **00-4117**

RICHARDSON, Maurice H[owe] (1851-1912)
Oration on surgery. When shall the physician distrust his own judgment in surgical matters. n. p., 1908. 15p. MH **00-4118**

RICHARDSON, Maurice H[owe] (1851-1912)
Remarks on paper by Dr. Gilman Osgood before the Massachusetts Medical Society, upon the relations of the country practitioner to the consultant. June 10, 1908. n. p., [1908?] 12p. MB **00-4119**

RICHARDSON, Maurice H[owe] (1851-1912)
On some of the difficulties and dangers in surgical operations upon the biliary tract. Richmond, 1908. 24p. MB **00-4120**

RICHEY, Stephen Olin
Eustachian catheterization. Chicago, 1900. 4p. DNLM **00-4121**

RICKARDS, Burton Ransom
A comparison of some of the more common liquid disinfectants. Boston, 1903. 6p. DNLM **00-4122**

RICKARDS, Burton Ransom
A consideration of some of the problems and difficulties of bacteriological diagnosis. Boston, [1906]. 12p. DNLM **00-4123**

RICKETTS, B[enjamin] Merrill (*b.* 1858)
Normal prophylactic appendectomy. St. Louis, 1900. 1 l. DNLM **00-4124**

RICKETTS, B[enjamin] Merrill (*b.* 1858)
Submucous ligature for rectal hemorrhoids and prolapse. [New York], 1900. 13p. DNLM **00-4125**

RICKETTS, B[enjamin] Merrill (*b.* 1858)
The appendix vermiformis and cecum. A comparative study. (1814-1901.) [*Also*:] Appendicectomy. Surgical history (1758-1888). Chicago, 1901. 14p. DNLM **00-4126**

RICKETTS, B[enjamin] Merrill (*b.* 1858)
Inguinal hernia. Philadelphia, 1901. 15p. DNLM **00-4127**

RICKETTS, B[enjamin] Merrill (*b.* 1858)
Nasal surgery. Cincinnati, 1901. 4p. DNLM **00-4128**

RICKETTS, B[enjamin] Merrill (*b.* 1858)
Some anomalies of the uterus: Uterus bicornis and uterus rudimentarius; uterus didelphys; clinical reports. Cincinnati, 1902. 15p. DNLM **00-4129**

RICKETTS, B[enjamin] Merrill (*b.* 1858)
Appendicitis. Cincinnati, 1902. 4p. DNLM **00-4130**

RICKETTS, B[enjamin] Merrill (*b.* 1858)
Ligation of arteries; cocaine anesthesia. St. Louis, 1902. 3p. DNLM **00-4131**

RICKETTS, B[enjamin] Merrill (*b.* 1858)
Surgical mélange. Cincinnati, 1902. 3p. DNLM **00-4132**

RICKETTS, B[enjamin] Merrill (*b.* 1858)
Surg. of heart. Bibliography. Ricketts, 1902. [593] leaves. ICJ [Manuscript sheets for the most part written on only one side of the leaf, typewritten copy, and manuscript and typewritten slips pasted on sheets. Printed, with additions, in Part I of his The surgery of the heart and lungs. New York: The Grafton Press, 1904.] **00-4133**

RICKETTS, B[enjamin] Merrill (*b.* 1858)
. . . Surgery of pancreas. General bibliography. Ricketts, 1902. [172] leaves. ICJ [Manuscript sheets for the most part written on only one side of the leaf, and typewritten slips pasted on sheets. Printed as p. [45]-74 of his Surgery of the prostate, pancreas, diaphragm, spleen, thyroid, and hydrocephalus. A historical review. Cincinnati, 1904.] **00-4134**

RICKETTS, B[enjamin] Merrill (*b.* 1858)
Surgery of the heart. St. Louis, 1903. 30p. DNLM
00-4135

RICKETTS, B[enjamin] Merrill (*b.* 1858)
Surgery of spleen. Bibliography to 1903. B. M. Ricketts, [1903]. [274] leaves. ICJ [Manuscript sheets and typewritten slips pasted on sheets. Printed as p. [92]-137 of his Surgery of the prostate, pancreas, diaphragm, spleen, thyroid, and hydrocephalus. A historical review. Cincinnati, 1904.]
00-4136

RICKETTS, B[enjamin] Merrill (*b.* 1858)
The lung: history and résumé of surgical conditions found therein and experimental and clinical research in lower animals with reference to pneumonotomy, pneumonectomy, and bronchiotomy. By [Benjamin Merrill Ricketts]. (34 illustrations.) [1903]. 2 v. plates. ICJ [Typewritten copy. Vol. 2 has t.-p.: Experimental research on the lung of the dog with reference to pneumonotomy, and pneumonectomy. By B. Merrill Ricketts, Ph.D., M.D., Cincinnati, Ohio, 1903. Printed in Part 2 of his The surgery of the heart and lungs. New York: The Grafton Press, 1904.] **00-4137-38**

RICKETTS, B[enjamin] Merrill (*b.* 1858)
The surgery of the heart and lungs. A history and résumé of surgical conditions found therein, and experimental and clinical research in man and lower animals, with reference to pneumonotomy, pneumonectomy, and bronchiotomy, and cardiotomy and cardiorrhaphy. New York: Grafton Press, 1904. 510p. 87 plates. DLC; ICJ; NcD; PPC
00-4139

RICKETTS, B[enjamin] Merrill (*b.* 1858)
Surgery of the prostate, pancreas, diaphragm, spleen, thyroid, and hydrocephalus. A historical review. . . . Cincinnati, 1904. 226p. 18 plates, illus. ICJ; IU-M; NcD **00-4140**

RICKETTS, B[enjamin] Merrill (*b.* 1858)
Surgery of hydrocephalus; a historic review. [Philadelphia, 1904.] 18p. illus. NIC **00-4141**

RICKETTS, B[enjamin] Merrill (*b.* 1858)
Villous papillomata of the rectum. New York, 1907. 28p. DNLM **00-4142**

RICKETTS, B[enjamin] Merrill (*b.* 1858)
Surgery of the ureter: an historical review. (1585-1905). Cincinnati, 1908. 244p. DNLM; ICJ
00-4143

RICKETTS, Howard T[aylor] (1871-1910)
Infection, immunity, and serum therapy in relation to the infectious diseases which attack man; wth considerations of the allied subjects of agglutination, precipitation, hemolysis, etc. Chicago: Amer. Medical Assoc. Press, 1906. 600p. DLC; DNLM; IU-M; OCIM **00-4144**

RICKETTS, Howard T[aylor] (1871-1910)
General report of an investigation of Rocky Mountain spotted fever, carried on during 1906 and 1907. [Helena: State Board of Health, 1908.] 46p. DNLM; IU-M
00-4145

RICKETTS, Howard T[aylor] (1871-1910)
Investigation of the cause and means of Rocky Mountain spotted fever carried on during 1907 and 1908. Helena: Montana State Board of Health, 1908. 114p. DLC; MH
00-4146

RICKETTS, Howard T[aylor] (1871-1910)
Contributions to medical science by Howard Taylor Ricketts, 1870-1910; published as a tribute to his memory by his colleagues under the auspices of the Chicago Pathological Society. Chicago, Ill.: The University of Chicago Press, 1910 [*c.* 1911]. 497p. plates. DLC; ICJ; NcD; PPC
00-4147

RICKETTS, Howard T[aylor] (1871-1910)
Infection, immunity and serum therapy in relation to the infectious diseases of man. . . . Second ed. Revised and enlarged by the author and by Geo. F. Dick, . . . with preface by Ludvig Hektoen. . . . Chicago: Amer. Medical Assoc. Press, 1910 [*c.* 1911]. 785p. DLC; ICJ; PPHa; PU
00-4148

RIDDELL, Newton N. (*b.* 1862)
Heredity and prenatal culture considered in the light of the new psychology. . . . Chicago: Child of Light Publishing Co., [1900]. 350p. DLC; ICJ; ICRM **00-4149**

RIDDELL, Newton (*b.* 1862)
A child of light; or, Heredity and prenatal culture considered in the light of the new psychology. . . . Chicago: Child of Light Publishing Co., 1900. 350p. DLC; ICJ
00-4150

RIDDELL, Newton H. (*b.* 1862)
Private lecture to women on health, strength and beauty. . . . Prenatal culture applied to the improvement of the race. . . . by Prof. N. N. Riddell. . . . [Raymond, Nev., 1901.] 39p. DLC [*c.* 1896. *vel subseq.*] **00-4151**

RIDDELL, Newton H. (*b.* 1862)
. . . Riddell's descriptive chart of human nature, for the use of practical phrenologists. New York: New York Phrenological Institute, 1902. 96p. DLC [*c.* 1896. *vel subseq.*]
00-4152

RIDDELL, Newton H. (*b.* 1862)
Child culture according to the laws of physiological psychology and mental suggestion. . . . Chicago, Ill.: Child of Light Publishing Co., [1902]. 129p. DLC; ICJ **00-4153**

RIDDELL, Newton H. (*b.* 1862)
Heredity and prenatal culture considered in the light of the new psychology. . . . Chicago: Riddell Publishing Co., [1903]. 350p. DLC; ICJ **00-4154**

RIDEAL, Samuel (1863-1929)
Sewage and the bacterial purification of sewage. . . . 2nd ed. New York: J. Wiley & Sons, 1901. 308p. plates. DLC; ICJ; MH; NN **00-4155**

RIDEAL, Samuel (1863-1929)
Water and its purification; a handbook for the use of local authorities, sanitary officers, and others interested in water supply . . . with numerous illustrations and tables. 2nd ed., rev. and extended. Philadelphia: J. B. Lippincott Co., 1902. 346p. fold. plate, tables, diags. DLC; ICJ; MB; NN
00-4156

RIDEAL, Samuel (1863-1929)
Disinfection and the preservation of food, together with an account of the chemical substances used as antiseptics and preservatives. . . . 3rd ed. New York: J. Wiley & Sons, 1903. 494p. DLC: ICJ; PP; PU **00-4157**

RIEGEL, Franz (1843-1904)
Diseases of the stomach . . . ed., with additions, by Charles G. Stockton . . . authorized translation from the German, under the editorial supervision of Alfred Stengel. . . . Philadelphia, New York, [etc.]: W. B. Saunders & Co., 835p. DLC; NNNAM; PPC; PU [American ed., Nothnagel's encyclopedia of practical medicine] **00-4158**

RIES, Emil (*b.* 1865)
The most rational method of operation for hemorrhoids. Detroit, 1903. 7p. DNLM **00-4159**

RIESMAN, David (1867-1940)
The urinary organs. Illus. Philadelphia, [1901]. 88p. MB **00-4160**

RIESMAN, David (1867-1940)
Albuminous expectoration following thoracocentesis. Philadelphia & New York, 1902. 11p. DNLM **00-4161**

RIESMAN, David (1867-1940)
Aneurysm of the aorta rupturing into the right bronchus; origin of the left vertebral artery directly from the aortic arch. Philadelhia, 1902. 4p. DNLM **00-4162**

RIESMAN, David (1867-1940)
Uremic aphasia. Chicago, 1902. 16p. DNLM **00-4163**

RIESMAN, David (1867-1940), A. C. WOOD, and G. E. PFAHLER
A case of gangrene of the lung cured by operation. Philadelphia & New York, 1903. 12p. DNLM **00-4164**

RIESMAN, David (1867-1940)
Pericarditis; its symptoms and diagnosis. Philadelphia & New York, 1904. 8p. DNLM **00-4165**

RIESMAN, David (1867-1940)
Some remarks on physical diagnosis. 1. Transmanual auscultation. 2. Ulnar palpation. Burlington, Vt., & New York, 1905. 7p. DNLM **00-4166**

RIESMAN, David (1867-1940)
Acute pulmonary oedema, with special reference to a recurrent form. Philadelphia & New York, 1907. 12p. DNLM **00-4167**

RIESMAN, David (1867-1940)
The development of cardiac murmurs during attacks of biliary colic. Chicago, 1907. 6p. DNLM **00-4168**

RIESMAN, David (1867-1940)
Hemorrhages in the course of Bright's disease; with especial reference to the occurrence of a hemorrhagic diathesis of nephritic origin. Philadelphia & New York, 1907. 8p. DNLM **00-4169**

RIESMAN, David (1867-1940)
Address to nurses; delivered at the graduation of nurses, Polyclinic Hospital Training School, November 11, 1908. New York, 1909. 6p. DNLM **00-4170**

RIGGS, Wilfred L.
Theory of osteopathy; by Wilfred L. Riggs. . . . Des Moines, Ia.: New Science Publishing Co., 1900. 218p. DLC; ICJ **00-4171**

RIGGS, Wilfred L.
A manual of osteopathic manipulations and treatment. . . . Elkhart, Ind.: New Science Publishing Co., 1901. 157p. DLC; DNLM; ICJ **00-4172**

RIGNANO, Eugenio (1870-1930)
Eugenio Rignano upon the inheritance of acquired characters: a hypothesis of heredity, development, and assimilation; authorized English translation by Basil C. H. Harvey . . . with an appendix upon the mnemonic origin and nature of the effective or natural tendencies. Chicago: The Open Court Publishing Co., 1910 [*c.* 1911]. 413p. DLC: ICJ; INC; NN **00-4173**

RIKER'S DRUG STORE (NEW YORK CITY)
Talks on rubber. Appliances and apparatus for medical purposes. . . . New York, 1900. 144p. NNNAM **00-4174**

RILEY, Cassius Marcellus (*b.* 1844)
Toxicology; the nature, effects and detection of poisons, with the diagnosis and treatment of poisoning. . . . [St. Louis]: The Author, 1901. 121p. DLC; DNLM; ICJ; PPC **00-4175**

RILEY, Cassius Marcellus (*b.* 1844)
Toxicology. The nature, effects and detection of poisons, with the diagnosis and treatment of poisoning. St. Louis: St. Louis Med. Book Pub. Co., 1902. 132p. DLC; ICJ; PPC **00-4176**

RILEY, Cassius Marcellus (*b.* 1844)
Toxicology. The nature, effects and detection of poisons, with the diagnosis and treatment of poisoning. 2nd ed. St. Louis: Matthews, 1904. 130p. DLC; ICJ; PPC **00-4177**

RILEY, Cassius Marcellus (*b.* 1844)
Toxicology; the nature, effects and detection of poisons, with the diagnosis and treatment of poisoning. . . . 3rd ed., rev. and enl. . . . Philadelphia: P. Blakiston's Son & Co., 1905. 215p. DLC; DNLM; ICJ; PPC **00-4178**

RINDFLEISCH, Eduard (1836-1908)
The elements of pathology. Transl. from the 1st German ed. by Wm. H. Mercur. . . . Rev. by James Tyson. . . . Philadelphia: P. Blakiston's Son & Co., 1901. [*c.* 1884]. 263p. DLC; ICJ; MH-M; PPC **00-4179**

RING, Arthur H.
Psychology in medicine. Boston, 1908. 7p. DNLM; MH **00-4180**

RING, Frank
How to examine for life insurance. St. Louis: D. Wilcox, 1901. 113p. DLC; ICJ **00-4181**

RING, Frank
How to examine for life insurance. St. Louis: The C. V. Mosby Medical Book & Pub. Co., [1906]. 112p. ICJ; OCIM **00-4182**

RISLEY, S[amuel] D[oty] (1845-1920) and E. A. SHUMWAY
Carcinomatous degeneration of a papilloma of the conjunctiva with infiltration of the eyelids. Philadelphia, 1901. 6p. DNLM; PPC **00-4183**

RISLEY, S[amuel] D[oty] (1845-1920)
A medical pilgrimage to the Republic of Panama, 1905, by Samuel D. Risley, M.D., and Roland G. Curtin, M.D. . . . [Philadelphia?], 1905. 43p. plates, fold. map. DLC; NN; PP; PPHa **00-4184**

RISLEY, S[amuel] D[oty] (1845-1920)
A medical pilgrimage to the Republic of Panama by Samuel D. Risley, M.D., and Roland G. Curtin, M.D. [Philadelphia?], 1905. 43p. plates. DLC: MH; NN; PPC **00-4185**

RITCHIE, John Woodside (*b.* 1871)
. . . Physiology and hygiene, with a chapter on physical exercise. . . . New York and Manila: World Book Co., 1906. 221p. col. plates. DLC; NIC; NN; PP [Philippine education series] **00-4186**

RITCHIE, John Woodside (*b.* 1871)
Human physiology; an elementary text-book of anatomy, physiology, and hygiene . . . illustrated by Mary H. Wellman. Yonkers-on-Hudson, N.Y.: World Book Co., 1908. 362p. DLC; ICJ; NIC; NN **00-4187**

RITCHIE, John Woodside (*b.* 1871)
Primer of sanitation for the tropics, by John Woodside Ritchie & Margaret Anna Purcell, with an introduction by Dr. David P. Barrows . . . and a chapter on opium by the Right Reverend Charles H. Brent. . . . Yonkers-on-Hudson, N.Y.: World Book Co., 1910. 182p. DLC; MH; NN; PU **00-4188**

RITCHIE, John Woodside (*b.* 1871)
. . . Primer of hygiene, by John W. Ritchie . . . and J. S. Caldwell . . . illustrated by Karl Hassmann and Hermann Heyer. Yonkers-on-Hudson, N.Y.: World Book Co., 1910. 144p. DLC; MH; NIC; NN **00-4189**

RITCHIE, John Woodside (*b.* 1871)
. . . Sanitation and physiology; being primar of sanitation and human physiology in one volume . . . illustrated by Karl Hassmann and Mary H. Wellman. Yonkers-on-Hudson, N.Y.: World Book Co., 1910. 2 pts. in 1 v. DLC; NIC; NN; PP [Each part also issued separately.] **00-4190**

RITTENHOUSE, William (*b.* 1852)
. . . The hygiene of childbearing. . . . Chicago, Ill.: Manhattan School of Preventive Medicine and Home Hygiene, 1908. 13p. DLC; ICJ **00-4191**

RITTER DENTAL MFG. CO. (NEW YORK)
Illustrated catalogue of dental furnishings. New York & Rochester, 1901. 675p. ICJ; NIC; NN **00-4192**

RITTER, Thomas Jefferson (*b.* 1855)
The people's home medical book. . . . Cleveland, O.: The R. C. Barnum Co., 1910. 478p. col. plates. DLC; ICJ; OCIM **00-4193**

ROBARTS, Heber (*b.* 1853)
Practical radium; the practical uses of radium in the treatment of obstinate forms of disease. . . . St. Louis, Mo.: Press of Nixon-Jones Printing Co., [1909]. 139p. DLC; ICJ; KU; PPC **00-4194**

ROBB, Hunter (1863-1940)
A clinical and pathological report of two cases of genital tuberculosis. [Cleveland, 1900.] 15p. DNLM **00-4195**

ROBB, Hunter (1863-1940)
The normal position of the uterus in the pelvis considered in relation to its physiologic mobility. Cleveland, 1900. 7p. DNLM **00-4196**

ROBB, Hunter (1863-1940)
The results of modern aseptic surgical technique, as demonstrated by a series of one hundred and fourteen consecutive, unselected abdominal sections without a death; with clinical and pathological reports. New York, 1900. 16p. DNLM **00-4197**

ROBB, Hunter (1863-1940)
The use of rubber gloves and gauntlets as a means of preventing infection. [Cleveland, 1900.] 2p. DNLM **00-4198**

ROBB, Hunter (1863-1940)
The advantages and disadvantages of drainage after abdominal operations. Chicago, 1901. 6p. DNLM **00-4199**

ROBB, Hunter (1863-1940)
Pus in abdominal operations. New York, 1901. 10p. DNLM **00-4200**

ROBB, Hunter (1863-1940)
Two cases of brain tumor in gynecological practice. New York: William Wood & Co., 1901. 7p. DNLM **00-4201**

ROBB, Hunter (1863-1940)
Aseptic surgical technique; with especial reference to gynaecological operations, together with notes on the technique employed in certain supplementary procedures . . . 2nd ed., rev. Philadelphia: J. B. Lippincott Co., 1902. 268p. col. plates. DLC; PPC; PPJ; PU **00-4202**

ROBB, Hunter (1863-1940)
Remarks on the writings of Louyse Bourgeois. . . . [Baltimore? 1903]. 19p. Illust. (port.) DLC; PPHa **00-4203**

ROBB, Hunter (1863-1940)
The mortality following operations for pus in the pelvis. Chicago, 1903. 7p. DNLM **00-4204**

ROBB, Hunter (1863-1940)
The vaginal incision in sepsis following abortion. New York, 1903. 7p. DNLM **00-4205**

ROBB, Hunter (1863-1940)
Conservation in pelvic surgery. New York: William Wood & Co., 1904. 9p. DNLM **00-4206**

ROBB, Hunter (1863-1940) and Winford H. SMITH
The streptococcus in gynecological surgery. New York: William Wood & Co., 1904. 5p. DNLM **00-4207**

ROBB, Hunter (1863-1940)
Aseptic surgical technique; with especial reference to gynaecological operations, together with notes on the technique employed in certain supplementary procedures. . . . 3rd ed. Philadelphia: J. B. Lippincott Co., [1904]. 268p. CtY-M; MBM; NNNAM; PU **00-4208**

ROBB, Hunter (1863-1940)
The early diagnosis of cancer of the fundus, with report of cases. New York: William Wood & Co., 1905. 10p. DNLM
00-4209

ROBB, Hunter (1863-1940)
Inflammatory conditions of the appendix accidentally brought to light in pelvic operations. New York, 1905. 5p. DNLM
00-4210

ROBB, Hunter (1863-1940)
A case of multiple gestation, ectopic and intrauterine. [Chicago, 1906.] 2 l. DNLM **00-4211**

ROBB, Hunter (1863-1940)
The immediate results of conservative operative measures on the tubes and ovaries. Philadelphia, 1906. 11p. DNLM
00-4212

ROBB, Hunter (1863-1940) ad Howard DITTRICK
Pulmonary complications following abdominal operations. Chicago, 1906. 6p. DNLM **00-4213**

ROBB, Hunter (1863-1940)
The treatment of nausea and vomiting following anaesthesia after abdominal operations. [1906.] 1 l. DNLM
00-4214

ROBB, Hunter (1863-1940)
Aseptic surgical technique, with especial reference to gynaecological operations, together with notes on the technique employed in certain supplementary procedures . . . 4th ed., rev. Philadelphia: J. B. Lippincott Co., 1906. 264p. col. plates. DLC; DNLM; NNNAM; PPC **00-4215**

ROBB, Hunter (1863-1940)
Bladder and bowel fistulae following an abdominal section; with report of a case. Cleveland, 1907. 4p. DNLM
00-4216

ROBB, Hunter (1863-1940)
Ectopic gestation with special reference to the treatment of tubal rupture. New York, 1907. 18p. DNLM
00-4217

ROBB, Hunter (1863-1940)
Ligatures and sutures in abdominal surgery. [1907.] 3p. DNLM **00-4218**

ROBB, Isabel Adams [Hampton] (1859-1910)
Nursing; its principles and practice. For hospital and private use. . . . [2nd ed.] rev. and enl. Philadelphia: W. B. Saunders Co., 1900. 3 fold. charts, 3 plates (incl. front.), illus. ICJ; NN
00-4219

ROBB, Isabel Adams [Hampton] (1859-1910)
Nursing; its principles and practice. For hospital and private use. By Isabel Adams Hampton. . . . Rev. and enl. . . . Cleveland: J. B. Savage, 1900. 512p. front., illus., plates, 3 fold. diags. ICJ **00-4220**

ROBB, Isabel Adams [Hampton] (1859-1910)
Nursing ethics; for hospital and private use. Cleveland: J. B. Savage, 1901. 273p. DNLM; ICJ; MB; OCIM
00-4221

ROBB, Isabel Adams [Hampton] (1859-1910)
Nursing; its principles and practice. For hospital and private use. . . . Rev. and enl. Cleveland: E. C. Koeckert, 1903. 512p. illus. DLC; NcD; PPC; PU **00-4222**

ROBB, Isabel Adams [Hampton] (1859-1910)
Nursing ethics for hospital and private use. Cleveland: E. C. Koeckert, 1906. 273p. ICJ; NN **00-4223**

ROBB, Isabel Adams [Hampton] (1859-1910)
Nursing; its principles and practice; for hospital and private use . . . 3rd ed. — rev. and enl. . . . Cleveland: E. C. Koeckert, 1906. 565p. plate, fold. charts. DLC; MB; PU
00-4224

ROBB, Isabel Adams [Hampton] (1859-1910)
Educational standards for nurses with other addresses on nursing subjects. . . . Cleveland: E. C. Koeckert, 1907. 266p. ICJ; PU **00-4225**

ROBBINS, F.
A peculiar case of infantile palsy of spinal origin. New York, 1906. 3p. DNLM **00-4226**

ROBBINS, Henry Alfred (1839-1911)
Hair and its anomalies. Chicago, 1900. 11p. DNLM
00-4227

ROBBINS, Henry Alfred (1839-1911)
Is leprosy the fourth stage of syphilis? St. Louis, 1902. 7p. DNLM **00-4228**

ROBBINS, Henry Alfred (1839-1911)
Syphilis of the vital organs. [St. Louis, 1907.] 6p. DNLM
00-4229

ROBBINS, Henry Alfred (1839-1911)
Chancre, chancroid, and bubo; a clinical lecture. St. Louis, 1908. 7p. DNLM **00-4230**

ROBBINS, Henry Alfred (1839-1911)
Evolution of the microscope; therapeutic action and dangers of the Roentgen and Becquerel rays; radium opsonic method of treatment of dermatological diseases. St. Louis, 1908. 7p. DNLM **00-4231**

ROBBINS, Henry Alfred (1839-1911)
Symptomatology of syphilis. Treatment of syphilis at the Hot Springs of Arkansas. St. Louis, 1908. 4p. DNLM
00-4232

ROBBINS, Henry Alfred (1839-1911)
Syphilis of the organs of sight, and hearing, and taste, and sense of smell, and the teeth, and accessory organs of digestion. St. Louis, 1908. 7p. DNLM **00-4233**

ROBBINS, Henry Alfred (1839-1911)
The therapeutic action of iodine and its compounds and mercury in diseases, especially exclusive of syphilis. [Washington, 1908.] 16p. DNLM **00-4234**

ROBERTS, Deering J. (1840-1925)
As to the proprietary medicines. Nashville, 1906. 7p. DNLM; PPHa **00-4235**

ROBERTS, Dudley
Hospital dietetics. New York, 1908. 7p. DNLM
00-4236

ROBERTS, George W.
The operative treatment of cancer of the rectum. New York, 1902. 12p. DNLM **00-4237**

ROBERTS, John B[ingham] (1852-1924)
The operative treatment of ugly ears. Philadelphia, 1900. 4p. DLC; DNLM **00-4238**

ROBERTS, John B[ingham] (1852-1924)
The surgical treatment of congenital and pathological disfigurements of the face. Abstract of the Mütter lectures of the College of Physicians of Philadelphia for 1900. Philadelphia: Philadelphia Med. Publ. Co., 1900. 53p. DLC: DNLM **00-4239**

ROBERTS, John B[ingham] (1852-1924)
The surgical treatment of disfigurements and deformities of the face. 2nd ed., with a chapter on the reconstruction of syphilitic noses. Philadelphia: Philadelphia Med. Publ. Co., 1901. 72p. DLC; DNLM **00-4240**

ROBERTS, John B[ingham] (1852-1924)
A case of gunshot wound of the kidney and stomach. Philadelphia, 1901. 3p. DLC; DNLM **00-4241**

ROBERTS, John B[ingham] (1852-1924)
The doctor's fee; a plea for honorable dealing. Philadelphia, 1901. 15p. DLC; DNLM **00-4242**

ROBERTS, John B[ingham] (1852-1924)
Suggestions for the reconstruction of syphilitic noses. Chicago, 1901. 8p. DLC; DNLM **00-4243**

ROBERTS, John B[ingham] (1852-1924)
Excision of the lumbar lymphatic nodes and spermatic vein in malignant disease of the testicle. Philadelphia: J. B. Lippincott, 1902. 11p. 1 plate. DLC; DNLM **00-4244**

ROBERTS, John B[ingham] (1852-1924)
The professional responsibility in accident cases involving litigation. New York, 1904. 2 l. DLC; DNLM **00-4245**

ROBERTS, John B[ingham] (1852-1924)
The doctor's duty to the state. New York, 1904. 28p. DLC; DNLM **00-4246**

ROBERTS, John B[ingham] (1852-1924)
The direct fixation of fractures. New York: A. R. Elliott Pub. Co., 1905. 7p. DLC; DNLM **00-4247**

ROBERTS, John B[ingham] (1852-1924)
A fatal case of bacillus pyocyaneus septicaemia after surgical operation. New York, 1905. 14p. DLC; DNLM **00-4248**

ROBERTS, John B[ingham] (1852-1924)
Some causes of inefficiency in medical practice. St. Louis, 1906. 7p. DLC; DNLM **00-4249**

ROBERTS, John B[ingham] (1852-1924)
Continuous passive hyperemia in delayed union of fractures and in hastening the consolidation of fractures. Philadelphia, 1907. 6p. DLC; DNLM **00-4250**

ROBERTS, John B[ingham] (1852-1924)
Improved methods in successful operative treatment of cleft palate. Philadelphia, 1907. 7p. DLC; DNLM **00-4251**

ROBERTS, John B[ingham] (1852-1924)
Modern methods in the repair of cleft palate. St. Louis, 1907. 7p. DLC; DNLM **00-4252**

ROBERTS, John B[ingham] (1852-1924)
Anesthesia peril in American hospitals. Detroit, 1908. 13p. DLC; DNLM **00-4253**

ROBERTS, John B[ingham] (1852-1924)
The doctor's duty to the state; essays on the public relations of physicians. . . . Chicago: American Medical Assoc. Press, 1908. 108p. DLC: ICJ; PP; PU **00-4254**

ROBERTS, John B[ingham] (1852-1924)
Gastric and duodenal ulcers secondary to wounds of the urinary bladder. Philadelhia, 1908. 24p. NN **00-4255**

ROBERTSON, F.
Home advice on health. . . . Janesville, Wis.: Recorder Printing Co., printers, [1901?] 80p. DLC; ICJ **00-4256**

ROBERTSON, John (*b.* 1854)
The confidential friend, a book for women of all ages and conditions. . . . Cincinnati: The New Method Cure Institute, 1901. 48p. col. plates. DLC: ICJ [*c.* 1890. *vel subseq.*] **00-4257**

ROBERTSON, William (*b.* 1865)
Meat and food inspection . . . with regulations governing meat inspection in the United States, by Maximilian Herzog. . . . Chicago: W. T. Keener & Co., 1908. 372p. 16 plates. plans. DLC; ICJ; ICU; NN **00-4258**

ROBINOVITCH, Louise G.
The genesis of epilepsy. New York: State Press, [1901]. 12p. DLC; NN **00-4259**

ROBINOVITCH, Louise G.
I. Resuscitation of subjects in a condition of apparent death, caused by chloroform, electrocution, etc. II. Electric anesthesia in laboratory surgery successfully applied during a period of three years. III. Resuscitation of a woman in profound syncope caused by chronic morphine poisoning. IV. Different effects of various electric currents. Choice of current for resuscitation. . . . V. Presentation of instruments for electric anesthesia and resuscitation. . . . VI. Jolyet's cannula modified by Dr. Robinovitch. . . . New York: Journal of Mental Pathology, 1909. 40p. DLC; NN **00-4260**

ROBINS, Charles R. (*b.* 1868)
Necessity for diagnosis as a preliminary step to gynecological operations. Richmond: Williams Printing Co., 1908. 6p. ICJ; ViRA **00-4261**

ROBINS, Charles R. (*b.* 1868)
Rupture of the uterus during labor. Charlotte, N.C., [1910?] 6p. DLC **00-4262**

ROBINS, William Littleton (*b.* 1869)
Medical inspection of schools. New York, 1900. 16p. DNLM **00-4263**

ROBINS, William Littleton (*b.* 1869)
A case of exhibitionism. New York, 1903. 5p. DNLM
00-4264

ROBINS, William Littleton (*b.* 1869)
Amyotrophic lateral sclerosis. Chicago, 1907. 4p. DNLM
00-4265

ROBINS, William Littleton (*b.* 1869)
Friedreich's disease. Report of a case; with a clinical digest of one hundred cases. . . . [Washington, 1907.] 9p. DNLM
00-4266

ROBINSON, A[ndrew] R[ose] (1845-1924)
Observations on the treatment of cancer. New York: Publisher's Printing Co. 1900. 19p. DNLM
00-4267

ROBINSON, A[ndrew] R[ose] (1845-1924)
Value of the Roentgen rays in cancer. [1902.] 14p. DNLM
00-4268

ROBINSON, A[ndrew] R[ose] (1845-1924)
Errors in the treatment of cutaneous cancers. New York, 1906. 19p. DNLM
00-4269

ROBINSON, Beverley (1844-1924)
Sanatoria for consumptives. St. Louis, 1900. 4p. DNLM
00-4270

ROBINSON, Beverley (1844-1924)
Clinical aspects of spa treatment. Philadelphia: J. B. Lippincott Co., 1901. 8p. DNLM
00-4271

ROBINSON, Beverley (1844-1924)
Essays on clincial medicine, being reprints of papers published at various times in the "American Journal of the Medical Sciences," by Beverley Robinson. Philadelphia: W. J. Dornan, 1903. [6, 9]-171p. CtY-M; ICJ; NN [Contents — Creosote as a remedy in phthisis pulmonalis. (January, 1889.) — On the course and treatment of certain uremic symptoms. (October, 1893.) — A contribution to the treatment of organic disease of the heart. (December, 1894.) — Etiology and treatment of certain kinds of cough. (November, 1895.) — Prognosis in heart disease. (December, 1899.) Minor forms of cardiac dilation. (August, 1900.) — Clinical study of acute myocarditis. (March, 1901.) — Chronic myocarditis and fatty degeneration of the heart. (June, 1901.) Angina pectoris. (February, 1902.) — Tuberculous pericarditis followed by Remarks upon paracentesis and incision. (June, 1902.) — A study of some cirrhoses of the liver. (February, 1903.)]
00-4272

ROBINSON, Beverley (1844-1924)
The community and tuberculosis. Philadelphia, 1903. 7p. DNLM
00-4273

ROBINSON, Beverley (1844-1924)
Some unsettled and important problems in the treatment of acute lobar pneumonia. New York, 1904. 12p. DNLM
00-4274

ROBINSON, Beverley (1844-1924)
General management and therapeutics of nephritis. New York, 1904. 12p. DNLM
00-4275

ROBINSON, Beverley (1844-1924)
Medicine as a science and medicine as an art; also, in view of this, a few words about specialist and general practitioner. Philadelphia, 1906. 2p. DNLM
00-4276

ROBINSON, Beverley (1844-1924)
Management of laryngeal phthisis. Philadelphia, 1907. 1 l. DNLM
00-4277

ROBINSON, Beverley (1844-1924)
Souvenirs of an old New York practitioner of medicine. [New York: William Wood & Co., 1908?] 15p. NNU-M
00-4278

ROBINSON, David Hamilton
The Latin grammar of pharmacy and medicine . . . with an introduction by L. E. Sayre . . . 4th ed., with elaborate vocabularies, thoroughly rev. by Hanna Oliver. . . . Philadelphia: P. Blakiston's Son & Co., 1903. 277p. DLC; DNLM; PPHa; PPJ
00-4279

ROBINSON, Ernest F.
Massage. A course of lessons. . . . Boston, Mass.: L. N. Cushman, 1903. 70p. plates. DLC; MH [Plates printed on both sides.]
00-4280

ROBINSON, [Frederick] Byron (1855-1910)
The peritoneum. . . . [2nd ed.] Chicago: Chicago Medical Book Co., 1901 [*c.* 1897]. 400, 103p. DLC; DNLM; PPHa
00-4281

ROBINSON, [Frederick] Byron (1855-1910)
Landmarks in gynecology. . . . 2nd ed., rev. and enl. . . . Chicago: E. H. Colegrove, 1901. 399p. DLC; ICJ; PPC; PPHa
00-4282

ROBINSON, [Frederick] Byron (1855-1910)
Arteria uterina ovarica. The utero-ovarian artery, or the genital vascular circle. Anatomy and physiology, with their application in diagnosis and surgical intervention. Chicago: E. H. Colegrove, 1903. 182p. DNLM; ICJ; IU-M; OCIM
00-4283

ROBINSON, [Frederick] Byron (1855-1910)
The elective line of renal incision; the natural division of the kidneys; Hyrtl's exsanguinated renal zone (Zona exsanguinata Hyrtlii). New York: A. R. Elliott Co., 1904. 4p. DNLM
00-4284

ROBINSON, [Frederick] Byron (1855-1910)
The abdominal and pelvic brain; with automatic visceral ganglia. . . . Hammond, Inc.: F. S. Betz, [1907]. 671p. DLC; ICJ; PPC
00-4285

ROBINSON, [Frederick] Byron (1855-1910)
The arteries of the gastro-intestinal tract with inoscultation circle, anatomy and physiology with application in treatment. . . . The function of the inosculation circle is to congest its peripheral viscus and to transport blood volume from one viscus to another. Chicago, Ill.: E. H. Colegrove, 1908. 222p. DNLM; ICJ; IU-M; PPC
00-4286

ROBINSON, George
The hospital ship in the war with Spain. A paper prepared and read before the Kansas commandery of the Military order of the loyal legion of the United States. [1901?] 12p. DLC
00-4287

ROBINSON, Samuel
Two cases of anatomical anomaly of the large intestine. Boston, 1905. 12p. DNLM **00-4288**

ROBINSON, Samuel
The Bennett fracture of the first metacarpal bone; diagnosis and treatment. Boston, 1908. 15p. 1 plate. DNLM **00-4289**

ROBINSON, Samuel
Progress in surgery. Thoracic surgery. [Boston, 1910.] 21p. MBM **00-4290**

ROBINSON, Tom (*d.* 1916)
Baldness and grayness, their etiology, pathology, and treatment. New York: William Wood & Co., 1903. 125p. DLC; ICJ; NN; PU [Reprinted out of Wood's Medical and Surgical Monographs, vol. 9, No. 3 (1891), pp. 725-796] **00-4291**

ROBINSON, William J[osephus] (1867-1936)
Robinson's materia medica. Organic materia medica, according to the U.S.P. 1893. Posology and toxicology, with definitions of botanical and medical terms. . . . For those preparing for the Board of Pharmacy examinations and for college students. New York: Press of G. Weinstein, 1901 [*c.* 1894]. 62p. tables. DLC; NN **00-4292**

ROBINSON, William J[osephus] (1867-1936)
A quiz-system of pharmacy and all the allied branches. For the use of teachers and board examiners and as a guide to home study. . . . New York: Critic Guide Co., 1903. 237p. DLC; NN **00-4293**

ROBINSON, William J[osephus] (1867-1936)
The Official State Journal vs. the Independent Medical Journal. [New York], 1906. 8p. DNLM **00-4294**

ROBINSON, Wilton Howarth (*b.* 1878)
Dermatology in abstract; a guide to the clinical study of diseases of the skin. . . . Pittsburgh, Pa.: Medical Abstract Publishing Co., [1909]. 175p. DLC; ICJ; PPC **00-4295**

ROBISON, John A.
Evidences that bovine tuberculosis is communicable to man by direct contact, or by food infection. Chicago, 1900. 16p. DNLM **00-4296**

ROBISON, John A.
Bone marrow in the treatment of various forms of anaemia. Chicago, [1900]. 11p. DNLM **00-4297**

ROBSON, A[rthur] W[illiam] Mayo (1853-1933) and Farquhar MACRAE
Diseases of the gall-bladder and bile-ducts, including gall-stones. 2nd ed. New York: William Wood & Co., 1900. 313p. DNLM; NNNAM **00-4298**

ROBSON, A[rthur] W[illiam] Mayo (1853-1933)
A guide to the instruments and appliances required in various operations . . . 2nd ed. . . . New York: Cassell & Co., 1900. 62p. DLC; ICJ **00-4299**

ROBSON, A[rthur] W[illiam] Mayo (1853-1933) and B. G. A. MOYNIHAN
Diseases of the stomach, and their surgical treatment. New York: William Wood & Co., 1901. 308p. DNLM; NNNAM **00-4300**

ROBSON, A[rthur] W[illiam] Mayo (1853-1933) and B. G. A. MOYNIHAN
Diseases of the pancreas and their surgical treatment. Philadelphia & London: W. B. Saunders & Co., 1902. 293p. 1 plate. DLC; DNLM; PPC; PU **00-4301**

ROBSON, A[rthur] W[illiam] Mayo (1853-1933) and B. G. A. MOYNIHAN
Diseases of the stomach, and their surgical treatment. 2nd ed. New York: William Wood & Co., 1904. 508p. DLC: DNLM; NNNAM **00-4302**

ROBSON, A[rthur] W[illiam] Mayo (1853-1933) and J. F. DOBSON
Diseases of the gall-bladder and bile-ducts, including gall-stones. 3rd ed. New York: William Wood & Co., 1904. 485p. 31 plates. DLC; DNLM; NNNAM **00-4303**

ROBSON, A[rthur] W[illiam] Mayo (1853-1933)
Cancer of the stomach. New York: William Wood & Co., 1907. 218p. 14 plates. DNLM; NNNAM **00-4304**

ROBSON, A[rthur] W[illiam] Mayo (1853-1933) and P. J. CAMMIDGE
The pancreas; its surgery and pathology. Philadelphia & London: W. B. Saunders & Co., 1907. 546p. 2 plates. DLC; DNLM; PPC; PU **00-4305**

ROBY, J[oseph]
Pasteurization; its advantages and disadvantages to the municipality. New York, 1907. 7p. DNLM **00-4306**

ROCHELLE, George I.
Clinical notes of a case of hyperchlorhydria successfully treated by mechanical vibratory stimulation. Philadelphia, 1903. 2 l. DNLM **00-4307**

THE ROCKEFELLER INSTITUTE FOR MEDICAL RESEARCH
Studies from the Rockefeller Institute for Medical Research. Reprints. New York, 1904. 2 v. DNLM; MH; NNNAM **00-4308**

THE ROCKEFELER INSTITUTE FOR MEDICAL RESEARCH
Studies on the pathology and on the etiology of variola and of vaccinia. Boston, [1904]. 361p. 29 plates. DNLM; MH; NN **00-4309**

THE ROCKEFELLER INSTITUTE FOR MEDICAL RESEARCH
Description of the buildings; addresses delivered at the opening of the laboratories in New York City, May 11, 1906. Lancaster, Pa.: New Era Ptg. Co., 1907. 50p. 14 plates. DLC; DNLM; NN; NNNAM **00-4310**

THE ROCKEFELLER INSTITUTE FOR MEDICAL RESEARCH. NEW YORK
. . . Tumors of animals. . . . New York: The Rockefeller Institute for Medical Research, 1910. 150p. plates. DLC; MH; NIC; NN **00-4311**

ROCKEFELLER SANITARY COMMISSION FOR THE ERADICATION OF HOOKWORM DISEASE. WASHINGTON, D.C.
. . . Annual report . . . [1st]-5th; 1910-14. Washington, D.C., 1910-15. 5 v. in 2. plates, maps. DLC; ICU; NIC; NN **00-4312**

ROCKEFELLER SANITARY COMMISSION FOR THE ERADICATION OF HOOKWORM DISEASE. WASHINGTON, D.C.
Publication[s] no. 1-9. Washington, D.C., 1910-15. 9 v. in 1. DLC; ICJ; MH; NN [No more published; the commission, which was organized Oct. 26, 1909, for a five-year period, went out of existence Dec. 31, 1914, and its unfinished work was assumed by the International Health Commission, an organization created by the Rockefeller Foundation in 1913.]
00-4313

ROCKWELL, Alfred E. P. (*b.* 1870)
Some phases of sectarian medicine. New York, 1906. 8p. DNLM **00-4314**

ROCKWELL, Alphonso D[avid] (1840-1925)
Diseases of the alimentary tract; diseases of the liver and kidney; gout and rheumatism. [Philadelphia, 1901.] 33p. MB
00-4315

ROCKWELL, Alphonso D[avid] (1840-1925)
The x-ray and the Finsen light in the treatment of lupus. New York: William Wood & Co., [1903]. 2p. NN
00-4316

ROCKWELL, Alphonso D[avid] (1840-1925)
The medical and surgical uses of electricity, including the X-ray, Finsen light, vibratory therapeutics, and high-frequency currents . . . with two hundred and fifty-two illustrations. New ed. New York: E. B. Treat & Co., 1903. 656p. DLC; DNLM; ICJ; NNNAM [A "New edition" of Beard and Rockwell's "A practical treatise on the medical and surgical uses of electricity," which "after passing through eight editions, was in 1896 thoroughly revised by the present writer. The old stereotyped plates were destroyed, all illustrations newly drawn, and much of the book rewritten. . . . Six chapters have been added."] **00-4317**

ROCKWELL, Alphonso D[avid] (1840-1925)
The medical and surgical uses of electricity, including the X-ray, photo-therapy, the Finsen light, vibratory therapeutics, high-frequency currents, and radio-activity . . . with two hundred and fifty-nine illustrations. New ed., rev. and enl. New York: E. B. Treat & Co., 1907. 676p. CtY-M; ICJ
00-4318

ROCKWELL, William Hayden (*b.* 1867)
. . . Anatomy. A manual for students and practitioners . . . illustrated with seventy engravings. Philadelphia and New York: Lea Bros. & Co., [1903]. 620p. DLC: DNLM; NNNAM; PPC **00-4319**

ROCKWELL, William Hayden (*b.* 1867)
Dissecting manual, based on Cunningham's anatomy. . . . New York: William Wood & Co., 1905. 306p. DLC: DNLM; MH-M; NNNAM **00-4320**

ROCKWOOD, Elbert William (*b.* 1860)
An introduction to chemical analysis, for students of medicine, pharmacy, and dentistry. . . . Philadelphia: P. Blakiston's Son & Co., 1901. 255p. DLC; DNLM; MH; PPC
00-4321

ROCKWOOD, Elbert William (*b.* 1860)
An introduction to chemical analysis, for students of medicine, pharmacy, and dentistry . . . 2nd rev. ed. . . . Philadelphia: P. Blakiston's Son & Co., 1904. 255p. DLC; ICJ; NN; PPC
00-4322

ROCKWOOD, Elbert William (*b.* 1860)
A laboratory manual of physiological chemistry . . . 2nd ed., rev. and enl., with one colored plate and three plates of microscopic preparations. Philadelphia: F. A. Davis Co., 1906. 229p. 4 plates. DNLM; NNNAM; PPC; PU
00-4323

ROCKWOOD, Elbert William (*b.* 1860)
A laboratory manual of physiological chemistry . . . 3rd ed., rev. and enl., with one colored plate and three plates of microscopic preparations. Philadelphia: F. A. Davis Co., 1910. 235p. 4 plates. DLC; ICJ; PPC; PPJ
00-4324

ROCKWOOD, Elbert William (*b.* 1860)
An introduction to chemical analysis, for students of medicine, pharmacy, and dentistry . . . 3rd rev. ed., with 20 illustrations. Philadelphia: P. Blakiston's Son & Co., 1910. 247p. DLC; ICJ; PPC; PU **00-4325**

RODERMUND, Matthew Joseph
Positive proofs that blood can circulate without the aid of the heart. Appleton, Wis.: Post Publishing Co., 1900 [*c.* 1899]. 15p. DNLM **00-4326**

RODERMUND, Matthew Joseph
The muderous fads in the practice of medicine, and the cause and prevention of disease. . . . Appleton, Wis., 1900. 654p. DLC; ICJ **00-4327**

RODERMUND, Matthew Joseph
Fads in the practice of medicine, and the cause and prevention of disease. This volume positively explains, for the first time in the world's history, the causes of yellow-fever, small-pox, diphtheria, scarlet fever, measles, consumption, etc. Chicago: Twentieth Century Pub. Co., 1901. 654p. port. DNLM
00-4328

RODERMUND, Matthew Joseph
"As it is." . . . Milwaukee, Wis.: [The Evening Wisconsin Printing Co.], 1907. 232p. DLC; DNLM; PPC ["My ambition is the desire and determination to bring out the truth, and present to the public and the medical profession the meaning of certain actions, expressions and phenomena of nature's laws and their relation to health and the cause and prevention of disease."—Pref.] **00-4329**

RODMAN, William Louis (1858-1916)
Influence of age and race in surgical affections. [Philadelphia, 1900.] 14p. Illus. MB **00-4330**

RODMAN, William Louis (1858-1916)
Diseases of the breast, with special reference to cancer . . . with 69 plates, of which 12 are printed in colors and 42 other illustrations. Philadelphia: P. Blakiston's Son & Co., 1908. 385p. DLC; ICJ; NcD; PPC **00-4331**

ROEMELE, E[ugene] C.
Ecthol, local and internal. St. Louis, 1903. 15p. DNLM
00-4332

ROGER, Georges Eugène Henri (1860-1946)
Introduction to the study of medicine. . . . Authorized translation by M. S. Gabriel, M D., with additions by the author. New York: D. Appleton & Co., 1901. 545p. DLC; DNLM; MH-M; NNNAM **00-4333**

ROGER, Georges Eugène Henri (1860-1946)
Infectious diseases, their etiology, diagnosis, and treatment . . . transl. by M. S. Gabriel, M.D., illustrated with forty-three engravings. New York and Philadelphia: Lea Bros. & Co., 1903. 874p. DLC; NNNAM; PPC; PU
00-4334

ROGER, Georges Eugène Henri (1860-1946)
Principles of medical pathology. Authorized transl. by M. S. Gabriel. With additions by the author. New York: D. Appleton & Co., 1905. 545p. CtY-M; DNLM; NNNAM; PPC
00-4335

ROGERS, Corydon Eugene
Lucotherapy; or, The therapeutic action of light, by . . . a practical treatise upon the principal methods of employing light rays in the treatment of all germ diseases. Seattle, Wash.: The Metropolitan Press, [1903]. 157p. plates. DLC; DNLM
00-4336

ROGERS, Corydon Eugene
A textbook on the therapeutic action of light, including the rho rays, solar and violet rays, electric arc light, the light cabinet . . . with original illustrations. [Chicago? Ill.]: The Author, [1910]. 323p. DLC; ICJ; PPJ; PU
00-4337

ROGERS, Edmund J[ames] A[rmstrong] (*b.* 1852)
Clinical reports: (1) Operation for carcinoma of the penis. (2) Operation for carcinoma of the anus. Denver, 1900. 2p. DNLM **00-4338**

[ROGERS, Geoge Adelmer] (*b.* 1852)
Skiascopy; a treatise on the shadow test in its practical application to the work of refraction, with an explanation in detail of the optical principles on which the science is based, with sixty-nine illustrations and four plates. Philadelphia: Pub. by the Keystone, 1901 [*c.* 1899]. 221p. plates. diags. DLC; ICJ; PP; PPC **00-4339**

[ROGERS, George Adelmer] (*b.* 1852)
The shadow test in ocular diagnosis, without prejudice as to method, mirror, distance or instrument. . . . Chicago: The Optic Press, [1905]. 110p. plates. DLC; ICJ
00-4340

ROGERS, J[ames] Frederick (*b.* 1870)
The effect of blowing upon wind musical instruments, with special reference to tuberculosis. New York: William Wood & Co., 1906. 25p. DNLM; NNNAM **00-4341**

ROGERS, J[ames] Frederick (*b.* 1870)
Life and health. . . . Philadelphia & London: J. B. Lippincott Co., 1910. 202p. DLC; DNLM; ICJ; MB
00-4342

ROGERS, John
The treatment of chronic obstruction in the larynx and trachea. Philadelphia: Lea Bros. & Co., 1905. 46p. DNLM
00-4343

ROGERS, John
The treatment of thyroidism by a specific serum. New York, 1906. 18p. DNLM **00-4344**

ROGERS, John and J. S. FERGUSON
The anatomy of the parathyroid glands. New York, 1906. 6p. DNLM **00-4345**

ROGERS, John and John C. TORREY
The treatment of gonorrheal infections by a specific antiserum. Chicago, 1907. 18p. DNLM **00-4346**

ROGERS, Joseph Goodwin (1841-1908)
A century of hospital building for the insane. Utica, N.Y., 1900. 19p. DNLM **00-4347**

ROGERS, Leonard (*b.* 1868)
The prevention of tropical abscess of the liver by the early diagnosis and treatment of the presuppurative stage of amebic hepatitis. Chicago, 1908. 7p. DNLM
00-4348

ROGERS, Loyal Dexter (*b.* 1856)
Asepsis; or, Surgical cleanliness, a manual for physicians, students and nurses. . . . Chicago: People's Health Journal Co., 1900. 80p. DLC; DNLM; ICJ **00-4349**

ROGERS, Loyal Dexter (*b.* 1856)
Homeopathy explained, with hints, indications, dose and directions for the use of fifty of the most commonly used homeopathic remedies. By L. D. Rogers . . . and Ida Wright Rogers. . . . Chicago: The People's Health Journal Co., 1901 [*c.* 1896]. 43p. ICJ **00-4350**

ROGERS, T. Avery
Prophylaxis in pregnancy and labor. New York, 1905. 14p. DNLM **00-4351**

ROGUES DE FURSAC, Joseph (*b.* 1872)
Manual of psychiatry. . . . Authorized translation from the French by A. J. Rosanoff . . . ed. by Joseph Collins . . . 1st ed. 1st thousand. New York: J. Wiley & Sons; [etc., etc.], 1905. 352p. DLC; ICJ; PPC; PPJ **00-4352**

ROGUES DE FURSAC, Joseph (*b.* 1872)
Manual of psychiatry . . . authorized translation from the French, by A. J. Rosanoff . . . 2nd American from the 2nd French ed. Rev. and enl. New York: J. Wiley & Sons; [etc., etc.], 1908. 406p. DLC; DNLM; ICJ; NNNAM
00-4353

ROHÉ, George Henry (1851-1899)
Text-book of hygiene; a comprehensive treatise on the principles and practice of preventive medicine from an American standpoint, by George H. Rohé . . . and Albert Robin . . . 4th rev. and enl. ed., with many illustrations and valuable tables. Philadelphia: F. A. Davis Co., 1908. 582p. plates. DLC; DNLM; NNNAM; PPC **00-4354**

ROHRER, Caleb W[yand] G[eeting] (*b.* 1873)
A contribution to the comparative anatomy of the prostate gland. . . . Baltimore, 1909. 124p. DLC; DNLM; ICJ; NcD
00-4355

ROHRER, Caleb W[yand] G[eeting] (*b.* 1873)
Symposium on the administration of the State Board of Health, Bureau of Communicable Diseases; paper read at the semi-annual meeting of the Medical and Chirurgical Faculty of Maryland, held at Annapolis on . . . September 12, 13 and 14, 1910. [Baltimore], 1910. 9p. NN **00-4356**

ROLLESTON, Humphry Davy (1862-1944)
Diseases of the liver, gall-bladder and bile-ducts. . . . Philadelphia, [etc.]: W. B. Saunders & Co., 1905 [1904]. 794p. col. plates. DLC; DNLM; PPC; PU **00-4357**

ROLLESTON, Humphry Davy (1862-1944)
Clinical lectures and essays on abdominal and other subjects. Philadelphia: P. Blakiston's Son & Co., 1904. 178p. CtY-M; DNLM; ICJ; PPC **00-4358**

ROMAN, C[harles] V.
When there is no physician there; or, Common sense in matters of health. . . . Dallas, Tex., [1901?] 106p. DLC; [*c.* 1896. *vel subseq.*] **00-4359**

ROMIG, J. H.
A medical handbook for missionaries in cold climates. . . . Philadelphia: Boericke & Tafel, 1904. 250p. DLC; PPC **00-4360**

ROOSA, Daniel Bennet St. John (1838-1908)
The old New York Hospital; an historical sketch. New York, 1900. 15p. 3 plates. DNLM; NNNAM **00-4361**

ROOSA, Daniel Bennet St. John (1838-1908)
Functional and paralytic strabismus. New York, 1902. 7p. DNLM **00-4362**

ROOSA, Daniel Bennet St. John (1838-1908)
Hand-book of the anatomy and diseases of the eye and ear, for students and practitioners, by D. B. St. John Roosa . . . and A. Edward Davis. . . . Philadelphia: F. A. Davis Co., 1904. 297p. DLC; DNLM; PPC: PPJ **00-4363**

ROOSA, Daniel Bennet St. John (1838-1908)
A text-book of the diseases of the ear, nose and pharynx, by D. B. St. John Roosa . . . and Beaman Douglass. . . . New York: The Macmillan Co.; London: Macmillan & Co., 1905. 621p. DLC; DNLM; MH-M; NNNAM **00-4364**

ROSE, A[chilles] (1839-1916)
A conspiracy to suppress the truth about living Greek. [New York: A. R. Elliott Publ. Co.], 1901. 6p. NN **00-4365**

ROSE, A[chilles] (1839-1916)
Greek in medicine. n. p., [1902]. 13p. DNLM; NNNAM **00-4366**

ROSE, A[chilles] (1839-1916)
Floating kidney; idoltry; a polemic. Chicago, 1902. 8p. DNLM; NNNAM **00-4367**

ROSE, A[chilles] (1839-1916)
Onomatologia gastrologica. [New York, 1905]. 14p. DNLM; NNNAM **00-4368**

ROSE, A[chilles] (1839-1916)
Carbonic acid in medicine. New York: Funk & Wagnalls Co., 1905. 259p. 3 port. DNLM; NNNAM **00-4369**

ROSE, A[chilles] (1839-1916) and Robert Coleman KEMP
Atonia gastrica (abdominal relaxation). New York: Funk & Wagnalls Co., 1905. 203p. 8 plates on 4 l. CtY-M; DLC; ICJ; PPC **00-4370**

ROSE, A[chilles] (1839-1916)
Is nervous dyspepsia a disease sui generis? New York: A. R. Elliott Co., 1906. 3p. DNLM; NNNAM **00-4371**

ROSE, A[chilles] (1839-1916)
Modern methods in the medical treatment of gastric diseases. New York, 1907. 8p. DNLM; NNNAM **00-4372**

ROSE, A[chilles] (1839-1916)
Barbarism in medical language. New York: A. R. Elliott Co., 1907. 7p. DNLM; NNNAM **00-4373**

ROSE, A[chilles] (1839-1916)
Memorial on medical language, presented for consideration to the rectoribus magnificis convening in Marburg, July 30, 1907. New York, 1907. 8p. DNLM; NNNAM **00-4374**

ROSE, A[chilles] (1839-1916)
Aetiology, pathology, and therapy of medical slang. Toledo, 1907. 2 l. DNLM; NNNAM **00-4375**

ROSE, A[chilles] (1839-1916)
Ancient Greek medicine. New York, 1908. 4p. DNLM; NNNAM **00-4376**

ROSE, A[chilles] (1839-1916)
Malaria in Greece. New York, 1908. 1 l. DNLM; NNNAM **00-4377**

ROSE, A[chilles] (1839-1916)
Medical Greek; collection of papers on medical onomatology and a grammatical guide to learn modern Greek. New York: Peri Hellados, 1908. 262p. DNLM; ICJ; NcD; NN **00-4378**

ROSE, A[chilles] (1839-1916)
Katharcuousa and scientific medical nomenclature. [Philadelphia], 1910. 11p. NN **00-4379**

ROSE, William (1847-1910) and Albert CARLESS
A manual of surgery for students and practitioners. 3rd ed. New York: William Wood & Co., 1900. 1182p. NNNAM **00-4380**

ROSE, William (1847-1910) and Albert CARLESS
A manual of surgery for students and practitioners. 4th ed. New York: William Wood & Co., 1901. 1182p. NNNAM; PPC; PU **00-4381**

ROSE, William (1847-1910) and Albert CARLESS
A manual of surgery for students and practitioners. 5th ed. New York: William Wood & Co., 1902. 1213p. 29 plates. DLC; DNLM; MBM; NNNAM **00-4382**

ROSE, William (1847-1910) and Albert CARLESS
A manual of surgery for students and practitioners. 6th ed. New York: William Wood & Co., 1905. 1330p. 30 plates. DLC; DNLM; ICJ; NNNAM **00-4383**

ROSE, William (1847-1910) and Albert CARLESS
A manual of surgery for students and practitioners. 7th ed. New York: William Wood & Co., 1908. 1376p. DLC; MH-M; NNC; PPC **00-4384**

ROSENAU, Milton J[oseph] (1869-1946)
. . . Laboratory course in pathology and bacteriology. . . . Washington: Government Printing Office, 1902. 56p. DLC; DNLM; NcD; NN **00-4385**

ROSENAU, Milton J[oseph] (1869-1946)
Disinfection and disinfectants; a practical guide for sanitarians, health and quarantine officers. . . . Philadelphia: P. Blakiston's Son & Co., 1902. 353p. plates. DLC; NcD; PPC; PU
00-4386

ROSENAU, Milton J[oseph] (1869-1946)
. . . The antiseptic and germicidal properties of glycerin. . . . Washington: Government Printing Office, 1903. 30p. DLC; DNLM; NcD; NN **00-4387**

ROSENAU, Milton J[oseph] (1869-1946)
. . . The bacteriological impurities of vaccine virus. An experimental study. . . . Washington: Government Printing Office, 1903. 50p. DLC; DNLM; MB; NN **00-4388**

ROSENAU, Milton J[oseph] (1869-1946)
. . . The immunity unit for standardizing diphtheria antitoxin (based on Ehrlich's normal serum). Official standard prepared under the act approved July 1, 1902. . . . Washington: Government Printing Office, 1905. 92p. DLC; DNLM; NcD; NN
00-4389

ROSENAU, Milton J[oseph] (1869-1946)
. . . A study of the cause of sudden death following the injection of horse serum. By M. J. Rosenau and John F. Anderson. Washington: Government Printing Office, 1906. 95p. DLC; MB; NcD; NN **00-4390**

ROSENAU, Milton J[oseph] (1869-1946)
. . . Studies upon hypersusceptibility and immunity, by M. J. Rosenau and John F. Anderson. Washington: Government Printing Office, 1907. 69p. DLC; MB; NcD; NN
00-4391

ROSENAU, Milton J[oseph] (1869-1946)
. . . The influence of antitoxin upon post-diphtheritic paralysis, by M. J. Rosenau and John F. Anderson. Washington: Government Printing Office, 1907. 34p. DLC; MB; NcD; NN
00-4392

ROSENAU, Milton J[oseph] (1869-1946)
. . . The thermal death points of pathogenic micro-organisms in milk. . . . Washington: Government Printing Office, 1908. 85p. DLC; MB; NcD; NN **00-4393**

ROSENAU, Milton J[oseph] (1869-1946)
. . . Further studies upon anaphylaxis, by M. J. Rosenau and John F. Anderson. Washington: Government Printing Office, 1908. 65p. DLC; DNLM; MB; NN **00-4394**

ROSENAU, Milton J[oseph] (1869-1946)
. . . Further studies upon the phenomenon of anaphylaxis, by M. J. Rosenau and John F. Anderson. Washington: Government Printing Office, 1909. 52p. DLC; MB; NcD; NN
00-4395

ROSENAU, Milton J[oseph] (1869-1946)
The role of animal experimentation and the diagnosis of disease. Chicago: American Medical Association, 1909. 6p. DNLM; PPC **00-4396**

ROSENBACH, Ottomar (1851-1907)
Physician versus bacteriologist. Transl. from the German by Achilles Rose. New York: Funk & Wagnalls Co., 1904. 462p. DLC; ICJ; NN; PU **00-4397**

ROSENBERG, Julius
My experience with photo-therapy; a preliminary report. New York, 1904. 7p. DNLM **00-4398**

ROSENBERG, Lionel
Some experience with tuberculin. New York, 1907. 8p. DNLM
00-4399

ROSENBERG, Lionel
Cause of premature separation of the placenta. New York, 1908. 2 l. DNLM **00-4400**

ROSENBERGER, Randle C.
The bacteriologic examination of clinical thermometers. Philadelphia, 1901. 6p. DNLM **00-4401**

ROSENBERGER, Randle C.
The identification of the colon bacillus by reactions produced in culture media containing neutral red; observations on reactions of other bacteria on the same media. Philadelphia, 1902. 12p. DNLM **00-4402**

ROSENBERGER, Randle C.
Notes from the pathologic laboratory of the Jefferson Medical College. Philadelphia, 1903. 7p. DNLM
00-4403

ROSENBERGER, Randle C. and Joseph W. ENGLAND
Lithiomercuric iodid. Philadelphia, 1904. 3p. DNLM
00-4404

ROSENBERGER, Randle C.
Hyaline bodies in tumors and kindred other conditions. Philadelphia, 1904. 12p. DNLM **00-4405**

ROSENBERGER, Randle C.
A case of acute lymphatic leukaemia. Philadelphia, 1904. 18p. DNLM **00-4406**

ROSENBERGER, Randle C.
The actual and comparative resistance of acid-fast bacilli. Detroit, 1904. 12p. DNLM **00-4407**

ROSENBERGER, Randle C.
A review of literature relating to serum diagnosis. Philadelphia, 1904. 27p. DNLM **00-4408**

ROSENBERGER, Randle C.
Bacteriology of the blood. Philadelphia, 1904. 24p. DNLM
00-4409

ROSENBERGER, Randle C.
The action of acid-fast bacilli when inoculated into the peritoneal cavity of white rats. Philadelphia, 1905. 10p. DNLM
00-4410

ROSENBERGER, Randle C.
The disinfection of catheters by the use of formalin. [Philadelphia, 1905.] 4p. DNLM **00-4411**

ROSENBERGER, Randle C.
A study of homogenized cultures of tubercle bacilli. Philadelphia, 1905. 5p. DNLM **00-4412**

ROSENBERGER, Randle C.
A study of the mesenteric glands in their relations to tuberculosis. Philadelphia, 1905. 6p. DNLM **00-4413**

ROSENBERGER, Randle C.
The use of the antitoxin of diphtheria in the treatment of cerebrospinal meningitis. [Philadelphia, 1905.] 4p. DNLM
00-4414

ROSENBERGER, Randle C.
The prognosis of pulmonary tuberculosis as determined by the morphology of the tubercle bacillus in the sputum. [Philadelphia, 1906.] 7p. DNLM **00-4415**

ROSENBERGER, Randle C.
The spirochaetae found in syphilis; a report of thirty-four cases. [Philadelphia, 1906.] 11p. DNLM
00-4416

ROSENBERGER, Randle C.
Bacteriologic studies of smegma. Burlington, Vt., & New York, 1907. 5p. DNLM **00-4417**

ROSENBERGER, Randle C.
The significance of tubercle bacilli in the feces. Philadelphia & New York, 1907. 12p. DNLM **00-4418**

ROSENBERGER, Randle C.
Noma, a bacteriological study of seven cases. New York, 1908. 10p. DNLM **00-4419**

ROSENBERGER, Randle C.
The present status of the aetiology of syphilis; the spirchaeta pallida; its biology and aetiological relation to the disease. New York, 1908. 32p. DNLM **00-4420**

ROSENOW, Edward C[arl]
On the association of stone and tumor of the urinary bladder, with report of a case. Philadelphia, 1902. 9p. DNLM
00-4421

ROSENSTIRN, Julius (*b.* 1850)
Post-operative hemorrhage twelve hours after vaginal hysterectomy; laparotomy under cocaine anaesthesia; hemorrhage from mesocaecum and mesoappendix. New York, 1901. 8p. DNLM
00-4422

ROSENSTIRN, Julius (*b.* 1850)
Operation for caries of the mastoid, secondary opening of the lateral sinus, and ligation of the internal jugular vein. New York: William Wood & Co., 1901. 11p. DNLM
00-4423

ROSENSTIRN, Julius (*b.* 1850)
Surgical interference in hypertrophic biliary cirrhosis of the liver. New York: William Wood & Co., 1903. 16p. DNLM
00-4424

ROSENTHAL, Edwin
The clinical value of purgative mineral waters. Philadelphia: Liberty Chemical Co., 1900. 6 l. DNLM
00-4425

ROSENTHAL, Edwin
The treatment of temperature by drugs. Chicago, 1901. 7p. DNLM **00-4426**

ROSEWATER, Charles
Some points bearing on the medicinal treatment of appendicitis. 1900. 6p. DNLM
00-4427

ROSEWATER, Nathan (*b.* 1854)
Enteroptosis relative to disorders of the digestive tract and circulation. Cleveland, 1900. 12p. DNLM
00-4428

ROSEWATER, Nathan (*b.* 1854)
A case of lithameic gangrene, a contribution to Haig's uric acid theory. New York: A. R. Elliott, 1905. 25p. DNLM; NNNAM **00-4429**

ROSS, James (1837-1892)
Aphasia: a contribution to the subject of the dissolution of speech from cerebral disease. New York: William Wood & Co., 1901. 155p. DLC; NIC; NNNAM; PU [Printed out of Wood's Medical & Surgical Monographs, vol. 6, No. 1 (1890), pp. 137-291] **00-4430**

ROSS, John W.
Lessons drawn from practical professional experience with trained women nurses in military service. [Carlisle, 1902.] 10p. DNLM **00-4431**

ROSS, Ronald (1857-1932)
Mosquito brigades and how to organize them. New York: Longmans, Green & Co., 1902. 100p. DLC; ICJ; MB
00-4432

ROSS, Ronald (1857-1932)
Malarial fever; its cause, prevention, and treatment. Containing full details for the use of travellers, sportsmen, soldiers, and residents in malarious places. 9th ed., revised and enlarged. New York: Longmans, Green & Co., 1902. 68p. 2 plates. DNLM; ICJ; MB; NNNAM **00-4433**

ROSS, Ronald, ed. (1857-1932)
Malarial diseases, influenza, and dengue. . . . By J. Mannaberg . . . O. Leichtenstern . . . edited with additions by Ronald Ross . . . J. W. Stephens . . . Albert S. Grünbaum. Philadelphia: W. B. Saunders & Co. 1905. 769p. DLC; ICJ; NNNAM; PU [American ed., Nothnagel's encyclopedia of practical medicine] **00-4434**

ROSS, Ronald (1857-1932)
The prevention of malaria, by Ronald Ross . . . with contributions by Professor L. O. Howard, United States; Colonel W. C. Gorgas, Panama . . . [and others]. New York: E. P. Dutton & Co., 1910. 609p. plates (part fold.), plan, diags. DLC; ICJ; MBM; NN **00-4435**

ROSS, William Frank
Mental healing, suggestion and magnetic healing. . . . Champaign, Ill.: W. F. Ross, 1900. 48p. DLC; ICJ
00-4436

ROSS, William Frank
Medical hygiene; or, Cures for all diseases without drugs. . . . St. Louis: W. F. Ross, [1901?] 200p. DLC
00-4437

ROSS, William Monroe (*b.* 1888)
My personal experience with tuberculosis. Stevens Point, Wis.: The Author, 1910. 64p. DLC **00-4438**

ROSS, William Monroe (*b.* 1888)
My personal experience with tuberculosis . . . [2nd ed., rev.] Stevens Point, Wis.: The Author, [1910]. 78p. DLC
00-4439

ROSSE, Irving C. (1847-1901)
Golf from a neurological view-point. . . . [Washington? 1900?] 4p. DLC **00-4440**

ROSSE, Irving C. (1847-1901)
Legal and judicial disagreement and the shortcomings of medical witnesses. Philadelphia, 1900. 7p. DNLM **00-4441**

ROSSE, Irving C. (1847-1901)
Contributions of Irving C. Rosse, Washington, D.C., 1871-1900. [Washington, 1900.] 8p. DLC; DNLM; MB **00-4442**

ROSSE, Irving C. (1847-1901)
Words not usually found in medical dictionaries. [Washington, 1901?] 8p. DLC; DNLM **00-4443**

ROTCH, Thomas Morgan (1849-1914)
A case of rhachischisis. New York, 1900. 9p. DNLM **00-4444**

ROTCH, Thomas Morgan (1849-1914)
The treatment of the proteids of cow's milk. Boston, 1900. 3p. DNLM **00-4445**

ROTCH, Thomas Morgan (1849-1914) and Maynard LADD
Pernicious anemia in infants; with a preliminary report of a case. New York, 1901. 20p. DNLM **00-4446**

ROTCH, Thomas Morgan (1849-1914)
Pediatrics; the hygiene and medical treatment of children . . . 3rd ed. rearranged and rewritten. . . . Philadelphia and London: J. B. Lippincott Co., 1901. 1021p. col. plates. DLC; DNLM; PPC; PU **00-4447**

ROTCH, Thomas Morgan (1849-1914)
The American methods in the modification of milk in the feeding of infants. New York, 1902. 46p. DNLM **00-4448**

ROTCH, Thomas Morgan (1849-1914)
Infantile scorbutus. New York, 1903. 8p. DNLM **00-4449**

ROTCH, Thomas Morgan (1849-1914)
Tubercular peritonitis in early life; with especial reference to its treatment by laparotomy. Chicago, 1903. 14p. DNLM **00-4450**

ROTCH, Thomas Morgan (1849-1914) and H. W. CUSHING
A case of decapsulation of both kidneys (Edebohls' operation) in a boy nine and one-half years old. New York, 1903. 3 l. DNLM **00-4451**

ROTCH, Thomas Morgan (1849-1914) and Charles Hunter DUNN
A case of pulmonary osteoarthropathy. New York, 1903. 4 l. DNLM **00-4452**

ROTCH, Thomas Morgan (1849-1914)
The study of pediatrics in its relation to medical education. An address delivered by request of the Chicago Pediatric Society, at a joint meeting of that society, and the Chicago Medical Society. Chicago: Amer. Med. Assoc. Press, 1903. 14p. NN **00-4453**

ROTCH, Thomas Morgan (1849-1914)
The hospital nurse in private nursing. Address to the graduating class of the Boston City Hospital Training School for Nurses. [1903.] 8p. MB **00-4454**

ROTCH, Thomas Morgan (1849-1914)
Pediatrics, the hygiene and medical treatment of children . . . 4th ed., rearranged and rewritten. . . . Philadelphia and London: J. B. Lippincott Co., 1903. 1021p. col. plates. CtY-M; DLC; NNNAM; PPC **00-4455**

ROTCH, Thomas Morgan (1849-1914)
Essential principles of infant feeding and the modern methods of applying them. Chicago, 1903. 31p. MB **00-4456**

ROTCH, Thomas Morgan (1849-1914)
The diarrheas of infancy and early childhood. Philadelphia, 1904. 24p. DNLM **00-4457**

ROTCH, Thomas Morgan (1849-1914)
Some considerations regarding substitute feeding during the first year. New York, 1904. 8 l. DNLM **00-4458**

ROTCH, Thomas Morgan (1849-1914) and Maynard LADD
Two operative cases of pyloric stenosis in infants. New York, 1905. 3 l. DNLM **00-4459**

ROTCH, Thomas Morgan (1849-1914)
Pediatrics; the hygiene and medical treatment of children . . . 5th ed., rearranged and rewritten; illustrated by numerous engravings in the text and by colored plates. Philadelphia and London: J. B. Lippincott Co., [1906]. 1060p. col. plates. DLC; IU-M; MBM; PPC **00-4460**

ROTCH, Thomas Morgan (1849-1914)
Disease and the prevention of disease in early life. Philadelphia, 1907. 18p. DNLM **00-4461**

ROTCH, Thomas Morgan (1849-1914) and Harry Chamberlain LOW
Some blood cultures in children and their significance. Chicago, 1907. 19p. DNLM **00-4462**

ROTCH, Thomas Morgan (1849-1914) and Fred Towsley MURPHY
Gastro-enteric obstruction in early infancy; general diagnosis and treatment, with a report of two cases of pyloric stenosis and one of volvulus, successfully treated by laparotomy. Boston, 1907. 41p. DNLM; MBM **00-4463**

ROTCH, Thomas Morgan (1849-1914)
An historical sketch of the development of percentage feeding. New York: A. R. Elliott Co., 1907. 17p. DNLM **00-4464**

ROTCH, Thomas Morgan (1849-1914)
The opsonic index in cerebrospinal meningitis in children. Philadelphia, 1907. 7p. DNLM **00-4465**

ROTCH, Thomas Morgan (1849-1914)
The Pasteurization of milk for public sale. Boston, 1907. 10p. DNLM **00-4466**

ROTCH, Thomas Morgan (1849-1914)
The Roentgen ray in pediatrics. [n. p.], 1907. 11p. 10 plates. DNLM **00-4467**

ROTCH, Thomas Morgan (1849-1914)
The necessity of a more uniform nomenclature of diseases for study, etc. [1907.] 10p. MB **00-4468**

ROTCH, Thomas Morgan (1849-1914) and Cleaveland FLOYD
The opsonic index and the tuberculin test; their relative value in the diagnosis and treatment of early tuberculosis in children. Chicago, 1907. 7p. DNLM **00-4469**

ROTCH, Thomas Morgan (1849-1914) and Wellington Arial GEORGE
A study of normal living anatomy in early life. Philadelphia, 1907. 8p. DNLM **00-4470**

ROTCH, Thomas Morgan (1849-1914) and Wellington Arial GEORGE
A study of the early conditions of osteomyelitis in young children by the Röntgen ray. New York, 1907. 4 l. DNLM **00-4471**

ROTCH, Thomas Morgan (1849-1914) and Wellington Arial GEORGE
The living pathology of tuberculosis of the bones in early life. [n. p., 1908.] 3p. 5 plates. DNLM **00-4472**

ROTCH, Thomas Morgan (1849-1914)
The development of milk laboratories in connection with the dispensing of food stuffs. A paper read before the Boston Obstetrical Society, Feb. 16, 1909. [St. Louis, 1909.] 8p. NN **00-4473**

ROTCH, Thomas Morgan (1849-1914)
The revision of the laws relating to child labor by means of the Roentgen ray. Delivered at the Jefferson Medical College, Philadelphia, Dec. 28, 1908. Philadelphia, 1909. 3p. NN **00-4474**

ROTCH, Thomas Morgan (1849-1914)
The position and work of the American Pediatric Society toward public questions. [Read before the 21st annual meeting of the American Pediatric Society, Lenox, Mass., May 27, 1909.[[Philadelhia, 1909.] 24p. NN **00-4475**

ROTCH, Thomas Morgan (1849-1914)
The cardinal principles for the successful feeding of infants. St. Louis: Interstate Medical Journal Co., 1910. 13p. DNLM; NN **00-4476**

ROTCH, Thomas Morgan (1849-1914)
The conditions pertaining to the safe-guarding of early life from a pediatric point of view. [New York, 1910.] 36p. NN **00-4477**

ROTCH, Thomas Morgan (1849-1914)
Living anatomy and pathology; the diagnosis of diseases in early life by the Roentgen method . . . three hundred and three illustrations. Philadelphia & London: J. B. Lippincott Co., [1910]. 225p. 264 plates. DLC; MB; PPJ **00-4478**

ROTH, Henry
Thrombosis of the cavernous sinus, with a report of three cases. New York, 1904. 10p. DNLM; NN **00-4479**

ROUS, F[rancis] Peyton (1879-1970)
Clinical studies of the cerebro-spinal fluid, with especial reference to pressure, protein-content, and the number and character of the cells. [1907.] 16p. NN **00-4480**

ROUTH, H[enry] F[elix] (1822-1909)
Infant feeding and its influence on life: or, The causes and prevention of infant mortality. . . . Third edition. New York: William Wood & Co., 1900. 270p. CtY-M; ICJ; PP; NN [First published in Wood's Library of Standard Medical Authors, 1879] **00-4481**

ROVINSKY, Alexander
The physician as a social factor. New York, 1901. 16p. DNLM **00-4482**

ROWE, George H[oward] M[alcolm] (1841-1916)
Observations on hospital organizaton. [Boston: S. J. Parkhill], 1902. 17p. DNLM **00-4483**

ROWE, George H[oward] M[alcolm] (1841-1916)
Observations on hospital organization. . . . [Detroit, Mich.? 1903?] 4 l. NN **00-4484**

ROWE, George H[oward] M[alcolm] (1841-1916)
The hospital unit. Boston: Rogers & Manson, 1904. 16p. DNLM **00-4485**

ROWE, George H[oward] M[alcolm] (1841-1916)
Historical description of the buildings and grounds of the Boston City Hospital, together with chronological tables, statistics of appropriations, cost, maintenance, etc. Boston, 1906. 102p. 2 maps. DNLM; MBM **00-4486**

ROWE, James William
A hand-book on the newly-born. Cincinnati, O., 1906. 132p. DLC **00-4487**

ROWE, J[ohn] T. W.
The causes of injuries among the insane. New York, 1906. 6p. DNLM **00-4488**

ROWELL, Hubert N.
Diabetes in childhood. New York, 1904. 3p. DNLM **00-4489**

ROWLEY, Mary W.
The occurrence of atypical phagocytic cells in the circulating blood. New York, 1907. 4p. DNLM **00-4490**

ROWLEY, Mary W.
A fatal anaemia with enormous numbers of circulating phagocytes. New York, 1908. 10p. 10 plates. DNLM **00-4491**

von RUCK, Karl (1849-1922)
Clinical report from the Winyah Sanitarium, giving the results in 225 cases of pulmonary tuberculosis treated in the institution from Jan. 1, 1899, to Dec. 31, 1900, with watery extract of tubercle bacilli; with an appendix of results obtained with this remedy by other physicians in private practice. Asheville, 1901. 51p. DNLM; NcD; PU **00-4492**

von RUCK, Karl (1849-1922)
A classification for cases of pulmonary tuberculosis and phthisis. New York: A. R. Elliott, 1905. 21p. DNLM; NcD; PU **00-4493**

von RUCK, Karl (1849-1922) and Silvio von RUCK
A clinical study of two hundred and sixty cases of pulmonary tuberculosis treated in the Winyah Sanitarium, Asheville, N.C., 1903 and 1904. Asheville: Hackney & Moale Co., 1905. 51p. DNLM **00-4494**

von RUCK, Karl (1849-1922) and Silvio von RUCK
A clinical study of two hundred and ninety-three cases of pulmonary tuberculosis treated at the Winyah Sanitarium, Asheville, N.C., in 1905 and 1906, with special reference to specific medication and its results. Asheville, N.C., 1907. 45p. DNLM **00-4495**

von RUCK, Karl (1849-1922) and Silvio von RUCK
A clinical study of three hundred and thirty-seven cases of pulmonary tuberculosis treated at the Winyah Sanitarium, Asheville, N.C., in 1907 and 1908. Asheville, N.C.: Hackney & Moale Co., 1909. 19p. DNLM **00-4496**

von RUCK MEMORIAL SANITORIUM, ASHEVILLE, N.C.
Advice to patients; rules and regulations. [1910?] 15p. NcD **00-4497**

von RUCK, Silvio (1874-1918)
The heart and circulation in the prognosis and management of pulmonary tuberculosis. New York, 1905. 15p. DNLM **00-4498**

von RUCK, Silvio (1874-1918)
The intercommunicability of human and bovine tuberculosis. Chicago, 1905. 23p. DNLM **00-4499**

von RUCK, Silvio (1874-1918)
The relation of pleurisy to tuberculosis. New York, 1905. 14p. DNLM **00-4500**

RUCKER, Samuel T.
The successful treatment of gonorrhea and all inflammatory diseases of the urethra by packing it with an antiseptic oil dressing. Chicago, 1902. 7p. DNLM **00-4501**

RUCKER, William Colby
The differential diagnosis of typhoid fever in its earliest stages. New York, 1904. 22p. DNLM **00-4502**

RUCKER, William Colby
The epidemiology of yellow fever. [1904.] 2 l. DNLM **00-4503**

RUDDIMAN, Edsel Alexander (*b.* 1864)
Incompatibilities in prescriptions. For students in pharmacy and medicine, and practicing pharmacists and physicians. . . . 2nd ed., rewritten. 1st thousand. New York: J. Wiley & Sons; [etc., etc.], 1900. 305p. DLC; NNNAM; PPC: PPJ **00-4504**

RUDDIMAN, Edsel Alexander (*b.* 1864)
Whys in pharmacy; a compilation of reasons underlying the principles of pharmacy, supplemented by a table of equations . . . 1st ed. 1st thousand. New York: J. Wiley & Sons; [etc., etc.], 1906. 196p. DLC; ICJ; MH; NNNAM **00-4505**

RUDDIMAN, Edsel Alexander (*b.* 1864)
A manual of materia medica especially designed for students of pharmacy. . . . Philadelphia and New York: Lea Bros. & Co., 1907. 453p. DLC; OCLloyd; PPC; PU **00-4506**

RUDDIMAN, Edsel Alexander (*b.* 1864)
Incompatibilities in prescriptions. For students in pharmacy and medicine and practicing pharmacists and physicians. . . . 3rd ed., partly rewritten. 1st thousand. New York: J. Wiley & Sons; [etc., etc.], 1908. 312p. DLC; ICJ; MH; NNNAM **00-4507**

RUDDOCK, Edward Harris (1822-1875)
The diseases of infants and children and their homoeopathic and general treatment. . . . 6th ed., revised and improved. London: The Homoeopathic Publishing Co.; New York and Philadelphia: Boericke & Tafel, 1901 [*c.* 1899]. 244p., illus. DLC; ICJ; NN ["For the present edition, the publishers are indebted to Dr. John H. Clarke . . . who has endeavoured to bring the work fully abreast with the times."—Pref. to the fifth edition. "In presenting a new edition . . . the publishers have thought it inadvisable to make any radical alteration."—Note on the sixth edition.] **00-4508**

RUDDOCK, Edward Harris (1822-1875)
Ruddock's stepping-stone to homeopathy and health, by E. H. Ruddock. . . . Revised for the American public by Reuben Ludlam. . . . With an appendix on the tissue remedies as used by Dr. Med. Schuessler . . . with practical suggestions by the publishers. 250th thousand. Chicago, St. Paul: Halsey Bros. Co., 1902. 262p. DLC **00-4509**

RUDDOCK, Edward Harris (1822-1875)
The stepping-stone to homoeopathy and health, by E. H. Ruddock . . . 4th American ed. Edited and enlarged with the addition of a chapter on diseases of women, and the tissue remedies, by Wm. Boericke. . . . Philadelphia: Boericke & Tafel, 1902. 256p. DLC **00-4510**

RUDDOCK, Edward Harris (1822-1875)
Ruddock's Family guide to homoeopathy and health, which includes "The stepping-stone" and the essential portions of "The lady's manual," by E. H. Ruddock . . . both of these books having been revised for the American public by Reuben Ludlam . . . with an appendix on the tissue remedies as used by Dr. Med. Schuessler . . . with practical suggestions by the publishers. 85th thousand. Chicago, St. Paul: Halsey Bros. Co., 1902. 408p. DLC **00-4511**

RUDDOCK, Edward Harris (1822-1875)
Ruddock's family doctor; a popular guide for the household, giving the history, causes, means of prevention and symptoms of all diseases of men, women and children, and the most approved methods of treatment. With plain instructions for the care of the sick, and full accurate directions for treating wounds, injuries, poisoning, etc., by E. Harris Ruddock. . . . With notes and additional chapters by James E. Cross. . . . Chicago: Halsey Bros. Co., 1903. 772p. NN **00-4512**

RUDDOCK, Edward Harris (1822-1875)
The stepping-stone to homeopathy and health. . . . By E. H. Ruddock. . . . Fifth American edition, edited and enlarged with the addition of a chapter on diseases of women, and the tissue remedies, by Wm. Boericke. . . . Philadelphia: Boericke & Tafel, 1906. 256p. DLC; NN **00-4513**

RUDDOCK, Edward Harris (1822-1875)
The diseases of infants and children and their homoeopathic and general treatment. 7th ed., rev. and imp. New York and Philadelphia: Boericke & Tafel, 1910. 243p. DLC: ICJ; PPC; PPHa **00-4514**

RUEDIGER, E. H.
Bacteriologic study of the blood in thirty cases of clinical typhoid fever, two of which proved to be para-typhoid and one doubtful. Chicago, 1903. 11p. DNLM **00-4515**

RUEDIGER, Gustav F[erdinand] (*b.* 1876)
A study of the bactericidal action of human and rabbit's serum on typhoid bacilli. Chicago, 1904. 7p. DNLM **00-4516**

RUEDIGER, Gustav F[erdinand] (*b.* 1876)
The effects on streptococci of sera of cold-blooded animals. Chicago, 1904. 4p. DNLM **00-4517**

RUEDIGER, Gustav F[erdinand] (*b.* 1876)
. . . The mechanism of natural and acquired streptococcus immunity. . . . Chicago, 1907. 27p. CtY-M; DLC; ICJ **00-4518**

RUEDIGER, William Carl (*b.* 1874)
The field of distinct vision with special reference to individual differences and their correlations. New York: Science Press, 1907. 67p. 8 tables. DLC; DNLM; NIC; NNNAM **00-4519**

RUGGLES, E. Wood
Monilethrix. New York, 1900. 7p. DNLM **00-4520**

RUGGLES, E. Wood
The management of genital sores. New York, 1904. 16p. DNLM **00-4521**

RUGGLES, E. Wood
The physician's relation to the social evil. New York: A. R. Elliott Co., 1907. 8p. DNLM **00-4522**

RUGH, J[ames] Torrance
An unpleasant experience with ethyl chloride. New York, 1907. 3p. DNLM **00-4523**

RUHL, J. H.
Outline of obstetrics. [Texas], J. Finck, 1901. 91p. NNNAM; LNT-M **00-4524**

RUHRÄH, John (1872-1935)
A manual of the diseases of infants and children. Philadelphia: W. B. Saunders & Co., 1905. 404p. 3 plates, 1 chart. DNLM; NNNAM; PPC; PU **00-4525**

RUHRÄH, John (1872-1935)
A manual of the diseases of infants and children. 2nd ed., thoroughly revised. Philadelphia & London: W. B. Saunders & Co., 1908. 423p. col. plates. CtY-M; DNLM; NNNAM; PPC **00-4526**

RUHRÄH, John (1872-1935)
A manual of the diseases of infants and children . . . .illustrated. 3rd ed., thoroughly rev. Philadelphia & London: W. B. Saunders & Co., 1910 [*c.* 1911]. 534p. col. plates. DLC; ICJ; PPHa; PPJ **00-4527**

RUMPEL, Oskar (*b.* 1872)
Cystoscopy as adjuvant in surgery, with an atlas of cystoscopic views and concomitant text for physicians and students. . . . Only authorized English translation by P. W. Shedd . . . with 85 illustrations in color on 36 plates and 22 textual figures. New York: Rebman Co., [1910]. 131p. mounted col. plates. DLC; ICJ; NNNAM; PU **00-4528**

RUPP, Adolph (1856-1907)
Antitoxine results and diphtheria definitions. New York, 1900. 10p. DNLM **00-4529**

RUSH, Benjamin (1745-1813)
Directions for preserving the health of soldiers, issued during the American Revolution by Benjamin Rush, M.D., with a biographical sketch and portrait of Surgeon Ebenezer Alden, by Major Henry P. De Forest. . . . [Washington, D.C.], 1908. 14p. DLC; PPC **00-4530**

RUSS, Raymond
Bennett's fracture. Chicago, 1906. 11p. DNLM **00-4531**

RUSS, Raymond
Surgical aspects of varix of the lower limbs. Chicago, 1908. 15p. DNLM **00-4532**

RUSS, Raymond
The magnetic splint; a new permanent surgical dressing. Chicago, 1908. 11p. DNLM **00-4533**

RUSSELL, John F[rancis] (*b.* 1855)
Weight and diet in pulmonary tuberculosis. New York, 1902. 11p. DNLM **00-4534**

RUSSELL, John F[rancis] (*b.* 1855)
The dispensary or home treatment of pulmonary tuberculosis. New York, 1902. 19p. DNLM **00-4535**

RUSSELL, John F[rancis] (*b.* 1855)
The management of exacerbations in the course of pulmonary tuberculosis. New York, 1903. 19p. DNLM **00-4536**

RUSSELL, John F[rancis] (*b.* 1855)
Report of the Annex of the Post-Graduate Hospital Dispensary for the Treatment of Pulmonary Tuberculosis from October 9th to June 30th, 1905. [New York, 1905.] 28p. DLC; NN **00-4537**

RUSSELL, John F[rancis] (*b.* 1855)
Report of fifty-five apparent cures of pulmonary tuberculosis occurring in working people who were treated at a dispensary without interruption to their work; being an appeal for systematic treatment of consumptive working people. New York, 1906. 127p. DNLM; NNNAM **00-4538**

RUSSELL, John F[rancis] (*b.* 1855)
Report of five more apparent cures of pulmonary tuberculosis occurring in working people who were treated at a dispensary without interruption to their work. New York, 1906. 17p. DNLM; NNNAM **00-4539**

RYERSON, George S[terling] (1855-1925)
Medical and surgical experiences in the South African War. Being addresses to the Toronto Clinical Society and Canadian Medical Association. [New York?], 1900. 23p. DNLM; ICJ; MH **00-4540**

RYERSON, George S[terling] (1855-1925)
Impressions of the medical side of the war in South Africa. [New York? 1900.] 16p. DLC; DNLM; MH **00-4541**

SABIN, Florence R[ena] (1871-1953)
On the anatomical relations of the nuclei or reception of the cochlear and vestibular nerves. [New York, 1900.] 17p. NN **00-4542**

SABIN, Florence R[ena] (1871-1953)
An atlas of the medulla and midbrain. A laboratory manual. Edited by Henry McE. Knower. Baltimore: Friedenwald Co., 1901. 146p. col. plates. DLC; MdU-D; PPC; PU
00-4543

SABIN, Florence R[ena] (1871-1953)
Tuberculous pericarditis, with effusion; repeated tappings; bacilli in the exudate; recovery. Philadelphia, 1902. 3p. DNLM
00-4544

SABIN, Oliver Corwin (1840-1914)
Christian science. What it is and what it does; or, Primary rules of metaphysical healing. How the sick are healed. Metaphysical healing explained. . . . Washington: Anderson Co., 1900 [*c.* 1899]. 64p. DLC **00-4545**

SABIN, Oliver Corwin (1840-1914)
Christology, science of health and happiness; or, Metaphysical healing exemplified through rules, formulas and incidents. . . . Washington, D.C.: News Letter Press, 1901. 315p. DLC [*vel subseq.*] **00-4546**

SABIN, Oliver Corwin (1840-1914)
Christology—science of health and happiness; or, Metaphysical healing exemplified—through rules, formulas and incidents. 6th ed. . . . Washington, D.C.: News Letter Press, 1903. 331p. DLC **00-4547**

SABIN, Oliver Corwin (1840-1914)
Sacred science, the highest thought cure. . . . 1st ed. Washington, D.C.: The News Letter Press, 1904. 131p. DLC
00-4548

SABIN, Oliver Corwin (1840-1914)
Christian science made plain; the science, how to overcome poverty and sickness plainly taught. . . . Washington, D.C.: The News Letter Press, [1905]. 172p. DLC
00-4549

SABOURAUD, Raimond J[acques] A[drien] (1864-1938)
Elementary manual of regional topographical dermatology. . . . English translation by C. F. Marshall. . . . With 231 illustrations in the text. New York, [etc.]: Rebman Co., 1906. 660p. CtY-M; DLC; ICJ; PPHa **00-4550**

SACHS, Bernard (1858-1944) and Harlow BROOKS
Progressive muscular dystrophy, with the report of an autopsy. [Philadelphia], 1901. 19p. DNLM **00-4551**

SACHS, Bernard (1858-1944)
Some unusual forms of acute myelitis. New York, 1904. 14p. DNLM; NNNAM **00-4552**

SACHS, Bernard (1858-1944)
A treatise on the nervous diseases of children, for physicians and students . . . 2nd ed., rev. New York: William Wood & Co., 1905. 571p. DLC; DNLM; ICJ; NNNAM
00-4553

SACHS, Theodore B[ernard] (*b.* 1868)
Tuberculosis in the Jewish district of Chicago. . . . Pub. by the Committee on the Prevention of Tuberculosis of the Visiting Nurse Association. . . . [Chicago, 1904.] 12p. charts on fold. l. DLC; ICJ **00-4554**

SACHSE, Helena Viola
How to cook for the sick and convalescent; arranged for the physician, trained nurse, and home use. . . . Philadelphia: J. B. Lippincott Co., 1901. 239p. DLC; MH; NIC; NN
00-4555

SADLER, William Samuel (*b.* 1875)
The science of living; or, The art of keeping well. . . . Chicago: A. C. McClurg & Co., 1910. 420p. plates, diags. DLC; ICJ; NN
00-4556

SADLER, William Samuel (*b.* 1875)
The cause and cure of colds. . . . Chicago: A. C. McClurg & Co., 1910. 147p. plates. DLC: ICJ; NN **00-4557**

SADTLER, Samuel Philip (1847-1923)
A text-book of chemistry. Intended for the use of pharmaceutical and medical students. By Samuel P. Sadtler . . . and Virgil Coblentz. . . . Being the 3rd rev. and enl. ed. of Sadtler and Trimble's Chemistry. . . . In two volumes. . . . Philadelphia, [etc.] : J. B. Lippincott Co., [1900]. 2 v. DLC: ICJ; MH-M; PU
00-4558

SADTLER, Samuel Philip (1847-1923) and Virgil COBLENTZ
A text-book of chemistry intended for the use of pharmaceutical and medical students. Being the 4th ed. of Sadtler and Coblentz's chemistry, revised and rewritten. Philadelphia & London: J. B. Lippincott Co., 1906. 794p. CtY-M; DNLM; PPC; PU **00-4559**

SAGE, Xenophon La Motte
. . . A correspondence course in personal magnetism, hypnotism, mesmerism, magnetic healing, suggestive therapeutics, psycho-therapeutics, etc., etc. . . . [Rochester, N.Y.]: New York Institute of Science, 1900. 81p. DLC
00-4560

SAGER, Daniel Showers (*b.* 1859)
The art of living in good health; a practical guide to well-being through proper eating, thinking, and living in the light of modern science. . . . New York: F. A. Stokes Co., [1907]. 353p. DLC; MH; NIC; NN **00-4561**

SAHLI, Hermann (1856-1933)
A treatise on diagnositic methods of examination . . . ed., with additions, by Francis P. Kinnicutt . . . and Nath'l Bowditch Potter. . . . Authorized translation from the 4th rev. and enl. German ed. Philadelphia and London: W. B. Saunders & Co., 1905. 1008p. col. plates. DLC; DNLM; NNNAM; PPC
00-4562

SAHLI, Hermann (1856-1933)
A treatise on diagnostic methods of examination . . . ed., with additions, by Nathaniel Bowditch Potter . . . 2nd ed., rev., authorized translation from the 5th rev. and enl. German ed. Philadelphia and London: W. B. Saunders & Co., 1910. 1229p. col plates. DLC; DNLM; NcD; PPC
00-4563

SAINSBURY, Harrington
Drugs and the drug habit . . . with eleven illustrations. New York: E. P. Dutton & Co., 1909. 307p. diags. DLC: MB; NIC; NN **00-4564**

SAJOUS, Charles E. de M. (1852-1929)
Sajous's analytical cyclopaedia of practical medicine, by Charles E. de M. Sajous, M.D., and one hundred associate editors, assisted by corresponding editors, collaborators and correspondents. . . . Rev. ed. Philadelphia: F. A. Davis Co., 1902. 6 v. illus. col. plates. DLC; DNLM; PPC; PPHa
00-4565

SAJOUS, Charles E. de M. (1852-1929)
The internal secretions and the principles of medicine. Philadelphia: F. A. Davis, 1903-7. 2 v. DLC; DNLM; PPC; PU **00-4566**

SAJOUS, Charles E. de M. (1852-1929)
Sajous's analytical cyclopaedia of practical medicine, by Charles E. de M. Sajous, M.D., and one hundred associate editors, assisted by corresponding editors, collaborators and correspondents. Illustrated with chromolithographs, engravings and maps. 2nd rev. ed. Philadelphia: F. A. Davis Co., 1903. 6 v. illus., plates (part col.), map. DLC; DNLM; PPHa
00-4567

SAJOUS, Charles E. de M. (1852-1929)
The vasomotor centre in inhibition of the heart. New York, 1904. 37p. DNLM; NNNAM **00-4568**

SAJOUS, Charles E. de M. (1852-1929)
Sajous's analytical cyclopaedia of practical medicine, by Charles E. de M. Sajous, M.D., and one hundred associate editors, assisted by coresponding editors, collaborators and correspondents. Illustrated with chrome lithographs, engravings and maps. 3rd rev. ed. Philadelphia: F. A. Davis Co., 1905. 6 v. illus., plates (part col.), map, tables. DLC; ICJ; NNNAM; PPC [Desk index to Sajous's analytical cyclopaedia of practical medicine. 3rd rev. ed. Philadelphia: F. A. Davis Co.], [1905]. **00-4569**

SAJOUS, Charles E. de M. (1852-1929)
The shortcomings of physiology as the chief obstacle to medical progress. The need of editorial intervention in such questions. Philadelphia, 1907. 8p. DNLM
00-4570

SAJOUS, Charles E. de M. (1852-1929)
The internal secretions and the principles of medicine. 2nd ed. Philadelphia: F. A. Davis Co., 1908. 2 v. 28 plates. DNLM; NNNAM; PPC; PPJ **00-4571**

SAJOUS, Charles E. de M. (1852-1929)
Analytical cyclopaedia of practical medicine. 5th rev. ed. Philadelphia: F. A. Davis, 1908. 6 v. illus. DLC; ICJ; MH-M; NNNAM [Desk index. 5th rev. ed., [1908?] 28p.
00-4572

SAJOUS, Charles E. de M. (1852-1929)
The internal secretions and the principles of medicine. 3rd ed. Philadelphia: F. A. Davis Co., 1909. 2 v. col. front., illus. (part col.) plates (part col.) DLC; ICJ; PPHa
00-4573

SAJOUS, Charles E. de M. (1852-1929)
Sajous's analytical cyclopaedia of practical medicine, by Charles E. de M. Sajous . . . and one hundred associate editors, assisted by corresponding editors, collaborators, and correspondents; illustrated with chromolithographs, engravings and maps. 6th rev. ed. . . . Philadelphia: F. A. Davis Co., 1910. 6 v. illus., col. plates. DLC; ICJ; MH-M; PPC
00-4574

SALEEBY, Caleb W[illiam] (*b.* 1878)
The cycle of life according to modern science; being a series of essays designed to bring science home to men's business and bosoms, by C. W. Saleeby, M.D., with diagrams by Richard Muir. New York and London: Harper & Bros., 1904. 342p. DLC; MH; NIC; NN **00-4575**

SALEEBY, Caleb W[illiam] (*b.* 1878)
The conquest of cancer, a plan of campaign; being an account of the principles and practice hitherto of the treatment of malignant growths by specific or cancrotoxic ferments. . . . New York: F. A. Stokes Co., [1907]. 361p. DLC; MB; NIC; NN **00-4576**

SALEEBY, Caleb W[illiam] (*b.* 1878)
Worry; the disease of the age. . . . New York: F. A. Stokes Co., [1907]. 311p. DLC; ICJ; ICU; NN **00-4577**

SALEEBY, Caleb W[illiam] (*b.* 1878)
Health, strength and happiness; a book of practical advice. . . . New York: M. Kennerley; [etc., etc.], 1908. 410p. DLC; ICJ; NIC; NN **00-4578**

SALEEBY, Caleb W[illiam] (*b.* 1878)
Parenthood and race culture; an outline of eugenics. . . . New York: Moffat, Yard & Co., 1909. 376p. DLC; MH; NIC; NN
00-4579

SALINGER, Julius Lincoln
Modern medicine, by Julius L. Salinger . . . and Frederick J. Kalteyer. . . . Philadelphia and London: W. B. Saunders & Co., 1900. 801p. col. plates. CtY-M; DLC; ICJ; PPC
00-4580

SALKOWSKI, Ernst Leopold (1844-1923)
A laboratory manual of physiological and pathological chemistry. For students in medicine. . . . Authorized translation from the 2nd rev. and enl. German ed. by W. R. Orndorff. . . . With ten figures and a colored plate of absorption spectra. 1st ed., 1st thousand. New York: J. Wiley & Sons; [etc., etc.], 1904. 263p. DLC; ICJ; MH; NN **00-4581**

SALTER, Jasper Colton (*b.* 1867)
A new idea in sanitation, the great menace to public health that covers every mile of railroad track in the United States and other countries, comp. by J. C. Salter. New York, 1910. 89p. DLC; NN **00-4582**

SAMPSON, John A[lbertson] (1873-1946)
Studies in gynecology presented in the form of illustrated problems for classroom work. . . . Albany, N.Y.: Brandow Printing Co., 1907. 442p. DLC; DNLM; ICJ; PPC
00-4583

SANDZEN, Carl
Vibratory massage as applied in myalgias, neuralgia and chronic constipation. . . . [Kansas City? Mo.], 1904. 8p. DLC
00-4584

SANDZEN, Carl
Physical diagnosis of diseases of the chest; a concise treatise designed as a practical aid for students in the physical indications of chest diseases. . . . Minneapolis, Minn.: The Burton Co., 1905. 82p. DLC; DNLM **00-4585**

SANFORD, Alexander E.
Pastoral medicine; a handbook for the Catholic clergy. . . . New York: J. F. Wagner, [1904]. 234p. DLC; NIC; NN
00-4586

SANFORD, Alexander E.
Pastoral medicine; a handbook for the Catholic clergy. . . . New ed., rev. and enl. by a chapter on The moment of death, by the Rev. Walter M. Drum, S.J. and by chapters on "The fifth commandment" and "Neurasthenia in its pastoral-psychiatric aspects." New York: J. F. Wagner, [1905]. 320p. DLC; MH; NIC; NN **00-4587**

SANGER, William W[allace] (1819-1872)
The history of prostitution: its extent, causes and effects throughout the world. New York: Medical Publishing Co., 1901 [*c.* 1895]. 709p. DLC; MH; NIC; PU **00-4588**

SANGSTER, Margaret Elizabeth (1838-1912)
Radiant motherhood; a book for the twentieth century mother. . . . Indianapolis: The Bobbs-Merrill Co., [1905]. 374p. DLC; MH; NIC; NN **00-4589**

SANTEE, Harris E[llett] (1864-1936)
Anatomy of the brain and spinal cord, with special reference to the grouping and chaining of neurones into conduction paths. For students and practitioners . . . with a preface by William T. Eckley . . . 2nd ed., rev. and enl. Chicago: E. H. Colegrove, 1902. 224p. DLC; DNLM; ICJ; IU-M **00-4590**

SANTEE, Harris E[llett] (1864-1936)
Anatomy of the brain and spinal cord, with special reference to the grouping and chaining of neurones into conduction paths; for students and practitioners. With a preface by William T. Eckley. 3rd ed., revised and enlarged. Chicago: E. H. Colegrove, 1903. 226p. 2 plates. DLC; DNLM; ICJ; PPC **00-4591**

SANTEE, Harris E[llett] (1864-1936)
Anatomy of the brain and spinal cord, with special reference to the grouping and chaining of neurones into conduction paths; for students and practitioners. With a preface by William T. Eckley. 4th ed., revised and enlarged. Philadelphia: P. Blakiston's Son & Co., 1907. 443p. DLC; DNLM; PPC; PU **00-4592**

SATTERLEE, George Reese (*b.* 1873)
Outlines of human embryology. A medical student's handbook of embryology. New York: J. Wiley & Sons, 1906. 164p., interleaved. DLC; DNLM; ICJ; NNNAM **00-4593**

SATTERTHWAITE, Thomas Edward (1843-1934)
Is internal antisepsis possible? New York, 1900. 5p. DNLM **00-4594**

SATTERTHWAITE, Thomas Edward (1843-1934)
Non-malignant gastric and duodenal ulcers; with illustrative cases. New York, 1900. 24p. DNLM **00-4595**

SATTERTHWAITE, Thomas Edward (1843-1934)
Superheated dry air in the treatment of rheumatic and allied affections. New York, 1900. 15p. DNLM **00-4596**

SATTERTHWAITE, Thomas Edward (1843-1934)
Fatty degeneration of the heart. New York, 1901. 19p. DNLM **00-4597**

SATTERTHWAITE, Thomas Edward (1843-1934)
Notes on some affections of the heart substance; with illustrative cases. New York, 1901. 16p. DNLM **00-4598**

SATTERTHWAITE, Thomas Edward (1843-1934)
The therapeutics of subacute and chronic heart disease. New York, 1901. 20p. DNLM **00-4599**

SATTERTHWAITE, Thomas Edward (1843-1934)
Nauheim methods in chronic heart disease, with American adaptations. Philadelphia: J. B. Lippincott Co., 1903. 14p. 4 plates. DNLM **00-4600**

SATTERTHWAITE, Thomas Edward (1843-1934)
Some recent advances in medical therapeutics. New York, 1903. 26p. DNLM **00-4601**

SATTERTHWAITE, Thomas Edward (1843-1934)
Diseases of the heart and aorta. . . . New York: E. R. Pelton, [1905]. 304p. plates. CtY-M; DLC: DNLM; NNNAM **00-4602**

SATTERTHWAITE, Thomas Edward (1843-1934)
The treatment of chronic valvular diseases of the heart. Richmond, Va., 1907. 31p. DNLM **00-4603**

SATTERTHWAITE, Thomas Edward (1843-1934)
The medical uses of carbonic acid. New York, 1908. 7p. DNLM **00-4604**

SAUR, Prudence B.
Maternity: a book for every wife and mother. Rev. and enl. By Mrs. P. B. Saur. . . . Chicago and Philadelphia: L. P. Miller & Co., 1901 [*c.* 1887]. 719p. DLC; ICJ; PP; PPC [In pocket: Plates illustrating Maternity; a book for every wife and mother. Chicago and Philadelphia: L. P. Miller & Co., 1888. [31] p. illus.] **00-4605**

SAUR, Prudence B.
Our mothers' guide book; a manual of health, beauty and happiness. A revised and enlarged edition of Maternity. . . . With a special introductory chapter by the celebrated Charles Pusheck. . . . Chicago, Ill.: A. B. Kuhlman & Co., 1902 [*c.* 1896]. 739p. DLC; ICJ; ICRM [In pocket: Plates illustrating Maternity; a book for every wife and mother. [31] p. illus.] **00-4606**

SAUR, Prudence B.
What every wife and mother should know. A revised and enlarged edition of Maternity. . . . With a special introductory chapter by the celebrated Charles Pusheck. . . . Philadelphia, Pa.: World Bible House, 1902 [*c.* 1896]. 739p. DLC; ICJ; NN; PPC **00-4607**

SAVAGE, George H[enry] (1842-1921)
Insanity and allied neuroses, practical and clinical, with the assistance of Edwin Goodall. New and enl. ed. Chicago: W. T. Keener & Co., 1907. 624p. ICJ; PPC **00-4608**

SAVAGE, George H[enry] (1842-1921)
Insanity and allied neuroses, practical and clinical, with the assistance of Edwin Goodall. New and enl. ed. New York: Funk & Wagnalls Co., 1910. 622p. NN; NNC: NNNAM **00-4609**

SAVAGE, Giles C[hristopher] (1854-1930)
Ophthalmic myology, a systematic treatise on the ocular muscles. Nashville, Tenn.: The Author, 1902. 589p. DLC; DNLM; ICJ; NN **00-4610**

SAVAGE, Giles C[hristopher] (1854-1930)
Ophthalmic neuro-myology. A study of the normal and abnormal actions of the ocular muscles from the brain side of the question. Nashville, Tenn.: The Author, 1905. 221p. DLC; DNLM; NcD; PPC **00-4611**

SAVAGE, Giles C[hristopher] (1854-1930)
Ophthalmic myology: a systematic treatise on the ocular muscles. [2nd ed.] Nashville: The Author, 1910-1911. 685p. textual illus., plates. DLC; ICJ; MBM; PU **00-4612**

SAVAGE, Thomas J[efferson] (*b.* 1855)
The mystery of alcoholism revealed . . . with an appendix containing brief extracts from the views of many modern authorities on the effects of alcoholics. . . . [Xenia, O.: The Aldine Press, 1903.] 163p. DLC **00-4613**

SAVAGE, William George (*b.* 1872)
The bacteriological examination of water-supplies. Philadelphia: P. Blakiston's Son & Co., 1906. 297p. DNLM; MH-M; PPC; PU **00-4614**

SAVILL, Thomas Dixon (1856-1910)
Clinical lectures on neurasthenia. 2nd ed. New York: William Wood & Co., 1902. 171p. CtY-M; DLC; DNLM; NNNAM **00-4615**

SAVILL, Thomas Dixon (1856-1910)
Clinical lectures on neurasthenia. 3rd ed. New York: William Wood & Co., 1907. 216p. DNLM; NNNAM; PPJ; PU **00-4616**

SAVILL, Thomas Dixon (1856-1910)
Clinical lectures on neurasthenia. [4th ed.] New York: William Wood & Co., 1909. 226p. DLC; DNLM; NNNAM; PPC **00-4617**

SAVILL, Thomas Dixon (1856-1910)
Lectures on hysteria and allied vasomotor conditions. New York: William Wood & Co., 1909. 262p. 21 plates. DNLM; ICJ; NNNAM; PU **00-4618**

SAWYER, James E[dward] H[ill] (*b.* 1874)
Physical signs of diseases of the thorax and abdomen. New York: William Wood & Co., 1908. 188p. CtY-M; DNLM; MBM; NNNAM **00-4619**

SAWYER, John P.
A comparison of methods of lavage with the siphon tube and Politzer bulbs. New York, 1905. 4p. DNLM **00-4620**

SAWYER, John P.
Incomplete forms of exophthalmic goitre in relation to gastro-intestinal disease. New York, 1907. 12p. DNLM **00-4621**

SAXE, G[eorge] A[lexander] De Santos (*b.* 1876)
Rational physical training for women. . . . [New York: D. Appleton & Co., 1900.] 28p. DLC; NN **00-4622**

SAXE, G[eorge] A[lexander] De Santos (*b.* 1876)
On determining the specific gravity of small volumes of urine, with a preliminary note on a special hydrometer (urinopyknometer) designed to work with a few cubic centimeters of fluid. New York, 1903. 17p. DNLM **00-4623**

SAXE, G[eorge] A[lexander] De Santos (*b.* 1876)
The psychical relations of tuberculosis in fact and fiction. [New York, 1903.] 29p. DLC: DNLM **00-4624**

SAXE, G[eorge] A[lexander] De Santos (*b.* 1876)
Examination of the urine. A manual for students and practitioners. Philadelphia: W. B Saunders & Co., 1904. 391p. 8 plates. DLC; DNLM; PPC; PU **00-4625**

SAXE, G[eorge] A[lexander] De Santos (*b.* 1876)
A study of sago bodies and other vesicular elements in massage urine in their relations to diagnosis. New York, 1907. 9p. DNLM **00-4626**

SAXE, G[eorge] A[lexander] De Santos (*b.* 1876)
A study of shreds in the urine in their relation to diagnosis and prognosis. New York: A. R. Elliott Co., 1907. 29p. DNLM; NNNAM **00-4627**

SAXE, G[eorge] A[lexander] De Santos (*b.* 1876)
Examination of the urine; a manual for students and practitioners . . . 2nd ed., rev. With text illustrations and colored plates, a number of them original. Philadelphia and London: W. B. Saunders & Co., 1909. 448p. DLC; NNNAM; PPC; PU **00-4628**

SAYRE, Lucius Elmer (1847-1925)
A manual of organic materia medica and pharmacognosy; an introduction to the study of the vegetable kingdom and the vegetable and animal drugs . . . 3rd ed., rev. With histology and microtechnique, by William C. Stevens. . . . With 377 illustrations, the majority of which are from original drawings and photomicrographs. Philadelphia: P. Blakiston's Son & Co., 1905. 692p. DLC; DNLM; OCLloyd; PPC **00-4629**

SAYRE, Lucius Elmer (1847-1925)
. . . Gelsemium; a study that embodies the recent work of Professor L. E. Sayre . . . together with fragments of a paper read by him before the American Pharmaceutical Association, Richmond, Virginia, 1910. Accompanied by a plate of physiological tracings by Professor H. W. Emerson. [Cincinnati: J. U. & C. G. Lloyd, 1910.] 11p. diags. DLC; DNLM; ICJ; PU **00-4630**

SCHACHNER, August (1865-1941)
The surgical aspects of the modern small-bore projectile. Philadelphia, 1900. 12p. DNLM **00-4631**

SCHACHNER, August (1865-1941)
New operating table and an improved bowl stand. Philadelphia, 1900. 7p. DNLM **00-4632**

SCHACHNER, August (1865-1941)
Foreign bodies accidentally left in the abdominal cavity. With report of one hundred and fifty-five cases. Philadelphia, 1901. 48p. DNLM **00-4633**

SCHACHNER, August (1865-1941)
Report of five cases of laparotomy for intestinal obstruction. Philadelphia: J. B. Lippincott Co., 1902. 7p. DNLM **00-4634**

SCHACHNER, August (1865-1941)
Hyperthyroidism and Basedow's disease. Cincinnati, 1909. 3p. DNLM **00-4635**

SCHAEFER, George H. A.
Diseases and their natural (anti-medical) treatment, by means of the new patented healing apparatus, "System Schaefer Bros." Buffalo, N.Y.: G. H. A. Schaefer, 1901 [*c.* 1898]. 74p. DLC **00-4636**

SCHAEFER, Theodore William
The contamination of the air of our cities with sulphur dioxid, the cause of respiratory disease. Boston, 1907. 15p. DNLM; NN **00-4637**

SCHAEFFER, Oskar (*b.* 1863)
Atlas and epitome of gynecology . . . authorized translation from the 2nd rev. and enl. German ed. Edited by Richard C. Norris. . . . With 207 colored illustrations on 90 plates, and 62 illustrations in the text. Philadelphia: W. B. Saunders & Co., 1900. 272p. DLC; ICJ; PPC; PU **00-4638**

SCHAEFFER, Oskar (*b.* 1863)
Anatomical atlas of obstetrics, with special reference to diagnosis and treatment. . . . Authorized translation from the 2nd rev. German ed.; edited by J. Clifton Edgar . . . with 122 figures on 56 lithographic plates, and 38 other illustrations. Philadelphia and London: W. B. Saunders & Co., 1901. 315p. DLC; ICJ; PPC; PU **00-4639**

SCHAEFFER, Oskar (*b.* 1863)
Atlas and epitome of labor and operative obstetrics . . . authorized translation from the 5th rev. German ed.; edited by J. Clifton Edgar. . . . Philadelphia and London: W. B. Saunders & Co., 1901. 112p. col. plates. DLC; ICJ; PPC; PU **00-4640**

SCHAEFFER, Oskar (*b.* 1863)
Atlas and epitome of operative gynecology . . . authorized translation from the German with editorial notes additions, ed. by J. Clarence Webster. . . . With 42 colored lithographic plates and many text-illustrations, some in colors. Philadelphia, New York [etc.]: W. B. Saunders & Co., 1904. 138p. DLC; ICJ; PPC; PU **00-4641**

SCHÄFER, Edward Albert (1850-1935)
Directions for class work in practical physiology, elementary physiology of muscle and nerve and of the vascular and nervous systems . . . with diagrams. New York: Longmans, Green & Co, 1901. 76p. DLC; DNLM; PP; PPJ **00-4642**

SCHÄFER, Edward Albert (1850-1935)
The essentials of histology, descriptive and practical. For the use of students. . . . 6th ed., rev. and enl. with 463 illustrations. Philadelphia and New York: Lea Bros. & Co., 1902. 416p. DLC; NNNAM; PPC; PU **00-4643**

SCHÄFER, Edward Albert (1850-1935)
The essentials of histology, descriptive and practical. For the use of students. . . . 7th ed. Philadelphia: Lea Bros. & Co., 1907. 507p. ICJ; NNC; PPJ **00-4644**

SCHÄFER, Edward Albert (1850-1935)
Aritifical respiration in its physiologic aspects. Chicago, 1908. 8p. DNLM **00-4645**

SCHÄFER, Edward Albert (1850-1935)
Albrecht von Haller. [n. p., 1908.] 3p. illus. CtY-M **00-4646**

SCHÄFER, Edward Albert (1850-1935)
The essentials of histology, descriptive and practical. For the use of students. . . . 8th ed. Philadelphia: Lea & Febiger, 1910. 571p. CtY-M; DNLM; ICJ; PPJ **00-4647**

SCHALEK, Alfred (*b.* 1865)
. . . Diseases of the skin. A manual for students and practitioners. . . . Philadelphia and New York: Lea Bros. & Co., [1902]. 225p. CtY-M; DLC; PPC; PU **00-4648**

SCHALEK, Alfred (*b.* 1865)
. . . Diseases of the skin; a manual for students and practitioners. . . . 2nd ed., thoroughly rev.; illustrated with 47 engravings. Philadelphia and New York: Lea & Febiger, [1910]. 255p. DLC; PPC; PPJ; PU **00-4649**

SCHAMBERG, Jay F[rank] (1870-1934)
. . . A compend of diseases of the skin . . . 2nd ed., rev. and enl. With 105 illustrations. . . . Philadelphia: P. Blakiston's Son & Co., 1900. 291p. DLC; ICJ; MH-M; PPC **00-4650**

SCHAMBERG, Jay F[rank] (1870-1934)
. . . A compend of diseases of the skin . . . 3rd ed., rev. and enl., with 106 illustrations. Philadelphia: P. Blakiston's Son & Co., 1903. 291p. DLC; NNNAM; PPC; PU **00-4651**

SCHAMBERG, Jay Frank (1870-1934)
Secondary eruptions in small-pox. New York: Grafton Press, 1903. 7p. 4 plates. DNLM **00-4652**

SCHAMBERG, Jay Frank (1870-1934)
. . . A compend of diseases of the skin . . . 4th ed., rev. and enl., with 108 illustrations. Philadelphia: P. Blakiston's Son & Co., 1905. 299p. CtY-M; DLC; IU-M; PPC **00-4653**

SCHAMBERG, Jay Frank (1870-1934)
Diseases of the skin and the eruptive fevers. Philadelphia & London: W. B. Saunders & Co., 1908. 534p. DLC: DNLM; NNNAM; PPC **00-4654**

SCHAMBERG, Jay Frank (1870-1934)
Vaccination and its relation to animal experimentation. Chicago, 1909. 50p. plates, charts. MB **00-4655**

SCHAMBERG, Jay Frank (1870-1934)
Diseases of the skin and the eruptive fevers . . . 2nd ed., thoroughly rev. Philadelpha and London: W. B. Saunders & Co., 1910 [*c.* 1911]. 573p. DLC; ICJ; MH-M; NNNAM **00-4656**

SCHAMBERG, Jay Frank (1870-1934)
Grain itch (acaro-dermatitis urticarioides): a study of a new disease in this country. . . . [New York, 1910.] 23p. plates. DLC; NNNAM; PU **00-4657**

SCHAMBERG, Jay Frank (1870-1934)
Vaccination and its relation to animal experimentation [by] Jay Frank Schamberg. . . . Chicago: American Medical Association, [1910?] 56p. DLC **00-4658**

SCHAMBERG, Jay Frank (1870-1934)
What vaccination has really done. Philadelphia, 1910? 48p. PPC **00-4659**

SCHAPPS, John C.
Pony, Montana, as a resort for cases of pulmonary tuberculosis. New York, 1900. 8p. DNLM **00-4660**

SCHENCK, Benjamin R[obinson] (1872-1920)
The prognosis of post-operative femoral phlebitis. New York, 1906. 15p. DNLM **00-4661**

SCHENCK, Friedrich Wilhelm Julius (1862-1916)
Outlines of human physiology, by F. Schenck, M.D., and A. Gürber . . . authorized translation from the 2nd German ed. by Wm. D. Zoethout; with a preface by Jacques Loeb. . . . New York: H. Holt & Co., 1900. 339p. diags. DLC; MH; NIC; PPJ **00-4662**

SCHENCK, Joseph H.
The lungs; the liver; the stomach. A plain, practical, household treatise on pulmonary consumption, dyspepsia and liver complaint. . . . [Philadelphia], 1901 [*c.* 1885]. 96p. DLC; PP [*vel subseq.*] **00-4663**

SCHENK, S[amuel] Leopold (1840-1902)
Schenk's theory. The determination of sex. Authorized translation. Chicago, Akron, O., [etc.]: The Werner Co., 1900 [*c.* 1898]. 222p. DLC; ICJ; ICU; NN **00-4664**

SCHEPPEGRELL, William (*b.* 1860)
The prevention of deafness. New York, 1907. 8p. DNLM **00-4665**

SCHERESCHEWSKY, Joseph Williams (1873-1940)
Problems of infant mortality, by J. W. Schereschewsky, M.D., of the Public Health and Marine Hospital, Washington, D.C. New York: Printed by the Child-helping Department of the Russell Sage Foundation [19-?] 27p. DLC **00-4666**

SCHERESCHEWSKY, Joseph Williams (1873-1940)
. . . The Fourth disease (Filatow-Dukes' disease). By Passed Asst. Surg. J. W. Schereschewsky, Public Heath and Marine Hospital Service. . . . Washington: Government Printing Office, 1907. 7p. DLC **00-4667**

SCHIMPF, Henry William (*b.* 1868)
A text-book of volumetric analysis, with special reference to the volumetric processes of the pharmacopoeia of the United States. Designed for the use of pharmacists and pharmaceutical students. . . . with sixty illustrations. 4th ed., rev. and enl. 1st thousand. New York: J. Wiley & Sons, 1903. 553p. DLC; ICJ; NIC; NN **00-4668**

SCHIMPF, Henry William (*b.* 1868)
Essentials of volumetric analysis. An introduction to the subject, adapted to the needs of students of pharmaceutical chemistry. Embracing the subjects of alkalimetry, acidimetry, precipitation analysis, oxidimetry, indirect oxidation, iodometry, assay processes for drugs, estimation of alkaloids, carbolic acid, sugars, theory, application and description of indicators. . . . 1st ed. 1st thousand. New York: J. Wiley & Sons; [etc., etc.], 1903. 227p. DLC; ICJ; NIC; PP **00-4669**

SCHIMPF, Henry William (*b.* 1868)
A systematic course of qualitative chemical analysis of inorganic and organic substances with explanatory notes. New York: J. Wiley & Sons, 1906. 156p. DNLM; MH; NIC; NN **00-4670**

SCHIMPF, Henry William (*b.* 1868)
A manual of volumetric analysis for the use of pharmacists, sanitary and food chemists, as well as for students in these branches . . . with one hundred and two illustrations. 5th ed., rev. and enl. 1st thousand. New York: J. Wiley & Sons; [etc., etc.], 1909. 725p. DLC; ICJ; PP; PU [The first four editions, 1894-1903, have title: A text-book of volumetric analysis.] **00-4671**

SCHIMPF, Henry William (*b.* 1868)
A systematic course of qualitative chemical analysis of inorganic and organic substances, with explanatory notes . . . 2nd ed. rev. 1st thousand. New York: J. Wiley & Sons; [etc., etc.], 1910. 150p. DLC; ICJ; MH; NN **00-4672**

SCHLEIF, William (*b.* 1868)
. . . Materia medica, therapeutics, medical pharmacy, prescription writing, and medical Latin. A manual for students and practitioners. . . . 2nd ed., rev. and enl. Philadelphia and New York: Lea Bros. & Co., [1902]. 389p. DLC; NNNAM; PPC; PPJ **00-4673**

SCHLEIF, William (*b.* 1868)
. . . Materia medica, therapeutics, pharmacology and pharmacognosy, including medical pharmacy, prescription writing and medical Latin; a manual for students and practitioners . . . 3rd ed., rev. and enl. Philadelphia and New York: Lea Bros. & Co., [1907]. 470p. DLC; IU-M; PPC; PU **00-4674**

SCHLEIP, Karl Friedrich Wilhelm (*b.* 1872)
Hematological atlas, with a description of the technic of blood examination, by Priv doz. Dr. Karl Schleip . . . English adaptation of text, by Frederic E. Sondern. . . . With 71 colored illustrations. New York: Rebman Co., [1908]. 256p. DLC; DNLM; ICJ; PPC **00-4675**

SCHMAUS, Hans (*b.* 1862)
A text-book of pathology and pathological anatomy. . . . Transl. from the 6th German ed., by A. E. Thayer. . . . Ed. with additions by James Ewing. . . . Illustrated with 351 engravings, including 35 colored inset plates. Philadelphia and New York: Lea Bros. & Co., 1902. 602p. DLC; ICJ; NNNAM; PU **00-4676**

SCHMIDT, Adolf (1865-1918)
The examination of the function of the intestines by means of the test-diet; its application in medical practice and its diagnostic and therapeutic value. . . . Authorized translation from the latest German ed., by Charles D. Aaron. . . . Philadelphia: F. A. Davis Co., 1906. 91p. DLC; DNLM; PPC; PPJ **00-4677**

SCHMIDT, Adolf (1865-1918)
The examination of the function of the intestines by means of the test diet; its application in medical practice and its diagnostic and therapeutic value . . . authorized translation from the 2nd rev. and enl. German ed. by Charles D. Aaron. . . . Philadelphia: F. A. Davis Co., 1909. 126p. plates. DLC; ICJ; PPC; PU **00-4678**

SCHMIDT, Louis E[rnst] (*b.* **1869)**
Genito-urinary and venereal diseases. A manual for students and practitioners. . . . Philadelphia and New York: Lea Bros. & Co., [1902]. 249p. DLC; NNNAM; PPC: PPJ
00-4679

SCHMIDT, Rudolph (*b.* **1875)**
Pain, its causation and diagnostic significance in internal diseases . . . transl. and ed. by Karl M. Vogel . . . and Hans Zinsser . . . Philadelphia & London: J. B. Lippincott Co., [1908]. 326p. plates. CtY-M; DLC; MH-M; PPC
00-4680

SCHMIDT, Rudolph (*b.* **1875)**
Pain, its causation and diagnostic significance in internal diseases . . . transl. and ed. from the 2nd enl. and rev. German ed. by Karl M. Vogel . . . and Hans Zinsser . . . 2nd ed. Philadelphia & London: J. B. Lippincott Co., [1910]. 358p. plates. DNLM; ICJ; PPC; PPJ **00-4681**

SCHMITT, Gustav
A brief necroscopy and its medico-legal relation, arranged by. . . . New York and London: Funk & Wagnalls Co., 1902. 186p. DLC; MH; NIC; NN **00-4682**

SCHMITZ, John P[eter]
Human physiology; analysis and digest. San Francisco: The Author, 1901 [*c.* 1894]. 347p. DLC **00-4683**

SCHMITZ, John P[eter]
Human physiology; analysis and digest. For the use of medical students and practitioners. By Prof. John P. Schmitz . . . 2nd ed. San Francisco: The Author, 1902 [*c.* 1899]. 347p. DLC
00-4684

SCHMITZ, John P[eter]
The microbe-producing disease theory inconsistent with the laws of nature. How diseases are produced. A new physiological law promulgated by Prof. J. P. Schmitz. . . . San Francisco, Cal.: Pub. by the Author, 1902. 50p. DLC
00-4685

SCHMITZ, John P[eter]
Over 3,000 questions on laws of the human body, or physiology; by Prof. J. P. Schmitz, M.D. San Francisco, Cal.: The Author, 1902. 121p. DLC **00-4686**

SCHNEIDER, Albert (1863-1928)
The limitations of learning, and other science papers. Chicago: Chicago Medical Book Co., 1900. 100p. DLC; ICJ
00-4687

SCHNEIDER, Albert (1863-1928)
Microscopy and micro-technique. Chicago: Chicago Medical Book Co., 1900 [*c.* 1899]. 189p. DLC; ICJ; NN
00-4688

SCHNEIDER, Albert (1863-1928)
General vegetable pharmacography. Chicago: Chicago Medical Book Co., 1900. 136p. DLC; ICJ **00-4689**

SCHNEIDER, Albert (1863-1928)
Powdered vegetable drugs. Pittsburgh: Calumet Publishing Co., 1902. 323p. DLC; OCLloyd **00-4690**

SCHNEIDER, Albert (1863-1928)
Literature on medical plants and drug plant culture. . . . Milwaukee: Pharmaceutical Review Publishing Co., 1908. 24p. ICJ **00-4691**

[SCHOEPF, Johann David] (1752-1800)
Materia medica americana potissimum regni vegetabilis. Erlangae, Sumtibus Io. Iac. Palmii, MDCCLXXXVII. [Cincinnati, O.: J. U. & C. G. Lloyd, 1903.] 170p. DLC; OCLloyd [Bulletin of the Lloyd library of botany, pharmacy and materia medica, no. 6. Reproduction series, no. 3]
00-4692

SCHOFIELD, Alfred T[aylor] (1846-1929)
The force of mind or the mental factor in medicine. Philadelphia: P. Blakiston's Son & Co., 1902. 309p. DLC; ICJ; NIC; PPC **00-4693**

SCHOFIELD, Alfred T[aylor] (1846-1929)
Nerves in disorder; a plea for rational treatment. New York: Funk & Wagnalls Co., 1903. 202p. DLC; ICJ; NNNAM; PU
00-4694

SCHOFIELD, Alfred T[aylor] (1846-1929)
Nerves in order; or, The maintenance of health. . . . New York: Funk & Wagnalls Co., [1905]. 291p. DLC; MH; NIC; NN **00-4695**

SCHOFIELD, Alfred T[aylor] (1846-1929)
Unconscious therapeutics; or, the personality of the physician. 2nd ed. Philadelphia: P. Blakiston's Son & Co., 1906. 317p. DLC; ICJ; PPC; PU **00-4696**

SCHOFIELD, Alfred T[aylor] (1864-1929)
The management of a nerve patient. Philadelphia: P. Blakiston's Son & Co., 1906. 267p. DLC; MH; PPC: PU
00-4697

SCHOFIELD, Alfred T[aylor] (1846-1929)
The unconscious mind. New York: Funk & Wagnalls Co., 1907 436p. DLC; MH; NN; PU **00-4698**

SCHOFIELD, Alfred T[aylor] (1846-1929)
The home life in order; or, Personal and domestic hygiene. . . . New York: Funk & Wagnalls Co., 1907. 345p. DLC; MB; PPC; PU **00-4699**

SCHOFIELD, Alfred T[aylor] (1846-1929)
Christian sanity. . . . With a preface by Dr. Handley Moule. . . . New York: A. C. Armstrong & Son, 1908. 165p. diag. DLC; MB; NIC; NN **00-4700**

SCHOFIELD, Alfred T[aylor] (1846-1929)
Functional nerve disease. New York: E. P. Dutton, 1908. 324p. CtY-M; ICU; NIC; NN **00-4701**

SCHOFIELD, Alfred T[aylor] (1846-1929)
The force of mind; or the mental factor in medicine. New York: Funk & Wagnalls Co., 1908. 309p. ICRM; MH; NBM; NcD **00-4702**

SCHOFIELD, Alfred T[aylor] (1846-1929)
Fit for work; or, Health in Christian service. . . . New York: A. C. Armstrong & Son, 1909. 212p. DLC; ICJ; NN; PPC
00-4703

SCHOFIELD, Alfred T[aylor] (1846-1929)
Mental and spiritual health. . . . New York: R. F. Fenno & Co., [1910]. 93p. DLC; MH; NIC; NN **00-4704**

SCHOFIELD, Alfred T[aylor] (1846-1929)
How to keep fit; an unconventional manual. . . . New York: Moffat, Yard & Co, [1910]. 90p. DLC; ICJ; MB; NN
00-4705

SCHOFIELD, Alfred T[aylor] (1846-1929)
Health for young and old; its principles and practice . . . an unconventional manual. New York and London: G. P. Putnam's Sons, 1910. 300p. DLC; DNLM; ICJ; NN
00-4706

SCHORER, Edwin Henry (*b.* 1879)
Vaccine and serum therapy, including also a study of infections, theories of immunity, openings and opsonic index. . . . St. Louis: C. V. Mosby Co., 1904. 131p. DLC
00-4707

SCHORER, Edwin Henry (*b.* 1879)
The opsonic index in erysipelas and its relation to treatment by inoculation of killed streptococci. Philadelphia & New York, 1907. 14p. DNLM **00-4708**

SCHRIEVER, James Boniface (*b.* 1868)
. . . Physicians' and surgeons' supplementary volume of the Complete self-instructing library of practical photography, comp. and ed. by J. B. Schriever and Thomas Harrison Cummings. Scranton, Pa.: American School of Art & Photography, 1909. 51p. plates. DLC [Plates printed on both sides.]
00-4709

SCHROEDER, Aimée Raymond
Health notes for young wives. New York: William Wood & Co., 1901. 210p. DLC; ICJ; IEN-M; NN [1st printing, 1895]
00-4710

SCHROEDER, John Henry (*b.* 1876)
Applied materia medica; a text book intended for the use of nurses in hospital training schools. . . . Cincinnati: The R. Clarke Co., 1904. 118p. DLC: OC; OCLloyd; PU
00-4711

SCHROEDER, John Henry (*b.* 1876)
Applied materia medica; a text book intended for the use of nurses in hospital training schools. Based upon the U.S. pharmacopoeia, eighth decennial revision, 1905. . . . 2nd ed. Cincinnati: The Robert Clarke Co., 1907. 113p. DLC; DNLM; ICJ; PU **00-4712**

SCHROEDER, John Henry (*b.* 1876)
A text book of chemistry, for the use of students of Cincinnati Veterinary College. . . . [Cincinnati? 1907.] 91p. DLC
00-4713

SCHROEDER, William
History of the ambulance system in Brooklyn, N.Y. Brooklyn, 1902. 49p. DLC; DNLM **00-4714**

SCHROEDER, William
Early history of medicine in Kings County. Brooklyn, 1903. 12p. DLC; DNLM **00-4715**

SCHROEDER, William
Historical résumé of clinical teaching. Brooklyn, 1904. 13p. DLC; DNLM **00-4716**

SCHROEDER, William
Honors that have come to the medical profession in America. Brooklyn, N.Y., 1906. 31, 18, 17, 13, 14p. DLC; DNLM
00-4717

SCHROEDER, William
Memorials in honor of the medical profession in America. Brooklyn: J. W. Palmer, 1906. 2p. 33 plates. DLC; DNLM
00-4718

SCHRYVER, Samuel Barnett (1869-1929)
Chemistry of the albumens. Ten lectures delivered in the Michaelmas term, 1904, in the physiological department of University College, London. . . . Published under the auspices of the University of London. Philadelphia: P. Blakiston's Son & Co., 1906. 192p. CtY-M; DLC; MBM; PPC
00-4719

SCHULTZE, Oskar Max Sigismund (1859-1930)
Atlas and text-book of topographic and applied anatomy . . . ed., with additions, by George D. Stewart. . . . With 25 colored illustrations on 22 lithographic plates, and 89 text-cuts, 60 in colors. Philadelphia and London: W. B. Saunders & Co., 1905. 189p. DLC; ICJ; PPC; PPHa
00-4720

DE SCHWEINITZ, George Edmund (1858-1938)
The comparative value of enucleation and the operations which have been substituted for it. [Philadelphia], 1900. 44p. DNLM **00-4721**

DE SCHWEINITZ, George Edmund (1858-1938)
Six notable American medical achievements. n. p., 1901. 16p. PU **00-4722**

DE SCHWEINITZ, George Edmund (1858-1938)
Uveitis. Symposium of papers read before the Ophthalmological section of the American Medical Association . . . Saratoga, N.Y., June 1902, by G. E. De Schweinitz, Hiram Woods, Harry Friedenwald, & others. Chicago: American Medical Association, 1902. 91p. PPJ; PPPH **00-4823**

DE SCHWEINITZ, George Edmund (1858-1938)
Diseases of the eye; a handbook of ophthalmic practice for student and practitioners . . . with 280 illustrations and six chromo-lithographic plates. 4th ed., thoroughly rev. Philadelphia and London: W. B. Saunders & Co., 1902. 773p. DLC; DNLM; NNNAM; PPC **00-4724**

DE SCHWEINITZ, George Edmund (1858-1938)
On the histology of bullous keratitis in glaucomatous eyes. n. p., 1903. 268p. DNLM; PU **00-4725**

DE SCHWEINITZ, George Edmund (1858-1938) and E. A. SHUMWAY
A note on the histology of vernal conjunctivitis (Frühjahr's catarrh). Philadelphia, 1903. 6p. DNLM
00-4726

DE SCHWEINITZ, George Edmund (1858-1938)
Relation of the cervical sympathetic to the eye; papers read before the . . . American Medical Association . . . May, 1903. Chicago: American Medical Association, 1904. 119p. illus. DLC; OC; PPJ **00-4727**

DE SCHWEINITZ, George Edmund (1858-1938)
The relation of the cervical sympathetic to the eye. Papers read before the section on ophthalmology of the American Medical Association. Chicago: American Medical Association, 1904. 149p. PPPH **00-4728**

DE SCHWEINITZ, George Edmund (1858-1938)
Diseases of the eye; a handbook of ophthalmic practice for students and practitioners. . . . With 313 illustrations and chromo-lithographic plates. 5th ed., thoroughly rev. Philadelphia and London: W. B. Saunders & Co., 1906. 894p. col. plates. DLC; DNLM PPC; PU **00-4729**

DE SCHWEINITZ, George Edmund (1858-1938)
The ocular symptoms of tumor of the cerebrum. Philadelphia, 1906. 20p. DNLM; PPC **00-4730**

DE SCHWEINITZ, George Edmund (1858-1938)
Pulsating exophthalmos, its etiology, symptomatology, pathogenesis, and treatment—being an essay based upon an analysis of sixty-nine case histories of this affection, by George E. de Schweinitz . . . and Thomas B. Holloway. . . . Philadelphia and London: W. B. Saunders & Co., 1908. 124p. tables. DLC; DNLM; ICJ; PPC **00-4731**

DE SCHWEINITZ, George Edmund (1858-1938)
Diseases of the eye; a handbook of ophthalmic practice for students and practitioners . . . with 351 illustrations and seven chromo-lithographic plates. 6th ed., thoroughly rev. Philadelphia and London: W. B. Saunders & Co., 1910. 945p. DLC; NNNAM; OCIM; PPC **00-4732**

SCHWYZER, Fritz
A contribution to the pathology of the elastic tissue of the aorta. [*Also*:] The pathogenesis of the aneurysmata of the aorta. New York, 1904. 36p. DNLM **00-4733**

SCHWYZER, Fritz
The construction of the valvular part of the aorta and the significance of its elastic and collagenous tissue. New York, 1904. 28p. DNLM **00-4734**

SCHWYZER, Fritz
Eructations in heart patients. [New York], 1907. 8p. DNLM **00-4735**

SCOTT, Franklin Waters (*b.* 1874)
Elementary materia medica for pupil nurses. . . . [New York? 1910.] 125p. DLC; NNNAM **00-4736**

SCOTT, George Dow (*b.* 1871)
The passing of the nusing mother. New York, 1906. 15p. DNLM **00-4737**

SCOTT, James F[oster] (*b.* 1863)
The sexual instinct, its use and dangers as affecting heredity and morals. 2nd ed., rev. and enl. New York: E. B. Treat & Co., 1908. 473p. DLC; ICJ; NN; PU [also appears under title: Heredity and morals as affected by the use and abuse of the sexual instinct. Essentials to the welfare of the individual and the future of the race.] **00-4738**

SCOTT, J[oseph] A[lison] (1865-1909)
A further study of perforation of the bowel of typhoid fever. New York: A. R. Elliott Co., 1907. 10p. DNLM; NNNAM **00-4739**

SCOTT, Lindley
The clinical examination of urine, with an atlas of urinary deposits. Philadelphia: P. Blakiston's Son & Co., 1900. 53p. 40 l., 41 plates. DNLM; ICJ; PPC; PU **00-4740**

SCOTT, N. Stone (*b.* 1863)
Spontaneous rupture of the uterus at three months. Cleveland, 1900. 3p. DNLM **00-4741**

SCOTT, N. Stone (*b.* 1863)
Results of operative procedures for mechanic obstruction of the pylorus. A contribution read before the Cleveland Medical Society, June 15, 1900. Cleveland, 1900. 7p. DNLM **00-4742**

SCOTT, N. Stone (*b.* 1863)
Ovarian pregnancy; is it an explanation of ovarian hematomata? [Cleveland], 1901. 10p. DNLM **00-4743**

SCOTT, R[ichard] J[ohn] E[rnst] (1863-1932)
Questions in anatomy set by the New York State Board of Medical Examiners from the foundation of the board to September 1901. . . . New York: Medical Review of Reviews, 1902. 47p. DLC; DNLM; NNNAM **00-4744**

SCOTT, R[ichard] J[ohn] E[rnst] (1863-1932)
. . . Questions in anatomy asked at the examinations held by the New York State Board of Medical Examiners, complete, with references and answers to every question. . . . New York and Philadelphia: Lea Bros. & Co., [1903]. 100p. DLC; NNNAM; PPC **00-4745**

SCOTT, R[ichard] J[ohn] E[rnst] (1863-1932)
. . . Questions in chemistry asked at the examinations held by the New York State Board of Medical Examiners, complete, with references and answers to every question. . . . New York and Philadelphia: Lea Bros. & Co., [1903]. 138p. DLC; NNNAM; PPC **00-4746**

SCOTT, R[ichard] J[ohn] E[rnst] (1863-1932)
. . . Questions in therapeutics, practice and materia medica asked at the examinations held by the New York State Board of Medical Examiners, complete, with references and answers to every question. . . . New York and Philadelphia: Lea Bros. & Co., [1903]. 119p. DLC; NNNAM; PPC: PPJ **00-4747**

SCOTT, R[ichard] J[ohn] E[rnst] (1863-1932)
. . . Questions in pathology and diagnosis asked at the examinations held by the New York State Board of Medical Examiners, complete, with references and answers to every question. . . . New York and Philadelphia: Lea Bros. & Co., [1903]. 148p. DLC; NNNAM; PPC; PU **00-4748**

SCOTT, R[ichard] J[ohn] E[rnst] (1863-1932)
. . . Questions in obstetrics, asked at the examinations held by the New York State Board of Medical Examiners, complete, with references and answers to every question. . . . New York and Philadelphia: Lea Bros. & Co., [1903]. 112p. DLC; DNLM; NNNAM **00-4749**

SCOTT, R[ichard] J[ohn] E[rnst] (1863-1932)
State medical practice laws. New York, 1904. 48p. DNLM; PPC **00-4750**

SCOTT, R[ichard] J[ohn] E[rnst] (1863-1932)
. . . Questions in surgery asked at the examinations held by the New York State Board of Medical Examiners, complete, with references and answers to every question. . . . New York and Philadelphia: Lea Bros. & Co., [1904]. 213p. DLC; NNNAM; PPC **00-4751**

SCOTT, R[ichard] J[ohn] E[rnst] (1863-1932)
. . . Questions in physiology and hygiene asked at the examinations held by the New York State Board of Medical Examiners, complete, with references and answers to every question. . . . New York and Philadelphia: Lea Bros. & Co., [1905]. 216p. DLC; NIC; NNNAM **00-4752**

SCOTT, R[ichard] J[ohn] E[rnst] (1863-1932)
State board examination questions and answers of twenty-three States. A valuable guide to the medical student, giving accurate answers that will prove helpful in passing State board examinations. New York: William Wood & Co., 1907. DNLM; NNNAM **00-4753**

SCOTT, R[ichard] J[ohn] E[rnst] (1863-1932)
State board examination questions and answers of thrity-four States. Edition of 1908. New York: William Wood & Co., 1908. 479p. DNLM; NNNAM **00-4754**

SCOTT, R[ichard] J[ohn] E[rnst] (1863-1932)
State medical practice laws. New York, 1909. 74p. DNLM **00-4755**

SCOTT, R[ichard] J[ohn] E[rnst] (1863-1932)
State board examinations; questions and answers of forty-one States and two Canadian Provinces; a practical work, giving authentic questions and authoritative answers that will prove helpful in passing State board examinations. 3rd ed. New York: William Wood & Co., 1910. 819p. DNLM **00-4756**

SCOVILLE, Wilbur Lincoln (1865-1942)
The art of compounding. A textbook for students and a reference book for pharmacists at the prescription counter. 3rd ed. revised and enlarged. Philadelphia: P. Blakiston's Son & Co., 1904. 237p. CtY-M; DNLM; PPC; PU **00-4757**

SCOVILLE, Wilbur Lincoln (1865-1942)
American pharmaceutical colleges and schools. [n. p.], 1905. 17p. DNLM **00-4758**

SCUDDER, Charles Locke (1860-1949)
The open or operative treatment of recent fractures; is it ever justifiable? With an analysis of the results of the present methods of treatment in one hundred and fifty-three fractures of the lower extremity and these unselected cases of fracture tabulated in order to show the results many years following treatment. Boston: Damrell & Upham, 1900. 17p. DNLM **00-4759**

SCUDDER, Charles Locke (1860-1949)
Surgery of the epiphyses. Philadelphia, 1900. 14p. DNLM **00-4760**

SCUDDER, Charles Locke (1860-1949)
Tumors of the breast; a series of cases illustrating certain clinical signs. St. Paul, Minn., 1900. 9p. DNLM **00-4761**

SCUDDER, Charles Locke (1860-1949)
The treatment of fractures. . . . Assisted by Frederic J. Cotton, M.D. With 585 illustrations. Philadelphia: W. B. Saunders, 1900. 433p. plates. DLC; DNLM; NNNAM; PPC **00-4762**

SCUDDER, Charles Locke (1860-1949)
Contusions of the abdomen. Boston, 1901. 26p. DNLM **00-4763**

SCUDDER, Charles Locke (1860-1949)
Gangrenous appendicitis; general peritonitis; multiple adhesions; gangrene of bowel wall; perforation of bowel; purulent and fecal abscesses; operation, drainage; autopsy. Boston, 1901. 6p. DNLM **00-4764**

SCUDDER, Charles Locke (1860-1949)
Ovarian cyst with twisted pedicle, acute symptoms; operation; recovery. Boston, 1901. 3p. DNLM **00-4765**

SCUDDER, Charles Locke (1860-1949)
Strangulation of the testis by torsion of the cord. A review of all recorded cases, together with the report of a recent case. Philadelphia, 1901. 15p. DNLM **00-4766**

SCUDDER, Charles Locke (1860-1949)
The treatment of fractures . . . assisted by Frederick J. Cotton, M.D. 2nd ed., rev. . . . Philadelphia and London: W. B. Saunders & Co., 1901. 457p. plates. DLC; DNLM; IU-M; NNNAM; PU **00-4767**

SCUDDER, Charles Locke (1860-1949)
Eight cases of tumor of the testicle; the clinical history, the pathologist's report, the end result. New York, 1902. 7p. DNLM **00-4768**

SCUDDER, Charles Locke (1860-1949)
The treatment of fractures . . . 3rd ed., thoroughly rev., with 645 illustrations. Philadelphia and London: W. B. Saunders & Co., 1902. 485p. plates. CU-M; DLC; DNLM; OCIM; PPC **00-4769**

SCUDDER, Charles Locke (1860-1949)
The treatment of fractures, with notes upon a few common dislocations . . . 4th ed., thoroughly rev. with 688 illustrations. Philadelphia, London [etc.]: W. B. Saunders & Co., 1903. 534p. plates. DLC; DNLM; MBM; PPC; ScCM **00-4770**

SCUDDER, Charles Locke (1860-1949)
Cholecystostomy and cholecystectomy; a study of a certain series of operations. Boston, 1904. 31p. DNLM **00-4771**

SCUDDER, Charles Locke (1860-1949)
A study of certain cases of sarcoma of the long bones from the Massachusetts General Hospital Clinic. Boston, 1904. 21p. DNLM **00-4772**

SCUDDER, Charles Locke (1860-1949)
The technique of resection of the cecum. Boston, 1904. 4p. 1 plate. **00-4773**

SCUDDER, Charles Locke (1860-1949)
Perforated duodenal and gastric ulcers; a report of two cases; operation; recovery. Boston, 1905. 8p. DNLM **00-4774**

SCUDDER, Charles Locke (1860-1949)
Volvulus of the jejunum. Philadelphia, 1905. 2p. 1 plate. DNLM **00-4775**

SCUDDER, Charles Locke (1860-1949)
The treatment of fractures, with notes upon a few common dislocations . . . 5th ed., thoroughly rev., with 739 illustrations. Philadelphia and London: W. B. Saunders & Co., 1905. 563p. plates. DLC; DNLM; LNT-M; MH-M; PU **00-4776**

SCUDDER, Charles Locke (1860-1949)
Stenosis of the pylorus in infancy. An analysis of one hundred and fifteen cases, [by] Charles L. Scudder . . . and William C. Quinby. . . . Boston, Mass., [1905?] 38p. DNLM; CtY-M; ICJ **00-4777**

SCUDDER, Charles Locke (1860-1949)
Stenosis of the pylorus in infancy, the report of a second case successfully operated upon; remarks. Boston, 1906. 3p. 1 plate. DNLM **00-4778**

SCUDDER, Charles Locke (1860-1949)
The treatment of fractures, with notes upon a few common dislocations . . . 6th ed., thoroughly rev. and enl., with 856 illustrations. Philadelphia and London: W. B. Saunders & Co., 1907. 628p. plates. DLC; DNLM; KyLoJM; MdBM **00-4779**

SCUDDER, Charles Locke (1860-1949)
Omentopexy to the intestine deprived of its mesentery. Boston, 1908. 3p. DNLM **00-4780**

SCUDDER, Charles Locke (1860-1949)
Papers upon surgical subjects. "Series C." [1908.] 21p. DNLM **00-4781**

SCUDDER, John M[ilton] (1829-1894)
The American eclectic materia medica & therapeutics. . . . 12th ed. Cincinnati: The Scudder Bros. Co., 1900 [*c.* 1898]. 748p. DLC; ICJ; PPJ **00-4782**

SCUDDER, John M[ilton] (1829-1894)
The principles of medicine. 7th ed. Cincinnati, O.: Scudder Bros. Co., 1900. 352p. DLC; ICJ **00-4783**

SCUDDER, John M[ilton] (1829-1894)
Principles of medicine. [7th ed.] Cincinnati: Wilstach, Baldwin & Co., 1900. 352p. OCLloyd; OCIM **00-4784**

SCUDDER, John M[ilton] (1829-1894)
Specific diagnosis: a study of disease, with special reference to the administration of remedies. . . . 10th ed. Cincinnati, O.: The Scudder Co., 1903. 387p. DLC; OCLloyd; OCIM **00-4785**

SCUDDER, John M[ilton] (1829-1894)
Specific diagnosis: a study of disease, with special reference to the administration of remedies. . . . 10th ed. Cincinnati, O.: The Scudder Co., 1903. 387p. DLC; OCLloyd; OCIM ["rev. ed."] **00-4786**

SEAMAN, Gilbert E[dmund] (*b.* 1869)
Diagnosis and treatment of some of the inflammatory conditions of the external ear. Milwaukee, 1904. 7p. DNLM **00-4787**

SEAMAN, Gilbert E[dmund] (*b.* 1869)
Cholesterin crystals in the vitreous with optic atrophy; report of a case. Chicago, 1906. 4p. DNLM **00-4788**

SEAMAN, Gilbert E[dmund] (*b.* 1869)
The diagnosis and treatment of injuries to the eye. Milwaukee, 1907. 11p. DNLM **00-4789**

SEAMAN, Louis Livingston (1851-1932)
The soldier's ration in the Tropics; its use and its abuse. New York, 1900. 15p. DNLM **00-4790**

SEAMAN, Louis Livingston (1851-1932)
Observations in China and the Tropics on the army ration and the post exchange or canteen. Carlisle, Pa., 1901. 23p. DNLM **00-4791**

SEAMAN, Louis Livingston (1851-1932)
Observations in China and the Tropics on the army ration and the post exchange or canteen. New York: Wynkoop Hallenbeck Crawford Co., 1901. 18p. DNLM **00-4792**

SEAMAN, Louis Livingston (1851-1932)
Observations on the medical features of the Russo-Japanese War. St. Louis, 1904. 31p. DNLM **00-4793**

SEAMAN, Louis Livingston (1851-1932)
Shall disease triumph in our army? A plea for the reorganization of the Medical Department of the United States Army, by Major Louis Livingston Seaman. . . . New York: American Defense Society, [1904]. 2 pts. in 1 v. illus. NIC; RPB **00-4794**

SEAMAN, Louis Livingston (1851-1932)
Military surgery. New York, 1904. 8p. DNLM **00-4795**

SEAMAN, Louis Livingston (1851-1932)
From Tokio through Manchuria with the Japanese. . . . New York: D. Appleton & Co., 1905 [1904]. 298p. plates. DLC; MB; NcD; PP **00-4796**

SEAMAN, Louis Livingston (1851-1932)
Observations in the Russo-Japanese War. Carlisle, Pa.: Cornman Co., 1905. 32p. DNLM **00-4797**

SEAMAN, Louis Livingston (1851-1932)
The real triumph of Japan; or, The conquest of the silent foe. [n.p., 1905?] 13p. DNLM **00-4798**

SEAMAN, Louis Livingston (1851-1932)
The real triumph of Japan. The conquest of the silent foe. New York: D. Appleton & Co., 1906. 291p. 31 plates. DLC; NIC; NN; PU **00-4799**

SEAMAN, Louis Livingston (1851-1932)
Shall disease triumph in our army? . . . New York: American Defense Society, [1906?] 1 v. illus. Various pagings. ICJ; NN **00-4800**

SEAMAN, Louis Livingston (1851-1932)
Some of the triumphs of scientific medicine in peace and war in foreign lands, with suggestions upon the necessity of important changes in the organization of the Medical Department of the United States Army. New York, 1908. 31p. DLC **00-4801**

SEARS, George G. (*b.* 1859)
Pregnancy and heart disease. St. Paul, Minn., 1900. 8p. DNLM **00-4802**

SEARS, George G. (*b.* 1859) and R. C. LARRABEE
An analysis of nine hundred and forty-nine cases of pneumonia. St. Paul, Minn., 1902. 15p. DNLM **00-4803**

SEARS, George G. (*b.* 1859) and Frederick T. LORD
The symptoms and treatment of hepatic cirrhosis in the light of seventy-eight autopsies. Boston: Damrell & Upham, 1902. 17p. DNLM **00-4804**

SEARS, George G. (*b.* 1859)
A note on pleurisy in typhoid fever. Boston, 1902. 7p. DNLM **00-4805**

SEARS, George G. (*b.* **1859)**
The prognosis of idiopathic pleurisy. Boston, 1904. 6p. DNLM
00-4806

SEARS, George G. (*b.* **1859)**
A case of diabetic coma, with recovery under alkaline treatment. [Boston, 1905.] 7p. DNLM
00-4807

SEARS, George G. (*b.* **1859)**
The results of medical treatment of peptic ulcer at the Boston City Hospital. Boston, 1905. 11p. DNLM
00-4808

SEARS, George G. (*b.* **1859)**
Accidents following thoracentesis; pneumothorax; sudden death from exploratory puncture. [Philadelphia], 1906. 7p. DNLM **00-4809**

SEARS, George G. (*b.* **1859)**
Exploratory puncture of the pericardium, with a report of three recent cases. Boston, 1906. 13p. DNLM
00-4810

SEARS, ROEBUCK & CO. (CHICAGO)
Surgical instruments and physicians' supplies. Chicago, 1906. 232p. DLC; ICJ; ICU **00-4811**

SEDGWICK, William T[hompson] (1855-1921)
Principles of sanitary science and the public health, with special reference to the causation and prevention of infectious diseases. New York: Macmillan Co., 1902. 368p. 4 plans. DNLM; ICJ; NIC; NNNAM **00-4812**

SEGNO, A. Victor (*b.* **1870)**
The law of mentalism; a practical, scientific explanation of thought or mind force; the law which governs all mental and physical action and phenomena: the cause of life and death. . . . Los Angeles, Cal.: American Institution of Mentalism, [1902]. 260p. DLC **00-4813**

SEGNO, A. Victor (*b.* **1870)**
The law of mentalism; a practical, scientific explanation of thought or mind force: the law which governs all mental and physical action and phenomena: the cause of life and death. . . . Los Angeles, Cal.: American Institute of Mentalism, [1902]. 208p. DLC **00-4814**

SEGNO, A. Victor (*b.* **1870)**
La ley del mentalismo; se expone una explicación práctica y cientifica del pensamiento ó fuerza del espíritu; la ley que gobierna todas las acciones morales y fisicas y los fenómenos; la causa de la vida y muerte. . . . Los Angeles, Cal.: Instituto Americano de Mentalismo, [1902]. 202p. DLC
00-4815

SEGNO, A. Victor (*b.* **1870)**
How to live 100 years and retain youth, health and beauty; a course of practical lessons in life culture. . . . Los Angeles, Cal.: The Life Culture Society, [1903]. 216p. DLC
00-4816

SEGUIN, Edward (1812-1880)
Idiocy: and its treatment by the physiological method. . . . Albany, N.Y.: Press of Brandow Printing Co., [1907]. 202p. DLC; MA; NcD; NN **00-4817**

SEIBERT, August (1854-1926)
Exclusive soup diet and rectal irrigations in typhoid fever. New York, 1900. 16p. DNLM **00-4818**

SEIBERT, August (1854-1926)
Scarlet fever in New York, and some of its therapeutical possibilities. New York: A. A. Elliott Co., 1904. 7p. DNLM
00-4819

SEIDELL, Atherton (*b.* **1878)**
A new standard for use in the colorimetric determination of iodine. New York, 1907. 3p. DNLM **00-4820**

SEIDELL, Atherton (*b.* **1878)**
Solubilities of inorganic and organic substances; a handbook of the most reliable quantitative solubility determinations. New York: D. Van Nostrand Co., 1907. 367p. DNLM; MH; NIC; NN **00-4821**

SEIDELL, Atherton (*b.* **1878)**
The solubilities of the pharmacopoeial organic acids and their salts. . . . Washington: Government Printing Office, 1910. 98p. DLC; DNLM; NcD; NN **00-4822**

SENATOR, Hermann, ed. (1834-1911)
Health and disease in relation to marriage and the marriage state. . . . Ed. by . . . Dr. H. Senator and Dr. Med. S. Kaminer. The only authorized translation from the German into the English language, by J. Dulberg. . . . New York: Rebman Co.; etc., etc. 1904-05. 2 v. DLC; ICJ; KU; PPC
00-4823

SENATOR, Hermann, ed. (1834-1911)
. . . Diseases of the kidneys and of the spleen, hemorrhagic diseases, by Dr. H. Senaor . . . and Dr. M. Litten . . . ed. with additions by James B. Herrick. . . . Authorized translation from the German, under the editorial supervision of Alfred Stengel. . . . Philadelphia and London: W. B. Saunders & Co., 1905. 815p. DLC; KU; NcD; NcU [Nothnagel's encyclopaedia of practical medicine, American ed.] **00-4824**

SENATOR, Hermann, ed. (1834-1911)
Marriage and disease, being an abridged edition of Health and disease in relation to marriage and the married state. Edited by H. Senator and S. Kaminer. Translated from the German by J. Dulberg. New York: Hoeber, 1909. 452p. DLC; OCIM; PP; PPJ **00-4825**

SENN, Emanuel John (*b.* **1869)**
Transplantation of omentum in the operative treatment of intestinal defects. A clinical and experimental contribution. Chicago, 1903. 7p. DNLM **00-4826**

SENN, Nicholas (1844-1908)
The pathology and surgical treatment of tumors . . . 2nd ed., rev. . . . Illustrated by 478 engravings, and 12 full-page plates in colors. Philadelphia: W. B. Saunders & Co., 1900. 718p. col. plates. DLC; DNLM; PPC; PU **00-4827**

SENN, Nicholas (1844-1908)
Medico-surgical aspects of the Spanish American War [by] Lieutenant-Colonel Dr. Nicholas Senn. . . . Chicago: American Medical Association Press, 1900. 379p. DLC; ICJ; NcD; NIC
00-4828

SENN, Nicholas (1844-1908)
A compact operating-case for military service; with a description of several new instruments for the same. Chicago, 1900. 8p. DNLM **00-4829**

SENN, Nicholas (1844-1908)
Compound fractures. (Address in surgery.) [Cleveland, 1900.] 30p. DNLM **00-4830**

SENN, Nicholas (1844-1908)
Medico-surgical aspects of the Spanish-American War. Chicago, 1900. 379p. 1 plan, 1 table. DLC; DNLM **00-4831**

SENN, Nicholas (1844-1908)
The physician as a scientist. Chicago, 1900. 8p. DNLM **00-4832**

SENN, Nicholas (1844-1908)
Restitution of the continuity of the tibia by transplantation of the patella into an extensive osteomyelitic defect. Philadelphia, 1900. 8p. DNLM **00-4833**

SENN, Nicholas (1844-1908)
The present status of the carcinoma question. Chicago, 1901. 36p. DNLM **00-4834**

SENN, Nicholas (1844-1908)
Principles of surgery . . . 3rd ed. Thoroughly rev. With 230 wood-engravings, half-tones, and colored illustrations. Philadelphia and Chicago: F. A. Davis Co., 1901. 699p. col. plates. DLC; DNLM; MBM; NNNAM; PPC **00-4835**

SENN, Nicholas (1844-1908)
Baccalaureate sermon delivered to the graduating class of Rush Medical College in affiliation with the University of Chicago, Sunday, June 1, 1901. . . . Notre Dame, Ind.: The Ave Maria, [1901]. 24p. DNLM; ICJ **00-4836**

SENN, Nicholas (1844-1908)
Practical surgery for the general practitioner. . . . With 650 illustrations, many of them in colors. Philadelphia and London: W. B. Saunders & Co., 1901. 1133p. col. plates. DLC; DNLM; IU-M; PPC; PU **00-4837**

SENN, Niholas (1844-1908)
A nurse's guide for the operating room. . . . Pub. under the direction of the Sisters of Charity, St. Joseph's Hospital . . . Chicago. Chicago: W. T. Keener & Co., [1902]. 127p. DLC: ICJ; IU-M **00-4838**

SENN, Nicholas (1844-1908)
Around the world via Siberia. . . . Chicago: W. B. Conkey Co., [1902]. 402p. plates. DLC: ICJ **00-4839**

SENN, Nicholas (1844-1908)
Life and work of the late Professor Christian Fenger. Memorial address delivered to the graduating class of Rush Medical College, April 4, 1902. . . . [Chicago, 1902.] 12p. ICJ **00-4840**

SENN, Nicholas (1844-1908)
Case of splenomedullary leukaemia successfully treated by the use of the Röntgen ray. New York, 1903. 7p. DNLM **00-4841**

SENN, Nicholas (1844-1908)
A comparison between foreign and American surgery. [Chicago, 1903.] 11p. DNLM **00-4842**

SENN, Nicholas (1844-1908)
Constantinople as a medical center. [Chicago, 1903.] 9p. DNLM **00-4843**

SENN, Nicholas (1844-1908)
Echoes from the Madrid International Medical Congress. [Chicago, 1903.] 13p. DNLM **00-4844**

SENN, Nicholas (1844-1908)
The first dressing on the battlefield. Carlisle, 1903. 40p. DNLM **00-4845**

SENN, Nicholas (1844-1908)
Glimpses of the practice of medicine and diseases in the West Indies. [Chicago, 1903.] 13, 13p. DNLM **00-4846**

SENN, Nicholas (1844-1908)
Hospital work of Carl Lauenstein. [Chicago, 1903.] 7p. DNLM **00-4847**

SENN, Nicholas (1844-1908)
The hospitals of Jerusalem. [Chicago, 1903.] 8p. DNLM **00-4848**

SENN, Nicholas (1844-1908)
Iodized catgut. Chicago, 1903. 6p. DNLM **00-4849**

SENN, Nicholas (1844-1908)
The medical institutions of Madrid. [Chicago, 1903.] 13p. DNLM **00-4850**

SENN, Nicholas (1844-1908)
Medical institutions of St. Petersburg. [Chicago, 1903.] 5p. DNLM **00-4851**

SENN, Nicholas (1844-1908)
Medical London in summer. [Chicago, 1903.] 10p. DNLM **00-4852**

SENN, Nicholas (1844-1908)
Medical Paris. [Chicago, 1903.] 4p. DNLM **00-4853**

SENN, Nicholas (1844-1908)
Medical practice in Cairo, and prevailing diseases of Egypt. [Chicago, 1903.] 9p. DNLM **00-4854**

SENN, Nicholas (1844-1908)
Medical and surgical notes from Asia. [Chicago, 1903.] 7p. DNLM **00-4855**

SENN, Nicholas (1844-1908)
The Pirogoff Museum, St. Petersburg. [Chicago, 1903.] 4p. DNLM **00-4856**

SENN, Nicholas (1844-1908)
Present surgical methods in the General Hospital, Hamburg-Eppendorf. [Chicago, 1903.] 14p. DNLM **00-4857**

SENN, Nicholas (1844-1908)
Professor Hoffa's orthopedic work. [Chicago, 1903.] 5p. DNLM **00-4858**

SENN, Nicholas (1844-1908)
Professor John Berg's surgical clinic. [Chicago, 1903.] 6p. DNLM **00-4859**

SENN, Nicholas (1844-1908)
Professor Nicoladoni's clinic, Gratz. [Chicago, 1903.] 8p. DNLM **00-4860**

SENN, Nicholas (1844-1908)
Professor Sonenburg and his appendicitis work at the Moabit Hospital. [Chicago, 1903.] 4p. DNLM
00-4861

SENN, Nicholas (1844-1908)
The proper perineal prostatectomy incision. Chicago, 1903. 7p. DNLM **00-4862**

SENN, Nicholas (1844-1908)
Renal surgery as practised by Professor James Israel. [Chicago, 1903.] 3p. DNLM **00-4863**

SENN, Nicholas (1844-1908)
The scalp face; a new plastic operation. New York, 1903. 16p. DNLM **00-4864**

SENN, Nicholas (1844-1908)
The seventh conference of the International Red Cross. [Chicago, 1903.] 3p. DNLM **00-4865**

SENN, Nicholas (1844-1908)
Subcutaneous drainage in the surgical treatment of hydrocephalus internus. St. Louis, 1903. 9p. 4 plates. DNLM
00-4866

SENN, Nicholas (1844-1908)
Surgical notes from four continents and the West Indies. [Twenty papers, paged separately. [Chicago, 1903.] DNLM
00-4867

SENN, Nicholas (1844-1908)
Surgical observations in Berlin; Professor Olshausen's gynecologic clinic; the Augusta Hospital. [Chicago, 1903.] 13p. DNLM **00-4868**

SENN, Nicholas (1844-1908)
The surgical treatment of traumatic hemorrhage of the spleen. Chicago: American Medical Assoc., 1903. 13p. DNLM
00-4869

SENN, Nicholas (1844-1908)
Surgical work of Professor von Mosetig-Moorhof in the Vienna Allgemeine Krankenhaus. [Chicago, 1903.] 10p. DNLM
00-4870

SENN, Nicholas (1844-1908)
The teaching and practice of surgery in the Vienna Allgemeine Krankenhaus. [Chicago, 1903.] 7p. DNLM
00-4871

SENN, Nicholas (1844-1908)
The therapeutic value of the Röntgen ray in the treatment of pseudoleucaemia. New York, 1903. 12p. DNLM
00-4872

SENN, Nicholas (1844-1908)
Tahiti from a medical standpoint. . . . Chicago: Press of the American Medical Assoc., 1904. 23p. ICJ
00-4873

SENN, Nicholas (1844-1908)
The needs and advantages of an international congress of military surgeons. Carlisle, 1905. 8p. DNLM
00-4874

SENN, Nicholas (1844-1908)
Father Damien, the leper hero. . . . Chicago: Press of the American Medical Assoc., 1905. 16p. DLC **00-4875**

SENN, Nicholas (1844-1908)
The surgical clinic of to-day; its status and methods of teaching. New York: A. R. Elliott Pub. Co., 1905. 16p. DNLM
00-4876

SENN, Nicholas (1844-1908)
Differential diagnosis between coxa vara and other static, inflammatory and traumatic affections of the hip joint. . . . Chicago: American Medical Assoc., 1905. 19p. ICJ
00-4877

SENN, Nicholas (1844-1908)
Address to the graduating class of the Mary Thompson Hospital Training School for Nurses. [Chicago], 1905. 48p. ICJ **00-4878**

SENN, Nicholas (1844-1908)
Around the world by way of India. A medical tour by Nicholas Senn. . . . Chicago: American Medical Assoc. Press, 1905. 347p. plates. ICJ **00-4879**

SENN, Nicholas (1844-1908)
First aid on the battlefield. Carlisle, 1906. 19p. DNLM
00-4880

SENN, Nicholas (1844-1908)
A plea for the international study of carcinoma. Chicago, 1906. 14p. DNLM; ICJ **00-4881**

SENN, Nicholas (1844-1908)
Fernand Henrotin. A commemorative address. [Chicago, 1907.] 8p. port. DNLM **00-4882**

SENN, Nicholas (1844-1908)
Tendon tissue versus catgut. Carlisle, Pa., 1907. 14p. DNLM
00-4883

SENN, Nicholas (1844-1908)
The choice of a profession. Address delivered before the graduating class of Omaha Medical College, Medical Depart. University of Nebraska May 23, 1907. 30p. ICJ
00-4884

SENN, Nicholas (1844-1908)
The etiology and classification of cystitis; paper read before the American Surgical Association. Philadelphia, [1908]. 39p. DNLM; PPC **00-4885**

SENN, Nicholas (1844-1908)
The scientific and practical value of hospital internship. . . . Chicago: American Medical Assoc., 1908. 7p. ICJ
00-4886

SENN, Nicholas (1844-1908)
Principles of surgery . . . 4th ed.—thoroughly rev. by Emanuel J. Senn . . . and Emanuel Friend. . . . With 231 wood-engravings, half-tones, and colored illustrations. Philadelphia: F. A. Davis Co., 1909. 706p. col. plates. DLC; NNNAM; OCIM; PPC **00-4887**

SEUFERT, Edward Constant (*b.* 1873)
Vade-mecum of treatment; a practical guide and index of treatment for the use of medical students and practitioners, by Edward C. Seufert . . . and John Stuart. . . . Chicago: W. T. Keener & Co, 1908. 332p. DLC; ICJ; IU-M; OCIM
00-4888

SEUFERT, Edward Constant (*b.* 1873)
Vade-mecum of treatment, a practical guide . . . for the use of medical students and practitioners, by Edward C. Seufert and John Stuart. [2nd ed.] Chicago: Chicago Medical Book Co., 1910. 454p. DLC; ICJ **00-4889**

SEWALL, Henry (1855-1936)
A preliminary note on the relation of the form of the tubercle bacillus to the clinical aspects of pulmonary tuberculosis. New York, 1901. 6p. DNLM **00-4890**

SEWALL, Henry (1855-1936)
Some relations of osmosis and ionic action in medicine. Philadelphia: J. B. Lippincott Co., 1901. 11p. DNLM **00-4891**

SEWALL, Henry (1855-1936)
Altitude in fact and fancy. Philadelphia, 1902. 6p. DNLM **00-4892**

SEWALL, Henry (1855-1936)
Physiological factors concerned in gallstone disease. Denver, 1903. 12p. DNLM **00-4893**

SEWALL, Henry (1855-1936)
Some considerations on the climatic treatment of consumption with especial reference to Denver as a health resort. Chicago, 1903. 4p. DNLM **00-4894**

SEWALL, Henry (1855-1936)
The effect upon edema of elaterium in non-purgative doses. Detroit: E. G. Swift, 1904. 10p. DNLM **00-4895**

SEWALL, Henry (1855-1936)
Some points in modern theories of immunity. Denver, 1904. 16p. DNLM **00-4896**

SEWALL, Henry (1855-1936)
Observations on the duty of the physician to his patients through the surgeon. Philadelphia, 1904. 7p. DNLM **00-4897**

SEWALL, Henry (1855-1936)
Experiments on venous blood pressure and its relations to arterial pressure in man. Chicago, 1906. 31p. DNLM **00-4898**

SEWALL, Henry (1855-1936)
An extraordinary case of anthracosis simulating thoracic aneurysm. [Philadelphia], 1906. 9p. DNLM **00-4899**

SEWALL, Henry (1855-1936) and S. B. CHILDS
The interpretation of X-ray pictures as an aid to the early diagnosis of thoracic aneurysm. Philadelphia, 1907. 11p. DNLM **00-4900**

SEWALL, Henry (1855-1936)
Observations on the failure of the radical pulse when the arms are elevated. Chicago, 1908. 15p. DNLM **00-4901**

SEWALL, Henry (1855-1936)
Safeguards of the heart-beat. Philadelphia & New York, 1908. 14p. DNLM **00-4902**

SEWALL, Henry (1855-1936)
A new and simple device for exploratory aspiration. Chicago, 1909. 3p. DNLM **00-4903**

SEWALL, Henry (1855-1936)
The origin of the "new leather" and "dry friction" sounds heard on auscultation. Philadelphia & New York, 1909. 3p. DNLM **00-4904**

SEYMOUR, William P[ierce] (1825-1893)
Seymour's key to psychology and electro-therapeutics. Rochester, N.Y.: [Morrison's Press], 1902. 2 pts. in 1 v. DLC **00-4905**

SEYMOUR, William P[ierce] (1825-1893)
Seymour's key to electro-therapeutics. Newark, N.J.: [Privately Printed], 1902. 87p. CtY-M; DLC; N **00-4906**

SHAFFER, Philip A[nderson] (*b.* 1881)
The excretion of kreatinin and kreatin in health and disease. Boston, 1908. 22p. DNLM **00-4907**

SHAFFER, Philip A[nderson] (*b.* 1881)
Metabolism in typhoid fever. Chicago, 1908. 11p. DNLM **00-4908**

SHALLER, John M. (1856-1931)
A therapeutic guide to alkaloidal dosimetric medication . . . 2nd ed., enl. and rev. Chicago: Clinic Pub. Co., 1904. 424p. DNLM; NcD **00-4909**

SHANAHAN, William T. (*b.* 1878)
Acute pulmonary oedema as a complication of epileptic seizures. New York, 1908. 10p. DNLM **00-4910**

SHANAHAN, William T. (*b.* 1878)
Why the marriage of defectives should be prevented when possible. . . . Brooklyn, N.Y.: Eagle Press, 1901. 7p. DLC; NN **00-4911**

SHANDS, Aurelius Rives (*b.* 1860)
Excision of the shoulder-joint. Richmond, 1900. 6p. DNLM **00-4912**

SHANDS, Aurelius Rives (*b.* 1860)
The treatment of supra condyloid fracture of the humerus. New York, 1900. 10p. DNLM **00-4913**

SHANDS, Aurelius Rives (*b.* 1860)
The early diagnosis and treatment of hip disease. New York, 1902. 7p. DNLM **00-4914**

SHANDS, Aurelius Rives (*b.* 1860)
Gant's femoral osteotomy. New York, 1902. 6p. DNLM **00-4915**

SHANDS, Aurelius Rives (*b.* 1860)
Pott's disease and some of its complications. Richmond, 1902. 15p. DNLM **00-4916**

SHANDS, Aurelius Rives (*b.* 1860)
Treatment of lateral curvature of the spine. New York, 1906. 17p. DNLM **00-4917**

SHANDS, Aurelius Rives (*b.* 1860)
Report of cases of unusual derangement of the knee-joint. Richmond, 1907. 16p. DNLM **00-4918**

SHARP & SMITH [CO.] (CHICAGO)
Catalogue of surgical instruments. . . . Chicago, [1900?]. 963p. ICJ **00-4919**

SHARP & SMITH [CO.] (CHICAGO)
. . . Catalogue of Sharp & Smith, importers, manufacturers, wholesale and retail dealers in surgical instruments, deformity apparatus . . . 18th ed. Chicago, [1901?] [275]-914p., 987-1014p. ICJ **00-4920**

SHARPE, Henry G[ranville] (*b.* 1858)
The provisioning of the modern army in the field. Kansas City: F. Hudson Co., 1905. 116p. 12 plates. DLC; DNLM; MH; NN **00-4921**

SHARPE, Henry G[ranville] (*b.* 1858)
The provisioning of the modern army in the field. . . . Rev. and rearranged by Captain Frank A. Cook . . . (2nd ed.) Kansas City, Mo.: F. Hudson Publishing Co., 1909. 96p. DLC: ICJ; NN **00-4922**

SHARPE, Norvelle W[allace]
Upon drainage of the abdominal cavity; with excerpts from the literature. St. Louis, 1900. 12p. DNLM **00-4923**

SHARPE, Norvelle W[allace]
Upon certain fractures. St. Louis, 1901. 24p. DNLM **00-4924**

SHASTID, Thomas H[all] (1866-1947)
Pterygium. Nashville, 1905. 12p. DNLM **00-4925**

SHASTID, Thomas H[all] (1866-1947)
A case of gratitude; spontaneous recovery. St. Louis, 1906. 7p. DNLM **00-4926**

SHASTID, Thomas H[all] (1866-1947)
How to suppress a malpractice suit, and other medical miscellanies. Marion. Marion Pub. Co., 1906. 128p. DNLM **00-4927**

SHASTID, Thomas H[all] (1866-1947)
The mastoid operations. Philadelphia, 1906. 12p. DNLM **00-4928**

SHASTID, Thomas H[all] (1866-1947)
Trials at the trial case. New York, 1906. 9p. DNLM **00-4929**

SHASTID, Thomas H[all] (1866-1947)
What is the primary cause of mal-legislation and non-legislation with regard to medical matters? Easton, 1907. 7p. DNLM **00-4930**

SHATTUCK, Frederick C[heever] (1847-1929)
Some thoughts on medical education. Boston: Damrell & Upham, 1900. 22p. DNLM **00-4931**

SHATTUCK, Frederick C[heever] (1847-1929)
Specialism in medicine. Chicago, 1900. 11p. DNLM **00-4932**

SHATTUCK, Frederick C[heever] (1847-1929)
Prognosis and treatment of tuberculous peritonitis as based on the experience of the Massachusetts General Hospital for the past ten years. Philadelphia, 1902. 16p. DNLM **00-4933**

SHATTUCK, Frederick C[heever] (1847-1929)
Prognosis and treatment of tuberculous peritonitis as based on the experience of the Massachusetts General Hospital for the past ten years. Philadelphia & New York, 1902. 12p. DNLM **00-4934**

SHATTUCK, Frederick C[heever] (1847-1929)
Anomalies of the thyroid secretion. Boston: Old Corner Book Store, 1904. 18p. DNLM **00-4935**

SHATTUCK, Frederick C[heever] (1847-1929)
The general management of diabetes. [New York, 1904.] 8p. DNLM **00-4936**

SHATTUCK, Frederick C[heever] (1847-1929)
The medical treatment of gastric ulcer and hyperchlorhydria. Boston, 1905. 14p. DNLM **00-4937**

SHATTUCK, Frederick C[heever] (1847-1929)
A case of hypernephroma. Boston, 1906. 3p. DNLM **00-4938**

SHATTUCK, Frederick C[heever] (1847-1929)
The clinics of the Harvard Medical School. [Boston], 1906. 6p. DNLM **00-4939**

SHATTUCK, Frederick C[heever] (1847-1929)
Depletion in heart disease. Boston, 1906. 5p. DNLM **00-4940**

SHATTUCK, Frederick C[heever] (1847-1929)
The dietetic treatment of nephritis. Chicago, 1906. 8p. DNLM **00-4941**

SHATTUCK, Frederick C[heever] (1847-1929)
How progress comes in medicine. Chicago, 1906. 9p. DNLM **00-4942**

SHATTUCK, Frederick C[heever] (1847-1929)
Method of instruction in the Harvard Medical School. Boston, 1906. 19p. DNLM **00-4943**

SHATTUCK, Frederick C[heever] (1847-1929)
The value of drugs in therapeutics. Boston, 1906. 11p. DNLM **00-4944**

SHATTUCK, Frederick C[heever] (1847-1929)
The past, present, and future of tuberculosis. Boston, 1907. 30p. DNLM **00-4945**

SHATTUCK, Frederick C[heever] (1847-1929)
The medical treatment of gastric ulcer and hyperchlorhydria. [1908.] 6p. MB **00-4946**

SHATTUCK, Frederick C[heever] (1847-1929)
Address to the candidates for degrees. University of Cincinnati, June 6, 1908. Cincinnati, 1908. 11p. DNLM **00-4947**

SHATTUCK, George B[rune] (1844-1923) and J. Collins WARREN, *et al.*
A study of twenty-four cases of typhoid fever with symptoms of peritoneal inspection; laparotomy. Boston: Damrell & Upham, 1900. 16p. DNLM; MBM **00-4948**

SHAW, Clara S.
A text-book of nursing, for the use of training schools, families, and private students . . . 3rd ed., thoroughly rev. and enl. New York: D. Appleton & Co., 1902. 397p. col. plate, fold. diag. DLC; MBM; NNNAM; PU
00-4949

SHAW, Harold Batty (*b.* 1866)
Organotherapy, or treatment by means of preparations of various organs. Chicago: W. T. Keener & Co., 1905. 256p. DNLM; ICJ; OCIM **00-4950**

SHAW, Harold Batty (*b.* 1866)
Organotherapy, or treatment by means of preparations of various organs. New York: Funk & Wagnalls Co., 1910. 256p. DLC; MH; NIC; NN **00-4951**

SHAW, John C[argyll] (1845-1900)
Essentials of nervous diseases and insanity; their symptoms and treatment. A manual for students and practitioners. 4th ed., thoroughly revised by Smith Ely Jelliffe. Philadelphia: W. B. Saunders & Co., 1904. 196p. DLC; DNLM; NNNAM; PPC
00-4952

SHAW-MACKENZIE John Alexander (*b.* 1857)
The nature and treatment of cancer. (Some methods of hypodermic medication in the treatment of inoperable cancer.) 3rd ed., revised and enlarged. New York: William Wood & Co., 1906. 99p. CtY-M; DNLM; NNNAM; PU
00-4953

SHEARER, James Y.
Quinine sulphate. New York, 1907. 8p. DNLM
00-4954

SHED, Zach
. . . A concise and rational course in hypnotism, personal magnetism, physical culture, health breathing, and magnetic bathing, together with complete instructions for the treatment of pain and disease by the use of magnetism. By Professor Zach Shed. . . . [Denver? Col.], 1900. 63p. DLC
00-4955

SHED, Zach
Mounte Bank, M.D. Member American medical trust. Member state medical trust. Member county medical trust. Member politico-religious trust. . . . Expose by Hon. Zach Shed. . . . Chicago: Association Independent Doctors (Incorporated), [1909]. 16p. DLC **00-4956**

SHEDD, Percy William (*b.* 1870)
The clinic repertory . . . including a repertory of time modalities, by Dr. Ide, of Stettin, Germany, transl. from the Berliner zeitschrift homöopathischer aerzte, band XXV., hefte 3 and 4. Philadelphia: Boericke & Tafel, 1908. 240p. DLC; DNLM; PPC; PPHa **00-4957**

SHEDD, Percy William (*b.* 1870)
Arsenicum; a challenging study. New York, 1906. 8p. NN
00-4958

SHEEDY, Bryan D[e F.]
Tonsil removal opsonic index, and immunity. New York: William Wood & Co., 1909. 8p. DNLM; NN
00-4959

SHEEDY, Bryan D[e F.]
Physiognomy; post-operative treatment of adenoid patients, deformity of nose corrected by the use of paraffin. New York, [1909]. 16p. DNLM; NN **00-4960**

SHEFFIELD, Herman B[ernard] (*b.* 1871)
Palatable medication. [New York, 1906.] 9p. DNLM
00-4961

SHEFFIELD, Herman B[ernard] (*b.* 1871)
Modern diagnosis and treatment of diseases of children; a treatise on the medical and surgical diseases of infancy and childhood, with especial emphasis upon clinical diagnosis and modern therapeutics. For practitioners and students of medicine . . . with one hundred and fifty original half-tone photoengravings and numerous smaller illustrations, some in colors. Philadelphia: F. A. Davis Co., 1910. 619p. DLC; ICJ; PPC; PPJ **00-4962**

SHEILD, A[rthur] Marmaduke (1858-1922)
Lectures on nasal obstruction. . . . With one coloured plate and 27 illustrations in the text. Philadelphia: P. Blakiston's Son & Co., 1901. 106p. CtY-M; ICJ; NNC; PU
00-4963

SHELDON, John G[lendon] (*b.* 1873)
The treatment of crushing injuries involving one articular surface of an interphalangeal joint. New York, 1904. 5p. DNLM; NN **00-4964**

SHELDON, John G[lendon] (*b.* 1873)
Biliary colic without gallstones. New York: A. R. Elliott Co., 1905. 6p. DNLM **00-4965**

SHELDON, John G[lendon] (*b.* 1873)
The indications for operative treatment, together with some suggestions as to surgical procedure. Designed to be a concise handbook for ready reference. Chicago: Cleveland Press, 1905. 423p. DLC; DNLM; ICJ; OCIM **00-4966**

SHELMERDINE, E. Kirkland
Ready methods of formulating modified milk mixtures. New York: A. R. Elliott Pub. Co., 1904. 13p. DNLM
00-4967

SHELMERDINE, E. Kirkland
Cream and whole milk calculation. New York, 1907. 4p. DNLM **00-4968**

SHELMERDINE, E. Kirkland
Winter diarrhoeas in infant feeding. New York, 1908. 4p. DNLM **00-4969**

SHEPARD, Charles Henry (1825-1910)
Hygiene of the Turkish bath. Brooklyn, N.Y., 1900. 32p. port. DNLM **00-4970**

SHEPARD, Charles Henry (1825-1910)
Turkish baths; the most important factor in personal hygiene. Brooklyn, 1900. 16p. 1 plate. DNLM
00-4971

SHEPARD, Charles Henry (1825-1910)
Insanity and the Turkish bath. Chicago, 1900. 7p. DNLM
00-4972

SHEPARD, Charles Henry (1825-1910)
Auto-intoxication and its treatment. Philadelphia, 1902. 10p. DNLM **00-4973**

SHEPARD, Charles Henry (1825-1910)
Ergoapiol in diseases of the female. New York, 1902. 8p. DNLM **00-4974**

SHEPARD, Charles Henry (1825-1910)
Shepard's Turkish baths, Russian and Roman, and massage. Brooklyn, 1905. 6 l. DNLM **00-4975**

SHEPARD, Hiram Hur (*b.* 1868)
Bacteria in foods; a treatise on the conservation of health; or the scientific preparation of pure food. . . . Chicago: A. Flanagan Co., [1910]. 32p. DLC; ICJ **00-4976**

SHEPHERD, Francis J[ohn] (1851-1924)
Rupture of the axillary vein in reducing an old dislocation of the shoulder. Philadelphia: J. B. Lippincott Co., 1902. 3p. DNLM **00-4977**

SHEPHERD, Francis J[ohn] (1851-1924)
Two cases of blastomycetic dermatitis, one of which was cured by iodid of potassium. New York, 1902. 6p. DNLM **00 4978**

SHEPHERD, Francis J[ohn] (1851-1924)
Note on a rapid method of diagnosis in leprosy. New York: Grafton Press, 1903. 3p. DNLM **00-4979**

SHERIDAN, J. P.
Four cases of diabetes mellitus. New York, 1900. 7p. DNLM **00-4980**

SHERIFF, Dewitt H.
The premature infant. New York, 1905. 13p. DNLM **00-4981**

SHERIFF, Dewitt H.
Concerning the first week of infant life. New York, 1908. 12p. DNLM **00-4982**

SHERMAN, Harry M[itchell] (*b.* 1854) and Thomas W. HUNTINGTON
Two cases of peripheral gangrene associated with localized disease of the arteries. Chicago, 1902. 5p. DNLM **00-4983**

SHERMAN, Harry M[itchell] (*b.* 1854) and G. J. McCHESNEY
Congenital dislocation of the hip. San Francisco, 1910. 9p. NN **00-4984**

SHERMAN, Harry M[itchell] (*b.* 1854)
The future of heart surgery. San Francisco, 1910. 8p. NN **00-4985**

SHERREN, James (*b.* 1872)
Injuries of nerves and their treatment. New York: William Wood & Co., 1908. 310p. ICJ; NcD; PPC; PPJ **00-4986**

SHERRINGTON, Charles Scott (1857-1952)
The integrative action of the nervous system. New Haven: Yale University Press, [*c.* 1906]. 141p. CtY-M; MH; NNC; PU [(Hepsa Ely Silliman memorial lectures)] **00-4987**

SHERRINGTON, Charles Scott (1857-1952)
The integrative action of the nervous system. . . . New York: C. Scribner's Sons, 1906. 411p. diags. CtY-M; DLC; DNLM; NNNAM **00-4988**

SHIELDS, A. W.
Observations in the treatment of irregular menstruation. New York, 1904. 8p. DNLM **00-4989**

SHIMER, Miles Herman (*b.* 1873)
Pennsylvania pharmacy laws, 1887-1905: a digest of the laws of Pennsylvania, regulating the sale of drugs and the practice of pharmacy, by Miles H. Shimer, Ph.G. Comp. and annotated by Walter Tresse Singer. . . . Philadelphia: Walther Printing House, 1905. 15p. DLC; PP; PPF **00-4990**

SHIVELY, Henry L.
The incidence of pulmonary tuberculosis in large families. New York, 1905. 7p. DNLM **00-4991**

SHIVELY, Henry L.
A clinical study of myoidema with especial reference to its occurrence in pulmonary tuberculosis. New York: A. R. Elliott Co., 1905. 15p. DNLM **00-4992**

SHIVELY, Henry L.
District nursing and extra diet in the treatment of tuberculous patients at the Presbyterian Hospital Dispensary. New York: A. R. Elliott Co., 1907. 10p. DNLM **00-4993**

SHIVELY, Henry L.
Experiences with the conjunctival and cutaneous tuberculin tests at the tube[r] culosis clinic of the Presbyterian Hospital. New York: William Wood & Co., 1908. 20p. NN **00-4994**

SHOBER, John B.
Recurrent tuberculous peritonitis after incomplete operation, with a report of such a case treated by the X-rays. New York, 1905. 7p. DNLM **00-4995**

SHOEMAKER, George Erety
Differences in the management of appendicitis and of salpingitis. New York, 1903. 6p. DNLM; NN **00-4996**

SHOEMAKER, George Erety
Significance and management of chronic uterine haemorrhage. New York: A. R. Elliott Pub. Co., 1905. 15p. DNLM; NN **00-4997**

SHOEMAKER, George Erety
Cases illustrating three methods of hysterectomy for different indications. Philadelphia, [1905]. 10p. DNLM; NN **00-4998**

SHOEMAKER, Harlan
Backward and defective children. New York, 1907. 9p. DNLM **00-4999**

SHOEMAKER, Harlan
Bacterial vaccines of staphylococci stains, a technique for their preparations. New York, 1908. 11p. DNLM **00-5000**

SHOEMAKER, Harlan
Observations on prophylactic inoculations against typhoid fever. New York, 1909. 7p. DNLM **00-5001**

SHOEMAKER, John V[ietch] (1852-1910)
. . . A practical treatise on materia medica and therapeutics, with especial reference to the clinical application of drugs; . . . 5th ed. Thoroughly rev. Philadelphia, New York, [etc.]: F. A. Davis Co., 1900. 766p. DLC; DNLM; NNNAM; PPC [Students' ed.] **00-5002**

SHOEMAKER, John V[ietch] (1852-1910)
. . . A practical treatise on materia medica and therapeutics, with especial reference to the clinical application of drugs; . . . 5th ed. Philadelphia: F. A. Davis Co., 1901. 1143p. DNLM; OCLloyd; PPC; PU **00-5003**

SHOEMAKER, John V[ietch] (1852-1910)
A practical treatise on diseases of the skin . . . 4th ed., rev. and enl. . . . New York: D. Appleton & Co., 1901. 892p. plates. DLC; NNNAM; NNU-M; OC **00-5004**

SHOEMAKER, John V[ietch] (1852-1910)
A clinical study of organic iron. Philadelphia, 1903. 8p. DNLM **00-5005**

SHOEMAKER, John V[ietch] (1852-1910)
A case of Hodgkin's disease. New York: A. R. Elliott Pub. Co., 1904. 16p. DNLM **00-5006**

SHOEMAKER, John V[ietch] (1852-1910)
A further contribution to the therapeutics of iron. [Chicago], 1905. 6p. DNLM **00-5007**

SHOEMAKER, John V[ietch] (1852-1910)
The practical value of some old remedies; scopolamine hydrobromide. New York: A. R. Elliott, 1905. 11p. DNLM **00-5008**

SHOEMAKER, John V[ietch] (1852-1910)
Rheumatic fever (acute articular rheumatism). New York, 1906. 10p. DNLM **00-5009**

SHOEMAKER, John V[ietch] (1852-1910)
The scientific foundation of modern treatment of disease. [New York], 1906. 7p. DNLM **00-5010**

SHOEMAKER, John V[ietch] (1852-1910)
A practical treatise on materia medica and therapeutics, with especial reference to the clinical application of drugs . . . 6th ed. Thoroughly rev. Philadelphia: F. A. Davis Co., 1906. 1164p. DLC; IEN-M; NNNAM; PPC **00-5011**

SHOEMAKER, John V[ietch] (1852-1910)
Raynaud's disease. [New York], 1907. 5p. DNLM **00-5012**

SHOEMAKER, John V[ietch] (1852-1910)
Clinical lecture on diphtheritic paralysis. St. Louis, 1908. 7p. DNLM **00-5013**

SHOEMAKER, John V[ietch] (1852-1910)
Health and beauty. Philadelphia: F. A. Davis Co., 1908. 476p. DLC; ICJ; PP; PU **00-5014**

SHOEMAKER, John V[ietch] (1852-1910)
Therapeutics in the light of ecology. Philadelphia, 1908. 10p. DNLM **00-5015**

SHOEMAKER, John V[ietch] (1852-1910)
A practical treatise on materia medica and therapeutics, with special reference to the clinical application of drugs . . . 7th ed. Rev. Philadelphia: F. A. Davis Co., 1908. 1255p. DLC; OCLloyd; PPC; PU **00-5016**

SHOEMAKER, John V[ietch] (1852-1910)
Sodium, lithium, calcium, and magnesium, and their action in the treatment of disease. New York, 1909. 15p. DNLM **00-5017**

SHOEMAKER, John V[ietch] (1852-1910)
A practical treatise on diseases of the skin . . . 5th ed., rev. and enl. Illustrated with 29 half-tone plates containing 40 figures, nearly all original. Philadelphia: F. A. Davis Co., 1909. 1012p. DLC; NNNAM; OCIM; PPC **00-5018**

SHOEMAKER, William T[oy] (*b.* 1869)
Binasal hemianopsia; a case of neuritic optic atrophy with binasal hemianopic fields. New York, 1905. 16p. DNLM **00-5019**

SHOEMAKER, William T[oy] (*b.* 1869)
Retinitis pigmentosa, with an analysis of seventeen cases occurring in deaf-mutes; being an essay for which was awarded the Alvarenga Prize of the College of Physicians of Philadelphia, July, 1908. by William T. Shoemaker. . . . Laboratory examinations of the blood and urine, by John M. Swan . . . with illustrations and three colored plates. . . . Philadelphia: J. B. Lippincott Co., [1909]. 106p. col. plates. DLC; ICJ; PPC; PPJ **00-5020**

SHRADY, John, ed. (1830-1914)
The College of Physicians and Surgeons, New York, and its founders, officers, instructors, benefactors and alumni; a history. . . . New York, Chicago: The Lewis Publishing Co., [*c.* 1903]. 2 v. DLC; NIC; NNC; PU **00-5021**

SHROYER, Samuel Grant
The science of health, holiness and happiness; a complete treatise on the practice and principles of divine healing. How to get well, and remain well, in a divinely natural way. The true plan of salvation. . . . Oklahoma City, 1901 [*c.* 1897]. 205p. DLC **00-5022**

SHUFELDT, R[obert] W[ilson] (1850-1934)
Havelock Ellis on sexual inversion. San Francisco, 1902. 9p. DNLM **00-5023**

SHUFELDT, R[obert] W[ilson] (1850-1934)
Wm. Lee Howard on the perverts. San Francisco, 1902. 8p. DNLM **00-5024**

SHUFELDT, R[obert] W[ilson] (1850-1934)
Impotency, medically and legally considered. San Francisco, 1905. 8p. DNLM **00-5025**

SHUFELDT, R[obert] W[ilson] (1850-1934)
The medico-legal consideration of perverts and inverts. San Francisco, 1905. 9p. DNLM **00-5026**

SHUFELDT, R[obert] W[ilson] (1850-1934)
The alienist in the courts of law. [n. p., 1907.] 8p. DLC; DNLM **00-5027**

SHUFELDT, R[obert] W[ilson] (1850-1934)
Studies of the human form for artists, sculptors and scientists. Philadelphia, Pa.: F. A. Davis Co., [1908]. 642p. illus. DLC; MB; NIC; NN [Title vignette.] **00-5028**

SHUMWAY, Edward A[dams] (*b.* 1870)
Carcinomatous degeneration of a papilloma of the conjunctiva with infiltration of the eyelids. [Philadelphia, 1901.] 6p. PU **00-5029**

SHUMWAY, Edward A[dams] (*b.* 1870)
Papilloma of the caruncle, with a report of a case. [Philadelphia, 1902.] 8p. PU **00-5030**

SHUMWAY, Edward A[dams] (*b.* 1870)
Note on the histology of vernal conjunctivitis, Fruehjahr's catarrh. [Philadelphia, 1903.] 6p. PU **00-5031**

SHUMWAY, Edward A[dams] (*b.* 1870)
Conjunctivitis nodos with histological examination. [Philadelphia, 1906.] 8p. PU **00-5032**

SHUMWAY, Edward A[dams] (*b.* 1870) and Mary BUCHANAN
Histological examination of the eyes in a case of amaurotic family idiocy. Philadelphia, 1906. 6p. DNLM **00-5033**

SHUMWAY, Edward A[dams] (*b.* 1870)
Carcinoma of the eyelids with secondary involvement of the eyeball, removal of the growth by extensive plastic operations; recurrence. [Philadelphia, 1907.] 3p. PU **00-5034**

SHURLY, Burt Russell (*b.* 1871)
Prolonged intubation tubes, with a method leading to their extraction. Chicago, 1903. 9p. DNLM **00-5035**

SHURLY, Ernest L[orenzo] (1849-1913)
A treatise on diseases of the nose and throat. . . . New York: D. Appleton & Co., 1900. 744p. col. plates. DLC; MBM; NNNAM; PPC **00-5036**

SHURLY, Ernest L[orenzo] (1849-1913)
Some reasons against the public registration or notification of cases of phthisis pulmonalis. New York, 1902. 9p. DNLM **00-5037**

SHURLY, Ernest L[orenzo] (1849-1913)
Disease of the thyroid gland as a cause of functional sensory disorders. Detroit, [1902]. 10p. DNLM **00-5038**

SHURLY, Ernest L[orenzo] (1849-1913)
The sanitorium treatment of phthisis pulmonalis. Detroit, 1903. 4p. DNLM **00-5039**

SHURLY, Ernest L[orenzo] (1849-1913)
The treatment of chronic nontuberculous inflammation of the lungs and pleura. Detroit & Ann Arbor, 1904. 6p. DNLM **00-5040**

SHURLY, Ernest L[orenzo] (1849-1913)
County sanatoria for tuberculosis and other chronic pulmonary affections. Detroit, 1905. 2p. DNLM **00-5041**

SHURLY, Ernest L[orenzo] (1849-1913)
Remarks on the problems connected with the study of pulmonary tuberculosis; and suggestions of a new plan for improving statistics relating to the disease. New York, 1905. 8p. DNLM **00-5042**

SHURLY, Ernest L[orenzo] (1849-1913)
The treatment of chronic pleuritis and empyema. Ann Arbor & Detroit, 1905. 8p. DNLM **00-5043**

SHURLY, Ernest L[orenzo] (1849-1913)
A treatise on diseases of the nose and throat . . . 2nd ed., rev.; two hundred and twenty-five illustrations in the text and six plates in colors. New York and London: D. Appleton & Co., 1905. 744p. DLC; LNT-M; NNNAM; PPC **00-5044**

SHURLY, Ernest L[orenzo] (1849-1913)
Address on climatology. [New York], 1906. 6p. DNLM **00-5045**

SHUTE, Daniel Kerfoot (*b.* 1858)
A first book in organic evolution. . . . Chicago: The Open Court Publishing Co.; [etc., etc.], 1901 [*c.* 1899]. 285p. col. plates. DLC. ICJ **00-5046**

SHUTE, Daniel Kerfoot (*b.* 1858)
. . . The philosophical foundations of charlatanry in medicine. . . . Washington, D.C.: The University, [1908]. 12p. DLC [George Washington University Publications] **00-5047**

SHUTE, Daniel Kerfoot (*b.* 1858)
. . . Reflex neuroses with particular reference to eyestrain. . . . Washington, D.C.: The University, [1908]. 6p. DLC [George Washington University Publications] **00-5048**

SHUTTLEWORTH, George E[dward] (1842-1928)
Mentally-deficient children; their treatment and training. 2nd ed. Philadelphia: P. Blakiston's Son & Co., 1900. 180p. CtY-M; DNLM; MH-M; PPC **00-5049**

SHUTTLEWORTH, George E[dward] (1842-1928)
Mentally-deficient children, their treatment and training, by G. E. Shuttleworth . . . and W. A. Potts . . . 3rd ed. Philadelphia: P. Blakiston's Son & Co., 1910. 236p. 18 plates, fold. table. DLC; MH; NIC; NN [Appendix: A. Public and charitable institutions in Great Britain and Ireland for mentally deficient children and adults. B. American state public institutions for "feeble-minded." C. Speaking exercises. D. Bibliography.] **00-5050**

SIDIS, Boris (1867-1923)
Psychopathological researches; studies in mental dissociation, with text figures and ten plates; Boris Sidis . . . director of the Psychological Laboratory. Pub. under the auspices of the trustees of the Psychopathic Hospital, department of the New York Infirmary for Women and Children. New York, [etc.]: G. E. Stechert, 1902. 329p. plates. DLC; ICJ; NNNAM; PU **00-5051**

SIDIS, Boris (1867-1923) and Morton PRINCE, *et al.*
A contribution to the pathology of hysteria based upon an experimental study of a case of hemianesthesia with clonic convulsive attacks simulating Jacksonian epilepsy. Boston, 1904. 15p. DNLM **00-5052**

SIDIS, Boris (1867-1923)
. . . An inquiry into the nature of hallucination. New York: The Macmillan Co., 1904. 47p. NNC
00-5053

SIDIS, Boris (1867-1923) and Simon P. GOODHART
Multiple personality. An experimental investigation into the nature of human individuality. New York: D. Appleton & Co., 1905. 462p. CtY-M; DLC; NN; ICJ
00-5054

SIDIS, Boris (1867-1923)
Studies in psychopathology. Boston: D. C. Heath & Co., 1907. 73p. ICU; MH **00-5055**

SIDIS, Boris (1867-1923)
Psychopathological researches; studies in mental dissociation, with text figures and ten plates. . . . Boston: R. G. Badger, 1908. 329p. MH; NIC; NN; PU **00-5056**

SIDIS, Boris (1867-1923)
An experimental study of sleep (from the physiological laboratory of the Harvard Medical School and from Sidis' laboratory). . . . Boston: R. G. Badger, 1909. 106p. DLC; ICJ; NIC; PU **00-5057**

SIHLER, Christian
The hydriatic treatment of typhoid fever, according to Brand, Tripier and Bouveret, and Vogl. . . . Cleveland, O.: C. Sihler, [1900?] 340p. diags., fold. forms. DLC; ICJ
00-5058

SILE, Ira S.
The value of differential leucocyte counts in medicine. New York: A. R. Elliott Co., 1907. 8p. DNLM
00-5059

SILL, Elisha Mather (*b.* 1873)
Infantile bronchitis. New York, 1904. 12p. DNLM
00-5060

SILL, Elisha Mather (*b.* 1873)
Adenoids, as seen from the paediatrist's standpoint; the frequency in childhood, and importance of early diagnosis and treatment. Observations based on 1,000 personal cases operated in. New York: A. R. Elliott Publ. Co., 1905. 10p. DNLM
00-5061

SILL, Elisha Mather (*b.* 1873)
The management of summer diarrhoea in infants and young children. Observations based on 5,000 cases, in private and dispensary practice. New York: A. R. Elliott, 1905. 11p. DNLM **00-5062**

SILL, Elisha Mather (*b.* 1873)
Is sterilized milk a safe food for infants? New York, 1908. 8p. DNLM **00-5063**

SIME, David
Rabies; its place amongst germ-diseases, and its origin in the animal kingdom. New York: G. P. Putnam's Sons, 1903. 290p. DLC; MH-M; NNNAM; PU **00-5064**

SIMMONS, Channing C. (*b.* 1877)
Osteogenesis imperfecta and idiopathic fragilitas ossium. Philadelphia, 1907. 11p. 2 plates. DNLM
00-5065

SIMON, Charles E[dmund] (1866-1927)
A manual of clinical diagnosis by means of microscopic and chemical methods, for students, hospital physicians, and practitioners. 3rd ed. Philadelphia & New York: Lea Bros. & Co., 1900. 558p. 18 plates. DLC; DNLM; NNNAM; PPC
00-5066

SIMON, Charles E[dmund] (1866-1927)
A text-book of physiological chemistry for students of medicine and physicians. Philadelphia & New York: Lea Bros. & Co., 1901. 453p. DLC; DNLM; NIC; PPJ
00-5067

SIMON, Charles E[dmund] (1866-1927)
A manual of clinical diagnosis by means of microscopic and chemical methods, for students, hospital physicians, and practitioners. 4th ed., thoroughly revised. New York: Lea Bros. & Co., 1902. 599p. 19 col. plates. DLC; NNNAM; PPC; PPJ
00-5068

SIMON, Charles E[dmund] (1866-1927)
A manual of clinical diagnosis by means of microscopic and chemical methods, for students, hospital physicians, and practitioners. 5th ed., thoroughly revised and enlarged. Philadelphia: Lea Bros. & Co., 1904. 695p. 25 plates. DLC; DNLM; NNNAM; PPC **00-5069**

SIMON, Charles E[dmund] (1866-1927)
A text-book of physiological chemistry for students of medicine and physicians. 2nd ed., revised and enlarged. New York & Philadelphia: Lea Bros. & Co., 1904. 500p. DLC; DNLM; PPC; PU **00-5070**

SIMON, Charles E[dmund] (1866-1927) and R. V. LAMAR
A method of estimating the opsonic content of blood and other fluids. [Baltimore, 1906.] 3p. DNLM
00-5071

SIMON, Charles E[dmund] (1866-1927)
A text-book of physiological chemistry for students of medicine and physicians. 3rd ed., thoroughly revised. Philadelphia & New York: Lea Bros. & Co., 1907. 490p. DLC; DNLM; NN; PU **00-5072**

SIMON, Charles E[dmund] (1866-1927)
The Bedford mineral water. [Baltimore, 1907.] 8p. DNLM
00-5073

SIMON, Charles E[dmund] (1866-1927)
A manual for clinical diagnosis by means of microscopic and chemical methods, for students, hospital physicians, and practitioners, 6th ed., thoroughly revised. Philadelphia & New York: Lea Bros. & Co., 1907. 682p. DLC; DNLM; MBM; PU **00-5074**

SIMON, Charles E[dmund] (1866-1927) and Walter S. THOMAS
On complement-fixation in malignant disease. New York, 1909. 17p. DNLM **00-5075**

SIMON, Charles E[dmund] (1866-1927)
A manual of clinical diagnosis by means of laboratory methods, for students, hospital physicians, and practitioners . . . 7th ed., enl. and thoroughly rev. Illustrated with 168 engravings and 25 plates. Philadelphia and New York: Lea & Febiger, 1910. 778p. DLC; ICJ; PPC; PPJ
00-5076

SIMON, William (1844-1916)
Manual of chemistry. A guide to lectures and laboratory work for beginners in chemistry. A text-book specially adapted for students of medicine, pharmacy, and dentistry . . . 7th ed., thoroughly rev. . . . Philadelphia and New York: Lea Bros. & Co., 1901. 613p. col. plates. DLC; NNNAM; PPC; PU
00-5077

SIMON, William (1844-1916)
History of the Baltimore College of Dental Surgery . . . [4th International Dental Congress, St. Louis, Mo., 1904] . . . . Philadelphia, 1904. 36p. MdU-D; PPC
00-5078

SIMON, William (1844-1916)
Manual of chemistry. A guide to lectures and laboratory work for beginners in chemistry. A text-book specially adapted for students of medicine, pharmacy, and dentistry . . . 8th ed., thoroughly rev. With sixty-six illustrations, one colored spectra plate, and eight colored plates representing sixty-four chemical reactions. Philadelphia and New York: Lea Bros. & Co., 1905. 643p. DLC; IU-M; MBM; PPC
00-5079

SIMON, William (1844-1916)
Manual of chemistry. A guide to lectures and laboratory work for beginners in chemistry. A text-book specially adapted for students of medicine, pharmacy, and dentistry. By W. Simon . . . and Daniel Base . . . 9th ed., thoroughly rev., with seventy-eight illustrations, one colored spectra plate, and eight colored plates representing sixty-four chemical reactions. Philadelphia and New York: Lea & Febiger, 1909. 716p. DLC; ICRM; NNNAM; PPC **00-5080**

SIMONS, Manning (*b.* 1846)
President's address (delivered before the South Carolina Medical Association), Spartanburg, S.C., April, 1903. Charleston: Walker, Evans & Cogswell Co., 1903. 14p. DNLM; ScMS **00-5081**

SIMPSON, Frank F. (*b.* 1868)
Some contraindications to intraperitoneal use of normal salt solution after abdominal section. New York, 1900. 10p. NN
00-5082

SIMPSON, Frank F. (*b.* 1868)
A catheter. New York: William Wood & Co., 1902. 1 l. DNLM
00-5083

SIMPSON, Frank F. (*b.* 1868)
Ice following abdominal section. New York: William Wood & Co., 1902. 10p. DNLM **00-5084**

SIMPSON, Frank F. (*b.* 1868)
Intra-abdominal but retroperitoneal shortening and anterior fixation of the round ligamets for posterior uterine displacements. Being a preliminary report concerning the technique, with a report of cases. New York: William Wood & Co., 1903. 8p. DNLM **00-5085**

SIMPSON, Frank F. (*b.* 1868)
Intra-abdominal but retroperitoneal shortening and anterior fixation of the round ligaments for posterior uterine displacements. New York, 1903. 8p. NN **00-5086**

SIMPSON, Frank F. (*b.* 1868)
A consideration of combined ectopic and intrauterine pregnancy, with report of a case. New York, 1904. 23p. NN
00-5087

SIMPSON, Frank F. (*b.* 1868)
A self-retaining abdominal retractor. New York, 1904. 2p. NN **00-5088**

SIMPSON, Frank F. (*b.* 1868)
One hundred consecutive abdominal sections in hospital practice without mortality. A review. Philadelphia, 1905. 15p. DNLM **00-5089**

SIMPSON, Frank F. (*b.* 1868)
Unusual dilation of cornual blood vessels: rupture into uterine cavity: hysterectomy: recovery: report of a case. New York, 1905. 4p. NN **00-5090**

SIMPSON, Frank F. (*b.* 1868)
Post-operative complications involving the alimentary tract. New York, 1907. 15p. NN **00-5091**

SIMPSON, Frank F. (*b.* 1868)
Deferred operation for ruptured ectopic gestation. New York, 1907. 8p. NN **00-5092**

SIMPSON, Frank F. (*b.* 1868)
The choice of time for operation for pelvic inflammation of tubal origin. New York, 1909. 17p. NN
00-5093

SIMPSON, Frederick T. (*b.* 1857)
A case of hydrophobia. New York, 1907. 5p. DNLM
00-5094

SIMPSON, G[eorge] A[ugustus] Garry (*b.* 1861)
Adenoid growths of the naso-parynx. Diagnosis, symptoms, and treatment. New York: William Wood & Co., 1905. 43p. 8 plates. DNLM; NNNAM; PPC; PPHa
00-5095

SIMPSON, William Kelly (1855-1914)
A case of laryngeal stenosis in the adult, successfully treated by intubation; continuous wearing of tube for four years. New York, 1909. 8p. DNLM; PPHa
00-5096

SINCLAIR, Daniel Alison (*b.* 1871)
Syphilis continuously treated by intramuscular injections of mercury salicylate. New York: A. R. Elliott Pub. Co., 1904. 9p. DNLM **00-5097**

SINEXON, Justus
Accidents and complications following operations on the nose and throat. New York, 1903. 10p. DNLM
00-5098

SINKLER, Wharton (1845-1910)
A case of acute poliomyelitis anterior in a youth seventeen years of age. New York, 1900. 4p. DNLM
00-5099

SINKLER, Wharton (1845-1910)
A note on aceton-chloroform (choleretone) in epilepsy. Philadelphia, 1901. 8p. DNLM **00-5100**

SINKLER, Wharton (1845-1910)
Use of hydrotherapy in neurasthenia and other nervous affections. Detroit, 1901. 5p. DNLM
00-5101

SINKLER, Wharton (1845-1910)
A case exhibiting the symptoms of both tabes and multiple sclerosis. Philadelphia, 1902. 4p. DNLM
00-5102

SINKLER, Wharton (1845-1910)
Myasthenia gravis (asthenic bulbar paralysis). Philadelphia, 1902. 10p. DNLM **00-5103**

SINKLER, Wharton (1845-1910)
Treatment of neurasthenia. Philadelphia, 1902. 2 l. DNLM
00-5104

SINKLER, Wharton (1845-1910)
The therapeutic status of the coal-tar products in neuralgia and other painful conditions. Detroit, 1903. 6p. DNLM
00-5105

SINKLER, Wharton (1845-1910)
Friedreich's ataxia, with a report of thirteen cases. New York, 1906. 24p. DNLM **00-5106**

SINKLER, Wharton (1845-1910)
A case of epilepsy of the family type. New York, 1907. 4p. DNLM **00-5107**

SINKLER, Wharton (1845-1910)
Address to the graduating class of nurses at the Orthopaedic Hospital and Infirmary for Nervous Diseases, November 14th, 1907. [Philadelphia, 1907.] 10p. PPC
00-5108

SINKS, Edward D. (*b.* 1877)
Pulmonary tuberculosis. Its diagnosis and course under favorable conditions. Carlisle, 1905. 17p. DNLM
00-5109

SKILLERN, Penn-Gaskell, Jr.
Anatomy of the central nervous system, eye and ear, cranial nerves (deep). . . . Philadelphia: E. P. Dolbey, [1909]. 107p. DLC; PP; PU **00-5110**

SKILLERN, Penn-Gaskell, Jr.
Descriptive anatomy. . . . Development. Microscopic anatomy. Bones. Philadelphia: Dolbey & Co., 1910. 295p. DLC; MH-M; PU **00-5111**

SKINNER, Clarence Edward (*b.* 1868)
A case of typhoid fever presenting some unusual features. New York, 1900. 15p. DNLM **00-5112**

SKINNER, Clarence Edward (*b.* 1868)
Dry hot air in therapeutics. New York, 1902. 16p. DNLM
00-5113

SKINNER, Clarence Edward (*b.* 1868)
X-light in therapeutics. New York, 1902. 24p. DNLM
00-5114

SKINNER, Clarence Edward (*b.* 1868)
X-light in the treatment of cancer. New York, 1902. 24p. DNLM **00-5115**

SKINNER, Clarence Edward (*b.* 1868)
Dry hot air in the treament of Bright's disease. New York, 1903. 25p. DNLM **00-5116**

SKINNER, Clarence Edward (*b.* 1868)
Dry superheated air in the treatment of septic infection. Philadelphia, 1903. 20p. DNLM **00-5117**

SKINNER, Clarence Edward (*b.* 1868)
Therapeutics of dry hot air. . . . New York: A. L. Chatterton & Co., [1903]. 200p. DLC; ICJ; NNNAM; PU
00-5118

SKINNER, Clarence Edward (*b.* 1868)
Dry superheated air in therapeutics. New York, 1904. 12p. DNLM **00-5119**

SKINNER, Clarence Edward (*b.* 1868)
A large fibro sarcoma treated by Roentgen radiation. Chicago, 1904. 7p. DNLM **00-5120**

SKINNER, Clarence Edward (*b.* 1868)
The present status of X-ray therapy in the management of cancer. New York, 1904. 8p. DNLM
00-5121

SKINNER, Clarence Edward (*b.* 1868)
The treatment of arthritis deformans. Chicago, 1904. 12p. DNLM **00-5122**

SKINNER, Clarence Edward (*b.* 1868)
Two cases of severe X-ray necrosis presenting some unusual features. Philadelphia, 1904. 12p. DNLM
00-5123

SKINNER, Clarence Edward (*b.* 1868)
Therapeutics of dry hot air . . . 2nd ed., enl. and thoroughly rev. New York: A. L. Chatterton & Co., [1905]. 262p. plates. DLC; DNLM; NNNAM; PP **00-5124**

SKINNER, Clarence Edward (*b.* 1868)
Roentgenization in the treatment of cancer, with an exhibition of cases in which the evidences of malignant disease have disappeared under Roentgen radiation. Chicago, 1906. 12p. DNLM **00-5125**

SKINNER, George A[lfred] (*b.* 1870)
Dysentery. St. Paul, 1903. 15p. DNLM **00-5126**

SKINNER, Robert P[eet] (*b.* 1866)
Yellow fever; its occurrence and quarantine management at the port of Marseille, France. Washington: Government Printing Office, 1902. 2p. DNLM **00-5127**

SKRAINKA, Philip
St. Louis: its history and ideals, prepared for the sixty-first annual session of the American Medical Association, June seventh, eighth, ninth and tenth, 1910, by Philip Skrainka, M.D. St. Louis: Lambert-Deacon-Hull Printing Co., 1910. 172p. illus. DLC; ICJ **00-5128**

SLADE, Charles Blount (*b.* 1874)
Physical examination and diagnositic anatomy. . . . Philadelphia and London: W. B. Saunders & Co., 1910. 146p. DLC; NNNAM; PPC; PU **00-5129**

SLADE, Walter W.
The making of a mechanical optician; a treatise on the equipment and mechanical work of optometrists and opticians. . . . Over two hundred illustrations. [New and enl. ed.] Philadelphia: The Keystone Publishing Co., [1910]. 188p. diags. DLC; MBM; NIC; NN **00-5130**

SLOCUM. Harris A. (*b.* 1857)
An operation for introversion: cuneiform shortening of the broad ligaments. New York, 1903. 6p. DNLM
00-5131

SLOCUM, Harris A. (*b.* 1857)
The use of the pessary. [New York], 1906. 10p. DNLM
00-5132

SLUDER, Greenfield (1865-1928)
The role of the splenopalatine (or Meckel's) ganglion in nasal headaches. New York, 1908. 5p. DNLM
00-5133

SLUSS, John William (*b.* 1867)
Emergency surgery, for the general practitioner . . . with 584 illustrations, some of which are printed in colors. Philadelphia: P. Blakiston's Son & Co., 1908. 602p. DLC; DNLM; NNNAM; PPC **00-5134**

SLUSS, John William (*b.* 1867)
Emergency surgery for the general practitioner . . . 2nd ed., rev. and enl., with 605 illustrations, some of which are printed in colors. Philadelphia: P. Blakiston's Son & Co., 1910. 748p. DLC; DNLM; MBM; PU **00-5135**

SMALL, William Bryant (1863-1905)
Preliminary treatment in minor gynecological surgery. New York, 1903. 7p. DNLM **00-5136**

SMALL-POX; its prevention, restriction and suppression. Issued by the Illinois State Board of Health, 1902. Springfield: Phillips Bros., 1903. 50p. DNLM; ICU
00-5137

SMART, Charles (1841-1905)
The germ of yellow fever. Philadelphia, 1900. 8p. DNLM
00-5138

SMART, Charles (1841-1905)
Handbook for the Hospital Corps of the U.S. Army and State military forces. Approved by the Surgeon-General of the Army. 3rd ed., revised and enlarged. New York: William Wood & Co., 1902. 413p. DLC; DNLM; ICJ; NNNAM
00-5139

SMART, Robert
Military hygiene; its theoretical and practical study in the Regular Army and militia forces. Carlisle, Pa., 1905. 15p. DNLM **00-5140**

SMART, Robert
The sterilization of patients, operators, assistants, instruments, dressings, etc. With brief résumé of after treatment, from notes taken while attending clinics at St. Mary's Hospital. Rochester: Minn. Surgeons' Club, [1906]. 13p. DNLM
00-5141

SMEDLEY, Emma
Institution recipes in use at the Johns Hopkins Hospital and Drexel Institute lunch room. . . . Philadelphia, Pa.: W. F. Fell Co., [1904]. 121p. DLC; MH; NIC; NN **00-5142**

SMEDLEY, Emma
. . . Dietary studies in public institutions in Philadelphia, Pa., by Miss Emma Smedley and R. D. Milner, and Dietary studies in public institutions in Baltimore, Md., by H. L. Knight, H. A. Pratt, and C. F. Langworthy. Washington: Government Printing Office, 1910. 98p. DLC: NN; PP; PU
00-5143

SMITH, Allen John (1863-1926)
Notes on the lectures of Prof. J. Guitéras, on general and special pathology, delivered before the students of the University of Pennsylvania. Arranged by A. J. Smith, A. Stengel, and F. S. Pearce. Philadlephia: Billstein & Sons, 1901? 170, 22, 28, 46p. NN [Inter-leaved with Ms. notes.]
00-5144

SMITH, Allen J[ohn] (1863-1926)
Lessons and laboratory exercises in bacteriology; an outline of technical methods introductory to the systematic study and identification of bacteria, arranged for the use of students. Philadelphia: P. Blakiston's Son & Co., 1902. 298p. diags. DLC; DNLM; PPC; PU **00-5145**

SMITH, Allen J[ohn] (1863-1926)
Syllabus on pathology. Ed. by W. P. Vail. [Philadelphia? 1905.] [unp.] DNLM; PPC **00-5146**

SMITH, Andrew H[eermance] (1837-1910)
Would it not be a gain to both pathology and practice if a direct interaction between the morbific agent (noxa) and the reparative effort were recognized and the conception of an intermediate, so-called inflammatory, process abandoned? Philadelphia, 1900. 11p. DNLM **00-5147**

SMITH, Andrew H[eermance] (1837-1910)
Reminiscences of Virchow. New York, 1902. 8p. DNLM
00-5148

SMITH, Andrew H[eermance] (1837-1910)
Specific medication. New York, 1902. 19p. DNLM
00-5149

SMITH, Andrew H[eermance] (1837-1910)
The past, present, and future of the New York Academy of Medicine. New York, 1902. 24p. DNLM
00-5150

SMITH, Andrew H[eermance] (1837-1910)
The young practitioner. New York, 1903. 9p. DNLM
00-5151

SMITH, Andrew H[eermance] (1837-1910)
Intramuscular hemorrhage from muscular action. New York: William Wood & Co., 1905. 11p. DNLM
00-5152

SMITH, Andrew H[eermance] (1837-1910)
President Garfield at Elberon. Philadelphia, 1905. 9p. DNLM
00-5153

SMITH, Andrew H[eermance] (1837-1910)
A perfect man. New York: The Author, 1909. 12p. NN
00-5154

SMITH, A[rchibald] D[elap] (*b.* 1876)
Infant feeding in summer, with a partial study of economic and sanitary conditions. [New York], 1905. 10p. DNLM
00-5155

SMITH, A[rthur] Lapthorn (*b.* **1855)**
Insanity in women from the gynecologic and obstetric point of view. St. Louis, 1901. 23p. DNLM
00-5156

SMITH, A[rthur] Lapthorn (*b.* **1855)**
Three cases of vaginal hysterectomy, with remarks on the future of hysterectomy for cancer. New York, [1902]. 2 l. DNLM **00-5157**

SMITH, A[rthur] Lapthorn (*b.* **1855)**
Ascites with abdominal tumors. Philadelphia, 1902. 3p. DNLM
00-5158

SMITH, A[rthur] Lapthorn (*b.* **1855)**
A change needed in our practice in dealing with cancer of the uterus and cancer of the breast. New York, 1902. 7p. DNLM
00-5159

SMITH, A[rthur] Lapthorn (*b.* **1855)**
Case of placenta praevia, with threatening uraemic convulsions; rapid manual dilatation of the os uteri; turning and delivery; recovery. [n. p.], 1902. 4p. DNLM **00-5160**

SMITH, A[rthur] Lapthorn (*b.* **1855)**
The outlook for hysterectomy for cancer. Boston, 1902. 3p. DNLM **00-5161**

SMITH, A[rthur] Lapthorn (*b.* **1855)**
The explosion of the theory of heredity. New York, 1908. 15p. DNLM **00-5162**

SMITH, D[avid] D.
Oral prophylaxis. Read before the Cincinnati Odontological Society, March 28, 1902. n. p., [1902]. 20p. DLC
00-5163

SMITH, D[avid] D.
Mouth infection due to natural teeth. Philadelphia, 1903. 12p. DNLM [*Also*: Philadelphia, 1903, 19p.]
00-5164

SMITH, D[avid] D.
Systemic infection, due to natural teeth conditions. Philadelphia, 1903. 12p. DLC **00-5165**

SMITH, Dean Tyler
Before and after surgical operations. A treatise on the preparations for, and the care of the patient after operations, including homoeopathic therapeutics. Written with special reference to the needs of the general practitioner and the hospital intern. . . . Philadelphia, Pa.: Boericke & Tafel, 1906. 260p. DLC; DNLM; ICJ; PPC **00-5166**

SMITH, Edgar F[ahs] (1854-1928)
Electrochemical analysis. 3rd ed., revised and enlarged. Philadelphia: P. Blakiston's Son & Co., 1902. 204p. CtY-M; DNLM; MBM; PU **00-5167**

SMITH, Edgar F[ahs] (1854-1928)
Electrochemical analysis. 4th ed. Philadelphia: P. Blakiston's Son & Co., 1907. 336p. DLC; DNLM; ICJ; PU
00-5168

SMITH, E[dward] Franklin
Text-book of anatomy, physiology, and hygiene. . . . New York: W. R. Jenkins, 1901 [*c.* 1898]. 198p. DLC: ICJ; NN; PP
00-5169

SMITH, E[lijah] W.
Electro-therapeutist. The modern treatment of stricture, prostatitis, urethritis, cystitis, fistula and ulceration of the rectum by electrolysis and cataphoresis. Terre Haute: Moore & Langen, 1902. 125p. 9 plates. DNLM
00-5170

SMITH, Ella Gertrude
A manual of the treatmnet of disease, by electricity and vital magnetism. How to get well. . . . Minneapolis, Minn.: The Aetna Co., 1901. 53p. DLC; DNLM
00-5171

SMITH, Ernest A[lfred]
A manual of dental metallurgy. 2nd ed. Philadelphia: P. Blakiston's Son & Co., 1903. 294p. DNLM; MdU-D; PPC; PU [1st ed., London: Churchill, 1898.]
00-5172

SMITH, Eugene A. (*b.* **1864)**
The early and late operations for appendicitis. Buffalo, 1900. 8p. DNLM **00-5173**

SMITH, Eugene A. (*b.* **1864)**
Report of a case of carcinoma of the cecum and a case of rupture of the sigmoid treated by intestinal anastomosis. Philadelphia, 1901. 3p. DNLM **00-5174**

SMITH, Eugene A. (*b.* **1864)**
Justifiableness of exploratory operations. Buffalo, 1904. 7p. DNLM **00-5175**

SMITH, Frederick C[harles] (*b.* **1874)**
The differential diagnosis of typhoid fever in its earliest stages. Carlisle, Pa., 1904. 41p. DNLM **00-5176**

SMITH, Frederick C[harles] (*b.* **1874)**
Pulmonary hemorrhage in the tuberculous at high altitude (6,200 feet); report of 56 deaths; frequency of associated heart disease. Washington: Government Printing Office, 1910. 9p. DLC; DNLM **00-5177**

SMITH, Frederick C[harles] (*b.* **1874)**
. . . The relation of climate to the treatment of pulmonary tuberculosis. . . . Prepared by direction of the Surgeon-General. Washington: Government Printing Office, 1910. 17p. DLC; NN
00-5178

SMITH, Frederick C[harles] (*b.* **1874)**
. . . Tuberculosis: its nature and prevention. . . . Prepared by direction of the Surgeon-General. Washington: Government Printing Office, 1910. 12p. DLC; NN
00-5179

SMITH, Frederick John (1857-1919)
Introduction to the outlines of the principles of differential diagnosis, with clincial memoranda. . . . New York: The Macmillan Co., 1900 [*c.* 1899]. 353p. DLC; ICJ; KU; NN
00-5180

SMITH, G[eorge] Carroll (*b.* **1853)**
Ménière's disease. Boston: Damrell & Upham, [1900?] 9p. DNLM **00-5181**

SMITH, G[eorge] Carroll (*b.* **1853)**
The psychic factor in disease. Boston, 1907. 22p. DNLM
00-5182

SMITH, G[eorge] Carroll (*b.* 1853)
What to eat and why. Philadelphia: W. B. Saunders & Co., 1910 [1911]. 310p. DLC; ICJ; PPC; PU
00-5183

SMITH, G. W.
How to control the sex of future offspring, embracing conception and prevention, and natural laws of sexual intercourse, promotion of healthful offspring, and natural parturition, by Prof. G. W. Smith, Ph.D. . . . Dallas, Tex.: G. W. Smith, 1900 [*c.* 1898]. 56p. DLC **00-5184**

SMITH, Harmon (1872-1934)
Paraffin injected subcutaneously for the correction of nasal and other deformities. Chicago, 1903. 11p. DNLM
00-5185

SMITH, Harmon (1872-1934)
Primary epithelioma of the uvula, with report of a case where recurrence took place after two operations for removal. New York, 1905. 7p. DNLM **00-5186**

SMITH, Harmon (1872-1934)
Laryngeal edema. New York, 1906. 14p. DNLM
00-5187

SMITH, Harmon (1872-1934)
Report of a case of radical operation for chronic otitis media suppurativa; operation for epidural abscess; death. New York, 1906. 7p. DNLM **00-5188**

SMITH, Harmon (1872-1934)
The accessory sinuses of the nose, from an operative standpoint. New York, 1908. 14p. DNLM
00-5189

SMITH, Henry Carlton (*b.* 1866)
Lecture notes on chemistry for dental students; including dental chemistry of alloys, amalgams, etc., such portions of organic and physiological chemistry as have practical bearing on the subject of dentistry, an inorganic qualitative analysis with specially adapted blowpipe and microscopical tests, and the chemical examination of urine and saliva . . . 1st ed. 1st thousand. New York: J. Wiley & Sons, [etc., etc.], 1906. 273p. plates, CtY-M; DLC; NNNAM; PU
00-5190

SMITH, Henry Lee (*b.* 1868)
Adam Thomson, the originator of the American method of inoculation for small-pox. Baltimore, 1909. 8p. DNLM
00-5191

SMITH, Homer E[rastus] (*b.* 1856)
Ametropia; its immediate and remote consequences. New York, 1907. 10p. DNLM **00-5192**

SMITH, J. C.
The animal parasite supposed to be the cause of yellow fever. New York, 1903. 11p. DNLM; NcD
00-5193

SMITH, J. C.
Discovery of yellow fever germ. [New Orleans], 1903. 6p. NcD **00-5194**

SMITH, Joseph T. (*b.* 1856)
Historical sketch of Elisha Perkins, inventor of the metallic tractors. Baltimore, 1910. 8p. DNLM; NN
00-5195

SMITH, Oliver C[otton] (*b.* 1859)
Two cases of Henoch's purpura; with remarks upon the gastro-intestinal lesions. New York, 1904. 8p. DNLM
00-5196

SMITH, Oliver C[otton] (*b.* 1859)
Accessory thyreoid on the posterior third of the tongue. New York: A. R. Elliott Pub. Co., 1904. 6p. DNLM
00-5197

SMITH, Oliver C[otton] (*b.* 1859)
A further report on the surgical treatment of hypertrophied prostate gland in the State of Connecticut. [Bridgeport, Conn.], 1904. 12p. DNLM **00-5198**

SMITH, Oliver C[otton] (*b.* 1859)
Advanced age as a contraindication to operation. New York, 1907. 11p. DNLM **00-5199**

SMITH, Oliver C[otton] (*b.* 1859)
Tumors of the caecum. Hartford, 1907. 18p. 3 plates. DNLM
00-5200

SMITH, Oliver C[otton] (*b.* 1859)
Notes on European surgical clinics. New York, 1908. 12p. DNLM **00-5201**

SMITH, Oliver C[otton] (*b.* 1859)
. . . The critical character of the age period from fourteen to sixteen. . . . [Hartford, 19—?] 8p. MBM
00-5202

SMITH, Peter (1753-1816)
The Indian doctor's dispensatory; being Father Smith's advice respecting diseases and their cure. . . . Cincinnati: Printed by Browne & Looker for the Author, 1812. [Cincinnati: J. U. & C. G. Lloyd, 1901.] 108p. DLC: ICJ; OCLloyd
00-5203

SMITH, Richard R[oot] (*b.* 1869)
Adenamatous hyperplasia of the cervical gland appendage of Gärtner's duct. New York, 1904. 7p. DNLM
00-5204

SMITH, Richard R[oot] (*b.* 1869)
Fibromymatous tumors of the vagina. New York: William Wood & Co., 1902. 30p. DNLM; NNNAM
00-5205

SMITH, Richard R[oot] (*b.* 1869)
Injuries to the axillary vessels occurring during operations for carcinoma of the breast. Philadelphia, 1904. 9p. DNLM
00-5206

SMITH, Robert Meade
Methods of studying the physiological action of drugs. Detroit: G. S. Davis, 1901 [*c.* 1884]. 20p. DLC: ICJ
00-5207

SMITH, S[eth] MacCuen (*b.* 1863)
The importance of cerebral lesions complicating suppurative otitis media. New York, 1909. 11p. DNLM
00-5208

SMITH, Stephen (1823-1922)
The ethics of nursing: an address, New York, December 7, 1900. New York: [Knickerbocker Press], 1900. 23p. NN
00-5209

SMITH, Stephen (1823-1922)
Diagnosing insanity at sight. New York, 1903. 4p. NN
00-5210

SMITH, Stephen (1823-1922), Robert F. WEIR and Louis A. LA GARDE
Treatment of gunshot wounds. New York, 1904. 47p. DNLM; NNNAM **00-5211**

SMITH, Stephen (1823-1922)
Curative Christianity. . . . An address delivered at the . . . American Medical Missionary College . . . June 21, 1904. [Battle Creek, Mich.: The College, 1904.] 28p. NN
00-5212

SMITH, Stephen (1823-1922)
Suggestions of a plan of organizing a hospital system for the City of New York. New York: William Wood & Co., 1907. 16p. NN **00-5213**

SMITH, Thomas C[roggon] (1842-1913)
The obstetrical and gynecological treasures of the Army Medical Museum. New York: William Wood & Co., 1900. 6p. DNLM **00-5214**

SMITH, Thomas C[roggon] (1842-1913)
Some interesting cases. New York, 1908. 4p. DNLM
00-5215

SMITH, William Johnson (*d.* 1911)
Nurses' guide to surgical bandaging and dressings. Philadelphia: J. B. Lippincott Co., [1904]. 167p. CtY-M; DNLM; PPC; PPJ
00-5216

SMITH, William Thayer (1839-1909)
Address delivered, May 17, 1901, at the annual meeting of the New Hampshire Medical Society by the retiring president. Concord, 1901. 10p. DNLM **00-5217**

SNOW, M[ary] L[ydia] H[astings]
Mechanical vibration and its therapeutic applications. New York: Scient. Authors Publ. Co., 1904. 297p. 9 plates. DNLM; ICJ; NNNAM; PU **00-5218**

SNOW, Sargent F.
Deafness from scarlet fever. Buffalo, 1901. 4p. DNLM
00-5219

SNOW, Sargent F.
Systemic factors in catarrhal diseases. Chicago, 1901. 7p. DNLM **00-5220**

SNOW, Sargent F.
Conservatism in the treatment of acute mastoiditis. Chicago, 1903. 7p. DNLM **00-5221**

SNOW, Sargent F.
Salient points in the treatment of catarrhal deafness. Buffalo, 1903. 4p. DNLM **00-5222**

SNOW, Sargent F.
Catarrhal deafness, with report of 400 chronic cases. [Syracuse, N.Y., 1905.] 4 l. DNLM
00-5223

SNOW, Sargent F.
Tic douloureux and other neuralgias from intra-nasal and accessory sinus pressures. New York, 1905. 8p. DNLM
00-5224

SNOW, Sargent F.
Modern possibilities in chronic catarrhal deafness. St. Louis, 1906. 8p. DNLM **00-5225**

SNOW, Sargent F.
Headaches from nasal causes. New York, 1907. 11p. DNLM
00-5226

SNOW, William B[enham] (1860-1930)
A manual of electro-static modes of application and therapeutics. . . . New York: A. L. Chatteron & Co., [1902]. 133p. DLC; ICJ; NNNAM **00-5227**

SNOW, William B[enham] (1860-1930)
A manual of electro-static modes of application, therapeutics, radiography, and radiotherapy. 2nd ed. . . . New York: A. L. Chatterton & Co., [1903]. 302p. plates. DLC; NcD; NNNAM; PPC **00-5228**

SNOW, William B[enham] (1860-1930)
A manual of electro-static modes of application, therapeutics, radiography, and radiotherapy. 3rd ed. New York: A. L. Chatterton & Co., 1904. 302p. 13 plates. DNLM; KU; NNNAM; PU **00-5229**

SNOW, William B[enham] (1860-1930)
High potential currents and currents of high frequency. New York, 1904. 11p. NN **00-5230**

SNOW, William B[enham] (1860-1930)
Currents of high potential of high and other frequencies. New York, 1905. 198p. 8 plates. DLC: DNLM; NNNAM
00-5231

SNOW, William B[enham] (1860-1930)
The static spark and its therapeutic indications. Read at the fifteenth annual meeting of the American Electro-Therapeutic Association, at New York, September 21, 1905. New York, 1906. 6p. NN **00-5232**

SNOW, William B[enham] (1860-1930)
The past, present, and future of physical therapeutics. New York, 1906. 10p. NN **00-5233**

SNOW, William B[enham] (1860-1930)
The employment of physical therapeutics by the general practitioner. New York, 1907. 11p. NN
00-5234

SNOW, William B[enham] (1860-1930)
New methods of treating diseases of the genito-urinary tract. New York, 1908. 11p. NN **00-5235**

SNOW, William B[enham] (1860-1930)
The treatment of arteriosclerosis and hypertension. [Read before the eighteenth annual meeting of the American Electro-Therapeutic Association, New York, September 21, 1908.] [New York, 1908.] 11p. NN **00-5236**

SNOW, William B[enham] (1860-1930)
Report of the committee of the American Electro-Therapeutic Association on static currents. New York, 1908. 15p. NN
00-5237

SNOW, William B[enham] (1860-1930)
Electromechanical and thermic removal of local statis. New York: William Wood & Co., 1908. 18p. NN
00-5238

SNOW, William B[enham] (1860-1930)
Physiological laws relating to the effects of physical measures as employed in therapeutics. New York, 1908. 22p. NN
00-5239

SNOW, William B[enham] (1860-1930)
The therapeutics of radiant light and heat and convective heat. . . . New York: Scientific Authors' Publishing Co., 1909. 119p. plates. DLC; ICJ; NNNAM; PU **00-5240**

SNOW, William B[enham] (1860-1930)
Treatment of hypertension resulting from alcoholic and other excesses by D'Arsonvalization. Read at the semi-annual meeting of the American Medical Society for the Study of Alcohol and other narcotics. Philadelphia, April 6 and 7, 1910. [New York, 1910.] 11p. NN **00-5241**

SNOW, William B[enham] (1860-1930)
Currents of high potenital of high and other frequencies. . . . 2nd ed. New York: Scientific Authors' Publishing Co., 1910. 275p. plates. DLC; ICJ; NN; PP **00-5242**

SNYDER, Sherwood Percy (*b.* 1879)
A treatise on foods, and their effects upon health and the physical and moral life; also a complete list of recipes and instructions for the hygienic preparation of the common food products. . . . [Dayton, O.: Press of the U. B. Publishing House, 1908.] 180p. DLC; ICJ **00-5243**

SNYDER, Sherwood Percy (*b.* 1879)
A treatise on foods and their effects upon health and the physical and moral life; also a complete list of recipes and instructions for the hygienic preparation of the common food products, with special lists of menus. 2nd ed., rev. and enl. . . . Dayton, O.: Health Publishing Co., 1910. 183p. DLC; ICJ **00-5244**

SNYDER, Walter Hamilton
Microphthalmos and cogenital ankylo-blepharon. Two cases. St. Louis, 1904. 3p. DNLM **00-5245**

SNYDER, Walter Hamilton
A new operative procedure for correction of badly placed canalicular cuts. Chicago, 1904. 1 l. DNLM
00-5246

SNYDER, Walter Hamilton
Epithelioma of the lid; removal by dissection and X-ray treatment. Chicago: Amer. Med. Assoc., 1905. 1 p. 1 plate. DNLM **00-5247**

SNYDER, Walter Hamilton
The physiological action of dionin. Chicago: Amer. Med. Assoc., 1905. 5p. DNLM **00-5248**

SNYDER, Walter Hamilton
My experience in treating diseases of the duct without operation. Chicago: Amer. Med. Assoc., 1906. 4p. DNLM
00-5249

SNYDER Walter Hamilton
Parlaysis of the fourth cranial nerve due to trauma, and the means used to overcome the resulting paralysis of the superior oblique muscle. New York, 1907. 5p. DNLM
00-5250

SNYDER, Walter Hamilton
The economic importance of the spread of trachoma in Ohio. Columbus, 1909. 3p. DNLM **00-5251**

SNYDER, Walter Hamilton
The relation of the medical profession to the public. Columbus, 1910. 7p. DNLM **00-5252**

SOBOTTA, Johannes (1869-1945)
Atlas and epitome of human histology and microscopic anatomy. . . . Ed., with extensive additions, by G. Carl Huber. . . . Authorized translation from the German. With 171 illustrations on 80 lithographic plates, and 68 text illustrations. Philadelphia and London: W. B. Saunders & Co., 1903. 248p. DLC; NNNAM; PPC; PU **00-5253**

SOBOTTA, Johannes (1869-1945)
Atlas and text-book of human anatomy . . . ed., with additions, by J. Playfair McMurrich. . . . Philadelphia and London: W. B. Saunders & Co., 1906-07. 3 v. col. plates. DLC; ICJ; MH-M; PPC ["The translation of the German text has been done by Dr. W. Hersey Thomas." — Editor's pref.]
00-5254

SODDY, Frederick (*b.* 1877)
The interpretation of radium: being the substance of six free popular experimental lectures delivered at the University of Glasgow, 1908. . . . New York: G. P. Putnam, 1909. 256p. plates, diags. NN; NNNAM; PPJ; PU [Published simultaneously in London: J. Murray, 1909, 256p.]
00-5255

SOLIS-COHEN, Myer
. . . Woman in girlhood, wifehood, motherhood; her responsibilities and her duties at all periods of life; a guide in the maintenance of her own health and that of her children . . . profusely illustrated with color plates, scientific drawings and half-tone engravings, with manikin chart printed in colors. . . . Philadelphia, Chicago, [etc.]: The J. C. Winston Co., [1906]. 443p. DLC; ICJ; NIC; NN **00-5256**

SOLIS-COHEN, Myer
. . . Life knowledge; or, Woman's responsibilities and duties at all periods of life, a guide in the maintenance of her own health and that of her children . . . profusely illustrated with color plates, scientific drawings and half-tone engravings, with manikin chart printed in colors. . . . Philadelphia: Uplift Publishing Co., [1909]. 469p. DLC; MH; NN; PP
00-5257

SOLIS-COHEN, Myer
The family health. . . . Philadelphia: The Penn Publishing Co., 1910. 267p. DLC; MdU-D; PP; PPL
00-5258

SOLIS-COHEN, Myer
The blue book for girl, wife and mother; a guide for women in all important periods of life. . . . Philadelphia: The John C. Winston Co., [1910]. 252p. DLC; NN; PP; PPL
00-5259

SOLLMANN, Torald H[ermann] (1874-1965)
Practical exercises in pharmacology; a synopsis of the laboratory course given in the Medical Department of Western Reserve University. [Cleveland: Faculty of the Medical College, 1900.] 40p. ICJ; NcD **00-5260**

SOLLMANN, Torald H[ermann] (1874-1965)
A text-book of pharmacology and some allied sciences (therapeutics, materia medica, pharmacy, prescription-writing, toxicology, etc.). Philadelphia & London: W. B. Saunders & Co., 1901. 894p. DNLM; MBM; NNNAM; PU **00-5261**

SOLLMANN, Torald H[ermann] (1874-1965)
The trend of pharmacological research. Cleveland, 1902. 7p. DNLM **00-5262**

SOLLMANN, Torald H[ermann] (1874-1965)
The teaching of therapeutics and pharmacology from the experimental standpoint. Chicago, 1902. 24p. DNLM **00-5263**

SOLLMANN, Torald H[ermann] (1874-1965)
Inhalation of gasolene vapors. Philadelphia, 1904. 4p. DNLM **00-5264**

SOLLMANN, Torald H[ermann] (1874-1965)
Intravenous injection of ergot; effects on the mammalian circulation. Chicago, 1905. 35p. DNLM **00-5265**

SOLLMANN, Torald H[ermann] (1874-1965)
A text-book of pharmacology and some allied sciences (therapeutics, materia medica, pharmacy, prescription-writing, toxicology, etc.). 2nd ed., thoroughly revised and greatly enlarged. Philadelphia & London: W. B. Saunders & Co., 1906. 1070p. CtY-M; DNLM; PPC; PU **00-5266**

SOLLMANN, Torald H[ermann] (1874-1965)
Some facts about digestive ferments. Chicago, 1907. 11p. DNLM **00-5267**

SOLLMANN, Torald H[ermann] (1874-1965)
A review of recent work on the mechanism of urine formation. [Chicago, 1907.] 26p. NN **00-5268**

SOMERS, G[eorge] H[orace]
Lecture notes in physical diagnosis and life insurance. . . . [Chicago?], 1900. 272p. DLC; ICJ **00-5269**

SOMERS, Lewis S[ummerl] (*b.* 1871)
Acute pharyngitis of the streptococcal type. Detroit: W. M. Warren, 1902. 8p. DNLM **00-5270**

SOMERS, Lewis S[ummerl] (*b.* 1871)
Urticaria of the upper respiratory tract. New York, 1902. 11p. DNLM **00-5271**

SOMMERFELD, Paul
Methods for the examination of milk; for chemists, physicians and hygienists . . . with a preface by . . . A. Baginsky . . . transl. by . . . A. T. Peters . . . and R. S. Hiltner. Chicago: A. Eger, 1901 [1900]. 100p. DLC; ICJ **00-5272**

SONDERN, Frederic E[wald] (1867-1947)
Genito-urinary tuberculosis: its diagnosis in the laboratory. [New York], 1906. 12p. MB; PU **00-5273**

SONDERN, Frederic E[wald] (1867-1947)
Value of the blood count in sepsis. [New York], 1906. 5p. DNLM **00-5274**

SONDERN, Frederic E[wald] (1867-1947)
General considerations in reference to blood examination in surgical diseases. New York: A. R. Elliott Co., 1907. 8p. DNLM **00-5275**

SOTHORON, Elmer (*b.* 1868)
The action of the uterus during labor. New York, 1903. 13p. DNLM **00-5276**

SOTHORON, Elmer (*b.* 1868)
The application of the forceps in contracted pelves. New York, 1905. 6p. DNLM **00-5277**

SOUCHON, Edmond (1841-1924)
True origin of the epidemic of yellow fever [1897]. . . . n. p., n. p. [1900?] 7p. LNT-M **00-5278**

SOUCHON, Edmond (1841-1924)
Surgical diseases and injuries of the face. Surgical diseases and injuries of the neck. Illus. New York, 1901. 45p. MB **00-5279**

SOUCHON, Edmond (1841-1924)
On the transmission of yellow fever by vessels, and its bearing upon quarantine regulations. New York: William Wood & Co., 1901. 8p. LNT-M; NN **00-5280**

SOUCHON, Edmond (1841-1924)
Treatment of vessels from yellow-fever ports; a reply to Drs. Reed and Carroll. New York: William Wood & Co., 1902. 22p. LNT-M; NN **00-5281**

SOUCHON, Edmond (1841-1924)
Reminiscences of Dr. J. Marion Sims in Paris. n. p., n. d. [1902?] 10p. MH **00-5282**

SOUCHON, Edmond (1841-1924)
The mosquito on board of vessels at quarantined ports as a factor in the transmission of yellow fever. New York: William Wood & Co., 1902. 4p. DNLM **00-5283**

SOUCHON, Edmond (1841-1924)
On the transportation of mosquitos by vessels. New York, 1902. 8p. DNLM **00-5284**

SOUCHON, Edmond (1841-1924)
Maritime quarantine without detention of non-infected vessels from ports quarantined against yellow fever. New York: William Wood & Co., 1903. 7p. DNLM **00-5285**

SOUCHON, Edmond (1841-1924)
A plea for a reform in medical education. New York: William Wood & Co., 1909. 4p. DNLM **00-5286**

SOUCHON, Edmond (1841-1924)
The Souchon Museum of Anatomy at Tulane University of Louisiana, New Orleans. New Orleans, 1910. 4 l. DNLM; LNT-M **00-5287**

SOUCHON, Edmond (1841-1924)
The philosophic anatomy of the liver. New York: William Wood & Co., 1910. 16p. NN **00-5288**

SOUTER, William Norwood (1861-1935)
The refraction and motility of the eye. For students and practitioners. . . . Illustrated with 101 engravings in the text and 4 plates in colors and monochrome. Philadelphia and New York: Lea Bros. & Co., 1903. 390p. col. plates. DLC; ICJ; MH; PPC
00-5289

SOUTER, William Norwood (1861-1935)
The refractive and motor mechanism of the eye . . . with 148 illustrations. Philadelphia: The Keystone Publishing Co., 1910. 353p. DLC; PPC; PU **00-5290**

SOUTHARD, E[lmer] E[rnest] (1876-1920)
Neuropathology; outline. Boston: J. L. Fairbanks & Co., 1904. 42p. DNLM; MBM **00-5291**

SOUTHARD, E[lmer] E[rnest] (1876-1920)
Outline of neuropathology. Boston: J. L. Fairbanks & Co., 1906. 92p. DNLM; MBM **00-5292**

SOUTHARD, E[lmer] E[rnest] (1876-1920)
Diffuse and focal lesions in a case of late epilepsy. [Boston, 1907.] 25p. DNLM; MBM **00-5293**

SOUTHARD, E[lmer] E[rnest] (1876-1920) and J. B. AYER
Dementia praecox, paranoid, associated with bronchiectatic lung disease and terminated by brain abscesses (micrococcus catarrhales). Boston, 1908. 24p. DNLM; MBM
00-5294

SOUTHWESTERN UNIVERSITY MEDICAL COLLEGE, DALLAS
Announcements of medical and pharmaceutical departments for sessions of 1905-06; 1907-08; 1909-10. Dallas, 1905-09. DNLM **00-5295**

SOUTHWICK, George R[inaldo] (1859-1930)
The prognosis of inoperable malignant diseases under treatment by X-rays. Boston, [1903]. 8p. DNLM
00-5296

SOUWERS, George F.
Venesection. New York, 1904. 25p. DNLM
00-5297

SOUWERS, George F.
Some notes on Riggs's disease and its treatment. New York: A. R. Elliott, 1904. 16p. DNLM **00-5298**

SOUWERS, George F.
The mephisto of the pale brotherhood of disease; a study of masked rheumatism, based, not on books, but experience. New York: A. R. Elliott, 1905. 64p. DNLM; NNNAM
00-5299

SOZINSKEY, Thomas S. (1852?-1889)
. . . Medical symbolism in connection with historical studies in the arts of healing and hygiene. Illustrated. . . . Philadelphia and London: F. A. Davis, 1901 [*c.* 1891]. 171p. DLC; ICJ; MH; NN **00-5300**

SPALDING, Heman (*b.* 1852)
Some facts about vaccination. Chicago, 1902. 8p. DNLM
00-5301

SPALDING, James A[lfred] (*b.* 1846)
Relations between medical practitioners and specialists in diseases of the eye. New York, 1906. 14p. DNLM
00-5302

SPALDING, James A[lfred] (*b.* 1846)
The friendship of Dr. Nathan Smith and Dr. Lyman Spalding. . . . [n. p., 1906.] 20p. DLC; DNLM
00-5303

SPALDING, James A[lfred] (*b.* 1846)
Jeremiah Barker, M.D., Gorham and Falmouth, Maine, 1752-1835. . . . Portland, Me. . . . [Portland? 1909.] 24p. ICJ; NN [Annual address before the Portland Medical Club, 1908.]
00-5304

SPALTEHOLZ, [Karl] Werner (1861-1940)
Hand atlas of human anatomy. By Werner Spalteholz . . . with the advice of Wilhelm His. . . . Transl. from the 3rd German edition by Lewellys F. Barker. . . . With a preface by Franklin P. Mall. . . . Leipzig: S. Hirzel; New York: G. E. Stechert, [etc., etc.], 1900-1903. 3 v. [paged continuously] ICJ; RPB
00-5305

SPALTEHOLZ, [Karl] Werner (1861-1940)
Hand-atlas of human anatomy . . . edited and transl. from the 3rd German ed. by Lewellys F. Barker. . . . With a preface by Franklin P. Mall . . . 3rd ed. Philadelphia and London: J. B. Lippincott Co., [1900-26?] 2 v. illus. (part col.) DLC; ICJ; MH; NN [Paged continuously. Printed by Fischer & Wittig, Leipzig. Vol. 3, 5th ed. in English] **00-5306**

SPALTEHOLZ, [Karl] Werner (1861-1940)
Hand atlas of human anatomy. Ed. and transl. from the 3rd German ed., by Lewellys F. Barker. Philadelphia: J. B. Lippincott, 1903. 3 v. illus. (part col.) DNLM; PPHa
00-5307

SPALTEHOLZ, [Karl] Werner (1861-1940)
Hand-atlas of human anatomy, ed. and transl. from fourth German ed. by Lewellys F. Barker, with preface by Franklin P. Mall. 2nd ed. in English. Philadelphia: J. B. Lippincott, 1906. 872p. illus. CtY-M; DNLM; IU-M
00-5308

SPALTEHOLZ, [Karl] Werner (1861-1940)
Hand-atlas of human anatomy . . . edited and transl. from the 4th German edition by Lewellys F. Barker . . . with a preface by Franklin P. Mall . . . 2nd ed. in English. Philadelphia and London: J. B. Lippincott Co., [1906?]. 3 v. DLC; ICJ; NN; PU **00-5309**

SPEAR, Edmund D[oe] (*b.* 1852)
Does a hole in the drumhead destroy the hearing? A popular delusion regarding the human ear. Boston, 1901. 7p. DNLM
00-5310

SPEAR, Edmund D[oe] (*b.* 1852)
The true undulatory theory of sound. [Boston, 1903.] 19p. MB **00-5311**

SPEAR, Raymond
Report on the Russian medical and sanitary features of the Russo-Japanese War to the Surgeon-General, U.S. Navy. . . . Washington, July 1, 1906. Washington: Government Printing Office, 1906. 84p. plates. DLC; DNLM
00-5312

SPEAR, Walter M. (*b.* **1871)**
Abscess of the spleen. Chicago, 1903. 7p. DNLM
00-5313

SPENCER, George W[icks] (*b.* **1870)**
Primary tuberculosis of the female breast, with a report of a recent case. Philadelphia, 1905. 8p. DNLM
00-5314

SPENCER, Selden (*b.* **1873)**
A case of aneurysm of the middle ear with intact drum head. New York, 1906. 5p. DNLM **00-5315**

SPENCER, Selden (*b.* **1873)**
A practical guide to the examination of the ear. With an introductory chapter by H. N. Spencer. St. Louis: C. V. Mosby, 1908. 66p. IEN-M; IU-M; MBM; MdBJ-W
00-5316

SPENCER, Walter G[eorge] (1858-1940)
Surgery of the stomach. Albany, 1900. 48p. DNLM
00-5317

SPENCER, Walter G[eorge] (1858-1940) and George Ernest GASK
The practice of surgery. Philadelpia: P. Blakiston's Son & Co., 1910. 1234p. 48 plates. CU-M; DNLM; MBM; PPC
00-5318

SPERRY, Lyman Beecher (1841-1923)
Husband and wife; a book of information and advice for the married and the marriageable. New York, Chicago, [etc.]: F. H. Revell Co., [1900]. 238p. DLC; NcD
00-5319

SPERRY, Lyman Beecher (1841-1923)
Physiology, fear and faith; a little book containing important facts and suggestions regarding the causes and the cure of disease, the employment of physicians, and the use of medicines. . . . Chicago, London, [etc.]: Fleming H. Revell Co., 1902. 79p. DLC; ICJ; MH; NN **00-5320**

SPIERS, Henry H.
Tuberculosis or consumption. . . . [2nd ed., enl.] [Ravenna, O., 1902.] 94p. DLC; DNLM; PPC **00-5321**

SPIERS, Henry H.
Tuberculosis or consumption. . . . [3rd ed., enl.] Ravenna? O., [1902]. 228p. DLC; DNLM; PPC **00-5322**

SPIERS, Henry H.
Tuberculosis or consumption. . . . [4th ed.] Ravenna? O., [1903]. 257p. port. DLC; PPC; PPHa; PPJ **00-5323**

SPILLER, William G[ibson] (1863-1940)
A case of cervical and bulbar tabes, with necropsy; microscopical study and comments. Philadelphia, 1901. 14p. DNLM
00-5324

SPILLER, William G[ibson] (1863-1940)
A case with the symptoms of cerebro-spinal meningitis, with intense and general alteration of the nerve cell-bodies, but with little evidence of inflammation. Philadelphia, 1901. 9p. DNLM **00-5325**

SPILLER, William G[ibson] (1863-1940) and William E. ROBERTSON, *et al.*
Cerebellar lesions without cerebellar symptoms. Philadelphia, 1901. 18p. 3 plates. DNLM **00-5326**

SPILLER, William G[ibson] (1863-1940)
Remarks on the importance of the so-called specific lesions of rabies. Philadelphia, 1901. 4p. DNLM
00-5327

SPILLER, William G[ibson] (1863-1940)
Renaut's bodies in a case of vesiculo-bullous dermatitis and gangrene. Philadelphia, 1901. 4p. DNLM
00-5328

SPILLER, William G[ibson] (1863-1940)
A case of complete absence of the visual system in an adult. Philadelphia, 1902. 7p. DNLM **00-5329**

SPILLER, William G[ibson] (1863-1940)
A case of primary degeneration of the pyramidal tracts. Philadelphia, 1902. 10p. DNLM **00-5330**

SPILLER, William G[ibson] (1863-1940)
The sensory segmental area of the umbilicus as determined by a case of fracture of the tenth thoracic vertebra, with complete compression of the spinal cord, and without knee-jerks and Babinski reflex. Philadelphia, 1902. 7p. DNLM
00-5331

SPILLER, William G[ibson] (1863-1940)
Two cases of partial internal hydrocephalus from closure of the intraventricular passages: with remarks on bilateral contractures caused by a unilateral cerebral lesion. Philadelphia, 1902. 12p. DNLM **00-5332**

SPILLER, William G[ibson] (1863-1940)
Case of external spinal pachymeningitis, implicating the entire ventral surface of the spinal dura. n. p., 1902. 8p. DNLM; PU
00-5333

SPILLER, William G[ibson] (1863-1940) and Charles H. FRAZIER
Division of the sensory root of the trigeminus for the relief of tic douloureux; an experimental, pathological and clinical study, with a preliminary report of one surgically successful case. Philadelphia, 1902. 12p. DNLM; PU
00-5334

SPILLER, William G[ibson] (1863-1940) and Charles H. FRAZIER
Further report upon the treatment of tic douloureux by division of the sensory root of the gasserian ganglion. n. p., 1902. 4p. DNLM; PU **00-5335**

SPILLER, William G[ibson] (1863-1940) and Theodore H. WEISENBURG
Partial paralysis of one upper limb, resulting from a vascular lesion of the lateral column and anterior horn on the corresponding side of the spinal cord. [n. p., 1903.] 7p. DNLM
00-5336

SPILLER, William G[ibson] (1863-1940), John H. MUSSER and Edward MARTIN
A case of intradural spinal cyst, with operation and recovery; with a brief report of eleven cases of tumor of the spinal cord or spinal column. Philadelphia, 1903. 22p. DNLM
00-5337

SPILLER, William G[ibson] (1863-1940)
A physiological, anatomical, and pathological study of the glossopharyngeus and vagus nerves in a case of fracture of the base of the skull. Philadelphia, 1903. 13p. 1 plate, 1 chart. DNLM **00-5338**

SPILLER, William G[ibson] (1863-1940)
Paralysis of all four limbs and of one side of the face. . . . n. p., 1903. 12p. DNLM; PU **00-5339**

SPILLER, William G[ibson] (1863-1940) and Charles H. FRAZIER
An experimental study on the regeneration of posterior spinal roots. [n. p., 1903.] 7p. DNLM; PU **00-5340**

SPILLER, William G[ibson] (1863-1940) and William F. HENDRICKSON
A report of two cases of multiple sarcomatosis of the central nervous system and of one case of intra-medullary primary sarcoma of the spinal cord. Philadelphia, 1903. 23p. DNLM **00-5341**

SPILLER, William G[ibson] (1863-1940)
A report of two cases of multiple sclerosis, with necropsy; with remarks on muscular atrophy, secondary degeneration, and loss of tendon reflexes, with increased muscular tonicity, occurring in this disease. Philadelphia, 1903. 13p. DNLM **00-5342**

SPILLER, William G[ibson] (1863-1940)
Traumatic lesions of the spinal cord with fracture of the vertebra. [n. p., 1903.] 11p. 1 plate. DNLM **00-5343**

SPILLER, William G[ibson] (1863-1940) and Charles H. FRAZIER
The treatment of cerebral palsies and athetosis by nerve anastomosis and transplantation. New York, 1905. 8p. DNLM; PU **00-5344**

SPILLER, William G[ibson] (1863-1940)
Congenital spastic rigidity of the limbs, congenital hypertonia, Little's disease, with report of two new cases of necropsy. Philadelphia, 1905. 16p. DNLM **00-5345**

SPILLER, William G[ibson] (1863-1940)
General or localized hypotonia of the muscles in childhood, myatonia congenita; report of a case with necropsy. Philadelphia, 1905. 12p. DNLM **00-5346**

SPILLER, William G[ibson] (1863-1940)
The importance in clinical diagnosis of paralysis of associated movements of the eyeballs (Blicklähmung), especially of upward and downward associated movements. [1905.] 57p. 4 l. DNLM **00-5347**

SPILLER, William G[ibson] (1863-1940)
The occasional clinical resemblance between caries of the vertebrae and lumbothoracic syringomyelia, and the location within the spinal cord of the fibres for the sensations of pain and temperature. Philadelphia, 1903. 23p. DNLM **00-5348**

SPILLER, William G[ibson] (1863-1940)
Primary degeneration of the pyramidal tracts; a study of eight cases, with necropsy. Philadelphia, 1905. 31p. DNLM **00-5349**

SPILLER, William G[ibson] (1863-1940)
Pseudo-sclerosis diffuse sclerosis with the report of a case with necropsy. n. p., 1905. 15p. DNLM; PU **00-5350**

SPILLER, William G[ibson] (1863-1940)
Chronic anterior polismyelitis. . . . n. p., 1905. 17p. DNLM; PU **00-5351**

SPILLER, William G[ibson] (1863-1940)
Abscess of the brain. Philadelphia, 1906. 24p. DNLM **00-5352**

SPILLER, William G[ibson] (1863-1940)
The earlier changes in arteriosclerosis of the nervous system. Philadelphia, 1906. 9p. DNLM **00-5353**

SPILLER, William G[ibson] (1863-1940)
Myopathy of the distal type and its relation to the neural form of muscular atrophy (Charcot-Marie, tooth type). [1906.] 17p. DNLM **00-5354**

SPILLER, William G[ibson] (1863-1940)
A pathologic study of amaurotic family idiocy. Philadelphia, 1906. 11p. DNLM **00-5355**

SPILLER, William G[ibson] (1863-1940) and Theodore H. WEISENBURG
Paraplegia dolorosa caused by vertebral carcinomata, spinal caries, and multiple neuritis. Philadelphia, 1906. 12p. DNLM **00-5356**

SPILLER, William G[ibson] (1863-1940) and Theodore H. WEISENBURG
Carcinoma of the nervous system, with the report of eleven cases. [n. p., 1906.] 25p. DNLM **00-5357**

SPILLER, William G[ibson] (1863-1940) and Charles H. FRAZIER
Cerebral decompression; palliative operations in the treatment of tumors of the brain based on the observation of fourteen cases. Philadelphia, 1906. 63p. DNLM; PU **00-5358**

SPILLER, William G[ibson] (1863-1940), Charles H. FRAZIER and J. J. A. VAN KAATHOVEN
Treatment of selected cases of cerebral, spinal and peripheral nerve palsies and athetosis by nerve transplantation, with report of a case of athetosis benefited by nerve transplantation. Philadelphia, 1906. 27p. DNLM; PU **00-5359**

SPILLER, William G[ibson] (1863-1940)
Physiologic extirpation of the ganglion of gasser, further report on division of the sensory root for tic douloureux based on the observations of four cases. n. p., 1906. 18p. DNLM; PU **00-5360**

SPILLER, William Gibson] (1863-1940) and Carl D. CAMP
Autochthonous sinus thrombosis of the cerebral dura; with a report of three cases. Philadelphia, 1906. 13p. DNLM **00-5361**

SPILLER, William G[ibson] (1863-1940) and Carl D. CAMP
Multiple sclerosis, with a report of two additional cases, with necropsy. Philadelphia, 1906. 12p. DNLM **00-5632**

SPILLER, William G. (1863-1940) and J. C. GITTINGS
Progressive muscular atrophy of cervicobulbar type occurring with cervical rib. [New York], 1906. 7p. DNLM **00-5363**

SPILLER, William G. (1863-1940) and Warfield T. LONGCOPE
Multiple motor neuritis, including Landry's paralysis and lead palsy, with reports of cases. [New York], 1906. 23p. DNLM **00-5364**

SPILLER, William G[ibson] (1863-1940)
Psychasthenic attacks simulating epilepsy. [Boston, 1906.] 13p. DNLM **00-5365**

SPILLER, William G[ibson] (1863-1940)
Separate sensory centers in the parietal lobe for the limbs. [New York, 1906.] 5p. DNLM **00-5366**

SPILLER, William G[ibson] (1863-1940)
Gliomatosis of the pia and metastasis of glioma. New York, 1907. 6p. DNLM **00-5367**

SPILLER, William G[ibson] (1863-1940)
Hemicraniosis and cure of brain tumor by operation. Chicago, 1907. 20p. DNLM **00-5368**

SPILLER, William G[ibson] (1863-1940) and Edward MARTIN
The occasional long duration of brain tumor; with the report of a case of Jacksonian epilepsy of eight years' duration as the only sign of a small cerebral glioma. Philadelphia, 1907. 9p. DNLM **00-5369**

SPILLER, William G[ibson] (1863-1940) and Alfred Reginald ALLEN
Internal hydrocephalus; with report of two cases, one resulting from occlusion of the aqueduct of Sylvius. Philadelphia, 1907. 8p. DNLM **00-5370**

SPILLER, William G[ibson] (1863-1940) and Carl D. CAMP
The clinical resemblance of cerebrospinal syphilis to disseminated sclerosis. Chicago, 1907. 8p. DNLM **00-5371**

SPINNEY, William Anthony
Health through self-control in thinking, breathing, eating. . . . Boston: Lothrop, Lee & Shepard Co., [1906]. 301p. DLC; MB; MH; NN **00-5372**

SPITZKA, Edward A[nthony] (1876-1922)
Is the central fissure duplicated in the brain of Carlo Giacomini, anatomist? [Philadelphia, 1901.] 4p. 1 plate. DNLM **00-5373**

SPITZKA, Edward A[nthony] (1876-1922)
The mesial relations of the inflected fissure; observations upon one hundred brains. New York, 1901. 13p. DNLM **00-5374**

SPITZKA, Edward A[nthony] (1876-1922)
A preliminary communication with projection-drawings, illustrating the topography of the paracoeles (lateral ventricles) in their relation to the surface of the cerebrum and the cranium. New York, 1901. 6p. DNLM **00-5375**

SPITZKA, Edward A[nthony] (1876-1922)
The redundancy of the preinsula in the brains of distinguished educated men. New York: William Wood & Co., 1901. 12p. DLC; DNLM **00-5376**

SPITZKA, Edward A[nthony] (1876-1922)
A rare fissural atypy in the brain of W. A., a New York assemblyman. [New York, 1902.] 2 l. DNLM **00-5377**

SPITZKA, Edward A[nthony] (1876-1922)
Three Eskimo brains, from Smith's Sound. [New York?, 1902.] 46p. NN **00-5378**

SPITZKA, Edward A[nthony] (1876-1922)
The brain-weight of the Japanese. New York, 1903. 3p. DNLM **00-5379**

SPITZKA, Edward A[nthony] (1876-1922)
The postorbital limbus; a formation occasionally met with at the base of the human brain. Philadelphia, 1903. 6p. DNLM **00-5380**

SPITZKA, Edward A[nthony] (1876-1922)
A study of the brain-weights of men notable in the professions, arts and sciences. [Philadelphia, 1903.] 14p. DLC; DNLM **00-5381**

SPITZKA, Edward A[nthony] (1876-1922)
A study of the brain of the late Major J. W. Powell. . . . Lancaster, Pa.: The New Era Printing Co., 1903. 58p. DLC; DNLM; NN **00-5382**

SPITZKA, Edward A[nthony] (1876-1922)
The execution and post-mortem examinations of the Van Wormer brothers at Dannemora, N.Y., October 1, 1903. New York, 1904. 4p. DNLM **00-5383**

SPITZKA, Edward A[nthony] (1876-1922)
. . . A study of the brains of six eminent scientists and scholars belonging to the American Anthropometric Society, together with a description of the skull of Professor E. D. Cope. . . . Philadelphia: The American Philosophical Society, 1907. 133p. DLC; NIC; PU **00-5384**

SPITZKA, Edward A[nthony] (1876-1922)
The resuscitation of persons shocked by electricity. Orange, 1909. 23p. DNLM **00-5385**

SPITZKA, Edward C[harles] (1852-1914)
The legal disabilities of natural children justified biologically and historically. St. Louis, 1900. 54p. DNLM [Continuation: 16p. (1900); 9p. (1901); 10p. (1901); 5p. (1901). DNLM] **00-5386**

SPITZKA, Edward C[harles] (1852-1914)
The Pathological Institute. [New York, 1900.] 16p. DLC; DNLM; NN **00-5387**

SPITZKA, Edward C[harles] (1852-1914)
The Czolgosz case. Philadelphia, 1901. 9p. DLC; DNLM; NN **00-5388**

SPITZKA, Edward C[harles] (1852-1914)
Fallacies of the Lombroso doctrine as evidenced in their application to the case of Musolino, the bandit. [New York, 1902.] 8 l. DLC; DNLM; NN **00-5389**

SPITZKA, Edward C[harles] (1852-1914)
A question of figures. [St. Louis, 1902.] 12p. DLC; DNLM; NN **00-5390**

SPITZKA, Edward C[harles] (1852-1914)
Mental diseases, forensic medicine. [New York, 1902.] 2 l. DLC; DNLM; NN **00-5391**

SPITZKA, Edward C[harles] (1852-1914)
Political assassins; are they all insane? [New York, 1902.] 32p. DLC; DNLM; NN **00-5392**

SPITZKA, Edward C[harles] (1852-1914)
A correspondence between Dr. Regis and Dr. Spitzka. Rejoinder to Dr. Regis' remonstrance. [Philadelphia, 1902.] 8p. DLC; DNLM; NN **00-5393**

SPITZKA, Edward C[harles] (1852-1914)
Remarks on the Czolgosz case and allied questions, as presented by Dr. Talbot. New York, 1902. 9p. DLC; DNLM; NN **00-5394**

SPITZKA, Edward C[harles] (1852-1914)
Regenticides not abnormal as a class; a protest against the chimera of degeneracy. [Philadelphia, 1902.] 24p. DNLM; NN **00-5395**

SPITZKA, Edward C[harles] (1852-1914)
Regicides, sane and insane. New York, 1903. 74p. DLC; DNLM; NN **00-5396**

SPIVAK, Charles D[avid] (1861-1927)
Autoinsufflation of the stomach; a new method. Philadelphia, 1900. 6p. DNLM **00-5397**

SPIVAK, Charles D[avid] (1861-1927)
Data and methods for diagnosis of diseases of the gastrointestinal tract; an epitome of lectures. Denver, 1900. 31p. DNLM **00-5398**

SPIVAK, Charles D[avid] (1861-1927)
Diet as a method of diagnosis. Philadelphia, 1900. 5p. DNLM **00-5399**

SPIVAK, Charles D[avid] (1861-1927)
The oesophagometer, or intragastric whistle, a new device for measuring the length of the oesophagus in the living. New York, 1901. 10p. DNLM **00-5400**

SPIVAK, Charles D[avid] (1861-1927)
Report of a case of carcinoma at the cardiac end of the esophagus, a distance of 21 inches from the incisor teeth! in a man 5 feet 3 inches tall. Burlington, Vt., & New York, 1901. 3p. DNLM **00-5401**

SPIVAK, Charles D[avid] (1861-1927)
The evolution of medical institutions in Colorado. Denver, 1902. 6p. DNLM **00-5402**

SPIVAK, Charles D[avid] (1861-1927)
Index medicus completum; a suggestion as to its realization. Burlington, Vt., & New York, 1902. 4p. DNLM **00-5403**

SPIVAK, Charles D[avid] (1861-1927)
The influence of biliary acids on surface tension; a preliminary report. [Chicago, 1902.] 4p. DNLM **00-5404**

SPIVAK, Charles D[avid] (1861-1927)
A new device for facilitating macroscopic and microscopic examination of feces. Burlington, Vt., & New York, 1902. 2p. DNLM **00-5405**

SPIVAK, Charles D[avid] (1861-1927)
Volvulus of the stomach. Burlington, Vt., & New York, 1903. 10p. DNLM **00-5406**

SPIVAK, Charles D[avid] (1861-1927)
A tent sanatorium for consumptives; the opening of a new Denver institution for the Jewish poor. [1904.] 2 l. DNLM **00-5407**

SPIVAK, Charles D[avid] (1861-1927)
Tympanites, eructation, merycism and aërophagia. Denver, 1904. 15p. DNLM **00-5408**

SPIVAK, Charles D[avid] (1861-1927)
Tubism; lavage habit. Burlington, Vt., & New York, 1904. 3p. DNLM **00-5409**

SPIVAK, Charles D[avid] (1861-1927)
Aërophagia and flatulence. New York, 1905. 24p. DNLM **00-5410**

SPIVAK, Charles D[avid] (1861-1927)
Benign strictures of the esophagus; report of cases. Burlington, Vt., & New York, 1905. 5p. DNLM **00-5411**

SPIVAK, Charles D[avid] (1861-1927)
A case of appendicitis simulating choleithiasis. Burlington, Vt., & New York, 1905. 1 l. DNLM **00-5412**

SPIVAK, Charles D[avid] (1861-1927)
Physicians in fiction; physicians as seen by Henry Fielding. Chicago, 1905. 8p. DNLM **00-5413**

SPIVAK, Charles D[avid] (1861-1927)
Physicians in fiction; physicians as seen by Oliver Wendell Holmes. New York, 1905. 16p. DNLM **00-5414**

SPIVAK, Charles D[avid] (1861-1927)
Habitual constipation, viewed from the standpoint of modern evolution of dietetics, is a physiological phenomenon. New York, 1906. 11p. DNLM **00-5415**

SPIVAK, Charles D[avid] (1861-1927)
The pelvic girdle for ptosis of the abdominal vicera; suggestion for its use in tuberculosis, etc. Burlington, Vt., & New York, 1906. 16p. DNLM **00-5416**

SPIVAK, Charles D[avid] (1861-1927)
The use of oxygen in asphyxia neonatorum. New York, 1906. 2p. DNLM **00-5417**

SPIVAK, Charles D[avid] (1861-1927)
Dietetics; a general consideration of its diagnostic and therapeutic value; monodiet. Denver, 1907. 16p. DNLM **00-5418**

SPIVAK, Charles D[avid] (1861-1927)
Iconoclastic revision of a classical case of diverticulum of the oesophagus. New York, 1910. 9p. DNLM **00-5419**

SPIVAK, Charles D[avid] (1861-1927)
Physicians in fiction; physicians as seen by Sara Orne Jewett. [New York, 1910.] 8p. DNLM **00-5420**

SPIVAK, Charles D[avid] (1861-1927)
Studies in feces; the use of carmine as an indicator in test-meals. Denver, 1910. 7p. DNLM **00-5421**

SPIVAK, Charles D[avid] (1861-1927)
The whistle in the stomach, who blew it first? A question of priority. [Chicago, 1910.] 3p. DNLM **00-5422**

SPRAGUE, Frank B[radford] (*b.* 1865)
Observations in two hundred cases of mastoid disease with operations. St. Louis, 1903. 14p. DNLM **00-5423**

SPRAGUE, Frank B[radford] (*b.* 1865)
Scarlatinal otitis. . . . [Philadelphia, New York: Lea Bros. & Co., 1905.] 9p. DLC **00-5424**

SPRAGUE, Frank B[radford] (*b.* 1865)
The blood-clot method of wound repair in aural surgery. St. Louis, 1906. 12p. DNLM **00-5425**

SPRATLING, William P[hilip] (1863-1915)
The Craig Colony for Epileptics at Sonyea in Livingston County, New York. Bulletin of general information concerning its origin, purposes and methods of work. [Buffalo], 1902. 53p. portrait, plates. MB **00-5426**

SPRATLING, William P[hilip] (1863-1915)
Epilepsy in its relation to crime. New York, 1902. 16p. DNLM **00-5427**

SPRATLING, William P[hilip] (1863-1915)
Epilepsy and its treatment. Philadelphia, New York & London: W. B. Saunders & Co., 1904. 522p. 30 plates. DNLM; MBM; NN; PU **00-5428**

SPRATLING, William P[hilip] (1863-1915)
Guides to the prognosis in epilepsy, with remarks on the curability of the disease, including reports of thirty-four cases. New York, 1904. 25p. DLC **00-5429**

SPRATLING, William P[hilip] (1863-1915)
The nonoperative relief of eyestrain for the possible cure of epilepsy as tested in 68 cases at the Craig Colony. Burlington, Vt., & New York, 1904. 14p. DLC **00-5430**

SPRATLING, William P[hilip] (1863-1915)
The psychological aspects of epilepsy. Detroit, 1904. 21p. DLC **00-5431**

SPRATLING, William P[hilip] (1863-1915)
List of food articles suitable for epileptics. [Sonyea, N.Y.: Craig Colony for Epileptics, 1904?] Folded sheet. MB **00-5432**

SPRINGER, Harold L. (*b.* 1881)
An analytical study of six hundred cases of anaesthesia. New York, 1908. 11p. DNLM **00-5433**

SPURZHEIM, Johann Gaspar (1776-1832)
Phrenology, or the doctrine of the mental phenomena; . . . With an introduction by Cyrus Elder. Rev. ed. from the 2nd American ed. . . . Philadelphia & London: J. B. Lippincott Co., 1908. 459p. plates. CtY-M; DLC; ICJ; PPC **00-5434**

SQUIBB, E[dward] H[amilton] (*b.* 1853)
Brief comments on the materia medica, pharmacy, and therapeutics of the year ending July 1, 1900. (Alphabetically arranged.) New York, 1901. 136p. DNLM; NNNAM **00-5435**

SQUIBB, Edward R[obinson] (1819-1900)
Semi-annual price list of standard pharmaceutical preparations and pharmacopoeial reagents. No. 84. [Brooklyn, N.Y., 1900.] DNLM [*Also*: No. 85, Brooklyn, N.Y., 1901; No. 86, Brooklyn, N.Y., 1901] **00-5436**

SQUIBB's . . . , Materia Medica. 1906 ed. A complete alphabetical list of all the Squibb products, embracing the articles in the U.S. pharmacopoeia (8th revision) and the national formulary, together with the non-official chemicals, pharmaceuticals and newer remedies in general use. . . . New York, Brooklyn: E. R. Squibb & Sons, [1906]. 394p. DLC; NNNAM; OCLloyd; PU **00-5437**

SQUIER, J[ohn] Bentley (1873-1948)
The significance of bladder symptoms in relation to some spinal cord lesions. New York: A. R. Elliott Co., 1907. 11p. DNLM **00-5438**

SQUIER, J[ohn] Bentley (1873-1948)
The bladder in tabes. New York, 1908. 6p. DNLM **00-5439**

SQUIER, J[ohn] Bentley (1873-1948)
Two unusual cystoscopic pictures. New York, 1908. 5p. DNLM **00-5440**

SQUIER, J[ohn] Bentley (1873-1948)
Suprapubic intra-urethral enucleation of the prostate. Boston: W. M. Leonard, 1910. 21p. NN **00-5441**

STACKHOUSE, Asa Matlack
. . . Maladies, remedies and physicians of colonial days in Burlington County, and other kindred topics. . . . Moorestown, N.J.: Settle Press Printing Co., 1908. 52p. DLC; ICJ; PPC; PU **00-5442**

STACPOOLE, Florence
Advice to women on the care of the health, before, during and after confinement. . . . New York: J. S. Ogilvie, 1900 [*c.* 1893]. 128p. DLC: MH; NIC; NN [*vel subseq.*] **00-5443**

STACY, Thomas Hobbs (*b.* 1850)
Rev. Otis Robinson Bacheler, M.D., D.D., fifty-three years missionary to India. . . . Boston, Mass.: The Morning Star Publishing House, 1904. 512p. plates. DLC; MB; MH; NN **00-5444**

STAFFORD, Ezra Hurlburt
Medicine, surgery and hygiene in the century. . . . Philadelphia, [etc.]: The Linscott Publishing Co., 1901. 527p. 6 port. (incl. front.) DLC; ICJ; MH; NN **00-5445**

STAFFORD, Ezra Hurlburt
. . . Medicine, surgery; and hygiene in the century. . . . Philadelphia, Detroit, [etc.]: The Bradley-Garretson Co., 1903. 527p. 5 port. (incl. front.) DLC; ICJ; NN; PU **00-5446**

STAINSBY, William
. . . Diseases and disease tendencies of occupation. The glass industry and the hatting industry. . . . Trenton, N.J.: [MacCrelish & Quigley, Printers], 1901. 55p. DLC; PU **00-5447**

STALL, Sylvanus (1847-1915)
What a man of forty-five ought to know. Philadelphia: The Vir Publishing Co., [1901]. 284p. port. DNLM; MH; NIC; NN
00-5448

STALL, Sylvanus (1847-1915)
. . . What a young man ought to know. . . . [New ed.] Philadelphia, [etc.] : The Vir Publishing Co., [etc., etc., 1904]. 269p. port. DLC; ICJ; NIC; NN **00-5449**

STALL, Sylvanus (1847-1915)
. . . What a young boy ought to know. . . . [New rev. ed.] Philadelphia: The Vir Publishing Co., [etc., etc., 1905]. 193p. port. DLC; MH; NIC; NN **00-5450**

STALL, Sylvanus (1847-1915)
The social peril. . . . Philadelphia, London: The Vir Publishing Co.; Toronto: W. Briggs, [1905]. 329p. port. DLC; ICU; MH; NN **00-5451**

STALL, Sylvanus (1847-1915)
. . . What a young husband ought to know. . . . [New rev. ed.] Philadelphia, [etc.] : The Vir Publishing Co., [1907]. 284p. port. DLC, ICJ; MH; NN **00-5452**

THE STANDARD Medical directory of North America, 1902. . . . Chicago: G. P. Englehard & Co., [1902. – Irregular] 924p. DLC; ICJ; ICU; MB [Includes a directory of practicing physicians in the U.S., Canada, Cuba, Mexico, and Central America; a list of Medical Colleges with a thumbnail historical sketch of each; directories of medical officers of the Armed services; summaries of the Medical Practice Acts of all the states and the Canadian provinces; list of all medicines & drugs then in use; list of sanitoria, medical springs, etc.]
00-5453

STANHOPE, Leonard E.
The science of magnetic healing, embracing hypnotism, vital magnetism, and mental science. Girard, Kansas: Appeal to Reason, 1900 [*c.* 1898]. 119p. DLC
00-5454

STANHOPE. Leonard E.
Magnetic healing explained. Nevada, Missouri, [1900?] 108p. DLC **00-5455**

STANISLAUS, Ignatius Valerius Stanley (*b.* 1870)
A short pharmaceutic chemistry, inorganic and organic, by I. V. Stanley Stanislaus . . . and Charles H. Kimberly . . . 2nd ed. Philadelphia: P. Blakiston's Son & Co., 1908. 610p. DLC; ICJ; NN; PPJ **00-5456**

STARKE, J.
Alcohol, the sanction for its use scientifically established and popularly expounded by a physiologist; transl. from the German of Dr. J. Starke. New York and London: G. P. Putnam's Sons, 1907. 317p. DLC; MH; NIC; NN
00-5457

STARKEY, Horace M[ann] (*b.* 1851)
A table of ocular extrinsic paralyses. Chicago, 1901. 8p. 1 table. DNLM **00-5458**

STARKEY, Horace M[ann] (*b.* 1851)
The use of mydriatic after the age of forty-five. Chicago, 1903. 18p. 1 table. DNLM
00-5459

STARLING, Ernest Henry (1866-1927)
Mercers' company lectures on recent advances in the physiology of digestion, delivered in the Michaelmas term, 1905, in the Physiological Department of University College, London. . . . Chicago: W. T. Keener & Co., 1906. 156p. DLC: ICJ; IU-M; OCIM **00-5460**

STARLING, Ernest Henry (1866-1927)
Elements of human physiology. . . . Eighth edition. Chicago: W. T. Keener & Co., 1907. 716p. illus. CtY-M; ICJ; NN; PPC
00-5461

STARLING, Ernest Henry (1866-1927)
The fluids of the body. Chicago: W. T. Keener & Co., 1909. 186p. illus. IU-M; NcD; PPC; PPJ [Herter lectures 1908]
00-5462

STARR, Louis (1849-1925)
Diseases of the digestive organs in infancy and childhood, with chapters on the diet and general management of children, and massage in pediatrics. . . . 3rd ed., rewritten and enl. . . . Philadelphia: P. Blakiston's Son & Co., 1901. 448p. plates. DLC; DNLM; PPC; PPJ **00-5463**

STARR, Louis (1849-1925)
Diets for infants and children in health and in disease. Philadelphia: W. B. Saunders, 1901. NNNAM; PPC; PU; PPJ [230 blanks (pocket-book size) perforated and bound in flexible morocco; the first series of blanks are prepared for the first seven months of infant life. Each blank indicates the *ingredients*, but not the *quantities*, of the food, the latter directions being left for the physician. After the seventh month, modifications being less necessary, the diet-lists are printed in full. Formulae for the preparation of diluents and foods are appended.] **00-5464**

STARR, Louis (1849-1925)
Hygiene of the nursery, including the general regimen and feeding of infants and children; massage, and the domestic management of the ordinary emergencies of early life. . . . 7th ed. With twenty-five illustrations. Philadelphia: P. Blakiston's Son & Co., 1906. 309p. DLC; DNLM; NNNAM; PPC **00-5465**

STARR, M[oses] Allen (1854-1932)
Organic nervous diseases. . . . Illustrated with 275 engravings in the text and 26 plates in colors and monochrome. New York and Philadelphia: Lea Bros. & Co., 1903. 751p. DLC; DNLM; NNNAM; PPC **00-5466**

STARR, M[oses] Allen (1854-1932)
Synopsis of lectures upon diseases of the nervous system; delivered at the College of Physicians and Surgeons, Medical Department of Columbia University, New York. New York: Doughtery, [*c.* 1904]. 99p. CtY-M; NNC **00-5467**

STARR, M[oses] Allen (1854-1932)
Organic and functional nervous diseases . . . 2nd ed., thoroughly rev., illustrated with 282 engravings in the text and 26 plates in colors and monochrome. New York and Philadelphia: Lea Bros. & Co., [1907]. 816p. DLC; DNLM; NNNAM; PPC
00-5468

STARR, M[oses] Allen (1854-1932)
Organic and functional nervous diseases; a textbook of neurology . . . 3rd ed., thoroughly rev., illustrated with 300 engravings in the text and 29 plates in colors and monochrome. New York and Philadelphia: Lea & Febiger, 1909. 911p. DLC; DNLM; NNNAM; PPC **00-5469**

STARRETT, Danvill William (*b.* **1859)**
Discoveries which make mental therapeutics and the transmission of mental communications an exact science. . . . Oakland, 1908. 78p. DLC; ICJ; NN **00-5470**

STARRETT, Danvill William (*b.* **1859)**
Mental therapeutics; or, How to cure all diseases with the mind. . . . San Francisco: [F. H. Abbott, printer], 1908. 84p. DLC; NN **00-5471**

STATE CHARITIES AID ASSOCIATION, NEW YORK
. . . Prevention of tuberculosis; proceedings of a public meeting held in Harmanus Bleecker Hall, Albany, January 27, 1908, and handbook of the campaign for the prevention of tuberculosis in New York State (outside of New York City) carried on by the State Charities Aid Association in co-operation with the New York State Department of Health, April 1, 1908. . . . New York, [1908]. 108p. incl. facsim., tables, plates, diags. DLC; NN **00-5472**

STATE CHARITIES AID ASSOCIATION, NEW YORK
. . . New hospitals needed in greater New York; recommendation by the Standing Committee on Hospitals of the State Charities Aid Association; with a report on present conditions and future needs by Mr. Phil P. Jacobs. . . . New York City, [1908]. 83p. incl. tables, 3 fold. maps. DLC; NN **00-5473**

STATE CHARITIES AID ASSOCIATION, NEW YORK
. . . Proceedings of the conference of the local committee on the prevention of tuberculosis of the State Charities Aid Association, Albany, New York, March 18-19, 1910. . . . [New York, 1910.] 248p. DLC; NN **00-5474**

STAVELY, Albert L[ivingston] (*b.* **1863)**
Acute and chronic gastro-mesenteric ileus, with cure in a chronic case by duodeno-jejunostomy. Baltimore, 1908. 11p. DNLM **00-5475**

STEARNS, Guy B[eckley] (*b.* **1870)**
Diseases of the middle ear and naso-pharynx. New York, 1904. 8p. DNLM **00-5476**

STEARNS, Guy B[eckley] (*b.* **1870)**
Apropos of radium, by. . . . [New York City, 19–.] 6p. NN **00-5477**

STEARNS, Guy B[eckley] (*b.* **1870)**
Treatment of influenza. [New York? 19–?] 10p. NN [For the Department of Materia Medica, New York Homoeopathic Medical College.] **00-5478**

STEDMAN, Henry R[ust] (1849-1926)
A case of moral insanity with repeated homicides and incendiarism and late development of delusions. Boston, 1904. 10p. 1 plate. DNLM **00-5479**

STEDMAN, Henry R[ust] (1849-1926)
The public obligations of the neurologist. Lancaster, Pa., 1906. 11p. DNLM **00-5480**

STEELE, J[ohn] Dutton (1868-1908)
Pathology of acquired heart disease in children. Philadelphia, 1900. 15p. PU **00-5481**

STEELE, J[ohn] Dutton (1868-1908)
The present aspects of the antitoxin treatment of diphtheria. Detroit, 1901. 14p. DNLM **00-5482**

STEELE, J[ohn] Dutton (1868-1908)
A case of chronic interstitial pancreatitis with involvement of the islands of Langerhans in a diabetic. Philadelphia, 1902. 6p. DNLM **00-5483**

STEELE, J[ohn] Dutton (1868-1908)
Gastroptosis and gastric motor insufficiency. Philadelphia, 1902. 24p. DNLM **00-5484**

STEELE, J[ohn] Dutton (1868-1908) and Albert Philip FRANCINE
An analysis of seventy cases of gastroptosis. Chicago, 1902. 20p. DNLM **00-5485**

STEELE, J[ohn] Dutton (1868-1908)
Experimental evidence of biliary obstruction in floating liver. Philadelphia, 1903. 25p. DNLM **00-5486**

STEELE, J[ohn] Dutton (1868-1908) and Albert Philip FRANCINE
Two years' experience in gastroptosis. Philadelphia, 1903. 36p. DNLM **00-5487**

STEELE, J[ohn] Dutton (1868-1908)
Pleural effusion in heart disease. Chicago, 1904. 15p. 1 table. DNLM **00-5488**

STEELE, J[ohn] Dutton (1868-1908)
Retroperitoneal sarcoma. Philadelphia, 1904. 28p. DNLM **00-5489**

STEELE, J[ohn] Dutton (1868-1908)
Two cases of scarlatina-morbilli and one case of the so-called scarlatiniform serum eruption in diphtheria. [Detroit], 1904. 17p. DNLM **00-5490**

STEELE, J[ohn] Dutton (1868-1908)
The detection of functional disturbances of digestion by the examination of the feces. New York, 1905. 19p. DNLM **00-5491**

STEELE, J[ohn] Dutton (1868-1908)
The tests for occult blood in the feces, and their clinical significance. Athens: W. G. Jordan, 1905. 7p. DNLM **00-5492**

STEELE, J[ohn] Dutton (1868-1908) and William R. BUTT
Occult blood in the feces, and its clinical significance. Philadelphia, 1905. 16p. DNLM **00-5493**

STEELE, J[ohn] Dutton (1868-1908)
The etiology and treatment of chronic constipation. [Philadelphia], 1906. 63p. DNLM **00-5494**

STEELE, J[ohn] Dutton (1868-1908)
Hyperesthesia of the gastric mucous membrane and its treatment. Detroit: E. G. Swift, 1906. 10p. DNLM **00-5495**

STEELE, J[ohn] Dutton (1868-1908)
Notes upon the clinical examination of the feces. [Philadelphia], 1906. 11p. DNLM **00-5496**

STEELE, J[ohn] Dutton (1868-1908)
The nucleus test in pancreatic disease. [Philadelphia], 1906. 17p. DNLM **00-5497**

STEELE, J[ohn] Dutton (1868-1908)
The relation of excessive gastric acidity to gastric symptoms. [Chicago], 1906. 8p. DNLM **00-5498**

STEELE, J[ohn] Dutton (1868-1908)
The therapeutical and prognostic value of occult hemorrhage in the stools. New York, 1906. 5p. DNLM **00-5499**

STEELE, J[ohn] Dutton (1868-1908)
Experimental observations upon the value of intestinal antiseptics. Philadelphia, 1907. 13p. DNLM **00-5500**

STEELE, J[ohn] Dutton (1868-1908)
The method of determining the total amount of the fecal bacteria by weight and its clinical significance. Chicago, 1907. 11p. DNLM **00-5501**

STEEVES, Alice M.
Is a medical education a necessary qualification for dental practice . . . read before the American Medical Association, section of stomatology, Atlantic City, N.J. June 5, 1900. [n.p.], 1900. 4p. DLC **00-5502**

STEIN, Sydney A.
The management of chronic endocarditis during the stage of compensation. New York, 1908. 8p. DNLM **00-5503**

STEINER, Walter Ralph (1870-1942)
Haemophilia in the negro. Baltimore, 1900. 8p. DNLM **00-5504**

STEINER, Walter Ralph (1870-1942)
Dermatomyositis, with report of a case which also presented a rare muscle anomaly but once described in man. Boston, 1901. 12p. DNLM **00-5505**

STEINER, Walter Ralph (1870-1942)
Report of a case of carcinoma diagnosed by means of paracentesis abdominis, with some remarks on the diagnositc value of examinations of serous effusions. Baltimore, 1901. 14p. DNLM **00-5506**

STEINER, Walter Ralph (1870-1942)
A contribution to the history of medicine in the Province of Maryland, 1636-71. Baltimore, 1902. 19p. DNLM **00-5507**

STEINER, Walter Ralph (1870-1942)
Peripheral venous thrombosis in pneumonia, with report of three cases and a review of those previously recorded. Abstract. Baltimore, 1902. 7p. DNLM **00-5508**

STEINER, Walter Ralph (1870-1942)
Governor John Winthrop, Jr., of Connecticut, as a physician. Baltimore, 1903. 26p. DNLM **00-5509**

STEINER, Walter Ralph (1870-1942)
Report on progress of medicine. New Haven, 1903. 13p. DNLM **00-5510**

STEINER, Walter Ralph (1870-1942)
The importance of blood examinations in medicine and surgery. New Haven, 1903. 7p. DNLM **00-5511**

STEINER, Walter Ralph (1870-1942)
Some early autopsies in the United States. Baltimore, 1903. 7p. DNLM **00-5512**

STEINER, Walter Ralph (1870-1942)
A case of typhoid fever presenting an arterial complication. Probably an arteritis. Philadelphia, 1904. 5p. DNLM **00-5513**

STEINER, Walter Ralph (1870-1942)
A contribution to the history of medicine in Maryland during the revolution, 1775. Baltimore, 1905. 23p. DNLM **00-5514**

STEINER, Walter Ralph (1870-1942)
Governor John Winthrop, Jr., of Connecticut, as a physician. (Second paper.) Baltimore, 1906. 10p. DNLM **00-5515**

STEINER, Walter Ralph (1870-1942)
The revered Gershom Bulkeley, of Connecticut, an eminent clerical physician. Baltimore, 1906. 14p. DNLM **00-5516**

STEINER, Walter Ralph (1870-1942)
Stokes-Adams disease, with report of three cases. Boston, 1906. 15p. DNLM **00-5517**

STEINER Walter Ralph (1870-1942)
Elisha North, one of Connecticut's most eminent medical practitioners. Baltimore, 1908. 19p. DNLM **00-5518**

STEINER, Walter Ralph (1870-1942)
The pathology of renal tuberculosis. New Haven, 1908. 4p. DNLM **00-5519**

STEINER, Walter Ralph (1870-1942)
Sporadic trichinosis, with report of a case. Boston, 1908. 12p. DNLM **00-5520**

STEINER, Walter Ralph (1870-1942) and Clarence B. INGRAHAM, Jr.
Epidemic cerebrospinal meningitis in Hartford, Connecticut, during 1904-5; with special references to the cases treated at the Hartford Hospital. Philadelphia, 1908. 15p. DNLM **00-5521**

STEINHARDT, Irving D[avid] (*b.* 1878)
Anterior poliomyelitis. New York, 1908. 15p. DNLM **00-5522**

STEINHARDT, Irving D[avid] (*b.* 1878)
Painful heels. New York, 1909. 7p. DNLM **00-5523**

STELLA, Antonio (1868-1927)
The effect of urban conditions on the Italian women and children. . . . New York: William Wood & Co., (1908). 36p. DLC **00-5524**

STELLA, Antonio (1868-1927)
The prevalence of tuberculosis among Italians in the United States, its causes and remedies. [Philadelphia, 1908?] 28p. MH **00-5525**

STELWAGON, Henry W[eightman] (1853-1919)
Address before the American Dermatological Association at the twenty-fourth annual meeting. [Chicago], 1900. 12p. DNLM **00-5526**

STELWAGON, Henry W[eightman] (1853-1919)
Phototherapy in cutaneous medicine; an account of a visit to Professor Finsen's Light-Institute at Copenhagen. Philadelphia, 1900. 8p. DNLM **00-5527**

STELWAGON, Henry W[eightman] (1853-1919)
A report of two cases of persistent exfoliation of the lips. Chicago, 1900. 8p. DNLM **00-5528**

STELWAGON, Henry W[eightman] (1853-1919)
Treatment of lupus by the concentrated light-rays. Philadelphia, 1900. 4p. DNLM **00-5529**

STELWAGON, Henry W[eightman] (1853-1919)
Treatment of skin cancers without operation. Chicago, 1900. 12p. DNLM **00-5530**

STELWAGON, Henry W[eightman] (1853-1919)
Report of a case of blastomycetic dermatitis. Philadelphia, 1901. 8p. DNLM **00-5531**

STELWAGON, Henry W[eightman] (1853-1919)
Treatise on diseases of the skin, for the use of advanced students and practitioners. . . . Philadelphia and London: W. B. Saunders & Co., 1902. 1175p. col. plates. DLC; DNLM; NNNAM; PPC **00-5532**

STELWAGON, Henry W[eightman] (1853-1919)
Treatise on diseases of the skin, for the use of advanced students and practitioners . . . 2nd ed., with 220 illustrations in the text, and 26 full-page lithographic and half-tone plates. Philadelphia and London: W. B. Saunders & Co., 1903. 1115p. DLC; DNLM; NNNAM; PPC **00-5533**

STELWAGON, Henry W[eightman] (1853-1919)
. . . Essentials of diseases of the skin, including syphilodermata; arranged in the form of questions and answers, prepared especially for students of medicine . . . 5th ed., thoroughly rev. . . . Philadelphia: W. B. Saunders & Co., 1903. 276p. plates. NNNAM; PU **00-5534**

STELWAGON, Henry W[eightman] (1853-1919)
Treatise on diseases of the skin, for the use of advanced students and practitioners . . . 3rd ed., with 220 illustrations in the text, and 26 full-page lithographic and half-tone plates. Philadelphia, London, [etc.]: W. B. Saunders & Co., 1904. 1115p. DLC; DNLM; MBM; PU **00-5535**

STELWAGON, Henry W[eightman] (1853-1919)
Treatise on the diseases of the skin, for the use of advanced students and practitioners . . . 4th ed., thoroughly rev. With 258 illustrations in the text, and 32 full-page lithographic and halftone plates. Philadelphia and London: W. B. Saunders & Co., 1905. 1136p. DLC; DNLM; NNNAM; PPC
00-5536

STELWAGON, Henry W[eightman] (1853-1919)
. . . Essentials of diseases of the skin, including the syphilodermata; arranged in the form of questions and answers, prepared especially for students of medicine . . . 6th ed., thoroughly rev. . . . Philadelphia, [etc.]: W. B. Saunders & Co., 1905. 274p. plates. DLC; PPC
00-5537

STELWAGON, Henry W[eightman] (1853-1919)
Treatise on diseases of the skin, for the use of advanced students and practitioners . . . 5th ed., thoroughly rev., with 267 illustrations in the text, and 34 full-page colored and half-tone plates. Philadelphia and London: W. B. Saunders & Co., 1907. 1150p. DLC; DNLM; LNT-M; PU
00-5538

STELWAGON, Henry W[eightman] (1853-1919)
. . . Essentials of diseases of the skin, including the syphilodermata, arranged in the form of questions and answers; prepared especially for students of medicine . . . 7th ed., thoroughly rev. . . . Philadelphia and London: W. B. Saunders & Co., 1909. 291p. plates. DLC; NNNAM; PPC
00-5539

STELWAGON, Henry W[eightman] (1853-1919)
Treatise on diseases of the skin, for the use of advanced students and practitioners . . . 6th ed., thoroughly rev. With 289 illustrations in the text, and 34 full-page colored and half-tone plates. Philadelphia and London: W. B. Saunders & Co., 1910. 1195p. DLC: DNLM; NNNAM; PPC
00-5540

STENGEL, Alfred (1868-1939)
A text-book of pathology . . . with 372 illustrations. 3rd ed., rev. Philadelphia and London: W. B. Saunders & Co., 1900. 873p. col. plates. DLC; DNLM; NNNAM; PPC
00-5541

STENGEL, Alfred (1868-1939)
Aneurism of the arch of the aorta, with rupture into the superior vena cava. Philadelphia, 1900. 9p. DNLM
00-5542

STENGEL, Alfred (1868-1939)
Some notes on the treatment of rheumatism. New York, 1900. 10p. DNLM **00-5543**

STENGEL, Alfred (1868-1939)
Progressive pernicious anemia. New York, 1900. 11p. DNLM **00-5544**

STENGEL, Alfred (1868-1939)
A review of the history of cardiac pathology, with especial reference to modern conceptions of myocardial disease. Philadelphia, 1900. 27p. DNLM **00-5545**

STENGEL, Alfred (1868-1939)
The treatment of typhoid fever. Pittsburgh, 1900. 7p. DNLM **00-5546**

STENGEL, Alfred (1868-1939)
Right-sided cardiac hydrothorax. Philadelphia, 1901. 24p. 1 plate. DNLM **00-5547**

STENGEL, Alfred (1868-1939) and C. Y. WHITE
The blood in infancy and childhood. Philadelphia, 1901. 36p. DNLM **00-5548**

STENGEL, Alfred (1868-1939)
Iodic purpura with fever. Detroit: W. M. Warren, 1902. 20p. DNLM **00-5549**

STENGEL, Alfred (1868-1939), C. Y. WHITE, and William PEPPER
Further studies on granular degeneration of the erythrocyte. Philadelphia, 1902. 8p. DNLM **00-5550**

STENGEL, Alfred (1868-1939)
Syphilis of the lungs simulating pulmonary tuberculosis. Philadelphia, 1903. 30p. DNLM **00-5551**

STENGEL, Alfred (1868-1939)
Sensations interpreted as live animals in the stomach. Philadelphia, 1903. 10p. DNLM **00-5552**

STENGEL, Alfred (1868-1939)
Articular rheumatism and some allied conditions. Philadelphia, 1903. 16p. DNLM **00-5553**

STENGEL, Alfred (1868-1939)
Diabetes as a complication of pregnancy. Philadelphia, 1903. 20p. DNLM **00-5554**

STENGEL, Alfred (1868-1939) and C. Y. WHITE
A report of a case of chronic acetanilid poisoning, with marked alterations in the blood. Philadelphia, 1903. 10p. 1 plate. DNLM **00-5555**

STENGEL, Alfred (1868-1939)
A text-book of pathology . . . with 394 illustrations in the text, many of them in colors, and 7 full-page chromolithographic plates. 4th ed., thoroughly rev. Philadelphia, [etc.] : W. B. Saunders & Co., 1903. 963p. CtY-M; DLC; DNLM; PPC **00-5556**

STENGEL, Alfred (1868-1939)
The clinical course and diagnosis of arteriosclerosis. Milwaukee, 1904. 18p. DNLM **00-5557**

STENGEL, Alfred (1868-1939)
The early diagnosis of arteriosclerosis. Philadelphia, 1904. 10p. DNLM **00-5558**

STENGEL, Alfred (1868-1939)
Varieties of splenic anaemia. Philadelphia, 1904. 40p. DNLM **00-5559**

STENGEL, Alfred (1868-1939) and W. B. STANTON
The heart and circulation in pregnancy and the puerperium. Philadelphia, 1904. 34p. DNLM **00-5560**

STENGEL, Alfred (1868-1939)
Aims and methods in medical diagnosis. Los Angeles, 1905. 8p. DNLM **00-5561**

STENGEL, Alfred (1868-1939)
The development of modern medical education. Philadelphia, 1905. 21p. DNLM **00-5562**

STENGEL, Alfred, ed. (1868-1939)
. . . Diseases of the blood, by Prof. Dr. P. Ehrlich . . . Prof. K. von Noorden . . . Dr. A. Lazarus . . . Dr. F. Pinkus . . . ed. with additions by Alfred Stengel. . . . Authorized translation from the German, under the editorial supervision of Alfred Stengel. . . . Philadelphia and London: W. B. Saunders & Co., 1905. 714p. col. plates. DLC; IU-M; NNNAM; PPC [American ed., Nothnagel's encyclopedia of practical medicine] **00-5563**

STENGEL, Alfred (1868-1939)
Albuminuria in nephritis and Bright's disease. Chicago, 1906. 7p. DNLM **00-5564**

STENGEL, Alfred (1868-1939)
Arteriosclerosis as a general disease. Burlington, Vt., & New York, 1906. 11p. DNLM **00-5565**

STENGEL, Alfred (1868-1939)
Chronic acetanilid poisoning. Report of two additional cases. Philadelphia, 1906. 7p. DNLM **00-5566**

STENGEL, Alfred (1868-1939)
The diagnosis and medical treatment of Graves' disease and hyperthyroidism. Athens, Pa., 1906. 6 l. DNLM **00-5567**

STENGEL, Alfred (1868-1939)
A fatal case of Stokes-Adams disease, with autopsy, showing involvement of auriculo-ventricular bundle of His. Philadelphia, 1906. 9p. DNLM **00-5568**

STENGEL, Alfred (1868-1939)
Mucocele of the appendix. With report of a case possibly carcinomatous in nature. Philadelphia, 1906. 15p. DNLM **00-5569**

STENGEL, Alfred (1868-1939)
A text-book of pathology. . . . With 399 illustrations in the text, many of them in colors, and 7 full-page chromolithographic plates. 5th ed., thoroughly rev. Philadelphia and London: W. B. Saunders & Co., 1906. 979p. DLC; DNLM; MBM; PU **00-5570**

STENGEL, Alfred (1868-1939)
The value of chemical and biological methods in medical diagnosis. Philadelphia, 1907. 40p. DNLM **00-5571**

STENGEL, Alfred (1868-1939), C. Y. WHITE, and Joseph S. EVANS
Cryptogenetic streptococcus infection with persistent cutaneous eruption, enlargement of the lymphatic glands, and fever, suggesting syphilis. Philadelphia, 1907-08. 18p. DNLM **00-5572**

STENGEL, Alfred (1868-1939)
Nervous manifestations of arteriosclerosis. Philadelphia & New York, 1908. 13p. DNLM **00-5573**

STENGEL, Alfred (1868-1939)
Some considerations of exophthalmic goitre from the medical standpoint. New York, 1908. 8p. DNLM **00-5574**

STENHOUSE, John (*b.* 1861)
. . . Pathology, general and special; a manual for students and practitioners. By John Stenhouse . . . and John Ferguson. . . . Illustrated with 16 engravings and a colored plate. Philadelphia and New York: Lea Bros. & Co., [1906]. 285p. CtY-M; DLC; ICJ; PPC **00-5575**

STEPHENS, Albert Franklin (*b.* 1860)
The essentials of medical gynecology according to the eclectic, or specific, practice of medicine in the treatment of disease. . . . Cincinnati: The Scudder Bros. Co., 1907. 428p. 3 col. plates. DLC; ICJ **00-5576**

STEPHENS, Margaret
Woman and marriage; a handbook; with a preface by Dr. Mary Scharlieb; and an introduction by Mrs. S. A. Barnett. New York: F. A. Stokes Co., [1910]. 294p. DLC; DNLM; MH; NN **00-5577**

STEPHENSON, Frank H[alleck] (*b.* 1856)
Multiple neuritis; a case resulting probably from morphine toxaemia. New York, 1904. 7p. DNLM **00-5578**

STERN, Heinrich (1868-1918)
Diabetes mellitus; its detection and successful treatment. [New York, 1900.] 14 l. 2 plates. DNLM **00-5579**

STERN, Heinrich (1868-1918)
A sulphosalt of the aliphatic creosote-esters, and its therapeutic usefulness. Chicago, 1900. 15p. DNLM **00-5580**

STERN, Heinrich (1868-1918)
The clinical importance of aërophagia. New York, 1904. 13p. DNLM **00-5581**

STERN, Heinrich (1868-1918)
The autoxicoses. Their theory, pathology and treatment. . . . Chicago: G. P. Engelhard & Co., 1906. 222p. ICJ; MH-M; PU **00-5582**

STERN, Walter Gustav (*b.* 1874)
Congenital dislocation of the hip-joint, with special reference to Lorenz's bloodless operation. Cleveland, 1901. 15p. DNLM **00-5583**

STERN, Walter Gustav (*b.* 1874)
Report of a case of paralytic club-foot. Cleveland, 1901. 2 l. DNLM **00-5584**

STERN, Walter Gustav (*b.* 1874)
The care and treatment of crippled and deformed children. Cleveland, 1903. 7p. DNLM **00-5585**

STERN, Walter Gustav (*b.* 1874)
Morton's painful disease of the toes. Burlington, Vt., & New York, 1904. 13p. DNLM **00-5586**

STERN, Walter Gustav (*b.* 1874)
The surgical treatment of paralytic deformities. Cleveland, 1904. 6p. DNLM **00-5587**

STERN, Walter Gustav (*b.* 1874)
A successful method of treating fracture of the femur in infancy. New York, 1905. 10p. DNLM **00-5588**

STERN, Walter Gustav (*b.* 1874)
Adult flat foot, symptoms and treatment. Cleveland, 1906. 6p. DNLM **00-5589**

STERN, Walter Gustav (*b.* 1874)
Plaster-of-Paris; the effect of various substances upon its rate of setting and the subsequent strength and durability of the cast. Philadelphia, 1907. 12p. DNLM **00-5590**

STERN, Walter Gustav (*b.* 1874) and
Emanual ROSENBERG
Plastic radiography; a preliminary communication. Chicago, 1907. 6p. DNLM **00-5591**

STERNBERG, George Miller (1838-1915)
. . . Disinfection and individual prophylaxis against infectious diseases. [Revised in December, 1899, by the author.] . . . . Columbus, O.: The Berlin Printing Co., 1900. 45p. DLC; DNLM; ICJ; PU **00-5592**

STERNBERG, George Miller (1838-1915)
A text-book of bacteriology. . . . Illustrated by heliotype and chromo-lithographic plates and two hundred engravings. 2nd rev. ed. New York: William Wood & Co., 1901. 706p. DLC; DNLM; NNNAM; PU **00-5593**

STERNBERG, George Miller (1838-1915)
The function of the Army Medical School. The address at the annual commencement of the Army Medical School, at Washington, April 4, 1902. Philadelphia, 1902. 14p. DNLM **00-5594**

STERNBERG, George Miller (1838-1915)
Infection and immunity, with special reference to the prevention of infectious diseases. . . . New York and London: G. P. Putnam's Sons, 1903. 293p. DLC; DNLM; NNNAM; NcU **00-5595**

STETTEN, De Witt (*b.* 1879)
The experiments of Sauerbruch in the field of oesophageal surgery. New York, 1905. 9p. DNLM **00-5596**

STETTEN, De Witt (*b.* 1879)
Two unusual cases of varix. New York, 1906. 11p. DNLM **00-5597**

STETTEN, De Witt (*b.* 1879)
The treatment of abscesses by puncture and disinfection without incision and drainage. Chicago, 1907. 3p. DNLM **00-5598**

STETTEN, De Witt (*b.* 1879)
The modern administration of general anaesthesia in mouth, nose and pharynx surgery. New York, 1908. 16p. DNLM **00-5599**

STETTEN, De Witt (*b.* 1879)
Musculo-spiral (radial) paralysis due to dislocation of the head of the radius, with especial reference to those cases complicating fracture of the ulna. New York, 1908. 18p. DNLM: NN **00-5600**

STETTEN, De Witt (*b.* 1879)
Idiopathic progressive curvature of the radius, or so-called Madelung's deformity of the wrist (carpus varus and carpus valgus). Chicago, 1909. 28p. DNLM **00-5601**

STETTEN, De Witt (*b.* 1879)
The radical extirpation of pharyngoesophageal pressure diverticula. [New York, 1910.] 19p. NN **00-5602**

STEVENS, Alviso Burdett (1853-1940)
Arithmetic of pharmacy. . . . Reprinted from Merck's Report. New York: Merck & Co., 1905. 85p. DLC; NNNAM; PPHa; PU **00-5603**

STEVENS, Alviso Burdett (1853-1940)
Arithmetic of pharmacy. Reprinted from Merck's Report. 2nd ed. New York: Merck & Co., 1908. 85p. DLC; NN; NNNAM; PU **00-5604**

STEVENS, Alviso Burdett (1853-1940)
A manual of pharmacy and dispensing . . . illustrated with 150 engravings. Philadelphia and New York: Lea & Febiger, 1909. 421p. DLC; DNLM; NNNAM; PPC **00-5605**

STEVENS, A[rthur] A[lbert] (1865-1944)
A manual of the practice of medicine, prepared especially for students. 6th ed., revised and enlarged. Philadelphia: W. B. Saunders & Co., 1903. 556p. DLC; DNLM; PPC; PU **00-5606**

STEVENS, A[rthur] A[lbert] (1865-1944)
Modern materia medica and therapeutics. 3rd ed., entirely rewritten. Philadelphia: W. B. Saunders & Co., 1903. 663p. DLC; DNLM; PU **00-5607**

STEVENS, A[rthur] A[lbert] (1865-1944)
A manual of the practice of medicine, prepared especially for students. 7th ed., revised. Philadelphia & London: W. B. Saunders & Co., 1905. 556p. DLC; DNLM; NNNAM; PPC **00-5608**

STEVENS, A[rthur] A[lbert] (1865-1944)
Modern materia medica and therapeutics. 4th ed., thoroughly revised in conformity with the 8th revision (1905) of the United States Pharmacopoeia. Philadelphia: W. B. Saunders & Co., 1905. 670p. DLC; DNLM; PPC; PU **00-5609**

STEVENS, A[rthur] A[lbert] (1865-1944)
A manual of the practice of medicine, prepared especially for students. 8th ed., revised. Philadelphia & London: W. B. Saunders & Co., 1907. 558p. DLC: DNLM; LNT-M; PPC **00-5610**

STEVENS, A[rthur] A[lbert] (1865-1944)
Modern materia medica and therapeutics. 5th ed. Philadelphia & London: W. B. Saunders & Co., 1909. 675p. DLC; DNLM; NNNAM; PU **00-5611**

STEVENS, A[rthur] A[lbert] (1865-1944)
A manual of the practice of medicine, prepared especially for students . . . 9th ed., rev. . . . Philadelphia and London: W. B. Saunders & Co., 1910. 573p. DLC; ICJ; MH-M; NNNAM **00-5612**

STEVENS, A. Jay (*b.* 1866)
. . . The star quizzer on pharmacy, chemistry and materia medica. . . . Carefully rev. and greatly enl. in conformity with the U.S. pharmacopoeia of 1900, issued in 1905. By A. Jay Stevens . . . and Chas. W. Mallory . . . [6th ed. . . .] Ada, O.: Stevens & Mallory, [1905] . 158p. DLC [*vel subseq.*] **00-5613**

STEVENS, George T[homas] (1832-1921)
A treatise on the motor apparatus of the eyes, embracing an exposition of the anomalies of the ocular adjustments and their treatment; with the anatomy and physiology of the muscles and their accessories. Philadelphia: F. A. Davis Co., 1906. 496p. port., plates. DLC; ICJ; PPC; PU **00-5614**

STEVENS, George T[homas] (1832-1921)
Studies of nervous affections in relation to the adjustments of the eyes. . . . [New York: A. R. Elliott Publishing Co., 1910.] 122p. [various pagings.] ICJ; NNNAM **00-5615**

STEVENS, Martin L. (*b.* 1864)
Quantitative changes in the blood in pulmonary tuberculosis. New York: William Wood & Co., 1902. 11p. DNLM; MB; PPHa **00-5616**

STEVENS, Martin L. (*b.* 1864)
Things every tuberculous patient should know. New York, 1903. 7p. DNLM **00-5617**

STEVENSON, Mark D[ellman] (*b.* 1876)
How to place lenses before eyes so that distance of their respective anterior foci shall be the same. Chicago, 1900. 4p. DNLM **00-5618**

STEVENSON, Mark D[ellman] (*b.* 1876)
The crossed cylinder and its uses. Chiago, 1902. 6p. DNLM **00-5619**

STEVENSON, Mark D[ellman] (*b.* 1876)
An adjustable lid speculum. Chicago, 1904. 4p. DNLM **00-5620**

STEVENSON, Mark D[ellman] (*b.* 1876)
The discharging eye. [Cincinnati] , 1904. 3p. DNLM **00-5621**

STEVENSON, Mark D[ellman] (*b.* 1876)
The eye and the digestive system. Philadelphia, 1904. 6p. DNLM **00-5622**

STEVENSON, Mark D[ellman] (*b.* 1876)
Granular lids; some general facts. Toledo, 1904. 3p. DNLM **00-5623**

STEVENSON, Mark D[ellman] (*b.* 1876)
A shade to protect the examiner's eyes from the bright light when working with the source of light close to the mirror in photoscopy (retinoscopy). Chicago, 1904. 1 l. DNLM **00-5624**

STEVENSON, Mark D[ellman] (*b.* 1876)
Description of an advancement suture. With collective suggestions regarding operations on the ocular muscles. [Chicago] , 1905. 14p. DNLM **00-5625**

STEVENSON, Mark D[ellman] (*b.* 1876)
A new needle holder for the ophthalmic surgeon. [Chicago] , 1905. 1 l. DNLM **00-5626**

STEVENSON, Mark D[ellman] (*b.* 1876)
Nonlocalized inflammation of the border of the lids. Toledo, 1905. 2 l. DNLM **00-5627**

STEVENSON, Mark D[ellman] (*b.* 1876)
The removal of foreign bodies and substances from the eyeball and inner surface of the lids. Detroit: E. G. Swift, 1905. 14p. DNLM **00-5628**

STEVENSON, Mark D[ellman] (*b.* 1876)
Simple eye conditions that should be familiar to every physician. [Cincinnati] , 1905. 5p. DNLM **00-5629**

STEVENSON, Mark D[ellman] (*b.* 1876)
The tear-passages and their diseases. [Cincinnati, 1905.] 5p. DNLM **00-5630**

STEVENSON, Mark D[ellman] (*b.* 1876)
Photoscopy (skiascopy or retinoscopy). Philadelphia & London: W. B. Saunders & Co., 1906. 126p. 2 plates. DNLM; PPC **00-5631**

STEWART, Acheson
Visceral surgery in abstract. . . . Pittsburgh, Pa.: Medical Abstract Publishing Co., [1909]. 176p. DLC; DNLM; ICJ **00-5632**

STEWART, Charles E. (*b.* 1869)
The influence of alcohol on the opsonic power of the blood. Battle Creek, Mich., 1907. 8p. DNLM
00-5633

STEWART, David Denison (1859-1905)
Acute splenic miliary tuberculosis. Philadelphia, 1901. 8p. DNLM **00-5634**

STEWART, David Denison (1859-1905)
The galvanic current in the treatment of saccular aneurism. Illus. Philadelphia, 1901. 24p. DNLM; NN; PU
00-5635

STEWART, David Denison (1859-1905)
Contributions to medicine. Philadelphia, 1905. 47p. PPC
00-5636

STEWART, F[rancis] Edward (1853-1941)
Proposed national bureau of materia medica. Chicago, 1901. 15p. DNLM **00-5637**

STEWART, F[rancis] Edward (1853-1941)
The proper introduction of materia medica products to science and brands of the same to commerce. Philadelphia, 1902. 26p. DNLM **00-5638**

STEWART, F[rancis] Edward (1853-1941)
The waters of the Glen Springs, Watkins, N.Y. Utica, N.Y.: Balch Bros. & West Co., [1902]. 11p. DNLM
00-5639

STEWART, F[rancis] Edward (1853-1941)
The waters of the Glen Springs, Watkins, N.Y. Utica, N.Y.: Balch Bros. & West Co., [1902?]. 11p. PPC
00-5640

STEWART, F[rancis] Edward (1853-1941)
. . . A compend of pharmacy. . . . Based upon Prof. Joseph P. Remington's "Text-book of pharmacy" and the United States pharmacopoeia, eighth revision (1905). 6th ed., rev. and enl., with a very complete index, and table for converting English measures into metric and the reverse. Philadelphia: P. Blakiston's Son & Co., 1906. 187p. DLC; DNLM; NNNAM; PU **00-5641**

STEWART, F[rancis] Edward (1853-1941)
. . . A compend of pharmacy. . . . Based upon Prof. Joseph P. Remington's "Text-book of pharmacy" and the U.S.P. eighth revision (1905). 7th ed., rev., in accordance with the additions and corrections made in the U.S.P. to comply with the new food and drug act, 1907. . . . Philadelphia: P. Blakiston's Son & Co., 1908. 187p. DLC; DNLM; OCLloyd; PPC
00-5642

STEWART, F[rancis] Edward (1853-1941)
. . . A compend of pharmacy. . . . Based upon Prof. Joseph P. Remington's "Text-book of pharmacy" and the U.S.P. eighth revision (1905). 8th ed. Philadelphia: P. Blakiston's Son & Co., 1910. 193p. DNLM; NNNAM; PPC; PPJ
00-5643

STEWART, Francis T[orrens] (1874-1920)
A manual of surgery, for students and physicians. . . . With 504 illustrations. Philadelphia: P. Blakiston's Son & Co., 1907. 778p. DLC; DNLM; NNNAM; PPC **00-5644**

STEWART, Francis T[orrens] (1874-1920)
A manual of surgery for students and physicians . . . 2nd ed., wih 553 illustrations. Philadelphia: P. Blakiston's Son & Co., 1910. 682p. DLC; ICJ; PPC; PPPH **00-5645**

STEWART, George N[eil] (1860-1930)
A manual of physiology. With practical exercises. For students and practitioners. 4th ed. Philadelphia: W. B. Saunders & Co., 1900. 894p. CU-M; NNNAM; PPC; PU
00-5646

STEWART, George N[eil] (1860-1930)
A manual of physiology. With practical exercises. For students and practitioners. 5th ed. Philadelphia: W. B. Saunders & Co., 1905. 911p. CtY-M; MBM; PPC; PPJ
00-5647

STEWART, George N[eil] (1860-1930)
A manual of physiology. With practical exercises. For students and practitioners. 6th ed. New York: William Wood & Co., 1910. 1064p. IU-M; NNNAM; NNU-M; PU
00-5648

STEWART, Morse (1818-1906)
Pocket therapeutics and dose-book, with classification and explanation of the actions of medicines; doses in troy weight with metric equivalents, genitive endings of all medicines and preparations given in italics; etc. 4th ed. Philadelphia & New York: W. B. Saunders & Co., 1910. 263p. DLC; DNLM; NNNAM; PU **00-5649**

STEWART, Netta
Gynaecological nursing. New York: William Wood & Co., 1903. 174p. DNLM; NNNAM; PPC: PPJ
00-5650

STEWART, Netta and James YOUNG
Practical gynaecology, a manual for nurses and students. New York: William Wood & Co., 1909. 327p. 4 plates. CtY-M; DNLM; NNC; NNNAM **00-5651**

STEWART, Thomas M.
Nasal fibroma; a case; operation and autopsy. New York, 1900. 3p. DNLM **00-5652**

STIEREN, Edward (*b.* 1873)
A case of Jamaica ginger amblyopia. Pittsburgh, 1900. 6p. DNLM **00-5653**

STIEREN, Edward (*b.* 1873)
A report of two cases of metastatic choroiditis occurring in children following measles. Pittsburgh, Pa., 1900. 8p. DNLM
00-5654

STIEREN, Edward (*b.* 1873)
Tubercular dacryoadenitis and conjunctivitis, containing the report of a probable case ending in spontaneous recovery and a review of the previous literature on tubercular dacryadenoitis. Baltimore, 1901. 10p. DNLM **00-5655**

STILES, Charles W[ardell] (1867-1941)
Report upon the prevalence and geographic distribution of hookworm disease (uncinariasis or anchylostomiasis) in the United States. Washington: Government Printing Office, 1903. 121p. DNLM **00-5656**

STILES, Charles W[ardell] (1867-1941)
Illustrated key to the trematode parasites of man. . . . Washington: Government Printing Office, 1904. 66p. DLC
00-5657

STILES, Charles W[ardell] (1867-1941)
. . . A statistical study of the prevalence of intestinal worms in man. By Charles Wardell Stiles and Philip E. Garrison. Washington: Government Printing Office, 1906. 77p. DLC
00-5658

STILES, Charles W[ardell] (1867-1941)
. . . Soil pollution and its relation to hookworm disease and typhoid fever. . . . Washington: Government Printing Office, 1909. 10p. illus. DLC **00-5659**

STILES, Charles W[ardell] (1867-1941)
. . . The treatment of hookworm disease. . . . Washington: Government Printing Office, 1909. 5p. DLC
00-5660

STILES, Charles W[ardell] (1867-1941)
Hookworm disease and the Negroes. . . . Hampton, Va.: The Press of the Hampton Normal and Agricultural Institute, 1909. 18p. DLC **00-5661**

STILL, Andrew Taylor (1828-1917)
The philosophy and mechanical principles of osteopathy. . . . Kansas City, Mo.: Hudson-Kimberly Pub. Co., 1902. 319p. DLC; DNLM; ICJ **00-5662**

STILL, Andrew Taylor (1828-1917)
Autobiography of Andrew T. Still—with a history of the discovery and development of the science of osteopathy; together with an account of the founding of the American School of Osteopathy; and lectures delivered before that institution. . . . rev. ed. Kirksville, Mo.: Published by the Author, 1908. 405p. illus., ports. CtY-M; DNLM; ICJ; KU
00-5663

STILL, Andrew Taylor (1828-1917)
Osteopathy, research and practice. . . . Kirksville, Mo.: The Author, 1910. 543p. DLC: DNLM **00-5664**

STILLÉ, Alfred (1813-1900)
Valuable miscellaneous library of the late Dr. A. Stillé of Philadelphia, comprising rare and scarce works in Americana, early French literature . . . to be sold . . . April 11 & 12, 1901. . . . Catalogue compiled and sale conducted by S. V. Henkels . . . auction rooms of Davis & Harvey. . . . [Philadelphia: Bicking Print, 1901.] 64p. NN; PPHa; PU
00-5665

STILLÉ, Alfred (1813-1900)
Table of comparison between typhus and typhoid fevers. [Transl. by Wm. Pepper.] Rufutations of A. F. Stewart's claims about typhus and typhoid fevers. Remarks on comencing the study of medicine. Philadelphia, 1904. 52p. DNLM; PPC **00-5666**

STILLMAN, Charles K[irtland] (*b.* 1879)
Postdelirious alcoholic stupor. New York, 1908. 14p. DNLM
00-5667

STILLMAN, John D.
The evolution of physiological and chemical science in a natural system of medicine, vs. the theories and fallacies of popular medicine. . . . St. Louis: The Mekeel Press, [1901?]. 69p. front. (port.) DLC **00-5668**

STIMSON, A[rthur] M[arston] (*b.* 1876)
Facts and problems of rabies. Washington: Government Printing Office, 1910. 90p. 4 plates. DLC: DNLM; NN
00-5669

STIMSON, G[eorge] W[illiam] (*b.* 1880)
Primary nasal diphtheria; with a report of several cases, one in an infant ten days old. New York, 1907. 12p. DNLM
00-5670

STIMSON, Julia Catherine (1881-1948)
Nurses handbook of drugs and solutions. . . . Boston: Whitcomb & Barrows, 1910. 82p. DLC: MBM; NcU; MH-M
00-5671

STIMSON, Lewis A[tterbury] (1844-1917)
A practical treatise on fractures and dislocations. 3rd ed. New York & Philadelphia: Lea Bros. & Co., 1900. 842p. 32 plates. DLC; DNLM; NNNAM; PU **00-5672**

STIMSON' Lewis A[tterbury] (1844-1917)
Cubitus varus; or "gunstock" deformity following fracture of the lower end of the humerus. Philadelphia, 1900. 8p. 4 plates. DNLM **00-5673**

STIMSON' Lewis A[tterbury] (1844-1917) and John ROGERS, Jr.
A manual of operative surgery. 4th revised ed. Philadelphia: Lea Bros. & Co., 1900. 586p. DLC: DNLM; NNNAM; PPC
00-5674

STIMSON, Lewis A[tterbury] (1844-1917)
Address. Ithaca, 1901. 19p. MB [Cornell University, Ithaca, N.Y. Medical College.] **00-5675**

STIMSON, Lewis A[tterbury] (1844-1917)
Cornell university. Address on teaching and research: distinct and indispensable functions of a university. Ithaca, New York: The University, [1903]. 16p. NN **00-5676**

STIMSON, Lewis A[tterbury] (1844-1917)
A practical treatise on fractures and dislocations. . . . 4th ed., rev. and enl. With 331 illustrations and 46 plates in monotint. New York and Philadelphia: Lea Bros. & Co., 1905. 844p. DLC; MBM; NNNAM; PPC **00-5677**

STIMSON, Lewis A[tterbury] (1844-1917)
A practical treatise on fractures and dislocations. . . . 5th ed., rev. and enl. With 352 illustrations and 52 plates in monotint. New York and Philadelphia: Lea Bros. & Co., 1907. 854p. DLC; LNT-M; NNNAM; PU **00-5678**

STIMSON, Lewis A[tterbury] (1844-1917)
A practical treatise on fractures and dislocations. . . . 6th ed., rev. and enl. With 361 illustrations and 65 plates in monotint. New York and Philadelphia: Lea & Febiger, 1910. 876p. DLC; GU; IU-M; PPC **00-5679**

STIRLING, William (1851-1932)
Outlines of practical physiology, being a manual for the physiological laboratory, including chemical and experimental physiology, with reference to practical medicine. . . . 3rd ed., rev. and enl. With 289 illustrations. Philadelphia: P. Blakiston's Son & Co., 1905. 402p. CtY-M; DLC; PPC; PU
00-5680

STIRLING, William (1851-1932)
Rudolph Albert von Kölliker, M.D., professor of anatomy in the University of Würzburg. [Washington, 1906.] 5p. DLC
00-5681

STITCHES and knots in surgery. Conshohocken, Pa.: J. Ellwood Lee Co., 1903. [unp.] DNLM **00-5682**

STITT, E[dward] R[hodes] (1867-1948)
Are there valid objections to the quinin prophylaxis of malaria? Chicago, 1908. 6p. DNLM **00-5683**

STITT, E[dward] R[hodes] (1867-1948)
Practical bacteriology, blood work, and animal parasitology, including bacteriological keys, zoological tables, and explanatory clinical notes. Philadelphia: P. Blakiston's Son & Co., 1909. 294p. 4 plates. DLC; DNLM; PPC; PU
00-5684

STITT, E[dward] R[hodes] (1867-1948)
Practical bacteriology, blood work, and animal parasitology, including bacteriological keys, zoological tables, and explanatory clinical notes. 2nd ed., rev. & enl., with 91 illustrations. Philadelphia: P. Blakiston's Son & Co., 1910. 345p. 4 plates. DNLM; MBM; NNNAM; PPC **00-5685**

STOCKHAM, Alice B[unker] (1833-1912)
Karezza; ethics of marriage. New and rev. ed. New York: Diehl, Landau & Pettit, [1903]. 140p. DLC; MH; NIC; NN
00-5686

STOCKHAM, Alice B[unker] (1833-1912)
Karezza; ethics of marriage. . . . New and rev. ed. Chicago: Stockham Publishing Co., [1903]. 141p. DLC; IEN-M; MH; NN **00-5687**

STOCKHAM, Alice B[unker] (1833-1912)
Tokology; a book for every woman. Chicago: A. B. Stockham & Co., 1905. 373p. DLC; ICJ; MB; NN [Book of plates in pocket on inside back cover.] **00-5688**

STOCKHAM, Alice B[unker] (1833-1912)
Tokology; a book for every woman. Chicago: Progress Publishing Co., 1909. 373p. 1 port. rev. ed. DLC; ICJ; NN [Pamphlet relating to book inserted in pocket on cover.]
00-5689

STOCKHAM, Alice B[unker] (1833-1912)
Tokology. A book for every woman. New York: R. F. Fenno, 1910. 373p. DLC: ICU; MH; NN [Includes a pamphlet of 8 color plates] **00-5690**

STOCKTON, Charles G. (1853-1931)
Hygiene of the digestive apparatus. Illus. Philadelphia, 1901. 42p. MB **00-5691**

STOCKTON, Charles G. (1853-1931)
Pernicious anemia and its relation to gastric digestion, based on twenty-five cases. Chicago, 1904. 14p. DNLM
00-5692

STOCKTON, Charles G. (1853-1931)
The delay of old age and the alleviation of senility. Chicago, 1905. 14p. DNLM **00-5693**

STOCKTON, Charles G. (1853-1931) and A. E. WOEHNERT
Thrombosis of the superior vena cava complicating Graves' disease. New York, 1908. 5p. DNLM **00-5694**

STOCKTON, George (*b.* 1854)
The relation of physical defects to mental development. New York, 1904. 12p. DNLM **00-5695**

STODDART, William Henry Butter (*b.* 1868)
Mind and its disorders; a text-book for students and practitioners. . . . Philadelphia: P. Blakiston's Son & Co., 1909. 488p. plates. DLC; ICJ; LNT–M; PPC
00-5696

STÖHR, Philipp (1849-1911)
Text-book of histology, including the microscopic technic . . . 3rd American from 8th German ed. Transl. by Dr. Emma L. Bilstein . . . edited, with additions by Dr. Alfred Schaper. . . . With 301 illustrations. Philadelphia: P. Blakiston's Son & Co., 1900. 432p. CtY-M; DLC; ICJ; PPC
00-5697

STÖHR, Philipp (1849-1911)
Text-book of histology, including the microscopic technic . . . 4th American based upon 9th German ed. Transl. by Dr. Emma L. Bilstein . . . ed., with additions by Dr. Alfred Schaper. . . . With 379 illustrations. Philadelphia: P. Blakiston's Son & Co., 1901. 503p. CtY-M; DLC; PPC; PU
00-5698

STÖHR, Philipp (1849-1911)
Text-book of histology, including the microscopic technic . . . 5th American from th 10th German ed., transl. by Dr. Emma L. Bilstein . . . ed., with additions by Dr. Alfred Schaper . . . with 353 illustrations. Philadelphia: P. Blakiston's Son & Co., 1903. 485p. DLC; NNNAN: PPC; PPJ
00-5699

STÖHR, Philipp (1849-1911)
Stohr's histology, arranged upon an embryological basis by Dr. Frederic T. Lewis. . . . From the 12th German ed. . . . 6th American ed., with 450 illustrations. Philadelphia: P. Blakiston's Son & Co., 1906. 2 v. CU-M; DNLM; PPC: PU
00-5700

STOKES, William (1804-1878)
William Stokes, his life and work by his son. New York: Longmans, Green & Co., 1900 [*c.* 1898]. 256p. DLC; ICJ; NIC; NN **00-5701**

STOKES, William Royal (*b.* 1870)
A case of sympus, or mermaid. Baltimore, 1902. 8p. DNLM
00-5702

STOKES, William Royal (*b.* 1870)
The pathology of smallpox. Baltimore, 1903. 18p. 10 plates. DNLM **00-5703**

STOKES, William Royal (*b.* 1870)
A study of the group actinomyces. Philadelphia & New York, 1904. 15p. DNLM **00-5704**

STOKES, William Royal (*b.* 1870)
Four great Anglo-American medical discoveries. Baltimore, 1905. 12p. 2 plates. DLC; MB; NN
00-5705

STOLL, Henry Farnum (*b.* 1878)
Osteoarthritis of the spine; report of a case. New York: A. R. Elliott, 1905. 4p. DNLM; NN
00-5706

STOLL, Henry Farnum (*b.* 1878)
Indigestion; its significance and diagnosis. New York: A. R. Elliott Co., 1907. 13p. DNLM; NN **00-5707**

STONE, Arthur K[ingsbury] (*b.* 1861)
Impressions of the British congress on tuberculosis. Boston, 1901. 5p. DNLM **00-5708**

STONE, Arthur K[ingsbury] (*b.* 1861)
Cardiac displacement. Boston, 1904. 30p. DNLM **00-5709**

STONE, Arthur K[ingsbury] (*b.* 1861)
The geographical distribution of tuberculosis in Boston in 1901-03 as compared with that of 1885-90. Boston: Old Corner Bk. Store, 1905. 12p. MBM **00-5710**

STONE, Arthur K[ingsbury] (*b.* 1861) and Cleaveland FLOYD
The daily care of consumptives at a general hospital as an aid to solving local tuberculosis problems. Boston, 1907. 17p. DNLM **00-5711**

STONE, I[saac] S[cott] (*b.* 1851)
Death after operation possibly due to unsuspected interstitial hepatitis. New York, 1900. 4p. DNLM **00-5712**

STONE, I[saac] S[cott] (*b.* 1851)
An improved method of treating prolapse of the uterus and bladder. New York, 1900. 7p. DNLM **00-5713**

STONE, I[saac] S[cott] (*b.* 1851)
The mortality resulting from abdominal section for pus in the pelvis. New York, 1900. 5p. DNLM **00-5714**

STONE, I[saac] S[cott] (*b.* 1851)
Supravaginal hysteromyomectomy. Boston, 1900. 5p. DNLM **00-5715**

STONE, I[saac] S[cott] (*b.* 1851)
The surgical and mechanical treatment of dysmenorrhea. New York, 1900. 7p. DNLM **00-5716**

STONE, I[saac] S[cott] (*b.* 1851)
The treatment of persistent fecal fistulae. New York, 1900. 5p. DNLM **00-5717**

STONE, I[saac] S[cott] (*b.* 1851)
So-called conservative treatment of appendicitis. Richmond, 1901. 8p. DNLM **00-5718**

STONE, I[saac] S[cott] (*b.* 1851)
Some recent operative work for the relief of the uterus and bladder. New York: William Wood & Co., 1901. 10p. DNLM **00-5719**

STONE, I[saac] S[cott] (*b.* 1851)
Iodoform and carbolic-acid intoxication. New York, 1902. 6p. DNLM **00-5720**

STONE, I[saac] S[cott] (*b.* 1851)
Some recent surgery for biliary obstructions. New York, 1902. 14p. DNLM **00-5721**

STONE, J[ames] S. (*b.* 1868)
Injuries about the shoulder at birth. Boston, 1900. 17p. DNLM **00-5722**

STONE, William Stephen (*b.* 1867)
Toxemia of pregnancy. Baltimore, [1903]. 32p. 1 plate. DNLM **00-5723**

STONE, William Stephen (*b.* 1867) and Ellice McDONALD
The gonococcus in the puerperium, with report of seventeen cases. Chicago, 1906. 12p. DNLM **00-5724**

STONEY, Emily M[arjory] A[rmstrong]
Bacteriology and surgical technique for nurses. . . . Philadelphia: W. B. Saunders & Co., 1900. 190p. plates. DLC; ICJ; PPC; PU **00-5725**

STONEY, Emily M[arjory] A[rmstrong]
Practical points in nursing, for nurses in private practice; with an appendix . . . by Emily A. M. Stoney . . . 3rd ed., thoroughly rev., illustrated with 79 engravings in the text and 8 colored and half-tone plates. Philadelphia, New York, [etc.]: W. B. Saunders & Co., 1903. 466p. DLC; DNLM; ICJ; PPC **00-5726**

STONEY, Emily M[arjory] A[rmstrong]
Practical materia medica for nurses; with an appendix containing poisons and their antidotes, with poison emergencies; mineral waters; weights and measures; dose list, and a glossary of the terms used in materia medica and therapeutics. 2nd ed., thoroughly revised. Philadelphia: W. B. Saunders & Co., 1904. 300p. DLC; DNLM; PPC; PU **00-5727**

STONEY, Emily M[arjory] A[rmstrong]
Bacteriology and surgical technic for nurses . . . 2nd ed., thoroughly rev. and enl. by Frederic Richardson Griffith. . . . Philadelphia-New York, [etc.]: W. B. Saunders & Co., 1905. 278p. DLC; NNNAM; PPC; PU **00-5728**

STONEY, Emily M[arjory] A[rmstrong]
Practical materia medica for nurses; with an appendix containing poisons and their antidotes, with poison emergencies; mineral waters; weights and measures; dose list, and a glossary of the terms used in materia medica and therapeutics. 3rd ed., thoroughly revised. Philadelphia & London: W. B. Saunders & Co., 1906. 300p. DLC; DNLM; PPC: PPJ **00-5729**

STONEY, Emily M[arjory] A[rmstrong]
Bacteriology and surgical technic for nurses . . . 3rd ed., thoroughly rev. and enl. by Frederic Richardson Griffith. . . . Philadelphia and London: W. B Saunders & Co., 1910. 311p. plates. DLC; NN; PPC; PU **00-5730**

STONEY, Emily M[arjory] A[rmstrong]
Practical points in nursing, for nurses in private practice; with an appendix containing rules for feeding the sick; recipes for invalid foods and beverages; weights and measures; dose list; and a full glossary of medical terms and nursing treatment . . . 4th ed., thoroughly rev., containing 97 text-illustrations and 8 colored and half-tone plates. Philadelphia and London: W. B. Saunders & Co., 1910. 495p. col. plates. DLC; NNNAM; PPC; PU **00-5731**

STORER, Malcolm (*b.* 1862) and M. T. THURBER
Repeated ectopic gestation in the same patient, with operation in each case. Boston: Damrell & Upham, 1900. 13p. DNLM **00-5732**

STORER, Malcolm (*b.* 1862)
On intermenstrual dysmenorrhea. Boston: Damrell & Upham, 1900. 16p. DNLM **00-5733**

STORER, Malcolm (*b.* 1862)
On some questions relative to extra-uterine pregnancy, with especial reference to tubal abortion. Boston, 1904. 17p. DNLM **00-5734**

STORER, Malcolm (*b.* 1862)
Bilateral torsion of the Fallopian tubes. Boston, 1906. 10p. DNLM **00-5735**

STOREY, Thomas Andrew (*b.* 1875)
Studies in voluntary muscular contraction. . . . Part I. — Some forms of apparatus devised for ergographic research. Part II. — Further observations upon the normal daily variation in the power of voluntary muscular contraction. . . . Stanford University, Calif.: University Press, 1904. 62p. DLC; MH; NIC; NN **00-5736**

STOUT, Emanuel J. (*b.* 1878)
Favus, with reports of two indigenous cases. New York, 1908. 4p. DNLM **00-5737**

STOVER, George H[enry] (1871-1915)
Report of X-ray therapeutics. Denver, 1903. 8 l. DNLM **00-5738**

STOVER, George H[enry] (1871-1915)
The therapeutic use of the X-ray. Denver, [1903]. 8p. DNLM **00-5739**

STOVER, George H[enry] (1871-1915)
The X-ray treatment of urethral carbuncle. Denver, 1904. 1 l. DNLM **00-5740**

STOVER, George H[enry] (1871-1915)
A frame for examining eye skiagrams. Chicago, 1905. 1 l. DNLM **00-5741**

STOVER, George H[enry] (1871-1915)
An improved X-ray for the study of bone injuries and foreign bodies. [Chicago], 1905. 4p. DNLM **00-5742**

STOVER, George H[enry] (1871-1915)
The Roentgen-ray treatment of carcinoma. [Boston], 1906. 8p. DNLM **00-5743**

STOVER, George H[enry] (1871-1915)
Two cases of cutaneous vaso-motor acurosis, with speculations thereupon. Denver, 1906. 4p. DNLM **00-5744**

STOVER, George H[enry] (1871-1915)
The treatment of glandular tuberculosis by the Roentgen-ray. New York, 1907. 6p. DNLM **00-5745**

STOW, Bond (*b.* 1865)
Congenital tricuspid stenosis complicated by mitral stenosis. Philadelphia & New York, 1905. 8p. DNLM **00-5746**

STOW, Bond (*b.* 1865)
The autopsy as a judge of our bedside conclusions; illustrated by a case of fatty heart, mistaken for valvular disease. New York, 1906. 10p. DNLM **00-5747**

STOW, Bond (*b.* 1865)
Organic heart diseases and immunity from pulmonary tuberculosis. Philadelphia & New York, 1906. 12p. DNLM **00-5748**

STOW, Bond (*b.* 1865)
Paraplegia caused by an aneurysm of the arch of the aorta. New York, 1907. 7p. DNLM **00-5749**

STOW, Bond (*b.* 1865)
Ureteritis cystica chronica (the clincal and autopsy records of a case with bilateral double ureters). New York, 1907. 16p. DNLM **00-5750**

STOWELL, William L.
The doctor outside of medicine. . . . [New York: D. Appleton & Co., 1900.] 22p. DLC; NN **00-5751**

STRASS, H.
The optic nerve and the accessory cavities of the nose: a contribution to the study of canalicular neuritis and atrophy of the optic nerves of nasal origin. Trans. [with additions] from A. Onodi. [New York, 1908.] 52p. 32 plates. DLC; NN **00-5752**

STRAUB, Paul Frederick (1865-1937)
Medical service in campaign; a handbook for medical officers in the field. . . . Prepared under the direction of the Surgeon-General, United States Army, and published by authority of the War Department. . . . Philadelphia: P. Blakiston's Son & Co., 1910. 164p. 2 fold. plates. CtY-M; DLC: ICJ; PPC **00-5753**

STRAUB, Paul Frederick (1865-1937)
Sanitation of the maneuver camp at San Antonio, Texas. By Major Paul F. Straub. . . . Washington: The Association of Military Surgeons, 1910. 23p. illus., diags. DLC **00-5754**

STRAUS, Nathan (1848-1931)
American solution of the milk problem, paper. . . . Second international Congrès des gouttes de lait Brussels, Sept. 12, 1907. [New York, 1907.] 11p. DLC; NN **00-5755**

STRAUS, Nathan (1848-1931)
America's latest contribution to the milk question; a review by Nathan Straus of the U.S. Government report "Milk and its relation to public health." (Published in Washington, D.C., 1908) [New York? 1908?] 15p. DLC; NN **00-5756**

STREMMEL, Samuel C[alhoun] (*b.* 1863)
When to operate for appendicitis. New York, 1904. 8p. DNLM **00-5757**

STRICKER, Louis (*b.* 1863)
The crystalline lens system; its embryology, anatomy, physiological chemistry, physiology, pathology, diseases, treatment, operations and after-changes, with a consideration of aphabia. [Cincinnati?], 1900 [*c.* 1899]. 599p. DLC; ICJ; MH; NN **00-5758**

STRICKER, Louis (*b.* 1863)
An original chart of the neuronic architecture of the visual apparatus; with explanation. Cincinnati, 1901. 10p. DNLM **00-5759**

STRONG, Frederick F[inch]
Technique and experiments with the "Hercules" high-frequency apparatus. . . . Boston: The Electro-radiation Co., [1905]. 21p. DLC; MH-M **00-5760**

STRONG, Frederick F[inch]
High-frequency currents. . . . With 183 illustrations in the text. New York: Rebman Co., 1908. 289p. DLC; ICJ; NNNAM; PU **00-5761**

STRONG, Frederick F[inch]
Essentials of modern electro-therapeutics; an elementary text-book on the scientific therapeutic use of electricity and radiant energy. . . . New York: Rebman Co., [1908]. 112p. diags. DLC; ICJ; NNNAM; PU **00-5762**

STRONG, Lawrence W[atson] (*b.* 1870)
Congenital tumors of the kidney; with a report of two cases. New York, 1903. 7 l. DNLM **00-5763**

STRONG, Richard P[earson] (1872-1948) and W. E. MUSGRAVE
The occurrence of Malta fever in Manila. Philadelphia, 1900. 12p. DNLM **00-5764**

STROUD, Bert B[renette]
A new head-rest for the removal of the human brain. Washington, D.C., 1900. 4p. DNLM **00-5765**

STROUD, Harrison E.
Report and clinic of cases of empyema. Phoenix, Arizona, 1902. 12p. 2 plates. DNLM **00-5766**

STRÜMPELL, Adolf von (1853-1925)
A text-book of medicine for students and practitioners . . . 3rd American ed., transl. by permission from the 13th German ed., by Herman F. Vickery . . . and Philip Coombs Knapp. . . . With editorial notes by Frederick C. Shattuck. . . . With one hundred and eighty-five illustrations in the text, and one plate. New York: D. Appleton & Co., 1901. 1242p. DLC; DNLM; NNNAM; PPC **00-5767**

STRÜMPELL, Adolf von (1853-1925)
A text-book of medicine for students and practitioners . . . 4th American ed., transl. by permission from the 17th rev. German ed., with editorial notes, additional chapters, and a section on mental diseases, by Herman F. Vickery . . . and Philip Coombs Knapp . . . with six plates three of which are in color, and two hundred and twenty-four illustrations in the text. . . . New York and London: D. Appleton & Co., 1910-1911. 2 v. DLC; ICJ; PPHa; PPC **00-5768**

STRUTHERS, Joseph
. . . Chemistry and physics. A manual for students and practitioners. By Joseph Struthers . . . D. W. Ward . . . and Charles H. Willmarth. . . . Philadelphia: Lea Bros. & Co., 1901 [*c.* 1893]. 288p. illus., diags. DLC; ICJ; NNNAM; PPC **00-5769**

STUBBERT, J[ames] Edward (*b.* 1859)
Statistics of the Loomis Sanatorium, at Liberty, N.Y. [Philadelphia, 1900.] 7p. DNLM **00-5770**

STUBBERT, J[ames] Edward (*b.* 1859)
The X-rays as a diagnostic agent in pulmonary diseases. Philadelphia, 1900. 13p. DNLM **00-5771**

STUBBERT, J[ames] Edward (*b.* 1859)
Subsequent histories of patients apparently cured under administration of antitubercle serum as an auxiliary to climatic treatment. New York, 1900. 15p. DNLM **00-5772**

STUBBERT, J[ames] Edward (*b.* 1859)
Sanitation in Panama. New York, 1907. 6p. DNLM **00-5773**

STUCKY, Joseph Addison (*b.* 1858)
Some displeasing results of the mastoid operation. New York, 1906. 8p. DNLM **00-5774**

STUDIES in the bacteriology and etiology of oriental plague . . . [by Edward Emil Klein (1844-1825)]. With 89 photographs. New York: Macmillan Co., 1906. 301p. DLC; DNLM; ICJ; PU **00-5775**

STUDIES in paranoia. Periodic paranoia and the origin of paranoid delusions, by Dr. Nikolaus Gierlich. . . . Contributions to the study of paranoia, by Dr. M. Friedmann. . . . Transl. and ed. by Smith Ely Jelliffe, M.D. New York: The Journal of Nervous and Mental Disease Publishing Co., 1908. 78p. DLC; MH; NIC; NN **00-5776**

STUDIES on the pathology and etiology of variola and of vaccinia, by W. T. Councilman, G. B. Magrath, W. R. Brinckerhoff [and others]. Boston, 1904. 29[31]p. plates and diags. MH; OCIM **00-5777**

STURGIS, Frederic R[ussell] (1844-1919)
Sexual debility in man. New York: E. B. Treat & Co., 1900. 432p. DLC; DNLM; NNNAM; PPJ **00-5778**

STURGIS, Frederic R[ussell] (1844-1919)
Prostitution: its suppression or control. New York: Stettiner Bros., 1901. 11p. NN **00-5779**

STURGIS, Frederic R[ussell] (1844-1919)
The student's manual of venereal diseases . . . 7th ed., revised by F. R. Sturgis and Follen Cabot. Philadelphia: P. Blakiston's Son & Co., 1901. 216p. DNLM; ICJ; PPC; PU **00-5780**

STURGIS, Frederic R[ussell] (1844-1919)
Should gonorrhea be considered as a local or constitutional affection? St. Louis, 1901. 15p. DNLM **00-5781**

STURGIS, Frederic R[ussell] (1844-1919)
Diagnostic points of difference between spermatorrhoea and seminal pollutions. New York, 1902. 3 l. DNLM **00-5782**

STURGIS, Frederic R[ussell] (1844-1919)
Of what clinical value is the gonococcus? New York, [1904]. 18p. DNLM **00-5783**

STURGIS, Frederic R[ussell] (1844-1919)
Notes and reflections on the causes which induce marital infelicity due to the relations of the sexes. Philadelphia, [1910?] 35p. DNLM **00-5784**

STURM, Meyer J[oseph] (*b.* **1872)**
The organization, construction and management of hospitals. By Meyer J. Sturm and Albert J[ohn] Ochsner. Chicago: Cleveland Press, 1907. 600p. DNLM; ICJ
00-5785

STURMER, Julius William (*b.* **1870)**
Course in pharmaceutical arithmetic including weights and measures. . . . Terre Haute, Ind.: Moore & Langen Printing Co., 1903. 155p. DLC; ICJ; NN; PPC **00-5786**

STURMER, Julius William (*b.* **1870)**
Rudiments of Latin; with special reference to the nomenclature of the U.S. Pharmacopoeia, the national formulary, and the text-books in materia medica and botany; including also prescription writing and notes on the nomenclature of the German Pharmacopoeia. Chicago: Marsh & Curtis, 1908. 92p. DLC; DNLM; IU-M; OCLloyd
00-5787

SUKER, George F. (*b.* **1869)**
Keratitis petrificans, the correct terminology for ribband-like keratitis. Chicago, 1900. 6p. DNLM **00-5788**

SUKER, George F. (*b.* **1869)**
The surgery of the superior cervical sympathetic ganglion. New York, 1900. 10p. DNLM **00-5789**

SUKER, George F. (*b.* **1869)**
On the employment of agar-agar in the formation of a stump after enucleation or evisceration. Chicago, 1901. 4p. DNLM
00-5790

SUKER, George F. (*b.* **1869)**
The value of excision of the superior cervical sympathetic ganglion in glaucoma. Chicago, 1901. 8p. DNLM
00-5791

SUKER, George F. (*b.* **1869)**
Chlorosis and its relation to the eye. Detroit, 1902. 10p. DNLM **00-5792**

SUKER, George F. (*b.* **1869)**
Is the dislocation of the lens into the vitreous ever justifiable? New York, 1902. 8p. DNLM **00-5793**

SUKER, George F. (*b.* **1869)**
A separate gumma of the caruncle and ocular conjunctiva. Report of a case, with a complete bibliography appertaining thereto. New York, 1902. 7p. DNLM
00-5794

SUKER, George F. (*b.* **1869)**
Thiosinamin. Clinical and experimental observations with reference to corneal opacities and other ocular lesions. Chicago, 1902. 12p. DNLM **00-5795**

SUKER, George F. (*b.* **1869)**
Concerning the terms antimetropia and anisometropia; brachymetropia and hypometropia in place of myopia; hypermetropia and hyperopia. A plea for the correct use of these terms in ophthalmology. Chicago, 1903. 16p. DNLM
00-5796

SUKER, George F. (*b.* **1869)**
Eye complications that at times attend measles. Detroit, 1903. 15p. DNLM **00-5797**

SUKER, George F. (*b.* **1869)**
A new and simple demonstration ophthalmoscope. Chicago, 1903. 4p. DNLM **00-5798**

SUKER, George F. (*b.* **1869)**
Can an ophthalmic examination aid the life insurance examiner in his work? Toledo, 1903. 4p. DNLM
00-5799

SUKER, George F. (*b.* **1869)**
Paraffin; its use in the formation of a stump after an enucleation. St. Louis, 1903. 4p. DNLM **00-5800**

SUKER, George F. (*b.* **1869)**
Paralysis and paresis of the muscle of accommodation. St. Louis, 1903. 25p. DNLM **00-5801**

SUKER, George F. (*b.* **1869)**
A consideration of the surgical treatment of chronic Bright's disease from the ophthalmic standpoint. New York, 1904. 7p. DNLM **00-5802**

SUKER, George F. (*b.* **1869)**
A criticism on the use and abuse of the lacrimal probe. New York, 1904. 6p. DNLM **00-5803**

SUKER, George F. (*b.* **1869)**
The molar teeth and the patellar reflex in hereditary syphilitic interstitial keratitis. Detroit, 1904. 15p. DNLM
00-5804

SUKER, George F. (*b.* **1869)**
Gonorrheal ophthalmia, with involvement of the anterior ethmoidal cells. A report of a case. St. Louis, 1905. 5p. DNLM **00-5805**

SUKER, George F. (*b.* **1869)**
Kuhnt's conjunctival flap (Schoeller-Kuhnt's conjunctival graft). Chicago, 1905. 8p. DNLM **00-5806**

SUKER, George F. (*b.* **1869)**
Diagnostic eye-findings in arteriosclerosis (angiosclerosis). [Cincinnati], 1906. 7p. DNLM **00-5807**

SUKER, George F. (*b.* **1869)**
Scopolamine and morphine anesthesia in ophthalmic surgery. Detroit: E. G. Swift, 1906. 12p. DNLM
00-5808

SUKER, George F. (*b.* **1869)**
Can a substitute for simple enucleation be employed in every instance? Milwaukee, 1908. 7p. DNLM
00-5809

SULTAN, Georg (*b.* **1865)**
Atlas and epitome of abdominal hernias . . . atuhorized transl. from the German; ed, by William B. Coley . . . with 119 illustrations, 36 of them in colors. Philadelphia and London: W. B. Saunders & Co., 1902. 277p. DLC; ICJ; PPC; PPJ
00-5810

SUMMERS, John E[dward] (*b.* **1858)**
Indications for the drainage in diseases of the biliary passages and the technic of operation. Philadelphia, 1900. 8p. DNLM
00-5811

SUMMERS, John E[dward] (*b.* 1858)
Double ureter. Report of a nephrectomy done upon a young child with this condition present. Philadelphia, 1901. 3p. 1 plate. DNLM **00-5812**

SUMMERS, John E[dward] (*b.* 1858)
Clean surgery versus mutilating and unscientific obstetric procedures as practiced upon the viable unborn infant. St. Joseph, 1901 6p. DNLM **00-5813**

SUMMERS, John E[dward] (*b.* 1858)
Endothelioma (adenoma) of the base of the tongue simulating a struma of the tongue. Lincoln, Neb., 1901. 11p. DNLM **00-5814**

SUMMERS, John E[dward] (*b.* 1858)
Intra-abdonimal lesions following traumatism. Des Moines, 1902. 13p. DNLM **00-5815**

SUMMERS, John E[dward] (*b.* 1858)
Personal experience with contused gunshot and stab wounds of the abdomen. Lincoln, Neb., 1902. 15p. DNLM **00-5816**

SUMMERS, John E[dward] (*b.* 1858)
The vermiform appendix as a cause of intestinal obstruction. Philadelphia, 1902. 3p. DNLM **00-5817**

SUMMERS, John E[dward] (*b.* 1858)
Report of two cases of acute intestinal obstruction following contusion of the abdominal walls. Chicago, 1903. 8p. DNLM **00-5818**

SUMMERS, John E[dward] (*b.* 1858)
The surgical aspect of prostatic hypertrophy. Omaha, 1903. 7p. DNLM **00-5819**

SUMMERS, John E[dward] (*b.* 1858)
The treatment of papilloma of the larynx in children. New York, 1903. 7p. DNLM **00-5820**

SUMMERS, John E[dward] (*b.* 1858)
The surgical aspect of prostatic hypertrophy. Omaha, 1903. 7p. DNLM **00-5821**

SUMMERS, John E[dward] (*b.* 1858)
The treatment of abdominal injuries with special reference to gunshot wounds of the liver. Carlisle, 1905. 11p. DNLM **00-5822**

SUMMERS, John E[dward] (*b.* 1858)
Invagination of limited annular gangrene of the small bowel versus resection. Chicago, 1908. 8p. DNLM **00-5823**

SUMMERS, John E[dward] (*b.* 1858)
Splenectomy in Banti's disease, followed by oedema of the large intestine with localized necrosis of its wall. Philadelphia, 1908. 6p. NN **00-5824**

SUMMERS, John E[dward] (*b.* 1858)
The cancer question. New York, 1909. 14p. DNLM **00-5825**

SUMMERS, John E[dward] (*b.* 1858)
Typhoidal cholecystitis. Read before the Western Surgical Association, Chicago, December 19, 1910. [New York: A. R. Elliott Publishing Co., 1910.] 9p. NN **00-5826**

SUMMERS, John E[dward] (*b.* 1858)
Some modifications of technic in the surgery of the gall-bladder and bile-ducts. Philadelphia, 1910. 4p. NN **00-5827**

SUMMERS, John E[dward] (*b.* 1858)
Peritonization in pelvic surgery, with special reference to the use of the sigmoid flexure of the colon. [Chicago, 1910.] 2p. 1 plate. NN **00-5828**

SUMMERS, John E[dward] (*b.* 1858)
The possible diagnosis and a technic in excision of a chronic indurated ulcer of the posterior wall of the stomach. Chicago: American Medical Association, 1910. 6p. illus. NN **00-5829**

[SUMNER, Albert E.]
Notes on physical diagnosis for use in the College of Physicians and Surgeons, Columbia University, New York: J. T. Dougherty, [1902]. 72p. DLC; NN **00-5830**

SURGERY two hundred years ago. . . . New York: F. T. Neely, [1901?] 48p. plates. DLC; NN **00-5831**

SUTCLIFFE, John A.
Report of two cases. Removal of a sole leather bougie from the male urethra, and a mulberry calculus from the bladder. Indianapolis, 1902. 4p. DNLM **00-5832**

SUTTON, Francis (1831-1917)
A systematic handbook of volumetric analysis, or the quantitative estimation of chemical substances by measure, applied to liquids, solids, and gases. Adapted to the requirements of pure chemical research, pathological chemistry, pharmacy, metallurgy, manufacturing chemistry, photography, etc., and for the valuation of substances used in commerce, agriculture, and the arts. 8th ed. Philadelphia: P. Blakiston's Son & Co., 1900. 640p. DNLM; MB; PPC; PU **00-5833**

SUTTON, Francis (1831-1917)
A systematic handbook of volumetric analysis; or, The quantitative determination of chemical substances by measure, applied to liquids, solids, and gases, adapted to the requirements of pure chemical research, pathological chemistry, pharmacy, metallurgy, manufacturing chemistry, photography, etc., and for the valuation of substances used in commerce, agriculture, and the arts. . . . 9th ed., rev., with 121 illustrations. Philadelphia: P. Blakiston's Son & Co., 1907. 617p. illus., tables. DLC; ICJ; LNT-M; PU **00-5834**

SUTTON, Howard A[nderson] and Cecil K. DRINKER
Osteology and syndesmology. Philadelphia: P. Blakiston's Son & Co., 1910. 225p. CtY-M; DNLM; PPC; PU **00-5835**

SUTTON, R[hoades] Stansbury (1841-1906)
Personal experiences in pelvic and abdominal surgery. Pittsburgh: Calumet Publ. Co., 1901. 378p. 5 plates, port. DNLM; PPC; PU **00-5836**

SUTTON, R. T.
Impetigo contagiosa. New York, 1908. 4p. DNLM **00-5837**

SWAIN, Henry L[aurence] (*b.* 1846)
Bronchial asthma; its relation to nasal disease. Waterbury, Conn., 1900. 15p. 3 plates. DNLM **00-5838**

SWAN, John M[umford] (*b.* **1870)**
A manual of human anatomy, arranged for first year students. Philadelphia: F. W. S. Langmaid, 1900. 276p. CtY-M; DNLM; PPC; PPHa **00-5839**

SWAN, John M[umford] (*b.* **1870)**
A manual of human anatomy . . . 2nd ed. Philadelphia: F. W. S. Langmaid, 1901-03. 3 v. DLC; DNLM; ICJ; PU [1st ed., 1898-1901. 2 v.] **00-5840**

SWAN, John M[umford] (*b.* **1870)**
A human embryonic vesicle showing early placenta formation. Philadelphia, 1904. 3p. DNLM **00-5841**

SWAN, John M[umford] (*b.* **1870)**
Visceral syphilis. Detroit, 1904. 14p. DNLM **00-5842**

SWAN, John M[umford] (*b.* **1870)**
A case of extensive arteriosclerosis simulating aneurysm of the arch of the aorta. Philadelphia, 1904. 12p. DNLM **00-5843**

SWAN, John M[umford] (*b.* **1870)**
Six lectures on diseases of the blood. New York: A. R. Elliott Publishing Co., 1905. 99p. DNLM; NNNAM **00-5844**

SWAN, John M[umford] (*b.* **1870)**
Report of a case of cyst of the cerebellum. New York, 1905. 7p. DNLM **00-5845**

SWAN, John M[umford] (*b.* **1870)**
A study of the metabolism of a vegetarian. Philadelphia, 1905. 7p. DNLM **00-5846**

SWAN, John M[umford] (*b.* **1870) and Howard T. KARSNER**
On the behavior of the eosinophile leucocytes in cases of pulmonary tuberculosis. New York: A. R. Elliott Publishing Co., 1907. 28p. DNLM; NNNAM **00-5847**

SWAN, John M[umford] (*b.* **1870)**
A clinical study of the Cammidge reaction in the urine. New York: A. R. Elliott Publishing Co., 1910. 52p. NN **00-5848**

SWAN, John M[umford] (*b.* **1870)**
Prescription writing and formulary. . . . Philadelphia: W. B. Saunders & Co., 1910. 185p. DLC; OCIM; PPC; PPJ **00-5849**

SWAN, John M[umford] (*b.* **1870)**
The hydrotherapeutic treatment of heart disease. St. Louis: Interstate Medical Journal Co., 1910. 9p. NN **00-5850**

SWAN, John M[umford] (*b.* **1870)**
The organic basis of neurasthenia. [Read before the Syracuse Academy of Medicine, Dec. 6, 1910.] [New York: A. R. Elliott Publishing Co., 1910.] 10p. NN; PPHa **00-5851**

SWAN, John M[umford] (*b.* **1870)**
Postanesthetic glycosuria of surgical patients. Chicago, 1910. 4p. DNLM **00-5852**

SWAN,John M[umford] (*b.* **1870)**
Tropical diseases and health in the United States. Philadelphia: American Academy of Political and Social Sciences, 1910. 17p. NN; NNC; PPHa **00-5853**

SWAN, John M[umford] (*b.* **1870)**
A résumé of the opinions upon the Nauheim treatment of chronic diseases of the heart. New York, 1910. 18p. DNLM **00-5854**

SWAN, John M[umford] (*b.* **1870)**
The hydrotherapeutic treatment of chronic diseases of the heart. New York, 1910. 22p. DNLM; PPHa **00-5855**

SWANZY, Henry Rosborough (1843-1913)
A handbook of the diseases of the eye and their treatment . . . 7th ed. . . . Philadelphia: P. Blakiston's Son & Co., 1900. 607p. fold. plate. DLC; DNLM; PPC; PU **00-5856**

SWANZY, Henry Rosborough (1843-1913)
A handbook of the diseases of the eye and their treatment . . . 8th ed., rev., with 168 illustrations and zephyr card of Holmgren's tests. Philadelphia: P. Blakiston's Son & Co., 1903. 580p. plates. DLC; NNNAM; PPC; PU **00-5857**

SWEENEY, Gilliford B. (*b.* **1861)**
Animal therapy in tuberculosis. New York, 1907. 4p. DNLM **00-5858**

SWEENEY, Gilliford B. (*b.* **1861)**
Animal therapy, its relation to immunity in the treatment of tuberculosis. Pittsburgh, 1907. 36p. 4 plates. DNLM **00-5859**

SWEENEY, Gilliford B. (*b.* **1861)**
Human and bovine tubercle bacilli. New York, 1909. 4p. DNLM **00-5860**

SWEET, Joshua E[dwin] (*b.* **1876)**
The artificial anastomosis between the portal vein and the vena cava inferior; Eck's fistula. New York, 1905. 10p. 3 plates. DNLM **00-5861**

SWEET, Joshua E[dwin] (*b.* **1876)**
Experimental observations on secretin; with special reference to diabetes and malnutrition. Philadelphia, 1908. 12p. DNLM; PU **00-5862**

SWEET, Joshua E[dwin] (*b.* **1876)**
Further studies on the influence of the ductless glands on the pancreas. By Joshua Edwin Sweet, and Ralph Pemberton. [1909.] 16p. DLC **00-5863**

SWEET, Paul P.
The diagnosis and treatment of tuberculous joints. New York, 1910. 10p. DNLM **00-5864**

SWINBURNE, George K[nowles] (*b.* **1858)**
Litholapaxy as an office operation, with report of cases. New York, 1908. 5p. DNLM **00-5865**

SWINBURNE, George K[nowles] (*b.* **1858)**
Some cases of kidney and ureteral stone. New York, 1908. 14p. DNLM **00-5866**

[SWINBURNE, John] (1820-1889)
A typical American; or incidents in the life of Dr. John Swinburne of Albany, the eminent patriot, surgeon, and philanthropist. Compiled and published by the Citizen's Association, Albany. [1901?] 350p. Frontisport. 4 plates. DLC; NIC; NNS [1st printing, 1888]
00-5867

SWITHINBANK Harold
Bacteriology of milk. New York: E. P. Dutton & Co., 1903. 605p. col. diags. DNLM: ICJ; MB; PU
00-5868

SYMONDS, Brandreth
Medical selection for life insurance. New Haven, 1904. 22p. CtY-M; MB **00-5869**

SYMONDS, Brandreth
Life insurance examinations; a manual for the medical examiner. . . . New York: G. P. Putnam's Sons, 1905. 214p. DLC; ICJ; MB; NN **00-5870**

SYMPOSIUM on gynecology, read before the Ann Arbor Medical Club, February 19, 1902. Detroit & Ann Arbor, 1902. 16p. DNLM **00-5871**

SYMS, Parker (*b.* 1860)
Strangulated hernia; some practical remarks concerning its diagnosis and its proper management. Chicago, 1900. 7p. DNLM **00-5872**

SYMS, Parker (*b.* 1860)
Perineal prostatectomy. Chicago, 1901. 7p. DNLM
00-5873

SYMS, Parker (*b.* 1860)
Diagnosis of cholecystitis and cholelithiasis. Chicago, 1904. 8p. DNLM **00-5874**

SYMS, Parker (*b.* 1860)
Prostatic obstruction to urination; when to operate and how to operate. Chicago, 1904. 16p. DNLM **00-5875**

SYMS, Parker (*b.* 1860)
Prostatic obstruction; indications for operation, with a description of a method of operating. [Burlington, 1910.] 10p. DNLM **00-5876**

SYMS, Parker (*b.* 1860)
Some surgical aspects of gastric ulcer. New York, 1910. 8p. DNLM **00-5877**

SYMS, Parker (*b.* 1860)
Tumor of the breast; prostatic obstruction; pyelitis; chronic appendicitis. New York, 1910. 19p. DNLM
00-5878

SYMS, Parker (*b.* 1860)
Exploratory laparotomy for abdominal tumor; cholelithiasis; calculous pyelonephritis; strangulated hemorrhoids. New York, 1910. 7p. DNLM **00-5879**

SYMS, Parker (*b.* 1860)
Results following perineal prostatectomy, based on fourteen years' experience with this method. [New York], 1910. 12p. DNLM; NN **00-5880**

SYNOPSIS of materia medica and therapeutics. New York: James T. Dougherty, [1900]. 151p. MBM; NNNAM; NNU-M
00-5881

A SYSTEM of electro-therapeutics. Physics of Roentgen rays. Skiagraphy. Practical applications of Roentgen rays. Physics of light and cautery. Scranton: International Correspondence Schools, [1903]. 94, 37, 108, 32, 18p. 39 plates and 74 text illustrations. DLC; ICJ **00-5882**

A SYSTEM of electrotherapeutics; electricity in diseases of the eye, ear, nose, and throat; electricity in genito-urinary diseases; therapeutics of static electricity; electricity in dentistry. Scranton: International Textbook Co., 1903. 2 v. DNLM; MdU-D; PPC **00-5883**

SZYMONOWICZ, Ladislaus (1869-1939)
A text-book of histology and microscopic anatomy of the human body, including microscopic technique . . . transl. and ed. by John Bruce MacCallum . . . illustrated with 277 engravings, including 57 plates in colors and monochrome. Philadelphia and New York: Lea Bros. & Co., 1902. 435p. DLC; DNLM; NNNAM; PPC **00-5884**

TABER, C[larence] Wilbur (*b.* 1870)
Suggestion: the secret of sex. Chicago: C. H. Kerr & Co., 1901? 96p. front. (port.) DLC; ICJ **00-5885**

TABER, C[larence] Wilbur (*b.* 1870)
Taber's medical dictionary for nurses . . . associate editor, Nicholas Senn. . . . Chicago: C. W. Taber, [1905]. 418p. DLC; ICJ; OCIM; PU **00-5886**

TABER, C[larence] Wilbur (*b.* 1870)
Taber's pocket encyclopedic medical dictionary . . . associate editor, Nicholas Senn. . . . Chicago: C. W. Taber, [1905]. 418p. DLC; ICJ; MB; NN **00-5887**

TABER, C[larence] Wilbur (*b.* 1870)
Taber's Family medical cyclopedia . . . associate editor, Nicholas Senn. . . . [White cross ed.] Chicago: C. W. Taber, [1905]. 418p. diags. DLC; ICJ; MH; NN
00-5888

TABOR, George R.
The 1903 epidemic of yellow fever in Texas, and the lesson to be learned from it. Austin, 1905. 22p. DLC
00-5889

TAIT, R[obert] Lawson (1845-1899)
On the discussion on vivisection at the church congress. . . . [Philadelphia: Reprinted by American Anti-vivisection Society, 1900?] 4p. DLC **00-5890**

TAIT, R[obert] Lawson (1845-1899)
The uselessness of vivisection upon animals as a method of scientific research. . . . Philadelphia: The American Anti-vivisection Society, 1901? 34p. DLC
00-5891

TAIT, R[obert] Lawson (1845-1899)
Lectures on ectopic pregnancy and pelvic haematocele. New York: William Wood & Co., 1901. 24p. DLC; ICJ; MH-M; NNNAM [Printed out of Wood's Medical & Surgical Monographs, Vol. 5, No. 2 (1890), pp. 463-585]
00-5892

TAKAKI, Kanehiro
Military hygiene of the Japanese army. . . . [New York: A. R. Elliott Pub. Co., 1906.] 22p. DLC; NN
00-5893

TALBOT, Clarence Weill (*b.* 1883)
Diseases of the eye and how recognized; a series of articles on the more common diseases with which the optician meets in his every-day work—the causes, symptoms, diagnosis and outlines of treatment. . . . New York: Frederick Boger Publishing Co., [1910]. 68p. DLC; ICJ; NN; NNNAM
00-5894

TALBOT, Clarence Weill (*b.* 1883)
Optometry quiz compend. . . . Kansas City, Mo.: Optometry Publ. Co., [19–]. 236p. illus. NNC
00-5895

TALBOT, Eugene S[olomon] (1847-1924)
Quiz compend on irregularities of the teeth. . . . 1st ed. Chicago: E. M. Clay & Co., 1901. 310p. DLC: ICJ; PU
00-5896

TALBOT, Eugene S[olomon] (1847-1924)
Fallacies of some of the old theories of irregularities of the teeth. . . . [Chicago, 1901?] 8p. PU **00-5897**

TALBOT, Eugene S[olomon] (1847-1924)
Degeneracy and political assassination. . . . [Detroit: William M. Warren, publisher], 1901. 24p. ICJ **00-5898**

TALBOT, Eugene S[olomon] (1847-1924)
Irregularities of the teeth and their treatment. . . . 4th ed. . . . Philadelphia: F. A Davis Co., 1901. 546p. DLC: MdU-D; PPC; PU **00-5899**

TALBOT, Eugene S[olomon] (1847-1924)
Irregularities of the teeth and their treatment. . . . 5th ed. Philadelphia: The S. S. White Dental Mfg. Co., 1903. 546p. 33 tables. ICJ; IU-M; PPC; PU **00-5900**

TALBOT, Eugene S[olomon] (1847-1924)
Developmental pathology. . . . Illustrations. First edition. Chicago, 1905. 454p. ICJ; PU **00-5901**

TALBOT, Eugene S[olomon] (1847-1924)
Developmental pathology: a study in degenerative evolution. Boston: R. G. Badger, The Gorman Press, 1910 [*c.* 1911]. 435p. DLC; MH; NIC; NN **00-5902**

TALBOT, Fritz B[radley] (*b.* 1873)
Casein curds in infants' stools. New York: E. B. Treat & Co., 1909. 3 l. DNLM **00-5903**

TALBOT, Fritz B[radley] (*b.* 1873)
Apparatus for metabolism experiments in male infants. Chicago, 1909. 4p. DNLM **00-5904**

TALBOT, Fritz B[radley] (*b.* 1873)
Chemical examination of the feces of infants and children after gastroenterostomy. Boston, 1909. 4p. DNLM
00-5905

TALBOT, Fritz B[radley] (*b.* 1873)
Casein curds in infants' stools; biologic proof of their casein origin. New York, 1910. 3 l. DNLM
00-5906

TALBOT, Fritz B[radley] (*b.* 1873)
Clinical significance of curds in infants' feces. Boston, 1910. 7p. DNLM **00-5907**

TALBOT, Fritz B[radley] (*b.* 1873)
A metabolism experiment on an infant after gastroenterestomy for congenital pyloric stenosis. Boston, 1910. 3p. DNLM
00-5908

TALCOTT, Selden H[aines] (1842-1902)
Mental diseases and their modern treatment. New York: Boericke & Runyon, 1901. 352p. DNLM; MH; N; PPHa
00-5909

TALMEY, B[ernard] S[imon] (1862-1926)
Woman; a treatise on the normal and pathological emotions of feminine love. New York: Stanley Press, 1904. 228p. DNLM; MH; NIC; NN **00-5910**

TALMEY, B[ernard] S[imon] (1862-1926)
Reflections concerning pretended therapeutic successes obtained by some practitioners of the ophthalmological specialty. New York: A. R. Elliott Pub. Co., 1905. 8p. DNLM
00-5911

TALMEY, B[ernard] S[imon] (1862-1926)
A case of cyst and hydrocele of the canal of Nuck. New York: A. R. Elliott, 1905. 3p. DNLM **00-5912**

TALMEY, B[ernard] S[imon] (1862-1926)
A case of tuboabdominal pregnancy secondary to an incomplete tubal abortion. New York, 1906. 3p. DNLM
00-5913

TALMEY, B[ernard] S[imon] (1862-1926)
A plea for the simple round-ligament ventrosuspension. New York, 1906. 9p. DNLM **00-5914**

TALMEY, B[ernard] S[imon] (1862-1926)
Woman; a treatise on the normal and pathological emotions of feminine love . . . for physicians and students of medicine. With twenty-two drawings in the text. New York: The Stanley Press Corporation, [1906]. 228p. plates. DLC; ICJ; N
00-5915

TALMEY, B[ernard] S[imon] (1862-1926)
A case of multilocular glandular cystoma complicating pregnancy. New York, 1907. 4p. DNLM
00-5916

TALMEY, B[ernard] S[imon] (1862-1926)
Notes on appendicitis. New York: A. R. Elliott Co., 1907. 7p. DNLM **00-5917**

TALMEY, B[ernard] S[imon] (1862-1926)
The law of beauty in human anatomy. [Philadelphia? 1908?] 14p. illus. NN **00-5918**

TALMEY, B[ernard] S[imon] (1862-1926)
Woman; a treatise on the normal and pathological emotions of feminine love . . . for physicians and students of medicine and jurisprudence; with twenty-three drawings in the text. 2nd enl. and improved ed. New York: Practitioners' Publishing Co., [1908]. 258p. DLC; MB; NN; PU [*vel subseq.*]
00-5919

TALMEY, B[ernard] S[imon] (1862-1926)
Woman; a treatise on the normal and pathological emotions of feminine love . . . for physicians and students of medicine and jurisprudence; with twenty-three drawings in the text. 3rd enl. and improved ed. New York: Practitioners' Publishing Co., [1908]. 258p. DLC; MH; NIC; NN **00-5920**

TALMEY, B[ernard] S[imon] (1862-1926)
Woman; a treatise on the normal and pathological emotions of feminine love . . . for physicians and students of medicine and jurisprudence; with twenty-three drawings in the text. 4th enl. and improved ed. New York: Practitioners' Publishing Co., [1908]. 258p. ICJ; NN; PPC **00-5921**

TALMEY, B[ernard] S[imon] (1862-1926)
Woman; a treatise on the normal and pathological emotions of feminine love . . . for physicians and students of medicine; with twenty-three drawings in the text. 5th enl. and rev. ed. New York: Practitioners' Publishing Co., [1908]. 260p. DLC; ICU; NIC; NN **00-5922**

TALMEY, B[ernard] S[imon] (1862-1926)
Neurasthenia sexualis; a treatise on sexual impotence in men and in women; for physicians and students of medicine . . . with nineteen drawings in the text. New York: The Practitioners' Publishing Co., [1910?] 196p. DLC; MH; NN; PP **00-5923**

TALMEY, B[ernard] S[imon] (1862-1926)
Woman; a treatise on the normal and pathological emotions of feminine love . . . for physicians and students of medicine; with twenty-three drawings in the text. 6th enl. and rev. ed. New York: Practitioners' Publishing Co., [1910]. 262p. DLC; NN; PPC **00-5924**

TALMEY, B[ernard] S[imon] (1862-1926)
Genesis; a manual for the instruction of children in matters sexual, for the use of parents, teachers, physicians and ministers . . . with nineteen cuts, forty-seven drawings, in the text. New York: The Practitioners' Publishing Co., [1910]. 194p. illus. DLC; ICJ; NN; NNNAM **00-5925**

TALMEY, Max (1867-1941)
Reflections concerning pretended therapeutic successes obtained by same practitioners of the ophthalmological specialty. [New York]: A. R. Elliott Publishing Co., 1905. 8p. NN **00-5926**

TALMEY, Max (1867-1941)
A contribution to the study of pseudoneuritis optica. New York, 1906. 6p. DNLM **00-5927**

TALMEY, Max (1867-1941)
Corneal burn by direct flame; report of a severe case, with remarks on the prognosis and treatment of corneal burns. New York, 1907. 8p. DNLM **00-5928**

TALMEY, Max (1867-1941)
Psyche. A concise and easily comprehensible treatise on the elements of psychiatry and psychology for students of medicine and law. New York: Med.-Leg. Publ. Co., 1910. 282p. DLC; DNLM; NN; OCIM **00-5929**

TALMEY, Max (1867-1941)
Manic depressive insanity or recurrent insanity? New York, 1910. 11p. DNLM **00-5930**

TANNER, Thomas Hawkes (1824-1871)
Memoranda on poisons . . . 8th rev. ed. By Henry Leffmann. . . . Philadelphia: P. Blakiston's Son & Co., 1901. 175p. DLC; DNLM; PPC; PU **00-5931**

TANNER, Thomas Hawkes (1824-1871)
Memoranda on poisons . . . 9th rev. ed. By Henry Leffmann. . . . Philadelphia: P. Blakiston's Son & Co., 1903 [1902]. 177p. DLC; DNLM; IU-M; PPC **00-5932**

TANNER, Thomas Hawkes (1824-1871)
Memoranda on poisons . . . 10th rev. ed. By Henry Leffmann. . . . Philadelphia: P. Blakiston's Son & Co., 1905. 177p. CtY-M; DLC; NNNAM; PPJ **00-5933**

TANNER, Thomas Hawkes (1824-1871)
Memoranda on poisons . . . 11th rev. ed. By Henry Leffmann. . . . Philadelphia: P. Blakiston's Son & Co., 1910. 167p. DLC; ICJ; KU; NNNAM **00-5934**

TANZI, Eugenio (*b.* 1856)
A textbook of mental diseases. Transl. from the Italian by W. Ford Robertson and T. C. Mackenzie. New York: Rebman Co., 1909. 808p. DLC; ICJ; NIC; NN **00-5935**

TASKER, Dain Loren (*b.* 1872)
Principles of osteopathy. . . . Los Angeles, Cal.: Baumgardt Publishing Co., 1903. 352p. DLC **00-5936**

TAUSSIG, Frederick Joseph (1872-1943)
The prevention and treatment of abortion . . . fifty-nine illustrations. St. Louis: C. V. Mosby Co., 1910. 180p. DLC; DNLM; ICJ; PPC **00-5937**

TAYLOR, Alonzo Englebert (*b.* 1871) and C. H. FRAZIER
The restitution of the blood-plasma following intravenous saline injections after hemorrhage. [Philadelphia, 1900.] 12p. DNLM **00-5938**

TAYLOR, Arthur N[elson] (*b.* 1867)
The law in its relations to physicians. New York: D. Appleton & Co., 1900. 550p. DNLM; MH; NN; NNNAM **00-5939**

TAYLOR, Arthur N[elson] (*b.* 1867)
The law in its relations to physicians. 2nd ed. New York: D. Appleton & Co., 1904. 559p. DNLM; ICJ; MB; NNNAM **00-5940**

TAYLOR, Charles Bell (1830-1909)
The fruits of vivisection. . . . [Philadelphia: American Anti-vivisection Society, 1901?] 2p. DLC **00-5941**

TAYLOR, Charles Chauncey
The druggists' English-German reference book. . . . Perrysburg: J. Timmons, general job printer, 1900. 31p. DLC [1884, *vel subseq.*] **00-5942**

TAYLOR, Charles Chauncey
Taylor's German lessons for druggists and drug clerks. . . . First[-fourth] term. . . . [Perrysburg, O., 1901?] 4 v. DLC **00-5943**

TAYLOR, Edward Wyllys (1866-1932)
Gumma of the oblongata. Boston, 1900. 8p. 1 plate. DNLM **00-5944**

TAYLOR, Edward Wyllys (1866-1932)
Poliomyelitis of the adult. New York, 1902. 32p. DNLM
00-5945

TAYLOR, Edward Wyllys (1866-1932) and George A. WATERMAN
Tumor in the region of the hypophysis. Boston, 1902. 7p. DNLM **00-5946**

TAYLOR, Edward Wyllys (1866-1932) and George A. WATERMAN
Two cases of so-called Landry's paralysis; autopsies. Boston, 1902. 11p. DNLM **00-5947**

TAYLOR, Edward Wyllys (1866-1932)
Unusual complications of tabes. I. Tabes with progressive muscular atrophy. II. Tabes with multiple sclerosis. Boston, 1902. 9p. DNLM **00-5948**

TAYLOR, Edward Wyllys (1866-1932) and George A. WATERMAN
Diffuse (combined) degeneration of the spinal cord. Boston, 1903. 17p. DNLM **00-5949**

TAYLOR, Edward Wyllys (1866-1932) and George A. WATERMAN
Sub-dural, cervical carcinoma, secondary to carcinoma of the breast. Boston, 1903. 8p. DNLM **00-5950**

TAYLOR, Edward Wyllys (1866-1932)
Polioencephalomyelitis and allied conditions. Boston, 1903. 27p. DNLM **00-5951**

TAYLOR, Edward Wyllys (1866-1932) and James Walker MYER
Notes from the Neurological Department, Massachusetts General Hospital. The relative frequency of multiple sclerosis. Boston, 1903. 5p. DNLM **00-5952**

TAYLOR, Edward Wyllys (1866-1932)
Sacral spina bifida, with reference to the skin representation of sacral nerve roots. Boston, [1904]. 10p. DNLM
00-5953

TAYLOR, Edward Wyllys (1866-1932) and Edward A. LINDSTRÖM
Experience in the treatment of tabes by co-ordinative exercises. Boston, 1907. 17p. illus. plates. MB
00-5954

TAYLOR, Edward Wyllys (1866-1932)
Diseases of the cerebral nerves. Philadelphia, 1910. 63p. DNLM
00-5955

TAYLOR, Edward Wyllys (1866-1932)
Case histories in neurology; a selection of histories setting forth the diagnosis, treatment and post-mortem findings in nervous disease. . . . Boston: W. M. Leonard, 1910. 305p. illus., diags. DLC; ICJ; NcD; PPJ **00-5956**

TAYLOR, Frederick (1847-1920)
A manual of the practice of medicine. 6th ed. Philadelphia: P. Blakiston's Son & Co., 1901. 1028p. CtY-M; DNLM; NNNAM; PPC [1st ed., London: J. & A. Churchill, 1890]
00-5957

TAYLOR, Frederick (1847-1920)
The practice of medicine . . . 9th ed. New York: The Macmillan Co., 1910. 1121p. DLC; ICJ; KU; PPJ **00-5958**

TAYLOR, Henry Lewis (*b.* 1855)
. . . Professional education in the United States. Prepared by Henry L. Taylor, Ph.D., under the direction of James Russell Parsons, Jr., M.A. Ed. for the Paris Exposition 1900. . . . Albany: University of the State of New York, 1900. 2 v. DLC; MH; NIC; NN **00-5959**

TAYLOR, Henry L[ing] (1857-1923)
Memoir of J. Henry Fruitnight. New York, 1901. 9p. DNLM
00-5960

TAYLOR, Henry L[ing] (1857-1923)
Retardation of growth as a cause of shortening after coxitis. Philadelphia, 1901. 6p. 1 table. DNLM
00-5961

TAYLOR, Henry L[ing] (1857-1923)
Chronic joint diseases in children. New York, 1902. 8p. DNLM
00-5962

TAYLOR, Henry L[ing] (1857-1923)
Surgery of rickets. Chicago, 1902. 8p. DNLM
00-5963

TAYLOR, Henry L[ing] (1857-1923)
Orthopedic surgery for practitioners. Assisted by Charles Ogilvy and Fred H. Albee. New York & London: D. Appleton & Co., 1909. 503p. DNLM; MH-M; NNNAM; PU
00-5964

TAYLOR, Hugh M[cGuire] (*b.* 1856)
Intestinal perforation in typhoid fever. New York: A. R. Elliott, 1905. 12p. DNLM **00-5965**

TAYLOR, Hugh M[cGuire] (*b.* 1856)
Popliteal aneurysm, its surgical treatment. New York, 1905. 4p. DNLM **00-5966**

TAYLOR, James (*b.* 1859)
Paralysis and other diseases of the nervous system in childhood and early life. Philadelphia: P. Blakiston's Son & Co., 1905. 512p. DNLM; NNNAM; PPC; PU **00-5967**

TAYLOR, J[ohn] Madison (*b.* 1855)
Nervous manifestations in the diseases of children. New York, 1900. 4p. DNLM **00-5968**

TAYLOR, J[ohn] Madison (*b.* 1855) and William H. WELLS
Manual of the diseases of children. 2nd ed. Philadelphia: P. Blakiston's Son & Co., 1901. 859p. 1 plate. DLC; MBM; NNNAM; PU **00-5969**

TAYLOR, J[ohn] Madison (*b.* 1855)
The amelioration of parlaysis agitans and other forms of tremor by systematic exercise. New York, 1901. 7p. DNLM
00-5970

TAYLOR, J[ohn] Madison (*b.* 1855)
Remarks on mechanotherapy, massage, bone setting, and osteopathy. New York, 1903. 16p. DNLM
00-5971

TAYLOR, J[ohn] Madison (*b.* 1855)
Respiratory education in the treatment of lung and heart disorders. New York, 1904. 13p. DNLM
00-5972

TAYLOR, J[ohn] Madison (*b.* 1855)
The principles of treatment in diseases of children. [New York], 1906. 16p. DNLM **00-5973**

TAYLOR, J[ohn] Madison (*b.* 1855)
The rational treatment of visceral ptoses. [New York], 1906. 16p. DNLM **00-5974**

TAYLOR, J[ohn] Madison (*b.* 1855)
Artificial supports for the viscera. New York, 1907. 9p. DNLM **00-5975**

TAYLOR, J[ohn] Madison (*b.* 1855)
Management of exhaustion states in men. Philadelphia, 1907. 15p. DNLM **00-5976**

TAYLOR, J[ohn] Madison (*b.* 1855)
Relief of nutritional disorders by developing the abdominal supports. New York, 1907. 10p. DNLM **00-5977**

TAYLOR, J[ohn] Madison (*b.* 1855)
Remarks on medical legislation. Philadelphia, 1907. 4p. DNLM **00-5978**

TAYLOR, J[ohn] Madison (*b.* 1855)
Treatment of writer's cramp. Professional spasm, occupation neurosis or scrivener's palsy, arm-pains, etc. Philadelphia, 1907. 4p. DNLM **00-5979**

TAYLOR, J[ohn] Madison (*b.* 1855)
What good can we get from consultation? Philadelphia, 1907. 4p. DNLM **00-5980**

TAYLOR, J[ohn] Madison (*b.* 1855)
The hand as a therapeutic agent. New York, 1908. 15p. DNLM **00-5981**

TAYLOR, J[ohn] Madison (*b.* 1855)
The medical treatment of tuberculosis as interpreted by Sajous. [Philadelphia], 1908. 5p. DNLM **00-5982**

TAYLOR, J[ohn] Madison (*b.* 1855)
The rational treatment of splanchnoptosis; displacements of viscera, both abdominal and thoracic. New York, 1908. 14p. DNLM **00-5983**

TAYLOR, J[ohn] Madison (*b.* 1855)
The curative powers in human milk. Philadelphia, 1909. 6p. DNLM **00-5984**

TAYLOR, J[ohn] Madison (*b.* 1855)
A few practical applications of the principles introduced by Dr. Sajous. Philadelphia, 1909. 6p. DNLM **00-5985**

TAYLOR, J[ohn] Madison (*b.* 1855)
The gospel of human efficiency; the conservation of vital energy by teaching right living essential to the highest achievement in any line of endeavor. New York, 1909. 8p. DNLM **00-5986**

TAYLOR, J[ohn] Madison (*b.* 1855)
A new era in medicine. New York, 1909. 15p. DNLM **00-5987**

TAYLOR, J[ohn] Madison (*b.* 1855)
Respiratory education; methods designed to amplify vital capacity by enhancing the mobility of the thorax, and thus contribute to the repair of disordered functions. New York, 1909. 8p. DNLM **00-5988**

TAYLOR, J[ohn] Madison (*b.* 1855)
Treatment of occupation neuroses and neuritis in the arms. Chicago, 1909. 7p. DNLM **00-5989**

TAYLOR, J[ohn] Madison (*b.* 1855)
Cases of chronic joint troubles (rheumatoid disease). With remarks on treatment. New York, 1910. 6p. DNLM **00-5990**

TAYLOR, John William
Result of research in mental science; or, The modern scientific phrenological and physiological register and self-instructor. . . . New York: Fowler & Wells Co., [1901?]. 108p. DLC; NN **00-5991**

TAYLOR, Lewis H. (*b.* 1850)
Non-medical therapeutics. Wilkes-Barre, 1901. 10p. DNLM **00-5992**

TAYLOR, Lewis H. (*b.* 1850)
The operation of couching performed by a mule. Chicago, 1901. 2p. DNLM **00-5993**

TAYLOR, Lewis H. (*b.* 1850)
Medical libraries in smaller cities. [n. p.], 1904. 7p. DNLM **00-5994**

TAYLOR, R[ichard] A[ugustus]
Tuberculosis, a clinical problem in the tenements. New York, 1908. 12p. DNLM; NN **00-5995**

TAYLOR, R[obert] Tunstall (1867-1929) and E[rnest] A. KNORR
A study of vaccines and the opsonic index in relation to orthopedic surgery. Boston, 1907. 20p. DNLM; MBM **00-5996**

TAYLOR, R[obert] Tunstall (1867-1929)
Orthopaedic surgery for students and general practitioners; preliminary considerations and diseases of the spine; 114 original illustrations. Baltimore: Williams & Wilkins Co., 1907. 241p. DLC; MdU-D; PPC; PU **00-5997**

TAYLOR, Robert W[illiam] (1842-1908)
A practical treatise on sexual disorders of the male and female. . . . 2nd ed., thoroughly revised. With 91 illustrations and 13 plates in color and monochrome. New York and Philadelphia: Lea Bros. & Co., 1900. 438p. DLC; NNNAM; PPC; PPJ **00-5998**

TAYLOR, Robert W[illiam] (1842-1908)
A practical treatise on genito-urinary and venereal diseases and syphilis. With 138 illustrations and 27 plates in colors and monotone. New York and Philadelphia: Lea Bros. & Co., 1900. 494p. col. plates. NNNAM; PPJ; PU; ScCM **00-5999**

TAYLOR, Robert W[illiam] (1842-1908)
A practical treatise on genito-urinary and venereal diseases and syphilis. . . . 2nd ed., thoroughly rev. With 138 illustrations and 27 plates in colors and monotone. New York and Philadelphia: Lea Bros. & Co., 1900. 722p. DLC; DNLM; MBM; PPC **00-6000**

TAYLOR, Robert W[illiam] (1842-1908)
A practical treatise on genito-urinary and venereal diseases and syphilis. . . . 3rd ed., thoroughly rev. With 163 illustrations and 39 plates in colors and monochrome. New York and Philadelphia: Lea Bros. & Co., [1904]. 757p. DLC; DNLM; NNNAM; PPC **00-6001**

TAYLOR, Robert W[illiam] (1842-1908)
A practical treatise on sexual disorders of the male and female. . . . 3rd ed., thoroughly rev. With 130 illustrations and 16 plates in colors and monochrome. New York and Philadelphia: Lea Bros. & Co., 1905. 525p. DLC; DNLM; NNNAM; PPC **00-6002**

TAYLOR, Robert W[illiam] (1842-1908)
Deformities of the penis due to syphilis, gonorrhoea, and other causes. New York, 1907. 31p. DNLM; NNNAM **00-6003**

TAYLOR, Robert W[illiam] (1842-1908)
Bone syphilis, hereditary and acquired. New York: A. R. Elliott Co., 1907. 42p. DNLM; NNNAM **00-6004**

TAYLOR, William Henry (1835-1917)
Outlines of medical jurisprudence, with reference to methods and practice chiefly. . . . Richmond: H. T. Ezekiel, printer, [1904]. 67p. DLC; ICJ; ViRA **00-6005**

TAYLOR, William Henry (1835-1917)
De quibus: discourse and essays. . . . Richmond, Va.: The Bell Book and Stationery Co., [1908]. 380p. DLC; ICJ; NcD; NN ["The largest and most important part of this book consists of courses addressed . . . to the classes of the Medical College of Virginia." Pref.] **00-6006**

TAYLOR, William J. (*b.* 1861) and William G. SPILLER
A case of multiple fibromata confined to the internal plantar nerve. Philadelphia, 1903. 3p. DNLM **00-6007**

TEASLEY, D[aniel] O[tis] (*b.* 1876)
Private lectures to mothers and daughters on sexual purity, including love, courtship, marriage, sexual physiology, and the evil effects of tight lacing. . . . Moundsville, W. Va.: Gospel Trumpet Co., 1904. 114p. DLC **00-6008**

TEASLEY, D[aniel] O[tis] (*b.* 1876)
Private lectures to men and boys. Including early training and sexual physiology, secret sins and sexual disorders, helps to purity, illicit intercourse and its attendant ills, and love, courtship and marriage. . . . Moundsville, W. Va.: Gospel Trumpet Co., 1905. 144p. DLC **00-6009**

TEMPLE COLLEGE, PHILADELPHIA, PA. DEPARTMENT OF MEDICINE
Annual announcements for the sessions of 1901-02 to 1910-11. Philadelphia, 1903-10. DNLM [Announcements for 1906-07 to 1910-11 contain list of students and graduates.] **00-6010**

TENNEY, Benjamin (*b.* 1863)
The anatomy and surgery of the internal derangements of the knee-joint. Philadelphia, 1904. 34p. 10 plates. DNLM **00-6011**

TENNEY, Benjamin (*b.* 1863)
Some conclusions based on a study of one hundred and thirty-four cases of calculus in the ureter. With a report of three new cases. Boston, 1904. 7p. DNLM **00-6012**

TENNEY, Benjamin (*b.* 1863)
The diagnosis of renal and ureteral calculi. Boston, 1905. 11p. DNLM **00-6013**

TENNEY, Benjamin (*b.* 1863)
Early diagnosis of surgical disease in the urinary organs. Boston, 1905. 15p. DNLM **00-6014**

TENNEY, Benjamin (*b.* 1863)
The satisfactory prostatectomy. Boston, 1905. 15p. DNLM **00-6015**

TENNEY, Benjamin (*b.* 1863) and Henry Melville CHASE
Mortality after prostatectomy. Chicago, 1906. 6p. DNLM **00-6016**

TENNEY, Benjamin (*b.* 1863)
The treatment of chronic urethral discharge. Boston, 1907. 9p. DNLM **00-6017**

TENNEY, Elmer S.
The sputum of typhoid fever patients as a possible source of infection. Boston, 1910. 14p. DNLM **00-6018**

TERRY, B[enjamin] T[aylor] (*b.* 1876)
The specific chemical therapy of the trypanosomiases and spirilloses. New York, 1909. 27p. DNLM; NNNAM **00-6019**

TERRY, Theodore Brainard (*b.* 1843)
How to keep well and live long. . . . Philadelphia, Pa.: The Farmer Co., [1909]. 227p. incl. illus., port. DLC; PP **00-6020**

THAYER, Alfred Edward
. . . Compend of general pathology. . . . Philadelphia: P. Blakiston's Son & Co., 1902. 322p. DLC; DNLM; PPC; PU **00-6021**

THAYER, Alfred Edward
A compend of pathology, general and special. A students' manual in one volume . . . 2nd ed., containing 131 illustrations. Philadelphia: P. Blakiston's Son & Co., 1903. 711p. DLC; DNLM; NNNAM; PU **00-6022**

THAYER, Alfred Edward
A study of deaths occurring in New York City. [New York, 1903.] 7p. NN **00-6023**

THAYER, C[armi] C[assander] (1840-1916)
Ovulation and menstruation not interdependent functions. Chicago, 1901. 8p. DNLM **00-6024**

THAYER, HENRY, & CO.
Net prices of medicinal extracts and all other pharmaceutical products. Latest ed. July 1, 1900. Cambridgeport, Mass.: H. Thayer & Co., 1900. 297p. illus. DLC; MH; MWA **00-6025**

THAYER, William S[ydney] (1864-1932)
Observations on the blood in typhoid fever. Baltimore, 1900. 61p. DLC; DNLM; ICJ; PPC **00-6026**

THAYER, William S[ydney] (1864-1932)
On recent advances in our knowledge concerning the etiology of malarial fever. New Haven, 1900. 12p. DNLM
00-6027

THAYER, William S[ydney] (1864-1932)
Bacteriology in health and disease. On recent advances in our knowledge concerng the aetiology of malarial fever. New Haven, 1900. 10p. MB **00-6028**

THAYER, William S[ydney] (1864-1932)
Observations on the blood in typhoid fever. Boston, 1900. 8p. DNLM **00-6029**

THAYER, William S[ydney] (1864-1932)
Obituary: Jesse William Lazear. [Baltimore, 1900.] 2 l. DNLM
00-6030

THAYER, William S[ydney] (1864-1932)
Observations on the frequency and diagnosis of the Flint murmur in aortic insufficiency. [Philadelphia, 1901.] 16p. DNLM **00-6031**

THAYER, William S[ydney] (1864-1932)
A case of aestivo-autumnal fever with unusually few parasites in the peripheral circulation. Baltimore, 1902. 8p. DNLM
00-6032

THAYER, William S[ydney] (1864-1932)
Remarks on the diagnosis of pancreatic disease. Philadelphia, 1902. 13p. DNLM **00-6033**

THAYER, William S[ydney] (1864-1932)
Laennec. Baltimore, 1902. 7p. DNLM
00-6034

THAYER, William S[ydney] (1864-1932)
Remarks on typhoid fever. St. Paul, 1902. 13p. DNLM
00-6035

THAYER, William S[ydney] (1864-1932)
Notes on a case of acute haemorrhagic poliomyelitis. Boston, 1902. 17p. DNLM **00-6036**

THAYER, William S[ydney] (1864-1932)
On the teaching of physical diagnosis. Boston, 1902. 19p. DNLM **00-6037**

THAYER, William S[ydney] (1864-1932)
Preliminary report of the Tuberculosis Commission of Maryland. Baltimore, 1903. 24p. DNLM
00-6038

THAYER, William S[ydney] (1864-1932)
On arteriitis and arterial thrombosis in typhoid fever. New York, 1903. 21p. DNLM **00-6039**

THAYER, William S[ydney] (1864-1932)
Bichat. Baltimore, 1903. 12p. DNLM
00-6040

THAYER, William S[ydney] (1864-1932)
Observations on the teaching of clinical medicine. Chicago, 1903. 9p. DNLM **00-6041**

THAYER, William S[ydney] (1864-1932)
Analysis of forty-two cases of venous thrombosis occurring in the course of typhoid fever. [New York], 1904. 10p. DNLM
00-6042

THAYER, William S[ydney] (1864-1932)
On the cardiac and vascular complications and sequels of typhoid fever. The Jerome Cochran lecture. Baltimore, 1904. 48p. DNLM **00-6043**

THAYER, William S[ydney] (1864-1932)
The problems of internal medicine. [New York, 1904.] 23p. DNLM **00-6044**

THAYER, William S[ydney] (1864-1932)
On the late effects of typhoid fever on the heart and vessels; a clinical study. Philadelphia, 1904. 31p. DNLM
00-6045

THAYER, William S[ydney] (1864-1932)
Observations on two cases of tuberculous pericarditis with effusion. Baltimore, 1904. 18p. DNLM
00-6046

THAYER, William S[ydney] (1864-1932) and Clinton Ethelbert BRUSH
The relation of acute Infections to arteriosclerosis. Chicago, 1904. 10p. DNLM **00-6047**

THAYER, William S[ydney] (1864-1932)
On some public duties of the physician. . . . Address delivered before the Medical and Chirurgical Faculty of Maryland at Deer Park, September 22, 1905. [Baltimore], 1905. 10p. NN
00-6048

THAYER, William S[ydney] (1864-1932)
Cotton Mather's rules of health. [Baltimore, 1905.] 21p. DNLM **00-6049**

THAYER, William S[ydney] (1864-1932)
Gonorrhoeal septicaemia and endocarditis. Chicago, 1905. 29p. DNLM **00-6050**

THAYER, William S[ydney] (1864-1932)
Observations on several cases of acute pancreatitis. [Baltimore, 1905.] 27p. DNLM **00-6051**

THAYER, William S[ydney] (1864-1932)
On the prophylaxis of typhoid fever. [Baltimore, 1906.] 9p. DNLM **00-6052**

THAYER, William S[ydney] (1864-1932)
An analysis of 808 cases of chorea with special reference to the cardiovascular manifestations. Chicago, 1906. 8p. DNLM
00-6053

THAYER, William S[ydney] (1864-1932)
Lines read at the dinner, given in honor of Dr. Robert Fletcher, Washington, Jan. 11, 1906. [Baltimore, 1906.] 2 l. DNLM
00-6054

THAYER, William S[ydney] (1864-1932)
The problems of internal medicine. Boston, 1906. 12p. MB
00-6055

THAYER, William S[ydney] (1864-1932)
On the importance of the simple physical and psychical methods of treatment. [New Orleans, 1907.] 16p. DNLM
00-6056

THAYER, William S[ydney] (1864-1932) and George Hoyt WHIPPLE
A hitherto undescribed disease characterized anatomically by deposits of fat and fatty acids in the intestinal and mesenteric lymphatic tissues. [Baltimore, 1907.] 26p. 6 plates. DNLM
00-6057

THAYER, William S[ydney] (1864-1932) and W. G. MacCALLUM
Experimental studies on cardiac murmurs. [Philadelphia, 1907.] 8p. 1 diag. DNLM **00-6058**

THAYER, William S[ydney] (1864-1932) and H. H. HAZEN
Calcification of the breast following typhoid fever. New York, 1907. 17p. 1 plate DNLM **00-6059**

THAYER, William S[ydney] (1864-1932) and Marshall FABYAN
The paravertebral triangle of dulness in pleural effusion (Grocco's sign). [Philadelphia, 1907.] 15p. DNLM
00-6060

THAYER, William S[ydney] (1864-1932) and Marshall FABYAN
Studies on arterio-sclerosis, with special reference to the radial artery. [Philadelphia, 1907.] 19p. DNLM
00-6061

THAYER, William S[ydney] (1864-1932)
On the early diastolic heart sound, the so-called third heart sound. Boston, 1908. 49p. DNLM **00-6062**

THAYER, William S[ydney] (1864-1932)
On some relations of the physician to the public. Duties and opportunities. Oration on medicine at the Fifty-ninth Annual Session of the American Medical Association at Chicago, June 2-5, 1908. . . . [Chicago: Amer. Medical Assoc., 1908.] 23p. NN **00-6063**

THAYER, William S[ydney] (1864-1932)
Note on pellagra in Maryland. [Baltimore, 1909.] 21p. 2 plates. DNLM **00-6064**

THAYER, William S[ydney] (1864-1932)
Further observations on the third heart sound. [Chicago, 1909.] 11p. DNLM **00-6065**

THAYER, William S[ydney] (1864-1932)
On two cases of intrathoracic tumor. [Richmond, 1910.] 14p. DNLM **00-6066**

THEISEN, Clement F[rank] (*b.* 1871)
Angina epiglottidea anterior. Report of three cases. [Albany, 1900.] 11p. 2 plates. DNLM **00-6067**

THEOBALD, Samuel (1846-1930)
A case of extensive detachment of the retina in myopic eye in which complete recovery followed rest in bed and the administration of pilocarpine. New York, 1900. 3p. DNLM
00-6068

THEOBALD, Samuel (1846-1930)
The evolution of the ophthalmoscope and what it has done for medicine. New York: A. R. Elliott Pub. Co., 1901. 26p. DNLM
00-6069

THEOBALD, Samuel (1846-1930)
Two new instruments. [Hartford, Conn.], 1901. 4p. DNLM
00-6070

THEOBALD, Samuel (1846-1930)
The ideal result to be kept in view in the operative treatment of convergent strabismus in children. Baltimore, 1902. 3p. DNLM **00-6071**

THEOBALD, Samuel (1846-1930)
Inflammation of the mastoid cells. New York, 1902. 13p. DNLM **00-6072**

THEOBALD, Samuel (1846-1930)
Observations upon recent methods of treating corneal ulcers, with especial reference to the use of carbolic acid as a not infrequent substitute for the actual cautery. Philadelphia, 1902. 4p. DNLM **00-6073**

THEOBALD, Samuel (1846-1930)
The importance of testing the ocular muscle balance for near as well as for distant vision. [Hartford, Conn., 1904.] 6p. DNLM **00-6074**

THEOBALD, Samuel (1846-1930)
The importance of testing the ocular muscle balance for near as well as for distant vision. Baltimore, 1905. 3p. DNLM
00-6075

THEOBALD, Samuel (1846-1930)
The genesis of sympathetic ophthalmia. Chicago, 1905. 11p. DNLM **00-6076**

THEOBALD, Samuel (1846-1930)
The success which at the present day attends the operation of cataract extraction and the causes that contribute to it. Philadelphia, 1906. 3p. DNLM **00-6077**

THEOBALD, Samuel (1846-1930)
A striking illustration of the efficacy of constitutional measures in controlling inflammation of the mastoid cells. [New Bedford], 1906. 4p. DNLM **00-6078**

THEOBALD, Samuel (1846-1930)
Prevalent diseases of the eye. A reference handbook, especially adapted to the needs of the general practitioner and the medical student. Philadelphia & London: W. B. Saunders & Co., 1906. 551p. 11 plates. CtY-M; DNLM; NNNAM; PPC
00-6079

THEOBALD, Samuel (1846-1930)
The conservative treatment of chronic suppuration of the middle-ear. Chicago, 1907. 4p. DNLM
00-6080

THEOBALD, Samuel (1846-1930)
Indications for the employment of adrenalin chlorid, in conjunction with cocain, in operations on the eye. Chicago, 1907. 3p. DNLM **00-6081**

THEOBALD, Samuel (1846-1930) and W. G. MacCALLUM
A case of intraocular tuberculosis with closely simulated glioma of the retina. Nashville, Tenn., 1907. 4p. 1 plate. DNLM **00-6082**

THEOBALD, Samuel (1846-1930)
A simplification of de Grandmont's operation for ptosis. Baltimore, 1908. 4p. DNLM **00-6083**

THOMAS, Henry M. (*b.* 1861)
Obstetrical paralysis, infantile and maternal. Baltimore, 1900. 9p. DNLM **00-6084**

THOMAS, Henry M. (*b.* 1861) and Harvey W. CUSHING
Exhibition of two cases of radicular paralysis of the brachial plexus, one from the pressure of a cervical rib with operation, the other of uncertain origin. Baltimore, 1903. 12p. DNLM **00-6085**

THOMAS, Henry M. (*b.* 1861)
The anatomical basis of the Argyll-Robertson pupil. Philadelphia & New York, 1903. 18p. DNLM **00-6086**

THOMAS, Henry M. (*b.* 1861)
A case of generalized lead paralysis, with a review of the cases of lead palsy seen in the hospital. Baltimore, 1904. 3p. DNLM **00-6087**

THOMAS, Henry M. (*b.* 1861) and Harry S. GREENBAUM
Multiple neuritis (nondiphtheritic) in children. Chicago, 1907. 10p. 1 chart. DNLM **00-6088**

THOMAS, Henry M. (*b.* 1861) and Harvey W. CUSHING
Removal of a subcortical cystic tumor at a second-stage operation without anesthesia. Chicago, 1908. 28p. DNLM **00-6089**

THOMAS, Henry M. (*b.* 1861)
Decussation of the pyramids; an historical inquiry. Baltimore, 1910. 29p. DNLM **00-6090**

THOMAS, Henry M. (*b.* 1861)
Diseases of the cerebral blood-vessels. Philadelphia, 1910. 90p. DNLM **00-6091**

THOMAS, J[ames] W. (*b.* 1866)
Gonorrheal peritonitis in the male. Seattle, 1907. 4p. DNLM **00-6092**

THOMAS, Jerome Beers (*b.* 1867)
A book of detachable diet lists for albuminuria, anemia and debility, constipation, diabetes . . . and a sick-room dietary . . . 2nd ed., rev. Philadelphia: W. B. Saunders & Co., 1900. 398p. DLC; MH-M; NNNAM; PPC [Contains 160 detachable (perforated) Diet Lists for Albuminuria, Anaemia and Debility, Constipation, Diabetes, Diarrhoea, Dyspepsia, Fevers, Gout or Uric-acid Diathesis, Obesity, and Tuberculosis; also 40 detachable sheets of Sick-Room Dietary, containing instructions for preparation of easily-digested food necessary for invalids. Each list is numbered only, the disease for which it is to be used in no case being mentioned,—an index key being reserved for the physician's private use.] **00-6093**

THOMAS, Jerome Beers (*b.* 1867)
Report of two cases of typhoid fever, with perforation and operation. . . . [Chicago: American Medical Association, 1905.] 7p. ICJ **00-6094**

THOMAS, John D. (*b.* 1868)
Nitrous oxide gas viewed from a practical standpoint. Philadelphia, [1901?]. 20p. CtY-M; DNLM; PPHa **00-6095**

THOMAS, John D. (*b.* 1868)
Abdominal signs of pulmonary diseaase in children. New York: William Wood & Co., 1907. 11p. DNLM **00-6096**

THOMAS, John J[enks] (*b.* 1861)
Five cases of injury of the cord resulting from fracture of the spine. Boston, 1900. 7p. 3 plates. DNLM **00-6097**

THOMAS, John J[enks] (*b.* 1861)
A case of myeloma of the spine with compression of the cord. Boston, 1901. 21p. DNLM **00-6098**

THOMAS, Joseph (1811-1891)
Lippincott's medical dictionary; a complete vocabulary of the terms used in medicine and the allied sciences, with their pronunciation, etymology, and signification . . . prepared on the basis of Thomas's Complete Medical Dictionary by Ryland W. Greene, with the editorial collaboration of John Ashhurst, Jr. . . . George A. Piersol . . . Joseph P. Remington. . . . Rev. ed. Philadelphia, [etc.]: J. B. Lippincott Co., [1905]. 1154p. 65 plates. DLC; NNNAM; PPC; PU **00-6099**

THOMAS, William I[saac] (1863-1947)
The medicine-man and the professional occupations. Chicago: Univ. of Chicago Press, 1903. 18p. DNLM; MB **00-6100**

THOMPSON, Joseph Ambrose
Hydrophobia and a remedy. Hyattsville, Md., [1906]. 2 l. DNLM **00-6101**

[THOMPSON, Joseph Ford] (1837-1917)
Complimentary dinner and presentation of loving cup to Joseph Ford Thompson, of Washington, D.C., on the fiftieth anniversary of his graduation in medicine at the University of Maryland, Thursday evening, March 7, 1907. Washington, 1907. [unp.] DNLM **00-6102**

THOMPSON, Millard F. (*b.* 1857)
Position in placenta previa. [Washington], 1905. 31p. DNLM **00-6103**

THOMPSON, Ralph L[eroy] (*b.* 1872)
An experimental study of the bacteriolytic complement content of the blood serum in normal, vaccinated, and variolated rabbits. Boston, 1903. 7p. DNLM **00-6104**

THOMPSON, Ralph L[eroy] (*b.* 1872)
The bacteriolytic complement content of the blood serum in variola. Boston, 1903. 15p. DNLM **00-6105**

THOMPSON, Ralph L[eroy] (*b.* 1872)
A clinical and experimental study of the bacteriolytic complement of the blood serum in variola. (In: Studies on the pathology . . . of variola. . . .) Boston, [1904]. 20p. DNLM **00-6106**

THOMPSON, Ralph L[eroy] (*b.* 1872)
Glimpses of medical Europe. Illustrated from photographs and from drawings by Tom Jones. Philadelphia & London: J. P. Lippincott Co., 1908. 236p. DNLM; ICU; NNNAM; PPC **00-6107**

THOMPSON, Silvanus Phillips
Optical tables and data for the use of opticians . . . 2nd ed., rev. New York: Spon & Chamberlain, 1907. 130p. illus., tables, diags. DLC; MB; NIC; NN **00-6108**

THOMPSON, W[illiam] Gilman (1856-1927)
A text-book of practical medicine. . . . Illustrated with seventy-nine engravings. New York and Philadelphia: Lea Bros. & Co., 1900. 1011p. DLC; DNLM; NNNAM; PPC
00-6109

THOMPSON, W[illiam] Gilman (1856-1927)
A text-book of practical medicine. . . . 2nd ed., rev. and enl. Illustrated with sixty-two engravings. New York and Philadelphia: Lea Bros. & Co., 1902. 1014p. DLC; DNLM; MBM; PU
00-6110

THOMPSON, W[illiam] Gilman (1856-1927)
Practical dietetics, with special reference to diet in diseases . . . 2nd ed., enl. and thoroughly rev. New York: D. Appleton & Co., 1902. 828p. DLC; DNLM; ICJ; NNNAM
00-6111

THOMPSON, W[illiam] Gilman (1856-1927)
The instruction of senior students in medicine. New York, 1903. 10p. DNLM **00-6112**

THOMPSON, W[illiam] Gilman (1856-1927)
Paroxysmal hematinuria (hémoglobinurie à frigore). New York, 1903. 22p. DNLM **00-6113**

THOMPSON, W[illiam] Gilman (1856-1927)
Illuminating gas poisoning. A clinical study of ninety cases. New York, 1904. 28p. DNLM **00-6114**

THOMPSON, W[illiam] Gilman (1856-1927)
The economic value of medical science. New York, 1904. 23p. DNLM **00-6115**

THOMPSON, W[illiam] Gilman (1856-1927)
Problems in dietetics. New York: William Wood & Co., 1904. 21p. DNLM **00-6116**

THOMPSON, W[illiam] Gilman (1856-1927)
A case of dibothriocephalus latus infection, causin pernicious anemia; with complete recovery. Philadelphia, 1905. 10p. DNLM **00-6117**

THOMPSON, W[illiam] Gilman (1856-1927)
Haematemesis from gastric ulcer; notes on over two hundred cases. Philadelphia, 1905. 8p. DNLM
00-6118

THOMPSON, W[illiam] Gilman (1856-1927)
Practical dietetics, with special reference to diet in disease . . . 3rd ed., enl. and thoroughly rev. New York and London: D. Appleton & Co., 1905. 846p. DLC; DNLM; NNNAM; PPC
00-6119

THOMPSON, W[illiam] Gilman (1856-1927)
The overtrained nurse. New York, 1906. 16p. DNLM
00-6120

THOMPSON, W[illiam] Gilman (1856-1927)
The relation of the visiting and house staff to the care of hospital patients. New York, 1906. 9p. DNLM
00-6121

THOMPSON, W[illiam] Gilman (1856-1927)
A clinical study of eighty cases of exophthalmic goitre. Philadelphia, 1906. 9p. DNLM **00-6122**

THOMPSON, W[illiam] Gilman (1856-1927)
The early diagnosis of gastric carcinoma; a clinical study. Columbus, 1907. 12p. DNLM **00-6123**

THOMPSON, W[illiam] Gilman (1856-1927)
Modern hospital construction. Chicago, 1907. 16p. DNLM
00-6124

THOMPSON, W[illiam] Gilman (1856-1927)
Street dirt and public health. New York, 1907. 8p. DNLM
00-6125

THOMPSON, W[illiam] Gilman (1856-1927)
Local thermotherapy. New York, 1907. 14p. DNLM
00-6126

THOMPSON, W[illiam] Gilman (1856-1927)
Fresh air treatment in hospital wards. New York, 1907. 12p. DNLM **00-6127**

THOMPSON, W[illiam] Gilman (1856-1927)
The treatment of pneumonia, especially by outdoor air. Philadelphia, 1908. 5p. DNLM **00-6128**

THOMPSON, W[illiam] Gilman (1856-1927)
A phenomenal aortic aneurysm. New York, 1908. 9p. DNLM
00-6129

THOMPSON, W[illiam] Gilman (1856-1927)
Address delivered at the fifty-third annual meeting of the Woman's Hospital in the State of New York, Wednesday, December 23, 1908. [New York, 1908.] 11p. DNLM
00-6130

THOMPSON, W[illiam] Gilman (1856-1927)
Practical dietetics, with special reference to diet in diseases . . . 4th ed., illustrated, enl. and completely rewritten. New York and London: D. Appleton & Co., 1909. 928p. DLC; DNLM; NNNAM; PPC **00-6131**

THOMPSON, W[illiam] Gilman (1856-1927)
Clinical experiments with homologous vaccines in the treatment of septic endocarditis and pyemia. Philadelphia, 1909. 14p. DNLM **00-6132**

THOMPSON, W[illiam] Gilman (1856-1927)
The scientific development of the Presbyterian Hospital. [New York, 1909.] 4 l. DNLM **00-6133**

THOMPSON, W[illiam] Gilman (1856-1927)
Visceral sarcomata; cases of sarcoma of the stomach, heart, mediastinum, etc. New York: William Wood & Co., 1910. 24p. DNLM **00-6134**

THOMPSON, W[illiam] Gilman (1856-1927)
Trichinosis; a clinical study of fifty-two sporadic cases. Philadelphia, 1910. 10p. DNLM **00-6135**

THOMPSON, W[illiam] Gilman (1856-1927)
The educational value of the trained nurse. New York, 1910. 4 l. DNLM **00-6136**

THOMPSON, W[illiam] Gilman (1856-1927)
Modern dietetic principles; their practical application. Boston: W. M. Leonard, 1910. 27p. DNLM; MBM
00-6137

THOMPSON, W[illiam] Gilman (1856-1927)
The great modern hospital. Present-day standards of organization and equipment. [New York], 1910. 13p. DNLM
00-6138

THOMSON, Alexis
General surgery. . . . Philadelphia: J. B. Lippincott Co., 1906. 2 v. DNLM; MBM; NNNAM; PU **00-6139**

THOMSON, Alexis and Alexander MILES
Manual of surgery. Philadelphia & London: J. B. Lippincott Co., 1906. 2 v. CtY-M; DNLM; NNNAM; PPC
00-6140

THOMSON, H[enry] Hyslop
Pulmonary phthisis; its diagnosis, prognosis and treatment. New York: William Wood & Co., 1906. 188p. DNLM; ICJ; NNNAM; PPC **00-6141**

THOMSON, H[erbert] Campbell (1870-1940)
Acute dilatation of the stomach. New York: William Wood & Co., 1902. 54p. CtY-M; DNLM; ICJ; NNNAM
00-6142

THOMSON, H[erbert] Campbell (1870-1940)
Diseases of the nervous system. Chicago: W. T. Keener Co., 1908. 480p. plates. CtY-M; MH; PPJ
00-6143

THOMSON, H[erbert] Campbell (1870-1940)
Diseases of the nervous system . . . With 8 coloured and 12 black-and-white plates, and 101 figures in the text. New York: Funk & Wagnalls Co., 1910. 480p. DLC: ICJ; IU-M; PU
00-6144

THOMSON, J[ohn] Arthur (1861-1933)
Progress of science in the century . . . Philadelphia, [etc.]: Linscott Publishing Co., 1903. 536p. DLC; MH; NIC; NN [Also: Philadlephia, Detroit: The Bradley-Garretson Co., 1903. 536p.] **00-6145**

THOMSON, J[ohn] Arthur (1861-1933)
Heredity. New York: G. P. Putnam's Sons, 1907. 608p. DLC; ICJ; NIC; NN **00-6146**

THOMSON, J[ohn] Arthur (1861-1933)
Darwinism and human life. New York: H. Holt, [1909?]. 245p. NN [The South African Lectures for 1909]
00-6147

THOMSON, St. Clair (1859-1943)
The cerebrospinal fluid; its spontaneous escape from the nose. With observations on its composition and function in the human subject. New York: William Wood & Co., 1901. 140p. DNLM; ICJ; NNNAM; PU **00-6148**

THOMSON, St. Clair (1859-1943)
Submucous excision of deviations and spurs of the nasal septum, with a report of 30 operations. [n. p., 1906?] 48p. DNLM **00-6149**

THOMSON, W[illiam] H[anna] (1833-1918)
Materialism and modern physiology of the nervous system. . . . New York, [etc.]: G. P. Putnam's Sons, 1901. 112p. plates. DLC; ICJ; MH; NN **00-6150**

THOMSON, W[illiam H[anna] (1833-1918)
Pathology and treatment of migraine. New York, 1901. 15p. DNLM **00-6151**

THOMSON, W[illiam] H[anna] (1833-1918)
Pathology and treatment of epilepsy. New York, 1902. 30p. DNLM **00-6152**

THOMSON, W[illiam] H[anna] (1833-1918)
Graves' disease with and without exophthalmic goitre. . . . New York: William Wood & Co., 1904. 143p. DLC; DNLM; ICJ; NNNAM **00-6153**

THOMSON, W[illiam] H[anna] (1833-1918)
Internal secretions. New York: A. R. Elliott Co., 1904. 39p. DNLM **00-6154**

THOMSON, W[illiam] H[anna] (1833-1918)
The true nature of functional nervous diseases. New York: A. R. Elliott, 1905. 13p. DNLM **00-6155**

THOMSON, W[illiam] H[anna] (1833-1918)
Brain and personality; or, The physical relations of the brain to the mind. . . . New York: Dodd, Mead & Co., 1906. 320p. DLC; DNLM; NN; NNC **00-6156**

THOMSON, W[illiam] H[anna] (1833-1918)
What is physical life? Its origin and nature. . . . New York: Dodd, Mead & Co., 1909. 206p. DLC; MH; NIC; NN
00-6157

THOMSON, W[illiam] H[anna] (1833-1918)
Asiatic cholera. New York: A. R. Elliott Co., 1909. 10p. DNLM **00-6158**

THOMSON, W[illiam] H[anna] (1833-1918)
Some wonders of biology. New York: Dodd, Mead & Co., 1909. 222p. DLC; NIC; NN; PU **00-6159**

THOMSON, W[illiam] H[anna] (1833-1918)
Life, death and immortality. . . . New York and London: Funk & Wagnalls Co., 1910. 117p. DLC; ICU; MB; NN
00-6160

THOMSON, W[illiam] Ross
The hot air treatment of acutely inflamed joints. New York: A. R. Elliott Pub. Co., 1905. 7p. DNLM
00-6161

THORINGTON, James (*b.* 1858)
Refraction and how to refract, including sections on optics, retinoscopy, the fitting of spectacles and eyeglasses, etc. . . . Two hundred illustrations, thirteen of which are colored. Philadelphia: P. Blakiston's Son & Co., 1900. 301p. DLC; ICJ; PPC; PPJ **00-6162**

THORINGTON, James (*b.* 1858)
Refraction and how to refract; including sections on optics, retinoscopy, the fitting of spectacles and eyeglasses, etc. . . . 2nd ed. Two hundred illustrations, thirteen of which are colored. Philadelphia: P. Blakiston's Son & Co., 1900. 301p. DLC; NNNAM; PPC; PU **00-6163**

THORINGTON, James (*b.* 1858)
Retinoscopy (or shadow test) in the determination of refraction at one meter distance, with the plane mirror . . . 4th ed., rev. and enl.; fifty-one illustrations, twelve of which are colored. Philadelphia: P. Blakiston's Son & Co., 1901. 89p. CtY-M; DLC; DNLM; PPC **00-6164**

THORINGTON, James (*b.* 1858)
Refraction and how to refract, including sections on optics, retinoscopy, the fitting of spectacles and eyeglasses, etc. . . . 3rd ed. Two hundred and fifteen illustrations, thirteen of which are colored. Philadelphia: P. Blakiston's Son & Co., 1904. 314p. DLC; DNLM; MBM; PU
00-6165

THORINGTON, James (*b.* 1858)
Retinoscopy (or shadow test) in the determination of refractions at one meter distance, with the plane mirror . . . 5th ed., rev. and enl. Fifty-four illustrations, ten of which are colored. Philadelphia: P. Blakiston's Son & Co., 1906. 67p. DLC; ICJ; DNLM; PPC **00-6166**

THORINGTON, James (*b.* 1858)
The ophthalmoscope and how to use it; with colored illustrations, descriptions, and treatment of the principal diseases of the fundus . . . 73 illustrations—12 colored plates. Philadelphia: P. Blakiston's Son & Co., 1906. 298p. DLC; DNLM; PPC; PU
00-6167

THORINGTON, James (*b.* 1858)
Refraction and how to refract, including sections on optics, retinoscopy, the fitting of spectacles and eyeglasses, etc. . . . 4th ed. Two hundred and twenty illustrations, thirteen of which are colored. Philadelphia: P. Blakiston's Son & Co., 1909. 324p. DLC; DNLM; NNNAM; PU
00-6168

THORINGTON, James (*b.* 1858)
Refraction and how to refract, including sections on optics, retinoscopy, the fitting of spectacles and eyeglasses, etc. . . . 5th rev. ed., two hundred and fifty-one illustrations, thirteen of which are colored. Philadlephia: P. Blakiston's Son & Co., 1910. 324p. DLC; DNLM; PPC; PPJ
00-6169

THORINGTON, James (*b.* 1858)
Retinoscopy (or shadow test) in the determination of refraction at one meter distance, with the plane mirror . . . 6th ed. rev. and enl. Sixty-one illustrations, ten of which are colored. Philadelphia: P. Blakiston's Son & Co., 1910. 71p. illus. (partly col.). DLC; ICJ; NNNAM; PPC
00-6170

THORNBURGH, Robert M.
The suprapubic operation for the radical cure of varicocele, with a report of 18 cases. New York: William Wood & Co., 1903. 8p. DNLM **00-6171**

THORNDIKE, Augustus (*b.* 1863)
A study of the amount of correction of deformity in Pott's disease obtained with plaster jackets. Boston, 1904. 7p. DNLM **00-6172**

THORNDIKE, Augustus (*b.* 1863)
Sacro-iliac disease in a young child. Boston, 1905. 4p. DNLM
00-6173

THORNDIKE, Augustus (*b.* 1863)
A modification of the back brace for Pott's disease. Boston, 1906. 4p. DNLM **00-6174**

THORNDIKE, Augustus (*b.* 1863)
A manual of orthopedic surgery. Philadelphia: P. Blakiston's Son & Co., 1907. 401p. DLC; DNLM; NNNAM; PPC
00-6175

THORNDIKE, Paul (*b.* 1863)
Clinical reports of cases of infection due to the bacillus aërogenes capsulatus of Welch. Boston, 1900. 24p. DNLM
00-6176

THORNDIKE, Paul (*b.* 1863) and John H. CUNNINGHAM
Hypernephroma. Boston, 1903. 14p. 6 plates. DNLM
00-6177

THORNDIKE, Paul (*b.* 1863)
When and how shall we operate for obstructing hypertrophy of the prostate gland? New York, 1904. 8p. DNLM
00-6178

THORNDIKE, Paul (*b.* 1863)
Notes on operations for renal and ureteral stone. Boston, 1905. 5p. 1 plate. DNLM **00-6179**

THORNDIKE, Paul (*b.* 1863)
Surgical treatment of nephritis; a résumé. Boston, 1905. 10p. DNLM **00-6180**

THORNDIKE, Paul (*b.* 1863) and L. R. G. CRANDON
Results of surgical treatment of movable kidney at the Boston City Hospital. Boston, 1905. 9p. DNLM
00-6181

THORNE, William Bezly (*d.* 1917)
The Schott methods of the treatment of chronic diseases of the heart, with an account of the Nauheim baths, and of the therapeutic exercises. 4th ed. Philadelphia: P. Blakiston's Son & Co., 1902. 138p. 4 plates, 8 diags. DNLM; ICJ; MBM; PPC
00-6182

THORNE, William Bezly (*d.* 1917)
The Schott methods of the treatment of chronic diseases of the heart, with an account of the Nauheim baths, and of the therapeutic exercises. 5th ed. Philadelphia: P. Blakiston's Son & Co., 1906. 140p. 9 plates. DNLM; ICJ; PPC; PU
00-6183

THORNTON, Augustus W.
Hysterical women; their trials, tears, tricks and tantrums. . . . Chicago: Donohue & Henneberry, 1901? 195p. incl. front. DLC; ICJ **00-6184**

THORNTON, Edward Quin (*b.* 1866)
The medical news pocket formulary revised for 1900. . . . Philadelphia and New York: Lea Bros. & Co., 1900. 272p. DLC; NNNAM; PPC; PU **00-6185**

THORNTON, Edward Quin (*b.* 1866)
Dose-book and manual of prescription-writing, with a list of the official drugs and preparations, and many of the newer remedies with their doses . . . 2nd ed., rev. and enl. Philadelphia and London: W. B. Saunders & Co., 1901. 362p. DLC; DNLM; NNNAM; PPC **00-6186**

THORNTON, Edward Quin (*b.* 1866)
The medical news pocket formulary for 1901 . . . 3rd ed., rev. and enl. Philadelphia and New York: Lea Bros. & Co., 1901. 272p. DLC; NNNAM; PPC; PU **00-6187**

THORNTON, Edward Quin (*b.* 1866)
The medical news pocket formulary for 1902. . . . 4th ed., rev. Philadelphia and New York: Lea Bros. & Co., 1902. 287p. DLC; NNNAM; PPC; PU **00-6188**

THORNTON, Edward Quin (*b.* 1866)
The medical news pocket formulary. . . . New (5th) ed., rev. Philadelphia and New York: Lea Bros. & Co., [1903]. 287p. DLC; MBM; NNNAM; PPC **00-6189**

THORNTON, Edward Quin (*b.* 1866)
The medical news pocket formulary. . . . New (6th) ed., rev. Philadelphia and New York: Lea Bros. & Co., [1904]. 287p. DLC; ICJ; PPC; PU **00-6190**

THORNTON, Edward Quin (*b.* 1866)
Dose-book and manual of prescription-writing, with a list of the official drugs and preparations, and many of the newer remedies with their doses . . . 3rd ed., rev. and enl. and adapted to the 8th revision (1905) of the United States pharmacopoeia. Philadelphia and London: W. B. Saunders & Co., 1905. 392p. plates. DLC; DNLM; NNNAM; PU **00-6191**

THORNTON, Edward Quin (*b.* 1866)
A pocket formulary. . . . New (7th) ed., rev. Philadelphia and New York: Lea Bros. & Co., [1906]. 287p. DLC; NNNAM; PPC; PU **00-6192**

THORNTON, Edward Quin (*b.* 1866)
A pocket formulary. . . . New (8th) ed. rev. Philadelphia and New York: Lea Bros. & Co., [1907]. 287p. DLC; NNNAM; PPC; PU **00-6193**

THORNTON, Edward Quin (*b.* 1866)
A pocket formulary. . . . 9th ed., rev. Philadelphia and New York: Lea & Febiger, [1909]. 287p. DLC; ICJ; NNNAM; PU **00-6194**

THORNTON, Edward Quin (*b.* 1866)
Dose-book and manual of prescription-writing, with a list of the official drugs and preparations, and many of the newer remedies with their doses . . . 4th ed., rev. and enl. and adapted to the eighth revision (1905) of the United States pharmacopoeia. Philadelphia and London: W. B. Saunders & Co., 1909. 410p. plates. DLC; DNLM; NNNAM; PPC **00-6195**

THORNTON, Edward Quin (*b.* 1866)
A manual of materia medica for medical students. . . . Philadelphia and New York: Lea & Febiger, 1910. 525p. DLC; ICJ; PPC; PPHa **00-6196**

THORNTON, G[ustavus] B. (*b.* 1835)
Annual address of the president of the Association of Medical Officers of the Army and Navy of the Confederacy. Memphis, 1910. 6p. DNLM; NN **00-6197**

THORPE, Burton L[ee] (*b.* 1871)
John Roach Spooner, discoverer of the use of arsenic for pulp devitalization and early experimenter in porcelain. Philadelphia: Dental Brief, 1906. 3p. DNLM **00-6198**

THORPE, Burton L[ee] (*b.* 1871)
Biographies of the founders, prominent early members and ex-presidents of the Missouri State Dental Association. . . . St. Louis, Mo.: E. E. Carreras, 1909. 142p. illus., ports. DNLM; ICJ; PU **00-6199**

THORPE, Burton L[ee] (*b.* 1871)
Biographies of pioneer American dentists and their successors. Fort Wayne, Ind.: National Art Publishing Co., 1910. 681p. DNLM; ICJ **00-6200**

THORPE, Eliza Jane Ellery
Speech defects: their causes and correction. . . . [Philadelphia: American Printing House], 1900 [*c.* 1890]. 24p. DLC; PLF; PP; PPAmP [*vel subseq.*] **00-6201**

THORPE, Eliza Jane Ellery
Speech hesitation. . . . New York: E. S. Werner Publishing & Supply Co., 1900. 75p. DLC; NN **00-6202**

THORPE, Francis N[ewton] (1857-1926)
A remarkable American: Dr. William Pepper. New York, 1901. 3p. port. CtY-M; DNLM **00-6203**

THORPE, Francis N[ewton] (1857-1926)
William Pepper, M.D., L.L.D., 1843-1898. Philadelphia & London: J. B. Lippincott Co., 1904. 555p. port., 10 plates. DNLM; NN; PPC; PU **00-6204**

THRESH, John C[lough] (1850-1932)
Water and water supplies. 2nd ed. Philadelphia: P. Blakiston's Son & Co., 1900. 438p. DNLM; PP; PPC; PPF **00-6205**

THRESH, John C[lough] (1850-1932)
Water and water supplies. 3rd ed. Philadelphia: P. Blakiston's Son & Co., 1901. 527p. DNLM; KU; PPF; PPL **00-6206**

THRESH, John C[lough] (1850-1932)
The examination of waters and water supplies. Philadelphia: P. Blakiston's Son & Co., 1904. 460p. 19 plates. DNLM; NN; PU; PPL **00-6207**

THRESH, John C[lough] (1850-1932)
Preservatives in food and food examination, by John C. Thresh . . . and Arthur E. Porter. . . . Philadelphia: P. Blakiston's Son & Co., 1906. 484p. incl. illus., 8 plates. ICJ; MB; NN; PU **00-6208**

TIFFANY, Flavel B[enjamin] (1846-1918)
Anomalies of refraction and of the muscles of the eye. . . . Author's 4th ed. Kansas City, Mo.: Hudson-Kimberly Publishing Co., 1900. 307p. col. plates. DLC; ICJ; NNNAM; PPC **00-6209**

TIFFANY, Flavel B[enjamin] (1846-1918)
Anomalies and diseases of the eye. . . . Author's ed. Kansas City, Mo.: Hudson-Kimberly Publishing Co., 1902. 619p. col. plates. DLC; ICJ; KU; NNNAM **00-6210**

TIFFANY, Flavel B[enjamin] (1846-1918)
Prosthetic surgery, with report of a case, illustrative. Kansas City, 1905. 15p. DNLM **00-6211**

TIFFANY, Flavel B[enjamin] (1846-1918)
Vacation memoirs, 1907. [Kansas City, Mo., 1907.] 23p. DNLM **00-6212**

TIFFANY, Flavel B[enjamin] (1846-1918)
Memoir. Kansas City, 1910. 50p. plate, port. DLC; ICJ; KU **00-6213**

TIGERSTEDT, Robert A[dolf] A[rmand] (1853-1923)
A text-book of human physiology . . . transl. from the 3rd German ed. and edited by John R. Murlin . . . with an introduction to the English ed. by Professor Graham Lusk. . . . New York and London: D. Appleton & Co., 1906. 751p. incl. illus. (part col.), col. plate. DLC; ICJ; MH-M; PU **00-6214**

TILDEN, John Henry (1851-1940)
The etiology of cholera infantum, typhoid fever and appendicitis, with the hygienic and dietetic treatment as applied. . . . Denver Col.: [The Merchants Publishing Co.], 1909. 114, 135, 123p. plates. CU-M; DLC
00-6215

TILDEN, John Henry (1851-1940)
Gonorrhoea and syphilis; a drugless treatment of venereal diseases. . . . [Denver: The Smith-Brooks Press, 1910.] *vel subseq.* 136p. DLC; DNLM **00-6216**

TILDEN, John Henry (1851-1940)
Diseases of women and easy childbirth. . . . [Denver: The Smith-Brooks Press, 1910.] *vel subseq.* 196p. DLC; ICJ
00-6217

TILDEN, John Henry (1851-1940)
Iconoclastic and constructive criticisms of the practice of medicine. Denver. Col.: The Author [cop. 1910]. unp. DNLM
00-6218

TILDEN, John Henry (1851-1940)
Food; its influence as a factor in disease and health. . . . 2nd ed., rev. Denver, Col.: J. H. Tilden, [1910. *vel subseq.*] 262p. ICJ **00-6219**

TILESTON, Wilder (*b.* 1875)
The blood in measles. Chicago, 1904. 36p. DNLM
00-6220

TILESTON, Wilder (*b.* 1875)
The blood in scarlet fever, by Wilder Tileston and Edwin A. Locke. Chicago, 1905. 36p. DNLM **00-6221**

TILESTON, Wilder (*b.* 1875)
Peptic ulcer of the oesophagus. Philadelphia, 1906. 27p. DNLM **00-6222**

TILESTON, Wilder (*b.* 1875)
The occurrence of occult hemorrhages in typhoid fever. Boston, 1906. 6p. DNLM **00-6223**

TILLINGHAST, Joseph Reynolds, Jr.
How can I cure my catarrh? . . . New York: The Contemporary Publishing Co., [1902]. 150p. DLC; NN
00-6224

TILLMANNS, R[obert] Hermann (1844-1927)
A text-book of surgery . . . transl. from the 7th German ed. by Benjamin T. Tilton . . . and John Rogers . . . ed. by Lewis A. Stimson. . . . New York: D. Appleton & Co., 1901-1904. 3 v. NNNAM; NNU-M; OCIM; PPC **00-6225**

TILLOTSON, H. John (*b.* 1857)
Diseases of men; cause and cure. . . . Rev. and enl. ed. . . . Chicago, Ill. [1905]. 128p. DLC; ICJ
00-6226

TINKER, Martin B[uel] (*b.* 1869)
The value of tuberculin in surgical diagnosis. [Baltimore, 1903.] 4p. MB **00-6227**

TINKER, Martin B[uel] (*b.* 1869)
A sketch of the lives of a German and an American master of surgery. [1906.] 6p. NN [Bernard R. C. von Langenbeck and Samuel D. Gross] **00-6228**

TIRARD, Nestor [Isidore Charles] (*b.* 1853)
A textbook of medical treatment, diseases and symptoms. Adapted to the United States Pharmacopoeia by E. Quin Thornton. Philadelphia & New York: Lea Bros. & Co., 1900. 632p. DNLM; NNNAM; PPC; PU **00-6229**

TODD, C[harles] H. (*b.* 1838)
Anesthetics. [Louisville], 1903. 1 l. DNLM
00-6230

TODD, James Campbell (1874-1928)
A manual of clinical diagnosis. . . . Philadelphia and London: W. B. Saunders & Co., 1908. 319p. col. plates. DLC; DNLM; NNNAM; PPC **00-6231**

TODD, John B. (*b.* 1855)
Alkaline beverages in the treatment of pneumonia. New York, 1905. 14p. DNLM **00-6232**

TODD, John B. (*b.* 1855)
Saline beverages in typhoid fever and their effects on heat dissipation. New York, 1906. 14p. DNLM
00-6233

TOLEDO UNIVERSITY, TOLEDO, OHIO. COLLEGE OF MEDICINE. COLLEGE OF PHARMACY
Annual announcements for the year 1909-10. Toledo, 1909. DNLM **00-6234**

TOMES, Charles Sissmore (1846-1928)
A manual of dental anatomy, human and comparative . . . 6th ed. Philadelphia: P. Blakiston's Son & Co., 1904. 636p. illus., tables. DNLM; ICJ; MH-M; NNNAM
00-6235

TOMES, John (1815-1895)
A system of dental surgery . . . 5th ed. Philadelphia: P. Blakiston's Son & Co., 1906. 780p. DNLM; MdU-D; PPC; PU
00-6236

TOMLINSON, H[arry] Ashton (1855-1913)
The puerperal insanities. Utica, N.Y., 1901. 10p. DLC
00-6237

TOMLINSON, H[arry] Ashton (1855-1913)
The history of typhoid fever in the Hospital at St. Peter during the past ten years. St. Paul, 1902. 6p. 1 chart. DNLM
00-6238

TOMLINSON, H[arry] Ashton (1855-1913)
The significance of parenchymatous change in the kidneys. New York, 1904. 24p. DNLM **00-6239**

TOMLINSON, H[arry] Ashton (1855-1913)
The general conditions associated with insanity; their connotations and certain deductions as to their significance. Chicago, 1906. 24p. DNLM **00-6240**

TOMLINSON, H[arry] Ashton (1855-1913)
Medicine, the physician and the public. St. Paul, Minn., 1907. 15p. DNLM **00-6241**

TOMPKINS, E[dmund] P[endleton] (1868-1952)
Pneumonia; one method of treatment. New York: A. R. Elliott Co., 1908. 5p. DNLM **00-6242**

TOOLEY, Sarah A.
The life of Florence Nightingale. New York: The Macmillan Co., 1905. 344p. ICU; MA; MH; NN **00-6243**

TOPLIFF, Cyrus L.
Immunity from consumption. Cause and treatment of consumption. Massage treatment for consumption. New York, 1904. 24p. DNLM; NNNAM **00-6244**

TOUSEY, Sinclair (*b.* 1864)
Radio-therapy in certain rectal diseases. [New York? 1903?] 2 l. NN **00-6245**

TOUSEY, Sinclair (*b.* 1864)
Hemorrhoids. . . . [New York? 1903?] 1 l. DNLM **00-6246**

TOUSEY, Sinclair (*b.* 1864)
An improvement in radiography; a print made by direct exposure and developed in half a minute without a dark room. New York, 1903. 4p. DNLM **00-6247**

TOUSEY, Sinclair (*b.* 1864)
The relation of the X-ray and radioactive solutions to examination of the stomach. New York, 1904. 11p. DNLM **00-6248**

TOUSEY, Sinclair (*b.* 1864)
Remarks on the results of X-ray treatment in several cases of carcinoma of the uterus. New York: A. R. Elliott, 1905. 10p. DNLM **00-6249**

TOUSEY, Sinclair (*b.* 1864)
The X-ray, ultraviolet ray, and high-frequency currents in diagnosis and therapy. New York, 1907. 14p. DNLM **00-6250**

TOUSEY, Sinclair (*b.* 1864)
The radiographic topography of the frontal sinus and other pneumatic sinuses of the face. New York, 1908. 12p. DNLM **00-6251**

TOUSEY, Sinclair (*b.* 1864)
The X-ray in dentistry. . . . [New York?], 1909. 12p. DLC **00-6252**

TOUSEY, Sinclair (*b.* 1864)
Demonstration of a simplified technique for X-ray localization of bullets in the thicker portions of the body. New York, 1910. 6p. DNLM **00-6253**

TOUSEY, Sinclair (*b.* 1864)
Medical electricity and Röntgen rays, with chapters on phototherapy and radium. Philadelphia & London: W. B. Saunders & Co., 1910. 1116p., 16 pl. DLC; DNLM; ICJ; PPC **00-6254**

TOUSEY, Sinclair (*b.* 1864)
Blotting-paper mold for obtaining crayons of carbonic-acid ice. Chicago: Amer. Medical Assoc., 1910. 3p. NN **00-6255**

TOWLE, Harvey P[arker] (*b.* 1867)
A review of the literature of the therapeutic use of the X-rays. Boston: Damrell & Upham, 1901. 18p. DNLM **00-6256**

TOWLE, Harvey P[arker] (*b.* 1867)
Vaccination eruptions. Boston, 1902. 9p. DNLM **00-6257**

TOWLE, Harvey P[arker] (*b.* 1867)
Pityriasis rosea. [New York, 1904.] 7p. DNLM **00-6258**

TOWLE, Harvey P[arker] (*b.* 1867)
The brown tail moth eruption. Boston, 1905. 6p. DNLM **00-6259**

TOWLE, Harvey P[arker] (*b.* 1867)
Gangraena cutis hysteria. New York, 1907. 27p. 1 plate. DNLM **00-6260**

TOWLES, William Beverley (1847-1893)
Descriptive anatomy. . . . Revised and enlarged by W. G. Christian. . . . [Charlottesville, Va.: Anderson Bros., 1901, *c.* 1898]. 540p. DLC; ICJ; PP **00-6261**

TOWN, Clara Harrison (*b.* 1874)
The train of thought; an experimental study of the insane. Philadelphia: Psychol. Clinic Press, 1909. 53p. DNLM; PPC **00-6262**

TOWN, Clara Harrison (*b.* 1874)
Two experimental studies of the insane. 1.—The train of thought. 2.—Some physiological conditions accompanying states of depression. . . . Philadelphia, Pa.: The Psychological Clinic Press, 1909. 84p. diags., tables, ICJ; PU **00-6263**

TOWNE, William Elmer (*b.* 1874)
Health and wealth from within; how to apply New thought to the attainment of health, success, and the solving of every-day problems. . . . Holyoke, Mass.: E. Towne, [1909]. 157p. front. (port.). DLC; MH **00-6264**

TOWNE, William Elmer (*b.* 1874)
The way to perfect healing; the power of the Word in ancient and modern spiritual healing. How to apply this power in self-healing. How to train the mind to realize health. . . . Holyoke, Mass.: W. E. Towne, [1910]. 80p. DLC; MH **00-6265**

TOWNSEND, Charles W[endell] (*b.* 1859)
Home modification of milk. Boston, 1900. 10p. DNLM **00-6266**

TOWNSEND, Charles W[endell] (*b.* 1859)
Cream for the home modification of milk. Boston, 1903. 8p. DNLM **00-6267**

TOWNSEND, Charles W[endell] (*b.* 1859)
An unusual case of tuberculosis in an infant. New York: E. B. Treat & Co., 1906. 6p. DNLM **00-6268**

TOWNSEND, Charles W[endell] (*b.* 1859)
Simplicity in infant feeding. Chicago, 1907. 7p. DNLM **00-6269**

TOWNSEND, Charles W[endell] (*b.* 1859)
The use of fat-free milk in infant feeding. Boston: D. C. Heath & Co., 1908. 8p. DNLM **00-6270**

TOWNSEND, David (*b.* 1873)
Day sanatorium for consumptives, Parker Hill, Boston. Boston, 1906. 9p. DNLM **00-6271**

TOWNSEND, David (*b.* 1873)
Mattapan day camp for consumptives, Boston, Mass. By D. Townsend . . . F. P. McCarthy and R. H. Houghton. Bsoton: D. C. Heath & Co., 1908. 19p. illus. NN **00-6272**

TOWNSEND, Terry M. (*b.* **1876)**
Prostatic gonococcal auto-reinfections of the urethra. New York: William Wood & Co., 1902. 12p. DNLM
00-6273

TOWNSEND, Terry M. (*b.* **1876)**
Emergency dilation of urethral stricture. [New York, 1902.] unp. DNLM; PPHa **00-6274**

TOWNSEND, Terry M. (*b.* **1876)**
Massage of prostate and stripping the seminal vesicles. [New York, 1903.] unp. PPHa **00-6275**

TRACY, Edward A[loysius] (*b.* **1863)**
A new spinal jacket. Boston, 1900. 4p. DNLM
00-6276

TRACY, Edward A[loysius] (*b.* **1863)**
A neglected case of Pott's disease of the spine under treatment with a new spinal brace. New York, 1900. 4p. DNLM
00-6277

TRACY, Edward A[loysius] (*b.* **1863)**
Tubercular disease of the knee-joint and hip-joint in children. Diagnosis and treatment. Chicago, 1901. 10p. DNLM
00-6278

TRACY, Edward A[loysius] (*b.* **1863)**
Treatment of broken collar bone. Chicago, 1902. 3 l. DNLM
00-6279

TRACY, Edward A[loysius] (*b.* **1863)**
The cure of tuberculosis of the joints, with report of cases. [New York], 1906. 10p. DNLM **00-6280**

TRACY, Edward A[loysius] (*b.* **1863)**
A note of surgical splinting. New York, 1907. 7p. DNLM
00-6281

TRACY, Martha (1876-1942)
Some micro-chemical reactions and their value in the study of cancer cells. Pt. I. Iron. [Boston], 1905. 11p. 2 plates. DNLM **00-6282**

TRACY, Samuel G[ately] (*b.* **1867)**
Radium in medicine. New York, 1903. 11p. DNLM
00-6283

TRACY, Samuel G[ately] (*b.* **1867)**
High frequency, high potential currents, and X radiations in the treatment of epilepsy. New York: A. R. Elliott, 1905. 11p. DNLM **00-6284**

TRACY, Samuel G[ately] (*b.* **1867)**
Radium, thorium and radioactivity. Illus. Philadelphia, 1905. 34p. MB **00-6285**

TRACY, Stephen E.
A study of the urinary analysis of operative cases and the treatment of complications arising from kidney insufficiency. [New York], 1907. 8p. DNLM **00-6286**

TRACY, Stephen E.
Report of a case operated on for advanced ectopic gestation associated with fibromyomata. New York, 1908. 4p. DNLM
00-6287

TRAINED nurses' directory; composed of names carefully selected by prominent physicians and surgeons . . . from their private lists. Compiled and edited by M. Louise Longway. . . . Buffalo and New York: The Matthews-Northrup Works, [1900–. Irregular] DLC **00-6288**

TRENTON, N.J. FREE PUBLIC LIBRARY
Catalogue of the medical collection in the Public Library. Trenton Medical Library Association. [Trenton], 1904. 54p. DLC **00-6289**

TREVES, Frederick (1853-1923)
Surgical applied anatomy. . . . New edition revised by the author, with the assistance of Arthur Keith. . . . Philadelphia: Lea Bros. & Co., [1901]. 571p., illus. ICJ; NNC; PPC; PPJ
00-6290

TREVES, Frederick (1853-1923)
Intestinal obstruction; its varieties with their pathology, diagnosis, and treatment. New and revised ed. New York: William Wood & Co., 1901. 565p. CtY-M; DNLM; NNNAM; PU ["The first edition of this work was published in 1884. It was in substance the essay to which the Jacksonian prize had been awarded by the Royal College of Surgeons of England."—Pref.] **00-6291**

TREVES, Frederick (1853-1923)
A manual of operative surgery. New ed., revised by the author and Jonathan Hutchinson, Jr. Philadelphia: Lea Bros. & Co., 1903. 2 v. 8 plates. DNLM; NNNAM; PPC; PU **00-6292**

TREVES, Frederick (1853-1923)
The student's handbook of surgical operations. New edition, rev. by the author and Jonathan Hutchinson. Chicago: W. T. Keener & Co., 1905. 486p. illus. CtY-M; ICRM; ICJ; NNNAM [Abridged from the author's "Manual of operative surgery."]
00-6293

TREVES, Frederick (1853-1923)
German-English dictionary of terms used in medicine and the allied sciences; ed. and completed by Bertram Abrahams. Philadelphia: P. Blakiston's Son & Co., 1905. 597p. DLC; ICJ; NN; PU **00-6294**

TREVES, Frederick (1853-1923)
Surgical applied anatomy. 5th ed., rev. by Arthur Keith. Philadelphia: Lea & Febiger, 1907. 640p. illus. (part col.) DLC; ICJ; KU; PPC **00-6295**

TREVES, Frederick (1853-1923)
Manual of operative surgery, by . . . and J. Hutchinson. New ed. Philadelphia: Lea & Febiger, 1908. 824p. CtY-M; DLC; PPC; PU **00-6296**

TREVES, Frederick (1853-1923)
A manual of operative surgery, by Sir Frederick Treves . . . and Jonathan Hutchinson . . . 3rd ed. with sixteen new coloured plates and many new illus. . . . In two volumes. . . . Philadelphia & New York: Lea & Febiger, 1910. 2 v. col. plates. DLC; ICJ; MH-M; PPC **00-6297**

TROPICAL medicine with special reference to the West Indies, Central America, Hawaii, and the Philippines, including a general consideration of tropical hygiene [by Thomas W. Jackson] . . . . One hundred and six illustrations. Philadelphia: P. Blakiston's Son & Co., 1907. 536p. DLC; ICJ; MBM; NNNAM [Some copies include Thomas W(right) Jackson's name as author on title page; others include name only at end of author's preface] **00-6298**

TRUAX, CHARLES, CO. (CHICAGO)
The mechanics of surgery, comprising detailed descriptions, illustrations, and lists of the instruments, appliances and furniture necessary in modern surgical art. Chicago, 1900 [*c.* 1899]. 1024p. ICJ; MBM; NNNAM; PU **00-6299**

TRUAX, Charles H[enry] (*b.* 1852)
Some classical allusions to medicine and surgery. [New York, 1900?] 12p. NN **00-6300**

TRUAX, GREENE & CO. (CHICAGO)
Price list of surgical instruments and hospital supplies. 7th ed. Chicago, [*c.* 1900]. 451p. PPC **00-6301**

TRUAX, GREENE & CO. (CHICAGO)
The physicians' manual. A handy reference book compiled expressly for our patrons from the most recent authentic sources. Containing new and popular remedies; dose list of official preparations; Latin terms used in prescriptions; poisons and antidotes; important incompatibles; therapeutic terms; medical water springs; urinary analysis; static machine and X-ray work; metric system; reference tables; etc., etc. Chicago: Truax, Greene & Co., 1901. 388p. ICJ; ICU **00-6302**

TRUAX, GREENE & CO. (CHICAGO)
. . . Catalogue of physicians' and hospital supplies. Truax, Greene & Co. (incorporated) . . . [6th ed.] Chicago, [1904]. 894p. DLC **00-6303**

TRUAX, GREENE & CO. (CHICAGO)
Catalogue of physicians' and hospital supplies. . . . Chicago: Truax, 1910. 640p. PPC **00-6304**

TRUDEAU, Edward L[ivingston] (1848-1915)
The treatment of experimental tuberculosis by Koch's tuberculin, Hunter's modification, and other products of the tubercle bacillus. 1900 [*c.* 1892]. 21p. 6 col. plates. NN **00-6305**

TRUDEAU, Edward L[ivingston] (1848-1915)
Experimental studies on the preparation and effects of antitoxins for tuberculosis. 1900 [*c.* 1899]. 36p. DLC **00-6306**

TRUDEAU, Edward L[ivingston] (1848-1915)
The sanitarium treatment of incipient pulmonary tuberculosis, and its results. New York, 1900. 17p. DNLM; MH **00-6307**

TRUDEAU, Edward L[ivingston] (1848-1915)
Recent research work on the chemistry of the tuberculosis bacillus. 1901. 3p. DLC **00-6308**

TRUDEAU, Edward L[ivingston] (1848-1915)
The history and work of the Saranac Laboratory for the Study of Tuberculosis. Baltimore, 1901. 12p. 1 plate. DNLM; MH **00-6309**

TRUDEAU, Edward L[ivingston] (1848-1915)
History of the tuberculosis work at Saranac Lake. 1903. 12p. DLC **00-6310**

TRUDEAU, Edward L[ivingston] (1848-1915)
Artificial immunity in experimental tuberculosis. New York, 1903. 19p. DLC **00-6311**

TRUDEAU, Edward L[ivingston] (1848-1915)
Two experiments in artificial immunity against tuberculosis. 1905. 10p. DLC **00-6312**

TRUDEAU, Edward L[ivingston] (1848-1915)
Studies from the Saranac Laboratory for the Study of Tuberculosis, 1900-1904. Boston, 1905. 94p. DNLM; MBM **00-6313**

TRUDEAU, Edward L[ivingston] (1848-1915)
Tuberculosis immunization in the treatment of pulmonary tuberculosis. 1907. 16p. DLC **00-6314**

TRUDEAU, Edward L[ivingston] (1848-1915)
Animal experimentation and tuberculosis. Chicago: American Medical Assoc. Press, 1909. 15p. DNLM **00-6315**

TRUDEAU, Edward L[ivingston] (1848-1915)
Anti-bacterial or antitoxic immunization in tuberculin treatment. 1909. 7p. DLC **00-6316**

TRUDEAU, Edward L[ivingston] (1848-1915)
The President's address. . . . The value of optimism in medicine. Read at Congress of American Physicians and Surgeons, May 4th, 1910. 7p. NNC **00-6317**

TRUDEAU, N.Y. SANATORIUM
[Circular of information, stating objects, etc., of the institution] [1904?] 2 l. DNLM **00-6318**

TSCHERNING, Marius Hans Erik (1854-1939)
Physiologic optics; dioptrics of the eye, functions of the retina, ocular movements and binocular vision . . . authorized translation from the original French ed., specially rev. and enl. by the author, by Carl Weiland. . . . With 212 illustrations. Philadelphia: The Keystone, 1900. 353p. DLC; MB; PPC; PU **00-6319**

TSCHERNING, Marius Hans Erik (1854-1939)
Physiologic optics, dioptrics of the eye, functions of the retina, ocular movements and binocular vision . . . authorized translation from the original French ed., specially rev. and enl. by the author, by C. Weiland. . . . Philadelphia: The Keystone, 1904. 358p. front. (port.) illus. DLC; ICJ; NN; PU **00-6320**

TUBERCULOSIS exhibitions; a catalogue of necessaries for their outfitting and maintenance. Providence: Educat. Exhib. Co., 1909. 24p. DNLM **00-6321**

[TUBERCULOSIS] A handbook on the prevention of tuberculosis. . . . New York: Charity Organization, 1903. 388p. MH; NN; NNNAM; PU **00-6322**

TUBERCULOSIS LEAGUE OF PITTSBURGH. DISPENSARY AID SOCIETY
Tuberculosis or consumption and how to avoid it; lessons for school children, provided by Dispensary Aid Society of Tuberculosis League of Pittsburgh. . . . [Pittsburgh: Tuberculosis League, [1910.] 47p. illus. DLC **00-6323**

TUCKER Beverley R[andolph] (1874-1945)
Epilepsy; the so-called idiopathic form. New York, 1908. 12p. DNLM **00-6324**

TUCKER, Edward Tobey (*b.* 1849)
Addresses by Edward T. Tucker, M.D., and John H. Dillingham, at the exercises held in the Friends Meeting House at Sandwich, Massachusetts, 10 mo. 10, 1907. On the 250th anniversary of the establishment of a meeting of the Society of Friends in Sandwich, the earliest meeting of that denomination in America. [New Bedford, Mass.: Printed at the office of the New Bedford Evening Standard, 1907?] 19p. incl. plate. DLC **00-6325**

TUCKER, Willis Gaylord (1849-1922)
Address delivered at the opening of the Albany College of Pharmacy, October 7, 1901. Albany, 1901. 19p. DNLM **00-6326**

TUCKER, Willis Gaylord (1849-1922)
Biographical sketch of the late Professor Maurice Perkins, M.D., of Schenectady, N.Y. Albany, 1901. 8p. 1 plate. DNLM **00-6327**

TUCKER, Willis Gaylord (1849-1922)
Food preservatives; their use and abuse. New York, 1903. 28p. DNLM **00-6328**

TUCKER, Willis Gaylord (1849-1922)
Educational democracy. Address delivered at the opening of the seventy-seventh session of the Albany Medical College, September 24, 1907. . . . [Albany, 1907.] 23p. DLC **00-6329**

TUCKER, Willis Gaylord (1849-1922)
On state licensing examination and state control in medicine. Easton, Pa., 1908. 10p. DNLM **00-6330**

TUCKER, Willis Gaylord (1849-1922)
On the character of the state board examinations and the competency of state medical examining boards. Albany, 1908. 4p. DNLM **00-6331**

TUCKER, Willis Gaylord (1849-1922)
Faraday. [Albany, 1910.] 23p. DNLM; NN **00-6332**

TUCKERMANN, L[ouis] B[ryant] (1850-1902)
Venereal disease as a factor in the moral evolution of the race. An address delivered before the Cleveland Council of Sociology, December 9, 1901. Cleveland: H. Carr, 1902. 25p. DNLM; OCIM **00-6333**

TUCKEY, C[harles] Lloyd (1855-1925)
Treatment by hypnotism and suggestion or psychotherapeutics. 4th ed. New York: G. P. Putnam's Sons, 1900. 376p. DLC; DNLM; NNNAM [Earlier editions in London (Baillière, Tindall and Cox, 1889–) under title, Psycho-Therapeutics] **00-6334**

TULEY, Henry Enos (1870-1923)
Obstetrical nursing for nurses and students; being an elaboration of the lectures in obstetrics to the pupils of the Training School for Nurses of the John N. Norton Memorial Infirmary and the City Hospital of Louisville. . . . Chicago: G. P. Engelhard & Co., 1902. 198p. front., illus., diag. DLC; ICJ; LNT-M; MH-M [Standard Monograph Series] **00-6335**

TULEY, Henry Enos (1870-1923)
. . . Pediatrics. A manual for students and practitioners. . . . Illustrated with thirty-three engravings. Philadelphia and New York: Lea Bros. & Co., [1904]. 266p. illus., diags. DLC: KU; NNNAM; PPC [The Medical Epitome Series] **00-6336**

TULEY, Henry Enos (1870-1923)
The diseases of children. . . . Baltimore: Southern Medical Publishing Co., 1909. 653p. front., illus., diags. DLC; GU; PPC; PPJ **00-6337**

TULEY, Henry Enos (1870-1923)
Obstetrical nursing, for nurses and students . . . with 73 illustrations. [2nd ed., rev. and rewritten] Louisville, Ky.: J. P. Morton & Co., 1910. 246p. front., illus. DLC; ICJ; KU; PPJ **00-6338**

TULEY, Henry Enos (1870-1923)
The diseases of children. . . . St. Louis: C. V. Mosby Co., 1910. 653p. illus., diags. DLC; ICJ; MH-M; PPC **00-6339**

TULL, Montrose Graham (*b.* 1859)
An unusually severe case of acute chorea successfully treated with apomorphine. New York: A. R. Elliott, 1905. 5p. DNLM **00-6340**

TUMORS of the cerebellum, by Charles K. Mills, M.D., Charles H. Frazier, M.D., George E. De Schweinitz, M.D., T. H. Weisenburg, M.D., Edward Lodholz, M.D. . . . New York: A. R. Elliott Publishing Co., 1905. 179p. incl. plates. DLC; MBM; NNNAM; PPC **00-6341**

TUMORS of the cerebrum, their focal diagnosis and surgical treatment; by Charles K. Mills, M.D., Charles H. Frazier, M.D., William G. Spiller, M.D., George E. De Schweinitz, M.D., Theodore H. Weisenburg, M.D. Philadelphia: E. Pennock, 1906. [293]p. illus., diags. DLC; ICJ; MH-M; PU **00-6342**

TUNIS, Joseph P[rice] (*b.* 1866)
Traumatic tetanus in a child; recovery. Philadelphia, 1902. 4p. 1 plate. DNLM **00-6343**

TUNIS, Joseph P[rice] (*b.* 1866)
The practical significance of a trace of albumin in the urine. Philadelphia, 1906. 10p. DNLM **00-6344**

TUNIS, Joseph P[rice] (*b.* 1866)
Inflammation of the sinus maxillaris, with special reference to empyema; the surgical pathology, diagnosis and treatment. St. Louis, 1910. 46p. 36 plates. DNLM; OCIM **00-6345**

TUNIS, Joseph P[rice] (*b.* 1866)
Alumni notes. [Medical Department of the University of Pennsylvania.] [Philadelphia, 1910.] 3p. DNLM **00-6346**

TURBAN, Karl (1856-1935)
The diagnosis of tuberculosis of the lung; with special reference to the early stages. Transl. by Egbert C. Morland. New York: William Wood & Co., 1906. 134p. DNLM; ICJ: NNNAM; PPC **00-6347**

TURCK, Fenton Benedict (1857-1932)
Further observation on the treatment of the abdominal viscera through the colon. Chicago, 1900. 15p. DNLM
00-6348

TURCK, Fenton Benedict (1857-1932)
Motivity of the stomach. Philadelphia, 1900. 10p. DNLM
00-6349

TURCK, Fenton Benedict (1857-1932)
The care of patients during surgical operations; with some methods of preventing shock and infection. Chicago, 1900. 30p. DNLM **00-6350**

TURCK, Fenton Benedict (1857-1932)
Necessity of a practical knowledge of dietetics, hydrotherapy and physico-mechanical therapeutics. Chicago, 1901. 14p. DNLM **00-6351**

TURCK, Fenton Benedict (1857-1932)
The gyromele in the diagnosis of stomach and intestinal diseases. Chicago, 1901. 30p. DNLM **00-6352**

TURCK, Fenton Benedict (1857-1932)
Treatment of atony of the stomach and colon. Philadelphia, 1901. 12p. DNLM **00-6353**

TURCK, Fenton Benedict (1857-1932)
The immediate and remote causes of death in operations on the stomach; treatment before, during and after operation. Chicago, [1903]. 12p. DNLM **00-6354**

TURCK, Fenton Benedict (1857-1932)
The expulsion method of obtaining stomach contents for diagnostic purposes. New York: A. R. Elliott, 1905. 12p. DNLM **00-6355**

TURCK, Fenton Benedict (1857-1932)
Ulcer of the stomach; pathogenesis and pathology. Experiments in producing artificial gastric ulcer and genuine induced peptic ulcer. Chicago, 1906. 31p. DNLM
00-6356

TURCK, Fenton Benedict (1857-1932)
Nonoperative treatment of gastric diseases. New York, 1907. 15p. DNLM **00-6357**

TURCK, Fenton Benedict (1857-1932)
The factors concerned in the healing of peptic ulcers. [n. p., 1907.] 4p. DNLM **00-6358**

TURNBULL, Charles Smith (1847-1918)
A consideration of the welfare of deaf children and the duty of the medical profession. . . . Read before the First International Congress in America on the Welfare of the Child, Washington, D.C., March 10 to 17, 1908. [Philadelphia: Printed by W. H. Pile's Sons, 1908.] 14p. DLC; DNLM; MH; NN
00-6359

TURNER, A[rthur] Logan (1865-1939)
The accessory sinuses of the nose, their surgical anatomy, and the diagnosis and treatment of their inflammatory affections. New York: Longmans, Green & Co., 1902. 211p. 40 plates. CtY-M; ICJ; NN; PU **00-6360**

TURNER, Dawson [Fryers Duckworth] (1857-1928)
A manual of practical medical electricity. 3rd ed. New York: William Wood & Co., 1902. 396p. DLC; DNLM; ICJ; NNNAM
00-6361

TURNER, Dawson [Fryers Duckworth] (1857-1928)
A manual of practical medical electricity. 4th ed. New York: William Wood & Co., 1904. 435p. DNLM; MB; NNNAM; PU
00-6362

TURNER, Dawson [Fryers Duckworth] (1857-1928)
Radium; its physics and therapeutics. . . . New York: William Wood & Co., 1910. 85p. illus., plates. DLC; ICJ; IU-M; NcU
00-6363

TURNER, John (*b.* 1876)
The physiology of the human body and hygiene. . . . For medical schools and college classes generally. Baltimore: The Sun Printing Office, 1902. 304p. DLC; MdU-D; PPC; PU
00-6364

TURNER, William Aldren (*b.* 1864)
A textbook of nervous diseases. Philadelphia: P. Blakiston's Son & Co., 1910. 607p. DNLM; MBM; MdU-D; PPC
00-6365

TUTTLE, Goerge M[arvine] (*b.* 1866)
Diseases of children. A manual for students and practitioners. . . . 2nd ed., rev. and enl. Illustrated with five plates in colors and monochrome. Philadelphia and New York: Lea Bros. & Co., [1906]. 392p. DLC; MH-M; PPC; PU
00-6366

TUTTLE, George T. (*b.* 1850)
Hallucinations and illusions. Baltimore, 1902. 11p. DNLM
00-6367

TUTTLE, George T. (*b.* 1850)
Hydrotherapeutics. Utica, 1904. 10p. DNLM
00-6368

TUTTLE, George T. (*b.* 1850)
The male nurse. Utica, 1906. 13p. DNLM
00-6369

TUTTLE, James P[ercival] (1857-1913)
A treatise on diseases of the anus, rectum, and pelvic colon . . . with eight colored plates and three hundred and thirty-eight illustrations in the text. New York: D. Appleton & Co., 1902. 961p. DLC; ICU; NcD; PPC **00-6370**

TUTTLE, James P[ercival] (1857-1913)
A treatise on diseases of the anus, rectum, and pelvic colon . . . with eight colored plates and three hundred and thirty-eight illustrations in the text. 2nd ed., rev. New York and London: D. Appleton & Co., 1905. 903p. DLC: ICJ; NNNAM; PU **00-6371**

TUTTLE, James P[ercival] (1857-1913)
Diarrhoea and its diagnositic significance. New York, 1906. 7p. DNLM **00-6372**

TUTTLE, James P[ercival] (1857-1913)
Mucous, mucomembranous, and membranous colitis. New York, 1907. 12p. DNLM **00-6373**

TUTTLE, James P[ercival] (1857-1913)
A treatise on diseases of the anus, rectum, and pelvic colon . . . with eight colored plates and three hundred and thirty-eight illustrations in the text. 2nd ed., rev. New York and London: D. Appleton & Co., 1907. 963p. DLC; MBM; NNNAM; PU **00-6374**

TUTTLE, James P[ercival] (1857-1913)
Acute flexures or angulations of the sigmoid and colon. New York, 1908. 24p. DNLM **00-6375**

TWEDDELL, Francis (*b.* 1863)
A mother's guide; a manual for the guidance of mothers and nurses. . . . New York: T. Dougherty, [1910]. 182p. DLC; MH; NIC; NN **00-6376**

TWITMYER, Edwin Burket (*b.* 1873)
. . . A study of the knee-jerk. Philadelphia: The John C. Winston Co., 1902. 36p. 1 plate. DLC; PU **00-6377**

TWOMBLY, Edward L[ambert] (*b.* 1859)
Conservative surgery of the uterine appendages with especial reference to the ovaries. Boston, 1904. 10p. DNLM **00-6378**

TYNDALE, J[ulius] Hilgard (*b.* 1843)
The skirmish line of incipient tuberculosis. Asheville, N.C., 1901. 3p. DNLM **00-6379**

TYRODE, Maurice Vejux (*b.* 1878)
Pharmacology; the action and uses of drugs. Philadelphia: P. Blakiston's Son & Co., 1908. 255p. CtY-M; DNLM; OCLloyd; PU **00-6380**

TYRODE, Maurice Vejux (*b.* 1878)
Pharmacology; action and uses of drugs . . . 2nd ed. Philadelphia: P. Blakiston's Son & Co., [1910?] 288p. DLC; MH-M; NNNAM; PPC **00-6381**

TYRRELL, Charles Alfred, ed. (*b.* 1846)
Vitality; how to acquire and conserve it. . . . Authors: Felix Oswald, M.D., Susanna W. Dodds, M.D., M. T. Holbrook, M.D., M. J. Rodermund, M.D., R. T. Trall, M.D., Paul von Boeckmann, R.S., and Charles A. Tyrrell, M.D., who has written an introduction to the book, and by whom it is compiled. . . . New York: The Health Publishing Co., [1905]. 278p. DLC; MH; NIC; NN **00-6382**

TYRRELL, Charles Alfred (*b.* 1846)
The royal road to health; or, The secret of health without drugs. . . . 45th ed., completely rev., enl. and illustrated. New York: Tyrrell's Hygienic Institute, 1907. 223p. front. (port.) illus. DLC; NN [Appeared originally as The royal road to health via, the J. B. L. cascade treatment, a treatise on hygiene. . . . New York, 1894. 166p. *vel subseq.*] **00-6383**

TYSON, James (1841-1919)
Founding of a hospital for consumptives: an address at the opening of the new wards of the Rush Hospital: May 15, 1899. With reports. [1900.] 6p. PHi **00-6384**

TYSON, James (1841-1919)
The practice of medicine. A text-book for practitioners and students with special reference to diagnosis and treatment. 2nd ed. Philadelphia: P. Blakiston's Son & Co., 1900. 1222p. 3 plates. DLC; DNLM; PPC: PU **00-6385**

TYSON, James (1841-1919)
The practice of medicine. A text-book for practitioners and students, with special reference to diagnosis and treatment. 2nd ed., thoroughly revised and in parts rewritten. Philadelphia: P. Blakiston's Son & Co., 1901. 1222p. 4 plates. DLC; MBM; NNNAM; PPC **00-6386**

TYSON, James (1841-1919)
Manual of physical diagnosis, for the use of students and physicians. . . . 4th ed., rev. and enl. . . . Philadelphia: P. Blakiston's Son & Co., 1901. 298p. col. plates. DLC; DNLM; NNNAM; PU **00-6387**

TYSON, James (1841-1919)
Memoir of the late William Pepper, M.D., LL.D. [Philadelphia], 1901. 21p. DNLM; PU **00-6388**

TYSON, James (1841-1919)
A guide to the practical examination of urine, for the use of physicians and students. . . . 10th ed. Rev. and cor. . . . Philadelphia: P. Blakiston's Son & Co., 1902. 297p. front. DLC; DNLM; MBM; PPC **00-6389**

TYSON, James (1841-1919)
The practice of medicine. A text-book for practitioners and students, with special reference to diagnosis and treatment. 3rd ed. Philadelphia: P. Blakiston's Son & Co., 1903. 1240p. 3 plates. DLC; DNLM; PPC; PPJ **00-6390**

TYSON, James (1841-1919)
Edebohls's operation of decapsulation of the kidney for the cure of chronic Bright's disease, and the indications for its performance. New York, 1903. 14p. DNLM **00-6391**

TYSON, James (1841-1919) and Charles H. FRAZIER
Report of a case of decapsulation of the kidney (Edebohls's operation) for the chronic parenchymatous nephritis. Philadelphia, 1903. 11p. DNLM **00-6392**

TYSON, James (1841-1919)
A treatise on Bright's disease and diabetes, with special reference to pathology and therapeutics 2nd ed., including a section on the ocular changes in Bright's disease and in diabetes by George E. de Schweinitz. Philadelphia: P. Blakiston's Son & Co., 1904. 381p. 7 plates. DNLM; NNNAM; PPC; PPJ **00-6393**

TYSON, James (1841-1919)
Hospital organization. St. Paul, 1904. 24p. DNLM **00-6394**

TYSON, James (1841-1919) and Edward MARTIN, *et al.*
Diffuse dilatation of the oesophagus due to cardiospasm. New York, 1904. 22p. DNLM **00-6395**

TYSON, James (1841-1919)
The practice of medicine. A text-book for practitioners and students, with special reference to diagnosis and treatment. 4th ed., revised and enlarged. Philadelphia: P. Blakiston's Son & Co., 1906. 1305p. 3 plates. DLC; DNLM; IU-M; PPC **00-6396**

TYSON, James (1841-1919)
Address of the president. Philadelphia, 1908. 5p. DNLM; PPC **00-6397**

TYSON, James (1841-1919)
Annual address of the president. Philadelphia, 1908. 5p. DNLM; PPC **00-6398**

TYSON, James (1841-1919) and Ralph PEMBERTON
Two cases of streptococcus infection which gave a typical Widal reaction. Philadelphia, 1908. 6p. DNLM **00-6399**

TYSON, James (1841-1919)
The practice of medicine. A text-book for practitioners and students, with special reference to diagnosis and treatment. 5th ed. Philadelphia: P. Blakiston's Son & Co., 1909. 1438p. 5 plates. DLC; DNLM; PPC; PU **00-6400**

UHLEIN, Stephen P.
Yellow fever and its treatment. New and successful plan. . . . Palatka, Fla.: Printed by the News Publishing Co., [1900?] 16p. DLC **00-6401**

ULTZMANN, Robert (1842-1889)
The neuroses of the genito-urinary system in the male with sterility and impotence. . . . Translated by Gardner W. Allen. Philadelphia: F. A. Davis, 1900. 167p. CtY-M; ICU; NNNAM; PU **00-6402**

ULTZMANN, Robert (1842-1889)
The neuroses of the genito-urinary system in the male with sterility and impotence. 2nd ed., revised, with notes and a supplementary article on nervous impotence by the translator, Gardner W. Allen. Philadelphia: F. A. Davis, 1902. 198p. DNLM; DLC; PPC; PPJ **00-6403**

UNDERHILL, Andrew F[indlay] (*b.* 1859)
Valid objections to so-called Christian Science. New York: E. S. Gorham, 1902. 49p. DLC; NN **00-6404**

UNDERHILL, Andrew F[indlay] (*b.* 1859)
Valid objections to so-called Christian Science. Yonkers, N.Y.: The Arlington Chemical Co., [1902]. 46p. MB; MH; NN **00-6405**

UNDERHILL, Andrew F[indlay] (*b.* 1859)
Valid objections to so-called Christian Science. 3rd ed. New York: Baker & Taylor, 1902. 62p. NN **00-6406**

UNDERHILL, Frank P[ell] (1877-1932)
Certain aspects of experimental diabetes. [New York, 1906.] 18p. DNLM **00-6407**

UNDERHILL, Frank P[ell] (1877-1932)
A consideration of some chemical transformations of proteins and their possible bearing on problems in pathology. . . . [Chicago: American Medical Association, 1910.] 26p. NN **00-6408**

UNDERWOOD, Arthur Swayne (1854-1916) and Douglas GABELL
Aids to dental surgery. 2nd ed. New York: William Wood & Co., 1907. 126p. DNLM; MdU-D; NNNAM; PU **00-6409**

UNDERWOOD, Arthur Swayne (1854-1916)
Aids to dental surgery. . . . New York: G. Putnam's Sons, 1909? 102p. DLC; NN **00-6410**

UNDERWOOD, Eugene C.
The treatment of secondary anaemia. Portland, Me., 1900. 4p. DNLM **00-6411**

U.S. COMMISSION ON THE BUBONIC PLAGUE IN SAN FRANCISCO
. . . Report of the Commission appointed by the Secretary of the Treasury for the investigation of plague in San Francisco, under instructions from the Surgeon-General, Marine Hospital Service. Washington: Government Printing Office, 1901. 50p. DLC; DNLM **00-6412**

UNITED STATES PHARMACOPOEIAL CONVENTION
Abstract of the proceedings of the National Convention of 1900 for Revising the United States Pharmacopoeia, May 2-4, 1900. Philadelphia: J. B. Lippincott Co., 1900. 54p. DLC; DNLM; PPC; PU **00-6413**

UPSHUR, John N[ottingham] (1848-1924)
The menopause. New York: A. R. Elliott Pub. Co., 1905. 12p. DNLM **00-6414**

UPSHUR, John N[ottingham] (1848-1924)
Medical reminiscences of Richmond during the past forty years. [Richmond, Va., 1906?] 24p. DLC; ViRA **00-6415**

UPSON, Henry Swift (*b.* 1859)
Hydrophobia, with report of three cases. Cleveland, 1901. 6p. DNLM **00-6416**

UPSON, Henry Swift (*b.* 1859)
Insomnia and nerve strain. New York & London: G. P. Putnam's Sons, 1908. 142p. 4 plates. DLC; DNLM; ICJ; NNNAM **00-6417**

VAIL, William Hooker (*b.* 1867)
Neurasthenia and insomnia. Philadelphia, 1901. 2 l. DNLM; PPHa **00-6418**

VAIL, William Hooker (*b.* 1867)
Clinical experience with hydroleine. [New York, 1902?] 4 l. DNLM **00-6419**

VAIL, William Hooker (*b.* 1867)
Uric acid solvent in gout. [Philadelphia, 1902?] 4p. PPHa **00-6420**

VAIL, William Penn, ed.
Syllabus on pathology. [Philadelphia?]: 1905. unp. DLC ["A syllabus on pathology as given by Dr. Allen J. Smith at the University of Pennsylvania."—Pref.] **00-6421**

VALE, Frank P[almer] (*b.* 1871)
Concerning shock. With a contribution to its pathology. New York: William Wood & Co., 1904. 24p. DNLM **00-6422**

VALE, Frank P[almer] (*b.* 1871)
The early diagnosis of Pott's disease. New York, 1904. 13p. DNLM **00-6423**

VALE, Frank P[almer] (*b.* 1871)
A brief note on the X-ray treatment of glandular tuberculosis. [New York: Lea Bros. & Co., 1904.] 7p. DNLM **00-6424**

VALE, Frank P[almer] (*b.* 1871)
Clinical and experimental experience with colloidal silver and virulent streptococcus. Philadelphia, 1906. 10p. DNLM **00-6425**

VALE, Frank P[almer] (*b.* 1871)
Has surgical treatment lessened the mortality from appendicitis. Providence. Snow & Farnham Co., 1908. 165p. DLC; DNLM; NNNAM; PPC **00-6426**

VALENTINE, Ferdinand C[arl] (1851-1910)
The irrigation treatment of gonorrhoea; its local complications and sequelae . . . illustrated by fifty-seven engravings. New York: William Wood & Co., 1900. 221p. DLC; DNLM; ICJ; NNNAM **00-6427**

VALENTINE, Ferdinand C[arl] (1851-1910)
Can the state suppress genito-urinary diseases? Chicago, 1900. 8p. DNLM **00-6428**

VALENTINE, Ferdinand C[arl] (1851-1910)
Gonococcal auto-reinfections of the urethra. Danbury, 1901. 16p. DNLM **00-6429**

VALENTINE, Ferdinand C[arl] (1851-1910)
Chronic gonorrhoea and post-gonorrhoeal urethritis. New York, 1901. 16p. DNLM **00-6430**

VALENTINE, Ferdinand C[arl] (1851-1910)
The urine from each kidney. New York: William Wood & Co., 1902. 15p. DNLM **00-6431**

VALENTINE, Ferdinand C[arl] (1851-1910)
Examination of a genito-urinary patient by the general practitioner. Chicago, 1902. 23p. DNLM **00-6432**

VALENTINE, Ferdinand C[arl] (1851-1910)
The morning drop; its treatment. New York, 1902. 17p. DNLM **00-6433**

VALENTINE, Ferdinand C[arl] (1851-1910)
The boy's venereal peril. Chicago, 1903. 35p. DNLM **00-6434**

VALENTINE, Ferdinand C[arl] (1851-1910)
Aids to cystoscopic practice. New York, 1903. 10p. DNLM **00-6435**

VALENTINE, Ferdinand C[arl] (1851-1910) and Terry M. TOWNSEND
Abnormal frequency of urination treated with epidural injections. New York, 1903. 20p. DNLM **00-6436**

VALENTINE, Ferdinand C[arl] (1851-1910) and Terry M. TOWNSEND
Vesical retention of urine. New York, 1904. 22p. DNLM **00-6437**

VALENTINE, Ferdinand C[arl] (1851-1910) and Terry M. TOWNSEND
How the general practitioner should treat gonorrhea. Chicago, 1904. 8p. DNLM **00-6438**

VALENTINE, Ferdinand C[arl] (1851-1910) and Terry M. TOWNSEND
On the treatment of gonorrhoea. Indianapolis: Barnes-Warner Co., 1905. 23p. DNLM **00-6439**

VALENTINE, Ferdinand C[arl] (1851-1910) and Terry M. TOWNSEND
Some forensic problems concerning venereal diseases. [Albany], 1905. 33p. DNLM **00-6440**

VALENTINE, Ferdinand C[arl] (1851-1910) and Terry M. TOWNSEND
The prevention of venereal diseases. Columbus, 1906. 14p. DNLM **00-6441**

VALENTINE, Ferdinand C[arl] (1851-1910) and Terry M. TOWNSEND
Urethral dilatations with expansible instruments. New York, 1906. 32p. DNLM **00-6442**

VALENTINE, Ferdinand C[arl] (1851-1910)
The American Urological Association. [New York], 1906. 8p. DNLM **00-6443**

VALENTINE, Ferdinand C[arl] (1851-1910) and Terry M. TOWNSEND
Education in sexual subjects. New York, 1906. 8p. DNLM **00-6444**

VALENTINE, Ferdinand C[arl] (1851-1910)
The venereal peril in its relation to the state. Burlington, Vt., 1906. 16p. DNLM **00-6445**

VALENTINE, Ferdinand C[arl] (1851-1910) and Terry M. TOWNSEND
The emergency dilatation of urethral stricture. New York, 1907. 14p. DNLM **00-6446**

VALENTINE, Ferdinand C[arl] (1851-1910) and Terry M. TOWNSEND
Urethral hemorrhage. New York, 1907. 15p. DNLM **00-6447**

VALENTINE, Ferdinand C[arl] (1851-1910) and Terry M. TOWNSEND
Massage of the prostate and stripping the seminal vesicles. New York: William Wood & Co., 1907. 16p. DNLM **00-6448**

VALENTINE, Ferdinand C[arl] (1851-1910) and Terry M. TOWNSEND
Presumedly cured gonorrhea and marriage. Chicago, 1908. 8p. DNLM **00-6449**

VALENTINE, Ferdinand C[arl] (1851-1910) and Terry M. TOWNSEND
The indications for and technique of internal urethrotomy. Cincinnati, 1909. 7p. DNLM **00-6450**

VALENTINE, Julius J[ohn]
The treatment of gonorrhoeal epididymitis. New York, 1907. 4p. DNLM **00-6451**

VALK, Francis (1845-1919)
Strabismus, or squint, latent and fixed. A supplement to the errors of refraction. New York: G. P. Putnam's Sons, 1904. 171p. 1 plate. DLC; DNLM; ICJ; NNNAM **00-6452**

VANCE, A[sbury] J. (*b.* 1856)
Treatment of obesity by the use of Vichy and Kissingen salts. Philadelphia: J. Wyeth & Bros., [1901]. 2 l. DNLM **00-6453**

VANCE, James (*b.* 1875)
The surgical treatment of fibroid tumors of the uterus complicated by pregnancy. New York, 1907. 21p. DNLM **00-6454**

VANCE, James (*b.* 1875)
How long shall the patient stay in bed after abdominal section? New York: A. R. Elliott Co., 1907. 10p. DNLM **00-6455**

VANDEGRIFT, George W[onson]
Notes on a few prevalent eye diseases. New York, 1910. 9p. DNLM **00-6456**

VANDER VEER, A[lbert] (1841-1929) and Arthur W. ELTING
Résumé of the subject of actinomycosis, with report of a case of actinomycosis abdominalis. Albany, 1902. 190. 4 plates. DNLM **00-6457**

VANDER VEER, A[lbert] (1841-1929)
. . . Requirements for admission to medical schools including the combined baccalaureate and medical course; a paper delivered at the 40th University convocation, July 1, 1902. . . . Albany: University of the State of New York, 1902. 9p. PPC **00-6458**

VANDER VEER, A[lbert] (1841-1929)
Surgery of the stomach, with report of cases. One case of gastrostomy. Two cases of gastrectomy. Albany, 1903. 10p. DNLM **00-6459**

VANDER VEER, A[lbert] (1841-1929)
Should the regents register college courses as the equivalent of the first year in a medical school? Albany, 1904. 16p. DNLM **00-6460**

VANDER VEER, A[lbert] (1841-1929)
Abstract of paper reporting six hundred and fifteen cases, with operations done at the Albany Hospital from March 1, 1902, to March 1, 1903. [Albany], 1904. 7p. DNLM **00-6461**

VANDER VEER, A[lbert] (1841-1929)
History of abdominal section in Albany with a report of seventy-five cases. [Albany, 1904?] 53p. PPHa; PU **00-6462**

VANDER VEER, A[lbert] (1841-1929) and Edgar A[lbert] VANDER VEER
Four cases of gangrene. One case of embolism of the anterior and posterior tibial arteries during an illness of typhoid fever; gangrene; amputation through middle third of left leg. Two cases of embolism of the brachial artery; amputation of the arm. One case of arterio-venous aneurism. following gunshot wound of the popliteal vessels; amputation of the thigh thirteen years after receipt of the injury. Albany, 1904. 8p. 4 plates. DNLM **00-6463**

VANDER VEER, A[lbert] (1841-1929)
End results in surgery of the kidney, based on a study of ninety cases, with one hundred and twenty-three operations. New York: A. R. Elliott Pub. Co., 1905. 34p. DNLM; NNNAM **00-6464**

VANDER VEER, A[lbert] (1841-1929)
Reciprocity in medical licensure. [New York], 1906. 8p. DNLM **00-6465**

VANDER VEER, A[lbert] (1841-1929)
Report of cases of uterine fibroids associated with gallstones. Chicago, 1906. 7p. DNLM **00-6466**

VANDER VEER, A[lbert] (1841-1929)
Organization, methods, and responsibilities in the study of medicine. Opening address, Albany Medical College, September 19, 1905. [Albany, 1906.] 12p. NN **00-6467**

VANDER VEER, A[lbert] (1841-1929)
Treatment of enlarged prostate. [Read at the meeting of the Onondaga County Medical Society . . . Syracuse, N.Y., May, 1908.] New York, 1908. 24p. NN **00-6468**

VANDER VEER, A[lbert] (1841-1929)
The ethics of our profession. [New York], 1909. 22p. NN **00-6469**

VANDER VEER, A[lbert] (1841-1929)
Some observations on gallstones, with reference to cancer of the gallbladder. New York: A. E. Elliott Pub. Co., 1910. 14p. NN **00-6470**

VANDER VEER, Edgar A[lbert] (*b.* 1879)
The early recognition of malignant growths. Albany, 1901. 8p. DNLM **00-6471**

VANDER VEER, Edgar A[lbert] (*b.* 1879)
Report of a case in which a scarf-pin was swallowed and passed per rectum on the seventh day. Albany, 1901. 4p. DNLM **00-6472**

VANDER VEER, Edgar A[lbert] (*b.* 1879)
An unusual case of abscess of the liver. Read before the Medical Society of the State of New York, January 29, 1901. Albany, 1902. 4p. DNLM **00-6473**

VANDER VEER, Edgar A[lbert] (*b.* 1879)
A case of ruptured intestine with artificial anus, fecal fistula and opening through the scrotum. Philadelphia, 1904. 4p. DNLM **00-6474**

VANDER VEER, James N[ewell] (*b.* 1877)
Some practical hints regarding medical post-graduate study in Berlin. Philadelphia, 1906. 10p. DNLM **00-6475**

VANDER VEER, James N[ewell] (*b.* 1877)
Report of cases treated by a modified Bier-Klapp method of passive hyperemia. Albany, 1906. 16p. DNLM **00-6476**

VANDER VEER, James N[ewell] (*b.* 1877)
The use of the Bier-Klapp methods of hyperemia in infections of children. [New York, 1907.] 7p. NN **00-6477**

VANDER VEER, James N[ewell] (*b.* 1877)
Clinical aspect of the enlarged prostate, with a review of 67 cases. [Read before the third district branch of the Medical Society of the State of New York, Oct. 27, 1908.] [Brooklyn: Eagle Press, 1909.] 13(1)p. NN. **00-6478**

VANDER VEER, James N[ewell] (*b.* 1877)
A lithopedion thirty-five years old, reported by J. N. Vander Veer and C. P. McCabe. **00-6479**

VANDER VEER, James N[ewell] (*b.* 1877)
Entire absence of kidney, ureter and blood vessels. [New York], 1910. 8p. NN **00-6480**

VAN DE WARKER, [Edward] Ely (1841-1910)
Woman's unfitness for higher coeducation. . . . New York: The Grafton Press, [1903]. 225p. DLC: ICJ; PP; PU **00-6481**

VAN DE WARKER, [Edward] Ely (1841-1910)
The surgery of the female urethra. [Philadelphia], 1904. 13p. DNLM **00-6482**

VAN DE WARKER, [Edward] Ely (1841-1910)
Gonorrhoea in its female pelvic relations. New York: A. R. Elliott, 1905. 14p. DNLM **00-6483**

VAN DOREN, De Witt T[almage]
Students' guide to health. . . . Asserting the debt of strength to weakness, of health to sickness, and addressed to all those who seek redemption for the body. . . . Norwalk, Conn.: The Author, 1901. 136p. DLC **00-6484**

VAN DOREN, De Witt T[almage]
Mental guide to health; not a theory, but a science . . . asserting the debt of strength to weakness, of health to sickness. . . . New York, London, [etc.]: The Abbey Press, [1902]. 204p. front. DLC; NN **00-6485**

VAN FLEET, Frank (*b.* 1860)
The attitude of the Medical Society of the State of New York toward the Dispensary and other medical bills that went before the legislature of 1898-99. [New York, 1900.] 23p. DLC; NN **00-6486**

VAN HARLINGEN, Arthur (1845-1936)
Report of three cases of creeping larvae in the human skin (hyponomoderma, Kaposi). New York, 1902. 6p. DNLM **00-6487**

VAN HARLINGEN, Arthur (1845-1936)
Text-book of diseases of the skin. 4th ed., thoroughly revised and rearranged. Philadelphia: P. Blakiston's Son & Co., 1907. 482p. DLC; DNLM; NNNAM; PU **00-6488**

VAN HOOK, Weller (*b.* 1862)
Surgery of the ureters. Philadelphia, 1901. 9p. MB **00-6489**

VAN HOOK, Weller (*b.* 1862)
Constitutional reactions to wounds and their infections. Aseptic wound fever; sapremia; septic intoxication; septicemia; pyemia; septicopyemia. Illus. plate. [1901?] 32p. MB **00-6490**

VAN HOOK, Weller (*b.* 1862)
Surgery of the intestines, but excluding the appendix, the rectum, and the anus; surgery of the omentum and the mesentery. Philadelphia, 1908. 97p. DNLM [with Allan B. Kanaval] **00-6491**

VAN LENNEP, William B. (1853-1919)
A few suggestive thoughts concerning the surgical treatment of cirrhotic ascites. Philadelphia, 1902. 4p. DNLM **00-6492**

VAN LENNEP, William B. (1853-1919)
Do we operate early enough in appendicitis? Philadelphia, 1902. 5p. DNLM **00-6493**

VAN LENNEP, William B. (1853-1919)
Appendicitis complicating pregnancy. Philadelphia, 1902. 10p. DNLM **00-6494**

VAN LENNEP, William B. (1853-1919)
Surgical clinics, Hahnemann Hospital, Phila., session of 1902-1903. [Philadelphia], 1903. 154p. PHi **00-6495**

VAN LENNEP, William B. (1853-1919)
The present status of the surgery of the stomach. Philadelphia, 1904. 19p. DNLM **00-6496**

VAN LENNEP, William B. (1853-1919)
A few thoughts concerning the surgery of the pancreas. Philadelphia, 1905. 7p. DNLM **00-6497**

VAN LENNEP, William B. (1853-1919)
The surgical treatment of prostatic hypertrophy. Philadelphia, 1905. 6p. DNLM **00-6498**

VAN LENNEP, William B. (1853-1919)
The teaching of surgery in our colleges. [Philadelphia], 1906. 10p. DNLM **00-6499**

VAN LENNEP, William B. (1853-1919)
Thoughts concerning surgical treatment of cirrhotic ascites. [Philadelphia, 1906?] 7p. PPHa **00-6500**

VAN LENNEP, William B. (1853-1919)
Surgical treatment prostatic hypertrophy. [Philadelphia, 1906?] 7p. PPHa **00-6501**

VAN LENNEP, William B. (1853-1919)
Surgical treatment of inflammation of right iliac fosea. [Philadelphia, 1906?] 7p. PPHa **00-6502**

VAN LENNEP, William B. (1853-1919)
Surgical clinics at Hahnemann Hospital. [Philadelphia, 1906?] 7p. PPHa **00-6503**

VAN LENNEP, William B. (1853-1919)
Surgery of the pancreas. [Philadelphia, 1906?] 7p. PPHa **00-6504**

VAN SCHAICK, George Gray (*b.* 1861)
Diseases of the blood in their relation to surgery, and their treatment. New York, 1900. 12p. DNLM **00-6505**

VAN SCHAICK, George Gray (*b.* 1861)
Regional minor surgery; describing the treatment of those conditions daily encountered by the general practitioner. . . . New York: International Journal of Surgery Co., [1902]. 226p. DLC; KU; MH-M; PU **00-6506**

VAN SCHAICK, George Gray (*b.* 1861)
Regional minor surgery. Describing the treatment of those conditions daily encountered by the general practitioner. [2nd ed.] New York: International Journal of Surgery Co., 1904. 226p. CtY-M; DNLM; ICJ; NNNAM **00-6507**

VASS CHEMICAL COMPANY, DANBURY, CONN.
A practical treatise on thialion, a laxative salt of lithia . . . 9th ed. Danbury, Conn.: The Vass Chemical Co., 1900. 176p. DLC; MH **00-6508**

VASS CHEMICAL COMPANY, DANBURY, CONN.
A practical treatise on uric acid poisoning in all its phases, including its treatment with thialion (a laxative salt of lithia). With a complete bibliography. 14th ed. Danbury, Conn.: The Vass Chemical Co., 1904. 265p. illus. DLC; MH **00-6509**

VAUGHAN, George Tully (1859-1948)
. . . The principles and practice of surgery, designed for students and practitioners. . . . Philadelphia & London: J. B. Lippincott Co., 1902. 569p. plates. DLC; DNLM; PPC; PU
00-6510

VAUGHAN, George Tully (1859-1948)
A case of volvulus with torsion of the entire mesentery; operation; recovery. New York, 1903. 5p. DNLM
00-6511

VAUGHAN, George Tully (1859-1948)
Nine cases of resection of the intestine. Philadelphia, 1903. 9p. DNLM **00-6512**

VAUGHAN, George Tully (1859-1948)
The treatment of anterior dislocation of the shoulder, with report of a case in which reduction was prevented by the detached greater tuberosity. New York, 1903. 5p. DNLM
00-6513

VAUGHAN, George Tully (1859-1948)
Intussusception. Report of a case reduced by operation. New York, 1903. 5p. DNLM **00-6514**

VAUGHAN, George Tully (1859-1948)
Volvulus of the small intestine. Its relation to hernia. Torsion of the entire mesentery. Report and résumé of cases. New York, 1903. 22p. DNLM **00-6515**

VAUGHAN, George Tully (1859-1948)
An analysis of twenty-five cases of strangulated hernia treated by operation. New York, 1904. 10p. DNLM
00-6516

VAUGHAN, George Tully (1859-1948)
Luxatio erecta. New York, 1904. 2p. DNLM
00-6517

VAUGHAN, George Tully (1859-1948)
Circumcision. Chicago, 1905. 3p. DNLM
00-6518

VAUGHAN, George Tully (1859-1948)
Patent urachus; a review of the cases reported; operation on a case complicated with stones in the kidneys; a note on tumors and cysts of the urachus. Philadelphia, 1905. 22p. DNLM
00-6519

VAUGHAN, George Tully (1859-1948)
Gunshot wounds of the ureter; two cases of ureterovesical anastomosis. Philadelpia, 1905. 4p. DNLM
00-6520

VAUGHAN, George Tully (1859-1948)
Remarks suggested by an experience of fifty operations for fracture of the skull. New York, 1906. 9p. DNLM
00-6521

VAUGHAN, George Tully (1859-1948)
Gunshot wounds of the abdomen; a review of fourteen cases, with remarks on the mortality and treatment. Philadelphia, 1906. 12p. DNLM **00-6522**

VAUGHAN, George Tully (1859-1948)
Volvulus of the intestine. New York, 1907. 5p. DNLM
00-6523

VAUGHAN, George Tully (1859-1948)
Aneurysmal varix; a case of pulsating exophthalmos and two cases of enormous dilatation on the cardiac side of the wound, and one case of moderate dilatation on the same side. Chicago, 1907. 5p. DNLM **00-6524**

VAUGHAN, George Tully (1859-1948)
Some rare forms of hernia. New York, 1907. 5p. DNLM
00-6525

VAUGHAN, George Tully (1859-1948)
The operative treatment of fractures, especially of the long bones. Philadelphia, 1907. 17p. DNLM
00-6526

VAUGHAN, George Tully (1859-1948)
Further remarks on the care of gunshot wounds of the abdomen, with especial reference to the treatment of wounds of the urinary bladder and the danger of abscess and fistula following wounds of the pancreas. Philadelphia, 1907. 4p. DNLM **00-6527**

VAUGHAN, George Tully (1859-1948)
Stone, tuberculosis of the kidney, and perinephric abscess. Chicago, 1908. 8p. DNLM **00-6528**

VAUGHAN, George Tully (1859-1948)
The uncertain results of suturing nerves. Philadelphia, 1908. 6p. DNLM **00-5629**

VAUGHAN, George Tully (1859-1948)
Aneurysmal varix; a case of pulsating exophthalmos and two cases of enormous dilatation on the cardiac side of the wound, and one case of moderate dilatation on the same side. Chicago, 1907. 5p. DNLM **00-6530**

VAUGHAN, J[ohn] W[alter] (*b.* 1880)
The comparative value of different methods of cancer treatment. New York, 1910. 18p. DNLM
00-6531

VAUGHAN, Paul Turner
Syphilitic manifestations in the nose and pharynx. New York: A. R. Elliott Pub. Co., 1904. 6p. DNLM
00-6532

VAUGHAN, Victor C[larence] (1851-1929)
Conclusions reached after a study of typhoid fever among the American soldiers in 1898; oration on state medicine before the fifty-first annual meeting of the American Medical Association at Atlantic City, N.J., June 5-8, 1900. [1900.] 31p. DLC
00-6533

VAUGHAN, Victor C[larence] (1851-1929)
Some bacteriological poisons in milk and milk products. New York, 1900. 7p. MB; PU **00-6534**

VAUGHAN, Victor C[larence] (1851-1929)
Physiological chemistry. . . . Ann Arbor, Mich.: F. A. Wagner, [1900?] 309 l. DLC ["Prepared for the special use of my own students. There is no intention of publishing this work."—Pref.] **00-6535**

VAUGHAN, Victor C[larence] (1851-1929)
Intoxications. [Philadelphia, 1901.] 46p. MB
00-6536

VAUGHAN, Victor C[larence] (1851-1929)
The toxin of the colon bacillus. Philadelphia, 1901. 6p. DNLM
00-6537

VAUGHAN, Victor C[larence] (1851-1929)
The bacterial toxins. Philadelphia, 1901. 12p. DNLM
00-6538

VAUGHAN, Victor C[larence] (1851-1929)
The etiology and spread of typhoid fever. Chicago, 1902. 29p. DNLM **00-6539**

VAUGHAN, Victor C[larence] (1851-1929)
Cellular toxins; or, The chemical factors in the causation of disease, by Victor C. Vaughan . . . and Frederick G. Novy . . . 4th ed., rev. and enl. Philadelphia and New York: Lea Bros. & Co., 1902. 495p. plates. DLC; DNLM; PPC; PU
00-6540

VAUGHAN, Victor C[larence] (1851-1929)
Some remarks on the present status of medical education in the United States. Chicago, 1903. 11p. DNLM
00-6541

[VAUGHAN, Victor C(larence)] (1851-1929)
Contributions to medical research, dedicated to Victor Clarence Vaughan, by colleagues and former students . . . on the twenty-fifth anniversary of his doctorate. Ann Arbor, Mich.: George Wahr, 1903. 620p. ICJ; OCIM
00-6542

VAUGHAN, Victor C[larence] (1851-1929)
The value of scientific research to the state. [Michigan] . n. p., 1904. 13p. MH; NN **00-6543**

VAUGHAN, Victor C[larence] (1851-1929)
The use of food preservatives. Chicago, 1905. 12p. DNLM
00-6544

VAUGHAN, Victor C[larence] (1851-1929)
A brief report on research in the writer's laboratory on bacterial toxins and immunity. Philadelphia, 1905. 11p. DNLM
00-6545

VAUGHAN, Victor C[larence] (1851-1929)
. . . A contribution to the chemistry of the bacterial cell and a study of the effects of some of the split products on animals. . . . Delivered at the annual meeting of the Massachusetts Medical Society, June 12, 1906. [1906.] 53p. diags. DLC; MH
00-6546

VAUGHAN, Victor C[larence] (1851-1929)
A contribution to the chemistry of the bacterial cell and a study of the effects of some of the split products on animals. [Ann Arbor, 1906?] 53p. illus. MBM; MH-M [Shattuck lectures, 1906] **00-6547**

VAUGHAN, Victor C[larence] (1851-1929) and May WHEELER
Experimental immunity to colon and typhoid bacilli. New York, 1907. 19p. DNLM **00-6548**

VEASEY, Clarence A[rchibald] (*b.* 1869)
Excision of the lachrymal sac and gland, followed by an unusual variety of neuroparalytic keratitis, markedly resembling clinically the so-called lattice-like keratitis. Philadelphia, 1900. 5p. DNLM **00-6549**

VEASEY, Clarence A[rchibald] (*b.* 1869)
A case of oculomotor paresis following indirect violence. Detroit: W. M. Warren, 1900. 2p. DNLM
00-6550

VEASEY, Clarence A[rchibald] (*b.* 1869)
A plea for the earlier recognition of squint in children by the family physician and the earlier application of the methods of treatment. Philadelphia, 1900. 4p. DNLM
00-6551

VEASEY, Clarence A[rchibald] (*b.* 1869)
A new portable sterilizer for eye instruments. Chicago, 1900. 2p. DNLM **00-6552**

VEASEY, Clarence A[rchibald] (*b.* 1869)
A case of monocular hysterical amaurosis in a girl eleven years old. New York, 1900. 3p. DNLM **00-6553**

VEASEY, Clarence A[rchibald] (*b.* 1869)
Gonorrheal conjunctivitis; conjunctivitis neonátorum; pseudo-membranous conjunctivitis. Charlotte, N.C., 1900. 12p. DNLM
00-6554

VEASEY, Clarence A[rchibald] (*b.* 1869)
Complete recovery from double neuroretinitis, clinically resembling albuminuric retinitis, in a case of prolonged hematuria with symptoms of Bright's disease. Chicago, 1901. 4p. DNLM **00-6555**

VEASEY, Clarence A[rchibald] (*b.* 1869)
Traumatic luxation of the crystalline lens; secondary glaucoma; extraction without loss of vitreous; recovery with normal vision. Nashville, 1901. 3p. DNLM **00-6556**

VEASEY, Clarence A[rchibald] (*b.* 1869)
Restoration of useful vision in a complicated case of acute inflammatory glaucoma of ten days' duration with visual acuity reduced to the perception of light. Philadelphia, 1901. 4p. DNLM **00-6557**

VEASEY, Clarence A[rchibald] (*b.* 1869)
Report of a case of complete right oculomotor and complete left trifacial paralysis. Philadelphia, 1901. 3p. DNLM
00-6558

VEASEY, Clarence A[rchibald] (*b.* 1869)
A case of endothelioma of the orbit. Detroit: W. M. Warren, 1902. 5p. DNLM **00-6559**

VEASEY, Clarence A[rchibald] (*b.* 1869)
Report of a case of spontaneous perforation of the cornea, in the center of a macula which had existed for more than six years, the perforation not closing until the twentieth day. Nashville, 1902. 1 l. DNLM **00-6560**

VEASEY, Clarence A[rchibald] (*b.* 1869)
A manual of diseases of the eye for students and general practitioners. Philadelphia: Lea Bros. & Co., 1903. 412p. 10 plates. DLC; MH-M; NNNAM; PPC
00-6561

VEASEY, Clarence A[rchibald] (*b.* 1869) and Edward A. SHUMWAY
Simple glaucoma in the young, with a report of two cases. Nashville, 1904. 7p. DNLM **00-6562**

VEASEY, Clarence A[rchibald] (*b.* 1869)
Brief report of a case of spring conjunctivitis resembling malignant growth of the corneal limbus. Philadelphia, 1904. 3p. DNLM **00-6563**

VEASEY, Clarence A[rchibald] (*b.* 1869)
Report of a case of congenital exophthalmos produced by orbital hemorrhage followed by metastatic choroiditis. Chicago, 1904. 4p. DNLM **00-6564**

VEASEY, Clarence A[rchibald] (*b.* 1869)
Observations on a case of bitemporal hemianopsia, with some unusual changes in the visual field. Philadelphia, 1905. 8p. DNLM **00-6565**

VEASEY, Clarence A[rchibald] (*b.* 1869)
Clinical and histologic observations on sympathetic ophthalmia. Chicago, 1905. 8p. DNLM **00-6566**

VEASEY, Clarence A[rchibald] (*b.* 1869)
Report of a case of papilloma of the lachrymal caruncle. Report of a case of leucosarcoma of the choroid with secondary involvement of the ciliary body. Chicago, 1905. 4p. DNLM **00-6567**

VEASEY, Clarence A[rchibald] (*b.* 1869)
Report of a case of fulminant retrobulbar neuritis. [Detroit], 1906. 8p. DNLM **00-6568**

VEASEY, Clarence A[rchibald] (*b.* 1869)
A case of keratitis disciformis. [Detroit], 1906. 3p. DNLM **00-6569**

VEASEY, Clarence A[rchibald] (*b.* 1869)
Primary melanotic spindle-cell sarcoma of the corneal limbus. Nashville, 1907. 8p. DNLM **00-6570**

VEASEY, Clarence A[rchibald] (*b.* 1869)
An instrument for testing the light-reflex of the pupil. Chicago, 1907. 4p. DNLM **00-6571**

VEASEY, Clarence A[rchibald] (*b.* 1869)
A case of unilateral mixed nystagmus benefited by treatment. Philadelphia, 1908. 3p. DNLM **00-6572**

VEASEY, Clarence A[rchibald] (*b.* 1869)
The treatment of trachoma. Detroit, 1908. 9p. DNLM **00-6573**

VEASEY, Clarence A[rchibald] (*b.* 1869)
Glaucoma in the young. New York, 1908. 3p. DNLM **00-6574**

VEASEY, Clarence A[rchibald] (*b.* 1869)
Rhythmical alterations in the width of the palpebral fissure of both eyes. probably produced by spasm of the levator palpebrae muscles. New York, 1908. 3p. DNLM **00-6575**

VEASEY, Clarence A[rchibald] (*b.* 1869)
The treatment of chronic simple glaucoma. Milwaukee, 1908. 19p. DNLM **00-6576**

VEASEY, Clarence A[rchibald] (*b.* 1869)
The importance of active cooperation between parents and teachers in order to promote and maintain the health of children's eyes during school life. Easton, Pa., 1908. 12p. DNLM **00-6577**

VEASEY, Clarence A[rchibald] (*b.* 1869)
Some unusual complications occurring during and following the extraction of cataract. Seattle, 1909. 14p. DNLM **00-6578**

VEASEY, Clarence A[rchibald] (*b.* 1869)
Report of a case of epibulbar sarcoma. Seattle, 1910. 4p. DNLM **00-6579**

VEASEY, Clarence A[rchibald] (*b.* 1869)
Large piece of wood embedded deeply in orbit of child, twenty-five months; removed with preservation of vision. Chicago, 1910. 1 l. DNLM **00-6580**

VECKI, Victor G. (1857-1938)
The pathology and treatment of sexual impotence . . . 3rd ed. Philadelphia: W. B. Saunders & Co., 1901. 329p. DLC; DNLM; NNNAM; PPC **00-6581**

VECKI, Victor G. (1857-1938)
The prevention of sexual diseases . . . with introduction by William J. Robinson. New York: The Critic and Guide Co., 1910. 132p. DLC; MH; NIC; NN **00-6582**

VEDDER, Edward Bright (1878-1952)
An examination of the stools of 100 healthy individuals with especial reference to the presence of entamoebae coli. Chicago, 1908. 8p. DNLM **00-6583**

VEDDER, Edward Bright (1878-1952)
The leucocytes in dengue. New York, 1907. 11p. DNLM **00-6584**

VEEDER, Major Albert (1848-1915)
Defective development and disease, with special reference to the curability of consumption and cancer. [Lincoln, Neb., 1900.] 12p. NN **00-6585**

VEEDER, Major Albert (1848-1915)
Note on fitting trusses. [Buffalo, N.Y., 1901.] 3p. NN **00-6586**

VEEDER, Major Albert (1848-1915)
Disinfection within and without the body in diphtheria. [Albany? 1901.] 7p. MH; NN **00-6587**

VEEDER, Major Albert (1848-1915)
. . . The relative importance of flies and water-supply in spreading disease. . . . New York: The Publishers Printing Co., [1901?]. 8p. DLC **00-6588**

VEEDER, Major Albert (1848-1915)
Typhoid fever from sources other than water supply. . . . New York: William Wood & Co., 1902. 15p. NN **00-6589**

VEEDER, Major Albert (1848-1915)
Why the open-air treatment of consumption succeeds. . . . New York: William Wood & Co., 1903. 11p. NN **00-6590**

VEEDER, Major Albert (1848-1915)
The dangers of hypnotism. New York: William Wood & Co., [1903?]. 3p. NN **00-6591**

VEEDER, Major Albert (1848-1915)
Faculties of the mind not understood and not used with special reference to the curability of epilepsy. [New York], 1904. 8p. DNLM; NN **00-6592**

VERHOEFF, Frederick Herman (*b.* 1874)
A simplified method of testing with trial prisms. Chicago, 1900. 2p. DNLM **00-6593**

VERHOEFF, Frederick Herman (*b.* 1874)
A secure stitch for advancement operations. Chicago, 1901. 3p. DNLM **00-6594**

VERHOEFF, Frederick Herman (*b.* 1874)
A theory of binocular perspective, and some remarks upon torsion of the eyes, the theory of the vicarious fovea, and the relation of convergence to the perception of relief and distance. St. Louis, 1902. 29p. DNLM **00-6595**

VERHOEFF, Frederick Herman (*b.* 1874)
A rare tumor arising from the pars ciliaris retinae (teratoneuroma) of a nature hitherto unrecognized, and its relation to the so-called glioma retinae. New York, 1904. 27p. 2 plates. DNLM **00-6596**

VERWORN, Max (1863-1921)
General physiology; an outline of the science of life . . . transl. from the 2nd German ed. and edited by Frederic S. Lee. . . . With two hundred and eighty-five illustrations. New York: The Macmillan Co., 1900 [*c.* 1899]. 615p. DLC: ICJ; MH; NN **00-6597**

[VESALIUS, Andreas] (1514-1564)
Andreas Vesalius, the reformer of anatomy [by James Moores Ball]. St. Louis: Medical Science Press, 1910. 149p. DLC; ICJ; MH; NN **00-6598**

VICKERS, George Morley, ed.
The education of sex; a compilation from the writings and teachings of many eminent physicians and authorities—whose names appear throughout the book—forming a text-book on the physiology of marriage, the phenomena of life, existing social evils and their needed reforms. Philadelphia and London: The Gravic Publishing Co., [1910]. 275p. illus. DLC; ICU; MH; NN **00-6599**

VIETH, H. and O. EHRMAN
Researches and observations on long known and on recently introduced balsams. New York, 1906. 8p. DNLM **00-6600**

VIETH, H.
Anthrasol. New York, 1908. 8p. DNLM **00-6601**

VINCENT, Ralph H[arry] (1870-1922)
The nutrition of the infant. New York: William Wood & Co., 1904. 295p. DNLM; ICJ; NNNAM; PPC **00-6602**

VINEBERG, Hiram N. (*b.* 1857)
Differential diagnosis of ectopic pregnancy with especial reference between it and that of early uterine pregnancy. Chicago, 1901. 10p. DNLM **00-6603**

VINEBERG, Hiram N. (*b.* 1857)
Clinical notes on a series of nine consecutive cases of ectopic gestation. New York: William Wood & Co., 1903. 19p. DNLM **00-6604**

VINEBERG, Hiram N. (*b.* 1857)
The treatment of puerperal sepsis. New York: William Wood & Co., 1903. 14p. DNLM **00-6605**

VINEBERG, Hiram N. (*b.* 1857)
Simultaneous uterine and extra-uterine pregnancy. Report of two cases. New York, 1906. 10p. DNLM **00-6606**

VINEBERG, Hiram N. (*b.* 1857)
Appendicitis in pregnancy. [New York], 1907. 15p. DNLM **00-6607**

VINEBERG, Hiram N. (*b.* 1857)
Pyelitis in pregnancy and the puerperium. New York: William Wood & Co., 1908. 21p. DNLM **00-6608**

[VIRGINIA]
The health resort of Virginia: Rawley Springs. Carbonate Protoxide Iron, Iron Tonic, Sulphur and Magnesia Water. [Harrisonburg, 1903.] 24p. DLC **00-6609**

VIRGINIA. MEDICAL COLLEGE OF VIRGINIA. RICHMOND
Annual catalogues and announcements for the sessions of 1860-61 (23.); 1878-79 (41.); 1886-87 to 1904-05 (49.-67.). Richmond, 1860-1904. DNLM [List of students and graduates for the years 1859-60; 1877-78; 1885-86 to 1902-03 in: Announcements for subsequent years. In 1897 a school of dentistry and a school of pharmacy were established in connection with the medical school.] **00-6610**

VIRGINIA. MEDICAL COLLEGE OF VIRGINIA. RICHMOND
Bulletins. Issued quarterly. Nos. 1-3, v. 1. Richmond, 1904. DNLM [Commenced March, 1904. For preceding documents, see Annual catalogues and announcements.] **00-6611**

VIVISECTION. Its barbarity. Its uselessness. Its wickedness. Some expert testimony. [Syracuse, N.Y.: C. A. Hamlin, 1901?] 4p. DLC **00-6612**

VIVISECTION REFORM SOCIETY
. . . Illustrations of human vivisection. . . . Chicago: Vivisection Reform Society, 1907. 31p. DLC: ICJ **00-6613**

VOAK, Asa F[leming] (*b.* 1875)
The household manual of medicine. . . . Cleveland, O.: The Manual Publishing Co., [1903]. 186p. DLC; OCIM **00-6614**

VOAK, Asa F[leming] (*b.* 1875)
Dr. Voak's pocket doctor; a condensed manual of valuable information concerning the more common diseases and their treatment. . . . General diseases, diseases of children, diseases of the eye . . . recipes for a number of useful and essential toilet preparations. [Cleveland, O.: A. F. Voak, 1910?] 94p. DLC; OCIM **00-6615**

WACHENHEIM, Frederick L. (*b.* 1870)
Notes on uremia, urea, and the urea tests. New York, 1904. 9p. DNLM **00-6616**

WACHENHEIM, Frederick L. (*b.* 1870)
Notes on the death rate of infants in the summer months. New York: A. R. Elliott, 1905. 7p. DNLM **00-6617**

WACHENHEIM, Frederick L. (*b.* 1870)
Late secondary haemorrhage following the removal of adenoids. New York, 1907. 5p. DNLM **00-6618**

WACHENHEIM, Frederick L. (*b.* **1870)**
The climatic treatment of children. . . . New York: Rebman Co., [1907]. 440p. DLC: ICJ; NNNAM; PU
00-6619

WACKERHAGEN, George
Aseptic and antiseptic preparations and treatment of emergencies after abdominal surgical operations. . . . New York: E. R. Pelton, 1904. 44p. DLC; ICJ; PPC; PU
00-6620

WACKERHAGEN, George
Intestinal anastomosis with the aid of accessory support to the intestinal wall, also a description of an operation for suturing the intestine without support. Brooklyn, N.Y., 1905. 15p. DNLM; NBM **00-6621**

WADE, J. Percy
On the use of a new, safe and efficient hypnotic in the treatment of the insane; chloretone. [New York, 1900.] 7p. DNLM **00-6622**

WADE, Martin Joseph (1861-1931)
A selection of cases on malpractice of physicians, surgeons and dentists. . . . St. Louis: Medico-Legal Publishing Co., 1909. 896p. DLC; ICJ; ICU; NN **00-6623**

WADSWORTH, Augustus B[aldwin] (*b.* **1872)**
On puerperal infection; with special reference to douching and the practical value of bacterial examinations. [New York, 1901.] 30p. DNLM; NNNAM **00-6624**

WADSWORTH, Augustus B[aldwin] (*b.* **1872)**
Studies on simple and differential methods of staining encapsulated pneumococci in smear and section. [Boston, 1906.] 8p. MB **00-6625**

WADSWORTH, William Scott (*b.* **1868)**
Injuries to the brain. [1901.] 6p. PU
00-6626

WADSWORTH, William Scott (*b.* **1868)**
Sudden death. [1903.] 8p. PU
00-6627

WADSWORTH, William Scott (*b.* **1868)**
Cerebellar lesions without cerebellar symptoms, by W. S. Wadsworth, W. A. Spiller and W. E. Robertson. [n. p., 1906.] 18p. PU **00-6628**

WADSWORTH, William Scott (*b.* **1868)**
The color sense. [St. Louis, Mod., 1908.] 10p. MH
00-6629

WADSWORTH, William Scott (*b.* **1868)**
Medicine in the colonies; a paper read before the Pennsylvania Society of the Order of the Founders and Patriots of America, January the fourteenth, nineteen hundred and ten. [n. p., 1910?] 16p. CtY-M; NN; NNC; PP **00-6630**

WAGNER, R. V., CO., CHICAGO
. . . Catalogue of electrical instruments for physicians and surgeons . . . [7th ed.] Chicago: R. V. Wagner Co., 1905. 160p. illus. DLC; ICJ **00-6631**

WAINWRIGHT, John William (*b.* **1850)**
Urinary diagnosis and treatment. . . . Chicago: G. P. Engelhard & Co., 1900. 134p. plates. DLC; ICJ; DNLM; OCIM
00-6632

WAINWRIGHT, J[ohn] W[illiam] (*b.* **1850)**
A syllabus of new remedies and theraputic measures, with chemistry, physical appearance and therapetuic application. . . . Chicago: G. P. Engelhard & Co., 1901. 224p. plates. DLC; DNLM; NNNAM; PU **00-6633**

WAINWRIGHT, J[ohn] W[illiam] (*b.* **1850)**
Theory of the action of inorganic and organic substances, and changes of substances in the organism. Philadelphia, 1901. 78p. DNLM; PU **00-6634**

WAINWRIGHT, J[ohn] W[illiam] (*b.* **1850)**
Secret poisons and their uses in ancient times. New York: William Wood & Co., 1903. 19p. DNLM
00-6635

WAINWRIGHT, J[ohn] W[illiam] (*b.* **1850)**
Animal remedial preparations. New York: William Wood & Co., 1905. 20p. DNLM **00-6636**

WAINWRIGHT, J[ohn] W[illiam] (*b.* **1850)**
A manual of acute poisoning, giving classification, varieties and individual substances usually met with in emergency poisoning, with special symptoms, simple tests, chemical antidotes, physiologic antagonists and treatment. Together with methods for use in first aid to the injured. . . . New York: E. R. Pelton, 1905. 96p. DLC; MH-M; NNNAM; PU
00-6637

WAINWRIGHT, J[ohn] W[illiam] (*b.* **1850)**
The medical and surgical kdnowledge of William Shakespeare; with explanatory notes. . . . [Author's ed.] New York: The Author, 1907. 78p. DLC; DNLM; MH-M; NNNAM
00-6638

WAINWRIGHT, Jonathan M[ayhew] (*b.* **1874)**
On the value of spinal analgesia in shock, a study in surgical physiology. Athens, Pa.: W. G. Jordan, 1905. 29p. DNLM
00-6639

WAINWRIGHT, Jonathan M[ayhew] (*b.* **1874)**
The Scranton typhoid epidemic. Preliminary note. New York: A. R. Elliott Co., 1907. 5p. DNLM **00-6640**

WAINWRIGHT, Jonathan M[ayhew] (*b.* **1874)**
The reduction of cancer mortality. New York, 1910. 10p. DNLM **00-6641**

WAINWRIGHT, Jonathan M[ayhew] (*b.* **1874) and Henry J. NICHOLS**
Hookworm disease and miners' anemia in the anthracite coal fields. New York: Lea Bros. & Co., 1904. 11p. DNLM
00-6642

WAINWRIGHT, Jonathan M[ayhew] (*b.* **1874) and Henry J. NICHOLS**
The relation between anthracosis and pulmonary tuberculosis. Philadelphia, 1905. 12p. DNLM **00-6643**

WAITE, Lucy
The element of truth in mental healing. New York: A. R. Elliott Pub. Co., 1905. 10p. DNLM
00-6644

WAKEFIELD, Homer (*b.* **1865)**
Some observations on modern cardio-therapy. New York, 1901. 28p. DLC; DNLM **00-6645**

WAKEFIELD, Homer (*b.* 1865)
The pathology of katabolism in relation to the etiology and pathology of cancer and allied states. Philadelphia, 1902. 66p. DLC; DNLM **00-6646**

WAKEFIELD, Homer (*b.* 1865)
The heart cure; its terminology, purposes and achievements including the etiology of fatty degeneration. New York, 1903. 28p. DLC; DNLM **00-6647**

WAKEFIELD, Homer (*b.* 1865)
The rational treatment of malignant tumors. Philadelphia, 1904. 29p. DNLM **00-6648**

WAKEFIELD, Homer (*b.* 1865)
Commentaries upon lues and leprosy as subcatabolic diseases. New York, 1904. 16p. DLC; DNLM **00-6649**

WAKEFIELD, Homer (*b.* 1865)
A dissertation on temperament, diathesis, dyscrasia, predisposition, cachexia, susceptibility, idiosyncrasy and heredity. Philadelphia, 1905. 69p. DNLM **00-6650**

WAKEFIELD, Homer (*b.* 1865)
A contribution to the etiology of malaria, and to the analysis of some relations of meteorology to chemical pathology. New York, 1905. 37p. DNLM **00-6651**

WAKEFIELD, Homer (*b.* 1865)
General suboxidation from prolonged unremitting effort, both physical and mental. Burlington, Vt., & N.Y., 1908. 12p. DNLM **00-6652**

WAKEFIELD, Homer (*b.* 1865)
The physiology and pathology of the emotions; the physical bases of mental etiology. New York, 1908. 19p. DNLM **00-6653**

WAKEFIELD, Homer (*b.* 1865)
Some serious lapses in administrative hygiene. New York, 1909. 14p. DNLM **00-6654**

WAKEFIELD, Homer (*b.* 1865)
The responsibility of departments of health for unwholesome foods and the high cost of living. New York, 1910. 16p. DNLM **00-6655**

WAKEFIELD, W. Francis B. (*b.* 1866)
The utero-sacral ligaments. San Francisco, 1904. 4p. DNLM **00-6656**

WALGREN, John Arvede (*b.* 1870)
The new health science; the art of positivism and psychic laws of healing. . . . Chicago, New York: Rand, McNally & Co., [1909]. 84p. DLC; ICJ **00-6657**

WALKER, Edwin (*b.* 1853)
Bilharzia hematobia. Chicago, 1900. 11p. DNLM **00-6658**

WALKER, Edwin (*b.* 1853)
Galvanism as a remedy for uterine hemorrhage. New York, 1901. 4p. DNLM **00-6659**

WALKER, Edwin (*b.* 1853)
The dry method in surgery. New York, 1901. 8p. DNLM **00-6660**

WALKER, Edwin (*b.* 1853)
Stricture of the esophagus. Louisville, 1901. 5p. DNLM **00-6661**

WALKER, Edwin (*b.* 1853)
Some experiences with the X-ray as a therapeutic agent. Report of the cure of a case of alveolar melanotic sarcoma. Chicago, 1903. 7p. DNLM **00-6662**

WALKER, George (*b.* 1869)
Remarkable cases of hereditary anchyloses or absence of various phalangeal joints, with defects of the little and ring fingers. Baltimore, 1901. 11p. 2 plates. DNLM **00-6663**

WALKER, H[enry] O. (1843-1912)
Abdominal vs. vaginal hysterectomy. [Detroit, 1902?] 8p. PPHa **00-6664**

WALKER, H[enry] O. (1843-1912)
Gastrojejunostomy with the McGraw elastic ligature, for the relief of gastroptosis. Chicago, 1903. 12p. DNLM **00-6665**

WALKER, H[enry] O. (1843-1912)
The aseptic technic of abdominal surgery, with the topographical and visceral anatomy of male and female abdomen. Detroit, 1904. 12p. DNLM **00-6666**

WALKER, H[enry] O. (1843-1912)
Surgery of the gall bladder. [Detroit], 1910. 12p. PPHa **00-6667**

WALKER, Holford
Report of a case of recurrent abscesses, associated with chronic pelvic and ileo-cecal inflammation, following typhoid. Treated by an old method in new costume. Philadelphia, 1904. 2 l. DNLM **00-6668**

WALKER, James (*b.* 1864) and Frank HUGH
Further report of a previously recorded case of blastomycosis of the skin; systemic infection with blastomyces; autopsy. Chicago, 1902. 12p. 1 chart. DNLM **00-6669**

WALKER, Jerome (*b.* 1845)
Anatomy of physiology and hygiene. New ed. Boston: Allyn & Bacon, 1900. 490p. DNLM; MA; MH; NN **00-6670**

WALKER, Jerome (*b.* 1845)
Summer resorts for the debilitated children of our cities. [New York, 1900?] 6p. NN **00-6671**

WALKER, J[ohn] M. (*b.* 1876)
Potassium iodide in mental diseases. New York, 1908. 10p. DNLM **00-6672**

WALKER, Norman (1862-1942)
An introduction to dermatology. 2nd ed. New York: William Wood & Co., 1902. 301p. 43 plates. CtY-M; DNLM; NNNAM **00-6673**

WALKER, Norman (1862-1942)
An introduction to dermatology. 3rd ed. New York: William Wood & Co., 1905. 284p. 49 plates. DNLM; NNNAM; PPC; PU **00-6674**

WALKER, Norman (1862-1942)
An introduction to dermatology. 4th ed. New York: William Wood & Co., 1908. 332p. 28 plates. DNLM; NNNAM; PPJ; PU
00-6675

WALKER, Norman (1862-1942)
An introduction to dermatology. . . . Fifth edition. With 43 coloured plates and 79 illustrations in the text. New York: William Wood & Co., 1910. 332p. DLC; ICJ; IU-M; NNNAM
00-6676

WALKER, W[illiam] K. (*b.* 1867)
A few general remarks regarding the essential nature of dementia praecox. New York, 1906. 15p. DNLM
00-6677

WALL & OCHS
Physicians' net price list of ophthalmological and laryngological apparatus. Philadelphia [*c.* 1900.] 24p. NNNAM
00-6678

WALL, Otto A[ugustus] (1846-1922)
Elementary lessons in Latin. . . . St. Louis, Mo.: A. Gast Bank-note and Litho. Co., 1900. 148p. DLC; PPC [Pharmaceutical Latin]
00-6679

WALL, Otto A[ugustus] (1846-1922)
Notes on pharmacognosy. 2nd ed., rev. and enl. . . . St. Louis, Mo.: Aug. Gast Bank Note and Litho. Co., 1902. 703p. DLC; ICJ
00-6680

WALLGREN, A[ndrew] B[ennett] (*b.* 1877)
Histology and bacteriology in abstract. Pittsburgh, Pa.: Medical Abstract Pub. Co., 1906. 207p. CtY-M; DNLM; ICJ
00-6681

WALLGREN, A[ndrew] B[ennett] (*b.* 1877)
Bacteriology in abstract . . . [2nd ed.] Pittsburgh, Pa.: Medical Abstract Pub. Co., [1910?]. 340p. DLC; ICJ; PPC; PPJ
00-6682

WALLIAN, Samuel S[pencer] (1836-1907)
Rhythmotherapy; a discussion of the physiologic basis and therapeutic potency of mechano-vital vibration, to which is added a dictionary of diseases, with suggestions as to the technic of vibratory therapeutics. . . . Chicago: The Ouellette Press, 1906. 210p. col. plates. DLC; ICJ; IU-M; OCIM
00-6683

WALLIS, Frederick Charles (1859-1912)
Surgery of the rectum. New York: William Wood & Co., 1907. 168p. DNLM; IEN-M; MBM; NNNAM
00-6684

WALSH, David
The Röntgen rays in medical work. Part I. Apparatus and methods, rewritten by Lewis Jones. Part II. Medical and surgical (brought up to date with an appendix). 3rd ed. New York: William Wood & Co., 1902. 316p. 33 plates. CU-M; DNLM; NNNAM; PPC
00-6685

WALSH, David
The Röntgen rays in medical work. Part I. Apparatus and methods, rewritten by Lewis Jones. Part II. Medical and surgical (brought up to date with an appendix). 4th ed. New York: William Wood & Co., 1907. 433p. 1 plate. CtY-M; DNLM; NNNAM; PU
00-6686

WALSH, David
The hair and its diseases including ringworm, greyness, and baldness; an introductory handbook. 2nd ed. Chicago: W. T. Keener, 1908. 94p. DNLM; ICJ; IU-M; PPC
00-6687

WALSH, Ferdinand C. (*b.* 1878)
Venereal diseases and marriage. St. Louis, 1910. 3p. DNLM
00-6688

WALSH, Ferdinand C. (*b.* 1878)
Prostatic calculi; report of a case. Nashville, 1910. 1 l. DNLM
00-6689

WALSH, Ferdinand C. (*b.* 1878)
Pyuria in latent genito-urinary lesions. St. Louis, 1910. 7p. DNLM
00-6690

WALSH, James J[oseph] (1865-1942)
Catholic churchmen in science; sketches of the lives of Catholic ecclesiastics who were among the great founders in science. . . . Philadelphia; American Ecclesiastical Review, 1906. 221p. ports. DLC; MH; NIC: NN
00-6691

WALSH, James J[oseph] (1865-1942)
The Irish school of medicine. [Baltimore: The Johns Hopkins Press, 1906.] 22p. DLC; NN
00-6692

WALSH, James J[oseph] (1865-1942)
The foundation of city hospitals. [New York, 1906?] 16p. DLC; NN
00-6693

WALSH, James J[oseph] (1865-1942)
Fauchard, the Father of Modern Dentistry. . . . New York, 1906? 16p. NN
00-6694

WALSH, James J[oseph] (1865-1942)
Makers of modern medicine. New York: Fordham Univ. Press, 1907. 362p. DNLM; NIC; NN; PU
00-6695

WALSH, James J[oseph] (1865-1942)
First picture of surgical operations extant. Chicago, 1907. 7p. DNLM
00-6696

WALSH, James J[oseph] (1865-1942)
Medieval medical education. St. Louis, 1907. 8p. DNLM
00-6697

WALSH, James J[oseph] (1865-1942)
History of the Medical Society of the State of New York. Brooklyn: Eagle Press, 1907. 208p. DNLM; MBM; NN; NNNAM
00-6698

WALSH, James J[oseph] (1865-1942)
The earliest modern law for the regulation of the practice of medicine. Chicago, 1908. 7p. DNLM
00-6699

WALSH, James J[oseph] (1865-1942)
The first American medical school. New York, 1908. 12p. DNLM
00-6700

WALSH, James J[oseph] (1865-1942)
A chapter in the history of quackery. Chicago, 1909. 8p. DNLM
00-6701

WALSH, James J[oseph] (1865-1942)
Catholic churchmen in science; sketches of the lives of Catholic ecclesiastics who were among the great founders in science. 2nd ed. Philadelphia: American Eccleciastical Review, 1910. 2 v. port. DLC; MB; NIC; NN **00-6702**

WALSH, Joseph (1870-1946)
Medication in tuberculosis. [Savannah], 1905. 8p. DNLM **00-6703**

WALSH, Joseph (1870-1946)
Prognosis in tuberculosis of the lungs. New York, 1906. 10p. DNLM **00-6704**

WALSH, Joseph (1870-1946)
The Pennsylvania Society for the Prevention of Tuberculosis. Report for year ending May 1, 1906. [Philadelphia, 1906.] 22p. DNLM **00-6705**

WALSH, Ralph (*b.* 1841)
The desk book of facts for physicians and pharmacists. Washington, 1909. 202p. DLC; PP; PPL **00-6706**

WALSHAM, Hugh
. . . The channels of infection in tuberculosis together with the conditions, original or acquired, which render the different tissues vulnerable; being the Weber-Parkes' prize essay 1903. . . . New York: William Wood & Co., 1905. 150p. 16 col. plates. DNLM; ICJ; NNNAM; PPC **00-6707**

WALSHAM, William J[ohnson] (1847-1903)
Surgery, its theory and practice. 7th ed. Philadelphia: P. Blakiston's Son & Co., 1900. 953p. 16 plates. CtY-M; DNLM; NNNAM; PPC **00-6708**

WALSHAM, William J[ohnson] (1847-1903)
Nasal obstruction: the diagnosis of the various conditions causing it, and their treatment. New York: William Wood & Co., 1901. 256p. DLC; ICJ; NNNAM; PU **00-6709**

WALSHAM, William J[ohnson] (1847-1903)
Surgery; its theory and practice . . . 8th ed., with 622 illustrations including 20 skiagram plates, by Walter George Spencer. . . . Philadelphia: P. Blakiston's Son & Co., 1903. 1227p. DLC; ICJ; NNNAM; PPC **00-6710**

WALTERS, Francis M[arion] (*b.* 1862)
The elements of physiology. Columbia, Mo.: E. W. Stephens, 1902. 185p. DLC **00-6711**

WALTON, George Edward (*b.* 1839)
Therapeutics of mineral waters. [Philadelphia, 1903?] 12p. PPHa **00-6712**

WALTON, George L[incoln] (1854-1941) and Walter Everard PAUL
Contribution to the study of the plantar reflex, based upon seven hundred examinations made with special reference to the Babinski phenomenon. [New York], 1900. 19p. DNLM **00-6713**

WALTON, George L[incoln] (1854-1941) and Walter Everard PAUL
The clinical value of astereognosis and its bearing upon cerebral localization. New York, 1901. 23p. DNLM **00-6714**

WALTON, George L[incoln] (1854-1941) and Walter Everard PAUL
Angina cruris (intermittent claudication) and allied conditions, including painful cramps. With remarks on the importance of examining the pedal arteries. Boston, 1902. 24p. DNLM **00-6715**

WALTON, George L[incoln] (1854-1941)
Contribution to the study of spinal fracture with special reference to the question of operative interference. New York, 1902. 22p. DNLM; MH; NN **00-6716**

WALTON, George L[incoln] (1854-1941)
The localization of the reflex mechanism. New York, 1902. 7p. DNLM; MH; NN **00-6717**

WALTON, George L[incoln] (1854-1941)
Contribution to the study of myospasm, myokymia, myoclonus multiplex, myotonia aquisita, intention spasm. New York, 1902. 16p. DNLM; MH; NN **00-6718**

WALTON, George L[incoln] (1854-1941)
Further observations on cervical dislocation and its reduction. Boston, 1903. 9p. DNLM; MH; NN **00-6719**

WALTON, George L[incoln] (1854-1941)
Worry and allied faulty mental habits. Boston, 1903. 16p. DNLM; MH; NN **00-6720**

WALTON, George L[incoln] (1854-1941) and Walter Everard PAUL
Contribution to the study of the Achilles-jerk and the front-tap. New York, 1903. 11p. DNLM **00-6721**

WALTON, George L[incoln] (1854-1941)
The prevailing conception of degeneracy and degenerate, with a plea for introducing the supplementary term deviation and deviate. Boston, 1904. 9p. DNLM; MH; NN **00-6722**

WALTON, George L[incoln] (1854-1941)
Brain tumors; a study of clinical and post-mortem records bearing on their operability and their symptomatology. New York, 1905. 10p. DNLM; MH; NN **00-6723**

WALTON, George L[incoln] (1854-1941)
Eyestrain, its importance and its limitations. Boston, [1905]. 23p. DNLM; MH; NN **00-6724**

WALTON, George L[incoln] (1854-1941)
The blood pressure in paresis. Chicago, 1906. 7p. DNLM; MH; NN **00-6725**

WALTON, George L[incoln] (1854-1941)
The cerebral element in the reflexes and its relation to the spinal element. New York, 1906. 11p. DNLM; MH; NN **00-6726**

WALTON, George L[incoln] (1854-1941)
Constitutional headaches. Chicago, 1906. 4p. DNLM; MH; NN **00-6727**

WALTON, George L[incoln] (1854-1941) and G. W. W. BREWSTER
Fracture of skull probably involing the base; recovery after operation; analysis of the aphasia. Also crush of cord from spinal fracture, by G. L. Walton. Boston, 1906. 11p. 1 plate. DNLM; MH; NN **00-6728**

WALTON, George L[incoln] (1854-1941)
Anterior poliomyelitis in the adult, with illustrative cases. Boston, 1907. 10p. DNLM; MH; NN **00-6729**

WALTON, George L[incoln] (1854-1941)
The classification of psycho-neurotics, and the obsessional element in their symptoms. Chicago, 1907. 8p. DNLM; MH; NN **00-6730**

WALTON, George L[incoln] (1854-1941)
Migraine, an occupation neurosis. Chicago, 1908. 8p. DNLM; MH; NN **00-6731**

WALTON, George L[incoln] (1854-1941)
Why worry? Philadelphia & London: J. B. Lippincott Co., 1908. 269p. DNLM; MH; NN **00-6732**

WALTON, George L[incoln] (1854-1941) and Walter Everard PAUL
Arteriosclerosis; a contribution to its clinical study. Chicago, 1908. 11p. DNLM **00-6733**

WALTON, George L[incoln] (1854-1941)
Distinction between the psychoneuroses not always necessary. Boston, 1909. 12p. DNLM; MH; NN **00-6734**

WALTON, George L[incoln] (1854-1941)
Those nerves. Philadelphia & London: J. B. Lippincott Co., 1909. 202p. DNLM; MH; NN **00-6735**

WARBASSE, James P[eter] (*b.* 1866)
On the co-operation of surgeons in the making of surgical history. Philadelphia, 1900. 7p. DNLM **00-6736**

WARBASSE, James P[eter] (*b.* 1866)
The treatment of delirium tremens by the intravenous infusion of saline solution. New York, 1901. 3p. DNLM **00-6737**

WARBASSE, James P[eter] (*b.* 1866)
Peritonitis of the duodenal region. Philadelphia, 1903. 7p. DNLM **00-6738**

WARBASSE, James P[eter] (*b.* 1866)
Some observations on perforating ulcer of the duodenum. Brooklyn, 1903. 15p. DNLM **00-6739**

WARBASSE, James P[eter] (*b.* 1866)
Observations of wounds of nerves. Carlisle, 1903. 11p. DNLM **00-6740**

WARBASSE, James P[eter] (*b.* 1866)
The treatment of fractures. Brooklyn, 1904. 24p. DNLM **00-6741**

WARBASSE, James P[eter] (*b.* 1866)
Memorial address. Brooklyn, 1904. 5p. DNLM **00-6742**

WARBASSE, James P[eter] (*b.* 1866)
Medicine in its relation to human progress. Brooklyn, 1904. 4p. DNLM **00-6743**

WARBASSE, James P[eter] (*b.* 1866)
Acute peritoneal infection and its relation to intestinal obstruction. Philadelphia, 1905. 6p. DNLM **00-6744**

WARBASSE, James P[eter] (*b.* 1866)
Ovarian transplantation. Philadelphia, 1905. 4p. DNLM **00-6745**

WARBASSE, James P[eter] (*b.* 1866)
Some observations on the treatment of fractures. Carlisle, 1905. 9p. DNLM **00-6746**

WARBASSE, James P[eter] (*b.* 1866)
The Medical Library Association of Brooklyn and its relation to the library of the Medical Society of the County of Kings. [New York, 1906.] 7p. DNLM **00-6747**

WARBASSE, James P[eter] (*b.* 1866)
Willard Parker and his medical library. Brooklyn, 1907. 3p. DNLM **00-6748**

WARBASSE, James P[eter] (*b.* 1866)
Cases of appendicitis which do not demand operation. Brooklyn, 1907. 3p. DNLM **00 6749**

WARBASSE, James P[eter] (*b.* 1866)
Doctors of Samuel Johnson and his court. Brooklyn, N.Y.: Huntington, 1908 [1907]. 56p. illus., ports. DNLM; NcD; NN **00-6750**

WARBASSE, James P[eter] (*b.* 1866)
Traumatism as an etiological factor in appendicitis. New York, 1908. 6p. DNLM **00-6751**

WARBASSE, James P[eter] (*b.* 1866)
Medical journalism; state journalism in particular; with especial reference to the New York State Journal of Medicine. New York, 1908. 8p. DNLM **00-6752**

WARBASSE, James P[eter] (*b.* 1866)
Some common injuries of the elbow. New York, 1909. 19p. DNLM **00-6753**

WARBASSE, James P[eter] (*b.* 1866)
Dislocations of cervical vertebrae. New York, 1909. 9p. DNLM **00-6754**

WARBASSE, James P[eter] (*b.* 1866)
The importance of the X-ray in the treatment of fractures. Brooklyn, N.Y., 1909. 12p. DNLM **00-6755**

WARBASSE, James P[eter] (*b.* 1866)
The treatment of fractures; some practical points. Chicago, 1909. 12p. DNLM **00-6756**

WARBASSE, James P[eter] (*b.* 1866)
Medical sociology. A series of observations touching upon the sociology of health and the relations of medicine to society. New York: D. Appleton & Co., 1909. 355p. DLC; MH; NIC; NN **00-6757**

WARBASSE, James P[eter] (*b.* 1866)
The conquest of disease through animal experimentation. New York & London: D. Appleton & Co., 1910. 175p. DLC; ICJ; NIC; NN **00-6758**

WARD, George Gray, Jr. (*b.* 1868)
A retrospect of forty cases of operative gynecology. New York, 1900. 23p. DNLM **00-6759**

WARD, George Gray, Jr. (*b.* **1868)**
Palpation of the uterine appendages. New York, 1901. 8p. DNLM **00-6760**

WARD, George Gray, Jr. (*b.* **1868)**
The prevention of post-operative adhesions of the peritoneum. New York: William Wood & Co., 1901. 18p. DNLM **00-6761**

WARD, George Gray, Jr. (*b.* **1868)**
Some recent methods of intestinal anastomosis. New York: William Wood & Co., 1903. 24p. DNLM **00-6762**

WARD, George Gray, Jr. (*b.* **1868)**
Intestinal resection and end to end anastomosis. New York, 1903. 6p. DNLM **00-6763**

WARD, Henry B[ascom] (*b.* **1876)**
Precision in the determination of human parasites. [Chicago], 1903. 15p. 1 table. DNLM **00-6764**

WARD, James W[illiam] (*b.* **1861)**
Why I am a homoeopathic physician. Presidential address before the California State Homoeopathic Medical Society, May 10, 1900. [n. p.], 1900. 35p. DLC; NN; PPHa **00-6765**

WARD, James W[illiam] (*b.* **1861)**
The agnositic in medicine. Presidential address delivered at the sixty-sixth annual session of the American Institute of Homoeopathy, held at Pasadena, Cal., July 11, 1910. San Francisco: Murdock Press, 1910. 21p. DNLM; ICJ: NcD; PU **00-6766**

WARD, Nathan G.
The preparation of the patient for nose and throat operation under local anaesthesia. New York, 1903. 6p. DNLM **00-6767**

WARD, Ralph Francis (*b.* **1877)**
Severe ivy poisoning. New York, 1908. 6p. DNLM **00-6768**

WARD, Ralph Francis (*b.* **1877)**
Some surgical considerations of non-malignant ovaries. New York, 1910. 4p. DNLM **00-6769**

WARD, Samuel B[aldwin] (*b.* **1842)**
Acute ulcerative endocarditis. Albany, 1903. 17p. 2 charts. DNLM **00-6770**

WARD, Samuel B[aldwin] (*b.* **1842)**
Erythema and urticaria, with a condition resembling angeioneurotic oedema, caused only by exposure to the sun's rays. New York, 1905. 7p. DNLM **00-6771**

WARD, W[illiam] D[ouglas] (*b.* **1874)**
Appendicitis; a plea for complete operations in pus cases. New York, 1906. 16p. DLC; DNLM **00-6772**

WARE, Martin W[iener] (*b.* **1869)**
Gonorrhoeal rheumatism. New York, 1906. 6p. DNLM **00-6773**

WARE, Martin W[iener] (*b.* **1869)**
Plaster of Paris and how to use it. New York: Surgery Pub. Co., 1906. 88p. DLC; DNLM; NNNAM; PU **00-6774**

WARE, Martin W[iener] (*b.* **1869)**
The diagnosis of unilateral tuberculous nephrocystitis, with a report of six operative cases. New York, 1908. 16p. DNLM **00-6775**

WARE, Martin W[iener] (*b.* **1869)**
Plaster of Paris and how to use it . . . 2nd ed., rev. and enl. Illustrated with 90 original drawings. New York: Surgery Publishing Co., 1910. 99p. DLC; NN; NNC; PU **00-6776**

WARK, David
Restoring lost health by growing new bodies. New York: Adipogen Co., [1900]. 16p. DLC **00-6777**

WARK, David
Pulmonary tuberculosis. [The successful treatment of pulmonary tuberculosis. Scientific principles stated] [New York: D. Wark, 1909.] 27p. NN **00-6778**

WARNER, L[ouis] H[enry] (*b.* **1857)**
Phosphaturia and its treatment with phosphoglycerate of lime. New York, 1901. 11 l. DNLM **00-6779**

WARNER, L[ouis] H[enry] (*b.* **1857)**
The therapeutical effect of iodine, demonstrated by physiological action and pathological demonstration. St. Louis, 1901. 1 l. DNLM **00-6780**

WARNER, L[ouis] H[enry] (*b.* **1857)**
Citrophen, antipyretic and antineuralgic. [New York, 1901.] 4 l. DNLM **00-6781**

WARNER, L[ouis] H[enry] (*b.* **1857)**
The anaemia and chlorosis of women. New York, [1902, *vel subseq.*] 11p. 5 plates on 3 l. DNLM **00-6782**

WARNER, WILLIAM R., AND CO.
(Philadelphia & N.Y.C.)
New therapeutic reference book, for physicians and students, by William R. Warner. Philadelphia: W. R. Warner, 1900. 237p. ICJ; PPC **00-6783**

WARNER, WILLIAM R., AND CO.
(Philadelphia & N.Y.C.)
Epitome of prices current, makers of fine pharmaceuticals. Philadelphia: Wm. R. Warner, 1900. 96p. PPC **00-6784**

WARNER, WILLIAM R., AND CO.
(Philadelphia & N.Y.C.)
. . . Epitome of prices current. Standard pharmaceutical preparations comprising: sugar and gelatin coated pills and granules, . . . , elixirs, wines, syrups, glycerin suppositories, filled and empty capsules, etc. manufactured by Wm. R. Warner & Co. . . . Philadelphia, 1901. [unp.] ICJ **00-6785**

WARREN, George W[ashington] (*b.* **1863)**
. . . A compend of dental pathology and dental medicine; containing the most noteworthy points upon the subjects of interest to the dental student and a section on emergencies . . . 4th ed. . . . Philadephia: P. Blakiston's Son & Co., 1903. 180p., illus. DLC; ICJ; PPC; PU **00-6786**

WARREN, George W[ashington] (*b.* 1863)
Electricity and its application to dental mechanics. [Philadelphia, 1904?] 10p. PPHa **00-6787**

WARREN, George W[ashington] (*b.* 1863)
A manual of mechanical dentistry and metallurgy . . . 2nd ed., rev. and in parts rewritten, with one hundred and seventy-nine illustrations. Philadelphia: P. Blakiston's Son & Co., 1905. 262p. DLC; DNLM; PPC; PU **00-6788**

WARREN, Henry S[tanley] (*b.* 1873)
A case of acute osteomyelitis of the cervical spine. Boston, 1903. 5p. DNLM; MH **00-6789**

WARREN, Ina R[usselle], ed.
The doctor's window: poems by the doctor, for the doctor, and about the doctor. Buffalo, N.Y.: C. W. Moulton, 1900 [*c.* 1898]. 288p. DLC; MH; NIC; NN [Also, Chicago, 1904. 288p.] **00-6790**

WARREN, J[ohn] Collins, ed. (1842-1927)
The international text-book of surgery, by American and British authors; ed. by J. Collins Warren . . . and A. Pearce Gould. . . . Philadelphia: W. B. Saunders & Co., 1900. 2 v. col. plates. DLC; MBM; NNNAM; PPC **00-6791**

WARREN, J[ohn] Collins (1842-1927)
The influence of anaesthesia on the surgery of the nineteenth century . . . ; being the address of the president before the American Surgical Association, [1897] Boston: Priv. print., 1900. 30p. facsim., plates, ports. NcD[One hundred copies printed. Unnumbered.] **00-6792**

WARREN, J[ohn] Collins (1842-1927)
Surgical pathology and therapeutics . . . 2nd ed., with an appendix containing an enumeration of the scientific aids to surgical diagnosis, together with a series of sections on regional bacteriology. Philadelphia: W. B. Saunders & Co., 1900. 873p. 11 col. plates, diags. DLC; DNLM; NNNAM; PPC **00-6793**

WARREN, J[ohn] Collins (1842-1927)
The radical cure of hernia. Boston: Damrell & Upham, 1900. 11p. DNLM; MH **00-6794**

WARREN, J[ohn] Collins (1842-1927)
A review of recent studies on the nature and origin of cancer. Boston: Damrell & Upham, 1900. 31p. DNLM; MH **00-6795**

WARREN, J[ohn] Collins (1842-1927)
The surgery of the spleen. St. Louis, 1901. 31p. 1 plate. DNLM; MH **00-6796**

WARREN, J[ohn] Collins (1842-1927)
Malignant disease of the breast. Boston, 1901. 24p. 4 plates. DNLM; MH **00-6797**

WARREN, J[ohn] Collins, ed. (1842-1927)
The international text-book of surgery, by American and British authors; ed. by J. Collins Warren . . . and A. Pearce Gould . . . 2nd ed., thoroughly rev. . . . Philadelphia and London: W. B. Saunders & Co., 1902. 2 v. col. plates. DLC; OCIM; NNC; PU **00-6798**

WARREN, J[ohn] Collins (1842-1927) and Charles J. WHITE
The treatment of rhinophyma. St. Paul, 1903. 10p. 2 plates. DNLM; MH **00-6799**

WARREN, J[ohn] Collins (1842-1927)
The operative treatment of umbilical hernia. Boston, 1903. 15p. DNLM; MH **00-6800**

WARREN, J[ohn] Collins (1842-1927)
Clinical lecture on epithelioma at the Massachusetts General Hospital. Boston, 1904. 14p. DNLM; MH **00-6801**

WARREN, J[ohn] Collins (1842-1927)
The surgeon and the pathologist. A plea for reciprocity as illustrated by the consideration of the classification and treatment of benign tumors of the breast. Chicago, 1905. 19p. DNLM; MH **00-6802**

WARREN, J[ohn] Collins (1842-1927)
The new classification of benign tumors of the breast, with an illustrative case. Boston, 1906. 10p. 1 plate. DNLM; MH **00-6803**

WARREN, J[ohn] Collins (1842-1927)
Abnormal involution of the mammary gland, with its treatment by operation. Philadelphia, 1907. 15p. DNLM; MH **00-6804**

WARREN, J[ohn] Collins (1842-1927)
Address on disinfection before the Massachusetts Medical Society. [1908.] 4 l. DNLM; MH **00-6805**

WARREN, J[ohn] Collins (1842-1927)
Surgery in London at the beginning of the nineteenth century, as observed by an American surgeon of the old school [i.e., Dr. Edward Reynolds]. Boston: W. M. Leonard, 1910. 28p. 1 plate, 1 port. NN **00-6806**

[WARREN, Joseph] (1741-1775)
Monument to Joseph Warren: its origin, history and dedication, 1894-1904. Boston: Municipal Printing Office, 1905. 110p. MBM; MH **00-6807**

WARREN, Stanley P[erkins] (*b.* 1846)
Technique of labor in private practice. New York: William Wood & Co., 1902. 14p. DNLM; NNNAM **00-6808**

WARREN, Stanley P[erkins] (*b.* 1846)
The principles of obstetrics. A practical manual for the student and general practitioner. New York: William Wood & Co., 1903. 373p. DLC; DNLM; MBM; NNNAM **00-6809**

WARREN, Stanley P[erkins] (*b.* 1846)
The prevalence of puerperal septicemia in private practice at the present time, contrasted with that of a generation ago. New York: William Wood & Co., 1905. 16p. DNLM; NNNAM **00-6810**

WARREN, Stanley P[erkins] (*b.* 1846)
Some comments on Dr. Reynolds's paper. New York, 1908. 8p. DNLM **00-6811**

WARTHIN, Alfred S[cott] (1866-1931)
Accessory adrenal body in the broad ligament; adrenal of Marchand. New York: William Wood & Co., 1900. 9p. DNLM **00-6812**

WARTHIN, Alfred S[cott] (1866-1931)
Multiple traumatic hemorrhages of the liver associated with multiple pulmonary emboli of liver-cells and giant cells resembling bone-marrow cells. Philadelphia, 1900. 31p. DNLM
00-6813

WARTHIN, Alfred S[cott] (1866-1931)
A case of primary adenocarcinoma of the gallbladder with secondaries in both adrenals, melanosis of skin (Addison's disease?) vitiligo, and hypertrophy of the pancreas. Philadelphia, 1900. 28p. DNLM **00-6814**

WARTHIN, Alfred S[cott] (1866-1931)
Multiple primary neoplasms in one individual (spindle-cell sarcoma of fore-arm, adenocarcinoma of pylorus, myomata of stomach-wall); treatment with Cole's mixture. Philadelphia, 1901. 7p. DNLM **00-6815**

WARTHIN, Alfred S[cott] (1866-1931) and William A. SPITZLEY
Disappearing tumors. New York, 1901. 14p. DNLM
00-6816

WARTHIN, Alfred S[cott] (1866-1931)
Adenoma of both adrenals in the newborn; associated with retrogressive changes in the adrenals of Marchand. New York: E. B. Treat & Co., 1901. 16p. DNLM **00-6817**

WARTHIN, Alfred S[cott] (1866-1931)
The changes produced in the hemolymph glands of the sheep and goat by splenectomy, hemolytic poisons, and hemorrhage. Boston, 1902. 20p. DNLM **00-6818**

WARTHIN, Alfred S[cott] (1866-1931)
The pathology of pernicious anaemia. Philadelphia, 1902. 45p. DNLM **00-6819**

WARTHIN, Alfred S[cott] (1866-1931)
An American medical student: James Jackson, Jr., 1810-1833. Ann Arbor & Detroit, 1903. 14p. DNLM
00-6820

WARTHIN, Alfred S[cott] (1866-1931)
A blank book for autopsy protocols . . . 3rd ed. Ann Arbor, 1903. unp. DLC **00-6821**

WARTHIN, Alfred S[cott] (1866-1931)
On the development of hemolymph nodes in adipose tissue. Philadelphia, 1903.15p. DNLM **00-6822**

WARTHIN, Alfred S[cott] (1866-1931)
Pseudomelanosis of the haemolymph glands. Philadelphia, 1904. 6p. DNLM **00-6823**

WARTHIN, Alfred S[cott] (1866-1931)
The neoplasm theory of leukemia, with report of a case supporting this view. Philadelphia, 1904. 12p. DNLM
00-6824

WARTHIN, Alfred S[cott] (1866-1931)
Two cases of accessory pancreas; omentum and stomach. Ann Arbor & Detroit, 1904. 17p. DNLM
00-6825

WARTHIN, Alfred S[cott] (1866-1931) and Herbert S. OLNEY
Pulmonary streptothricosis; notes on a case with clinical picture of pulmonary tuberculosis; sputum containing an acid-resisting streptothrix; no tubercle bacilli. Philadelphia, 1904. 13p. DNLM **00-6826**

WARTHIN, Alfred S[cott] (1866-1931)
An experimental study of the effects of Röntgen rays upon the blood-forming organs. n. p., [1905?]. 12p. NN
00-6827

WARTHIN, Alfred S[cott] (1866-1931)
Primary basal-celled carcinoma of the appendix; report of a new case with some observations bearing upon its histogenesis. [Philadelphia], 1906. 8p. DNLM **00-6828**

WARTHIN, Alfred S[cott] (1866-1931)
Two cases of sudden death associated with hypertrophy of the thymus. One case with universal enlargement of the lymph nodes, the other without. [Philadellphia], 1906. 16p. DNLM
00-6829

WARTHIN, Alfred S[cott] (1866-1931)
A case of lymphatic leukaemia with histological picture resembling that of Hodgkin's disease. [Philadelphia], 1906. 10p. DNLM **00-6830**

WARTHIN, Alfred S[cott] (1866-1931)
Inflammation. . . . [New York: William Wood & Co., 1906.] 74p. ICJ; NN **00-6831**

WARTHIN, Alfred S[cott] (1866-1931)
Disseminated focal necroses due to tubercle bacilli (tuberculosis without tubercle formation). A preliminary report. [Philadelphia, 1907.] 4p. DNLM **00-6832**

WARTHIN, Alfred S[cott] (1866-1931)
Experimental ligation of splenic and portal veins, with the aim of producing a form of splenic anemia. [Philadelphia, 1907.] 4p. DNLM **00-6833**

WARTHIN, Alfred S[cott] (1866-1931)
An experimental study of effects of Roentgen rays upon the blood-forming organs, with especial reference to the treatment of leukemia. [Philadelphia, 1907.] 45p. 13 plates. DNLM
00-6834

WARTHIN, Alfred S[cott] (1866-1931)
Localized tuberculosis of the liver. (A preliminary report.) [Philadelphia, 1907.] 3p. DNLM **00-6835**

WARTHIN, Alfred S[cott] (1866-1931)
The changes produced in the kidneys by Roentgen irradiation. [Philadelphia], 1907. 11p. DNLM **00-6836**

WARTHIN, Alfred S[cott] (1866-1931)
A comparison of the value of Roentgen irradiation and the administration of arsenic in the treatment of leukaemia. Philadelphia: J. B. Lippincott Co., 1907. 15p. DNLM
00-6837

WARTHIN, Alfred S[cott] (1866-1931)
The organization of a state anti-tuberculosis association. Detroit, 1908. 4 l. DNLM **00-6838**

WARTHIN, Alfred S[cott] (1866-1931)
The University and the anti-tuberculosis campaign. [Ann Arbor, 1908.] 4p. DNLM **00-6839**

WARTHIN, Alfred S[cott] (1866-1931)
A blank book for autopsy-protocols . . . 10th ed. Ann Arbor: G. Wahr, 1908. 104p. DNLM **00-6840**

WARTHIN, Alfred S[cott] (1866-1931)
Acute pylephlebogenous miliary tuberculosis of the liver, with clinical picture of acute infectious jaundice; primary tuberculosis of mesenteric glands. [New York], 1909. 4p. DNLM **00-6841**

WARTHIN, Alfred S[cott] (1866-1931)
Hyperplasia of the hemolymph nodes. [Philadelphia], 1909. 8p. DNLM **00-6842**

WARTHIN, Alfred S[cott] (1866-1931)
The pathology of thymic hyperplasia and the status lymphaticus. New York, 1909. 2p1. DNLM **00-6843**

WARTHIN, Alfred S[cott] (1866-1931)
The needs of Michigan in the fight against tuberculosis. Detroit, 1909. 3 l. DNLM **00-6844**

WARTHIN, Alfred S[cott] (1866-1931)
Practical pathology; a manual of autopsy and laboratory technique for students and physicians . . . 2nd ed., rewritten and enl. . . . 55 figures. Ann Arbor: G. Wahr, 1910. 321p. illus. DLC; ICJ; PPC; PU **00-6845**

WARWICK, Francis James
First aid to the injured; plain and simple rules to be followed in cases of accident or emergency as well as in the first stages of illness. . . . Philadelphia: The Penn Publishing Co., 1904 [1903]. 235p. illus. DLC; MH; NN; PU **00-6846**

WASDIN, Eugene (1869-1911)
Yellow fever; its nature and cause. Chicago, 1900. 24p. DNLM **00-6847**

WASDIN, Eugene (1869-1911)
The etiology of yellow fever. Philadelphia, 1900. 9p. DNLM **00-6848**

WASDIN, Eugene (1869-1911)
Toxicity versus septicity in the infectious pathogenic bacteria. New York, 1900. 16p. DNLM **00-6849**

WASHBURN, Frederick A[ugustus] (*b.* 1869)
Open-air treatment of patients at the Massachusetts General Hospital and the Children's Hospital of Boston. [Boston], 1906. 16p. DNLM; MBM **00-6850**

WASHINGTON, D.C. FREEDMEN'S HOSPITAL
Course of nurse training at the Freedmen's Hospital, Washington, D.C. Approved by the Secretary of the Interior October 27, 1909. Washington: Government Printing Office, 1909. 6p. DLC **00-6851**

WASHINGTON, D.C. FREEDMEN'S HOSPITAL
Regulations of the Freedmen's Hospital, Washington, D.C. Approved by the Secretary of the Interior September 18, 1909. Washington: Government Printing Office, 1909. 67p. DLC **00-6852**

WASHINGTON POST-GRADUATE MEDICAL SCHOOL, WASHINGTON, D.C.
Schedule of clinics, laboratory work and lectures for the session of 1903. [Jan. to May.] [Washington, 1902.] 4 l. DNLM **00-6853**

WASHINGTON POST-GRADUATE MEDICAL SCHOOL, WASHINGTON, D.C.
Schedule of clinics, laboratory work and lectures of the Washington Post-Graduate Medical School. . . . [Washington, 1903.] [8]p. DLC **00-6854**

WASHINGTON, D.C. SIBLEY MEMORIAL HOSPITAL
Sibley Memorial Hospital. . . . [Washington, D.C.: Press of B. S. Adams, 1903?] [16]p. illus. DLC **00-6855**

WASHINGTON UNIVERSITY, ST. LOUIS, MO.
Quarterly Bulletin, Medical Department of Washington University, St. Louis. v. 2, nos. 2-4; v. 3-6; v. 7, no. 1, Oct. 1903-Dec., 1908. St. Louis, 1903-08. DNLM **00-6856**

WASSERMANN, A[ugust] von (1866-1925)
Immune sera haemolysins, cytotoxins, and precipitins; authorized translation by Charles Bolduan. New York: J. Wiley & Sons, 1904. 77p. DNLM; NNNAM; PPC; PU **00-6857**

WASSERMANN, A[ugust] von (1866-1925)
Several new points concerning the theory and practice of immunity. New York: A. R. Elliott Pub. Co., 1904. 6p. DNLM **00-6858**

WATERMAN, Moses W. (1849-1907)
A rational treatment for narcotic inebriety. . . . New York: The Trow Press, 1907. 148p. DLC; DNLM; ICJ; MH-M **00-6859**

WATERS, Bertram H[oward] (*b.* 1867)
The modern management of tuberculosis. New York, 1907. 8p. DNLM **00-6860**

WATERS, Yssabella
Visiting nursing in the United States; containing a directory of the orgnizations employing trained visiting nurses, with chapters on the principles, organization and methods of administration of such work. . . . New York: Charities Publication Committee, 1909. 367p. front. (map) plates, forms. DLC; ICJ; MH; NN **00-6861**

WATERS, Yssabella
Visiting nursing in the United States, containing a directory of the organizations employing trained visiting nurses . . . [2nd ed.]. New York: Charities Publication Committee, 1910? 377p. illus. DNLM; KU; NIC; PU **00-6862**

WATHEN, John R[oach] (*b.* 1872)
. . . Normal histology. A manual for students and practitioners. . . . illustrated with one hundred and fourteen engravings. Philadelphia and New York: Lea Bros. & Co., [1903]. 229p. DLC; DNLM; NNNAM; PPC **00-6863**

WATHEN, William H[udson] (1846-1913)
A brief report of some interesting surgical cases. Louisville, 1900. 16p. DNLM **00-6864**

WATHEN, William H[udson] (1846-1913)
Minimum requirements for admission to a medical college. Philadelphia, 1903. 9p. DNLM **00-6865**

WATHEN, William H[udson] (1846-1913)
Timely operation in primary appendicitis. New York, 1903. 10p. DNLM **00-6866**

WATHEN, William H[udson] (1846-1913)
Doctorate address. Relation of academic to medical education; the typical physician. Louisville, 1903. 11p. DNLM
00-6867

WATHEN, William H[udson] (1846-1913)
Intraligamentous and retroperitoneal tumors of uterus. [Philadelphia, 1904?] 8p. PPHa **00-6868**

WATKINS, Robert Lincoln (*b.* 1863)
Diagnosis by means of the blood; illustrated by 154 photomicrographs of specimens of blood, as observed in general practice, showing products that are found in definite diseases. . . . New York and London: The Physicians' Book Pub. Co., 1902. 388p. DLC; ICJ; MB; NN **00-6869**

WATKINS, Robert Lincoln (*b.* 1863)
Catechism of haematology. . . . New York and London: The Physicians' Book Publishing Co., 1908. 31p. DLC; ICJ; NNNAM **00-6870**

WATKINS, T[homas] J[ames] (*b.* 1863)
Vaginal section and drainage for pelvic abscess with report of cure. [New York, 1905.] 8p. DNLM; NN
00-6871

WATKINS, T[homas] J[ames] (*b.* 1863)
. . . Gynecology. . . . Chicago, Ill.: Manhattan School of Preventive Medicine and Home Hygiene, 1910. 8p. DLC; ICJ
00-6872

WATKINS, V[ictor] E.
Neurasthenia among blondes in the Southwest. [New York], 1905. 3p. DNLM; NN **00-6873**

WATSON, Francis S[edgwick] (1853-1942)
Some observations upon the value of the phloridzin test for estimating the functional capacity of the kidneys; renal sufficiency. Boston: Damrell & Upham, 1902. 14p. DNLM; MBM
00-6874

WATSON, Francis S[edgwick] (1853-1942)
Subparietal injuries of the kidney. Boston: Damrell & Upham, 1903. 49p. DNLM; MBM **00-6875**

WATSON, Francis S[edgwick] (1853-1942)
Diseases and surgery of the genito-urinary system, by Francis S. Watson . . . assisted by John H. Cunningham, Jr. . . . Philadelphia and New York: Lea & Febiger, 1908. 2 v. col. plates. DLC; DNLM; NNNAM; PPC **00-6876**

WATSON, Francis S[edgwick] (1853-1942)
A day with the specialists; or, Cured at last; a tragic farcelet. . . . New York: The Grafton Press, 1910. 51p. CtY-M; MH; PU ["One hundred copies of this book have been printed for private distribution."] **00-6877**

WATSON, Harry G. (*b.* 1869)
Syphilis communicated in assault and battery. New York, 1908. 6p. DNLM **00-6878**

WATSON, Harry G. (*b.* 1869)
A morning at Bier's clinic in Berlin. [Philadelphia], 1910. 4 l. illus. NN **00-6879**

WATSON, J[ames] K[enneth]
A handbook for nurses. American ed. under the supervision of A. A. Stevens. Philadelphia: W. B. Saunders & Co., 1900. 413p. DNLM; PPC: PPJ; PU **00-6880**

WATSON, John (1850-1907)
A doctor of the old school [*pseud.,* Ian MacLaren] with illustrations by Frederick C. Gordon. New York: Dodd, Mead & Co., 1900 [*c.* 1895]. 208p. DLC; NIC; NN; PU
00-6881

WATSON, Leigh F[estus] (*b.* 1884)
Local anaesthesia in general surgery. New York, 1910. 27p. DNLM; NN **00-6882**

WATTLES, Wallace D.
The new science of living and healing . . . with commentary by Elizabeth Towne. . . . Holyoke, Mass.: E. Towne, [1907]. 94p. DLC; MH **00-6883**

WATTLES, Wallace D.
The science of being well. . . . Holyoke, Mass.: Elizabeth Towne, 1910. 155p. front. (port.) DLC; MH
00-6884

WAUGH, William F[rancis] (1849-1918)
The diseases of the respiratory organs, acute and chronic; arranged in two parts and interleaved for supplemental notes. . . . Chicago: The Clinic Publishing Co., 1901. 146p. DLC; ICJ; IEN-M; PPHa **00-6885**

WAUGH, William F[rancis] (1849-1918)
The diseases of the respiratory organs, acute and chronic. Arranged in two parts. . . . Chicago: G. V. Engelhard & Co., 1901. 221p. DLC; ICRM; ICU; PU **00-6886**

WAUGH, William F[rancis] (1849-1918)
A textbook of alkaloidal therapeutics; being a condensed résumé of all available literature on the subject of the active principles added to the personal experience of the authors, by W. F. Waugh, M.D. and W. C. Abbott, M.D. . . . Chicago: The Clinic Publishing Co., 1904. 405p. DLC; ICRM; PPC; PPJ
00-6887

WAUGH, William F[rancis] (1849-1918)
A text-book of alkaloidal therapeutics; being a condensed résumé of all available literature on the subject of the active principles added to the personal experience of the authors, by W. F. Waugh, M.D., and W. C. Abbott, M.D., with the collaboration of E. M. Epstein, M.D. 2nd ed. Chicago: The Clinic Publishing Co., 1907. 477p. DLC; GU; IEN-M; PU
00-6888

WAUGH, William F[rancis] (1849-1918)
A text-book of alkaloidal practice; this new "treatment of the sick," with especial reference to the use of the active principles and other positive definite medicaments, not only contains the living essentials of Dr. Waugh's old book, whatever has stood the test of time and progress, but the very latest . . . in modern medicine. . . . By William F. Waugh, M.D. [and] Wallace C. Abbott, M.D. Chicago: The Clinic Publishing Co., 1907. 822p. DLC; ICRM; IEN-M; PU **00-6889**

WAUGH, William F[rancis] (1849-1918)
The treatment of the sick; a system of applied therapeutics; 3rd ed., rev., with additions. . . . Chicago, [1910?]. 546p. DLC; ICJ; IU-M; PU **00-6890**

WEAVER, B[enjamin] F[ranklin] (*b.* 1839)
Physical atlas, or, Practical family doctor book, containing 300 modern and up-to-date recipes for treating both general and special diseases. . . . Bucyrus, O.: The Author, 1902. 36p. DLC; DNLM; ICJ; OCIM **00-6891**

WEAVER, B[enjamin] F[ranklin] (*b.* 1839)
The lightning doctor; a self-diagnostician and practical doctor book for private families, students, and physicians . . . with thirty-two illustrations (four etchings and twenty-eight photo-engravings from life) and 1,554 modern and up-to-date recipes for treating both general and special diseases of men, women, and children. Akron, O., New York, [etc.]: The Saalfield Publishing Co., 1905. 484p. DLC; ICJ; NN
00-6892

WEAVER, B[enjamin] F[ranklin] (*b.* 1839)
Physical chart of pains, aches and tender spots. An up-to-date family doctor book. . . . With nine illustrations and 400 modern and up-to-date recipes for treating both general and special diseases of men, women, and children. Bucyrus, O.: Northern Ohio Publishing Co., 1907. 46p. DLC; DNLM; ICJ; NN **00-6893**

WEAVER, George H[owitt] (*b.* 1866)
Bacteriological studies of the skin and throat in cases of scarlatina. Philadelphia, 1903. 6p. DNLM
00-6894

WEAVER, George H[owitt] (*b.* 1866)
A study of streptococcus immunization [by] George H. Weaver and Ruth Tunnicliff. . . . Chicago, 1908. 18p. ICJ
00-6895

WEAVER, George H[owitt] (*b.* 1866)
The effects of injections of killed streptococci. . . . n. p., 1910. 5p. ICJ **00-6896**

WEAVER, H[enry] B[ascom] (1851-1914)
Immunity in tuberculosis; how shall we induce it? Asheville, 1900. 12p. DNLM **00-6897**

WEBB, Gerald Bertram (1871-1948)
Reports of two cases of cured Graves's disease. New York: A. R. Elliott, 1905. 6p. DNLM **00-6898**

WEBB, Walter D.
Appendicostomy and cecostomy in the treatment of chronic dysentery. [New York], 1910. 7p. DNLM
00-6899

WEBBER, Samuel Gilbert (1838-1926)
Additional contribution to cases of multiple sclerosis, with autopsies. [New York, 1905.] 5p. DNLM
00-6900

WEBSTER, David (*b.* 1842)
An operation for divergent strabismus. New York, 1900. 3p. DNLM **00-6901**

WEBSTER, David (*b.* 1842)
Enucleation of the eye. New York, 1900. 4p. DNLM
00-6902

WEBSTER, David (*b.* 1842) and Edgar S. THOMSON
A case of acute glaucoma with subhyaloid haemorrhage supervening upon uniocular retinitis albuminurica. New York, 1900. 6p. DNLM **00-6903**

WEBSTER, George W[ashington] (*b.* 1857)
Report of the curricula of American medical colleges. New York, 1904. 9p. DNLM; PPHa **00-6904**

WEBSTER, J[ohn] Clarence (1863-1950)
Human placentation. An account of the changes in the uterine mucosa and in the attached fetal structures, during pregnancy. Chicago: W. T. Keener & Co., 1901. 126p. 30 plates. DNLM; ICJ; OCIM; PU **00-6905**

WEBSTER, J[ohn] Clarence (1863-1950)
A text-book of obstetrics. Philadelphia: W. B. Saunders & Co., 1903. 767p. 11 plates. DNLM; ICJ; PPC; PU **00-6906**

WEBSTER, J[ohn] Clarence (1863-1950)
Some fundamental problems in obstetrics and gynecology. St. Louis, 1904. 18p. MB **00-6907**

WEBSTER, J[ohn] Clarence (1863-1950)
A text-book of diseases of women. Philadelphia & London: W. B. Saunders & Co., 1907. DNLM; NNNAM; PPC; PU
00-6908

WEBSTER, J[ohn] Clarence (1863-1950)
Harrington Lectures: progress in obstetrics and gynecology. Buffalo: University of Buffalo, 1910. 29p. DNLM; NN
00-6909

WEBSTER, Ralph W[aldo] (1873-1930)
A contribution to the physical analysis of the phenomena of absorption of liquids by animal tissues. Chicago, 1903. 32p. DNLM **00-6910**

WEBSTER, Ralph W[aldo] (1873-1930) and Waldemar KOCH
A laboratory manual of physiological chemistry. Chicago, 1903. 107p. DNLM; ICJ **00-6911**

WEBSTER, Ralph W[aldo] (1873-1930)
Modern conceptions of the metabolism of the diabetic. De Kalb, Ill, 1906. 7p. DNLM **00-6912**

WEBSTER, Ralph W[aldo] (1873-1930)
Metabolic aspects of over-feeding and of under-feeding. St. Louis, 1906. 15p. DNLM **00-6913**

WEBSTER, Ralph W[aldo] (1873-1930)
The pathology and treatment of nephritis. Philadelphia, 1907. 16p. DNLM **00-6914**

WEBSTER, Ralph W[aldo] (1873-1930)
Toxemia from the standpoint of perverted metabolism. Philadelphia, 1908. 9p. DNLM **00-6915**

WEBSTER, Ralph W[aldo] (1873-1930)
Value and limitations of blood examinations. Chicago, 1908. 11p. DNLM **00-6916**

WEBSTER, Ralph W[aldo] (1873-1930)
General observations on acute and chronic rheumatism. St. Louis, 1908. 14p. DNLM **00-6917**

WEBSTER, Ralph W[aldo] (1873-1930)
Diagnostic methods, chemical, bacteriological and microscopical. Philadelphia: P. Blakiston's Son & Co., 1909. 641p. 37 plates. DLC; DNLM; PPC; PU **00-6918**

WECHSELMANN, Wilhelm
The treatment of syphilis with salvarsan, by Sanitätsrat Dr. Wilhelm Wechselmann . . . with an introduction by Professor Dr. Paul Ehrlich. . . . Only authorized translation, by Abr. L. Wolbarst . . . with 15 textual figures and 16 coloured illustrations. New York: Rebman Co.; [etc., etc., 1910]. 175p. DLC; ICJ; MH-M; PU **00-6919**

WEEKS, John Elmer (1853-1949)
Pathology of the cervical sympathetic. Chicago, 1904. 10p. MB **00-6920**

WEEKS, John Elmer (1853-1949)
What stage in the development of the cataract, particularly senile cataract, is the most suitable for its removal by extraction? New York, 1907. 8p. DNLM **00-6921**

WEEKS, John Elmer (1853-1949)
A treatise on diseases of the eye . . . with 528 engravings and 25 full-page plates in color. New York and Philadelphia: Lea & Febiger, 1910. 944p. illus., 25 plates (part col.) DLC: ICJ; PPJ; PU **00-6922**

WEGENER, Hans (*b.* 1869)
We young men . . . ; the sexual problem of an educated young man before marriage; purity, strength and love. Introduction by Sylvanus Stall. Philadelphia, Pa.: The Vir Publishing Co.; [etc., etc., 1910]. 204p. DLC; PP; NN **00-6923**

WEIL, Henry
Puerperal sepsis. New York, 1909. 13p. DNLM **00-6924**

WEIL, Richard (1876-1917)
Clinical examination of the stools. New York, 1906. 18p. DNLM **00-6925**

WEINBURGH, Harry Bennett
Perfect health. An exhaustive treatise on natural laws that make and maintain perfect health and perfect human development. Written from experience—not theory. . . . New York: P. Eckler, [1903]. 330p. front. (port.). DLC; NN **00-6926**

WEINGARTEN, Fred[erick] S[eymour]
The influence of internal hemorrhage on chemical changes in the organism, with particular reference to protein catabolism, by Fred S. Weingarten in collaboration with Burrill B. Crohn. . . . New York, 1908. 37p. DLC; NN **00-6927**

WEINSTEIN, Harris (*b.* 1869)
The early diagnosis of gastric carcinoma. New York, 1906. 4p. DNLM; NN **00-6928**

WEINSTEIN, Harris (*b.* 1869)
Gastroptosis a causative factor of tachycardia. New York: A. R. Elliott Co., 1907. 4p. DNLM; NN **00-6929**

WEINSTEIN, Harris (*b.* 1869)
Silver nitrate in gastric diseases. New York, 1907. 7p. DNLM; NN **00-6930**

WEINSTEIN, Harris (*b.* 1869)
Treatment of chronic indigestion. New York, 1907. 6p. DNLM; NN **00-6931**

WEINSTEIN, Harris (*b.* 1869)
Neurasthenia ventriculi and gastroptosis. New York, 1908. 7p. DNLM; NN **00-6932**

WEINSTEIN, J[ulius] W[illiam]
Dr. Beard's theory in the crucible of test; an experimental study of the trypsin treatment in cancer. New York, 1908. 8p. DNLM; NN **00-6933**

WEINZIRL, John (1870-1935)
The action of a high, dry climate in the cure of tuberculosis. Albuquerque, N.M., 1908. 4p. DNLM **00-6934**

WEIR, Robert F[ulton] (1838-1927)
Perforating duodenal ulcers. New York, 1900. 47p. DNLM **00-6935**

WEIR, Robert F[ulton] (1838-1927)
Black-board headings used in the lectures on surgery, by Robert F. Weir . . . Edited by Abraham L. Wolbarst . . . and George Alexander Saxe . . . 2nd rev. ed. New York: Doughtery, 1901. 79p. NNC; PPC [1st ed., New York: Evening Post Job Print., 1898. 72p. DLC; DNLM] **00-6936**

WEIR, Robert F[ulton] (1838-1927)
An improved method of treating high-seated cancers of the rectum. New York, 1902. 13p. DNLM **00-6937**

WEIR, Robert F[ulton] (1838-1927)
A point in the technique of breast amputation for cancer. New York, 1906. 4p. DNLM **00-6938**

WEIR, William H[awksley] (*b.* 1870)
Torsion of a hydrosalpinx resulting in infarction. New York: William Wood & Co., 1901. 6p. DNLM **00-6939**

WEIR, William H[awksley] (*b.* 1870)
Rupture of the posterior wall of the cervix uteri without involvement of the external os, occurring during abortion at the fourth month; escape of the fetus through the laceration. New York, 1902. 3p. DNLM **00-6940**

WEIR, William H[awksley] (*b.* 1870)
A report in gynecological pathology. New York: William Wood & Co., 1902. 14p. DNLM **00-6941**

WEIR, William H[awksley] (*b.* 1870)
Eosinophilia in pelvic lesions and in the vermiform appendix. Philadelphia, 1903. 12p. DNLM **00-6942**

WEIR, William H[awksley] (*b.* 1870)
Subclavian thrombophlebitis following abdominal section. Cleveland, 1908. 5p. DNLM **00-6943**

WEISENBURG, T[heodore] Herman (1876-1934)
Partial paralysis of one upper limb, resulting from a vascular lesion of the lateral column and anterior born on the corresponding side of the spinal cord. n. p., 1903. 7p. DNLM **00-6944**

WEISENBURG, T[heodore] Herman (1876-1934)
Uremic hemiplegia with changs in the nerve cells of the brain and cord and recent primary degeneration of one central motor tract. Philadelphia, 1904. 9p. DNLM **00-6945**

WEISENBURG, T[heodore] Herman (1876-1934)
Further study on the sensory segmental zone of the umbilicus. n. p., 1904. 683. PU [with W. G. Spiller] **00-6946**

WEISENBURG, T[heodore] Herman (1876-1934)
Pseudobulbar palsy; report of three cases with necropsy and of three cases without necropsy. Philadelphia, 1905. 39p. DNLM **00-6947**

WEISENBURG, T[heodore] Herman (1876-1934)
Bulbar symptoms occurring with carcinoma of parts other than the nervous system, and resulting from intoxication. Philadelphia, 1905. 6p. DNLM **00-6948**

WEISENBURG, T[heodore] Herman (1876-1934)
The pathology of cerebellar tumors. [Nw York]: A. R. Elliott, 1905. 26p. DNLM **00-6949**

WEISENBURG, T[heodore] Herman (1876-1934)
Subdivision of the representation of cutaneous and muscular sensibility and of stereognosis in the cerebral cortex. n. p., 1906. 34p. DNLM **00-6950**

WEISENBURG, T[heodore] Herman (1876-1934)
Advances in the surgery of the nervous system considered from the standpoint of the neurologist. [New York], 1906. 18p. DNLM **00-6951**

WEISENBURG, T[heodore] Herman (1876-1934)
Hysteria simulating brain tumor, with a report of two cases. Philadelphia, 1906. 5p. DNLM **00-6952**

WEISENBURG, T[heodore] Herman (1876-1934)
Conjugate deviation of the eyes and head and disorders of the associated ocular movements in tumors and other lesions of the cerebrum. [Philadelphia, 1906.] 32p. DNLM
00-6953

WEISENBURG, T[heodore] Herman (1876-1934)
Carcinoma of the nervous system, with the report of eleven cases. n. p., 1906. 25p. PU **00-6954**

WEISENBURG, T[heodore] Herman (1876-1934)
Paraplegia dolorsa caused by vertebral carcinomata, spinal carus and multiple neuritis. n. p., 1906. 12p. PU **00-6955**

WEISENBURG, T[heodore] Herman (1876-1934)
Sensory and motor disturbances in parts above the distribution involved by definite organic lesions of the spinal cord. Philadelphia, 1907. 13p. DNLM **00-6956**

WEISENBURG, T[heodore] Herman (1876-1934)
Neurologic teaching in America; chairman's address before the section on nervous diseases, Chicago, 1908. Chicago, 1908. 14p. DNLM **00-6957**

WEISENBURG, T[heodore] Herman (1876-1934)
Meningism. Serous meningitis and hydrocephalus. . . . Philadelphia, 1908. 10p. DNLM **00-6958**

WEISMANN, August [Friedrich Leopold] (1834-1914)
On germinal selection as a source of definite variation. Transl. from the German by Thomas J. McCormack. 2nd ed. Chicago: Open Court Pub. Co., 1902. 87p. DNLM; ICJ; NIC; PPC
00-6959

WEISMANN, August [Friedrich Leopold] (1834-1914)
The germ-plasm, a theory of heredity . . . transl. by W. Newton Parker . . . and Harriet Rönnfeldt. . . . New York: C. Scribner's Sons, 1902. 477p. DLC; ICJ; MH; NN **00-6960**

WEISSE, Faneuil Dunkin (1842-1915)
Practical human anatomy; working-guide for students of medicine and a ready-reference for surgeons and physicians. 4th ed., "Atlas" form, by Faneuil D. Weisse. Illustrated by 222 lettered plates containing 321 figures. . . . New York: James T. Dougherty, 1900. [13]-31p. 222 plates. DLC; NN **00-6961**

WELCH, John Edgar
Normal human blood serum as a curative agent in hemophilia neonatorum; a preliminary report with suggestions for its use in other conditions. Philadelphia, 1910. 16p. DNLM
00-6962

[WELCH, Thomas B.]
Some plain facts regarding the teeth; with suggestions concerning their character; their treatment during eruption; their preservation and restoration to health when diseased. . . . Philadelphia: Printed by J. B. Lippincott Co., 1900. 73p. illus. DLC; PU [Text also in the phonetic alphabet.]
00-6963

WELCH, William H[enry] (1850-1934)
Argument against . . . the anti-vivisection bill. [1900.] 28p. DLC; MB **00-6964**

WELCH, William H[enry] (1850-1934)
Remarks on the present mild type of smallpox. Philadelphia, 1900. 18p. DNLM **00-6965**

WELCH, William H[enry] (1850-1934)
The material needs of medical education. [1900.] 10p. NN
00-6966

WELCH, William H[enry] (1850-1934)
Relations of laboratories to public health. [1900.] 28p. DLC
00-6967

WELCH, William H[enry] (1850-1934)
A course of lectures on pathology, by William H. Welch and Simon Flexner. Medical School, The Johns Hopkins Hospital. Baltimore, 1900 [*c.* 1899]. 280 l. MdBJ-W; NNC
00-6968

WELCH, William H[enry] (1850-1934)
The material needs of medical education. [Baltimore, 1900.] 10p. MH **00-6969**

[WELCH, William H(enry)] (1850-1934)
Contributions to the science of medicine, dedicated by his pupils to William Henry Welch on the 25th anniversary of his doctorate. Baltimore: Johns Hopkins Press, 1900. 1066p. ICJ; MB; NcU; NN [38 papers by Cushing, Mall, Hemeter, MacCallum, L. F. Barker, F. Sabin, T. S. Cullen, H. H. Young, S. Flexner, Halsted and others] **00-6970**

WELCH, William H[enry] (1850-1934)
The relation of Yale to medicine. New Haven, 1901. 35p. port. CtY-M; DNLM; PPJ **00-6971**

WELCH, William H[enry] (1850-1934)
The origin and aims of the new section of physiology and experimental medicine. [1903.] 6p. DLC
00-6972

WELCH, William H[enry] (1850-1934)
The origin and aims of the new section (K) of the physiology and experimental medicine of the American Association for the Advancement of Science; address delivered Dec. 29, 1902. Lancaster, Pa.: Press of the New Era Printing Co., 1906. 8p. DLC **00-6973**

WELCH, William H[enry] (1850-1934)
The unity of the medical sciences. [Chicago], 1906. 8p. DNLM
00-6974

WELCH, William H[enry] (1850-1934)
The endowment for medical research. [1906.] 7p. DLC
00-6975

WELCH, William H[enry] (1850-1934)
Some of the conditions which have influenced the development of American medicine, especially during the last century. . . . 1907. 20p. NNC **00-6976**

WELCH, William H[enry] (1850-1934)
The relation of the hospital to medical education and research. [1907.] 15p. DLC **00-6977**

WELCH, William H[enry] (1850-1934)
The interdependence of medicine and other sciences of nature. [Chicago], 1908. 15p. DNLM **00-6978**

WELCH, William H[enry] (1850-1934)
A consideration of the introduction of surgical anaesthesia. [Address delivered at the Massachusetts General Hospital on the sixty-second anniversary of Ether Day] Boston: The Barta Press, [1908]. 24p. DNLM; MB; NcD; NN
00-6979

WELCH, William H[enry] (1850-1934)
Fields of usefulness of the American Medical Association. Chicago, 1910. 20p. DNLM **00-6980**

WELCH, William H[enry] (1850-1934)
In honour of William H. Welch. 2 April, 1910. [Baltimore, 1910.] 57p. DLC; ICJ; MH; NN [Presentation of medallion to Dr. Welch. Includes poem for occasion by S. Weir Mitchell, and a cartoon by Max Broedel.] **00-6981**

WELCH, William M[iller] (*b.* 1837)
Acute contagious diseases by William M. Welch and Jay F. Schamberg. Illustrated with 109 engravings and 16 full-page plates. Philadelphia and New York: Lea Bros. & Co., 1905. 781p. DLC; IEN-M; NNNAM; PPC **00-6982**

WELKER, William H[enry]
A contribution to our knowledge of the effects of urinary preservatives on urinary analysis. New York, 1907. 3p. DNLM
00-6983

WELLMAN, Frederick C[reighton] (1871-1960)
Fatal case of blackwater fever supervening on amebic dysentery, and showing malarial parasites in the blood. Chicago, 1905. 3p. DNLM **00-6984**

WELLMAN, Frederick C[reighton] (1871-1960)
Relapsing fever; its occurrence in the Tropics and its relation to tick fever in Africa. Philadelphia, 1905. 11p. DNLM
00-6985

WELLMAN, Frederick C[reighton] (1871-1960)
Notes on the tropical diseases of the Angola highlands. New York: A. R. Elliott, 1905. 49p. DNLM
00-6986

WELLMAN, Frederick C[reighton] (1871-1960)
On Ornithodoros moubata, Murray: A disease-bearing African tick. 1905. 16p. DNLM **00-6987**

WELLMAN, Frederick C[reighton] (1871-1960)
The study of tropical medicine; its aim, its method, and its scope. [n. p.], 1905. 8p. DNLM
00-6988

WELLMAN, Frederick C[reighton] (1871-1960)
Report on the insanitary condition of various towns in the colony of Angola. New York, 1906. 4p. DNLM
00-6989

WELLMAN, Frederick C[reighton] (1871-1960)
Bite of the ombuta (Clotho arietans, Gray) treated with potassium permanganate; recovery. New York, 1906. 4p. DNLM **00-6990**

WELLMAN, Frederick C[reighton] (1871-1960)
The African poison test as observed in the Portuguese colony of Angola, West Africa. [n. p., 1906.] 11p. DNLM
00-6991

WELLMAN, Frederick C[reighton] (1871-1960)
Some medical plants of Angola, with observations on their use by natives of the province. Philadelphia, 1906. 20p. DNLM
00-6992

WELLMAN, Frederick C[reighton] (1871-1960)
Studies in tropical medicine. Philadelphia, 1906. 10p. DNLM
00-6993

WELLMAN, Frederick C[reighton] (1871-1960)
Interim report on trypanosomiasis in Portuguese Southwest Africa. Burlington, Vt., & New York, 1907. 13p. DNLM
00-6994

WELLMAN, Frederick C[reighton] (1871-1960)
Report on a peculiar disease of tropical Africa called "onyalai." [n. p.], 1907. 8p. DNLM **00-6995**

WELLMAN, Frederick C[reighton] (1871-1960)
List of the cutaneous affections observed in Angola, West Africa. St. Louis, [1907]. 16p. DNLM **00-6996**

WELLMAN, Frederick C[reighton] (1871-1960)
Clinical charts of a case of quartan malarial fever observed in West Africa, with commentary. New York, 1908. 7p. DNLM
00-6997

WELLMAN, Frederick C[reighton] (1871-1960)
Diseases in the Tropics. New Orleans, 1910. 47p. DNLM
00-6998

WELLMAN, Frederick C[reighton] (1871-1960)
A list of the tropical diseases observed in the region of San Francisco Bay. New York, 1910. 9p. DNLM
00-6999

WELLMAN, Frederick C[reighton] (1871-1960) and Edward von ADELUNG
A case of filarial hematochyluria treated after the method of Wherry and McDill with apparent recovery. Chicago, 1910. 8p. DNLM **00-7000**

WELLMAN, Frederick C[reighton] (1871-1960) and Finley M. EASTMAN
The relation of mosquitoes to filariasis in the region of San Francisco Bay. Chicago, 1910. 3p. DNLM
00-7001

WELLS, Charlotte Fowler
. . . Some account of the life and labors of Dr. Francois Joseph Gall, founder of phrenoloyy. . . . New York: Fowler & Wells Co.; [etc., etc., 1901] [*c.* 1896]. 154p. front., illus. (incl. ports.). DLC; ICJ; MB; NN **00-7002**

WELLS, David Washburn (*b.* 1862)
Sight and hearing of school children, examination of the public schools of Wellesley, Mass. [n. p., 1900.] 20p. DNLM
00-7003

WELLS, David Washburn (*b.* 1862)
Eye strain notwithstanding acute vision. Boston, 1901. 13p. DNLM **00-7004**

WELLS, David Washburn (*b.* 1862)
Eye strain from unbalanced muscles. Boston, 1902. 9p. DNLM
00-7005

WELLS, David Washburn (*b.* 1862)
Ocular analgesics. New York, 1903. 6p. DNLM
00-7006

WELLS, David Washburn (*b.* 1862)
The therapeutic value of training the fusion faculty with discussion by W. R. King. New York, 1904. 14p. DNLM
00-7007

WELLS, David Washburn (*b.* 1862)
A practical method of testing the sight and hearing of school children. Boston, 1904. 8p. DNLM **00-7008**

WELLS, David Washburn (*b.* 1862)
The problem of eye strain. New York, 1906. 9p. DNLM
00-7009

WELLS, David Washburn (*b.* 1862)
Psychology applied to medicine. Philadelphia: F. A. Davis Co., 1907. 141p. DLC; DNLM; PPC **00-7010**

WELLS, David Washburn (*b.* 1862)
The psychic element in the practice of medicine. Boston, 1907. 8p. DNLM **00-7011**

WELLS, H[arry] Gideon (1875-1943)
Studies in fat necrosis. Chicago, 1903. 27p. DLC; DNLM; ICJ; NN **00-7012**

WELLS, H[arry] Gideon (1875-1943)
. . . Studies in fat necrosis. . . . Chicago: The University of Chicago Press, 1903. 27p. DLC; MB; NIC; PPL
00-7013

WELLS, H[arry] Gideon (1875-1943)
Chemical pathology; being a discussion of general pathology from the standpoint of the chemical processes involved. . . . Philadelphia and London: W. B. Saunders & Co., 1907. 549p. DLC; DNLM; PPC; PU **00-7014**

WELLS, S. M.
The electropathic guide: prepared with particular reference to home practice; containing hints on the care of the sick, the treatment of disease, and the use of electricity: with full directions for treating over 100 diseases. . . . 10th ed. Rev. New York: J. H. Bunnell & Co., 1900. [*c.* 1895]. 96p. DLC; NN [First ed., and *vel subseq.*: The electropathic guide: prepared with particular reference to home practice; containing hints on the care of the sick, the treatment of disease, and the use of electricity; with full directions for treating over 100 cases. . . . Chicago: Horton & Leonard, 1867. 90p. DLC]
00-7015

WELLS, Walter A[ugustine] (*b.* 1870)
On sounding and irrigating the frontal sinus through the natural opening. St. Louis, 1901. 8p. DNLM **00-7016**

WELLS, Walter A[ugustus] (*b.* 1870)
Report of a case of thyroid gland tumor in the larynx. St. Louis, 1902. 12p. DNLM **00-7017**

WELLS, Walter A[ugustus] (*b.* 1870)
Medical education and the state. Chicago, 1902. 21p. DNLM
00-7018

WELLS, Walter A[ugustus] (*b.* 1870)
Two cases of objective aural tinnitus due to the action of tubo-palatal muscles. [Chicago], 1905. 11p. DNLM
00-7019

WELLS, Walter A[ugustus] (*b.* 1870)
A new septotome. [Chicago], 1905. 1 l. DNLM
00-7020

WELLS, Walter A[ugustus] (*b.* 1870)
The intranasal route in operating upon the nasal accessory sinuses. [St. Louis], 1905. 19p. DNLM
00-7021

WELLS, Walter A[ugustus] (*b.* 1870)
The choice of operation in the treatment of maxillary sinus suppuration. St. Louis, 1906. 20p. DNLM
00-7022

WELLS, Walter A[ugustus] (*b.* 1870)
Button twelve years in external auditory canal. [n. p., 1906.] 1 l. DNLM **00-7023**

WELLS, Walter A[ugustus] (*b.* 1870)
Some clinical considerations of frontal sinusitis. [Richmond, 1907.] 12p. DNLM **00-7024**

WELLS, Walter A[ugustus] (*b.* 1870)
Invading the labyrinth. St. Louis, 1907. 4p. DNLM
00-7025

WELLS, Walter A[ugustus] (*b.* 1870)
Aural vertigo and Ménière's syndrome. New York, 1907. 12p. DNLM **00-7026**

WELLS, Walter A[ugustus] (*b.* 1870)
Remarks on diphtheria, croup and allied affections, with special reference to intubation. Washington, 1907. 15p. DNLM
00-7027

WELLS, Walter A[ugustus] (*b.* 1870)
The significance of vertigo occurring in connection with diseases of the ear. St. Louis, 1970. 6p. DNLM
00-7028

WELLS, Walter A[ugustus] (*b.* 1870)
The voice as affected by general conditions. Richmond, 1908. 16p. DNLM **00-7029**

WELLS, Walter A[ugustus] (*b.* 1870)
Diseases of the ear complicating measles and scarlatina. Richmond, 1909. 14p. DNLM **00-7030**

WELLS, Walter A[ugustus] (*b.* 1870)
Danger signals in inflammation of the ear. New York, 1909. 12p. DNLM **00-7031**

WELLS, Walter A[ugustus] (*b.* 1870)
On the various affections of the voice and their local causation. St. Louis, 1909. 12p. DNLM
00-7032

WELLS, Walter A[ugustus] (*b.* 1870)
Suppuration of the anthrum of Highmore. New York, 1910. 11p. DNLM **00-7033**

WELLS, Walter A[ugustus] (*b.* 1870)
The hygienic, economic, and sociologic aspect of the throat. St. Louis, 1910. 15p. DNLM **00-7034**

WELLS, William H[ughes] (1859-1919)
. . . Compend of gynecology . . . 3rd ed., rev., enl., with 145 illustrations. Philadelphia: P. Blakiston's Son & Co., 1903. 293p. DLC; MH-M; PPC; PU **00-7035**

WELLS, William H[ughes] (1859-1919)
. . . Compend of gynecology . . . 4th ed., rev. and enl., with 153 illustrations. Philadelphia: P. Blakiston's Son & Co., 1910. 290p. illus. DLC; ICU; NNNAM; PPC **00-7036**

WELTMER, Ernest
The practice of suggestive therapeutics; a manual of the theory and technic of the practice of suggestive therapeutics, with a brief study of the most important auxiliary disciplines; for the use of students and practitioners of suggestive therapeutics. . . . Nevada, Mo.: The Weltmer Institute of Suggestive Therapeutics Co., 1910? 655p. illus, col. plates. DLC **00-7037**

WELTMER, S[idney] A[bram] (*b.* 1858)
Suggestion simplified. [Nevada, Mo., 1900.] 117p. front. (port.) pl. DLC **00-7038**

WELTMER, S[idney] A[bram] (*b.* 1858)
The real man, by Prof. S. A. Weltmer. . . . Nevada, Mo., 1901. 46p. port. DLC **00-7039**

WELTMER, S[idney] A[bram] (*b.* 1858)
Regneration; a discussion of the sex question, from a new and scientific standpoint. . . . Nevada, Mo.: Southwest Mail Printing Co., [1901?]. 126p. front. (port.) DLC **00-7040**

WELTMER, S[idney] A[bram] (*b.* 1858)
Regeneration; a scientific discussion of the sex principle. . . . Rev. and enl. . . , 24th ed., 132nd thousand. Inspirational section added. . . . [Nevada, Mo.: Weltmer Institute of Suggestive Therapeutics Co., 1908.] 156p. port. DLC **00-7041**

WENTWORTH, A[rthur] H[oward] (*b.* 1864)
A consideration of the principal objections to "section teaching," together with some of its advantages. Boston: Damrell & Upham, 1900. 4p. DNLM **00-7042**

WENTWORTH, A[rthur] H[oward] (*b.* 1864)
A system of clinical instruction; for simultaneous instruction in small sections of a large number of students. Boston, 1900. 4p. DNLM **00-7043**

WENTWORTH, A[rthur] H[oward] (*b.* 1864)
The association of anaemia with chronic enlargement of the spleen. Boston, 1901. 67p. DNLM **00-7044**

WENTWORTH, A[rthur] H[oward] (*b.* 1864)
The importance of milk analysis in infant feeding. Boston: Damrell & Upham, 1902. 9p. DNLM **00-7045**

WENTWORTH, A[rthur] H[oward] (*b.* 1864)
A consideration of the etiology and dietetic treatment of infantile atrophy. Chicago, 1905. 20p. DNLM **00-7046**

WENTWORTH, A[rthur] H[oward] (*b.* 1864)
A description of "Pfeiffer's disease" (glandular fever), with a report of two cases. Boston, 1905. 7p. DNLM **00-7047**

WENTWORTH, A[rthur] H[oward] (*b.* 1864)
A study of the metabolism of atrophic infants and children. Chicago, 1905. 27p. DNLM **00-7048**

WENTWORTH, A[rthur] H[oward] (*b.* 1864)
A case of acute yellow atrophy of the liver in a child five years of age. New York, 1906. 8p. DNLM **00-7049**

WENTWORTH, A[rthur] H[oward] (*b.* 1864)
The cause of infantile atrophy deduced from a study of secretion in normal and atrophic infants. Chicago, 1907. 20p. DNLM **00-7050**

WENTWORTH, A[rthur] H[oward] (*b.* 1864)
The estimation of chlorids in the stomach contents from normal and from atrophic infants. Chicago, 1910. 11p. DNLM **00-7051**

WENTWORTH, A[rthur] H[oward] (*b.* 1864)
The absorption of fat by the intestines in infantile atrophy. Boston, 1910. 3p. DNLM **00-7052**

WENTWORTH, A[rthur] H[oward] (*b.* 1864)
The utilization of milk-fat by an atrophic infant. Chicago, 1910. 7p. DNLM **00-7053**

WEST, Charles I. (*b.* 1868)
Re-displacement in adjusted Colles' deformity. [Philadelphia], 1910. 4 l. DNLM **00-7054**

WEST, Hamilton Atchison (1859-1903)
Therapeutics of the glycerophosphates. New York, 1902. 8p. DNLM **00-7055**

WESTBROOK, Frank Fairchild (1868-1918)
Rabies in Minnesota. St. Paul, Minnesota. 1900. 10p. DLC **00-7056**

WESTBOOK, Frank Fairchild (1868-1918)
Problems in the laboratory study of diphtheria. Detroit: W. M. Warren, 1903. 13p. DNLM **00-7057**

WESTBROOK. Frank Fairchild (1868-1918)
The relationship of the Minnesota State Board of Health to water supply. St. Paul, 1904. 9p. DNLM **00-7058**

WESTBROOK, Frank Fairchild (1868-1918)
Co-ordinated specialism in public health work. Chicago, 1905. 19p. DNLM **00-7059**

WESTBROOK, Frank Fairchild (1868-1918)
Diphtheria infection in Minnesota. Recent experiences with the disease in school children and in institutional epidemics. Chicago, 1905. 11p. DNLM **00-7060**

WESTBROOK, Frank Fairchild (1868-1918)
Cooperation of state and local sanitary officers in the prevention and management of outbreaks of infectious diseases. Albany, 1905. 23p. DNLM **00-7061**

WESTBROOK, Frank Fairchild (1868-1918)
Correlation of medical teaching. Philadelphia, 1906. 12p. DNLM **00-7062**

WESTBROOK, Frank Fairchild (1868-1918)
The public health laboratory; its function and relation to general medicine and modern social and industrial activity. Philadelphia, 1906. 13p. DNLM **00-7063**

WESTERN RESERVE UNIVERSITY. MEDICAL DEPARTMENT. CLEVELAND, OHIO
Annual catalogues for the sessions 1901-02 to 1911-12. With announcements for 1902-03 to 1912-13. Cleveland, 1902-13. DNLM **00-7064**

WESTLAND, Albert (1853-1915)
Tocology for mothers; a medical guide to the care of their health, and the management of children. American reprint ed. Prepared for publication by E. B. Foote, Jr. New York: Murray Hill Publishing Co., 1901. 292p. DLC; DNLM; NNNAM; PPC [*vel subseq.*] **00-7065**

WESTLAND, Albert (1853-1915)
Tocology for mothers: a medical guide to the care of their health and the management of children. American reprint edition prepared for publication. . . . By E. B. Foote, Jr. New York: Murray Hill Publishing Co., 1902. 1244p., illus. DLC; DNLM; MH; NN [Issued with E. B. Foote, New plain home talk on love, marriage and parentage] **00-7066**

WETHERILL, Henry Emerson (*b.* 1871)
Blood, urine, feces and moisture. A book of tests. Philadelphia: C. P. Pilling & Sons, [1904]. 7 l. 5 plates. DNLM [Test papers in pockets.] **00-7067**

WETHERILL, Henry Emerson (*b.* 1871)
Hygromedry. Philadelphia: W. E. Johnson & Co., 1906. 82p. DNLM; ICJ; PPC; PU **00-7068**

WETTERSRAND, Otis G[eorge] (*b.* 1845)
Hypnotism and its application to practical medicine. . . . Authorised transl. (from the German ed.) by Henrik G. Petersen . . . together with medical letters on hypno-suggestion by Henrik G. Petersen. New York: G. P. Putnam's Sons, 1901 [*c.* 1897]. 186p. diags. DLC; MH; NIC; NN **00-7069**

WHARTON, Henry R[edwood] (1853-1925)
The practice of surgery; a treatise on surgery for the use of practitioners and students, by Henry R. Wharton . . . and B. Farquhar Curtis . . . 3rd ed. Philadelphia and London: J. B. Lippincott Co., 1902. 1241p. col. plates. DLC; DNLM; PPC; PU **00-7070**

WHARTON, Henry R[edwood] (1853-1925)
Minor surgery and bandaging; including the treatment of fractures and dislocations, the ligation of arteries, amputations, excisions and resections, intestinal anastomosis, operations upon nerves and tendons, tracheotomy, intubation of the larynx, etc. . . . 5th ed., enl., and thoroughly rev. . . . Philadelphia and New York: Lea Bros. & Co., 1902. 621p. DLC; ICJ; NNNAM; PPC **00-7071**

WHARTON, Henry R[edwood] (1853-1925)
Minor and operative surgery, including bandaging . . . 6th ed., enl. and thoroughly rev., with 532 illustrations. Philadelphia and New York: Lea Bros. & Co., 1905. 650p. DLC; DNLM; PPC; PU **00-7072**

WHARTON, Henry R[edwood] (1853-1925)
Minor and operative surgery including bandaging . . . 7th ed., enl. and thoroughly rev., with 555 illustrations. Philadelphia and New York: Lea & Febiger, 1909. 683p. CtY-M; DLC; DNLM; PPC **00-7073**

WHEATE, Justus M.
Some unpublished observations on endemic neuritis, with a review of the researches and opinions of some recent investigators. New York, 1907. 34p. DNLM; NNNAM **00-7074**

WHEATLAND, Marcus Fitzherbert (*b.* 1868)
The value of electricity in gynecological work of the general practitioner. New York, 1902. 7p. DNLM **00-7075**

WHEATON, Clarence L. (*b.* 1873)
The climatic treatment of tuberculosis, with special reference to Colorado. [Philadelphia], 1905. 8p. DNLM **00-7076**

WHEATON, Clarence L. (*b.* 1873)
Sanatoria in the United States and Canada for the treatment of tuberculosis. Chicago, [1906]. 8 l. DNLM **00-7077**

WHEATON, Clarence L. (*b.* 1873)
Integument atrophy, a sign of diagnostic importance in early pulmomary tuberculosis; preliminary report. Chicago, 1910. 1 l. DNLM **00-7078**

WHEELER, Alexander (*d.* 1903) and William R. JACK
Handbook of medicine and therapeutics. 2nd ed., revised and enlarged by William R. Jack. New York: William Wood & Co., 1903. 512p. DNLM; ICJ; NNNAM; PPC **00-7079**

WHEELER, Alexander (*d.* 1903) and William R. JACK
Handbook of medicine and therpeutics. 3rd ed., revised and enlarged by William R. Jack. New York: William Wood & Co., 1908. 512p. NNNAM; PPJ; PPC; PU **00-7080**

WHEELER, Marianna (*b.* 1856)
The baby, his care and training. . . . New York and London: Harper & Bros., 1901. 183p. front., illus., plates. DLC; ICJ; MH; NN **00-7081**

WHEELER, Marianna (*b.* 1856)
Plain hints for busy mothers . . . illustrated by F. M. Miller. New York: E. B. Treat & Co., 1903. 200p. DLC: NN **00-7082**

WHEELER, William I[reland] De Courcy (1879-1945)
Student's handbook of operative surgery. New York: William Wood & Co., 1906. 300p. DNLM; ICJ; NNNAM; PU **00-7083**

WHEELOCK, Kent Kane (*b.* 1857)
Ocular symptoms of gout, illustrated by clinical reports. New York: A. R. Elliott Pub. Co., 1905. 6p. DNLM **00-7084**

WHELPLEY, Henry Milton (1861-1926)
Therapeutic terms for pharmacists and physicians. 2nd ed., rev. and enl. St. Louis: The Author, 1900. 89p. ICJ
00-7085

WHELPLEY, Henry Milton (1861-1926)
A few notes on the microscope in the drug store. [St. Louis, 1900.] 1 l. DNLM **00-7086**

WHELPLEY, Henry Milton (1861-1926)
New wine in old bottles. [St. Louis, 1902.] 2 l. DNLM
00-7087

WHELPLEY, Henry Milton (1861-1926)
A sample examination for the average state board of pharmacy. [St. Louis, 1903?] fol. DNLM; ICJ
00-7088

WHELPLEY, Hnery Milton (1861-1926)
How can the pharmacopoeia be made more popular? [St. Louis, 1903?] 1 l. DNLM; ICJ **00-7089**

WHELPLEY, Henry Milton (1861-1926)
A duty pharmacists owe their unregistered apprentices. [St. Louis, 1903?] 1 galley sheet. DNLM; ICJ
00-7090

WHELPLEY, Henry Milton (1861-1926)
Suggestions for the use of board of pharmacy members in preparing and conducting their examinations. [St. Louis, 1903?] 1 galley sheet. DNLM; IJC **00-7091**

WHELPLEY, Henry Milton (1861-1926)
The metric system in medical colleges. [St. Louis, 1903?] 1 l. DNLM; ICJ **00-7092**

WHELPLEY, Henry Milton (1861-1926)
A course in microscopical technology for colleges of pharmacy. [Philadelphia, 1903?] 3p. DNLM; ICJ
00-7093

[Ma] WHINNEY, Elgin
A series of lectures on special pathology and therapeutics delivered to the senior class, Northwestern University Dental School. Session 1901-1092. . . . Chicago, 1902. 317p. ICJ
00-7094

[Ma] WHINNEY, Elgin
Oral pathology and therapeutics; a systematic presentation of the subject from the standpoint of modern therapeutics. With 116 illustrations. . . . New York: The Consolidated Dental Mfg. Co.; London: C. Ash & Sons (Limited), 1905. 233p. DLC; ICJ; NNNAM; PU **00-7095**

WHIPPLE, George C[handler] (1866-1924)
The microscopy of drinking water. 2nd ed., revised. New York: J. Wiley & Sons, 1905. 323p. 19 plates. DNLM; MH; NNNAM; PU **00-7096**

WHIPPLE, George C[handler] (1866-1924)
The value of pure water. New York: J. Wiley & Sons, 1907. 84p. DNLM; MH; NNNAM **00-7097**

WHIPPLE, George C[handler] (1866-1924)
Typhoid fever; its causation, transmission and prevention; with an introductory essay by William T. Sedgwick. 1st ed. New York: J. Wiley & Sons, 1908. 407p. DNLM; ICJ; NNNAM; PU
00-7098

WHIPPLE, George C[handler] (1866-1924)
Stream pollution and sanitation of natural ice; an address. . . . New York: Natural Ice Association of America, [191-?] 8p. NIC **00-7099**

WHIPPLE, George Hoyt (*b.* 1878)
The pathology of blackwater fever. Mobile, 1910. 6p. DNLM
00-7100

WHIPPLE, Guy Montrose
. . . Questions in school hygiene. . . . Syracuse, N.Y.: C. W. Bardeen, 1909. 88p. DLC; MH; NIC; NN
00-7101

WHIPPLE, Leander Edmund (*d.* 1916)
The philosophy of mental healing; a practical exposition of natural restorative power. . . . 3rd ed. New York: The Metaphysical Publishing Co., 1901. 234p. DLC; ICJ; NN
00-7102

WHIPPLE, Leander Edmund (*d.* 1916)
The philosophy of mental healing; a practical exposition of natural restorative power . . . 4th ed. New York: The Philosophic Co., 1902. 234p. NN **00-7103**

WHIPPLE, Leander Edmund (*d.* 1916)
Mental healing . . . 5th ed.—rev. and enl., with portrait of the author. New York: The Metaphysical Publishing Co., 1905. 280p. DLC; NN **00-7104**

WHIPPLE, Leander Edmund (*d.* 1916)
Practical health. . . . New York: The Metaphysical Publishing Co., 1907. 316p. NN **00-7105**

WHIPPLE, Leander Edmund (*d.* 1916)
Mental healing . . . 6th ed. . . . New York: Metaphysical Publishing Co., [etc.], 1907. 280p. CtY-M; DNLM; NN; PPC
00-7106

WHITACRE, Horace J. (*b.* 1869)
Notes on the ear. New York, 1900? 11p. illus. DNLM
00-7107

WHITACRE, Horace J. (*b.* 1869)
Notes on the larynx and brain. New York, 1900. 50p. illus. DNLM **00-7108**

WHITACRE, Horace J. (*b.* 1869)
The pathology and treatment of diabetic gangrene of the lower extremity. New York, 1905. 23p. DNLM
00-7109

WHITACRE, Horace J. (*b.* 1869)
Scopolamine-morphine-chloroform anaesthesia. New York, 1906. 15p. DNLM **00-7110**

WHITALL, James Dawson (*b.* 1883)
Case of a sesamoid bone of the knee. New York, 1910. 2 l. DNLM **00-7111**

WHITALL, James Dawson (*b.* 1883)
Report of a case of pelvic peritonitis complicated by post-operative hysteria. New York, 1910. 3p. DNLM
00-7112

WHITE, Charles J[ames] (*b.* 1868)
The role of the staphylococcus in skin diseases. Boston, 1901. 14p. MB **00-7113**

WHITE, Charles J[ames] (*b.* 1868)
The clinical study of four hundred and eighty-five cases of nail disease. Boston, 1902. 6p. DNLM **00-7114**

WHITE, Charles J[ames] (*b.* 1868)
Colloid degeneration of the skin. New York, 1902. 9p. DNLM **00-7115**

WHITE, Charles J[ames] (*b.* 1868)
Erythrodermie pityriasique en plaques disséminées. New York, 1903. 6p. 1 plate. DNLM **00-7116**

WHITE, Charles J[ames] (*b.* 1868)
Recurrent, progressive, bullous dermatitis in an hysterical subject. [New York, 1903.] 14p. 1 plate. DNLM **00-7117**

WHITE, Charles J[ames] (*b.* 1868)
Fordyce's disease. New York, 1905. 18p. 2 plates. DNLM **00-7118**

WHITE, Charles J[ames] (*b.* 1868)
Vegetable parasites of the skin and modern methods of culture. Boston, 1905. 12p. DNLM **00-7119**

WHITE, Charles J[ames] (*b.* 1868)
The evolution of a case of mycosis fungoides under the influence of Roentgen rays. New York, 1906. 16p. 5 plates. DNLM **00-7120**

WHITE, Charles J[ames] (*b.* 1868)
Some statistics of indigestion in dermatological patients. Boston, 1907. 6p. DNLM **00-7121**

WHITE, Charles J[ames] (*b.* 1868)
Syringocystoma. New York, 1907. 10p. 4 plates. DNLM **00-7122**

WHITE, Charles J[ames] (*b.* 1868)
The evolution of a case of mycosis fungoides under the influence of Roentgen rays. Boston, 1907. 22p. plates, chart. MB **00-7123**

WHITE, Charles S[tanley] (*b.* 1877)
Iodized catgut. New York, 1904. 4p. DNLM **00-7124**

WHITE, Charles S[tanley] (*b.* 1877)
The necessity of a reliable sign of complete anaesthesia. New York, 1904. 4p. DNLM **00-7125**

WHITE, Charles S[tanley] (*b.* 1877)
The relation of conception and birth to season and hour. New York: William Wood & Co., 1905. 6p. DNLM **00-7126**

WHITE, Charles S[tanley] (*b.* 1877)
A case of foreign body in the rectum. [New York], 1905. 2p. DNLM **00-7127**

WHITE, Charles S[tanley] (*b.* 1877)
Cerebral contusion. New York, 1908. 12p. DNLM **00-1728**

WHITE, Courtland Y[ardley] (1872-1938)
Blood in infancy and childhood. . . . [n. p., 1901.] 36p. PU **00-7129**

WHITE, Courtland Y[ardley] (1872-1938)
Observations of blood changes following celiotomy. Philadelphia, 1901. 16p. DNLM; PU **00-7130**

WHITE, Courtland Y[ardley] (1872-1938) and William PEPPER
Granular degeneration of the erythrocyte. Philadelphia, 1901. 8p. 1 plate. DNLM; PU **00-7131**

WHITE, Courtland Y[ardley] (1872-1938)
Further studies of granular degeneration of the erythrocyte. [n. p., 1902.] 8p. PU **00-7132**

WHITE, Courtland Y[ardley] (1872-1938)
Karyokinesis in the macroblast. Philadelphia, 1903. 8p. DNLM; PU **00-7133**

WHITE, Courtland Y[ardley] (1872-1938)
Report of a case of chronic acetanilla poisonina, with marked alterations in the blood. [n. p., 1905.] 10p. PU **00-7134**

WHITE, Courtland Y[ardley] (1872-1938)
Methods of clinical examinations: embodying the practical course given to the third year students of the University of Pennsylvania. [Philadelphia, 1905?] 40p. PU [Alternate pages blank.] **00-7135**

WHITE, Courtland Y[ardley] (1872-1938)
Diagnosis by means of the formed elements of the blood. Philadelphia, 1906. 8p. DNLM; PU **00-7136**

WHITE, Courtland Y[ardley] (1872-1938)
Sarcoma of the large intestine. [n. p., 1907.] 22p. DNLM; PU **00-7137**

WHITE, Franklin W[arren] (*b.* 1869)
Observations on milk coagulation and digestion. Boston, 1900. 13p. 1 plate. DNLM **00-7138**

WHITE, Franklin W[arren] (*b.* 1869) and Maynard LADD
Whey-cream modification in infant feeding. Philadelphia, 1901. 17p. DNLM **00-7139**

WHITE, Franklin W[arren] (*b.* 1869)
An apparent case of diphtherial infection from well persons carrying diphtheria bacilli. Boston, 1901. 5p. DNLM **00-7140**

WHITE, Franklin W[arren] (*b.* 1869) and Howard H. SMITH
Heart complications in diphtheria. A clinical study of 946 cases. Boston, 1904. 25p. DNLM **00-7141**

WHITE, Franklin W[arren] (*b.* 1869)
The after-effects of diphtheria on the heart. Chicago, 1905. 15p. DNLM **00-7142**

WHITE, Franklin W[arren] (*b.* 1869)
Achylia gastrica. [Boston, 1906.] 28p. DNLM **00-7143**

WHITE, Franklin W[arren] (*b.* 1869)
Cancer of colon. Boston, 1907. 13p. DNLM **00-7144**

WHITE, Franklin W[arren] (*b.* 1869)
Value of tests for invisible hemorrhage in diagnosis and treatment of diseases of the digestive organs. Chicago, 1907. 29p. DNLM **00-7145**

WHITE, George Burbidge
An important advance in iron therapy. St. Louis, 1904. 7p. DNLM **00-7146**

WHITE, James C[larke] (1833-1916)
Case of Brocq's érythrodermie pityriasique en plaques disséminées. New York, 1900. 12p. DNLM **00-7147**

WHITE, James C[larke] (1833-1916)
Dermatitis venenata; a supplemental list. Read before the 27th annual meeting of the American Dermatological Association, Washington, D.C., May 12-14, 1903. [Boston], 1903. 16p. DNLM **00-7148**

WHITE, James C[larke] (1833-1916)
Meralgia paresthetica. New York, 1904. 4p. DNLM **00-7149**

WHITE, James C[larke] (1833-1916)
Some notes concerning domestic remedies formerly used in skin diseases. New York, 1904. 6p. DNLM **00-7150**

WHITE, James W[illiam] (1826-1891)
Taking impressions of the mouth. . . . Taking the bite by W. Storer How. To which is added a catalogue of impression trays, bite-plates, materials and appliance. . . . 6th ed. Philadelphia: The S. S. White Dental Mfg. Co., 1902. 120p. ICJ; MdU-D; PPC; PU [*vel subseq.*] **00-7151**

WHITE, James W[illiam] (1826-1891)
Taking impressions of the mouth; to which is added a catalog of impression trays, articulators, materials and appliances. [8th ed.] Philadelpia, 1908. 76p. DNLM; ICJ; MdU-D; PPC [*vel subseq.*] **00-7152**

WHITE, J[ames] William (1850-1916)
Genito-urinary surgery and venereal diseases. By J. William White . . . and Edward Martin. . . . Illustrated with two hundred and forty-three engravings and seven colored plates. 4th ed. Philadelphia, [etc.]: J. B. Lippincott Co., [1900]. 1061p. CtY-M; DLC; DNLM; PPC **00-7153**

WHITE, J[ames] William (1850-1916)
Two cases of interscapulo-thoracic amputation. Philadelphia, 1900. 12p. DNLM **00-7154**

WHITE, J[ames] William (1850-1916)
The topical treatment of focal and Jacksonian epilepsy. Philadelphia, 1901. 12p. DNLM **00-7155**

WHITE, J[ames] William (1850-1916)
Genito-urinary surgery and venereal diseases, by J. William White . . . and Edward Martin . . . illustrated with two hundred and forty-four engravings and seven colored plates. 5th ed. Philadelphia and London: J. B. Lippincott Co., 1902. 1068p. DLC; DNLM; IEN-M; PU **00-7156**

WHITE, J[ames] William (1850-1916)
Genito-urinary surgery and venereal diseases, by J. William White . . . and Edward Martin . . . illustrated with three hundred engravings and fourteen colored plates. 6th ed. Philadelphia and London: J. B. Lippincott Co., [1905]. 1002p. DLC; DNLM; OCIM; PPC **00-7157**

WHITE, J[ames] William (1850-1916)
Genito-urinary surgery and venereal diseases, by J. William White . . . and Edward Martin . . . illustrated with three hundred engravings and fourteen colored plates. 7th ed. Philadelphia and London: J. B. Lippincott Co., [1906]. 1076p. DLC; DNLM; NNNAM; PU **00-7158**

WHITE, J[ames] William (1850-1916)
Genito-urinary surgery and venereal diseases. by J. William White . . . and Edward Martin . . . illustrated with three hundred engravings and fourteen colored plates. 8th ed. Philadelphia and London: J. B. Lippincott Co., [1907]. 1076p. DLC; DNLM; MH-M; PPC **00-7159**

WHITE, J[ames] William (1850-1916)
Cryptogenetic streptococcus infection with persistent cutaneous eruption, enlargement of the lymphatic glands and fever suggesting syphilis. n. p., 1908. 18p. PU **00-7160**

WHITE, J[ames] William (1850-1916)
Genito-urinary surgery and venereal diseases, by J. William White . . . and Edward Martin . . . illustrated with three hundred engravings and fourteen colored plates. 9th ed. Philadelphia and London: J. B. Lippincott Co., [1910]. 1092p. DLC; DNLM; NNC; PPJ **00-7161**

WHITE, J[ames] William (1850-1916)
Rules governing the treatment of appendicitis: clinical lecture delivered at the hospital of the University of Pennsylvania. [1910?] 13p. PU **00-7162**

WHITE, John Vernon (*b.* 1858)
Diet in tuberculosis. New York, 1907. 7p. DNLM **00-7163**

WHITE, John Vernon (*b.* 1858)
A few facts concerning the causes of failures in adenoidectomies. New York, 1910. 7p. DNLM **00-7164**

WHITE, Joseph H[ill] (*b.* 1859)
Fallacy to quarantine against freight. New Orleans, 1905. 1 sheet. DNLM **00-7165**

WHITE, Joseph H[ill] (*b.* 1859)
A partial résumé of the prophylaxis of tropical disease. New York, 1907. 15p. DNLM **00-7166**

WHITE, Joseph H[ill] (*b.* 1859)
Yellow fever and the mosquito. [Washington, 1908.] 12p. DLC **00-7167**

WHITE, Leon Edward (*b.* 1867)
Resection of the nasal septum, with report of fifteen cases. Boston, 1904. 14p. DNLM **00-7168**

[WHITE, L. M.]
The old druggist's medical recipe book; or, Fifty choice recipes by an old druggist. . . . Bloomsburg, Penn.: L. M. White, 1901? [*c.* 1894]. 31p. DLC **00-7169**

WHITE, Mark Johnston (*b.* 1875)
Pathological characters, diagnosis and epidemiology of bubonic plague. New York, 1905. 36p. DNLM; NNNAM **00-7170**

WHITE, S. S. DENTAL MANUFACTURING CO. (PHILADELPHIA)
Descriptive list of teeth of S. S. White's manufacture. Philadelphia, 1901? 36p. PPHa [commentary by Charles James Essig, 1841-1901] **00-7171**

WHITE, S. S. DENTAL MANUFACTURING CO. (PHILADELPHIA)
The selection and adaption of porcelain teeth, with a catalogue of porcelain teeth manufactured by the S. S. White Dental Mfg. Co., Philadelphia [*c.* 1903]. 174p. illus. DLC; ICJ **00-7172**

WHITE, S. S. DENTAL MANUFACTURING CO. (PHILADELPHIA)
A catalog of the world's premium porcelain teeth, showing all the molds, classified for ready comparison. Together with . . . special papers for prosthetic dentists. Philadelphia, [1905]. 196p. illus. DLC; ICJ **00-7173**

WHITE, Theodore H[arrison] (*b.* 1875)
. . . Dr. Theodore H. White's higher courses and complete system of occult science. A correspondence course in spiritualism, hypnotism, personal magnetism, mental healing, magnetic healing, planetary readings and white and black art . . . 3rd ed. Baltimore, Md., 1905. 208p. illus. DLC; MH; NN **00-7174**

WHITE, William A[lanson] (1870-1937)
The definition of insanity. New York, 1906. 13p. DNLM **00-7175**

WHITE, William A[lanson] (1870-1937)
Outlines of psychiatry. . . . New York: The Journal of Nervous and Mental Disease Publishing Co., 1907. 232p. DLC; ICJ; NN; PPC **00-7176**

WHITE, William A[lanson] (1870-1937)
Expert testimony and the alienist. New York, 1908. 16p. DNLM **00-7177**

WHITE, William A[lanson] (1870-1937)
The theory of the complex. St. Louis, 1909. 15p. DNLM **00-7178**

WHITE, William A[lanson] (1870-1937)
Outlines of psychiatry. 2nd ed., revised and enlarged. New York: The Journal of Nervous and Mental Disease Publishing Co., 1909. 232p. DLC; ICJ; NN; PU **00-7179**

WHITE, William A[lanson] (1870-1937)
Some thoughts on heredity. Brooklyn, 1909. 8p. DLC; NN **00-7180**

WHITE, William A[lanson] (1870-1937)
The theory, methods, and psychotherapeutic value of psychoanalysis. St. Louis, 1910. 15p. DLC; NN **00-7181**

WHITE, William A[lanson] (1870-1937)
. . . Mental mechanisms. . . . New York: The Journal of Nervous and Mental Disease Publishing Co., 1910. 151p. CtY-M; DLC; NN; PU **00-7182**

WHITE, William A[lanson] (1870-1937)
. . . Outlines of psychiatry . . . 3rd ed., rev. and enl. New York: The Journal of Nervous and Mental Disease Publishing Co., 1910. 272p. illus., diags. DLC; MH-M; NNNAM; PU **00-7183**

WHITE, William Charles (*b.* 1874) and F. PROESCHER
On the presence of spirochaeta in pseudoleucaemia, acute lymphatic leucaemia, and lymphosarcoma. New York, 1908. 8p. DNLM **00-7184**

WHITEHEAD, Richard Henry (1865-1916)
The anatomy of the brain; a text-book for medical students . . . illustrated with forty-one engravings. Philadelphia, New York, [etc.]: F. A. Davis Co., 1901. 96p., illus. DLC; MH-M; NNNAM; PU **00-7185**

WHITEHEAD, Richard Henry (1865-1916)
Evolution of medical education in America. Charlottesville, 1907. 12p. PP **00-7186**

WHITEHEAD, William H. (*b.* 1855)
Gonorrhea; a rational, rapid and efficient remedy; with later remarks by Dr. Whitehead. Detroit, 1903. 13p. DNLM **00-7187**

WHITEIS, W. R.
The correction of nasal deformities. Iowa City: Republican Printing, 1901. 29p. DLC **00-7188**

WHITESIDE, George S[hattuck] (*b.* 1873)
Twenty cases of acute gonorrheal urethritis treated with injections of one per cent argyrol. St. Paul, 1903. 4p. DNLM **00-7189**

WHITESIDE, George S[hattuck] (*b.* 1873)
A case of gumma of the Fallopian tube. [Boston, 1903.] 6p. DNLM **00-7190**

WHITESIDE, George S[hattuck] (*b.* 1873)
The Casper-Hirschmann demonstration and photographic cystoscope. Boston, 1904. 5p. 1 plate. DNLM **00-7191**

WHITESIDE, George S[hattuck] (*b.* 1873)
The measurements of the trigone. Portland, Oreg., 1904. 8p. DNLM **00-7192**

WHITESIDE, George S[hattuck] (*b.* 1873)
Teaching cystoscopy. New York, 1904. 6p. DNLM **00-7193**

WHITESIDE, George S[hattuck] (*b.* 1873)
Concerning genito-urinary tuberculosis, with the report of five cases. Portland, Oreg., 1905. 7p. DNLM **00-7194**

WHITESIDE, George S[hattuck] (*b.* 1873)
The care and treatment of the urinary function in locomotor ataxia. Portland, Oreg., 1905. 4p. DNLM **00-7195**

WHITESIDE, George S[hattuck] (*b.* 1873)
Some untoward results of perineal prostatectomy. New York, 1905. 16p. DNLM **00-7196**

WHITESIDE, George S[hattuck] (*b.* 1873)
What should we teach the public regarding venereal disease? Chicago, 1906. 7p. DNLM **00-7197**

WHITESIDE, George S[hattuck] (*b.* 1873)
The importance of functional diagnosis in renal disease. Portland, Oreg., 1906. 7p. DNLM **00-7198**

WHITING, Arthur J[ohn] (1865-1941)
Aids to medical diagnosis. New York: William Wood & Co., 1907. 152p. CtY-M; DNLM; ICJ; NNNAM
00-7199

WHITING, Frederick
The modern mastoid operation . . . illustrated by twenty-five half-tone and twenty-three key plates made from original drawings. Philadelphia: P. Blakiston's Son & Co., 1905. 353p. illus. 25 plates (incl. front.), fold. tab., diags. CtY-M; DLC; DNLM; PPC **00-7200**

WHITMAN, Royal (1857-1946)
Clinical lessons in orthopaedic surgery . . . to the students of the College of Physicians and Surgeons of Columbia University. Ed. by George Alexander Saxe and Abraham L. Wolbarst. New York: James T. Dougherty, 1900. 107p. CtY-M; DLC; NNC; NNNAM **00-7201**

WHITMAN, Royal (1857-1946)
A treatise on orthopaedic surgery. . . . Illustrated with four hundred and forty-seven engravings. Philadelphia and New York: Lea Bros. & Co., 1901. 650p. DLC; DNLM; NNNAM; NNU-M **00-7202**

WHITMAN, Royal (1857-1946)
A treatise on orthopedic surgery . . . 2nd ed., rev. and enl., illustrated with five hundred and seven engravings. Philadelphia and New York: Lea Bros. & Co., 1903. 848p. DLC; DNLM; MdBJ-W; PPC **00-7203**

WHITMAN, Royal (1857-1946)
A treatise on orthopedic surgery . . . 3rd ed., rev. and enl. Illustrated with five hundred and fifty-four engravings. Philadelphia and New York: Lea Bros. & Co., 1907. 871p. DLC; DNLM; NBM; PU **00-7204**

WHITMAN, Royal (1857-1946)
A treatise on orthopedic surgery . . . 4th ed., rev. and enl., illustrated with six hundred and one engravings. Philadelphia and New York: Lea & Febiger, 1910. 908p. CtY-M; DLC; DNLM; MBM **00-7205**

WHITNEY, Charles M[elville] (*b.* 1862)
The etiology and modern methods of treatment of chronic urethritis. Boston, 1904. 21p. DNLM
00-7206

WHITNEY, Charles M[elville] (*b.* 1862)
The etiology and diagnosis of spermatocele, with a report of three cases. New York, 1907. 23p. 2 plates. DNLM; NNNAM
00-7207

WHITNEY, E[dward] L. (*b.* 1870) and Clyde A. CLAPP
Urine changes in pregnancy and puerperal eclampsia. New York, 1903. 60p. DNLM; NNNAM **00-7208**

WHITNEY, E[dward] L. (*b.* 1870) and Clyde A. CLAPP
A laboratory manual of clinical pathology and pharmacology. By E. L. Whitney and C. A. Clapp. Baltimore: G. W. King Print Co., 1907. 103p. illus. CtY-M; DLC [Blank leaves for notes interleaved with text] **00-7209**

WHITNEY, William F[iske] (1850-1921)
Statistics of cancer in Massachusetts. [Boston, 1900.] 23p. MB **00-7210**

WHITNEY, William F[iske] (1850-1921)
The alleged increase of cancer in Massachusetts. Boston, 1901. 34p. DNLM; MBM **00-7211**

WHITNEY, William F[iske] (1850-1921)
A comparative study of the death rates for the state of Massachusetts for the years, 1850, 1875, 1900. [Boston, 1904.] 12p. MH **00-7212**

WHITNEY, William F[iske] (1850-1921)
A study of the birth-rates, general death-rates, and death-rates from cancer for the New England States for the year 1900. Boston, 1905. 8p. DNLM **00-7213**

WHITNEY, William F[iske] (1850-1921)
Varicose veins of the papilla of the kidney. A cause for persistent hematuria. n. p., [1908]. 8p. MH
00-7214

WHITNEY, William F[iske] (1850-1921)
The Warren Anatomical Museum of the Harvard Medical School and the arrangement of its collection. [Boston?], 1910. 18p. plate. MB; NNC **00-7215**

WHITTAKER, N. T.
Christian science, is it safe? Boston: J. H. Earle, 1900. 32p. DLC; MH **00-7216**

WHITWORTH, A[lbert] J[ames] (*b.* 1858)
Bed chamber secrets; or, The revelations of a doctor. By a retired physician, surgeon and specialist. . . . [McComb, Miss.: Press of the Journal, 1910.] 192p. illus. DLC
00-7217

WHITWORTH, A[lbert] J[ames] (*b.* 1858)
The Hot Springs specialist, by A. J. Whitworth . . . assisted by J. M. Byrd . . . giving, in plain English, the treatment and prescriptions in full, used for many years by these two physicians and surgeons; the knowledge gained by experience in their life-time study and treatment of acute and chronic diseases. . . . [Memphis: Press of S. C. Toof & Co., 1910.] 189p. ports. DLC **00-7218**

WIDE, Anders G[ustaf] (*b.* 1854)
Hand-book of medical and orthopedic gymnastics. . . . With a frontispiece, and 94 illustrations in the text. Fourth revised edition in English. New York and London: Funk & Wagnalls Co., 1909. 373p. DLC; ICJ; PPHa; PP
00-7219

WIEDER, Henry S. (*b.* 1881)
Attempted suicide by potassium cyanide. Detroit, Mich., 1904. 3p. DNLM **00-7220**

WIEDER, Henry S. (*b.* 1881)
Brain injury. 1. Loss of one quarter of brain substance with consciousness and ability to talk retained until death. 2. Fracture of the skull with porencephalia. Philadelphia, 1904. 4p. DNLM **00-7221**

WIEDER, Henry S. (*b.* 1881)
Intrahepatic gall-bladder. Philadelphia, 1905. 9p. DNLM
00-7222

WIEDER, Henry S. (*b.* 1881) and Harold L. SPRINGER
Uraemia with pericarditis; clinical and pathological reports. New York, 1905. 4p. DNLM **00-7223**

WIEDER, Henry S. (*b.* 1881) and Harold L. SPRINGER
Tuberculous meningitis with congenital stricture of the rectum. New York, 1905. 4p. DNLM **00-7224**

WIEDER, Henry S. (*b.* 1881)
Sarcoma of the eyelid, with the report of a case in an infant seven weeks old. New York, 1907. 11p. DNLM **00-7225**

WIEDER, Henry S. (*b.* 1881)
Treatment of local infections. Detroit, Mich., 1907. 16p. DNLM **00-7226**

WIEDER, Henry S. (*b.* 1881)
A primer on the administration of ether. Detroit, Mich., 1907. 15p. DNLM **00-7227**

WIEDER, Henry S. (*b.* 1881)
Regeneration of bone. Philadelphia, 1907. 176p. DNLM **00-7228**

WIENER, Alfred (*b.* 1865)
Some remarks on the drainage method in the treatment of acute middle-ear disease. New York, 1907. 11p. DNLM **00-7229**

WIENER, Alfred (*b.* 1865)
Report upon three interesting cases of sinusitis associated with serious eye complications. New York, 1908. 10p. DNLM **00-7230**

WIENER, Alfred (*b.* 1865)
Case of acute mastoiditis with some unusual features. Chicago, 1908. 8p. DNLM **00-7231**

WIENER, Alfred (*b.* 1865)
Chronic otitis media purulenta. New York, 1908. 6p. DNLM **00-7232**

WIENER, Joseph (1828-1904)
Executor's sale. Catalogue of the library of the late Dr. Joseph Wiener. To be sold at acution, Monday, Tuesday and Wednesday, May 22, 23, 24, 1905. New York: Merwin-Clayton Sales Co., 1905. 90p. NN **00-7233**

WIENER, Joseph (1828-1904)
The diagnosis and treatment of prostatic hypertrophy. New York, 1907. 12p. DNLM **00-7234**

WIENER, Joseph (1828-1904)
General surgical considerations of joint and bone tuberculosis. New York, 1908. 12p. DNLM **00-7235**

WIGGERS, Carl J[ohn] (1883-1963)
The relations of physiology to dentistry. . . . Opening lecture in physiology before the junior class of the Department of Dentistry, University of Michigan. Philadelphia, 1909. 4p. PU **00-7236**

WIGGERS, Carl J[ohn] (1883-1963)
Studies in inaccessible internal hemorrhage. Chicago, 1909. 20p. DNLM **00-7237**

WIGGERS, Carl J[ohn] (1883-1963)
The prognostic significance of pulse-pressure changes during hemorrhage. Chicago, 1910. 11p. DNLM **00-7238**

WIGGERS, Carl J[ohn] (1883-1963)
A brief text of physiology for dental, pre-medical, and college students. . . . 47 illustrations. Ann Arbor: G. Wahr, [1910]. 207p. diags. DLC; ICJ; PU **00-7239**

WIGGIN, Frederick H[olme] (1853-1911)
President's address; the past and present needs of the medical profession. New York, 1903. 16p. DNLM **00-7240**

WIGGIN, Frederick H[olme] (1853-1911)
Abdominal pain of intestinal origin. New York, 1904. 11p. DNLM **00-7241**

WIGGIN, Frederick H[olme] (1853-1911)
Some practical points in abdominal surgery, with special reference to a simple technic for appendicectomy and intestinal anastomosis. Philadelphia, 1904. 25p. DNLM **00-7242**

WIGGIN, Twing Brooks (*b.* 1865)
Lectures on general pathology . . . [n. p., 1901.] 116p. DLC; DNLM; ICJ; NN **00-7243**

WIGGINS, John H. (1854-1907)
The untrained nurse; her legitimate field and her opportunity for self-improvement. New York, 1907. 8p. DNLM **00-7244**

WIGGINS, Theodore C. (*b.* 1855)
Some results following the use of the magnetic wave. New York, 1908. 4 l. DNLM **00-7245**

WIGHT, Jarvis Sherman, Jr. (*b.* 1874)
Acute primary dilatation of the heart; report of a case. New York, 1906. 7p. DNLM **00-7246**

WIGHT, Jarvis Sherman, Jr. (*b.* 1874)
Excision of the wrist joint; report of a case. New York, 1907. 9p. DNLM **00-7247**

WIGHT, Jarvis Sherman, Jr. (*b.* 1874)
Postoperative treatment of malignant disease of the buccal cavity. New York, 1907. 5p. DNLM **00-7248**

WILBERT, Martin I[nventius] (1865-1916)
John Michael Maisch, an ideal pharmacist. . . . Philadelphia, 1903. 26p. illus., ports. DLC; PPAmP; PPG **00-7249**

WILBERT, Martin I[nventius] (1865-1916)
John Morgan; the founder of the first medical school and the originator of pharmacy in America. Philadelphia, 1901. 15p. port. DNLM; PPAmP; PHi; PU **00-7250**

WILBERT, Martin I[nventius] (1865-1916)
College of pharmacy degrees. New York, 1905. 11p. DNLM **00-7251**

WILBUR, Cressy L[ivingston] (1865-1928)
A uniform classification for health statistics. [Lansing, 1900.] 1 l. DLC **00-7252**

WILBUR, Cressy L[ivingston] (1865-1928)
The collection and registration of vital statistics. Lansing, Mich., 1904. 6p. DNLM **00-7253**

WILBUR, Cressy L[ivingston] (1865-1928)
The international classification; its advantages, defects, and deficiencies. New York, 1908. 16p. DNLM
00-7254

WILCOX, Reynold W[ebb] (1856-1931)
The treatment of influenza in adults. New York, 1900. 7p. DLC; DNLM **00-7255**

WILCOX, Reynold W[ebb] (1856-1931)
Internal antisepsis. New York, 1900. 14p. DLC; DNLM
00-7256

WILCOX, Reynold W[ebb] (1856-1931)
Belladonna vs. scopolia. New York, 1901. 8p. DLC; DNLM
00-7257

WILCOX, Reynold W[ebb] (1856-1931)
A review of the progress of therapeutics for the preceding 12 months. New York, 1901. 12p. DLC; DNLM
00-7258

WILCOX, Reynold W[ebb] (1856-1931)
A review of the progress of therapeutics for the last twelve months. New York, 1902. 22p. DLC; DNLM
00-7259

WILCOX, Reynold W[ebb] (1856-1931)
Purinemia; a clinical study. Philadelphia, 1904. 14p. DLC; DNLM **00-7260**

WILCOX, Reynold W[ebb] (1856-1931)
The present status of iron therapy. St. Louis, 1904. 8p. DLC; DNLM **00-7261**

WILCOX, Reynold W[ebb] (1856-1931)
A manual of fever nursing. . . . Philadelphia: P. Blakiston's Son & Co., 1904. 236p. DLC; DNLM; PPC; PU
00-7262

WILCOX, Reynold W[ebb] (1856-1931)
Pharmacology and therapeutics . . . 6th ed., based on the 5th ed. of White and Wilcox's "Materia medica and therapeutics." Philadelphia: P. Blakiston's Son & Co., 1905. 1010p. DLC; DNLM; NNNAM; PU **00-7263**

WILCOX, Reynold W[ebb] (1856-1931)
The newer preparations of bismuth. New York, 1905. 8p. PPHa **00-7264**

WILCOX, Reynold W[ebb] (1856-1931)
Modern use of synthetics. New York, 1905. 12p. PPHa
00-7265

WILCOX, Reynold W[ebb] (1856-1931)
Materia medica and pharmacy . . . 6th ed., based on the 5th ed. of White and Wilcox's "Materia medica and therapeutics." Philadelphia: P. Blakiston's Son & Co., 1905. 624p. DLC; OCLloyd; PPC; PU **00-7266**

WILCOX, Reynold W[ebb] (1856-1931)
Modern iron therapy. Baltimore, 1906. 8p. DNLM
00-7267

WILCOX, Reynold W[ebb] (1856-1931)
Purinemia. A clinical study. New York, 1906. 12p. PPHa
00-7268

WILCOX, Reynold W[ebb] (1856-1931)
The treatment of disease; a manual of practical medicine. . . . Philadelphia: P. Blakiston's Son & Co., 1907. 911p. DLC; DNLM; NNNAM; PPC **00-7269**

WILCOX, Reynold W[ebb] (1856-1931)
The treatment of disease; a manual of practical medicine . . . 2nd ed., rev. Philadelphia: P. Blakiston's Son & Co., 1908 [1907]. 932p. DLC; DNLM; MBM; PU
00-7270

WILCOX, Reynold W[ebb] (1856-1931)
Materia medica and pharmacy . . . 7th ed., rev. Philadelphia: P. Blakiston's Son & Co., 1907. 490p. DLC; DNLM; OCLloyd; PPC **00-7271**

WILCOX, Reynold W[ebb] (1856-1931)
Pharmacology and therapeutics . . . 7th ed., rev., with index of symptoms and diseases. Philadelphia: P. Blakiston's Son & Co., 1907. 885p. DLC; ICRM; NNNAM; PU
00-7272

WILCOX, Reynold W[ebb] (1856-1931)
A manual of fever nursing . . . 2nd ed., rev. . . . Philadelphia: P. Blakiston's Son & Co., 1908. 229p. DLC; DNLM; PPC; PPJ **00-7273**

WILCOX, Reynold W[ebb] (1856-1931)
The therapeutics of old age. New York, 1909. 17p. NN
00-7274

WILCOX, Reynold W[ebb] (1856-1931)
The treatment of disease; a manual of practical medicine . . . 3rd ed., thoroughly rev. and enl. Philadelphia: P. Blakiston's Son & Co., 1910. 1023p. illus. (charts). DLC; ICJ; NNNAM; PU **00-7275**

WILCOX, Sidney F[reeman]
Surgery of childhood. . . . New York and Philadelphia: Boericke & Runyon, 1909. 395p. DLC; MBM; PPC; PPHa
00-7276

WILCOX, Starling S[ullivant] (*b.* 1864)
. . . Essentials of genito-urinary and venereal diseases, arranged in the form of questions and answers; prepared especially for students of medicine. . . . Philadelphia and London: W. B. Saunders & Co., 1906. 313p. DLC; DNLM; NNNAM; PPC
00-7277

WILCOX, Starling S[ullivant] (*b.* 1864)
Lectures on venereal diseases. Columbus, O.: Lawrence Press Co., 1906? 164p. DLC; ICJ **00-7278**

WILCOX, Starling S[ullivant] (*b.* 1864)
. . . Essentials of genito-urinary and venereal diseases, arranged in the form of questions and answers, prepared especially for students of medicine . . . 2nd ed., thoroughly rev. Philadelphia and London: W. B. Saunders & Co., 1909. 321p. DLC; DNLM; PPC; PPJ **00-7279**

WILDER, Alexander (1823-1908)
History of medicine. A brief outline of medical history and sects of physicians, from the earliest historic period; with an extended account of the new schools of the healing art in the nineteenth century, and especially a history of the American eclectic practice of medicine, never before published . . . 1st thousand. New Sharon, Me.: New England Eclectic Publishing Co., 1901. 946p. port. DLC; DNLM; MBM; NNNAM
00-7280

WILDER, Alexander (1823-1908)
History of medicine. A brief outline of medical history from the earliest historic period with an extended account of the various sects of physicians and new schools of medicine in later centuries. . . . Latest edition. Augusta, Me., 1904. 946p. front. (port.). DLC **00-7281**

WILDER, Burt Green (1841-1925)
Revised interpretation of the central fissures of the educated suicide's brain, exhibited [at twenty-sixth meeting of the American Neurological Association] to the association in 1894. [New York, 1900.] 5p. DNLM **00-7282**

WILDER, Burt Green (1841-1925)
Anatomic nomenclature; an open letter to Professor Llewellys F. Barker. New York, 1906. 2p. DNLM **00-7283**

WILDER, Burt Green (1841-1925)
The medical profession and simplified spelling. Buffalo, 1907. 4p. DNLM **00-7284**

WILDER, Burt Green (1841-1925)
The brain of the American Negro. [New York, 1909.] 66p. DNLM; NNNAM; NNS; NNU-M **00-7285**

WILDER, Harris H[awthorne] (1864-1928)
History of the human body. New York: Henry Holt & Co., 1909. 573p. DLC; ICJ; NIC; NN **00-7286**

WILDER, William H[amlin] (*b.* 1860)
On the prevalence of trachoma in the State of Illinois. Nashville, Tenn., 1901. 8p. 1 chart. DNLM **00-7287**

WILDER, William H[amlin] (*b.* 1860)
The influence of resection of the cervical sympathetic ganglia in glaucoma. Chicago, 1904. 47p. illus. plates. MB **00-7288**

WILE, Ira S[olomon] (1877-1943)
Preliminary notice of a new and simplified double stain for bacillus tuberculosis. New York, 1905. 2 l. DNLM **00-7289**

WILE, Ira S[olomon] (1877-1943)
Carsickness. New York, 1908. 9p. DNLM **00-7290**

WILE, Ira S[olomon] (1877-1943)
Blood examination in surgical diagnosis; a practical study of its scope and technic. . . . New York: Surgery Publishing Co., 1908. 101p. plates. DLC; MH-M; NNNAM; PU **00-7291**

WILE, Ira S[olomon] (1877-1943)
Clinical statistics. New York, 1910. 11p. DNLM **00-7292**

WILE, Udo J[ulius] (*b.* 1882)
Anaemic infarction of the adrenal with thrombosis of the veins. New York, 1907. 5p. DNLM **00-7293**

WILE, Udo J[ulius] (*b.* 1882)
Tuberculosis among medical students and its possible prevention. New York, 1908. 6p. DNLM **00-7294**

WILEY, Harley R[upert]
A treatise on pharmacal jurisprudence, with a thesis on the law in general. San Francisco: Hick-Judd Co., 1904. 262p. DLC; DNLM; PPC; PU **00-7295**

WILEY, Harvey W[ashington] (1844-1930)
. . . In memory of Emil Alexander de Schweinitz. Memorial meeting under auspices of Columbian University, March 5, 1904. Washington, D.C.: [Washington, Judd & Detweiler, 1904?] 12p. DLC **00-7296**

WILEY, Harvey W[ashington] (1844-1930)
. . . Influence of food preservatives and artificial colors on digestion and health. I. Boric acid and borax. By H. W. Wiley and the collaboration of W. D. Bigelow . . . and others. Washington: Government Printing Office, 1904. 477p. DLC **00-7297**

WILEY, Harvey W[ashington] (1844-1930)
. . . General results of the investigations showing the effect of salicylic acid and salicylates upon digestion and health . . . [Washington: Government Printing Office, 1906.] 12p. incl. diag. DLC **00-7298**

WILEY, Harvey W[ashington] (1844-1930)
Foods and their adulteration; origin, manufacture, and composition of food products; description of common adulterations, food standards and national food laws and regulations. . . . With eleven colored plates and eighty-six other illustrations. Philadelphia: P. Blakiston's Son & Co., 1907. 623p. incl. illus., tables. 11 col. plates. DLC; MBM; NN; PU **00-7299**

WILEY, Harvey W[ashington] (1844-1930)
Foods and their adulteration; origin, manufacture, and composition of food products; infants' and invalids' foods; detection of common adulterations, and food standards. . . . With eleven colored plates and eighty-seven other illustrations. 2nd ed., rev. and enl. Philadelphia: P. Blakiston's Son & Co., 1910. 641p. illus., 11 col. plates. DLC; MH; NIC; NN **00-7300**

WILKINSON, A[lonzo] D. (*b.* 1857)
Abortion. Lincoln, Nebr., 1900. 61p. DNLM **00-7301**

WILKINSON, Oscar (*b.* 1870)
Astigmatic accommodation, a clinical study of its relative frequency in 100 asthenopic cases. [Washington, 1905?] 55p. illus. DNLM **00-7302**

WILKINSON, Oscar (*b.* 1870)
A case of keratitis nodosa. St. Louis, 1905. 3p. DNLM **00-7303**

WILKINSON, Oscar (*b.* 1870)
A clinical study of the relative actions of atropine and homatropine as cycloplegics. Detroit, 1905. 12p. DNLM **00-7304**

WILKINSON, Oscar (*b.* 1870)
The preventive treatment of senile cataract. New York, 1906. 12p. DNLM **00-7305**

WILKINSON, Oscar (*b.* 1870)
Headaches. Richmond, 1906. 8p. DNLM **00-7306**

WILKINSON, Oscar (*b.* **1870)**
The early and preventive treatment of acute otitis media. New York, 1906. 8p. DNLM **00-7307**

WILKINSON, Oscar (*b.* **1870)**
History of the ocular treatment of migraine and headache. Chicago, 1906. 14p. DNLM **00-7308**

WILKINSON, Oscar (*b.* **1870)**
How should we determine errors of refraction, and what is their actual relation to general conditions? Richmond, 1909. 13p. DNLM **00-7309**

WILKINSON, Oscar (*b.* **1870)**
Exophoria; its symptoms, significance, and treatment. Chicago, 1909. 5p. DNLM **00-7310**

WILLARD, De Forest (1846-1910) and Wm. G. SPILLER
Cystic pelvic tumor appearing below Poupart's ligament and containing numerous peculiar loose bodies. Philadelphia, 1900. 11p. DNLM **00-7311**

WILLARD, De Forest (1846-1910)
Deformities, congenital multiple; arms and legs; femurs deficient. Philadelphia, 1900. 8p. DNLM **00-7312**

WILLARD, De Forest (1846-1910)
Technique employed in the children's orthopedic department of the University Hospital. Philadelphia, 1900. 4p. DNLM **00-7313**

WILLARD, De Forest (1846-1910)
1. Coxa vara. 2. Ankylosis of the hip. Philadelphia, 1900. 5p. DNLM **00-7314**

WILLARD, De Forest (1846-1910)
Aneurism of the thoracic aorta of traumatic origin; treatment by introduction of wire and electricity. [St. Louis], 1901. 13p. DNLM **00-7315**

WILLARD, De Forest (1846-1910)
Aneurism of the thoracic aorta of traumatic origin; treatment by introduction of wire and electricity. Philadelphia, 1901. 17p. DNLM **00-7316**

WILLARD, De Forest (1846-1910)
Congenital deformity of wrist; osteotomy of radius. Philadelphia, 1901. 4p. DNLM **00-7317**

WILLARD, De Forest (1846-1910)
Joint tuberculosis. Chicago, 1901. 6p. DNLM **00-7318**

WILLARD, De Forest (1846-1910)
Removal of foreign bodies from the air passages. Chicago, 1901. 16p. DNLM **00-7319**

WILLARD, De Forest (1846-1910)
Spinal caries paraplegia; forcible reduction in a long-standing case; immediate benefit and rapid recovery. Philadelphia, 1901. 2p. DNLM **00-7320**

WILLARD, De Forest (1846-1910)
Treatment of lateral curvature of the spine. Detroit: W. M. Warren, 1901. 8p. DNLM **00-7321**

WILLARD, De Forest (1846-1910)
Presidential address. Philadelphia, 1902. 8p. DNLM [American Surgical Association] **00-7322**

WILLARD, De Forest (1846-1910)
Gonorrheal arthritis; treatment by early irrigation of joint. Philadelphia, 1902. 8p. DNLM **00-7323**

WILLARD, De Forest (1846-1910)
Traumatic rupture of the gall-bladder without injury to the liver; sixty-four ounces of bile in abdominal cavity; recovery. New York, 1902. 7p. DNLM **00-7324**

WILLARD, De Forest (1846-1910)
Club-foot; astragalectomy for relapsed and inveterate cases. A clinical lecture delivered at the University Hospital. Philadelphia, 1902. 5p. 3 plates. DNLM **00-7325**

WILLARD, De Forest (1846-1910)
Medical articles, 1869-1902. Philadelphia, 1902. 31p. PP; PPC; PPL **00-7326**

WILLARD, De Forest (1846-1910)
Surgery of tubercular cavities of the apex of the lung. Chicago, 1902. 24p. 1 table. DNLM **00-7327**

WILLARD, De Forest (1846-1910)
Sunshine and fresh air vs. the Finsen ultra-violet rays and the Roentgen-rays in tuberculosis of the joints and bones. Chicago, 1903. 13p. DNLM **00-7328**

WILLARD, De Forest (1846-1910)
Widener Memorial Industrial Training School for Crippled Children. Philadelphia, 1903. 4p. DNLM **00-7329**

WILLARD, De Forest (1846-1910)
Old unreduced dislocations. Chicago, 1904. 16p. DNLM **00-7330**

WILLARD, De Forest (1846-1910)
Empyema. [Philadelphia], 1904. 9p. DNLM **00-7331**

WILLARD, De Forest (1846-1910)
Knee ankylosis. Athens, 1905. 5p. DNLM **00-7332**

WILLARD, De Forest (1846-1910)
Knee injuries, and how to manage them. Burlington, Vt., and New York, 1905. 10p. DNLM **00-7333**

WILLARD, De Forest (1846-1910)
Joint diseases, especially those of children. New York: A. R. Elliott & Co., 1906. 20p. DNLM **00-7334**

WILLARD, De Forest (1846-1910)
Fracture of neck of femur. Detroit, 1906. 4p. DNLM **00-7335**

WILLARD, De Forest (1846-1910) and W. H. ANDRUS
Ostitis deformans. [Philadelphia], 1904. 13p. DNLM **00-7336**

WILLARD, De Forest (1846-1910) and A. Bruce GILL
The Widener Memorial Industrial Training School for Crippled Children. Philadelphia, 1903. 6p. 2 plates. DNLM **00-7337**

WILLARD, De Forest (1846-1910)
Joint diseases versus rheumatism. Athens, 1910. 2 l. DNLM
00-7338

WILLARD, De Forest (1846-1910)
The surgery of childhood, including orthopaedic surgery. Philadelphia and London: J. B. Lippincott Co., 1910. 800p. 17 plates. DLC; ICJ; NNNAM; PPC
00-7339

WILLARD, De Forest (1846-1910) and Benjamin L. SINGER
Multiple hand and foot deformities in the third, fourth, seventh and ninth children of the same family; the others being normal and the parents normal. Philadelphia, 1910. 8p. DNLM **00-7340**

WILLARD, De Forest (1846-1910)
Address at the opening of the one hundred and forty-fifth session of the Medical School of the University of Pennsylvania. Philadelphia, 1910. 14p. PPC **00-7341**

WILLARD, De Forest (1846-1910)
List of medical and surgical articles from 1869 to 1910. [Philadelphia, 1910.] 31p. PPC **00-7342**

WILLETTS, Joseph E. (*b.* 1860)
Corneal corpuscular activity. [Chicago, 1900.] 6p. DNLM
00-7343

WILLETTS, Joseph E. (*b.* 1860)
Analytical description of the eye as an end organ. Athens, Pa.: W. G. Jordan, 1909. 19p. DNLM; PPC
00-7344

WILLIAMS, Charles (*d.* 1907)
The bibliography of the "Religio medici." Norwich, 1905. 15p. DNLM **00-7345**

WILLIAMS, Charles (*d.* 1907)
The bibliography of the "Religio medici." 2nd ed. Norwich: Goose & Son, 1907. 20p. DNLM **00-7346**

WILLIAMS, Charles (*d.* 1907)
Souvenir of Sir Thomas Browne. With twelve illustrations and notes. . . . Norwich: Jarrold & Sons, 1905. 11 l. 12 plates. DNLM **00-7347**

WILLIAMS, Charles D[ickins] (*b.* 1871)
Pathological report of the gynecological service of the Lakeside Hospital, 1901 and 1902. Cleveland, 1908. 22p. DNLM; OCIM
00-7348

WILLIAMS, Charles D[ickins] (*b.* 1871)
Etiology of ectopic gestation. [Chicago], 1908. 16p. DNLM
00-7349

WILLIAMS, Charles M[allory] (*b.* 1872)
Four cases of chancre of the lip. New York, 1905. 5p. DNLM
00-7350

WILLIAMS, Charles M[allory] (*b.* 1872)
The treatment of acne. New York, 1905. 14p. DNLM
00-7351

WILLIAMS, Charles M[allory] (*b.* 1872)
X-ray treatment of cutaneous epithelioma. Philadelphia, 1905. 9p. DNLM **00-7352**

WILLIAMS, Charles M[allory] (*b.* 1872)
The contagiousness of gumma. New York, 1906. 42p. DNLM
00-7353

WILLIAMS, Charles M[allory] (*b.* 1872)
Some results which have been obtained in the experimental inoculation of syphilis. [New York, 1907.] 7p. DNLM
00-7354

WILLIAMS, Chisholm (1866-1928)
High-frequency currents in the treatment of some diseases. New York: Rebman Co., 1903. 222p. DLC; ICJ; IEN-M; NNNAM **00-7355**

WILLIAMS, Daniel H[ale] (1858-1931)
An unusual case of molluscum fibrosum. [Philadelphia, 1900.] 4p. DNLM **00-7356**

WILLIAMS, Daniel H[ale] (1858-1931)
The need of hospitals and training schools for the colored people of the South. [Detroit, 1900.] 6p. DNLM
00-7357

WILLIAMS, Daniel H[ale] (1858-1931)
A report of two cases of Caesarean section under positive indications, with termination in recovery. New York: William Wood & Co., 1901. 8p. DNLM **00-7358**

WILLIAMS, Daniel H[ale] (1858-1931)
Ovarian cysts in colored women, with notes on the relative frequency of fibromata in both races. Chicago, [1901]. 12p. DNLM **00-7359**

WILLIAMS, Dawson (*b.* 1854)
Medical diseases of infancy and childhood . . . 2nd ed., rev., with additions by Frank Spooner Churchill. . . . Illustrated with 72 engravings and 2 colored plates. Philadelphia and New York: Lea Bros. & Co., 1900. 542p. illus., 2 col. plates. CtY-M; DLC; NNNAM; PPC **00-7360**

WILLIAMS, Edward T[ufts] (*b.* 1844)
Tettenhamer on eosinophiles. Philadelphia, 1902. 4p. DNLM
00-7361

WILLIAMS, Edward T[ufts] (*b.* 1844)
Marrow and spleen cells, considered in their relation to the blood-cells. Philadelphia, 1902. 6p. DNLM
00-7362

WILLIAMS, Edward T[ufts] (*b.* 1844)
Studies on the leucocytes. Boston, 1903. 63p. DNLM
00-7363

WILLIAMS, Edward T[ufts] (*b.* 1844)
The demonstration of nucleated red blood corpuscles in animal spleens. Philadelphia, 1903. 5p. DNLM
00-7364

WILLIAMS, Edward T[ufts] (*b.* 1844)
A comparative study of animal blood. Philadelphia, 1904. 2p. DNLM **00-7365**

WILLIAMS, Edward T[ufts] (*b.* 1844)
Additional papers on the blood; a sequel to Studies on the leucocytes. Boston, 1904. 30p. DLC; ICJ
00-7366

WILLIAMS, Edward T[ufts] (*b.* **1844)**
The pathology of leukemia. Philadelphia, 1904. 2p. DNLM **00-7367**

WILLIAMS, Edward T[ufts] (*b.* **1844)**
The alleged destruction of red blood-corpuscles in the spleen. Philadelphia, 1905. 6p. DNLM **00-7368**

WILLIAMS, Edward T[ufts] (*b.* **1844)**
The office of the spleen. An essay in comparative physiology. Philadelphia, 1905. 2p. DNLM **00-7369**

WILLIAMS, Edward T[ufts] (*b.* **1844)**
Blood studies. [3rd series.] Boston: Puritan Press, 1905. 32p. DNLM **00-7370**

WILLIAMS, Edward T[ufts] (*b.* **1844)**
The use of stearin as a food preservative. Boston, 1906. 6p. DNLM **00-7371**

WILLIAMS, Edward T[ufts] (*b.* **1844)**
The edibility of animal spleens. Philadelphia, 1906. 4p. DNLM **00-7372**

WILLIAMS, Ennion G[ifford] (1874-1931)
X-ray therapy, with a report of a case. Richmond, 1903. 7p. DNLM **00-7373**

WILLIAMS, Ennion G[ifford] (1874-1931)
Gelatine treatment in aneurism. Richmond, 1903. 4p. 1 plate. DLC **00-7374**

WILLIAMS, Ennion G[ifford] (1874-1931)
The regulation of the duration of exposure and the distance from the tube in X-ray therapy. [1904.] 5p. DLC **00-7375**

WILLIAMS, Ennion G[ifford] (1874-1931)
Some observations on the possibilities of X-ray therapy. [1904.] 4p. DLC **00-7376**

WILLIAMS, Ennion G[ifford] (1874-1931)
Principles governing the technic of Roentgen ray therapy. [1905.] 5p. DLC **00-7377**

WILLIAMS, Ennion G[ifford] (1874-1931)
Illustrations of the X-ray treatment of malignant growth. [1906.] 7p. DLC **00-7378**

WILLIAMS, Ennion G[ifford] (1874-1931)
Regulation and measurement of the therapeutic dose of the Roentgen ray. [1906.] 7p. DLC **00-7379**

WILLIAMS, Ennion G[ifford] (1874-1931)
A few remarks on the proper value of the X-ray in therapeutics. [1906.] 5p. DLC **00-7380**

WILLIAMS, Ennion G[ifford] (1874-1931)
The X-ray treatment of malignant growths. [1906.] 8p. DLC **00-7381**

WILLIAMS, Ennion G[ifford] (1874-1931)
A few remarks on the principles governing Roentgen therapy. [1906.] 4p. DLC **00-7382**

WILLIAMS, Ennion G[ifford] (1874-1931)
The tube in Roentgen therapy. [1907.] 8p. DLC **00-7383**

WILLIAMS, Ennion G[ifford] (1874-1931)
The postoperative treatment of malignant disease. [1907.] 4p. DLC **00-7384**

WILLIAMS, Ennion G[ifford] (1874-1931)
Reply of Dr. Ennion G. Williams to the statements of Mr. Mark Gunat, in opposition to plan to build a city hospital. Richmond: O. Fianhart Printing Co., 1907. 9p. DLC **00-7385**

WILLIAMS, Ennion G[ifford] (1874-1931)
Report of one hundred and seven (107) cases of cancer treated with the X-ray, with comments thereon. [1907.] 4p. DLC **00-7386**

WILLIAMS, Ennion G[ifford] (1874-1931)
A general city hospital and the new colored almshouse. A statement presented for consideration to the committee on relief of the poor, by Councilman Ennion G. Williams, Feb. 19, 1907. [Richmond]: Richmond Press, [1907]. 10p. DLC **00-7387**

WILLIAMS, Francis H[enry] (1852-1936)
Some cases of cancer treated by the X-rays. Boston, 1901. 7p. plates. MB **00-7388**

WILLIAMS, Francis H[enry] (1852-1936)
The reduction of temperature in fevers by evaporation bath, warm water being used for baths. Chicago, 1901. 8p. DNLM **00-7389**

WILLIAMS, Francis H[enry] (1852-1936)
The Roentgen rays in medicine and surgery as an aid in diagnosis and as a therapeutic agent. Designed for the use of practitioners and students. New York: Macmillan Co., 1901. 658p. DNLM; ICJ; MH; NNNAM **00-7390**

WILLIAMS, Francis H[enry] (1852-1936)
The Roentgen rays in medicine and surgery, as an aid in diagnosis and as a therapeutic agent; designed for the use of practitioners and students. 2nd ed., with enl. appendix. New York: Macmillan Co., 1902 [*c.* 1901]. 704p. DNLM; ICJ; NcD; PPC **00-7391**

WILLIAMS, Francis H[enry] (1852-1936)
The Roentgen rays in medicine and surgery as an aid in diagnosis and as a therapeutic agent; designated for the use of practitioners and students . . . with four hundred and twenty-eight illustrations. 3rd ed. With enl. appendix. New York: Macmillan Co., 1903. 757p. illus., diags. DLC; ICJ; NcD; PPHa **00-7392**

WILLIAMS, Francis H[enry] (1852-1936)
A case of transfusion after intestinal hemorrhage in typhoid fever. [1904?] 5p. DNLM **00-7393**

WILLIAMS, Frederic A[llen]
Eye troubles . . . their cause, symptoms and treatment. . . . [Boston? Mass.], 1903. 62p. DLC; MBM **00-7394**

WILLIAMS, H[enry] Smith (1863-1943)
Alcohol; how it affects the individual, the community, and the race. New York: The Century Co., 1909. 151p. DNLM; ICU; KU; NN **00-7395**

WILLIAMS, Henry T. (*b.* 1858)
Abdominal hysterectomy for fibroid tumor of the uterus complicated with pregnancy and prolonged retention of a foetus and placenta. New York, 1906. 2p. 1 plate. DNLM
00-7396

WILLIAMS, Herbert U[pham] (*b.* 1866)
The morbid anatomy and etiology of fat-necrosis. Buffalo: Baker, Jones & Co., 1900. 61p. 5 plates. DNLM; NNNAM
00-7397

WILLIAMS, Herbert U[pham] (*b.* 1866)
A critical summary of recent literature on plasmacells and mast-cells. [Philadelphia, 1900.] 8p. DNLM
00-7398

WILLIAMS, Herbert U[pham] (*b.* 1866)
A manual of bacteriology. . . . With eight-nine illustrations. 2nd ed., rev. and enl. Philadelphia: P. Blakiston's Son & Co., 1901. 290p. DLC; DNLM; PPC; PU
00-7399

WILLIAMS, Herbert U[pham] (*b.* 1866)
A manual of bacteriology . . . with ninety-nine illustrations. 3rd ed., rev. and enl. Philadelphia: P. Blakiston's Son & Co., 1903. 351p. CtY-M; DLC; DNLM; NNNAM; PU
00-7400

WILLIAMS, Herbert U[pham] (*b.* 1866)
A manual of bacteriology . . . rev. by B. Meade Bolton . . . with 108 illustrations. 4th ed., rev. and enl. Philadelphia: P. Blakiston's Son & Co., 1905. 357p. DLC; DNLM; MBM; PPC **00-7401**

WILLIAMS, Herbert U[pham] (*b.* 1866)
A manual of bacteriology . . . rev. by B. Meade Bolton . . . with 113 illustrations. 5th ed., rev. and enl. Philadelphia: P. Blakiston's Son & Co., 1908. 466p. DLC; DNLM; LNT-M; PPC **00-7402**

WILLIAMS, Herbert U[pham] (*b.* 1866)
The epidemic of the Indians of New England, 1616-1620, with remarks on native American infections. [n. p., 1909.] 29p. MH; MHi **00-7403**

WILLIAMS, Howard J.
Osteomyelitis. New York, 1904. 24p. DNLM
00-7404

WILLIAMS, Hugh
A case of gunshot wound of the stomach; operation; recovery. Boston: Old Corner Book Store, 1903. 7p. DNLM
00-7405

WILLIAMS, John R[alston] (*b.* 1874)
On the occurrence of indican, albumin, and casts in the urine. New York, 1907. 3p. DNLM **00-7406**

WILLIAMS, John T[homas] (*b.* 1881)
The relation of carcinoma of the corpus uteri to fibroids. Boston, 1908. 15p. DNLM; MBM **00-7407**

WILLIAMS, John T[homas] (*b.* 1881)
Cancer of the cervix complicating pregnancy. Boston: D. C. Heath & Co., 1909. 28p. DNLM; MBM
00-7408

WILLIAMS, J. Whitridge (1866-1931)
Pelvic indications for the performance of Caesarean section. [Philadelphia], 1901. 17p. DNLM **00-7409**

WILLIAMS, J. Whitridge (1866-1931)
Obstetrics; a text-book for the use of students and practitioners . . . with eight coloured plates and six hundred and thirty illustrations in the text. New York and London: D. Appleton & Co., 1903. 845p. DLC; DNLM; NNNAM; PPC **00-7410**

WILLIAMS, J. Whitridge (1866-1931)
A sketch of the history of obstetrics in the United States up to 1860. [n. p., 1903?] 55p. DNLM; KU; NN
00-7411

WILLIAMS, J. Whitridge (1866-1931)
Indications for and most satisfactory methods of bringing about premature labor and accouchement forcé. New York, 1903. 18p. 1 plate. DNLM **00-7412**

WILLIAMS, J. Whitridge (1866-1931)
The introduction of clinical teaching of obstetrics in the United States. New York, 1904. 19p. DNLM
00-7413

WILLIAMS, J. Whitridge (1866-1931)
Subperitoneal hematoma following labor not associated with lesions of the uterus. [Philadelphia], 1904. 18p. DNLM
00-7414

WILLIAMS, J. Whitridge (1866-1931)
Toxemic vomiting of pregnancy. Philadelphia, 1906. 12p. DNLM **00-7415**

WILLIAMS, J. Whitridge (1866-1931)
The induction of premature labor and accouchement forcé in the first 5,000 labors in the obstetrical department of the Johns Hopkins Hospital. [Philadelphia, 1906.] 18p. DNLM
00-7416

WILLIAMS, J. Whitridge (1866-1931)
Obstetrics; a text-book for the use of students and practitioners . . . 2nd enl. and rev. ed., with sixteen plates and six hundred and sixty-six illustrations in the text. New York and London: D. Appleton & Co., 1908. 950p. DLC; DNLM; NNNAM; ScCM **00-7417**

WILLIAMS, J. Whitridge (1866-1931)
Is pubiotomy a justifiable operation? New York, 1908. 30p. DNLM **00-7418**

WILLIAMS, J. Whitridge (1866-1931)
The clinical significance of glycosuria in pregnant women. Philadelphia, 1909. 26p. DNLM **00-7419**

WILLIAMS, J. Whitridge (1866-1931)
Frequency, etiology and practical significance of contractions of the pelvic outlet. Chicago, 1909. 20p. DNLM
00-7420

WILLIAMS, J. Whitridge (1866-1931)
Ligation or excision of thrombosed veins in the treatment of puerperal pyemia. New York: William Wood & Co., 1909. 32p. DNLM **00-7421**

WILLIAMS, J. Whitridge (1866-1931)
Is pubiotomy a justifiable operation? New York, 1910. 32p. DNLM **00-7422**

WILLIAMS, J. Whitridge (1866-1931), Edwin Bradford CRAGIN and Franklin S. NEWELL
Report on the employment of vaccine therapy in gynecology and obstetrics. Chicago, 1910. 8p. DNLM
00-7423

WILLIAMS, J. Whitridge (1866-1931)
. . . What the obstetrician can do to prevent infantile mortality. [n. p., 1910.] 12p. NN **00-7424**

WILLIAMS, Linsly R[udd] (1875-1934)
The physical reconstruction of school children by means of fresh air. New York, 1907. 12p. DNLM
00-7425

WILLIAMS, Linsly R[udd] (1875-1934)
A review of the recent efforts to improve New York City's milk supply. New York, 1907. 7p. DNLM
00-7426

WILLIAMS, Linsly R[udd] (1875-1934)
The value of the social worker and the visiting nurse to the dispensary patient. New York, 1908. 16p. DNLM
00-7427

WILLIAMS, M[ilan] B[ertrand]
Sex problems, as related to health and disease, morality and religion, heredity and environment, both in the individual and society at large. . . . Chicago, New York, [etc.]: F. H. Revell Co., 1901. 252p. DLC; ICJ; NN [*vel subseq.*]
00-7428

WILLIAMS, M[ilan] B[ertrand]
Sex problems as related to health and disease, morality and religion, heredity and environment, both in the individual and society at large. . . . New and rev. ed. 7th ed. New York, Chicago, [etc.]: Fleming H. Revell Co., [1910]. 251p. DLC; ICJ; NN **00-7429**

WILLIAMS, Robert F[indlater] (*b.* 1869)
Notes on materia medica. . . . Richmond, Va.: Whittet & Shepperson, 1902. 174p. DLC **00-7430**

WILLIAMS, Robert F[indlater] (*b.* 1869)
Food and diet in health and disease. . . . Philadelphia and New York: Lea Bros. & Co., 1906. 392p. DLC; MBM; NNNAM; PPC **00-7431**

WILLIAMS, Tom A[lfred] (*b.* 1870)
The role of the doctor in producing or maintaining the maladies derived from the imagination. Burlington, Vt., New York, 1908. 13p. DNLM **00-7432**

WILLIAMS, Tom A[lfred] (*b.* 1870)
Recent advances regarding hysteria in relation to traumatic neurosis. Philadelphia, 1908. 3p. DNLM
00-7433

WILLIAMS, Tom A[lfred] (*b.* 1870)
The French clinics in neurology and psychiatry. Burlington, Vt., and New York, 1908. 14p. DNLM
00-7434

WILLIAMS, Tom A[lfred] (*b.* 1870)
The pathogenesis of tabes dorsalis. Philadelphia, 1908. 20p. DNLM **00-7435**

WILLIAMS, Tom A[lfred] (*b.* 1870)
The differential diagnosis of functional from organic palsies; hemiplegia, paralysis agitans, occupation and habit cramps and spasms. New York, 1908. 6p. DNLM **00-7436**

WILLIAMS, Tom A[lfred] (*b.* 1870)
A few hints from personal experience. Philadelphia, 1908. 3p. DNLM **00-7437**

WILLIAMS, Tom A[lfred] (*b.* 1870)
The physiological basis of inebriety; its aetiological and social factors; remedies. [n. p., 1908, *vel subseq.*] 12p. DNLM
00-7438

WILLIAMS, Tom A[lfred] (*b.* 1870)
The so-called gastric neuroses. [n. p., 1908, *vel subseq.*] 6p. DNLM **00-7439**

WILLIAMS, Tom A[lfred] (*b.* 1870)
The treatment of a case of hysteria. [n. p., 1908, *vel subseq.*] 5p. DNLM **00-7440**

WILLIAMS, Tom A[lfred] (*b.* 1870)
The importance for research and treatment of distinguishing clinical types among the psycho-neuroses. Boston, 1909. 1p. DNLM **00-7441**

WILLIAMS, Tom A[lfred] (*b.* 1870)
The trend of the clinicians' concept of hysteria. Boston, 1909. 18p. DNLM **00-7442**

WILLIAMS, Tom A[lfred] (*b.* 1870)
The rational treatment of tabes dorsalis in relation to its pathogenesis. New York, 1909. 8p. DNLM
00-7443

WILLIAMS, Tom A[lfred] (*b.* 1870)
The importance of modifications of the sensibility in the diagnosis of disease. Philadelphia, 1909. 7p. DNLM
00-7444

WILLIAMS, Tom A[lfred] (*b.* 1870)
The present status of hysteria. New York, 1909. 16p. DNLM
00-7445

WILLIAMS, Tom A[lfred] (*b.* 1870)
The psychological basis of inebriety. New York, 1909. 23p. DNLM **00-7446**

WILLIAMS, Tom A[lfred] (*b.* 1870)
The clarification of our concepts concerning hysteria. Philadelphia, 1909. 4p. DNLM **00-7447**

WILLIAMS, Tom A[lfred] (*b.* 1870)
The more recent conceptions regarding hysteria, and their relation to the traumatic neurosis. Chicago, 1909. 3p. DNLM
00-7448

WILLIAMS, Tom A[lfred] (*b.* 1870)
The differential diagnosis of functional from organic forms of motor disability. Mobile, 1909. 10p. DNLM
00-7449

WILLIAMS, Tom A[lfred] (*b.* 1870)
. . . Psychoprophylaxis in childhood. . . . [Cincinnati, 1909?] 9p. DLC **00-7450**

WILLIAMS, Tom A[lfred] (*b.* 1870)
Modern neurology on spiritualism and possession. New York, 1910. 8p. DNLM **00-7451**

WILLIAMS, Tom A[lfred] (*b.* 1870)
The psychogenesis of some "reflex" neuroses. New York, 1910. 3p. DNLM **00-7452**

WILLIAMS, Tom A[lfred] (*b.* 1870)
Intra-cranial neoplasms; remarks on diagnosis and indications for treatment. Cincinnati, 1910. 14p. DNLM **00-7453**

WILLIAMS, Tom A[lfred] (*b.* 1870)
Poliomyelitis; new facts concerning its etiology, early diagnosis and treatment. Philadelphia, 1910. 7p. DNLM **00-7454**

WILLIAMS, Tom A[lfred] (*b.* 1870)
The treatment of "parasyphilis" of the nervous system in the light of recent research; paresis and tabes dorsalis. Philadelphia, 1910. 8p. DNLM **00-7455**

WILLIAMS, Tom A[lfred] (*b.* 1870)
Diagnosis of disorders of the cerebellar apparatus. New York, 1910. 11p. DNLM **00-7456**

WILLIAMS, Tom A[lfred] (*b.* 1870)
Facial spasm and tic; torticollis; diagnosis and treatment. Philadelphia, 1910. 7p. DNLM **00-7457**

WILLIAMS, Tom A[lfred] (*b.* 1870)
The pathological prodromes of taboparesis; syphilis; meningitis; the genesis of the cranial nerve implications. New York, 1910. 27p. DNLM **00-7458**

WILLIAMS, Tom A[lfred] (*b.* 1870)
So-called reflex neurotic symptoms, and the psychic factor. New York, 1910. 3p. DNLM **00-7459**

WILLIAMS, Tom A[lfred] (*b.* 1870)
"Nervousness" and education. The role of the teacher. . . . [Toledo, 1910.] 11p. ICJ **00-7460**

WILLIAMS, Tom A[lfred] (*b.* 1870)
"Nervousness" and education. The role of the teacher. [Springfield], 1910. 7p. NN **00-7461**

WILLIAMS, Tom A[lfred] (*b.* 1870)
The psychological basis of inebriety: its aetological and social factors; remedies. [Washington, 191-?] 12p. NN **00-7462**

WILLIAMS, W[illiam] Roger
Uterine tumours; their pathology and treatment. New York: William Wood & Co., 1901. 359p. DNLM; NNNAM; PPC **00-7463**

WILLIAMS, W[illiam] Roger
Cancer. (Theories of the parasitic origin.) New York, 1903. 38p. MB **00-7464**

WILLIAMS, W[illiam] Roger
Essentials of the practice of medicine, prepared especially for students of medicine. Philadelphia: W. B. Saunders & Co., 1905. 460p. CU-M; DNLM; NNNAM; PPC **00-7465**

WILLIAMS, W[illiam] Roger
The natural history of cancer. With special reference to its causation and prevention. . . . New York: William Wood & Co., 1908. 519p. tables. MB; ICJ; NcU; PPJ **00-7466**

WILLIAMSON, A[llan] N[eale]
Observations on the treatment of epilepsy. New London, Conn.: E. E. Darrow, 1900. 15p. DNLM; NN **00-7467**

WILLIAMSON, A[llan] N[eale]
Observations on the treatment of epilepsy. Dobbs Ferry, N.Y., 1902. 14p. DNLM **00-7468**

WILLIS, [Achille] Murat (*b.* 1878)
Appendicitis; methods of treatment; report of two hundred and six cases with four deaths. Charlotte, N.C., 1908. 7p. DNLM **00-7469**

WILLIS, [Achille] Murat (*b.* 1878)
The factor of mortality in the operation of hysterectomy. Atlanta, Ga., 1908. 3p. DNLM **00-7470**

WILLIS, [Achille] Murat (*b.* 1878)
The treatment of the appendix stump after appendectomy. St. Louis, 1908. 5p. DNLM **00-7471**

WILLIS, Byrd C. (*b.* 1880)
Congenital union of spleen and liver. Richmond, 1910. 3p. DNLM **00-7472**

WILLIS, WM. V., & CO. (PHILADELPHIA)
. . . Illustrated catalogue of high-grade surgical instruments, invalid articles and hospital supplies. Philadelphia: W. V. Willis & Co., [1901]. 325p. illus. DLC; ICJ; PP **00-7473**

WILLMAN, Reinhold (*b.* 1855)
The errors of mind healing compared with the miracles of Christ and His disciples in the healing of the afflicted as viewed by a physician. . . . Saint Joseph, Mo.: The Advocate Publishing Co., [1909]. 179p. DLC; ICJ; OC **00-7474**

WILLMS, CHARLES SURGICAL INSTRUMENT CO.
Illustrated and descriptive catalog of surgical instruments, orthopaedic appliances, trusses, microscopes, static machines, hospital supplies. . . . Baltimore, [*c.* 1900]. 506p. MdBM; NNNAM **00-7475**

WILLS, William Le Moyne (*b.* 1853)
Vicarious menstruation or hysterical dysmenorrhea—which? [San Francisco], 1900. 12p. DNLM **00-7476**

WILLS, William Le Moyne (*b.* 1853)
Ununited fractures of the lower extremity. San Francisco, 1903. 14p. DNLM **00-7477**

WILLS, William Le Moyne (*b.* 1853)
Impacted fractures of the neck of the femur. Report of two interesting cases. Chicago, 1904. 7p. DNLM **00-7478**

WILLSON, Prentiss (*b.* 1882)
Snake poisoning in the United States; a study based on an analysis of 740 cases. Chicago, 1908. 59p. DNLM **00-7479**

WILLSON, Robert Newton (1873-1916)
The contagiousness of pneumonia. New York, 1904. 12p. DLC; DNLM **00-7480**

WILLSON, Robert Newton (1873-1916)
The American boy and the social evil. From a physician's standpoint. Philadelphia: J. C. Winston Co., 1905. 159p. DLC; DNLM **00-7481**

WILLSON, Robert Newton (1873-1916)
The social evil in university life. A talk with the students of the University of Pennsylvania. Philadelphia, 1905. 58p. DLC; DNLM **00-7482**

WILLSON, Robert Newton (1873-1916)
Syphilis with late or absent secondary eruption. New York, 1905. 13p. DLC; DNLM **00-7483**

WILLSON, Robert Newton (1873-1916)
Memoir of Charles Stewart Wurts. [1830-1907.] [Philadelphia, 1909.] 6p. DLC; DNLM **00-7484**

WILLSON, Robert Newton (1873-1916) and Randle C. ROSENBERGER
The duration of the actively infectious stage of tuberculosis. Chicago, 1909. 19p. DLC; DNLM **00-7485**

WILLSON, Robert Newton (1873-1916)
Medical men in the time of Christ. Philadelphia: Sunday School Times Co., 1910. 157p. 6 plates. DNLM; ICJ; NN **00-7486**

WILLYOUNG, ELMER G. [COMPANY] (PHILADELPHIA)
Price list of induction coils, x-ray machines and accessory apparatus. 2nd ed. Philadelphia, 1900. 32p. NNNAM; PU [1st ed., 1895. 123p.] **00-7487**

WILLYOUNG, ELMER G. [COMPANY] (PHILADELPHIA)
Catalogue W. Electrical and scientific instruments and apparatus. November 20th, 1899. New York, [1900?]. 175p. illus. DLC **00-7488**

WILLYOUNG, ELMER G. [COMPANY] (PHILADELPHIA)
Condensers and their applications; Jas. G. Biddle, ed. Philadelphia, [1901?]. 40p. PU **00-7489**

WILNER, Anna S. (*b.* 1879)
Primary nasal diphtheria; a plea for its early recognition, and a report of three cases. New York, 1904. 26p. DNLM; NNNAM **00-7490**

WILNER, Anna S. (*b.* 1879)
A case of paralysis of the abducent nerve following influenza. New York, 1907. 6p. DNLM **00-7491**

WILSON, Daniel S.
The sexual anatomy, and its adaptations. 4th ed. Nashville, Tenn., 1900? [*c.* 1898]. DLC [3rd ed., Nashville, Tenn., 1896. 179p., illus. DLC] **00-7492**

WILSON, Edmund B[eecher] (1856-1939)
. . . The cell in development and inheritance . . . 2nd ed., rev. & enl. . . . New York: The Macmillan Co.; London: Macmillan & Co., 1900. 483p. illus. DLC; MH; NIC; NN **00-7493**

WILSON, Edmund B[eecher] (1856-1939)
Biology [a lecture delivered at Columbia University in the series on science, philosophy and art, November 20, 1907]. . . . New York: The Columbia University Press, 1908. 24p. DLC; NN **00-7494**

WILSON, Ezra H[erbert] (1858-1905)
Anti-typhoid inoculations. Carlisle, 1903. 8p. DNLM **00-7495**

WILSON, Frank C[aruthers] (*b.* 1841)
A plea for more humane treatment of advanced cases of tuberculosis. St. Louis, 1907. 2p. DNLM **00-7496**

WILSON, Frederick M. (*b.* 1851) and Edgar S. THOMSON
Case of glioma retinae and brain metastases, with autopsy and review of literature. New York, 1900. 10p. 1 plate. DNLM **00-7497**

WILSON, Harry A[ugustus] (1853-1919)
Pus in the pelvis as a result of bone or joint necrosis; diagnosis and treatment. Philadelphia, 1902. 5p. DNLM **00-7498**

WILSON, Harry A[ugustus] (1853-1919)
Tuberculous joint disease. New York, 1902. 13p. DNLM **00-7499**

WILSON, Harry A[ugustus] (1853-1919), J. Torrance RUGH and W. M. L. COPLIN
Congenital dislocation of the hip; report of a bloodless reposition, followed by death, with an analysis of twenty-three cases in process of treatment. Philadelphia, 1903. 19p. DNLM **00-7500**

WILSON, Harry A[ugustus] (1853-1919)
Apparently unavoidable errors in the diagnosis of psoas abscess. Wilkes-Barre, 1905. 10p. DNLM **00-7501**

WILSON, Harry A[ugustus] (1853-1919)
The ocular factors in the aetiology of spinal curvatures. New York, 1906. 11p. DNLM **00-7502**

WILSON, Harry A[ugustus] (1853-1919)
Out-door life versus confinement in the treatment of bone tuberculosis. Pittsburgh, 1906. 16p. DNLM **00-7503**

WILSON, Harry A[ugustus] (1853-1919)
Modern tendencies in the treatment of bone tuberculosis. Philadelphia, 1907. 12p. DNLM **00-7504**

WILSON, Harry A[ugustus] (1853-1919)
The clinical significance of the so-called acute stage of bone tuberculosis. Pittsburgh, 1907. 4p. DNLM **00-7505**

WILSON, Harry A[ugustus] (1853-1919)
Treatment of ununited fractures of the neck of the femur by the use of coin silver nails. Boston, 1908. 15p. DNLM **00-7506**

WILSON, Harry B.
Haunts of health and pleasure along the Jersey coast; a descriptive guide and souvenir of the summer resorts located on the "northern shore." New York: L. Weiss & Co., [1900]. 171p. illus. DLC; NN **00-7507**

WILSON, J[ames] C[ornelius] (1847-1934)
Memoir of J. M. Da Costa. . . . Read before the College of Physicians of Philadelphia, November 5, 1902. [Philadelphia: Dornan, printer], 1902. 20p. port. DLC; PPC
00-7508

WILSON, J[ames] C[ornelius] (1847-1934)
Brief account of the disease known as osteitis deformans. n. p., [1902]. 4p. NN **00-7509**

WILSON, J[ames] C[ornelius] (1847-1934)
The complete medical pocket-formulary and physician's vade-mecum: containing upwards of 2500 prescriptions. . . . Collated for the use of practitioners . . . 3rd rev. ed. Philadelphia: J. B. Lippincott Co., [1903]. 307p. DLC; NNNAM; PPC; PU
00-7510

WILSON, J[ames] C[ornelius] (1847-1934) and Frederick J. KALTEYER
Report of a case of sarcomatosis cutis, together with an analytical study of fifty other cases collected from recent literature. New York, 1903. 18p. DNLM
00-7511

WILSON, J[ames] C[ornelius] (1847-1934)
. . . Fever-nursing: designed for the use of professional and other nurses, and especially as a text-book for nurses in training . . . 4th ed., rev. and enl. Philadelphia, London: J. B. Lippincott Co., [1904]. 246p. fold. charts. DLC; MBM; NNNAM; PU **00-7512**

WILSON, J[ames] C[ornelius] (1847-1934)
Cases of enteric fever complicated by polyuria. [New York, 1904.] 4p. NN **00-7513**

WILSON, J[ames] C[ornelius] (1847-1934)
An address delivered at the unveiling of a monument erected by the American Medical Association to the memory of Benjamin Rush in Washington, D.C., June 11, 1904. . . . [Philadelphia: Press of J. B. Lippincott Co., 1904.] 20p. DLC; ICJ; NN; PPJ **00-7514**

WILSON, J[ames] C[ornelius] (1847-1934)
Borderline between medicine and surgery. n. p., [1904]. 6p. NN **00-7515**

WILSON, J[ames] C[ornelius] (1847-1934)
. . . Infectious diseases . . . an authorized translation from "Die deutsche klinik" under the general editorial supervision of Julius L. Salinger, M.D. With two colored plates and sixty illustrations in the text. New York and London: D. Appleton & Co., 1905. 925p. DLC; ICJ; NNNAM; PU
00-7516

WILSON, J[ames] C[ornelius] (1847-1934)
Cerebrospinal fever. [Chicago, 1905.] 6p. NN
00-7517

WILSON, J[ames] C[ornelius] (1847-1934)
The symptomatology and diagnosis of atypical forms of pneumonia. New York, 1905. 10p. DNLM
00-7518

WILSON, J[ames] C[ornelius] (1847-1934)
Concerning the diagnosis of acute haemorrhagic pancreatitis. New York, 1905. 9p. DNLM **00-7519**

WILSON, J[ames] C[ornelius] (1847-1934)
Chylous and chyliform effusions into the serous sacs. n. p., [1905]. 8p. NN **00-7520**

WILSON, J[ames] C[ornelius] (1847-1934)
The complete medical pocket-formulary and physician's vade-mecum: containing upwards of 2500 prescriptions . . . for the use of practitioners . . . 4th ed., thoroughly rev. by F. J. Kalteyer, M.D. Philadelphia: J. B. Lippincott Co., [1906]. 310p. DLC; NNNAM; PPC; PPJ **00-7521**

WILSON, J[ames] C[ornelius] (1847-1934)
The practitioner's part in the movement against tuberculosis. Chicago, 1906. 6p. DNLM **00-7522**

WILSON, J[ames] C[ornelius] (1847-1934)
. . . Fever-nursing: designed for the use of professional and other nurses, and especially as a text-book for nurses in training . . . 5th ed., rev. and enl. Philadelphia and London: J. B. Lippincott Co., [1907]. 248p. fold. charts. DLC; IU-M; KyLoJM; PPC **00-7523**

WILSON, J[ames] C[ornelius] (1847-1934)
The complete medical pocket-formulary and physician's vade-mecum: containing upwards of 2500 prescriptions. . . . Collated for the use of practitioners . . . 5th ed., thoroughly rev. by F. J. Kalteyer, M.D. Philadelphia: J. B. Lippincott Co., [1907]. 271p. DLC; OCLloyd; NNC; PPC **00-7524**

WILSON, J[ames] C[ornelius] (1847-1934)
A handbook of medical diagnosis . . . for the use of practitioners and students . . . 408 text illustrations and 14 full page plates. . . . Philadelphia & London: J. B. Lippincott Co., [1909]. 1435p. col. plates. DLC; NNNAM; PPC; PU
00-7525

WILSON, J[ames] C[ornelius] (1847-1934)
Clinical diagrams. Designed for the graphic representation of clinical phenomena for preservation with the notes of cases. Philadelphia: J. B. Lippincott Co., 1909. DLC; DNLM [Twenty-five perforated sheets with 150 figures, in manila envelope.] **00-7526**

WILSON, J[ames] C[ornelius] (1847-1934)
A handbook of medical diagnosis . . . for the use of practitioners and students . . . 408 text illustrations and 14 full page plates . . . [2nd ed.] Philadelphia & London: J. B. Lippincott Co., [1910]. 1436p. col. plates. CtY-M; CU-M; DLC; PPC
00-7527

WILSON, J[ames] C[ornelius] (1847-1934)
. . . Fever-nursing: designed for the use of professional and other nurses, and especially as a text-book for nurses in training. . . . 6th ed., rev. and enl. Philadelphia and London: J. B. Lippincott Co., [1910]. 259p. plates. DLC; LNT-M; MH-M; PPC **00-7528**

WILSON, J[ames] C[ornelius] (1847-1934)
. . . Infectious diseases. . . . An authorized translation from "Die deutsche klinik" under the general editorial supervision of Julius L. Salinger, M.D. With two colored plates and sixty illustrations in the text. New York and London: D. Appleton & Co., 1910. 933p. DLC; ICJ; NNNAM; PPC
00-7529

WILSON, J[ames] C[ornelius], ed. (1847-1934)
. . . Infectious diseases. . . . An authorized translation from "Die deutsche klinik" under the general editorial supervision of Julius L. Salinger, M.D. With two colored plates and sixty illustrations in the text. New York and London: D. Appleton & Co., 1910. 979p. DLC; MH-M; NNNAM; PPC
00-7530

WILSON, J[ames] C[ornelius] (1847-1934)
A handbook of medical diagnosis . . . for the use of practitioners and students . . . 418 text illustrations and 14 full page plates. 3rd ed., thoroughly rev. . . . Philadelphia and London: J. B. Lippincott Co., [1910]. 1438p. DLC; KU; MBM; PU **00-7531**

WILSON, Robert
High frequency oscillating and high periodicity pulsating currents in medicine. New York, 1906. 15p. DNLM
00-7532

WILSON, Samuel J[erome] (*b.* 1850)
Microbes and health. . . . [Lansing], Mich.: Pub. by the Author, 1901. 230p. DLC **00-7533**

WILSON, Samuel J[erome] (*b.* 1850)
Christian science and disease. . . . The knowledge of to-day. Chicago: The Clinic Publishing Co., 1901. 217p. DLC; ICJ **00-7534**

WILSON, Samuel J[erome] (*b.* 1850)
Comparative therapeutics. . . . Detroit, Mich.: Raynor & Taylor, 1910? 320p. DLC; ICJ **00-7535**

WILSON, W[illiam] Reynolds (*b.* 1863)
A reference handbook of obstetric nursing. Philadelphia & London: W. B. Saunders & Co., 1907. 258p. DLC; DNLM; NNNAM; PPC **00-7536**

WILSON, W[illiam] Reynolds (*b.* 1863)
A reference handbook of obstetric nursing. 2nd ed., thoroughly rev. Philadelphia & London: W. B. Saunders & Co., 1910. 256p. DLC; ICJ; PPJ; PU **00-7537**

WINBIGLER, Charles F[remont] (1857-1925)
Christian science and kindred superstitions; their facts and fallacies. . . . With an introduction by Rev. J. Herndon Garnett. New York, London, [etc.]: The Abbey Press, [1901]. 168p. DLC; MH; NIC; NN **00-7538**

WINBIGLER, Charles F[remont] (1857-1925)
Suggestion, its law and application; or, The principle and practice of psycho-therapeutics . . . 1st ed. Washington, D.C.: S. A. Lewis Co., 1909. 472p. front. (port.) diag. DLC
00-7539

WINDSOR, Lilla D.
The way to heal yourself; or, The road to health and happiness. . . . [Washington]: The Author, [1900?] 25p. incl. front., illus., port. DLC **00-7540**

WINFIELD, J[ames] Macfarlane (*b.* 1859)
Pemphigus and bullous dermatoses, and notes on some personally observed cases. [New York, 1908.] 12p. DNLM
00-7541

WINFIELD, J[ames] Macfarlane (*b.* 1859)
The treatment of eczema in infants and young children. New York, 1908. 14p. DNLM **00-7542**

WINFIELD, J[ames] Macfarlane (*b.* 1859)
Some of the cutaneous manifestations of diseased ductless glands and the application of animal therapy in certain skin diseases. St. Louis, 1909. 3 l. DNLM **00-7543**

WINFIELD, J[ames] Macfarlane (*b.* 1859)
Osteopathies of quaternary syphilis (Gaucher); a report of the examination of forty-six orthopaedic cases for evidences of inherited syphilis. New York, 1909. 4p. DNLM
00-7544

WINFIELD, J[ames] Macfarlane (*b.* 1859)
Cutaneous manifestations of diseased ductless glands and animal therapy in skin diseases. [Philadelphia, 1909.] 12p. PPHa **00-7545**

WINSLOW, Charles-Edward A[mory] (1877-1957)
The case for vaccination. New York & Lancaster, Pa., 1903. 7p. DNLM **00-7546**

WINSLOW, Charles-Edward A[mory] (1877-1957)
The sanitary dangers of certain occupations. Boston, 1904. 9p. DNLM **00-7547**

WINSLOW, Charles-Edward A[mory] (1877-1957)
Elements of applied microscopy. A text-book for beginners. New York: J. Wiley & Sons, 1905. 183p. DNLM; ICJ; NNNAM; PU **00-7548**

WINSLOW, Charles-Edward A[mory] (1877-1957)
The systematic relationships of the *coccaceae* with a discussion of the principles of bacterial classification. New York: John Wiley & Sons, 1908. 300p. DLC; ICJ; MH; NN
00-7549

WINSLOW, John R[andolph] (*b.* 1866)
A case of membranous synechia of the vocal chords due to intubation of the larynx; laryngo-fissure cure. [Baltimore, 1905.] 4p. DNLM **00-7550**

WINSLOW, John R[andolph] (*b.* 1866)
A case of radical mastoidectomy performed under unusual indications. [Baltimore, 1905.] 4p. DNLM
00-7551

WINSLOW, Kenelm (*b.* 1863)
Nervous diseases, woman and child, the heart, the stomach and bowels, common abdominal pains. [Circulation and digestion.] New York: Review of Reviews Co., 1907. 270p. 6 plates. DLC; NIC; NN [Home Medical Library, v. 3]
00-7552

WINSLOW, Kenelm (*b.* 1863)
Personal hygiene, family medicines. . . . Exercise, by D. A. Sargent. Long life, by Sir H. Thompson. Practical kitchen science, by J. M. Hill. New York: Review of Reviews Co., 1907. 268p. 1 port. illus. DLC; NN [Home Medical Library, v. 4] **00-7553**

WINSLOW, Kenelm (*b.* 1863)
The home medical library . . . with the cooperation of many medical advising editors and special contributors. . . . New York: The Review of Reviews Co., 1907. 6 v. col. plates. DLC; ICJ; NNNAM; PU **00-7554**

WINSLOW, Kenelm (*b.* 1863)
The production and handling of clean milk. . . . New York: W. R. Jenkins Co., [1907]. 207p. plates. DLC; ICJ; NN; PU
00-7555

WINSLOW, Kenelm (*b.* 1863)
The production and handling of clean milk, including practical milk inspection, by Kenelm Winslow . . . and Essentials of milk bacteriology, by H. W. Hill . . . [2nd ed.] New York: W. R. Jenkins Co., [1909]. 367p. DLC; NN; NNC; PU
00-7556

WINSLOW, Randolph (*b.* 1852)
Penetrating wounds of the abdomen. Chicago, 1905. 20p. DNLM **00-7557**

WINTERNITZ, Milton C[harles] (*b.* 1885) and F. C. AINLEY
The catalytic activity of the blood in the toxemias of pregnancy. New York, 1910. 14p. DNLM **00-7558**

WINTERNITZ, Milton C[harles] (*b.* 1885) and Thomas R. BOGGS
A unique coincidence of multiple subcutaneous haemangio-endothelioma, multiple lymphangio-endothelioma of the intestinal tract and multiple polypi of the stomach undergoing malignant changes; associated with generalized vascular sclerosis and cirrhosis of the liver. Baltimore, 1910. 26p. 21 plates. DNLM; MdBJ-W **00-7559**

WINTERNITZ, Wilhelm (1835-1917)
. . . Hydrotherapy, thermotherapy, heliotherapy, and phototherapy by Dr. Wilhelm Winternitz . . . assisted by Dr. Alois Strasser . . . and Dr. B. Bauxbaum . . . and Balneology and crounotherapy by Dr. E. Heinrich Kisch . . . transl. by Augustus A. Eshner. . . . Philadelphia: P. Blakiston's Son & Co., 1902. 570p. DLC; ICJ; NNNAM; PU
00-7560

WINTERS, Joseph E[deil] (*d.* 1922)
The feeding of infants. Home guide for modifying milk. New York: E. P. Dutton & Co., 1901. 47p. DNLM; NNNAM
00-7561

WINTERS, Joseph E[deil] (*d.* 1922)
The food factor as a cause of health and disease during childhood, or the adaptation of food to the necessities of the growing organism. New York: William Wood & Co., 1902. 19p. DNLM; NNNAM **00-7562**

WINTERS, Joseph E[deil] (*d.* 1922)
Feeding in early infancy. Formulae for feeding. New York, 1903. 24p. DNLM; NNNAM **00-7563**

WINTERS, Joseph E[deil] (*d.* 1922)
Treatment of croupous pneumonia in children. [New York, 1906.] 16p. DNLM; NNNAM **00-7564**

WINTERS, Joseph E[deil] (*d.* 1922)
Feeding in the first year of infancy. [New York, 1906.] 16p. DNLM; NNNAM **00-7565**

WINTERS, Joseph E[deil] (*d.* 1922)
Etiology of rheumatism. Diet in rheumatism. Relation of chorea and rheumatism and of tonsillitis and rheumatism. [New York? 1907.] 16p. NIC ["Read before the Society of Alumni of Bellevue Hospital, Nov. 6, 1907."]
00-7566

WINTERS, Joseph E[deil] (*d.* 1922)
Practical infant feeding; feeding formulas. . . . New York, [*c.* 1909?]. 23p. CtY-M **00-7567**

WINTERS, Joseph E[deil] (*d.* 1922)
Metabolism in rheumatism. The food factor in rheumatism. Prevention of heart disease. Feeding in rheumatism. [New York, 1910?]. 8p. NIC **00-7568**

WINTERS, Joseph E[deil] (*d.* 1922)
Intestinal infections in children; treatment of diarrhea. [n. p., 1910?] 16p. DNLM [Read before the Cleveland Academy of Medicine, April 15, 1910, and before the Medical Association of Greater New York, May 16, 1910.]
00-7569

WINTSCH, Carl Herman
Some of the needs of the medical profession and homoeopathy. . . . [Newark, N.J., 1910.] 15p. DLC
00-7570

WIRT, William E[dgar]
Two cases of extreme genu-valgum corrected by supracondyloid osteotomy. Cleveland, 1900. 7 l. DNLM
00-7571

WIRT, William E[dgar]
Tuberculous disease of bone and joints. Cleveland, 1901. 15p. DNLM **00-7572**

WISCONSIN MEDICAL INSTITUTE
The home private medical adviser in plain language for the young people, the unmarried and the married. By the master specialist . . . and president of the Wisconsin Medical Institute. Milwaukee, [1902?]. 187p. DLC **00-7573**

WISCONSIN. STATE BOARD OF HEALTH
. . . The powers and duties of boards of health. Laws relating to the organization of the state and local health boards, nuisances, offenses against public health, water supplies and sewerage systems, general public health regulations and the law providing for the collection of vital statistics. Rules and regulations for the control of communicable diseases, transportation rules and rules for the use of the state hygienic laboratory. Book of instructions and laws issued to health boards and health officers by the Wisconsin State Board of Health. 7th ed., 1909. [Madison, 1909.] 144p. DLC; ICJ
00-7574

WISE, Peter M[anuel] (1851-1907)
The State of New York and the pathology of insanity. New York, 1900. 31p. DNLM; NNNAM **00-7575**

WISE, Peter M[anuel] (1851-1907)
Results of five years experience with co-operation between state hospitals for the insane: may it be profitably extended to other charitable institutions? [Albany, 1900.] 19p. PPC
00-7576

WISE, Peter M[anuel] (1851-1907)
A textbook for training schools for nurses, including physiology and hygiene, and the principles and practice of nursing. New York: G. P. Putnam's Sons, 1900 [*c.* 1896]. 2 v. DLC; MBM; MH; NN **00-7577**

WISHART, Charles A.
A diagnositic point in the third nerve paralysis. Nashville, 1900. 2p. DNLM **00-7578**

WISTAR INSTITUTE OF ANATOMY AND BIOLOGY, PHILADELPHIA
. . . List of biological series, exclusive of botany, in the libraries of Philadelphia. Philadelphia: Press of the John C. Winston Co., 1909. 61p. DLC; MB; PP; PPAmP **00-7579**

WISTAR INSTITUTE OF ANATOMY AND BIOLOGY, PHILADELPHIA
Style brief, a guide for authors in preparing copy and correcting proof of professional papers and for the use of editors and printer, adopted as the standard of the journals published by the Wistar Institute of Anatomy and Biology, Philadelphia. 1st ed., December, 1910. . . . Baltimore, Md.: The Waverly Press, [1910]. 32p. illus., 7 plates on 5 l. (part col.). DLC; PHi; PP; PPL **00-7580**

WITHERSPOON, Thomas C[asey] (*b.* 1868)
An operation to reach the lower ureter by an extra-peritoneal route. New York, 1904. 9p. DNLM **00-7581**

WITHERSPOON, Thomas C[asey] (*b.* 1868)
Anatomy of the inguinal region. Chicago, 1906. 15p. DNLM **00-7582**

WITHINGTON, Charles F[rancis] (1852-1917)
A clinical study of one hundred and thirty-five cases of empyema based upon the bacteriologic findings in the exudate. [Philadelphia], 1902. 20p. DNLM **00-7583**

WITHINGTON, Charles F[rancis] (1852-1917)
Addison's disease, with and without adrenal tuberculosis. New York, 1904. 24p. DNLM **00-7584**

WITHINGTON, Charles F[rancis] (1852-1917)
Renal suppurations in typhoid fever. Philadelphia, 1909. 20p. DNLM **00-7585**

WITHINGTON, Charles F[rancis] (1852-1917)
Some observations on human rabies. [Boston, 1909.] 16p. DNLM **00-7586**

WITTHAUS, R[udolph] A[ugust] (1846-1915)
The medical student's manual of chemistry . . . 5th ed. New York: William Wood & Co., 1902. 678p. DLC; DNLM; NNNAM; PU **00-7587**

WITTHAUS, R[udolph] A[ugust] (1846-1915)
A laboratory guide in urinalysis and toxicology. 5th ed. New York: William Wood & Co., 1903. 115 l. 1 plate. DNLM; ICJ; NNNAM; PU **00-7588**

WITTHAUS, R[udolph] A[ugust] (1846-1915)
The medical student's manual of chemistry . . . 6th ed. New York: William Wood & Co., 1906. 820p. DLC; DNLM; NNNAM; PPC **00-7589**

WITTHAUS, R[udolph] A[ugust] (1846-1915)
Medical jurisprudence, forensic medicine and toxicology, by R. A. Witthaus . . . and Tracy C. Becker . . . with the collaboration of August Becker, Esq.; Chas. A. Boston, Esq.; Hon. Goodwin Brown [and others] . . . 2nd ed. New York: William Wood & Co., 1906-11. 4 v. plates. CtY-M; DLC; NNNAM; PPC **00-7590**

WITTHAUS, R[udolph] A[ugust] (1846-1915)
Essentials of chemistry and toxicology, for the use of students in medicine . . . 13th ed., rev. by R. J. E. Scott. . . . New York: William Wood & Co., 1907. 306p. DLC; DNLM; NNNAM; PU **00-7591**

WITTHAUS, R[udolph] A[ugust] (1846-1915)
Manual of toxicology . . . reprinted from Witthaus' and Becker's Medical jurisprudence, forensic medicine and toxicology. 2nd ed. New York: William Wood & Co., 1910. 1261p. illus. DLC; DNLM; KU; PPJ **00-7592**

WODEHOUSE, Robert E[lmer] (*b.* 1882)
Results obtained from use of diphtheria antitoxine refined and concentrated by Gibson's method. New York, 1908. 6p. DNLM **00-7593**

WODEY, Jean
The determination of sex. Chicago: Wodey Pub. House, 1900. 76p. DLC; ICJ **00-7594**

WOLBARST, Abraham L[eo] (*b.* 1872)
The rôle of the prostate affections of the urinary tract. New York, [1905]. 8p. DLC; NN **00-7595**

WOLBARST, Abraham L[eo] (*b.* 1872)
The problem of venereal prophylaxis; some remedial suggestions relating to it. Boston, [1906]. 11p. DLC; NN **00-7596**

WOLBARST, Abraham L[eo] (*b.* 1872)
The three-glass catheter test; an improved method for the identification and separation of urethral and bladder detritus in urethritis. New York, 1906. 4p. DLC; NN **00-7597**

WOLBARST, Abraham L[eo] (*b.* 1872)
Sarcoma of the testicle. Chicago, 1907. 8p. DLC; NN **00-7598**

WOLBARST, Abraham L[eo] (*b.* 1872)
A brief study of the prostate with reference to the curability of gonorrhoea. New York, 1908. 8p. DLC; NN **00-7599**

WOLBARST, Abraham L[eo] (*b.* 1872)
Pyuria; its causes, and the methods of determining them. New York, 1908. 18p. DLC; NN **00-7600**

WOLBARST, Abraham L[eo] (*b.* 1872)
A contribution to the subject of syphilitic prophylaxis by the use of calomel ointment; report of a case. New York, 1908. 4p. DLC; NN **00-7601**

WOLBARST, Abraham L[eo] (*b.* 1872)
Sexual neurasthenia as a sequel to gonorrhea. New York, 1909. 5p. DLC; NN **00-7602**

WOLBARST, Abraham L[eo] (*b.* 1872)
A further contribution to the study of the prostate, with reference to the curability of gonorrhoea. New York, 1909. 13p. DLC; NN **00-7603**

WOLBARST, Abraham L[eo] (*b.* 1872)
The prevalence of venereal disease among recently arrived immigrants, with special reference to intermarital infection. New York: A. R. Elliott Pub. Co., 1909. 10p. DLC; NN **00-7604**

WOLBARST, Abraham L[eo] (*b.* 1872)
A study of 329 cases of gonorrhea in the male, with particular reference to the therapeutic value of arhovin. New York: Schering & Glatz, 1909. 8p. DLC; NN **00-7605**

WOLBARST, Abraham L[eo] (*b.* 1872)
The value of microscopical examination of the prostato-vesicular secretion in the diagnosis and prognosis of gonococcus infection. New York, 1909. 14p. DLC; NN
00-7606

WOLBARST, Abraham L[eo] (*b.* 1872)
The proper attitude of the general practitioner toward the venereal diseases. Philadelphia, 1910. 15p. DLC; NN
00-7607

WOLBARST, Abraham L[eo] (*b.* 1872)
Ehrlich's arsenobenzol; its technique and indications for general use. New York, 1910. 7p. DLC NN
00-7608

WOLBARST, Abraham L[eo] (*b.* 1872)
A case of accidental cauterization of the male urethra with a concentrated silver nitrate solution; complete recovery. New York, 1910. 8p. DLC; NN **00-7609**

WOLBARST, Abraham L[eo] (*b.* 1872)
Gonococcus urethritis in male children. New York, 1910. 10p. DLC; NN **00-7610**

WOLBARST, Abraham L[eo] (*b.* 1872)
Personal observations on the Ehrlich-Hata 606. New York, 1910. 9p. DLC; NN **00-7611**

WOLDERT, Albert (*b.* 1867)
A preliminary investigation of the theory of the inoculation of malarial fever through the agency of mosquitoes. Chicago, 1900. 19p. 1 plate. DNLM **00-7612**

WOLDERT, Albert (*b.* 1867)
The importance of a correct diagnosis in the treatment of diseases of the stomach; with a summary of 30 consecutive cases. Philadelphia, 1904. 8p. DNLM
00-7613

WOLDERT, Albert (*b.* 1867)
Some personal observations made in Pennsylvania and in Texas regarding malarial fever and the Anopheles mosquito. Philadelphia, 1906. 17p. DNLM **00-7614**

WOLDERT, Albert (*b.* 1867)
Malarial fever. Shreveport, 1906. 18p. 1 plate. DNLM
00-7615

WOLDERT, Albert (*b.* 1867)
Résumé of the complete gastric analyses in sixty-one consecutive cases of indigestion. Chicago, 1907. 11p. DNLM
00-7616

WOLDERT, Albert (*b.* 1867)
An original investigation of an epidemic of grippe, followed by a large number of cases of pneumonia. New York, 1907. 20p. DNLM **00-7617**

WOLDERT, Albert (*b.* 1867)
Malarial fever and its expense to the people of Texas. Austin, Texas, 1908. 27p. DNLM **00-7618**

WOLF, Charles G[eorge] L[ewis] (*b.* 1872)
A laboratory hand book of urine analysis and physiological chemistry. Philadelphia & London: W. B. Saunders & Co., 1901. 203p. 2 plates. CU-M; DNLM; PPC; PU
00-7619

WOLF, Charles G[eorge] L[ewis] (*b.* 1872)
The chemistry of toxaemias in pregnancy. New York, 1906. 8p. DNLM **00-7620**

WOLF, Heinrich F[ranz] (*b.* 1872)
Artificial hyperaemia, with special reference to Bier's method. New York, 1907. 10p. DNLM **00-7621**

WOLF, Heinrich F[ranz] (*b.* 1872)
The present status of the methods of physical therapeutics, and their importance for medical schools and practicing physicians. New York, 1907. 10p. DNLM
00-7622

WOLF, Henry J. (*b.* 1861)
Malaria as a complicating factor in the diagnosis of appendicitis. New York, 1902. 7p. DNLM **00-7623**

WOLFF, Bernard
Practical dermatology; a condensed manual of diseases of the skin; designed for the use of students and practitioners of medicine. . . . Chicago: Cleveland Press, 1906. 278p. illus. DLC; ICJ **00-7624**

WOLFF, Lawrence (1845?-1901)
. . . Essentials of medical chemistry, organic and inorganic, containing also, questions of medical physics, chemical philosophy, analytical processes, toxicology, etc., prepared especially for students of medicine . . . 6th ed., thoroughly rev. by A. Ferree Witmer. . . . Philadelphia and London: W. B. Saunders & Co., 1904. 225p. DLC; MH-M; PPC; PU
00-7625

WOLFF, Lawrence (1845?-1901)
. . . Essentials of medical chemistry, organic and inorganic; containing also questions of medical physics, chemical philosophy, analytical processes, toxicology, etc., prepared especially for students of medicine . . . 7th ed., rev., by A. Ferree Witmer. . . . Philadelphia and London: W. B. Saunders & Co., 1908. 225p. DLC; MBM; PPC; PPJ **00-7626**

WOLLSTEIN, Martha (*b.* 1868)
The dysentery bacillus in a series of cases of infantile diarrhea. Boston, 1903. 8p. DNLM; MH **00-7627**

WOLLSTEIN, Martha (*b.* 1868)
A study of the bacteriology of pertussis, with special reference to the agglutination of the patient's blood. [New York, 1906.] 8p. DNLM **00-7628**

WOOD, Alfred C. (*b.* 1863)
A jack-stone inthe esophagus located by the fluoroscope, and removed after performing gastrotomy. Philadelphia, 1903. 6p. DNLM **00-7629**

WOOD, Alfred C. (*b.* 1863)
Cholelithiasis with special reference to surgical treatment. Charlotte, 1904. 19p. DNLM **00-7630**

WOOD, Alfred C. (*b.* 1863) and Augustus A. ESHNER
Actinomycosis (streptothricosis) in man; with the report of a case of pulmonary involvement. New York, 1910. 28p. DNLM; NNNAM **00-7631**

WOOD, Casey A[lbert] (1856-1942)
Address on an exhibit of early (prior to 1860) British and American ophthalmic literature. [Chicago, 1902.] 28p. MB; PPHa **00-7632**

WOOD, Casey A[lbert], ed. (1856-1942)
. . . The eye, ear, nose and throat, ed. by Casey A. Wood . . . Albert H. Andrews, M.D., T. Melville Hardie. . . . Chicago: The Year Book Publishers, [1902]. 346p. plates. DLC; ICJ; NN **00-7633**

WOOD, Casey A[lbert] (1856-1942)
Exophthalmic goitre; its etiology, symptoms and treatment. Buffalo, 1902. 10p. DNLM **00-7634**

WOOD, Casey A[lbert] (1856-1942)
The various methods of preserving and mounting gross-eye preparations. Chicago, 1903. 26p. DNLM **00-7635**

WOOD, Casey A[lbert], ed. (1856-1942)
. . . The eye, ear, nose and throat; ed. by Casey A. Wood . . . Albert H. Andrews, M.D., Gustavus P. Head, M.D. December, 1903. Chicago: The Year Book Publishers, [1903]. 332p. plates. DLC; ICJ; OCIM **00-7636**

WOOD, Casey A[lbert] (1856-1942)
The commoner diseases of the eye, how to detect and how to treat them. For students of medicine; with 250 illustrations, many of them original, of which seven are colored plates. By Casey A. Wood . . . and Thomas A. Woodruff. . . . Chicago: G. P. Engelhard & Co., 1904. 490p. 2 col. plates. DLC; DNLM; OCIM; PU **00-7637**

WOOD, Casey A[lbert] (1856-1942)
The commoner diseases of the eye, how to detect and how to treat them. For students of medicine; with 250 illustrations, many of them original, of which seven are colored plates. By Casey A. Wood . . . and Thomas A. Woodruff [2nd ed.] Chicago: G. P. Engelhard & Co., 1904. 499p. ICJ; OCIM; NN **00-7638**

WOOD, Casey A[lbert] (1856-1942)
Poisoning by wood or methyl alcohol and its preparations as a cause of death and blindness; a supplementary report. New York: A. R. Elliott Co., 1905. 24p. DNLM **00-7639**

WOOD, Casey A[lbert] (1856-1942)
Some forms of hereditary cataract. Chicago, 1906. 12p. DNLM **00-7640**

WOOD, Casey A[lbert] (1856-1942)
The sanitary regulation of the schoolroom with reference to vision. [n. p.], 1906. 10p. DNLM **00-7641**

WOOD, Casey A[lbert], ed. (1856-1942)
. . . The eye, ear, nose and throat; ed. by Casey A. Wood . . . Albert H. Andrews, M.D., Gustavus P. Head. . . . Chicago: The Year Book Publishers, [1906]. 368p. plates. DLC: ICJ; NN **00-7642**

WOOD, Casey A[lbert] (1856-1942)
A medical career and the intellectual life. Easton, Pa., 1907. 10p. DNLM **00-7643**

WOOD, Casey A[lbert] (1856-1942)
The common diseases of the eye, how to detect and how to treat them. For students of medicine: with 280 illustrations (many original) and 8 colored plates, by Casey A. Wood . . . and Thomas A. Woodruff . . . 3rd ed., enl. and improved, with index. Chiago: W. T. Keener & Co., 1907. 598p. CtY-M; DLC; DNLM; NNNAM **00-7644**

WOOD, Casey A[lbert], ed. (1856-1942)
. . . The eye, ear, nose and throat; ed. by Casey A. Wood . . . and Albert H. Andrews, M.D., Gustavus P. Head. . . . Chicago: The Year Book Publishers, [1907]. 353p. plates. DLC; ICJ **00-7645**

WOOD, Casey A[lbert] (1856-1942)
A system of ophthalmic therapeutics; being a complete work on the non-operative treatment, including the prophylaxis, of diseases of the eye. Ed. and chiefly written by Casey A. Wood. . . . Illustrated and completely indexed. Chicago: Cleveland Press, 1909. 926p. DLC; DNLM; OCIM; PPC **00-7646**

WOOD, Casey A[lbert], ed. (1856-1942)
. . . The eye, ear, nose and throat, ed. by Casey A. Wood . . . Albert H. Andrews, M.D., Gustavus P. Head. . . . Chicago: The Year Book Publishers, [1909]. 366p. plates. DLC; ICJ; IU-M **00-7647**

WOOD, Casey A[lbert], ed. (1856-1942)
. . . The eye, ear, nose and throat, ed. by Casey A. Wood . . . Albert H. Andrews . . . Gustavus P. Head. . . . Chicago: The Year Book Publishers, 1910. 367p. plates. DLC; OCIM; PPC **00-7648**

WOOD, C[harles] E.
The public health plank. New York, 1908. 16p. DNLM **00-7649**

WOOD, Eugene H[alsey]
The quest of the germ: with observations thereanunt . . . Milwaukee, Wis.: The Author, 1906. 229p. front., illus. DLC; ICJ **00-7650**

WOOD, Francis C[arter] (1869-1951)
Laboratory guide to clinical pathology. New York: J. T. Dougherty, 1901. 284p. DLC; NN **00-7651**

WOOD, Francis C[arter] (1869-1951)
Laboratory guide to clinical pathology. New York: [Theo. Gaus' Sons], 1904. 284p. illus. CtY-M; DLC; NN; NNNAM **00-7652**

WOOD, Francis C[arter] (1869-1951)
The mixed tumors of the salivary glands. Philadelphia, 1904. 72p. 12 plates. DNLM; PPC **00-7653**

WOOD, Francis C[arter] (1869-1951)
Chemical and microscopical diagnosis. New York: D. Appleton & Co., 1905. 745p. 9 plates. DLC; DNLM; PPC; PPJ **00-7654**

WOOD, Francis C[arter] (1869-1951)
The viability of the pneumococcus after drying; a study of one of the factors in pneumonic infection. [New York, 1906.] 34p. DNLM; NNNAM **00-7655**

WOOD, Francis C[arter] (1869-1951)
Chemical and microscopical diagnosis . . . 2nd ed., with one hundred and ninety-two illustrations in the text and nine colored plates. New York and London: D. Appleton & Co., 1909. 767p. DLC; PPC; PPJ; PU **00-7656**

WOOD, George Bacon (1871-1954)
The lymphatic drainage of the faucial tonsils. Philadelphia, 1905. 12p. DNLM **00-7657**

WOOD, George Bacon (1797-1879)
The dispensatory of the United States of America, by Dr. Geo. B. Wood and Dr. Franklin Bache. 19th ed. Thoroughly rev., largely rewritten, and based upon the eighth decennial revision of the United States pharmacopoeia. By H. C. Wood . . . Joseph P. Remington . . . and Samuel P. Sadtler . . . assisted by Albert B. Lyons . . . and Horatio C. Wood, Jr. . . . Philadelphia: J. B. Lippincott Co., [1907]. 1947p. DLC; NNNAM; OCLloyd; PU **00-7658**

WOOD, George P.
Vitalogy; or, Encyclopedia of health and home . . . [by] G. P. Wood, M.D., E. H. Ruddock, M.D. . . . New York, Chicago: Northern Publishing House, 1900. 2 v. fronts., illus., plates (part col.) ports. DLC; ICJ [1st ed., Vitalogy, adapted for home and family use. . . . Embracing food remedies for the cure and prevention of all diseases. . . . [By] Geo. P. Wood, M.D., E. H. Ruddock, M.D. Chicago, Ill.: I. N. Reed, 1896. 1250p. DLC] **00-7659**

WOOD, George P.
Vitalogy; or, Encyclopedia of health and home . . . from the most authentic sources in this country, Europe and Japan. 2 v. in 1. New York and Chicago: Northern Pub. House, 1900. 1268p. DLC **00-7660**

WOOD, George P.
Vitalogy; or, Encylcopedia of health and home, adapted for home and family use . . . [by] Geo. P. Wood, M.D., E. H. Ruddock. . . . Chicago, New York: Vitalogy Association, 1907. 971p. DLC; ICJ [Part of the colored plates are superimposed.] **00-7661**

WOOD, George P.
Vitalogy; or, Encyclopedia of health and home, adapted for home and family use . . . [by] Geo. P. Wood, M.D., E. H. Ruddock. . . . Chicago, New York: Vitalogy Association, 1907. 2 v. fronts., illus., plates (partly col.) ports. DLC; ICJ **00-7662**

WOOD, Harold B[acon] (*b.* 1878)
Scarlatinal epidemic from infected milk bottles. New York, 1908. 4p. DNLM **00-7663**

WOOD, Horatio C. (1841-1920)
Therapeutics: its principles and practice. . . . 11th ed. Remodelled and in greater part rewritten by Horatio C. Wood, and Horatio C. Wood, Jr. . . . Philadelphia and London: J. B. Lippincott Co., 1900. 850p. DLC; DNLM; NNNAM; PU **00-7664**

WOOD, Horatio C. (1841-1920)
Therapeutics: its principles and practice. . . . 12th ed. Thoroughly rev. and adapted to the eighth (1905) edition of the United States pharmacopoeia by Horatio C. Wood and Horatio C. Wood, Jr. . . . Philadelphia and London: J. B. Lippincott Co., 1905. 907p. DLC; DNLM; OCLloyd; PPC **00-7665**

WOOD, Horatio C. (1841-1920)
Therapeutics: its principles and practice. By Horatio C. Wood . . . and Horatio C. Wood, Jr. . . . 13th ed. Thoroughly rev. and adapted to the 8th (1905) ed. of the United States pharmacopoeia. Philadelphia and London: J. B. Lippincott Co., 1906. 963p. DLC: DNLM; NNNAM; PPC **00-7666**

WOOD, Horatio C. (1841-1920)
Bibliographical record 1860-1900, Horatio C. Wood. [n. p., 1907?] 24p. DLC; DNLM; NN **00-7667**

WOOD, Horatio C. (1841-1920)
Therapeutics: its principles and practice . . . thoroughly rev. and rewritten by Horatio C. Wood, Jr. . . . 14th ed. Philadelphia and London: J. B. Lippincott Co., [1908]. 778p. DLC; DNLM; NNNAM; PU **00-7668**

WOOD, Horatio C. (1841-1920)
The scientific evidence of the possibility of intestinal antisepsis; read before the Philadelphia County Medical Society, November 9, 1910. Detroit: E. G. Swift, 1910. 10p. NN **00-7669**

WOOD, Horatio C. (1841-1920)
The comparative danger of ethyl chlorid as an anaesthetic. [Chicago: American Medical Association, 1910.] 3p. NN **00-7670**

WOOD, James C[raven] (*b.* 1858)
Cystic distension of the appendix vermiformis, with a review of the literature of the subject. New York, 1900. 11p. DNLM **00-7671**

WOOD, James C[raven] (*b.* 1858)
Appendicitis associated with diseased conditions of the female pelvic organs. Chicago, 1901. 16p. 1 table. DNLM **00-7672**

WOOD, James C[raven] (*b.* 1858)
Cleveland alumni banquet of U. of M., February 8, 1901. The college professor. Chicago, 1901. 6p. DNLM **00-7673**

WOOD, James C[raven] (*b.* 1858)
The use of the spray in the local treatment of gynecological diseases. New York, 1901. 5p. DNLM **00-7674**

WOOD, James C[raven] (*b.* 1858)
Present status of homoeopathy, being the presidential address delivered before the fifty-eighth session of the American Institute of Homoeopathy, Cleveland, Ohio . . . 1902. [unp.] PPHa **00-7675**

WOOD, James C[raven] (*b.* 1858)
Profound lesions within the pelvis resulting from gonorrhea, giving rise to distressing indigestion, malnutrition, etc. [Cleveland, 1904, *vel subseq.*] 3p. DNLM **00-7676**

WOOD, James C[raven] (*b.* 1858)
The surgical aspect of indigestion and so-called gastralgia. [Cleveland, 1904.] 12p. DNLM **00-7677**

WOOD, James C[raven] (*b.* 1858)
Pudenal hematocele. Philadelphia, 1904. 3p. DNLM **00-7678**

WOOD, James C[raven] (*b.* 1858)
A clinical case, with comments. [Rahway, N.J., 1904.] 4p. DNLM **00-7679**

WOOD, James C[raven] (*b.* 1858)
Celiotomy during pregnancy; six clinical cases. [New York, 1906.] 8p. DNLM **00-7680**

WOOD, James C[raven] (*b.* 1858)
Two cases of appendicitis associated with retroflexion of the uterus and displacement of the ovaries; description of the internal "Alexander" operation. [Rahway, N.J., 1906.] 6p. DNLM **00-7681**

WOOD, James C[raven] (*b.* 1858)
The tragedy of the gonococcus. New York, 1909. 8p. MH; NN **00-7682**

WOOD, James C[raven] (*b.* 1858)
Gastro-intestinal auto-intoxication and mucous enterocolitis from the viewpoint of surgery, with illustrative cases. Chicago, 1910. 16p. 1 plate. DNLM **00-7683**

WOOD, Joseph R[emington] (*b.* 1872)
Tablet manufacture, its history, pharmacy and practice. Philadelphia and London: J. B. Lippincott Co., 1906. 224p. plates. DLC; DNLM; ICJ; PU **00-7684**

WOOD, Nathan E[lliott]
Dollars to doctors: or diplomacy and prosperity in medical practice. Chicago: The Lion Publishing Co., 1903. 272p. DLC; ICU; NN; PU **00-7685**

WOOD, William C.
One hundred years of publishing (1804-1904). A brief historical account of the house of William Wood and Company. New York: William Wood & Co., 1904. 29p. DLC; MH; NNNAM; NN **00-7686**

WOODBURY, Frank T[hompson] (*b.* 1875)
Report of a case of puerperal convulsions for which Caesarean section was required. New York: A. R. Elliott Pub. Co., 1905. 8p. DNLM **00-7687**

WOODBURY, Frank T[hompson] (*b.* 1875)
Iodine, the ideal surgical antiseptic. New York, 1910. 10p. DNLM **00-7688**

WOODHEAD, G[erman] Sims (1855-1921)
Some phase of the evolution of modern preventive medicine, as illustrated by the present campaign against tuberculosis. New York, 1910. 30p. DNLM; NNNAM **00-7689**

WOODHULL, Alfred A[lexander] (1837-1921)
Notes on military hygiene, for officers of the line. A syllabus of lectures formerly delivered at the U.S. Infantry and Cavalry School. . . . 3rd ed., rewritten. 1st thousand. New York: J. Wiley & Sons; [etc., etc.], 1904. 238p. DLC; DNLM; NIC; NNNAM **00-7690**

WOODHULL, Alfred A[lexander] (1837-1921)
(a) Hygienic instruction of Army medical officers; (b) their powers and duties; (c) needed improvements; (d) camp sanitation; (e) sanitation of an army en route. [Columbus, O., 1906.] 8p. DNLM **00-7691**

WOODHULL, Alfred A[lexander] (1837-1921)
Personal hygiene, designed for undergraduates. New York: J. Wiley & Sons, 1906. 221p. DNLM; NNNAM **00-7692**

WOODHULL, Alfred A[lexander] (1837-1921)
Military hygiene, for officers of the line . . . 4th ed., rewritten and greatly enl. New York: J. Wiley & Sons; [etc., etc.], 1909. 384p. DLC; DNLM; NIC; NNNAM **00-7693**

WOODHULL, Alfred A[lexander] (1837-1921)
A suggestion for field sanitary study. [n. p., 1908, *vel subseq.*] 5p. DNLM **00-7694**

WOODHULL, Alfred A[lexander] (1837-1921)
Direct responsibility for military health and sanitation. Columbus: Miller Co., 1910. 14p. DNLM **00-7695**

WOODRUFF, Charles E[dward] (1860-1915)
An anthropological study of the small brain of civilized man and its evolution. Utica, 1901. 77p. DNLM **00-7696**

WOODRUFF, Charles E[dward] (1860-1915)
The military importance of mild typhoid infections, such as mountain fever. [Philadelphia], 1904. 12p. DNLM **00-7697**

WOODRUFF, Charles E[dward] (1860-1915)
Alcohol in the tropics. New York, 1904. 35p. DNLM **00-7698**

WOODRUFF, Charles E[dward] (1860-1915)
The effects of tropical light on white men. New York & London: Rebman Co., 1905. 358p. DLC; LNT-M; MH-M; NN **00-7699**

WOODRUFF, Charles E[dward] (1860-1915)
Complexions of the insane. New York, 1905. 7p. DLC **00-7700**

WOODRUFF, Charles E[dward] (1860-1915) and Frank Thomas WOODBURY
The prevention of disease in the Army, and the best method of accomplishing that result. Carlisle, 1906. 37p. DLC; ICJ **00-7701**

WOODRUFF, Charles E[dward] (1860-1915)
The dangers of excessive sunlight in tuberculosis. New York, 1908. 22p. DLC **00-7702**

WOODRUFF, Thomas A[dams] (*b.* 1865)
Prevention of blindness [Philadelphia, 1902?] 12p. PPHa **00-7703**

WOODRUFF, Thomas A[dams] (*b.* 1865)
Diaphoretics in ophthalmic therapeutics. [Philadelphia, 1902?] 6p. PPHa **00-7704**

WOODRUFF, Thomas A[dams] (*b.* 1865)
The treatment of certain non-specific lesions of the uveal tract with pilocarpin and sweat baths. [Chicago, 1902.] 6p. MB **00-7705**

WOODRUFF, Thomas A[dams] (*b.* 1865)
The treatment of recent trachoma. Chicago: American Medical Assoc. Press, 1907. 7p. DNLM **00-7706**

WOODRUFF, William L[awrence] (*b.* 1860)
Therapeutics of vibration, the healing of the sick an exact science. . . . Los Angeles, Cal.: J. F. Elwell Publishing Co., [1907]. 144p. 2 plates, 2 fold. tables. DLC **00-7707**

WOODS, Hiram (1857-1931)
Use of diaphoresis and diaphoretic agents in ophthalmic therapeutics . . . and Diaphoretics and diaphoresis in ophthalmic therapeutics, by T. A. Woodruff. Chicago, 1905. 11p., 7p. DNLM; MH; NN; PPHa **00-7708**

WOODS, Richard F. (*b.* 1873)
The after treatment of a series of forty-four laparotomies. New York, 1908. 8p. DNLM **00-7709**

WOODS, Walter V.
Health, how to get and keep it. The hygiene of press, food, exercise, rest, bathing, breathing, and ventilation. . . . Philadelphia: The Penn Publishing Co., 1905. 196p. DLC; MH; NN; PU **00-7710**

WOODWARD, Alfred W. (1839-1902)
Constitutional therapeutics. "The patient, not the disease." . . . Philadelphia: Boericke & Tafel, 1903. 557p. DLC; ICJ; PPC; PPHa **00-7711**

WOODWARD, Alfred W. (1839-1902)
Report of provings. [Philadelphia, 1903?] 12p. PPHa **00-7712**

WOODWARD, Charles (*b.* 1845)
An original and comprehensive method of intra-uterine medication for the treatment of the various forms of uterine diseases, presenting a course which, in the author's experience of nearly thirty years, has proven successful far beyond that claimed for any other method. . . . Chicago: The Woodward Co., 1904. 208p. illus. DLC; ICJ **00-7713**

WOODWARD, J[ulius] H[ayden] (*b.* 1858)
The ocular complications of mumps. New York, 1904. 7p. DNLM **00-7714**

WOODWARD, J[ulius] H[ayden] (*b.* 1858)
Five illustrative cases of primary melanosarcoma of the choroid. [New York, 1910.] 12p. 5 plates. NN **00-7715**

WOODY, Samuel E[lisha] (*b.* 1854)
Essentials of medical chemistry and urinalysis. 4th ed., rev. and enl. Philadelphia: P. Blakiston's Son & Co., 1900. 243p. DLC; DNLM; ICJ; PPC **00-7716**

WOOLF, Charles H[yatt], ed.
The optical dictionary; an optical and ophthalmological glossary of English terms, symbols and abbreviations, together with the English equivalents of some French and German terms . . . to which are added a number of general and mathematical expressions. . . . Philadelphia: P. Blakiston's Son & Co., 1904. 166p. DLC; ICJ; MH; NN **00-7717**

WOOLLEY, Paul G[erhard] (*b.* 1875)
A case of primary malignant tumor of the thyroid composed of adenocarcinoma and perithelial hemangiosarcoma (sarcocarcinoma). Philadelphia, 1902. 3p. DNLM **00-7718**

WOOLLEY, Paul G[erhard] (*b.* 1875)
Some observations on disease in Manila. New York, 1906. 19p. DNLM **00-7719**

WOOLSEY, George (*b.* 1861)
Applied surgical anatomy, regionally presented for the use of students and practitioners of medicine. Philadelphia: Lea Bros. & Co., 1902. 521p. 59 plates. DLC; DNLM; PPC; PU **00-7720**

WOOLSEY, George (*b.* 1861)
Applied surgical anatomy, regionally presented, for the use of students and practitioners of medicine . . . 2nd ed., enl. and thoroughly rev. With 200 illustrations, including 59 plates, mostly colored. New York and Philadelphia: Lea & Febiger, 1908. 601p. DNLM; NNNAM; OCIM; PPC **00-7721**

WOOTON, A. C. (*d.* 1910)
Chronicles of pharmacy. New York: Macmillan Co., 1910. 2 v. DLC; ICJ; NN; PU **00-7722**

WORCESTER, Alfred (1855-1951)
Addresses, relative to the Cambridge School of Nursing, before the Cambridge Medical Improvement Society, the Colonial Club of Cambridge, and the students of Radcliffe College. Waltham, Mass., 1905. 28p. DNLM; MH **00-7723**

WORCESTER, Alfred (1855-1951)
Addresses, relative to the Waltham Training School for Nurses. Dr. Alfred Worcester, President Charles W. Eliot. Report of the meeting held at 85 Mt. Vernon St., Boston, December 31, 1906. [Boston], 1906. 25p. MB **00-7724**

WORCESTER, Elwood (1862-1940), S. McCOMB and Isador CORIAT
Religion and medicine, the moral control of nervous disorders. New York: Moffat, Yard & Co., 1908. 427p. DLC; DNLM; NIC; NN **00-7725**

WORTH, Claud (1869-1936)
Squint; its causes, pathology, and treatment. Philadelphia: P. Blakiston's Son & Co., 1903. 229p. DNLM; PPC; PPJ; PU **00-7726**

WORTH, Claud (1869-1936)
Squint; its causes, pathology and treatment. 2nd ed. Philadelphia: P. Blakiston's Son & Co., 1905. 231p. CtY-M; DLC; NNNAM; PPC **00-7727**

WORTH, Claud (1869-1936)
Squint; its causes, pathology, and treatment. 3rd ed. Philadelphia: P. Blakiston's Son & Co., 1906. 234p. IU-M; NNNAM; OCIM; PPC **00-7728**

WOSE, A[lfred] M[illard] (*b.* 1876)
Renal distention. New York: A. R. Elliott, 1905. 17p. DNLM **00-7729**

WRIGHT, Adam H[enry] (*b.* 1846)
A text-book of obstetrics. New York: D. Appleton & Co., 1905. 501p. CU-M; DNLM; NNNAM; PPC **00-7730**

WRIGHT, Almroth E[dward] (1861-1947)
Principles of microscopy; being a handbook to the microscope. . . . New York: The Macmillan Co., 1907. 250p. illus. DLC; MB; NIC; PU **00-7731**

WRIGHT, Almroth E[dward] (1861-1947)
Studies on immunization and their application to the diagnosis and treatment of bacterial infections. New York: William Wood & Co., 1910. 490p. 1 plate. CU-M; CtY-M; NNNAM; PU **00-7732**

WRIGHT, Barton L[isle] (*b.* 1870)
Malaria; a summary of recent progress in the knowledge of its etiology and prophylaxis. Philadelphia, 1902. 9p. DNLM **00-7733**

WRIGHT, Barton L[isle] (*b.* 1870)
The treatment of tuberculosis by the administration of mercury at the U.S. Naval Hospital, New Fort Lyon, Colorado. New York, 1908. 16p. DLC; DNLM
00-7734

WRIGHT, Barton L[isle] (*b.* 1870)
The treatment of tuberculosis by the administration of mercury; being a compilation of a preliminary report and a second paper on the subject. Washington, 1908. 63p. DLC; ICJ; NN **00-7735**

WRIGHT, Clarence A[lfred] [Joseph]
Notes on instrumentation. Published in connection with the English translation of radio-therapy by Leopold Freund. New York: Rebman Co., 1904. 59p. DNLM; ICJ; NNNAM; PPC
00-7736

WRIGHT, G[eorge] A[rthur] (1851-1922) and Charles H[enry] PRESTON
Handbook of surgical anatomy. Philadelphia: P. Blakiston's Son & Co., 1904. 202p. CtY-M; DNLM; PPC; PU
00-7737

WRIGHT, Hiram A. (*b.* 1863)
The pathology of paretic dementia. New York, 1905. 12p. DNLM **00-7738**

WRIGHT, James H[omer] (1869-1928) and Arthur K. DRAKE
A case of extreme malformation of the heart. Philadelphia, 1903. 3p. 2 plates. DNLM **00-7739**

WRIGHT, James H[omer] (1869-1928)
The biology of the microorganism of actinomycosis. Boston, 1905. 56p. 10 plates. DNLM **00-7740**

WRIGHT, James H[omer] (1869-1928)
The origin and nature of the blood plates. Boston, 1906. 10p. 1 plate. DNLM **00-7741**

WRIGHT, James H[omer] (1869-1928)
A method for the differential staining of blood plates. Boston, 1906. 2p. DNLM **00-7742**

WRIGHT, James H[omer] (1869-1928) and Oscar RICHARDSON
Treponemata (spirochaetae) in syphilitic aortitis; five cases, one with aneurism. Boston, 1909. 7p. 1 plate. DNLM
00-7743

WRIGHT, James H[omer] (1869-1928)
The histogenesis of the blood platelets. Philadelphia, 1910. 16p. 2 plates. DNLM **00-7744**

WRIGHT, J[ohn] A. (*b.* 1854)
Medical progress. New York, 1905. 18p. DNLM; NNNAM
00-7745

WRIGHT, John S[hepard] (*b.* 1870)
Pharmacology of the fluid extracts in common use; a brief account of the derivation, the most important constituents and the chief physiological effects produced by the drugs employed in their preparation, with incidental mention of their therapeutic uses. . . . Indianapolis, Ind.: From the Research Department of E. Lilly & Co., 1905. 225p. DLC; ICJ
00-7746

WRIGHT, John S[hepard] (*b.* 1870)
A guide to the organic drugs of the United States Pharmacopoeia 1900 and a few of the more commonly used unofficial drugs. Containing, in addition to the brief accounts of organic drugs, a conspectus of the families of the plants mentioned, a glossary of the botanical and therapeutical terms used and an index of botanical synonyms. . . . Rev. with the assistance of Arthur L. Walters. 2nd revision, with app. . . . Prepared for students of pharmacy. Indianapolis, Ind.: Botanical Dept. of E. Lilly & Co., 1906. 186p. DLC; ICJ
00-7747

WRIGHT, John W[estley] (1842-1935)
A text-book of ophthalmology. 2nd ed. Philadelphia: P. Blakiston's Son & Co., 1900. 378p. DNLM; NNNAM; PPC; PPJ **00-7748**

WRIGHT, John W[estley] (1842-1935)
A text-book of ophthalmology. 3rd ed., thoroughly rev. Philadelphia: P. Blakiston's Son & Co., 1909. 398p. DLC; ICJ; PPC; PU **00-7749**

WRIGHT, Jonathan, ed. (1860-1928)
A treatise on diseases of the nose, throat, and ear. For students and practitionrs. By various authors. . . . Volume II of A treatise on diseases of the eye, nose, throat, and ear. Ed. by William Campbell Posey and Jonathan Wright. Philadelphia and New York: Lea Bros. & Co., [*c.* 1902]. [689]-1199p. illus., plates (part col.). DLC; IU-M; NNC; PPJ
00-7750

WRIGHT, Jonathan (1860-1928)
The nose and throat in medical history. . . . St. Louis, Mo.: L. S. Matthews & Co., 1904. 244p. DLC; ICJ; ICU; PU
00-7751

WRIGHT, Jonathan (1860-1928)
Cysts in lymphoid tissue, an exceptional manifestation of tonsillar retrogression. St. Louis, 1905. 4p. DNLM
00-7752

WRIGHT, Jonathan (1860-1928)
The difference in the behavior of dust from that of bacteria in the tonsillar crypts. New York, 1906. 16p. 1 plate. DNLM
00-7753

WRIGHT, Jonathan (1860-1928)
The fat content of the tonsils and its relation to the processes of metabolism and infection. New York, 1906. 16p. DNLM
00-7754

WRIGHT, Jonathan (1860-1928)
The primordial nature of the forces exerted against the penetration of bacteria beneath the surface of the body. New York, 1906. 14p. DNLM **00-7755**

WRIGHT, Jonathan (1860-1928)
A nasal sporozoon (rhinospiridium kinealyi). New York, 1907. 12p. DNLM **00-7756**

WRIGHT, Jonathan (1860-1928)
The physical processes of immunity and infection. New York, 1907. 51p. DNLM **00-7757**

WRIGHT, Jonathan (1860-1928)
The mechanico-biological standpoint in medical problems. New York, 1908. 22p. DNLM **00-7758**

WRIGHT, Jonathan (1860-1928)
The tonsil from an evolutionary point of view. New York, 1908. 16p. DNLM **00-7759**

WULLING, Grederick J[ohn] (*b.* 1866)
An elementary course in inorganic pharmaceutical and medical chemistry. . . . Rev., and reprinted from the Pharmaceutical record. 1st ed. First thousand. New York: J. Wiley & Sons, 1901 [*c.* 1894]. 311p. DLC; MH; NN; PU **00-7760**

WUNDERLICH, Karl R[heinhold] A[ugust] (1815-1877)
Medical thermometry, and human temperature. By C. A. Wunderlich . . . and Edward Seguin, M.D. New York: William Wood & Co., 1900 [*c.* 1871]. 208p. DLC; CU-M; ICJ; PPC [First German ed. of pt. 1 published in 1868 with title: Das verhalten der eigenwarme in krankheiten. *Contents* — pt. 1. On the temperature in diseases . . . by C. A. Wunderlich. Abridged by Edward Seguin. — pt. 2. Suggestions on thermometry and human temperature, by Edward Seguin.] **00-7761**

WUNDT, Wilhelm M[ax] (1832-1920)
Outlines of psychology . . . translated with the cooperation of the author, by Charles Hubbard Judd . . . 2nd rev. English ed., from the 4th rev. German ed. Leipzig: W. Engelmann; New York: G. E. Stechert; [etc., etc.], 1902. 390p. DLC; MH; NIC; NN [1st American ed., New York: G. E. Stechert, 1897. 342p.] **00-7762**

WYETH, John A[llan] (1845-1922)
Sarcoma of the undescended testes. New York: A. R. Elliott Pub. Co., 1905. 3p. DNLM **00-7763**

WYETH, John A[llan] (1845-1922)
Water as a local anaesthetic. New York, 1906. 2p. DNLM **00-7764**

WYETH, John A[llan] (1845-1922)
A synopsis of the histories of seven cases of appendicitis, with comments. New York, 1907. 8p. DNLM **00-7765**

WYETH, John A[llan] (1845-1922)
Surgery . . . with 864 illustrations. New York City: M. S. Wyeth & Co., 1908. 816p. DLC; NNNAM **00-7766**

WYETH, John A[llan] (1845-1922)
Memorial address on Doctor Robert Koch. By J. A. Wyeth and A. Knopf. New York: William Wood & Co., [1910]. 11p. illus. NN **00-7767**

WYETH, JOHN, & BROTHER. PHILADELPHIA
Physician's pocket-list, John Wyeth & Brother, manufacturing chemists, Philadelphia. January 2, 1901. [Philadelphia, 1901.] 252p. CtY-M; DLC; ICJ; PPC [*vel subseq.*] **00-7768**

WYETH, JOHN, & BROTHER. PHILADELPHIA
An epitome of therapeutics with special reference to the laboratory products of John Wyeth & Brother. Philadelphia: John Wyeth & Brother, 1901. 371p. DLC; ICJ; PPC **00-7769**

WYETH, JOHN, & BROTHER. PHILADELPHIA
Therapy of the glycero-phosphates, with special reference to elixir glycero-phosphates of soda and lime. [Philadelphia]: J. Wyeth & Bros., 1901. 7p. DNLM **00-7770**

WYETH, JOHN, & BROTHER. PHILADELPHIA
The new antipyretics, antiseptics and analgesics. [Philadelphia, 1902.] 11p. DNLM **00-7771**

WYETH, JOHN, & BROTHER. PHILADELPHIA
Clinical excerpts; sevetol. Philadelphia, [1902]. 10p. DNLM **00-7772**

WYETH, JOHN, & BROTHER. PHILADELPHIA
An epitome of therapeutics, with special reference to the laboratory products of John Wyeth & Brother. . . . Philadelphia: J. Wyeth & Brother, 1906. 375p. CtY-M; DLC; ICJ; MH **00-7773**

WYETH, JOHN, & BROTHER. PHILADELPHIA
Physicians' pocket-list. John Wyeth & Brother . . . manufacturing chemists, Philadelphia. [Philadelphia], 1908. 318p. ICJ **00-7774**

WYETH, JOHN, & BROTHER. PHILADELPHIA
Remedies for influenza, with brief notes for their employment. Philadelphia, [190-?] 10p. MB **00-7775**

WYLIE, Samuel M. (*b.* 1855)
Nicholas Senn, an appreciation. [Chicago? 1908.] 27p. DNLM; ICJ; IU-M **00-7776**

WYMAN, Walter (1848-1911)
. . . The health of the nation. . . . [New York? 1905.] 11p. DLC **00-7777**

WYMAN, Walter (1848-1911)
How to prevent yellow fever—No mosquitoes, no yellow fever. . . . [Washington: Government Printing Office, 1905.] 2 l. DLC **00-7778**

WYMAN, Walter (1848-1911)
. . . The present organization and work for the protection of health in the United States, by Walter Wyman, Surgeon-General, United States Public Health and Marine-Hospital Service. Washington: Government Printing Office, 1910. 16p. DLC **00-7779**

WYNTER, W[alter] Essex (1860-1945)
Minor medicine; a treatise on the nature and treatment of common ailments. New York: D. Appleton & Co., 1908. 275p. DLC: ICJ; NNNAM; PPC **00-7780**

XEROFORM (tribromphenol-bismuth). The ideal substitute for iodoform in surgery, gynaecology and dermatology, being a powerful antibacterial, desiccating and deodorizing agent which is odorless, non-poisonous and non-irritating. [New York, 1900?] 11p. NN **00-7781**

YAGER, Willard E.
The Oneota; medicine in the forest. . . . Oneonta, N.Y.: Oneonta Herald Pub. Co., 1910. 84p. illus. DLC [Indians of North America—Medicine.] **00-7782**

YALE, Arthur W[ells] (*b.* 1875)
The use of picric acid in the treatment of pelvic inflammations. Philadelphia, 1902. 4p. DNLM **00-7783**

YALE, Arthur W[ells] (*b.* 1875)
Mucous membranes; their pathologic conditions and treatment. Philadelphia: J. Wyeth & Bros., 1903. 7p. DNLM; PPC **00-7784**

YALE, Arthur W[ells] (*b.* **1875**)
Adjuvant treatment of tuberculosis. [Philadelphia, 1903?] 4p. PPHa **00-7785**

YALE, Leroy M[ilton] (1841-1906)
Nursery problems, ed. by. . . . New and enl. ed. New York: The Contemporary Publishing Co., 1900 [*c.* 1897]. 340p. DLC; DNLM; MB; PPL [1st ed., 1893]. **00-7786**

YALE, Leroy M[ilton] (1841-1906)
Overstudy. New York, 1900. 6p. DNLM **00-7787**

YALE, Leroy M[ilton] (1841-1906) and Gustav POLLAK
The Century book for mothers. A practical guide in the rearing of healthy children. New York: The Century Co., 1901. 461p. DNLM; MH; NIC; NN **00-7788**

YALE UNIVERSITY. SHEFFIELD SCIENTIFIC SCHOOL
Biographical record, classes from eighteen hundred and sixty-eight to eighteen hundred and seventy-two of the Sheffield Scientific School. [New Haven]: Class Secretaries' Bureau, Yale University, 1910. 254p. CtY-M; DNLM; MH **00-7789**

YANKAUER, Sidney (*b.* **1872**)
An unusual case of empyaema of the antrum of Highmore. New York, 1903. 3p. DNLM **00-7790**

YANKAUER, Sidney (*b.* **1872**)
Submucous resection of the deviated nasal septum. New York, 1905. 8p. DNLM **00-7791**

YARROW, Thomas J. and Arthur P. HITCHENS
On the clinical estimation of the quantity of hemoglobin in the human blood. Philadelphia, [1900]. 9p. DNLM **00-7792**

YARROW, Thomas J.
Injuries of the kidney and traumatic (parenchymatous) nephritis, with clinical report of an illustrative case accompanied by haematoidinuria and albumosuria, terminating in complete recovery. New York, 1900. 16p. DNLM; NN **00-7793**

YARROW, Thomas J.
Chronic carbon monoxid poisoning and carbonyl hemoglobinuria; the latter a hitherto undescribed condition. Philadelphia, 1902. 16p. DNLM; NN **00-7794**

YARROW, Thomas J.
The albumoses; their clinical significance viewed from a modern standpoint; their detection and distinction from the other proteids found in the urine as a means of lowering the death rate in obscure suppurative and other diseases. Philadelphia, 1903. 29p. DNLM; NN **00-7795**

YELLIN, David
Maimonides. By David Yellin and Israel Abraham. Philadelphia: Jewish Publication Society, 1903. 239p. DNLM; ICJ; MH; NN **00-7796**

YELLOW fever statistics during years 1878, 1897, and 1905. New Orleans: Merchants Printing Co., [1905]. 1 galley sheet. DNLM; LNT-M **00-7797**

YEO, I[saac] Burney (1835-1914)
Food in health and disease. 8th ed. Chicago: W. T. Keener & Co., [1901]. 592p. DLC; DNLM; ICJ; OCIM **00-7798**

YEO, I[saac] Burney (1835-1914)
A manual of medical treatment or clinical therapeutics . . . 10th edition . . . Vol. I-[II]. Chicago: W. T. Keener & Co., 1902. 2 v. DLC: ICJ; MH-M; PPC **00-7799**

YEO, I[saac] Burney (1835-1914)
A manual of medical treatment or Clinical therapeutics. . . . New and revised edition. Eleventh edition . . . Vol. I-[II]. Chicago: W. T. Keener & Co., 1903. 2 v. DLC: ICJ; IU-M; PPJ **00-7800**

YEO, I[saac] Burney (1835-1914)
A manual of medical treatment and clinical therapeutics. [Rev. ed.] Chicago: W. T. Keener & Co., 1904. 2 v. DNLM; ICJ; PU **00-7801**

YEO, I[saac] Burney (1835-1914)
A manual of medical treatment; or, Clinical therapeutics. New and rev. ed. 12th ed. Chicago: W. T. Keener & Co., 1905. 2 v. DLC; IU-M; NNNAM; PU **00-7802**

YEO, I[saac] Burney (1835-1914)
A manual of medical treatment and clinical therapeutics. Revised ed., with formulae adapted to the standard of strength of preparations employed in America, by Oscar Oldberg. 14th ed. Chicago: W. T. Keener & Co., 1906. 2 v. DNLM; ICJ; NNNAM **00-7803**

YEO, I[saac] Burney (1835-1914)
A manual of medical treatment and clinical therapeutics. New ed., revised by Raymond Crawford and E. Farquhar Buzzard. New York: William Wood & Co., 1909. 2 v. DLC; DNLM; NNNAM **00-7804**

YEO, I[saac] Burney (1835-1914)
The therapeutics of mineral springs and climates. New York: Funk & Wagnalls, 1910. 760p. CtY-M; DLC; ICJ; NN [Contains dictionary of health resorts.] **00-7805**

YONGE, Eugene S[tephen]
Hay fever and paroxysmal sneezing (Vasomotor Rhinitis). New York: William Wood & Co., 1910. 150p. DNLM; ICJ; PPC; NN **00-7806**

[YONKERMAN CONSUMPTION CURE CO., KALAMAZOO, MICH.]
Tuberculozyne (Yonkerman) . . . cures consumption. [Kalamazoo, Mich.: Yonkerman Consumption Cure Co., 1904.] 199p. DLC; DNLM **00-7807**

[YONKERMAN CONSUMPTION CURE CO., KALAMZOO, MICH.]
Tuberculozyne (Yonkerman) . . . cures consumption. [Kalamazoo, Mich.: Yonkerman Consumption Cure Co., 1905.] 205p. DLC **00-7808**

YONKERMAN CONSUMPTION REMEDY COMPANY, KALAMAZOO, MICH.
Consumption; its diagnosis, treatment and cure. Kalamazoo, Mich., [1907]. 197p. DLC; DNLM **00-7809**

[YONKERMAN, D. P.]
Consumption. Its diagnosis, treatment and cure. Kalamazoo: Yonkerman Consumption Remedy Co., 1909. 197p. DLC **00-7810**

YORKE-DAVIS, Nathaniel Edward (*b.* 1844)
Foods for the fat: a treatise on corpulency and a dietary for its cure. . . . American ed. Edited by Charles W. Greene. . . . Philadelphia: J. B. Lippincott Co., 1900. 138p. DLC; NNNAM; PPC; PU **00-7811**

YOUNG, Adelbert A.
The vermiform appendix and appendicitis. Buffalo, 1901. 7p. DNLM **00-7812**

YOUNG, Albion G. (*b.* 1843)
Tuberculosis; infection, heredity, prevention, hygienic treatment. Augusta, Me., 1900. 157p. 11 plates. DLC **00-7813**

YOUNG, Albion G. (*b.* 1843)
Formaldehyde as a milk preservative. Augusta, Me., 1900. 9p. PP **00-7814**

YOUNG, Albion G. (*b.* 1843)
Infant feeding and milk for infant feeding. Augusta, [Me.], 1902. 102p. DLC **00-7815**

YOUNG, Albion G. (*b.* 1843)
. . . How typhoid fever is spread, and notes on dysentery and cholera. 1906. Reprinted from its fourteenth report by the State Board of Health of Maine. [Augusta? 1906.] 67p. DLC **00-7816**

YOUNG, Antonio D. (*b.* 1873)
Diagnosis of tabes in the preataxic stage. New York, 1906. 3p. DNLM **00-7817**

YOUNG, Antonio D. (*b.* 1873)
The proper method of administering ether. New York, 1910. 9p. DNLM **00-7818**

YOUNG, Bicknell
Christian science; its principle and method: a lecture delivered in the Royal Albert Hall, London, England, April 23, 1907. . . . Boston, Mass.: The Christian Science Publishing Co., 1909. 31p. DLC; MH **00-7819**

YOUNG, Bicknell
Christian science, deren prinzip und methode; ein vortrag, gehalten in der "Royal Albert Hall," London, England, am 23, april 1907. . . . Boston, Mass.: The Christian Science Publishing Society, 1909. 38p. DLC; MH **00-7820**

YOUNG, D. Hastings
First aid to the child; a guide to the feeding and treatment of infants in health and disease. . . . New York: E. P. Dutton & Co., 1910. 317p. DLC; NN **00-7821**

YOUNG, D. Hastings
First aid to the sick; or diseases, their description, and treatment; a work of reference for the home, written in plain language. . . . New York: E. P. Dutton & Co., [1910]. 280p. DLC; ICJ; NN **00-7822**

YOUNG, Ernest Boyen (1869-1923)
Supernumerary breasts and nipples, with report and photograph of a case. Boston, 1904. 8p. DNLM **00-7823**

YOUNG, Ernest Boyen (1869-1923)
The intra-abdominal rupture of ovarian cysts. With report of a case. Boston, 1904. 19p. DNLM **00-7824**

YOUNG, Ernest Boyen (1869-1923)
A cyst of Gärtner's duct extending from the vagina into the parametrium. Boston, 1905. 9p. 2 plates. DNLM **00-7825**

YOUNG, Ernest Boyen (1869-1923)
The effect of tubal abscess upon the position of the ureter. Boston, 1905. 11p. DNLM **00-7826**

YOUNG, Ernest Boyen (1869-1923)
The efficacy of serum treatment in streptococcus puerperal septicemia. Boston, 1905. 13p. DNLM **00-7827**

YOUNG, Ernest Boyen (1869-1923)
An analysis of twenty-one cases of pelvic abscess treated by vaginal section. Boston: D. C. Heath, 1907. 11p. DNLM **00-7828**

YOUNG, Frank Philip (*b.* 1870)
Surgery from an osteopathic standpoint, by F. P. Young . . . collaborated by Charles E. Still . . . with one hundred and fifty-six illustrations in etchings and halftones. Quincy, Ill.: Volk, Jones & McMein Co., printers, 1904. 438p. plates. DLC; ICJ **00-7829**

YOUNG, Frank P[hilip] (*b.* 1870)
Surgery from an osteopathic standpoint. Collaborated by Charles E. Still. . . . Quincy, Ill.: Volk, Jones & McMein Co., 1904. [unp.] IEN-M; IU-M; OCIM **00-7830**

YOUNG, George B.
The proposed enlarged National Public Health Organization; a discussion of plans for its organization. Chicago, 1910. 31p. DNLM; ICJ; MH; NN **00-7831**

YOUNG, Hugh H[ampton] (1870-1945)
Treatment of stricture of the urethra and review of the literature [with J. T. Geraghty]. [Philadelphia, 1906.] 58p. DLC; MdBJ-W **00-7832**

YOUNG, Hugh H[ampton] (1870-1945)
. . . Studies on hypertrophy and cancer of the prostate. . . . Baltimore: Johns Hopkins Press, 1906. 626p. MdBJ-W; NNC; PPJ; PU **00-7833**

YOUNG, Hugh H[ampton] (1870-1945)
Operative treatment of vesical diverticula with report on 4 cases. [Philadelphia, 1906.] 46p. DLC: MdBJ-W **00-7834**

YOUNG, Hugh H[ampton] (1870-1945)
Chronic prostatitis. An experimental and clinical study with an analysis of 358 cases. [Philadelpia, 1906.] 114p. ICJ; MH-M; PPC; PU **00-7835**

YOUNG, Hugh H[ampton] (1870-1945)
The early diagnosis and radical cure of carcinoma of the prostate. . . . [Philadelpia, 1906.] 50p. MdBJ-W; NNC; OC; PPC **00-7836**

YOUNG, Hugh H[ampton] (1870-1945)
After fifteen years; a glance at the recent progress in medicine and surgery. Address delivered before the alumni of the University of Virginia, June 15, 1909. Charlottesville, Va.: Michie Co., [1909]. 14p. NcD **00-7837**

YOUNG, Hugh H[ampton] (1870-1945)
Perineal prostatectomy. . . . [Troy, New York: The Southworth Co., *c.* 1910.] 38 l. NN **00-7838**

YOUNG, James K[elly] (1862-1923)
Orthopedic apparatus. Illus. Philadelphia, 1904. 36p. MB **00-7839**

YOUNG, James K[elly] (1862-1923)
Synopsis of human anatomy; being a complete compend of anatomy, including the anatomy of the viscera and numerous tables, by James K. Young . . . 2nd ed., rev. and enl. With 171 engravings, some in colors. Philadelphia: F. A. Davis Co., 1905. 402p. DLC; NNNAM; OCIM; PPC **00-7840**

YOUNG, James K[elly] (1862-1923)
Handbook of anatomy; being a complete compend of anatomy, including the anatomy of the viscera and numerous tables. 2nd ed., rev. & enl. Philadelphia: F. A. Davis Co., 1905. 402p. illus. DNLM; MH; NN; PU **00-7841**

YOUNG, James K[elly] (1862-1923)
A manual and atlas of orthopedic surgery, including the history, etiology, pathology, diagnosis, prognosis, prophylaxis, and treatment of deformities . . . illustrated with over seven hundred photographs and line drawings, mostly from original sources. Philadelphia: P. Blakiston's Son & Co., 1905. 942p. DLC; ICRM; PPC; PU **00-7842**

YOUNG, James K[elly] (1862-1923)
Handbook of anatomy; being a complete compend of anatomy, including the anatomy of the viscera and numerous tables . . . 3rd ed., rev. and enl. With 172 engravings, some in colors. Philadelphia: F. A. Davis Co., 1909. 402p. DLC; NNNAM; PPC; PU **00-7843**

YOUNG, J[ohn] Van Doren (*b.* 1864)
Sacral suspension of the uterus, a new technic. New York, 1909. 13p. DNLM **00-7844**

ZAHORSKY, John (*b.* 1871)
A few clinical studies of cardiac diseases in infancy and childhood. New York, 1900. 15p. DNLM; NN **00-7845**

ZAHORSKY, John (*b.* 1871)
Baby incubators. A clinical study of the premature infant, with especial reference to incubator institutions conducted for show purposes. . . . St. Louis, Mo.: Courier of Medicine Co., 1905. 136p. incl. illus., tables, diags., front. (port.) CtY-M; DNLM; ICJ **00-7846**

ZAHORSKY, John (*b.* 1871)
. . . Golden rules of prediatrics; aphorisms, observations and precepts on the science and art of pediatrics: giving practical rules for the diagnosis and prognosis, the essentials of infant feedings, and the principles of scientific treatment. . . . With an introduction by E. W. Saunders. . . . St. Louis: The C. V. Mosby Medical Book Co., 1906. 362p. DLC; OCIM; PU; ScC **00-7847**

ZAHORSKY, John (*b.* 1871)
Golden rules of pediatrics; aphorisms, observations, and precepts on the science and art of pediatrics . . . [2nd ed.] St. Louis: C. V. Mosby Medical Book Co., 1910. 284p. DNLM; ICJ; MH-M; PU **00-7848**

[ZAKRZEWSKA, Marie Elizabeth] (1829-1902)
Marie Elizabeth Zakrzewska, 1829-1902. A memoir. Boston: New England Hospital for Women and Children, 1903. 30p. MBM; MH **00-7849**

ZAPFFE, Frederick C[arl] (*b.* 1873)
. . . Bacteriology. A manual for students and practitioners . . . illustrated with one hundred and forty-six engravings and seven colored plates. Philadelphia and New York: Lea Bros. & Co., [1903]. 350p. 7 plates. DLC; DNLM; PPC; PPHa **00-7850**

ZEIT, Frederick R[obert] (*b.* 1864)
Effect of direct, alternating Tesla currents and X-ray on bacteria. Chicago, 1901. 32p. DNLM **00-7851**

ZEIT, Frederick R[obert] (*b.* 1864)
The pathology and bacteriology of uretero-intestinal anastomosis. New York, 1901. 38p. DNLM; NN **00-7852**

ZELLER, George Anthony (*b.* 1858)
Pellagra: some clinical and other features of the disease. . . . St. Louis: Interstate Medical Journal Co., 1910. 15p. illus. DLC **00-7853**

ZELLER, George Anthony (*b.* 1858)
The spread of pellagra throughout the United States. . . . Philadelphia: J. B. Lippincott Co., 1910. 9p. plates, map. DLC **00-7854**

ZELLER, George Anthony (*b.* 1858)
Diet and pellagra. A warning against ill-advised attacks on foodstuffs. . . . Chicago: American Medical Association, 1910. 6p. DLC **00-7855**

ZENNER, Philip (*b.* 1852)
Education in sexual physiology and hygiene: a physician's message. Cincinnati: R. Clarke Co., 1910. 126p. DLC; DNLM; ICJ; NNC **00-7856**

ZENTMAYER, William (*b.* 1864)
Some unusual ocular manifestations of arteriosclerosis. Chicago, 1906. 13p. DNLM **00-7857**

ZENTMAYER, William (*b.* 1864)
Keratitis disciformis. Seattle, 1907. 3p. DNLM **00-7858**

ZENTMAYER, William (*b.* 1864)
A case of bitemporal hemianopsia with an unusual clinical history. St. Louis, 1910. 5p. 3 plates. DNLM **00-7859**

ZENTMAYER, William (*b.* 1864)
The present status of the etiology of squint. Chicago, 1910. 3p. ICJ **00-7860**

ZIEGEL, Hermann F[red] L[ange] (*b.* 1876)
The medical climatology of Southern California. New York, 1906. 20p. DLC; NN **00-7861**

ZIEGEL, Hermann F[red] L[ange] (*b.* 1876)
Precocious tertiary syphilis; report of a case with manifold manifestations. New York, 1909. 6p. DNLM
00-7862

ZIEGEL, Hermann F[red] L[ange] (*b.* 1876)
Balanic hypospadias complicated with simultaneous intra-urethral chancre and gonorrhoea, and idiopathic low specific gravity of the urine. New York, 1910. 5p. DNLM
00-7863

ZIEGEL, Hermann F[red] L[ange] (*b.* 1876)
On the affections clinically simulating typhoid fever, with especial reference to and reports of cases of Brill's disease. New York, 1910. 14p. 1 chart. DNLM **00-7864**

ZIEGEL, Hermann F[red] L[ange] (*b.* 1876)
Brill's disease. New York: William Wood & Co., 1910. 14p. DNLM **00-7865**

ZIEGEL, Hermann F[red] L[ange] (*b.* 1876)
An analysis of twenty cases belonging to the unclassified group of affections clinically resembling typhoid fever. New York: William Wood & Co., [1910?] 4p. DNLM **00-7866**

ZIEGLER, Ernst (1849-1905)
General pathology; or, the science of the causes, nature and course of the processes of disease. Transl. from the 10th revised German ed. (G. Fischer, Jena, 1901) and edited by Aldred Scott Warthin. New York: William Wood & Co., 1903. 760p. CtY-M; DLC; DNLM; NNNAM **00-7867**

ZIEGLER, Ernst (1849-1905)
General pathology; or, the science of the causes, nature and course of the processes of disease. Transl. from the 11th revised German ed. Edited and brought up to date by Aldred Scott Warthin. New York: William Wood & Co., 1908. 781p. DLC; DNLM; GU; NNNAM **00-7868**

ZIEGLER, S[amuel] L[ewis] (1861-1926)
Reflex neuroses arising from ocular and nasal abnormalities. [New York, 1908.] 8p. NN **00-7869**

ZIEGLER, S[amuel] L[ewis] (1861-1926)
Oration in ophthalmology. Reflex neuroses arising from ocular and nasal abnormalities. [New York, 1908.] 23p. NN
00-7870

ZIEGLER, S[amuel] L[ewis] (1861-1926)
History of iridotomy. [Chicago, 1909.] 12p. ICJ; NN
00-7871

ZIEHEN, Theodor (*b.* 1862)
Introduction to physiological psychology. . . . Transl. by C. C. van Liew . . . and Otto W. Beyer. . . . With 21 illustrations. New York: The Macmillan Co., 1909. 305p. incl. diags. DLC; ICJ; NIC; NN **00-7872**

ZIEMSSEN, Hugo W[ilhelm] von (1829-1902)
Neurasthenia and its treatment. New York: William Wood & Co., 1900. 26p. DNLM; NN [Reprinted out of Wood's Medical & Surgical Monographs, vol. I (1889), 529-555]
00-7873

ZIEMSSEN, Hugo W[ilhelm] von (1829-1902)
Antipyresis and antipyretic methods of treatment. New York: William Wood & Co., 1901. 22p. DNLM; NN [Reprinted out of Wood's Medical & Surgical Monographs, vol. II (1889), 559-582] **00-7874**

ZIEMSSEN, Hugo W[ilhelm] von (1829-1902)
The etiology, diagnosis, and treatment of tuberculosis. New York: William Wood & Co., 1902. 75p. NN; ICJ [Reprinted out of Wood's Medical & Surgical Monographs, vol. I (1889), 643-717] **00-7875**

ZIEMSSEN, Hugo W[ilhelm] von (1829-1902)
The pathology and treatment of scarlet fever. New York: William Wood & Co., 1903. 35p. NN [Reprinted out of Wood's Medical & Surgical Monographs, vol. IV (1889), 683-718]
00-7876

ZIMMERMANN, Charles (*b.* 1856)
On ocular affections in puerperal eclampsia. New York, 1900 [*c.* 1898]. 9p. DNLM **00-7877**

ZINKE, [Ernst] Gustav (1846-1922)
The out-door obstetric clinic of the Medical College of Ohio. . . . Cincinnati, 1900. 136p. illus. DLC; OC; OCIM
00-7878

ZINKE, [Ernst] Gustav (1846-1922)
Diagnosis of the attitude of the fetus in utero by external examination. Columbus: Columbus Med. Pub. Co., 1900. 10p. DNLM **00-7879**

ZINKE, [Ernst] Gustav (1846-1922)
The practice of obstetrics. Chicago, 1901. 10p. DNLM
00-7880

ZINKE, [Ernst] Gustav (1846-1922)
Is Caesarean section justifiable in the treatment of placenta praevia? New York: J. D. Emmet, 1901. 13p. DNLM; NNNAM
00-7881

ZINKE, [Ernst] Gustav (1846-1922)
A case of extra- and intra-uterine pregnancy, with tabulated record of eighty-eight cases. New York: William Wood & Co., 1902. 24p. DNLM; NNNAM **00-7882**

ZINKE, [Ernst] Gustav (1846-1922)
The limitation of Caesarean section. New York: William Wood & Co., 1903. 8p. DNLM; NNNAM **00-7883**

ZINKE, [Ernst] Gustav (1846-1922)
The work of Downes' electrothermic angiotribe in two abdominal and two vaginal hysterectomies; in one large ovarian cyst complicating a six months' pregnancy; in three bilateral salpingo-oöphorectomies; in one of epithelioma of the external genitalia and in two cases of external hemorrhoids. New York: William Wood & Co., 1903. 8p. DNLM; NNNAM
00-7884

ZUNKERKANDL, Otto (1861-1921)
Atlas and epitome of operative surgery. . . . Ed. by J.Chalmers da Costa . . . with 24 col. plates and 217 illustrations in the text. Philadelphia: W. B. Saunders & Co., 1900 [*c.* 1898]. 395p. DLC; MBM; NNNAM; PPC **00-7885**

ZUNKERKANDL, Otto (1861-1921)
Atlas and epitome of operative surgery. . . . Ed. by J. Chalmers da Costa . . . 2nd ed., rev. and enl. Philadelphia: W. B. Saunders & Co., 1902. 410p. 40 col. plates. DLC; NNNAM; OCIM; PPC
00-7886

APPENDIX:
WOOD'S LIBRARY OF STANDARD MEDICAL AUTHORS: A CHECKLIST

WOOD'S LIBRARY OF STANDARD MEDICAL AUTHORS A CHECKLIST AND BIBLIOGRAPHICAL GUIDE

Introduction

In the last third of the 19th century, William Wood & Co. of New York City established a reputation as one of the preeminent American medical publishers, challenging even the redoubtable Philadelphia publishing firm founded by Mathew Carey in 1785, whose Lea imprints were acknowledged as the leading medical publications of the time. The Wood firm's origins went back to 1804 when its founder, Samuel Wood, established a general publishing house which he conducted with great success for some forty years. After Samuel Wood's death in 1844, the business was continued by his sons, Samuel S. Wood and William Wood. After William Wood's retirement in 1868 (Samuel S. Wood died in 1861), his son William H. S. Wood assumed control of the company, and with Isaac F. Wood, a grandson of the founder, continued the firm as William Wood & Company.

In the early 1860's the house turned its attention to medical publication, and by the mid-1870's its efforts were almost exclusively devoted to medical publishing. Its entry into the medical field and the house's growing attention to medicine were most likely encouraged by its success with a number of medical periodicals which were very well received. In 1866 the firm launched *The Medical Record* (edited from 1866 to 1904 by George F. Shrady, Secretary of the New York Pathological Society), at first published semi-monthly, but soon changed to a weekly; and in 1869, William Wood & Company undertook to sponsor the *American Journal of Obstetrics and Diseases of Women and Children*, edited for many years by Paul F. Mundé, President of the American Gynecological Society; and these journals were joined by *New Remedies* in 1872, a pharmaceutical trade journal.

The shift to medical publishing was largely due to William H. S. Wood's efforts. A brief centennial history (*One Hundred Years of Publishing [1804-1904], A Brief Historical Account of the House of William Wood & Company, 1904*), speaks to the point: "From the time of his admission to the firm Wm. H. S. Wood advocated further specialization in the direction of medical publications, and proceeded, with characteristic energy and good judgment, to develop the business in this line. The wholesale handling of general stationery supplies was abandoned, as was also the sale of religious and miscellaneous literature, and scientific and medical publications became the chief concern of the house. Numerous medical books by American authors were published, while a complete stock of medical literature in the English language was carried, and sold at wholesale and retail" (pp. 16-17); and in the same centennial memorial (attesting the firm's eventual virtually exclusive medical publishing program), notice is made of one of the truly great feats of 19th centural medical publishing: "In 1874 the house commenced the publication of the largest medical work hitherto issued in the English language, a translation of Ziemssen's *Cyclopedia of the Practice of Medicine*, in twenty-two royal octavo volumes. By special arrangement with the German publishers, advance sheets were sent to this country and translated under the supervision of Dr. Albert H. Buck. This great collection of treatises marked the most important advance in the history of medicine up to this time. In another way the series was remarkable, in that it was sold only by subscription, being the first medical work to be marketed in this way either here or abroad. Through a systematically organized canvass the work was offered to the medical profession not only in the United States, but also to English-speaking physicians throughout the world. It had a very remarkable success." (pp. 24-26)

It is against this background that the genesis of "Wood's Library of Standard Medical Authors" is best understood. The *Library* decisively marked the inauguration of subscription methods of bookselling as applied to medical works, an old and venerable practice in general publishing. The *Library* was begun January 1, 1879, and "involved the monthly issue of important cloth-bound octavo medical books, in yearly sets of twelve volumes. The issue of these series was continued for eight years, and their sale was enormous." (*One Hundred Years . . .*, p. 26)

Actually, the *Library* was continued until October, 1887 when its final volume appeared, appropriately entitled an *Index to Wood's Library of Standard Medical Authors, Complete in One Hundred Volumes*. The *Index*, essentially a subject index, included no bibliographical data on any of the volumes (author's full name; date of original publication in the *Library*; pagination, etc.). Actually, the *Index* was a clever merchandising effort intended to promote sales of complete *Library* sets.

The language of the Index's prefatory note is unashamedly enthusiastic (and not without cause) about the success of the *Library* and its value: "The wonderfully low price at which they have been sold has always been astonishing to all—that the publishers have been enabled to continue this library until it now comprises ONE HUNDRED VOLUMES is due to the quick and continued appreciation of the medical profession, and the consequent practical support it has received. It may not be out of place to state in this prefatory note that, as originally published, the hundred volumes of this series, even if it were possible to obtain them all, would cost nearly six times as much as they are sold for in this 'Library,' exclusive of the handsomely-finished bookcase which accompanies each complete set. In this Index, probably the most compact and still complete of any covering so large a number of volumes, every expedient to condense, without injury, has been adopted, and it is believed it will be found indispensable to all who possess the Library and really desire to avail themselves of its wonderful richness and wealth of practical knowledge. The names of the authors will be found printed in small capitals, and at the same time the consecutive number of the volume in heavy-face type, as stamped on the back of each, is given."

The *Library* continued to sell phenomenally both in and out of its "handsomely-finished book-case" well into the early 1900's.* Its success prompted William Wood & Company to issue still another subscription series, *Wood's Medical and Surgical Monographs, Consisting of Original Treatises and Reproductions, in English, of Books and Monographs Selected from the Latest Literature of Foreign Countries* . . . , but this series lasted only three years (vols. 1-12; January, 1889–December, 1891), and its failure may well lie in the indomitable competition ironically afforded by the larger *Library* whose 100 volumes literally overwhelmed the medical marketplace.

The long history of William Wood & Company ended with its purchase in 1932 by the Williams & Wilkins Company of Baltimore. The Wood firm had come on the market only by reason of the death of the last member of the Wood family associated with the business.

The acquisition of William Wood & Company added 386 active titles to the Williams & Wilkins list, an indication of the vigor and strength of the Wood imprint in medical publishing. Many of the Wood titles, in new editions, continue in the Williams & Wilkins list, and the Baltimore firm is the first to recognize the importance of the Wood acquisition. "Acquisition of the Wood Company immediately added 386 titles to our list. Most of these were of English origin because importation had been a Wood specialty for many years. But there were also many titles of American origin, including quite a few used as text-books in medical schools. The astonishing vitality of the list is emphasized by the fact that 62 of these titles are still, after a full generation, in new editions in the catalog. Some of the most widely known are May's *Diseases of the Eye*, Cabot's (now Adams') *Physical Diagnosis*, Bailey's *Textbook of Histology*, Stedman's *Medical Dictionary*, Bailey's *Physical Signs in Clinical Surgery*, and Topley and Wilson's *Principles*

*Unfortunately, the William Wood & Company ledgers and ancillary records have not survived, and no extended notice of the firm exists beyond the brief 1904 centennial history. The volumes in the *Library* continued to be reprinted until the stereotyped plates, no longer usable, were probably melted down, sometime before 1910. In all, between 1879 and 1910 (?), I estimate that the total print-run in the *Library* exceeded 700,000 volumes.

of Bacteriology and Immunity. One title, not on the present list, went out in a blaze of glory in 1942, when a special printing of 20,000 copies was made for the U.S. Government. This was Tuttle's *Handbook for the Medical Soldier*." (*Three Quarters of a Century Plus Ten: 1890-1975*. Baltimore: Williams & Wilkins Co., 1975, p. 25)

In this bibliographical checklist of "Wood's Library of Standard Medical Authors," I have listed the volumes by the numbers assigned to each of them by the publisher (for this the *Index*, itself Volume 100, is the guide). For each volume, I have furnished comprehensive bibliographical data: author(s)' full name(s); complete title; original year of publication (*i.e.*, in or out of the *Library* by William Wood & Co.); major pagination; and any other relevant details. I have also cited locations for each of the volumes, limited to four libraries for each entry. Given the enormous sale, the volumes of the *Library* are not rare, but they are (like most 19th century medical textbooks) less frequently encountered.

It must be remembered that Wood did not initially number the volumes of the *Library*. Many of the volumes (with the ornamentally distinct title, "Wood's Library of Standard Medical Authors" embossed on their covers) are without numbers on their spines. The commercial success of the *Library* prompted Wood's clever merchandising with numbered volumes for a *One Hundred Volume Library* in "a handsomely-finished bookcase." There is, therefore, no chronological order in the numbering of the volumes truly congruent with their publication dates in the *Library*. Wood's volume-numbering was, at best, idiosyncratic, and probably convenient to the publisher's needs and intentions.

WOOD'S LIBRARY OF STANDARD MEDICAL AUTHORS

[Volumes 1, 2]

ELLIS, George Viner (1812-1900) and G. H. FORD
Illustrations of dissections in a series of original colored plates the size of life, representing the dissection of the human body. 2nd ed. New York: William Wood & Co., 1882. 2 v. DNLM; NNNAM; PPC; PU

[Volumes 3, 4, 5]

ZIEGLER, Ernst (1849-1905)
A text-book of pathological anatomy and pathogenesis. Transl. and edited for English students by Donald MacAlister. New York: William Wood & Co., 1883-7. 2 pts. in 3 v. DNLM; NNNAM; PPC; PU

[Volume 6]

HOLDEN, Luther (1815-1905)
Human osteology comprising a description of the bones with delineations of the attachments of the muscles, the general and microscopic structure of bone and its development. . . . Assisted by James Shuter. . . . 6th ed. New York: William Wood & Co., 1885. 276p. DLC; NNNAM; PPC; PU

[Volume 7]

RANNEY, Ambrose Loomis (1848-1905)
Practical medical anatomy. A guide to the physician in the study of the relations of the viscera to each other in health and disease and in the diagnosis of the medical and surgical conditions of the anatomical structures of the head and neck. New York: William Wood & Co., 1882. 339p. DLC; DNLM; ICJ; PPC

[Volumes 8, 9]

KIRKES, William Senhouse (1823-1864)
Manual of physiology. . . . Edited by W. Morrant Baker and Vincent Dormer Harris. 11th ed. New York: William Wood & Co., 1885. 2 v. 1 plate. DNLM; NNNAM; OClM; PU

[Volumes 10, 11]

PARKES, Edmund Alexander (1819-1876)
A manual of practical hygiene. . . . Ed. by F. S. B. François de Chaumont. . . . From the last [6th] London ed. With an appendix giving the American practice in matters relating to hygiene, prepared by and under the supervision of Frederick N. Owen. New York: William Wood & Co., 1884. 2 v. in 1. 9 plates, maps, diags. DLC; NNNAM; PPC; PU

[Volume 12]

PAVY, Frederick William (1829-1911)
A treatise on food and dietetics physiologically and therapeutically considered . . . 2nd ed. New York: William Wood & Co., 1881. 402p. DLC; DNLM; NNNAM; PU

[Volume 13]

BELL, Agrippa Nelson (1820-1911)
. . . Climatology and mineral waters of the United States. . . . New York: William Wood & Co., 1885. 386p. maps. DLC; DNLM; NNNAM; OClM

[Volumes 14, 15]

CARPENTER, William Benjamin (1813-1885)
The microscope and its relations. 6th ed. New York: William Wood & Co., 1883. 2 v. CtY-M; NNNAM; OClM; PPC

[Volume 16]

WITTHAUS, Rudolph August (1846-1915)
Essentials of chemistry, inorganic and organic, for the use of students in medicine. . . . New York: William Wood & Co., 1879. 257p. DLC; DNLM; NNNAM; PU

[Volume 17]

LYMAN, Henry M[unson] (1835-1904)
. . . Artificial anaesthesia and anaesthetics. . . . New York: William Wood & Co., 1881. 338p. DLC; NNNAM; PPC; PU

[Volume 18]

KEETLEY, C[harles] R[obert] B[ell] (1848-1909)
An index of surgery; being a concise classification of the main facts and theories of surgery, for the use of senior students and others. . . . New York: William Wood & Co., 1882. 320p. DLC; DNLM; NNNAM; PPC

[Volume 19]

CLARKE, W[illiam] Fairlie (1833-1884)
A manual of the practice of surgery. From the last London edition. New York: William Wood & Co., 1879. 316p. CtY-M; NNNAM; OClM; PPC

[Volumes 20, 21]

POULET, Alfred
A treatise on foreign bodies in surgical practice. New York: William Wood & Co., 1880. 2 v. IU-M; KyLoJM; NNNAM; PU

[Volume 22]

PILCHER, Lewis Stephen (1845-1934)
The treatment of wounds: its principles and practice; general and specific. . . . With one hundred and sixteen wood engravings. New York: William Wood & Co., 1883. 391p. DLC; NNNAM; PPC; PPJ

[Volume 23]

BARWELL, Richard (1827-1916)
A treatise on diseases of the joints. 2nd ed. New York: William Wood & Co., 1881. 463p. CtY-M; NNNAM; OClM; PPC

[Volume 24]

HILTON, John (1804-1878)
On rest and pain: a course of lectures on the influence of mechanical and physiological rest in the treatment of accidents and surgical diseases and the diagnostic value of pain. Delivered at the Royal College of Surgeons of England in the years 1860, 1861, and 1862. Edited by W. H. A. Jacobson. 2nd ed. New York: William Wood & Co., 1879. 299p. DNLM; NNNAM; OClM; PPC

[Volume 25]

GUTTMANN, Paul (1834-1893)
A handbook of physical diagnosis, comprising the throat, thorax, and abdomen. Transl. from the 3rd German ed. by Alex. Napier. New York: William Wood & Co., 1880. 344p. 1 col. plate. CtY-M; DNLM; NNNAM; PPC

[Volume 26]

SAVAGE, Henry (*d.* 1900)
The surgery, surgical pathology, and surgical anatomy of the female pelvic organs, in a series of plates taken from nature with commentaries, notes and cases. 3rd ed., rev. and greatly enl. New York: William Wood & Co., 1880. 129p. + 32 plates. IU-M; NNNAM; OClM; PPC

[Volume 27]

VERRIER, Eugène (1824-1910)
Practical manual of obstetrics. 4th ed., with the four obstetric tables of Prof. Pajot. 1st American ed., with revision and annotations by Edward L. Partridge. New York: William Wood & Co., 1884. 395p. CtY-M; DNLM; MBM; PPC

[Volume 28]

MUNDÉ, Paul F[ortunatus] (1846-1902)
Minor surgical gynecology: a manual of uterine diagnosis and the lesser technicalities of gynecological practice; for the use of the advanced student and general practitioner. New York: William Wood & Co., 1880. 381p. DLC; DNLM; NNNAM; PPC

[Volumes 29, 30]

HART, David Berry and A. H. BARBOUR
Manual of gynecology. New York: William Wood & Co., 1883. 2 v. DNLM; MH-M; NNNAM; PU

[Volume 31]

TAIT, [Robert] Lawson (1845-1899)
Diseases of women. New York: William Wood & Co., 1879. 192p. DNLM; MBM; NNNAM; PU

[Volume 32]

FRITSCH, Heinrich (1844-1915)
The diseases of women. . . . Transl. by Isidor Furst. New York: William Wood & Co., 1883. 355p. DLC: ICJ; MBM; NNNAM

[Volume 33]

TILT, Edward [John] (1815-1893)
A handbook of uterine therapeutics. New York: William Wood & Co., 1881. 328p. ICJ; NNNAM; OClM; PU

[Volume 34]

ELLIS, Edward
A practical manual of the diseases of children, with a formulary. 3rd ed. New York: William Wood & Co., 1879. 213p. DNLM; NNNAM; OClM; PPC

[Volume 35]

HENOCH, Eduard Heinrich (1820-1900)
. . . Lectures on diseases of children: a handbook for physicians and students. . . . New York: William Wood & Co., 1882. 357p. DLC; NNNAM; OClM; PPC

[Volume 36]

SMITH, Eustace (1835-1914)
A practical treatise on disease in children. . . . New York: William Wood & Co., 1884. 844p. DLC; NNNAM; OClM; PU

[Volume 37]

ROUTH, Charles Henry Felix (1822-1909)
Infant feeding and its influence on life; or, The causes and prevention of infant mortality. . . . Third edition. New York: William Wood & Co., 1879. 270p. CtY-M; ICJ; PP; NN

[Volumes 38, 39, 40]

PHILLIPS, Charles Douglas Fergusson (1830-1904)
Materia medica and therapeutics. . . . New York: William Wood & Co., 1879-1882. 3 v. DLC; NNNAM; PPC; PU

[Volumes 41, 42, 43]

TROUSSEAU, Armand (1801-1867)
Treatise on therapeutics, transl. by D. F. Lincoln, M.D., from the French of A. Trousseau . . . and H. Pidoux . . . 9th ed., rev. and enl., with the assistance of Constantine Paul. . . . New York: William Wood & Co., 1880. 3 v. DLC; DNLM; NNNAM; PPC

[Volume 44]

JOHNSON, Laurence (1845-1893)
A medical formulary based on the United States and British pharmacopoeias, together with numerous French, German and unofficinal preparations. . . . New York: William Wood & Co., 1881. 402p. DLC; DNLM; NNNAM; OCLloyd

[Volume 45]

EDES, Robert T[haxter] (1838-1923)
Therapeutic handbook of the United States pharmacopoeia, being a condensed statement of the physiological and toxic action, medicinal value, methods of administration and doses of the drugs and preparations in the latest ed. of the United States pharmacopoeia (apothecaries' and metric system) with some remarks on unofficinal preparations. . . . New York: William Wood & Co., 1883. 397p. DLC; OCLloyd; NNNAM; PU

[Volume 46]

ERB, Wilhelm H[einrich] (1840-1921)
Handbook of electro-therapeutics. Transl. by L. Putzel. New York: William Wood & Co., 1883. 366p. IEN-M; LNT-M; NNNAM; PPC

[Volume 47]

AMORY, Robert (1842-1910)
A treatise on electrolysis and its applications to therapeutics and surgical treatment in disease. New York: William Wood & Co., 1886. 307p. DLC; DNLM; NNNAM; PU

[Volume 48]

JOHNSON, Laurence (1845-1893)
. . . A manual of the medical botany of North America. . . . New York: William Wood & Co., 1884. 292p. 9 col. plates. DLC; DNLM; NNNAM; OCLloyd

[Volumes 49, 50]

HIPPOCRATES
The genuine works of Hippocrates. Transl. from the Greek with a preliminary discourse and annotations by Francis Adams. New York: William Wood & Co., 1886. 2 v. 8 plates. DLC; MH; NIC; NN

[Volumes 51, 52]

HOOPER, Robert (1775-1835)
. . . Hooper's Physician's vade-mecum: a manual of the principles and practice of physic; with an outline of general pathology, therapeutics, and hygiene. 10th ed. Rev. by William Augustus Guy . . . and John Harley. . . . New York: William Wood & Co., 1884. 2 v. CtY-M; ICJ; NIC; PP

[Volumes 53, 54, 55, 56]

EICHHORST, Hermann Ludwig (1849-1921)
Handbook of practical medicine. . . . New York: William Wood & Co., 1886. 4 v. DLC; MBM; NNNAM; PPC

[Volume 57]

STERNBERG, George M[iller] (1838-1915)
Malaria and malarial diseases. New York: William Wood & Co., 1884. 329p. DLC; DNLM; ICJ; NNNAM

[Volume 58]

WENDT, Edmund C[harles] (1857-1903)
A treatise on Asiatic cholera, edited and prepared by Edmund Charles Wendt . . . in association with Drs. John C. Peters . . . Ely McClellan . . . John B. Hamilton . . . and Geo. M. Sternberg. . . . New York: William Wood & Co., 1885. 403p. maps. DLC; MH-M; NNNAM; PU

[Volume 59]

CHARCOT, Jean Martin (1825-1893)
Clinical lectures on the diseases of old age. . . . Transl. by Leigh H. Hunt. . . . With additional lectures by Alfred L. Loomis. . . . New York: William Wood & Co., 1881. 280p. 3 plates. DLC; DNLM; NNNAM; PPC

[Volume 60]

WILSON, James Cornelius (1847-1934)
A treatise on the continued fevers. . . . With an introduction by J. M. Da Costa. New York: William Wood & Co., 1881. 365p. diags. DLC; DNLM; MBM; NNNAM

[Volume 61]

SALTER, Henry H. (1823-1871)
Asthma, its pathology and treatment. New York: William Wood & Co., 1882. 284p. IU-M; MBM; NNNAM; PPC

[Volume 62]

MACLAGAN, Thomas John (1838-1903)
Rheumatism; its nature, its pathology, and its successful treatment. New York: William Wood & Co., 1886. 277p. CtY-M; DNLM; NNNAM; PPC

[Volume 63]

LONGSTRETH, Morris (1846-1914)
Rheumatism, gout, and some allied disorders. New York: William Wood & Co., 1882. 280p. DNLM; MH-M; NNNAM; PU

[Volume 64]

DIDAY, Paul (1812-1894)
A treatise on syphilis in new-born children and infants at the breast. . . . Transl. by G. Whitley, M.D. With notes and an appendix by F. R. Sturgis. . . . New York: William Wood & Co., 1883. 310p. col. front. plate. DLC; NNNAM; OClM; PPC

[Volume 65]

KEYS, E[dward] L[awrence] (1843-1924)
The venereal diseases, including stricture of the male urethra. New York: William Wood & Co., 1880. 348p. DLC; DNLM; NNNAM; PPC

[Volume 66]

MILTON, John Laws (1820-1898)
On the pathology and treatment of gonorrhoea. 5th ed. New York: William Wood & Co., 1884. 306p. DNLM; IU-M; NNNAM; PPC

[Volume 67, 68]

ROSENTHAL, Moritz (1833-1889)
A clinical treatise on the diseases of the nervous system. . . . With a preface by Professor Charcot; transl. from the author's rev. and enl. ed. by L. Putzel. New York: William Wood & Co., 1879. 2 v. DLC; NNNAM; OClM; PU

[Volume 69]

GRIESENGER, Wilhelm (1817-1868)
Mental pathology and therapeutics. Transl. from the German (2nd ed.) by C. Lockhart Robertson and J. Rutherford. New York: William Wood & Co., 1882. 375p. DNLM; NNNAM; PPC; PU

[Volume 70]

GOWERS, William R[ichard] (1845-1915)
Epilepsy and other chronic convulsive diseases; their causes, symptoms, and treatment. New York: William Wood & Co., 1885. 255p. DNLM; IU-M; NNNAM; PPC

[Volume 71]

BRAMWELL, Byrom (1847-1931)
The diseases of the spinal cord. New York: William Wood & Co., 1882. 300p. 40 plates. DNLM; IU-M; NNNAM; PPC

[Volume 72]

PUTZEL, Leopold
A treatise on common forms of functional nervous diseases. . . . New York: William Wood & Co., 1880. 256p. DLC; DNLM; MBM; NNNAM

[Volume 73]

BLANDFORD, G[eorge] Fielding (1829-1911)
Insanity and its treatment; lectures on the treatment, medical and legal, of insane patients. 3rd ed., together with, Types of insanity, an illustrated guide in the physical diagnosis of mental disease, by Allan McLane Hamilton. New York: William Wood & Co., 1886. 379p. CtY-M; DNLM; LNT-M; NNNAM

[Volume 74]

GOWERS, William R[ichard] (1845-1915)
Diagnosis of diseases of the brain and of the spinal cord. New York: William Wood & Co., 1885. 293p. DNLM; IEN-M; NNNAM; PU

[Volume 75]

NOYES, Henry Drury (1832-1900)
. . . A treatise [on] diseases of the eye. . . . New York: William Wood & Co., 1881. 360p. 2 col. plates, diags. DLC; DNLM; NNNAM; PPC

[Volume 76]

BUCK, Albert Henry (1842-1922)
Diagnosis and treatment of ear diseases. . . . New York: William Wood & Co., 1880. 411p. DLC; DNLM; NNNAM; PPC

[Volumes 77, 78]

MACKENZIE, Morell (1837-1892)
A manual of diseases of the throat and nose, including the pharynx, larynx, trachea, oesophagus, nose, and naso-pharynx. New York: William Wood & Co., 1880. 440p. [vol. 2: William Wood & Co., 1884. 400p.] DLC; DNLM; NNNAM; PPC

[Volume 79]

JAMES, Prosser
The therapeutics of the respiratory passages. New York: William Wood & Co., 1884. 316p. CtY-M; DNLM; NNNAM; PPC

[Volume 80]

PAUL, Constantin [Charles T.] (1833-1896)
. . . Diagnosis and treatment of diseases of the heart. . . . Transl. from the French. New York: William Wood & Co., 1884. 335p. diags. DLC; DNLM; NNNAM; PPC

[Volume 81]

POWELL, Richard Douglas (1842-1925)
On diseases of the lungs and pleurae, including consumption. 3rd ed. New York: William Wood & Co., 1886. 34p. 2 plates. DNLM; NNNAM; PPC; PU

[Volume 82]

SEE, Germain
Diseases of the lungs (of a specific not tuberculous nature). Acute bronchites; infectious pneumonia; gangrene, syphilis, cancer and hydatid of the lungs. Transl. by E. P. Hurd, with appendices by Geo. M. Sternberg [and] Dujardin Beaumetz. New York: William Wood & Co., 1885. 398p. CtY-M; DNLM; NNNAM; PPC

[Volumes 83, 84, 85]

FRERICHS, Friedrich [Theodor] (1819-1885)
A clinical treatise on diseases of the liver. Transl. by Charles Murchison. New York: William Wood & Co., 1879. 3 v. CtY-M; NcD; NN; PPJ

[Volume 86]

DUJARDIN-BEAUMETZ, Georges Octave (1833-1895)
Diseases of the stomach and intestines; a manual of clinical therapeutics for the student and practitioner. Transl. from the 4th French ed. by E. P. Hurd. New York: William Wood & Co., 1886. 389p. 1 chart. DLC; DNLM; NNNAM; PPC

[Volume 87]

BRISTOWE, John Syer (1827-1895)
Diseases of the intestines and peritoneum. By John Syer Bristowe, J. R. Wardell, J. W. Begbie, S. O. Habershon, T. B. Curling, W. H. Ransom. New York: William Wood & Co., 1879. 243p. DLC; MBM; OClM; NNNAM

[Volume 88]

DICKINSON, W[illiam] H[owship]
A treatise on albuminuria. New York: William Wood & Co., 1881. 300p. 11 plates. CtY-M; DNLM; NNNAM; OClM

[Volume 89]

DICKINSON, W[illiam] H[owship]
On renal and urinary affections. In three parts. Part III. Miscellaneous affections of the kidneys and urine. New York: William Wood & Co., 1885. 343p. DNLM; OClM; PPC; PU [This edition differs from the original (London, 1885) in that detail reports of cases are omitted.]

[Volume 90]

BELFIELD, William Thomas (1856-1929)
. . . Diseases of the urinary and male sexual organs. . . . New York: William Wood & Co., 1884. 351p. DLC; DNLM; NNNAM; PPJ

[Volume 91]

COULSON, William (1802-1877)
. . . Coulson on the diseases of the bladder and prostate gland. 6th ed., rev. by Walter J. Coulson. . . . New York: William Wood & Co., 1881. 393p. DLC; NNNAM; OClM; PPC

[Volume 92]

KELSEY, Charles Boyd (1850-1917)
Diseases of the rectum and anus. . . . New York: William Wood & Co., 1882. 299p. DLC; DNLM; NNNAM; PPC

[Volume 93]

PIFFARD, Henry Granger (1842-1910)
A treatise on the materia medica and therapeutics of the skin. New York: William Wood & Co., 1881. 351p. DLC; DNLM; NNNAM; OCLloyd

[Volumes 94, 95]

BLYTH, Alexander Wynter (1844-1921)
Poisons, their effects and detection; a manual for the use of analytical chemists and experts, with an introductory essay on the growth of modern toxicology. . . . New York: William Wood & Co., 1885. 2 v., fold. tab. DLC; ICJ; NNNAM; PU

[Volumes 96, 97, 98]

TIDY, Charles Meymott (1843-1892)
Legal medicine. New York: William Wood & Co., 1882-1884. 3 v. DNLM; ICJ; NNNAM; PU

[Volume 99]

KIRBY, F. O., ed.
Veterinary medicine and surgery in diseases and injuries of the horse. Compiled from standard and modern authorities and edited by F. O Kirby. Illus. by four colored plates and one hundred and sixty-eight wood engravings. New York: William Wood & Co., [1883]. 332p. col. plates. CtY-M; DNLM; ICJ; PPC [Each plate has descriptive letterpress, not included in pagination.]

[Volume 100]

WOOD, WILLIAM & CO. New York
Index to Wood's library of standard medical authors, complete in one hundred volumes. New York: William Wood & Co., 1887. 568p. DLC; ICJ; NNNAM; PPC

INDEX OF NAMES

REFERENCES ARE TO ENTRY NUMBERS

	CHRONOLOGICAL SCHEMA	ENTRY NUMBERS
I.	American Medical Imprints, 1820-1829	20-0001 - 20-0645
II.	American Medical Imprints, 1830-1839	30-0001 - 30-0976
III.	American Medical Imprints, 1840-1849	40-0001 - 40-1406
IV.	American Medical Imprints, 1850-1859	50-0001 - 50-2042
V.	American Medical Imprints, 1860-1869	60-0001 - 60-2061
VI.	American Medical Imprints, 1870-1879	70-0001 - 70-4148
VII.	American Medical Imprints, 1880-1889	80-0001 - 80-7070
VIII.	American Medical Imprints, 1890-1899	90-0001 - 90-10,378
IX.	American Medical Imprints, 1900-1910	00-0001 - 00-7886

INDEX

References are to entry numbers.

INDEX

INDEX

INDEX

INDEX

INDEX